D0022758

Foundations of Nursing

Third Edition

DEDICATIONS

Lois White:
To my beloved husband, John, who is on his last great adventure and learning experience.

Gena Duncan:
To my husband, who gives me unconditional love and brings balance, calmness, and excitement to my life.
To Lois White, who modeled the role of an author and committed much of her life to this textbook.
To Wendy Baumle, for her hard work and dedication in developing this textbook. Thanks.
To future nurses who are caring and competent.

Wendy Baumle:
This book is dedicated to my beloved family—Patrick, Taylor, Madeline, Blair, Connor, Janet, and Robert—for their love and support, to Juliet Steiner for inspiring me and for making a difference in my life, to Gena Duncan for her guidance and friendship, and to my friends, colleagues, and students for their support and valuable insight into today's nursing education.

Foundations of Nursing

Third Edition

Lois White, RN, PhD
Former Chairperson and Professor, Department of Vocational Nurse Education, Del Mar College, Corpus Christi, Texas

Gena Duncan, RN, MSEd, MSN
Former Associate Professor of Nursing, Ivy Tech Community College, Fort Wayne, Indiana

Wendy Baumle, RN, MSN
James A. Rhodes State College, School of Nursing, Lima, Ohio

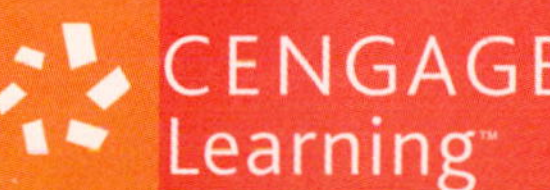

Australia • Brazil • Japan • Korea • Mexico • Singapore • Spain • United Kingdom • United States

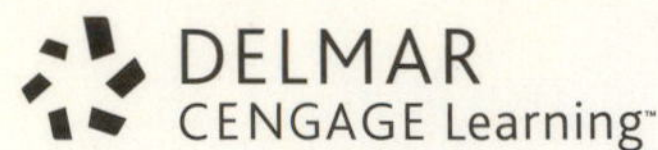

Foundations of Nursing, **Third Edition**
Lois White, RN, PhD, Gena Duncan, RN, MSEd, MSN, and Wendy Baumle, RN, MSN

Vice President, Career and Professional Editorial: Dave Garza

Director of Learning Solutions: Matt Kane

Executive Editor: Steven Helba

Managing Editor: Marah Bellegarde

Senior Product Manager: Juliet Steiner

Editorial Assistant: Meghan E. Orvis

Vice President, Career and Professional Marketing: Jennifer Ann Baker

Marketing Director: Wendy Mapstone

Senior Marketing Manager: Michele McTighe

Marketing Coordinator: Scott Chrysler

Production Director: Carolyn Miller

Production Manager: Andrew Crouth

Senior Content Project Manager: James Zayicek

Senior Art Director: Jack Pendleton

Technology Project Manager: Mary Colleen Liburdi

Production Technology Analyst: Patricia Allen

Production Technology Analyst: Ben Knapp

© 2011, 2005, 2001 Delmar Cengage Learning

ALL RIGHTS RESERVED. No part of this work covered by the copyright herein may be reproduced, transmitted, stored, or used in any form or by any means graphic, electronic, or mechanical, including but not limited to photocopying, recording, scanning, digitizing, taping, Web distribution, information networks, or information storage and retrieval systems, except as permitted under Section 107 or 108 of the 1976 United States Copyright Act, without the prior written permission of the publisher.

For product information and technology assistance, contact us at
Cengage Learning Customer & Sales Support, 1-800-354-9706
For permission to use material from this text or product,
submit all requests online at **www.cengage.com/permissions.**
Further permissions questions can be e-mailed to
permissionrequest@cengage.com

Library of Congress Control Number: 2010920753
ISBN-13: 978-1-4283-1773-4
ISBN-10: 1-4283-1773-2

Delmar
5 Maxwell Drive
Clifton Park, NY 12065-2919
USA

Cengage Learning is a leading provider of customized learning solutions with office locations around the globe, including Singapore, the United Kingdom, Australia, Mexico, Brazil, and Japan. Locate your local office at: **international.cengage.com/region**

Cengage Learning products are represented in Canada by Nelson Education, Ltd.

To learn more about Delmar, visit **www.cengage.com/delmar**

Purchase any of our products at your local college store or at our preferred online store **www.CengageBrain.com**

Notice to the Reader

Publisher does not warrant or guarantee any of the products described herein or perform any independent analysis in connection with any of the product information contained herein. Publisher does not assume, and expressly disclaims, any obligation to obtain and include information other than that provided to it by the manufacturer. The reader is expressly warned to consider and adopt all safety precautions that might be indicated by the activities described herein and to avoid all potential hazards. By following the instructions contained herein, the reader willingly assumes all risks in connection with such instructions. The publisher makes no representations or warranties of any kind, including but not limited to, the warranties of fitness for particular purpose or merchantability, nor are any such representations implied with respect to the material set forth herein, and the publisher takes no responsibility with respect to such material. The publisher shall not be liable for any special, consequential, or exemplary damages resulting, in whole or part, from the readers' use of, or reliance upon, this material.

Printed in the United States of America
1 2 3 4 5 6 7 13 12 11 10

CONTENTS

CHAPTER 2: HOLISTIC CARE / 32

CHAPTER 3: NURSING HISTORY, EDUCATION, AND ORGANIZATIONS / 44

CHAPTER 8: CLIENT TEACHING / 143

CHAPTER 9: NURSING PROCESS/ DOCUMENTATION/INFORMATICS / 161

UNIT 4

Developmental and Psychosocial Concerns / 197

CHAPTER 10: LIFE SPAN DEVELOPMENT / 198

CHAPTER 11: CULTURAL CONSIDERATIONS / 229

CHAPTER 12: STRESS, ADAPTATION, AND ANXIETY / 257

CHAPTER 13: END-OF-LIFE CARE / 273

UNIT 5

Health Promotion / 299

CHAPTER 14: WELLNESS CONCEPTS / 300

CHAPTER 15: SELF-CONCEPT / 315

CHAPTER 16: SPIRITUALITY / 326

CHAPTER 17: COMPLEMENTARY/ ALTERNATIVE THERAPIES / 342

CHAPTER 18: BASIC NUTRITION / 363

CHAPTER 19: REST AND SLEEP / 403

CHAPTER 20: SAFETY / HYGIENE / 416

UNIT 7

Fundamental Nursing Care / 483

CHAPTER 24: FLUID, ELECTROLYTE, AND ACID–BASE BALANCE / 484

CHAPTER 25: MEDICATION ADMINISTRATION AND IV THERAPY / 515

CHAPTER 26: ASSESSMENT / 552

CHAPTER 27: PAIN MANAGEMENT / 573

CHAPTER 28: DIAGNOSTIC TESTS / 601

UNIT 8

Nursing Procedures / 657

CHAPTER 29: BASIC PROCEDURES / 658

CHAPTER 30: INTERMEDIATE PROCEDURES / 809

CHAPTER 31: ADVANCED PROCEDURES / 925

Section II
Adult Health Nursing / 953

UNIT 9

Essential Concepts / 953

CHAPTER 32: ANESTHESIA / 954

CHAPTER 33: SURGERY / 967

CHAPTER 34: ONCOLOGY / 996

UNIT 10

Nursing Care of the Client: Oxygenation and Perfusion / 1021

CHAPTER 35: RESPIRATORY SYSTEM / 1022

CHAPTER 36: CARDIOVASCULAR SYSTEM / 1071

CHAPTER 37: HEMATOLOGIC AND LYMPHATIC SYSTEMS / 1115

UNIT 11

Nursing Care of the Client: Digestion and Elimination / 1147

CHAPTER 38: GASTROINTESTINAL SYSTEM / 1148

CHAPTER 39: URINARY SYSTEM / 1190

UNIT 12

Nursing Care of the Client: Mobility, Coordination, and Regulation / 1227

CHAPTER 40: MUSCULOSKELETAL SYSTEM / 1229

CHAPTER 41: NEUROLOGICAL SYSTEM / 1257

CHAPTER 42: SENSORY SYSTEM / 1311

CHAPTER 43: ENDOCRINE SYSTEM / 1340

UNIT 13

Nursing Care of the Client: Reproductive and Sexual Health / 1381

CHAPTER 44: REPRODUCTIVE SYSTEM / 1382

CHAPTER 45: SEXUALLY TRANSMITTED INFECTIONS / 1433

UNIT 14

Nursing Care of the Client: Body Defenses / 1451

CHAPTER 46: INTEGUMENTARY SYSTEM / 1452

CHAPTER 47: IMMUNE SYSTEM / 1495

CHAPTER 49: SUBSTANCE ABUSE / 1569

UNIT 16

Nursing Care of the Client: Older Adult / 1597

CHAPTER 50: THE OLDER ADULT / 1598

UNIT 17

Nursing Care of the Client: Health Care in the Community / 1629

CHAPTER 51: AMBULATORY, RESTORATIVE, AND PALLIATIVE CARE IN COMMUNITY SETTINGS / 1630

UNIT 18

Applications / 1649

CHAPTER 52: RESPONDING TO EMERGENCIES / 1650

CHAPTER 53: INTEGRATION / 1677

Section III
Maternal & Pediatric Nursing / 1683

UNIT 19

Nursing Care of the Client: Childbearing / 1683

CHAPTER 54: PRENATAL CARE / 1684

CHAPTER 55: COMPLICATIONS OF PREGNANCY / 1712

CHAPTER 56: THE BIRTH PROCESS / 1752

CHAPTER 57: POSTPARTUM CARE / 1789

CHAPTER 58: NEWBORN CARE / 1817

UNIT 20

Nursing Care of the Client: Childrearing / 169

CHAPTER 59: BASICS OF PEDIATRIC CARE / 1852

CHAPTER 60: INFANTS WITH SPECIAL NEEDS: BIRTH TO 12 MONTHS / 1871

CHAPTER 61: COMMON PROBLEMS: 1 TO 18 YEARS / 1914

CONTRIBUTORS

Joy E. Ache-Reed, RN, MS
Assistant Professor of Nursing
Indiana Wesleyan University
Marion, IN
Chapter 11, Cultural Considerations

Carol A. Fetters Andersen, RN, MSN
Director of Mental Health Services
St. Anthony Regional Hospital and Nursing Home
Carroll, IA
Chapter 50, The Older Adult

Carma Andrus, RN, MN, CNS
Dauterive Primary Care Clinic
St. Martinville, LA
Chapter 42, Sensory System

Diane R. Behrens, RNCS, MA, MSEd
Instructor
University of Saint Francis
Fort Wayne, IN
Chapter 47, Immune System

Susan L. Bredemeyer, RN, MS
Assistant Professor
Lutheran College of Health Professions
Fort Wayne, IN
Chapter 26, Assessment

Ali Brown, RN, MSN
Assistant Professor
College of Nursing
University of Tennessee
Knoxville, TN
Chapter 9, Nursing Process/Documentation/Informatics

Gyl A. Burkhard, RN, BSN, MS
Instructor
OCM BOCES
Syracuse, NY
Chapter 39, Urinary System

Donna J. Burleson, RN, MS
Chair of Health Occupations
Cisco Junior College
Abilene, TX
Chapter 1, Student Nurse Skills for Success

Anne H. Cary, RN, PhD, MPH, A-CCC
Professor and Coordinator, PhD in Nursing Program
College of Nursing and Health Sciences
George Mason University
Fairfax, VA
Chapter 3, Nursing History, Education, and Organizations

Diana L. Case, RN, MA, FNP
Family Nurse Practitioner
Fort Wayne, IN
Chapter 33, Surgery

Judy Conlon
Chapter 20, Safety/Hygiene

Jan Corder, RN, DNS
School of Nursing
Northeast Louisiana University
Monroe, LA
Chapter 9, Nursing Process/Documentation/Informatics

Julie Coy, RNC, MS
Pain Consultation Service
The Children's Hospital
Denver, CO
Chapter 19, Rest and Sleep
Chapter 27, Pain Management

Janice Eilerman, MSN, RN
Rhodes State College
Lima, OH
Chapter 46, Integumentary System

Jennifer Einhorn, MS, RN
Nursing Instructor
Chamberlain College of Nursing
Addison, IL
Chapter 57, Postpartum Care
Chapter 58, Newborn Care

Mary Elias, RNC, BSN, CCE
Instructor
Family Nurse Practitioner
Fort Wayne, IN
Chapter 44, Reproductive System

Cheryl Erickson, RN, BSN, MA
Associate Professor
University of Saint Francis
Fort Wayne, IN
Chapter 26, Assessment

Mary Ellen Zator Estes, RN, MSN, FNP, APRN-BC, NP-C
Family Nurse Practitioner in Internal Medicine
Fairfax, VA
and
Adjunct Faculty
School of Health Professions
Marymount University
Arlington, VA
Chapter 26, Assessment

Michael A. Fiedler, CRNA, MS
Assistant Professor
Applied Health Sciences
University of Alabama at Birmingham
Birmingham, AL
Chapter 32, Anesthesia

Nancy Fieldhouse, MSN, RNBC
Assistant Professor, School of Health Sciences
Ivy Tech Community College Northeast
Fort Wayne, IN
Chapter 51, Ambulatory, Restorative, and Palliative Care in Community Settings

Lynn Franck, MS, RN
Assistant Professor
Rhodes State College
Lima, OH
Chapter 43, Endocrine System

Mary Frost, RN, BSN
Covington, LA
Chapter 17, Complementary/ Alternative Therapies

Norma Fujise, RN, C, MS
School of Nursing
University of Hawaii
Honoloulu, HI
Chapter 46, Integumentary System

Cathy Greer, RN, MS
Instructor
Lutheran College of Health Professions
Fort Wayne, IN
Chapter 33, Surgery

Margaret L. Griffin, RN, BSN, MS
Former Director of Associate Degree Program
University of Saint Francis
Fort Wayne, IN
Chapter 46, Integumentary System

Susan Halley, RN, MS, FNP
Geriatric Nurse Practitioner
Fort Wayne, IN
Chapter 4, Legal and Ethical Responsibilities

Mary Jane Hamilton, RN, C, PhD
Professor of Nursing
Texas A&M University-Corpus Christi
Corpus Christi, TX
Chapter 59, Basics of Pediatric Care

Beverly F. Hidebrand, RN, BSN, MS
Former Health Occupations Coordinator
Washington, Saratoga, Warren, Hamilton & Essex Counties BOCES
Saratoga, NY
Chapter 39, Urinary System

Lucille Joel, RN, EdD, FAAN
Professor
College of Nursing
Rutgers, The State University of New Jersey
Newark, NJ
Chapter 5, The Health Care Delivery System

Janet Leah Joost, RN, BSN
Director of Nursing Education Program
Front Range Community College
Boulder, CO
Chapter 35, Respiratory System

Denise M. Jordan, RN, BSN, MA
Chair of Nursing Program
IT Technical Institute
Fort Wayne, IN
Chapter 4, Legal and Ethical Responsibilities

Janet E. Keith, RN, MSEd
Former Instructor, Practical Nursing Program
Ivy Tech State College
Fort Wayne, IN
Chapter 40, Musculoskeletal System

Vicki L. Khouli, RN, BSN, MA, IBCLC
Instructor
Practical Nursing Program
Ivy Tech State College
Fort Wayne, IN
Chapter 45, Sexually Transmitted Infections

Mary E. A. Laskin, RN, CS, MN
Clinical Nurse Specialist
Surgical/Orthopedic Services
Kaiser Permanente
San Diego, CA
Chapter 27, Pain Management

Celinda Kay Leach, RN, BS, MPH
Program Chair
Practical Nursing Program
Ivy Tech State College
Bloomington, IN
Chapter 34, Oncology

Sandra Liming, RN, MN
Nursing Instructor
North Seattle Community College
North Seattle, WA
Chapter 44, Reproductive System

Patricia Lokken, RN, MSN, CNP
Family Nurse Practitioner
Clearwater Health Services
Bagley, MN
Chapter 51, Ambulatory, Restorative, and Palliative Care in Community Settings

Judy Martin, RN, MS, JD
Nurse Attorney
Louisiana Department of Health and Hospitals
Health Standards Section
Baton Rouge, LA
Chapter 4, Legal and Ethical Responsibilities

Kim Martz
Instructor
Department of Nursing
Boise State University Department of Nursing
Boise, ID
Chapter 16, Spirituality

Carla McCuan, MS, RN
Sanford Brown College
St. Peters, MO
Chapter 54, Prenatal Care

Linda McCuistion, RN, PhD
Assistant Professor
School of Nursing
Our Lady of Holy Cross College
New Orleans, LA
Chapter 9, Nursing Process/Documentation/Informatics

Cheryl McGaffic, RN, PhD
Clinical Instructor
College of Nursing
The University of Arizona
Tucson, AZ
Chapter 47, Immune System

Robin Theresa McKenzie, RN, MSN, CCRN
Assistant Chairman
Navy Medical Center
San Diego, CA
Chapter 42, Sensory System

Betty Miller
Staff Development Coordinator
Meadowcrest Hospital
Gretna, LA
Chapter 13, End-of-Life Care

David K. Miller, RNC, BSN, MSEd
ICU/Medical-Surgical Manager
W.S. Major Hospital
Shelbyville, IN
Chapter 47, Immune System

Barbara S. Moffett, RN, PhD
Associate Professor of Nursing
School of Nursing
Southeastern Louisiana University
Hammond, LA
Chapter 9, Nursing Process/Documentation/Informatics

Mary Anne Mordcin-McCarthy, RN, PhD
Associate Professor and Director of the Undergraduate Program
College of Nursing
University of Tennessee–Knoxville
Knoxville, TN
Chapter 9, Nursing Process/Documentation/Informatics

Barbara Morvant, RN, MN
Louisiana State Board of Nursing
Metairie, LA
Chapter 4, Nursing History, Education, and Organizations

Joan Fritsch Needham, RNC, MS
Director of Education
DeKalb County Nursing Home
DeKalb IL
Chapter 6, Arenas of Care
Chapter 13, End-of-Life Care

Rebecca Osterhaut
Chapter 2, Holistic Care

Brenda Owens, RN, PhD
Associate Professor
School of Nursing
Louisiana State University Medical Center
New Orleans, LA
Chapter 25, Medication Administration and IV Therapy

Raymond Phillips, RN, MS, CCRN
Clinical Nurse Specialist
Staff Development Coordinator
U.S. Naval Hospital
Rota, Spain
Chapter 42, Sensory System

Demetrius Porche, RN, CCRN, DNS
Associate Professor and Director
Bachelor of Science in Nursing Program
Nicholsa State University
and
Adjunct Assistant Professor
Tulane University
School of Public Health and Topical Medicine
New Orleans, LA
Chapter 20, Safety/Hygiene
Chapter 21, Infection Control/Asepsis
Chapter 22, Standard Precautions and Isolation

Susan Reinhart, RN, MS
Assistant Professor
Department of Registered Nurse Education
Del Mar College
Corpus Christi, TX
Chapter 48, Mental Illness

Suzanne Riche, RN
Charity School of Nursing
Delgado Community College
New Orleans, LA
Chapter 9, Nursing Process/Documentation/Informatics

Kathy Rockwell, BSN, MA, MSN, PNP
Professor
Department of RN Education
Del Mar College Corpus Christi, TX
and
Supervisor, Surgical Services
94th General Hospital
Seagoville, TX
Chapter 52, Responding to Emergencies

Martha Ann Rust, RN, BSN, MSN
Renaissance Village
Fort Wayne, IN
Chapter 41, Neurological System

Mary Kay Schultz, RN, MSN, ANP
Instructor
Department of Nursing
Regis University
Denver, CO
Chapter 43, Endocrine System

Leslee R. Sinn, RN, BSN
Instructor
Front Range Community College
Boulder, CO
Chapter 38, Gastrointestinal System

Russlyn A. St. John, RN, MSN
Associate Professor & Coordinator
Practical Nursing
St. Charles Community College
St. Peters, MO
Chapter 43, Endocrine System

Maureen Straight, RN, BSN, MSEd
Regents College
Albany, NY
Chapter 1, Student Nurse Skills for Success

Susan Stranahan, RN, PhD
Shell Point Retirement Community
Fort Meyers, FL
Chapter 11, Cultural Considerations

Patricia Sunderhaus, MSN, RN
Senior Instructor, Nursing
Brown Mackie College
Cincinnati, OH
Chapter 59, Basics of Pediatric Care
Chapter 61, Common Problems: 1 to 18 Years

Leonie Sutherland, RN, PhD
Assistant Professor
Department of Nursing
Boise State University
Boise, ID
Chapter 16, Spirituality

Patricia R. Teasley, MSN, RN, APRN, BC
Nursing Program Coordinator/Professor
Central Texas College
Killeen, TX
Chapter 23, Bioterrorism

Patricia Tutor, PhD
Riverside Community College
Riverside, CA
Chapter 38, Gastrointestinal System

Donna Jean White, RN, MS
Rhodes State College
Lima, OH
Chapter 50, The Older Adult

John M. White, PhD
Former Chairperson, Professor
Biology Department
Del Mar College
Corpus Christi, TX
Chapter 24, Fluid, Electrolyte, and Acid-Base Balance

Donna Wofford, RN, PhD
Professor, Department of RN Education
Del Mar College
Corpus Christi, TX
Chapter 60, Infants with Special Needs: Birth to 12 Months
Chapter 61, Common Problems: 1 to 18 Years

Lorrie Wong, RN, MS
School of Nursing
University of Hawaii
Honolulu, HI
Chapter 46, Integumentary System

Zayda Yeoh, RN, MSN
Practical Nursing Department Chair
Brown Mackie College
Fort Wayne, IN
Chapter 60, Infants with Special Needs: Birth to 12 Months

Rothlyn Zahourek, RN, CS, MS
Certified Clinical Nurse Specialist
Amherst, MA
Chapter 17, Complementary/Alternative Therapies

PROCEDURE CONTRIBUTORS

Gaylene Bouska Altman, RN, PhD
Director, Learning Lab
Faculty, School of Nursing
University of Washington
Seattle, WA

Sharon Aronovitch, RN, PhD, CETN
Regents College
Albany, NY

Dale D. Barb, MHS, PT
Academic Coordinator of Clinical Education
Department of Physical Therapy
Wichita State University
Wichita, KS

Theresa A. Barenz, RN, MN

Susan Weiss Behrend, RN, MSN
Fox Chase Cancer Center
Philadelphia, PA

Patricia Buchsel, RN, MSN, FAAN
Clinical Instructor
School of Nursing
University of Washington
Seattle, WA

Bethaney Campbell, RN, MN, OCN
University of Washington Medical Center
Seattle, WA

Curt Campbell
Integrated Health Services of Seattle
Seattle, WA

Jung-Chen (Kristina) Chang, RN, MN, PhD
University of Washington
School of Nursing
Seattle, WA

Eileen M. Collins, MN, ARNP, CNOR
University of Washington
School of Nursing
Seattle, WA

Cheryl L. Cooke, RN, MN
Student Services Coordinator
University of Washington
School of Nursing
Seattle, WA

Valerie Coxon, RN, PhD
Affiliate Assistant Professor
University of Washington
School of Nursing
Seattle, WA
and
Chief Executive Officer
NRSPACE Software, Inc.
Bellevue, WA

Gayle C. Crawford, RN, BSN,
Staff Nurse
University of Washington Medical Center
Seattle, WA

Eleonor U. de la Pena, RN, BS
Northwest Asthma and Allergy Center
Seattle, WA

Tom Ewing, RN, BSN
Hematology-Oncology
University of Washington Medical Center
Seattle, WA

Amy Fryberger, RN, MN, ONC

Karrin Johnson, RN
Health Care Project Manager
NRSPACE Software, Inc.
Bellevue, WA

Kimberly Sue Kahn, RN, MSN, FNP-C, CS, AOCN
University of Virginia
Portsmouth, VA

Catherine H. Kelley, RN, MSN, OCN
Chimeric Therapies, Inc.
Palatine, IL

Carla A. Bouska Lee, PhD, ARNP, FAAN
Clarkston College
Omaha, NE

Kathryn Lilleby, RN
Clinical Research Nurse
Fred Hutchinson Cancer Research Center
Seattle, WA

Joan M. Mack, RN, MSN, CS
Nebraska Medical Center
Omaha, NE

Marianne Frances Moore, RN, MSN
Clarkson Hospital
Omaha, NE

Susan Randolph, RN, MSN, CS
Manager, Transplant Services
Coram Healthcare
Parkersburg, WV

Susan Rives, RN, BSN, OCN
CARE Center Coordinator
Martha Jefferson Hospital
Charlottesville, VA

Barbara Sigler, RN, MNEd, CORLN
Technical Publications Editor
Oncology Nursing Press, Inc.
Formerly:
Clinical Nurse Specialist in Otolaryngology—Head and Neck Surgery
University of Pittsburgh Medical Center
Pittsburgh, PA

Pam Talley, MN, PhD
University of Washington
School of Nursing
Seattle, WA

Hsin-Yi (Jean) Tang, RN, MS, PhD
University of Washington
School of Nursing
Seattle, WA

Robi Thomas, MS, RN, AOCN
Clinical Nurse Specialist for Oncology and the Pain Center
St. Mary's Mercy Medical Center
Grand Rapids, MI

Chandra VanPaepeghem, RN, BSN
University of Washington Medical Center
Seattle, WA

REVIEWERS

Charlene Bell, RN, MSN, NCSN
Instructor
Associate Degree Nursing Program
Southwest Texas Junior College
Uvalde, TX

Donna Burleson
Chair of Nursing Department
Cisco Junior College
Abilene, TX

Dotty Cales, RN
Instructor
North Coast Medical Training Academy
Kent, OH

Carolyn Du, BSN, MSN, NP, CDe
Director of Education
Pacific College
Costa Mesa, CA

Janice Eilerman, MSN, RN
Rhodes State College
Lima,OH

Jennifer Einhorn, RN, MS
Nursing Instructor
Chamberlain College of Nursing
Addison, IL

Patricia Fennessy, RN, MSN
Education Consultant
Connecticut Technical High School System
Middletown, CT

Carol Greulich, CS, RN, MSN
Assistant Professor
University of Saint Francis
Fort Wayne, IN

Helena L. Jermalovic, RN, MSN
Assistant Professor
University of Alaska
Anchorage, AK

Lee Klopfenstein, MD, CMD
Family Physician
Long Term Care Medical Director
Van Wert, OH

Leon Klopfenstein, ASN
Emergency Department
Van Wert, OH

Sharon Knarr, RN
Clinical Instructor
LPN Program
Northcoast Medical Training Academy
Kent, OH

Christine Levandowski, RN, BSN, MSN
Director of Nursing
Baker College
Auburn Hills, MI

Wendy Maleki, RN, MS
Director
Vocational Nursing Program
American Career College
Ontario, CA

Deborah McMahan, MD
Health Commissioner of Allen County
Fort Wayne, IN

Katherine C. Pellerin, RN, BS, MS
Department Head, LPN Program
Norwich Technical High School
Norwich, CT

Jennifer Ponto, RN, BSN
Faculty
Vocational Nursing Program
South Plains College
Levelland, TX

Cheryl Pratt, RN, MA, CNAA
Regional Dean of Nursing
Rasmussen College
Mankato, MN

Cherie R. Rebar, RN, MSN, MBA, FNP
Chair, Associate Professor, Nursing Program
Kettering College of Medical Arts
Kettering, OH

Timm Reed, RRT, RN, BS, MSN, MBA
Assistant Professor
University of Saint Francis
Fort Wayne, IN

Patricia Schrull, RN, MSN, MBA, MEd., CNE
Director, Practical Nursing Program
Lorain County Community College
Elyria, OH

Laura Spinelli
Keiser Career College
Miami Lakes, FL

Frances S. Stoner, RN, BSN, PHN
Instructor, NCLEX Coordintor
American Career College
Anaheim, CA

Tina Terpening
Associate Nursing Faculty
University of Phoenix, Southern California Campus

Lori Theodore, RN, BSN
Orlando Tech
Orlando, FL

Kimberly Valich, RN, MSN
Nursing Faculty, Department Chairperson
South Suburban College
South Holland, IL

Sarah Elizabeth Youth Whitaker, DNS, RN
Nursing Program Director
Computer Career Center
El Paso, TX

Shawn White, RN, BSN
Clinical Coordinator, Nursing Instructor
Griffin Technical College
Griffin, GA

Christina R. Wilson, RN, BAN, PHN
Faculty, Practical Nursing Program
Anoka Technical College
Anoka, MN

MARKET REVIEWERS AND CLASS TEST PARTICIPANTS

Deborah Ain
Nursing Professor
College of Southern Nevada
Las Vegas, NV

Mary Ann Ambrose, MSN, FNP
Program Director
Cuesta Community College Vocational Nursing Program
Paso Robles, CA

Jennie Applegate, RN, BSN
Practical Nursing Instructor
Keiser Career College
Greenacres, FL

Charlotte A. Armstrong, RN, BSN
Instructor
Northcoast Medical Training Academy
Kent, OH

Camille Baldwin
High Tech Central
Fort Myers, FL

Priscilla Burks, RN, BSN
Practical Nursing Instructor
Hinds Community College
Pearl, MS

Virginia Chacon
Colorado Technical University
Pueblo, CO

Sherri Comfort, RN
Practical Nursing Instructor Department Chair
Holmes Community College
Goodman, MS

Brandy Coward, BNS, MA
Director of Nursing
Angeles Institute
Lakewood, CA

Scott Coward, RN
Campus Director
Angeles Institute
Lakewood, CA

Jennifer Decker
Clinical Instructor
College of Eastern Utah
Price, UT

C. Kay Devereux
Professor
Department Chair, Vocational Nurse Education
Tyler Junior College
Tyler, TX

Carolyn Du, BSN, MSN, NP, CDe
Director of Education
Pacific College
Costa Mesa, CA

Laura R. Durbin, RN, BSN, CHPN
Instructor
West Kentucky Community and Technical College
Paducah, KY

Robin Ellis, BSN, MS
Nursing Faculty
Provo College
Provo, UT

Suzanne D. Fox, RN
Practical Nursing Instructor
Arkansas State University Technical Center
Marked Tree, AR

Judie Fritz, RN, MSN
Instructor
Keiser Career College
Miami Lakes, FL

Edith Gerdes, RN, MSN, BHCA
Associate Professor of Nursing
Ivy Tech Community College
South Bend, IN

Juanita Hamilton-Gonzalez
Professor
Coordinator – Practical Nursing Program
City University of New York – Medgar Evers
Brooklyn, NY

Jane Harper
Assistant Professor
Southeast Kentucky Community & Technical College
Pineville, KY

Angie Headley
Nursing Instructor
Swainsboro Technical College
Swainsboro, GA

Lillie Hill
Clinical Coordinator/Instructor
Practical Nursing
Durham Technical Community College
Durham, NC

Michelle Hopper
Sanford-Brown College
St. Peters, MO

Karla Huntsman, RN, MSN
Instructor
Nursing Program
AmeriTech College
Draper, UT

Connie M. Hyde, RN, BSN
Practical Nursing Instructor
Louisiana Technical College
Lafayette, LA

Denise Isackila
Instructor
North Coast Medical Training Academy
Kent, OH

Kimball Johnson, RN, MS
Nursing Professor
College of Eastern Utah
Price, UT

Sandy Kamhoot, BSN
Faculty
Santa Fe College
Gainesville, FL

Juanita Kaness, MSN, RN, CRNP
Nursing Program Coordinator
Lehigh Carbon Community College
Schnecksville, PA

Mary E. Kilbourn-Huey, MSN
Assistant Professor
Maysville Community and Technical College
Maysville, KY

Gloria D. Kline, RN
Practical Nursing Instructor
Hinds Community College
Vicksburg, MS

Christine Levandowski, RN, BSN, MSN
Director of Nursing
Baker College
Auburn Hills, MI

Mary Luckett, RN, MS
Professor Vocational Nursing
Level 1 Coordinator
Houston Community College
Coleman College for Health Sciences
Houston, TX

Wendy Maleki, RN, MS
Director
Vocational Nursing Program
American Career College
Ontario, CA

Luzviminda A. Malihan
Assistant Professor
Hostos Community College
Bronx, NY

Vanessa Norwood McGregor, RN, BSN, MBA
Practical Nursing Instructor
West Kentucky Community and Technical College
Paducah, KY

Kristie Oles, RN, MSN
Practical Nursing Chair
Brown Mackie College
North Canton, OH

Beverly Pacas
Department Head/Instructor
Practical Nursing
Louisiana Technical College
Baton Rouge, LA

Debra Perry, RN, MSN
Instructor
Lorain County Community College
Elyria, OH

Cheryl Pratt, RN, MA, CNAA
Regional Dean of Nursing
Rasmussen College
Mankato, MN

Charlotte Prewitt, RN, BSN
Practical Nursing Instructor
Meridian Technology Center
Stillwater, OK

Stephanie Price
Faculty, Practical Nursing
Holmes Community College
Goodman, MS

Patricia Schrull, RN, MSN, MBA, MEd, CNE
Director, Practical Nursing Program
Lorain County Community College
Elyria, OH

Margi J. Schutlz, RN, MSN, PhD
Director, Nursing Division
GateWay Community College
Phoenix, AZ

Sherie A. Shupe, RN, MSN
Director of Nursing
Computer Career Center
Las Cruces, NM

Sherri Smith, RN
Chairwoman
Arkansas State University Technical Center
Jonesboro, AR

Cheryl Smith, RN, BSN
Practical Nursing Instructor
Colorado Technical University
North Kansas City, MO

Laura Spinelli
Keiser Career College
Miami Lakes, FL

Jennifer Teerlink, RN, MSN
Nursing Faculty
Provo College
Provo, UT

Dana L. Trowell, RN, BSN
LPN Program Director
Dalton State College
Dalton, GA

Racheal Vargas, LVN
Clinical Liaison
Medical Assisting/Vocational Nursing
Lake College
Reading, CA

Sarah Elizabeth Youth Whitaker, DNS, RN
Nursing Program Director
Computer Career Center
El Paso, TX

Shawn White, RN, BSN
Clinical Coordinator, Nursing Instructor
Griffin Technical College
Griffin, GA

Sharon Wilson
Program Director/Instructor, Practical Nursing
Durham Technical Community College
Durham, NC

Vladmir Yarosh, LVN, BS
Program Coordinator —Vocational Nurse Program
Gurnick Academy of Medical Arts
San Mateo, CA

DiAnn Zimmerman
Director, Instructor
Dakota County Technical College
Rosemount, MN

PREFACE

Foundations of Nursing, third edition, is designed to cover the six cores of a practical/vocational nursing curriculum (Fundamentals; Medical-Surgical/Adult Health; Maternal-Newborn; Pediatrics; Mental Health; and Leadership). There is a strong emphasis on life span development, older adult needs, and professional adjustments. on bioterrorism, spirituality, and self-concept chapters enhance the student's learning of current nursing issues. Since the entire curriculum is covered, the student can see how subject matter across different areas is interrelated. Students will also find this text helpful by having all information in one book.

Although a systems approach is presented, the concept of holistic care is fundamental to this text. Throughout the book, boxes highlight special topics regarding critical thinking questions, memory tricks, life span development, client teaching, cultural considerations, professional tips, community/home health care, safety, and infection control.

Each medical/surgical chapter begins with an anatomy and physiology review. Pharmacology basics, medication administration, and diagnostic testing are presented. The concept of critical thinking, presented in the first chapter, lays the foundation for the entire nursing process, presented in great detail and incorporating current NANDA diagnoses and NIC/NOC references. The student is provided with opportunities to demonstrate knowledge and develop critical thinking skills by completing Case Studies included in many of the chapters. Concept Maps and Concept Care Maps challenge the student to incorporate the interrelatedness of nursing concepts in preparation for clinical practice. The student has the opportunity to assess knowledge and critical thinking of essential nursing concepts by answering NCLEX®-style review questions at the end of each chapter.

Health care settings are changing, multifaceted, challenging, and rewarding. Critical thinking and sound nursing judgments are essential in the present health care environment. Practical/Vocational nursing students confront and adapt to changes in technology, information, and resources by building a solid foundation of accurate, essential information. A firm knowledge base also allows nurses to meet the changing needs of clients. This text was written to equip the LPN/VN with current knowledge, basic problem-solving and critical thinking skills to successfully pass the NCLEX®-PN exam and meet the demanding challenges of today's health care.

ORGANIZATION

Foundations of Nursing, third edition, consists of 61 chapters grouped into 3 sections: Basic Nursing, Adult Health Nursing, and Maternal & Pediatric Nursing. These 3 sections altogether are grouped into 20 units.

Basic Nursing

- **Unit 1:** FOUNDATIONS—discusses student nurse skills for success (including critical thinking, time management, study skills, and life organizing skills); holistic care; nursing history, education, and organizations; and legal and ethical responsibilities.
- **Unit 2:** THE HEALTH CARE ENVIRONMENT—describes the health care delivery system and arenas of care, focusing on the various settings in which practical/vocational nurses practice.
- **Unit 3:** COMMUNICATION—addresses the process of communication, how communication is used in the nurse/client relationship; generational differences; and technical and legal aspects of documentation. Each component of the nursing process is explained in a clear, concise manner. Electronic medical records and technological information is incorporated throughout the chapters. The client teaching process is presented as a major nursing intervention for clients throughout the life span.
- **Unit 4:** DEVELOPMENTAL AND PSYCHOSOCIAL CONCERNS — describes the growth and development changes throughout the life span; cultural aspects and considerations; stress, adaptation, and anxiety; grief and end-of-life care.

- **Unit 5:** HEALTH PROMOTION—addresses self-concept, spirituality, and complementary/alternative therapies. Wellness concepts, basic nutrition, rest and sleep, and safety/hygiene are presented as methods of promoting health.
- **Unit 6:** INFECTION CONTROL—presents the chain of infection, describes various types of pathogenic microorganism, presents the concepts of asepsis and aseptic technique along with Standard Precautions and isolation measures, and discusses issues regarding bioterrorism.
- **Unit 7:** FUNDAMENTAL NURSING CARE—discusses fluid, electrolyte and acid-base balance. Medication administration and IV therapy are presented in nursing process format. Also included are legal considerations, dose equivalents, and dosage calculations. Assessment is covered in great detail, including head-to-toe physical assessment, nursing history, and functional assessment. Pain management is detailed in causes of pain, transmission and perception, assessment methods, and nursing interventions for pain relief. Nursing care for a client encountering diagnostic tests is thoroughly covered. The most commonly-ordered diagnostic tests are presented in tables that provide the normal results and nursing considerations.
- **Unit 8:** NURSING PROCEDURES—basic, intermediate, and advanced procedures follow the nursing process format and are presented in step-by-step fashion. Rationale is given for each step, and figures add to the clarity of the procedures.

Adult Health Nursing

- **Unit 9:** ESSENTIAL CONCEPTS—discusses the various types of anesthesia and the nursing care required for each. Surgery describes the perioperative care of clients. The Oncology chapter covers the various types of cancer, the usual treatments, and the nursing care required.

The chapters in Units 10 through 14 each include an anatomy and physiology review and a presentation of each disorder, with medical/surgical management, nursing management, pharmacological, dietary, and activity aspects of treatment. The nursing process identifies subjective and objective data with health history questions, possible nursing diagnoses, outcomes, interventions, and evaluation. A sample nursing care plan is found in each chapter in these units. New client case studies have also been added throughout.

- **Unit 10:** NURSING CARE OF THE CLIENT: OXYGENATION AND PERFUSION— includes the respiratory system, cardiovascular system, and hematological and lymphatic systems.
- **Unit 11:** NURSING CARE OF THE CLIENT: DIGESTION AND ELIMINATION— discusses the gastrointestinal system and urinary system.
- **Unit 12:** NURSING CARE OF THE CLIENT: MOBILITY, COORDINATION, AND REGULATION—covers the musculoskeletal system, neurological system, sensory system, and endocrine system.
- **Unit 13:** NURSING CARE OF THE CLIENT: REPRODUCTIVE AND SEXUAL HEALTH—includes the male and female reproductive systems and sexually transmitted infections.
- **Unit 14:** NURSING CARE OF THE CLIENT: BODY DEFENSES—discusses the integumentary system and the immune system.
- **Unit 15:** NURSING CARE OF THE CLIENT: PHYSICAL AND MENTAL INTEGRITY— addresses substance abuse and the care of clients with common mental illnesses. Substance abuse describes substances that are commonly abused, the signs and symptoms of abuse, and treatments available.
- **Unit 16:** NURSING CARE OF THE CLIENT: OLDER ADULT—explains nursing care for the older adult. Physiological changes of aging are presented for each body system.
- **Unit 17:** NURSING CARE OF THE CLIENT: HEALTH CARE IN THE COMMUNITY— defines the role of the nurse in ambulatory, restorative, and palliative care in community settings. Discusses appropriate client assessments and nursing interventions in each healthcare setting.
- **Unit 18:** APPLICATIONS—describes how nursing knowledge is applied in emergencies. Specific information is provided for common emergencies. A number of scenarios describing clients with multisystem problems assist students to see the integration of the body.

Maternal & Pediatric Nursing

- **Unit 19:** NURSING CARE OF THE CLIENT: CHILDBEARING—covers preconception education, prenatal care, fetal development, complications of pregnancy, the birth process, postpartum care, and care of the newborn.
- **Unit 20:** NURSING CARE OF THE CLIENT: CHILDREARING—presents the basics of pediatric care. The two chapters in this unit, *Infants with Special Needs: Birth to 12 Months* and *Common Problems: 1 to 18 Years*, address the major situations of pediatric care.

FEATURES

Each chapter includes a variety of learning aids designed to help the reader further a basic understanding of key concepts. Each chapter opens with a **Making the Connection** box that guides the reader to other key chapters related to the current chapter. This highlights the integration of the text material. Procedures used for the care of clients with medical/surgical disorders are identified as appropriate. **Learning Objectives** are presented at the beginning of each chapter as well. These help students focus their study and use their time efficiently. A listing of **Key Terms** is provided to identify the terms the student should know or learn for a better understanding of the subject matter. These are bolded and defined at first use in the chapter. Each medical/surgical chapter has a brief review of anatomy & physiology to review the organs and functions of the system being discussed.

The content of each chapter is presented in nursing process format. Where appropriate, a **Sample Nursing Care Plan** is provided in the chapter. These serve as models for students to refer to as they create their own care plans based on case studies. **Case Studies** are presented at the conclusion of most chapters. These call for students to draw upon their knowledge base and synthesize information to develop their own solutions to realistic cases. **Nursing Diagnoses, Planning/Outcomes**, and **Interventions** are presented in a convenient table format for quick reference. **Concept Maps** and **Concept Care Maps** are visual pictures of interrelated concepts as they relate to nursing.

A bulleted **Summary** list and multiple-choice **NCLEX®-style Review Questions** at the end of each chapter assist the student in remembering and using the material presented.

References/Suggested Readings allow the student to find the source of the material presented and also to find additional information concerning topics covered. **Resources** are also listed and provide names and internet addresses of organizations specializing in a specific area of health care.

Boxes used throughout the text emphasize key points and provide specific types of information. The boxes are:

- **CRITICAL THINKING:** encourages the student to use the knowledge gained to think critically about a situation.
- **MEMORY TRICK:** provides an easy to remember saying or abbreviation to assist the student in remembering important information presented.
- **LIFE SPAN CONSIDERATIONS:** provides information related to the care of specific age groups during the life span.
- **CLIENT TEACHING:** identifies specific items that the client should know related to the various disorders.
- **CULTURAL CONSIDERATIONS:** shares beliefs, manners, and ways of providing care, communication, and relationships of various cultural and ethnic groups as a way to provide holistic care.
- **PROFESSIONAL TIP:** offers tips and technical hints for the nurse to ensure quality care.
- **SAFETY:** emphasizes the importance of and ways to maintain safe care.
- **COMMUNITY/HOME HEALTH CARE:** describes factors to consider when providing care in the community or in a client's home, and adaptation in care that may be necessary.
- **DRUG ICON:** highlights pharmacological treatments and interventions that may be appropriate for certain conditions and disorders.
- **COLLABORATIVE CARE:** mentions members of the care team and their roles in providing comprehensive care to clients.
- **INFECTION CONTROL:** indicates reminders of methods to prevent the spread of infections.

The back matter includes a **Glossary of Terms**. The appendices include **NANDA-International Nursing Diagnoses**; **Recommended Childhood, Adolescent, and Adult Immunization Schedules**; **Abbreviations, Acronyms** and **Symbols**; and **English/Spanish Words and Phrases. Standard Precautions** are found on the inside back cover.

NEW TO THIS EDITION

Added 4 new chapters:

- **Chapter 15**, *Self-Concept*, presents a global understanding of the dimensions, formation, and factors affecting self-concept to facilitate client coping and promote overall physical and mental wellness.
- **Chapter 16**, *Spirituality*, provides understanding of the basic human need for spirituality and prepares the nurse to integrate the spiritual aspect of each client into the care provided.
- **Chapter 23**, *Bioterrorism*, discusses the major agents of bioterrorism, protective measures prior to and following a terrorist attack, and delineates the roles of the nurse, various levels of government, and each person in the event of a terrorist attack.
- **Chapter 51**, *Ambulatory, Restorative, and Palliative Care in Community Settings*, defines the role of the nurse, explains the legal issues when providing nursing care, and discusses appropriate client assessments and nursing interventions in each healthcare setting.

Extensively updated chapters:

- **Chapter 13**, *End-of-Life Care*, includes sections on fluids and nutrition, palliative care and hospice care, and pain management.
- **Chapter 27**, *Pain Management*, features an improved section on patient controlled analgesia (PCA) and oral patient controlled analgesia, medication on demand (MOD®); a discussion of gate control theory of pain; and a presentation of the Joint Commission standards for pain management and the World Health Organization's (WHO) pain management guidelines.
- **Chapter 33**, *Surgery*, now contains additional robotic and minimally invasive surgeries.
- **Chapter 36**, *Cardiovascular System*, has improved anatomy and physiology and assessment sections, explanations of cuttingedge diagnostic tests, and extensively updated content on implantable cardioverter-defibrillator, pacemaker, cardiac valve management, angina, minimally invasive surgery, ventricular assist device, and pharmacological care.
- **Chapter 53**, *Integration*, includes more in-depth case studies to use as appropriate throughout educational experience.

Updated content within chapters:

- Additional coverage of learning disabilities.
- Information on preparing for exams and test-taking tips.
- Coverage of Scientology beliefs in the Cultural Considerations chapter.
- Dietary recommendations follow the new recommended food pyramid, MyPyramid.
- Updates to the assessment chapter include assessing client using complementary/alternative therapy and assessment of edema.
- Updates to the neurological system chapter include intrathecal chemotherapy, chemotherapy disk-shaped wafers, Stroke Risk Scorecard, diet therapy, position emission

tomography scanning and ablation procedures for Parkinson's disease; sniff test to diagnose Alzheimer's disease, Parkinson's disease, and other neurodegenerative disorders.
- Thorough updating of the basic, intermediate, and advanced procedure chapters with new photos for the visual learner.
- Thorough updating of Diagnostic Tests chapter with addition of new current diagnostic testing procedures.
- Added older adult content to Lifespan Development chapter and emphasized geriatric content in Life Span Considerations boxes.
- Updated Maternal & Pediatric chapters to include current nursing trends.

Other additions:

- Added case studies to all chapters as appropriate; case studies have a mixture of critical thinking and nursing process questions.
- Added concept maps to several chapters so the student can link facts with real life clinical practice.
- Added concept care maps to chapters as appropriate for visual picture of the nursing process.
- Increased number of challenging and applicable critical thinking questions.
- Cultural considerations updated and cultural content included throughout the text.
- Added Adult Immunization Schedule along with Childhood and Adolescent Immunization Schedules.
- Added objective and subjective assessment guidelines to medical-surgical chapters for student use in clinical settings.
- Cited research articles in understandable manner for easy application of evidence-based practice.
- Added current NANDA diagnoses according to NANDA-International (2010) *Nursing Diagnoses, 2009-11 Edition: Definitions and Classification (NANDA-/Nursing Diagnosis).*
- Added new NCLEX®-style review questions at the end of chapters to help students challenge their understanding of content while gaining practice with this important question style.
- Added Memory Tricks for ease of student recall of pertinent information.
- Numerous new photos and illustrations for improved presentation of concepts.
- New free StudyWARE™ CD-ROM provides interactive games, animations, videos, heart and lung sounds, and much more to augment the learning experience and support mastery of concepts.

EXTENSIVE TEACHING/ LEARNING PACKAGE

The complete supplements package for *Foundations of Nursing*, third edition, was developed to achieve two goals:

1. To assist students in learning the information and procedures presented in the text.
2. To assist instructors in planning and implementing their programs for the most efficient use of time and other resources.

INSTRUCTOR RESOURCES

Foundations of Nursing Instructor's Resource, third edition

ISBN-10: 1-4283-1780-5
ISBN-13: 978-1-4283-1780-2

The Instructor's Resource has four components to assist the instructor and enhance classroom activities and discussion.

Instructor's Guide

- **Instructional Approaches:** Ideas and concepts to help educators manage different presentation methods. Suggestions for approaching topics with rich discussion topics and lecture ideas are provided.
- **Student Learning Activities:** Ideas for activities such as classroom discussions, role play, and individual assignments designed to encourage student critical thinking as they engage with the concepts presented in the text.
- **Resources:** Additional books, videos, and resources for use in developing and implementing your curriculum.
  - **Web Activities:** Suggestions for student learning experiences online, including specific websites and accompanying activities.
  - **Suggested Responses to the Case Study:** Case studies located throughout the core book challenge student critical thinking with questions about nursing care, with suggested responses provided herein.
  - **Answers to Review Questions**: Answers and rationales for all end-of-chapter NCLEX® style questions are provided.

Computerized Testbank

- Includes a rich bank of questions that test students on retention and application of material in the text.
- Many questions are now presented in NCLEX® style, with each question providing the answer and rationale, as well as cognitive levels.
- Allows the instructor to mix questions from each of the didactic chapters to customize tests.

Instructor Slides Created in PowerPoint

- A robust offering of instructor slides created in PowerPoint outlines the concepts from text in order to assist the instructor with lectures.
- Ideas presented stimulate discussion and critical thinking.

Image Library

A searchable Image Library of more than 800 illustrations and photographs that can be incorporated into lectures, class materials, or electronic presentations.

Student Resources

Foundations of Nursing Study Guide

ISBN-10: 1-4283-1777-5
ISBN-13: 978-1-4283-1777-2

A valuable companion to the core book, this student resource provides additional review on all 61 chapters of *Foundations of Nursing* with Key Terms matching review questions, Abbreviation Review Exercises, Self-Assessment Questions, and other Review Exercises and Activities. Answers to questions are provided at the back of the book, making this an excellent resource for self-study and review.

Foundations of Nursing Procedures Checklist

ISBN-10: 1-4283-1784-8
ISBN-13: 978-1-4283-1784-0

This excellent resource helps students evaluate their comprehension and execution of all the basic, intermediate and advanced procedures covered in the core book.

Foundations of Nursing Online Companion

ISBN-10: 1-4283-1779-1
ISBN-13: 978-1-4283-1779-6

The Online Companion gives online access to all the components in the Instructor's Resource as well as additional tools to reinforce the content in each chapter and enhance classroom teaching. Multimedia animations, Concept Care Map Model, and Physical Assessment Guide are just some of the many resources found on this robust site. To access the site for *Foundations of Nursing*, third edition, simply point your browser to http://www.delmar.cengage.com/companions. Select the nursing discipline and then select *Foundations of Nursing*, third edition.

CL eBook to accompany *Foundations of Nursing*, third edition

Printed access code ISBN-10: 1-4354-8793-1
Printed access code ISBN-13: 978-1-4354-8793-2
Instant access code ISBN-10: 1-4354-8792-3
Instant access code ISBN-13: 978-1-4354-8792-5

Foundations of Nursing WebTutor Advantage on Blackboard

ISBN-10: 1-4283-1781-3
ISBN-13: 978-1-4283-1781-9

Foundations of Nursing WebTutor Advantage on WebCT

ISBN-10: 1-4283-1782-1
ISBN-13: 978-1-4283-1782-6

- A complete online environment that supplements the course provided in both Blackboard and WebCT format.
- Includes chapter overviews, chapter outlines, and competencies.
- Useful classroom management tools include chats and calendars, as well as instructor resources such as the instructor slides created in PowerPoint.
- Multimedia offering includes video clips and 3D animations.
- Comprehensive Audio Glossary with all terms and definitions from this text in downloadable audio format.

ABOUT THE AUTHORS

Lois Elain Wacker White earned a diploma in nursing from Memorial Hospital School of Nursing, Springfield, Illinois; an Associate degree in Science from Del Mar College, Corpus Christi, Texas; a Bachelor of Science in Nursing from Texas A & I University—Corpus Christi, Corpus Christi, Texas; a Master of Science in Education from Corpus Christi State University, Corpus Christi, Texas; and a Doctor of Philosophy degree in education administration—community college from the University of Texas, Austin, Texas.

She has taught at Del Mar College, Corpus Christi, Texas, in both the Associate Degree Nursing program and the Vocational Nursing program. For 14 years, she was also chairperson of the Department of Vocational Nurse Education. Dr. White has taught fundamentals of nursing, mental health/mental illness, medical-surgical nursing, and maternal/pediatric nursing. Her professional career has also included 15 years of clinical practice.

Dr. White has served on the Nursing Education Advisory Committee of the Board of Nurse Examiners for the State of Texas and the Board of Vocational Nurse Examiners, which developed competencies expected of graduates for each level of nursing.

Gena Duncan has worked as an RN for 36 years in the clinical, community health, and educational arenas. This has equipped Mrs. Duncan with a wide range of nursing experiences and varied skills to meet the educational needs of today's students. She has a MSEd and MSN.

During her professional career, Mrs. Duncan served as a staff nurse, an assistant head nurse of a medical-surgical unit, a continuing education instructor, an associate professor in an LPN program, and director of an Associate degree nursing program. She has taught LPN, ADN, BSN, and MSN nursing students. As a faculty member, she taught many nursing courses and served on a statewide curriculum committee for a state college. As director of an Associate degree nursing program, she was instrumental in starting and obtaining state board approval of an LPN-RN nursing program.

Her master's research thesis was entitled, "An Investigation of Learning Styles of Practical and Baccalaureate Students." The results of the study are published in the *Journal of Nursing Education*. She has coauthored two textbooks, a medical-surgical textbook, and a transitions text for LPN to RN students. She has been an active member of Sigma Theta Tau.

Wendy Baumle is currently a nursing instructor at James A. Rhodes State College in Ohio. She has spent 19 years as a clinician, educator, school district health coordinator, and academician. Mrs. Baumle has taught fundamentals of nursing, medical-surgical nursing, pediatrics, obstetrics, pharmacology, anatomy and physiology, and ethics in health care in practical nursing and associate nursing degree programs. She has previously taught at Lutheran College, Fort Wayne, Indiana, at Northwest State Community College, Archbold, Ohio, and at James. A. Rhodes State College in Lima, Ohio. Mrs. Baumle earned her Bachelor of Science degree in Nursing from The University of Toledo, Toledo, Ohio and her Master's degree in Nursing from The Medical College of Ohio, Toledo, Ohio. Mrs. Baumle is a member of a number of professional nursing organizations, including Sigma Theta Tau, the American Nurses Association, the National League for Nursing, and the Ohio Nurses Association.

ACKNOWLEDGMENTS

Many people must work together to produce any textbook, but a comprehensive book such as this requires even more people with various areas of expertise. We would like to thank the contributors for their time and effort to share their knowledge gained through years of experience in both the clinical and academic settings. Nancy Emke, clinical nurse oncology specialist at Parkview Health Comprehensive Cancer Center, contributed content to Chapter 2, Holistic Care.

To the reviewers, we thank you for your time spent critically reading the manuscript, expertise, and valuable suggestions that have added to this text.

We would like to acknowledge and sincerely thank the entire team at Delmar Cengage Learning who has worked to make this textbook a reality. Juliet Steiner, senior product manager, receives a special thank you. She has kept us on track and provided guidance with humor, enthusiasm, sensitivity, and expertise. We extend a special thank you to Steve Helba, executive editor, for his vision for this text, calm demeanor, and patience. Other members on the team—Marah Bellegarde, managing editor, James Zayicek, senior content product manager, Jack Pendleton, senior art director, and Meghan Orvis, editorial assistant, have all worked diligently for the completion of this textbook. Thank you to all.

HOW TO USE THIS TEXT

This text is designed with you, the reader, in mind. Special elements and feature boxes appear throughout the text to guide you in reading and to assist you in learning the material. Following are suggestions for how you can use these features to increase your understanding and mastery of the content.

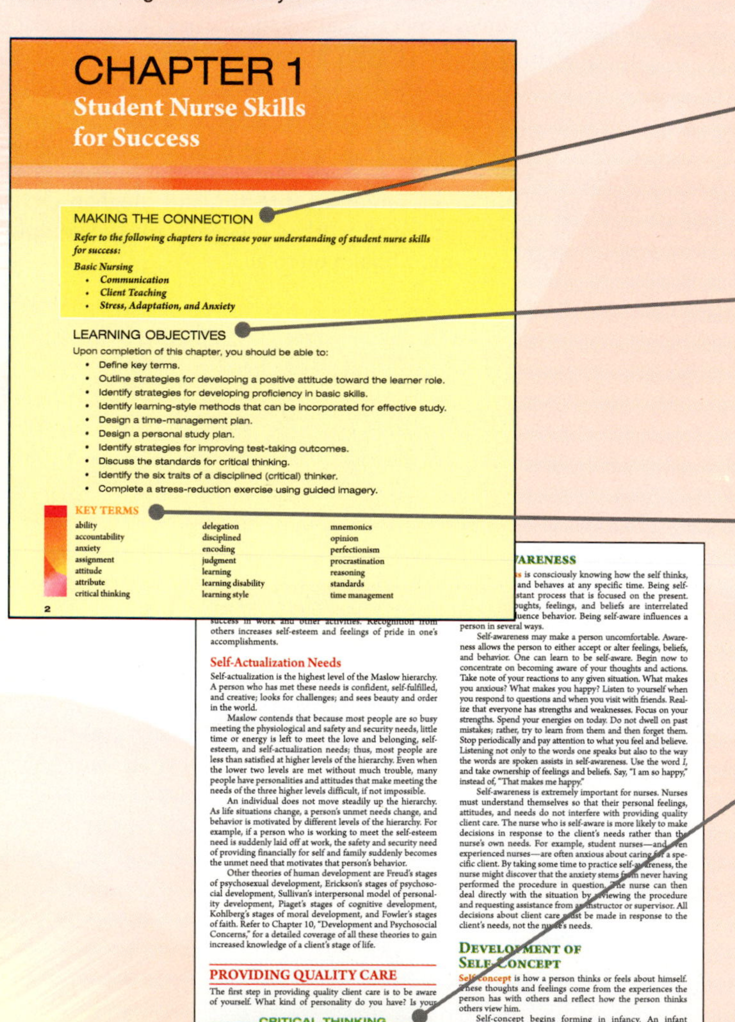

CHAPTER 1
Student Nurse Skills for Success

MAKING THE CONNECTION

Refer to the following chapters to increase your understanding of student nurse skills for success:

Basic Nursing
- ***Communication***
- ***Client Teaching***
- ***Stress, Adaptation, and Anxiety***

LEARNING OBJECTIVES

Upon completion of this chapter, you should be able to:
- Define key terms.
- Outline strategies for developing a positive attitude toward the learner role.
- Identify strategies for developing proficiency in basic skills.
- Identify learning-style methods that can be incorporated for effective study.
- Design a time-management plan.
- Design a personal study plan.
- Identify strategies for improving test-taking outcomes.
- Discuss the standards for critical thinking.
- Identify the six traits of a disciplined (critical) thinker.
- Complete a stress-reduction exercise using guided imagery.

KEY TERMS

ability
accountability
anxiety
assignment
attitude
attribute
critical thinking
delegation
disciplined
encoding
judgment
learning
learning disability
learning style
mnemonics
opinion
perfectionism
procrastination
reasoning
standards
time management

2

others increases self-esteem and feelings of pride in one's accomplishments.

Self-Actualization Needs

Self-actualization is the highest level of the Maslow hierarchy. A person who has met these needs is confident, self-fulfilled, and creative; looks for challenges; and sees beauty and order in the world.

Maslow contends that because most people are so busy meeting the physiological and safety and security needs, little time or energy is left to meet the love and belonging, self-esteem, and self-actualization needs; thus, most people are less than satisfied at higher levels of the hierarchy. Even when the lower two levels are met without much trouble, many people have personalities and attitudes that make meeting the needs of the three higher levels difficult, if not impossible.

An individual does not move steadily up the hierarchy. As life situations change, a person's unmet needs change, and behavior is motivated by different levels of the hierarchy. For example, if a person who is working to meet the self-esteem need is suddenly laid off at work, the safety and security need of providing financially for self and family suddenly becomes the unmet need that motivates that person's behavior.

Other theories of human development are Freud's stages of psychosexual development, Erickson's stages of psychosocial development, Sullivan's interpersonal model of personality development, Piaget's stages of cognitive development, Kohlberg's stages of moral development, and Fowler's stages of faith. Refer to Chapter 10, "Development and Psychosocial Concerns," for a detailed coverage of all these theories to gain increased knowledge of a client's stage of life.

PROVIDING QUALITY CARE

The first step in providing quality client care is to be aware of yourself. What kind of personality do you have? Is your

CRITICAL THINKING

Health and Wellness

What are your attitudes about health and wellness?

…ARENESS

…s is consciously knowing how the self thinks, … and behaves at any specific time. Being self-… …stant process that is focused on the present. …oughts, feelings, and beliefs are interrelated …luence behavior. Being self-aware influences a person in several ways.

Self-awareness may make a person uncomfortable. Awareness allows the person to either accept or alter feelings, beliefs, and behavior. One can learn to be self-aware. Begin now to concentrate on becoming aware of your thoughts and actions. Take note of your reactions to any given situation. What makes you anxious? What makes you happy? Listen to yourself when you respond to questions and when you visit with friends. Realize that everyone has strengths and weaknesses. Focus on your strengths. Spend your energies on today. Do not dwell on past mistakes; rather, try to learn from them and then forget them. Stop periodically and pay attention to what you feel and believe. Listening not only to the words one speaks but also to the way the words are spoken assists in self-awareness. Use the word *I*, and take ownership of feelings and beliefs. Say, "I am so happy," instead of, "That makes me happy."

Self-awareness is extremely important for nurses. Nurses must understand themselves so that their personal feelings, attitudes, and needs do not interfere with providing quality client care. The nurse who is self-aware is more likely to make decisions in response to the client's needs rather than the nurse's own needs. For example, student nurses—and even experienced nurses—are often anxious about caring for a specific client. By taking some time to practice self-awareness, the nurse might discover that the anxiety stems from never having performed the procedure in question. The nurse can then deal directly with the situation by reviewing the procedure and requesting assistance from an instructor or supervisor. All decisions about client care must be made in response to the client's needs, not the nurse's needs.

DEVELOPMENT OF SELF-CONCEPT

Self-concept is how a person thinks or feels about himself. These thoughts and feelings come from the experiences the person has with others and reflect how the person thinks others view him.

Self-concept begins forming in infancy. An infant whose needs are met feels satisfied and good. Experiences, both positive and negative, influence a person's self-concept (Figure 2-5). Interactions with significant others, such as parents, extended family, and friends, have a great impact on self-concept. This is true not only during the developing years but also throughout life. Because of its influence on client care, it is important for the nurse to be aware of how

MAKING THE CONNECTION

Read these boxes before beginning a chapter to link material across the holistic care continuum and to tie new content to the material you have already encountered.

LEARNING OBJECTIVES

Read the chapter objectives before reading the chapter to set the stage for learning. Revisit the objectives when preparing for an exam to see which entries you can respond to with "Yes, I can do that."

KEY TERMS

Review this list before reading the chapter to familiarize yourself with the new terms and to revisit those terms you already know to link them to the content in the new chapter.

CRITICAL THINKING

Visit these boxes after reading the entire chapter to check your understanding of the concepts presented.

HOW TO USE THIS TEXT (Continued)

PROFESSIONAL TIP

Use these boxes to increase your professional competence and confidence, and to expand your knowledge base.

COMMUNITY/HOME HEALTH CARE

Read these boxes before making a home visit to a client with a given disorder.

CULTURAL CONSIDERATIONS

Test your sensitivity to cultural and ethnic diversity by scanning these boxes and using the guidelines and suggestions in your practice. You may also want to ask yourself what biases or preconceptions you have about different cultural practices before reading a chapter and then read these boxes for information that may help you be more sensitive in your nursing care and approach to clients.

MEMORY TRICK

Use the mnemonic devices provided in the new Memory Trick feature to help you remember the correct steps or proper order of information when working with clients.

HOW TO USE THIS TEXT (Continued)

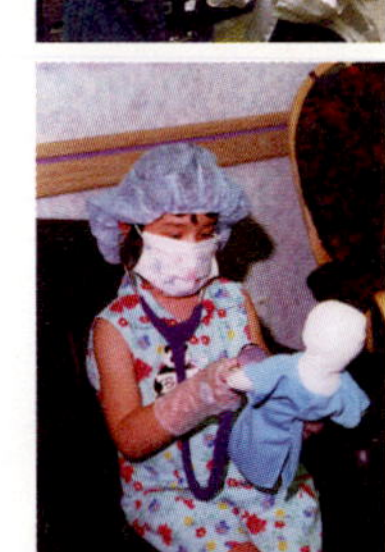

COLLABORATIVE CARE

These boxes explain which other health care professionals may be involved in the comprehensive care offered to clients. Review these boxes and ask yourself if you understand how your role as a nurse will complement the care provided by others on the health care team.

DRUG ICONS

These symbols draw attention to information relating to the pharmacological management available for certain disorders. Review these sections to understand the pharmacological treatments appropriate for your clients' conditions.

INFECTION CONTROL

When reading a chapter, stop and pay attention to these features and ask yourself, "Had I thought of that? Do I practice these precautions?"

LIFE SPAN CONSIDERATIONS

Use these boxes to increase your awareness of variations in care based on client age; this will help you deliver more effective and appropriate care.

CLIENT TEACHING

Read these boxes to gain insight into client learning needs related to the specific disorder or condition. You may want to make your own index cards or electronic notes listing these teaching guidelines to use when you are working with clients.

HOW TO USE THIS TEXT (Continued)

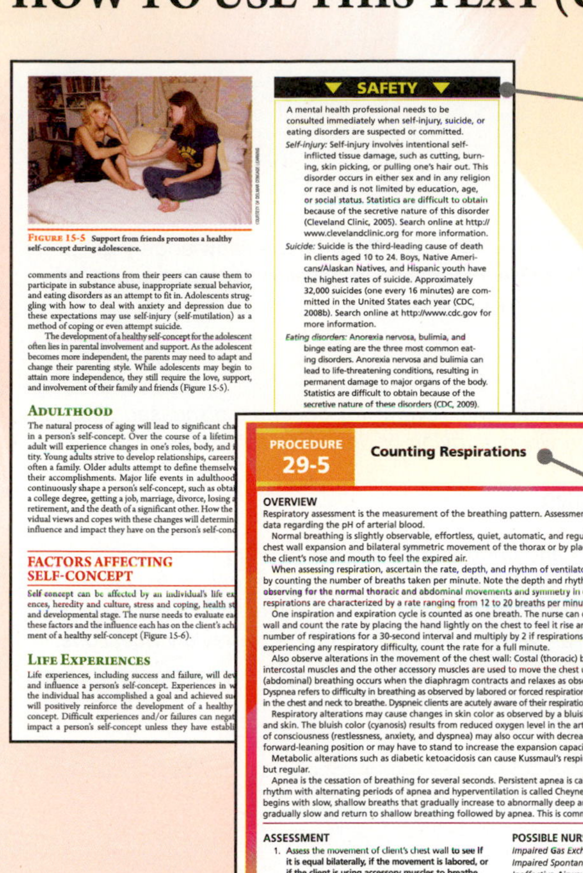

SAFETY

Pause while reading to consider these elements and quiz yourself, "Do I take steps such as these to ensure my own and the client's safety? Do I follow these guidelines in every practice encounter?"

PROCEDURES

Reference the procedures as you read the chapters. Study the techniques, review the figures, and be prepared for your clinical days with questions of clarification for your instructor.

SAMPLE NURSING CARE PLAN

Use this feature to test your understanding and application of the content presented. Ask yourself, "Would I have come up with the same nursing diagnoses? Are these the interventions that I would have proposed? What other interventions would be appropriate?"

CONCEPT CARE MAPS

Review these graphical tools to help incorporate the interrelatedness of nursing concepts in preparation for clinical practice.

HOW TO USE THIS TEXT (Continued)

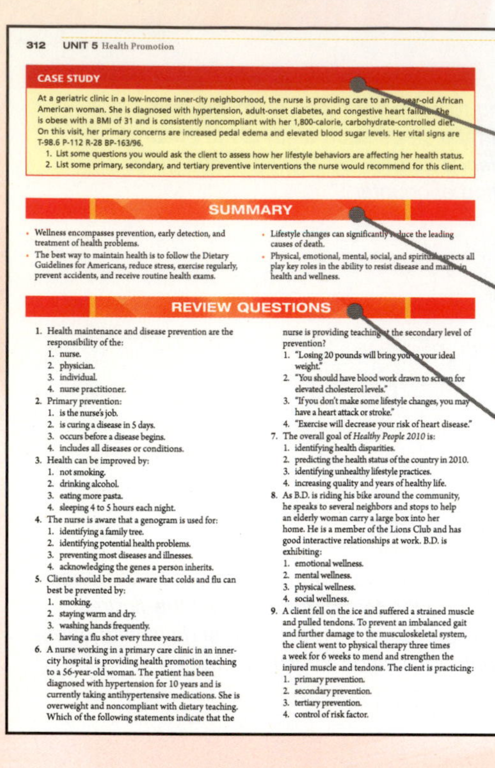

312 UNIT 5 Health Promotion

CASE STUDY

At a geriatric clinic in a low-income inner-city neighborhood, the nurse is providing care to an [illegible]-year-old African American woman. She is diagnosed with hypertension, adult-onset diabetes, and congestive heart failure. She is obese with a BMI of 31 and is consistently noncompliant with her 1,800-calorie, carbohydrate-controlled diet. On this visit, her primary concerns are increased pedal edema and elevated blood sugar levels. Her vital signs are T-98.6 P-112 R-28 BP-163/96.

1. List some questions you would ask the client to assess how her lifestyle behaviors are affecting her health status.
2. List some primary, secondary, and tertiary preventive interventions the nurse would recommend for this client.

SUMMARY

- Wellness encompasses prevention, early detection, and treatment of health problems.
- The best way to maintain health is to follow the Dietary Guidelines for Americans, reduce stress, exercise regularly, prevent accidents, and receive routine health exams.
- Lifestyle changes can significantly reduce the leading causes of death.
- Physical, emotional, mental, social, and spiritual aspects all play key roles in the ability to resist disease and maintain health and wellness.

REVIEW QUESTIONS

1. Health maintenance and disease prevention are the responsibility of the:
   1. nurse.
   2. physician.
   3. individual.
   4. nurse practitioner.
2. Primary prevention:
   1. is the nurse's job.
   2. is curing a disease in 5 days.
   3. occurs before a disease begins.
   4. includes all diseases or conditions.
3. Health can be improved by:
   1. not smoking.
   2. drinking alcohol.
   3. eating more pasta.
   4. sleeping 4 to 5 hours each night.
4. The nurse is aware that a genogram is used for:
   1. identifying a family tree.
   2. identifying potential health problems.
   3. preventing most diseases and illnesses.
   4. acknowledging the genes a person inherits.
5. Clients should be made aware that colds and flu can best be prevented by:
   1. smoking.
   2. staying warm and dry.
   3. washing hands frequently.
   4. having a flu shot every three years.
6. A nurse working in a primary care clinic in an inner-city hospital is providing health promotion teaching to a 56-year-old woman. The patient has been diagnosed with hypertension for 10 years and is currently taking antihypertensive medications. She is overweight and noncompliant with dietary teaching. Which of the following statements indicate that the nurse is providing teaching at the secondary level of prevention?
   1. "Losing 20 pounds will bring you to your ideal weight."
   2. "You should have blood work drawn to screen for elevated cholesterol levels."
   3. "If you don't make some lifestyle changes, you may have a heart attack or stroke."
   4. "Exercise will decrease your risk of heart disease."
7. The overall goal of *Healthy People 2010* is:
   1. identifying health disparities.
   2. predicting the health status of the country in 2010.
   3. identifying unhealthy lifestyle practices.
   4. increasing quality and years of healthy life.
8. As B.D. is riding his bike around the community, he speaks to several neighbors and stops to help an elderly woman carry a large box into her home. He is a member of the Lions Club and has good interactive relationships at work. B.D. is exhibiting:
   1. emotional wellness.
   2. mental wellness.
   3. physical wellness.
   4. social wellness.
9. A client fell on the ice and suffered a strained muscle and pulled tendons. To prevent an imbalanced gait and further damage to the musculoskeletal system, the client went to physical therapy three times a week for 6 weeks to mend and strengthen the injured muscle and tendons. The client is practicing:
   1. primary prevention.
   2. secondary prevention.
   3. tertiary prevention.
   4. control of risk factor.

CASE STUDY

Read over these boxes within the text. Draw on the knowledge you have gained and synthesize information to develop your own educated responses to the case study challenges.

SUMMARY

Carefully read the bulleted list to review key concepts discussed. This is an excellent resource when studying or preparing for exams.

REVIEW QUESTIONS

Test your knowledge and understanding by answering the NCLEX®-style review questions with each chapter. These are an excellent way to test your mastery of the concepts covered in the chapter, and a good opportunity to become familiar with answering NCLEX®-style review questions.

HOW TO USE STUDYWARE™ TO ACCOMPANY FOUNDATIONS OF NURSING, THIRD EDITION

Minimum System Requirements

- Operating systems: Microsoft Windows XP w/SP 2, Windows Vista w/ SP 1, Windows 7
- Processor: Minimum required by Operating System
- Memory: Minimum required by Operating System
- Hard Drive Space: 500 MB
- Screen resolution: 1024 x 768 pixels
- CD-ROM drive
- Sound card & listening device required for audio features
- Flash Player 10. The Adobe Flash Player is free, and can be downloaded from http://www.adobe.com/products/flashplayer/

Setup Instructions

1. Insert disc into CD-ROM drive. The StudyWare™ installation program should start automatically. If it does not, go to step 2.
2. From My Computer, double-click the icon for the CD drive.
3. Double-click the *setup.exe* file to start the program.

Technical Support

Telephone: 1-800-648-7450
8:30 A.M.–6:30 P.M. Eastern Time
E-mail: delmar.help@cengage.com

StudyWARE™ is a trademark used herein under license.

Microsoft® and Windows® are registered trademarks of the Microsoft Corporation.

Pentium® is a registered trademark of the Intel Corporation.

Getting Started

The StudyWARE™ software helps you learn terms and concepts in *Foundations of Nursing*, third edition. As you study each chapter in the text, be sure to explore the activities in the corresponding chapter in the software. Use StudyWARE™ as your own private tutor to help you learn the material in your *Foundations of Nursing*, third edition textbook.

Getting started is easy! Install the software by following the installation instructions provided above. When you open the software, enter your first and last name so the software can store your quiz results. Then choose a chapter or section from the menu to take a quiz or explore media and activities.

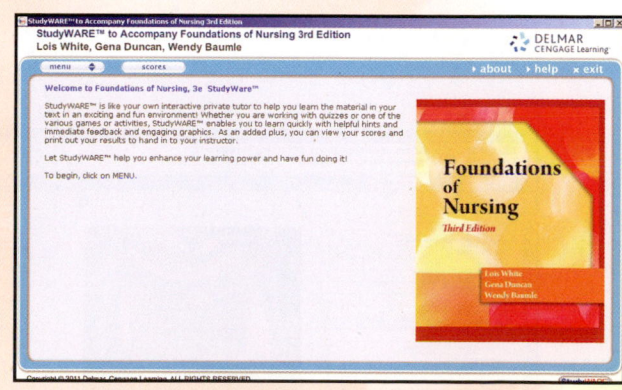

HOW TO USE STUDYWARE™ (Continued)

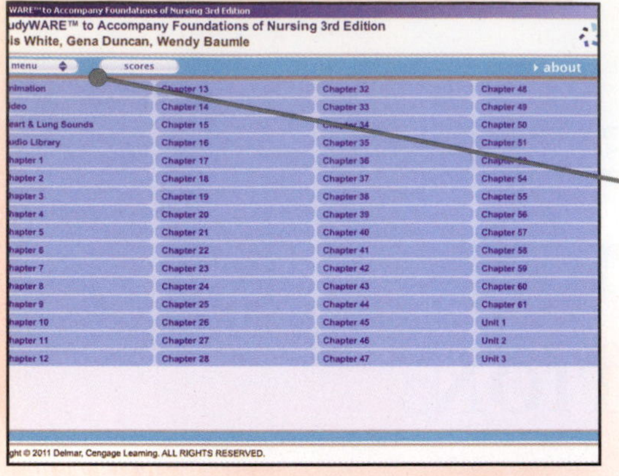

MENU

You can access the menu from wherever you are in the program. The Menu includes Animations, Video, Heart & Lung Sounds, Chapter activities for all didactic chapters, and NCLEX®-Style Quizzes for each major unit. You can also access your scores from the button to the right of the main menu button.

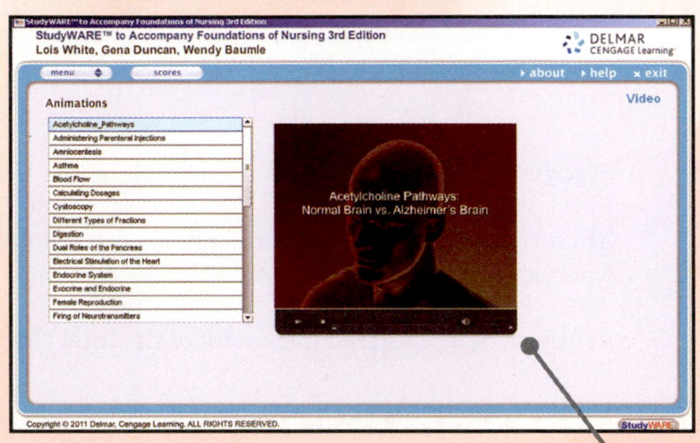

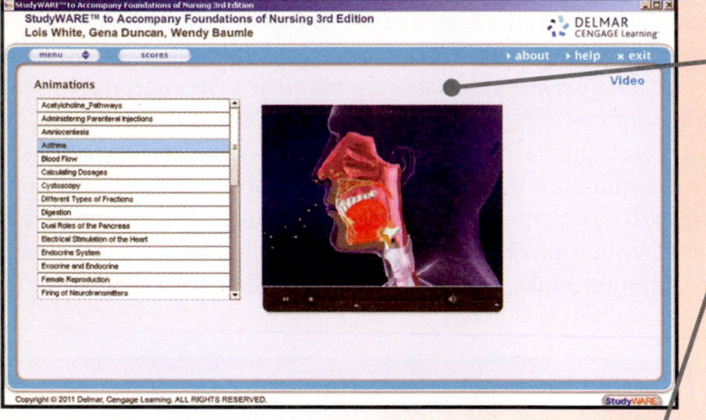

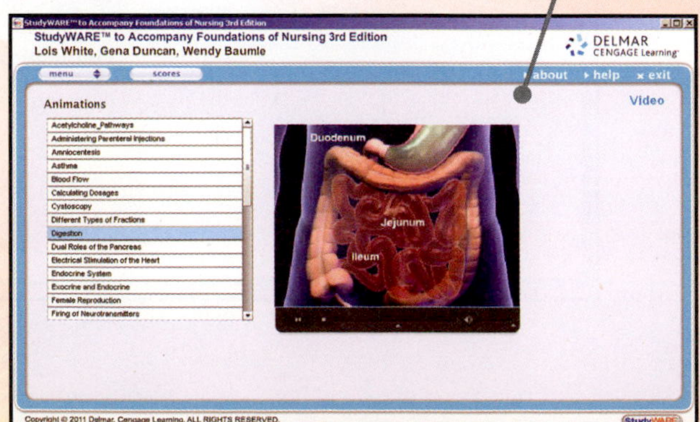

ANIMATION

This section on your StudyWARE™ CD-ROM provides 35 multimedia animations of biological, anatomical, and pharmacological processes. These animations visually explain some of the more difficult concepts and are an engaging resource to support your understanding.

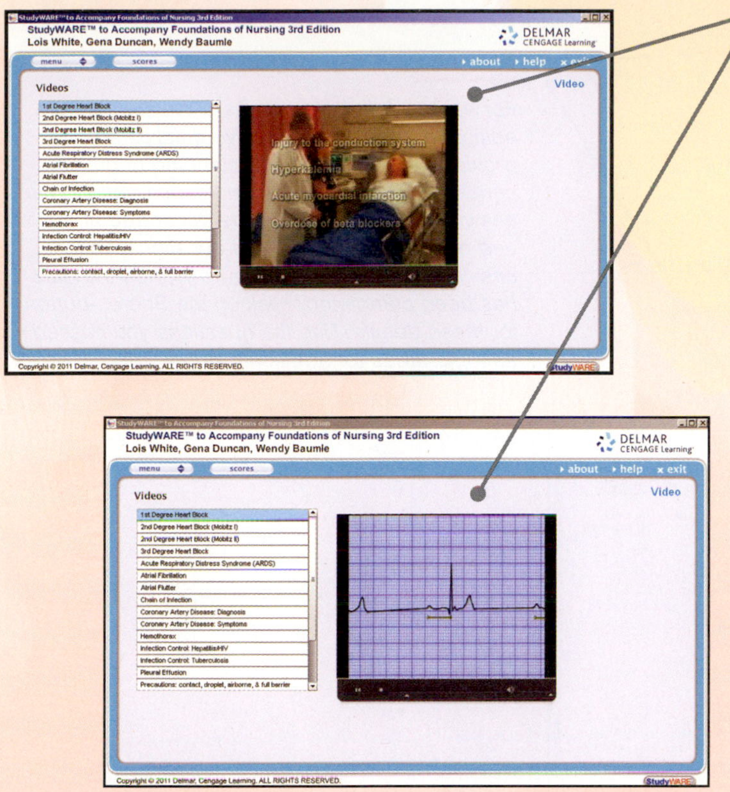

VIDEO

A selection of 20 high quality video clips on topics ranging from infection control to the cardiovascular and respiratory systems has been provided. Click on the clip you would like to view, then click on the play button on the media viewer in the center of the screen. These video clips, many of which were developed by Concept Media, are a wonderful resource to help visualize difficult processes and skills.

HEART & LUNG SOUNDS

This searchable multimedia program provides a comprehensive library of audio files for different heart and lung sounds that will be encountered by nurses. Sounds can be viewed according to category or specific sounds can be found by using the alphabetical term search function. In addition to hearing the sounds, related information about etiology and auscultation is provided.

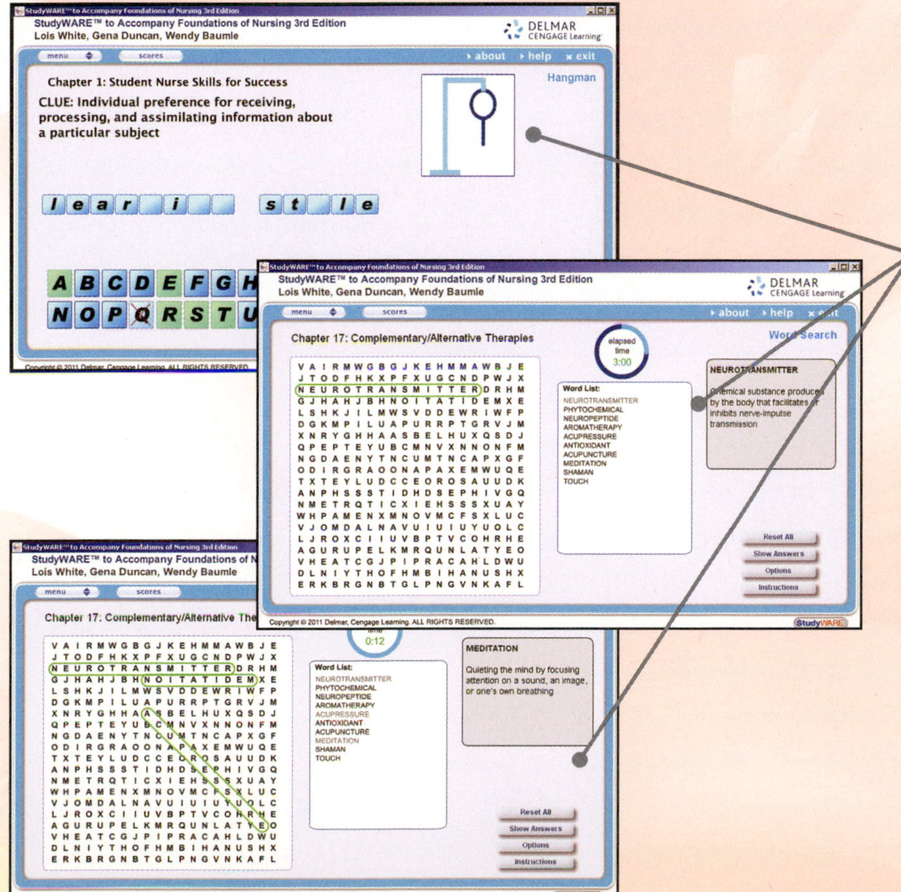

CHAPTER ACTIVITIES

For each chapter from Foundations of Nursing, third edition, that contains glossary terms, games and activities are provided to help you master the terminology in a fun and interesting way. Concentration is a memory game that asks you to flip cards to match definitions with their terms. Flash Cards allow you to test your knowledge of a term by reading the term, thinking about the definition, then checking the actual definition. Hangman follows the traditional hangman game format and can be played by one or two players, challenging you to fill in the blanks for a term before the puzzle is completed. Crossword Puzzles provide definitions of key terms as clues so you can fill in the the appropriate term and clear the board.

HOW TO USE STUDYWARE™ (Continued)

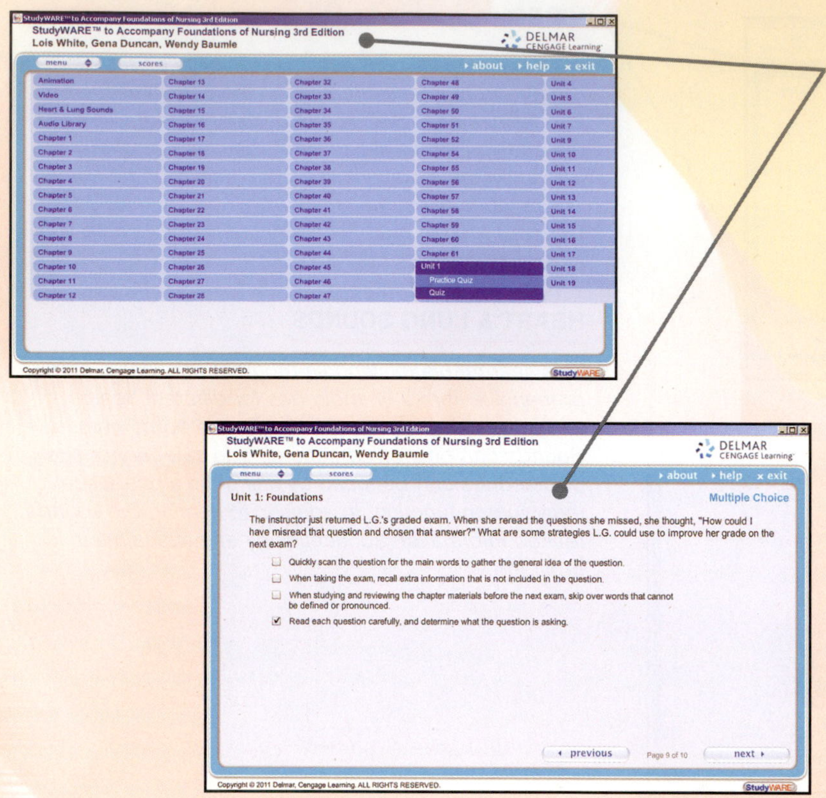

QUIZZES

For each unit in Foundations of Nursing, third edition, both practice and live quizzes are provided to test your understanding of critical concepts. The quiz program keeps track of your answers and a report can be generated at the end of the quiz outlining the questions, your answer, and the correct answer. Once the quiz has been completed, click on the Scores button for these details. Use the questions you missed as topic areas for additional study.

SECTION I

Basic Nursing

UNIT 1 Foundations

CHAPTER 1
Student Nurse Skills for Success

MAKING THE CONNECTION

Refer to the following chapters to increase your understanding of student nurse skills for success:

Basic Nursing

- ***Communication***
- ***Client Teaching***
- ***Stress, Adaptation, and Anxiety***

LEARNING OBJECTIVES

Upon completion of this chapter, you should be able to:

- Define key terms.
- Outline strategies for developing a positive attitude toward the learner role.
- Identify strategies for developing proficiency in basic skills.
- Identify learning-style methods that can be incorporated for effective study.
- Design a time-management plan.
- Design a personal study plan.
- Identify strategies for improving test-taking outcomes.
- Discuss the standards for critical thinking.
- Identify the six traits of a disciplined (critical) thinker.
- Complete a stress-reduction exercise using guided imagery.

KEY TERMS

ability
accountability
anxiety
assignment
attitude
attribute
critical thinking
delegation
disciplined
encoding
judgment
learning
learning disability
learning style
mnemonics
opinion
perfectionism
procrastination
reasoning
standards
time management

INTRODUCTION

Welcome to practical/vocational nursing. You have chosen one of life's rewarding careers. The next few months of your life will be challenging, exhilarating, frustrating, and full of new experiences. When you consider the difficulty of the nursing program's admission process, being a member of this nursing class is no small achievement. The fact that you have survived the admissions process demonstrates that you are capable of overcoming the challenges that lie ahead. Balancing family, community, and school responsibilities will require self-discipline.

LEARNING

Learning is defined as the act or process of acquiring knowledge and/or skill in a particular subject. An individual never stops learning. This is especially true in the field of nursing and health care. The amount of information within the health care domain has expanded exponentially in just the past several years. Consider, for example, the advances in drug therapies, complementary/alternative therapies, and genetics. By graduation, some of the information learned in the beginning of the program will have been displaced by new information and discoveries. We are living in the information age and have constant access to thousands of pieces of information through various media, including television and the Internet. Knowledge is never static. Learning also is not static but, rather, is a lifelong process.

Individuals seek knowledge to effect some type of change. As a student, you are seeking knowledge to learn skills and to prepare yourself for a career in nursing. Referring to yourself as a learner implies that you are an active participant in the learning process, as opposed to a passive recipient of information. You bring to this new adventure yourself, your past experiences, your abilities, and your motivation to master the knowledge necessary to reach your goals. You have already learned much in your lifetime and are ready to continue the process. It is important that you take some time to think about the competencies needed for the role of learner. It is equally important to realize that *you* are in charge of developing the competencies that will enable you to learn.

The learning you are seeking will afford you the knowledge and skills necessary to become a nurse and, thus, to demonstrate your ability to competently provide care to clients who seek your professional talents. Nursing education is different from many other college majors in the turnaround time allowed for learning. Few other disciplines require the student to apply on Thursday that which was acquired on Monday. Nursing students must acquire a greater depth of understanding in a shorter amount of time; to achieve this, basic learning processes will need to be well developed.

This chapter addresses *how* you learn rather than *what* you learn. It focuses on competencies necessary to master the learning process: attitude, basic skills, learning style, time management, study strategies, critical thinking, and test-taking strategies. Assessing which habits you already practice and which ones you have yet to incorporate, internalize, and utilize will assist you in improving your process of learning. As you do so, your potential for attaining your goals will increase.

> **PROFESSIONALTIP**
>
> **Learning**
>
> The key to your success is not how you are taught but how you decide to learn.

DEVELOP A POSITIVE ATTITUDE

Attitude is defined as a manner, feeling, or position toward a person or thing. In order to effect change in your behavior, you must first develop a positive attitude about the experience you are about to begin. You are in charge of setting yourself up for success. This is your opportunity to acquire the knowledge and skills that will make it possible for you to reach the goal of becoming a licensed practical/vocational nurse. Start by developing a positive attitude toward yourself as a person and a learner as well as a genuine desire to learn. To maintain this attitude late at night when you are struggling over the names of the latest drugs and writing client assessments, you must be convinced that you have the capability to complete your task, that some intrinsic factor will be able to support you in the pursuit of your goal. This positive self-attitude sustains the question "Why am I doing this?" Among the strategies you can practice to help you build a positive attitude are the following:

- Create positive self-images and visualize yourself attaining your goals.
- Recognize your abilities.
- Identify realistic expectations.

Create Positive Self-Images

To create a positive self-image, you must know those attributes that are unique to you. An **attribute** is a characteristic, either positive or negative, that belongs to you. For instance, some positive attributes that are typical to nurses include caring and compassion. Attributes are sometimes referred to as strengths and weaknesses. Whatever you call them, you must actively engage in listing and recalling these qualities about yourself. Divide a paper into two columns, with one headed positive and the other negative. List as many words describing your attributes as you can.

Which side has more entries? Did you start with the negative list? It is unfortunate that sometimes we can recall the negatives faster than the positives. We often speak about ourselves in negative terms, which creates negative self-images. For example, you may recall thinking some of the following: "I wish I were thinner . . . ," "I hope I can do this, I'm not very good at math." Neither of these statements draws a positive image of the speaker. You may need to lose 10 pounds or improve your math skills, but these are not the total measure of your attributes. If they are the only qualities you recall, they might become the overall image you see of yourself. Regardless of where you started, you must concentrate on the positive side of the chart. You must actively recall your positive side at least as often as you recount the things that could be improved.

Begin to speak of yourself in positive terms and accept compliments from yourself! When an assignment is particularly difficult, you can refocus from "I hope I can do this. I have never been good at math" to "I can read and follow the chapter instructions on how to complete the problems." This simple restatement can sometimes make the difference between success or failure at attempts to acquire new knowledge.

The list does not have to stop at just the words you write today. Continue to practice and do periodic self-assessments. You will add more and more words to the positive side and begin to complement yourself more often. When things go awry, you will be able to draw on these positive attributes and know that you have these strengths.

Recognize Your Abilities

Recognizing your abilities is also an attitude builder. **Ability** can be defined as competence in an activity. An ability is something you can learn; competency is proficiency in a task. Your degree of competence as a nurse will depend on such factors as prior exposure, motivation, how often and with whom you practice, expectations of those things that you should be doing, and a willingness to laugh at attempts and learn from mistakes.

You have abilities and skills that you perform well. To acquire these skills took courage, discipline, and hard work. Recalling these abilities and the ways you developed competency in them not only adds to your positive self-image, but also showcases your strengths. Begin by making a four-column chart with the headings "I am really good at . . ."; "Skills I currently have to be 'really good' . . ."; "I avoid doing . . ."; and "Skills I need to be 'really good'. . . ." In the second column, list the skills you presently have to be "really good." In the third column, write the things you tend to avoid doing. Finally, in the fourth column, list the skills you need to acquire to be "really good" at the tasks you "avoid doing" (refer to Table 1-1).

For example, perhaps you wrote, "I am really good at cooking." Some skills you could have written are the following:

- *Arithmetic:* You must have an understanding of fractions and the relationships of parts to the whole.
- *Reading:* You must comprehend the words in the recipe in order to follow all the steps.
- *Prioritizing:* You must know with what items to start in order to have all of the food ready at the same time.
- *Risk taking:* You may worry about whether your guests will like your dish, but you persist, confident in your ability to turn the raw ingredients into a delicious meal.

Now look at the third column. Maybe you wrote math. Mathematics is an ability you must develop in order to safely administer medications to your clients. If you view this skill only as something to avoid, you begin with a negative attitude toward an ability you will need. You are creating a negative image of yourself completing this task. Instead, look to your past experiences for your strengths; you may realize that you already possess much of the mathematical knowledge you need to correctly compute medication dosages. Realizing this puts a positive slant on this ability.

Now you must develop mathematical competency. Begin by listing the skills needed to perform mathematical operations. You must pay attention to details, understand the way parts relate to the whole, and have solid skills in arithmetic (addition, subtraction, division, and multiplication). Mathematics requires you to choose appropriate formulas to solve a variety of real-world problems. For example, to give the correct dose of medication to your client, you must know the correct formula to use for the calculation. This is a real-world problem for which you must both choose the correct formula and understand it. You must then accurately perform the arithmetic operations.

Identify Realistic Expectations

As mentioned earlier, developing a positive self-image is of primary importance to learning. Your expectations regarding how you will perform in the role as a learner affects your attitude toward both yourself and learning. You have an expectation about the way you will progress through the nursing program. Ideally, you will attend all classes, pass all exams, and graduate. Further, your current life responsibilities will cooperate with and support this plan. You will likely, however, encounter at least some obstacles. When you hit that first "speed bump" to your plan, your ability to look at the reality of your expectations will be important in regaining a positive focus. Consider the following example:

> G. is a 25-year-old female enrolled full time in a nursing program for the fall. She did well in high school and has already attended a college part time prior to this program. G. expects that she will get grades in the B and A range, as she did in prior course work. She works full time and has a 4-year-old daughter. When the class schedule is published, the times conflict with one of the days that she works. This will cause her to be 20 minutes late to work on that day. She has not shared with her employer that she is attending school. She has child care for her daughter, but the need to arrive at the clinical site at 7 A.M. means that she must rearrange her child care and that she will be 30 minutes late for clinical on Fridays. She does not tell her instructors of her time constraints for child care. She has always needed quiet time for study and is a morning person. G. finds her reading assignments take twice as long as she had planned. With all her other responsibilities, her only time for study is after her daughter goes to bed. She has a family that lives close by, but she does not like to burden them with

Table 1-1 Recognizing Your Abilities

"I AM REALLY GOOD AT . . ."	SKILLS I HAVE TO BE "REALLY GOOD . . ."	"I AVOID DOING . . ."	SKILLS I NEED TO BE "REALLY GOOD. . ."
Cooking	Arithmetic	Math	Attention to details
	Reading		Understanding the way parts relate to the whole
	Prioritizing		Solid skills in addition, subtraction, division, and multiplication
	Risk taking		

COURTESY OF DELMAR CENGAGE LEARNING

baby-sitting. She has always found a way to do things on her own in the past.

G. is a capable person, but her expectation of being able to control all the various facets of her life in perfect harmony is unrealistic. Maintaining a positive attitude while in the midst of the stress of completing all the tasks at hand is difficult, if not impossible, and the plan is often abandoned. In G.'s case, abandoning the plan may mean abandoning her plans for school. G.'s reality is that she cannot increase her time commitment by 30 hours of school work and keep everything else she does at the same level. She must set priorities with regard to the demands on her time, and she must identify realistic expectations for those things that she can accomplish.

When everything on your "to do" list cannot be completed, change the way you approach the list and realign your expectations. One way to do this is to ask for help. Asking for help is not a weakness, it is a success strategy. The most successful people are typically those who know when to ask for help and who have devised a plan to structure that help. In the previous example, G. needs to remove some of the stress related to work, child care, and school commitments by informing her employer and instructors of her situation and asking for their help in guiding her to manage the many demands. Help may mean something as simple as talking to the employer about coming in 20 minutes late and working 20 minutes longer and asking a family member to take her daughter to the child care place on Fridays.

If you do not set realistic expectations for yourself, you may fall victim to a positive attitude's biggest enemy, perfectionism. **Perfectionism** is an overwhelming expectation of being able to get everything done in a flawless manner. This is a setup for failure because it is a standard no one can achieve. Table 1-2 suggests some behaviors of perfectionists versus those of pursuers of excellence. Which list describes you most accurately? Remember to strive to be as realistic with your expectations as possible; be patient with yourself and ask for help when needed.

DEVELOP YOUR BASIC SKILLS

Reading, arithmetic and mathematics, writing, listening, and speaking are skills basic for success in academics and life. When you consider the importance of these basic skills, you must have a strong foundation in them to advance your knowledge beyond the level of memorization to comprehension and application. If you are struggling with these basic skills, you will have difficulty advancing. Developing these skills is basic to the habits of successful learners.

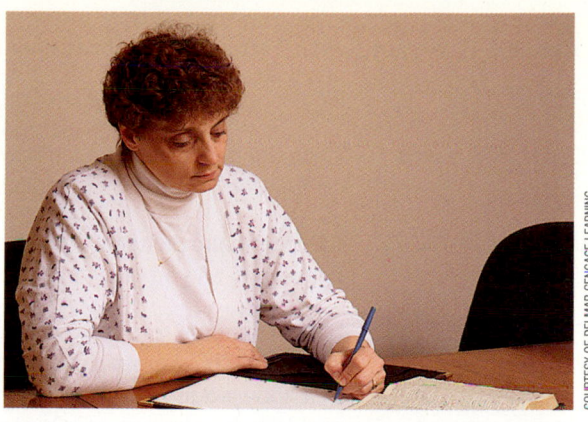

COURTESY OF DELMAR CENGAGE LEARNING

FIGURE 1-1 Keep a notebook of new terms to expand your vocabulary. Review your notebook and try to use the words in practice daily.

READING

A large percentage of your program is in written format. To study effectively, you must be highly adept in the basic skill of reading. To be competent in reading, you must be able to locate, understand, and interpret written information; determine the main idea or essential message; find the meanings for unknown or technical words; and judge the accuracy and plausibility of the writers.

Strategies to effectively improve your reading skills include vocabulary building, comprehension, and reading level. Your basic skill of reading encompasses vocabulary building, which includes the skill of identification and understanding of both English and medical terminology. Investing in quality medical and English dictionaries is a good step to understanding both these languages. When reading assignments, take the time to look up the words you do not know (Figure 1-1).

The primary reason for building a strong medical vocabulary is that words are the tools for thinking about and understanding your world, and you are entering the new world of nursing: You must therefore take the time to learn its language. Developing the habit of vocabulary building takes time initially, but as you persist in practicing this skill, your comprehension of the material will increase.

TABLE 1-2 Behaviors of Perfectionists and Pursuers of Excellence

PERFECTIONISTS	PURSUERS OF EXCELLENCE
Reach for impossible goals	Enjoy meeting high standards within reach
Value themselves for what they do	Value themselves for who they are
Get depressed and give up	Experience disappointment but keep going
Are devastated by failure	Learn from failure
Remember mistakes and dwell on them	Correct mistakes, then learn from them
Can only live with being number one	Are pleased with knowing they did their best
Hate criticism	Welcome criticism
Have to win to maintain high self-esteem	Do not have to win to maintain high self-esteem

COURTESY OF DELMAR CENGAGE LEARNING

Table 1-3 Strategies to Improve Comprehension

Reread	Do this after reading one section of the text or even after one paragraph.
Define new words	Write the definitions of each new word in new words the margin of your text and then reread the paragraph. Use a small notebook to build your own glossary. Make your own flashcards for further study.
Visualize	Create mental pictures of the material you are reading. You may even want to draw a simple stick figure, and as you continue to read, adjust the picture.
Research	Many times the reason you are unable to comprehend the material presented is that you have insufficient background in the subject. A solution may be to consult another text that is specific to that knowledge base. Use a dictionary, anatomy and physiology text, general subject text (like a psychology text), or a nursing journal to increase your background knowledge in a subject area (Meltzer & Marcus-Palau, 1997).
Summarize	Use your own words to "tell" yourself what you just read and how this connects to what you are going to be doing. Ask yourself, "Why might I need to know this material?"

COURTESY OF DELMAR CENGAGE LEARNING

Comprehension goes beyond rote memorization. One sign of true comprehension is the ability to summarize the writer's message. When you summarize, state the material in your own words. Unless you understand the words you have read, you will not be able to advance your level of knowledge from rote memorization to comprehension. When you are actively reading your nursing textbook and you realize that you are not understanding what you have read, you may find it helpful to use one, some, or all of the five strategies outlined in Table 1-3.

Reading level is another element of your reading skills. Reading level is not related to what you can understand but, rather, refers to the length of the words and the sentences used in a text to explain, describe, and convey information. It does not have anything to do with your intelligence, but it has a great deal to do with the length of time it takes you to read.

Arithmetic and Mathematics

A skill in which you must develop competency is arithmetic and mathematics. To be competent in this skill, you must be able to perform basic computations using whole numbers, percentages, fractions, and decimals, and choose the appropriate formula to use. You will be responsible for correctly calculating dosages and safely administering medications to your clients. You must be able to recognize whether your calculations are correct and logical. In nursing, your mastery of mathematical basic skills cannot be overemphasized. According to a research study, approximately 7,000 deaths annually are due to medication errors (Sakowski et al. 2005). Hughes and Edgerton (2005) state:

> The most common calculations involve fractions, percentages, decimals, and ratios. In mathematical tests, new interns and nurses have been found to have poor mathematical skills. . . . The inability to calculate the correct therapeutic volume of a drug dose accounts for the majority of pediatric medication errors. Research has found that the major problems behind many of these miscalculations are associated with an inability to conceptualize the right calculation to be performed and understand the mathematical process leading to the solution. . . . Misplacement of the decimal point is a common dosing error than can lead to a tenfold error in overdosing or underdosing. . . . Some errors of this type have been linked to performance on calculation tests because those who perform poorly on such tests are more likely to make a mistake in practice, especially when fatigued or distracted. (p. 81)

Give yourself a reality check on your competency in mathematics and commit to improving those areas where you are weakest. You may want to investigate a resource such as the learning services center at your school, enlist the assistance of a tutor, or use a programmed-learning text to refresh your skills. There are also numerous texts written to assist nursing students in developing these essential skills. Consider also using computer-assisted instruction (CAI) programs or self-paced study modules to hone your math skills. Whatever means you use, an honest assessment of your competency in mathematics and a commitment to improvement is essential to your practice in the nursing profession.

Writing

In your role as a student and as a professional, you will need writing skills. To be competent in writing, you must be able to communicate thoughts and information clearly and completely using proper grammar, spelling, and punctuation. Contrary to popular opinion, the influx of the computer into health care has not removed the need for this skill. You will be writing client assessments, transfer summaries, discharge summaries, and client-teaching plans. The skill of writing can be practiced and improved.

Listening

The old saying "I know you can hear me, but are you listening?" can be applied to all of us. You must be listening, understanding, and processing information, as opposed to just hearing, when you are in class, as well as when you begin working with clients. To be competent in listening you must receive, interpret, and respond to verbal messages and other cues such as body language while attempting to both comprehend the information and evaluate the speaker. You may need to polish up on ways that you can improve listening and evaluation skills to make the most of your class time. Listening effectively can make efficient use of the class period to increase your comprehension of the content.

Among the many strategies that can be used to improve listening skills are the following:

- *Be interested in the subject.* Make a connection with the reason you are going to this lecture. What is the connection between the information and your need for the information? Have you read the material and come with questions about the subject?
- *Be open to the information.* When you hear a topic and immediately react with your instinct, you often miss the point and some aspect of the presentation you had not considered before. Listening does not automatically mean you will change your mind on topics, but it will allow you to evaluate and incorporate those aspects that are beneficial to you.
- *Focus on the message, not the messenger.* The speaker may not be a member of a theatrical company that entertains you. The speaker's role is to impart information. You can concentrate on the information that you need to know and apply it properly.
- *Concentrate on the information.* Be attentive to the lecture. If you find yourself falling asleep, do muscle flexes or breathe deeply to try to stay alert and aware. Imagine test questions that might be asked on the information.
- *Evaluate the information.* Not every word is critical. Relate the information to what you know, where you may use it, and whether you agree with what is said. If you have difficulty with what is being said, use the next strategy to maintain your concentration.
- *Write down questions as you listen.* This allows you to follow the speaker to the end, and many of your questions may have been answered. If not, you have them written down and can refer later to the list. This promotes concentration on the information presented. You will not be distracted trying to remember questions you wanted to ask.

Speaking

You have entered one of the most "speaking"-oriented professions. You will communicate daily with clients, their families, instructors, peers, ancillary staff members, and the multiple members of the health care team. To be competent in speaking, organize your ideas and communicate them using verbal language in a tone, style, and level of complexity appropriate to the listener.

Many students will not ask questions during a lecture specifically because they believe themselves incapable of speaking clearly and identifying exactly the information they need. There is a saying, "There is no stupid question"; believe it. Develop the confidence to speak up when you have a question. There are potential serious consequences to your clients if you fail to clarify a medical order or question a procedure that is unclear.

The following strategies may help when you want to ask a question:

- *Understand why you are asking the question.* Instead of saying, "I don't understand," say, "I was with you on the physiology of the kidney until you reached the Bowman's capsule. Can you connect this particular part of the kidney with osmosis for me?" This puts you and the speaker in a positive light; you have not attacked the speaker's explanation, and you acknowledge your skill in listening. You are communicating what you need and asking the speaker to help by connecting the two concepts for you.
- *Know when to ask the question.* Writing down those topics on which you need further information may help you decide the correct time to ask a question. If the instructor begins by saying, "Today we will be speaking about pharmacokinetics," and you do not understand the word, stopping her before she has a chance to define the word may not be the most effective strategy. If instead you write down, "What does pharmacokinetics mean?" and listen for the meaning of that word in the context of the lecture, you will most likely hear clues as to the word's meaning. The instructor will use other words, such as *absorption, distribution, metabolism,* and *excretion* to describe what happens to a drug as it goes through the body. When an appropriate time in the presentation comes, review those things that have been said and clarify: "So, Prof. Z., am I correct when I say that pharmacokinetics has to do with the movement of drugs through all the systems of the body?" You will get your answer, and your instructor will know from your question that you have been listening.

Speak clearly and articulate your needs as you attend classes; listen to your instructors; listen to your clients; and transmit information to instructors, colleagues, support staff, doctors, and allied health care team members. Practice both the skills of listening and speaking equally and keep asking questions.

DEVELOP YOUR LEARNING STYLE

The term **learning style** refers to the ways you best receive, process, and assimilate information (knowledge) about a

> **PROFESSIONALTIP**
>
> **Speaking**
>
> Thorough preparation is an important strategy for speaking. Formulating multiple examples is one way of increasing your comfort level with the given information. For example, if you are asked to explain the way the pancreas produces insulin, you might draw the organ and indicate where the islets of Langerhans are. Or you may use a lock and key to explain the way insulin works to open the channels for glucose to enter the cells. You may trace a cracker as it travels through the body from teeth to cells and indicate just where and when insulin is utilized. Regardless of the specifics, creating multiple examples will assist you in thoroughly learning a topic and creating a feeling of comfort about your knowledge of the subject.

particular subject. In your life as a student, you have probably had both of the following experiences:

> You attend class with Professor A for Course 100. The professor arranges the room casually in small groupings and breaks up class time to alternate short lectures with small-group work. There is time for a hands-on demonstration of the principle along with actual work-related items used as examples. Professor A allows for student–teacher interchange of ideas and gives credence to experiences of the students during the class discussions. You leave the class exhilarated and with ideas, aware that this content connects with your desired outcome. You plan a review of the notes with a fellow student you met in your class group. You continue to prepare throughout the course and prior to the final, on which you get a B.
>
> The next day you attend Course 200 with Professor B. The room is arranged in rows. Professor B puts up the class outline on the overhead, lectures for 40 minutes, then allows 10 minutes at the end for questions. If you hand him a written question, he will answer it during the next class. You dread his boring presentation and wish that Professor B was more like Professor A. You really do not know anyone in the class with whom to study, you cannot understand the text, and your grades are in the low C to D range. You know you need this class for your major. You try to do your part, but you just cannot "get into it."

Think about Professor A, who presents information in a variety of methods—short lecture, small group, hands-on demonstration. As a student, you can grasp the information from whichever method appeals to you. You come away feeling connected to the subject and your classmates and want to continue learning about the subject. You are rewarded for your efforts through the academic grade system.

Now consider Professor B, who knows just as much about the subject as does Professor A but who presents it using only one method—lecture. Lecture is not your preferred learning style, and your ability to clarify your understanding through questions is limited by the class format. Your outcomes on tests are less rewarding, and you begin to avoid putting time into studying the subject all together. You end up thinking that you really do not do well in that subject and consider changing your major.

The difference in the outcomes of the two examples lies in the perceived role of the learner. In these examples, the student relied heavily on the *teacher's* ability to present material in the student's preferred learning style. Remember, *you* are in charge of your learning. Teacher presentations vary in ways that may not appeal to your primary learning style, but you can still learn the information. You must take charge of developing your abilities, increasing your awareness of your preferred learning styles, and implementing some simple strategies to enhance those styles. As you increase your skills in your preferred methods and strengthen those in your weaker ones, your outcomes will change.

PROFESSIONALTIP

Learning Disabilities

According to the National Center for Learning Disabilities (2008), 15 million children, adolescents, and adults have some form of learning disability. **Learning disability** is a generic term that refers to a heterogeneous group of disorders manifested as significant difficulties in the acquisition and use of listening, speaking, reading, writing, reasoning, or mathematical abilities.

Having a learning disability will not prohibit your success; you must, however, understand your different abilities. Find out the types of accommodations that will enhance your learning capabilities, and ask for those things that you need. Accommodations in postsecondary programs are mandated by the federal government; however, the onus to disclose, provide documentation, and request accommodations is on the student. Accommodations are determined on a case-by-case basis. Reasonable accommodations in the classroom may be as simple as having the instructor wear a microphone, being able to use a tape recorder or note taker, or requesting textbook tapes. In the clinical area, all reasonable accommodations are made within the confines of client safety and essential skills needed to participate in a nursing program. A quiet work area and ear protectors provide quiet for students who are hypersensitive to background noise. Using a computer for writing assignments, note taking in class, and studying may assist students who have difficulty writing. Getting a tutor who is skilled at working with students with learning disabilities is another intervention to consider.

Whatever you suspect your needs to be, getting professional testing to ascertain whether you have a disability and to determine any specific accommodations you need is crucial. Seek the assistance of your instructors, student service personnel, learning center personnel, or call the special education coordinator at the nearest high school. These resources will help you locate an accredited testing agency to provide you with further resources and documentation.

Classification of Learning Styles

Learning styles are cognitive (mental) functions. They refer to the ways you perceive, remember, think, and solve problems: Their focus is *how* you learn as opposed to *what* you learn. Your preference for one style over another can be argued to be both genetic and developmental. Regardless, your awareness of the ways you best learn will affect your learning outcomes.

Learning styles are classified in many different ways. One classification method focuses on the route by which students best perceive and remember information: visual, auditory, or kinesthetic. These divisions are not mutually exclusive; we possess all three, and we use all of them to acquire information. Visual learners make up approximately 65% of the population, auditory learners approximately 30%, and kinesthetic learners approximately 5% (Mind Tools, 2008).

Visual learners think in pictures. No matter how information is obtained (reading, hearing, or seeing), it is stored as visual images. This person says "I see" or "I get the picture." Auditory learners relate best to the spoken word and prefer class discussion and oral presentations. This person says "That sounds right" or "I hear you." Kinesthetic learners process and remember information well if they touch, imitate, and practice what they are studying. All of us have the capacity to learn in all three modes. You naturally gravitate to one over the others based on which style has led to your greatest learning successes.

Another way to classify learning styles is according to brain-hemisphere dominance. The left hemisphere of the brain is associated with analytical activities, such as logic, structure, speech, reasoning, numbers, verbal expression, verification of data, and analysis of parts of the whole. The right side is associated with creativity and synthesizing parts to form a whole idea. The right side is also considered the more emotional side and links to insight, intuition, daydreams, visualization, music, rhythm, and color visualization.

We need both sides of the brain to function and learn. Numerous studies demonstrated that individuals with left-brain dominance are primarily auditory learners and those with right-brain dominance are primarily visual. Additional studies show that right-brain–dominant learners process, recall, and retain more from information presented in computer-assisted instructional programs, whereas left-brain–dominant learners derive more success from a lecture format. To overlook or use one style to the exclusion of the other is using only part of your overall potential learning ability.

Strategies for Learning

You can determine your preferred learning style by going to one of the following Web sites, doing a search for learning-style test, and taking the test (www.Vmentor.com; www.mindtools.com; and www.vark-learn.com). You can also check the Web site resources at the end of the chapter for more learning-style information. By determining your preferred learning style, you will adopt strategies to enhance that style when you study. You want to effectively move the required information into long-term memory and increase your knowledge level from memorization to comprehension and, finally, to application. To accomplish this you must know which strategies work with which learning styles. Refer to Table 1-4 and note all the strategies listed that you consistently use in your study routine. Start with the style you previously ascertained to be your preferred learning style.

Are there strategies listed under your preferred style that you currently do not use? To enhance your acquisition of material, begin to incorporate these into your study plan. Are there strategies listed under any of the other styles that you could use when the material you are learning is especially difficult for you?

One way to incorporate more than one learning style into your study program is to employ a CAI program. Many texts now come with an accompanying disk designed to enhance learning style. Such disks may contain the total text along with testing materials, exercises that accompany the text, and/or resource material for the text. For example, several medical terminology packages come as program-instruction texts with disks and provide audio pronunciation in the computer programs. The student can read the text, manipulate the information on the computer, and hear the correct pronunciation.

When faced with a particularly difficult passage or concept, incorporate more than one style and one strategy to process the information. The more action you put into your learning methods, the more effective your time and outcomes will be. **Mnemonics**, words or phrases used to aid memory, may help. For example, ABC reminds you of airway, breathing, and circulation. You will find several examples of mnemonics to illustrate concepts in Memory Trick boxes throughout the text.

DEVELOP A TIME-MANAGEMENT PLAN

Somewhere in your decision-making process to go to school, you decided you would have the time to do so. You now must make that a reality by actively engaging in a time-management plan. **Time management** is a system to help meet goals through problem solving. Practicing time-management strategies will not eliminate the need to perform tasks you do not like, but it will make doing so more manageable. Active application of time-management strategies will make a difference in what you can accomplish in the time you have.

Strategies for time management include the following:

- Analyzing your time commitments
- Knowing yourself
- Clarifying your goals
- Setting priorities and identifying one or two valued goals to achieve
- Disciplining yourself to adhere to the plan through changes and until the goal is reached

Table 1-4 Sample Learning Strategies

VISUAL LEARNER	AUDITORY LEARNER	KINESTHETIC LEARNER
Takes notes in class	Reads aloud	Takes notes and rewrites them to condense
Writes notes in margin of books	Reads into a tape recorder and plays it back to self	Expresses self with hands, even while reading
Looks for reference books with pictures, graphs, and charts	Discusses ideas about class content with others	Handles visual aids during class
Draws own illustrations	Requests explanations of illustrations	Requests to do a demonstration

COURTESY OF DELMAR CENGAGE LEARNING

Analyze Time Commitments

To analyze your time commitments, start by listing them. Provide yourself with both a big-picture plan and a daily plan. Creating a year-at-a-glance calendar that lists all of your important time commitments can provide a quick illustration of the way the months ahead will be used. Start by putting in your graduation date in red capital letters. This will give you an instant visual reminder of your current goal. Next, using a pencil, insert all important dates, including holidays, birthdays, work, and organizational obligations. Remember to also include activities for those in your household that will require your participation, such as carpooling, special school programs, after-school activities, and child care. Use your academic program calendar as the source for the dates that classes, as well as vacations, begin and end, financial aid forms and tuition payments are due, and the like. Use your individual class schedules as the sources for dates of exams, special review or clinical days, field trips, or any other time commitments you must meet in order to complete the courses. This exercise will give you a big-picture view of your time commitments and will also point out any conflicts.

Conflicts are not impossible obstacles. Knowing about them in advance will allow you to take steps now to prioritize and reschedule. When prioritizing, think about delegating some tasks to other people. Do not always solve a conflict by removing those tasks you enjoy or that will renew you. Taking care of yourself during this time is very important. Never give up the time you need to refresh and renew, even if it is just a hot bath, a brisk 15-minute walk, or a dinner out with family and friends. Place yourself near the top of the priority list to complete your goal.

Each learner's big-picture map will differ. The challenge is to mesh your map with your other relationships and keep yourself toward the top of the list. One strategy is to prominently display your big-picture calendar in an area where all of the members of your household can see it—including and especially you. Everyone will then have the opportunity to see that he is on the list and that he contributes to helping you reach your goal.

The next step is daily planning. Using a week-at-a-glance planner helps illustrate more concrete expectations of those things you plan to do and the amount of time you actually have (Figure 1-2). You should include time to sleep, eat, drive, work, attend class, and study.

You may find that you must rearrange your schedule. This does not mean continuing to do all of the things you have listed but just on different days; rather, it means choosing two valued goals on which to work. *One goal must be to be a learner. The other will be unique to you.* This does not mean that you replace all other goals with these two valued goals. Rather, it means that these goals must take precedence when choosing ways to use your time. If you choose child care and learner as your most valued goals, you could refine them even further to complement each other. For example, you may opt to keep driving the carpool but negotiate to drive every morning because doing so will afford you 2 hours to study prior to class. You may then have to make child care arrangements for after school, which might mean asking your neighbor or contracting with an after-school program. You may also have to set aside 1 hour each evening to get everything laid out for the next day, a task you might ask someone else in the household to do each night so that you can gain an extra hour of study time. That extra hour, in turn, might mean that you dedicate Saturdays for nothing but family commitments. Regardless of the way you choose to solve such problems, the solutions must be designed to help you reach your goals.

Know Yourself

To develop your system, you must know yourself. You must be honest with yourself about your work habits and preferences. Consider the time of day when you are at your intellectual best. Is it early in the morning, or do you come alive at 10 P.M.? You must be able to focus and concentrate when you are studying. Deciding you are going to carpool in the morning to get to school early to study will not be effective if you cannot concentrate until after noon. If this is the case, it would be better to do the more mechanical and less intellectually demanding tasks, such as the shopping or laundry, in the 2 hours before class. Are you a person who is more left-brain oriented (logical, orderly, structured, and plays by the rules)? Then writing out lists of tasks and crossing them off may be your time-management strategy to stay on track. Perhaps you are a more right-brain personality (creative, resists rules, has own sense of time)? Scheduling your task within a specific time frame that has a time-sensitive goal/reward at the end may assist you to use your available time more effectively.

	Monday	Tuesday	Wednesday	Thursday	Friday	Saturday	Sunday
7 AM	Work	Carpool	Carpool	Carpool	Clinical	House	
9 AM	Work	Class	Class	Class		House	Sunday school
11 AM	Work	Class	Class	Class		Chores	Church
1 PM	Work	Class	Class	Class			
3 PM	Work				Work	Work	
5 PM	Carpool Dinner				Work	Work	
7 PM	Study	Study	Study	Study	Work	Work	

COURTESY OF DELMAR CENGAGE LEARNING

Figure 1-2 Week-at-a-Glance Calendar

PROFESSIONALTIP

Time Wasters

Are you a time waster? We all sometimes behave in ways that sabotage the best of plans. Following are some examples of time wasters along with some strategies for helping you reclaim those wasted hours.

1. *Clutter:* Wisdom holds that you can save 1 hour each day by just clearing your work area of clutter and keeping it clean. This time can be put to good use in the form of study. Organize your study area so that when you arrive it is ready for work and take a few minutes at the end of your session to prepare your area for the next session.
2. *Interruptions:* Intrusions into your study or work hours (from either people or things) can be real time wasters. Try the following:
   - Learn to say "no." You do not have to agree to every request. Learn to pick your involvements carefully and according to those that are most important to you reaching your goals.
   - Put your answering machine on, and turn the phone's ringer off. Delegate a time to listen and respond to messages after studying.
   - Open your mail over the garbage can. Respond, delegate, or throw it out.
   - Organize your papers. For instance, have a folder for each child's paper/notes. Keep your class notebooks, your calendar, and phone lists in one three-ring binder so you have all your essentials together.
3. *Procrastination:* This refers to intentionally putting off or delaying something that should be done. **Procrastination** is a time waster because it does not afford effective use of time. Time management is not necessarily finishing everything at one sitting, but, rather, scheduling time to return to the task until you complete it; whereas procrastination is intentionally delaying the task without good cause or a plan to complete it in a time-efficient manner. Breaking the task down into manageable segments and rewards will encourage you to return to it again and again until it is complete.
4. *Perfectionism:* Very often we do not stick to a plan because it does not give us results immediately or does not give the results we expected. Perfectionism affects your time-management plan by prohibiting you from accepting anything less than perfection; it also damages your positive attitude of yourself by setting unrealistic expectations. Focus on your positive accomplishments, look for ways to improve, accept your failures, and build on your experiences.

CLARIFY GOALS

Without setting goals, we cannot know whether we are making any progress. Goals are like grocery lists. Think about when you go to the store without a list. You may purchase many items, but when you get home you often discover that you did not get all the things you needed. If the next time you go to the store you make a list, you will likely get all the items you want.

Just like the grocery list, goals must be written down. They must be based on reality and broken down into manageable parts. Say your goal is to provide study time each week that will allow you to be successful in each unit exam of your program. This time will comprise the time you need to prepare and review material, prepare for clinical assignments, view information in the library, and practice new skills in the lab. As a rule, you will need 1 to 2 hours of study time for each hour you spend in class. If you are in class 12 hours per week, you will thus need to find 24 more hours to study; and if you are in clinical 6 hours 3 days per week for a total of 18 hours, you will need to fit in 36 hours of study. As a rough estimate, this would mean 12 class hours plus 24 study hours plus 18 clinical hours plus 36 preparation hours for a total of 90 hours per week (30 class hours plus 60 study hours) for the ideal study week and 30 hours (class attendance only) for a week without any study. So now you know what amount of time you are aiming for. You can now take this goal of 60 study hours per week and compare it to your written schedule and calendar to determine how to best arrange the demands on your time in order to meet your goals.

SET PRIORITIES

Another part of setting goals is prioritizing tasks into general categories. Look at your daily calendar and list the general categories. Some examples might be as follows:

- Work
- Study
- Personal (eating, sleeping)
- Household chores (shopping, budget)
- Transportation (self, others)
- Supervising children
- Decision making (planning, outside organizational responsibility, time for self, time for spouse, friends, and children)

Next, rank these general categories in order of priority, keeping in mind that not everything is a primary priority. If you uncover conflicts, try to further clarify which items take top priority.

Another way to prioritize is to group tasks according to the time frame in which you wish them to be accomplished. To do this, divide a sheet of paper into three parts. Label the first part column A, the second, column B, and the third, column C. Under column A, write "I must work on these tasks now." This list includes your priority tasks that need immediate attention. Under column B, write "I can do these after A is done." Under

A	B	C
I must work on these tasks now	I can do these after A is done	I can delay, eliminate, or delegate until after B is done
school/study	supervise children	organization
child care		shopping
self-care		
work		

COURTESY OF DELMAR CENGAGE LEARNING

FIGURE 1-3 Prioritizing Tasks

column C, write "I can delay, eliminate, or delegate these until after B is done" (Figure 1-3).

If you placed your entire list under column A, go back to your original two goals—one of which includes your new role as learner—and rethink your list. You must prioritize your activities in order to reach your goal. You cannot be all things at all times to all people. You also must know how to work smarter, not longer or harder, to remain focused on the priority task.

Discipline Yourself

The hardest strategy to commit to may be discipline of self. The idea that you must actively engage in using the plan sounds simple. In practice, the plan will not always work. When this happens, you may be tempted to abandon the plan instead of changing it. If the plan is not working, you must ascertain the reasons. Maybe you lack resources, have not scheduled enough time, or need to revisit and reevaluate your goals. Build time to plan into your weekly schedule. If you really want to use a time-management system, your ability to go back to the plan and revise it is very important.

DEVELOP A STUDY STRATEGY

Developing a study plan involves more than just buying a textbook and reading it. Several strategies that will assist you to study more efficiently and effectively follow.

Set Up the Environment

Where and when you study are as important as how. The fact that you assign a specific behavior to your study space will set you up for success. The space should fit your style. Do you like everything organized in neat spaces, or do you just need it near you? What type of lighting, seating, or noise level will assist or detract from your concentration? Consider your preferred learning style when setting up your study space. If you are a kinesthetic learner, you may want to put motion into your space by, for instance, using a treadmill in your study plan. You may want to spend a percentage of your study time sitting to read and take notes and then switch to walking or running on the treadmill to recite and reflect on the material. You will be increasing comprehension and making connections, all while walking 2 miles! Regardless of the way you arrange your space, take into consideration the type of learner you are and your biological and personality preferences.

Gather Your Resources

Your resources should all be easily accessible from your study space. In some homes, the kitchen table serves as the study space. If your study space serves more than one function, as would the kitchen table, consider keeping your study resources in a milk crate or box, so they are portable yet readily at hand when needed.

Gathering your resources is your start to building a library of textbooks, which will serve you throughout your program. These resources become a reference library for you when you study. Some general resources to keep on hand include the following:

- A recent edition of an unabridged dictionary
- A medical dictionary
- An anatomy and physiology text

Additional resources you will need as you progress through your program may include texts on pharmacology, nutrition, and the nursing process. Depending on your personal knowledge base, you may need further resources in the foundation sciences—biology, psychology, and sociology. These areas serve as the knowledge base for your future profession.

Keeping your learning style in mind, consider purchasing accompanying workbooks or other study aids that come with the text and research CAI or videotapes available in your nursing program library. Using varied and multiple resources enhances your knowledge base and will increase your comprehension of the content. You must go beyond memorization, beyond amassing facts, to comprehension of this knowledge base in order to answer the questions on the exams. Keep in mind that you are studying for the program examination, the National Council Licensure Examination (NCLEX-PN®), and, ultimately, to apply your knowledge base to provide safe, effective care to your clients.

Remember to use journals as resources. The articles and related client situations can assist you in understanding the application of content to the clinical area. Your ultimate goal is to apply your content information to client care. Consider getting a subscription to your nursing journal, *Journal of Practical*

Nursing or *Practical Nursing Journal*. Nursing organizations such as the National Federation of Licensed Practical Nursing or the National Association for Practical Nurse Education and Service are also valuable resources, and many have Web sites that you can visit.

Whatever resources you ultimately choose, gathering them and having your resources readily at hand are simple strategies that will make the time you have allotted for study more efficient and effective.

Minimize Interruptions

Interruptions to your study time decrease the actual time you can focus on the material and affect your concentration. Interruptions may also become your procrastination "triggers." If you allow your study time to be constantly interrupted, you will soon be doing something other than studying. At the very least, these interruptions minimize your efficient use of time. When you plan your time to study, do not set yourself up for interruptions. Look realistically at your time schedule and do not schedule your study time around the household's naturally busy times of the day—typically mornings, mealtimes, early evenings, and bedtimes.

This is where you put the strategies listed in the section on time management to work. If you have set aside a time and a space for study, make it known that you are not to be interrupted unless there is an emergency. Hang a sign on the door that reads, "Think before you knock." Studying in 1- or 1½-hour blocks is also a way to cut down on interruptions. This is a reasonable time period for you to put the world on hold in order to accomplish your task.

Get to Know the Textbook

Your textbook is not intended to be read like the latest mystery novel, from beginning to end in one sitting. It has directions on the way to use it (introduction, preface) and built-in references (glossary, appendix, summary questions). It is arranged in sections, each dealing with a major topic, and then subdivided into the parts (chapters) that make up the sum of that topic. Getting to know your textbook and its resources and the author's approach to writing may constitute the first part of your study plan. Having this information gives you some insight into the way the material has been grouped and connected.

Another author may have written the book in totally stand-alone chapters and may encourage students to review the table of contents and start anywhere they feel they need to. Self-instruction modules or texts in math often give students instructions to first take all of the post-tests in the chapters and, as long as a certain score is reached, to go on. This is a means of giving students credit for knowledge already learned and facilitating recall of knowledge in preparation for new learning.

Take a look at various parts of this text. How is the information organized? What built-in references can assist you? Consider the cues given about the way to use this text to help you organize the big picture.

Set Up the Study Plan

Each time you enter your study space, your study plan should be with you. You should have a plan or a specific goal for that time. Each time you enter the space, bring a positive attitude toward reaching that goal. Your nursing course outline will drive your study plan. You will have a certain amount of material to cover in a specific time span. You first must know those things that are expected of you. Your course outline, curriculum, and instructors will give you this information.

As an example, consider a unit on vital signs, which is assigned to be completed in 1 week. The components of the unit include understanding the theory base about vital signs as well as learning the psychomotor skills involved in actually measuring these indicators. You are expected to acquire the knowledge by reading the chapter in the text, attending the lecture and demonstration, and practicing in the lab. You will be tested on your ability to apply your knowledge through a pencil-and-paper test and a redemonstration of your psychomotor skills. Now that you know the information you must cover, the sources of the information, and the way you will be tested, you can map out a study plan. Consider the following steps:

1. *Preview the material to be studied.* Your assigned reading from the text on the content of the unit may be contained in one chapter or may span several chapters. Always preview the assigned chapter(s). Often, the student reads only the pages assigned, thinking that this is the most efficient way to study. By not spending the 5 or 10 minutes to preview the entire chapter, the connections between the content may be lost. Previewing can be done very quickly by scanning the chapter headings, art, and tables.
2. *Consider the chapter heading.* The material about vital signs may be contained in a chapter labeled "Baseline Assessment" or "Measurement of Baseline Values" or "Physiologic Functions of the Body." All of these give you a cue as to what you are about to study.
3. *Read the objectives for the chapter.* The objectives list those things you should be able to do when you are finished learning the content of the chapter.
4. *Scan the vocabulary section and the end-of-chapter summary and questions.* Read the key terms and the summary and questions at the chapter's end. Doing so gives you an overview of the scope of the reading you will need to do and should take no more than 5 to 10 minutes.
5. *Set up your questions.* Beginning at the chapter objectives, write down those things you already know, questions about those things you must learn for each objective, and some additional resources that you think you should check. For example, in a chapter about vital signs, the initial page may look like the one in Figure 1-4. Jot down your current knowledge and your questions. The resources note relates to the reasons you are trying to learn this material. Connecting the material to your role in the profession is most important. You are now ready to read the chapter critically for the answers to your questions. You may uncover more and have more questions at the end; but you have a plan and can move on to the next step.
6. *Read and take notes.* Answer your questions and check your vocabulary knowledge as you read.
7. *Reread when necessary.* Remember your basic skills and concentration.

The Measurement of Vital Signs

At the completion of this chapter, you should be able to:

1. Describe the physiologic mechanisms controlling temperature, pulse, respiration, and blood pressure.

   Temp = ?, Pulse = heart, Respiration = lungs, Blood pressure = arteries need to find out about temp.

2. Identify the normal range for vital sign measurements.

   For adults? Children?

3. Select the appropriate equipment used to take vital signs.

   Thermometer, stethoscope, blood pressure cuff

4. Demonstrate the correct psychomotor technique used in measuring vital signs.

   I do this in the lab/get procedure from book or instructor? Ask in class.

5. Document the normal findings of the measurement of blood pressure.

   Temp = 98.6, p = 60–80, bp = 120/80; I need to know this to be able to tell if the client is normal or having trouble.

COURTESY OF DELMAR CENGAGE LEARNING

FIGURE 1-4 Start with the chapter objectives and devise questions and answers to determine the things you know and the things you need to give more attention.

8. *Reflect on the connections you can make between the material and client care.* Identify the reasons the information is important and the way you will use it.
9. *Recite or create your individual style cues.* This is where you will put your individual unique learning styles to work. Make up songs. Create mnemonics. Design flash cards for items that must be memorized. Try to create a logical connection when recalling information.
10. *Review or summarize the information.* Answer the objectives. Use your own words to answer your initial questions. Do you have more questions? Must you consult a second resource to answer them?
11. *End the session with a critical thinking question.* What would the client look like if his temperature were 103°F? What other body systems would be affected? What nursing measures might I use to support the client with this level temperature (e.g., monitor the client's fluid intake and output because the body would be losing fluid as a result of the thermoregulation [sweating and evaporation that would reduce the temperature]), and why? Write these questions down in your notes. You will soon have a collection of "client scenarios" that you will be able to build on as you increase your knowledge base.

The preceding 11 study plan steps require skill in five areas: reading, rereading, reflecting, reciting, and review. With each step, you are engaging in the process of encoding the material. **Encoding** is thought of as actually laying down tracks in the areas of your brain. Each time you read, reread, reflect, recite, and review, you increase the depth of the tract, and your ability to recall and utilize the information increases. You move the information from short-term to long-term memory, and you increase your level of knowledge. The more senses and action you put into your study plan, the more you are able to utilize the information.

You move your level of knowledge from the memorization of a group of facts to the comprehension of the facts in a logical, organized fashion that allows you to apply the information to the client's situation to whom you will provide care. Each time you sit down to study, make your goal the application of knowledge to the client's condition. You can preview, question, and quickly outline the major points in the chapters before class. Listen to the lecture and take notes. Approach new material with the read, reread, reflect, recite, and review steps before moving on to the next topic.

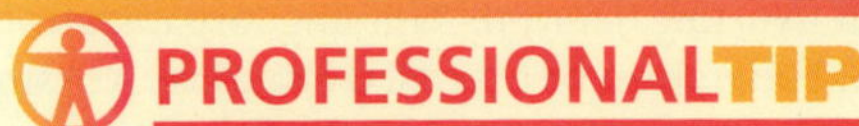

Mnemonics

Create your own mnemonics to group the steps of a procedure. A mnemonic is simply a method for helping your association and recall; it consists of a memorable word or phrase created from the letters of the list of items you are trying to recall. For example, to remember all of the areas to include when assessing a client to whom a cast has been applied (pulse, circulation, sensation, movement, and temperature), you might make up a silly sentence to help you remember, such as "**P**aul **C**an **S**hine ***M***y **T**uba." This type of statement will help you group these facts together (pulse, circulation, sensation, movement, temperature) and assist you in recalling them. You could sing this also. Do whatever you can to be active in moving material from short-term to long-term memory.

NOTE TAKING

Note taking is an action that connects you to the content of written material or a lecture presentation and will assist you in identifying the main ideas and their connection to the overall topic.

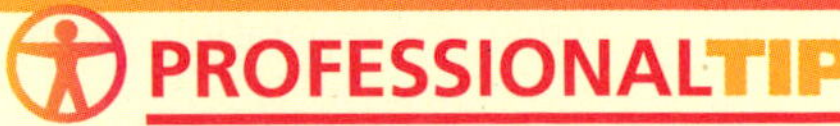

Attending Class

In general, the best strategies for getting the most from classes are to:

- Get to class on time.
- Get a front row seat.
- Listen attentively with a pencil in your hand and take notes.

Keep materials for each of your classes or topics in a separate three-ring binder. Take notes on loose-leaf paper and write on one side only because this allows you to arrange your preview notes and lecture notes chronologically. You can also insert handouts from the class in the appropriate order as you receive them. Using this method, you can also review notes against additional information you have from other resources to assist you when it is time to review for the examinations.

When you are taking notes from the text, read with a pencil in your hand to put yourself in the action mode. You will thus be ready to receive and process information. You may also take notes from text readings on your computer, which facilitates editing and rearranging material.

Before class, preview your chapter material and divide your paper, leaving a 3-inch border on the left side. From the assigned reading, identify the main topic to be covered, list the main section and the subheadings, and summarize the information in the left column. Then write your questions in this column. This prepares you for more active participation in the lecture; use the right column to take notes from the lecture.

Regardless of the way you choose to take notes, note taking while you study sets you up for connecting with the content. It positions you as an active participant in the learning process, and any time you increase your active participation in the learning process, you increase your learning.

When taking notes in class, listen attentively, lean forward, and concentrate on the information the speaker is imparting (Figure 1-5). Take notes on the following:

- The topic, as stated by the speaker; write it on the top of the page
- The main ideas and the details that support the topic
- The most important points, based on the speaker's organization and emphasis
- Other students' questions and the responses from the speaker, which are often the very questions you had

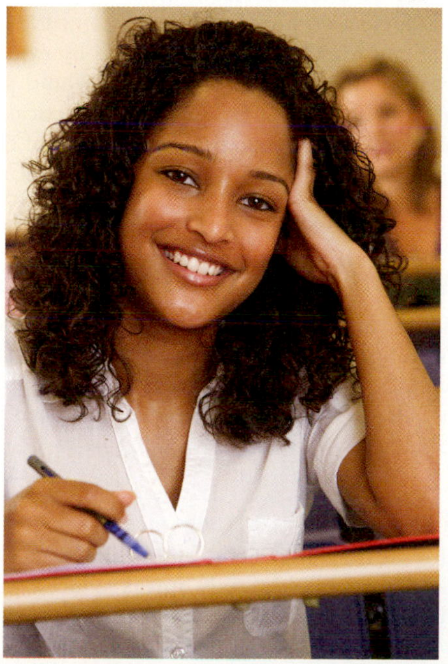

PHOTO COURTESY OF SHUTTERSTOCK

FIGURE 1-5 **Note taking is an important component of increasing your comprehension of the material.**

Look for visual and auditory cues from the speaker, for example, if the speaker says, "This is important," or writes steps on the board. Do not form an opinion of what is being said until you have heard the entire lecture. As stated earlier, a good strategy is to write your questions as you think of them. They may be answered by the time the lecture is over.

The purpose of note taking during a lecture is not to create a transcript of the information imparted but, rather, to record what you understand. The combination of attending lecture, listening, and note taking can provide you with much knowledge that you will not have to learn elsewhere. Previewing the material to be covered further contributes to this dynamic. When taking notes, consider the following guidelines to make your note taking efficient and effective:

- Do not take notes with the intent of writing them over. This is a waste of time, and, contrary to what you may expect, it does not improve recall.
- If your handwriting is sloppy, print or use a laptop computer.
- Condense the amount of actual writing you do by using symbols and abbreviations and leaving out everything but necessary words. For instance, instead of writing "If the client's blood pressure reading is greater than 140 systolic and 90 diastolic, . . ." write "If BP >140/90. . . ."
- Write definitions and mathematical formulas exactly as you heard them in lecture.
- In mathematics and science lab courses, write the process step by step exactly as explained. Indicate which formulas are used with which problems, for example:

  "Use ratio/proportion for word problems."
- Pick an abbreviation system and stick to it.
- Review the notes as soon as possible after class. Many studies have demonstrated that even a brief review of notes after class increases retention of the material by 50%.

PREPARE FOR EXAMS

The final plus of having a study plan is the ability to review for exams. Reviewing for exams is not studying all of the material over from the beginning. You will already have studied the subject matter you are going to cover on the exam; now, you are reviewing and recalling it through a series of exercises designed to increase your comprehension and facilitate application. Some nursing examinations are written at the comprehension or recall level. The NCLEX-PN® is written at the application level. On the NCLEX-PN® exam you will not see many questions about naming where the pulse points are (comprehension, recall). You will instead find questions about which of the pulse points of the body are most appropriate for assessing an infant (application). Making decisions about which fact or groups of principles you have learned will be the basis for most nursing examination questions.

Depending on the curriculum, you may have examinations every week or every month, a weekly quiz, a midterm, and a final. Regardless, you will know the schedule, and you must set aside review time for preparation. If you are to have weekly quizzes, you must build a time for review into your daily study plan. One way to do so is to set aside the last 30 minutes of each study session for review. Take each objective of your course outline and, without looking at your notes or text, turn them into questions and then answer them. If you are weak in one area, refer to your notes and devise a technique for recall, such as the use of flash cards, rhythms, mnemonics, pictures, or graphic drawings. Work through each of the objectives for the content that is covered.

If your examinations are by unit, you must divide the material up over the time you will need to cover it, leaving at least 2 days for review and recall before the examination. Each of these review sessions will also serve as preparation for both your final examination and the NCLEX-PN®. As you are successful in each of your examinations and continue to see further connections in your clinical application, your depth as well as breadth of content mastery will increase.

Participate in Test Reviews

Test reviews vary from one instructor or class to another but are a great way to review your level of knowledge and ability to succeed within a class and the nursing profession. As nurses, our final evaluation and rite-of-passage for nursing practices is the NCLEX-PN® exam. It is a computerized multiple-choice exam, and it is only by successfully passing the exam that a nurse begins a nursing career. So it is imperative that nursing students learn to successfully take exams. A test review is a great way to identify common mistakes or patterns of mistakes on exams. Some students learn that they frequently change from the right answer to a wrong answer. Others eliminate all but two answers and then struggle choosing the right one. Changing these patterns could make the difference between succeeding and failing in nursing school (DePew, 2008).

Learn from Mistakes

Some nursing student's mistakes might be failing an exam, skipping class, or choosing not to complete an assignment. The ability to learn from one's mistakes provides an opportunity to turn failure into success. A challenge after each exam might be to understand each missed question so that if a student sees those question concepts again, he would understand the concept and get that question correct. If pertinent information is missed from class because of an absence, then next time it is important to contact the instructor and peers to ensure that no information covered or provided in class is omitted. A mistake might occur in the clinical setting, and the clinical instructor offers time to review and relearn the skill. Mistakes are opportunities to learn and grow and are important not to repeat, since a nurse's mistakes could impact another human life. Taking time to learn from one's mistakes will lead to success in nursing care and nursing practice (DePew, 2008).

Talk with Instructors

Many people are available to discuss experiences and concerns with a nursing student. Some of these people are instructors, advisors, and peers. It is important to remember the value in talking with peers. Share with each other what is working and what is not working in class. Explore ideas that might help or hinder success in the class and nursing school.

If you feel you are not achieving the desired results and you are unable to identify ways to correct a class problem, ask to meet with the instructor. Instructors are often available before and after a class, or have specific office hours available to discuss student concerns. Instructors are great resources for explaining or clarifying class specific information and details. They also hold the key to what has worked for former students and assignments in the past. Collaboration between student and faculty is a very important part of a student's success when accompanied by a trusting relationship (Sayles, Shelton & Powell, 2003). Remember these resources when evaluating and modifying for success in nursing school. These tips help identify the resources needed to succeed (DePew, 2008).

PRACTICE CRITICAL THINKING

Most of this chapter thus far has been devoted to presenting strategies for the effective and efficient acquisition of knowledge. Your ultimate goal is to be able to use this knowledge to provide safe client care. To do so, you must go beyond the initial stage of simply acquiring information. In delivering nursing care, facts alone do not constitute a sufficient knowledge base for making sound decisions about client care. You must internalize these facts and be able to use them when presented with new situations.

In considering which actions you may need to take in a new situation, you must consider past experience and principles of care, postulate possible outcomes from a variety of interventions, and seek additional information from colleagues, clients, and resource materials. This process is called critical thinking, and it is what you will be expected to do with the knowledge you are acquiring.

The first step is to develop an understanding of **critical thinking**. A comprehensive definition is the **disciplined** (taught by instruction and exercise) intellectual process of applying skillful **reasoning** (use of the elements of thought to solve a problem or settle a question), imposing intellectual **standards** (a level or degree of quality), and self-reflective thinking as a guide to a belief or an action (Heaslip, 1994; Paul, 1995).

Many students find the process of becoming responsible for their own thinking painful. You, along with many other students, may be uncomfortable when asked to defend your **opinions** (subjective beliefs) and **judgments** (conclusions based on sound reasoning and supported by evidence) or to decide what is important. Probably you would prefer to be told what you need to know. Because practical/vocational nurses must make many decisions in the care of their clients, knowing how to make good decisions is essential.

Skills of Critical Thinking

Your abilities in the four basic skills of critical reading, critical listening, critical writing, and critical speaking can be measured by how well you achieve the universal intellectual standards (UIS). These standards are discussed in the next section: Standards of Critical Thinking.

Critical Reading

Reading for the meaning of concepts is basic to the acquisition of knowledge from books. Study time is reduced, and information will be retained, leading to better results on tests. Use of a highlighter to mark the main ideas is often helpful. Those who do not read critically usually mark most of the page. Form a study group to compare the main ideas marked in the assigned material. When reviewing tests, note when misreading or misinterpretation was the cause of your incorrect answer. Make a conscious effort to identify your weaknesses.

As you prepare your assignments, have a dialogue with yourself:

- Before beginning to read, preview the material and ask yourself: What is it about; how is it related to what I already know; how it is organized; and are other resources required?
- As you are reading, ask yourself: Does it make sense; are all terms familiar or should I look them up; how is this related to what I already know; and can I summarize this section?
- After reading, ask yourself: Do I understand the main points; can I outline the main points; how will I use or apply this information; does something need to be clarified; and what questions are likely to be on the exam?

Critical Listening

Communication skills, especially listening skills, are greatly emphasized in the nursing curriculum. Many students do not have effective listening skills. Many persons have developed the habit of tuning in only occasionally to what is said, resulting in lost communication. Improve your listening skills by restating the points made in a discussion with another student and ask that student to give feedback about how accurately you have restated her position. As you listen, focus on what the speaker is saying, listen for key points, and make a note of anything that seems confusing to you (Figure 1-6).

Critical listening requires a conscious commitment to focus on the topic of discussion. Recognize things that distract your attention. Attempting to take word-for-word notes, daydreaming, and focusing on the mannerisms or appearance of the speaker are common distractors. A good thinker is not afraid to identify weaknesses and strengths in order to improve.

Critical Speaking

Disciplined speaking is perhaps the most neglected skill. Examples of clear, logical, and accurate spoken communication are seldom heard. Oral communication is usually more spontaneous than written communication and must be carefully presented. Ambiguous statements are misleading, and personal biases influence what the other person hears. Small group practice followed by feedback from the listeners can help a student assess and improve speaking skills.

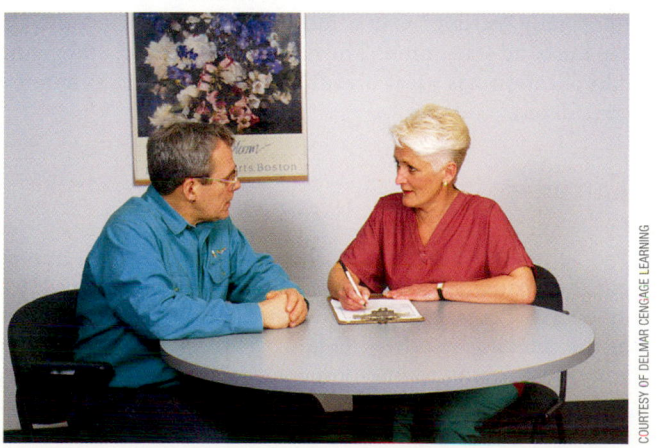

FIGURE 1-6 Effective listening skills are essential to all client interactions.

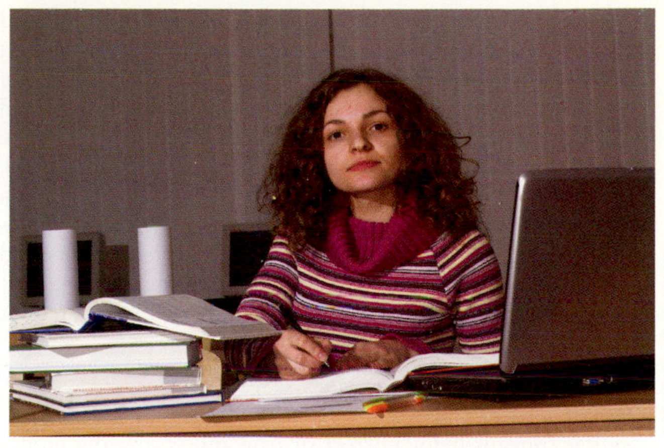

FIGURE 1-7 Effective writing skills are integral to critical thinking.

Critical Writing

Basic to good thinking skills is the ability to state one's thoughts coherently, clearly, and concisely. Many students arrive at college unable to write well. The quality of thinking is improved by the discipline required to write well. Many students feel that writing is too revealing and are afraid to write down their thoughts. Writing is important for the improvement of thinking because it can be reviewed using the standards for critical thinking to evaluate the quality of the thinking reflected in the writing (Figure 1-7). The standards for critical thinking are discussed next.

Standards for Critical Thinking

Critical thinking relies on the use of intellectual standards for checking the quality of thinking (Elder & Paul, 2008). The first requirement is to become familiar with the Universal Intellectual Standards developed at The Center for Critical Thinking. These are used in this discussion because they provide a valid and reliable measure for the quality of thinking. Whether you are reading, listening, writing, answering test questions, or speaking, the standards of clarity, accuracy, precision, relevance, consistency, logic, depth, breadth, and fairness should be applied.

Clarity

Fundamental to quality thinking is the ability to think clearly. Clarity of thought means placing facts and ideas into a logical and coherent framework. The standard is the degree to which others can understand your position. Pay particular attention to the exact meaning of words. There will be many new terms and concepts in your nursing curriculum. Practice the proper use of these terms and apply concepts appropriately to improve clarity of thought and increased retention of content.

Think about the word *clarity*. There are several shades of meaning in the dictionary. Look up the word for yourself and decide which definition applies to the use of clarity in describing a standard for critical thinking.

Think about expressions you use frequently. Would someone from another part of the country understand them? The term *this evening* is common in some parts of the country. When would you expect someone who told you that she would visit "this evening?" In some places, the person might arrive in the early afternoon; in other places, at night. When speaking to clients, families, and other health team members, be sure that the words used clearly express the intended message. Do not assume that you understand a term; take time to verify the meaning. When a statement is unclear, it cannot be determined whether it is accurate or relevant.

Accuracy

Accuracy means being correct or true and within the proper parameters. The need for accurate calculation of a drug dose or accurate measurement of blood pressure can readily be understood. In the same way, the collection and interpretation of data must be accurate. Being accurate implies the use of some measuring instrument. Accuracy in thinking may be hard to conceptualize. When a person uses the term *hypertension* to mean someone who is anxious and very active instead of the actual meaning, an elevation of blood pressure above the accepted normal maximum, the standard of accuracy is not met. Students can improve their accuracy in thinking by writing new information in their own words and asking another student to interpret what was written. Inaccurate information will become evident.

Accurate documentation of client care is essential to quality care. There are degrees of accuracy. For example, you might measure a client's temperature using a thermometer that can measure to the 0.01 degree, but this degree of accuracy is not necessary. On the other hand, when figuring a pediatric dosage, a difference of 0.01 is very important. A challenge to you is to learn the degree of accuracy required in given nursing situations.

Precision

Sometimes, students learn enough about a subject to be "in the ballpark" but not enough to hit a home run. The result is a general idea about a fact or idea, but not enough understanding to apply it. Precise thinking means that there is enough detail and specificity for a concept or word to be clearly understood in terms of its relationship to other concepts or words.

Relevance

Relevance refers to information connected to the issue as opposed to information that is not. Students may get sidetracked from the purpose of an exercise by failing to limit their discussion to the issue at hand. Their responses are not relevant. When studying, ask yourself how a particular concept is relevant to client care. It is also important to be able to recognize when sufficient relevant information is not available.

Consistency

Consistency is the appropriate use of principles and concepts. For instance, a particular nursing diagnosis based on specified indicators should be used when those indicators are present and never used when the indicators are not present.

Knowing the basic actions of epinephrine enables the nurse to predict client responses to the administration of the drug. It also helps the nurse understand that the client will have the same response when an increased secretion of epinephrine is released by the client's adrenal medulla.

Logic

Thinking brings a variety of thoughts together in some order. Logic asks the question "Does this make sense?" Symptoms exhibited by clients can usually be understood based on knowledge of normal physiology and those changes produced by the client's disease or condition. For example, a client with a gallstone blocking the common bile duct is concerned because his stool is very light gray in color. Bile is the substance that colors the stool brown, so it follows that if there is no bile, the stool will not be brown. These two items make sense in combination.

When calculating a medication dosage, the standard of logic is extremely important. If the calculation answer is to give the client 200 pills of a certain medication, this is not logical; it does not make sense. Most likely, there is a missing decimal point, with the correct answer being two pills.

Depth

Students are often tempted to rely on the specific learning objectives as an indicator of which material they must master. This may result in a superficial understanding of the material. The ability to recognize the depth to explore concepts and ideas can be learned. Students should ask themselves, "What are the most significant factors; and what are the complexities in this situation; and what other problems may be involved?" These questions will guide the student to see other aspects that also need to be explored for a thorough understanding. Your instructor and the learning aids within your textbook are useful guides for identifying relevant information and the appropriate depth of knowledge required to make good clinical decisions.

Breadth

Breadth of thinking entails considering another point of view and asking if there is another way to look at the question or problem. Consider a pregnant woman, with a 6-year-old son, who has been told she must stay in bed because of complications. The problem is broader than just the complication of the pregnancy. Who will care for the son, take him to school? Who will do the cooking, cleaning, laundry? Is this financially feasible? Can a mother or friend help out? Can the husband stay home? The narrow problem of a pregnancy complication has great breadth when the entire situation is considered.

Fairness

Everyone has a set of beliefs, opinions, and points of view. People tend to believe that what they think is true. Improving the quality of your thinking depends on your ability to identify the biases in your thinking and those biases present in the thinking of others. Following the standard of fairness will lead a person to question conclusions based on personal bias. When a nurse who responds to pain in a stoic manner assesses a person who responds to pain emotionally, the nurse may allow personal values to influence the assessment, with the result that the nurse provides inadequate pain relief for the client.

Reasoning and Problem Solving

Although reasoning involves thinking, all thinking is not reasoning. Thinking is occurring when a person daydreams, jumps to conclusions, or decides to listen to music. However, these activities cannot be called reasoning. In order to effectively use reasoning, to figure things out, or to problem-solve, the student must become familiar with the components of reasoning. These components are purpose, the question at issue, assumptions, point of view, data and information, concepts, inferences and conclusions, and implications and consequences.

Purpose

All reasoning is directed toward some specific purpose. This is one aspect where reasoning is different from daydreaming. For the nursing student, the purpose of reasoning is to use the information learned in class to effectively solve client care problems.

The Question at Issue

The purpose of the reasoning process is to figure something out, answer a question, or solve some problem. This problem or question must be clearly stated. At the beginning of a study period, state clearly the problems presented by this particular material. Good clinical judgment begins with a clear statement of problems presented by each client.

Assumptions

Assumptions are ideas or things that are taken for granted. They are accepted as being true without examination. Assumptions may be helpful in problem solving, but recognize them for what they are. An example of an assumption is that nursing makes a difference in the outcome of a client's illness. This is a necessary assumption for nurses to make in order to engage in problem-solving related to client care needs.

Assumptions that have proven reliable can help in decision making, while faulty assumptions may cause you to draw faulty conclusions and may lead to inadequate problem-solving. Learn to recognize your own assumptions and those of others. Never be afraid to challenge your own assumptions or to ask others to clarify the assumptions they are using.

Point of View

Each person reasons from his own point of view, which is influenced by previous experience, available information, the quality of thinking already acquired, and many other factors. All together these factors give each person a unique perspective and a unique way of thinking. Seek other points of view and evaluate their strengths and weaknesses. Each person sees things differently. An individual's point of view will determine what facts and information will be noticed, the importance given to the information, and even the acceptable solutions to the problem. Identify your own point of view and its limitations and acknowledge the right of others to have their own points of view (Figure 1-8).

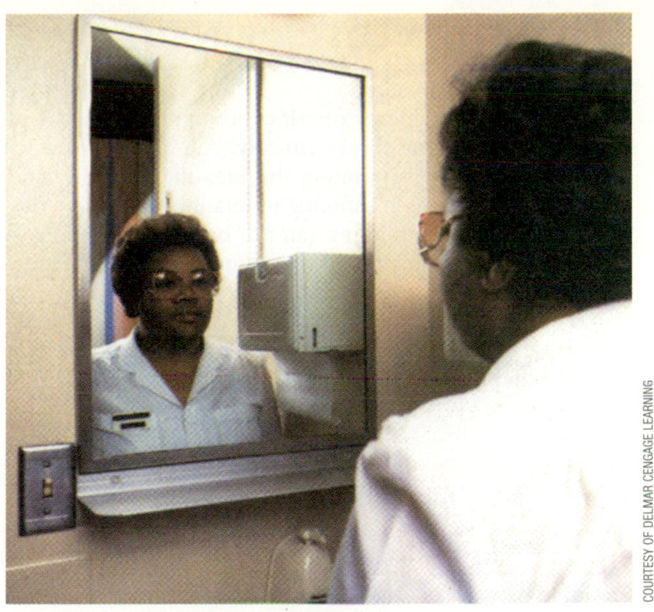

COURTESY OF DELMAR CENGAGE LEARNING

Figure 1-8 To be effective problem-solvers and critical thinkers, nurses must first take a good look at their own point of view.

Data and Information

Data and information are the basic materials of reasoning. Be sure that all information and data are clear, accurate, and relevant to the question or problem at issue. Search for information that not only supports your position but also refutes it. Make conclusions supported by the data you have collected.

Concepts

Identify concepts needed to explore the problem and the implications of each. The concepts (such as asepsis, pain, adaptation, and so on) important to nursing care must be part of the evidence supporting a nursing judgment.

Inferences and Conclusions

Reasoning requires interpretation of facts and information. The interpretation must be justified by the relevant facts. It must be supported by the data and information. Many times, students state opinions as judgments or inferences. This happens when inferences are based on assumptions and personal preferences rather than on the information.

Properly drawing judgments or inferences is basic to thinking well. For example, when the body's temperature goes above 98.6 degrees, the body's metabolic rate increases. Increased metabolism requires more oxygen for the tissues. More oxygen can be delivered to the tissues by increasing the heart rate. From these facts, it is inferred that an elevated body temperature results in an increased heart rate.

The product of reasoning is a conclusion regarding the problem. It is the answer to the question that began the process. The conclusion must be logical.

Implications and Consequences

The reasoning process usually produces more than one solution. Now it is necessary to examine the implications of each solution by thinking about the ease with which a solution can be applied, the ability of a person to carry out the required actions, or the risks involved. Look for both positive and negative consequences.

Consequences can result from action or inaction. It may not be possible to predict all consequences, but the possible outcomes should be examined as completely as possible.

Traits of a Disciplined Thinker

Reading the requirements of critical thinking in this chapter will not make anyone think critically. You can improve your own thinking by incorporating the idea that thinking about the quality of your own thinking in relation to UIS is a desirable goal. Improved thinking can not be acquired in a day or two. It takes time, effort, and disciplined practice. The result is well worth it, however. Consistent efforts to improve your thinking can result in the acquisition of the traits of a disciplined person (Center for Critical Thinking, 2008). These traits, or habitual ways of thinking, can be recognized by others and enable a person to compete successfully in the high-tech world (Table 1-5).

Critical Thinking and the Nursing Process

A nursing education program is intended to help students develop the logic of nursing. In other words, you will learn to think like a nurse. The method nurses have adopted to implement the practice of nursing is called the nursing process. The nursing process applies the problem-solving process to the practice of nursing and requires critical thinking. When you find the relationship between the content of the textbooks

Table 1-5 Traits of a Disciplined Thinker

TRAIT	DESCRIPTION
Faith in reason	Confident that interests of humankind are best served by giving free play to reason Values reasoning in self and others Has faith that people can learn to think for themselves, think coherently and logically, and come to reasonable conclusions
Intellectual humility	Aware of how much he does not know Sensitive to bias, prejudice, and limitations of own viewpoint Willing to examine beliefs and conclusions based on new evidence Respects thoughts and ideas of others Continually learning and improving own thinking
Intellectual courage	Addresses ideas, beliefs, or viewpoints causing strong negative emotions that have not received a serious hearing Recognizes that ideas considered dangerous are sometimes jusitified Willing to take unpopular positions based on reasoning
Intellectual integrity	Is true to own thinking Consistent in intellectual standards applied and does not change to suit circumstances or personal bias Admits discrepancies and inconsistencies in own thoughts and actions Practices what he advocates for others
Intellectual perseverance	Uses intellectual insights and truths despite difficulties and frustrations Pursues question or problem until conclusion is reached Adheres to rational principles Willing to struggle with confusion and unsettled questions over an extended time period to achieve deeper meaning
Intellectual empathy	Imaginatively puts self in place of others to genuinely understand them Able to reconstruct accurately the viewpoints and reasoning of others Remembers past occasions when he was wrong despite intense conviction of being right
Fair-mindedness	Considers all viewpoints Adheres to intellectual standards Is impartial

COURTESY OF DELMAR CENGAGE LEARNING

and the logic of nursing, the study of nursing will be an exciting and challenging process. Using the nursing process will improve the quality of your thinking, and using reasoning will enhance your use of the nursing process.

DEVELOP TEST-TAKING SKILLS

Testing is not studying; however, the skills you need for testing are similar to those needed for studying. The task involved in taking a test is not to pass it; to pass the test is the *outcome*. You cannot achieve the outcome if you do not perform the task. The task is to read the question, understand what the question is asking, and make a decision about a correct response.

To hone your test-taking behaviors, you must first perform a personal analysis with regard to your attitudes, preparation methods, and behaviors related to a testing situation. Only after you have identified these variables can you initiate strategies to improve your outcomes.

Attitude and Expectations

If you are like most students, you may feel quite anxious about taking a test. You may think of each test as the final chance to show your worth. Or you may consider receiving less than an A on an examination as being the same as failing. Neither of these is a reasonable expectation for testing. Testing is a useful tool for both measuring your level of knowledge and showing what you still need to learn. Have you ever considered that receiving a grade of C on an examination usually indicates that you know 75% of all of the knowledge that was tested? And the knowledge on any given test does not represent all the knowledge you possess. Your attitude toward testing is very important if you are to improve your outcome. Maintain a reasonable expectation about both the purpose of the test and the meaning of your grade. This is often a key factor in improving your test performance.

Preparation

In analyzing your preparation for test taking, you must critically examine your study habits. Review the section in this chapter on study strategies and consider whether you are on task when it comes to your study habits. There may be some areas where you can improve. If you know of an area of weakness, make a conscious effort to develop this part of your preparation. Be reasonable in your expectations and do not expect to see results overnight. Building your study habits takes time and persistence. Persevere and your outcome on tests will improve.

Next, consider the way you review for an examination. Do you cram the night before, or are you consistently planning for questions in your study plan and adding time for review of material before the examination? One strategy is to use the technique of note mapping to help you organize the material into manageable parts. (See the Professional Tip: Note Mapping.) Taking each part and developing a more detailed one-page outline that you can take with you to review for 15 to 20 minutes at a time is another method to try. Another suggestion is to change your study place and times. Instead of 1-hour sessions, break your review sessions into 30-minute recall sessions. You must draw an imaginary line between studying and reviewing. Studying is the learning of new knowledge; reviewing comprises recall, organization, and summary of information.

Do not study only just before the test. This is a poor technique. Approaching preparation in this manner serves only to put a few facts into short-term memory. Better to spend the time before the examination relaxing with a good book or good friends or at the spa or gym. You must be confident and rested and come to the testing area with that good feeling that results from doing something you like.

PROFESSIONALTIP

The 30-Second Vacation

For those of you who need an "anxiety buster," consider a "30-second vacation." The 30-second vacation is based on a guided imagery technique that is used often in the client care arena. This technique takes practice. Start by doing the following:

Sit in a comfortable spot where you will not be disturbed, close your eyes, and think of an event or a place that evokes a feeling of calmness (not necessarily happiness). This is an event or place that made you feel like everything was right with the world and with you. It can be from any time in your life.

It may take some time to settle on the right event or place. Relax and take a few minutes now and think.

Once you have it, don't tell anyone! This is your secret place, your place of peace, and when you go there, no one can find you.

Once you have selected this event or place, start to give it "life." To do this, you must begin to recall this event or place regularly. Practice doing so at the beginning of your study sessions, when you are stuck in traffic, when you are at the dentist, when you have something difficult to do, at the beginning of your test-taking exercises, or at the beginning of your real tests.

Each time you recall your event or place, give it more "life." Recall the time of day, the setting, the colors of that day. Was it raining, was it sunny, was it snowing? If it was raining, was it a summer rain or an autumn rain? Recall what you were wearing and what colors you had on. Were you alone or with others? Were you eating something? What did the food smell like?

Consider the rest you get the night before the examination. Physical stamina is needed for concentration. If you cram for a test by "pulling an all-nighter," you are setting yourself up for possible errors on the examination. Be reasonable, revisit your study plan, and get adequate rest.

Next, consider whether you have enough energy to take the test. You can eat what you want, but eat. The cells of the brain require glucose to function; this glucose is supplied in the calories you consume. Try not to increase caffeine intake immediately before a test because doing so may make you jittery.

Finally, ask yourself whether surrounding yourself with positive people helps keep you focused, or whether talking to students before a test only makes you more anxious. If the latter is the case, you should arrive with just enough time to walk into the testing room and you should not speak to anyone.

Minimize Anxiety

Anxiety is the physiologic response of the autonomic nervous system to a perceived stressful situation. As the situation becomes more stressful, the body's response increases. This affects the ability to process information and make rational choices. People are often not good at identifying what they are feeling and are often unaware of the degree to which stress affects the ability to take tests.

Develop a plan to deal with anxiety. Anxiety about performance is always present. Past experience with testing often contributes to the development of test anxiety. If the expectation regarding performance on a test is not mirrored in the grade we receive, our confidence in our ability is shaken, and we approach the whole experience with more and more anxiety.

To deal with anxiety, consciously develop an activity to counter the feeling that anxiety evokes. Some people listen to music, pace, or do deep breathing to combat feelings of stress and anxiety. All of these are good strategies, even if all of them cannot be done *while you are actually taking the test.*

Improve Test-Taking Skills

How do you improve your test-taking skills? You practice, practice, practice and analyze, analyze, analyze. Consider the following:

> *Treat every wrong answer as a treasure. Examine it and discover the secret of why you got it wrong.*

This is the only way to know which errors you are making. Always request to review your examinations, and track your incorrect responses using the analysis worksheet presented in Figure 1-9. Initially, when you review your tests, do not concern yourself with the content of the questions. Simply write the number of the question in the row that indicates the reason you got that question incorrect. You will also notice that there is a heavy black line before the last row of the worksheet. The first four rows represent what are known as *mechanical errors*; these can be eliminated by developing positive habits and revising current practices. You will notice after three or four quizzes that a pattern starts to emerge. Imagine that you just took a 100-question test and received a score of 60/100. You then use the worksheet to categorize your incorrect responses.

Of the 40 incorrect answers you provided, you see that 10 of them fell in "did not read carefully," 2 in "did not know the vocabulary," 7 in "inferred additional data," 4 in "identified priorities incorrectly," and 7 in "did not know the material." If you could eliminate the bad habits that resulted in the first 23 errors, this would improve your test score immediately. Your grade would be 83/100. More important, tests would truly represent only what you did not know, not areas where bad habits resulted in poor test scores.

After you have identified your error patterns, you can work on developing the counterhabits that will eliminate them. Work first on the one that is the most glaring.

Test Question Analysis Worksheet

Reason for Incorrect Response	Test 1 Date	Test 2 Date
Did not read carefully (missed details, missed key words)		
Did not know the vocabulary (medical terminology, English vocabulary)		
Inferred additional data (made assumptions, "read into the question")		
Identified priorities incorrectly (placed events in wrong order)		
Did not know the material		
Marked the correct answer and then changed it (changed answer instead of going with first choice)		

COURTESY OF DELMAR CENGAGE LEARNING

FIGURE 1-9 Test Question Analysis Worksheet

Read Carefully

Reading carefully is a test-taking behavior that must be practiced. The section on study strategies noted the value of scanning in looking for important words when you read. When you are reading a test question, however, you must *never* scan. Many students choose incorrect responses because they miss key words, scan the question for familiar terms, infer what the question is, or misinterpret words they read too quickly. Incorrect responses resulting from any of these actions represent poor reading habits rather than a substandard knowledge base. The following exercise will help improve your reading habits.

Exercise for Improving Your Literal Reading Skills

You will need:

- A timer (stove)
- An NCLEX-PN® review text or any comparable question and answer book. It is important that you have the answers and the rationales for each answer in a review text.
- Two sheets of paper: one to take the test on and one to make your analysis worksheet
- Pencil or pen
- Dictionary

PROFESSIONALTIP

Note Mapping

Note mapping is taking conventional notes and organizing them into a picture that allows one to see connections and links between ideas and concepts. A note map is similar to the concept maps within this text. When a note map is developed, one thinks through complex problems, fuses together the information, summarizes the content, and displays the information in a way that is easy to recall. More of the brain is engaged in assimilating and connecting the facts, so one can easily recall information because one can easily recall the shape and structure of the note map. The advantage of note mapping over conventional notes is that one can see the informational links and recall the basic facts within the notes. All the pages of notes are fit onto one page, so the note map is easy to carry and study in spare minutes. Here is an example of a note map for the section you are reading, "Develop Test-Taking Skills."

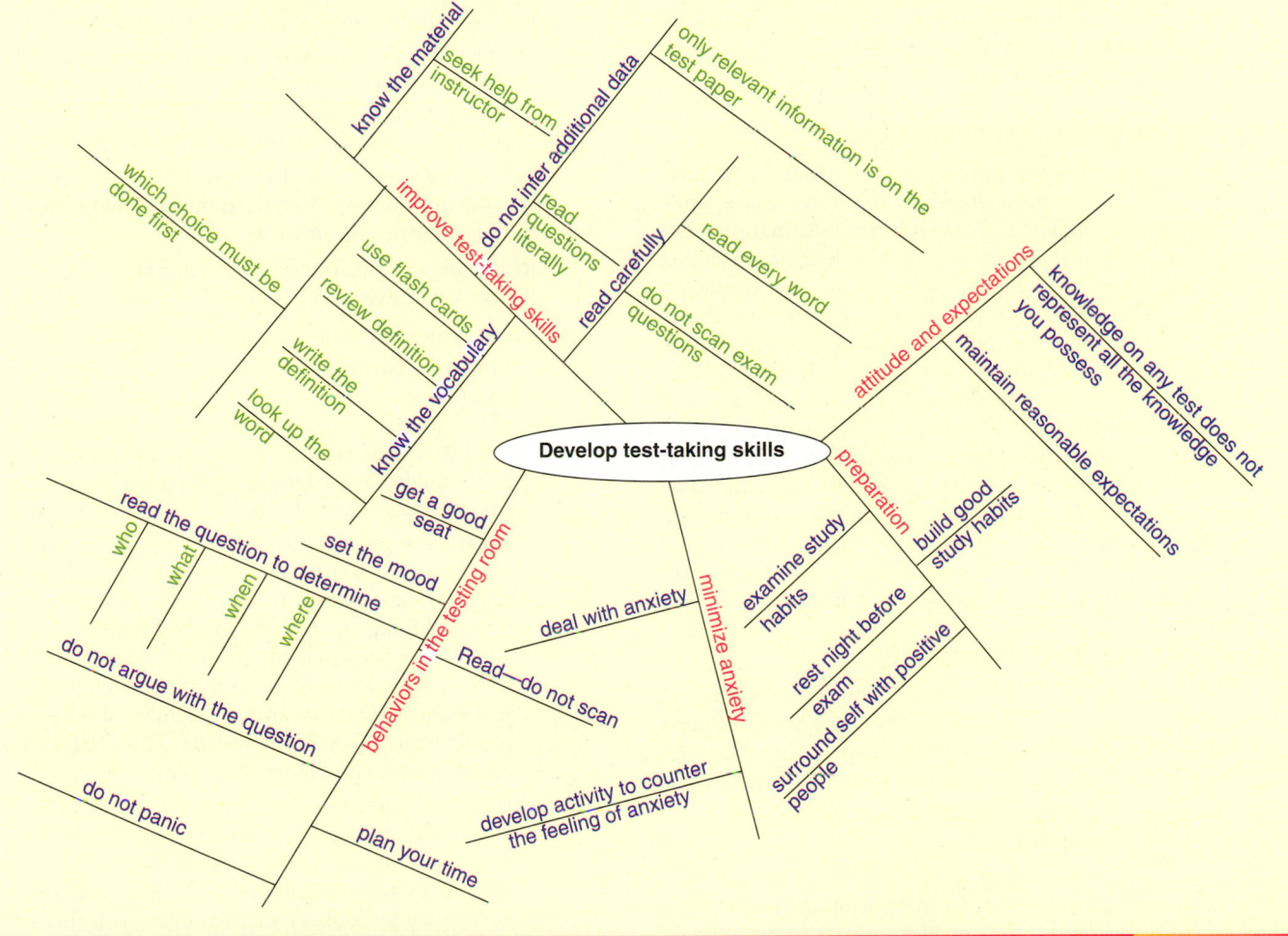

1. Pick a time and a place where there will be no interruptions for 20 minutes. You may neither speak to anyone nor get up to use any other resources. You are taking a test.
2. Randomly pick a page of the review book and choose five questions from that page. It does not matter whether you have studied the content in your program.
3. Set the timer for 5 minutes.
4. Start the test. Read each question out loud.
   a. If you read "over" a word, stop reading, make a mark next to that word, and begin again from the beginning.
   b. If you mispronounce a word, stop reading, make a mark next to that word, and begin again from the beginning.
   c. If you do not know the meaning of a word (English or medical), stop and look it up.
5. At the end of the question, restate what is being asked of you.
6. Read the choices, connect each to the question, and choose the most correct answer.
7. When the timer goes off, score your questions.
8. Analyze why you got questions correct or incorrect. You can use the test question analysis worksheet and your personal critical thinking skills to analyze the answers.

9. Repeat this exercise with five different questions three or four times a week.

The object of this exercise is not to finish all the questions, nor is it even to get all the answers right. Rather, the object is to consciously practice reading every word literally. Each time you do this exercise, you must treat it as a test—no food, no talking, no music, no interruptions. You must associate this type of reading with taking a test so that each time you take a test, this literal reading habit is instinctual.

Know the Vocabulary

If vocabulary is your weak area, there is only one thing to do-learn the vocabulary. Look up the word (English and medical) in the appropriate dictionary, write the definition on the back of your analysis sheet and review the definition during your next study session. Add additional time in your study plan for vocabulary building. Use additional modes of learning, such as audio or flashcards to master your vocabulary skills.

Do Not Infer Additional Data

The more experiences you have in life, the easier it is to infer additional data in any given situation. You must realize, however, that for the moment, the only relevant information is the information on the test paper—no more, no less. Based on that information alone and the given choices, you must decide on the correct responses. You base your decision on those things you have learned about the topic, on standards of care, on the nursing process, and on your knowledge base. If you read into the question, you have in essence rewritten it and may not choose the correct answer. One strategy for overcoming this habit is to recognize when you begin to interject information into a question. In any such instance, you must stop, take some physical action to call your attention to the fact that you are adding information, and clear your mind—take a breath, clear your throat, or wear a rubber band and snap it! Then start over again, concentrating on reading the question literally.

Identify Priorities Correctly

When questions concern priorities, ask yourself which of the given choices would result in serious consequences if not done first. When you are being questioned about procedural tasks, ask which of the given choices must be done before the others.

Know the Material

Not knowing the material represents a lack of knowledge base. Write down the content area of each of the questions you miss, then go back and review the concept or facts in question. If the same content areas are problematic over several tests, seek additional assistance from your instructor. You need clarification regarding your understanding of both the information and the questions.

Go with the First Answer

Have you ever found yourself reading a test question and then eliminating all but two choices? Finally you choose one of the answers. You start to go to the next question but then second-guess yourself and change the answer. When the exam is returned, you find your first choice was the correct answer.

Generally, a student's first choice is correct. Unless you have the thought, "Oh, my goodness, why did I choose that answer?" do not change the answer. That thought indicates you recalled or found information that made the second choice incorrect. Unless you know the answer is definitely wrong, go with your first intuition. Often the first choice is correct.

Behaviors in the Testing Room

Setting yourself up in the testing room for a positive experience can make a difference in your outcome. Be sure to practice the following behaviors:

1. *Get a good seat.* Unless your seat is assigned, sit in an area that is quiet and, has good light, and where you can "zone in" on the test and "zone out" the rest of the room. If you are a student who gets anxious when you are the last one left in the room, pick a seat in the front row and farthest from the door and turn your seat slightly toward the wall. You will be less apt to notice as people leave.
2. *Set the mood.* As you wait for the test to be passed out, take your 30-second vacation. Adopt the most positive attitude possible. Identify the task ahead of you. Take a breath and repeat the following:

   "I have prepared. I am able to read the questions, process the information, and, from the choices given, make the best choice and move on."
3. *Read—do not scan.* You must read literally every word in the question. Every word counts!
4. *Read the question to determine the following:*
   - *Who is the question about?* This will affect your chosen answer. If you automatically assume that all of the questions relate to the nurse, you may miss a question that asks you to decide those things the father might say to demonstrate his understanding of the discharge instructions, for example.
   - *What is the question about?* You must determine to which part of the knowledge base the question refers. Is the question about the way to teach a 9-year-old diabetic to check his blood glucose? To answer this question, you must consider the learning style of the 9-year-old, his cognitive development and manual dexterity, and any significant others who should be involved in the session. The correct choice must support all of these principles.
   - *When is the question about?* The time frame of the question is also significant in terms of the client's continuum of care. Is this the acute session? Is this a client who has had diabetes for 20 years and is now developing pulmonary vascular disease? Is this a new mother with her first child or a new mother with her fifth? Are you in the assessment phase of the nursing process, are you in the planning stage, or are you evaluating the effects of a treatment or a drug?
   - *Where is the question about?* The focus of the nurse in the acute care institution is different from that of the nurse in the community clinic. This will affect your choice.
5. *Do not argue with the question.* Whether you agree with the question is irrelevant. The task is to read the question, put your mind to the question and, given the choices offered, make your choice based on principles and the application of your knowledge base.
6. *Plan your time.* Do not spend an inordinate amount of time on one question. There are some things you will

not know, and if you spend so much time on one question, you can sabotage your success on others. You can come back to any question, but you must be able to clear your mind of this question before moving on to tackle another. This is a good place for a 30-second vacation to put you back on task! If you cannot let a question go, you will be unable to concentrate on the next few questions and, very likely, will get several questions in a row incorrect. It is best to read, choose, and move on. Going back may work for paper-and-pencil tests during the nursing program, but the NCLEX-PN®, which you will take on computer for licensure upon completion of the nursing program, does not allow going back. Each question must be answered in the order presented.

7. *Do not panic.* When you come to a question that you cannot immediately answer, do not panic. Use your 30-second vacation to counter your anxiety and facilitate your ability to process. Recite again, "I have prepared, I am able to read, process, choose, and move on." (See Memory Trick.) Remember, the answer is on the paper.

YOUR PROGRAM IS ALMOST COMPLETED

Additional skills for success are required when you leave the protection of your nursing program. These include scope of practice/competence, tasks of the unlicensed assistive personnel (UAP), delegation, prioritizing care, and the nursing team.

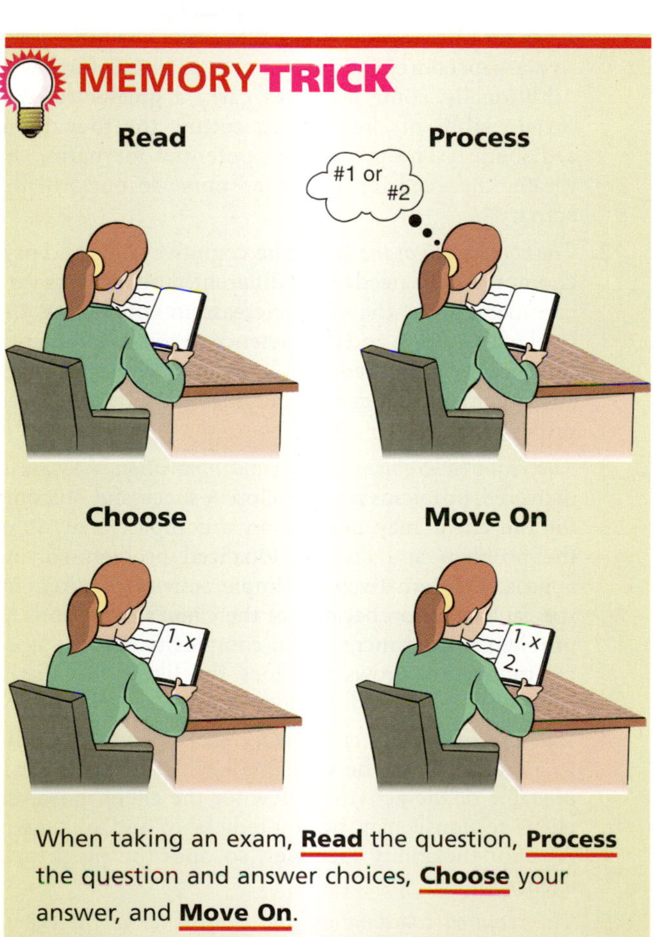

When taking an exam, **Read** the question, **Process** the question and answer choices, **Choose** your answer, and **Move On**.

PROFESSIONALTIP

LP/VN Services

Any time nursing services are provided by an LP/VN, the supervising RN must be on the premises or immediately available by telephone. Being available by an answering machine or service does not fall within the definition of "immediately available." The amount of supervision is a function of the setting. In home health care or long-term care settings, it is common practice for the supervising RN to be available by telephone rather than on the premises.

Scope of Practice/Competence

Registered nurses (RNs) and licensed practical/vocational nurses (LP/VNs) are individually licensed. Although some overlap exists in the scopes of practice of the LP/VN and the RN, there are also some significant differences. LP/VNs are dependent practitioners, meaning that an RN, doctor, dentist, or some other health care provider must supervise them. Most often the supervisor is an RN.

In addition to a scope of practice, LP/VNs and RNs have scopes of competence. Within the scope of practice, there are tasks and responsibilities the individual may or may not be competent to implement. For example, it is within the scope of practice for the LP/VN to perform phlebotomy, but this task does not fall within the scope of competence of every LP/VN. The scope of competence expands as new skills are acquired, but all skills must fall within the scope of practice.

LP/VNs are qualified to care for clients with common illnesses and to provide basic and preventive nursing procedures. LP/VNs can participate in data collection, planning, implementation, and evaluation of nursing care in all settings. In most states, some specific activities are considered beyond the scope of practice of the LP/VN. These activities, with some variances by state, include the following:

- Client assessments (can collect data but not perform physical assessments)
- Independent development of the nursing care plan
- Triage, case management, or mental health counseling
- Intravenous chemotherapy
- Administration of blood and blood products
- Administration of initial doses of any intravenous medication
- Any procedures involving central lines

Tasks of the UAP

Unlicensed assistive personnel do not have a scope of practice. A task that falls within the protected scope of practice of any licensed profession (including registered nursing and licensed practical/vocational nursing) *cannot* be performed by a UAP. These personnel can perform only those health-related activities for which they have been determined competent to perform. These activities include the following:

- Activities of daily living (feeding, grooming, toileting, ambulating, dressing)
- Vital signs
- Venipuncture
- Glucometer use
- Mouth care and oral suctioning
- Care of hair, skin, and nails
- Electrocardiogram measurements
- Applying clean dressings without assessment
- Nonnursing functions (clerical work, transport, cleaning)

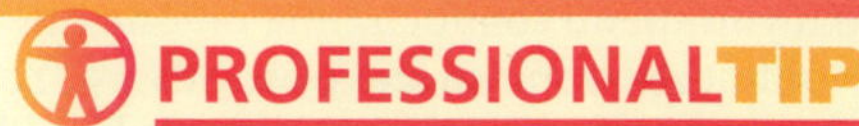

Unlicensed Personnel

Much controversy surrounds the role of UAP. Concerns have been raised that unlicensed personnel are functioning as de facto licensed nurses in violation of Nursing Practice Acts. Further, serious questions exist about the cost savings and quality of care in light of increased reliance on UAP and a corresponding reduction in licensed nurses. Understanding the role and limitations of UAP is critical.

DUTY DELEGATION

Delegation is the process of transferring to a competent individual the authority to perform a select task in a select situation. State provisions for the delegation of nursing tasks vary. Some states allow for the delegation of nursing tasks by an RN to both LP/VNs and UAP. In some states, LP/VNs may delegate certain nursing tasks to other LP/VNs or to UAP. Other states restrict delegation to licensed personnel only. It is *most* important to know what is allowed in your state. The National Council of State Boards of Nursing (NCSBN) Web site keeps a current listing of the address, telephone number, and Web site for each state board of nursing at www.ncsbn.org.

The licensed nurse retains accountability for the delegation. **Accountability** is defined as responsibility for actions and inactions performed by oneself or others. **Assignment**, another term frequently used to describe the transfer of activities from one person to another, involves the downward or lateral transfer of both responsibility and accountability for an activity.

At least one state differentiates between *delegating* nursing tasks to licensed nurses and *assigning* tasks to UAP. In New York, a nurse is not legally responsible for the process or outcome of care delegated to another licensed nurse. The nurse does remain responsible for tasks assigned to UAP, however. As an LP/VN, you are responsible for the decisions you make to delegate or assign tasks. Your knowledge of the client, activity, and worker will help you make sound decisions.

PROFESSIONALTIP

LP/VN Supervision

As defined in the Nursing Practice Acts, or in the state nursing board's rules and regulations, an LP/VN works under the direction of an RN, physician, or dentist. These are the professionals who directly supervise the LP/VN. In some states, the language of the law indicates that "other health care providers" can supervise the LP/VN. The question is, who are the other health care providers? In your state, do you follow orders written by a physician's assistant? A nurse practitioner? A physical therapist? The answers vary by state. It is critical that you know who can direct your nursing activities.

In most settings, RNs decide which nursing activities can be delegated or assigned to other licensed nurses (RNs or LP/VNs) and to UAP. Registered nurses and LP/VNs must consider five factors when making the decision to delegate or assign duties:

1. *The potential for harm.* Certain nursing activities carry a risk for harming the client. Generally, the more invasive a procedure, the greater the potential for harm. Additionally, some activities carry a greater risk for certain kinds of clients (e.g., cutting the toenails of a diabetic). The greater the potential for harm, the greater the need for a licensed nurse to perform the activity.
2. *The complexity of the task.* The cognitive skills and psychomotor skills needed for different nursing tasks vary considerably. As the skills increase in complexity, the level of education and competence becomes more critical. Some activities require a level of nursing assessment and judgment that can be provided only by a licensed professional.
3. *The required problem solving and innovation.* As care is delivered, problems may develop. A successful outcome for the client may depend on a complex analysis of the problem and an individualized problem-solving approach. Alternatively, a simple activity may require special adaptation because of the client's condition. As problem solving increases in complexity and the need for innovation grows, so does the likelihood that a licensed nurse should provide the care.
4. *The unpredictability of the outcome.* A client's response to an activity may be very predictable. If the client is unstable or the activity is new for the client, however, client response may be unpredictable and unknown. As unpredictability increases, so does the need for a licensed nurse.
5. *The required coordination and consistency of the client's care.* Effective planning, coordination, and evaluation of

client care requires the nurse to have direct client contact. The more stable the client and the more common the medical diagnosis, the more care can generally be delegated to support personnel. The need for a licensed nurse increases as the required coordination needed to deliver quality care increases.

The five rights of delegation provide further direction in making appropriate decisions about delegation. They are as follows:

1. *Right task:* The nurse must determine whether the task should be delegated for a specific client.
2. *Right circumstance:* Factors to consider include the client setting, availability of resources, client's condition, and other considerations.
3. *Right person:* The nurse must ask the question, "Is the right person delegating the right task to the right person to be performed on the right client?"
4. *Right direction/communication:* A clear, concise description of the task should be conveyed, including all expectations for accomplishing the task.
5. *Right supervision:* Appropriate monitoring, implementation, evaluation, and feedback must be provided.

Registered nurses are frequently responsible for delegating care and assigning clients to the other nursing staff. In some settings, however, LP/VNs make these decisions. LP/VNs should use the same guidelines to make decisions regarding delegating an activity to another LP/VN or assigning the task to UAP.

PRIORITIZING CARE

Establishing priorities requires an understanding of the importance of different problems to the nurse, the client, the family, and other health care providers. For example, a client may be impatient to bathe because family is scheduled to visit. The nurse, however, does not want to remove the client's dressing for a bath until the physician has been able to examine the wound. Providing quality care while balancing such competing demands and ensuring completion of all tasks is challenging.

Information obtained during the change-of-shift report is needed to appropriately establish priorities. This information can be useful in creating a worksheet identifying a list of tasks and target times for accomplishing these tasks. The time allotted for activities varies based on the condition of the client, the availability of support personnel, the availability of supplies, and a number of other factors. The effective use of time is important whether caring for one client, caring for a group of clients, or supervising the activities of others providing care.

Although it is useful to get an overview of the day's activities, the clinical setting can change quickly and frequently. This is especially true in acute care settings. The nurse must be flexible and continually evaluate and reorder the priorities of care.

Given the same assignment, nurses will not necessarily establish the priorities of care in exactly the same way. If working closely with an RN, you should determine the priorities as she views them. When supervising UAP, you must be clear about your priorities and expectations. Among the factors that can be examined when establishing priorities are the following:

- *Safety:* You should ascertain whether a safety situation must be addressed immediately. A client experiencing a cardiac arrest, a fall, an insulin reaction, and other situations presenting an imminent threat must be tended to first.
- *Timing:* Medications, tests, and vital signs are frequently ordered at specific times. Often, there is very little flexibility in shifting the times. In hospitals, medications, for example, must be given within a specified time frame, usually half an hour before or after the established time.
- *Interdependence of events:* You must ascertain whether some activity must occur before another activity can take place. For example, a fasting blood sugar must be completed before the client receives either insulin or food; blood is drawn a specified time after the medication is given to ascertain the peak level of gentamyacin.
- *Client requests:* Quality care depends on meeting client needs. Some events—showers, bed changings, enema administration, and so on—can be scheduled after consulting with the client regarding personal preferences.
- *Availability of help:* If two people are needed to turn a client, ambulate a client, or provide other care, coordination of the health care team is essential for effective utilization of time. Ascertain which activities require assistance, then consult with coworkers about their availability.
- *Client's status:* Clients vary in the extent to which they can participate in their care. This factor influences the order of executing tasks and the length of time a task takes. A semi-independent client can be performing a task (e.g., bathing) with minimal assistance while the nurse attends to some other need.
- *Availability of resources:* If six clients are supposed to get out of bed and sit in chairs, and only two chairs are available, the clients clearly cannot get out of bed at the same time. Geri-chairs, wheelchairs, and other equipment are sometimes limited. Additionally, tasks may need to be delayed because supplies must be obtained from central supply.

Effectively organizing and establishing priorities with regard to care takes practice. Obtaining answers to certain questions when looking back at the day's events can help you hone this skill: Did you lack information that would have helped you prioritize more effectively? Did you fail to or inaccurately consider the client's status, the availability of help, or other factors? Did you establish priorities and set a schedule without getting client input? Did you fail to coordinate with coworkers? You will learn from experience. Both client and nurse feel the positive benefits of a day that flowed smoothly.

THE NURSING TEAM

Within the nursing staff are different team members. Nursing staff includes nursing UAP, certified nurse assistants (CNAs), LP/VNs, RNs, and nurse practitioners (NPs). The roles, levels of education, skills, levels of independence, and lengths of education vary considerably (Figure 1-10). Familiarizing yourself with the roles of other nursing staff will help ensure that your practice conforms to the scope of practice as outlined by law.

Nursing UAP can have a number of different titles including UAP, patient care technician, clinical technician, and nursing assistant. These persons provide hands-on care to clients in addition to performing other duties. None of

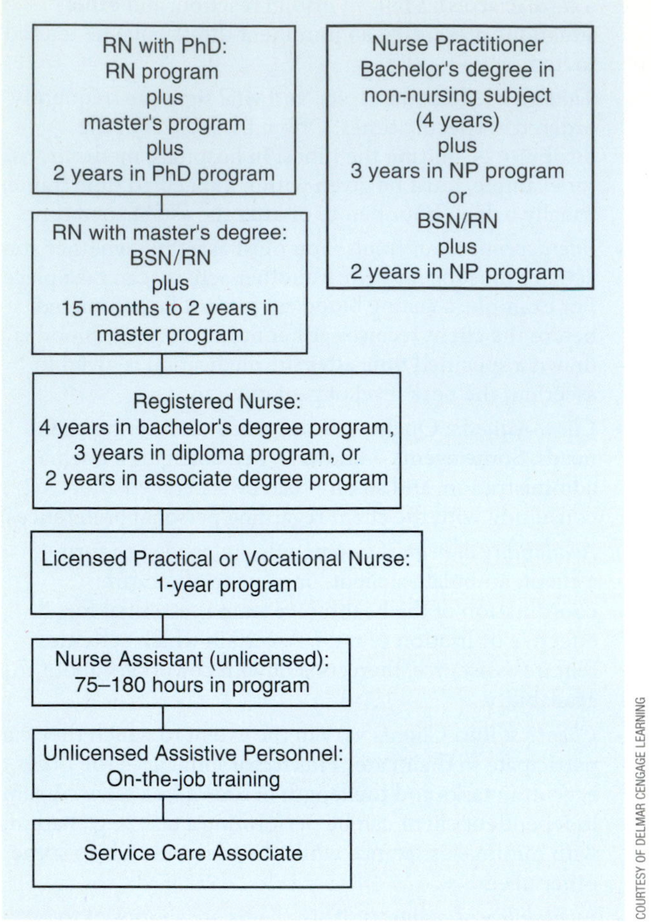

FIGURE 1-10 Workplace Hierarchy

these personnel has a license to practice. Rather, training is provided by the employer and may last from 2 to 10 weeks. The tasks they are expected to perform are designated by the employer.

A CNA is also unlicensed. In contrast to other UAP, however, the curriculum and length of training to become a CNA are prescribed. As part of health care reforms in the long-term care setting, the primary employment setting of CNAs, a set curriculum of a minimum of 100 hours duration must be completed to be certified.

LP/VNs work very closely with registered nurses. The LP/VN attends a 1-year program and must pass the NCLEX-PN®. The RN is educated in a 3-year hospital-diploma program, a 2-year college associate-degree program, or a 4-year college baccalaureate program and must pass the NCLEX-RN®.

An NP is an RN who has obtained additional education (usually a master's degree) and is certified by the state. The role of the NP typically includes diagnosis and treatment of commonly occurring medical conditions. Outpatient clinics frequently employ NPs. Increasingly, they are also found working in hospitals, long-term care facilities, and rehabilitation centers.

FROM STUDENT TO LP/VN

You have completed the LP/VN educational program. Through formal education and clinical supervision, you have studied and learned the skills necessary to become competent in providing client care. Now you are ready to graduate and begin your career as a nurse.

Your first task as a graduate practical nurse is to take and pass the NCLEX-PN® and obtain your nursing license. After you have obtained your license, you can begin the search for a job. The effort required in the period of time between the job search and employment can be considered a job in and of itself. There are many tasks to complete and skills to master to land your first job as an LP/VN.

EXAMINATION AND LICENSURE

In some states, you can begin work as a graduate LP/VN. A graduate LP/VN has completed the educational requirements and either is waiting to take the NCLEX-PN® or to receive test results and a license. Check with your state board of nursing to learn both the requirements for a temporary license to practice nursing as a graduate LP/VN and any restrictions put on your practice while working under this status. For most students, however, the time after graduation is used to prepare for the licensure exam.

The NCLEX-PN®

The examination that all practical/vocational nurses must pass in order to be licensed is the NCLEX-PN®. The NCLEX® tests the skills and knowledge required for entry-level practice. The state boards use the results of this examination to determine whether a license will be issued to the graduate. Figure 1-11 lists the steps each graduate must follow in order to take the examination. The NCLEX® tests knowledge of client needs such as physiologic and psychological needs, safety, and health promotion, as well as the nursing process, including data collection, planning, and implementation. The test is administered via a computer using a method called

1. The candidate applies for licensure in the state or territory in which he wishes to be licensed and meets their eligibility requirements.
2. Candidate gets an NCLEX® Examination Candidate Bulletin from the board of nursing, National Council of State Boards of Nursing (www.ncsbn.org), or on the NCLEX® Candidate website (www.vue.com/nclex).
3. The candidate receives registration confirmation from Pearson VUE.
4. The board of nursing with which you desire licensure sends eligibility to take the examination.
5. Pearson VUE sends an Authorization to Test (ATT) to the candidate.
6. After receiving the ATT, an appointment to test can be made through the Web (www.pearsonvue.com/nclex) or by telephone to Pearson VUE.
7. On the appointed day, the candidate takes the test at a Pearson Professional Center. The candidate presents an approved form of identification and the ATT at the testing center.
8. Test results from the board of nursing to which you applied are sent within one month of taking the examination.

COURTESY OF DELMAR CENGAGE LEARNING

FIGURE 1-11 NCLEX® Examination Process (Data from NCSBN, 2008c) computerized adaptive testing (CAT), wherein the computer selects the test questions as you take the examination. You must answer all of the questions as they are presented to you, and you may not skip questions. Most of the questions are four-option multiple choice in format.

In April 2003, alternate item formats were added to the NCLEX®. These alternate item formats include multiple choice requiring more than one response, fill-in-the-blank (must be spelled correctly), and identifying an area on a picture or graphic. The answers will be either correct or incorrect; no partial credit will be given (National Council of State Boards of Nursing [NCSBN], 2007).

All LP/VN candidates answer a minimum of 85 questions and a maximum of 205 questions during the maximum 5-hour testing period (NCSBN, 2008b). The results are mailed to the candidate by the state board 1 month or less after the examination. Candidates may retake the examination; however, the National Council requires a wait of at least 91 days between testings. Your state board may have other policies related to retaking the exam.

Your License

After you have successfully passed the NCLEX®, you will be issued your nursing license from your state board. It is your responsibility to maintain your license according to your state's standards and inform your state board of any changes in name, address, and employment. Once licensed, you are ready to practice.

SUMMARY

- Developing a positive attitude enhances your learning experience.
- Strategies for developing a positive attitude include creating a positive self-image, recognizing your abilities, and identifying realistic expectations for meeting those goals.
- Competency in the basic skills of reading, arithmetic and mathematics, writing, listening, and speaking is necessary.
- It is important to build your vocabulary and comprehension of medical terminology to better enable you to meet your clients' learning needs.
- Identifying your preference for a particular learning style will help you identify the strategies you need to be a successful student.
- Organizing your study space and decreasing interruptions will increase your efficiency and facilitate your sticking to your study plan.
- Several methods can be used to take notes. Note taking in lectures and from your text is a strategy to help you retain the information presented.
- Critical thinking is the ability to apply your knowledge base.
- Critical thinking is a disciplined way of thinking that the nursing student can begin to develop. The effective use of the nursing process depends on the ability to think well.
- Four basic intellectual skills are essential to quality thinking: critical reading, critical listening, critical writing, and critical speaking.
- Reasoning is the process of applying critical thinking to some problem to find an answer or to figure something out. Therefore, reasoning has a purpose.
- When students begin to be aware of their own thinking and begin to assume responsibility for it, they will begin to use their own logic to discover the logic of nursing. The result will be better learning and the ability to make high-quality decisions related to client care.
- Consistent attention to improving the quality of thinking will produce the traits of an educated person.
- Developing a strategy to minimize anxiety when taking tests will improve your performance.
- To successfully complete a test, read each question thoroughly, do not infer additional information, and identify priorities.

REVIEW QUESTIONS

1. The sign of true comprehension of material is:
   1. the ability to repeat a paragraph word for word.
   2. memorization of the material.
   3. the ability to recite the material.
   4. the ability to summarize the material using your own words.
2. If you suspect you have a learning disability, it is important that you:
   1. ignore it; you will be able to work around it on your own.
   2. be tested to determine the assistance you will need to compensate for the disability.
   3. keep it to yourself; you will not be able to pass the program if you tell anyone about it.
   4. use it as an excuse to put less work into the program.
3. The best way to study is to:
   1. read only the assigned material.
   2. take notes in the lecture only.
   3. read, reread, reflect, recite, and review.
   4. read and attend lectures.
4. The best way to deal with any anxiety you may experience during a test is:
   1. jogging.
   2. listening to music.
   3. practicing deep breathing and imagery.
   4. asking for more time to take the test.

5. The person who has the ability to separate needed information from information not needed at the present time is practicing the standard for critical thinking called:
   1. logic.
   2. relevance.
   3. adequacy.
   4. significance.
6. To improve test-taking skills, one should: (Select all that apply.)
   1. quickly scan the question and answers and choose a response.
   2. connect each choice to the question to determine correctness.
   3. write definitions of unfamiliar words and study them prior to the exam.
   4. relate to life experiences and weave them into the answers.
   5. when determining priorities decide what choice would have the most serious consequences if not done first.
   6. not waste time reviewing the wrong answers on an exam.
7. The best strategy to decrease test anxiety is to:
   1. sit by the door so I can see all the students leave after taking their exam.
   2. postpone reviewing test content until the night before the exam.
   3. take a 30-second vacation right before the exam.
   4. use self-talk such as, "This is only one of the four exams in this course."
8. The instructor just returned L.G.'s graded exam. When she rereads the questions she missed, she thought, "How could I have misread that question and chosen that answer?" What is a strategy L.G. could use to improve her grade on the next exam?
   1. Stay up late the night before the next exam reviewing her notes.
   2. When she takes the exam, recall extra information that is not included in the question.
   3. Skip over words that she cannot define or pronounce as she reads the chapter.
   4. Read each question carefully and determine what the question is asking.
9. On the first clinical day, the nurse asks P.W., a new student nurse, to give P.L., the client in room 423, her medication because she is so busy. What right of delegation is the nurse violating?
   1. Right task
   2. Right circumstance
   3. Right person
   4. Right direction/communication
10. Note mapping is
    1. strategically placing class notes in visible places throughout the house.
    2. cramming the night before the final exam.
    3. putting class notes on flash cards to review in spare minutes.
    4. organizing notes into a picture to see connections and links between concepts.

REFERENCES/SUGGESTED READINGS

American Nurses Association. (2008). Unlicensed assistive personnel. Retrieved August 19, 2008, from http://www.nursingworld.org/MainMenuCategories/HealthcareandPolicyIssues/ANA Position

Browne, M., & Keeley, S. (2006). *Asking the right questions: A guide to critical thinking* (8th ed.). Upper Saddle River, NJ: Prentice Hall College Division.

Center for Critical Thinking. (2008). Valuable intellectual traits. Retrieved August 21, 2008, from http://www.criticalthinking.org/page.cfm?PageID=528&CategoryID=68

Center for New Discoveries in Learning, Inc. (2007). Personal Learning Style Inventory. Retrieved August 21, 2008, from http://www.howtolearn.com/lsinventory_student.html

Chaffee, J. (2006). *Thinking critically* (8th ed.). Boston: Houghton Mifflin College.

Chopra, D. (1997, May–June). How can I keep up? *Natural Health*, 208.

DePew, R. (2008). Successfully mastering medical-surgical content. Manuscript submitted for publication.

Duncan, G., & DePew, R. (2011). *Transitioning from LPN/VN to RN: Moving ahead in your career.* Clifton Park, NY: Delmar Cengage Learning.

Elder, L., & Paul, R. (2008). Universal intellectual standards. Retrieved August 18, 2008, from http://www.criticalthinking.org/articles/universal-intellectual-standards.cfm

Ham, K. (2001). *From LPN to RN—Bridges for role transitions.* Philadelphia: W. B. Saunders.

Heaslip, P. (1994, November). Defining critical thinking. *Dialogue: A Critical Thinking Newsletter for Nurses*, 3.

Higbee, K. (2001). *Your memory: How it works and how to improve it* (2nd ed.) Indianapolis, IN: Macmillan.

Holkeboer, R., & Walker, L. (2003). *Right from the start: Taking charge of you college success* (4th ed.). Belmont, CA: Wadsworth.

Hughes, R., & Edgerton, E. (2005). Reducing pediatric medication errors: Children are especially at risk for medications errors. *American Journal of Nursing*, 105(5), 79–84.

Korchek, N., & Sides, M. (1998). *Successful test-taking: Learning strategies for nurses* (3rd ed.). Philadelphia: Lippincott Williams & Wilkins.

Lesar, T. (1998). Errors in the use of medication dosage equations. *Archives of Pediatric Adolescent Medicine*, 152(4), 340–344.

Martin, C. (2002). The theory of critical thinking of nursing. *Nursing Education Perspectives*, 23(5), 243–247.

Meltzer, M., & Marcus-Palau, S. (1997). *Learning strategies in nursing: Reading, studying and test taking* (2nd ed.). Philadelphia: W. B. Saunders Company.

Mind mapping. (2008). Retrieved October 27, 2008, from http://www.achieve-goal-setting-success.com/mind-mapping.html

Mind Tools. (2008). Mind maps a powerful approach to note taking related variants: Spray diagrams, spider diagrams, spidograms, spidergrams and mindmaps. Buzan Organization. Retrieved October 31, 2008, from http://www.mindtools.com/pages/article/newISS01.htm

Mind Tools. (2008, August 15). Use of Mnemonics. Retrieved August 15, 2008, from http://www.mindtools.com/mnemlstylo.htm

National Center for Learning Disabilities, Inc. (NCLD) January 24, 1999 [Online]. Available. http://www.ncid.org

National Center for Learning Disabilities. (2008, August 18). Retrieved August 18, 2008, from http://www.guidestar.org/pqShowGsReport.do?partner+justgive&npoId=67112

National Council of State Boards of Nursing (NCSBN). (2007) Fast facts about alternative item formats and the NCLEX examinations. Retrieved August 21, 2008, from https://www.ncsbn.org/01_08_04_Alt_Itm.pdf

National Council of State Boards of Nursing (2008a). The NCLEX process. Retrieved August 20, 2008, from https://www.ncsbn.org/NCLEX_Process_public.ppp

National Council of State Boards of Nursing (2008b). 2008 NCLEX examination candidate bulletin. Retrieved August 20, 2009, from https://www.ncsbn.org/2008_NCLEX_Candidate_Bulletin.pdf

National Council of State Boards of Nursing (2008c). The eight steps of the NCLEX examination process. Retrieved August 20, 2008, from https://www.ncsbn.org/Eight_Steps_of_NCLEX.pdf

Nosich, G. (2008) *Learning to think things through: A guide to critical thinking across the curriculum* (3rd ed.). Upper Saddle River, NJ: Prentice Hall.

Nugent, P., & Vitale, B. (2000). *Test taking techniques for beginning nursing students* (3rd ed.). Philadelphia: F. A. Davis.

Paul, R. (1995) *Critical Thinking: How to Prepare Students for a Rapidly Changing World* (3rd ed.). Dillon Beach, CA: Foundation for Critical Thinking, http://www.criticalthinking.org/resources/books/how-to-prepare-students.cfm

Paul, R., & Elder, L. (2002). *Critical thinking: Tools for taking charge of your professional and personal life* (2nd ed.). Upper Saddle Rive, NJ: Prentice Hall.

Rubenfeld, M., & Scheffer, B. (1998). *Critical thinking in nursing: An interactive approach* (2nd ed.). Philadelphia: Lippincott Williams & Wilkins.

Sakowski, J., Leonard, T., Colburn, S., Michaelsen, B., Schiro, T., Schneider, J., & Newman, J. (2005). *Using a bar-coded medication administration system to prevent medication errors.* American Society of Health-System Pharmacists, 62(24), 2619–2625.

Saucier, B., Stevens, K., & Williams, G. (2000). Critical thinking outcomes of computer-assisted instruction versus written nursing process. *Nursing and Health Care Perspectives,* 21(5), 240–246.

Sayles, S., Shelton, D., & Powell, H. (2003). Predictors of success in nursing education. *ABNF Journal,* 14(6), 116–120.

Schank, R. (2000). *Dynamic memory revisited* (2nd ed.). Cambridge, UK: Cambridge University Press.

Scriven, M., & Paul, R. (2008) Defining Critical Thinking. Retrieved August 21, 2008, from http://www.criticalthinking.org/page.cfm?CategoryID=51

Sheehan, J. (2001). Delegating to UAPs—A practical guide. *RN,* 64(11), 65–66.

Smith, G., Davis, P., & Dennerll, J. T. (1999). *Medical terminology: A programmed systems approach* (8th ed.). Clifton Park, NY: Delmar Cengage Learning.

VARK: A guide to learning styles. (2006). Learning style quiz. Retrieved August 20, 2008, from http://vark-learn.com/english/index.asp

VMentor. (2006). Identifying your learning style strategies to help you be a better student. Retrieved August 20, 2008, from http://www.Vmentor.com/docs/learning_styles_module.pdf

Walter, T., Knudsvig, G., & Smith, E. (2002). *Critical thinking: Building the basics,* (2nd ed.). Belmont, CA: Wadsworth.

RESOURCES

Center for Critical Thinking at Sonoma State University, http://www.criticalthinking.org

Indentifying Your Learning Style Strategies to Help www.vmentor.com

Insight Assessment, http://www.calpress.com

LD Resources, http://www.ldresources.org/

Mind Tools, http://www.mindtools.com

National Association for Practical Nurse Education and Service, Inc., www.napnes.org/

National Center for Learning Disabilities, Inc., www.ncld.org

Socratic Arts, http://socraticarts.com

Vark a Guide to Learning Styles, http://www.vark-learn.com/

CHAPTER 2
Holistic Care

MAKING THE CONNECTION

Refer to the following chapters to increase your understanding of holistic care:

Basic Nursing
- ***Legal and Ethical Responsibilities***
- ***Life Span Development***
- ***Cultural Considerations***
- ***Stress, Adaptation, and Anxiety***
- ***Self-Concept***
- ***Spirituality***
- ***Complementary/Alternative Therapies***
- ***Basic Nutrition***
- ***Safety/Hygiene***
- ***Standard Precautions and Isolation***
- ***Fluid, Electrolyte, and Acid-Base Balance***

Basic Procedures
- ***Hand Hygiene***
- ***Proper Body Mechanics***

LEARNING OBJECTIVES

Upon completion of this chapter, you should be able to:

- Define key terms.
- Define health as it relates to the whole person.
- List and discuss the five aspects of total wellness.
- List and discuss Maslow's Hierarchy of Needs.
- Describe self-awareness and why it is important to nurses.
- Describe self-concept.
- Discuss the concept of personal responsibility for one's own illness.
- Discover personal attitudes about health and illness and take responsibility for personal well-being.
- Identify the components of a healthy lifestyle.

KEY TERMS

attitude
body mechanics
culture
healing
health
health continuum
holistic
homeostasis
intellectual wellness
Maslow's Hierarchy of Needs
physical wellness
psychological wellness
self-awareness
self-concept
sociocultural wellness
spiritual wellness
spirituality
wellness

INTRODUCTION

As a nurse, you will be a professional caregiver. Your intimate contact with clients allows you the opportunity not only to provide physical and emotional support but also to teach ways to take an active role in maintaining health.

You may have contact with hundreds of clients, each needing specialized treatment and care. The care you provide will vary from routine to critical to emergency. You will be part of a multidisciplinary team of caregivers that includes registered nurses, physicians, nursing assistants, physical therapists, respiratory therapists, laboratory technicians, dietitians, and social workers. All caregivers work together to promote and maintain client health.

Because the caregiver's goal is promoting and maintaining health, understanding the concept of health is paramount. Health is "the condition of being sound in body, mind, or spirit" (Merriam-Webster Online Dictionary, 2008).

INTERRELATED CONCEPTS OF HEALTH

In 1948, the World Health Organization (WHO) was founded. The WHO, which functions as an arm of the United Nations, places particular emphasis on combating communicable diseases, educating health care workers, and improving the health of all people of the world. The WHO defines **health** as follows: "Health is a state of complete physical, mental, and social well-being and not merely the absence of disease or infirmity" (WHO, 1974).

Many people believe that health or wellness is only the absence of disease. Health, in holistic terms, is more than the absence of disease. It is a state of well-being on a physical, emotional, and spiritual level while having a sense of fulfilling one's mission in life (Telstar Innovations, Inc., 2000). In its truest form, health refers to the total well-being of the whole person.

Holistic is a term derived from the Greek word *holos*, meaning "whole." Holistic health views the physical, intellectual, sociocultural, psychological, and spiritual aspects of a person's life as an integrated whole. These five aspects cannot be separated or isolated; anything that affects one aspect of a person's life also affects the other aspects. The environment within which a person lives and the manner whereby the person interacts with that environment are also considerations. Figure 2-1 illustrates the holistic perspective.

Healing means to be or become whole (Quinn, 2005). It is a state of harmony or balance in the body, mind, and spirit connection. **Homeostasis** is the balance or stability that the body strives to achieve among these aspects of a person's life by continuous adaptation.

The goal of holistic nursing is the "enhancement of healing the whole person from birth to death" (American Holistic Nurses Association [AHNA], 2004). Nurses must understand the integration of these aspects of a person's life in order to help clients through healing processes. Healing is often different from curing. Although curing a disease may or may not be possible, healing is always possible. A major component of healing is caring. Thus, the goal in holistic care is to heal.

Holistic Care

The AHNA is the professional nursing organization dedicated to the promotion of holism and healing. It supports the belief that health involves the harmonious balance of body, mind, emotions, and spirit within an ever-changing environment. The AHNA serves as a bridge between the conventional medical model and complementary and alternative healing practices. The AHNA supports an integrative model, which involves integration of both complementary and alternative modalities and conventional therapies, enabling the client to benefit from all available therapies. The National Institutes of Health (NIH) established the National Center for Complementary and Alternative Medicine to investigate holistic modalities. The NIH defines holistic care as care that "considers the whole person, including physical, mental, emotional, and spiritual aspects." The final goal of investigating holistic modalities is to allow the validated therapies to be further integrated into general client care.

Success in using holistic modalities in client care requires an awareness of a fundamental principle of holism: The nurse *facilitates* the client in attaining the best state for healing to occur. Among the holistic modalities most frequently used in nursing are the following:

- Biofeedback
- Exercise and movement
- Goal setting
- Humor and laughter
- Imagery
- Journaling
- Massage
- Play therapy
- Prayer
- Therapeutic touch

Nurses must be open to new ideas and must not allow holistic modalities to become just another technology. According to the AHNA, the holistic nurse is "an instrument of healing and a facilitator in the healing process (AHNA, 2004). Nurses develop personal healing qualities and become more aware of

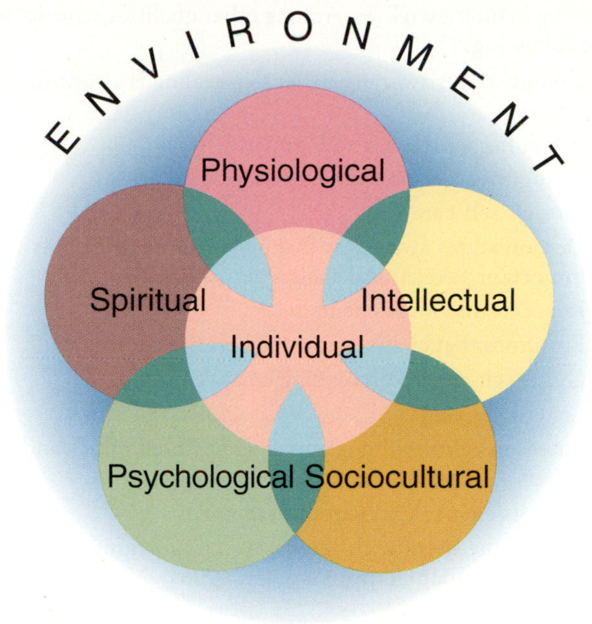

COURTESY OF DELMAR CENGAGE LEARNING

FIGURE 2-1 Holistic View of an Individual

healing in their own lives. Among other qualities, a healer does the following:

- Demonstrates awareness that self-healing is a continual process
- Is familiar with self-development
- Recognizes personal strengths and weaknesses
- Models self-care
- Demonstrates awareness that personal presence is as important as technical skills
- Respects and loves clients
- Presumes that clients know the best life choices
- Guides clients in discovering creative options
- Listens actively
- Shares insights without imposing personal values and beliefs
- Accepts client input without judgment
- Views time spent with clients as an opportunity to serve and share (adapted from Dossey, 1998)

Nursing the Whole Person

Nursing the whole person, or holistic health care, is a comprehensive approach to health care. It considers physical, intellectual, sociocultural, psychological, and spiritual aspects; the response to illness; and the effect of illness on a person's ability to meet self-care needs. Also taken into account is the individual's responsibility for personal well-being. Teaching preventive care is always a focus.

Nurses work with people throughout life to promote wellness and prevent illness (Figure 2-2). The highest level of wellness should be the goal of each nurse and every client.

Wellness

Wellness is a responsibility, a choice, a lifestyle design that helps maintain the highest potential for personal health (Hill & Howlett, 2005). The **health continuum** is a way to visualize the range of an individual's health, from highest health potential to death (Figure 2-3).

An individual's place on the continuum may change daily or even hourly depending on what is happening to that individual. Constant effort is required to balance all aspects of life and to maintain the highest level of health. A person at the highest level of wellness is one who demonstrates good

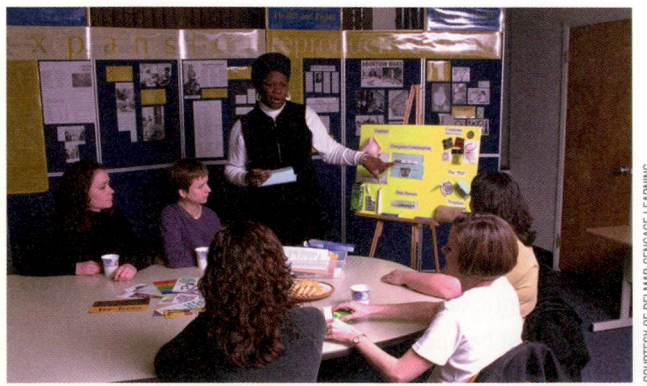

Figure 2-2 Nurses work with clients of all age-groups to encourage health and wellness.

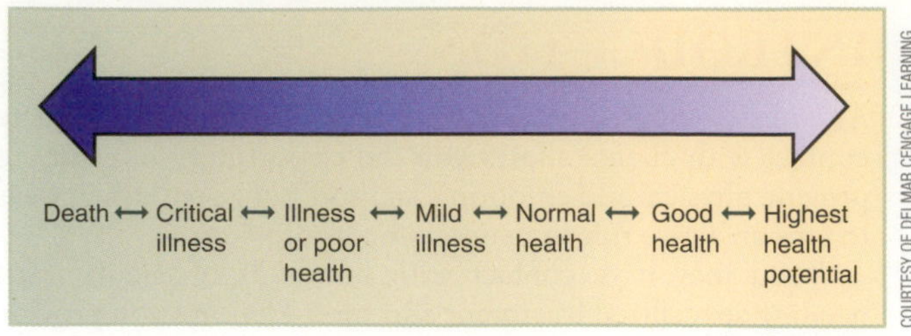

Figure 2-3 Health Continuum

physical self-care, emotional well-being, creative expression, and positive relationships with others.

Wellness incorporates physical, intellectual, sociocultural, psychological, and spiritual wellness. To provide holistic care, all aspects of the individual's wellness must be addressed.

Maslow's Hierarchy of Needs

Abraham Maslow developed a theory of behavioral motivation based on needs. This theory is often referred to as **Maslow's Hierarchy of Needs**. There are five levels in this hierarchy. The basic physiological needs must be met to maintain life. The rest of the needs are related to quality of life. They are safety and security, love and belonging, self-esteem, and self-actualization. The needs of the lower levels must be met before a person is motivated to meet the needs of the next higher level (Figure 2-4).

Many nursing programs use Maslow's Hierarchy of Needs as a basis for planning the care of clients. This ensures that basic physiological needs as well as the other needs are assessed and addressed in individualized care plans.

Physiological Needs

Although Maslow (1987) did not specifically identify the physiological needs, they are generally accepted to be the needs of oxygen, water, food, elimination, rest (sleep)/activity (exercise), and sex. With the exception of sex, all of these needs must be met for the life of the individual to be maintained. Satisfying the sexual need, while not necessary for individual survival, is necessary for survival of the human race. The basic physiological needs must be met before higher-level needs become motivators of behavior. For example, a person who is truly hungry is motivated by that need, and behavior is focused on getting food.

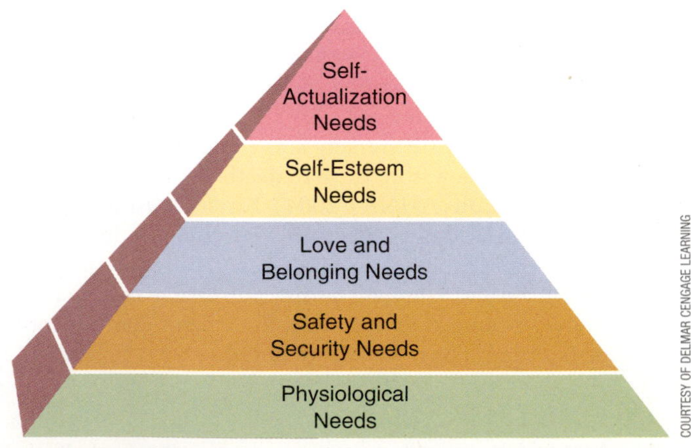

Figure 2-4 Maslow's Hierarchy of Needs

Safety and Security Needs

The next level, safety, encompasses the needs for shelter, stability, security, physical safety, and freedom from undue anxiety. Safety needs include both physical and emotional aspects. Illness is often a threat to safety because the stability of life is disrupted.

Love and Belonging Needs

The third level of the hierarchy, love and belonging, incorporates not only giving but also receiving affection. Having friends and participating with others in groups and organizations are two ways to meet these needs. Meeting these needs is extremely important for mental health.

Self-Esteem Needs

The needs of the self-esteem level are met by achieving success in work and other activities. Recognition from others increases self-esteem and feelings of pride in one's accomplishments.

Self-Actualization Needs

Self-actualization is the highest level of the Maslow hierarchy. A person who has met these needs is confident, self-fulfilled, and creative; looks for challenges; and sees beauty and order in the world.

Maslow contends that because most people are so busy meeting the physiological and safety and security needs, little time or energy is left to meet the love and belonging, self-esteem, and self-actualization needs; thus, most people are less than satisfied at higher levels of the hierarchy. Even when the lower two levels are met without much trouble, many people have personalities and attitudes that make meeting the needs of the three higher levels difficult, if not impossible.

An individual does not move steadily up the hierarchy. As life situations change, a person's unmet needs change, and behavior is motivated by different levels of the hierarchy. For example, if a person who is working to meet the self-esteem need is suddenly laid off at work, the safety and security need of providing financially for self and family suddenly becomes the unmet need that motivates that person's behavior.

Other theories of human development are Freud's stages of psychosexual development, Erickson's stages of psychosocial development, Sullivan's interpersonal model of personality development, Piaget's stages of cognitive development, Kohlberg's stages of moral development, and Fowler's stages of faith. Refer to Chapter 10, "Development and Psychosocial Concerns," for a detailed coverage of all these theories to gain increased knowledge of a client's stage of life.

PROVIDING QUALITY CARE

The first step in providing quality client care is to be aware of yourself. What kind of personality do you have? Is your self-concept positive, or do you have self-doubts and lack self-confidence? What are your beliefs and attitudes? Knowing the answers to such questions will help you in your role as caregiver.

The next step is taking care of your own needs (see the preceding section on Maslow's Hierarchy of Needs). When you attend to the needs in your own life, you are then free to concentrate on caring for others. Your example of self-care inspires clients to have confidence that you will provide quality care. Thus, self-care is a factor in your effectiveness as a caregiver.

> **CRITICAL THINKING**
>
> **Health and Wellness**
>
> What are your attitudes about health and wellness?

SELF-AWARENESS

Self-awareness is consciously knowing how the self thinks, feels, believes, and behaves at any specific time. Being self-aware is a constant process that is focused on the present. A person's thoughts, feelings, and beliefs are interrelated and greatly influence behavior. Being self-aware influences a person in several ways.

Self-awareness may make a person uncomfortable. Awareness allows the person to either accept or alter feelings, beliefs, and behavior. One can learn to be self-aware. Begin now to concentrate on becoming aware of your thoughts and actions. Take note of your reactions to any given situation. What makes you anxious? What makes you happy? Listen to yourself when you respond to questions and when you visit with friends. Realize that everyone has strengths and weaknesses. Focus on your strengths. Spend your energies on today. Do not dwell on past mistakes; rather, try to learn from them and then forget them. Stop periodically and pay attention to what you feel and believe. Listening not only to the words one speaks but also to the way the words are spoken assists in self-awareness. Use the word *I*, and take ownership of feelings and beliefs. Say, "I am so happy," instead of, "That makes me happy."

Self-awareness is extremely important for nurses. Nurses must understand themselves so that their personal feelings, attitudes, and needs do not interfere with providing quality client care. The nurse who is self-aware is more likely to make decisions in response to the client's needs rather than the nurse's own needs. For example, student nurses—and even experienced nurses—are often anxious about caring for a specific client. By taking some time to practice self-awareness, the nurse might discover that the anxiety stems from never having performed the procedure in question. The nurse can then deal directly with the situation by reviewing the procedure and requesting assistance from an instructor or supervisor. All decisions about client care must be made in response to the client's needs, not the nurse's needs.

DEVELOPMENT OF SELF-CONCEPT

Self-concept is how a person thinks or feels about himself. These thoughts and feelings come from the experiences the person has with others and reflect how the person thinks others view him.

Self-concept begins forming in infancy. An infant whose needs are met feels satisfied and good. Experiences, both positive and negative, influence a person's self-concept (Figure 2-5). Interactions with significant others, such as parents, extended family, and friends, have a great impact on self-concept. This is true not only during the developing years but also throughout life. Because of its influence on client care, it is important for the nurse to be aware of how

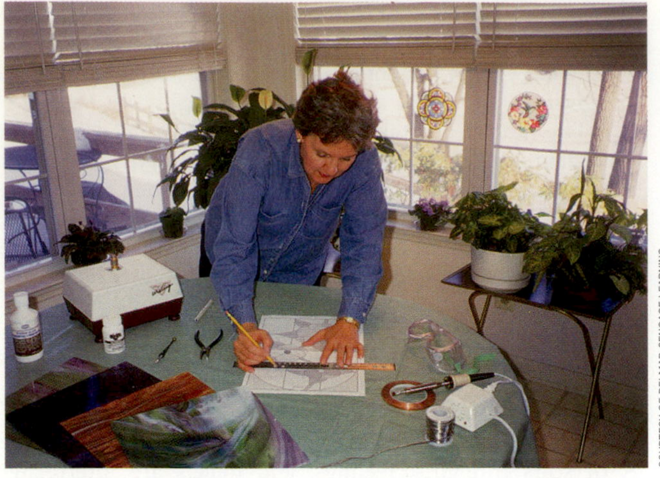

COURTESY OF DELMAR CENGAGE LEARNING

FIGURE 2-5 Self-concept and self-esteem can be enhanced by learning new skills.

her own self-concept has developed. Self-concept develops through feedback from others. The nurse is responsible for providing feedback that will not negatively affect the client's self-concept.

An individual who is constantly ignored or who receives messages such as "Don't bother me," "Can't you do anything right?" or "You don't have any sense" may very well begin to view himself in these terms, with the likely result being a negative self-concept. On the other hand, a person who is shown caring and who hears messages such as "Let me help you in a minute," "Let's try it this way," or "Have you thought about . . . ?" will move toward a positive self-concept.

SELF-CARE AS A PREREQUISITE TO CLIENT CARE

The most effective means to teach wellness is by positive example. By first practicing good health habits as a nursing student, you will become, by example, an important factor in your clients' overall well-being and good health. Remind yourself and your clients that health is a personal choice and that each person has control over his or her own wellness.

You will be helping clients recognize how their own actions can prevent many of the conditions that cause illness. Choosing to exercise regularly, to eat a balanced diet, to eat breakfast each day, to control fat content, and to select from the basic food groups are good rules for wellness. Choosing to not smoke, to practice moderation in the use of alcohol, to avoid all nontherapeutic drugs, and to practice safe sex can help prevent many of the conditions that cause disease and death.

While emphasizing health promotion and client education, the nurse must also encourage and respect the client's responsibility for wellness. This respect allows the client to become an active partner in, rather than a passive recipient of, health care. It is not enough to tell a client *what* can be done to improve health; the nurse must also be prepared to explain *why*. If a client understands the reason behind an action, the likelihood of compliance increases.

Just as you are aware of yourself as a whole person with many components, help your clients see themselves and their health care as more than physical health. Help clients understand how physical, intellectual, sociocultural, psychological, and spiritual health are all related and can lead to an overall sense of well-being. This is the full meaning of holistic care.

PHYSICAL WELLNESS

Physical wellness refers to a healthy body that functions at an optimal level. To achieve physical wellness, a person must practice good grooming; use proper body mechanics; have good posture; refrain from smoking and the use of drugs and alcohol; and have adequate nutrition, sleep, rest, relaxation, and exercise.

Grooming

The nurse communicates a message of health and well-being by being clean and neatly dressed (Figure 2-6). A daily bath or shower and the use of a deodorant form the basis of good grooming. Hair should be clean, combed, and neatly styled. Perfume should not be worn because some clients may have allergies, and it may be offensive to other clients. Frequent brushing, regular dental checkups, and avoiding refined sugars helps control dental caries.

While important for client safety, good hand hygiene is also crucial to the nurse's wellness. Antiseptic hand lotion can be used to prevent cracked, dry skin. Fingernails should be kept short because long nails not only harbor dirt and microorganisms but also can scratch clients.

Standard Precautions have been established by the Centers for Disease Control and Prevention in Atlanta, Georgia. These precautions are designed to protect all health care workers and their clients from the transmission of communicable disease. Good hand hygiene is an integral part of Standard Precautions. As soon as you have been taught the skill of hand hygiene, practice it. Make it a part of your daily life. Encourage your clients to establish good hand hygiene habits.

Jewelry, which can harbor bacteria, and excessive makeup are both inappropriate for the nurse in uniform. Clothing should be clean and free of stains and wrinkles. Clients will have confidence in the nurse who maintains a professional appearance and who practices good hygiene.

Body Mechanics

Wellness involves more than just good grooming practices. It also requires proper **body mechanics** (i.e., using the body in the safest and most efficient way to move or lift objects). The use of proper body mechanics is very important because many

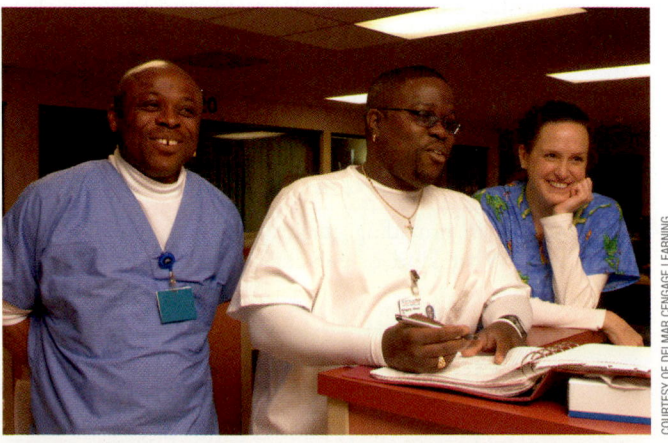

COURTESY OF DELMAR CENGAGE LEARNING

FIGURE 2-6 Holistically healthy nurses' positive attitudes are contagious.

of the skills and tasks you will perform as a nurse involve lifting or moving clients or objects. Bending, lifting, or stooping can cause injury if done incorrectly. One of the first skills you will study involves the practice of proper body mechanics to prevent physical disability, including safe methods for bending, lifting, and moving.

Posture

Good posture is the basis for proper body mechanics. Good posture means the ability to carry oneself well and in correct body alignment. Posture can also send messages about a person. A person who stands with feet spread apart and with hands on hips, for example, may be perceived as aggressive or authoritative, whereas one who holds the arms tightly folded over the chest may be viewed as closed minded.

Observe those around you as they communicate with others. Notice the differences in posture. Does the person who stands in good alignment, with shoulders back and head up, convey self-confidence and capability? Does the individual whose shoulders are drooped and head bowed convey depression, sadness, or lack of self-confidence?

As you continue your studies and begin client care, you will realize that clients appreciate having nurses who appear confident in their own abilities and decision making. When you are with clients, you must be particularly careful of the way you stand. Remember that your posture sends messages about your attitude and feelings. The client should feel that you are confident, caring, relaxed, and willing to listen.

Smoking

Smoking contributes to many health hazards and illnesses. It may also be personally offensive to clients. The odor of smoke on clothing or the breath (halitosis) may precipitate allergic reactions or lead to a feeling of nausea in some clients. Most health care facilities have strict rules about smoking. Many facilities are "smoke free." The nurse should never smoke in a client's room. Furthermore, great care should be taken to ensure that no offensive tobacco odors remain if the nurse uses or is in close proximity to tobacco products. In each situation, every effort should be made to enforce all safety rules for clients and visitors. "No smoking" signs should be posted and strictly enforced when oxygen is in use.

Drugs and Alcohol

A frightening trend in the United States is the increasing rate of alcohol and drug abuse. Drug abuse has become so widespread within the health professions that impaired caregiver programs have been implemented. Many states now provide access to treatment for the impaired nurse through the state board of nursing. Drug abuse can begin very insidiously when a nurse says to herself, "I'll borrow a pill just this once for my headache." The second time is easier, and the downward spiral begins.

A nurse should never give or make a drug available to anyone without the written order of a physician or other person who can legally prescribe medications, such as a nurse practitioner. Approximately 10% of nurses have a substance abuse problem (Dunn, 2005). If you believe that a colleague is abusing drugs, you have an obligation to let your supervisor know so that the colleague can receive help through the impaired nurse program in your state. If you become addicted, you have a duty to your clients, your peers, and yourself to accept help through a recovery program.

Nutrition

Nursing is emotionally, mentally, and physically demanding. Nurses must be able to think clearly and work efficiently. A balanced diet, including fruits and vegetables, whole grains and cereals, milk and milk products, and meats or other protein foods, is required for optimal body function.

Nursing students may be tempted to skip meals, omit breakfast, eat snacks, and follow fad diets. This is never a wise practice. While you are in school, your success depends on your functioning at your best. Skipping meals, especially breakfast, leaves a person tired, weak, and hungry. It is impossible to think efficiently when hungry. Remember Maslow's Hierarchy of Needs: The need for food must be satisfied before you will be motivated to meet the need to learn or to study.

Always eat a balanced breakfast. Pastries and coffee, although satisfying in the moment, elevate the blood sugar level only for a short while before the level plummets. This reaction leaves a person drained, irritable, and hungrier than before. Try to avoid snacking on junk foods, which contain empty calories, or those having very little nutritional value. Instead, plan to eat fruit or high-protein snacks.

Plan a routine for mealtimes and stick to it. Doing so helps prevent the urge to binge on unhealthy snacks. Also, drink plenty of water. Water is the body's most important nutrient (Figure 2-7). A human being can survive for weeks without food but only for a few days without water. By weight, approximately 60% of the adult body is water. In order to maintain proper fluid balance and to facilitate the elimination of body wastes, it is necessary to drink plenty of fluids.

LIFE SPAN CONSIDERATIONS

Nutrition

- Children's appetites vary with their growth spurts and growth plateaus.
- Healthy eating habits should be established during childhood.
- The amount of food eaten generally declines in the elderly person.
- Proper food choices are more important than quantity for the elderly person.

CLIENT TEACHING

Tips on Maintaining Proper Nutrition

- Read product labels.
- Avoid foods high in fat, sugar, and salt.
- Work to maintain or attain your ideal weight.
- If you drink alcohol, do so in moderation.
- Always eat breakfast.
- Make between-meal snacks healthy, such as raw fruits and vegetables.

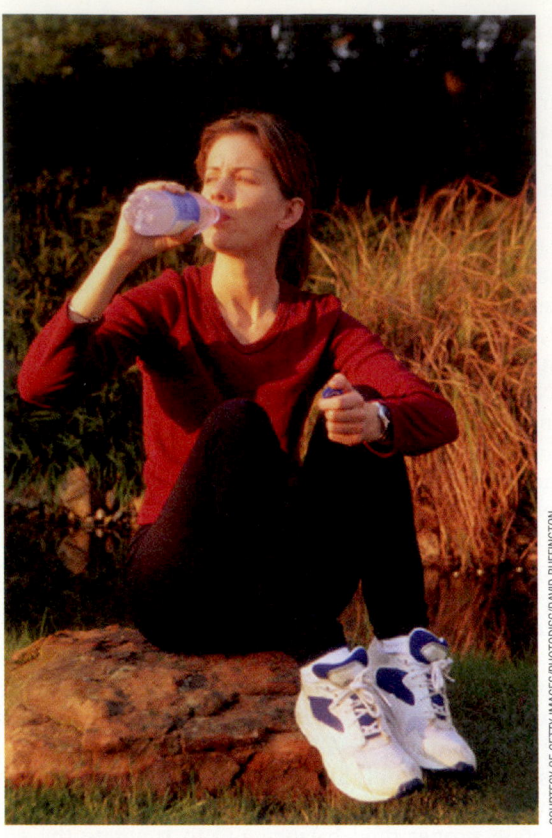

FIGURE 2-7 **Drinking plenty of water is an important element of proper nutrition.**

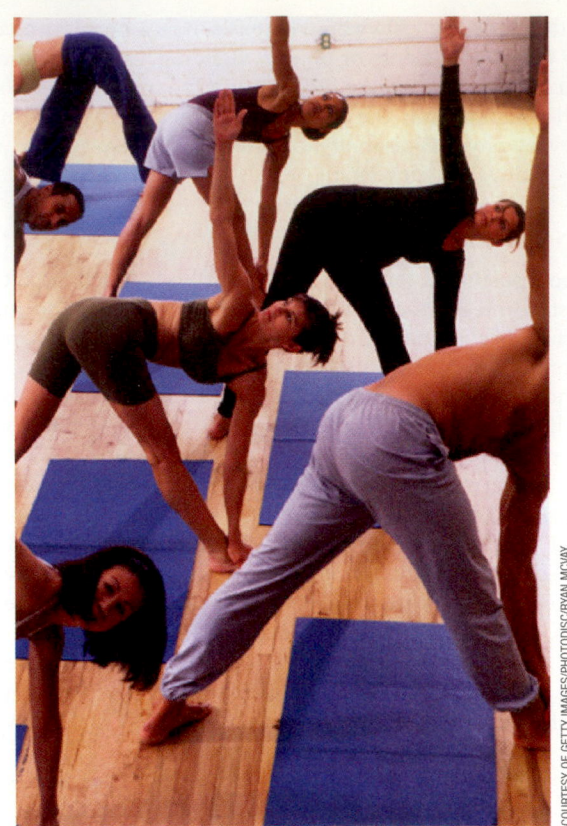

FIGURE 2-8 **Exercise is an essential ingredient for wellness because it improves physiological functioning and increases ability to concentrate.**

Most authorities agree that the average adult needs six to eight (8-ounce) glasses of water each day. It is important to maintain a balance in the diet for optimal wellness.

Sleep, Rest, Relaxation, and Exercise

Wellness implies more than eating balanced meals, avoiding harmful substances, and practicing good grooming. Wellness also means taking time to enjoy yourself. It means making time for sleep, rest, relaxation, and exercise.

Sleep is time for the body to replenish its energy reserves and to heal itself. The amount of time needed may vary with the individual or even with the day. One person may need 8 hours of sleep after a heavy workday but need only 6 hours after a less strenuous day. An infant, of course, needs more sleep than does a young adult. Sleep is necessary to allow the body's organs to function at their most minimal levels. This period of rejuvenation for the body is necessary for total wellness.

Rest, meaning conscious freedom from activity and worry, is just as important as sleep. Rest is a time of inner quiet and physical inactivity. Only when a person is relaxed and at inner peace can that person rest.

Relaxation means doing something for the fun of it. That which is relaxing to one person may not be relaxing to another. Examples of relaxation activities include reading a novel, reading to children, playing cards or other games, fishing, painting, or sewing or other handwork.

Many experts agree that the best rest follows planned exercise. During exercise, heart rate and breathing increase, circulation improves, and muscles stretch. Exercise is also a time to free the mind of anxiety-producing thoughts. Sometimes after a day's work, a brisk walk frees the mind and allows the body to relax in preparation for rest.

Whichever form of exercise, rest, and relaxation is best for you, make time for it in each day (see Figure 2-8). Rest and relaxation as well as regular sleep and exercise are essential ingredients for wellness and result in reduced fatigue and irritability and possibly increased resistance to colds, flu, and serious infections. Furthermore, the capacity to concentrate increases, which should make a significant difference in your studies.

INTELLECTUAL WELLNESS

Intellectual wellness is the ability to function as an independent person capable of making sound decisions. Such decisions are based on the individual's needs but at the same time take into account the needs of others. Clear thinking, problem-solving skills, good judgment, and the desire to continually learn are all qualities found in the person who is intellectually well.

Nursing requires making many decisions, some of which may mean life or death to the client. The nurse must have intellectual wellness to make the best decisions possible with regard to client care.

SOCIOCULTURAL WELLNESS

Sociocultural wellness is the ability to appreciate the needs of others and to care about one's environment and the inhabitants of it. As a nurse, you will care for clients of all ages and races who speak different languages and come from various cultural groups. Each client's **culture** (behavior, customs, and beliefs of the family, extended family, tribe, nation, and society) influences the way that person views wellness and responds to illness.

It is important that the nurse understand that while everyone's basic needs are the same, the ways that those needs are met may vary based on the client's culture. Today's population is working, playing, and contributing to society for more years than ever before. People are more health conscious, better educated, and more involved in making health choices than perhaps any previous generation. Nurses should encourage such involvement and work to dispel discrimination by accepting each person as an individual.

Psychological Wellness

Psychological wellness encompasses the enjoyment of creativity, the satisfaction of the basic need to love and be loved, the understanding of emotions, and the ability to maintain control over emotions. Emotions are an integral part of the balance sought in life and are important factors in the way a person relates to others. They are measures of inner thoughts and feelings and are apparent in actions or behaviors.

Wellness requires that individuals recognize emotions and control their reactions in various situations. By controlling their emotions, nurses help create a therapeutic environment within which to help clients.

Another aspect of emotional wellness is a positive attitude. An **attitude** is a feeling about people, places, or things that is evident in the way one behaves. It can be positive or negative. Many books and hundreds of studies have described the role that a positive attitude plays in helping conquer illness. Many authorities believe that having a positive attitude is at least as important as having the best treatment for an illness.

Nursing requires that you see the best in people during the worst of times. In order to survive and function well, the nurse needs to see life as a challenge and as a gift to cherish and enjoy.

Because a positive attitude is so important when caring for your clients, it is vital that you share yours with them. An attitude can become a habit. If you repeatedly think positively, soon you will unconsciously find yourself seeing the positive aspects in any given situation. For example, you may find yourself at work when the usual number of staff does not show up. You can say to yourself at the beginning of your shift, "There is no way I will ever finish my work on time," or you can tell yourself, "This is the perfect opportunity to get organized early and work together as a team." Either way, you will have the same number of staff members. But whereas having a negative attitude will increase your chances of being miserable and unsuccessful, having a positive attitude will help the day go smoother and increase the likelihood of your coworkers being cheerful and willing to help.

Having a positive attitude will also help you in your studies. It will help open your mind and will spill into your daily life, making life more enjoyable.

CULTURAL CONSIDERATIONS

Sociocultural Wellness

Nurses and nursing students come from various cultural backgrounds and are thus excellent resources for you to learn about cultural variations.

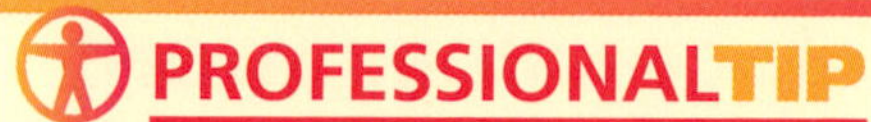

PROFESSIONAL TIP

Self-Nurturing

- Develop activities that recharge the body, mind, and spirit.
- Make time for fun. Any activity that brings happiness or joy is beneficial.
- Schedule a few minutes each day to do at least one fun thing.

Spiritual Wellness

Spiritual wellness manifests as inner strength and peace. **Spirituality** is a broad concept incorporating more than a client's religious affiliation. It encompasses the beliefs that a person has that give meaning and purpose to their existence (Fitchett, 2002). It encompasses values, purpose, caring, love, honesty, wisdom, and imagination (Roberts, 2005), and it may also reflect a belief in the existence of a higher power or guiding spirit outside of the client's self (Burkhardt & Jacobson, 2005). Spirituality manifests as meaningful work, creative expression, familiar rituals, and religious practices (Wright, 1998). It involves finding meaning in everything, including life, illness, and death. Spiritual needs include love, meaning in life, forgiveness, and hope. The human spiritual dimension is a major healing force. It can mean the difference between life and death and wellness and illness (Dossey, Keegan, & Guzzetta, 2004).

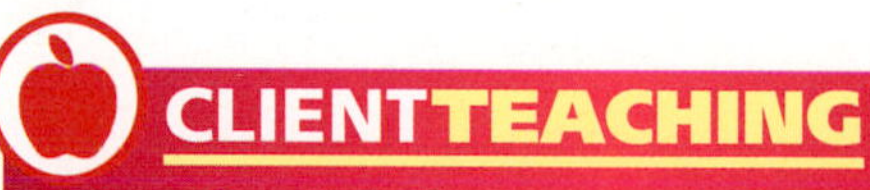

CLIENT TEACHING

Tips for Wellness

Encourage clients to adopt the following tips for wellness:

- Eat healthy meals and healthy snacks.
- Eat breakfast.
- Do not use tobacco products.
- Exercise regularly.
- Do not use drugs.
- Do not drink alcoholic beverages or drink only in moderation.
- Focus on one problem at a time.
- Get enough sleep every night.
- Practice having a positive attitude.
- Think before speaking.
- Make a list of goals for each day.

LIFE SPAN CONSIDERATIONS

Older Adult's Spiritual Wellness

As the older adult experiences life and all the challenges that are presented, spirituality is evolving. Spiritual needs and expressions of spirituality may change. The older adult may find new meaning to life. On the other hand, if confronted with many age-related changes and losses that seem insurmountable, the older adult may believe that there is no longer any meaning to life and that life is not worth living. The older adult may experience closeness to a higher power that has never been previously experienced. Older adults may become angry at a higher power because of all the losses they have endured. Age-related changes may have resulted in the older adult becoming bitter about "the golden years." A realistic goal to assist the older adult in achieving a spiritual sense of harmony is to encourage the person to discuss her feelings about spirituality (Brill & Anderson, 2003).

Florence Nightingale spoke boldly about the importance of the spiritual aspect of client care. Dossey and Dossey (1998) state that the richness of a person's interactions with others correlates with positive health outcomes and that practice of any religion correlates with greater health and increased longevity.

CRITICAL THINKING

Personal Well-Being

What are you doing or what can you do to take responsibility for your well-being?

Nurses are not asked to take over the role of spiritual counselors. Clark (2004) proposes that nurses ask simple, open-ended questions, such as asking the client to tell a story about the struggles in his journey to wholeness. The nurse encourages the client to explain what spirituality means to him. The nurse asks the client if he has thoughts about the purpose and meaning of his life and if he could share it. In addition, the nurse assesses if the client has ever felt "lost in life" and, if so, if anything has helped him find his way or if he is still feeling lost.

Because nurses play a key role in helping clients find hope and meaning in life, it is important that nurses understand spirituality. For many, religious practices are an expression of their spirituality. An important function for the nurse is to respect the religious beliefs of clients, provide clients with privacy to practice those beliefs, and make spiritual guidance available through the client's minister, priest, rabbi, or other representative, when requested.

NURTURE YOURSELF

The worthy and challenging profession of nursing requires unselfish caring for others. Those who select nursing as a

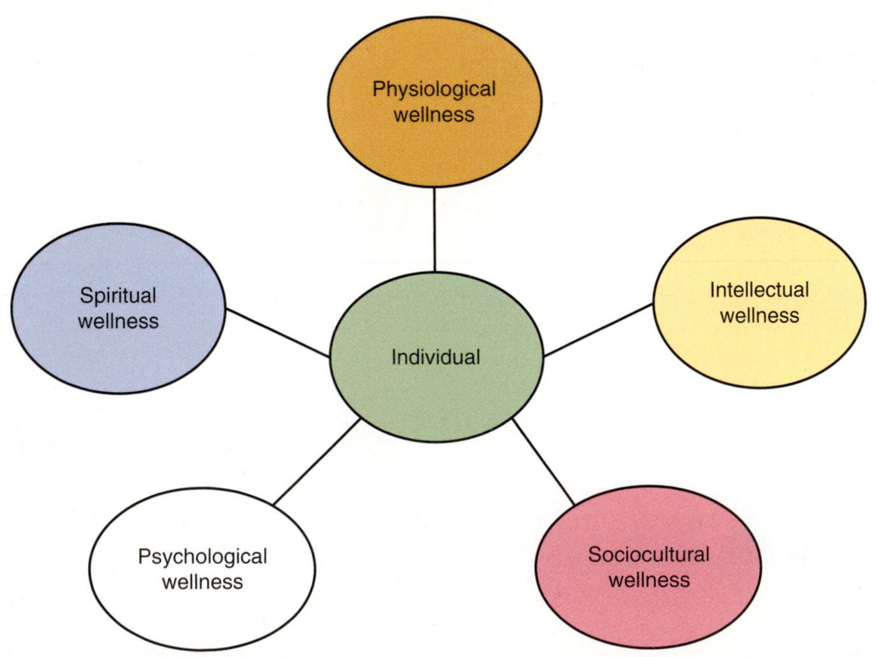

COURTESY OF DELMAR CENGAGE LEARNING

CONCEPT MAP 2-1 **Student Wellness Activity**

1. Read the chapter content for physiological, intellectual, sociocultural, psychological, and spiritual wellness.
2. Inside each wellness balloon, list areas of wellness that apply to the designated wellness category.
3. Highlight the listed areas where you are "whole" or "well."
4. How can you take responsibility to improve the areas that are not highlighted?

career generally want to make a difference in people's lives. The demands of clients, employers, and coworkers can cause stress for the nurse. The nurse's personal life may also be a source of stress. Many caregivers do not know how to care for themselves. Those who do not nurture themselves will suffer stress symptoms and illnesses (American Holistic Health Association, 2007).

Persons who are well physically, intellectually, socioculturally, psychologically, and spiritually lead productive, creative lives. They are better able to meet life's challenges and to control their stressors. For nurses, wellness means practicing wellness habits daily. Nurses are excellent role models when they are holistically healthy individuals.

CASE STUDY

H.B. is a 52-year-old woman who presents to the nurse practitioner with a 3-week history of right-sided abdominal pain. The pain first started infrequently at night, but H.B. has noticed that it is now happening during the daytime, and that the frequency has increased. H.B. states that the pain occurs a few hours after eating but is not associated with eating any particular types of food. She rates the pain as a 7 to 8 on a 0 to 10 scale. She is not having pain at the time of her appointment with the nurse practitioner.

H.B. is perimenopausal—experiencing "mild" hot flashes and periodic episodes of "feeling very edgy and not herself"—and she describes her menstrual cycles as being "normal" for her. She had a right oophorectomy for a benign cyst 20 years ago. She is allergic to ragweed, for which she takes Rhinecort and Singular.

As H.B. describes her pain, she becomes tearful and admits that this is the last thing that she needs. She admits to being fearful of what this pain could indicate. She states that she is "overwhelmed" by all the demands that she has going on with her life. She "doesn't have time for herself" to do the things that she enjoys.

When asked about her life struggles, H.B. admits that she has had a "rough" time. She married into an abusive relationship. She divorced at a young age, and despite having two small children at the time, she went to college and earned a degree in food science management. She is very active in her church and finds this to be a source of support. She admits that she has had to decrease her involvement over the past few years. She admits that she is just "living day to day . . . just trying to survive."

H.B. is a single mother with two teenage daughters. The youngest is having difficulties adjusting to middle school and is having behavior problems. H.B. has elderly parents who live nearby. They have multiple health problems, and H.B. is worried about their ability to live independently. H.B. is employed as a manager of a restaurant, often working 12-hour days and taking calls on the weekend.

The following questions will guide your development of a nursing care plan for the case study.

1. Assess H.B.'s physical, intellectual, sociocultural, psychological, and spiritual wellness.
2. Review your assessment and develop a plan written as a measurable goal of how H.B. could become "whole."
3. What are some steps (interventions) H.B. could take to improve her wholeness?
4. According to the plan and interventions you developed, how would you know if H.B. is becoming "well" or "whole"?

SUMMARY

- Wellness includes physical, intellectual, sociocultural, psychological, and spiritual health.
- The keys to wellness are prevention and education.
- Each individual learns to accept responsibility for his or her own wellness.
- The most effective means to reinforce teachings of wellness is by positive example.
- There are five levels in Maslow's Hierarchy of Needs: physiological, safety and security, love and belonging, self-esteem, and self-actualization.
- Self-awareness is important for nurses so their own needs do not interfere with providing quality client care.
- Nurses should get to know themselves by becoming aware of their thoughts, actions, and reactions to situations.
- Good posture is necessary for personal and client safety.
- Dental health is necessary for overall wellness and professionalism.
- Wellness tips include exercising regularly, getting enough sleep, and finding a quiet time each day for relaxing.
- A positive attitude is helpful in looking for the best in everyone.
- All nurses should learn to laugh at themselves and enjoy life's little pleasures.

REVIEW QUESTIONS

1. Rest is defined as:
   1. sleeping.
   2. physical inactivity.
   3. playing games with family or friends.
   4. conscious freedom from activity and worry.
2. What responsibility does the nurse have who believes a colleague is abusing drugs?
   1. Report it to the supervisor.
   2. Ignore it; it is not the nurse's concern.
   3. Tell the colleague to stop or the nurse will call the police.
   4. Assist the nurse to receive help through the local drug treatment program.
3. What can be the result when breakfast is omitted?
   1. The person loses weight faster.
   2. The person is left tired, weak, and hungry.
   3. The person eats more at the noon and evening meals.
   4. The person's mind is sharper, and study time is more productive.
4. Positive or negative feelings about people, places, or things are called:
   1. culture.
   2. empathy.
   3. symptoms.
   4. attitudes.
5. The aspects of total wellness are:
   1. rest, exercise, and good grooming.
   2. physical, psychological, spiritual, intellectual, and sociocultural.
   3. self-awareness; rest; balanced, nutritious diet; good grooming; dental care.
   4. physiological; safety and security; love and belonging; self-esteem; self-actualization.
6. The goal of holistic nursing is:
   1. curing the client of disease.
   2. assessing, planning, intervening, and evaluating the client.
   3. assisting the client to heal.
   4. collaborating with the client.
7. Spirituality includes: (Select all that apply.)
   1. the client's religious affiliation.
   2. beliefs that give meaning and purpose to life.
   3. values such as honesty, wisdom, and caring.
   4. a belief in the existence of a higher power.
   5. feeling "lost in life."
   6. telling a story of sustaining hope during a struggle toward wholeness.
8. A nurse desires a healthy lifestyle. What activities will contribute to her healthy lifestyle? (Select all that apply.)
   1. Choosing foods low in fat and high in vitamins, minerals, and nutrients for her and her family.
   2. The nurse refuses to forgive a colleague for a statement that hurt her deeply.
   3. The nurse sees working overtime once a week and having to rearrange daycare for her children as a challenge and opportunity.
   4. The nurse takes a class on the values and beliefs of other cultures.
   5. The nurse works all the overtime she can and averages 4 to 5 hours of sleep per night.
   6. The nurse stands in good alignment with her shoulders back and head up.
9. Holistic assessments consist of the following:
   1. physiologic, psychological, and spiritual aspects.
   2. psychological and physiological aspects.
   3. spiritual, social, psychological, and physiological aspects.
   4. environmental, social, spiritual, psychological, and physiological aspects.
10. A nurse establishes a therapeutic relationship by: (Select all that apply.)
    1. focusing on the client and her family.
    2. imposing personal values and beliefs on the client.
    3. establishing a foundation of trust with the client.
    4. actively listening and caring.
    5. collaboratively working with the client as an active partner.
    6. assessing the client's past and current relationships.

REFERENCES/SUGGESTED READINGS

American Holistic Nurses Association. (1994). AHNA philosophy. *Journal of Holistic Nursing, 12*(3), 350–351.

American Holistic Nurses Association. (2004) Standards of holistic practice. Retrieved April 10, 2007, from http://www.ahna.org

American Holistic Health Association. (2007). Wellness from within: The first step. Retrieved April 10, 2007, from http://www.ahha.org

Brill, C., & Anderson, M. (2003). Common clinical problems: Psychological. In M. A. Anderson (Ed.), *Caring for older adults holistically* (pp. 212–231). Philadelphia: F. A. Davis.

Burkhardt, M., & Jacobson, M. G. (2005). Spirituality and health. In B. Dossey, D. Guzzetta, & L. Keegan (Eds.), *Holistic nursing: A handbook for practice* (pp. 135–172). Sudbury, MA: Jones and Bartlett.

Cerrato, P. (1998a). Spirituality and healing. *RN, 61*(2), 49–50.

Cerrato, P. (1998b). Understanding the mind/body link. *RN, 61*(1), 28–31.

Clark, C. (2004). *The holistic nursing approach to chronic diseases.* New York: Springer Publishing.

Diluzio, J., & Spillane, E. (2002). Holistic nursing: Is it right for you? *RN, 65*(8), 32–35.

Dossey, B. (1997). *Core curriculum for holistic nursing.* Gaithersburg, MD: Aspen.

Dossey, B. (1998). Holistic modalities and healing moments. *American Journal of Nursing, 98*(6), 44–47.

Dossey, B. (2000). *Florence Nightingale: Mystic, visionary, healer.* Springhouse, PA: Springhouse.

Dossey, B., & Dossey, L. (1998). Attending to holistic care. *American Journal of Nursing, 98*(8), 35–38.

Dossey, B., Keegan, L., & Guzzetta, C. (2004). *Holistic nursing: A handbook for practice* (4th ed.). Sudbury, MA: Jones and Bartlett.

Dunn, D. (2005). *Substance abuse among nurses—Defining the issue* (PMID: 16370231). Wayne, NJ: St. Joseph's Wayne Hospital. Retrieved February 1, 2009, from http://www.ncbi.nlm.nih.gov/pubmed/16370231?ordinalpos=1&itool=EntrezSystem2.PEntr

Dyer, E. (1998, April 6). Faith and healing. *Corpus Christi Caller-Times.*

Edlin, G. (2004). *Health and wellness* (8th ed.). Sudbury, MA: Jones and Bartlett.

Fitchett, G. (2002). *Assessing spiritual needs: A guide for caregiver.* Lima, OH: Academic Renewal Press.

Frisch, N., Dossey, B., Guzzetta, C., Fristh, N., & Quinn, J. (2000). *AHNA standards of holistic nursing practice: Guidelines for caring and healing.* Gaithersburg, MD: Aspen.

Hill, S., & Howlett, H. (2005). Success in practical nursing: Personal and vocational issues (5th ed.). Philadelphia: W. B. Saunders.

Hughs, C. (1997). Prayer and healing: A case study. *Journal of Holistic Nursing, 15*(3), 318.

Ivker, R. (2002). Comparing holistic and conventional medicine. Retrieved August 28, 2008, from http://ahha.org/articles/ivker.htm

Jerome, A., & Ferraro-McDuffie, A. (1992). Nurse self-awareness in therapeutic relationships. *Pediatric Nursing, 18*(2), 153–156.

Kahn, S., & Saulo, M. (1995). *Healing yourself.* Clifton Park, NY: Delmar Cengage Learning.

Kurzen, C. (2000). *Contemporary practical/vocational nursing* (4th ed.). Philadelphia: Lippincott Williams & Wilkins.

Maslow, A. (1987). *Motivation and personality* (3rd ed.). New York: HarperCollins.

Merriam-Webster Online Dictionary. (2008). Health. Retrieved August 28, 2008, from http://www.merriam-webster.com/dictionary/health

National Institutes of Health. (2000). Complementary and alternative medicine at the NIH. Available: http://nccam.nih.gov/nccam/ne/newsletter/spring2000

Quinn, J. (2005). Transpersonal human caring and healing. In B. Dossey, D. Guzzetta, & L. Keegan (Eds.), *Holistic nursing: A handbook for practice* (pp. 39–54). Sudbury, MA: Jones and Bartlett.

Rivera-Andino, J., & Lopez, L. (2000). When culture complicates care, *RN, 63*(7), 47–49.

Roberts, D., Taylor, S., Bodell, W., Gostick, G. Silkstone, J., Smith, L., Phippen, A., Lyons, B., Denny, D., Norris, A., & McDonald, H. (2005). Development of a holistic admission assessment: An integrated care pathway for the hospice setting. *International Journal of Palliative Nursing,* 11, 322–332.

Selye, H. (1978). *The stress of life* (2nd ed.). New York: McGraw-Hill.

Taber's Cyclopedic Medical Dictionary (20th ed.). (2005). Philadelphia: F. A. Davis.

Telstar Innovations, Inc. (2000). Retrieved April 8, 2007, from http://www.findhealer.com

Walter, S. (1999). Holistic health. Available: http://ahha.org/rosen.htm

Waughfield, C. (2002). *Mental health concepts* (5th ed.). Clifton Park, NY: Delmar Cengage Learning.

World Health Organization. (1974). *Chronicle of WHO.* Geneva: Organization Interim Commission.

Wright, K. (1998). Professional, ethical, and legal implications for spiritual care in nursing. *Image: Journal of Nursing Scholarship, 30*(1)81–83.

RESOURCES

American Holistic Health Association, http://ahha.org

American Holistic Nurses' Association, http://www.ahna.org

National Center for Complementary and Alternative Medicine (NCCAM), http://nccam.nih.gov

Nurse Healers—Professional Associates International, Inc., http://www.therapeutic-touch.org

CHAPTER 3
Nursing History, Education, and Organizations

MAKING THE CONNECTION

Refer to the following chapters to increase your understanding of nursing history, education, and organizations:

Basic Nursing

- ***Legal and Ethical Responsibilities***

LEARNING OBJECTIVES

Upon completion of this chapter, you should be able to:

- Define key terms.
- Define nursing as an art and a science.
- Identify major historical and social events that have shaped current nursing practice.
- Describe Florence Nightingale's impact on current nursing practice.
- Discuss the contributions of early nursing leaders in the United States.
- Discuss the impact of selected landmark reports on nursing education and practice.
- Define the role of the RN.
- Define the role of the LP/VN.
- Describe select nursing organizations and their purposes and functions.
- Differentiate between program approval and program accreditation.

KEY TERMS

accreditation
autonomy
clinical
didactic
empowerment
health maintenance organizations (HMOs)
morbidity
mortality
nursing
primary care providers
primary health care
staff development

INTRODUCTION

Nursing is the art and science of promoting, restoring, and maintaining the health of clients founded on a knowledge base supported by evidence-based theory. Nursing has developed into a scientific profession resulting in change from mystical beliefs to sophisticated technology and caring. Nursing uses caring behaviors, critical thinking skills, and scientific knowledge.

Nursing focuses on the client's *response* to illness rather than on the illness. Nursing promotes health and assists clients move to a higher level of wellness, including assistance during a terminal illness with the maintenance of comfort and dignity during the final stage of life.

In this chapter, the development of nursing is traced through its rich history and the social forces that affected it. Nursing education and nursing organizations are also discussed.

HISTORICAL OVERVIEW

A basic knowledge about the history of nursing is necessary to understand what nursing is today. The study of nursing history helps the nurse better understand the issues of **autonomy** (being self-directed), unity within the profession, education, supply and demand, salary, and current practice. Learning from the role models of history, nurses can increase their capacity to make positive changes in the present and set goals for the future.

The major reason for studying history is to learn from the past. By applying the lessons learned from history, nurses will continue to be a vital force in the health care system.

By studying nursing history, nurses learn how the profession has advanced from its beginnings. The process of enabling others to do for themselves is called **empowerment**. Today, magnet hospitals encourage the autonomy of nurses (Summers, 2008). When nurses are empowered, they are autonomous. Historically, it has been difficult for nurses to achieve autonomy.

Empowerment and autonomy are necessary for nursing to bring about positive changes in health care today. Personal power comes to individuals who are clear about what they want from life and who see their work as essential to the contributions they wish to make.

Evolution of Nursing

Nursing has evolved alongside human civilization. Although it is not possible to present a complete history of nursing and health care within the scope of this text, it is necessary for all nurses to have some understanding of their profession's heritage and of those pioneers who led the way on the path to modern nursing. Table 3-1 is a chronological listing of events in the evolution of nursing.

Early Civilizations

Nursing dates back to 4000 B.C. to the primitive societies where mother–nurses worked with priests. The use of wet nurses in Babylonia and Assyria is recorded in 2000 B.C.

Ancient Greece

Temples to honor Hygiea, the goddess of health, were built by the ancient Greeks. These temples, religious institutions governed by priests, were more like health spas than hospitals. Priestesses (who were not nurses) attended to those visiting the temples. Nursing was done by women in the homes.

Hippocrates, a Greek physician born in 460 B.C., is considered the father of medicine. He used a system of physical assessment, observation, and record keeping in his care of the sick. Hippocrates wrote about many aspects of medicine, including anatomy, physiology, pathology, diagnosis, prognosis, mental illness, gynecology, obstetrics, surgery, client-centered care, bedside observation, hygiene, and professional ethics. Case histories that he wrote are still used as examples today. His emphasis on the importance of caring for the client laid a foundation for nursing. The Hippocratic Oath, taken by physicians today, is based on his principles.

Roman Empire

The first hospitals were established in the Eastern Roman Empire (Byzantine Empire). Fabiola, disciple of St. Jerome, was responsible for introducing hospitals in the West. These were primarily religious and charitable institutions sheltered in monasteries and convents. The caregivers who volunteered their time to nurse the sick had no formal training in therapeutic modalities.

Middle Ages

Hospitals in large Byzantine cities of the medieval era were staffed primarily by paid male assistants and male nurses. This was not true in the rural parts of the Eastern Roman Empire and in the West, where nursing was viewed as a natural nurturing job for women.

In Western Europe, medical practices remained basically unchanged until the 11th and 12th centuries. At that time, formal medical education for physicians was required in a university setting, but other caregivers were not required to receive any formal education.

Renaissance

Interest in the arts and sciences emerged during the Renaissance (A.D. 1400–1550). This was also the time of many geographic explorations by Europeans, which resulted in the expansion of the world.

Universities were established because of a renewed interest in science, but there were no formal nursing schools. Social status and customs encouraged women to stay at home and attend to the traditional role of nurturer/caregiver.

Industrial Revolution

The Industrial Revolution led to a proliferation of factories, where conditions for the workers were deplorable. Grueling work, long hours, and unsafe conditions prevailed in the workplace, and the health of laborers received little attention.

The Royal College of Surgeons in London and other medical schools were founded in 1800. Male barbers in France also functioned as surgeons by performing leeching, giving enemas, and extracting teeth.

It was still considered unseemly in the mid-1800s for women to be nurses, even though some hospitals (almshouses) relied on women to bathe the poor, make beds, and scrub floors. Most nursing care was still performed in the home by female relatives of the ill.

TABLE 3-1 Historical Events Influencing the Evolution of Nursing

DATE	EVENT
4000 B.C.	Primitive societies
2000 B.C.	Babylonia and Assyria
800–600 B.C.	Health religions of India
700 B.C.	Greece: source of modern medical science
460 B.C.	Hippocrates
3 B.C.	Ireland: pre-Christian nursing
A.D. 390	Fabiola: first hospital founded
390–407	Early Christianity, deaconesses
711	Field hospital with nursing, Spain
1096–1291	Military Nursing Orders (Knights Hospitalers of St. John in Jerusalem)
1100	Ambulatory clinics, Spain (Muslims)
1440	First Chairs of Medicine, Oxford and Cambridge
1500–1752	Deterioration of hospitals and nursing, "dark ages of nursing"
1633	Founded: Daughters of Charity
1820	Florence Nightingale born
1836	Kaiserswerth, Lutheran Order of Deaconesses reestablished
1841	Founded: Nursing Sisters of the Holy Cross
1848	Women's Rights Convention, Seneca Falls, New York
1854–1856	Crimean War
1859	Nightingale's *Notes on Nursing* published in England
1860	Founded: first Nightingale School of Nursing, St. Thomas Hospital, London
1861–1865	Civil War, United States
1861	Dorothea Dix appointed Superintendent of the Female Nurses of the Army
1871	Founded: New York State Training School for Nurses, Brooklyn Maternity, Brooklyn, New York
1872	New England Hospital for Women's one-year program for nurses yields America's first educated nurse, Linda Richards
1873	Founded: first three Nightingale schools in United States: Bellevue Hospital School of Nursing (New York City), Connecticut Training School (New Haven, CT), and Boston Training School (Boston, MA)
1881	Founded: American Red Cross, by Clara Barton
1892	Founded: Ballard School at YWCA Brooklyn, NY; first practical nursing school
1893	Founded: American Society of Superintendents of Training Schools for Nurses
1899	Founded: International Council of Nurses (ICN)
1900	*American Journal of Nursing* (*AJN*) established
1903	New York: efforts fail to pass a nurse licensing law
	North Carolina: first state nurse registration law passes
	Founded: Army Nurse Corps
1907	Thompson Practical Nursing School in Brattleboro, VT established
1910	Flexner report
1911	Founded: American Nurses Association (ANA), formerly the Associated Alumnae
1912	Founded: National League of Nursing Education, formerly the Superintendents' Society
1914	Mississippi is first state to license practical nurses
1917	Smith-Hughes Act passes (provided federal funds for practical nursing programs in vocational schools)
1918	Household Nursing Association School of Attendant Nursing in Boston, MA, established
1920s	First prepaid medical plan established, Pacific Northwest Hospitals offer a prepaid plan Baylor Plan (prototype of Blue Cross) established
1921	Women get the right to vote
1923	Goldmark Report: Nursing and Nursing Education in the United States
1935	Social Security Act passes
1941	Founded: Association of Practical Nursing Schools
1942	Association of Practical Nursing Schools becomes National Association of Practical Nurse Education (NAPNE)
	Practical nursing curriculum planned and advocated across United States

TABLE 3-1 Historical Events Influencing the Evolution of Nursing (Continued)

DATE	EVENT
1944	U.S. Department of Vocational Education commissions intensive study to differentiate tasks of the practical nurse
1945	New York only state to have mandatory licensure law for practical nurses
1948	Brown Report: Future of Nursing
1949	Founded: National Federation of Licensed Practical Nurses (NFLPN)
1952	National League of Nursing Education changes name to National League for Nursing (NLN)
1955	Practical nursing established under (Title III) Health Amendment Act
	All states pass licensure laws affecting practical/vocational nursing
1959	National Association of Practical Nurse Education (NAPNE) changes name to National Association for Practical Nurse Education and Service (NAPNES)
1960s	Established: Medicare and Medicaid
1961	National League for Nursing establishes a Council for Practical Nursing Programs
	Surgeon General's Consultant Group
1965	First nurse practitioner program, pediatric
	ANA position paper on entry into practice
1966	Educational opportunity grants for nurses
1970	Secretary's commission to study extended roles for nurses
1973	Health Maintenance Organization Act
1977	Rural Health Clinic Service Act
1979	U.S. Surgeon General Report *Healthy People*
1980	Omnibus Budget Reconciliation Act (OBRA)
1980	National Commission on Nursing
1982	Budget cut to Health Maintenance Organization Act
	Tax Equity Fiscal Responsibility Act (TEFRA)
1983	Institute of Medicine Committee on Nursing and Nursing Education study
1987	Secretary's Commission on Nursing
1990s	Health care reform
1991	U.S. Department of Health and Human Services *Healthy People 2000*
1996	Certification Examination for Practical and Vocational Nurses in Long-term Care
1997	Established: NLN Accrediting Commission (NLNAC)
2000	U.S. Department of Health and Human Services *Healthy People 2010*
2002	Nurse Reinvestment Act of 2002 (PL 107-205)

COURTESY OF DELMAR CENGAGE LEARNING

RELIGIOUS INFLUENCES

Religion had a strong influence on the development of nursing beginning in India in 800–600 B.C. The religious influence prospered in Greece and Ireland in 3 B.C. with male nurse–priests.

Theodor Fleidner, a pastor in Kaiserswerth, Germany in 1836, revived the Lutheran Order of Deaconesses to care for the sick in a hospital he had founded. He established the first real school of nursing to educate the deaconesses in the care of the sick. These deaconesses of Kaiserswerth became famous because they were the only ones formally educated in nursing. Pastor Fleidner had a profound influence on nursing through Florence Nightingale, who received her nursing education at the Kaiserswerth Institute.

Religious orders were established by the Catholic Church to care for the sick and poor. Only nurses who functioned within a religious order were approved by society. The need for nurses in the mid-19th century and changing social conditions set the stage for Florence Nightingale's reforms.

The order of the Nursing Sisters of the Holy Cross was founded in LeMans, France, by Father Bassil Moreau in 1841. Also in 1841, four sisters were brought to Notre Dame in South Bend, Indiana, by a Father Sorin. These sisters established St. Mary's Academy in Bertrand, Michigan, in 1844. In 1855, the school was moved to Notre Dame and became known as Saint Mary's College, which later had a strong influence on the emerging role of women (Wall, 1993).

FLORENCE NIGHTINGALE

The founder of modern nursing is Florence Nightingale (1820–1910), who grew up in a wealthy, upper-class family in England. Unlike other young women of her era, Nightingale was educated in Greek, Latin, mathematics, history, and philosophy. She always had an interest in relieving suffering and caring for the sick, but social mores of her time made it impossible for her to consider caring for others because she was not a member of a religious order. After receiving encouragement from a family visitor, Dr. Samuel Gridley Howe, however, she became a nurse over the objections of society and her family.

On completion of a 3-month course of study at Kaiserswerth Institute, Nightingale worked to reform health care.

CRITICAL THINKING

Florence Nightingale's Characteristics

Florence Nightingale has been described as being strong-minded and assertive. In what ways would it be helpful for you to develop such characteristics?

Britain's war in the Crimea presented her with the opportunity to volunteer with 38 other nurses to serve in the battle-site hospital (Figure 3-1). The physicians in charge assigned the nurses to nonclient care duties. Florence Nightingale persisted in advocating cleanliness, good nutrition, and fresh air. When battle casualties mounted, the nurses had a chance to prove their worth. They worked around the clock, caring for the wounded and carrying oil lamps to light their way in the darkness. The symbol of the oil lamp is still used today in nursing and is the reason Florence Nightingale is called the "Lady with the Lamp." The implementation of her principles in the areas of nursing practice and environmental modifications resulted in reduced **morbidity** (illness) and **mortality** (death) rates during the war.

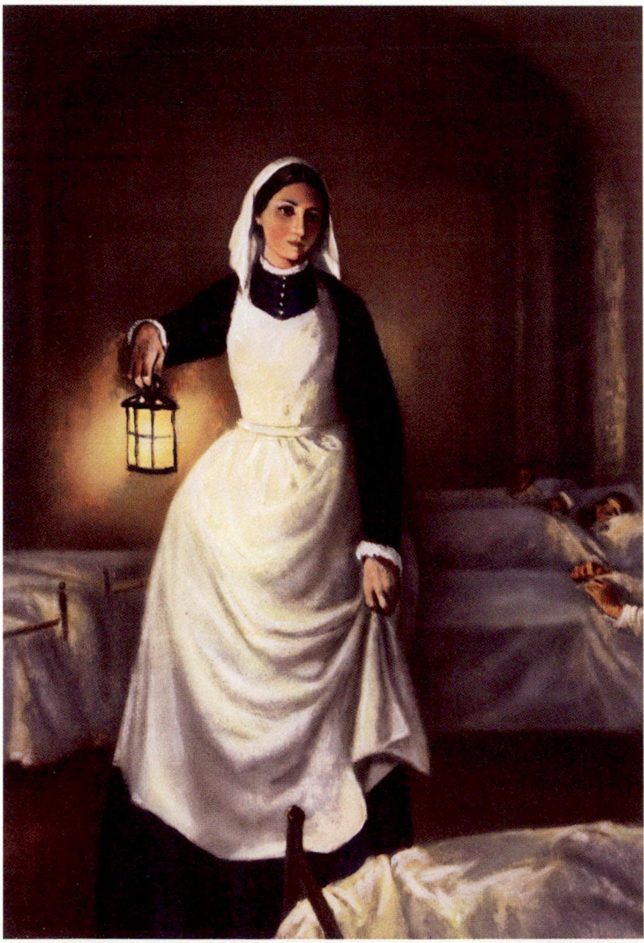

FIGURE 3-1 Florence Nightingale in the Crimea (*Reprinted with permission from Bettmann/Corbis.*)

Nightingale worked to further develop the public's awareness of the need for educated nurses and forged the future of nursing education as a result of her experiences in educating nurses to care for British soldiers. At St. Thomas' Hospital in London, she established the Nightingale Training School of Nurses. This was the first school for nurses providing both theory-based knowledge and clinical experience. She fundamentally changed both the public's perception of nursing and the method for educating nurses. Some of Nightingale's unique beliefs about nursing and nursing education were the need for the following:

- A holistic framework inclusive of illness and health
- A theoretical basis for nursing practice
- A liberal education as a foundation of nursing practice
- An environment that promotes healing
- A body of nursing knowledge distinct from medical knowledge (Macrae, 1995)

She introduced many other concepts that are still used today, although they were unique in her day. Specifically, Nightingale recommended (a) a systematic method of assessing clients, (b) individualized care based on the client's needs and preferences, and (c) confidentiality.

Recognizing the influence of environmental factors on health, she recommended that clean surroundings, fresh air, and light would improve the quality of care (Nightingale, 1969). She believed that nurses should be formally educated and function as client advocates (Selanders, 1994). She is credited with being the originator of modern nursing because many of these beliefs and concepts are still advocated in nursing schools today.

THE CIVIL WAR AND NURSING

During the Civil War (1861–1865), America's need for nurses increased dramatically. The Sisters of the Holy Cross were the first to respond to the need for nurses, with 12 sisters caring for wounded soldiers. By the end of the war, 80 sisters had cared for soldiers in Illinois, Missouri, Kentucky, and Tennessee (Wall, 1993).

Nursing care was also provided by the Sisters of Mercy, Daughters of Charity, Dominican Sisters, and the Franciscan Sisters of the Poor. These sisters, although influenced by the roles assigned to women during the 19th century, were willing to take risks when human rights were threatened (Wall, 1993). Other women also volunteered to care for the soldiers of both the Union and the Confederate armies. These women implemented sanitary conditions in field hospitals and performed various other duties.

Dorothea Dix (1802–1887) was the first woman ever appointed to an administrative position by the federal government when she was made superintendent of the female nurses of the army in 1861. Her recruitment efforts procured more than 2,000 women to care for the sick in the Union army. Following the Civil War, she concentrated on reforming the treatment of the mentally ill (Mohr, 2005).

Clara Barton (1821–1912), who volunteered her nursing services during the Civil War, organized the Red Cross in the United States in 1881.

Blanche E. Oberle was a World War I Red Cross Army Nurse. According to Oberle, nurses were not allowed to take blood pressures in 1918. Only a physician could take a client's blood pressure. However, registered nurses mixed sterile water into powdered medications that was injected into clients.

Men in Nursing

Males impacted nursing even though their involvement is overshadowed by female nurses. During the Middle Ages, men provided nursing care in the military and religious and lay orders, including the Knights Hospitalers, the Teutonic Knights, the Tertiaries, the Knights of St. Lazarus, and the Hospital Brothers of St. Anthony. St. Camillus was from this era and he originated the red cross symbol that is still used today and developed the first ambulance service (Kauffman, 1978). Male nurses served on both sides during the Civil War, but female nurses received more recognition as Union volunteers. The Confederate army had 30 men per regiment who were designated to care for the wounded (Pokorny, 1992). Male nursing schools—Mills School for Nursing and St. Vincent's Hospital School for Men—were started in 1888 in New York (Wilson et al., 2009). Male nurses served on a U.S. Navy hospital ship, the U.S.S. *Solace*, during the Spanish-American War (Navsource.com, 2007). Today, men are a vital component in the nursing profession.

The Women's Movement

The beginnings of social unrest started in 1848 with the Women's Rights Convention in Seneca Falls, New York. Women were not considered equal to men, women did not have the right to vote, and society did not value education for women. With suffrage, the rights of women and the nursing profession were advanced. More women were being accepted into colleges and universities by the mid-1900s, but there were only a few university-based nursing programs available.

Nursing Pioneers and Leaders

The contributions of many outstanding nurses through the years made nursing what it is today. Nursing pioneers and leaders established public health nursing, rural health care services, and advanced nursing education.

Linda Richards

In 1873, Linda Richards (1841–1930) was awarded the first diploma from an American school educating nurses. She established numerous hospital-based schools for nurses and introduced the practice of keeping nurses' notes and physicians' orders as part of medical records. She also instituted the practice of nurses' wearing uniforms. While working as the first superintendent of nurses at Massachusetts General Hospital, she showed that educated nurses gave better care than nurses without formal nursing education.

Mary Mahoney

Mary Mahoney (1845–1926) was America's first African American professional nurse (Figure 3-2). She was a noted nursing leader who encouraged respect for cultural diversity. Today, the American Nurses Association (ANA) bestows the Mary Mahoney Award to recognize individuals who have made significant contributions toward improving relationships among the various cultural groups.

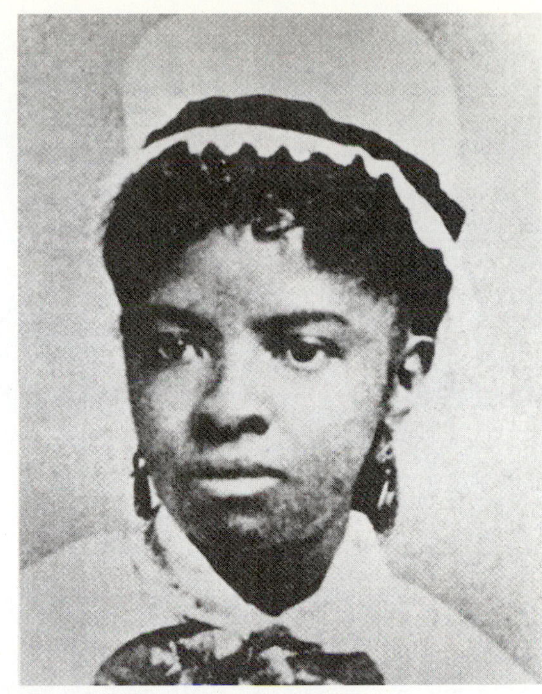

FIGURE 3-2 Mary Mahoney (*Photo courtesy of the American Nurses Association.*)

Adelaide Nutting

As a nursing educator, historian, and scholar, Adelaide Nutting (1858–1947) actively campaigned for the university education of nurses. She was the first nurse appointed as a university professor.

Lavinia Dock

Another influential leader in nursing education, Lavinia Dock (1858–1956) graduated from Bellevue Training School for Nurses in 1886. She worked at the Henry Street Settlement House in New York City, caring for the indigent. Dock wrote one of the first nursing textbooks, *Materia Medica for Nurses*. Also, she was the first editor of the *American Journal of Nursing* (*AJN*) and wrote many other books.

Isabel Hampton Robb

Isabel Hampton Robb (1860–1910) was the founder of the Superintendents' Society in 1893 and the Nurses' Associated Alumnae of the United States and Canada in 1896. She knew it was important for nurses to participate in professional organizations and to work for unity across the profession on important issues. She worked to establish both the ANA and the National League of Nursing Education, the predecessor of the National League for Nursing (NLN). As an early supporter of the rights of nursing students, she urged that there be shorter working hours and stressed the role of the nursing student as a learner instead of an employee.

Lillian Wald

Lillian Wald (1867–1940) spent her life providing nursing care to poor people. She founded public health nursing with the establishment of the Henry Street Settlement Service in 1893 (Figure 3-3) in New York City (Silverstein, 1994). Wald was the first community health nurse and also established a school of nursing. As a tireless reformer, she worked to:

- Improve housing conditions in tenement districts
- Establish education for the mentally challenged

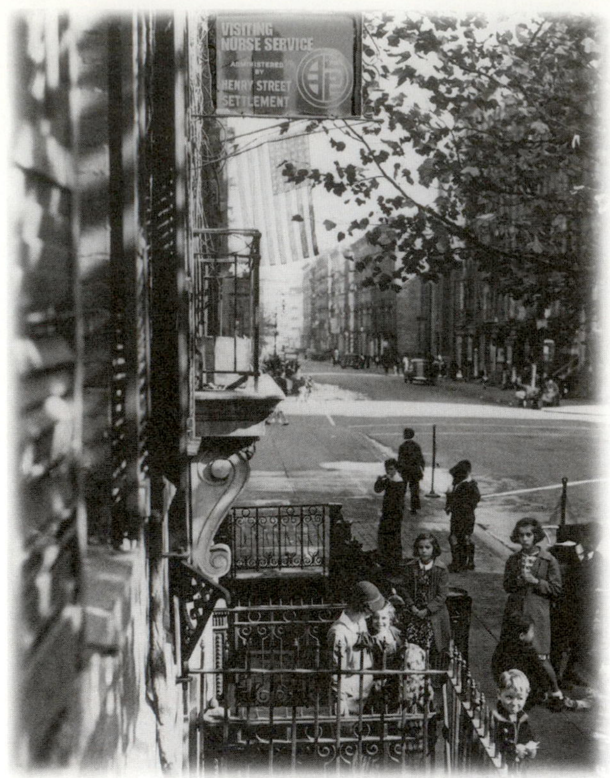

FIGURE 3-3 Nurses at the Henry Street Settlement in New York City (*Photo courtesy of Visiting Nurses Service of New York.*)

- Pass more lenient immigration regulations
- Initiate change of child labor laws and founded the Children's Bureau of the U.S. Department of Labor

Mary Breckenridge

In 1925, Mary Breckenridge (1881–1965) introduced a decentralized system of delivering health care to rural America. This system for providing primary nursing care services in the Kentucky Appalachian Mountains, called the Frontier Nursing Service, lowered the childbirth mortality rate in Leslie County, Kentucky, from the highest in the nation to below the national average.

Mamie Hale

The Arkansas Health Department hired Mamie Hale (1911–1968?) in 1942 to upgrade the educational programs for midwives. A graduate of Tuskegee School of Nurse-Midwifery, she gained the support of public health nurses, granny midwives, and obstetricians. Through education, she decreased illiteracy and superstition among those functioning as midwives. Hale's efforts improved mortality rates for both infants and mothers (Bell, 1993).

PRACTICAL NURSING PIONEER SCHOOLS

Women who cared for others but who had no formal education often called themselves "practical nurses." Formal education for practical nursing began in the 1890s. The first schools were the Ballard School, the Thompson Practical Nursing School, and the Household Nursing Association School of Attendant Nursing.

Ballard School

In 1892, the Ballard School, funded by Lucinda Ballard, was opened in New York City by the YWCA. It offered several courses for women, one of which was practical nursing. The 3-month course in simple nursing care focused on the care of infants, children, elders, and disabled persons in their own homes. The course included cooking, nutrition, basic science, and basic nursing procedures. When the YWCA was reorganized in 1949, the school closed.

Thompson Practical Nursing School

Thomas Thompson of Brattleboro, Vermont, left money in his will to help women who were making shirts for the army and were receiving only $1 per dozen. His executor, Richard Bradley, saw the need for nursing service and, in 1907, established a practical nursing school in Brattleboro. It is still operating today and is accredited by the NLN.

Household Nursing School

In 1918, a group of women in Boston were concerned about providing nursing care for people who were sick at home. After talking with Richard Bradley, they opened the Household Nursing Association School of Attendant Nursing. The name was later changed to the Shepard-Gill School of Practical Nursing. It closed in 1984.

NURSING IN THE TWENTIETH CENTURY

The beginning of the twentieth century brought about changes that have greatly influenced contemporary nursing. Several landmark reports about medical and nursing education, early insurance plans, the establishment of visiting nurse associations and their use of protocols, and health care initiatives are discussed next.

Flexner Report

In 1910, Abraham Flexner, supported by a Carnegie grant, visited the 155 medical schools in the United States and Canada. The goal of the resulting Flexner report, which was based on his findings, was to impose accountability for medical education. Flexner's study resulted in the closure of inadequate medical schools, consolidation of schools with limited resources, creation of nonprofit status for remaining schools, and establishment of medical education in university settings that was based on standards and strong economic resources.

Seeing the value and impact of the Flexner report on medical education, Adelaide Nutting, together with colleagues from the Superintendents' Society, presented a proposal to the Carnegie Foundation in 1911 to study nursing education. That study was never done.

In 1906, Richard Olding Beard established a 3-year diploma school of nursing at the University of Minnesota under the College of Medicine.

Early Insurance Plans

At the turn of the twentieth century, the concepts of third-party payments and prepaid health insurance were instituted. Third-party payment is the payment by someone other than the recipient of health care (usually an insurance company) for the health care services provided. Prepaid medical plans were started in lumber and mining camps of the Pacific Northwest, where employers contracted for medical services, for which they paid a monthly fee. As the first president of the National Organization for Public Health Nursing, Lillian Wald suggested that a national health insurance plan be established.

Visiting Nurses Associations

In 1901, Lillian Wald suggested that Metropolitan Life Insurance Company enter into an agreement with the Henry Street Settlement to provide visiting nursing services to its policyholders. One form of managed care began as Wald worked with Metropolitan to expand the services of the Henry Street Settlement to other cities.

Nurses providing care in the home had experienced greater autonomy of practice than did hospital-based nurses (Figure 3-4). This led to discord among physicians regarding the scope of medical practice versus the scope of nursing practice. Some physicians encouraged nurses to do whatever was necessary to care for the sick at home, whereas other physicians believed nurses were going to take over their practice.

In 1912, the Chicago Visiting Nurse Association developed a list of standing orders for nurses to follow when providing home care. When the nurse did not have specific orders from a physician, these orders were to direct the nursing care of clients. This established the groundwork for nursing protocols.

Blue Cross and Blue Shield

The main impetus for the growth of insurance plans was the Depression. The philosophy in the United States of health care for all further contributed to the growth of insurance plans. In 1920, American hospitals offered a prepaid hospital plan, which became the prototype for Blue Cross.

The American Hospital Association laid the groundwork for an insurance company to provide benefits to subscribers when hospitalized. This eventually became Blue Cross. The American Medical Association developed Blue Shield to provide subscribers reimbursement for medical services.

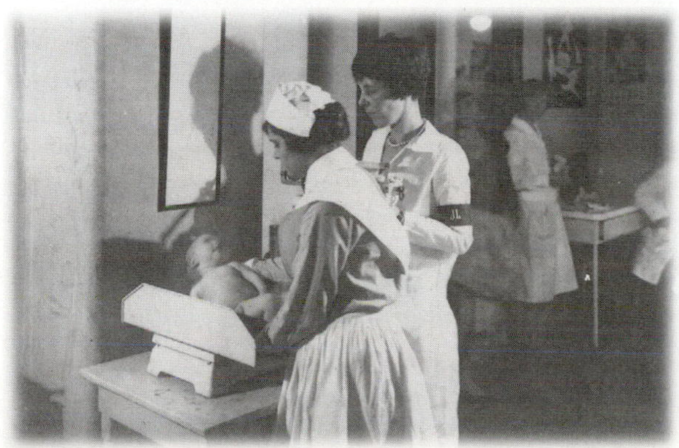

FIGURE 3-4 A baby being weighed by a student nurse and a Junior League volunteer in 1929. (*Photo courtesy of Touro Infirmary Archives, New Orleans, LA.*)

The federal government became involved in health care delivery in 1935 when the Social Security Act was passed. It provided for benefits for elderly persons, child welfare, and federal funding for educating health care personnel, among other things. During World War II, the U.S. government extended the benefits of military personnel to include their dependents and health care for veterans.

Landmark Reports in Nursing Education

Several reports were issued concerning nursing education and practice during the first half of the twentieth century. Three reports that had a profound impact on nursing education are the Goldmark, the Brown, and the Institute of Research and Service in Nursing Education.

Goldmark Report

In 1918, Adelaide Nutting approached the Rockefeller Foundation for support of nursing education reform. They provided funding, and, in 1919, the Committee for the Study of Nursing Education was established to investigate the education of public health nurses. A social worker, Josephine Goldmark, served as the secretary to the committee and developed the method of collecting data and the analysis for a small sampling of the 1,800 schools of nursing then in existence.

The Goldmark report, titled *Nursing and Nursing Education in the United States*, was published in 1923. Goldmark identified that the major weakness of the hospital-based education programs was that the needs of the institution (service delivery) were put before the needs of the student (education). The apprenticeship form of education along with nursing tradition put the needs of the client before the learning needs of the student.

Limited resources, low admission standards, poorly educated instructors, lack of supervision, and failure to correlate clinical practice with theory were identified by the study as major inadequacies in nursing education. The report concluded that nursing education should take place in the university setting if nursing was to be on equal footing with other disciplines.

Brown Report

In 1948, the social anthropologist Esther Lucille Brown published *Nursing for the Future and Nursing Reconsidered: A Study for Change*. The Brown report, published 26 years after the Goldmark report, identified many of the same problems in hospital nursing education, including the fact that nursing students were still being used for service by the hospitals, resources were inadequate, and authoritarianism still prevailed.

Brown understood that the proper intellectual climate for educating professional nurses would be the university setting. Visionary nurse educators were securing libraries, laboratories, and clinical facilities as necessary learning resources. Nurse leaders were implementing professional endeavors such as research and publication.

Institute of Research and Service in Nursing Education Report

The 1950s addressed different aspects of nursing. After World War II, a deficit in the supply of nurses coincided with an increased demand for nursing services. Hospitals were closed as a result of the nursing shortage. Other factors contributing to the scarce supply of nurses were the long hours combined with a heavy workload, low esteem of nursing as a profession, and low salaries.

The Institute of Research and Service in Nursing Education Report resulted in the establishment of practical nursing under Title III of the Health Amendment Act of 1955. There was a proliferation of practical nursing schools in the United States following this report.

Other Health Care Initiatives

In the 1960s, health care services were provided to the elderly and the indigent populations through the federal programs of Medicare and Medicaid.

The Nurse Training Act was passed in 1964 to provide federal funds to expand the enrollment in schools of nursing. Federal funds were made available to construct nursing schools and provide student loans and scholarships to nursing students.

The Health Maintenance Organization Act of 1973 provided an alternative to the private health insurance industry. **Health maintenance organizations (HMOs)** are prepaid health plans that provide primary health care services for a preset fee and focus on cost-effective treatment methods. **Primary health care** refers to the client's point of entry into the health care system and includes assessment, diagnosis, treatment, coordination of care, education, preventive services, and surveillance.

In 1977, the National Commission for Manpower Study resulted in amendments to Title XVIII of the Social Security Act, which provided payment for rural health clinic services. Anne Zimmerman, former president of the ANA, had the bill amended to substitute the term **primary care providers** (health care providers whom a client sees first for health care) for *physician extenders*, which allowed nurse practitioners to be paid directly for their services. This represented the first time that nurses could be directly reimbursed for care they rendered.

Costs and Quality Controls

During the 1970s, the rapid escalation of health care expenditures made the cost-control systems of various federal health programs inadequate. The 1982 Tax Equity Fiscal Responsibility Act (TEFRA) was passed in response to the $287 billion spent on health care in 1981. At the same time that the federal government was trying to control costs with TEFRA and prospective payment legislation, concern was also growing regarding the quality of health care.

Although business and industry embraced quality control systems in the 1940s and 1950s, the health care industry failed to see the need for such controls until the 1980s. The Joint Commission on Accreditation of Healthcare Organizations (formerly JCAHO, now the Joint Commission) in the late 1980s emphasized monitoring for quality of outcomes rather than process. This changed the system from a static quality assurance system to a dynamic quality improvement program. The Joint Commission (2008) views quality of care as an ongoing process that continuously looks for ways to improve the care provided.

CRITICAL THINKING

Learning from Experience

By studying nursing history, we gain a better understanding of autonomy, professionalism, advancements in nursing education, and nursing care. Think of some lessons you have learned from the past. Can you identify some life experiences that taught you something? List two things you learned from these experiences or situations.

Health Care Reform

With an ever-increasing number (over 60 million) of Americans being uninsured or underinsured, health care access and costs became a major focus of attention in the 1990s (Edelman & Mandle, 2002). Children are especially at risk for having their health care neglected, with one in five children in the United States being uninsured (Baker, 1994).

Nursing as a profession has made great strides in affecting federal and state health care legislation (Figure 3-5). Hospitals are moving away from the controlling, bureaucratic entities they once were and instead are more often being characterized by an environment of shared governance where nurses have a voice in both clinical and administrative decision making. Nurses now serve as case managers and collaborate with physicians and other health care providers. Advocates are working to obtain prescriptive privileges for all advanced practitioners.

Nurses are seeking to improve their scientific knowledge and client outcomes by developing evidence-based practice. Evidence-based practice is "the integration of best research evidence with clinical expertise, and patient values" (Sackett, Straus, Richardson, Rosenberg, & Haynes, 2000, p. 1). Evidence-based practice ensures best practice and best client outcomes.

NURSING EDUCATION

Educational programs that prepare graduates to take a licensing examination must be approved by a state board of nursing.

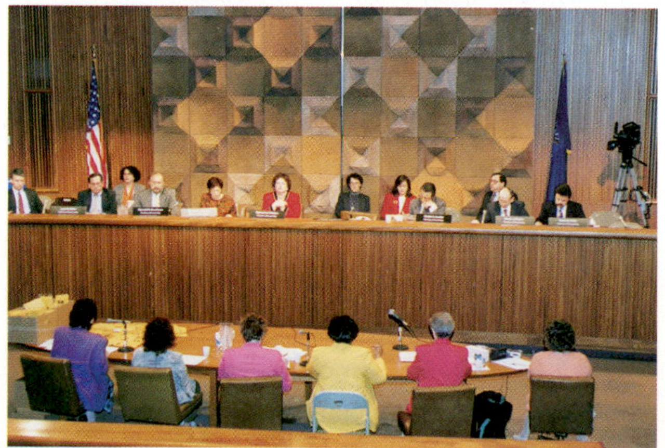

FIGURE 3-5 Nurses making a presentation before a state legislature. (*Photo courtesy of the New York State Nurses Association.*)

These boards approve entry-level programs to ensure the safe practice of nursing by setting minimum educational requirements and guaranteeing that graduates of the program are eligible candidates to take a licensing examination. Candidates in the United States must pass the National Council Licensure Examination (NCLEX®) before a state board of nursing will issue a license to practice nursing.

Types of Programs

There are two types of entry-level nursing programs available in the United States: licensed practical or vocational nurse (LPN or LVN) and registered nurse (RN). An entry-level educational program is one that prepares graduates to take a licensing examination. Graduates of licensed practical/vocational programs take the NCLEX® for practical nurses (NCLEX-PN®), and graduates of registered nurse programs take the NCLEX® for registered nurses (NCLEX-RN®).

Postgraduate programs prepare nurses to practice in various roles as advanced-practice registered nurses (APRNs). Statutory provisions for APRNs vary from state to state.

Licensed Practical/Vocational Nursing

Licensed practical nurses (LPNs) or licensed vocational nurses (LVNs, as they are called in Texas and California) work under the supervision of an RN or other licensed provider such as a physician or dentist. The LP/VN, like the RN, was first educated in hospitals. The Smith Hughes Act passed by Congress in 1917 gave impetus to the formation of vocational school–based practical nursing programs. In 2006, there were 11,172 students enrolled in practical nursing programs in the United States (National League for Nursing Accreditation Commission [NLNAC], 2008). In 2006, 8,047 new graduates entered the nursing workforce from practical nursing programs (NLNAC, 2008).

Programs are state approved and in some cases also have accreditation by the NLN. **Accreditation** is a process by which a voluntary, nongovernmental agency or organization appraises and grants accredited status to institutions and/or programs or services that meet predetermined structure, process, and outcome criteria. These educational programs are generally 1 year in length and provide both **didactic** (systematic presentation of information) and **clinical** (observing and caring for living clients) experience. The education is focused on basic nursing skills and direct client care. Although most clinical experience is in hospitals, long-term care facilities, physicians' offices, home health agencies, and ambulatory care facilities are also used.

Admission generally requires a high school diploma or General Education Development (GED) certificate. Schools may require a preentrance examination that assesses such skills as math, reading, and writing.

Once licensed, the LP/VN is prepared to work in structured settings such as hospitals, long-term care, home health, medical offices, and ambulatory care facilities. Just as the RN has been delegated duties previously considered the domain of the physician, the LP/VN has been assigned duties once considered the domain of the RN. Many hospitals offer programs that provide levels of advancement for the LP/VN.

The National Federation of Licensed Practical Nurses has written standards of nursing practice for the LP/VN. They are listed in Table 3-2.

Registered Nursing

Registered nurses are graduates of state-approved and, in many cases, NLN-accredited programs. They are prepared for entry into practice in one of three ways: hospital diploma programs, associate degree nursing programs, or baccalaureate degree nursing programs.

Diploma Program Diploma nursing programs are offered by hospitals and are typically 3 years in length. Most are now affiliated with colleges or universities that grant college credit for select courses. Graduates of these programs receive a diploma from the hospital rather than a college degree.

Program content historically prepared the graduate in basic nursing skills particularly suitable for hospitalized clients. Now, however, most diploma schools also use community-based settings such as physicians' offices, visiting nurse services, clinics, and health departments for clinical experiences.

Although prominent in the early history of nursing education, the number of diploma nursing programs in the United States has decreased. In 2006, 4% of all entry-level nursing programs in the United States were diploma programs with 11,266 students enrolled (ANA, 2008a; NLNAC, 2008). In 2006, 3,600 graduates or 8% of all new graduates eligible to enter the nursing workforce came from diploma programs (NLN, 2008a; NLNAC, 2008).

Associate Degree Program Associate degree programs are offered through community colleges and are typically 2 years in length. They may also be offered as an option at 4-year degree-granting universities. The graduate receives an associate degree in nursing (ADN). In 2006, 58.9% of all entry-level nursing programs in the United States were ADN programs with 139,008 students enrolled (ANA, 2008a; NLNAC, 2008). In 2006, 49,878 or 59% of all new graduates eligible to enter the nursing workforce came from ADN programs (NLN, 2008a; NLNAC, 2008). Traditionally, program content reflects basic skill preparation and emphasizes clinical practice in the hospital setting. Because of a decreasing use of hospital beds, however, students are now likely to spend a higher number of clinical hours in community-based institutions (e.g., ambulatory settings, clinics, or schools).

Baccalaureate Degree Program Baccalaureate degree programs are offered through colleges and universities and are typically 4 years in length. The graduate receives a bachelor of science in nursing (BSN). These programs emphasize a broader preparation for practice, not only in hospital settings but also for autonomous and collaborative practice. In 2006, 38% of all entry-level nursing programs in the United States were baccalaureate programs with 52,481 students enrolled (ANA, 2008a; NLNAC, 2008). In 2006, 14,233 graduates or 38% of all new graduates eligible to enter the nursing workforce came from baccalaureate programs (NLN, 2008a; NLNAC, 2008).

Continuing Education and Staff Development

Once a nurse is in practice, both continuing education and staff development are used to maintain the needed knowledge and skills for continuing practice.

Nurses are responsible for their own continuing education. Continuing education offers both personal and professional growth to the nurse and constitutes an essential dimension of

TABLE 3-2 Nursing Practice Standards for the Licensed Practical/Vocational Nurse

Education

The licensed practical/vocational nurse:

1. Shall complete a formal education program in practical nursing approved by the appropriate nursing authority in a state.
2. Shall successfully pass the National Council Licensure Examination for Practical Nurses.
3. Shall participate in initial orientation within the employing institution.

Legal/Ethical Status

The licensed practical/vocational nurse:

1. Shall hold a current license to practice nursing as an LP/VN in accordance with the law of the state wherein employed.
2. Shall know the scope of nursing practice authorized by the Nursing Practice Act in the state wherein employed.
3. Shall have a personal commitment to fulfill the legal responsibilities inherent in good nursing practice.
4. Shall take responsible actions in situations wherein there is unprofessional conduct by a peer or other health care provider.
5. Shall recognize and commit to meet the ethical and moral obligations of the practice of nursing.
6. Shall not accept or perform professional responsibilities that the individual knows (s)he is not competent to perform.

Practice

The licensed practical/vocational nurse:

1. Shall accept assigned responsibilities as an accountable member of the health care team.
2. Shall function within the limits of educational preparation and experience, as related to the assigned duties.
3. Shall function with other members of the health care team in promoting and maintaining health, preventing disease and disability, caring for and rehabilitating individuals who are experiencing an altered health state, and contributing to the ultimate quality of life until death.
4. Shall know and utilize the nursing process in planning, implementing, and evaluating health services and nursing care for the individual patient or group.
   a. Planning: The planning of nursing includes:
      1) assessment/data collection of health status of the individual patient, the family, and community groups
      2) reporting information gained from assessment/data collection
      3) the identification of health goals
   b. Implementation: The plan for nursing care is put into practice to achieve the stated goals and includes:
      1) Observing, recording, and reporting significant changes that require intervention or different goals
      2) Applying nursing knowledge and skills to promote and maintain health, to prevent disease and disability, and to optimize functional capabilities of an individual patient
      3) Assisting the patient and family with activities of daily living and encouraging self-care as appropriate
      4) Carrying out therapeutic regimens and protocols prescribed by an RN, physician, or other persons authorized by state law
   c. Evaluation: The plan for nursing care and its implementations are evaluated to measure the progress toward the stated goals and will include appropriate persons and/or groups to determine:
      1) The relevancy of current goals in relation to the progress of the individual patient
      2) The involvement of the recipients of care in the evaluation process
      3) The quality of the nursing action in the implementation of the plan
      4) A reordering of priorities or new goal setting in the care plan
5. Shall participate in peer review and other evaluation processes.
6. Shall participate in the development of policies concerning the health and nursing needs of society and in the roles and functions of the LP/VN.

Continuing Education

The licensed practical/vocational nurse:

1. Shall be responsible for maintaining the highest possible level of professional competence at all times.
2. Shall periodically reassess career goals and select continuing education activities that will help to achieve these goals.
3. Shall take advantage of continuing education opportunities that will lead to personal growth and professional development.
4. Shall seek and participate in continuing education activities that are approved for credit by appropriate organizations, such as the NFLPN.

Specialized Nursing Practice

The licensed practical/vocational nurse:

1. Shall have had at least one year's experience in nursing at the staff level.
2. Shall present personal qualifications that are indicative of potential abilities for practice in the chosen specialized nursing area.
3. Shall present evidence of completion of a program or course that is approved by an appropriate agency to provide the knowledge and skills necessary for effective nursing services in the specialized field.
4. Shall meet all of the standards of practice as set forth in this document.

(Reprinted with permission of the National Federation of Licensed Practical Nurses, Inc.)

lifelong learning. In some states, license renewal depends on acquiring continuing education units (CEUs) according to the board of nursing's rules. Lifelong learning is essential to career development and competency achievement in nursing practice.

Staff development generally occurs in the setting of employment and is described as the delivery of instruction to assist nurses to achieve the goals of the employer. It is guided by the accreditation standards of the Joint Commission and ANA's *Standards for Nursing Staff Development* (ANA, 1990).

Orientation is an important organizational tool for both recruitment and retention. The sessions typically occur at the beginning of employment and whenever positions or roles change. The sessions include information unique to the institution of employment, such as philosophy, goals, policies and procedures, role expectations, facilities, resources and special services, and assessment and development of competency with equipment and supplies used in the work setting.

In-service education occurs after orientation and throughout employment. It supports the nurse in acquiring, maintaining, and increasing skills to fulfill assigned responsibilities.

The American Nurses Credentialing Center (ANCC) is an international credentialing program that certifies registered nurses and advanced-practice nurses in specialty practice areas. The ANCC certification exams validate a "nurse's skills, knowledge, and abilities" (ANCC, 2009, p. 1). NAPNES provides certification for LPNs in long-term care that covers not only geriatrics but also chronic illnesses for all age-groups (NAPNES, 2009). For more information on certification for LPNs go to www.napnes.org and search for "Certifications for LPN/LVNs."

Trends in Nursing Education

Trends in nursing education reflect issues in nursing, nursing education, delivery of care, and the public's health. At the heart of many of these trends are two fundamental issues: competency development and delivery of care.

Competency Development

The debate about multiple education levels for entry into nursing practice will continue. Demonstration of basic competency by all entry-level graduates regardless of education is likely to gain great support from nursing. It allows for not only consensus about the outcome (competency) but also diversity (innovation) about the process. Many changes in nursing education are being stimulated by competency development.

Delivery of Care

The demand for nursing care will continue to be driven by a larger aging population that uses long-term care and home health services. Other changes will include expansion of primary and preventive care to focus on health promotion and wellness; an increased use of ambulatory care services because they are less expensive; increased complexity of health care delivery, which requires well-educated nurses; and increased demand to provide health services such as prenatal care, well-child clinics, adolescent clinics, and neighbor care clinics to underserved populations (such as inner-city residents).

Managed care arrangements are the delivery systems of the future. They emphasize wellness, health promotion, and disease prevention. More and more factors contributing to disease point to health behaviors as preventive interventions. The Healthy People 2010 goals, focus areas, and leading health indicators can be found on the Web at www.health.gov.

NURSING ORGANIZATIONS

Nursing organizations exist for LP/VNs and RNs. Some organizations also welcome as members those who are interested in nursing but who are not nurses. There are also many specialty nursing organizations.

All nurses are encouraged to maintain membership in a nursing organization. The organizations represent the nurses to the public; to legislative bodies, both state and national; to federal agencies; and to all health care facilities. Through these organizations, nurses' concerns about workplace issues are addressed, high standards of practice are fostered, ethics codes are established, continuing education programs are certified and provided, and nurses' general welfare is protected. It is a professional opportunity to be a participating member of a nursing organization. It is an option to present a strong unified voice regarding nursing issues. Table 3-3 provides pertinent information about selected nursing organizations.

National League for Nursing

The original organization, established in 1893, was named the American Society of Superintendents of Training Schools for Nurses. The last name change, National League for Nursing, was made in 1952. Because of the growth of practical/vocational nursing programs, the NLN established a Department of Practical Nursing Programs (now called Council of Practical Nursing Programs [CPNP]) in 1961. The NLN offers accreditation services to all nursing programs through an independent subsidiary called the National League for Nursing Accrediting Commission (NLNAC) (NLN, 2008b).

National Association of Practical Nurse Education and Service

Originally called the Association of Practical Nurse Schools, this organization was dedicated exclusively to practical nursing. The multidisciplinary membership planned the first standard curriculum for practical nursing. In 1959, the name was changed to the National Association of Practical Nurse Education and Service (NAPNES, 1998).

PROFESSIONALTIP

Professional Memberships

Every nurse is encouraged to be involved in a nursing organization. Membership means more political clout for passing legislation to improve health care for all citizens and to improve the profession of nursing.

Nursing students have an opportunity to stay abreast of current issues and meet with local nursing leaders to discuss health care reform, alternative health care delivery models, and other issues. Then as graduates, they can share this information with both the public and legislators.

Table 3-3 Selected Nursing Organizations

ORGANIZATION	DESCRIPTION
National League for Nursing (NLN)	Established: 1893 as The American Society of Superintendents of Training Schools for Nurses. 1952 name changed to National League for Nursing. Purpose: To advance quality nursing education that prepares the nursing workforce to meet the needs of diverse populations in an ever-changing health care environment Activities: • Accredit (through voluntary participation from schools) nursing education programs • Conduct surveys to collect data on education programs • Provide continuing-education programs • Offer testing services, including: Achievement tests for use in nursing schools Preadmission testing for potential nursing students Membership: • Open to any individual (nurse or nonnurse) or agency interested in improving nursing services or nursing education Publications: • *Nursing Education Perspectives* • *The Scope and Practice for Academic Nurse Educators©* • *National Study of Faculty Role Satisfaction©* • *The NLN Report* • *NLN Member Update* • *Professional Development Bulletin* • *Nursing Education Policy*
National Association for Practical Nurse Education and Service, Inc. (NAPNES)	Established: 1941 Purpose: To improve the quality, education, and recognition of nursing schools and LP/VNs in the United States Activities: • Provide workshops, seminars, and continuing-education programs • Evaluate and certify continuing-education programs of others • Provide individual student professional liability insurance program • Inform legislatures and public on LP/VN issues • Authorize those who pass the Certification Examination for Practical and Vocational Nurses in Long-term Care (CEPN-LTC)™ to use the initials *CLTC* Membership: • LP/VNs • RNs, physicians, and caregivers in all fields • Practical/vocational nursing students Publications: • *Journal of Practical Nursing* • *NAPNES Forum*
National Federation of Licensed Practical Nurses, Inc. (NFLPN)	Established: 1949 Purpose: • Provide leadership for LP/VNs • Foster high standards of practical/vocational nursing education and practice • Encourage continuing education • Achieve recognition for LP/VNs • Advocate effective utilization of LP/VNs • Interpret role and function of LP/VNs • Represent practical/vocational nursing • Serve as central source of information on practical/vocational nursing education and practice Activities: • Promote continuing education of LP/VNs; evaluate programs for CEU credit • Offer IV and gerontology certification

Table 3-3 Selected Nursing Organizations (Continued)

ORGANIZATION	DESCRIPTION
	• Establish principles of ethics • Offer members an opportunity to participate in activities of the organization • Keep members informed on matters of interest and concern • Offer members best type of low-cost insurance • Represent and speak for LP/VNs in Congress • Encourage fellowship among LP/VNs • Develop mutual understanding and good will among members, other allied health groups, and the general public Membership: • Three-tier concept of local, state, and national enrollment • LP/VNs • Practical/vocational nursing students • Affiliate (person who has an interest in the work of NFLPN but is neither an LP/VN nor an LP/VN student) Publication: • *Practical Nursing Journal*
American Nurses Association (ANA)	Established: 1911 Purpose: To work for the improvement of health standards and availability of health care service for all people, foster high standards for nursing, stimulate and promote the professional development of nurses, and advance their economic and general welfare. Activities: • Establish standards for nursing practice • Establish a professional code of ethics • Develop educational standards • Promote nursing research • Oversee a credentialing system • Influence legislation affecting health care • Protect the economic and general welfare of registered nurses • Assist with the professional development of nurses (i.e., by providing continuing education programs) Membership: • Registered nurses only • Federation of state nurses' associations • Individual, by joining respective state nurses' association Publications: • *American Nurse Today* • *The American Nurse*
National Council of State Boards of Nursing, Inc. (NCSBN)	Established: 1978 Purpose: Provide an organization through which boards of nursing act and counsel together on matters of common interest and concern affecting the public health, safety, and welfare, including the development of licensing examinations in nursing Activities: • Develop and administer licensure examinations for registered nurse and licensed practical/vocational nurse candidates • Conduct job analyses that provide data required to support the NCLEX® examinations and the test development process • Maintain a national disciplinary data bank • Monitor and analyze issues and trends in public policy, nursing practice, and nursing education that impact nursing regulation • Serve as the national clearinghouse of information on nursing regulation • Offer educational conferences and regional meetings

(*Continues*)

Table 3-3 Selected Nursing Organizations (Continued)

ORGANIZATION	DESCRIPTION
	Membership: • Boards of nursing in the 50 states, the District of Columbia, and four United States territories • No individual membership Publications: • *Education Issues* • *NCLEX-PN® Program Reports* • *NCLEX-RN® Program Reports* • *NCLEX-PN® Detailed Test Plan* • *NCLEX-RN® Detailed Test Plan*

Data from About ANA (online), by American Nurses Association, 2008a, http://www.nursingworld.org/FunctionalMenuCategories/AboutANA.aspx; History of NAPNES by National Association for Practical Nurse Education and Service, Inc., 1998, Silver Spring, MD: Author; About Us (online), by National Association for Practical Nurse Education and Service, 2008, http://www.napnes.org/about/index.html; About NFLPN (online), by National Federation of Licensed Practical Nurses, 2008, http://www.nflpn.org/about.html; Bylaws, by National League for Nursing, 1995, New York: Author; About the NLN (online), by National League for Nursing, 2008, http://www.nln.org/aboutnln/index.htm; About NCSBN (online), by National Council of State Boards of Nursing, Inc., 2008a, https://www.ncsbn.org/about.htm.

National Federation of Licensed Practical Nurses

The National Federation of Licensed Practical Nurses (NFLPN) was founded in 1949 by a group of LPNs who recognized that to gain status and recognition in the health field and to have a channel through which they could officially speak and act for themselves, they needed an organization of their own. Since 1991, affiliate membership (lacking the rights to vote and hold office) has been available to anyone who is interested in the work of NFLPN but who is neither a practicing LP/VN nor an LP/VN student. The NFLPN is the official organization for LP/VNs (NFLPN, 2008).

American Nurses Association

The ANA represents registered nurses through its constituent state organizations. The ANA fosters high standards of nursing practice, promotes the economic and general welfare of nurses in the workplace, projects a positive and realistic view of nursing, and lobbies Congress and regulatory agencies on health care issues affecting nurses and the public (ANA, 2008a).

National Council of State Boards of Nursing

The National Council of State Boards of Nursing (NCSBN) was established in 1978 to assist member boards, collectively and individually, to promote safe and effective nursing practice in the interest of protecting public health and welfare. They have developed the NCLEX-PN® and NCLEX-RN® to test the entry-level nursing competence of candidates for licensure as LP/VNs and RNs.

In 1996, they began administration of the first large-scale, national certification examination available to LP/VNs. It is named the Certification Examination for Practical and Vocational Nurses in Long-Term Care (CEPN-LTC™). Those who pass the examination are certified in long-term care and are authorized by NAPNES to use the initials CLTC to signify their new status (Washington State Department of Health: The Nursing Commission Newsletter, 1999).

CASE STUDY

C.J. is a new nursing student. One of his first assignments is to read a chapter on nursing history. C.J. thinks that history is boring and considers skipping the assignment. However, he desires to make good grades and is a dedicated nursing student, so he reads the chapter.

1. How will knowing nursing history affect C.J.'s view of nursing?
2. What is presently happening in nursing that will become part of the nursing history archives in 10 years?
3. What is presently happening in nursing or legislation that will change the face of nursing in 5 years?

SUMMARY

- Nursing is the art and science of assisting people in learning to care for themselves whenever possible and of caring for them when they are unable to meet their own needs.
- By studying nursing history, the nurse is better able to understand such issues as autonomy, unity within the profession, supply and demand, salary, education, and current practice and can thus promote the empowerment of nurses.
- Nursing's early history was heavily influenced by religious organizations and the need for nurses to care for soldiers during wartime.
- Florence Nightingale forged the future of nursing practice and education as a result of her experiences in educating nurses to care for soldiers.
- Early American leaders, professional organizations, and landmark reports of nursing determined the infrastructure of current nursing practice.
- Influential nursing leaders such as Lillian Wald, Isabel Hampton Robb, Adelaide Nutting, and Lavinia Dock were instrumental in the advancement of nursing education and practice.
- Other nursing leaders such as Mary Breckenridge, Mary Mahoney, and Linda Richards made important contributions to both nursing education and practice.
- In 1923, the Goldmark Report concluded that for nursing to be on equal footing with other disciplines, nursing education should occur in the university setting.
- The Brown Report (1948) addressed the need for nurses to demonstrate greater professional competence by moving nursing education to the university setting.
- Title III of the Health Amendment Act of 1955 resulted in the establishment of practical nursing.
- The Health Maintenance Organization Act of 1973 provided an alternative to the private health insurance industry.
- Types of programs that currently prepare nurses for entry-level practice are practical/vocational, diploma, associate degree, and baccalaureate degree.

REVIEW QUESTIONS

1. The founder of modern nursing is considered to be:
   1. Lillian Wald.
   2. Dorothea Dix.
   3. Florence Nightingale.
   4. The Nursing Sisters of the Holy Cross.
2. The first practical nursing school was:
   1. Ballard School.
   2. Thompson Practical Nursing School.
   3. Bellevue Training School for Nurses.
   4. Household Nursing Association School of Attendant Nursing.
3. Practical nursing was established under:
   1. Bureau of Medical Services, 1908.
   2. Health Maintenance Organization Act of 1973.
   3. Title III of the Health Amendment Act of 1955.
   4. Nursing and Nursing Education in the United States, 1923.
4. A nursing organization that accredits schools of nursing is:
   1. ANA.
   2. NLN.
   3. NFLPN.
   4. NAPNES.
5. The National Council of State Boards of Nursing began administering a national certification examination available to the LP/VN. It is for:
   1. licensure.
   2. acute care.
   3. accreditation.
   4. long-term care.
6. The science of nursing is evidenced by: (Select all that apply.)
   1. critical thinking skills.
   2. using scientific knowledge.
   3. caring behaviors.
   4. using evidence-based practice.
   5. providing comfort and dignity in death.
   6. evidence-based practice.
7. The official organization to speak and act for the LPN/VN is the:
   1. National Council of State Boards of Nursing.
   2. American Nurses Association.
   3. National League of Nursing.
   4. National Federation of Licensed Practical Nurses.
8. A nurse desires to join a nursing organization because such organizations: (Select all that apply.)
   1. protect the nurse's welfare.
   2. stress best standards of nursing practice.
   3. establish the nurse's code of conduct and practice.
   4. develop curricula for nursing education programs.
   5. oversee and discipline nursing misconduct.
   6. leave continuing education programs to hospitals.
9. Studying nursing history: (Select all that apply.)
   1. gives the nurse a sense of autonomy.
   2. encourages nurses to make a positive impact on present nursing events.
   3. serves only to give a view of previous nursing events.
   4. enhances the present view of current practice.
   5. has little relevance to current nursing practices.
   6. increases understanding of advances in nursing education.

10. Nursing as a science: (Select all that apply.)
    1. promotes restores, and maintains the health of clients.
    2. is founded on evidence-based research.
    3. uses nursing principles based on scientific theory.
    4. is demonstrated in skillful caring acts.
    5. is individualized care based on the client's needs and preferences.
    6. is the application of data collection (research) in client care.

REFERENCES/SUGGESTED READINGS

American Nurses Association. (1990). Standards for nursing staff development. Kansas City, MO: Author.

American Nurses Association. (2008a). About ANA. Retrieved September 29, 2008, from http://www.nursingworld.org/FunctionalMenuCategories/AboutANA.aspx

American Nurses Association. (2008b). About nursing. Retrieved September 29, 2008, from http:/www.nursingworld.org/MainMenuCategories/CertificationandAccreditaition/AboutN

American Nurses Association. (2008c). ANA bylaws. Retrieved September 29, 2008, from http://www.nursingworld.org/DocumentVault/MemberCenter/ANABylaws2006PDF.aspx

American Nurses Association. (2008d). ANA's statement of purpose. Retrieved September 29, 2008, from http://www.nursingworld.org/FunctionalMenuCategories/AboutANA/WhoWeAre/ANAsStatementofPurpose.aspx

American Nurses Association. (2009). What is nursing? Retrieved February 7, 2009, from http://www.nursingworld.org/EspeciallyForYou/StudentNurses/WhatisNursing.aspx

American Nurses Credentialing Center. (2009). About ANCC. Retrieved February 7, 2009, from http://www.nursecredentialing.org/FunctionalCategory/AboutANCC.aspx

Anglin, L. (2000). Historical perspectives: Influences of the past. In J. Zerwekh (Ed.), *Nursing today: Transitions and trends* (3rd ed.). Philadelphia: W. B. Saunders.

Baker, C. (1994). School health: Policy issues. *Nursing and Health Care, 15*(4), 178–184.

Bell, P. (1993). "Making do" with the midwife: Arkansas' Mamie O. Hale in the 1940s. *Nursing History Review*, 155–169.

Calhoun, J. (1993, March). The Nightingale pledge: A commitment that survives the passage of time. *Nursing and Health Care, 14*(3), 130–136.

Cushing, A. (1995, Summer). A historical note on the relationship between nursing and nursing history. *International History Nursing Journal, 1*(1), 57–60.

Department of Health and Human Services: Centers for Disease Control and Prevention. (2008). Health people 2010. Retrieved September 29, 2008, from http://www.cdc.gov/nchs

Dossey, B. (1995). Endnote: Florence Nightingale today. *Critical Care Nursing, 15*(4), 98.

Edelman, C., & Mandle, C. (2002). *Health promotion throughout the lifespan* (5th ed.). St. Louis, MO: Mosby.

Estabrooks, C. (1995). Lavinia Lloyd Dock: The Henry Street years. *Nursing History Review, 3,* 143–172.

Guide to Nursing Organizations. (2000). *Nursing2000, 30*(5), 54–56.

Humphreys, K. (2002). Guide to 2002 nursing organizations. *Nursing 2002, 32*(5), 46–48.

Joint Commission on the Accreditation of Healthcare Organizations. (2008). Principles respecting joint commission core performance measurement activities. Retrieved September 29, 2008, from http://www.jointcommission.org/NR/rdonlyres/A2C1C8AF-D879-41DD-A4DF-E6D9CCA21362/0/AttachAPMPrinciplesFinalWebVersion.pdf

Kauffman, C. (1978). *The ministry of healing.* New York: Seabury Press.

Macrae, J. (1995). Nightingale's spiritual philosophy and its significance for modern nursing. *Image: Journal of Nursing Scholarship, 27*(1), 8–10.

Mason, D., & Leavitt, J. (1995). The revolution in health care: What's your readiness quotient? *American Journal of Nursing, 95*(6), 50–54.

Mohr, W. (2005). *Psychiatric-mental health nursing* (6th ed.). Philadelphia: Lippincott Williams & Wilkins.

National Association for Practical Nurse Education and Service. (1998). *History of NAPNES.* Silver Spring, MD: Author.

National Association for Practical Nurse Education and Service. (2008). About us. Retrieved September 29, 2008, from http://www.napnes.org/about/index.html

National Association for Practical Nurse Education and Service. (2009). Certifications for LPN/LVNs. Retrieved February 7, 2009, from http://www.napnes.org/certifications.htm

National Council of State Boards of Nursing. (2008a). About NCSBN. Retrieved September 29, 2008, from https://www.ncsbn.org/about.htm

National Council of State Boards of Nursing. (2008b). What is NCLEX? Retrieved September 29, 2008, from https://www.ncsbn.org/1200.htm

National Federation of Licensed Practical Nurses. (2008). About NFLPN. Retrieved September 29, 2008, from http://www.nflpn.org/about.html

National League for Nursing. (1995). *Bylaws.* New York: Author.

National League for Nursing. (1998). Research Department Communication. New York: Author.

National League for Nursing. (2000, August 15). *Unofficial, unpublished data from 1998.* Research Department Communication.

National League for Nursing. (2008a). About the NLN. Retrieved September 29, 2008, from http://www.nln.org/aboutnln/index.htm

National League for Nursing. (2008b). Number of nursing school graduates—Including ethnic and racial minorities—On the rise. Retrieved September 29, 2008, from http://www.nln.org/newsreleases/data_release_03032008.htm

National League for Nursing Accrediting Commision. (2008). NLNAC 2008 report to constituents. Retrieved September 29, 2008, from http://www.nlnac.org/reports/2008.htm

Navsource.com. (2007). NavSource online: Service ship photo archive. Retrieved on February 9, 2009, from http://www.navsource.org/archives/09/12/1202.htm

Nightingale, F. (1969). *Notes on nursing: What it is and what it is not.* New York: Dover.

Ogren, K. (1994). The risk of not understanding nursing history. *Holistic Nursing Practice, 8*(2), 10.

Pokorny, M. (1992). An historical perspective of confederate nursing during the Civil War, 1861–1865. *Nursing Research, 41*(1), 29.

Sackett, D., Straus, S., Richardson, W., Rosenberg, W., & Haynes, R. (2000). *Evidence-based medicine: How to practice and teach EBM* (2nd ed.). Edinburgh: Churchill Livingstone.

Secretary's Commission on Nursing. (1988). *Final report.* Washington, DC: Department of Health and Human Services.

Selanders, L. (1994). *Florence Nightingale: An environmental adaptation theory.* Newbury Park, CA: Sage.

Silverstein, N. (1994). Lillian Wald at Henry Street, 1893–1895. In P. L. Chinn (Ed.), *Developing the discipline: Critical studies in nursing history and professional issues*. Gaithersburg, MD: Aspen.

Summers, S. (2008). What is magnet status and how's that whole thing going? Retrieved September 10, 2008, from http://www.nursingadvocacy.org/faq/magnet.html

U.S. Department of Health and Human Services. (1996). The registered nurse population. Washington, DC: Author.

Washington State Department of Health: The Nursing Commission Newsletter. (1999). Self directed care. Retrieved September 29, 2008, from https://fortress.wa.gov/doh/hpqa1/hps6/Nursing/documents/nwsltr_f99.pdf

Wall, B. (1993). Grace under pressure: The nursing sisters of the Holy Cross, 1861–1865. *Nursing History Review*, 71–88.

Wilson, Sprouse, D., Gause, G., Jr., Tallent, D., Ahlfield, R., Holbrook, B. (2009). The story of men in American nursing. Retrieved February 9, 2009, from http://www.geocities.com/Athens/Forum/6011/sld002.htm

Wolf, P. (2003). Guide to nursing organizations. *Nursing 2003, 33*(5), 50–52.

RESOURCES

American Association of the History of Nursing (AAHN), http://www.aahn.org

American Nurses Association (ANA), http://www.ana.org

National Association for Practical Nurse Education and Service (NAPNES), http://www.napnes.org

National Council of State Boards of Nursing (NCSBN), http://www.ncsbn.org

National Federation of Licensed Practical Nurses (NFLPN), http://www.nflpn.org

National League for Nursing (NLN), http://www.nln.org

National League for Nursing Accrediting Commission (NLNAC), http://www.nlnac.org

CHAPTER 4
Legal and Ethical Responsibilities

MAKING THE CONNECTION

Refer to the following chapters to increase your understanding of legal and ethical responsibilities:

Basic Nursing

- ***Student Nurse Skills for Success***
- ***Nursing Process/Documentation/ Informatics***
- ***Cultural Considerations***
- ***End-of-Life Care***
- ***Safety/Hygiene***

LEARNING OBJECTIVES

Upon completion of this chapter, you should be able to:

- Define key terms.
- Describe the difference between public law and civil law.
- State the purpose and identify various sources of standards of practice.
- Discuss the difference between intentional and unintentional torts.
- Discuss ways that informed consent impacts nursing practice.
- Discuss the concept of advance directives.
- Describe the purpose and correct utilization of an incident report.
- Discuss ways the nurse can reduce personal liability.
- Identify the benefits of having one's own malpractice insurance policy.
- List steps to be taken when suspecting a colleague of being impaired by drugs or alcohol.
- Describe the major ethical principles that have an impact on health care.
- Explain the link between ethics and values and the process involved in reconciling the potential conflicts between them.
- Relate the ethical code developed by the National Federation of Licensed Practical Nurses daily nursing practice.
- Identify the rights of the client as established by the American Hospital Association.
- Discuss the roles of the nurse as client advocate and whistle-blower in the delivery of ethical nursing care.

KEY TERMS

active euthanasia
administrative law
advance directive
assault
assisted suicide
autonomy
battery
beneficence
bioethics
civil law
client advocate
confidential
constitutional law
contract law
criminal law
defamation
deontology
durable power of attorney for health care (DPAHC)
ethical dilemma
ethical principles
ethical reasoning
ethics
euthanasia
expressed contract
false imprisonment
felony
fidelity
formal contract
fraud
Good Samaritan laws
impaired nurse
implied contract
incident report
informed consent
justice
law
liability
libel
living will
malpractice
material principle of justice
misdemeanor
negligence
nonmaleficence
nursing practice act
passive euthanasia
peer assistance programs
privacy
public law
restraint
slander
standards of practice
statutory law
teleology
tort
tort law
utility
value system
values
values clarification
veracity
whistle-blowing

INTRODUCTION

Nursing, which embodies a concern for the client in every aspect of life, encompasses a great responsibility—one that requires knowledge, skill, care, and commitment. As society and technology change, the issues affecting nursing practice also change. We continue to recognize the importance of the right to decide what is best for oneself, informed consent, and belief in the client's bill of rights; however, difficult issues, such as advance directives, do-not-resuscitate (DNR) orders, and impaired nurses, now must be faced by the nursing profession. The delivery of ethical health care is becoming an increasingly difficult and confusing issue in contemporary society. Nurses are committed to respecting their clients' rights in terms of providing health care and treatment. This desire to maintain clients' rights, however, often conflicts with professional duties and institutional policies. Nurses must thus learn to balance these potentially conflicting perspectives to achieve the primary objective—the care of the client. This chapter provides a general overview of many legal and ethical concepts that affect nursing.

BASIC LEGAL CONCEPTS

Because it is useful to have working definitions of some basic legal concepts before applying them to a health care setting, a discussion of pertinent legal concepts follows.

Definition of Law

Laws are decisions about conduct that guide the interactions of people. Laws are necessary, binding, and enforceable so people can live and work together. When laws are broken, a penalty is incurred.

The word **law** is derived from an Anglo-Saxon term meaning "that which is laid down or fixed." The two types of law are **public law**, which deals with the individual's relationship to the state, and **civil law**, which deals with relationships among individuals.

Sources of Law

The four sources of public law at the federal and state levels are constitutional, statutory, administrative, and criminal. At the federal and state levels, the three sources of civil law are contracts, torts, and protective/reporting laws.

Public Law

Constitutional law, set forth in the U.S. and state constitutions, defines and limits the powers of government. **Statutory law** is enacted by legislative bodies. State boards and professional practice acts, such as nursing practice acts, are created and governed under statutory laws.

Administrative law (regulatory law) is developed by those persons appointed to governmental administrative agencies. These persons are entrusted with enforcing the statutory laws passed by the legislature. Administrative law gives state boards of nursing the power to make rules and regulations governing nursing as set forth in the nursing practice acts. In these administrative rules, nursing boards delineate the specific processes for educational programs, licensure, grounds for disciplinary proceedings, and the establishment of fees for services and for penalties rendered by the board.

Criminal law, the most common example of public law, addresses acts or offenses against the safety or welfare of

Table 4-1 Types of Public Law

TYPE	FEDERAL EXAMPLES	STATE EXAMPLES
Constitutional law	U.S. Constitution Civil Rights Act	State constitutions
Statutory law	None	Various state boards and professional practice acts
Administrative law	Social Security Act National Labor Relations Act	Rules and regulations of various state boards
Criminal law	Controlled Substance Act Homicide	Criminal codes (defining manslaughter, murder, criminal negligence, rape, illegal possession of drugs, fraud, theft, assault, and battery)

COURTESY OF DELMAR CENGAGE LEARNING

the public. Under criminal law, there are two types of crime: **felony** (a crime of a serious nature that is usually punishable by imprisonment at a state penitentiary or by death or a crime violating a federal statute that involves punishment of more than 1 year incarceration) and **misdemeanor** (offense less serious than a felony that may be punishable by a fine or a sentence to a local prison for less than 1 year). Table 4-1 outlines the types of public law.

Civil Law

Civil law addresses crimes against a person(s) in matters such as contracts, torts, and protective/reporting law (Table 4-2). Most cases of malpractice fall under the civil law of torts (Flight, 2004).

Contract law is the enforcement of agreements among private individuals. The three essential elements in a legal contract are:

- Promise(s) between two or more legally competent individuals that state what each individual must do or not do
- Mutual understanding of the terms and obligations the contract imposes on each individual
- Compensation for lawful actions performed

Contract terms may be agreed on in writing or orally; however, a **formal** (written) **contract** cannot be changed legally by an oral agreement. An **expressed contract** gives, in writing, the conditions and terms of the contract. An **implied**

Table 4-2 Types of Civil Law

TYPE	FEDERAL EXAMPLES	STATE EXAMPLES
Contract law	None	Business contracts with clients Employment contracts
Torts	Federal Torts Claims Act	State Torts Claims Act (allows claims against the state) Assault Battery Defamation (libel and slander) Fraud False imprisonment Invasion of privacy Negligence (common law claim) Malpractice statutes (professional liability)
Protective/reporting laws	Child Abuse Prevention and Treatment Act Privacy Act of 1974	Good Samaritan law Abuse statutes (domestic violence, child, elderly) Age of consent statutes (medical treatment, drugs, sexually transmitted disease) Americans with Disabilities Act Living will legislation Involuntary Hospitalization Act Abortion statute

COURTESY OF DELMAR CENGAGE LEARNING

PROFESSIONALTIP

Good Samaritan Laws

Good Samaritan laws vary in coverage from state to state and may be amended periodically by legislation. It is the responsibility of caregivers to know the law for their respective jurisdictions.

contract acknowledges a relationship between parties for services.

In accord with U.S. Contract Law, the nurse is legally required to:

- Follow the employer's policies and standards unless they conflict with state or federal law
- Complete the terms of contracted service with the employer
- Respect the rights and responsibilities of other health care providers, especially to promote continuity of client care

Along with these legal responsibilities, the nurse has a right to expect:

- Adequate and qualified assistance in providing care
- Reasonable and prudent conduct from the client
- Compensation from the employer for services rendered
- A safe work environment with the necessary resources to render services
- Prudent, reasonable conduct from other health care providers

A **tort** is a civil wrong committed by a person against another person or property (Zerwekh & Claborn, 2003). **Tort law** is the enforcement of duties and rights among individuals independent of contractual agreements.

The protective/reporting law may be considered criminal law, depending on classification by the state. Two examples of protective law are the Americans with Disabilities Act (ADA) and the Good Samaritan laws.

The ADA was passed by the U.S. Congress in 1990. It prohibits discrimination in employment, public services, and public accommodations on the basis of disability. The ADA defines a disability as a physical or mental impairment that substantially limits one or more of the major life activities.

All 50 states and the District of Columbia have enacted **Good Samaritan laws**, which protect health care providers by ensuring immunity from civil **liability** (obligation one has incurred or might incur through any act or failure to act).

The Good Samaritan law applies only in emergency situations, usually those outside the hospital setting. It stipulates that the health care worker must not be acting for an employer or receive compensation for care given. In most states, health care professionals are not required to stop at the scene of accidents. If they do stop, however, they are held to higher standards than is a layperson. Health care professionals are expected to use their specialized body of knowledge when providing care. They are expected to act as would most other professionals with the same background and education.

THE LAW AND NURSING PRACTICE

Nursing practice falls under both public law and civil law. In all states, nurses are bound by rules and regulations stipulated by the **nursing practice act** as determined by the legislature.

Public laws are designed to protect the public. When these laws are broken by a nurse, while either on or off duty, she can be punished by paying a fine, losing her license, or being incarcerated. For example, a nurse guilty of diverting drugs, which is a crime against the state, could lose her license to practice and could be sent to jail. There is a common misconception that this only applies to the nurse's work behavior or that marijuana is not included.

Civil laws deal with problems occurring between a nurse and a client. For example, if a nurse catheterizing a client perforates the bladder, the client has sustained injury. No law affecting the population as a whole has been broken, but the client may bring a civil suit against the nurse. The client may receive compensation for injuries, but the nurse receives no jail time.

Multistate nursing practice has become a pressing issue with telehealth, transporting of clients across state lines, and employment by staffing companies operating in several states (Ventura, 1999b). The National Council of State Boards of Nursing (NCSBN), in 1997, endorsed a model of nursing regulations for RNs and LP/VNs now called the Nurse Licensure Compact that allows nurses licensed in one of the compact states to practice in any of the compact states. Nurses are licensed in their state of residence. When necessary, disciplinary action may be taken by any of the compact states against a nurse, even when licensed by another compact state. The 15 states that have passed the legislation and have implemented this compact are Arizona, Arkansas, Delaware, Idaho, Iowa, Maine, Maryland, Mississippi, Nebraska, North Carolina, North Dakota, South Dakota, Texas, Utah, and Wisconsin. Three states—Indiana, New Jersey, and Tennessee—are writing their rules for implementation (NCSBN, 2002).

STANDARDS OF PRACTICE

State boards of nursing have the responsibility of regulating nursing practice and setting educational guidelines for the programs. They stipulate who may practice nursing in their respective states through licensure. The related criteria usually involve graduating from a state-approved program, passing the National Council Licensure Exam (NCLEX)®, and meeting certain legal and moral standards. The boards have authority to bring disciplinary action against a nurse for violation of its rules and regulations. Disciplinary action may include revocation or suspension of the nurse's license and/or a fine.

PROFESSIONALTIP

Nursing Practice Act

Nursing practice acts state those things that the nurse can and cannot do. The nurse is responsible to know the state practice act for any state that she practices in.

From the nursing practice acts, guidelines have been developed to direct nursing care. These guidelines are called **standards of practice** or standards of care.

Standards of practice are also derived from other sources. Professional organizations such as the American Nurses Association (ANA) for the registered nurse (RN) and the National Federation of Licensed Practical Nurses (NFLPN) for the LP/VN have also developed standards of practice. Nursing care planning books, especially for specialized areas, are other resources for practice standards.

Policy and procedure manuals also represent standards of practice. Each facility has identified specific ways of performing procedures such as collecting specimens, passing medications, and inserting catheters. Nurses employed by the facility are expected to follow the guidelines in the policy and procedure manuals. For situations not covered in the policy and procedure manuals, the nurse is expected to exercise good judgment. In other words, the nurse is expected to act in a reasonable and prudent manner.

What is meant by reasonable and prudent? In nursing, it means that the nurse is expected to act as would other nurses at the same professional level and with the same amount of education or experience. If most nurses respond to a particular situation in a certain way, and the nurse in question does too, the nurse is acting in a reasonable and prudent manner; however, if most nurses respond differently than the nurse in question, the nurse is not be behaving in a reasonable and prudent manner and can be held responsible or liable for damages. Liability is determined by whether the standards of practice were adhered to.

Legal Issues in Practice

Many aspects relating to nursing practice and areas of nursing are subject to liability, including physician's orders, floating, inadequate staffing, critical care, and pediatric care. Nurses are held accountable to the stricter of either the state practice act or the policies of the facility of employment.

Physician's Orders

The physician is in charge of directing the client's care, and nurses are to carry out the physician's orders for care, unless the nurse believes that the orders are in error or would be harmful to the client. In this case, the physician must be contacted to confirm and/or clarify the orders. If the nurse still believes the orders to be inappropriate, the nursing supervisor should be immediately contacted and why the orders are not being carried out put in writing. A nurse who carries out an erroneous or inappropriate order may be held liable for harm experienced by the client. *Nurses are responsible for their actions regardless of who told them to perform those actions.*

Floating

Nurses sometimes are asked to "float" to an unfamiliar nursing unit. The supervisor should be informed about a float nurse's lack of experience in caring for the type of clients on the new nursing unit. The nurse should be given an orientation to the new unit and will be held to the same standards of care as are the nurses who regularly work on that unit.

Inadequate Staffing

The Joint Commission on Accreditation of Healthcare Organizations (JCAHO) has established guidelines for determining the number of staff needed for any given situation (staffing ratios) (JCAHO, 2008). When there are not enough nurses to meet the staffing ratio and provide competent care, substandard care may result, placing clients at physical risk and the nurse and institution at legal risk. The nurse in this situation should provide nursing administration with a written account of the situation. *A nurse who leaves an inadequately staffed unit could be charged with client abandonment.*

Critical Care

Because the monitors used in critical care units are not infallible, constant observation and assessment of clients are required. This makes a 1:1 or a 1:2 nurse–client ratio imperative. Furthermore, equipment must be checked regularly and on a schedule by the biomedical department.

Pediatric Care

Legislation in each state requires that suspected child abuse or neglect be reported. Legal immunity is provided to the person who makes a report in good faith. When suspected child abuse or neglect is not reported by health care providers, legal action, civil or criminal, may be filed against them.

NURSE–CLIENT RELATIONSHIP

Situations can develop between a nurse and a client that may require legal intervention. The types of torts that may arise are discussed following.

Torts

When a case is brought against a nurse, it is usually a civil action that falls under tort law. Torts can be intentional or

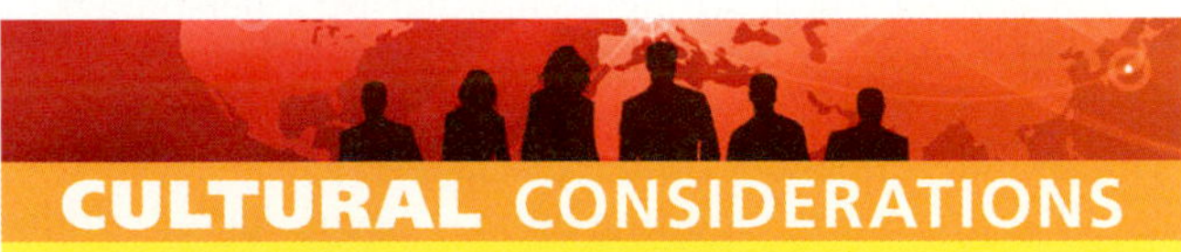

CULTURAL CONSIDERATIONS

Assault and Battery Charges

To prevent assault and battery charges, note the following:

- Respect the client's cultural values, beliefs, and practices with regard to "touching."
- African Americans sometimes view touching another person's hair as offensive.
- Asian Americans usually do not touch others during conversations. Touching someone on the head is considered disrespectful because the head is considered sacred.
- European Americans employ handshakes for formal greetings.
- Hispanic Americans are very tactile and may embrace and shake hands when greeting one another.
- Native Americans prohibit touching a dead body. This may leave the offender open to charges of assault.

TABLE 4-3 Selected Torts: Definitions and Examples

TYPE OF TORT	DEFINITION	EXAMPLE
Intentional		
Assault	Threaten or attempt to touch another person.	Tells client he will be tied in bed if he tries to get out.
Battery	Unconsented touching.	A treatment is performed against the client's will.
False imprisonment	Unwarranted restriction of the freedom of an individual.	A client who is of sound mind and is not in danger of inflicting injury on self or another is restrained.
Quasi-intentional		
Invasion of privacy	All individuals have the right to privacy and may bring charges against any person who violates this right.	Information is disclosed about a client that is considered private or photographs taken without client consent.
Defamation (libel and slander)	Verbal (slander) or written (libel) remarks that may cause the loss of an individual's reputation.	A statement is made that could either ruin the client's reputation or cause the client to lose his or her job.
Unintentional		
Negligence	Failure to use such care as a reasonably prudent person would use under similar circumstances, which leads to harm.	Client's property is lost. A medication error occurs. A client is burned from the improper use of equipment. A change in the client's condition is not observed and/or reported. Inaccurate count of sponges in the operating room is taken.
Malpractice	Failure of a professional to use such care as a reasonably prudent member of the profession would use under similar circumstances, which leads to harm.	An inaccurate nursing diagnosis is made and the wrong treatment is implemented. Physician's orders are not followed. Physician's clearly erroneous order is not questioned.

COURTESY OF DELMAR CENGAGE LEARNING

unintentional (Table 4-3). The person who commits an intentional tort violates the civil rights of another individual knowingly and willfully. Examples of intentional torts are assault and battery, defamation (libel and slander), fraud, false imprisonment, and invasion of privacy. Unintentional torts are those actions that cause harm to the client resulting from carelessness or negligence by the nurse. If found liable, the nurse generally must pay monetary damages. Prison terms are rare.

Intentional Torts

Assault and battery, defamation, fraud, false imprisonment, and invasion of privacy are types of intentional torts.

Assault and Battery **Assault** and **battery** are in fact two separate terms. Assault is the threat to do something that may cause harm or be unpleasant to another person. Battery is the unauthorized or unwanted touching of one person by another.

The key elements in assault are fear and intimidation. The person assaulted must believe that the threat can and will be carried out; for example, a client confined to a wheelchair is told, "If you do not finish your meal, you are going to sit there all night." The client complies because he believes the health care worker will leave him to sit there. The client knows the worker is in a position to carry out this threat.

Consent is the key factor in battery. People have the right to be free of unwanted handling of their person. Striking a client, performing a procedure without the client's consent, and forcing a person to take medication he does not want are all battery. Any unwanted touching can be construed as battery.

Defamation **Defamation** is using words to harm or injure the personal or professional reputation of another person. If the words are written down, they constitute **libel**. If the information is communicated verbally to a third party, it constitutes **slander**.

Negative or derogatory comments that are untrue leave the nurse no defense against charges of defamation. If comments are true, the relevance of the information is important. The most common examples of this tort are giving out inaccurate or inappropriate information from the medical record; discussing clients, families, or visitors in public areas; or speaking negatively about coworkers (Zerwekh & Claborn, 2003).

Fraud **Fraud** is a wrong that results from a deliberate deception intended to produce unlawful gain. Common forms of fraud in health care include deceit in obtaining or attempting to obtain a nursing license and illegal billing.

False Imprisonment **False imprisonment** refers to making the client wrongfully believe that she cannot leave a place. Any means used to confine a client or to restrict movement can be considered a restraint and a form of false imprisonment. This includes threats, physical restraints such as wrist or vest restraints, locked doors, side rails, geriatric chairs, and psychotropic drugs. A common example of this tort is telling a client not to leave the hospital until the bill is paid (Zerwekh & Claborn, 2003).

A dilemma arises when a client decides to leave the health care facility and no discharge order has been written. If the health care problem has not been resolved, the nurse may feel that it is not in the best interest of the client to leave. A client of sound mind has the right to make this decision, regardless of what others think is best. Detaining the individual could bring charges of false imprisonment.

Documentation is very important in these situations, including the client's reasons for leaving the facility and any teaching or interventions related to the situation. Facility policy usually requires that the client sign a form indicating that he is leaving against medical advice (AMA), which releases the facility of any liability. If the client refuses to sign the AMA form, the client's refusal should be documented, and the nursing supervisor and the client's physician should be notified.

Any device used to restrict movement is called a **restraint**. To prevent possible charges of false imprisonment, carefully assess the situation and include the client or significant other in the care planning process. If it is decided that a restraint is needed, the purpose and use of the restraint should be explained, including how the restraint fits into the plan of care, the length of time the restraint may be necessary, and the expected outcome. Document the planning session in the client's medical record. Documentation must show that the client is toileted, receives food and water, and has position changes.

In acute care settings, restraints can generally be applied temporarily as a nursing measure for client safety; however, in most states, a physician's order must be immediately obtained. In long-term care settings, a physician's order is required before utilizing any restraints.

Invasion of Privacy **Privacy** includes the right to be left alone, to choose care based on personal beliefs, to govern body integrity, and to choose when and how sensitive information is shared. People are entitled to **confidential** (nondisclosure of information) health care. All information gathered from working with a client or from his medical records must be kept confidential. Therefore, a client's health status may not be discussed with a third party, unless either the client is present and has given verbal permission or permission has been obtained in writing. This does not apply to nurses discussing a client's health status with other health care workers involved in the care of the client.

Invasion of privacy occurs when a person's private affairs become public knowledge without the person's permission. Photographing a client without his consent is an invasion of privacy, as is failure to pull curtains to shield the client when performing personal or intimate care.

Discussing clients in public areas is a common mistake made by health care personnel. When talking in the cafeteria or in the elevator, it is difficult to know who may overhear what is said. The client's job or family situation may be compromised, depending on the nature of the information. For example, news of an abortion, positive HIV status, or venereal disease may be socially damaging. *Clients or their health care status should never be discussed in public areas or with anyone not directly involved in the care of the client.*

To protect the client's privacy, permission should be obtained before going through a client's belongings, doors should be kept closed and curtains pulled when providing personal care, and people not involved in the performance of a procedure should not be invited to watch unless the client has given permission. Clients cannot be photographed or videotaped without their permission, and a release form must be signed. Nursing students should never use a client's full name on care plans, case studies, or other assignments. Only initials should be used to protect the client's privacy in case the papers are lost. The client's chart and other materials should not be left lying around, allowing a client's private information to become public knowledge.

Since the time of Florence Nightingale, nurses have been practicing and advocating clients' basic right to privacy and confidentiality. Now there is a federal regulation covering these aspects. On April 14, 2003, the Health Insurance Portability and Accountability Act (HIPAA) privacy regulations went into effect. Protected health information (PHI) includes all health care information that can be traced to or identified with a specific individual (Ziel & Gentry, 2003).

The rules now protect how client health care information is stored and transferred and prescribe to whom it can be revealed. Also, clients are given the right to access their health care records, amend health care information, and obtain a list of who has seen their health care records (Frank-Stromborg & Ganschow, 2002; Trossman, 2003). Clients must be given a written notice by hospitals, physicians, pharmacies, and other covered entities of their privacy practices (Frank-Stromborg & Ganschow, 2002; Ziel & Gentry, 2003). When a state's law is more stringent than HIPAA regulations, the state's law will prevail.

Unintentional Torts

Negligence and malpractice are considered unintentional torts.

Negligence **Negligence** is a general term referring to negligent or careless acts on the part of an individual who is not exercising reasonable or prudent judgment. All nurses, including student nurses, are expected to use good judgment when providing client care. For example, side rails should not be left down on confused clients' beds, and puddles and spills should be cleaned up immediately to prevent falls rather than waiting for housekeeping. Any person, even without the specialized knowledge required for nursing, could make these judgments. When a nurse fails to protect a client in such a situation or in one requiring similar judgment, the nurse could be found negligent.

Malpractice Negligent acts on the part of a professional can be termed **malpractice**, or professional negligence. Malpractice relates to the conduct of a person while acting in a professional capacity.

Not meeting the standards of care, not doing what a reasonable and prudent nurse would do in similar circumstances, results in negligent or careless acts on the part of a nurse. A nurse can be charged with malpractice for acts committed or acts omitted. Failing to properly assess a client or act on the assessment information are examples of omission. Giving a client the wrong medication and improperly performing a procedure resulting in client injury are acts of commission.

Malpractice differs from negligence in that anyone can be accused of negligence; only professionals can be accused of malpractice. Several factors must hold true for a nurse to be found guilty of malpractice (professional negligence):

- The nurse owed a special duty to the client; that is, a nurse–client relationship existed.
- The nurse failed to meet the standards of care.
- The injury occurred as a direct result of the nurse's action or inaction.
- Damage such as physical or emotional pain, suffering, monetary losses, or medical expenses must be proved. If there is not damage, the plaintiff is not entitled to an award (Lee, 2000).

The prudent nurse is protected by adhering to facility policy and procedure and attempting to meet the standards of care at all times.

Legal Risk

Nurses today are more likely to have problems for violating statutes (i.e., laws and regulations) than to be sued for malpractice (Infante, 2000). Two common sources of statutory liability are federal antifraud laws and state reporting requirements. Statutory liability may lead to criminal charges rather than just civil penalties (Infante, 2000). The best protection against statutory liability is to learn about the federal and state laws and regulations that apply to the nurse's particular practice setting. A good resource is the facility's risk manager.

Federal Antifraud Laws

The federal government has:

- Expanded the list of activities that constitute fraud
- Imposed new criminal sanctions on violators
- Increased the budget for investigating and prosecuting these activities

Infante (2000) lists as examples of fraudulent activities the following:

- Billing for services either unnecessary or not provided
- Falsifying care plans
- Forging physician's signature
- Filing false cost reports
- Falsifying or omitting information about a client's condition to obtain reimbursement

State Reporting Requirements

Nurses are required to report cases of suspected child abuse or neglect in every state (Infante, 2000). Most states also require nurses to report cases of suspected elder abuse and neglect. Infante (2000) identifies some criminal acts that must be reported. Many states require that:

- Police are notified of known or suspected cases of rape
- Reports of gunshot or stab wounds are made

Some states require that clients who have taken narcotics or who have a blood alcohol level higher than the legal limit for driving be reported.

These laws are not only for the general public but also for health care providers. If a suspected abuser is a health care provider, many states require that the event be reported to the agency that licenses that professional. Also, many states require nurses to report *any* provider who acts unprofessionally or is incompetent (Infante, 2000).

Professional Discipline

More than 5,000 nurses (RNs and LP/VNs) are annually disciplined for professional misconduct in the United States (LaDuke, 2000). That is, the nurses are found to have violated existing laws or regulations that govern a nurse's practice. LaDuke (2000) suggests that a nurse:

- Should *immediately* seek representation by an attorney specializing in professional misconduct and discipline if under investigation
- Is not obligated to talk to *any* investigator without an attorney present
- Know and understand the applicable state nursing practice act and established standards of care
- Look closely at the disciplinary process and ask questions to promote understanding

Sanctions

Boards of nursing determine and issue sanctions for nurses found to have demonstrated professional misconduct. Monetary damages are not generally awarded to consumers. A sample of sanctions from which boards of nursing may choose includes:

- Warn, censure, or reprimand the licensees.
- Impose a fine.
- Place on probation or set a condition of licensure.
- Limit the license.
- Suspend the license.
- Revoke the license.
- Dismiss the complaint.

Disciplinary Data Banks

The NCSBN maintains a Disciplinary Data Bank (DDB), as do many other professional organizations. The purpose of these data banks is to facilitate the communication of information about unsafe practitioners. In 1990, Congress created the National Practitioner Data Bank (NPDB) to improve the quality of health care by encouraging the identification and discipline of health care professionals (mostly physicians and dentists) who engage in incompetent and unsafe behavior.

As part of the HIPAA of 1996, the Healthcare Integrity and Protection Data Bank (HIPDB) was implemented in 2000. This data bank collects and discloses certain final adverse actions taken against nurses at all levels of practice, other licensed practitioners, and unlicensed persons who provide health care services or are involved in the health insurance business. The Data Banks' Proactive Disclosure Service Prototype (PDS) went online in 2007. PDS offers health care providers and facilities the opportunity to query enrolled practitioners. Health care practitioners and facilities that subscribe to PDS receive notification within 24 hours of the Data Banks' receipt of a report on any of its enrolled practitioners. PDS saves time and money when compared to the traditional method of querying the Data Banks (Health Resources and Services Administration, 2008).

DOCUMENTATION

The source of information regarding the client's clinical history is the medical record, or the chart. The chart should accurately reflect diagnosis, treatment, testing, clinical course, nursing assessment, and intervention. According to the law, "If it was not charted, it was not done." When a chart ends up in court, this is the standard the jury applies in determining what happened and who is at fault.

Medications should not be charted before they are given. This constitutes a direct violation of the standards of practice for documentation and medication administration. The standard of practice is that medications are documented *after* they are administered. All client care, including treatments, is documented after being provided.

Documentation must be objective and accurate. The nurse should describe what is seen and done. Nurses' notes should reflect facts, not inferences or opinions, about the client. It is not enough to chart nursing assessment or identified problems; any actions taken, including nursing interventions and physician's orders implemented, must also be documented.

Entries must be neat, legible, spelled correctly, written clearly, and signed or initialed. It is illegal to change a chart.

INFORMED CONSENT

Informed consent refers to a competent client's ability to make health care decisions based on full disclosure of the benefits, risks, potential consequences of a recommended treatment plan, and alternate treatments, including no treatment, and the client's agreement to the treatment as indicated by the client's signing a consent form. This detailed explanation, provided by the physician, lets the client make intelligent decisions about treatment options. Consent to treatment also protects health care workers from unwarranted charges of battery (Figure 4-1) (Delaune & Ladner, 2006).

Nurses must obtain consent for nursing procedures. Each client, on admission, signs a general care consent form. The nurse is obligated to explain what is to be done to the client and to receive at least implied consent, as indicated by lack of objection on the part of the client. Individuals who are declared incompetent are assigned a guardian or someone

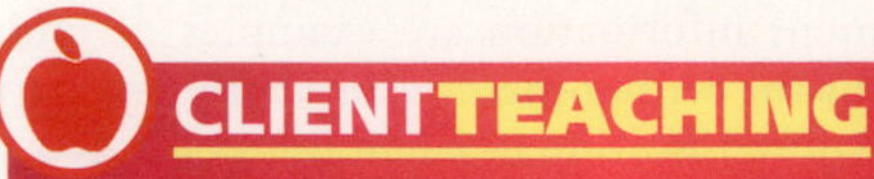

Informed Consent

Consent may be withdrawn, either verbally or in writing, at any time.

who has power of attorney to make heath care decisions and give consent for treatment. The physician is responsible for obtaining consent for medical or surgical treatment. The discussion about the risks and benefits of treatment generally takes place when the nurse is not present, often in the physician's office. The client usually decides on the basis of the discussion whether to accept the treatment recommendation. Confusion arises, however, because nurses are often delegated the duty of collecting the signature on the informed consent form. *Student nurses should neither ask the client to sign a consent form nor witness a consent form.*

When a nurse has a client sign the informed consent form, the nurse is verifying the following three things:

1. The client's signature is authentic.
2. The client has the mental capacity to understand what was discussed with the physician.
3. The client was not coerced into signing the form.

The client should not sign the form if the client still has questions or if the nurse is unsure about the client's understanding. The nurse should document the client's lack of understanding and contact the physician. Further clarification must come from the physician.

Clients older than age 18 may give consent for their own health care. Parents or guardians give consent for minor children. In most states, minors who live on their own, are married, become pregnant, or require treatment for sexually transmitted infections, substance abuse, or mental illness may give consent for themselves.

Complex situations occur when minors refuse treatments to which parents have consented or parents refuse consent or treatment that has been deemed medically necessary for their minor children. The court has had to intervene in such cases. In situations such as these, the child may be made a ward of the court and decision making temporarily taken away from the parents. An example would be the child of Jehovah's Witnesses who needs a blood transfusion but whose parents refuse treatment on the basis of religious beliefs.

A typical consent form (Figure 4-2) is used to obtain client permission for the performance of invasive medical, surgical, or diagnostic procedures, such as surgery, cardiac

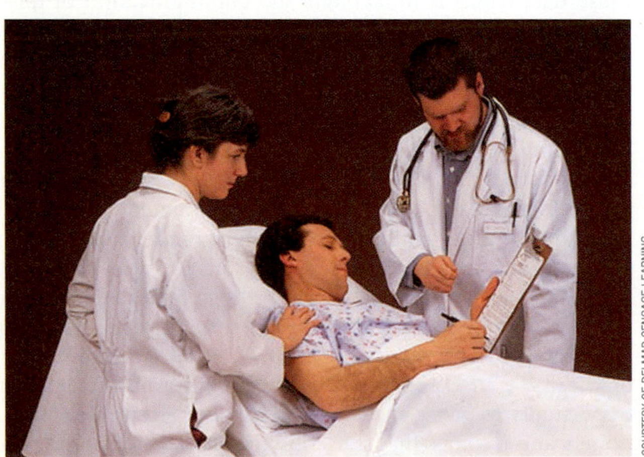

COURTESY OF DELMAR CENGAGE LEARNING

FIGURE 4-1 A nurse is witnessing the signing of a consent form after the physician has fully informed the client about the proposed treatment.

PROFESSIONAL TIP

Consent in Emergencies

- Consent is implied when immediate action is necessary to save a life or to prevent permanent physical harm. Written consent is waived.
- After the emergency is over, consent must be obtained for further care.

TO THE PATIENT: You have the right as a patient to be informed about your condition and the recommended surgical, medical, or diagnostic procedure to be used so that you may make the decision whether or not to undergo the procedure after knowing the risks and hazards involved. This disclosure is not meant to scare or alarm you, but is simply an effort to make you better informed so you may give or withhold your consent to the procedure. Any questions or concerns you may have with respect to the proposed procedure, its risks, complications, or benefits should be directed to your treating physician.

I (we) voluntarily request Dr. ______________ as my physician, and such associates, technical assistants and other health care providers as they may deem necessary to treat my condition, which has been explained to me as: ______________

____

I (we) understand that the following surgical, medical, and/or diagnostic procedures are planned for me, and I (we) voluntarily consent and authorize these procedures: ______________

____

I (we) understand that my physician may discover other or different conditions which require additional or different procedures than those planned. I (we) authorize my physician, and such associates, technical assistants, and other health care providers, to perform such procedures which are advisable in their professional judgment.

I (we) [DO] [DO NOT] consent to the use of blood and blood products as deemed necessary.

I (we) understand that no warrant or guarantee has been made to me as a result or cure.

Just as there may be risks and hazards in continuing my present condition without treatment, there are also risks and hazards related to the performance of the surgical, medical, and/or diagnostic procedures planned for me. I (we) realize that common to surgical, medical, and/or diagnostic procedures is the potential for infection, blood clots in veins and lungs, hemorrhage, allergic reactions, and even death. I (we) realize that the following risks and hazards may occur in connection with this particular procedure:

____

____

____

(Additional Consent Information On Back.)

INITIAL: ______________

3025

CHRISTUS SPOHN HEALTH SYSTEM

DISCLOSURE AND CONSENT
MEDICAL AND SURGICAL PROCEDURES
PATIENT CARE SERVICES

2704980 NEW: 05/82
REVISED: 10/99

I (we) understand that anesthesia involves additional risks and hazards, but I (we) request the use of anesthetics for the relief and protection from pain during the planned and additional procedures. I (we) realize the anesthesia may have to be changed, possibly without explanation to me (us).

I (we) understand that certain complications may result from the use of any anesthetic, including respiratory problems, drug reaction, paralysis, brain damage, or even death. Other risks and hazards which may result from the use of general anesthetics range from minor discomfort to injury to vocal cords, teeth, or eyes. I (we) understand that other risks and hazards resulting from spinal or epidural anesthetics include headache, chronic pain, remote possibility of nerve injury, hematoma, infection, septic and aseptic meningitis, nausea, vomiting, itching, and urinary retention.

I (we) consent to the photographing of the operations or procedures to be performed, including appropriate portions of the body, for medical, scientific, or educational purposes, provided my identity is not revealed by descriptive texts accompanying the picture.

I (we) consent to the disposition by hospital authorities of any tissues or parts which may be removed.

I (we) have been given the opportunity to ask questions about my conditions, alternative forms of anesthesia and treatment, risks of non-treatment, the procedures to be used, and the risks and hazards involved, and I (we) believe that I (we) have sufficient information to give this informed consent.

My physician has discussed the alternatives, risks and benefits, of the proposed procedures. I (we) certify that this form has been fully explained to me; that I (we) have read it or have had it read to me; that the blank spaces have been filled in, and that I (we) understand its contents.

____
PHYSICIAN'S SIGNATURE

DATE: ______________ TIME: ______________ A.M./P.M.

____
Witness (Signature of witness/print name of witness)

____
Patient/Other Legally Responsible Person
(Minor patient and parent/guardian signature)

FIGURE 4-2 Disclosure and Consent—Medical and Surgical Procedures (*Courtesy of CHRISTUS Spohn Health System, Corpus Christi, TX.*)

CRITICAL THINKING

Informed Consent

How would you address a situation in which a 17-year-old client is adamantly refusing to have surgery but the parents sign the consent form anyway?

catheterization, or HIV testing. Consent for procedures that are not invasive can be either given verbally or implied. Consent is implied when the client cooperates with the procedure offered. For example, if the orderly says, "Mr. Garza, I am here to take you for your hand x-ray," and Mr. Garza gets into the wheelchair, consent is implied by Mr. Garza's cooperation.

ADVANCE DIRECTIVES

An **advance directive** is a written instruction for health care, recognized under state law, related to the provision of care when the individual is incapacitated. Advance directives emphasize the client's right to self-determination. These instructions about health care preferences regarding life-sustaining measures may indicate who is to make health care decisions for the client if he becomes unable to do so for himself.

A client of sound mind has the right to make all health care decisions and even reverse previous decisions. When a situation arises and the person becomes incapable of making decisions, advance directives guide family members concerning those kinds of treatment that should or should not be allowed. Advance directives permit those involved in the decision-making process to know what the client prefers. Although these instructions are best put in writing, this is not always done. Sometimes, health care preferences are shared verbally with family members or friends. Verbal instructions can be interpreted differently by different people, creating difficulty for all involved—the physician, the health care facility, and the family. Thus, it is best to get this information in writing. When an advance directive indicates that the client does not wish to have cardiopulmonary resuscitation (CPR) performed in the event of cardiac arrest, the physician must write a DNR order, also referred to as a "No Code."

Health care facilities that receive Medicaid or Medicare monies are required to offer the opportunity to complete advance directives to all competent clients on admission. The client should be told about the availability and purpose of a living will and durable power of attorney for health care (discussed following). If desired, assistance in completing these documents is to be offered to the client. The medical record must show that the client was offered the opportunity to complete these documents, and documentation must indicate decisions made or not made at that time. Clients cannot be discriminated against for not signing an advance directive, nor can they be coerced into signing an advance directive.

PROFESSIONAL TIP

Consent in Special Situations

- If a client is unable to consent and the family is too far away, consent may be received over the telephone, according to agency policy. (Usually, two persons must hear the consent being given.)
- A client who has already received preoperative or preprocedure medication is not competent to sign a consent. When this situation arises, the surgery or procedure may have to be postponed.
- For blood transfusions, some facilities require that a denial form be signed if the client indicates *No* on the consent form.

CLIENT TEACHING

Advance Directives

- Advance directives should be discussed with the family and physician so that everyone understands the client's wishes and conflicts are less likely to occur at a later time.
- An advance directive may be changed by the client as long as the client is competent.

DURABLE POWER OF ATTORNEY FOR HEALTH CARE

A **durable power of attorney for health care (DPAHC)** is a legal document designating who may make health care decisions for a client when that client is no longer capable of decision making. This health care representative, appointed by the client, is expected to act in the best interests of the client. This appointment can be revoked any time the competent client chooses.

For example, if a client becomes comatose and the prognosis is poor, the health care representative having DPAHC can either give consent for certain types of treatment or withhold consent for treatment, even if the lack of treatment results in the client's death. Only when the client is no longer competent to make health care decisions is the DPAHC activated.

The person who has a regular power of attorney does not have the same authority about health care issues. The right to make health care decisions must be specified in the power of attorney agreement, or a DPAHC must be signed (Figure 4-3). A person who stands to benefit from the client's estate cannot be appointed health care representative.

CRITICAL THINKING

Advance Directives

You observe a coworker coercing a new nursing home resident into signing an advance directive. How would you handle this? What are the client's rights in this situation?

Part I. Durable Power of Attorney for Health Care

• If you do NOT wish to name an agent to make health care decisions for you, write your initials in the box [Initials]

This form has been prepared to comply with the "Durable Power of Attorney for Health Care Act" of Missouri.

It is suggested that only one Agent be named. However, if more than one Agent is named, anyone may act individually unless you specify otherwise.

1. Selection of agent. I appoint:
Name:____________________
Address:____________________
____
Telephone:____________________
as my Agent.

2. Alternate Agents. Only an Agent named by me may act under this Durable Power of Attorney. If my Agent resigns or is not able or available to make health care decisions for me, or if an Agent named by me is divorced from me or is my spouse and legally separated from me, I appoint the person(s) named below (in the order named if more than one):

First Alternate Agent	Second Alternate Agent
Name:____________	Name:____________
Address:____________	Address:____________
____________	____________
Telephone:____________	Telephone:____________

This is a Durable Power of Attorney, and the authority of my Agent shall not terminate if I become disabled or incapacitated.

Part I. Durable Power of Attorney for Health Care (Continued)

3. Effective date and durability. This Durable Power of Attorney is effective when two physicians decide and certify that I am incapacitated and unable to make and communicate a health care decision.

• If you want ONE physician, instead of TWO, to decide whether you are incapacitated, write your initials in the box to the right. [Initials]

4. Agent's powers. I grant to my Agent full authority to:

A. Give consent to, prohibit, or withdraw any type of health care, medical care, treatment, or procedure, even if my death may result;

• If you wish to AUTHORIZE your Agent to direct a health care provider to withhold or withdraw artificially supplied nutrition and hydration (including tube feeding of food and water), write your initials in the box to the right. [Initials]

• If you DO NOT WISH TO AUTHORIZE your Agent to direct a health care provider to withhold or withdraw artificially supplied nutrition and hydration (including tube feeding of food and water), write your initials in the box to the right. [Initials]

B. Make all necessary arrangements for health care services on my behalf, and to hire and fire medical personnel responsible for my care;

C. Move me into or out of any health care facility (even if against medical advice) to obtain compliance with the decisions of my Agent; and

D. Take any other action necessary to do what I authorize here, including (but not limited to) granting any waiver or release from liability required by any health care provider, and taking any legal action at the expense of my estate to enforce this Durable Power of Attorney.

5. Agent's Financial Liability and Compensation. My Agent acting under this Durable Power of Attorney will incur no personal financial liability. My Agent shall not be entitled to compensation for services performed under this Durable Power of Attorney, but my Agent shall be entitled to reimbursement for all reasonable expenses incurred as a result of carrying out any provision hereof.

Part II. Health Care Directive

• If you DO NOT WISH to make a health care directive, write your initials in the box to the right, and go to Part III. [Initials]

I make this HEALTH CARE DIRECTIVE ("Directive") to exercise my right to determine the course of my health care and to provide clear and convincing proof of my wishes and instructions about my treatment.

If I am persistently unconscious or there is no reasonable expectation of my recovery from a seriously incapacitating or terminal illness or condition, I direct that all of the life-prolonging procedures which I have initialed below be withheld or withdrawn.

I want the following life-prolonging procedures to be withheld or withdrawn:

• artificially supplied nutrition and hydration (including tube feeding of food and water) .... [Initials]

• surgery or other invasive procedures. .... ______ Initials
• heart-lung resuscitation (CPR) .... ______ Initials
• antibiotic. .... ______ Initials
• dialysis. .... ______ Initials
• mechanical ventilator (respirator). .... ______ Initials
• chemotherapy. .... ______ Initials
• radiation therapy. .... ______ Initials
• all other "life-prolonging" medical or surgical procedures that are merely intended to keep me alive without reasonable hope of improving my condition or curing my illness or injury. .... ______ Initials

However, if my physician believes that any life-prolonging procedure may lead to significant recovery, I direct my physician to try the treatment for a reasonable period of time. If it does not improve my condition, I direct the treatment be withdrawn even if it shortens my life. I also direct that I be given medical treatment to relieve pain or to provide comfort, even if such treatment might shorten my life, suppress my appetite or my breathing, or be habit forming.

IF I HAVE NOT DESIGNATED AN AGENT IN THE DURABLE POWER OF ATTORNEY, THIS DOCUMENT IS MEANT TO BE IN FULL FORCE AND EFFECT AS MY HEALTH CARE DIRECTIVE.

Part III. General Provisions Included in the Directive and Durable Power of Attorney

YOU MUST SIGN THIS DOCUMENT IN THE PRESENCE OF TWO WITNESSES.
IN WITNESS WHEREOF, I have executed this document this__________day of __________, year____.

____
Signature

Print name ____________________
Address ____________________

The person who signed this document is of sound mind and voluntarily signed this document in our presence. Each of the undersigned witnesses is at least eighteen years of age.

Signature____________	Signature____________
Print name ____________	Print name ____________
Address ____________	Address ____________

ONLY REQUIRED FOR PART I — DURABLE POWER OF ATTORNEY

STATE OF MISSOURI)
) as
________OF ______)

On this ________day of ____________, year_______, before me personally appeared to me known to be the person described in and who executed the foregoing instrument and acknowledged that he/she executed the same as his/her free act and deed.

IN WITNESS WHEREOF, I have hereunto set my hand and affixed my official seal in the County of ____________, State of Missouri, the day and year first above written.

____
Notary Public

My Commision Expires:

FIGURE 4-3 Durable Power of Attorney for Health Care and Health Care Directive (*Reprinted with permission of the Missouri Bar.*)

Living Will

A **living will** is a legal document that allows a person to state preferences about the use of life-sustaining measures in case she is unable to make her wishes known. These preferences can be expressed either with a living will or a Life-Prolonging Procedure Declaration. These documents allow the client to specify, in advance, those life-sustaining measures that are to be done or not done. Food, fluids, and comfort measures are generally continued, and the person is not abandoned; however, artificial means of sustaining life, such as ventilators or feeding tubes, are not to be used.

Although not all states currently recognize living wills, the client's requests should be given due weight when making health care decisions. The nurse must be knowledgeable about living will legislation in her state. A sample living will is shown in Figure 4-4.

A Life-Prolonging Procedure Declaration stating that the person wants all possible procedures done to delay the dying process, including the use of ventilators, is available in some places.

Sample Living Will

Declaration made this ____ day of __________, year_____.
I, ______________________, willfully and voluntarily make known my desire that my dying not be artificially prolonged under the circumstances set forth below, and I do hereby declare:

If at any time I have a terminal condition and if my attending or treating physician and another consulting physician have determined that there is no medical probability of my recovery from such condition, I direct that life-prolonging procedures be withheld or withdrawn when the application of such procedures would serve only to prolong artificially the process of dying, and that I be permitted to die naturally with only the administration of medication or the performance of any medical procedure deemed necessary to provide me with comfort care or to alleviate pain.

It is my intention that this declaration be honored by my family and physician as the final expression of my legal right to refuse medical or surgical treatment and to accept the consequences for such refusal.

In the event that I have been determined to be unable to provide express and informed consent regarding the withholding, withdrawal, or continuation of life-prolonging procedures, I wish to designate, as my surrogate to carry out the provisions of this declaration:

Name: ______________________
Address: ______________________
______________________ Zip Code: __________
Phone: ______________________

I wish to designate the following person as my alternate surrogate, to carry out the provisions of this declaration should my surrogate be unwilling or unable to act on my behalf:

Name: ______________________
Address: ______________________
______________________ Zip Code: __________
Phone: ______________________

Additional instructions (optional):

I understand the full importance of this declaration, and I am emotionally and mentally competant to make this declaration.
Signed: ______________________

Witness 1:
Signed: ______________________
Address: ______________________

Witness 2:
Signed: ______________________
Address: ______________________

Figure 4-4 Sample Living Will (*Reprinted by permission of Partnership for Caring, 1620 Eye Street NW, Suite 202, Washington, DC 20006.*)

INCIDENT REPORTS

An **incident report** is a risk management tool used to describe and report any unusual event that occurs to a client, visitor, or staff member. It is used by the facility to identify or track problem areas and to alert the legal department to possible lawsuits. An incident report is not a punitive device, although it is often perceived that it is.

Incident reports are completed to document such events as falls, medication errors, forgotten treatment, injuries—anything that happens out of the ordinary. An incident report may also be called a variance report or an occurrence report. The following three examples illustrate the types of occurrences that should be documented in an incident report.

- R.D. had blood drawn for various laboratory tests. It was later discovered that the laboratory work had been ordered on F.T., not R.D. The requisition had been stamped with the wrong name.
- C.S. was given Lasix 20 mg po at 9 A.M. When reviewing the physician's orders, the evening nurse discovered that Losec 20 mg had been ordered. C.S. received the wrong medication.
- M.C. was visiting her daughter, who had just given birth to the family's first grandchild. While walking down the hall, M.C. slipped and fell, injuring her right hip.

The previous examples are incidents or variances that occur in health care settings. For each situation, an incident report must be completed and channeled to the risk management department. Risk management convenes representatives from various departments, such as nursing administration, dietary services, environmental safety, and others, to review the incident reports. This group tries to identify those factors, if any, that contributed to the incident. Examples of questions asked include "Can the causal factors be eliminated or reduced?," "Does the possibility of a lawsuit exist as a result of the incident?" and "What can be done to prevent this incident from occurring again?"

Incident reports are filed by the person who was responsible for, who discovered, or who witnessed the incident. The report should state what was observed, as opposed to what is supposed. It should be concise and factual. In the third example given previously, if the nurse did not witness the actual fall, the correctly worded report would read, "M.C. found lying on floor outside room 222. Several puddles of liquid found under and around her; paper cup lying nearby." An incorrect, presumptuous, and potentially damaging report might read, "M.C. tripped and fell outside room 222. She slipped in a puddle of water." M.C. may have spilled the cup of water she was carrying during the fall; however, this second note implies that M.C. slipped in water that was already on the floor, thus implicating the facility.

Incident reports should include a description of the care given to the client or individual and the name of the physician who was notified. The incident should be charted in the client's medical record, but the incident report should not be referred to in any way. Although the incident report is not a part of the medical record, the details described in the medical record and in the incident report should be the same.

When completing an incident report, the nurse should be sure to include the date and time of the incident as well as assessments and interventions. The time that family members and physicians were notified should also be included. The nurse should refer to nursing administration policy and procedure regarding follow-up documentation.

LIABILITY INSURANCE

Many nurses assume the insurance provided by their employer is adequate and they do not need their own malpractice or liability insurance. This attitude may leave a nurse vulnerable both professionally and personally (LaDuke & Biondo, 2003).

Nurses assert they are knowledgeable and competent health care providers. Health care consumers hold nurses accountable for their actions, resulting in nurses being named as defendants in malpractice suits. Under the doctrine of *Respondeat Superior*, employers are responsible for the actions of their employees; however, if policy was violated and the employer has to pay damages, the employer has the right to sue the nurse to recover the loss. Also, this responsibility stops when the employee leaves work.

A professional liability policy provides the nurse with an attorney who will represent that nurse in court. The needs of an individual nurse will be secondary to an attorney representing the facility or a group of employees. The individual nurse is better represented in court by private counsel.

Friends and family members ask nurses for assistance and advice in health care matters. They seek this advice because of their experience and knowledge. Family members or friends might bring a law suit against the nurse later depending on the results of the advice. The nurse is accountable for the advice given even though no money was exchanged for information or services.

The nurse needs legal representation if the situation ends up in court, which is costly as are judgments against the nurse. The nurse is protected with a professional liability insurance policy that provides legal representation and pays the judgments.

Liability protection comes in two forms: the claims made policy and the occurrence policy. The claims made policy covers claims made while the policy is in effect. The nurse is not covered if a claim is made after the policy is terminated. An occurrence policy protects the nurse for events taking place during the active period of the policy even if a claim is filed after the policy is terminated. The occurrence policy seems to provide better protection for the nurse. Check if there is coverage for disciplinary claims (Sloan, 2002a).

Whether nurses should carry individual liability insurance is often debated. Some health care professionals and attorneys believe this practice encourages lawsuits. The benefits and cost of buying professional liability insurance must be compared against the loss of personal assets and cost of potential legal fees. When buying liability insurance the company's reputation should be investigated. Many nursing organizations offer group professional liability insurance. Sloan (2002a) suggests that nurses must assess their liability risk by considering their employment status (employee, independent contractor, or borrowed servant [agency nurse]); employer (well financed, having financial hardship, government); and area of specialty (ED, critical care, and obstetrics are considered high-risk settings).

IMPAIRED NURSE

A sensitive issue in nursing today is the impaired nurse. By definition, an **impaired nurse** is a nurse who is habitually intemperate or is addicted to the use of alcohol or habit-forming drugs. Although job performance may not be immediately compromised, substance abuse does eventually interfere with clinical judgment and performance. The chemical dependency rate among nurses is no higher than in the general population (Trinkoff et al., 2000).

In cases of impaired health care workers, the primary concern is client care. As a client advocate, the nurse cannot let loyalties to coworkers interfere with duty to the client. It is difficult reporting a coworker. No one wants to be a squealer. In many states, however, the board of nursing requires nurses to report impaired coworkers. Nurses suspected of being under the influence of drugs or alcohol must be reported to the proper authority at the place of employment. The second consideration is getting help for the impaired nurse and taking action to correct the problem.

When a coworker is suspected of diverting drugs or abusing alcohol, the nurse should:

1. Document the dates, times, and observed behavior. It is critical to be specific and descriptive of what was observed. For example:

   March 10, 2010. C.D. working 3–11 shift. Client A and Client B verbalized unrelieved postoperative pain. Documentation by C.D. stated both clients were comfortable after administration of Demerol 75 mg IM to each client. Narcotic count at shift change satisfactory.

   March 11, 2010. Client C and Client D verbalized unrelieved pain. Documentation by C.D. indicated both clients stated pain was relieved after administration of Demerol 100 mg IM. Narcotic count at shift change okay.

   March 12, 2010. Narcotic count listed 1 Demerol 100-mg syringe as broken and 1 Demerol 75-mg syringe as wasted, "client changed her mind." C.D. signed the narcotic sheet.

   or

   April 13, 2010. S.L. working the night shift. Strong odor of alcohol on his breath.

   April 14, 2010. S.L. observed walking with unsteady gait, speech is slurred, strong odor of alcohol on breath.

2. Report concerns to the supervisor and provide a copy of the documentation about the incidents. The supervisor is responsible for confronting the suspected employee. Intoxication requires immediate removal from the clinical area. In other situations, the supervisor will devise a plan before confronting the nurse.
3. Do not approach or confront the coworker yourself. The impaired coworker may become defensive and deny the problem or make threats. Also, once aware that someone is suspicious, the nurse may become more secretive, making detection less likely. Frequently, the nurse will leave one facility and go to another, repeating the same pattern.

Some employers offer an employee assistance program to rehabilitate the impaired nurse. In addition, most states have **peer assistance programs** (rehabilitation programs designed to provide an impaired nurse with referrals, professional and peer counseling support groups, and assistance and monitoring for reentry into nursing). These peer assistance programs operate under the guidance of the state nurses association in conjunction with the board of nursing. The goals of assistance programs are to protect the public from impaired nurses, provide the needed assistance to the impaired nurse, and assist the nurse to reenter nursing by monitoring the nurse's compliance. The peer counselor helps the impaired nurse develop a contract for treatment. Compliance is monitored, and confidentiality is ensured. Successful completion of the program allows the nurse to return to the practice setting.

Participation in these programs is optional. A nurse choosing not to cooperate, however, may be terminated, and the board of nursing may impose sanctions, including revoking the license to practice.

CONCEPT OF ETHICS

Ethics is the branch of philosophy concerned with determining right from wrong on the basis of knowledge rather than on opinions. Ethics deals with one's responsibilities (duties and obligations) as defined by logical argument. It is *not* a religious dogma. Ethics looks at human behavior—what people do in what circumstances. But ethics is *not* merely philosophical in nature; ethical persons put their beliefs into action.

HEALTH CARE AND ETHICS

Bioethics is the application of general ethical principles to health care. Every area of health care, including direct care of clients, utilization of staff, and allocation of finances is affected by ethics.

Ethics raises questions but does not provide easy answers. Ethical practice has more importance in health care today for several reasons. Some of these reasons are:

- An increase in technology. Advanced technology creates situations involving complicated issues, such as:
  - Newborns are surviving at earlier gestational ages, and many have serious health problems.
  - People are living much longer than ever before.
  - Organ transplants and use of bionic body parts are becoming more common.
- Changing of our society. Family structure is moving to more single-parent families and nonrelated groups living together as families.
- Clients are more knowledgeable about their health and health care, resulting in a consumer-driven system.

TABLE 4-4 Overview of Ethical Principles

PRINCIPLE	EXPLANATION
Autonomy	Respect individual's right to self-determination; respect individual liberty
Nonmaleficence	Cause or do no harm to another
Beneficence	Do good to others and maintain a balance between benefits and harms
Justice	Distribute equitable potential benefits and risks
Veracity	Tell the truth
Fidelity	Do what one has promised

COURTESY OF DELMAR CENGAGE LEARNING

ETHICAL PRINCIPLES

Ethical principles are widely accepted codes generally based on the humane aspects of society that direct or govern actions. Ethical decisions reflect what is best for the client and society. Table 4-4 summarizes the major ethical principles. Each principle is discussed in detail in the following paragraphs.

The nurse can become more systematic in solving ethical conflicts by using ethical principles. They can be used as guidelines in analyzing dilemmas and can serve as justification (rationale) for resolving ethical problems.

AUTONOMY

The principle of **autonomy** refers to the individual's right to choose and the individual's ability to act on that choice. Each person's individuality is respected. This respect is a dominant value in U.S. society.

Nurses must respect the client's right to decide and must protect those clients who are unable to decide for themselves. The ethical principle of autonomy respects the individual's right to self-determination for a competent person. The right to autonomy rests on the client's competency to decide; however, the legal definition of competency varies among states.

Informed consent is based on the client's right to make choices. Respecting autonomy means the nurse accepts client choices, even choices not in the client's best interests or choices that conflict with the nurse's values. Examples of autonomous client behavior that can hinder recovery or treatment include:

- Smoking after a diagnosis of emphysema or lung cancer
- Refusing to take medication
- Continuing to drink alcohol after being diagnosed with cirrhosis of the liver
- Refusing to receive a blood transfusion because of religious beliefs

PROFESSIONALTIP

Autonomy

- Competent clients have a right to self-determination, even if their decisions may result in self-harm.
- Probably one of the most difficult things for nurses to accept is that clients are ultimately responsible for themselves; they will do what they want to do.

COMMUNITY/HOME HEALTH CARE

Client Autonomy

With the increased acuity level of clients cared for in the home setting, home health nurses face ever-increasing ethical challenges because they have less control over what the client does on a day-to-day basis at home.

Nonmaleficence

Nonmaleficence is the obligation to cause no harm to others. Harm can be physiological, psychological, financial, social, and/or spiritual. Included are both the risk of harm and intentional harm. The principle of nonmaleficence when guiding treatment decisions asks the question "Will this treatment modality cause more harm or more good to the client?" There may not be a clear-cut answer. Consider these factors when choosing a treatment:

- A reasonable expectation of benefit
- Lack of excessive pain, expense, or other inconvenience

The nurse practices according to professional and legal standards of care when following the principle of nonmaleficence. Nonmaleficence is considered a fundamental duty of health care providers. The Practical Nurse's Pledge (Box 4-1) and the Nightingale Pledge (Box 4-2) profess similar philosophies of nursing care. Some clinical examples of nonmaleficence are:

- Preventing medication errors (including drug interactions)
- Being aware of potential risks of treatment modalities
- Removing hazards (e.g., obstructions or water on the floor that might cause a fall)

Beneficence

Beneficence is the duty to promote good and to prevent harm. Beneficence is often viewed as the core of nursing practice. The nurse nurtures the client and incorporates the desires of the client into the plan of care. Sometimes, it is difficult to determine what is "good," especially when doing good causes the client discomfort. For example, a client who has had a serious stroke may resist performing range-of-motion exercises and become angry at the nurse for insisting. The nurse knows the long-term value of these exercises yet perceives the client's physical and psychological pain.

Justice

The principle of **justice** is based on the concept of fairness extended to each individual. The major health-related issues of justice involve the way people are treated and the way resources are distributed.

This principle directs that unless there is a justification for unequal treatment, all people must be treated equally. The **material principle of justice** is the rationale for determining those times when there can be unequal allocation of scarce

BOX 4-1 PRACTICAL NURSE'S PLEDGE

Before God and those assembled here, I solemnly pledge:

To adhere to the code of ethics of the nursing profession.

To cooperate faithfully with the other members of the nursing team and to carry out faithfully and to the best of my ability the instructions of the physician or the nurse who may be assigned to supervise my work.

I will not do anything evil or malicious and I will not knowingly give any harmful drug or assist in malpractice.

I will not reveal any confidential information that may come to my knowledge in the course of my work.

And I pledge myself to do all in my power to raise the standards and the prestige of practical nursing.

May my life be devoted to service, and to the high ideals of the nursing profession.

Reprinted with permission of the National Association for Practical Nurse Education and Services, Inc., Silver Spring, MD.

BOX 4-2 NIGHTINGALE PLEDGE

I solemnly pledge myself before God and in the presence of this assembly: To pass my life in purity and to practice my profession faithfully.

I will abstain from whatever is deleterious and mischievous, and will not take or knowingly administer any harmful drug.

I will do all in my power to maintain and elevate the standards of my profession, and will hold in confidence all personal matters committed to my keeping, and all family affairs coming to my knowledge in the practice of my profession.

With loyalty will I endeavor to aid the physician in his work, and devote myself to the welfare of those committed to my care.

resources. This concept specifies that resources may be allocated according to:

- Need
- Individual effort
- The individual's merit (ability)
- The individual's contribution to society

The Veterans Affairs (VA) Medical Centers are an example of the application of the material principle of justice (according to the individual's contribution to society). Only those who served their country by joining the military are eligible to receive health care through the VA in acute care, ambulatory, and psychiatric facilities.

VERACITY

Veracity means truthfulness (neither lying nor deceiving others). There are many forms of deception: intentional lying, partial disclosure of information, or nondisclosure of information. Veracity often is difficult to achieve. Telling the truth may not be hard, but deciding how much truth to tell may be very hard. Exceptions to truth-telling are sometimes upheld by the principle of nonmaleficence, when the truth does greater harm than good. The act of giving placebo medications is an example of when telling the truth does greater harm than good.

FIDELITY

Fidelity, which is the ethical foundation of nurse–client relationships, means faithfulness and keeping promises.

Clients have a right to expect nurses to act in their best interests. The nurse's function as a **client advocate** (a person who speaks up for or acts on behalf of the client) upholds the principle of fidelity. Fidelity is demonstrated when nurses:

- Share the client's wishes with other members of the health care team
- Keep their own personal values from influencing their advocacy for clients
- Support the client's decision, even if it conflicts with their own preferences

Within the nurse–client relationship, nurses are to be loyal to their responsibilities, maintain privacy, keep promises, and meet clients' reasonable expectations. Nurses also have a duty to be faithful to themselves. The nurse may question who is owed fidelity when conflict between commitments occurs. Remaining client centered may help clarify the question, but it may not resolve the conflict. For example, if the mother of a frightened teenage girl tried to pressure the nurse into revealing the results of the daughter's pregnancy test after the daughter had already requested that her mother not be told, although the nurse may believe that the mother has the girl's best interests at heart, the nurse must protect the client's right to privacy.

ETHICAL THEORIES

Ethical theories have been debated since the time of Plato and Aristotle. Ethical theories can be used to analyze ethical problems, but no theory by itself can provide the "correct" answer to any ethical conflict. Common ethical theories include teleology, deontology, situational theory, and caring-based theory.

CULTURAL CONSIDERATIONS

Smoke-Free Facilities

- Declaring health care facilities "smoke free" results in the most benefit and least harm for everyone.
- The minority group of smokers and the individual's right to smoke are ignored.

TELEOLOGY

Teleology is an ethical theory that states that the value of a situation is determined by its consequences. The criterion for determining the value of an action is the outcome of an action, not the action itself. An example would be immunizations—receiving an injection is not "good," but preventing the illness is.

A basic concept of teleology is the principle of **utility**, which states that an act must result in the greatest positive benefit for the greatest number of people involved. Thus, any act can be ethical if it delivers positive results. All alternatives are assessed for potential outcomes, both negative and positive. The action selected results in the most benefits and the least harm for all involved. Minority and individual rights may be ignored for the benefit of the masses.

DEONTOLOGY

Deontology is an ethical theory that considers the intrinsic significance of an act itself as the criterion for determination of good. A person must consider the motives of the individual performing the act, not the consequences of the act. For example, health care researchers might risk the well-being of a person participating in an experimental procedure for the sake of finding a drug that will save many people from suffering.

SITUATIONAL THEORY

The situational theory holds that there are no set norms, rules, or majority-focused results. Each situation must be considered individually, with an emphasis on the uniqueness of the situation and a respect for the person involved. Decisions made in one situation cannot be generalized to another situation (Pappas, 2000).

SAFETY

Immunizations

- The outcome of immunizations is the prevention of given illnesses in the individual and, thus, the prevention of the spread of those illnesses to the community.
- The greatest good for the greatest number of persons is achieved with immunizations.

Caring-Based Theory

Caring-based theory is founded on the idea that ethical decisions are not made based on principles but are made with respect to relationships, communication, caring, responsiveness, and a desire not to hurt others. Caring-based theory focuses on emotions, feelings, and attitudes. The ethical concept of caring is viewed by society as the core of the nurse's role (Daniels, Nosek, & Nicoll, 2007; Fry & Johnstone, 2002).

ETHICS AND VALUES

Ethics and values are closely related, both enlightening and complicating the nurse's balancing the ethical principles of the client with those of the health care profession. Nurses must understand their own values in order to practice ethically. **Values** influence the development of beliefs and attitudes rather than behaviors, although they often indirectly influence behaviors. A **value system** is an individual's collection of inner beliefs that guides the way the person acts and helps determine the choices the person makes in life. Although nearly nothing in life is value free, the impact of values on decisions and resultant behaviors is often not considered. Values are similar to the act of breathing; one does not think about them until a problem arises.

Nurses often care for clients whose value systems conflict with their own. For example, a client with a value system of "grin and bear it" may be insulted by a nurse's attempts to offer pain medications. In order to ascertain those things that are meaningful to the client, the nurse must have an understanding of the client's value system (Figure 4-5). Furthermore, nurses must be aware of their own values, especially when they conflict with the values of clients to prevent any personal values from influencing or interfering with client care.

Values Clarification

Values clarification is the process of analyzing one's own values to better understand those things that are truly important. Values clarification can increase nurses' self-awareness and help them better care for clients whose values differ from their own. Raths, Harmin, and Simon's (1978) classic work *Values and Teaching* explained their theory of values clarification and three-step process of valuing as follows:

- *Choosing:* Beliefs are chosen freely (without coercion).
- *Prizing:* The beliefs selected are cherished.
- *Acting:* The selected beliefs are demonstrated consistently through behavior.

Because values are individual and not universal, the nurse should not impose personal values on clients. Providing ethical nursing care is directly related to the nurse's values. For example, the nurse who strongly values the sanctity of life may experience an ethical conflict when caring for a terminally ill client who refuses treatment that might extend life for a short time.

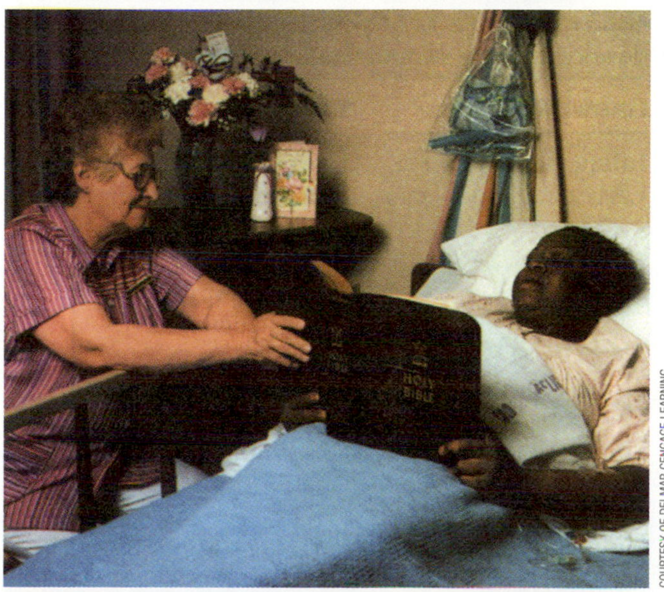

COURTESY OF DELMAR CENGAGE LEARNING

FIGURE 4-5 **Clients' values determine those things that are meaningful to them.**

> **PROFESSIONALTIP**
>
> **Values Clarification**
>
> It is the nurse's responsibility to make known to the supervisor any personal values that may influence or interfere with client care. For instance, a nurse who believes abortions should not be performed would find a conflict in working on a unit where abortions are performed. The nurse with this belief should make her values known to the employer before employment so that an assignment to that unit would not be made.

CODES OF ETHICS

Professions determine ethical behavior for their members. Several nursing organizations have developed codes as guidelines for ethical conduct. The Code for Licensed Practical/Vocational Nurses, developed by the National Federation of Licensed Practical Nurses, Inc. (NFLPN), is presented in Table 4-5. This code, providing motivation for establishing, maintaining, and elevating professional standards, was adopted by NFLPN in 1961 and revised in 1979 and in 1998. Each LP/VN entering the profession inherits the responsibility to adhere to the standards of ethical practice and conduct as set forth in this code.

A Code for Nurses was developed by both the International Council of Nurses (ICN) and the American Nurses Association (ANA) for the ethical conduct of registered nurses (See the ANA website for their code at http://www.nursingworld.org/ethics/chcode.htm). A code of ethics identifies broad principles for determining and evaluating nursing care but is not legally binding. Most state boards of nursing have authority to reprimand nurses for unprofessional conduct resulting from violation of the ethical code.

CLIENT RIGHTS

Culture defines rights and obligations. The dominant culture in the United States, however, holds the ethnocentric perspective that our rights and values are shared globally.

TABLE 4-5 The Code for Licensed Practical/Vocational Nurses

1. Know the scope of maximum utilization of the LP/VN as specified by the nursing practice act and function within this scope.
2. Safeguard the confidential information acquired from the source about the patient.
3. Provide healthcare to all patients regardless of race, creed, cultural background, disease, or lifestyle.
4. Uphold the highest standards in personal appearance, language, dress, and demeanor.
5. Stay informed about issues affecting the practice if nursing and delivery of health care and, where appropriate, participate in government and policy decision.
6. Accept the responsibility for safe nursing by keeping oneself mentally and physically fit and educationally prepared to practice.
7. Accept responsibility for membership in NFLPN and participate in its efforts to maintain the established standards of nursing practice and employment policies which lead to quality patient care.

From Nursing Practice Standards for the Licensed Practical/Vocational Nurse, by National Federation of Licensed Practical Nurses, Inc. (NFLPN), 2003, Garner, NC: Author. Copyright 2003 by Author. Reprinted with permission.

Clients have certain rights that apply regardless of the setting for delivery of care. These rights include, but are not limited to, the right to:

- Make decisions regarding their care (Figure 4-6)
- Be actively involved in the treatment process
- Be treated with dignity and respect

MEMORY TRICK

RIGHTS

An easy memory trick to use when learning about clients' rights is the acronym **RIGHTS**. Clients have a right to:

R = Review their medical records
I = Inclusion in making decisions regarding their care
G = Give consent or decline to participate in treatment or care
H = Have an advanced directive
T = Treatment with respect and dignity
S = Sensitivity to their cultural, religious, age, gender, or other differences

COMMUNITY/HOME HEALTH CARE

The Client's Rights

The client's rights (Figure 4-8) should be respected regardless of the setting for delivery of care. For care delivered in the home environment, for instance, the home health care nurse should discuss the client's rights with the client during the initial assessment (Figure 4-7).

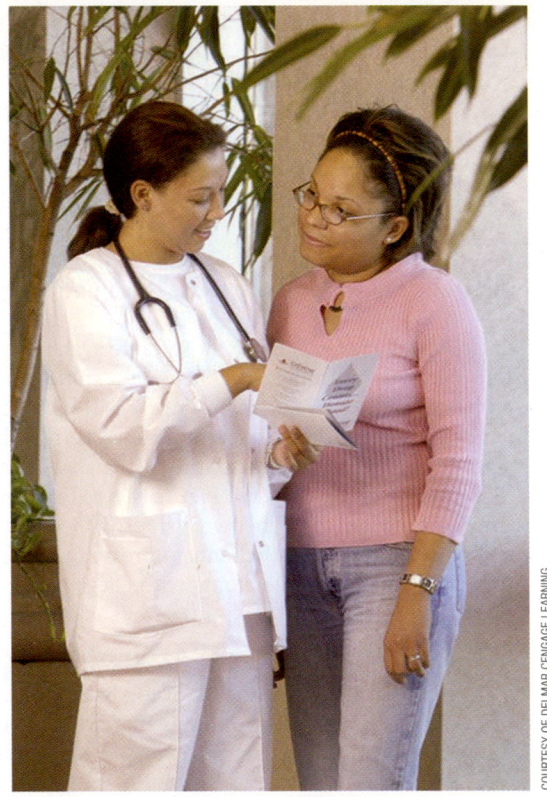

COURTESY OF DELMAR CENGAGE LEARNING

FIGURE 4-6 Clients have the right to information that will enable them to make decisions regarding their care.

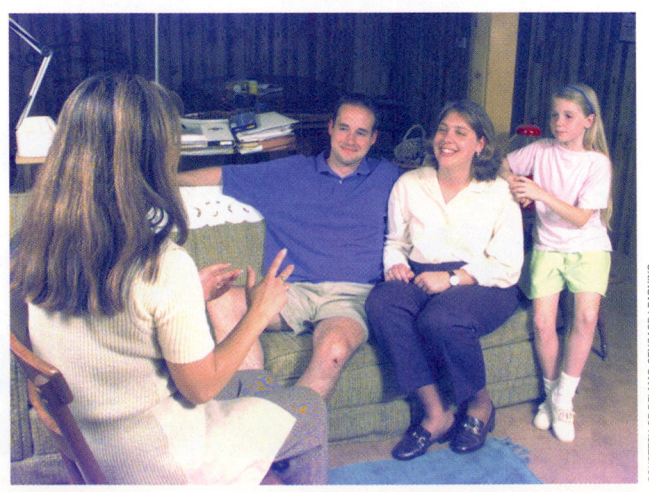

COURTESY OF DELMAR CENGAGE LEARNING

FIGURE 4-7 A home health nurse explains a client's rights.

Clients in short-term acute care agencies or extended care facilities are entitled to certain rights. The American Hospital Association (AHA) adopted *A Patient's Bill of Rights* in 1973. It identifies the rights and responsibilities of clients receiving care in hospitals. In 2003, this document was replaced by a brochure called *The Patient Care Partnership* (AHA, 2003) (Figure 4-8).

ETHICAL DILEMMAS

When two or more ideals or values are in conflict, there is an **ethical dilemma**. In an ethical dilemma, a choice is to be made between the conflicting ideals or values. Questions remain in some cases, even after the dilemma seems to have been settled. Areas where ethical dilemmas frequently occur are euthanasia, refusal of treatment, and scarcity of resources.

EUTHANASIA

The word *euthanasia* comes from the Greek word *euthanatos*, which literally means "good, or gentle, death." In current times, **euthanasia** refers to intentional action or lack of action that causes the merciful death of someone suffering from a terminal illness or incurable condition.

Active euthanasia refers to taking specific action to hasten a client's death, such as removing a client who is in a vegetative state from a respirator. **Passive euthanasia** is working with the client's dying process. An example is not putting in a feeding tube to provide nourishment when the client cannot or will no longer eat.

Assisted suicide is a form of active euthanasia where another person provides a client with the means to end his own life. Some nurses look on assisted suicide as violating ethical principles on which the practice of nursing is based, whereas other nurses see assisted suicide as an ethical dilemma. For example, in answer to the question "Does assisted suicide violate the principle of autonomy?" it might be argued that *refusing* to assist a suicide violates a client's autonomy.

Oregon and Washington allow physician-assisted suicide with laws that were adopted through ballot initiatives (Blesch, 2009). In 1997, Oregon enacted the *Death with Dignity Act*, which allows terminally-ill state residents to end their lives voluntarily by self-administration of a lethal medication that has been prescribed by a physician for that specific purpose (Oregon State Public Health, 2007). For more information regarding the *Death with Dignity Act*, visit *http://www.oregon.gov/DHS/ph/pas/faqs.shtml*. In November 2008, Washington state voters adopted physician-assisted dying in accordance with *Initiative 1000*. Washington Department of Health proposed rules similar to Oregon's in January 2009 that would govern *Initiative 1000* (O'Reilly, 2009a).

Montana is the third state that legalized physician-assisted suicide. In December 2008, a lower-court state judge ruled in the case *Baxter v. Montana* that terminally-ill clients have a constitutional right to physician-assistance in dying (O'Reilly, 2009b).

REFUSAL OF TREATMENT

The principle of autonomy is the basis of a client's right to refuse treatment. Only after treatment methods and their consequences have been explained can the client refuse treatment. The values of most health care providers are challenged when a client refuses treatment.

> Honoring the refusal of treatments that a patient does not desire, that are disproportionately burdensome to the patient, or that will not benefit the patient is ethically and legally permissible. (Curtin, 1995)

One possible ethical dilemma in this area relates to the use of ventilators for clients who would otherwise die. These clients continue to breathe as long as they are connected to the machine. What are the physical, emotional, psychological, and fiscal costs? What quality of life is prolonged by technology?

SCARCITY OF RESOURCES

The use of expensive services is being closely examined because of the emphasis on containing health care costs. For example, the length of a hospital stay and the number of office visits allowed for individual clients are already set by many third-party payers. The availability of goods (such as organs) contributes to a scarcity of resources.

Clients often wait extended periods to receive donated organs. Allocating scarce resources is a major ethical dilemma: Who should receive the benefit of such a scarce and precious resource as a living organ? How should the determination be made? Currently, organ recipient selection is based on objective criteria such as blood type, tissue type, size of the organ, medical urgency of the client, time on the waiting list, and distance between donor and recipient (Organ Procurement and Transplantation Network, 2009). Should only objective criteria be used in determining who receives a donated organ, or should moral judgments also be made?

ETHICAL DECISION MAKING

Ethical questions (dilemmas) are not easy to answer. **Ethical reasoning** is the process of examining the issue in a methodical manner. Ethical decisions should not be made based on emotions. Ethical decision making is used in situations where conflicts of rights and duties exist.

PROFESSIONAL TIP

Providing Ethical Care

- Find out about the client's wishes. Listen more than talk. (For example, it might be helpful to ask "If your heart stopped, would you want us to try to start it again?")
- Assess the client's understanding of the illness and treatment options available.
- Allow time for the client to explore values and to communicate.
- Facilitate communication of the client's desires to family and other health care providers.

AMERICAN HOSPITAL ASSOCIATION PATIENT CARE PARTNERSHIP

The Patient Care Partnership: Understanding Expectations, Rights and Responsibilities

When you need hospital care, your doctor and the nurses and other professionals at our hospital are committed to working with you and your family to meet your health care needs. Our dedicated doctors and staff serve the community in all its ethnic, religious and economic diversity. Our goal is for your and your family to have the same care and attention we would want for our families and ourselves.

The sections explain some of the basics about how you can expect to be treated during your hospital stay. They also cover what we will need from you to care for you better. If you have questions at any time, please ask them. Unasked or unanswered questions can add to the stress of being in the hospital. Your comfort and confidence in your care are very important to us.

What to Expect During Your Hospital Stay

◎ **High quality hospital care.** Our first priority is to provide you the care you need, when you need it, with skill, compassion, and respect. Tell your caregivers if you have concerns about your care or if you have pain. You have the right to know the identity of doctors, nurses and others involved in your care, and you have the right to know when they are students, residents or other trainees.

◎ **A clean and safe environment.** Our hospital works hard to keep you safe. We use special policies and procedures to avoid mistakes in your care and keep you free from abuse or neglect. If anything unexpected and significant happens during your hospital stay, you will be told what happened, and any resulting changes in your care will be discussed with you.

◎ **Involvement in your care.** You and your doctor often make decisions about your care before you go to the hospital. Other times, especially in emergencies, those decisions are made during your hospital stay. When decision-making takes place, it should include:

- Discussing your medical condition and information about medically appropriate treatment choices. To make informed decisions with your doctor, you need to understand:
  - — The benefits and risks of each treatment.
  - — Whether your treatment is experimental or part of a research study.
  - — What you can reasonably expect from your treatment and any long-term effects it might have on your quality of life.
  - — What you and your family will need to do after you leave the hospital.
  - — The financial consequences of using uncovered services or out-of-network providers.

Please tell your caregivers if you need more information about treatment choices.

- Discussing your treatment plan. When you enter the hospital, you sign a general consent to treatment. In some cases, such as surgery or experimental treatment, you may be asked to confirm in writing that you understand what is planned and agree to it. This process protects your right to consent to or refuse a treatment. Your doctor will explain the medical consequences of refusing recommended treatment. It also protects your right to decide if you want to participate in a research study.

- Getting information from you. Your caregivers need complete and correct information about your health and coverage so that they can make good decisions about your care. That includes:
  - — Past illnesses, surgeries or hospital stays.
  - — Past allergic reactions.
  - — Any medicines or dietary supplements (such as vitamins and herbs) that you are taking.
  - — Any network or admission requirements under your health plan.

- Understanding your health care goals and values. You may have health care goals and values or spiritual beliefs that are important to your well-being. They will be taken into account as much as possible throughout your hospital stay. Make sure your doctor, your family and your care team know your wishes.

- Understanding who should make decisions when you cannot. If you have signed a health care power of attorney stating who should speak for you if you become unable to make health care decisions for yourself, or a "living will" or "advance directive" that states your wishes about end-of-life care; give copies to your doctor, your family and your care team. If you or your family need help making difficult decisions, counselors, chaplains and others are available to help.

(Continues)

FIGURE 4-8 A Patient's Bill of Rights (*Reprinted with permission of the American Hospital Association, copyright 2003. All rights reserved.*)

AMERICAN HOSPITAL ASSOCIATION PATIENT CARE PARTNERSHIP (continued)

What to Expect During Your Hospital Stay (continued)

- **Protection of your privacy.** We respect the confidentiality of your relationship with your doctor and other caregivers, and the sensitive information about your health and health care that are part of that relationship. State and federal laws and hospital operating policies protect the privacy of your medical information. You will receive a Notice of Privacy Practices that describes the ways that we use, disclose and safeguard patient information and that explains how you can obtain a copy of information from our records about your care.
- **Preparing you and your family for when you leave the hospital.** Your doctor works with hospital staff and professionals in your community. You and your family also play an important role in your care. The success of your treatment often depends on your efforts to follow medication, diet and therapy plans. Your family may need to help care for you at home.

  You can expect us to help you identify sources of follow-up care and to let you know if our hospital has a financial interest in any referrals. As long as you agree that we can share information about your care with them, we will coordinate our activities with your caregivers outside the hospital. You can also expect to receive information and, where possible, training about the self-care you will need when you go home.
- **Help with your bill and filing insurance claims.** Our staff will file claims for you with health care insurers or other programs such as Medicare and Medicaid. They also will help your doctor with needed documentation. Hospital bills and insurance coverage are often confusing. If you have questions about your bill, contact our business office. If you need help understanding your insurance coverage or health plan, start with your insurance company or health benefits manager. If you do not have health coverage, we will try to help you and your family find financial help or make other arrangements. We need your help with collecting needed information and other requirements to obtain coverage or assistance.

While you are here, you will receive more detailed notices about some of the rights you have as a hospital patient and how to exercise them. We are always interested in improving. If you have questions, comments, or concerns, please contact______________________.

Reprinted with permission of the American Hospital Association, copyright 2003. All rights reserved.

FIGURE 4-8 *(Continued)*

Kinsella (2001) identifies eight steps to guide ethical decision making:

1. Recognize the ethical dimension of the issue.
2. Identify the parties involved, their relationships to each other, and their rights and responsibilities.
3. Examine the values involved, what ideals or principles are at issue.
4. Compare benefits and burdens (positives and negatives) for each option.
5. Evaluate similar cases or ask colleagues about situations of ethical decision making.
6. Discuss, if possible, the issue with the relevant others.
7. Check legal and organizational policies so the decision meets legal, professional, and organizational standards.
8. Assess your comfort level with the decision, if uncomfortable reconsider.

CRITICAL THINKING

Ethical Decision

An 80-year-old woman is in a persistent vegetative state as a result of a cardiovascular accident. She has always talked about "someday" signing a living will requesting that heroic measures not be taken, but her family wants "everything to be done that can be done." Whose wishes should prevail? What ethical principles would come into play in this decision process?

NURSING AND ETHICS

Because nurses are accountable for protecting the interests and rights of the client, quality nursing practice involves making ethical decisions. Each practice setting has its own set of ethical concerns. Nurses must balance their ethical responsibilities to each client with their professional obligations.

ETHICS COMMITTEES

Providing ethical health care requires both dialogue among health care providers and self-examination by each care provider. Many health care agencies now recognize the need for a systematic manner for discussing ethical concerns (Figure 4-9). Multidisciplinary committees (also referred to as institutional ethics committees) constitute one arena for dialogue regarding ethical dilemmas. Ethics committees can serve as a forum for discussion of ethical issues and lead to policies and procedures for preventing and resolving dilemmas.

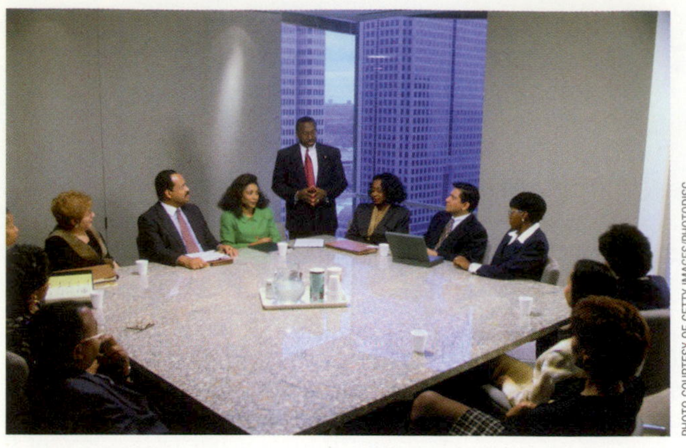
PHOTO COURTESY OF GETTY IMAGES/PHOTODISC

FIGURE 4-9 Ethics Committee Meeting

Nurse as Client Advocate

The nurse's first step in acting as a client advocate is to develop a meaningful relationship with the client. The nurse is then able to make decisions with the client based on the strength of the relationship. The nurse's primary ethical responsibility is to protect clients' rights to make their own decisions.

Nurse as Whistle-Blower

Whistle-blowing refers to calling public attention to the unethical, illegal, or incompetent actions of others. The ethical principles of veracity and nonmaleficence are the basis for whistle-blowing. Professionals are expected to monitor coworkers' abilities to perform their duties safely. Although nurses are expected to "blow the whistle" on incompetent health care providers, many are reluctant to do so because there are inherent risks in whistle-blowing. Haddad (1999) identifies some of the questions a person should consider before reporting unethical or incompetent behavior:

- Has the behavior in question created or is it likely to create serious harm?
- Have I gathered all appropriate information, and am I competent to judge this behavior?
- Do others confirm my information and judgment?
- Have all internal resources been exhausted to resolve the problem?
- Is it likely that past wrongdoing will be corrected or future damage prevented after the problem is reported?
- Is the harm created by whistle-blowing likely to be less than the harm done by the behavior in question?

The False Claims Act (FCA) encourages whistle-blowers to report evidence of fraud against the federal government (Sloan, 2002b).

Protection of privacy to whistle-blowers is provided by federal law and state laws (to varying degrees). The fear of reprisal and the inclination to protect one's coworkers may keep a nurse from fulfilling the ethical obligation to report substandard behaviors.

CASE STUDY

An alert and oriented 62-year-old client was diagnosed with colon cancer. Surgery was recommended, and she agreed to surgical excision of the tumor. Postoperatively, she experienced serious complications and remained in the surgical intensive care unit for 2 months. During that time, she experienced cardiac failure, temporary respiratory failure, and renal failure and required multiple surgical procedures.

One day she was asked to sign a consent form for surgical revision of her colostomy. She refused, stating that she could no longer tolerate any procedures and that she was ready to die a peaceful death. The nurse informed the resident of the client's decision. The resident called the attending physician, who ordered a stat dose of Valium 10 mg IM for the client. He then stopped by the nurses' desk and asked that the client be prepped for surgery.

1. Identify three elements needed to ensure informed consent.
2. Did this client give informed consent?
3. Identify which of the elements of informed consent were met or not met. Be sure to include your rationale.
4. What type of ethical dilemma does this case study present?
5. Which ethical principle pertains to this situation?
6. Explain the deontological view of this ethical dilemma.

SUMMARY

- Laws are rules that guide personal interaction. They are derived from several sources and can be classified as public or civil.
- Within most states, the nursing practice act indicates the scope of practice for nurses. Standards have been developed to guide nursing practice.
- The nurse must be familiar with client rights. Care must be taken not to falsely imprison a client or violate the client's right to privacy.
- The client's chart is a legal document and should accurately reflect client status and care. Entries should be neat and timely.

- Informed consent is more than just signing a form. It requires a competent client understanding the risks, benefits, and alternatives to treatment.
- Whether to purchase malpractice insurance is a personal decision, but having one's own policy provides both coverage off the job and individual legal counsel.
- Incident reports are a risk management tool. They are not meant to be used for punitive purposes.
- Advance directives are instructions about health care preferences. They both protect the rights of the client and guide the family through difficult decisions.
- Ethics examines human behavior—those things that people do under a given set of circumstances.
- There is a connection between acts that are legal and acts that are ethical. Nursing actions are to be both legal and ethical.
- Ethical decisions are based on principles such as autonomy, nonmaleficence, beneficence, justice, veracity, and fidelity.
- Because ethics and values are so closely associated, nurses must explore their own values in order to acknowledge the value systems of their clients.
- Ethical codes that have been developed by nursing organizations such as the NFLPN, the ICN, and the ANA establish guidelines for the ethical conduct of nurses with clients, coworkers, society, and the nursing profession.
- The Patient's Bill of Rights is designed to guarantee ethical care of clients.
- The roles of client advocate and whistle-blower enable nurses to protect their clients' rights and ensure the ethical and competent actions of their peers within the nursing profession.

REVIEW QUESTIONS

1. The nurse is providing care for a 25-year-old male client. His health is deteriorating, but he remains alert and oriented. His sister, an RN, asks to see his chart. What should the nurse do initially?
   1. Ask the client's permission.
   2. Ask the client's physician's permission.
   3. Deny her access to his chart.
   4. Provide her a private place to review the chart.

2. The nurse enters the room and tells the client that he has to take the medication, including an injection. The client refuses the medication, but the nurse continues to administer the medications. This action is an example of the intentional tort of:
   1. battery.
   2. invasion of privacy.
   3. libel.
   4. malpractice.

3. The nurse finds a client obnoxious and totally disapproves of the client's behavior. She writes on the chart that the client "is obnoxious and leads an immoral lifestyle, which has resulted in hospitalization." This is referred to as:
   1. assault.
   2. slander.
   3. libel.
   4. a supported statement.

4. Even though the nurse may obtain the client's signature on a form, obtaining informed consent for a medical treatment is the responsibility of the:
   1. client.
   2. physician.
   3. student nurse.
   4. supervising nurse.

5. Nurses would use the Code for Licensed Practical/Vocational Nurses to: (Select all that apply.)
   1. solve an ethical dilemma.
   2. establish a guideline for ethical conduct.
   3. develop a nursing care plan.
   4. seek answers to a client care problem.
   5. understand the professional expectations of them.
   6. establish, maintain, and elevate professional standards.

6. The nurse is working the night shift with a colleague who has been his friend for several years. He discovers that his colleague is routing drugs regularly and is taking them herself. When confronted, the colleague tells the nurse that she needs the drugs to cope and that she cannot lose her job because she is a single parent of three young children. Which of the following is the most appropriate response by the nurse?
   1. "It will be alright. I can get help for you."
   2. "This must be a very difficult time for you. Would you like to talk about this?"
   3. "How long have you been doing this?"
   4. "This is illegal, and I must report this to the supervisor."

7. A nursing student is learning about client rights. Which of the following statements made by the student nurse indicates that further teaching is required?
   1. "My client can make her own decisions regarding her care."
   2. "I need to treat clients with dignity and respect."
   3. "I should do as much as possible for the client."
   4. "My client should be informed of the side effects of new medication."

8. A client is at risk for invasion of privacy when which of the following actions occur? (Select all that apply.)
   1. Photographing a client.
   2. Writing the client's allergies on the chart.
   3. Talking about the client during lunch break.
   4. Clarifying a physician's illegible written order.
   5. Closing the door to give an injection.
   6. E-mailing the client's HIV lab results.

9. Which of the following is an example of an ethical dilemma?
   1. A young couple seeking marriage counseling.
   2. A terminally ill client refusing treatment.
   3. A client signing an advanced directive.
   4. A client donating a kidney to his son.
10. A 17-year-old Jehovah's Witness is brought to the ED after passing out at the mall. It is determined that she is suffering from an ulcer that has perforated her stomach wall. The bleeding is severe, and she is in need of a blood transfusion to save her life. The client is refusing the blood transfusion. What is the most appropriate nursing intervention for this client?
    1. Administer the blood transfusion immediately.
    2. Contact the hospital's ethical advisory committee.
    3. Contact the client's parents.
    4. Follow the client's decision.

REFERENCES/SUGGESTED READINGS

American Hospital Association. 2003. The patient care partnership. Retrieved November 28, 2008, from http://www.aha.org/aha/issues/Communicating-With-Patients/pt-care-partnership.html

American Nurses Association. (2005). Code of ethics for nurses with interpretive statements. Retrieved November 28, 2008, from http://nursingworld.org/ethics/code/protected_nwcoe813.htm

Bandman, E., & Bandman, B. (2001). *Nursing ethics through the life span* (4th ed.). Norwalk, CT: Appleton-Lange.

Bemis, P. (2008). Nurses in the legal field. *RN, 71*(6), 20–21.

Blesch, G. (2009). Montana court hears arguments on physician-assisted death. Retrieved September 27, 2009 from http://www.modernhealthcare.com/article/20090902/REG/309029935

Brooke, P. (2003). How good a SAMARITAN should you be? *Nursing 2003, 33*(6), 46–47.

Burkhardt, M., & Nathaniel, A. (2008). *Ethics and issues in contemporary nursing* (3rd ed.). Clifton Park, NY: Delmar Cengage Learning.

Curtin, L. (1995). Nurses take a stand on assisted suicide. *Nursing Management, 26*(5), 71–76.

Daniels, R., Nosek, L., & Nicoll, L. (2007). *Contemporary medical-surgical nursing*. Clifton Park, NY: Delmar Cengage Learning.

Douglas, R., & Brown, H. (2002). Attitudes toward advance directives. *Journal of Nursing Scholarship, 34*(1), 61–65.

Flick, C. (2002). Organ donation: A delicate balance. *RN, 65*(12), 43–46.

Flight, M. (2004). *Law, liability, and ethics* (4th ed.). Clifton Park, NY: Delmar Cengage Learning.

Flores, J. (2002). What if you're named in a lawsuit? *RN, 65*(12), 65–68.

Frank-Stromborg, M., & Ganschow, J. (2002). How HIPAA will change your practice. *Nursing2002, 32*(9), 54–57.

Fry, S., & Johnstone, M. (2002). *International Council of Nurses Ethics in nursing practice: A guide to ethical decision-making*. Malden, MA: Blackwell.

Gebbie, K. (2001). Privacy: The patient's right. AJN, 101(6), 69–73.

Grace, P., & Hardt, E. H. (2008). Ethical issues: When a patient refuses assistance. *American Journal of Nursing, 108*(8), 36–38.

Haddad, A. (1999). Ethics in action. *RN, 62*(1), 23–26.

Health Resources and Services Administration. (2008). Practitioner data banks: National practitioner data bank. Retrieved November 28, 2008, from http://bhpr.hrsa.gov/dqa

Helm, A., & Kihm, N. (2001). Is professional liability insurance for you? *Nursing2001, 31*(1), 48–49.

Higginbotham, E. (2003). Does error 1 injury 5 negligence? *RN, 66*(5), 67–68.

Hill, S., & Howlett, H. (2001). *Success in practical nursing: Personal and vocational issues* (4th ed.). Philadelphia: W. B. Saunders.

Infante, M. (2000). Malpractice may not be your biggest legal risk. *RN, 63*(7), 67–73.

Joint Commission on Accreditation of Healthcare Organizations. (2008). Health care at the crossroads. Retrieved November 28, 2008, from http://www.jointcommission.org/NR/rdonlyres/5C138711-ED76-4D6F-909F-B06E0309F36D/0/health_care_at_the_crossroads.pdf

Kinsella, L. (2001). Truth telling in patient care: Resolving ethical issues. *Nursing2001, 31*(12), 52–55.

LaDuke, S. (2000). The effects of professional discipline on nurses. *American Journal of Nursing, 100*(6), 26–33.

LaDuke, S., & Biondo, T. (2003). Protect your future with personal liability insurance. *Nursing2003, 33*(2), 52–53.

Lee, N. (2000). Proving nursing negligence. *American Journal of Nursing, 100*(11), 55–56.

Maltz, A. (2001). Keeping pace with new patient privacy rules. *RN, 64*(9), 71–74.

McCurdy, D. (2008). Ethical spiritual care at the end of life. *American Journal of Nursing, 108*(5), 11.

Mock, K. (2001). Keep lawsuits at bay with compassionage care. *RN, 64*(5), 83–86.

National Council of State Boards of Nursing, Inc. (2000). NCSBN welcomes two more states to the nurse licensure compact. Available: http://www.ncsbn.org.public/nurselicensurecompact/nurselicensurecompact_index.htm

National Council of State Boards of Nursing, Inc. (2000). Why disciplinary databanks? Why the National Practitioner Data Bank (NPDB)? Available: http://www.ncsbn.org/files/publications/issues/vol171/ddb.171

National Council of State Boards of Nursing, Inc. (2002). What boards of nursing do . . . and what you can do. Available: http://www.ncsbn.org/public/regulation/boards_of_nursing.htm

Oregon State Public Health. (2007). FAQs about the Death With Dignity Act. Retrieved September 27, 2009 from http://www.oregon.gov/DHS/ph/pas/faqs.shtml

O'Reilly, K. (2009a). Montana judge rejects stay of physician-assisted suicide ruling. Retrieved September 27, 2009 from http://www.ama-assn.org/amednews/2009/01/26/prsd0129.htm

O'Reilly, K. (2009b). 5 people die under new Washington physician-assisted suicide law. Retrieved September 27, 2009 from http://www.ama-assn.org/amednews/2009/07/06/prsc0706.htm

Organ Procurement and Transplantation Network. (2009). Donor matching system. Retrieved June 21, 2009 from http://optn.transplant.hrsa.gov/about/transplantation/matchingProcess.asp

Pappas, A. (2000). Ethical issues. In J. Zerwekh & J. Claborn (Eds.), *Nursing today: Transitions and trends* (3rd ed.). Philadelphia: W. B. Saunders.

Raths, L., Harmin, M., & Simon, S. (1978). *Values and teaching* (2nd ed.). Columbus, OH: Merrill.

Roman, L. (2007). How to stay out of legal water. *RN, 70*(1), 26–31.

Sloan, A. (2002a). Liability insurance: Is your coverage adequate? *RN, 65*(10), 69–72.

Sloan, A. (2002b). Whistleblowing: Proceed with caution. *RN, 65*(1), 67–70.

Sloan, A., & Vernarac, E. (2001). Impaired nurses: Reclaiming careers. *RN, 64*(2), 58–63.

Trinkoff, A., Zhou, Q., et al. (2000). Workplace access, negative proscriptions, job strain, and substance use in registered nurses. *Nursing Research, 49*(2), 83.

Trossman, S. (2003). Protecting patient information. *American Journal of Nursing, 103*(2), 65–68.

U.S. Department of Health and Human Services. (2001). National standards to protect the privacy of personal health information. Available: http://www.hhs.gov/acr/hipaa

Ventura, M. (1999a). Staffing issues. *RN, 62*(2), 26–30.

Ventura, M. (1999b). The great multistate licensure debate. *RN, 62*(5), 58–62.

Ventura, M. (1999c). When information must be revealed. *RN, 62*(6), 61.

White, L., & Duncan, G. (2002). *Medical surgical nursing: An integrated approach* (2nd ed.). Clifton Park, NY: Delmar Cengage Learning.

Zerwekh, J., & Claborn, J. C. (2003). *Nursing today: Transitions and trends* (4th ed). Philadelphia: W. B. Saunders.

Ziel, S., & Gentry, K. (2003). Ready? HIPAA's here. *RN, 66*(2), 67–70.

RESOURCES

Partnership for Caring,
http://www.partnershipforcaring.org

The Living Bank International,
http://www.livingbank.org

Living Wills, Films for the Humanities and Sciences,
http://ffh.films.com

National Association for Practical Nurse Education and Service, Inc. (NAPNES),
http://www.napnes.org

National Federation of Licensed Practical Nurses, Inc. (NFLPN), http://www.nflpn.org

United Network for Organ Sharing (UNOS),
http://www.unos.org

UNIT 2 The Health Care Environment

CHAPTER 5
The Health Care Delivery System

MAKING THE CONNECTION

Refer to the following chapters to increase your understanding of the health care delivery system:

Basic Nursing

- ***Legal and Ethical Responsibilities***
- ***Arenas of Care***
- ***Wellness Concepts***

LEARNING OBJECTIVES

Upon completion of this chapter, you should be able to:

- Define key terms.
- Describe the three levels of service in the U.S. health care delivery system.
- Identify the members of the health care team and their respective roles.
- Describe the differences among financial programs for health care services and reimbursement.
- Explain the factors that influence health care delivery.
- Identify the challenges to providing care.
- Describe nursing's role in meeting the challenges within the health care system.
- Discuss the emerging trends and issues for the health care delivery system.

KEY TERMS

capitated rates
comorbidity
exclusive provider organizations (EPOs)
fee-for-service
health care delivery system
health maintenance organizations (HMOs)
managed care
Medicaid
medical model
Medicare
Medigap insurance
preferred provider organizations (PPOs)
prescriptive authority
primary care
primary care provider
primary health care
prospective payment
secondary care
single-payer system
single point of entry
tertiary care

INTRODUCTION

A **health care delivery system** is a method for providing services to meet the health needs of individuals. The U.S. health care delivery system is experiencing dramatic change. The once economically thriving health care institutions now search for ways to survive. Health care providers seek cost-effective ways to deliver a larger range of services to consumers, who are demanding greater accessibility to quality affordable health care services. The increase in consumerism is fueled by the Internet, regulatory changes, the rising popularity of nontraditional therapies, and frustration of clients and their families feeling they have been mistreated by the system (Haugh, 1999).

Because nursing is a major component of the U.S. health care delivery system, nurses must understand the changes occurring within the system and nursing's role in shaping those changes. This chapter explores the levels of health care services available, the settings offering those services, and the members of the health care team. The economics of health care, the challenges within the health care delivery system, and nursing's role in meeting those challenges are also addressed.

LEVELS OF HEALTH CARE SERVICES

Health care services are classified into three levels: primary, secondary, and tertiary. Table 5-1 provides an overview of the levels of care. The trend is toward holistic care (i.e., care of the entire person, including physiological, psychological, social, intellectual, and spiritual aspects).

CRITICAL THINKING

Levels of Health Care

A nurse is providing care for a 72-year-old female client diagnosed with terminal breast cancer. Which level of health care service will the client utilize? What is the purpose of this level of care? What would be an appropriate goal for this client?

Primary Care

The major purposes of **primary care** are to promote wellness and prevent illness or disability. Care is coordinated by the office of the primary care provider, usually a family practice physician, pediatrician, internal medicine physician, or family nurse practitioner. The U.S. health care system traditionally focused on treating illness rather than promoting wellness. Now, however, the focus is on health-promoting behaviors such as regular exercise, reducing fat in the diet, monitoring cholesterol level, and managing stress. Direct wellness promotion activities toward the individual, the family, or the community.

Under the traditional **medical model**, our health care delivery system was not a *health* care system at all but rather an *illness* care system. Services were directed toward care after disease or disability developed rather than preventive aspects of care. Today, however, there is more of an emphasis on the holistic promotion of wellness and on the preventive aspects of care.

Secondary Care

Services within the realm of **secondary care**—diagnosis and treatment—occur after the client exhibits symptoms of

TABLE 5-1 Levels of Health Care Services

TYPE OF CARE	DESCRIPTION	EXAMPLES
Primary	*Goal:* To decrease the risk to a client (individual or community) for disease or dysfunction *Explanation:* General health promotion Protection against specific illnesses	Teaching Lifestyle modification for health (e.g., smoking cessation, nutrition counseling) Referrals Immunization Routine screenings Promotion of a safe environment (e.g., sanitation, protection from toxic agents)
Secondary	*Goal:* To alleviate disease and prevent further disability *Explanation:* Early detection and intervention	Diagnostic testing Acute care Various therapies Surgery
Tertiary	*Goal:* To minimize effects and permanent disability associated with chronic or irreversible conditions *Explanation:* Restorative and rehabilitative activities to attain optimal level of functioning	Education and retraining Provision of direct care Environmental intervention (e.g., advising on necessity of wheelchair accessibility for a person who has experienced a cerebrovascular accident [stroke])

COURTESY OF DELMAR CENGAGE LEARNING

illness. Acute treatment centers (hospitals) still constitute the predominant site for the delivery of these health care services, but there is a growing movement to provide diagnostic and therapeutic services in locations that are more easily accessed by the population. These are often satellite care centers of a major hospital, where holistic care is promoted.

Tertiary Care

Restoring an individual to the state of health that existed before the development of an illness is the purpose of **tertiary** (rehabilitative) **care**. When a person is unable to regain previous functional abilities, the rehabilitation goal is to reach the optimal level of health possible. For example, a client regains partial use of an arm after experiencing a stroke. Restorative care is holistic in that the physiological, psychological, social, and spiritual aspects of the person are all addressed in the provision of care.

HEALTH CARE DELIVERY SYSTEM

The intricate U.S. health care delivery system involves many providers, consumers, settings, personnel, and services.

Providers/Consumers

Health care services in the United States are delivered by public (including official and voluntary), public/private, and private sectors. Consumers are the individuals who receive the health care services.

Public Sector

Tax monies fund public agencies, and these agencies are accountable to the public. Official (or governmental) agencies and voluntary agencies make up the public sector.

The U.S. Public Health Service (USPHS), the major agency that oversees the actual delivery of care services, is administered by the U.S. Department of Health and Human Services (USDHHS). Table 5-2 lists the USPHS agencies and their purposes. The Veterans Administration (VA), also financed by tax monies, has hospitals and clinics providing services to veterans of the armed services.

The states vary in the public health services provided. Generally, activities of local health departments are coordinated by a state department of health. Local services provide immunizations, maternal–child care, and control of infectious and chronic diseases.

Voluntary agencies also constitute an important part of the public sector of the health care delivery system. These not-for-profit agencies (e.g., the National Federation of Licensed Practical Nurses [NFLPN], the American Nurses Association [ANA], the National League for Nursing [NLN], and the American Medical Association [AMA]) can exert significant legislative influence. Other voluntary agencies, such as the American Diabetes Association and the American Heart Association, provide educational resources to health care providers and the general public. Voluntary agencies receive

Table 5-2 Agencies of the U.S. Public Health Service

AGENCY	PURPOSE
Health Resources and Services Administration (HRSA)	Furnish health-related information; control programs of health care for the homeless; people with human immunodeficiency virus (HIV) and acquired immunodeficiency syndrome (AIDS); rural health care; organ transplants; and employee occupational health
Food and Drug Administration (FDA)	Protect the public from unsafe drugs, food, and cosmetics
Centers for Disease Control and Prevention (CDC)	Study and control the transmission of communicable diseases
National Institutes of Health (NIH)	Conduct research and education about specific illnesses
Alcohol, Drug Abuse, and Mental Health Administration (ADAMHA)	Serve as clearinghouse for information on substance abuse and mental health issues
Agency for Toxic Substances and Disease Registry (ATSDR)	Keep registry of certain diseases Provide information on toxic agents Study mortality and morbidity on defined population groups
Indian Health Service (IHS)	Furnish health care services to Native Americans, including health promotion, nutrition, maternal–child health, disease prevention, alcoholism, suicide prevention, and substance abuse
Agency for Health Care Research and Quality (AHRQ)	Serve as main source of federal support for research related to quality of health care delivery

COURTESY OF DELMAR CENGAGE LEARNING

funds from individual contributions, membership dues, and corporate philanthropy.

Public/Private Sector

A blending of the public and private sectors in many areas of health care has gradually occurred following the inception of Medicare and the diagnosis-related groups (DRGs), discussed in an upcoming section. Federal regulations guide both the care provided to clients in private nonprofit and for-profit agencies by private physicians and the reimbursement to both the agencies and the physicians.

Private Sector

The private sector of the health care delivery system is composed mainly of independent health care agencies and providers who are reimbursed on a **fee-for-service** basis (the recipient directly pays the provider for services as they are provided). Fee-for-service clients may have private insurance or use their own financial resources to pay for the services.

Settings

The various settings where health care is delivered include acute care hospitals, extended care facilities, outpatient settings, home health care agencies, schools, and hospice, which are discussed in Chapter 6, "Arenas of Care."

Personnel and Services

Many personnel and services exist within the various health care settings. Large hospitals provide the greatest number of services. Other health care settings may provide some but not all of these same services. The service departments most commonly found in the various settings include nursing units, specialized client care units, diagnostic departments, therapy departments, and support services.

HEALTH CARE TEAM

Health care services are delivered by a multidisciplinary team (Figure 5-1). Table 5-3 lists the various health care team members, their educational requirements, and their roles. Nurses work daily with other team members, so they must understand the role of each team member.

Nurses have various roles when assisting clients to meet their needs. Table 5-4 identifies the most common nursing roles. Nurses function in independent, interdependent, and dependent roles. In the independent role, the nurse requires no direction or order from another health care professional (e.g., in deciding that a client's edematous arm should be elevated). In the interdependent role, the nurse works in collaboration with other health care professionals (e.g., in a client care conference where several members of the health care team together plan ways to meet the client's needs). In the dependent role, the nurse requires direction from a physician or dentist (e.g., medications must be ordered by a physician or dentist before a nurse may administer them to the client). The degree of autonomy nurses experience is related to client needs, nurse expertise, and practice setting.

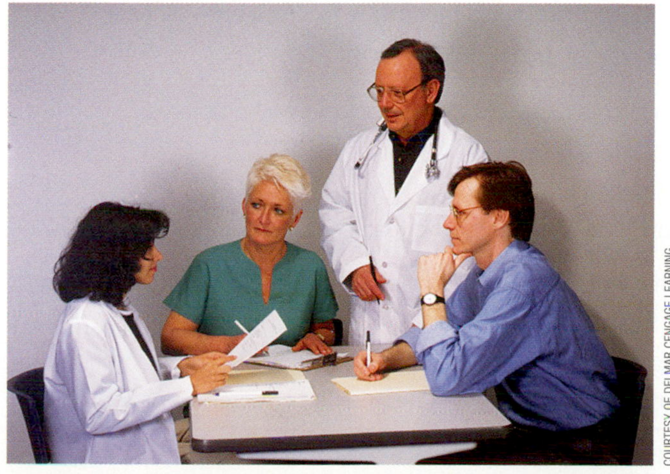

COURTESY OF DELMAR CENGAGE LEARNING

Figure 5-1 **Members of the health care team work together for the benefit of the client.**

HEALTH CARE ECONOMICS

Cost has been the primary motivation of the reform movement in health care. Control of costs has shifted from the health care providers to the insurers, with the result being increasing constraints on reimbursement. The predominant method of paying health care costs was for years fee for service, with little incentive for cost-effective delivery of care. All that is changing.

The U.S. health care system's financial base is composed of both public and private funding, resulting in administrative costs for health care reimbursement that are higher in this country than in countries with a **single-payer system** (a model wherein the government is the only entity to reimburse health care costs, such as in Canada). Despite the enormous expenditure of public funds, the United States has not found a way to provide health care coverage for all its citizens. Figure 5-2 shows the sources of the nation's health dollars in 2007.

Private Insurance

The private insurance model is the basis for the system of financing health care services in the United States. Private insurance companies constitute one of the largest sectors of the health care system. Payment rates to health care providers vary among insurance companies.

In the United States, insured individuals pay substantial monthly premiums for insurance coverage having high deductibles for health care services. For many, these costs may prove barriers to procuring necessary insurance coverage and health services. In addition, insurers will no longer pay for services that *they* deem unnecessary, effectively taking client care decisions out of the hands of physicians. The quality of care provided is now being monitored not only by providers (physicians) but also by third-party payers (insurance companies) and, ever increasingly, by consumers.

Medigap insurance to pay for costs not covered by Medicare is purchased from private insurance companies. As of 2006, an estimated 18% of Medicare beneficiaries were covered by a Medigap policy (Henry J. Kaiser Family Foundation, 2006). Nursing home care costs are covered 39% by private insurance, about 10% by Medicare, and 48% by Medicaid (CMS, 2002a). Long-term care insurance benefits vary greatly depending on the insurance company.

TABLE 5-3 Health Care Team Members

TEAM MEMBER	EDUCATION	FUNCTION/ROLE
Nurse (LP/VN, RN, and APRN)	LP/VN: 1 year RN: 2 to 4 year APRN (Advanced Practice Registered Nurse): 1 to 3 years post-RN	Emphasize health (wellness) promotion Use a holistic approach to assist clients in coping with illness or disability by providing nursing care, health and health care education, and discharge planning Formulate nursing diagnoses to guide plan of care Address the needs of the client (individual, family, or community) Assist physician Functions may vary by state and specialization
Physician (medical doctor [MD])	8+ years	Formulate medical diagnoses and prescribe therapeutic modalities Perform medical and surgical procedures
Dentist (both doctor of dental surgery [DDS] and doctor of dental medicine [DMD])	8+ years	Diagnose and treat conditions affecting the mouth, teeth, and gums Perform preventive measures to promote dental health
Registered pharmacist (Rph)	5 to 6 years	Prepare and dispense drugs for therapeutic use May be involved in client education
Physician's assistant (PA)	2 years (plus a master's degree for PA licensure, required in many states)	Provide medical services under the supervision of a physician
Registered dietitian (RD)	4+ years	Plan diets to meet special needs of clients Promote health through nutrition education and counseling May supervise preparation of meals
Social worker (SW)	4 years	Assist clients with psychosocial problems (e.g., financial, housing, marital) Make referrals to other facilities and support groups May assist with discharge planning
Respiratory therapist (RT)	2 years	Provide various therapeutic treatments for respiratory illnesses Administer pulmonary function tests
Physical therapist (PT)	4 years	Work with clients experiencing musculoskeletal problems Assess client's strength and mobility Perform therapeutic measures (e.g., range of motion, massage, application of heat and cold) and teach new skills (e.g., crutch walking)
Occupational therapist (OT)	4 years	Work with clients who have functional impairment to teach skills for activities of daily living
Speech therapist	4 years	Assist clients who have speech impairments to speak understandably or to learn another method of communication
Chaplain	8 years	Assist clients in meeting spiritual needs Provide individual counseling and support to families Conduct religious services

COURTESY OF DELMAR CENGAGE LEARNING

TABLE 5-4 Nursing Roles

Caregiver: LP/VN and RN	Traditional and most essential role Function as nurturer Provide direct care Be supportive Demonstrate clinical proficiency Promote comfort of client
Teacher: LP/VN and RN	Provide information Serve as counselor Seek to empower clients in self-care Encourage compliance with prescribed therapy Promote healthy lifestyles Interpret information
Advocate: LP/VN and RN	Protect the client Provide explanations in client's language Act as change agent Support client's decision
Manager: LP/VN and RN	Make decisions Coordinate activities of others Allocate resources Evaluate care and personnel Serve as a leader Take initiative
Expert: RN	Advanced practice clinician Conduct research Teach in schools of nursing Develop theory Contribute to professional literature Provide testimony at governmental hearings and in court
Case manager: RN	Track client's progress through the health care system Coordinate care to ensure continuity
Team member: LP/VN and RN	Collaborate with others Use excellent communication skills

COURTESY OF DELMAR CENGAGE LEARNING

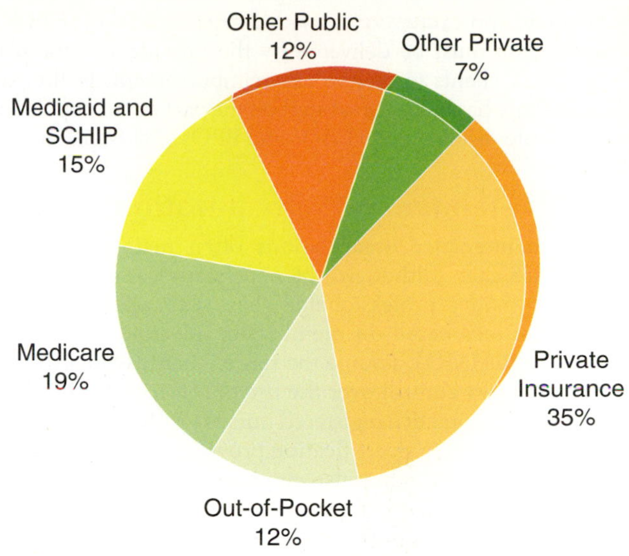

FIGURE 5-2 Source of the Nation's Health Dollar in 2007 *(Note: "Other Public" included workers' compensation, public health activity, Department of Defense, Department of Veterans Affairs, Indian Health Service, state and local hospital subsidies, and school health. "Other Private" includes industrial in-plant, privately funded construction, and nonpatient revenues, including philanthropy.) (Courtesy of Centers for Medicare and Medicaid Services, Office of the Actuary, National Health Statistics Group, 2009.)*

MANAGED CARE

Managed care is a system of providing and monitoring care wherein access, cost, and quality are controlled before or during delivery of services. Delivering services in the most cost-efficient manner possible is the goal of managed care. Managed care organizations combine financing and delivery of health care and try to control costs by monitoring delivery of services and restricting access to expensive procedures and providers.

Managed care was designed to provide coordinated services emphasizing prevention and primary care. The rationale behind managed care is to give consumers preventive services delivered by a **primary care provider** (a health care provider whom a client sees first for health care, typically a family practitioner, internist, or pediatrician). The primary care provider is responsible for managing or coordinating all care of a client when illness makes referrals necessary. This approach is supposed to result in less expensive interventions.

Although managed care has existed for years, only within the past 20 years has it enjoyed national prominence. In 1973 the Health Maintenance Organization Act implemented two mandates. First, federal grants and loans were made available to **health maintenance organizations (HMOs)** (prepaid health plans that provide primary health care services for a preset fee and that focus on cost-effective treatment measures) that complied with strict federal regulations instead of the less restrictive state requirements. Second, large employers were required to provide employees with an HMO option for health care coverage. From the beginning, HMOs have been a viable alternative to the traditional fee-for-service system.

Managed care is not a place but, rather, an organizational structure with several variations. One such variation is the HMO, which is both provider and insurer. Other variations are **preferred provider organizations (PPOs)**, wherein members must use providers within the system in order to obtain full reimbursement but may use other providers for lesser reimbursement, and **exclusive provider organizations (EPOs)**, wherein care must be delivered by the providers in the plan in order for clients to receive any reimbursement. In the past decade, there has been a great shift on the part of the population from private insurance to HMOs and PPOs (Feldstein, 2005).

Health Maintenance Organizations

Health maintenance organizations often maintain primary health care sites (although not necessarily) and commonly employ provider professionals. They use **capitated rates** (preset flat fees based on membership in, not services provided by, the HMO), assume the risk of clients who are heavy users, and exert control over the use of services. HMOs have used advanced practice registered nurses (APRNs) as primary care providers and precertification programs to limit unnecessary hospitalization. They also emphasize client education for health promotion and self-care.

Another common feature of HMOs is the practice of **single point of entry** (entry into the health care system through a point designated by the plan), through which primary care is delivered. **Primary health care** is the client's point of entry into the health care system and includes assessment, diagnosis, treatment, coordination of care, education, preventive services, and surveillance. It covers all the services provided by a family practitioner (nurse or physician) in an ambulatory setting. Primary care providers (PCPs) are "gatekeepers" to the health care system by deciding which, if any, referrals to specialists are needed by the client. HMOs purposely limit direct access to specialists to reduce costs. Managed care plans assume much of the risk of providing health care and, therefore, encourage wise use by both providers and consumers. In 1976, there were 175 HMOs in the United States; by 2002 there were 650 (Centers for Education and Research on Therapeutics [CERTS], 2003).

Preferred Provider Organizations

The most common managed care systems are PPOs. A PPO is a contractual relationship between providers, hospitals, insurers, employers, and third-party payers forming a network wherein providers negotiate with group purchasers to provide health services for a specific population at a preset cost (Feldstein, 2005). Care received within the network is associated with the highest reimbursement; care received outside the network is associated with lower reimbursement, with the client paying the difference. Preferred provider organizations have been very popular in the United States. In fact, the number of PPOs has increased from fewer than 10 in 1981 to more than 670 PPOs and over 55 PPO chains in 2008 (First Mark, 2008).

Exclusive Provider Organizations

Exclusive provider organizations create a network of providers (such as physicians and hospitals) and offer the incentive of consumer services for little or no copayment if the network providers are used exclusively. If a member receives treatment outside the network, no benefit is paid. For instance, a member who becomes ill and receives treatment while visiting relatives in another state would receive no benefits for the treatment.

FEDERAL GOVERNMENT PLANS

With the advent of Medicare and Medicaid in 1965, the federal government became a third-party payer for health care services. The Health Care Financing Administration (HCFA) is a federal agency that regulates Medicare, Medicaid, and Children's Health Insurance Program (CHIP) expenditures.

With the ultimate goal of curtailing spending for hospitalized Medicare recipients, the federal government created DRGs to categorize the average cost of care for each diagnosis. A prospective payment system was then created based on the DRGs. **Prospective payment** is a predetermined rate paid for each episode of hospitalization based on the client's age and principal diagnosis and on the presence or absence of surgery and **comorbidity** (simultaneous existence of more than one disease process in an individual). Hospitals are reimbursed the predetermined amount regardless of the actual cost of providing services to the client. The prospective payment system, originally designed for Medicare, has been adopted by other agencies and insurance companies.

Medicare

In 1965, **Medicare** (Title XVIII) was signed into law as an amendment to the Social Security Act. It was originally intended to protect those older than 65 years from excessive health care costs. In 1972, Medicare was modified to also cover permanently disabled individuals and those with end-stage renal disease. The federal government through the Centers for Medicare and Medicaid Services (CMS) administers Medicare. Medicare Part A covers inpatient hospital care, home health care, and hospice care. It may pay for care in a skilled nursing facility, but there are many restrictions, and coverage criteria changes frequently. Medicare Part B partially covers costs for physician services, outpatient rehabilitation, and certain services and supplies not covered by Part A.

Limited skilled care and rehabilitation services in certified long-term care facilities may be paid if the client and the services provided meet specific criteria. Intermittent visits for skilled health care by a registered nurse may be reimbursed to certified home health care agencies. In 2006, the total expenditures for Medicare were $408.3 billion (U.S. Social Security Administration, 2007).

PROFESSIONALTIP

Impact of Prospective Payment System and DRGs

- Decreased length of client stay in hospitals
- More emphasis on preventive care
- Increased concern about consumer's (client's) response to care
- Increased number of critically ill clients in hospitals
- Clients sicker upon discharge from hospital
- Increase in outpatient care
- Client and family more responsible for care
- Greater need for home health care
- Mergers or closures of hospitals because of inordinate competition

Medicaid

Medicaid (Title XIX) pays for health services for low-income families with dependent children, the aged poor, and the disabled (Abrams et al., 2000). It is financed by both federal and state funds but is administered by the states. Each state determines who is "medically indigent" and qualifies for public monies, so services provided vary from state to state. Medicaid is the primary health financing program for disabled individuals and low-income families. This means-tested program provides funds only when all other financial resources have been exhausted. Services covered include physician services, inpatient and outpatient hospital care, diagnostic services, skilled nursing care, rural health clinic services, and home health services. States may choose to cover other services, such as dental, vision, and prescription drugs. Medicaid will spend an estimated $339 billion between 2007 and 2008 (CMS, 2007). It is the principal source of financial assistance for long-term care and pays for skilled home health care in all states. The optional benefit of personal care in the home is also covered in 29 states. There are 50 million estimated beneficiaries enrolled in Medicaid (CMS, 2007). Medicaid benefits spending is estimated to be $4.9 trillion over the next 10 years (CMS, 2007).

State Children's Health Insurance Program

The State Children's Health Insurance Program (CHIP, formerly SCHIP) was created in 1997 as part of the Balanced Budget Act. The program is designed to provide health care to uninsured children, many of whom are members of working families that earn too little to afford private insurance on their own but earn too much to be eligible for Medicaid. It is a partnership between the federal and state governments to cover previously uninsured children. The states administer the program.

FACTORS INFLUENCING HEALTH CARE

Despite cost-containment efforts (such as DRGs, established by the federal government, and managed care, established by the insurers), the U.S. health care system still has problems with issues of access, cost, and quality. These issues are important for nurses to understand and are integral to any effort toward health reform.

Cost

Cost is a driving force for change in the health care system, as shown by the number of managed care plans, greater use of outpatient services, and shorter hospital stays. Maximum profits with minimum costs are the market forces dominating the current changes in the health care system.

The cost of providing health care has risen dramatically during the past 15 years. The U.S. government spends more on health care per person than does any other country. The use of federal funds for health care means that resources are not available for other areas of need, such as education, housing, and social services (Grace, 2001). Figure 5-3 illustrates health care expenditures.

The most cost-efficient programs in terms of administration are Medicare and Medicaid (HCFA, 1998). Private agencies and organizations are subcontracted to administer these programs. In contrast, some private small business plans use more than 40 cents of each dollar for administration. The cost of employee health care benefits is thus an expensive commitment for small businesses.

MEMORY TRICK

The memory trick **COST** identifies changes in the health care system due to the dramatic cost of health care:

- **C** = Concept of maximum profit for minimum cost
- **O** = Outpatient services are accessed more
- **S** = Shorter hospital stays
- **T** = The increase in managed care plans

Three major factors increase the cost of health care: (a) an oversupply of specialized providers (fees are raised to maintain provider income in light of fewer clients), (b) a surplus of hospital beds (empty beds are a cost liability), and (c) the passive role assumed by most consumers (when someone else pays the bill, consumers typically are less concerned about cost) (Feldstein, 2005). Other factors contributing to the high cost of health care are the aging population, the increased number of people with chronic illnesses, and the proliferation of health-related lawsuits and the associated use of unnecessary services (e.g., additional diagnostic testing). Advanced technology has allowed more people to survive formerly fatal illnesses.

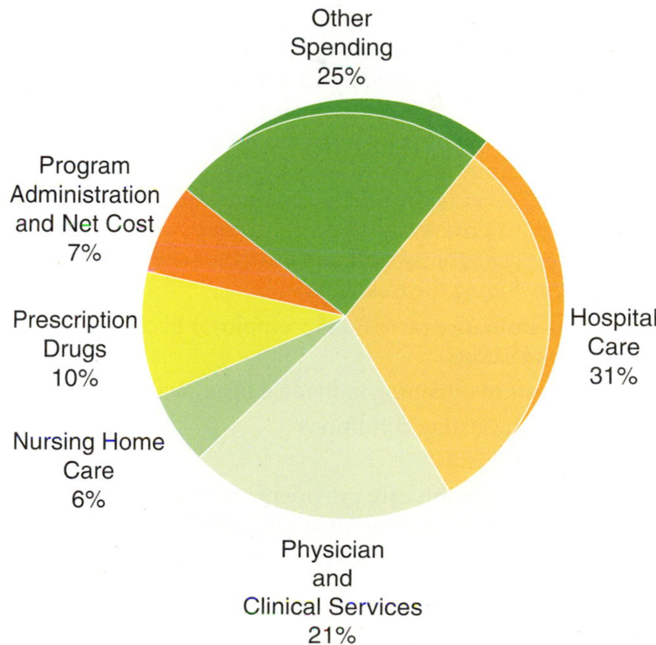

FIGURE 5-3 **Health Care Expenditures in 2007** (*Note: "Other Spending" included dentist services, other professional services, home health, durable medical products, over-the-counter medicines and sundries, public health, other personal health care, research, and structures and equipment.*) (*Courtesy of Centers for Medicare and Medicaid Services, Office of the Actuary, National Health Statistics Group, 2009.*)

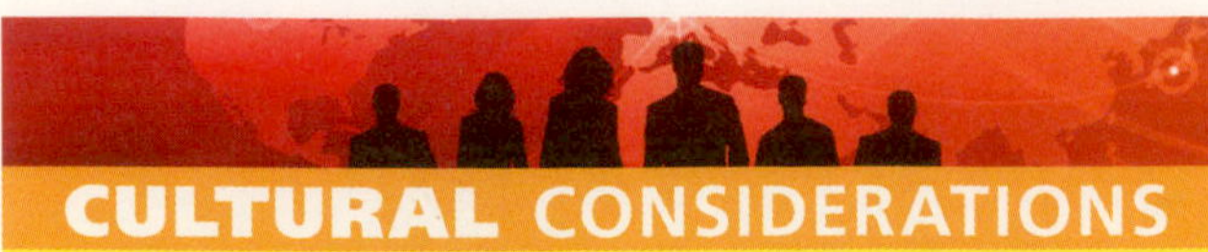

CULTURAL CONSIDERATIONS

Barriers to Health Care Services

Certain cultural beliefs and values may prevent individuals from seeking health care. These may include the following:

- Belief in divine healing
- Refusal of care on holy days
- Belief that the individual taking the ill person to a health care facility is responsible for the ill person for the rest of that person's life after recovery
- Belief that illness is a result of sins committed in previous life
- View of prayer as a tool for deliverance from illness
- Belief that illness is God's punishment

ACCESS

Related to the issue of cost is that of access to health care services, which carries serious implications for the functioning of the health care system. Health care for many people is crisis oriented and fragmented because of the high costs. Numerous people in the United States are unable to gain access to health care services because of inadequate or no insurance; thus, illness among these people may progress to an acute stage before intervention is sought. Their access is typically through emergency departments during acute illnesses. Emergency room and acute care services are very expensive compared to prevention and early intervention. According to Hoffman (2007), more than 46 million Americans had no health insurance at some point in 2005. Having health insurance could reduce mortality for the uninsured by 10% to 15% (Hoffman, 2007).

Medicare covers only a small portion of the medically indigent. The many underinsured individuals are neither poor nor old but are those who have jobs lacking adequate health care benefits or middle-class unemployed Americans. In addition to poverty and unemployment, other factors can hinder a person's ability to obtain insurance and/or health care services, including the following:

- Lack of insurance provision by employer because of prohibitive costs
- High costs of obtaining individual insurance
- Certain preexisting conditions
- Cultural barriers
- Shortages of health care providers in some geographic areas (especially rural or inner-city areas)
- Limited access to ancillary services (e.g., child care and transportation)
- Status as single-parent or two-income family, making it difficult for parents to take time from work to transport children to health care providers

QUALITY

Lee, Soffel, and Luft (1997) report that 30% to 40% of diagnostic and medical procedures performed in this country are unnecessary. This inappropriate use of resources can be traced to several factors, including:

- The litigious environment and resultant tendency toward defensive practice (e.g., ordering all possible tests instead of only those that the provider deems truly necessary)
- The widely held American belief that more is better
- Lack of access to and continuity of services and the subsequent misuse of acute care services

Quality may be sacrificed in an attempt to provide universal access to services in a cost-effective manner. For example, hospitals that reduce the number of nurses (downsizing) risk endangering quality. Safety and quality are often compromised by inappropriately substituting unqualified personnel for LP/VNs and RNs in direct client care. The quality of care in hospitals decreases with cross training of staff, greater use of unlicensed personnel, and reduction of full-time positions for nurses.

CHALLENGES WITHIN THE HEALTH CARE SYSTEM

The major challenges facing the U.S. health care delivery system, which also impact the control of costs, include the public's disillusionment with providers, consumers' and providers' loss of control over health care decisions, changing practice settings, decreased use of hospitals, vulnerable populations, and ethical issues.

DISILLUSIONMENT WITH PROVIDERS

Greed and waste have been identified as major problems of the U.S. health care system (Maraldo, 2001). The cause of these problems is irrelevant to the public. Reform success means starting with public expectations of eliminating the greed of providers and the waste in the health care system. Furthermore, people in the United States have become suspicious of health care providers. The high level of esteem in which medicine has traditionally been held has eroded over the past few years. Consumers, increasingly tired of paying the high cost of care, are questioning medical practices and fees (Zerwekh & Claborn, 2008); however, the public is not as disillusioned with nurses. As reported in the *American Journal of Nursing* (*AJN*), a November 1999 Gallup poll reported that almost three-quarters of those surveyed rated the honesty and ethics of nurses as "high" or "very high" (Health Care News, 2000). Nursing received higher ratings than any other profession, including other health care professionals. *Nurse Week* and Sigma Theta Tau International commissioned another survey. It revealed that 92% of the public trusts health information provided by registered nurses.

CRITICAL THINKING

Perception of Nurses

What factors do you think have contributed to a positive perception of nurses? A negative perception? What can you do specifically to promote positive images of nursing to the public?

Positive Perception of Nurses

Nurses are viewed as part of the solution, not the problem. If nurses were allowed to use their skills, the public believes they would significantly enhance quality and reduce costs. One survey (ANA, 1993) asked consumers about receptivity to nurses' having expanded responsibilities. Respondents supported *prescriptive authority* (legal recognition of the ability to prescribe medications) for RNs and endorsed the role of nurses in performing physical examinations and managing minor acute illnesses. Nurses should expand their focus on holistic care and spend as much time as possible on prevention of illness and wellness issues.

Loss of Control

Consumers express feeling terrorized by the health care delivery system. They feel they have lost personal control over their health care. Many stay in their current jobs because of their health care benefits or give up employment mobility out of fear of being denied a new policy because of preexisting conditions.

Providers feel they have lost control over the care they provide to their clients. Increasingly, the insurance companies or the managed care organizations decide which care can and cannot be provided to the client.

Changing Practice Settings

Most nurses practice in hospitals and will continue to do so in the future. The increasing presence of severely ill clients requires that nurses who work in hospitals possess technical expertise, critical thinking skills, and interpersonal competence. Outside the hospital setting, there is an ever-increasing need for nurses in different areas of practice. Home health services, in particular, will need to continue expanding in order to meet the growing needs of the steadily increasing elderly population. Social and political changes are affecting nurses by creating the need for expanded services and settings. More nurses will be needed in the future because:

- The increasing elderly population requires more health care services.
- Admissions to nursing homes is increasing.
- The number of homeless individuals is increasing rapidly.

Reforms may displace some nurses from their current jobs. The demand for greater access to health care services will create many more jobs. More nurses will be needed for primary care, extended care, home care, and public health.

Decreased Hospital Use

In the early 20th century, hospital focus was providing care to those who had no caregivers in the family or community. These early institutions provided care, not cure (Grace, 2001). In the mid-1940s the focus of hospitals changed because of technology and the 1946 Hill–Burton Act, which funded the renovation and construction of hospitals. This resulted in sizable oversupply of hospital beds. To keep the hospital beds occupied, everyone was put in the hospital, for everything from a complete physical examination to specific diagnostic testing to acute care or surgery, and health care costs escalated.

The demand for hospital beds steadily increased from 1945 to 1982. After 1982, there was a steady decline in hospital admissions and the average length of stay (Grace, 2001). In 1995, there were 23.7% fewer inpatient days than in 1985 (Feldstein, 2005). Many small hospitals have closed because they could no longer compete with the large hospitals.

Hospitals are still the center of the U.S. health care system. They employ a majority of health care workers. Fewer clients are in hospitals today because of earlier discharge and the large number of procedures performed in outpatient settings. Clients hospitalized today need more nursing care because of their complex needs and severity of illness. Additional factors that have contributed to the decreased hospital population include:

- Greater availability of outpatient facilities and services
- Advances in technology
- Expectations/demands of third-party payers

The changes in reimbursement practices resulted in hospital restructuring (also referred to as redesigning and reengineering). Examples include mergers with larger institutions; development of integrated systems that provide a full range of services focusing on continuity of care, such as preadmission, outpatient, acute inpatient, long-term inpatient, and home care; and the substitution of multiskilled workers for nurses.

Vulnerable Populations

Meeting the health care needs of underserved populations is especially challenging. Groups that may be unable to gain access to health care services include children, the elderly, people with AIDS, rural residents, and the homeless and others living in poverty. Increasing poverty strains hospitals because Medicaid can no longer meet the needs of the medically indigent.

Our current health care system neglects the overall needs of children who are more likely than adults to be uninsured or underinsured. Children who are covered by health insurance have a greater degree of well-being.

Many parents have their children immunized only when the children are ready to start school because immunization is a requirement for entry into the public school system. Preventive health care emphasizing early immunization should be encouraged and made available to children of all ages.

Rural areas have fewer health care providers and facilities than urban areas. Many people in rural areas have no health insurance because they tend to be self-employed or work for small businesses.

The Centers for Disease Control and Prevention (CDC) estimated that in 2006, 1,106,400 persons in the United States were living with an HIV infection (CDC, 2008). It is estimated that at least 56,300 persons were newly infected with HIV in 2006 (CDC, 2008). It is spreading most rapidly among women, children, and intravenous drug users and their sexual partners. Additional funding is necessary, and outpatient care

COMMUNITY/HOME HEALTH CARE

Cost of Home Health Care

- Since the advent of Medicare and Medicaid, home health care has grown rapidly. Because it is much less costly to provide home care, clients are sent home to recuperate.
- Expenditures for health care in the home are greatly increasing.

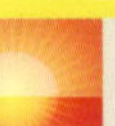

LIFE SPAN CONSIDERATIONS

Health Care for Children

- Approximately one-third of the 71,731,000 children younger than age 18 who live in poverty are younger than 6 years of age (U.S. Census Bureau, 2002).
- There are 9 million uninsured children in the United States (Agency for Healthcare Research and Quality [AHRQ], 2008).
- An estimated 2.3 million children with insured parents are uninsured (AHRQ, 2008).
- Six out of 10 parents whose children may qualify for Medicaid or State Children's Health Insurance Program (SCHIP) do not believe these programs apply to them (RWJF, 2001).
- Belief that their children do not qualify is highest in households where both parents work or when annual income is $25,000 or more (Robert Wood Johnson Foundation, 2001).
- By 1996, 90% or more of toddlers had received the most critical doses of vaccines for children by age 2 (CDC, 2002b).
- Nine percent fewer poor children complete the full series of immunizations (National Academies, 2002).
- Each day 11,000 babies are born who will need immunizations (National Academies, 2002).
- Federal funds supporting the immunization network are shrinking (CDC, 2002b).

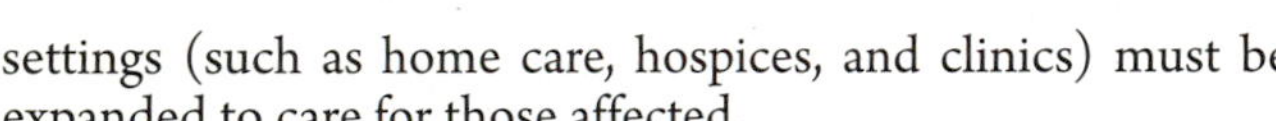

settings (such as home care, hospices, and clinics) must be expanded to care for those affected.

The homeless and others living in poverty are often mobile, having no permanent address. They may not know which services are available to them or how to access the system except through inner-city hospitals. This creates a significant financial burden on these health care agencies. Illegal aliens, because of fears of being arrested and deported, may enter emergency departments under false identities and in acute distress, receive treatment, and then disappear.

ETHICAL ISSUES

The United States is struggling with the ethical issue of cost containment versus compassionate care. According to Hicks and Boles (1997), no country can provide all citizens with every health care service they need or desire. The U.S. health care delivery system has a dilemma of needs being greater than available resources. Difficult choices must be made to determine which needs are met and which remain unmet.

The national mentality, reflected in the expectation that everything must be done to save a dying person, has created an enormous drain on health care resources. There will be much debate about the ethics of decisions made about how scarce resources are to be allocated. Nurses must strongly advocate for just and ethical distribution of resources.

NURSING'S RESPONSE TO HEALTH CARE CHALLENGES

The United States will continue to seek ways to reform health care. There will be increasing implications for nursing. Some nurses feel threatened, but others are excited about changing the health care system into something better. The nursing profession responded to these challenges by proposing a plan for reform.

NURSING'S AGENDA FOR HEALTH CARE REFORM

In 1991, in response to high cost, limited access, and eroding quality affecting the U.S. health care system, the nursing community wrote a public policy agenda that was endorsed by more than 70 organizations. *Nursing's Agenda for Health Care Reform* (ANA, 1991) provides a framework for health care policy changes and establishes a legislative program through which to implement these changes. A major aspect of the proposal is that health care services be delivered in familiar, easily accessible, and consumer-friendly environments. Another essential aspect is that consumers are empowered in the area of self-care. The health care system continues to be costly and fragmented with unequal distribution of services (ANA, 2009). The *ANA's Health Care Agenda 2005* represents the ANA's commitment to the principle that all Americans are entitled to quality, accessible, and affordable health care services. ANA's updated *Health System Reform Agenda* (ANA, 2009) continues to represent ANA's role as a leading advocate for health care reform in the current national health care debate. For more information on ANA's health care agenda and reform, visit the ANA's website at *http://nursingworld.org/default.aspx.*

STANDARDIZATION OF CARE

A move toward standardization of care is another approach to the challenges of the health care delivery system. The Agency for Health Care Policy and Research (AHCPR) was established in December 1990 with the specific charge of reaching consensus within the medical/ health care community about the diagnosis and treatment of certain illnesses and diseases. The AHCPR aspires to identify standards of diagnosis and treatment for high-volume, expensive disease conditions to which the health care community can be held. Currently, 18

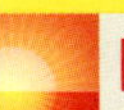

LIFE SPAN CONSIDERATIONS

Rural Elders

Health care barriers experienced by elderly persons living in rural areas include the following:

- Lower Medicare reimbursement rates for rural hospitals than for urban hospitals contributed to the closure of some rural hospitals
- Fewer health care providers available
- Greater travel distances to obtain services

AHCPR-published guidelines are available to the public and should be integral to nursing practice.

Advanced Practice

Advanced-practice nursing developed as nursing became more complex and specialized. Nurse practitioners (NPs), clinical nurse specialists (CNSs), certified nurse midwives (CNMs), and other advanced practice registered nurses (APRNs) have provided primary health care services to individuals since the late 1960s. Many of these individuals would have had inadequate or no access to services (Boyd, Lowes, Guglielmo, & Slomski, 2000). The APRN has advanced skills and in-depth knowledge in specific areas of practice. Although there are differences among various advanced-practice roles, all APRNs are experts who work with clients to promote health and prevent disease.

Advanced-practice nurses are moving toward independent practice. Advanced-practice nurses prescribe less expensive diagnostic tests, have client visits comparable in length to that of physicians, and charge less for services because of the lower cost of professional liability insurance (Boyd et al., 2000). The single biggest obstacle to APRN practice is that most people are unaware of what APRNs can offer.

Currently, all states award APRNs some type of prescriptive authority (Pearson, 2000). In 10 states, this authority is complete and unrestricted and includes all classes of drugs (Pearson, 2000). According to the American Academy of Nurse Practitioners (2007), in 2007 there were approximately 120,000 NPs with an estimated 6,000 new graduates each year from 325 colleges and universities in the United States.

Public vs. Private Programs

The competition between the public and private sectors has encouraged quality and progress. Each setting has benefits as well as obstacles for health care recipients.

Public dollars are needed to help the poor and those who have no health care benefits through the workplace. To prevent the health care system from becoming a two-tiered process based on personal resources, both the poor and nonpoor and the privileged and nonprivileged should be enrolled in the same programs. Minimal national standards should be set, but local planning and implementation should be promoted.

The U.S. philosophy of states' rights is an obstacle to having national standards. Some consistency in the cost of services from coast to coast is needed with some local adjustments allowed.

CRITICAL THINKING

Health Care System

Even with the advantages of technology, biomedical research, and state-of-the-art clinical equipment and facilities, many consider the U.S. health care system to be in crisis. From your perspective, is the health care system in a state of strength or weakness? Explain your response.

LIFE SPAN CONSIDERATIONS

Meeting the Needs of Homeless Elderly Clients

The Health Resources and Services Administration (2003) listed recommendations from providers who serve elderly people who are homeless to assist in meeting their health care needs.

- Provide homeless elderly persons with a comprehensive multiservice center all under one roof
- Bring together the skills of different providers to provide comprehensive assessment and evaluation
- Develop health care resources for homeless persons 55 to 64 years old who are not eligible for benefits such as Medicare
- Provide outreach services to elderly persons who may be living alone, homeless, or living in a shelter who are at risk for depression and other health problems

Public Health

In the past decade, public health has visibly deteriorated. Immunizations, environmental concerns (conditions that may affect health), prenatal care, and analysis of the prevailing disease patterns in a community are included in public health services. Current public health problems include:

- Prevalence of overweight population
- Emergence of drug-resistant strains of tuberculosis and other infections
- Presence of toxic environmental conditions

Community Health

Prevention and primary care are the focus of community-based care. Nursing has a rich legacy of contributing community aid, as demonstrated by the work of pioneers such as Mary Breckenridge and Lillian Wald.

ISSUES AND TRENDS

As various trends appear, the delivery of health care services will continue to change. The challenge is to improve the nation's delivery of health care services by preserving nursing integrity. Nursing must be involved from the beginning of any change. Factors that will continue to shape reform of the health care delivery system include:

- Aging of the U.S. population
- Increasing population diversity
- More single-parent families and children living in poverty
- Growth of outpatient care and a greater demand for primary care providers
- Technological advances resulting in more services in outpatient settings (including the home)

- More states using managed care to provide the medically indigent with services
- Incentives for those participating in preventive activities
- Federal funds for health care provider education requiring service to underserved populations and areas
- Managed care dominating service delivery
- Focus on quality improvement

CASE STUDY

A 45-year-old male client is diagnosed with lung cancer. In the past month, he has lost his job and his health insurance. He shares with you his concerns regarding his lack of income and insurance and his worries about providing for his wife and two young children.

1. What health care options are available for him? For his family?
2. What health care services could he be eligible to receive? His family?
3. As his nurse, what are your roles in providing care for him?
4. What level of care does he need?

SUMMARY

- The three levels of health care services are classified as primary, secondary, and tertiary.
- Health care services are financed and delivered by the public (official, voluntary, and nonprofit agencies), public/private, and private sectors.
- The health care team is composed of nurses, nurse practitioners, physicians, physician's assistants, pharmacists, dentists, dietitians, social workers, various therapists, and chaplains.
- Managed care organizations seek to control health care costs by monitoring the delivery of services and restricting access to costly procedures and providers.
- The primary federal government insurance plans are Medicare, which provides health care coverage for elderly persons and disabled persons; Medicaid, which is administered with the states to provide health care services for the poor; and CHIP, which provides health care to uninsured children.
- To achieve equity for all Americans, health care reform must address the three critical issues of cost, access, and quality of health care services.
- The challenges that the health care delivery system must overcome are the public's disillusionment with providers, provider and consumer loss of control over health care decisions, the decreased use of hospitals, the change in practice settings, ethical issues, and the health care needs of vulnerable populations.
- The Agency of Health Care Policy and Research aims to identify therapeutic standards to which the health care community can be held.
- A primary goal of the nursing profession is to provide health care services emphasizing prevention and primary health care, which will help reduce costs and increase the quality of health care.

REVIEW QUESTIONS

1. A nursing student is taught about the three levels of health care service in the United States. Which of the following statements made by the nursing student indicates that further teaching is needed?
   1. "A health care delivery system is a method for providing services to meet the health needs of individuals."
   2. "An example of primary care is when a parent takes her 6-month-old infant to the health department for immunizations."
   3. "Secondary care is when a client regains partial use of an arm after experiencing a stroke."
   4. "A client who is utilizing rehabilitation services is participating in tertiary care."
2. Which of the following is not considered a major challenge facing the U.S. health care delivery system?
   1. Changing practice settings.
   2. Ethical issues.
   3. Vulnerable populations.
   4. Health care teams.
3. As various issues and trends appear in health care, which of the following are factors that will shape the reform of the health care delivery system? (Select all that apply.)
   1. Aging of the U.S. population.
   2. More single-parent families.
   3. Fewer children living in poverty.
   4. Decreasing population diversity.
   5. Focus on quality improvement.
   6. Fewer states using managed care.

4. When a nurse tracks a client's progress through the health care system, this role is known as:
   1. caregiver.
   2. expert.
   3. case manager.
   4. team member.
5. A 64-year-old client asks the nurse, "What is the difference between Medicare and Medicaid?" The most appropriate response by the nurse is:
   1. "Medicare was originally intended to protect those older than 65 years from excessive health care costs, and Medicaid pays for health services for low-income families with dependent children, the aged poor, and the disabled."
   2. "Medicare covers the cost for low-income families with dependent children, and Medicaid pays for those older than 65 years of age."
   3. "Medicare is the primary health financing program for disabled individuals and low-income families, and Medicaid was modified to cover permanently disabled individuals and those with end-stage renal disease."
   4. "Medicare is for individuals that are over the age of 65, and Medicaid is for the wealthy that can afford it."
6. The major agency that oversees the actual delivery of care services is:
   1. U.S. Public Health Service.
   2. Medicare.
   3. American Medical Association.
   4. National Institutes of Health.
7. Factors that hinder a person's ability to obtain insurance and/or health care services include which of the following? (Select all that apply.)
   1. Certain preexisting conditions.
   2. Cultural barriers.
   3. High costs of obtaining individual insurance.
   4. Multiple surgical procedures.
   5. Upper-middle-class status.
   6. Shortages of health care providers.
8. As the homeless elderly population is increasing in numbers, the United States is facing the challenge of caring for this group of individuals. The best intervention to assist these individuals is:
   1. provide homeless elderly persons with a comprehensive multiservice center all under one roof.
   2. develop health care resources for homeless elderly persons who are not eligible for benefits such as Medicare.
   3. identify therapeutic standards to which the health care community is held.
   4. restrict access to costly procedures and providers.
9. A single working mother with three young children earns too little to afford private insurance and too much to be eligible for Medicaid. The nurse knows that which of the following is the best option for the client's children?
   1. Enroll the family in Medicare.
   2. Contact the States Children's Health Insurance Program (CHIP).
   3. Contact the local health department.
   4. Register for the Low-Income State Family Insurance Program.
10. A newly diagnosed diabetic client is being discharged home later today. The most important role for the nurse at this time is:
    1. teacher.
    2. advocate.
    3. caregiver.
    4. team member.

REFERENCES/SUGGESTED READINGS

Abrams, W. B., Beers, M. H., & Berkow, R. (Eds.). (2000). *The Merck manual of geriatrics* (3rd ed.). Whitehouse Station, NJ: Merck Research Laboratories.

Agency for Healthcare Research and Quality. (2008). More than 2 million children with uninsured parents are uninsured; most are low to middle income. Retrieved November 11, 2008, from http://www.ahrq.gov/news/press/pr2008/childuninspr.htm

American Academy of Nurse Practitioners. (2007). Why choose a nurse practitioner as your healthcare provider? Retrieved November 15, 2008, from http://www.npfinder.com/faq.pdf

American Nurses Association. (1991). *Nursing's agenda for health care reform*. Kansas City, MO: Author.

American Nurses Association. (1993, September). *Consumers willing to see a nurse for routine "doctoring" according to Gallup poll* [news release]. Washington, DC: Author.

American Nurses Association. (1995). Managed care: Challenges and opportunities for nursing. *Nursing facts* (Item PR-27). Washington, DC: Author.

American Nurses Association. (2009). Health system reform agenda. Retrieved September 27, 2009 from http://nursingworld.org/MainMenuCategories/HealthcareandPolicyIssues/HealthSystemReform/Agenda.aspx

Boyd, L., Lowes, R., Guglielmo, W., & Slomski, A. (2000). Advanced practice nursing today. *RN, 63*(9), 57–62.

Centers for Disease Control and Prevention. (2002). IOM Report—Calling the shots: Immunization finance policies and practice. Available: www.cdc.gov/nip/registry/ss/irc-2001p24.pps

Centers for Disease Control and Prevention. (2006). HIV/AIDS surveillance report: Cases of HIV infection and AIDS in the United States and dependent areas. Retrieved on November 5, 2008, from http://www.cdc.gov/hiv/topics/surveillance/resources/factsheets/prevalence.htm

Centers for Education and Research on Therapeutics. (2003). Annual report. Available: http://certs/hhs/gov/aboutcerts/annualreports/year2/y2certs.pdf

Centers for Medicare and Medicaid Services (2000). The state of the Children's Health Insurance Program. Available: www.cms.hhs.gov/schip/wh0700.pdf

Centers for Medicare and Medicaid Services. (2002a). Program information, June 2002, ed. Available www.cms.hhs.gov/chart/series/sec1.pdf

Centers for Medicare and Medicaid Services. (2002b). Program information, June 2002, ed. Available: www.cms.hhs.gov/chart/series/sec2.pdf

Centers for Medicare and Medicaid Services. (2007). Medicaid spending projected to rise much faster than the economy: Cumulative spending on Medicaid benefits projected to reach $ 4.9 trillion over 10 years. Retrieved November 11, 2008, from http://www.cms.hhs.gov/apps/media/press/release.asp?Counter=3311&intNumPerPage=10&checkDate=&checkKey=&srchType=1&numDays=350

Dochterman, J., & Grace, H. K. (Eds.). (2001). Current issues in nursing (6th ed.). St. Louis, MO: Mosby.

Feldstein, P. J. (2005). *Health care economics* (6th ed.). Clifton Park, NY: Delmar Cengage Learning.

First Mark. (2008). Preferred provider organizations list. Available: http://www.firstmark.com/fmkcat/ppo.htm

Grace, H. K. (2001). Can medical costs be contained? In J. Dochterman & H. K. Grace (Eds.), *Current issues in nursing* (6th ed.). St. Louis, MO: Mosby.

Grace, H. K., & Brock, R. M. (2001). Solving the health care dilemma: What will work? In J. Dochterman & H. K. Grace (Eds.), *Current issues in nursing* (5th ed.). St. Louis, MO: Mosby.

Haugh, R. (1999). The new consumer. *Hospital Health Network,* 73(12), 30–34, 36.

Health Care Financing Administration. (1998). Medicare and Medicaid expenses, 1997. Available: http://www.hcfa. gov/pubforms/finance/97/ch2n1216.htm

Health Care Financing Administration. (2002). The nation's healthcare dollar: 2000. Available: http://www.hcfa.gov/stats/nhe-oact/tables/chart.htm

Health Care News. (2000). Maryland group shows universal coverage can work. *American Journal of Nursing, 100*(8), 20.

Health Resources and Services Administration. (2003). Homeless and elderly: Understanding the special health care needs of elderly persons who are homeless. Retrieved November 15, 2008, from http://bphc.hrsa.gov/policy/pal0303.htm

Henry J. Kaiser Family Foundation. (2006). Examining sources of coverage among Medicare beneficiaries: Supplemental insurance, Medicare advantage, and prescription drug coverage. Retrieved November 11, 2008, from http://www.kff.org/medicare/upload/7801.pdf

Hicks, L. L., & Boles, K. E. (1997). Why health economics? In C. Harrington & C. L. Estes (Eds.), *Health policy and nursing: Crisis and reform in the U.S. health care delivery system* (2nd ed.). Boston: Jones & Bartlett.

Hoffman, C. B. (2007). Simple truths about America's uninsured. *American Journal of Nursing, 107*(1), 40–47.

Lee, P. R., Soffel, D., & Luft, H. (1997). Costs and coverage: Pressures towards health care reform. In P. Lee, C. Estes, & N. Ramsay (Eds.), *The nation's health* (5th ed.). Boston: Jones & Bartlett.

Maraldo, P. J. (2001). Nursing's agenda for health care reform. In J. Dochterman & H. K. Grace (Eds.), *Current issues in nursing* (6th ed.). St. Louis, MO: Mosby.

National Academies. (2002). Strengthening America's vaccine safety net. Available: http://www.national-academies. org/includes/shots.htm

National Information Center on Health Services Research and Health Care Technology. (2008). The nation's health dollar: 2000. Retrieved November 11, 2008, from http://www.nlm.nih.gov/nichsr/edu/healthecon/02_he_07.html

News. (2000). High public esteem for nurses. *American Journal of Nursing, 100*(1), 26.

Pearson, L. J. (2000). Annual legislative update: How each state stands on legislative issues affecting advanced nursing practice. *Nurse Practitioner, 25*(1), 16.

Peck, S. P. (2001). Community nursing centers: Implications for health care reform. In J. Dochterman & H. K. Grace (Eds.), *Current issues in nursing* (6th ed.). St. Louis, MO: Mosby.

Robert Wood Johnson Foundation. (2001). About covering kids. Available: http://www.coveringkids.org/ about

Stafford, M., & Appleyard, J. (2001). Clinical nurse and nurse practitioners. In J. Dochterman & H. K. Grace (Eds.), *Current issues in nursing* (6th ed.). St. Louis, MO: Mosby.

U.S. Census Bureau. (2002). Poverty 2000. Available: http://www.census.gov/hhes/poverty/poverty00/tables00.html

U.S. Social Security Administration. (2007). Annual statistical supplement. Retrieved November 12, 2008, from http://www.ssa.gov/policy/docs/statcomps/supplement/2007/medicare.pdf

Vrabec, N. J. (1995). Implications of U.S. health care reform for the rural elderly. *Nursing Outlook, 43*(6), 260–265.

Zerwekh, J., & Claborn, J. C. (2008). *Nursing today: Transitions and trends* (5th ed.). Philadelphia: W. B. Saunders.

Zerwic, J. J., Simmons, B., & Zerwic, M. J. (2007). Helping hands health center: Chicago-area volunteers respond to the uninsured. *American Journal of Nursing, 107*(1), 48–50.

RESOURCES

American Academy of Ambulatory Care Nursing (AAACN), http://www.aaacn.org

American Nurses Association (ANA), http://www.nursingworld.org

National Federation of Licensed Practical Nurses (NFLPN), http://www.nflpn.org

CHAPTER 6
Arenas of Care

MAKING THE CONNECTION

Refer to the following chapters to increase your understanding of areas of care:

Basic Nursing
- ***Legal and Ethical Responsibilities***
- ***Cultural Considerations***
- ***End-of-Life Care***
- ***Assessment***
- ***Pain Management***

Adult Health Nursing
- ***The Older Adult***

LEARNING OBJECTIVES

Upon completion of this chapter, you should be able to:

- Define key terms.
- List three reasons for the growth in nonacute care services.
- Distinguish among licensure, certification, and accreditation.
- Describe the role of the LP/VN as a member of the interdisciplinary health care team in various health care settings.
- Discuss the types of clients that would benefit from participation in a rehabilitation program.
- Identify the responsibilities of the LP/VN in acute care, rehabilitation, long-term care, home care, and hospice.
- List the various types of long-term care services.

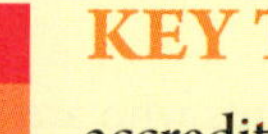

KEY TERMS

accreditation
adult day care
assisted living
certification
hospice
licensure
long-term care facility
rehabilitation
respite care
subacute care

INTRODUCTION

The traditional arenas for providing care have been physicians' offices and acute care hospitals. Many nonacute arenas of health care are now available, including long-term care, outpatient settings, home health care, and hospice, with rehabilitation provided in any of these. Most of these facilities must be licensed and certified, and some have accreditation.

AGENCY LICENSURE, CERTIFICATION, AND ACCREDITATION

Several methods have been designed to ensure that the agency, facility, or service meets minimal standards of care. Three of the methods are agency licensure, certification, and accreditation.

Licensure

Licensure is a mandatory system of granting licenses according to specified standards and is regulated by each state. All health care facilities must be licensed. A designated agency (often the department of public health) is responsible for licensing health care facilities in each state. Annually each facility is visited by a team of surveyors to determine if the facility complies with the rules and regulations of the state. Any area of noncompliance results in severe sanctions and financial penalties for the institution. A limited amount of time is given to the facility to correct any deficiencies. The facility may lose its license to operate if residents' lives or well-being are threatened.

Certification

Certification is a voluntary process that establishes and evaluates compliance with rules and regulations but is required for any provider who seeks reimbursement from government funds, Medicare, and Medicaid. Because government funding is regulated by the federal government, certification rules are generated by the federal government.

State agencies perform this function under contract with centers for Medicare and Medicaid services. In some states, the long-term care survey for licensure and certification is done concurrently. The states have generally adopted the federal regulations but in some cases exceed federal regulations. Facilities not complying with regulations are not granted certification, resulting in no reimbursement from Medicare or Medicaid.

Accreditation

Accreditation is an additional confirmation of quality and generally indicates that the delivery of care and service is above minimum standards. Accreditation is a voluntary (not required by law) process. Standards are issued by accrediting organizations, whereas rules and regulations are issued by state/federal licensure and certification agencies. The Joint Commission (JCAHO) has long been accrediting hospitals and skilled nursing facilities. The Commission on Accreditation of Rehabilitation Facilities (CARF) has been accrediting comprehensive inpatient rehabilitation programs since 1966. Rehabilitation facilities may seek accreditation from both groups.

ACUTE CARE HOSPITAL

Large acute care hospitals provide the greatest number of services. Other health care settings may provide some but not all of these services. The service departments most commonly found in acute care hospitals include nursing units, specialized client care units, diagnostic departments, therapy departments, and support services.

Nursing Units

Nursing units are composed of client rooms, where most nursing care is provided. Units often serve one particular type of client, such as cardiac, orthopedic, diabetic, surgical, pediatric, or obstetric. The nurse responsible for the unit may be called by several different titles, such as unit coordinator, nurse manager, or head nurse. Registered nurses (RNs), licensed practical/vocational nurses (LP/VNs), and nursing assistants provide the nursing care.

Specialized Client Care Units

Specialized units provide nursing care for specific needs of the clients. The LP/VN may work in these areas depending on experience, education, the size and location of the hospital, and the number of RNs available. Examples of specialized units include the following:

- Emergency department (ED): Provides care to clients involved in all types of accidents and those confronted with medical emergencies such as heart attack or stroke
- Intensive care unit (ICU): Provides care to critically ill clients until they are stabilized and can be managed with routine nursing interventions on a regular nursing unit
- Coronary care unit (CCU): Provides care to clients who have had a heart attack or who have had heart surgery such as coronary artery bypass or valve replacement
- Mental health unit: Provides care to clients who are having difficulty with relationships, coping with everyday demands, or dealing with a crisis
- Psychiatric unit: Provides care to clients diagnosed as having mental illness
- Rehabilitation unit: Provides care to clients who must learn to regain the highest level of self-care possible following injury, accident, or illness
- Dialysis unit: Provides care to clients who need dialysis because of renal failure
- Hospice unit: Provides both care to clients who are dying and support to their families; may be a unit in a hospital or a freestanding unit
- Outpatient unit: Provides care to clients when admission to the hospital is unnecessary
- Home care: Provides care to clients in their homes when professional supervision and/or minimal care is required; has been added to many hospitals to provide continuity of care
- Client education unit: Provides teaching to clients, either individually or in groups, about specific client conditions or other health-related issues

Surgical Units

Care of the client just before, during, and after surgery is performed by the operating room (OR) and recovery room (RR) personnel. In addition to the main surgical unit, many hospitals also have a day surgery/ambulatory surgery unit. Clients come in a couple of hours before their scheduled surgeries and leave when recovered from the anesthesia. Total length of stay is shorter than 24 hours.

Diagnostic Departments

Diagnostic departments provide specialized tests that assist the physician in making a diagnosis.

Clinical Laboratory

Clinical laboratory personnel examine specimens of tissues, feces, and body fluids, such as blood, sputum, urine, amniotic fluid, and spinal fluid. Testing assesses values of normal components and of any abnormal components of these specimens.

Radiology (Nuclear Medicine)

X-ray studies are performed in the radiology department, along with positron emission tomography (PET) scans, computed tomography (CT) scans, mammography, ultrasound, arteriograms, venograms, echocardiograms, and magnetic resonance imaging (MRI).

Other Diagnostic Services

Other diagnostic services may include the following:

- Sleep center: Provides observation, testing, and monitoring of clients as they sleep to identify sleep-related problems
- Electroencephalography (EEG): Records brain waves and ascertains electrical activity in the brain
- Electrocardiogram (EKG): Records electrical activity in the heart
- Electromyogram (EMG): Records electrical activity in body muscles

Therapy Departments

The function of the various therapy departments is to provide specialized treatments and/or rehabilitation services to clients to improve functional level in a specific area. Most hospitals have respiratory therapy and physical therapy departments. Some large teaching hospitals also have occupational therapy and speech therapy departments.

Support Services

Support services meet various other needs in providing care to clients. Pharmacists mix and dispense medications to the various client care units. Nurses then administer the medications to the clients. Dietitians supervise food preparation for all clients. They specifically choose the foods and calculate the amounts for special diets and provide client teaching for those clients on special diets. Social workers help clients deal with psychosocial problems, providing assistance in areas such as housing, finances, and referrals to support groups. Chaplains provide individual counseling to clients and support to families and assist clients in meeting spiritual needs. The admission department handles the admission process by preparing necessary paperwork and ensuring that the ordered preadmission laboratory testing and x-rays are performed. The business office oversees insurance and financial affairs on client discharge from the health care agency. Medical records, also called health information systems, maintains and stores all medical records for every client cared for by the health care agency. Housekeeping and maintenance keep the physical facilities and equipment clean, in good repair, and in proper working order.

Role of the LP/VN

Depending on the geographical location within the nation and nursing shortages, LP/VNs may have limited opportunities in acute care hospitals because of the high acuity level of clients in these facilities. Generally, in an acute care facility, LP/VNs provide direct client care on the general nursing units. This may include assisting with personal hygiene and ambulation, checking vital signs, and administering medications and IV therapy. LP/VNs perform client assessments and work with RNs to formulate nursing diagnoses and write plans of care. Each state has a scope of practice for the LP/VN. It is the LP/VN's responsibility to know the scope of practice for the state in which he or she is practicing. In some states, an LP/VN performs a partial assessment while another state allows full assessments. The Nurse Practice Act distinguishes between assessment data collection and assessment of the data. Generally, the LP/VN collects data, and then an RN assesses the data and determines the course of client care with the LP/VN's input (JCAHO, 2001). After some years of experience and additional education in specific areas, LP/VNs may work in specialized client care units, such as ICU, CCU, dialysis, and home care, as previously described.

Clients are transferred to rehabilitation centers and subacute facilities because of the short stays within an acute care facility. Some hospitals incorporate subacute units within the acute care facilities. Many LP/VNs are hired in rehabilitation centers and subacute facilities.

LONG-TERM CARE

Long-term care refers to the various services provided to individuals having an ongoing need for health care. Traditionally, long-term care has meant a community-based nursing home licensed for skilled or intermediate care. The rights of residents of long-term care facilities are regulated by the Omnibus Budget Reconciliation Act (OBRA) of 1987 (Table 6-1). There is a great demand for this level of care, and there is also a market for other levels of long-term care. It is estimated that by 2030, more than 8 million seniors will be residing in nursing homes It is estimated that by 2050, the older adult population will more than double to 87 million persons (Hollinger-Smith, 2005). Currently, 1.6 million persons live in 17,000 nursing homes. Of those residents, 90% are older than age 65, with almost half older than age 85 (Info USA & U.S. Department of State, 2008).

The growing population of elderly persons has caused tremendous changes in health care delivery. Various housing options are now part of the package of services available. The least restrictive level of care, appropriate for the client's needs, is generally the most cost effective. The Joint Commission has established standards for pain assessment and treatment in long-term care facilities (JCAHO, 2004; JCAHO, 2007).

TABLE 6-1 Residents' Rights—Long-Term Care

This is an abbreviated version of the Resident's Rights as set forth in the Omnibus Budget Reconciliation Act. This document must be given to all residents and/or their families prior to admission to any long-term care facility.

1. **The resident has the right to free choice, including the right to:**
   - choose an attending physician
   - full advance information about changes in care or treatment
   - participate in the assessment and care planning process
   - self-administration of medications
   - consent to participate in experimental research
2. **The resident has the right to freedom from abuse and restraints, including freedom from:**
   - physical, sexual, mental abuse
   - corporal punishment and involuntary seclusion
   - physical and chemical restraints
3. **The resident has the right to privacy including privacy for:**
   - treatment and nursing care
   - receiving/sending mail
   - telephone calls
   - visitors
4. **The resident has the right to confidentiality of personal and clinical records.**
5. **The resident has the right to accommodation of needs including:**
   - choices about life
   - receiving assistance in maintaining independence
6. **The resident has the right to voice grievances.**
7. **The resident has the right to organize and participate in family and resident groups.**
8. **The resident has the right to participate in social, religious, and community activities including the right to:**
   - vote
   - keep religious items in the room
   - attend religious services
9. **The resident has the right to examine survey results and correction plans.**
10. **The resident has the right to manage personal funds.**
11. **The resident has the right to information about eligibility for Medicare/Medicaid funds.**
12. **The resident has the right to file complaints about abuse, neglect, or misappropriation of property.**
13. **The resident has the right to information about advocacy groups.**
14. **The resident has the right to immediate and unlimited access to family or relatives.**
15. **The resident has the right to share a room with the spouse if they are both residents in the same facility.**
16. **The resident has the right to perform or not perform work for the facility if it is medically appropriate for the resident to work.**
17. **The resident has the right to remain in the facility except in certain circumstances.**
18. **The resident has the right to personal possessions.**
19. **The resident has the right to notification of change in condition.**

(As determined by Omnibus Budget Reconciliation Act [OBRA] of 1987)

LONG-TERM CARE FACILITIES

A **long-term care facility** may be licensed for either intermediate care or skilled nursing care. Long-term care facilities provide services to individuals who have continuing health care needs but are not acutely ill yet cannot function independently at home. Intermediate care facilities (ICFs) may be certified for Medicaid funding but are not certified for reimbursement from Medicare. Skilled nursing facilities (SNFs) are eligible to be certified by both Medicare and Medicaid, but not all facilities choose to do so. These facilities were formerly called rest homes, nursing homes, or convalescent centers. An *extended care facility* (ECF) is any facility that provides care for a long period of time and could refer to either an intermediate or a skilled facility. Every facility that receives government funds from any source is required by law to comply with OBRA regulations. It is estimated that 60% of persons over age 65 will need long-term care at some time in their lives (Info USA & U.S. Department of State, 2008).

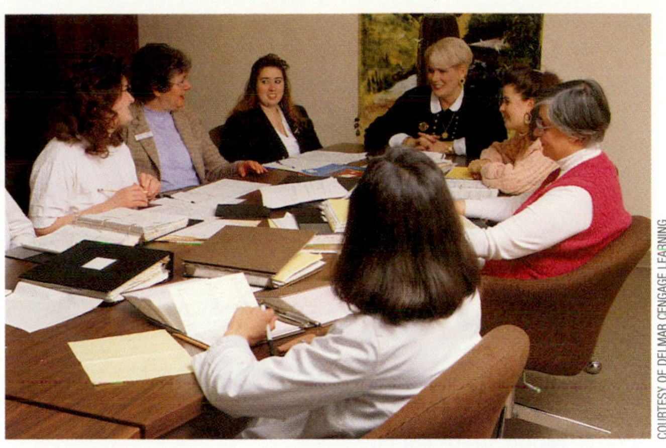

COURTESY OF DELMAR CENGAGE LEARNING

FIGURE 6-1 **An interdisciplinary team plans a client's care with the client's family as part of the team.**

Today's restorative philosophy of care directs the interdisciplinary team, which emphasizes assisting the client (usually called resident) to attain and maintain the highest level of physical, mental, and psychosocial function. The approach is holistic with family members part of the care team (see Figure 6-1).

Many facilities have special units for the care of residents with specific problems, such as Alzheimer's, diabetes, and respiratory disorders.

SUBACUTE CARE

Subacute care is a concept designed to provide services for clients who are out of the acute stage of their illnesses but who still require ongoing treatments, skilled nursing, and monitoring. The clients have complex medical needs. It is intended to fill the gap between the acute care hospital and the traditional long-term care facility (Cheek, Tumlinson, & Blum, 2005).

Subacute care facilities are usually part of a freestanding long-term care facility. Services may include intensive rehabilitation therapies, postsurgical services, wound and pain management, care for clients with acquired immunodeficiency syndrome (AIDS), oncology care, peritoneal dialysis, ventilator care, intravenous therapy, nutritional support, and cardiac monitoring. Many subacute care units specialize in one or two of these areas. Clients stay from 20 to 30 days. Thorough discharge planning with client teaching are essential components to the plan of care.

CONTINUING CARE RETIREMENT COMMUNITIES

Continuing Care Retirement Communities (CCRCs) are designed to provide continuous care as the individual's health care needs change. Such levels are the following:

- Independent living apartments on the premises with housekeeping services and meals provided.
- **Assisted living**—a combination of housing and services for those who need help with ADLs.
- Full care—short-term for persons recovering from a temporary disorder or permanent for long-term illnesses such as Alzheimer's disease; the CCRC health care facility may be licensed as either intermediate or skilled.

Usually, a fee is charged on entry and then a monthly fee. The client must show proof of adequate financial resources for acceptance into the system. The residents are secure knowing that they will receive care for the rest of their lives. Most CCRCs want individuals to enter the system when they can live independently in the apartments. The CCRC health care facility may be certified for Medicaid for clients who exhaust their financial resources; it may also be certified for Medicare for clients qualified to receive such services. Neither Medicaid nor Medicare will pay for the independent living or assisted living areas of a CCRC.

ASSISTED LIVING

Assisted living provides housing and services for those who require assistance with activities of daily living (ADLs). No nursing care is provided. These persons cannot live alone but do not need 24-hour care. The individual's independence and freedom of choice are maintained. This care may be available in a freestanding facility or as part of a long-term care facility or CCRC as previously described. The monthly fee covers meals, rent, utilities, housekeeping services, assistance with ADLs, health promotion, medication management, exercise programs, and transportation (Assisted Living Federation of America [ALFA], 2008a).

There are an estimated 20,000 assisted living residences in the United States with more than a million residents (ALFA, 2008a). The typical resident is a female (single or widowed) in her 80s (ALFA, 2008a). Assisted living residences are licensed by the state. The average cost is $3,241 per month and is paid mainly from personal funds (AFLA, 2008b). Some residents have financial assistant programs that aid with the cost. The Department of Veterans Affairs assists with assisted living costs for veterans and their widows if the veteran served in wartime.

ADULT DAY CARE

Adult day care centers may be freestanding, located in a private home or as a separate part of a long-term care facility. It is a protective setting for adults who are unable to stay alone but who do not need 24-hour care. A variety of services are provided. The centers are usually open 5 days a week and serve two or three meals. The daily or hourly fee does not include meals. Services may be comprehensive offering nursing care and some rehabilitation or limited to socialization. Working persons whose spouse or parent living with them cannot be left alone often use these services. Fifty-two percent of day care clients have some degree of cognitive impairment (National Adult Day Services Association, 2008).

RESPITE CARE

Respite care may be offered by long-term care facilities, adult day care centers, or private homes. It provides a break to caregivers for a few hours a week, for an occasional weekend, or for longer vacations. Supervision, meals, and planned activities are included.

FOSTER CARE

Foster homes for individuals unable to live independently yet who do not require care in a health care facility are being investigated in some states. These homes are similar to the foster home concept for children.

Role of the LP/VN

Long-term care facilities probably offer more career opportunities for the LP/VN than any other type of health care described in this chapter. Small facilities may use the LP/VN as supervisor during the evening or night shift according to the LP/VN scope of practice within the state. The LP/VN might have charge of one unit with an RN as house supervisor in larger facilities. The nurse needs good assessment skills and the ability to make nursing judgments based on assessment findings. The LP/VN may also be expected to coordinate and supervise the work of nursing assistants. LP/VNs may take the Certification Examination for Practical and Vocational Nurses in Long-Term Care (CEPN-LTC™ given by the National Council of State Boards of Nursing (NCSBN). Those who pass the examination are certified in long-term care and may use the initials "CLTC" to signify their certification.

OUTPATIENT CARE

Outpatient care includes services provided without actually admitting the client to a health care facility. Same-day surgery (in and out within 24 hours) may be found as a unit in an acute care hospital or as a freestanding facility. Various clinics and treatment centers offer diagnostic testing, chemotherapy, physical therapy, and other services.

Role of the LP/VN

The major role of LP/VNs is preparing the client for the treatment or procedure, checking vital signs, answering questions, and doing discharge teaching. They may also assist with the test or procedure.

HOME HEALTH CARE

Home care is the fastest-growing segment of health care and encompasses many services delivered to persons in their homes. Clients may receive IV therapy, chemotherapy, ventilator care, and parenteral nutrition at home. Nurse specialists often care for complicated cases involving wounds, diabetes, and respiratory or cardiac problems.

Medicare-certified agencies (7,747 in 1999) provide intermittent care to persons meeting the criteria for care (National Association for Home Care and Hospice (NAHC), 2008a). A registered nurse calls on the client a certain specified number of times each week to assess the client's condition, deliver skilled nursing care, and supervise the work of LP/VNs and unlicensed workers. Nursing assistants give personal care, check vital signs, and do positioning, transfers, and passive range-of-motion exercises. In addition, the agency may provide therapists and social workers to serve their clients, also on an intermittent basis. These services are time limited by Medicare and are not reimbursable if the client does not require skilled care.

The home health agency may provide homemaker services for light housekeeping tasks, companion services, transportation for outpatient care, and pain management. The home health nurse must be aware of the availability of respite care for family members needing a break from the rigors of caregiving and may need to encourage them to do so. Client rights and responsibilities are listed in Table 6-2.

Table 6-2 Client Rights and Responsibilities—Home Care

Clients receiving home health care services or their families possess basic rights and responsibilities. These include:

The right to:

1. be treated with dignity, consideration, and respect.
2. have their property treated with respect.
3. receive a timely response from the agency to requests for service.
4. be fully informed on admission of the care and treatment that will be provided, how much it will cost, and how payment will be handled.
5. know in advance if they will be responsible for any payment.
6. be informed in advance of any changes in care.
7. receive care from professionally trained personnel, to know their names and responsibilities.
8. participate in planning care.
9. refuse treatment and to be told the consequences of this action.
10. expect confidentiality of all information.
11. be informed of anticipated termination of service.
12. be referred elsewhere if denied services solely based on ability to pay.
13. know how to make a complaint or recommend a change in agency policies and services.

The responsibility to:

1. remain under a doctor's care while receiving services.
2. provide the agency with a complete health history.
3. provide the agency all requested insurance and financial information.
4. sign the required consents and releases for insurance billing.
5. participate in care by asking questions, expressing concerns, stating whether information is not understood.
6. provide a safe home environment in which care is given.
7. cooperate with the doctor, the staff, and other caregivers.
8. accept consequences for any refusal of treatment.
9. abide by agency policies that restrict duties the staff may perform.
10. advise agency administration of any dissatisfaction or problems with care.

COURTESY OF DELMAR CENGAGE LEARNING

PROFESSIONALTIP

Sharps Injuries in the Home

- A recent study found that 34.9% of home health care nurses had a sharps injury during their career. In analyzing the data from 2001–2007, no safety sharp was used in 65% of the sharp injury incidences (Quinn et al., 2008).
- OSHA cannot regulate private homes.
- Home health employers are responsible for meeting OSHA requirements that are not site specific, including sharps with built-in injury protection.

Role of the LP/VN

The role of the LP/VN in home care is expanding, with 56,610 LP/VNs working in home health care. Also, there are 126,453 RNs, 458,685 home care aids, 21,196 physical therapists, 12,564 social workers, and 6,272 occupational therapists working in home care (NAHC, 2008a). The LP/VN responsibilities vary among agencies. All nurses working in home care must have excellent assessment skills and a keen ability to identify actual and potential problems. Working with the family may be a greater challenge than meeting client needs. A major responsibility for the home health nurse is teaching the client and family. Clients with chronic health problems have ongoing needs after home health care is discontinued. They and their family caregivers must be taught the following:

The disease process

- Complications that may occur
- How to prevent complications
- Signs and symptoms of complications
- How to reduce risk factors, such as dietary adaptations and exercise programs

Medications

- Actions of medications
- Special administration guidelines, such as timing related to meals
- Side effects

Special skills

- Drawing up and administering insulin or other injectables
- Using a blood glucose monitor
- Changing dressings
- Monitoring vital signs
- Using special client care equipment, adaptive devices, and assistive devices

Documentation and communication

- How to keep records for nurse or physician visit, for example, blood glucose, blood pressure, and weight
- How and when to contact the home health nurse
- How and when to contact the physician
- How and when to contact emergency services

HOSPICE

Hospice is humane, compassionate care provided to clients who can no longer benefit from curative treatment and have 6 months or less to live. The special care is designed to provide sensitive support, allowing clients to be alert and pain free and have other symptoms managed so that the last days are spent with dignity and quality of life at home or in a homelike setting. This is sometimes referred to as palliative care.

The first hospice in the United States began in 1974. Today, there are 3,257 Medicare participating hospices, and in 2006, there were a total of 4,500 hospice programs. In 2006, 964,614 Medicare clients and their families received hospice services (Hospice Foundation of America [HFA], 2008).

The primary physician must refer the client to hospice. Care and support are provided to both client and family by a team consisting of the physician, nurses, counselors, therapists, social worker, aides, and volunteers. The team regards dying as a normal process and does nothing to hasten or postpone death. Relief of pain and other distressing symptoms is provided. The client is supported to live as actively as possible until death. The family is supported to help them cope during the client's illness and in their bereavement after the client's death. Health care workers may also need support because the task of caring for the dying is often quite stressful but can be fulfilling because most of the time the care encompasses all aspects of pure nursing care.

Benefits for hospice are included in most private health care insurance, HMOs, and managed care; Medicare; and in 43 states plus the District of Columbia by Medicaid. Forty-four states have licensure laws for hospice programs. Some programs are certified voluntarily by Medicare and accredited by the JCAHO or Community Health Accreditation Program (CHAP) (HFA, 2008).

Other health care environments include schools, community nursing centers, adult day care centers/programs, rural primary care hospitals, and industrial clinics. Table 6-3 describes arenas of care, services provided, and the nurse's role.

PROFESSIONALTIP

Hospice Settings

Hospice care may be implemented in a variety of settings: the client's home, a special area of hospitals or nursing homes, or freestanding inpatient facilities. Most clients receive care at home. In 2006, approximately 36% of all deaths in the United States were given care by hospice personnel (National Hospice and Palliative Care Organization, 2007).

CRITICAL THINKING

Working in Various Facilities

What are the pros and cons related to working for an acute care hospital, home health agency, hospice, or long-term care facility?

TABLE 6-3 Health Care Arenas

ARENA	SERVICES PROVIDED	NURSE'S ROLE
Acute care hospital	Diagnosis and treatment of illnesses (chronic and acute) Acute inpatient services Diagnostic procedures Surgical interventions Ambulatory care services Critical (intensive) care Rehabilitative care	Provide ongoing assessment Caregiver and educator Maintain client safety Coordinate care and collaborate with other health care providers Initiate discharge planning
Extended-care (long-term care) facilities (e.g., nursing homes, skilled nursing facilities)	Intermediate and long-term care for people who have chronic illnesses and are unable to care for themselves Restorative and rehabilitative care until client is ready for discharge home	Plan and coordinate care Provide care directed toward meeting basic needs (e.g., nutrition, hydration, comfort, elimination) Administer medications, treatments, and other therapeutic modalities Provide teaching and counseling
Outpatient (clinics, physician's offices, ambulatory treatment centers)	Treatment of illness (acute and chronic) Diagnostic testing Select surgical procedures	*Traditional role:* Prepare client for examination Check vital signs Assist with diagnostic tests *Expanded role:* Perform physical (or mental status) examination Provide teaching and counseling In some settings, advanced practice registered nurses (APRNs) act as primary care providers
Home health care agencies	Wide range of services, including curative and rehabilitative	Provide skilled nursing care Coordinate health-promotion activities (e.g., education)
Hospice	Care of individuals who have terminal illnesses Improve the quality of life until death	Promote comfort measures Provide pain control Support grieving families Educate family/client
Schools (school-based clinics [SBCs])	Federally funded to provide physical and mental health services in middle and high schools	Coordinate health-promotion and disease prevention activities Provide health education Treat minor illnesses
Community nursing centers	Direct access to professional services	Promote health and wellness Treat client's responses to health problems
Adult daycare centers/ programs	Maintain safety for clients Provide social experiences Monitor health	Provide safe environment Encourage socialization Health assessment and promotion
Rural primary care hospitals (RPCHs)	Stabilize clients until they are physiologically able to be transferred to more skilled facilities	Perform assessments and provide emergency care
Industrial clinics	Maintain safety and health of workers	Conduct ongoing screenings Provide preventive services (e.g., tuberculosis testing) Coordinate health-promotion activities Provide education for safety Provide urgent care as needed Maintain health records

COURTESY OF DELMAR CENGAGE LEARNING

REHABILITATION

Rehabilitation is the process of helping individuals reach their optimal level of physical, mental, and psychosocial functioning. This is accomplished by modifying the effects of the disability, preventing complications, and increasing independence. The individual's self-esteem is increased, thus improving the quality of life. Rehabilitation works to increase the client's ability to complete the basic ADLs and the instrumental activities of daily living (IADLs). ADLs include grooming and hygiene, dressing, eating, mobility, and toileting. IADLs include higher-level tasks such as using the telephone, household and money management, and driving a car. The goal is to teach clients to manage their own care when there is limited potential for regaining total independence.

The Interdisciplinary Health Care Team

An interdisciplinary health care team (IHCT) is the essential component to the rehabilitation process. Client and family are the focus and are encouraged to participate in the planning of care. The client determines the amount of family participation. The professional members of the team are selected based on the needs of the client. The physician, rehabilitation nurses, social workers, dietitians, physical and occupational therapists, a speech-language pathologist, recreational therapists, and mental health professionals are usually required to provide services (see Figure 6-2).

Each discipline completes an assessment and shares this information at the care planning conference so that a consensus among members (including the client and family) can be reached. This avoids both duplication of services and fragmented care. A holistic approach is used so that the client's physical, mental, and psychosocial needs are identified.

Functional Assessment and Evaluation for Rehabilitation

Clients who need rehabilitation are screened before admission to a program. Assessments are completed by health care professionals whose services may be required by the client. The purpose of screening is to select the best setting for services. Criteria for admission to a program usually require that the client be the following:

- Medically stable
- Able to learn
- Able to sit supported for at least 1 hour per day and to actively participate in the program

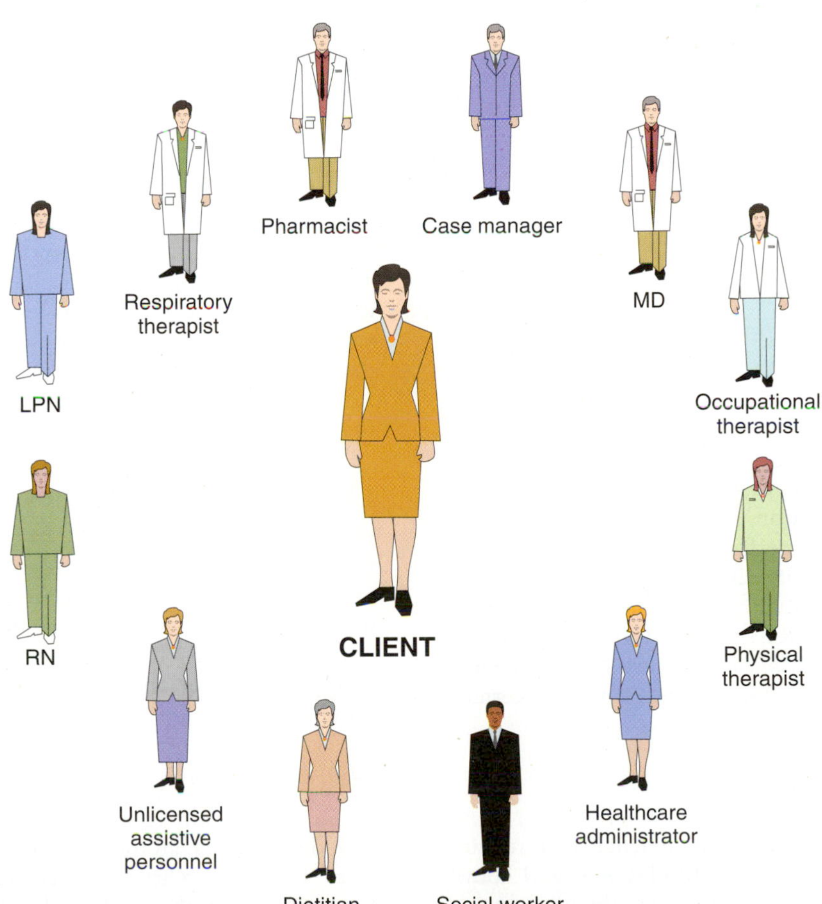

COURTESY OF DELMAR CENGAGE LEARNING

FIGURE 6-2 The Interdisciplinary Health Care Team

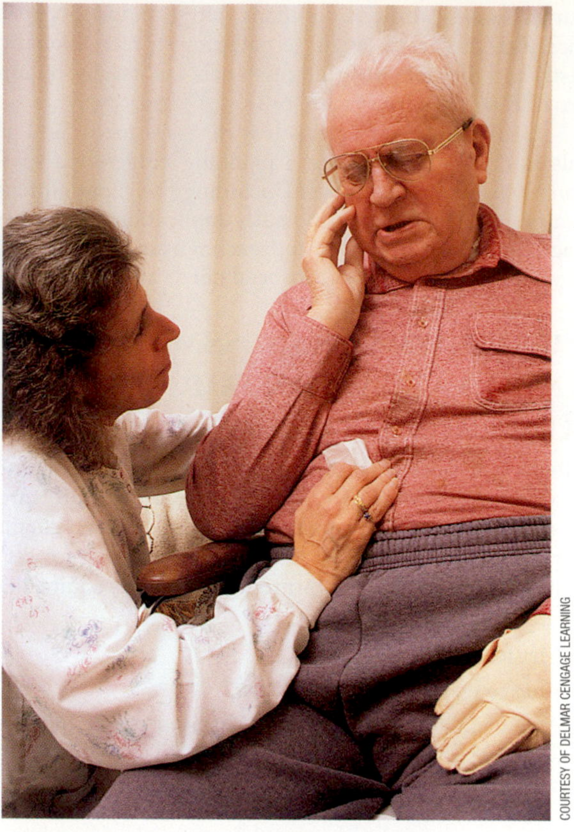

FIGURE 6-3 **The role of a rehabilitative nurse is caregiver, client advocate, counselor, and coordinator of care.**

Interdisciplinary programs may stipulate that the client has disabilities in two or more areas of function:

- Mobility
- Performance of ADLs
- Bowel and bladder control
- Cognition
- Emotional function
- Pain management
- Swallowing
- Communication

Several standardized assessment instruments are designed to evaluate cognition, speech and language, motor function, mobility, and the performance of ADLs. There are additional tools that identify the client's risk for pressure ulcer formation and potential for bowel and bladder management for incontinence. Refer to the AHCPR publication *Post-Stroke Rehabilitation, Clinical Guideline Number 16* for a complete description of assessment instruments (Kernich, 1996).

Role of the LP/VN

Rehabilitation nursing is a specialty practice that requires specialized knowledge, skills, and attitudes. A sound knowledge base in the anatomy and physiology of the neurological, musculoskeletal, gastrointestinal, and urological systems is a prerequisite. The nurse must have excellent clinical skills in the areas of therapeutic positioning, range-of-motion exercises, transfers, ambulation, and ADLs. The nurse is responsible for planning measures to prevent complications, such as impaired skin integrity and contractures, and to implement interventions for dysphagia, incontinence, and other identified problems.

The nurse, as a member of the interdisciplinary team, may function as caregiver, client advocate, counselor, and coordinator of care (see Figure 6-3). The nurse needs to understand the roles and responsibilities of each discipline and how to relate to each discipline.

Rehabilitation Settings

Rehabilitation takes place in a variety of settings. It begins during the acute stage of illness when the client's medical condition stabilizes. Rehabilitative services are often needed after discharge from acute care, necessitating transfer to a hospital inpatient program, an outpatient rehabilitation program, a home rehabilitation program, or a skilled nursing facility. Entry into a rehabilitation program should reflect a consensus among the client, family or significant others, physician, and the rehabilitation program.

Hospital Inpatient Program

Hospitals may have a separate rehabilitation unit, or services may be available in a freestanding hospital specializing in rehabilitation services. The hospitals are staffed by a full range of rehabilitation professionals with RNs and a physician skilled in rehabilitation (physiatrist) available 24 hours a day.

Skilled Nursing Facility

The skilled nursing facility offering rehabilitation services may be hospital based or community based. Programs are similar to those offered in hospital settings, with a full range of services and health care professionals. Physician coverage varies, but professional nursing care is provided 24 hours a day. Families should research the services available to make sure their loved ones are receiving the best rehabilitation for their situation.

Outpatient Rehabilitation

Outpatient services offered by hospital-based rehabilitation programs range from occasional visits to three or four visits per week. Day hospital programs are another form of outpatient services but require the client to spend several hours per day for 3 to 5 days per week at the hospital. Availability of transportation is a prerequisite for all outpatient programs.

Home Rehabilitation

Some home health agencies provide a full scope of services, including nursing, all therapies, rehabilitation, and social services. The accessibility of services varies greatly depending on the availability of therapists in the area.

SAMPLE NURSING CARE PLAN

The Client Requiring Rehabilitation

M.J., 65 years old, was admitted to a skilled nursing facility following hospitalization for a right cerebral hemisphere stroke. He is unable to purposefully change position without assistance. His gag reflex is weakened, swallowing is delayed, and there is coughing after swallowing. M.J. has smoked for 50 years and is still doing so. Rehabilitation was initiated in the hospital. A feeding tube was put in place with the goal to assist M.J. to regain his swallowing ability so the tube can be removed. M.J. frequently expresses his discouragement with his dependency on the staff. He is married and lives in the community with his wife. M.J. had been retired for 1 year before the stroke. His wife, A.J., works full time. Two adult children live in other states. A.J. hopes that her husband will regain adequate mobility skills so she can eventually take him home.

NURSING DIAGNOSIS 1 *Impaired Physical Mobility* related to musculoskeletal, neuromuscular, and sensoriperceptual impairments as evidenced by inability to purposefully change position of body without assistance

Nursing Outcomes Classification (NOC)
Ambulation: Walking
Body Positioning: Self-Initiated

Nursing Interventions Classification (NIC)
Exercise Therapy: Ambulation
Positioning

PLANNING/OUTCOMES	NURSING INTERVENTIONS	RATIONALE
M.J. will maintain current level of range of motion in all joints.	Change position at least every 2 hours. Do passive range-of-motion exercises twice a day on affected extremities.	Prevents contracture formation and pressure ulcers. Hemiplegic limbs are flaccid immediately after stroke and then become spastic.
M.J. will remain free of contractures.	Assist with active range-of-motion exercises on unaffected extremities. Teach to do self-range-of-motion exercises when condition permits.	Maintains joint mobility and prevents contracture formation, also increases strength and endurance.
M.J. will begin program of progressive mobilization.	Teach M.J. to move in bed: • Begin in supine position with the knees bent and feet flat in bed. • Raise the hips by pressing his heels down. • Stabilize the affected limb by nurse exerting pressure downward through the thigh just above the knee while assisting the client to lift the pelvis clear of the bed.	Increases the client's bed mobility. The recovery of a client with a stroke is dependent on the cooperative efforts of several interdisciplinary team members.
	Consult with physical therapist about program for progressive mobilization.	The physical therapist is an expert in mobility.

EVALUATION

Range of joint motion is preserved. No contractions noted. Progress in mobilization is achieved; movement in bed, transfers with 1 to 2 assists.

(*Continues*)

SAMPLE NURSING CARE PLAN (Continued)

NURSING DIAGNOSIS 2 *Impaired **S**wallowing* related to neuromuscular impairment as evidenced by weakened gag reflex, delayed swallowing, and coughing after swallowing

Nursing Outcomes Classification (NOC)
Swallowing Status

Nursing Interventions Classification (NIC)
Swallowing Therapy

PLANNING/OUTCOMES	NURSING INTERVENTIONS	RATIONALE
M.J. will swallow without aspirating.	Consult with speech-language pathologist regarding video-recorded fluoroscopy for swallowing evaluation.	Makes a definitive diagnosis of impaired swallowing and is the basis for intervention.
	Serve semisolid foods of medium consistency. Use a commercial thickener for liquids. Avoid milk, citrus juices, and water.	Requires less manipulation in the mouth and allows concentration on swallowing rather than chewing. Liquids are more manageable when thickened. Milk and citrus juices stimulate production of saliva.
	Allow rest period before eating. Position client at 60- to 90-degree angle before, during, and for 1 hour after eating.	Decreases risk of aspiration.
	Maintain head in midline with neck slightly flexed.	Facilitates the passage of food through the pharynx.
	Face M.J., avoid haste.	Allows feeder to evaluate the eating process.
	Minimize distractions, keep conversation minimal.	Focuses the client's attention on eating.
	Allow M.J. to see and smell food. Give verbal descriptions. Use regular metal teaspoon, give one-half teaspoon at a time.	Sensory cues promote awareness of eating.
	Place food on unaffected side of mouth. Teach to hold food in mouth, think about swallowing, and then swallow twice.	Buccal pocketing of food in the cheek on the affected side is common after a stroke.

EVALUATION
There are no signs of aspiration.

NURSING DIAGNOSIS 3 *Situational Low **S**elf-Esteem* related to the functional impairments of inability to move and delayed swallowing as evidenced by verbal expression of discouragement

Nursing Outcomes Classification (NOC)
Grief Resolution
Psychosocial Adjustment: Life Change

Nursing Interventions Classification (NIC)
Grief Work Facilitation
Coping Enhancement

SAMPLE NURSING CARE PLAN (Continued)

PLANNING/OUTCOMES	NURSING INTERVENTIONS	RATIONALE
M.J. will verbalize acceptance of self, situation, and lifestyle changes.	Assess for signs of severe or prolonged grieving.	May indicate need for counseling.
	Assess client's interactions with significant others.	Others may reinforce the concepts of helplessness and invalidism.
	Listen in nonjudgmental fashion to comments about situation.	Builds trust and encourages verbalization of thoughts.

EVALUATION

M.J. is progressing through all rehabilitation therapies and presents no signs of prolonged grieving.

SUMMARY

- There has been a significant increase in the growth of nonacute care settings.
- Medicare (federal funds) and Medicaid (state and federal funds) are major sources of health care payment, especially for the elderly and permanently disabled.
- Rehabilitation can be provided in a variety of settings.
- There is a need for the services and skills of the LP/VN in all health care services. Experience and additional education may be required for employment in special care settings.

REVIEW QUESTIONS

1. Subacute care is most often provided:
   1. in a step-down unit of the hospital.
   2. in a special care unit of a skilled care facility.
   3. for clients who are terminally ill.
   4. for clients who require life support.
2. Which of the following clients would be most likely to benefit from rehabilitation services?
   1. Mr. J, 64 years old, had a stroke, is responsive and stable.
   2. Mrs. B, 89 years old, has Alzheimer's disease in the fourth stage.
   3. Miss Z, 26 years old, is recovering from pneumonia.
   4. Mr. K, 56 years old, has terminal cancer of the lung.
3. As a member of the interdisciplinary health care team, the LP/VN must be able to:
   1. participate in the planning of client care.
   2. plan the appropriate diet for clients.
   3. teach the new amputee how to walk with a prosthesis.
   4. provide alternative methods of communication for the client with recent stroke.
4. In the home health care setting, it is essential that the LP/VN possess skills in:
   1. advanced intravenous therapy.
   2. respiratory therapy treatments.
   3. physical assessment.
   4. planning and providing speech therapy.
5. In a long-term care facility, the LP/VN may serve as the:
   1. charge nurse of a unit.
   2. physical therapist.
   3. clinical nurse specialist.
   4. social worker.
6. Agency certification: (Select all that apply.)
   1. is regulated by the state.
   2. is required for government reimbursement.
   3. rules are generated by federal government.
   4. establishes and evaluates compliance with rules and regulations.
   5. assures that delivery of care and service is above minimum standards.
   6. is a voluntary process.
7. Long-term care services include: (Select all that apply.)
   1. assisted living.
   2. acute care hospital.
   3. subacute care.
   4. hospice.
   5. outpatient care facility.
8. The nurse's roles, as a member of the interdisciplinary team, are: (Select all that apply.)
   1. instruct in ambulation techniques.
   2. provide care.
   3. evaluate home environment.
   4. order medications.
   5. advocate for the client.
   6. coordinate client care.

9. The goal of rehabilitation is to:
   1. improve quality of life.
   2. assist the client to reach optimal physical, mental, and psychosocial level.
   3. restore the client's activities of daily living only.
   4. regain total independence.
10. Nonacute arenas of health care includes a(n): (Select all that apply.)
   1. acute care hospital.
   2. school-based clinic.
   3. industrial clinic.
   4. adult day care center/program.
   5. skilled nursing home.
   6. home health care agency.

REFERENCES/SUGGESTED READINGS

American Association of Retired Persons. (1998). *A profile of older Americans*. Washington, DC: U.S. Department of Health and Human Services.

Assisted Living Federation of America (ALFA). (2003). What is assisted living? Retrieved September 13, 2008 from http://www.hospicefoundation.org/hospiceInfo/dearabby/default.asp

Assisted Living Federation of America. (2008a). About assisted living. Retrieved September 13, 2008, from http://www.alfa.org/i4a/pages/Index.cfm?pageid=3285

Assisted Living Federation of America. (2008b). As costs continue rising, assisted living remains the more affordable care choice. Retrieved September 13, 2008, from http://www.alfa.org/i4a/pages/Index.cfm?pageIC=4706

Assisted Living Info. (2003). What is assisted living? Retrieved on 5-17-09 at http://www.assistedlivinginfo.com/alserve.html

Barker, E. (1999). Life care planning. *RN, 62*(3), 58–61.

Boon, T. (1998). Don't forget the hospice option. *RN, 61*(2), 30–33.

Bral, E. (1998). Caring for adults with chronic cancer pain. *American Journal of Nursing, 98*(4), 26–32.

Bulecheck, G., Butcher, H., McCloskey, J., & Dochterman, J., eds. (2008). *Nursing Interventions Classification (NIC)* (5th ed.). St. Louis, MO: Mosby/Elsevier.

Cheek, M., Tumlinson, A., & Blum, J. (2005). American health keeping pace—Trends, options and opportunities in long term care. Retrieved September 12, 2008, from http://www.ahcancal.org/research_data/funding/Documents/Avalere_TrendsOptionsAndOpportunitiesInLTC.pdf

Feldkamp, J. (2002). The legal landscape of long-term care. *RN, 65*(4), 61–62.

Ferrell, B., & Coyle, N. (2002). An overview of palliative nursing care. *American Journal of Nursing, 102*(5), 26–31.

Ferrell, B., & Coyle, N. (Eds.). (2005). *Textbook of palliative nursing* (2nd ed.). Oxford: Oxford University Press.

Grove, N. (1997). Helping families select a nursing home. *RN, 60*(3), 37–40.

Haddad, A. (2003). When should you suggest hospice? *RN, 66*(5), 27–30.

Hollinger-Smith, L. (2005). Averting a care crisis. *Extended Care Product News, 98*(2), 18–23.

Hospice Foundation of America. (2008). What is hospice? Retrieved September 13, 2008, from http://www.hospicefoundation.org/hospiceInfo/dearabby/default.asp

Info USA & U.S. Department of State. (2008). What is long-term care? Retrieved September 12, 2008, from http://usinfo.state.gov/infousa/government/social/longtermcare.html

Joint Commission. (2001). LPN's performing assessment. Retrieved September 12, 2008, from http://www.jointcommission.org/AccreditationPrograams/Hospitals/Standards/FAQs/Provis

Joint Commission. (2004). Nutritional, functional, and pain assessments and screens. Retrieved September 12, 2008, from http://www.joint commission.org/AccreditationPrograms/Hospitals/Standards/FAQs/Provis

Joint Commission. (2007). Provision of care, treatment, and services. Retrieved September 12, 2008, from http://www.jointcommission.org/NR/rdpm;ures/D315C586-0D2B-4DB4-A9E4-FFC7681A55CC/0/LTC2008PCChapter.pdf

Kennison, M. (1999). A case study in care. *RN, 62*(1), 46–48.

Kernich, C. (1996). Post-stroke rehabilitation: Clinical practice guideline, number 16. *Journal of Neuroscience Nursing, 4*, 1–248.

Kovner, C., & Harrington, C. (2003). Nursing care in assisted living facilities. *American Journal of Nursing*, 102(1), 97–98.

Lattanzi-Licht, M. E. (1998). *The hospice choice: In pursuit of a peaceful death*. New York: Simon and Schuster/Fireside.

Loeb, J., & Pasero, C. (2000). JCAHO standards in long-term care. *American Journal of Nursing, 100*(5), 22–23.

Mitty, E. (2003). Assisted living and the role of nursing, *American Journal of Nursing, 103*(8), 32–43.

Moorhead, S., Johnson, J., & Mass, M. (2004). *Nursing Outcomes Classification (NOC)* (3rd ed.). St. Louis, MO: Mosby.

National Adult Day Services Association. (2008). Adult day services: Overview and facts. Retrieved September 13, 2008, from http://www.nadasa.org/adsfacts/default.asp

National Association for Home Care and Hospice. (2008a). Basic statistics about home care. Retrieved September 13, 2008, from http://www.nahc.org/home.html

National Association for Home Care and Hospice. (2008b). Hospice facts and statistics. Retrieved September 13, 2008, from http://www.nahc.org/facts

National Center for Assisted Living. (2006). Assisted living resident profile. Retrieved September 13, 2008, from http://www.ncal.org/about/resident.cfm

National Hospice and Palliative Care Organization. (2007). NHPCO facts and figures: Hospice care in America. Retrieved September 13, 2008, from http://www.nhpco.org/files/public/Statistics_Research/NHPCO_facts-and-figures_Nov2007.pdf

NewsHour. (2008). Today's nursing homes. Retrieved September 12, 2008, from http://www.pbs.org/newshour/health/nursinghomes

Puopolo, A. (1999). Gaining confidence to talk about end-of-life care. *Nursing99, 29*(7), 49–51.

Quinn, M., Markkanen, P., Galligan, C., Chalupka, S., Kim, H., Gore, R., et al. (2008). *Risk of sharps injuries and blood exposures among home health care workers* (182600). San Diego, CA: American Public Health Association.

Resnick, B., & Fleishell, A. (2002). Developing a restorative care program: A five-step approach that involves the resident. *American Journal of Nursing, 102*(7), 91–95.

Skokal, W. (2000). IV push at home? *RN, 63*(10), 26–29.

Ufema, J. (1999). Reflections on death and dying. *Nursing99, 29*(6), 56–59.

RESOURCES

American Association of Homes and Services for the Aging (AAHSA), http://www.aahsa.org

American Association of Retired Persons (AARP), http://www.aarp.org

American Health Care Association (AHCA), http://www.ahca.org

American Hospital Association (AHA), http://www.ahcanca.org

Assisted Living Federation of America (ALFA), http://www.alfa.org

Association of Rehabilitation Nurses (ARN), http://www.rehabnurse.org

Department of Health and Human Services (DHHS), http://www.hhs.gov

Home Healthcare Nurses Association (HHNA), http://www.hhna.org

Hospice Association of America (HAA), http://www.nahc.org/HAA

Hospice Education Institute, http://www.hospiceworld.org

Hospice Foundation of America (HFA), http://www.hospicefoundation.org

National Adult Day Services Association, Inc. (NADSA), http://www.nadsa.org/ncoa

National Association for Home Care (NAHC), http://www.nahc.org

National Center for Assisted Living (NCAL), http://www.ncal.org

National Citizens' Coalition for Nursing Home Reform (NCCNHR), http://www.nccnhr.org

National Hospice and Palliative Care Organization (NHPCO), http://www.nhpco.org

National Rehabilitation Association, http://www.nationalrehab.org

National Rehabilitation Information Center (NARIC), http://www.naric.com

UNIT 3 Communication

CHAPTER 7
Communication

MAKING THE CONNECTION

Refer to the following chapters to increase your understanding of communication:

Basic Nursing

- ***Student Nurses Skills for Success***
- ***Legal and Ethical Responsibilities***
- ***Nursing Process/Documentation/ Informatics***
- ***Cultural Considerations***
- ***End-of-Life Care***
- ***Self-Concept***
- ***Complementary/Alternative Therapies***
- ***Assessment***

LEARNING OBJECTIVES

Upon completion of this chapter, you should be able to:

- Define key terms.
- Discuss the process of communication and factors that influence it.
- Compare and contrast between verbal and nonverbal communication.
- Utilize therapeutic communication.
- Describe the psychosocial aspects of communication.
- Demonstrate proper telephone communication.
- Communicate effectively with clients and families.
- Communicate with special clients who are visually impaired, hearing impaired, speech impaired, unconscious, and non–English speaking.
- Communicate effectively with terminally ill clients and their families.
- Communicate effectively with other members of the health care team.

KEY TERMS

active listening
aphasia
communication
congruent
dysarthria
dysphasia
empathy
feedback
hearing
interpersonal communication
intrapersonal communication
listening
nonverbal communication
professional boundaries
proxemics
rapport
shift report
telehealth
telemedicine
telenursing
therapeutic communication
verbal communication

INTRODUCTION

Why study communication? Students in a nursing program have generally had a minimum of 17 years of communicating. Have you ever told another person a story and then heard the story repeated by someone else? Or have you ever played the game "telephone," where a message is whispered from one person to another and the last one states the message out loud? In both situations, when you hear the story or message again, it typically has changed from the original. When communicating with a client, family, or another member of the health care team, it is important that the message be sent and received accurately.

This chapter addresses the process of communication; methods of communicating, including verbal and nonverbal communication; and factors that influence communication, such as age, culture, education, language, attention, emotions, and surroundings. Techniques that promote effective (therapeutic) communication are also described, as are barriers to communication, and examples of both are presented. Also explored are psychosocial aspects of communication, such as style, gestures, meaning of time, meaning of space, cultural values, and political correctness, and their importance to the health care system. Finally, communication with the client, family, and health care team as well as self-communication is discussed.

PROCESS OF COMMUNICATION

Communication is the process by which information is exchanged between the sender and receiver. The six aspects of communication are sender, message, channel, receiver, feedback, and influences.

Sender

The person who has a thought, idea, or emotion to convey to another person is called the sender. Messages stem from a person's need to relate to others, to create meanings, and to understand various situations.

Message

The thought, idea, or emotion one person sends to another person is called the message. It is a stimulus produced by the sender and responded to by the receiver. A person's perception (the meaning that the individual assigns to any sensory input) can alter the message.

Channel

The person sending the message must decide how to send the message. The method by which a message may be transmitted is verbal or nonverbal (Table 7-1).

Receiver

The physiological component involves auditory, visual, and kinesthetic processes. The person's psychological processes may enhance or hinder the receiving of messages. For example, anxiety may cause an individual to experience alterations in **hearing** (act or power of perceiving sounds), vision, or feeling.

The cognitive element is the "thinking" part of receiving. It involves interpreting stimuli and converting them into meaning, as in **listening** (interpreting sounds heard and attaching meaning to them).

Feedback

Feedback is a response from the receiver that enables the sender to verify that the message received was the message sent. When these are not the same, more messages are sent and received until the receiver understands the message sent by the sender.

Table 7-1 Methods of Communication

SENDING	RECEIVING	DESCRIPTION	EXAMPLE
Verbal Speaking	Auditory • Hearing • Listening	Receives auditory stimulus Interprets sounds heard and attaches meaning to them	Hears the client say, "My head hurts" Hears loud moaning in a client's room, and nurse checks if the client is in pain
Nonverbal or Verbal Writing Gestures Facial Expressions Body Posture Eye Contact Physical Appearance	Visual • Sight • Reading • Observation • Perception	Receives a visual stimulus Interprets a visual stimulus by noting accompanying sounds Assigns meaning to a visual event	Sees reddened area on heels Documents on client's record Makes note of moaning sounds when client turns to side and concludes that client has pain Decides client has pain when grimaces
Nonverbal Touch	Kinesthetic • Procedure sensation • Caring sensation	Performs nursing care Conveys emotional support	Gives the client a back rub Places hand on client's shoulder

COURTESY OF DELMAR CENGAGE LEARNING

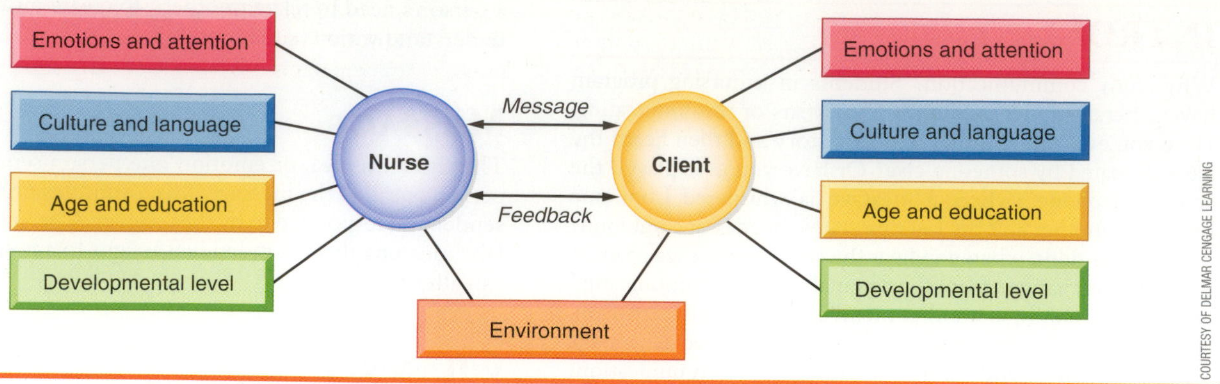

FIGURE 7-1 Concept Map representing the communication process with influences identified.

INFLUENCES

Culture, age, emotions, language, and attention influence both the sender and receiver as well as the situation within which they find themselves. All of these elements together are called a person's frame of reference. These influences sometimes help communication, and sometimes they hinder communication. Figure 7-1 shows the process of communication with the influences affecting both the sender and receiver.

METHODS OF COMMUNICATION

There are two methods of communicating: verbally and nonverbally. Which is better? The answer is neither, or, more accurately, it depends on what the sender is trying to communicate. Nonverbal aspects accompany virtually every spoken message. Since nonverbal communication is usually conveyed unconsciously by the sender, it is believed to be more honest than is verbal communication.

VERBAL COMMUNICATION

Verbal communication is the use of words, either spoken or written, to send a message. Methods of verbal communication include speaking, listening, writing, and reading.

Speaking/Listening

Speaking is usually thought of as verbal communication, but the receiver of a spoken message must listen. For communication to take place, both speaking and listening must occur. Have you ever spoken to someone in the same room with you and received a nonmeaningful, senseless response from that person or no response at all? The other person probably was only hearing words but not listening to the message.

Communication experts say that people speak at a rate of 125 to 150 words per minute (WPM) but hear at a rate of 400 to 800 WPM. This extra time allows for distractions. Listeners are generally distracted because they are not concentrating on what is being said. Listening is one of the most difficult skills to learn and execute well.

Intonation

Tone of voice has been estimated to convey 23% of the context of a message. When the same words are said in different tones of voice, they can have very different meanings. Tone of voice might be pleasant, sincere, sorrowful, sarcastic, joyful, or angry.

Writing/Reading

The other method of verbal communication is writing. The receiver of the written message reads the words. The reader must understand the words and then attach meaning to them. With a written message, there is generally no opportunity for immediate feedback. Therefore, great care should be taken to ensure clarity when composing a written message. A good example is charting. The physician may read the caregivers' notes after they have gone home, allowing no opportunity for immediate feedback. In such an instance, if the notes read that a client was "uncooperative," the physician would have little idea exactly what the caregiver meant. An entry of "refused to eat lunch, refused to get out of bed and sit in chair," however, is far more exact, illustrating the clarity in writing that is essential to good communication.

NONVERBAL COMMUNICATION

Nonverbal communication, or body language, is a method of sending a message without using speech or writing. Communication without words is done in many ways, including gestures, facial expressions, posture and gait, tone of voice, touch, eye contact, body position, and physical appearance.

Nonverbal communication, which is part learned behavior and part instinct, is generally unconscious. Feelings are believed to be most honestly expressed nonverbally because there is little conscious control over nonverbal communication.

Clients are particularly sensitive to nonverbal messages and seem to believe them. Nurses must therefore make every effort to be aware of the nonverbal messages they may be sending to clients. Consider, for example, the nursing skills that are not pleasant yet must be done. How would the client feel if the nurse had a facial expression of disgust or revulsion when emptying a bedpan?

Nurses must also be aware of and sensitive to the client's nonverbal messages. Many clients do not want to bother "busy" nurses, so they say they are fine or do not need anything when in fact they do. The perceptive nurse will observe nonverbal signs, such as clenched fists, stiff posture, or a frowning expression, and know that something is not right. The nurse would then proceed with further assessment to determine the reason the client is sending those nonverbal clues.

Gestures

Gestures are often referred to as "talking with hands." Gestures may be used to help clarify a verbal message, to emphasize an idea, to hold another's attention, or to relieve stress. Fingertapping, fidgeting, or ring twisting generally indicates tension, nervousness, or impatience. Shaking a fist indicates anger, whereas pointing may be used to clarify directions.

Facial Expressions

Although some people have very expressive faces, others do not. A big smile is easily interpreted as indicating happiness. Eyebrows can be very expressive, showing surprise, worry, thoughtfulness, or displeasure. The manner in which the forehead is wrinkled also sends a message.

Nurses must be very aware of their own facial expressions, especially when caring for a client under "unpleasant" conditions, such as when a client is vomiting or suffering from bowel incontinence. An expression of displeasure manifested as a "curled-up" nose or disgust is easily identified by the client. The client, often already embarrassed at requiring such care, will be reassured and comforted by a nurse's facial expression indicating caring, concern, and empathy.

Posture and Gait

Good posture, with the head held up, and a purposeful gait are usually interpreted as meaning self-confidence, competence, and a positive self-image. Stooped shoulders, a downward-held head, and a shuffling gait generally convey low self-esteem, depression, lack of confidence, or apathy.

Touch

Touch is a simple yet powerful form of nonverbal communication that even a newborn infant can understand. Touch can communicate caring, understanding, encouragement, warmth, reassurance, or affection. Of course, touch can also communicate anger, displeasure, or a lack or caring and understanding.

Many nursing tasks involve touching the client (i.e., bathing, dressing changes, ambulating). Touch, along with other nonverbal communication such as facial expression, posture, eye contact, and tone of voice, will convey the nurse's caring and acceptance. Most clients accept touch as an integral part of nursing care when it is done appropriately and professionally.

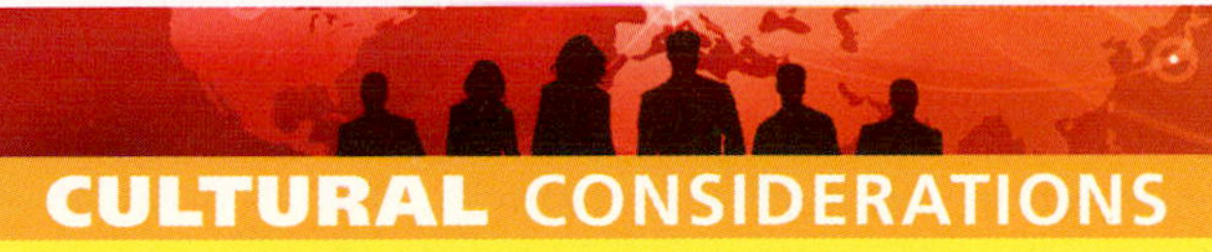

CULTURAL CONSIDERATIONS

Eye Contact

In some Asian cultures, it is considered rude or disrespectful to make direct eye contact.

Eye Contact

Eyes, it is said, mirror the soul. Have you ever seen joy, sadness, pain, or laughter in someone's eyes? It is very difficult to control these messages of the eyes.

Eye contact is generally interpreted as indicating interest and attention, whereas lack of eye contact is thought to indicate avoidance, disinterest, or discomfort.

Body Position

Body position is often a good indicator of a person's attitude. For example, crossed arms generally indicate withdrawal, although the person could just be cold. The nurse needs to be cautious not to misinterpret the client's body language. Open body positions, with the arms held freely at the sides, are usually taken to mean a receptive attitude.

Physical Appearance

A person's physical appearance says a great deal about that person. A clean, neat, appropriately dressed individual conveys a positive self-image, knowledge, and competence. A dirty, sloppy, or inappropriately dressed person conveys the message of "I don't care how I look," with the potential implication of "maybe I am not too knowledgeable or competent" or "I am sloppy in what I do."

It is very important for every nurse to be clean, neat, and professionally dressed. Clients and families understand the nonverbal message that appearance conveys. Appearance does influence communication.

INFLUENCES ON COMMUNICATION

Communication involves more than just sending and receiving verbal and nonverbal messages. How a person sends or receives a message is influenced by such factors as age, education, emotions, culture, and language. Attention to the message and the surroundings are other influences. These factors must be taken into account for accurate communication to take place.

AGE

Factors related to age affect communication. For instance, communicating with a child is different from communicating with an adult and depends on the child's age. Nonverbal communication, particularly touch, and facial expression can be understood by infants. Before learning to understand words, a child can interpret tone of voice and gestures. Preschool children respond well to communication involving toys or play situations. They should be allowed some choices, but no more than two alternatives should be offered. As the child's vocabulary increases, more verbal communication can take place.

Elderly persons may have some degree of hearing loss or a slowed response time. The nurse should face the elderly client when speaking and allow time for a response. The client should be addressed as "Mr." or "Ms." unless he or she asks to be called by his or her first name. These measures reflect respect to the individual from the caregiver.

Generational categories are determined by a person's age. By understanding the characteristics of the four main generations (traditional, baby boomers, Generation X, and Generation Y), communication between the nurse and the client, family members, coworkers, and others will be enhanced (Box 7-1).

Developmental Level

Age and developmental level do not necessarily go hand in hand. Individuals with mental retardation or developmental delays will communicate at their level of development, not at what is usually expected for their chronological age.

Education

Education is another strong influence on communication. Vocabulary generally increases as does the ability to discuss and understand concepts and abstract ideas.

Emotions

A person's emotional state greatly influences how messages are sent or received. Someone who is very anxious or upset, for example, may not hear what is said or may interpret the message differently than the sender intended. This same person typically speaks in an abrupt manner, loudly, and in harsh tones. The depressed person, on the other hand, typically says very little, speaking only one or two words or in very short sentences.

Box 7-1 CHARACTERISTICS OF THE FOUR MAIN GENERATIONS

Traditional

(1922–1945)

This generation is known for surviving the Great Depression, developing the space program, creating vaccines, developing suburbia, and pursuing equality through the civil rights movement.

Values

Respect authority and rules
Defined sense of right and wrong
Honor loyalty

Attributes

Disciplined
Detailed oriented
Dislike conflict
Learn from history to plan for the future

Work Style

Command-and-control leadership style
Prefer hierarchical organization
Uniformity and consistency

Medical

Chronic diseases common to the age group: chronic obstructive pulmonary disease, diabetes, osteoporosis, high blood pressure, and cardiovascular disease. Compliance to treatment depends on ability to afford medical care and medication. Least likely to seek mental health services (i.e., depression) because of embarrassment and the stigma attached to it.

Communication

Given this generation's respect for authority, communication needs to be respectful, direct, and in person or by phone. The client will most likely follow the health care provider's orders out completely and not question them.

Baby Boomers

(1946–1964)

This generation is known for the civil rights movement, the women's movement, an equal opportunity workplace, increased educational and financial opportunities, space exploration, and prosperity for many Americans.

Values

Health and wellness
Prosperity
Community involvement
Self-actualizing
Individual choice
Ownership

Attributes

Adaptive
Goal oriented
Positive attitude
Focus on individual choices and freedom

Work Style

Avoid conflict
Team building
Group decision making
Collaborative

Medical

Chronic diseases common to this age group include diabetes, high cholesterol, high blood pressure, and heart and lung disease. Cosmetic advancements have helped this generation try to delay the aging process. Lifestyle issues include obesity, certain forms of cancer (i.e., lung cancer from smoking), and liver problems from alcohol consumption. This generation feels an added stress by not only raising their own children but also caring for and managing the health care for their aging parents. This age group participates in self-improvement services and preventive health care.

Communication

Given this generation's respect for individual choice, the client will prefer to be a part of the decision-making process. This age group prefers to be called on the phone or to meet in person to discuss important topics. The client will expect to hear all of his or her health care options and for health care to be a collaborative effort.

(*Continues*)

Box 7-1 CHARACTERISTICS OF THE FOUR MAIN GENERATIONS (continued)

Generation X (Boomerang)

(1965–1980)

This was an era of emerging technology, autonomy, self-reliance, economic decline, and political and institutional issues, such as Watergate, Three Mile Island, and the Iranian hostage crisis. This is the first generation to be recognized as "latchkey" kids because of parents working and the rise in divorce.

Values

Autonomy
Feedback and recognition
Time with manager
Contribution

Attributes

Multitasking
Independence
Adaptability

Work Style

High-quality end results
Productivity
Free agent
Independent (Don't look over my shoulder)
Flexible work hours/job sharing appealing
Balance between work and life—work to live, not live to work
Sees self as marketable commodity
Technically competent
Ethnic diversity

Medical

Typically, this generation has waited to marry and begin having children at an older age than previous generations because of careers. Medical issues affecting this age group include pregnancy, smoking, depression, anxiety, and eating disorders.

Communication

Phone calls and e-mails are the preferred methods of communication for this age group. Given this generation's respect for independence and feedback, the client will prefer making his or her own health care decisions, obtaining second opinions, confidentiality, and prompt feedback from health care providers regarding health care (i.e., diagnostic testing results). This client will extensively research health issues on the Internet and bring the findings with him or her to physician appointments.

Generation Y (Millennial)

(1980–1995)

This was the era of technology; self-expression; being a team player; the Columbine High School shootings; the attacks of September 11, 2001; "a village raising a child"; and "No Child Left Behind." This age group has been nurtured and protected by their parents and is now entering the workforce with expectations of wanting everything instantly because of parental upbringing and technology.

Values

Self-expression is more important than self-control
Marketing and branding self is important
Violence is an acceptable means of communication
Fear living a poor lifestyle
Respect must be earned; it is not freely granted based on age, authority, or title

Attributes

Adapt rapidly/create constantly
Crave change and challenge/exceptionally resilient
Committed and loyal when committed to an idea or cause
Accept others of diverse backgrounds easily and openly
Global in perspective

Work Style

Seek work in teams/virtual problem solving
Prefer flexible work hours and dress code
View their work as an expression of themselves, not a definition of themselves
Want to know how what they do fits into the big picture and need to understand how everything fits together
Exceptional at multitasking (need more than one activity happening at a time)
Feeling of entitlement/wanting everything instantly
Seek to balance work and lifestyle, with more focus on lifestyle

Medical

This age group is young with few medical issues. Common health care issues include motor vehicle accidents, pregnancy, depression, anxiety, asthma, acne, drug experimentation, and binge drinking. Visits to the emergency room are more common for this generation than making an appointment to see the family physician, as it provides more immediate care.

Communication

This generation prefers communication via technology including cell phone, texting, e-mail, pagers, blogging, skyping, Facebook, chat rooms, and Webcams. It is common for parents to be present with the client during a health care appointment.

Adapted from www.ValueOptions.com, 2009.

Culture

Each culture has its own standards of communication, especially with regard to nonverbal behavior. In the United States, for example, eye contact is considered a sign of openness and honesty. Those of Spanish heritage, however, believe eye contact to be disrespectful. Similarly, in many parts of Europe, a kiss on the cheek between two men is accepted. People from other parts of the world, however, may look suspiciously on this behavior.

Language

Language certainly influences communication. Speaking the same language assists people in understanding each other, although regional accents or dialects of a language can inhibit communication and understanding. When verbal communication comes to a standstill, nonverbal communication is often employed to assist. Any nurse who works in an area where there is a predominant second language should learn a few words or phrases in that language to help put clients at ease and to facilitate their understanding. Most health care facilities are required to have certified language interpreters for consultation.

Attention

The amount of attention each individual focuses on a given communication greatly affects the outcome. In selective listening, the receiver hears only what he wants or expects to hear. Pain or discomfort, physical or mental, may result in preoccupation, limiting the attention given to the communication.

Surroundings

Most people do not want to talk about the intimate details of their health care concerns in public (Figure 7-2). Thus, privacy should be provided. If the client occupies a room alone, the nurse should close the door; if the client shares a room, the nurse should take the client to a conference room or to another private place, if possible, to discuss personal information.

The nurse should respect the client's current "home" (e.g., the hospital room) as she would any person's home, knocking on the door before entering the room, not sitting on the bed without permission, and asking before moving any personal articles. These simple courtesies show respect for the client as a person. When the client feels respected, communication is enhanced.

CONGRUENCY OF MESSAGES

It is important that verbal and nonverbal communications are in agreement, or **congruent**. Saying, "I really appreciate what you just did," in a pleasant tone of voice while smiling is congruent and clear; saying the same words in a disgusted tone of voice while frowning is incongruent and, thus, potentially unclear. The receiver may not know whether the sender is genuinely pleased with what was done or is displeased and being sarcastic. Messages such as these can confuse the receiver, who then may require feedback in order to correctly interpret the message.

It is important for the nurse to watch for congruency between verbal and nonverbal messages and to ask for clarification when incongruity exists.

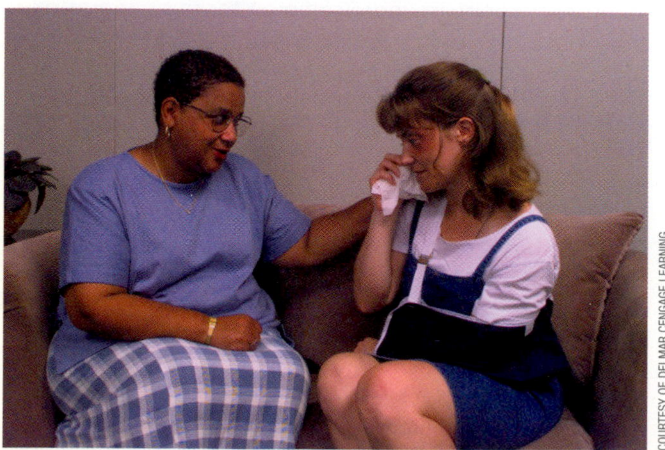

COURTESY OF DELMAR CENGAGE LEARNING

FIGURE 7-2 Provide privacy when discussing personal or intimate health concerns with clients.

LISTENING/OBSERVING

Listening and observing are two of the most valuable skills a nurse can have. These two skills are used to gather the subjective and objective data for the nursing assessment. Because the nursing diagnoses and nursing interventions are based on the assessment, it is imperative that the assessment be accurate.

The term **active listening** has been used to describe the behavior of listening and observing; it reflects the process of hearing spoken words and noting nonverbal behavior. It is listening for the meaning behind the words. This takes energy and concentration. To show undivided attention to the client, the nurse should be at eye level with the client, lean slightly forward toward the client, and make eye contact. In this position the nurse will be able to listen and observe more accurately. Responses from the nurse such as "go on," "yes," "tell me more," "mmhm," or "what else?" communicate that the nurse is really listening and encourage the client to continue.

PSYCHOSOCIAL ASPECTS OF COMMUNICATION

The psychosocial aspects of communication are important for nurses to understand and then apply when caring for individual clients. Consideration of these aspects makes communication more effective.

The psychosocial aspects of communication include gestures, style, meaning of space, meaning of time, cultural values, and political correctness. These aspects are based on individuality and culture and influence the nurse–client relationship.

Gestures

Gestures are movements of the body to reflect a thought, feeling, or attitude. Some gestures are known globally, such as applause to indicate approval. Some gestures, however, have entirely different meanings in various countries. The nurse must be sensitive to cultural variances and exercise good judgment when caring for clients of different backgrounds and heritages.

Style

Each person has a style of communication reflecting the personality and self-concept of that person. According to Jack (2000), there are three common types of style: passive, aggressive, and assertive. Remember that a person's style of communication is learned and has been reinforced over the years. Because communication style is learned, it can be changed.

PROFESSIONALTIP

When Clients Block Communication

In instances when clients block communication, keep the following things in mind:

- The client may not wish to discuss the topic introduced by the nurse or may not wish to talk at all. Everyone needs time alone to think.
- Accept and respect the client's desires to not communicate at a particular time.
- Let the client know that you are ready to listen whenever the client is ready to talk.

The stress, fear, and anxiety associated with being a client in the health care system may change a client's style to passive or aggressive.

Passive

The person using the passive style of communication is not able to share feelings or needs with others, has difficulty asking for help, does not stand up for himself, and is hurt and angry when others take advantage of him. This person has a weak, soft voice; uses apologetic words; makes little eye contact; and is often fidgety. The person with a passive style of communication will often go along with others without expressing a personal desire for an alternate plan of action. The client who is generally very compliant, asks for nothing, and gets little attention has a passive style of communication.

Aggressive

The person using the aggressive style of communication puts his own needs and feelings first. Communication is done in a haughty or angry manner. The voice is often demanding. This person works to control or manipulate others, shows no concern for anyone else's feelings, and has an attitude of superiority.

CULTURAL CONSIDERATIONS

Gestures

The meaning of gestures is not universal. For instance, in many places, a small circle made with the thumb and forefinger means "okay." This is not true in Japan and France, however, where this gesture means "money" and "zero," respectively. And in Brazil and Turkey, this gesture is a symbol for female genitalia and is considered an insult.

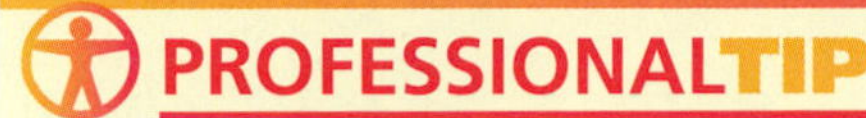

Being Assertive

"I" messages—I think . . . , I expect . . . , I feel . . . , I need . . .—are excellent ways to begin practicing assertive communication. Such messages indicate ownership of the thought, feeling, or need—a fact with which no one can argue.

Assertive

The assertive person stands up for himself without violating the basic rights of others. True feelings are expressed in an honest, direct manner, and others are not allowed to take advantage of him. The voice is firm and confident, and appropriate eye contact is made. Such a person also respects the rights, needs, and feelings of others; takes responsibility for the consequences of his actions; and behaves in a manner that enhances self-respect.

A person using the assertive style of communication effectively lets others know his thoughts, feelings, and needs. He also listens to and acknowledges the other person's thoughts, feelings, and needs. If the thoughts, feelings, or needs of the persons communicating are in conflict, a compromise acceptable to both can usually be worked out.

Meaning of Space

For many years Edward T. Hall (1959) studied **proxemics**, the study of space between people and its effect on interpersonal behavior. Hall says that like other animals, humans are territorial. Consider the following examples of human territoriality: People on a beach mark territory with a towel or blanket; space is marked in waiting rooms with a hat, jacket, luggage, or newspaper; and students in a classroom generally sit in the same place and expect others to respect that space.

How much space do you prefer between yourself and another person? This distance usually varies with the person and the situation. The distance at which one person is comfortable with another person is influenced by age, gender of those interacting, and cultural values. Hall (1959) categorizes these comfort zones as intimate, personal, social, and public space, defined as follows:

- Intimate—touch to 18 inches; usually limited to family and close friends; necessary when performing most nursing procedures
- Personal—18 inches to 4 feet; used with friends and coworkers; effective for many nurse–client interactions involving interviewing or data gathering
- Social—4 to 12 feet; preferred distance with casual acquaintances
- Public—12 feet or more; generally used with strangers in public places

Comfort zone distances vary from person to person. While some people are comfortable being very close to the person with whom they are interacting, others prefer a greater distance. Nurses should always be aware of the client's spatial comfort level (Figure 7-3).

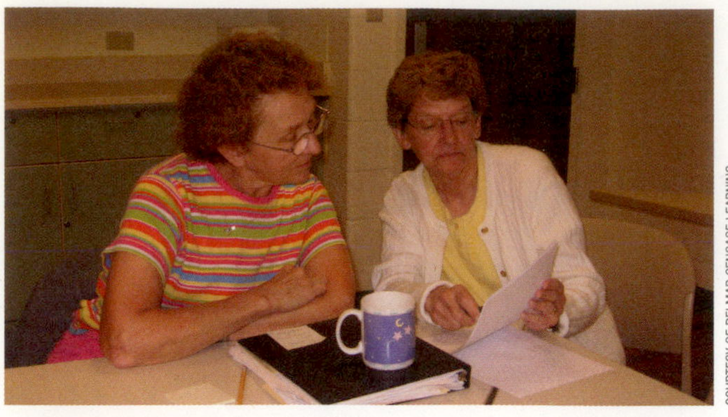
COURTESY OF DELMAR CENGAGE LEARNING

FIGURE 7-3 Personal space (18 inches to 4 feet) is used by friends and coworkers.

Much of nursing care involves touching the client, yet on admission the nurse and client generally do not know each other. The nurse must move from the client's public space to the client's intimate space in a very short span of time to provide care. When care is given competently and professionally, it helps the client feel more comfortable as the nurse occupies the client's intimate space.

Meaning of Time

In the United States, great emphasis is placed on schedules and being on time. Time is money. The clock is watched, so individuals know where they are to be every hour of the day and night. When scheduled appointments are kept, the person is considered to be dependable.

Some cultures do not have an instrument for telling time. They have other ways of perceiving and dividing time. Some cultures know a day has passed because the sun has risen, has set, and is rising again. Scheduling in these cultures often means "when we get around to it."

Cultural Values

It is important that the nurse be familiar with the cultural values of the people in the nurse's region of employment, especially when those values differ from the values of the dominant culture. For example, optimal health for all is the focus of the dominant U.S. culture. In some cultures, however, health is not a major concern, and little financial or political effort is dedicated to health. Likewise, individualism is stressed in our culture. In many other cultures, however, the social group, not the individual, is the primary focus.

As another example, consider that a number of cultural groups have learned to enjoy what they have and do not feel the need to keep working for some goal or material object. This contrasts with the dominant U.S. culture, where persons must work hard, achieve, and keep busy in order to be considered successful. Finally, in the dominant U.S. culture, cleanliness is closely related to optimal health and is a dominant value. Few cultural groups emphasize cleanliness in the way the U.S. culture does.

> **PROFESSIONALTIP**
>
> **Time Orientation**
>
> Be sensitive to the fact that clients of different cultural backgrounds may value time differently than you do. Do not jump to conclusions that the client who is always late is lazy or inconsiderate of schedules.

Political Correctness

Politically correct communication uses language that shows sensitivity to those who are different from oneself. It is intended to avoid the use of language that offends and to help eliminate prejudice. Terms that suggest inferior status for members of minority groups and terms that exclude older people, women, and those with handicaps are replaced by politically correct language. Prejudice and false ideas, which often lead to violence, are perpetuated by racist and bigoted language.

THERAPEUTIC COMMUNICATION

Therapeutic communication, sometimes called effective communication, is purposeful and goal directed, creating a beneficial outcome for the client. The focus of the conversation is the client, the client's problems, or the client's needs, not the problems or needs of the nurse.

Goals of Therapeutic Communication

Therapeutic communication has several goals or purposes. One or more of these goals guides each therapeutic communication between the nurse and client. The goals are to develop trust, obtain or provide information, show caring, and explore feelings.

Develop Trust

Clients and nurses are generally strangers when they first meet. The nurse then works to establish trust with each client. Examples of ways to build trust include answering questions honestly, responding to call lights promptly, and following through. When caring is shown, trust develops faster. Mutual trust established between client and nurse is termed **rapport**.

Obtain or Provide Information

The nurse obtains information from the client about general health and specific health problems. With this information, the nurse can make an accurate assessment and plan of care.

The nurse provides information to the client from admission to discharge, beginning with the orientation of a new client to the hospital policies and routines. Sharing of information continues throughout the hospital stay as the nurse explains procedures, treatments, and tests; teaches the client self-care; clarifies instruction from other health care workers; and answers client questions. The discharge instructions constitute the final stage of information provision.

Show Caring

Two ways to show caring are offering a drink of water without being asked or fluffing a pillow. Knocking on the room door

TABLE 7-2 Ways to Show Caring

ACTIVITY	STATEMENTS TO USE WITH ACTIVITY
Cover the client with a blanket.	"It feels chilly in here. Perhaps this blanket will help."
Assist the client to dress.	"I noticed you're having a little trouble getting your robe on. Perhaps I can help."
Serve a tray to the client.	"It's time to eat. I hope you're hungry because it really looks good."
Offer assistance.	"Here, let me help you. Perhaps together we can arrange these flowers."
Ask when leaving the room.	"Is there anything more I can do for you before I go?" or "I'm leaving now, but I'll be back in 20 minutes."
Move the client up in bed.	"You look so uncomfortable. Let me move you up in bed."
Make the client's bed.	"Now you have a nice fresh bed."
Regulate environmental temperature.	"It seems very warm in here. Perhaps if I turn the air conditioner up, it will help."
Turn the client in bed.	"Changing position really makes a difference, doesn't it?"
Straighten a pillow.	"Let me straighten your pillow for you."

COURTESY OF DELMAR CENGAGE LEARNING

before entering and taking time to always greet the client by name are additional ways to show caring.

Explore Feelings

After rapport is established, the nurse can encourage the client to explore feelings. Many clients are anxious about their illness. Some have anxiety about being in the hospital, and some fear the results of diagnostic tests. Some individuals will not admit they are anxious or fearful. The nurse is often able to help the client talk about feelings and reduce anxiety by using therapeutic communication techniques. Sometimes, only a clarifying statement is needed to alleviate fear or anxiety. Other times, fear and anxiety are reduced by allowing the client to talk.

BEHAVIORS/ATTITUDES TO ENHANCE COMMUNICATION

Behaviors and attitudes that enhance therapeutic communication include warmth, active listening, caring, genuineness, empathy, acceptance and respect, and self-disclosure.

Caring

Caring is an attitude that enhances communication as well as a goal of therapeutic communication. Caring is the basis of a nurse–client relationship and makes the client feel important. The client can easily identify a caring attitude. Table 7-2 gives some examples of ways to show caring.

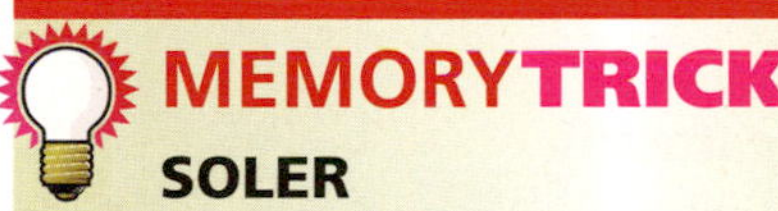

MEMORYTRICK

SOLER

The nurse should use the memory trick **SOLER** when talking with a client:

- **S** = Sit upright
- **O** = Open arms
- **L** = Lean forward
- **E** = Eye contact
- **R** = Relax

Warmth

Warmth, expressed predominantly by nonverbal communication, makes the client feel relaxed, welcomed, and unjudged.

While touch is an important method to show warmth, it must be used appropriately. Society dictates the touching that is appropriate in various situations. Communication may be greatly enhanced by holding a client's hand or putting a hand on the shoulder. This touching provides a connection between the nurse and the client. Remember that touch may not always be welcomed by the client.

Active Listening

As implied, listening is an active process requiring energy and concentration. It involves listening to the spoken words as well as being attentive to the nonverbal messages.

Responses from the nurses indicate that the nurse is really listening to the client. It is important that the nurse concentrate on the interaction at hand and not become distracted by other thoughts (Figure 7-4).

Genuineness

Effective communication is genuine. The nurse must be honest about personal feelings. Sometimes it is appropriate to cry with a client.

Genuineness means being truthful and not attempting to answer a question when the answer is not known. After admitting not knowing, the nurse should offer to find the answer and then do so. Knowing that being genuine builds trust, the nurse must use good judgment about confronting a family member, client, or another health care worker or expressing negative thoughts.

Empathy

Empathy, the capacity to understand another person's feelings or perception of a situation, is an objective awareness of or a sensitivity to another person's feelings and thoughts. Although the nurse is not involved in the thoughts and feelings of the

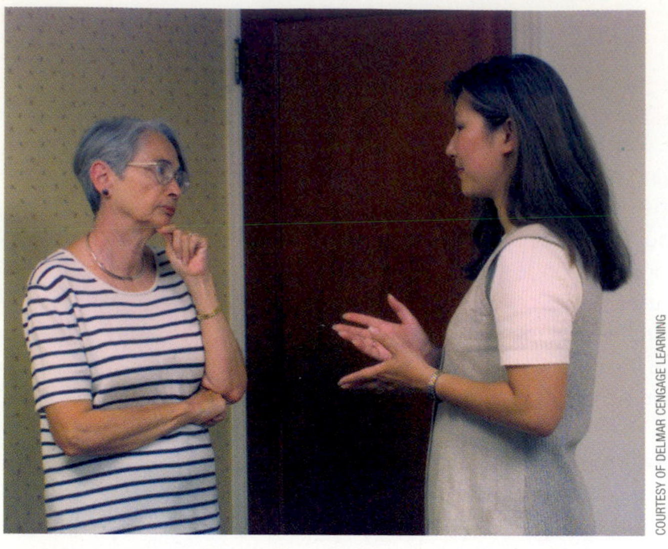
COURTESY OF DELMAR CENGAGE LEARNING

FIGURE 7-4 Active listening, concentrating on the interaction with the client, enhances communication.

client, through empathy the nurse is able to understand and accept the feelings and thoughts of the client. Sympathy is different from empathy. In sympathy, the nurse shares in the feelings and thoughts of the client. These feelings and thoughts are generally related to a loss.

Acceptance and Respect

Acceptance of clients as individuals with values and beliefs of their own is an attitude that enhances communication. Nurses must accept the fact that clients may have different values and beliefs. It is called being nonjudgmental when a client is accepted at face value.

Acceptance is shown by not expressing differing beliefs or values and by simply accepting the statements or complaints of clients. Clients then feel free to communicate and cooperate in their care.

After acceptance comes respect. In order to understand clients as unique individuals, they must be accepted in a nonjudgmental way. Acceptance and respect by the nurse lets clients know that they can be themselves and that they will still receive quality nursing care even though they have different values and beliefs than the nurse. Respect is shown when the nurse introduces herself and also addresses the client by name (preceded by "Mr.," "Mrs.," or "Ms.").

Self-Disclosure

Sharing something about yourself such as thoughts, expectations, feelings, or ideas is termed self-disclosure. It does not mean sharing personal problems. A nurse who shares something, such as personal future goals in nursing, is trusting the client with that knowledge. The client who feels trusted will trust the nurse, and therapeutic communication is augmented.

Techniques of Therapeutic Communication

Certain techniques promote therapeutic communication. These techniques should be learned and incorporated into the nurse's manner of communicating.

Clarifying/Validating

Clarifying or validating are used when the nurse is not sure of the meaning of a message. Clarifying is the technique used to understand verbal messages, such as the following:

"Do you mean . . . ?"

Validating is used to establish truth or accuracy. It is used for nonverbal as well as verbal messages. Examples are as follows:

"Are you saying that you did not get your medication today?"

"You are holding your side. Are you having pain there?"

Open-Ended Questions

Open-ended questions encourage clients to express their own thoughts and feelings. *How, when, where,* and *what* are words with which to begin an open-ended question. Open-ended questions cannot typically be answered with "yes" or "no" or with just one or two words, such as the following:

"How has this medication affected your vision?"

"What did the doctor tell you about going home?"

Open-Ended Statements

An open-ended statement calls for a response from the client. Because it is a statement and not a question, the client does not feel quizzed. Open-ended statements allow the client to determine the direction of the conversation, thus helping the client maintain a feeling of independence. Examples of open-ended statements are as follows:

"Tell me about your physical therapy today."

"You were telling me about . . ."

Reflecting

Reflecting is repeating all or part of a message back to the sender. Often, reflecting focuses on feelings and helps the sender "hear" the message from the receiver. This allows the sender a chance to clarify the message and shows that the listener is trying to understand the message. Reflecting can be a very useful technique if not overused. Examples include the following:

Client: "I'm really nervous about my surgery tomorrow. My friend got an infection after her surgery. I'm very frightened."

Nurse: "You are anxious about your surgery and afraid of getting an infection?"

Paraphrasing/Restating

Paraphrasing is restating the message in the receiver's own words. This lets the sender know how the receiver interpreted the message. Clarification can then be done if necessary. The sender is aware that the receiver is listening and trying to understand the message, as in the following:

Nurse: "You are afraid that you might have complications from your surgery?"

Summarizing

Summarizing is stating in a sentence or two the major points of a conversation to let the sender know what was heard.

The sender can then add more information or clarify what was originally heard. An example might be as follows:

"Let me see, we have discussed . . ."

Focusing

Keeping communication focused on the topic being discussed can sometimes be difficult. Clients may wander off to other topics, or the topic may shift to the nurse. It is important to keep the focus on the client and not the nurse. For example, the nurse could say the following:

"We can discuss that in a minute, right now I'd like to discuss . . ."

"A minute ago you mentioned that you'd had an upset stomach after taking your medication. Tell me more about that."

Silence

Silence is one of the most difficult but effective techniques to use. In the dominant U.S. culture, most people are uncomfortable with silence and feel the need to fill the gap by saying something. Silence can be a valuable therapeutic technique, allowing the client time to gather thoughts or check emotions. Silence also gives the nurse a chance to decide how best to continue the interaction. If the nurse employs behaviors to enhance communication during the silence, the client will often verbalize thoughts or feelings.

Barriers to Communication

Employing behaviors and attitudes to enhance communication will be of little use if the nurse also employs barriers to communication. Although the communication process is intense, it should not be threatening. The purpose in learning about things that block communication is to enable the nurse to identify them and avoid using them. Many mistakes can be corrected when identified. A simple "I'm sorry, I shouldn't have said that" will often take care of the situation. Practice helps sharpen communication skills. The most common barriers are discussed in the following sections.

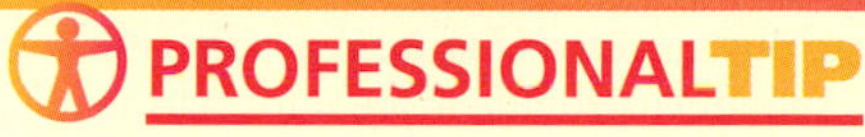

Improve Communication Skills

Communication skills can be improved by the following:

- Minimizing distractions
- Making eye contact
- Listening
- Being patient
- Not interrupting
- Checking congruency of words spoken with non-verbal cues
- Using clear, easy-to-understand terminology and explaining medical terms when used
- Asking client to paraphrase important information

PROFESSIONALTIP

Therapeutic Communication

Practice the techniques of therapeutic communication with family, classmates, friends, and instructors. This may seem artificial and uncomfortable at first, but it will become easier with practice. If you begin using the techniques of therapeutic communication now, you will have incorporated them into your manner of communication by the time you begin clinical experience.

Closed Questions

Questions that can be answered with "yes" or "no" or with only one or two words are considered closed. After the one- or two-word answer, communication is usually ended; there is no other avenue for the communication to follow. This type of question is appropriate in certain circumstances, however, such as when taking a health history or in an emergency. Examples of closed questions are as follows:

"Is the pain gone?"

"Did you sleep well?"

Clichés

Clichés are overused, trite phrases that are almost meaningless. They are impersonal and often used when individuals are at a loss for anything better to say. They are used without thinking of the impact on the other person and often seem disrespectful of the client's individual circumstances. Examples include the following:

"Hang in there; tomorrow is another day."

"It could be worse."

False Reassurance

False reassurance about the outcome of a situation is often used in an effort to cheer up the client regardless of the facts. False reassurance can be especially traumatic to a terminally ill client who may be desperate to believe assurances even if they are not founded in reality. An example of false reassurance is as follows:

"Don't worry, I'm sure everything will be fine."

Judgmental Responses

Judgmental responses are based on the nurse's personal value system and imply right or wrong. Such responses allow no room for further discussion, such as the following:

"You shouldn't feel that way."

"You ought to do . . ."

Agreeing/Disagreeing or Approving/Disapproving

Whether the nurse is agreeing/approving or disagreeing/disapproving, offering an opinion implies that one belief is right and the other wrong. Clients are thus prevented from sharing their feelings and may feel pressured to express the same values and opinions as the nurse. One example is as follows:

"I wouldn't do it that way."

Giving Advice

Giving advice involves offering personal rather than professional opinion. When the nurse does this, the client's responsibility for making decisions is diminished. Furthermore, some clients may end up feeling unable to make their own choices and may therefore become more dependent on the nurse. One example might be the following:

"I think you should . . ."

Stereotyping

Stereotyping occurs when individual differences are ignored and a person is automatically put into a specific category because they have certain characteristics. Examples might be the following:

"Someone your age shouldn't worry about that."

"Boys aren't supposed to cry."

Belittling

Belittling conveys to a person that his thoughts or feelings really have no value, that it is silly to think or feel a certain way, or that he is no different from other individuals in similar circumstances. Examples include the following:

"Many people have it much worse."

"Yes, everyone feels like that."

Defending

Defending is a response to a feeling of being directly or indirectly threatened. The nurse may make statements in defense of self, another nurse, a doctor, or the health care facility. Defending implies that the client is not permitted to criticize or express feelings. This may be one of the most difficult communication barriers to overcome. No one likes to be criticized or to hear coworkers criticized. A natural first response is to defend why something was said, done, or not done. An example of defending is as follows:

"No one on this unit would say that."

Requesting an Explanation

It can be very intimidating for a client when a nurse asks for an explanation of behaviors, feelings, or thoughts. Often, the client does not know the "why." The usual results are increased anxiety, becoming defensive, and an end to communication. Examples are as follows:

"Why did you do that?"

"Why do you feel that way?"

Changing the Subject

An abrupt change of subject by the nurse generally indicates to the client that the nurse is uncomfortable or anxious about the topic under discussion. It often is used to avoid listening to a client's fear, distress, or problems and is interpreted by the client as a lack of interest:

Client: "I don't think I'll ever get well."

Nurse: "Isn't it a beautiful day?"

PROFESSIONAL BOUNDARIES

All communication with clients must take place within **professional boundaries** (the limits of the professional relationship that allow for a safe, therapeutic connection between the professional and the client). The nurse must abstain from obtaining personal gain at the expense of the client and refrain from inappropriate involvement in the client's personal relationships.

NURSE–CLIENT COMMUNICATION

One of the most important aspects of nursing care is communication. Good communication skills are essential whether the nurse is gathering admission information, taking a health history, teaching, or implementing care. **Interpersonal communication** is an exchange of information between the nurse and the client. This basic level of communication occurs between 2 or more people in a small group and is the most common form of communication in nursing.

Nurses have both an ethical and a moral responsibility to use any information gathered from the client in the client's best interest. Information that affects the health status or care of the client should be shared with other members of the health care team. All information concerning a client is confidential and should never be discussed in elevators, the cafeteria, the hallways, or other public places outside the health care facility.

Nurses' competence is often judged by their communication skills. Client satisfaction is increased by good communication, and increased client satisfaction leads to better compliance with the therapeutic regimen.

A key factor in the client's perception and evaluation of the health care services provided is communication.

Formal/Informal Communication

Formal communication is purposeful and is employed in a structured situation, such as information gathering on admission or scheduled teaching sessions (Figure 7-5). Specific items covered in a planned sequence provide more information in the shortest amount of time.

Informal communication does not follow a structured approach, although it often reveals information that is pertinent to the client's care. For instance, a client may comment that the tape holding her bandage in place is irritating to her skin. This would lead the nurse to assess the wound area and take action to correct the problem. This interaction, although not planned or structured, was nonetheless helpful in ensuring quality nursing care.

CRITICAL THINKING

Communication Barriers

Can you identify communication barriers you may have seen in the past? If so, list them and discuss ways to eliminate these communication barriers.

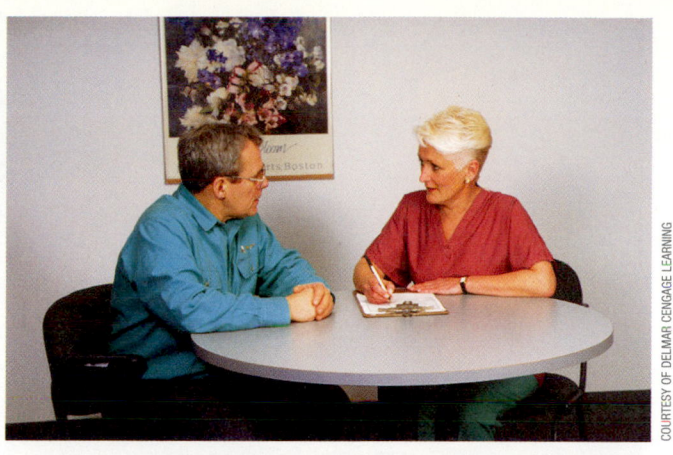
COURTESY OF DELMAR CENGAGE LEARNING

FIGURE 7-5 Formal Interaction, Admission Interview

SOCIAL COMMUNICATION

Everyday conversations with friends, family, and acquaintances are called social communication. Topics usually are those of interest to both parties and reflect the social relationship of the persons involved. Both people share information, feelings, and thoughts. Social communication provides a way to get acquainted with clients to learn about each other and to begin a nurse–client relationship.

Although social communication is not considered therapeutic communication, it is used in the nurse–client relationship. It is nonthreatening and puts the client at ease, allowing the nurse to get to know the client and what is important to the client. Social communication is often interpreted by clients as expressions of caring on the part of the nurse—that is, the nurse cares enough about the client to spend time communicating as a person rather than as a nurse.

INTERACTIONS

Nurse–client interactions and relationships progress through three phases. The purpose of the interaction dictates the amount of time spent on each phase.

Introduction Phase

The introduction phase of any interaction is usually fairly short. After greeting the client by name, the nurse should introduce himself and define his role. Then expectations of the interaction are clarified, and mutual goals are set. A good format might be as follows:

> "Good morning, Mrs. Ishdu. My name is Lorenzo Lopez. I am a student practical (vocational) nurse. I will be caring for you today and tomorrow. During this time, I will be teaching you some leg exercises that you will have to do after your surgery tomorrow."

Working Phase

The working phase generally constitutes the major portion of any interaction and is used to accomplish the goal or objective defined in the introduction. Feedback should always be asked for to ensure understanding on the part of the client. In the previously presented scenario, the client's demonstrating the leg exercises and verbalizing why the exercises are necessary would indicate understanding.

Termination Phase

The termination phase is the final phase of any interaction. Seldom do nurses have unlimited time to spend with one client, and there are several ways for the nurse to indicate the end of an interaction. The nurse may ask whether the client has any questions about the topic discussed. Summarizing the topic is another good way for the nurse to indicate closure.

FACTORS AFFECTING NURSE–CLIENT COMMUNICATION

As mentioned previously, factors such as age, education, emotions, culture, language, attention, and surroundings affect both parties in a communication. In nurse–client communications, additional factors relating to both the nurse and the client also come into play. The nurse must be sensitive to these factors and avoid personal biases in order to provide appropriate nursing care.

Nurse

Many factors pertaining to the nurse influence nurse–client communication. The nurse's state of health, home situation, workload, staff relations, and past experiences as a nurse can all impact the attitude, thinking, concentration, and emotions of the nurse. These all influence the way a nurse sends and receives messages. Self-awareness (an awareness of all these factors) is very important for the nurse when communicating.

Client

Factors related to the client that must be considered include social factors, religion, family situation, visual ability, hearing ability, speech ability, level of consciousness, language proficiency, and state of illness. The National Institute on Deafness and Other Communication Disorders (NIDCD, 2008) estimates that more than 46 million Americans suffer from a communication disorder and that approximately 36 million Americans have some degree of hearing loss (NIDCD, 2008a).

Hearing Ability If a hearing-impaired person is able to read, writing may be the easiest method of communication; however, many hearing-impaired persons have learned to speech read at least to some degree. This was formerly known as lip-read. Communicating with a client who is hearing impaired requires time and patience.

The client may experience frustration when communicating. Such frustration generally stems more from trying to understand others rather than from trying to be understood. Face the client and speak slowly and deliberately using slightly exaggerated word formation. Gesturing can also be very effective. Check to see whether the client has a hearing aid and, if so, encourage its use during the communication.

Speech Ability Dysphasia, the impairment of speech, and **aphasia**, the absence of speech, are most commonly seen as the result of a stroke, although both can result from a brain lesion. Other neurological diseases such as Parkinson's disease may also cause **dysphasia**. A dysfunction of the muscles used for speech is termed **dysarthria**, which makes a person's speech difficult, slow, and hard to understand. Dysphasia, aphasia, and dysarthria create communication problems.

LIFE SPAN CONSIDERATIONS

Communication

With Older Client

- Assess for sensory disturbances.
- Face the client when speaking.
- Have patience; response may be slow.
- Show respect and be considerate of the older client's personal dignity.

With Children

- Be at eye level with the child.
- Use vocabulary appropriate for the child's level of development.

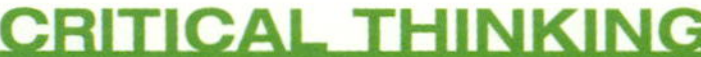

CRITICAL THINKING

Communication and the Unconscious Client

Why should you communicate with an unconscious client?

How can you communicate with an unconscious client?

The person with dysphasia has difficulty putting thoughts and feelings into words and sending messages. It should be noted, however, that seldom does the person with dysphasia have difficulty receiving and interpreting messages; thus, explanations should be given before doing anything. If the client can write, paper and pencil can be used for communication. A picture board, word board, letter board, or computer may also be employed. A person with speech impairments may feel frustrated and helpless. Establishing some method of communication for the client provides hope and maintains self-esteem while minimizing or preventing feelings of depression, anger, and hostility.

Level of Consciousness True communication cannot be accomplished with unconscious or comatose clients. It should be remembered, however, that unconscious or comatose clients may be able to hear even though they cannot respond. Caregivers should speak to these clients just as they would to alert clients. Always greet the client by name, identify yourself, and explain why you are in the room (i.e., what you are going to do). Then let the client know when you are leaving and, if possible, when you will return. Although one sided, this interaction is critical to the client's care.

Language Proficiency The client's ability to communicate effectively through spoken language also influences the nurse–client interaction. Clients who do not speak English generally come from another culture. Learning about the other culture, especially about the values and beliefs, will help prevent the nurse from violating those values and beliefs.

A family member who speaks English could be used as an interpreter, as shown in Figure 7-6. When another health care worker on the nursing unit speaks the same language as does the client, that person could also be used as an interpreter as long as it does not interfere with his or her work. Speak directly to the client whether an interpreter is present or not. Make eye contact with the client and speak slowly and clearly. Use simple words and avoid slang and medical jargon. The nurse may recommend a professional interpreter when obtaining informed consent.

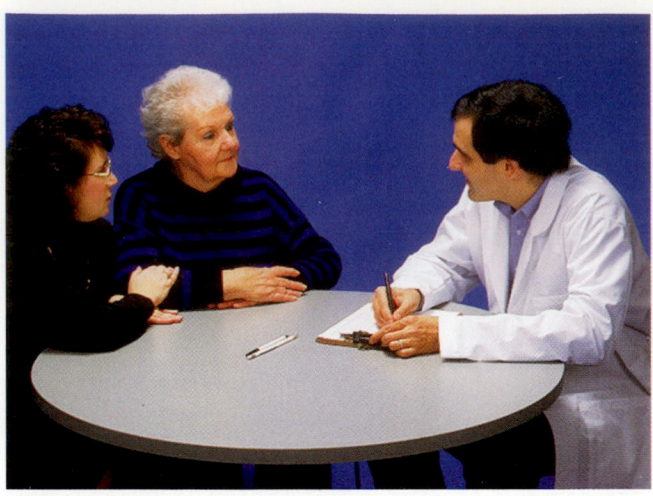

COURTESY OF DELMAR CENGAGE LEARNING

FIGURE 7-6 **A family member interprets communication with a non–English-speaking client.**

Pictures or a two-language dictionary are often helpful. When another language is prevalent in the community, nurses should learn some phrases in that language to use in client assessment and care. *Remember, gestures, facial expressions, and other nonverbal communication send messages without the use of language.*

Social Factors Socially acceptable health concerns, such as having the gallbladder or appendix removed or having the flu, are easy to discuss. It may be more difficult to communicate with a woman who is having a breast removed. The symbolic meaning of the breast may make it difficult for the client to accept its removal and may influence how she relates to others. A person who is HIV positive or has another sexually transmitted infection may be very reluctant to discuss the illness.

Stage of Illness The stage of a client's illness may influence the client's desire to communicate with the nurse. Clients in the early stages of illness may be eager to learn all they can about the illness or may express anger and resentment at their current state of health.

Terminally ill clients may pose special challenges for the nurse. Most terminally ill clients know they are dying and are concerned about those whom they love. It is thus important for the nurse to have the client identify those persons the client considers to be "family." Family and nurses often struggle with effective communication techniques when speaking with one who is dying. Death is not a prime subject for discussion, as it is often considered a defeat by health care workers. *Remember that silence and listening are both part of communication and can relay caring, compassion, and acceptance.*

Whenever a client begins talking about death, the nurse must be willing to listen and take part in the conversation. Many times nurses hesitate to communicate with the terminally ill for fear they will say the wrong thing. The client who wishes to talk needs a good listener. Allow the client to guide

PROFESSIONALTIP

Caring for the Client Who Is Hearing Impaired

- Check to see whether the client wears a hearing aid. Be sure it is in working order and turned on.
- Make every effort to move the client to a setting with minimal background noise.
- Always face the client.
- Speak in a normal tone and at a normal pace.
- Determine whether the client uses sign language. If signing is used, enlist the assistance of an interpreter.
- Pay particular attention to nonverbal cues of the client and to your own nonverbal behavior.
- Provide a pen and paper to facilitate communication, if necessary.

the conversation. Listen and accept what the client says. Trying not to give advice may be very difficult to do.

The nurse and the family must work together to understand the ways that the terminally ill client communicates. It can take persistence and insight to identify and decipher some messages. "Listening" to the client's gestures and facial expressions helps facilitate understanding of messages.

Religion Communication can be difficult when religious beliefs conflict with those of the health care team. Members of some religions seek healing only through faith and not through conventional medical services, including not receiving blood transfusions. When a client has a minister, priest, or rabbi visit, privacy should be provided if at all possible.

Family Situation Illness often unites family members around the client, but communication between the family and client may be strained if the family has not been close to or supportive of the client before the illness. The nurse must be careful not to discuss aspects of the client's condition or treatment in front of family members. It is usually best to ask family members to step out of the room when any nursing care is being given. This maintains the client's right to privacy and confidentiality.

If the client asks for a specific person to remain in the room, it is usually allowed unless specifically contraindicated.

Visual Ability Communicating with clients who are visually impaired may not seem to be a challenge at first; however, because the nonverbal part of any message, such as facial expressions, gestures, and other body language, is not able to be observed, an important part of every message is lost to the client.

Generally, persons who are visually impaired speak only when spoken to. Their speech is often loud when they are not sure where the other person is. Silence makes them uncomfortable.

When orienting a new client who cannot see, the nurse must include an explanation of "hospital sounds." Describe the room in detail and guide the client around the room if possible. Always speak and identify yourself when entering the room. Each step of a procedure as well as any touching should be described before it is initiated. To prevent startling a client, always inform the visually impaired client before touching.

PROFESSIONALTIP

Caring for the Client Who Is Visually Impaired

- Look directly at the client when speaking.
- Use a normal tone and volume of voice.
- Advise the client when you are entering or leaving the room.
- Orient the person to the immediate environment; use clock hours to indicate positions of items in relation to the client.
- Ask for permission before touching the client.

PROFESSIONALTIP

Objectivity

The nurse must remain objective and nonjudgmental when the client's idea of family is different from the nurse's idea of family.

CULTURAL CONSIDERATIONS

Family Interaction Patterns

- In some families, the male members make all the decisions.
- In some families, decisions are made jointly, with all members (or all adults) participating.
- In some families, unrelated persons such as godparents or special friends are involved in decision making.

COMMUNICATING WITH THE HEALTH CARE TEAM

Because providing care to clients is a team effort, effective communication is necessary. This communication between team members may be oral or written, individual, group, or on computer.

ORAL COMMUNICATION

Oral communication takes place among all health care team members. To provide continuity of care to the client, all persons who provide that care communicate orally concerning that care.

Nurse–Student Nurse

Student nurses communicate not only with their clinical instructor but with the staff nurses too. How well staff nurses interact with student nurses depends on the experiences the staff nurses have had with other student nurses and also on how the staff nurses were treated as students. Student nurses are present in the clinical facility for very specific learning experiences that are selected by the instructor and relate to classroom discussion. They will review client records, communicate with and care for their clients, and, when possible, observe others performing procedures. Depending on how far they have progressed through the nursing curriculum, students may be limited in their nursing activities. Communication between student nurses and staff nurses is essential because staff nurses are responsible for the care of clients even though clients are assigned to students. Usually, a helping relationship develops between staff nurses and nursing students.

Nurse–Nursing Assistant

The nurse is responsible for assigning duties to the nursing assistants. A relationship of trust and mutual respect is established by answering questions and providing reasons for specific activities requested.

Nursing assistants are often much more comfortable and confident in providing bedside care. Therefore, they can be of considerable assistance to the new graduate (whether an LP/VN or RN). They often have creative solutions to problems and should be included in planning care.

Nurse–Nurse

Nurse–nurse communications can be either peer–peer or superior–subordinate communication. Peer–peer communication takes place many times every day. When each nurse uses effective communication with peers as well as clients, the unit runs more efficiently, and client care will be more effective. Superior–subordinate communication often occurs when the superior discusses client care to be performed by the subordinate. The way this communication is handled affects both the attitude of the subordinate and the client care given.

Nurse–Physician

Nursing education and expertise have evolved over the years to a professional level. Nurses are responsible for their own actions even when under the direction of a physician. Nurses have a duty to secure physician clarification of any order that is illegible, that is unclear, or that violates hospital policy or procedure.

Nurses must communicate openly and honestly with physicians, demonstrating competence in assessments, nursing skills, provision of quality care, reporting change in client status, and accurate documentation.

Nurse–Other Health Professionals

Communicate with professionals in other departments on a peer-to-peer basis. The focus of communication should be clarification of goals for each client and ways to meet those goals. Top-quality care is provided to clients by listening to those in other departments and establishing mutual respect for each other's area of expertise.

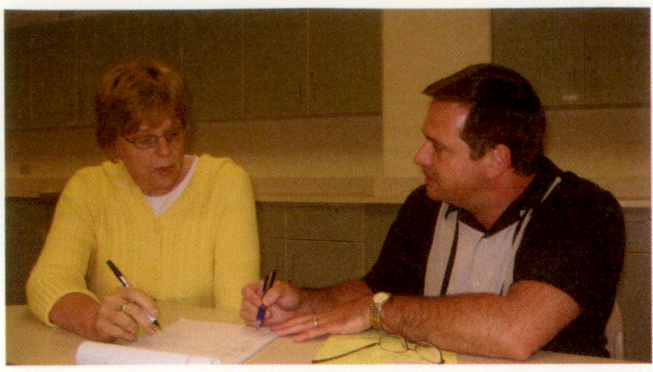

COURTESY OF DELMAR CENGAGE LEARNING

FIGURE 7-7 Nurses work together to plan client care.

Group Communication

Client care conferences may be scheduled whenever the need arises or on a regular basis. Some conferences may be only for the staff of a specific nursing unit; others may include some members of other departments. Only persons directly involved with client care should be invited (Figure 7-7).

The objectives of the conference are established by the conference leader, who makes all necessary arrangements. The meeting site should be a conference room or other private place. One person should record the discussion. When the conference is about a particular client, only facts are to be documented on the client's chart. When the topic is general and not related to any one client, only a record of the discussion is needed.

Telephone

When a student nurse takes a telephone call, the call should be answered with the name of the department or floor and the student's full name and position (i.e., student nurse). If a message is taken, the student nurse should write it down and read it back to the caller, asking for the caller's name and for the caller to spell out his or her name. The student nurse must never give out any information about clients.

Shift Report

Vital to continuity of client care is the **shift report** (report about each client between shifts). An oral report is the most common. The charge nurse of the outgoing shift may report to all members of the incoming shift or only to the incoming charge nurse who, in turn, shares the information with the appropriate caregivers on the incoming shift.

Sometimes, the report is put on a tape recorder for the next shift. This allows no chance for feedback, which can be a disadvantage.

Another method is a "walking report." The outgoing nurse reports to the oncoming nurse on each client as they walk from bed to bed. This way the client is included and aware of the information provided to the next shift.

The shift report about each client should be complete and concise no matter which method is used. The report should be focused on the clients and given in an orderly manner. This is not the time for social conversation.

Written Communication

Most written communication relates to the client's chart. All aspects of a client's care are recorded on that client's chart.

PROFESSIONALTIP

Client Information for Shift Report

- Name, room and bed, age, sex
- Physician, diagnosis, admission date, any surgery
- Diagnostic tests (results if available) or treatments in past 24 hours
- General status, significant changes in condition
- Changed or new physician's orders
- Nursing diagnoses with nursing orders
- Evaluation of nursing interventions
- Last PRN medication given, IV fluids left hanging and amount given
- Any concerns about the client or family

Requisitions to x-ray or to physical or respiratory therapy and requests for laboratory services for a client are all forms of written communication. The reports resulting from these requests become part of the client's chart.

One type of written communication not pertaining to a specific client is the interdepartmental memo requesting equipment, supplies, maintenance, or housekeeping. Documents such as this are necessary to keep the nursing unit functioning efficiently and effectively.

Electronic Communication

Computers are being used extensively in the business offices of health care agencies and have been so for years. The introduction of computers into the departments of direct client care has been slower, however. Nonetheless, in many places, computers are used by client care departments to send requisitions to other departments and to receive test results. Some hospital pharmacies use computer programs that show safe dosages and drug interactions. There are also programs to aid physicians in diagnosing and treating some conditions. Some acute care and long-term facilities have implemented full online documentation, including nursing notes, nursing care plans, and the medication administration record MAR.

Hing, Burt, and Woodwell (2007) studied the use of electronic medical records (EMR) by office-based physicians throughout the United States as well as plans to install new EMR systems or replace current systems within the next 3 years. Approximately 29% of physicians reported using full or partial EMR systems. This represents a 22% increase since 2005 and a 60% increase since 2001. With the expanding use of computers in health care and the corresponding potential for increased use, it is important for all health care workers to have some knowledge about computers.

Telehealth

According to Hutcherson (2001), **telehealth** is using telecommunication equipment and communication networks to transfer health care information between participants at different locations. It can be used in almost every area of health care.

Telenursing, an element of telehealth, permits nurses to provide care through a telecommunication system. The simplest form has been used for years—the telephone. **Telemedicine**, another element of telehealth, permits physicians to provide care through a telecommunication system. Recognized subspecialties include teledermatology, teleoncology, telepathology, and teleradiology.

Two issues related to telehealth that are especially important to nursing include licensure and standards of practice. The National Council of State Boards of Nursing (NCSBN) developed a plan for multistate licensure through legal agreement (interstate compacts) between a group of states. In these agreements, a nurse is licensed in one state but can practice nursing in any of the states in the compact. Before multistate licensure, nurses could participate in telenursing only within the state of their licensure. Practice standards for telenursing are in the process of being established. To assist nurses when providing telenursing care, the American Nurses Association (ANA) has developed some core principles for telehealth (ANA, 1999) and telehealth protocols (ANA, 2001).

The use of two-way video allows the client and health care provider to see, hear, and talk to each other. A stethoscope or otoscope (called peripherals) can be included in the hookup so that the sounds and visual images can be transmitted (Granade, 1997). This allows physician specialists in large medical centers to examine a client many miles away.

COMMUNITY/HOME HEALTH CARE

Use of Telenursing

- From the office, a home health nurse can watch a client at home change a dressing or self-administer insulin.
- During a video consult, a home health nurse might assist by manipulating the peripherals or actually performing a physical assessment.

PROFESSIONALTIP

Cell Phones in Health Care

According to C. Peter Waegermann, CEO, Medical Records Institute (Waegemann, 2007). "A healthcare revolution is on the horizon. The new capabilities of modern cell phones, smart phones, PDAs, and others . . . are creating new possibilities for healthcare." Physicians and nurses are using cell phones to load client information to be synchronized with the hospital's IT system at the end of the shift. Clients are downloading their medical records on their cell phones, PDAs, and so on to have on hand for easy retrieval in case of an emergency and to share with health care providers. Cell phones with e-mail capabilities can send images and diagnostic testing results to physicians as well as the client. The use of cell phones is an exciting development in the health care telecommunications industry.

Nurses should document all activities, assessment findings, information provided by the client, and any instructions given to the client. All data transmissions (e.g., telemetry printouts or videotapes) should be stored in the client's record. Most telemedicine laws require that existing confidentiality rules be maintained.

COMMUNICATING WITH YOURSELF

People talk to themselves every day whether they admit it or not. **Intrapersonal communication** is internal thoughts and discussion with oneself. This self-talk is what people say to themselves, thus influencing their personalities and how they interact with others. Self-talk may be positive or negative.

Positive Self-Talk

The practice of positive self-talk is key to positive self-concept. You can send positive thoughts to yourself about yourself, but, better yet, say the thoughts out loud. Thinking, saying, and hearing positive statements about oneself reinforces a positive self-concept. When you have had a difficult day, whether in the classroom or clinical area, remind yourself of your good attributes and accomplishments. Every day, tell yourself out loud what you learned or what good care you gave to your client(s).

The desire to succeed is reinforced by positive self-talk. When things are not going well and frustration sets in, memories of success can serve as positive influences.

Positive affirmation is a positive thought or idea on which a person consciously focuses to produce a desired result. Positive affirmation can be used to change negative inner messages to positive messages. For instance, say, "I know I can pass this test" instead of saying, "I don't know if I can pass this test." Of course, positive affirmation cannot be a substitute for studying and preparing for the test. Positive affirmation merely serves to modify your attitude about the test—or about any other situation.

Negative Self-Talk

Whenever you say to yourself, "I can't do . . . ," you are decreasing your self-concept with the negative self-talk. Negative self-talk may originate within you or may be a replay of things that others have said about you. Negative self-talk is self-destructive. Your self-image is lowered by your own criticism, and you begin to see yourself as a failure.

CASE STUDY

Self-Talk

A student nurse is sitting in a preconference meeting with her peers and clinical instructor preparing for the first day of clinical to begin. She begins to think to herself, "Oh, I'm so nervous. I can't do this. I am terrible at meeting and talking with people. How am I ever going to go into my client's room and introduce myself?"

1. This is an example of which type of self-talk? Explain.
2. List three positive thoughts or ideas that the student nurse could tell herself.
3. What other positive affirmations could the student nurse use to increase her self-concept?
4. What affect does negative self-talk have on a person's self-concept?

SUMMARY

- Communication is influenced by factors such as age, education, emotions, culture, language, attention, surroundings, and past experience.
- Nonverbal messages are generally more accurate in communicating a person's feelings.
- Verbal and nonverbal messages must be congruent for clear communication to take place.
- Techniques of therapeutic communication should be practiced and incorporated into the nurse's communication.
- Barriers to communication should be identified and avoided when communicating.
- People have four comfort zones of closeness: intimate, personal, social, and public.
- Therapeutic communication is purposeful and goal directed.
- Psychosocial aspects of communication may hinder or aid communication.
- Most nurse–client interactions should involve therapeutic communication.
- Nurse–client communication is influenced by both the client and the nurse.
- The nurse is many times a role model for the family in terms of communicating with the terminally ill client.
- Accurate communication among the health care team is necessary for continuity of client care.

REVIEW QUESTIONS

1. B.R. is in the bathroom with the door partially closed. A nurse enters his room and says, "You will not be able to eat or drink after supper because of tests tomorrow," and then leaves. Did communication take place?
   1. No, there was no feedback.
   2. No, there was no eye contact.
   3. Yes, Mr. George had to hear the message.
   4. Yes, there was a sender, receiver, and message.
2. Which of the following are all examples of verbal communication?
   1. Singing, dancing, smiling.
   2. Reading, writing, listening.
   3. Shaking hands, reading, grimacing.
   4. Whispering, making eye contact, answering.
3. When a client says, "I'm not sure how I'll handle all this," which response of the nurse represents clarification?
   1. "Handle all this?"
   2. "Well, you can ask your sister to help."
   3. "Oh, you'll be able to handle things. You're an intelligent person."
   4. "I'm not sure I understand what it is you're concerned about being able to handle."
4. A critically ill client denies there is anything wrong and talks constantly about going home. The nurse should:
   1. listen but say nothing.
   2. acknowledge the client's wishes and hopes.
   3. advise the client that it will be impossible to go home.
   4. assist the client in planning when to return home.
5. A client tells the nurse that she would rather die than have chemotherapy. The nurse should report this communication to:
   1. the physician only.
   2. all nurses on the unit.
   3. the physician and charge nurse.
   4. no one; it is a confidential communication.
6. The nurse is establishing a helping relationship with a new client on the unit. In addressing the client, the nurse should:
   1. gently touch the client on the shoulder right away.
   2. ask the client why he or she is in the hospital.
   3. call the client by his or her first name.
   4. knock before entering the client's room.
7. In using communication skills with clients, the nurse evaluates which response as being the most therapeutic?
   1. "Don't worry, I'm sure everything will be fine."
   2. "I noticed that you didn't take your medication this morning. Is something wrong?"
   3. "I think you should try the medication first before having surgery."
   4. "Why do you feel that way?"
8. The nurse asks the client, "What did the physician tell you about going home?" This is an example of:
   1. an open-ended question.
   2. a confrontational question.
   3. a closed question.
   4. a double-barreled question.
9. The client informs the nurse of her concerns that she might be experiencing depression due to her sad feelings, lack of energy, and daily episodes of crying. She states that she has thoroughly researched depression on the Internet and has brought the information to discuss with the physician. The client is most likely in which generation?
   1. Traditional.
   2. Baby boomer.
   3. Generation X.
   4. Generation Y.
10. The student nurse stated, "I think that Mr. Smith is showing improvement because his vital signs are stable today." This is an example of which type of communication?
    1. Passive.
    2. Assertive.
    3. Aggressive.
    4. Congruent.

REFERENCES/SUGGESTED READINGS

American Nurses Association. (1999). Core principles on telehealth. Retrieved September 3, 2008, from http://www.nursingworld.org

American Nurses Association. (2001). Developing telehealth protocols: A blueprint for success. Retrieved September 3, 2008, from http://www.nursingworld.org

Barry, P., & Farmer, S. (2000). *Mental health and mental illness* (7th ed.). Philadelphia: Lippincott Williams & Wilkins.

Bush, K. (2001). Do you really listen to patients? *RN, 64*(3), 35–37.

Calloway, S. D. (2001). Preventing communication breakdowns. *RN, 64*(1), 71–74.

Deering, C., & Jennings, D. (2002). Communicating with children and adolescents. *American Journal of Nursing, 102*(3), 34–41.

Estes, M. E. Z. (2010). *Health assessment and physical examination* (4th ed.), Clifton Park, NY: Delmar Cengage Learning.

Frisch, N. C, & Frisch, L. E. (2011). *Psychiatric Mental Health Nursing* (4th ed.). Clifton Park, NY: Delmar Cengage Learning.

Granade, P. (1997). The brave new world of telemedicine. *RN, 60*(7), 59–62.

Gravely, S. (2001). When your patient speaks Spanish—And you don't. *RN, 64*(5), 65–67.

Hall, Edward T. (1959). *The silent language*. New York: Doubleday.

Hing, E. S., Burt, C. W., & Woodwell, D. A. (2007). *Electronic medical record use by office-based physicians and their practice: United States, 2006*. Atlanta: Centers for Disease Control and Prevention.

Hutcherson, C. (2001, September 30). Legal considerations for nurses practicing in a telehealth setting. *Online Journal of Issues in Nursing, 6*(3), manuscript 3. Available: http://www.nursingworld.org/onjin/topic16/tpc16_3.htm

Kübler-Ross, E. (1969). *On death and dying*. New York: Macmillan.

Kübler-Ross, E. (1975). *Death: The final stage of growth*. Englewood Cliffs, NJ: Prentice Hall.

Kübler-Ross, E. (1978). *To live until we say good-bye*. Englewood Cliffs, NJ: Prentice Hall.

Lyon, B. (2000). Conquering dysfunctional anxiety: What you say to yourself matters. *Reflections on Nursing Leadership, 26*(4), 33–35.

Milliken, M. (2004). *Understanding human behavior* (7th ed.). Clifton Park, NY: Delmar Cengage Learning.

National Institute on Deafness and Other Communication Disorders. (2008). Mission. Retrieved September 3, 2008, from http://www.nidcd.nih.gov/about/learn/mission.asp

National Institute on Deafness and Other Communication Disorders. (2008a). Quick statistics. Retrieved September 3, 2008, from http://www.nidcd.nih.gov/health/statistics/quick.htm

North American Nursing Diagnosis Association International. (2010). *NANDA-I nursing diagnoses: Definitions and classification 2009-2011*. Ames, IA: Wiley-Blackwell.

Rochman, R. (2000). Are computerized patient records for you? *Nursing2000, 30*(10), 61–62.

Tamparo, C., & Lindh, W. (2007). *Therapeutic communications for health professionals* (3rd ed.). Clifton Park, NY: Delmar Cengage Learning.

Thomas, N., & Thompson, J. (2003). Tomorrow's nurses need your help today. *RN, 66*(6), 51–53.

Waegemann, C. P. (2007). The next big wave is m-health: Smart phones in healthcare. Retrieved September 3, 2008, from http://www.medrecinst.com/cellphone/articles.html

Waughfield, C. (2002). *Mental health concepts* (6th ed.). Clifton Park, NY: Delmar Cengage Learning.

RESOURCES

American Health Information Management Association, http://www.ahima.org

American Nurses Association, http://www.nursingworld.org

Health Resources and Services Administration, http://telehealth.hrsa.gov

Language Line Services, http://www.languageline.com

National Council of State Boards of Nursing, http://www.ncsbn.org

ValueOptions, http://www.valueoptions.com

CHAPTER 8
Client Teaching

MAKING THE CONNECTION

Refer to the following chapters to increase your understanding of client teaching:

Basic Nursing

- ***Legal and Ethical Responsibilities***
- ***Communication***
- ***Nursing Process/Documentation/Informatics***
- ***Life Span Development***
- ***Cultural Considerations***
- ***Stress, Adaptation, and Anxiety***

LEARNING OBJECTIVES

Upon completion of this chapter, you should be able to:

- Define key terms.
- Explain the importance of client education in today's health care climate.
- Relate principles of adult education to client teaching.
- Identify common barriers to learning.
- Explain the ways that learning varies throughout the life span.
- Discuss the nurse's professional responsibilities related to teaching.
- Relate the teaching–learning process to the nursing process.
- Describe teaching strategies that make learning meaningful to clients.

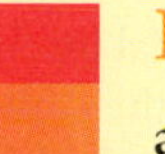

KEY TERMS

affective domain
auditory learner
cognitive domain
formal teaching
informal teaching
kinesthetic learner
learning
learning plateau
learning style
motivation
psychomotor domain
readiness for learning
teaching
teaching–learning process
teaching strategies
visual learner

INTRODUCTION

Client education is an integral part of nursing care. The nurse is responsible to help the client identify learning needs and resources that will restore and maintain that client's optimal level of functioning. This chapter discusses the teaching–learning process, including barriers and responsibilities, and relates it to the nursing process.

THE TEACHING–LEARNING PROCESS

The **teaching–learning process** is a planned interaction that promotes behavioral change that is not a result of maturation or coincidence. **Teaching** is an active process wherein one individual shares information with another to facilitate learning and thereby promote behavioral changes. A teacher is someone who uses a variety of goal-directed activities to promote change by assisting the learner to absorb new information.

Learning is the process of assimilating information, resulting in behavior change. Knowledge is power. By sharing knowledge with clients, the nurse helps them achieve their maximum level of wellness. The teaching–learning process has the same basic steps as the nursing process: assessment, identification of learning needs (nursing diagnosis), planning, implementation of teaching strategies, and evaluation of learner progress and teaching efficacy. These steps are discussed in greater detail later in this chapter.

Edelman and Mandle (2002) describe the goal of health education as helping individuals achieve optimal states of health through their own actions. Often, deficient knowledge about the course of illness and/or self-care practices hinders the client's recovery or in practicing health-promoting behaviors. The nurse's role is to help bridge the gap between those things a client knows and those things a client needs to know to achieve optimal health.

Client teaching is done for a variety of reasons, including to:

- Promote wellness
- Prevent illness
- Restore health
- Facilitate coping abilities

Client education focuses on the client's ability to practice healthy behaviors. The client's ability to care for self is enhanced by effective education. Client education may:

- Improve quality of care
- Decrease length of hospital stays
- Decrease chance of hospital readmission
- Improve compliance with treatment regimens

These benefits are enhanced through nurses' continued active participation as client educators.

Formal teaching is planned and goal directed, but informal teaching can occur in any setting at any time.

FORMAL TEACHING

Formal teaching takes place at a specific time, in a specific place, and on a specific topic. It is planned and goal directed (Figure 8-1). The teacher prepares the information and/or activities related to the topic. Formal teaching may take place in a class setting with several learners, or it may be performed one-on-one. For example, many health care facilities provide formal classes related to diabetes. The same basic information is necessary for all clients with diabetes.

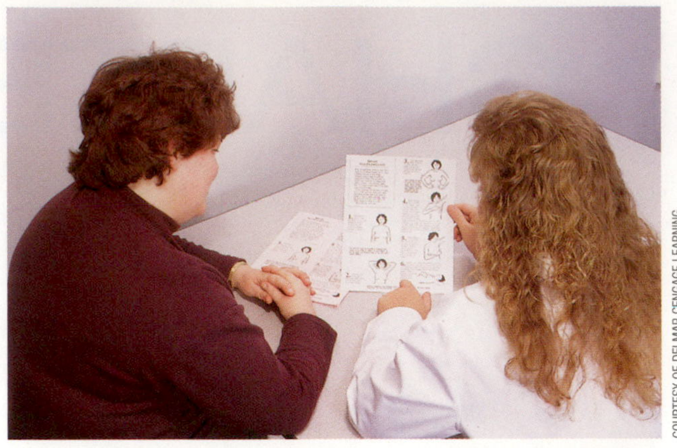

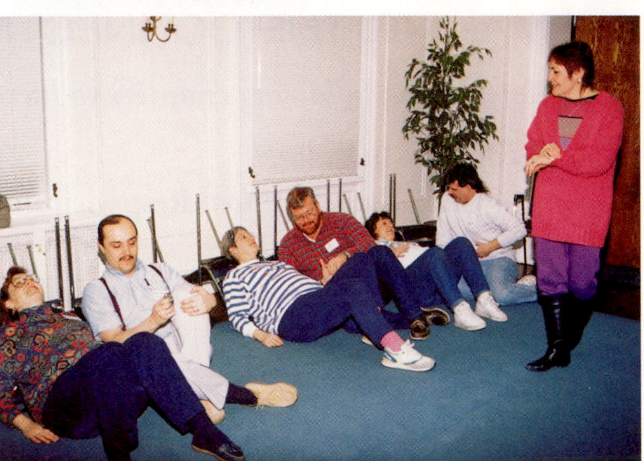

FIGURE 8-1 Nurses engage in formal teaching with both individual and groups clients. (*Bottom photo courtesy of Bellevue Woman's Hospital, Niskayuna, NY.*)

INFORMAL TEACHING

Informal teaching takes place any time, any place, whenever a learning need is identified. While providing nursing care, nurses have many opportunities for informal teaching, such as answering the clients' questions and explaining care being given to the client. Informal teaching may also occur in the midst of formal teaching. A comment or question from a learner in a formal setting may trigger some informal teaching in response. For example, during a class on diet for the diabetic client, a question about dietary cholesterol may be asked. The response would be considered informal teaching because it was not the planned topic.

An understanding of learning domains, learning principles, learning styles, learning barriers, and teaching methods is helpful. These topics are discussed as follows.

LEARNING DOMAINS

In his classic work, Bloom (1977) identifies three areas or domains wherein learning occurs: the **cognitive domain**, which involves intellectual understanding; the **affective domain**, which involves attitudes, beliefs, and emotions; and the **psychomotor domain**, which involves the performance of motor skills. Information is processed in each domain.

TABLE 8-1 Learning Domains

DOMAIN	DEFINITION	EXAMPLE
Cognitive	Learning involving the acquisition of facts and data; used in decision making and problem solving	Client states the symptoms of possible complications
Affective	Learning involving attitude, emotion, and belief changing; used in making judgments	Client begins to accept the lifestyle changes required
Psychomotor	Learning involving gaining motor skills; used in physical application of knowledge	Client uses glucose monitor

COURTESY OF DELMAR CENGAGE LEARNING

TABLE 8-2 Teaching Strategies for the Learning Domains

COGNITIVE	AFFECTIVE	PSYCHOMOTOR
Lecture or discussion	Role playing	Demonstration
Audiovisual materials	Discussion group	Return demonstration
Printed materials	Support group	Audiovisual materials
Programmed instruction	Role modeling	Discovery
Computer-assisted learning	Printed materials	Skill repetition
Independent study	One-on-one counseling	Printed materials

From *Teaching the Client and Family*, by R. Smith, 2008, manuscript submitted for publication, adapted from *Community Based Nursing* (2nd ed.), by R. Hunt, 2001, Philadelphia: Lippincott.

Table 8-1 briefly outlines the three learning domains and provides clinical examples.

Nurses must be sensitive to all three learning domains when developing effective teaching plans and must use **teaching strategies**, or techniques to promote learning, that will tap into each of the domains. For instance, teaching a diabetic client how insulin works in the body falls within the cognitive domain; helping the same client learn how to use a glucose monitor falls within the psychomotor domain; and encouraging the client to view diabetes as only one aspect of the individual falls within the affective domain. Table 8-2 gives examples of teaching strategies for each learning domain.

LEARNING PRINCIPLES

Fundamental principles of learning can be used when teaching clients. Knowles, Holton, and Swanson (2005) cite four basic assumptions about adult learners, which are applicable to client education:

- *Assumption 1:* Personality develops in an orderly fashion from dependence to independence. *Nursing application:* Plan teaching–learning activities promoting client participation. This encourages independence and increases client control and self-care.
- *Assumption 2:* Learning readiness is affected by developmental stage and sociocultural factors. *Nursing application:* Conduct a psychosocial assessment before planning teaching–learning activities.
- *Assumption 3:* Previous learning experiences are a foundation for further learning. *Nursing application:* Perform a complete assessment to ascertain what the client already knows and build on that knowledge base.
- *Assumption 4:* Immediacy reinforces learning. *Nursing application:* Provide opportunities for immediate application of knowledge and skills and incorporate feedback as part of each nurse–client interaction.

Learning principles include relevance, motivation, readiness, maturation, reinforcement, participation, organization, and repetition.

Relevance

The material to be learned must be meaningful to the client, easily understood by the client, and related to previously learned information. Individuals must believe that they need to learn the information before learning can occur. If an individual sees the information as being personally valuable, the information is more likely to be learned. Because relevance is individually determined, the nurse must assess the personal meaning of learning for each client.

Motivation

One of the most critical indicators of the potential success of a teaching session is the client's motivation level. Redman (2006) describes **motivation** as forces acting on or within an organism that initiate, direct, and maintain behavior. Motivation is complex and constantly changing dependent on positive or negative influences in life (Smith, 2008). To maximize motivation, the nurse must keep the teaching–learning goals realistic by breaking the content down into small, achievable steps. For example, the cardiac client must see value in information about exercise, such as that the heart will be strengthened and the client will have more energy.

Readiness

The client should be able and willing to learn. Readiness is closely related to growth and development. For example, the

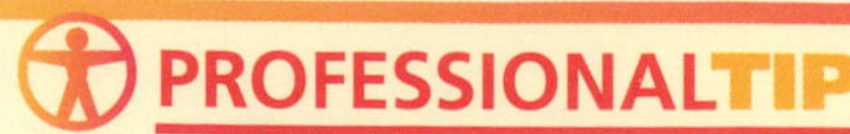

Checking Literacy

"Lscean uyro sdhna. Seu yver dloc rweat."

The preceding is what some clients see when given printed educational materials. Avoid making assumptions about client literacy. Check comprehension through return explanation of the written material.

client must have the requisite cognitive and psychomotor skills for learning a particular task, and the client must comprehend the information. One indicator of learning readiness is if clients ask questions; another is if clients become involved in learning activities, such as participating in return demonstration of a dressing change. Some indicators of lack of client readiness are anxiety, avoidance, denial, and lack of participation in discussion, demonstration, or self-care activities.

Maturation

The client should be developmentally able to learn and have requisite cognitive and psychomotor abilities. Assess the client for characteristics that will hinder or facilitate learning, such as developmental stage. Assess the client's developmental stage. Do not automatically assume that a 34-year-old client has mastered the developmental tasks of earlier stages.

Maturity level greatly influences the client's ability to learn information. Each developmental stage is characterized by unique skills and abilities affecting the response to various teaching tools. Developmental stage greatly determines the type of data taught, the method(s), the vocabulary, and the location of teaching. In addition to developmental stage, the nurse should also evaluate the client's cognitive skills, problem-solving abilities, and attention span.

Reinforcement

Feedback provided to the learner should be immediate and positive to reinforce the client's motivation and readiness to learn. For example, the client who is learning to apply a sterile dressing to an open wound should be told during the application of the dressing that it is being done correctly (if it is) and should be praised upon completion for learning so quickly (or whatever is appropriate). If some aspect of the dressing application is lacking, the nurse must maintain a positive approach in guiding the client to correctly perform the application.

Participation

The client's active involvement in the learning process promotes and enhances learning. Client involvement is relatively easy to monitor when a psychomotor skill is learned, as the client is actively involved in practicing a physical skill. Learning that takes place in the cognitive or affective domain is also most effective when active involvement of the client is encouraged. For example, the client who is on a low-fat diet can be involved in learning to self-regulate with regard to diet by reading labels of foods and planning menus of low-fat meals.

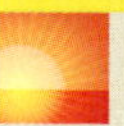

LIFE SPAN CONSIDERATIONS

Ability to Learn

Remember that age is not always synonymous with developmental level; observation of behavior provides the clearest picture of developmental level.

Organization

The material to be learned should incorporate previously learned information and be presented in sequence from simple to complex and from familiar to unfamiliar. Again using the example of the client learning about a low-fat diet, the nurse begins the teaching session by finding out what the client knows about the nutrient content of foods and then proceed by helping the client learn to read food labels, then plan a meal, and plan a menu for a day and a week, and so forth.

Repetition

Retention of material is reinforced with practice, repetition, and presentation of the same material in a variety of ways. The more often the learner hears or sees the material, the greater the chance of retention.

It is good to keep in mind that a **learning plateau**, or peak in the effectiveness of teaching and depth of learning, will occur in relation to the client's motivation, interest, and perception of relevance of the material. Frequent reinforcement of learning through immediate feedback and continual reassessment of effectiveness will enhance the value of the learning process for both the teacher and the learner. Making the information-acquisition process as user friendly as possible also increases satisfaction and success. This can be done by making learning as creative and interesting as possible and by adopting a flexible approach to allow the learning process to be dynamic.

CRITICAL THINKING

Learning

Will knowledge acquisition alone result in learning (behavioral change)? Why? Why not?

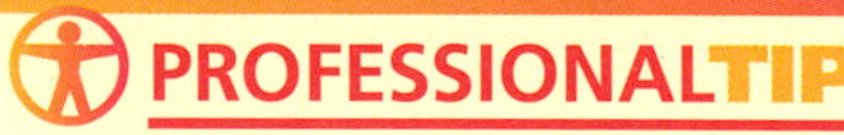

Beliefs about Learning

- Each individual has the capacity to learn, but learning ability varies.
- The pace of learning varies from person to person.
- Learning occurs throughout the life span.
- Learning occurs in formal and informal settings.
- Learning is an individualized process.
- Learning new information is based on previous knowledge and experiences.
- Motivation and readiness are necessary prerequisites for learning.
- Prompt feedback facilitates learning.

Learning Style

Each individual has a unique way of processing information. The manner whereby an individual takes in new information and processes the material is called **learning style**. Some people learn by processing information visually (**visual learner**), others by listening to the words (**auditory learner**), and others by experiencing the information or by touching, feeling, or doing (**kinesthetic learner**). According to Reed (2007), approximately 40% to 65% of students are visual learners, and 10% to 30% are kinesthetic learners. Use a variety of techniques, such as lecture, discussion, role play, modeling, games, return demonstration, imitation, problem solving, and question-and-answer sessions, to match various learning styles of clients. A good way to discover learning style is by asking the client, "What helps you learn?" or "What kinds of things do you enjoy doing?" Then teaching strategies can be matched to the client's learning style. Web sites with tools to determine an individual's learning style are listed in the "Resources" section at the end of the chapter. Table 8-3 gives suggestions for teaching–learning methods and study methods for each learning style. Students may use these to assist in personal study habits and when teaching clients.

Barriers to the Teaching–Learning Process

The giving and receiving of information does not, in and of itself, guarantee that learning will occur. Several barriers can impede the teaching–learning process. In a nursing

Table 8-3 Teaching–Learning Methods and Study Methods for Learning Styles

STYLE OF LEARNING	TEACHING–LEARNING METHODS	STUDY METHODS
Visual	Printed outline for student to follow PowerPoint slides Supplemental reading/articles Pictures/visual display (charts, graphs, diagrams) Demonstration with return demonstration Brainstorming with ideas written on whiteboard Short lecture with opportunity to try new methods Guided imagery Games	Workbooks Lab manuals Computer-aided instruction Assembly kits Videos Reading material
Auditory	Lecture Discussion Problem solving Question and answer Brainstorming Interactive video Guided imagery Verbally explain how to solve math problems Verbally explain any slides, charts, graphs, diagrams	Videos verbal explanation CDs Study with background music Read out loud
Kinesthetic	Role playing Modeling Games Demonstration/return demonstration Writing assignments Hold and play with pen or other object when reading or listening to lecture Take notes during lecture Field trips Experiential situations Short lecture with opportunity to try new methods	Workbooks Lab manuals, computer-aided instruction Assembly kits Hold and play with squeeze toys when reading

Adapted from "An Investigation of Learning Styles of Practical and Baccalaureate Nursing Students," by G. Duncan, 1996, *Journal of Nursing Education*, 35(1); "A New Definition for Individual: Implications for Learning and Teaching," by A. Gregorc and H. Ward, 1977, *NASSP Bulletin*; and Learning Your Way, by S. Reed, 2007, from www.presentations.com/msg/content_display/training/e3i7639605670451237f7bf2bea3bf8bad3.

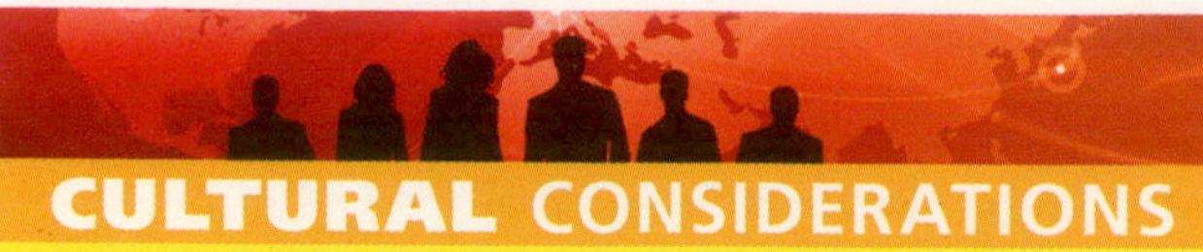

CULTURAL CONSIDERATIONS

Overcoming Sociocultural Barriers

- Use pictures whenever possible.
- Provide written material in the appropriate language.
- Use a culturally sensitive interpreter or a family member who understands health care terminology.
- Avoid the use of clichés, jargon, or value-laden terms.
- Learn about the client's cultural norms.
- Be aware of your own values.
- Tailor teaching (information and questions) to the client's ability to read and write.
- Have the client verbalize his understanding from the teaching–learning session.

situation, the nurse, the client, or both may encounter one or more of these barriers. Learning barriers can be classified as either internal (psychological or physiological) or external (environmental or sociocultural). Examples of these barriers are listed in Table 8-4. To facilitate the learning process, the nurse must assess for the presence of learning barriers. Specific assessment information is presented later in this chapter.

Environmental Barriers

Both the nurse and client are subject to environmental barriers. As part of planning for a teaching session, the nurse ensures necessary privacy and minimizes interruptions and extraneous stimuli.

TABLE 8-4 Barriers to Learning

EXTERNAL BARRIERS	INTERNAL BARRIERS
Environmental • Lack of privacy • Extraneous stimuli • Interruptions	Psychological • Anxiety • Anger • Fear • Depression
Sociocultural • Language • Level of education • Values	Physiological • Pain • Oxygen deprivation • Fatigue • Hunger

COURTESY OF DELMAR CENGAGE LEARNING

Sociocultural Barriers

When language is a barrier to the teaching–learning process, several steps can be taken to ensure that learning takes place, such as using pictures, providing printed material in the appropriate language, or using an interpreter. Even when the nurse and client both speak the same language, a language barrier may exist when clichés, health care jargon, or value-laden terms are used. Furthermore, the meanings that the nurse and client attach to specific types of body language may differ depending on cultural influences. Nurses must be aware of their own value systems but focus client teaching within the client's value system. The client's level of education is kept in mind and words tailored to the client's educational level without "talking down" to the client.

Psychological Barriers

Nurses may be anxious about client teaching. Knowing the client's learning needs and adequate preparation related to content, environmental and sociocultural aspects, and developmental ability of the client alleviates some of this anxiety. What little anxiety is left will likely make the nurse more alert and sensitive.

Clients and families are often upset about the health situation. They may be anxious, angry, fearful, or depressed. In addition to the client's words, the nurse should pay attention to body language and behavior. If clients or family members are obviously angry, the nurse should acknowledge the anger by saying something like "You appear to be very angry about something. Tell me what you are feeling." Allowing clients and family members to express their emotions clears the air and allows learning to take place.

PROFESSIONALTIP

Overcoming Psychological Barriers

- Recognize your own emotions related to client teaching.
- Assess for psychological barriers to learning.
- Acknowledge the client's emotions but do not respond in kind.

PROFESSIONALTIP

Physiological Comfort and Learning

- Administer pain medication, as appropriate, before a teaching session to enable the client to concentrate on the information presented.
- Plan teaching sessions when the client is not fatigued, as might be the case after a physical therapy session, for example.
- Ensure that the client is in a comfortable position and does not have to go to the bathroom.

CRITICAL THINKING

Barriers to Learning

A 56-year-old male is admitted to the ER with epigastric discomfort, pain radiating from the chest down the right arm, weakness, pallor, diaphoresis, and shortness of breath. He is an executive with a large corporation and has a wife and two adolescent children. His wife is at his bedside and is very anxious and upset over his condition. He is also anxious and believes that he is having a heart attack. The client states that his father died of a massive heart attack at age 56. What barriers to learning would be affecting this client? How could the nurse's approach help overcome these barriers?

Physiological Barriers

The physiological situation affects the client's ability to learn. The client who is struggling to breathe, for example, is unable to pay attention to any teaching. A teaching session should be planned for a time when the client is rested and free from pain.

Teaching Methods

Many different teaching methods can be used depending on the client's learning need and the applicable learning domain.

Teaching Methods Applicable in the Cognitive Domain

Effective methods for promoting cognitive learning include discussion, formal lecture, question-and-answer sessions, role play, and games/computer activities.

Discussion Discussions may involve the nurse and one or several clients who need to learn the same information. Active participation in the discussion is promoted. Group discussions allow peer support.

Formal Lecture In formal lectures, the teacher presents the information to be learned, and learner participation is usually minimal.

Question-and-Answer Sessions Question-and-answer sessions can take two forms. In one, the client's concerns are addressed by the client asking the questions and the nurse providing answers. In the other, the nurse assists the client in applying the knowledge learned by asking the client questions that the client then answers (Figure 8-2).

Role Play Role play provides the client an opportunity to apply knowledge in a safe, controlled environment. In role play, the nurse and client each assume a certain role in order to play out different possible scenarios. For instance, the nurse teaching a client sex education information intended for an adolescent may have the client assume the role of parent, while

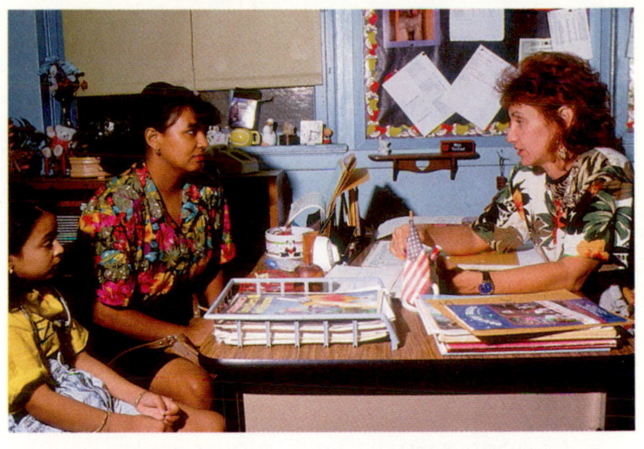

COURTESY OF DELMAR CENGAGE LEARNING

FIGURE 8-2 A Question-and-Answer Session with School Nurse, Mother, and Child

the nurse assumes the role of the teenager. The two can then engage in practice discussion sessions to prepare the client for the actual parent–teen discussion.

Games/Computer Activities Games and computer activities can be used to teach clients at a level that is appropriate for them. These methods allow the client to use the new information in various situations and to have fun while learning.

Teaching Methods Applicable in the Affective Domain

Role play and discussion are both effective methods for stimulating affective learning.

Role Play Role play allows expression of feelings, attitudes, and values in a safe, controlled environment. The client can try out different attitudes and values.

Discussion One-on-one discussion between nurse and client is effective for personal or sensitive topics related to values, feelings, attitudes, and emotions.

Teaching Methods Applicable in the Psychomotor Domain

Demonstration, supervised practice, and return demonstration assist the client to learn psychomotor skills.

Demonstration In demonstration, the nurse presents in a step-by-step manner the skill or procedure to be learned, explaining what is done and why. In this way, the client sees not only the equipment and the way it is used, but also the nurse's attitude and behaviors.

Supervised Practice In supervised practice, the client uses the equipment and performs the skill or procedure while the nurse watches. The nurse gives suggestions or corrects the client as the practice proceeds. Repetition can continue until the client feels confident in performing the skill or procedure.

Return Demonstration In return demonstration, the client performs the skill or procedure without any coaching from the nurse. Upon completion of the task, the nurse provides feedback and reinforcement to the client.

LIFE SPAN CONSIDERATIONS

Teaching Children

- Ensure that the child is comfortable.
- Encourage participation of caregiver.
- Assess the child's developmental level, learning readiness, and motivation. Do not equate age with developmental level.
- Assess the child's psychological status.
- Determine self-care abilities of the child.
- Use play, imitation, and role play.
- Use various visual stimuli, such as books, chalkboards, and videos, to share information and assess understanding.
- Use terms easily understood by the client and caregiver.
- Provide frequent repetition and reinforcement.
- Develop realistic goals consistent with developmental level.
- Remember that the goals of educating children are to improve cooperation, prevent excessive anxiety, and hasten the recovery process.

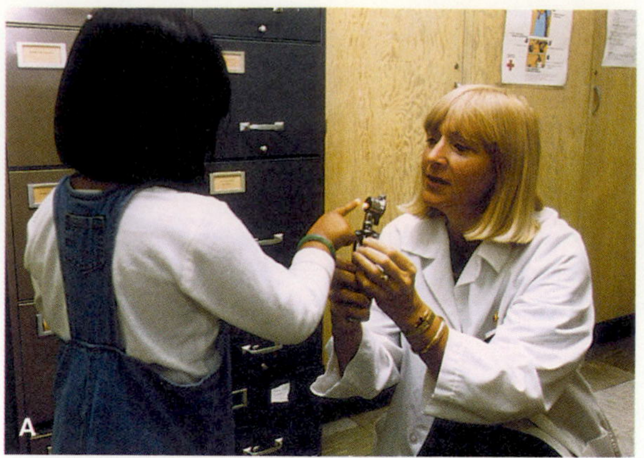

COURTESY OF DELMAR CENGAGE LEARNING

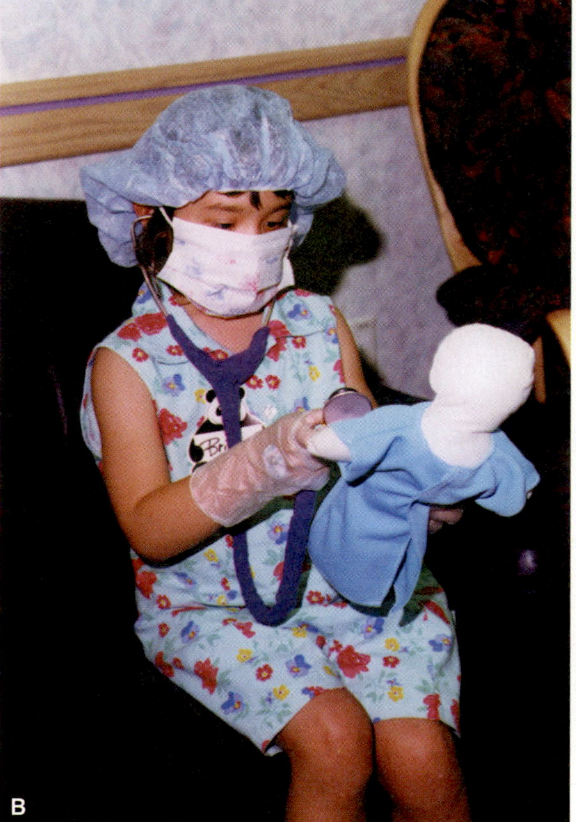

COURTESY OF DELMAR CENGAGE LEARNING

FIGURE 8-3 ***A,*** **The nurse is at the child's level, while the child learns about the instrument to be used in the examination;** ***B,*** **Role playing with a doll decreases a child's anxiety and enhances teaching opportunities.**

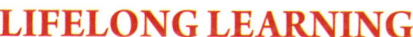

LIFELONG LEARNING

One basic assumption underlies teaching: *All people are capable of learning.* However, the ability to learn varies from person to person and from situation to situation. Learning needs and learning abilities change throughout life. The client's developmental stage and chronological age greatly influence the ability to learn. The principles of learning discussed earlier in this chapter are relevant to learners of all ages. Teaching approaches must be altered depending on the client's developmental stage and level of understanding. Specific information for children, adolescents, and older adults is described in the following sections.

CHILDREN

Readiness for learning (evidence of willingness to learn) varies during childhood depending on maturation level. The nurse must work closely with the child's caretaker, especially when caring for young children.

Young children learn primarily through play. Incorporating play into teaching activities for children can therefore enhance learning (Figure 8-3). Puppets, coloring books, and toys can be effective teaching tools for the young child. Encourage the young child to be an active participant in the learning process.

Older children can also benefit from the use of art materials to express their emotions and their understanding of those things that are or will be happening to them. Using medical supplies (such as medicine cups or bandages), the child may play at giving medicine to a doll or putting a bandage on the doll like the bandage that will be put on the

CLIENT TEACHING

Do As I Do

- Individuals learn from examples set by role models.
- Adolescents are very sensitive to any discrepancy between words and actions.
- Encourage parents to model the behaviors they wish their children to develop.

child. While the child is involved in play, the nurse is both teaching the child what to expect regarding treatment procedures and alleviating anxiety.

ADOLESCENTS

Individuals approaching adolescence are able to understand relationships between things. Usually, reading and comprehension ability have advanced, and the adolescent understands more complex information. Because one of the strongest influences on the adolescent is peer support, group meetings are often useful in teaching. The nurse can be a potent teacher as a role model.

OLDER ADULTS

Many physiological changes accompany aging. These changes cause some older adults to experience perceptual impairments in vision and hearing. The nurse assesses for these changes and adjusts teaching materials accordingly. For example, providing large-print written material and verifying that the client hears all instructions and directions are strategies helpful in teaching older clients.

LIFE SPAN CONSIDERATIONS

Teaching Adolescents

- Respect the adolescent.
- Boost their confidence by seeking their input and opinions on health care matters.
- Encourage exploration of their own feelings.
- Be sensitive to peer pressure.
- Help adolescents identify and build on their positive qualities.
- Use language that is clear yet appropriate to the health care setting.
- Encourage independent and informed decision making by engaging them in problem-solving activities.

PROFESSIONAL RESPONSIBILITIES OF TEACHING

The nurse empowers clients in their self-care abilities through teaching. Teaching provides information to clients about health-promoting behaviors, specific disease processes, and treatment methods. Although each state has its own definition of nursing practice, teaching is a required function of nurses in most states. Redman (2006) cites National League for Nursing documents dating back to 1918 as stating that "the nurse is essentially a teacher and an agent of health."

Providing client education is an expected role of all nurses. However, because of the nursing shortage and personal time constraints, some nurses are omitting the important responsibility of client teaching. If nurses give up their

LIFE SPAN CONSIDERATIONS

Teaching Older Adults

- Ensure that the client is comfortable. Fatigue, pain, a full bladder, or hunger can hinder learning.
- Assess the client's developmental level, motivation, and learning readiness.
- Assess the client for depression, anxiety, or denial, which can interfere with learning.
- Determine client's ability for self-care.
- Use words easily understood by the client.
- Avoid talking down to the client; a condescending, paternalistic manner hinders learning.
- Find the time of day when the client is most alert.
- Present material slowly using examples.
- Encourage client participation.
- Ask for feedback and listen actively.
- Provide feedback frequently.
- Assess for perceptual impairments and individualize teaching strategies accordingly:

For memory-impaired clients:

- Repeat material.
- Use different cues (spoken words, pictures, written materials, and symbols).

For visually impaired clients:

- Use large-print materials.
- Furnish a magnifying glass.
- Be sure prescription eyeglasses are worn.
- Arrange adequate lighting and reduce glare.

For hearing-impaired clients:

- Face the client when speaking.
- Use short sentences with words that are easily understood.
- Use gestures and demonstrate to reinforce verbal information.
- Eliminate distractions (activities or noises in the environment) as much as possible.

role as client educators to spend time performing additional tasks, nursing's worth to the health care system could greatly diminish. Client teaching requires the depth of information that only nurses possess; as such, it is one of the truly independent functions of nursing practice.

Client teaching is also required by several accrediting bodies, including the Joint Commission (2008). The American Hospital Association's *Patient Care Partnership* (2009) calls for the client's understanding of health status and treatment approaches. Only clients who are well informed can give informed consent. Nurses assess clients' level of understanding about treatment methods and correct any knowledge deficits. The nurse often serves as an interpreter for the client by explaining, clarifying, and referring.

Teaching supports behavioral changes that lead to positive adaptation by the client. Teaching decreases the fear of change by reducing anxiety and anticipation stresses.

Client teaching is an essential nursing function in every practice setting. All clients require information about disease prevention, growth and development, safety, first aid, nutrition, and hygiene. The hospitalized client needs information about his condition, the expected treatment, and the environment of the health care facility. By the time of discharge, clients must also have information about postdischarge care related to medications, dietary modifications, activity, complication prevention, and rehabilitation plans.

Clients recovering at home and their families also have significant learning needs. A primary role of the home health nurse is to teach the client about caring for himself at home. This often involves teaching family members ways to provide care (Figure 8-4) and information about their illness, accident, or injury. They should also be taught ways to achieve and maintain a maximum state of wellness. Accurate teaching plans for the home-based client and family are established by assessing many factors, such as:

Support system

- Individuals available to help give care
- Caregivers' knowledge about necessary care

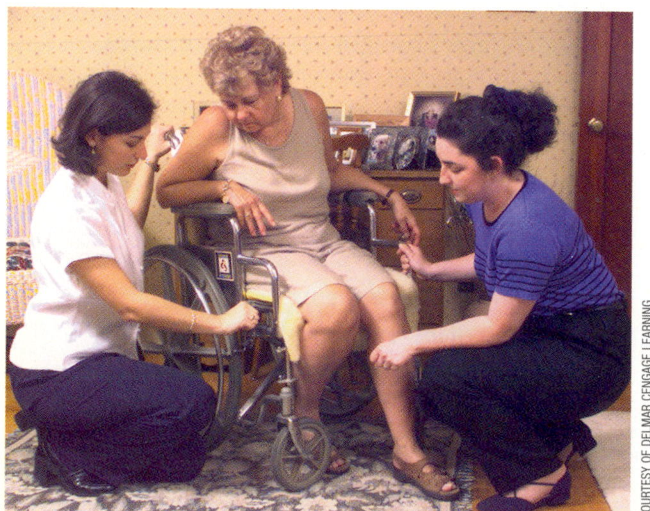

FIGURE 8-4 **The nurse teaches a family member how to provide care.**

COMMUNITY/HOME HEALTH CARE

Client Teaching Considerations

- Preparation of the client and family for home care begins at the time of hospital admission, not at the time of discharge.
- Discharge planning should consider current and potential learning needs of clients and caregivers.
- Teach about community resources.

Environmental

- Home accessibility
- Space to meet special needs of the client
- Need for and availability of equipment and supplies
- Need for assistance with self-care activities
- Need for information about environmental cleanliness related to health

Economic

- Ability to purchase medications, equipment, and supplies
- Available financial assistance

Community resources

- Area resources
- Awareness of and access to support services
- Respite availability for the family

SELF-AWARENESS

Several characteristics of nurses influence the outcome of the teaching–learning process. Nurse self-awareness with regard to the concepts discussed in the following sections is an all-important first step in teaching.

Knowledge Base

It is impossible for nurses to teach if they lack the knowledge or skills that are to be taught. Staying both current in knowledge and proficient in skills is the first step to maintaining efficacy and credibility as a teacher. Although it is impossible for one individual to be an expert in every area of nursing, knowing when to refer the client to others for teaching is an important critical-thinking skill.

Interpersonal Skills

Effective teaching is based on the nurse's ability to establish rapport with the client. The empathic nurse shows sensitivity to the client's needs and preferences. An atmosphere in which the client feels free to ask questions promotes learning. Activities that help establish an environment conducive to learning include:

- Showing genuine interest in the client
- Including the client in *every* step of the teaching–learning process
- Employing a nonjudgmental approach
- Communicating at the client's level of understanding

CRITICAL THINKING

Teaching Ethics

Is it ethical for a nurse to attempt to change a client's beliefs under the guise of teaching? Should a nurse "teach" a client the "right" attitude or belief?

PROFESSIONALTIP

Medical Jargon and Teaching

- Consider the language used by most nurses; think of the terms nurses take for granted. When a client is asked to "void," for example, does the client understand what is meant?
- These frequently used terms can easily be misunderstood by clients and families: *ambulate, defecate, dangle, NPO, vital signs,* and *contraindicated.*
- How can you communicate without using professional jargon?

DOCUMENTATION

The standard is for nurses to document client education. From a legal perspective, if the nurse teaches a client but does not document it, the teaching never occurred. Documentation of teaching facilitates accurate communication to other health care colleagues and promotes continuity of care.

Many different approaches are used to document client teaching. Figure 8-5 is an example of a documentation form related to client teaching in an inpatient setting.

Because client education is a standard and essential component of nursing practice, each nurse must document the teaching interventions used and the client's response. Elements to be documented in all practice settings include:

- Content
- Teaching methods
- Learner(s) (e.g., client, family member, other caretaker)
- Client/family response to teaching activities

TEACHING–LEARNING AND THE NURSING PROCESS

The teaching–learning process and the nursing process are interdependent. Both are dynamic and comprise the same phases: assessment, diagnosis, planning, implementation, and evaluation.

ASSESSMENT

Primary (client) and secondary (family or significant other) sources are used by nurses to assess learning needs. Communication is the foundation of assessment related to learning. Factors to be considered include:

- Actual learning needs
- Potential learning needs
- Ability and readiness to learn
- Client strengths and limitations
- Previous experiences

Actual Learning Needs

Everyone who receives health care services has some need for learning. Client teaching may be indicated when a client:

- Asks for information to make decisions
- Requires new skills
- Desires to make lifestyle changes
- Is in an unfamiliar environment

The client's knowledge about the content to be taught must be evaluated. Previous knowledge can be used as a foundation for new concepts. The client's learning needs can be determined in a variety of ways, including:

- Asking the client directly
- Observing client behaviors
- Asking the client's family or significant others

The nurse first addresses the client's immediate need for knowledge. For example, preoperative clients are taught deep breathing exercises and leg exercises before surgery so that they are able to perform those exercises after surgery and thereby prevent potential complications. As soon as possible after surgery, begin teaching incision care so that the client is ready to care for the incision when discharged.

Potential Learning Needs

Potential learning needs are also assessed so that anticipatory planning can be done to prevent a relapse in the recovery process or to maintain wellness. Following are two scenarios with related potential learning needs noted:

- N.L. is pregnant for the first time. *Potential learning need:* Infant care
- T.A. has diabetes and has just been told that he must take insulin daily. *Potential learning need:* Self-administration of insulin

PROFESSIONALTIP

Learning Needs Assessment

Assess the client's learning needs by answering the following:

- Is the client uncertain about an upcoming procedure?
- Does the client know about medications, purposes, and side effects?
- Can the client describe necessary lifestyle modifications?
- Is the client able to correctly perform treatment procedures (e.g., colostomy irrigations, injections, blood glucose monitoring)?

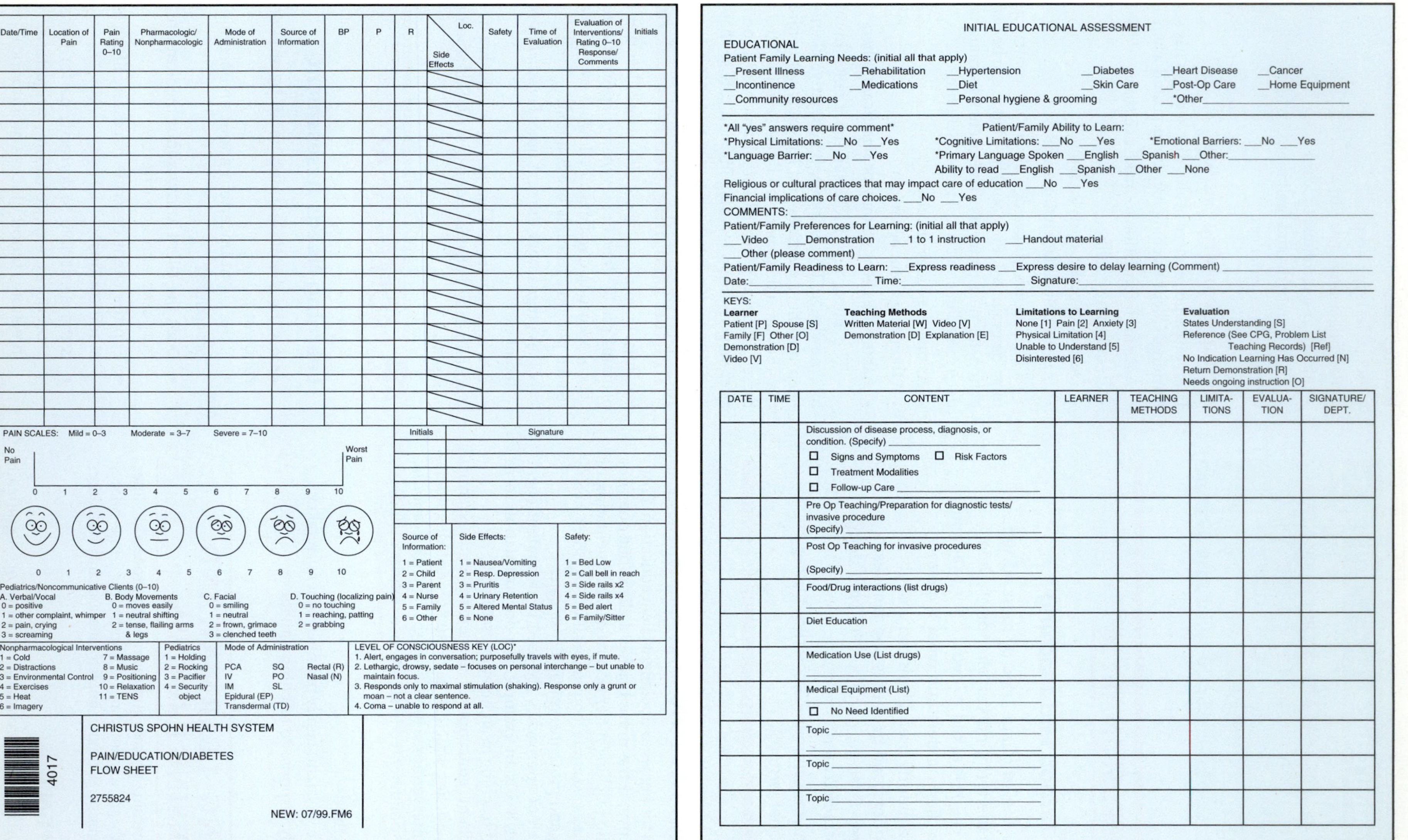

Date/Time	Location of Pain	Pain Rating 0–10	Pharmacologic/ Nonpharmacologic	Mode of Administration	Source of Information	BP	P	R	Loc. / Side Effects	Safety	Time of Evaluation	Evaluation of Interventions/ Rating 0–10 Response/ Comments	Initials

PAIN SCALES: Mild = 0–3 Moderate = 3–7 Severe = 7–10

No Pain 0 1 2 3 4 5 6 7 8 9 10 Worst Pain

0 1 2 3 4 5 6 7 8 9 10

Initials	Signature

Pediatrics/Noncommunicative Clients (0–10)

A. Verbal/Vocal
0 = positive
1 = other complaint, whimper
2 = pain, crying
3 = screaming

B. Body Movements
0 = moves easily
1 = neutral shifting
2 = tense, flailing arms & legs

C. Facial
0 = smiling
1 = neutral
2 = frown, grimace
3 = clenched teeth

D. Touching (localizing pain)
0 = no touching
1 = reaching, patting
2 = grabbing

Source of Information:	Side Effects:	Safety:
1 = Patient	1 = Nausea/Vomiting	1 = Bed Low
2 = Child	2 = Resp. Depression	2 = Call bell in reach
3 = Parent	3 = Pruritis	3 = Side rails x2
4 = Nurse	4 = Urinary Retention	4 = Side rails x4
5 = Family	5 = Altered Mental Status	5 = Bed alert
6 = Other	6 = None	6 = Family/Sitter

Nonpharmacological Interventions
1 = Cold 7 = Massage
2 = Distractions 8 = Music
3 = Environmental Control 9 = Positioning
4 = Exercises 10 = Relaxation
5 = Heat 11 = TENS
6 = Imagery

Pediatrics
1 = Holding
2 = Rocking
3 = Pacifier
4 = Security object

Mode of Administration
PCA SQ Rectal (R)
IV PO Nasal (N)
IM SL
Epidural (EP)
Transdermal (TD)

LEVEL OF CONSCIOUSNESS KEY (LOC)*
1. Alert, engages in conversation; purposefully travels with eyes, if mute.
2. Lethargic, drowsy, sedate – focuses on personal interchange – but unable to maintain focus.
3. Responds only to maximal stimulation (shaking). Response only a grunt or moan – not a clear sentence.
4. Coma – unable to respond at all.

4017

CHRISTUS SPOHN HEALTH SYSTEM

PAIN/EDUCATION/DIABETES
FLOW SHEET

2755824

NEW: 07/99.FM6

INITIAL EDUCATIONAL ASSESSMENT

EDUCATIONAL
Patient Family Learning Needs: (initial all that apply)
__Present Illness __Rehabilitation __Hypertension __Diabetes __Heart Disease __Cancer
__Incontinence __Medications __Diet __Skin Care __Post-Op Care __Home Equipment
__Community resources __Personal hygiene & grooming __*Other________

All "yes" answers require comment Patient/Family Ability to Learn:
*Physical Limitations: ___No ___Yes *Cognitive Limitations: ___No ___Yes *Emotional Barriers: ___No ___Yes
*Language Barrier: ___No ___Yes *Primary Language Spoken ___English ___Spanish ___Other:________
Ability to read ___English ___Spanish ___Other ___None
Religious or cultural practices that may impact care of education ___No ___Yes
Financial implications of care choices. ___No ___Yes
COMMENTS: ________
Patient/Family Preferences for Learning: (initial all that apply)
___Video ___Demonstration ___1 to 1 instruction ___Handout material
___Other (please comment) ________
Patient/Family Readiness to Learn: ___Express readiness ___Express desire to delay learning (Comment) ________
Date:________ Time:________ Signature:________

KEYS:

Learner
Patient [P] Spouse [S]
Family [F] Other [O]
Demonstration [D]
Video [V]

Teaching Methods
Written Material [W] Video [V]
Demonstration [D] Explanation [E]

Limitations to Learning
None [1] Pain [2] Anxiety [3]
Physical Limitation [4]
Unable to Understand [5]
Disinterested [6]

Evaluation
States Understanding [S]
Reference (See CPG, Problem List Teaching Records) [Ref]
No Indication Learning Has Occurred [N]
Return Demonstration [R]
Needs ongoing instruction [O]

DATE	TIME	CONTENT	LEARNER	TEACHING METHODS	LIMITA-TIONS	EVALUA-TION	SIGNATURE/ DEPT.
		Discussion of disease process, diagnosis, or condition. (Specify) ________ ☐ Signs and Symptoms ☐ Risk Factors ☐ Treatment Modalities ☐ Follow-up Care ________					
		Pre Op Teaching/Preparation for diagnostic tests/ invasive procedure (Specify) ________					
		Post Op Teaching for invasive procedures (Specify) ________					
		Food/Drug interactions (list drugs) ________					
		Diet Education ________					
		Medication Use (List drugs) ________					
		Medical Equipment (List) ________ ☐ No Need Identified					
		Topic ________					
		Topic ________					
		Topic ________					

(Continues)

FIGURE 8-5 Documentation Form for Client Teaching: Inpatient Setting (*Courtesy of CHRISTUS Spohn Health System, Corpus Christi, TX.*)

DATE	TIME	CONTENT	LEARNER	TEACHING METHODS	LIMITA-TIONS	EVALUA-TION	SIGNATURE/ DEPT.
		Rehabilitation (Describe) PT ______ TR ______ OT ______ Speech ______					
		Special Treatments (Describe)					
		Community Resources (Specify) ______					
		Diabetes Teaching ☐ DM Medication ☐ Insulin Adm. Techniques ☐ Diet Guidelines ☐ Hypoglycemia–Sx., Tx, Prev. ☐ Foot Care ☐ Sick Day Guidelines Referred to OP Diabetes Class					
		Explanation of safety program, level precautions, and wristband					
		Topic: Pain Management Information Sheet					
		Topic ______					
		Topic ______					
		Topic ______					
		Topic ______					
		Topic ______					
		Topic ______					
		Topic ______					
		Topic ______					
		Topic ______					
		Topic ______					

Initial/Signatures

1.____ / ______	8.____ / ______	15.____ / ______
2.____ / ______	9.____ / ______	16.____ / ______
3.____ / ______	10.____ / ______	17.____ / ______
4.____ / ______	11.____ / ______	18.____ / ______
5.____ / ______	12.____ / ______	19.____ / ______
6.____ / ______	13.____ / ______	20.____ / ______
7.____ / ______	14.____ / ______	21.____ / ______

DIET: ______

INJECTION SITE:
RA – Right Arm
LA – Left Arm
RT – Right Thigh
LT – Left Thigh
RG – Right Gluteal
LG – Left Gluteal
RQ – Right Abdominal Quadrant
LQ – Left Abdominal Quadrant

For Documentation of Routine Blood Sugar Results i.e. BID, TID or AC and HS

DATE		AC Break-fast	AC Lunch	AC Dinner	AC HS Snack	2 AM	COMMENTS	DATE		AC Break-fast	AC Lunch	AC Dinner	AC HS Snack	2 AM	COMMENTS
	Bld Glu								Bld Glu						
	Meter #								Meter #						
	Insulin Admin.								Insulin Admin.						
	Bld Glu								Bld Glu						
	Meter #								Meter #						
	Insulin Admin.								Insulin Admin.						
	Bld Glu								Bld Glu						
	Meter #								Meter #						
	Insulin Admin.								Insulin Admin.						
	Bld Glu								Bld Glu						
	Meter #								Meter #						
	Insulin Admin.								Insulin Admin.						

Int.	#	Problem	Goal	Exp. Date of Resol.	Date Comp. Int.	Int.	#	Problem	Goal	Exp. Date of Resol.	Date Comp. Int.
		Alteration in Comfort	Comfort maintained					Impaired Skin Integrity	Regain Skin Integrity		
		Injury Potential	Safety Maintained					Pot. For Skin Impairment	Skin Integrity Maintained		
		Fever	Temp. within Normal Limits					Activity Intolerance	Maintain/Increase Activity		
		Anxiety/Fear	Reduced Anxiety/Fear					Impaired Mobility	Imp. Function/ Mobility		
		Knowledge Deficit	Increased Understanding					Self Care Deficit	Improve ADL's		
		Infection	Minimized/Absent Signs					Altered Thought Process	Reduced Disorientation		
		Body Image Disturbance	Acknowledge Change					Impaired Communication	Improve Communication		
		Fluid/Lyte Imbalance	Main. Fluid/Lyte Bal.					Constipation	Bowel Elim. With WNL		
		Impaired Gas Exchange	Main./Increase Gas Ex.					Diarrhea	Bowel Elim. With WNL		
		Ineffective Airway Clearance	Maintain Patient Airway					Incontinence	Maintain Bowel Integrity		
		Ineffective Breathing Pattern	Maintain Patient Airway					Impaired Swallowing/ Chewing	Optimal Nutrition Status		
		Altered Tissue Perfusion	Optimal Tissue Perfusion					Alteration in Nutrition	Optimal Nutrition Status		

Pain-Ed-Diabetes.FM6 09/16/99

FIGURE 8-5 *(Continued)*

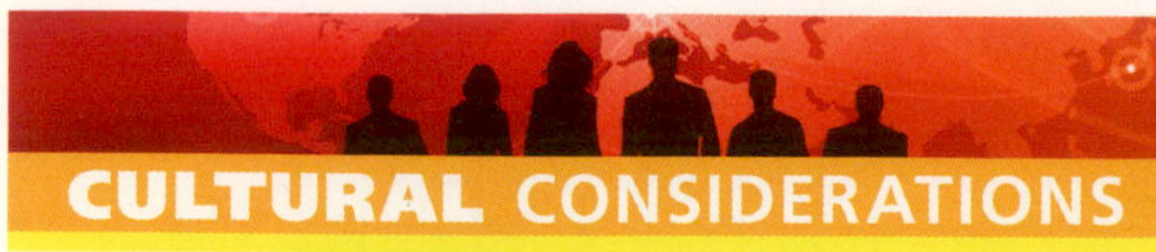

CULTURAL CONSIDERATIONS

Learning and Culture

- Culture plays an important role in knowledge acquisition.
- Attitudes, which are derived from a cultural context, toward what is appropriate to learn and who should teach may require alterations in the nurse's approach.
- Sensitivity to cultural values affects every aspect of the teaching–learning process.

Ability and Readiness to Learn

Assess the client for factors that will hinder or facilitate learning. Age does not determine developmental level. Behavior provides the best indication of developmental level. The client's cognitive skills and attention span, along with developmental level, all indicate a client's ability to learn.

Readiness to learn is influenced by the client's ability to learn, the client's comfort, and the client's motivation (or lack of) to learn.

Client Strengths and Limitations

Identification of the client's strengths and limitations is the foundation for realistic expectations. Understanding the client's strengths and limitations allows the nurse to plan successful teaching–learning experiences. Determining a client's strengths assists the nurse to select appropriate teaching methods. For example, a client who has limited vision should not be given pamphlets or other reading material in small print from which to learn the intended information.

Previous Experiences

The client's knowledge base acquired from life experiences affects the client's attitude about learning and perception of the importance of the information to be learned. A client who has had several experiences of hospitalization will have both a basis of knowledge and feelings (positive and negative) about those experiences. Current attitudes about this hospitalization are influenced by prior hospital experiences.

Nursing Diagnosis

Several nursing diagnoses are pertinent to the learning process. When lack of knowledge is the primary learning need, the diagnosis of *Deficient **K**nowledge (specify)* is applicable. For example:

- A client who is to use crutches for assisted ambulation may have the diagnosis of *Deficient **K**nowledge: Crutchwalking,* R/T lack of exposure AEB many questions and hesitancy to walk.
- A client who must give self-insulin and will be discharged soon may have a diagnosis of *Deficient **K**nowledge: Insulin Injection,* R/T lack of exposure AEB many questions.

*Deficient **K**nowledge* may also be a component of many other nursing diagnoses that encompass risk or impaired ability. For instance, *Risk for **C**onstipation* may relate to a client's compromised health status; this risk may be modified or reduced through certain dietary changes and client education. A client having a diagnosis of *Feeding **S**elf-Care Deficit* may need both assistance in cutting the food and opening containers related to present physical ability.

Planning

Learning does not just happen by chance—it is planned. An important part of planning is goal setting. The client and family or significant others be involved in setting goals. Specific learning goals include the following elements:

- Measurable behavioral change
- Time frame
- Methods and intervals for evaluation

Teaching–learning goals must be realistic (i.e., based on the abilities of the learner and the teacher).

Establishing teaching–learning goals involves setting priorities. One way to set priorities with regard to goals is to teach "need-to-know" content (that which is necessary for survival) before moving on to "nice-to-know" content. For example, Mrs. Stone, who is in her first trimester of pregnancy, must be taught guidelines for diet and exercise ("need-to-know" content); information about infant care ("nice-to-know" content at this time) can be given later in the pregnancy.

Planning involves considering the following:

- Why teach?
- What should be taught?
- How should teaching be done?
- Who should teach and who should be taught?
- When should teaching occur?
- Where should teaching occur?

Why Teach?

Client need is *why* teaching is done. The client may realize the need for knowledge about a given subject and ask for information or ask questions about the subject. The nurse recognizes the client's need for knowledge even when the client does not recognize that need. For example, the nurse recognizes that a preoperative client needs to know how to do deep breathing exercises and leg exercises after surgery. The nurse then plans teaching for that purpose.

What Is Taught?

Determination of *what* to teach is accomplished through comprehensive assessment. The content to be taught depends greatly on the client's knowledge base, current health status, and readiness to learn.

How Is Teaching Done?

Deciding *how* to teach involves deciding which teaching strategies are best for the content and the client's learning style and abilities. The effective teacher uses methods that capture the client's interest. Teaching methods are often influenced by the teaching location. For example, videos can often be used effectively in inpatient settings; however, the same information may need to be presented with flip charts or brochures in the home setting.

Who Teaches and Who Is Taught?

Planning includes deciding *who* will teach the client. The nurse is the coordinator of the health care team's teaching activities. Responsibility for a comprehensive teaching approach rests with the nurse. The teaching plan greatly affects continuity of care. The "who" part of planning also relates to who will be taught. The nurse must determine who in addition to the client (e.g., family members, significant others) will receive the teaching.

When Does Teaching Occur?

When to teach should be carefully considered. The nurse should recognize that every interaction with the client is an opportunity for teaching. When a client asks a question, it is an opportunity for teaching. These opportunities for teaching must be used. A client's motivation to learn is quickly destroyed when comments such as "Ask your doctor that" or "We'll talk about that later. Right now, take your medicine" are made. The best time for teaching is when the client is comfortable—physically and psychologically.

Where Does Teaching Occur?

Where teaching occurs must also be well planned. The location of teaching affects the quality of learning. Some factors to be considered in determining the location of teaching include privacy and equipment availability.

> **PROFESSIONALTIP**
>
> **Guidelines for Effective Client Teaching**
>
> - Assess the client's needs and knowledge.
> - Organize content from the simple to the complex, building on what the client already knows.
> - Be creative.
> - Ensure a comfortable environment.
> - Maintain a flexible approach.
> - Use a variety of teaching methods.
> - Relate material to client's prior knowledge.
> - Encourage the client's active participation.
> - Reinforce learning frequently.
> - Provide immediate feedback.
> - Provide for immediate application of knowledge or skill.
> - Emphasize oral instructions with the written word and pictures.
> - Expect learning plateaus.

IMPLEMENTATION

Katz (1997) suggests several strategies to achieve successful client teaching, as outlined in the following sections.

Get and Keep the Client's Attention

Begin a teaching session by telling the client what will be taught and why it is important to the client. The client's interest is held by varying the tone of voice and using assorted teaching methods to present the material. Making the abstract concrete by using realistic examples from the client's experience also keeps the client's attention.

Stick to the Basics

Because the average adult remembers only five to seven points at a time, the nurse is specific about what the client is to learn. Simple, everyday language is used, and the most critical information presented first.

Use Time Wisely

The nurse incorporates teaching into client care by providing information during each nurse–client interaction. Involving the client's family and friends, allowing them to discuss the material with the client, is also helpful. The nurse considers supplementing teaching with written material for the client and/or family to read; this provides time for the learners to review the material and then ask questions to clarify understanding.

Reinforce Information

Repetition creates habits; the nurse takes advantage of this by reviewing the material with the client and serving as a role model. For example, when teaching a client a procedure, the nurse takes care to do it correctly each time and to avoid taking shortcuts. The nurse rewards the client by giving positive reinforcement such as a smile, a nod, or a few words of praise.

EVALUATION

Evaluation of teaching–learning is a twofold process:

1. Determining what the client has learned
2. Assessing the nurse's teaching effectiveness

Evaluation of Client's Learning

In performing the continual process of evaluating what the client has learned, the nurse determines whether a behavior

> **PROFESSIONALTIP**
>
> **Evaluation of Learning**
>
> - Did the client meet the goals and objectives?
> - Can the client demonstrate skills?
> - Did the client's attitude change?
> - Can the client cope better?
> - Does the family understand how to help?

PROFESSIONALTIP

Evaluation of Teacher Effectiveness

- Were learning objectives stated in behavioral terms (i.e., easy to evaluate)?
- Was content presented clearly and at the client's level of comprehension?
- Did the nurse show interest in the client and in the material?
- Were a variety of teaching aids used?
- Were the teaching aids appropriate for the client and the content?
- Was the client encouraged to participate?
- Did the nurse give frequent feedback and allow for immediate return demonstration?
- Was the nurse supportive?

change has occurred, whether the behavior change is related to learning activities, whether further change is necessary, and whether continued behavior change will promote health. The following strategies are used to evaluate client learning:

- Asking questions
- Observation
- Return demonstration
- Written follow-up (e.g., questionnaires)

Evaluation of Teaching Effectiveness

A major purpose of evaluation is to assess the effectiveness of the teaching activities and to decide which modifications, if any, are necessary. If learning objectives are not met, teaching–learning activities are reassessed and modified. Goals that are measurable and specific facilitate evaluation. Evaluating teaching effectiveness is accomplished through:

- Feedback from the learner
- Feedback from colleagues
- Self-evaluation

CASE STUDY

The nurse admitted a 46-year-old male who has recently been diagnosed with stage II colon cancer. He has a wife and two school-age children and has just started his own construction company in the past year. The client is scheduled for a colon resection with a colostomy in 2 days. The nurse is assessing him and his wife for preoperative teaching. They are verbalizing a significant amount of distress and anxiety over the diagnosis and pending surgery.

1. What assessment data would you need to collect before initiating teaching?
2. What barriers would you expect to encounter in the teaching and learning process?
3. What would be two teaching goals for the session?
4. Identify two prioritized nursing diagnoses for this client?
5. Identify teaching strategies you might utilize in this teaching session?
6. How would you evaluate the teaching goals?

SUMMARY

- The teaching–learning process is a planned interaction that promotes behavioral change that is not a result of maturation or coincidence.
- Learning is the process of assimilating information that results in behavioral change.
- Three domains of learning are the cognitive (intellectual), the affective (emotional), and the psychomotor (motor skills).
- Learning readiness is affected by developmental and sociocultural factors.
- Elements of documenting client education include the content taught, the teaching methods used, the person(s) taught, and the response of the learners.
- Evaluation of the teaching–learning process involves: determining what the client has learned and assessing teacher efficacy.

REVIEW QUESTIONS

1. Bloom identified three areas wherein learning occurs: the psychomotor domain, the affective domain, and the:
   1. attitude domain.
   2. cognitive domain.
   3. emotional domain.
   4. knowledge domain.

2. A clinical example of psychomotor learning is when a client:
   1. changes the dressing on a leg ulcer.
   2. states an acceptance of a chronic illness.
   3. states the name and purpose of a medication.
   4. chooses to change the type of exercise performed.

3. When teaching a client, the nurse is aware that learning needs:
   1. change daily.
   2. are the same for everyone.
   3. change throughout the life span.
   4. change as teaching approaches are modified.
4. Nurses are required to provide teaching by:
   1. all state nursing practice acts.
   2. the National League for Nursing.
   3. the American Hospital Association.
   4. the Joint Commission.
5. Because age is not synonymous with developmental level, the nurse, when preparing to teach a client, must:
   1. teach everyone the same way.
   2. set the goals for the client.
   3. observe the client's behavior.
   4. ask the client about self-efficacy.
6. The nurse is providing discharge teaching to a 65-year-old male who is newly diagnosed with adult-onset diabetes. He is being discharged on an 1,800-calorie American Diabetes Association diet, oral hypoglycemic medications, and blood glucose checks four times a day using a glucometer. What learning domain is the nurse addressing when teaching the client how to perform blood glucose checks?
   1. Affective.
   2. Psychomotor.
   3. Cognitive.
   4. Social.
7. The nurse is teaching a 48-year-old female who was recently diagnosed with breast cancer. The nurse observes that she is an avid reader while in the hospital. What teaching strategies would be most effective in helping her understand her disease and the treatment process?
   1. Pamphlets, pictures, and written materials.
   2. Support group, discussion, and audiotapes.
   3. Videos, role modeling, and games.
   4. Examples, discovery, and explanation.
8. The nurse is caring for a 55-year-old Hispanic woman who was recently diagnosed with renal failure and placed on a protein-restricted diet. When the nurse enters the room, the client is observed eating shredded beef with refried beans that the family brought from home. Which of the following responses indicate that the nurse is aware of the client's dietary restrictions and is sensitive to her cultural needs?
   1. "I see your family brought in some home-cooked food. I'm glad you are able to enjoy this."
   2. "Those foods you are eating are all high in protein. You will not be able to eat them anymore."
   3. "The meal you are eating is too high in protein for your diet. Substituting beans and eating a smaller amount of meat in your tortilla would satisfy your diet restrictions."
   4. "The foods you are eating are too high in protein. I will have the dietitian bring you a list of acceptable foods for your diet."
9. The nurse is providing care to a 15-year-old female who is a newly diagnosed diabetic. When planning diabetic teaching for this client, what developmental considerations could guide the nurse's choice of teaching strategies?
   1. Adolescents respond well to authority figures, so the client will be very attentive to what the nurse says.
   2. The reading level of an adolescent may be low, so written materials are not used.
   3. Family involvement is not encouraged because as an adolescent she is striving for independence.
   4. Adolescents identify with their peer group and often respond well to peer-led support groups.
10. A 76-year-old female is discharged home from a subacute nursing facility. She has a history of osteoarthritis and underwent a right-knee replacement about 2 weeks ago. The teaching goal of the nurse at discharge is that the client will gradually increase weight bearing to the right knee to the point that she is able to support full weight bearing in 3 weeks. What client statement indicates that the teaching goal is met?
    1. "Until the pain improves, I will take it easy on my knee."
    2. "I can't wait to get home so I can walk without this walker."
    3. "I will increase the weight on my knee a little each day while continuing to use my walker."
    4. "Exercise is not helpful in my rehabilitation."

REFERENCES/SUGGESTED READINGS

American Hospital Association. (1998). A patient's bill of rights. Chicago: Author. Retrieved November 30, 2008, from http://www.patienttalk.info/AHA-Patient_Bill_of_Rights.htm

American Hospital Association. (2009). The patient care partnership. Retrieved June 18, 2009, from http://www.aha.org/aha/issues/Communicating-With-Patients/pt-care-partnership.html

Bandura, A. (1977). Social learning theory. Englewood Cliffs, NJ: Prentice Hall.

Beare, P., & Myers, J. (1998). *Principles and practice of adult health nursing* (3rd ed.). St. Louis, MO: Mosby.

Bloom, B. (1977). *Taxonomy of educational objectives: The classification of educational goals, handbook I: Cognitive domain.* New York: Longman.

Bruccoliere, T. (2000). How to make patient teaching stick. *RN, 63*(2), 34–38.

Clark, M. (2003). *Community health nursing: Caring for populations* (4th ed.). Upper Saddle River, NJ: Prentice Hall.

Doak, C., Doak, L., & Root, J. (1996). *Teaching patients with low literacy skills* (2nd ed.). Philadelphia: Lippincott Williams & Wilkins.

Duffy, B. (1997). Using creative teaching process with adult patients. *Home Healthcare Nurse, 15*(2), 102–108.

Duncan, G. (1996). An investigation of learning styles of practical and baccalaureate nursing students. *Journal of Nursing Education, 35*(1), 40–42.

Edelman, C., & Mandle, C. (2002). *Health promotion throughout the lifespan* (5th ed.). St. Louis, MO: Mosby.

Freda, M. (1997). Don't give it away. *MCN—The American Journal of Maternal/Child Nursing, 22*(6), 330.

Gregorc, A., & Ward, H. (1977). A new definitions for individual: Implications for learning and teaching. *NASSP Bulletin,* 20–26.

Hunt, R. (2001). *Community based nursing* (2nd ed.). Philadelphia: Lippincott.

Joint Commission. (2008). Healthcare organization survey activity guide. Retrieved November 30, 2008, from http://www.jointcommission.org/NR/rdonlyres/481CE5EA-D02C-46C3-AA5F-DF328FE13174/0/08_HCO_SAG_3.pdf

Joint Commission for Accreditation of Healthcare Organizations. (2002). *Accreditation manual.* Chicago: Author.

Jubeck, M. (1994). Teaching the elderly: A commonsense approach. *Nursing94, 24*(5), 70–71.

Katz, J. (1997). Back to basics: Providing effective patient teaching. *American Journal of Nursing, 97*(5), 33–36.

Knowles, M., Holton, E., & Swanson, R. (2005). *The adult learner: The definitive classic in adult education and human resource development* (6th ed.). St. Louis, MO: Elsevier Science and Technology Books.

Mayer, G., & Rushton, N. (2002). Writing easy-to-read teaching aids. *Nursing2002, 32*(3), 48–49.

Messner, R. (1997). Patient teaching tips from the horse's mouth. *RN, 60*(8), 29–31.

Meyers, D. (1998). *Client teaching guides for home health care* (2nd ed.). New York: Aspen.

Muma, R., Lyon, B., & Newman, T. (Eds.). (1996). *Patient education: A practical approach.* New York: McGraw-Hill.

Redman, B. (2006). *The practice of patient education: A case study approach* (10th ed.). St. Louis, MO: Elsevier Science.

Reed, S. (2007). Learning your way. Retrieved June 20, 2009, from http://www.presentations.com/msg/content_display/training/e3i7639605670451237f7bf2bea3bf8bad3

Ruholl, L. (2003). Tips for teaching the elderly. *RN, 66*(5), 48–52.

Seley, J. (1994). 10 strategies for successful patient teaching. *American Journal of Nursing, 94*(11), 63–65.

Smith, R. (2008). *Teaching the client and family.* Manuscript submitted for publication.

Sodeman, W., Jr., & Sodeman, T. (2005). *Instructions for geriatric patients* (3rd ed.). St. Louis, MO: Elsevier Health Sciences.

VARK a Guide to Learning Styles. (2009). Research and statistics. Retrieved June 20, 2009, from http://www.vark-learn.com/english/page.asp?p=research

Weissman, M., & Jasovsky, D. (1998). Discharge teaching for today's times. *RN, 61*(6), 38–40.

Winslow, E. (2001). Patient education materials: Can patients read them, or are they ending up in the trash? *American Journal of Nursing, 101*(10), 33–38.

RESOURCES

Center for Research on Learning and Teaching, http://www.crlt.umich.edu/index.php

Gregorc Associates, Inc., http://gregorc.com

The Learning Web, http://www.thelearningweb.net

VARK, http://www.vark-learn.com

CHAPTER 9
Nursing Process/Documentation/Informatics

MAKING THE CONNECTION

Refer to the following chapters to increase your understanding of the nursing process:

Basic Nursing

- ***Holistic Care***
- ***Legal and Ethical Responsibilities***
- ***The Health Care Delivery System***
- ***Communication***
- ***Assessment***

LEARNING OBJECTIVES

Upon completion of this chapter, you should be able to:

- Define key terms.
- Explain the nursing process.
- Describe the components of assessment.
- Describe the three types of nursing diagnoses.
- Discuss planning and outcome identification.
- Discuss the types of skills that nurses must possess in order to perform the nursing interventions during the implementation step of the nursing process.
- Identify factors that may influence evaluation.
- Explain how critical thinking and problem solving are related to the nursing process.
- Use the nursing process to provide safe, effective client care.
- Discuss the purposes of documentation in health care.
- Explain the principles of effective documentation.
- Describe various methods of documentation.
- Identify various types of documentation records.
- Document client care accurately and completely.

KEY TERMS

actual nursing diagnosis
analysis
assessment
assessment model
charting by exception (CBE)
collaborative problems
comprehensive assessment
critical pathways
data clustering
defining characteristics
dependent nursing interventions
discharge planning
documentation
etiology
evaluation
expected outcome
focus charting
focused assessment
goal
health history
implementation
incident reports
independent nursing interventions
initial planning
interdependent nursing interventions
Kardex
long-term goal
medical diagnosis
narrative charting
nursing care plan
nursing diagnosis
nursing intervention
Nursing Interventions Classification (NIC)
Nursing Minimum Data Set (NMDS)
Nursing Outcomes Classification (NOC)
nursing process
objective data
ongoing assessment
ongoing planning
planning
point-of-care charting
primary source
Problem, Intervention, Evaluation (PIE) charting
problem-oriented medical record (POMR)
risk nursing diagnosis
secondary sources
short-term goal
SOAP
source-oriented charting
subjective data
synthesis
wellness nursing diagnosis

INTRODUCTION

The nursing process and documentation depend on each other for providing safe and effective client care. The nursing process lays out a plan of care that guides not only the care provided but also the accurate recording of that care. Documentation provides a legal record that all aspects of the nursing process were properly carried out and that professional standards of care, regulatory standards, and agency policies were met.

Every day, individuals process information and take steps that lead to goal attainment. For example, when a meal is prepared, the cook goes through a process of obtaining the food, then preparing the meal for the ultimate goal of eating good food. In deciding what to wear, an individual goes through a process of considering the weather for appropriate clothing, then choosing matching clothes for the goal of looking attractive in the chosen outfit. Nursing has a process, called the nursing process, that provides quality care to a client. There are several steps in the nursing process that a nurse takes to provide effective care.

This chapter first explains the nursing process in general and then each step individually. The legal aspects, methods, and forms for documenting are explained. Many examples are provided throughout the chapter.

NURSING PROCESS HISTORY

The first reference to nursing as a "process" was in a 1955 journal article by Lydia Hall, yet the term *nursing process* was not widely used until the late 1960s (Edelman & Mandle, 2002). Johnson (1959), Orlando (1961), and Wiedenbach (1963) referred to the nursing process as a series of three steps: assessment, planning, and evaluation. Yura and Walsh (1967) identified four steps in the nursing process:

1. Assessing
2. Planning
3. Implementing
4. Evaluating

The term *nursing diagnosis* was first used by Fry (1953). After the first meeting of the group now called NANDA-International in 1974, nursing diagnosis was added as a separate step in the nursing process. Now, the steps of the nursing process are:

1. Assessment
2. Diagnosis
3. Planning and outcome identification
4. Implementation
5. Evaluation

THE NURSING PROCESS

A **process** is a series of steps or acts that lead to accomplishing some goal or purpose. According to Bevis (1989), "processes have three characteristics: (1) inherent purpose, (2) internal organization, and (3) infinite creativity." These characteristics are found in the nursing process. The **nursing process** is a systematic method for providing care to clients. The purpose is to provide individualized, holistic, effective

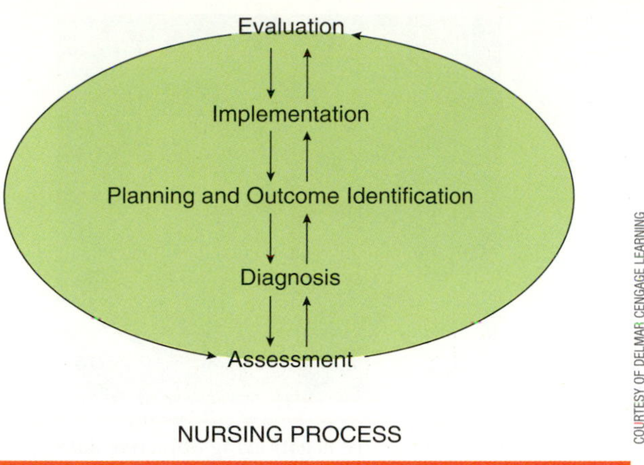

FIGURE 9-1 Five Components of the Nursing Process: Assessment, Diagnosis, Planning and Outcome Identification, Implementation, and Evaluation. The arrows going down represent revisions.

client care efficiently. Although the steps of the nursing process build on each other, they are not linear. Each step overlaps with the previous and subsequent steps (Figure 9-1).

The nursing process is dynamic and requires creativity in its application. The steps are the same for each client situation, but the correlation and results will be different. The nursing process is used with clients of all ages and in any care setting. It is also the organizing system for the National Council Licensure Examination for both practical/vocational nurses (NCLEX-PN®) and registered nurses (NCLEX-RN®).

Assessment

Assessment, the first step in the nursing process, includes systematic collection, verification, organization, interpretation, and documentation of data. The completeness and correctness of this data relate directly to the accuracy of the steps that follow. Assessment involves the following steps:

- Data collection from a variety of sources
- Data validation
- Data organization
- Data interpretation
- Data documentation

In some states, LPN/VNs do not perform complete assessments but collect data. For safe practice, LPN/VNs follow the Standards of Practice in their state of employment.

Purpose of Assessment

The purpose of assessment is to organize a database regarding a client's physical, psychosocial, and emotional health so that health-promoting behaviors and actual and/or potential health problems can be identified. The nurse ascertains the client's functional abilities, the absence or presence of dysfunction, normal activities of daily living, and lifestyle patterns through assessment. Identifying the client's strengths gives the nurse information about the abilities, behaviors, and skills the client can use during the treatment and recovery process. Assessment also provides an opportunity to form a therapeutic interpersonal relationship with the client. During assessment, the client can discuss health care concerns and goals with the nurse.

PROFESSIONALTIP

The Nursing Process

- The nursing process involves overlapping steps.
- The steps are explained one after the other for ease of understanding, but in actual practice, there may not be a definite beginning or ending to each step.
- Work in one step may begin before work in the preceding step is completed.

Types of Assessment

The information needed for assessment is usually determined by the health care setting and needs of the client. Three types of assessment are comprehensive, focused, and ongoing. A comprehensive assessment is most desirable when first determining a client's need for nursing care. Time limits or special circumstances may require an abbreviated data collection, as shown in a focused assessment. The assessment database can then be broadened through ongoing assessment.

Comprehensive Assessment A **comprehensive assessment** provides baseline client data including a complete health history and current needs assessment. It is usually completed upon admission to a health care agency. Changes in the client's health status can be measured against this database. It includes assessment of the client's physical and psychosocial health, perception of health, presence of health risk factors, and coping patterns.

Focused Assessment A **focused assessment** is limited to potential health care risks, a particular need, or health care concern. They are not as detailed as comprehensive assessments and are often used when short stays are anticipated (e.g., outpatient surgery centers and emergency departments), in specialty areas such as mental health settings, labor and delivery, or for screening for specific problems or risk factors (e.g., well-child clinics).

Ongoing Assessment When problems are identified during a comprehensive or focused assessment, follow-up is required. An **ongoing assessment** includes systematic monitoring of specific problems. This type of assessment broadens the database and allows the nurse to confirm the validity of data obtained during the initial assessment. Systematic monitoring allows the nurse to determine the client's response to nursing interventions and to identify any other problems.

Sources of Data

Although data are collected from a variety of sources, the client is considered the **primary source** of data (the major provider of information about a client). As much information as possible should be gathered from the client, using both interview techniques and physical examination skills. Sources of data other than the client are considered **secondary sources** and include family members, other health care providers, and medical records.

LIFE SPAN CONSIDERATIONS

Assessment and Interventions for Hearing Impairment

Approximately 30% of those over 65 have a hearing impairment. According to Wallhagen, Pettengill, and Whiteside (2006), studies show that hearing is not a routine assessment in older adults, even those in nursing homes. Some observational assessment techniques that may assist a nurse in determining hearing impairment are:

- Does the client cup her hand behind her ear?
- Does she tilt her head or lean into you as you speak?
- Is the volume higher than normal on the television?
- Does she misunderstand questions or respond inappropriately?

If you notice these signs in a client, use these interventions to improve communication and nursing care:

- State the client's name, pause, and then ask a question or make a statement.
- Speak in a normal tone and enunciate clearly without exaggerating lip movements.
- Keep your mouth visible to the client (e.g., avoid placing hand over mouth when speaking or turning face away from the client).
- Make sure the hearing aids are in place and that the batteries are correctly operating.
- Restate a phrase rather than repeat the same phrase.

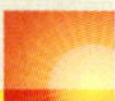

Types of Data

Two types of information are collected through assessment: subjective and objective. **Subjective data** are data from the client's (sometimes family's) point of view and include perceptions, feelings, and concerns. The primary method of collecting subjective data (also called symptoms) is the interview. The **health history**, a review of the client's functional health patterns prior to the current contact with the health care agency, provides much of the subjective data.

Objective data (also called signs) are observable and measurable data that are obtained through both standard assessment techniques performed during the physical examination (Figure 9-2) and the results of laboratory and diagnostic testing. Table 9-1 provides examples of both subjective and objective data.

PROFESSIONALTIP

Clients Who Were Adopted

Remember that clients who were adopted will have varying degrees of knowledge about their biological parents. Sensitivity to this issue is critical in gaining client trust during the interview process.

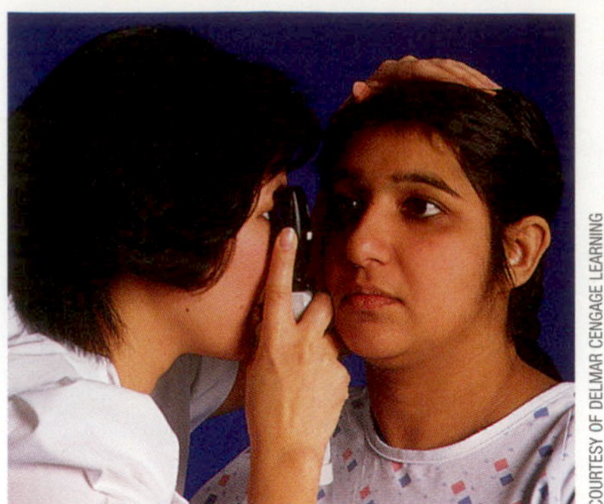

FIGURE 9-2 The nurse is gathering objective data by examining retinal structures.

Validating the Data

Objective data may add to or validate subjective data. Validation is a critical step that prevents misunderstandings, omissions, and incorrect inferences and conclusions (Figure 9-3). This process is particularly important if data sources are considered unreliable, such as when a client is confused or unable to communicate. If two sources provide conflicting data, further information or clarification must be sought. Findings should also be compared with norms, and grossly abnormal findings should be rechecked and confirmed.

Organizing the Data

Collected data must be organized so as to be useful to the health care professional collecting the data and to others involved in the client's care. After being organized into categories, the data are clustered into groups of related pieces. **Data clustering** is the process of putting data together in order to identify areas of the client's problems and strengths. Many health care agencies use an admission assessment format, which assists the nurse in collecting and organizing data.

An **assessment model** is a framework providing a systematic way to organize data. A few of the many assessment models available to nurses are described in the next sections.

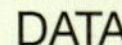

TABLE 9-1 Types of Data

DATA

An African American male, age 79, comes to the emergency room because he cannot move his left arm. The client states, "It happened about an hour ago when my headache got worse. Now I am nauseated and dizzy."

The nurse takes his vital signs—T 99, P 100, R 28, BP 200/102—and observes that he cannot move his left arm and his face is flushed.

SUBJECTIVE	OBJECTIVE
Headache	T 99, P 100
Nausea	R 28, BP 200/102
Dizziness	Cannot move left arm Flushed face

COURTESY OF DELMAR CENGAGE LEARNING

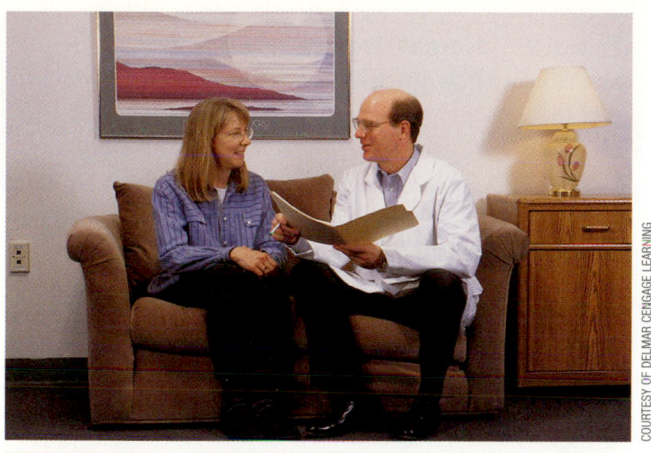

FIGURE 9-3 **The nurse is validating information collected from the client during assessment.**

Hierarchy of Needs Maslow's Hierarchy of Needs proposes that an individual's basic needs (physiological) must be met before higher-level needs can be met. An initial assessment of all physiological needs followed by assessment of the higher-level needs is necessary when using this model.

Body Systems Model The body systems model organizes data collection according to tissue and organ function in the various body systems (e.g., respiratory, cardiovascular, gastrointestinal). Physicians frequently use this model, so it is sometimes called the "medical model."

Functional Health Patterns Gordon's Functional Health Patterns (Gordon, 1998) provides a framework for data collection focusing on 11 functional health patterns. These functional health pattern areas cluster information about a client's habitual patterns and any recent changes to determine if the client's current response is functional or dysfunctional. For example, the elimination pattern is assessed for a client who now has diarrhea several times a week. Data collection would be focused on elimination habits, diet, and fluid intake before the diarrhea began and the effect of any changes on the client's functional ability and lifestyle. The 11 patterns are:

- Health perception/health management pattern
- Nutritional/metabolic pattern
- Elimination pattern
- Activity/exercise pattern
- Cognitive/perceptual pattern
- Sleep/rest pattern
- Self-perception/self-concept pattern
- Role/relationship pattern
- Sexuality/reproductive pattern
- Coping/stress-tolerance pattern
- Value/belief pattern (Gordon, 1998)

Theory of Self-Care Orem (2001) developed the theory of self-care based on a client's ability to perform self-care activities. Self-care, learned behavior with deliberate actions responding to need, includes activities an individual performs to maintain health. This theory focuses on the assessment of the client's ability to meet self-care needs and identifying existing self-care deficits. This theory is concerned primarily with illness states. The self-care essentials are:

- Maintenance of a sufficient intake of air
- Maintenance of a sufficient intake of water
- Maintenance of a sufficient intake of food
- Provision of care associated with elimination processes and excrements
- Maintenance of a balance between activity and rest
- Maintenance of a balance between solitude and social interaction
- Prevention of hazards to human life, human functioning, and human well-being
- Promotion of human functioning and development within social groups in accord with human potential, known human limitations, and the human desire to be normal (Orem, Taylor, and Renpenning, 2001)

Interpreting the Data

After data is collected, the nurse can begin developing impressions or inferences about the meaning of the data. Organizing data in clusters helps the nurse recognize patterns of response or behavior. When data are placed in clusters, the nurse can:

- Distinguish between relevant and irrelevant data.
- Determine whether and where there are gaps in the data.
- Identify patterns of cause and effect.

Documenting the Data

Assessment data must be recorded and some reported. The nurse must decide which data should be immediately reported to the head nurse and/or physician and which data can just be recorded. Data reflecting a significant change from the normal (e.g., BP 180/100, severe difficulty in breathing, or a high level of anxiety) would need to be reported as well as recorded. Data that need only be recorded include the fact that prescribed medication relieved a headache and that an abdominal dressing is dry and intact.

It is essential for accurate and complete recording of assessment data to communicate information to other health care team members. The basis for determining quality of care is documentation, which includes data to support identified problems.

Diagnosis

The second step in the nursing process involves further **analysis** (breaking down the whole into parts that can be examined) and **synthesis** (putting data together in a new way) of the collected data. A list of nursing diagnoses is the result of this process. According to NANDA-International, a **nursing diagnosis**

> is a clinical judgment about individual, family, or community responses to actual or potential health problems/life processes. A nursing diagnosis provides the basis for selection of nursing interventions to achieve outcomes for which the nurse is accountable. (NANDA-I, 2010, p. 419)

The nursing diagnoses provide the basis for client care through the remaining steps. Clients have both medical and nursing diagnoses. Table 9-2 compares the two categories of diagnoses. It is important to have a clear understanding of the nature of a nursing diagnosis as compared to a **medical diagnosis** (clinical judgment by the physician that identifies or determines a specific disease, condition, or pathological state). Table 9-3 compares selected nursing and medical diagnoses.

TABLE 9-2 Comparison of Nursing and Medical Diagnoses

NURSING DIAGNOSIS	MEDICAL DIAGNOSIS
Recognizes situations that the nurse is licensed and qualified to treat	Recognizes conditions the physician is licensed and qualified to treat
Concentrates on the client's responses to health problems or life processes	Concentrates on injury, illness, or disease processes
Varies as the client's responses and/or health problems change	Stays the same until a cure is realized or client dies
Example: ***N**ausea* *Acute **P**ain* *Acute **P**ain* *Impaired Physical **M**obility*	Example: Choleithiasis Exploratory surgery Cholecystectomy

COURTESY OF DELMAR CENGAGE LEARNING

TABLE 9-3 Comparison of Select Nursing and Medical Diagnoses

NURSING DIAGNOSIS	MEDICAL DIAGNOSIS
*Decreased **C**ardiac Output* *Ineffective **B**reathing Pattern* *Risk for Imbalanced **F**luid Volume*	Congestive heart
*Impaired Physical **M**obility*	Ménierè's disease
*Death **A**nxiety*	Lung cancer
*Ineffective **A**irway Clearance* *Ineffective **B**reathing Pattern* ***A**nxiety*	Chronic obstructive pulmonary disease

COURTESY OF DELMAR CENGAGE LEARNING

The nurse uses critical-thinking and decision-making skills in developing nursing diagnoses. These skills are discussed later in the chapter. The LPN/VN's role in developing nursing diagnoses varies from state to state. For safe practice, the LPN/VN must be familiar with the Standards of Practice in the state of employment.

Components of a Nursing Diagnosis

The nursing diagnosis may be stated as a two-part statement or a three-part statement. The two-part statement is NANDA-International approved and used by most nurses because it is brief and precise. The three-part statement is often required of nursing students and is preferred by nurses who desire the diagnostic statement to include specific manifestations. Refer to the appendices for the list of NANDA-International approved nursing diagnoses.

Two-Part Statement The first part, the actual nursing diagnosis, is a problem statement or diagnostic label describing the client's response to an actual or risk health problem or a wellness condition.

The second part is the **etiology**, the related cause or contributor to the problem, which is identified in the complete NANDA-International diagnosis description. The diagnostic label and etiology are linked by the term *related to* (R/T). Because the NANDA-International list of nursing diagnoses is constantly evolving, there may be times when no etiology is provided. In such cases, the nurse attempts to describe likely contributing factors to the client's condition. Examples of a two-part nursing diagnosis statement are *Disturbed **B**ody Image* R/T loss of left lower extremity and *Activity Intolerance* R/T decreased oxygen-carrying capacity of cells.

Three-Part Statement In a three-part statement, the first two parts are the diagnostic label and the etiology. The third part consists of **defining characteristics** (collected data, also known as signs and symptoms, subjective and objective data, or clinical manifestations). The third part is joined to the first two parts with the connecting phrase *as evidenced by* (AEB). An example of a three-part nursing diagnosis statement is *Ineffective Breathing Pattern* R/T pain AEB respiratory rate less than 11 and use of accessory muscles. Table 9-4 provides other examples.

Types of Nursing Diagnoses

Analysis of the collected data leads the nurse to make a diagnosis in one of three categories:

- An **actual nursing diagnosis** indicates that a problem exists; it is composed of the diagnostic label, related factors, and signs and symptoms. An example of an actual diagnosis is *Situational Low Self-Esteem* R/T loss (first chair trumpet in band) AEB self-negating verbalization "I'm no good anymore."

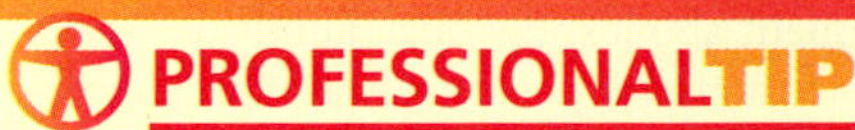

Benefits of Nursing Diagnosis

- Nursing diagnosis is unique because it focuses on a client's *response* to a health problem rather than on the problem.
- Nursing diagnosis provides a way for effective communication.
- Holistic care is facilitated through the use of nursing diagnosis.

PROFESSIONALTIP

Nursing Diagnosis

- The nursing diagnosis must evolve from the data, never the other way around.
- Never try to fit a client to a nursing diagnosis; select the appropriate diagnosis based on the data presented by the client. Failing to do this may result in errors in nursing diagnoses.

TABLE 9-4 Examples of Nursing Diagnoses Written as Two- and Three-Part Statements

TWO-PART STATEMENT	THREE-PART STATEMENT
*Toileting **S**elf-Care Deficit* R/T neuromuscular impairment	*Toileting **S**elf-Care Deficit* R/T neuromuscular impairment, right sided AEB inability to ambulate to the bathroom
*Impaired **S**wallowing* R/T mechanical obstruction	*Impaired **S**wallowing* R/T/mechanical obstruction AEB presence of tracheostomy tube
*Impaired **U**rinary Elimination* R/T urinary tract infection	*Impaired **U**rinary Elimination* R/T urinary tract infection AEB frequency and dysuria
*Impaired **M**emory* R/T fluid and electrolyte imbalance	*Impaired **M**emory* R/T fluid and electrolyte imbalance AEB inability to recall recent or past events
*Impaired **H**ome Maintenance* R/T individual/family member disease or injury	*Impaired **H**ome Maintenance* R/T individual/family member disease or injury AEB repeated lice infestations

COURTESY OF DELMAR CENGAGE LEARNING

- A **risk nursing diagnosis** (potential problem) indicates that a problem does not yet exist but that specific risk factors are present. A risk diagnosis begins with the phrase *Risk for* followed by the diagnostic label and a list of the risk factors. An example of a risk diagnosis is *Risk for Situational Low **S**elf-Esteem*; risk factors include unrealistic self-expectations AEB receiving "B" in two college courses while working full-time (expected "A").
- A **wellness nursing diagnosis** denotes the client's statement of a desire to attain a higher level of wellness in some area of function. It begins with the phrase *Readiness for Enhanced* followed by the diagnostic label. For example, a wife who has been caring for her husband who had a stroke two months ago asks the nurse about meeting with other wives who are/have been in a similar situation. The nurse would make a wellness diagnosis of *Readiness for Enhanced Family **C**oping*.

Examples of the three types of diagnoses are shown in Table 9-5.

After formulation, the nursing diagnoses is discussed with the client, but if this is not possible, the diagnoses is discussed with family members. The list of nursing diagnoses is recorded on the client's record, and the remainder of the client's care plan is completed. The list of nursing diagnoses is dynamic, changing as more data are collected and as client goals and responses to interventions are evaluated.

Carpenito (2009) discusses situations in which nurses intervene in collaboration with other disciplines. She defines **collaborative problems** as "certain physiologic complications that nurses monitor to detect onset or changes in states. Nurses manage collaborative problems using physician-prescribed and nursing-prescribed interventions to minimize the complications of the events." She has identified 52 specific collaborative problems grouped under nine generic problem categories. For example, under the generic collaborative problem category of *Potential Complication (PC): Respiratory* are the specific collaborative problems of "PC: Hypoxemia, PC: Atelectasis/pneumonia, PC: Tracheobronchial Constriction, and PC: Pneumothorax."

The collaborative problem statement *always* begins with *Potential Complication* or PC. This differentiates it from a nursing diagnosis. A benefit of using collaborative problem statements is that they identify, and thus keep the nurses aware of, the potential complications a client may encounter. As in the previous example, the specific potential complication for a client with a respiratory problem would be listed on the care plan.

TABLE 9-5 Types of Nursing Diagnoses

TYPE	EXAMPLE
Actual diagnosis	*Perceived **C**onstipation* R/T faulty appraisal AEB expectation of passage of stool at same time every day
Risk diagnosis	*Risk for **A**spiration* R/T decreased cough and gag reflexes
Wellness diagnosis	*Readiness for Enhanced **S**piritual Well-Being*

COURTESY OF DELMAR CENGAGE LEARNING

PLANNING AND OUTCOME IDENTIFICATION

Planning and outcome identification are the third step of the nursing process and include both establishing guidelines for the proposed course of nursing action to resolve the nursing diagnoses and developing the client's plan of care. After the nursing diagnoses and the client's strengths have been identified, planning begins.

The planning occurs in three phases: initial, ongoing, and discharge. **Initial planning** involves development of a preliminary plan of care by the nurse who performs the admission assessment and gathers the comprehensive admission assessment data. Progressively shorter stays in the hospital make initial planning very important to ensure resolution of the problems. **Ongoing planning** updates the client's plan of care. New information about the client is collected and evaluated and revisions made to the plan of care. **Discharge planning** involves anticipation of and planning for the client's needs after discharge.

The planning phase involves several tasks:

- Prioritizing the nursing diagnoses
- Identifying and writing client-centered long- and short-term goals and outcomes (outcome identification)
- Identifying specific nursing interventions
- Recording the entire nursing care plan in the client's record

Prioritizing the Nursing Diagnoses

Prioritizing the nursing diagnoses involves deciding which diagnoses are the most important and require attention first. Maslow's hierarchy of needs is one of the most common methods of selecting priorities. After basic physiological needs (e.g., respiration, nutrition, temperature, hydration, and elimination) are met to some degree, the nurse can then consider needs on the next level of the hierarchy (e.g., safe environment, stable living condition, affection, and self-worth) and so on up the hierarchy until all the nursing diagnoses have been prioritized.

Alfaro-LeFevre (2008) suggests a three-level approach to prioritizing client problems (nursing diagnoses):

- **First-level priority problems (immediate):**
  Airway problems
  Breathing problems
  Signs (vital sign problems)
- **Second-level priority problems (immediate, after treatment for first-level problems is initiated):**
  Mental status change
  Acute pain
  Acute urinary elimination problems
  Untreated medical problems requiring immediate attention (e.g., a diabetic who has not had insulin)
  Abnormal lab values
  Risks of infection, safety, or security (for client or others)
- **Third-level priority problems:**
  Health problems that do not fit in the above categories

She also proposes that *sometimes* the priority order may change. For example, if acute pain causes breathing problems, managing the pain may have the higher priority; if abnormal lab values are life threatening, then they have a higher priority. Table 9-6 illustrates the prioritizing process.

Table 9-6 Prioritizing Nursing Diagnoses

NURSING DIAGNOSIS	PRIORITIZING METHOD	PRIORITY
*Decreased **C**ardiac Output* R/T altered heart rate rhythm	Maslow, physiologic	High
	Alfaro-LeFevre, cardiac/circulatory	High
***D**iarrhea* R/T travel	Maslow, physiologic	High
	Alfaro-LeFevre, untreated medical problem	Moderate
***R**elocation Stress Syndrome* R/T isolation from family/friends	Maslow, safety and security	Moderate
	Alfaro-LeFevre, risk to security	Moderate
*Disturbed **S**leep Pattern* R/T daytime activity pattern	Maslow, safety and security	Moderate
	Alfaro-LeFevre, other health problems	Low
*Ineffective **C**oping* R/T inadequate resources available	Maslow, self-esteem	Low
	Alfaro-LeFevre, other health problems	Low

COURTESY OF DELMAR CENGAGE LEARNING

Identifying Outcomes

Outcome identification includes establishing goals and expected outcomes, which together provide guidelines for individualized nursing interventions and establish evaluation criteria to measure the effectiveness of the nursing care plan.

Goals A **goal** is an aim, intent, or end. Goals are broad statements that describe the desired or intended change in the client's condition or behavior. Client-centered goals are established in collaboration with the client when possible. Goal statements refer to the diagnostic label (or problem statement) of the nursing diagnosis. Client-centered goals ensure that nursing care is individualized and focused on the client.

A **short-term goal** is a statement that profiles the desired resolution of the nursing diagnosis over a short period of time, usually a few hours or days (less than a week). It focuses on the etiology part of the nursing diagnosis. A **long-term goal** is a statement that profiles the desired resolution of the nursing diagnosis over a longer period of time, usually weeks or months. It focuses on the problem part of the nursing diagnosis. Table 9-7 provides examples of short-term and long-term goals.

Expected Outcomes After the goals have been established, the expected outcomes can be identified based on those goals. An **expected outcome** is a detailed, specific statement describing the methods to be used to achieve the goal. It includes direct nursing care, client teaching, and continuity of care. Outcomes must be measurable, realistic, and time limited. Several expected outcomes may be required for each goal (Table 9-8). Then nursing interventions are formulated to enable the client to reach the goals.

Table 9-7 Short- and Long-Term Goals

Nursing Diagnosis: *Disturbed **B**ody Image* R/T Surgery for Breast Cancer

Short-Term Goals (focus on etiology)	**Long-Term Goals** (focus on problem)
Will verbalize loss of breast	Will verbalize acceptance of change in physical self
Will identify negative feelings about body	
Will touch chest where breast was	

COURTESY OF DELMAR CENGAGE LEARNING

TABLE 9-8 Goal and Expected Outcomes

Nursing Diagnosis: *Impaired Urinary Elimination* R/T Urinary Tract Infection AEB Frequent Urination in Small Amounts	
GOAL	**EXPECTED OUTCOMES**
Client will have improved urinary elimination.	Client will take antibiotic as ordered. By next visit, client will identify three factors to prevent a urinary tract infection. In 2 days, client will have a plan to increase water intake. By next visit, client will be urinating at least 150 mL at 2-hour or longer intervals.
Nursing Diagnosis: ***Powerlessness*** R/T Illness-Related Regimen AEB Nonparticipation in Care or Decision Making When Opportunities Are Provided	
GOAL	**EXPECTED OUTCOMES**
Client will participate in care and decision making.	In 2 days, client will participate in one aspect of own care each day. Client will state preference in decision making situation within 1 week.

COURTESY OF DELMAR CENGAGE LEARNING

Identifying Specific Nursing Interventions

A **nursing intervention** is an action performed by the nurse that helps the client achieve the results specified by the goals and expected outcomes. Nursing interventions refer directly to the related factors or the risk factors in nursing diagnoses. Nursing interventions that reduce or remove the related factors and risk factors resolve or prevent the problem.

There may be a number of nursing interventions for each nursing diagnosis. Nursing interventions are stated in specific terms. Examples of nursing interventions are as follows:

- Assist client to turn, cough, and deep breathe q 2 h beginning at 0800, 4/15
- Teach cord care at 1000, 6/20
- Weigh client at 0700 each day

Interventions formulated for each diagnosis are recorded on the client's care plan. The list of interventions is also dynamic and may change as the nurse interacts with the client, assesses responses to interventions, and evaluates those responses.

CRITICAL THINKING

Goals and Outcomes

How are goals and outcomes different?

CRITICAL THINKING

Nursing Interventions

Differentiate among the three categories of nursing interventions: independent, interdependent, and dependent.

Categories of Nursing Interventions

Nursing interventions are classified into one of three categories: independent, interdependent, or dependent. **Independent nursing interventions** are initiated by the nurse and do not require direction or an order from another health care professional. Most states' nursing practice acts allow independent nursing interventions for activities such as daily living, health education, health promotion, and counseling. An example of an independent nursing intervention is elevating a client's edematous extremity.

Interdependent nursing interventions are implemented collaboratively by the nurse in conjunction with other health care professionals. For example, the nurse may assist a client to perform an exercise taught by the physical therapist.

Dependent nursing interventions require an order from a physician or another health care professional. Administration of a medication is an example of a dependent intervention. This intervention requires specific nursing knowledge and responsibilities, but it is not within the realm of legal practice for LP/VNs to prescribe medications. The nurse is responsible for knowing the classification, normal dosage, pharmacological action, contraindications, adverse effects, and nursing implications of the drug. Dependent nursing interventions must be governed by appropriate knowledge and judgment.

Recording the Nursing Care Plan

The **nursing care plan** is a written guide of strategies to implement to help the client achieve optimal health. Nursing care plans usually include components such as assessment, nursing diagnoses, goals and expected outcomes, and nursing interventions. The care plan is begun on the day of admission and is continually updated until discharge.

Care plans may be standardized, institutional, or computerized.

The standardized care plan is a printed guide for the care of clients with common needs. This care plan usually follows the nursing process format. It may be individualized by including handwritten notes for unusual problems.

Institutional nursing care plans are concise documents that become a part of the client's medical record after discharge. This care plan may simply include the nursing diagnoses, nursing interventions, and evaluation. Figure 9-4 provides an example of an institutional care plan.

Computers can generate both standardized and individualized nursing care plans. Appropriate diagnoses are selected from a menu, which lists possible goals and nursing interventions. Figure 9-5 is an example of a computerized nursing care plan.

IMPLEMENTATION

The fourth step in the nursing process is **implementation**, the performance of the nursing interventions identified during the planning phase. It also involves the delegation (process of transferring a select nursing task to a licensed individual who is

Nursing Diagnosis	Nursing Interventions	Evaluation
Ineffective Breastfeeding R/T deficient knowledge AEB inability to latch on to the maternal breast correctly	1. Teach various breastfeeding positions and techniques to encourage the infant. 2. Stay with mother during feeding and assist as needed.	1. Client tried the various positions and techniques. 2. Client able to assist infant to latch on to breast correctly.
Risk for Constipation R/T abdominal muscle weakness and hemorrhoids	1. Assess daily for bowel movement frequency and consistency. 2. Encourage more fluid and fiber intake.	1. Bowel movement daily, very firm consistency. 2. Asking for fruit between meals; drinking 8 oz water every 2 hours when awake.

COURTESY OF DELMAR CENGAGE LEARNING

FIGURE 9-4 Handwritten Institutional Care Plan

competent to perform that specific task) of some nursing interventions to staff members or assigning a specific nursing task to assistive (unlicensed) personnel capable of competently performing the task. The nurse is accountable for appropriate delegation and supervision of care provided by unlicensed personnel.

Requirements for Effective Implementation

Implementation involves many skills, including assessing the client's condition before, during, and after each nursing intervention. Positive responses add information to the database to use when evaluating the intervention. Negative responses must be dealt with immediately.

Psychomotor, interpersonal, and cognitive skills are also needed to perform the planned nursing interventions. Psychomotor skills are used when handling medical equipment and performing skills such as changing dressings, giving injections, and helping a client perform range-of-motion (ROM) exercises.

Interpersonal skills are used when collecting data, providing information in teaching sessions, and offering support in times of grief.

Cognitive skills enable the nurse to make appropriate observations, understand the rationale for the activities performed, ask appropriate questions, and make decisions about those things that need to be done. Critical thinking is an important element within the cognitive domain. It helps the nurse analyze data, organize observations, and apply prior knowledge and experiences to current client situations.

Orders for Nursing Interventions

Nursing interventions are written as orders in the care plan and may be initiated by nurses or physicians or from collaboration with other health care professionals. Interventions can be implemented on the basis of specific orders, standing orders, or protocols.

A **specific order** is an order written in a client's medical record by a physician or nursing care plan by the nurse especially for that individual client; it is not used for any other client.

A **protocol** is a series of standing orders or procedures that should be followed under certain specific conditions. It defines interventions that are permitted and circumstances under which the nurse can implement the measures. Health care agencies or individual physicians often use standing orders or protocols for preparing clients for diagnostic tests or for immediate interventions in life-threatening circumstances. Protocols prevent needlessly writing the same orders for different clients, saving valuable time.

Documenting and Reporting Interventions

The implementation step also involves documentation and reporting. Data to be recorded include the client's condition before the intervention, the specific intervention performed, the client's response to the intervention, and client outcomes. Documentation provides valuable communication among health care team members to ensure continuity of care and evaluate progress toward expected outcomes. Written documentation also provides data necessary for reimbursement.

Verbal communication between nurses generally occurs at the change of shift, when care responsibility changes. Nursing students must report relevant information to the nurse responsible for their clients when they leave the unit. Information that should be shared in the verbal report includes:

- Completed activities and those not completed
- Status of current relevant problems
- Assessment changes or abnormalities
- Results of treatments
- Diagnostic tests scheduled or completed (and results)

Both written and verbal communication must be objective, descriptive, and complete. It must include observations, not opinions and be stated or written to show an accurate picture of the client's condition. Communication of implementation activities is basic to client care and evaluation of progress toward goals.

EVALUATION

Evaluation, the fifth step in the nursing process, determines whether client goals have been met, partially met, or not met. When a goal is met, the nurse decides whether nursing interventions should stop or continue for the status to be maintained. When a goal is partially met or not met, the nurse reassesses the situation. The reasons the goal is not met and modifications to the plan of care are determined by more data collection. Reasons that goals are not met or are only partially met include:

- Initial assessment data were incomplete.
- Goals and expected outcomes were unrealistic.

Client Name: J. W. **Sex:** Female

Age: 77 **Temp:** 101.5 **BP:** 168/74 **Pulse:** 124 **O_2 Sat:** 89%

Client Health History

J.W. has smoked two to three packs of cigarettes a day for the past 60 years. She was diagnosed with COPD 4 years ago and has required supplemental oxygen at 2 L/min for the past 18 months. Her chief complaints are increasing dyspnea on exertion and a cough, which is sometimes productive, yielding thick, green-yellow sputum. She states, "I don't know why I'm coughing up this awful stuff."

Assessment Findings

Respiratory Rate 38

Sonorous and sibilant wheezes on expiration in the posterior lung fields with superimposed coarse crackles heard in the right posterior lower lung field.

Unable to ambulate to the bathroom or complete other ADLs because of dyspnea

Nursing Diagnosis: *Ineffective **B**reathing Pattern* R/T diseased lungs, infection, and increased secretions AEB severe dyspnea, elevated blood pressure, and increased pulse

Goal: J.W. will have an effective respiratory rate.

Outcomes: J.W. will:

1. Have a respiratory rate of 12–20 within 1 week.
2. Have clear lung sounds within 1 week.
3. Complete ADLs within 1 week.
4. Increase oral fluid intake to 2 L within 1 day.

Planning and Intervention

Intervention	Rationale
1. Assist client in assuming a high Fowler's position	Maximizes thoracic cavity space, decreases pressure from diaphragm and abdominal organs, facilitates use of accessory muscles
2. Provide humidified, low flow (2 L/min) oxygen, as ordered	Provides some supplemental oxygen to improve oxygenation and makes secretions less viscous
3. Administer bronchodilators, as ordered	Reduces bronchospasm and improves air flow
4. Administer IV fluids and increase oral fluids (2000–3000 mL/day as tolerated), as ordered	Improves hydration, decreases secretions
5. Administer expectorants, as ordered	Decreases secretions of previously ineffective cough
6. Administer antibiotics, as ordered	Eradicates respiratory infection or pneumonia and reduces secretions and end inflammation
7. Administer xanthines (aminophylline, theophylline), as ordered	Decreases smooth muscle spasm and edema of the mucosa
8. Administer non-narcotic cough suppressants, as ordered	Coughing can lead to fatigue. It is important for COPD clients to get adequate rest and not become fatigued with coughing

Evaluation:

Client's breathing is eupenic with a respiratory rate of 16

Client is able to cough up secretions

Client is able to ambulate to bathroom and complete ADLs

Client is drinking at least 2000 mL/day of water

Nursing Diagnosis: *Impaired **G**as Exchange* R/T lower airway (alveolar) wall destruction preventing adequate exchange of gases of respiration and airway obstruction (secretions) preventing adequate oxygenation AEB severe dyspnea, tachypnea, elevated blood pressure, increased pulse, and decreased oxygen saturation

Goal: J.W. will have improved gas exchange in her lungs.

Outcomes: J.W. will:

1. Have O_2 saturation of 95% within 1 week.
2. Have vital signs within normal ranges within 1 week.

Planning and Interventions

Intervention	Rationale
1. Assist client in assuming a high Fowler's position	Decreases the work of breathing (at least through crisis period)
2. Administer medications to loosen secretions, as ordered	Loosens secretions of previously ineffective cough
3. Provide humidified, low flow (2 L/min) oxygen, as ordered	Improves oxygenation, moistens thick secretions

Evaluation:

Client's O_2 saturation is 94%.

Client's vital signs are within normal ranges—T 98.6 P 80 R 20 BP 120/74.

COURTESY OF DELMAR CENGAGE LEARNING

FIGURE 9-5 Computer-Generated Nursing Care Plan

- Time frame was not adequate.
- Nursing interventions were not appropriate for the client or situation.

Evaluation is a fluid process that depends on all the other components of the nursing process. As shown in Figure 9-6, evaluation affects and is affected by the other four parts. Table 9-9 shows how evaluation is woven into every component of the nursing process. Ongoing evaluation is essential for the nursing process to be implemented appropriately. As Alfaro-LeFevre (2003) states,

> When we evaluate early, checking whether our information is accurate, complete, and up-to-date, we're able to make corrections *early*. We avoid making decisions based on outdated, inaccurate, or incomplete information. Early evaluation enhances our ability to act safely and effectively. It improves our *efficiency* by helping us stay focused on priorities and avoid wasting time continuing useless actions.

THE NURSING PROCESS AND CRITICAL THINKING

Many skills are necessary when nurses use the nursing process as a framework for providing client care. Critical thinking is one. Critical thinkers ask questions, identify assumptions,

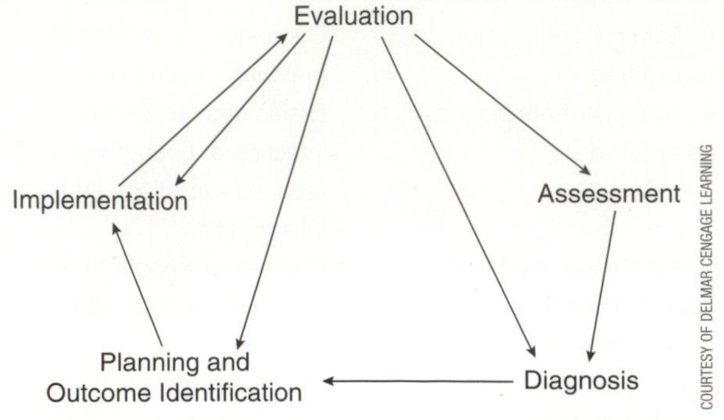

FIGURE 9-6 Relationship of Evaluation to the Other Components of the Nursing Process: Evaluation Impacts Every Component

evaluate evidence, examine alternatives, and seek to understand various points of view.

Critical thinking can be learned, just as other skills are learned. The skill of critical thinking is an especially vital tool for the nurse but is useful in all aspects of a person's life.

COMMUNITY/HOME HEALTH CARE

Effectiveness of Care

In the home, the nurse can use the following questions to evaluate client achievement of expected outcomes:

- Were the goals realistic for client abilities and the time frame?
- Did external variables (e.g., finances, housing problems, impaired family dynamics) prevent goal achievement?
- Did the family have resources (e.g., money, transportation) necessary to meet the goals?
- Was care appropriately coordinated with other providers?

Examples of questions the nurse, as critical thinker, might ask at each step in the nursing process are listed in Table 9-10.

TABLE 9-9 Interaction of Other Components of the Nursing Process with Evaluation

NURSING PROCESS COMPONENTS	EVALUATION QUESTIONS
Assessment	Are data relevant to client needs?
	Are data obtained appropriately?
	Are data collected from many, varied sources?
	Is a systematic, organized method used to collect data?
	Is data collection complete?
Diagnosis	Are diagnoses based on the data collected?
	Is each nursing diagnosis complete?
	Are nursing diagnoses client centered and relevant?
	Do nursing diagnoses guide planning and implementation of care?
	Are nursing diagnoses prioritized?
Planning and Outcome Identification	Are expected outcomes relevant to nursing diagnoses?
	Are outcomes realistic?
Implementation	Are resources (also team members) used effectively and efficiently?
	Are care plans documented?
	Is care plan revised according to the client's needs?
	Is plan of care followed by all team members?
	Are necessary resources available?
	Do nursing actions assist client in meeting expected outcomes?
	Are expected outcomes achieved?
	Does documentation reflect client status and responses to nursing interventions?

COURTESY OF DELMAR CENGAGE LEARNING

Table 9-10 Use of Critical Thinking with the Nursing Process

STEP OF NURSING PROCESS	SAMPLE CRITICAL THINKING QUESTIONS
Assessment	What data are necessary to prevent, anticipate, or detect health problems? What data are necessary to manage or eliminate a client's health problems? From what other sources can data be obtained? How does the client view his health situation? How efficient is care delivery? What assumptions or biases does the nurse have?
Diagnosis	How can the data be put together and analyzed? Are there any gaps in the data? What health problems can be identified? What are the underlying causes of risk factors for the health problems? What are the client's strengths and resources? Which satisfactory aspects of the client's health could be improved?
Planning and Outcome Identification	What are the specific desired outcomes for this client? What interventions will detect or prevent health problems? Which interventions will manage the client's health problems? What interventions will promote optimum wellness and independence for the client? How can the desired outcomes be achieved in a cost-effective, timely manner? Who is best qualified to carry out the interventions? How much does the client wish to be involved?
Implementation	How ready is the health care giver to perform the interventions? What are the critical steps of this intervention? How can the intervention be altered to meet this client's needs yet maintain principles of safety? How does the client respond during and after the intervention? What is to be documented to monitor the client's progress toward the goals and outcomes?
Evaluation	Were the specific desired goals and outcomes met? If all were met, can these goals and outcomes be eliminated? If not met, how should the plan be modified (revised)? If revision of the plan, goals, or outcomes is necessary, what ongoing, continuous assessments (data) are required? Were assumptions or biases missed that affected the interventions? What other nursing diagnosis(es) may be appropriate? What additional outcomes and interventions should be considered?

COURTESY OF DELMAR CENGAGE LEARNING

THE NURSING PROCESS AND DECISION MAKING

Every day, nurses make decisions. These decisions should be the best decisions possible based on reliable information, and made using critical thinking. Each step of the nursing process requires decisions.

Each decision, resulting from critical thought and reliable information, leads to appropriate nursing interventions for the client.

THE NURSING PROCESS AND HOLISTIC CARE

The broad base of nursing knowledge is derived from many fields, including natural science, social science, behavioral science, arts and humanities, and nursing science. With this broad knowledge base, the nurse interacts with the client in a holistic manner. Referral and collaboration among nurses and other health care professionals contribute to holistic achievement of client goals.

In some settings, the traditional nursing care plan formulated solely by nurses has been replaced by plans that are developed by a multidisciplinary team and referred to as critical pathways. Critical pathways are comprehensive, standard plans of care for specific conditions.

DOCUMENTATION

The methods of recording and reporting information relevant to client care have developed as a response to standards of practice, legal and regulatory standards, institutional standards and policies, and society's norms.

Recording and reporting are the major ways health care providers communicate. The client's medical record is a legal document of all activities regarding client care.

Documentation is any printed or written record of activities. In health care it should include:

- Changes in the client's condition
- The administration of tests, treatments, procedures, and client education, with the results of or client's response to them
- The client's response to an intervention
- The evaluation of expected outcomes
- Complaints from client or family

Purposes of Documentation

The two primary reasons for documentation are professional responsibility and accountability. The professional responsibility of all health care practitioners, documentation provides evidence of the practitioner's accountability to the client, the institution, the profession, and society. Other reasons are communication, legal and practice standards, education, reimbursement, research, and auditing.

Communication

Documentation is a communication method that confirms the care provided to the client and clearly outlines all important information regarding the client. Thorough documentation provides:

- Accurate data to plan care and ensure continuity of care
- Communication to health care team members involved in the client's care
- Evidence of things done to or for the client, the client's response, and revisions made in the plan of care
- Evidence of compliance with professional practice standards
- Evidence of compliance with accreditation criteria (e.g., those of the Joint Commission)
- A resource for reimbursement, education, and research and audit
- A written legal record to protect the client, institution, and practitioner

The client's medical record contains documents for recordkeeping. The type of documents that constitute the medical record in a given health care institution is determined by that institution. Table 9-11 outlines the content of the documents generally found in a client's record.

Practice and Legal Standards

Thoroughly documenting care in the medical record provides legal evidence that the care provided meets approved standards of care (Ferrel, 2007). *The medical record is a legal document, and in a lawsuit, it is the record that serves as the description of exactly what happened to a client.* In 80% to 85% of client care lawsuits, the determining factor in providing proof of

TABLE 9-11 Documents of the Client Medical Record

DOCUMENT	CONTENT
Face Sheet	*Demographic Data:* name, client's identifying number, address, telephone number, date of birth, place of birth, sex, race, marital status, religion, name and address of closest relative, social security number, admission date and hour, type of admission *Financial Data:* expected payer(s), insured's name and sex, client relationship to insured, employer's name and location, group name, insurance group number, insured's policy number *Clinical Data:* admitting diagnosis, admitting diagnosis-related group (DRG), client's advance directive (if has one) *Discharge Data* (to be entered by the physician on discharge of client): name of attending physician, discharge date and hour, principal diagnosis and other diagnoses, external cause of injury code, procedures and dates, operating physician(s), disposition of client
Medical History and Physical Examination	Client's description of chief complaint, present and past illnesses, personal and family histories, and review of systems as elicited by the physician, findings of physician's assessment of all body systems
Nursing Admission Assessment	Data from interview and physical assessment performed by the nurse
Prescriber's Orders	Physician's written or verbal orders to admit, to direct client's diagnostic and therapeutic course, and to discharge
Consultation Report	Findings of a physician whose opinion or advice is requested by another physician for evaluation and/or treatment of a client
Physician's Progress Notes	Provides a pertinent, chronologic report of the client's course in the hospital and reflects any changes in condition and response to treatment. May also contain notes by other members of the health care team (e.g., dietary or social service)
Laboratory Reports	Results from laboratory tests ordered by the physician
Radiology Reports	Radiologists interpretation of radiologic and fluoroscopic diagnostic services
Nuclear Medicine	Describes diagnostic studies and therapeutic procedures performed using radiopharmaceutical agents
Graphic Sheet	Various client parameters, most commonly: T, P, R, and BP. May also include weight, diet, I&O
Client Care Plan (Nursing Plan of Care)	Treatment plan including nursing diagnoses or problem list, client goals, nursing actions, and evaluation
Nurse's Progress Notes	Details care and treatments provided, client's response to care and treatments, achievement of expected outcomes that do not duplicate information on Flow Sheet (if used)

TABLE 9-11 Documents of the Client Medical Record (Continued)

DOCUMENT	CONTENT
Flow Sheet	All routine interventions that can be indicated by a check mark or other simple descriptor
Medication Administration Record (MAR)	Contains all medications administered orally, topically, by injection, inhalation, and infusion in one place; includes date, time, dosage, route of administration, and name of professional administering the drug. Routine, PRN, and single dose orders generally have separate sections
Consent Forms	*Admission:* gives the institution and physician permission to treat *Surgical:* explains the reason for and nature of the treatment, the risks, complications, alternate forms of treatment, no treatment, consequences of treatment or procedure. Sometimes surgical and anesthesia consents are separate so that responsibility is placed appropriately *Blood Transfusion:* gives specific permission to administer blood or blood products *Other:* procedure specific consent forms, participate in research project, photography
Client Education Record	Describes the nurse's teaching to the client, family, or other caregiver and the learner's response
Health Care Team Record	Used by respiratory, physical therapy, dietary when physician's progress are used only by physicians
Nursing Discharge Summary	Contains brief summary of care provided, medications, teaching, and other instructions (e.g., return appointment, referrals), discharge status, and mode of discharge
Discharge Plan and Summary	Review of events describing the client's illness, investigation (diagnostic studies), treatment, response, and condition at discharge. Instructions to the client and plans for follow-up care as included
Advance Directive	Both a living will and a durable power of attorney for health care are considered advance directives. Federal law requires that all clients be given written information about their rights so they can make decisions concerning medical care. An advance directive is not required to be in a client's medical record
Other Documents	These may or may not be in a client's medical record: Operative report, Anesthesia report, Pathology report, Transfusion record, Rehabilitation report, Critical pathway, Restraint record, and Autopsy report

COURTESY OF DELMAR CENGAGE LEARNING

significant events is the medical record (Iyer & Camp, 2005). The legal aspects of documentation require:

- Writing, legible and neat
- Spelling and grammar, properly used
- Authorized abbreviations
- Time-sequenced, and factual descriptive entries

State Nursing Practice Acts State nursing practice acts establish guidelines to ensure safe practice and to demonstrate accountability to society. The standards of care set forth in the practice acts are based on the nursing process components and require documentation as evidenced of compliance. Nurses must be familiar with the practice act of the states in which they work.

The Joint Commission The Joint Commission surveys health care facilities that voluntarily apply for accreditation to measure compliance with its standards for providing safe health care. Eligibility for Medicare, Medicaid, and private funding reimbursement depends on Joint Commission accreditation.

The Joint Commission requires documented evidence of an individualized plan of care (Joint Commission, 2008). The Joint Commission standards require:

- The involvement of the client or family in the development of the plan, which must be documented in the medical record
- Interdisciplinary planning and implementation of all aspects of care

The reviewers during an accreditation survey look for evidence of an organized and systematic method of monitoring and evaluating client care by checking documentation in medical records. Documenting the steps of the nursing process ensures compliance with the Joint Commission's plan of care requirements.

Confidentiality The client record is **confidential** and is to be read only by those health care providers directly involved in the care of that client. The record should not be left where just anyone has access to it. Keep it in its proper storage place when not being used.

Informed Consent Informed consent is a competent client's ability to make health care decisions based on full disclosure of the benefits, risks, and potential consequences of a recommended treatment plan and of alternative treatments, including no treatment, and the client's agreement to the treatment. Informed consent can be given either orally or in writing. A written informed consent document records the process of informed consent and is invaluable in the event of a lawsuit. The physician who will perform the procedure is responsible for obtaining the client's informed consent, but the nurse is often the one who actually has the client sign the form.

PROFESSIONALTIP

The Importance of Communication

Important assessment information needing immediate intervention should be documented and communicated orally to the other practitioners involved in the client's care. Time must direct decision making when critical information is obtained.

The nurse's signature as a witness on an informed consent form is vouching that the client or appropriate surrogate is the person signing and that the person signing is making an autonomous, noncoerced informed decision to have the procedure, treatment, or research completed. It is the nurse's responsibility to assess if the client is adequately informed, especially if the procedure has potential, serious consequences, and to advocate for the client to receive additional explanation as needed from the physician (Grace & McLaughlin, 2005; White, 2000).

Advance Directives An advance directive (i.e., living will and durable power of attorney for health care) is written instructions about an individual's health care preferences regarding life-sustaining measures to guide family members and health care professionals as to those treatment options that should or should not be considered when the individual is no longer able to decide. This allows competent clients to make end-of-life decisions and to choose the types of life-sustaining procedures they wish to be performed.

Reimbursement

The federal government requires peer review organizations (PROs) to monitor and evaluate the quality and appropriateness of care provided. Medical records are reviewed for documentation of intensity of services and severity of illness.

The diagnosis-related group (DRG) classification system changed the reimbursement process from a cost-per-case to a prospective payment system (PPS). With PPS, the medical record must have documentation supporting the DRG and the appropriateness of care. It also must show evidence of client and family education and discharge planning.

From the agency's perspective, when information in the medical record shows compliance with Medicare and Medicaid standards, reimbursement is maximized. Failure to document equipment or procedures used daily (e.g., feeding pump; daily weight, intake and output; intravenous therapy; drug additives) can result in reimbursement being denied.

PROFESSIONALTIP

Consent from Sedated Clients

Sedated clients should never be asked or allowed to sign an informed consent. If the client is not capable of understanding the nature of and risks associated with the procedure, the consent is invalid, and the nurse and institution are legally at risk. Either wait for the client to be competent and free of sedation (usually 4 hours after administration of medication that alters the level of consciousness) or have a legally acceptable family member sign.

COMMUNITY/HOME HEALTH CARE

Documentation

Home health agencies also keep client medical records. They must also comply with state and federal regulations affecting health care, documentation, and reimbursement.

Education

Health care students use the medical record as a tool to learn about disease processes, medical and nursing diagnoses, complications, and interventions. The results of laboratory and diagnostic testing and physical examinations provide valuable information about specific diagnoses and interventions.

Nursing students can enhance their critical-thinking skills by examining and analyzing the records of the health care team's plan of care, including the way the care plan was developed, implemented, and evaluated. All health care professionals including students must maintain confidentiality when reading any client's chart.

Research

The client's medical record is used by researchers to determine whether a client meets the research criteria for a study. Documentation can also indicate a need for research. For example, if documentation shows an increased rate of falls on certain nursing units, researchers can look for and study the variables associated with the increased fall rate.

Nursing Audit

A **nursing audit** is a method of evaluating the quality of care provided to clients. A nursing audit can focus on implementation of the nursing process, on client outcomes, or on both in order to evaluate the quality of care provided. The nursing audit is follow-up evaluation that not only evaluates the quality of care of an individual client but also provides an evaluation of overall care given in that health care facility. During a nursing audit, the evaluators look for documentation of all five components of the nursing process in the client records.

Each health care facility has an ongoing nursing audit committee to evaluate the quality of care given. The nursing audit committee reviews client records after discharge of the clients. They examine the records for data related to:

- Safety measures
- Treatment interventions and client responses to them
- Expected outcomes as basis for interventions
- Client teaching
- Discharge planning
- Adequate staffing

EFFECTIVE DOCUMENTATION PRINCIPLES

The health care facility (hospital, nursing home, home health agency), the setting within the facility (e.g., emergency room,

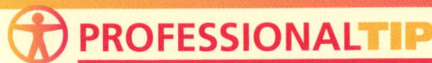

Follow the Nursing Process

Document according to the nursing process to ensure compliance with nursing practice acts and with reimbursement and accreditation criteria.

perioperative unit, medical-surgical unit), and the specific client population (e.g., obstetric, pediatric, geriatric) determine different documentation requirements. Even so, the documentation of the client care provided must reflect the nursing process. General documentation guidelines are listed in Table 9-12.

Follow the Nursing Process

Nursing notes must be logical, focused, and relevant to care, and the outcomes must represent each phase in the nursing process.

Table 9-12 General Documentation Guidelines

- Ensure that you have the correct client record or chart and that the client's name and identifying information are on every page of the record.
- Document as soon as the client encounter is concluded to ensure accurate recall of data (follow agency guidelines on frequency of charting).
- Date and time each entry.
- Sign each entry with your full legal name and with your professional credentials, per your institutional policy.
- Do not leave space between entries.
- If an error is made while documenting, use a single line to cross out the error, then date, time, and sign the correction (follow institutional policy); avoid erasing, crossing out, or using correction fluid.
- Never change another person's entry, even if it is incorrect.
- The first entry of the shift should be made early (e.g., at 7:30 A.M. for the 7–3 shift, as opposed to 11:30 A.M. or 12 P.M.). Chart at least every 2 hours, or per institutional policy.
- Use quotation marks to indicate direct client responses (e.g., "I feel lousy").
- Document in chronological order; if chronological order is not used, state why.
- Write legibly.
- Use a permanent-ink pen (black is usually preferable because it photocopies well).
- Document in a complete but concise manner by using phrases and abbreviations as appropriate.
- Document all telephone calls that you make or receive that are related to a client's case.

Adapted from *Health Assessment & Physical Examination* (4th ed.), by M. Estes, Clifton Park, NY: Delmar Cengage Learning.

Nursing documentation based on the nursing process facilitates effective care because client needs can be traced from assessment, through identification of the problems to the care plan, implementation, and evaluation. A brief outline of the elements of the nursing process as they relate to documentation follows:

- *Assessment:* Assessment data related to an actual or potential health care need are summarized without duplication. With reassessment, any new findings or any changes in the client's condition (e.g., increased pain) are highlighted.
- *Nursing diagnosis:* NANDA-International terminology is used to identify the client's problem or need.
- *Planning and outcome identification:* The expected outcomes and goals of client care, as discussed with the client and communicated to members of the multidisciplinary team, should be documented on the care plan or critical pathway rather than in the progress notes.
- *Implementation:* After an intervention has been performed, observations, treatments, teaching, and related clinical judgments should be documented on the flow sheet and progress notes. Client teaching should include learning needs, teaching plan content, methods of teaching, who was taught, and the client's response.
- *Evaluation:* The effectiveness of the interventions in terms of the expected outcomes is evaluated and documented: progress toward goals; client response to tests, treatments, and nursing interventions; client and family response to teaching and significant events; and questions, statements, or complaints voiced by the client or family.
- *Revisions of planned care:* The reasons for the revisions along with the supporting evidence and client agreement are documented.

Effective Documentation Elements

If documenting on paper forms, the elements for effective documentation are:

- Document accurately, completely, and objectively including any errors that occurred
- Note date and time
- Use appropriate forms
- Identify the client
- Write in ink (Usually all charting is written with black ink, but each agency determines protocol.)
- Use standard abbreviations
- Spell correctly
- Write legibly
- Correct errors properly
- Write on every line
- Chart omissions
- Sign each entry

If documenting electronically, the guidelines are the same in documenting accurately, completely, and objectively. However, many of the issues of paper charting are completed automatically on an electronic health record, such as not needing to use ink to chart, writing legibly, and signing each entry. A nurse cannot obtain a client's electronic health record without logging on to the computer, which automatically signifies the writer, date, time, and entry.

NURSE'S PROGRESS RECORD

DATE	HOUR	PROGRESS NOTES
2/3/10	0815	Client verbalizes severe abdominal pain (8 on a 0-10 pain
		scale). Lying on Right side. States "I don't want to take a
		bath, and I don't want any breakfast". Abdomen distended.
		No bowel sounds asculatated. Acute Pain R/T no flatus
		passed since surgery. ——— L. White, RN
2/3/10	0820	Administered Prostigmin Injection 0.5 mg (1 mL of 1:2000
		solution) given IM in Right gluteus maximus. Assisted to Left
		side (Sim's position). ——— L. White, RN
2/3/10	0900	Client states "I passed some gas, the pain is much less now,
		about a 4 (on 0-10 pain scale). ——— L. White, RN

COURTESY OF DELMAR CENGAGE LEARNING

FIGURE 9-7 Accurate, Complete, Objective Documentation

Accurate, Complete, and Objective

Record just the facts—exactly what you see, hear, and do. For example, "Two 4 × 4s completely soaked with yellow-green drainage in 20 minutes" is more accurate than "large amount of drainage." Never record opinions or assumptions. Chart relevant information relating to client care and reflecting the nursing process (Figure 9-7). *Remember, if it is not charted, it was not done.* It is difficult to prove in court that an aspect of client care was provided if it was not documented.

Document information promptly; the information is more likely to be accurate and complete. Important details may be forgotten if charting is left until the end of the shift, and those details may later become a legal issue. Chart medications immediately *after* administration. This prevents errors such as another nurse administering pain medication when the first dose was not charted.

Avoid subjective statements such as "client is uncooperative." Record the client's exact words using quotation marks, for example, *Client stated, "I don't want to take a bath, and I don't want any breakfast."*

Date and Time

Be sure each entry is dated and has a specific time. Especially note the exact time of sudden changes in a client's condition, nursing actions, and other significant events. Do not chart in blocks of time, such as 7 A.M. to 11 A.M. This is vague and sounds like the client has had no attention during that time frame.

When military time is used, there is no confusion between A.M. and P.M. entries. For this reason, many facilities use military time (Figure 9-8).

If documentation cannot be done in a timely manner, explain the delay. For example, "chart in x-ray with client." When an entry must be added after notes are completed, follow the facility's policy for recording a late entry. Generally, the practice is to enter the date and time and note "Late Entry."

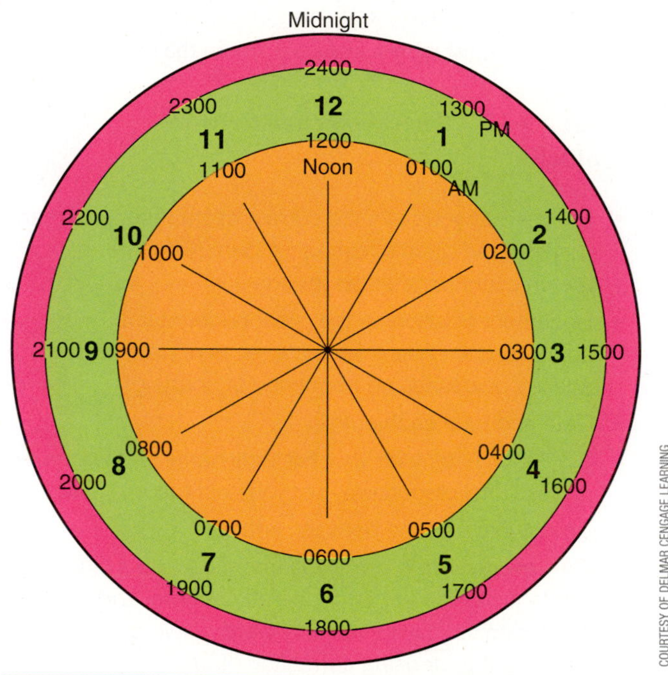

FIGURE 9-8 Military time uses a 24-hour clock.

This indicates that the entry is out of sequence. Then the date and time the entry should have been made is followed by the information to be recorded (Figure 9-9). A nurse charts a late entry on the electronic health record by changing the time notation as needed on all entries during her shift.

Use Appropriate Forms

Use the appropriate forms as required by the facility's policy manual. The forms used are not the same in every facility. Some facilities use flow sheets instead of progress notes.

NURSE'S PROGRESS RECORD

DATE	HOUR	PROGRESS NOTES
2/3/10	1100	Late Entry (2/3/10—0900) Client crying after talking to
		mother on the telephone. ——— L. White, RN

COURTESY OF DELMAR CENGAGE LEARNING

FIGURE 9-9 Recording a Late Entry

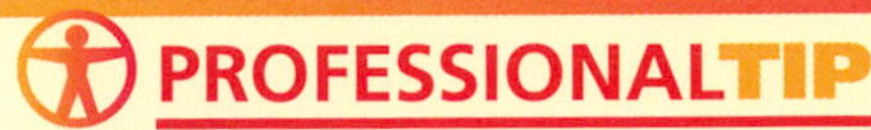

Abbreviations

Avoid abbreviations that can be misunderstood (Figure 9-10). For example, what does the abbreviation *Pt* mean? Does it refer to the patient, prothrombin time, physical therapy, or part time? Refer to your institution's approved abbreviations listing.

Identify the Client

Each page of the client's record should have the client's name on it. This aids in preventing confusion and helps ensure that information is charted on the correct record. Many facilities use the addressograph to stamp the client's name on each page. When charting electronically, make sure the correct client document is on the screen before making an entry.

Write in Ink

The client's record is a permanent document, and information should be charted in ink or printed out from a computer. Only black ink should be used because it will photocopy well. Felt-tipped pens are not to be used, especially on forms with carbons, because they do not hold up under pressure to make a clear copy. Also, they often bleed through the paper.

Use Standard Abbreviations

Each health care facility has a list of approved abbreviations and symbols for documenting information on its client records. This is to meet the Joint Commission standards and the regulations in many states. Such a list prevents confusion. The use of some abbreviations causes ambiguity that could be misleading and endanger a client's health (Figure 9-10). Appendix C lists commonly used abbreviations and terms that the Joint Commission officially lists as "Do not to use" terms.

Spell Correctly

Misspelled words on client records may be confusing and certainly convey a sense of unprofessionalism. They may generate questions about the quality of the care provided, increase the chance of liability, and produce a loss of the writer's credibility. When you are unsure of how to spell a word, *look it up*. Most units in a health care facility have a dictionary and other books to use as references. If these resources are not available and if spelling correctly is difficult, carry a small pocket dictionary and use it as needed.

Write Legibly

Legible handwriting is imperative for effective documentation. Sloppy writing hinders communication, and errors in client care can occur. Trying to decipher illegible writing wastes time. Illegible handwriting also creates a poor impression of the person who did the writing and damages that person's credibility. Print rather than use cursive writing; it is usually easier to read.

Correct Errors Properly

Promptly correct any error you make in documenting on a client's record. Know and follow your facility's policy for correcting errors. Generally, it is acceptable to draw a single line through the mistaken entry so that what was written can still be read. Above it carefully write "Mistaken Entry" followed by your initials and the date (Brooke, 2002; Dumpel, James, & Phillips, 1999; Pethtel, 2000). The original entry must still be readable. *NEVER scratch out, erase, or use correction fluid (white-out)* on a mistaken entry. Using these methods makes it look as if something is trying to be hidden. Be sure the mistaken entry is still readable (Figure 9-11).

Write on Every Line

Fill each line completely. Leave no blank lines or partially blank lines. Draw a line through the empty part of the line (see Figure 9-12). This prevents others from inserting information later that may change the meaning of the original documentation. On forms, when information requested does not apply to a particular client, write "NA" (not applicable) or draw a line through the space. This indicates that every item on the form has been addressed.

NURSE'S PROGRESS RECORD

DATE	TIME	ORDER
11/18/10	1400	Give MS 2 mg I.V. every 4 hours Dr. D. Ledbetter

Does the MS stand for morphine sulphate, or magnesium sulfate?

COURTESY OF DELMAR CENGAGE LEARNING

FIGURE 9-10 Misleading Abbreviation

NURSE'S PROGRESS RECORD

DATE	HOUR	PROGRESS NOTES
2/3/10	0600	Client verbalizes severe abdominal pain (8 on a 0–10 pain
		scale) when lying on ~~Left side~~ (Mistaken Entry LW 2/3/10) Right side.—L. White, RN

COURTESY OF DELMAR CENGAGE LEARNING

FIGURE 9-11 Mistaken Entry

NURSE'S PROGRESS RECORD

DATE	HOUR	PROGRESS NOTES
2/3/10	0900	Abdominal dressing not changed. Client in x-ray for a flat
		plate of the abdomen.——————L. White, RN

COURTESY OF DELMAR CENGAGE LEARNING

FIGURE 9-12 Charting an Omitted Part of the Care Plan

NURSE'S PROGRESS RECORD

DATE	HOUR	PROGRESS NOTES
2/3/10	1300	to assess client's knowledge of diabetes (Continued on next
		page)——————L. White, RN

NURSE'S PROGRESS RECORD

DATE	HOUR	PROGRESS NOTES
2/3/10	1300	(Continued from previous page) on the 3rd or 4th day
		post op——————L. White, RN

COURTESY OF DELMAR CENGAGE LEARNING

FIGURE 9-13 Entry Continues on Another Page

Chart Omissions

Charting is supposed to show implementation of the medical and nursing plans of care. Whenever a part of the plan is omitted, document the reason for the omission. For example, a treatment is not provided or medication is not administered because the client was in x-ray (Figure 9-12).

Sign Each Entry

Each entry on the nurse's notes (progress notes) is to be signed with your first name or initial, full last name, and professional licensure (i.e., LVN, LPN, RN). The signature should be at the end of the entry on the far right side. When there is not enough room on the last line of the documentation, draw a line from the last word to the end of the line and on the next line, leaving enough room to sign the entry at the far right.

For a long entry that will conclude on another page, record "(Continued on Next Page)" and sign your name. Begin the next page with "(Continued from Previous Page)", finish the entry, and sign your name (Figure 9-13).

Documenting a Medication Error

An incident report is required for all medication errors (discussed later). The medication given in error should be recorded on the Medication Administration Record (MAR) and in the nurse's progress notes. Remember, the purpose of the medical record is to report any care or treatment the client receives; this includes any errors made. Document in the nurse's notes the name and dosage of the medication, time it was given, client's response to the medication, time and name of the practitioner notified of the error, nursing interventions or medical treatment to counteract the error, and client's response to treatment. Do not mention that an incident report was completed.

Some health care facilities are now using a specific medication incident (variance) report for situations related to medications (Figure 9-14). This provides the facility with specific information to possibly change policies or procedures that will work to prevent medication incidents.

SYSTEMS OF DOCUMENTATION

Systems of recording and reporting data pertinent to client care have evolved primarily in response to demands that health care practitioners be held to societal norms, professional standards of practice, legal and regulatory standards, and institutional policies and standards. The documentation systems used today reflect specific needs and preferences of the many health care agencies.

Among the many systems used for documentation are the following:

- Narrative charting
- Source-oriented charting
- Problem-oriented charting
- PIE charting
- Focus charting
- Charting by exception
- Computerized documentation
- Critical pathways

Addressograph | CHRISTUS Health | *Addressograph*

CHRISTUS Health
QUALITY COMMITTEE
Medication Safety And Quality Report
Adverse Drug Event(Errors/Reactions)
Medical Record #:
Γ Male Γ Female
Name:

Address:

Medication Error: any preventable event that may cause or lead to inappropriate medication use or patient harm, including prescribing, order communication, product labeling, packaging, compounding, dispensing, distribution, administration and use. (adapted from USP); any variance from the established process.

Instructions: Person discovering event completes Sections 1 through 13 according to facility policy and procedure. Forward to manager for additional review and investigation. Manager or analyst completes sections 14 through 19.

Event Number: ____________ **(# assigned by Risk Management)** **1. Diagnosis:**

2. FACILITY NAME ____________

3. Date of Occurrence: ___/___/___ Time ___:___ AM PM

Check if event occurred on: ☐Holiday ☐Weekends

4. Event Type: Variance Occurred to: ☐ Patient(01) ☐ Other(OT)

5. Type/Event Indicator:

☐ Adverse Drug Reaction	(70.10)	☐ Monitoring Error	(70.60)	☐ Wrong Rate	(77.10)
☐ Deteriorated Drug Errors (dispensing expired drug)	(70.20)	☐Clinical (lab, vital signs)	(70.61)	☐Too Fast	(71.11)
☐ Dose Omission	(70.30)	☐Documented Allergy	(70.62)	☐Too Slow	(71.12)
☐ Improper Dose	(70.40)	☐Drug-Disease Interaction	(70.63)	☐ Wrong Route of Administration	(71.20)
☐Extra Dose	(70.41)	☐Drug-Drug Interaction	(70.64)	☐ Wrong Strength/Concentration	(71.30)
☐Frequency	(70.42)	☐Drug-Food/ Interaction	(70.65)	☐ Wrong Technique	(71.40)
☐Resulting in Overdosage	(70.43)	☐ Narcotic Discrepancy	(71.60)	☐ Wrong Time	(71.50)
☐Resulting in Under Dosage	(70.44)	☐ Wrong Dosage Form	(70.70)	☐ Other	(79.99)
☐ IV Infiltration/Extravasation	(70.50)	☐ Wrong Drug	(70.80)		
		☐ Wrong Duration	(70.90)		
		☐ Wrong Patient	(70.00)		

6. Setting of initial event:(Dept. or unit)

7. Setting where event discovered: (Dept or unit)

8. Medication as Ordered: (Name, Dose, Route, Frequency)

9. Medication as Dispensed or Administered:

10. DESCRIPTION OF EVENT:

11. Patient Outcome: (Errors or reactions with ** to left of description require physician notification and notification of Risk Management according to facility policy and procedure)

☐ No Error, but circumstances, policies or procedures that could lead to error	(31.0)
☐ Error occurred but medication did not reach patient.(i.e. dispensing error, caught in pharmacy or on delivery to unit)	(32.1)
☐ Error or reaction that reaches patient	(32.2)
☐ Medication reaches the patient but not administered	(32.4)
☐ ** Medication reaches the patient and is administered, no additional treatment, monitoring or intervention	(32.3)
☐ **Increased patient monitoring only(more frequent vital signs, laboratory tests ordered)	(32.5)
☐ **Treatment or intervention required(meds ordered, procedures required)	(33.1)
☐ **Initial or prolonged hospitalization	(33.2)
☐ **Permanent patient harm	(33.3)
☐ **Near-death event (e.g., anaphylaxis, cardiac arrest)	(33.4)
☐ **Death	(34.0)

12. Reported By: ____________ **Date:** ___/___/___ **Time:** ___:___ AM PM **Risk Mgmt notified?** ☐Yes ☐No

13. Physician Notified ☐Yes ☐No **By:** ____________ **Date:** ___/___/___ **Time:** ___:___ AM PM

THIS IS A COMMITTEE DOCUMENT & IS PRIVILEGED AND CONFIDENTIAL.

Sections 14 through 19 to be completed by Manager

14. Persons Involved (include name and phone, if appropriate, for purpose of followup or participation in possible root cause analysis)

Ordered Med: ____________ ☐ Intern (A1) ☐ Resident(A2) ☐ Other Physician(A3) ☐ Nurse Practitioner/Advanced Practice (C1)

Prepared/Administered Med: ____________ ☐ Registered Nurse(C2) ☐ Licensed Practical Nurse(C3) ☐Pharmacy Technician (E) ☐ Pharmacist (B) ☐ Other(H) ____________

Dispensed Med ____________ ☐ Pharmacist (B) ☐ Other(H) ____________

15. System Breakdown Points: Were any of the following items identified during error investigation? Check all that apply

☐ Administration not documented	(C1)	☐ Location(adjacent medications)	(C27)
☐ Allergy information not in chart	(C2)	☐ Look alike/Sound alike product name/packaging	(C28)
☐ Allergy information not on MAR/Kardex	(C3)	☐ Look alike/Sound alike patient name	(C29)
☐ Armband/name not checked	(C4)	☐ MAR/Kardex incorrect, misleading or unclear	(C30)
☐ Abbreviations	(C5)	☐ Medication not available at scheduled admin time	(C31)
☐ Automated dispensing device	(C6)	☐ Medication stored in wrong drawer/location	(C32)
☐ Calculation error in pharmacy	(C7)	☐ Multiple orders for same medication	(C33)
☐ Calculation error on nursing unit	(C8)	☐ Order entry error (user error)	(C18)
☐ Change of shift	(C9)	☐ Order not sent to/received by pharmacy	(C34)
☐ Computer system down	(C10)	☐ Order overlooked/missed by pharmacy	(C35)
☐ Computer system functionality	(C50)	☐ Order overlooked/missed by nursing	(C36)
☐ Decimal error(NOT Leading/Trailing Zeros)	(C11)	☐ Order misinterpreted by pharmacy	(C37)
☐ Delayed dose	(C12)	☐ Order misinterpreted by nursing	(C49)
☐ Documentation	(C17)	☐ Order stamped/labeled for wrong patient	(C19)
☐ Error in stocking/restocking/cart fill/floor stock etc	(C13)	☐ Order unclear or ambiguous	(C38)
☐ Handwriting	(C14)	☐ Patient off unit	(C39)
☐ Illegible fax or NCR order copy	(C15)	☐ Patient with stated allergy to medication given	(C40)
☐ Incomplete order	(C16)	☐ Policy/procedure not followed	(C41)
☐ Insufficient staff	(C20)	☐ Prepared in patient care area	(C42)
☐ Inexperienced staff	(C21)	☐ Pump programmed incorrectly	(C43)
☐ Fatigue or extended shift	(C22)	☐ Pump/Equipment failure	(C44)
☐ Lack of training	(C23)	☐ Transfer patient /orders	(C45)
☐ Leading/Trailing zeros	(C24)	☐ Transcription error	(C46)
☐ Labeling of drug incorrect or misleading	(C25)	☐ Verbal order	(C47)
☐ Lack of knowledge	(C26)	☐ Other (Explain in section 16)	(C48)

16. Notes regarding investigation, action, recommendations for system improvement:

17. Nature of Injury: (Check all that apply)				
☐ Abscess (04)	☐ Blood Disorder (62)	☐ Hearing Disorder (39)	☐ Respiratory Disorder/ Asphyxia/Choking (43)	☐ Tissue Damage (61)
☐ Amputation (06)	☐ Circulatory Impairment (11)	☐ Heart Attack (41)	☐ Rupture (59)	☐ Visual Impairment (40)
☐ Anoxia (44)	☐ Dermatitis/Skin Disorder(29)	☐ Hematoma (51)	☐ Seizure (22)	☐ Other (99) ________
☐ Blister (50)	☐ Deterioration in Condition(14)	☐ Infection (31)	☐ Shock (Non-Electrical) (37)	
	☐ Fever (24)	☐ Inflammation (27)	☐ Stroke (45)	☐ No Injury Noted (48)
	☐ Headache (52)	☐ Phlebitis (19)		

18. Does this injury involve one of these outcomes... (Check only one)				
	☐ Amputation (01)	☐ Burn (04)	☐ Loss of Hearing (13)	☐ Residual Paralysis (18)
	☐ Birth Injury (02)	☐ Events Resulting in Disability (06)	☐ Loss of Eyesight (12)	☐ Septicemia After Admission (19)
	☐ Brain Damage (03)	☐ Kidney Failure (11)	☐ Loss of Sensation (14)	☐ Unexpected Death (20)

19. Manager Review: ____________ Date:

20. Director/Administrator Review: ____________ Date:

THIS IS A COMMITTEE DOCUMENT & IS PRIVILEGED AND CONFIDENTIAL.

FIGURE 9-14 Medication Incident Report (*Courtesy of CHRISTUS Spohn Hospital Shoreline, Corpus Christi, TX.*)

NURSE'S PROGRESS RECORD

DATE	HOUR	PROGRESS NOTES
2/3/10	1630	Client 6 hours post op; awakens easily, oriented x 3.
		Abdominal dressing dry and intact. Denies pain but stated he
		felt nauseated and immediately vomited 50 mL of clear fluid.
		Attempted to ambulate to bathroom with assistance, but felt
		dizzy. Assisted to lie down in bed. Voided 250 mL clear, yellow
		urine in urinal. Client encouraged to turn in bed, cough, and
		deep breathe.——————L. White, RN
2/3/10	1650	Continues to feel nauseated. Zofran 4 mg IV given
		——————L. White, RN
2/3/10	1730	States he is no longer nauseated. Remains pain free.
		Properly demonstrated coughing and deep breathing.——
		——————L. White, RN

COURTESY OF DELMAR CENGAGE LEARNING

FIGURE 9-15 Narrative Charting

NARRATIVE CHARTING

Narrative charting, the traditional method of nursing documentation, is a chronologic account written in paragraphs that describe client status, interventions and treatments, and the client's response to treatments. This was the only method for documenting care before the advent of flow sheets.

Narrative documentation is the most flexible of all systems and is usable in any clinical setting. The relationship between nursing interventions and client's responses is clearly shown (Figure 9-15).

However, subjectivity is a common problem. Client problems may be difficult to track because the same information may not be consistently documented. The client's progress may be difficult to identify. Narrative charting often fails to reflect the nursing process.

SOURCE-ORIENTED CHARTING

Source-oriented charting is a narrative recording by each member (source) of the health care team on separate documents. Each discipline uses a separate record, often resulting in fragmented care and time-consuming communication between disciplines.

PROBLEM-ORIENTED CHARTING

Problem-oriented medical record (POMR) employs a structured, logical format and focuses on the client's problem. There are four critical components of POMR:

- Database (assessment data)
- Problem list (client's problems numbered according to when identified)
- Initial plan (outline of goals, expected outcomes, and learning needs and further data, if needed)
- Progress notes (charting based on the **SOAP**, SOAPIE, or SOAPIER format)

The format in which progress notes are written includes SOAP, SOAPIE, or SOAPIER:

- S: subjective data (what the client or family states)
- O: objective data (what is observed/inspected)
- A: assessment (conclusion reached on the basis of data formulated as client problem or nursing diagnosis)
- P: plan (expected outcomes and actions to be taken)

SOAPIE and SOAPIER refer to formats that add the following:

- I: implementation
- E: evaluation
- R: revision

An entry need not be made for each component of SOAP(IER) at every documentation (Figure 9-16); however, each problem must have a complete note every 24 hours if unresolved or whenever the client's condition changes.

Continuity of care is shown when the plan of care and interventions performed are documented together. Figure 9-16 shows an example of SOAPIE charting. Some physicians use this format when writing progress notes.

PIE CHARTING

After the SOAP format gained popularity, the **Problem, Intervention, Evaluation (PIE) charting** system was developed to streamline documentation. The main parts of this system are an integrated plan of care, assessment flow sheets, and nurse's progress notes. Figure 9-17 shows an example of PIE charting.

FOCUS CHARTING

Focus charting is a documentation system using a column format to chart Data, Action, and Response (DAR) (Smith, 2000c) (Figure 9-18). Usually the focus is a nursing diagnosis, but it may also be:

- A sign or symptoms (e.g., abnormal vaginal bleeding)
- An acute change in the client's condition (e.g., sudden increase in blood pressure)
- A patient behavior (e.g., crying after talking on the phone)
- A treatment of procedure (e.g., dressing change with wound drainage)
- A special need (e.g., a discharge referral) (Smith, 2000a)

Focus charting reflects the stages of the nursing process. Data are the subjective and objective information describing

NURSE'S PROGRESS RECORD

DATE	HOUR	PROGRESS NOTES
2/3/10	0730	#1 Pain
		S: Client states "The pain in my hip is so bad."
		O: Client states pain is 9 (0–10 scale); skin warm, moist,
		pale. Lying stiffly in bed with fists clenched.
		A: Acute Pain, needs medication for relief
		P: Check orders for analgesia; check vital signs; if within
		normal limits give analgesia as ordered; then recheck in 30
		minutes for response.——L. White, RN
2/3/10	0740	#1 Pain
		O: BP 142/86, P 110, R 28
		I: meperidine 75 mg IM in right gluteus maximus.——L. White, RN
2/3/10	0810	#1 Pain
		S: Client states "The pain is better."
		O: Client states pain now 4 (0–10 scale); skin warm, dry,
		normal color. Lying relaxed in bed.
		A: Pain relieved
		P: Continue to monitor for pain
		E: Analgesic effective——L. White, RN
2/3/10	0810	#2 Anxiety
		S: Client states "I'm still worried about the surgery onmy
		hip."
		O: Client clutching sheet
		A: Anxiety R/T surgery the next day
		P: Encourage verbalization of concerns and feelings. Involve
		family in discussion of concerns, if client agreeable.——
		——L. White, RN

COURTESY OF DELMAR CENGAGE LEARNING

FIGURE 9-16 SOAPIE Charting

NURSE'S PROGRESS RECORD

DATE	HOUR	PROGRESS NOTES
2/3/10	0830	P #1: Disturbed Body Image R/T bilateral mastectomy——
		I #1: Encourage verbalization of feelings and concerns and
		remain alert for client's comments about body changes;
		encourage looking at surgical site when ready——
		E #1: Glanced at chest during dressing change. Continue
		encouraging client's involvement in dressing changes.——
		——L. White, RN
2/3/10	0830	P #2: Ineffective Breathing Pattern R/T musculoskeletal
		impairment following mastectomy——
		I #2: Encourage use of incentive spirometer every 2 hours
		increasing level each day; assess breath sounds, rate, and
		quality of respirations every 4 hours; monitor O_2 saturation
		with pulse oximeter——
		E #2: Using incentive spirometer every 2 hours when
		awake. Breath sounds normal, respirations 20 shallow, O_2
		saturation 93%.——L. White, RN

COURTESY OF DELMAR CENGAGE LEARNING

FIGURE 9-17 PIE Charting

NURSE'S PROGRESS RECORD

DATE	HOUR	FOCUS	PROGRESS NOTES
2/3/10	1300	Deficient	D: Client states that she does not
		Knowledge R/T	understand why she has to take three
		medications	medications. "I don't like to take pills."
			A: Reason for each medication explained,
			dosages, and side effects.———
			R: Client verbalizes action and side effects
			of her medications.———L. White, RN
2/3/10	1600	Abnormal	D: Client states that her period just
		vaginal bleeding	started and she is passing clots.
			A: One maxi pad saturated in 30 minutes.
			BP 110/68, P 100, R 20. No clotsseen.
			Status reported to Dr. Medoffer and
			orders received. IV started with 20 G
			catheter, 1000 mL normal saline hung at
			100 mL/h. Continue monitoring bleeding
			and vital signs. Dr. Medoffer will see
			client in 1 hour.
			R: Client states reason for IV.——
			———L. White, RN

COURTESY OF DELMAR CENGAGE LEARNING

FIGURE 9-18 Focus Charting

the focus. The data information corresponds to assessment in the nursing process. Action is the nursing interventions and mirrors the planning and implementation stages of the nursing process. Response is the client's response to the interventions reflecting the evaluation stage of the nursing process (Smith, 2000a). The column format of this system is used within the progress notes but is easily distinguished from other entries.

Charting by Exception

Charting by exception (CBE) is a documentation system using standardized protocols stating what the expected course of the illness is, and only significant findings (exceptions) are documented in a narrative form. It assumes that client care needs are routine and predictable and that the client's responses and outcomes are also routine and predictable.

The rule of thumb related to charting "if it is not charted, it was not done" is replaced in CBE by the presumption that unless documented otherwise, all standardized protocols have been met and no further documentation is needed. Time spent by nurses documenting client care may be reduced. Murphy (2003) states that when CBE is designed and implemented properly within a facility and when charting follows state or local requirements, CBE is not illegal. However, Guido (2001), states, "Charting by exception may make it impossible to show the attentiveness of the nursing staff to patients" and "may not assist nurses in being able to defend themselves, because even they cannot recreate what was done and not done" (p. 183).

Computerized Documentation

Health care facilities have been using computers for many years to order diagnostic tests and medications and to receive results of diagnostic tests. Using a totally computerized client record is slowly being adopted. In terms of both time and finances, it is a huge commitment for a facility to plan for and make the change to computerized client records.

Issues to be addressed when considering computerized client records include data standards, vocabularies, security, legal issues, and costs.

- Data standards—include length of fields, how dates and times are shown, and ASCII or binary data
- Vocabularies—the most commonly used are the combination of the NANDA-International nursing diagnoses, Nursing Interventions Classification (NIC) nursing interventions, and **Nursing Outcomes Classification (NOC)** nursing outcomes
- Security—includes privacy, confidentiality, who has access to which data, how errors are to be corrected, and protection against data loss
- Legal issues—electronic signatures
- Costs—include planning, hardware, software, and training for all users

Nursing information systems (NIS) are various software programs that allow nursing documentation in an electronic record. These systems generally follow the components of the nursing process. The NIS works in conjunction with the

CRITICAL THINKING

Systems for Charting

Why are there so many systems for charting? Of what value is each?

hospital information system (HIS). Each NIS can be customized to fit a facility's documentation forms.

Decision-support systems are available to alert nurses, physicians, and pharmacists of client drug incompatibility, appropriate antibiotics based on culture and antibiotic susceptibility results, and adverse drug reactions. Another decision-support system uses assessment data to suggest possible nursing diagnoses, goals and outcome criteria, and interventions from which the nurse selects those appropriate for a specific client. A medical spell check is also available.

Bedside computer terminals allow the nurse to immediately document client assessments, medications given, and interventions performed; the nurse can also check care plans and revise if necessary, check test results, and many other functions. Timeliness, completeness, and the quality of nursing documentation are improved.

Voice-activated systems are available in some facilities. The nurse speaks into a special telephone handset, and the words appear on the computer screen. These are generally located at a central place rather than at the bedside.

Besides reducing documentation time and increasing accuracy, computerized charting increases legibility, stores and retrieves information quickly and easily, helps link diverse sources of client information, and uses standardized terminology, thus improving communication among health care departments. Planners for health care, researchers, lawyers, and third-party payers can quickly and easily retrieve information for their respective jobs.

Problems with computerized charting may occur if used incorrectly, and client information may be mixed up. When security measures are neglected, client confidentiality may be compromised. Users (e.g., nurses, physicians) should never share computer ID numbers or passwords with anyone. Many systems keep a record of what each user has done in the system.

To prevent these problems, users must also remember to log off to prevent unauthorized access by others. Users should also follow facility protocol for correcting errors and keep monitors and print versions of client information where others cannot see the information.

Information is temporarily unavailable when the computer system is "down" either for routine servicing or an unexpected failure. Processing time may be slow during peak usage times when too few terminals are available.

Point-of-Care Charting

Point-of-care charting is a computerized documentation system allowing health care providers to have immediate access to client information. The system permits input and retrieval of client data at the bedside with a handheld portable computer. This is especially useful for nurses working in home health care.

The advantages of point-of-care charting are related to the computer system efficiency, through which the following can be achieved:

- Operating costs are controlled.
- Existing information systems are complemented.
- Redundant data entry is eliminated.
- The practitioner has more one-on-one time for client care.
- Crucial client information is available to all health care providers in a timely fashion.

Point-of-care charting enhances continuity of care by providing each health care practitioner with client data. It also fosters compliance with accreditation and regulatory standards.

Critical Pathway

A **critical pathway** (care map) is a comprehensive preprinted interdisciplinary standard plan of care reflecting the ideal course of treatment for the average client with a given diagnosis or procedure, especially those with relatively predictable outcomes. They are generally not written for extremely complex client situations with less predictable outcomes.

The overall goal for critical pathways is to improve the quality and efficiency of client care. The sequence and timing of interdisciplinary activities is established, including assessments, consultations, diagnostic tests, nutrition, medications, activities, treatments, therapeutics, education, and discharge planning. Although nursing diagnoses as such are not generally included in a critical pathway, a nurse may identify nursing diagnoses and interventions for a specific client.

Health care facilities develop their own critical pathways. An interdisciplinary team, including nurses, physicians, dietary, rehabilitative services, social services, and others when needed, develops the critical pathway through consensus about the management of the identified case situation. This is a time-consuming task, but once written, a critical pathway can be revised based on a review of the variances.

Goals not met or interventions not performed within the established time frame are called **variances**. The nurse documents on a variance form why a goal is not met or an intervention is not performed. Documentation becomes complicated when clients have more than two diagnoses or variations. Additional documentation forms are needed to complement the pathway.

FORMS FOR DOCUMENTATION

Forms for recording data include Kardex, flow sheets, nurse's progress notes, and discharge summaries. They are designed to facilitate record keeping and allow quick, easy access to information.

Kardex

A **Kardex** is a brief worksheet with basic client care information that traditionally is not part of the medical record. The Kardex is used as a reference throughout the shift and during change-of-shift reports. It comes in various sizes, shapes, and types, including computer-generated. The Kardex usually contains the following information:

- Client name, age, marital status, religious preference, physician, family contact with phone number
- Medical diagnoses: listed by priority
- Nursing diagnoses: listed by priority
- Allergies
- Medical orders: diet, medications, intravenous (IV) therapy, treatments, diagnostic tests and procedures (including dates and results), consultations, DNR (do-not-resuscitate) order (when appropriate)

COMMUNITY/HOME HEALTH CARE

Home Health Kardex

The home health Kardex also contains information related to family contacts, practitioners (physician), other services, and emergency referrals.

- Activities permitted: functional limitations, assistance needed in activities of daily living, and safety precautions

Some facilities are eliminating the Kardex in favor of keeping all data at fingertips on the computer.

Flow Sheets

Flow sheets, with vertical or horizontal columns for recording date, time, and assessment data and intervention information, make it easy to track the client's changes in condition. Special equipment used in client teaching and IV therapy are other parts of the flow sheet. These forms usually contain legends identifying the approved abbreviations for charting data because they have small spaces for recording (Figure 9-19). Flow sheets must be completely filled out because blank spaces imply that something was not recognized, attempted, or completed.

Because they decrease the redundancy of charting in the nurse's progress notes, flow sheets are used as supplements in many documentation systems. They do not, however, replace the progress notes. Nurses still must document observations, client responses and teaching, detailed interventions, and other significant data in the progress notes.

Nurse's Progress Notes

Nurse's progress notes are used to document the client's condition, problems, and complaints; interventions; the client's response to interventions; and achievement of outcomes. Documents falling under the general heading of nurse's progress notes includes nurse's notes, personal care flow sheets, MAR, teaching records, vital sign records, intake and output forms, and specialty forms (e.g., diabetic flow sheet or neurologic assessment form). Progress notes can be either narrative or incorporated into a standardized flow sheet (Figure 9-19) to complement SOAP(IE), PIE, focus charting, and other documentation systems.

Discharge Summary

The client's illness and course of care are highlighted in the discharge summary. A narrative discharge summary in the progress notes includes:

- Client status on admission and discharge
- A brief summary of the client's care
- Intervention and education outcomes
- Resolved problems and continuing care needs for unresolved problems, including referrals
- Client instructions about medications, diet, food-drug interactions, activity, treatments, follow-up, and other special needs

Many facilities have a form itemizing discharge and client instructions. The form has a duplicate copy for the client, with the original being placed in the medical record. Figure 9-20 is an example of this form.

DOCUMENTATION TRENDS

Computerized charting is one of the most widespread trends in nursing documentation; however, computerized nursing documentation can demonstrate the quality, effectiveness, and value of the services nurses provide only if standardized databases are developed that ensure accuracy and precision of the information. The need to define and develop standard terminology for nursing data, nursing diagnoses, nursing interventions, and nursing outcomes is continually evolving.

Nursing Minimum Data Set

In 1985, Werley and Lang convened an invitational working conference to identify the elements that should be included in a **Nursing Minimum Data Set (NMDS)** (elements that should be in clinical records and abstracted for studies on the effectiveness and costs of nursing care) (Werley & Lang, 1988). The three categories into which the 16 identified elements were grouped are:

1. *Demographics:* personal identification, date of birth, gender, race and ethnicity, and residence
2. *Service:* unique facility or service agency number, episode admission or encounter date, discharge or termination date, disposition of client, expected payer, unique health record number of client, and unique number of principal registered nurse provider
3. *Nursing care:* nursing diagnosis, nursing intervention, nursing outcome, and intensity of nursing care (Werley & Lang, 1988)

The development of standard terminology for the four nursing care categories: diagnoses, interventions, outcomes, and intensity is challenging. For example, automated information systems must be able to support cost-effective nursing practice with efficient, comprehensive documentation. The consistent use of a taxonomy promoting validity and reliability is basic to standardizing databases. The NMDS, however, does not specify for any of the four elements a taxonomy such as NANDA-International nursing diagnoses, Nursing Interventions Classification (NIC), Nursing Outcomes Classification (NOC), or acuity ratings. Nursing must find consensus in terminology so clinical data can be included in the nursing care elements of an NMDS.

Nursing Diagnoses

NANDA-International is recognized as the pioneer in diagnostic classification in nursing. The NANDA-International definition of a nursing diagnosis is: "A nursing diagnosis is a clinical judgment about individual, family, or community responses to actual or potential health problems or life processes" (NANDA-International, 2010). Currently, there are approximately 188 approved nursing diagnoses classified into 47 classes and 13 domains.

Many diagnostic labels (nursing diagnoses) now have new descriptors. The word *altered* has been removed and a more specific term used. This allows for more specific documentation and for the nursing diagnoses to be linked to NIC and NOC. The nursing diagnoses are now listed in alphabetical order by the diagnostic concept, not by the first word of the nursing diagnosis (NANDA-International, 2010). For example: *Excess **Fluid** Volume* is found under "fluid." The entire listing can be found in Appendix A.

Each diagnosis has a label, definition, major and minor defining characteristics, and related factors. The diagnoses identify client states which can then be used to select interventions that are intended to achieve the desired outcomes.

In 1992, the NANDA-International terms were accepted into the Unified Medical Language System (UMLS). The UMLS was begun in 1986 by the National Library of Medicine as a way to help health professionals and researchers retrieve and integrate electronic biomedical information from a variety of sources (National Library of Medicine, 2006).

Date:

Nutrition:	Hygiene:	7-3			3-11			11-7		
Diet ☐ NPO ☐ Hyperal ☐ Tube Fed ☐	Bath ☐ Sitz ☐ Shower ☐	self ☐ assist ☐ total refused ☐			self ☐ assist ☐ total refused ☐			self ☐ assist ☐ total refused ☐		
Breakfast: All ☐ >1/2 ☐ <1/2 ☐ 0 ☐	Oral Care	self ☐	assist ☐	Total	self ☐	assist ☐	Total	self ☐	assist ☐	Total
	Shave	self ☐	assist ☐	Total	self ☐	assist ☐	Total	self ☐	assist ☐	Total
	Peri Care	self ☐	assist ☐	Total	self ☐	assist ☐	Total	self ☐	assist ☐	Total
Lunch: All ☐ >1/2 ☐ <1/2 ☐ 0 ☐	Other:									
	Comments:									
Dinner: All ☐ >1/2 ☐ <1/2 ☐ 0 ☐										
Snacks: All ☐ >1/2 ☐ <1/2 ☐ 0 ☐										

Tube Feeding Residuals		Intake						Output			
Time	Amount	7-3	PO	IV	NG & Flush	Enteral	Other	Urine	Ng/Emesis	Stool	Drains
		7-3 Total									
Weight		3-11									
Today:											
Previous:											
Vital/Signs											
Time / T / P / R / B/P / P/S		3-11 Total									
		11-7									
		11-7 Total									
		24 / Total									

4010

CHRISTUS SPOHN HEALTH SYSTEM

FLOW SHEET - 24 HOUR RECORD
PATIENT CARE SERVICES

2705066

REV. 06/00

	Date:	7-3 Time:	3-11 Time:	11-7 Time:
Neuro	Normal: alert, oriented to time, place, person, follows command, speech clear	WNL: ☐ *	WNL: ☐ *	WNL: ☐ *
Respiratory	Normal: Regular, unlabored symmetrical respirations, no abnormal lung sounds	WNL: ☐ *	WNL: ☐ *	WNL: ☐ *
Cardiovascular	Normal: Heart rhythm regular, peripheral pulses easily palpable and strong bilaterally, no edema, capillary refill brisk	WNL: ☐ *	WNL: ☐ *	WNL: ☐ *
Musculo-Skeletal	Normal: Full ROM of All joints, no weakness, steady balance and gait, handgrips equal	WNL: ☐ *	WNL: ☐ *	WNL: ☐ *
Nutrition	Normal: Consumes greater than 1/2 of solid food meals	WNL: ☐ *	WNL: ☐ *	WNL: ☐ *
G.I.	Normal: Abdomen soft, bowel sounds present all 4 quadrants, no nausea/ vomiting, diarrhea/constipation Last BM:	WNL: ☐ *	WNL: ☐ *	WNL: ☐ *
G.U.	Normal: Voiding without difficulty, clear urine, no bladder distention	WNL: ☐ *	WNL: ☐ *	WNL: ☐ *
Skin	Normal: Skin warm, dry, intact, tugor elastic, oral cavity moist and intact Date of Last EZ Graph ______ Site: ______	WNL: ☐ *	WNL: ☐ *	WNL: ☐ *
Psychosocial	Normal: Thought processes logical, memory intact, behavior appropriate for situation	WNL: ☐ *	WNL: ☐ *	WNL: ☐ *
Incision	Normal: Incision clean, no redness, drainage Site: ______	WNL: ☐ *	WNL: ☐ *	WNL: ☐ *
Wound	Normal: Dry, no drainage, no odor Site: ______	WNL: ☐ *	WNL: ☐ *	WNL: ☐ *

Safety Assessment

STATUS: MENTAL/PHYSICAL

D E N
☐☐☐ (5) Confused/judgement impaired
☐☐☐ (5) Sensory impairment
☐☐☐ (5) Combative/aggressive
☐☐☐ (5) "Sundowners" syndrome
☐☐☐ (5) Noncompliance/uncooperative
☐☐☐ (5) Paralysis/amputee
☐☐☐ (5) Urgent/frequent elimination needs
☐☐☐ (10) Restraints in use
☐☐☐ (5) Weakness/debilitation/mobility impaired

MEDICATIONS

D E N
☐☐☐ (5) Diuretics
☐☐☐ (5) Laxatives/G.I. preps
☐☐☐ (3) Antihypertensives
☐☐☐ (3) Antiseizures
☐☐☐ (5) Sedative/hypnotics
☐☐☐ (3) Analgesics
☐☐☐ (3) Antipsychotics/ antidepressants

HISTORY

D E N
☐☐☐ (5) Age greater than 60
☐☐☐ (5) History of previous falls
☐☐☐ (3) From nursing home
☐☐☐ (3) Has had sitter/ companion at home

SAFETY LEVEL

D E N
☐☐☐ Level 1 (0-17)
☐☐☐ Level 2 (18-24)
☐☐☐ Level 3 (25 or greater)

TOTAL D ______ E ______ N ______

FIGURE 9-19 Assessment and Intervention Flow Sheet (*Courtesy of CHRISTUS Spohn Health System, Corpus Christi, TX.*)

(Continues)

EDUCATION REASSESSMENT

Have the Education needs of the patient changed in past 24 hours? ☐ Yes ☐ No
Is the patient scheduled for any new test or procedure today? ☐ Yes ☐ No
Explanation given? ☐ Yes ☐ No
Patient/significant other verbalizes understanding: ☐ Yes ☐ No
Patient desires/requires education on: ____________________

Have Discharge Planning needs changed in past 24 hours? ☐ Yes ☐ No
If yes, send consult to Social Services and document changes below.

ALL EDUCATION MUST BE DOCUMENTED ON THE MULTIDISCIPLINARY EDUCATION FORM

TIME	PROBLEM #	PROGRESS NOTES

TIME	PROBLEM #	PROGRESS NOTES

PLAN OF CARE VERIFICATION		______ RN	______ Time
IV SITE ASSESSMENT	7-3 Time:	3-11 Time:	11-7 Time:
Normal: IV Patent; No redness, drainage or edema — Site #1: Start Date:	WNL: ☐ *	WNL: ☐ *	WNL: ☐ *
# of IVAC's in use ___ — Site #2: Start Date:	WNL: ☐ *	WNL: ☐ *	WNL: ☐ *

IV Site Care per hospital standard ☐ Time: *
IV Tubing Change per hospital standard ☐ Time: *

IV Start:	Time	Attempts	Site	Needle Size	S	U
					☐	☐
					☐	☐
Site prep per Standard ☐					☐	☐

INITIALS	SIGNATURE	INITIALS	SIGNATURE

FIGURE 9-19 *(Continued)*

Tulane
UNIVERSITY
Medical Center

COORDINATION OF DISCHARGE CARE

DISCHARGE ASSESSMENT

DESCRIPTION				COMMENT	DESCRIPTION				COMMENT	DESCRIPTION				COMMENT
LOC	NL	AB			respiration quality	NL	AB			Foley removed/voided	N	Y	NA	
pupils	NL	AB			lung auscultation	NL	AB			bladder habit problems	N	Y		
range of motion	NL	AB			heart sounds	NL	AB			sleep problems	N	Y	UTO	
extremity strength	NL	AB			telemetry removed	N	Y	NA		IV removed and intact	N	Y	NA	
appetite	NL	AB	UTO		peripheral pulses	NL	AB			break in skin integrity	N			
swallowing difficulty	N	Y	UTO		bowel sounds	NL	AB			discomfort/pain	N	Y	UTO	
feeds self	N	Y			bowel habit problems	N	Y		Date Last BM					

Signature RN Date Time

DISCHARGE MEDICATIONS

☐ None Medication	Dosage	Route	Schedule	Special Instructions ▼medication instruction sheets given food/drug interaction sheet given▼	RX given
				☐ ☐	
				☐ ☐	
				☐ ☐	
				☐ ☐	
				☐ ☐	
				☐ ☐	
				☐ ☐	
				☐ ☐	

HOME ROUTINE

Activity: ☐ As tolerated ☐ Restrictions________________

Diet: ☐ Regular ☐ Modified

Special Instructions: (document discharge sheet given to patient)

Social Services:

(SIGNATURE)

Physical Therapy ☐ Exercise Program ☐ Equipment

☐ Gait Instruction

(SIGNATURE)

Occupational Therapy:

(SIGNATURE)

Nutrition Care:

(SIGNATURE)

Other Services:

(SIGNATURE)

FOLLOW-UP CARE

Your MD is: To Contact Call: In An Emergency Call:

☐ No Appointment ☐ Appointment(s) made:

Name clinic/floor date/time phone #

Name clinic/floor date/time phone #

Appointment(s) not made:

Call phone # ext. for an appointment in days/weeks with MD

Call phone # ext. for an appointment in days/weeks with MD

I understand the above instructions.

Patient or Guardian's Signature Date Time of Discharge Nurse's Signature & Title

FIGURE 9-20 Discharge Summary *(Reprinted with permission of Tulane University Hospital & Clinic, New Orleans, LA.)*

Nursing Interventions Classification

The **Nursing Interventions Classification (NIC)** is a comprehensive standardized language for nursing interventions organized in a three-level taxonomy. This taxonomy sorts, labels, and describes interventions used by nurses for various diagnostic categories. Initiated by a research team (Iowa Intervention Project, 1993) at the University of Iowa in 1987, the three-level taxonomy now comprises 7 domains, 30 classes, and 542 interventions. The seven domains are:

1. Physiological: basic
2. Physiological: complex
3. Behavioral
4. Safety
5. Family
6. Health system
7. Community

A nursing intervention is any direct care treatment that a nurse performs using clinical judgment and knowledge to improve a client's outcomes (University of Iowa College of Nursing, 2008a). These treatments include nurse-initiated treatments resulting from nursing diagnoses, physician-initiated treatments resulting from medical diagnoses, and performance of the daily essential functions for the client who cannot do these. NIC interventions address physiological and psychological needs and include illness treatment, illness prevention, and health promotion.

Each nursing intervention has a label, a definition, a set of activities to carry out the interventions and a list of references. *Activities are not interventions and should not be identified as such in nursing information systems* (Bulecheck, Butcher, & Dochterman, 2008).

Although continuing to evolve, this classification system already provides assistance in choosing interventions based on nursing diagnoses or problems. The NIC interventions have been incorporated into health care data sets and the computerized client medical record. The NIC is included in the *National Library of Medicine's Metathesaurus*, one of four knowledge sources for the UMLS.

Nursing Outcomes Classification

An outcome is a measurable individual, family, or community state, behavior, or perception that is measured along a continuum and is responsive to nursing interventions (University of Iowa College of Nursing, 2008b).

The Iowa Outcomes Project being conducted at the University of Iowa has developed a taxonomy of client outcomes for nursing care, called **Nursing Outcomes Classification (NOC)**. This classification system now comprises 330 outcomes grouped into 31 classes and 7 domains (Moorhead, Johnson, & Maas, 2008). The seven domains are:

1. Functional health
2. Physiologic health
3. Psychosocial health
4. Health knowledge and behavior
5. Perceived health
6. Family health
7. Community health

Each NOC outcome has the outcome label, the outcome definition, a list of indicators for measurement, an outcome rating, identification of data source, a 5-point measurement scale, and a list of references (University of Iowa College of Nursing, 2008b). The NOC includes 311 individual, 10 family, and 9 community outcomes. The NOC is included in the *National Library of Medicine's Metathesaurus for a Unified Medical Language* (NIH: United States National Library of Medicine, 2009AA).

REPORTING

Reporting summarizes the current critical information pertinent to clinical decision making and continuity of care. Reporting, like recording, is based on the nursing process, standards of care, and legal and ethical principles. To verbally report in a well-organized efficient manner, the nurse should consider the following questions:

- What to say
- Why to say it
- How to say it

Another critical element of reporting is listening. Reports require everyone present to participate. When receiving a report, enhance listening skills by eliminating distractions, putting thoughts and concerns aside, concentrating on those things being said, and not anticipating the presenter's next statements. The reporting process is integral to promoting continuity of client care. Some facilities tape record the end-of-shift report. Summary reports, walking rounds, telephone reports and orders, and incident reports are all types of reporting.

Summary Reports

Information pertinent to the client's needs and identified by the nursing process is outlined in summary reports. Summary reports commonly occur either at the change of shift when new caregivers arrive or when the client is transferred to

PROFESSIONALTIP

Information for Shift Report

1. Client name, room and bed, age, and gender
2. Physician, admission date and diagnosis, and any surgery
3. Diagnostic tests or treatments performed in the past 24 hours; results, if available
4. General status, any significant change in condition
5. New or changed physician's orders
6. Nursing diagnoses and suggested nursing orders
7. Evaluation of nursing interventions
8. Intravenous fluid amounts
9. Administration time of last PRN medication
10. Concerns about the client

another area. A summary report should include the following information in the order indicated:

1. Background data obtained from client interactions and assessment of the client's functional health patterns
2. Prioritized medical and nursing diagnoses
3. Identified client risks
4. Recent changes in condition or in treatments (e.g., new medications, elevated temperature)
5. Effective interventions or treatments of priority problems, inclusive of laboratory and diagnostic results (e.g., client's response to pain medication)
6. Progress toward expected outcomes
7. Adjustments in the plan of care
8. Client or family complaints

This logical and time-sequenced format follows the nursing process and thus provides structure and organization to the data. In order to provide continuity of care, the new caregiver must receive an accurate, concise report about those things that happened during the previous shift. Because client and family complaints usually generate questions and discussion, they should be addressed last.

Walking Rounds

Walking rounds can take the form of nursing rounds, instructor–student rounds, physician–nurse rounds, or multidisciplinary rounds. **Walking rounds** is when the members of the care team walk to each client's room and discuss progress and care with each other and with the client, as shown in Figure 9-21.

Nursing rounds are used most frequently by charge nurses as their method of report. The oncoming nurse is introduced to the client and the offgoing nurse discusses with the client and the oncoming nurse any changes in the plan of care. This is more time consuming than a summary report, but gives the nurses and the client time to evaluate the effectiveness of care together.

Nursing rounds are also used for teaching when the instructor introduces the client to the student and they discuss the client's care together. The student's observation, communication, and decision-making skills can also be assessed by the instructor.

Nurse–physician rounds involve the physician and either staff nurse or the charge nurse. These rounds usually occur daily and allow the nurse, the physician, and the client to evaluate the effectiveness of care.

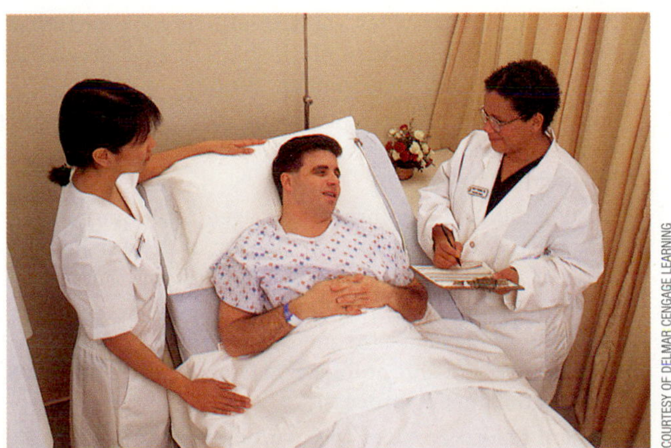

COURTESY OF DELMAR CENGAGE LEARNING

FIGURE 9-21 Nursing Rounds

Multidisciplinary rounds involving all disciplines occur less frequently than other types of rounds, primarily because it is difficult to schedule everyone. Multidisciplinary rounds are done most commonly to discuss discharge planning or to supplement case conferences.

Telephone Reports and Orders

Nurses are expected to exhibit courtesy and professionalism when using the telephone. When initiating a phone call, the nurse organizes the information to be reported or received. For example, the nurse:

- Ensures that all lab results are back; if they are not, identify those that are missing and telephone the lab or check the computer to ascertain whether the results are available. Spell the client's name and provide the client's medical record number when calling the lab to minimize the chances of receiving results for the wrong client. Write down the tests and the results.
- Has the client's assessment data available, especially any significant data related to abnormal results.
- Minimizes the chance of being interrupted during the call by informing the charge nurse or someone else at the nurses' station of the call.

State the reason for the call, for example, "I am calling Dr. Wojtal regarding the blood culture results for Mrs. Beacon." Be brief, listen carefully, and verify the test results and any orders received by repeating them back to the physician.

The date and time the phone call was placed, the client data reported by the nurse, the name of the person with whom the nurse spoke, and whether an order was obtained is recorded accurately in the client's record. Telephone orders are charted and the nurse's progress notes updated immediately after the call to prevent another caregiver from writing an entry before the telephone orders are written.

Figure 9-22 shows how to write a telephone order on the physician's order sheet: the entry is dated and timed; the order as given by the physician is recorded; the order is signed beginning with t.o. (telephone order); the physician's name is written; and the nurse's name is signed. If another nurse witnesses the phone order, that nurse's signature follows the first nurse's signature.

The physician must countersign the order within a time frame specified by the facility's policy. The use of fax machines and computers has decreased the need for lengthy or complicated telephone orders, saving time and minimizing errors. The physician is phoned to confirm the physician's identity as the initiator of the fax orders. The physician countersigns the fax orders according to agency policy.

PROFESSIONALTIP

Documenting an Incident

The incident should be factually documented in the nurse's notes, but the notes should not say "incident report filed."

PHYSICIAN'S ORDER SHEET

DATE	HOUR	ORDERS
2/3/10	1420	Give Demerol 50 mg IM stat.
		——————T.O. Dr. Weng/L. White RN

COURTESY OF DELMAR CENGAGE LEARNING

FIGURE 9-22 Documenting a Telephone Order

INCIDENT REPORTS

Incident reports, also called occurrence reports or variance reports, document any unusual occurrence or accident in the facility. Incident reports are not a means of punishment, but ethical practice requires that an incident report be filed to protect the individual involved.

Incident reports are not only an internal device for the facility; they are required by federal, national, and state accrediting agencies. For legal reasons, nurses are often advised not to document the filing of an incident report in the nurse's notes.

An incident report serves two functions:

1. It informs the facility's administration of the incident and allows risk management personnel to consider ways to prevent similar occurrences in the future.
2. It alerts the facility's insurance company to a potential claim and the possible need for investigation.

Incident report forms vary from one facility to another, but the following information must be recorded on the report:

- The date, exact time, and place the nurse discovered the occurrence.
- The person(s) involved in the occurrence, including witnesses.
- The exact occurrences witnessed by the nurse (e.g., "Found the client sitting on the floor, client stated that . . . ," rather than "Client fell").
- The exact details and time sequence of what happened and the consequences for the persons involved.
- The nurse's actions to provide care and the results of the nurse's assessment for injuries and client complaints.
- The supervisor on duty who was notified and the time and name of the physician notified; if telephone orders were received from the physician, these should be documented as previously discussed and the orders implemented.
- Never record personal opinions, assumptions, judgments, or conclusions about what happened; point blame; or suggest ways to prevent similar occurrences. Forward the incident report to the designated person defined in the facility's policy.

Iyer and Camp (2005) suggest writing a brief, accurate description of the incident and keeping it at home. The description should include details of the incident and the names of the people who were involved. Because lawsuits may take several years until the case goes to court, personal notes will help accurate recall of the incident. The notes may be read by the plaintiff's attorney and should reflect the same elements as the incident report.

SUMMARY

- The nursing process composed of five steps: assessment, diagnosis, planning and outcome identification, implementation, and evaluation, is an organized way to plan and deliver nursing care.
- The nurse uses the assessment process to establish a database about the client, to form an interpersonal relationship with the client, and to provide the client with an opportunity to discuss health care concerns.
- The second step in the nursing process involves further analysis and synthesis of the data and results in a list of nursing diagnoses.
- Nursing diagnoses identify knowledge unique to nursing, improve communication among nurses and other health care professionals, and promote individualized client care.
- Planning and outcome identification, the third step in the nursing process, involves prioritizing nursing diagnoses, identifying and writing goals and client outcomes, developing nursing interventions, and recording the plan of care in the client's record.
- The implementation step of the nursing process is directed toward meeting client needs, resulting in health promotion, prevention of illness, illness management, or health restoration.
- Evaluation, the fifth step in the nursing process, measures the effectiveness of nursing interventions by the examination of the goals and expected outcomes, which provide direction for the plan of care and serve as standards against which the client's progress is measured.
- Critical-thinking, decision-making, and holistic skills are important in the nursing process.
- Documentation provides a system of written records that reflect client care provided on the basis of assessment data and the client's response to interventions.
- Nurses are responsible for assessing and documenting that the client has an understanding of the treatment prior to the intervention.
- Accreditation and reimbursement agencies require accurate and thorough documentation of the nursing care rendered and the client's response to interventions.
- Effective documentation requires clear, concise, accurate recording of all client care and other significant events in an organized and chronological fashion representing each phase of the nursing process.
- Incident reports are used to document any unusual occurrence in a health care facility.

REVIEW QUESTIONS

1. M. R. was admitted to the unit 2 hours ago. The following data are recorded on her chart. Which data are objective?
   1. Temperature 102°F.
   2. Nausea.
   3. Headache.
   4. Pain in abdomen.
2. The nursing care plan includes:
   1. collected documentation of all team members providing care for the client.
   2. physician orders, demographic data, and medication administration and rationales.
   3. client's nursing diagnoses, goals, expected outcomes, nursing interventions, and evaluation.
   4. client assessment data, medical treatment regimen and rationales, and diagnostic test results and significance.
3. Systematic documentation is critical because it:
   1. is done every hour.
   2. shows the care given by all health care providers.
   3. identifies the planning and implementation phases.
   4. presents in a logical fashion the care provided by nurses.
4. The person responsible for ensuring that the client understands the procedure or intervention and has signed the informed consent is the:
   1. nurse.
   2. physician.
   3. social worker.
   4. admission officer.
5. Documentation of the nursing care the client receives must:
   1. never have an error.
   2. be neatly spaced out.
   3. reflect the nursing process.
   4. be signed at the end of each shift.
6. A nurse is giving oxygen at 2 L/min per nasal cannula. What phase of the nursing process is the nurse's action an example?
   1. Assessment.
   2. Planning and Outcome Identification.
   3. Implementation.
   4. Evaluation.
7. A 78-year-old woman fell and broke three ribs with one of the ribs puncturing her lung. She arrives in the emergency room short of breath and anxious. She is on Plavix, so she has multiple bruises over her entire body with possible internal hemorrhaging. After the nurse assesses her, she finds she also is blind and hard of hearing and has difficulty empting her bladder. Of the listed symptoms, what is the priority problem that the nurse needs to address?
   1. Difficulty breathing.
   2. Internal hemorrhaging.
   3. Difficulty with urination.
   4. Blindness and difficulty hearing.
8. Of the following medical and nursing diagnoses, which ones are nursing diagnoses? (Select all that apply.)
   1. Chronic obstructive pulmonary disease.
   2. Congestive heart failure.
   3. Nausea.
   4. Acute pain.
   5. Ineffective breathing.
   6. Parkinson's disease.
9. During and after a nursing assessment, the nurse organizes data to identify areas of the client's problems and strengths. The charting form that assists the nurse to cluster data is:
   1. flow sheet.
   2. client care plan or nursing plan of care.
   3. assessment sheet following an assessment model.
   4. client education record.
10. What type of nursing diagnoses is the nursing diagnosis *Decreased* **C***ardiac Output* R/T altered heart rhythm AEB irregular pulse, cyanosis, weak pedal pulse, and weakness?
    1. Data cluster.
    2. Actual nursing diagnosis.
    3. Risk nursing diagnosis.
    4. Wellness nursing diagnosis.

REFERENCES/SUGGESTED READINGS

Alfaro-LeFevre, R. (2009). *Applying nursing process: A tool for critical thinking* (7th ed.). (5th ed.). Philadelphia: Lippincott Williams & Wilkins.

Alfaro-LeFevre, R. (2008). *Critical thinking and clinical judgment: A practical approach to outcome-focused thinking* (4th ed.). Philadelphia: W. B. Saunders.

American Nurses Association. (1991). *Standards of nursing practice.* Kansas City, MO: Author.

Bevis, E. (1989). *Curriculum building in nursing: A process* (3rd ed., Publication No. 15-2277). New York: National League for Nursing.

Beyea, L. (1996). *Critical pathways for collaborative nursing care.* Menlo Park, CA: Addison-Wesley Nursing.

Brooke, P. (2002). Legal questions: Documentation errors. *Nursing 2002, 32*(1), 67.

Bulechek, G., Butcher, H., McCloskey, J., & Dochterman, J., eds. (2008). *Nursing Interventions Classification (NIC)* (5th ed.). St. Louis, MO: Mosby-Elsevier.

Calloway, S. (2001). Preventing communication breakdowns. *RN, 64*(1), 71–74.

Carpenito, L. (2009). *Nursing diagnosis: Application to clinical practice* (13th ed.). Philadelphia: Lippincott Williams & Wilkins.

Celia, L. (2002). Keep electronic records safe! *RN, 65*(6), 69–71.

Chaffee, M. (1999). A telehealth odyssey. *American Journal of Nursing, 99*(7), 26–32.

Charting Tips. (1999a). Documenting discharges and transfers in long-term care. *Nursing99, 29*(6), 17.

Charting Tips. (1999b). Easy as PIE. *Nursing99, 29*(4), 24.

Clark, M. (1998). Implementation of nursing standardized languages NANDA, NIC, and NOC. *Online Journal of Issues in Nursing 2*(2). Available: http://www.nursingworld.org

DeWitt, A. (2000). *Documentation: Legal principles of good charting, Penumbra Seminars LLC.* Available: http://www.respiratorycase-online.com/doc_handoutPDF

Dumpel, H., James, M., & Phillips, T. (1999). Charting by exception. *California Nurse*, June/July 1999, 9.Dykes, P., & Wheeler, K. (Eds.) (1997). *Planning, implementing, and evaluating critical pathways.* New York: Springer Publishing.

Edelman, C., & Mandle, C. (2002). *Health promotion throughout the lifespan* (5th ed.). St. Louis, MO: Mosby.

Estes, M. (2010). *Health assessment and physical examination* (4th ed.). Clifton Park, NY: Delmar Cengage Learning.

Ferrel, K. (2007). Documentation, part 2: The best evidence of care. *American Journal of Nursing, 107*(7), 61–64

Fry, V. (1953). The creative approach to nursing. *American Journal of Nursing, 53*(3), 301–302.

Gardner, P. (2002). *Nursing process in action.* Clifton Park, NY: Delmar Cengage Learning.

Gordon, M. (1998). Nursing nomenclature and classification system development. *Online Journal of Issues in Nursing.* Retrieved November 20, 2008, from http://www.nursingworld.org/MainMenuCategories/ANAMarketplace/ANAPeriodicals/OJIN/TableofContents/Vol31998/No2Sept1998/NomenclatureandClassification.aspx

Gordon, M. (2002). *Manual of nursing diagnoses* (10th ed.). St. Louis, MO: Mosby.

Grace, P., & McLaughlin, M. (2005). When consent isn't informed enough: What's the nurse's role when a patient has given consent but doesn't fully understand the risks? *American Journal of Nursing, 105*(4), 79–84.

Grane, N. (1995). Documenting a "harmless" medication error. *Nursing95, 25*(4), 80.

Gregory, K. (2000). Nurse the patient! *RN, 63*(9), 52–54.

Grulke, C. (1995). Seven ways to help a student nurse. *American Journal of Nursing, 96* (60), 24L.

Guido, G. (2001). *Legal and ethical issues in nursing* (3rd ed.). Upper Saddle River, NJ: Prentice Hall.

Heery, K. (2000). Straight talk about the patient interview. *Nursing2000, 30*(6), 66–67.

Humphrey, C. (1998). *Home care nursing handbook* (3rd ed.). Gaithersburg, MD: Aspen.

Iowa Interventions Project. (1993). The NIC taxonomy structure. *Image: Journal of Nursing Scholarship, 25*(3), 187–192.

Iyer, P., & Camp, N. (2005). *Nursing documentation: A nursing process approach* (4th ed.). Fleminiton, NJ: Medical League Support Services.

Johnson, D. (1959). A philosophy for nursing diagnosis. *Nursing Outlook, 7,* 198–200.

Johnson, M., & Maas, M. (1998). Implementing the nursing outcomes classification in a practice setting. *Outcomes Management for Nursing Practice, 2*(3), 99–104.

Johnson, M., Bulechek, G., Dochterman, J., Maas, M., & Moorhead, S. (2001). *Nursing diagnoses outcomes and interventions, NANDA, NOC and NIC linkages.* St. Louis, MO: Harcourt Health Sciences.

Joint Commission. (2008, November 10). Table of contents (standard PC.4.10). Retrieved November 17, 2008, from http://www.jointcommission.org/NR/rdonlyres/6530941D-98AD-4AC7-8944-9DSE1116E503/0/OBS_Standards_Sampler_2007_final.pdf

Joint Commission on Accreditation of Healthcare Organizations. (1998). *1998 Hospital accreditation standards.* Oakbrook Terrace, IL: Author.

Klenner, S. (2000). Mapping out a clinical pathway. *RN, 63*(6), 33–36.

LaDuke, S. (2000). Spotlight: What you really do with this powerful documentation tool. *Nursing2000, 30*(6), 68.

Malestic, S. (2003). A quick guide to verbal reports. *RN, 66*(2), 47–49.

McCloskey, J., & Bulechek, G. (1995). Validation and coding of the NIC taxonomy structure. *Image: Journal of Nursing Scholarship, 27*(1), 43–49.

McCloskey, J., & Maas, M. (1998). Interdisciplinary team: The nursing perspective is essential. *Nursing Outlook, 46*(4), 157–163.

McConnell, E. (1999). Charting with care. *Nursing99, 29*(10), 68.

Moorhead, S., Johnson, M., & Maas, M. (Eds.). (2008). *Nursing outcomes classification (NOC)* (4th ed.). St. Louis, MO: Mosby.

Murphy, E. (2003). Charting by exception—OR nursing law. *AORN Journal, 11.* Retrieved November 19, 2008, from http://findarticles.com/p/articles/mi_m0FSL/is_5_78/ai_111011830/print?tag=artBody;coll

National Institutes of Health (NIH): United States National Library of Medicine. (2009AA). Appendix to the License Agreement for Use of the UMLS® Metathesaurus. Retrieved July 29, 2009 from http://www.nlm.nih.gov/research/umls/metaa1.html

National Library of Medicine. (2006). Fact sheet: Unified medical language system®. Retrieved June 22, 2009, from http://www.nlm.nih.gov/pubs/factsheets/umls.html

North American Nursing Diagnosis Association International. (2010). *NANDA-I nursing diagnoses: Definitions and classification 2009–2011.* Ames, IA: Wiley-Blackwell.

Oermann, M., & Huber, D. (1999). Patient outcomes: A measure of nursing's value. *American Journal of Nursing, 99*(9), 40–47.

Olson-Chavarriaga, D. (2000). Informed consent: Do you know your role? *Nursing2000, 30*(5), 60–61.

Orem, D., Taylor, S., & Renpenning, K. (2001). *Nursing: Concepts of practice* (6th ed.). St. Louis, MO: Mosby.

Orlando, I. (1961). *The dynamic nurse–patient relationship.* New York: Putnam.

Pethtel, P. (2000). *Nursing documentation.* Available: http://garnet.indstate.edu/ppethtel/chartingforweb

Raymond, L. (2001). How to chart for peer review. *RN, 64*(6), 67–70.

Raymond, L. (2002). Documenting for the "PROs." *Nursing2002, 32*(3), 50–53.

Roberts, D. (2002). How to keep electronic health records private. *Nursing2002, 32*(10), 95.

Rochman, R. (2000). Are computerized patient records for you? *Nursing2000, 30*(10), 61–62.

Seaback, W. (2001). *Nursing process: Concepts and application.* Clifton Park, NY: Delmar Cengage Learning.

Sheehan, J. (2001). Delegating to UAPs—A practical guide. *RN, 64*(11), 65–66.

Smith, L. (2000a). Charting tips. Nursing2002. Retrieved November 18, 2008, from http://findarticles.com/p/articles/mi_qa3689/is_200005/ai_n8880050/print?tag+artBody;c

Smith, L. (2000b). How to use focus charting. *Nursing 2000, 30*(5), 76.

Smith, L. (2000c). Safe computer charting. *Nursing 2000, 30*(9), 85.

Smith, L. (2002). How to chart by exception. *Nursing 2002, 32*(9), 30.

Springhouse. (2005). *Charting made incredibly easy.* Springhouse, PA: Author.

Stewart, K. (2001). Charting tips: Documenting adverse incidents. *Nursing2001, 31*(3), 84.

Sullivan, G. (2000). Keep your charting on course. *RN, 63*(5), 75–79.

Thede, L. (2003). *Informatics and nursing: Opportunities and challenges* (2nd ed.). Philadelphia: Lippincott Williams & Wilkins.

Thompson, C. (1995, May). Writing better narrative notes. *Nursing95, 25*(5), 87.

Tucker, S., Canobbio, M., Paquette, E., & Willis, M. (2000). *Patient care standards: Collaborative planning and nursing interventions* (7th ed.). St. Louis, MO: Mosby.

United States National Library of Medicine. (2006). Fact sheet: Unified medical language system®. Retrieved June 22, 2009 from http://www.nlm.nih.gov/pubs/factsheets/umls.html

University of Iowa College of Nursing. (2008a). Nursing Interventions Classification (NIC): Overview of NIC. Retrieved November 19, 2008, from http://www.nursing.uiowa.edu/excellence/nursing_knowledge/clinical_effectiveness/nicoverview.htm

University of Iowa College of Nursing. (2008b). Nursing Outcomes Classification (NOC): Overview of NOC. Retrieved November 19, 2008, from http://www.nursing.uiowa.edu/excellence/nursing_knowledge/clinical_effectiveness/nocoverview.htm

Wallhagen, M., Pettengill, E., & Whiteside, M. (2006). Sensory impairment in older adults: Part 1: Hearing loss. *American Journal of Nursing, 106*(10), 40–48.

Werley, H., & Lang, N. (1988). The consensually derived nursing minimum data set: Elements and definitions. In H. H. Werley & N. M. Lang (Eds.), *Identification of the nursing minimum data set* (pp. 402–411). New York: Springer Publishing.

White, G. (2000). Informed consent. *American Journal of Nursing, 100*(9), 83.

Wiedenbach, E. (1963). The helping art of nursing. *American Journal of Nursing, 63*(11), 54–57.

Wilkinson, J. (2004). *Prentice Hall nursing diagnosis handbook: With NIC interventions and NOC outcomes* (8th ed.). Upper Saddle River, NJ: Prentice Hall.

Wilkinson, J. (2006). *Nursing process and critical thinking* (4th ed.). Upper Saddle River, NJ: Prentice Hall.

Yocum, R. (2002). Documenting for quality patient care. *Nursing2002, 32*(8), 58–63.

Yura, H., & Walsh, M. (1967). *The nursing process.* Washington, DC: Catholic University of America Press.

RESOURCES

American Health Information Management Association, http://www.ahima.org

American Nursing Informatics Association (ANIA), http://www.ania.org

Center for Nursing Classification, http://www.nursing.uiowa.edu

NANDA International, http://www.nanda.org

UNIT 4 Developmental and Psychosocial Concerns

CHAPTER 10
Life Span Development

MAKING THE CONNECTION

Refer to the following chapters to increase your understanding of the life span:

Basic Nursing

- ***Communication***
- ***End-of-Life Care***
- ***Self-Concept***
- ***Spirituality***
- ***Basic Nutrition***
- ***Safety/Hygiene***

Adult Health Nursing

- ***Sexually Transmitted Infections***
- ***Mental Illness***
- ***The Older Adult***

Maternal & Pediatric Nursing

- ***Prenatal Care***

LEARNING OBJECTIVES

Upon completion of this chapter, you should be able to:

- Define key terms.
- Discuss the basic concepts and principles of growth and development.
- Identify the factors influencing growth and development.
- Compare the major developmental theories.
- Discuss the importance of growth and development as a holistic framework for assessing and promoting health.
- Describe the important milestones for each developmental period.
- Discuss the specific nursing interventions relevant to each developmental stage.

KEY TERMS

accommodation
adaptation
adolescence
assimilation
bonding
critical period
development
developmental tasks
embryonic phase
fetal alcohol syndrome (FAS)
fetal phase
germinal phase
growth
infancy
learning
maturation
menarche
middle adulthood
moral maturity
neonatal stage
older adulthood
polypharmacy
preadolescence
prenatal stage
preschool stage
puberty
school-age stage
self-concept
spirituality
teratogenic substance
toddler stage
young adulthood

INTRODUCTION

Individuals constantly change from conception to death. Physical growth; emotional maturation; psychological, cognitive, and moral development; and spiritual growth occur throughout life. Progress through each developmental stage influences health status. Quality nursing practice depends on a thorough understanding of developmental concepts. This chapter presents the eleven life span stages.

BASIC CONCEPTS OF GROWTH AND DEVELOPMENT

Development occurs continuously through the life span. Adults continue to have transition periods during which growth and development occur.

Growth is the measurable changes in the physical size of the body and its parts. Examples of growth are the changes in height, weight, bone density, and dental structure. Growth patterns can be predicted even though growth is not a steady process. The rate varies from periods of rapid growth to periods of slower growth. Rapid growth is most common in the prenatal, infant, and adolescent stages.

Development is the behavioral changes in skills and functional abilities. Thus, developmental changes are not as easily measured. **Maturation,** the process of becoming fully grown and developed, applies to the individual's physiological and behavioral aspects. It depends on biological growth, behavioral changes, and **learning** (assimilation of information resulting in a behavior change). During each life span stage, certain goals (**developmental tasks**) must be accomplished. These developmental tasks are the foundation for future learning.

The time of most rapid growth or development in a stage of the life span is called the **critical period**. An individual is most vulnerable to stressors during a critical period.

Growth, development, maturation, and learning are interdependent processes. The individual must be mature enough to grasp the concepts and make required behavioral changes for learning to occur. Physical growth is essential for many types of learning; for example, a child must have the physical ability to reach the door knob before learning to open the door. Likewise, cognitive maturation precedes learning.

MEMORYTRICK

GROWTH

- **G** = Goals (developmental tasks) must be accomplished in each life span stage.
- **R** = Rapid growth occurs during the "critical period."
- **O** = Observe for changes in bone density and dental structure.
- **W** = Weight changes will occur throughout the life span stages.
- **T** = Time routine wellness checks throughout the life span to monitor growth.
- **H** = Height changes are expected during the process of aging.

PRINCIPLES OF GROWTH AND DEVELOPMENT

Individual abilities and talents contribute to each person's development as a unique entity. *The exact rate of development for any given individual cannot be predicted.* There are a few general principles relating to growth and development of all humans (Table 10-1).

The sequence of development is predictable, but performance of specific skills varies with each person. For example, not all infants roll over at the same age, but most roll over before they crawl.

FACTORS THAT INFLUENCE GROWTH AND DEVELOPMENT

Many factors such as heredity, health status, life experiences, and culture influence growth and development. A person's choices about health behaviors are also determined by these factors.

Heredity

Genetic information is passed from parents to children. An individual's genetic makeup determines not only physical characteristics such as skin color, facial features, hair texture, and body structure but also a predisposition to certain diseases (i.e., sickle cell anemia, Huntington's disease). Heredity is the genetic blueprint for an individual's growth and development. The role of heredity is complex and not yet fully understood.

Health Status

Individuals experiencing wellness progress through the life span as expected. Achievement of developmental milestones can be delayed by illness or disability. Individuals with a chronic condition may meet developmental milestones but later.

Life Experiences

The rate of growth and development can be influenced by life experiences. For example, a child whose family has few resources for food, shelter, and health care has a higher risk of lagging in physical and mental growth and development than a child whose family has plenty of resources.

Culture

Individuals are expected to master certain skills at each developmental period, but the age for mastery is determined partly by culture. For instance, some cultures expect mate selection at age 12 or 13, with the birth of a child soon after.

DIMENSIONS AND THEORIES OF HUMAN DEVELOPMENT

Nurses need to thoroughly understand growth and development so they can provide individualized care. Remember, *chronological age and developmental age are not the same.* An overview of the dimensions and major theories of human development follows.

TABLE 10-1 Principles of Growth and Development

PRINCIPLE	EXAMPLE
Growth and development are orderly and predictable, occurring from:	Everyone goes through the same processes.
• *cephalocaudal* (head to toe)	Head larger at birth in relation to body. Head controlled before crawling, and sitting occurs before walking.
• *proximodistal* (functions near midline develop before those distant)	Arm movements controlled before finger movements.
• *general to specific*	Sounds and noises made before words are spoken. Walking occurs before hopping or skipping.
Rate of growth and development:	Rapid growth in infancy and adolescence.
• is not consistent	Slower growth in school age and young adulthood.
• is individual	Slower-growing child will be smaller than others of the same age.
Each stage has specific characteristics.	Infants depend on others for survival. Adolescents search for their own identity.
Certain tasks must be accomplished in each stage.	Infants must develop trust so as adolescents they can establish individual identity.
Some stages are more critical than others.	First few weeks of pregnancy are critical for embryonic development.

COURTESY OF DELMAR CENGAGE LEARNING

CRITICAL THINKING

Heredity or Life Experiences

What is most important in determining a person's behavior: the person's genetic predisposition or the response of other people and socialization?

CULTURAL CONSIDERATIONS

Growth and Development

The time for mastery of such developmental tasks as speaking and toilet training is as dependent on cultural norms as it is on physiological development. In Japan, toilet training begins at a later age (Norimatsu, 2006). In 1990, 22% of mothers with an 18-month-old child had not started toilet training. In 2000, that percentage increased to 52%. Japanese consumers purchase approximately 5 million big-size diapers a month for recommended ages of 3 to 7 years (Connell, 2005).

PHYSIOLOGICAL DIMENSION

The physiological dimension of growth and development consists of physical size and functioning of the individual. It is influenced by the interaction of genetic predisposition, nutrition, the central nervous system (CNS), and the endocrine system.

PSYCHOSOCIAL DIMENSION

Growth and development's psychosocial dimension consists of feelings and interpersonal relationships. A positive **self-concept** (perception of one's self, including body image, self-esteem, and ideal self) is an important part of a person's happiness and success. Characteristics of an individual with a positive self-concept include:

- Self-confident
- Willing to take risks
- Able to accept criticism and not become defensive
- Able to adapt to stressors
- Has innovative problem-solving skills

People with a positive self-concept believe in themselves and set goals they can achieve. Achieving the goals reinforces their positive self-concept.

An individual with a negative or poor self-concept, on the other hand, is likely to have low self-esteem, a lack of confidence, and difficulty setting and achieving goals. A person with a positive self-concept is more likely to change unhealthy habits (such as smoking and sedentary lifestyle) to promote health than someone with a negative self-concept.

Various psychosocial theories have been put forth to explain the development of self-concept. A discussion of various theories of personality development follows.

Theorists

Two major theorists of personality development are Sigmund Freud and Erik Erikson. Freud's theory is called the psychosexual theory (Table 10-2). He identified sexuality (anything that gives bodily pleasure) as the underlying motivation for behavior. He believed that all behaviors have meaning and that repressed sexual problems in childhood cause problems later in life. Excessive gratification or excessive frustration at any stage, he thought, may cause a fixation (preoccupation with the pleasures of that stage).

Erikson (1968) theorized that psychosocial development proceeds throughout life. His theory is known as the psychosocial theory. Erikson believed that each stage has a task to be mastered. His eight developmental stages of life are described in Table 10-2.

Cognitive Dimension

The way a person thinks and understands the world shapes that person's perception, memory, attitude, action, and judgment and is the basis of cognitive theory. It develops as an individual progresses through life. Cognition is an adaptive process. Intelligent beings are able to change behavior in response to the demands of an ever-changing environment.

Jean Piaget (1963) studied the differences in children's thinking patterns at various ages and how they used intelligence to answer questions and solve problems. He theorized that children learn to think by playing.

Piaget (1963) lists four stages of intellectual development: sensorimotor, preoperational, concrete operations, and formal operations. Table 10-2 describes these stages. Each stage is characterized by the ways that the child interprets and uses the environment. There is great variation in age for each phase; ages are approximate.

Individuals learn by interacting with the environment using three processes: assimilation, accommodation, and adaptation. **Assimilation** is the process of taking in new experiences or information. **Accommodation** allows for adjustment of thinking to take in new information and increase understanding. **Adaptation** is the change resulting from assimilation and accommodation.

Moral Dimension

The moral dimension is a person's value system, which helps one differentiate right and wrong. Closely related to emotional and cognitive development is **moral maturity** (the ability to independently decide for oneself what is "right"). Lawrence Kohlberg (1977) described a framework for understanding how individuals decide on a moral code.

According to Kohlberg, there are six stages of moral development. Each stage is built on the previous stage and becomes the foundation for the next stage. Moral development evolves relative to cognitive development. Individuals who think at higher levels have the reasoning skills on which to base moral decisions. Table 10-2 provides an overview of Kohlberg's stages of moral development. Kohlberg indicates that individuals move through the six stages sequentially, but not everyone reaches stages five and six (Kohlberg, 1977).

Spiritual Dimension

The spiritual dimension is described as a sense of personal meaning. The term *spirit* is derived from the Latin word meaning breath, air, and wind. Thus, spirit refers to whatever gives life to a person. **Spirituality** refers to relationships with oneself, others, and a divine source or a higher power. It does not refer to a specific religion. Spirituality is developed throughout life.

The work of Erikson, Piaget, and Kohlberg all influenced Fowler's theory of spiritual development. Fowler's theory has a prestage and six distinct stages of faith development (Fowler, 1995). The sequence of stages remains the same, although the age at which individuals experience each stage varies. Table 10-3 outlines Fowler's theory.

Some clients seem to be unaware of their spiritual natures. The understanding of a client's spirituality is basic to nursing. Caring for the whole person is the distinguishing characteristic of a holistic nurse. Table 10-2 (shown on page 202) provides a summary of the ages and stages of the developmental theories.

HOLISTIC FRAMEWORK FOR NURSING

A basic concept of nursing is to provide care to the whole person. So it is essential for nurses to know growth and development concepts. Nursing interventions must be appropriate to each client's stage of development. Nursing's holistic perspective recognizes that an individual's development progresses throughout life. Progress, or lack thereof, in one dimension affects the other dimensions of development. Figure 10-1 shows the holistic nature of individuals.

Knowledge of growth and development is useful as a guideline for assessment. When developmental milestones are not met, prompt identification and comprehensive intervention is essential. For example:

- The infant who does not roll over, sit, or walk at expected times
- The adolescent girl who has not experienced menarche by the expected time
- The adult who fails to adjust to physiological changes

LIFE SPAN STAGES

Eleven developmental stages will be discussed: prenatal, neonatal, infancy, toddler, preschooler, school-age, preadolescent, adolescent, young adult, middle adult, and older adult. The indications of growth and development in the physiological, psychosocial, cognitive, moral, and spiritual dimensions are discussed for each stage, along with pertinent nursing implications.

Prenatal Stage

The **prenatal stage** (development beginning with conception and ending with birth) is a critical time in growth and

TABLE 10-2 Summary of Ages and Stages Developmental Theories

STAGE/AGE	PIAGET'S COGNITIVE STAGES	FREUD'S PSYCHOSEXUAL STAGES	ERIKSON'S PSYCHOSOCIAL STAGES	KOHLBERG'S MORAL STAGES
1. **Infancy** Birth to 1 year	**Sensorimotor** (birth to 2 years): Begins to acquire language, develops sense of cause and effect Task: Object permanence	**Oral:** Pleasure from exploration with mouth, tongue, and through sucking Task: Weaning	**Trust vs. Mistrust:** Establish a sense of trust Task: Trust Socializing agent: Mothering person Central process: Mutuality Ego quality: Hope	
2. **Toddler** 1 to 3 years	**Sensorimotor** continues **Preoperational** (2 to 7 years) begins: Use of representational thought (symbolism) and imagination Task: Use language and mental images to think and communicate	**Anal:** Control of elimination muscles Task: Toilet training	**Autonomy vs. Shame and Doubt:** Do things for self Task: Autonomy Socializing agent: Parents Central process: Imitation Ego quality: Self-control and willpower	**Preconventional Level:** (birth to 9 years) 1. **Morality Stage:** Avoid punishment by not breaking rules of authority figures
3. **Preschool** 3 to 6 years	**Preoperational** continues	**Phallic:** Attracted to opposite-sex parent Task: Resolve Oedipus/Electra complex	**Initiative vs. Guilt:** Iniate activities and moral responsibility Task: Initiative and moral responsibility Socializing agents: Parents Central process: Identification Ego quality: Direction, purpose, and conscience	2. **Individualism, Instrumental Purpose, and Exchange Stage:** "Right" is relative, follow rules when in own interest
4. **School Age** 6 to 12 years	**Preoperational** continues **Concrete Operations** (7 to 12 years) begins: Engage in inductive reasoning and concrete problem solving Task: Learn concepts of conservation and reversibility	**Latency:** Identify with same-sex parent Task: Identify with same-sex parent, and test and compare own capabilities with peer norms	**Industry vs. Inferiority:** Develop self-esteem, social and scholastic skills Task: Industry, self-assurance, self-esteem Socializing agents: Teachers and peers Central process: Education Ego quality: Competence	**Conventional Level:** (9 to 13 years) 3. **Mutual Expectations Relationships, and Confirmity to Moral Norms Stage:** Need to be "good" in own and others' eyes, believe in rules and regulations

5. Adolescence 12 to 18 years	**Formal Operations** (12 years to adulthood): Engage in abstract reasoning and analytical problem solving Task: Develop a workable philosophy of life	**Genital:** Develops sexual relationships Task: Establish meaningful relationship for lifelong pairing	**Identity vs. Role Confusion:** Seek sense of identity and values Task: Self-identity and concept Socializing agents: Society of peers Central process: Role experimentation and peer pressure Ego quality: Fidelity and devotion to others, personal and sociocultural values	**4. Social System and Conscience Stage:** Uphold laws because they are fixed social duties
6. Young Adult 18 to 30 years	**Formal Operations** continues		**Intimacy vs. Isolation:** Choose career and develop intimate relationships Task: Intimacy Socializing agent: Close friends, partners, lovers, spouse Central process: Mutuality among peers Ego quality: Intimate affiliation and love	**Postconventional Level:** (13+ years) **5. Social Contract or Utility and Individual Rights Stage:** Uphold laws in the interest of the greatest good for the greatest number; uphold laws that protect universal rights
7. Early Middle Age 30 to 50 years			**Generativity vs. Stagnation:** Become productive and establish a family (30 to 65 years) Task: Generativity Socializing agent: Spouse, partner, children, sociocultural norms Central process: Creativity and person-environment fit Ego quality: Productivity, perserverence, charity, and consideration	
8. Late Middle Age 50 to 70 years			**Generativity vs. Stagnation** continues	**6. Universal Ethical Principles Stage:** Support universal moral principles regardless of the price for doing so
9. Late Adult 70 years to death			**Ego Integrity vs. Despair:** Accept one's life (65 years to death) Task: Ego integrity Socializing agent: Significant others Central process: Introspection Ego quality: Wisdom	

Adapted from *Health Assessment and Physical Examination* (4th ed.), by M. E. Estes, 2010, Clifton Park, NY: Delmar Cengage Learning.

TABLE 10-3 Fowler: Stages of Faith

STAGE	AGE	CHARACTERISTICS
Prestage: *undifferentiated faith*	Infant	Trust, hope, and love compete with environmental inconsistencies or threats of abandonment.
Stage 1: *intuitive-projective faith*	Toddler and preschooler	Has no understanding of spiritual concepts but imitates parents' behaviors and attitudes about religion and spirituality.
Stage 2: *mythical-literal faith*	School-age child	Accepts existence of a deity. Religious and moral beliefs are symbolized by stories. Accepts concept of reciprocal fairness.
Stage 3: *synthetic-conventional faith*	Adolescent	Questions values and religious beliefs while attempting to form own identity.
Stage 4: *individuative-reflective faith*	Late adolescent and young adult	Assumes responsibility for own attitudes and beliefs.
Stage 5: *conjunctive faith*	Adult	Integrates other perspectives about faith into own definition of truth.
Stage 6: *universalizing faith*	Adult	Makes concepts of love and justice tangible.

Data from *Stages of Faith: The Psychology of Human Development and the Quest for Meaning*, by J. W. Fowler, 1995, New York: Harper & Row. Copyright 1995 by Harper & Row; *Psychiatric-Mental Health Nursing: Evidence-Based Concepts, Skills and Practices* (7th ed.), by W. Mohr, 2009, Philadelphia: Lippincott Williams & Wilkins. Copyright 2009 by Lippincott Williams & Wilkins.

development and consists of three phases: germinal, embryonic, and fetal. The **germinal phase** begins with conception and lasts approximately 10 to 14 days. Rapid cell division and implantation of the fertilized egg in the uterine wall delineates this stage. In this very early stage, the central nervous system (CNS) is already forming.

The **embryonic phase** (weeks 2 to 8 after conception) is marked by rapid differentiation of cells, development of the body systems, and growth. In this period, the embryo is most vulnerable for a spontaneous abortion (i.e., miscarriage).

The **fetal phase** (the intrauterine developmental period from 8 weeks to birth) is characterized by rapid growth and differentiation of body systems and parts.

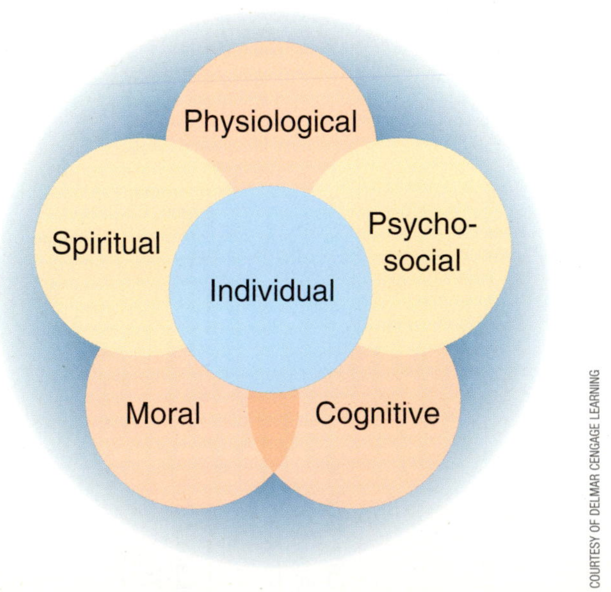

FIGURE 10-1 Holistic Nature of Individuals

Significance for Nursing

Early prenatal care is essential for a positive pregnancy outcome, with physical examinations and screenings throughout pregnancy.

Enhancing Wellness The primary environment affecting prenatal growth and development is the uterus.

The mother must provide a sufficient supply of nutrients. Women who consume an insufficient amount of protein during pregnancy have a high rate of preterm and low birth weight infants. Teaching must emphasize that vitamin supplements are not substitutes for adequate food intake. Other ways to promote prenatal health include:

- Screening (blood pressure, urine glucose, and albumin)
- Teaching (e.g., nutrition, self-care)
- Assisting economically disadvantaged clients to obtain prenatal care

Safety Concerns Any substances consumed by the mother affect the fetus, whether they are wholesome nutrients or deadly toxins. Cigarette toxic substances, including nicotine, cross the placenta and interfere with oxygen transport to the fetus. These toxins may result in fetal death, premature birth, retarded growth, and learning difficulties.

SAFETY

Use of Tobacco and Alcohol During Pregnancy

No cigarette smoking is advised during pregnancy. All pregnant women should abstain from drinking alcohol, because a "safe" amount of alcohol consumption has not been determined.

Alcohol use during pregnancy can result in **fetal alcohol syndrome (FAS)**, a condition wherein fetal development is impaired, resulting in physical and intellectual problems. Alcohol consumption is most dangerous during the first 3 months of pregnancy, when the embryo's brain and other vital organs are developing. The effects of alcohol on the fetus are permanent. Fetal alcohol syndrome is considered to be the leading cause of mental retardation among infants, and the incidence continues to increase (Hockenberry & Wilson, 2007).

There are many other teratogenic substances in addition to nicotine and alcohol. A **teratogenic substance** is anything that crosses the placenta and impairs normal growth and development. The Food and Drug Administration (FDA) requires that all manufactured drugs list the potential for causing birth defects. Illegal drug use by pregnant women is a very serious threat to the unborn.

Neonatal Stage

The **neonatal stage** (the first 28 days of life following birth) is a time of major adjustment to extrauterine life. The neonate (newborn) focuses energy on achieving equilibrium by stabilizing major body systems. Table 10-4 outlines neonatal development.

The neonate's activities are reflexive, consisting mainly of sucking, crying, eliminating, and sleeping. Reflexes play a major role in the neonate's ability to survive. The neonate progresses developmentally from a mass of reflexes to behavior that is more purposeful.

Adjusting to the parental figure(s) is the major psychological task of neonates. **Bonding**, the attachment between parent and child, begins when the parent and neonate make initial eye contact. Parent–neonate bonding is the foundation for trust necessary when developing future interpersonal relationships.

Significance for Nursing

A thorough assessment of the neonate is performed immediately after delivery. The neonate's reflexes should be evaluated at the same time or when the neonate is physiologically stable.

Soon after birth, encourage the parents to cuddle the newborn, explain the neonate's interactive abilities, and encourage mutual eye contact between neonate and parents by showing parents how to hold the child in a position facing them.

CLIENT TEACHING

Pregnancy and Medications

Pregnant women should check labels of *all* medicines, especially over-the-counter, about potential effects on the fetus. Expectant mothers should question their practitioner about the safety of any drug taken during pregnancy.

CRITICAL THINKING

Changes in the Family

What are the typical changes that occur in a family after the birth of a new baby?

Enhancing Wellness The most important nursing activity in promoting neonatal wellness is teaching. Other nursing interventions enhancing neonatal wellness are:

- Continually assess physiological status
- Provide a warm environment
- Monitor nutritional status
- Provide a clean environment; teach parents that neonates need a clean environment, not a sterile one
- Conduct screening tests; for example, the blood test for phenylketonuria (PKU)
- Promote *early* parent–neonate interaction

Safety Concerns Because neonates depend totally on others to meet their needs, safety is a primary concern. One important method to prevent neonatal accidents is to teach parents about using infant car seats. Under current federal law, neonates and infants must be secured in an approved infant car seat each time the child travels in a motor vehicle.

According to the World Health Organization (WHO, 2008a), the primary causes of neonatal deaths in the world are premature birth, low birth weight, and infections. Infections are a serious health risk to the neonate. Newborns should not be near anyone who has an infectious disease. It is essential that the neonate's skin integrity be maintained. Teach parents the importance of skin cleanliness. Diaper rash, a common skin problem for newborns and infants, is caused by the ammonia found in urine, which can burn and irritate the skin. In addition to changing wet diapers promptly, bathing and protective creams may be useful in preventing skin breakdown.

Infancy Stage

Infancy (development from the end of the first month to the end of the first year of life) is a period of continued adaptation,

SAFETY

Car Seats

A neonate should never be sent home from the hospital in a car unless an infant seat is available for the trip.

TABLE 10-4 Neonatal Stage: Growth and Development

DIMENSION	CHARACTERISTICS	NURSING CONSIDERATIONS
Physiological	Heart takes over circulatory function from umbilical cord.	Accurately assess neonate's cardiovascular status.
	Gas exchange shifts from placenta to lungs.	Immediately after birth, hold the neonate's head lower than body to allow fluids that may block respiratory passages to drain.
	Respiratory reflexes are activated within seconds of birth.	Resuscitate immediately if spontaneous respirations do not occur.
	Neck and shoulder muscles are weak.	Support the neonate's head.
	Temperature-regulating mechanism is immature.	To conserve heat: • Dry neonate immediately after birth and place in a warmed bassinet and • Place a stockinette cap on neonate's head.
	Ossification (process of cartilage changing to bone) is incomplete.	Protect the anterior fontanel on neonate's skull.
	Visual acuity is poor, and visual focus is generally rigid.	Teach parents to be directly in front of the neonate (about 9–12 inches from child's face) when communicating.
Motor	Reflexes direct the majority of movement.	Teach parents to recognize neonate's protective reflexes.
	The full-term neonate has some limited ability to hold the head erect and is able to lift the head slightly when lying prone.	Support neonate's neck and head when lifting.
Psychosocial	Crying is the neonate's way of communicating. There is a reason for crying.	Teach parents about the dynamics of crying so that they neither label the neonate as "fussy" nor develop the misconception that they are inadequate caregivers.
	The bonding process begins shortly after birth.	Encourage parents to distinguish the various cries.
		Encourage parents to interact with the neonate during every contact (feeding, bathing, changing, cuddling).
Cognitive	Neonates learn through sensory experiences. Learning is enhanced in an environment providing stimuli without bombarding the neonate. Learning occurs by repeated exposure to stimuli.	Encourage parents to provide frequent sensory stimuli (touching, talking, looking the neonate in the eyes).

Data from *Health Assessment: A Nursing Approach* (3rd ed.), by J. Fuller and J. Schaller-Ayers, 2000, Philadelphia: Lippincott Williams & Wilkins. Copyright 2000 by Lippincott Williams & Wilkins; *Health Promotion Strategies through the Life Span* (8th ed.), by R. B. Murray and J. P. Zentner, 2008, Upper Saddle River, NJ: Prentice Hall. Copyright 2008 by Prentice Hall; *Wong's Nursing Care of Infants and Children* (8th ed.), by M. J. Hockenberry and D. Wilson, 2007, St. Louis, MO: Mosby Elsevier. Copyright 2007 by Mosby Elsevier.

CLIENT TEACHING

Parents and Newborn

Parents need information about:

- Basic newborn needs
- Nutrition
- Infection control (especially hand hygiene and hygienic diaper changing practices)
- Care of the umbilicus
- Incorporating the newborn into the family unit
- Growth and development milestones in order to provide appropriate stimulation and have realistic expectations for their newborn

with rapid physiological growth and psychosocial development (Figure 10-2). Table 10-5 provides an overview of infant development.

Significance for Nursing

The nurse providing care to an infant must focus on safety, prevention of infection, and teaching parents about incorporating the child into the family. It is essential for parents and other caregivers to know the developmental milestones. Nursing care involves providing information, support, and reassurance to the parents.

Enhancing Wellness Nurses enhance infant wellness by teaching growth and development concepts to parents. Knowing the behavior to expect at certain ages both guides and reas-

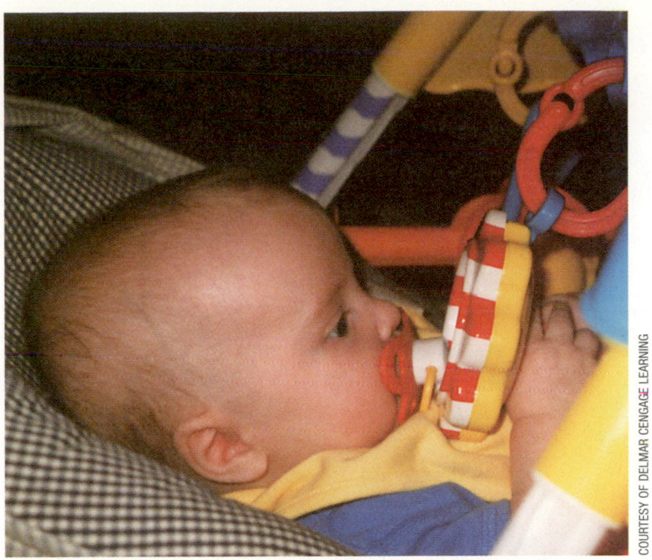
COURTESY OF DELMAR CENGAGE LEARNING

FIGURE 10-2 This infant is exploring his world and is developing in both the physiological and cognitive dimensions.

CULTURAL CONSIDERATIONS

Choice of Infant Feeding Method

There are some cultural sanctions against breastfeeding, and some cultures view bottle-feeding as a status symbol. The changing role of women in American society has impacted breastfeeding practices. Modern-day parenting practices discourage breastfeeding and influence women to not breastfeed for social reasons. Formula feeding in the United States has become a sign of affluence, sophistication, modernity, and freedom (Spangler, 2009). Be sensitive to the client's cultural background and norms when discussing infant feeding.

TABLE 10-5 Infancy Stage: Growth and Development

DIMENSIONS	CHARACTERISTICS	NURSING CONSIDERATIONS
Physiological	Physical growth is rapid. Birth weight usually triples by age 1 and length increases approximately 9 inches.	Teach parents the developmental norms.
	All body systems move toward maturation.	Encourage parents to have recommended "well-baby" checkups.
	Teeth eruption begins at 4–6 months.	
	Brain grows rapidly (reaching approximately half the adult size).	
	Eyes begin to focus.	Provide visual stimulation.
Motor	Physical maturation allows for development of motor skills.	Teach parents anticipated ages for various motor skills to develop.
	Primitive reflexes are replaced by movement that is more voluntary and goal directed.	
	Motor skills develop rapidly: • 6 months: rolls over voluntarily • 8–10 months: crawls • 8 months: sits alone	
	Grasping of objects, reflexive for the first 2–3 months, gradually becomes voluntary.	
Psychosocial	***Freud:*** oral stage	Encourage parents to provide toys and objects for sucking and teething.
	Seeks immediate gratification of needs.	
	Receives pleasure and comfort through mouth, lips, and tongue.	
	Erikson: trust vs. mistrust stage	Encourage parents to feed promptly and consistently (feed on demand rather than a fixed schedule).
	A sense of self begins to develop.	
	Responds to caregiver's voice.	Promote trust by providing warmth, diapering, and comforting.
	Separation anxiety develops at approximately 6 months.	

(*Continues*)

TABLE 10-5 Infancy Stage: Growth and Development (Continued)

DIMENSIONS	CHARACTERISTICS	NURSING CONSIDERATIONS
Cognitive	***Piaget:*** sensorimotor stage Infant learns by interacting with the environment.	Encourage parents to provide a variety of sensory stimuli: visual, sensory, auditory, and tactile (e.g., colorful mobiles; musical toys; soft, plush animals; rubbing, patting, and stroking of the infant's skin).
	Language development includes babbling, repetition, and imitation. 8–10 months says "mama" and "dada."	Encourage caregivers to talk to the infant and to name objects that are the focus of the infant's attention.
Moral	***Kohlberg:*** preconventional stage	Parents should start teaching (by role modeling) the difference between "right" and "wrong."
Spiritual	***Fowler:*** stage of undifferentiated faith	Encourage caregivers to model the values they want the infant to learn.

Data from *Health Promotion Strategies through the Life Span* (8th ed.), by R. B. Murray and J. P. Zentner, 2008, Upper Saddle River, NJ: Prentice Hall. Copyright 2008 by Prentice Hall; *Wong's Nursing Care of Infants and Children* (8th ed.), by M. J. Hockenberry and D. Wilson, 2007, St. Louis, MO: Mosby Elsevier. Copyright 2007 by Mosby Elsevier.

sures parents. Parents often need guidance about nutrition, protection from infection, and promotion of sleep.

An important factor enhancing infant wellness is providing adequate nutrients in a loving, consistent manner. Special formulas are available for infants who have PKU, are hypersensitive to protein, or experience fat malabsorption. Soy-based formulas are available for the infant who is lactose intolerant or allergic to regular formula. Infants who are formula fed usually have more subcutaneous fat. Whole cow's milk is not recommended for infants younger than 1 year of age. Human milk and commercially prepared formula are more easily digested.

Solid foods are usually introduced at 3 to 4 months of age. Rice cereal is the first solid food of choice because it causes the fewest allergic responses.

Infants are especially vulnerable to infections because the immune system is not fully matured.

Immunizations are important for infants. Nurses should advocate the administration of all recommended immunizations, which now include pneumococcal conjugate vaccine (PCV) to prevent invasive pneumococcal infections (WHO, 2008b), and

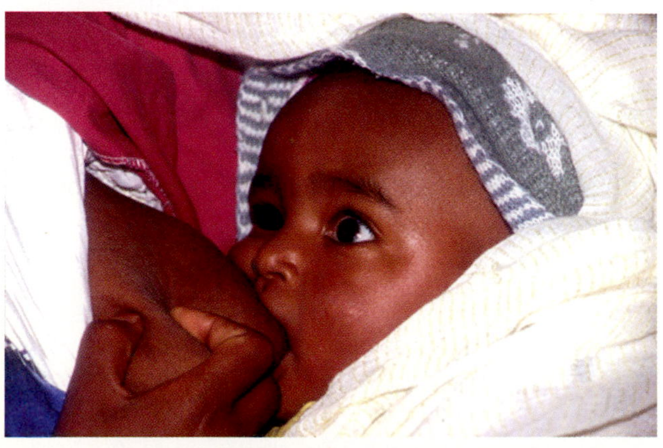

FIGURE 10-3 Breast milk is easily digested and the preferred nutrition for an infant in the first year of life. (*Courtesy of WHO/P. VIROT.*)

INFECTION CONTROL

Hand Hygiene and Infant Care

Hand hygiene is important to prevent the transmission of microorganisms. This is especially true when caring for infants, whose immune systems are still immature.

should confirm those received by the infant. Refer to the appendices for a recommended schedule for immunizations.

Information about normal sleep patterns of infants and how those patterns change with maturation is often needed by parents. To promote sleep, parents should:

- Provide a quiet room for the infant.
- Schedule feedings and other care activities during periods of wakefulness rather than drowsiness.
- Develop awareness to the unique sleep and rest periods of the infant.
- Provide comfort and security measures (e.g., rocking, singing).
- Establish routine times for sleep.

Safety Concerns Most infant injuries and deaths are related to motor vehicle accidents. The consistent and proper use of infant car seats is one of the most effective measures to ensure the infant's safety.

TODDLER STAGE

The **toddler stage** begins at 12 to 18 months of age, when a child begins to walk alone, and ends at approximately 3 years of age. The family promotes language development and teaches toileting skills. The child becomes more independent, and temper tantrums often result when attempts at autonomy

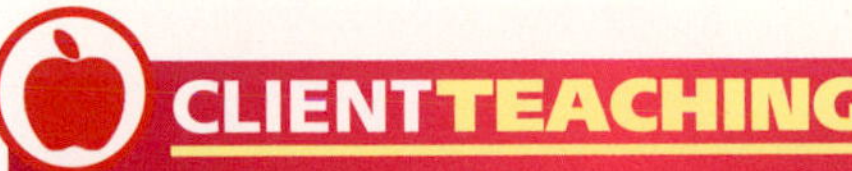

CLIENT TEACHING

Bottle-Feeding

- Assume a comfortable position and place the baby in a semireclining position, cradled close to your body.
- Never prop a bottle; choking may result.
- Use care if heating bottles. Do not warm bottles in the microwave; the hot liquid may burn the mouth and throat.
- Avoid using the bottle as a pacifier; this may result in tooth decay and may set the stage for overeating in the future.

are prevented. This stage is often called "the terrible twos." The toddler's frequent use of the word *no* is an expression of developing autonomy.

Nurses greatly influence the quality of parent–child interaction when teaching parents developmental concepts. This information helps parents have realistic expectations of the toddler's behavior. Using firm limits consistently applied helps the toddler learn and provides parameters for safe, socially acceptable behavior. Table 10-6 outlines the toddler's growth and development.

Significance for Nursing

Nurses working with toddlers must be sensitive that children this age are often anxious and fearful in the presence of strangers. Establishing rapport by playing with the child helps alleviate stranger anxiety.

Fear and anxiety can make a hospital experience a negative one. The major stressor is separation from the parents. The unfamiliar environment is also a stressor for the toddler. Nurses can help reduce stress by teaching both the child and parents about procedures. Anxiety is lessened through play.

Regular health examinations and immunizations are an essential part of health care for toddlers. Involve parents during examinations and immunizations. They can alleviate the toddler's stress by holding the child and talking calmly when the health care provider is present.

Enhancing Wellness Teaching involves both toddlers and their parents. Use play to establish an effective relationship with the child. Play is a valuable process for toddlers because it is the primary way they learn and socialize. When teaching, the nurse should be at the toddler's eye level and use words she can understand.

Respiratory infections are common health problems for toddlers. Parasitic diseases are also fairly common. Teach parents about preventive measures such as frequent hand washing with antibacterial soaps. The nurse should also verify which immunizations are needed.

As the rate of growth slows, nutritional needs change. Toddlers need fewer calories than do infants. The required amounts of protein and fluids (Hockenberry & Wilson, 2007) also decrease. Most toddlers become picky about the foods they will eat, so it may be difficult to provide enough calcium and iron. Toddlers should consume an average of 2 to 3 cups of milk per day to ensure adequate calcium intake. Drinking more than a quart of milk per day increases the risk of developing anemia, because the child will be "full" and may not eat other foods (Hockenberry & Wilson, 2007). Nurses can play a key role in nutritional counseling for toddlers.

CLIENT TEACHING

Preventing Infant Accidents

- To prevent vehicular accidents: Use infant seats and keep infants out of the paths of automobiles and other vehicles.
- To prevent burns: Keep infants away from open heaters, fireplaces, hot stoves, and matches.
- To protect from falls: Keep crib rails up at all times, never leave the infant lying unattended on furniture, and use protective gates and barriers to block stairways.
- To prevent drowning: Never leave the infant unattended near water (buckets, bathtubs, swimming pools).
- To prevent electrocution: Keep electrical cords out of the infant's reach and use plastic safety plugs to cover all electrical outlets.
- To prevent choking: Closely monitor the infant exploring the environment. During this oral phase, the infant tests out the environment and seeks pleasure through the mouth. Aspiration accidents are common, with infants choking on objects such as buttons and coins.

SAFETY

Aiding a Choking Infant

Never use the Heimlich maneuver on a choking infant. Instead, use alternating back blows and chest compressions to dislodge the object.

PROFESSIONAL TIP

Health Care for Toddlers

- Explain what is being done in a calm voice.
- Alleviate anxiety with play (e.g., demonstrate a procedure on a doll or teddy bear; allow the child to handle equipment, such as a stethoscope, before using it on the child).
- Provide simple, short directions.
- Comfort the child after a painful procedure.
- Encourage active participation of parents.

TABLE 10-6 Toddler Stage: Growth and Development

DIMENSIONS	CHARACTERISTICS	NURSING CONSIDERATIONS
Physiological	Overall rate of growth slows. By 24 months of age, weight is usually four times that at birth.	Instruct parents on need for vitamin D, calcium, and phosphorus.
	Brain grows rapidly.	
	Bones in extremities grow in length. Physiological readiness for bowel and bladder control develops.	Explain timing for toilet training and need for consistency and patience.
Motor	Learns to walk, run, climb stairs, jump, ride a tricycle, and throw a ball.	Have parents assess home environment for safety.
Psychosocial	*Freud:* anal stage	Have parents avoid overemphasis on toilet training.
	Receives pleasure from contraction and relaxation of sphincter muscles.	
	Erikson: autonomy vs. shame and doubt stage	Teach parents to encourage toddler's attempts at independence (e.g., trying to feed and dress self).
Cognitive	*Piaget:* preoperational stage	
	Can follow simple directions.	Instruct parents to give only one direction at a time.
	Thought processes are concrete.	
	Able to anticipate future events.	Use a calendar to show today's date and the number of days until a significant event.
	Child has short attention span.	
	Child comprehends self as a separate entity.	Teach caregivers importance of calling child by name.
	Language: At approximately 1 year of age, the child can make two-syllable sounds (e.g., ma-ma, da-da)	Have caregivers talk to child frequently but avoid "baby talk."
	By age 3, the child can form short sentences and has a vocabulary of approximately 900 words.	
Moral	*Kohlberg:* preconventional stage	Parents should be consistent in setting limits.
	Child learns to distinguish right from wrong.	Emphasize the significance of modeling desired behavior to the child.
Spiritual	*Fowler:* intuitive-projective stage of faith	Instruct parents to provide simple answers to questions related to religion, God, and church. Instruct on the importance of incorporating religious rituals and ceremonies into daily life.

Data from *Health Promotion Strategies through the Life Span* (8th ed.), by R. B. Murray and J. P. Zentner, 2008, Upper Saddle River, NJ: Prentice Hall. Copyright 2008 by Prentice Hall; *Wong's Nursing Care of Infants and Children* (8th ed.), by M. J. Hockenberry and D. Wilson, 2007, St. Louis, MO: Mosby Elsevier. Copyright 2007 by Mosby Elsevier.

Safety Concerns Accidents (especially those involving automobiles) are a frequent cause of disability and death among toddlers (Figure 10-4) (Edelman & Mandle, 2010). The information regarding use of car seats for neonates and infants also applies to toddlers.

Another common type of accident among toddlers involves toys. As children gain new skills (Figure 10-5), parents must reassess the safety of toys and the environments where the toddler might play.

With their increased mobility and curiosity, toddlers are especially prone to accidental poisoning. Parents should thus childproof the home and carefully observe the toddler.

SAFETY

Toys for Toddlers

Parents should check toys for:

- Age appropriateness
- Sharp pieces or corners
- Small parts that can be swallowed
- Poisonous paint (e.g., lead-based paint)
- Flammable or toxic materials
- Manner in which toys are used

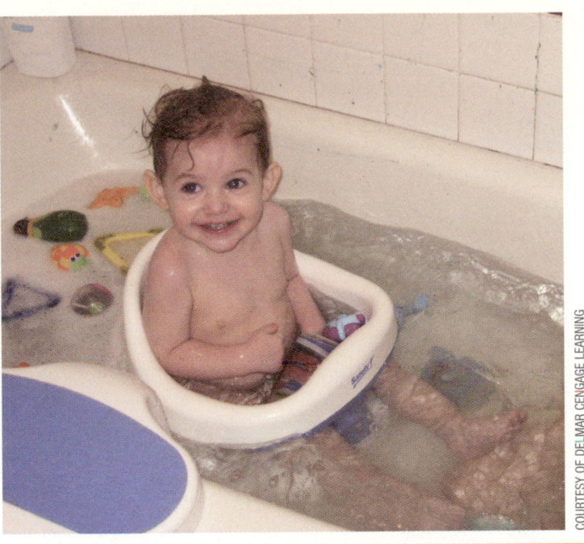

COURTESY OF DELMAR CENGAGE LEARNING

FIGURE 10-4 **Parents should carefully observe toddlers and childproof their home to prevent accidents, as shown here with the use of a bath safety seat.**

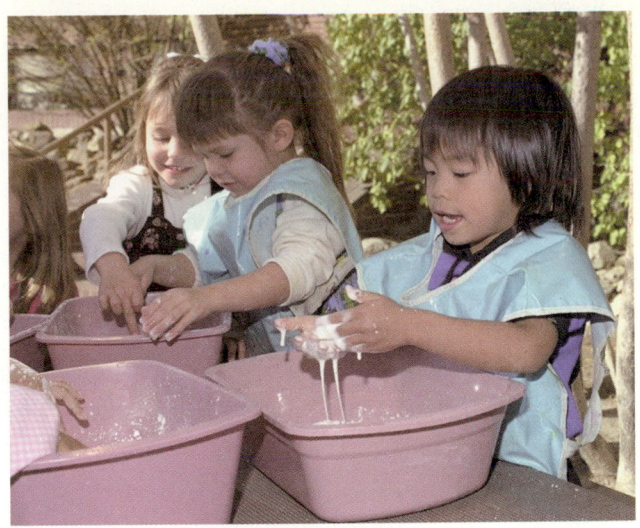

COURTESY OF DELMAR CENGAGE LEARNING

FIGURE 10-5 **Parents must ensure that all materials a child plays with are safe, nontoxic, and nonflammable.**

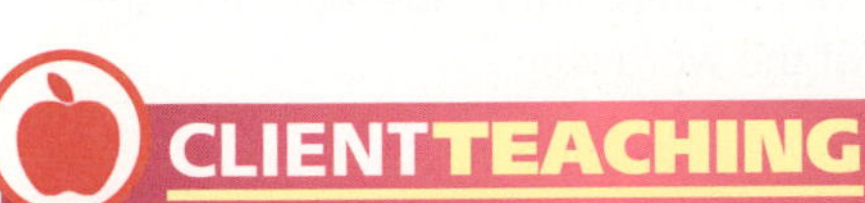

Toddler Nutrition

- Avoid using food as a reward because doing so encourages overeating.
- Do not serve large helpings; it may overwhelm the child, possibly resulting in a refusal to eat.
- Expect sporadic eating patterns (eating a lot one day and very little the next, or enjoying one food for several days and then suddenly refusing to eat that food).
- Avoid power struggles related to meals. It is counterproductive to establishing healthy eating habits to force a child to eat.
- Establish a mealtime routine and follow it; toddlers like rituals.
- Provide nutritional snacks to meet dietary requirements.

CRITICAL THINKING

Male/Female Stereotypes

Our society labels certain characteristics as "masculine" or "feminine." How do you think these stereotypes influence the development of young boys and girls in our society?

PRESCHOOL STAGE

Development from ages 3 to 6 years is called the **preschool stage.** During this stage, physical growth slows, and psychosocial and cognitive development accelerate. Table 10-7 outlines preschool development in detail.

During this period, curiosity increases, and the child is better able to communicate. Parents should be taught that the child's frequent use of the word *why* is necessary for normal psychosocial and cognitive development.

The child's world continues to expand outside the immediate home environment. The preschooler uses play to both learn about and develop relationships.

Significance for Nursing

Play is a tool that can be used by nurses to help reduce fear and anxiety in the preschooler. Play helps preschoolers reduce tension, learn about the environment, and incorporate socially defined expectations for behavior (Figure 10-6).

Enhancing Wellness It is important to communicate at the child's level of comprehension yet not talk down to the child. Include the child in decisions and activities as much as possible. During the preschool years, the child begins showing an interest in health. To promote the development of lifelong health-promoting lifestyles, the astute nurse capitalizes on this by making health education fun. Immunizations are a major wellness intervention for preschoolers. At each checkup the nurse should verify that immunizations are up to date.

Safety Concerns Accidents are the leading cause of death among young children. Cognitive immaturity coupled with an eagerness to explore the environment lead to the preschooler's risk for accidents. Parents must understand the importance of teaching young children the meaning of the word *no*.

Common accidents among preschoolers include automobile accidents, falls, burns, animal bites, drowning, and ingestion of poisonous substances.

The nurse should emphasize parental education about protecting preschoolers from potential hazards. The safety practices learned as a preschooler will be lifelong. Accident prevention can be best taught through modeling. Parents who always buckle their seatbelts in a car protect themselves and teach their children an important accident prevention measure.

TABLE 10-7 Preschooler Stage: Growth and Development

DIMENSION	CHARACTERISTICS	NURSING CONSIDERATIONS
Physiological	Physical growth slows; average weight at age 5 years is 45 pounds. Head size approximates that of an adult. Deciduous teeth come in fully; these "baby teeth" start to fall out about age 6 and will be replaced by permanent teeth.	Eats a variety of foods and larger meals.
Motor	Fine motor skills develop (e.g., can skip, throw a ball overhand, use scissors, tie shoelaces).	Emphasize providing a safe environment for play and exploration. Praise attempted independent activities.
Psychosocial	*Freud:* phallic stage Oedipal conflict leads to development of superego (conscience). *Erikson:* initiative vs. guilt stage	Self-control is learned by interacting with others.
Cognitive	*Piaget:* preoperational stage Vocabulary over 2,000 words. Play more reality based. Increased ability to communicate, increases socialization with peers.	Tell parents that children of this age learn through frequent use of the word *why.*
Moral	*Kohlberg:* preconventional stage A conscience begins to develop. Fears wrongdoing, and seeks parental approval.	Encourage parents to teach the child basic values, ideally by modeling. Encourage parents to provide consistent praise and acceptance of child.
Spiritual	*Fowler:* intuitive-projective stage of faith Not yet able to understand spiritual concepts but imitates parent's behaviors.	Teaching by example is the best approach for a child of this age.

Data from *Health Promotion Strategies through the Life Span* (8th ed.), by R. B. Murray and J. P. Zentner, 2008, Upper Saddle River, NJ: Prentice Hall. Copyright 2008 by Prentice Hall; *Wong's Nursing Care of Infants and Children* (8th ed.), by M. J. Hockenberry and D. Wilson, 2007, St. Louis, MO: Mosby Elsevier. Copyright 2007 by Mosby Elsevier.

CLIENT TEACHING

Promoting Wellness

- Encourage healthy lifestyles (nonsedentary activities, nutritious meals).
- Teach children appropriate hygienic measures.
- Schedule regular checkups.
- Keep immunizations up to date.
- Schedule dental checkups and encourage daily brushing and flossing.
- Teach safety precautions.
- Establish sleep patterns.
- Report any symptoms of illness to the health care provider.

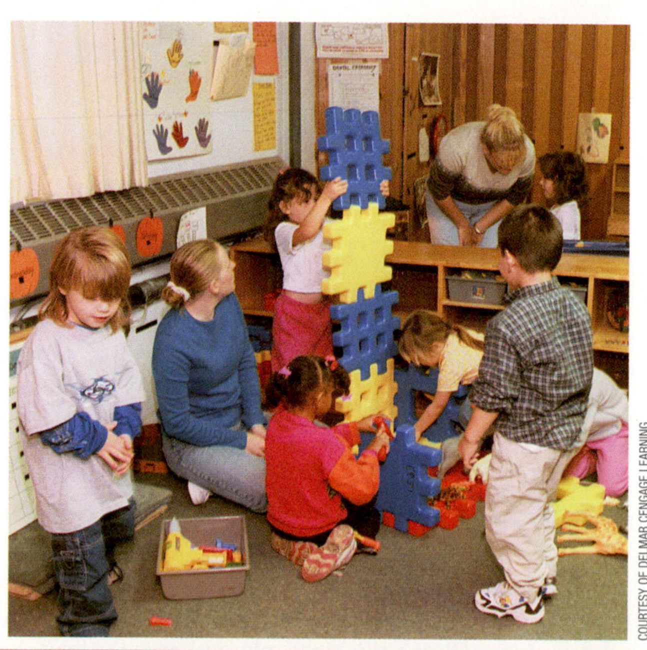

COURTESY OF DELMAR CENGAGE LEARNING

FIGURE 10-6 Play is an important vehicle for socialization among preschoolers.

School-Age Stage

During the **school-age stage** (development from the ages of 6 to 10 years), physical changes are slow, even, and continuous. Table 10-8 gives an overview of growth and development of the school-age child.

The world of a school-age child expands greatly. Participating in school activities, team sports, and play enlarges their social network. As they mature, play becomes more structured and less spontaneous. Communication increases, and an expanded vocabulary allows the expression of thoughts, needs, and feelings.

The school-age child's cognitive abilities expand, and academic, sporting, and social activities stimulate creativity.

Significance for Nursing

Common health problems among school-age children are minor illnesses such as upper respiratory infections and accidents. Teaching health promotion is a major role when caring for school-age children.

Enhancing Wellness Nurses can promote healthy lifestyles among children in schools. This is a cost-effective way to teach wellness behaviors.

Table 10-8 School-Age Stage: Growth and Development

DIMENSION	CHARACTERISTICS	NURSING CONSIDERATIONS
Physiological	Steady physical growth (approximately 3–6 pounds and 2–3 inches per year).	Emphasize to parents the need for a balanced diet to sustain growth requirements.
	Body has an overall slimmer shape.	
	CNS maturation is nearly complete. By age 12, all permanent teeth (except second and third molars) are present.	Need daily dental hygiene (brushing and flossing) and regularly scheduled visits to the dentist. Change toothbrush every 3 months.
Motor	Motor control continues to develop.	Encourage participation in physical activities.
	Less dependent on parents for activities of daily living.	Praise independent activities.
Psychosocial	*Freud:* latency stage	To develop a sense of confidence, encourage child to:
	Same-gender companions are preferred.	• Participate in group and individual activities
	Erikson: industry vs. inferiority stage	
	Develops initiative and high self-esteem as manifested in school and sports.	Encourage parents to praise child's efforts.
	Less dependent on family.	
Cognitive	*Piaget:* concrete operations stage	
	Ability to cooperate with others and to see other points of view leads to more meaningful communication.	Encourage group activities.
	Reasoning now logical and rational.	
	Abstract thinking is not fully developed.	Remember child's level of comprehension.
	The concept of time develops: • Knows difference between past and present • Begins to learn to tell time	
	Able to categorize, classify, and order objects.	
	Relationships between objects seen.	
Moral	*Kohlberg:* conventional stage	Encourage parents to provide consistent limits.
	Understands what is unacceptable behavior but may need assistance to choose between right and wrong.	Emphasize modeling appropriate behavior. Praise appropriate behavior.
Spiritual	*Fowler:* mythical-literal stage	Encourage parents to discuss their beliefs.
	Accepts deity existence.	Stories reinforce understanding of spiritual concepts.
	Beliefs are symbolized through stories.	

Data from *Health Promotion Strategies through the Life Span* (8th ed.), by R. B. Murray and J. P. Zentner, 2008, Upper Saddle River, NJ: Prentice Hall. Copyright 2008 by Prentice Hall; *Health Promotion throughout the Lifespan* (7th ed.), by C. L. Edelman and C. L. Mandle, 2010, St. Louis, MO: Mosby Elsevier. Copyright 2010 by Mosby Elsevier.

SAFETY

Accidents and Abductions

- Children must learn safety rules for riding toys (e.g., use of protective equipment, see Figure 10-7).
- Parents must frequently remind children of the danger of playing near traffic.
- Teach children to use caution with strangers because of the possibility of abduction.

Safety Concerns School-age children often experience accidents during play. Common injuries relate to the use of trampolines, skates, skateboards, and bicycles.

Preadolescent Stage

Preadolescence (development from the ages of 10 to 12 years) is marked by rapid physiological changes having psychological and social implications. The child begins to experience hormonal changes that will result in the onset of **puberty** (the emergence of secondary sex characteristics). Girls generally experience puberty at a younger age than do boys—approximately 9 to 10 years of age, as compared to 10 to 11 years of age for boys (Edelman & Mandle, 2010). Table 10-9 provides an overview of preadolescent development.

In girls, breast development begins between the ages of 10 and 11. The release of estrogen during puberty stimulates further breast development. **Menarche** (onset of the first menstrual period) occurs about 2 years after breast buds appear. The first menstrual periods are usually scant, irregular, and ovulation may or may not occur. The average age of menarche has declined over the past century in the United States and is now 12.8 years. This decline is probably caused by improved general health status (Hockenberry & Wilson, 2007).

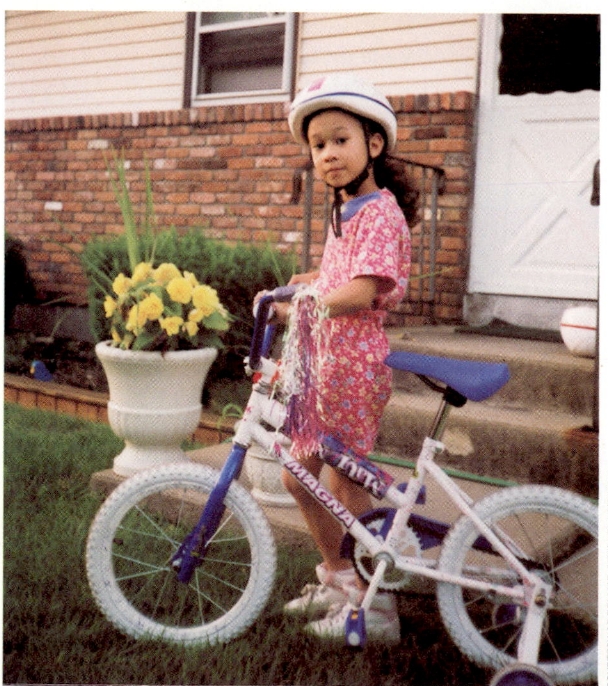

COURTESY OF DELMAR CENGAGE LEARNING

Figure 10-7 Safety equipment such as helmets helps protect school-age children from injury.

The menstrual cycle has physiological and psychological changes occurring monthly. A girl's cycle usually is established in a regular pattern after the first 6 to 12 months. Nurses must remember that some girls may receive incorrect or inadequate information regarding menstruation. Client teaching should emphasize the physiological changes, emotional changes, and personal hygiene.

In preadolescent boys, the first signs of puberty are:

- Testicles enlarge
- Penis enlarges
- Scrotum becomes redder and thins
- Pubic hair grows

Significance for Nursing

Sensitivity is essential in working with the preadolescent. To increase sensitivity, the nurse should use a nonjudgmental approach and attend to the preadolescent's body language.

Enhancing Wellness Information about nutrition, activity and rest, and physiological changes is needed by the preadolescent. This client should be taught about the dramatic growth spurt, the sexual changes, and the psychosocial changes that characterize this life stage (Figure 10-8). Preparing the preadolescent for upcoming changes promotes physical and emotional health. Confirm that immunizations are current.

Safety Concerns The preadolescent is at risk for injury during play and sports activities.

Other areas in which to promote safety are development of healthy lifestyle, substance abuse prevention, and sex education.

Adolescent Stage

Adolescence (development from the ages of 13 to 20 years) begins with the onset of puberty. The individual undergoes the transition from child to adult as many physiological changes and rapid growth occur. The rapid changes occurring are not only physical; many psychosocial adjustments must also be made. Friendships become very important (Figure 10-9). Establishing a sense of personal identity takes up a great amount of the adolescent's psychic energy. Questions such as "Who am I?" and "What is really important?" are common ones among adolescents.

Most adolescents are very concerned with their appearance. The importance of physical attractiveness may cause eating disorders, such as anorexia nervosa (self-imposed starvation that results in a 15% loss of body weight), bulimia nervosa (episodic binge-eating followed by purging), or obesity (weight that is 20% or more above ideal body weight).

PROFESSIONAL TIP

Preadolescent–Nurse Relationship

To encourage the preadolescent to ask questions about health-related concerns, the nurse must establish a trusting relationship with the preadolescent.

TABLE 10-9 Preadolescent and Adolescent Stage: Growth and Development

DIMENSION	CHARACTERISTICS	NURSING CONSIDERATIONS
Physiological	*Physiological changes:* Physical growth accelerates and is accompanied by changes in body proportion. Extremities grow first, then trunk and hips.	Teach child and parents to expect growth spurts.
	Endocrine changes: Hypothalamus stimulates pituitary to secrete gonadotropins, causing reproductive maturity. Primary and secondary sex characteristics develop. Beginning of puberty is evidenced in girls by: • Breasts develop. • Pubic and axillary hair grows. • Menarche (onset of menses). • Height increases. Beginning of puberty is evidenced in boys by: • Genitals develop. • Facial, pubic, and axillary hair grows. • Ejaculations occur at night. • Height increases. • Voice deepens.	Provide information and support about sexual changes.
	Musculoskeletal changes: Bones ossify. Muscle mass and strength increase.	Encourage physical activities and adequate intake of calcium.
	Dental changes: Last four molars erupt.	Continue daily dental hygiene.
	Integumentary changes: Skin becomes thicker and tougher. Activation of sebaceous glands may lead to acne. Pubic hair appears.	Encourage sunscreen use and to avoid prolonged sunlight exposure. Support preadolescent experiencing acne.
Motor	Completely independent in performing self-care activities.	Encourage parents to allow some freedom of expression and choice.
Psychosocial	*Freud:* genital stage *Erikson:* identity vs. role diffusion stage The major task is to develop a sense of identity. A new body image develops.	
	Intimacy with members of opposite gender is established. Primary support is the peer group.	Provide sex education.
	Often rebels against adult authority.	Educate parents that rebellion is a normal developmental experience.
Cognitive	*Piaget:* formal operations stage Approach to thinking is logical, organized, and consistent. Most adolescents think in terms of cause and effect.	False sense of immunity ("It can't happen to me" attitude) has an impact on health behaviors.
	Sees self as exceptional, special, and unique, and views self as being immune to problems. Tends to be extremely idealistic. Egocentric (self-centered) thinking is common, as is a view of self as omnipotent.	Educate about safety in: • Sex practices • Driving practices (no driving with alcohol use)

(*Continues*)

TABLE 10-9 Preadolescent and Adolescent Stage: Growth and Development (Continued)

DIMENSION	CHARACTERISTICS	NURSING CONSIDERATIONS
Moral	*Kohlberg:* postconventional stage The adolescent tends to support the morality of law and order in determining right from wrong. Adolescents begin to question and discard the status quo and to choose different values. Moral maturity depends on the context of the situation and the relationship. Own moral reasoning may be overcome by peer pressure.	Teach parents that questioning of values is normal. Teach assertiveness skills preadolescent can use when communicating with peers.
Spiritual	*Fowler:* synthetic-conventional stage The adolescent questions values and beliefs.	Curiosity about other religious beliefs is normal.

Data from *Health Promotion throughout the Lifespan* (7th ed.), by C. L. Edelman and C. L. Mandle, 2010, St. Louis, MO: Mosby Elsevier. Copyright 2010 by Mosby Elsevier.

Significance for Nursing

Support the adolescent by providing information about the many bodily changes experienced during this developmental stage. Encourage adolescents to share health concerns with parents, but honor the adolescent's choice to keep sensitive information from parents. The confidentiality of the client as well as of those in a relationship with the client (sexual partners) must be protected.

Enhancing Wellness The adolescent's wellness is enhanced primarily through teaching. Areas to emphasize in health education for adolescents include nutrition, hygiene, developmental changes, sex education, and substance abuse prevention. Information is available from the American Academy of Pediatrics (AAP, 2008a).

Teaching adolescents about the physical changes they are undergoing is often done by school nurses.

Safety Concerns Unhealthy behaviors contribute to the three major causes of adolescent death: accidents, homicide, and suicide. The adolescent's risk for accidents increases because of:

- Impulsive behavior
- Feeling invulnerable to accidents
- Testing limits
- Rebelling

As a result, many adolescents engage in unhealthy behaviors such as smoking, consuming alcohol and other drugs, reckless driving, unprotected sexual activity, and violence.

Many adolescent health problems relate to sexual behaviors. For example, consider the following facts:

- The CDC estimates that approximately 19 million new sexually transmitted infections occur each year, almost half of them among young people ages 15 to 24. Young females aged 15 to 19 had the highest Chlamydia rate (CDC, 2007).
- Approximately one-third of girls in the United States get pregnant before age 20. In 2006, a total of 435,427 infants were born to mothers aged 15 to 19 years (CDC, 2008c).

COURTESY OF DELMAR CENGAGE LEARNING

FIGURE 10-8 Preadolescence is a time of gender role discovery and increasing independence.

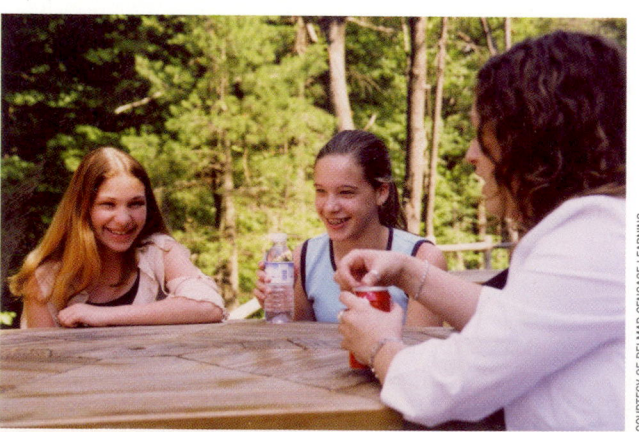

COURTESY OF DELMAR CENGAGE LEARNING

FIGURE 10-9 Adolescence is a time of developing peer group relationships.

PROFESSIONALTIP

Working with Adolescents

- Use a nonjudgmental attitude to establish rapport when working with adolescents.
- Treat every adolescent in a respectful, dignified manner.
- Avoid using a condescending attitude when communicating with the adolescent.
- To form a collaborative partnership, treat the adolescent as an active participant in health care.
- Answer all questions honestly.
- Be sensitive to nonverbal clues. Adolescents are often too embarrassed to initiate discussion.
- Remember that the peer group is of major importance to the adolescent; use group settings.
- Demonstrate acceptance of the adolescent even when limits must be established.
- Questioning adult authority is a normal part of adolescence. Do not personalize such behavior. Nurses who do so become defensive and lose their interpersonal effectiveness and credibility with adolescents.

Teen pregnancy has a great effect on families and communities. Social programs providing resources to meet the needs of pregnant adolescents are decreasing. Many pregnant teens become trapped in a cycle of school failure (or dropout), limited employment opportunities, and poverty.

The pregnant adolescent needs information, expert prenatal care, and a supportive environment. Teaching must emphasize preventing STIs because the pregnancy is evidence of high-risk (i.e., unprotected) sexual activity. According to the AAP (2007), 47.8% of youth (grades 9–12) have engaged in sexual intercourse, and 61.5% used a condom during their most recent sexual intercourse. Nurses teaching safe-sex practices must be sensitive to cultural influences on sexual activity.

A high risk of suicide is a major health problem during adolescence. The rate is higher among adolescent males than females. Suicide is often thought to be the only alternative to an overwhelming situation. Suicidal behavior can be traced to low self-esteem, lack of maturity, and resultant impulsive behaviors.

Assessment for suicide potential should always be direct questions about plans for harming or killing themselves. The following are signs of suicide risk in adolescents:

- Change in eating and sleeping habits
- Writing suicide notes
- Discussion of suicide
- Aggressive behavior
- Substance abuse
- Loss of interest in pleasurable activities
- Preoccupation with death
- Neglect of personal hygiene
- The giving away of treasured objects
- Marked personality change

SAFETY

Suicide Prevention

- Never leave the suicidal adolescent alone.
- The best deterrent to suicide is close observation.

- Verbal cues (e.g., "You won't have to worry about me much longer.")
- Fatigue, headache, stomachache
- Social withdrawal

When someone exhibits signs of suicide risk, contact a health care professional *immediately*. Most communities have a special suicide-prevention telephone line available.

Another significant health problem for many adolescents is substance abuse. A common maladaptive way to cope with the stressors of adolescence is using alcohol or other drugs.

Nurses can help adolescents make responsible, informed decisions before experimenting with drugs.

Young Adulthood Stage

Physical growth stabilizes during **young adulthood** (development from the ages of 21 years through approximately 40 years). The young adult still experiences physical and emotional changes, but at a slower rate than the adolescent. Table 10-10 outlines the development of young adults. This is a time of transition from adolescence to adulthood. According to Estes (2010), this time of separation and independence leads to new commitments and responsibilities in work, social, and family roles and relationships (Figure 10-10).

Pregnancy is experienced by many young adults. It is a time of transition and lifestyle adjustments. Women experience changes in self-concept during pregnancy and may need reassurance that this is normal.

Significance for Nursing

Young adulthood is usually the healthiest time in a person's life. Consequently, concern for health is low, and wellness is taken for granted. Preventive measures fall into two categories:

- Developing health-promoting behaviors (e.g., lifestyle modification)
- Avoiding accident, injury, and violence

By teaching and counseling, the nurse plays an important role in each of these areas of health promotion. Other

CRITICAL THINKING

Sexually Active Adolescents

How would you provide care to sexually active adolescents if you think their behavior is immoral or "wrong"? Is it ethical for you to try to change their values so they become congruent with yours? Should you change your values to be congruent with those of the client?

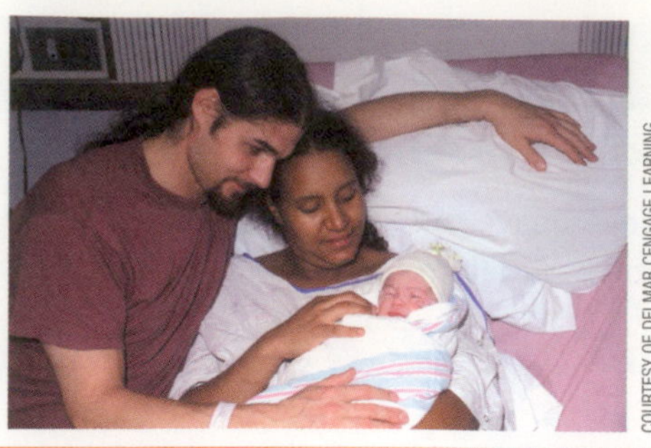

FIGURE 10-10 Young adulthood is a time for new responsibilities and commitments, including the beginning of a new family.

developmentally appropriate topics for the nurse to address are vocational counseling and relationship establishment.

Enhancing Wellness Decision making by young adults affects their health status. Young adults often take excessive risks, making them at greater risk for accidents, suicide, or homicide (Edelman & Mandle, 2010). Reckless driving, driving while intoxicated, and unprotected sex are examples that demonstrate a lack of fear by many young adults. Sexually transmitted infections often result in reproductive dysfunction. Nurses should teach women how to perform a breast self-examination (BSE) monthly, and men must learn how to perform a testicular self-examination (TSE). The nurse should confirm currency of tetanus/diphtheria (Td) immunization.

Safety Concerns A health risk to many young adults is sunbathing. Exposure to the radiation resulting from direct sunlight or the lighting used in tanning salons is directly linked to skin cancer. According to the American Cancer Society (2008), more than 1 million new cases of squamous and basal cell skin cancer are diagnosed every year. Nurses can teach and model safe behaviors related to sunbathing.

MIDDLE ADULTHOOD STAGE

Middle adulthood (development from the ages of 40 to 65 years) is characterized by productivity and responsibility. Many physiological changes occur during middle adulthood. Table 10-11 lists the major changes experienced by the middle-aged person. Most activity revolves around family and work with success measured by family life and career accomplishments.

The major developmental task of middle adulthood concerns the conflict of generativity (a sense that one is making a contribution to society) versus stagnation (a sense of nonmeaning in one's life). An individual who successfully resolves this developmental conflict is usually accepting of age-related changes.

TABLE 10-10 Young Adulthood: Growth and Development

DIMENSION	CHARACTERISTICS	NURSING CONSIDERATIONS
Physiological	*Physiological changes:* Physical growth stabilizes. Physical functioning is at an optimum and therefore less likely to be concerned with own health. Maturation of body systems is complete. *Cardiovascular changes:* Men are more likely to have an increased cholesterol level than are women. *Gastrointestinal changes:* After age 30, digestive juices decrease. *Musculoskeletal changes:* At approximately age 25, skeletal growth is complete. *Reproductive changes:* *Women:* Ages 20–30 are optimal years physically for reproduction. *Men:* Beginning at approximately age 24, male hormones slowly decrease (does not affect reproductive ability).	Teach importance of health-promoting behaviors. Encourage a healthy lifestyle.
Psychosocial	*Erikson:* intimacy vs. isolation stage Engages in productive work. Develops intimate relationships.	Emphasize need for social support as the person assumes new roles. Provide sex education information, including information on prevention of STIs.
Cognitive	*Piaget:* formal operations stage Problem-solving abilities are realistic. Manifests less egocentricism. Many engage in formal education.	

TABLE 10-10 Young Adulthood: Growth and Development (Continued)

DIMENSION	CHARACTERISTICS	NURSING CONSIDERATIONS
Moral	*Kohlberg:* postconventional stage Right and wrong are defined in terms of personal beliefs and principles.	Respect the person's value system and beliefs.
Spiritual	*Fowler:* individuative-reflective faith stage Assumes responsibility for own beliefs.	Encourage use of spiritual support system.

Data from *Health Promotion throughout the Lifespan* (7th ed.), by C. L. Edelman and C. L. Mandle, 2010, St. Louis, MO: Mosby Elsevier. Copyright 2010 by Mosby Elsevier.

TABLE 10-11 Middle Adulthood: Growth and Development

DIMENSION	CHARACTERISTICS	NURSING CONSIDERATIONS
Physiological	*Cardiovascular changes:* Decreased capacity for physical activity. Blood vessels lose elasticity. Hypertension (high blood pressure), coronary artery disease, and cerebral vascular accidents ("strokes") may appear.	Encourage to remain physically active. Teach lifestyle modifications related to cardiovascular health: • Quit smoking. • Avoid secondary tobacco smoke. • Practice good nutrition (low fat, low cholesterol). • Engage in physical activity.
	Neurological changes: Impaired sensation of heat and cold.	Explain age-related changes. Teach safety precautions regarding: • Exposure to sunlight • Sensitivity to heat stroke and frostbite
	Gastrointestinal changes: Slower gastrointestinal motility results in constipation.	Teach to: • Increase high-fiber food intake; drink more fluid • Maintain physical activity
	Genitourinary changes: Nephron units diminish in number and size; blood supply to kidneys diminishes.	Teach signs indicating dehydration. Educate to maintain adequate fluid intake.
	Integumentary changes: Wrinkles develop. Hair may thin and turn gray.	Assess for body image alterations. Employ nonjudgmental listening.
	Musculoskeletal changes: Bone mass and density decreases. Slight loss of height (1–4 inches) may occur.	Educate about: • Need for increased calcium intake • Decreasing caffeine and alcohol consumption • Effects of sedentary lifestyle on osteoporosis
	Generalized decrease in muscle tone; appearance becomes "flabby," and agility lessens, leading to an increased risk of injury.	Instruct about need for proper posture (especially when sitting), exercise, and adequate fluid intake. Educate about need for physical activity.
	Endocrine changes: Reduced production of enzymes and increased hydrochloric acid, leading to acid indigestion and belching.	Instruct client to: • Eat foods that are not spicy or fried. • Avoid eating within 2 hours of bedtime.
	Reproductive changes: *Women:* Estrogen and progesterone production cease at menopause. Secondary sex characteristics regress (decreased breast size, loss of pubic hair). Vaginal secretions decrease.	Teach age-related sexual/reproductive changes.

(*Continues*)

TABLE 10-11 Middle Adulthood: Growth and Development (Continued)

DIMENSION	CHARACTERISTICS	NURSING CONSIDERATIONS
Physiological (Continued)	*Men:* Testosterone level decreases as does the amount of viable sperm. Sexual energy declines, and it takes longer to achieve an erection, but it is sustained longer. Adapting to chronic diseases and sexual problems may diminish self-esteem.	Encourage responsible sexual behavior. Teach prevention of sexually transmitted infections.
Psychosocial	*Erikson:* generativity vs. stagnation stage Those who have achieved generativity feel good about themselves and comfortable with their lives. Become involved in altruistic acts (volunteer work). Family roles may change (become caregiver to aging parents, become grandparent).	Provide support as aging occurs. Encourage involvement in community activities. Explain the need to care for self while caring for others.
Cognitive	*Piaget:* Uses all stages, depending on the task. Able to reflect on the past and anticipate the future. Reaction time diminishes. Learning ability remains for motivated person.	Encourage clients who return to school or participate in other intellectually stimulating activities.
Moral	*Kohlberg:* postconventional stage	Be nonjudgmental when discussing values.
Spiritual	*Fowler:* conjunctive faith stage The middle-aged adult is able to appreciate others' belief systems. Middle-aged adults are less dogmatic about own beliefs. Religion is often a source of comfort.	Encourage use of spiritual support. Refer to clergy if desired by client.

Data from *Health Promotion throughout the Lifespan* (7th ed.), by C. L. Edelman and C. L. Mandle, 2010, St. Louis, MO: Mosby Elsevier. Copyright 2010 by Mosby Elsevier; *Health Assessment: A Nursing Approach* (3rd ed.), by J. Fuller and J. Schaller-Ayers, 2000, Philadelphia: Lippincott Williams & Wilkins.

Evaluation of one's life may lead to a midlife crisis, especially if the individual feels that little has been accomplished or self-expectations have not been met.

Significance for Nursing

Middle-aged adults constitute almost half the U.S. population (Edelman & Mandle, 2010). The baby-boom generation has entered this stage, and more nurses will be required to care for them.

Assist middle-aged clients in improving their health by identifying risk factors and providing early intervention. The major risk factors are primarily behavioral and environmental for adults in the middle years, so they can be changed. In assisting the middle-aged client to change unhealthy behaviors, the nurse can work on either a one-on-one or group basis.

Enhancing Wellness Encourage middle-aged adults to assume more responsibility for their own health by receiving influenza and pneumococcal immunizations as recommended by their physicians. Confirm currency of tetanus/diphtheria (Td) immunization.

Safety Concerns Middle adulthood is the time when lifelong unhealthy practices, such as smoking, being sedentary, and overuse of alcohol, begin to exhibit their adverse effects. Reversing these practices can greatly improve one's health status. Occupational health hazards are another significant problem.

Most middle-aged individuals have more leisure time for jogging, tennis, golf, or boating, resulting in an increased risk of injuries (Figure 10-11).

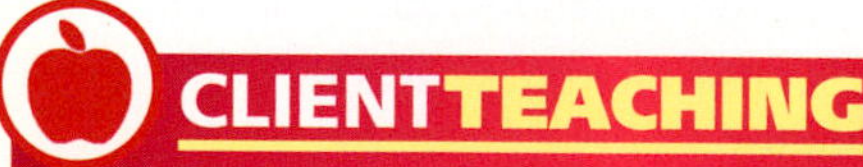

Self-Care for Middle Adulthood

Self-care topics for the middle-aged adult include:

- Nutrition, exercise, and weight control
- Managing stress
- Recommendations for health screening (cholesterol, prostate exam, mammogram, Pap test)
- Changes related to aging

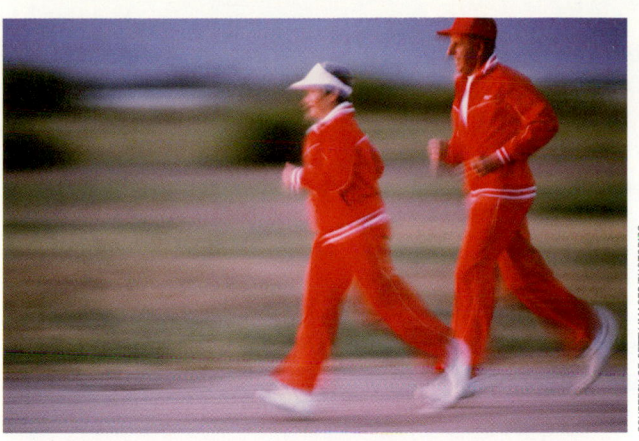
COURTESY OF GETTY IMAGES/PHOTODISC

FIGURE 10-11 **Healthy activities such as jogging enhance wellness in the middle-aged adult.**

OLDER ADULTHOOD STAGE

Older adulthood is development occurring from age 65 until death. Table 10-12 provides an overview of growth and development in the older adult. Table 10-13 lists common disorders of the older adult.

The CDC (2008) estimates that by 2030, the number of American older adults will more than double to 71 million people. This will be roughly 20% of the U.S. population. The CDC (2008b) states, "An enhanced focus on promoting and preserving the health of older adults is essential if we are to effectively address the health and economic challenges of the aging society" (p. 1). The demands associated with long-term care will pose one of the greatest challenges for both personal/family resources and public resources (CDC, 2003).

Older adults have several psychosocial tasks to accomplish, including:

- Accepting own life as it is (refer to Concept Map 10-1)
- Finding meaningful activities

TABLE 10-12 Older Adulthood: Growth and Development

DIMENSION	CHARACTERISTICS	NURSING CONSIDERATIONS
Physiological	*Respiratory changes:*	
	Respiratory muscles become less flexible resulting in decreased vital capacity of the lungs. Effectiveness of cough mechanism lessons. Alveoli thicken and decrease in size and number. Less effective gas exchange. Structural changes in the chest skeleton such as kyphosis can decrease diaphragmatic expansion.	Educate about the importance of obtaining a pneumovaccine and influenza vaccine. Assess lung sounds, effectiveness of cough mechanism, pulse oximetry, and need for oxygen therapy. Monitor for any signs of respiratory distress.
	Cardiovascular changes:	
	Cardiac output declines. Heart rate slows. Blood flow to all organs decreases. Arterial elasticity decreases causing increased peripheral resistance and a slight increase in systolic and diastolic blood pressure.	Arrange for and encourage regular blood pressure checks. Monitor for signs of fluid retention, and arterial and venous insufficiency. Assess apical and peripheral pulses. Educate the client about limiting dietary intake of fat, cholesterol, sodium, and alcohol. Recommend a smoking cessation program.
	Neurovascular changes:	
	Neurons in brain decrease in number. Decreased production of neurotransmitters. Cerebral blood flow and oxygen utilization decrease.	Monitor general health status. Assess client for cognitive changes. Assess for risk factors for stroke.
	Sensory changes:	
	Vision:	
	Lacrimal glands secrete less fluid causing dryness and itching. The lens becomes less pliable causing presbyopia and yellows resulting in distorted color perception. Accommodation of pupil size decreases. Vitreous humor changes cause blurred vision.	Encourage regular examination by an ophthalmologist. Ensure clients have their glasses on when needed.
	Hearing:	
	Cerumen (earwax) production increases. The number of neurons in the cochlea decrease and the blood supply lessons causing the cochlea and the ossicles to degenerate.	Encourage regular hearing testing by an audiologist. Assess for ear pain, drainage, and impacted cerumen. Ensure clients have their hearing aids in when needed.

(*Continues*)

Table 10-12 Older Adulthood: Growth and Development (Continued)

DIMENSION	CHARACTERISTICS	NURSING CONSIDERATIONS
Physiological (Continued)	*Gastrointestinal changes:*	
	Periodontal disease rate increases and tooth enamel thins. Effectiveness of gag reflex lessons. Esophageal peristalsis slows and hiatal hernia may occur. Gastric emptying slows and peristalsis decreases. Liver size and enzymes decrease, slowing drug metabolism.	Inspect the mouth regularly for signs of dental disorders. Assess nutritional status and gag reflex. Educate the client to avoid the overuse of laxatives. Discuss the importance of dietary fiber and exercise for regular bowel elimination.
	Urinary changes:	
	Glomerular filtration rate decreases resulting in decreased renal clearance of drugs. Bladder capacity decreases. Sodium conserving ability diminishes. Bladder and perineal muscles weaken. Prostate may enlarge.	Monitor fluid intake and output. Complete an assessment for bladder management and implement an appropriate bladder management program as needed. Teach and encourage client to empty the bladder every 3 to 4 hours. Offer absorbent incontinent pads or briefs.
	Integumentary changes:	
	Skin becomes thinner and less elastic. Wrinkles develop. Melanocytes diminish ability to produce even pigmentation, resulting in "age spots." Eccrine, apocrine, and sebaceous glands decrease in size, numbers, and function resulting in dry itchy skin. Body temperature regulation diminishes. Capillary blood flow decreases. Melanin production decreases causing gray-white hair. Facial hair growth occurs on upper lip and chin.	Ensure adequate intake of protein and fluids to promote good skin integrity. Assess client for risk of pressure ulcer formation.
	Musculoskeletal changes:	
	Bone demineralization occurs. Joints undergo degenerative changes. Muscle mass and elasticity diminish.	Assess dietary intake of calcium, protein and vitamin D. Teach, encourage, and assist clients to establish exercise programs appropriate to their capabilities. Teach the client and caregivers about measures to reduce the risk of falling and sustaining fractures.
	Endocrine changes:	
	Alterations occur in the production and reception of hormones. Thyroid changes lower the basal metabolic rate. Blood glucose levels may increase related to the slowing of insulin release by the beta cells of the pancreas.	Monitor for signs and symptoms of hypo-/hyperthyroidism. Assess for signs and symptoms of hypo-/hyperglycemia.
	Reproductive changes: *Women:*	
	Estrogen production decreases with the onset of menopause (the cessation of menses). Uterus, ovaries, and cervix decrease in size. Vaginal lining thins and vaginal secretions decrease. Breast tissue diminishes.	Teach and encourage monthly breast self-exams. Encourage annual gynecological examinations with primary care provider.
	Men:	
	Testosterone production decreases. Sperm count and viscosity of seminal fluid decreases. Prostate gland may enlarge. Impotency may occur.	Teach and encourage monthly testicular self-exams, and yearly digital rectal examinations of the prostate gland by a primary care provider.

TABLE 10-12 Older Adulthood: Growth and Development (Continued)

DIMENSION	CHARACTERISTICS	NURSING CONSIDERATIONS
Psychosocial	*Erikson:* integrity vs. despair stage Accepts own life as it is. A sense of worth is gained from helping others.	Seek the older person's advice. Identify and use the older adult's strengths. Advocate reminiscence. Encourage socialization with peers.
Cognitive	*Piaget:* formal operations stage No decline in IQ is associated with aging. Reaction time slows. *Memory:* *Short-term:* Capacity for recall decreases. *Long-term:* Capacity remains unchanged.	Allow time for responses. Watch for medication-induced confusion.
Moral	*Kohlberg:* postconventional stage Makes moral decisions to fit own principles and beliefs.	Support decision making. Respect values even when different from own.
Spiritual	*Fowler:* universalizing stage Generally satisfied with own spiritual beliefs and tends to act on beliefs.	Listen carefully to determine spiritual needs. Acknowledge losses and encourage appropriate grieving.

Data from Women's Health: *Health Promotion throughout the Lifespan* (7th ed.), by C. L. Edelman and C. L. Mandle, 2010, St. Louis, MO: Mosby Elsevier. Copyright 2010 by Mosby Elsevier; *Health Promotion Strategies through the Life Span* (8th ed.), by R. B. Murray and J. P. Zentner, 2008, Upper Saddle River, NJ: Prentice Hall. Copyright 2008 by Prentice Hall.

TABLE 10-13 Common Disorders of the Older Adult

Respiratory	Respiratory tract infection (RTI) Chronic obstructive pulmonary disease (COPD) Pulmonary tuberculosis (TB)
Cardiovascular	Peripheral vascular disease (PVD) Hypertension Chronic congestive heart failure (CHF)
Neurovascular	Dementia Alzheimer's Depression Transient ischemic attack (TIA)
Sensory	Presbyopia Cataract Glaucoma Hearing impairment
Gastrointestinal	Dental disorders Constipation Dehydration Over/undernutrition
Urinary	Incontinence Urinary tract infections
Integumentary	Skin cancer Pressure ulcers Herpes zoster (shingles)
Musculoskeletal	Osteoporosis Degenerative arthritis Fractured hip
Endocrine	Diabetes mellitus type 2 Hypo/Hyperthyroidism
Reproductive	*Women:* Breast cancer Uterine prolapse *Men:* Benign prostatic hypertrophy (BPH) Impotence

COURTESY OF DELMAR CENGAGE LEARNING

Client Scenerio

65-year-old male with Schizophrenia needs to achieve growth and development tasks for age

Assessment

Does client accept own life as it is?
Proud of current job and role in family
Does client express a sense of worth in helping others?
Minimal contact with others except through employment
Does client participate in meaningful activities?
Attends church, holds job, can read and write
Does client express adjustment to health issues?
Physical decline impacting ability to maintain employment and care for self
How does client cope with changes and losses?
No longer feels safe in own home
Has client planned for own death?
Unknown
Has IQ changed?
Unknown, sister assists with some tasks
Has reaction time slowed?
May need to retire related to physical decline
Assess short- and long-term recall
No identified changes noted
Does client express consistent moral principles and beliefs?
Attends church regularly
Does client express satisfaction with spiritual beliefs?
Attends church regularly
Is home environment safe?
Recently injured during mugging, verbalizes does not feel safe, lives in area with increased crime rate

Nursing Diagnosis

At risk for alteration in achieving age-related growth and development task related to declining physical ability.

Outcome

Growth and developmental tasks achieved as evidenced by:

1. Accepts life as is
2. Maintains current level of physical and cognitive health
3. Maintains current moral principle and beliefs
4. Maintains spiritual beliefs

Evaluation

1. Outcomes met
2. Maintains pride in current abilities including job, spiritual beliefs, and ability to read and write
3. Identifies methods to promote personal safety, attends medical appointments, and utilizes social agencies appropriately

Nursing Interventions

1. Explore with client/significant other (sister) physiological, psychosocial, cognitive, moral, and spiritual characteristics for age that may alter client's ability to achieve growth and developmental tasks.
2. Explore with client/significant other alternative solutions to identified actual or potential alterations in normal growth and developmental tasks.

Activities

1. Identification of risk factors

Activities

1. Compare alternative solutions
2. Refer client to health care providers or social agencies to facilitate achievement of growth and developmental tasks

CONCEPT MAP 10-1

COMMUNITY/HOME HEALTH CARE

Home Safety for Older Adults

Encourage the elderly client to make the home environment safe by:

- Ensuring adequate lighting
- Removing all throw or loose rugs
- Clearing all walking paths
- Having a handrail on all stairs
- Installing hand-holds in tubs and showers

- Adjusting to age- and health-related changes
- Coping with changes and losses
- Making preparations for death

Significance for Nursing

Nursing care is important in assisting the aging person to develop a sense of well-being (Eliopoulos, 2004). Nurses working with elderly clients must be aware of their own attitudes, feelings, and beliefs about aging and understand how these may affect care provided to these clients.

CRITICAL THINKING

Retirement

What factors affect an older adult's adjustment to retirement?

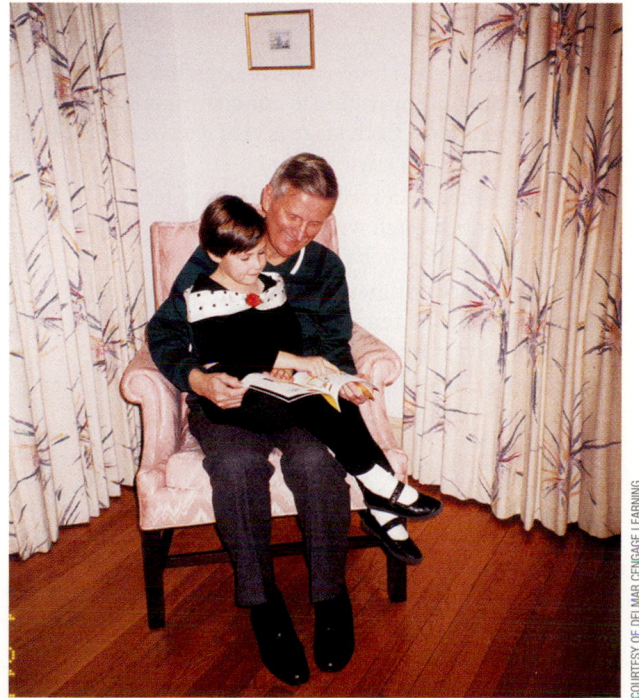

COURTESY OF DELMAR CENGAGE LEARNING

FIGURE 10-12 Older adults often experience more free time to participate in enjoyable and satisfying activities.

LIFE SPAN CONSIDERATIONS

Urinary Tract Infections in Older Adults

The older adult frequently does not present with the usual signs and symptoms of a urinary tract infection (UTI). Falling or signs of acute confusion (more than usual) may often be the major clinical manifestations.

Older adults assume new roles such as grandparents. They enjoy spending time with family and friends sharing stories, family history, and wisdom with the younger generation (Figure 10-12).

Assessment of the older adult should include the client's background, family history, work history, achievements, sense of self-worth (refer to Chapter 15 Self-Concept), and hobbies. Encourage clients to talk about their life experiences. Care is more likely to be individualized when the client's unique experiences and assets are recognized.

The issue of caregiving for the older adult has become a national health concern. The 2004 *Caregiving in the U.S.* report (CDC, 2008a) estimated that 44 million men and women provided unpaid care to an older adult family member, friend, or neighbor, resulting in an estimated economic value of $306 billion. Caregivers should be encouraged to respect the client's values, support decision making, encourage the client's socialization with peers, and assist the older adult in accomplishing psychosocial tasks within their developmental stage.

When clients express dissatisfaction and regrets about the past, listen in a nonjudgmental manner. Help older clients put disappointments into perspective by reviewing with them their achievements and accomplishments. Encourage family members to reminisce with the older client. Many nursing interventions for the older adult include introspection and reflection on their lives. Life review (or reminiscence therapy) promotes a positive self-concept in older people.

Enhancing Wellness Health-promotion activities should focus on maintaining functional independence

PROFESSIONAL TIP

Polypharmacy

A challenge for many older adults is that side effects from one medication are often treated with another prescription medication. If a client then goes to a different physician, he may prescribe even more medication to address the same or other health concerns. This is called **polypharmacy,** the problem of clients taking numerous prescription and over-the-counter medications for the same or various disease processes, with unknown consequences from the resulting combinations of chemical compounds and cumulative side effects.

and maximizing abilities and strengths. Independent, older adults are generally healthier. Specific topics for discussion with older clients are regular physical activity, use of leisure time, increased socialization, maintaining a positive mental attitude, and adequate nutrition. Encourage the client to obtain influenza and pneumococcal immunizations as recommended and confirm currency of Td immunization.

Safety Concerns Falls pose a major health threat to elderly persons. Teach ways to minimize risk of falling. Confusion with complicated medication regimens causes problems for many elderly. Emerging technology is producing many assistive devices related to safe medication administration.

CRITICAL THINKING

Driving Issues

A 92-year-old female client informs you that her family is planning on moving her into an assisted living apartment. She is alert and oriented and in good physical health. Her family insists that she sell her car before moving. The client adamantly wants to take her car with her, and the assisted living apartment has parking spaces available for residents. Should the client take her car with her to the assisted living apartment? Why or why not? What factors should be taken into consideration when making this decision? How would you handle this situation if the client were your mother?

CASE STUDY

C.W., a 68-year-old female, was admitted to the skilled care facility for rehabilitation following an open reduction internal fixation (ORIF) of the left hip. C.W. had fallen while going down the porch steps in front of her home, suffering a fracture of the left femur. She has no recollection of what caused her to fall. She is widowed and volunteers part time at the local library. While in the hospital, C.W. exhibited signs of disorientation and confusion.

Her family reports that she has never had this problem before and has been in good health until the fall. C.W. and her family agree that she will return home after rehabilitation is complete.

1. Write a nursing diagnosis and goal for C.W.
2. List three nursing interventions related to altered mental status.
3. List two outcomes for C.W.
4. Develop a teaching plan for C.W.

SUMMARY

- Growth is the measurable changes in physical size, and development refers to behavioral changes in functional abilities and skills.
- Growth and development of an individual are influenced by heredity, life experiences, health status, and cultural expectations.
- Maturation is the process of becoming fully grown and developed both physically and behaviorally.
- Certain developmental tasks must be achieved during each developmental stage for normal development to occur.
- According to Freud, repressed sexual problems in childhood cause problems later in life.
- Erikson explains that psychosocial development is a series of conflicts occurring during eight stages of life.
- Piaget's theory cites four stages of cognitive development: sensorimotor, preoperational, concrete operations, and formal operations. Each stage is characterized by how the child interprets the environment.
- Kohlberg's theory describes six stages of moral development through which individuals develop a moral code to guide their behavior.
- Fowler's theory outlines six distinct stages of faith development. The sequence remains the same, but the age at which each stage is experienced varies.
- Promoting the health and safety of individuals at each stage of life is an important role for nurses.

REVIEW QUESTIONS

1. The nurse has assessed four children of varying ages. Which one requires further evaluation?
   1. A 5 month old who eats rice cereal.
   2. A 2 year old who is not potty trained.
   3. A 7 year old with a casted broken leg from skateboarding.
   4. A 15 year old who is neglecting personal hygiene.

2. Nursing interventions that enhance neonatal wellness include: (Select all that apply.)
   1. conducting screening tests.
   2. providing a warm environment.
   3. limiting visitation by siblings.
   4. providing a sterile environment.
   5. promoting early parent–neonate interaction.
   6. monitoring nutritional status.
3. The nurse is teaching safety information to the mother of a 22-month-old toddler. Which of the following actions by the mother indicates understanding of the safety needs of a toddler?
   1. Placing a gate at the top of the stairs.
   2. Securing the seat belt properly across the toddler's lap.
   3. Placing all medication on the top shelf of the medication cabinet.
   4. Checking toys for lead-based paint.
4. When a school-aged child experiences changes in height, weight, bone density, and dental structure, this is known as:
   1. accommodation.
   2. critical period.
   3. growth.
   4. assimilation.
5. During this stage of cognitive development, the client's imagination flourishes, thinking begins using representational thought, and events are interpreted in relation to the client's self:
   1. sensorimotor.
   2. preoperational.
   3. formal operational.
   4. concrete operational.
6. During the admission health history, the 22-year-old client informs the nurse that he has been having "safe sex" with his girlfriend for 2 years. This indicates that the client is in which stage of Freud's psychosexual development?
   1. Anal.
   2. Phallic.
   3. Latency.
   4. Genital.
7. A client who graduated from law school and who is beginning her career as a lawyer is in which stage of Erikson's psychosocial development?
   1. Identity vs. role confusion.
   2. Industry vs. inferiority.
   3. Intimacy vs. isolation.
   4. Integrity vs. despair.
8. Respecting authority, believing in rules, seeking approval of others through actions, and maintaining cordial interpersonal relationships occurs in which level of Kohlberg's moral development theory?
   1. Conventional.
   2. Preconventional.
   3. Postconventional.
   4. Preoperational.
9. A 70-year-old client has noticed that his short-term memory recall has decreased, but IQ and long-term memory recall have remained unchanged. Which stage of Piaget's theory is this client in?
   1. Formal operational.
   2. Concrete operational.
   3. Latency operational.
   4. Integrity operational.
10. An 81-year-old client is informed that she has terminal cancer. When her physician leaves the room, she begins to cry and expresses dissatisfaction and regrets about her past to the nurse. Appropriate nursing interventions at this time include all the following except:
    1. listening in a nonjudgmental manner.
    2. contacting hospice to make arrangements for impending death.
    3. providing uninterrupted time for the client to discuss her concerns.
    4. offering to contact the client's religious counselor.

REFERENCES/SUGGESTED READINGS

American Academy of Child and Adolescent Psychiatry. (2008a). Teenagers with eating disorders. Available: http://www.aacap.org/publications/factsfam/eating.htm

American Academy of Child and Adolescent Psychiatry. (2008b). Teen suicide. Available: http://www.aacap.org/publications/factsfam/suicide.htm

American Academy of Pediatrics. (2007). Adolescent health: critical adolescent health issues—Sexual health. Retrieved November 30, 2008, from http://www.aap.org/sections/adolescenthealth/sexualhealth.cfm

American Academy of Pediatrics. (2008a). Adolescent health. Available: http://www.aap.org/advocacy/washing/chiah/htm

American Academy of Pediatrics (AAP). (2008b). Puberty—Ready or not expect some changes. Available: http://www.aap.org/healthtopics/stages.cfm#adol

American Cancer Society. (2003). *Cancer facts and figures 2003.* Atlanta: Author.

American Cancer Society. (2008). What are the key statistics about squamous and basal cell skin cancer? Retrieved August 30, 2009 from http://www.cancer.org/docroot/CRI/content/CRI_2_4_1X_What_are_the_key_statistics_for_skin_cancer_51.asp?sitearea=

Beare, P. & Myers, J. (1998). *Adult health nursing* (3rd ed.). St. Louis, MO: Mosby.

Bradley-Springer, L. (2001). HIV prevention: What works? *American Journal of Nursing, 101*(6), 45–48.

Centers for Disease Control and Prevention. (2002). AIDS falls from top ten causes of death; teen births, infant mortality, homicides all decline; Updated November 30, 2008. Available: http://www.cdc.gov/od/oc/media/pressrel/r981007.htm

Centers for Disease Control and Prevention. (2003). Public health and aging: Trends in aging—United States and worldwide. *Morbidity and Mortality Weekly Report, 52*(06), 101–106. Retrieved December 14, 2008, from http://www.cdc.gov/mmwr/preview/mmwrhtml/mm5206a2.htm

Centers for Disease Control and Prevention. (2007). Trends in reportable sexually transmitted diseases in the United States, 2006. Retrieved November 30, 2008, from http://www.cdc.gov/std/stats/trends2006.htm

Centers for Disease Control and Prevention. (2008a). Assuring healthy caregivers, a public health approach to translating research into practice: The RE-AIM framework. Retrieved December 14, 2008, from http://www.cdc.gov/aging/caregiving/index.htm

Centers for Disease Control and Prevention. (2008b). The state of aging and health in America 2007 report. Retrieved December 14, 2008, from http://www.cdc.gov/aging/saha.htm

Centers for Disease Control and Prevention. (2008c). Teen pregnancy. Retrieved November 30, 2008, from http://www.cdc.gov/reproductivehealth/AdolescentReproHealth

Connell, R. (2005). Japan messes up with potty training. Retrieved June 21, 2009, from http://www.deeker.com/Articles/japan_messes_up_with_potty_training.html

Edelman, C. & Mandle, C. (2010). *Health promotion throughout the lifespan* (7th ed.). St. Louis, MO: Mosby Elsevier.

Eliopoulos, C. (2004). *Gerontological nursing* (6th ed.). Philadelphia: Lippincott Williams & Wilkins.

Erikson, E. (1968). *Childhood and society.* New York: Norton.

Estes, M. (2010). *Health assessment and physical examination* (4th ed.). Clifton Park, NY: Delmar Cengage Learning.

Firth, P. & Watanabe, S. (1996). *Women's health: Instant nursing assessment.* Clifton Park, NY: Delmar Cengage Learning.

Fowler, J. (1995). *Stages of faith: The psychology of human development and the quest for meaning.* New York: Harper & Row.

Freud, S. (1961). *Civilization and its discontents.* New York: Norton.

Fuller, J. & Schaller-Ayers, J. (2000). *Health assessment: A nursing approach* (3rd ed.). Philadelphia: Lippincott Williams & Wilkins.

Guyton, A. & Hall, J. (2002). *Textbook of medical physiology* (10th ed.). Philadelphia: W. B. Saunders.

Hockenberry, M. & Wilson, D. (2007). *Wong's nursing care of infants and children* (8th ed.). St. Louis, MO: Mosby Elsevier.

Kimbell, S. (2001). Before the fall: Keeping your patient on his feet. *Nursing2001, 31*(8), 44–45.

Kohlberg, L. (1977). *Recent research in moral development.* New York: Holt, Rinehart and Winston.

Levinson, D. (1978). *The seasons of a man's life.* New York: Knopf.

Mayo Clinic. (2008). Children's snacks: 20 tips for healthier snacking. Retrieved December 17, 2008, from http://www.mayoclinic.com/health/childrens-health/HQ00419

Mohr, W. (2009). *Psychiatric-mental health nursing* (7th ed.). Philadelphia: Lippincott Williams & Wilkins.

Murray, R. & Zentner, J. (2008). *Health promotion strategies through the life span* (8th ed.). Upper Saddle River, NJ: Prentice Hall.

Norimatsu, H. (2006). Development of child autonomy in eating and toilet training: One to-three-year-old Japanese and French children. *Early Development and Parenting,* 2(1), 39–50. Retrieved June 22, 2009, from http://www3.interscience.wiley.com/journal/112465782/abstract

Overman, B. (2009). *Older adult concept care map.* Lima, OH.

Piaget, J. (1963). *The origins of intelligence in children.* New York: Norton.

Spangler, A. (2009). Breastfeeding in a bottle-feeding culture. Retrieved June 21, 2009, from http://www.breastfeeding.com/reading_room/bottle_culture.html

World Health Organization. (2008a). The global burden of disease: 2004 update. Retrieved November 30, 2008, from http://www.who.int/child_adolescent_health/media/causes_death_u5_neonates_2004.pdf

World Health Organization. (2008b). Vaccines to prevent pneumonia and improve child survival. Retrieved November 30, 2008, from http://www.who.int/bulletin/volumes/86/5/07-044503/en/index.html

RESOURCES

American Academy of Pediatrics, http://www.aap.org

American Association of Retired Persons, http://www.aarp.org

American Foundation for Suicide Prevention, http://www.afsp.org

American Society on Aging, http://www.asaging.org

Centers for Disease Control and Prevention (CDC), http://www.cdc.gov

Gerontological Society of America, http://www.geron.org

National Institute of Child Health and Human Development, http://www.nichd.nih.gov

Zero to Three: National Center for Infants, Toddlers and Families, http://www.zerotothree.org

CHAPTER 11
Cultural Considerations

MAKING THE CONNECTION

Refer to the following chapters to increase your understanding of cultural considerations and nursing:

Basic Nursing

- ***Holistic Care***
- ***Legal and Ethical Responsibilities***
- ***Communication***
- ***Wellness Concepts***
- ***Spirituality***
- ***Complementary/Alternative Therapies***
- ***Pain Management***

LEARNING OBJECTIVES

Upon completion of this chapter, you should be able to:

- Define key terms.
- Describe the characteristics and components of culture.
- Discuss the impact of cultural beliefs on illness and health.
- Compare and contrast diverse health beliefs of major cultural groups in the United States.
- Describe cultural differences in relation to time and space.
- Identify nutritional preferences held by various cultural groups.
- Identify the general beliefs that account for the differences among religions.
- Describe the way that the nurse's religious beliefs or lack thereof influences nursing care.
- Discuss the nurse's role in meeting the spiritual needs of the client and family.
- Analyze personal values and cultural beliefs.
- Perform a cultural assessment.

KEY TERMS

acculturation
agnostics
atheists
cultural assimilation
cultural diversity
culture
dominant culture
ethnicity
ethnocentrism
minority group
oppression
race
religious support system
spiritual care
spiritual needs
stereotyping
yin and yang

INTRODUCTION

Every aspect of a person's life—including attitudes, values, and beliefs—is influenced by that person's culture. Behavior, including behavior affecting health, is culturally determined. Recognition of cultural differences and their impact on health care becomes even more critical as the population of the United States continues to diversify. Because nurses provide health care to culturally diverse client populations in various settings, knowledge of culturally relevant information is essential for delivery of competent nursing care. This chapter discusses the various concepts related to culture, the influence of culture on health, the relationships between culture and health beliefs, cultural aspects and the nursing process, and illnesses associated with ethnic groups.

CULTURE

Each individual is culturally unique. A person's culture, as influenced by life experiences, education, and creative thought, is the lens through which a person sees everything. The nurse needs a thorough understanding of cultural concepts to provide holistic care.

In society, **culture** refers to an integrated dynamic structure of knowledge, attitudes, behaviors, beliefs, ideas, habits, customs, languages, values, symbols, rituals, and ceremonies that are unique to a particular group of people. This structure provides the group of people with a general design for living.

Individuals often acquire cultural beliefs unconsciously throughout the process of growth and maturation (Giger & Davidhizar, 2004). People are exposed to culture at an early age through the observance of traditions (established customary patterns of thought and behavior). Cultural beliefs, values, customs, and behaviors are transmitted from one generation to another through interaction, daily activities, and celebrations. For instance, the birth of a child is celebrated according to the family's cultural norms and customs, which may include prayers, blessings, special naming ceremonies, religious rites, and so forth. Parents, grandparents, and other elders all teach children cultural norms and expectations through demonstration, discussion, and role modeling (Figure 11-1).

Culture is not static, nor is it uniform among all members within a given cultural group. Culture represents adaptive dynamic processes learned through life experiences. Diversity among and within cultural groups results from individual perspectives and practices. Consider, for example, the way that a family deals with a crisis. A crisis may cause a family that is part of a culture with a strong sense of responsibility to family and blood relatives to become closer; conversely, the same situation may cause a family that is from a culture that values independence and individuality to withdraw and create distance among its members. These reactions are rooted in the family's cultural background and heritage.

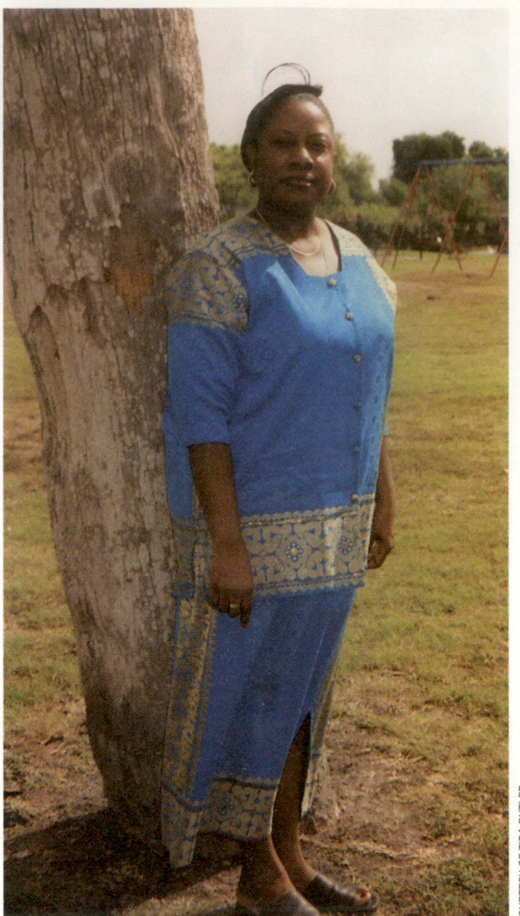

COURTESY OF TIRA BUTLER

FIGURE 11-1 This woman celebrates her African American heritage when wearing this ethnic dress.

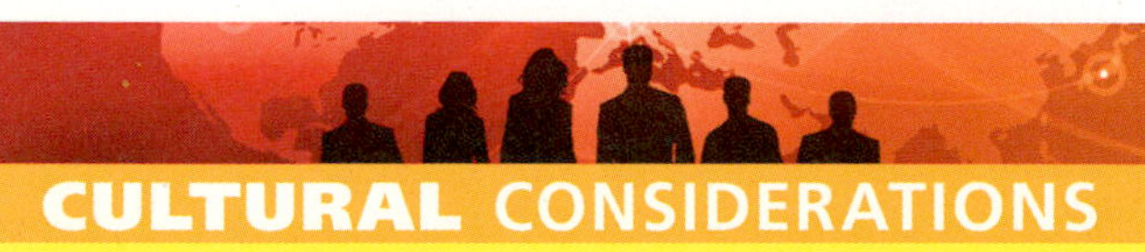

CULTURAL CONSIDERATIONS

Sharing Culture

Cultural messages are transmitted in a variety of settings, such as homes, schools, religious organizations, and communities. The various media, such as radio and television, are also powerful transmitters and shapers of culture.

ETHNICITY AND RACE

Ethnicity is a cultural group's perception of itself, or a group identity. Ethnicity is a common social heritage providing a sense of belonging that is passed from one generation to the next. Members of an ethnic group display their sense of identity through common traits and customs. Ethnic identity can be expressed in many ways, including dress; for instance, many African Americans display ethnic pride by choosing clothing that highlights their ethnic origin and shared heritage.

Race is a group of people with biological similarities. Members of a racial group have similar physical characteristics, such as facial features and color of hair, eyes, and skin. Racial and ethnic groups often overlap because the cultural and biological commonalities support one another (Giger & Davidhizar, 2004). The similarities of racial and ethnic group members reinforce a sense of identity and cohesiveness.

CULTURAL DIVERSITY

Cultural diversity refers to the differences among people resulting from ethnic, racial, and cultural variations. A variety of rich cultural heritages exists within the United States. The sociopolitical climate is enriched by this vast potential of human resources with divergent viewpoints and behaviors. A diverse population provides varied ideas, viewpoints, and problem-solving approaches and an expectation of increased tolerance.

Living and working in such a culturally diverse society has some disadvantages. Problems arise when differences between and within cultural groups are not understood. Apprehension and turmoil often accompany people's expectations of others.

Some cultural groups have historically experienced prejudice or bias in the form of racism (discrimination based on race and biological differences). Individuals may experience sexism (discrimination based on gender) and classism (prejudice based on perceived social class). Society perpetuates these biases consciously or unconsciously. The underlying premise is that one way is superior and that every other way is inferior. **Ethnocentrism**, the assumption of cultural superiority and inability to accept another culture's ways, results in oppression. When the rules, values, and ideals of one group are imposed on another group, it is termed **oppression**. Oppression is based on cultural biases, which stem from beliefs, expectations, and traditions.

Stereotyping is the belief that all people within the same ethnic, racial, or cultural group will act the same way, sharing the same beliefs and attitudes. Stereotyping results in labeling people according to cultural preconceptions, thereby ignoring individual identity.

The group whose values prevail within a given society is the **dominant culture**. The dominant culture of the United States is composed of white, middle-class Protestants of European ancestry. The European values have greatly influenced U.S. culture.

These dominant values may conflict with the values of minority groups. A **minority group** is a group of people constituting less than a numerical majority of the population. Such groups are often labeled and treated differently from others in the society. Minority groups are generally considered to have less power than the dominant group (Giger & Davidhizar, 2004).

CULTURAL CONSIDERATIONS

Individuality

Remember that each person is first and foremost an individual and second a member of a cultural group. Although similarities may exist within an ethnic or culture group, individual differences are respected.

When people assume the characteristics of the dominant culture, it is called **acculturation** (the process of learning beliefs, norms, and behavioral expectations of a group). **Cultural assimilation** happens when members of a minority group are absorbed by the dominant culture, taking on the characteristics of the dominant culture.

CULTURE'S COMPONENTS

Stewart identified five components of culture that establish the way people think about life (as cited in Lock, 1992):

- *Perception of self and the individual:* Refers to personal identity, respect for individuals, and value
- *Motivation:* Explains the methods and value of achievement
- *Activity:* Identifies the ways people organize and value work
- *Social relations:* Explains the structure and importance of gender roles, friendships, and class
- *Perception of the world:* Indicates the explanation of religious beliefs and life events

These concepts are particularly helpful to the nurse when planning care for a client from another cultural group. Self-identity, social relationships, work, success, and religion influence the cultural group's definition of health and illness and the response to health events. For example, if a culture values relationships more than work, the culture may sanction an extended period of illness and a lengthy time away from the employment site; however, if a culture measures achievement by output at work, illness may be interpreted negatively. Members of the latter culture may deny illness and delay seeking appropriate health care.

CULTURE'S CHARACTERISTICS

Leninger (2002) has identified certain characteristics shared by all cultures:

- Culture is "learned behavior." Behavior patterns are picked up as children imitate adults and develop actions and attitudes acceptable in society.
- Culture is a "reflection of shared beliefs." Cultural beliefs are widely known and adopted. The beliefs and values of the group "guide human thought and action."
- Culture defines acceptable behavior. Behavioral patterns are not individually defined but rather are defined, accepted, and practiced by everyone who belongs to the cultural group. Everyone in the cultural group understands acceptable behavior.
- Culture is dynamic. New ideas experienced by each generation may lead to different standards of behavior.
- Culture is an observance of traditions. Traditional observances, ceremonies, and food festivities connect the family and bind group relationships.

CULTURAL INFLUENCES ON HEALTH CARE BELIEFS AND PRACTICES

Culture influences health care decisions and practices and determines the way we react to illness and pain. In cultures where raw foods are not consumed, for instance, the

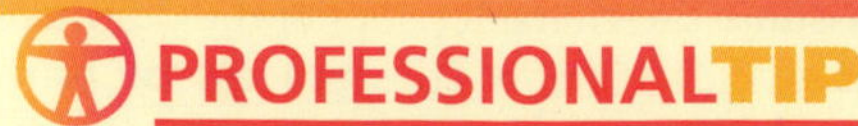

Cultural Sensitivity

Nurses who are culturally competent provide culturally appropriate care to a diverse population of clients. Cultural diversity presents special challenges for nurses who provide care that is incongruent with personal beliefs and values. Culturally sensitive nurses caring for clients who differ from themselves remember to find out how the client views the event (illness), including the significance (meaning) that the client assigns the event. The culturally diverse nurse honors individual differences.

incidence of shigellosis may be lower than cultures where consumption of raw meat and fish is common. On the other hand, cultural taboos against eating protein during pregnancy have a harmful or destructive effect on fetal development. Cultural values define human responses to illness and determine whether an individual will seek professional care when ill and comply with prescribed treatment.

Beliefs and patterns of behavior affect attitudes about various aspects of health. Beliefs about the definition of health, etiology (cause and origin of disease), health promotion and protection practices, and health practitioners and remedies are all influenced by cultural background. Clients tend to define wellness and illness in the context of their own culture.

Definition of Health

The most widely accepted definition of health, developed by the World Health Organization (WHO), states that health is not only the absence of disease but also complete physical, mental, and social wellness. While this definition of health is broad enough to be global, the physical, mental, and social dimensions are culturally defined. Any deviation from that which is culturally understood to be normal health is considered illness. For example, a biological disease of immediate etiology might not be interpreted as an illness by some cultures; intestinal parasites are so common in some areas in Africa that the presence of ascaris in stools is considered normal. If a cultural group does not perceive certain symptoms or behaviors as illness, members are not likely to seek medical care when these symptoms appear. In this situation, disease conditions may persist untreated, resulting in permanent damage or even death.

Etiology

The noted medical anthropologist Peter Morley presents four views of the origin of disease: supernatural, nonsupernatural, immediate, and ultimate (Morley & Wallis, 1978). The supernatural view of disease traces diseases to metaphysical forces such as witchcraft, sorcery, and voodoo. An individual with this view might attribute illness to evil spirits or to a curse by a powerful spiritual person. The nonsupernatural view holds that diseases have an accepted cause-and-effect relationship, even though that relationship may lack scientific rationale. For example, people of many cultures believe that colic in an infant is caused by breast milk rendered impure when a nursing mother has sexual relations. In such cultures, sexual relations are prohibited for nursing mothers. The immediate view of disease traces diseases to known pathogenic agents, such as chickenpox being caused by *Herpes varicella*, and the ultimate view describes determinates for diseases, such as smoking resulting in lung cancer. Most cultural groups support a multietiologic origin, believing there may be three or four explanations as to why and how diseases occur.

Health Promotion and Protection

Strategies for achieving and maintaining good health vary by cultural group. For example, the dominant U.S. culture has come to endorse a low-fat, high-fiber diet; regular exercise; and appropriate immunizations as means to promote and protect health. Other cultures may place greater value on prayer, meditation, and restored relationships, particularly in those cultures where disease prevention and health maintenance are closely linked to beliefs about disease etiology. For example, disease prevention may require paying homage to ancestral spirits to avoid offending them and seeking their revenge through illness.

Practitioners and Remedies

Variety in health/illness care providers is a natural extension of culturally diverse concepts of etiology and definitions of health and illness. Standard medicine may not be accepted as treatment when a scientific rationale for the etiology of disease is not accepted by a cultural group. Alternative remedies and practitioners are often found in culturally diverse groups. In order to enhance client compliance with treatment regimens, health care providers must make efforts to base therapy and prescribe treatments that respect culturally traditional remedies. Clients who trace disease etiology to a supernatural cause are more likely to seek interventions from spiritual leaders or traditional healers.

The folk medicine system categorizes illnesses as either natural or unnatural (Giger & Davidhizar, 2004). The classification of an illness determines the type of treatment and healer used. Because the folk medicine system (also referred to as alternative medicine) can present challenges to nurses caring for clients from diverse cultures, knowledge of basic beliefs about illness, factors contributing to illness, and home remedies is necessary.

Folk healers are knowledgeable about cultural norms and customs (Edelman & Mandle, 2005). Table 11-1 lists the various healers within the five dominant cultural groups in the United States (European American, African American, Hispanic American, Asian American, and Native American) and the common folk healing practices within these cultures. Nurses must be able to relate care and treatment to the client's cultural context and incorporate informal caregivers, healers, and other members of the client's support system as allies in treatment.

TABLE 11-1 Cultural Groups in Communication, Relationships, Health Values and Beliefs, and Health Practices

CULTURAL GROUP	COMMUNICATIONS STYLES	FAMILY, SOCIAL, AND WORK RELATIONSHIPS	HEALTH VALUES AND BELIEFS	HEALTH CUSTOMS AND PRACTICES
Asian-American				
Chinese	Nonverbal and contextual cues important. Silence after a statement is used by a speaker who wishes the listener to consider the importance of what is said. Self-expression repressed. Value silence. Touching limited. May smile when do not understand. Hesitant to ask questions.	Hierarchical, extended family pattern. Deference to authority figures and elders. Both parents make decisions about children. Value self-reliance and self-restraint. Important to preserve family's honor and save face. Value working hard and giving to society.	Health viewed as gift from parents and ancestors and the result of a balance between the energy forces of *yin* (cold) and *yang* (hot). Illness caused by an imbalance. Blood is the source of life and cannot be regenerated. Lack of blood and chi (innate energy) produces debilitation and long illness. Respect for the body and belief in reincarnation dictates that one must die with the body intact. Believe a good physician can accurately diagnose an illness by simply examining a person using the senses of sight, smell, touch, and listening.	May use medical care system in conjunction with Chinese methods of acupuncture (a *yin* treatment consisting of the insertion of needles to meridians to cure disease or relieve pain) and moxibustion (a *yang* treatment during which heated, pulverized wormwood is applied to appropriate meridians to assist with labor and delivery and other yin disorders). Medicinal herbs, e.g., ginseng, are widely used. Fear painful, intrusive diagnostic tests, especially the drawing of blood. May refuse intrusive surgery or autopsy. May be distrustful of physicians who order and use painful or intrusive diagnostic tests. Accept immunizations as valid means of disease prevention. Heavy use of condiments such as mono-sodium glutamate and soy sauce.
Japanese	Attitude, action, and feeling more important than words. Tend to listen empathically. Touching limited. Direct eye contact considered a lack of respect. Stoic, suppress overt emotion. Value self-control, politeness, and personal restraint.	Close, interdependent, intergenerational relationships. Individual needs subordinate to family's needs. Will endure great hardship to ensure success of next generation. Belonging to right clique or society important to status and success. Obligation to kin and work group. Education highly valued.	Believe illness caused by contact with polluting agents (e.g., blood, skin diseases, corpses), social or family disharmony, or imbalance from poor health habits. Cleanliness highly valued.	Tend to rely on Euro-American medical system for preventive and illness care. Oldest adult child responsible for care of elderly. Care of disabled is a family's responsibility. Take pride in good health of children. Believe in removal of diseased areas. Practice of emotional control may make pain assessment more difficult. When visiting ill, often bring fruit or special Japanese foods.

(*Continues*)

TABLE 11-1 Cultural Groups in Communication, Relationships, Health Values and Beliefs, and Health Practices (Continued)

CULTURAL GROUP	COMMUNICATIONS STYLES	FAMILY, SOCIAL, AND WORK RELATIONSHIPS	HEALTH VALUES AND BELIEFS	HEALTH CUSTOMS AND PRACTICES
Vietnamese	Respect and harmony most important values. Disrespectful to question authority figures. Avoid direct eye contact. Strong focus on respect through use of titles and terms indicating family and generational relationships. Modesty of speech and action valued. Relaxed concept of time; punctuality less significant than propriety. Use Ya to indicate listening, not understanding. Avoid asking direct questions.	Family close, multigenerational, and primary social network. Filial piety of primary importance. Father is family decision maker. Individual needs are subordinate to family's needs. Training of children shared by extended family. Behavior of individual reflects on total family. Education highly valued.	Believe illness caused by naturalistic (bad food, water), supernaturalistic (punishment for displeasing a deity), metaphysical (imbalance of hot and cold) forces, or from contamination by germs.	Often use both folk and some parts of the scientific health care system such as drugs. Family orally transmits folk medicine information. Health care regarded as family responsibility. Use medicinal herbs, therapeutic diets, hygienic measures to promote health, prevent illness, and treat illness. All means and resources available to family are tried before seeking outside help. Folk care practices include cao gio (rubbing skin with coin) for respiratory illnesses, bat gil (skin pinching) for headaches, inhalation of aromatic oils and liniments for respiratory and gastrointestinal illnesses. May consult priest, astrologer, shaman, or fortune-teller for prediction or instruction about health, or use hot and cold foods and substances to restore balance.
Filipinos	Personal dignity and preserving self-esteem highly valued. Nonverbal communication important. Eye contact avoided. Avoid direct expressions of disagreement, particularly with authority figures. Sex, socioeconomic status, and tuberculosis too personal to discuss. Need to engage in "small talk" before discussing more serious matters.	Multigenerational matrifocal family with strong family ties. Avoid behavior that shames family. Defer to elderly. Individual interests subordinate to family's interests. Value interpersonal relationships over current events.	Tend to believe illness is related to natural (unhealthy environment), supernatural (God's will and providence), and metaphysical (imbalance between hot and cold) forces. Tend to be fatalistic in outlook on life.	If accessible, may use both folk and scientific medical systems. Folk practices include flushing (stimulating perspiration, vomiting, bowel evacuation), heating (hot and cold substances to maintain internal body temperature), and protection (use of amulets, good luck pieces, religious medals, pictures, statues). Tend to be stoic; believe pain is God's will and He will give one the strength to bear it.

Black Americans				
African Americans	Many have high level of caution or distrust of majority group. Expressive use of nonverbal behavior and speech. Many use an English dialect: "black English." Very sensitive to lack of congruence between verbal and nonverbal messages. Value direct eye contact. May "test" health professionals before submitting self to decisions and care of the majority group's health care providers.	Strong kinship bonds in extended family. 50% patriarchical; 50% matriarchical families. Large social networks of family and unrelated members. Elderly members respected, particularly maternal grandparents. Strong sense of peoplehood; come to aid of others in crisis. Black minister a strong influence in community. Women protect health of family. Worth of education is judged by its "usability in living."	Illness is a collective event that disrupts the total family system. Illness believed to be a natural event resulting from conflict or disharmony in one's life, failure to protect oneself from cold air, pollution, food, and water, or sent by God as punishment. Those more assimilated to dominant culture perceive illness to be due to preventable injury or pathology.	Health is maintained by proper diet, rest, clean environment. Self-care and folk medicine (usually religious in origin) very prevalent. Individuals from more rural backgrounds are more likely to use folk practitioners. Attempt home remedies first; may not seek help from the medical establishment until illness serious; often will elect to retain dignity rather than seek care if values and sensibilities are demeaned. Prayer is common means for prevention and treatment. When ill or hospitalized, visits by family minister are sought, expected, and valued to help cope with illness and suffering.
Haitians	New immigrants and older persons often speak only Haitian Creole. Hand gesturing and tone of voice frequently used to complement speech. Smiling and nodding often do not indicate understanding. Direct eye contact used in formal and casual conversations. Unassertve—will not ask questions if health care provider appears busy or rushed.	Two-class social system: wealthy and poor. Rural and poor families tend to be matriarchical. Children taught unquestioning obedience to adults. Child-rearing shared by parents and older siblings. Tend to be status conscious, thus parents often choose children's mate to increase family status.	Illness believed to be caused by supernatural forces (angry spirits, enemies, or the dead) or natural forces (irregularities of blood volume, flow, viscosity, purity, color or temperature [hot and cold]; gas [*gaz*]; movement and consistency of mother's milk; hot/cold imbalance in the body; bone displacement). Believe health is a personal responsibility.	Use medical care and folk medicine simultaneously. Health maintained by good dietary and hygienic habits. Adherence to prescribed treatments directly related to perceived severity of illness; resist dietary and activity restrictions. Hot and cold and light and heavy properties of food are used to gain harmony with one's life cycle and bodily states. Natural illnesses are first treated by home remedies.

(*Continues*)

TABLE 11-1 Cultural Groups in Communication, Relationships, Health Values and Beliefs, and Health Practices (Continued)

CULTURAL GROUP	COMMUNICATIONS STYLES	FAMILY, SOCIAL, AND WORK RELATIONSHIPS	HEALTH VALUES AND BELIEFS	HEALTH CUSTOMS AND PRACTICES
Haitians *continued*	Touch is perceived as comforting, sympathetic, and reassuring.			Supernatural illnesses treated by healers; herbalist or leaf doctor (*dokte fey*), midwife (*fam saj*), or voodoo priest (*houngan*) or priestess (*mambo*). Use amulets and prayer to protect against supernatural illnesses.
Hispanic Americans				
Mexicans	Most bilingual; may use nonstandard English. Introductory embrace common. Tend to revert to native language in times of stress. Consider prolonged eye contact disrespectful but value direct eye contact. Appreciate "small talk" before initiating actual conversation topic. Appreciate a nondirective approach with open-ended questions. Hesitant to talk about sex but may do so more freely with nurse of same sex. Father should be present when speaking with a male child.	Strong kinship bonds among nuclear and extended families including *compadres* (godparents). Strong need for family group togetherness. Respect wisdom of elders. Children highly desired and valued; accompany family everywhere. Entire family contribute to family's financial welfare. Homes frequently decorated with statues, medals, and pictures of saints. Children often reluctant to share communal showers in schools. Relaxed concept of time.	Illness can be prevented by: being good, eating proper foods, and working proper amount of time; also accomplished through prayer, wearing religious medals or amulets, and sleeping with relics at home. Some believe illness is due to: body imbalance between *caliente* (hot) and *frio* (cold) or "wet" and "dry"; dislocation of parts of the body (*empacho*—ball of food stuck to the stomach wall or *caida de la mollera*—more serious, depression of fontanelle in infant); magic or supernatural (*mal ojo* [evil eye] or punishment from God); strong emotional state (*susto*—soul loss following an extreme fright); or *envidio* (success leads to envy by others resulting in misfortune). More concerned with present than with future and therefore may focus on immediate solutions rather than long-term goals. May view hospital as place to go to die.	Magico-religious practices common. Usually seek help from older women in family before going to a Jerbero, who specializes in the use of herbs and spices to restore balance/health, or curandero or curandera (holistic healers) with whom they have a uniquely personal relationship and share a common worldview. Prevent and treat illness with "hot" and "cold" food prescriptions and prohibitions. For severe illness, use scientific medical system but also make promises, visit shrines, use medals and candles, offer prayers—elements of Catholic and Pentecostal rituals and artifacts. Extreme modesty; may avoid seeking medical care and open discussions of sex. Children and adults expected to and do endure pain stoically.

Puerto Ricans	Older, newly moved to the mainland often speak only Spanish; others usually bilingual. May use nonstandard English. Personal and family privacy valued. Consider questions regarding family disrespectful and presumptuous. Tend to have a relaxed sense of time.	Paternalistic, hierarchical family; father is family provider and decision maker. Family of central importance. Families usually large. Parents demand absolute obedience and respect from children. Women in family tend to all ill members and dispense all medicines. Children valued—seen as gift from God.	Many believe illness is caused by imbalance of hot and cold, evil spirits, and forces. Many believe in spirits and spiritualism, having visions, and hearing voices. Accept many idiosyncratic behaviors; often perceive behavioral disturbances as symptoms of illness that need to be treated rather than judged. Suspicious and fearful of hospitals.	Use folk practitioners and medical establishment or both. When ill; first seek advice from women in family; if not sufficient, seek help from a senoria (woman especially knowledgeable about causes and treatment of common illnesses); if unable to help, consult an *espiritista*, *curandera*, or *santeria* (if psychiatric problem) who listens nonjudgmentally; often use herbs, lotions, salves, and massage and *caliente* (hot), *fresco* (cool), and *frio* (cold) treatments; if no relief, may go to a medical physician; if not satisfied, may return to any of the preceding.
Cuban American	Most new immigrants are bilingual. Expect some social talk before getting to actual reason for discussion.	Strong family and maternal and paternal kinship ties. Mother tends to explain and reason constantly to obtain child's conformity to family norms. Elderly cared for at home. Mother primary health care provider in home and must be included in all health education programs for family members. Children often supported and assisted by parents long after becoming adults. Extensive network of support for family and family members from social institutions such as schools, health clinics, and social clubs. Ambitious and take advantage of any opportunity to be successful in their work.	Believe good health results from prevention and good nutrition. Believe plump babies and young children are most healthy and admirable.	Combine use of medical practitioners with religious and nonreligious folk practitioners. Tend to be eclectic in health-seeking practices and, in some instances, may seek assistance of *santeros* (Afro-Cuban healers) and *espiritista* to complement treatment by medical practitioners. Parents very concerned about eating habits of their children; may spend a considerable part of the family budget on food.

(*Continues*)

TABLE 11-1 Cultural Groups in Communication, Relationships, Health Values and Beliefs, and Health Practices (Continued)

CULTURAL GROUP	COMMUNICATIONS STYLES	FAMILY, SOCIAL, AND WORK RELATIONSHIPS	HEALTH VALUES AND BELIEFS	HEALTH CUSTOMS AND PRACTICES
American Indians	Most speak their Indian language and English. Nonverbal communication important. Unwavering eye gaze viewed as insulting. Tend to take time to form an opinion of health professionals. Consider silence essential to understanding and respecting another. A pause following a question signifies that the question is important enough to be given thoughtful consideration. Hesitant to discuss personal affairs until trust is developed, which can take some time. Believe it is ethically wrong to speak for another person. Hesitant to talk about sex but may do so more freely with a nurse of the same sex. Sensitive about having their words and behavior written down.	Strong extended family and kinship structure—usually including relatives from both sides of the family. Believe family members are responsible for one another. Elder members greatly respected and assume leadership roles. Children valued. Children taught respect for traditions and to honor wisdom and those who possess it.	Medicine and religion strongly interwoven. Believe health results from being in harmony with nature and universe. Reject germ theory as cause of illness; believe every sickness and pain is a price to be paid for something that occurred in the past or will happen in the future. May carry object believed to guard against witchcraft.	Use total immersion in water, sweat lodges, and special rituals in the gathering, preparation, and use of herbs to regain harmony and thus health. Diviner-diagnosticians determine cause of illness, recommend treatment, and refer to a specific medicine man—diagnose but do not have powers or skill to implement medical treatment. Medicine man—traditional healer in whom most faith placed—uses herbs and special chants and rituals to cure illness. Singers effect cures by laying on of hands and by the power of the songs they obtain from supernatural beings.
Middle Eastern	Men and women do not shake hands or touch each other in any manner outside immediate family or marital relationship. Touching and embracing on arrival and on departure are common among same sex.	Providing family care and support is an important responsibility. Male-dominated. Eldest male is the decision maker. Male children valued more than females.	Magico-religious; follow will of Allah—passive role is norm. Various beliefs about the causes of disease coexist: "hot" and "cold" and "evil eye." Physically robust person considered healthier.	Use magico-religious, folk, self-care, and medical science. Use amulets inscribed with verses of the Koran, turquoise stones, charm of a hand with five fingers to enhance protective powers against evil eye.

Middle Eastern continued	Use silence to show respect for another.	Adult male must not be alone with any female except wife.	Emotional distress expressed as "heart disease." Obligation and responsibility to visit the sick, help others when they are ill, especially children and elderly. Expect immediate pain relief from health professionals.	Male health professionals prohibited from touching or examining a female patient. May refuse to have female health professionals care for males. The dead must be buried with the body intact. May perform female circumcision to ensure Muslim females become "good wives" and are accepted by other women in the family and community.
White Americans				
Euro-Americans (middle class)	Often separate into male and female groups at social events unless the activity is for couples. Nod to denote understanding or indicate agreement. Tend to maintain a "neutral" facial expression in public. Tolerate hugs and embraces among intimates and close friends. Pat on shoulder denotes camaraderie; firm handshake symbolic of goodwill. Good social manners include smiling, speaking pleasantly and warmly to put the other person at ease. Insist on own personal space.	Nuclear family professed norm. Two primary family goals: encourage and nurture each individual, produce healthy, autonomous children. Power more egalitarian. Socialize primarily with work-related and neighborhood friends. Generosity in time of crisis. Espouse the Protestant work ethic; work and plan for the future. Competitive and achievement oriented. Value education and knowledge from books as well as from experience.	Generally future oriented and believe one's internal and external environments can be controlled. Expect the most modern medical technology to be used when ill. Believe good health is a personal responsibility. Accept the germ theory and perceive illness to be the result of injury or pathology that can usually be prevented or contained through individual lifestyle and community health efforts.	Engage in self-care practices; strive for balanced diet, rest and activity, and work and leisure. Utilize self-care over-the-counter remedies for minor illnesses. Utilize medical health care system and health professionals for health screening, illness care, and follow-up. Intolerant of delays in health care services and of health professionals whose practices they believe are out of date. Read and access other media sources to increase understanding of risk factors, health promotion practices, and treatment techniques. Want to be consulted by health professionals before treatment is initiated but tend to accept health professionals' medical and health care judgments.

(*Continues*)

TABLE 11-1 Cultural Groups in Communication, Relationships, Health Values and Beliefs, and Health Practices (Continued)

CULTURAL GROUP	COMMUNICATIONS STYLES	FAMILY, SOCIAL, AND WORK RELATIONSHIPS	HEALTH VALUES AND BELIEFS	HEALTH CUSTOMS AND PRACTICES
Appalachian	Avoid answering questions related to income, children's school attendance, the affairs of others in the household and of neighbors. May consider direct eye contact impolite or aggressive. Uncomfortable with the impersonal and bureaucratic orientation of the American health system. May evaluate health professional on basis of interpersonal skills rather than on professional competence.	Community interdependence. Stay near home for protection. Keep ties with kin. Guard against strangers and outsiders. Kindness to others valued. Do more for others, less for self.	Disability an inevitable part of life and aging. Severity of illness perceived in terms of degree of dependency it necessitates during the period of illness. Believe cold and lack of personal care cause illness. Frugal; always use home remedies first. The hospital is "the place where people die."	Use folk practices "first and last." Rule for primary prevention: "eat right, take fluids, keep the body strong, stay warm when it's cold." Self-care for minor illnesses. Medical care for serious illnesses. Help from kin as needed for primary care. Help from family members and extended family expected and accepted.

Note: Used by permission from Estes, M., *Health Assessment & Physical Examination*, 4th edition (2010). Clifton Park, NY: Delmar Cengage Learning. Compiled from information in *Transcultural Nursing: Assessment and Intervention* (4th ed.), by J. N. Giger and R. E. Davidhizar, 2004, Baltimore: Mosby; *Transcultural Nursing: Concepts. Theory, Research, and Practice* (3rd ed.), by M. M. Leininger and M. McFarland, 2002, New York: McGraw-Hill Professional; *Pocket Guide to Cultural Assessment* (3rd ed.), by E. M. Geissler, 2003, Baltimore: Mosby-Year Book; *Cultural Diversity in Health and Illness* (6th ed.), by R. Spector, 2003, Norwalk, CT: Appleton & Lange; *Wong's Nursing Care of Infants and Children* (7th ed.), by D. L. Wong, M. J. Hockenberry, D. Wilson, M. L. Winkelstein, and N. E. Kline, 2003, Philadelphia: Mosby; *Transcultural Health Care: A Culturally Competent Approach* (2nd ed.), by L. Purnell and F. Paulanka, 2003, Philadelphia: F. A. Davis.

Beliefs of Select Cultural Groups

While the population of the United States encompasses innumerable ethnic groups, European Americans, African Americans, Hispanic Americans, Asian Americans, and Native Americans together represent a majority. These groups form the basis for the following brief discussion of specific health beliefs influenced by culture.

European American

In 2000, Americans of European descent represented 71% of the U.S. population (U.S. Census Bureau, 2001). The prevailing value system for many European Americans is based on what is referred to as the white, Anglo-Saxon, Protestant (WASP) ethic (Sue & Sue, 2007). This ethnic group traces its origins to the Caucasian Protestants who came to this country from northern Europe more than 200 years ago. Values that still dominate the Caucasian American middle-class ethic include independence, individuality, wealth, comfort, cleanliness, achievement, punctuality, hard work, aggression, assertiveness, rationality, orientation toward the future, and mastery of one's own fate (Andrews & Boyle, 2008; Edmission, 1997).

Traditionally, most Caucasian Americans have wanted to be recognized as individuals rather than as members of groups. Thus, Caucasian Americans, unlike members of many other cultures, tend to be competitive rather than cooperative with each other. Mainstream American culture also values the nuclear family and its traditions (Luckmann, 2000).

African American

The African American population in 2000 represented 12% of the U.S. population (U.S. Census Bureau, 2001). African American ancestors came to North America from various African countries and the Caribbean as either free immigrants or slaves. The heterogeneous (different) cultural practices among African Americans today may be explained by the diverse countries of origin, disparate educational levels, income, occupations, and religious beliefs.

Traditional African societies may believe that disease is caused by disharmony in relationships. Discord may occur between a client and evil spirits, living relatives, or ancestral spirits. Restoration of harmony may be achieved through prayer, meditation, or other activities, such as wearing a charm, offering a gift, or confessing a wrong, leading to healing.

Disease may be viewed as sent by God or another higher power as a punishment for a serious infraction. Evil forces may be thought to account for illness in other cases. Healing may be found in home remedies and herbs, consultation with a local healer, or prayer.

CULTURAL CONSIDERATIONS

Subculture

Many Caucasian Americans do not belong to the mainstream culture but instead belong to ethnic subcultures that hold strong values of their own (e.g., Irish, Jewish, German, Italian, Norwegian, Appalachian, and Amish subcultures).

Hispanic American

Hispanic Americans also represented 12% of the U.S. population in 2000 (U.S. Census Bureau, 2001). The majority of this group has origins in Mexico, Puerto Rico, and Cuba. Although the Spanish language is common to most Hispanics, cultural patterns vary according to the different countries of origin. The Hispanic American usually belongs to a large extended family system within which females are seen as subservient to males but as having a major role in family cohesiveness (Giger & Davidhizar, 2004).

In Hispanic populations the influence of religion on culture is particularly evident. Most Hispanic Americans have roots in Catholicism blended with traditional Indian beliefs. Illness may be viewed as "an act of God" as punishment for sin, as the result of witchcraft or a curse by an enemy, or as having a natural cause. Diseases may be traced to an imbalance between "hot" and "cold" or "wet" and "dry" forces. Treatment depends on the cause. Western medicine is believed to be appropriate for some diseases, whereas the native healer (curandera) may be called on to intervene for illnesses having supernatural causes. The elders of the community are valued for folk care knowledge, sometimes taking precedence over professional health care advice. Families have an obligation to care for the ill person. Treatment may consist of religious ceremonies, herbal potions, or diets based on hot and cold foods. If the Hispanic client wears an amulet, he believes that the removal of it precedes certain death. The amulet is believed to protect the person from external evils, and the person is reluctant to remove it.

Asian American

Asian Americans, representing 4% of the U.S. population in 2000 (U.S. Census Bureau, 2001), have origins in the Pacific Rim countries: China, Japan, Korea, Vietnam, Laos, the Philippines, and Cambodia. Generalization of a specific Asian culture is not possible; however, certain similarities do exist. Family relations are traced through males. Males as the head of household are the decision makers. Elders are revered and respected. Only physical complaints are acceptable, and maintaining eye contact is considered disrespectful (Estin, 1999).

Asians believe in yin (cold) and yang (hot) as etiology of disease. **Yin and yang** are opposing forces that yield health when in balance. An imbalance in these forces causes illness. Foods are identified as either hot or cold and are used in treatment. For example, if yang is overpowering yin, hot foods are avoided until balance is restored. Illness may be thought to be caused by supernatural powers such as God, ancestral spirits, or evil spirits. In this situation, healing is sought through prayer or treatment by a traditional healer. Many Asian Americans rely on acupuncture, herbal remedies, and cupping and burning. In cupping, the inside and rim of a cup are heated with a candle flame. Then the rim of the cup is applied directly to the client's skin. Blood is drawn to the surface of the skin as the cup cools, causing a bruised appearance. Cupping is used to draw out evil or illness in order to restore yin and yang. The nurse, aware of these cultural practices, views them not as abusive but as an important cultural custom.

Native American

Native Americans represented 1% of the U.S. population in 2000 (U.S. Census Bureau, 2001). These peoples form a very diverse group, descending from more than 200 different tribes across the United States. Although many Native Americans have assumed Euro-American practices with regard to health, some still use traditional practices. Health is believed to result from a harmonious relationship with nature and the universe. Illness is frequently traced to a supernatural origin and discord with the forces of nature. Using witchcraft is believed to cause illness, and treatment may require the exorcism of evil spirits. Disease prevention may be achieved through prayer, charms, and fetishes (objects having power to protect or aid the owner). "Medicine men" are persons believed to have supernatural powers of healing. Health may be restored through herbal drinks, prayers, rituals, and ceremonies.

CULTURAL AND RACIAL INFLUENCES ON CLIENT CARE

Clients' cultural backgrounds and preferences influence the manner whereby they interact with other people and with the world around them. In an unfamiliar situation, such as admission to a health care setting, cultural differences may seem even greater. In these instances of stress, most people hold tightly to that which is familiar in order to protect themselves from the unknown. The nurse can show caring in such a situation by acknowledging the expression of these differences and encouraging the client to retain what is familiar. Providing opportunities for decisions in their care decreases the stress of unfamiliar situations.

The influences of culture and race can be viewed through the phenomena of communication, space and time orientation, social organization, and biological variations.

Communication

Although language is common to all human beings, not everyone shares the same language. This cultural difference can lead to misunderstanding and frustration. The nurse must realize that a client who speaks a different language or with an accent simply has a different means of expressing needs. When communication is restricted because of language differences, alternative methods of communication, such as gestures and flash cards, can be used.

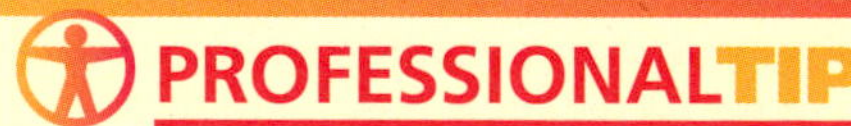

Nonnative Speakers

When interacting with someone who does not understand English well, many people will try to compensate for the lack of understanding by speaking loudly. Speaking slowly, distinctly, and in a normal volume; making eye contact; and avoiding slang and medical jargon are effective measures to ensure communication.

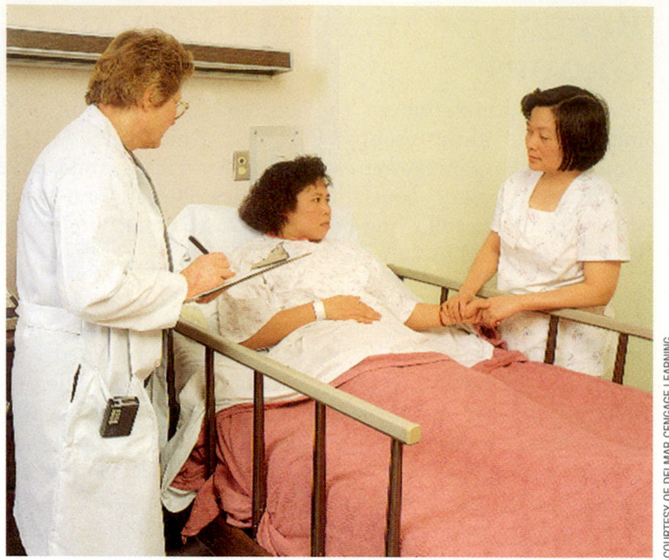

COURTESY OF DELMAR CENGAGE LEARNING

FIGURE 11-2 Family members may serve as interpreters to help clients who do not speak English understand procedures and instructions, and to communicate the client's thoughts and questions to the nurse.

The client's family may be able to assist when there is a block in communication. Family members can interpret procedures and instructions for the client and communicate the client's thoughts and questions to the nurse (Figure 11-2). If no family members are available, the hospital social worker may be able to find an interpreter. Often hospitals will have a pool of staff or people within the community whom they can request to interpret for different clients as needed.

Orientation to Space and Time

Orientation with regard to space and time represents two other culturally influenced variables that may affect a client's attitude toward care. Territoriality, or interpretation of personal space, is a pattern of behavior resulting from an individual's belief that certain spaces and objects belong to that person. The distance that a person prefers to maintain from another is determined by one's culture. In general, people of Arabic, southern European, and African origin frequently sit or stand relatively close to each other (0–18 inches), whereas people of Asian, northern European, and North American origin are more comfortable with a larger personal space (more than 18 inches).

Affection and caring behaviors are not communicated by touch in some cultures. For instance, among Asians, adults seldom touch one another, and the head is believed to be sacred. The nurse should thus not touch an Asian client's head without permission to do so. When working with clients from cultures where personal touch is viewed negatively, the nurse should use the universal sign of caring and acceptance: the smile.

People in U.S. society tend to be future oriented: They plan for the future, establish long-term goals, and, increasingly, are concerned with prevention of future illnesses. In daily life, they are oriented to time of day, constantly referring to clock time for everything from mealtime to time of appointments with health care professionals as well as other obligations. The nurse must also be very attentive to time. Medications are given at scheduled times, and work begins and ends at specified times. Other groups that tend to be future oriented are Japanese, Jews, and Arabs. These groups tend to view time as a commodity for achieving future goals.

Not all cultural groups are future oriented, however. People of some cultures (e.g., Asians) may be oriented to the past. For Asians, this orientation is reflected in the roles that ancestor worship and Confucianism play in the present. Members of other cultural groups, such as Native Americans, tend to be present oriented. Many Native Americans do not own clocks, and they live one day at a time, showing little concern for the future (Giger & Davidhizer, 2004). Mexican Americans and African Americans often value relationships with people in the present more than in the future. African Americans tend to be present oriented in health care behaviors as well. They often express the fatalistic belief that "it's going to happen anyway, so why bother" and fail to seek medical attention until a disabling condition occurs. The African American culture often teaches flexible attention to schedules; whatever is happening currently is most important. Explanations about the necessity of time scheduling (e.g., the need for strict schedules for medication requiring therapeutic blood level maintenance) must be given to the client.

An individual's orientation to time may affect promptness or attendance at health care appointments, compliance with self-medication schedules, and reporting the onset of illness or other health concerns. Clients might not see the necessity for preventive health care measures if they experience no difference in their health today when they follow a special diet or exercise program. The nurse teaches clients when timing is critical in health care situations and practices patience when working with people whose background differs from that of the dominant culture.

Social Organization

Social organization refers to the ways that cultural groups determine rules of acceptable behavior and roles of individual members. Examples of social organization include family structure, gender roles, and religion.

Family Structure

The definition of family has changed dramatically through the years. Until 1920, the norm was the "institutional family," which was organized around economic production and the kinship network. Marriage was not a romantic relationship but a functional one. Family loyalty and tradition were more important than individual romantic interests or goals. Responsibility was the chief value.

From 1920 to 1960, the norm was the "psychological family." Affairs were more private and less tied to the extended family. Family was based on fulfillment of the individual members and personal satisfaction in a nuclear, two-parent arrangement. Satisfaction was the chief value (Figure 11-3).

The social changes of the 1960s caused modifications in the family, including gender equality and personal freedom. The increased divorce rate may have resulted from the sexual revolution and the attitude that the individual deserves more and owes less to the family.

Today, no single family arrangement has a monopoly. Many types of families have emerged and are accepted. Flexibility is the chief value. Family no longer necessarily implies biological relation but rather has come to mean members of

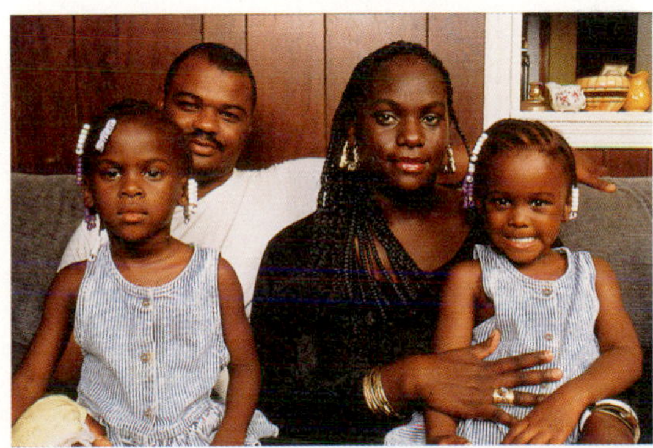
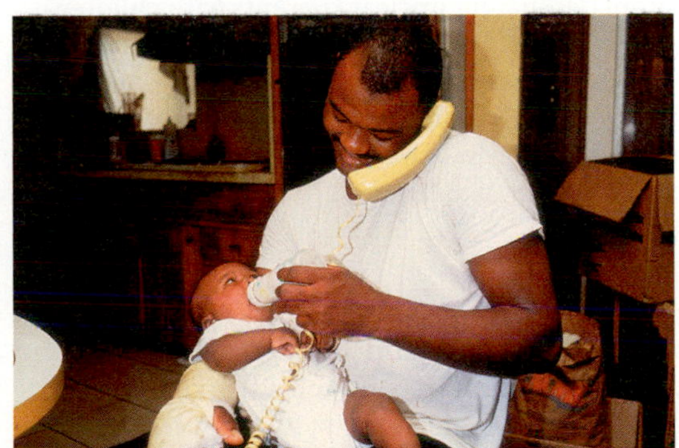
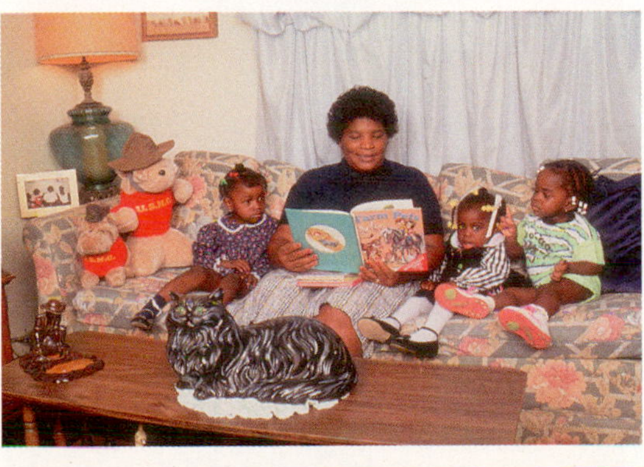
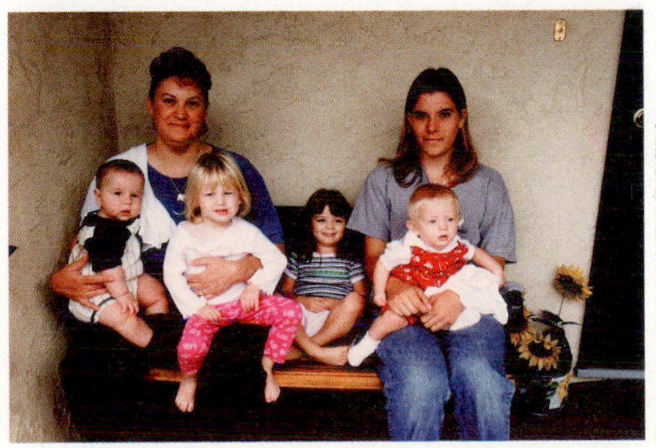

PHOTOS COURTESY OF DELMAR CENGAGE LEARNING

FIGURE 11-3 Family structures are diverse.

PROFESSIONAL TIP

Families

Each individual defines family differently. These definitions are shaped by personal experience and observation of other families. Nurses must remain objective and nonjudgmental when the client's family is different from their idea of family. The client should identify family members so that the nurse knows exactly who the client considers to be family.

a shared household who have similar values and participate in shared goals. Fawcett (1993) cites the following characteristics of family:

- Love and affection
- Caring and compassion
- Sense of belonging and connectedness
- History and linkage to posterity
- Rituals of rejoicing
- Sense of place
- Acceptance of members, including shortcomings
- Honor of elders
- System of earning and spending money
- Competent manner of parenting or caretaking
- Division of chores and labor

Systems theory states that families are considered to be interacting, interdependent individuals related by marriage, birth, or mutual consent. Examples of families with varying lifestyles today are two-parent nuclear (parents with children), attenuated (single parent with children), blended (through remarriage), extended (including grandparents), incipient (married couple with no children), cohabitating (couple having never married), gay or lesbian, divorced, adoptive, multiadult, and mixed or interracial families.

Gender Roles

Gender roles vary according to cultural context (Figure 11-4). For example, in families organized around a patriarchal structure (with the man being the head of the household and chief authority figure), the husband/father is the dominant member. Such expectations are typically the cultural norm in Latino, Hispanic, and traditional Muslim families. The husband/father is the one who makes decisions regarding health care for all family members. Also, in such cultures, the wife is responsible for child care and household maintenance, whereas the father's role is to protect and support the family members.

Religion

Anthropologists have identified the strength of the influence of religion on culture. In many cases, culture and tradition have been maintained and preserved through religious beliefs. Religion often is the formal organizational structure for social behavior.

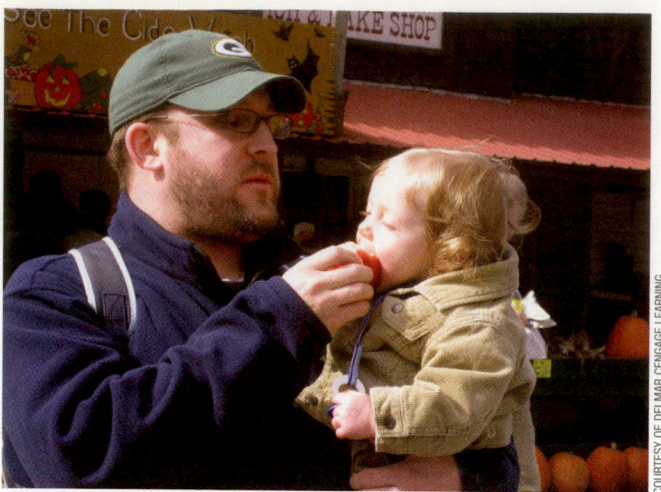

FIGURE 11-4 **Fathers assuming more responsibility in caring for children is one example of shifting gender roles.**

Religious and spiritual beliefs are important in many individuals' lives. These beliefs can influence attitudes, lifestyle, and feelings about life, pain, and death. Some religions specify practices about diet, birth control, and appropriate medical care. Often, spiritual beliefs assume a greater significance at the time of illness than at other times in a person's life. These

COMMUNITY/HOME HEALTH CARE

Culturally Sensitive Care

To provide culturally sensitive care in the home:

- Remember that the setting for care is controlled not by the health care provider but by the client and family.
- Be aware that the nurse is often viewed as a guest by the client and family. Social communication may be necessary to facilitate rapport.
- Be nonjudgmental about the home (e.g., presence of clutter and disarray).
- Display consideration and respect for the client. For example:
  —Before entering the home, wipe your feet.
  —Before washing your hands, ask permission to use the sink or bathroom.
  —Before moving the client's belongings, ask permission, then replace items when finished.
- Benefit from the home environment by assessing cultural values and norms. Clues to cultural values may include:
  —Possessions and decor on display in the home
  —Family roles and task assignment
  —Interactions among family members
  —Value placed on privacy and possessions

beliefs assist some people in accepting their illnesses and help explain illness for others. Religion can both help people live fuller lives and console or strengthen people during suffering and in preparation for death. Religion, by providing meaning to life and death, can supply the client, the family, and the nurse with a sense of security and strength during a time of need.

Spiritual needs are identified as an individual's desire to find purpose and meaning in life, pain, and death. To provide holistic care, the nurse must be attentive to the spiritual dimension of each client and assist the client in meeting spiritual needs (Figure 11-5).

While spiritual needs are recognized by many nurses, **spiritual care** (recognition of and assistance toward meeting spiritual needs) is often neglected. Spirituality is defined as an individual's search to find purpose and meaning in life. The goal of spiritual nursing care is to empower clients to identify and utilize their spiritual beliefs to cope with a health crisis. Among reasons that nurses give for failing to provide spiritual care are:

- Spirituality is a private matter.
- They are uninformed about the religious beliefs of others.
- They have not identified their own spiritual beliefs.
- Meeting the spiritual needs of the client is a family or clergy responsibility, not a nursing responsibility.

Spiritual nursing care is appropriate when the nurse cares about the client's emotional, physical, and psychosocial health. The nursing diagnosis of *Spiritual Distress* can be apparent in a client who is unable to practice religious or spiritual rituals because of illness or confinement in a health care institution.

The **religious support system** is a group of ministers, priests, nuns, rabbis, shamans, mullahs, or laypersons who are able to meet clients' spiritual needs. The nurse is responsible for working with these individuals and including them in the client care team.

Be aware of the general philosophies of clients' spiritual beliefs and also be aware that some individuals do not believe in a higher being or practice a specific religion. **Agnostics** believe that the existence of God cannot be proved or disproved, whereas **atheists** do not believe in God or any other deity.

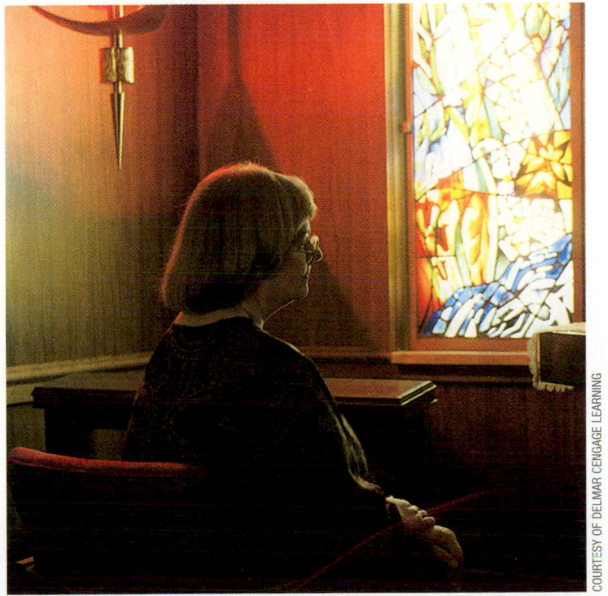

COURTESY OF DELMAR CENGAGE LEARNING

FIGURE 11-5 Spiritual needs often increase when individuals are sick.

It is important to identify particular beliefs from various religions that can influence client care activities. Some of these beliefs concern holy day practices, dietary restrictions, birth, death, and organ donation.

Protestant Many separate denominations (more than 1,200) constitute the group known as Protestant. Protestant groups include such denominations as Baptist, Episcopal, Lutheran, Methodist, Presbyterian, and Seventh-Day Adventist. The majority worship on Sunday, and their primary written reference is the Holy Bible.

Baptist Baptists believe that baptism is performed only after the believer reaches an age of understanding and confesses a personal acceptance of Jesus' saving work. Communion is a spiritual act symbolizing the suffering, death, and resurrection of the Lord.

Episcopal Episcopalians have a number of sacraments, including baptism, confession, communion, and anointing of the sick (Holy Unction). Holy Unction is most often given as a healing sacrament. They believe that a dying infant should be baptized, and a nurse may perform the rite. Usually, an Episcopal priest administers these sacraments.

Lutheran Traditionally, Lutherans baptize infants and adults by sprinkling. Any baptized Christian may perform an emergency baptism. The Lutheran churches recognize two sacraments: baptism and Holy Communion. Holy Communion is understood to be the body and the blood of Jesus. It is often administered to the ill or those awaiting surgery. Central to Lutheran doctrine is the belief in "justification by faith." People are redeemed by God solely on the basis of God's grace, which they receive through faith in what God has done for them.

Methodist Methodists practice both infant and adult baptism. For them, religion is a matter of personal belief, and the conscience is used as a guide for living.

Presbyterian Presbyterians also practice baptism and communion, which is a remembering of the death of Jesus Christ for them. Salvation is believed to be a gift from God.

Seventh-Day Adventist Seventh-Day Adventists baptize individuals only after they reach an age of accountability. Some dietary restrictions are followed. Sunset on Friday to sunset on Saturday is observed as their Sabbath. Jobs or worldly pleasures are not pursued during this time.

Roman Catholic Priests perform various rites known as Sacraments (sacred) at various times in the life of the Catholic. Sacraments that might be encountered in the health care setting are baptism, the Eucharist (Communion), confession, and sacrament of the sick. Baptism, administered only once in the life of a Catholic, is believed to be absolutely necessary for salvation. A client preparing for communion is generally asked to abstain from food or drink an hour before the rite. Water and medications are allowed at any time. Confession is a sacrament for forgiveness of sins. It should be respected as a very private matter. The Sacrament of the Sick, in which the client is anointed with holy oil, was formerly given to someone near death and was called the "last rites."

Orthodox Orthodox churches show their love of God through worship liturgies. It is important that followers remain faithful to the teachings of the ancient church. Holy Unction, anointing the body with oil, is used for healing of both bodily and spiritual infirmities. Baptism is important, so in life-threatening situations an unbaptized child should have an emergency baptism.

Jehovah's Witness Receiving any blood or blood products, including plasma, is prohibited. Also, they will not eat anything containing blood. Blood volume expanders that are not derivatives of blood are permissible. To receive blood when a medical condition requiring blood transfusion is life threatening, children have been made wards of the court. They hold a special observance of the Lord's Supper.

Mormon (Church of Jesus Christ of the Latter-Day Saints) Mormons baptize at the age of 8 years. When necessary, baptism of the dead is performed for adults. Mormons wear a special undergarment that symbolizes dedication to God. This may be worn under the hospital gown.

Christian Science Christian Scientists believe that illness will be eliminated through prayer and spiritual understanding. A critically ill Christian Scientist client may wish to have a Christian Science practitioner contacted to provide treatment through prayer. They usually do not use medicine, do not agree to surgical procedures, and do not accept blood transfusions.

Scientology is a study of the interactions of the spirit with itself, others, and life (Church of Scientology International, 2009). The fundamental truths of the scientology religion are that man is an immortal, spiritual being with unlimited capabilities that allow him to solve problems, accomplish goals, gain lasting happiness, and gain higher awareness and abilities (Church of Scientology International, 2009). Man consists of the spirit, called thetan (thought or spirit); mind; and body. The mind is a means of communication between himself and his environment. The body is not the person. The thetan is the most important component making up the spirit or individuality of a person. A main principle of scientology is the ARC Triangle, which guides interpersonal relationships and understanding (Church of Scientology International, 2009). The ARC Triangle consists of affinity, reality, and communication. Affinity is the emotional response of affection or lack of affection. Reality is the real objects in life. Communication is the interchange of ideas. For communication to occur, there must be agreement and affinity. To improve communication, persons find something on which they agree and improve affinity by talk or contact and tangible touch.

An individual applies principles of Scientology through a process called auditing (Church of Scientology International, 2009). During an auditing session, the auditor helps an individual explore and rid oneself of damaging spiritual conditions and thereby improve awareness and ability.

American Indian Religions That all life is sacred and all things are interconnected is the central belief of the various religions. Community importance is emphasized. The individual who is able to communicate with the spirits or the Great Spirit is the spiritual leader. There are no written religious books. Religious traditions are passed on orally and through participation in ceremonies and festivals. Illness may be the result of a sin or a spirit or god who is unhappy.

Judaism Judaism is both an ethnic identity and a religious faith. The religion is based on the five books of Moses called the Torah. Religion and culture are deeply interwoven in the Jewish faith, resulting in ritual, tradition, religious ceremony, and social laws.

There are three groups of Judaism: Orthodox, Conservative, and Reformed. They vary in how strictly they follow the traditions, but all share the fundamental teachings of Judaism. Orthodox Jews strictly observe all traditional practices. The Conservative group observes many of the traditional practices, and the Reformed group loosely interprets the traditions. The spiritual leader of the Jewish congregation is the rabbi and the person to be informed when a client requests it. The Jewish Sabbath, or day of worship, begins at sunset on Friday and ends at sunset on Saturday. Circumcision is performed on the male infant 8 days after birth. It may be done by the pediatrician or by the Mohel, who may also be a rabbi.

Islam Islam is the religion of Muslims. Allah is the supreme deity, and Mohammed, the founder of Islam, is the chief prophet. The Muslim's day of worship lasts from sunset on Thursday to sunset on Friday. Some Muslims pray five times a day (after dawn, at noon, at mid-afternoon, after sunset, and at night). A bed or chair may be positioned facing southeast (in the continental United States) when a client requests that he face Mecca, the holy city of Islam. Muslim clients may wear an article of writing from the Koran on a piece of string around the neck, waist, or arm. This should not be removed or allowed to get wet. Rules of cleanliness involve eating with the right hand and cleansing self with the left hand after defecating or urinating. Hand medications or other materials to the Muslim client with the right hand so as not to offend them.

Some Islamic females wish to be clothed from head to ankle. They may prefer to undress one body part at a time during a physical examination and may refuse to be cared for by male nurses or physicians.

Buddhism Buddhism is a general term indicating a belief in Buddha, "the enlightened one." Nirvana, a state of greater spontaneity and inner freedom, is the goal of existence. When one achieves Nirvana, the mind has supreme purity, strength, and peace. Buddhism does not dictate any specific sacraments or practices. There are no special holy days or religious restrictions for therapy. Buddhists believe in reincarnation but not in healing through faith. The religious support system for the sick is the priest. Figure 11-6 shows the inside of a Buddhist temple.

Hindu Hinduism has no common doctrines or creeds that keep Hindus together. They are free to worship one or more of their 320,000 gods. The Vedas are the Scripture of Hinduism. Reincarnation is central in Hindu thought. Freedom from the cycle of rebirth and death and entrance into what the Hindus, like the Buddhists, call Nirvana is the goal of existence. Hindu temples are dwelling places of deities and where offerings are

CRITICAL THINKING

Religion and Culture

Describe your religious support system.

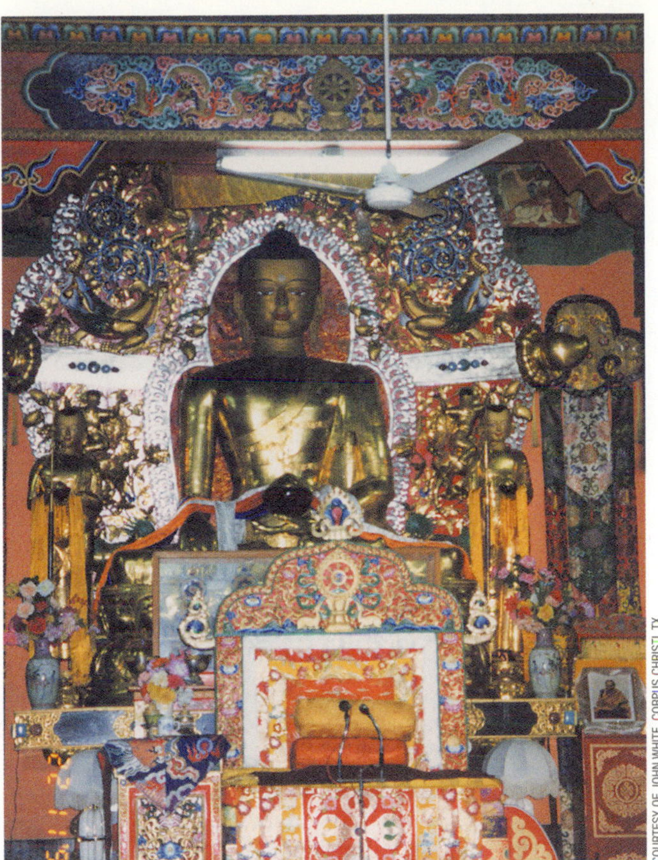
COURTESY OF JOHN WHITE, CORPUS CHRISTI, TX.

FIGURE 11-6 The inside of a Buddhist temple.

brought. Some Hindus believe that illness is God's way of punishing a person for sins; others believe in faith healing.

BIOLOGICAL VARIATION

Biological variations distinguish one racial or cultural group from another. Easily identified biological variations include skin color, hair texture, eye shape, thickness of lips, and body structure (Degazon, 2000). Less obvious biological variations include enzyme differences and susceptibility to disease (Andrews & Boyle, 2008; Giger & Davidhizar, 2004). Enzyme differences account for varied responses of some groups to dietary and drug therapy (Table 11-2).

According to Kudzma (1999), drug metabolism is genetically determined, and race seems to affect the response. A drug is more efficient in clients who metabolize the drug rapidly. Sometimes it may be metabolized too quickly for the full clinical effect to be achieved. When a drug is metabolized slowly, it is less effective, and the client experiences greater drug toxicity.

CULTURAL ASPECTS AND THE NURSING PROCESS

Each individual comes from a cultural background that, in some way, influences behavior and attitudes about health and illness. Personal attitudes and behaviors determine not only the ways that clients interpret health events and utilize health care but also the ways that nurses interpret health events and

TABLE 11-2 Biological Variations

Cultural Group	Biological Variation
European American	• Liver enzyme differences cause caffeine to be metabolized and excreted faster. • Increased susceptibility for breast cancer, heart disease.
African American	• Isoniazid (drug used to treat tuberculosis) is metabolized rapidly, thereby becoming quickly inactive; occurs in approximately 60% of population. • Increased susceptibility for keloid formation, hypertension, lactose intolerance, sickle cell disease. • Higher doses of antihypertensive drugs (e.g., propranolol) must be administered to produce same effects as in European Americans.
Hispanic American	• Increased susceptibility for diabetes, hypertension, lactose intolerance.
Asian American	• Isoniazid is metabolized rapidly, thereby becoming quickly inactive; occurs in approximately 85% to 90% of population. • Alcohol is rapidly metabolished resulting in excessive facial flushing and other vasomotor symptoms. • Increased susceptibility for hypertension, liver and stomach cancer, lactose intolerance. • Chinese men require half as much propranolol (antihypertensive drug) to produce same effects as in European American men.
Native American	• Isoniazid is metabolized rapidly, thereby becoming quickly inactive; occurs in approximately 60% to 90% of population. • Increased susceptibility for tuberculosis, diabetes, cirrhosis of the liver, heart disease. • Rapid metabolism of alcohol results in excessive facial flushing and other vasomotor symptoms

Data compiled from *Transcultural Concepts in Nursing Care*, by M. Andrews and J. Boyle, 2003, Philadelphia: Lippincott Williams & Wilkins; *Transcultural Nursing: Assessment and Intervention* (4th ed.), by J. Giger and R. Davidhizar, 2004, St. Louis, MO: Mosby-Year Book; Cultural Diversity and Community Health Nursing, by C. Degazon, in *Community Health Nursing* (5th ed.), by M. Stanhope and J. Lancaster (Eds.), 2000, St. Louis, MO: Mosby-Year Book; and *Transcultural Concepts in Nursing Care* (5th ed.), by M. M. Andrews and J. S. Boyle, 2008, Philadelphia, PA: Lippincott Williams & Wilkins.

PROFESSIONALTIP

Culturally Diverse Coworkers

Many nursing units have a mix of nationalities and cultures. While such a mix has the potential of improving nursing care, in practice it often leads to conflict and poor teamwork. The same cultural differences discussed in relation to clients may also be found among coworkers. Ways to successfully manage diversity in the workplace include:

- Be aware of your own biases and strive to avoid stereotyping others.
- Be aware of the way in which the things you do and say affect others.
- Help others be more sensitive and help correct misconceptions.
- Learn to welcome different opinions and viewpoints.
- Be open to feedback.

Nurses must cultivate a cultural consciousness. There must be a heightened sensitivity and awareness of the uniqueness and diversity of perspective each individual has to offer. Cultural awareness is essential in the process of providing appropriate, effective care (Mullins, 1999). As health care professionals, even if we cannot understand or accept particular cultural practices, it is important to show respect for them. This directly reflects how we value our own beliefs and practices.

their personal views about health and illness before assessing and caring for clients from other cultural groups.

Assessment

Culturally sensitive nursing care begins with an examination of one's own culture and beliefs. It is followed by an assessment of the client's cultural beliefs and background.

Personal Cultural Assessment

Spradley and Allender (2001) suggest five areas to be examined when assessing one's culture and the influence it has on personal beliefs about health care:

- Influences from racial/ethnic background
- Usual verbal and nonverbal communication patterns
- Cultural norms and values
- Religious practices and beliefs
- Health practices and beliefs

They suggest that the nurse identifies information on each issue and then validates this information with another person(s) from the same cultural group.

CRITICAL THINKING

Culture and Health Practices

How has your culture influenced your beliefs about health practices?

If a client put an amulet (religious icon and necklace) around her newborn's neck, how would you approach the client to discuss your concern about the risk of strangulation?

Client Cultural Assessment

After examining one's own culture and the influences it had in developing personal beliefs about health and sickness, then assess the client's cultural background (Figure 11-7). Data about various cultures may be collected from members of the culture to be studied, from others familiar with the culture, or from the local library.

Six categories of information necessary for a comprehensive cultural assessment of the client are suggested by Spradley and Allender (2001):

- *Ethnic or racial background.* Where did the client group originate, and how does that influence the status and identity of group members?
- *Language and communication patterns.* What is the preferred language spoken, and what are the culturally based communication patterns?
- *Cultural values and norms.* What are the beliefs, values, and standards regarding education, roles, leisure, family functions, child rearing, work, aging, death and dying, and rites of passage?
- *Biocultural factors.* Are there genetic or physical traits unique to the ethnic or racial group that predispose group members to certain conditions or illnesses?
- *Religious beliefs and practices.* What are the religious beliefs, and how do they influence roles, life events, health, and illness?
- *Health beliefs and practices.* What are the beliefs and practices regarding treatment, causes, and prevention of illnesses?

Nursing Diagnosis

Any nursing diagnosis may be appropriate for a client of any cultural group. When cultural variables are identified during assessment, the nurse should be as specific as possible when asking questions and determining appropriate nursing diagnoses so that interventions can be individualized with respect to the client's cultural beliefs. For instance, *Decreased Cardiac Output* may be viewed by the nurse or physician as having a medical or physical cause, whereas the client may attribute the origin to an imbalance of yin and yang. Table 11-3 lists select nursing diagnoses that are most likely to have cultural implications.

Planning/Outcome Identification

Cultural variables must be taken into consideration when establishing goals and planning interventions. Care will be

Cultural Assessment Guide

Name: ______

Nickname or other names or special meaning attributed to your name: ______

Primary language:

When speaking ______

When writing ______

Date of birth: ______

Place of birth: ______

Educational level or specialized training: ______

To which ethnic group do you belong? ______

To what extent do you identify with your cultural group? ______

Who is the spokesperson for your family? ______

Describe some of the customs or beliefs that you have about the following:

Health ______

Life ______

Illness ______

Death ______

How do you learn information best?

- ☐ Reading
- ☐ Having someone explain verbally
- ☐ Having someone demonstrate

Describe some of your family's dietary habits and your personal food preferences. ______

Are there any foods forbidden from your diet for religious or cultural reasons? ______

Describe your religious affiliation. ______

What role do your religious beliefs and practices play in your life during times of good health and poor health? ______

Who/what is your primary source of information about your health? ______

On whom do you rely for health care services or healing? ______

Of what cultural health practices are you aware, and which do you utilize? ______

Are there cultural restrictions that your caregiver should know? ______

Describe your current living arrangements. ______

How do members of your family communicate with each other? ______

Describe your strengths. ______

Is there anything else that is important about your cultural beliefs that you would like to share? ______

(Adapted from Daniels, Grendell, & Wilkins, 2010, *Nursing Fundamentals: Caring and Clinical Decision Making*, Delmar Cengage Learning.)

FIGURE 11-7 Cultural Assessment Guide

TABLE 11-3 Nursing Diagnoses With Cultural Implications

Anxiety
*Disturbed **Body** Image*
*Ineffective **Breastfeeding***
*Impaired Verbal **Communication***
*Decisional **Conflict*** (specify)
*Ineffective **Coping***
*Compromised Family **Coping***
Fear
*Anticipatory **Grieving***
*Ineffective **Health** Maintenance*
***Health**-Seeking Behaviors* (specify)
Noncompliance
*Imbalanced **Nutrition**: More than Body Requirements*
Pain
*Ineffective **Role** Performance*
*Disturbed **Sleep** Pattern*
*Impaired **Social** Interaction*
***Spiritual** Distress*

COURTESY OF DELMAR CENGAGE LEARNING

CLIENTTEACHING

Culturally Sensitive Teaching Guidelines

Consider the following guidelines for teaching clients from diverse cultures:

- Identify the client's cultural background.
- Evaluate the client's current knowledge by asking the client to state what he knows about the topic.
- Identify the perception of need by asking the client and family what they need and want to learn.
- Observe interactions between the client and family to determine family roles and authority figures. Ask the client which family member they would like included in teaching and care sessions.
- Use language easily understood by the client, avoiding jargon and complex medical terms.
- Clarify your verbal and nonverbal messages with the client.
- Ask the client to repeat the information. Ask the client to do a return demonstration of the material taught.

most effective when the client and family are active participants in planning care and when cultural preferences are respected. Suggested goals to consider when cultural factors are involved include:

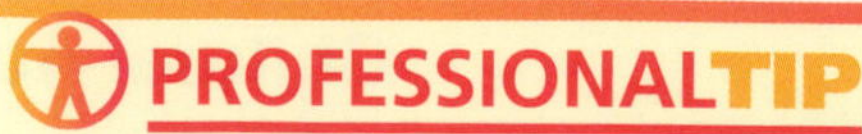

Culturally Appropriate Care

- Respect clients for their beliefs.
- Be sensitive to behaviors and practices different from your own.
- Accommodate differences if they are not detrimental to the client's health. For example, a client might believe that eating onions will resolve his respiratory infection. While eating onions may not be therapeutic, it is also not likely to cause any health problems.
- Listen for cues in the client's conversation that relay a unique ethnic belief about prevention, etiology, transmission, or some other aspect of disease. For example, a client might say, "I knew I would be sick today. I heard an owl last night."
- Use the occasion to teach positive health habits if the client's practices are deleterious to good health. For example, when asked about her diet, a pregnant woman might reply that she never eats meat or eggs while pregnant because she believes that gaining too much weight will increase her risk of a difficult delivery. This situation offers the nurse an opportunity to provide nutritional instruction.

- Client will express health care needs to family and caregiver.
- Client will maintain cultural health practices as appropriate.
- Client and family will understand the effect that health care beliefs have on health status.

IMPLEMENTATION

Cultural aspects are always a factor in a nursing care plan, and effective communication and client education are important nursing responsibilities that can enhance cultural understanding and appreciation. Interventions should be carried out in a manner that will respect, to the degree possible, the preferences and desires of the client. When a client does not speak or understand the native language well, the nurse should arrange to have an interpreter present to explain procedures and tests.

EVALUATION

Evaluation includes feedback from the client and family to determine their reaction to the interventions. Revisions to the plan of care are made with client and family input and alternative sources and resources brought in when needed to enhance communication and exchange of information. Culturally competent nurses perform self-evaluations to identify their attitudes toward caring for clients from diverse cultures.

CASE STUDY

M.G. brings her Catholic, 18-year-old sister, R.G., to the hospital emergency room with a high temperature, chills, vomiting, and complaint of right lower quadrant pain. M.G. brings her three children, ages 3, 2, and 1 year old, with her. M.G. understands and speaks broken English, but R.G. is fluent in Spanish only. The nurse directs M.G. to the waiting room with her children and then takes R.G. to the examination room. R.G. is examined by a male nurse who promptly complains at the nurse's station about how uncooperative R.G. was during the physical examination. R.G. is admitted for inpatient care with a diagnosis of appendicitis requiring emergency surgery. M.G. is left in the waiting room unaware of the difficulty that the nursing staff has had communicating with her sister. R.G. is taken upstairs to her room to prepare her for surgery. M.G. is notified that she can go upstairs for a few minutes but then must leave because her children do not meet the age requirement for visitor privileges. A hospital volunteer was asked to watch the children until M.G. returned. M.G. finds R.G. weeping and nearly hysterical. The nurse informs M.G. that R.G. will not sign the surgical permit form. Tearfully, M.G. tells her sister that the "nurse took my amulet, and she won't let me wear it to surgery." The physician walks in and asks M.G. why she waited so long to bring R.G. in for treatment. He informs her that R.G.'s appendix was close to rupturing and that treatment should have been started 3 days ago when her symptoms began. M.G. informs him that she had taken R.G. to the curandero, who had given her some herbal tea to drink, but when it did not help, she brought R.G. to the hospital.

The following questions will guide your development of a nursing care plan for the case study.

1. Why was communication between M.G., R.G., and the health care professionals a problem?
2. What Hispanic cultural diversities were not addressed by the health care professionals? As a result, what needs of M.G. and R.G. were ignored by the health care professionals?
3. Write three individualized culturally sensitive nursing diagnoses and goals for R.G.
4. Recall the diagnoses and goals identified in question 3 and list pertinent nursing interventions for R.G.
5. List at least three successful client outcomes for R.G.

SAMPLE NURSING CARE PLAN

The Family with Ineffective Coping

M.W., an 82-year-old Asian American housewife, is in the hospital with severe nausea and vomiting related to recurrent breast cancer with bone metastasis treatment. Her appetite is decreasing, although she is able to drink some fluids.

At M.W.'s insistence, her husband of 61 years and their two grown daughters remain at her bedside. She does not bother the nurses for her basic care and insists that the oldest daughter bathe her and walk her to the bathroom. Mr. W. leaves only to go home and shower. Both daughters remain when he goes home.

Mr. W. looks exhausted and appears to have lost weight. The daughters try to relieve their father at night, but he insists on remaining at the bedside.

M.W. has her husband and daughters constantly massaging her back but never voices discomfort. She changes position slowly and grimaces with each movement. M.W. lets her family talk for her. When questioned by the nurse, she denies pain, but she complains of pain to her family. She does not sleep well.

M.W.'s treatment plan is supportive. The hospital staff suggested the idea of hospice care when M.W. stated that she wants to go home.

NURSING DIAGNOSIS 1 *Compromised Family Coping* related to prolonged disease or disability progression that exhausts the supportive capacity of significant people as evidenced by Mr. W.'s looking exhausted

Nursing Outcomes Classification (NOC)
Caregiver Emotional Health
Caregiver Stressors
Family Normalization
Self-Esteem

Nursing Interventions Classification (NIC)
Emotional Support
Family Support
Family Therapy
Normalization Promotion

(Continues)

SAMPLE NURSING CARE PLAN (Continued)

PLANNING/OUTCOMES	NURSING INTERVENTIONS	RATIONALE
Family will plan a rotation schedule to meet each one's needs for rest and support while caring for M.W.	Provide empathy and support for the husband and daughters. Provide family with unlimited visitation, adequate space for members who stay overnight, and privacy.	Family is very important in the life of the Asian American. A sense of obligation to intervene and assist is highly valued. Casual help from strangers is avoided.
	Assess family members for signs of fatigue or overexertion.	Self-control and self-sufficiency are highly valued. Asking for help would mean loss of face and dignity.
	Explore with husband and daughters other support persons who would be willing and accepted by M.W. to keep her company.	Prolonged periods of unrelieved vigil will exhaust family members.
	Develop trusting and respectful relationships with M.W. and family members.	Asian Americans tend to be reserved with those whom they view as being in authority.
Client and family will maintain open communication.	Encourage Mr. W. to discuss realistic plans and expectations of daughters, including health care providers as needed.	Asians traditionally value authoritarian styles of leadership, where the father makes unilateral family decisions.
Family will provide care without compromising their own physical and emotional health.	Assess if basic physical and emotional needs of M.W. and family are being met focusing on nonverbal clues.	Silent communication and stoic reactions to pain and other uncertain situations is common. Direct expression of negative feelings is unusual.
	Monitor ability of family members to carry out treatment plan and provide safe care.	Care is provided by family members who are exhausted, which is a safety issue.

EVALUATION

Husband and eldest daughter remain at bedside during daytime hours. Youngest exchanges places with the father and eldest sister at night. M.W. is agreeable. The entire family meets with the primary care nurse to discuss the plan of care. Mr. W. and his daughters continue to provide the physical care for M.W. The daughters express gratefulness that their father is stronger and has taken on the leadership role.

(Continues)

SAMPLE NURSING CARE PLAN (Continued)

NURSING DIAGNOSIS

Impaired Communication related to cultural misunderstandings and lack of communication

NOC: *Communication Ability*
NIC: *Communication Enhancement*

CLIENT GOAL

M.W. will communicate personal needs as evidenced by verbally sharing needs with family and nurses by the next day.

NURSING INTERVENTIONS

1. Express that tiredness and loss of weight is noted in family members.
2. State that you notice she is grimacing and moving slowly and offer pain medication.
3. Explain pain physiology and state the benefits of taking pain medication on a routine basis and as needed.
4. State the benefits of accepting medication for nausea and vomiting and offer medication.

SCIENTIFIC RATIONALES

1. When a person does not get the proper rest and nutrition, it may be evidenced by tiredness and loss of weight.
2. Some cultures do not encourage persons to freely express pain.
3. If the pain threshold is not kept under control, it is very difficult to keep the client comfortable and relaxed. Regular assessment and administration of medication keeps the client's pain below a 2 on a 0-10 scale with 0 being no pain and 10 is the most pain one has experienced.
4. If the nausea and vomiting is controlled with medication, the client has more energy for other needed tasks.

EVALUATION

Is the client verbalizing personal needs to family and nursing staff?

CONCEPT CARE MAP 11-1

SUMMARY

- Culture is composed of beliefs about relationships, motivation, activities, perception of the world, and self.
- Culture is learned, shared, integrated, unspoken, and dynamic.
- Beliefs about concepts of health, disease etiology, health promotion and protection, and practitioners and remedies are influenced by culture.
- Unlike opinions, preferences, and attitudes, which can change, cultural characteristics are deeply rooted and are thus difficult to change. Clients reflect their cultural and ethnic heritage every time they interact with the world around them.
- Culture is influenced by religion, which also affects practices and beliefs about health and illness.
- Spiritual and religious beliefs are important in many people's lives. They can influence lifestyle, attitudes, and feelings about illness and death.
- Individuality exists among all peoples; nurses should not make assumptions based on the client's religious and cultural affiliations.
- The focus of nursing care is to help clients maintain their own beliefs when in a health care crisis. Those personal beliefs can be used to strengthen coping patterns.
- It is an important aspect of nursing to understand client differences.
- Response to health and illness varies depending on cultural origin.
- Providing culturally appropriate care begins with an understanding of the nurse's own cultural beliefs.
- Prerequisite to providing appropriate nursing care is performing a cultural assessment.

REVIEW QUESTIONS

1. A mother is observed breastfeeding her 4-year-old son, a client in the hospital. The nurses talk in the nursing station about why a mother would continue to breastfeed a 4-year-old. They state that the American way is better. The nurses are expressing:
   1. stereotyping.
   2. ethnocentrism.
   3. acculturation.
   4. cultural diversity.
2. The nurse knows that the religious group teaching that physical healing comes exclusively through prayers and readings is:
   1. Hindu.
   2. Roman Catholic.
   3. Christian Science.
   4. Seventh-Day Adventist.
3. A blood transfusion would most likely be refused by:
   1. Buddhist.
   2. Orthodox.
   3. American Indian.
   4. Jehovah's Witness.
4. The nursing diagnosis that might be used for a client who is hospitalized and has religious practices that conflict with hospital procedure is:
   1. *Religious Guilt.*
   2. *Guilt and Misery.*
   3. *Spiritual Distress.*
   4. *Spiritual Depression.*
5. If a client says to the nurse, "I need to pray with my group leader to get well," the most appropriate response for the nurse is:
   1. "May I call your group leader for you and ask her to visit you?"
   2. "The medications and treatment will make you well."
   3. "Why do you think your group leader is needed to make you well?"
   4. "When you are released from the hospital, you can go to your group leader and pray."
6. An Egyptian Muslim comes to the emergency room. The examination reveals a diagnosis of pneumonia. The nurse taking care of the client approaches his bed with Tylenol. Holding his hand with her right hand to read his patient ID band, she hands him the Tylenol with her left hand. As the nurse turns to pick up the water glass to hand to the client, she sees him throw the Tylenol away in the bedside wastebasket. How do you explain his behavior?
   1. He does not like taking medication from a female. It is demeaning to him.
   2. He regards the left hand as unclean and refuses to swallow a medication that he feels is contaminated.
   3. He is a fatalist and believes that nothing can be done to reverse the infectious process in his lungs.
   4. He hates European Americans and is unwilling to accept anything that the Caucasian nurse has touched.
7. An Asian American woman is being treated for new-onset diabetes mellitus. The nurse caring for her is attempting to teach her how to inject insulin. The nurse becomes increasingly frustrated because the client will not engage in the lesson. She refuses to look at the nurse's face when she talks to her, and she does not respond quickly to the questions that the nurse asks her. Why will this client not look at the nurse when she is communicating with her?
   1. The client is being defiant.
   2. The client has low self-esteem.
   3. Engaging in eye contact is considered disrespectful.
   4. The client is not ready to learn.
8. A Korean American is being discharged today from the hospital. The nurse is at the bedside giving discharge instructions and also has several prescriptions that the client needs to take home with her. The nurse reviews the instructions and pharmacy orders and extends the papers to the client. She accepts the paperwork initially but then tries to hand them back to the nurse. When you consider cultural perspectives, what could be an explanation for this behavior?
   1. The client does not agree with the doctor's home-going instructions.
   2. The client is trying to communicate to the nurse that she needs to give home-going instructions and prescriptions to the head of the family, her husband.
   3. The client does not work, and she has no money to purchase the prescriptions.
   4. The client thought that the nurse gave her the hospital bill, and she assumed that medical care would be free for her since it was in her home country.
9. A Haitian American is brought to the emergency room with acute stomach pains. She is brought by her supervisor at the grocery store where she works. The examining physician determines that the client has appendicitis and needs surgery immediately. The doctor telephones the client's husband to obtain permission for the surgery. The husband replies that he will come to the hospital as soon as possible. On arrival, the husband refuses to sign the consent form for the operation. He wants his wife discharged immediately so that he can take her home. He promises to bring her back later. The emergency room staff is puzzled. How is this behavior explained?
   1. The couple cannot afford to pay for surgery, but the husband is too embarrassed to say so.

2. The husband does not trust the hospital staff, so he wants to take his wife to their private physician instead.
3. The husband wants to consult the hungan (voodoo priest) to rule out the possibility of spiritual causes for the abdominal pain.
4. The husband wants to give his wife some cold cucumber soup before her surgery.

10. A Chicano (Mexican American) student from Texas volunteers at the gift shop in the hospital. A nurse from the hospital encounters the Mexican student on the street pushing a stroller with a year-old baby. The baby is friendly, smiling and appears well nourished. The student informs the nurse that the baby is her sister. The nurse compliments the student on her solicitous care of her sister "the baby is a beautiful, adorable little girl isn't she?" Without responding, the student immediately turns the carriage away from the nurse, and after a strained moment of silence states, "I must get home to help my mother." How would you explain the student's behavior?

1. The student does not feel that it is respectful to take up the nurse's time, so she feels that she should leave.
2. Seeing the nurse reminds the student that she needs to get ready to volunteer at the gift shop.
3. The student needs to go home to help her mother.
4. The student is afraid that the baby has been given the evil eye, and she wants to tell her mother about it as soon as possible.

REFERENCES/SUGGESTED READINGS

Andrews, M. (2008). Religion, culture, and nursing. In M. M. Andrews & J. S. Boyle (Eds.), *Transcultural concepts in nursing care* (5th ed.). Philadelphia: Lippincott Williams & Wilkins.

Andrews, M., & Boyle, J. (2008). *Transcultural concepts in nursing care* (4th ed.). Philadelphia: Lippincott Williams & Wilkins.

Boyle, J. (2008). Culture, family, and community. In M. M. Andrews & J. S. Boyle (Eds.), *Transcultural concepts in nursing care* (5th ed.). Philadelphia: Lippincott Williams & Wilkins.

Bulechek, G., Butcher, H., McCloskey, J., & Dochterman, J., eds. (2008). *Nursing Interventions Classification (NIC)* (5th ed.). St. Louis, MO: Mosby/Elsevier.

Church of Scientology International. (2009). Introduction to scientology. Retrieved February 12, 2009, from http://www.scientology.org/religion/presentation/pg006.html

Clark, M. (1999). *Community health nursing handbook.* New York: Prentice Hall.

Daniels, R., Grendell, R., & Wilkins, F. (2010). *Nursing fundamentals: Caring and clinical decision making* (2nd ed.). Clifton Park, NY: Delmar Cengage Learning.

Davidhizar, R., Dowd, S., & Giger, J. (1998). Educating the culturally diverse health care student. *Nurse Educator, 23*(2), 38–42.

Degazon, C. (2000). Cultural diversity and community health nursing practice. In M. Stanhope & J. Lancaster (Eds.), *Community and public health nursing* (5th ed.). St. Louis, MO: Mosby.

Doherty, W. (1992). Private lives, public values. *Psychology Today, 25*(3), 27–32.

Doswell, W., & Erlen, J. (1998). Multicultural issues and ethical concerns in the delivery of nursing care interventions. *Nursing Clinics of North America, 33*(2), 353–361.

Edelman, C., & Mandle, C. (2005). *Health promotion throughout the lifespan* (6th ed.). St. Louis, MO: Elsevier/Mosby.

Edmission, K. (1997). Psychosocial dimensions of medical–surgical nursing. In J. M. Black & E. Matassarin-Jacobs (Eds.), *Medical surgical nursing: Clinical management for continuity of care* (5th ed.). Philadelphia: W. B. Saunders.

Estes, M. (2010). *Health assessment and physical examination* (4th ed.). Clifton Park, NY: Delmar Cengage Learning.

Estin, P. (1999). Spotting depression in Asian patients. *RN, 62*(4), 39–40.

Fawcett, C. (1993). *Family psychiatric nursing.* St. Louis, MO: Mosby.

Giger, J., & Davidhizar, R. (2004). *Transcultural nursing: Assessment and intervention* (4th ed.). St. Louis, MO: Mosby-Year Book.

Gonzalez, R. (1999). ANA advocates more diversity in nursing. *American Journal of Nursing, 99*(11), 24.

Gravely, S. (2001). When your patient speaks Spanish—and you don't. *RN, 64*(5), 65–67.

Grossman, D. (1996). Cultural dimensions in home health nursing. *American Journal of Nursing, 96*(7), 33–36.

Kelz, R. (1997). Delmar's English–Spanish pocket dictionary for health professionals. Clifton Park, NY: Delmar Cengage Learning.

Kelz, R. (1999). *Conversational Spanish for health professionals* (3rd ed.). Clifton Park, NY: Delmar Cengage Learning.

Kirkpatrick, M., Brown, S., & Atkins, T. (1998). Using the internet to integrate cultural diversity and global awareness. *Nurse Educator, 23*(2), 15–17.

Kudzma, E. (1999). Culturally competent drug administration. *American Journal of Nursing, 99*(8), 46–51.

Lee, E. (Ed.). (2000). *Working with Asian Americans: A guide for clinicians.* New York: Guilford Press.

Leininger, M., & McFarland, M. (2002).*Transcultural nursing: Concepts, theories, research, and practice* (3rd ed.). New York: McGraw-Hill.

Lock, D. (1992). *Increasing multicultural understanding: A comprehensive model.* Newbury Park, CA: Sage.

Louie, K. (1999). Health promotion interventions for Asian American Pacific Islanders. In L. Zhan (Ed.), *Asian voices* (pp. 3–13). Boston: Jones & Bartlett.

Luckmann, J. (2000). *Transcultural communication in nursing.* Clifton Park, NY: Delmar Cengage Learning.

Malone, B. (1998). Diversity, divisiveness and divinity. *American Nurse, 30*(1), 5.

Marrone, S. (2008). Factors that influence critical care nurses' intentions to provide culturally congruent care to Arab Muslims. *Journal of Transcultural Nursing, 19*(1), 8–15.

Mazanec, P., & Tyler, M. (2003). Cultural considerations in end-of-life care. *American Journal of Nursing, 103*(3), 50–57.

McCaffery, M., & Pasero, C. (1999). Pain control. *American Journal of Nursing, 99*(8), 18.

Miller, J., Leininger, M., Leuning, C., Andrews, M., Ludwig-Beymer, P., & Papadopoulos, I. (2008). Commentary: Transcultural Nursing Society Position Statement on Human Rights. *Journal of Transcultural Nursing, 19*(1), 5–7.

Moorhead, S., Johnson, M., & Maas, M. (2007). *Nursing Outcomes Classification (NOC)* (4th ed.). St. Louis, MO: Mosby.

Morley, P., & Wallis, R. (Eds.). (1978). *Culture and curing: Anthropological perspectives on traditional medical beliefs and practices.* Pittsburgh, PA: University of Pittsburgh Press.

Mullins, M. (1999). Cultural awareness. *OB/GYN Nurse Forum, 7,* 3.

NewsWatch. (2000). Delay in seeking MI treatment is tied to social factors. *RN, 63*(10), 20.

North American Nursing Diagnosis Association International. (2010). *NANDA-I nursing diagnoses: Definitions and classification 2009–2011.* Ames, IA: Wiley-Blackwell.

Competent Care. (2001, September). *Travel Nursing Today* (A supplement to *RN*), 26–32.

Purnell, L., & Paulanka, B. (2008). *Transcultural health care: A culturally competent approach* (3rd ed.). Philadelphia: F. A. Davis.

Rivera-Andino, J., & Lopez, L. (2000). When culture complicates care. RN, 63(7), 47–49.

Shelley, J. (2000). Spiritual care: A guide for caregivers. Downers Grove, IL: Inter Varsity.

Simpson, J., & Carter, K. (2008). Muslim women's experiences with health care providers in a rural area of the United States. *Journal of Transcultural Nursing, 19*(1), 16–23.

Smith, L. (1998). Concept analysis: Cultural competence. *Journal of Cultural Diversity, 5*(1), 4–10.

Spector, R. (2000). *Cultural care: Guides to heritage assessment and health traditions* (2nd ed.). Upper Saddle River, NJ: Prentice Hall.

Spector, R. (2008). *Cultural diversity in health and illness* (5th ed.). Upper Saddle River, NJ: Prentice Hall.

Spradley, B., & Allender, J. (2001). *Community health nursing: Concepts and practice* (5th ed.). Philadelphia: Lippincott Williams & Wilkins.

Stanhope, M., & Knollmueller, R. (2000). *Handbook of community-based and home health nursing practice* (3rd ed.). St. Louis, MO: Mosby.

Stanhope, M., & Lancaster, J. (2003). *Community and public health nursing* (6th ed.). St. Louis, MO: Mosby.

Sue, D., & Sue, D. (2007). *Counseling the culturally diverse: Theory and practice* (5th ed.). New York: Wiley.

U.S. Census Bureau. (2001). Population estimates. Available: http://www.census.gov/population/estimates/nation/intfile3-1.txt

U.S. Department of Commerce, U.S. Census Bureau. (2007). *Statistical abstract of the United States: 2008* (127th ed.). Washington, DC: U.S. Government Printing Office.

RESOURCES

Transcultural Nursing Society, http://www.tcns.org

CHAPTER 12
Stress, Adaptation, and Anxiety

MAKING THE CONNECTION

Refer to the following chapters to increase your understanding of stress, adaptation, and anxiety:

Basic Nursing
- ***Holistic Care***
- ***Communication***
- ***Complementary/Alternative Therapies***
- ***Rest and Sleep***
- ***Infection Control/Asepsis***
- ***Pain Management***

LEARNING OBJECTIVES

Upon completion of this chapter, you should be able to:

- Define key terms.
- Describe how stress, adaptation, and anxiety affect health.
- Identify factors that contribute to the stress response.
- Describe the general adaptation syndrome.
- Detail the effects of stress on the whole individual.
- Explain intrinsic stressors in the change process.
- Describe the role of the nurse as a change agent.
- Discuss nursing interventions that promote positive adaptation to stress.
- Develop an individualized plan for managing stress.

KEY TERMS

adaptation
adaptive energy
adaptive measures
anxiety
burnout
catharsis
change
change agent
cognitive reframing
conditioning
crisis
crisis intervention
defense mechanisms
depersonalization
distress
endorphin
eustress
fight-or-flight response
general adaptation syndrome (GAS)
homeostasis
local adaptation syndrome (LAS)
maladaptive measures
stress
stressor

INTRODUCTION

Stress and anxiety are universal experiences that can be either a catalyst for positive change or a source of discomfort and pain. Nurses help clients cope with the stress of illness, disability, injury, or treatment approaches. Caring for clients experiencing a high level of anxiety can also be stressful for the nurse. Successful stress management is necessary for everyone's well-being. This chapter discusses the major concepts related to stress and anxiety, including strategies for coping with stress.

STRESS

According to Hans Selye (1974), **stress** is a nonspecific response to any demand made on the body. Selye termed such demands **stressors**. Any situation, event, or agent that produces stress is a stressor. A stressor is a stimulus that evokes the need to adapt. Stressors can be internal or external. For example, pain is an internal stressor, whereas loss of a job is an external stressor.

Even pleasant events can be stressful when they evoke the need to adapt. Stressors themselves are neutral, neither good nor bad. It is the individual's *perception* of the stressor that determines whether the effect is positive or negative. Any event can be stressful, depending on how the person views the event.

Responses to Stress

Adaptive energy is the term Selye coined to describe the inner force an individual uses to respond or adapt to stress. All persons have adaptive energy, but the amount of adaptive energy varies. When an individual has used all of his adaptive energy, illness, disease, or even death may result, as he is no longer able to adapt. Reactions to stress are typically categorized as either general (affecting the entire body) or local (affecting only the involved body part).

General Adaptation Syndrome

Stressors cause structural and chemical changes in the body as the body attempts to maintain **homeostasis**, which is the balance or equilibrium among the physiologic, psychological, sociocultural, intellectual, and spiritual needs of the body. Selye called these responses to stressors the **general adaptation syndrome (GAS)**.

Selye divided the GAS into three stages, as illustrated in Figure 12-1. In the first stage, crisis or alarm, the body readies itself to handle the stressors. The physiologic changes may result in symptoms such as cool, pale skin; shivering; and sweating of the palms and soles of the feet. Severe stress may cause dilated pupils, dry mouth, pounding heart, nausea, and diarrhea.

> **PROFESSIONALTIP**
>
> **Anticipatory Stress**
>
> Thoughts can be stressors that trigger the GAS, such as a person worrying about a situation. The body responds as if the person were *actually* experiencing the event, and the individual may feel ill, sweaty, nauseous, or very jittery.

During the second stage, adaptation or resistance, the body attempts to defend against the stressor through the **fight-or-flight response**. The body becomes physiologically ready to defend itself by either fighting or fleeing from the stressor.

The third stage, exhaustion, occurs if adaptive energy is inadequate to deal with prolonged or overwhelming stress.

The physiologic reactions of the body are essentially the same no matter what the source of the stress. For example, an imagined stressor will have the same physiologic response (GAS) as if the stressor had actually been experienced. According to Selye (1976), all stress reactions exhibit similar physiologic reactions.

Local Adaptation Syndrome

Selye also described the **local adaptation syndrome (LAS)**, which is the physiologic response to a stressor (e.g., trauma, illness) on a specific part of the body. For example, if a person cuts a hand, the LAS is initiated, inducing localized inflammation. The classic symptoms of inflammation (redness, swelling, and warmth) occur at the injured site. The LAS is usually a temporary process that resolves when the traumatized area is restored to its preinjury state; however, if the inflammation does not resolve with the LAS, the individual then experiences the GAS as the entire body becomes affected.

Signs and Symptoms of Stress

The signs and symptoms of stress are many and affect every dimension of a person. Common signs and symptoms of stress are outlined in Table 12-1.

Outcomes of Stress

Experiencing stress provides the individual with two possibilities: (a) an opportunity for personal growth or (b) the risk of disorganization and distress. When stressors are handled appropriately, adaptation is attained, and the body returns to normal.

The term **eustress** describes a type of stress resulting in positive outcomes. Consider for example, students who have an examination scheduled the following week. The stress over the impending test motivates them to study early, and they pass the examination. This stress was positive because it motivated them to study (an example of growth) and resulted in positive or desired outcomes.

Stressors evoking an ineffective response cause **distress**. For example, students who have a scheduled examination the next day put studying off until the last minute. They "cram" all night, do not know the material, are not alert, and fail the examination; they experience distress.

ADAPTATION

Adaptation is an ongoing process whereby individuals adjust to stressors and change. The nurse's goal is to identify and support the client's positive adaptive responses. Adaptation is a holistic response that involves all dimensions of an individual. Individuals seek to maintain a steady state in all dimensions of life: physiologic, psychological, cognitive, social, and spiritual. Wellness is an adaptive state; that is, the well person is one who is coping effectively with stressors and thus maintains a high level of wellness. Adaptation may be physiologic, psychological, cognitive, social, or spiritual.

Physiologic adaptation is the way the body responds to stressors affecting the functioning of the body. It may involve the

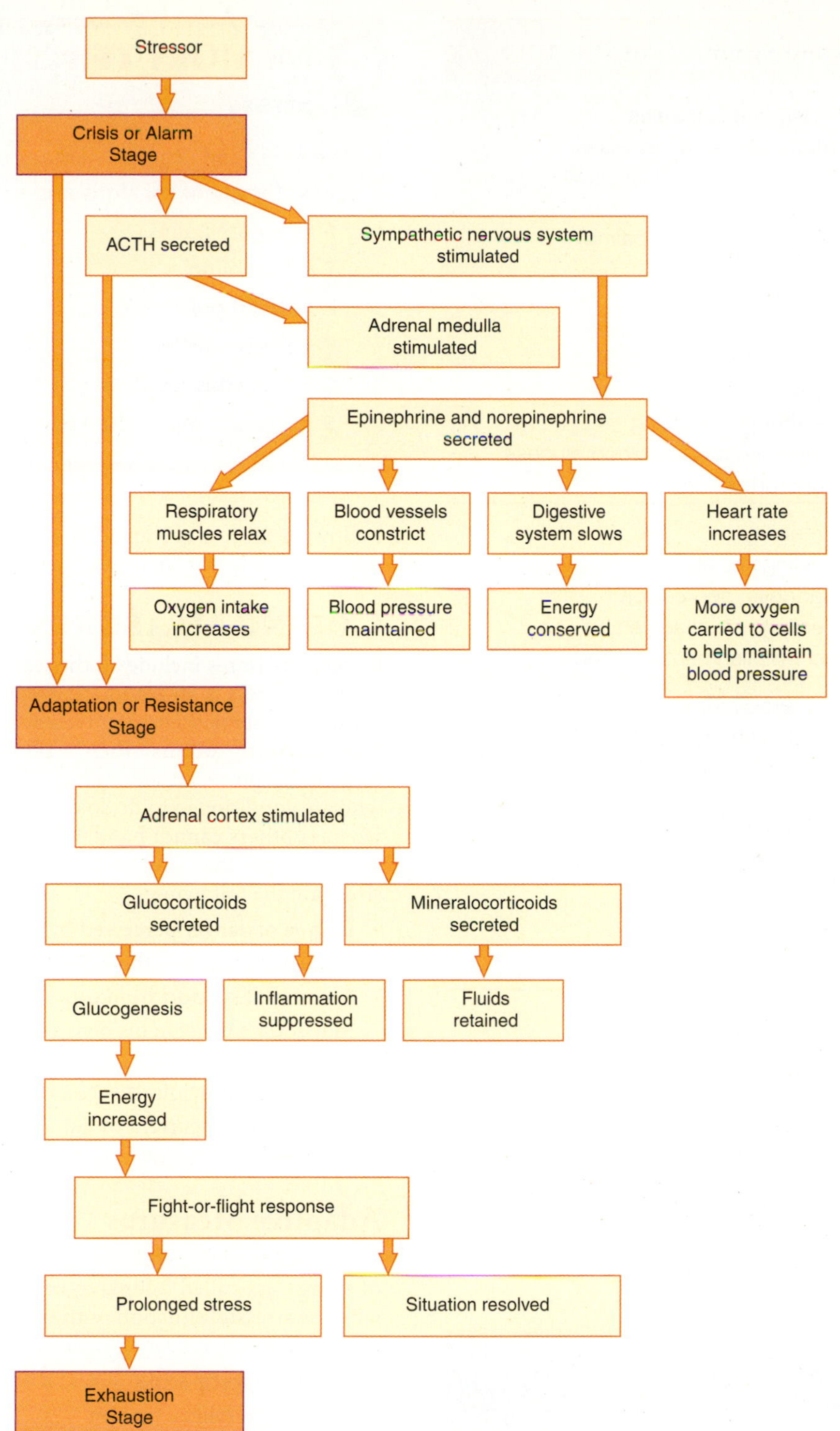

COURTESY OF DELMAR CENGAGE LEARNING

FIGURE 12-1 **Physiological Effects of the General Adaptation Syndrome (GAS)**

entire body (GAS) or only a specific area (LAS). An individual who lives in the mountains (high elevation) produces more red blood cells to carry enough oxygen to meet the body's needs. The chest also enlarges to allow the lungs to expand to accommodate the needed exchange of oxygen and carbon dioxide.

Psychological adaptation involves the use of defense mechanisms and learning to mentally accept new situations. A 55-year-old worker who suddenly finds himself unemployed will need to learn to adapt psychologically to the new situation and decide which steps to take next.

Cognitive adaptation involves education, communication, problem-solving ability, and perception of people and the world. A person gains these methods throughout life. For example, the high school student will have a different perspective of the world and different problem-solving abilities than will this same individual as a college graduate.

Social adaptation involves social relationships with family, friends, and coworkers who may provide support in times of stress (Figure 12-2). A person unable to cope may withdraw socially. An example of social adaptation would be a family

TABLE 12-1 Signs and Symptoms of Stress

Physiologic	• Pulse rate increases • Blood pressure increases • Breathing is rapid, shallow • Blood thickens • Dizziness, sweaty palms • Headache • Pupils dilate • Nausea, change in appetite • Constipation or diarrhea • Increased urination • Twitching, trembling • Increased level of blood glucose and cortisol
Psychological	• Irritability • Feelings easily hurt • Sadness, depression • Feelings of pleasure and accomplishment reduced
Cognitive	• Impaired memory and judgment • Confusion, unable to concentrate • Poor decision making • Altered perceptions, delayed response
Behavioral	• Pacing, rapid speech • Insomnia • Withdrawal • Easily startled
Spiritual	• Alienation, social isolation • Feeling of emptiness

COURTESY OF DELMAR CENGAGE LEARNING

moving to a new town and making new friends and modifying relationships with existing friends.

Spiritual adaptation involves beliefs about a supreme being and a positive sense of life's purpose and meaning. These beliefs are a personal resource for coping with stressors.

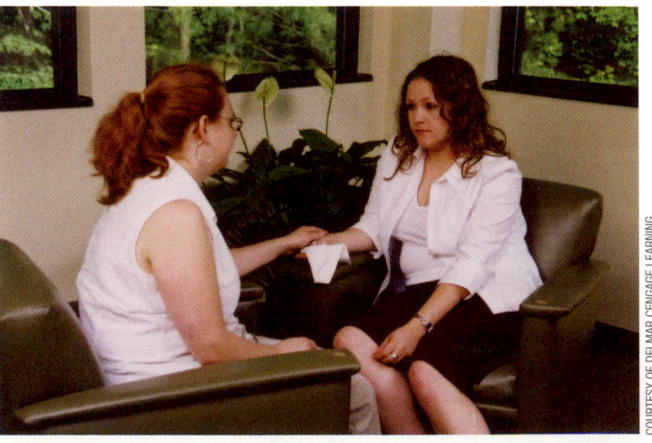

COURTESY OF DELMAR CENGAGE LEARNING

FIGURE 12-2 A coworker providing support is an example of social adaptation.

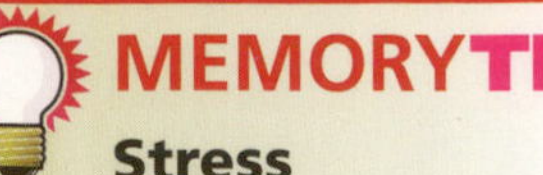

MEMORYTRICK

Stress

The nurse can use the memory trick **STRESS** to assess the client for signs and symptoms of stress:

- **S** = Sweaty palms
- **T** = Trembling
- **R** = Rapid pulse rate
- **E** = Easily startled
- **S** = Speech is rapid
- **S** = Shallow rapid respirations

Following the loss of a loved one, for instance, a family's spirituality and sense of faith may undergo changes.

COPING MEASURES

Coping measures include all the ways an individual may react to stress. Stress is an automatic response, but individuals can learn to conserve their adaptive energy through conditioning. **Conditioning** occurs when a person is taught a behavior until it becomes an automatic response. Some individuals who are conditioned to do so can handle a great deal of stress, whereas others cannot handle even a small amount of stress. Other factors that affect an individual's ability to cope with stress are the following:

- Degree of danger perceived by the individual
- Immediate needs of the individual
- Amount of support from others
- Individual's belief in his own ability to handle the stressful situation
- Individual's previous successes and failures in coping
- Number of concurrent or cumulative stresses being handled by the individual (Waughfield, 2002)

Adaptive Measures

Measures for coping with stress that require a minimal amount of energy are called **adaptive measures**. They deal directly with the stressful situation or the symptoms thereof. Adaptive measures useful in dealing with stressful situations include:

- Using support people
- Relaxing to relieve tension
- Changing behavior
- Developing more realistic goals
- Solving problems

Defense Mechanisms

Just as the body has physiologic mechanisms (e.g., the immune system, the inflammatory response) to defend against infection and disease, the mind has psychological protective mechanisms. Most **defense mechanisms** are unconscious functions protecting the mind from anxiety. They are used to gain and maintain psychological homeostasis. The individual does not consciously decide to use a defense mechanism; it happens automatically.

LIFE SPAN CONSIDERATIONS

Coping Ability

An individual's ability to cope with stressors depends in part on age and developmental level.

Everyone uses defense mechanisms. Their use does not imply mental illness or psychosocial imbalance. Defense mechanisms are considered maladaptive only when they are the only way an individual responds to a threat or when they limit the individual's ability to function. Table 12-2 describes and gives examples of various defense mechanisms.

Maladaptive Measures

Measures used to avoid conflict and stress are considered **maladaptive measures** because they prevent the individual from making progress toward resolving and accepting stress. They may include somatic disorders (transferring stress to an organ as pain), rituals, excessive use of alcohol or drugs, excessive eating, or withdrawal from reality.

Crisis

A crisis occurs when stressors surpass the ability to cope. A **crisis** (an acute state of disorganization) occurs when the usual coping mechanisms are no longer adequate. Crisis is characterized by extreme anxiety, disorganized behavior, and inability to function. A crisis is time limited because no one can stay in acute disequilibrium for a long time and experi-

CULTURAL CONSIDERATIONS

Adaptive Measures

Nurses must be sensitive to the fact that culture and ethnicity may influence an individual's choice of coping mechanisms. For instance, moaning and chanting may be an expected response to stress in some cultures; the nurse must be careful to view this behavior not as maladaptive but as a culturally healthy response to a stressor.

TABLE 12-2 Defense Mechanisms

DEFENSE MECHANISM	DESCRIPTION	EXAMPLE
Denial	Refusal to acknowledge the reality of threatening situations despite factual evidence	A person with heart disease continues to eat fatty foods and fried foods despite medical advice to the contrary.
Displacement	Transfer of feelings or reactions from one object to another object, usually one that is "safer"	A husband who is angry with his wife yells at the dog instead of dealing with his anger at his wife.
Projection	Attribution of one's own thoughts, feelings, or impulses to others	An adolescent who does not want to go with the crowd states, "My parents won't let me go."
Rationalization	Intellectual explanation or justification of ideas, feelings, or behavior	A student responds after failing a test that "The test had many trick questions on it; I really know the material."
Reaction formation	Expression of a feeling that is the opposite of one's real feeling	A client brings a gift to a nurse with whom he is really angry.
Regression	A return to a previous developmental level	A child who has not sucked her thumb in 2 years starts to do so again when admitted to the hospital.
Repression	The unconscious blocking from awareness of material that is painful or threatening	Adult's claim, despite evidence, that "I never got angry with my parents; we lived in love and harmony."
Suppression	A conscious or unconscious attempt to keep threatening or unpleasant material out of consciousness	Failure to remember a house fire during childhood.
Sublimation	Channeling of socially unacceptable impulses into socially acceptable activities	A young man who deals with aggression by playing football.

Adapted from *Psychiatric Mental Health Nursing* (4th ed.), by N. Frisch and L. Frisch, 2010. Clifton Park, NY: Delmar Cengage Learning.

PROFESSIONALTIP

Defense Mechanisms

The nurse who is unfamiliar with defense mechanisms may be judgmental about clients who do not respond as the nurse expects. If the nurse tries to break through a client's denial (defense mechanism) too quickly by presenting reality, the client may be overwhelmed by anxiety and will panic.

ence the great discomfort. Given the time-limited nature of crisis, a client in crisis needs immediate intervention for a successful resolution. Crisis intervention is discussed later in this chapter.

Crisis can be a negative experience, but it can also present an opportunity for growth and learning. The outcome depends on each individual's perception and coping abilities. Nurses can guide clients to discover opportunities in the crisis and adapt in positive, healthy ways.

Stressful events do not always result in a crisis. A crisis is *not* a mental illness, even though persons experiencing the acute anxiety and discomfort fear for their sanity. Each crisis is unique to the individual; however, crises have common characteristics (Table 12-3).

ANXIETY

Anxiety is a subjective response that occurs when a person experiences a real or perceived threat to well-being; it is a diverse feeling of dread or apprehension. There is a close relationship between anxiety and stress. Anxiety is the psychological response to a threat, such as the worry that results when oversleeping on a workday. This worry can translate into stress (the person's physiologic response to a stimulus) by rushing, perspiring, and becoming careless. Anxiety can be an activator of stress *and* a response to stress: It is usually activated by stress and may lead to more stress. Anxiety is a major component of mental health disturbances.

TABLE 12-3 Crisis Characteristics

- A loss, actual or perceived, is a part of every crisis.
- A crisis occurs suddenly.
- A crisis has a known precipitating event.
- The situation is seen as overwhelming or life threatening.
- Communication becomes impaired.
- Usual coping skills cannot resolve the situation.
- Intervention is required to reestablish equilibrium.

Data from *Contemporary Psychiatric-Mental Health Nursing*, by H. S. Wilson, C. R. Kneisl, and E. Trigoboff, 2004, Upper Saddle River, NJ: Prentice Hall. Copyright 2004 by Prentice Hall.

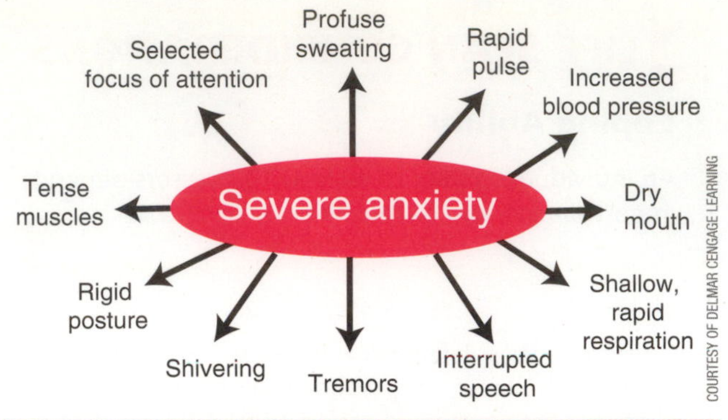

FIGURE 12-3 Physical and Mental Responses to Severe Anxiety

The most common emotional (affective) response to stress is anxiety. Individuals feel anxious when they are threatened, even if the threat is only perceived. Anxiety occurs on a continuum; some degree of anxiety is beneficial as a motivator. A high level of anxiety, however, can overpower a person and diminish the ability to function and think. The person is less able to function as the level of anxiety increases (Figure 12-3). Table 12-4 describes the levels of anxiety.

EFFECTS OF AND ON ILLNESS

Anxiety often increases during illness and recovery. It is often difficult to determine whether illness or stress came first. Illness occurs when adaptive attempts are unsuccessful. Also, an ill person has fewer usable adaptive resources to cope with stressors. Some stressors may not directly cause disease, but stress is a substantial aspect in the onset and progress of many illnesses. Some disorders commonly associated with stress include:

- Arrhythmias
- Asthma
- Back pain
- Decreased libido
- Diabetes
- Eating disorders
- Eczema
- Emphysema
- Fertility problems
- Headache
- Hives
- Hypertension
- Impotence
- Irritable bowel syndrome
- Menstrual disorders
- Periodontal disease
- Psoriasis
- Sleep disturbance
- Ulcers
- Viral activation, herpes, or HIV
- Weight gain or loss

The immune system is impaired during prolonged periods of stress. Steroid production increases as the body fights

COMMUNITY/HOME HEALTH CARE

Reducing Stressors

Remember, as a home health or visiting nurse, you are a guest in the client's home. If changes must be made in the home or the way it is kept, provide suggestions that are directly related to the client or the care of the client. Never criticize the home itself or the way it is kept.

TABLE 12-4 Levels of Anxiety

ANXIETY LEVEL	CHARACTERISTICS OF THE ANXIOUS PERSON	NURSING CONSIDERATIONS
Mild	• Increased degree of alertness • Increased vigilance • Increased motivation • Readiness for action • Slight increase in vital signs	• Best time for client teaching.
Moderate	• Subjective distress (tension) • Decreased perception and attention • Alert only to specific information • Possible tendency to complain or argue • Possible headache, diarrhea, nausea, or vomiting	• Assist client in determining cause and effect between stressor and anxiety.
Severe	• Increased subjective distress • Feeling of impending danger • Selective attention • Distorted communication • Distorted perception • Feelings of fatigue	• Encourage verbalization. • Encourage motor activity (walking, exercise). • Give specific directions.
Panic	• Major perceptual distortion • Immobilization; inability to function • Feelings of terror • Possible harm to self and others	• Provide guidelines and limits. • Maintain client safety (both physical and psychological).

Data from *Interpersonal Relations in Nursing*, by H. E. Peplau, 1952, New York: Putnam; *The Interpersonal Theory of Psychiatry*, by L. S. Sullivan, 1953, New York: Norton.

the perceived or actual threat. Steroids reduce the immune system's ability to function, and the body is less able to protect itself from disease.

All clients in a health care facility have a change in their routine that may cause anxiety and stress. The unfamiliar environment, loss of control over their schedule, and dependence on others for care are issues with which these clients must cope. Each issue is a stressor requiring adaptation by the client to maintain homeostasis. Some clients do not have the adaptive energy to cope with the many changes and cope with their illness. Cues that a person may not be coping well to hospitalization include:

- Increased stress response
- High level of anxiety
- Increased use of coping mechanisms
- Inability to function
- Disorganized behavior

The person having "minor" surgery at an outpatient center, the adolescent being treated by the school nurse, or the employee being treated at an industrial clinic for a work-related injury may also experience client role stressors. Even clients who are treated in their homes may experience stressors from having a health care provider in their personal environment.

The greater the threat (or perceived threat), the higher the level of anxiety. Nurses must be sensitive to stress and many changes caused by illness. This reduces the risk of depersonalizing the client.

Depersonalization is the process of treating an individual as an object instead of a person. It takes away a client's individuality by treating him as a thing. Nursing interventions focus on assisting the client to lessen feelings of loss of control.

CHANGE

Change, a dynamic process whereby an individual's response to a stressor leads to an alteration in behavior, is an inevitable part of life. Whether change is planned or unplanned, it is inevitable and constant. Change can be stressful to individuals and activate the GAS. Characteristics of change are that it:

- May be stressful or distressful
- Can be externally imposed or self-initiated
- Can occur abruptly or have a gradual onset
- Requires energy to effect as well as to resist

CRITICAL THINKING

Stress and Illness

How would you explain the relationship between stress and illness to a client?

PROFESSIONALTIP

Promoting Client Control

- *Communicate clearly.* Avoid using medical jargon.
- *Thoroughly answer questions.* Validate the level of understanding.
- *Teach relaxation techniques,* such as progressive muscle relaxation and guided imagery.
- *Instruct clients how to use* **cognitive reframing** (the individual changes a negative perception of a situation to a less-threatening perception).
- *Provide support and reassurance.* The most therapeutic way to alleviate client anxiety is the nurse's therapeutic use of self (Figure 12-4).

All health care providers should know how to initiate and cope with change. Critical thinking and problem-solving skills are needed to effectively initiate and cope with change.

Types of Change

Change may be unplanned or planned. Unplanned change is unpredictable and may be imposed by others or by uncontrollable events (e.g., losing one's home in a fire). Planned change is a specific effort to modify a situation. A marriage is an example of a planned change. In addition to planned change and unplanned change, there are other types of change.

Developmental changes are physical and emotional alterations occurring at different stages of life. These are usually predictable and occur in a certain order. For instance, a baby will first learn to roll over, then crawl, then walk. The exact age will vary, but the sequence usually does not.

Accidental or reactive changes are adaptive responses to change imposed by others. This may include a change in one's working hours or a child's baseball game being rescheduled.

Covert changes are often subtle and occur without a person's conscious awareness. These might include a gradual shifting of responsibilities as new skills are acquired or developed at work.

Overt changes are obvious and identifiable, and an individual is aware they are occurring. They are usually not under an individual's direct control, such as the restructuring of one's place of employment, but must be adapted to and accepted in order to continue functioning effectively.

Resistance to Change

People tend to resist change because of the energy required to adapt, although energy is also required to resist change, or to maintain the status quo. The ability to tolerate (or even thrive on) change differs in individuals. There are no guarantees that change will lead to a positive outcome. Uncertainty regarding outcome is a major barrier to change.

It is risky to challenge one's own ideas or those of others by initiating change. Questioning is one of the first signs of the need for change. The nurse who wonders "Why?" "What if?" or "Why not?" will likely risk initiating change. Successful risk takers consider the costs and benefits of their ideas and the outcomes relative to available resources.

Because change is inevitable, nurses must learn ways to deal with change. Resistance looks like the individual is rejecting proposed new ideas without critically thinking about the proposal. Nurses must take time to research ideas and make informed decisions as to whether change is worthwhile. Coping with change calls for adaptability, flexibility, and resilience.

Nurse as Change Agent

The nurse often serves as a **change agent** (a person who intentionally creates and implements change). Change agents seek ways to make improvements using critical thinking to develop innovative, creative solutions.

Change should be planned by individuals who are proactive. The proactive individual initiates action rather than waiting for others to solve problems, make decisions, or become rescuers. Reactive persons, on the other hand, respond only to externally imposed change. Proactive nurses are change agents who often affect the entire health care system as well as individual clients.

Change agents work toward a positive outcome. Client education is a powerful tool for initiating change. The client is provided with an opportunity to change when taught a disease process, a treatment modality, or a lifestyle alteration. Learning results in behavioral changes. The change process is similar to the nursing process in that change involves assessment, planning, decision making, implementation, and evaluation.

NURSING PROCESS

Nurses can be instrumental in helping clients both understand their anxiety and learn measures to cope with and control their feelings of stress.

Assessment

The nurse must first ascertain the anxious client's perception of the situation. This is accomplished by directly asking the client and then listening carefully to the client's response (Figure 12-4). Nurses must be aware of their own body language because the nurse's nonverbal behavior can affect the client's anxiety level. Anxiety is a subjective experience and

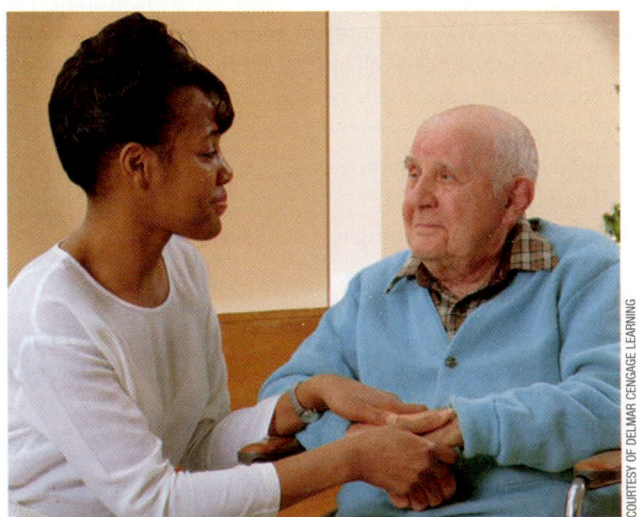

Figure 12-4 **Through talking, listening, and touch, the nurse can help relieve the client's feelings of anxiety.**

cannot be directly observed. The nurse must therefore look for signs of anxiety (refer back to Table 12-4).

A thorough assessment of stress and anxiety levels includes asking the client about:

- Types or patterns of stressors
- Usual response to stressful situations
- Cause-and-effect relationships among stressors and thoughts, feelings, and behaviors
- History of successful coping

The client's coping abilities can be assessed in various ways. Open-ended questions can be used to ascertain previously used coping mechanisms. Some sample questions are:

- What is the problem?
- What have you tried before?
- How well did it work?

Appropriate nursing diagnoses and an effective plan of care can be established by identifying the client's coping abilities. Assessment provides the data necessary for identifying nursing diagnoses.

Nursing Diagnosis

Several nursing diagnoses may apply to clients experiencing anxiety; the most common of these are ***A**nxiety*, *Ineffective **C**oping*, *Ineffective **D**enial*, and ***P**owerlessness*. Additional North American Nursing Diagnosis Association International (NANDA-I, 2010) diagnoses that may also apply include:

- *Impaired **A**djustment*
- *Ineffective **R**ole Performance*
- *Disturbed **T**hought Processes*
- *Defensive **C**oping*
- ***F**ear*
- ***P**ost-Trauma Syndrome*
- *Impaired **S**ocial Interaction*
- ***S**piritual Distress*
- ***H**opelessness*
- ***F**atigue*
- *Disturbed **S**leep Pattern*

Planning/Outcome Identification

Involving clients in planning care is essential because helping clients learn to cope successfully is part of the empowerment process. Planning means exploring with the client self-responsibility issues. A major goal for working with an anxious client is to reduce anxiety so problem solving and learning can occur.

There may be many expected outcomes (goals) appropriate for clients experiencing stress or anxiety. A few basic goals are for the client to:

- Identify situations when stress and anxiety increase.
- Describe ways to decrease the effects of usual stressors.
- Identify positive and negative stressors in the client's life.
- Group stressors into categories: ones that can be eliminated, ones that can be controlled, and ones that cannot be controlled directly by self.
- Demonstrate correct use of select stress-management exercises (e.g., progressive muscle relaxation, guided imagery, thought stopping).
- Describe the plan for managing stress, including lifestyle modifications.

> **SAFETY**
>
> **The Client Experiencing Panic**
>
> Never leave a panic-stricken client alone. The client with panic-level anxiety may harm herself. Stay with this client or have someone else do so.

Implementation

Teaching is part of holistic nursing practice. Stress-management methods can be taught to clients of every age and developmental stage in all health care settings.

A major step in improving self-care is to teach clients how to reduce their own stress level. Education gives clients options. Clients who understand their options can make informed decisions (Figure 12-5). Some of the many interventions that may assist the anxious client follow.

Meet Basic Needs

Stress and basic physiologic needs are closely related. Anything interfering with basic needs being met elicits the stress response, causing anxiety. Clients who are in pain, cold, or hungry have a higher anxiety level than when comfortable. The perception of pain increases with a higher level of anxiety. The nurse actually improves the potential for recovery by reducing client anxiety.

Minimize Environmental Stimuli

An individual's immediate environment can influence stress levels. The nurse should decrease environmental stimuli that may cause anxiety. Environmental stimuli can be reduced by:

- Closing the client's room door
- Turning the television off
- Reducing loudness of the telephone ringer or disconnecting the phone, if feasible

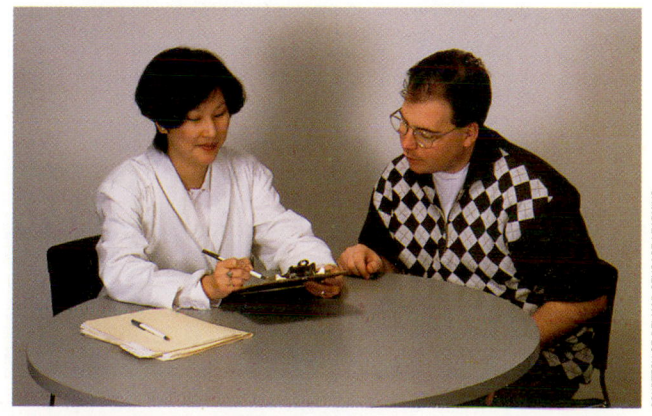

COURTESY OF DELMAR CENGAGE LEARNING

FIGURE 12-5 The nurse discusses the options for care and provides the client with the information needed to plan effective lifestyle changes.

- Dimming the lights or closing the blinds
- Limiting the number of visitors (unless isolation increases the client's anxiety)

Verbalize Feelings

Encouraging clients to express their feelings is especially helpful to reduce stress. Freud (1959) described the process of talking out one's feelings as a **catharsis**. People seem to instinctively know the value of "getting things off their chest." Verbalizing promotes relaxation because (a) a verbalized feeling becomes real and an identified problem can be dealt with, and (b) the activity of talking uses energy and reduces anxiety.

Involve Family/Significant Others

The type of intervention for managing stress is influenced by the client's developmental stage. Children need and rely on their parents or caretakers for security and support. Because families provide essential support for clients, it is important to include the entire family in the care of the client whenever possible (Figure 12-6) to decrease the stress level of everyone involved.

Family members who are anxious may have a negative impact on the client's health status. One way nurses must often help family members relax is to provide information and explanations. Researchers have concluded that both the client and family benefit from family presence during invasive procedures and resuscitation (Meyers et al., 2000).

Several national organizations, such as the American Heart Association, the Society of Critical Care Medicine, the American Association of Critical-Care Nurses, and the Emergency Nurses Association, have developed guidelines and practice statements to advocate family presence during invasive procedures and CPR. Studies have indicated that "family presence doesn't usually interfere with medical interventions when the focus is on a patient's survival" (Briguglio, 2007).

Use Stress-Management Techniques

A variety of stress-management techniques can easily be taught to clients, families, and significant others. Some of the most common approaches for managing stress are discussed next.

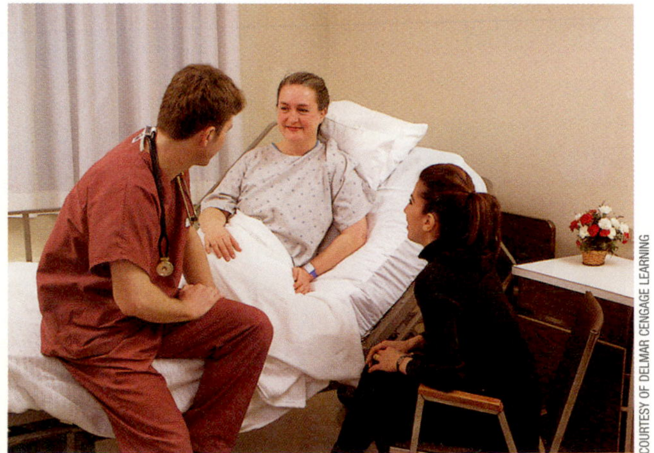
COURTESY OF DELMAR CENGAGE LEARNING

FIGURE 12-6 The nurse encourages interaction between the client and family members and significant others. This involvement helps ease the client's anxiety and keeps the family informed about the client's cares.

Exercise A powerful way to reduce anxiety is physical exercise. The need for incorporating exercise into one's lifestyle should be emphasized in client teaching. To establish an exercise program:

- Explore the different exercise programs available
- Ask a health care provider about the safety of a specific exercise program
- Set realistic goals
- Select a routine allowing warm-up and cool-down periods
- Take up activities that increase heart rate for a period of time

If exercise is to reduce anxiety, it must be done on a regular, ongoing basis. Physiologic benefits of regular exercise are listed in Table 12-5 and include:

- Feelings of well-being are enhanced
- Concentration and memory improve
- Depression is lessened
- Insomnia is lessened
- Dependence on external stimulants or relaxants is reduced
- Self-esteem increases
- Sense of self-control over anxiety is renewed

Relaxation Techniques Several techniques can help individuals relax (Figure 12-7). Complementary and alternative interventions such as progressive muscle relaxation and guided imagery are useful in helping clients learn to relax. Meditation and hypnosis can also be very effective in inducing relaxation and relieving stress.

Cognitive Reframing or Thought Stopping Cognitive reframing is a technique based on Beck's (1976) theory that a person's emotional response to an event is determined by the meaning attached to it. For example, the client is likely to feel anxious if an event is perceived as threatening. The client will be less anxious if the interpretation of the event can be modified. Reframing is used to alter one's perceptions and interpretations by changing one's thoughts.

Crisis Intervention

Some clients will be in an acute crisis state and require **crisis intervention**, a specific technique to help a person regain equilibrium. Crisis intervention views individuals as capable of personal growth and able to influence and control their own lives (Kneisl & Riley, 1996). The five steps of crisis intervention are:

1. Identify the specific problem, including the underlying issues.
2. Identify all possible options.
3. Examine possible outcomes for each option and select an option.
4. Implement the selected option.
5. Evaluate the overall effectiveness of the plan.

Clients sometimes need more assistance than the nurse is able to provide. Prompt consultation with or referral to other health care providers is necessary, such as:

- Psychiatric clinical nurse specialists
- Nurse psychotherapists

TABLE 12-5 Physiological Benefits of Exercise

EFFECT OF EXERCISE	PHYSIOLOGICAL BENEFIT
Promotes metabolism of adrenalin and thyroxine	• Minimizes autonomic arousal and hypervigilance
Reduces musculoskeletal tension	• Decreases feelings of being tense and "uptight"
Improves circulation, resulting in better oxygenation of the brain	• Increases alertness and concentration, and leads to enhanced problem-solving ability
Stimulates **endorphin** (a group of opiate-like substances produced naturally by the brain) production	• Raises the body's pain threshold, and promotes a sense of well-being
Reduces cholesterol level	• Decreases the risk of atherosclerosis
Reduces blood pressure	• Decreases the risk of myocardial infarction (heart attack) and cerebral vascular accident (CVA) (stroke)
Stimulates elimination (through lungs, skin, bowels)	• Reduces toxin buildup in the body

Data from "Nutrition, Exercise, and Movement," by L. Keegan, 2000, in B. Dossey, L. Keegan, and C. Guzzetta (Eds.), *Holistic Nursing: A Handbook for Practice* (3rd ed.), Gaithersburg, MD: Aspen; "Health Promotion and the Individual," by C. Mandle and R. Gruber-Wood, 2002, in C. Edelman and C. Mandle (Eds.), *Health Promotion throughout the Lifespan* (5th ed.), St. Louis, MO: Mosby.

- Psychologists
- Psychiatrists
- Social workers
- Clergy or other counselors

EVALUATION

Evaluation of the client's coping abilities must include client input. The nurse must evaluate client outcomes as well as nursing care. The family can also be a valuable source of information about the effectiveness of the stress-reduction approaches.

STRESS MANAGEMENT FOR THE NURSE

There are many stressors in nursing. It is essential that nurses learn to cope successfully with the stressors (Figure 12-8). Nurses must cope successfully with stress to maintain their own wellness and to model healthy behaviors. Nurses must first be able to manage their own stress before helping clients learn to manage theirs.

High stress levels among nurses often lead to **burnout**, a state of physical and emotional exhaustion occurring when caregivers use up their adaptive energy. In an article by Fink

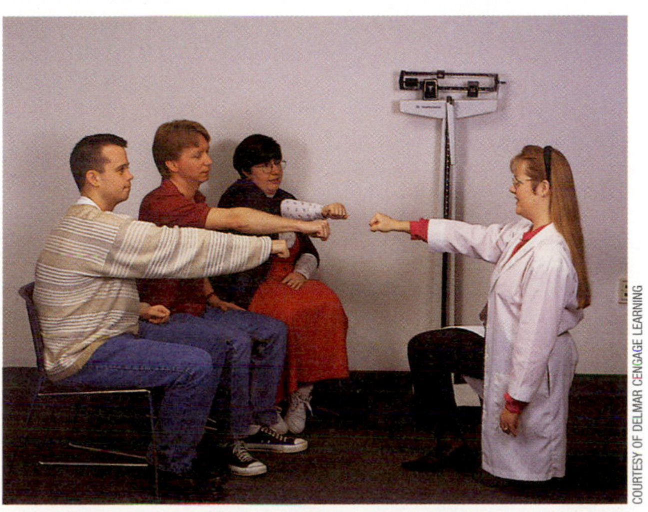
COURTESY OF DELMAR CENGAGE LEARNING

FIGURE 12-7 The nurse demonstrates the technique of progressive muscle relaxation in a client-education program.

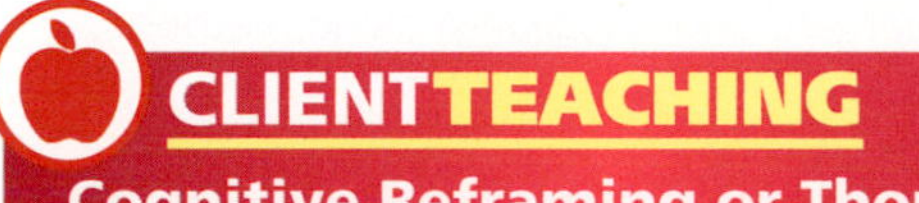

Cognitive Reframing or Thought Stopping

- Listen to self-talk (thoughts).
- Identify negative self-talk.
- Do something physical when a negative thought is detected to stop the train of thought, such as clapping your hands or snapping a rubber band on your wrist.
- Replace the negative thought with one that is both realistic and positive.

Like all other relaxation exercises, thought stopping becomes more effective with repetition.

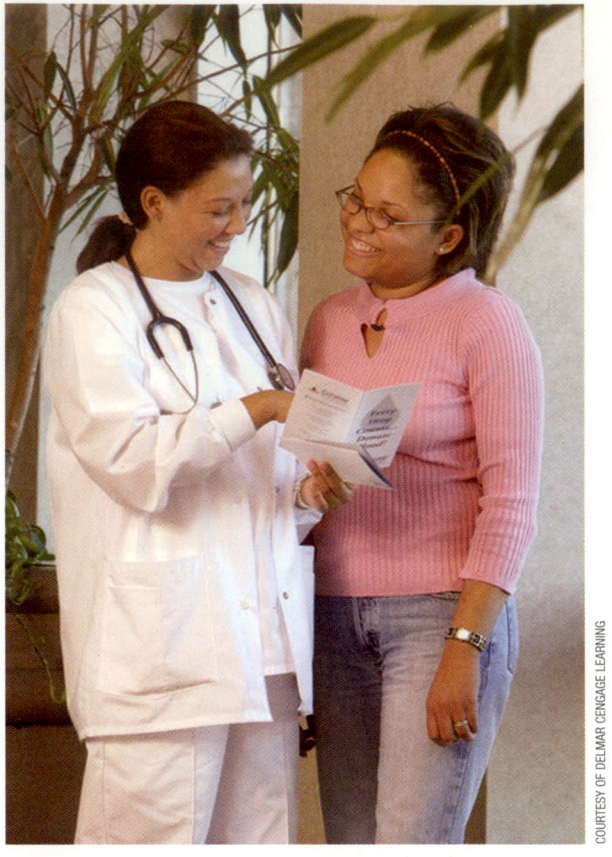

COURTESY OF DELMAR CENGAGE LEARNING

FIGURE 12-8 Sharing a light and humorous moment with a friend is a wonderful way to relieve stress and regain perspective.

(2005), she discussed a recent study of nurses in five countries in which 30% to 40% stated that they felt burned out. The nurses at highest risk of experiencing burnout were the best and brightest who set high standards for themselves. Nurses experiencing such an overwhelming degree of stress often treat clients in a depersonalizing manner. These nurses also lack feelings of personal accomplishment. Burnout imposes a high price on individual nurses and on the profession as highly qualified professionals leave nursing. The quality of care declines as a result.

Several work-related factors can contribute to burnout:

- Heavy workload (critically ill clients)
- Interpersonal conflict in the work environment
- Mandatory overtime and "floating" to other units
- Little work-related social support

Stress management is the key to burnout prevention and recovery. A stress-management plan begins with self-awareness. It is a continuous process, not the occasional use of a technique or exercise. Nurses often fail to take care of themselves, but it is essential that nurses learn to care for themselves.

CRITICAL THINKING

Burnout

A client is exhibiting panic-level anxiety and should not be left alone. You are experiencing severe burnout because of very long work hours and recent stressful situations. Your stress level is so high that you feel you cannot stay in the room with this client. If you leave the room to find another nurse to stay with him, he may injure himself; if you stay, you risk your own emotional well-being. How do you deal with this situation?

TABLE 12-6 Strategies for Managing Professional Stress

STRATEGY	RATIONALE
Develop active support systems at work and away from work.	Non–health care provider friends help maintain a balance in life.
Use time management and decision-making methods.	Viewing personal needs as a priority encourages one to schedule time to meet those needs. Breaking down large tasks into small, realistic ones prevents being overwhelmed.
Focus on accomplishments.	Increases self-esteem.
Know personal limits.	Helps separate the important from the less important.
Avoid harmful substances.	Smoking, overeating, and intake of caffeine, alcohol, or other substances often increase stress and anxiety in the long run.
Nourish the body with healthy diet, exercise, and sleep.	A healthy mind and body is better able to handle stress.
Practice slow, focused breathing.	Muscle tension is alleviated with more oxygen in the blood.
Vary tasks between mental and physical activities.	Conserves energy, reduces fatigue, and maintains a sense of balance.
Maintain a sense of humor.	Helps keep a positive outlook; can be used to reframe a situation.

COURTESY OF DELMAR CENGAGE LEARNING

CRITICAL THINKING

Stressors

Reflect on the past month. List some of the stressors that you have experienced during that time. How did you respond to the stressors? Would you now respond differently in similar situations? If so, what would you change?

There are many strategies to help nurses manage professional and personal stress, as outlined in Table 12-6.

Nurses who cultivate the hardiness factor will likely be resilient to stress. Kobasa (1979) put forth the concept of hardiness in the late 1970s. Hardiness consists of a set of attitudes, beliefs, and behaviors that make individuals more resilient (or hardy) to the negative effects of stress. The three components to stress hardiness are:

- *Commitment:* Become involved in what one is doing
- *Challenge:* Perceive change as an opportunity for growth instead of an obstacle or threat
- *Control:* Believe that one is directing what happens to oneself rather than feeling victimized and helpless

According to studies (Kobasa, 1979; Kobasa, Maddi, & Kahn, 1982), persons having higher degrees of hardiness are healthier than those with low degrees of hardiness. When experiencing multiple stressors, such people develop fewer illnesses.

Many nurses must learn when to stop working and relearn the value of play. Nursing students, spending many hours working and studying, may need to schedule playtime. The student nurse doing so is making a start on managing stress.

SAMPLE NURSING CARE PLAN

The Client Experiencing Severe Anxiety

S.H. is a 38-year-old female in the emergency department of the local hospital. She paces, wrings her hands, and is tearful. She says she has chest pressure, palpitations, and shortness of breath. She is diaphoretic and her hands are trembling. Her blood pressure is 140/90, pulse 110, and respirations 30 and shallow. She says that her husband left her a month ago. She states, "I feel like I'm going crazy! My heart is racing and I can't sit still."

Assessment reveals autonomic hyperactivity (rapid pulse and respirations, elevated blood pressure), verbalized feelings of apprehension, restlessness, and going crazy.

NURSING DIAGNOSIS *Anxiety* related to situational crisis, threat to self-concept, and change in role status as evidenced by statement "I feel like I'm going crazy" and the fact that her husband left her a month ago

Nursing Outcomes Classification (NOC)
Anxiety Control
Coping
Psychosocial Adjustment: Life Change

Nursing Interventions Classification (NIC)
Anxiety Reduction
Coping Enhancement
Simple Relaxation Therapy

PLANNING/OUTCOMES	NURSING INTERVENTIONS	RATIONALE
S.H. will identify effective coping mechanisms.	Establish a trusting relationship.	Reduces anxiety.
	Have S.H. identify and describe physical and emotional feelings.	Is the first step in coping with anxiety.
	Help S.H. relate cause-and-effect relationship between stressors and anxiety.	Enhances S.H.'s sense of power and control over the situation.
	Encourage S.H. to use previously successful coping mechanisms.	Builds confidence in own coping abilities.

(*Continues*)

SAMPLE NURSING CARE PLAN (Continued)

PLANNING/OUTCOMES	NURSING INTERVENTIONS	RATIONALE
S.H. will report that anxiety has lessened and is manageable.	Using therapeutic communication techniques, encourage S.H. to talk about what has been happening in her life.	Clarifies situation by talking about it.
S.H. will demonstrate relaxation skills.	Teach S.H. relaxation techniques (such as cognitive reframing and imagery).	Counters the physiologic effects of the stress response (lower blood pressure, decreased heart rate, and respirations).

EVALUATION

S.H. looks relaxed. Vital signs are within normal limits. S.H. verbalizes that she feels calmer and no longer afraid that she is "going crazy."

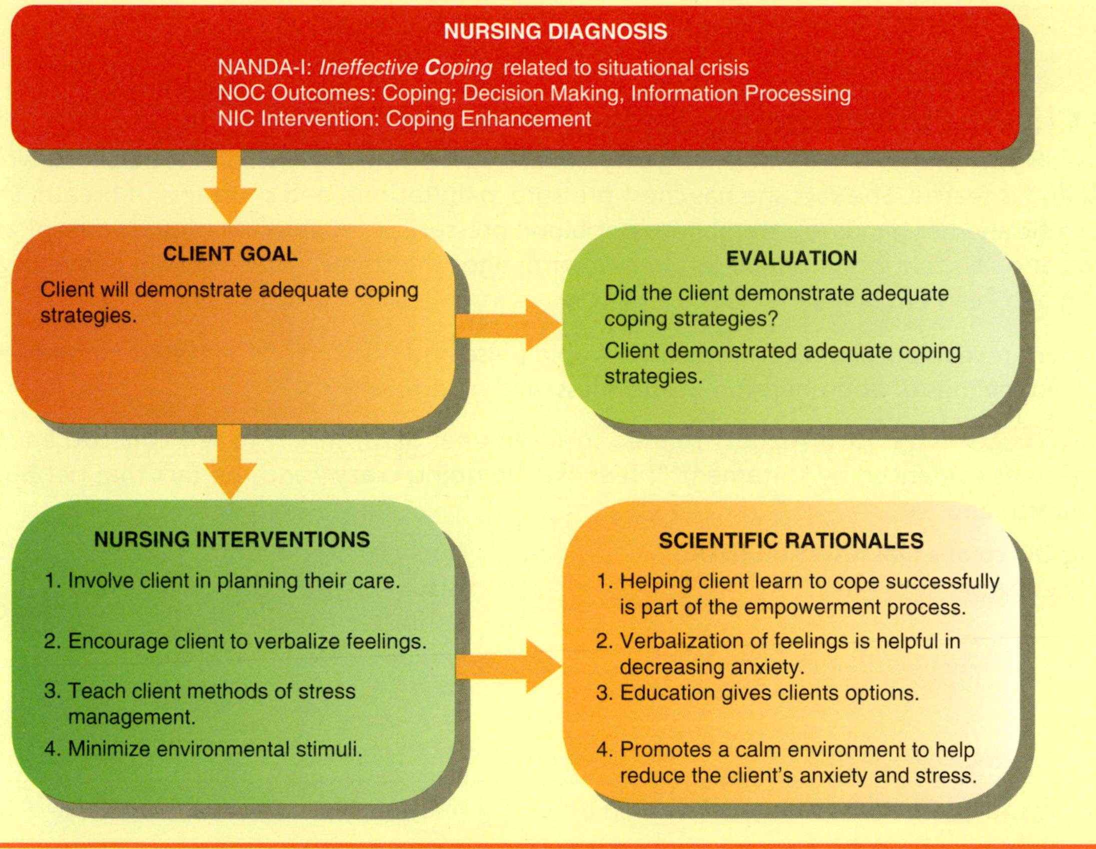

NURSING DIAGNOSIS
NANDA-I: *Ineffective **Coping*** related to situational crisis
NOC Outcomes: Coping; Decision Making, Information Processing
NIC Intervention: Coping Enhancement
CLIENT GOAL
Client will demonstrate adequate coping strategies.
EVALUATION
Did the client demonstrate adequate coping strategies?
Client demonstrated adequate coping strategies.
NURSING INTERVENTIONS
1. Involve client in planning their care.
2. Encourage client to verbalize feelings.
3. Teach client methods of stress management.
4. Minimize environmental stimuli.
SCIENTIFIC RATIONALES
1. Helping client learn to cope successfully is part of the empowerment process.
2. Verbalization of feelings is helpful in decreasing anxiety.
3. Education gives clients options.
4. Promotes a calm environment to help reduce the client's anxiety and stress.

Concept Care Map 12-1

SUMMARY

- Stress is an individual's physiologic response to a demand made on the body.
- Individuals experiencing prolonged periods of stress risk developing stress-related diseases.
- Anxiety, the psychological response to a real or perceived threat to the health and well-being of an individual, activates the stress response.
- An individual seeks equilibrium through adaptation. When adaptation is effective, homeostasis is maintained.
- The general adaptation syndrome (GAS), the physiologic response to stress, consists of three stages: alarm, resistance, and exhaustion. The GAS is the same whether the stressor is actual or imagined, present or potential.

- Major stressors for clients and their families are illness and hospitalization. To alleviate the stress of hospitalization, nursing interventions should reduce the client's feelings of unfamiliarity and loss of control.
- Change can be perceived as stressful because of a fear of failure, a threat to security, or a potential for loss of self-esteem.
- Burnout occurs when the nurse is overwhelmed by stress, resulting in physical, emotional, and behavioral dysfunction, including decreased productivity.
- A stress-management plan for nurses involves maintaining support systems, using time-management and decision-making skills, maintaining a sense of humor, and knowing personal limits.

REVIEW QUESTIONS

1. The client is in an acute crisis state and requires crisis intervention. The nurse recognizes that the client needs more assistance than the nurse is able to provide. Prompt consultation/referral to other health care providers is necessary and would include:
   1. psychologist, psychiatrist, social worker.
   2. family physician, midwife, social worker.
   3. social worker, respiratory therapist, nursing supervisor.
   4. psychologist, nursing supervisor, pharmacist.
2. The general adaptation syndrome (GAS) is the:
   1. behavioral response to stress.
   2. sociocultural response to stress.
   3. psychological response to stress.
   4. physiologic response to stress.
3. The nurse tells her unit supervisor that she is feeling burned out and not sure that she wants to be a nurse anymore. Which of the following work-related factors can contribute to her burnout? (Select all that apply).
   1. Heavy workload.
   2. Mandatory overtime.
   3. Recently divorced.
   4. Little work-related social support.
   5. Child care issues.
   6. Interpersonal conflict in the work environment.
4. The purpose of the first stage of the GAS is to:
   1. alert the individual to danger.
   2. determine the cause of the danger.
   3. mobilize energy needed for adaptation.
   4. prevent the individual from having an unpleasant experience.
5. Which of the following statements is correct when teaching the client about the degree and duration of stress?
   1. A large number of stressors at one time will increase the severity of stress.
   2. The longer a stress lasts, the less severe it becomes for a person.
   3. A large amount of stress will improve performance.
   4. Many persons under severe stress go through life without any psychological effect.
6. While assisting the client with his morning care, the nurse notes that the client is quieter than yesterday and appears to be very anxious. To determine the level of anxiety that the client is experiencing, the nurse should ask which of the following questions?
   1. "You seem worried about something. Would it help to talk about it?"
   2. "Would you like for me to call a family member to come and give you support?"
   3. "Would you like to go down the hall and talk with another client who had the same surgery?"
   4. "How serious do you think your illness is?"
7. A 68-year-old client is in a rehabilitative facility after having had a cerebrovascular accident. The client is noncommunicative, heart rate increases, blood pressure is maintained, and respirations are becoming increased and labored. Which of the stages of the GAS is the client experiencing?
   1. Resistance stage.
   2. Alarm reaction.
   3. Exhaustion stage.
   4. Reflex pain response.
8. A factory worker cuts his arm while trimming a piece of steel, and it bleeds profusely. He quickly applies pressure to his arm and causes a cessation of the bleeding within minutes. Shortly afterward, the factory worker bumps the arm again. The bleeding begins again and will not stop. Which stage of the GAS would the factory worker have experienced if the blood loss continued and he could not obtain assistance?
   1. Stage of alarm reaction.
   2. Stage of resistance.
   3. Stage of exhaustion.
   4. Stage of distress.
9. A client who has been newly diagnosed with a terminal illness and is hospitalized for the first time is exhibiting signs that she is not coping well, which include all of the following except:
   1. increase in stress response.
   2. increased use of coping mechanisms.
   3. inability to function.
   4. increased organizational behavior.
10. Coping mechanisms to avoid dealing directly with stress are called:
    1. adaptive measures.
    2. maladaptive measures.
    3. nonadaptive measures.
    4. progressive measures.

REFERENCES/SUGGESTED READINGS

Aguilera, D. C. (1998). *Crisis intervention: Theory and methodology* (8th ed.). St. Louis, MO: Mosby.

Alfaro-LeFevre, R. (2009). *Critical thinking and clinical judgment* (4th ed.). Philadelphia: W. B. Saunders.

American Institute of Stress. (2002a). America's #1 health problem. Available: http://www.stress.org/problem.htm

American Institute of Stress. (2002b). Job stress. Available: http://www.stress.org/job.htm

American Institute of Stress. (2002c). Stress. Available: http://www.stress.org

Badger, J. M. (1995). Tips for managing stress on the job. *American Journal of Nursing, 95*(9), 31–33.

Beck, A. (1976). *Cognitive therapy and emotional disorders.* New York: International Universities Press.

Briguglio, A. (2007). Should the family stay? *RN, 70*(5), 42–48.

Bulechek, G., Butcher, H., McCloskey, J., & Dochterman, J., eds. (2008). *Nursing Interventions Classification (NIC)* (5th ed.). St. Louis, MO: Mosby/Elsevier.

Cullen, A. (1995). Burnout: Why do we blame the nurse? *American Journal of Nursing, 95*(11), 23–27.

Delaune, S. C., & Ladner, P. K. (2006). *Fundamentals of Nursing Standards & Practice* (3rd ed.)., Clifton Park, NY: Delmar Cengage Learning.

Fink, J. L. W. (2005). Burned out? Here's help. *Nursing, 35*(4), 53.

Freud, S. (1959). Inhibitions, symptoms and anxiety. In J. Strachey (Trans.), *The standard edition of the complete psychological works of Sigmund Freud* (Vol. 20). London: Hogarth.

Frisch, N., & Frisch, L. (2010). *Psychiatric mental health nursing* (4th ed.). Clifton Park, NY: Delmar Cengage Learning.

Keegan, L. (2000). Nutrition, exercise, and movement. In B. M. Dossey, L. Keegan, & C. E. Guzzetta (Eds.), *Holistic nursing: A handbook for practice* (3rd ed.). Gaithersburg, MD: Aspen.

Kneisl, C. R., & Riley, E. (1996). Crisis intervention. In H. S. Wilson & C. R. Kneisl (Eds.), *Psychiatric nursing* (5th ed., pp. 711–731). Menlo Park, CA: Addison-Wesley.

Kobasa, S. C. (1979). Stressful life events, personality and health: An inquiry into hardiness. *Journal of Personality and Social Psychology, 37*(1), 1–11.

Kobasa, S. C., Maddi, S. R., & Kahn, S. (1982). Hardiness and health: A prospective study. *Journal of Personality and Social Psychology, 45*(4), 839–850.

Lyon, B. L. (2000). Situational anger and self-empowerment. *Reflections on Nursing Leadership, 26*(3), 36–37.

Mandle, C. L., & Gruber-Wood, R. (2002). Health promotion and the individual. In C. L. Edelman & C. L. Mandle (Eds.), *Health promotion throughout the lifespan* (5th ed.). St. Louis, MO: Mosby.

Mayo Clinic. (1999). Stress patrol: Stop tension in its tracks. Available: http://www.mayohealth.org/mayo/9912/ htm/stress_patrol.htm

Mayo Clinic. (2000a). Dealing with co-worker conflict. Available: http://www.mayohealth.org/mayo/9704/ htm/stre_1sb.htm

Mayo Clinic. (2000b). Workplace stress: Can you control it? Available: http://www.mayohealth.org/mayo/9704/ htm/stress.htm

Meyers, T. A., Eichhorn, D. J., Guzzetta, C. E., Clark, A. P., Klein, J. D., Taliaferro, E., et al. (2000). Family presence during invasive procedures and resuscitation. *American Journal of Nursing, 100*(2), 32–40.

Moorhead, S., Johnson, M., Maas, M., & Swanson, E. (2007). *Nursing Outcomes Classification (NOC)* (4th ed.). St. Louis, MO: Mosby.

North American Nursing Diagnosis Association International. (2010). *NANDA-I nursing diagnoses: Definitions and classification 2009–2011.* Ames, IA: Wiley-Blackwell.

Page, K. (2002). Panic attack. *Nursing2002, 32*(1), 88.

Peplau, H. (1952). *Interpersonal relations in nursing.* New York: Putnam.

Selye, H. (1974). *Stress without distress.* New York: New American Library.

Selye, H. (1976). *Stress in health and disease* (Rev. ed.). Boston: Butterworths.

Sullivan, H. S. (1953). *The interpersonal theory of psychiatry.* New York: Norton.

Talbott, S. W. (1997). Political analysis: Structure and process. In D. J. Mason, S. W. Talbott, & J. K. Leavitt (Eds.), *Policy and politics for nurses* (2nd ed., pp. 129–148). Philadelphia: W. B. Saunders.

U.S. Preventive Services Task Force. (2002). Screening for depression: Recommendations and rationale. *Annals of Internal Medicine, 136*(10), 760.

Waughfield, C. (2002). *Mental health concepts* (5th ed.). Clifton Park, NY: Delmar Cengage Learning.

Wilson, H. S., & Kneisel, C. R. (1996). *Psychiatric nursing* (5th ed.). Menlo Park, CA: Addison-Wesley.

Wilson, H. S., Kneisel, C. R., & Trigoboff, E. (2004). *Contemporary psychiatric-mental health nursing.* Upper Saddle River, NJ: Prentice Hall.

RESOURCES

American Holistic Nurses Association, http://www.ahna.org

American Institute of Stress, http://www.stress.org

International Stress Management Association UK, http://www.isma.org.uk

CHAPTER 13
End-of-Life Care

MAKING THE CONNECTION

Refer to the following chapters to increase your understanding of loss, grief, and death:

Basic Nursing

- ***Legal and Ethical Responsibilities***
- ***Arenas of Care***
- ***Life Span Development***
- ***Cultural Considerations***
- ***Spirituality***
- ***Complementary/Alternative Therapies***

LEARNING OBJECTIVES

Upon completion of this chapter, you should be able to:

- Define key terms.
- Discuss the various losses that affect individuals at different stages of the life span.
- Identify characteristics of an individual experiencing grief.
- Compare and contrast adaptive grief and pathological grief.
- Discuss the stages of the normal grieving process.
- Describe the holistic needs of the dying person and family.
- Plan care for a dying client.
- Describe nursing responsibilities when a client dies.
- Discuss ways that nurses can cope with their own grief.

KEY TERMS

advance directive
algor mortis
anticipatory grief
autopsy
bereavement
breakthrough pain
Cheyne-Stokes respirations
complicated grief
death rattle
disenfranchised grief
dysfunctional grief
end-of-life care
grief
Health Care Surrogate Law
hospice
life review
liver mortis
loss
maturational loss
mortuary
mourning
palliative care
postmortem care
resuscitation
rigor mortis
shroud
situational loss
traumatic imagery
uncomplicated grief

INTRODUCTION

Individuals are constantly experiencing loss. Episodes of personal crisis, natural disaster, and terrorism result in the experience of loss. The nurse must be aware of the many ways individuals react and adapt to losses.

Individuals are faced with losses throughout the life cycle. Growth and development would not continue to progress without some losses.

Nurses encounter clients every day who are responding to grief associated with losses. An understanding of the major concepts related to loss and grieving is necessary for each nurse. Many people consider loss only in terms of death and dying. Because nurses also care for dying clients, this chapter includes information on meeting the special needs of terminally ill clients and their families.

LOSS

Loss is any situation, either potential, actual, or perceived, wherein a valued object or person is changed or is not accessible to the individual. Everyone experiences losses because change is a major constant in life. Loss can be actual (e.g., a child is lost in the woods) or anticipated (a diabetic client is faced with having a foot amputated). The loss can be tangible or intangible. For example, when a person is not selected for a job, the tangible loss is income, and the intangible loss is self-esteem.

Losses also occur as a person moves from one developmental stage to another. An example of such a **maturational loss** is the toddler who loses the bottle after learning to drink from a glass. A **situational loss** takes place in response to external events generally beyond the individual's control, such as losing a job when the company is bankrupt.

The four major categories of loss are loss of significant other, loss of aspects of self, loss of external objects, and loss of a familiar environment.

Loss of Significant Other

Losing a loved one is a very significant loss. Such a loss can result from moving to a different area, separation, divorce, or death.

Loss of Aspect of Self

Loss of an aspect of self can be physiological or psychological. Physiological loss includes loss of physical function or loss resulting from disfigurement or disappearance of a body part, as is the case with amputation or mastectomy. Loss of a physical aspect of self can result from trauma, illness, or a treatment methodology such as surgery. Psychological aspects of self that may be lost include a sense of humor, ambition, or enjoyment of life. These feelings of loss may result from life events such as losing a job or failing at a task that the individual deems important.

Loss of an External Object

Whenever an object that a person highly values is changed or damaged or disappears, loss occurs. The type and amount of grieving depends on the significance of the lost object to the individual. For instance, an individual who loses a family heirloom in a fire may react not only to the lost financial value of the piece but also to the lost sense of history and heritage that the piece represented.

Loss of Familiar Environment

The loss of a familiar environment occurs when a person moves away from familiar surroundings, for instance to another home or a different community, to a new school, or to a new job. A client who is hospitalized or institutionalized may also experience loss when faced with new surroundings. This type of loss evokes anxiety related to fear of the unknown.

GRIEF

Grief is a series of intense psychological and physical responses occurring after a loss. These responses are necessary, normal, natural, and adaptive responses to the loss. Loss moves the individual to the adaptive process of **mourning**, the period during which grief is expressed and integration and resolution of the loss occur. **Bereavement** is the period of grief that follows the death of a loved one (Figure 13-1).

Stages of Grief

Three stages of grief generally recognized are shock, reality, and recovery.

Shock Stage

The period of shock may last from only days to a month or more. The person may describe feeling "numb." It is an emotional numbness rather than a physical one.

Reality Stage

A painful experience begins when the individual consciously realizes the full meaning of the loss. Anger, guilt, fear, frustration, and/or helplessness may be the expressed reactions.

Recovery Stage

During the last stage, recovery, the loss is integrated into the reality of the individual's life. The person exhibits adaptive

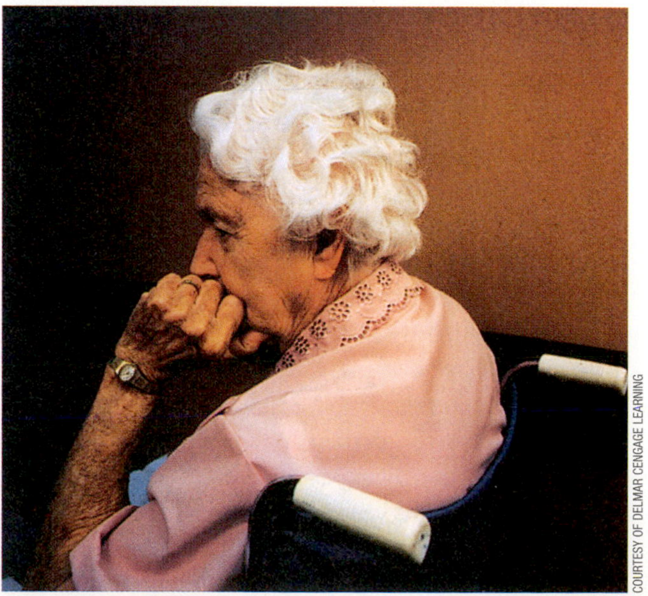
COURTESY OF DELMAR CENGAGE LEARNING

FIGURE 13-1 Older adults may grieve intensely over the loss of a person or situation that has been a part of their lives for many years.

MEMORY TRICK

A memory trick to recall the grief stages is "**SRR**":

S = Shock

R = Reality

R = Recovery

behaviors and begins to live again, doing things that were formerly enjoyed.

Types of Grief

Grief is a normal, universal, response to loss. Grief drains people, both physically and emotionally, and relationships often suffer. Different types of grief include uncomplicated ("normal"), anticipatory, dysfunctional, and disenfranchised grief.

Nurses assist many individuals to understand the normal grieving process. Nurses who understand all types of grief are better prepared to assist others.

Uncomplicated Grief

Uncomplicated grief is what many individuals would refer to as *normal grief*. Engle (1961) proposed the term **uncomplicated grief** to describe the grief reaction normally following a significant loss. Uncomplicated grief has a fairly predictable course that ends with relinquishing the lost object and resuming the duties of life.

The grieving person may feel angry, hopeless, or sad and may express feelings of depression. A person who is grieving may experience loss of appetite, weight loss, insomnia, restlessness, indecisiveness, impulsivity, and inability to concentrate or carry out daily activities.

Anticipatory Grief

Anticipatory grief is the occurrence of grief before an expected loss actually occurs. Anticipatory grief may be experienced by both the person's family and the terminally ill person. This process promotes early grieving, freeing emotional energy for adapting once the loss has occurred. Although anticipatory grieving may be helpful in adjusting to the loss, it also has some potential disadvantages. For example, in the case of the dying client, the family members may distance themselves and not be available for support. Also, if the family members have separated themselves emotionally from the dying client, they may seem cold and distant and, thus, not meet society's expectations of mourning behavior. This response can, in turn, prevent the mourners from receiving their own much-needed support from others (Pritchett & Lucas, 1997b).

PROFESSIONAL TIP

Successful Grieving

The person experiencing successful grieving will:

- Consciously recognize that a significant loss has occurred.
- Progress through the stages of grief.
- Use adaptive coping behaviors, such as interacting with others, participating in and completing tasks, and having a positive attitude.

PROFESSIONAL TIP

Identifying Dysfunctional Grief

Normal and dysfunctional grief are differentiated in that the person experiencing dysfunctional grief is unable to adapt to life without the deceased person.

Dysfunctional grief can take several forms, specifically chronic grief, delayed grief, exaggerated grief, or masked grief.

Chronic grief is the inability to conclude grieving.

Delayed grief occurs when grief work does not take place at the time of loss.

Exaggerated grief describes the situation when grief is experienced as overwhelming.

Masked grief occurs when grief is covered up by maladaptive behaviors such as apathy, irritability, and unstable moods or a physical symptom such as loss of libido, with the person being unaware of the connection to the loss and grief.

Dysfunctional Grief

Dysfunctional grief is a demonstration of a persistent pattern of intense grief that does not result in reconciliation of feelings. The person experiencing dysfunctional (or pathological) grief does not progress through the stages of grief. The dysfunctionally grieving person cannot reestablish a routine. The professional caregiver must be aware of these behaviors and refer the pathologically grieving person to professional counseling.

Disenfranchised Grief

Disenfranchised grief is described as grief not openly acknowledged, socially sanctioned, or publicly shared. When an individual either is reluctant to recognize the sense of loss and develops guilt feelings or feels pressured by society to "get on with life," grief can become disenfranchised. An example of disenfranchised grief is extreme sadness over the loss of a pet when this mourning might be viewed by others as excessive or inappropriate. A mother's sadness over a miscarriage might also be considered disenfranchised grief because a lengthy period of mourning may not be publicly expected despite the mother's intense feelings of loss and despair.

Factors Affecting Loss and Grief

Variables affecting the intensity and duration of grieving are:

- Developmental stage
- Religious and cultural beliefs

- Relationship with the lost object
- Cause of death

Developmental Stage

Depending on the client's place on the age/development continuum, the grief response to a loss will be experienced differently. For example, a pregnant woman will, to some degree, experience loss after delivery of a first child (loss of freedom, independence, and self-focused life), even when the child is normal and healthy. Certain kinds of loss at key developmental points may have a profound effect on a person's ability to both work through the resulting grief and achieve the tasks of the given developmental stage. For example, an adolescent who has lost a parent may have difficulty forming an intimate relationship with members of the opposite sex.

Childhood Children vary in their reactions to loss and in the ability to comprehend the meaning of death. It is important to understand the way a child's concept of death evolves because the concept varies with developmental level and may affect mastery of developmental tasks (Table 13-1).

Children who are grieving need honest explanations about death using terms they can understand.

Adolescence Physical attractiveness and athletic abilities are valued by most adolescents. Because adolescents seek approval of their peer group, when the adolescent suffers the loss of a body part or function, grief includes fear of being rejected. After a disfiguring accident, grief is usually very intense. Even though they have an intellectual understanding of death, adolescents believe themselves to be invulnerable and, thus, immune to death; they reject the possibility of their own mortality.

Early Adulthood In the young adult, grief is often precipitated by loss of role or status. For example, significant grief may be caused by unemployment or the breakup of a relationship. The concept of death in this age-group reflects primarily spiritual beliefs and cultural values (Figure 13-2).

Middle Adulthood The potential for experiencing loss increases during middle adulthood. The death of parents often occurs during this developmental phase. As an individual ages, it can be especially threatening when peers die, because these deaths force acknowledgment of one's own mortality.

Late Adulthood Most individuals recognize the inevitability of death during late adulthood. It is challenging for elders to experience the death of age-old friends or to find themselves the last one of their peer group left living. Older adults often turn to their children and grandchildren as sources of comfort and companionship. Cultivating friendships in all age-groups helps prevent loneliness and depression.

TABLE 13-1 Perception of Death by Children and Adolescents

DEVELOPMENTAL STAGE	PERCEPTION	POTENTIAL DEVELOPMENTAL DISRUPTIONS
Infancy, toddlerhood	• Unaware of death • Aware of changes in normal routine • Reacts to family's expressions of grief	• Death of primary caregiver during the first 2 years of life may have significant long-lasting psychosocial implications.
Preschool	• Believes death is a temporary separation • Reacts to the gravity of death as they see parents or others react	• Loss of either parent may have significant psychosocial implications, especially between ages 4 and 6 years (because of magical thinking, wherein children may believe death is their fault). • Problems with development of sexual identity, depending on the gender of the parent lost, the child's identification with that parent, and the child's present state of sexual identity.
School age	• Comprehends that death is inevitable and final • Conjectures about and is inclined to personify death ("the boogie-man")	• Potential nightmares. • Potential death-avoidance behaviors (e.g., hiding under the covers, leaving the lights on, closing closet doors). • Possible intense guilt and a sense of responsibility for the death.
Preadolescence and adolescence	• Acknowledges that death is final • Comprehends that death is inevitable • *Preadolescents:* may worry about dying; *adolescents:* seem to deny that they could die	• Loss of a parent may cause difficulty in forming an intimate relationship with members of the opposite sex.

COURTESY OF DELMAR CENGAGE LEARNING

LIFE SPAN CONSIDERATIONS

Talking with Children about Death

- *Avoid the* use of euphemisms. For example, if a child is told that the deceased person has "gone away," the child may believe that the dead person will return. Also, a child may develop sleep phobia if told that the deceased is "asleep."
- *Do not overexplain.* Keep explanations concise and factual; do not offer lengthy explanations of medical conditions.
- *Use simple, concrete terms.* Young children are not able to conceptualize abstract ideas, such as "grandma is in a better place now."
- *Show them.* Many young children understand something only when they see it. Take them to the funeral service and cemetery.

From *National Directory of Bereavement Support Groups and Services* (3rd ed.), by M. Wong, 1998, New York: ADM Publishing.

Religious and Cultural Beliefs

An individual's grief experience is significantly affected by religious and cultural beliefs. Every culture has rituals for care of the dying and beliefs about the significance of death. Other beliefs regarding an afterlife, redemption of the soul, a supreme being, and reincarnation can assist the individual in grief work.

Relationship with the Lost Person or Object

Generally, the grief experienced is more intense the more intimate the relationship was with the deceased. The risk for dysfunctional grieving is particularly great after the death of a child.

The death of a child is generally thought to be exceptionally painful because it upsets the natural order of things; parents do not expect their children to die before them.

Parents experiencing grief usually have intense responses and reactions (Figure 13-3). Parental grief is unique in that it encompasses both the loss of the perceived potential of that child and the loss of parental hopes for the child. Table 13-2 suggests some characteristics of parents of infants who have died.

CRITICAL THINKING

Perceptions of Death

Find a classmate from a different cultural background than yours. How does your classmate's perception of death differ from yours?

The death of a sibling or parent can be a major challenge for children. Adults failing to understand the child's need to mourn may not recognize the child's feelings. Normal reactions of a child when a sibling dies as an infant, and nursing responses to these reactions, are given in Table 13-3.

Cause of Death

The intensity of the grief response also varies depending whether the cause of death was unexpected, traumatic, or a suicide.

Unexpected Death The bereaved have particular difficulty in achieving closure when the loss occurs as a result of an unexpected death. Survivors are shocked and bereaved after an unanticipated death, such as an aneurysm, heart attack, or stroke. Usually, the bereaved can work through the grieving process without complications.

Traumatic Death **Complicated grief** is associated with traumatic death such as death by accident, violence, or homicide. Survivors are not necessarily predisposed to complications in mourning but often have more intense emotions than those associated with normal grief.

Following a violent death, the bereaved may undergo **traumatic imagery** (imagining the feelings of horror felt by the victim or reliving the terror of the incident). Traumatic imagery is a common occurrence in cases of traumatic death. Such thoughts, coupled with intense grief, can lead to posttraumatic stress disorder (PTSD) in the survivors. Nurses' awareness of the possibility of PTSD and alertness for the presence of symptoms is important. Symptoms may include:

- Chronic anxiety
- Psychological distress
- Sleep disturbances, such as recurrent, terror-filled nightmares

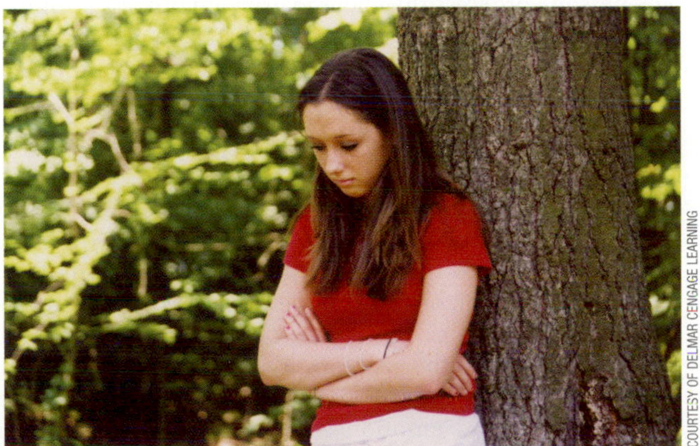
COURTESY OF DELMAR CENGAGE LEARNING

FIGURE 13-2 Young adults usually grieve loss of a role, such as employment or the breakup of a relationship.

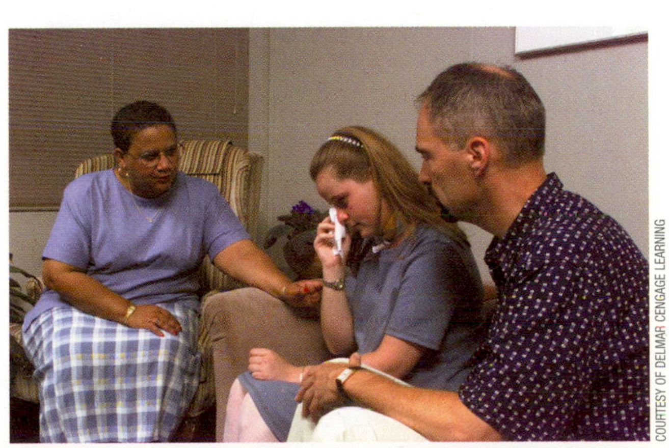
COURTESY OF DELMAR CENGAGE LEARNING

FIGURE 13-3 The couple discusses grief over the loss of a child.

TABLE 13-2 Characteristics of Parents When a Child Dies

TYPE OF DEATH	PARENTAL CHARACTERISTICS
Spontaneous abortion (miscarriage) and stillbirth	• The mother, especially, may have feelings of intense sadness, guilt, or anger. If the loss occurs in early weeks of pregnancy, the death may be inadequately recognized by others. • The death may be regarded as a personal failure. • Parents may blame themselves or others. • Previous miscarriages may be relived and grieved. • If the condition of the infant was known, anticipatory grief may occur. • Grief may increase if ambivalent about being pregnant. • Despair may be greatest when the parents leave the hospital or birthplace without the baby.
Neonatal death	• Similar reactions as with stillbirth. • The bond between parents and infant intensifies the grief. • Both parents may have intense grief.
Sudden infant death syndrome (SIDS)	• Parents are in a state of shock. • Lack of knowledge and misinformation increases pain. • Because SIDS usually occurs during the first 6 months of life, parental bonding is complete. • May feel guilt. • Grief is acute; parents are not prepared for the loss. • May be engrossed with the details of the death.
Induced Abortion	• Secrecy, guilt, and shame may accompany grief. • May have ambivalent feelings. • May find little support or comfort from others. • Feelings of despair and depression may be present when relief was expected. • If child was not wanted, no guilt may be felt.

From *Healing and the Grief Process*, by S. Roach and B. Nieto, 1997, Clifton Park, NY: Delmar Cengage Learning.

Only when this problem is identified and the survivors are encouraged to express their intense feelings will they be able to move through the normal, adaptive grieving process.

Suicide The loss of a loved one to suicide is frequently compounded by feelings of guilt by the survivors for failing to recognize clues that may have permitted the victim to receive help. The feelings of guilt and self-blame can change into anger at the victim for inflicting such pain. Having a suicide in the family may evoke feelings of shame. Survivors may be prohibited from successfully resolving their grief by the negative stigma of suicide.

Nursing Care of the Grieving Client

Rodebaugh, Schwindt, and Valentine (1999) suggest that grief be thought of as a journey through four broad categories titled reeling, feeling, dealing, and healing. Clients are reeling when experiencing shock or disbelief. Feelings are expressed in various emotions and behaviors. Dealing occurs when they begin to adapt to the loss. Things do not necessarily get better; they just get different. Healing is when the loss becomes part of them, and the acute anguish lessens; it does not mean forgetting. People are changed by grief. Self-esteem is affected, new ways of coping are developed, and a new lifestyle without the deceased is begun. Although it is a painful process, clients must resolve the loss in their own way. As the client moves through the process of mourning, nurses can assist by providing support. The nurse asks the client what he can do to help and listens for needs expressed.

Nurses can assist people to grieve by encouraging them to experience their feelings to the fullest in order to work through them. Providing support and explaining to the bereaved that it will take time to grieve the loss and to gain some closure to the relationship are both important nursing responsibilities.

After the loved one dies, the caregiver feels grief and relief. Caregivers often feel guilty for feeling relieved. Assure them these feelings are very normal, as caregiving is exhausting, leaving one with little emotional and physical reserve. The nurse assists the caregiver to find ways to fill his life with meaningful activities.

Assessment

Determining the personal meaning of the loss is the beginning of a thorough assessment of the grieving client and family. The person's progress through the grieving process is another key assessment area. The stages of grieving are not necessarily mastered sequentially, but instead individuals may move back and forth through the stages of grief.

Nursing Diagnosis

The North American Nursing Diagnosis Association International (NANDA-I) defines *Dysfunctional **G**rieving* as "extended, unsuccessful use of intellectual and emotional responses by which individuals, families, communities attempt to work through the process of modifying self-concept based upon the perception of loss" (NANDA, 2010). The other grieving diagnosis is *Anticipatory **G**rieving*, defined as "intellectual and emotional responses and behaviors by which individuals, families, communities work through the process of modifying self-concept based on the perception of potential loss" (NANDA, 2010).

Table 13-3 Reactions of Siblings after Infant Death

NORMAL REACTION	NURSING RESPONSE
• Fear loss of and separation from parents	• Reassure that parents will not leave them
• Guilt, because of feelings of jealousy and anger related to wishing that the infant would go away	• Reassure siblings that they did not influence the cause of death by providing information (at the appropriate level of understanding)
• Fear that parents' intense reactions will hinder parents' ability to take care of them	• Provide assurance that life will go on by continuing routine activities
• Fear of dying soon and concern over own health	• Persuade parents to avoid being overprotective, which will reinforce children's fears

Data adapted from "Supporting Families after Sudden Infant Death," by M. McClain and S. Shaefer, 1996, *Journal of Psychosocial Nursing and Mental Health Services, 34*(4), 30–34.

Planning/Outcome Identification

When planning care for the grieving client, it is important to clarify the expected outcomes. Some expected goals for the person experiencing grief are:

- Accept the loss
- Verbalize feelings of grief
- Share grief with significant others
- Renew activities and relationships

Some of these expected outcomes will take a long time to achieve, and some must be achieved before others are mastered. For example, to accept the loss, the person must begin to share grief with others by verbalizing those feelings. Two of the expected outcomes are discussed below.

Acceptance of the Loss Individuals are able to reach some acceptance and resolution of feelings about the loss only by going through grief work. Often, people try to find some meaning in their situations. This search involves introspection, for which spiritual support may be therapeutic.

Renewal of Activities and Relationships The basis of grief work revolves around accepting the fact that the needs met by key people in life can be met by other people in other ways. Knowing that the deceased cannot be replaced, healing must occur so that new relationships may begin.

Implementation

Basic to therapeutic nursing care is an understanding of the significance of the loss to the client. The nurse must spend time listening to understand the client's perspective. Even if the client does not respond according to the nurse's belief system or expectations, the nurse must demonstrate acceptance. The nurse's nonjudgmental, accepting attitude is essential during the bereaved's expression of all feelings, including anger and despair. The nurse avoids personalizing and using defensive behaviors by communicating an understanding of the client's anger. The expression of grief is not only appropriate but also essential for therapeutic resolution of the loss.

Grieving people need reassurance, support, and counseling. One mechanism of support on a long-term basis is support groups. The nurse must be informed about the availability of such groups within the community in order to make appropriate referrals. Members of support groups have experienced similar losses. Discussions in support groups decrease the feelings of loneliness and social isolation that are so common in the grief experience.

Evaluation

People follow their own time schedule for grief work. Because it takes months or years for grief resolution, nurses usually do not have the opportunity to know when the bereaved family completes its grief work. The nurse does have a unique opportunity to lay the foundation for adaptive grieving by encouraging the family to verbalize their experience and share their feelings with significant others. The foundation for evaluation is the goals mutually established with client and family. It is important for nurses to teach grieving individuals that resolution of the loss is generally a process of lifelong adjustment.

DEATH

Historically, death has been considered as natural as birth, as simply the last stage of life. Significant changes in the perception of death have occurred in the past three decades. In some cases, dying and death are no longer simple matters but are issues involving ethical concerns and, in some cases, legal intervention by the court system.

Each person dies a unique death, just as each person lives a unique life. Death may be sudden and unexpected, caused by accident or heart attack, for example, or death may be prolonged, coming after a distressing long-term illness. For the older person who dies during sleep, death comes quietly. Those who choose to die on their own terms by suicide plan their deaths.

Health care workers must understand the ethical and legal issues surrounding dying and death. Understanding the stages

PROFESSIONALTIP

Adaptive Grieving

How long does the process of adaptive grieving take? The length of time necessary for grief resolution is as individual as the person experiencing it and depends on the intensity of the grief. Grief is considered to be a "long-term process" (Corless, Germino, & Pittman, 2006). Grief work takes time. There are no definite time frames within which grief should occur. Each person grieves in his own way and at his own pace.

CULTURAL CONSIDERATIONS

Cultural Diversity and Death

Cultural Group	Role of Family	Display of Emotion	Care of Dying in Home
African American	Health care providers should communicate with the oldest family member about the dying client.	Expected	Families frequently care for dying elders in the home.
Chinese American	Family may prefer dying client not be told of terminal illness or imminent death or may prefer a family member tell the client.	Express sorrow at parents' funeral; the first son is in mourning for 72 days and cannot wear red clothing or marry during that time.	Some believe bad luck will occur if client dies in the home and others think the client's spirit will get lost if death occurs in the hospital. Family may use amulets or cloths.
Filipino American	Health care providers should communicate with the head of the family and not in the presence of the client.	Expected	Dying client may desire to die in the home.
Hispanic or Latino American	Extended families care for the dying client. Families share information and decision making.	Wailing shows respect for the dead client.	Some believe the spirit will get lost if the client dies in the hospital. Use of amulets, rosary beads, and prayers are common.

Data from "Cultural Considerations in End-of-Life Care" by P. Mazanec and M. Tyler, 2003, *American Journal of Nursing*.

of death and dying and the signs of impending death will help prepare the nurse to render sensitive, effective care, both to the client and family and to the client's body after death. Nurses must also come to terms with their own mortality and feelings about death if they are to provide comfort to dying clients and their families. Health care workers can learn a great deal about life from the dying client.

LEGAL CONSIDERATIONS

The *Patient Self-Determination Act* (PSDA) is part of the Omnibus Budget Reconciliation Act (OBRA) of 1990. This act provides a legal means for individuals to specify the circumstances under which life-sustaining measures should or should not be rendered to them. The individual's choices are identified in advance directives. An **advance directive** is any written instruction recognized under state law, including a durable power of attorney, for health care or living will. The act applies to hospitals, home health agencies, long-term care facilities, hospice programs, and certain health maintenance organizations (HMOs). According to the PSDA, all clients entering the health care system through any of these organizations must be given information and the opportunity to complete advance directives if they have not already done so. In many states, just signing these documents may not be adequate for carrying out client wishes. They may also need to indicate their desires regarding intubation, artificial feeding, blood transfusions, chemotherapy, surgery, and transfer to the hospital (for residents in skilled care facilities).

Although a durable power of attorney for health care and living will are legal documents, they do not prevent **resuscitation** (support measures to restore consciousness and life). The medical record must have a written do-not-resuscitate (DNR) order from a physician if this is in agreement with the client's wishes and with the advance directives. In the absence of such an order, resuscitation will be initiated.

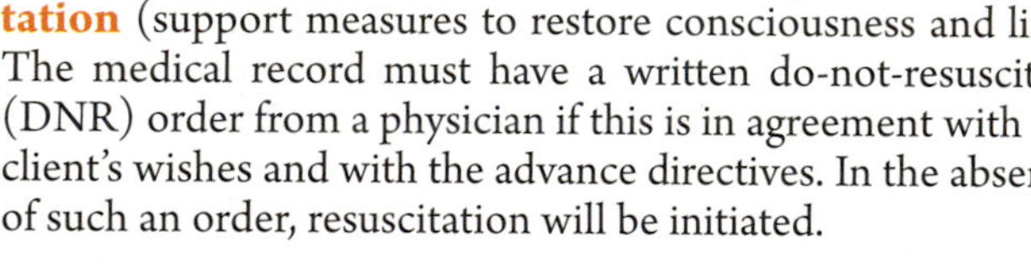

PROFESSIONALTIP

Care of the Dying Client

Dying was once considered to be a normal part of the life cycle. Today, it is often considered to be a medical problem that should be handled by health care providers. Technological advances in medicine have led to depersonalized and mechanical care of those who are dying. Our highly technological world calls for application of high-touch interventions with the dying. In other words, appropriate care of the dying is administered by compassionate nurses who are both technically competent and able to demonstrate caring. Huizdos (2000) learned that death is not the enemy—lack of caring is.

In many states a **Health Care Surrogate Law** is implemented when there is no advance directive. This law varies from state to state but basically provides a legal means for certain individuals to make decisions for the client when the client cannot do so. The spouse is the first person who would act in the interests of the client. Then children in the event there is no spouse.

Ethical Considerations

Death is often fraught with ethical dilemmas that occur almost daily in health care settings. Ethics committees in many health care agencies develop and implement policies to deal with end-of-life issues. These committees are interdisciplinary and may have clergy and attorneys as well as health care providers as members. Ethical decision making is a complex issue. Determining the difference between killing and allowing someone to die by withholding life-sustaining treatment methods is one of the most difficult dilemmas.

The American Nurses Association (ANA) distinguishes mercy killing (euthanasia or assisted suicide) and relieving pain. Euthanasia is viewed as unethical, whereas pain relief is a central value in nursing. The ANA's position is that increasing doses of medication to control pain in terminally ill clients is ethically justified, even at the expense of maintaining life (ANA, 1996, 2008).

Stages of Dying and Death

Elizabeth Kübler-Ross (1997a, 1997d) identified in her classic works five stages of dying that are experienced by clients and their families (Table 13-4). Every client does not move through each stage sequentially. These stages are experienced for varying lengths of time and in varying degrees. The client may express denial and then, a few minutes later, express acceptance of the inevitable and then anger. An important value of Kübler-Ross's work is that it has increased sensitivity to the dying client's needs.

Table 13-4 Kübler-Ross's Stages of Dying and Death

STAGE	EXAMPLE
Denial	*Verbal:* "No, I don't believe that." *Behavioral:* Client diagnosed with leukemia and refuses to consider treatment options.
Anger	*Verbal:* "Why me, why?" *Behavioral:* Client is demanding and demonstrates aggressive behavior.
Bargaining	*Verbal:* Client prays, "Please, just let me live to see my new grandbaby." *Behavioral:* Client makes deals with caregivers or god.
Depression	*Verbal:* "I just want to be alone." *Behavioral:* Client turns away and closes eyes.
Acceptance	*Verbal:* "I am ready. I feel at peace now." *Behavioral:* Client gets legal and financial affairs in order and says goodbye to family and friends.

Data from *On Death and Dying*, by E. Kübler-Ross, 1997a, New York: Macmillan. Copyright 1969 by Macmillan.

Denial

During the first stage of dying, the initial shock can be very overwhelming, making denial a useful tool of coping. It is an essential, protective mechanism that may last for only a few minutes or may manifest for months.

In some clients, denial manifests as "doctor shopping" (not to imply that second opinions are not sometimes necessary) or insisting that there must have been a mix-up or mistake in the diagnostic tests. In other clients, denial manifests as simply avoiding the issue. Their daily routines are the same as though nothing in their lives has changed. Given time, most people will eventually move past the stage of denial.

Clients may choose to be selective in the use of denial. For example, clients try to protect certain family members or friends from the truth by using denial. Clients may also use denial from time to time to set aside thoughts of illness and death in order to focus on living.

Anger

Anger often follows the initial stage of denial. The client's security is threatened by the unknown, with the normal daily routines becoming disrupted. This stage is typically very difficult for family and caregivers because they often feel useless in terms of helping their loved one through the situation. Since the client has no control over the situation, anger is the response. The anger may be directed at self, God, others, the environment, and the health care system. In the client's eyes, whatever is done is not the right thing. Family members may be greeted with silence or with outbursts of anger. Their response, in turn, may be anger, guilt, or despair.

Bargaining

The client attempts to postpone or reverse the inevitable by bargaining. The client's bargaining represents an attempt to

LIFE SPAN CONSIDERATIONS

Reactions to Impending Death

- Persons of all ages generally experience the same feelings and emotions as they progress through a terminal illness.
- Persons of any age who have endured a long illness may view death as a release from their suffering.
- Persons of any age may find it difficult to reach acceptance if they have unfinished business.
- Many people receive satisfaction from **life review** (a form of reminiscence wherein a client attempts to come to terms with conflict or to gain meaning from life and die peacefully).
- Elderly clients may welcome death, especially if they have outlived everyone who was near and dear to them.

MEMORYTRICK

A memory trick for the stages of dying and death is "**DA-B-DA**":

D = Denial

A = Anger

B = Bargaining

D = Depression

A = Acceptance

postpone death and usually has self-imposed limitations. For example, a client may ask to live long enough to see the first grandchild in exchange for giving money to a charity. Most clients bargain in silence or in confidence with their spiritual leader. It is not uncommon for a client to live long enough for some special event (a wedding or birth), then die shortly afterward.

Depression

Depression resulting from the realization that death can no longer be delayed is different from dysfunctional depression because it helps the client detach from life and makes it easier to accept death. Depression in this sense is a therapeutic experience for the dying person. Clients sometimes feel abandoned, as persons who were once friends begin to visit less and less, sometimes severing ties with the client even before death; this may compound the client's feelings of depression and hopelessness.

Acceptance

Every dying client may not reach the final stage, acceptance. Peace and contentment comes with acceptance. The client often expresses feeling that all that could be done has been done. It is important to reinforce the client's feelings and sense of personal worth. Many clients will make an effort to get all of their personal and financial affairs in order.

Sleep is required to fill a physical and emotional need, not to avoid reality. The client may limit visitors to those people with whom he feels comfortable and safe. The most significant forms of communication at this time are touch and moments of silence.

END-OF-LIFE CARE

End-of-life care is nursing care of the terminally ill that focuses on meeting the physical and psychosocial needs of the client and his family. Attention is directed to the control of symptoms, identification of client needs, the promotion of interaction between the client and significant others, and the facilitation of a peaceful death. The nurse focuses on improving the quality of life for the dying client during the final stage of life and ensures a dignified and peaceful death. As a member of the interdisciplinary team responsible for providing end-of-life care, the nurse plays a critical role in identifying client needs and in supporting family members through the end-of-life experience (Hull, 2008).

The decision to abandon aggressive treatment should not be regarded as a sign of "immediate death." Palliative and hospice care evolved over the years to bridge the gap between cure-focused treatments to end-of-life care. Both approaches serve as coordinated, multidisciplinary efforts developed purposefully to address the needs of the client and family facing a terminal illness (Hull, 2008).

Palliative Care

Terminally ill clients are often given **palliative care**, or care that relieves symptoms, such as pain, but does not alter the course of disease. Palliative care is an approach that focuses on the seriously ill client and family and is most often provided in the home, hospital setting, or long-term facilities (Hull, 2008).

In palliative care, the goal is to ensure the highest possible quality of life for the client and family (Hull, 2008). A primary aim is to help the client feel comfortable, safe, and secure. The nurse can do much to increase the client's feelings of safety by being available when needed. Holding the client's hand and listening are therapeutic measures.

Care delivered by an interdisciplinary team emphasizes the management of psychological, social, and spiritual problems experienced by clients and families during end of life. The nurse addresses pain control and the management of other physical problems (Hull, 2008). The client needs to know that he has the nurse's support as an advocate for his care and well-being.

Hospice Care

Hospice is care for the terminally ill founded on the concept of allowing individuals to die with dignity surrounded

CULTURAL CONSIDERATIONS

Rituals Following Death

- Judaism practices burial of the dead within 24 hours. A 7-day period of mourning, called Shiva, begins the day of the funeral.
- In the Islamic faith, men wash the body of a man and women wash the body of a woman after death.
- Buddhists believe that after death, the body should not be disturbed by movement, talking, or crying.
- Hindus pour holy water into the mouth of the dying person. The eldest son arranges for the funeral and cremation within 24 hours of death. Embalming is forbidden.
- Jehovah's Witnesses believe that the soul dies with the body, but 144,000 will be resurrected at the end-time and will be born again as spiritual sons of God.
- Native Americans believe that the spirit lives on after death. Ancestor worship is practiced.

by those who love them. Clients enter hospice care either at home or in a hospice center when aggressive medical treatment is no longer an option or when the client refuses further medical care. Hospice care is based on the belief that meaningful life can be achieved during terminal illness and that care of the dying is best supported in the home setting or hospice center, free from technological interventions to prolong physiologic dying (Hull, 2008).

Hospice is a coordinated program of interdisciplinary services provided by professional caregivers and volunteers. Hospice care does not hasten life, nor does it prolong death through artificial means. Instead, it assists the client and family in understanding the death process and how best to enjoy life until the end (Hull, 2008).

Differentiating Palliative Care and Hospice Care

Although used interchangeably, the terms *palliative care* and *hospice care* are different in several ways. For example, palliative care can start much earlier in the disease process than hospice care, which is usually offered in the last 6 months of life. Table 13-5 explains the two approaches in end-of-life care (Hull, 2008).

Nursing Care of the Dying Client

Despite health care advances, care of the terminally ill client remains a challenging and rewarding reality for many nurses. The death process is typically a very emotional time for clients and their families; compassionate and sensitive nursing care that respects clients' wishes and that meets their physical needs can help bring peace and dignity to this natural process.

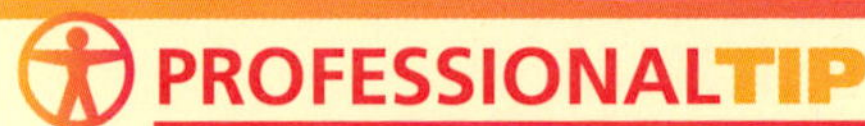

Information Gathered in Assessment of the Dying Client

- Client and family goals and expectations
- Client's awareness that illness is terminal
- Client's stage of dying
- Identification of support systems
- History of positive coping skills
- Client perception of unfinished business to be completed

Adapted from "Death and Dying," by K. Pritchett and P. Lucas, 1997a. In *Psychiatric–Mental Health Nursing: Adaptation and Growth* [4th ed., pp. 206–207], by B. S. Johnson [Ed.], Philadelphia: Lippincott Williams & Wilkins.

Assessment

A thorough assessment of the client's holistic needs is the basis for nursing interventions. Assessment of the dying client includes an ongoing collection of data regarding the strengths and limitations of the dying person and the family.

Nursing Diagnoses

The nurse's assessment of the dying client may lead to several diagnoses. One NANDA-I-approved nursing diagnosis that is applicable for many dying clients is ***Powerlessness***, that is, "the perception that one's own action will not significantly affect an outcome; a perceived lack of control over a current situation or

Table 13-5 Approaches in End-of-Life Care

DIMENSIONS	PALLIATIVE CARE	HOSPICE CARE
Recipient of care	Anyone with a serious illness regardless of life expectancy	Life expectancy of 6 months or less
Services provided	Symptom management Physical therapy Client and family counseling Spiritual care	Symptom management Provision of medications, medical supplies, and equipment Coverage for short-term inpatient care Grief support Volunteer services
Care settings	Home care Ambulatory/outpatient Acute care Long-term care	Inpatient care Home care
Third-party coverage	Some treatments and medications may be covered by Medicare, Medicaid, and private insurers	Medicare Hospice Benefit Medicaid Hospice Benefit Some private insurers

Data from *Palliative and End of Life Care*, by E. Hull, 2008. Manuscript submitted for publication.

PROFESSIONAL TIP

Planning Care for the Dying Client

- Schedule time to spend with the client.
- Identify areas of special concern to the client and make referrals when appropriate (e.g., social worker consult for information on equipment rental).
- Promote and protect individual self-esteem and self-worth.
- Balance the client's needs for assistance and independence.
- Meet the physiological needs of the client and family.
- Respect the client's confidentiality.
- Provide factual information to the client and family and answer all questions.
- Offer to contact clergy or other spiritual leader.

Adapted from "Death and Dying," by K. Pritchett and P. Lucas, 1997a. In *Psychiatric–Mental Health Nursing: Adaptation and Growth* (4th ed., p. 208), by B. S. Johnson (Ed.), Philadelphia: Lippincott Williams & Wilkins.

immediate happening" (NANDA-I, 2010). Another response that is often experienced by the dying is described by the diagnosis ***Hopelessness***, "a subjective state in which an individual sees limited or no alternatives or personal choices available and is unable to mobilize energy on own behalf" (NANDA-I, 2010). The client may also exhibit *Death* ***Anxiety***, "apprehension, worry, or fear related to death or dying" (NANDA-I, 2010).

Planning/Outcome Identification

The major goals of nursing care are the physical, emotional, and mental comfort of the client. The goals of nursing care for the dying client are the same as those goals developed for all clients who are unable to meet their own needs. The dying client should be treated as a unique individual worthy of respect instead of a diagnosis to be cured. Many dying clients do not fear death but are anxious about a painful death or dying alone.

Promoting optimal quality of life includes treating the client and family with respect and providing a safe environment for expressing their feelings. Planning should focus on meeting the client's and family's holistic needs, as specified in the Dying Person's Bill of Rights (Figure 13-4). It is as relevant today as when it was written in 1975. When planning care, the nurse should make every effort to be sensitive to the rights of the dying client.

Implementation

The first priority is to communicate caring to the client and family. Powell (1999) found that the presence of a comforting nurse made a tremendous difference to the client. LaDuke (2001) suggests holding a client's or family member's hand and saying "I will not leave you." This assurance of the nurse's presence is a powerful way to show caring.

The nurse should approach the client in denial with understanding and the knowledge that moving between the stages of dying is enhanced by a trusting nurse–client relationship.

The Dying Person's Bill of Rights

- I have the right to be treated as a living human being until I die.
- I have the right to maintain a sense of hopefulness, however changing its focus may be.
- I have the right to be cared for by those who can maintain a sense of hopefulness, however challenging this might be.
- I have the right to express my feelings and emotions about my approaching death in my own way.
- I have the right to participate in decisions concerning my care.
- I have the right to expect continuing medical and nursing attention even though "cure" goals must be changed to "comfort" goals.
- I have the right not to die alone.
- I have the right to be free from pain.
- I have the right to have my questions answered honestly.
- I have the right not to be deceived.
- I have the right to have help from and for my family in accepting death.
- I have the right to die in peace and dignity.
- I have the right to retain my individuality and not be judged for my decisions, which may be contrary to beliefs of others.
- I have the right to discuss and enlarge my religious and/or spiritual experiences, whatever these may mean to others.
- I have the right to expect that the sanctity of the human body will be respected after death.
- I have the right to be cared for by caring, sensitive, knowledgeable people who will attempt to understand my needs and will be able to gain some satisfaction in helping me face my death.

FIGURE 13-4 The Dying Person's Bill of Rights (*From The Dying Person's Bill of Rights, by A. Barbus, 1975, American Journal of Nursing, 75[1].*)

Establishing rapport facilitates the client's verbalization of feelings (Figure 13-5). A safe environment established by the nurse allows the client to express those feelings being experienced. Nurses must understand that clients are not angry with them but, rather with the situation they are experiencing.

Physiological Needs Physiological needs are essential for existence, according to Maslow's hierarchy of needs. Therefore, they must be met before all other needs. Areas that are often problematic for the terminally ill client are respirations; fluids and nutrition; mouth, eyes, and nose; mobility; skin care; and elimination.

Respirations Oxygen is frequently ordered for the client experiencing labored breathing. Suctioning may be needed to remove secretions that the client is unable to swallow.

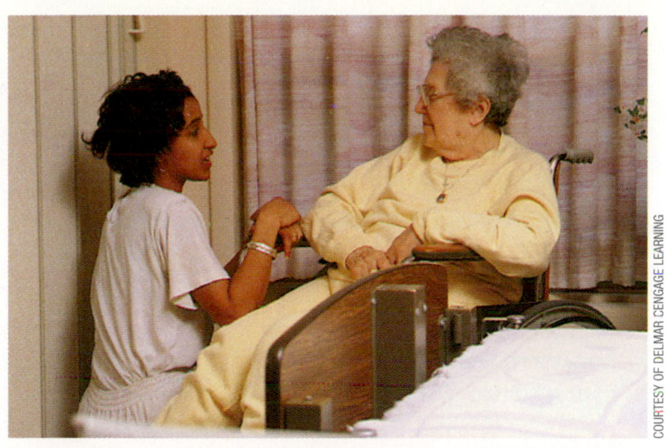
COURTESY OF DELMAR CENGAGE LEARNING

FIGURE 13-5 **Establishing a caring and trusting relationship helps the client come to terms with a terminal illness.**

Fluids and Nutrition Dying clients are rarely hungry and gradually stop eating and drinking. Refusal of food and fluids is a natural part of the dying process. A study of clients dying of cancer found the clients did not feel hunger or thirst (Robert Wood Johnson Foundation, 2004). In fact, hospice workers found that clients who are not given artificial nutrition and hydration are more comfortable than those who receive it (Robert Wood Johnson Foundation, 2004). When artificial nutrition and hydration are withheld, symptoms of nausea, vomiting, abdominal pain, loss of bladder control, and shortness of breath decrease. Artificial nutrition often increases the client's agitation and risk of aspiration pneumonia. When clients are nearing death and artificial nutrition and hydration are stopped, the client dies within 3 to 14 days. Health care personnel noticed that the dying process was peaceful and that the clients did not experience pain or distress (Robert Wood Johnson Foundation, 2004).

The client's wishes must always take precedence in every situation. Family members must be given truthful and accurate information when a comatose client has not previously made his wishes known. The American Dietetic Association, the American Medical Association, and the ANA agree that it is ethically, legally, and professionally acceptable to discontinue nutritional support if that is the terminally ill client's request.

Mouth, Eyes, and Nose The administration of oxygen and mouth breathing increase the need for meticulous oral care. Saliva substitutes and moisturizers can be used to alleviate discomfort. Regular use of toothpaste and a toothbrush may be adequate. The tongue should be gently brushed. Offer ice chips and sips of favorite beverages frequently. Apply petroleum jelly to the lips to prevent dryness. To maintain the client's comfort, give oral care every 2 to 3 hours.

If the client's eyes remain open, apply an ophthalmic lubricating gel to the conjunctiva every 3 to 4 hours or artificial tears or physiologic saline solution every 15 to 30 minutes. A cotton ball is used to gently wipe the eye from inner to outer canthus (one wipe per cotton ball) to remove any discharge.

The nares may become dry and crusted. Oxygen given by cannula can further irritate the nares. A thin layer of water-soluble jelly applied to the nares alleviates discomfort. The elastic strap of the oxygen cannula is not applied too tightly, lest it cause discomfort. If oxygen tubing is placed behind the ears, the area is assessed for irritation.

Mobility Mobility decreases as the client's condition deteriorates. The client requires more assistance as he becomes less able to move about in bed or get out of bed. Physical dependence increases the risk of complications related to immobility, such as atrophy and pressure ulcers. These complications, which increase both cost of care and client discomfort, can be prevented by attentive nursing care.

Reposition the client at least every 2 hours. Remember that the client may have other disorders that contribute to discomfort related to mobility, such as arthritis or lung disease. Maintain body alignment with the use of pillows and other supportive equipment and use positioning techniques to facilitate ease of breathing. Perform passive range-of-motion exercises at least twice a day to prevent stiffness and aching of the joints. The client may wish to be in a reclining type of chair several times a day. Use a wheelchair to increase the client's environmental space and give the client more mobility, control, and independence.

Skin Care Prevention of pressure ulcers is a priority. They are painful, can cause secondary complications, and are costly to treat. Two preventive measures are passive range-of-motion exercises every 1 to 2 hours and regular repositioning every hour to hour and a half. Turning the client with the use of a draw sheet decreases pain and prevents skin shearing. The use of air mattresses or air beds reduces pressure to all body surfaces. In addition, keeping the skin clean and moisturized will promote healthy tissue. Inspect the skin once or twice daily, with special attention paid to pressure points and areas where skin surfaces rub together. Gentle massages with soothing lotion are comforting and decrease skin breakdown by improving circulation. Areas of nonblanching erythema or actual skin breakdown should not be massaged. Apply hydrocolloid dressings to bony prominences to protect them from pressure and skin breakdown. Bed baths are adequate if the client cannot get into the tub or sit in a shower chair.

Elimination Side effects of pain medications and a lack of physical activity may cause constipation. For clients with adequate oral intake, foods with high-fiber content and fluids can be effective preventive measures. Constipation can also be alleviated by administering suppositories, if necessary, and maintaining a scheduled time for bowel elimination. A commode with padded arms can be more comfortable than a toilet.

The client may become incontinent of bowel and bladder. After each incontinent episode, clean the skin with peri-washes, and apply a moisture barrier. Urine and fecal material on the skin will quickly lead to excoriation and skin breakdown.

Indwelling catheters are not a first choice for bladder management; however, for some clients, the discomfort of

PROFESSIONALTIP

Adjuvant Therapy

Adjuvant therapy may be effective. Nonsteroidal anti-inflammatory agents are beneficial for bone metastases, tricyclic antidepressants and antiseizure medications for neurogenic pain, antidepressants for terminally ill clients, and steroids for headaches related to cerebral edema. Nonpharmacological techniques can be used along with medication. Relaxation techniques, guided imagery, massages, and repositioning may enhance the action of the medications.

using a bedpan, getting out of bed to use the toilet or commode, or the need for frequent cleaning may cause agonizing pain. The benefits of a urinary catheter greatly outweigh the risks in such circumstances.

Comfort The primary activities for promoting physical comfort include pain relief, keeping the client dry and clean, and providing a safe, nonthreatening environment. The nurse who has a caring, respectful attitude increases the client's psychological comfort. Fear of a painful death is almost universal. Pain is a subjective, personal experience, and the client is the best judge of the severity of the pain. Many, but not all, dying clients experience pain. The ANA states in its position statement on pain relief for the terminally ill that promotion of comfort is the major goal of nursing care (ANA, 1996, 2008). Comfort is to be maximized by managing pain and other causes of discomfort.

The client must know that caregivers accept and believe complaints of pain and that they will intervene to alleviate or prevent the pain. Ask the client to rate the pain on a scale from 0 to 10, with 0 being no pain and 10 being severe pain. Pain is defined as what the client states it is, and the nurse administers pain medication according to the client's statement of need.

To maintain therapeutic blood level, medication must be given around the clock and not "as needed." A nonnarcotic analgesic may be effective in early stages for mild, intermittent pain. As the pain increases, the client may need to start on morphine, titrated at increments until adequate pain relief is achieved without severe side effects. Finding the lowest dose and the longest interval that will relieve pain is called titrating the dose. The dosage that should be used is the one that controls the pain to the satisfaction of the client and that causes minimal side effects. The dose is individual and continually assessed to remain therapeutic in controlling pain.

The World Health Organization (WHO) has a three-step ladder that guides pain administration and titration. Clients with mild pain are given acetaminophen (Tylenol) or nonsteroidal anti-inflammatory drugs (NSAIDs); for moderate pain, a weak opioid or combination agents, such as oxycodone/hydrocodone and acetaminophen or tramadol (Ultram); and for severe pain, strong longer-acting opioids, such as morphine, hydromorphone hydrochloride (Dilaudid), fentanyl (Duragesic), or oxycodone (OxyContin) (Webster & Dove, 2007). Figure 13-6 shows some long- and short-acting opioids. Treatment starts at the level of the client's pain and does not have to start at the first step.

Guidelines for administering pain medication in palliative care are:

- Assess the client's pain and note how it affects quality of life
- Give sustained-release medications around the clock
- Treat breakthrough pain with immediate-release medications
- Monitor pain status frequently
- Treat adverse effects as needed
- Know drug–drug and drug–disease interactions
- Reassess pain on a regular basis (Panke, 2002)

When the client cannot verbalize his pain, note the nonverbal behavior. Nonverbal clues of pain are decreased activity or restlessness, furrowed brow, grimacing, crying, moaning, withdrawal from others, guarded or stiffened posture, irritability, elevated blood pressure, and increased pulse. If the furrowed brow comes and goes, it may indicate mental activity of dreams and hallucinations. Assess other nonverbals to obtain the total pain picture.

Opioids	
Long Acting	**Short Acting**
fentanyl transdermal system (Duragesic)	Codeine sulfate
methadone hydrochloride (Metadol)	hydrocodone bitartrate and acetaminophen (Vicodin)
buprenorphine hydrochloride (Buprenex)	hydromorphone hydrochloride (Dilaudid)
Morphine sulfate	Morphine sulfate
oxycodone hydrochloride (Roxicodone)	oxycodone hydrochloride (Roxicodone)
oxymorphone hydrochloride (Numorphan)	Tramadol (Ultram)

FIGURE 13-6 Long-Acting and Short-Acting Opioids *(Adapted from Optimizing Opioid Treatment for Breakthrough Pain, by L. Webster and M. Dove, 2007, Retrieved October 14, 2007, from http://www.medscape.com.)*

Monitor the client's responses with regard to pain rating and respiratory rate. For example, 30 mg of morphine sulfate given orally may provide pain relief, but if the respiratory rate drops from 12 to 6 per minute, adjust or change the medication. If the same dose given to another client provides minimal relief and the client is alert and displays no change in respirations, the next dose is increased (Webster & Dove, 2007).

Pain medication is given by the least invasive route of administration, preferably oral or buccal mucosa, then IV or subcutaneous, with intramuscular rarely used. The rectal route is also used when medication cannot be given orally (Panke, 2002). If the dying client has diminished liver or renal function, continuous administration of morphine causes an accumulation of active metabolites leading to terminal delirium. Fentanyl is the drug of choice at this point because it has no active metabolites to accumulate and cause toxicity (Webster & Dove, 2007).

Monitor the client for **breakthrough pain**, or sudden, acute, temporary pain that is usually precipitated by a treatment, a procedure, or unusual activity of the client. A supplemental dose of medication is then required. If the precipitating factor is known (e.g., dressing changes), give medication 30 to 60 minutes before the procedure. Table 13-6 describes care given to a client during end-of-life care.

Physical Environment The client's comfort can be significantly increased by a soothing physical environment. Soft lighting may enhance vision. Complying with the client's request for a nightlight is also helpful in creating a pleasant and nonthreatening environment. If possible, the client should be offered the opportunity to have the bed or a chair near a window to increase the range of the environment. Since body temperature falls as circulation becomes more sluggish, a lightweight comforter will increase warmth without adding much weight. Help eliminate environmental odors by ensuring adequate ventilation, daily cleaning of the room, removal of leftover food, and frequent linen changes.

Table 13-6 Nursing Management during End-of-Life Care

PHYSIOLOGIC RESPONSE	CONTRIBUTING FACTORS	NURSING INTERVENTIONS
Pain	Terminal illness Fear and anxiety	Assess for pain frequently and thoroughly Administer pain medications in a timely manner and around the clock Address break through pain in a timely manner Do not delay or deny pain medication for the terminally ill client Evaluate effectiveness of pain medication frequently
Dyspnea	Fear and anxiety Primary lung tumors Lung metastases Pleural effusion Restrictive lung disease	Assist with relaxation techniques Administer prescribed medications to relieve dyspnea (anxiolytic, bronchodilators, corticosteroids, diuretics, opioids) Administer prescribed oxygen therapy Teach client and family energy conservation techniques For home or hospice care, offer electric bed, lift chair, and bedside commode
Anorexia	Fear and anxiety Treatment Complications of disease process	Feed the client when hungry Assess for nausea and vomiting Offer culturally appropriate foods Provide frequent mouth care, especially following vomiting episodes
Weakness fatigue	Terminal illness Treatment Change in metabolic demands	Assess loss of tolerance for activities Provide frequent rest periods Time nursing interventions to conserve energy
Constipation	Medications Immobility Dehydration	Encourage foods high in fiber Increase fluid intake as tolerated Encourage activity
Nausea and vomiting	Complications of disease process Medications	Encourage the client to avoid eating if nauseated Suggest small meals of cool nonodorous foods Encourage the client to eat slowly
Delirium	Use of opioids and steroids	Reorient to time, place, and person frequently Ensure frequent nursing rounds Provide a quiet, well-lit room Administer sedatives and benzodiazepines

Data from *Palliative and End of Life Care,* by E. Hull, 2008, Manuscript submitted for publication.

Noise can be distracting and anxiety provoking, so the nurse and visitors should comply with the client's wishes with regard to the use of radio and television. The telephone can be removed from the room if the client finds the ringing disturbing.

Psychosocial Needs Death presents a threat to one's psychological integrity as well as to one's physical existence. The dying person is often tethered to tubes and electronic gadgetry in an intensive care unit. The client is held captive in a tangle of technology and is kept at a distance from the supportive presence and touch of family and friends.

Technology cannot replace concern, touch, compassion, or human companionship. By their presence, nurses and family can humanize the dying person's environment. Invite and encourage families to participate in the client's care if they desire to do so and the client is willing.

For many clients, maintaining a well-groomed appearance is important. When the client can no longer make requests or give directions for care, caregivers should presume that the

COMMUNITY/HOME HEALTH CARE

Equipment to Increase Client Comfort

The following equipment can be rented and may qualify for payment by Medicare or private insurance:

- An electric hospital bed with overhead trapeze allows the client some control of the environment.
- A commode promotes the client's independence in elimination.
- A lifting device eases getting the dependent client out of bed.
- Handheld shower and chair for the bathtub or shower are helpful.
- Devices such as cushions for chairs and special mattresses for the bed provide comfort.
- An overbed table for eating and other activities is useful.
- Comfortable chairs close to the bed facilitate visits of friends and family.

client would prefer to maintain the same grooming habits as were previously preferred. Shaving the male client's beard or cleaning and trimming the client's fingernails and toenails, for instance, will help the client maintain a well-groomed appearance and will also promote client dignity. Combing and brushing the hair not only improves appearance but is also a comforting and relaxing activity for many clients.

Dressing and undressing may become a cumbersome, frustrating, and fatiguing activity. The client who spends time up and about may choose attractive pajamas, housecoats, dusters, or exercise suits. Advise individuals who may be purchasing clothing for the client to select items that are loose fitting, have few fasteners, and are washable.

Spiritual Needs Dying persons may experience confusion, anger at their god, crises of faith, or other types of spiritual distress. Nurses have the opportunity to play a major role in promoting the dying client's spiritual comfort.

Yet a survey on end-of-life care by Ferrell, Virani, Grant, Coyne, and Uman (2000) showed that fewer than 35% of nurses described grief/bereavement support and the attention to spiritual needs as effective; however, 66% of nurses said that care of the dying was better than 5 years prior.

Dying clients are most vulnerable. The moral health and integrity of the broader community can be measured in part by the way we respond to their needs.

Dying is a personal and often a lonely process. Table 13-7 provides information on the views of various religions with regard to withdrawal of life support, death, and organ donation. Listen as a client expresses values and beliefs related to death. Therapeutic nursing interventions that address the spiritual needs of the dying client include:

- Using touch
- Playing music
- Praying with the client
- Communicating empathy
- Contacting clergy if requested by the client
- Reading religious literature aloud at the client's request

Support for the Family The presence of the nurse is extremely important. It shows support and caring not only for the client but for the family as well. Family members may have increased guilt because of feelings of helplessness. The nurse encourages family members to speak to, touch, read to, sing to, pray with, or just sit with the client. This can give family members a sense of purpose, ease feelings of helplessness, and provide more pleasant memories in the future.

Each family group has its unwritten rules, its leaders and followers, and its methods for coping with crises. The family's equilibrium is threatened by the impending death. If family members have limited coping skills and inadequate support systems, they need assistance and guidance from the caregivers. Nurses must remember that the rules and coping mechanisms used by the family may not always coincide with the values and beliefs of the staff and that the client's and family's wishes must be respected to the extent possible.

The relationship with the family does not always end with the client's death. Staff members may attend visitations, funerals, or memorial services. If a hospice was involved, the family may participate in a bereavement support program. If the client was a resident in a long-term care facility, family members may return to visit other residents with whom they became acquainted.

Learning Needs The nurse's role is to provide the client and family members with support and information. For example, they may not realize that the dying person should conserve energy. Family activities are best scheduled early in the morning or following a period of rest by the client. The nurse may need to point out to the family this type of commonsense approach, as simple interventions such as these can be overlooked during this highly charged emotional time.

Client and family learning needs may relate to:

- Information about physical condition and treatment regimen
- Anticipating a medical crisis
- Inexperience with the personal threat of death
- Unfamiliarity with what to do in case of an emergency outside the hospital

CLIENT TEACHING

Guidelines for Teaching a Family Caregiver

- Use adult-education principles.
- Frequently reinforce material.
- Provide information about the nature and extent of the disease process.
- Explain the purpose of palliative care yet maintain a sense of realistic hope.
- Reassure client and family by informing them of available community resources; tell them that they are not alone.
- Discuss steps for caregiver to follow if an emergency arises at home by providing written instructions, including persons to be contacted and important telephone numbers.

TABLE 13-7 Religions and Death and Dying Issues

RELIGION	LIFE SUPPORT WITHDRAWAL IN TERMINAL ILLNESS	DEATH	ORGAN DONATION
Judaism	Allowed under the right circumstances (when life support is serving only to impede a natural death).	• Suicide is forbidden. • Burial should occur within 24 hours. • Cremation is forbidden. • Autopsy is permitted if it will save future lives.	• Permitted because the procedure saves life. • Rejected by Orthodox Jews.
Islam	Permitted if only serving to prolong death or if client's condition is medically hopeless.	• Suicide is forbidden. • Relatives and friends are present. • Autopsy is permitted to solve a crime or provide further medical knowledge.	• Permitted.
Catholicism/ Orthodoxy	Controversial; permitted if client's condition is hopeless.	• Prayers are offered at time of death. • Burial and cremation are permitted. • Autopsy is permitted.	• Permitted.
Protestantism	Permitted if client's condition is hopeless.	• Prayers are offered at time of death. • Burial and cremation are permitted. • Autopsy is permitted.	• Permitted, although may be rejected by some Baptists or Pentecostals.
Jehovah's Witness	Permitted if serving only to prolong death or if quality of life is nonexistent.	• Suicide is not approved. • Autopsy is permitted if legally necessary.	• Individual choice.
Buddhism	Acceptable for those on threshold of death.	• Suicide is criticized. • Cremation is common.	• Controversial.
Hinduism	Supported to allow a natural death.	• Prefer to die at home. • Embalming is forbidden. • Autopsy is discouraged. • Suicide is forbidden.	• Discouraged because of disturbing the body after death.
Mormons	A client or family decision.	• Cremation is discouraged. • Autopsy is a family decision.	• A family decision.
Native Americans	Life support is viewed as unnatural and, therefore, unnecessary.	• Complex beliefs about death and treatment of the body; some are forbidden to touch a dead body. • Ancestral worship. • Often believe the spirit of the person continues to live.	• Discouraged because of death and burial practices.
Christian Science	Most have advance directives to avoid medical treatment; however, no illness is seen as hopeless.	• Practitioner should always be notified at death. • Autopsy is permitted. • Cremation is usual practice.	• Do not donate or receive organs because the spiritual cause of organ failure is not treated with an organ transplant.
Unitarian	Support withdrawal of life support when quality of life is poor and suffering is great.	• Suicide is a tragedy. • Autopsy is permitted as needed.	• Permitted.

Data from *Health Assessment and Physical Examination* (4th ed.), by M. Estes, 2010, Clifton Park, NY: Delmar Cengage Learning. Copyright 2010 by Delmar Cengage Learning.

CRITICAL THINKING

Caring for a Dying Client

Think about caring for a dying client. How can you prepare to care for a dying client?

Impending Death

There is no way to predict how long a client may be in the terminal stages of illness. A client may have signs of impending death and then rally to live several more days. Clients often live until a family member arrives for a last good-bye. The client who has had a long illness and is ready to die may need "permission" to die from a loved one, who says, "It's okay, you can go now." Some clients may not wish to die when anyone is present and will wait to take the last breath until alone in the room.

It is never easy for the family, even when death is expected. The family should be simply and thoroughly informed about what will happen before and after the client's death, including:

- Physical changes that occur just before and following death
- Death pronouncement
- Postmortem care
- Body removal

Impending death is signaled by a series of irrevocable events (Hull, 2008):

- The lungs become unable to provide adequate gas diffusion.
- The heart and blood vessels become unable to maintain adequate tissue perfusion.
- The brain ceases to regulate vital centers.

Cheyne-Stokes respirations (breathing characterized by periods of apnea alternating with periods of dyspnea) most often herald pulmonary system failure. Secretions accumulate in the larynx and trachea, causing noisy respirations, often called the **death rattle**.

COMMUNITY/HOME HEALTH CARE

When the Client Dies at Home (Preparing for an Expected Death)

Have the family prepare:

- A list of names and telephone numbers they wish to notify of the death including the name and telephone number of the funeral director.

Instruct the family:

- Whom to call (physician or hospice nurse or funeral director).
- Whom *not* to call (ambulance and emergency services).
- To record the time of death, last medications given, the condition of the client during the last few hours, and the last time the client was seen by the nurse.

The heart fails in its pumping function, resulting in poor perfusion, ischemia, and cell death. The skin becomes cool and, possibly, very pale, cyanotic, jaundiced, or mottled. The pulse becomes rapid, irregular, weak, and thready. Death is several hours away if a peripheral pulse is strong and easily palpated. Cold, cyanotic extremities and irregular respirations indicate that death is imminent.

Inadequate cerebral perfusion hinders the brain's ability to integrate vital functions. The client may be confused and lethargic and may respond only to direct visual, auditory, or tactile stimulation. Pupils no longer react to light and become fixed. The client may "talk" to dead loved ones. A frown or tight facial muscles may indicate pain or discomfort. A client in a coma will move only in response to deep pain. Analgesics should not be withdrawn from a conscious client in a coma.

The care of the client does not cease during this final stage of life. The nursing actions previously described should be continued. Tell the client in brief, simple terms what is happening as care is rendered. The family should be allowed and encouraged to continue their participation if that is their wish. Caution family members that the dying client can hear even in the absence of verbal response, so all comments and conversation should continue to be respectful.

There may be other indications that death is near. The client may report seeing someone who has died or angels or hearing someone or beautiful music (Pitorak, 2003). These experiences should be accepted as a natural step in the process of dying. When the final breath is taken, the heart stops beating. Within a few minutes, cerebral death (the point at which brain cells die) occurs, and brain activity ceases.

Physical signs of death are:

- Absence of a heartbeat
- Cessation of respirations
- Mottling of skin or skin that is cool to the touch
- Eyelids remain slightly open
- Jaws relaxed and mouth slightly open
- No response to name, touch, or environmental sounds
- Eyes fixed on a certain spot
- No eye blinking in response to touch or air movement over the eyes
- Release of bowel and bladder contents (Hull, 2008)

Care after Death

Meeting the needs of the grieving family and caring for the deceased body are nursing responsibilities. Treat the body of the deceased with respect by maintaining privacy and preventing damage to the body. **Postmortem care** is given immediately after death but before the body is moved to the mortuary (see Professional Tip: Postmortem Care).

After death, several physiological changes occur. Body temperature decreases, resulting in a lack of skin elasticity (**algor mortis**). In order to avoid skin breakdown, the nurse must therefore use caution when removing tape from the body. **Liver mortis**, a bluish-purple discoloration of the skin, is a by-product of red blood cell destruction. It usually begins within 20 minutes of death (Harvey, 2001). This discoloration occurs in dependent areas of the body; the nurse should therefore elevate the head of the bed 30 degrees to prevent discoloration of the head and neck. If the body is moved on a stretcher, keep the head elevated on two pillows. **Rigor mortis**, the natural stiffening of muscles after death, begins about 4 hours after death. The funeral director

PROFESSIONALTIP

Postmortem Care

- Treat the body with dignity and respect.
- Bathe and put a clean gown on the body—and place an incontinent pad under the client's hips.
- Remove dressings and tubes, unless these must remain in place for an autopsy.
- Place the body in alignment with the head elevated.
- Place dentures in a denture cup and send with the body.
- Comb the client's hair.

will have the best results if embalming is completed before rigor mortis sets in (Harvey, 2001). Position the body in a natural position.

When preparing the body for family viewing, endeavor to make the body look natural and comfortable. This means preparing and positioning the body as previously described. According to Harvey (2001), if the client wore dentures, they should not be put in the deceased person's mouth. Jaw muscles relax after death, so dentures often fall out and are lost or broken. Put them in a hospital denture cup without water and send them with the body to the funeral director. After the family has viewed the body, place identification tags on the body's toe and wrist. Sometimes the body is placed is a plastic or fabric **shroud** (a covering for the body after death) and tagged. Next, transport the body to the morgue according to the agency's policy, where it is kept until it is transported to a **mortuary** (funeral home). In some institutions, the body is kept in the room until the funeral director arrives. The nurse is also responsible for returning the deceased's possessions, such as jewelry, eyeglasses, clothing, and all other personal items, to the family.

Information for Funeral Director

Harvey (2001) explains information that is important to the funeral director when preparing the body. The cause of death influences which procedures are used. For example, a client with liver or renal failure has a high level of ammonia in the body. A special solution will have to be used because the ammonia neutralizes the formaldehyde generally used. If the client had tuberculosis (TB) or any other communicable disease, special procedures will be followed to prevent spreading the disease. If the client weighed more than 300 pounds (136 kg), the funeral director will need extra staff for transferring the body.

Legal Aspects

The physician is legally responsible for determining the cause of death and signing the death certificate in most states. In certain situations, the RN may be responsible for certifying the death. Some institutions require two nurses to certify death. Nurses must know their legal responsibilities as defined by their respective state boards of nursing.

Autopsy

An **autopsy** is the examination of the body after death by a pathologist to determine the cause of death. It is mandated in situations where an unusual death has occurred. For example, a violent death or an unexpected death is a circumstance necessitating an autopsy. For an autopsy to be performed in other situations, families must give consent. The funeral director must know whether an autopsy is to be performed.

Organ Donation

Organ donation for transplantation requires sensitivity and compassion from the health care team. Health care facilities must have a policy regarding the referral of a potential organ donor to appropriate organ procurement agencies. The Centers for Medicare and Medicaid Services requires hospitals to notify a local organ-procurement organization (OPO) of a client in imminent death or who has died so that the person who initially approaches the family is an OPO representative or "designated requestor" (Truog, 2008). When an organ(s) is donated, the OPO representative coordinates the entire process, including finding organ recipients (OrganDonor.Gov, 2008).

The organs and tissues that can be transplanted are:

- Liver
- Lungs
- Heart
- Kidneys
- Pancreas
- Skin
- Bones (middle ear bones and long bones)
- Corneas

The average waiting time is 230 days for a heart, 1,068 days for a lung, 796 days for a liver, 1,121 days for a kidney, and 501 days for a pancreas. Transplantation must occur within 4 to 6 hours for heart and lungs, 12 to 24 hours for liver and pancreas, and 48 to 72 hours for kidneys (OrganDonor.Gov, 2008).

Care of the Family

The nurse provides invaluable support to the family of the deceased at the time of death. It is extremely important to inform the family of the circumstances surrounding the death. The nurse offers information about viewing the body and contacts support people (e.g., other relatives, clergy). The nurse may even help the family with decisions regarding transportation, a funeral home, and removal of the deceased's belongings. Sensitive and compassionate interpersonal skills are essential when providing information and support to families. Providing coffee, tissues, and light snacks are small gestures that convey sensitivity to the family and friends and are appreciated.

Nurse's Self-Care

Working with dying clients can evoke both a personal and a professional threat in the nurse. Grief is a common experience for nurses because many nurses are confronted with death and loss daily. Smith-Stoner and Frost (1998) describe a part of the psyche called the shadow self, where stresses are stored. Unresolved sadness is called shadow grief. Everyone has a shadow self and may have some shadow grief. Nurses often have a great deal of shadow grief, which, if not released, may

PROFESSIONALTIP

Care for Yourself during Grief

- Do what nurses do well: care. Help the family and your feelings of helplessness will diminish.
- Plan time for your own grieving.
- Allow for crying to help ease the pain.
- Learn when to ask your coworkers for help.
- Express your feelings of grief to someone you can trust.
- Find support within your facility from counselors, support groups, and clergy.
- Use rituals to say good-bye to the deceased client and bring closure.

From "Please Cry with Me: Six Ways to Grieve," by C. D. Reese, 1996, *Nursing96, 26*(8), 56.

cause illness and burnout. Frequent exposure to death can interfere with the nurse's effectiveness because of subsequent anxiety and denial.

Nurses are at particular risk for experiencing negative effects from caring for the dying, whether working in a hospital, a hospice, a long-term care facility, or the home. They may not wish to confront their grief and will often use some of the common defense mechanisms against grieving, such as being strong, keeping busy, and suffering in silence. Nurses must talk about the intense emotions associated with caregiving instead of pretending that they do not experience grief. According to Smith-Stoner and Frost (1998), shadow grief may be staring to overwhelm a person if that person experiences the following:

- A loss of energy, spark, joy, and meaning in life
- Detachment from surroundings
- A feeling of being powerless to make a difference
- Increased smoking or drinking
- Unusual forgetfulness
- Constant criticism directed toward others
- Consistent inability to get work done
- Uncontrolled outbursts of anger
- Perception of clients and their families as objects
- Surrender of hobbies or interests

To effectively cope with their own grief, nurses need education, support, and assistance when coping with the death of clients. The focus of staff education should be on ways to seek support, decreasing staff anxiety when working with grieving clients and families, and ways to provide support to coworkers. Smith-Stoner and Frost (1998) suggest the following ways to cope:

- Take time to cry with and for clients
- Get physical: run, walk, bike, play tennis
- Ask colleagues to help with tasks; do not try to be "Supernurse"
- Connect to a place of worship; pray
- Look for joy in work—laughter is a great healer
- Create a caring circle of friends
- Listen to music

The nurse's own fears and doubts about death may surface and cause anxiety about feelings of mortality. Caring for the dying client and the client's family is emotionally draining, so nurses must remember to care for themselves.

SAMPLE NURSING CARE PLAN

The Client with a Terminal Illness/Cancer of the Lung

V.P., an 84-year-old widow, was diagnosed with cancer of the right lung 6 months ago. After a right lower lobectomy, she was discharged to a local skilled-care facility and planned to go home after completing her radiation therapy. After completing the treatments, V.P.'s condition began deteriorating. She did not want to go home, so discharge plans were discontinued. Now she is frequently short of breath, has dyspnea, requires pain medication, and needs some assistance with activities of daily living because of fatigue. She frequently grimaces and says, "I hurt." Her nutritional intake is very little because of swallowing difficulties. V.P. gets up only to use the commode. Her two adult children and four grandchildren live nearby and visit often. They want to assist their mother to get her affairs in order, but she resists their efforts. The family is trying to make V.P.'s remaining time as serene and comfortable as possible, but V.P. often defies their attempts.

NURSING DIAGNOSIS 1 *Chronic* ***Pain*** related to disease progression as evidenced by verbal statements, body language, and the need for pain medication

Nursing Outcomes Classification (NOC)	Nursing Interventions Classification (NIC)
Pain: Disruptive Effects	*Pain Management*
Pain: Psychological Response	*Analgesic Administration*
Pain Control	*Coping Enhancement*

(*Continues*)

SAMPLE NURSING CARE PLAN (Continued)

PLANNING/OUTCOMES	NURSING INTERVENTIONS	RATIONALE
V.P. will verbalize relief from pain.	Give analgesics as ordered.	Administering regular doses of analgesics is more effective than waiting until the pain begins.
	Have client rate pain on a scale of 0 to 10, with 0 being no pain and 10 being severe pain, to assess the need for morphine. Give morphine as ordered, titrated at increments until adequate pain relief is achieved.	The client should be given analgesics when pain is experienced. Morphine is the drug of choice for severe pain associated with cancer.
	Monitor for signs of breakthrough pain. If the precipitating factor is known, give medication 30 to 60 minutes before the event. Medicate as soon as possible for unpredictable breakthrough pain.	Breakthrough pain is often precipitated by activity or stress and supplemental medication is required.
	Assure V.P. that the nurses will help her manage the pain and keep it under control. Reposition frequently and give back massages for comfort. Assist with relaxation techniques if client agreeable.	Needs reassurance that everything possible will be done to manage the pain. Promotes psychological comfort.
	Monitor bowel elimination.	Pain medication often causes constipation.

EVALUATION

V.P.'s body language and verbal statements indicate freedom from pain

NURSING DIAGNOSIS 2 *Ineffective Coping* related to terminal illness as evidenced by inability to communicate effectively with family members and to accept their help

Nursing Outcomes Classification (NOC)
Coping
Self-Esteem
Social Interaction Skills

Nursing Interventions Classification (NIC)
Coping Enhancement
Counseling
Emotional Support

PLANNING/OUTCOMES	NURSING INTERVENTIONS	RATIONALE
V.P. will express her feelings openly.	Consult V.P. on all aspects of care. Give complete information. Provide opportunities to express feelings. Acknowledge V.P.'s feelings and let her know that crying and grieving are beneficial.	Allows V.P. to express her feelings and validates those feelings as being normal and expected.

(*Continues*)

SAMPLE NURSING CARE PLAN (Continued)

PLANNING/OUTCOMES	NURSING INTERVENTIONS	RATIONALE
	Listen for clues indicating unfinished business that needs to be completed. Encourage the process of life review.	Life review is a process of reflection and pondering of one's past and accepting one's life as being meaningful and valuable.
V.P. will maintain a satisfying relationship with her family.	Encourage family visits. Provide privacy.	Families need privacy in order to feel free to express their emotions.

EVALUATION

V.P. still resists family's assistance.

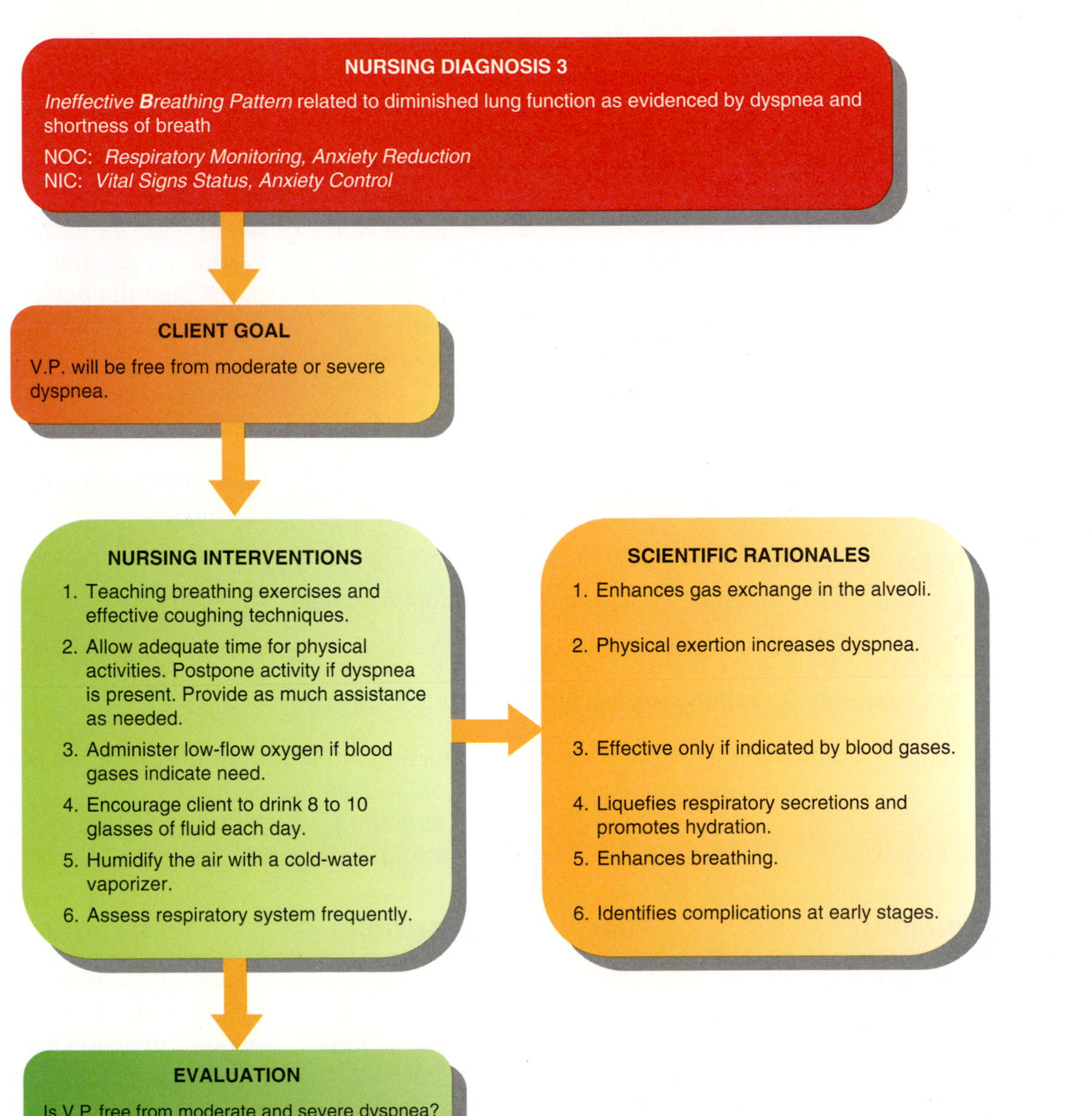

NURSING DIAGNOSIS 3
Ineffective Breathing Pattern related to diminished lung function as evidenced by dyspnea and shortness of breath
NOC: Respiratory Monitoring, Anxiety Reduction
NIC: Vital Signs Status, Anxiety Control
CLIENT GOAL
V.P. will be free from moderate or severe dyspnea.
NURSING INTERVENTIONS
1. Teaching breathing exercises and effective coughing techniques.
2. Allow adequate time for physical activities. Postpone activity if dyspnea is present. Provide as much assistance as needed.
3. Administer low-flow oxygen if blood gases indicate need.
4. Encourage client to drink 8 to 10 glasses of fluid each day.
5. Humidify the air with a cold-water vaporizer.
6. Assess respiratory system frequently.
SCIENTIFIC RATIONALES
1. Enhances gas exchange in the alveoli.
2. Physical exertion increases dyspnea.
3. Effective only if indicated by blood gases.
4. Liquefies respiratory secretions and promotes hydration.
5. Enhances breathing.
6. Identifies complications at early stages.
EVALUATION
Is V.P. free from moderate and severe dyspnea?

Concept Care Map 13-1

SUMMARY

- Loss is when someone (or something) of value is no longer available. It is a universal response.
- Grief is a psychological response to loss evidenced by deep sorrow and mental anguish.
- The difference between pathological and normal grief is the inability of the individual to adapt to life without the loved one.
- Kübler-Ross identified five psychological stages of the dying process: denial, anger, bargaining, depression, and acceptance.
- Complicated grief is associated with traumatic death such as suicide, accident, or homicide.
- Each person dies a unique death.
- Hospice care is an alternative to hospitalization when aggressive medical treatment is no longer an option.
- After death, the nurse's focus is on supporting the family and caring for the deceased body.
- Nurses must care for themselves in order to provide compassionate, quality care to the dying person and family.

REVIEW QUESTIONS

1. S.R., age 11 years, was left with a distant relative 2 weeks ago. Her parents have not returned or called. S.R. is experiencing a/an:
   1. physical loss.
   2. situational loss.
   3. maturational loss.
   4. anticipational loss.
2. A defining characteristic of the NANDA-I nursing diagnosis *Anticipatory **G**rieving* is:
   1. prolonged denial or depression.
   2. unsuccessful adaptation to loss.
   3. social isolation or withdrawal from others.
   4. an expression of distress at potential loss.
3. The purpose of the Patient Self-Determination Act is to:
   1. serve as an order for "do not resuscitate."
   2. designate a guardian for an incompetent client.
   3. provide a means, instead of a will, to designate what is to be done with a person's property, money, and personal possessions.
   4. provide a legal means for individuals to state those circumstances under which life-sustaining treatment should or should not be provided to them.
4. One of the major goals of hospice care is:
   1. freedom from pain and other symptoms.
   2. free care for all dying clients and their families.
   3. to cure the client using very aggressive medical treatment.
   4. to transfer all dying clients to the hospital when death is imminent.
5. A client is in the last stages of dying. The nurse assesses for the signs of impending death that include:
   1. flushed warm skin.
   2. very slow regular pulse rate.
   3. inability to hear.
   4. Cheyne-Stokes respirations.
6. Nursing care of a grieving client includes: (Select all that apply.)
   1. telling the grieving client that he will feel better soon.
   2. assuring the grieving client that feeling relief after a long illness is normal.
   3. exploring ways to fill his life with meaningful activities.
   4. encouraging him to feel his feelings to the fullest so that he can work through the feelings.
   5. leaving him alone so that he can work through the feelings on his own.
   6. explaining that each person works through grief in his own way and in his own timing.
7. A dying client tells God that he will become a pastor if he is healed. The nurse knows that the client is experiencing what stage of death and dying?
   1. Denial
   2. Anger
   3. Bargaining
   4. Depression
8. A client is in hospice care. To meet the physiological comfort needs of the client, the nurse: (Select all that apply.)
   1. accepts and believes the client's expressions of pain.
   2. cleans the skin and applies a moisture barrier after urination.
   3. reads scripture passages as requested by the client.
   4. provides soft lighting in the room.
   5. applies petroleum jelly to the lips.
   6. listens as the client shares his fears.
9. A terminally ill client is agitated and keeps stating, "I want to talk to my children, all of my children!" The nurse's best response is:
   1. "I know you are upset. Let me reposition you and make you more comfortable."
   2. "You seem agitated. Tell me the reason you want to speak with your children."
   3. "I know you want to talk with your family. Tell me how I can help you speak to your children."
   4. "It is late at night, and your children are in bed. Try to go to sleep."

10. A terminally ill client enters the hospital and the daughter presents the client's advanced directive papers and states she is the durable power of attorney. The client has not signed a do-not-resuscitate (DNR) form. The daughter leaves the hospital and the client codes. The nursing staff:
    1. starts resuscitation because there is no DNR order from a physician.
    2. does not start resuscitation because the client is terminal.
    3. does not start resuscitation but places a call to the daughter for her decision regarding resuscitation desires.
    4. starts resuscitation but then stops when no DNR order is found.

REFERENCES/SUGGESTED READINGS

American Nurses Association. (1996). Promotion of comfort and relief of pain in dying patients. In *Compendium of ANA position statements.* Washington, DC: Author.

American Nurses Association. (2008). Communique: The newsletter of the Center for Ethics and Human Rights 5(2). Retrieved October 10, 2008, from http://198.65.150.241/readroom/cmqfw97.htm

Andreas, L. (1998). Controlling pain: Keeping a dying patient comfortable. Nursing98, 28(1), 70.

Backer, B., Hannon, N., & Russell, N. (1994). *Death and dying: Understanding and care* (2nd ed.). Clifton Park, NY: Thomson Delmar Learning.

Barbus, A. (1975). The dying person's bill of rights. *American Journal of Nursing, 75*(1), 99.

Boon, T. (1998). Don't forget the hospice option. *RN, 61*(2), 30–33.

Boss, P. (2000). *Ambiguous loss: Learning to live with unresolved grief.* Cambridge, MA: Harvard University Press.

Bowlby, J. (1982). *Attachment and loss: Vol. 2. Separation anxiety and anger.* New York: Basic Books.

Bral, E. (1998). Caring for adults with chronic cancer pain. *American Journal of Nursing, 98*(4), 27–32.

Bulechek, G., Butcher, H., McCloskey, J., & Dochterman, J., eds. (2008). *Nursing Interventions Classification (NIC)* (5th ed.). St. Louis, MO: Mosby/Elsevier.

Caring Connections. (2008). Supporting a grieving caregiver. Retrieved from http://www.caringinfo.org/GrievingALoss/GriefSupport/SupportingAGrieving Caregiver.htm

Castillo, L., & Phoummarath, M. (2009). Culturally competent school counseling with Asian American adolescents. Retrieved April 14, 2009, from http://www.jsc.montana.edu/articles/v4n20.pdf

Cerrudo, J. (1998). Letting go of Abuelo. *American Journal of Nursing, 98*(8), 53.

Corless, I., Germino, B., & Pittman, M. (Eds.). (2006). *Dying, death, and bereavement: A challenge for living* (2nd ed.). New York: Springer Publishing.

Corr, C., Nabe, C., & Corr, D. (2000). *Death and dying, life and living* (3rd ed.). Belmont, CA: Wadsworth.

Dineen, K. (2002). Gift of presence. *Nursing2002, 32*(7), 76.

Durham, E., & Weiss, L. (1997). How patients die. *American Journal of Nursing, 97*(12), 41–46.

Edelman, C., & Mandle, C. (2002). *Health promotion throughout the lifespan* (5th ed.). St. Louis, MO: Mosby.

Egan, K., and Arnold, R. (2003). Grief and bereavement care. *American Journal of Nursing, 103*(9), 42–52.

Emanuel, L., Ferris, F., vonGunten, C., & Roenn, J. (2007). The last hours of living: Practical advice for clinicians. Retrieved April 22, 2008, from http://www.medscape.com/viewprogram/5808_pnt

Engle, G. L. (1961). Is grief a disease? *Psychosomatic Medicine, 23,* 18–22.

Estes, M. (2010). *Health assessment and physical examination* (4th ed.). Clifton Park, NY: Delmar Cengage Learning.

Ferrell, B. (1998a). End-of-life care. *Nursing98, 28*(9), 58.

Ferrell, B. (1998b). How can we improve care at the end of life? *Nursing Management, 29*(9), 41–43.

Ferrell, B., & Coyle, N. (2005). *Textbook of palliative nursing* (2nd ed.). New York: Oxford University Press.

Ferrell, B., Virani, R., Grant, M., Coyne, P., & Uman, G. (2000). End-of-life care: Nurses speak out. *Nursing2000, 30*(7), 54–57.

Forbes, V. (1998). The dying game. *American Journal of Nursing,* 98(9), 50.

Frisch, N., & Frisch, L. (2005). *Psychiatric mental health nursing* (3rd ed.). Clifton Park, NY: Delmar Cengage Learning.

Furman, J. (2000). Taking a holistic approach to the dying time. *Nursing2000, 30*(6), 46–49.

Furman, J. (2001). Living with dying: How to help family caregivers. *Nursing2001, 31*(4), 36–41.

Furman, J. (2002). What you should know about chronic grief. *Nursing2002, 32*(2), 56–57.

Harvey, J. (2001). Debunking myths about postmortem care. *Nursing2001, 31*(7), 44–45.

Haynor, P. (1998). Meeting the challenge of advance directives. *American Journal of Nursing, 98*(3), 27–32.

Hellwig, K. (2000). A family lesson in dying. *RN, 63*(12), 32–33.

Hooks, F., & Daly, B. (2000). Hastening death: Is a natural death always best? *American Journal of Nursing, 100*(5), 56–63.

Huizdos, D. (2000). The tie that binds: Hanging on by a shoelace. *American Journal of Nursing, 100*(7), 25.

Hull, E. (2008). *Palliative and end of life care.* Manuscript submitted for publication.

Kübler-Ross, E. (1989). *To live until we say good-bye.* Upper Saddle River, NJ: Prentice Hall Trade.

Kübler-Ross, E. (1995). *Death is of vital importance: On life, death, and life after death.* Barrytown, NY: Station Hill.

Kübler-Ross, E. (1997a). *On death and dying.* New York: Macmillan.

Kübler-Ross, E. (1997b). *Death, the final stage of growth.* Old Tappan, NJ: Simon & Schuster.

Kübler-Ross, E. (1997c). *Meaning of our suffering.* Barrytown, NY: Barrytown, Ltd.

Kübler-Ross, E. (1997d). *Questions and answers on death and dying.* New York: Macmillan.

Kübler-Ross, E., & Kessler, D. (2001). *Life lessons: Two experts on death and dying teach us about the mysteries of life and living.* Carmichael, CA: Touchstone Books.

Kübler-Ross, E., & Kessler, D. (2007). *On grief and grieving: Finding the meaning of grief through the five stages of loss.* New York: Scribner.

Kubler-Ross, E., & Myss, C. (2008). *On life after death.* Berkeley, CA: Celestial Arts.

Kubler-Ross, E., & Warshaw, M. (1992). *To live until we say good-bye.* New York: Simon & Schuster.

LaDuke, S. (2001). Terminal dyspnea and palliative care. *American Journal of Nursing,* 101(11), 26–31.

Lindemann, E. (1944). Symptomatology and management of acute grief. *American Journal of Psychiatry, 101*, 141–148.

Lynn, J., Schuster, J., & Kabcenell, A. (2000). *Improving care for the end of life: A sourcebook for health care managers and clinicians*. New York: Oxford University Press.

Mazanec, P., & Tyler M. (2003). Cultural considerations in end-of-life care. *American Journal of Nursing, 103*(3), 50–58.

McCaffery, M., & Pasero, C. (1999). *Pain: Clinical manual for nursing practice* (2nd ed.). St. Louis, MO: Mosby.

McClain, M., & Shaefer, S. (1996). Supporting families after sudden infant death. *Journal of Psychosocial Nursing and Mental Health Services, 34*(4), 30–34.

McGowan, D. (1998). The right to say goodbye. *RN, 61*(5), 84.

Moorhead, S., Johnson, M., Swanson, E., & Maas, M. (2007). *Nursing Outcomes Classification (NOC)* (4th ed.). St. Louis, MO: Mosby.

North American Nursing Diagnosis Association International. (2010). *NANDA-I nursing diagnoses: Definitions and classification 2009–2011*. Ames, IA: Wiley-Blackwell.

OrganDonor.Gov. (2008). The matching process—Waiting list. Retrieved October 16, 2008, from http://www.organdonor.gov/transplantation/matching_process.htm

Paice, J. (2002). Managing psychological conditions in palliative care. *American Journal of Nursing, 102*(11), 36–42.

Panke, J. (2002). Difficulties in managing pain at the end of life. *American Journal of Nursing, 102*(7), 26–34.

Pitorak, E. (2003). Care at the time of death: How nurses can make the last hours of life a richer, more comfortable experience. *American Journal of Nursing, 103*(7), 42–51.

Popernack, M. (2000). Are we overlooking a hidden source of organs? *Nursing2000, 30*(1), 44–47.

Powell, C. (1999). Near death: A nurse reflects. *RN, 62*(4), 43–44.

Pritchett, K., & Lucas, P. (1997a). Death and dying. In B. S. Johnson (Ed.), *Psychiatric–mental health nursing: Adaptation and growth* (4th ed., pp. 206–207). Philadelphia: Lippincott Williams & Wilkins.

Pritchett, K., & Lucas, P. (1997b). Grief and loss. In B. S. Johnson (Ed.), *Psychiatric–mental health nursing: Adaptation and growth* (4th ed., pp. 199–218). Philadelphia: Lippincott Williams & Wilkins.

Puopolo, A. (1999). Gaining confidence to talk about end-of-life care. *Nursing99, 29*(7), 49–51.

Reese, C. D. (1996). Please cry with me: Six ways to grieve. *Nursing96, 26*(8), 56.

Robert Wood Johnson Foundation. (2004). When patients cannot eat or drink. Retrieved October 8, 2008 from http://www.rwjf.org/common/templates/printallfriendly.jsp?id+2093&referer+http%3A//

Rodebaugh, L., Schwindt, R., & Valentine, F. (1999). How to handle grief with wisdom, *Nursing99, 29*(10), 52–53.

Scanlon, C. (2003). Ethical concerns in end-of-life care. *AJN, 103*(1), 48–55.

Simmons, S. (1999). Multicultural interview—Grief in the Chinese culture. Grief in a family context—HPER F460F560. Retrieved April 14, 2009, from http://www.indiana.edu/~famlygrf/culture/simmons.html

Slade, J., & Lovasik, D. (2002). Understanding brain death criteria. *Nursing2002, 32*(12), 68–69.

Smalkin, P. (2001). Facing a mother's death. *Nursing2001, 31*(7), 51.

Smith-Stoner, M., & Frost, A. (1998). Coping with grief and loss: Bringing your shadow self into the light. *Nursing98, 28*(2), 49–50.

Smith-Stoner, M., & Frost, A. (1999). How to build your "hope skills." *Nursing99, 29*(9), 49–51

Spicer, T. (2003). Coping with grief when a patient dies. *Nursing2003, 33*(3), 32hn6.

Taylor, M. (1995). Benefits of dehydration in terminally ill clients. *Geriatric Nursing, 16*(6), 271–272.

Thompson, G. (2002). Taking the measure of a father's grief. *Nursing2002, 32*(3), 46–47.

Truog, R. (2008). Consent for organ donation—Balancing conflicting ethical obligations. *New England Journal of Medicine, 358*(12), 1209–1211.

Tutka, M. A. (2001). Near-death experiences: Seeing the light. *Nursing2001, 31*(5), 62–64.

Ufema, J. (1995a). How to help dying clients feel "safe." *Nursing95, 25*(9), 59.

Ufema, J. (1995b). Insights on death and dying. *Nursing95, 25*(11,12), 19, 22–23.

Ufema, J. (1999). Reflections on death and dying. *Nursing99, 29*(6), 56–59.

Ufema, J. (2000a). Death and dying: Bedside vigils. *Nursing2000, 30*(7), 26.

Ufema, J. (2000b). Death and dying: Seeking closure. *Nursing2000, 30*(8), 28.

Ufema, J. (2000c). Death and dying: Setting goals, withholding nutrition, will to die. *Nursing2000, 30*(9), 66–67.

Ufema, J. (2002). Insights on death and dying. *Nursing2002, 32*(10), 28–30.

Vanderbeek, J. (2000). Till death do us part: A firsthand account of family presence. *American Journal of Nursing, 100*(2), 44.

Virani, R., & Sofer, D. (2003). Improving the quality of end-of-life care. *American Journal of Nursing, 103*(5), 52–60.

Webster, L., & Dove, M. (2007). Optimizing opioid treatment for breakthrough pain. Retrieved October 14, 2007, from http://www/medscape.com/viewprogram/7869_pnt

Wong, M. (1996). *The 1996 national directory of bereavement support groups and services*. Forest Hills, NY: ADM.

Wong, M. (2001). *Understanding your grieving heart after a loved one's death*. Forest Hills, NY: ADM.

Zerwekh, J. (2003). End-of-life hydration—Benefit or burden? *Nursing2003, 33*(2), 32hn1–32hn3.

RESOURCES

American Nurses Association Center for Ethics and Human Rights, http://www.nursingworld.org

Americans for Better Care of the Dying, http://www.abcd-caring.org

Association for Death Education and Counseling, http://www.adec.org

Compassion in Dying Federation, http://www.compassionindying.org

Hospice Foundation of America, http://www.hospicefoundation.org

Last Acts, http://www.lastacts.org

National Hospice and Palliative Care Organization, http://www.nhpco.org

Partnership for Caring: America's Voices for the Dying, http://www.partnershipforcaring.org

TransWeb, The Northern Brewery, http://www.transweb.org

United Network for Organ Sharing, http://www.unos.org

UNIT 5 Health Promotion

CHAPTER 14
Wellness Concepts

MAKING THE CONNECTION

Refer to the following chapters to increase your understanding of wellness concepts:

Basic Nursing
- ***Cultural Considerations***
- ***End-of-Life Care***

Adult Health Nursing
- ***Reproductive System***
- ***The Older Adult***

LEARNING OBJECTIVES

Upon completion of this chapter, you should be able to:

- Define key terms.
- Explain the importance of *Healthy People 2010*.
- Discuss the scope of prevention.
- Describe the benefits of using a genogram.
- Teach and follow the guidelines for healthy living.
- Make a teaching plan to promote and maintain wellness.

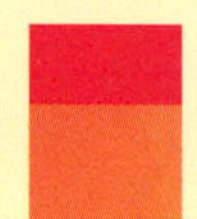

KEY TERMS

genogram
health
prevention
primary prevention
secondary prevention
tertiary prevention
wellness

INTRODUCTION

Individual adults have the responsibility for maintaining their own health, and parents are also responsible for maintaining their children's health and teaching them a healthy lifestyle. Health maintenance includes prevention of disease and early detection and treatment of disease, requiring constant effort focusing on all aspects of a person's life.

In 1896, Dr. Wood Hutchinson wrote in the *Journal of the American Medical Association* that "our system's philosophy might be condensed in the motto 'millions for health care and not a penny for prevention.'" More than 100 years have passed, and still less than 3 cents of each health dollar is spent on prevention and education.

The United States is 31st among nations in life expectancy yet is the world leader in medical science and education (CNN, 2008a). In 2008, the United States reportedly spent more than $2,500 per person per year for health care (CNN, 2008b). In 2005, the average spent on prescription drugs was $1,141 per person (CNN, 2008b). In 1960, the United States ranked 12th in infant mortality, and in 2004, the ranking dropped to 29th (*Harris*, 2008). Yet the United States spends more for health care than any other country. One of the major reasons for these statistics is that many doctors need to move preventive medicine from the sidelines to the forefront of their practice (CNN, 2008b; Cohen, Davis, & Mikkelsen, 2000). The focus is treating the disease rather than preventing the disease.

There is no profit in prevention. Insurance pays for diagnosis and treatment of illnesses, not health maintenance, but often will not pay for preventive testing and treatment. Paying for clinical care makes illness the priority, not wellness.

HEALTH

The generally accepted definition of **health** from the World Health Organization (WHO) defines health as a state of complete physical, mental, and social well-being, not merely the absence of disease or infirmity.

Another concept of health focuses on motivation. The individual is motivated by joy and self-fulfillment and believes that health is the realization of potential, and illness is an obstacle in that realization.

Those who have an adaptive view of health are motivated by altering the risks in self or the environment through diet and exercise or by reducing exposure to environmental hazards. When the individual is unable to cope with the stresses and risks of daily life, illness results.

Some individuals are motivated by being able to meet responsibilities at home, at work, at play, and in the community: Their health focus is role performance. Health is considered achieved when the individual fulfills the responsibilities and obligations to family, job, and community.

Other individuals are motivated by the absence of disease: Theirs is a clinical health focus. As long as no disease is present, the individual considers himself healthy. A person's definition of health influences personal health decisions and life choices.

WELLNESS

Wellness is defined as a state of optimal health wherein an individual maximizes human potential, moves toward integration of human functioning, has greater self-awareness and self-satisfaction, and takes responsibility for health. Floyd, Mimms, and Yelding-Howard (1995), Hoeger, Turner, and Hafen (2001), and Seiger, Kanipe, Vanderpool, and Barnes (2000) describe the behaviors exhibited by individuals in a state of wellness. These researchers outline seven areas of wellness: emotional, mental, intellectual, vocational, social, spiritual, and physical wellness. Various areas of wellness overlap and none is mutually exclusive.

Emotional Wellness

Emotions bridge the gap between body and mind. The individual who is emotionally well understands his own feelings and knows when to express them appropriately. This person accepts limitations, copes with stress in healthy ways, has the ability to adjust to change, is optimistic and happy, enjoys life, and shows respect and affection to others.

Mental Wellness

The person who is mentally well is alert, curious, clear thinking, open-minded, creative, logical, and accepting of others. This person also has a good memory, common sense, and a desire for continual learning.

Intellectual Wellness

Intellectual wellness is revealed by an ability to think, process information, and solve problems. The intellectually well person questions and evaluates information and situations; is creative, flexible, and open to new ideas; and learns from life experiences.

Vocational Wellness

The individual who is satisfied in school and/or job and who works in harmony with others enjoys vocational wellness (Figure 14-1).

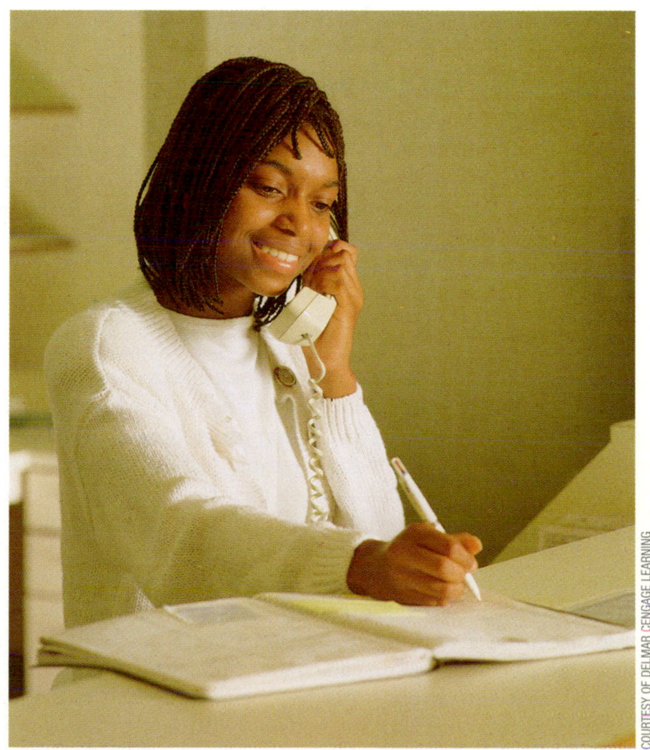

COURTESY OF DELMAR CENGAGE LEARNING

FIGURE 14-1 Vocational wellness means being content and satisfied with your occupation.

CLIENT TEACHING

Suppressed Anger in Women

Research has shown that women who suppress anger and who have hostile attitudes may be at greater risk for developing cardiovascular disease and physical problems (Meyers, 2008). Nurses can help such women minimize this risk by encouraging them to learn to express negative feelings constructively, to talk calmly about their feelings, to find other women who may share some of the same concerns and stressors, and to engage in regular exercise routines to relieve stress and tension. Encourage the person to change her perception of the situation to lessen the impact on her thoughts and feelings. Learning and using assertive communication allows the person to express her feelings and increase control of the situation. Maintaining positive relationships provides upbeat input into one's life.

Social Wellness

The person who shows affection, fairness, concern, and respect for others; communicates effectively; has satisfying relationships; and interacts well with others enjoys social wellness. This person has a network of friends and family, is a member of various organizations, and enjoys working together. Other behaviors exhibited are confidence, loyalty, honesty, and tolerance.

Spiritual Wellness

Spiritual wellness gives direction, meaning, and purpose to life through values, morals, and ethics. The spiritually healthy person has optimism, faith, and high self-esteem.

Physical Wellness

Physical wellness is seen in individuals who exercise regularly, eat a well-balanced diet, and have regular physical examinations. They avoid risky sexual behavior, try to limit exposure to environmental contaminants, and restrict the intake of alcohol, tobacco, caffeine, and drugs (Figure 14-2).

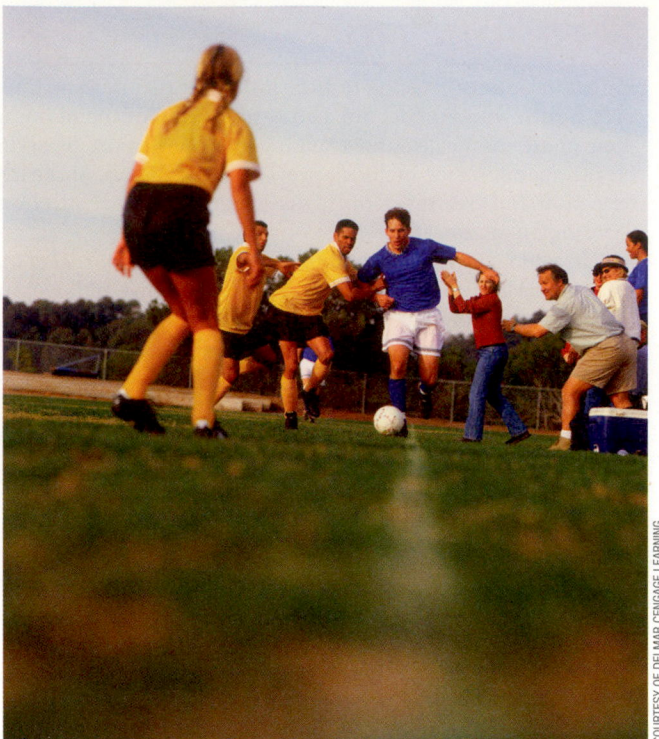

COURTESY OF DELMAR CENGAGE LEARNING

FIGURE 14-2 A person maintains physical wellness by exercising, eating a well-balanced diet, having a regular physical exam, and avoiding at risk behaviors.

HEALTH PROMOTION

Health promotion is more than preventing illness: It means assisting individuals to better health, functioning, and well-being and to maximize their potential. Health promotion focuses on choosing healthy behaviors rather than on escaping illness. The goal is for individuals to control and improve their health. Health promotion is appropriate for the individual and the entire population.

The concept of self-responsibility is important to health promotion. No one else can make a person live a healthy life; self-responsibility is the only way to make changes. An individual can be given information relating to health and wellness, but only that person can change unhealthy or destructive habits. With the exception of small children, each individual must take responsibility for behaviors leading to health and wellness (Figure 14-3). Objectives for healthy living are outlined in the *Healthy People 2000* and *Healthy People 2010* documents issued by the federal government.

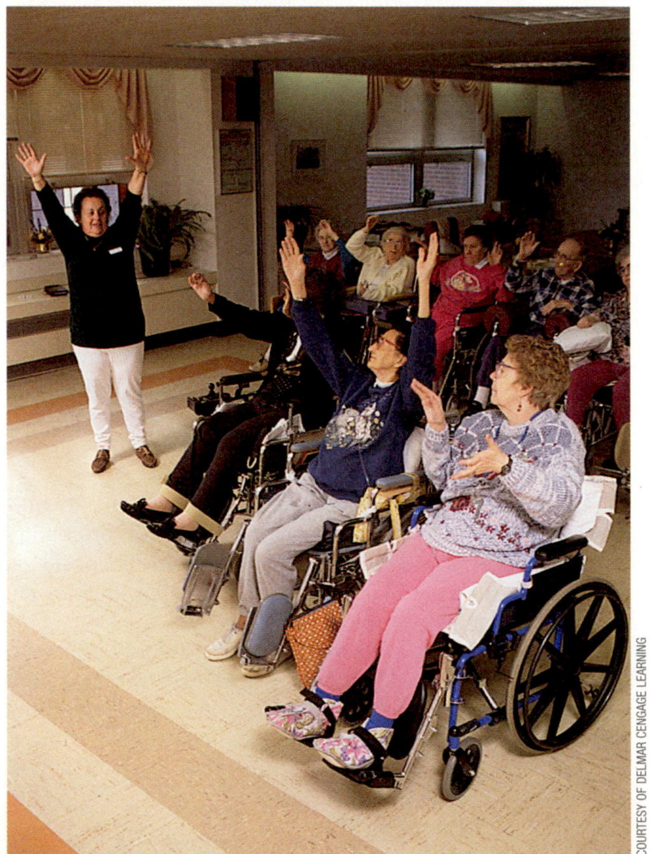

COURTESY OF DELMAR CENGAGE LEARNING

FIGURE 14-3 Individuals must learn to achieve physical wellness in a manner that accommodates their lifestyles and physical abilities.

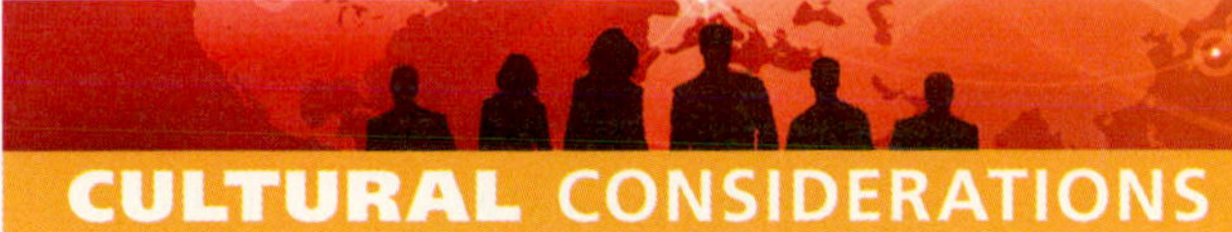

CULTURAL CONSIDERATIONS

Spiritual Well-Being

According to a study by Hall (2006), weekly attendance at religious services add 2 to 3 additional years of life. Stibich (2007) suggests increased social contacts, prayer, and spiritual reflection as possible reasons for longevity. This underscores the importance of religion and spiritual wellness to an individual's overall state of health.

HEALTHY PEOPLE 2000

In 1980 and again in 1990, the U.S. Department of Health and Human Services (DHHS) released a list of objectives for disease prevention and health promotion in 22 priority areas (DHHS, 1990). More than 10,000 individuals representing 300 national organizations met in 1990 to develop the health objectives for the year 2000. More than 300 health objectives were drafted for the nation to achieve by the year 2000. These objectives were published in a document titled *Healthy People 2000: National Health Promotion and Disease Prevention Objectives*, which addresses three important issues:

- *Personal responsibility:* Each individual must be health conscious and must practice informed, responsible, health behaviors (Figure 14-4).
- *Health benefits for all people:* Everyone must have health benefits for the nation to be healthy.
- *Health promotion and disease prevention:* Health care must change from a treatment focus to a prevention focus to increase the quality of life and to cut costs.

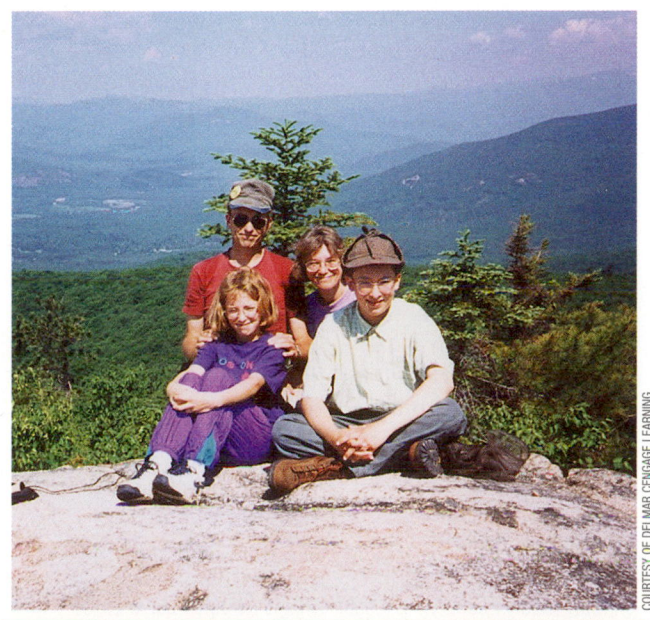

FIGURE 14-4 **Families can engage in activities together to achieve wellness.**

LIFE SPAN CONSIDERATIONS

Older Adults and Exercise

Health promotion activities in the older client have been shown to contribute to improving the quality if not the quantity of life (Resnick, 2001). Maintaining some type of physical activity benefits the musculoskeletal, cardiac, and respiratory systems for the older adult (Carethers, 1992). Other benefits include decreased bone loss, improved glucose tolerance, improved lipid profile, decreased body fat, and increased self-esteem and cognitive status (Carethers, 1992).

The Agency for Healthcare Research and Quality (AHRQ) suggests that older people can benefit the most from regular physical exercise because they are more at risk of the health problems that exercise prevents (Marshall & Altpeter, 2005). Physical activity improves muscle strength, flexibility, gait, and balance. These positive effects decrease the risk of falls for the older client. More than one-third of adults over the age of 65 fall each year in the United States, and falls are the leading cause of injury and injury-related deaths in the older population (Centers for Disease Control and Prevention, 2006).

The extent of exercise prescribed for the elderly client is dependent on the client's health status. The client with several risk factors for cardiovascular disease or with diagnosed cardiac disease will need to be evaluated by a physician before initiating an exercise program (Resnick, 2001). The level of fitness necessary to produce health benefits in the elderly can be attained through low-intensity activities, including walking, cycling, and swimming (Carethers, 1992). Elderly with functional disabilities can also receive benefits from physical activity, such as range-of-motion exercises, wheelchair push-ups, and isotonic exercises (Carethers, 1992). These activities will prevent joint contractures and muscle atrophy.

There are many exercise programs and gyms that offer programs geared to the exercise needs of the older client. These programs usually combine weight training with aerobic exercise. Encouraging older clients to participate in an exercise program will provide them with a variety of physical and psychosocial benefits and may contribute to an increased quality of life (Smith, in press).

The overall goals included:

- Increasing the span of healthy life for Americans
- Reducing health disparities among Americans
- Achieving access to preventive services for all Americans

PROFESSIONALTIP

Predictors of Healthy Aging

The most consistent predictors of healthy aging are low serum glucose, normal blood pressure, avoidance of smoking, and maintenance of target weight for height (Reed, 1998). To prevent disease in later years, young adults and even adolescents must keep these four factors in check. It is never too late to modify these four factors to improve health.

HEALTHY PEOPLE 2010

Healthy People 2010 is a document developed by the federal government to serve as a "road map" for improving the health of American citizens for the first decade of the 21st century. It is the third such document developed by the DHHS. The underlying premise of *Healthy People 2010* is that the health of the individual is almost inseparable from the health of the larger community (Hunt, 2008). Health care providers in all settings are using this document to guide them in developing programs of care. The DHHS is currently creating *Healthy People 2020,* a document that will address the major health issues of the next decade. They expect to have the framework of the document completed by early 2009 and to have the objectives completed by January 2010. Updates on the progress of the document and ways to provide input to the document can be accessed through the *Healthy People 2010* Web site at http://www.healthypeople.gov.

Overview and General Goals

Healthy People 2010 has two broad goals that it hopes to achieve: to increase the quality and years of healthy life and to eliminate health disparities. The 467-page document was developed with input from a national consortium of health care professionals, citizens, and private and public government agencies (Hunt, 2008). It contains demographic, statistical, and disease-related information that describes current health trends in the country. It is divided into four areas: (a) promoting healthy behaviors, (b) promoting healthy and safe communities, (c) improving systems for personal and public health, and (d) preventing and reducing diseases and disorders (Potter & Perry, 2009).

Healthy People 2010 identifies 10 leading health indicators (LHIs) that are major health issues for the nation. These LHIs include physical activity, overweight and obesity, tobacco use, substance abuse, responsible sexual behavior, mental health, injury and violence, environmental quality, immunization, and access to health care. The document states that improving health behaviors in these areas will move the nation toward an increased level of wellness and achievement of the document's broad goals.

Focus Areas and Specific Goals

Healthy People 2010 identifies 28 focus areas that the country should target to improve its health status. Box 14-1 lists these focus areas. Each focus area has specific goals related to that topic area. For example, two goals related to the focus area of diabetes include:

Goal 5-1: Increase the proportion of persons with diabetes who receive formal diabetes education.

Goal 5-5: Reduce the diabetes death rate.

Most focus areas have at least 15 stated goals, and most goals are statistically measurable. Current statistical information related to each goal is included in the document so that change toward achievement of the goal can be measured (Smith, 2008).

ILLNESS PREVENTION

Prevention (obstructing, thwarting, or hindering a disease or illness) incorporates both new and old ideas. The dietary laws, taboos, and traditions of various ethnic, cultural, and religious groups were begun for a reason. There is no reason not to practice the old ways if scientific research has not proven them incorrect or harmful. New methods of illness prevention emerge as technology expands and health awareness increases.

Preventive health should be practiced in all stages of life, beginning before conception with healthy parents and

Box 14-1 *HEALTHY PEOPLE 2010* FOCUS AREAS

1. Access to quality health services
2. Arthritis, osteoporosis, and chronic back conditions
3. Cancer
4. Chronic kidney disease
5. Diabetes
6. Disability and secondary conditions
7. Education and community-based programs
8. Environmental health
9. Family planning
10. Food safety
11. Health communication
12. Heart disease and stroke
13. Human immunodeficiency virus (HIV)
14. Immunization and infectious disease
15. Injury and violence prevention
16. Maternal, infant, and child health
17. Medical product safety
18. Mental health
19. Nutrition and obesity
20. Occupational safety and health
21. Oral health
22. Physical activity and fitness
23. Public health infrastructure
24. Respiratory diseases
25. Sexually transmitted diseases
26. Substance abuse
27. Tobacco use
28. Vision and hearing

From Healthy People 2010 (2005). What Is Healthy People 2010? Retrieved April 21, 2009, from http://www.healthypeople.gov/About/hpfact.htm

continuing through prenatal care and the life span. Interventions for disease prevention range from lifestyle changes that cost little or nothing to high-tech procedures that are very expensive.

Major changes are needed in health care delivery, funding, and insurance coverage before the full impact of illness prevention can be discovered. The health care system must insist on more research relating to prevention and must then apply the results of the research to insurance practices. Prevention practices must be supported and funded by the health care system in order for a change from illness treatment to illness prevention to occur. Enhanced health, longer life expectancy, and a population that functions better, feels better, and looks better will be the rewards of such a shift.

Types of Prevention

There are three types of prevention: primary, secondary, and tertiary. Primary prevention has not historically been supported by our health care system, whereas secondary and tertiary prevention have been and still are the main focus. They are also the most expensive.

Primary Prevention

Primary prevention includes all practices designed to keep health problems from developing. Primary prevention includes following recommended childhood immunization schedules, eating calcium-rich foods to prevent osteoporosis, and not smoking to prevent lung cancer. Every individual and health care provider should focus on primary prevention. It is usually the least expensive intervention and provides the greatest benefits.

Secondary Prevention

Secondary prevention includes activities related to early identification and treatment of disease processes. At this level of prevention, when taking the client's history, the nurse would focus on identification of family history, risk factors, and signs and symptoms of possible disease in the client. The client would also be screened for a variety of conditions as appropriate for age and evidence of risk. For example, all adults are screened for hypertension on every physician visit, and school-age children are screened for hearing and vision problems. The American Cancer Society has determined the age and frequency that certain cancer screenings should occur in adults. It is recommended that women over the age of 40 have a baseline mammography and then have a clinical breast examination and mammography yearly thereafter. If it was determined that the client has a strong family history of breast cancer, these screening recommendations may be increased to detect a problem at an earlier age. Secondary preventive activities often result in early detection of disease and the ability to obtain a quick and effective resolution of the illness (Smith, in press).

Tertiary Prevention

Tertiary prevention focuses on maximizing recovery after an illness or injury and preventing long-term complications. Rehabilitative and educational activities are common at this level of prevention. The client who has experienced a stroke usually undergoes intensive physical rehabilitation to promote independence with activities of daily living. They may learn how to utilize adaptive equipment, such as a quad cane or splint to improve mobility. They may also benefit from a stroke support group to help cope with the psychosocial issues they are facing as a result of their current illness (Smith, in press).

Prevention Health Care Team

The individual assisted by nurses, the nurse practitioner, and the primary physician make up the prevention health care team.

Individual

The center of the prevention health care team is the individual. The individual must combine the knowledge of preventive health care with behavioral changes necessary to live a healthier life.

Individuals should decide those things that they want and expect from health care. Clients must be honest with self, the nurses, and physician; be assertive and ask questions of the physicians and nurses; and be active, informed health care consumers. Ultimately, responsibility for health care rests with the individual.

Nurses

Nurses, especially nurse practitioners, often do the initial health screening in clinics and physicians' offices. This provides a great opportunity to inquire about the preventive health habits and

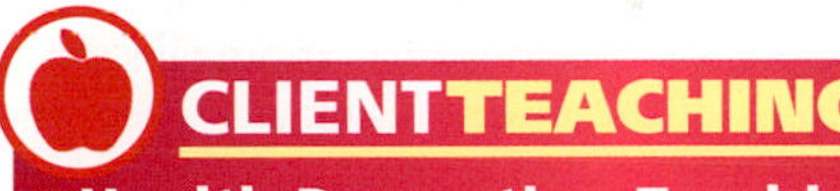

Health Promotion Teaching

- Infancy: Teach parents about healthy lifestyle during prenatal period, infant feeding, basic infant care, and infant safety.
- Childhood: Teach parents about immunizations, nutrition, growth and development, building self-esteem in children, and childhood safety.
- Adolescence: Teach parents and adolescents about sexual health; avoidance of drug, alcohol, and tobacco use; motor vehicle safety and other adolescent safety issues; support of mental health; and prevention of suicide.
- Adulthood: Teach adults about nutrition, physical activity, stress management, sexual health, avoidance of tobacco and substance abuse, recommended cancer screenings, and risk factor reduction for heart disease, stroke, and cancer.
- Older Adults: Teach older adults about changing nutritional requirements, exercise, stress management, safety issues related to mobility and sensory changes, promotion of independence and self-esteem, and prevention of suicide.

From Nettina, S. (2001) *The Lippincott Manual of Nursing Practice*. Philadelphia: Lippincott.

lifestyle of the client. Nurses can use their excellent listening skills to give clients time to discuss health care habits and ask questions. Nurses are also great teachers of preventive health habits and health promotion activities.

Primary Physicians

Primary physicians usually are family practitioners, internists, or pediatricians. These are the family doctors seen on a regular basis. They have the opportunity and obligation to discuss and inquire about preventive health habits. They refer clients to specialists for specific problems when necessary. When the problem is resolved, the client returns to the primary physician for further care.

FACTORS AFFECTING HEALTH

The many factors affecting health can be categorized into four broad topics:

- Genetics and human biology
- Environmental influences
- Personal behavior
- Health care

Genetics and Human Biology

Inherited traits and the way the human body functions have an impact on an individual's state of health and wellness. An individual's genetic makeup may include inherited disorders, such as sickle-cell anemia, or chromosomal anomalies, such as Down syndrome. Both of these may ultimately affect the individual's quality of life and level of health.

Human biology affects health because normal body functioning prevents some illnesses and makes us more susceptible to others.

Environmental Influences

Environmental factors that may influence health are numerous, can be natural or man-made, and vary depending on geographic location and living conditions. Exposure to or ingestion of certain natural biological irritants can cause disease, such as results from exposure to poison ivy, and even death, such as results from ingestion of poisonous mushrooms. Exposure to chemicals such as asbestos in older buildings, lead paint in older houses, and mercury in polluted water sources also are health hazards. Radiation from the sun and some types of machinery can be harmful; extreme, prolonged exposure to solar radiation can even result in death. Natural disasters, such as hurricanes, floods, volcanic eruptions, droughts, heat waves, blizzards, and other extreme weather conditions, pose health risks, as do man-made environmental crises, including wars, bombings, pollution, and overpopulation.

Personal Behavior

Personal behavior is the area with the most factors affecting health and wellness, and they are controlled entirely by the individual. It is the individual's decision to use or not to use these factors to promote health and wellness. Factors typically deemed to be under the individual's control include diet, exercise, personal care, sexual relationships, level of stress, tobacco and drug use, alcohol use, and safety.

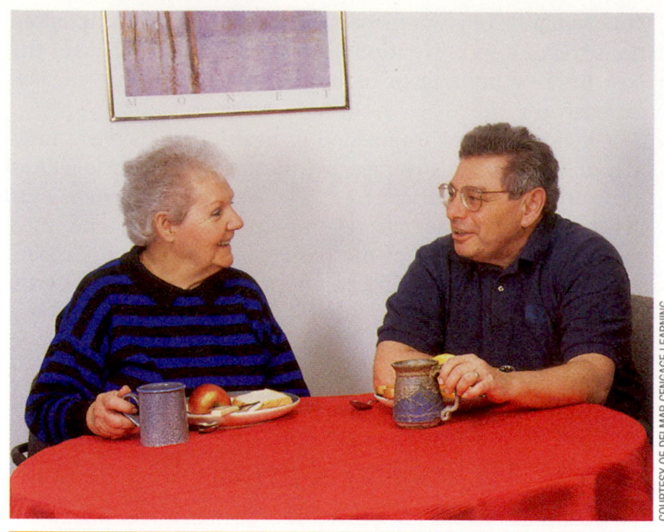

COURTESY OF DELMAR CENGAGE LEARNING

FIGURE 14-5 Sharing meals together is a wonderful means of meeting both physical and interpersonal needs.

Diet

Healthy eating habits and a proper diet greatly enhance an individual's overall state of health and well-being. Eating both fulfills the basic biological needs of sustenance, nutrition, and hydration and allows individuals to meet social and interpersonal needs (Figure 14-5). All of these factors contribute to overall wellness.

Exercise

Integrating physical activity into daily life is one of the best ways of promoting health. Exercise improves muscle strength, circulation, and emotional well-being; increases endurance; lowers blood pressure; and reduces the chances of heart attack, osteoporosis, and stroke. The individual who exercises regularly feels better and looks healthier.

Health clubs are used by many people in an effort to meet their need for exercise. Health clubs are a wonderful place for regular exercise but also can be a source of disease. For example, perspiration on exercise machines is a prime source of impetigo. Clients should be made aware of such dangers so that they can practice safety precautions, such as wearing thigh-length shorts and always keeping a towel between the body and the exercise equipment.

Personal Care

The skin works with the immune system to defend the body against harmful allergens, bacteria, fungi, and viruses by protecting the body from outside elements. Regular skin, hair, and nail care will enhance wellness and foster self-esteem. Personal care also includes such wellness habits as proper posture, proper body mechanics, adequate sleep, and dental hygiene.

Sexual Relationships

Establishing intimacy and a sexual relationship with another person is a natural step in growth and development. To maintain health and wellness, the individual will use values, ethics, and morals to guide the development of the relationship. A healthy sexual relationship is based on mutual satisfaction of the parties, a consensual approach to pleasurable activities, and mutual respect for preferences and personal choices.

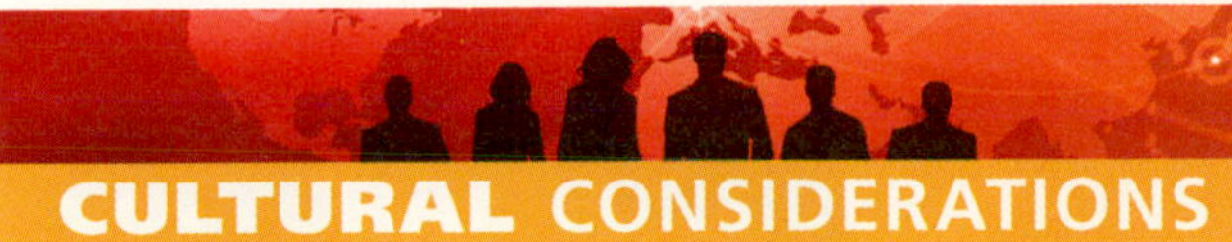

CULTURAL CONSIDERATIONS

Parents' Beliefs about Feeding Children

Many parents:

- Believe that milk alone will not satisfy their babies' hunger, so they begin feeding cereal and other solid foods earlier than recommended.
- Use food to console children.
- Believe that a plump child is a healthier child.
- View a heavy infant or toddler as evidence of parental competence (Baughcum, 1998).

Nurses can work with these clients by respecting their cultural beliefs while enforcing the notion that a healthy child is a child who is satisfied following a meal and who shows a healthy, normal physical and emotional growth pattern. These factors, not plumpness, are indicators of wellness.

One role of the nurse is to educate the client on ways to prevent sexually transmitted infections.

Level of Stress

Not all stress is harmful. Limited stress raises one's energy level and makes one more alert. The way one responds to or copes with stressors dictates whether the situation is healthy or harmful. For instance, one individual may enjoy the challenge of balancing work and family, while another may feel torn by these seemingly conflicting demands and will experience undue stress. Stress results not from an individual's life situation but from that individual's reaction to and perception of the life situation.

Tobacco and Drug Use

Refraining from tobacco use is a strong step toward health promotion and maintenance. Even when a longtime smoker gives up the habit, the health risks begin to decrease at once, although it will take 10 to 15 years to eliminate all the effects of smoking from the lungs. The person who smokes exhales secondhand smoke, which presents a health risk to those who do not smoke. According to the Office of the Surgeon General (2007), exposure to secondhand smoke at home or work increased one's risk of developing heart disease by 25% to 30% and lung cancer by 20% to 30%.

Abuse of both illegal and prescription drugs is a serious medical and social problem in our society. Drugs prescribed by a physician are abused if they are not taken as directed or if they are taken by anyone other than the client for whom they were prescribed. If not taken as directed, many prescribed drugs can be addictive. Health can be maintained when clients understand the effects, indications, side effects, and interactions of the prescription medications they are taking.

Alcohol Use

The decision to consume alcohol is a personal choice that can influence an individual's state of health. The amount of alcohol consumed will affect sobriety, decision-making ability, and, in many instances, safety. The use of alcohol can play a prominent role in drownings, suicides, traffic fatalities, adult fire deaths, and falling fatalities.

CLIENT TEACHING

Dietary Guidelines for Americans

- Consume a sufficient amount of fruits and vegetables while staying within energy needs. Two cups of fruit and 2½ cups of vegetables per day are recommended for persons consuming a 2,000-calorie intake.
- Choose a variety of fruits and vegetables each day. In particular, select from all five vegetable subgroups (dark green, orange, legumes, starchy vegetables, and other vegetables) several times a week.
- Consume three or more ounce equivalents of whole-grain products per day, with the rest of the recommended grains coming from enriched or whole-grain products. In general, at least half the grains should come from whole grains.
- Consume 3 cups per day of fat-free or low-fat milk or equivalent milk products.
- Include lean meats, poultry, fish, beans, eggs and nuts in your diet.
- Limit saturated fats, trans fats, cholesterol, sodium and added sugars.

From Office of Disease Prevention and Health Promotion. (2006). *Dietary Guidelines for Americans 2005.* Retrieved December 2, 2006, from http://www.odphp.osophs.dhhs.gov

Safety

Personal choices concerning safety affect many areas of an individual's life and can be viewed collectively more as a lifestyle

CLIENT TEACHING

Preventing Food-Borne Diseases

Share the following tips with clients to educate them in ways to prevent food-borne diseases:

- Allow cooked foods to sit at room temperature for no more than 2 hours.
- Date leftovers, refrigerate, and eat within 2 to 3 days.
- Wash dirty dishes in hot (120°F) water, as dirty dishes are an ideal place for bacteria to multiply.
- Keep dishcloths and sponges clean and allow to dry between uses.
- Use a bleach solution to clean cutting boards and countertops.
- Wash all fruits and vegetables in a diluted bleach solution (a bleach to water ratio of 1:100).

PROFESSIONALTIP

Moderate Exercise Reduces Stroke Risk

- Individuals who burn 1,000 to 1,999 calories per week by exercising moderately have a 24% lower risk of suffering a stroke than do those who burn less.
- Individuals who burn 2,000 to 2,999 calories per week by exercising moderately have a 46% lower risk.
- Burning over 2,999 calories a week through moderate exercise lowered the risk of having a stroke by only 20%.
- Moderate exercise includes activities such as brisk walking, dancing, and cycling (Krarup et al., 2008; Lee & Paffenbarger, 1998).

choice than individually as separate acts to promote safety. For example, individuals who embrace safety as a fundamental element of health and well-being will ensure safety in their homes by having smoke detectors, fire extinguishers, carbon monoxide detectors, practiced escape plans, locked medicine cabinets, and gates blocking dangerous stairways. These individuals will also most likely buckle their car seat belts, secure their children in child car seats, and obey speed limits when driving. All these elements of safety support a healthy lifestyle.

Health Care

Most people use the health care system to treat their illness or condition. However, health promotion and disease prevention are a more effective use of the health care system. Routine physical examinations with minimal testing are beneficial for preventing disease and maintaining health (Figure 14-6). Healthy adults should consider health care services based on family health history, personal habits, or personal health history. The presence of symptoms will alter the time frame for suggested health care services.

Physical Exam

The physical examination begins with a review of family health history, personal health history, personal habits (sexual practices, tobacco, alcohol, and drug use), and concerns or questions the client may have. The client should write down questions and concerns before visiting the physician so that none will be forgotten. Between the ages of 20 and 39 years, individuals should have a complete physical exam every 1 to 3 years; those 40 to 49 years of age, every 1 to 2 years; and those older than 50 years of age, every year.

Immunizations

Adults who did not have the recommended immunizations as children should discuss this with their primary physicians. The physician may recommend having the immunizations as an adult based on the client's risk factors.

Every adult should have a tetanus booster every 10 years for life. Health care workers and college students; those with

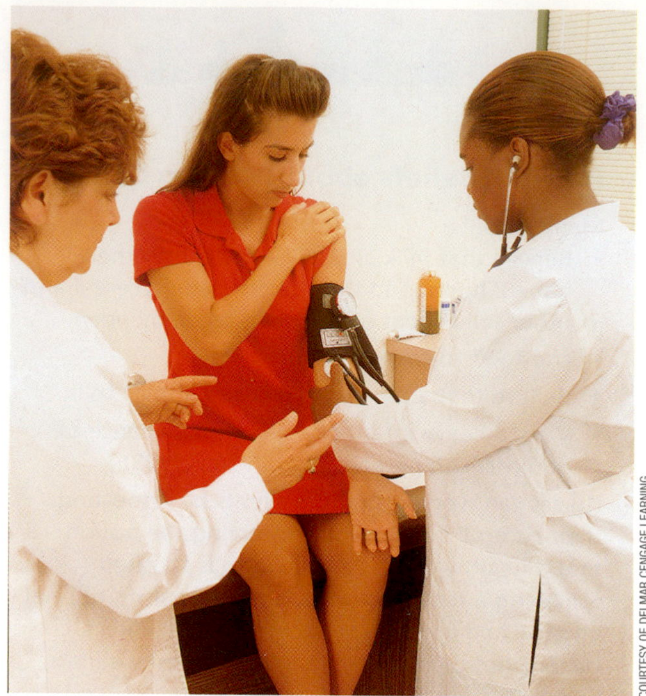
COURTESY OF DELMAR CENGAGE LEARNING

FIGURE 14-6 **Routine physical examinations are essential to maintaining health and preventing disease.**

high risk of exposure; those with chronic heart, pulmonary, or kidney disease; those with diabetes; and those 65 years of age and older should have an influenza immunization every year and a pneumococcal pneumonia immunization every 6 years.

Tests

The following tests should be done with every physical exam: complete blood count, blood sugar, cholesterol, urinalysis, stool for blood, and, for women, a Papanicolau (Pap) smear. An electrocardiogram (EKG or ECG) should be done at ages 20 and 40 and every 5 years thereafter (yearly if the client is at high risk). Women should have a breast exam with every physical exam and a baseline mammogram (Figure 14-7) at age 40 and yearly thereafter. Men should have a testicular exam and a rectal exam to check the prostate with every physical exam after age 40. A breast self-exam should be done by every woman after each menstrual period. A testicular self-exam should be done monthly by every male.

PROFESSIONALTIP

Mammograms

The Centers for Disease Control and Prevention (2005) reports that in 2002, 68.4% of women, age 40 and older, at less than $15,000 annual income, had a mammogram, as did 75.3% with annual incomes of $15,000 to $34,999 and 82.5% with annual incomes of $50,000 or more. Women with less than a high school education, never being married, and with no health insurance had fewer mammograms than those who were college graduates, married, and had health insurance.

PROFESSIONALTIP

Hepatitis B Vaccine

Health care personnel who may be exposed to blood and body fluids are at risk for contracting the hepatitis B virus. Health care employers are required by law to offer the hepatitis B vaccination without cost to employees who are in direct care positions. Employees have the option of having or refusing this immunization. The vaccine is not contraindicated during pregnancy, and there are no apparent adverse effects to developing fetuses; however, the vaccine may cause shock in individuals who are allergic to baker's yeast.

Dental Exam

Throughout life, a dental exam, prophylaxis, and needed treatment should be performed every 6 to 12 months.

Eye Exam

An eye exam, including tonometry for glaucoma, should be performed every 2 to 3 years from ages 40 to 49 years and every 1 to 2 years after the age of 50.

MAKING A GENOGRAM

A **genogram** is a way to visualize family members, their birth and death dates or ages, and specific health problems. At least four generations should be included: the individual, the parents, the grandparents, and the children. Then it is easy to follow health problems through the generations. Health problems that may be encountered can be identified and steps taken to prevent them. Figure 14-8 shows a sample genogram.

GUIDELINES FOR HEALTHY LIVING

Because of their education and training, nurses are in a unique position to practice healthy living habits themselves and to promote such habits in their clients. Table 14-1 identifies the top 9 causes of death and the controllable factors that most contribute to these types of deaths. While it is important to remember that certain health variables such as gender and race cannot be controlled or changed, others, such as diet and tobacco use, result from individual choice. These lifestyle choices are based on individual preference, and nurses can help clients make the

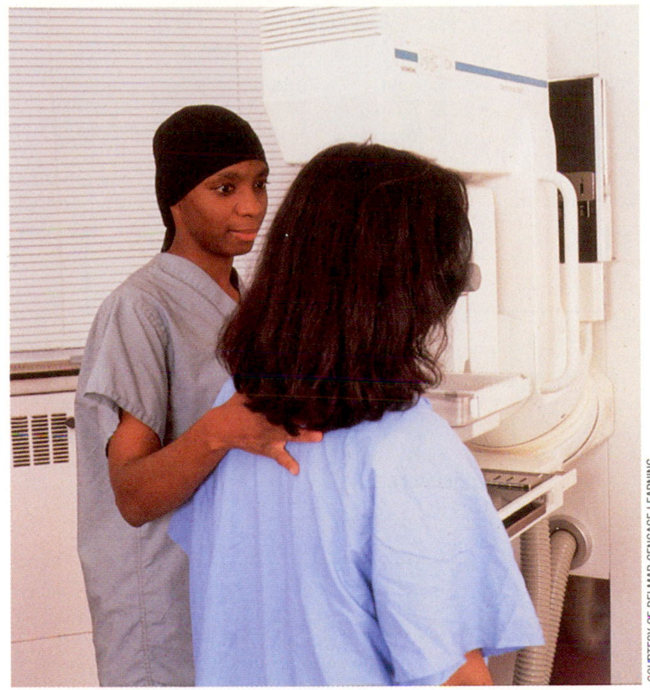

FIGURE 14-7 Mammograms are a key element to wellness promotion for all women older than 40 years of age.

CRITICAL THINKING

Wellness

How can you assist clients to assess their state of wellness?

What preventive health care should be received by a person 20 years old, 42 years old, and 65 years old?

How does the nurse's state of wellness affect client care?

CLIENTTEACHING

Crucial Health Practices

Simon (1992) states that all the medical progress in the United States from 1900 to 1990 increased the life span of an average adult by 4 years but that simple lifestyle changes increased the life span of an average adult by 11 years. His 10 crucial health practices are still applicable today:

- Use no tobacco or drugs.
- Consume no more than 2 ounces of alcohol per day.
- Eat a diet low in fat, cholesterol, and salt but high in fiber, fruits, vegetables, and fish.
- Exercise regularly—1 hour each week is helpful, 3 is ideal.
- Stay lean.
- Drive cars with air bags and wear seat belts; drive prudently, and never drink before driving.
- Avoid excessive stress.
- Minimize exposure to radiation, ultraviolet rays, chemical pollutants, and other environmental hazards.
- Protect self from sexually transmitted diseases.
- Obtain regular medical care including immunizations and screening tests.

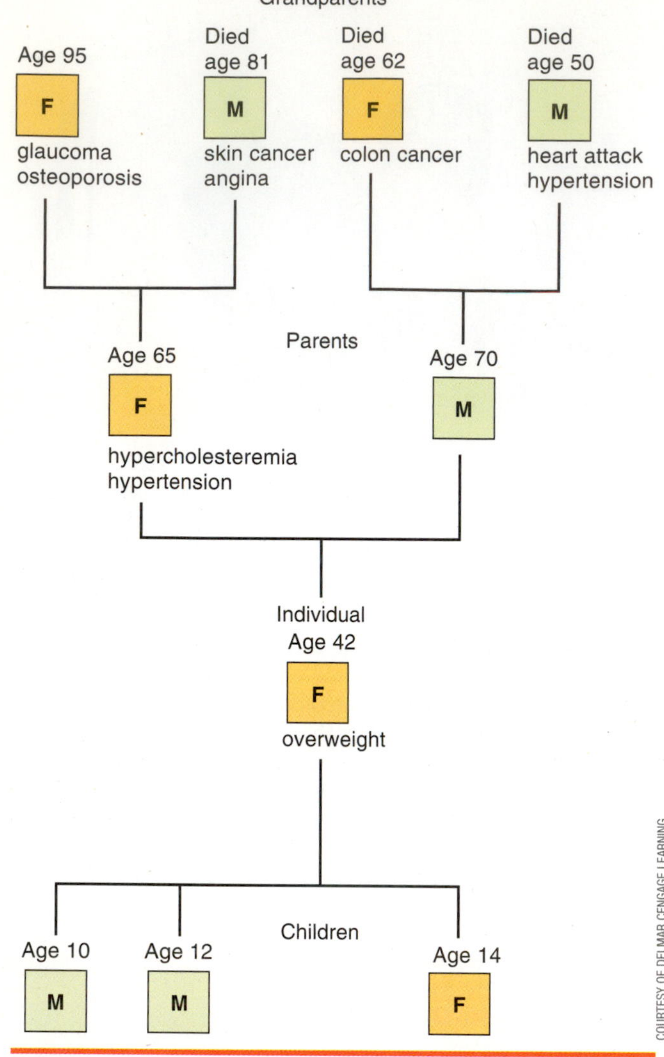

FIGURE 14-8 Sample Genogram

best choices to promote wellness and optimal functioning. Following is a list of select guidelines, for nurses and their clients, to promote healthy living and wellness in daily life.

Heart Disease:

- Eat a diet low in fat and cholesterol and high in fiber.
- Exercise regularly, 30 minutes three to five times a week (walking, swimming, cycling).
- Quit smoking or do not start to smoke.
- Reduce stress; use relaxation or meditation.
- Do not use caffeine or alcohol excessively.
- Maintain appropriate height-to-weight ratio.
- Maintain normal blood pressure.
- Have a physical exam regularly.

Osteoporosis:

- Throughout life, eat a balanced diet and calcium-rich foods (milk and milk products).
- Get plenty of exercise.
- Discuss with the primary care physician the need for a calcium supplement and estrogen replacement therapy (females).
- Do not smoke.

Cancer:

- Do not smoke.
- Avoid unnecessary exposure to radiation.
- Protect skin from ultraviolet rays; use sunscreen.
- Avoid exposure to harmful chemicals.
- Minimize exposure to pesticides, herbicides, and poisons.
- Limit alcohol intake.
- Eat a well-balanced diet with adequate fiber.
- Exercise regularly.
- Practice safe sex.
- Have cancer screening tests—mammogram, Pap smear, rectal exam—fecal occult blood test with each physical exam.

Low-Back Pain:

- Exercise regularly.
- Practice good posture and proper body mechanics.

Colds and Flu:

- Wash hands frequently.
- Use paper tissues and dispose of properly.
- Have flu shots yearly.
- Eat a balanced diet.
- Drink plenty of fluids.

Breast Cancer:

- Eat a diet low in fat.
- Exercise regularly.
- Limit alcohol and caffeine intake.
- Perform monthly breast self-examinations.
- Have mammograms as recommended by the American Cancer Society.

Sexually Transmitted Infections:

- Practice monogamous sex between noninfected individuals.
- Use latex condoms.

Tuberculosis (especially for health care workers):

- Take a Mantoux test.
- Receive isoniazid preventive therapy; any newly exposed and infected individual should take a full course of therapy.

Urinary Tract Infections:

- Drink plenty of water.
- Empty bladder frequently, especially before and after sexual intercourse.
- Wear cotton-crotch underwear.
- Wipe from front to back.
- Drink cranberry juice.
- Avoid bubble bath, douches, and colored or scented toilet paper.

Sickle-Cell Anemia and Thalassemia:

- Request genetic screening and counseling if a high-risk group.

Cataracts:

- Wear a brimmed hat and sunglasses.
- Eat a well-balanced diet.
- Do not smoke.

Glaucoma:

- Have tonometry performed.
- Have an optic nerve exam.

TABLE 14-1 Controllable Risk Factors for Top 9 Causes of Death

CAUSE OF DEATH	CONTROLLABLE RISK FACTORS
Heart disease	Tobacco use, high blood pressure, high cholesterol, lack of exercise, excessive stress, diabetes, obesity
Cancer	Tobacco use, radiation, alcohol abuse, improper diet, environmental exposure
Stroke	Tobacco use, high blood pressure, high cholesterol, lack of exercise
Chronic lung disease	Tobacco use, environmental exposures
Accidents	Alcohol abuse, drug abuse, tobacco use, failure to use seat belts, fatigue, stress, recklessness
Diabetes	Obesity, improper diet, lack of exercise, excessive stress
Alzheimer's disease	Prevent head injuries by wearing seat belts, helmets, and decreasing fall risks; control heart disease risk factors as there is a link between heart damage and vascular disease and Alzheimer's; stay socially involved; exercise mind and body; avoid tobacco and excess alcohol use; maintain healthy weight
Pneumonia and influenza	Chronic lung disease, environmental exposures, tobacco use, alcohol abuse, lack of immunizations
Kidney disease	Blood pressure and blood sugar control as a diabetic; maintain blood pressure within normal limits; avoid urinary system blockages; limit use of nonsteroidal anti-inflammatory drugs (NSAIDs) and acetaminophen (Tylenol); avoid heroin and cocaine use; promptly treat *Streptococcus* infections

From Risk factors. By Alzheimer's Association, 2008. Retrieved April 21, 2009, from http://www.alz.org/alzheimers_disease_causes_risk_factors.asp; National vital statistics report, vol. 15, no. 5. By National Center for Health Statistics, 2001. Retrieved April 21, 2009, from http://www.cdc.gov/nchs/data/nvsr/nvsr51/nvsr51_05.pdf; National vital statistics report, vol. 57, no. 14. By National Center for Health Statistics, 2001. Retrieved April 21, 2009, from http://www.cdc.gov/nchs/products/nvsr.htm#vol57

Sunburn:

- Always wear suncreen (with a minimum SPF of 15) when out in the sun.

Dental Caries and Periodontal Disease:

- Floss daily and brush after each meal.
- Use toothpaste with fluoride.
- Have a professional cleaning twice a year.
- Have a dental exam yearly.

Home Safety:

- Lock cupboards containing medicines and cleaning materials.
- Keep smoke alarms and fire extinguishers working.
- Use a carbon monoxide alarm in the presence of gas appliances and heaters.
- Plan escape routes in case of fire and have fire drills.
- Safety-proof home against falls.
- Know water safety rules.

Work Safety:

- Follow safety regulations at work.
- Report unsafe practices or equipment.

Travel Safety:

- Wear seat belts.
- Do not drive and drink.
- Drive defensively and safely.
- Use infant and child seats and restraints.
- Wear a helmet when riding a motorcycle or bicycle.
- Never swim alone.

Weight:

- Follow the Dietary Guidelines for Americans for a balanced diet.
- Exercise daily for 30 minutes.
- If overweight, eat the least number of servings recommended and use raw fruits or vegetables as snacks between meals.
- If underweight, eat the largest number of servings recommended and eat a nutritious snack between meals.

Stress:

- Identify sources of stress.
- Establish realistic expectations and goals.
- Try to be flexible.
- Express feelings and thoughts.
- Do not use alcohol or drugs for relaxation.
- Exercise regularly.
- Practice muscle relaxation and deep breathing.
- Get enough sleep.
- Have a sense of humor—laugh.
- Obtain professional help when needed.

After reading this chapter and especially the "Guidelines for Healthy Living," list three behaviors you could change to improve your health. What actions could you take to improve these behaviors? Write three specific measurable goals to achieve improved health. At the end of the semester, evaluate your achievement.

CASE STUDY

At a geriatric clinic in a low-income inner-city neighborhood, the nurse is providing care to an 80-year-old African American woman. She is diagnosed with hypertension, adult-onset diabetes, and congestive heart failure. She is obese with a BMI of 31 and is consistently noncompliant with her 1,800-calorie, carbohydrate-controlled diet. On this visit, her primary concerns are increased pedal edema and elevated blood sugar levels. Her vital signs are T-98.6 P-112 R-28 BP-163/96.

1. List some questions you would ask the client to assess how her lifestyle behaviors are affecting her health status.
2. List some primary, secondary, and tertiary preventive interventions the nurse would recommend for this client.

SUMMARY

- Wellness encompasses prevention, early detection, and treatment of health problems.
- The best way to maintain health is to follow the Dietary Guidelines for Americans, reduce stress, exercise regularly, prevent accidents, and receive routine health exams.
- Lifestyle changes can significantly reduce the leading causes of death.
- Physical, emotional, mental, social, and spiritual aspects all play key roles in the ability to resist disease and maintain health and wellness.

REVIEW QUESTIONS

1. Health maintenance and disease prevention are the responsibility of the:
   1. nurse.
   2. physician.
   3. individual.
   4. nurse practitioner.
2. Primary prevention:
   1. is the nurse's job.
   2. is curing a disease in 5 days.
   3. occurs before a disease begins.
   4. includes all diseases or conditions.
3. Health can be improved by:
   1. not smoking.
   2. drinking alcohol.
   3. eating more pasta.
   4. sleeping 4 to 5 hours each night.
4. The nurse is aware that a genogram is used for:
   1. identifying a family tree.
   2. identifying potential health problems.
   3. preventing most diseases and illnesses.
   4. acknowledging the genes a person inherits.
5. Clients should be made aware that colds and flu can best be prevented by:
   1. smoking.
   2. staying warm and dry.
   3. washing hands frequently.
   4. having a flu shot every three years.
6. A nurse working in a primary care clinic in an inner-city hospital is providing health promotion teaching to a 56-year-old woman. The patient has been diagnosed with hypertension for 10 years and is currently taking antihypertensive medications. She is overweight and noncompliant with dietary teaching. Which of the following statements indicate that the nurse is providing teaching at the secondary level of prevention?
   1. "Losing 20 pounds will bring you to your ideal weight."
   2. "You should have blood work drawn to screen for elevated cholesterol levels."
   3. "If you don't make some lifestyle changes, you may have a heart attack or stroke."
   4. "Exercise will decrease your risk of heart disease."
7. The overall goal of *Healthy People 2010* is:
   1. identifying health disparities.
   2. predicting the health status of the country in 2010.
   3. identifying unhealthy lifestyle practices.
   4. increasing quality and years of healthy life.
8. As B.D. is riding his bike around the community, he speaks to several neighbors and stops to help an elderly woman carry a large box into her home. He is a member of the Lions Club and has good interactive relationships at work. B.D. is exhibiting:
   1. emotional wellness.
   2. mental wellness.
   3. physical wellness.
   4. social wellness.
9. A client fell on the ice and suffered a strained muscle and pulled tendons. To prevent an imbalanced gait and further damage to the musculoskeletal system, the client went to physical therapy three times a week for 6 weeks to mend and strengthen the injured muscle and tendons. The client is practicing:
   1. primary prevention.
   2. secondary prevention.
   3. tertiary prevention.
   4. control of risk factor.

10. What statements describe *Health People 2010*? (Select all that apply.)
    1. The basis of *Healthy People 2010* is healthy individuals make a healthy larger community and finally a nation.
    2. *Healthy People 2010* is a grassroots organization that mandates healthy behavior of all in the community.
    3. *Healthy People 2010* identified leading health indicators that are major health issues in the United States.
    4. *Healthy People 2010* singles out groups with poor health and pays them to try activities to improve their health.
    5. *Healthy People 2010* is a nationalized health care plan that goes into effect in 2010.
    6. *Healthy People 2010* attempts to eliminate health inequalities within the nation.

REFERENCES/SUGGESTED READINGS

Alzheimer's Association. (2008). Risk factors. Retrieved April 21, 2009, from http://www.alz.org/alzheimers_disease_causes_risk_factors.asp

Baughcum, A. (1998). Mom's beliefs may cause child obesity. *Archives of Pediatric and Adolescent Medicine, 152,* 1010–1014.

Browder, S. (1998). Attention, women over 50. Available: http://www.seniornews.com/new-choices/article593.html

Carethers, M. (1992). Health promotion in the elderly. *American Family Physician, 45*(5), 2253–2260.

Centers for Disease Control and Prevention. (2005). Breast cancer screening and socioeconomic status—35 metropolitan areas, 2000 and 2002. *Morbidity and Mortality Weekly Report, 54*(39), 981–985. Retrieved on October 22, 2008, from http://www.cdc.gov/mmwr/preview/mmwrhtml/mm5439a2.htm

Centers for Disease Control and Prevention. (2006). Falls among older adults: An overview. Retrieved December 19, 2006, from http://www.cdc.gov/ncipc/factsheets/adultfalls.htm

Cerrato, P. (1999). A radical approach to heart disease. *RN, 62*(4), 65–66.

Chopra, D., & Simon, D. (2001). *Grow younger, live longer.* New York: Harmony Books.

CNN. (2008a). U.S. life expectancy still trails 30 countries. Retrieved October 21, 2008, from http://cnn.site.printthis.clickability.com/pt/cpt?action=cpt&title=U.S.+life+expectancy+st

CNN. (2008b). WHO slams global health care, calls for universal coverage. Retrieved October 21, 2008, from http://cnn.site.printthis.clickability.com/pt/cpt?action=cpt&title=WHO+slams+global+he

Cohen, L., Davis, R., & Mikkelsen, L. (2000, March/April). Comprehensive prevention: Improving health outcomes through practice. *Minority Health Today.* Retrieved October 20, 2008, from http://preventioninstitute.org/minorityhealth.html

Edlin, G., Golanty, E., & McCormack-Brown, K. (1999). *Essentials for health and wellness.* Boston: Jones & Bartlett.

Floyd, P., Mimms, S., & Yelding-Howard, C. (1995). *Personal health: A multicultural approach.* Englewood, CO: Morton.

Hall, D. (2006). Religious attendance: More cost-effective than Lipitor? *Journal of the American Board of Family Medicine, 19,* 103–109.

Harris, G. (2008, October 16). Infant deaths drop in U.S., but rate is still high. *New York Times.* Retrieved October 20, 2008, from http://www.nytimes.com/2008/10/16/health/16infnat.html?_r=1&em=&oref+slogin&pag

Healthy People 2010. (2005). What is Healthy People 2010? Retrieved April 21, 2009, from http://www.healthypeopel.gov/About/hpfact.htm

Hoeger, W., & Hoeger, S. (2000). *Lifetime physical fitness and wellness* (5th ed.). Belmont, CA: Wadsworth.

Hoeger, W., Turner, L., & Hafen, B. (2001). *Wellness: Guidelines for a healthy lifestyle* (3rd ed.). Belmont, CA: Wadsworth.

Hoffman, E. (1996). *Our health, our lives.* New York: Pocket Books.

Hunt, R. (2008). *Introduction to Community-Based Nursing* (4th ed.). Philadelphia: Lippincott Williams & Wilkins.

Krarup, L. et al. (2008). Prestroke physical activity is associated with severity and long-term outcome from first ever stroke. *Neurology, 71*(17), 1313–1318.

Lee, I., & Paffenbarger, R. (1998). Exercise can cut stroke risk 50%. *Stroke, 29,* 2049–2054.

Lifeoptions. (2009). Risk factors for CKD. Retrieved April 21, 2009, from http://www.lifeoptions.org/kidneyinfo/ckdinfo.php?page=3

Lyon, B. (2000). Conquering stress. *Reflections on Nursing Leadership, 26*(1), 22–23, 43.

Malaty, H. (1998). Twin study: *H. pylori* tied to hygiene. *American Journal of Epidemiology, 148,* 793–797.

Marshall, V., & Altpeter, M. (2005) Cultivating social work leadership in health promotion and aging: Strategies for active aging interventions. *Health and Social Work, 30*(2), 135–145.

Matthews, K. (1998). Suppressed anger hard on women's hearts. *Psychosomatic Medicine, 60,* 633–638.

Maville, J., & Huerta, C. (2002). *Health promotion in nursing.* Clifton Park, NY: Delmar Cengage Learning.

McEwen, M. (2002) *Community-based nursing: An introduction* (2nd ed.). Philadelphia: W. B. Saunders.

Meyers, S. (2008). Anger and health—An update. Retrieved October 21, 2008, from http://www.extension.umn.edu/distribution/familydevelopment/components/7269ai.html

National Center for Health Statistics. (2001a). National vital statistics report, vol. 51, no. 5. Retrieved April 21, 2009, from http://www.cdc.gov/nchs/data/nvsr/nvsr51/nvsr51_05.pdf

National Center for Health Statistics. (2001b). National vital statistics report, vol. 57, no. 14. Retrieved April 21, 2009, from http://www.cdc.gov/nchs/products/nvsr.htm#vol57

Nettina, S. (2001) *The Lippincott manual of nursing practice.* Philadelphia: Lippincott.

Office of Disease Prevention and Health Promotion. (2006). Dietary guidelines for Americans 2005. Retrieved December 2, 2006, from http://www.odphp.osophs.dhhs.gov

Office of the Surgeon General. (2007). The health consequences of involuntary exposure to tobacco smoke: A report of the surgeon general, U.S. Department of Health and Human Services—6 major conclusions of the surgeon general report. Retrieved October 22, 2008, from http://www.surgeongeneral.gov/library/secondhandsmoke/factsheets/factsheet6.html

Oman, D., & Reed, D. (1998). Religious elderly tend to live longer. *American Journal of Public Health, 88,* 1469–1475.

Payne, W., & Hahn, D. (2000). *Understanding your health* (6th ed.). New York: McGraw-Hill.

Poliafico, F. (1999). Abstinence is not the only answer. *RN, 62*(1), 58–60.

Potter, P., & Perry, A. (2009). *Fundamentals of nursing* (7th ed.). St Louis, MO: Mosby.

Reed, D. (1998). Four factors predict "healthy aging." *American Journal of Public Health, 88,* 1463–1469.

Reichler, G., & Burke, N. (1999). *Active wellness: A personalized 10 step program for a healthy body, mind and spirit.* Richmond, VA: Time Life.

Resnick, B. (2001). Geriatric health promotion. *Topics in Advanced Practice Nursing eJournal.* Retrieved October 20, 2008, from http://www.medscape.com/viewarticle/408406

Seiger, L., Kanipe, D., Vanderpool, K., & Barnes, D. (2000). *Fitness and wellness strategies* (2nd ed.). New York: McGraw-Hill.

Simmerman, J. M., & Mauzy, C. (2001). Finally! Babies can get this vaccine. *RN, 64*(7), 28–32.

Simon, H. (1992). *Staying well.* Boston: Houghton Mifflin.

Smith, C., & Maurer, F. (1999). *Community health nursing: Theory and practice* (2nd ed.) Philadelphia: W. B. Saunders.

Smith, R. (in press). *Promoting health and wellness.*

Stibich, M. (2007). Religion might add years to your life. Retrieved October 21, 2008 from http://longevity.about.com/od/longevityboosters/a/religion_life.htm?p=1

U.S. Department of Agriculture, U.S. Department of Health and Human Services. (2000). *Home and Garden Bulletin No. 232* (5th ed.).

U.S. Department of Health and Human Services. (1990). *Healthy People 2000: National health promotion and disease prevention objectives* (DHHS Publication No. [PHS] 91-50212). Washington, DC: Author.

U.S. Department of Health and Human Services, Public Health Service. (1998). Healthy People 2000: National health promotion and disease prevention objectives and first draft Healthy People 2010: National health promotion and disease prevention objectives. Available: http://web.health.gov/healthypeople

U.S. Department of Health and Human Services, Public Health Service. (2000a). Healthy People 2010: National health promotion and disease prevention objectives. Available: http://web.health.gov/healthypeople

U.S. Department of Health and Human Services, Public Health Service. (2000b). *1998–1999 progress review.* Available: http://odphp.osophs.dhhs.gov/pubs/hp2000

Wash your hands (to help prevent colds). (1996, January). *Consumer Reports on Health, 2*(1).

Weil, A. (1998). *Natural health, natural medicine* (2nd ed.). Boston: Houghton Mifflin.

Weil, A. (2001). *Eating well for optimum health: The essential guide to bringing health and pleasure back to eating.* Camperdown, New South Wales, Australia: Quill.

Weil, A., & Daley, R. (2002). *The healthy kitchen: Recipes for a better body, life and spirit.* Westminster, MD: Knopf.

RESOURCES

Aerobics and Fitness Association of America, http://www.afaa.com

American Dietetic Association, http://www.eatright.org

American Health Care Association, http://www.ahcancal.org

American Heart Association, http://www.ahs.org

American Holistic Nurses' Association, http://www.ahna.org

Center for Science in the Public Interest, http://www.cspinet.org

Centers for Disease Control and Prevention, http://www.cdc.gov

Environmental Protection Agency, http://www.epa.gov

Food and Drug Administration, http://www.fda.gov

Food and Nutrition Information Center, http://www.nal.usda.gov

Healthy People 2010, http://www.cdc.gov/nchs/hphome.htm

Medic Alert Foundation International, http://www.medicalert.org

National Highway Traffic Safety Administration, http://www.nhtsa.dot.gov

National Institute for Occupational Safety and Health, http://www.cdc.gov/niosh

National Institute on Aging, http://www.nih.nia.gov

National Institutes of Health, http://www.nih.gov

National Safety Council, http://www.nsc.org

National Wellness Institute, http://www.nationalwellness.org

National Women's Health Network, http://www.nwhn.org

U. S. Consumer Product Safety Commission, http://www.cpsc.gov

U.S. Department of Agriculture, http://www.usda.gov

U.S. Department of Health and Human Services, http://www.hhs.gov

World Health Organization, http://www.who.int

CHAPTER 15
Self-Concept

MAKING THE CONNECTION

Refer to the following chapters to increase your understanding of self-concept:

Basic Nursing

- ***Communication***
- ***Life Span Development***
- ***Stress, Adaptation, and Anxiety***
- ***End-of-Life Care***
- ***Spirituality***
- ***Complementary/Alternative Therapies***

Adult Health Nursing

- ***Surgery***
- ***Oncology***
- ***Mental Illness***

LEARNING OBJECTIVES

Upon completion of this chapter, you should be able to:

- Define key terms.
- Discuss the development of self-concept throughout the life span.
- Describe four major components of self-concept.
- Identify factors affecting self-concept.
- Delineate nursing interventions that promote self-concept.

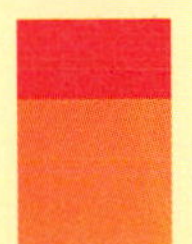

KEY TERMS

body image
empowerment
ideal self
identity
public self
real self
role
role performance
self-awareness
self-concept
self-esteem

SELF-CONCEPT

Self-concept is the way people think about themselves. It is unique, dynamic, and always evolving. This mental image of oneself influences a person's identity, self-esteem, body image, and role in society. As a global understanding of oneself, self-concept shapes and defines who we are, the decisions we make, and the relationships we form (Figure 15-1). Self-concept is perhaps the basis for all motivated behavior (Franken, 1994).

COMPONENTS OF SELF-CONCEPT

Self-concept is an individual's perception of self, including self-esteem, body image, and ideal self. A person's self-concept is often defined by self-description such as "I am a mother, a nurse, and a volunteer." Client self-descriptive statements such as these help the nurse gain insight into the client's perception of self. The nurse should be observant for self-descriptive statements when assessing the client's self-concept. A healthy self-concept is necessary for overall physical and mental wellness.

Three basic components of self-concept are the ideal self, the public self, and the real self (Figure 15-2). The **ideal self** is the person the client would like to be, such as a good, moral, and well-respected person. Sometimes, this ideal view of how a client would like to be conflicts with the **real self** (how the client really thinks about oneself, such as "I try to be good and do what's right, but I'm not well respected"). This conflict can motivate a client to make changes toward becoming the ideal self. However, the view of the ideal self needs to be realistic and obtainable, or the client may experience anxiety or be at risk for alterations in self-concept. **Public self** is what the client thinks others think of him and influences the ideal and real self. Positive self-concept and good mental health results when all three components are compatible.

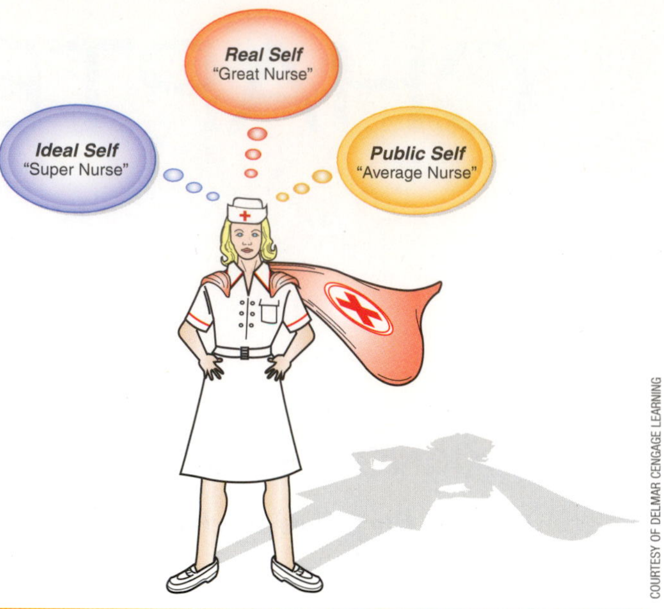

FIGURE 15-2 Example of how a nurse may view her ideal self, real self, and public self.

A positive self-concept is an important part of a client's happiness and success. Individuals with a positive self-concept have self-confidence and set goals they can achieve. Achieving their goals reinforces their positive self-concept. A client with a positive self-concept is more likely to change unhealthy habits (such as sedentary lifestyle and smoking) to promote health than a client with a negative self-concept.

A person's self-concept is composed of evolving subjective conscious and unconscious self-assessments. Physical attributes, occupation, knowledge, and abilities of the person will change throughout the life span, contributing to changes in one's self-concept. Memory Trick 15-1 lists nursing interventions to promote positive self-concept.

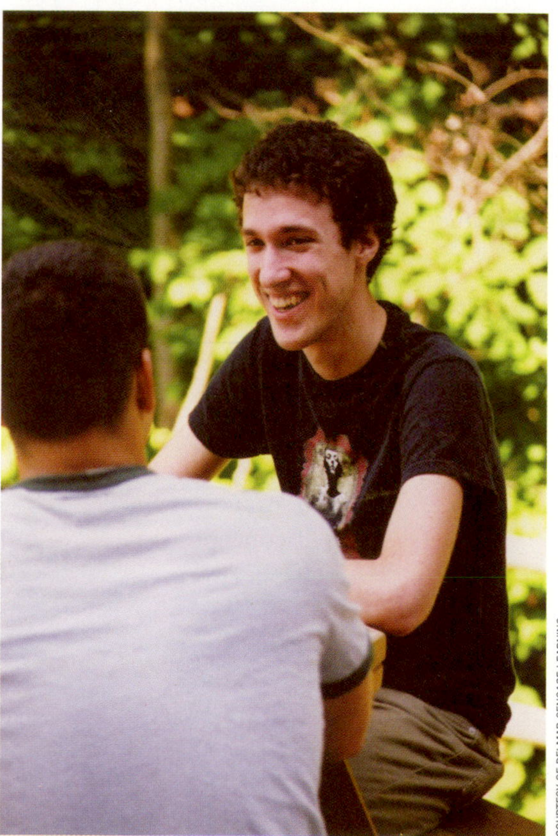

FIGURE 15-1 A positive self-concept enhances healthy relationships.

PROFESSIONALTIP

Characteristics of a Positive Self-Concept

Characteristics of a client with a positive self-concept include:

- Self-confidence
- Ability to accept criticism and not become defensive
- Setting obtainable goals
- Willingness to take risks and try new experiences

MEMORY TRICK

I LIKE ME

The memory trick **I LIKE ME** lists nursing interventions to promote a positive self-concept in clients:

- **I** = Identify client's strengths.
- **L** = Listen to the client's self-description.
- **I** = Involve the client in decision making.
- **K** = Keep goals realistic.
- **E** = Encourage client to think positively.
- **M** = Maintain an environment conducive to client self-expression.
- **E** = Explain to the client how to use positive self-talk instead of negative self-talk.

CLIENT TEACHING

Positive Self-Talk

Positive self-talk can be used to change negative inner messages to positive ones.

1. Send yourself positive thoughts.
2. Say the positive thoughts out loud.
3. Remind yourself of your positive attributes and accomplishments.
4. Recall memories of success.
5. Tell yourself out loud something new that you learned or something good that you did today.

Identity

Identity is an individual's conscious description of who he is. A client's identity is assessed by asking the person to describe oneself. This description of oneself provides the nurse with insight into whether the client is comfortable with one's identity. A client who uses positive self-descriptions will exhibit a healthy self-identity.

An individual's identity is developed over time, constantly evolving, and influenced by self-awareness. **Self-awareness** involves consciously knowing how the self thinks, feels, believes, and behaves at any specific time (Figure 15-3). According to Burkhardt and Nathaniel (2008), we can enhance self-awareness by developing the ability to step back and look at any situation while being aware of ourselves and how we are reacting to the situation. A client needs to be able to identify one's personal and emotional feelings of a situation without judging oneself.

Body Image

An individual's perception of physical self, including appearance, function, and ability, is known as one's **body image**.

PROFESSIONAL TIP

Emotional Intelligence

Emotional intelligence (EI) refers to the ability to perceive, understand, control/manage, and evaluate emotions. A number of quizzes and testing instruments have been developed to measure EI. To take a fun and quick quiz to learn more about your emotional intelligence, go to http://psychology.about.com and search for Emotional Intelligence Test.

Normal growth and developmental changes may influence and alter body image, such as the physical and hormonal changes that occur during puberty and adolescence. The onset of puberty involves the emergence of secondary sex characteristics in the female and male client. While these are normal expected physical changes that occur during the adolescent stage, these changes will impact an adolescent's body image, thus affecting self-concept.

In later adulthood, physical and hormonal changes present as thinning and graying of hair, wrinkling and loss of skin elasticity, weight gain, decrease in hearing and vision, and decrease in mobility. While some adults accept these changes as the normal process of aging, others may find themselves resisting or feeling negatively about them. These changes will naturally cause the adult to reevaluate the image they have of their body and how they feel about it. A person's body image will continue to change throughout the growth and developmental life span stages.

Health-related factors that may affect body image include stroke, spinal cord injury, amputation, mastectomy, burns, surgical and/or procedural scarring, and loss of a body part or function. Other common physical changes that affect body image involve the development of acne and weight gain and/or loss. According to the Centers for Disease Control and Prevention (CDC, 2007), approximately 66% of American adults are overweight or obese. These physical issues may add stress and anxiety on the client, lowering their self-esteem and self-confidence.

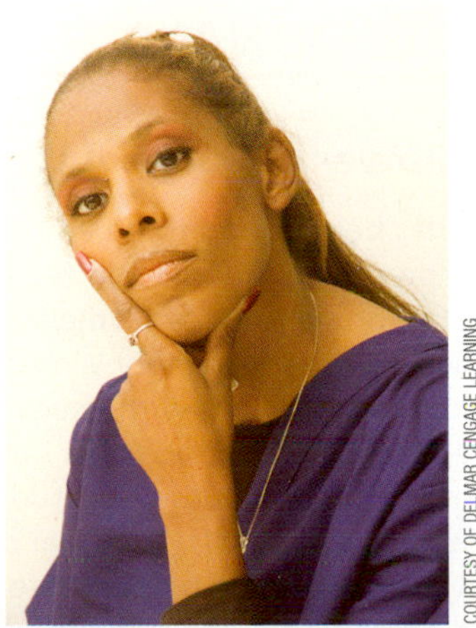

COURTESY OF DELMAR CENGAGE LEARNING

FIGURE 15-3 Self-awareness involves reflecting on feelings, thoughts, and reactions to situations.

CRITICAL THINKING

Body Image versus Self-Esteem

What are the differences between body image and self-esteem? How do they affect each other?

Self-Esteem

Self-esteem is a personal opinion of oneself and is shaped by individuals' relationships with others, experiences, and accomplishments in life. A healthy self-esteem is necessary for mental well-being and a positive self-concept. This is achieved by setting attainable goals and successfully accomplishing the goals, resulting in an increase in self-confidence, assertiveness, and feeling valued. Since self-esteem impacts all aspects of life, it is important to establish a healthy, realistic view of oneself (Mayo Clinic, 2009).

Individuals with low self-esteem put little value on themselves and their accomplishments. They feel that they are not good enough and that they are worth less than others and often feel ashamed of themselves. They engage in negative self-talk, frequently apologize, and seek constant reassurance. Often this type of person is a perfectionist who struggles with failure.

One method of improving an individual's low self-esteem is for the nurse to empower the client. Burkhardt and Nathaniel (2008) define **empowerment** as "a helping process and partnership, enacted in the context of love and respect for self and others, through which individuals and groups are enabled to change situations, and are given skills, resources, opportunities, and authority to do so" (p. 542). Chamberlin (2008) recognized that empowerment has elements in common with concepts of self-esteem and self-efficacy. As a client becomes more empowered, one will feel more confident in one's ability to manage one's life, resulting in improved self-esteem and self-image. Box 15-1 lists the elements of empowerment that nurses may teach clients to use to increase their self-esteem.

Research and assessment has been conducted on self-esteem for several decades. The Rosenberg Self-Esteem Scale was originally developed to assess self-esteem among adolescents (Rosenberg, 1965). This self-report consists of statements related to feelings of self-worth or self-acceptance to measure global self-esteem. The scale has been validated to be used with male and female adolescents, adults, and elderly populations and remains in use today.

PROFESSIONALTIP

Healing Power of Journal Writing

Journaling has been found to be a powerful way to bridge a person's thoughts and feelings. Merrill Devito at Stanford University formed a support group of women titled "Hungry Women Writing" to assist women struggling with issues of food, confidence, and self-image to learn how to use journal writing to explore their attitudes toward their bodies (Hanson, 2004). The goal of each participant is to overcome his negative thoughts and to feel empowered and self-confident about himself and his body image.

CRITICAL THINKING

Feelings of Empowerment

1. Consider a situation in which you felt empowered. List and describe factors that contributed to your feelings of empowerment.
2. Reflect on a situation in which you felt disempowered. What would have helped you feel more empowered?

Role

We experience many roles in our lifetime. As we pass from birth to death, we will become a child, teenager, friend, worker, and perhaps spouse or parent. Many of our roles are defined by our success, education, relationships, and career. An individual's **role** is defined as an ascribed or assumed expected behavior in a social position or group. Specific behaviors that a person exhibits within each role make up **role performance**.

Illness, injury, and aging can lead to alterations in a person's role. Additional alterations may include pregnancy, loss of a job, retirement, or death of a significant other. How the individual views these changes or losses will determine the impact on one's self-concept. Individuals who view these alterations negatively are at risk for ineffective role performance and a decreased self-concept.

DEVELOPMENT OF SELF-CONCEPT

Various psychosocial theories have been developed to explain the development of self-concept. A discussion of Erikson's

BOX 15-1 ELEMENTS OF EMPOWERMENT

A client's self-esteem will increase when using the following elements:

- Having decision-making power
- Having access to information and resources
- Having a range of options from which to make choices
- Using assertiveness skills
- Feeling that oneself can make a difference
- Feeling part of a group, not alone
- Effecting change in one's life and one's community
- Learning skills that the individual defines as important
- Self-initiated growth and change
- Increasing one's positive self-image

From A Working Definition of Empowerment. By J. Chamberlin, 2008. Retrieved February 1, 2009, from http://www.power2u.org/articles/empower/working_def.html

CLIENT TEACHING

Activities That Increase Self-Esteem

The following are activities that the nurse can teach the client to engage in to increase one's self-esteem:

- Taking good care of self
- Taking time to do enjoyable activities
- Journaling
- Getting something done that has been put off
- Spending time with people that make you feel good about yourself
- Learning something new
- Forgiving yourself
- Doing something nice for someone else
- Positive self-talk
- Giving yourself rewards

theory of psychosocial development related to self-concept follows.

Erikson's Theory

Erikson's (1963) psychosocial theory states that an individual's development proceeds throughout life. Each of his eight developmental stages includes psychosocial tasks that need to be mastered (see Chapter 10, "Life Span Development").

Newborn and Infant

At birth, the newborn does not differentiate itself from the parents. As the parents begin to care for the newborn, their feelings and attitudes toward the newborn will begin to develop the baby's self-concept. The parents will experience a change in their own self-concept. Parental roles are being established, body images are formed in the mother before and after giving birth, and emotional changes will affect the parents' self-concept.

The nurse will need to teach the family about the infant's emotional needs in developing a trusting relationship to promote the infant's feelings of security and trust in the parents. A sense of security and trust is especially important for the infant if it becomes ill and is hospitalized. Parents need to be encouraged to spend as much time as possible with the infant and provide routine care and developmental interventions for the infant to facilitate the continued healthy development of self-concept.

Toddler and Preschooler

The toddler needs a supportive environment for body image and self-esteem to develop positively. The parents should provide the toddler with an environment to practice his newly learned skills. The toddler needs to be encouraged to try his skills again (such as learning to walk or potty training) if not successful at first. Praising the toddler for mastery of learning his new skill is important in developing a positive self-concept.

Preschoolers begin to exhibit a sense of sexual curiosity. As they hear the names and functions of their body parts, they may ask a lot of questions. How the parents answer a preschooler's questions may have an impact on his self-concept and body image. As preschoolers develop their self-concept, they will often imitate parents and siblings.

School Age and Adolescence

The school experience has a major impact on a child's development of self-concept, identity, body image, self-esteem, and role. Parents, teachers, and peers have a direct influence on the child's developing feelings, views, and sense of self. Children compare their physical appearance, academic and athletic abilities, and social status to those of their peers and seek approval and acceptance from this group. Bullying by verbal, emotional, or technological methods (e-mail, chatting, blogging, texting, or twittering) is common in this age group and negatively affects a child's developing self-concept. The school-age child places importance on receiving acceptance and approval by one's peer group to feel included and positive about oneself.

Adolescence marks numerous physical and hormonal changes, including in the female the onset of menses, pubic and axillary hair growth, breast development, and an increase in height, and in the male a slow, progressive deepening of the voice; pubic, axillary, and chest hair growth; enlargement of the testicles and penis; and thinning and reddening of the scrotum. The development of acne and body odor will also occur at this age. These changes influence the adolescent's view of one's body and oneself. Adolescents look to their peers, parents, role models, and the media to view what is expected of them (Figure 15-4).

Many adolescents are experiencing issues with the image of their body weight, shape, size, hair, acne, or height. Negative

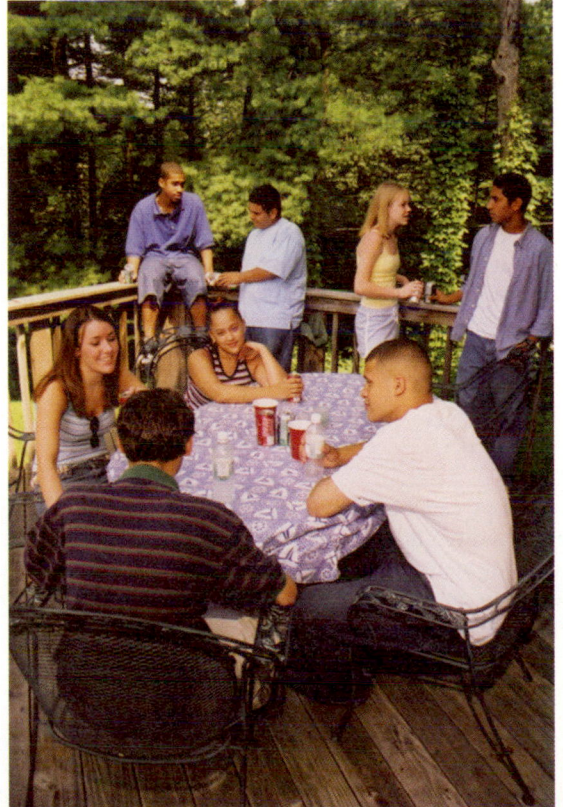

COURTESY OF DELMAR CENGAGE LEARNING

FIGURE 15-4 Peer relationships are important during adolescence.

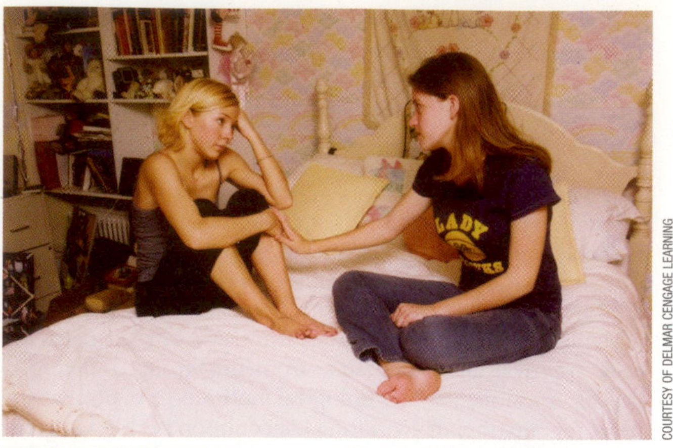
COURTESY OF DELMAR CENGAGE LEARNING

FIGURE 15-5 Support from friends promotes a healthy self-concept during adolescence.

comments and reactions from their peers can cause them to participate in substance abuse, inappropriate sexual behavior, and eating disorders as an attempt to fit in. Adolescents struggling with how to deal with anxiety and depression due to these expectations may use self-injury (self-mutilation) as a method of coping or even attempt suicide.

The development of a healthy self-concept for the adolescent often lies in parental involvement and support. As the adolescent becomes more independent, the parents may need to adapt and change their parenting style. While adolescents may begin to attain more independence, they still require the love, support, and involvement of their family and friends (Figure 15-5).

ADULTHOOD

The natural process of aging will lead to significant changes in a person's self-concept. Over the course of a lifetime, an adult will experience changes in one's roles, body, and identity. Young adults strive to develop relationships, careers, and often a family. Older adults attempt to define themselves by their accomplishments. Major life events in adulthood will continuously shape a person's self-concept, such as obtaining a college degree, getting a job, marriage, divorce, losing a job, retirement, and the death of a significant other. How the individual views and copes with these changes will determine the influence and impact they have on the person's self-concept.

FACTORS AFFECTING SELF-CONCEPT

Self-concept can be affected by an individual's life experiences, heredity and culture, stress and coping, health status, and developmental stage. The nurse needs to evaluate each of these factors and the influence each has on the client's achievement of a healthy self-concept (Figure 15-6).

LIFE EXPERIENCES

Life experiences, including success and failure, will develop and influence a person's self-concept. Experiences in which the individual has accomplished a goal and achieved success will positively reinforce the development of a healthy self-concept. Difficult experiences and/or failures can negatively impact a person's self-concept unless they have established coping strategies to deal effectively with these challenges to their self-concept. Coping strategies are learned as a person encounters and deals with various situations in life.

SAFETY

A mental health professional needs to be consulted immediately when self-injury, suicide, or eating disorders are suspected or committed.

Self-injury: Self-injury involves intentional self-inflicted tissue damage, such as cutting, burning, skin picking, or pulling one's hair out. This disorder occurs in either sex and in any religion or race and is not limited by education, age, or social status. Statistics are difficult to obtain because of the secretive nature of this disorder (Cleveland Clinic, 2005). Search online at http://www.clevelandclinic.org for more information.

Suicide: Suicide is the third-leading cause of death in clients aged 10 to 24. Boys, Native Americans/Alaskan Natives, and Hispanic youth have the highest rates of suicide. Approximately 32,000 suicides (one every 16 minutes) are committed in the United States each year (CDC, 2008b). Search online at http://www.cdc.gov for more information.

Eating disorders: Anorexia nervosa, bulimia, and binge eating are the three most common eating disorders. Anorexia nervosa and bulimia can lead to life-threatening conditions, resulting in permanent damage to major organs of the body. Statistics are difficult to obtain because of the secretive nature of these disorders (CDC, 2009). Search online at http://www.cdc.gov for more information.

HEREDITY AND CULTURE

Individuals typically grow up learning and integrating their family's heredity and culture into their life. Beginning at birth, heredity and culture shape and influence a person's self-concept. Individuals who have integrated their heredity and culture into their life tend to have a healthier self-identity and self-concept (Figure 15-7).

STRESS AND COPING

Everyone experiences stress at some level each day. Common stressors include financial, work-related, relationship, and health issues. Individuals react and deal with stress in different ways depending on their past experiences and success and failure with dealing with stress. Individuals who learn and use effective coping strategies to deal with stress will most likely develop a positive self-concept. People who become overwhelmed with stress may feel hopeless and powerless, leading to a feeling of low self-confidence and self-esteem (Figure 15-8). The nurse may need to teach the client effective coping strategies and techniques for handling stress.

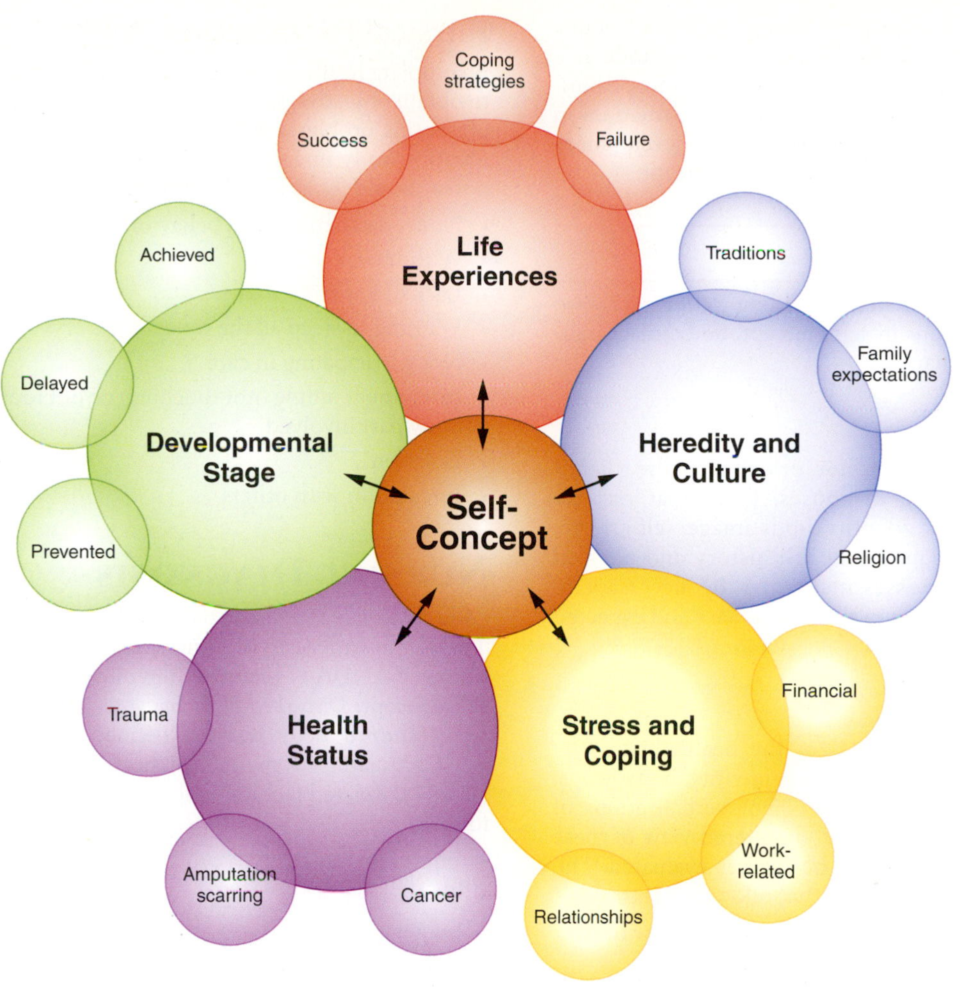

FIGURE 15-6 Concept Map Depicting Factors That Affect Self-Concept

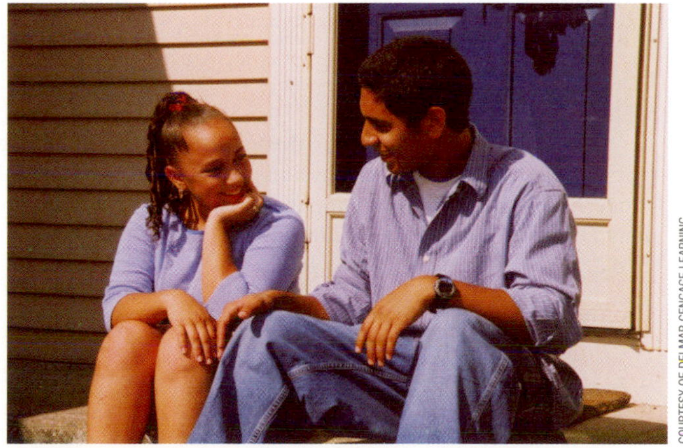

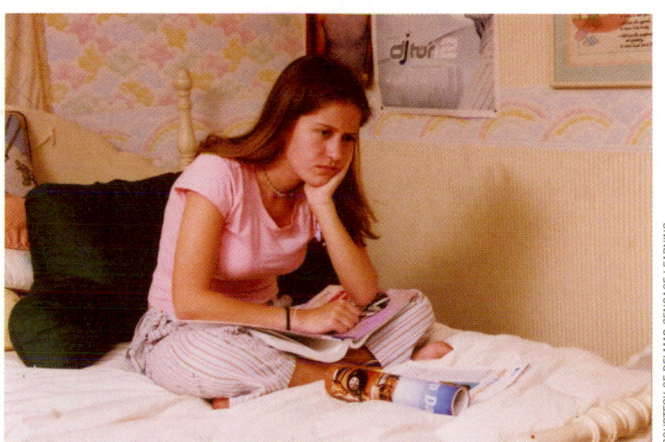

FIGURE 15-7 Self-concept is influenced by an individual's heredity and culture.

FIGURE 15-8 Ineffective coping and stress may lead to feelings of low self-confidence and self-esteem.

HEALTH STATUS

People tend to take their good health for granted. When they become ill, their altered health status can change their self-identity and self-concept. Alterations in body image can result from such health issues as amputation, cancer, mastectomy, trauma, or scarring. The nurse needs to monitor for changes in the client's self-concept due to alterations in their health status.

DEVELOPMENTAL STAGE

Growth and development begins at birth and continues into adulthood. Typically a person will achieve specific developmental tasks as one passes through each stage of life. The successful accomplishment of each task will influence and reinforce the development of a healthy self-concept. Individuals who experience developmental delays or situations in life that prevent or delay the accomplishment of developmental tasks can have an altered or negative self-concept.

NURSING PROCESS

The nursing process facilitates providing nursing care to clients at risk for alterations in self-concept, body image, self-esteem, and role performance.

ASSESSMENT

Assessment data are the basis for prioritizing the client's problems and the nursing diagnoses. Clients at risk for alterations in self-concept, identity, body image, self-esteem, and role performance require a health history and physical examination. Frequent reassessment may be necessary to facilitate appropriate changes in the plan of care and expected outcomes.

Health History

The nurse begins gathering data for the health history by assessing the client's perception of their identity, body image, self-esteem, and role performance. Client verbalizations of feelings and perceptions that reflect an altered view of these areas of self-concept will need to be further evaluated. The nursing history should elicit data in the following areas:

- Feelings or perceptions that reflect the client's view of oneself
- Client report of any changes in body image, self-esteem, or role
- Feelings of powerlessness and/or hopelessness related to any of these changes

BOX 15-2 QUESTIONS TO USE IN OBTAINING A HEALTH HISTORY

Obtaining a Client History of Self-Concept

- How would you describe yourself?
- How do others describe you?
- What has been your greatest accomplishment?
- How does this make you feel?
- When you receive praise, do you feel worthy of it?
- What do you admire most about yourself?
- How do you react when you experience failure?
- How do you cope with failure?
- Have you experienced past or recent changes in body image, self-esteem, or role performance?
- Have you experienced feelings of powerlessness or hopelessness?
- Who do you consider your support group?
- What do you do to make yourself laugh or feel good about yourself?

Physical Examination

A complete health assessment includes a physical examination to obtain objective data relative to the client's health status and presenting problems. When assessing the client's self-concept, identity, body image, self-esteem, and role performance, the nurse should focus the physical examination on:

- Nonverbal actions and behaviors
- Withdrawal
- Lack of appetite
- Wanting to sleep all the time
- Not participating in care
- Intentional hiding, not touching, or not looking at the body part involved
- Isolation
- Interaction with others

NURSING DIAGNOSIS

After data collection and analysis, identify a nursing diagnosis. The North American Nursing Diagnosis Association International (NANDA-I) identifies the nursing diagnosis related to self-concept: *Disturbed **B**ody Image.*

*Disturbed **B**ody Image* is defined by NANDA-I (2010) as "Confusion in mental picture of one's physical self" (p. 197). Related factors to disturbances in body image are as follows:

- Injury
- Trauma
- Surgery
- Illness
- Illness treatment
- Perceptual
- Cognitive
- Spiritual
- Cultural
- Psychosocial
- Developmental changes
- Biophysical

Clients who are at risk for disturbances in body image may have other associated physiological and psychological concerns. The common nursing diagnoses that often accompany *Disturbed **B**ody Image* include:

*Readiness for Enhanced **S**elf-Concept*
*Situational Low **S**elf-Esteem*
*Chronic Low **S**elf-Esteem*
*Ineffective **R**ole Performance*
*Social **I**solation*
***P**owerlessness*
***H**opelessness*
*Disturbed Personal **I**dentity*
*Risk for Compromised Human **D**ignity*
*Risk for **L**oneliness*
*Readiness for Enhanced **P**ower*

The list identifies related diagnoses for alterations in self-esteem and role performance that must be considered when planning care for a client at risk for alterations in self-concept.

Planning/Outcome Identification

Holistic nursing care requires collaborating with each client to identify goals for each nursing diagnosis. Planning and outcome identification for the client focuses on promoting a healthy self-concept or facilitating change in an altered self-concept. These individualized goals should reflect the client's abilities and limitations.

Nursing interventions are selected and prioritized to support the client's achievement of expected outcomes based on the goals. For example, if the client states that she considers herself overweight, unattractive, and undesirable to others, this leads to a nursing diagnosis of *Disturbed **B**ody Image*, and the goals might include expressing positive feelings about herself and integrating a realistic body image.

Implementation

Several interventions can promote a positive healthy self-concept in clients; they are as follows:

- Encourage client to list past and current accomplishments
- Ask client to describe how they and others would describe them
- Assess the client's report of changes in their self-concept, body image, self-esteem, or role performance
- Encourage verbalization of the positive and negative feelings and perceptions of the changes that have occurred to their self-concept, body image, self-esteem, or role
- Acknowledge normalcy of changes in the emotional response and grieving stages to changes
- Assist client in incorporating the necessary changes into their daily life
- Assist the client in identifying methods of coping that have been useful in the past
- Assist client in contacting appropriate support groups and/or counseling as needed

Evaluation

Evaluation of the effectiveness of nursing care is based on the achievement of goals and expected outcomes. The plan of care must be updated on a regular basis with additional interventions used as needed.

SAMPLE NURSING CARE PLAN

The Client with Alterations in Self-Concept

T.H., a 38-year-old male, had surgery for placement of a cardiac pacemaker. Two days postoperatively, T.H. refused to participate in his care and appeared quiet and withdrawn. When the nurse asked T.H. if he would like to talk about it, he replied, "I don't want to look at it or touch it. I will never be able to take my shirt off in the summer again. Why did the scar have to be so big?"

NURSING DIAGNOSIS *Disturbed **B**ody Image* related to scarring from surgical pacemaker placement

Nursing Outcomes Classification (NOC)
Body Image
Self-Esteem

Nursing Interventions Classification (NIC)
Body Image Enhancement
Grief Work Facilitation
Coping Enhancement

PLANNING/OUTCOMES	NURSING INTERVENTIONS	RATIONALE
T.H. will be able to look at, touch, and talk about the surgical scar on his chest where the cardiac pacemaker was inserted.	Encourage T.H. to verbalize his feelings and perceptions regarding the scar on his chest.	Verbalizing feelings and perceptions may help T.H. express and identify his concerns.
	Assist T.H. to identify effective coping strategies.	Identifying coping strategies may assist T.H. to deal effectively with his body image issues.
	Acknowledge T.H.'s emotional response to the changes in the appearance of his chest.	Acknowledging a client's emotional response promotes trust and is validating their feelings and thoughts.
	Provide empathy and support to T.H.	Providing empathy and support are necessary to facilitate a positive nurse–client helping relationship.

EVALUATION

T.H. states that he does not like the scar on his chest, but he can live with it. He has participated in his activities of daily living and washed and dried his chest during morning hygiene care.

SUMMARY

- A positive self-concept is important in achieving happiness, success, and a healthy self-identity.
- The four main components of self-concept are identity, body image, self-esteem, and role performance.
- A variety of activities are available for the nurse to teach the client to promote a positive self-concept.
- Body image continuously changes throughout an individual's growth and developmental life stages.
- Self-esteem is shaped by relationships with others, experiences, and accomplishments in life.
- A variety of factors affecting self-concept include life experiences, heredity and culture, values and beliefs, stress and coping, health status, and developmental stage.

REVIEW QUESTIONS

1. A 16-year-old female client tells the nurse, "I am fat, ugly, and stupid." This statement best reflects the client's:
   1. ideal self.
   2. real self.
   3. public self.
   4. other self.

2. The nurse knows that a positive self-concept is an important part of a client's happiness and success. Individuals with a positive self-concept exhibit all of the following except:
   1. difficulty accepting criticism.
   2. setting goals they can achieve.
   3. changing unhealthy habits.
   4. self-confidence.

3. A 78-year-old male client presents with thinning and graying of hair, wrinkling and loss of skin elasticity, weight gain, decrease in hearing and vision, and a decrease in mobility. These data are describing which component of self-concept?
   1. Self-esteem.
   2. Body image.
   3. Role performance.
   4. Identity.

4. The nurse knows that activities to promote and enhance a client's self-esteem include: (Select all that apply.)
   1. empowering the client.
   2. encouraging negative self-talk.
   3. providing support and counseling as needed.
   4. using passive skills.
   5. including the client in decision making.
   6. proving information and resources as needed.

5. A 43-year-old male client tells the nurse, "In the last year, my wife has divorced me, my father passed away from cancer, and now last week I lost my job because of downsizing in the company. I really don't know who I am anymore." This statement best reflects a change in the client's:
   1. role.
   2. body image.
   3. self-esteem.
   4. self-awareness.

6. A 12-year-old female client experiencing the onset of menses, pubic and axillary hair growth, breast development, and an increase in height would be identified as being in which of Erikson's stages of development?
   1. Trust versus mistrust.
   2. Autonomy versus shame.
   3. Identity versus role confusion.
   4. Integrity versus despair.

7. A 65-year-old retired schoolteacher states that she is enjoying retirement by traveling and playing more with the grandchildren. According to Erikson's theory, she would be in the stage of:
   1. trust versus mistrust.
   2. autonomy versus shame.
   3. identity versus role confusion.
   4. integrity versus despair.

8. While the nurse is completing a physical exam on a 15-year-old male client, he notices unusual straight razorlike cuts on his forearm. On questioning, the client informs the nurse that he has been cutting himself for the past 6 months because of "unbearable stress" in his life. Which of the following nursing diagnoses is appropriate for the client?
   1. Hopelessness.
   2. Powerlessness.
   3. Disturbed personal identity.
   4. All of the above.

9. A 52-year-old female client has recently been diagnosed with breast cancer. The factor most likely to affect the client's self-concept is:
   1. her health status.
   2. her developmental stage.
   3. her culture.
   4. her ethnicity.

10. The nurse is obtaining a health history on self-concept for a 45-year-old male client who has recently lost his job. Which of the following questions is the most appropriate to ask the client when gathering data regarding self-concept?
   1. "When did you lose your job?"
   2. "Why did the company terminate your work position?"
   3. "How would you describe yourself?"
   4. "How many years did you work there?"

REFERENCES/SUGGESTED READINGS

Bulechek, G., Butcher, H., McCloskey, J., & Dochterman, J. (2008). *Nursing Interventions Classification (NIC)* (5th ed.). St. Louis, MO: Mosby/Elsevier.

Burkhardt, M., & Nathaniel, A. (2008). *Ethics and issues.* Clifton Park, NY: Delmar Cengage Learning.

Cappeliez, P. (2008). An explanation of the reminiscence bump in dreams of older adults in terms of life goals and identity. *Self and Identity, 7*(1), 25–33.

Centers for Disease Control and Prevention. (2005). Self-injury. Retrieved February 7, 2009, from http://www.clevelandclinic.org/disorders/self-injury/hic_self-injury.aspx

Centers for Disease Control and Prevention. (2007). Fastfacts a to z: Overweight. Retrieved February 1, 2009, from http://www.cdc.gov/nchs/fastats/overwt.htm

Centers for Disease Control and Prevention. (2008a). NCHS data on adolescent health. Retrieved February 7, 2009, from http://www.cdc.gov/nchs/data/infosheets/infosheet_adoleshealth.htm

Centers for Disease Control and Prevention. (2008b). Suicide prevention: youth suicide. Retrieved February 7, 2009, from http://www.cdc.gov/ncipc/dvp/suicide/youthsuicide.htm

Centers for Disease Control and Prevention. (2009). College health and safety. Retrieved February 7, 2009, from http://www.cdc.gov/family/college

Chamberlin, J. (2008). A working definition of empowerment. Retrieved February 1, 2009, from http://www.power2u.org/articles/empower/working_def.html

Classen, S., Velozo, C., & Mann, W. (2007). The Rosenberg self-esteem scale as a measure of self-esteem for the noninstitutionalized elderly. *Clinical Gerontologist, 31*(1), 77–93.

Daniels, R., Grendell, R., & Wilkins, F. (2010). *Nursing fundamentals: Caring and clinical decision making* (2nd ed.). Clifton Park, NY: Delmar Cengage Learning.

Delaune, S., & Ladner, P. (2006). *Fundamentals of nursing: Standards and practice* (3rd ed.). Clifton Park, NY: Delmar Cengage Learning.

Erikson, E. (1963). *Childhood and society* (2nd ed.). New York: W. W. Norton

Franken, R. (1994). *Human motivation* (3rd ed.). Pacific Grove, CA: Brooks/Cole.

Hanson, K. (2004). Battling the burden of body image: The healing power of journal writing. Retrieved February 2, 2009, from http://daily.stanford.edu/article/2004/11/17/battlingTheBurdenOfBodyImageTheHealingPowerOfJournalWriting

Hermann, A., & Lucas, G. (2008). Individual differences in perceived esteem across cultures. *Self and Identity, 7*(2), 151–167.

Koch, E., & Shepperd, J. (2008). Testing competence and acceptance explanations of self-esteem. *Self and Identity, 7*(1), 54–74.

Maslow, A. (1987). *Motivation and personality* (3rd ed.). New York: Harper & Row.

Mayo Clinic. (2009). Self-esteem check: Too low, too high or just right? Retrieved February 1, 2009, from http://www.mayoclinic.com/health/seelf-esteem/MH00128

Moorhead, S., Johnson, M., Maas, M., & Swanson, E. (2007). *Nursing Outcomes Classification (NOC)* (4th ed.). St. Louis, MO: Mosby.

National Institutes of Health. (2007). NIH news in health: Stressed out? Stress affects both body and mind. Retrieved February 1, 2009, from http://newsinhealth.nih.gov/2007/January/docs/01features_01.htm

North American Nursing Diagnosis Association International. (2010). *NANDA-I nursing diagnoses: Definitions and classification 2009–2011.* Ames, IA: Wiley-Blackwell.

Rosenberg, M. (1965). *Society and the adolescent self-image.* Princeton, NJ: Princeton University Press.

Wilburn, V., & Smith, D. (2005). Stress, self-esteem, and suicidal ideation in late adolescence. *Adolescence, 40*(157), 33.

RESOURCES

National Alliance on Mental Illness (NAMI), http://www.nami.org

National Empowerment Center, http://www.power2u.org

National Institute of Mental Health, http://www.nimh.nih.gov

National Mental Health Consumers' Self-Help Clearinghouse, http://www.mhselfhelp.org

SAMHSA's National Mental Health Information Center, http://mentalhealth.samhsa.gov

CHAPTER 16
Spirituality

MAKING THE CONNECTION

Refer to the following chapters to increase your understanding of the health care delivery system:

Basic Nursing

- ***Cultural Considerations***
- ***Complementary/Alternative Therapies***

LEARNING OBJECTIVES

Upon completion of this chapter, you should be able to:

- Define key terms.
- Discuss spiritual health concepts.
- List the defining characteristics of spiritual distress.
- Assess the spiritual needs of clients utilizing spiritual assessment models.
- Contribute to a plan of care for a client experiencing spiritual distress.
- Evaluate client outcomes for attainment of spiritual health.

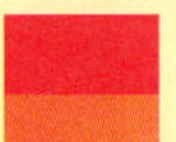

KEY TERMS

faith
hope
meditation
prayer
religion
spiritual distress
spirituality
transcendence
values

INTRODUCTION

Spirituality has come to the forefront of nursing as an important aspect of client care. A growing body of evidence suggests a connection between spirituality and health (Hay, 2002; Park, 2007). **Spirituality** is the core of a person's being, a higher experience or **transcendence** (a state of being or existence above and beyond the limits of material experience) of oneself. The medical advances can make nursing seem more science and technology based (Cavendish et al., 2004). But over the past few years, an increasing number of nurses are advocating care involving the whole person. Assessing and meeting a client's spiritual needs has long been an inherent part of nursing. Incorporating a client's spiritual and religious values in the planning and delivering of care encompasses the art of nursing: caring and being there for the client.

The ever-increasing diverse and mobile society exposes nurses to different values, beliefs, and health care practices. Nurses can find themselves faced with clients who may speak different languages, eat different foods, and believe in healing practices far removed from Western medicine. This diversity may also result in a range of values and beliefs that are vastly different from what nurses believe. Nurses need to find ways to provide nursing care that respects a client's values and offers health care options that will enhance the client's wellness, provide care and comfort during times of illness, and protect and respect the client's choices.

Caring for clients whose values and beliefs are considerably different may pose a dilemma for the nurse if there is conflict with what the nurse believes. Even if there is little conflict, it may be difficult for the nurse to understand or support choices that seem different. In order to provide care that is respectful of beliefs and values, it may be helpful for the nurse to take her personal beliefs and values into consideration. Having a clear understanding of personal principles and convictions will enable the nurse to put the client's beliefs into perspective. Providing spiritual care requires the nurse to have a comfort level with this type of care and also requires conscientious thought and personal reflection.

SPIRITUALITY

For many years, scholars have been attempting to define spirituality. It is difficult to put into words something that cannot be seen, touched, or heard. According to Wilt and Smucker (2001), "The spiritual dimension is one beyond and yet somehow within, the physical and material world" (p. 4). People may have spiritual experiences or feel spiritual, and the experience or feeling is different for every person. Although the word "spirit" may be used in everyday conversation, many nurses find it difficult to describe how spirituality is an integral part of their client's being. Spirituality is often represented in pictures and paintings as a light in the sky (see Figure 16-1).

CRITICAL THINKING

Disclosure

When would it be an appropriate situation for the nurse to disclose her personal values and beliefs to a client?

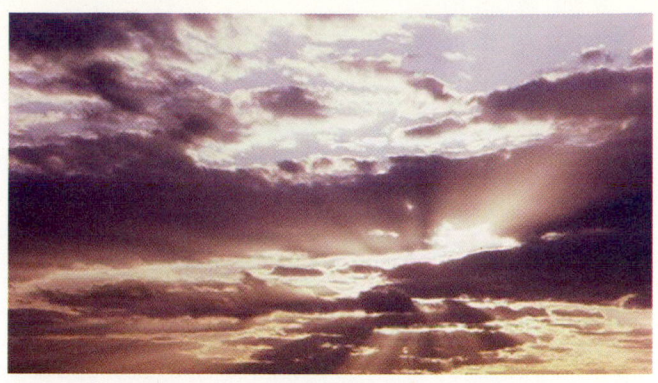

COURTESY OF PHOTO DISC

FIGURE 16-1 **An abstract concept like spirituality is sometimes depicted as the sky, indicating a higher power.**

Over the past 30 years, many nursing authors have defined spirituality. Most agree that spirituality applies to all persons. However, more complex definitions of spirituality have been developed. Table 16-1 lists some of the definitions of spirituality taken from the nursing literature. While there are some differences within the definitions, there is general agreement within the nursing profession regarding spirituality.

For practicing nurses, however, it is important to remember that spirituality is at the core of a person's being and includes the feelings and thoughts that bring purpose and meaning to that person's life. If a nurse can come to understand the client's purpose and meaning, nursing care can support the needs specific for that person. Providing individualized care that is in harmony with the client's spirituality may result in a health care experience that is positive for both the client and the nurse.

SPIRITUAL HEALTH CONCEPTS

A variety of spiritual health concepts are used in describing an individual's spirituality. Nurses need an understanding of these various concepts to better understand their client's personal views of spiritual health.

Faith

The concept of **faith** is closely linked to beliefs. Faith is a confident belief in the truth, value, or trustworthiness of a person, idea, or thing. Faith allows people to hold beliefs that cannot be observed (Mauk & Schmidt, 2004). A client may have faith that God will heal the injury or have faith that the physician will make a correct diagnosis. Faith is frequently referred to in terms of religion such as "faith in God." For the nurse, it is important to note that there are beliefs linking spirituality to health.

LIFE SPAN CONSIDERATIONS

Spirituality in Older Adults

Several research studies have shown that older people believe having a relationship with God supports their psychological well-being (Barton, Grudzen, & Zielske, 2003; Mackenzie, Rajagopal, Meilbohn, & Lavizzo-Mourney, 2000).

Table 16-1 Definitions of Spirituality

LITERATURE SOURCE	DEFINITION
(Macrae, 1995)	In her manuscript "Suggestions for Thought," Nightingale attempted to integrate science and mysticism. She wrote that the universe is the incarnation of a divine intelligence that regulates all things through law. For Nightingale, the laws of science are the "Thoughts of God."
(Burkhardt & Jacobson, 2000)	Spirituality is known and experienced relationships. (p. 95)
(Friesen, 2000)	Spirituality is described as one's quest for vision, meaning, insight, or inspiration. It is the way one sees the world, lives in the world, and derives meaning from the world. Each person's spiritual journey is a highly personalized experience that is different from another's. (p. 13)
(Dossey & Guzzetta, 2000)	Spirituality is a unifying force of a person; the essence of being that permeates all of life and is manifested in one's being, knowing, and doing; the interconnectedness with self, others, nature and God/life. (p. 7)
(Wilt & Smucker, 2001)	Spirituality is the recognition or experience of a dimension of life that is invisible and both within us yet beyond our material world, providing a sense of connectedness and interrelatedness with the universe.
(Carson & Koenig, 2004)	Spirituality is relational even in its focus on meaning and purpose. When people ask questions such as "Why me?," "Why now?," or "What does it mean?," they are attempting to define the relationship of their lives to ultimate truth and reality. (p. 74)
(Galek, Flannelly, Vane, & Galek, 2005)	The Eight Gates of Zen provide a comprehensive model of spirituality including meditation, study with a teacher, academic study, liturgy, right action, art practice, body practice, and work practice. All Zen paths are interrelated: together they provide a more balanced spiritual life. (p. 64)

COURTESY OF DELMAR CENGAGE LEARNING

Prayer

Prayer is defined as a human being's communication with spiritual and divine entities (Gill, 1987). Since prayer is intended for divine beings, humans have very different conceptions of what prayer is and how it should be enacted. Figure 16-2 demonstrates a prayer enactment by showing a spiritual counselor praying with an older adult. However, prayer can occur within and outside a religious context. Thus, a person not affiliated with **religion** (a system of organized beliefs, rituals, and practices with which a person identifies and wishes to be associated) can still engage in prayer (Taylor, 2002). Nurses may be asked to pray with a client, yet prayer can also benefit the nurse in promoting spiritual health.

When questioned about how they cope with the difficulties of illness, many clients report that prayer and faith is what gets them through (Taylor, 2002). Hence, it may also benefit nurses to encourage their own spiritual health. Whether prayer is done in private or communally with a body of believers, the purpose for the nurse is to find the connectedness and meaning for spiritual health.

CRITICAL THINKING

Faith

How can a client's faith help or hinder her recovery from an illness episode?

Meditation

To some, meditation may seem similar to prayer. The main distinguishing feature is that prayer is directed toward a divine entity, whereas **meditation** is an activity that brings the mind and spirit in focus on the present (Mauk & Schmidt, 2004). Meditation also provokes a sense of peace, relaxation, and self-awareness (see Figure 16-3). Meditation has been practiced for thousands of years in many different forms. Taylor (2002) has some introductory suggestions for an individual who is new to meditation (see Box 16-1). It is important to remember that the purpose of using meditation is to help the nurse develop a connectedness to the universe and to experience peacefulness and relaxation.

Values

Values are principles, standards, or qualities considered worthwhile or desirable. Individuals may not always be aware of their values, yet each person has a core set of personal values. Values can encompass a wide range of situations with common values involving such matters as the belief in hard work and punctuality. At the other end of the spectrum are psychological values, such as self-reliance, concern for others, and harmony of purpose (Posner, 2006). The way a person behaves or spends time or money can be indicative of the

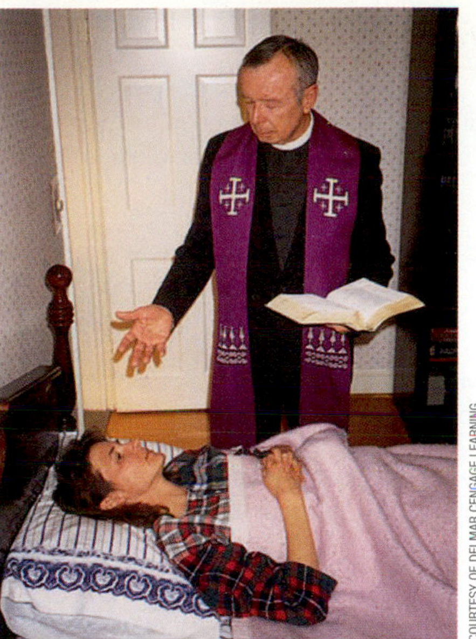

FIGURE 16-2 Today, spiritual counselors freely pray with their clients as part of providing spiritual care.

values he holds. Thus, someone who claims to value the environment can be expected to endorse recycling programs.

Values are formed over a person's lifetime and at first are learned from parents. Over the years, these can change as a child is exposed to friends, school, the media, and the community. Simon, Howe, and Kirschenbaum (1978) identified four ways parents and adults may transmit values to their children (see Table 16-2).

When a person needs to make an important decision, personal values help determine what choice the person will make. Awareness of the client's values will help the nurse

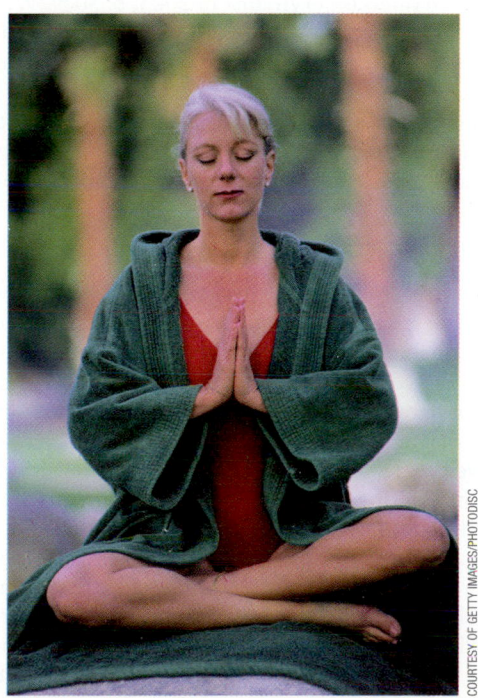

FIGURE 16-3 Developing Self-Awareness in Quiet Meditation

Box 16-1 Introductory Suggestions for Meditation

- Select a short phrase to repeat during the meditation. Some people select a prayer or verse that is meaningful.
- Assume a comfortable position.
- Close the eyes.
- Relax the muscles.
- Maintain a passive attitude.
- Develop an awareness of breathing and concentrate on a slow and rhythmic pattern.

provide care that will be supportive of the client's decisions. Moreover, the nurse's awareness of her own values will add a stronger dimension of understanding regarding the client's choices. A nurse who has gone through the process of becoming aware of her values, like embracing diversity, will be able to better understand her client's reluctance to be cared for by a nurse whose ethnicity is different from the client's.

THE JOINT COMMISSION SPIRITUAL CARE CRITERIA

The Joint Commission, a major accrediting agency for hospitals, includes spiritual care criteria in their accreditation criteria. Specifically, the Joint Commission recommends that "healthcare organizations 1) acknowledge patient's rights to spiritual care and 2) provide for these needs through pastoral care and a diversity of services that may be offered by certified, ordained, or lay individuals" (La Pierre, 2003, p. 219). Nursing organizations have also crafted statements reflecting the need to incorporate spiritual care in everyday practice. The International Council of Nurses (2006), a federation of national nurse's organizations, include spiritual care in their code of ethics stating that, "in providing care, the nurse promotes an environment in which the human rights, values, customs and spiritual beliefs of the individual, family and community are respected." Furthermore, the American Association of Colleges of Nursing (1995) advocates teaching students how to conduct spiritual care assessments, nursing diagnoses, interventions, and outcomes. For these reasons, developing spiritual awareness can be a key step toward providing care that encompasses the client's need for the search for meaning during times of illness.

AMERICAN NURSES ASSOCIATION CODE OF ETHICS

The American Nurses Association (ANA, 2005) *Code of Ethics* clearly states the ethical responsibility for providing spiritual care. Specifically, the code states, "An individual's lifestyle, value system and religious beliefs should be considered in planning health care with and for each patient. Such consideration does not suggest that the nurse necessarily agrees with or condones certain individual choices, but that the nurse respects the patient as a person" (ANA, 2005, Provision 1:1.2). Furthermore, the code also addresses spirituality by stating,

TABLE 16-2 Four Ways Parents Transmit Values to Children

Moralizing	From an early age, some parents teach their own moral values to their children in the hopes of preparing them to lead productive lives. Moralizing instills the values without giving the recipient an opportunity to compare different values.
Laissez-faire	This attitude allows the child to explore different values without parental or adult intervention. Children, however, may become confused and conflicted as they attempt to make sense of the different values they encounter.
Modeling	Children learn values from those who exhibit the behavior associated with the value. Modeling can lead to both socially acceptable and socially unacceptable behavior.
Values clarification	Helps young people develop their own value system by answering questions that may be confusing. Values clarification assists by providing a mechanism by which adolescents can make decisions when faced with conflicting values.

COURTESY OF DELMAR CENGAGE LEARNING

"The measures nurses take to care for the patient enable the patient to live with as much physical, emotional, social and spiritual well-being as possible" (Provision 1:1.3). Thus, nurses are ethically bound to provide care for the spiritual well-being of the client. It is then up to the nurse to ensure that spiritual assessment and interventions are provided for the client's well-being. Under no circumstances should nurses engage in the promotion of personal religious beliefs. Any act that resembles proselytizing is an unethical practice and should be avoided at all times.

As stated previously, the ANA's (2005) *Code of Ethics* explicitly deals with the provision of spiritual care. The code also provides nurses with a guide for managing diversity of beliefs and values. "The nurse strives to provide patients with opportunities to participate in planning care, assures that patients find the plans acceptable and supports the implementation of the plan" (Provision 2:2.1). Furthermore, the code states, "Nurses must examine the conflicts arising between their own personal and professional values, the values and interests of others who are also responsible for patient care and health care decisions, as well as those of patients. Nurses strive to resolve such conflicts in ways that ensure patient safety, guard the patient's best interests and preserve the professional integrity of the nurse" (Provision 2:2.2). Key in this section is the reference to protecting the patient's interests while preserving one's own professional integrity.

An example of how the *Code of Ethics* can help a nurse is illustrated with the birth process. A Hmong family may participate in spiritual practices designed to protect their children from evil spirits. One of these consists of tying strings on a child's wrist to bind the child's soul to the body. Over time, these strings may become soiled (Fadiman, 1997). The nurse believes this practice is not appropriate and wants to cut them off, believing circulation could be impaired. This then results in a conflict between the family and the nurse. A review of the *Code of Ethics* reveals that the nurse's responsibility is to examine the conflict and then to resolve it with the client. An assessment of the family's beliefs related to the behavior is of utmost importance to resolve this conflict. When the nurse begins to understand the rationale behind the religious practice, the differences between the nurse and the client can be managed in a way that respects the client.

SPIRITUAL DISTRESS

Many clients experience spiritual distress when faced with a health care crisis. This spiritual distress causes various responses in many areas of the client's life, including physical, mental, psychosocial, and spiritual.

DEFINITION

Spiritual distress is defined as "disruption in the life principle that pervades a person's entire being and that integrates and transcends one's biologic and psychosocial nature" (Cox et al., 2002, p. 683) A similar definition of spiritual distress suggests an "impaired ability to experience and integrate meaning and purpose in life through a person's connectedness with self, others, art, music, literature, nature, or a power greater than oneself" (Wilkinson, 2005, p. 507). While somewhat different, these two definitions share the notion that a client in this situation may have a troubled, fragmented, or possibly disintegrating spirit (Wilt & Smucker, 2001). Given the relationship between health and spirituality, expedient diagnosis and intervention for a client experiencing spiritual distress may possibly enhance recovery and promote wellness.

DESCRIPTION

Over the past 30 years, nurses have been developing ways in which to help clients with their spiritual needs. Recognizing that spirituality is personal and not necessarily grounded in religion, the North American Nursing Diagnosis Association International (NANDA-I) first developed spirituality-related nursing diagnoses in 1979 (Mauk & Schmidt, 2004). These diagnoses were labeled "spiritual concerns," "spiritual distress," and "spiritual despair." Over the years, these labels have been refined, and today, "spiritual distress" is the accepted label for addressing the needs of the client. Another way of describing this diagnosis is distress of the human spirit, essentially conveying the idea that there are factors causing disequilibrium for the client. The factors can be the response to disease, family altercations, self-doubt, or reasons a client might lose sight of personal meaning. Nurses now routinely assess the client's spirit, and spiritual care needs are addressed as part of holistic nursing care.

Defining Characteristics

A client experiencing spiritual distress will most likely exhibit signs and symptoms indicating distress. Just as a client with impaired gas exchange may exhibit signs of cyanosis or confusion and symptoms of dyspnea, the client experiencing spiritual distress will show evidence of the distress. Box 16-2 summarizes the defining characteristics of spiritual distress.

The defining characteristics related to spiritual distress stem from both subjective and objective data. Thus, clients may verbally express concerns such as conflicting feelings about previously held religious beliefs. Furthermore, the nurse may be the one to whom the client turns, as she may feel uncomfortable talking to a family member about these conflicts. Other signs of spiritual distress may be evident as behavior that will require additional assessment as to the cause.

When dealing with clients who may be experiencing spiritual distress, the nurse needs to use all manner of assessment skills since the signs and symptoms may be subtle. A client may initiate the discussion by asking the nurse, "Why is this happening to me? Why must I suffer so much?" An opening statement such as this is like an invitation for the nurse to further explore the client's illness experience from a spiritual perspective. Other cues, however, are not as straightforward and may require the nurse to be attuned to subtle innuendos. For example, a client experiencing spiritual distress may complain only of sleeplessness and not feeling rested. A nurse who suggests the client take a sleeping aid may be missing an opportunity to assist the client through a difficult period.

Box 16-2 Spiritual Distress: Defining Characteristics

- Expresses lack of acceptance
- Expresses lack of courage
- Expresses lack of hope
- Expresses lack of love
- Expresses lack of meaning in life
- Expresses lack of purpose in life
- Expresses lack of serenity (e.g., peace)
- Guilt
- Poor coping
- Displacement of anger toward religious representative
- Expresses anger toward God

From *Nursing Diagnoses: Definitions and Classification 2009–2011*, by North American Nursing Diagnosis Association International, 2010, Ames IA: Wiley-Blackwell.

NURSING PROCESS

The nursing process is used in the same way as for other client problems. One of the major differences is in the data collection methods and tools used. Conducting a spiritual care assessment requires sensitivity and compassion.

ASSESSMENT

To assess the person's spirit requires a consideration of both subjective and objective data. While the objectivedata may seem unrelated, subtle objective signs may be evident and would cue the nurse that additional assessment may be necessary. For example, a client who has been communicative and outgoing in the past may show episodes of silence and disinterest. The spiritually aware nurse, seeing the change in behavior, can explore the client's feelings using a spiritual assessment tool. At times it may be difficult for the nurse not to feel intrusive. However, nurses have a moral responsibility to address and manage all aspects of client care.

Spiritual Assessment Models

Various authors and researchers have developed models that can assist the nurse to assess spirituality. A comprehensive spiritual assessment tool provides a valuable mechanism to address these sometimes sensitive issues. Novice nurses are encouraged to use these tools until they find a way that works well for them in actual practice. There are many spiritual care models available, with many originating from the fields of psychology and pastoral care. Assessment guides developed from these models can be a valuable tool to help the nurse gather relevant spirituality data. Limiting spiritual care assessments questions to religious preference restricts the focus of spirituality. Therefore, making use of a spiritual care model will allow the nurse to conduct a comprehensive spiritual assessment leading to identification and management of client needs (Taylor, 2002). The following models provide useful tools for nurses conducting spiritual assessments.

CASE STUDY: FAMILY EXPERIENCING SPIRITUAL DISTRESS

M.B., a 73-year-old widow, has been admitted to the intensive care unit with the diagnosis of a massive cerebrovascular accident. She is experiencing both dysphagia and dysphasia. Over the past 3 days, her condition has deteriorated, and the family has decided to stop all heroic measures. M.B. has four daughters, and at least two have been at her bedside around the clock. At 9:00 A.M., the cardiac monitor shows a bradycardia with subsequent asystole. All four daughters are present, tearfully saying good-bye to their mother. A nurse enters the room, places her hand on one daughter's shoulder, and begins to sing the hymn "Amazing Grace." The daughter angrily shrugs off the nurse's hand and tells her to leave the room.

The following questions will guide your development of contributions to the nursing care plan for the case study.

1. After making these observations, what nursing diagnosis and goals might the nurse identify for M.B.'s family?
2. List the nursing interventions to be performed in caring for M.B.'s family.

Stoll (1979) developed one of the first nursing spiritual care models for nursing. This model is predicated on the notion that not all clients have clearly identified and articulated religious beliefs, and some may find the discussion threatening. The model has four distinct dimensions and suggests guiding questions to elicit the information. Spiritual issues can be burdened with emotions, so conducting the assessment at the latter part of the nursing interview may be more comfortable for both the client and the nurse (Stoll, 1979).

Another spiritual assessment model uses the acronym FICA to guide assessment questions (Puchalski & Romer, 2000). This basic model allows the health care practitioner to incorporate the spiritual assessment questions in the initial client interview. Additionally, the model provides an avenue for the client to be in control of the way in which her spiritual issues are addressed. The FICA model is straightforward to use and provides a method to document the results simply and straightforward. Moreover, the acronym is easy to remember and gives the nurse the ability to conduct a spiritual assessment when a sudden opportunity arises (Mauk & Schmidt, 2004).

Another spiritual assessment tool incorporates the dimensions of meaning and purpose, inner strengths, and interconnections (Dossey, 1998). Although not a specific model, the dimensions of this tool provide ways to elicit client information regarding spirituality. Relying heavily on the concept of holistic nursing, the tool focuses on determining how a person makes sense of meaning in her life. While there is some focus on divinity, this tool may be especially useful for clients who are not affiliated with a formal religion. Furthermore, using these questions, the nurse can easily perform a spiritual self-assessment (see Table 16-3).

MEMORY TRICK

FICA represents the following:

F = Faith or beliefs
What is your faith? Do you consider yourself religious? What gives meaning to your life?

I = Importance and influence
Is it important in your life? What influence does it have on how you take care of yourself? Have your beliefs influenced your behavior during this illness? What role do your beliefs play in regaining your health?

C = Community
Are you part of a spiritual or religious community? Is this a support to you and how? Are there people who support you or are really important to you?

A = Address
How would you like me to address these issues in your nursing care?

A model developed for use by physicians is also useful for nursing. Created by Maugans (1996), the model utilizes the acronym SPIRIT. The acronym makes this model easy to remember and may afford the nurse the opportunity to implement this when the opportunity presents itself. Using this model, the nurse can ask questions appropriate to the client's developmental level and specific situation (Maugans, 1996;

TABLE 16-3 Spiritual Assessment Tool

The following reflective questions may assist you in assessing, evaluating, and increasing spirituality in yourself and others.

Meaning and Purpose These questions assess a person's ability to seek meaning and fulfillment in life, manifest hope, and accept ambiguity and uncertainty.	• What gives your life meaning? • Do you have a sense of purpose in life? • Does your illness interfere with your life goals? • Why do you want to get well? • How hopeful are you about obtaining a better degree of health? • Do you feel that you have a responsibility in maintaining your health? • Will you be able to make changes in your life to maintain your health? • Are you motivated to get well? • What is the most important or powerful thing in your life?
Inner Strengths These questions assess a person's ability to manifest joy and recognize strengths, choices, goals, and faith.	• What brings you joy and peace in your life? • What can you do to feel alive and full of spirit? • What traits do you like about yourself? • What are your personal strengths? • What choices are available to you to enhance your healing? • What life goals have you set for yourself? • Do you think that stress in any way caused your illness? • How aware were you of your body before you became sick? • What do you believe in? • Is faith important in your life? • How has your illness influenced your faith? • Does faith play a role in recognizing your health?

(*Continues*)

Table 16-3 Spiritual Assessment Tool (Continued)

Interconnections These questions assess a person's positive self-concept, self-esteem, and sense of self; sense of belonging in the world with others; capacity to pursue personal interests; and ability to demonstrate love of self and self-forgiveness.	• How do you feel about yourself right now? • How do you feel when you have a true sense of yourself? • Do you pursue things of personal interest? • What do you do to show love for yourself? • Can you forgive yourself? • What do you do to heal your spirit?
These questions assess a person's ability to connect in life-giving ways with family, friends, and social groups and to engage in the forgiveness of others.	• Who are the significant people in your life? • Do you have friends or family in town who are available to help you? • Who are the people to who you are the closest? • Do you belong to any groups? • Can you ask people for help when you need it? • Can you share your feelings with others? • What are some of the most loving things that others have done for you? • What are the loving things that you do for other people? • Are you able to forgive others?
These questions assess a person's capacity for finding meaning in worship or religious activities and a connectedness with a divinity.	• Is worship important to you? • What do you consider the most significant act of worship in your life? • Do you participate in any religious activities • Do you believe in God or a higher power? • Do you think that prayer is powerful? • Have you ever tried to empty your mind of all thoughts to see what the experience might be? • Do you use relaxation or imagery skills? • Do you meditate? • Do you pray? • What is your prayer? • How are your prayers answered? • Do you have a sense of belonging in this world?
These questions assess a person's ability to experience a sense of connectedness with life and nature, an awareness of the effects of the environment on life and well-being, and a capacity or concern for the health of the environment.	• Do you ever feel a connection with the world or universe? • How does your environment have an impact on your state of well-being? • What are your environmental stressors at work and at home? • What strategies reduce your environmental stressors? • Do you have any concerns for the state of your immediate environment? • Are you involved with environmental issues such as recycling environmental resources at home, work, or in your community? • Are you concerned about the survival of the planet?

From Holistic Modalities and Healing Moments, by B. Dossey, 2008, *American Journal of Nursing, 98*(6), 44–47.

Mauk & Schmidt, 2004). Although this model is focused primarily on religious affiliation, it can provide a starting point for a spiritual assessment. Once this information has been gathered, the nurse can conduct a more in-depth assessment addressing life meaning, connectedness, and client strength.

Cultural Differences When conducting assessments, the nurse should include the cultural uniqueness of the client. Culture, religion, and spirituality are closely related in that these concepts frequently are intertwined in a client's life. Thus, religion, health, spirituality, and healing are highly interdependent and require compassionate attention when caring for clients from different cultures. Sensitivity in matters concerning religion and healing is necessary in order to protect the client's autonomy. Moreover, it is important for nurses to recognize that addressing religious issues during times of

MEMORYTRICK

Spiritual assessment using the **SPIRIT** model:

S = Spiritual belief system

P = Personal spirituality

I = Integration and involvement in a spiritual community

R = Ritualized practices and restrictions

I = Implications for medical (nursing) care

T = Terminal events planning (advance directives)

health crisis may not be beneficial for the client. Instead, it may be more appropriate to engage the help of the client's spiritual leader (Mauk & Schmidt, 2004).

Determining spiritual needs from clients from other cultures is not much different from the basic spiritual assessment. Special attention to the client's environment may provide information that religion is part of the person's spiritual makeup. Religious items, get-well cards, or special clothing can alert the nurse to focus the assessment. Client behavior and verbalization also may indicate the presence of religion or spirituality in the client's life. Special attention may need to be given to health situations, such as death and bereavement, which include spiritual and religious components (Andrews & Boyle 2003; Spector, 2004).

Nursing Diagnoses

Once the assessment has been completed, the nurse analyzes the subjective and objective data to determine if a spiritual problem exists. Based on the assessment, the nurse selects either *Spiritual well-being, Spiritual Distress, or Risk for Spiritual Distress.*

For clients who are spiritually healthy, there are actions the nurse can take to increase spiritual well-being. The appropriate nursing diagnosis is *Spiritual well-being, readiness for enhanced,* and is defined as "the ability to experience and integrate meaning and purpose in life through a person's connectedness with self, others, art, music, literature, nature, or a power greater than oneself" (Wilkinson, 2005, p. 513).

Wilkinson (2005) divides the defining characteristics of this nursing diagnosis into four categories: connections to self; connections with art, music, literature, and nature; connections with others; and connections with power greater than self. The descriptions under each category may be helpful for the nurse in determining if the client is ready for enhanced spiritual well-being (see Concept Map 16-1).

At times it may be difficult to differentiate between the diagnoses. It may help to remember that spiritual distress is an actual problem occurring at the time of the assessment. Clients with spiritual distress exhibit characteristics that can cue the nurse. A review of the defining characteristics can help the nurse sort through the assessment data to make the clinical judgment.

Clients who are at risk for spiritual distress may not state or indicate that they have a disruption of the spirit. These clients are experiencing situations where spiritual distress may occur. Thus nurses must be aware of their client's circumstances and behavior and note when spiritual distress may occur. The diagnosis of risk for spiritual distress will allow the nurse to intervene and assist the client to avert actual spiritual distress. Table 16-4 illustrates the differences between *Spiritual Distress* and *Risk for Spiritual Distress.*

Clients can respond to illness experiences in a variety of ways. The psychosocial responses may be difficult to categorize and treat. The following are diagnoses related to spiritual distress:

- *Ineffective individual coping*
- *Anxiety*
- *Chronic sorrow*
- *Decisional conflict*
- *Powerlessness*

Individuals sometimes have difficulty coping with the effects of illness. If this is the case, a more appropriate diagnosis would be *Ineffective Individual Coping* (Cox et al., 2002; Wilkinson, 2005). A diagnosis that may be more appropriate to the client's situation is anxiety, especially if the situation is related to death and dying. *Chronic Sorrow and Decisional Conflict* are two more diagnoses that may be used with clients who are having difficult illness experiences (Wilkinson, 2005). Another diagnosis that may be used is *Powerlessness.* Client's may feel powerless during illness but express this in terms of disruption of the spirit.

Planning/Outcome Identification

Contributing to the plan of care requires careful thought and design. Matters of the spirit are personal, and the nurse needs to ensure that goals and interventions are acceptable to the client. As such, some of the suggested goals and interventions are intended to place the nurse in the role of a supporter.

If the nurse has conducted an empathetic assessment and used sound clinical judgment in determining the nursing diagnosis, the client will most likely be in agreement with the plan of care. The goal should be client focused and realistic. Since clients may be believe that all people have a spirit, some expressing this through formal religion and others through connectedness with the universe, a wide variety of possible outcomes exist. Table 16-5 depicts some outcomes that would be appropriate to manage spiritual distress.

As can be seen, the goals or outcomes for managing spiritual distress are not necessarily measurable or time limited. That is because spirituality is dynamic, and change may take months or even years. Wilkinson (2005) suggests short-term or immediate goals that are appropriate for the hospitalized client (see Box 16-3).

For clients experiencing spiritual distress, these goals can seem more realistic and easier to attain. Once the client feels comfortable with these smaller steps, she may be ready to address spirituality on a more long-term basis.

Implementation

The second step for contributing to a plan of care is designing the interventions. There is a vast difference between interventions for a biological problem and interventions for a spiritual problem. For spiritual care, the nurse uses a different type of intervention. This is due to the very unique nature of spirituality. If a client has no **hope** (to look forward to with confidence or expectation), the nurse cannot give a client hope. Instead, the nurse can support the hoping abilities of the client.

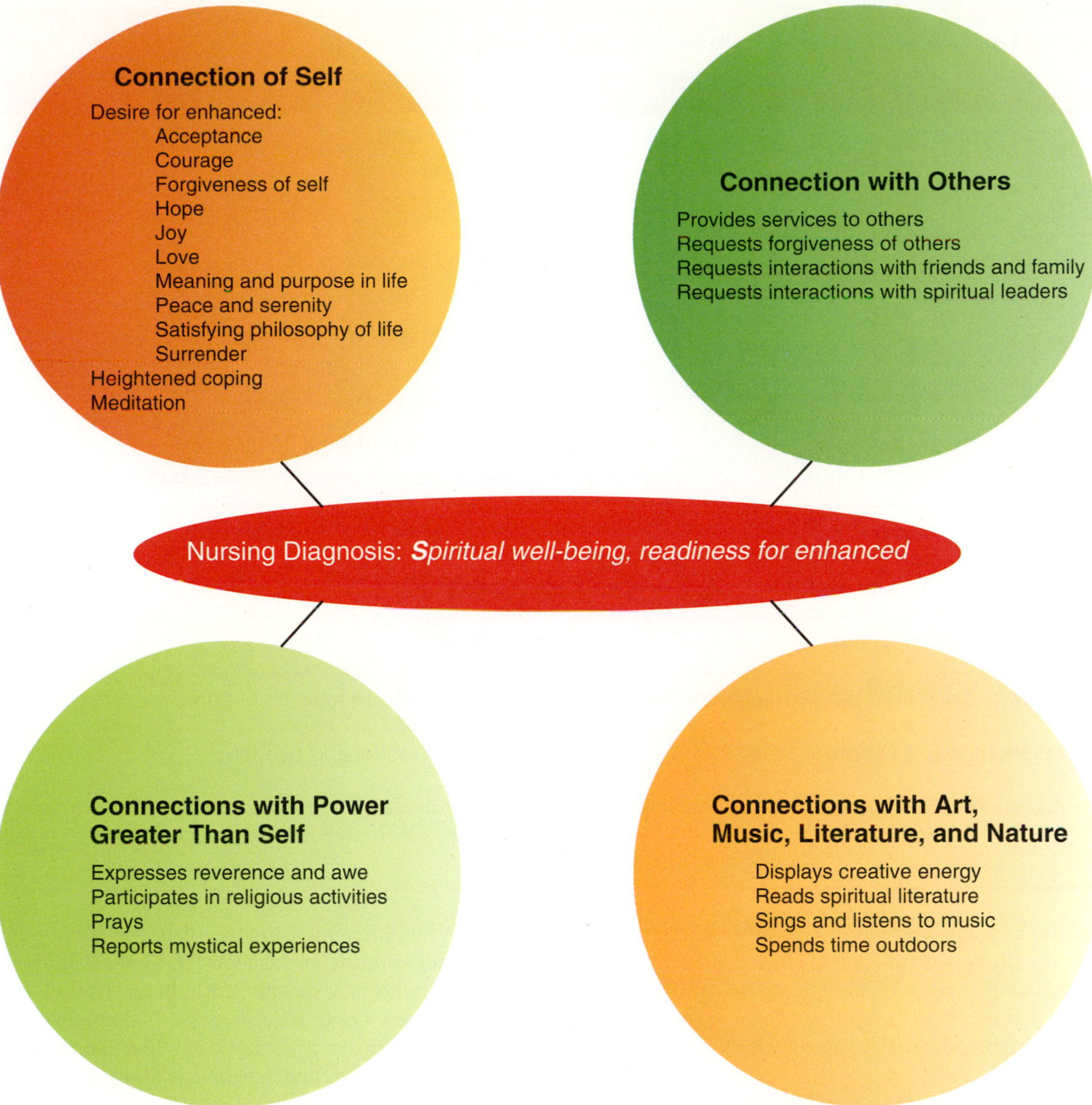
Connection of Self
Desire for enhanced:
Acceptance
Courage
Forgiveness of self
Hope
Joy
Love
Meaning and purpose in life
Peace and serenity
Satisfying philosophy of life
Surrender
Heightened coping
Meditation
Connection with Others
Provides services to others
Requests forgiveness of others
Requests interactions with friends and family
Requests interactions with spiritual leaders
Nursing Diagnosis: Spiritual well-being, readiness for enhanced
Connections with Power Greater Than Self
Expresses reverence and awe
Participates in religious activities
Prays
Reports mystical experiences
Connections with Art, Music, Literature, and Nature
Displays creative energy
Reads spiritual literature
Sings and listens to music
Spends time outdoors

CONCEPT MAP 16-1

TABLE 16-4 Differences Between Spiritual Distress and Risk for Spiritual Distress

SPIRITUAL DISTRESS	RISK FOR SPIRITUAL DISTRESS
T.M., a 33-year-old married woman, is recovering from a total abdominal hysterectomy. She has a 12-year-old son. She is crying and says to the nurse, "I signed the form saying I know I won't be able to have more children. Everyone tells me how to recover from surgery. But no one has talked to me about what I feel like. I wanted more children, and now that's impossible. I feel like part of what I am as a woman is missing."	P.B. had a total prostatectomy 5 years ago. Two years ago, he underwent radiation treatment for a rise in prostate-specific antigen (PSA). After 18 months of a stable PSA, he has just been told that the latest PSA level has risen to 2.6. He tells the nurse, "I just don't understand it; I have done everything right. I had routine PSA screenings, my surgery was done in a timely manner, I underwent radiation, and I eat right and exercise. What else could I have done? I am so frustrated. The next treatment will be so much worse. What else do I have to do to keep this cancer from coming back?"
Diagnosis statement: ***S****piritual Distress* related to questioning about the meaning of her role in life.	*Diagnosis statement:* ***S****piritual Distress,* risk for, related to recurring elevated PSA levels and future uncertainty.

COURTESY OF DELMAR CENGAGE LEARNING

Table 16-5 Goals and Evaluation Criteria: Spiritual Distress

GOAL	EVIDENCE
• Demonstrate hope	• Expression of faith • Meaning in life • Inner peace
• Demonstrate spiritual well-being	• Meaning and purpose in life • Spiritual world view • Serenity, love, and forgiveness • Prayer, worship, or meditation • Interaction with spiritual leaders • Connectedness with inner self • Connectedness with others to share thoughts, feelings, and beliefs
• Describe support systems	• Access during times of spiritual crisis
• Decreased sense of anxiety regarding . . .	• Verbalization
• Decreased dissatisfaction with . . .	• Verbalization
• Movement toward increased positive regard for God	• Verbalizes decreased feelings of anger
• Decreased feelings of sadness	• Appears more restful and peaceful

From *Clinical Applications of Nursing Diagnosis: Adult, Child, Psychiatric, Gerontic, and Home Health Considerations* (4th ed.), by H. Cox et al., 2002, Philadelphia: F. A. Davis; *Spiritual Care, Nursing Theory, Research, and Practice,* by E. Taylor, 2002, Upper Saddle River, NJ: Prentice Hall; *Nursing Diagnosis Handbook,* by J. Wilkinson, 2005, Upper Saddle River, NJ: Prentice Hall.

The traditional nursing intervention definition suggests that nurses "do" something for the client. However, with spiritual care, the nurse should "be" with the client (Mayer, 1992). The nurse strives to establish an environment where the client can share concerns, be heard, and be supported.

General Interventions and Activities

Some of the interventions useful for managing spiritual care are those designed to "boost the spirit" (Taylor, 2002). These interventions are used with other nursing diagnoses, such as ***P**owerless, Chronic **S**orrow, and **A**nxiety*. General interventions should be used by nurses as part of standardized nursing care since these are the hallmark of caring (see Box 16-4).

Box 16-3 Appropriate Goals for the Hospitalized Client

These goals or outcomes suggest that the client will do the following:

- Acknowledge that illness is a challenge to belief system
- Acknowledge that treatment conflicts with belief system
- Demonstrate coping techniques to deal with spiritual distress
- Express acceptance of limited religious or cultural ties
- Discuss spiritual practices or concerns

When implementing the plan, the nurse must make sure the interventions are acceptable to the client. For example, a client who is a devout Catholic and relies on prayer and worship services to meet her spiritual needs may find guided imagery offensive and think it is part of New Age religion. Sensitivity to the client's beliefs is of utmost importance.

Role of Prayer

Some nurses may question whether they should pray with a client. Prayer is a very personal and private act and should be approached with respect. If a client requests that the nurse pray, it is important to determine what the client's prayer habits are. A Muslim client may not appreciate a Christian nurse's prayer to Jesus. Some religious traditions support ritualized prayer, while others incorporate a conversational style. A nurse can offer to pray with a client, but permission should be obtained first.

Seeking out peers with more experience can be beneficial for the novice nurse. For example, a novice nurse was caring for an elderly client who asked her to pray with him. The novice nurse asked, "What religion are you?" The client responded by saying he was Catholic. The novice nurse had no idea what kind of prayer Catholics used, so she solicited the help of a

PROFESSIONALTIP

Today, spiritual care is a recognized nursing activity. One key point for nurses to remember is that every person experiences spirituality in a unique way.

Box 16-4 General Interventions

General interventions used by nurses include the following:

- Active listening
- Caring touch
- Guided imagery
- Use of humor
- Meditation
- Client involvement in care and decision making
- Calm environment

fellow nurse who was a practicing Catholic. Both nurses came to the client's bedside, and while the Catholic nurse prayed, the other held the client's hand and listened. Even though the novice nurse had little experience, she was able to use her caring concern to provide spiritual care to the client.

Being Present

A new nurse may find attending to spiritual needs daunting. One intervention that requires no special training is being present. Presence can be defined as a giving of one's self in the present moment. It also includes listening with full awareness of the privilege of being there for a person—to be available with all the self in a way that is meaningful to another person (Pettigrew, 1990). Presence is an active intervention and suggests more than a physical presence. The nurse who makes eye contact while listening instead of writing notes on the clipboard is exhibiting presence. The client is the one who can most accurately identify nurses who are present.

PROFESSIONALTIP

The history of nursing demonstrates strong support for spiritual care as an integral part of nursing care. The past 20 years have shown a renewed interest in spiritual care. This renewed interest is based on the results from nursing research that demonstrates the positive outcomes when nurses engage in spiritual care (Taylor, 2002).

PROFESSIONALTIP

Most hospitals have a spiritual care or similar department frequently staffed by someone who has had formal or informal spiritual training. The hospital chaplain may be the most immediate resource available to the nurse. Before any professionals are notified, it is important for the nurse to ask the client if he or she wishes a visit from a clergy of their choice.

Evaluation

At times, it may be difficult to evaluate the outcomes of spiritual distress. Evaluating the outcome for airway clearance is objective: either the airway is clear or it is not. However, Mauk and Schmidt (2004) point out that a person cannot truly observe the spirit. It is therefore imperative that the nurse first involve the client when writing the outcome statements. This will allow the client to state whether the goal was met.

Family Involvement

Up to now, the recommended resources for spiritual care have been personnel trained in spiritual care. Clergy, spiritual leaders, and parish nurses can provide valuable assistance for the client in spiritual distress. However, the family can also be included as spiritual care resources. The family may understand the client's situation and the client's religious and spiritual preferences and share the rituals and celebrations of faith. Family can pray with the client, be present, and provide love and empathy. The nurse's role can be to encourage family participation. The nurse can also be the one who can arrange the client's activities to include private time for prayer and reflection. Keeping the client at the center of concern, the nurse can help the family continue to provide the support they wish to give.

SAMPLE NURSING CARE PLAN

The Client with Spiritual Distress

R.G. is a 53-year-old man diagnosed with colon cancer. He was admitted with severe rectal bleeding, and tests showed that surgery needed to be done soon. R.G. has been married to his wife for 12 years. They have one daughter. This is R.G.'s first marriage but his wife's second. She has two sons from a previous marriage who no longer live at home. Both R.G. and his wife are practicing Catholics. His wife's first marriage was conducted by a priest in the Catholic Church. When that marriage broke up, she chose not to ask for annulment, believing it was in the best interest of her children. Six years later, she met and married R.G. However, because she was a divorced woman, they were not allowed to marry in the Church.

(Continues)

SAMPLE NURSING CARE PLAN (Continued)

Over the past 12 years, they have attended Sunday mass and taken communion. According to Catholic Church doctrine, couples like R.G. and his wife may not receive communion. The couple has decided that since the church is large, they could just quietly do so anyway. Now R.G. is facing a serious surgery, and he wants the priest to bring him communion. The church they attend is very strict and follows the rules and regulations prescribed by the Church in Rome. Although they will send a priest to visit, the senior priest will not allow R.G. to take communion. R.G. is devastated and tells his primary nurse that he just doesn't understand. He believes in the Catholic Church with all his heart yet believes he has done nothing wrong marrying his wife. After all, it is his first marriage. "How can they deny me access to God?" he asks.

NURSING DIAGNOSIS *Spiritual Distress* related to separation from religious practices

Nursing Outcomes Classification (NOC)
Hope
Spiritual
Emotional Support

Nursing Interventions Classification (NIC)
Spiritual Support
Well-Being Coping Enhancement

PLANNING/OUTCOMES	NURSING INTERVENTION	RATIONALE
R.G. and his family will demonstrate spiritual well-being as evidenced by prayer.	Conduct a focused assessment regarding R.G.'s faith, prayer life, relationship to spiritual leaders, and receptiveness to a visit from the hospital chaplain.	Obtaining assessment data that are pertinent to R.G. specific to his religion or spiritual beliefs and practices will improve the nurse's understanding of the client's needs.
R.G. and his family will discuss spiritual concerns with a spiritual leader.	Conduct an indirect assessment of R.G.'s spiritual status by observing R.G.'s concept of God through books, exploring R.G.'s meaning in life, determining R.G.'s source of hope and strength, asking "Who is most important to you?" and observing for signs of prayer and meditation.	Obtaining indirect assessment data will improve the nurse's understanding of the client's needs.
	Request spiritual consultation.	During a time of crisis, R.G. may not have the inner strength to call for spiritual consultation without assistance.
R.G. and his family will verbalize connectedness to God.	Involve his wife in spiritual care conferences.	This facilitates communication between R.G. and his wife, may reduce the feeling of isolation, and may facilitate a resolution of the spiritual distress that he is feeling.
	Encourage his wife to pray and be with R.G.	This faciliates communication and interaction between R.G. and his wife and may facilitate a resolution of the spiritual distress.
	Be open to R.G.'s expressions of anger and disappointment.	Allowing R.G. to express his emotions creates a supportive climate and demonstrates caring.
	Assure R.G. you will be available for support.	Being present and allowing the opportunity to express emotions creates a supportive climate and sends a message of caring.

(*Continues*)

SAMPLE NURSING CARE PLAN (Continued)

EVALUATION

Evidence of R.G.'s progress toward relieving spiritual distress is his verbalization of a closer relationship with God. He might also indicate that he would like to visit with a spiritual leader, such as the hospital chaplain. A continued close relationship with his wife indicates that he does not blame her.

SUMMARY

- Spirituality is the core of a person's being, the dimension of life that is invisible, and brings meaning to one's life.
- Research studies have shown that spirituality is closely related to health.
- Values and beliefs are closely connected to spirituality: the search for meaning and making sense of life.
- Beliefs and spirituality may have strong ties to religion.
- Religion is not necessary for spirituality.
- Nurses should be sensitive to clients experiencing spiritual distress.
- Several spiritual care models exist that can help nurses conduct a spiritual assessment.
- A trusting nurse–client relationship is necessary and provides an environment where the client feels free and safe to share private thoughts and feelings.
- Family involvement can be beneficial for the client experiencing spiritual distress.

REVIEW QUESTIONS

1. Which of the following statements is correct regarding spirituality?
   1. A growing body of evidence does not suggest a connection between spirituality and health.
   2. Spirituality is the core of a person's being, a higher experience or transcendence of oneself.
   3. Assessing and meeting a client's spiritual needs is a new concept in nursing.
   4. The Four Gates of Zen provide a comprehensive model of spirituality.
2. When discussing spirituality with a client, the nurse knows that the definition of values is/are:
   1. principles, standards, or qualities considered worthwhile or desirable.
   2. a confident belief in the truth, value, or trustworthiness of a person, idea, or thing.
   3. human communication with divine and spiritual entities.
   4. an activity that brings the mind and spirit in focus on the present.
3. The nurse is assessing a client for spiritual distress. Defining characteristics indicative of spiritual distress in the client include: (Select all that apply.)
   1. lack of hope.
   2. poor coping.
   3. anger toward God.
   4. displacement of anger toward family.
   5. maintaining feelings of love and courage.
   6. lack of purpose in life.
4. A 33-year-old married female client is recovering from a total abdominal hysterectomy. She states, "I wanted more children and now that's impossible. I feel like part of what I am as a woman is missing." Which of the following nursing diagnoses is the most appropriate for the client?
   1. Anxiety related to ineffective individual coping and lack of spousal support.
   2. Decisional conflict related to powerlessness and inability to make decisions.
   3. Spiritual distress related to questioning about the meaning of her role in life.
   4. Ineffective coping related to anxiety and powerlessness due to a total abdominal hysterectomy.
5. Appropriate assessment questions for the nurse to ask a client include: (Select all that apply.)
   1. Are there any religious practices that are important to you?
   2. Who is an important person to you?
   3. Why do you pray?
   4. What religious books or symbols are helpful to you?
   5. Why are you refusing to speak with the hospital chaplain?
   6. What is your source of hope or strength?
6. The nurse observes a terminally ill client crying as she reads from her Bible. Which of the following interventions is the most appropriate?
   1. Contact the client's family.
   2. Provide quiet uninterrupted time.
   3. Contact the client's clergy.
   4. Provide a distraction.

7. A client has recently been in a serious car accident in which his wife and two children were killed. He tells the nurse that he does not understand why God has done this to him and that he feels like God has abandoned him. Which of the following nursing diagnoses is the most appropriate for this client?
   1. Chronic sorrow.
   2. Readiness for enhanced religiosity.
   3. Readiness for enhanced spiritual well-being.
   4. Spiritual distress.
8. Specific nursing actions to promote spiritual well-being in a client who has recently been diagnosed with a terminal illness include all the following except:
   1. make referrals to clergy when appropriate.
   2. respect the client's beliefs.
   3. listen actively to the client's concerns.
   4. provide sympathy to the client and family.
9. Which of the following need interferences would receive the highest priority when providing care to a client experiencing spiritual distress?
   1. The client has difficulty falling asleep.
   2. The client has disturbed body image.
   3. The client has a decreased appetite.
   4. The client has suicidal thoughts.
10. A recently hospitalized client states, "I believe that God and my doctor will heal my injury and make me all better." This is an example of:
   1. hope.
   2. values.
   3. faith.
   4. wellness.

REFERENCES/SUGGESTED READINGS

American Association of Colleges of Nursing. (1995). A model for differentiated nursing practice. Retrieved September 23, 2006, from http://www.aacn.nche.edu/Publications/pdf/DIFFMOD.PDF.

American Nurses Association. (2005). Code of ethic for nurses with interpretive statements. Retrieved October 25, 2008, from http://www.nursingworld.org/ethics/ecode.htm

Andrews, M. M., & Boyle, J. S. (2003). *Transcultural concepts in nursing care*. Philadelphia: Lippincott Williams & Wilkins.

Barton, J., Grudzen, M., & Zielske, R. (2003). *Vital connections in long-term care: Spiritual resources for staff and residents*. Baltimore: Health Professions Press.

Burkhardt, M., & Jacobson, M. (2000). Spirituality and health. In B. M. Dossey, L. Keegan & C. E. Guzzetta (Eds.), *Holistic Nursing: A handbook for practice* (pp. 91–121). Gaithersburg: Aspen.

Carson, V., & Koenig, H. (2004). *Spiritual caregiving: Healthcare as ministry*. Philadelphia: Templeton Foundation Press.

Cavendish, R., Kraynyak-Luise, B., Russo, D., Mitzeliotis, C., Bauer, M., McPartlan-Bajo, M., et al. (2004). Spiritual perspectives of nurses in the United States relevant for education and practice. *Western Journal of Nursing Research, 26*(2), 196–212.

Cox, H., Hinz, M., Lubno, M., Scott-Tilley, D., Newfield, S., Slater, M., et al. (2002). *Clinical applications of nursing diagnosis: Adult, child, psychiatric, gerontic, and home health considerations* (4th ed.). Philadelphia: F. A. Davis.

Dossey, B. (1998) Holistic modalities and healing moments. *American Journal of Nursing, 98*(6), 44–47.

Dossey, B., & Guzzetta, C. E. (2000). Holistic nursing practice. In B. M. Dossey, L. Keegan & C. E. Guzzetta (Eds.), *Holistic nursing practice: A handbook for practice* (pp. 5–26). Rockville: Aspen.

Fadiman, A. (1997). *The spirit catches you and you fall down*. New York: Farrar, Straus & Giroux.

Friesen, M. (2000). *Spiritual Care for Children Living in Specialized Settings*. Binghamton: Haworth Press.

Galek, K., Flannelly, K., Vane, A., & Galek, R. (2005). Assessing patient's spiritual needs. *Holistic Nursing Practice, 19*(2), 62–69.

Gill, S. (Ed.). (1987). *Prayer*. New York: Macmillan.

Hay, D. (2002). The spirituality of adults in Britain: Recent research. *Scottish Journal of Healthcare Chaplaincy, 5*(1), 4–8.

International Council of Nurses. (2006). The ICN code of ethics for nurses. Retrieved September 23, 2006, from http://www.icn.ch/icncode.pdf

La Pierre, L. (2003). JCAHO safeguards spiritual care. *Holistic Nursing Practice, 17*(4), 219.

Mackenzie, E., Rajagopal, D., Meilbohn, M., & Lavizzo-Mourney, R. (2000). Spiritual support and psychological well-being: Older adults' perceptions of religion and health connection. *Alternative Therapies in Health and Medicine, 6*(6), 37–45.

Macrae, J. (1995). Nightingale's spiritual philosophy and its significance for modern nursing. *Image: The Journal of Nursing Scholarship, 27*(1), 8–10.

Maugans, T. (1996). The SPIRITual history. *Archives of Family Medicine, 5*(1), 11–16.

Mauk, K., & Schmidt, N. (2004). *Spiritual care in nursing practice*. Philadelphia: Lippincott Williams & Wilkins.

Mayer, J. (1992) Wholly responsible for a part, or partly responsible for a whole? The concept of spiritual care in nursing. *Second opinion, 17*(3), 26–55.

Park, C. (2007). Religiousness/spirituality and health: A meaning systems perspective. *Journal of Behavioral Medicine, 30*, 319–328.

Pettigrew, J. (1990) Intensive nursing care: Four ways of being there. *Critical Care Nursing Clinics of North America, 2*, 503–508.

Posner, R. (2006). The power of personal values. Retrieved July 13, 2006, from http://gurusoftware.com/Gurunet/Personal/Topics/Values.htm

Puchalski, C., & Romer, A. L. (2000). Taking a spiritual history allows clinicians to understand patients more fully. *Journal of Palliative Medicine, 3*(1), 129–137.

Simon, S., Howe, L., & Kirschenbaum, H. (1978). *Values clarification: A handbook of practical strategies for teachers and students*. New York: Hart.

Spector, R. (2004). *Cultural diversity in health and illness*. Upper Saddle River, NJ: Prentice Hall.

Stoll, R. (1979). Guidelines for spiritual assessment. *American Journal of Nursing, 79*(9), 1574–1577.

Taylor, E. (2002). *Spiritual care, nursing theory, research, and practice*. Upper Saddle River, NJ: Prentice Hall.

Wilkinson, J. (2005). *Nursing diagnosis handbook*. Upper Saddle River, NJ: Prentice Hall.

Wilt, D. & Smucker, C. (2001). *Nursing the spirit*. Washington, DC: American Nurses Association.

RESOURCES

American Academy of Family Physicians, http://www.aafp.org

Duke University Center for Spirituality, Theology and Health, http://www.dukespiritualityandhealth.org

Johns Hopkins Medicine, http://www.hopkinsmedicine.org

Mayo Clinic, http://www.mayoclinic.com

MedlinePlus, http://www.medlineplus.gov

National Cancer Institute, http://www.cancer.gov

National Center for Complementary and Alternative Medicine, http://www.nccam.nih.gov

Spirituality & Practice, http://www.spiritualityandpractice.com

University of Minnesota Center for Spirituality and Healing, http://www.csh.umn.edu

WholeHealthMD, http://www.wholehealthmd.com

CHAPTER 17
Complementary/Alternative Therapies

MAKING THE CONNECTION

Refer to the following chapters to increase your understanding of complementary/alternative therapy:

Basic Nursing
- ***Holistic Care***
- ***Cultural Considerations***
- ***Wellness Concepts***
- ***Spirituality***
- ***Rest and Sleep***

LEARNING OBJECTIVES

Upon completion of this chapter, you should be able to:

- Define key terms.
- Describe the influences of history on current complementary/alternative modalities.
- Discuss the connection between mind and body and how this affects a person's health.
- Explain the concept of the nurse as an instrument of healing.
- Identify the various mind-body, body-movement, energy healing, spiritual, nutritional, and other modalities that can be used as complementary therapies in client care.
- Discuss the use of complementary/alternative modalities.

KEY TERMS

acupressure
acupuncture
allopathic
alternative therapies
antioxidant
aromatherapy
biofeedback
bodymind
complementary therapies
curing
energy therapy
free radicals
healing
healing touch
hypnosis
imagery
meditation
neuropeptides
neurotransmitters
phytochemicals
psychoneuroimmuno-endocrinology (PNIE)
shaman
shamanism
therapeutic massage
therapeutic touch
touch

INTRODUCTION

Our Western society generally equates health and healing with medicine, surgery, and other technological interventions. Many other cultures, however, promote healing through faith, ritual, magic, and other nonmedical approaches.

The use of **complementary therapies** (therapies used *in conjunction with* conventional medical therapies) and **alternative therapies** (therapies used *instead of* conventional or mainstream medical modalities) is becoming more prevalent among the general public (National Center for Complementary and Alternative Medicine [NCCAM], 2008a).

This chapter addresses complementary/alternative (C/A) treatment methods that are currently being used in holistic nursing practice. Nurses must think critically before recommending or implementing any of these therapies. Whether simply discussed with clients or performed, nurses should understand the ramifications. The abbreviation C/A will be used in this chapter.

LEGAL ASPECTS

Because more and more states are regulating C/A therapies, nurses must know the laws that govern these therapies in the states in which they work. Some states have outlawed certain therapies or consider them experimental procedures, whereas other states require licensure or certain educational standards before allowing practitioners to perform C/A therapies. Nurses who perform C/A therapies not in accordance with the laws of their respective states could have legal charges filed against them (Lorenzo, 2003).

Employer policy and the nurse's job description must also be checked to confirm that performing C/A therapies is within the nurse's scope of practice at that agency. Employer malpractice insurance policies typically do not cover situations where a client is injured as a result of a C/A therapy. The financial risk of any nurse who engages in C/A therapies will be lowered by having insurance that specifically covers those therapies.

HISTORIC FOUNDATION

People have tried to relieve pain and cure ills throughout history. Early cave drawings depict healers. Primitive healers believed that magic and superstition caused diseases, resulting in the intertwining of religious beliefs and health practices. Practices and remedies based in ancient traditions are being rediscovered and used. A brief look at ancient Greek, Far Eastern, Indian, and shamanistic practices will highlight their influences on modern C/A modalities.

ANCIENT GREECE

In the ancient Greek culture, health was perceived as maintaining balance in all dimensions of life. In Greek mythology, Asclepius was the god of healing. Temples (called Ascleipions) were beautiful places for people (regardless of ability to pay) to worship, rest, and restore themselves. Their system of healing used symbols, myths, and rites administered by specially trained priest-healers. Illnesses were treated by restoring balance to a person's life through baths, massage, music, laughter, art, herbs, and simple surgery (Keegan, 1994). Many of our current therapies, such as massage, art therapy, and herbal therapy, have origins in ancient Greek traditions.

THE FAR EAST

Healing systems of the Far East have traditionally integrated body, mind, and spirit into a system balancing energy between the individual and the universe. The practices of traditional Chinese medicine (TCM) have been used for centuries and are not considered to be an alternative therapy in Asia. It is a lived philosophy of health and well-being. Restoring and maintaining a balance of vital energy is the goal of TCM. Life energy *qi* (pronounced "key") or *chi* (pronounced "chee") are the words used to describe the vital energy that is the focus of the philosophical principles of TCM. Fundamental elements include balancing opposing forces of *yin* and *yang* (e.g., light–dark, cold–hot, and female–male). Assessment and diagnostic techniques of the TCM practitioner are very different from the **allopathic** (traditional medical and surgical treatment) approach of Western medicine. The five senses are used to assess the client by looking, listening, feeling, smelling, and tasting (if needed).

Chinese medicine is used to treat a range of human diseases and illnesses, such as allergies, asthma, headaches, infertility, and cancer. The nurse's role in care of the client who may integrate TCM with allopathic medicine for treatment of disease is to be sure that the client is aware of potential interactions of prescribed medications and treatments with prescribed herbs.

Herbs are an important part of traditional Chinese healing practice. A discussion of the use of herbs in contemporary health practices appears later in this chapter.

Traditional Chinese healing techniques are being studied and used by contemporary Western health care providers. **Acupuncture**, one technique of traditional Chinese medicine, applies needles and heat to various points on the body to alter the energy flow (Figure 17-1). The Mayo Clinic (2007) acknowledged the efficacy of acupuncture in treating pain and nausea after surgery, low back pain, headaches, fibromyalgia, migraines, osteoarthritis, postoperative dental pain, chemotherapy-induced nausea and vomiting, chronic menstrual cramps, and tennis elbow. Acupuncture may not be safe for clients with bleeding disorders or those taking anticoagulants.

INDIA

For more than 5,000 years, the people of India have practiced Ayurvedic medicine emphasizing "certain lifestyle interventions and natural therapies to regain a balance between the

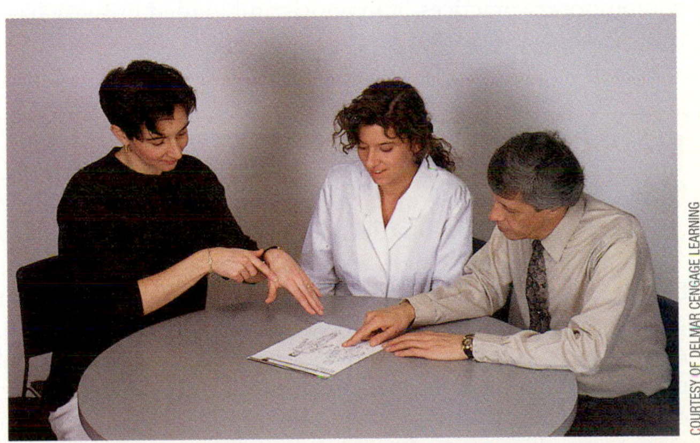

COURTESY OF DELMAR CENGAGE LEARNING

FIGURE 17-1 Acupuncturist, Nurse, and Client

body, mind, and the environment" (Bloomington Hospital, 2008a). The term *ayurveda* ("the science of life") refers to India's traditional medicine, which has an underlying spiritual basis. The life energy (prana) is moved through the body by a "wind," or Vata, which regulates every type of movement.

Vata, Kapha, and Pitta are the three metabolic principles (doshas) that "express particular patterns of energy-unique blends of physical, emotional, and mental characteristics" (Chopra, 2008). Kapha is the energy responsible for body structure. Pitta is the transformative process between Vata and Kapha. Each person is born with a unique balance of the three doshas. The dominant dosha determines temperament, body type, and susceptibility to certain illnesses.

The areas of energy concentration in the body are called chakras. Like the Chinese pathways (or meridians), these areas can become blocked and stagnant, causing illness. Ayurvedic healers try to activate chakra energy for self-healing.

The primary goals in the Ayurvedic system are preventing illness and restoring health by inner searching and spiritual growth. In contemporary practice, Ayurvedic intervention may consist of yoga, herbs, diet, and exercise; methods to cleanse the body, such as steam baths, cathartics, and detoxifying massage; and nasal purging.

Shamanistic Practices

Part of being human is a need to understand and explain life processes (i.e., birth, health, illness, and death). In many cultures, both modern and ancient, ritualized practices have been used to keep peace with the great spirits, to harness their power, to promote power, and to prevent death.

Shamanism refers to the practice of entering an altered state of consciousness with the intent to help others. The **shaman** is a folk healer–priest who uses natural and supernatural forces to help others and who is skilled in many forms of healing, has an extensive knowledge of herbs, and serves as guardian of the spirits. Illness is believed to be the result of spirit loss. Shamans work with the spirits to encourage their full return to the individual. The shaman functions as both priest and healer and has access to the supernatural.

Seeking wisdom about the universe, establishing a relationship with the creator, and avoiding death are all feats accomplished through ritualized processes performed by the shaman. The shaman uses special objects, such as power animals, fetishes, and totems, as well as dances, ritual songs, food, and clothing. Ritual chants, imagery, drumming, and hallucinogenic drugs may be used to create a trancelike state through which the shaman contacts the spirit world. The contemporary practices of hypnosis and guided imagery have roots in shamanistic traditions.

CURRENT TRENDS

The public perception of C/A treatment methods has been changing over the past few decades. In the late 1960s and early 1970s, the "natural," "new age," and "self-help" movements began to attract followers, first among consumers and later among health care practitioners. During that time period, there was a growing trend toward rejection of traditional medicine because of its perceived invasiveness, painfulness, cost, and ineffectiveness. A rekindled interest in Eastern religions, lifestyle, and medicine has fueled the development of contemporary holistic, C/A modalities.

In 1992, the U.S. government established the Office of Alternative Medicine (OAM) at the National Institutes of Health and allocated \$2 million to disseminate information about complementary and alternative medicine to practitioners and the public. Congress increased the OAM's budget to \$20 million for fiscal year 1998 (NCCAM, 2002).

Then in late 1998, Congress established the National Center for Complementary and Alternative Medicine (NCCAM), which replaced the OAM. Its budget for fiscal year 2002 was \$104.6 million (NCCAM, 2008a). The NCCAM has the added responsibility of conducting and supporting basic and applied research and research training on C/A therapies. The NCCAM (2000) reported that as many as 42% of the U.S. population in 1997 used some type of C/A therapy, with a conservative estimate of spending \$21.2 billion on these therapies.

In 2008, the NCCAM reported that 36% of American adults are using some form of C/A. When prayer and megavitamin therapy are included, that number rises to 62%. The profession of nursing is evolving from a traditional Western medical model of client care to an integrative model that incorporates healing tools from cultures and customs other than our own (Fontaine, 2005). Current nursing practice is advancing toward a holistic approach to healing the whole person through integration of complementary and alternative practices with conventional medical treatments into client health care for individuals, families, and communities (Dossey, Keegan, & Guzzetta, 2004; Falsafi, 2001).

Mind/Body Research

Traditional medicine is founded on the belief that the body, mind, and spirit are separate entities. A relatively new field of science, called **psychoneuroimmunoendocrinology (PNIE)**, describes the connection of thought with physical reactions. This word envelops the relationship of neural messages from thoughts, emotions, feelings, and attitudes into molecular responses from the immune and endocrine systems (Dossey et al., 2004). The power of thought is the basis of mindfulness-based healing therapies.

All body cells have receptor sites for **neuropeptides**, amino acids produced in the brain and other sites in the body that act as chemical communicators. Neuropeptides are released when **neurotransmitters** (chemical substances produced by the body that facilitate nerve-impulse transmission) signal emotions in the brain. Pert, of the National Institutes of Health, wrote in 1986 that "the more we know about neuropeptides, the harder it is to think in the traditional terms of a mind and a body. It makes more sense to speak of a single integrated entity, a 'body-mind'" (Pert, 1986).

Cells can be directly affected by emotions. This means that people can affect their health by what they feel and think. There are many examples of terminally ill persons hanging on to life until the occurrence of a specific event, such as a child coming to visit or a grandchild's graduation or marriage.

This complex, intermeshed system of psyche and body chemistry is now called the **bodymind**, an inseparable connection and operation of thoughts, feelings, and physiological functions.

Holism and Nursing

The growing acceptance of the concept that body, mind, and spirit are interconnected is the basis for the expansion of the holistic health movement. The physiological, psychological, sociocultural, intellectual, and spiritual aspects of each individual are considered in holism. Holistic nursing has been described by the American Holistic Nurses' Association (AHNA) as embracing "all nursing practice which has healing the whole person as its goal" (Dossey et al., 2004). Nurses who embrace their personal and professional lives within a holistic perspective are aware that their presence, attention, and intention are essential elements of wholeness and healing. Living within the framework of holism, nurses use their knowledge, nursing concepts and theories, expertise, and intuition to discover patterns of health for themselves and their clients that promote health and well-being. As the nurse and client become therapeutic partners, wholeness and healing is achieved for the client, family, group, and community.

Nurses as holistic caregivers may use C/A techniques to promote clients' well-being. The focus of care in these practices is healing as opposed to curing. The word **healing** comes from the Anglo-Saxon word *hael*, meaning "to make whole, to move toward, or to become whole." It is important to understand that healing is not **curing** (ridding one of disease) but is instead a process activating the individual's forces from within. The nurse as a healing facilitator enters into a relationship with the client to assist the client by being a guide. The objective is to assist the client in releasing inner resources for healing.

CRITICAL THINKING

Alternative Methods

A close friend has AIDS and is experiencing a great deal of pain and discouragement. She wants to find alternative methods to ease the pain. She confides to you that she believes there may be a cure available at the holistic health center. How do you best help your friend in this situation?

Nurses have an important role to educate clients about nontraditional interventions throughout the life span (Table 17-1).

COMPLEMENTARY/ ALTERNATIVE THERAPIES

Many C/A therapies are used in holistic nursing practice. These interventions are categorized as mind/body, spiritual, manipulative and body based, energy therapies, biologically based, and other methodologies.

TABLE 17-1 Suggested Complementary Therapies through Life

STAGE OF LIFE	SUGGESTED COMPLEMENTARY THERAPIES	
Infants	• Massage (modified) • Movement (rocking)	• Music
Young Children	• Massage • Music • Play	• Humor • Imagery • Art/drawing
School-Age Children	• Massage • Music • Play • Humor • Animal-assisted therapy	• Imagery • Aromatherapy • Yoga • Tai chi
Adolescents	All therapies discussed in this chapter, as appropriate to the condition	
Adults	All therapies discussed in this chapter, as appropriate to the condition	
Older Adults	• Massage (lighter pressure and other modifications for body's status) • Animal-assisted therapy • Aromatherapy (with precautions) • Any other therapy discussed in this chapter, as appropriate to the condition and with precautions	
Terminally Ill	• Massage • Reflexology • Energy therapies • Music	• Prayer • Any other therapies discussed in this chapter, as appropriate to the condition and with precautions

COURTESY OF DELMAR CENGAGE LEARNING

CASE STUDY

Complementary Therapies

A female client is diagnosed with stage 3 breast cancer. She is considering surgery to remove the tumor and cancer therapy options, yet she would like to know more about complementary therapies (CT) for health recovery and health promotion. Her medical team is not familiar with complementary and alternative therapies.

1. As the nurse on the health care team for this client, what interventions can be provided to promote support for this client during this time?
2. How can the nurse create a more informed health care team when clients ask about CT?

Mind/Body Interventions

Mind/body interventions are methods by which an individual can, independently or with assistance, consciously control some sympathetic nervous system functions (e.g., heart rate, respiratory rate, and blood pressure). When the client is learning the way to perform these techniques, an assistant is involved; later, however, the client can perform them independently. Self-regulatory techniques include meditation, relaxation, imagery, biofeedback, and hypnosis.

Meditation

Meditation, a quieting of the mind by focusing attention on a sound or image or one's own breathing, is an ancient art. The person is no longer aware of worries or preoccupations, and stress is reduced. Health benefits from reduced stress include decreased respiration, heart rate, and oxygen consumption; improved mood; spiritual calm; and heightened awareness.

Nurses can assist clients with meditation by explaining what it is and answering any questions. When the client is in a comfortable position, instruct in a calm voice to concentrate on inhaling and exhaling. If the client's mind wanders, a refocus on breathing is needed. This should be practiced every day for 15 minutes.

PROFESSIONAL TIP

Use of Complementary/Alternative (C/A) Therapy

Nurses wanting to use C/A therapies should:

- Ask the client if he or she is currently using C/A and, if so, which therapy, the purpose of using the therapy, and the outcome.
- Educate the client about C/A prior to using it.
- Create a supportive environment of healing conducive to C/A therapy.
- Obtain the necessary training, certification, or licensure.
- Be aware of the potential risks.
- Provide nonjudgmental supportive counsel.

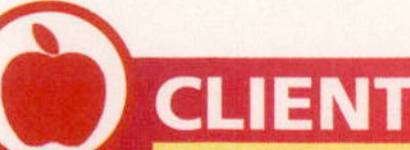

CLIENT TEACHING

Progressive Muscle Relaxation

Explain the purpose and process of progressive muscle relaxation, then have the client:

- Assume a comfortable position in a quiet environment.
- Close eyes and keep them closed until the exercise is completed.
- Breathe in deeply to a count of 4.
- Hold breath for a count of 4.
- Breathe out to a count of 4.
- Continue to breathe slowly and deeply.
- Tense both feet until muscle tension is felt.
- Hold a gentle state of tension in both feet for a count of 5.

Tighten the muscles only until tense, but not painful.

- Slowly release the tension from the feet.
- Recognize the difference between tension and relaxation.
- Repeat the previous three steps.
- Gently tense the muscles of both lower legs.
- Continue the process with all muscle groups in a toe-to-head direction.
- After tensing and releasing all muscle groups, take in a few more deep relaxing breaths and scan your body for any areas that remain tense. Concentrate on tensing and relaxing the muscles in those areas.
- Breathe in deeply to a count of 4.
- Hold breath for a count of 4.
- Breathe out to a count of 4.
- Resume your usual breathing pattern.
- Slowly stretch and open your eyes.

This takes approximately 20 to 30 minutes and is most effective with repetition.

Meditation has proved particularly beneficial for clients in labor.

Relaxation

Progressive muscle relaxation (PMR) is one method for achieving relaxation. It employs the alternate tensing and relaxing of muscles. Clients are instructed to concentrate on a certain body area (the jaw, for instance), tense the muscles for a count of 5, then relax the muscles for a count of 5. This process is repeated for muscle groups over the entire body until the client has achieved a state of overall relaxation. Nurses can use relaxation techniques to reduce pain and stress in clients.

Imagery

Imagery is a technique of using the imagination to visualize a pleasant, soothing image. The client is encouraged to use as

BOX 17-1 GUIDED IMAGERY

- Allow 10 to 20 minutes for this exercise.
- Provide a quiet comfortable environment.
- Set a goal for the session such as "pain relief" or "relaxation."
- Assess the client by asking him [or her] to describe a relaxing setting.
- Allow the client to use sensory details of the setting that include a visual image, the feeling (e.g., temperature, wind, sun), and the scents (e.g., evergreen, ocean breeze, lavender). Add music or be quiet for the auditory sense.
- Once the client is in a comfortable position. soften your voice to say:

  Bring your attention to the rhythm of your breathing. As you breathe in and out, allow an image to develop of a comfortable setting. In this setting you are relaxed and feel a sense of peace. Bring to mind the colors of the setting, the feel of the environment, the details of the setting as they surround you, and any comforting scents or aromas that allow you to feel at peace. Take a moment to enjoy this image.

  When you are ready, allow yourself to image the pain or areas of tension as a round ball of light. Bring your awareness to this light. Then, become aware of your ability to dim this light, slowly turning the light down to release the pain and tension. (Allow 2–3 minutes of quiet.)

  When you are ready, allow yourself to create a memory of this feeling of relaxation and comfort. As you rest, bring your awareness to areas of your body that need healing. Allow this feeling to facilitate healing throughout your body.

Downey, M. (2009). *Understanding Complementary and Alternative Therapies.* Manuscript submitted for publication.

many of the senses as possible to enhance the formation of vivid images. Table 17-2 presents examples of using all five senses in imagery.

Nurses can use guided imagery with clients capable of hearing and understanding the nurse's suggestions. For example, show and explain a chart of the stages of bone healing to a client who has suffered a fracture and ask the client to imagine this sequential activity in his body.

With guided imagery, the nurse can promote a sense of well-being in clients and help them change their perceptions about their disease, treatment, and healing ability (Dossey, 1999a). Research has shown positive effects of imagery when used with guidance from a trained health care practitioner (Dossey et al., 2004). Although imagery and visualization are effective complementary therapies for health and healing, contraindications should be noted for clients with mental disorders who are sensitive to traumatic images.

TABLE 17-2 Using All Five Senses in Imagery

SENSE	IMAGERY
Visual	See the white, fluffy clouds.
Auditory	Hear the waves on the beach.
Kinesthetic	Feel yourself floating in the water.
Gustatory	Taste the tartness of the lemonade.
Olfactory	Smell the hotdogs cooking on the grill.

COURTESY OF DELMAR CENGAGE LEARNING

BIOFEEDBACK

Biofeedback measures physiological responses, which assist individuals to improve their health by using signals from their own bodies. The biological functions commonly measured are muscle tension, skin temperature, heart rate, sweat gland activity, and brain wave activity. Biofeedback works by teaching clients to "recognize how their bodies are functioning and to control patterns of physiological functioning" (Association for Applied Psychophysiology and Biofeedback [AAPB], 2008). Biofeedback is effective for migraine and tension headaches, urinary incontinence, hypertension, chronic pain, sleeping problems, epilepsy, and Raynaud's disease (AAPB, 2008).

Hypnosis

The practice of hypnosis was once overshadowed by mystery and misconception. Today, with the expanding knowledge of the human mind, hypnosis is being used more. Therapeutic **hypnosis** induces an altered state of consciousness or awareness resembling sleep and during which the person is more receptive to suggestion. Hypnosis does not magically cure anything. Nurses desiring to use hypnosis in their practices must be aware of their scope of practice as defined by their respective state boards of nursing.

Spiritual Therapies

A state of health depends on one's relationship not only to the physical and interpersonal environments but also to the spiritual part of self. The idea of a relationship between spirituality and health is not new. "From the earliest time of the shaman we have witnessed the mysterious spiritual element of healing . . . the connection of the healer with the divine" (Keegan, 1994).

Many cultures accept the inseparable link between the state of one's soul (life energy or spirit) and the state of one's health. Scientists (especially psychoneuroimmunologists) are beginning to validate that individuals have inner mechanisms of healing. Many religions have ideologies about health, illness, and healing.

Faith Healing At the heart of spiritual or faith healing is the belief that practitioners must purify themselves and reach a state of unity with God or a higher power before faith healing can occur. This process is usually accomplished through prayer. When preparing for healing, the practitioner adapts a passive and receptive mood to be a channel for divine power. The ill person's belief enhances but is not necessary for healing.

Healing Prayer When praying, people believe they are communicating directly with God or a higher power. Prayer, an integral part of a person's spiritual life, can affect well-being. Florence Nightingale recognized that prayer helps connect individuals to nature and the environment (Nightingale, 1969). Medical research is currently investigating the effects of prayer on physical health.

Shamanism Shamanism was discussed earlier in this chapter.

MANIPULATIVE AND BODY-BASED METHODS

Body-based methods use techniques of manipulating or moving various body parts to achieve therapeutic outcomes. Movement/exercise, yoga, tai chi, and chiropractic treatment are discussed in the following sections.

Movement/Exercise

The therapeutic intervention and health-promoting activity of movement is associated with athletic exercise, dance, celebration, and healing rituals. The primary goal of exercise is fitness (muscle strength, endurance, flexibility, and cardiovascular and respiratory health). There are many other positive outcomes of exercise, such as sleeping better and having more energy.

Nurses can help clients use movement as therapy through range-of-motion exercises, stretching exercises, and physical therapy. Movement is an effective method through which people of all ages can improve their level of functioning.

Yoga/Yoga Therapy

Yoga (meaning "union" in Sanskrit) integrates mental, physical, and spiritual energies to promote health and wellness. The basic elements of yoga are proper breathing, posture, and movement. The breathing is believed to promote relaxation and enhance the flow of prana (vital energy). Yoga develops proprioception (an awareness of where the body is in space and time) and an awareness of movement, weight distribution, and position (Davis, 2002).

Traditional yoga has always been primarily concerned with healthy individuals and promoting health by maintaining the balance and flow of life forces.

Yoga therapy is an effort to integrate traditional yogic concepts and techniques with Western medical and psychological knowledge (Feuerstein, 1998). The focus of yoga therapy is to holistically treat various psychological or somatic dysfunctions ranging from back problems to emotional distress. Both yoga and yoga therapy are based on the understanding that the human being is an integrated body/mind system that best functions in a state of dynamic balance (Feuerstein, 1998). Yoga is used for a variety of health conditions, including depression, high blood pressure, stress, and asthma. Research suggests that yoga may reduce heart rate and blood pressure, increase lung capacity, positively affect specific brain or blood chemical levels, and improve body composition and muscle relaxation (NCCAM, 2008b). Yoga improves overall strength, flexibility, and fitness.

Tai Chi

The philosophy of looking for harmony with nature and the universe through complementary (yin and yang) balance is the basis for tai chi. When there is perfect harmony, everything functions spontaneously, effortlessly, perfectly, and according to the laws of nature. If one moves to the right, one must also move to the left. Tai chi is a series of slow, graceful, nonaerobic movements with controlled rhythmic breathing (Bloomington Hospital, 2008b).

Those who regularly practice tai chi believe that it enhances agility, stamina, and balance and that it boosts energy and bestows a sense of well-being. The entire tai chi form can take as little as 7 minutes or as long as an hour to practice. Tai chi has been shown to decrease blood pressure; increase muscle tone, stamina, and flexibility; and improve balance, muscle mass, posture, and strength in older people (Bloomington Hospital, 2008b).

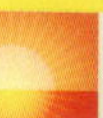

LIFE SPAN CONSIDERATIONS

Tai Chi Chih

A research trial conducted by the University of California (Irwin, Olmstead, & Motivala, 2008) concluded that tai chi chih can improve sleep quality in older adults ages 59 to 86 years with moderate sleep complaints. Tai chi chih can be considered a useful nonpharmacological approach to improve sleep quality in older adults.

Chiropractic Therapy

Chiropractic therapy is based on the principle that the brain sends vital energy to every organ in the body via the nerves originating in the spinal column. Disease, body disharmony, or malfunction results from vertebral subluxation complex (spinal nerve stress). The body is rebalanced and realigned using chiropractic "spinal adjustment" techniques.

The goal of chiropractic care is to awaken the client's own natural healing ability by correcting any areas of vertebral subluxation complex. Vitality, strength, and health are thus promoted. The Chiropractic Arts Center (2007) reports case histories of clients recovering from heart trouble, hyperactivity, fatigue, digestive problems, and many other conditions.

Stedman (1999) explains that chiropractic practitioners fall into one of two groups: the "straights" and the "mixers." The straights believe in the chiropractic therapy just described. The mixers use spinal adjustments mainly to relieve back pain, neck stiffness, and headaches, conditions that have sometimes been shown to be alleviated by chiropractic therapy. Most mixers are willing to work closely with a client's medical doctor.

Chiropractic services have gained increasing acceptance in the United States. Insurance coverage for chiropractic services is extensive. All state workers' compensation systems and many health maintenance organizations and private health insurance companies provide coverage for chiropractic therapy

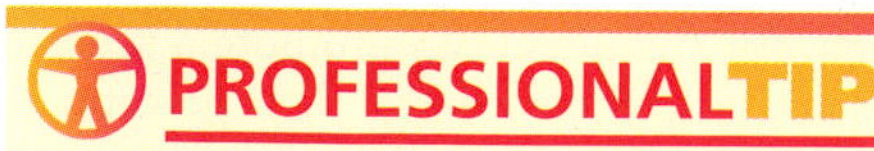

PROFESSIONALTIP

Preparing for Chiropractic Therapy

Encourage clients considering the use of chiropractic services to first undergo a comprehensive health assessment to rule out any contraindications.

(NCCAM, 2007). The client should check with their insurance company prior to seeking treatment to verify coverage.

Energy Therapies

One category of C/A therapies incorporated into nursing practice in the past 25 years is the **energy therapies**, or the use of the hands to direct or redirect the flow of the body's energy fields and enhance balance within those fields. These therapies are effective for many problems and can restore harmony in all aspects of health. These therapies can be used with persons of all ages and all stages of wellness and illness.

Energy therapies have their roots in traditional Chinese, ancient Eastern, and Native American philosophies. The fundamental concept is that individuals have a life force, energy not confined to physical skin boundaries. Figure 17-2 illustrates the energy field that extends beyond a person's physical body.

An individual's energy field consists of energy layers in constant flux. They can be reduced or otherwise adversely affected by any type of trauma, illness, or distress. The energy system can also be positively affected intentionally by the use of a practitioner's hands. The primary focus is to restore the optimal flow of life energy through the energy fields.

Many energy therapies are being used by nurses today, such as touch, therapeutic massage, therapeutic touch, and healing touch. Other therapies are acupressure and reflexology, both of which involve deep-tissue body work and require advanced training for the practitioners.

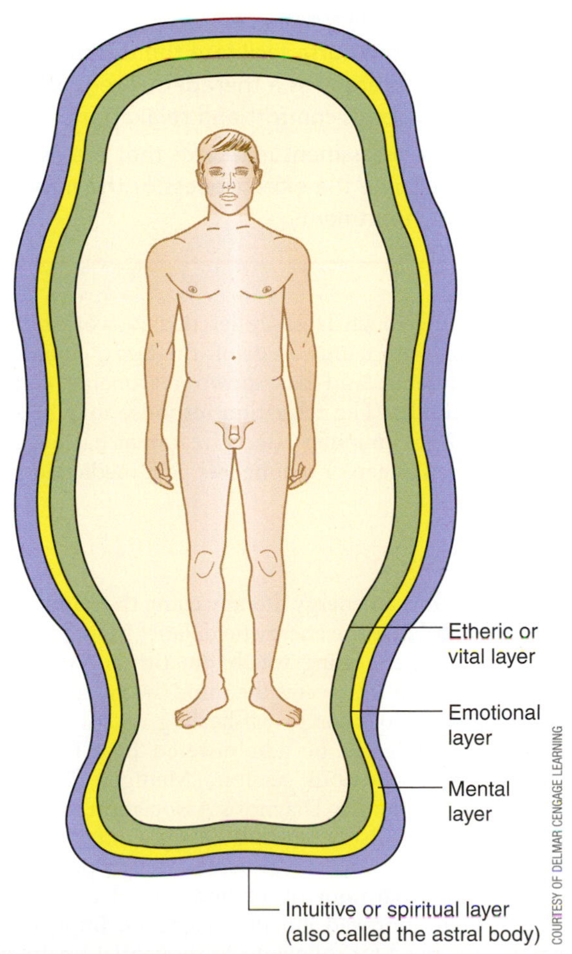

Figure 17-2 Layers of the Human Energy Field Extending Beyond the Physical Boundaries

CULTURAL CONSIDERATIONS

Touch

- Ask permission before touching a client.
- Tell the client what is going to happen.
- The meaning of touch and the body areas acceptable to touch vary from culture to culture.

Touch

The most universal C/A therapy is touch. **Touch** is the means of perceiving or experiencing through tactile sensation. Although it was used in all ancient cultures and shamanistic traditions for healing, the advent of scientific medicine and Puritanism led many healers away from the purposeful use of touch. It should be noted that touch carries with it taboos and prescriptions that are culturally dictated. Some cultures are very comfortable with physical touch; others specify that touch may be used only in certain situations and within specified parameters.

The nurse must be sure to convey positive intentions when touching. If in doubt, the nurse should not touch until establishing effective communication with the client. Touch is important in nursing practice, because it:

- is an integral part of assessment.
- promotes bonding between nurse and client (Figure 17-3).
- is an important means of communication, especially when other senses are impaired.
- assists in soothing, calming, and comforting.
- helps keep the client oriented.

Therapeutic Massage

Therapeutic massage is the application of hand pressure and motion to improve the recipient's well-being. It involves rubbing, kneading, and using friction.

Massage therapy is recognized as highly beneficial and is prescribed by many physicians. Many states now have licensing requirements for massage practitioners.

Traditionally, back rubs were given by nurses to provide comfort to hospitalized clients. Massage techniques can be used with all age-groups and are especially beneficial to those

PROFESSIONALTIP

Contraindications for Touch

It is important to know when *not* to touch.

- It may be difficult for persons who have been neglected, abused, or injured to accept touch therapy.
- Touching those who are distrustful or angry may increase negative behaviors.
- Persons with burns or overly sensitive skin may not benefit from touch.

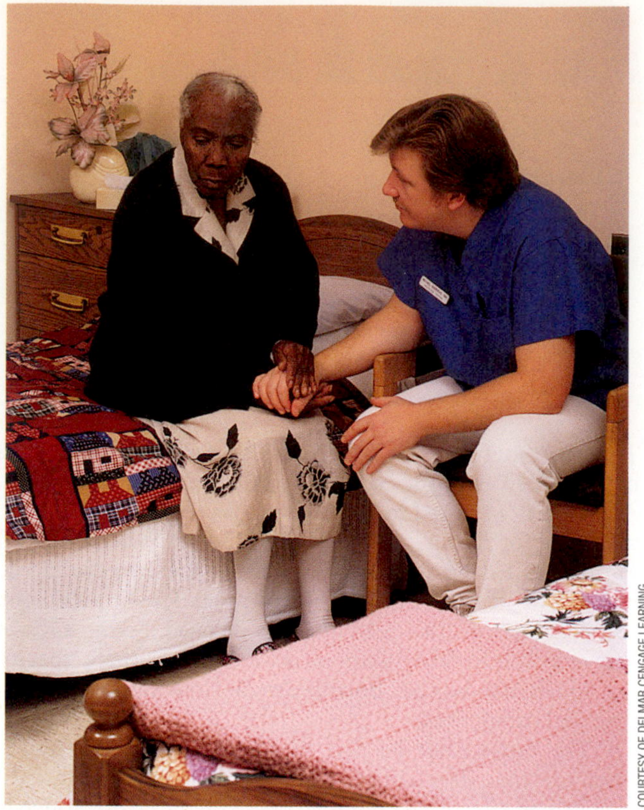

FIGURE 17-3 Touch promotes bonding between nurse and client.

who cannot move. A back rub or massage results in relaxation, increased circulation of the blood and lymph, and relief from musculoskeletal stiffness, spasm, and pain (Figure 17-4).

Therapeutic Touch

Therapeutic touch, based on the ancient practice of the laying on of hands, consists of finding alterations in a person's energy field and using the hands to direct energy to achieve a balanced state. Therapeutic touch is based on four assumptions:

- A human being is an open energy system.
- Anatomically, a human being is bilaterally symmetrical.
- Illness is an imbalance in an individual's energy field.
- Human beings have natural abilities to transform and transcend their conditions of living (Krieger, 1993).

SAFETY

Precautions for Massage

- Increased circulation may be harmful in people with heart disease, diabetes, hypertension, or kidney disease.
- Never attempt massage in areas of circulatory abnormality, such as aneurysm, varicose veins, phlebitis, thrombus, or necrosis, or in areas of tissue injury, inflammation, open wounds, dermatitis, joint or bone injury, recent surgery, or sciatica.

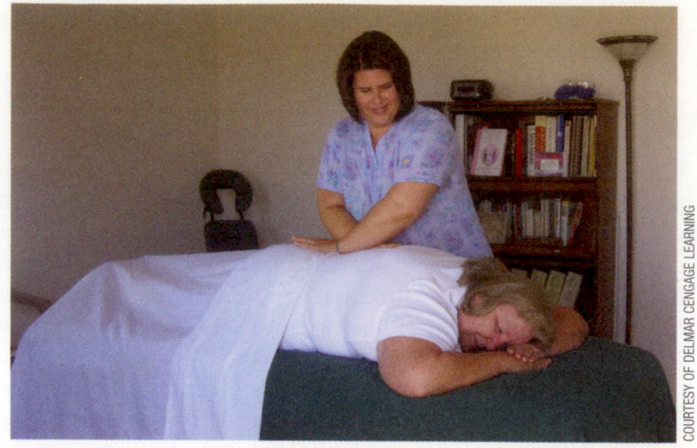

FIGURE 17-4 Therapeutic massage promotes relaxation, health, and well-being for the client.

CASE STUDY

Massage Therapy

A 42-year-old male is admitted to the cardiovascular observation unit prior to his fourth cardiac bypass surgery. He is experiencing a great deal of anxiety in anticipation of his postoperative pain related to this procedure. The client proposes that he be given massage therapy along with the customary preoperative medications.

1. How can the nurse facilitate the use of massage therapy as a therapeutic regimen for this client's comfort and relaxation?
2. Describe assessment measures that are used to determine the effectiveness of the massage therapy treatments.

Therapeutic touch is easily learned in workshops, can be done either with hands on or off the body, complements medical treatments, and has shown reasonably consistent and reliable results. The relaxation response may be seen in the client in 2 to 5 minutes after a treatment has begun, and some clients fall asleep or require less pain medication after a treatment.

Healing Touch

Healing touch is an energy therapy using the hands to clear, energize, and balance the energy field. Janet Mentgen, a nurse, developed it. The healing touch practitioner realigns the energy flow, which reactivates the mind/body/spirit connection to eliminate blockages to self-healing.

Healing touch can be administered in a few minutes or, ideally, in a one-hour session (Mentgen, 2002). The North American Nursing Diagnosis Association International (NANDA-I, 2010) lists *Disturbed Energy Field*, defined as "a disruption of the flow of energy surrounding a person's being that results in disharmony of the body, mind, and/or spirit," as one of their approved nursing diagnoses. Implicit in this therapy is the need for follow-up or sequential treatments as well as discharge planning and referral to assist the client in adequately meeting goals.

CRITICAL THINKING

Reflexology

A client asks the nurse to rub his foot in a particular spot because that is where his reflexologist rubs to relieve his abdominal pain. How should the nurse handle this situation?

Acupressure and Shiatsu

Both acupressure and shiatsu are based on the Chinese meridian theory, which states that the body is divided into meridian channels through which qi, or energy, flows. Cold, damp, fire, bacteria, or viruses may block the flow of qi, causing disease in the body. **Acupressure** is a technique of releasing blocked energy within an individual when specific points (Tsubas) along the meridians are pressed or massaged by the practitioner's fingers, thumbs, and heel of the hands. When the blocked energy is freed, the disease subsides. Shiatsu, a Japanese form of acupressure, also uses the forearm, elbow, knee, and foot to activate the points. Both acupressure and Shiatsu relieve tension and many stress-related ailments. Contraindications include venous stasis, phlebitis, and traumatic and deep-tissue injuries (Sutherland, 2000).

Shiatsu treatment is holistic, with the aim of aiding the whole body to heal rather than focusing on the area where symptoms are most obvious. The aim is for the Shiatsu practitioner to assist the client's body to naturally heal by encouraging the client's energy to move into a more balanced state (Shiatsu Society, 2008).

Reflexology

Reflexology is a noninvasive complementary modality that involves the application of pressure by the use of the practitioner's hands, fingers, and thumb to the client's feet, hands, and ears with specific thumb, finger, and hand techniques. The fundamental concept of reflexology divides the body into 10 equal, longitudinal zones running the length of the body, from the top of the head to the tip of the toes. These 10 zones correspond to the 10 fingers and toes. The foot is viewed as a microcosm of the entire body (Figure 17-5). Reflexology theory states that illness is evident as calcium deposits and acids in the corresponding part of the person's feet. Pressing certain points on the feet brings an autonomic nervous system response or reflex. Reflexology induces an optimal state of relaxation, which is conducive to healing. It promotes health by relieving pressures and accumulation of toxins in the corresponding body part.

Reflexology can be used as a complementary therapy for chronic conditions such as asthma, sinus infections, migraines, irritable bowel syndrome, constipation, and kidney stones.

Biologically Based Therapies

In the past 20 to 30 years, nutritional interventions for prevention and treatment of disease have generated increasing interest among consumers and health care providers. This section addresses the C/A nutritional and herbal approaches.

Phytochemicals

Currently, certain foods are being studied for their medicinal value. **Phytochemicals** are "non-nutritive plant chemicals that have protective or disease preventive properties"

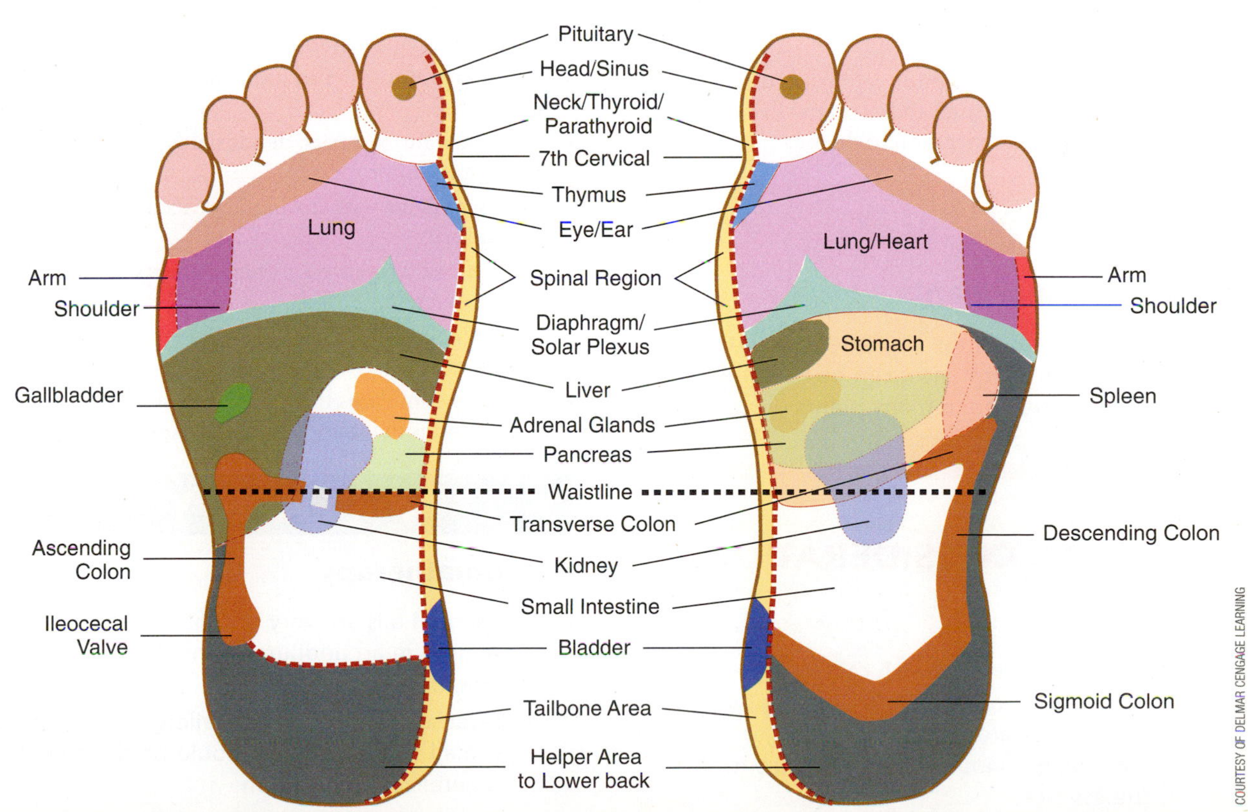

FIGURE 17-5 Foot reflexology chart indicates points on the foot that reflexively correspond to other areas of the body.

(Phytochemicals, 2008). *Phyto* is the Greek word for "plant." Therefore, phytochemicals are plant chemicals. These chemicals have several functions, including storage of nutrients and provision of structure, aroma, flavor, and color. Phytochemicals protect against cancer and prevent heart disease, stroke, and cataracts. Phytochemicals are found in fruits and vegetables.

No single fruit or vegetable contains all phytochemicals. The consumption of a wide variety of fruits and vegetables provides the best supply. The major sources of phytochemicals are onions, garlic, leeks, chives, carrots, sweet potatoes, squash, pumpkin, cantaloupe, mango, papaya, tomatoes, citrus fruits, grapes, strawberries, raspberries, cherries, legumes, soybeans, tofu, and the cruciferous vegetables (broccoli, cauliflower, brussels sprouts, and cabbage). Nurses can use this information to encourage clients to eat more fruits and vegetables.

Antioxidants

Antioxidants are substances that prevent or inhibit oxidation, a chemical process whereby a substance is joined to oxygen. In the body, antioxidants prevent tissue damage related to **free radicals**, which are unstable molecules that alter genetic codes and trigger the development of cancer growth in cells. Vitamins C and E, beta-carotene (which is converted to vitamin A in the body), and selenium are antioxidants. Antioxidants may prevent heart disease, some forms of cancer, and cataracts. Other vitamins, minerals, trace elements, and enzymes are being investigated for their possible therapeutic value. Phytosterols (plant sterols) are structurally similar to cholesterol and act in the intestine to decrease cholesterol absorption. Research has shown that phytosterols effectively reduce low-density-lipoprotein (LDL) cholesterol when given as supplements (Ostlund, 2004). Increasing the intake of phytosterols may reduce coronary heart disease with minimum risk.

Herbs

Herbs and plants have been used for centuries in the care of the sick. Many of the drugs used today originally were plant remedies passed from one generation to the next.

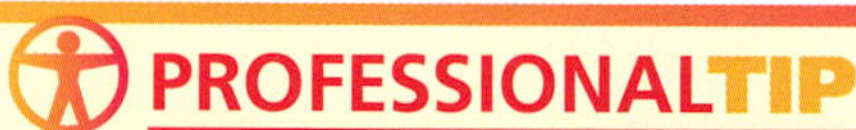

Use of Medicinal Plants

Be cautious in the casual use of plants to treat self or others. "Natural" substances can be harmful if not processed properly, and many plants (including some herbs) can be poisonous.

LIFE SPAN CONSIDERATIONS

Essential Oils

Essential oils should be used with caution in elderly persons. These clients are usually more sensitive to essential oils than are adults and teenagers and thus require smaller amounts and less concentrated forms of the essence.

Although herbs may have medicinal value (Table 17-3), some can cause potentially harmful herb–drug interactions when used with prescribed medications. It is important to ask during assessment specifically about the client's use of herbal and vitamin supplements. Feverfew, ginseng, and garlic prolong the clotting time. Encourage clients to reveal the use of herbs to their primary care provider.

OTHER METHODOLOGIES

Iridology, aromatherapy, humor, animal-assisted therapy, music therapy, and play therapy are also used by holistic practitioners.

Iridology

According to Caradonna (2008), iridology began more than 100 years ago when two physicians began observing eyes and organizing their findings. Iridology is the study of the iris, or colored part, of the eye. It is theorized that the fibers and pigmentation of the iris reflects information about a person's physical and psychological makeup.

Aromatherapy

Aromatherapy is the therapeutic use of concentrated essences or essential oils extracted from plants and flowers. Essential oils diluted in oil for massage or in warm water for inhalation may be stimulating, relaxing, or soothing. According to the National Association for Holistic Aromatherapy (NAHA, 2008b), the top 10 essential oils are the following:

- *Peppermint* is useful in treating headaches, muscle aches, and digestive disorders.
- *Eucalyptus* boosts the immune system, relieves muscle tension, and treats respiratory problems.
- *Ylang-ylang* aids in relaxation and depression.
- *Geranium* balances hormones and skin.
- *Lavender* promotes relaxation and is used to treat wounds and burns.
- *Lemon* has antibacterial, deodorizing, anti-infective, and antidepressant properties.
- *Clary sage* helps with insomnia, relaxation, and pain/discomfort.
- *Tea tree* is said to have antifungal effects and boosts the immune system.
- *Roman chamomile* decreases anxiety, promotes relaxation, and treats infections.
- *Rosemary* stimulates the digestive system and immune system and is mentally stimulating and uplifting.

SAFETY

Aromatherapy

- Essential oils are very potent and should never be used in an undiluted form, be used near the eyes, or be ingested orally.
- Because some people are allergic to certain oils, a small skin-patch test should be done before generalized application.

Table 17-3 Common Herbs for Health Promotion

HERB	REPORTED USES	ADMINISTRATION/ AVAILABILITY	CAUTIONS/INTERACTIONS	CLINICAL CONSIDERATIONS AND ASSESSMENTS
Aloe (*Aloe vera*)	Used topically to treat minor burns, sunburn, cuts, abrasions, acne, and stomatitis. Internally used as a stimulant laxative (little evidence base). Possible antidiabetic action related to the thromboxane inhibitor (TXA2) effects.	Capsules, cream, extract, gel, jelly, and juice. Teach client to use aloe internally only under the supervision of a qualified herbalist.	Internal administration of dried aloe juice is contraindicated for pregnancy and lactation and for children under 12 years of age. Avoid with kidney and cardiac disease and bowel obstruction. Aloe may enhance the effects of cardiac medications, diuretics, and steroids. Hypersensitivity (allergy) to garlic, onions, or tulips may indicate sensitivity to aloe.	• Assess clients for cardiac or renal disease/medications, steroids, and diuretics. • Assess for pregnancy and lactation. • Assess fluid and electrolyte balance. • Assess for allergy (see contraindications).
Bilberry (*Vaccinium myrtillus*)	Improvement of night vision, prevention of cataracts, macular degeneration, diabetic retinopathy, myopia, and glaucoma. Treatment of varicose veins, hemorrhoids, and postoperative hemorrhage.	Bilberry can be taken orally in the form of capsules, tinctures, fluid extract, and fresh berries.	Contraindicated for pregnancy, lactation, and children. Interactions: Anticoagulants (heparin, warfarin), antiplatelet agents (aspirin), nonsteroidal anti-inflammatory drugs (NSAIDs), insulin, and oral antidiabetics.	• Assess clients for use of anticoagulants, antidiabetics, and antiplatelets. • Assess and monitor vision changes. • Monitor blood glucose. • Assess for pregnancy and lactation.
Black cohosh (*Cimicifuga racemosa*)	Used as a smooth-muscle relaxant, antispasmodic, diuretic, antidiarrheal, astringent, antitussive, and antiarthritic; more commonly known for hormone balance in perimenopause and for dysmenorrhea. Possible decreased uterine spasms in first trimester of pregnancy and, for children, as an antiasthmatic.	Capsules, extract, powdered extract, and tincture. Standardized products should be used for administration of black cohosh.	Contraindicated for use in pregnancy after first trimester because of uterine stimulation. This herb should not be used during lactation and for children. Interactions: Black cohosh may interfere with antihypertensive and hormone replacement therapies.	• Assess for menopausal and menstrual irregularities: duration of cycle, flow, pain, and hot flashes. • Assess history of client for fibroids and ovarian cysts. • Assess use of other hormonal products such as estrogen, progesterone, and oral contraceptives.

(Continues)

Table 17-3 Common Herbs for Health Promotion (Continued)

HERB	REPORTED USES	ADMINISTRATION/ AVAILABILITY	CAUTIONS/INTERACTIONS	CLINICAL CONSIDERATIONS AND ASSESSMENTS
Capsicum (cayenne, chili, or hot peppers) (*Capsicum annum*)	Capsicum (peppers) can be used topically for treatment of arthritis, diabetic neuropathy, herpes zoster, peripheral circulation, psoriasis, and Raynaud's disease. Internal use for promotion of cardiovascular health, arthritic and muscular pain, gastric protection for peptic ulcers, and cold and flu symptoms.	Capsules, tablets, and tincture, topical cream/gel/lotion (0.025%–0.075% concentration) for approximately 2 weeks for pain relief (up to q.i.d.).	Minimal research has been done to support the use of capsicum during pregnancy and lactation or for children. Hypersensitivity (allergic reaction) is a contraindication. Capsicum in any form should not be used on open wounds, on abrasions, and near the eyes. Interactions: For internal application, avoid concurrent use with alpha-adrenergic blockers, clonidine, monoamine oxidase inhibitors (MAOIs), and methyldopa.	• Assess for use of alpha-adrenergic blocking agents, clonidine, MAOIs, and methyldopa. • Assess for improvement of symptoms in topical use such as psoriasis, peripheral vascular effects, diabetic neuropathy, or herpes zoster. • Assess for gastrointestinal conditions such as peptic ulcers and irritable bowel syndrome.
Chamomile (*Matricaria chamomilla*)	Used to treat anxiety and insomnia, as a digestive aid and an anti-inflammatory, and to promote wound healing.	Capsules, cream, fluid extract, lotion, tea, and tinctures.	Contraindicated for pregnancy and lactation. Allergies to sunflowers, ragweed, or asters (echinacea, feverfew, milk thistle) may cause hypersensitivity to chamomile. Asthmatics should avoid chamomile. Interactions: Avoid using alcohol, anticoagulants, and sedatives when taking chamomile because of the enhanced effects of these substances when used with this herb.	• Assess for hypersensitivity (see contraindications). • Assess client's sleeping patterns if taking chamomile. • Assess for use of alcohol, sedatives, and anticoagulants before administering this herb.
Cinnamon (*Cinnamomum*)	Used as an antifungal, analgesic, appetite stimulant, and antidiarrheal. Cinnamon is also reported to treat the common cold, abdominal pain, passive internal bleeding, hypertension, and bronchitis.	Essential oil, fluid extract, powder, and tincture. Dosage for passive bleeding is to use the essential oil in combination with Erigeron oil, diluted in carrier oil.	Contraindicated for pregnancy, lactation, and small children. No known drug interactions.	• Assess for hypersensitivity in the form of wheezing or a rash. Discontinue this herb if these symptoms are present and administer an antihistamine.

Echinacea purpura (*Echinacea angustifolia*)	Primarily used as an immune support for the common cold, influenza, and bacterial infections. Echinacea may be used to promote wound healing, bruises, burns, scratches, and leg ulcers.	Capsules, fluid extract, juice, powder, sublingual tablets, tea, and tincture. For prevention of colds and infections, the root tincture is recommended at ½ teaspoon b.i.d. Do not use this herb longer than 8 weeks.	Contraindicated for pregnancy, lactation, and children under 2 years of age. Caution should be used for persons with autoimmune diseases (HIV/AIDs), lupus erhythematosus, multiple sclerosis, tuberculosis, and hypersensitivity. Interaction: Echinacea may decrease the action of econazole vaginal cream.	• Assess for hypersensitivity to this herb and to daisies. • Teach clients not to use this herb longer than 8 weeks.
Feverfew (*Chrysanthemum parthenium*)	Used to treat arthritis, fever, menstrual irregularities, and threatened miscarriages. It may be effective for prevention of migraine headaches.	Capsules, fresh herb, extract, tablets, and tinctures.	Contraindicated for pregnancy, lactation, and children. Avoid if hypersensitive to feverfew. Interactions: None known.	• Assess client for hypersensitivity to feverfew. • Assess for effects of this herb. • Assess for side effects such as mouth ulcers and muscle and joint pain.
Garlic (*Allium sativum*)	Cholesterol-lowering effects for decreasing low-density lipoprotein (LDL) and triglycerides raises high-density lipoproteins (HDL). It may regulate blood sugar and decrease blood pressure and platelet aggregation.	Capsules, extract, fresh garlic bulbs, oil, powder, and syrup.	Do not use with anticoagulants because of prolongation of bleeding. Because of potentiation of insulin and oral antidiabetics when taking garlic, insulin dosages may need to be adjusted. Garlic may stimulate labor and cause colic in infants and is contraindicated for pregnancy and lactation. Persons with hyperthyroidism should avoid consuming garlic because of the side effect of reducing iodine uptake. Garlic increases clotting time and should be avoided for persons undergoing surgery.	• Assess client for hypersensitivity to garlic. • Assess lipid levels if used for lipid lowering or cholesterol reduction. • Assess client's diabetic regimen (insulin or oral antidiabetics). • Assess coagulation studies and CBC. • Assess for use of anticoagulants.

(*Continues*)

TABLE 17-3 Common Herbs for Health Promotion (Continued)

HERB	REPORTED USES	ADMINISTRATION/ AVAILABILITY	CAUTIONS/INTERACTIONS	CLINICAL CONSIDERATIONS AND ASSESSMENTS
Ginger root (*Zingiber officinale*)	Prevents nausea and vomiting and acts as a digestive aid, peripheral circulatory stimulant, and antioxidant. May treat migraine headaches and induce platelet aggregation.	Capsules, extract, fresh and dried root, powder, tablets, tea, and tincture.	Contraindicated for pregnancy, lactation, and hypersensitivity reactions. Not recommended for persons with cholelithiasis. Interactions: It may potentiate bleeding if used with anticoagulants and antiplatelets.	• Assess client for allergies to ginger. • Assess for use of anticoagulants and antiplatelets. • Assess for effectiveness of ginger for intended use (i.e., nausea).
Ginkgo (*Ginkgo biloba*)	An antioxidant that may improve peripheral vascular circulation. Used to reduce peripheral vascular insufficiency and cerebral dysfunction in Alzheimer's disease. Also used for treatment of arthritis, mild depression, dizziness, headaches, and intermittent claudication.	Capsules, fluid extract, tablets, tea, and tincture.	Ginkgo is contraindicated for pregnancy, lactation, and children. Avoid use in persons with coagulation disorders and hemophilia or with allergies to ginkgo. Interactions: This herb may increase bleeding. Use with anticoagulants, platelet inhibitors, and MAOIs should be avoided.	• Assess clients for allergic reaction to this herb. • Assess for use of anticoagulants, platelet inhibitors, and MAOIs.
Horse chestnut (*Aesculus hippocastanum*)	Decreases capillary permeability. Used to treat venous insufficiency, phlebitis, and varicose veins. Possible effectiveness for edema, hemorrhoids, inflammation, and prostate enlargement.	Standard forms of horse chestnut include extract and tincture.	Contraindicated for pregnancy, lactation, and children. May cause hepatotoxicity and renal dysfunction in high doses. Interactions: Anticoagulants, aspirin, and salicylates.	• Assess client for allergic reaction. • Assess for bleeding tendencies. • Assess lab values for hepatic (AST, ALT, and bilirubin levels) and renal (BUN and creatinine) functioning.
Kava kava (*Piper methystium*)	Sedative and sleep enhancer. Used for anxiety, stress, restlessness, depression, and muscle relaxation. Possible effectiveness as an antiepileptic and antipsychotic.	Beverage, capsules, extract, tablets, and tinctures.	Do not combine with alcohol or central nervous system (CNS) depressants. Persons with Parkinson's disease, allergies, and major depressive disorders should not use this herb. Kava is contraindicated for pregnancy, lactation, and children under 12 years of age. Interactions: Sedatives, CNS depressants, antiparkinsonians.	• Assess clients for allergies. • Assess for use of alcohol, antidepressants, barbiturates, Parkinson's medications, benzodiazepines, sedatives, and CNS depressants.

Milk thistle (*Silybum marianum*)	Used for treatment of liver toxicity due to poisonous mushrooms, cirrhosis of the liver, chronic hepatitis C, and liver transplantation.	Tincture.	Contraindicated for pregnancy, lactation, and children. Avoid use with allergies to herbs and plants from the aster family. Interactions: Drugs that are metabolized via the liver.	• Assess client for allergies to this herb. • Monitor liver lab values (AST, ALT, and bilirubin). • Assess for use of drugs that are metabolized by the liver.
St. John's Wort (*Hypericum perforatum*)	Used to treat mild to moderate depression and anxiety. Used topically as an anti-inflammatory for hemorrhoids, vitiligo, and burns.	Capsules (sublingual), cream, and tincture.	Contraindicated for pregnancy, lactation, and children. Avoid use with allergies to this herb. Interactions: Alcohol, amphetamines, immunosuppressants, antiretroviral agents, MAOIs, selective serotonin reuptake inhibitors (SSRIs), sedatives, and tricyclics.	• Assess for allergies to St. John's Wort. • Assess for use of antidepressants, antiretrovirals, and sedatives.
Saw palmetto (*Sabal serralata*)	Reports of effectiveness for chronic cystitis and to increase breast size, sperm count, and sexual potency are related to saw palmetto use. Most notably, this herb is used for treatment of benign prostatic hypertrophy (BPH).	Berries, capsules, extract, tablets, and tea.	Contraindicated for pregnancy, lactation, and children. Interactions: Anti-inflammatories, hormones, immunostimulants.	• Assess for allergic reaction. • Assess for urinary retention, frequency, urgency, and nocturia. • Assess client's use of anti-inflammatory drugs, hormones, and immunostimulants.

Adapted from *Understanding Complementary and Alternative Therapies,* by M. Downey, 2009, manuscript submitted for publication.

Aromatherapists have used oils to treat specific ailments. Some essential oils have antibacterial properties and are used in a variety of pharmaceutical preparations. These oils should be used intelligently and with caution.

A growing phenomenon in aromatherapy is called Raindrop Therapy (NAHA, 2008a). This type of aromatherapy uses seven single undiluted oils that are dripped onto the spinal area of a client's back. The therapist uses his fingertips to work the oil into the skin. These treatments have become common in homes and spas, and clients have claimed a variety of healing properties from their use. However, there is controversy and warning regarding the use of Raindrop Therapy because of the possibility of serious skin rashes, irritation, and burns from the undiluted oils.

Humor

Therapeutic humor includes any intervention that promotes health and wellness by stimulating a playful discovery, expression, or appreciation of the absurdity or incongruity of life's situations (Association for Applied and Therapeutic Humor, 2008). It is probably the least understood but the easiest to do.

To avoid giving offense, it is important to determine the client's perception of what is humorous. Whether a given situation is considered humorous or offensive will vary greatly from culture to culture and person to person. Good taste and common sense should serve as guides.

Nurses can promote humor in various ways. A humor cart (cart filled with cartoon and joke books, silly noses, and magic tricks) allows clients to select their own humor tools. A "humor room" may be made available where clients can watch comedy videos or play fun games with visitors or other clients.

Humor has many therapeutic outcomes. Norman Cousins, former chairperson of the Task Force in Psychoneuroimmunology at the School of Medicine at UCLA, tells how his recovery from an incurable connective tissue disorder, ankylosing spondylitis, was enhanced by watching films and movies that made him laugh daily (Cousins, 1979). Humor can effectively relieve anxiety, improve respiratory function, promote relaxation, enhance immunological function, and decrease pain by stimulating endorphin production.

Animal-Assisted Therapy

Animals were used in England in 1792 at York Retreat, where psychiatric clients cared for rabbits and poultry (McConnell, 2002). It was 1944 before animals were used in a therapeutic setting in the United States.

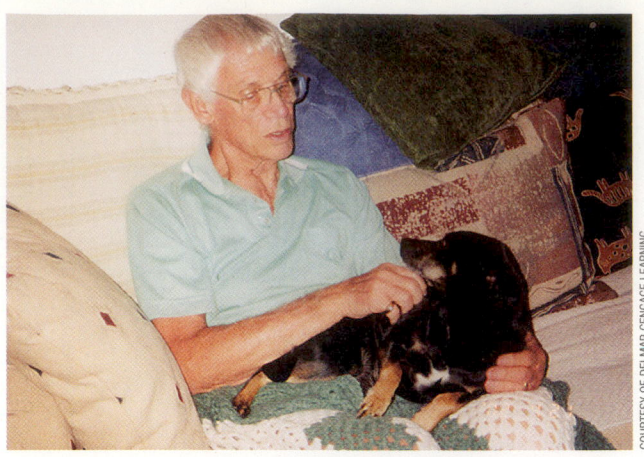

COURTESY OF DELMAR CENGAGE LEARNING

FIGURE 17-6 Pet therapy provides health benefits.

In animal-assisted therapy (AAT), a prepared handler and trained animal work one-on-one with a client toward identified short- and long-term goals.

Currently, AAT is used as a complementary therapy for people in both acute and long-term care settings (Figure 17-6).

Dogs are the animals most often used in AAT. Cats are less predictable, and many people are allergic to cat dander (Miller & Connor, 2000). Animal-assisted therapy has many applications, including overcoming physical limitations, improving mood, lowering blood pressure, and improving socialization skills and self-esteem.

Music Therapy

Therapeutic use of music consists of playing music to elicit positive changes in behavior, emotions, or physiological response. Music encourages clients to actively participate in their health care and recovery and complements other treatment modalities.

Music is good to use with imagery, as it enhances the relaxation response and heightens images. All music influences human behavior by triggering brain processes that affect a client's cognitive, emotional, and physical functions. Music radiates throughout society and culture and is easily accessible (Center for Music Therapy, 2007).

A CD player, iPod, or MP3 player with headphones playing music can be a useful tool for immobilized clients, those

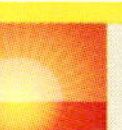

LIFE SPAN CONSIDERATIONS

Creative Therapies

Modalities such as aromatherapy, music therapy, art therapy, humor, and pet therapy are among the group of creative and sense-complementary interventions in health care. These therapies are therapeutic in a variety of clinical situations and especially for children and elderly who may have difficulty verbally expressing their feelings.

CULTURAL CONSIDERATIONS

Music and Culture

- Each culture and each generation within each culture has its own preferred type of music.
- Music that is soothing to one client may be irritating to another.
- Either ask which type of music the client would prefer or allow the client to bring music.

waiting for diagnostic tests, or those waiting for surgery. Some facilities allow clients to choose the type of music played while they undergo procedures such as cardiac catheterization. Pleasurable sound and music can reduce stress, perception of pain, anxiety, and feelings of isolation. Music can be very useful to help adolescents relax.

Play Therapy

Play therapy is especially useful with children. Toys are used to allow children to learn about what will be happening to them and to express their emotions and their current situations. Drawing and artwork also provide a way for children to share their experiences. When language ability is reduced or not yet well developed, play therapy and drawings constitute a method for children to communicate their needs and feelings to care providers.

CRITICAL THINKING

Comfort Therapies

In the hospice setting, it is common for family members to ask about comfort therapies that they may be able to provide for the client.

1. What complementary therapies can a nurse teach family members?
2. What precautions would the nurse include in the teaching of these complementary therapies?
3. What evaluative measures can the nurse teach the family members to determine whether the complementary therapy that is provided is effective for the client?

SUMMARY

- More and more health care consumers are using nontraditional treatment modalities.
- Healing is not curing. It is regaining balance and finding harmony and wholeness as changes take place within the individual.
- No one can heal another, but a nurse can act as a guide and support system for the client.
- Some of the mind/body modalities used by nurses are meditation, relaxation, imagery, biofeedback, and hypnosis.
- Body-movement modalities include movement and exercise and chiropractic therapy.
- Energy therapies can be used with clients of all ages and in various stages of illness and wellness.
- Nutritional/medicinal therapies include the use of antioxidants and herbal therapy.
- Other modalities such as aromatherapy, humor, animal-assisted therapy, music therapy, and play therapy are valuable adjuncts to conventional treatment.

REVIEW QUESTIONS

1. Therapies that are used instead of mainstream medical practice are called:
   1. alternative therapies.
   2. contemporary therapies.
   3. complementary therapies.
   4. nontraditional therapies.
2. When assessing a client's use of complementary and alternative therapies for pain management, the nurse would gain more information from the client when asking which of the following questions in the interview?
   1. Which pain medications have you used in the past?
   2. What therapies are most effective for managing your pain?
   3. Have you discussed acupuncture with your medical physician?
   4. What is your experience with traditional Chinese medicine?
3. A 40-year-old female client is being treated for high blood pressure and diabetes. She tells the nurse that she has read about herbal preparations that may enhance metabolism of insulin in the body. The nurse's response should be:
   1. "There is no evidence that this herbal therapy is effective for diabetes."
   2. "You must consult your physician about this herb."
   3. "The type of diabetes that you have is controlled only with diet, exercise, and insulin injections."
   4. "You should search for studies that investigate the effects of this herb on diabetes management."
4. One of the most universal complementary/alternative modalities is:
   1. touch.
   2. massage.
   3. nutrition.
   4. faith healing.
5. A 17-year-old male is admitted to the emergency department following a skateboarding accident. He sustained a fractured pelvis and possible skull fracture. The physician has requested low doses of pain medication until the client's neurological status is stable. The client is restless and complaining of pain at a 9/10. Which of the following methods of relaxation

can the nurse use to complement the effects of the pain medication and increase the client's comfort?
   1. Imagery, gentle massage to nontraumatized areas, and music.
   2. Herbs, Ayurvedic medicine, and biofeedback.
   3. Chiropractic, craniosacral therapy, and yoga.
   4. Hypnosis, prayer, and naturopathy.
6. In contemporary practice, Ayurvedic interventions include: (Select all that apply.)
   1. antibiotics.
   2. herbs.
   3. detoxifying massage.
   4. nasal purging.
   5. chemotherapy.
   6. yoga.
7. The nurse explains the basic elements of yoga to a client who is considering taking a yoga class. Which of the following statements indicates that the client needs further teaching?
   1. "Yoga integrates mental, physical, and spiritual energies to promote my health and wellness."
   2. "The basic elements are proper breathing, posture, and movement."
   3. "Yoga can holistically treat my back problems and emotional distress."
   4. "The nurse will use her hands to redirect my energy flow."
8. A client informs the nurse that he would like to use aromatherapy in treating his headaches. The most appropriate response from the nurse is:
   1. "Lavender is useful in treating headaches, muscle aches, and digestive disorders."
   2. "I encourage you to inform your physician that you are considering using aromatherapy to treat your headaches."
   3. "Aromatherapy has not been scientifically proven to work."
   4. "You will want to try eucalyptus and clary sage, as they work well together to treat headaches."
9. The nurse knows that which of the following complementary and alternative therapies should not be performed on a client who is diagnosed with a deep-vein thrombosis?
   1. Massage.
   2. Music therapy.
   3. Hypnosis.
   4. Aromatherapy.
10. Chamomile tea is contraindicated in which of the following clients?
   1. A client with a stage 3 decubitus ulcer.
   2. A client who has insomnia.
   3. A client who is 7-months pregnant.
   4. A client who has a history of heartburn.

REFERENCES/SUGGESTED READINGS

Achterberg, J. (2002). *Imagery in healing: Shamanism and modern medicine*. Boston: Shambhala.

Achterberg, J., Dossey, B., & Kolkmeier, L. (1994). *Rituals of healing: Using imagery for health and wellness*. New York: Bantam.

Association for Applied Psychophysiology and Biofeedback. (2008). Potential clients. Retrieved August 26, 2008, from http://www.aapb.org

Association for Applied and Therapeutic Humor. (2008). Purpose. Retrieved August 26, 2008, from http://www.aath.org

Astin, J. (1998). Why patients use alternative medicine: Results of a national study. *Journal of the American Medical Association, 279*(19), 1248.

Avis, A. (1999). Aromatherapy in practice. *Nursing Standard, 13*(24), 14–15.

Benson, H. (1975). *The relaxation response*. New York: Morrow.

Bloomington Hospital. (2008a). Ayurveda: What is it? Retrieved August 28, 2008, from http://www.bloomingtonhospital.org

Bloomington Hospital. (2008b). Body movement. Retrieved August 26, 2008, from http://www.bloomingtonhospital.org

Brett, H. (1999). Aromatherapy in the care of older people. *Nursing Times, 95*(33), 56–57.

Brown, H., Cassileth, B., Lewis, J., & Renner, J. (1994, June 15). Alternative medicine—Or quackery? *Patient Care*, 80–98.

Byers, D. (2001). *Better health with foot reflexology* (10th ed.). St. Petersburg, FL: Ingham.

Byrd, C., & Sherrill, J. (1995). The therapeutic effects of intercessory prayer. *Journal of Christian Nursing, 12*(1), 21–23.

Caradonna, B. (2008). Iridology: An introduction. Available: http://www.iridologyassn.org/index.php?page=2887

Carpenter, D. (2008). Basic iridology. Available: http://www.iridologyassn.org/index.php?page=2889

Center for Music Therapy. (2007). Center for Music Therapy philosophy. Retrieved August 29, 2008, from http://www.centerformusictherapy.com

Cerrato, P. (1998). Aromatherapy: Is it for real? *RN, 61*(6), 51–52.

Cerrato, P. (1999a). A radical approach to heart disease. *RN, 62*(4), 65–66.

Cerrato, P. (1999b). Tai chi: A martial art turns therapeutic. *RN, 62*(2), 59–60.

Cerrato, P. (2000). Diet and herbs for BPH? *RN, 63*(2), 63–64.

Cerrato, P. (2002). Complementary therapies update. *RN, 65*(9), 23.

Chiropractic Arts Center. (2007). Frequently asked questions. Available: http://www.chiroarts.com/faqs.html

Chopra, D. (1998). *Ageless body, timeless mind*. New York: Harmony.

Chopra, D. (2008). The wisdom of Ayurveda. Retrieved August 25, 2008, from http://www.chopra.com

Cousins, N. (1979). *Anatomy of an illness*. New York: Norton.

Davis, J. (2002). Yoga finds new twists in the U.S. Available: http://aolsvc.health.webmed.aol.com/content/article/1668.51358?SRC=aolkw&K W=yoga

Dossey, B. (Ed.). (1997). *Core curriculum for holistic nursing*. Gaithersburg, MD: Aspen.

Dossey, B. (1999a). Imagery: Awakening the inner healer. In B. Dossey, L. Keegan, C. Guzzetta, & L. Kolkmeier (Eds.), *Holistic nursing: A handbook for practice* (3rd ed.). Gaithersburg, MD: Aspen.

Dossey, B. (1999b). The psychophysiology of bodymind healing. In B. Dossey, L. Keegan, C. Guzzetta, & L. Kolkmeier (Eds.), *Holistic nursing: A handbook for practice* (3rd ed.). Gaithersburg, MD: Aspen.

Dossey, B., Keegan, L., & Guzzetta, C. (2004). *Holistic nursing: A handbook for practice.* (4th ed.). Boston: Jones & Bartlett.

Dossey, L. (1997). *Healing words: The power of prayer and the practice of medicine.* San Francisco: Harper.

Dossey, L. (1999). *Prayer, healing, and medicine: An evening with Larry Dossey.* Arvada, CO: Lutheran Medical Center Community Foundation, Arvada Center.

Dossey, L. (2003). *Healing beyond the body: Medicine and the infinite reach of the mind.* Boston: Shambhala.

Dossey, L., Polkinghorne, J., & Benson, H. (2002). *Healing through prayer: Health practitioners tell the story.* Toronto: Anglican Book Centre.

Downey, M. (2009). *Understanding Complementary and Alternative Therapies.* Manuscript submitted for publication.

Evans, B. (1999). Complementary therapies and HIV infection. *American Journal of Nursing, 99*(2), 42–45.

Falsafi, N. (2001). The use of holistic concepts in professional practice. *Journal of Holistic Nursing, 19*(4), 390–392.

Feuerstein, G. (1998). Yoga and yoga therapy. Available: http://members.aol.com/yogaresearch/yogatherapy.htm

Floyd, J., & Fernandes, J. (2003). Making a place for CAM in the ICU. *RN, 66*(7), 44–47.

Fonnesbeck, B. (1998). Are you kidding? *Nursing98, 28*(3), 64.

Fontaine, K. (2005). *Complementary and alternative therapies for nursing practice* (2nd ed.). Upper Saddle River, NJ: Prentice Hall.

Frisch, N. (1997). Changing of the guard. *Beginnings, 17*(1), 1, 11.

Frisch, N., & Frisch, L. (2010). *Psychiatric mental health nursing* (4th ed.). Clifton Park, NY: Delmar Cengage Learning.

Gates, R. (1997). Legal issues in alternative medicine. *Alternative Therapies in Clinical Practice, 4*(4), 143.

Geiter, H. (2002). The spiritual side of nursing, *RN, 65*(5), 43–44.

Geller, U. (2002). *Mind medicine: The secret of powerful healing.* Boston: Element Books.

Guinness, A. (1993). *Family guide to natural medicine: How to stay healthy the natural way.* Pleasantville, NY: Reader's Digest.

Hatcher, T. (2001). The proverbial herb. *American Journal of Nursing, 101*(2), 36–43.

Herbert-Ashton, M. (2002, September). Getting a handle on herbals. *Travel Nursing Today* (Supplement to *RN*), September, 16–24.

Hodge, P., & Ullrich, S. (1999). Does your assessment include alternative therapies? *RN, 62*(6), 47–49.

Hover-Kramer, D. (2002). *Healing touch: A resource for health care professionals* (2nd ed.). Clifton Park, NY: Delmar Cengage Learning.

Hutchison, C. (1999). Healing touch: An energetic approach. *American Journal of Nursing, 99*(4), 43–48.

Irmin, M., Olmstead, R., & Motiva, S. (2008). Improving sleep quality in older adults with moderate sleep complaints: A randomized controlled trial of tai chi chih. *Sleep, 31*(7), 1001–1008.

Japsen, B. (1995, August 21). Cost-conscious providers take to holistic medicine. *Modern Healthcare*, 138–142.

Kane, J. (2001). *The healing companion: Simple and effective ways your presence can help people heal.* San Francisco, CA: Harper.

Keegan, L. (1994). *The nurse as healer.* Clifton Park, NY: Delmar Cengage Learning.

Keegan, L. (1998). Alternative and complementary therapies. *Nursing98, 28*(4), 50–53.

Keegan, L. (1999a). Nutrition, exercise, and movement. In B. Dossey, L. Keegan, C. Guzzetta, & L. Kolkmeier (Eds.), *Holistic nursing: A handbook for practice* (3rd ed., pp. 257–285). Gaithersburg, MD: Aspen.

Keegan, L. (1999b). Touch: Connecting with the healing power. In B. Dossey, L. Keegan, C. Guzzetta, & L. Kolkmeier (Eds.), *Holistic nursing: A handbook for practice* (3rd ed.). Gaithersburg, MD: Aspen.

Keegan, L. (2001). *Healing with complementary and alternative therapies.* Clifton Park, NY: Delmar Cengage Learning.

King, M., Pettigrew, A., & Reed, F. (1999). Complementary, alternative, integrative: Have nurses kept pace with their clients? *Medsurg Nursing, 8*(4), 249–56.

Klein, A. (2001). How can you laugh at a time like this? Available: http://aath.org/art_klein.html

Kolkmeier, L. (1999). Relaxation: Opening the door to change. In B. Dossey, L. Keegan, C. Guzzetta, & L. Kolkmeier (Eds.), *Holistic nursing: A handbook for practice* (3rd ed.). Gaithersburg, MD: Aspen.

Krieger, D. (1993). *Accepting your power to heal: The personal practice of therapeutic touch.* Santa Fe, NM: Bear.

Levin, J. (2001). *God, faith and health: Exploring the spirituality-healing connection.* Hoboken, NJ: Wiley.

Lorenzo, P. (2003). Complementary therapies—They're not without risk. *RN, 66*(1), 65–68.

Marwick, C. (1995). Should physicians prescribe prayer for health? Spiritual aspects of well-being considered. *Journal of the American Medical Association, 273*(20), 1561–1562.

Mason, J. (1999). Massage: The nursing touch. In C. Hutchinson, Healing touch: An energetic approach. *American Journal of Nursing, 99*(4), 44.

Maxwell, J. (1997). The gentle power of acupressure. *RN, 60*(4), 53–56.

Mayo Clinic. (2007). Acupuncture: Can it help? Retrieved August 25, 2008, from http://www.mayoclinic.com

McConnell, E. (2002). Myths and facts about animal-assisted therapy. *Nursing2002, 32*(3), 76.

McGhee, P. (1998). Rx: Laughter. *RN, 69*(7), 50–53.

McGhee, P. (1999). *Health, healing, and the amuse system* (3rd ed.). Dubuque, IA: Kendall/Hunt.

Mentgen, J. (2002). The clinical practice of healing touch. In D. Hover-Kramer (Ed.), *Healing touch: A resource for health care professionals* (2nd ed.). Clifton Park, NY: Delmar Cengage Learning.

Miller, J., & Connor, K. (2000). Going to the dogs . . . for help. *Nursing2000, 30*(11), 65–67.

Mills, E. M. (1994). The effect of low-intensity aerobic exercise on muscle strength, flexibility, and balance among sedentary elderly persons. *Nursing Research, 43,* 206–211.

Moyers, B. (1995). *Healing and the mind.* New York: Doubleday.

National Association for Holistic Aromatherapy. (2008a). *Aromatherapy undiluted—Safety and ethics.* Retrieved August 28, 2008, from http://www.naha.org

National Association for Holistic Aromatherapy. (2008b). Top 10 essential oils. Retrieved August 28, 2008, from http://www.naha.org

National Center for Complementary and Alternative Medicine. (2002). Funding: Appropriations history. Available: http://nccam.nih.gov/about/appropriations/index.htm

National Center for Complementary and Alternative Therapy. (2007). Insurance coverage. Retrieved August 26, 2008, from http://www.ncaam.nih.gov

National Center for Complementary and Alternative Medicine. (2008a). The use of complementary and alternative medicine in the United States. Retrieved August 25, 2008, from http://nccam.nih.gov/news/camsurvey_fs1.htm

National Center for Complementary and Alternative Medicine. (2008b). Yoga for health: An introduction. Retrieved August 26, 2008, from http://www.nccam.nih.gov

Nightingale, F. (1969). *Nursing: What it is and what it is not.* New York: Dover.

Nontraditional Choices. (2001a). Discovering yoga. *Nursing2001, 31*(2), 20.

Nontraditional Choices. (2001b). Potentially dangerous herbs. *Nursing2001, 31*(10), 92.
Nontraditional Choices. (2001c). Trying therapeutic massage. *Nursing2001, 31*(6), 26.
Nontraditional Choices. (2001d). When patients ask about . . . reflexology. *Nursing2001, 31*(9), 68.
Nontraditional Choices. (2002a). Learning about acupuncture. *Nursing2002, 32*(1), 28–29.
Nontraditional Choices. (2002b). Learning about tai chi chuan. *Nursing2002, 32*(12), 86.
Nontraditional Choices. (2002c). Practicing meditation. *Nursing2002, 32*(4), 70.
Nontraditional Choices. (2002d). Understanding biofeedback. *Nursing2002, 32*(6), 88–90.
Nontraditional Choices. (2003a). Putting imagery to work for your patient. *Nursing2003, 33*(6), 73.
Nontraditional Choices. (2003b). Understanding echinacea. *Nursing2003, 33*(1), 76.
North American Nursing Diagnosis Association International. (2010). *NANDA-I nursing diagnoses: Definitions and classification 2009–2011*. Ames, IA: Wiley-Blackwell.
Ostlund, R. Jr. (2004). Phytosterols and cholesterol metabolism. *Current Opinion in Lipidology*, 15(1), 37–41.
Payne, M. (2002). Power of touch. *Nursing2002, 32*(6), 102.
Pert, C. (1986). The wisdom of the receptors: Neuropeptides, the emotions, and bodymind. *Advances, 3,* 8–16.
Phytochemicals. (2008). What are phytochemicals? Retrieved August 30, 2008, from http://www.phytochemicals.info
Renner, J., Dillard, J., & Edelberg, D. (1999). Should the FDA regulate alternative medicines? *Hospital Health Network,* 73(10), 24.
Rosing, M. (2001). Warm hands, warm heart. *Nursing2001, 31*(12), 32.
Schroeder-Shecker, T. (1994). Music for the dying. *Journal of Holistic Nursing, 12*(1), 83–99.
Shiatsu Society. (2008). Frequently asked questions. Retrieved August 29, 2008, from http://www.shiatsusociety.org
Smith, M., Kemp, J., Hemphill, L., & Vojir, C. (2002). Outcomes of therapeutic massage for hospitalized cancer patients. *Journal of Nursing Scholarship, 34*(3), 257–262.
Snyder, J. R. (1999). Therapeutic touch in hospice care. In C. Hutchison, Healing touch: An energetic approach. *American Journal of Nursing, 99*(4), 46.
Spencer, J., & Jacobs, J. (Eds.) (1999). *Complementary/alternative medicine: An evidence-based approach*. St. Louis, MO: Mosby.
Stanley-Hermanns, M., & Miller, J. (2002). Animal-assisted therapy. *American Journal of Nursing, 102*(10), 69–76.
Stedman, M. (1999). Alternatives: You'd better shop around. *Health, 13*(1), 60–66.
Sutherland, J. (2000). Getting to the point. *American Journal of Nursing, 100*(9), 40–43.
Trevelyan, J. (1993). Aromatherapy. *Nursing Times, 89*(25), 38–40.
Vacca, V. (1998). Back to high touch. *RN, 69*(7), 88.
Weil, A. (1998). *Natural health, natural medicine: A comprehensive manual for wellness and self-care* (Rev. ed.). New York: Houghton Mifflin.
Weil, A. (2000). *Spontaneous healing: How to discover and enhance your body's natural ability to maintain and heal itself.* New York: Ivy Books.

RESOURCES

Acupressure Institute, http://www.acupressureinstitute.com
American Academy of Medical Acupuncture (AAMA), http://www.medicalacupuncture.org
American Holistic Nurses Association (AHNA), http://www.ahna.org
American Massage Therapy Association (AMTA), http://www.amtamassage.org
Association for Applied Psychophysiology and Biofeedback (AAPB), http://www.aapb.org
Association for Applied and Therapeutic Humor (AATH), http://www.aath.org
Healing Touch International, Inc., http://www.healingtouchinternational.org
International Iridology Practitioners Association, http://www.iridologyassn.org
National Center for Complementary and Alternative Medicine, National Institutes of Health, http://www.nccam.nih.gov
Tai Chi Association, http://www.tai-chi-association.com
Yoga Research and Education Foundation (YREF), http://www.yref.org

CHAPTER 18
Basic Nutrition

MAKING THE CONNECTION

Refer to the following chapters to increase your understanding of nutrition:

Basic Nursing
- ***Life Span Development***
- ***Cultural Considerations***
- ***Diagnostic Tests***

Basic Procedures
- ***Hand Hygiene***
- ***Measuring Intake and Output***

Intermediate Procedures
- ***Feeding and Medicating via Enteral Tube***

LEARNING OBJECTIVES

Upon completion of this chapter, you should be able to:

- Define key terms.
- Describe the role of the nurse in promoting proper nutrition.
- Explain how the body uses nutrients.
- Compare the six types of nutrients for functions, sources, digestion, absorption, storage, and signs of deficiency and excess.
- Describe factors affecting kilocalorie needs.
- Explain the food guide pyramid.
- Explain the purposes of the Dietary Guidelines for Americans and the recommended dietary allowances (RDAs).
- Discuss factors influencing nutrition.
- Explain the dietary needs and nutritional assessments for infancy, childhood, adolescence, older adulthood, pregnancy, and lactation.
- Explain the relationship between health and nutrition.
- Discuss weight management.
- Explain how to determine energy (kcal) needs.
- Describe three ways to promote food safety.
- Describe the standard hospital diets: regular, soft, liquid, mechanical, and pureed.

- Cite the proper procedure for serving a meal tray.
- List important points to follow when feeding a client.

KEY TERMS

absorption
anabolism
anthropometric measurements
atherosclerosis
basal metabolism
body mass index
calorie
catabolism
cholesterol
chyme
complete proteins
deglutition
dehydration
diet therapy
dietary prescription/order
digestion
enriched
enteral nutrition
euglycemia
excretion
extracellular fluid
fat-soluble vitamins
fortified
gluconeogenesis
glycogenesis
glycogenolysis
hyperglycemia
hypoglycemia
incomplete proteins
ingestion
insensible water loss
insulin
interstitial fluid
intracellular fluid
ketosis
kilocalories
kwashiorkor
lipids
marasmus
mastication
metabolic rate
metabolism
monounsaturated fatty acids
nutrition
obesity
oxidation
parenteral nutrition
peristalsis
phospholipids
polyunsaturated fatty acids
satiety
sensible water loss
triglycerides
vitamins
water-soluble vitamins

INTRODUCTION

Nutrition encompasses all of the processes involved in consuming and utilizing food for energy, maintenance, and growth. These processes are ingestion, digestion, absorption, metabolism, and excretion. Much of the discussion throughout this chapter focuses on ingestion because this is the process that the individual can control and with which the nurse can be of assistance to the client. Basic information is presented about proper nutrition and the role of the nurse in assisting clients to meet their nutritional needs. Topics covered include specific nutrients and their functions in the body; phytochemicals; promoting proper nutrition; factors influencing nutrition; nutritional needs during the life cycle; nutrition and health; weight management; food labeling, quality, and safety; food allergies; and nutrition and the nursing process.

PHYSIOLOGY OF NUTRITION

Five processes are involved in the body's use of nutrients: ingestion, digestion, absorption, metabolism, and excretion.

INGESTION

Nutrition begins with **ingestion**, taking food into the digestive tract, generally through the mouth. In special circumstances, ingestion occurs directly into the stomach, through a feeding tube; this situation is discussed later in the chapter.

DIGESTION

Digestion refers to the mechanical and chemical processes that convert nutrients into a physically absorbable state. Mechanical digestion includes **mastication** (chewing), breaking food into fine particles and mixing it with enzymes in saliva, and **deglutition** (swallowing food), the peristaltic waves and mucus secretions that move the food down the esophagus.

> **PROFESSIONALTIP**
>
> **Role of the LP/VN in Meeting Nutritional Needs**
>
> There are several aspects to the role of the licensed practical/vocational nurse (LP/VN) in meeting a client's nutritional needs. These are discussed throughout the chapter and are summarized as follows:
>
> - Teach clients ways to meet their nutritional needs.
> - Receive and implement physician's orders.
> - Help clients understand their diets.
> - Assist clients with eating their meals.
> - Report and record observations about nutrient intake and the nutritional status of clients.
> - Act as a communication link between the client, the physician, and the dietitian.

Chemical digestion is the process whereby enzymes, gastric and intestinal juices, bile, and pancreatic juices change food into the individual nutrients that can be used by the body.

Digestion begins in the stomach (except in the case of some starches, for which digestion begins in the mouth) and is completed in the intestines. **Peristalsis** (rhythmic, coordinated, serial contractions of the smooth muscles of the GI tract) forces **chyme** (an acidic, semifluid paste) through the small and large intestines. Only carbohydrates, proteins, and fats require chemical digestion to make the nutrients available for absorption. Figure 18-1 illustrates the basic elements and functions of the digestive system.

Absorption

Absorption is the process whereby the end products of digestion (i.e., individual nutrients) pass through the epithelial membranes in the small and large intestines and into the blood or lymph systems. The nutrients are absorbed and taken to the parts of the body that need them. Most nutrients are water soluble and can be absorbed directly through the villi (fingerlike projections that line the small intestine) and into the blood. Fats, which are not water soluble, are absorbed first into the lymph system and eventually enter the circulatory system.

Metabolism

The conversion of nutrients into energy by the body is called **metabolism**; this process is the sum total of all the biological and chemical processes in the body as they relate to the use of nutrients in every body cell. Metabolism involves two processes: anabolism and catabolism. **Anabolism** is the constructive process of metabolism, wherein new molecules are synthesized and new tissues are formed, as in growth and repair. This process requires energy. **Catabolism** is the destructive process of metabolism, wherein tissues or substances are broken into their component parts. This process releases energy. During metabolism, energy is also produced by the process of **oxidation**, which is the chemical process of combining nutrients with oxygen. The energy produced by the body is used in a number of ways: electrical energy for brain and nerve activities, chemical energy for metabolism, mechanical energy for muscle contractions, and thermal energy to keep the body warm.

Metabolic rate is the rate of energy utilization in the body; it is expressed in units called calories. One **calorie** is the amount of heat required to raise the temperature of one gram of water by 1° Celsius. Because of the large quantity of energy released during metabolism, the energy is expressed in **kilocalories** (kcal), each of which is equal to 1,000 calories.

Basal metabolism is the amount of energy needed to maintain essential physiologic functions, when a person is at *complete* rest. It is the lowest level of energy expenditure.

The major factor affecting basal metabolism is body composition. Lean muscle tissue has a higher metabolic rate and thus produces more energy than does fatty tissue. Generally, women have a lower metabolism than men because they

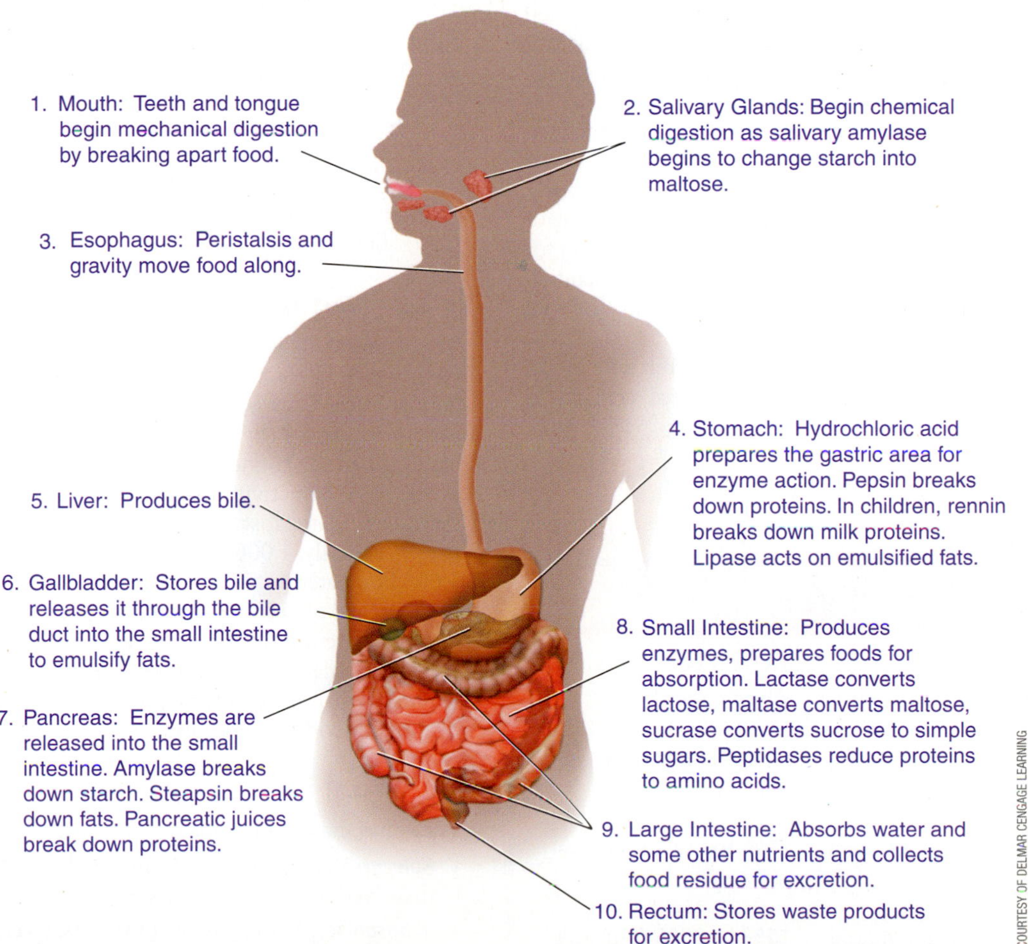
1. Mouth: Teeth and tongue begin mechanical digestion by breaking apart food.
2. Salivary Glands: Begin chemical digestion as salivary amylase begins to change starch into maltose.
3. Esophagus: Peristalsis and gravity move food along.
4. Stomach: Hydrochloric acid prepares the gastric area for enzyme action. Pepsin breaks down proteins. In children, rennin breaks down milk proteins. Lipase acts on emulsified fats.
5. Liver: Produces bile.
6. Gallbladder: Stores bile and releases it through the bile duct into the small intestine to emulsify fats.
7. Pancreas: Enzymes are released into the small intestine. Amylase breaks down starch. Steapsin breaks down fats. Pancreatic juices break down proteins.
8. Small Intestine: Produces enzymes, prepares foods for absorption. Lactase converts lactose, maltase converts maltose, sucrase converts sucrose to simple sugars. Peptidases reduce proteins to amino acids.
9. Large Intestine: Absorbs water and some other nutrients and collects food residue for excretion.
10. Rectum: Stores waste products for excretion.
COURTESY OF DELMAR CENGAGE LEARNING

Figure 18-1 Functions of the Digestive System

have a higher percentage of fat tissue; however, metabolism increases during menstruation, pregnancy, and lactation. Age is also an influence because growth periods increase metabolism. Glandular activity, especially of the thyroid gland, affects metabolism. The rate of metabolism is governed primarily by the hormones triiodothyronine (T3) and thyroxine (T4). Hypothyroid activity, a decrease in the secretion of thyroid hormones, causes a lower rate of metabolism, whereas hyperthyroid activity, an increase in the secretion of thyroid hormones, causes a higher rate of metabolism.

Excretion

Excretion is the process of eliminating or removing waste products from the body. Dietary fiber and other indigestible materials, salts, and other products such as bile and water are formed into feces and excreted from the body as solid waste. Other excretory organs that aid the digestive system in the elimination of wastes include the kidneys, bladder, sweat glands, skin, and lungs. Most liquid waste is sent through the kidneys and bladder to be excreted as urine. Some liquid waste is removed through the sweat glands of the skin as perspiration. Gaseous waste is eliminated through the lungs.

NUTRIENTS

The body must have six types of nutrients to function efficiently and effectively. These are water, carbohydrates, fats, proteins, vitamins, and minerals. If a person eats a well-balanced diet, all the nutrients the body requires are provided by the food. Table 18-1 offers an overview of the first four nutrients in relation to their fuel value (the amount of energy they supply) and their daily requirements.

Nutrients are classified as energy nutrients, organic nutrients, and inorganic nutrients, as shown in Table 18-2.

Energy nutrients release energy for use by the body. Organic nutrients build and maintain body tissues and regulate body processes. Inorganic nutrients provide a medium for the body's chemical reactions, transport materials, maintain body temperature, promote bone formation, and conduct nerve impulses.

The functions of the nutrients are interrelated. Intake changes in one nutrient may lead to functional changes in another. Some examples of interrelated functions include that (a) iron is better absorbed when vitamin C is present and that (b) calcium absorption depends on the presence of vitamin D.

Table 18-1 Nutrients, Fuel Values, and Daily Requirements

NUTRIENT	FUEL VALUE	DAILY REQUIREMENTS
Water	0	1,000 mL/ 1,000 kcal eaten
Carbohydrates	1 g = 4 kcal	50% to 60% total kcal per day
Fats	1 g = 9 kcal	25% to 30% total kcal per day
Protein	1 g = 4 kcal	15% to 20% total kcal per day

COURTESY OF DELMAR CENGAGE LEARNING

Table 18-2 Classification of Nutrients

CLASSES	NUTRIENTS
Energy nutrients	Carbohydrates Fats (Lipids) Proteins
Organic nutrients	Carbohydrates Fats (Lipids) Proteins Vitamins
Inorganic nutrients	Water Minerals

COURTESY OF DELMAR CENGAGE LEARNING

Water

Water is the most important nutrient. It is more vital to life than is food. Virtually all body functions require water. An individual may live for weeks without food but for only approximately 10 days without water.

Water is the major constituent in every cell of the body. Approximately 55% to 65% of an adult's weight is water, and approximately 70% to 75% of an infant's weight is water. The body's water content decreases with age.

Approximately two-thirds of the water in the body is **intracellular fluid** (ICF), fluid within the cells. The other one-third is **extracellular fluid** (ECF), fluid outside the cells, including plasma fluid, lymph, cerebrospinal fluid, **interstitial fluid** (fluid in tissue spaces around each cell), and GI fluids.

Daily Requirements

The amount of water needed by the body varies based on environmental factors, such as temperature and humidity, and physical factors, such as activity level, metabolic need, functional losses (urine and feces), age, respiratory rate, and state of health. Higher environmental temperatures and vigorous physical activity cause more water loss as perspiration increases. Water lost must be replaced to maintain metabolism. Generally, 1,000 mL of water is needed to process every 1,000 kcal eaten.

A state of relative water balance exists when the body has adequate fluid distributed appropriately as ICF and ECF. A person's daily water intake and output should be equal (Figure 18-2). Excessive intake of fluids is not a problem in a healthy individual; more intake simply causes more output.

Functions

Water has many functions in the body:

- *Solvent:* Water is the liquid in which many substances are dissolved to form solutions.
- *Transporter:* Water carries nutrients, wastes, and other materials throughout the body and to and from each cell via blood, tissue fluids, and body secretions.

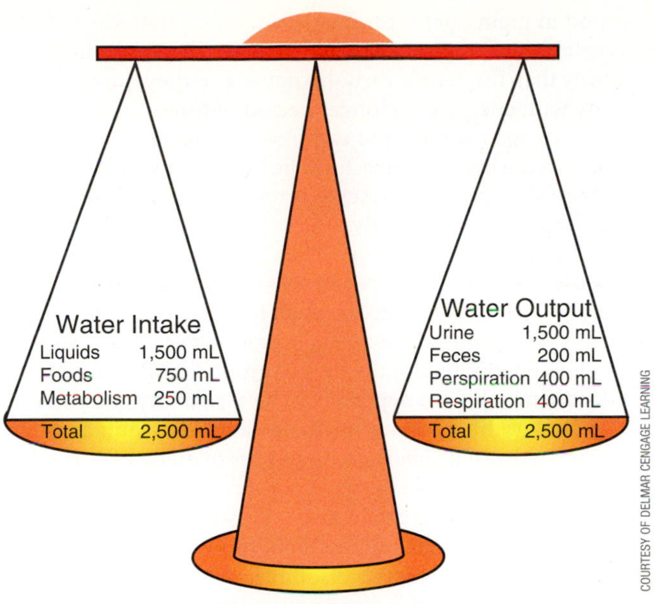

COURTESY OF DELMAR CENGAGE LEARNING

FIGURE 18-2 Body Water Balance (Approximate Figures for a Sedentary Adult)

- *Regulator of body temperature:* Water is excreted as perspiration when the temperature goes up. Evaporation of perspiration cools the body.
- *Lubricant:* Water is a component of fluid within the joints, called synovial fluid, which provides smooth movement of the many joints in the body.
- *Component of all cells:* Water gives structure and form to the body.
- *Hydrolysis:* Water breaks apart substances, especially in metabolism.

Classification and Sources

There are three sources of water for the body:

- Liquids consumed, including water, coffee, juice, tea, milk, and soft drinks
- Foods consumed, especially vegetables and fruits
- Metabolism, which produces water when oxidization occurs

Digestion, Absorption, and Storage

Water is not digested but, rather, is absorbed and used by the body as we drink it. It is not stored by the body and is excreted daily. Water losses are classified as **sensible**, the person is aware of the loss, or **insensible**, the person is not generally aware of the loss. There are four ways the body normally loses water:

- *Urine:* accounts for the greatest amount of water lost from the body (sensible loss)
- *Feces:* contains a small amount of water (insensible loss, except in cases of diarrhea)
- *Perspiration:* varies with temperature, but some fluid is always lost (insensible or sensible loss)
- *Respiration:* releases moisture with every breath (insensible loss)

> **LIFE SPAN CONSIDERATIONS**
>
> **Dehydration**
>
> Infants, small children, and elderly persons are more susceptible to dehydration. For them, dehydration occurs more rapidly and is more severe.

Signs of Deficiency and Excess

Abnormal water losses from the body include profuse sweating, vomiting, diarrhea, hemorrhage, wound drainage (burns), fever, and edema. With edema, the water is still in the body but is not usable.

A deficiency of water is called **dehydration**. Prolonged dehydration results in death. Some conditions cause an excessive accumulation of fluid in the body. This condition is called *positive water balance.* It occurs when more water is taken in than is used and excreted, and edema results. Hypothyroidism, congestive heart failure, hypoproteinemia (low amounts of protein), some infections and cancers, and some renal conditions can cause water retention because sodium is not being excreted normally.

CARBOHYDRATES

Carbohydrates are made of the elements carbon, hydrogen, and oxygen. In nutrition, the first letters of these three elements are used as the abbreviation: CHO.

Carbohydrates constitute the chief source of energy for all body functions. They are also the major food source for all people because they are the least expensive and the most abundant foods.

> **PROFESSIONALTIP**
>
> **Signs and Symptoms of Dehydration**
>
> - Health history reveals inadequate intake of fluids.
> - Urine output is decreased.
> - Urine specific gravity is greater than 1.035.
> - Weight loss (% body weight) is 3% to 5% for mild, 6% to 9% for moderate, and 10% to 15% for severe dehydration.
> - Eyes appear sunken; tongue displays increased furrows and fissures.
> - Oral mucous membranes are dry.
> - Skin turgor is decreased.
> - Venous filling and emptying times are delayed (longer than 3 to 5 seconds).
> - In infants, fontanels are sunken.
> - Changes in neurological status may occur with moderate to severe dehydration.
>
> (From *Health Assessment and Physical Examination* [4th ed.], by M. E. Z. Estes, 2010, Clifton Park, NY: Delmar Cengage Learning.)

Daily Requirements

It is recommended that carbohydrates make up 50% to 60% of an individual's kcal intake per day. For example, if an individual's total energy requirement is 2,000 kcal, 50% of this number is 1,000; this number is then divided by 4 (the number of kcal in each gram of carbohydrate; Table 18-1), for an estimated carbohydrate requirement of 250 g/day. It is estimated that current U.S. diets contain only 45% of their kcal from carbohydrates (Roth, 2006).

Functions

Carbohydrates constitute the primary source of energy for the body. The body must maintain a constant supply of energy; therefore, it stores approximately one-half a day's supply of carbohydrates in the liver and muscles for use as needed. A sufficient supply of carbohydrates spares proteins from being used for energy, thus allowing proteins to perform their primary function of building and repairing body tissues. Carbohydrates are needed to oxidize fats completely and for synthesis of fatty acids and amino acids. The central nervous system and erythrocytes rely solely on carbohydrates for energy.

Classification and Sources

Carbohydrates are classified as either simple or complex. Simple carbohydrates are single sugars (monosaccharides) such as glucose, fructose, and galactose found in fruits, honey, and corn syrup. Monosaccharides require no digestion, are quickly absorbed, and are either used for energy or stored as glycogen.

Double sugars (disaccharides), such as sucrose, maltose, and lactose, are two single sugars joined together. They are found in milk, sweeteners, sugar, and molasses. Before they can be absorbed by the body, disaccharides must be separated into monosaccharides through digestion.

Complex carbohydrates (polysaccharides) are composed of many single sugars joined together. Those important in nutrition are starch, glycogen, and dietary fiber (cellulose). The most significant of these in the diet is starch, which is found in grains, grain products, legumes, potatoes, and other vegetables. Complex carbohydrates are digested much more slowly than the simple carbohydrates, and they thus supply the body with energy for a longer period of time.

Glycogen is a form of carbohydrate made by the liver and stored in the liver and muscles. The body keeps a 12- to 48-hour store of glycogen. This reserve is used between meals and during sleep to maintain **euglycemia** (normal blood glucose level) for body functions. **Glycogenesis** is the process of converting glucose to glycogen. **Glycogenolysis** is the process of changing the glycogen back to glucose when it is needed by the body for energy. **Insulin** is a pancreatic hormone necessary for cells to produce energy and for the liver to produce and store glycogen. Glucose metabolism depends on the availability of insulin.

Dietary fiber has no nutritive value: The human body is unable to digest it. There are two types of dietary fiber: soluble and insoluble. Soluble dietary fiber slows gastric emptying and binds bile acids and cholesterol. This fiber provides **satiety** (a feeling of adequate fullness from food) and lowers the cholesterol level in the blood. Insoluble dietary fiber holds water, which increases fecal bulk and stimulates peristalsis for better elimination. Good sources of both kinds of dietary fiber are whole grains, whole-grain products, legumes, and fruits and vegetables with their skins.

> **PROFESSIONALTIP**
>
> **Insulin Levels and the Client Who Is Diabetic**
>
> When the secretion of insulin is impaired or absent, the glucose level in the blood becomes excessively high. This condition is called **hyperglycemia** and is usually a symptom of diabetes mellitus. If control by diet is ineffective, insulin injections or an oral hypoglycemic must be used to control blood sugar. When insulin is given, the client's intake of carbohydrates must be carefully controlled to balance the prescribed dosage of insulin. **Hypoglycemia** occurs when blood glucose levels are unusually low. A mild form of hypoglycemia may occur if one waits too long between meals or if the pancreas secretes too much insulin. Symptoms include fatigue, shaking, sweating, and headache.

Digestion, Absorption, and Storage

Digestion of cooked starches begins in the mouth, when the salivary enzyme ptyalin mixes with the starch in food during chewing. Little digestion takes place in the stomach. Carbohydrate digestion is completed in the small intestine by pancreatic and intestinal enzymes present there. Carbohydrates leave no waste for the kidneys to eliminate.

Glucose and other monosaccharides, the final products of carbohydrate digestion, are absorbed into the blood through the capillaries in the villi of the intestinal mucosa. Fructose and other monosaccharides are converted to glucose in the liver.

Glucose not needed for immediate energy is converted to glycogen by the liver and stored there and in the muscles. Any remaining glucose is then converted to fatty acids and stored as adipose tissue (fat). The body has no way to rid itself of excess carbohydrates; they are either used or stored.

Signs of Deficiency and Excess

A mild deficiency of carbohydrates can result in weight loss and fatigue. A diet seriously deficient in carbohydrates causes

> 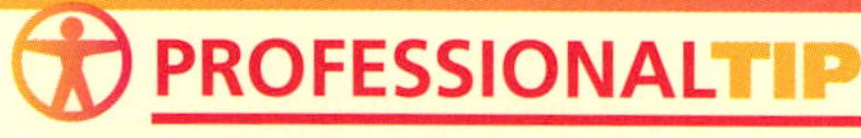
>
>
> **Lactose Intolerance**
>
> Many adults are unable to digest lactose and suffer from bloating, abdominal cramps, and diarrhea after drinking milk or consuming milk-based food products such as processed cheese. This reaction is called lactose intolerance. It is caused by insufficient lactase, the enzyme required for digestion of lactose. Special low-lactose milk products can be used instead of regular milk. Lactase-containing products are also available.

extra fat to be metabolized to meet the body's energy needs. Without carbohydrates, fat is incompletely oxidized, producing ketones, an acid by-product, which accumulates in the blood and urine causing **ketosis**. Ketosis can result from uncontrolled insulin-dependent diabetes mellitus, starvation, or diets extremely low in carbohydrates. It can lead to coma and even death.

Excess carbohydrate consumption is one of the most common causes of obesity. Although some of the surplus carbohydrate is changed to glycogen, the major part of any surplus becomes adipose tissue. Too many carbohydrates may cause tooth decay, irritate the lining of the stomach, or cause flatulence.

Fats

Fats constitute the most concentrated source of energy in the diet, providing 9 kcal per gram of fat. People in developed countries tend to eat diets relatively high in fat. Although fat is an essential nutrient, too much fat is a hazard to good health. *Lipids* is the descriptive word for fats of all kinds. **Lipids** are organic compounds that are insoluble in water but soluble in organic solvents, such as ether and alcohol, and include true fats and fatlike compounds such as lipoids and sterols. Fats provide slightly more than twice the calorie content of carbohydrates. Like carbohydrates, fats are composed of carbon, hydrogen, and oxygen, but they have a substantially lower proportion of oxygen.

Daily Requirements

It is recommended that fats make up no more than 25% to 30% of an individual's caloric intake per day. For example, assuming that one's total energy requirement is 2,000 kcal/day, one-quarter (25%) of this would be 500 kcal. Dividing 500 kcal by 9 (the number of kcal in each gram of fat; Table 18-1) yields an estimated fat requirement of 55.5 g/day.

Functions

Fat has many functions in the body. It:

- Provides a concentrated source of energy (more than twice the kcal of carbohydrates)
- Assists in the absorption of fat-soluble vitamins
- Is a major component of cell membranes and myelin sheaths
- Improves the flavor of food and delays the stomach's emptying time, providing a feeling of satiety

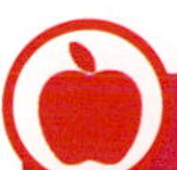

CLIENT TEACHING

Fats

The average American fat intake has decreased to 33% of the total daily caloric intake. The total fat intake should be less than 30% of an individual's daily caloric intake with no more than 10% of total kcal as saturated fats, 10% polyunsaturated fats, and 10% monounsaturated fats. For example, if an individual consumes 2,000 calories a day, she should eat no more than 65 grams of fat, or about 600 calories of fat (University of Iowa Health Care, 2006).

- Protects and helps hold organs in place
- Insulates the body, thus assisting in temperature maintenance

Classification and Sources

Fat is formed by one molecule of glycerol being joined to one, two, or three fatty-acid molecules. The most important lipids are:

- **Triglycerides** (true fats), composed of one glycerol molecule attached to three fatty-acid molecules. Most dietary fat and body fat are triglycerides.
- **Phospholipids** (lipoids), composed of glycerol, fatty acids, and phosphorus. They are structural components of cells, for example, myelin (insulating covering of many nerves) and lecithin (a part of cell membranes).
- **Cholesterol** (a sterol), not essential in the diet because the liver manufactures approximately 1,000 mg every day. Cholesterol is found in all cell membranes, in brain and nerve tissue, and in blood, and it is excreted in bile. Cholesterol is required to produce several hormones, including estrogen, testosterone, adrenalin, and cortisone. The intake of dietary cholesterol from animal food products may affect the serum (blood) cholesterol level.

Fats can also be classified by source, visibility, and saturation. The source of fats can be either animal or plant (vegetable). Examples of animal fat are lard, butter, milk, cream, egg yolks, and the fat in meat, poultry, and fish. Examples of plant fat are oils (corn, safflower, olive, cottonseed, peanut, palm, and coconut), nuts, and avocado.

Fats are either visible or invisible. Visible fats are easy to identify, such as butter, oils, margarine, lard, shortening, bacon, salt pork, and the fat around beef. Examples of invisible fats are those in egg yolks, whole milk and whole-milk

CLIENT TEACHING

Blood Cholesterol

- Blood cholesterol level should not exceed 200 mg of cholesterol/dL of blood.
- To decrease the blood cholesterol level, the client should follow a diet low in saturated fat.
- Weight loss and exercise also help lower blood cholesterol level.
- A diet high in saturated fat increases the blood cholesterol by 15% to 25%.

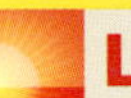

LIFE SPAN CONSIDERATIONS

Children and Cholesterol

If children are not fed high-cholesterol foods on a regular basis, their chance of overusing these foods as adults lessens, as does their risk of heart attack and stroke.

products, cheeses, nuts, seeds, olives, avocados, many desserts, and baked goods.

The saturation of a fat refers to its chemical composition. When fatty acids, the main building blocks of fats, contain all the hydrogen ions possible in the molecule, they are said to be saturated. Saturated fats tend to be solid at room temperature. Generally, animal fats are saturated. Plant fats that are saturated are coconut, palm kernel, and palm oils. Unsaturated fats are missing a hydrogen ion at one or more places in the molecule. They tend to be soft or liquid at room temperature. Plant fats are generally unsaturated, with the exceptions already mentioned. Unsaturated fats are subdivided into monounsaturated and polyunsaturated fats. **Monounsaturated fatty acids** are those that form glycerol esters with one double or triple bond; foods in this category are nuts, fowl, and olive oil. **Polyunsaturated fatty acids** form glycerol esters that have many carbons unbonded to hydrogen atoms. Foods such as fish, corn, sunflower seeds, soybeans, cottonseeds, and safflower oil contain polyunsaturated fat.

There are three essential fatty acids (linoleic, linolenic, and arachidonic) necessary for growth, cholesterol metabolism, and heart action. They are found primarily in vegetable oils, egg yolks, and poultry.

Digestion, Absorption, and Storage

No chemical breakdown of fats occurs in the mouth, and very little fat digestion takes place in the stomach. When fat reaches the small intestine, digestion begins. The digestive agents for fat are bile, from the gallbladder, and enzymes, from the pancreas and the small intestine. The final products of fat digestion are fatty acids and glycerol. Approximately 95% of dietary fat is absorbed in the small intestine.

Fats not immediately needed by the body are stored as adipose tissue. Approximately 5 g of fat are excreted daily in the feces.

Signs of Deficiency and Excess

Deficiency symptoms occur when fats provide less than 10% of the total daily kcal requirement. Gross deficiency may result in eczema (inflamed and scaly skin condition), retarded growth, and weight loss.

Excess fat in the diet can lead to overweight and heart disease. In addition, studies point to an association between high-fat diets and cancers of the colon, breast, uterus, and prostate.

An elevated level of cholesterol in the blood is thought to be a contributing factor in heart disease, because hypercholesterolemia (high serum cholesterol) is common in clients with atherosclerosis. **Atherosclerosis** is a cardiovascular disease wherein plaque (fatty deposits containing cholesterol and other substances) forms on the inside of artery walls, reducing the space for blood flow.

LIFE SPAN CONSIDERATIONS

Proteins

By the age of 4 years, body protein content reaches the adult level of approximately 18% of body weight.

PROTEIN

Proteins are made of the elements carbon, hydrogen, oxygen, and nitrogen. In nutrition, the first letters of these four elements are used as the abbreviation: CHON.

Protein is the only nutrient that can build, repair, and maintain body tissues. An adequate supply of proteins in the daily diet is essential. All tissues and fluids in the body, with the exception of bile and urine, contain some protein. The basic building materials of protein are amino acids.

Daily Requirements

Daily protein requirement is determined by size, age, gender, and physical and emotional condition. A large person has more body cells to maintain than does a small person. A growing child, a pregnant woman, or a woman who is breastfeeding needs more protein for each pound of body weight than does the average adult. When digestion is inefficient, fewer amino acids are absorbed by the body; consequently, the protein requirement is higher. This is sometimes thought to be the case with elderly clients. Extra proteins are usually required after surgery or severe burns or during infections to replace lost tissue and manufacture antibodies. In addition, emotional trauma can cause the body to excrete more nitrogen than it normally does, thus increasing the need for protein-rich foods.

The National Research Council of the National Academy of Sciences considers the average adult's daily requirement to be 0.8 g of protein for each kilogram of body weight. Daily protein requirement is determined by multiplying body weight in kilograms (weight in pounds divided by 2.2) by 0.8. For instance:

$$\begin{aligned} 130 \text{ lb. woman} \div 2.2 \text{ lb/kg} &= 59.1 \text{ kg} \times 0.8 \text{ g/kg} \\ &= 47.3 \text{ g protein/day} \end{aligned}$$

Functions

The primary function of protein in the diet is to provide the amino acids necessary for the synthesis of body proteins, which are used to build, repair, and maintain the body tissues. Protein composes most of the muscles, skin, hair, nails, brain, nerves, and internal organs.

Another function of protein is to assist in regulating fluid balance. Proteins are a vital part of enzymes, hormones, and blood plasma. Many body processes are regulated by enzymes and hormones. Plasma proteins help control water balance between the circulatory system and surrounding tissues. Protein is also used to build antibodies, which help defend the body against disease and foreign substances.

In the event of insufficient stores of carbohydrate and fat (the body's primary and secondary sources of energy), protein, in the form of amino acids, can be converted into glucose and used for energy. This process is called **gluconeogenesis**; however, when protein is used for energy, it is not available for its primary function. Using protein for energy also results in waste products that are difficult for the kidneys to excrete.

Classification and Sources

Protein is classified by source and completeness. Animal sources include meat, fish, poultry, eggs, milk, and dairy products. Plant sources are grains, legumes, nuts, and seeds. The completeness of a protein refers to its quality. Of the 22 amino acids, nine are called essential amino acids (i.e., they must be present in the diet because the body cannot synthesize them). **Complete proteins** contain all nine essential amino acids. All animal proteins, with the exception of gelatin, are complete proteins; the only complete plant protein is soybeans.

Plant proteins (with the exception of soybeans) are **incomplete proteins** (i.e., one or more of the essential amino acids are missing). Because all plant proteins do not lack the same essential amino acids, they can be combined in various ways to provide all the essential amino acids. When two plant protein foods are combined to provide the essential amino acids, they are said to be complementary. Some of the common complementary plant proteins are rice and beans (legumes), corn and beans, wheat bread and beans, toast and pea soup, and rice and lentils. Complementary proteins are a very important part of planning a healthy vegetarian diet.

Digestion, Absorption, and Storage

Chemical digestion of protein begins in the stomach, when hydrochloric acid activates the enzyme pepsin; however, most of the digestion takes place in the small intestine with the action of pancreatic and intestinal enzymes. The end product of protein digestion is amino acids. The body can then combine the amino acids to build, repair, and maintain body tissues.

The amino acids are absorbed into the blood by the capillaries in the villi of the intestinal mucosa. Amino acids not used to build proteins are converted to glucose, glycogen, or fat and are stored.

Signs of Deficiency and Excess

When people are unable to obtain an adequate supply of protein for an extended period, muscle wasting occurs, and arms and legs become very thin. At the same time, albumin (protein in blood plasma) deficiency causes edema, resulting in an extremely swollen appearance. The edema decreases when sufficient protein is eaten. Clients with edema become lethargic and depressed. These signs are seen in grossly neglected children or in the elderly poor or incapacitated. Children who lack sufficient protein do not grow to their potential size. Infants born to mothers eating insufficient protein during pregnancy can have permanently impaired mental capacities (Roth, 2006).

Two deficiency diseases that affect children are caused by a grossly inadequate supply of protein, energy, or both. **Marasmus**, a condition resulting from severe malnutrition, afflicts very young children who lack both energy and protein foods as well as vitamins and minerals. The infant with marasmus appears emaciated but does not have edema; hair is dull and dry, and the skin is thin and wrinkled. **Kwashiorkor** results when there is a sudden or recent lack of protein-containing food (such as during a famine). This disease results in edema, painful skin lesions, and changes in the pigmentation of skin and hair (Roth, 2006).

It is easy for people living in the developed parts of the world to ingest more protein than the body requires. This should be avoided because the saturated fats and cholesterol common to complete protein foods may contribute to heart disease and provide more kcal than needed. Some studies indicate a connection between long-term high-protein diets and colon cancer and high calcium excretion, which depletes the bones of calcium and may contribute to osteoporosis. People who eat excessive amounts of protein-rich foods may ignore essential fruits and vegetables, and excess protein intake may put more demands on the kidneys than they can handle (Roth, 2006).

PROFESSIONALTIP

Daily Allowance of Protein

The National Research Council recommends that protein intake represent no more than 15% to 20% of one's daily kcal intake and not exceed double the amount given in the table of Recommended Dietary Allowances.

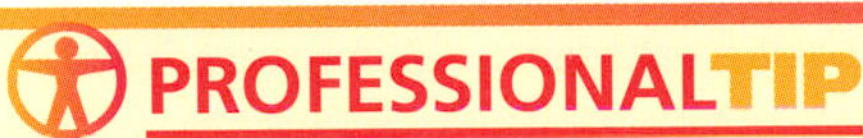

Vegetarians and Protein

It is essential that clients following vegetarian diets carefully calculate the types and amount of protein in their diets to prevent protein deficiency.

VITAMINS

Vitamins are organic compounds essential to life and health. They regulate body processes and are needed in very small amounts. They have no fuel value but are required for the metabolism of fats, carbohydrates, and proteins.

Daily Requirements

The Food and Nutrition Board of the National Academy of Sciences—National Research Council prepared a list of recommended dietary allowances for the 11 vitamins for which it considers current scientific research to be adequate for determining daily recommendations. Vitamin allowances are given by weight in milligrams (mg) or micrograms (mcg).

Vitamins taken in addition to the diet are called vitamin supplements. Lifestyle choices may affect the need for vitamin supplementation (Table 18-3).

Functions

The functions of vitamins are unique to each individual vitamin. Tables 18-4 and 18-5 list the functions of each type of vitamin.

TABLE 18-3 Supplements for Lifestyle Choices

LIFESTYLE CHOICE	SUGGESTED SUPPLEMENT
Restricted diets	B_{12} (cobalamin)
Extensive exercise program	Riboflavin
Oral contraceptives	Pyridoine, niacin, vitamin C
Smoking	Vitamin C
Alcohol	Thiamine, folate
Caffeine	B vitamins, vitamin C

COURTESY OF DELMAR CENGAGE LEARNING

TABLE 18-4 Fat-Soluble Vitamins

VITAMIN	FUNCTION	SOURCES	DEFICIENCY	TOXIC EFFECTS
A	• Aids in night vision • Promotes growth of bones and teeth • Maintains skin and mucous membranes	• Fish oils • Carrots • Sweet potatoes • Broccoli • Cantaloupe • Green leafy vegetables	• Night blindness • Dry, scaly skin • Diarrhea • Respiratory infections	• From supplementation: anorexia, diarrhea, hair loss, bone pain, liver damage
D	• Stimulates absorption of calcium and phosphorus for good bone mineralization	• Yeast • Fish liver oils • Fortified milk and cereals	• Rickets • Malformed teeth • Bone deformities	• Hypercalcemia • Kidney stones • Cardiovascular damage
E	• Acts as an antioxidant • Maintains cell membrane integrity • Protects red blood cells (RBCs) from hemolysis	• Vegetable oils • Leafy vegetables • Wheat germ	• Increased RBC hemolysis • Rare, except in cases of fat malabsorption	• Depression • Fatigue • Diarrhea • Cramps • Headaches
K	• Responsible for synthesis of prothrombin, needed for normal blood clotting	• Dark-green leafy vegetables • Made by intestinal bacteria	• Rare, except in newborns • Delayed blood clotting	• No toxic effects

COURTESY OF DELMAR CENGAGE LEARNING

TABLE 18-5 Water-Soluble Vitamins

VITAMIN	FUNCTION	SOURCES	DEFICIENCY	TOXIC EFFECTS
C (asorbic acid)	• Builds and maintains strong tissues • Promotes wound healing • Aids in resisting infection • Enhances iron absorption	• Citrus fruits • Green and red peppers • Tomatoes • Melons • Cabbage • Broccoli • Strawberries	• Scurvy • Easy bruising • Delayed wound healing • Swollen, inflamed gums • Secondary infections	• Megadoses: excessive iron absorption • Nausea • Diarrhea
B_1 (thiamine)	• Promotes CHO metabolism • Ensures normal nervous system functioning	• Enriched grains and cereals • Pork • Legumes	• Beriberi • Mental confusion • Anorexia • Fatigue • Muscle weakness	• None known
B_2 (riboflavin)	• Promotes CHO, protein, and fat metabolism • Promotes deoxyribonucleic acid (DNA) synthesis • Aids in protein synthesis	• Milk and milk products • Meat, poultry, fish • Enriched grains and cereals	• Oral lesions • Dermatitis • Cheilosis • Red, swollen tongue • Reddening of cornea	• None known

(*Continues*)

TABLE 18-5 Water-Soluble Vitamins (Continued)

VITAMIN	FUNCTION	SOURCES	DEFICIENCY	TOXIC EFFECTS
Niacin (nicotinic acid)	• Aids in oxidation • Promotes CHO, protein, and fat metabolism • Aids tissue protein building	• Meat, poultry, fish • Legumes • Enriched grains • Peanuts	• Pellegra • Anorexia • Apathy • Weakness • Dermatitis • Diarrhea • Dementia	• Large doses: flushing, itching, hypotension, tachycardia
B_6 (pyridoxine)	• Is necessary for amino acid metabolism • Promotes blood formation • Maintains nervous tissue	• Chicken, fish, pork • Eggs • Whole grains	• Depression • Dermatitis • Abnormal brain wave patterns • Convulsions • Anemia	• Clumsiness • Nerve degeneration
B_{12} (cobalamin)	• Promotes normal function of all cells, especially those of the nervous system • Promotes blood formation • Promotes CHO, protein, and fat metabolism • Aids in synthesis of ribonucleic acid (RNA) and DNA • Is necessary for folate metabolism	• Fresh shrimp, oysters, meats, milk, eggs, and cheese	• Pernicious anemia • Anorexia • Indigestion • Paresthesia of hands and feet • Poor coordination • Depression	• None known
Folate (folic acid)	• Is necessary for synthesis of RNA and DNA • Promotes amino acid metabolism, RBC and white blood cell (WBC) formation • Prevents neural tube defects	• Green leafy vegetables • Milk • Eggs • Yeast	• Glossitis • Diarrhea • Macrocytic anemia	• None known
Pantothenic acid	• Promotes CHO, protein, and fat metabolism	• Animal tissues • Whole-grain cereals • Legumes • Milk	• Not observed in humans	• None known
Biotin	• Promotes CHO and fat metabolism • Is necessary for glycogen formation	• Egg yolk • Yeast • Milk • Soy flours • Cereals • Legumes • Made by intestinal bacteria	• Only induced with long-term total parenteral nutrition (TPN)	• None known

COURTESY OF DELMAR CENGAGE LEARNING

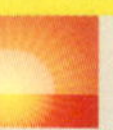

LIFE SPAN CONSIDERATIONS

Vitamins

Vitamin needs vary with the life cycle. Vitamin supplements are generally needed for pregnant or lactating women and for infants, and elders.

Classification and Sources

Vitamins are commonly grouped according to solubility. Vitamins A, D, E, and K are fat soluble, and vitamin C and the B-complex vitamins are water soluble.

Fat-Soluble Vitamins The **fat-soluble vitamins** (A, D, E, and K) require the presence of fats for their absorption from the GI tract into the lymphatic system and for cellular metabolism. They must attach to protein carriers to be transported through the blood. The body's stored reserve makes daily intake unnecessary. In fact, the reserve can result in toxic levels if large supplemental doses are taken, especially in the case of vitamin A. Deficiencies can occur in conditions that interfere with fat absorption.

Water-Soluble Vitamins The **water-soluble vitamins** (C and the B-complex vitamins) require daily ingestion in normal quantities because they are not stored in the body. They are absorbed by the capillaries in the intestinal villi directly into the circulatory system. Deficiency symptoms develop quickly in response to inadequate intake. Foods should be cooked in the least amount of water possible, because the water-soluble vitamins are released into the cooking water: when the water is discarded, the vitamins are lost.

MEMORYTRICK

Fat-Soluble Vitamins

To remember the fat soluble vitamins A, D, E, and K, memorize "Fat ADEK," as in "fat addict."

CLIENTTEACHING

Natural or Synthetic Vitamins

Some people believe that natural vitamins are superior in quality to synthetic vitamins. According to the U.S. Food and Drug Administration (FDA), however, the body cannot distinguish between a vitamin of plant or animal origin and one manufactured in a laboratory. The two types of the same vitamin are chemically identical.

CRITICAL THINKING

Vitamin Supplements

What recommendations should be made to a client regarding vitamin supplements?

Digestion, Absorption, and Storage

Vitamins do not require digestion. Fat-soluble vitamins are absorbed into the lymphatic system, whereas water-soluble vitamins are absorbed directly into the circulatory system. Excess amounts of fat-soluble vitamins cannot be excreted but are stored in the liver and adipose tissue. Water-soluble vitamins are excreted through urine, when excess amounts are taken into the body.

Signs of Deficiency or Excess

Vitamin deficiencies can occur and result in disease. Those persons inclined to vitamin deficiencies because they do not eat balanced diets include alcoholics, the poor, incapacitated elders, clients with serious diseases that affect appetite, mentally retarded persons, and young children who receive inadequate care. Deficiencies of fat-soluble vitamins occur in clients with chronic malabsorption diseases such as cystic fibrosis, celiac disease, and Crohn's disease.

Vitamins consumed in excess amounts can be toxic to the body (Tables 18-4 and 18-5).

MINERALS

Minerals are inorganic elements that help regulate body processes and/or serve as structural components of the body. Like vitamins, they have no fuel value.

Chemical analysis shows that the human body is made up of specific chemical elements. Four of these elements—oxygen, carbon, hydrogen, and nitrogen—make up 96% of body weight. All the remaining elements are minerals, making up 4% of body weight. Nevertheless, these minerals are essential for good health.

Daily Requirements

Major minerals are required in amounts greater than 100 mg/day. Trace minerals are those required in amounts less than 100 mg/day. See list of major and trace minerals in Table 18-6.

Functions

The functions of minerals are unique to each individual mineral. Table 18-7 outlines the functions, sources, deficiencies, and toxic effects of each mineral.

Classification and Sources

Minerals are generally classified as major minerals and trace elements. Minerals are found in water and in natural (unprocessed) foods, together with proteins, carbohydrates, fats, and vitamins. Minerals in the soil are absorbed by growing plants. Humans obtain minerals by eating plants grown in mineral-rich soil or by eating animals that have eaten such plants.

TABLE 18-6 Major Minerals and Trace Elements

MAJOR MINERALS	TRACE ELEMENTS	
	Essential	Questionable
Calcium (Ca)	Iron (Fe)	Arsenic (As)
Phosphorus (P)	Iodine (I)	Boron (B)
Sodium (Na)	Zinc (Zn)	Cadmium (Cd)
Potassium (K)	Selenium (Se)	Nickel (Ni)
Magnesium (Mg)	Copper (Cu)	Silicon (Si)
Chlorine (Cl)	Manganese (Mn)	Tin (Sn)
Sulfur (S)	Fluorine (Fl)	Vanadium (V)
	Chromium (Cr)	
	Molybdenum (Mo)	
	Cobalt (Co)	

COURTESY OF DELMAR CENGAGE LEARNING

Highly processed or refined foods such as sugar and white flour contain almost no minerals. Iron, together with the vitamins thiamin, riboflavin, niacin, and folate, is commonly added back to some flour and cereals, which are then labeled enriched.

Most minerals in food occur as salts, which are soluble in water. Therefore, the minerals leave the food and remain in the cooking water when foods are cooked in water. Foods should be cooked in as little water as possible or, preferably,

LIFE SPAN CONSIDERATIONS

Mineral Supplements

- During adolescence, calcium may be needed if the diet is insufficient.
- Pregnant and lactating women require added calcium, phosphorus, and iron.

TABLE 18-7 Minerals

MINERAL	FUNCTION	SOURCES	DEFICIENCY	TOXIC EFFECTS
Calcium (Ca)	• Aids in bone and teeth formation • Promotes muscle contraction and relaxation • Aids blood clotting • Aids in nerve transmission • Promotes normal heart rhythm • Needs vitamin D for Absorption	• Milk • Cheese • Sardines • Salmon • Green, leafy vegetables • Whole grains	• Rickets • Osteoporosis • Tetany • Poor tooth formation	• Kidney stones • Deposits in joints and soft tissue • May inhibit iron and zinc absorption
Phosphorus (P)	• Aids in bone and teeth formation • Involved in energy metabolism • Regulates acid–base balance • Ensures structure of cell membranes • Is part of nucleic acids	• Fish, beef, pork, poultry • Cheese • Legumes • Milk • Carbonated beverages	• Rickets • Osteoporosis • Poor tooth formation • Disturbed acid base balance	• Low serum calcium • Kidney stones
Sodium (Na)	• Helps regulate fluid balance and acid–base balance • Regulates cell membrane irritability • Regulates nerve Transmission	• Table salt • Milk • Meat • Processed foods • Carrots • Celery	• Hyponatremia • Nausea • Headache • Mental confusion • Hypotension • Anxiety • Muscle spasms	• Hypernatremia • Hypertension • Cardiovascular disturbance • Edema

(Continues)

Table 18-7 Minerals (Continued)

MINERAL	FUNCTION	SOURCES	DEFICIENCY	TOXIC EFFECTS
Potassium (K)	• Maintains fluid balance • Maintains acid–base balance • Regulates muscle activity • Aids in protein synthesis • Aids in CHO metabolism	• Fruits, especially oranges, bananas, and prunes • Red meats • Vegetables • Milk and milk products • Coffee	• Hypokalemia • Fluid and electrolyte imbalances • Tissue breakdown • Cardiac weakness • Muscle cramps	• Hyperkalemia • Muscle weakness • Severe dehydration • Mental confusion • Hypotension • Cardiac arrest
Magnesium (Mg)	• Is necessary for muscle–nerve action • Regulates CHO, CHON, and fat metabolism • Activates enzymes • Aids in bone formation	• Green, leafy vegetables • Whole grains • Legumes	• Hypomagnesemia • Tremors • Spasms • Convulsions	• Hypermagnesemia • Central nervous system (CNS) depression • Coma • Hypotension
Chlorine (Cl)	• Helps regulate fluid balance and acid–base balance • Aids digestion as part of hydrochloric acid in stomach	• Table salt • Milk • Meat • Processed foods	• Rare	• Rare
Sulfur (S)	• Serves as component of amino acids • Aids vitamin, enzyme, and hormonal activity • Is part of skin, hair, nails, and soft tissue	• Cheese • Eggs • Poultry • Fish	• None specific	• None specific
Iron (Fe)	• Aids in formation of hemoglobin • Aids in antibody formation	• Meat • Whole grains • Egg yolk • Legumes • Prunes • Raisins • Apricots	• Iron deficiency • Anemia	• Hemochromatosis • GI cramping • Vomiting • Nausea • Shock • Convulsions • Coma
Iodine (I)	• Is a component of thyroid hormones	• Iodized salt • Seafood (salt water) • Milk	• Cretinism • Goiter	• Hyperthyroidism • Fatal in large amounts
Zinc (Zn)	• Is a component of DNA and RNA • Aids in physical and sexual development • Helps ensure normal taste and smell • Aids in wound healing	• Meats, oysters • Eggs • Milk • Whole grains	• Poor wound healing • Decreased taste and smell • Growth retardation	• Muscle incoordination • Vomiting • Diarrhea • Renal failure

(*Continues*)

TABLE 18-7 Minerals (Continued)

MINERAL	FUNCTION	SOURCES	DEFICIENCY	TOXIC EFFECTS
Selenium (Se)	• Acts as an antioxidant • Works with vitamin E	• Seafoods • Meats	• Muscle weakness • Cardiomyopathy	• Selenosis • Nausea • Peripheral neuropathy • Fatigue
Copper (Cu)	• Aids in bone and blood formation • Promotes iron absorption • Is part of myelin sheath	• Seafood • Nuts • Legumes	• Iron-deficiency anemia • Hypocholesterol-emia	• None known
Manganese (Mn)	• Aids bone growth • Aids reproduction • Acts as enzyme activator	• Whole-grain cereals • Legumes • Tea	• Unknown	• Unlikely
Fluorine (Fl)	• Protects against dental caries • Contributes to bone formation and integrity	• Fluoridated water • Tea • Seafood	• Dental caries	• Mottled stains on teeth
Chromium (Cr)	• Associated with glucose metabolism	• Whole grains • Brewers yeast	• Insulin resistance • Impaired glucose tolerance	• Dietary: unlikely
Molybdenum (Mo)	• Helps ensure normal body metabolism	• Milk • Legumes • Whole grains	• Decreased production of uric acid	• Interferes with copper metabolism
Cobalt (Co)	• Is a component of vitamin B_{12} • Aids in RBC formation	• Meat, as B_{12}	• Associated with vitamin B_{12} deficiency	• Unknown

COURTESY OF DELMAR CENGAGE LEARNING

steamed, and any cooking liquid should be saved to be used in soups, gravies, and white sauces. Using this liquid improves the flavor as well as the nutrient content of foods to which it is added.

Supplemental minerals may be required during growth periods and in some clinical situations. Individuals with iron-deficiency anemia require extra iron. Persons taking potassium-losing diuretics need a potassium supplement.

Digestion, Absorption, and Storage

Minerals are absorbed in their ionic forms (i.e., carrying a positive or negative electrical charge). The amount of a mineral absorbed by the body is influenced by three factors:

- *Type of food:* Minerals in foods that come from animals are more readily absorbed than those in foods that come from plants.
- *Need of body:* If there is a deficiency of a mineral in the body, more will be absorbed.
- *Health of absorbing tissue:* If absorbing tissue (intestine) is affected by disease, less will be absorbed.

Signs of Deficiency and Excess

Because it is known that minerals are essential to good health, some people think "more is better." More can be hazardous to one's health when it comes to minerals. In a healthy individual eating a balanced diet, there will be some normal mineral loss through perspiration and saliva, and amounts in excess of body needs will be excreted in urine and feces. When concentrated forms of minerals are taken regularly over a period of time, however, they become more than the body can handle, and toxicity develops. An excessive amount of one mineral sometimes causes a deficiency of another mineral. Excessive amounts of minerals can cause hair loss and changes in the blood, hormones, bones, muscles, blood vessels, and nearly all tissues. Concentrated forms of minerals should be used only on the advice of a physician. Refer to Table 18-7 for specific signs of deficiency and toxicity of each mineral.

PROFESSIONALTIP

Vitamins, Minerals, and Herbs

Since July 1994, the federal Food and Drug Administration has placed limitations on marketing claims for vitamins, minerals, and herbs. The rules are aimed at deterring false or unproven health claims and require that companies selling these products make only claims that are substantiated by broad scientific consensus. Labeling requirements of dietary supplements began in July 1995.

PROMOTING PROPER NUTRITION

Through the years, various ways to promote proper nutrition have been devised. The best known are the four food groups, the food guide pyramid, the *Dietary Guidelines for Americans*, the recommended daily allowances, and the dietary reference intakes.

Four Food Groups (Historical)

For many years, the four food groups assisted people in eating a well-balanced diet. Eating foods from the four groups—milk, meat, fruit/vegetable and bread/cereal—provided most nutrients required in a daily diet. The minimum number of servings yielded approximately 1,200 kcal. Additional servings were to be added depending on the individual's age and activity level.

Food Guide Pyramid

In 2005, the U.S. Department of Agriculture (USDA) created the new MyPyramid and recommended the food pyramid in Figure 18-3 for a person with regular dietary needs. Each bandwidth represents a guide to the proportion of food from that group. The stepping person in the pyramid represents the importance of balancing the diet with activity. The steps in the pyramid represent the activity of an individual and recommend that the amount consumed, balance the physical activity of the person. The new pyramid has six categories of food groups represented by the six colored bands (Mathew, 2008).

Each food group of the food guide pyramid provides some but not all of the nutrients needed each day. Foods in one group cannot replace foods in another group. No one group is more important than another: all are needed.

The Orange Band: Grains or Carbohydrates

The orange band represents grains or carbohydrates and includes whole-grain bread, cereal, crackers, rice, and pasta. The nutrients contributed by this group are complex carbohydrates, incomplete protein, the B vitamins, and iron, if the product is whole grain or **enriched** (nutrients that are removed during processing are added back) with iron. Six to 11 servings a day should come from this group. Examples of serving sizes from this group are one slice of bread, one tortilla, 1 ounce (1 cup) dry cereal, and ½ cup cooked cereal, rice, or pasta.

The Green Band: Vegetables

The nutritional contributions of vegetables are carbohydrates, vitamins, minerals, water, and very small amounts of proteins and fats. Dietary fiber, important for elimination, is found in the skin of many foods in this group. Three to five servings a day from the vegetable group are suggested. Among the vegetables eaten daily, one should be a dark-green (collards

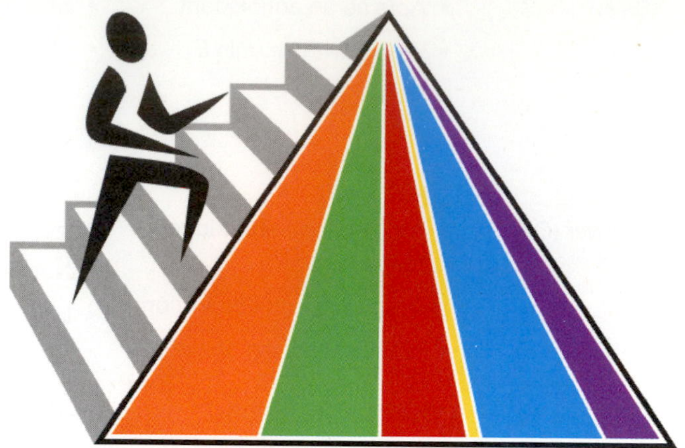

WHAT COUNTS AS A SERVING?

Bread, Cereal, Rice, and Pasta Group (Grains Group)—whole grain and refined
- 1 slice of bread
- About 1 cup of ready-to-eat cereal
- 1/2 cup of cooked cereal, rice, or pasta

Vegetable Group
- 1 cup of raw leafy vegetables
- 1/2 cup of other vegetables—cooked or raw
- 3/4 cup of vegetable juice

Fruit Group
- 1 medium apple, banana, orange, pear
- 1/2 cup of chopped, cooked, or canned fruit
- 3/4 cup of fruit juice

Milk, Yogurt, and Cheese Group (Milk Group)*
- 1 cup of milk** or yogurt**
- 1 1/2 ounces of natural cheese** (such as Cheddar)
- 2 ounces of processed cheese** (such as American)

Meat, Poultry, Fish, Dry Beans, Eggs, and Nuts Group (Meat and Beans Group)
- 2–3 ounces of cooked lean meat, poultry, or fish
- 1/2 cup of cooked dry beans# or 1/2 cup of tofu counts as 1 ounce of lean meat
- 2 1/2-ounce soyburger or 1 egg counts as 1 ounce of lean meat
- 2 tablespoons of peanut butter or 1/3 cup of nuts counts as 1 ounce of meat

NOTE: Many of the serving sizes given above are smaller than those on the Nutrition Facts Label. For example, 1 serving of cooked cereal, rice, or pasta is 1 cup for the label but only 1/2 cup for the Pyramid.

* This includes lactose-free and lactose-reduced milk products. One cup of soy-based beverage with added calcium is an option for those who prefer a non-dairy source of calcium.

** Choose fat-free or reduced-fat dairy products most often.

Dry beans, peas, and lentils can be counted as servings in either the meat and beans group or the vegetable group. As a vegetable, 1/2 cup of cooked, dry beans counts as 1 serving. As a meat substitute, 1 cup of cooked, dry beans counts as 1 serving (2 ounces of meat).

FIGURE 18-3 Daily appropriate intake of nutrition and exercise makes one healthy. MyPyramid (*Courtesy of United States Department of Agriculture [USDA, 2008] and United States Department of Health and Human Services [HHS]. Nutrition and your health: Dietary guidelines for American, 2000. Food Guide Pyramid, A Guide to Daily Food Choices [Home and Garden Bulletin No. 232]. Washington, DC: U.S. Department of Agriculture and U.S. Department of Health and Human Services*).

and spinach) or orange vegetable (sweet potato or carrot) to provide vitamin A. Sample serving sizes from the vegetable group include 1 cup of raw leafy vegetables, ½ cup of cooked or chopped raw vegetables, or ¾ cup of vegetable juice.

The Red Band: Fruits

The red band represents fruits and includes fresh, frozen, canned, or dry fruits limiting the amount of fruit juices. The nutritional contributions of fruits are carbohydrates, vitamins, minerals, and fiber. Each person should have two or four servings of fruit every day. Citrus fruits, melons, and berries should be eaten regularly, as they are high in vitamin C. Examples of serving sizes from the fruit group are one medium-sized apple, pear, banana, or orange; ½ cup of cooked, chopped, or canned fruit; or ¾ cup of fruit juice.

The Yellow Band: Oils

The yellow band represents oils. Consume most of the daily calories from plant foods (grains, fruits, and vegetables). The recommended fat sources are fish, nuts, and vegetable oils, limiting butter, margarine, shortening, and lard.

The Blue Band: Milk, Yogurt, and Other Milk Products

The blue band represents calcium-rich food, such as low-fat or fat-free milk and dairy products. The nutritional contributions of the milk group are calcium, protein, riboflavin, fat, carbohydrates, phosphorus, sodium, vitamin B_{12}, and vitamin A. If skim milk or skim milk products are used, there is no fat and significantly fewer kcal. All commercial milk products are **fortified** (a nutrient not naturally occurring in a food is added to the food) with vitamin D. Vitamin D, not naturally found in milk, is added because the calcium provided by milk is better absorbed when vitamin D is present.

Two to three servings a day are suggested from the milk group. Eight ounces of milk is considered one serving. Other milk products and their serving sizes to provide the equivalent nutrients of 8 ounces of milk are 1½ ounces of cheese, 1 cup of yogurt, 1½ cups of cottage cheese, and 1½ cups of ice cream. The kcal content of these foods varies, with ice cream containing more kcal than the other foods in the milk group.

The Purple Band: Meat and Beans

The purple band represents meat and beans, which include lean meats or poultry, fish, beans, peas, nuts, or seeds. The meat and beans group contributes complete protein, fats, iron, most other minerals, and the B vitamins. Cheese and bacon are not considered part of this group: cheese has too little iron and bacon has too much fat.

The suggested number of servings from the meat group is two to three each day. A serving size is 2 to 3 ounces of meat, fish, or poultry. Other foods that can be substituted for one serving of meat are two eggs, 4 tablespoons of peanut butter, or 1 cup cooked beans or peas (legumes). Legumes such as dried peas, beans, or lentils can be used instead of meat because of their high protein content. Peanuts as well as many other nuts are high in protein, but they are also high in fats and should be used sparingly.

Number of Servings

The number of servings for an individual depends on the number of calories the individual needs. The number of calories needed by a person depends on age, gender, size, and activity. Almost everyone should have the minimum number of servings for each group. The serving recommendations for three general calorie levels are listed in Table 18-8.

The Vegetarian Diet

There are several vegetarian diets. The common factor among them is that they do not include red meat. When carefully planned, these diets can be nutritious. They can even contribute to a reduction in obesity, high blood pressure, heart disease, some cancers, and, possibly, diabetes (Roth, 2006). They must be carefully planned so they include all the needed nutrients.

Lacto-ovo vegetarians use dairy products and eggs but no meat, poultry, or fish. Lacto vegetarians use dairy products but no meat, poultry, or eggs. Vegans avoid all animal foods.

TABLE 18-8 How Many Servings Do You Need Each Day?

FOOD GROUP	CHILDREN AGES 2 TO 6 YEARS, WOMEN, SOME OLDER ADULTS (ABOUT 1,600 CALORIES)	OLDER CHILDREN, TEEN GIRLS, ACTIVE WOMEN, MOST MEN (ABOUT 2,200 CALORIES)	TEEN BOYS, ACTIVE MEN (ABOUT 2,800 CALORIES)
Bread, Cereal, Rice, and Pasta Group (Grains Group)—especially whole grain	6	9	11
Vegetable Group	3	4	5
Fruit Group	2	3	4
Milk, Yogurt, and Cheese Group (Milk Group)—preferably fat free or low fat	2 or 3*	2 or 3*	2 or 3*

(*Continues*)

Table 18-8 How Many Servings Do You Need Each Day? (Continued)

FOOD GROUP	CHILDREN AGES 2 TO 6 YEARS, WOMEN, SOME OLDER ADULTS (ABOUT 1,600 CALORIES)	OLDER CHILDREN, TEEN GIRLS, ACTIVE WOMEN, MOST MEN (ABOUT 2,200 CALORIES)	TEEN BOYS, ACTIVE MEN (ABOUT 2,800 CALORIES)
Meat, Poultry, Fish, Dry Beans, Eggs, and Nuts Group (Meat and Beans Group)—preferably lean or low fat	2, for a total of 5 ounces	2, for a total of 6 ounces	3, for a total of 7 ounces

* The number of servings depends on your age. Older children and teenagers (ages 9 to 18 years) and adults over the age of 50 need 3 servings daily. Others need 2 servings daily. During pregnancy and lactation, the recommended number of milk group servings is the same as for nonpregnant women.

Adapted from U.S. Department of Agriculture, Center for Nutrition Policy and Promotion, The Food Guide Pyramid, Home and Garden Bulletin Number 252, 1996. United States Department of Agriculture (USDA) and United States Department of Health and Human Services (HHS). Nutrition and your health: Dietary guidelines for Americans (Home and Garden Bulletin No. 232, 2000).

They use soybeans, chickpeas, meat analogues, and tofu. It is important that their meals be carefully planned to include appropriate combinations of the essential amino acids. For example, beans served with corn or rice, or peanuts eaten with wheat, are complementary proteins. Vegans can show deficiencies of calcium; vitamins A, D, and B_{12}; and, of course, proteins.

Dietary Guidelines

The *Dietary Guidelines* developed by the U.S. Department of Agriculture and the U.S. Department of Health and Human Services were last revised in 1990. They are now stated in positive terms (i.e., "eat . . ."; "consume . . .") instead of negative terms ("avoid . . ."). These guidelines attempt to prevent overnutrition by incorporating some of the concepts of the food guide pyramid (Table 18-9).

Recommended Dietary Allowances

Recommended dietary allowances (RDAs) of essential nutrients are the recommended intake levels judged adequate to meet the known nutrient needs of practically all healthy people. Recommendations are grouped according to infants, children, males, females, and pregnant/ lactating women, and are subdivided within those groups according to age. The RDAs are compiled by the Food and Nutrition Board of the National Academy of Sciences and are periodically revised.

Dietary Reference Intakes

The dietary reference intakes (DRIs) are nutrient-based reference values for use in planning and assessing diets. They are intended to replace the old RDAs. The DRIs focus on decreasing the risk of chronic disease through nutrition, rather than on protecting against deficiency diseases, as do the RDAs.

The DRIs encompass four categories:

- *Estimated average requirement* (EAR) is the amount that meets the estimated nutrient need of 50% of the individuals in a specific group.
- *Recommended dietary allowance* (RDA) is the amount that meets the nutrient need of almost all (97% to 98%) healthy individuals in a specific age and gender group. It is the EAR plus an increase, based on scientific evidence, to account for variation within the specific group. The RDA should be used to achieve adequate nutrient intake aimed at decreasing the risk of chronic disease.
- *Adequate intake* (AI) is set when there is insufficient scientific evidence to estimate an average requirement. It is derived through experimental or observational data that show a mean intake that appears to sustain a desired indicator of health, such as calcium retention in bone.
- *Tolerable upper intake level* (UL) is the maximum intake by an individual that is unlikely to pose risks of adverse health effects in almost all healthy individuals in a specified group. It is not intended to be a recommended level of intake. There is no established benefit for individuals to consume nutrients at levels above the RDA or AI.

FACTORS INFLUENCING NUTRITION

Many factors influence nutrition. Some of the major factors are culture, religion, socioeconomics, fads, and superstitions.

Culture

A person's culture encompasses a total way of life including values, attitudes, and practices. Food practices are a substantial part of a culture. These food habits are based on availability of foods, preparation techniques, methods of serving, and the personal meaning of food (Figure 18-4). American cuisine (cooking style) is a marvelous composite of countless national, regional, cultural, and religious food customs. Consequently, categorizing a client's food habits can be difficult. People who are ill commonly have little interest in food, and sometimes foods that were familiar to them during their childhood and youth are more tempting than other types. The following section briefly discusses some food patterns typical of various cultures, regions, and countries. Of course, there can be and usually are enormous variations within any one classification.

Native American

It is thought that approximately one-half of the edible plants commonly eaten in the United States today originated with the Native Americans. Examples are corn, potatoes, squash, cranberries, pumpkin, peppers, beans, wild rice, and cocoa beans. In addition, wild fruits, game, and fish were used. Foods were

TABLE 18-9 Dietary Guidelines for Americans

	DIETARY GUIDELINES	EXPLANATION
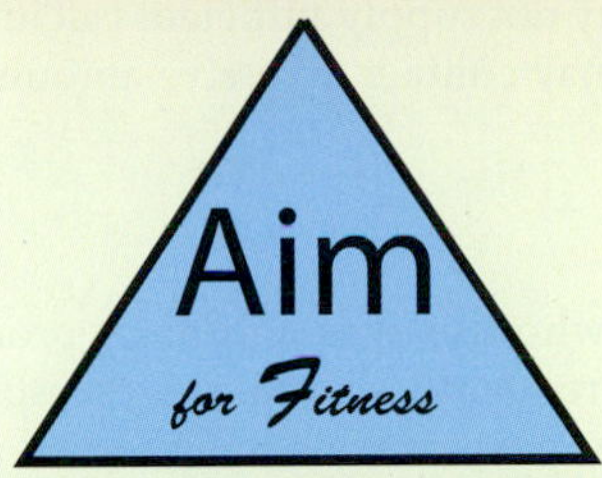	• Aim for a healthy weight. • Be physically active each day.	Following these two guidelines will help keep you and your family healthy and fit. Healthy eating and regular physical activity enable people of all ages to work productively, enjoy life, and feel their best. They also help children grow, develop, and do well in school.
 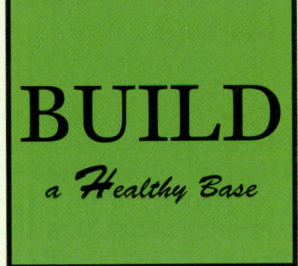	• Use the food guide pyramid to make your food choices. • Choose a variety of grains daily, especially whole grains. • Choose a variety of fruits and vegetables daily. • Keep food safe to eat.	Following these four guidelines builds a base for healthy eating. Let the food guide pyramid guide you so that you get the nutrients your body needs each day. Make grains, fruits, and vegetables the foundation of your meals. This forms a base for good nutrition and good health and may reduce your risk of certain chronic diseases. Be flexible and adventurous, try new choices from these three groups in place of some less nutritious foods or in place of higher calorie foods that you usually eat. Whatever you eat, always take steps to keep your food safe to eat.
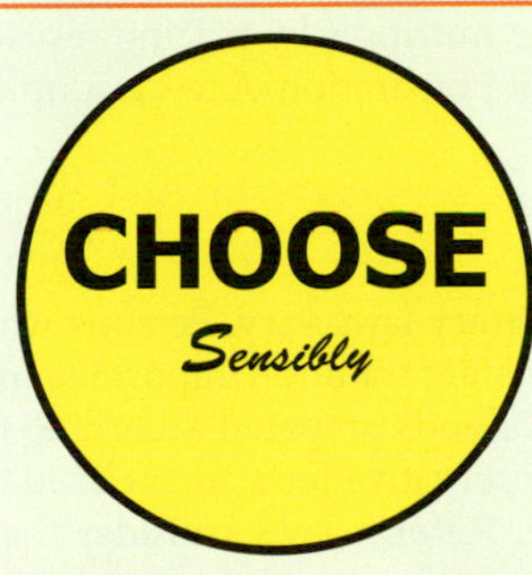	• Choose a diet that is low in saturated fat and cholesterol and moderate in total fat. • Choose beverages and foods to moderate your intake of sugars. • Choose and prepare foods with less salt. • If you drink alcoholic beverages, do so in moderation.	These four guidelines help you make sensible choices that promote health and reduce the risk of certain chronic diseases. You can enjoy all foods as part of a healthy diet as long as you do not overdo it on fat (especially saturated fat), sugars, salt, and alcohol. Read labels to identify foods that are higher in saturated fats, sugars, and salt (sodium).

From U.S. Department of Agriculture (USDA) and U.S. Department of Health and Human Services (HHS), 2000. *Nutrition and your Health: Dietary Guidelines for Americans* (Home and Garden Bulletin No. 232, 5th ed). Washington, DC: USDA.

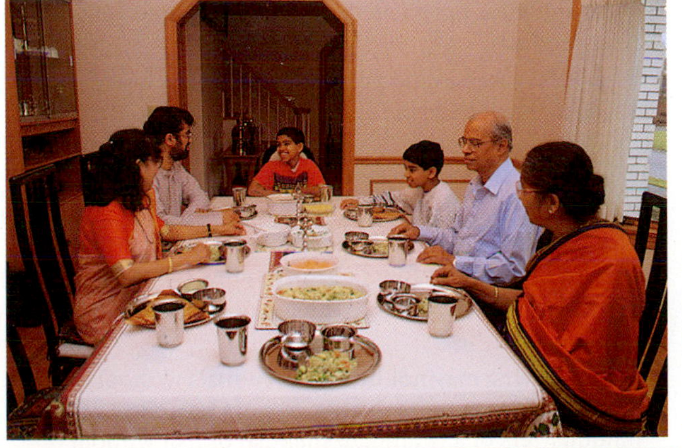

FIGURE 18-4 Family and cultural values often affect diet.

commonly prepared as soups and stews or were dried. The original Native American diets were probably more nutritionally adequate than current diets. Native American diets today may be deficient in calcium, vitamins A and C, and riboflavin (Roth, 2006).

U.S. Southern

Hot breads such as corn bread and baking powder biscuits are common in the U.S. South because the wheat grown in this area does not make good-quality yeast breads. Grits and rice are also popular carbohydrate foods. Favorite vegetables include sweet potatoes, squash, green beans, and lima beans. Watermelon, oranges, and peaches are popular fruits. Fried fish is served often, as are barbecued and stewed meats and poultry. These diets have a great deal of carbohydrate and fat and limited amounts of protein in some cases. Iron, calcium, and vitamins A and C may be deficient (Roth, 2006).

Mexican

Mexican food is a combination of Spanish and Native American foods. Beans, rice, chili peppers, tomatoes, and corn meal are favorites. Meat is often cooked with a vegetable, as in chili con carne. Cornmeal or flour is used to make tortillas, which are served as bread. The combination of beans and corn makes a complete protein. Corn tortillas filled with cheese (called enchiladas) provide some calcium, but the use of milk should be encouraged. Additional green and yellow vegetables and vitamin C–rich foods would also make these diets more well-balanced.

Puerto Rican

Rice is the basic carbohydrate food in Puerto Rican diets. Vegetables commonly used include beans, plantains, tomatoes, and peppers. Bananas, pineapple, mangoes, and papayas are popular fruits. Favorite meats are chicken, beef, and pork. Additional milk would make a more balanced diet (Roth, 2006).

Italian

Pastas with various tomato or fish sauces and cheese are popular Italian foods. Fish and highly seasoned foods are common southern Italian cuisine; whereas meat and root vegetables are common northern cuisine. The eggs, cheese, tomatoes, green vegetables, and fruits in Italian diets provide excellent sources of many nutrients. Added fat-free milk and low-fat meat would make the diet more complete (Roth, 2006).

Northern and Western European

Northern and Western European diets are similar to those of the U.S. Midwest, but with a greater use of dark breads, potatoes, and fish, and fewer green-vegetable salads. Beef and pork are popular, as are various cooked vegetables, breads, cakes, and dairy products. The addition of fresh vegetables and fruits would add vitamins, minerals, and fiber to these diets.

Central European

Citizens of Central Europe obtain the greatest portion of their calories from potatoes and grain, especially rye and buckwheat (Roth, 2006). Pork is a popular meat. Cabbage cooked in many ways is a popular vegetable, as are carrots, onions, and turnips. Eggs and dairy products are used abundantly. Limiting the number of eggs consumed and using fat-free or low-fat dairy products would reduce the fat content in this diet. Adding fresh vegetables and fruits would increase vitamins, minerals, and fiber.

Middle Eastern

Grains, wheat, and rice provide energy in Middle Eastern diets. Chickpeas in the form of hummus are popular. Lamb and yogurt are commonly used, as are cabbage, grape leaves, eggplant, tomatoes, dates, olives, and figs. Black, very sweet coffee is a popular beverage. There may be insufficient protein and calcium in this diet, depending on the amounts of meat and calcium-rich foods eaten. Fresh fruits and vegetables should be added to the diet to increase vitamins, minerals, and fiber.

Chinese

The Chinese diet is varied. Rice is the primary energy food and is used in place of bread. Vegetables are lightly cooked, and the cooking water is saved for future use. Soybeans are used in many ways, and eggs and pork are commonly served. Soy sauce is extensively used, but it is very salty and could present a problem for clients needing low-salt diets. Tea is a common beverage, but milk is not. This diet is typically low in fat (Roth, 2006).

Japanese

Japanese diets include rice, soybean paste and curd, vegetables, fruits, and fish. Food is frequently served tempura style, which means fried. Soy sauce (shoyu) and tea are commonly used. Current Japanese diets have been greatly influenced by Western culture. Japanese diets may be deficient in calcium, given the near-total lack of milk in the diet (Roth, 2006). Although fish is eaten with bones, this may not supply sufficient calcium to meet needs. Japanese diets may contain excessive amounts of salt.

Indian

Many Indians are vegetarians who use eggs and dairy products. Rice, peas, and beans are frequently served. Spices, especially curry, are popular. Indian meals are generally served as one course with many dishes.

Thai, Vietnamese, Laotian, and Cambodian

Rice, curries, vegetables, and fruit are popular in Thailand, Vietnam, Laos, and Cambodia. Meats and fish are used in small amounts. The wok (a deep, round fry pan) is used for sautéing many foods. A salty sauce made from fermented fish is commonly used. Thai, Vietnamese, Laotian, and Cambodian diets may be deficient in protein and calcium (Roth, 2006).

RELIGION

Religious beliefs often influence nutrition by placing restrictions on the foods eaten and their preparation. A few examples follow.

Jewish

Interpretations of the Jewish dietary laws vary. Persons who adhere to the Orthodox view consider tradition important and always observe the dietary laws. Foods prepared according to these laws are called kosher. Conservative Jews are inclined to observe the rules only at home. Reform Jews consider their dietary laws to be essentially ceremonial and thus minimize their significance. Essentially the laws require the following (Roth, 2006):

- Slaughtering must be done by a qualified person and in a prescribed manner.
- Meat and meat products may not be prepared with milk or milk products.
- The dishes used in the preparation and serving of meat products must be kept separate from those used for dairy foods.
- Dairy products and meat may not be eaten together. Six hours must elapse after eating meat before eating dairy products, and at least 30 minutes to 1 hour must elapse after eating dairy products before eating meat.
- The mouth must be rinsed after eating fish and before eating meat.
- The following may not be eaten: animals without cloven (split) hooves or animals that do not chew their cud, hindquarters of any animal, shellfish or fish without scales or fins, birds of prey, creeping things and insects, and leavened (containing ingredients that cause it to rise) bread during Passover.

There are prescribed fast days: Passover Week, Yom Kippur, and Feast of Purim. Chicken and fresh smoked and salted fish are popular, as are noodles, eggs, and flour dishes. These diets can be deficient in fresh vegetables and milk.

Roman Catholic

Although the dietary restrictions of the Roman Catholic religion have been liberalized, meat is not allowed on Ash Wednesday and Fridays during Lent.

Eastern Orthodox

The Eastern Orthodox religion includes Christians from the Middle East, Russia, and Greece. Although interpretations of the dietary laws vary, meat, poultry, fish, and dairy products are restricted on Wednesdays and Fridays and during Lent and Advent.

Seventh-Day Adventists

In general, Seventh-Day Adventists are lacto-ovo vegetarians, meaning that they use milk products and eggs, but no meat, fish, or poultry. Nuts, legumes, meat analogues (substitutes), and tofu (made from soybeans) may be used. Coffee, tea, and alcohol are considered to be harmful.

Mormon (Latter-Day Saints)

The only dietary restriction observed by the Mormons is the prohibition of coffee, tea, and alcoholic beverages.

Islamic

Adherents of Islam are called Muslims. Dietary laws prohibit the use of pork and alcohol, and other meats must be slaughtered according to specific laws. During the month of Ramadan, Muslims do not eat or drink during daylight hours.

Hindu

To the Hindus, all life is sacred, and animals contain the souls of ancestors. Consequently, most Hindus are vegetarians and do not use eggs in food preparation because eggs represent life.

Socioeconomics

The amount of money available to purchase food certainly influences nutrition. More money, however, does not always mean better nutrition. Persons with less money often plan their meals and buy food more carefully than do those with higher incomes. Expensive food does not mean better nutrition. Many times, persons with no monetary worries eat what they want, when they want, without paying attention to nutritional value, thereby shortchanging themselves nutritionally.

Fads

Food fads are beliefs that persist for a period of time about certain foods and that generally have no scientific basis. Often, these fads are translated into diets that can be harmful if basic nutrients are missing or are in excess. One of the most popular diets some years ago was the grapefruit and egg diet. One of the more recent fads was the liquid-protein diet. This diet overloaded the body with protein, yet other nutrients were lacking. The excessive amount of protein damaged the kidneys of many people. Indeed, some people died from this fad diet (American Heart Association, 1999).

High-protein, low-carbohydrate diets, such as the Atkins diet, have been around for over a century. An individual can lose weight very quickly on the diet, but it is not the diet of choice in the long run, as individuals usually prefer to revert to more varied and desirable choices. Once carbohydrates are reintroduced into the diet, weight gain returns. High-protein diets are not recommended for clients with liver or kidney conditions and may leave the person with depleted glycogen stores. The long-term issues encountered with this diet are uncertain at this point (Brown, 2005).

Superstitions

Superstitions are irrational beliefs about a food that are generally passed down from generation to generation. The nurse should be aware of the beliefs and the facts that contradict them so as to be knowledgeable and respectful. Examples of such superstitions are:

- *Superstition:* Toast is less fattening than bread.
- *Fact:* Only moisture is removed during toasting.
- *Superstition:* "Cravings" during pregnancy should be satisfied, or the infant will be marked or deformed.
- *Fact:* Foods eaten or not eaten by the mother do not directly affect the infant; only the nutrients or lack thereof affect the unborn child.

NUTRITIONAL NEEDS DURING THE LIFE CYCLE

As a person grows and develops from birth to old age, nutritional needs change. These changes generally are based on growth needs, energy needs, and utilization of nutrients. A nutritional assessment should be conducted to ascertain the nutritional needs of the individual.

Infancy

Food and its presentation are extremely important during the baby's first year. Physical and mental development depend on the food itself, and psychosocial development is affected by the time and manner whereby the food is offered.

Although babies have been fed according to prescribed time schedules in the past, it is preferable to feed infants on demand. Feeding on demand prevents the frustrations that hunger can bring and helps the child develop trust in people. The newborn may require more frequent feedings, but, normally, the demand schedule averages approximately every 4 hours by the time the baby is 2 or 3 months old (Roth, 2006).

Nutritional Requirements

The first year of life is a period of the most rapid growth in one's life. A baby doubles its birth weight by 6 months of age and triples it within the first year. This explains why the infant's energy, vitamin, mineral, and protein requirements are higher per unit of body weight than are those of older children or adults.

PROFESSIONALTIP

Nutritional Needs of Infants

It is important to remember that growth rates vary from child to child. Nutritional needs depend largely on a child's growth rate.

During the first year, the normal child needs approximately 100 kcal per kilogram of body weight each day. This is approximately two to three times the adult requirement. Infants who have suffered from low birth weight, malnutrition, or illness require more than the normal number of kcal per kilogram of body weight.

The nutritional status of infants is reflected in many of the same characteristics as those of adults.

The American Academy of Pediatrics recommends breast milk for the first 12 months of life, although parents must decide on the method of feeding based on their lifestyle, values, and personal feelings (Gartner et al., 2005).

Breast Milk Breastfeeding is nature's way of providing a good diet for the baby. It is, in fact, used as the guide by whom nutritional requirements of infants are measured.

Mother's milk provides the infant with temporary immunity to many infectious diseases. It is sterile, easy to digest, and usually does not cause GI disturbances or allergic reactions. Breastfed infants grow more rapidly during the first few months of life than do formula-fed babies, and they typically have fewer infections (especially ear infections). Because breast milk contains less protein and minerals than infant formula, it reduces the load on the infant's kidneys. Breastfeeding also promotes oral motor development in infants because sucking requires more and different muscles than does bottle-feeding (Roth, 2006).

One can be quite confident the infant is getting sufficient nutrients and kcal from breastfeeding if (a) there are six or more wet diapers per day, (b) there is normal growth, (c) there are one or two mustard-colored bowel movements per day, and (d) the breast becomes soft during nursing.

CLIENT TEACHING

Breastfeeding

If the mother works and cannot be available for every feeding, breast milk can be expressed earlier, refrigerated or frozen, and used at the appropriate time, or a bottle of formula can be substituted. Never warm the breast milk in a microwave oven because the antibodies will be destroyed. Instead, warm a cup of water and place the bag of breast milk in the water to heat it.

CLIENT TEACHING

Cow's Milk

Infants younger than 1 year of age should not be given regular cow's milk. Its protein is more difficult and slower to digest than that of human milk and can cause GI blood loss. The kidneys are challenged by its high protein and mineral content, and dehydration and even damage to the CNS can result. In addition, the fat is less bioavailable, meaning it is not absorbed as efficiently as that in human milk (Roth, 2006).

Formula If the baby is bottle-fed, the pediatrician provides information on commercial formulas and feeding instructions. Formulas are usually based on cow's milk because it is abundant and easily modified to resemble human milk in nutrient and kcal values.

When an infant is extremely sensitive or allergic to infant formulas, a synthetic formula made from soybeans may be given. Formulas with predigested proteins are used for infants unable to tolerate all other types of formulas (Roth, 2006).

Formulas are available in ready-to-feed, concentrated, or powdered forms. Sterile water must be mixed with the concentrated and powdered forms. The most convenient type is also the most expensive.

If the type purchased requires the addition of water, it is essential that the amount of water added be correctly measured. Too little water will create too heavy a protein and mineral load for the infant's kidneys; too much water will dilute the nutrient and kcal value such that the infant will not thrive.

Solid Foods Introducing solid foods before the age of 4 to 6 months is not recommended. The child's GI tract and kidneys are not sufficiently developed to handle solid food before that age. Furthermore, it is thought that the early introduction of solid foods may increase the likelihood of overfeeding and the possibility of food allergies developing, particularly in children whose parents suffer from food allergies.

An infant's readiness for solid foods will be demonstrated by (a) the physical ability to pull food into the mouth rather than always pushing the tongue and food out of the mouth, (b) a willingness to participate in the process, (c) the ability to sit up with support, (d) having head and neck control, and (e) the need for additional nutrients. An infant drinking more than 32 ounces of formula or nursing 8 to 10 times in 24 hours should be started on solid food.

CLIENT TEACHING

Honey

Honey should never be given to an infant under 12 months because it could be contaminated with *Clostridium botulinum* bacteria.

CLIENT TEACHING

Nursing Bottle Syndrome

Infants should not be put to bed with a bottle. Saliva, which normally cleanses the teeth, diminishes as the infant falls asleep. The milk then bathes the upper front teeth, causing tooth decay. Also, the bottle can cause the upper jaw to protrude and the lower to recede. The result is known as the baby bottle mouth, or nursing bottle syndrome. It is preferable to feed the infant the bedtime bottle, cleanse the teeth and gums with some water from another bottle or cup, and then put the infant to bed.

Solid foods must be introduced gradually and individually. One food is introduced and then no other new food for 4 or 5 days. If there is no allergic reaction, another food can be introduced, a waiting period allowed, then another, and so on. The typical order of introduction begins with cereal, usually iron-fortified rice, then oat, wheat, and mixed cereals. Cooked and pureed vegetables follow, then cooked and pureed fruits, egg yolk, and, finally, finely ground meats. Avoid giving infants egg whites before 1 year of age. Between 6 and 12 months, toast, zwieback, teething biscuits, and Cheerios can be added.

When the infant learns to drink from a cup, juice can be introduced. Juice should never be given from a bottle because babies will fill up on it and not get enough calories from other sources. Pasteurized apple juice is usually given first. Only 100% juice products are recommended because they are nutrient dense (Roth, 2006).

By the age of 1 year, most babies are eating foods from all the food guide pyramid's groups and may have most any food that is easily chewed and digested; however, until the age of 2, precautions must be taken to avoid offering foods that might cause the child to choke. Examples include hotdogs, nuts, whole peas, grapes, popcorn, small candies, and small pieces of tough meat or raw vegetables. Cautiously introduce nuts, as these cause severe allergic responses in some people. Foods should be selected according to the advice of the pediatrician.

CHILDHOOD

Although specific nutritional requirements change as children grow, nutrition always affects physical, mental, and emotional growth and development. Studies indicate that the mental ability and size of an individual are directly influenced by nutrition during the early years.

Eating habits develop during childhood. Once developed, poor eating habits are difficult to change. They can exacerbate emotional and physical problems such as irritability, depression, anxiety, fatigue, and illness. Good eating habits formed in early childhood will generally last a lifetime (Figure 18-5).

Parents should be aware that children's appetites vary. The rate of growth is not constant. As the child ages, the rate of growth actually slows. The approximate weight gain of a child during the second year of life is only 5 pounds. Children between the ages of 1 and 3 years learn to feed themselves.

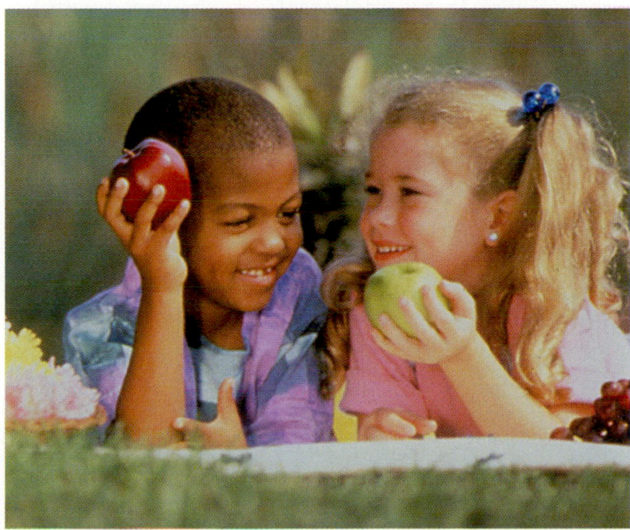

FIGURE 18-5 Good health radiates from these two children. (*Photo by Keith Weller, ARS.USDA.*)

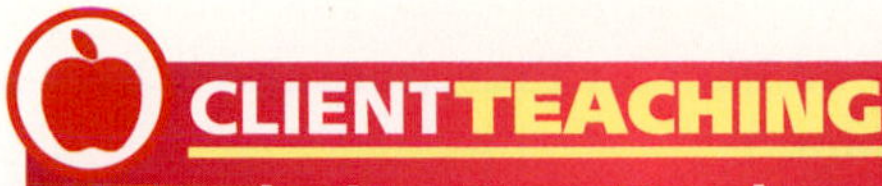

CLIENT TEACHING

Introducing New Foods

Allowing the child to assist in purchasing and preparing a new food is often a good way of arousing interest in the food and a desire to eat it.

As children continue to grow and develop, their likes and dislikes may change. New foods should be introduced gradually, in small amounts, and as attractively as possible.

Children should be offered nutrient-dense foods because the amount eaten will be small. Fats should not be limited before the age of 2 years, but meals and snacks should not be fat laden either. Whole milk is recommended until the age of 2, but low fat or fat free should be served from 2 years on. The guideline for fat intake after the age of 2 is the same as that for adults. Children should not salt their food at the table or have foods prepared with a lot of salt (Roth, 2006).

Children are especially sensitive to and reject hot (temperature) foods, but they like crisp textures, mild flavors, and familiar foods. They are wary of foods covered by sauce or gravy. Parents should set realistic goals and expectations as to the amount of food a child needs. A good rule of thumb for preschool children is one tablespoon of new food for each year of age. Table 18-10 details serving sizes according to age.

PROFESSIONAL TIP

Snacks

A child needs a snack every 3 to 4 hours for continued energy. Children often prefer finger foods for snacks. Snacks should be nutrient dense and as nutritious as food served at mealtimes. Cheese, saltines, fruit, milk, and unsweetened cereals make good snacks.

CLIENT TEACHING

Preventing Choking

Instruct parents to:

- Avoid the use of foods that may cause choking in infants and small children (up to 3 years old), such as corn, nuts, raw peas and carrots, celery, small candies, hotdogs, popcorn, and any other small, hard food.
- Offer peanut butter only on bread or a saltine.
- Stress the importance of sitting upright while eating.
- Prohibit running with food or objects in the mouth.

TABLE 18-10 Food Plan for Preschool and School-Age Children Based on the Food Guide Pyramid

		APPROXIMATE SERVING SIZE*			
FOOD GROUP	NUMBER OF SERVINGS	AGES 1–2	AGES 3–4	AGES 5–6	AGES 7–12
Milk, yogurt, and cheese	3	½ to ¾ cup or 1 oz	¾ cup or 1½ oz	1 cup or 2 oz	1 cup or 2 oz
Meat, poultry, fish, dry beans, eggs, and nuts	2 or more	1 oz or 1 to 2 Tbsp	1½ oz or 3 to 4 Tbsp	1½ oz or ½ cup	2 oz or ½ cup
Vegetables	3 or more	1 to 2 Tbsp	3 to 4 Tbsp	½ cup	½ cup
Fruits	2 or more	1 to 2 Tbsp or ½ cup juice	3 to 4 Tbsp or ½ cup juice	½ cup or ½ cup juice	½ cup or ½ cup juice
Bread, cereal, rice, and pasta	6 or more	½ slice or ½ cup	1 slice or ½ cup	1 slice or ¾ cup	1 slice or ¾ cup

*Use as a starting point. Increase serving size as energy yields dictate, but maintain variety in the diet by making sure all food groups are still appropriately represented.

Adapted from Food and Nutrition Services, U.S. Department of Agriculture: *Meal Plan Requirements and Offer versus Serve Manual*, FNS-265, 1990.

Calorie needs depend on rate of growth, activity level, body size, metabolism, and health.

Nutritional Requirements

The rate of growth diminishes from the age of 1 year until about age 10; thus, the kcal requirement per pound of body weight also diminishes during this period. For example, at 6 months, a girl needs approximately 54 kcal per pound of body weight, but by age 10, she will require only 35 kcal per pound of body weight.

Nutrient needs, however, do not diminish. From the age of 6 months to 10 years, nutrient needs actually increase because of the increased body size. Therefore, it is especially important that young children are given nutritious foods they will eat.

In general, the young child will need 2 to 3 cups of milk each day, or the equivalent in terms of calcium; however, excessive use of milk should be avoided because it can crowd out other iron-rich foods and possibly cause iron deficiency. The number of servings of the other food groups is the same as for adults, but the sizes will be smaller. The use of sweets should be minimized because children generally prefer them to nutrient-rich foods. Sweetened fruit juices should especially be avoided. Children also need water and fiber in their diets. They need to drink 1 mL of water for each kcal. If 1,200 kcal is eaten, five 8-ounce glasses of water are needed. Fiber needs are calculated according to age. After age 3 years a child's fiber needs are "age + 5g" and no more than "age + 10g." A child eating more fiber than that might be too full to eat enough other foods providing the kcal needed for growth and development. Fiber should be added slowly, if not already in the diet, with fluids also increased. Childhood is a good time to develop the lifelong good habit of getting enough dietary fiber to prevent constipation and diseases such as colon cancer and diverticulitis (Roth, 2006).

ADOLESCENCE

Adolescence is a period of rapid growth that causes major physiologic changes. The growth rate may be as much as 3 inches per year for girls and 4 inches for boys; nutrition plays a role in overall healthy adolescent development. Bones grow and gain density, muscle and fat tissue develop, and blood volume increases (Roth, 2006).

Adolescents typically have enormous appetites. When good eating habits have been established during childhood and there is nutritious food available, the teenager's food habits should present no serious problem. Peer pressure is great at this time, and good eating habits may be forgotten. Many adolescents skip breakfast and/or lunch and then eat at fast-food places (Figure 18-6). Adolescents are concerned with body

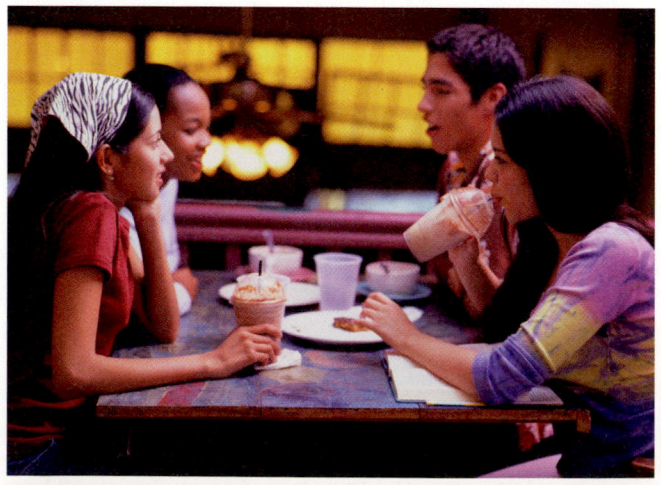
COURTESY OF GETTY IMAGES/PHOTODISC

FIGURE 18-6 Adolescents are vulnerable to peer pressure.

image and often compare their bodies to those of peers and popular media figures. They may restrict food intake, leading to inadequate nutrient intake.

Nutritional Requirements

Because of adolescents' rapid growth, kcal requirements naturally increase. Boys' kcal requirements tend to be greater than girls' because boys are generally bigger, tend to be more physically active, and have more lean muscle mass than do girls (Roth, 2006).

Except for vitamin D, nutrient needs increase dramatically at the onset of adolescence. Because of menstruation, girls have a greater need for iron than do boys. The RDAs for vitamin D, vitamin C, vitamin B_{12}, calcium, phosphorus, and iodine are the same for both sexes. The RDAs for the remaining nutrients are higher for boys than they are for girls (Roth, 2006).

Young and Middle Adulthood

The period of young adulthood ranges from approximately 18 years to 40 years of age. They appear to have boundless energy for both social and professional activities and are usually interested in exercise for its own sake, often participating in athletic events.

The middle adulthood period ranges from approximately 40 years to 65 years of age. This is a time when the physical activities of young adulthood typically begin to decrease, resulting in lowered kcal requirement for most individuals. During these years, people seldom have young children to supervise, and the strenuous physical labor of some occupations may be delegated to younger people. Middle-age people may tire more easily than they did when they were younger. They may not get as much exercise as they did in earlier years. Because appetite and food intake may not decrease, there is a common tendency toward weight gain during this period (Roth, 2006).

Nutritional Requirements

Physical growth is usually complete by the age of 25 years. Consequently, except during pregnancy and lactation, the essential nutrients are needed only to maintain and repair body tissue and to produce energy. During these years, the nutrient requirements of healthy adults change very little.

Despite men's generally larger size, only 11 of the given RDAs are greater for men than for women. Six of the RDAs are the same for both sexes. The iron requirement for women throughout the childbearing years remains higher than that for men. Extra iron is needed to replace blood loss during menstruation and to help build both the infant's and the extra maternal blood needed during pregnancy. After menopause, this requirement for women matches that of men (Roth, 2006).

The kcal requirement begins to diminish after the age of 25 years, as basal metabolism is reduced by approximately 2% to 3% per decade. This is a small amount each year, but, after 25 years, a person will gain weight if the total kcal value of the food eaten is not reduced accordingly. An individual's actual need, of course, will be determined primarily by activity and amount of lean muscle mass. Those who are more active will require more kcal than those with a high proportion of fat tissue.

A normal healthy adult should eat a variety of foods as shown on the food guide pyramid. This, along with following the *Dietary Guidelines for Americans*, should provide a healthy diet for the adult.

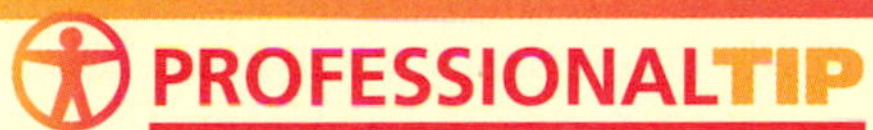

Preventing Eating Disorders

- Encourage healthy dietary habits and adequate exercise.
- Emphasize a healthy lifestyle over physical appearance and weight loss.
- Encourage increased self-esteem and stress a positive self-worth.
- Avoid pressuring children to achieve perfection or perform beyond their abilities.
- Recognize signs and symptoms of eating disorders, and seek professional help when suspected.

(From *Health Assessment and Physical Examination* [4th ed.], by M. E. Z. Estes, 2010, Clifton Park, NY: Delmar Cengage Learning.)

Older Adulthood

Physical changes of aging affect nutrition in several ways. The body's functions slow with age, and its ability to replace worn cells likewise diminishes. Metabolic rate slows; bones become less dense; lean muscle mass lessens; eyes do not focus on nearby objects as they once did, and some grow cloudy from cataracts; poor dentition is common; the heart and kidneys become less efficient; and hearing, taste, and smell are less acute.

Digestion is affected because the secretion of hydrochloric acid and enzymes diminishes. This, in turn, decreases the intrinsic factor synthesis, which may lead to a vitamin B_{12} deficiency. The tone of the intestines is reduced, possibly resulting in constipation or, in some cases, diarrhea (Roth, 2006).

Healthy eating habits throughout life, an exercise program suited to one's age, and enjoyable social activities can prevent or delay physical deterioration and depression during the senior years. They give purpose to the day, joy to the heart, and zest to the appetite. Nutrition and lifestyle should be carefully reviewed in any elderly client suspected of having depression.

Food–drug interactions must be monitored closely in the elderly client. Frequently, specific foods will prevent, decrease, or enhance the absorption of a particular drug.

Drug–drug interactions as well as food–drug interactions can contribute to decreased nutritional status. These interactions could affect both appetite and the absorption of nutrients from the food eaten. Careful monitoring is recommended.

Nutritional Requirements

In general, most elderly persons decrease their activity; thus their kcal needs also decrease.

The kcal requirement decreases approximately 2% to 3% per decade because both metabolism and activity slow. If kcal intake is not reduced, weight will increase. Additional weight increases the work of the heart and puts increased stress on the skeletal system. An exercise plan appropriate to one's age and health can be helpful in burning excess kcal and in toning and strengthening the muscles.

PROFESSIONALTIP

Food–Drug Interactions

Dairy products should not be consumed within 2 hours of taking the antibiotic tetracycline or the drug will not be absorbed. A person taking a blood clot–reducing drug such as warfarin sodium (Coumadin) must consume vitamin K–rich food in moderation, as this vitamin counteracts blood thinners. Even vitamin supplements can cause interactions. The antioxidant vitamins are not to be taken with blood clot–reducing medications, because they also have a tendency to thin the blood (Roth, 2006).

CLIENTTEACHING

Special Dietary Considerations for the Elderly

- Give special attention to water needs, regardless of physical activity, because the thirst mechanism is less responsive than in younger people.
- Decrease the kcal requirements in relation to activity: 10% for ages 51 to 75 and 20% to 25% for ages 75 and older. Bedridden and immobilized persons need a further reduction in kcal. Limit the quantities of empty-kcal foods (e.g., sugars, sweets, fats, oils, and alcohol).
- Maintain protein requirements, with 12% to 14% of kcal intake being derived from protein food (meat, eggs, poultry, milk, and cheese).
- Ensure adequate consumption of unsaturated fats, to provide a source of energy, provide the essential fatty acids, utilize the fat-soluble vitamins, and serve as a lubricating agent.
- Select carbohydrates as follows: limit concentrated sweets; use moderate amounts of simple sugars (candy, sugar, jams, jellies, preserves, and syrups); select most sources from complex carbohydrates (fruits, vegetables, cereals, and breads).
- Ensure adequate amounts of vitamin D, calcium, and phosphorus to maintain bone integrity (fortified milk is a good source).
- Consume high-fiber foods (dried fruits, whole-grain cereals, nuts, fresh fruit, and vegetables) to increase satiety and maintain intestinal motility and thereby prevent constipation.
- Maintain a safe, adequate intake of sodium, avoiding canned foods and salted or cured meats high in sodium content for those with cardiac problems and hypertension.
- Include foods from the food guide pyramid in the amounts that meet the RDAs for ages 51 and older.

Protein needs remain the same or may increase during illness. A well-balanced diet of a variety of foods should supply adequate amounts of vitamins and minerals. An increase in water and dietary fiber is often needed to maintain proper elimination.

Pregnancy and Lactation

Good nutrition during the 38 to 40 weeks of a normal pregnancy is essential for both mother and child. In addition to her normal nutritional requirements, the pregnant woman must provide nutrients and kcals for the fetus, the amniotic fluid, the placenta, and the increased blood volume and breast, uterine, and fat tissue.

The pregnant woman who follows a nutritionally adequate diet is more apt to feel better, retain her health, and bear a healthy infant than one who chooses her foods thoughtlessly (Roth, 2006).

Studies have shown a relationship between the mother's diet and the health of the baby at birth. It is also thought that the woman who consumes a nutritious diet before pregnancy is more apt to bear a healthy infant than one who does not. Malnutrition of the mother is believed to cause growth and mental retardation in the fetus. Infants with low birth weight (less than 5.5 pounds) have a higher mortality (death) rate than those of normal birth weight.

Nutritional Requirements

Despite the saying, the pregnant woman is not "eating for two." No increase in kcal is required during the first 12 weeks of pregnancy. After that time, an extra 300 kcal/day is recommended. This increase can almost be accomplished by drinking two *extra* 8-ounce glasses of 2% milk each day, which supplies 240 kcal. Those two extra glasses of milk also supply the extra calcium, protein, and vitamin D required during pregnancy. The other nutrients that should be increased during pregnancy are folic acid and iron. Folic acid is necessary to prevent neural tube deformities in the fetus. Folic acid has been approved as a supplement for pregnant women. Good sources of folic acid are beef, legumes, wheat germ, and eggs. Good sources of iron are red meat, dried fruit, egg yolk, and whole-grain products.

To ensure that the nutritional requirements of pregnancy are met, vitamin supplements may be prescribed in addition to an iron supplement; however, it is not advisable for the mother to take any unprescribed nutrient supplement, as an excess of vitamins or minerals can be toxic to mother and infant. Excessive vitamin A, for example, can cause birth defects (Roth, 2006).

The mother's kcal requirement increases during lactation. The kcal requirement depends on the amount of milk produced. Approximately 85 kcal are required to produce 100 mL (3⅓ oz) of milk. During the first 6 months, average daily milk production is 750 mL (25 oz), and for this, the mother requires approximately 640 extra kcal a day. During the second 6 months, when the baby begins to eat food in addition to breast milk, average daily milk production slows to 600 mL (20 oz), and the kcal requirement reduces to approximately 510 extra kcal a day.

NUTRITION AND HEALTH

An individual who embraces good nutrition is more likely to have good health than is someone who does not follow good nutritional practices. Of course, all situations of disease or ill health cannot be prevented by good nutrition.

The nutrients in the food we eat may be thought of as the building materials, fuel, and regulators necessary to keep the body functioning. When the body is supplied with nutrients in the proper amounts, it is most likely to function efficiently and effectively. The body is very adaptable and keeps functioning, although less effectively, even when not supplied with the proper amounts of nutrients. In this situation, however, the body is more susceptible to some diseases.

Primary Nutritional Disease

A primary nutritional disease occurs when nutrition is the cause of the disease. Usually, there is an inadequate intake of one or more nutrients. Some examples of such diseases are scurvy, from inadequate intake of vitamin C; rickets, from insufficient intake of vitamin D; and anemia, from a deficiency of iron in the diet.

Excesses of nutrients can also cause illness. These, however, occur when nutrient supplements are taken in excess, rather than from food intake. For instance, excess vitamin D may cause nausea, diarrhea, weight loss, and calcification of the renal tubules, blood vessels, and bronchi. Excess niacin may cause flushing, itching, and hypotension.

Secondary Nutritional Disease

Most nutritional diseases are secondary diseases; that is, they are a complication of another disease or condition. The original disease or condition interferes with digestion or absorption, or there is an increased need for one or more nutrients. For instance, in pregnancy, the body's need for iron increases. Not receiving the increased amount may cause anemia in the mother. In malabsorption disorders, the body is unable to absorb sufficient amounts of certain nutrients. The amount ingested may be adequate, but the body is unable to use it. Rapid excretion from the body, as in diarrhea, does not allow the nutrients to be absorbed and utilized. Uncontrolled diarrhea can lead to dehydration along with electrolyte and acid–base imbalance.

WEIGHT MANAGEMENT

Maintaining weight at a desired level can be very difficult for some people. Weight management is based on the relationship between the intake and use of kcal. When these two elements are balanced, weight is maintained at a steady level. A range of 10% over or under the desired weight is considered appropriate.

Determining Caloric Needs

The number of kcal needed to achieve or maintain a desired weight is based on two factors: basal energy needs and total energy requirements.

Basal Energy Needs

Basal energy need refers to the number of kcal required to keep an individual alive when at rest. There are two ways to determine basal energy (kcal) needs. One is based on the person's desired weight (Table 18-11), the other on the person's actual weight.

Calculation using desired weight is as follows:

Basal energy needs = desired weight × 10

Table 18-11 Determining Desired Weight

BUILD	WOMEN	MEN
Medium	100 lb for 5 ft of height, plus 5 lb for each additional inch	106 lb for 5 ft of height, plus 6 lb for each additional inch
Small	Subtract 10%	Subtract 10%
Large	Add 10%	Add 10%

COURTESY OF DELMAR CENGAGE LEARNING

Examples

Female: 5 ft 5 in tall
5 ft = 100 lb
5 in = 25 lb
125 lb desired weight
125 × 10 = 1,250
Basal energy needs = 1,250 kcal

Male: 5 ft 9 in tall
5 ft = 106 lb
9 in = 54 lb
160 lb desired weight
160 × 10 = 1,600
Basal energy needs = 1,600 kcal

Calculation using actual weight is as follows:

Female weight in kg × 0.9 × 24 = basal kcal
Male weight in kg × 1 × 24 = basal kcal
(Weight in lb ÷ 2.2 = weight in kg)

Examples

Female weighs 130 lb
130 ÷ 2.2 = 59.1 kg
59.1 kg × 0.9 × 24 = 1,276.6
Basal energy needs = 1,276.6 kcal

Male weighs 170 lb
170 ÷ 2.2 = 77.3 kg
77.3 kg × 1 × 24 = 1,855.2
Basal energy needs = 1,855.2 kcal

Total Energy Requirements

People do not live their lives at rest. They are active! Kilocalories must be added to the basal metabolic requirement in order to meet the needs of activity. All activity is not equal in kcal needed, however. A person's overall activity level can be divided into sedentary (light, such as watching television), moderate (such as playing tennis), or strenuous (such as running a marathon). The following formulas can be used to determine the number of kcal to add given the activity level:

Sedentary: basal kcal × 1.3 = total kcal
Moderate: basal kcal × 1.5 = total kcal
Strenuous: basal kcal × 2.0 = total kcal

Example: The 125-lb woman in the preceding example who is planning on running a marathon would need the following:

1,250 (basal kcal) × 2 = 2,500 kcal

Factors in addition to activity that have an effect on the total kcal need are state of health and climate. A person who is ill needs more kcal to repair tissue. A cold climate requires a person to take in more kcal to provide more thermal energy to maintain body temperature.

OVERWEIGHT

A person is considered to be overweight when 11% to 19% above the desired weight. **Obesity** is considered present in a person who is 20% or more above the desired weight. Overweight conditions can become serious health hazards by placing increased strain on the heart, lungs, muscles, bones, and joints. Overweight and obese people are more susceptible to diabetes and hypertension and tend to have a shorter life span.

According to the Centers for Disease Control and Prevention (CDC, 2006), obesity is a major problem in the United States, with an increase of overweight and obesity in children and adults throughout the world. In the United States, children between the ages of 2 and 19 years are 17.1% overweight. Among adults, 32.2% are overweight with almost 5% extremely obese.

Causes

There is no single cause of obesity. Genetic, physiologic, biochemical, and psychological factors may all contribute to overweight conditions. Most often, the cause of being overweight or obese is an energy imbalance. That is, more kcal are being taken in than are being used. When this occurs, the body stores the excess kcal as adipose tissue. Hypothyroidism is a possible but rare cause of obesity. In this condition, basal metabolism is low, thereby reducing the number of kcal needed for energy. Unless corrected, this condition can result in excess weight (Roth, 2006).

Treatment

Treatment for an overweight person involves two parts: revised eating habits and exercise. Revised eating habits include reducing daily kcal intake at mealtime, limiting between-meal snacks to fresh fruits or vegetables, and restricting or eliminating empty calories.

One pound of body weight equals 3,500 kcal. Therefore, to lose 1 pound per week, a person must reduce kcal intake by 500 kcal each day. Weight loss should be limited to 1 to 2 pounds per week, unless the client is under strict medical supervision. Diets should be planned according to the minimum servings of the food guide pyramid and should not be reduced to below 1,200 kcal/day in order for the dieter to receive adequate nutrients to sustain health.

Attention should also be given to food preparation. Frying adds many kcal from fat to a food item. Broiling, grilling, baking, roasting, boiling, and poaching are healthy ways to prepare foods. Vegetables should be eaten raw or steamed; the addition of butter, margarine, or sauces should be avoided. Eating habits may be adapted to decrease the amount eaten and yet provide satisfaction: place food on a smaller plate, cut food into smaller bites, chew each bite at least 12 times, and place the fork on the plate between bites.

Exercise, particularly aerobic exercise, is an excellent adjunct to any weight-loss program. Aerobic exercise uses energy from the body's fat reserves, as it increases the amount of oxygen the body takes in. Examples of aerobic exercise are dancing, jogging, bicycling, skiing, rowing, and power walking. Such exercise helps tone the muscles, burns kcal, increases the basal metabolism so that food is burned faster, and is fun for the participant. Any exercise program must begin slowly and increase over time so that no physical damage occurs.

> **CRITICAL THINKING**
>
> **Weight Loss**
>
> What should the nurse know about nutrition in order to help an obese client lose weight?

Exercise alone can only rarely replace the need to be mindful of diet, however. The dieter should be made aware of the number of kcal burned by specific exercises to avoid overeating after the workout.

UNDERWEIGHT

Persons are considered to be underweight when their weight is 10% to 15% below the desired weight. An underweight person is more likely to have nutritional deficiencies because of the decreased intake of food. For women, this can cause complications during pregnancy. Being underweight may lower a person's resistance to infection. Being severely underweight may even cause death.

Causes

There are several possible causes of being underweight, such as an inadequate intake of food, excessive exercise, poor absorption of nutrients, or severe infection. Occasionally, hyperthyroidism may be the cause. After the adequacy of food intake and the appropriate activity level are ascertained, specific diagnostic tests must be done to determine whether poor absorption, infection, or hyperthyroidism are present.

Treatment

Dietary treatment for an inadequate intake of food is to gradually increase the amount of food eaten. Also, higher-kcal foods can be eaten. Between-meal snacks and a bedtime snack can help increase the intake of food.

If the individual is to gain 1 pound per week, 3,500 kcal in addition to the individual's basic normal weekly kcal requirement are prescribed. This means an extra 500 kcal must be taken in each day. If a weight gain of 2 pounds per week is required, an additional 7,000 kcal each week, or an additional 1,000 kcal per day, are necessary. This diet cannot be immediately accepted at full kcal value. Time will be needed to gradually increase the daily kcal value by increasing intake of foods rich in carbohydrates, some fats, and protein. Vitamins and minerals are supplied in adequate amounts. If there are deficiencies of some vitamins and minerals, supplements are prescribed (Roth, 2006).

FOOD LABELING

In 1990, Congress passed the Nutrition, Labeling and Education Act (NLEA). This was the first legislation on labeling since the 1970s. Before this newest legislation, labeling was required only if a nutrient was added or a nutritional claim was made about the product. Now labeling is required on virtually all retail food products, including bulk foods, fresh produce, and seafood. The nutrition information for fresh produce and seafood is to be displayed or made available at the point of purchase through counter cards, booklets, loose-leaf binders, signs, or tags.

The labels must follow the approved uniform format and use standard serving sizes and household measurements.

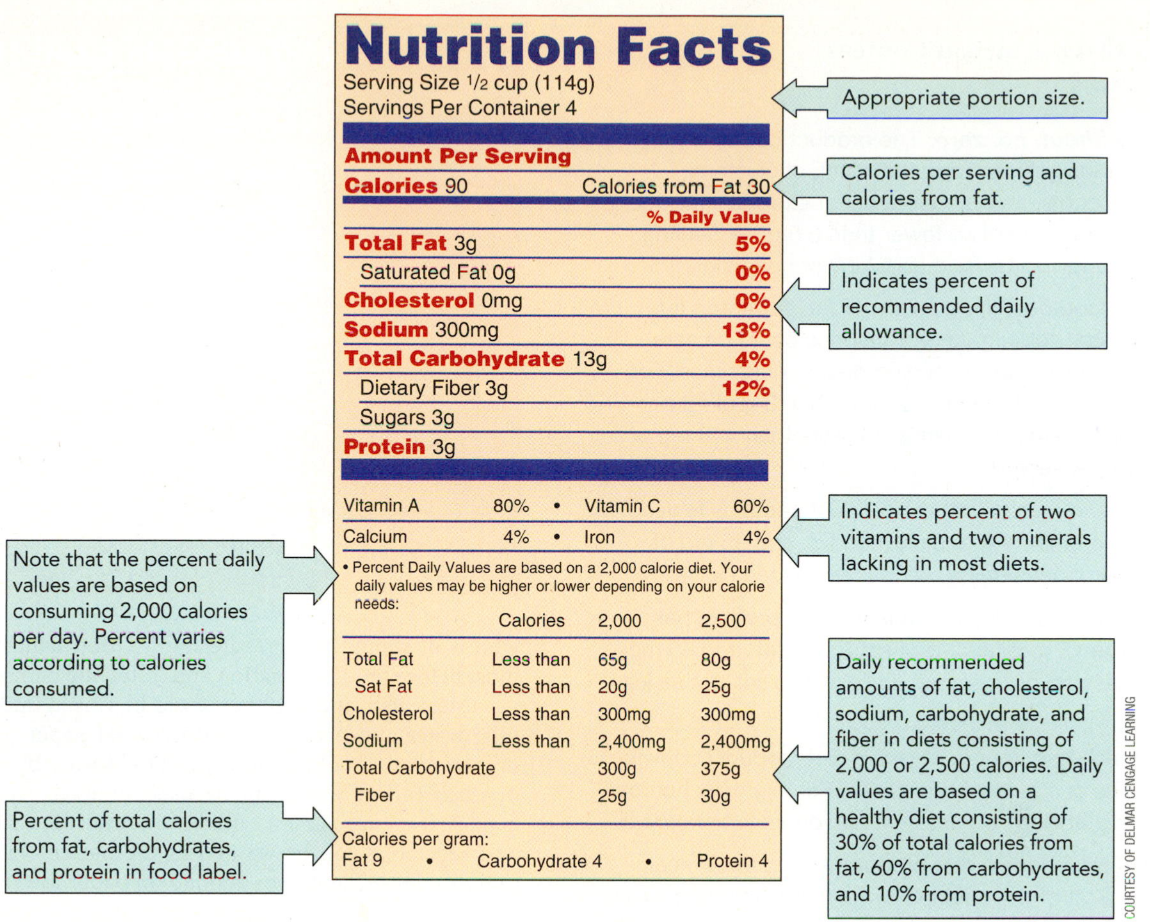

FIGURE 18-7 Sample Food Label

Information on the label includes calories per serving; calories from fat; total fat, saturated fat, and cholesterol; total sodium; total carbohydrate, dietary fiber, and sugar; amount of protein; and percentages of vitamins A and C, calcium, and iron. A sample food label is shown in Figure 18-7.

Words used to describe nutrient content, such as low, light, lean, or reduced, now have specific, consistent definitions (Table 18-12).

The standardized label and word definitions make it easier for the consumer not only to know the amount of specific nutrients in a food or food product, but also to easily compare foods and food products.

FOOD QUALITY AND SAFETY

When planning an adequate diet, the quality and safety of the food is considered in addition to the types of foods and serving sizes. To ensure the quality (nutrient content) and safety of food, proper storage, preparation, sanitation, and cooking are necessary; such measures prevent or reduce the risk of food-borne illnesses.

CRITICAL THINKING

Evaluating Food Labels

Evaluate the health value of the food described in Figure 18-7. For example, calculate the serving size, read the total fat content, and decide if the food is a good value or lesser value to eat.

Quality of Food

Foods usually begin to lose nutrients when they are harvested, so they are best purchased when fresh in appearance and of bright color. Dates should be checked on all processed foods such as dairy products, lunch and other processed meats, crackers, and breads; all foods should be used before their expiration dates. All produce should be cooked until tender and thoroughly done, in the smallest amount of water possible to prevent loss of vitamins. Cooking meats via stewing increases mineral loss, so cooking methods that retain the most nutrients should be used instead; these include stir-frying, steaming, microwaving, or pressure cooking.

Safety of Food

There are three aspects to food safety: proper storage, proper sanitation, and proper cooking.

Proper Storage

Foods must be properly stored before and after purchase. Packages and jars should be tightly sealed, and cans should not leak or bulge. Any foods that look or smell unusual or show signs of mold or deterioration should be discarded. Hot foods should be kept hot—above 140°F—and cold foods should be kept below 40°F. Foods allowed to stand at temperatures

Table 18-12 Nutrient Content Descriptors

- ***Free, without, no, zero:*** The product contains only a tiny or insignificant amount of fat, cholesterol, sodium, sugar, and/or calories. For example, *fat-free* and *sugar-free* contain fewer than 0.5 g per serving. *Calorie-free* has fewer than 5 kcal per serving.
- ***Low:*** A food described as *low* in fat, saturated fat, cholesterol, sodium, and/or calories could be eaten fairly often without exceeding dietary guidelines. For instance, *low-fat* means no more than 3 g of fat per serving; *low-sodium* means no more than 140 mg of sodium per serving.
- ***Lean:*** *Lean* means that the product contains fewer than 10 g of fat, 4 g of saturated fat, and 95 mg of cholesterol per serving. *Lean* is not as lean as is *low.*
- ***Extra lean:*** *Extra lean* means that the product has fewer than 5 g of fat, 2 g of saturated fat, and 95 mg of cholesterol per serving. *Extra lean* is still not as lean as is *low.*
- ***Reduced, less, fewer:*** Means a diet product contains 25% less of a nutrient or calories. For example, hotdogs might be labeled *25% less fat than our regular hotdogs.*
- ***Light/lite:*** Means a diet product with ⅓ fewer kcal or ½ the fat of the original. *Light in sodium* means a product with ½ the usual sodium.
- ***More:*** A food in which one serving has at least 10% more of the daily value of a vitamin, mineral, or fiber than usual.
- ***Good source of:*** One serving contains 10% to 19% of the daily value for a particular nutrient.
- ***High:*** One serving contains 20% or more of the daily value for a particular nutrient.
- ***Trans fat free:*** Indicates that the product has less than 0.5 grams of trans fat and less than 0.5 grams of saturated fat.
- ***Healthy:*** *Healthy* means that the serving does not have more than 60 milligrams of cholesterol, 3 grams of fat, 1 gram of saturated fat, 360 milligrams or less of sodium, and more than 10% of the daily value of vitamin A, vitamin C, iron, calcium, protein, or fiber.

COURTESY OF DELMAR CENGAGE LEARNING

between 40°F and 140°F provide an ideal breeding ground for pathogens. Leftovers must be refrigerated promptly and not allowed to cool before refrigerating.

Proper Sanitation

Proper sanitation means that all cooking utensils, pots, pans, and cutting boards, as well as the cook's hands, have been washed with soap and hot water before preparation begins. To prevent contamination of one food by another, cutting boards, utensils, and the cook's hands should be washed well with soap and hot water between preparation of different foods. A person who is ill should not prepare food. Good hand hygiene is a must before food preparation and following bathroom use.

Meat, fish, and poultry should be rinsed under cold running water and patted dry with several paper towels before preparing and cooking. A capful of chlorine bleach in a sink one-half full of water can be used to wash fruits and vegetables: leafy vegetables, cauliflower, broccoli, and other fruits and vegetables can be washed in the bleach water for a few minutes, rinsed, and then drained on paper towels.

COMMUNITY/HOME HEALTH CARE

Resources for Meal Preparation

Ensure that the family has:

- Hot and cold running water
- A working refrigerator
- A working oven and range
- A clean, pest-free kitchen
- Fresh perishables stored in the refrigerator
- Adequate food supplies (including canned goods and staples, such as milk and bread), safely stored
- Appropriate adaptive equipment, if needed, such as low countertops that facilitate wheelchair access

Data from "Home Health Nutrition" by M. Costello, 1996, *MedSurg Nursing 5*(4), 229–238.

Proper Cooking

Meats, fish, shellfish, and eggs should be cooked well done to ensure that harmful microorganisms are destroyed (Figure 18-8).

Food-Borne Illnesses

When proper storage, sanitation, or cooking are not maintained, food-borne illnesses often occur. These illnesses range in severity from fairly mild (such as staphylococcal food poisoning) to potentially fatal (such as botulism and *E. coli*). The important thing to remember is that food-borne illness is highly preventable with proper handling, preparation, and storage of food.

Nutrition involves the appropriate kinds and amounts of a variety of available foods so that a properly functioning body can digest and use the nutrients in the foods. If the foods are unsafe, they cannot adequately nourish the body.

NURSING PROCESS

Collection of subjective and objective data regarding the client's nutrition serves as the basis for determining the type of nutritional care the client requires.

Assessment

Proper assessment allows the health care team to determine the degree to which the client's nutritional needs are met. Assessment must be performed logically and should include a nutritional history, physical examination, and the results of laboratory tests.

Age and pregnancy determine some specific items to be included in the nutritional assessment.

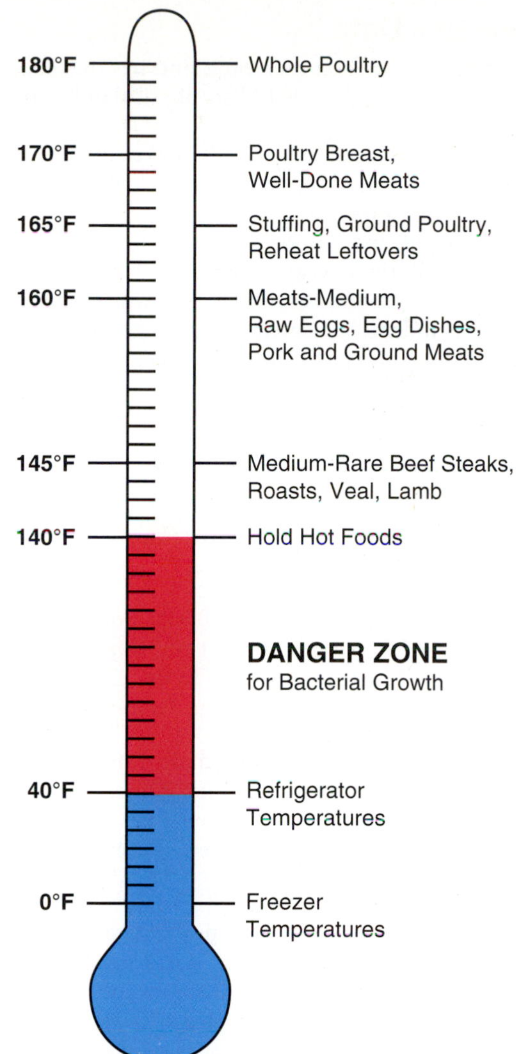

FIGURE 18-8 **Bacterium can increase from one to 2,097,152 bacteria within one hour at temperatures between 40 and 140° F. Cook foods at temperatures as indicated on the thermometer.** *(From United States Department of Agriculture [USDA] and United States Department of Health and Human Services [HHS], 2000. Nutrition and your health: Dietary guidelines for Americans [Home and Garden Bulletin, No. 232, 5th ed.]. Washington, DC: U.S. DA and HHS.)*

Nutritional assessment for an infant should include:

- Height and weight
- Sleeping habits
- Type of feeding (breast- or bottle-fed)
- If breastfeeding, the mother's nutritional status and use of alcohol, tobacco, caffeine, and drugs; infant's feeding schedule (how often fed and for how long)
- If formula feeding, type, frequency, and method of preparation and storage; feeding schedule; amount taken at each feeding
- Use of vitamin/mineral supplements
- If on solid foods, age at introduction, and any reactions or allergies
- Family attitudes about eating, food, and weight

The basic nutritional assessment for everyone over 1 year old should include:

- Nutritional status
- Height and weight
- Meal and snack pattern (food record or 24-hour recall)
- Adequacy of intake based on the food guide pyramid
- Food allergies
- Physical activity
- Cultural, ethnic, and family influences
- Use of vitamin/mineral supplements

In addition to the basic nutritional assessment, during childhood dental health is also assessed.

In addition to the basic nutritional assessment, the following is assessed for the adolescent client:

- Use of alcohol, tobacco, caffeine, and drugs
- Use of fad diets
- Family attitude toward thinness and the adolescent's weight

In addition to the basic nutritional assessment, the following is assessed for the adult client:

- Use of alcohol, tobacco, caffeine, and drugs
- Use of fad diets
- Prescribed restricted diet

In addition to the basic nutritional assessment, the following is assessed for elderly clients:

- Undesirable change in weight
- Dentition and swallowing
- Appetite
- Vision
- Hand–eye coordination
- Adequacy of daily intake of food
- Ability to self-feed
- Prescribed restricted diet
- Use of alcohol, tobacco, caffeine, and drugs

In addition to the basic nutritional assessment, the following is assessed for the pregnant client:

- Weight and rate of weight gain
- Diet changes in response to pregnancy
- Cravings for foods or nonfoods (pica)
- Intake of supplemental vitamins/minerals
- Feeding plans (breast or formula)
- Use of alcohol, caffeine, tobacco, or drugs

Subjective Data

Subjective data are obtained through a nutritional history by asking clients questions. Several methods are used in collecting these subjective data: 24-hour recall, food-frequency questionnaire, food record, and diet history. Although the history data may indicate adequate nutrition, clients must be reassessed periodically to prevent nutritional problems.

24-Hour Recall The 24-hour recall requires client identification of everything consumed in the previous 24 hours. It is performed easily and quickly by asking pertinent questions; however, clients may be unable to accurately recall their intake or anything atypical in the diet. Family members can often assist with these data, if necessary.

PROFESSIONAL TIP

Nutritional History

Food preferences are an expression of an individual's likes and dislikes. They may be related to the texture of food, how it is prepared, or what was served to the individual during childhood; however, preferences can also be an expression of the person's economic, ecological, ethical, or religious beliefs.

Peer pressure often dictates what teenagers eat. Stress, depression, and alcohol abuse alter the appetite. Medications can alter food absorption and excretion and affect the taste of food. Gastrointestinal disorders can cause anorexia, nausea, vomiting, diarrhea, constipation, discomfort, and pain, all of which may alter eating habits and food preferences.

Food-Frequency Questionnaire The food-frequency method gathers data relative to the number of times per day, week, or month that the client eats particular foods. The nurse can tailor the questions to particular nutrients, such as cholesterol and saturated fat. This method validates the accuracy of the 24-hour recall and provides a more complete picture of foods consumed.

Food Record The food record provides quantitative information regarding all foods consumed, with portions weighed and measured for three consecutive days. This method requires full client or family member cooperation.

Diet History The diet history elicits detailed information regarding the client's nutritional status, general health pattern, socioeconomic status, and cultural factors. This method incorporates information similar to that collected by the 24-hour recall and food-frequency questionnaire. The history may require more than one interview because of the amount of data to be collected.

Objective Data

A physical examination may elicit findings that suggest nutritional imbalance. Table 18-13 lists physical indicators of nutritional status.

The measurement of a client's intake and output and daily weight are critical assessments, especially for hospitalized clients. **Anthropometric measurements** (measurement of the size, weight, and proportions of the body) are indicative of the client's calorie–energy expenditure balance, muscle mass, body fat, and protein reserves. The measurements used are body mass index (calculated using weight and height), skinfolds, and limb and girth circumferences.

Body Mass Index **Body mass index** (BMI) is a measurement that determines whether a person's weight (in kilograms) is appropriate for height (in meters). It is calculated using a simple formula:

$$\text{BMI} = \frac{\text{weight (kg)}}{[\text{height (m)}]^2}$$

A BMI of 27 or greater indicates obesity. For example, a person who weighs 65 kilograms and is 1.6 meters tall would have a BMI of 65 kg/(1.6)2, or 25.4. Go to the CDC's Web site for a body mass index calculator at http://www.cdc.gov.

Skinfold Measurement Skinfold measurement indicates the amount of body fat. The skinfold is measured by grasping the subcutaneous tissue and taking a reading using a special caliper. Measurements can be taken of the tricep, subscapular, bicep, and suprailiac skinfolds.

Other Measurements Mid–upper-arm circumference serves as an index of skeletal muscle mass and protein reserve. Abdominal-girth measurement serves as an index as to whether the abdomen is increasing, decreasing, or remaining the same. Both of these measurements should be made repeatedly over a span of time, for best assessment.

TABLE 18-13 Physical Indicators of Nutritional Status

BODY AREA	GOOD NUTRITION	INADEQUATE NUTRITION
General	Alert, responsive, sleeps well, energetic, seldom ill	Apathetic, easily fatigued, looks tired, often ill
Weight	Appropriate for age, height, body build	Overweight, underweight
Skeleton	Good posture, no malformations	Poor posture
Skin	Good color, no rashes or swelling, smooth, moist, good turgor	Rough, dry, pale, poor turgor
Muscles	Firm, good tone	Flaccid, poor tone
Nails	Pink, firm	Pale, brittle
Eyes	Clear, bright, moist	Dull, pale, dry
Hair	Shiny, smooth	Dull, dry, brittle
Elimination	Regular, soft	Diarrhea or constipation

COURTESY OF DELMAR CENGAGE LEARNING

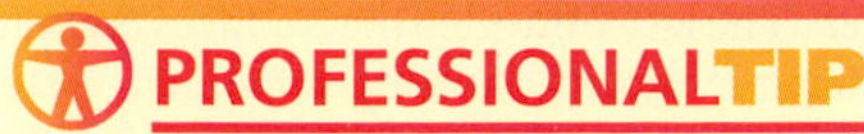

Creatinine Excretion

Record the client's height and gender on the laboratory request for a creatinine excretion test because the normal values are standardized on the basis of these variables.

Laboratory Tests Several laboratory tests provide information about a client's nutritional status. These include the protein indices of serum albumin, prealbumin, and serum transferrin; hemoglobin; total lymphocyte count; blood urea nitrogen (BUN); and urine creatinine. The serum albumin blood test is used to measure prolonged protein depletion that occurs in chronic malnutrition, liver disease, and nephrosis. The prealbumin test indicates protein depletion in acute conditions such as trauma and inflammation. Serum transferrin also measures the protein level as indicated by iron stores. Hemoglobin is a measurement of the oxygen- and iron-carrying capacity of the blood. Total lymphocyte count may reflect protein-calorie malnutrition, which inhibits lymphocyte synthesis. Blood urea nitrogen is a nitrogen balance study that indicates the degree to which protein is being depleted or replaced, and urine creatinine excretion indicates the amount of creatinine eliminated by the kidneys.

Nursing Diagnosis

Nursing diagnoses (NANDA-I, 2010) related specifically to nutrition include:

*Imbalanced **Nutrition**: Less Than Body Requirements*
*Imbalanced **Nutrition**: More Than Body Requirements*
*Risk for Imbalanced **Nutrition**: More Than Body Requirements*

Other possible nursing diagnoses related to nutritional problems include the following:

*Disturbed **Body** Image*
*Ineffective **Breastfeeding***
*Impaired **Dentition***
*Deficient **Knowledge*** (specify)
*Impaired **Oral** Mucous Membrane*
*Acute **Pain**, Chronic **Pain***
*Feeding **Self**-Care Deficit*
*Chronic Low **Self**-Esteem*
*Risk for Impaired **Skin** Integrity*

Planning/Outcome Identification

A plan should be formulated by the nurse and client to achieve mutually agreed-upon goals. The plan is individualized to meet the client's specific needs. These needs may include achieving desired weight, correcting nutritional deficiencies, maintaining a special diet, preventing nutritional disorders secondary to a particular therapy, or improving nutrition to promote health and prevent disease.

Goals for clients with nutritional alterations might be as follows:

Client will maintain intake and output balance.
Client will comply with diet therapy, avoiding high-sodium foods.
Client will gain 2 pounds in 4 weeks.

Implementation

The nurse and client actually carry out the plan through specific actions. Interventions to accomplish the goals may include diet therapy, assistance with meals, weight and intake monitoring, and nutritional support.

Diet Therapy

Diet therapy is the treatment of a disease or disorder with a special diet. A **dietary prescription/order** is an order written by the physician for food, including liquids. This is similar to a medication prescription written for medications a client receives. A client must not be given anything to eat or drink without an order. The dietary prescription is written for one or more of the following purposes:

- Provide the client with nutrients needed for maintenance or growth
- Prepare a client for diagnostic tests
- Treat the client with a disease or condition

When the dietary prescription has been received, the dietary department is notified so that the proper food is sent to the client.

Many times a client needs some help in understanding changes in the diet and the reasons the changes are necessary. A basic knowledge of nutrition and diet therapy contributes to the nurse's ability to competently answer the client's questions about nutrition and diet. It is important, however, for the nurse to recognize when to refer questions to the dietitian.

The dietary prescription may be for nothing by mouth, a standard diet, or a special diet.

Nothing by Mouth Nothing by mouth (nil per os, NPO) status is a type of diet modification as well as a fluid restriction. This is often prescribed before surgery and certain diagnostic procedures, to rest the GI tract, or when the client's nutritional problem has not been identified.

Standard Diets Each health care agency has standard or house diets. The standard diets include general (sometimes called regular), soft, clear liquid, full liquid, mechanical soft, and pureed.

General or Regular Diet The general or regular diet is planned according to the food guide pyramid. There are no restrictions of any kind. It is an adequate diet providing approximately 2,000 kcal a day.

Soft Diet A soft diet provides foods that are easy to chew and swallow, thus promoting mechanical digestion of foods. Foods avoided on this diet include nuts, seeds (tomatoes and berries with seeds), raw fruits and vegetables, fried foods, and whole grains. The food guide pyramid is the basis for this diet, although fewer kcal, usually approximately 1,800, are provided.

Clear-Liquid Diet The clear-liquid diet, also called the surgical liquid diet, is ordered as preparation for diagnostic tests or as the first meal or two after surgery. It consists mostly of water and carbohydrates, providing approximately 500 kcal/day. This is a very nutritionally inadequate diet but does relieve thirst, aids in hydration, and mildly stimulates peristalsis.

Liquids included are water; clear, fat-free broth; tea; coffee; clear and strained fruit juices; jello; popsicles; and carbonated drinks such as lemon-lime soda.

Full-Liquid Diet A full-liquid diet provides approximately 800 to 1,000 kcal per day. It includes all foods that are liquid at room temperature. In addition to the liquids on a clear-liquid diet, milk; milk drinks; cream soups; strained, cooked cereals; ice cream; puddings; all fruit and vegetable juices; and custard are included.

Mechanical Soft or Edentulous Diet A mechanical soft or edentulous diet consists of food fixed especially for a person who has no teeth or has difficulty chewing. The food is either ground or chopped into very small pieces and cooked very soft, to ease the work of chewing.

Pureed Diet A pureed diet uses foods that have been blended to a smooth consistency. It is prescribed for clients who have difficulty swallowing.

Special Diets A special diet restores or maintains a client's nutritional status. These diets are variations of the general diet; however, they still must provide all the nutrients of the general diets. Special diets may provide specific amounts of nutrients or may increase or restrict certain foods. Low-residue, high-fiber, liberal bland, fat-controlled, and sodium-restricted are types of special diets.

Low-Residue Diet The low-residue diet of 5 to 10 g of fiber a day reduces the normal work of the intestines by reducing food residue. Some low-residue diets limit tough or coarse meats, milk, and milk products. The low-residue diet is prescribed to decrease GI mucosal irritation in clients with diverticulitis, ulcerative colitis, and Crohn's disease. Foods to be avoided include raw fruits (except bananas), vegetables, seeds, plant fiber, and whole grains. Dairy products are limited to two servings per day.

High-Fiber Diet A high-fiber diet contains 25 to 35 g or more of dietary fiber. A high-fiber diet is an integral part of the treatment regimen for diverticulosis because it increases the forward motion of the indigestible wastes through the colon. This diet prevents constipation, hemorrhoids, and colon cancer, along with helping to treat diabetes mellitus and atherosclerosis.

The recommended foods for this diet include coarse and whole-grain breads and cereals, bran, all fruits, vegetables (especially raw), and legumes. This nutritionally adequate diet must be introduced gradually to prevent the formation of gas and the discomfort that accompanies it. Eight 8-oz glasses of water also must be consumed along with the increased fiber.

Liberal Bland Diet A liberal bland diet eliminates chemical and mechanical food irritants such as fried foods, alcohol, and caffeine. This diet is prescribed for clients with gastritis and ulcers because it reduces GI irritation.

PROFESSIONALTIP

Opening a Food Tray

Remove the tray cover before moving the over-bed table in front of the client. The concentration of odors when the lid is first removed can be nauseating to the client.

Fat-Controlled Diet The fat-controlled diet reduces the total fat ingested by replacing saturated fats with monounsaturated and polyunsaturated fats and restricting cholesterol. This diet is prescribed for clients with atherosclerosis, heart disease, and obesity. Saturated-fat foods to be avoided include animal fats, gravies, sauces, chocolate, and whole-milk products.

Sodium-Restricted Diet Sodium-restricted diets tailor the level of sodium to mild (2 to 3 g), moderate (1,000 mg), strict (500 mg), or severe (250 mg). This diet is prescribed for clients with fluid volume excess, hypertension, heart failure, myocardial infarction, or renal failure.

Assistance with Meals

Assisting with meals consists of preparing the client, preparing the environment, serving the tray, and assisting with eating.

Preparing the Client Before taking a meal tray into a client's room, the nurse must ensure that the client is ready to eat: face and hands are washed, oral hygiene completed, and, if necessary, the bladder emptied. The nurse should help the client into a comfortable eating position; this must be individualized to each client, as not everyone is allowed or able to sit up to eat a meal.

Preparing the Environment The nurse should make every effort to see that the physical environment is as conducive to a pleasant mealtime atmosphere as possible. This may necessitate cleaning and clearing the over-bed table so that the tray can be placed on it, tidying the room to remove offensive sights and smells, and brightening the room.

Serving the Tray The nurse checks that the tray contains the diet ordered, that everything on the tray is appropriate for the diet, and that nothing has spilled. For example, if a low-sodium diet tray has a salt packet, the packet is removed. The nurse checks the client's ID band against the name on the tray; it is very important that the correct meal is served to each client. The nurse prepares the food by opening cartons or cutting food, if necessary.

Assisting with Eating The client who needs assistance in eating is served last. This way, the nurse will have ample time and not have to hurry the client through the meal (Figure 18-9).

PROFESSIONALTIP

Feeding a Client

- Position yourself at the same level as the client (stand if the bed is high, sit if the bed is low).
- Allow time for prayer, if the client wishes.
- Protect the client's clothing with a napkin.
- Allow time for chewing (do not hurry the client).
- Give bite-size portions.
- Warn about hot foods (do not blow on food to cool).
- Use a separate straw for each liquid.
- Allow the client to choose the order in which the food is eaten.
- Offer pleasant conversation.

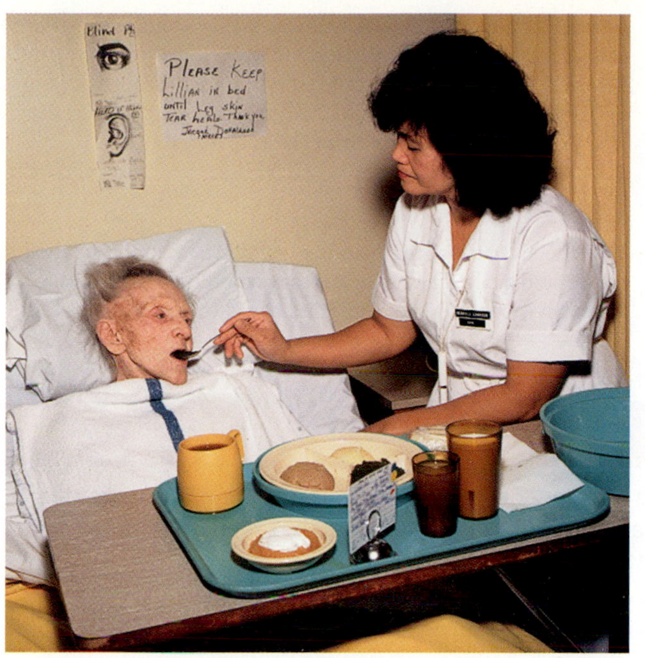

COURTESY OF DELMAR CENGAGE LEARNING

FIGURE 18-9 Older adults may have health problems that affect their ability to self-feed.

Weight and Intake Monitoring

Measuring weight daily or weekly and measuring the amount of food and fluid intake monitors therapy effectiveness.

Recording and Reporting

After the client has finished eating, the tray is promptly removed. The amount of food eaten is recorded, usually as the percentage of the meal eaten. When a client with diabetes does not eat all the food on the tray, both the charge nurse and the dietitian must be notified so that a supplemental feeding is sent later. If the client is on intake and output (I&O), the amount of fluids consumed during the meal is recorded. Any problems or difficulty in eating as well as likes and dislikes are reported and documented on the client's medical record.

Nutritional Support

There are two ways nutritional support for adult clients are delivered: enteral nutrition and parenteral nutrition. **Enteral nutrition** includes both the ingestion of food orally and the delivery of nutrients through a GI tube, but is generally used to mean the latter. **Parenteral nutrition** refers to nutrients bypassing the GI system and entering the blood directly.

Enteral Nutrition When clients cannot or will not take food by mouth, but their GI tracts are working, they are given tube feedings (TF). Sometimes, this may be necessary because of unconsciousness, surgery, stroke, severe malnutrition, or extensive burns. Tube feedings maintain the structural and functional integrity of the GI tract, enhance the utilization of nutrients, and are a safe, economical way to provide nutrients.

Usually, for periods that do not exceed 6 weeks, tube feeding is administered through a nasogastric (NG) tube inserted through the nose and into the stomach or small intestine. When the tube cannot be placed in the nose or when tube feedings are required for more than 6 weeks, an opening called an ostomy is surgically created into the esophagus (esophagostomy), the stomach (gastrostomy), or the intestine (jejunostomy) (Figure 18-10). The physician selects the route and type of feeding tube. The tubes used for these feedings are soft, flexible, and as small as they can be and still allow the feeding to pass through. Numerous commercial formulas are available, with varying types and amounts of nutrients.

There are three methods for administering tube feedings: intermittent, bolus, and continuous. Usually, tube feedings are administered by the continuous infusion method, preferably with a pump. This means the feeding is continuous over a 18- to 24-hour period. Sometimes, the formula is given at half

PROFESSIONALTIP

The Visually Impaired Client and Eating

Clients with impaired vision need an explanation of what is on the plate. For example, using the face of a clock, describe where each food is located. The plate should have a raised edge so the food can be scooped to the outside of the plate. Serving liquids in either a glass or a cup with a lid and straw is helpful to prevent spills.

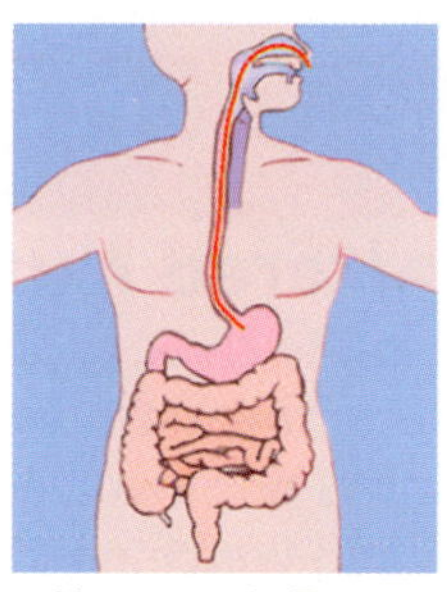
Nasogastric Route

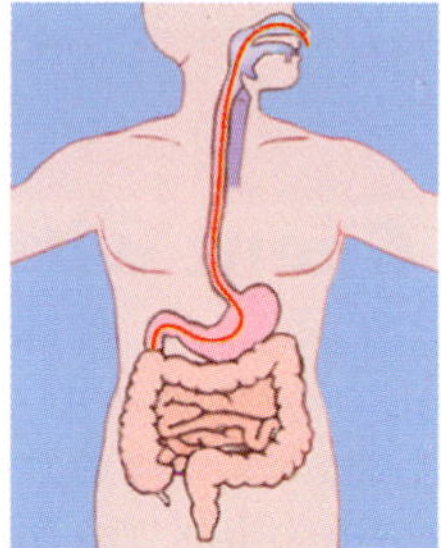
Nasoduodenal Route

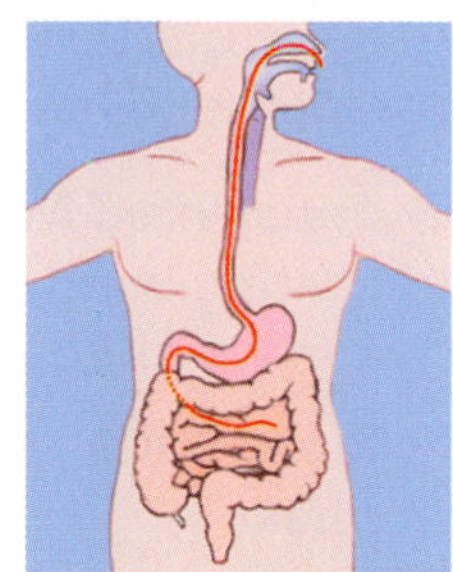
Nasojejunal Route

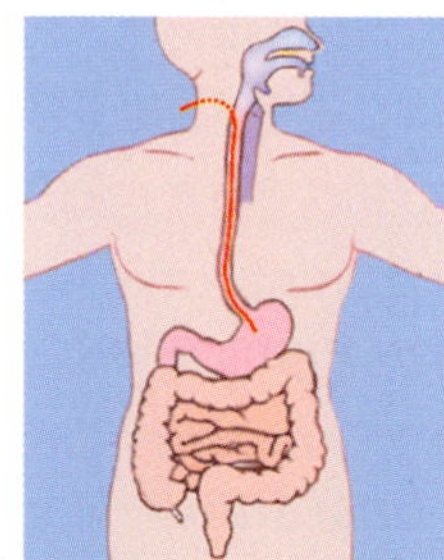
Esophagostomy Route

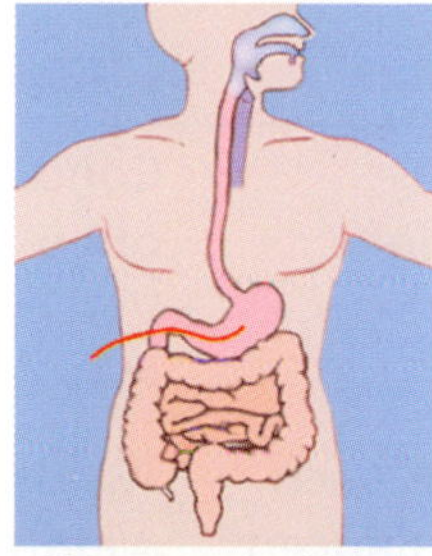
Gastrostomy Route

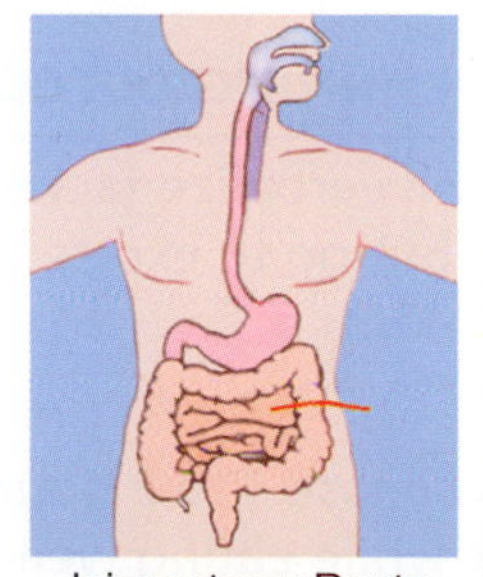
Jejunostomy Route

COURTESY OF DELMAR CENGAGE LEARNING

FIGURE 18-10 Enteral Feeding Routes

strength at a rate of 30 to 50 mL per hour. This rate may be increased by approximately 25 mL every 4 hours until tolerance has been established. As soon as the client tolerates the half-strength formula, a full-strength formula is initiated at the appropriate rate. When clients are ready to return to oral feedings, the transfer must be done gradually.

Parenteral Nutrition Parenteral nutrition is the infusion of a solution of nutrients directly into a vein to meet the client's daily requirements. It is used if the GI tract is not functional or if normal feeding is not adequate for the client's needs. Formerly called hyperalimentation, it is now generally referred to as total parenteral nutrition (TPN). The solution used in this intravenous infusion contains dextrose, amino acids, fats, essential fatty acids, vitamins, and minerals. Administration of TPN is generally a function of the registered nurse.

EVALUATION

The effectiveness of the plan is evaluated in relation to attaining the desired goals. The nurse assesses whether the goals were met. The plan is continued or modified based on the evaluation.

CASE STUDY

L.J. is an 18-year-old female brought in by her parents with a history of steady weight loss, failing in school, poor interest with social groups, and increasingly staying home and spending time alone. L.J. is 5 feet 3 inches tall and weighs 80 pounds. L.J. lost more than 10 pounds in the past several months.

1. Calculate L.J.'s BMI.
2. Identify risk factors for an eating disorder in L.J.
3. Write a nursing diagnosis for L.J.
4. What are other nursing diagnoses for clients with malnutrition?
5. Write a nursing goal for L.J.
6. List nursing interventions with rationales for L.J.

SAMPLE NURSING CARE PLAN

The Client with Altered Nutrition

V.B., age 58 years, is seen in the clinic for her yearly physical examination. She says, "I hardly have the energy to get up and dress in the morning. Cleaning the house and doing the laundry make me exhausted." She does not work and is not involved in community activities. Her daily routine involves cooking for her husband, reading, and watching TV for 6 to 8 hours. She loves to bake fresh breads and pastry. She has a history of being overweight and does not exercise. She says, "I eat because I have nothing else to do." Assessment reveals: height, 5′3″; weight, 166 pounds; weight gain, 14 pounds in the past year; sedentary lifestyle; eats in response to having nothing to do.

NURSING DIAGNOSIS *Imbalanced Nutrition: More Than Body Requirements*, related to excess intake of high-calorie foods, eating in response to boredom, and sedentary lifestyle as evidenced by height–weight relationship and weight gain

Nursing Outcomes Classification (NOC)
Nutritional Status: Nutrient Intake
Weight Control

Nursing Interventions Classification (NIC)
Nutrition Management
Weight Reduction Assistance

PLANNING/OUTCOMES	NURSING INTERVENTIONS	RATIONALE
V.B. will verbalize factors contributing to excess weight.	Conduct a dietary history, using open-ended questions to assist V.B. in exploring factors that may contribute to excess eating.	Encourages client trust and honesty.
V.B. will lose 1 to 2 pounds each week while eating well-balanced meals.	Assess V.B.'s motivation to lose weight.	Will influence success.

(Continues)

SAMPLE NURSING CARE PLAN (Continued)

	Suggest methods to adapt eating habits to decrease amount of intake (smaller servings, taking small bites and chewing each bite 12 times, placing the fork on the plate between bites, drinking water with meals, eating only at mealtime, chewing sugar-free gum when watching TV).	Helps the client eat to satisfy hunger, not boredom.
	Ask V.B. to maintain a daily dietary intake log: time, food, and amount.	Helps the client recognize her eating patterns and note healthy and unhealthy behaviors.
	Provide and review the food guide pyramid and *Dietary Guidelines*; plan with V.B. a diet for 1 week, taking into consideration food preferences.	Ensures that the client has information necessary to plan healthy meals within recommended guidelines.
V.B. will engage in 20 to 30 minutes of exercise three times a week.	Review with V.B. age-appropriate exercises; emphasize the need for walking.	Increases self-esteem, burns calories, increases energy level, and decreases boredom.
V.B. will explore outside interests to decrease boredom and increase feelings of self-worth.	Review with V.B. community interests outside the home, unrelated to cooking and eating.	Helps the client focus on activities not involving food, thereby decreasing boredom and increasing self-esteem.

EVALUATION

V.B. verbalized boredom as the main reason for eating. V.B. is drinking water with meals, chewing her food slowly, and chewing gum while watching TV. She has lost 1.5 pounds in 1 week. V.B. now walks 30 minutes 4 days a week. V.B. will begin volunteering 2 hours three times a week at the church's child care center.

SUMMARY

- The LP/VN plays an important role in promoting proper nutrition.
- The six types of nutrients are water, carbohydrates, fats, protein, vitamins, and minerals.
- Water is the most vital nutrient.
- There must always be a balance between water intake and output to maintain health.
- Nutrients build, repair, and maintain body tissue; provide energy; and regulate body processes.
- The food guide pyramid identifies the five food groups for a well-balanced diet along with a range of servings to meet varying kcal needs.
- Nutritional needs vary as an individual moves through the life cycle.
- Nutrition is influenced by culture, religion, socioeconomics, fads, superstitions, age, and health.
- The kcal needs of an individual are based on basal energy needs plus activity.
- Weight management is based on the relationship between the intake and the use of kcal.
- Food safety is based on proper storage, proper sanitation, and proper cooking.
- Food-borne illnesses can be fairly mild or fatal.

REVIEW QUESTIONS

1. The role of the LP/VN in meeting the nutritional needs of the client includes:
   1. writing the diet order.
   2. preparing food for clients.
   3. preparing a complete diet plan.
   4. answering questions about nutrition.
2. Which of the following would most likely be on a clear liquid diet?
   1. Milkshake.
   2. Tomato soup.
   3. Orange juice.
   4. Cranberry juice.
3. Which of the following is the best source of dietary fiber?
   1. Popcorn.
   2. Chicken.
   3. Tomato juice.
   4. Macaroni and cheese.
4. Cholesterol:
   1. is made in the body.
   2. has no function in the body.
   3. is not important in any disease.
   4. should not be included in the diet.
5. Why should the nurse advise a client to take an iron supplement with orange juice?
   1. To prevent heartburn.
   2. To prevent constipation.
   3. To improve absorption of the iron.
   4. To improve digestion of the orange juice.
6. R.E. is a 45-year-old woman whose weight has been steadily rising over the past 12 years since the birth of her two children. She currently suffers from arthritis in both knees. Her BMI based on her height and weight is 35, placing her in class II obesity. R.E. is concerned about her weight and arthritis. R.E. eats a balanced diet and walks regularly. She enjoys eating out one or two nights a week. She would most likely benefit from:
   1. skipping a meal a day.
   2. eliminating eating out.
   3. exercising every day.
   4. decreasing the amount of food consumed during meals.
7. A positive outcome of management of a client with malnutrition is demonstrated when the client:
   1. states that "I am feeling better."
   2. eats an increased amount of food.
   3. has a steady increase in weight.
   4. expresses a concern over weight gain.
8. An excessively overweight client expressing a desire to lose weight must be advised initially to:
   1. follow a weight-loss diet and increase activity level.
   2. start a treatment combination of exercise, drugs, and weight-loss diet.
   3. consider a referral for surgical intervention.
   4. participate in vigorous exercise.
9. A client with severe malnutrition is admitted to an acute care unit exhibiting many clinical manifestations of malnutrition. While planning a meal for this client, the nurse understands that:
   1. the patient must be given total parenteral nutrition.
   2. the patient must be on a high-calorie, high-protein diet.
   3. allowed to plan own meal and provided privacy to eat.
   4. the nurse and nutritionist must plan the diet for the patient.
10. D.G., a 76-year-old with Parkinson's disease, has difficulty swallowing and handling utensils because of tremors. When preparing to feed D.G., the nurse: (Select all that apply.)
    1. offers a urinal to D.G. and leaves it on the bedside rail after use.
    2. pushes items to one end of the over-bed table with the meal tray.
    3. assists with washing face and hands and oral hygiene prior to eating.
    4. checks that the tray has the diet ordered.
    5. cuts the meat since he is on a pureed diet.
    6. checks his ID band against the name on the tray.

REFERENCES/SUGGESTED READINGS

American Heart Association. (1999). Non-AHA-approved diets. Retrieved October 18, 1999 from http://www.deliciousdecisions.org/ff/tsd_nondiets_fad.html

American Heart Association. (2002). Delicious decisions. Available: http://www.deliciousdecisions.org

Brown, J. (2005). *Nutrition now* (4th ed.). Belmont, CA: Thomson Wadsworth.

Bulechek, G., Butcher, H., McCloskey, J., & Dochterman, J., eds. (2008). *Nursing Interventions Classification (NIC)* (5th ed.). St. Louis, MO: Mosby/Elsevier.

Centers for Disease Control and Prevention. (1997). Update: Prevalence of overweight among children, adolescents, and adults—United States, 1988–1994. *Morbidity and Mortality Weekly Report, 46*(9), 199.

Centers for Disease Control and Prevention. (2002). Body mass index Web calculator. Available: http://www.cdc.gov/nccdphp/dnpa/bmi/calc-bmi.htm

Centers for Disease Control and Prevention. (2006). Obesity still a major problem. Retrieved December 6, 2008, from http://www.cd.gov/nchs/pressroom/06facts/obesity03-04.htm

Cerrato, P. (1999). When food is the culprit. *RN, 62*(6), 52–56.

Cobb, M. (1997). Improving your patient's nutritional status. *Nursing97, 27*(6), 32hhr, 32hh6.

Collins, J. (2002). Helping an older patient eat well to stay well. *Nursing2002, 32*(11), 32hn6–32hn8.

Costello, M. (1996). Home health nutrition. *MedSurg Nursing, 5*(4), 229–238.

Craig, W. (1997). Phytochemicals: Guardians of our health. *Journal of the American Dietetic Association, 97*(10, Suppl. 2), S199–S204.

Dudek, S. (2000). Malnutrition in hospitals: Who's assessing what patients eat? *American Journal of Nursing, 100*(4), 36–42.

Dudek, S. (2006). *Nutrition essentials for nursing practice* (5th ed.). Philadelphia: Lippincott Williams & Wilkins.

Estes, M. (2010). *Health assessment and physical examination* (4th ed.). Clifton Park, NY: Delmar Cengage Learning.

Gartner, L., Eidelman, A., Morton, J., Lawrence, R., Naylor, A., O'Hare, D., et al. (2005) Breastfeeding and the use of human milk. *Pediatrics, 115*(2), 496–506.

Gartner, L., & Greer, F. (2003). Prevention of rickets and vitamin D deficiency: New guidelines for vitamin D intake. *Pediatrics, 111* (4, Pt. 1), 908.

Goldrick, B. (2003). Foodborne diseases. *American Journal of Nursing, 103*(3), 105–106.

Institute of Medicine & Food and Nutrition Board. (1997). *Dietary reference intakes for calcium, phosphorus, magnesium, vitamin D, and fluoride.* Washington, DC: National Academies Press. Available: http://www.nap.edu/books/0309063507/html/index.html

Institute of Medicine & Food and Nutrition Board. (2000a). *Dietary reference intakes for thiamin, riboflavin, niacin, vitamin B6, folate, vitamin B12, pantothenic acid, biotin, and choline.* Washington, DC: National Academies Press. Available: http://www.nap.edu/books/0309065542/html/index.html

Institute of Medicine & Food and Nutrition Board. (2000b). *Dietary reference intakes for vitamin C, vitamin E, selenium, and carotinoids.* Washington, DC: National Academies Press. Available: http://www.nap.edu/books/0309069351/html

Institute of Medicine & Food and Nutrition Board. (2002). *Dietary reference intakes for vitamin A, vitamin K, arsenic, boron, chromium, copper, iodine, iron, manganese, molybdenum, nickel, silicon, vanadium, and zinc.* Washington, DC: National Academies Press. Available: http://www.nap.edu/books/0309072694/html

Kohn-Keeth, C. (2000). How to keep feeding tubes flowing freely. *Nursing2000, 30*(3), 58–59.

Kurtzwell, P. (1998). Staking a claim to good health. Available: http://www.fda.gov/fdca/features/1998/698_labl.html

Loan, T., Magnuson, B., & Williams, S. (1998). Debunking six myths about enteral feeding. *Nursing98, 28*(8), 43–48.

Mathew, L. (2008). *Caring for clients with lower gastrointestinal disorders.* Manuscript submitted for publication.

McConnell, E. (1998). Administering parenteral nutrition. *Nursing98, 28*(7), 18.

McConnell, E. (2001). Administering total parenteral nutrition. *Nursing2001, 31*(11), 17.

McConnell, E. (2002). Measuring fluid intake and output. *Nursing2002, 32*(7), 17.

Metheny, N., & Titler, M. (2001). Assessing placement of feeding tubes. *American Journal of Nursing, 101*(5), 36–45.

Moorhead, S., Johnson, M., Maas, M., & Swanson, E. (2007). *Nursing Outcomes Classification (NOC)* (4th ed.). St. Louis, MO: Elsevier, Health Sciences Division.

North American Nursing Diagnosis Association International. (2010). *NANDA-I nursing diagnoses: Definitions and classification 2009-2011.* Ames, IA: Wiley-Blackwell.

National Academy of Sciences. (1989). *Recommended dietary allowances: 10th edition.* Washington, DC: National Academies Press. Available: http://bob.nap.edu.books/0309046335/html

Nix, S. (2008).*Williams' basic nutrition and diet therapy* (13th ed.). St. Louis, MO: Mosby.

Obarzanek, E., Kimm, S., Barton, B.,Horn, L., Kwiterovich, P., Simons-Morton, D. (2001). Long-term safety and efficacy of a cholesterol-lowering diet in children with elevated low-density lipoprotein cholesterol: Seven-year results of the Dietary Intervention Study in Children (DISC). *Pediatrics, 107*(2), 256.

Roth, R. (2006). *Nutrition and diet therapy (8th ed.).* Clifton Park, NY: Delmar Cengage Learning.

Sheff, B. (2002). Salmonella. *Nursing2002, 32*(7), 81.

Simons, S. (1997). *Vegetables and fruits: Natural "phyters" against disease.* College Station, TX: Texas Agriculture Extension Service.

Stanfield, P., & Hui, Y. (2003). *Nutrition and diet therapy* (4th ed.). Sudbury, MA: Jones and Bartlett.

U.S. Department of Agriculture. (1996). *The food guide pyramid* (Home and Garden Bulletin, No. 252). Washington, DC: U.S. Department of Agriculture, Center for Nutrition Policy and Promotion. Available: http://www.usda.gov/cnpp/pyrabklt.pdf

U.S. Department of Agriculture. (2008). *Inside the pyramid.* Retrieved December 5, 2008, from http://www.mypyramid.gov/pyramid/index.html

U.S. Department of Agriculture & U.S. Department of Health and Human Services. (2000). *Nutrition and your health: Dietary guidelines for Americans* (Home and Garden Bulletin No. 232) (5th ed.). Washington, DC: U.S. Department of Agriculture and U.S. Department of Health and Human Services. Retrieved December 4, 2008, from http://www.cnpp.usda.gov/Publications/DietaryGuidelines/2000/2000DGProfessionalBooklet.pdf

U.S. Food and Drug Administration. (1999). The food label. Available: http://www.fda.gov/opacom/backgrounders/foolaabel/newlabel.html

University of Iowa Health Care. (2006). Fat makes you fat. Iowa City: University of Iowa Hospitals and Clinics. Retrieved December 5, 2008, from http://www.uihealthcare.com/topics/weightcontrol/weig5290.html

Washington, H. (1998). The vitamin revolution. *Health, 12*(6), 104–110.

Wilkes, G. (2000). Nutrition: The forgotten ingredient in cancer care. *American Journal of Nursing, 100*(4), 46–51.

Williams, S. (2001). *Basic nutrition and diet therapy* (11th ed.). St. Louis, MO: Mosby.

RESOURCES

American Dietetic Association, http://www.eatright.org
Food and Nutrition Board, http://www.iom.edu
Food and Nutrition Information Center, http://www.nal.usda.gov
Nestlé Nutrition, http://www.nestle-nutrition.com
U.S. Department of Agriculture, MyPyramid.gov, http://mypyramid.gov

CHAPTER 19
Rest and Sleep

MAKING THE CONNECTION

Refer to the following chapters to increase your understanding of rest and sleep:

Basic Nursing

- ***Communication***
- ***Client Teaching***
- ***Nursing Process/Documentation/Informatics***
- ***Stress, Adaptation, and Anxiety***
- ***Complementary/Alternative Therapies***
- ***Pain Management***

LEARNING OBJECTIVES

Upon completion of this chapter, you should be able to:

- Define key terms.
- Describe the phases and stages of sleep.
- Identify factors that affect normal sleep.
- Discuss age-related sleep variations.
- State the outcomes of sleep deprivation.
- Delineate nursing interventions that promote rest and sleep.

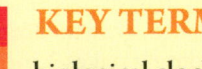

KEY TERMS

biological clock
bruxism
cataplexy
chronobiology
circadian rhythm
hypersomnia
insomnia
narcolepsy
parasomnia
REM movement disorder
rest
restless leg syndrome (RLS)
sleep
sleep apnea
sleep cycle
sleep deprivation
sleep hygiene
somnambulism

INTRODUCTION

The quality of rest and sleep can have a significant impact on a person's health, including physical well-being, mental status, and coping effectiveness. This chapter discusses the importance of rest and sleep and nursing care to assist clients to maintain optimal health when disturbances in rest and sleep occur.

REST AND SLEEP

Rest and sleep are basic to health well-being. Age, developmental level, health status, activity level, and cultural norms influence the need for rest and sleep. **Rest** is a state of mental and physical relaxation and calmness. Rest can take place when lying down, reading a book, or taking a quiet walk. The nurse should try to ascertain which activities and places the client finds restful (Figure 19-1).

Sleep is a state of altered consciousness during which a person has minimal physical activity, changes in level of consciousness, and a slowing of physiologic processes. Sleep is cyclical, usually lasting for several hours. Disruptions in the usual sleep routine can be distressing to clients and often prevent further sleep. Sleep is a restorative function needed for physiologic and psychological healing. It is important that health care providers, clients, and their significant others understand the normal sleep–wake cycle and how sleep affects healing and mood.

PHYSIOLOGY OF SLEEP

Centers in the brain control the cycles of wakefulness and sleep, which are influenced by environmental factors and routines. An individual's biological clock helps determine the specific cycles of wakefulness and sleep.

Phases and Stages of Sleep

The stages of sleep are identified by electroencephalograph (EEG) patterns, eye movements, and muscle activity. Sleep phases are classified as non–rapid eye movement (NREM) and rapid eye movement (REM) sleep (see Box 19-1).

NREM Sleep The first phase of sleep is called non– rapid eye movement, or NREM, sleep and consists of four stages. *Stage 1 sleep* is a light sleep, in which muscles relax and brain waves are rapid and irregular. In adults with normal sleep patterns, stage 1 sleep usually lasts 10 minutes or so. During this stage, it is easy to awaken a sleeper.

Stage 2 sleep is still fairly light sleep. Brain waves become larger with bursts of electrical activity. Half of normal adult sleep may be spent in stage 2. After 20 minutes or so in stage 2 sleep, a deep sleep is entered.

Stage 3 and *stage 4* sleep are usually discussed together because they are difficult to identify and separate. Stage 3 is a medium-deep sleep, and stage 4 is the deepest sleep. Each stage lasts 15 to 30 minutes. During these stages large, slow waves are seen on the EEG. Vital signs are significantly lower than when awake. It is difficult to awaken a person in this stage of sleep.

Stages 3 and 4 sleep are thought to have restorative value, needed for physical recovery. Human growth hormone is secreted mainly at night, especially during stages 3 and 4 sleep, near the beginning of a sleep period. Growth hormone is necessary for growth and also for normal tissue repair in individuals of all ages. About 75% of sleep is NREM sleep.

REM Sleep After the first 60 to 90 minutes of NREM sleep in adults, the individual enters rapid eye movement, or REM, sleep. The brain waves are almost the same as when awake. This is a highly active time with rapid eye movements, heart rate, respiratory rate, and blood pressure similar to when awake; large muscle tone is decreased, and the person is "virtually paralyzed" (American Academy of Sleep Medicine, 2005; Harvard Medical School, 2007); and muscles are flaccid, making the body paralyzed. This is the time when dreams occur. Dreams are ways for individuals to consolidate memories, solve problems, adapt behaviors, and clarify thoughts and

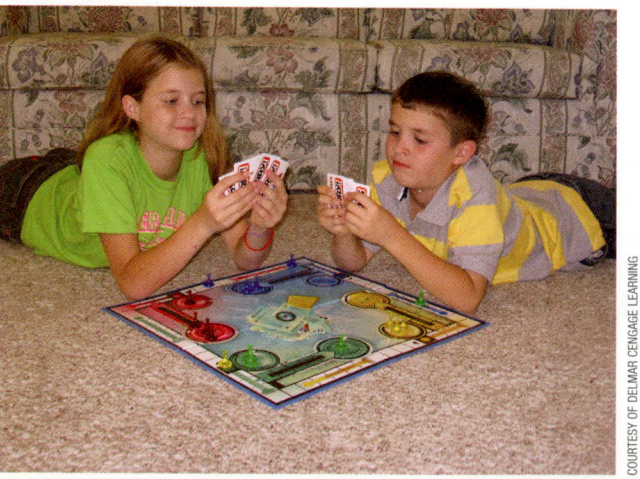
COURTESY OF DELMAR CENGAGE LEARNING

FIGURE 19-1 **Playing a quiet board game can be a relaxing activity for children.**

BOX 19-1 STAGES OF SLEEP

NREM Stage 1
- The lightest stage of sleep.
- Client is easily aroused by light or noise.

NREM Stage 2
- This stage is deeper than stage 1.
- Client is still easily aroused.
- Blood pressure and respirations decrease.

NREM Stage 3
- Beginning of deep sleep.
- Muscles relax.
- Blood pressure and respirations continue to decrease.

NREM Stage 4
- The deepest and most restful stage of sleep.
- Physical and mental restoration occurs during this stage.
- Sleepwalking and enuresis may occur.

REM
- Vivid, full-color dreaming (dreaming may occur in all other stages but not as vivid).
- REM stage occurs at the end of each NREM cycle.
- Eyes dart rapidly under closed eyelids.

emotions. About 25% of sleep is REM sleep, with REM-sleep periods becoming longer as the night goes on.

Sleep Cycle

The **sleep cycle** is the sequence of sleep beginning with the four stages of NREM sleep, a return to stage 3 and then stage 2 (the first phase), followed by the first REM sleep (Figure 19-2). The duration of a sleep cycle is usually 60 to 90 minutes, and the sleeper will generally go through four to six sleep cycles during a sleep period of 7 to 8 hours.

The length of the NREM and REM periods of sleep change as the sleep period progresses, and dreams during REM sleep may become more vivid and intense. Whenever the sleep cycle is broken, a new sleep cycle starts, beginning again at NREM sleep stage 1.

Biological Clock

The **biological clock** is an internal mechanism in a living organism capable of measuring time. It controls the daily variations in hundreds of physiologic processes, including body temperature, respiratory rate, alertness, performance, and the level of several hormones. According to Coleman (1986), the major characteristics of biological clocks are:

- They are internal physiologic systems that measure the passage of time.
- They have their own daily cycle length, which is close to, but not exactly, 24 hours.
- When exposed to normal environmental cues, such as the day–night cycle, they adapt to a 24-hour day.
- When free of environmental cues, such as the day–night cycle, the organism's internal cycle length determines its behavior.

When external time cues such as day–night, mealtimes, and sleep–wake are inconsistent, a desynchronization of the circadian biological rhythms occurs. This internal desynchronization disrupts the timing of physiologic and behavioral activity, which, in turn, causes disrupted sleep patterns, chronic fatigue, and decreased performance and coping abilities. An example of desynchronization is shift workers who try to sleep in the daytime when activities around them and their own biological clock tell them to be awake.

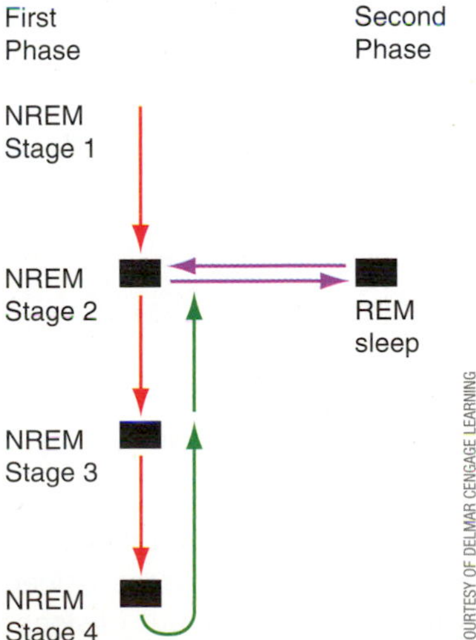

Figure 19-2 The two phases and four stages of the sleep cycle.

> **PROFESSIONALTIP**
>
> **Biorhythms**
>
> **Chronobiology** is a relatively new branch of science that studies the rhythms controlled by our biological clocks, or biorhythms. The **circadian rhythms**, those that cycle on a daily basis, such as the sleep–wake cycle, are the most widely studied. Other biological rhythms include:
>
> - **Ultradian:** those lasting much shorter than a day, such as the milliseconds it takes for a neuron to fire
> - **Infradian:** those lasting a month or more, such as the monthly menstrual cycle
> - **Circannual:** those requiring approximately 1 year to complete, such as seasonal affective disorder, which causes depression in susceptible people during the short days of winter

Factors Affecting Rest and Sleep

Several factors can influence the quality and quantity of both rest and sleep. Often, sleep problems result from a combination of many factors.

Physical Factors

Comfort is a very subjective experience. The nurse must make sure the client's physical and psychological needs are met. When basic needs are not met, the person encounters discomfort, which leads to physiologic tension and anxiety and, possibly, disturbed rest and sleep. For example, a client

> **PROFESSIONALTIP**
>
> **Assessing the Effect of Pain on Sleep**
>
> Questioning clients about the effect pain has on their sleep habits will help clarify the intensity of the pain and its effect on the clients' patterns of daily living. The nurse should ask the client whether the pain:
>
> - Prevents the client from falling asleep
> - Makes finding a comfortable sleeping position difficult
> - Wakes the client from a sound sleep
> - Keeps the client from falling back asleep once awakened
> - Leaves the client feeling tired and unrefreshed after a sleeping session (White & Duncan, 2002)

experiencing hunger or pain may become restless and irritable and will focus on getting these needs met instead of getting restful sleep.

Some physical problems can interfere with the ability to fall asleep or stay asleep. Conditions that cause discomfort or pain, such as arthritis, make it difficult to sleep well, as can breathing disorders such as sleep apnea and asthma. Hormonal changes that cause premenstrual syndrome (PMS) or menopause with its hot flashes can disrupt sleep. Even pregnancy, especially during the last few weeks, may make sleeping difficult.

Psychological Factors

An active mind and restless body interfere with the ability to sleep. Many individuals have intrusive thoughts or muscle tension, which interferes with rest and sleep. Anxiety related to family demands, work pressures, and other stressors does not necessarily cease when an individual tries to go to sleep and often results in difficulty falling or staying asleep. Usually, sleep problems disappear when the stressful situation is resolved.

Environment

Temperature, lighting, ventilation, odors, and noise level can interrupt sleep when different from the person's usual sleep environment. The comfort and size of the bed, firmness of the pillow, and habits (snoring or movements) of a sleep partner may all interfere with sleep.

Sleep is especially disrupted when a person is hospitalized. Some factors associated with hospitalization that lead to sleep impairment include:

- Physical or emotional pain
- Unfamiliar surroundings
- Change in routine
- Fear of the unknown
- Timing of assessments, procedures, and treatments
- Intrusive lighting or equipment
- Noise level (especially unfamiliar noises)
- Lack of privacy

Lifestyle Stressors

A fast-paced life with many stressors may result in a person being unable to relax easily or fall asleep quickly. Relaxation precedes healthy sleep. Vigorously exercising within an hour of going to bed or performing mentally intense activities just before or after getting into bed often work against getting a good night's sleep.

A work schedule that does not fit with an individual's biological clock (e.g., working at times other than the day shift) may interfere with sleep. More than 15 million Americans are shift workers (National Sleep Foundation [NSF], 2008c). Individuals who frequently change work shifts or travel across several times zones face a real challenge in trying to stabilize their biological rhythms and rest comfortably.

Diet

Foods high in caffeine, such as coffee, colas, and chocolate, are stimulants and often delay sleep. Consuming a large, spicy, or heavy meal just before bedtime may cause indigestion, which often interferes with sleep. Going to bed when hungry can also delay sleep because the individual will be focused on food and hunger pangs instead of on sleep.

CRITICAL THINKING

Client Assessment

During morning report, the night nurse tells the day nurse that the client "slept through the night." However, during the morning assessment, the client tells the nurse that she didn't sleep well and is very tired. What are some possible explanations for the discrepancy between what the night nurse and the client told the day nurse?

CLIENT TEACHING

Methods to Reduce Anxiety

Teach clients the following methods to relieve anxiety:

- Progressive muscle relaxation
- Guided imagery
- Deep breathing
- Thought stopping
- Meditation
- Therapeutic massage

SAFETY

Medications and Sleep

Some medications used to treat high blood pressure, asthma, or depression may cause sleeping difficulties. For instance, captopril (Capoten) and theophylline (Theomar), used to treat high blood pressure and asthma, respectively, may cause insomnia, whereas trazodone (Desyrel), an antidepressant, can either induce drowsiness or cause insomnia.

CULTURAL CONSIDERATIONS

Expectations Affecting Sleep

Some people perceive sleep as a luxury to be indulged in when they are not too busy with "important" activities. Others view sleep as an absolute necessity. The amount of sleep that a person considers necessary is partially determined by the attitudes of family and culture.

CRITICAL THINKING

Age-Related Sleep Variations

What age-related sleep variations should be considered when assessing the sleep habits of neonates, infants, toddlers, school-age children, adolescents, and elders?

Medications and Other Substances

Many medications, both prescription and over-the-counter, list fatigue, restlessness, sleepiness, agitation, or insomnia as side effects. A small amount of alcohol may help some people fall asleep; however, alcohol may interrupt sleep later in the night. Nicotine, a stimulant, also delays sleep.

Age/Aging

Some sleep variations are based on age.

The neonate (birth–1 month) sleeps 16 to 20 hours per day in 3- to 4-hour intervals. The newborn usually sleeps very soundly and with little activity occurring during sleep ("sleeping like a baby"). There is often no difference in day and night sleep patterns.

As the infant gets older, the amount of sleep needed decreases. When infants begin to sleep through the night, they will usually have two or three naps during the day.

Toddlers typically sleep 10 to 12 hours at night with one or two daytime naps (Figure 19-3). Bedtime rituals such as a bath, brushing teeth, and reading books help establish expectations and provide nighttime security.

During preschool years, daytime napping decreases or ceases, and vivid dreams and nightmares may occur at night. These often awaken the child several times during the night.

School-age children need 10 to 12 hours of sleep daily but may resist bedtime as they struggle for independence. They may develop a fear of the dark and need reassurance and a system to cope with this fear.

Adolescents need 8 to 10 hours of sleep per day. Irregular sleeping habits often become the norm as their high activity level often interferes with regular sleep patterns.

The young adult requires about 8 hours of sleep per day. Sleep may be interrupted by their young children or by work responsibilities. Lifestyle stressors cause difficulties in falling or staying asleep.

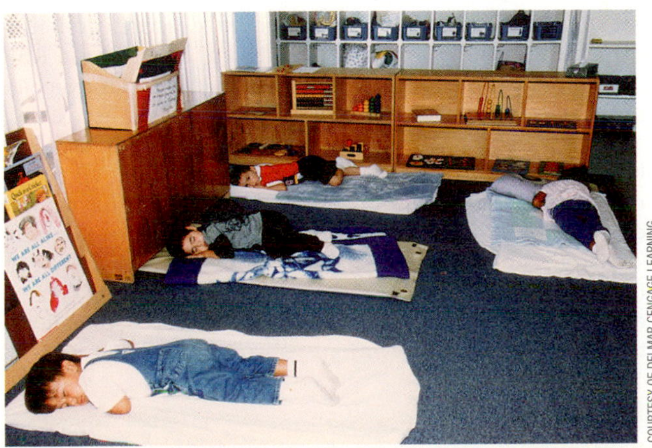

COURTESY OF DELMAR CENGAGE LEARNING

FIGURE 19-3 Young children require naps and rest periods throughout the day.

CRITICAL THINKING

Caffeine

Which foods and beverages have the most and least caffeine? Check out the National Sleep Foundation's (NSF) Caffeine Calculator on its Web site at www.sleepfoundation.org.

LIFE SPAN CONSIDERATIONS

Sleep and Aging

- Sleep needs do not decline with age but stay fairly constant at 7 to 9 hours per day.
- Middle-aged and elderly clients are more likely to experience sleep apnea, restless leg syndrome, and periodic limb movement disorder (NIA, 2007).

Most middle-age adults sleep 6 to 8 hours each day. Daily stressors may result in insomnia and the use of sleep-inducing medications.

Most older adults sleep less at one time than do those who are younger, although overall sleep needs remain constant at 7 to 9 hours (National Institute on Aging, 2007). They may go to sleep earlier, wake up more often, get less deep sleep, and rise earlier (NSF, 2003). Often, a daytime nap is taken. The quality of sleep may diminish because of frequent waking and physical discomfort. The percentage of REM sleep remains fairly constant.

SLEEP PATTERN ALTERATIONS

Sleep disturbances are varied and are quite common. Sleep pattern alterations are either primary sleep disorders (those where the fundamental problem is the sleep alteration) or secondary sleep disorders (those where a medical or clinical cause results in or contributes to the sleep alteration). The most common sleep alterations include insomnia, hypersomnia, narcolepsy, sleep apnea/snoring, sleep deprivation, parasomnias, restless leg syndrome, and periodic limb movement disorder.

Insomnia

Insomnia refers to difficulty falling asleep or staying asleep (American Academy of Sleep Medicine [AASM], 2008). According to NSF (2008a), approximately 30 million American adults are affected by chronic insomnia each year. Insomnia is not a disease, but it may be a manifestation of many illnesses. Causes may include stress, depression, medical problems, caffeine, alcohol, pain, poor sleep habits, or changes in sleep patterns related to travel or shift work. The person experiencing insomnia often gets caught up in a vicious cycle of not being able to sleep, trying harder to fall asleep, and experiencing increasing anxiety about not sleeping, which, in turn, increases the inability to fall asleep.

Symptoms of insomnia include difficulty falling asleep, waking frequently during the night, waking very early and not being able to go back to sleep, feeling unrested in the morning and/or tired during the day, and becoming anxious and restless as bedtime arrives. Many who have insomnia actually sleep significantly more than they think they do.

Often, insomnia may occur only for a night or two. If it continues or is viewed as very disturbing or disruptive by the individual, a health care provider should be consulted for relief. Treatment is best focused on modifying the factors or behaviors causing it.

Hypersomnia

Hypersomnia is characterized by excessive sleep, especially in the daytime. Persons with hypersomnia often feel they do not sleep enough at night, so they sleep late into the morning and nap several times during the day. Causes of hypersomnia can be physical (such as a disease or medication) or psychological (such as a self-imposed short sleep time); treatment must address the underlying cause.

Narcolepsy

Narcolepsy is a sudden, irresistible urge to fall asleep during the daytime. Approximately 1 in 2,000 people have narcolepsy (National Institute of Neurological Disorders and Stroke, 2008). These "sleep attacks" can occur during a conversation or while driving, and last from a few seconds to more than 30 minutes. The hallmark symptom of narcolepsy is **cataplexy**, a sudden loss of muscle tone without loss of consciousness, which may cause the person to fall (Stansberry, 2001).

Individuals with narcolepsy often sleep adequately at night. There is no cure, but symptoms may be controlled by taking scheduled daytime naps, waking at the same time each morning, and avoiding caffeine, food, and alcohol after 8:00 P.M. (Stansberry, 2001).

Sleep Apnea/Snoring

Apnea is a Greek word meaning "without breath." **Sleep apnea** is a period, during sleep, of not breathing following a period of loud snoring. People with untreated sleep apnea may stop breathing hundreds of times for up to 60 seconds or more. Sleep apnea affects 18 million people in the United States (NSF, 2008a) and is most common in obese, middle-aged men (NSF, 2002).

There are three types of apnea: obstructive, caused by relaxation of muscles in the back of the throat that block the airway; central, caused by a failure of the brain to signal the muscles to breathe; and mixed, a combination of the two (American Sleep Apnea Association, 2008).

The unaware sleeper stops breathing repeatedly during sleep and as frequently as 100 times per hour, often for a minute or longer. Usually, those with sleep apnea have no idea that they are not breathing or that they are continually waking up (AASM, 2008).

Sleep apnea results in REM-sleep deprivation, manifesting as excessive daytime sleepiness. Sleep apnea can cause hypertension and an increased risk of heart attack or stroke. A nasal continuous positive airway pressure (CPAP) device, which maintains airflow with a small compressor, may give relief. Dental appliances that reposition the tongue may also help. With some individuals, surgical intervention is required to correct the cause of the apnea.

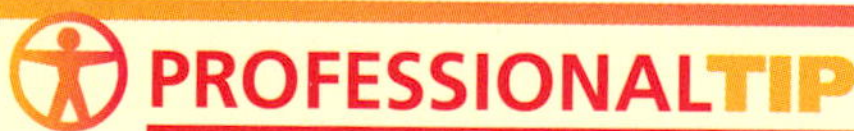

Sleep Apnea

There are a number of factors that increase the risk for sleep apnea. These risk factors include having a small upper airway (or large tongue, tonsils, or uvula); being overweight; having a recessed chin, a small jaw, or a large overbite; having a large neck size (17 inches or greater in a man or 16 inches or greater in a woman); smoking and alcohol use; being age 40 or older; and ethnicity (African Americans, Pacific Islanders, and Hispanics) (NSF, 2005).

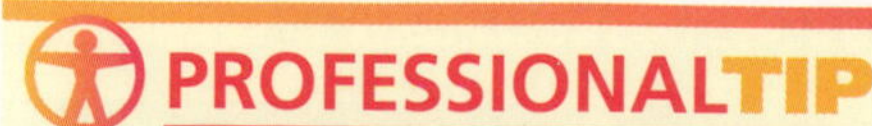

Sleep Deprivation

Sleep deprivation can be deadly, and the price tag is staggering. According to the National Sleep Foundation (NSF, 2001), the costs of drowsy drivers are estimated to be $12.5 billion per year. Drowsy drivers are blamed for 100,000 police-reported crashes and kill more than 1,500 Americans each year.

The person who is deprived of restful sleep is less alert, less attentive, less able to perform even simple tasks, and more irritable and has poorer concentration and judgment and mood problems that make relationships with family, friends, and coworkers difficult. No matter the cause of sleep deprivation, inadequate sleep reduces the quality of life and is harmful to health.

Sleep Deprivation

Sleep deprivation is a term used to describe prolonged inadequate quality and quantity of sleep, either of the REM or of the NREM type. Sleep deprivation can result from age, prolonged hospitalization, drug and substance use, illness, and frequent changes in lifestyle patterns. Sleep and dreaming have a restorative value necessary for mental and emotional recovery, and they appear to enhance the ability to cope with emotional problems. Therefore, sleep deprivation can cause symptoms ranging from irritability, hypersensitivity, and confusion to apathy, sleepiness, and diminished reflexes. Treating or minimizing the factors that cause the sleep deprivation is the most effective intervention.

Parasomnia

Parasomnia refers to disorders that intrude on sleep in very active ways. **Somnambulism** (sleepwalking), sleep talking, night terrors, REM movement disorder, bed-wetting, and

bruxism (teeth grinding) are the most common parasomnias; the first four are discussed in more detail in the following. Treatment for parasomnias varies, and the client and family should be helped to understand the disorder and its potential safety problems.

Somnambulism Sleepwalking, done mostly by children, is typically not remembered by the individual the next morning. The sleepwalker usually moves around furniture very safely. Doors and windows must be kept locked at night to protect the sleepwalker from harm. Sleepwalkers are difficult to rouse during an episode and if awakened are often confused and without any specific recall of events that led to their behavior. Sleepwalking tends to run in families and usually stops at puberty.

Sleep Talking Sleep talking can occur at any age. It may be a word or two or a long speech, sometimes understandable and sometimes gibberish. The person has no memory of talking, but the sleep partner may have been awakened.

Sleep Terrors Sleep terrors are more common in children and seldom continue into adulthood. The child suddenly appears to awaken, thrashes about, sweats, and may even cry. This can last anywhere from 1 minute to approximately 15 minutes. The child remembers nothing in the morning. Reassurance by the parents during the episode is the only treatment; the child will eventually outgrow the behavior.

REM Movement Disorder **REM movement disorder** results when the normal paralysis of REM sleep is absent or incomplete and the sleeper acts out the dream. It is most common among older men. Violent behavior and injuries may result. The person can remember the dream in the morning. Medication usually is effective in controlling the physical movements.

Restless Leg Syndrome

Restless leg syndrome (RLS) is the uncomfortable sensations of tingling or crawling in the muscles and twitching, burning, prickling, or deep aching in the foot, calf, or upper leg when at rest. The sensations return in seconds or minutes. The legs frequently jump involuntarily if they are not moved. Symptoms worsen at night. If sleep does come, the leg movements awaken the person frequently.

Although the cause is unknown, some cases of RLS have been linked to iron deficiency, dialysis treatment, peripheral neuropathy, pregnancy, excessive caffeine intake, alcohol dependence, and smoking. The disorder is more common among women who have passed middle age. Avoiding or reducing smoking, caffeine, and alcohol intake may help. Symptoms may be relieved by opiates, benzodiazepines, or L-dopa.

Periodic Limb Movements in Sleep

Periodic limb movements in sleep (PLMS) is a condition of repetitive leg movements every 20 to 40 seconds throughout the night. It is typically not uncomfortable for the affected person but may be distressing to the sleep partner. Multiple sleep interruptions occur, leading to daytime sleepiness and nighttime insomnia.

The disorder is quite common in persons older than age 65 years. Approximately 35% of elders have at least a mild form of PLMS, which occurs only during sleep and is not as uncomfortable as RLS (NSF, 2008a).

Nocturnal Sleep-Related Eating Disorder

Nocturnal sleep-related eating disorder (NSRED) is rapid and chaotic eating when partially or fully awake with variable recall of the episode. An estimated 4 million people have this disorder, with two-thirds being women (Montgomery, Haynes, & Garner, 2002). This combination sleep and eating disorder may be misdiagnosed as anorexia, bulimia, or depression.

Clients gain weight with only moderate daytime eating, are not hungry in the morning, and are chronically tired. They typically eat food high in calories and fat at night, often foods they do not eat in the daytime. A spouse, partner, or family member may be able to shed light on the situation.

NURSING PROCESS

All standardized nursing history tools include questions related to a client's rest and sleep patterns. Care of the client who is diagnosed with a sleep disorder is collaborative, with the nurse participating in an interdisciplinary team providing treatment. Concept Map 19-1 identifies key components of the nursing process for clients with a *Disturbed **Sleep** Pattern.*

ASSESSMENT

The nursing assessment includes a history of sleep and rest patterns; **sleep hygiene**, or the client's personal habits in preparing for sleep; and a physical exam. Sleep survey tools such as the Pittsburgh Sleep Quality Index can be administered by the nurse to assess for sleep disturbances or deficits (Smyth, 2008). The client with a sleep disturbance should be thoroughly assessed to determine the types of disturbance, sleep alterations, and impact of sleep problems. Usually, the client is a reliable source for this information,

> **PROFESSIONALTIP**
>
> **Sleep History**
>
> To help detect a sleep disorder, ask the client:
>
> - What time do you usually go to bed?
> - How long does it take to fall asleep?
> - What wakes you up in the morning?
> - What time do you wake up in the morning?
> - Do you take a nap during the day? When? How long?
> - How much food do you eat in the evening?
> - Do you drink caffeinated beverages? How much? In the evening?
> - Do you drink alcohol? How much? In the evening?
> - Do you take medications or herbal supplements to help you sleep?

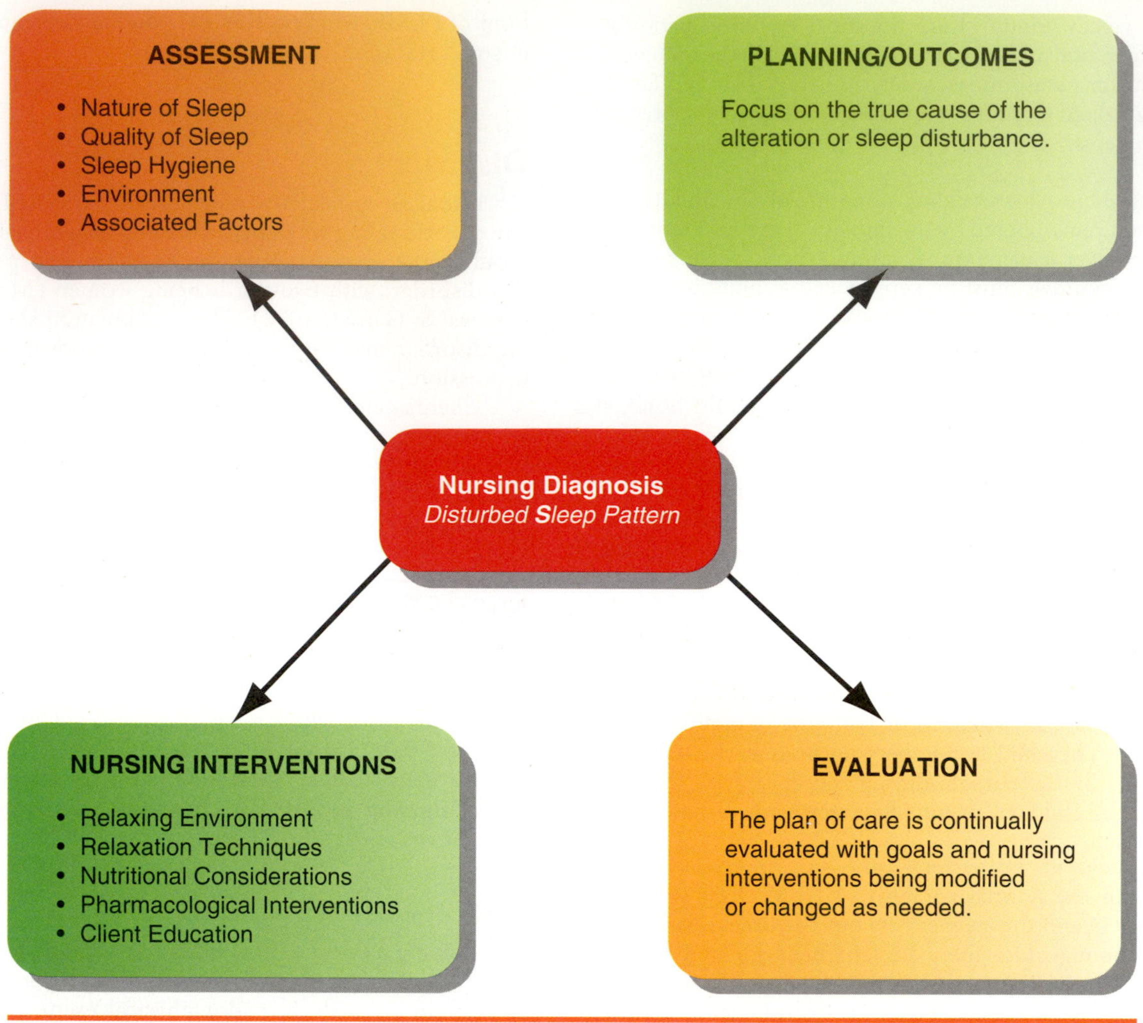

CONCEPT MAP 19-1 Nursing Process for Clients with a *Disturbed Sleep Pattern*

but a spouse or partner sharing sleeping arrangements may add valuable information to the client's report. Questions regarding the client's usual sleep patterns should focus on the following:

- Nature of sleep (restful, uninterrupted)
- Quality of sleep (feeling on waking)
- Sleep environment (description of room, temperature, noise level)
- Associated factors (bedtime routines, use of sleep medications or any other sleep inducers)
- Opinion of sleep (adequate, inadequate, problematic)

To discover information about altered sleep patterns, ask questions about:

- Type of problem (inability to fall asleep, difficulty remaining asleep, inability to fall asleep after awakening, restless sleep, daytime sleepiness)
- Quality of the problem (number of hours of sleep versus number of hours spent trying to sleep, duration and frequency of naps, number of awakenings per sleep period)
- Environmental factors (lighting, bed, noise level, surrounding stimulation, sleep partner)
- Other factors (relation to meals eaten, activity before retiring, life stressors, work stressors, anxiety level, pain, recent illness or surgery)
- Alleviating factors (mild diet, warm drink before retiring, reading, listening to quiet music, taking a hot bath)
- Effect of problem (fatigue, irritability, confusion)

A daily journal of their sleep patterns may be helpful for clients whose sleep problems are not well defined. Other factors, such as age, medical diagnosis, occupation, allergies, and psychiatric disorders, must also be considered when assessing sleep problems.

NURSING DIAGNOSIS

After information about the sleep impairment has been collected, the data must be analyzed to formulate appropriate nursing diagnoses. Alterations in sleep can manifest as verbal complaints on the part of the client, physical signs such as yawning or dark circles under the eyes, or alterations in mood, such as apathy or irritability. The primary diagnosis for individuals experiencing sleep problems is *Disturbed **S**leep Pattern*. Another diagnosis related to rest and sleep is ***S**leep Deprivation*

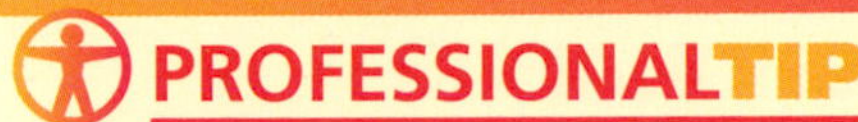

Communicating with the Client Who Is Sleep-Impaired

- Thoroughly explain procedures before implementation.
- Encourage the client and significant others to verbalize feelings and ask questions.
- Answer questions honestly and completely.
- Identify and support coping mechanisms of the client and family.
- Spend adequate time with the client to facilitate communication.
- Assess and incorporate the client's preferences as much as possible into the plan of care.

(North American Nursing Diagnosis Association International, 2009).

If the client has problems in addition to a sleep disturbance, think about the possibility that the sleep disturbance is the cause (not the effect) of another problem. For example, a client may be experiencing *Activity Intolerance* related to lack of sleep as evidenced by verbal complaint, extreme fatigue, disorientation, confusion, and lack of energy.

Planning/Outcome Identification

Client input should be incorporated into the plan and goals. The plan of care and the goals must focus on the true cause of the alteration or sleep disturbance. For example, if the client is experiencing *Disturbed Sleep Pattern* because of bed-wetting, the bed-wetting should be the focus of intervention.

Many sleep disturbances require long periods of time (weeks or months as opposed to days) to correct. Sleep is by nature habitual and part of the person's lifestyle patterns. When planning care, the nurse should time procedures and treatments so they do not disturb sleep time.

Implementation

Several interventions can promote rest and sleep in clients; these are discussed next.

Trusting Nurse–Client Relationship

The client's ability to rest and sleep can be enhanced by the quality of the nurse–client relationship. Knowing that the nurse is trustworthy and genuinely cares about the client allows the client to relax and feel secure. Anxiety can be minimized by the nurse's use of therapeutic communication skills. The therapeutic use of self helps allay client anxiety.

Relaxing Environment

A place to sleep should be inviting. The immediate surroundings should be arranged to promote sleep for the sleep-impaired client. The nurse should ascertain what environment the client finds relaxing, then try to provide this environment in the inpatient setting or help the client establish this type of environment in the home setting.

CLIENT TEACHING

Managing Sleep Disturbance

To facilitate rest and sleep, the client should be encouraged to:

- Select regular times for going to bed and awakening and try to observe them.
- Drink a warm cup of milk before bed.
- Eat a light healthy snack at bedtime.
- Take a warm bath before going to bed.
- Avoid stimulating activities, such as strenuous exercise or demanding intellectual activity, during the hour before bedtime and use the time instead to wind down with relaxing activities such as taking a warm bath, reading a book, or sitting by the fire.
- Use bedtime rituals on a consistent basis.
- Void before going to bed.
- Use the bed only for sleeping.
- Avoid caffeine, spicy foods, and heavy meals in the several hours before bedtime.

PROFESSIONAL TIP

Noise Control in Health Facilities

- Keep the door to the client's room closed.
- Reduce the volume of paging and telephone systems, especially at night.
- Ensure that unused equipment in the client's room is turned off.
- Turn off or lower the volume on radios and televisions.
- Workers should keep noises to a minimum, especially at night.
- Hold discussions and conferences away from the client's room.

Relaxation Techniques

The client's mood before sleep is very important. Believing that one can and will sleep affects both sleep quality and quantity. The calm, relaxed client is likely to fall asleep quickly and stay asleep all night. Relaxation techniques are useful sleep aids (Figure 19-4). Progressive muscle relaxation may be helpful for the person who has tense muscles. A warm bath may be relaxing.

Nutritional Considerations

Some foods enhance sleep. Tryptophan, an amino acid in milk, promotes sleep by stimulating the brain's production of serotonin. Scientific data support the old wives' tale that drinking warm milk promotes sleep. Other ways to promote sleep are to avoid caffeine after noon, avoid large or heavy meals close to bedtime, and refrain from eating foods that cause gastrointestinal distress.

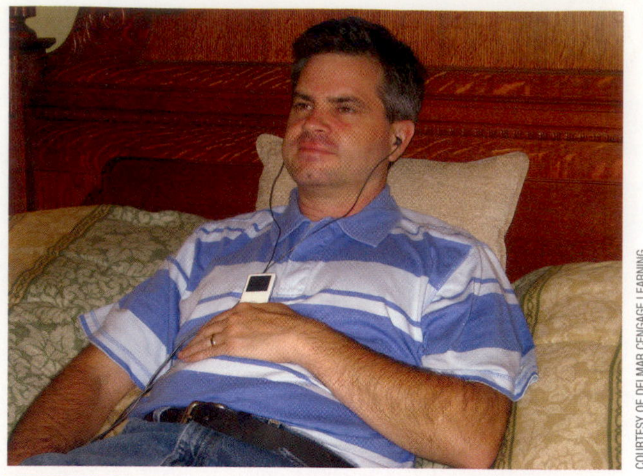
COURTESY OF DELMAR CENGAGE LEARNING

FIGURE 19-4 Listening to favorite music can be very relaxing before going to bed.

Pharmacologic Interventions

If pain is a reason for sleep disturbance, interventions should first focus on pain management. Some nonpharmacologic relaxation and imagery interventions may be effective.

Pharmacologic agents such as tricyclic antidepressants, antihistamines, and short-acting hypnotics may be helpful for clients with sleep disturbances (McCaffery & Pasero, 1999). The tricyclic antidepressant amitriptyline (Elavil) improves the client's ability to fall asleep and stay asleep by causing sedation when given 1 to 3 hours before bedtime; doses are significantly less than those given for depression.

If given at bedtime, antihistamines such as hydroxyzine (Vistaril, Atarax) and diphenhydramine (Benadryl) have mild sedative effects that can promote sleep.

The last group are the short-acting hypnotics. These are not recommended for long-term or routine use, as they may cause insomnia; however, for short-term treatment they may be effective. When used, a hypnotic with a short half-life is recommended.

Client Education

Educating the client about sleep-promoting activities is a good investment of the nurse's time. The nurse can use the memory trick "**REST**" to teach the client interventions that promote rest and sleep. By providing clients with ways of promoting good sleep habits, the nurse helps them gain a sense of control over their sleep disturbances and boosts their confidence so that they can successfully meet their sleep and rest needs.

EVALUATION

The plan of care must be updated on a regular basis with additional interventions used as needed.

PROFESSIONALTIP

Variables to Consider in Evaluation

When evaluating the care of the client experiencing a sleep disorder, consider the following questions:

- Were the client's basic needs met?
- Did client education include the family or significant others?
- Was an environment conducive to rest maintained?
- Were therapeutic activities balanced with the client's need for rest and sleep?
- Were the client's bedtime rituals followed as closely as possible?
- Were anxiety-reduction techniques used appropriately?

MEMORYTRICK

REST stands for:

R = Read a relaxing book

E = Enjoy listening to soothing music

S = Sip a warm glass of milk

T = Take a warm bath

SAMPLE NURSING CARE PLAN

The Client with Trouble Sleeping

Six-year-old C.R. is brought to your clinic by his father, who states that C.R. has trouble sleeping at night. In the evenings after a dinner of hotdogs, corn or baked beans, and chocolate milk, C.R. reads some books, then watches his favorite superhero video. Afterward, he runs and plays, mimics the actions he sees in the video, and refuses to take a bath or cooperate when getting ready for bed. After being put to bed at 9:00 P.M., he is up several times for any number of reasons and often is not asleep until midnight. When his father wakes him at 7:00 A.M. for school, C.R. is disagreeable, tired, and difficult to get moving.

NURSING DIAGNOSIS *Disturbed **S**leep Pattern* (less than age-normal total sleep time) related to environmental factors (excessive stimulation) and parental lack of knowledge of sleep-promoting behaviors as evidenced by parental complaint, ineffective bedtime rituals, and insufficient hours of sleep for developmental age

SAMPLE NURSING CARE PLAN (Continued)

Nursing Outcomes Classification (NOC)
Rest
Sleep

Nursing Interventions Classification (NIC)
Sleep Enhancement
Energy Management

PLANNING/OUTCOMES	NURSING INTERVENTIONS	RATIONALE
C.R. and his family will determine those sleeping behaviors they would like to achieve.	Explain that the normal sleep requirement for a child of C.R.'s age is 10 to 12 hours each day.	Helps family understand C.R.'s sleep requirements.
C.R. and his family will develop bedtime rituals to help C.R. wind down from the day.	Teach the family about the effect that certain foods can have on digestion and sleep habits and identify with them those foods that are good choices for dinner.	Informs family about potential adverse effects of certain foods and allows them to plan meals more appropriately.
	Discuss those bedtime activities that can be detrimental to sleep induction.	Assists the family in modifying pre-bedtime behaviors.
	Suggest appropriate bedtime rituals such as taking a bath, brushing the teeth, reading a book, or listening to calming music.	Helps the body and mind prepare for bedtime.
C.R. and his family will identify behaviors that are helpful before bedtime.	Explain that overstimulation close to bedtime, such as watching superhero movies and engaging in rowdy play, prevents the body and mind from slowing down and preparing for sleep.	Helps the family in choosing more appropriate bedtime activities.
	Emphasize the importance of establishing a calming bedtime routine that is followed every night, especially for the school-age child.	Helps C.R. know what is expected of him by practicing appropriate bedtime routines.
	Describe an appropriate sleep environment for C.R., such as a calm room kept at a comfortable temperature and lit only by a night-light.	Such an environment promotes sleep and does not interfere with falling back asleep once awake.

EVALUATION

C.R. and his family have decided they would like C.R. to cooperate in getting ready for bed and to be asleep in 30 minutes. Together they have established a bedtime ritual that begins with playing quietly, followed by taking a warm bath, reading two books, brushing teeth, and then going to bed. The behaviors identified as helpful include no watching of stimulating videos after 7:00 P.M. and engaging in quiet play such as reading, arts and crafts, or writing. Some modification to C.R.'s diet is planned for the next few weeks.

SUMMARY

- Sleep has two phases: non–rapid eye movement (NREM) and rapid eye movement (REM).
- The biological clock controls the daily variations of many physiologic processes.
- Nonpharmacologic interventions should be used in promoting rest and sleep.
- The amount of sleep required differs according to developmental stage.
- Pharmacologic agents can be therapeutic for clients experiencing sleep pattern disturbances. However, the medications should not be the only interventions used.

REVIEW QUESTIONS

1. The nurse is teaching the client interventions to promote sleep. Which of the following interventions are appropriate for the nurse to teach a client? (Select all that apply.)
   1. Drink a warm cup of milk before bed.
   2. Eat a light healthy snack at bedtime.
   3. Exercise within 2 hours of going to bed to relax muscles.
   4. Take a brief nap during the day.
   5. Take a warm bath at bedtime.
   6. Void before going to bed.
2. Which of the following questions is the least appropriate to ask a client when gathering subjective data regarding sleep disturbances?
   1. Why are you having difficulty sleeping?
   2. What are your bedtime rituals?
   3. Can you describe your pain to me?
   4. Do you have frequent dreams or nightmares?
3. What stage of sleep is occurring when a client falls asleep and experiences a decrease in large muscle tone and becomes virtually paralyzed?
   1. REM
   2. NREM stage 2
   3. NREM stage 3
   4. NREM stage 4
4. A client informs the nurse that he is having difficulty falling asleep at night and does not understand why. The nurse asks the client to share which activities he uses to promote relaxation and sleep. Which of the following statements made by the client indicates that he needs further teaching?
   1. "I go for a walk after dinner to relax and unwind from the day."
   2. "I sit on a park bench in the evening and watch the sunset."
   3. "I drink a cup of hot tea and read my favorite relaxing book."
   4. "I always try to go to bed at the same time every night."
5. A client's wife informs the nurse that her husband will sometimes stop breathing for up to 30 seconds in his sleep and then begins snoring so loudly that she cannot sleep. This is an example of:
   1. hypersomnia.
   2. bruxism.
   3. cataplexy.
   4. apnea.
6. A client informs the nurse that she has not been able to sleep for 3 days. Which of the following objective assessment findings supports the client's statement?
   1. The client states that she needs a prescription for sleeping medication.
   2. The client informs the nurse that she is exhausted.
   3. The client yawns frequently and has red puffy eyes.
   4. The client appears calm and coordinated with clear speech.
7. To facilitate rest and sleep, the client should be encouraged to:
   1. practice relaxation techniques.
   2. watch television while lying in bed.
   3. eat a big meal to prevent hunger in the night.
   4. perform a daily exercise workout.
8. Which of the following factors affect the quality and quantity of rest and sleep? (Select all that apply.)
   1. Work schedule.
   2. Age.
   3. Room ventilation.
   4. Nicotine.
   5. Muscle tension.
   6. Hormonal changes.
9. Individuals have several rhythms controlled by their biological clocks. The circadian rhythm cycle occurs:
   1. daily.
   2. every year.
   3. every month or so.
   4. several times a day.
10. A new sleep cycle for a client who is awakened during stage 4 NREM sleep will begin in:
    1. REM sleep.
    2. stage 1 sleep.
    3. stage 2 sleep.
    4. stage 3 sleep.

REFERENCES/SUGGESTED READINGS

American Academy of Sleep Medicine. (2005). *Sleep as we grow older* [Brochure]. Westchester, IL: Author.

American Academy of Sleep Medicine. (2008). Insomnia. Available: http://www.aasmnet.org

American Sleep Apnea Association. (2008). Information about sleep apnea. Available: http://www. sleepapnea.org/geninfo.html

Bulechek, G., Butcher, H., McCloskey, J., & Dochterman, J., eds. (2008). *Nursing Interventions Classification (NIC)* (5th ed.). St. Louis, MO: Mosby/Elsevier.

Coleman, R. (1986). *Wide awake at 3:00 a.m.: By choice or by chance?* New York: Freeman.

Coren, S. (1997). *Sleep thieves: An eye-opening exploration into the science and mysteries of sleep*. New York: Free Press.

Harvard Women's Health Watch (2007). Repaying your sleep debt. Harvard Medical School, *14*(11).

Hogstel, M. (2001). *Gerontology: Nursing care of the older adult* (4th ed.). Clifton Park, NY: Delmar Cengage Learning.

McCaffery, M., & Pasero, C. (1999). *Pain: Clinical manual* (2nd ed.). St. Louis, MO: Mosby.

Merritt, S. (2000). Putting sleep disorders to rest. *RN, 63*(7), 26–30.

Montgomery, L., Haynes, L., & Garner, L. (2002). An unusual sleep disorder. *RN, 65*(4), 41–43.

Moorhead, S., Johnson, M., Maas, M., & Swanson, E. (2007). *Nursing Outcomes Classification (NOC)* (4rd ed.). St. Louis, MO: Mosby.

National Institute on Aging. (2007). Sleep and aging. Retrieved August 23, 2008, from http://www.nia.nih.gov/HealthInformation/Publications/sleep.htm

National Institute of Neurological Disorders and Stroke. (2008). Narcolepsy fact sheet. Retrieved August 23, 2008, from http://www.ninds.nih.gov/disorders/narcolepsy/detail_narcolepsy.htm

National Sleep Foundation. (2001). Sleep facts and stats. Retrieved August 23, 2008, from http://www.sleepfoundation.org/site/c.huIXKjM0IxF/b.2419253/k.7989/Sleep_Facts_and_Stats.htm

National Sleep Foundation. (2002). Sleep apnea—An unknown epidemic? Retrieved August 23, 2008, from http://www.sleepfoundation.org/site/apps/nlnet/content3.aspx?c=huIXKjM0IxF&b=2464479&content_id=%7BA9D2F632-83A5-405D-98E2-63F389C095BF%7D¬oc=1

National Sleep Foundation. (2003). Health and aging: The experts speak. Retrieved August 23, 2008, from http://www.sleepfoundation.org/site/c.huIXKjM0IxF/b.2419293/k.23CA/Health_and_Aging_The_Experts_Speak.htm

National Sleep Foundation. (2005). Sleep apnea basics. Retrieved August 23, 2008, from http://www.sleepfoundation.org/site/c.huIXKjM0IxF/b.2464479/apps/nl/content3.asp?content_id=%7B3E9E479E-4C8E-4C35-9564-363A6918C391%7D¬oc=1

National Sleep Foundation. (2008a). Facts about PLMS. Retrieved August 23, 2008, from http://www.sleepfoundation.org/site/apps/nlnet/content3.aspx?c=huIXKjM0IxF&b=2464461&content_id=%7BB0211B38-4864-49EA-A322-E511477EFE71%7D¬oc=1

National Sleep Foundation. (2008b). Sleeping smart. Retrieved August 23, 2008, from http://www.sleepfoundation.org/site/c.huIXKjM0IxF/b.4389513/k.9A3E/Sleeping_Smart.htm

National Sleep Foundation. (2008c). Strategies for shift workers. Retrieved August 17, 2008, from http://www.sleepfoundation.org/site/c.huIXKjM0IxF/b.2421189/k.DF93/Strategies_for_Shift_Workers.htm

North American Nursing Diagnosis Association International. (2010). *NANDA-I nursing diagnoses: Definitions and classification 2009-2011.* Ames, IA: Wiley-Blackwell.

Penland, K. (2009). Caring for clients with sleep disorders. Manuscript submitted for publication.

Smyth, C. (2008). Evaluating sleep quality in older adults. *American Journal of Nursing, 108*(5), 42–45.

Sorrell, J. (1999). Taking steps to calm restless legs syndrome. *Nursing99, 29*(9), 60–61.

Stansberry, T. (2001). Narcolepsy: Unveiling a mystery. *American Journal of Nursing, 101*(8), 50–53.

Tate, J., & Tasota, F. (2002). More than a snore: Recognizing the danger of sleep apnea. *Nursing2002, 32*(8), 46–49.

White, L., & Duncan, G. (2002). *Medical-surgical nursing: An integrated approach* (2nd ed.). Clifton Park, NY: Delmar Cengage Learning.

RESOURCES

American Sleep Apnea Association, http://www.sleepapnea.org

American Academy of Sleep Medicine, http://www.aasmnet.org

Narcolepsy Network, http://www.narcolepsynetwork.org

National Sleep Foundation, http://www.sleepfoundation.org

Restless Legs Syndrome Foundation, Inc., http://www.rls.org

CHAPTER 20
Safety/Hygiene

MAKING THE CONNECTION

Refer to the following chapters to increase your understanding of safety/hygiene:

Basic Nursing

- ***Holistic Care***
- ***Legal and Ethical Responsibilities***
- ***Communication***
- ***Nursing Process/Documentation/Informatics***
- ***Cultural Considerations***
- ***Stress, Adaptation, and Anxiety***
- ***Wellness Concepts***
- ***Self-Concept***
- ***Complementary/Alternative Therapies***
- ***Infection Control/Asepsis***
- ***Standard Precautions and Isolation***
- ***Assessment***
- ***Diagnostic Tests***

Adult Health Nursing

- ***The Older Adult***

Basic Procedures

- ***Hand Hygiene***
- ***Assisting with Crutches, Cane, or Walker***
- ***Bed Making: Unoccupied Bed***
- ***Bed Making: Occupied Bed***
- ***Bathing a Client in Bed***
- ***Perineal Care***
- ***Oral Care***
- ***Eye Care***
- ***Giving a Back Rub***
- ***Shaving a Client***
- ***Application of Restraints***

LEARNING OBJECTIVES

Upon completion of this chapter, you should be able to:

- Define key terms.
- Describe the kinds of accidents that can occur in health care settings.
- Describe the importance of and procedure for correctly identifying clients.
- Identify safety factors to be considered before using equipment.
- Recount safety measures related to the use of protective restraints.
- Detail safety measures related to preventing fire when oxygen is in use.
- Discuss the factors influencing a client's personal hygiene practices.
- Explain how assessment maintains a safe environment.
- Describe the modifications that can be used to resolve environmental hazards in institutional and home settings.

KEY TERMS

body image
chemical restraints
dental caries
gingivitis
halitosis
hygiene
perineal care
physical restraints
poison
pyorrhea
restraints
self-care deficit
sensory overload
stomatitis

INTRODUCTION

Safety is basic to the care of all clients. Nurses are responsible for providing professional, quality nursing care to the client in a safe environment. This involves both safety precautions and hygiene assistance. The nurse's role in these areas is described in this chapter.

SAFETY

Safety is the number-one priority when providing client care. The first step is to raise nurses' awareness regarding risk factors because prevention is the key to safety. Nurses must be aware of those factors that have the potential to endanger a client's safety. Constant attention to these factors enables the nurse to maintain a safe environment for the client.

A safety committee is required in all health care facilities, with the purpose of maintaining an overall safe facility for clients, employees, and visitors. The committee is composed of representatives from all departments of the facility. Responsibilities range from analyzing environmental safety in the facility to researching illness rates.

Safety is associated with health promotion and illness prevention. A safe environment reduces the risk of accidents and subsequent alterations in health and lifestyle; it also helps contain the cost of health care services (Figure 20-1). Many factors in the environment can threaten safety.

FACTORS AFFECTING SAFETY

Client safety and health are influenced by several factors, including age, lifestyle/occupation, mobility, sensory and perceptual alterations, and emotional state.

Age

Injury risk varies with chronological age and developmental stage. Education about preventive measures can prevent injury among clients of various ages.

The potential for injury increases as infants mature. Most accidents occur as infants, toddlers, and preschoolers explore the environment. These can be prevented with careful adult supervision.

The risk for injury increases when school-age children explore the environment outside the home. During this stage, preventive measures should focus on stranger awareness; traffic safety rules; bicycle, skating, and swimming safety; protective equipment; and avoidance of substance abuse.

While good physical health is usually enjoyed by adolescents and young adults, their lifestyle may put them at risk for injury. Because this age-group spends much time away from home, educational efforts of parents, schools, and community health care providers must focus on environmental safety. High-risk factors for injury and death are automobile accidents, substance abuse, violence, unwanted pregnancies, and sexually transmitted diseases.

The injury risk for adults is usually related to lifestyle, behaviors, and work practices. Preventive measures for adults emphasize exercise, nutrition, and occupational safety. High-risk factors for this age-group include anxiety, fatigue, caregiver role strain, sleep pattern disturbances, and altered health maintenance.

The older adult is prone to falls, especially in the bathroom, bedroom, and kitchen because of poor vision and mobility; loss of muscle strength and flexibility; changes in the inner ear that upset the sense of balance; effects of medications; and chronic diseases such as osteoarthritis, Parkinson's disease, and Alzheimer's disease. Preventive measures for older adults include good lighting, using hand rails, changing

> **PROFESSIONALTIP**
>
> **Workplace Safety**
>
> **EMPLOYEE RIGHT-TO-KNOW LAWS**
>
> Under the authority of the Occupational Safety and Health Administration (OSHA) of the Department of Labor and Industry, several states have passed employee right-to-know laws, which state that employees are legally entitled to information regarding hazardous substances or harmful agents in the workplace. Such substances include skin and eye irritants, flammables, poisons, carcinogens, pathogens, and harmful rays (radiation).
>
> **REGULATIONS RELATING TO HAZARDOUS MATERIALS**
>
> OSHA also outlines and enforces regulations that all health care facilities must follow with regard to employees' exposure to and handling of potentially infectious materials.
>
> **MATERIAL SAFETY DATA SHEET**
>
> As part of conforming to OSHA regulations, all facilities must have a material safety data sheet (MSDS) for each hazardous substance. The MSDS describes the substance in question, including the associated dangers. Protective equipment, safe handling techniques, and first-aid information are also given. The MSDSs for toxic materials must be kept on site for no fewer than 30 years. All employees must know how to use the MSDS.

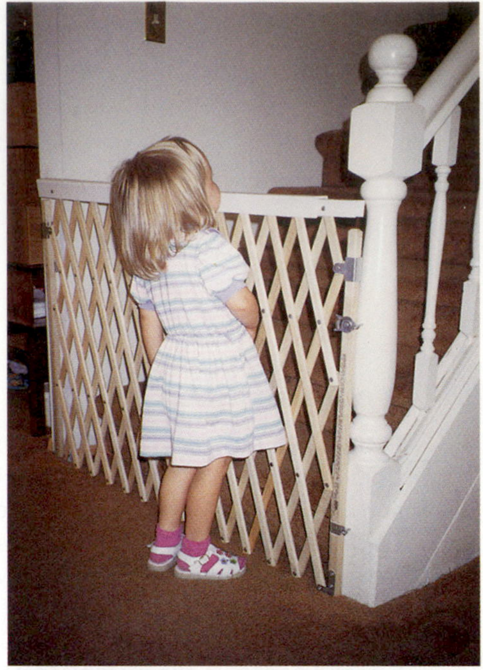

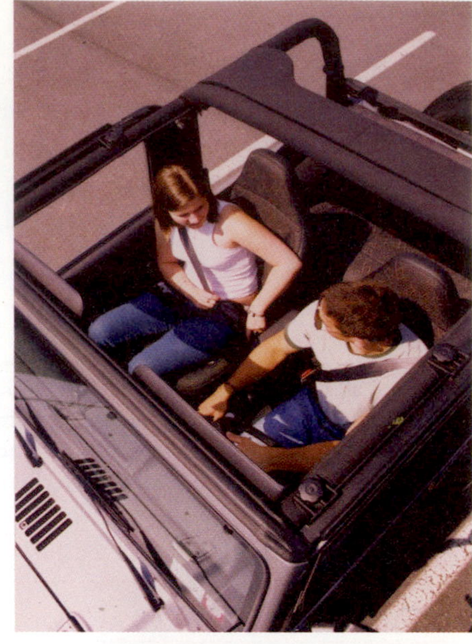

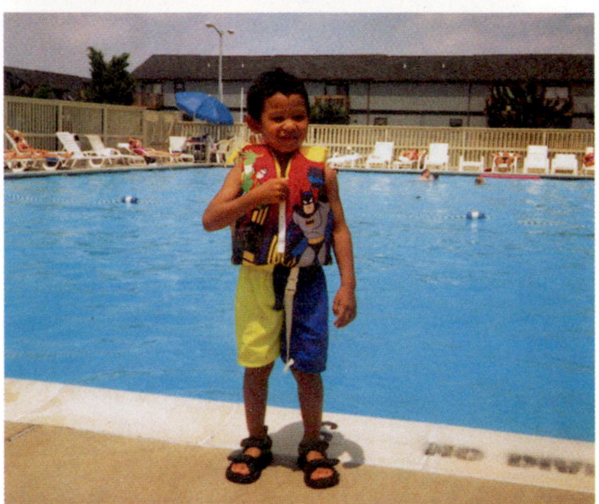

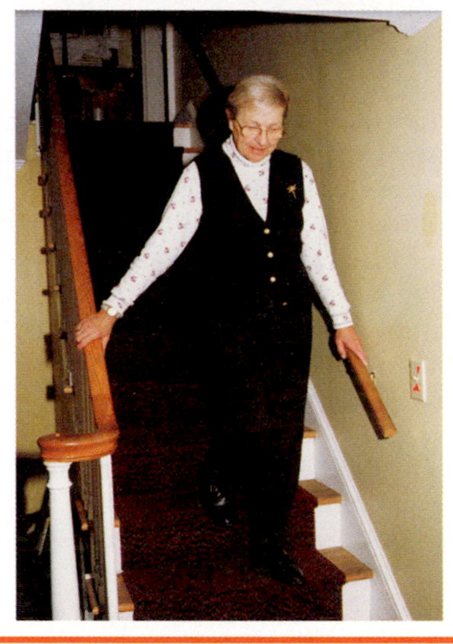

PHOTOS COURTESY OF DELMAR CENGAGE LEARNING

FIGURE 20-1 Use of stair gates, life vests, seat belts, and hand rails minimizes safety risks.

position slowly, skidproof mats in bathtub or shower, and removing throw rugs and loose carpets.

According to the Centers for Disease Control and Prevention (CDC, 2002a), one in three adults older than age 65 falls each year. The CDC (2008) states that in 2005, 15,800 people 65 and older died from injuries related to unintentional falls, and about 1.8 million people 65 and older were treated in emergency departments for nonfatal injuries from falls. More than 433,000 of these patients were hospitalized.

Lifestyle/Occupation

Lifestyle practices, reflecting an individual's personal choices about activities or habits to pursue, can increase a person's risk for injury and potential for disease. For instance, individuals who operate machinery; experience excessive stress, anxiety, and fatigue; use alcohol and drugs (prescription and non-prescription); and live in high-crime neighborhoods are at increased risk for injury and alterations to health. Risk-taking behaviors, such as participating in daredevil activities, driving vehicles at high speeds, and not wearing seat belts, are factors that pose a threat to an individual's safety and well-being. Unlike other factors such as age, however, lifestyle/occupation practices are modifiable.

The National Institute for Occupational Safety and Health (2002) reports that an average of 9,000 U.S. workers sustain disabling injuries each day, costing $145 billion each year. Compare this cost to $33 billion for AIDS and $170.7 billion for cancer.

Sensory/Perceptual Changes

Sensory functions are essential for environmental safety. Clients having visual, hearing, smell, taste, communication, or touch impairments have an increased risk for injury because they may not be able to perceive a potential danger.

Mobility

A client with impaired mobility has an increased risk for injury, especially from falls. Impaired mobility may result from poor balance or coordination, muscle weakness, or paralysis. Immobility may lead to physiologic and emotional complications such as pressure ulcers and depression.

PROFESSIONALTIP

Accidents in the Health Care Setting

In the health care setting, accidents are categorized by their causative agent: client behaviors, therapeutic procedures, or equipment:

- **Client behavior accidents** result from the client's behavior or actions. Examples include poisonings, burns, and self-inflicted cuts and bruises.
- **Therapeutic procedure accidents** result from the delivery of medical or nursing interventions. Examples include medication errors, client falls during transfers, contamination of sterile instruments or wounds, and improper performance of nursing activities.
- **Equipment accidents** result from the malfunction or improper use of medical equipment such as electrocution and fire. National and institutional policies establish safety standards with regard to equipment. For example, a facility may attempt to minimize the risk of equipment accidents by requiring the biomedical engineering department to check equipment before use.

All accidents and incident reports must be fully documented according to institutional protocol.

Emotional State

Emotional states such as depression and anger affect the perception of environmental hazards and the degree of risk associated with certain behaviors. These emotional states alter a person's thinking patterns and reaction time. During periods of emotional stress, usual safety precautions may be forgotten.

HYGIENE

Hygiene is the study of health and ways of preserving health. Hygiene provides comfort and relaxation, improves self-image, and promotes cleanliness and healthy skin. Client hygiene is part of client safety in that proper hygiene protects the client against disease. The body's first line of defense, the skin and mucous membranes, is kept healthy by proper hygiene. Nurses are responsible for ensuring that client hygiene needs are met. The care provided depends on the client's needs, ability, and practices.

Factors Influencing Hygiene Practices

Hygiene practices are unique to each client. Nurses provide individualized care based on needs and these practices. Hygiene practices are influenced by body image, personal preferences, social and cultural practices, knowledge, and socioeconomic status.

CULTURAL CONSIDERATIONS

Hygiene

- Some cultures do not permit women to submerge their bodies in water during menstruation because of a fear that the woman may drown.
- In North America, people typically bathe daily and use deodorant products.
- In Europe, many people do not bathe daily, nor do they use deodorant products. They do not consider the smell of human perspiration offensive.

Body Image

Body image is the individual's perception of physical self, including appearance, function, and ability. Body image is linked to the person's attitude, mood, emotions, and values. Body image directly affects the practice of personal hygiene, which may change if the client's body image is altered because of surgical procedures or illness. At these times, the nurse should assist the client to maintain the client's preillness level of hygiene and personal preferences.

Personal Preferences

Personal preferences include the timing of bathing, products used for bathing, and how bathing is performed. For example, some men shave before bathing, whereas others shave after bathing; some people bathe in the morning, whereas others bathe at bedtime to encourage relaxation and sleep. The client should be permitted to practice usual routines and to use preferred hygiene products unless the client's health is adversely affected. Individualized nursing care incorporates the client's personal hygiene preferences.

Social and Cultural Practices

Social and cultural practices and beliefs come from family, religious, and personal values developed during maturation. Clients learn hygiene practices in early childhood. Later, hygiene practices are influenced by socialization outside the family. For example, teenagers often follow the trends in personal hygiene accepted by their peers.

Clients from various cultural backgrounds have differing hygiene practices. A nonjudgmental attitude must be maintained when assessing or providing hygiene care to clients from different social or cultural backgrounds.

Knowledge

The client's understanding of the hygiene and health relationship is influenced by knowledge. For clients to practice basic hygiene, however, they must have more than knowledge; they must be motivated and believe that they are capable of self-care.

An illness or surgical procedure frequently results in a knowledge deficit about the correct hygiene procedure or type of hygiene that can be used. Providing the necessary education about hygiene during an illness is the nurse's responsibility. The nurse may have to perform all hygiene care for a client during an illness until the client is able to do so again.

Socioeconomic Status

A client's hygiene practices may also be influenced by socioeconomic status. Limited economic resources may affect the frequency, extent, and type of hygiene practiced. Some clients may not be able to afford soap, shampoo, toothpaste, and deodorants. The nurse can advocate for the client by contacting social services for referrals to community agencies providing assistance to needy persons.

NURSING PROCESS

The nursing process facilitates providing nursing care to clients at risk for injury or a self-care deficit.

Assessment

Assessment data are the basis for prioritizing the client's problems and the nursing diagnoses. Clients at risk for injury require frequent reassessment, so appropriate changes can be made in the plan of care and expected outcomes.

The health history and physical examination data correlated with laboratory data identify those clients at risk for problems relating to safety or hygiene. Appropriate risk appraisals may be incorporated into the nursing health history interview.

Subjective Data

The nursing health history interview provides the client's subjective account of specific health data. It is important for the nurse to gather complete, pertinent, and relevant information at this point.

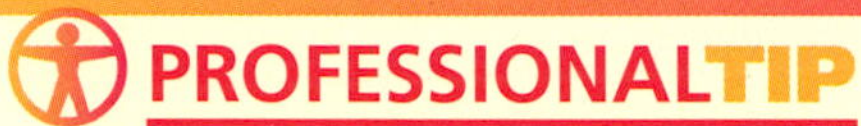

Key Interview Questions about Safety and Hygiene

- What do you do to stay healthy?
- How do you usually spend the day (e.g., home or work)?
- What health care concerns do you have?
- Do you need assistance with bathing and dressing?
- How often do you visit the dentist and eye doctor?
- How often do you use dental floss?
- Do you wash your hands before preparing food?
- Do you keep meats and dairy products refrigerated until ready to use?
- Is there a smoke detector and fire extinguisher in your home?
- Are emergency phone numbers readily available?

Health History Key elements of relevant data regarding the client at risk for injury and infection are obtained in the health history. A health history questionnaire may be used, but depending on the client's status, the nurse may have to perform an interview to obtain these data. When the client cannot provide the subjective data, the nurse must specify, either on the questionnaire or in the nursing progress notes, who provided the information.

During the nursing health history interview, the client's general health perception and management status should be assessed to ascertain how the client manages self-care. This information will provide data regarding the client's routine self-care and health-promotion needs.

Objective Data

Objective data are gathered through the physical examination and the diagnostic and laboratory findings.

Physical Examination When assessing the client specifically for the level of risk for injury and hygiene deficits, the nurse should focus on the following areas and signs:

- Level of consciousness: The Glasgow Coma Scale (GCS) is an objective measurement tool (Neurological System chapter).
- Range of motion: Immobilization of an extremity and/or limited mobility are risk factors for developing skin breakdown, joint contractures, and muscle atrophy.
- Secretions or exudate of the skin or mucous membranes.
- Condition of the skin: Skin condition provides data about a client's nutritional and hydration status, skin integrity, hygiene practices, and overall physical abilities.

Risk Appraisals Specifically developed risk assessment tools appraise the client for potential risks. The client's self-care abilities are appraised during the health history. An analysis of relevant risk factors identifies actual or possible risks. For instance, the risk of impaired skin integrity increases when a person is placed on bed rest. A skin integrity risk appraisal (Table 20-1) should be completed to assist with planning care.

Client in an Inpatient Setting Inpatient clients should be assessed for skin and fall risk factors. The client's risk of falling is identified after gathering specific assessment data, as shown in Table 20-2. Each of these indicators carries a specific weight to determine the client's risk. Special safety measures are implemented as required.

The client should be assessed for safety risks every shift or according to institutional policy. Nurses ensure a safe environment by leaving the bed in low position, side rails up, nurse call light and personal belongings within easy reach, and assistive devices (e.g., a walker) nearby, as shown in Figure 20-2.

Client in the Home Injuries in the home result primarily from falls, poisonings, fires, suffocation, and malfunctioning household equipment (Stanhope & Knollmueller, 2000). Home health nurses may use a safety risk appraisal to determine the client's level of safety knowledge.

The safety risk data assessed in the home direct the nurse's planning for the client's and caregiver's education. Assessment, teaching, and outcome evaluation of the safety hazards can take several home visits.

Diagnostic and Laboratory Data Appraising the client's risk for injury also involves evaluating laboratory findings related to an abnormal blood profile (e.g., anemia, infection). Malnourished clients are at risk for injury.

TABLE 20-1 Skin Breakdown Potential Checklist

	Score	Description
_____	(1)	Fair: Major underlying disease, controlled
_____	(2)	Poor: Uncontrolled underlying disease
Mental Status		
_____	(1)	Lethargic: Listless
_____	(2)	Confused: Inappropriate communication
_____	(4)	Comatose: Unresponsive
Mobility/Activity		
_____	(2)	Minor Deficit: Some limitation in movement Needs assistance with ADLs
_____	(4)	Major Deficit: Movement requires assistance
_____	(6)	Immobile: No voluntary movement
Incontinence		
_____	(1)	Mild: Stress incontinence, 1 BM per day
_____	(4)	Frequent: No bladder control, BMs >2–4 per day
_____	(6)	Total: No bladder control, frequent/continuous BM
Nutrition		
_____	(2)	Fair: Intake < body requirements, eats 75% or less
_____	(3)	Poor: Eats 50% or less, started on TPN or tube feeding
_____	(4)	Compromised: No intake, dehydrated
Skin Integrity		
_____	(2)	Fair: Single stage I or II
_____	(4)	Poor: More than one break in skin integrity
_____		TOTAL SCORE OF 8 OR ABOVE, ENTER SKIN INTEGRITY POTENTIAL ON PCP PROBLEM LIST, INITIATE PREVENTATIVE ADLs

Excerpt from Patient Admission Data Base, *Courtesy of CHRISTUS Spohn Health System, Corpus Christi, TX.*

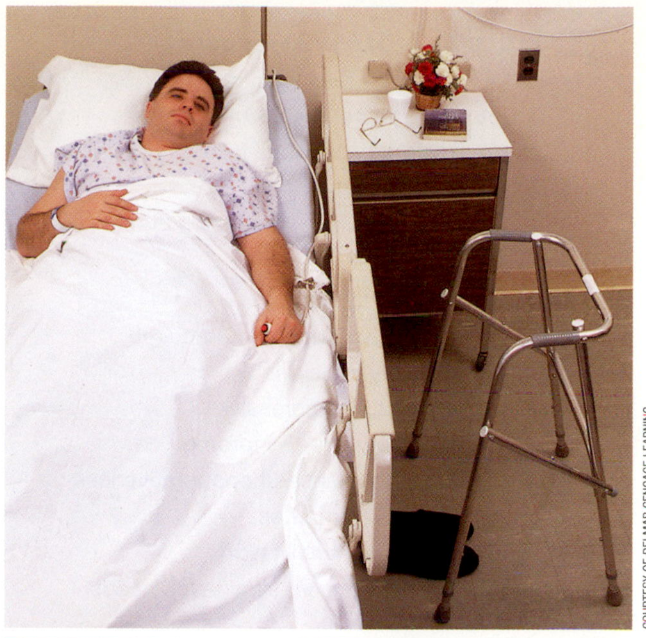

COURTESY OF DELMAR CENGAGE LEARNING

FIGURE 20-2 This client's safety risk has been assessed and responded to through the measures shown here.

NURSING DIAGNOSIS

Following data collection and analysis, the nurse formulates a nursing diagnosis. The main nursing diagnoses that relate to safety and hygiene deficits are *Risk for **I**njury* and the ***S**elf-Care Deficit* diagnoses.

Risk for Injury

The primary nursing diagnosis *Risk for **I**njury* exists when the client is "at risk of injury as a result of environmental conditions interacting with the individual's adaptive and defensive resources" (North American Nursing Diagnosis Association International [NANDA-I], 2010). Although this diagnostic label has no defining characteristics set forth by NANDA, it is categorized as having either internal or external risk factors. An internal biochemical risk factor for a client with impaired vision would be stated as *Risk for **I**njury* related to the risk factor of sensory dysfunction (visual). In contrast, medications on a nightstand in a home with a toddler present should be identified by a home health nurse as creating an external chemical risk factor for the toddler; the nursing diagnosis would be stated as *Risk for **I**njury* related to the risk factor of medications in the environment.

Examples of the other risk nursing diagnoses that may be a risk factor for *Risk for **I**njury* are:

*Risk for **A**spiration:* **risk for entry of gastrointestinal secretions, oropharyngeal secretions, or solids or fluids into the tracheobronchial passages**

*Risk for **D**isuse Syndrome:* **at risk for deterioration of body systems as the result of prescribed or unavoidable musculoskeletal inactivity**

*Risk for **F**alls:* **increased susceptibility to falling that may cause physical harm**

*Risk for Latex **A**llergy Response:* **at risk for allergic response to natural latex rubber products**

*Risk for **P**oisoning:* **at accentuated risk of accidental exposure to, or ingestion of, drugs or dangerous products in doses sufficient to cause poisoning**

*Risk for **S**uffocation:* **accentuated risk of accidental suffocation (inadequate air available for inhalation)**

*Risk for **S**uicide:* **at risk for self-inflicted, life threatening injury**

*Risk for **T**rauma:* **accentuated risk of accidental tissue injury (e.g., wound, burn, fracture)**

These eight nursing diagnoses allow specific nursing interventions to be related to the diagnosed problem. For example, the specific nursing diagnosis for the toddler encountering medications on a nightstand in the home would be *Risk for **P**oisoning*, related to the risk factor of medications accessible to children. The level of risk would be higher if the medications were in open containers or if the closed containers did not have childproof caps. This diagnosis points to specific nursing interventions directed toward the need for client teaching.

TABLE 21-2 Safety Assessment

- ❑ (5) Age greater than 60
- ❑ (5) History of previous falls
- ❑ (3) From nursing home
- ❑ (3) Has had sitter/companion at home

Status: Mental/Physical

- ❑ (5) Confused/judgement Impaired
- ❑ (5) Sensory impairment
- ❑ (5) Combative/aggressive
- ❑ (5) "Sundowners" Syndrome
- ❑ (5) Noncompliance/uncooperativeness
- ❑ (5) Paralysis/amputee
- ❑ (5) Weakness/debilitation
- ❑ (5) Urgent/frequent elimination needs

Medications

- ❑ (5) Diuretics
- ❑ (5) Laxatives/G.I. preps
- ❑ (3) Antihypertensives
- ❑ (3) Antiseizures
- ❑ (5) Sedative/hypnotics
- ❑ (3) Analgesics
- ❑ (3) Antipsychotics/antidepressants

- ❑ LEVEL 1 (0–17)
- ❑ LEVEL 2 (18–24)
- ❑ LEVEL 3 (25 or greater)

____ TOTAL

- ❑ Safety precautions implemented
- ❑ Restraints per protocol
- ❑ Patient/family instructed
- ❑ Color coded band on

Excerpt from Patient Admission Data Base (*Courtesy of CHRISTUS Spohn Health System, Corpus Christi, TX.*)

Self-Care Deficits

A **self-care deficit** exists when an individual is not able to perform one or more activities of daily living (ADLs). Three self-care deficits related to hygiene practices are identified by NANDA-I (2010). These nursing diagnoses, definitions, defining characteristics, and related factors are presented in Table 20-3.

Other Nursing Diagnoses

The client at risk for injury or having a self-care deficit may have other associated physiologic or psychological problems. The following nursing diagnoses may also be appropriate:

*Imbalanced **Nutrition**:* less than body requirements
*Imbalanced **Nutrition**:* more than body requirements
*Ineffective **Protection***
*Impaired **Tissue** Integrity*
*Impaired **Skin** Integrity*
***Social** Isolation*
*Risk for **Loneliness***
*Ineffective **Coping***
*Impaired Bed **Mobility***
*Impaired Physical **Mobility***
*Impaired Wheelchair **Mobility***
Hopelessness
Powerlessness
*Deficient **Knowledge** (specify)*
*Acute **Pain***
Anxiety
Fear

PLANNING/OUTCOME IDENTIFICATION

The primary nursing goal is to provide safe care by identifying actual or potential risks and implementating safety measures. The nurse reviews assessment data with the client and records what the client indicates are needs for change and health teaching. These findings, when incorporated into the plan of care, reflect the individualized needs of each client. Identified outcomes provide direction for nursing care implemented to reduce the risk of injury.

Another important part of the care plan is client/caregiver education related to identifying potential risks and health-promotion practices. The nursing care plan should include educating the client about preventive actions and changes for an unsafe environment.

IMPLEMENTATION

Implementation involves continual assessment of client health risks and prioritization of nursing interventions aimed at risk reduction, such as:

- Promoting adequate rest and exercise
- Teaching client about health risks
- Administering prescribed medications
- Providing balanced nutritional intake

Implementation of safety measures may require an alteration in the physical environment, as identified by agency fall prevention protocol.

Identify Client

In order to provide safe care, it is essential that nurses correctly match clients with the activity, medication, diet, or treatment

TABLE 20-3 Self-Care Deficits Related to Hygiene Practices

NURSING DIAGNOSIS AND DEFINITION	DEFINING CHARACTERISTICS	RELATED FACTORS
*Bathing/Hygiene **S**elf-Care Deficit:* Impaired ability to perform or complete bathing/hygiene activities for oneself	Inability to get bath supplies, wash body or body parts, obtain or get to water source, regulate the temperature or flow of bath water, get in and out of bathroom, dry body	Decreased or lack of motivation; weakness and tiredness; severe anxiety; inability to perceive body part or spatial relationship; perceptual or cognitive impairment; pain; neuromuscular impairment; musculoskeletal impairment; environmental barriers
*Dressing/Grooming **S**elf-Care Deficit:* Impaired ability to perform or complete dressing and grooming activities for oneself	Inability to choose clothing, use assistive devices, use zippers, remove clothes, put on socks, put clothing on upper body, maintain appearance at a satisfactory level, put clothing on lower body, pick up clothing; put on shoes, impaired ability to put on or take off necessary items of clothing, obtain or replace articles of clothing, fasten clothing	Decreased or lack of motivation; pain; severe anxiety; perceptual or cognitive impairment; neuromuscular impairment; musculoskeletal impairment; discomfort; environmental barriers; weakness or tiredness
*Toileting **S**elf-Care Deficit:* Impaired ability to perform or complete own toileting activities	Inability to manipulate clothing, carry out proper toilet hygiene, sit on or rise from toilet or commode, get to toilet or commode, flush toilet or commode	Environmental barriers; weakness or tiredness; decreased or lack of motivation; severe anxiety; impaired mobility status; impaired transfer ability; musculoskeletal impairment; neuromuscular impairment; pain; perceptual or cognitive impairment

From *Nursing Diagnoses: Definitions and Classification 2009–2011*, by North American Nursing Diagnosis Association, 2009, Indianapolis, IN: Wiley-Blackwell.

ordered for them. The client's well-being is placed in jeopardy by administering unordered care.

The identification (ID) band or bracelet is the primary means of correctly identifying a client. It lists the client's name, room number, bed number, hospital number, and doctor and may include other information such as age, sex, and religion.

This band is placed on the client's wrist on admission to the hospital. Each time care is given, the band must be checked against the assignment sheet, order sheet, diet card, and medication and treatment sheet or card (Figure 20-3). The client's identity should always be further verified by one other method, such as stating the client's name, asking the client to state his name, or obtaining a positive identification from another person. None of these methods is safe when used alone but, when used with the ID band, can help the nurse verify identity.

If a client is discovered without an ID band, care should be withheld until positive identification is made. A new ID band should be placed on the client's wrist as soon as identity is verified.

Most nursing home residents also wear ID bands. Some, however, do not, and other methods of identification, such as photographs, are used. Nurses working in such long-term care facilities must learn to safely use the identification system. Whatever the system, client identification is essential before rendering any care.

Increase Safety Awareness

In all settings, nurses must show an awareness of safety hazards and teach clients accordingly. Clients must be made aware of safety precautions such as specific information about the use of heating devices, oxygen, intravenous equipment, and automatic bed controls.

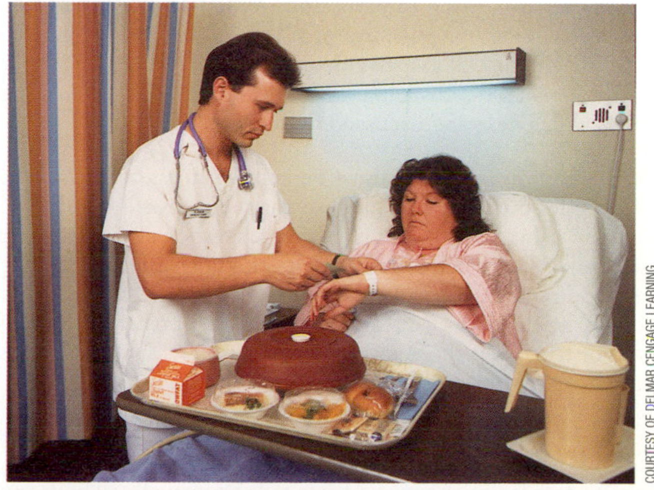

COURTESY OF DELMAR CENGAGE LEARNING

FIGURE 20-3 Checking the client's ID band ensures that the correct person receives care.

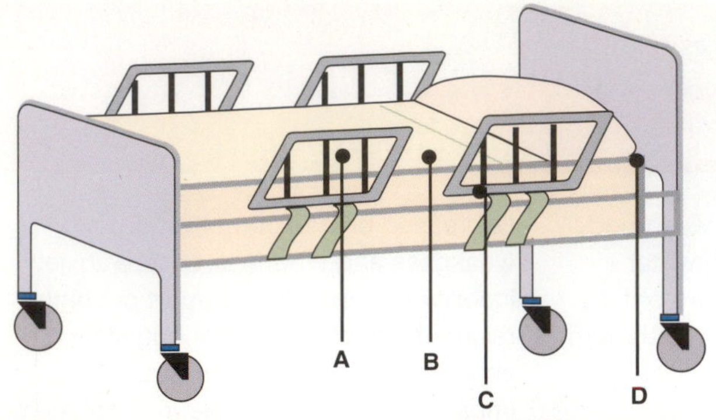

FIGURE 20-4 Entrapment Hazards Associated with Hospital Bed Side Rails; *A,* Between the Bars of the Side Rail; *B,* Between two Side Rails; *C,* Between the Side Rail and Mattress; *D,* Between the Headboard or Footboard, Side Rail, and Mattress (*Source: Food and Drug Administration, Safety Alert, August 1996.*)

A 2008 Food and Drug Administration (FDA) safety alert discussed entrapment hazards related to side rails on hospital beds. The FDA received 772 reports of head and body entrapment incidents resulting in 460 deaths, 136 injuries, and 176 entrapments without injury (FDA, 2008). These incidents occurred in private homes, hospitals, and long-term care facilities. Entrapment hazards associated with hospital bed side rails are illustrated in Figure 20-4.

Prevent Falls

Most falls occur when clients are weak, uncoordinated, fatigued, confused, paralyzed, or disoriented. The data obtained from the safety risk appraisal identifies those clients requiring special measures to prevent falls. The risk for falls can be reduced by:

- Properly supervising clients
- Orienting clients to the environment and the call system
- Providing ambulatory aids (e.g., a wheelchair or walker)
- Keeping personal items and call light in easy reach
- Keeping beds in lowest position and side rails up
- Using rubber mats in shower and tub
- Having adequate lighting

Specific nursing interventions aimed at preventing falls include wiping up spills, use of side rails, applying restraints, encouraging use of assistive devices for walking, using proper body mechanics, ensuring adequate lighting, and removing obstacles. These are discussed following.

Wipe Up Spills Floors must be kept clean and free of spills. Although the housekeeping department usually does the actual washing of floors, it is the nurse's responsibility to either wipe up a spill when it occurs or mark the area as a safety hazard and notify the appropriate person for immediate cleanup. Wet or sticky floors can easily cause a weak, unsteady client to slip or trip. Even those unimpaired by illness, such as visitors and hospital personnel, are at risk.

Use Side Rails Side rails have been used to prevent falls from hospital beds for more than 50 years. Since the 1970s, health care facilities have had side rails on virtually all beds and written policies for the routine use of side rails with all clients. Side rails may be full length, half length, or one-third length.

Clients use side rails to help turn from side to side in bed or to sit up on the edge of the bed and as a support when standing (Figure 20-5). Some clients feel more secure in a strange bed and environment with the side rails up.

Injuries and deaths have occurred with side rail use when clients try to get out of bed by climbing over the rails or when the client becomes entrapped in the rail or between the rail, mattress, and bed frame (Figure 20-4). Many cognitively impaired or older clients feel that they are "in jail" or being "treated like a child" and resist the use of side rails.

The Centers for Medicare and Medicaid Services (CMS) have identified that if the client cannot easily remove or release a side rail, it is considered a restraint and must meet the requirements for restraints (discussed in the next section) (CMS, 2008).

Talerico and Capezuti (2001) suggest safe alternatives to side rail use, including low-height beds, motion sensors, hip pads, floor mats alongside the bed, full-length body pillows, adequate nighttime pain control, individualized nighttime toileting rounds, bed alarms, treating depression and sleep disorders, and individualized sleep regimens. Choosing the appropriate alternative to restrictive side rails (restraint) requires a thorough client assessment. *Clients at risk for falls must always be closely monitored.*

Use Restraints **Restraints** are devices used to limit the physical activity of a client or to immobilize a client or extremity. Restraints are used to protect the client from falls, protect a body part, keep the client from interfering with therapies (e.g., pulling out tubes, disconnecting intravenous setups, or removing wound coverings), and reduce the risk of injury to self and others. Restraints should *never* be used as a substitute for close observation and supervision by nursing personnel.

Before using restraints, find the cause of the problem and then intervene appropriately. Alternatives to restraints may include assessing for pain or other discomfort, using diversional activities, reducing stimuli, coordinating care to minimize sleep interruptions, adjusting room temperature, providing extra pillows and blankets, lowering bed to lowest level, placing call bell within client's reach, having a clock with large numbers and a calendar with large print at the bedside, reintroducing yourself each time you enter the room, providing bathroom breaks every 2 hours, and keeping fluids available and within reach (unless contraindicated) (Napierkowski, 2002; Sweeney-Calciano, Solimene, & Forrester, 2003).

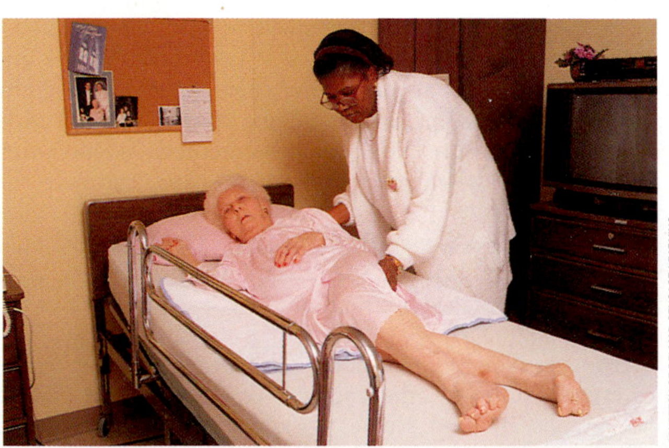
COURTESY OF DELMAR CENGAGE LEARNING

FIGURE 20-5 The use of side rails can contribute to a safe and secure environment.

PROFESSIONALTIP

Key Elements of Restraint Documentation

- Reason for using a restraint
- Type of restraint
- Explanation given to client and family
- Date and time of and client's response to application
- Length of time restraint used
- Frequency of monitoring and client's response
- Safety (release from the restraint along with periodic, routine exercise and assessment for circulation and skin integrity)
- Assessment for continued need of restraint
- Outcome of restraint use

Restraint use is very controversial because of client injuries related to these devices. The Omnibus Budget Reconciliation Act (OBRA) of 1987 defines clients' rights and choices and gives the following as acceptable reasons for using physical restraints:

- Restraints are part of the medical treatment.
- All other interventions have been tried first.
- Other disciplines have been consulted for assistance with the problem.
- Supporting documentation has been provided.

The Joint Commission has also updated its guidelines on physical restraints. Citing studies, the Joint Commission stated that the use of restraints may violate clients' rights and cause "physical and psychological harm, loss of dignity . . . and even death" (Joint Commission, 2001).

Since 1999, the CMS has had regulations regarding the use of restraints. A physician or other licensed independent practitioner (LIP) must conduct a face-to face assessment of the client before writing a restraint order. Each order has a maximum limit of 4 hours for adults, 2 hours for children ages 9 to 17, and 1 hour for clients younger than age 9. They can be written for a shorter time frame. Nurses must continually assess, monitor, and reevaluate the client so that the restraint can be removed at the earliest possible time. The physician or LIP may be telephoned for an order renewal based on the nurse's most recent assessment. The physician or LIP must perform another face-to-face assessment every 24 hours if the restraint is still used (CMS, 2008).

Once restrained, clients are rendered less able to care for their own basic needs; thus, the nurse's responsibility in meeting these needs increases. Facility policy regarding use of restraints, care of the client in restraints, and method of documentation must be followed precisely.

Restraints can be physical or chemical. **Physical restraints** reduce the client's movement through the application of a device (Figure 20-6). **Chemical restraints** are medications used to control the client's behavior. Anxiolytics and sedatives are commonly used chemical restraints.

The nursing plan of care should include safety measures to reduce the potential for injury from restraints. Additional safety measures to observe when using restraint devices are as follows:

SAFETY

Restraints

- Placing a jacket or belt restraint too tightly on the diaphragm will inhibit lung expansion.
- To avoid accidental injury in the event that the side rail is released, the restraint strap should be secured to the bed frame, not to the side rail.

- Restraints should never interfere with a treatment (e.g., intravenous therapy) or intensify the client's health problem.
- At least once every 2 hours, the nurse must assess the color, temperature, sensation, motion, and capillary refill in the area distal to the restraint and perform range-of-motion exercises.
- The client and significant others should be provided psychological support, as needed.

Use Assistive Devices for Walking Devices used to assist walking include canes, crutches, walkers, and wheelchairs.

Canes Canes are curved walking devices that provide support to the weak side of the body. Three common types of canes are the single stick, the tripod (three footed), and the quad (four footed). All types should have a sturdy grip and rubber tips. The tips should be checked frequently for signs of wear.

Canes should be held on the strong side of the body (Figure 20-7). The affected side and the cane should move simultaneously while the weight is supported on the strong side. The strong side is moved while the weight is supported on the cane and the weaker side.

Crutches Crutches are wooden or metal staffs used either temporarily or permanently to increase mobility. There are two types of crutches: the axillary crutch and the Lofstrand, or forearm, crutch. The axillary crutch, the type most commonly used, fits under the axilla, with the weight being placed on the handgrips. The Lofstrand crutch has a handgrip and a metal cuff that fits around the arm. This type of crutch is more convenient but not as stable as the axillary crutch.

CRITICAL THINKING

Restraints

An 83-year-old widow fractured her hip when she fell in the bathtub. She had hip replacement surgery yesterday. Tonight she is very confused and is trying to dislodge the bandage and stitches. She is now being restrained for her protection. What other nursing activities could have been implemented before use of restraints? Do you think restraints will affect her mental status? If so, in what way(s)? What are some other effects she may experience as a result of being restrained?

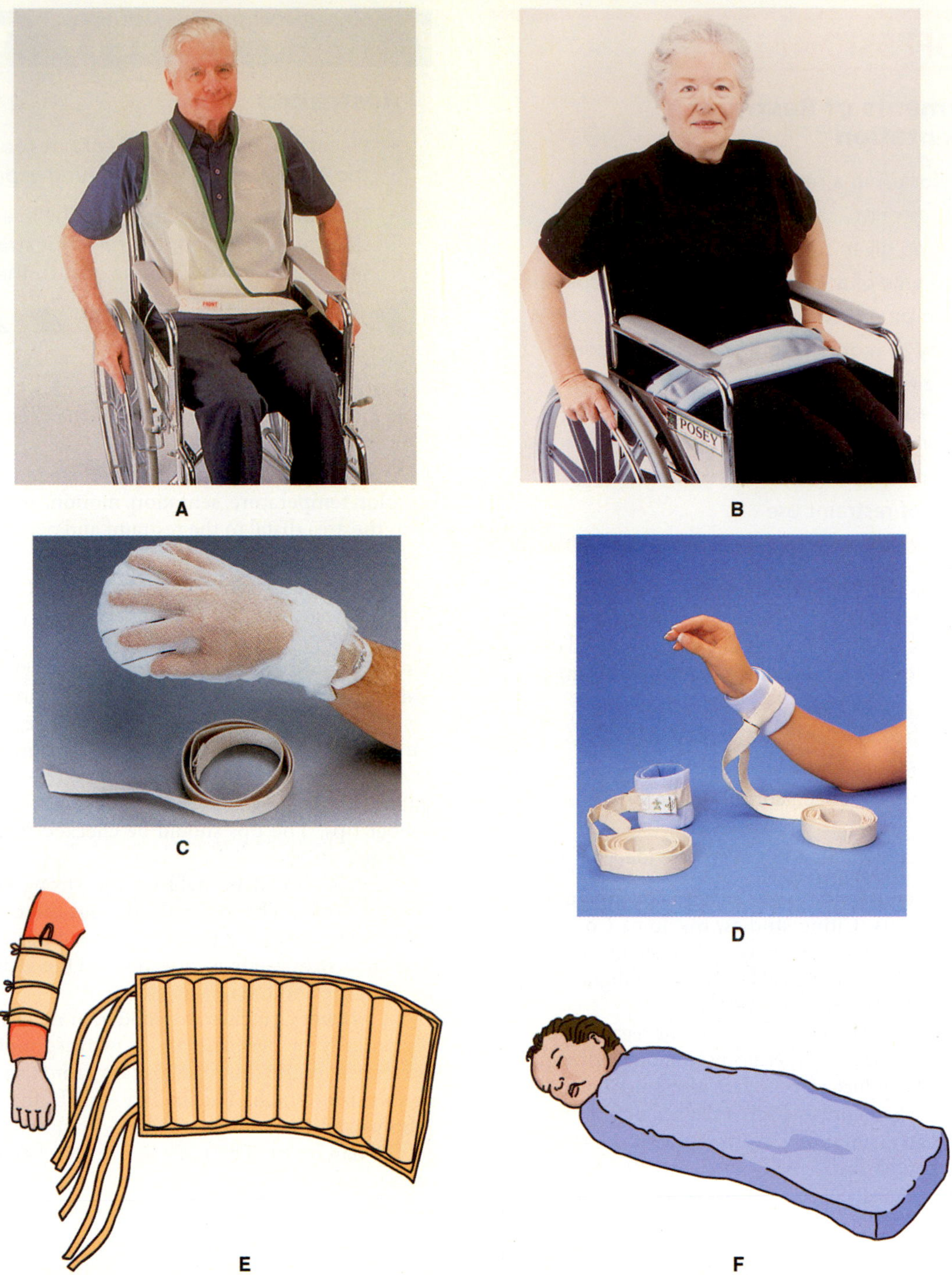

FIGURE 20-6 Types of Restraints: *A*, Jacket or Vest Restraint; *B*, Belt Restraint for Chair; *C*, Mitten or Hand Restraint; *D*, Limb or Extremity Restraint; *E*, Elbow Restraint; *F*, Mummy Restraint (*Images A and B courtesy of J. T. Posey. All others courtesy of Delmar Cengage Learning.*)

To prevent slipping, crutches have rubber tips, which must be kept dry. The tips should also be inspected regularly. If tips become loose or worn, they must be replaced immediately. The structure of the crutch must also be inspected regularly. The person's weight will not be properly dispersed if there are cracks or bends in the crutch.

Walkers A walker is a waist-high metal tubular device with a handgrip and four legs. Some walkers have wheels on the front two legs, whereas other walkers have rubber tips on all four legs. Walkers give a sense of security and extra support, as well as independence, to clients. The client first moves the walker forward and then takes a step while balancing weight on the walker.

Wheelchairs A wheelchair is a means of ambulation for clients who are unable to support their weight while standing. The nurse should instruct the client in the safe use of a wheelchair by reminding the client to keep the wheelchair locked when not moving and to lift the footrests out of the way when getting in or out of the wheelchair. The wheelchair should be pushed slowly from behind and should be backed into doorways and into and out of elevators.

Use Proper Body Mechanics The human body is able to move in many different ways, some more efficient than others. The most effective, safest way of lifting and moving things is

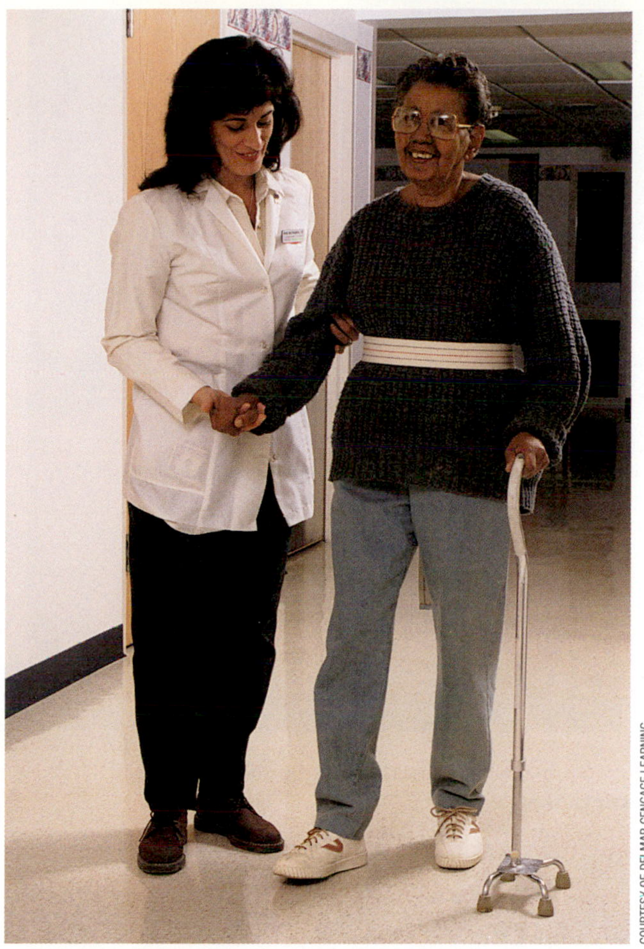
COURTESY OF DELMAR CENGAGE LEARNING

FIGURE 20-7 A nurse ensures the safety of a client using the quad cane.

by using the principles of body mechanics, including center of gravity, base of support, and body alignment.

Center of Gravity The center of gravity is located in the center of the body, in the pelvic area. Body weight is approximately equal above and below this area. All movement should pivot around this central point. This keeps the weight over the base of support, making it easier to stay balanced. Keeping the back straight and bending at the knees and hips helps maintain the center of gravity in the pelvic area. If the center of gravity shifts, the body tends to fall.

Base of Support Feet are the base of support. The feet should be kept wide apart when lifting heavy items because it is easier to stay balanced with a wide base of support. Furthermore, one foot should be kept a little forward of the other to give stability from front to back. Keeping the knees slightly bent allows for quick movement and for jolts to the body to be absorbed. When turning, the feet rather than the body should be moved, in order to prevent injury to the back.

Body Alignment Proper body alignment requires that the various parts of the body be kept in proper anatomic relationship to each other.

Ensure Adequate Lighting Adequate lighting helps people see environmental hazards. Rooms should have adequate light so the client can safely perform ADLs and health care providers can perform procedures.

Remove Obstacles Obstacles in heavily traveled areas represent a risk to the client's safety. Older adults and persons unfamiliar with the environment have the greatest risk of injury from obstacles.

SAFETY

Body Mechanics

- Stoop to lift objects from the floor: bend at the hips and the knees, keeping the back straight and base of support wide. The large muscles of the legs can then be used to straighten the body and lift the object.
- Avoid bending from the waist because doing so strains the lower back muscles.
- To prevent undue stress and strain on the back when caring for clients, adjust the height of the bed to one of comfort and ease.
- Carry objects close to the midline of the body.
- Avoid stretching to reach objects.

Reduce Bathroom Hazards

Bathrooms pose a threat to the client because of the presence of water. Accidents common to the bathroom are falls, scalds,

COMMUNITY/HOME HEALTH CARE

Preventing Fires and Burns

- Turn handles of pots and pans toward the center of the stove to prevent children from pulling them down and burning themselves.
- Keep matches in a metal can and in a place where children cannot reach them.
- Be aware of loose, flowing clothing when cooking, especially over an open flame.
- Avoid using candles for light or heat and never leave a burning candle unattended.
- Install smoke alarms near bedrooms and check batteries twice a year.
- Do not place portable heaters near curtains, which can easily catch on fire.
- Allow only certified electricians to work on wiring in the home.
- Do not place electrical cords under carpeting.
- Do not use multiple-plug outlets.
- Do not stick anything into appliances that are plugged in (e.g., a fork in the toaster).
- Teach family members routes of escape from the house, pick a place to meet outside to verify that everyone is safe, and conduct practice fire drills.
- Teach *stop, drop, and roll* to extinguish fire on clothing.

or burns. Accidents can be reduced by using grab bars near the tub, shower, and toilet; nonslip mats in the tub and shower; and a secured bathroom rug near the tub or shower; always check the temperature of the water before entering the tub or shower. Medications should be stored in a locked cabinet, out of reach of children and disoriented or confused adults.

Prevent Fire

Fire is a potential danger in institutional and home environments. Fire requires the interaction of three elements: sufficient *heat* to ignite the fire, combustible material (*fuel*), and *oxygen* to support the fire.

Immobilized or incapacitated clients are at great risk during a fire. Common causes of fire are smoking in bed, discarding cigarette butts in trash cans, and faulty electrical equipment. Because smoking is a health hazard, most health care facilities are now smoke free.

Goals regarding fire are twofold: fire prevention and client protection during a fire. Interventions to prevent or reduce the risk of fire are:

- Make sure fire exits are clearly marked.
- Identify the locations and demonstrate the operation of fire extinguishers.
- Practice fire evacuation procedures.
- Post emergency phone numbers near all telephones.
- Keep open spaces and hallways clear of obstacles.
- Check electrical cords for exposed or damaged wires.
- Teach clients about fire hazards.

When there is a fire, follow institutional policy and procedures for fire containment and evacuation (Figure 20-8). During a fire, nursing interventions are focused on protecting the client from injury and containing the fire. When a fire occurs, nurses should ensure client safety, immediately report the exact location and type of fire, and evacuate if necessary. Nurses should know the locations and operation of fire extinguishers (Figure 20-9). The four types of fire extinguishers are water, carbon dioxide, dry chemical, and Halon. Each type of fire extinguisher is used for a specific class of fire, as outlined in Table 20-4.

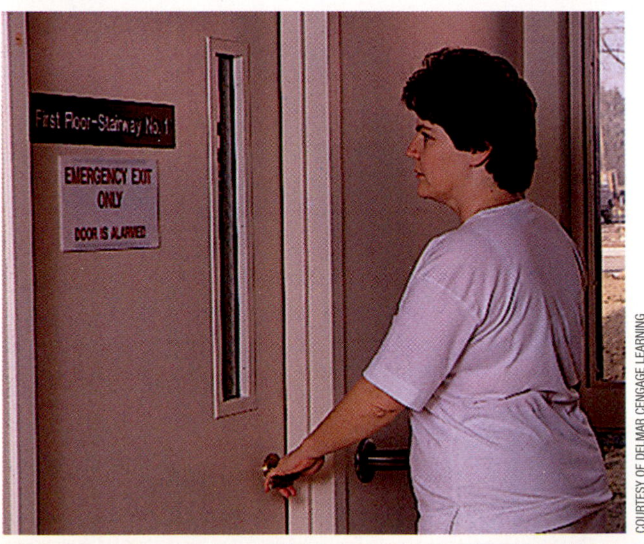

COURTESY OF DELMAR CENGAGE LEARNING

FIGURE 20-8 **All personnel should be familiar with the evacuation plan and emergency exits.**

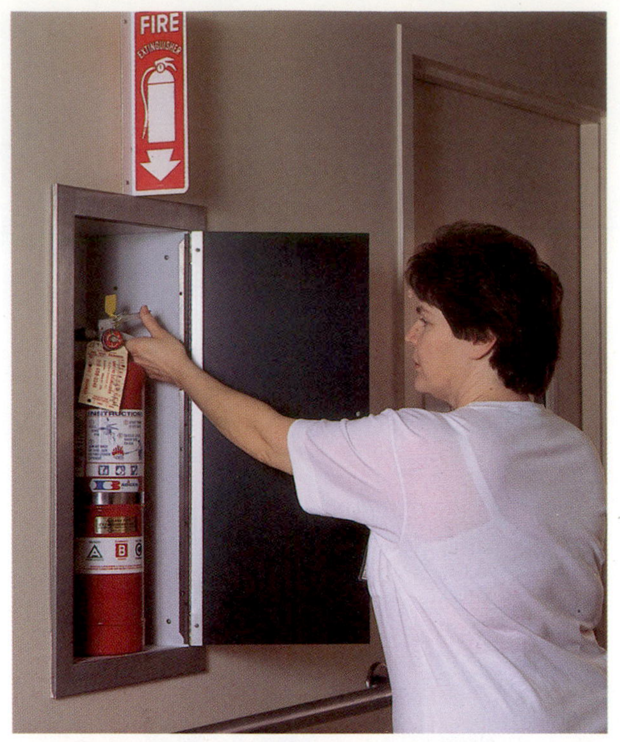

COURTESY OF DELMAR CENGAGE LEARNING

FIGURE 20-9 **Know the location and use of fire extinguishers.**

MEMORYTRICK

RACE

If you discover a fire or see flame or smoke, follow the **RACE** procedures:

R = Rescue individuals directly threatened by the fire

A = Activate alarm and call 911 or have someone call 911

C = Confine the fire by closing doors

E = Evacuate/Extinguish the fire

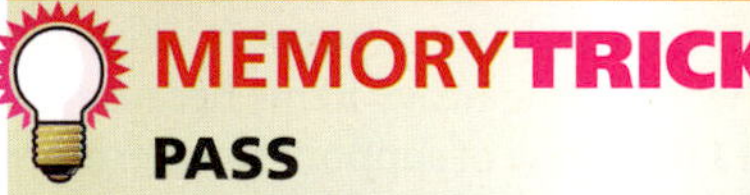

PASS

By using the memory trick **PASS**, a nurse will know how to correctly use a fire extinguisher when needed (U.S. Department of Energy, 2001):

P = Pull the pin at the top of the fire extinguisher

A = Aim the nozzle of the fire extinguisher at the base of the fire while standing approximately 8 feet away

S = Squeeze the handle to discharge the fire extinguisher

S = Sweep the nozzle back and forth aiming at the base of the fire

TABLE 20-4 Fire Extinguishers

NEW LABEL		OLD LABEL
	Class A: Puts out ordinary combustibles such as wood, paper, and cloth.	A Ordinary Combustibles
	Class B: Used on fires of flammable liquids such as grease, gasoline, and oil.	B Flammable Liquids
	Class C: Suitable for electrical fires.	C Electrical Equipment
NONE	Class D: For flammable metals, specific for the type of metal.	D Combustible Metals

Extinguishing Agents	Use
Water	Class A
Carbon Dioxide	Class B & C
Dry Chemical	Class A, B & C
Halon (leaves no residue on valuable electrical equipment)	Class C

Data from *HFD: All You Ever Wanted to Know about Fire Extinguishers*, 2001, U.S. Department of Energy, available: http://www.hanford.gov/fire/safety/extingrs.htm, and *Types of Fire Extinguishers*, 2007, Occupational Safety and Health Administration, available: http://www.osha.gov/SLTC/etools/evacuation/portable_about.html#Types.

Ensure Equipment Safety

Checking all equipment and supplies carefully before use and refusing to use any damaged goods or equipment can prevent many accidents. A good rule to follow is *never use any piece of equipment that is damaged in any way or not working properly.* If a wheel comes off an over-bed table, do not attempt to prop the table up but remove it from the room and send it to the appropriate area for repair. The same holds true for smaller supplies given to or used on clients. The safety of clients must always come first.

Glass and Plastic Glass and plastic equipment and supplies should be inspected for cracks and chips before use. The nurse should also check that there are no rough edges that may injure clients.

Disposable Sterile Supplies When using disposable sterile supplies, the nurse should first always check that the package is intact. Any break in or wetness of the wrapper renders it unsterile. Expiration dates should also be verified before use.

Electrical Equipment The hospital environment has a variety of electrical equipment such as bed controls and intravenous and patient-controlled analgesia (PCA) pumps. Each piece of electrical equipment should have a three-pronged, grounded electrical plug. A grounded plug transmits any stray electrical current from equipment to ground. To protect the client from electrical injury, the nurse should read the warning labels on all equipment, check for frayed electrical cords, use only grounded electrical equipment, avoid overloading circuits, and report any shocks received from equipment to the biomedical department (Figure 20-10).

Personal electrical appliances that the client is allowed to keep at the bedside, such as shavers, hair dryers, or curling irons, should be safety checked by the biomedical department before being used.

If a client receives an electrical shock, the electricity should be turned off before touching the client. Then the client's pulse should be checked; if no pulse, CPR should be initiated. The nurse should assess vital signs, mental status, and skin integrity for burns on the client with a pulse. The physician should be notified of the event, and an incident report filled out.

Reduce Exposure to Radiation

Injury from radiation can occur to clients during diagnostic testing and therapeutic interventions if overexposure or exposure to untargeted tissues occurs. Dislodged radiation implants can result in exposure to untargeted tissues. Time, distance, and shielding are the basis of radiation exposure and protection. Protection from radiation therapy involves the following:

- Minimize the time spent in contact with the radiation source (implant or client).
- Maximize the distance from the radiation source (implant or client).
- Use appropriate radiation shields.
- Monitor radiation exposure with a film badge.
- Label all potentially radioactive material.
- Never touch dislodged implants or the body fluids of a client receiving radiation therapy.

The client's risk for injury can be reduced by following all instructions and precautions. The nurse's risk for injury can be

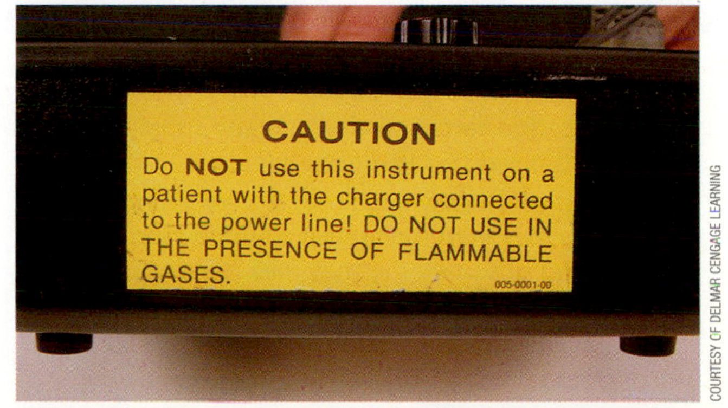
CAUTION
Do NOT use this instrument on a patient with the charger connected to the power line! DO NOT USE IN THE PRESENCE OF FLAMMABLE GASES.
005-0001-00
COURTESY OF DELMAR CENGAGE LEARNING

FIGURE 20-10 Heed warning labels on electrical equipment.

SAFETY

Locked Cabinets

Locked cabinets should be used to store all poisonous substances away from children or mentally confused persons.

reduced by observing all radioactive labels, wearing gloves when handling radioactive body discharges, wearing a lead apron, washing hands, disposing of radioactive substances in special containers, reducing the length of client contact, and wearing a badge that measures the amount of radiation exposure.

Prevent Poisoning

A **poison** is any substance that, when taken into the body, interferes with normal physiologic functioning. Poisons may be inhaled, injected, ingested, or absorbed into the body. Many substances can be poisonous if taken in sufficient quantity.

Dangerous chemicals may be found in any workplace, but some are specific to the health care industry, such as radioactive isotopes, laboratory dyes, antiseptics, irrigating solutions, disinfectants, and therapeutic drugs. The nurse must ensure that potentially dangerous materials are never left unattended in clients' rooms. Alcohol and other antiseptics or medications used for dressing changes or other procedures must be removed from the client's room after use.

On admission, clients are asked whether they have brought any medications to the facility. If so, these medications must be either removed to a safe place or sent home with the client's family. Family members sometimes bring in remedies that the client used at home. The nurse should be observant for potentially harmful substances in client rooms.

When poisoning is suspected, the poison control center should be notified. The number can generally be found on the inside cover or first few pages of the telephone book. The person reporting the poisoning should know the amount and type of poison inhaled, ingested, or injected and the client's age and symptoms. Anyone ingesting poison should be turned on the side to prevent aspiration while awaiting further treatment (Stanhope & Knollmueller, 2000).

SAFETY 

Medication and Cleaning Carts

- Medication carts and cleaning and supply carts should never be left unattended.
- Confused, visually impaired, or very young clients may help themselves to something harmful or something they may use in a harmful way.
- Medication cupboards and carts must be kept locked when not in use.

PROFESSIONALTIP

Oxygen Use

Special precautions must always be taken when oxygen is in use. Because one of the three elements essential to starting a fire is oxygen, the presence of pure oxygen can transform the tiniest spark into a tremendous hazard.

When oxygen is being used, "No Smoking" signs must be posted in the room and on the outside of the door to the room. It is vital that all visitors and other clients understand that the rule applies to everyone in the room, not just to the person receiving the oxygen. Because many critically ill clients use oxygen, it is also necessary for the nurse to caution clergy not to use open flames or candles in any religious rites.

Woolen and nylon blankets should not be used, as they can cause static electricity and thus pose a fire risk in an atmosphere of pure oxygen. Cotton blankets are recommended.

Electrical appliances such as radios and razors are generally not used in the presence of oxygen. Oil should not be used on oxygen equipment because it is flammable. Hospital policy, as well as equipment itself, must be checked to determine what is safe to be used in a room where oxygen is being used.

Whenever tank oxygen is used, the cylinders must be securely strapped to a holder or cart to prevent the tank from tipping over and knocking off the valve, which could in turn cause a spark that would quickly ignite in the presence of oxygen.

Prevent Choking

To prevent choking on food, special techniques are used when feeding clients in at-risk categories. Nothing should ever be given by mouth to an unconscious client because the epiglottis does not function, and choking and suffocation are likely. Likewise, to prevent aspiration of vomitus, food and drink are usually withheld before the induction of general anesthesia. After some tests, such as a bronchoscopy, food and drink are withheld until the gag reflex returns.

LIFE SPAN CONSIDERATIONS

Vitamins and Minerals

Adult iron preparations are especially poisonous to young children and should be stored in a locked cabinet out of the reach of children.

COMMUNITY/HOME HEALTH CARE

Proper Storage and Use of Medications

Teach clients about:

- Childproofing cupboards where medications are stored.
- The proper use and dosages of medications.
- The use of special medication containers that are divided into days and times (to help prevent the client from duplicating a medication dose).

CLIENT TEACHING

Prevent Accidental Poisonings

- Store medications in child-resistant containers.
- Do not take medications in front of children.
- Never call medicine "candy."
- Place toxic substances in a locked cabinet.
- Keep labels on containers.
- Never put poisonous substances in food or beverage containers.
- Place poison stickers on toxic substances.
- Display poison control center phone numbers near telephones.

Prevent Suffocation

Smothering can be prevented by proper nursing observation of at-risk clients such as infants, those who are impaired with regard to ADLs, and paralyzed or unconscious clients. Such clients should be repositioned frequently and checked for a patent (open) airway. Soft pillows, mattresses, and comforters, in which they might bury their faces, should not be used. In the presence of oral secretions, the client's head should be turned to the side to prevent choking. Monitors that beep if breathing ceases should be used for at-risk clients.

Prevent Drowning

Infants, young children, and weak or confused clients are most at risk for drowning. These clients should never be left alone in the bathtub. If the nurse must leave for any reason, either the client must be removed from the tub or another member of the health care team must stay with the client until the nurse returns or the bath is completed.

Clients should be instructed in the use of call systems installed in tub and shower rooms. Clients should also be instructed to first pull the plug in the tub and then call the nurse should they feel weak or faint.

Reduce Noise Pollution

Noise pollution, an uncomfortable noise level, often occurs in health care facilities from visitor traffic, personnel, and medical equipment. It can result in sensory overload and a disorganized environment. **Sensory overload** is an increased rate and intensity of auditory and visual stimuli. Sensory overload can alter a client's recovery by increasing or causing anxiety, paranoia, hallucinations, and depression.

SAFETY

Noise Pollution

- Maintain a quiet environment.
- Control traffic.
- Provide earplugs.

Provide for Client's Bathing Needs

An essential component of nursing care is bathing clients. The nurse is responsible for ensuring that the hygiene needs of the client are met whether the nurse performs the bath or delegates the activity to another health care provider. The purpose of the bath and the client's self-care abilities determine the type of bath provided. The two general types of baths are cleansing and therapeutic.

Cleansing Baths Cleansing baths are routine client care for personal hygiene. The five types of cleansing baths are shower, tub bath, self-help bath, complete bed bath, and partial bath.

Shower Most ambulatory clients are capable of taking a shower. Clients with physical limitations can use a waterproof chair in the shower. The nurse may provide some assistance with the shower.

Tub Bath Some clients may prefer and enjoy a tub bath. Tub baths can also be therapeutic. Clients with physical limitations should be assisted when entering and exiting the tub.

Self-Help Bath A self-help bed bath provides hygiene care to clients confined to bed. The nurse prepares the bath equipment and assists in washing difficult-to-reach body areas such as the back, legs, feet, and perineal area.

Complete Bed Bath A complete bed bath is provided for dependent clients who are confined to bed. The nurse washes the client's entire body.

SAFETY

Tub Bath

Water temperature must be checked in the bathtub before allowing the client to enter.

PROFESSIONAL TIP

Bathing

- Baths are an excellent time to assess the skin.
- Bathing provides time to meet the client's psychosocial needs through assessment and counseling and to educate the client on basic and special hygiene needs.

Partial Bath In a partial bath, only those body areas that would cause discomfort or odor are cleansed. These areas are the face, hands, axillae, and perineal area. The client or nurse may perform a partial bath, depending on the client's self-care abilities. Partial baths may be performed with the client in bed or standing at the sink.

Therapeutic Baths A physician's order is required for therapeutic baths, stating the type of bath, body surface to be treated, temperature of the water, and type of medicated solutions to be used. A therapeutic bath is usually taken in a tub and lasts approximately 20 to 30 minutes. They are classified as hot, warm, tepid, or cool; soak or sitz; and oatmeal (Aveeno), cornstarch, or sodium bicarbonate.

Hot- or warm-water tub baths reduce muscle spasms, soreness, and tension but can cause skin burns. Cool or tepid baths relieve tension and lower body temperature. To prevent chilling and rapid temperature fluctuations during a tepid or cool bath, the nurse must not leave the client in the tub too long.

A soak is usually limited to a body part but can involve the entire body. Water, with or without a medicated solution, is applied to reduce irritation, pain, or swelling or to soften or remove dead tissue.

Sitz baths reduce inflammation and cleanse the perineal and anal areas. Sitz baths are usually used for hemorrhoids or anal fissures and after perineal or rectal surgery. Skin irritations can be soothed with oatmeal (Aveeno), cornstarch, or sodium bicarbonate baths.

Provide Clean Bed Linens

Clean linens are placed on the bed to promote comfort after a bath. Clients able to be out of bed can sit in a chair while the nurse makes the bed.

If the client cannot be out of bed, the nurse will make an occupied bed. If the client cannot be turned or is in traction, assistance will be needed. Care must be taken to avoid disturbing any traction weights.

Provide Perineal Care

Perineal care is the cleansing of the external genitalia, the perineum, and surrounding area. Perineal care may be called *peri-care*. Perineal care prevents or eliminates infection and odor, promotes healing, removes secretions, and provides comfort. Perineal care can be provided as part of the bath or separately.

Offer Back Rubs

Back rubs and massages stimulate the client's circulation, relieve muscle tension, and relax muscles and give the nurse an opportunity to assess the skin. Cream and lotion facilitate the rubbing and skin lubrication during a back rub or massage.

The client lies either on the side or prone. The nurse uses friction and pressure when rubbing the hands on the client's skin. Friction creates heat, which dilates the peripheral blood vessels and increases the blood supply to the skin. Pressure stimulates the muscle fibers, which relaxes the muscles. The nurse must check for contraindications before giving a back rub or massage. Be cautious when massaging limbs, especially the lower limbs. A thrombus (blood clot) might be dislodged, resulting in an embolus (circulating blood clot). Bony prominences should be massaged lightly to prevent damage to underlying tissue.

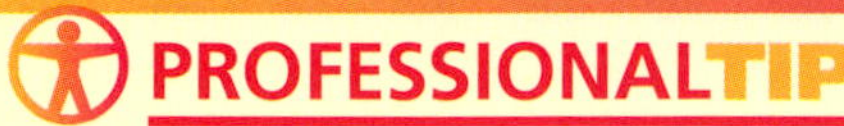

PROFESSIONALTIP

Perineal Care

Perineal care may be embarrassing for both the client and the nurse, especially if the client is of the opposite sex. In this situation, the nurse may provide the client with warm water, a moistened washcloth, soap, a dry towel, and privacy. The nurse is responsible for providing perineal care in a professional and private manner if the client is unable to do so.

CRITICAL THINKING

Perineal Care

What is the best way to approach providing perineal care to someone of the opposite sex or of your similar age?

Provide Foot and Toenail Care

Proper foot and toenail care are necessary for standing and ambulation. Often, foot and toenail care are ignored until problems arise. Foot and toenail problems may result from poorly fitted shoes, inadequate foot and toenail hygiene, incorrect nail trimming, and exposure to harsh chemicals. These problems may cause a loss of skin integrity and potential for infection.

Pain or tenderness is usually the first sign of foot and toenail problems. These symptoms may result in limping, causing strain to certain muscle groups. Clients with diabetes mellitus have changes in circulation predisposing them to foot problems requiring special foot and toenail care.

Foot and toenail care prevents infection and soft tissue trauma from ingrown or jagged nails and eliminates odor. Hygiene care of feet and toenails includes regular cleansing, rinsing, and drying the feet and toenails; trimming the toenails; cleaning under the toenails; and wearing properly fitted shoes.

Soaking facilitates cleansing dirty or thickened toenails. Use an orangewood stick to clean under the toenails because a metal instrument roughens the nail and causes harboring of dirt. The nail clipper is the safest instrument to trim the toenails; however, some people think that cutting the nails makes them brittle. The client who chooses not to cut the nails should file them straight across with an emery board. The

PROFESSIONALTIP

Foot and Toenail Care

- Soak feet in warm water and wash with soap.
- Clean under the nails with an orangewood stick.
- Cut or file the nails straight across.
- Trim the cuticles when needed.
- Dry feet and between toes.
- Apply lotion or cream.

areas between the toes should be carefully dried. An emollient, such as cold cream, helps keep toenails and cuticles soft.

Callused areas should never be cut. Lotion applied to the feet maintains moisture and softens callused areas. Soaking also facilitates callus removal. If the client's feet are excessively moist (sweat), water-absorbent powder can be applied between the toes.

Everyone should wear clean, properly fitted shoes. Shoes should not be too tight but should be snug enough to provide support to the feet and have arch supports. Shoes should be half an inch longer than the longest toe.

Provide Oral Care

The oral cavity takes in food, chews it, secretes mucus to moisten and lubricate the food, and secretes a digestive enzyme. Common problems occurring in the oral cavity include:

- Bad breath (**halitosis**)
- Cavities (**dental caries**)
- Inflammation of the gums (**gingivitis**)
- Inflammation of the oral mucosa (**stomatitis**)
- Periodontal disease (**pyorrhea**)
- Plaque

Poor oral hygiene and loss of teeth affects a person's social interaction, body image, and nutritional intake. Daily oral care is vital to maintain the integrity of the mucous membranes, gums, teeth, and lips. Preventive measures can preserve the oral cavity and teeth. Preventive oral care consists of flossing, brushing, and rinsing with fluoride.

Fluoride Research has determined that fluoride can prevent dental caries so communities add fluoride to their water supplies. Fluoride is common in toothpastes and mouthwashes, but persons with very dry or irritated mucous membranes should not use commercial mouthwashes because the alcohol content further dries the mucous membranes.

Infants can be given fluoride drops as early as 2 weeks of age to prevent dental caries. Nurses should inform clients that excessive fluoride can darken the color of tooth enamel. Fluoride should be administered with a dropper directed toward the back of the throat to prevent discoloration of the tooth enamel.

Flossing Flossing should be done daily before brushing the teeth. Flossing prevents the formation of plaque and removes plaque and food debris between the teeth. Regular flossing can prevent dental caries and periodontal disease.

Brushing Brushing promotes blood circulation in the gums and removes plaque and food debris. Tooth brushing should follow flossing. Brush teeth after each meal using a dentifrice (toothpaste) containing fluoride. Brush the tongue to remove bacteria and prevent halitosis. Dentures are brushed the same way as teeth. The oral cavity of a client who wears dentures must also be cleansed. Dentures should be kept moist by putting back in the mouth or immersing in water after cleansing.

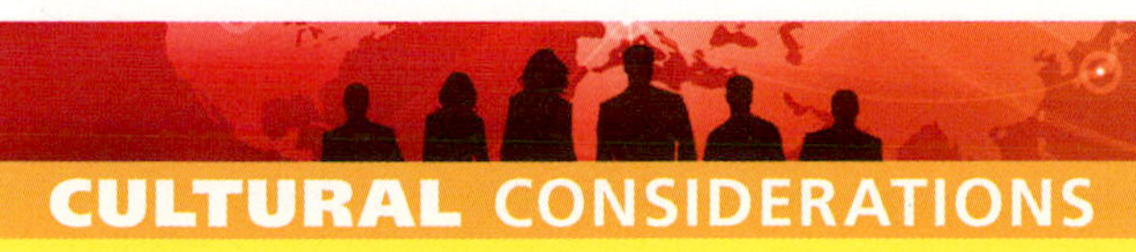

CULTURAL CONSIDERATIONS

Influences on Hygiene

- All self-care and hygiene practices are influenced by the client's cultural values and background.
- Ask clients about preferences before performing care and show sensitivity about those practices that may differ from your own.

PROFESSIONALTIP

Oral Care for the Unconscious Client

Special care should be taken when doing oral care for the unconscious client to prevent both client aspiration and injury to the nurse (from the client biting because of the gag reflex).

- Never use your fingers to hold a client's mouth open; use a bite block or padded tongue blade.
- Assess for gag reflex.
- Turn the client's head to one side with a basin under the mouth.
- Use only a small amount of liquid and oral suctioning to facilitate removal of secretions.
- Brush the teeth and tongue in the usual manner. Exercise caution to prevent aspiration.

Provide Hair Care

Hair affects a person's appearance and body image. Hair maintains body temperature and is a receptor for the sense of touch. Hair texture, growth, and distribution provide information on a person's general health status. Common hair problems include hair loss, dandruff, tangled or matted hair, and infestations such as lice. Daily hair care can reduce hair problems and promote hair growth; prevent hair loss, infections, or infestations; promote circulation to the scalp; evenly distribute oils along hair shafts; and maintain the client's physical appearance. Hair care consists of brushing and combing, shampooing, shaving, and mustache and beard care.

Brushing and Combing Hair should be brushed or combed daily in the client's preferred manner. A clean brush or comb should be used to brush from the scalp toward the hair ends. Be gentle when brushing or combing sensitive scalps.

Some clients may have tangled or matted hair. Prevent pain when combing tangled or matted hair by holding the tangled hair near the scalp while combing. The hair can be loosely braided to prevent tangling or matting if the client permits. Tight braids may cause pain and hair loss. Written informed consent must be received before cutting a client's hair.

Shampooing Hair should be shampooed according to the client's usual routine. Shampooing removes soil from the hair, stimulates scalp circulation, and facilitates brushing and combing. Depending on the client's abilities and preferences, hair can be shampooed in the tub, in the shower, at the sink, or in the bed.

Hair can be shampooed with water or with shampoos not requiring water. Use the fingertip pads to gently massage the scalp. Thoroughly rinse and dry with an absorbent towel, comb and style as the client desires.

SAFETY

Shaving

- Review the client's medical record and the facility's policy regarding the use of razors for shaving.
- Clients prone to bleeding should use only electrical razors for shaving.
- The nurse should wear gloves unless using an electric razor.

Shaving Shaving is the removal of hair from the skin surface. Men often shave to remove facial hair, and women may shave to remove leg and/or axillary hair. Operative procedures may also require shaving an area of the body.

Shaving may be performed before, during, or after the bath. The area should be washed with soap and warm water to soften the hair before shaving. Apply shaving cream or mild soap to the area to ease hair removal. Pull the skin taut, hold the razor at a 45-degree angle, and move the razor over the skin in firm, short strokes in the direction of hair growth. Care should be taken to avoid cutting the skin. Wash, rinse, and pat the skin dry following shaving.

Mustache and Beard Care Mustaches and beards need daily care to keep the hair clean, trimmed, and combed. They can be washed with soap or shampoo but often require only gentle wiping with a moist washcloth. A mustache or beard should never be shaved off by the nurse without written informed consent from the client.

Provide Eye, Ear, and Nose Care

Eye, ear, and nose care should be included in routine hygiene care.

Eye Care Eyes are continually cleansed by tears and the movement of the eyelids over the eyes. Eyelids should be washed daily with a warm washcloth and from the inner to the outer canthus.

Eyelashes prevent foreign material from entering the eyes and conjunctival sacs. Eyelashes and eyebrows should be washed with the face.

Although some artificial eyes (prosthetics) are permanently implanted, others may require daily removal and cleaning: The eye is removed from the eye socket and washed.

Comatose clients lack a blink reflex and need special eye care. Lubricants or eyedrops should be frequently instilled to prevent corneal abrasions.

INFECTION CONTROL

Eye Care

In order to prevent the transfer of pathogens, a new, clean corner of the washcloth should be used for each eye and with each stroke.

PROFESSIONALTIP

Eye Care for the Comatose Client

- At least every 4 hours, use a warm washcloth to cleanse eyelids, eyelashes, and eyebrows. Clean from the inner to the outer canthus.
- Liquid tear solutions should be instilled to prevent corneal drying and ulcerations if eyes remain open and the blink reflex is absent.
- If eye patches or shields are used, they should be removed at least every 4 hours to assess the eyes and provide eye care.

Clients who can insert, remove, and manage the care of their contact lenses require little assistance from the nurse. The client who also has corrective eyeglasses may wish to wear eyeglasses during hospitalization. There are hard and soft types of contact lenses. Each type requires different cleansing and care. The lenses should be removed during emergency situations and placed in the appropriate solution.

Ear Care Foreign material or wax in the external ear canal can affect hearing. Cleansing the ears involves cleansing the external ear canal and auricles. No objects should be inserted into the ear canal. Excess wax or foreign material may be removed with a warm washcloth while pulling the ear up and back in the adult client. The ear is pulled down and back in children under the age of 3. Irrigation of the ear may be necessary to remove dried wax; this will require a physician's order.

Hearing aids amplify sound. Hearing aids should be cleansed regularly to ensure proper functioning.

If the hearing aid is not functioning properly, the nurse should check the on–off switch and volume control, the battery (and replace as necessary), the plastic tubing for cracks and loose connections, and the telephone switch, which should be in the off position unless the client is using the phone. Hearing aids should be handled carefully because bumping or dropping them can damage their delicate mechanisms. The hearing aid should be stored in a container when not in use because dust and dirt can damage the mechanism.

Nose Care The nose is the organ of smell, which humidifies inhaled air, facilitates breathing, and prevents entrance of foreign material into the respiratory tract. Excessive or dried secretions may impair nasal function. If the client cannot blow the nose, insert a cotton-tip applicator moistened with water or saline into the nostrils but not beyond the cotton tip. A suction bulb can remove excessive nasal secretions in infants. The client with a nasogastric tube should receive meticulous skin care to the nose area to prevent skin breakdown.

Evaluation

Evaluation looks for achievement of goals and expected outcomes.

The client should be not only kept free of injury during hospitalization but also helped to develop an awareness of the factors increasing the risk for injury. In the home, modifications to ensure a safe environment serve as evidence for the home health nurse that learning has taken place.

The therapeutic value of hygiene is greatest when the client participates and is free from infection and changes in skin integrity. Evaluation identifies the client's level of functioning in self-care activities. At the time of discharge, appropriate referrals can be made to home health care agencies to assist the client in safety and hygiene practices.

CASE STUDY

K.H., an 80-year-old male, was involved in a motor vehicle accident (MVA) 1 month prior to being admitted to a rehabilitation facility. The MVA resulted in chest contusions from the seat belt and injury to the lungs, which resulted in general muscle weakness and a medical diagnosis of pneumonia. Before coming to the rehabilitation facility, K.H. lived independently at home and plans on returning home on discharge. When assessed by the nurse, he was alert; oriented to person, place, and time; wheelchair dependent; and ambulating 60 feet once a day with assistance from physical therapy. K.H.'s hand grasp, pedal push/pull, and muscle strength are grade 3. K.H. stated, "I feel so weak. I need to strengthen my muscles if I want to be able to go home."

1. What would be an appropriate nursing diagnosis for this client?
2. What goal/outcome would be appropriate for K.H.?
3. List four nursing interventions and provide rationale for each intervention.
4. When evaluating the plan of care, what data support that the goal/outcome criteria was met?

SAMPLE NURSING CARE PLAN

The Client at Risk for Injury

M.S., age 75 years, presents with coronary heart disease (CHD) on being admitted to the hospital. He has a family history of CHD. He smokes two packs of cigarettes per day, has diabetes mellitus, and is obese. He has gained 7 pounds in the past month and exhibits diminished visual acuity, decreased bladder tone, weakness, and syncope. His blood cholesterol is 320 mg/dL, and his high-density lipoprotein (HDL) level is 28 mg/dL. On the Glasgow Coma Scale (GCS), he received a score of 12 (15 is fully oriented; 7 is comatose). His blood pressure is 186/116.

NURSING DIAGNOSIS 1 *Risk for Injury* related to failure to adapt to sensory dysfunctions as evidenced by diminished visual acuity and a GCS score of 12

Nursing Outcomes Classification (NOC)
Risk Control: Cardiovascular Health
Neurological Status

Nursing Interventions Classification (NIC)
Surveillance
Surveillance: Safety

PLANNING/OUTCOMES	NURSING INTERVENTIONS	RATIONALE
M.S. will be protected from injury during hospitalization.	Initiate fall-prevention protocol.	Identifies and reduces the risk for injury.
	Place M.S. in a room as close as possible to the nurses' station.	Facilitates faster response time to the client's needs.
	Place fall-alert signs on M.S.'s door and head of bed.	Alerts other health care workers to the client's risk status.
	Turn the bed alarm on.	Helps monitor client status and facilitates prompt response if the client tries to get out of bed unassisted.
	Monitor M.S. and the environment every 2 hours and whenever a caregiver passes by his room.	Provides information on status, progress, and needs of the client; encourages team approach to client care.

(*Continues*)

SAMPLE NURSING CARE PLAN (Continued)

PLANNING/OUTCOMES	NURSING INTERVENTIONS	RATIONALE
	Reassess M.S.'s status every 4 hours.	Identifies changes and, thus, the need to modify the plan of care.
	Instruct all caregivers to respond promptly to the call light.	Ensures rapid response to the client's needs.
	Teach M.S. to use the call light; reinforce teaching each time before leaving him alone.	Ensures that the client has the means and knowledge to call for assistance if necessary.

EVALUATION

The fall prevention protocol was implemented. When discharged on the third day of hospitalization, M.S. was free of injury.

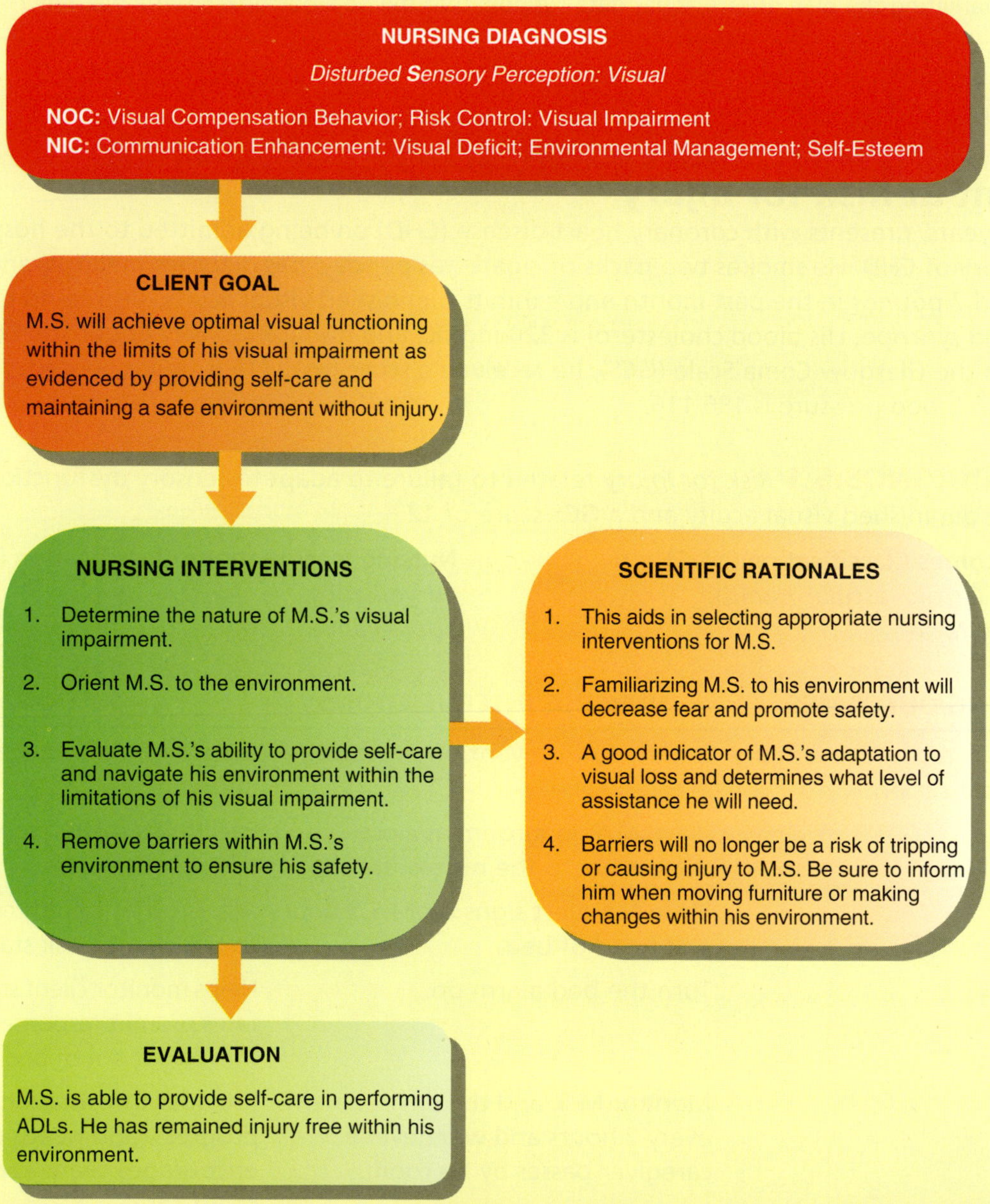

NURSING DIAGNOSIS

Disturbed Sensory Perception: Visual

NOC: Visual Compensation Behavior; Risk Control: Visual Impairment
NIC: Communication Enhancement: Visual Deficit; Environmental Management; Self-Esteem

CLIENT GOAL

M.S. will achieve optimal visual functioning within the limits of his visual impairment as evidenced by providing self-care and maintaining a safe environment without injury.

NURSING INTERVENTIONS

1. Determine the nature of M.S.'s visual impairment.
2. Orient M.S. to the environment.
3. Evaluate M.S.'s ability to provide self-care and navigate his environment within the limitations of his visual impairment.
4. Remove barriers within M.S.'s environment to ensure his safety.

SCIENTIFIC RATIONALES

1. This aids in selecting appropriate nursing interventions for M.S.
2. Familiarizing M.S. to his environment will decrease fear and promote safety.
3. A good indicator of M.S.'s adaptation to visual loss and determines what level of assistance he will need.
4. Barriers will no longer be a risk of tripping or causing injury to M.S. Be sure to inform him when moving furniture or making changes within his environment.

EVALUATION

M.S. is able to provide self-care in performing ADLs. He has remained injury free within his environment.

CONCEPT CARE MAP 20-1

SUMMARY

- Maintaining a safe environment for clients must be the highest priority for nurses.
- The best way to ensure safety is to recognize hazards and eliminate them. Prevention is the best safety measure.
- Clients having a high risk factor for injury must be provided extra protection measures.
- Factors influencing client safety are age, lifestyle, sensory and perceptual alterations, mobility, and emotional state.
- Accidents occurring in health care settings are related to client behavior, therapeutic procedures, and equipment.
- A safety risk appraisal is part of an assessment of a safe environment.
- Nurses can help clients maintain a safe environment by eliminating hazards related to falls, lighting, obstacles, the bathroom, fire, electricity, radiation, poisoning, and noise pollution.
- Safety precautions should be explained thoroughly to clients and/or families.
- Hygiene practices are influenced by personal preference, social and cultural practices, body image, socioeconomic status, and knowledge.
- Basic hygiene practices include bathing, skin care, perineal care, back rubs, foot and nail care, oral care, hair care, and eye, ear, and nose care.

REVIEW QUESTIONS

1. A 60-year-old diabetic client had his left leg amputated. He is in a semiprivate room with another client who is receiving oxygen. What sign should be posted on the door?
   1. "Amputee"
   2. "No Visitors"
   3. "No Smoking"
   4. "Regular Diet"
2. A client, just admitted to the hospital, is overweight, unsteady on her feet, and visually impaired. Her two daughters enter the room as the nurse puts the side rails up on the bed. The client begins to cry. The daughters accuse her of being a baby. The best nursing intervention would be to:
   1. tell the daughters to leave until their mother has calmed down.
   2. explain to the daughters that they are making their mother feel worse.
   3. explain to the client that side rails must be used to protect her from falling out of bed.
   4. explain to the client and her daughters both the purpose of the side rails and the facility's alternate policy.
3. Hygiene is considered a safety measure because:
   1. it changes a person's self-image.
   2. the same thing is done for all clients.
   3. it rids the body of all microorganisms.
   4. it promotes the health of the body's first line of defense.
4. A 42-year-old client is admitted to the hospital with mental changes, a headache, and shakiness. The nurse knows that the priority for nursing care is:
   1. safety.
   2. timeliness.
   3. one-to-one care.
   4. the execution of procedures exactly as written.
5. The nurse's place of employment has recently conducted a seminar for all staff on the use of side rails. After attending the seminar, the nurse knows that the use of side rails:
   1. is needed only at night.
   2. is required for all clients.
   3. has caused injury to clients.
   4. relieves the nurse from checking on the client as frequently.
6. Nursing measures to prevent falls in elderly clients include: (Select all that apply.)
   1. providing good lighting.
   2. placing rugs on the floor to prevent client from slipping.
   3. orienting client to the environment.
   4. keeping bed in the lowest position.
   5. not using restraints.
   6. placing a call light within reach.
7. The nurse is teaching a client about safety and asks the client to identify four factors that affect client safety. Which of the following factors identified by the client indicates that further teaching is needed?
   1. Age.
   2. Body image.
   3. Occupation.
   4. Sensory changes.
8. Which nursing intervention is the most appropriate to utilize at night for a client who uses a walker and is taking diuretics?
   1. Keep side rails up.
   2. Check on client periodically.
   3. Use a night-light.
   4. Place commode at bedside.
9. The nurse is making rounds and discovers a fire in a client's room. Her first action would be to:
   1. pull the nearest fire alarm.
   2. extinguish the fire following the "PASS" method.
   3. close doors on the unit to confine the fire.
   4. evacuate clients in immediate danger.

10. A 55-year-old female client with cancer has recently received a radiation implant. The nurse knows that protection from radiation therapy involves all of the following except:
    1. using appropriate radiation shields.
    2. minimizing the time spent in contact with the client while the implant is in place.
    3. monitoring radiation exposure with a film badge.
    4. immediately placing the radiation implant into a lead-lined bag if it becomes dislodged.

REFERENCES/SUGGESTED READINGS

Association for Professionals in Infection Control and Epidemiology, Inc. (2003). *The use of hand sanitizers in the healthcare setting.* Available: http://www.apic.org/pdf/FINALHandSanitizers.pdf

Bulechek, G., Butcher, H., McCloskey, J., & Dochterman, J., eds. (2008). *Nursing Interventions Classification (NIC)* (5th ed.). St. Louis, MO: Mosby/Elsevier.

Carpenito-Moyet, L. N. (2007). *Handbook of nursing diagnosis* (12th ed). Philadelphia: Lippincott Williams & Wilkins.

Centers for Disease Control and Prevention. (2008). Falls among older adults: An overview. Retrieved November 16, 2008, from http://www.cdc.gov/ncipc/factsheets/adultfalls.htm

Centers for Disease Control and Prevention, National Center for Injury Prevention and Control. (2002a). The costs of fall injuries among older adults. Available: http://www.cdc.gov/ncipc/factsheets/fallcost.htm

Centers for Disease Control and Prevention, National Center for Injury Prevention and Control. (2002b). Preventing falls. Available: http://www.cdc.gov/ncipc/ duip/spotlite/falls.htm

Centers for Medicare and Medicaid Services. (2008). CMS guidance document: Revised interpretative guidelines for restraint or seclusion. Retrieved November 22, 2008, from http://cms.hhs.gov/EOG/downloads/EO%200306.pdf

Converso, A., DeMass Martin, S. L., & Markle-Elder, S. (2007). Health and safety: Is your hospital safe? *American Journal of Nursing, 107*(2), 37.

Guyton, A. C., & Hall, J. (2005). *Textbook of medical physiology* (11th ed.). Philadelphia: W. B. Saunders.

Jasniewski, J. (2006). Healthier aging: Take steps to protect your patient from falls. *Nursing2006, 36*(4), 24–25.

Joint Commission. (2001). *Comprehensive accreditation manual for hospitals.* Oakbrook Terrace, IL: Author.

Kimbell, S. (2001). Before the fall: Keeping your patient on his feet. *Nursing2001, 31*(8), 44–45.

Larson, E. (2002). The "hygiene hypothesis": How clean should we be? *American Journal of Nursing, 102*(1), 81–89.

Moorhead, S., Johnson, M., Maas, M. L., & Swanson, E. (2007). *Nursing Outcomes Classification (NOC)* (4th ed.). St. Louis, MO: Mosby.

Napierkowski, D. (2002). Using restraints with restraint. *Nursing2002, 32*(11), 58–62.

National Institute for Occupational Safety and Health. (2002). *About NIOSH research and services.* Available: http://www.cdc.gov/niosh/about.html

National Institute for Occupational Safety and Health. (2008). NIOSH safety and health topic: Traumatic occupational injuries. Retrieved November 16, 2008, from http://www.cdc.gov/niosh/injury/#data

North American Nursing Diagnosis Association International. (2010). *NANDA-I nursing diagnoses: Definitions and classification 2009-2011.* Ames, IA: Wiley-Blackwell.

Occupational Safety and Health Administration. (2009) Types of fire extinguishers. Retrieved May 16, 2009, from http://www.osha.gov/SLTC/etools/evacuation/portable_about.html#Types

Parini, S., & Myers, F. (2003). Keeping up with hand hygiene recommendations. *Nursing2003, 33*(92), 17.

Ramponi, D. (2001). Eye on contact lens removal. *Nursing2001, 31*(8), 56–57.

Schweon, S., & Novatnack, E. (2003). Don't underestimate Group A strep. *RN, 66*(8), 28–32.

Stanhope, M., & Knollmueller, R. (2000). *Handbook of community-based and home health nursing practice: Tools for assessment, intervention, and education* (3rd ed.). St. Louis, MO: Mosby.

Swauger, K., & Tomlin, C. (2002). Moving toward restraint free patient care. *Journal of Nursing Administration, 30*(6), 325–329.

Sweeney-Calciano, J., Solimene, A., & Forrester, D. (2003). Finding a way to avoid restraints. *Nursing2003, 33*(5), 32hn1–32hn4.

Talerico, K., & Capezuti, E. (2001). Myths and facts about side rails. *American Journal of Nursing, 101*(7), 43–48.

U.S. Department of Energy (Hanford Fire Department). (2001). HFD: All you ever wanted to know about fire extinguishers. Available: http://www.hanford.gov/fire/safety/extingrs.htm

U.S. Department of Labor. (2002). Workplace fire safety. Available: http://www.cdc.gov/nasd/docs/d000701-0000800/d000737/d000737.html

U.S. Food and Drug Administration. (1996). FDA safety alert: Entrapment hazards with hospital bed side rails. Available: http://www.fda.gov/cdrh/bedrails.html

U.S. Food and Drug Administration. (2008). A guide to bed safety bed rails in hospitals, nursing homes and home health care: The facts. Retrieved November 22, 2008, from http://www.fda.gov/cdrh/beds/bed_brochure.html

Walker, B. (1998). *Injury prevention for the elderly: Preventing falls.* Gaithersberg, MD: Aspen.

Walker, B. (1998). Preventing falls. *RN, 61*(5), 40–42.

Yoneyama, T., et al. (2002). Oral care reduces pneumonia in older patients in nursing homes. *Journal of the American Geriatric Society, 50*(3).

RESOURCES

Association for Professionals in Infection Control and Epidemiology, Inc., http://www.apic.org

Centers for Medicare and Medicaid Services, http://www.cms.hhs.gov

Environmental Protection Agency, http://www.epa.gov

Food and Drug Administration, http://www.fda.gov

Joint Commission, http://www.jointcommission.org

National Institute for Occupational Safety and Health, http://www.cdc.gov.niosh

U.S. Consumer Product Safety Commission, http://www.cpsc.gov

UNIT 6 Infection Control

CHAPTER 21
Infection Control/Asepsis

MAKING THE CONNECTION

Refer to the following chapters to increase your understanding of infection control/ asepsis:

Basic Nursing
- ***Basic Nutrition***
- ***Safety/Hygiene***
- ***Standard Precautions and Isolation***
- ***Fluid, Electrolyte, and Acid–Base Balance***

Adult Health Nursing
- ***Surgery***

Basic Procedures
- ***Hand Hygiene***
- ***Use of Protective Equipment***

Intermediate Procedures
- ***Surgical Asepsis: Preparing and Maintaining a Sterile Field***
- ***Performing Open Gloving***
- ***Applying a Dry Dressing***

LEARNING OBJECTIVES

Upon completion of this chapter, you should be able to:

- Define key terms.
- Describe the chain of infection.
- Discuss the body's nonspecific and specific immune defenses.
- Describe the stages of the inflammatory process.
- Discuss the stages of the infectious process.
- Identify the signs and symptoms of inflammation and infection.
- Explain the principles of medical and surgical asepsis.
- Provide client care maintaining the principles of medical and/or surgical asepsis.

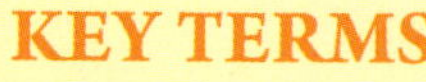

KEY TERMS

acquired immunity
agent
airborne transmission
antibodies
asepsis
aseptic technique
bactericides
biological agents
carriers
chain of infection
chemical agents
clean objects

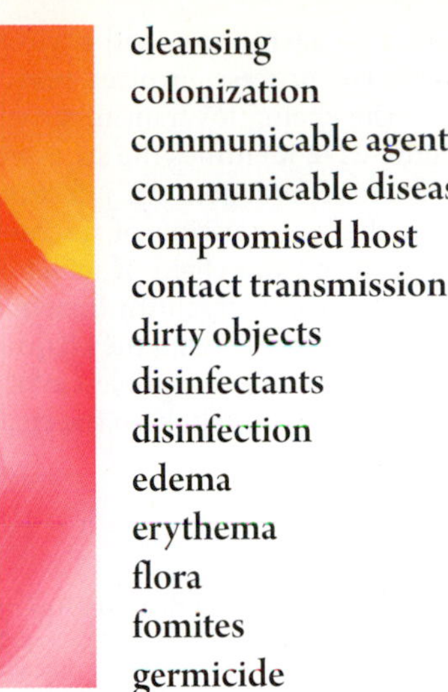

cleansing
colonization
communicable agents
communicable disease
compromised host
contact transmission
dirty objects
disinfectants
disinfection
edema
erythema
flora
fomites
germicide
hand hygiene
hospital-acquired infection
host
humoral immunity
immunization
infection
infectious agents
inflammation
localized infections
medical asepsis
mode of transmission
pathogens
pathogenicity
physical agents
portal of entry
portal of exit
purulent exudate
reservoir
resident flora
sterilization
surgical asepsis
susceptible host
systemic infection
transient flora
vaccination
vector-borne transmission
vehicle transmission
virulence

INTRODUCTION

Nurses are responsible for providing quality care that incorporates infection-control principles. These principles are a major component of a safe environment. This chapter discusses infection-control principles. including naturally occurring microorganisms, pathogens, infection and colonization, chain of infection, body defenses, stages of the infectious process, and hospital-acquired infections. Discussion of the nurse's role in controlling infections is emphasized.

FLORA

Flora are microorganisms that occur or have adapted to live in a specific environment, such as intestinal, skin, vaginal, or oral flora. There are two types of flora: resident and transient. **Resident** (normal) **flora** are microorganisms that are always present, usually without altering the client's health; an example would be *propionibacterium* on the skin. Resident flora prevent the overgrowth of harmful microorganisms; only when the balance is upset does disease result. **Transient flora** are microorganisms that are episodic (of limited duration); an example would be *staphylococcus aureus*. They attach to the skin for a brief period of time but do not continually live on the skin. Transient flora are usually acquired from direct contact with the microorganisms on environmental surfaces.

PATHOGENICITY AND VIRULENCE

Although most microorganisms found in the environment do not cause disease and infection, some do. Disease-producing microorganisms are called **pathogens**; **pathogenicity** refers to the ability of a microorganism to produce disease. **Virulence** refers to the frequency with which a pathogen causes disease. The factors affecting virulence are the strength of the pathogen to adhere to healthy cells, the ability of a pathogen to damage cells or interfere with the body's normal regulating systems, and the ability of a pathogen to evade the attack of white blood cells (WBCs).

Five types of microorganisms can be pathogenic: bacteria, viruses, fungi, protozoa, and *rickettsia*.

BACTERIA

Bacteria are small, one-celled microorganisms that lack a true nucleus or mechanism to provide metabolism. Therefore, bacteria need an environment that will provide food for survival. Bacteria can be spherical, rodlike, spiral, or curving in shape, usually appearing as single cells, pairs, chains, or groups. Although most bacteria multiply by simple cell division, some forms of bacteria produce spores, a resistant stage that withstands unfavorable environments. When proper environmental conditions return, spores germinate and form new cells. Spores are difficult to kill because of their resistance to heat, drying, and disinfectants. The growth rate of bacteria is affected by environmental factors such as changes in temperature and nutrition. The optimal temperature for pathogenic bacteria is 98.6°F.

Bacteria can be found in all environments, yet not all bacteria are harmful or cause disease. Only a small percentage of bacteria are actually pathogenic. Common bacterial infections include diarrhea, pneumonia, sinusitis, urinary tract infections, cellulitis, meningitis, gonorrhea, otitis media, and impetigo.

VIRUSES

Viruses are organisms that can live only inside cells. They cannot get nourishment or reproduce outside cells. Viruses contain a core of deoxyribonucleic acid (DNA) or ribonucleic acid (RNA) surrounded by a protein coating. Some viruses have the ability to create an additional coating called an envelope, which helps protect the cell from attack by the immune system. Viruses damage the cells they inhabit by blocking the normal protein synthesis of the cells and by using the cell's mechanism for metabolism to reproduce.

The same viral infection may cause different symptoms in different individuals, based on the individual's immune response to the invading virus. Some viruses will immediately trigger a disease response, whereas others may remain latent for many years. Common viral infections include influenza, measles, common cold, chickenpox, hepatitis B, genital herpes, and HIV.

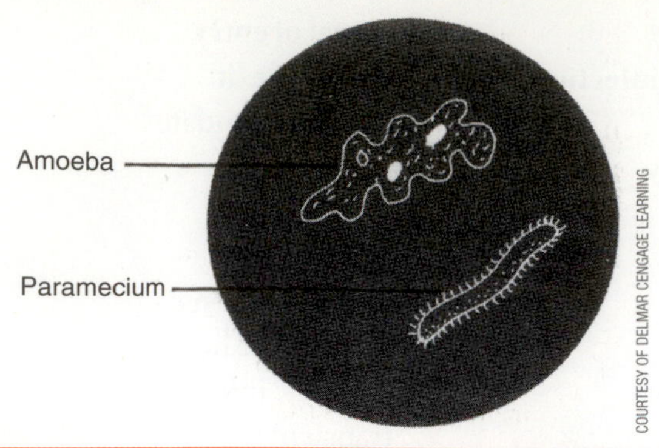

FIGURE 21-1 Protozoa

FUNGI

Fungi grow in single cells, as in yeast, or in colonies, as in molds. Fungi obtain food from dead organic matter or from living organisms. Most fungi are not pathogenic and make up many of the body's normal flora. Disease from fungi is found mainly in individuals who are immunologically impaired. Fungi can cause infections of the hair, skin, nails, and mucous membranes.

PROTOZOA

Protozoa are single-celled parasitic organisms with the ability to move (Figure 21-1). Most protozoa obtain their nourishment from dead or decaying organic matter. Infection is spread through ingestion of contaminated food or water or through insect bites. Common protozoan infections include malaria, gastroenteritis, and vaginal infections.

RICKETTSIA

Rickettsia are intracellular parasites that need to be in living cells to reproduce. Infection from *rickettsia* is spread through fleas, ticks, mites, and lice. Common *rickettsia* infections include typhus, Rocky Mountain spotted fever, and Lyme disease.

COLONIZATION AND INFECTION

Colonization is the multiplication of microorganisms on or within a host that does not result in cellular injury; an example of colonization is the normal flora (microorganisms) in the intestines. However, if host susceptibility increases or the microorganism's virulence increases, colonized microorganisms on a host may be a potential source of infection.

Infection is the invasion and multiplication of pathogenic microorganisms in body tissue that results in cellular injury; an example is strep throat. These microorganisms are called **infectious agents**. Infectious agents capable of being transmitted to a client by direct or indirect contact, through a vehicle (or vector) or airborne route are called **communicable agents**. Diseases produced by these agents are referred to as **communicable diseases**.

CHAIN OF INFECTION

Neither a susceptible host nor the presence of a pathogen means that an infectious process will occur. The **chain of infection** describes the development of an infectious process. An interactive process involving an agent, host, and environment is required. This interactive process involves several essential elements, or "links in the chain," for transmission of microorganisms to occur. Figure 21-2 identifies the six essential links (elements) in the chain of infection. An infectious process cannot occur without the transmission of microorganisms. Therefore, knowledge about the chain of infection facilitates control or elimination of microorganism transmission by breaking the links in the chain. Breaking the chain of infection is achieved by altering the interactive process of the agent, host, and environment. Each of the six links in the chain of infection is discussed following.

AGENT

An **agent** is an entity that is capable of causing disease. Agents that cause disease may be as follows:

- **Biological agents**: Living organisms that invade the host, causing disease, such as bacteria, viruses, fungi, protozoa, and rickettsia
- **Chemical agents**: Substances that can interact with the body, causing disease, such as food additives, medications, pesticides, and industrial chemicals
- **Physical agents**: Factors in the environment that are capable of causing disease, such as heat, light, noise, and radiation

In the chain of infection, the main concern is biological agents and their effect on the host.

RESERVOIR

The **reservoir** is a place where the agent can survive. Colonization and reproduction take place while the agent is in the reservoir. A reservoir that promotes growth of pathogens must contain the proper nutrients (such as oxygen and organic matter), maintain proper temperature, contain moisture, maintain a compatible pH level (neither too acidic nor too alkaline), and maintain the proper amount of light exposure. The most common reservoirs are:

- Humans
- Animals
- Environment
- **Fomites** (objects contaminated with an infectious agent, such as bedpans, urinals, bed linens, instruments, dressings, specimen containers, and other equipment)

Humans and animals can have symptoms of the infectious agents or can be strictly carriers of the agent. **Carriers** have the infectious agent but are symptom free. The agent can be spread to others in both instances.

PORTAL OF EXIT

The **portal of exit** is the route by which an infectious agent leaves the reservoir to be transferred to a susceptible host. The agent leaves the reservoir through body secretions including:

- Sputum, from the respiratory tract
- Semen, vaginal secretions, or urine, from the genitourinary tract
- Saliva and feces, from the gastrointestinal tract
- Blood
- Draining wounds
- Tears

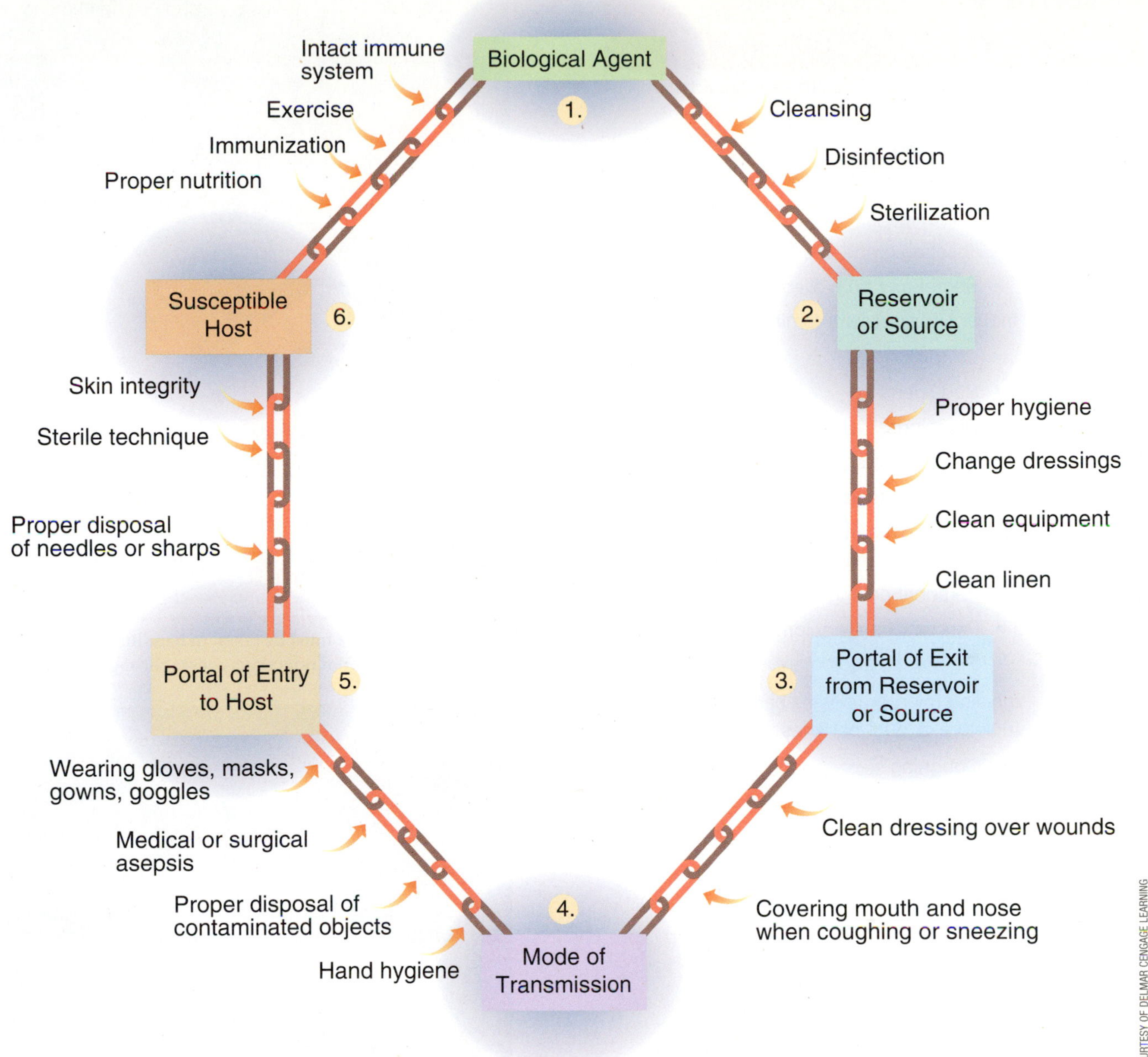

FIGURE 21-2 The Chain of Infection: Preventive Measures Follow Each Link of the Chain

MODES OF TRANSMISSION

The **mode of transmission** is the process of the infectious agent moving from the reservoir or source through the portal of exit to the portal of entry of the susceptible "new" host. Most infectious agents have a usual or primary mode of transmission, but some microorganisms may be transmitted by more than one mode (Table 21-1). Depending on the agent, almost anything in the environment can become a potential mode of transmission.

Contact Transmission

The most important and frequent mode of transmission is **contact transmission**. This involves the transfer of an agent from an infected person to a host by direct contact with the infected person, indirect contact with the infected person through a fomite, or close contact with contaminated secretions (Figure 21-3). Sexually transmitted diseases are spread by direct contact. Common viral infections (cold, measles, flu) are spread by close contact with contaminated secretions.

Airborne Transmission

Airborne transmission occurs when a susceptible host contacts droplet nuclei or dust particles that are suspended in the air. Particle size influences the length of time that the organism can remain airborne. The longer the particle is suspended, the greater the chance it will find an available port of entry to the human host. A disease that relies on airborne transmission is measles. Contaminated droplets containing the measles virus are in the spray from sneezing. The droplet can find a portal of entry through the mucous membranes or conjunctiva.

Vehicle Transmission

Vehicle transmission occurs when an agent is transferred to a susceptible host by contaminated inanimate objects such as

TABLE 21-1 Modes of Transmission

MODE	EXAMPLES
Contact	Direct contact of health care provider with client: • Touching • Bathing • Rubbing • Toileting (urine and feces) • Secretions from client Indirect contact with fomites: • Clothing • Bed linens • Dressings • Health care equipment • Instruments used in treatments • Specimen containers used for laboratory analysis • Personal belongings • Personal care equipment • Diagnostic equipment
Airborne	Inhaling microorganisms carried by moisture or dust particles in air: • Coughing • Talking • Sneezing
Vehicle	Contact with contaminated inanimate objects: • Water • Blood • Drugs • Food • Urine
Vector-borne	Contact with contaminated animate hosts: • Animals • Insects

COURTESY OF DELMAR CENGAGE LEARNING

water, food, milk (Figure 21-4), drugs, and blood. Cholera is transmitted through contaminated drinking water, and salmonellosis is transmitted through contaminated meat.

Vector-Borne Transmission

Vector-borne transmission occurs when an agent is transferred to a susceptible host by animate means such as mosquitoes, fleas, ticks, lice, and other animals (Figure 21-5). Lyme disease, malaria, and West Nile virus are examples of diseases spread by vectors.

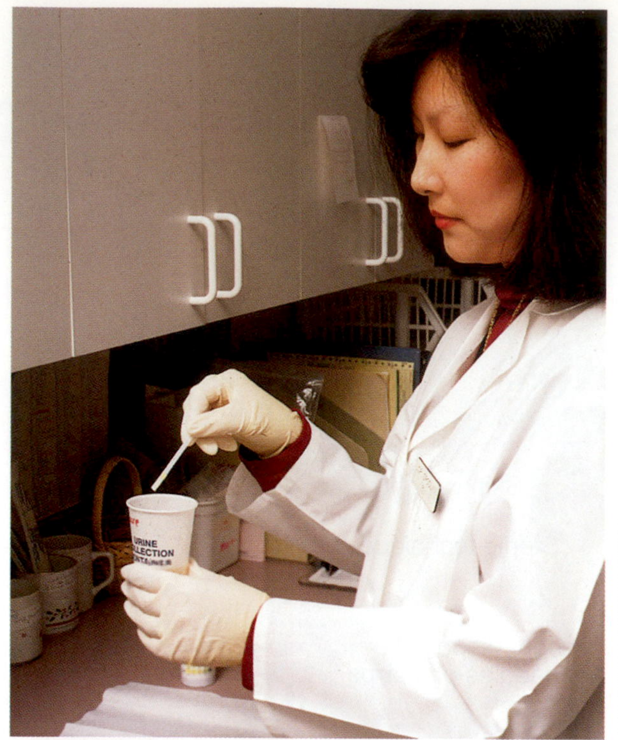

COURTESY OF DELMAR CENGAGE LEARNING

FIGURE 21-3 Care must be taken in handling bodily fluids to prevent the transfer of infectious agents through contact.

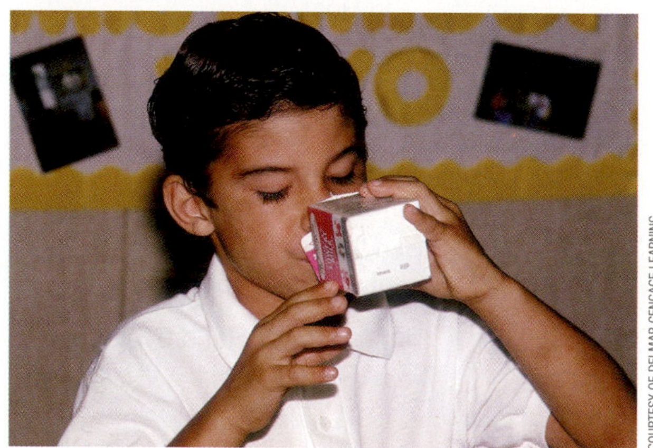
COURTESY OF DELMAR CENGAGE LEARNING

FIGURE 21-4 Vehicle transmission occurs through contamination of inanimate objects, such as milk.

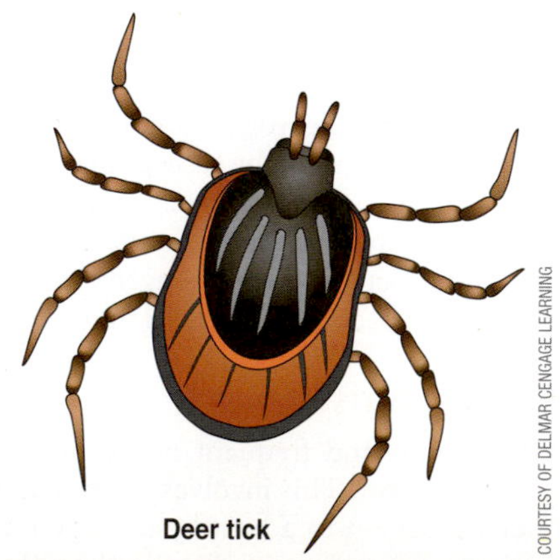

COURTESY OF DELMAR CENGAGE LEARNING

FIGURE 21-5 Lyme disease and other infections are caused by the bite of a tick.

Portal of Entry

A **portal of entry** is the route by which an infectious agent enters the host. Portals of entry include the following:

- *Integumentary system,* through a break in the integrity of the skin or mucous membranes (e.g., infections of surgical wounds)
- *Respiratory tract,* by inhaling contaminated droplets (such as cold, influenza, measles)
- *Genitourinary tract,* through contact with infected vaginal secretions or semen (as in sexually transmitted diseases)
- *Gastrointestinal tract,* by ingesting contaminated food or water (e.g., typhoid, hepatitis A)
- *Circulatory system,* through the bite of insects (such as mosquito bites resulting in malaria)
- *Transplacental,* through transfer of microorganisms from mother to fetus via the placenta and umbilical cord (including HIV, hepatitis B)

Host

A **host** is an organism that can be affected by an agent. A human being is usually considered a host. A **susceptible host** is a person who has no resistance to an agent and thus is vulnerable to disease. For example, an individual who has not received the measles vaccine is more likely to contract the infection because of the lack of immunity to the infectious agent. A **compromised host** is a person whose normal body defenses are impaired and is therefore susceptible to infection. For example, a person with a common cold or superficial burns is at greater risk for infection because of the impaired state of the body system mechanisms.

Characteristics of the host influence the susceptibility to and severity of infections. These include:

- *Age.* As a person ages, immunity declines, thus increasing susceptibility to infection.
- *Concurrent diseases.* The existence of comorbid diseases indicates an environment susceptible to infection.
- *Stress.* An individual experiencing a compromised emotional state may have altered or decreased immune system response.
- *Immunization/vaccination status.* Individuals who are not fully immunized are at greater risk for infection.
- *Lifestyle.* Lifestyle practices such as having multiple sex partners or sharing intravenous drug needles increase an individual's potential for illness.
- *Occupation.* Forms of employment that involve an increased exposure to pathogens might include dealing with chemical agents (such as asbestos) or handling sharp instruments (such as scalpels).
- *Nutritional status.* Individuals who maintain targeted weight for height and body frame are less prone to illness.
- *Heredity.* Some individuals are naturally more susceptible to infection than others.

Interaction between agent and host occurs in the environment, which is everything other than the agent and host. Many of the conditions promoting transmission of microorganisms reflect changes in the relationship between humans and their environments.

PROFESSIONALTIP

Infectious Diseases

Berlinguer (1992) notes that the causes of most emerging infectious diseases are the same today as throughout recorded history: the transfer and dissemination of existing agents to new host populations (a process called "global microbial traffic"). For instance, cholera probably originated in Asia in ancient times; in the 19th century, it spread to Europe and the New World because of increased global travel. Cholera entered South America for the first time in 1992 through the possible contaminated bilge water released from a Chinese freighter. West Nile virus was unknown in the United States until 1999 (APIC, 2004). The causes of emerging infectious diseases and outbreaks require careful consideration of changes in relationship between humans and their environments.

BREAKING THE CHAIN OF INFECTION

Nurses focus on breaking the chain of infection by applying proper infection-control practices to interrupt the transmission of microorganisms. Specific strategies can be directed at breaking or blocking the transmission of infection from one link in the chain to the next. A discussion regarding each of the six links follows (refer back to Figure 21-2).

Between Agent and Reservoir

The first link in the chain of infection is between the agent and the reservoir. The keys to eliminating infection at this point in the chain are cleansing, disinfection, and sterilization. These practices prevent the formation of a reservoir where infectious agents can live and multiply.

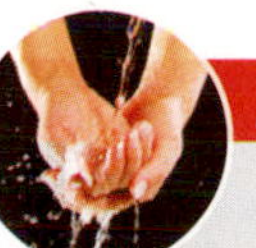

INFECTION CONTROL

First Line of Defense

Hand hygiene is the first line of defense against infection and is the single most important practice in preventing the spread of infection.

CRITICAL THINKING

Chain of Infection

How is the chain of infection applicable in everyday life in a person's home?

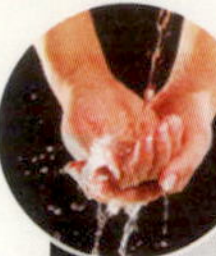

INFECTION CONTROL

Cleansing

Cleansing is a potential hazard to the nurse from the splashing of contaminated material onto the body. Nurses should wear gloves, masks, and goggles during cleansing.

Cleansing

Cleansing is the removal of soil or organic material from instruments and equipment used in providing client care. Nurses often cleanse instruments after assisting or performing invasive procedures. To reduce the amount of contamination and loosen the material on reusable objects, the objects are cleansed before sterilization or disinfection. Cleansing involves the use of water, mechanical action, and, sometimes, a detergent. Contaminated objects are cleansed using a soft-bristled brush to scrub the surface. The steps for proper cleansing are:

1. Wet the object with *cold* water; warm water coagulates the proteins in organic material and makes them stick.
2. Apply detergent and scrub the object under running water using a soft-bristled brush.
3. Rinse the object under warm running water.
4. Dry the object before sterilization or disinfection.

Disinfection

Disinfection is the elimination of pathogens, except spores, from inanimate objects. **Disinfectants** are chemical solutions used to clean inanimate objects. The U.S. Environmental Protection Agency (EPA) licenses intermediate and low-level disinfectants. The Food and Drug Administration (FDA) regulates high-level disinfectants. Common disinfectants are alcohol, sodium hypochlorite, quaternary ammonium, and phenolic solutions.

A **germicide** is a chemical that can be applied to both animate (living) and inanimate objects to eliminate pathogens. Antiseptic preparations such as alcohol and silver sulfadiazine are germicides.

Sterilization

Sterilization is destroying all microorganisms including spores. Equipment that enters normally sterile tissue or blood vessels must be sterilized. Methods of achieving sterilization are moist heat (steam), dry heat, and ethylene oxide gas. The method of sterilization depends on the object to be sterilized and the kind and amount of contamination.

COMMUNITY/HOME HEALTH CARE

Disinfection

In the home, Lysol and bleach are common disinfectants capable of eliminating some pathogens. The recommended concentration of bleach solution is one part bleach to nine parts water (CDC, 2007a).

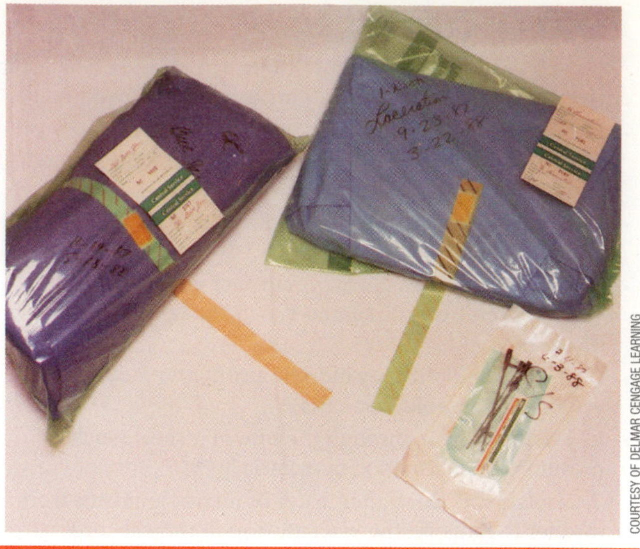

COURTESY OF DELMAR CENGAGE LEARNING

FIGURE 21-6 Sterilized packages. The strips below each package show the way they looked before sterilization. The strips on the packages have changed color because they have been sterilized.

Autoclaving sterilization, which uses moist heat or steam, is the most common sterilization technique used in the hospital setting (Figure 21-6). Boiling water is not an effective sterilization measure because some viruses and spores can survive boiling water.

BETWEEN RESERVOIR AND PORTAL OF EXIT

Promoting proper hygiene, changing dressings and linens, and ensuring that clean equipment is used in client care are ways to break the chain of infection between the reservoir and the portal of exit. The goal is to eliminate the reservoir for the microorganism before a pathogen can escape to a susceptible host.

Proper Hygiene

Educate clients on the importance of maintaining the cleanliness and integrity of the skin and the mucous membranes. Clean skin, hair, and nails maintain the body's normal flora and eliminate transient flora from the client's system. Bathing and hand hygiene are important ways to eliminate the potential for infection. Clients should be encouraged to practice daily bathing and teeth brushing. Clients who are unable to perform these activities independently should be assisted.

COMMUNITY/HOME HEALTH CARE

Sterilization at Home

The CDC (2008) recommends boiling water as the preferred way to kill harmful bacteria and parasites. Bringing water to a rolling boil for 1 full minute will kill most organisms. Chemical contaminants in water will not be removed by boiling.

PROFESSIONALTIP

The Client Who Is Bedridden

Be alert to the formation of pressure ulcers in clients who are bedridden. Open ulcers are a possible source for infection if left untreated.

Change Dressings

Any open injury or other break in skin integrity represents a potential reservoir for infectious agents and portal of exit for a pathogen to be transferred to another individual. Dressings on open or oozing wounds must be changed regularly. To protect both yourself and the client from infection, follow proper aseptic technique when changing dressings. This technique is discussed in detail later in this chapter.

Clean Linens

Bed linens, gowns, and towels are catchalls for bodily secretions. Infectious agents can be easily transferred from one individual to the next through contact with a client's linens. Linens must be changed regularly, and soiled linens must be properly disposed. When changing linens, take care to keep the soiled articles from contact with your uniform. This will prevent being infected from the soiled linens or passing the infection on to other clients.

Clean Equipment

All equipment used in the care of a client must be cleansed and disinfected after each use. Although many items such as disposable gowns can be discarded after use, items such as beds must be thoroughly cleansed after each use. Clients should be instructed never to share care items. Any nondisposable equipment used in an invasive procedure (such as equipment used in the operating room [OR]) must be sterilized before being used again. Wear gloves and masks when cleansing equipment to avoid being splashed with contaminated waste products or secretions.

Between Portal of Exit and Mode of Transmission

The goal in breaking the chain of infection between the portal of exit and the mode of transmission is to prevent the exit of the infectious agents. Clean dressings must be maintained on all wounds. Clients should be encouraged to cover their mouths and noses when sneezing or coughing, and the nurse must do so as well. Gloves must be worn when caring for a client who may have infectious secretions, and care must be taken to properly dispose of any contaminated article.

Between Mode of Transmission and Portal of Entry

To break the chain of infection between the mode of transmission and the portal of entry, asepsis must be ensured and barrier protection worn when the care of clients involves contact with body secretions. Gloves, masks, gowns, and goggles are barrier protection that can be used. Proper hand hygiene and proper disposal of contaminated equipment and linens are ways to prevent transmission of microorganisms to other clients and health care workers. A thorough discussion of asepsis and disposal of contaminated items is included later in this chapter.

Between Portal of Entry and Host

Maintaining skin integrity and using sterile technique for client contacts are methods of breaking the chain of infection between portal of entry and host. Avoiding needle sticks by properly disposing of sharps also reduces the potential for infection by denying a portal of entry. The goal at this point in the chain is to prevent the transmission of infection to a client or health care worker who is not infected.

Between Host and Agent

Breaking the chain of infection between host and agent means eliminating infection before it begins. There are many ways to reduce the risk of acquiring infection: Proper nutrition, exercise, adequate rest and sleep, and immunizations allow an individual to maintain an intact immune system, thus preventing infection.

Proper Nutrition

Proper nutrition assists the body's immune system to function properly. Clients need adequate amounts of protein in their diets to maintain and repair tissue as well as to produce the antibodies needed to fight infection. A balanced diet also allows the body to maintain appropriate acid–base balance.

Exercise

Exercise maintains the body's metabolic rate and, therefore, allows the body to maintain the antibodies and energy necessary to ward off infection.

Rest and Sleep

Rest and sleep are basic to a client's health and well-being. The quality of rest and sleep can have a significant impact on a person's health. Adequate levels of rest and sleep provide a restorative function needed for physiological and psychological healing.

Immunization

Immunization is the process of creating immunity, or resistance to infection, in an individual. Many immunizations are given in early childhood (e.g., measles, mumps, and rubella). Immunization for the flu must be given every year and for tetanus every 10 years.

BODY DEFENSES

A host's immune system is a defense against infectious agents. The immune system is able to recognize "self" and "nonself"; that is, the immune system recognizes what is not consistent with the genetic composition of the host (self). These agents are called antigens (nonself). An immune response against an antigen protects the body from infection.

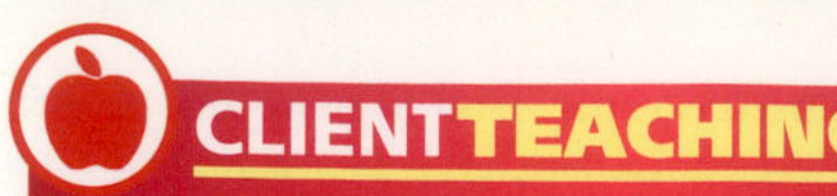

Inappropriate Use of Antibiotics

- Do not pressure the physician or nurse practitioner to prescribe antibiotics for every illness. Antibiotics are not always appropriate. They are not effective against viruses.
- When antibiotics are prescribed, the client should take all of the medication as directed.
- Antibiotics taken only until the client feels better allow the microorganisms to become resistant to the antibiotic, and the antibiotic will no longer be effective.
- Antibiotics also destroy normal flora microorganisms, and other illnesses may ensue.

Nonspecific Immune Defense

The nonspecific immune defense protects the host from all microorganisms; it does not depend on prior exposure to an antigen. Nonspecific immune defenses are skin and normal flora; mucous membranes; coughing, sneezing, and tearing reflexes; elimination and acidic environment; and inflammation.

Skin and Normal Flora

The skin, the first line of defense against infection, serves as a physical barrier to infectious agents. Skin cells, shed daily, remove potentially harmful microorganisms. Sebum, a substance produced by the skin, contains fatty acids that kill some bacteria. The normal flora residing on the skin and in the body compete with pathogenic flora for food and inhibit pathogen multiplication. The balance of normal flora may become disrupted, allowing pathogenic organisms to proliferate, causing infection or superinfection.

Mucous Membranes

Mucous membranes also are a physical barrier to infectious agents. Mucus produced by these membranes entraps infectious agents and inhibits bacterial growth. For example, the cilia of the respiratory tract trap and propel mucus and microorganisms away from the lungs, thereby reducing the potential for infection.

Coughing, Sneezing, and Tearing Reflexes

The cough and sneeze reflexes forcibly expel mucus and microorganisms from the respiratory tract. Tears protect the eyes by continually flushing away microorganisms. Tears also contain **bactericides**, which are bacteria-killing chemicals.

Elimination and Acidic Environment

Elimination and an acidic environment usually prevent growth of pathogenic organisms. Resident flora of the large intestines prevent the growth of pathogens. The mechanical process of defecation removes microorganisms with the feces. Urine acidity prevents microbial growth. Urination flushes and cleans the bladder neck and urethra of microorganisms and prevents microorganisms from ascending into the urinary tract.

Normal vaginal flora prevent growth of several pathogens. At puberty, lactobacilli ferment and produce sugars in the vagina that lower the pH to an acidic range. The acidic environment of the vagina prevents pathogenic growth.

Inflammation

Inflammation is a nonspecific cellular response to tissue injury. Tissue injury caused by bacteria, trauma, chemicals, heat, or any other occurrence releases substances, producing dramatic secondary changes in the injured tissue. This entire complex of tissue changes in response to injury is called the *inflammatory process* (Table 21-2). The body's response to injury produces characteristic local and systemic signs of inflammation.

Inflammation, while not necessarily the result of invading microorganisms, does have signs and symptoms similar to those of an infection. The primary signs of inflammation and infection are as follows:

- Redness (**erythema**) results from increased blood flow to the area.
- Heat results from increased blood flow and metabolism in the area.

Table 21-2 Stages of the Inflammatory Process

STAGE	DESCRIPTION	RESULT
1	Initial injury causes release of chemicals: histamine, bradykinin, serotonin, prostaglandins, and lymphokines.	Initiates the inflammation process
2	Blood flow increases to the injured area.	Produces characteristic redness and warmth
3	Increased capillary permeability leaks large amounts of plasma into the damaged tissue; tissue spaces and lymphatics are blocked by fibrinogen clots.	"Walls off" infection; results in nonpitting edema
4	Leukocytes infiltrate damaged tissue and engulf the bacteria and necrotic tissue. After several days, these leukocytes die and form a cavity of necrotic tissue and dead leukocytes.	Produces purulent exudate (pus)
5	Destroyed tissue cells are replaced by identical or similar structural and functioning cells and/or fibrous tissue.	Promotes tissue healing or the formation of fibrous (scar) tissue, which may reduce the functional capacity of the tissue

COURTESY OF DELMAR CENGAGE LEARNING

- Pain results from increased pressure on pain sensors in the area.
- Swelling (**edema**, a detectable accumulation of increased interstitial fluid) results from fluid and leukocytes entering the tissues from the circulatory system.
- Loss of function results from both pain and swelling and is the body's way of resting the injured part.
- Pus (**purulent exudate**), resulting from infection, is a secretion made up of white blood cells, dead cells, bacteria, and other debris.

The inflammatory process intensity is usually in proportion to the degree of tissue injury.

Specific Immune Defense

The specific immune defense is a response specific to the invading antigen. It is activated when phagocytes fail to completely destroy the antigen. This causes production of T lymphocytes (T cells), which regulate the immune response by activating other cells. The T cells move to the injured area and release chemical substances called lymphokines. Lymphokines attract other phagocytes and lymphocytes to the injured area and assist in antigen destruction.

The T cells also stimulate the production of B cells, which become plasma cells, producing antibodies specific to the antigen. **Antibodies** are protein substances that destroy the antigen. The stimulation of B cells and the production of antibodies are collectively known as **humoral immunity**.

Memory B cells are formed to remember the antigen and prepare the host for future antigen invasion. When the antigen enters the body again, the immune response occurs faster by rapidly producing antibodies. The formation of these antibodies is referred to as **acquired immunity**, which protects the individual against future invasions of already experienced antigens such as lethal bacteria, viruses, toxins, and even foreign tissues.

The process of **vaccination** (inoculation with a vaccine to produce immunity against specific diseases) provides acquired immunity. There are three types of vaccines:

1. Dead organisms that are no longer capable of causing disease but still have their chemical antigens, such as typhoid, whooping cough, and diphtheria
2. Toxins that have been chemically treated so their toxic nature is destroyed but their antigens are still intact, such as for tetanus and botulism
3. Live organisms that have been attenuated (rendered incapable of causing the disease yet still have the specific antigen), such as for poliomyelitis, yellow fever, measles, smallpox, and many other viral diseases (Guyton & Hall, 2005)

TYPES AND STAGES OF INFECTIONS

Infection is the result of tissue invasion and damage by an infectious agent. There are two types of infections:

1. **Localized infections** are limited to a defined area or single organ with symptoms that resemble inflammation (redness, tenderness, and swelling), such as a cold sore.
2. **Systemic infections** affect the entire body and involve multiple organs, such as AIDS.

All infections progress through four stages: incubation, prodromal, illness, and convalescence.

SAFETY

Incubation Period

Always verify the incubation period of a suspected infection. Remember that a client may be able to transmit the infection to another person before the onset of symptoms.

Incubation Stage

The incubation period is the time between entry of an infectious agent in the host and the onset of symptoms. During this time, the infectious agent invades the tissue and multiplies to produce an infection. The client is typically infectious to others during the latter part of this stage. For example, the incubation period for varicella (chickenpox) is 2 to 3 weeks; the infected person is contagious from 5 days before any skin eruptions to no more than 6 days after the skin eruptions appear.

Prodromal Stage

The prodromal stage is the time from the onset of nonspecific symptoms until specific symptoms begin to manifest. The infectious agent continues to invade and multiply in the host. A client may also be infectious to other persons during this time period. In the client with chickenpox, a slight elevation in temperature will occur during this stage, followed within 24 hours by eruptions on the skin.

Illness Stage

The illness stage is the time when the client has specific signs and symptoms of an infectious process. The client with chickenpox will experience a further rise in temperature and continued outbreaks of skin eruptions for at least 2 to 3 more days.

Convalescent Stage

The convalescent stage is from the beginning of the disappearance of acute symptoms until the client returns to the previous state of health. The client with chickenpox will see the skin eruptions and irritation begin to resolve during this stage.

HOSPITAL-ACQUIRED INFECTIONS

A **hospital-acquired infection** is an infection acquired in a hospital or other health care facility that was not present or incubating at the time of the client's admission. They also include those infections that become symptomatic after the client is discharged and infections passed among medical personnel. Hospital-acquired infections are also called *nosocomial infections* or health care–associated infections. These types of infections typically fall into four categories: urinary tract, surgical wounds, pneumonia, and septicemia.

Most hospital-acquired infections are transmitted by health care personnel who fail to practice proper hand hygiene or who fail to change gloves between client contacts.

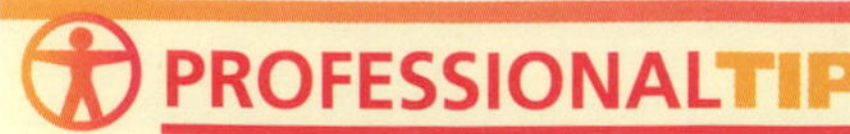

Health Care–Associated Infections

Each year, 1.7 million health care–associated infections occur in the United States. Further, the client's length of stay is increased, costing nearly $20 billion annually for the associated extended care and treatment (Wright, 2008).

CRITICAL THINKING

Hospital-Acquired Infections

Why are hospital-acquired infections such a huge problem?

The hospital environment provides exposure to a variety of organisms to which the client has not typically been exposed in the past. Therefore, the client has no resistance to these organisms. Illness impairs the body's defenses.

NURSING PROCESS

Quality nursing care requires the reduction of microorganism transmission in the health care environment. Infection-control practices are directed at controlling or eliminating sources of infection in the health care agency or home. Nurses are responsible for protecting clients and themselves by using infection-control practices.

Assessment

Assessment data guides the prioritization of the client's problem and identification of appropriate nursing diagnoses. Clients at risk for infection require frequent reassessment followed by appropriate changes in the plan of care, goals, and nursing interventions.

The health history and physical examination data correlated with the laboratory results identify those clients at risk for infection. Appropriate risk appraisals may be incorporated into the nursing health history interview.

Subjective Data

Relevant data regarding the client at risk for infection are obtained in the health history. A comprehensive assessment also involves appraising the client's environment to detect potential hazards and the client's self-care abilities. Reviewing such factors as work environment, immunization status, and other health-related issues may help identify actual or possible infection risks.

Objective Data

Objective data are gathered through the physical examination and the diagnostic and laboratory findings.

Physical Examination A complete health assessment includes a systematic physical examination, generally conducted from head to toe, to obtain objective data relative to the client's health status and presenting problems. When assessing the client to determine the level of risk for infection, focus the physical examination on:

- Range of motion and mobility (A client with limited mobility is at risk for developing joint contractures, skin breakdown, and muscle atrophy.)
- Localized redness, warmth, swelling, pain, and loss of use in a specific body part
- Fever with an increase in pulse and respirations; weakness; anorexia, nausea, vomiting, and/or diarrhea; enlarged and/or tender lymph nodes
- Secretions or exudate of the skin or mucous membranes; hydration status
- Auscultation of the lungs for crackles or wheezes

Diagnostic and Laboratory Data The laboratory indicators for an infection are:

- An elevated leukocyte (white blood cell [WBC]) and WBC differential:

  Neutrophils: Increased in acute, severe inflammation

  Lymphocytes: Increased in chronic bacterial and viral infections

  Monocytes: Increased in some protozoan and rickettsial infections and TB

  Eosinophils and basophils: Unaltered in an infectious process
- An elevated erythrocyte sedimentation rate (ESR): increased in the presence of inflammation
- An elevated pH of involved body fluids (gastric, urine, or vaginal secretions): indicative of microorganism presence
- Positive cultures of involved body fluids (blood, sputum, urine, or other drainage): indicative of microorganism growth (Guyton & Hall, 2005)

Nursing Diagnosis

After data collection and analysis, identify a nursing diagnosis. The North American Nursing Diagnosis Association International (NANDA-I) identifies one nursing diagnosis related to infection: *Risk for Infection.*

Risk for infection is an increased risk for being invaded by pathogenic organisms (NANDA-I, 2010). The risk factors that increase a client's susceptibility to infections are as follows:

- Inadequate primary defenses (broken skin, traumatized tissue, decrease in ciliary action, stasis of body fluids, change in pH of secretions, and altered peristalsis)

PROFESSIONALTIP

Questions Related to Infection Control

- What do you do to stay healthy?
- What health care concerns do you have?
- Have you recently been in contact with someone who has an infectious disease?
- When do you wash your hands?
- Have you traveled out of the country, especially to Third World countries, in the past 6 months?

MEMORYTRICK

Infection

A nurse can use the memory trick **INFECTION** to remember signs and symptoms of infection and important nursing assessment skills to use when assessing a client for an actual or potential infection:

I = Inflammation (swelling) is a sign of infection

N = Need to auscultate lungs for crackles or wheezes

F = Feels warm or hot (skin) to the touch

E = Erythema (redness) appears at the site of the infection

C = Check client's temperature for a fever

T = Tender (sore or painful) at the site of the infection

I = Inspect site of infection for secretions or exudates

O = Observe and practice proper hand hygiene protocol

N = Need to report abnormal lab values to the physician

- Inadequate secondary defenses (decreased hemoglobin, leukopenia, suppressed inflammatory response)
- Inadequate acquired immunity
- Immunosuppression
- Tissue destruction and increased environmental exposure
- Chronic disease
- Malnutrition
- Invasive procedures
- Pharmaceutical agents
- Trauma
- Rupture of amniotic membranes
- Insufficient knowledge to avoid exposure to pathogens (NANDA-I, 2010)

Clients who are at risk for infection may have other associated physiologic and psychological concerns. The common nursing diagnoses that often accompany *Risk for **I**nfection* include:

- *Imbalanced **N**utrition: Less Than Body Requirements* or *More Than Body Requirements*
- *Ineffective **P**rotection*
- *Impaired **T**issue Integrity*
- *Impaired **O**ral Mucous Membrane*
- *Impaired **S**kin Integrity*
- *Deficient **K**nowledge* (specify)

This list indicates several related problems that must be considered when planning care for the client at risk for infection.

PLANNING/OUTCOME IDENTIFICATION

The nurse collaborates with the client and other health care providers to determine goals, outcomes, and interventions to reduce the risk of infection. Outcomes provide direction for nursing care to reduce the risk of infection. Client and caregiver education about identifying potential hazards and health-promotion practices is another critical element of the care plan.

IMPLEMENTATION

Nurses are responsible for providing the client with a safe environment, including prevention of hospital-acquired infections. Nursing interventions to reduce the risk of infection center around ensuring asepsis and properly disposing of infectious materials to reduce or eliminate infectious agents. **Asepsis** refers to the absence of microorganisms. **Aseptic technique** is the infection-control practice used to prevent the transmission of pathogens. The use of aseptic technique decreases the risk and spread of hospital-acquired infections. There are two types of asepsis: medical and surgical.

Medical Asepsis

The term **medical asepsis** refers to those practices used to reduce the number, growth, and spread of microorganisms. It is also called *clean technique*. In medical asepsis, objects are generally referred to as "clean" or "dirty." **Clean objects** are considered to have the presence of some microorganisms that are usually not pathogenic. **Dirty** (soiled) **objects** are considered to have a high number of microorganisms, some being potentially pathogenic. Common medical aseptic measures used for clean or dirty objects are hand hygiene, daily changing of linens, and daily cleansing of floors and hospital furniture.

Hand Hygiene **Hand hygiene** is a general term that includes *hand washing* (using plain soap and water), *antiseptic hand wash* (using

COMMUNITY/HOME HEALTH CARE

Clients at Risk for Infection

Clients at risk for infection should have follow-up visits by the home health nurse to measure the effectiveness of client teaching and to assess resources in the home to prevent the transmission of infections.

INFECTION CONTROL

Hand Hygiene

- Wash hands before and after every client contact.
- The most common cause of hospital-acquired infections is contaminated hands of health care providers.
- When in doubt, *wash your hands.*

antimicrobial substances and water), *antiseptic hand rub* (using alcohol-based hand rub), and *surgical hand antisepsis* (using antiseptic hand wash or antiseptic hand rub preoperatively by surgical personnel to eliminate transient and reduce resident hand flora). Perform hand hygiene after arriving at work, before leaving work, before and after each client contact, after removing gloves, when hands are visibly soiled, before eating, after excretion of body waste (urination and defecation), after contact with body fluids, and after handling contaminated equipment. When hands are visibly dirty, wash hands with soap (plain or antimicrobial) and water. If hands are not visibly soiled, an alcohol-based hand rub may be used. If soap and water are not available, an alcohol-based wipe or hand gel may be used (Centers for Disease Control and Prevention [CDC], 2009a).

Hand washing is the rubbing together of all surfaces and crevices of the hands using plain soap and water, followed by rinsing in a flowing stream of water. Friction physically removes soil and transient flora, and a flowing stream of water rinses it all away. To remove transient flora from the hands, a washing time of 20 to 30 seconds is recommended. High-risk areas such as nurseries usually require a hand wash of approximately 2 minutes' duration. Soiled hands usually require more time. Hand washing is the most basic infection-control measure to prevent and control the transmission of infectious agents. According to the CDC (2009b), alcohol-based hand rubs (foam or gel) are more effective in killing bacteria than soap and water.

Antiseptic hand rub uses an alcohol-containing preparation designed to reduce the number of viable microorganisms on the hands. In the United States, these preparations usually contain 60% to 95% ethanol or isopropanol. Apply product to palm of one hand and rub hands together, covering all surfaces of hands and fingers, until hands are dry. Follow the manufacturer's recommendation for the amount of product to use.

Surgical Asepsis

Surgical asepsis, or sterile technique, consists of those practices that eliminate all microorganisms and spores from an object or area. Surgical asepsis relates to surgical hand washing, establishing and maintaining sterile fields, donning surgical attire (caps, masks, and eyewear), and sterile gloves, gowning, with closed gloving.

Surgical asepsis is practiced in the OR, in labor and delivery, and for many therapeutic and diagnostic interventions at the client's bedside. Common nursing procedures requiring sterile technique are:

- All invasive procedures, either entry into a bodily orifice (tracheobronchial suctioning, insertion of a urinary catheter) or intentional perforation of the skin (injections, insertion of intravenous needles or catheters)
- Nursing interventions when there is a disruption of skin surfaces (changing a surgical wound or intravenous site dressing) or destruction of skin layers (trauma and burns)

Surgical Hand Antisepsis Surgical hand antisepsis scrub removes soil and microorganisms from the skin. Workers in the OR do surgical hand antisepsis to minimize the client's risk for infection. The skin on the hands and arms should be intact (free of lesions). Agency policy determines the method and timing for the scrub.

Sterile Field and Equipment Establish and maintain a sterile field when performing procedures that require sterile technique, such as inserting a urinary catheter or changing wound dressings. Before preparing the sterile field, review the agency's policy and gather all the necessary supplies.

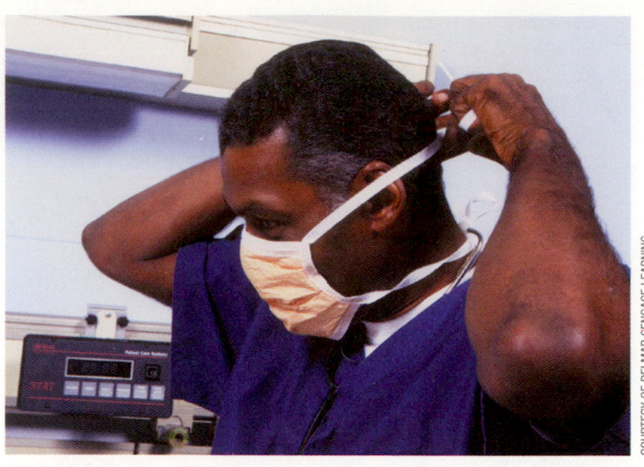
COURTESY OF DELMAR CENGAGE LEARNING

FIGURE 21-7 Putting on a Surgical Mask

Donning Surgical Attire Surgical nurses are required to wear a surgical mask (Figure 21-7) and a clean cap covering all of the hair. Protective eyewear (glasses or goggles) is worn during all procedures posing a threat of body fluids splashing into the eyes. Masks, caps, eyewear, gowns, and gloves are considered barrier precautions because they are a physical impediment to the spread of microorganisms.

Donning Sterile Gloves There are two methods of applying sterile gloves: open and closed. The open method is used when performing procedures requiring sterile technique, such as dressing changes. The closed method is used when the nurse wears a sterile gown, as in the OR.

Gowning with Closed Gloving When donning a sterile gown, nurses in the OR and special procedure areas such as cardiac cath labs use the closed gloved method. After the surgical scrub, don the sterile gown and gloves using the closed method. The sterile gown serves as a barrier to decrease the risk of wound contamination and also allows the nurse to move freely in the environment of sterile fields.

Disposal of Infectious Materials All health care facilities must have guidelines for the disposal of infectious-waste materials as required by the OSHA Act of 1991. The types of materials included are:

- Laboratory wastes
- All body fluids including blood, blood products
- Client care items (soiled bed linen and protection pads, urinals, and bedpans)
- Disposable instruments
- Medication and soiled treatment items
- Surgical wastes

All health care workers must be diligent in observing the biological hazard symbol and handling all infectious materials as hazardous.

CRITICAL THINKING

Medical and Surgical Asepsis

How are medical asepsis and surgical asepsis the same? How are they different?

When disposing of infectious waste, all personnel must be sure to:

- Wear gloves.
- Use the proper containers (red or one labeled with the biological hazard symbol as required by the facility), sharps containers for needles, scalpels, and other sharp instruments or devices; and leakproof plastic bags for waste from client areas (soiled dressings, gloves, linen).
- Ensure that all infectious waste is properly labeled.
- Carefully handle plastic bags to avoid punctures and tearing.
- Disinfect carts used to carry infectious waste.
- Dispose of waste only in designated areas.
- Wash hands after disposing of hazardous materials.

Containers for contaminated sharps should be readily accessible to personnel and maintained in an upright position.

The CDC (2003) reports that health care workers who have received the hepatitis B virus (HBV) vaccine and who have developed immunity to the virus are at virtually no risk for infection after an occupational exposure. For a health care worker who has not been immunized for HBV, the risk of infection after an occupational exposure ranges from 6% to 30%. The number of HBV occupational infections has decreased 95% since the HBV vaccine began being administered in 1982. The risk for a hepatitis C virus (HCV) infection after an occupation exposure is approximately 1.8%, and the risk for a human immunodeficiency virus (HIV) infection postexposure is 0.3% (CDC, 2003).

INFECTION CONTROL

Needle Disposal

- Used needles should not be recapped, bent, or broken.
- Needles should be placed in a puncture-resistant, marked or color-coded container close to the work site.
- Correct disposal decreases the risk of needle punctures to caregivers.

EVALUATION

Evaluation of the effectiveness of nursing care is based on the achievement of goals and expected outcomes. Keeping the client free from infection requires frequent reassessment followed by timely adjustments made in the plan of care in order for nursing interventions to be effective. It is important for the client to remain free of infection during hospitalization as well as develop a true awareness of the factors that increase the risk for infection.

SAMPLE NURSING CARE PLAN

The Client at Risk for Infection

F.S., a 38-year-old homeless person, was struck and dragged by a speeding car as he crossed the street. He was taken to the hospital by ambulance. His left leg is broken, and there are lacerations and abrasions on his right side, arm, and leg. The left leg is in a cast and the lacerations have been sutured. F.S. grimaces when he tries to move his legs, but he does not verbalize pain. F.S. is very thin and says that he has not eaten for 2 days.

NURSING DIAGNOSIS 1 *Risk for Infection* related to inadequate primary defenses as evidenced by lacerations and abrasions

Nursing Outcomes Classification (NOC)
Tissue Integrity: Skin & Mucous Membranes
Nutritional Status

Nursing Interventions Classification (NIC)
Wound Care
Nutrition Management

PLANNING/OUTCOMES	NURSING INTERVENTIONS	RATIONALE
F.S. will not have developed an infection in the lacerations and abrasions at discharge.	Use proper hand hygiene before and after caring for F.S.	Reduces microorganisms on hands.
	Use sterile technique when caring for lacerations and abrasions.	Prevents introduction of microorganisms into lacerations and abrasions.
	Apply antibiotic ointment on abrasions, as ordered.	Promotes healing of abrasions.
	Keep bed linens clean and dry.	Removes any drainage that may harbor microorganisms.
	Administer oral antibiotics, as ordered.	Prevents or cures infection.

(*Continues*)

SAMPLE NURSING CARE PLAN (Continued)

EVALUATION

F.S. has some redness around one laceration.

NURSING DIAGNOSIS 2 *Acute **P**ain* related to physical injury as evidenced by facial grimacing

Nursing Outcomes Classification (NOC)	Nursing Interventions Classification (NIC)
Pain Control	*Pain Management*
Symptom Severity	*Analgesic Administration*
Memory	*Hope Instillation*

PLANNING/OUTCOMES	NURSING INTERVENTIONS	RATIONALE
F.S. will experience increased comfort and will verbalize that pain is under control within 24 hours.	Use pain scale to determine level of discomfort.	Provides objective measure of pain.
	Assist client to a position of comfort and elevate extremities.	Reduces pain and swelling by increasing blood return to the heart.
	Administer analgesics, as ordered.	Provides comfort.

EVALUATION

F.S. states that he is experiencing less discomfort by 16 hours but that he still desires pain medication.

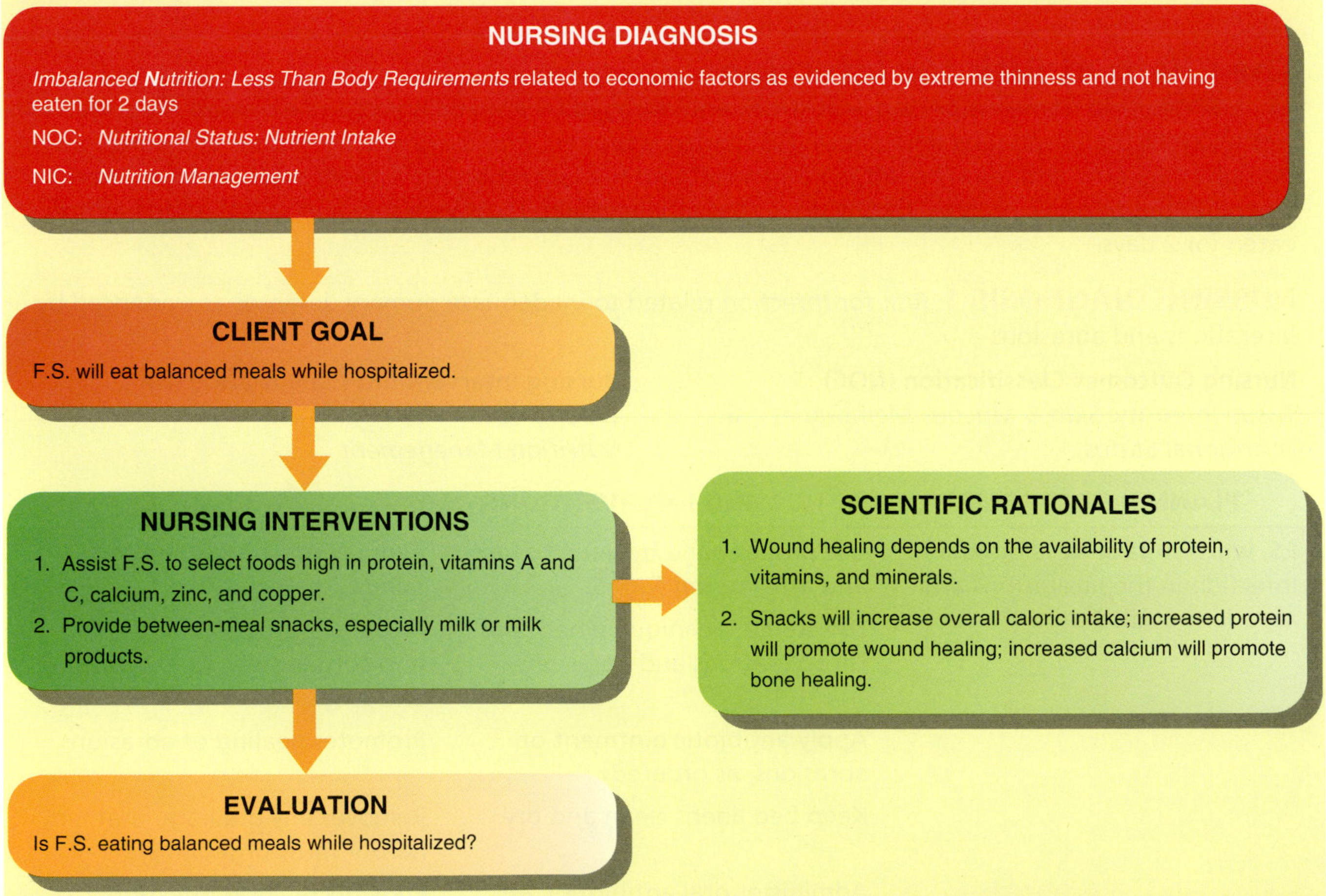

NURSING DIAGNOSIS

*Imbalanced **N**utrition: Less Than Body Requirements* related to economic factors as evidenced by extreme thinness and not having eaten for 2 days

NOC: *Nutritional Status: Nutrient Intake*

NIC: *Nutrition Management*

CLIENT GOAL

F.S. will eat balanced meals while hospitalized.

NURSING INTERVENTIONS

1. Assist F.S. to select foods high in protein, vitamins A and C, calcium, zinc, and copper.
2. Provide between-meal snacks, especially milk or milk products.

SCIENTIFIC RATIONALES

1. Wound healing depends on the availability of protein, vitamins, and minerals.
2. Snacks will increase overall caloric intake; increased protein will promote wound healing; increased calcium will promote bone healing.

EVALUATION

Is F.S. eating balanced meals while hospitalized?

CONCEPT CARE MAP 21-1

SUMMARY

- Flora are microorganisms that occur or have adapted to live in a specific environment.
- Pathogens are microorganisms that cause disease; they include bacteria, viruses, fungi, protozoa, and *rickettsia*.
- The elements of the chain of infection include the agent, the reservoir, the portal of exit, the modes of transmission, the portal of entry, and the host.
- The body has two primary defenses: the nonspecific immune defense, protecting the host from all microorganisms regardless of previous exposure, and the specific immune defense, reacting to a specific antigen that the body has previously experienced.
- Infections progress through four stages: incubation, prodromal, illness, and convalescence.
- Hand hygiene must be done before and after every client contact and after removing gloves. It is the most important procedure for preventing hospital-acquired infections.
- Other means of preventing the spread of infection include cleansing equipment, cleansing soiled linen, changing dressings over wounds, practicing barrier precautions, maintaining skin integrity, and receiving all appropriate immunizations.
- The OSHA regulations mandate that sharps be properly disposed of immediately after use.

REVIEW QUESTIONS

1. When caring for a client who is postoperative for a bowel resection, the nurse knows that which of the following procedures requires surgical aseptic technique?
   1. Administering PO medication.
   2. Removal of intravenous catheter.
   3. Insertion of Foley catheter.
   4. Disposal of surgical wound dressing.
2. The nurse is caring for a client with lower abdominal pain. Which of the following is the most effective infection-control measure to prevent and control the transmission of infectious agents?
   1. Sterilizing.
   2. Hand hygiene.
   3. Disinfecting.
   4. Use of bactericides.
3. A client with chickenpox will exhibit a slight elevation in body temperature followed within 24 hours by eruptions on the skin during which stage of infection?
   1. Incubation.
   2. Prodromal.
   3. Illness.
   4. Convalescent.
4. When disposing of infectious waste, all personnel must be sure to: (Select all that apply.)
   1. inform the Infectious Waste Department.
   2. write the client's name, room number, and allergies on the container.
   3. wear gloves.
   4. use proper biohazard containers.
   5. carefully handle biohazard plastic bags.
   6. disinfect carts used to carry infectious waste.
5. Which of the following is not a risk factor that increases a client's susceptibility to infection?
   1. Noninvasive procedure.
   2. Chronic disease.
   3. Malnutrition.
   4. Rupture of amniotic membranes.
6. A client is being discharged home, and prevention of infection is part of his treatment plan. Which of the following statements made by the client regarding prevention of infection indicates that further teaching is needed by the nurse?
   1. "I need to keep my bed linens clean and dry."
   2. "I need to take my antibiotic as ordered."
   3. "I need to wash my hands only before I change my dressings because I will be wearing gloves."
   4. "I need to keep my dressings clean and dry."
7. A client with an infected abdominal incision is brought to the primary care clinic. Which of the following assessments will the nurse be able to make?
   1. Pinpoint pupils, hypothermia, and elevated blood pressure.
   2. Decreased respirations, low blood pressure, and constricted pupils.
   3. Clammy skin, dilated pupils, slow pulse, and low blood pressure.
   4. Fever, localized redness, warmth, swelling, and pain.

8. The nursing care plan of a client who is at risk for an infection is likely to include:
   1. use clean gloves for all procedures.
   2. take a daily multivitamin.
   3. use proper hand hygiene before and after providing care.
   4. administer intravenous antibiotic.
9. A client with a sinus infection blows his nose in a facial tissue and asks the nurse to dispose of it. The nurse puts on gloves before touching the used facial tissue because she knows that the facial tissue is identified as which of the following links in the chain of infection?
   1. Portal of entry.
   2. Mode of transmission.
   3. Portal of exit.
   4. Susceptible host.
10. An AIDS client is admitted to the hospital with renal insufficiency, elevated liver enzymes, jaundice, pneumonia, elevated WBC, fever, and diarrhea. Which of the following types of infection is the client experiencing?
    1. Systemic infection.
    2. Humoral infection.
    3. Localized infection.
    4. Transient infection.

REFERENCES/SUGGESTED READINGS

Association for Professionals in Infection Control and Epidemiology. (2002a). Infection control—A few ounces of prevention. Available: http://www.apic.org/cons/icdesc.cfm

Association for Professionals in Infection Control and Epidemiology. (2002b). Infection control tips on handwashing. Available: http://www.apic.org/cons/washtips.cfm

Association for Professionals in Infection Control and Epidemiology. (2002c). West Nile virus: Consumer information. Available: http://www.apic.org/cons/westnile.cfm

Association for Professionals in Infection Control and Epidemiology. (2004). West Nile virus: General information. Retrieved October 20, 2008, from http://www.apic.org/Content/NavigationMenu/PracticeGuidance/Topics/WestNileVirus/West_Nile_Virus.htm#General_Information

Bender, K., & Thompson, F. (2003). West Nile Virus: A growing challenge. *American Journal of Nursing, 103*(6), 32–39.

Berlinguer, G. (1992). The interchange of disease and health between the old and new worlds. *American Journal of Public Health, 82*(10), 1407–1414.

Bulechek, G., Butcher, H., McCloskey, J., & Dochterman, J., eds. (2008). *Nursing Interventions Classification (NIC)* (5th ed.). St. Louis, MO: Mosby/Elsevier.

Centers for Disease Control and Prevention. (2003). *Exposure to blood: What healthcare personnel need to know* [Brochure], 1–10.

Centers for Disease Control and Prevention. (2007a). Appropriate disinfectants: Bleach. Retrieved October 20, 2008, from http://www.cdc.gov/healthyswimming/bodyfluidspill.htm

Centers for Disease Control and Prevention. (2007b). Preventing occupational HIV transmission to healthcare personnel. Retrieved October 5, 2008, from http://www.cdc.gov/hiv/resources/factsheets/hcwprev.htm

Centers for Disease Control and Prevention. (2008). Fact sheet: Keep food and water safe after a disaster or power outage. Retrieved October 20, 2008, from http://emergency.cdc.gov/disasters/foodwater/facts.asp

Centers for Disease Control and Prevention. (2009a). Hand hygiene interactive education. Retrieved May 9, 2009, from http://www.cdc.gov/handhygiene/training/interactiveEducation/frame.htm

Centers for Disease Control and Prevention. (2009b). An ounce of prevention keeps the germs away. Retrieved May 9, 2009, from http://www.cdc.gov/ounceofprevention/docs/oop_brochure_eng.pdf

Centers for Disease Control and Prevention/Hospital Infection Control Practices Advisory Committee. (2007). Type and duration of precautions recommended for selected infections and conditions. Retrieved October 8, 2008, from htp://www.cdc.gov/ncidod/dhqp/pdf/guidelines/Isolation2007.pdf

Czark, G., & Mattys, A. (2008). Nation's top healthcare organizations announce strategies to prevent deadly healthcare-associated infections. Retrieved October 12, 2008, from http://www.apic.org

Daniels, R. (2010). *Delmar's guide to laboratory and diagnostic tests,* 2nd edition. Clifton Park, NY: Delmar Cengage Learning.

Delahanty, K. M., & Myers, F. E., III. (2007). Nursing2007 infection control survey report. *Nursing2007, 37*(6), 28–36.

Dochterman, J., & Bulechek, G. (2004). *Nursing Interventions Classification (NIC)* (4th ed.). St. Louis, MO: Mosby.

Goldrick, B., & Goetz, A. (2003). Keeping West Nile Virus at bay. *Nursing2003, 33*(8), 44–47.

Guyton, A. & Hall, J. (2005). *Textbook of medical physiology* (11th ed.). Philadelphia: W. B. Saunders.

Hadaway, L. C. (2006). Keeping central line infections at bay. *Nursing2006, 36*(4), 58–63.

Hass, J. & Larson, E. (2008). Compliance with hand hygiene guidelines: Where are we in 2008? *American Journal of Nursing, 108*(8), 40–44.

Infection Control. (2002). "Hand hygiene" news. *Nursing2002,* 32(5), 32hn6.

Leung-Chen, P. (2008). Emerging infections: Everybody's crying MRSA. *American Journal of Nursing, 108*(8), 29.

Moorhead, S., Johnson, M., Maas, M., & Swanson, E. (2008). *Nursing Outcomes Classification (NOC)* (4th ed.). St. Louis, MO: Mosby.

National Center for Infectious Disease. (2002). Sterilization or disinfection of medical devices: General principles. Available: http://www.cdc.gov/ncidod/hip/sterile/sterilgp.htm

National Foundation for Infectious Diseases. (2008). Call to action: Influenza immunization among health care personnel. Retrieved October 12, 2008, from http://www.nfid.org/pdf/publications/fluhealthcarecta08.pdf

North American Nursing Diagnosis Association International. (2010). *NANDA-I nursing diagnoses: Definitions and classification 2009-2011.* Ames, IA: Wiley-Blackwell.

Occupational Safety and Health Administration. (2001). Occupational exposure to bloodborne pathogens; needlestick and other sharps injuries; final rule, 29 CFR Part 1910 66:5317–5325. Retrieved

October 5, 2008, from http://www.osha.gov/pls/oshaweb/owadisp.show_document?p_table=FEDERAL_REGISTER&p_id=16265

Occupational Safety and Health Administration. (2003). Model plans and programs for the OSHA bloodborne pathogens and hazard communications standards. Retrieved October 5, 2008, from http://www.osha.gov/Publications/osha3186.html

Oriola, S. (2006). *C. difficile*: A menace in hospitals and homes alike. *Nursing2006, 36*(8), 14–15.

Schweon, S. (2003). West Nile virus: Get ready for its return. *RN, 66*(4), 56–60.

Siegel, J. Rhinehart, E., Jackson, M., Chiarello, L., & the Healthcare Infection Control Practices Advisary Committee. (2006). Management of multidrug-resistant organisms in healthcare settings, 2006. Retrieved on October 12, 2008, from http://www.cdc.gov/ncidod/dhqp/pdf/ar/mdroGuideline2006.pdf

Siegel, J. Rhinehart, E., Jackson, M., Chiarello, L., & the Healthcare Infection Control Practices Advisory Committee. (2007). Guideline for isolation precautions: preventing transmission of infectious agents in healthcare settings 2007. Retrieved on October 3, 2008, from http://www.cdc.gov/ncidod/dhqp/pdf/isolation2007.pdf

Wilson, M. (2003). The traveler and emerging infections: Sentinel, courier, transmitter. *Journal of Applied Microbiology, 94*(Suppl.), 1S–11S.

Wright, D. (2008). HHS efforts to reduce healthcare-associated infections. Retrieved October 20, 2008, from http://www.apic.org/AM/Template.cfm

Yokoe, D. & Classen, D. (2008). Supplement article: Introduction. Improving infection control: A new healthcare imperative. *Infection Control and Hospital Epidemiology, 29,* S3–S11.

RESOURCES

Association for Professionals in Infection Control and Epidemiology (APIC), http://www.apic.org

Centers for Disease Control and Prevention (CDC), http://www.cdc.gov

National Foundation for Infectious Diseases (NFID), http://www.nfid.org

Occupational Safety and Health Administration (OSHA), http://www.osha.gov

Society for Healthcare Epidemiology of America (SHEA), http://info@shea-online.org

CHAPTER 22
Standard Precautions and Isolation

MAKING THE CONNECTION

Refer to the following chapters to increase your understanding of Standard Precautions and isolation:

Basic Nursing
- ***Infection Control/Asepsis***

Adult Health Nursing
- ***Surgery***

Basic Procedures
- ***Hand Hygiene***
- ***Initiating Strict Isolation Precautions***

Intermediate Procedures
- ***Performing Open Gloving***

LEARNING OBJECTIVES

Upon completion of this chapter, you should be able to:

- Define key terms.
- Describe each of the eleven aspects of Standard Precautions.
- Identify the three transmission-based precautions and when each is to be used.
- Apply Standard Precautions in providing appropriate client care.

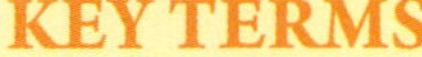

KEY TERMS

Airborne Precautions
aseptic technique
barrier precautions
Contact Precautions
Droplet Precautions
endemic
epidemic
hospital-acquired infection
infection
isolation
nosocomial infections
reverse isolation
Standard Precautions
Transmission-Based Precautions

INTRODUCTION

For more than 120 years, health care facilities and their personnel have struggled to prevent the spread of infections among their clients. This chapter reviews some of the historical methods as well as the current methods used to prevent the spread of infection.

HISTORICAL PERSPECTIVE

A hospital handbook published in 1877 recommended placing clients with infectious diseases in a separate facility (Lynch, 1949). These facilities became known as infectious-disease hospitals. Yet, **hospital-acquired infections**, **infections** acquired in the hospital that were not present or incubating at the time of the client's admission (**nosocomial infections**), continued in these facilities because the infected clients were not separated according to disease, and **aseptic technique** (infection-control practices used to prevent the transmission of pathogens) was seldom, if ever, practiced. To combat the continuing problem of nosocomial infections in the infectious-disease hospitals, personnel began to set aside a floor or ward for clients with similar diseases (Gage, Landon, & Sider, 1959).

Nursing has always been at the forefront of preventing the spread of infections among clients and personnel. Infectious-disease hospital personnel began practicing aseptic technique as recommended in nursing textbooks published from 1890 to 1900 (Lynch, 1949). Isolation practices and the use of infectious-disease hospitals were altered in 1910 when the cubicle system of isolation was introduced in U.S. hospitals (Gage et al., 1959). The cubicle system of **isolation** (separation from other persons, especially those with infectious diseases) placed clients in multiple-bed wards, with hospital personnel using a separate gown when caring for each client, washing their hands in an antiseptic solution after contact with each client, and disinfecting objects contaminated by any client. These nursing procedures were known as *barrier nursing*. Barrier nursing was aimed at preventing transmission of pathogenic organisms to other clients and to health care personnel. The cubicle system of isolation, including the barrier nursing procedures, gave the clients the alternative of receiving care in general hospitals instead of the infectious-disease hospitals (Centers for Disease Control and Prevention [CDC]/Hospital Infection Control Practices Advisory Committee [HICPAC], 1997).

During the 1950s, infectious-disease hospitals closed, with the exception of the tuberculosis (TB) hospitals, which closed in the 1960s. Thus, by the end of the 1960s, clients with infectious diseases were cared for in general hospitals.

In 1970, the CDC published *Isolation Technique for Use in Hospitals*, a revised edition of which was released in 1975 (CDC, 1975). This manual introduced and recommended seven categories of isolation: Strict Isolation, Respiratory Isolation, Protective Isolation, Enteric Precautions, Wound and Skin Precautions, Discharge Precautions, and Blood Precautions. By the mid-1970s, 93% of U.S. hospitals had adopted the recommendations of this book (Haley & Shachtman, 1980).

By 1980, **endemic** (occurring continuously in a particular population and having low mortality) and **epidemic** (infecting many people at the same time, in the same geographic area) nosocomial infections were surfacing. Some of these infections were caused by multidrug-resistant (MDR) microorganisms, others by newly identified pathogens. Both types required isolation precautions different from those specified in any of the seven isolation categories. As Schaffner (1980) describes, isolation precautions needed to be directed more specifically at nosocomial transmission in special-care units rather than at community-acquired infectious diseases being spread within the hospital.

In 1983, the CDC replaced the 1975 isolation manual with the *Guideline for Isolation Precautions in Hospitals* (Garner & Simmons, 1983). One of the most important changes was the emphasis on decision making by the users as to which guideline was appropriate in a particular situation (Garner, 1984; Haley, Garner, & Simmons, 1985).

Another change was to rename Blood Precautions, primarily used for clients who were chronic carriers of hepatitis B virus (HBV), to Blood and Body Fluid Precautions, which now were to apply to clients with acquired immunodeficiency syndrome (AIDS); body fluids other than blood, such as semen and vaginal secretions; amniotic, cerebrospinal, pericardial, peritoneal, pleural, and synovial fluids; and any other body fluid visibly contaminated with blood. It did not apply to feces, nasal secretions, sputum, sweat, tears, urine, or vomitus unless blood was visible in them.

Until 1985, clients placed in isolation either had a confirmed diagnosis or were suspected of having an infectious disease. Mainly because of the human immunodeficiency virus (HIV) epidemic and those other blood-borne infections often yet unrecognized in a client, it was decided that Blood and Body Fluid Precautions were to be applied universally to all clients, regardless of their presumed infection status (CDC, 1985). Thus, the new name became Universal Precautions.

A new system of isolation called Body Substance Isolation (BSI) was proposed in 1987 as an alternative to the diagnosis-driven isolation system of the 1983 *Guideline for Isolation Precautions in Hospitals*. BSI focused on isolating all moist and potentially infectious body substances (blood, feces, urine, sputum, saliva, wound drainage, and other body fluids) from all clients. The use of gloves was the primary method of isolating infectious agents; however, BSI did not contain adequate provisions to prevent droplet transmission, direct or indirect contact transmission, or true airborne transmission of infections. Also, BSI recommended hand washing after removal of gloves only if the hands were soiled (Lynch, Jackson, Cummings, & Stamm, 1987), whereas Universal Precautions recommended hand washing after every removal of gloves (CDC, 1987, 1988).

In 1991, the HICPAC was established to provide advice and guidance to the secretary and assistant secretary of the U.S. Department of Health and Human Services (USDHHS), the director of the CDC, and the director of the National Center for Infectious Diseases (CDC/HICPAC, 1997). The committee also provides advice to the CDC about updating guidelines and other policy statements related to the prevention of nosocomial infections.

The CDC, with the assistance of HICPAC, revised the *Guideline for Isolation Precautions in Hospitals* in 1996. The new guideline combined the major features of Universal Precautions and Body Substance Isolation into a single set of Standard Precautions, and the specific isolation categories into three Transmission-Based Precautions.

The CDC recommendations are not subject to legal enforcement; however, regulations of the Occupational Safety and Health Administration (OSHA) must be followed by all health care facilities. These regulations, laws enforced through the Department of Labor (OSHA, 1991, 2001), ensure that Standard Precautions and Transmission-Based Precautions are followed. According to OSHA regulations, all health care facilities must:

- Determine which employees have occupational exposure
- Provide hepatitis B vaccine free of charge to all employees with occupational exposure
- Provide personal protective equipment (e.g., gowns, gloves, masks, goggles) for all employees with occupational exposure
- Provide adequate hand-washing facilities and supplies
- Provide training regarding these rules to all employees with occupational exposure, both at hire and then annually
- Provide evaluation and follow-up for any employee who experiences an exposure incident
- Provide appropriate, properly labeled containers for contaminated sharps
- Provide and prominently display an exposure control plan for staff to follow

STANDARD PRECAUTIONS

Standard Precautions, listed on the inside back cover of this book, are preventive practices to be used in the care of all clients in hospitals regardless of diagnosis or presumed infection status. These guidelines are designed to reduce the risk of microorganism transmission from both recognized and unrecognized sources of infection in hospitals.

Standard Precautions apply to:

- Blood
- All body fluids, secretions, and excretions except sweat, regardless of whether those fluids contain visible blood
- Nonintact skin
- Mucous membranes

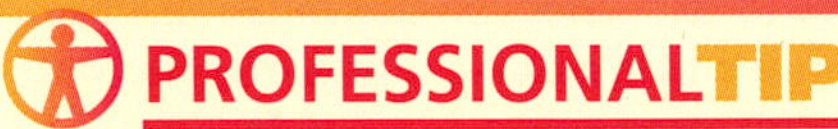

Exposure Incident

- Immediately report all exposure incidents to the proper person in the health care facility.
- The OSHA regulations require initial screening and follow-up care.

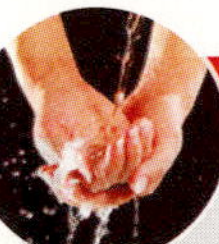

INFECTION CONTROL

Standard Precautions

- Standard Precautions must be practiced with all clients.
- Standard Precautions represent the most effective means of decreasing the risk of infection among clients and caregivers.

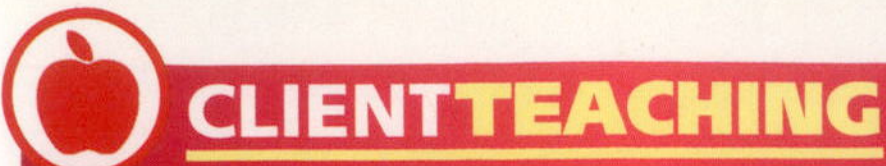

Standard Precautions

- Assist the client to understand that the techniques and procedures associated with Standard Precautions are designed to prevent the transmission of microorganisms and not to isolate the client.
- Explain why each technique and procedure is used.

Barrier precautions, used to minimize the risk of exposure to blood and body fluids, involve the use of personal protective equipment, such as masks, gowns, and gloves, to create a barrier between the person and the microorganism and thus prevent transmission of the microorganism. *Hand hygiene, however, is the most basic aspect of Standard Precautions.* The other aspects of Standard Precautions are gloves; mask, eye protection, and face shield; gown; client-care equipment; environmental control; linen; occupational health and bloodborne pathogens; and client placement.

HAND HYGIENE

Refer to hand hygiene in Chapter 21, "Infection Control/Asepsis." To prevent cross contamination of different body sites on one client, hand hygiene may be necessary between tasks and procedures on that client.

GLOVES

Clean, nonsterile gloves are to be worn when touching blood, body fluids, secretions, excretions, and contaminated items. Clean gloves should be put on just before touching mucous membranes and nonintact skin. Gloves must be changed between tasks and procedures being performed on one client if material that may contain microorganisms in high concentrations is touched. Gloves must be removed promptly after use, and hands must be cleansed immediately before touching uncontaminated items or providing care to another client.

SAFETY

Latex Allergies

- Standard Precautions include the use of gloves when there is a possibility of contact with client body fluids.
- Be alert that health care personnel or the client may be allergic to the latex gloves. Reactions range from an eczematous contact dermatitis to anaphylactic shock.
- Before touching clients when wearing latex gloves, ask whether they have a known allergy to latex products. If they do, use nonlatex gloves for those clients.

Mask, Eye Protection, Face Shield

A mask and eye protection or a face shield should be worn to protect the mucous membranes of the eyes, nose, and mouth when procedures and client-care activities are likely to generate splashes or sprays of blood, body fluids, secretions, or excretions.

Gown

A clean, nonsterile gown should be worn to protect the skin and prevent soiling of clothing during procedures and client-care activities that are likely to generate splashes or sprays of blood, body fluids, secretions, or excretions. A gown that is appropriate for the activity and potential amount of fluids should be selected. A soiled gown should be removed as promptly as possible and the hands cleansed to prevent transfer of microorganisms to other clients or environments.

Client-Care Equipment

Client-care equipment soiled with blood, body fluids, secretions, or excretions must be handled in a manner to prevent skin and mucous membrane exposure, clothing contamination, and microorganism transfer to other clients or environments. Reusable equipment must not be used in the care of another client until it has been cleansed and sterilized appropriately. All single-use items must be properly discarded.

Environmental Control

The hospital must have adequate procedures for the routine care, cleansing, and disinfection of environmental surfaces, beds, bed rails, bedside equipment, and other frequently touched surfaces. All personnel must ensure that these procedures are followed.

Linen

Linen that is soiled with blood, body fluids, secretions, or excretions must be handled, transported, and processed in a manner to prevent skin and mucous membrane exposure, clothing contamination, and microorganism transfer to other clients and environments. Follow agency policy.

Occupational Health and Blood-Borne Pathogens

Care must be taken to prevent injury when using needles, scalpels, and other sharp instruments and when handling, cleansing, and disposing of such items after use. The OSHA regulations state that "contaminated (used) sharps shall be discarded immediately or as soon as feasible in containers that are closable, puncture-resistant, leakproof on the sides and bottom and are labeled or color coded" (OSHA, 1991, 2001) (Figure 22-1).

Used needles should never be recapped by using both hands. A one-handed "scoop" method is acceptable. Used needles should never be removed from disposable syringes by hand, nor should they be bent, broken, or otherwise manipulated by hand. Disposable syringes and needles, scalpel blades, and other sharp items should be placed in designated puncture-resistant containers.

In areas where the need for resuscitation is predictable, mouth pieces, resuscitation bags, or other ventilation devices should be used instead of the direct mouth-to-mouth resuscitation method.

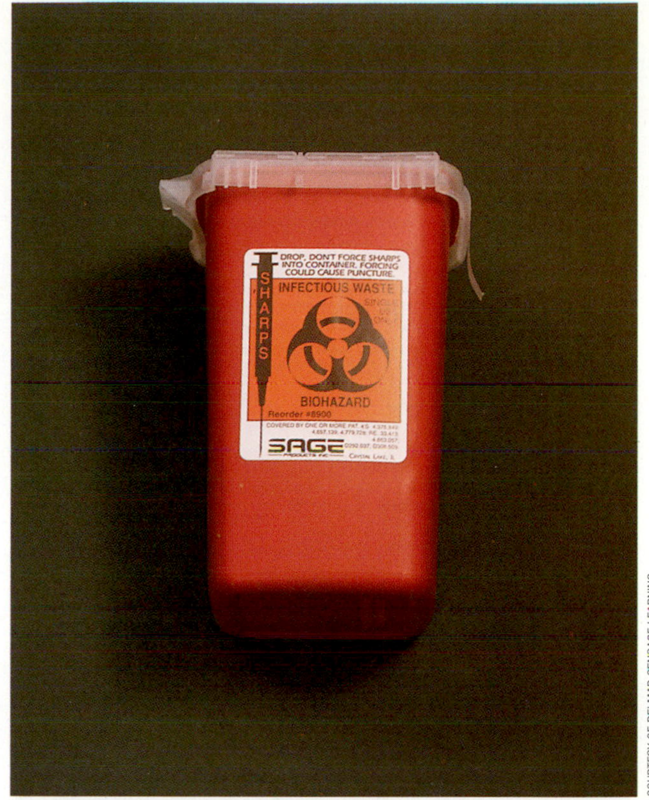

Figure 22-1 Sharps-Disposal Container

> **CRITICAL THINKING**
>
> **Standard Precautions**
>
> When, where, and why are Standard Precautions to be implemented?

Client Placement

Any client who contaminates the environment or who does not or cannot be expected to assist with maintaining appropriate hygiene or environment control should be placed in a private room. When a private room is unavailable, infection-control professionals must be consulted.

ISOLATION

The 1996 CDC guideline eliminated the previous category-specific isolation precautions and condensed the former disease-specific precautions into three sets of precautions based on the route of transmission: airborne (Figure 22-2), contact (Figure 22-3), or droplet (Figure 22-4). These new, Transmission-Based Precautions are to be used *in addition to* the Standard Precautions. **Transmission-Based Precautions** are practices designed for clients documented as or suspected of being infected with highly transmissible or epidemiologically important pathogens for which additional precautions beyond the Standard Precautions are required to interrupt transmission in hospitals (Table 22-1).

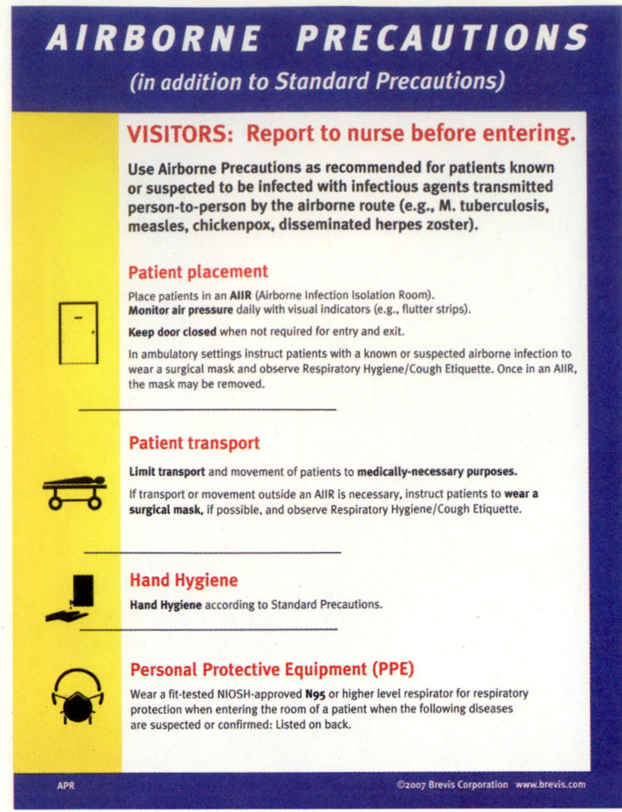

FIGURE 22-2 **Transmission-Based Precautions: Airborne Precautions** (© 2007. *Reprinted with permission from Brevis Corporation, http://www.brevis.com.*)

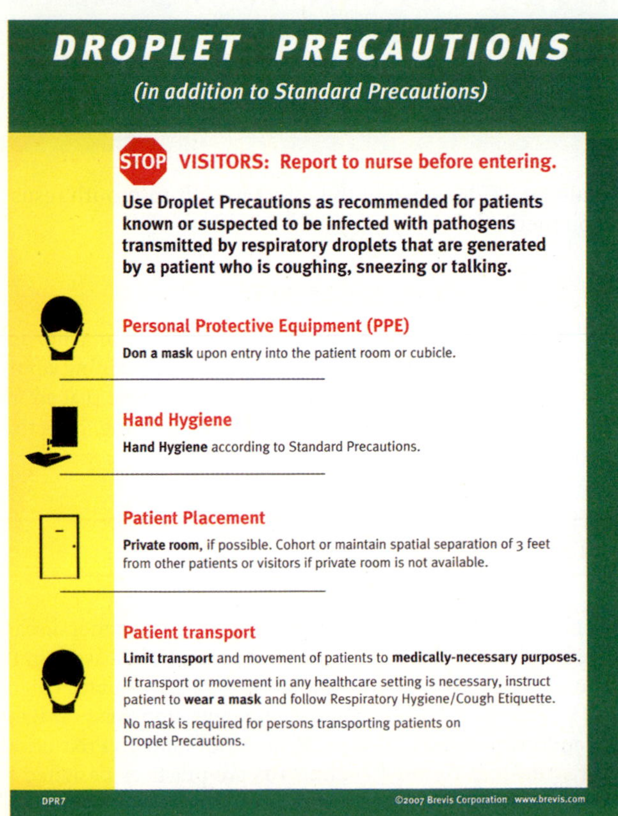

FIGURE 22-4 **Transmission-Based Precautions: Droplet Precautions** (© 2007. *Reprinted with permission from Brevis Corporation, http://www.brevis.com.*)

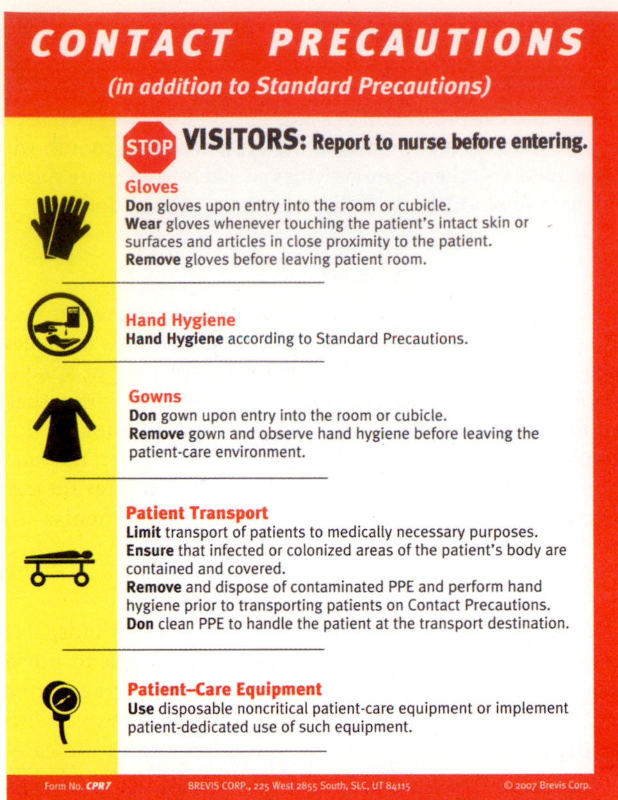

FIGURE 22-3 **Transmission-Based Precautions: Contact Precautions** (© 2007. *Reprinted with permission from Brevis Corporation, http://www.brevis.com.*)

CRITICAL THINKING

Transmission-Based Precautions

How are the three Transmission-Based Precautions the same? How are they different?

The Transmission-Based Precautions are also to be used in addition to the Standard Precautions in the event of suspicious infections and with clients who are immunosuppressed either from disease or chemotherapy. More than one of the transmission-based precautions is used at the same time for clients with certain infections or conditions.

Isolation precautions are usually ordered by the physician; however, nurses may initiate these precautions whenever a nursing diagnosis related to the infectious process is identified, for example, *Risk for Infection* related to decreased resistance of immune system. Most agencies require nurses to obtain a culture from a draining body area and to initiate isolation precautions when positive cultures are reported. After isolation precautions have been instituted, visitors and all personnel should comply with the agency's policy regarding isolation precautions. Signs should be posted in a prominent location outside the client's room. The signs should indicate the type of isolation precautions and preparation required before entering the room (Figure 22-5). The necessary supplies should be readily available.

Clients requiring isolation should be placed in a private room with adequate ventilation and should have their own supplies. Personal belongings should be kept to a minimum, and health care providers should use disposable supplies and

TABLE 22-1 Precautions Related to the Type of Disease

PRECAUTION	TYPE OF DISEASE
Standard Precautions	All clients, regardless of disease or condition
Airborne Precautions	In addition to Standard Precautions, used for clients known to have or suspected of having serious illnesses spread by airborne droplet nuclei, including: • Measles • Varicella • Tuberculosis
Contact Precautions	In addition to Standard Precautions, used for clients known to have or suspected of having serious illnesses easily spread by direct client contact or contact with fomites, including: • Wound infections • Gastrointestinal infections • Respiratory infections • Skin infections including: Herpes simplex Impetigo Major abscesses, cellulitis, or pressure ulcers Pediculosis Scabies Varicella (Zoster) • Viral hemorrhagic infections (Ebola)
Droplet Precautions	In addition to Standard Precautions, used for clients known to have or suspected of having illnesses spread by large particle droplets, including: • Meningitis • Adenovirus • Pneumonia • Influenza • Diphtheria • Mumps • Pertussis • Rubella • Scarlet fever • Parvovirus B19

From *Table I: Synopsis of Types of Precautions and Patients Requiring Precautions*, by Centers for Disease Control and Prevention (CDC)/Hospital Infection Control Practices Advisory Committee (HICPAC), 2002; *Guideline for Isolation Precautions: Preventing Transmission of Infectious Agents in Healthcare Settings 2007,* by CDC/HICPAC, 2007, available: http://www.cdc.gov/ncidod/dhqp/pdf/guidelines/Isolation2007.pdf.

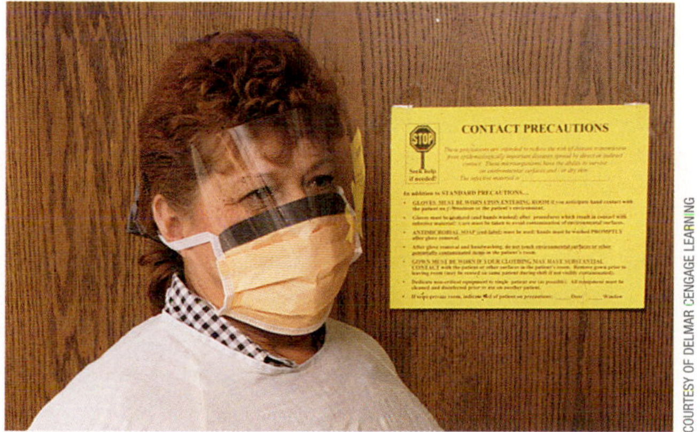

COURTESY OF DELMAR CENGAGE LEARNING

FIGURE 22-5 The sign on the door to the client's room indicates the type of isolation precaution and preparation needed before entering the room.

equipment whenever possible. All articles leaving the room, such as soiled linen and collected specimens, should be labeled and either placed in impermeable bags or double bagged.

Reverse isolation, also known as protective isolation, is a barrier protection designed to prevent infection in clients who are severely compromised and highly susceptible to infection. This includes clients who:

- are taking immunosuppressive medications
- are receiving chemotherapy or radiation therapy
- have diseases such as leukemia, which depress resistance to infectious organisms
- have extensive burns, dermatitis, or other skin impairments that prevent adequate coverage with dressings

These clients are at increased risk for infection from their own microorganisms, contact with health care workers whose hands have not been properly cleansed, and exposure to improperly disinfected and nonsterile items such as air, food, water, and equipment. Nursing responsibilities toward these clients include ensuring that everyone entering the client's room has completed meticulous hand hygiene and is properly attired in gown, gloves, and mask; ensuring that the client's environment is as clear of pathogens as possible; and knowing the institutional policy regarding caring for clients requiring reverse isolation.

COMMUNITY/HOME HEALTH CARE

Isolation

- Provide the client and family with appropriate written isolation instructions relative to the specific precautions.
- Provide necessary supplies or suggest a list of those things to buy and places to purchase the supplies.

MEMORYTRICK

ALONE

The nurse should use the memory trick **ALONE** when providing nursing care for a client in isolation:

A = Always post an isolation precaution sign on the client's door to notify individuals entering the room.

L = Listen to the client's feelings and concerns about being in isolation.

O = Observe isolation procedures to make sure they are accurately being followed.

N = Need to convey a sense of empathy, understanding, and support to the client.

E = Explain the pertinent isolation procedures to the client.

CLIENT RESPONSES TO ISOLATION

Isolation precautions are for the client's protection; however, clients who are placed on isolation precautions may experience psychological discomfort (Figure 22-6). Symptoms of anxiety, depression, rejection, guilt, or loneliness may be found in isolated clients. Clients should be educated on those isolation precautions that will be practiced and their purposes. Clients should be encouraged to verbalize their feelings regarding the isolation precautions and should be provided with intellectual stimulation and diversional activities such as paperback books, crossword puzzles, music, radio, or television. Visitors should be encouraged as a method to alleviate the client's feelings of isolation and loneliness. Wearing appropriate barrier precautions, visitors can safely enter an isolated client's room.

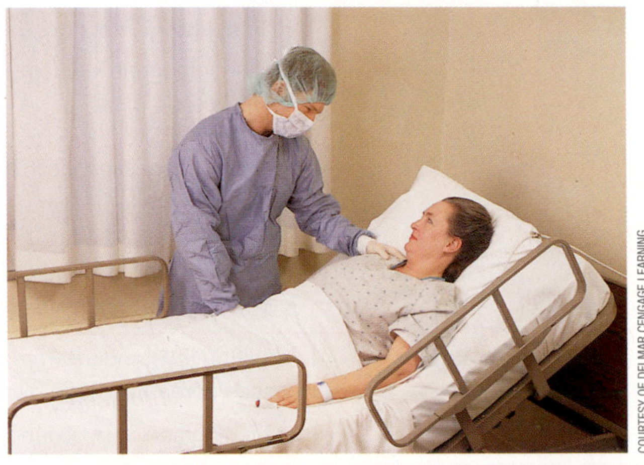

COURTESY OF DELMAR CENGAGE LEARNING

FIGURE 22-6 Nurse Interacting with Client Requiring Isolation Precautions

SUMMARY

- Standard Precautions are to be used when caring for *every* client.
- Airborne Precautions are to be used when caring for clients who have or may have serious illnesses spread by airborne droplet nuclei.
- Contact Precautions are to be used when caring for clients who have or may have serious illnesses spread by direct client contact or fomite contact.
- Droplet Precautions are to be used when caring for clients who have or may have serious illnesses spread by large-particle droplets.

REVIEW QUESTIONS

1. In 1996, the revised *Guideline for Isolation Precautions in Hospitals* combined Universal Precautions and Body Substance Isolation into:
   1. Barrier Precautions.
   2. Contact Precautions.
   3. Standard Precautions.
   4. Transmission-Based Precautions.
2. The use of masks, gowns, and gloves is termed:
   1. Droplet Precautions.
   2. Barrier Precautions.
   3. Contact Precautions.
   4. Standard Precautions.
3. The nursing action most basic to Standard Precautions is:
   1. gloving.
   2. gowning.
   3. hand hygiene.
   4. wearing a face mask.
4. Airborne Precautions require:
   1. paper masks.
   2. a private room.
   3. the wearing of gloves.
   4. the wearing of a gown.

5. Those precautions to be used in the care of all clients in hospitals regardless of diagnosis or presumed infection status are called:
   1. Standard Precautions.
   2. Airborne Precautions.
   3. Universal Precautions.
   4. Body Substance Isolation.
6. Nursing responsibilities for a client in reverse isolation include which of the following? (Select all that apply.)
   1. Ensuring that client's environment is as clear of pathogens as possible.
   2. Knowing institutional policies regarding caring for clients requiring reverse isolation.
   3. Discouraging visitation from family and friends.
   4. Observing that everyone entering the client's room is properly attired in gown, gloves, and mask.
   5. Encouraging the client to verbalize his or her feelings regarding isolation.
   6. Educating the client on the purpose of isolation.
7. A client has recently received a heart transplant and has been prescribed immunosuppressive medication. In which of the following types of isolation will the client be placed?
   1. Reverse.
   2. Institutional.
   3. Universal.
   4. Aseptic.
8. A nursing student is learning about clients placed in airborne precautions. Which of the following statements made by the student nurse indicates that further teaching is required?
   1. "The client needs to wear an N95 respirator mask when being transported to medically necessary purposes."
   2. "I need to keep the client's door closed when not required for entry and exit."
   3. "Visitors must report to the nurse before entering the client's room."
   4. "I need to wear a surgical mask when I enter the client's room."
9. Nursing responsibilities when caring for a client placed in contact isolation include:
   1. donning gloves when entering the client's room.
   2. hand hygiene according to standard precautions.
   3. removing gloves before leaving the client's room.
   4. all of the above.
10. The nurse observes a client in isolation crying. Which of the following responses made by the nurse is the most appropriate?
    1. "You will be alright. This will last only a week."
    2. "Don't worry. Lots of clients go through the same thing that you are."
    3. "You seem upset. Would you like to talk about it?"
    4. "Why are you crying? I can help you."

REFERENCES/SUGGESTED READINGS

Centers for Disease Control and Prevention. (1975). *Isolation techniques for use in hospitals* (2nd ed.) (HHS [CDC] Publication No. 80-8314). Washington, DC: U.S. Government Printing Office.

Centers for Disease Control and Prevention. (1985). Recommendations for preventing transmission of infection with human T-lymphotropic virus type III/lymphadenopathy-associated virus in the workplace. *Morbidity and Mortality Weekly Report, 34*, 681–686, 691–695.

Centers for Disease Control and Prevention. (1987). Recommendations for prevention of HIV transmission in health-care settings. *Morbidity and Mortality Weekly Report, 36*(2S), 1S–18S.

Centers for Disease Control and Prevention. (1988). Update: Universal precautions for prevention of transmission of human immunodeficiency virus, hepatitis B virus, and other blood borne pathogens in health-care settings. *Morbidity and Mortality Weekly Report, 37*(24), 377–382, 387–388. Available: http://www.cdc.gov/mmwr/preview/mmwrhtml/00000039.htm

Centers for Disease Control and Prevention. (2002). Guideline for hand hygiene in health care settings. Available: http://www.cdc.gov/mmwr/preview/mmwrhtml/rr5116a1.htm

Centers for Disease Control and Prevention. (2007a). Airborne precautions. Retrieved October 5, 2008, from http://www.cdc.gov/ncidod/dhqp/gl_isolation_airborne.html

Centers for Disease Control and Prevention. (2007b). Contact precautions. Retrieved October 5, 2008, from http://www.cdc.gov/ncidod/dhqp/gl_isolation_contact.html

Centers for Disease Control and Prevention. (2007c). Droplet precautions. Retrieved October 5, 2008, from http://www.cdc.gov/ncidod/dhqp/gl_isolation_droplet.html

Centers for Disease Control and Prevention. (2007d). Standard precautions. Retrieved October 5, 2008, from http://www.cdc.gov/ncidod/dhqp/gl_isolation_standard.html

Centers for Disease Control and Prevention. Preventing occupational HIV transmission to healthcare personnel. Retrieved October 5, 2008, from www.cdc.gov/hiv/resources/factsheets/hcwprev.htm

Centers for Disease Control and Prevention. (2009a). Hand hygiene interactive education. Retrieved May 9, 2009, from http://www.cdc.gov/handhygiene/training/interactiveEducation/frame.htm

Centers for Disease Control and Prevention. (2009b). An ounce of prevention keeps the germs away. Retrieved May 9, 2009, from http://www.cdc.gov/ounceofprevention/docs/oop_brochure_eng.pdf

Centers for Disease Control and Prevention/Hospital Infection Control Practices Advisory Committee (HICPAC). (1997). Part I: Evolution of isolation practices. Available: http://www.cdc.gov/ncidod/hip/isolat/isopart1.htm

Centers for Disease Control and Prevention/Hospital Infection Control Practices Advisory Committee. (2002). Table I. Synopsis of types of precautions and patients requiring precautions. Available: http://www.cdc.gov/ncidod/hip/isolat/isotab_1.htm

Centers for Disease Control and Prevention/Hospital Infection Control Practices Advisory Committee. (2007). Table 2. Clinical syndromes or conditions warranting empiric transmission-based precautions in addition to standard precautions in addition to standard precautions pending confirmation of diagnosis. Retrieved October 5, 2008, from http://www.cdc.gov/ncidod/dhqp/pdf/guidelines/Isolation2007.pdf

Centers for Disease Control and Prevention/Hospital Infection Control Practices Advisory Committeee. (2007a). Table 4. Recommendations for application of standard precautions for the care of all patients in all healthcare settings. Retrieved October 5, 2008, from http://www.cdc.gov/ncidod/dhqp/pdf/guidelines/Isolation2007.pdf

Centers for Disease Control and Prevention/Hospital Infection Control Practices Advisory Committeee. (2007b). Type and duration of precautions recommended for selected infections and conditions. Retrieved October 5, 2008, from http://www.cdc.gov/ncidod/dhqp/pdf/guidelines/Isolation2007.pdf

Delahanty, K. & Myers, F., III (2007). Nursing2007 infection control survey report. *Nursing2007, 37*(6), 28–36.

Gage, N. Landon, J. & Sider, M. (1959). *Communicable disease.* Philadelphia: F. A. Davis.

Garner, J. S. (1984). Comments on CDC guideline for isolation precautions in hospitals, 1984. *American Journal of Infection Control, 12,* 163.

Garner, J., & Simmons, B. (1983). *CDC Guideline for isolation precautions in hospitals* (HHS [CDC] Publication No. 83-8314). Atlanta: U.S. Department of Health and Human Services, Public Health Service, Centers for Disease Control. *Infection Control* (1983) 4:245–325; and *American Journal of Infection Control* (1984) 12:103–163.

Haley, R., & Shachtman, R. (1980). The emergence of infection surveillance and control programs in U.S. hospitals: An assessment, 1976. *American Journal of Epidemiology, 111,* 574–591.

Haley, R., Garner, J., & Simmons, B. (1985). A new approach to the isolation of patients with infectious diseases: Alternative systems. *Journal of Hospital Infection, 6,* 128–138.

Hass, J., & Larson, E. (2008). Compliance with hand hygiene guidelines: Where are we in 2008? *American Journal of Nursing, 108*(8), 40–44.

Hospital Infection Control Practices Advisory Committee. (1995). Recommendations for preventing the spread of Vancomycin resistance. *Infection Control and Hospital Epidemiology, 16*(2), 105–113.

Infection Control. (2002). "Hand hygiene" news. *Nursing2002, 32*(5), 32hn6.

Jagger, J. (2002). Avoiding blood and body fluid exposures. *Nursing2002, 32*(8), 68.

Jarvis, W. (2001). Infection control and changing health-care delivery systems. *Emerging Infectious Diseases, 7*(2). Available: http://www.cdc.gov/ncidod/eid/vol7no2/jarvis.htm

Lynch, P., Jackson, M. Cummings, J., & Stamm, W. (1987). Rethinking the role of isolation practices in the prevention of nosocomial infections. *Annals of Internal Medicine, 107,* 243–246.

Lynch, T. (1949). *Communicable disease nursing.* St. Louis, MO: Mosby.

Occupational Safety and Health Administration. (2001). Occupational exposure to bloodborne pathogens; needlestick and other sharps injuries; final rule, 29 CFR Part 1910 66:5317–5325. Retrieved October 5, 2008, from http://www.osha.gov

Occupational Safety and Health Administration. (2003). Model plans and programs for the OSHA Bloodborne Pathogens and Hazard Communications Standards. Retrieved October 5, 2008, from http://www.osha.gov

Perry, J. (2001). The bloodborne pathogens standard, 2001. *Nursing2001, 31*(6), 32hn16.

Porche, D. (1998). Nursing management of adults with immune disorders. In P. Beare & J. Myers (Eds.), *Adult health nursing* (3rd ed.). St. Louis, MO: Mosby.

Schaffner, W. (1980). Infection control: Old myths and new realities. *Infection Control, 1,* 330–334.

Siegel, J., Rhinehart, E., Jackson, M., Chiarello, L., & the Healthcare Infection Control Practices Advisory Committee. (2007). Guideline for isolation precautions: Preventing transmission of infectious agents in healthcare settings 2007. Retrieved October 3, 2008, from http://www.cdc.gov/ncidod/dhqp/pdf/isolation2007.pdf

RESOURCES

Association for Professionals in Infection Control and Epidemiology, Inc. (APIC), http://www.apic. org

Centers for Disease Control and Prevention (CDC), http://www.cdc.gov

Occupational Safety and Health Administration (OSHA), http://www. osha.gov

CHAPTER 23
Bioterrorism

MAKING THE CONNECTION

Refer to the following chapters to increase your understanding of the nursing process:

Basic Nursing

- ***Stress, Adaptation, and Anxiety***
- ***Infection Control/Asepsis***

LEARNING OBJECTIVES

Upon completion of this chapter, you should be able to:

- Identify and discuss major agents of bioterrorism.
- Define terminology pertinent to bioterrorism.
- Review the history of bioterrorism.
- Delineate the roles of each person in a potential or real terrorist attack.
- Delineate the roles of the various levels of government in a potential or real terrorist attack.
- Discuss protective measures, both prior to and following a terrorist attack.
- Describe the various components of the Centers for Disease Control and Prevention, including the Strategic National Stockpile, and its role in emergency preparedness.
- Describe the role of the nurse as a health care professional.
- List various agencies that have been designated as having a role in terrorist preparation or response.

KEY TERMS

anthrax
bioterrorism
Centers for Disease Control and Prevention (CDC)
Chemical, Biological, Radiological/Nuclear, and Explosive Enhanced Response Force Package (CEREPs)
chemical warfare agents
Expeditionary Medical Support (EMEDS)
first responders
nerve agents
plague
radiation sickness
ricin
sarin
smallpox
terrorism
zoonotic disease

INTRODUCTION

Terrorism consists of using any product or weapon or of the threat of using a harmful act or substance to kill or injure a large number of people. **Bioterrorism** is the purposeful use of a biological agent for the purposes of harming, killing, and/or instilling fear in large numbers of people. People who are intent on harming many others or causing death to large numbers of people at one time have used various bioterrorism methods for hundreds of years. Early humans used plants for bioterrorism attacks. Modern-day humans use substances manufactured in a laboratory, many of which have been adapted from the plants used hundreds or even thousands of years ago. Terrorism and bioterrorism are not new to the national or international scene. Sometimes the threat of an attack is all that is needed because a society becomes so afraid of what might happen that it becomes crippled and its members incapable of leading normal lives. Cities, counties, states, and the federal government, have plans in place to increase preparation and to deal with actual terrorism and bioterrorism attacks. Nurses and other health care professionals must also be prepared to respond.

UNDERSTANDING BIOTERRORISM

Following the World Trade Center attack on September 11, 2001, many terroristic and bioterroristic preparations were put into place, and *Bacillus anthracis* was one of the first threats against the American people. Anthrax spores were mailed to several locations around the country in a subsequent bioterroristic act causing illness and death. The spores were released into the air, resulting in the pulmonary form of anthrax. Five people lost their lives, at least 22 others were infected, and numerous postal workers were threatened (Centers for Disease Control and Prevention [CDC], 2007a). There were many reports of a mysterious white powder found in envelopes and packages in several areas of the country. This was assumed to be intentional bioterrorist activity. The public was instructed not to open any suspicious envelopes or packages but rather to take them to a safe place and notify the local police so that proper action could be taken. The packages were examined, and most were found to have an innocuous powder, but the perpetrators of these acts accomplished what they set out to do: instill fear in the people of the United States.

The **Centers for Disease Control and Prevention (CDC)** is an agency of the federal government whose goal is to promote health and quality of life by preventing and controlling disease, injury, and disability. Through programs of education and service, it has categorized infectious agents used by bioterrorists into three groups: biological, chemical, and nuclear radiation.

CRITICAL THINKING

September 11, 2001, Attack

Recall your feelings on September 11, 2001. Where were you when the planes crashed into the Twin Towers of the World Trade Center in New York City? What was your first thought? Feeling? Action?

BIOLOGICAL BIOTERRORISTIC AGENTS/DISEASES

Biological agents are bacteria, viruses, fungi, and toxins that are cultivated to cause harm to humans. These agents cause a variety of responses from mild, allergic reactions to serious infectious diseases resulting in death. The organisms in biologics are found in the natural environment, such as water, soil, plants, and animals. Specific agents may be plant or animal diseases that are readily available, highly virulent or lethal, and easy to aerosolize and disseminate without harming the terrorists themselves.

The CDC has three categories of biological agents classified as category A, category B, and category C (see columns titled "Category of Biological Agents" and "Examples" in Table 23-1 for categorized biological agents). The biological agents in these categories produce serious infectious diseases. The CDC divided the infectious diseases on the basis of their ability to disseminate or be disseminated to large numbers of persons. See Table 23-1 for an adaptation of that information. More complete information on emerging infectious diseases can be obtained at http://www.cdc.gov.

Biologics have certain advantages over other substances when used as a weapon. They are easy to obtain, are inexpensive to produce, do not need a large area for production, and do not need specialized equipment. The potential for widespread dissemination exists. In addition, it is easy to create mass public panic because biologics are colorless and odorless and people cannot be certain if they were exposed. Just the threat of a biologic being released into the air will cause large numbers of persons to panic. Biologics can easily overwhelm available medical services when large groups of persons have been exposed to a biological substance in a short period of time. These persons do not have to demonstrate symptoms but will seek medical care because they have been exposed or believe they have been exposed. The final advantage is that the person who released the substance can easily escape detection. It is not necessary to have a large quantity of the substance, so no one would be suspicious of someone transporting a large package. It would take no special equipment to disseminate the substance, so again suspicion would not be aroused. Knowing which agents bioterrorists are most likely to use helps plan appropriate action for public health preparedness. Several biologic bioterrorism agents exist, but the four potential biologic agents are anthrax (bacterial), botulism (toxin), plague (bacteria), and smallpox (virus). All these are lethal biologic weapons. The untreated mortality of anthrax is more than 90%, for pneumonic plague more than 90%, and for bubonic plague more than 60% (Ohio Department of Health [ODH], 2005). Any of the following bacteria or viruses can cause infectious diseases and could conceivably be used to unleash a massive bioterrorist attack on the people of the world.

ANTHRAX

Anthrax is an acute infectious disease caused by a spore-forming gram-positive bacterium, *Bacillus anthracis*. It normally affects domestic animals, mainly cattle, goats, and sheep. Horses,

Table 23-1 Categories of Biological Agents and Infectious Diseases

CATEGORY OF BIOLOGICAL AGENTS	DISSEMINATION	MORTALITY/ MORBIDITY RATES	IMPACT ON PUBLIC	ACTION NEEDED	EXAMPLES
A	Agents that can be easily disseminated person to person	High mortality	Potential for major public health impact with public panic and social disruption	Special, for public health preparedness	Anthrax (*Bacillus anthracis*) Smallpox (*Variola major*) Plague (*Yersinia pestis*) Botulism (*Clostridium botulinum* toxin) Viral hemorrhagic fevers (filoviruses [e.g., Ebola, Marburg] and arenaviruses [e.g., Lassa, Machupo]) Tularemia (*Francisells tularensis*)
B	Moderately easy to disseminate	Moderate morbidity; low mortality	Potential for major health impacts	Enhancement of CDC's diagnostic capacity and disease surveillance	Brucellosis (*Brucella* species) Glanders (*Burkolderia mallei*) Psittiacosis (*Chlamydia psittaci*) Ricin toxin from *Ricinus communis* (castor beans) Epsiolon toxin of *Clostridium perfringens* Food safety threats (e.g., *Salmonella* species, *Escherichia coli* O157:H7, *Shigella*) *Staphylococcal enterotoxin B* Typhus fever (*Rickettsia prowazekii*) Viral encephalitis (*Alphaviruses* [e.g., Venezuelan equine encephalitis, eastern equine encephalitis, western equine encephalitis]) Water safety threats (e.g., *Vibio cholerae*, *Crytosporidium parvum*) Melioidosis (*Burkholderia pseudomallei*) Q fever (*Coxiella burnetii*)
C	Could be specifically engineered for mass dissemination	Potential for high morbidity and high mortality	Potential for major health impacts	Watchfulness; awareness of possibility; vigilance for new infectious agents	Hantavirus (*Sin Nombre* virus) Yellow fever Tick-borne encephalitis viruses (TBEV) Multi-drug-resistant tuberculosis (MDR TB)

From Biological and chemical terrorism: Strategic plan for preparedness and response. By CDC, 2000a, *Morbidity and Mortality Weekly Report, 49*(RR04), 1–14; Bioterrorism. By CDC, 2008a, retrieved November 5, 2008, from http://emergency.cdc.gov/agent/agentlist-category.asp; Public health preparedness report—Appendix 6. By CDC, 2008e, retrieved November 5, 2008, from http://emergency.cdc.gov/publications/feb08phprep/appendix/appendix6.asp.

donkeys, and pigs are also affected. Wild animals, such as elephants, lions, antelopes, and the American bison, can become infected. Three forms of human anthrax infection exist: pulmonary, cutaneous, and gastrointestinal. The infection depends on the route of exposure. *Bacillus anthracis* enters the human body through contaminated food, by inhalation, or through an open wound. Person-to-person transmission of inhalation type anthrax does not occur, but inhalation of the anthrax bacterium causes a serious form of the disease in humans. Bioterrorists use the spores as an inhalant (ODH, 2005). However, anthrax is usually acquired when a break in the skin comes into direct contact with infected animals and their hides. Direct contact with secretions from cutaneous anthrax lesions may cause a cutaneous infection.

A real problem surrounding *B. anthracis* is that it has the ability to form spores, which can remain viable in soil for at hundreds, perhaps thousands, of years. These spores appear to be resistant to heat, drying, and some harsh chemicals. The spores pose a public health problem because they are responsible for producing inhalation anthrax. If treatment is not immediate and aggressive, the infected person will die. The person may develop tissue necrosis, hemorrhage, edema, or meningitis. Anthrax spores also can be made into a fine powder that is difficult to detect and then spread onto almost any surface.

Diagnosis

Pulmonary or inhalation anthrax is diagnosed with a chest x-ray. If the x-ray shows mediastinal widening, indicating hemorrhaging in the mediastinum, mortality is 90% (ODH, 2005) (Figure 23-1). A blood culture shows the presence of gram-positive bacilli. Enzyme-linked immunosorbent assay (ELISA) and polymerase chain reaction (PCR) tests determine the presence of anthrax.

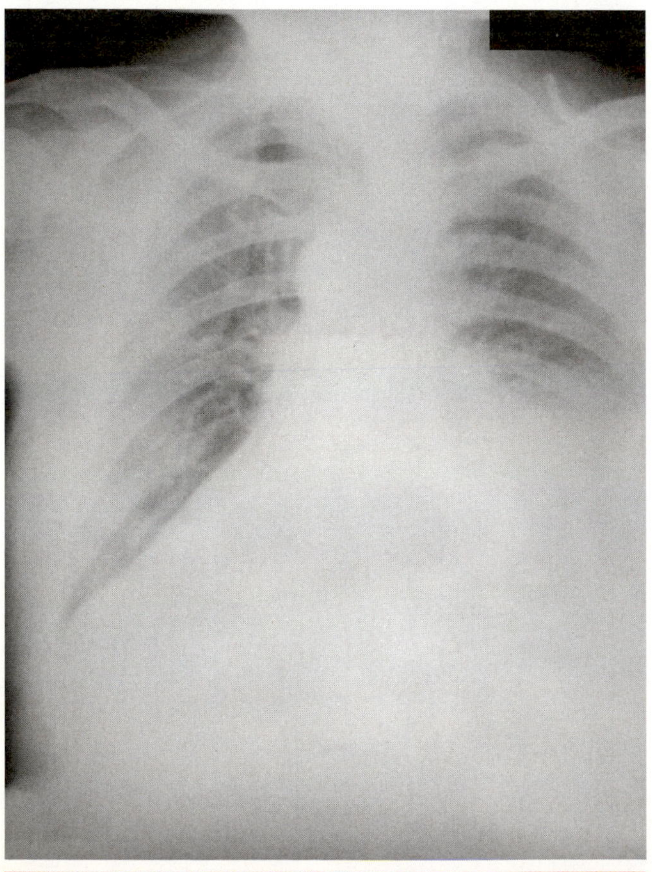

FIGURE 23-1 PA Chest Radiograph of Anthrax, Fourth Day of Illness (*Courtesy of Centers for Disease Control and Prevention.*)

Symptoms of Exposure

The incubation period for pulmonary anthrax is 1 to 5 days, but it can last up to 60 days (CDC, 2006b). Pulmonary anthrax disease has two phases. The first phase presents with flu-like symptoms of sore throat, low-grade fever, nonproductive cough, malaise, fatigue, profound sweats, chest discomfort, and muscle aches. One to 3 days of improvement may follow this phase of symptoms. The second phase, 1 to 5 days after the onset of initial symptoms, is an acute phase of respiratory failure and toxemia. The serious symptoms are pulmonary flu-like symptoms (dyspnea, stridor, and cyanosis) and acute hemorrhagic mediastinitis (CDC, 2006b; ODH, 2005). Shock and death may occur within 24 to 36 hours of the later symptoms.

The incubation period for skin or cutaneous anthrax is 1 to 7 days following exposure. Cutaneous anthrax occurs when skin comes into direct contact with spores or bacilli. The first symptoms of cutaneous anthrax are localized itching followed by skin reactions resembling ulcerated papular lesions that become vesicular, which then forms a dark scab within 7 to 10 days surrounded by brawny edema.

Preventing Exposure

A vaccination for anthrax has been available in the United States for more than 30 years. It has not been widely used because anthrax was not a problem in this country prior to 2001. Controversy surrounds the issue of how protective and how safe the vaccine is. The CDC does not recommend widespread vaccination programs for anthrax. The only persons it recommends get the anthrax vaccination are military members who travel to high-risk areas, laboratory workers who come into contact with anthrax, and persons who deal with animal products imported from high-risk areas (CDC, 2000b, 2002b).

Medical Treatment

Only two antibiotics have been proven to be effective in treating anthrax: doxycycline hydrochloride (Doxylin) and ciprofloxacin (Cipro). Doxylin is approved by the Food and Drug Administration for naturally occurring anthrax (ODH, 2005). However, Cipro is recommended for a bioterrorist attack because a penicillin-resistant strain of anthrax is used.

Nursing Care

After exposure, remove contaminated clothing with minimal handling and place them in a labeled plastic bag. Decrease contamination by having the client shower with soap and water. Postexposure prophylactic treatment is antibiotic therapy for 8 weeks. The exposed person can also receive a vaccination of three doses. One dose is given on exposure followed with other doses in 2- and 4-week intervals. Antibiotic therapy is reduced to 4 weeks with a vaccination. Environmental surfaces or fomites are washed with an Environmental Protection Agency–registered, facility-approved sporicidal/germicidal agent or 0.5% hypochlorite solution (1:9 ratio of household bleach to water) (CDC, 1999).

When a client is diagnosed with anthrax, care is initiated as soon as possible to save his life. Treatment includes medication, supportive care, and prevention of spreading cutaneous anthrax to other persons, including health care workers. Health care personnel should maintain standard precautions (ODH,

2005). When the client is discharged, stress the importance of client adherence to antibiotic therapy.

Smallpox

Smallpox, or variola (a highly contagious viral disease in which humans are the only reservoir for the virus), is considered to be a potential biohazard. Even though the CDC and other governmental agencies throughout the world consider naturally occurring smallpox as eradicated, it was discovered that the virus is stored in some research laboratories in various countries (CDC, 2007a). The last known case of smallpox in the United States was in 1949 (CDC, 2007b), and the last known case of smallpox in the world was in 1977 in Somalia (CDC, 2007b). The occurrence of smallpox is well known throughout history.

Routine immunizations of American citizens stopped in 1972 because smallpox was eradicated in the United States (CDC, 2007c). In 1980, the World Health Organization stated that smallpox was eradicated because of a worldwide vaccination program (Casey et al., 2005). Individuals immunized prior to these dates may retain some degree of immunity, but the population as a whole is susceptible to smallpox. The Advisory Committee on Immunization Practices recommends that states establish and maintain immunized smallpox response teams and that acute care facilities identify and vaccinate designated health care workers to provide screening for or direct medical care to suspected smallpox clients in the event of a terrorist attack (CDC, 2002a).

Smallpox is highly contagious and potentially fatal. Two varieties exist: variola minor and variola major. Variola minor is a mild disease and is less common, with a 1% mortality rate [CDC, 2007b]. Variola major occurs in 90% of smallpox cases and has approximately a 30% mortality rate [CDC, 2007b]. Infection occurs when a very small amount of virus is inhaled and then travels from lungs to regional lymph nodes, where the virus replicates.

LIFE SPAN CONSIDERATIONS

Immunization Protection

Each of us must make a proactive choice to be as protected as possible against biological attack. The only way to do this is for children and adults to become immunized and keep all immunizations up to date. The adult population is the group that is the least protected against some diseases. We refer to diseases that can be protected against by immunizations as diseases of childhood and forget that adults can also contract them. The CDC publishes recommended immunization schedules and updates them annually (see Appendix B: Recommended Childhood and Adolescent Immunization Schedule [CDC, 2009b] and Appendix C: Recommended Adult Immunization Schedule [CDC,2009a]). Each of us must keep abreast of new developments and see to it that we and our children, relatives, and acquaintances are protected. This is the only way that we can be active in protecting ourselves against the illnesses and possible death following a terrorist attack.

Transmission

Smallpox is spread person to person as an aerosol or a droplet or by contact with contaminated objects, such as clothing or bedding. Only a very small amount of viral particles is needed to cause infection. Animals or plants are not a reservoir for the smallpox virus. It is estimated that as many as one-third of persons could die if the virus is unleashed into an unvaccinated population (ODH, 2005).

Symptoms of Exposure

The symptoms of smallpox include fever, prostration, and a vesicular, pustular rash. A papular rash appears on the face 2 to 3 days later, spreading to the extremities, including the palms of the hands and soles of the feet. The rash then becomes vesicular, painful, and pustular (Figure 23-2). A person experiences the onset of headache, high fever, and myalgias 10 to 17 days following airborne or droplet virus inhalation or contact with an infected person who has bleeding lesions. Death may follow the appearance of symptoms. The patient is contagious from the onset of the rash until the scabs separate, about a 3-week period.

Preventing Exposure

The U.S. government has stockpiled an adequate supply of smallpox vaccine to vaccinate every person in the United States.

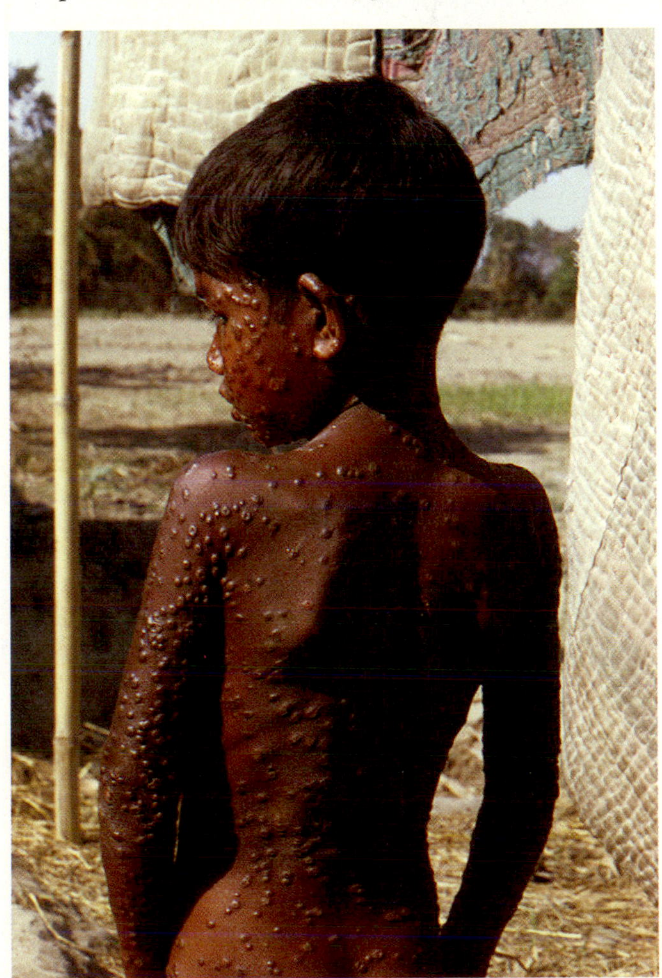

Figure 23-2 Young Child with Smallpox (*Courtesy of Centers for Disease Control and Prevention/photo by Jean Roy.*)

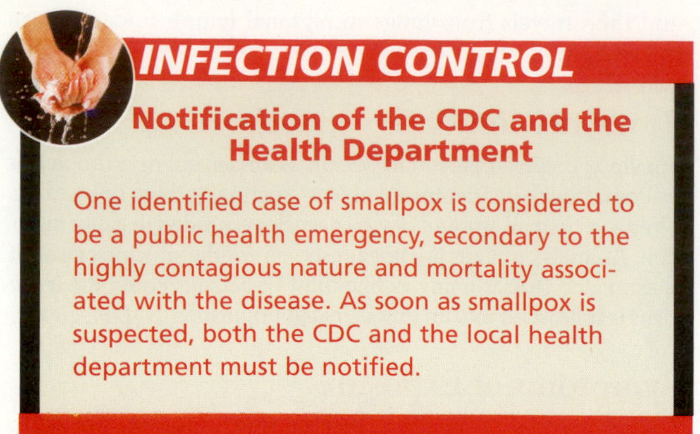

INFECTION CONTROL

Notification of the CDC and the Health Department

One identified case of smallpox is considered to be a public health emergency, secondary to the highly contagious nature and mortality associated with the disease. As soon as smallpox is suspected, both the CDC and the local health department must be notified.

The vaccine will protect an individual if given prior to exposure or up to 3 days following exposure. The U.S. government has been reluctant to order mass vaccination programs because of the side effects associated with the smallpox vaccination, including death (CDC, 2007c).

Medical Treatment

No effective treatments for smallpox exist. The only recommendations are vaccinations within 2 to 3 days of exposure and immediate initiation of airborne isolation procedures. Figure 23-3 shows a smallpox vaccination reaction.

Nursing Care

Nursing care must begin as soon as a diagnosis of smallpox is suspected. Standard contact and airborne precautions must be initiated for any patient with a vesicular rash. Supportive care is provided to the patient, and symptoms are treated accordingly. Nurses and other personnel caring for the patient with suspected or confirmed smallpox must be extremely careful to avoid contact with the organism while providing care to the patient. This includes wearing protective clothing, including gown, gloves, and a special mask.

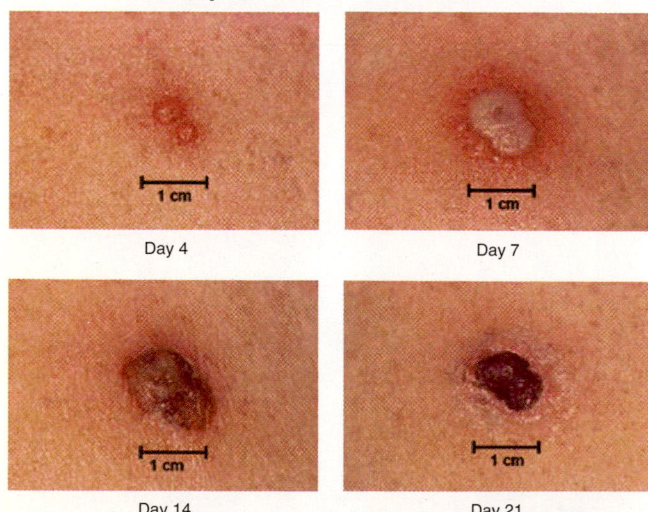

FIGURE 23-3 Smallpox Vaccination Reaction: Day 1 Papule, Days 7 to 14 Pustule, and Day 21 Scab (*Redrawn from data courtesy of Centers for Disease Control and Prevention.*)

PLAGUE

Plague is a disease caused by the bacterium *Yersinia pestis*. It is a **zoonotic disease**, a disease of animals that can be directly transmitted to humans by the animals that have the disease. Two types of plague exist: bubonic plague and pneumonic plague. The transmission and symptoms of the two types of plague are different. Humans acquire bubonic plague from the bite of a flea feeding on a rat or other rodent infected with *Y. pestis* or when an open wound is exposed to the bacterium. If bubonic plague is not treated, the bacterium enters the bloodstream and invades the lungs, causing pneumonic plague. A person can also acquire pneumonic plague by breathing in *Y. pestis* particles from the air. Pneumonic plague is less common but highly contagious and frequently fatal. Pneumonic plague is transmitted from person to person by droplets containing the plague bacterium. Bubonic plague is not transmitted from person to person. Bioterrorists could release *Y. pestis* as an aerosol weapon, causing many people to develop pneumonic plague within 1 to 6 days. The plague could also spread to those who come in close contact with those first exposed. One exposure advantage of *Y. pestis* is that it is destroyed by sunlight and drying and survives up to 1 hour when released into the air.

Diagnosis

Bubonic plague is diagnosed by blood cultures and lymph gland samples. Pneumonic plague is diagnosed by blood cultures and sputum specimens. If plague is present, all cultures and samples contain *Y. pestis*.

Symptoms of Exposure

A client becomes ill within 2 to 6 days of exposure. The main symptom of bubonic plague is a painful, swollen, tender lymph gland in the groin, armpit, or neck. The swollen gland is called a "bubo" (thus "bubonic plague"). Other symptoms are fever, chills, headache, malaise, and extreme exhaustion. Bubonic plague can progress to septicemia (septicemic plague), shock and death, or pneumonic plague.

The incubation period for pneumonic plague, if the client is exposed by intentional aerosol release or by close or direct contact, is 1 to 6 days (CDC, 2005). The first signs of pneumonic plague are fever, headache, weakness, chest pain, cough, and sometimes bloody or watery sputum. Pneumonia develops quickly with shortness of breath (CDC, 2004). Other symptoms that may occur are nausea, vomiting, and abdominal pain. If antibiotic treatment is not started within 24 hours after symptom onset, the disease progresses to respiratory failure, shock, and rapid death.

DRUGS

Antibiotics for Pneumonic Plague

The antibiotics of choice for pneumonic plague are streptomycin sulfate (Streptomycin), gentamicin sulfate (Garamycin), tetracyclines, and chloramphenicol (Chloromycetin). Antibiotics must be given within 24 hours of the first symptoms to prevent respiratory failure, shock, and death. Do not start antibiotic therapy until all cultures and specimens are obtained.

Preventing Exposure

Researchers are working on developing an oral vaccine to protect against plague, cholera, and anthrax, but it will not be available for several more years. Military personnel will be the first ones to receive this vaccine when it becomes available. Immunity is expected to occur in a matter of days (Fox, 2008). Persons in contact with infected clients are placed on antibiotics for 7 days. Caregivers should also wear a close-fitting surgical mask to prevent inhalation of the *Y. pestis* bacterium (CDC, 2004).

Medical Treatment

The treatment for bubonic plague includes antibiotics, supportive care, isolation, and surgical drainage of any lesions in the neck, groin, or axilla. The most important treatment component is preventing the spread of disease to others. With pneumonic plague as well, preventing its spread to others is of prime importance. Since pneumonic plague results in bronchopneumonia, the patient is treated as any patient with bronchopneumonia, with the addition of isolation being instituted immediately on suspicion of the disease.

The antibiotic of choice for bubonic plague is streptomycin. Gentamicin is used if streptomycin is contraindicated. Tetracyclines and chloramphenicol can also be used.

If a client acquires pneumonic plague by close contact with an infected person, antibiotics should be started within 7 days of exposure and taken for at least 7 days. To prevent death from intentional aerosol release, start antibiotics within 24 hours of the first symptoms. Effective oral antibiotics are doxycycline (Vibramycin) and ciprofloxacin (Cipro) and, for injection or intravenous use, streptomycin sulfate or gentamicin sulfate (Garamycin).

Nursing Care

Nursing care of the client with plague includes droplet precautions until 72 hours after initiating antibiotic therapy. Contact precautions are necessary until decontamination is complete, especially if many people are suspected or known to have been contaminated. Standard precautions are recommended if the patient has lesions that have been incised.

CHEMICAL BIOTERRORIST AGENTS

Bioterrorists could also use **chemical warfare agents**, including gases, liquids, or solids that cause injury or death to people, animals, and plants. The extent of injury depends on the chemical and the amount and length of exposure. The chemical categories are nerve, blood, choking or vomiting, and blister or vesicant agents. Chemical agents include nerve agents, blood agents, choking or vomiting agents,

MEMORYTRICK

Antibiotic Therapy for Pneumonic Plague

For close contact acquired pneumonic plague, give antibiotics 7/7—within 7 days of exposure and for at least 7 days.

COMMUNITY/HOME HEALTH CARE

Plans for a Terrorist Attack

The United States is now focused on how to recognize possible terrorist attacks and how to treat those who have been exposed regardless of the form of the attack—biological, chemical, or nuclear. Researchers are attempting to develop antidotes and vaccinations against biological agents. Possible chemical and nuclear agents are being identified and studied. Government agencies have banded together to plan for the aftermath of terrorist attacks. Not only have plans been made, but mock attacks are routinely held so that each person is aware of his role following an attack. Each person is given information on how to protect himself, one's family, and also one's role in the community should an attack occur. It is far better to be prepared and never need to put the plans into action than to be attacked and not have a well-planned response.

and blister or vesicant agents. The most common chemical agents are sulfur mustard (mustard gas), sarin, and VX (nerve agents). **Nerve agents** are powerful acetylcholinesterase inhibitors, altering cholinergic synaptic transmission at neuroeffector junctions (muscarinic effects), at skeletal myoneural junctions and autonomic ganglia (nicotinic effects), and in the central nervous system. Death can occur within 15 minutes if one drop to a few milliliters of a nerve agent come in contact with the skin (Agency for Toxic Substances and Disease Registry [ATSDR], 2008). Table 23-2 provides examples of each category of chemical bioterrorist agent.

Chemical agents have been available since World War I. Most chemical agents were designed to create one of two situations: to kill as many persons as possible or to make the soldiers and others so sick that they would be unable to continue fighting.

RICIN

Ricin is one of the newest chemicals identified as a nerve agent. It is a poison made from the waste products of processing castor beans into castor oil. According to the CDC (2008b), ricin has some potential medical uses, such as bone marrow transplants and as a treatment to kill cancer cells. Accidental exposure is extremely unlikely. It would take a deliberate act of terrorism to make ricin and use it as a poison. Ricin can be a powder, a mist, a pellet, or a weak acid preparation. Humans are poisoned by breathing in ricin as a mist or powder. Ricin can also be put into food or dissolved in water and then swallowed. A final way to poison someone with ricin is to dissolve it and then inject it into a person's body. Ricin poisoning is not contagious and cannot be spread from person to person through casual contact.

Ricin enters the cells of a human body and prevents the cells from making necessary proteins. Without these proteins, the cells die. Eventually, this is harmful to the entire body, and death may occur.

TABLE 23-2 Examples of Each Category of Chemical Agent

CATEGORY OF CHEMICAL AGENT	EXAMPLES	FORM(S)	SYMPTOMS OF EXPOSURE
Nerve agents	Sarin (GB) Soman (GD) Tabun (GA) VX	Gaseous liquid	Runny nose, sweating, blurred vision, headache, difficulty breathing, drooling, nausea, vomiting, muscle cramps and twitching, confusion, convulsions, paralysis, coma, and death
Blood agents	Hydrogen cyanide	Liquid	Headache, dizziness, confusion, nausea, shortness of breath, convulsions, vomiting, weakness, anxiety, irregular heartbeat, tightness in chest, and unconsciousness
	Cyanogen chloride	Gas	Rhinorrhea, sore throat, drowsiness, confusion, nausea, vomiting, cough, unconsciousness, and edema
Choking/vomiting agents	Phosgene	Gas	Coughing, burning sensation in throat and eyes, tearing, blurred vision, difficulty breathing, nausea, vomiting Skin contact: frostbite or burn-type lesions Pulmonary edema occurs within 2 to 6 hours of exposure.
	Adamsite—vomiting agent	Crystalline dispensed in aerosol	Rapid onset; irritation of the eyes, skin, and upper airway; nausea; vomiting; spasmodic blinking; corneal necrosis; burning in throat; chest tightness and pain; uncontrollable and violent coughing and sneezing; increased nasal secretions; abdominal cramps; diarrhea; malaise; headache; mental depression; and chills
Blister/vesicant agents	Distilled mustard (HD) Mustard gas (H) Lewisite Mustard/lewisite Mustard/T Nitrogen mustard Phosgene oxime Sesqui mustard Sulfur mustard	Liquid or crystalline	**Respiratory exposure:** rhinorrhea, nasal irritation and pain, sore throat, cough, dyspnea, chest tightness, tachypnea, and hemoptysis **Skin exposure:** itching and erythema Immediate blanching with phosgene oxime Blisters (within 1 hour with phosgene oxime, 2 to 12 hours with lewisite, and 2 to 24 hours with mustards) Necrosis and eschar in 7 to 10 days **Eye exposure:** conjunctivitis, lacrimation, eye burning and pain, photophobia, blurred vision, eyelid edema, corneal ulceration, and blindness **Gastrointestinal ingestion exposure:** abdominal pain, nausea and vomiting, hematemesis, and diarrhea (possibly bloody) **High-dose exposure:** hypotension, atrioventricular block with cardiac arrest, tremors, convulsions, ataxia, and coma

From Medical management guidelines for nerve agents: Tuban (GA); sarin (GB); soman (GD); and VX. By Agency for Toxic Substances and Disease Registry, 2008, Department of Health and Human Services, retrieved September 9, 2008, from http://www.atsdr.cdc.gov/MHMI/mmg166.html; NIOSH emergency response card: Cyanogen chloride (ERC506-77-4). By CDC, 2005, retrieved November 14, 2008, from http://emergency.cdc.gov/agent/cyanide/erc506-77-4.pr.asp; Facts about Phosgene. By CDC, 2006a, retrieved November 14, 2008, from http://emergency.cdc.gov/agent/phosgene/basics/facts.asp; NIOSH emergency response card: Hydrogen cyanide (ERC74-90-8). By CDC, 2006c, retrieved November 14, 2008, from http://emergency.cdc.gov/agent/cyanide/erc74-90-8.asp; Toxic syndrome description: Vesicant/blister agent poisoning. By CDC, 2006e, retrieved November 13, 2008, from http://www.bt.cdc.gov/agent/vesicants/tsd.asp

Symptoms of Exposure

The symptoms of ricin poisoning depend on whether ricin was inhaled, ingested, or injected. A large dose may affect many organs. Symptoms begin to appear within 8 hours after ricin inhalation. Following inhalation, symptoms include respiratory distress, fever, cough, nausea, and tightness in the chest. Diaphoresis and pulmonary edema follow. Cyanosis becomes apparent. Severe hypotension and respiratory failure occur, leading to death. Powder or mist forms of ricin cause redness and pain of the skin and eyes. Symptoms usually appear within 6 hours of ingesting ricin. The symptoms include vomiting and diarrhea (that may become bloody) and severe dehydration, followed by hypotension. Hallucinations, seizures, and hematuria occur. Within several days, kidney, hepatic, and spleen failure also occur; if this happens, the person will likely die. Death may occur within 36 to 72 hours following exposure to ricin, depending on the route and the amount of exposure. If the person is still alive after 3 to 5 days, recovery is likely.

Preventing Exposure

The most important preventive factor is avoiding exposure to ricin. No antidote is available, only supportive care. If exposure occurred, it is important to get the ricin out of or off of the body as quickly as possible.

Medical Treatment

If exposed to ricin, get away from the area of exposure or get outside. Remove clothing, wash the entire body with large amounts of soap and lukewarm (not hot) water, and then seek medical attention. Do not let soap get into the eyes during the shower. Do not remove clothing by taking it over the victim's head and re-exposing them to ricin; instead, cut the clothing off the person. Clothing and anything that comes into contact with the clothing is double bagged. Notify emergency health care personnel of bagged items so that they can properly dispose of the bag. Eyeglasses are washed with soap and water, dried, and then put back on. Contacts must be disposed of with the contaminated clothing and not put back into the eyes. Client care may be as simple as rinsing out the eyes or as complicated as ventilatory assistance and administering medications to raise the blood pressure or control seizures.

Nursing Care

A nurse or **first responder**, the first people who will spring into action when a terrorist attack occurs, must be extremely careful to avoid contact with anything that may have been exposed to ricin when assisting a client. The health care provider wears rubber gloves and does not handle clothing and other articles with bare hands. Other nursing care is based on the needs of the patient and the medical orders given. Much emotional support is needed both for the patient and for the family members. Education is also important since ricin exposure is a new and previously unknown condition to most people.

MEMORY TRICK

Ricin Exposure

If a person is exposed to ricin, remember **GROWS**:

G = Get away from the exposed area.

R = Remove clothing and all personal items (i.e., eyeglasses, contacts).

O = Over the head; cut it **O**ff.

W = Wash eyes with water.

S = Seek medical help.

CRITICAL THINKING

First Responders

Why is it of major importance to protect the first responders in a bioterrorist attack?

Sarin

Sarin GB (O-isopropyl methylphosphonofluoridate) is a dangerous nerve agent that has been available since World War II (CDC, 2006d). During the rush hour on March 20, 1995, a Japanese cult, Aum Shinrikyo, released a liquid form of sarin in five cars of three different Tokyo subway lines that joined at the Kasumigaseki station, the location of several government ministries. Twelve people were killed, and approximately 6,000 sought medical care. This attack shows how easy it is for a small terrorist group to plan and launch a chemical warfare terrorist attack (Council on Foreign Relations, 2008; Salmon, 2008).

Sarin is a clear, colorless, odorless, and tasteless gas and is the most toxic and fastest acting of all the chemical agents. Sarin is also the most volatile nerve agent, meaning that it can easily and rapidly evaporate from a liquid form into a vapor and spread rapidly through the environment. Extremely small amounts (0.01 mg/kg) of sarin can kill a person. Food and water can also be contaminated; sarin mixes easily with water. Sarin is slightly heavier than air, and it hovers close to the ground when released. People are exposed to liquid forms of sarin through skin or eye contact or by breathing air containing sarin vapors. Sarin vapors are absorbed through the skin only at very high concentrations. It is not necessary to come into contact with the liquid form of the agent. Exposure to sarin vapor can and does cause serious symptoms of exposure. Sarin is released from clothing in approximately half an hour after it comes in contact with sarin vapor.

Symptoms of Exposure

Sarin is a powerful acetylcholinesterase inhibitor, producing muscarinic and nicotinic effects. Sarin exposure symptoms include loss of consciousness, seizures, paralysis, and respiratory failure, leading to death within seconds to minutes of exposure. Three factors determine the amount of poisoning caused by exposure to sarin: the amount of sarin to which a person was exposed, how the exposure occurred, and the length of time the exposure lasted. For specific symptoms of exposure to small amounts of sarin, see Table 23-3.

Preventing Exposure

The best prevention is to avoid exposure to sarin. If exposure cannot be prevented, then treatment must be started as soon as possible following exposure.

TABLE 23-3 Symptoms of Sarin and Other Nerve Agent Exposure

MUSCARINIC EFFECTS	NICOTINIC EFFECTS
Pinpoint pupils	Skeletal muscle twitching, cramping, and weakness
Blurred or dim vision	Tachycardia
Conjunctivitis	Hypertension
Eye and head pain	
Hypersecretion of salivary, lacrimal, sweat, and bronchial glands	
Bronchial restriction	
Nausea	
Vomiting	
Diarrhea	
Abdominal cramping	
Urinary and fecal incontinence	
Bradycardia	

COURTESY OF DELMAR CENGAGE LEARNING

Medical Treatment

Treatment of sarin exposure and other nerve agents involves removing the sarin from the body as soon as possible and providing supportive care.

Nursing Care

After exposure to sarin, if possible, move to an area where there is fresh air; this action is effective in decreasing the possibility of death from sarin exposure. Move to the highest ground available since the sarin vapor will stay in low-lying areas. If the sarin was released indoors, then the persons exposed should move outside as quickly as possible. Any clothing that has liquid sarin on it must be removed and double bagged in plastic bags. If the nurse is assisting other people to remove contaminated clothing, avoid touching any areas contaminated with liquid sarin. If the person complains of any burning of the eyes or blurred vision, assist in rinsing the eyes with plain water for 10 to 15 minutes. Immediately wash liquid sarin from the body with copious amounts of soap and water. If sarin has been swallowed, do not induce vomiting or give any fluids by mouth. Atropine sulfate, an acetylcholine inhibitor, and pralidoxime chloride (pyridine-2-aldoxime methochloride and 2-PAM chloride) are the only known antidotes for sarin poisoning. Persons with mild or moderate exposure to sarin usually recover completely. Persons with severe exposure are not expected to survive. Neurological problems should not last longer than 1 to 2 weeks. As soon as the previously mentioned measures have been completed and emergency personnel notified, take the client to the emergency room. Emergency personnel must protect themselves against exposure before getting near the client (Figure 23-4).

CRITICAL THINKING

Sarin

Why is sarin so dangerous as a biological weapon?

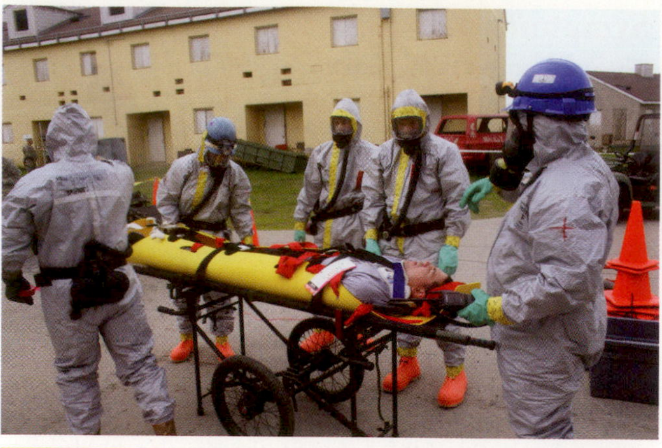

FIGURE 23-4 First responders and emergency personnel must take appropriate precautions to protect themselves during an attack. (*Courtesy U.S. Army/photo by Lt. Col. Richard Goldenberg.*)

Specific care depends on the client's symptoms. A patent airway must be established and maintained. Administer antidotes of atropine sulfate and pralidoxime chloride (Protopam Chloride) as soon as possible. If seizures are present, administer diazepam (Valium) as needed. Cardiac manifestations are treated as they appear.

NUCLEAR RADIATION BIOTERRORIST AGENT

Radiation sickness, or, more properly, acute radiation syndrome (an abnormal condition resulting from exposure to ionizing radiation), is dependent primarily on the dose of radiation that a person receives. Radiation sickness can occur hours or days after high doses of radiation exposure.

Symptoms of Exposure

The first symptoms are nausea, vomiting, and diarrhea. Later symptoms include anorexia, fatigue, weight loss, and bone marrow suppression. Persons who live through the acute exposure are at high risk for developing certain cancers, especially leukemia, secondary to bone marrow suppression.

Preventing Exposure

Unfortunately, exposure to nuclear radiation cannot be prevented. One is not aware of potential exposure until a bomb is dropped and exposure has already occurred. If a person is working with nuclear radiation, prevent accidents that lead to exposure.

Medical Treatment

Little to no effective treatments exist for radiation exposure. The best treatment available is to treat the symptoms. Administration of potassium iodide (KI) tablets following radiation exposure prevents up to 100% of the radioactive iodine released by a nuclear explosion from entering the thyroid gland and damaging the thyroid cells. KI should be taken prior to or immediately following exposure to radiation but is effective if taken as long as 3 to 4 hours following exposure. KI protects only the thyroid gland; it does not protect any other body structures.

Nursing Care

Initial care of external radiation exposure involves removing all clothing and properly disposing of it, cleansing the skin, and initiating isolation procedures to protect others. Initial care of a person who has inhaled or ingested radioactive material should follow protocols for anyone who has been exposed to chemical poisons. Body wastes are checked for radiation levels. If a wound is present, extra care is taken to prevent cross contamination of exposed surfaces. Any and all emergency lifesaving techniques must be done at the same time to avoid the spread of the radiation effects. Nursing staff and others caring for the patient must wear surgical gowns, gloves, and caps.

BIOTERRORISM PREPAREDNESS

In the event of a covert bioterrorist attack, nurses and other health care professionals will be the first ones to see the victims after the first responders. Victims appear in emergency rooms, physician offices, clinics, or school health settings. Since nurses staff these areas and are the first persons who see and evaluate potential clients, they must be able to identify symptoms, unusual happenings, trends in client symptoms, and other significant events.

Nurses must be aware of the emergency response system at local, state, and federal levels. They also are aware of their role in emergency response and emergency preparations. Nurses are vital committee members in developing, maintaining, and evaluating emergency response plans for health care facilities and communities. Hospitals have emergency plans in place to care for clients involved in bioterrorism acts and other emergency situations.

Government Agency Involvement

Many government agencies are available to assist with planning for disasters. Two of the older agencies are the U.S. Department of Defense and the CDC. Although their primary functions are very different, they join in efforts to combat terrorism. Their common goals are to inform, educate, and prepare U.S. citizens for unusual disease outbreaks.

Department of Health and Human Services

The Department of Health and Human Services is the main agency of the U.S. government tasked with protecting the health of all Americans and providing essential human services, especially to those who are least able to provide for themselves. This department works closely with state and local governments.

One of the branches of the Department of Health and Human Services is the Coordinating Office for Terrorism Preparedness and Emergency Response. The mission of this branch is to protect the health and enhance the potential for living at the highest possible level across the life span of all people in all communities related to community preparedness and response. It works with the CDC and maintains response operations, including the Strategic National Stockpile (SNS). The SNS is a program managed by the CDC that is designed to ensure that essential medical supplies are sent immediately to a community that has sustained a large-scale chemical or biological attack.

Federal Emergency Management Agency

The Federal Emergency Management Agency (FEMA) was established by a law passed in 1974, PL 93-288, the Disaster Relief Act. FEMA's mission is to decrease the loss of life and property and to protect the United States from all hazards, including natural disasters, acts of terrorism, and other man-made disasters.

The intent of Congress was to provide an orderly and continuing means of assistance by the federal government to state and local governments in carrying out their responsibilities to citizens, specifically to alleviate suffering and damage resulting from disasters. The Stafford Act expanded the scope of existing disaster relief programs. Among its provisions are encouraging the development of comprehensive disaster preparedness and assistance plans and programs by state and local governments, encouraging all entities to obtain insurance coverage that would supplement or replace government assistance, and providing federal assistance programs for both private and public losses incurred as a result of disasters.

The administrator of FEMA is appointed by the president and reports directly to the secretary of Homeland Security. The administrator may be called on by the president to serve as a member of the cabinet in the event of a disaster or an act of terrorism.

CDC

The CDC expanded its programs to inform all Americans of the new threats against health and life. One of its functions is managing the SNS, which ensures that a community that has experienced a massive chemical or biological attack will have immediate necessary supplies. Some of the materials included are antibiotics, vaccines, chemical antidotes, antitoxins, bandages, airways, and intravenous equipment. The SNS has two divisions. One division consists of large prepackaged emergency supplies that are stored in various places throughout the country. Each storage site was chosen so that no site is more than 12 hours away from every community in the country. The 50-ton packaged supplies are stored in a climate-controlled warehouse.

The second division of the SNS is a vendor-managed inventory (VMI), which consists of materials that are more specific to certain biological preparations. They arrive at a site that has experienced a bioterroristic attack after the agent used is identified and within 24 to 36 hours after the attack occurs. Because of the SNS, individuals or even individual communities should not attempt to store materials in preparation for an attack because the materials would most likely become outdated before the need would arise.

National Guard Medical Services Branch

The National Guard established two programs to promptly provide supplies to emergency situations: the **Expeditionary Medical Support (EMEDS)** and the **Chemical, Biological, Radiological/Nuclear, and Explosive Enhanced Response Force Package (CERFPs)**. The EMEDS is a total package that includes everything necessary to screen and treat clients who need outpatient care. It also releases clients that need more than outpatient care to other facilities for longer-term care. EMEDS used in civilian settings provides emergency care while local facilities gear up to provide necessary care. EMEDS has enhanced packages, called EMEDS + 10 or EMEDS + 25, that include up to 25 critical care beds.

A medical component to CERFP is similar to an EMEDS and can be expanded to the same contents and capabilities of an EMEDS. This component can be deployed alone without the rest of the CERFP. It can also include a surgical suite if needed. The CERFP can respond rapidly following a call by the governor to a state adjutant general and be at the scene of a disaster, ready to function in 6 hours (Figure 23-5). It can also respond to disasters outside the home state, but the governor can deny the request if an emergency exists in that state.

The Joint Commission

The Joint Commission, previously known as the Joint Commission on the Accreditation of Healthcare Organizations, has had emergency preparedness as part of its core components for many years. Until recently, the Joint Commission focused on preparing for natural disasters, such as floods and tornados, rather than man-made ones. In today's world, facilities prepare to handle natural disasters as well as man-made situations. Facilities must have written plans for dealing with the situation at hand, for being sure that their usual functions are completed, and for returning to normal functioning once the situation has been resolved. All employees must be aware of these plans and know where the written plans are located.

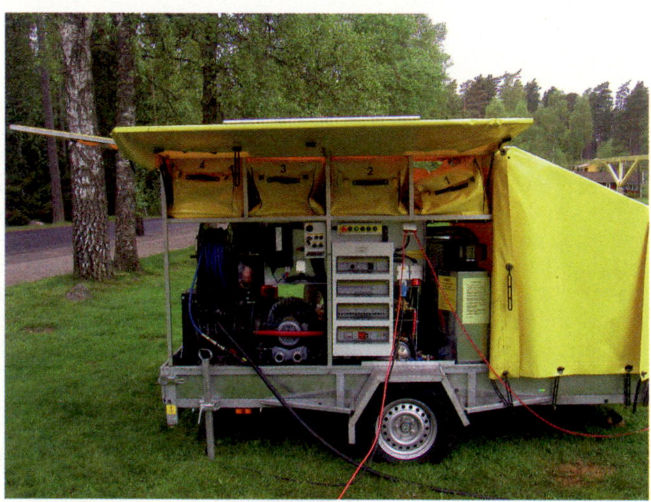

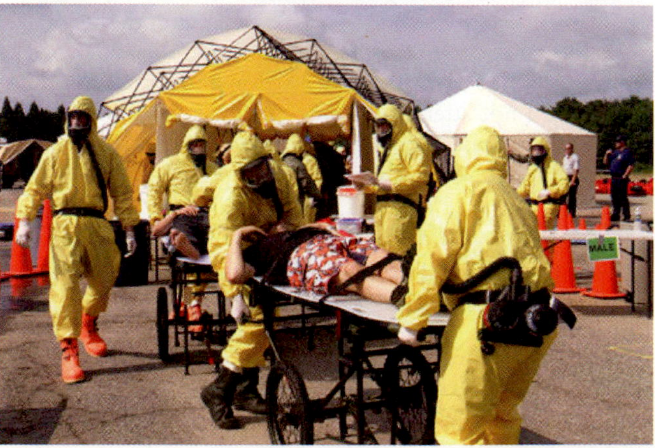

FIGURE 23-5 EMEDS and CERFP respond to bioterrorist sites with trailers, vehicles, and tents to treat emergency situations. (*Images courtesy of SEDAB and National Guard.*)

The Joint Commission sets standards ensuring that health care facilities provide a safe environment for both clients and health care workers. Disaster planning falls under these standards in the section titled "Environment of Care" (Joint Commission, 2007).

Each facility should have an emergency operations plan (EOP). The EOP contains information on when to activate a response and who will be notified first, both internally and within the community. Once the emergency plan has been activated, protection of the facility environment takes priority. This will most likely be accomplished by security personnel. Persons already within the facility, such as employees, clients, and other people, are protected from infection or contamination by suspected victims. These victims are kept in an area away from the general occupants of the facility. If a bioterrorism attack occurs or is suspected to have occurred, standard precautions in addition to disease-specific precautions are instituted. If the agent is unknown, efforts are made to identify it so that disease-specific precautions can be instituted.

After the previous steps are completed, a decontamination protocol is followed. The published protocol for decontamination includes guidelines for handling contaminated clients, facilities availability, and specific measures to complete, depending on the type of contamination that occurred.

An agency has an EOP to prevent chaos in the event of a disaster. Practice drills are conducted on a regular basis so that everyone knows their expected role.

EMERGENCY RESPONSE TEAMS

A group of persons are identified as those who will be **first responders** in case of a terrorist attack. They are nurses, emergency room personnel, EMS personnel, public health personnel, primary care providers, and other persons, such as law enforcement, animal control officers, firefighters, and veterinarians. Communities around the country are asked to identify and train persons who are designated as first responders should the need for them arise.

PROFESSIONALTIP

Terrorist Attack

The possibility of a terrorist attack exists on a day-to-day basis in the United States. Nurses, especially those employed in an emergency room setting, must be aware of the symptoms of exposure to chemical agents. They recognize the symptoms and are prepared to take immediate steps to protect themselves, other persons who are nearby, and the client. It is better to err on the side of caution and to institute actions if the client's symptoms indicate exposure to a chemical agent than to ignore such symptoms or deny that an attack can happen.
A bioterrorist attack can occur, and health care personnel must be prepared to act competently and quickly.

Nurse need to understand the rationale for preparing for the possible consequences of any disaster or attack. Many thousands of people could be injured or killed and many more people could suffer long-term effects following the occurrence, both physical and psychological. Nurses have a responsibility to get involved in disaster planning and disaster awareness programs. Part of this involvement is knowing which agents may be used, effects of various agents, emergency care needed by the victims, and personal protection precautions. Many web sites sponsored by the CDC and other official groups provide information about biological warfare and bioterrorism preparation. The web sites provided in the "Resources" section at the end of the chapter are informative resources for the nurse to use professionally and as a resource for clients.

CASE STUDY

A licensed practical nurse works for a physician who is employed by the Indian Health Service at a Navajo reservation. The nurse and physician are not Native American but have worked in the clinic for 8 years and know most of the residents. They have a trusting relationship with the tribal elders and, through them, with the people, many of whom are elderly. Within the past 36 hours, 37 persons have come into the clinic with the following symptoms: vomiting, diarrhea that has become bloody in some cases, dehydration, hallucinations, and fainting. The persons who initially showed symptoms now have hematuria. Two of the first persons who demonstrated symptoms died. The elders are concerned because their people are generally healthy and not had any flu outbreaks or other mass illness in many years. The nurse suspects ricin poisoning.

1. What symptoms led the nurse to her conclusion?
2. What assessment questions would the nurse ask the clients and elders?
3. What precautions would the nurse, physician, and other health care personnel take in caring for the clients?
4. What interventions would the nurse and physician continue for those who are ill?
5. What interventions can be done to prevent others (including health care workers) from becoming ill with the same symptoms?
6. What reassurances could the nurse give to the tribal elders?

SUMMARY

- The three forms of terrorist attacks are biological, chemical, and nuclear.
- Government agencies have expanded and new agencies formed in planning and preparing for the possibility of terrorist attacks.
- Agencies from the federal government to a community hospital prepare for bioterrorists attacks.
- The CDC is one of the major agencies involved in bioterrorist attack preparedness.
- The Joint Commission incorporated terrorist attack preparedness in its survey criteria for health care facilities.
- The major biologic substances expected in terroristic attacks are variola (smallpox), plague, sarin, and ricin.
- Nurses are aware of the symptoms of bioterroristic agents and the emergency care for clients exposed to agents.
- First responders are well trained and know how to protect themselves against contamination and care for the victims of an attack.

REVIEW QUESTIONS

1. The top priority for a first responder following a terrorist attack is:
   1. protecting oneself from contamination.
   2. identifying the agent that was used.
   3. removing uncontaminated persons from the site.
   4. cordoning off the immediate area.
2. The federal agency designated to lead the overall planning effort to upgrade the ability of the United States to respond in a bioterrorist attack is the:
   1. Center for Domestic Preparedness.
   2. U.S. Department of Health and Human Services.
   3. Centers for Disease Control and Prevention.
   4. U.S. Army Corps of Engineers.
3. Biologic agents may be more successful than other types of agents in a terrorist attack because they:
   1. are very effective in small quantities.
   2. are readily available.
   3. are manufactured of volatile ingredients.
   4. provide no protection with immunizations.
4. Clients who receive priority care immediately following a terrorist act are those clients who:
   1. are important to the local governmental structure.
   2. are most seriously injured.
   3. have the greatest chance for survival.
   4. have jobs and contribute positively to society as a whole.

5. The first priority action when a person is exposed to ricin vapors is to:
   1. rinse eyes with plain water.
   2. remove all clothing.
   3. move away from the exposed area.
   4. seek medical assistance.
6. An agency's emergency operations plan must include information about: (Select all that apply.)
   1. who will notify the community agencies involved.
   2. what agent was used in the attack.
   3. notifying family members of a relative's deaths.
   4. how people will be prevented from leaving or entering the agency.
   5. decontamination of any staff needing it.
   6. managing the Strategic National Stockpile.
7. The first priority action when a person is exposed to sarin is to:
   1. remove all clothing and double bag them in a plastic bag.
   2. wash the body with copious amounts of soap and water.
   3. notify the emergency personnel and take the victim to an emergency room.
   4. move to the highest ground where there is fresh air.
8. A bioterrorist released an aerosol in a Chicago subway. Two days later, a client enters the emergency room with a fever and a pustular rash on his face, hands, and soles of the feet. The nurse suspects that the client has smallpox. Her first action is to:
   1. don protective clothing, including gown, gloves, and a special mask.
   2. obtain an order for atropine sulfate.
   3. remove the clothing and wash the client with soap and water.
   4. request an order for smallpox vaccine.
9. A sheep rancher came to the emergency room with a cut on his hand that he received while shearing his sheep 5 days ago. The man stated that the area around the cut has "itched awfully" for the past 3 days. He states that the cut has changed in appearance today. When the nurse exams the cut, he notices that the cut is an ulcerated papular lesion. He suspects the man has:
   1. plague.
   2. been exposed to ricin.
   3. smallpox.
   4. anthrax.
10. The local hospital does not need to stock up on supplies in case of a bioterrorist attack because:
    1. EMEDS is a total package that includes everything necessary to screen and treat clients who need outpatient care.
    2. each facility has an emergency operations plan that would immediately be put into effect to cover the emergency situation.
    3. the Strategic National Stockpile has prepackaged emergency supplies that are stored 12 hours away from every community in the country.
    4. a bioterrorist attack will not occur in the United States with all the security precautions presently in place.

REFERENCES/SUGGESTED READINGS

Agency for Toxic Substances and Disease Registry. (2008) Medical management guidelines for nerve agents: Tuban (GA); sarin (GB); soman (GD); and VX. Department of Health and Human Services. Retrieved September 9, 2008, from http://www.atsdr.cdc.gov/MHMI/mmg166.html

Casey, C., Iskander, J., Roper, M., Mast, E., Wen, X., Torok, T., et al. (2005). Adverse events associated with smallpox vaccination in the United States, January–October 2003. *Journal of the American Medical Association, 294*(21), 2734–2743.

Cava, M., Fay, K., Beanlands, H., McCay, E., & Wignall, R. (2005). Risk perception and compliance with quarantine during the SARS outbreak. *Journal of Nursing Scholarship, 37*(4), 343–347.

Centers for Disease Control and Prevention. (1999). Bioterrorism readiness plan: A template for healthcare facilities. Retrieved November 6, 2008, from http://www.cdc.gov/ncidod/dhqp/pdf/bt/13apr99APIC-CDCBioterrorism.PDF

Centers for Disease Control and Prevention. (2000a, April 21). Biological and chemical terrorism: Strategic plan for preparedness and response. *Morbidity and Mortality Weekly Report, 49*(RR04), 1–14.

Centers for Disease Control and Prevention. (2000b, December 15). Use of anthrax vaccine in the United States. *Morbidity and Mortality Weekly Report, 49*(RR15), 1–20.

Centers for Disease Control and Prevention. (2002a). Message from HHS: Smallpox vaccination. Retrieved November 7, 2008, from http://www.bt.cdc.gov/training/smallpoxvaccine/reactions/message.htm

Centers for Disease Control and Prevention. (2002b, November 15). Notice to readers: Use of anthrax vaccine in response to terrorism: Supplemental recommendations of the advisory committee on immunization practices. *Morbidity and Mortality Weekly Report, 51*(45), 1024–1026.

Centers for Disease Control and Prevention. (2004). Facts about pneumonic plague. Retrieved August 25, 2008, from http://emergency.cdc.gov/agent/plague/factsheet.asp

Centers for Disease Control and Prevention. (2005). NIOSH emergency response card: Cyanogen chloride (ERC506-77-4). Retrieved November 14, 2008, from http://emergency.cdc.gov/agent/cyanide/erc506-77-4pr.asp

Centers for Disease Control and Prevention. (2006a). Facts about Phosgene. Retrieved November 14, 2008, from http://emergency.cdc.gov/agent/phosgene/basics/facts.asp

Centers for Disease Control and Prevention. (2006b). Fact sheet: Anthrax information for health care providers. Retrieved November 8, 2008, from http://www.bt.cdc.gov/agent/anthrax/anthrax-hcp-factsheet.asp

Centers for Disease Control and Prevention. (2006c). NIOSH emergency response card: Hydrogen cyanide (ERC74-90-8). Retrieved November 14, 2008, from http://emergency.cdc.gov/agent/cyanide/erc74-90-8.asp

Centers for Disease Control and Prevention. (2006d). Sarin (GB). Retrieved January 20, 2007, from http://www.bt.cdc.gov/agent/sarin

Centers for Disease Control and Prevention. (2006e). Toxic syndrome description: Vesicant/blister agent poisoning. Retrieved November 13, 2008, from http://www.bt.cdc.gov/agent/vesicants/tsd.asp

Centers for Disease Control and Prevention. (2007a). The history of bioterrorism [Video]. Retrieved November 7, 2008, from http://emergency.cdc.gov/training/historyofbt

Centers for Disease Control and Prevention. (2007b). Smallpox fact sheet: Smallpox disease overview. Retrieved November 7, 2008, from http://emergency.cdc.gov/agent/smallpox/overview/disease-facts.asp

Centers for Disease Control and Prevention. (2007c). Smallpox fact sheet: Vaccine overview. Retrieved November 7, 2008, from http://emergency.cdc.gov/agent/smallpox/vaccination/facts.asp

Centers for Disease Control and Prevention. (2008a). Bioterrorism agents/diseases. Retrieved November 5, 2008, from http://emergency.cdc.gov/agent/agentlist-category.asp

Centers for Disease Control and Prevention. (2008b, March 3). CDC fact sheet: Facts about ricin. Retrieved August 25, 2008, from http://www.bt.cdc.gov/agent/ricin/facts.asp

Centers for Disease Control and Prevention. (2008c). MMWR quick guide: Recommended adult immunization schedule—United States, October 2007–September 2008. Retrieved August 21, 2008, from http://www.cdc.gov/mmwr/pdf/wk/mm5641-Immunization.pdf

Centers for Disease Control and Prevention. (2008d, February 29). Official CDC health advisory: CDC alert on ricin. Retrieved April 24, 2008, from http://www.cdcinfo@cdc.gov

Centers for Disease Control and Prevention. (2008e). Public health preparedness report—Appendix 6. Retrieved November 5, 2008, from http://emergency.cdc.gov/publications/feb08phprep/appendix/appendix6.asp

Center for Disease Control and Prevention. (2009a). Adult immunization schedule. Retrieved June 8, 2009 from http://www. cdc.gov/vaccines/recs/schedules/adult-schedule.htm

Center for Disease Control and Prevention. (2009b). Child and adolescent immunization schedules. Retrieved June 8, 2009 from http://www.cdc.gov/vaccines/recs/schedules/child-schedule.htm#printable

Chettle, C. (2007). Are you prepared for a flu pandemic? *NurseWeek; South Central edition*, 16–19.

Council on Foreign Relations. (2008). Aum Shinrikyo. Retrieved November 13, 2008, from http://www.cfr.org/publication/9238

Department of Homeland Security. (2007, October 9). Fact sheet: National strategy for homeland security. Retrieved April 23, 2008, from http://www.whitehouse.gov/deptofhomeland/analysis

Desenclos, J., & Guillemot, D. (2004, April 23). Consequences of bacterial resistance to antimicrobial. Retrieved August 25, 2008, from http://www.cdc.gov/nicod/EID/index.htm

Eckert, S. (2006). Preparing for disaster: How to plan for the unthinkable. *American Nurse Today, 1*(1), 34–37.

Fauci, A. (2005) Emerging and re-emerging infections diseases: The perpetual challenge. *Academic Medicine, 80*, 1079–1085.

Fox, M. (2008, January 22). Avant works on oral vaccine for plague, anthrax. Retrieved August 25, 2008, from http://www.ph.ucla.edu/epi/bioter/avantoralvaccine.html

Guillemin, J. (2005). *Biological weapons: From the invention of state-sponsored programs to contemporary bioterrorism.* New York: Columbia University Press.

Ignatavicius, D., & Workman, M. (2006). *Medical-surgical nursing: Critical thinking for collaborative care* (5th ed.). St. Louis, MO: Elsevier/Saunders.

Johnson, C. (2003, December 3). Emergency preparedness and bioterrorism fact sheets: Sarin as a chemical terrorist agent. Retrieved August 25, 2008, from http://webserver.health.state.pa.us/health/cwp/view.asp%3Fa%3D171%26Q%3D233572

Joint Commission. (2007). Joint Commission Resources: Environment of Care, Inc. Retrieved August 26, 2008, from http://www.jcrinc.com/26632

Nursing World. (2002, June 30). ANA, HHS establish national nurses response team. Retrieved August 25, 2008, from http://nursingworld.org/Functional MenuCategories/MediaResources/PressReleases/2006

Ohio Department of Health. (2005). Health care facilities and bioterrorism preparedness. Retrieved November 5, 2008, from http://www.odh.ohio.gov/search/search.asp?SearchString=bioterrorism

Pilch, R., & Zilinskas, R. (Eds.). (2005). *Encyclopedia of bioterrorism defense.* Hoboken, NJ: Wiley-Liss.

Salmon, A. (2008). *1995:* Aum Shinrikyo Tokyo subway gas attack. Retrieved November 9, 2008, from http://terrorism.about.com/od/originshistory/a/AumShinrikyo.htm

U.S. Department of Labor. (2008). Biological agents. Retrieved November 5, 2008, from http://www.osha.gov/SLTC/biologicalagents/index.html

Washington State Department of Health. (2008) Chemical agents (DOH Publication No. 821-019). Olympia: Author. Retrieved November 9, 2008, from http://www.doh.wa.gov/phepr/handbook/hbk_pdf/chemical.pdf

RESOURCES

American Nurses Association, http://www.nursingworld.org

American Red Cross, http://www.redcross.org

Centers for Disease Control and Prevention, http://www.cdc.gov

Department of Defense, http://www.defenselink.mil

Department of Homeland Security, http://www.whitehouse.gov/deptofhomeland

Federal Emergency Management Agency, http://www.fema.gov

National Disaster Medical System, http://ndms.dhhs.gov

National Institutes of Health, http://www.nih.gov

National Nurses Response Team, http://nursingworld.org

U.S. Army Medical Research Institute of Chemical Defense, http://chemdef.apgea.army.mil

U.S. Army Surgeon General, http://www.surgeongeneral.gov

U.S. Department of Health and Human Services, http://www.dhhs.gov

UNIT 7 Fundamental Nursing Care

CHAPTER 24
Fluid, Electrolyte, and Acid–Base Balance

MAKING THE CONNECTION

Refer to the following chapters to increase your understanding of fluid, electrolyte, and acid–base balance:

Basic Nursing
- ***Assessment***
- ***Diagnostic Tests***

Adult Health Nursing
- ***Respiratory System***

Basic Procedures
- ***Measuring Intake and Output***

LEARNING OBJECTIVES

Upon completion of this chapter, you should be able to:

- Define key terms.
- Discuss the importance of pH regulation in the body.
- Describe the three buffer systems of the body.
- Describe and give examples in the body of diffusion, osmosis, and filtration.
- Name the fluid compartments, the fluids contained in them, and the function of those fluids.
- Describe the way the kidneys work to maintain fluid and electrolyte balance.
- Describe the way the lungs work to maintain pH in the body.
- Detail causes, assessment data, nursing interventions, and criteria for evaluating effectiveness of care for clients with a nursing diagnosis of *Deficient Fluid Volume* or *Excess Fluid Volume*.
- Detail causes, assessment data, nursing diagnoses, nursing interventions, and criteria for evaluating the effectiveness of nursing care for clients with sodium, potassium, calcium, and magnesium imbalances.
- Relate principles of nursing management for clients receiving fluids and electrolytes via oral supplements, intravenous solutions, enteral feedings, and total parenteral nutrition.

- Differentiate the causes, assessment data, and nursing management of metabolic and respiratory acidosis and alkalosis.
- Use the nursing process to plan care for a client experiencing a fluid, electrolyte, and/or acid–base imbalance.

KEY TERMS

acid
acidosis
alkalosis
anion
arterial blood gases (ABGs)
atom
base
buffer
cation
compound
crenation
decomposition
dehydration
dialysis
diffusion
edema
electrolyte
element
extracellular fluid (ECF)
filtration
hemolysis
homeostasis
hydrostatic pressure
hypertonic solution
hypotonic solution
hypoxemia
infiltration
interstitial fluid
intracellular fluid (ICF)
intravascular fluid
intravenous (IV) therapy
ion
isotonic solution
isotope
matter
mixture
molecule
osmolality
osmolarity
osmosis
osmotic pressure
oxidized
permeability
potential hydrogen (pH)
salt
selectively permeable membrane
semipermeable membrane
synthesis
turgor

INTRODUCTION

The external environment within which we live undergoes continual changes, both small and large. For example, the daily and seasonal temperatures may fluctuate over a wide range. The light intensity is bright on sunny days and less so on cloudy days. The humidity may be either high or low. These are just a few of the many factors that constantly change in the external environment. Our bodies must continually adjust to such changes in the external environment. In order for life to continue, however, our internal environment—the one inside our bodies—must remain relatively constant, varying only slightly within narrow ranges. This internal environment consists of the various body fluids such as the fluid inside cells, the blood, tissue fluids that bathe the cells, and other fluids. Maintenance of the internal environment within very narrow limits is termed **homeostasis** (equilibrium).

HOMEOSTASIS

Homeostasis is an ongoing process; that is, the body simply does not reach a state of equilibrium and remain there. Small changes constantly occur in response to physiologic processes. The body must therefore continuously make subtle adjustments to maintain the constancy of the internal environment within a normal range.

Homeostasis is accomplished by various physiologic processes and the coordinated activities of the organ systems. Some examples are as follows:

- The gastrointestinal (GI) system changes large, complex molecules of ingested food to simpler, less complex molecules that can be utilized by the cells of the body to produce the energy necessary for life.
- The respiratory system supplies the cells with the constant source of oxygen required to release the energy from the products of digestion. It also eliminates carbon dioxide, the waste product produced by the cells as a result of energy production.
- The blood acts as a transport mechanism, carrying the products of digestion along with hormones and oxygen to the cells, where these substances are utilized.
- It also transports carbon dioxide from the energy-releasing processes of the cells to the lungs, where it will be eliminated.
- All the activities of the various organ systems are integrated and coordinated through the nervous system and the endocrine system.

When the body loses the ability to maintain homeostasis and the internal environment changes, the physiologic processes can be interrupted or changed, leading to disease, disorder, or death. In essence, then, maintaining homeostasis is essential to life. Because the processes of homeostasis involve many chemical and physical processes, it is necessary to examine some of these before studying homeostasis in more detail.

CHEMICAL ORGANIZATION

The human body is highly organized. This organization exists in increasing levels of complexity. Most basic is the chemical level. To understand the higher levels of organization, it is necessary to know something about basic chemical and physical principles.

ELEMENTS

The cell consists of living matter. **Matter** is anything that occupies space and possesses mass. All matter has certain physical properties such as color, odor, hardness, and density. Matter also has extensive properties such as size, shape, and weight. Matter is composed of basic substances called **elements**. Elements are made of tiny units called atoms. Atoms of each element are alike. Different elements have different kinds of atoms. Presently, 112 elements are recognized. Some examples are iron, gold, carbon, hydrogen, oxygen, nitrogen, and copper. Many of the elements occur in the human body in varying amounts. Some are present in large amounts, and others are found in only trace amounts. The four elements oxygen, carbon, hydrogen, and nitrogen constitute more than 95% of the total body weight of the elements. Some of the elements and their function in the body are presented in Table 24-1.

TABLE 24-1 Elements Occurring in the Human Body

ELEMENT	APPROXIMATE % OF BODY WEIGHT	FUNCTION
Major Elements		
Oxygen (O)	65.0	Found in both organic and inorganic compounds; as a gas, is necessary in metabolizing glucose and other chemical compounds into energy
Carbon (C)	18.5	Found in all organic compounds such as carbohydrates, protein, lipids, and nucleic acids; necessary for cellular respiration
Hydrogen (H)	9.5	Found in many organic and inorganic compounds; in ionic form, involved in pH; component of water; necessary for life
Nitrogen (N)	3.2	Important in proteins, which are the body's building blocks, an energy source, and a component of hormones
Calcium (Ca)	1.5	Important element in bone and tooth composition; involved in nerve conduction, muscle contraction, and blood clotting
Phosphorus (P)	1.0	Found in bones, teeth, the high-energy carrying compound adenosine triphosphatase (ATP), some proteins, and nucleic acid
Potassium (K)	0.4	Major electrolyte in intracellular fluid; important in muscle contraction and transmission of nerve impulses; activates enzymes; influences cellular osmotic pressure; involved in kidney function and acid–base balance
Sulfur (S)	0.3	Found in some proteins, nucleic acids, and some vitamins and hormones
Sodium (Na)	0.2	Constitutes major electrolyte in extracellular fluid; important in osmoregulation and acid–base balance; necessary for nerve transmission and muscle contraction
Chlorine (Cl)	0.2	Found in extracellular fluid; important in water balance, acid–base balance, and production of hydrochloric acid in the stomach
Magnesium (Mg)	0.1	Important to muscle and nerve function and bone formation and in some coenzymes
Essential Trace Elements		
Present in the human body in minimal amounts, constituting approximately 0.1% of body weight; have known functions		
Cobalt (Co)		Important component of vitamin B_{12}
Copper (Cu)		Necessary for formation of hemoglobin and for bone development
Chromium (Cr)		A cofactor involved with enzymes for fat, cholesterol, and glucose metabolism
Fluorine (F)		Gives hardness to teeth and bones
Iodine (I)		Necessary for synthesis of thyroid hormone
Iron (Fe)		Necessary for transportation of oxygen by hemoglobin
Manganese (Mn)		Necessary in activating some enzymes
Selenium (Se)		Acts with vitamin E as an antioxidant; component of teeth
Zinc (Zn)		Found in some enzymes; needed for protein metabolism and carbon dioxide transport
Other Trace Elements		
Have probable, but as yet undetected, functions		
Aluminum (Al) Nickel (Ni) Arsenic (As) Tin (Sn) Boron (B) Silicon (Si) Cadmium (Cd) Vanadium (V)		

COURTESY OF DELMAR CENGAGE LEARNING

Atoms

An **atom** is the smallest unit of chemical structure, and no chemical change can alter it. Atoms are made up of three basic particles: protons, neutrons, and electrons. Protons and neutrons are similar in size, but whereas protons have a positive electrical charge, neutrons have no charge. Together, they form the nucleus of the atom. Because the protons have a positive charge and the neutrons are neutral, the nucleus of an atom has a positive charge. The electrons have a negative charge and move in an orbit around the nucleus. There are as many electrons as protons, rendering the overall atom neutral. The number of protons in an atom is called its atomic number. The simplest element is hydrogen. It has an atomic number of 1. One proton with a positive charge forms the nucleus, and one electron moves in an orbit around the nucleus. Hydrogen atoms may or may not have a neutron. A hydrogen atom is illustrated in Figure 24-1.

Depending on the element, other atoms may have more than one proton and one electron and may have neutrons. The number of protons and neutrons in the nucleus is approximately equal to the atomic weight. Thus, hydrogen has an atomic weight of 1.

Isotopes

The number of protons in the nucleus is the same for all atoms of a given element, but the number of neutrons may vary in atoms of the same element. For instance, all hydrogen atoms have one proton and one electron; however, some hydrogen atoms have one neutron in the nucleus, while others have two (Figure 24-2). Atoms of the same element that have different atomic weights (i.e., have a different number of neutrons) are called **isotopes**. All the isotopes of a given element react the same way chemically.

Some isotopes, called radioactive isotopes, have an unstable nucleus, which decomposes and gives off energy in the form of radiation. This radiation can be in the form of alpha, beta, or gamma rays. All are damaging to cells. Alpha radiation is the least harmful, and gamma radiation is the most harmful. Iodine, oxygen, and cobalt are examples of elements having radioactive isotopes. Some of the radioactive isotopes are useful as biological markers and can be used to track metabolic pathways of food. Others such as iodine^{131} can be injected into the body and used to track the circulation of blood. Still others such as cobalt^{60} are used in cancer treatment.

Molecules and Compounds

Atoms of the same element can unite with each other to form a **molecule**. For example, atoms of hydrogen unite to form a

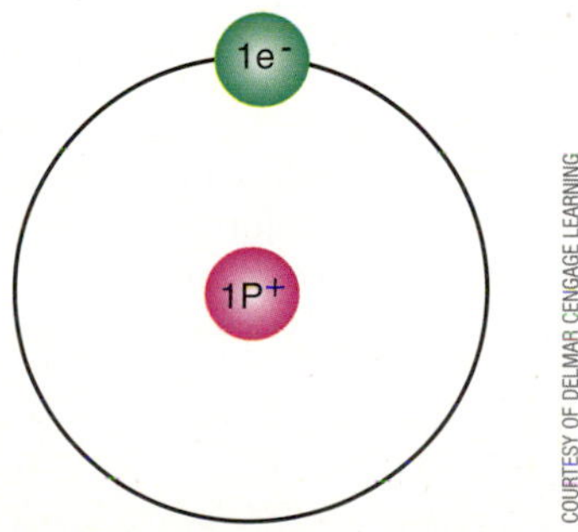

FIGURE 24-1 Hydrogen Atom Showing Positively Charged Proton in the Nucleus and Negatively Charged Electron in Orbit

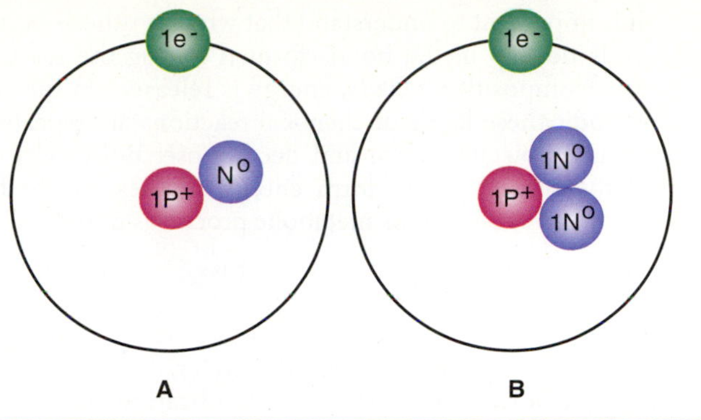

FIGURE 24-2 Isotopes of Hydrogen; *A,* Deuteridium has one positively charged proton and one neutron in the nucleus and one electron in orbit; *B,* Tritium has one positively charged proton and two neutrons in the nucleus and one electron in orbit.

hydrogen molecule. This can be expressed in a chemical equation using the chemical symbol for hydrogen:

$$H + H \rightarrow H_2$$

In this reaction, the atoms on the left are the reactants, the arrow is read as "yield," and the last symbol is the product—a molecule of hydrogen. A chemical equation uses the chemical symbols of elements and shows the ratios by which they combine. Because atoms of elements always combine in the same ratio under similar conditions, it is possible to predict the nature of a chemical change.

When atoms of two or more different elements combine (react), they form a **compound**. For example, if one atom of sodium (Na) and one atom of chlorine (Cl) react, they form a molecule of the compound called sodium chloride. This is expressed in the following equation:

$$Na + Cl \rightarrow NaCl$$

Compounds can be divided into two groups. Those without carbon are inorganic compounds, and those with carbon are organic compounds. By using chemical equations, chemical changes, called reactions, can be shown. Sometimes, different substances are combined in no specific way, and the components do not have a definite ratio every time. For instance, water, sugar, and table salt mixed without being measured will yield different results depending on the ratio of each substance. Such a combination is called a **mixture**. Its composition may vary each time the components are mixed.

Chemical reactions occur whenever atoms join together or separate. They join together by forming bonds, and they separate by breaking bonds. Either way, new combinations result. When two or more atoms (reactants) bond and form a more complex molecular product, the reaction is called **synthesis**. A sample equation would be as follows:

$$\underset{\text{hydrogen and}}{2H} + \underset{\text{oxygen}}{O} \underset{\text{yields}}{\rightarrow} \underset{\text{water}}{H_2O}$$

When the bonding between the atoms in a molecule is broken and simpler products are formed, the reaction is called **decomposition**. If a molecule of sodium chloride is decomposed, it forms sodium and chlorine. This can be expressed as follows:

$$\underset{\text{sodium chloride}}{NaCl} \underset{\text{yields}}{\rightarrow} \underset{\text{sodium and}}{Na} + \underset{\text{chloride}}{Cl}$$

(decomposition)

It is important to understand that when synthesis occurs, energy is tied up in the bonds formed during the reaction. When decomposition occurs, energy is released. In the cells of the body, these kinds of chemical reactions are repeatedly occurring: Molecules form and decompose. Body cells can utilize these reactions to form energy sources and to free energy to drive the various metabolic processes of the cells.

IONS

When some compounds are placed in water, they decompose, or ionize. The result is an **ion**, an atom bearing an electrical charge. An ion with a positive charge is called a **cation**; an ion with a negative charge is termed an **anion**. For example, sodium chloride in water dissociates to form sodium ions bearing a positive charge and chloride ions bearing a negative charge (Figure 24-3). Because the atoms in this combination are charged, they will conduct electricity. The reaction can be shown as follows:

NaCl	→	Na^+	+	Cl^-
sodium chloride	yields	sodium (cation)	and	chloride (anion)

A compound that dissociates into ions in water is called an **electrolyte**. Many electrolytes are extremely important in body chemistry.

WATER

Water constitutes approximately 60% of the total body weight of an adult and is involved in many of the physical and physiological processes of the body. Because water is so integral to the body's processes, fluctuations in the amount of water in the body can have harmful or even fatal consequences.

Water is the major component of blood. Approximately 92% of the body's organic and inorganic compounds dissolve in this water into less complex molecules and atoms and then are transported throughout the body. Necessary substances such as oxygen and nutrients from the GI system are carried to the cells, where they are utilized. Cellular waste products such as carbon dioxide, urea, and excessive minerals are carried by water to sites of elimination: carbon dioxide to the lungs and urea and minerals to the kidneys.

Water also absorbs heat resulting from muscle contractions and distributes this heat over the body. Water in the form of perspiration released from sweat glands in the skin can cool the body by evaporation. Water also can break apart the bonds in large molecules such as starches to form smaller molecules in the digestive process. This type of reaction is called *hydration*.

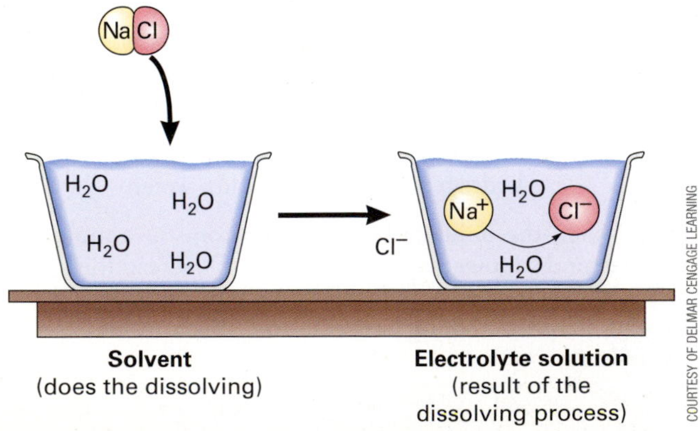

FIGURE 24-3 Dissociation of Electrolytes

> **LIFE SPAN CONSIDERATIONS**
>
> **Body Water and Body Size**
>
> The amount of body water is inversely proportional to body size. The smaller the body, the higher the water content:
>
> | | |
> |---|---|
> | Embryo: | 97% |
> | Infant: | 70% to 80% |
> | Child: | 60% to 77% |
> | Adult: | 60% |
> | Older Adult: | 45% to 55% |
>
> Body water diminishment in older adults is related to tissue loss.

GASES

Two important gases in the body are oxygen (O_2) and carbon dioxide (CO_2). Because these elements are gases, their molecules are free and can move swiftly in all directions. Oxygen enters the body through the lungs and is transported by the red blood cells throughout the body to the cells. The cells use oxygen in the release of energy from glucose and other molecules. This energy is needed by the cells to carry out their activities. As a result of the energy-releasing processes, carbon dioxide is produced by the cells and transported in the blood to the lungs, where it is eliminated.

ACIDS, BASES, SALTS, AND pH

Other chemical substances important for life are acids, bases, and salts; pH is the measure of acid and base strength.

ACIDS

An **acid** is any substance that in solution yields hydrogen ions bearing a positive charge. As an example, hydrochloric acid (HCl) in water dissociates as shown following:

HCl	→	H^+	+	Cl^-
hydrochloric acid	yields	hydrogen	and	chloride

The hydrogen ion characterizes this as an acid. Important acids in the body are hydrochloric acid, produced in the stomach, and carbonic acid, formed when the carbon dioxide released from cells reacts with some of the water in the extracellular fluid (all body fluids except for those contained within the cells).

BASES

A **base** is a substance that when dissociated produces ions that will combine with hydrogen ions. For example, when sodium hydroxide dissociates in water, it forms a sodium ion bearing a positive charge and a hydroxyl ion bearing a negative charge as shown following:

NaOH	→	Na^+	+	OH^-
sodium hydroxide	yields	sodium	and	hydroxyl

The hydroxyl ion is capable of combining with a hydrogen ion to form water. Sodium bicarbonate is an example of a base found in the body.

SALTS

A **salt** is formed when an acid and a base react with each other. Salts result from the neutralization of an acid by a base, as illustrated by the following reaction:

HCl	+	NaOH	→	H_2O	+	NaCl
hydrochloric acid	and	sodium hydroxide	yields	water	and	sodium chloride

The hydrochloric acid reacts with the sodium hydroxide to form a molecule of water and a molecule of a salt—sodium chloride. When salts are placed in water, they dissociate into a cation and an anion. For instance, in water, the sodium chloride would dissociate into Na^+ and Cl^-. One reason salts are of great biological importance is that many of the compounds that dissociate into ions in living cells are salts. For example, sodium and chlorine ions are present in great amounts in body fluids. Many other salts occur in lesser amounts.

PH

Acid and bases are classified as either strong or weak by the number of hydrogen ions or hydroxyl ions they produce when they dissociate. Strong acids release many hydrogen ions; weak acids release relatively few. The same is true of hydroxyl ions in strong and weak bases. The acidity or alkalinity of a solution is determined by the concentration of hydrogen ions in the solution. **Potential hydrogen (pH)** indicates the hydrogen ion concentration in a solution, expressed as a number from 0 to 14. A solution with a pH of 7 is neutral (i.e., it is neither an acid nor a base). A solution with a pH greater than 7 is a base, or alkaline. A solution with a pH less than 7 is an acid. The higher above 7 the pH, the more alkaline the solution; the lower below 7 the pH, the more acid the solution. pH is of great biological importance. The human body can tolerate only very slight changes in pH. For example, the pH of human blood ranges from 7.35 to 7.45 (Figure 24-4). Blood pH above or below this range can cause severe or even fatal physiological problems.

Although small amounts of acids may enter the body through food intake, the greatest source of acids—and thus H^+ ions—is cellular metabolism, resulting in products including lactic acid, phosphoric acid, pyruvic acid, and many fatty acids. When blood pH falls below 7.35 as a result of an elevated concentration of H^+ ions, **acidosis** occurs. Rarely does blood pH fall to 7 or become acidic because death will usually occur first. As acidosis increases, the central nervous system (CNS) becomes involved, and the client may become unconscious. The heartbeat may become weak and irregular, and blood pressure may decrease or even disappear.

When blood pH increases above 7.45, **alkalosis** occurs. Alkalosis is a condition characterized by an excessive loss of hydrogen ions. This happens less often than does acidosis. Symptoms of alkalosis include a heightened state of nervous system activity, resulting in spasmodic muscle contractions, convulsions, and even death.

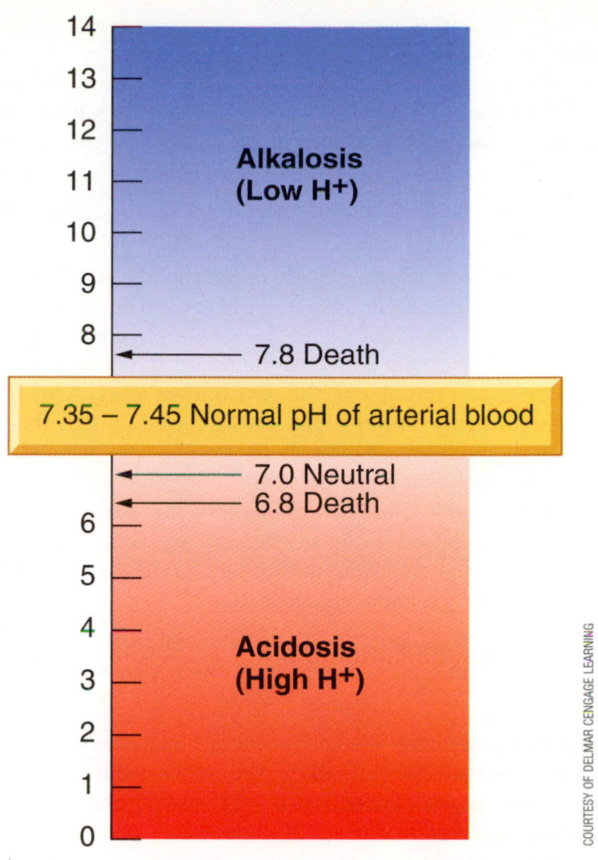

FIGURE 24-4 The pH of human blood ranges from 7.35 to 7.45.

BUFFERS

Buffers are substances that attempt to maintain pH range, or H^+ ion concentration, in the presence of added acids or bases. Buffers usually occur in pairs in the body fluids. They act to keep the pH of body fluids within normal range. If body fluids become acidic, buffers in the body fluids combine with the excess hydrogen ions and restore normal pH. Likewise, if the body fluids become alkaline, other buffers in the blood combine with the strong bases, converting them to weak bases and restoring normal pH.

Three important buffer systems occur in body fluids: the bicarbonate buffer system, the phosphate buffer system, and the protein buffer system. Because a change in pH of one fluid may bring corresponding changes in the pH of other fluids, an interplay between buffer systems acts to maintain the body's pH. The buffer systems react quickly to prevent excessive changes in the hydrogen ion concentration.

BICARBONATE BUFFER SYSTEM

The bicarbonate buffer system is found in both the extracellular and intracellular fluids and is the body's primary buffer system. It has two components: carbonic acid (H_2CO_3) and sodium bicarbonate ($NaHCO_3$). When a strong acid such as hydrochloric acid is added to this buffer system, the acid will react with the sodium bicarbonate and form a weaker acid (carbonic acid) and a salt (sodium chloride).

HCl	+	$NaHCO_3$	→	H_2CO_3	+	NaCl
hydrochloric acid	and	sodium bicarbonate	yields	carbonic acid	and	sodium chloride

The strong acid is converted into a weak acid, and the pH is raised toward normal.

If a strong base such as sodium hydroxide is added to this buffer system, the carbonic acid will react with it to form a weak base (sodium bicarbonate) and water.

$NaOH$	$+$	H_2CO_3	$\rightarrow$	$NaHCO_3$	$+$	H_2O
sodium hydroxide	and	carbonic acid	yields	sodium bicarbonate	and	water

The strong base, which initially raised the pH, is converted to a weak base, which will lower the pH toward normal. It is vital to note that hydrochloric acid and sodium hydroxide are substances not normally added to the blood. They are used here only as good examples of the way buffers work. This buffer system normally buffers organic acids found in body fluids.

In the body, bicarbonate helps stabilize pH by combining reversibly with hydrogen ions. Most of the body's bicarbonate is produced in red blood cells, where the enzyme carbonic anhydrase accelerates the conversion of carbon dioxide to carbonic acid. The production of bicarbonate is illustrated in the following reversible equation:

CO_2	$+$	H_2O	$\leftrightarrow$	H_2CO_3	$\leftrightarrow$	H^+	$+$	HCO_3^-
carbon dioxide		water		carbonic acid		hydrogen		bicarbonate

When the hydrogen ion concentration increases in the extracellular (outside the cell) space, the reaction shifts toward the left. A decreased concentration of hydrogen ions drives the reaction to the right.

Phosphate Buffer System

The phosphate buffer system is involved in regulating the pH of intracellular fluid and the fluid of the kidney tubules. It has two phosphate compounds: sodium monohydrogen phosphate ($NaHPO_4$) and sodium dihydrogen phosphate (NaH_2PO_4). In the presence of a strong acid such as hydrochloric acid, the sodium monohydrogen phosphate reacts with the acid to form a weak acid (sodium dihydrogen phosphate) and a salt (sodium chloride), thus raising the pH.

HCl	$+$	$NaHPO_4$	$\rightarrow$	NaH_2PO_4	$+$	$NaCl$
hydrochloric acid	and	sodium monohydrogen phosphate	yields	sodium dihydrogen phosphate	and	sodium chloride

When sodium dihydrogen phosphate encounters a strong base such as sodium hydroxide, a weak base (sodium monohydrogen phosphate) and water are formed.

$NaOH$	$+$	NaH_2PO_4	$\rightarrow$	$NaHPO_4$	$+$	H_2O
sodium hydroxide	and	sodium dihydrogen phosphate	yields	sodium monohydrogen phosphate	and	water

Protein Buffers

Proteins are complex substances formed when amino acids bond. Each amino acid contains a carboxyl group (COOH) and an amino group (NH_2). The carboxyl group can ionize and release hydrogen, thus acting as an acid. The amino group can accept hydrogen, thus acting as a base. This ability allows proteins to act as a buffer system. The protein buffer system is found inside cells, especially in the hemoglobin of red blood cells, where the proteins can act to maintain the pH inside the cell. They are also found in the plasma.

SUBSTANCE MOVEMENT

Substances must be able to both enter and leave cells. For example, oxygen and various end products of digestion must enter a cell through the cell membrane for use by the cell. Waste products from cellular processes must be eliminated from the cell. Various ions must also both enter and leave cells. Everything that enters and leaves the cell must pass through the cell membrane. Thus, the cell membrane serves not only as an envelope around the cell but also as a gatekeeper, regulating which substances can enter and leave the cell. The cell membrane is a very thin and delicate, but complex and living, elastic covering around each cell. It consists of an inner and outer layer of phospholipids in which protein molecules are embedded. Many small channels pass through the membrane. These channels allow some water molecules and some water-soluble substances to pass through the membrane. The ability of a membrane to permit substances to pass through it is called **permeability**. Because a cell membrane allows passage of only certain substances, it is called a **selectively permeable membrane**. An artificial membrane such as cellophane is known as a **semipermeable membrane** (Kee, Paulanka, & Polek, 2010).

Some substances can pass through the cell membrane without energy expenditure on the part of the cell. This is called passive transport. The passage of other substances requires an expenditure of energy by the cell. This is called active transport.

Passive Transport

There are several types of passive transport: diffusion, osmosis, and filtration.

Diffusion

Diffusion is the tendency of molecules of either gases, liquids, or solids to move from a region of higher molecular concentration to a region of lower molecular concentration until an equilibrium is reached. This movement is caused by the kinetic energy in molecules. Kinetic energy causes the molecules to move constantly, colliding with one another and knocking each other about, thus causing them to move farther apart. An example is a drop of black ink placed in a glass of water; over time, the glass of water will turn a uniform black color because of diffusion, as shown in Figure 24-5.

In the body, oxygen moves by diffusion from the lungs to the bloodstream because the oxygen concentration is higher in the lungs and lower in the blood. Carbon dioxide moves by diffusion from the bloodstream, where the concentration of carbon dioxide is higher, to the lungs, for elimination. The size of

CRITICAL THINKING

Substance Movement: Class Activity

During class, place a tea bag into a glass of warm water. Allow time for the students to record their observations. Ask the students to write an explanation of which type(s) of substance movement occurred using the correct terminology (Science Spot, 2009). For more class activity ideas, visit http://sciencespot.net/index.html.

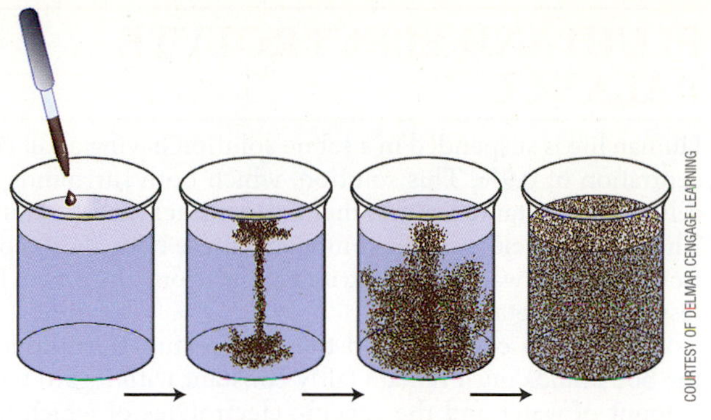

FIGURE 24-5 Diffusion is the spreading of particles from an area of greater concentration to an area of lesser concentration. Dye put into a beaker of water gradually spreads throughout the water.

the channels in the cell membrane can prevent large molecules from passing through the membrane. Some substances, such as glucose molecules, combine with carrier molecules, which carry them into the interior of the cell, where they are released.

The term **dialysis** is used when diffusion is employed to separate molecules out of a solution by passing them through a semipermeable membrane. Dialysis is the process used in the artificial kidney. As blood from a client circulates through a machine, small, toxic waste molecules such as urea leave the blood and pass through the semipermeable membrane by diffusion and out into the surrounding fluid. The blood, thus cleaned, is then returned to the body.

Osmosis

Osmosis is the diffusion of water through a semipermeable membrane from a region of higher water concentration to a region of lower water concentration. In a solution undergoing osmosis, only the water (solvent) molecules move through the membrane; the dissolved molecules do not (Figure 24-6).

If a cell, having both a membrane that will not allow sodium chloride to pass through and a molecular concentration of 10% sodium chloride, were placed in a container with a 5% sodium chloride solution, the cell would contain 10% sodium chloride and 90% water, and the 5% solution in which it was placed would contain 5% dissolved sodium chloride and 95% water. There would be more water outside than inside the cell; thus, water would pass through the membrane into the cell. Because the cell membrane is elastic, the cell would increase in size as a result of the water accumulation within it facilitated by the process of osmosis. The pressure exerted against the cell membrane by the water inside the cell is called **osmotic pressure**.

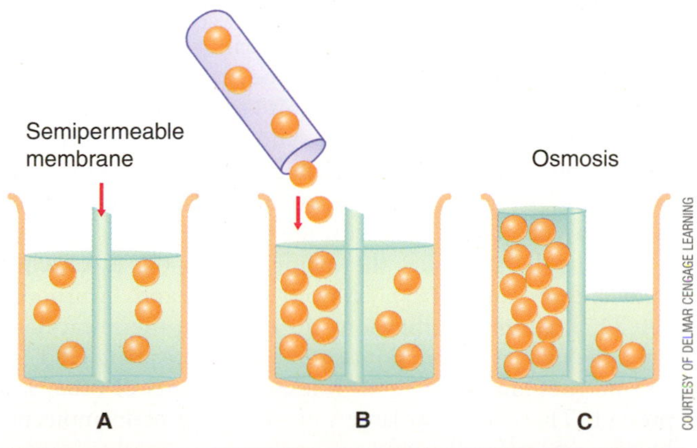

FIGURE 24-6 The process of osmosis.

A solution that has the same molecular concentration as the cell is called an **isotonic solution**. It neither increases nor decreases the size of the cell. A solution that has a lower molecular concentration than the cell is called a **hypotonic solution**. Placing cells in a hypotonic solution causes them to swell, possibly to the point of eventual rupture. The rupture of red blood cells due to osmosis is called **hemolysis**. As red blood cells swell, the hemoglobin contained within passes to the outside of the cell and into the solution surrounding the cell, rendering the blood cells no longer capable of carrying oxygen. A solution that has a higher molecular concentration than the cell is called a **hypertonic solution**. When placed in such a solution, water leaves the cell, and the cell decreases in size. In the case of red blood cells, they shrivel and become wrinkled. This shrinkage, called **crenation**, leaves the cells incapable of functioning.

In persons who have lost large volumes of blood, it is sometimes necessary to administer additional fluids to maintain blood pressure. Generally, normal saline can be used. This 0.9% sodium chloride solution has approximately the same osmotic concentration as blood. Because it is isotonic, it will not damage the cells. Figure 24-7 shows osmosis in cells with different solution concentrations.

Filtration

In **filtration**, fluids and the substances dissolved in them are forced through cell membranes by **hydrostatic pressure**—the pressure the fluid exerts against the membrane. The molecules passing through the membrane are determined by

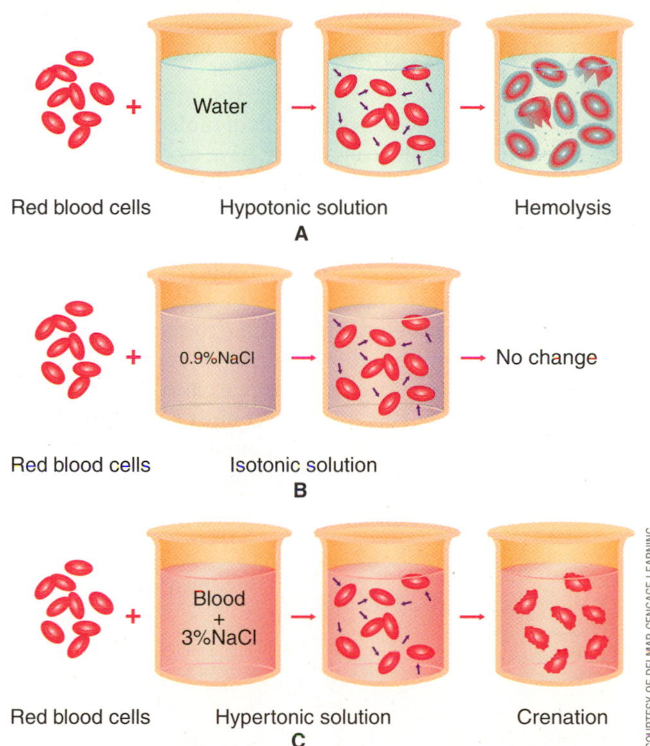

FIGURE 24-7 Osmosis is the movement of water through a membrane from an area of lower concentration to one of higher concentration. *A,* In a hypotonic solution, the water moves into the cells, causing them to swell and burst. *B,* In an isotonic solution, cells are normal in size and shape because the same amount of water is entering and leaving the cells. *C,* In a hypertonic solution, cells are losing water because water moves from an area of lower concentration (inside the cell) to an area of higher concentration (outside the cell).

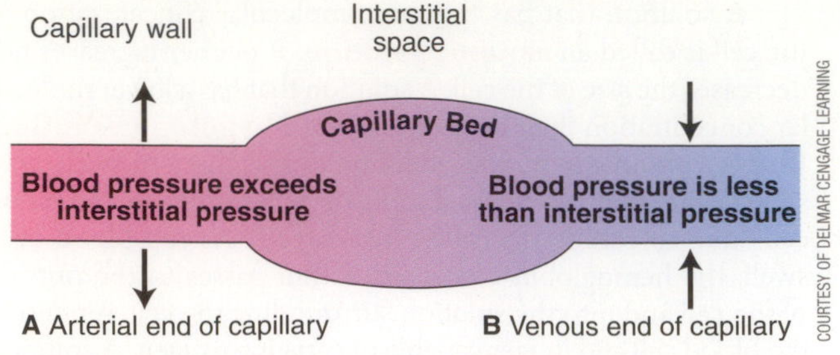

FIGURE 24-8 Filtration; *A,* Pressure in the arteriole is greater then interstitial (between the cells) pressure, causing fluid with dissolved substances to move out of capillaries. *B,* Pressure in venules is less than interstitial fluid pressure, causing fluid and waste products to move back into the capillaries.

the size of the pores in the membrane. Tissue fluids are formed by filtration. As blood passes through the capillaries, hydrostatic pressure exerted by the pumping action of the heart causes some of the liquid fraction of the blood (but not the cells) to pass out of the capillaries, resulting in formation of the tissue fluid (Figure 24-8). As the blood circulates through the capillaries of the kidneys, the hydrostatic pressure of the blood causes many materials to leave the blood through the filtration process. These materials pass into the tubules of the kidneys, where the toxic waste products are removed to form urine. The urine is then eliminated from the body.

ACTIVE TRANSPORT

In the processes discussed thus far, the movement of molecules depends on the concentration of molecules or on pressure. In other words, the cells do not have to expend energy to move the molecules in or out of the cell. In active transport, the cell must use energy to move the molecules. For instance, in the body, sodium ions are in higher concentration in the fluids surrounding the cell than inside the cell. Although some sodium ions can diffuse into the cell, the cell actively transports them through the membrane to the outside. Active transport is accomplished by means of carrier molecules, which can latch onto specific molecules and transport them in or out of the cell. This process requires an expenditure of cellular energy (Figure 24-9). Examples of important ions transported by this process are calcium, sodium, potassium, and magnesium.

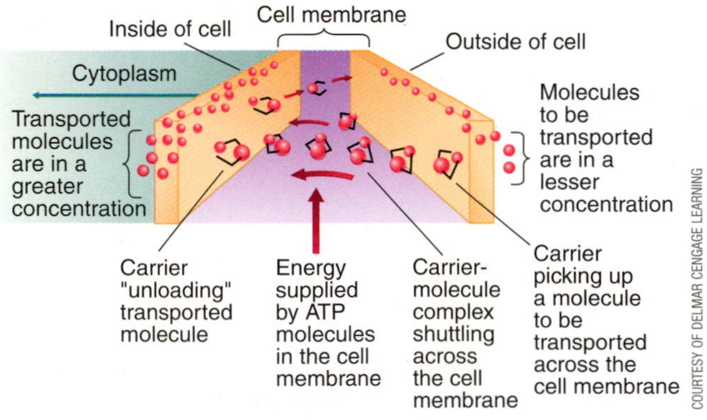

FIGURE 24-9 Active Transport of Molecules from an Area of Lesser Concentration to an Area of Greater Concentration

FLUID AND ELECTROLYTE BALANCE

Human life is suspended in a saline solution having a salt concentration of 0.9%. This solution, which both surrounds the cells and is contained within them, constitutes the body fluids. The water and electrolytes composing these body fluids come from ingested water and nutrients, and from the water that results from metabolism.

For life to continue and the cells to function properly, the body fluids must remain fairly constant with regard to the amount of water and the specific electrolytes of which they are composed. Water is essential because it is the basic component of all the body fluids. Water is involved in many of the metabolic processes in the body and is a by-product of some of these reactions. The various electrolytes all have essential roles in cellular physiological processes. If some of either is lost, it must be replaced, and if either water or an electrolyte is in excess, it must be removed. Maintaining the consistency of this fluid environment is homeostasis.

For cells to survive and carry out their multitude of physiologic functions, they need both a continuing source of water, nutrients, and oxygen and a mechanism to remove cellular wastes. These physiologic processes affect the amount of water, the pH, and the ions both inside and outside the cells. A balance must be maintained between the components of the fluids inside and outside the cell. Because the ions are dissolved in water, these two components are tied together: Anything affecting the amount of water in the body will affect the ion concentration.

BODY FLUIDS

Much of the body weight of an average adult is due to the water in the body fluids surrounding the cells and contained within them. The fluid around the cells cushions them and serves as the medium of exchange. Everything that enters or leaves the cells must pass through this fluid layer.

There are two kinds of body fluids. They can be thought of as being contained within two separate containers, called compartments. The **intracellular fluid (ICF)** compartment contains all the water and ions inside the cells. By far the largest amount of water in the body, approximately 65%, is found within this compartment.

The extracellular fluid compartment contains the remaining body fluids, called **extracellular fluid (ECF)**, or fluid outside the cells. These can be further subdivided into interstitial, intravascular, and other fluids. **Interstitial fluid** is the fluid in the tissue spaces around each cell. The **intravascular fluid** is the plasma in the blood vessels and the lymph in the lymphatic system (Figure 24-10). There are also small amounts of other specialized body fluids such as synovial fluid, cerebrospinal fluid, serous fluid, aqueous and vitreous humor, and the endolymph and perilymph. The proportions of extracellular fluid and intracellular fluid vary with age.

Generally speaking, the major ions in the extracellular fluid are sodium (Na^+), chloride (Cl^-), and bicarbonate (HCO_3^-), although other ions do occur. In the intracellular fluid, the major ions are potassium (K^+), phosphate (PO_4^{--}), and magnesium (Mg^{++}), with lesser amounts of other ions present. There are also large numbers of protein molecules bearing a negative charge.

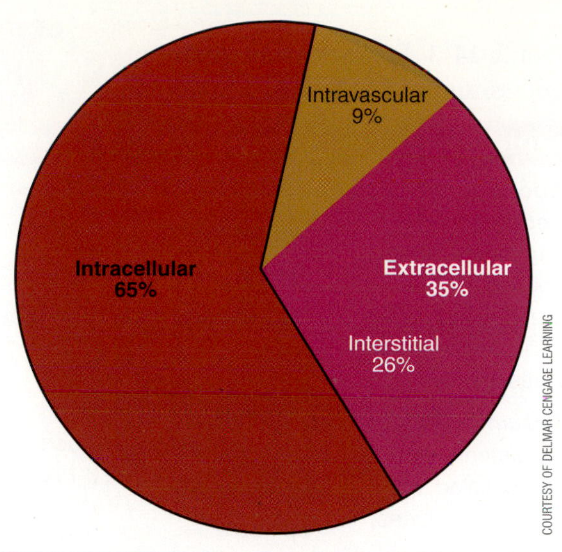

FIGURE 24-10 Body Fluid Compartments of an Adult

Exchange between the Extracellular and Intracellular Fluids

Water and ions moving between the extracellular and intracellular fluids must first pass through the selectively permeable cell membrane. This movement is governed primarily by osmosis. Diffusion and active transport also play a role.

The difference in the ion concentration inside the cell and outside the cell is due primarily to the cell's ability to pump some ions inside and pump others out. If the intracellular fluid becomes hypertonic to the extracellular fluid, water from the extracellular fluid will move by osmosis into the cell to restore the balance and vice versa.

A fluid balance also occurs between the interstitial fluid and the plasma. This balance is regulated primarily by hydrostatic pressure (blood pressure) and osmotic pressure. When the circulating blood passes from the arterioles into the capillaries, the pressure in the capillaries is higher than that in the interstitial fluid. This forces some of the water from the plasma out of the capillaries and into the interstitial fluid. Because of osmotic pressure, some of the water in the interstitial fluid is forced back into the capillaries in the area where they join the venules. Some water is also returned to the bloodstream through the lymphatic system. If the amount of interstitial fluid returned to the circulatory system lessens and the fluid accumulates in the tissue spaces, the tissues become swollen. This condition is called **edema**. Several conditions can cause edema, including kidney or liver disease and heart disorders. Many of these conditions can have serious consequences.

When more water is lost from the body than is replaced, **dehydration** occurs. Among the various causes of dehydration are water deprivation, excessive urine production, profuse sweating, diarrhea, and extended periods of vomiting. As water is lost, the amount of water in the interstitial fluid decreases. Water then moves from the cells to the tissue spaces by osmosis, causing an electrolyte imbalance. Circulatory impairment occurs, which in turn affects the kidney's ability to function normally. This condition is corrected by supplying water and the appropriate electrolytes.

Regulators of Fluid and Electrolyte Balance

There must be a balance in the amounts of fluids and electrolytes consumed and lost daily. Under typical conditions, the average adult loses some water through the skin, lungs, and GI tract and loses the largest amount of water through urine production. This can amount to a per-day fluid loss of approximately 2,500 mL, depending on conditions.

Skin

In the average adult, an estimated water loss of 300 to 500 mL per day occurs by diffusion through the skin. Because the person is not aware of this water loss, it is called *insensible loss*. Water is also lost through the skin by perspiration. The total amount of water lost through perspiration varies depending on environmental factors and body temperature.

Lungs

In the average adult, an estimated insensible water loss of 400 to 500 mL per day occurs with expired air, which is saturated with water vapor. This amount varies with the rate and depth of respirations.

Gastrointestinal Tract

Although a large amount of fluid—approximately 8,000 mL per day in the average adult—is secreted into the gastrointestinal tract, almost all of this fluid is reabsorbed by the body. In adults, approximately 200 mL of water are lost per day in feces. Severe diarrhea can cause a fluid and electrolyte deficit because the GI fluids contain a large amount of electrolytes.

Kidneys

The kidneys play a major role in maintaining fluid balance by excreting 1,000 to 1,500 mL of water per day in the average adult. The excretion of water by healthy kidneys is proportional to the fluid ingested and the amount of waste or solutes excreted.

When an extracellular fluid volume deficit occurs, hormones play a key role in restoring the extracellular fluid volume. Release of the following hormones into circulation causes the kidneys to conserve water:

- *Antidiuretic hormone (ADH)*. Released by the posterior pituitary gland; acts on the distal tubules of the kidneys to reabsorb water.
- *Aldosterone*. Produced in the adrenal cortex; causes the reabsorption of sodium from the renal tubules, leading to water retention in the extracellular fluid, thereby increasing its volume.
- *Renin*. Released by the juxtaglomerular cells of the kidneys; promotes vasoconstriction and the release of aldosterone.

The interaction of these hormones with regard to renal functions serves as the body's compensatory mechanism to maintain homeostasis.

Sodium is the main electrolyte that promotes the retention of water. An intravascular water deficit causes the renal tubules to reabsorb more sodium into circulation. Because water molecules go with the sodium ions, the intravascular water deficit is corrected by this action of the renal tubules.

TABLE 24-2 Average Fluid Losses and Gains in 24 Hours

INTAKE		OUTPUT	
Oral liquids	1,300 mL	Urine	1,000 mL – 1,500 mL
Water in food	1,000 mL	Stool	200 mL
Water from metabolism	300 mL	Insensible losses	
		Lungs	400–500 mL
		Skin	300–500 mL
Total	2,600 mL	Total	2,600 mL (average)

Adapted from: Roth, R. (2007). *Nutrition and Diet Theray* (9th ed.). Clifton Park, New York: Delmar Cengage Learning.

Fluid and Food Intake

Fluids must be replaced in the amounts lost. The primary source of fluid replacement is water consumption. Approximately 60% may be obtained in this way, with an additional 30% being obtained from foods and 8% to 10% being a product of metabolism (metabolic water), for a total of 2,600 mL. Table 24-2 illustrates fluid balance.

Thirst

Water consumption usually occurs in response to the sensation of thirst. This mechanism is poorly understood. It is generally believed to be brought about by the loss of body fluids, which in turn causes a dryness in the mouth and the thirst sensation. Replacing the lost fluids by water consumption causes the sensation to diminish. The thirst mechanism appears to be regulated by the hypothalamus in the brain.

Dehydration is one of the most common and most serious fluid imbalances that can result from poor monitoring of fluid intake. One nursing goal is to ensure that all clients understand both the role that water plays in health and the way to maintain adequate hydration.

DISTURBANCES IN ELECTROLYTE BALANCE

In health, normal homeostatic mechanisms function to maintain electrolyte balance. In illness, one or more of the regulating mechanisms may be affected, or an imbalance may become too great for the body to correct without treatment. Electrolytes are measured by laboratory analysis of a blood sample. Table 24-3 lists foods rich in sodium, potassium, and calcium. Table 24-4 lists the types, causes, signs and symptoms, and nursing interventions for electrolyte imbalances.

SODIUM

Sodium (Na^+) is the major electrolyte in extracellular fluid. It regulates fluid balance through osmotic pressure that results

TABLE 24-3 Foods Rich in Sodium, Potassium, and Calcium

SODIUM	POTASSIUM	CALCIUM
Processed/prepared foods: canned vegetables, soups, luncheon meats, frozen foods, potato chips, snack foods, olives, pickles *Sodium-containing condiments:* soy sauce, salad dressings, sauces, dips, ketchup, mustard, relishes *Natural foods:* meat, poultry, dairy, vegetables	Banana Orange Apricot Cantaloupe Dried fruit Avocado Raw carrots Baked potato Spinach Milk Yogurt Meat Fish	Milk Yogurt Cheese Tofu/soybeans Almonds Broccoli Spinach

COURTESY OF DELMAR CENGAGE LEARNING

from water following sodium in the body. Sodium stimulates conduction of nerve impulses and helps maintain neuromuscular activity. Excretion occurs primarily via the kidneys. The normal serum sodium for an adult is 135 to 145 mEq/L. Critical values are <130 or >160 mEq/L (Daniels, 2010; Daniels, Nosek, & Nicoll, 2007).

Hyponatremia

A subnormal serum sodium value indicates hyponatremia. The cause is either a sodium deficit or a water excess. A hypo-osmotic state exists: The water moves out of the vascular space, into the interstitial space, and then into the intracellular space, causing edema. Hyponatremia may be caused by prolonged vomiting, diarrhea, or gastric or intestinal suctioning. This can be life threatening.

Hypernatremia

An elevated serum sodium level indicates hypernatremia. Excess sodium or a loss of water causes a rise in the extracellular osmotic pressure and pulls water out of the cells and into the extracellular space.

POTASSIUM

Potassium (K^+) is the major electrolyte in intracellular fluid. Its concentration inside cells is approximately 150 mEq/L. The normal value range of extracellular (serum) potassium is narrow: 3.5 to 5.3 mEq/L. Critical values are <3.5 or >5.3 mEq/L (Kee et al., 2010). Consequently, the slightest changes can dramatically affect physiological functions. Potassium maintains normal nerve and muscle activity, especially of the heart, and osmotic pressure within the cells. It also assists in the cellular metabolism of carbohydrates and proteins. The kidneys prefer to retain sodium and excrete potassium, even when both electrolytes are depleted. When potassium is lost from cells, sodium and hydrogen move into the cells. This aids

TABLE 24-4 Electrolyte Imbalances

ELECTROLYTE AND TYPE OF IMBALANCE	CAUSES OF IMBALANCE	SIGNS AND SYMPTOMS	NURSING INTERVENTIONS
Sodium			
Hyponatremia *(serum sodium level <135 mEq/L)*	• Sodium deficit • Water excess • Prolonged vomiting, diarrhea, excessive perspiration, burns, or gastric or intestinal suctioning • Syndrome of inappropriate ADH (SIADH) • Diuretics	Hypotension, tachycardia, edema, headache, lethargy, confusion, muscle weakness and twitching, abdominal cramps, dry mucous membranes, dry skin	Monitor serum sodium lab results. Assess for physical manifestations. Encourage foods and fluids high in sodium if ordered. Monitor I&O. Teach the client about sodium rich foods. Administer IV solution as ordered.
Hypernatremia *(serum sodium level >145 mEq/L)*	• Excess sodium • Loss of water • Decreased renal function	Muscle twitching, tremor, hyperreflexia, agitation, restlessness, stupor, increased body temperature, tachycardia	Monitor serum sodium lab results. Limit foods and fluids high in sodium if ordered. Assess for physical manifestations. Monitor I&O.
Potassium			
Hypokalemia *(serum potassium level <3.5 mEq/L)*	• Excessive loss of gastric fluids • Use of diuretics	Muscle weakness, paralytic ileus, polyuria, polydipsia, EKG changes, elevated blood glucose level	Teach the client about potassium rich foods. Administer oral potassium replacement as ordered. Administer IV potassium as ordered. Monitor and assess heart rate, rhythm, and EKG readings. Monitor serum potassium lab results. Monitor I&O. Assess for physical manifestations. Encourage foods and fluids high in potassium if ordered.
Hyperkalemia *(serum potassium level >5.3 mEq/L)*	• Renal disease • Extensive trauma • Insulin deficiency	Anxiety, irritability, diarrhea, abdominal cramping, EKG changes, cardiac arrest	Be prepared to administer IV calcium gluconate. May need to prepare client for dialysis and/or the administration of Kayexalate. Monitor serum potassium lab results. Monitor I&O. Assess for physical manifestations. Monitor and assess heart rate, rhythm, and EKG readings.
Calcium			
Hypocalcemia *(total serum calcium <8.5 mg/dL)*	• Hypoalbuminemia • Renal failure • Chronic diarrhea • Hormonal and electrolyte influence	Anxiety, irritability, tetany, abdominal and muscle cramps, positive Chvostek's sign, positive Trousseau's sign, weak heart contractions, fractures	Teach the client about calcium-rich foods. Monitor serum calcium lab results. Monitor I&O. Assess for physical manifestations. Monitor and assess heart rate, rhythm, and EKG readings. Administer oral calcium replacement as ordered. Encourage foods and fluids high in calcium if ordered.

(Continues)

Table 24-4 Electrolyte Imbalances (Continued)

ELECTROLYTE AND TYPE OF IMBALANCE	CAUSES OF IMBALANCE	SIGNS AND SYMPTOMS	NURSING INTERVENTIONS
Hypercalcemia *(total serum calcium >10.5 mg/dL)*	• Increased use of calcium supplements • Renal dysfunction • Diuretics • Use of steroids • Hyperparathyroidism	Depression, signs of heart block, pathological fractures, kidney stones	Monitor serum calcium lab results. Monitor I&O. Assess for physical manifestations. Monitor and assess heart rate, rhythm, and EKG readings.
Magnesium			
Hypomagnesemia *(serum magnesium level <1.5 mEq/L)*	• Diarrhea, • Steatorrhea • Chronic alcoholism • Diabetes mellitus malnutrition • Chronic use of laxatives acute renal failure • Acute myocardial infarction	Hyperirritability, tetany-like symptoms, increased tendon reflexes, hypertension, cardiac dysrhythmias	Monitor serum magnesium lab results. Monitor I&O. Assess for physical manifestations.
Hypermagnesemia *(serum magnesium level >2.5 mEq/L)*	• Renal insufficiency • Laxatives and antacids with magnesium • Severe dehydration • Diabetic ketoacidosis	Bradycardia, cardiac arrest, hypotension, EKG changes, muscle weakness, paralysis, CNS depression, confusion, flushing	Monitor serum magnesium lab results. Monitor I&O. Assess for physical manifestations. Monitor and assess heart rate, rhythm, and EKG readings.
Phosphate			
Hypophosphatemia *(serum phosphorus level <2.5 mg/dL)*	• Malnutrition • Chronic alcoholism • TPN administration vomiting • Chronic diarrhea • Hyperparathyroidism • Burns • Diuretics • Aluminum-containing antacids • Respiratory alkalosis	Muscle weakness, fatigue, tremors, bone pain, seizures, coma, weak pulse, anorexia, bone changes	Use safety precautions to prevent falls or injury. Monitor serum phosphorus lab results. Monitor I&O. Assess for physical manifestations.
Hyperphosphatemia *(serum phosphorus level >4.5 mg/dL)*	• Chemotherapy • Renal insufficiency • Hypoparathyroidism • Metabolic and respiratory acidosis	Tetany, hyperreflexia, flaccid paralysis, muscle weakness, tachycardia, abdominal cramps	Monitor serum phosphorus lab results. Monitor I&O. Assess for physical manifestations.

Table 24-4 Electrolyte Imbalances (Continued)

ELECTROLYTE AND TYPE OF IMBALANCE	CAUSES OF IMBALANCE	SIGNS AND SYMPTOMS	NURSING INTERVENTIONS
Chloride			
Hypochloremia *(serum chloride level <95 mEq/L)*	• Prolonged diarrhea or diaphoresis • Vomiting • Gastric surgery • Gastric suctioning	Tremors, twitching, hypotension, slow, shallow breathing	Monitor serum chloride lab results. Monitor I&O. Assess for physical manifestations.
Hyperchloremia *(serum chloride level >108 mEq/L)*	• Dehydration • Hypernatremia • Metabolic acidosis	Weakness, deep and rapid breathing, lethargy	Monitor serum chloride lab results. Monitor I&O. Assess for physical manifestations.

COURTESY OF DELMAR CENGAGE LEARNING

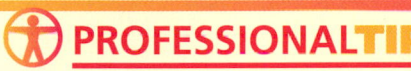

Hypokalemia

Hypokalemia can cause cardiac arrest when:

- The potassium level is <2.5 mEq/L.
- The client is taking digitalis (a drug that strengthens the contraction of the myocardium and slows down the heart rate). *Hypokalemia enhances the action of digitalis, causing toxicity.*

in regulating acid–base balance. Intracellular potassium deficit may coexist with an excess of extracellular potassium.

Hypokalemia

A low serum potassium level indicates hypokalemia. Excessive loss of gastric fluids and the use of diuretics can place the client at risk for hypokalemia and an acid–base imbalance (metabolic alkalosis). Potassium-wasting diuretics, such as furosemide (Lasix) or chlorothiazide (Diuril) can cause hypokalemia.

SAFETY

Potassium Chloride

- Use IV route only when hypokalemia is life threatening or when oral replacement is not feasible.
- Always dilute potassium chloride in a large amount of IV solution.
- Never administer more than 10 mEq/L of IV potassium chloride (KCl) per hour; the normal dose of IV KCl is 20 to 40 mEq/L infused over an 8-hour period.
- Never give KCl intramuscularly (IM) or as an IV bolus; potentially fatal hyperkalemia may result.
- Monitor the IV site frequently for early signs of infiltration, as potassium is caustic to the tissues.

Hyperkalemia

An elevated serum potassium level indicates hyperkalemia. Clients with renal disease develop hyperkalemia because potassium cannot be excreted adequately by the kidneys. Extensive trauma causes potassium to be released from the cells and enter the bloodstream, leading to hyperkalemia. Hyperkalemia inhibits the action of digitalis. This condition is much more critical than is hypokalemia.

Calcium

Calcium (Ca^{++}) plays an essential role in bone and teeth integrity, blood clotting, muscle functioning, and nerve impulse transmission. Vitamin D is required for absorption of calcium from the GI tract. Only 1% of the body's calcium is found in the blood plasma (serum). Normally, 50% of the serum calcium is ionized (physiologically active), with the remaining 50% being bound to protein. Free, ionized calcium is needed for cell membrane permeability. The calcium that is bound to plasma protein cannot pass through the capillary wall and, therefore, cannot leave the intravascular compartment. Total serum calcium concentration measures both the ionized calcium and the calcium bound to albumin. The normal value range of total serum calcium concentration for an adult is 8.5 to 10.5 mg/dL. Critical values are <7.0 or >12 mg/dL. Values for the older adult are slightly lower (Daniels, 2010; Daniels et al., 2007).

PROFESSIONALTIP

Serum Calcium

Approximately 50% of serum calcium is bound to protein. When evaluating laboratory results, correlate the serum calcium level with the serum albumin level. *Any change in serum protein will result in a change in the total serum calcium.*

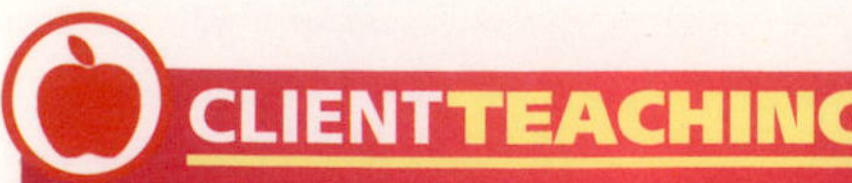

Calcium and Vitamin D

Vitamin D is necessary for the absorption of calcium from the GI tract. Clients who do not get adequate exposure to the sun or who use sunscreen (which is needed to prevent skin cancer) may not make enough vitamin D to support adequate calcium absorption. Advise these clients to consult their physicians regarding a vitamin D supplement.

Hypocalcemia

Hypocalcemia is indicated by a low serum calcium level. Alkalosis, elevated serum albumin, and the rapid administration of citrated blood increase the activity of calcium binders, thereby decreasing the amount of free calcium.

Hypercalcemia

An elevated total serum calcium level indicates hypercalcemia. Generally, three separate evaluations of either total serum calcium or ionized serum calcium are performed before a diagnosis of hypercalcemia is made. Hypercalcemia is often a symptom of an underlying disease such as metastatic bone tumors, Paget's disease, acromegaly, and hyperparathyroidism, which all increase bone reabsorption and, thereby, foster the release of calcium into circulating blood. Calcium-containing antacids and excess calcium from the diet may also cause hypercalcemia.

Magnesium

Most magnesium (Mg^{++}) is found in intracellular fluid and in combination with calcium and phosphorus in bone, muscle, and soft tissue. Blood serum contains only approximately 1%. Magnesium plays an important role as a coenzyme, in the metabolism of carbohydrates and proteins, and as a mediator, in neuromuscular activity. It is the only cation that is found in higher concentration in cerebrospinal fluid than in extracellular fluid. When a magnesium deficiency develops, the body conserves magnesium at the expense of excreting potassium. A close relationship exists between magnesium, calcium, and potassium in the intracellular fluid: A low level of one results in low levels of the other two. The normal serum magnesium level for an adult is 1.5 to 2.5 mEq/L (Kee et al., 2010).

Hypomagnesemia

A serum magnesium level of $<$1.5 mEq/L indicates hypomagnesemia (Daniels, 2010), which most commonly results from chronic alcoholism. Increased renal excretion is associated with prolonged diuretic therapy or use of gentamicin (Garamycin), cyclosporin (Sandimmune), or cisplatin (Platinol).

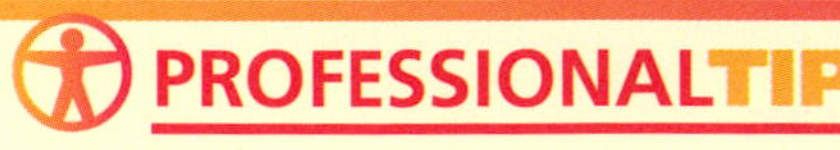

Hyperalimentation

Total parenteral nutrition (TPN) provided continuously (hyperalimentation) and without a magnesium supplement can cause hypomagnesemia.

SAFETY

Magnesium Level

When the serum magnesium level reaches 10 to 15 mEq/L, respiratory paralysis may occur.

Hypermagnesemia

A serum magnesium level of $>$2.5 mEq/L indicates hypermagnesemia (Daniels, 2010). This condition rarely occurs if kidney function is normal. An increased magnesium level is associated with uncontrolled diabetes (ketoacidosis), renal failure, and ingestion of magnesium antacids (Maalox, Mylanta) or laxatives (milk of magnesia [MOM], magnesium citrate [Citromal]).

Phosphate

Phosphate (PO_4^{--}) is the main intracellular anion. It appears as phosphorus in the serum, where the normal value range is 2.5 to 4.5 mg/dL (Kee et al., 2010). Phosphorus is critical for normal cell functioning. Most phosphorus is found combined with calcium in teeth and bones. Phosphate and calcium exist in an inverse relationship (i.e., as one increases the other decreases).

Hypophosphatemia

A client with a low serum phosphorus level has hypophosphatemia. Rarely does this condition result from decreased dietary intake. More commonly, it stems from respiratory alkalosis. Intense, prolonged hyperventilation can cause severe hypophosphatemia.

Hyperphosphatemia

A client with an elevated serum phosphorus level has hyperphosphatemia. This condition most commonly results from renal failure with resultant decreased renal phosphorus excretion. Excessive use of phosphate-containing laxatives or phosphate enemas may cause hyperphosphatemia.

Chloride

Chloride (Cl^-) is the major anion in extracellular fluid. Chloride functions in combination with sodium to maintain

PROFESSIONAL TIP

Hyperphosphatemia

A client with hyperphosphatemia generally remains asymptomatic unless hypocalcemia results, in which case the client may describe both tingling sensations around the mouth and in the fingertips as well as muscle cramps.

CRITICAL THINKING

Vomiting

A client has been vomiting for 3 days and is unable to keep anything down. Besides fluid volume deficit, what other problems would you expect to find?

osmotic pressure. It also assists in maintaining acid–base balance. When the carbon dioxide level increases, bicarbonate shifts from the intracellular compartment to the extracellular compartment. Chloride, in an effort to maintain homeostasis, then moves into the intracellular compartment. The kidneys selectively excrete chloride or bicarbonate ions depending on the acid–base balance. The normal serum chloride range is 95 to 108 mEq/L (Kee et al., 2010).

Hypochloremia

A low serum chloride level indicates hypochloremia. Excess losses of chloride may result from prolonged diarrhea or diaphoresis. Loss of hydrochloric acid related to vomiting, gastric suctioning, or gastric surgery may cause hypochloremia.

Hyperchloremia

An elevated serum chloride level indicates hyperchloremia, which usually occurs in conjunction with dehydration, hypernatremia, or metabolic acidosis.

ACID–BASE BALANCE

As described earlier, the body maintains a normal pH within the relatively narrow range of 7.35 to 7.45. Body pH is maintained by the buffer systems, the respiratory system, and the kidneys. A pH below 7.35 is termed acidosis, and a pH above 7.45 is termed alkalosis. Either of these conditions can be brought about by respiratory or metabolic changes.

Regulators of Acid–Base Balance

The body has three main control systems that regulate acid–base balance to counter acidosis or alkalosis: the buffer systems, respirations, and renal control of hydrogen ion concentration. These systems vary in their reaction times in regulating and restoring balance to the hydrogen ion concentration.

Buffer Systems

The buffer systems bicarbonate, phosphate, and protein were previously discussed. They react quickly to prevent excessive changes in the hydrogen ion concentration.

Respiratory Regulation of Acid–Base Balance

The respiratory system helps maintain acid–base balance by controlling the content of carbon dioxide in extracellular fluid. The *rate of metabolism* determines the formation of carbon dioxide. Various intracellular metabolic processes continuously form carbon dioxide in the body. The carbon in foods is **oxidized** (joined with oxygen) to form carbon dioxide.

It takes the respiratory regulatory mechanism several minutes to respond to changes in the carbon dioxide concentration of extracellular fluid. With the increase of carbon dioxide in extracellular fluid, respiration increases in rate and depth so that more carbon dioxide is exhaled. As the respiratory system removes carbon dioxide, less carbon dioxide is present in the blood to combine with water to form carbonic acid. Likewise, if the blood level of carbon dioxide is low, respirations decrease to maintain a normal ratio between carbonic acid and basic bicarbonate.

Renal Control of Hydrogen Ion Concentration

The kidneys control extracellular fluid pH by eliminating either hydrogen ions or bicarbonate ions from body fluids. If the bicarbonate concentration in the extracellular fluid is greater than normal, the kidneys excrete more bicarbonate ions, making the urine more alkaline. Conversely, if more hydrogen ions are excreted in the urine, the urine becomes more acidic. The renal mechanism for regulating acid–base balance cannot readjust the pH within seconds, as can the extracellular fluid buffer system, nor within minutes, as can the respiratory compensatory mechanism, but it can function over a period of several hours or days to correct acid–base imbalance.

Diagnostic and Laboratory Data

The biochemical indicators of acid–base balance are assessed by measuring the **arterial blood gases (ABGs)**. The arterial blood gas test measures the levels of oxygen and carbon dioxide in arterial blood. The test assesses pH, partial pressure of oxygen (PO_2 or PaO_2), partial pressure of carbon dioxide (PCO_2 or $PaCO_2$), saturation of oxygen (SaO_2), and bicarbonate (HCO_3). pH has already been discussed.

The PO_2 or PaO_2 expresses the amount of oxygen that can combine with hemoglobin to form oxyhemoglobin, the form in which oxygen is transported through the body. At sea level, the normal range is 80 to 100 millimeters of mercury (mm Hg). The rate at which the oxygen/hemoglobin reaction occurs is influenced by pH. The rate decreases as the pH value decreases.

The PCO_2 or $PaCO_2$ in the blood is a reflection of the efficiency of gaseous exchange in the lungs. At sea level, the normal range is 35 to 45 mm Hg. If the alveoli are obstructed or damaged by disease, carbon dioxide cannot be eliminated and will combine with water to form carbonic acid, which in turn causes acidosis. Conversely, in a person who

PROFESSIONALTIP

Pulse Oximeter Reading

Warming a client's cold hand will provide more accurate results from a pulse oximeter.

is hyperventilating, too much carbon dioxide is eliminated, which may trigger alkalosis.

The SaO_2 is the percentage of oxygen that combines with hemoglobin in the blood. The normal range is 95% to 100% saturation. This value, along with the PO_2 and hemoglobin levels, indicates the degree to which the tissues are receiving oxygen. Oxygen saturation can also be measured with a pulse oximeter, a noninvasive technique.

Determining the amount of bicarbonate (HCO_3) in the blood is important because, along with carbonic acid, bicarbonate is a major buffer in the blood. The two substances occur in a ratio of 20 parts bicarbonate to 1 part carbonic acid. Regardless of the carbonic acid and bicarbonate values, the pH of the blood will remain in the normal range as long as the ratio remains 20:1. The normal range for HCO_3 at sea level is 24 to 28 mEq/L. The carbonic acid level is always 3% of the PCO_2 level.

DISTURBANCES IN ACID–BASE BALANCE

The acid–base imbalances are respiratory acidosis and alkalosis and metabolic acidosis and alkalosis. In determining whether the acid–base imbalance is caused by a respiratory or a metabolic alteration, the key indicators are bicarbonate and carbonic acid levels (Figure 24-11). Table 24-5 lists those changes in laboratory values that indicate the various acid–base imbalances.

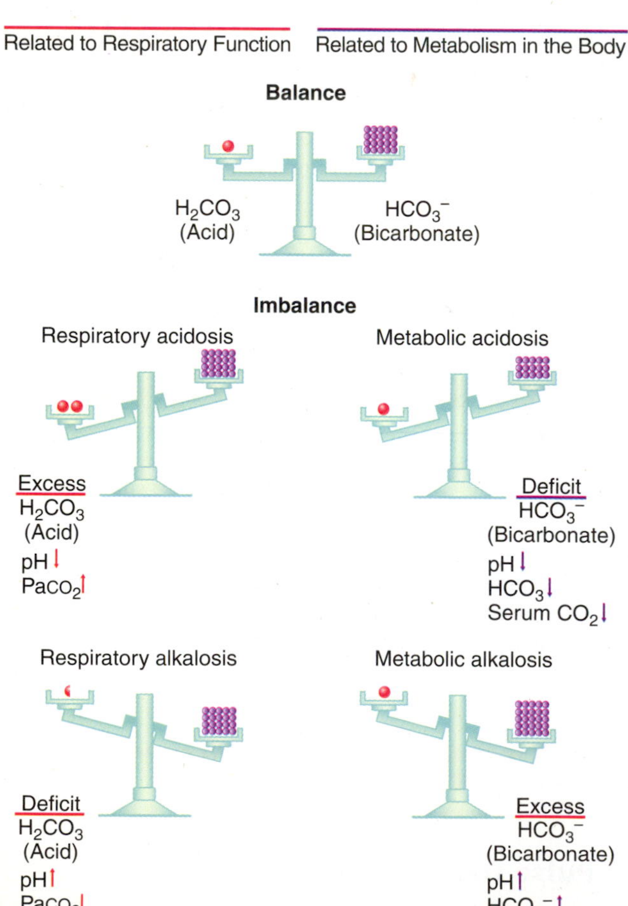

FIGURE 24-11 Acid-Base Balance and Imbalance

TABLE 24-5 Laboratory Values in Acid–Base Imbalances

SITUATION	pH	PCO_2	HCO_3
Normal parameters	7.35 to 7.45	35 to 45 mm Hg	24 to 28 mEq/L
Respiratory acidosis			
Acute	<7.35	>45 mm Hg	Normal
Chronic	<7.35	>45 mm Hg	>28 mEq/L
Respiratory alkalosis	>7.45	<35 mm Hg	Normal
Metabolic acidosis	<7.35	Normal	<24 mEq/L
Metabolic Alkalosis	>7.45	Normal	>28 mEq/L

COURTESY OF DELMAR CENGAGE LEARNING

RESPIRATORY ACIDOSIS

When carbon dioxide is not eliminated by the lungs as fast as it is produced by cellular metabolism, the amount of carbon dioxide increases in the blood. It then reacts with water and forms excess hydrogen ions, as shown in the following reaction:

$$CO_2 + H_2O \rightarrow H^+ + HCO_3$$

In respiratory acidosis, there is an increased concentration of hydrogen ions (a blood pH below 7.35), an increased PCO_2 level (greater than 45 mm Hg), and an excess of carbonic acid. It is caused by hypoventilation or any condition that depresses ventilation. Hypoventilation can be caused by brain injury, chest injuries, emphysema, and chronic obstructive pulmonary disease (COPD). When the respiratory rate and the amount of oxygen supplied to the lungs suddenly lessen, acute respiratory acidosis can occur. This condition can be life threatening, and it must be recognized and corrected quickly. Chronic respiratory acidosis occurs when the respiratory rate is continually depressed.

Clients with respiratory acidosis experience neurological changes as a result of the cerebrospinal fluid and brain cells acidity. Hypoventilation causes **hypoxemia** (decreased oxygen in the blood), which in turn causes further neurological impairment. Hyperkalemia may accompany acidosis.

PROFESSIONALTIP

Electrolyte Shift

An electrolyte shift occurs in metabolic acidosis. Hydrogen and sodium ions move into the cells, and potassium moves into the extracellular fluid. Hyperkalemia may cause ventricular fibrillation and death.

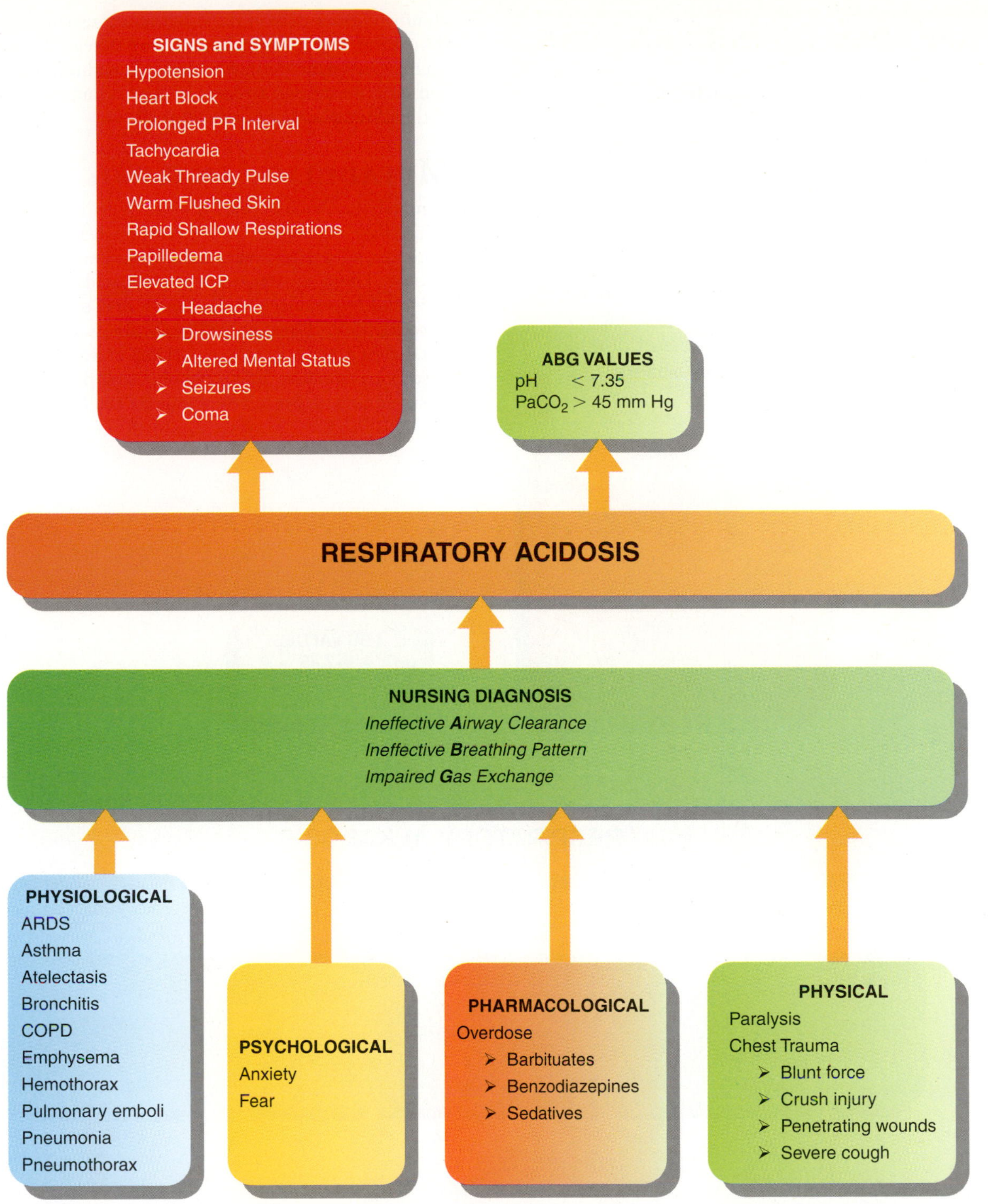

CONCEPT MAP: Respiratory Acidosis (*Courtesy of Leon Klopfenstein and Eric Mason: Lima, Ohio.*)

RESPIRATORY ALKALOSIS

In respiratory alkalosis, there is a decreased concentration of hydrogen ions (a blood pH above 7.45) and a below-normal PCO_2 level (lower than 35 mm Hg). It is caused by hyperventilation (excessive exhalation of carbon dioxide) resulting in hypocapnia (decreased arterial carbon dioxide concentration). As the breathing rate increases, the amount of carbon dioxide in the blood decreases, which in turn increases the pH of the blood.

Hyperventilation can be triggered by anxiety, fear, fever, pain, rapid mechanical ventilation, and hypoxia at high altitudes. This condition is usually self-correcting. As the breathing returns to normal, the carbon dioxide level in the blood increases, and the normal pH is restored. Other causes of hyperventilation, which involves overstimulation of the respiratory center, include salicylate poisoning, brain tumors, meningitis, encephalitis, and pulmonary embolus.

METABOLIC ACIDOSIS

In metabolic acidosis there is an increased concentration of hydrogen ions (blood pH below 7.35) or a decrease in bicarbonate concentration. Such a change may be brought about by kidney disease when the mechanism to excrete excess hydrogen ions is compromised. Diarrhea, diabetes mellitus, and, sometimes, diuretics may also be responsible. The lungs

LIFE SPAN CONSIDERATIONS

Risk for Respiratory Acidosis

Older adults are at greater risk for development of respiratory acidosis because of the increased incidence of chronic lung diseases such as COPD. As the population increases in age, the incidence of complications related to chronic illnesses also increases. Older adults are at risk for respiratory distress or respiratory failure because of the increase in age-related or seasonal illnesses, such as pneumonia or influenza. This increases their chances of developing the complication of respiratory acidosis.

eliminate more carbon dioxide but are usually ineffective in decreasing acids. The kidneys try to increase the pH and the excretion of hydrogen by exchanging sodium ions for hydrogen ions. Metabolic acidosis is most common in individuals with kidney disease or diabetes mellitus.

METABOLIC ALKALOSIS

In metabolic alkalosis there is a loss of acid from the body or a gain in base (increased level of bicarbonate). Blood pH is above 7.45. Excessive ingestion of antacids and milk may cause a gain in base. These substances neutralize acids, resulting in alkalosis and hypercalcemia. Excessive oral or parenteral intake of sodium bicarbonate or other alkaline salts (e.g., sodium or potassium acetate, lactate, or citrate) increases the amount of base in extracellular fluid. Loss of gastric fluids from vomiting or suctioning may result in metabolic alkalosis.

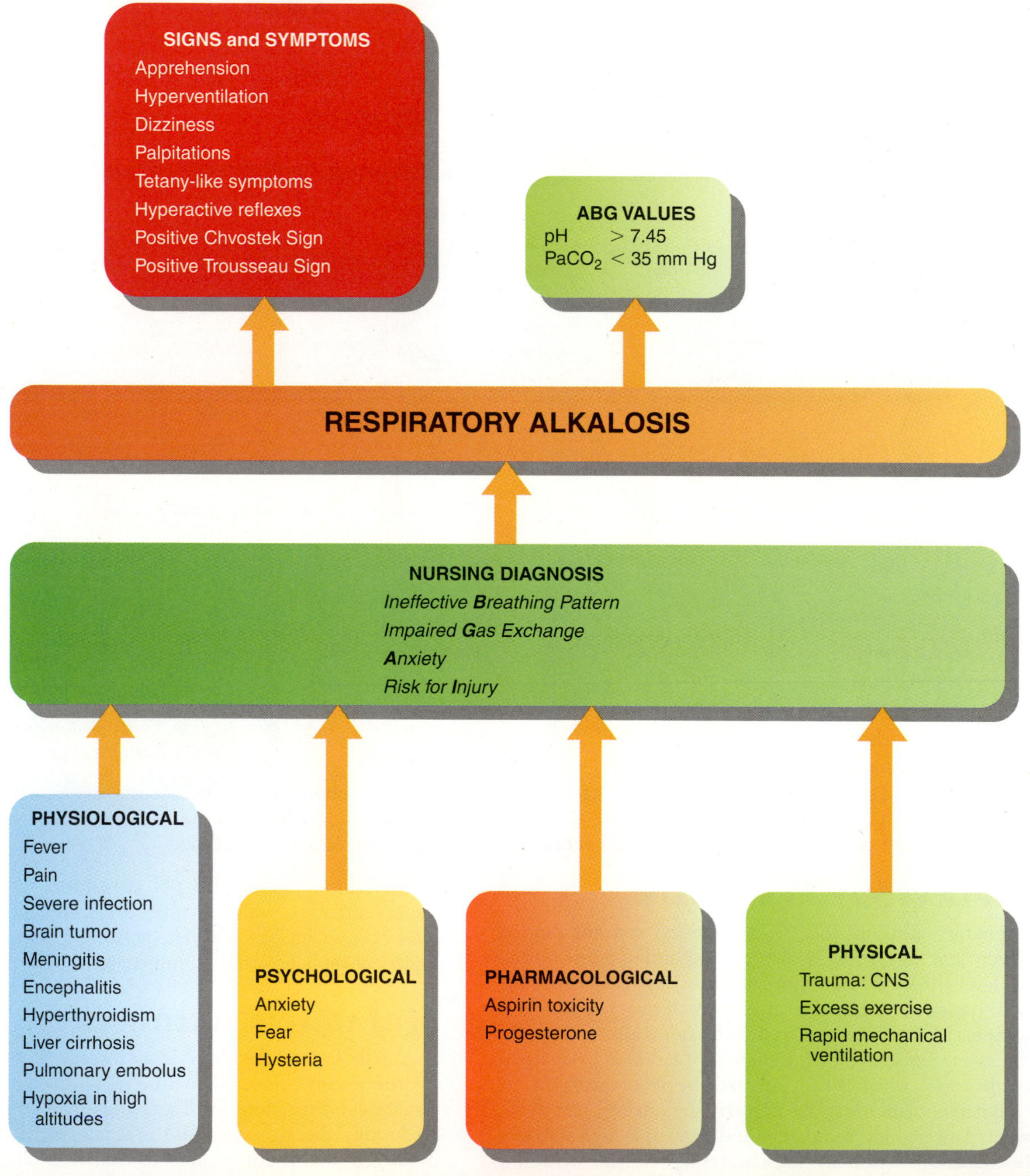

CONCEPT MAP: Respiratory Alkalosis

PROFESSIONALTIP

Metabolic Alkalosis

The following clinical conditions can place clients at risk for metabolic alkalosis:

- Vomiting and nasogastric suctioning or lavage cause a loss of hydrochloric acid and chloride. With the loss of the hydrogen and chloride ions, bicarbonate ions are absorbed, unneutralized, into the bloodstream, and the pH of the extracellular fluid rises (alkalosis).
- Diarrhea and steroid or diuretic therapy can cause excessive loss of potassium, chloride, and other electrolytes. The potassium deficit causes the kidneys to exchange hydrogen ions (instead of potassium ions) for sodium ions, which promotes the loss of hydrogen, thereby increasing bicarbonate level.

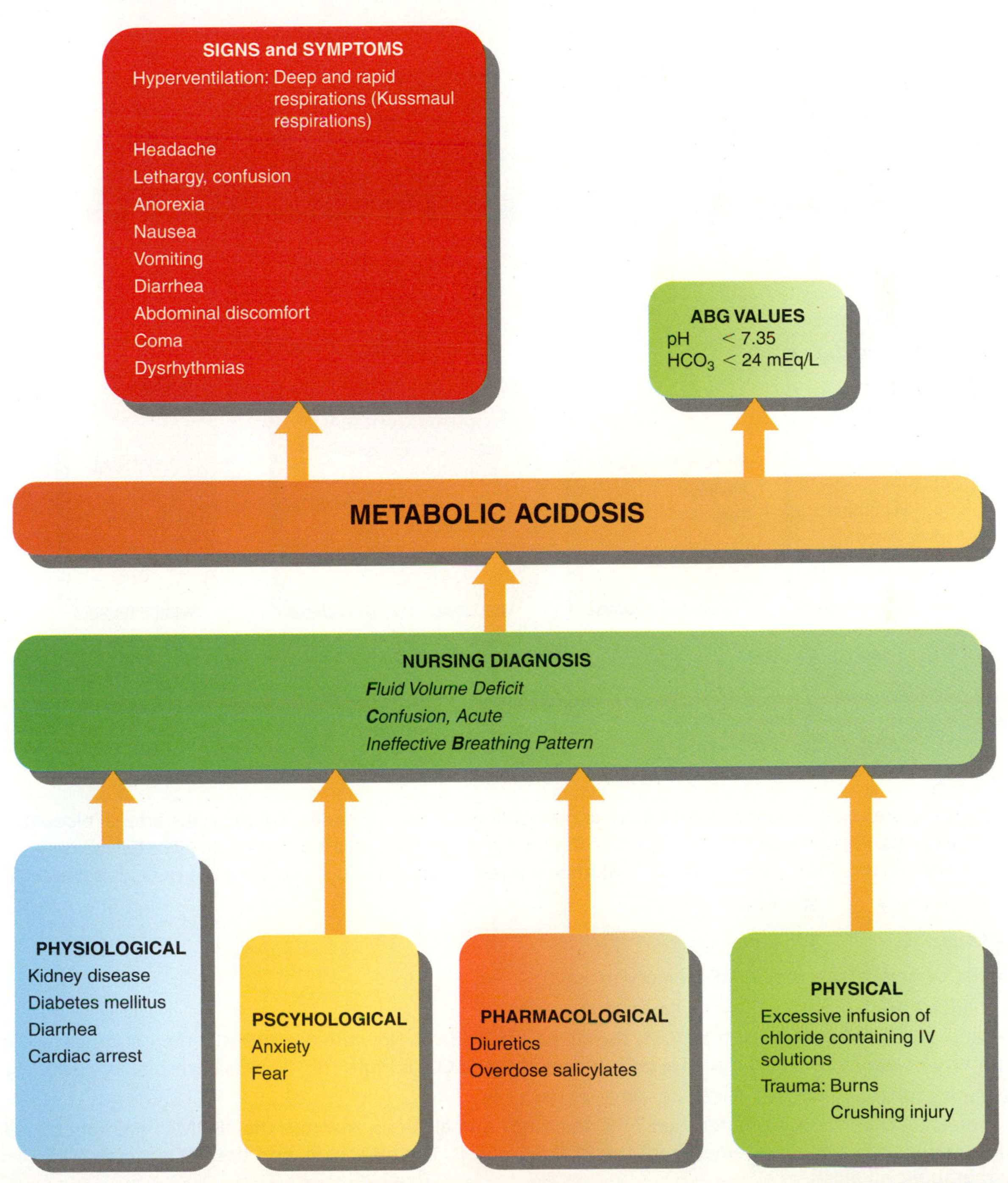

CONCEPT MAP: Metabolic Acidosis (*Courtesy of Kami L. Fox, MS, CNP.*)

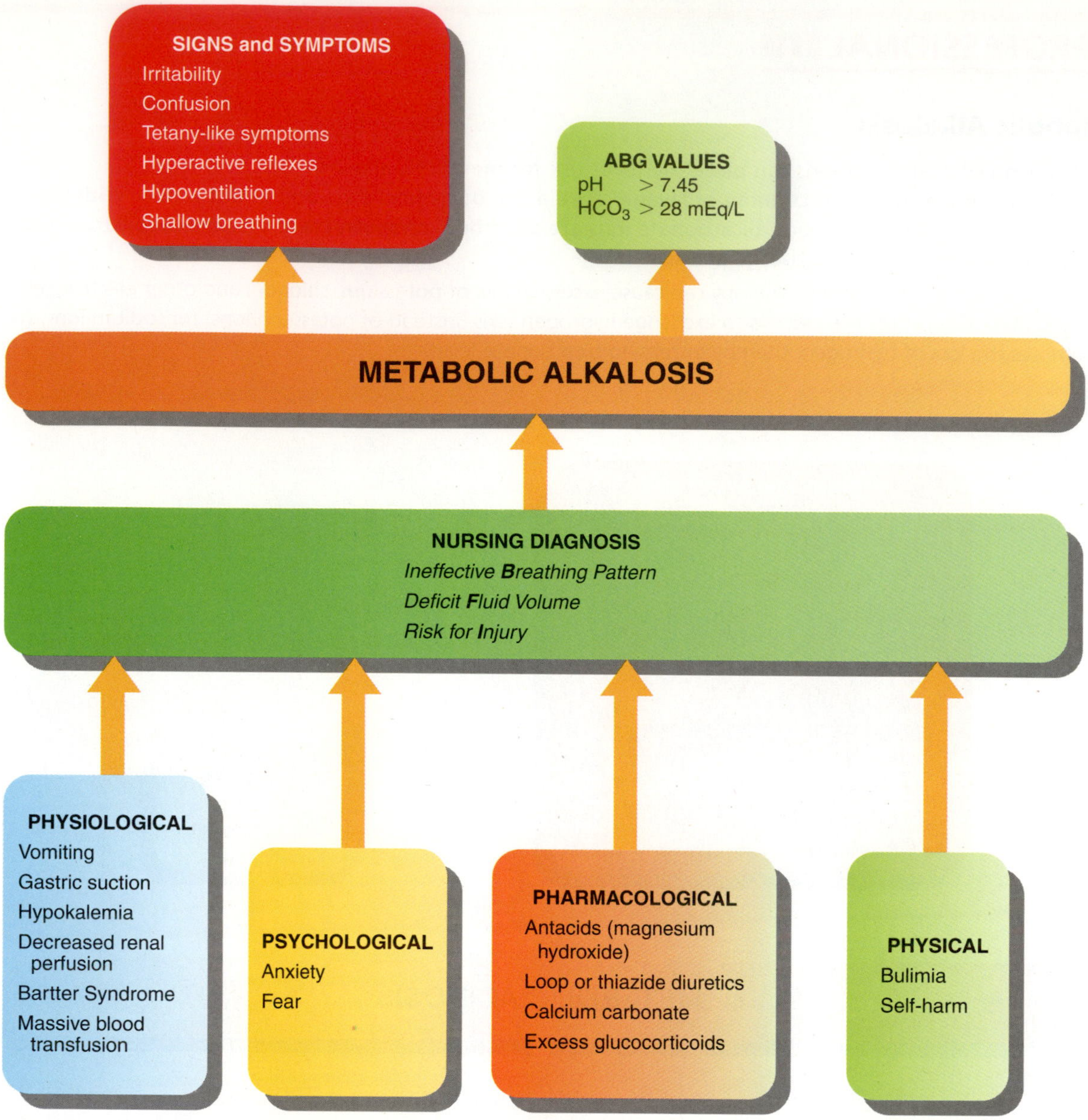

SIGNS and SYMPTOMS
Irritability
Confusion
Tetany-like symptoms
Hyperactive reflexes
Hypoventilation
Shallow breathing

ABG VALUES
pH > 7.45
HCO_3 > 28 mEq/L

METABOLIC ALKALOSIS

NURSING DIAGNOSIS
*Ineffective **B**reathing Pattern*
*Deficit **F**luid Volume*
*Risk for **I**njury*

PHYSIOLOGICAL
Vomiting
Gastric suction
Hypokalemia
Decreased renal perfusion
Bartter Syndrome
Massive blood transfusion

PSYCHOLOGICAL
Anxiety
Fear

PHARMACOLOGICAL
Antacids (magnesium hydroxide)
Loop or thiazide diuretics
Calcium carbonate
Excess glucocorticoids

PHYSICAL
Bulimia
Self-harm

CONCEPT MAP: Metabolic Alkalosis

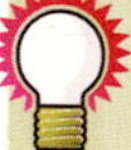

MEMORY TRICK

ROME

A nurse can figure out if a client is in respiratory or metabolic acidosis/alkalosis depending on the arterial blood gas (ABG) laboratory results. An easy way to decide whether it is respiratory or metabolic is by using the "ROME" memory trick. If the pH is opposite the $PaCO_2$ (either high or low), then it is respiratory. If the pH is equal to the HCO_3, it is metabolic.

R = Respiratory **M** = Metabolic

O = Opposite **E** = Equal

Examples of how to use the ROME memory trick:

1. A client's ABGs are pH 7.31, $PaCO_2$ 54, HCO_3 24, PaO_2 62
   Because the client's pH is less than 7.35, the client is in acidosis. Now use the "ROME" memory trick. Is the pH opposite of the $PaCO_2$? Yes, it is. The pH is low, and the $PaCO_2$ is high. This client is in respiratory acidosis.
2. A client's ABGs are pH 7.49, $PaCO_2$ 40, HCO_3 42, PaO_2 80
   Because the client's pH is greater than 7.45, the client is in alkalosis. Now use the "ROME" memory trick. Is the pH equal to (following the same trend) the HCO_3? Yes, it is. The pH is high, and the HCO_3 is high. This client is in metabolic alkalosis.

The renal and respiratory compensatory mechanisms respond to an increased bicarbonate/carbonic acid ratio. In an effort to retain carbon dioxide, the rate and depth of respirations decreases. To counter the pH imbalance of metabolic alkalosis, the arterial carbon dioxide concentration rises, creating respiratory acidosis.

A normal serum potassium level is necessary for renal compensation. When potassium ions enter the cells in exchange for hydrogen ions, in alkalosis hypokalemia results. The kidneys cannot function as a compensatory mechanism when hypokalemia is present; they continue to excrete hydrogen, and bicarbonate excess continues.

NURSING PROCESS

The nursing process assists the nurse in planning client care.

ASSESSMENT

Assessment data are used to identify clients who have potential or actual alterations in fluid volume. Electrolyte and acid-base imbalances are identified primarily with laboratory data, while fluid balances are identified primarily with the health history and physical examination.

Health History

The nursing history should elicit data in the following areas:

- Lifestyle (sociocultural and economic factors, stress, exercise)
- Dietary intake (recent changes in the amount and types of fluid and food, increased thirst)
- Weight (sudden gain or loss)
- Fluid output (recent changes in the frequency or amount of urine output)
- Gastrointestinal disturbances (prolonged vomiting, diarrhea, anorexia, ulcer, hemorrhage)
- Fever and diaphoresis
- Burns, trauma, draining wounds
- Disease conditions that can upset homeostasis (renal disease, endocrine disorders, neural malfunction, pulmonary disease)
- Therapeutic programs that can produce imbalances (special diets, medications, chemotherapy, IV fluid or total parenteral nutrition [TPN] administration, gastric or intestinal suction)

Table 24-6 lists health history assessment questions to ask a client experiencing a fluid, electrolyte, and/or acid–base imbalance.

TABLE 24-6 Health History Assessment Questions

- What recent illnesses have you experienced?
- What prescription medications are you currently taking?
- Do you have any chronic illnesses which affect the way you breathe? If so, please describe the illnesses.
- What over-the-counter medications including herbs are you currently taking?
- Have you recently traveled outside of the continental United States? If so, where?
- What type of work do you do regularly?
- What types of environmental allergies do you have?
- Have you been diagnosed with diabetes? If so, what are your last several blood glucose readings?
- Have you or anyone else noticed a difference in the odor of your breath?
- Have you had any recent changes in your kidney function?
- What types of respiratory illnesses have you experienced recently?
- Have you experienced any changes in your appetite recently?
- What types of foods including fruits do you eat on a regular basis?
- Have you noticed any difference in the way your heart feels?
- Have you experienced any unusual muscle weakness or loss of strength?
- Have you recently experienced diarrhea, vomiting, headache, or dehydration?

COURTESY OF DELMAR CENGAGE LEARNING

Physical Examination

Because fluid alterations may affect any body system, the nurse performs a complete physical examination and identifies all abnormalities.

Daily Weight Changes in the body's total fluid volume are reflected in body weight. For instance, each liter (1,000 mL) of fluid gained or lost is equivalent to 1 kilogram (2.2 lb) of weight.

Vital Signs The client with an elevated temperature is at risk for dehydration related to an increased loss of body fluid. Changes in the pulse rate, strength, and rhythm may indicate fluid alterations. Fluid volume changes may cause the following pulse changes:

- *Fluid volume deficit.* Increased pulse rate and weak pulse strength
- *Fluid volume excess.* Increased pulse strength and third heart sound

Inspect chest wall movement, count the respiratory rate, and auscultate the lungs to assess respiratory changes. Rate and depth changes may cause respiratory acid–base imbalances or may indicate a compensatory response to metabolic acidosis or alkalosis.

The degree of fluid volume deficit can be assessed by blood pressure measurements. Fluid volume deficit can lower the blood pressure. A narrow pulse pressure (lower than 20 mm Hg) may indicate severe hypovolemia (fluid volume deficit).

Intake and Output The client's I&O should be measured and recorded for a 24-hour period to assess for an actual or potential imbalance. A minimum intake of 1,500 mL is essential to balance urinary output and the body's insensible water loss. All liquids taken by mouth (e.g., soup, ice cream, gelatin, juice, and water) and liquids administered through tube feedings (nasogastric or jejunostomy) and parenterally (IV fluids and

SAFETY

Fluid Measurements

To protect both the nurse and the client from transfer of microorganisms, Standard Precautions are always followed during fluid administration and output measurement.

CRITICAL THINKING

Pitting Edema

Nursing assessment reveals a client with new onset (+2) pitting edema of both hands and (+4) pitting edema of both ankles. What nursing action is warranted for (+2) pitting edema? What nursing action is warranted for (+4) pitting edema?

blood or its components) are included. Output includes urine, vomitus, diarrhea, and drainage from tubes such as gastric suction or surgical drains.

Thirst Thirst is the most common indicator of fluid volume deficit. The hypothalamus triggers a thirst response when there is a decrease in extracellular fluid volume or an increase in plasma osmolality.

Food Intake Ingested food also helps maintain extracellular fluid volume. One-third of the body's fluid needs are met

Skin Edema and skin turgor are two important indicators of fluid, electrolyte, and acid–base balances.

Edema The main symptom of fluid volume excess is edema. It may be confined to a specific area (localized) or occur throughout the body (generalized). The skin is taut, shiny, smooth, and pale in localized edema. Assess and palpate edematous areas for color, tenderness, and temperature. Firmly press your thumb against the edematous area or a dependent portion of the client's body (hands, arms, feet, ankles, legs, or sacrum) for 5 seconds. Release pressure and observe for indentation on the skin (Estes, 2010). Edema is not normally present (Daniels et al., 2007). Pitting edema is rated on a 4-point scale, as follows:

- +0: no pitting
- +1: 0 to ¼ inch pitting (mild)
- +2: ¼ to ½ inch pitting (moderate)
- +3: ½ to 1 inch pitting (severe)
- +4: greater than 1 inch pitting (severe)

Turgor Skin **turgor** refers to the normal resiliency of the skin, a reflection of hydration status. When skin is pinched and released, it springs back to a normal position because the cells and interstitial fluid exert outward pressure. To measure the client's skin turgor, use the thumb and forefinger to grasp and raise and then release a small section of skin (Figure 24-12). Dehydration is the main cause of decreased skin turgor, which manifests as lax skin that returns slowly to the normal position. Increased skin turgor, which occurs in conjunction with edema, manifests as smooth, taut, shiny skin that cannot be grasped and raised.

Buccal (Oral) Cavity The nurse should inspect the buccal cavity. With fluid volume deficit, saliva decreases, causing sticky, dry mucous membranes and dry, cracked lips. The tongue has longitudinal furrows.

Eyes The eyes should be inspected for sunkenness, dry conjunctiva, and decreased or absent tearing, all signs of fluid volume deficit. Puffy eyelids (periorbital edema or papilledema) are signs of fluid volume excess. The client may have a history of blurred vision.

Jugular and Hand Veins Circulatory volume is assessed by measuring venous filling of the jugular and hand veins. With the client in a low Fowler's position:

1. Palpate the jugular (neck) veins. Fluid volume excess causes a distention in the jugular veins (Figure 24-13).
2. Place the client's hand below heart level and palpate the hand veins. Fluid volume deficit causes decreased venous filling (flat hand veins).

Neuromuscular System Fluid and electrolyte imbalances may cause neuromuscular alterations. The muscles lose tone, becoming soft and flabby, and reflexes diminish. Calcium and magnesium imbalances cause an increase in neuromuscular irritability. To assess for neuromuscular irritability, the tests for Chvostek's sign and Trousseau's sign are performed. Other neurological signs of fluid, electrolyte, and acid–base imbalances include inability to concentrate, confusion, and emotional lability.

Diagnostic and Laboratory Data

Laboratory tests can reveal imbalances before clinical symptoms are evident in the client; however, unless clients are having the tests for some other reason, symptoms are detected first.

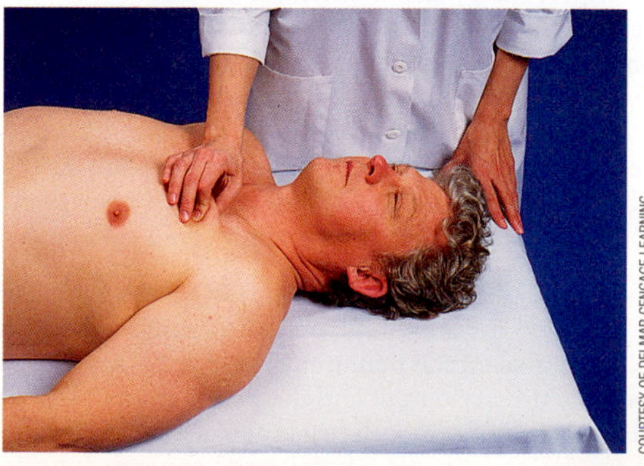
COURTESY OF DELMAR CENGAGE LEARNING

FIGURE 24-12 Assessing Skin Turgor

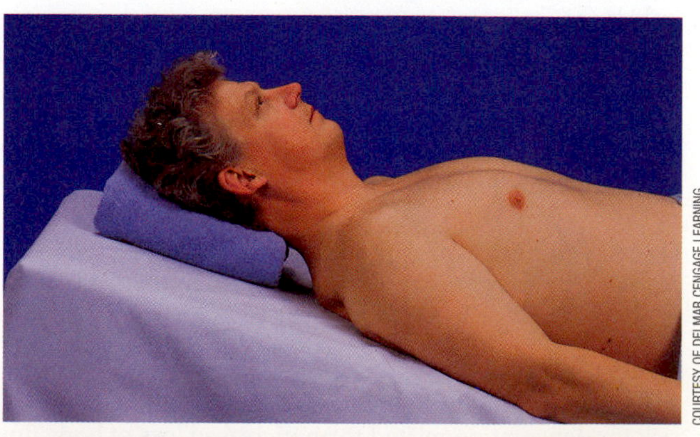
COURTESY OF DELMAR CENGAGE LEARNING

FIGURE 24-13 Client Position when Assessing Jugular Vein Distention

Hemoglobin and Hematocrit Indices The hemoglobin (Hgb) level decreases in the event of severe hemorrhage. Hematocrit (Hct) is affected by changes in plasma volume. For instance, with severe dehydration and hypovolemic shock, hematocrit increases. Conversely, overhydration decreases hematocrit.

Osmolality **Osmolality** is a measurement of the total concentration of dissolved particles (solutes) per kilogram of water. Osmolality measurements are performed on both serum and urine samples to identify changes in fluid and electrolyte balance.

Serum Osmolality Serum osmolality is a measurement of the total concentration of dissolved particles per kilogram of water in serum, recorded in milliosmoles per kilogram (mOsm/kg). The particles measured in serum osmolality include electrolyte ions (i.e., sodium and potassium), and electrically inactive substances (i.e., glucose and urea). Water and sodium are the main entities controlling the osmolality of body fluids. Serum sodium is responsible for 90% of the serum osmolality (Daniels, 2010). The normal range of serum osmolality is 280 to 300 mOsm/Kg (Daniels, 2010). The value increases with dehydration and decreases with water excess.

In clinical practice, the terms *osmolality* and **osmolarity** (the concentration of solutes per liter of cellular fluid) are often used interchangeably to refer to the concentration of body fluid; however, these terms actually have different meanings, in that osmolality refers to the concentration of solutes in the total body water rather than in cellular fluid. The appropriate term to use in conjunction with IV fluid therapy is *osmolarity*.

Urine Osmolality Urine osmolality measures the number of solute particles in a defined amount of solution. The particles measured are nitrogenous waste (creatinine, urea, and uric acid), with urea being predominant. Urine osmolality varies greatly with diet and fluid intake and reflects the kidney's ability to concentrate urine. The normal range of urine osmolality is 500 to 800 mOsm/kg (Daniels, 2010).

Urine pH The measurement of urine pH reveals the hydrogen ion concentration in the urine, indicating the urine's acidity or alkalinity. The pH of the urine should be within normal range (4.5 to 8.0) when the kidney buffering system is compensating for either metabolic acidosis or alkalosis. This is considered a sign of normal function; however, when the renal compensatory function fails to respond to the blood pH, the urine pH will either increase, with acidosis, or decrease, with alkalosis.

Nursing Diagnosis

The North American Nursing Diagnosis Association-International (NANDA-I, 2010) identifies the primary nursing diagnoses for clients with fluid imbalances as *Deficient **Fluid** Volume, Excess **Fluid** Volume, Risk for Deficient **Fluid** Volume,* and *Risk for Imbalanced **Fluid** Volume.* Numerous secondary nursing diagnoses may also apply.

> **PROFESSIONALTIP**
>
> **Urine Osmolality**
>
> Urine osmolality is more accurate than urine specific gravity as an indicator of hydration. Some medications and the presence of glucose and protein solutes in urine can give a false high specific gravity reading.

Deficient Fluid Volume

*Deficient **Fluid** Volume* is defined as "decreased intravascular, interstitial, and/or intracellular fluid. This refers to dehydration, water loss alone without change in sodium" (NANDA-I, 2010). The many causes of fluid volume deficit include:

- Excessive fluid loss resulting from diaphoresis, vomiting, diarrhea, hemorrhage, burns, ascites, wound drainage, indwelling tubes, or suction
- Diabetes insipidus
- Diabetes mellitus
- Addison's disease (adrenal insufficiency)
- Gastrointestinal fistula or draining abscess
- Intestinal obstruction

Assessment findings in the client with fluid volume deficit include thirst and weight loss of an amount consistent with the degree of dehydration. Marked dehydration manifests as dry mucous membranes and skin; poor skin turgor; low-grade temperature elevation; tachycardia; respirations of 28 or greater; decreased (10 to 15 mm Hg) systolic blood pressure; slowed venous filling; decreased urine output (less than 25 mL/hr); concentrated urine; elevated Hct, Hgb, and BUN; and acidic blood pH (less than 7.4).

Severe dehydration is characterized by the symptoms of marked dehydration plus a flushing of the skin. Systolic blood pressure continues to drop (60 mm Hg or below), and behavioral changes (restlessness, irritability, disorientation, and delirium) occur. The signs of fatal dehydration are anuria and coma, leading to death.

Excess Fluid Volume

*Excess **Fluid** Volume* is defined as "increased isotonic fluid retention" (NANDA-I, 2010). Fluid volume excess is related to excess fluid in either the tissues or the extremities (peripheral edema) or the lung tissues (pulmonary edema). The several causes of excess fluid volume include:

- Excessive fluid intake (e.g., IV therapy, sodium)
- Excessive loss or decreased intake of protein (chronic diarrhea, burns, kidney disease, malnutrition)
- Compromised regulatory mechanisms (kidney failure)
- Decreased intravascular movement (impaired myocardial contractility)
- Lymphatic obstruction (cancer, surgical removal of lymph nodes, obesity)
- Medications (steroid excess)
- Allergic reactions

The client with fluid volume excess will exhibit acute weight gain; decreased serum osmolality (lower than 275 mOsm/Kg), Hgb, Hct; protein and albumin, blood urea nitrogen (BUN); increased central venous pressure (greater than 12 to 15 cm H2O); and signs and symptoms of edema. The clinical expressions of edema are relative to the area of involvement, either pulmonary or peripheral (Table 24-7).

Risk for Deficient Fluid Volume

*Risk for Deficient **Fluid** Volume* is defined as "at risk for experiencing vascular, cellular, or intracellular dehydration" (NANDA-I, 2010). The many factors that place a client at risk for fluid volume deficit were listed previously.

TABLE 24-7 Clinical Manifestations of Edema

PULMONARY EDEMA	PERIPHERAL EDEMA
Cough	Pitting edema in extremities
Pink, frothy sputum	Edematous area: tight, smooth, dry
Dyspnea	Shiny, pale, cool skin
Cold, clammy skin	Puffy eyelids
Engorged neck and hand veins	Weight gain
Crackles and wheezes in lungs	
Tachypnea	
Tachycardia	

COURTESY OF DELMAR CENGAGE LEARNING

Risk for Imbalanced Fluid Volume

*Risk for Imbalanced **F**luid Volume* is defined as "at risk for a decrease, increase, or rapid shift from one to the other of intravascular, interstitial, and/or intracellular fluid. This refers to body fluid loss, gain, or both" (NANDA-I, 2010). The greatest risk factor is a client undergoing a major invasive procedure.

Other Nursing Diagnoses

In clients with a fluid imbalance, the relationship between the primary nursing diagnoses previously discussed and the secondary nursing diagnoses is reciprocal: The primary nursing diagnoses influence and are influenced by the secondary nursing diagnoses. Some commonly identified secondary nursing diagnoses include:

- *Impaired **G**as Exchange*
- *Decreased **C**ardiac Output*
- *Ineffective **B**reathing Pattern*
- ***A**nxiety*
- *Disturbed **T**hought Processes*
- *Risk for **I**njury*
- *Risk for **I**nfection*
- *Impaired **Oral** Mucous Membrane*
- *Deficient **K**nowledge* (specify)

PLANNING/OUTCOME IDENTIFICATION

Holistic nursing care requires collaborating with each client to identify goals for each nursing diagnosis. These individualized goals should reflect the client's abilities and limitations.

PROFESSIONAL TIP

Loss of Gastric Juices

Clients who lose excessive amounts of gastric juices, either through vomiting or suctioning, are prone to not only fluid volume deficit but also metabolic alkalosis, hypokalemia, and hyponatremia. Gastric juices contain hydrochloric acid, pepsinogen, potassium, and sodium.

CRITICAL THINKING

Student Activity

Review the chart of a client who has been receiving IV fluids for at least 48 hours for the following information: vital signs, subjective and objective assessment findings, intake and output records, lab results, and medications administered. What conclusions can you make about the client's fluid, electrolyte, and acid–base balance?

Nursing interventions are selected and prioritized to support the client's achievement of expected outcomes based on the goals. For example, if vomiting and diarrhea along with dry mucous membranes and a 5% weight loss led to a nursing diagnosis of *Deficient **F**luid Volume*, the goals might include to relieve vomiting and diarrhea and achieve the proper balance of intake and output.

IMPLEMENTATION

The nurse has a responsibility to collaborate with and advocate for clients to ensure they receive appropriate and ethical care based on practice standards. The data obtained from the history serve as the basis for formulating expected outcomes and selecting nursing interventions appropriate to the client's natural patterns as revealed in their history.

Interventions related to changes in fluid, electrolyte, or acid–base balance are based on the goal of maintaining homeostasis and regulating and maintaining essential fluids and nutrients. Clients' adaptive capabilities are kept in mind when selecting interventions based on the clients' perceptions of their support systems, strengths, and options.

The nurse is responsible for performing frequent assessments and monitoring for adverse effects of fluid and electrolyte therapy to prevent complications.

Nursing activities related to assessment and implementation often involve the same measurements (e.g., weight and vital signs). Common interventions that promote reaching expected outcomes for restoring and maintaining homeostasis are discussed following.

Monitor Daily Weight

One of the main indicators of fluid and electrolyte balance is weight. The accurate measuring and recording of the client's daily weight is a vital responsibility. This information along with other clinical findings determine fluid therapy requirements for the client.

Measure Vital Signs

The client's acuity level and clinical situation determine the frequency of vital sign measurement. For example, vital signs are taken every 15 minutes until stable on the typical postoperative client, whereas vital signs should be monitored continuously on the client in shock or hemorrhaging. Vital signs and other clinical data are used to determine the amount and type of fluid therapy.

Measure Intake and Output

Intake and output (I&O) measurements monitor the client's fluid status over a 24-hour period. Agency policy for I&O may vary regarding:

- Times for charting (e.g., every 8 hours versus every 12 hours)
- Time when 24-hour totals are calculated
- Definition of "strict" I&O

PROFESSIONALTIP

"Strict" I&O

- "Strict" I&O measurement usually involves accounting for incontinent urine, emesis, and diaphoresis and might require weighing soiled bed linens.
- *Gloves should always be worn when handling soiled linen.*

Review the client's 24-hour I&O calculations to evaluate fluid status. Intake should exceed output by 500 mL to offset insensible fluid loss. Intake and output and daily weight are critical interventions because they are used to evaluate the effectiveness of rehydration or diuretic therapy.

Having an accurate I&O requires the efforts of the client and family. The client and family must be taught how to measure and record the I&O.

Provide Oral Hygiene

Providing oral hygiene that promotes both client comfort and the integrity of the buccal cavity is an important responsibility. The condition of the client's buccal cavity and the type of fluid imbalance dictates the frequency of oral hygiene.

Initiate Oral Fluid Therapy

Depending on the client's clinical situation, oral fluids may be totally restricted, commonly referred to as *nothing by mouth* (NPO, which is from the Latin *non per os*), or they may be restricted or forced.

COMMUNITY/HOME HEALTH CARE

Considerations for Measuring I&O

- Ask for client and family input to select household items for intake measurement.
- Provide containers for measuring output, adapting the urinary container to home facilities, and teach client and family about proper washing and storage of the containers.
- Teach proper hand hygiene.
- Provide written instructions on what is to be measured.
- Leave sufficient I&O forms to last until the nurse's next visit.
- Identify the parameters for evaluating a discrepancy between the intake and the output and for notifying the nurse or physician.

SAFETY

Remove Gloves Before Charting

To prevent the transfer of microorganisms when the I&O form is removed from the client's room, remove gloves and wash hands before recording the amount of drainage on the form.

PROFESSIONALTIP

Mouthwashes

Mouthwashes with alcohol or glycerin and swabs with lemon or glycerin may feel refreshing, but these ingredients dry the mucous membranes.

Nothing by Mouth Clients are designated NPO as prescribed by the physician. Based on agency policy and clarification from the physician, the client may be allowed small amounts of ice chips when designated NPO. The NPO status may be required to:

- Avoid aspiration in unconscious, perioperative, and preprocedural clients who will receive anesthesia or conscious sedation
- Rest and heal the GI tract when there is severe vomiting or diarrhea or a GI disorder (inflammation or obstruction)
- Prevent more loss of gastric juices in clients on nasogastric suctioning

Clients who are NPO should receive oral hygiene every 1 to 2 hours or as needed to prevent alterations of the mucous membranes and for comfort.

Restricted Fluids Fluid intake is commonly restricted when treating fluid volume excess related to heart and renal failure. Intake may be restricted to 200 mL in a 24-hour period.

The way fluids are limited should be determined in collaboration with the client. For example:

- Half of the allowed fluid might be divided between breakfast and lunch, and
- The remaining half might be divided between the evening meal and before bedtime, unless the client must be awakened during the night for medication.

Forced Fluids "Forcing" or encouraging the intake of oral fluids, mainly water, is sometimes done when treating clients who are at risk for dehydration or who have renal and urinary problems (kidney stones). Compliance is obtained through client education and honoring client preferences of timing and type of liquids. A client might, for example, be requested to consume 2,000 mL over a 24-hour period. Explain that this is only eight glasses or one glass every 2 hours. Also tell the client that ice, gelatin, soups, and ice cream all count as liquid.

Maintain Tube Feeding

The client who cannot ingest oral fluids but has a normal GI tract can have fluids and nutrients administered through a feeding tube as prescribed by a physician.

PROFESSIONALTIP

Temperature of Fluids

Clients should drink room-temperature fluids. Hot or cold fluids may increase peristalsis and abdominal cramping.

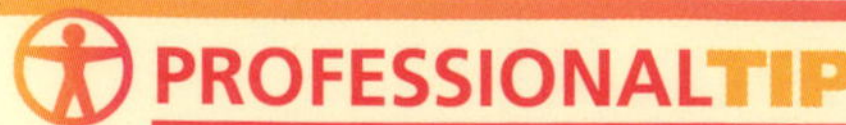

Fluid Replacement

Fluid replacement is based on weight loss. A 2.2-pound (1 kg) weight loss is equivalent to 1 liter (1,000 mL) of fluid loss.

Monitor Intravenous Therapy

Fluid volume is replaced parenterally when fluid loss is severe or the client cannot tolerate oral or tube feedings. **Intravenous (IV) therapy** is the administration of fluids, electrolytes, nutrients, or medications by the venous route. The physician prescribes IV therapy to prevent or treat fluid, electrolyte, or nutritional imbalances. There are specific nursing responsibilities during IV therapy. Specifically, the nurse must:

- Know why the IV fluid is prescribed
- Document client understanding
- Select, according to agency policy, the appropriate equipment
- Obtain the correct prescribed solution
- Assess the client for allergies to iodine, tape, ointment, or antibiotic preparations used for skin preparation of the venipuncture site
- Administer the fluid at the prescribed rate
- Observe for signs of **infiltration** (seepage of the fluid into the interstitial tissue as a result of accidental dislodgement of the needle from the vein) and other complications that are fluid specific
- Document in the client's medical record the implementation of the prescribed IV therapy

Evaluation

Evaluation is an ongoing process. When evaluating whether the time frames and expected outcomes are realistic (such as whether the intake and output are within 200 to 300 mL of each other), the focus should be on the client's responses such as vital signs within normal limits, the IV infusion rate maintains the client's hydration, and the IV site remains free from erythema, edema, and purulent drainage. The nursing care plan should be modified as necessary to support the client's expected outcomes.

CASE STUDY

J.M. is a 71 year old man diagnosed with type II diabetes 10 years ago with an average blood sugar of 220 mg/dl. In addition, J.M. was diagnosed with congestive heart failure 15 years after his 5 vessel coronary artery bypass grafts (CABG). The cardiac history is a result of the untreated hypertension he suffered from for 12 years before his bypass surgery. Physical assessment data reveals: oral temperature 98.4 F, respiratory rate 10 bpm, apical pulse 128 bpm, blood pressure 186/96 mm Hg, and pulse oximetry is 80%, and crackles scattered throughout all lung fields. J.M. complains of shortness of breath (SOB) with activity, denies pain, is able to perform ADLs, states problems with swallowing thin liquids, and requests to be placed in high Flower's position. Respiratory pattern is irregular and shallow. J.M. is alert and oriented to person and place, and skin is cool, moist, and pale. Bowel sounds are active in all 4 quadrants, and the abdomen is semi hard and slightly distended. J.M. has (+2) pitting edema to the lower extremities.

The following questions will guide your development of a nursing care plan for the case study.

1. List subjective and objective assessment data.
2. What acid-base imbalance does the nurse suspect?
3. Select 3 priority nursing diagnoses for J.M.'s acid-base imbalance.
4. Choose the priority nursing diagnosis and develop an appropriate client centered goal.
5. What nursing interventions should the nurse implement to assist J.M.?

SAMPLE NURSING CARE PLAN

The Client with Excess Fluid Volume

When brought to the emergency department by his granddaughter, R.W., a 68-year-old widower, stated, "I can't breathe." R.W. has a history of hypertension and heart disease, and he is obese. The practitioner ordered a stat chest x-ray, CBC, and electrolytes, which revealed pulmonary congestion (x-ray), decreased Hct, and decreased Hgb. The physical assessment results were as follows: Wt 162; TPR 97.6, 98, 30 (labored); BP 186/114; shortness of breath, crackles; constant cough; pitting edema (ankles); and engorged neck veins. R.W. stated, "I thought I could stop taking the heart medication and eat what I wanted when I felt good again."

NURSING DIAGNOSIS 1 *Excess Fluid Volume* related to a compromised regulatory mechanism as evidenced by edema, shortness of breath, crackles, decreased Hgb and Hct, and jugular vein distention

Nursing Outcomes Classification (NOC)
Cardiac Pump Effectiveness
Respiratory Status: Ventilation
Fluid Balance

Nursing Interventions Classification (NIC)
Fluid Management
Medication Management
Fluid Monitoring

SAMPLE NURSING CARE PLAN (Continued)

PLANNING/OUTCOMES	NURSING INTERVENTIONS	RATIONALE
R.W. will have a balanced I&O for 2 days.	Measure and document hourly I&O; restrict fluids as ordered.	Monitors fluid status.
	Administer diuretics as ordered and document response.	Increases excretion of fluids and electrolytes.
R.W. will identify a specific amount of weight to lose over the next 6 months.	Weigh daily at the same time, with the same scale, and with R.W. wearing the same clothing.	Allows weight to be compared from one day to another.
	Discuss with R.W. the need for weight loss.	Allows R.W. to voice his thoughts about weight loss and provides an avenue to determine number of pounds to be lost.
R.W. will show normal hydration status before discharge.	Measure and document vital signs every hour until shortness of breath subsides, then every 2 hours.	Monitors R.W.'s response to therapy.
	Hourly assess heart sounds; breath sounds; rate, rhythm, and depth of respirations; and the position R.W. takes to relieve the shortness of breath.	Provides information for use in modifying the plan of care.

EVALUATION

Output for the first 3 hours was 2,020 mL; on day 2, I&O indicated fluid balance. R.W. identified the need to lose 30 pounds over the next 6 months. R.W. demonstrated normal hydration status, as shown by normal levels of Hct and Hgb, BP 156/92, normal breath sounds, and absence of shortness of breath, jugular engorgement, and peripheral edema.

NURSING DIAGNOSIS 2 *Deficient **K**nowledge* related to information misinterpretation as evidenced by R.W.'s statement "I thought I could stop taking the heart medication and eat what I wanted when I felt good again."

Nursing Outcomes Classification (NOC)
Knowledge: Disease Process
Communication: Receptive Ability
Memory

Nursing Interventions Classification (NIC)
Teaching: Disease Process
Teaching: Prescribed Medication
Medication Management

PLANNING/OUTCOMES	NURSING INTERVENTIONS	RATIONALE
R.W. will demonstrate an understanding of the causes of fluid excess and the role of heart medications, foods, and exercise in assisting with weight reduction.	Assess R.W.'s knowledge of hypertension; decreased cardiac output; digitalis; the effects of a large abdominal girth on breathing; and foods low in sodium, fats, and carbohydrates.	Provides a basis for educating R.W. about causes, aggravating and alleviating factors, and effects of fluid excess.

EVALUATION

R.W. was unable to verbalize understanding of how weight, high-sodium diet, and failure to take his heart medications caused the fluid excess. He was referred to home health for client teaching.

(Continues)

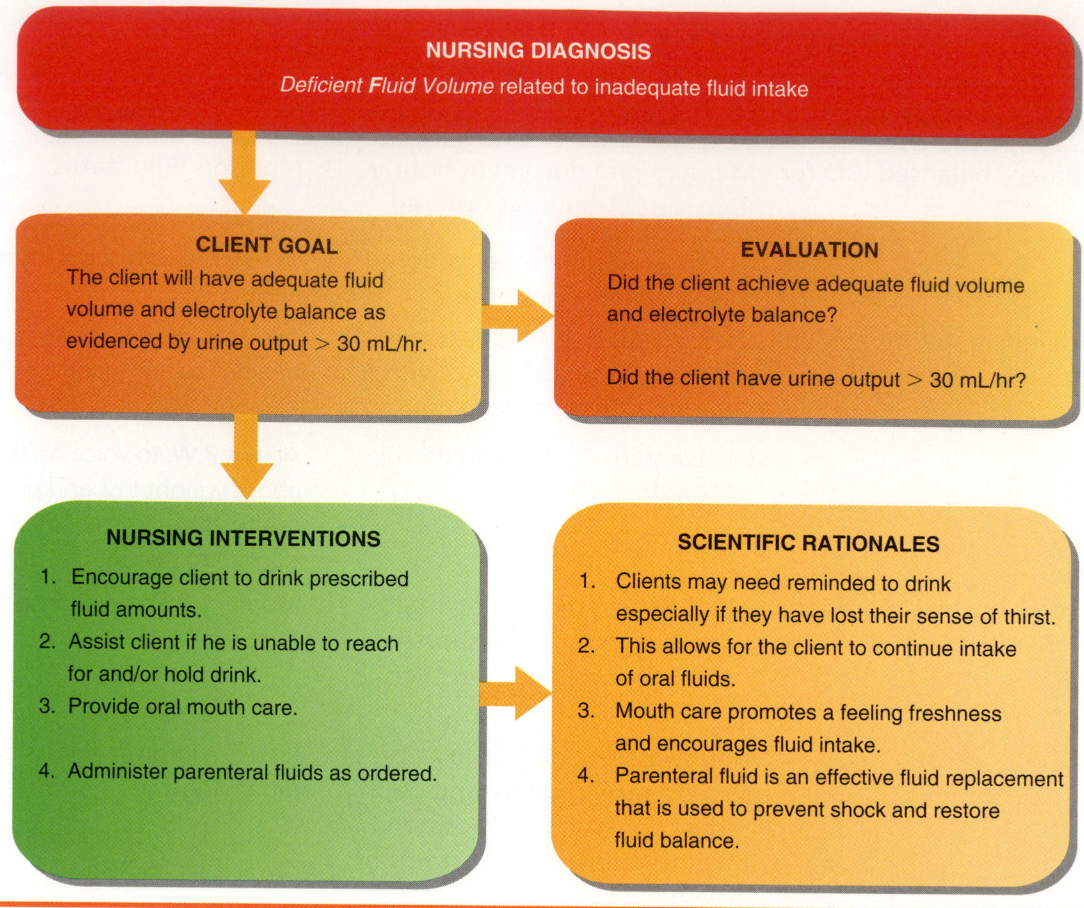

Concept Care Map 24-1 Deficit Fluid Volume (*Courtesy of Janice Eilerman, RN, MSN, Lima, Ohio.*)

SUMMARY

- Homeostasis is the maintenance of the body's internal environment within a narrow range of normal values. It is an ongoing process, with changes constantly occurring in the body.
- Compounds that ionize in water are called electrolytes.
- The normal range of blood pH is 7.35 to 7.45. A decrease or increase beyond this range can cause severe or even fatal physiologic problems.
- The bicarbonate buffer system works to regulate pH in both intracellular and extracellular fluids.
- The phosphate buffer system works to regulate the pH of intracellular fluid and fluid in kidney tubules.
- Protein buffers work to regulate pH inside cells, especially red blood cells.
- Substances move in and out of cells by the passive transport methods of diffusion, osmosis, and filtration and by active transport.
- The kidneys regulate fluid and electrolyte balance.
- Sodium is the main electrolyte that promotes the retention of water.
- The slightest decrease or increase in electrolyte levels can cause serious, adverse, or life-threatening effects on physiologic functions.
- Hospitalized clients, especially elderly clients, are at risk for developing dehydration.
- Clients receiving IV therapy require constant monitoring for complications.

REVIEW QUESTIONS

1. A nurse is assessing a 77-year-old postoperative client using a morphine sulfate PCA pump for pain control. The assessment data reveals a respiratory rate of 8 bpm and irregular. The client is lethargic and confused. The nurse is updating the client's care plan and selects which nursing diagnosis as top priority?
   1. Risk for injury related to regulatory function.
   2. Impaired gas exchange related to inadequate ventilation.

3. Ineffective airway clearance related to viscosity of secretions.
4. Rest and sleep disturbance related to ineffective breathing pattern.

2. The nurse determines that which of the following clients is at greatest risk for developing a decrease in pH?
   1. 39-year-old client diagnosed with pneumonia.
   2. 89-year-old client prescribed Vasotec 5mg, IV push.
   3. 45-year-old client diagnosed with asthma
   4. 64-year-old client diagnosed with irritable bowel syndrome
3. A nurse is caring for a client receiving mechanical ventilation treatment for respiratory failure. The nurse suspects that the ventilator rate is set too high, causing hyperventilation. What acid–base problem could result from the ventilator rate being set too high?
   1. Metabolic acidosis
   2. Respiratory acidosis
   3. Metabolic alkalosis
   4. Respiratory alkalosis
4. Acidosis and alkalosis are identified by changes in the pH. Which of the following statements is true?
   1. A pH above 7.45 is called acidosis.
   2. A pH above 7.45 is called alkalosis.
   3. A pH increase caused by an increase of bicarbonate in the blood is metabolic acidosis.
   4. A pH decrease caused by an accumulation of carbonic acid results in respiratory alkalosis.
5. A nurse is taking a health history from a client who admits to using an excessive amount of base-containing antacids every day. The nurse's best response to client is:
   1. "Antacids can decrease the risk of alkalosis."
   2. "The more antacids you take, the greater risk you have for developing alkalosis."
   3. "You should not take antacids."
   4. "Acidosis is increased when an excessive amount of antacids are used."
6. Which client is at greatest risk for developing metabolic acidosis?
   1. 29-year-old client with broken ribs.
   2. 41-year-old client with hypertension.
   3. 63-year-old client positive for ketones.
   4. 58-year-old client with hypokalemia.
7. The nurse is teaching a client with a serum potassium level of 3.2 mEq/L about foods that are rich in potassium. The client correctly identifies all the following foods as potassium rich except:
   1. dinner roll.
   2. raw carrots.
   3. baked potato.
   4. apricot.
8. A client experiencing fever, pain, and rapid, shallow respirations is brought to the emergency department for treatment. Assessment findings include hyperactive reflexes, a positive Chvostek's sign, and muscle tremors. The ABG results are pH 7.50 and $PaCO_2$ 28 mm Hg. This client is at risk for:
   1. respiratory acidosis.
   2. respiratory alkalosis.
   3. metabolic acidosis.
   4. metabolic alkalosis.
9. Which of the following arterial blood gas values would the nurse document as respiratory acidosis?
   1. pH = 7.31; $PaCO_2$ = 50; HCO_3 = 30
   2. pH = 7.32; $PaCO_2$ = 39; HCO_3 = 25
   3. pH = 7.42; $PaCO_2$ = 29; HCO_3 = 19
   4. pH = 7.50; $PaCO_2$ = 35; HCO_3 = 22
10. When the intracellular fluid (ICF) compartment develops an osmolality greater than the extracellular fluid (ECF) compartment, water shifts from the ECF into the ICF compartment. This fluid shift is known as:
    1. active transport.
    2. osmosis.
    3. diffusion.
    4. filtration.

REFERENCES/SUGGESTED READINGS

Bulechek, G., Butcher, H., McCloskey, J., & Dochterman, J., eds. (2008). *Nursing Interventions Classification (NIC)* (5th ed.). St. Louis, MO: Mosby/Elsevier.

Chernecky, C., Macklin, D., & Murphy-Ende, K. (2001). *Fluids and electrolytes.* Philadelphia: W. B. Saunders.

Daniels, R. (2010). *Delmar's guide to laboratory and diagnostic tests* (2nd ed.) Clifton Park, NY: Delmar Cengage Learning.

Daniels, R., Nosek, L. J., & Nicoll, L. H. (2007). *Contemporary medical-surgical nursing.* Clifton Park, NY: Delmar Cengage Learning.

Eilerman, J. (2009). *Concept care map: Deficient Fluid Volume.* Lima, OH.

Estes, M. E. Z. (2010). *Health assessment and physical examination* (4th ed.). Clifton Park, NY: Delmar Cengage Learning.

Fox, K. (2009). *Concept map: Metabolic acidosis.* Lima, OH.

Hadaway, L. (2002). I.V. infiltration: Not just a peripheral problem. *Nursing2002, 32*(8), 36–42.

Hamilton, S. (2001). Detecting dehydration and malnutrition in the elderly. *Nursing2001, 31*(12), 56–57.

Hogstel, M. (2001). *Nursing care of the older adult* (4th ed.). Clifton Park, NY: Delmar Cengage Learning.

Incredibly Easy! (2002). Understanding hypokalemia. *Nursing2002, 32*(3), 56.

Incredibly Easy! Understanding hypokalemia. (2000) *Nursing2000, 30*(11), 74–76.

Josephson, D. L. (2004). *Intravenous infusion therapy for nurses: Principles and practice* (2nd ed.). Clifton Park, NY: Delmar Cengage Learning.

Kee, J. L., Paulanka, B. J., & Polek, C. (2010). *Fluids and electrolytes with clinical applications: A programmed approach* (8th ed.). Clifton Park, NY: Delmar Cengage Learning.

Klopfenstein, L. (2009). *Concept map: Respiratory acidosis.* Lima, OH.

Krueger, D., & Tasota, F. (2003). Keeping an eye on calcium levels. *Nursing2003, 33*(6), 68.

Mader, S. (2001). *Understanding human anatomy and physiology* (4th ed.). Boston: McGraw-Hill College Division.

Marieb, E. (2002). *Essentials of human anatomy and physiology* (7th ed.). Redwood City, CA: Cummings.

Martini, F., & Welch, K. (2001). *Fundamentals of anatomy and physiology* (5th ed.). Englewood Cliffs, NJ: Prentice Hall.

Mason, E. (2009). *Caring for clients with acid-base imbalances.* Manuscript submitted for publication.

McConnell, E. (2002). Measuring fluid intake and output. *Nursing2002, 32*(7), 17.

Moorhead, S., Johnson, M., Maas, M., & Swanson, E. (2007). *Nursing Outcomes Classification (NOC)* (4th ed.). St. Louis, MO: Mosby.

North American Nursing Diagnosis Association International. (2010). *NANDA-I nursing diagnoses: Definitions and classification 2009-2011.* Ames, IA: Wiley-Blackwell.

Scanlon, V., & Sanders, T. (2003). *Essentials of anatomy and physiology* (4th ed.). Philadelphia: F. A. Davis.

Schmidt, T. C., & Williams-Evans, S. A. (2000). How to recognize hypokalemia. *Nursing2000, 30*(2), 22.

Science Spot. (2009). *Biology lesson plans.* Retrieved June 26, 2009, from http://sciencespot.net/Pages/classbio.html

Senisi-Scott, A., & Fong, E. (2009). *Body structures and functions* (11th ed.). Clifton Park, NY: Delmar Cengage Learning.

White, L., & Duncan, G. (2002). *Medical-surgical nursing: An integrated approach* (2nd ed.). New York: Delmar Cengage Learning.

RESOURCE

Infusion Nurses Society, http://www.ins1.org

CHAPTER 25
Medication Administration and IV Therapy

MAKING THE CONNECTION

Refer to the following chapters to increase your understanding of medication administration and IV therapy:

Basic Nursing

- ***Legal and Ethical Responsibilities***
- ***Nursing Process/Documentation/Informatics***
- ***Basic Nutrition***
- ***Infection Control/Asepsis***
- ***Standard Precautions and Isolation***
- ***Diagnostic Tests***

Basic Procedures

- ***Administering an Enema***
- ***Measuring Intake and Output***

Intermediate Procedures

- ***Administering an Oral, Sublingual, and Buccal Medication***
- ***Withdrawing Medication from an Ampule***
- ***Withdrawing Medication from a Vial***
- ***Administering an Intradermal Injection***
- ***Administering a Subcutaneous Injection***
- ***Administering Intramuscular Injections***
- ***Administering Eye and Ear Medications***

Advanced Procedures

- ***Performing Venipuncture (Blood Drawing)***
- ***Preparing an IV Solution and Starting an IV***
- ***Setting the IV Flow Rate***
- ***Administering Medications via Secondary Administration Sets (Piggyback)***
- ***Assessing and Maintaining an IV Insertion Site***

LEARNING OBJECTIVES

Upon completion of this chapter, you should be able to:

- Define key terms.
- Describe how drug standards and legislation influence medication administration.
- Explain pharmacokinetics, including absorption, distribution, metabolism, and excretion of drugs.

- Describe factors that can affect a drug's action.
- Explain the different types of medication orders, when each is used, and the nurse's responsibilities for each type.
- Identify principles of safe medication administration.
- Discuss potential liabilities for the nurse administering medications.
- Develop teaching guidelines for clients regarding medication administration in the home.
- Explain procedures for the various methods of medication administration, including the choice of route and site.

KEY TERMS

absorption
angiocatheter
aspiration
bioavailability
butterfly needles
chemical name
distribution
drug allergy
drug incompatibilities
drug interaction
drug tolerance
enteral instillation
excretion
extravasation
flashback
flow rate
generic name
half-life
hypervolemia
idiosyncratic reaction
implantable port
infiltration
intracath
intradermal (ID)
intramuscular (IM)
intravenous (IV)
IV push (bolus)
metabolism
onset of action
parenteral
patency
peak plasma level
pharmacokinetics
phlebitis
piggybacked
plateau
stock supplied
subcutaneous
toxic effect
trade (brand) name
unit dose
vesicant

INTRODUCTION

Managing medications requires collaboration of many health care providers. Medications are prescribed by a physician, dentist, or other authorized prescriber such as advanced practice registered nurses as determined by individual state licensing boards. Medications are prepared and dispensed by pharmacists. Nurses are responsible for administering medications. Dietitians may be involved in identifying possible food–drug interactions.

Medication administration requires specialized knowledge, judgment, and nursing skills based on the principles of pharmacology. This chapter focuses on assisting students to apply knowledge of pharmacology and to acquire safe administration of medications skills. The nursing process directs nursing decisions about safe drug administration and ensures compliance with standards of practice.

DRUG STANDARDS AND LEGISLATION

A drug is a chemical substance intended to have a specific effect. Nurses assume, before administering any medication, that the drug will be safe for the client if the dose, route, and frequency are within the therapeutic range for that drug. This assumption is implied by standards ensuring drug uniformity in strength, purity, efficacy, safety, and **bioavailability** (readiness to produce a drug effect).

Standards

Standards ensure drug uniformity for predictable effects. The *United States Pharmacopeia* and the *National Formulary* (USP and NF) are books of drug standards used in the United States. The USP and NF list drugs recognized for compliance with legal standards of purity, quality, and strength.

The USP has been providing standards for pharmaceutical preparations since its first edition was published in 1851. The American Pharmaceutical Association first published the NF in 1898 to provide a list of drugs complying with established standards.

Legislation

The USP and the NF were designated by the Pure Food and Drug Act of 1906 as the official bodies to establish drug standards. The authority to enforce these standards was given to the federal government. The federal Food, Drug, and Cosmetic Act of 1938 authorized the Food and Drug Administration (FDA) to test all new drugs for toxicity before giving approval to market a drug. In 1952, the federal Food, Drug, and Cosmetic Act of 1938 was amended to differentiate prescription (legend) drugs from nonprescription (over-the-counter) drugs and to regulate prescription dispensing. Drug effectiveness testing came with the Kefauver-Harris Act of 1962 (Lehne, 2006).

In 1914, the Harrison Narcotic Act classified habit-forming drugs as narcotics and began regulating them. This law and other drug abuse laws were replaced with the Comprehensive Drug Abuse Prevention and Control Act (Controlled Substance Act) in 1970. This act defines a *drug-dependent person* in terms of physical and psychological dependence and provides for strict regulation of narcotics and other controlled drugs such as barbiturates with the five categories of scheduled drugs (Table 25-1). Records must be kept by the dispensing pharmacist for all controlled substances. Pharmacists employed by the Drug Enforcement Agency (DEA) inspect records and prescriptions to discover illicit distribution of these substances.

All states must adhere to the schedule of controlled substances as minimum standards; however, individual states can pass stricter controls of these substances. For example, the Controlled Substance Act has antitussives with codeine as a schedule V drug, but an individual state may place this drug in the more restrictive schedule II category.

DRUG NOMENCLATURE

The terms *medication, medicine,* and *drug* are used interchangeably by laypersons and health care providers.

Drugs are identified by a chemical, generic, official, or trade name. The **chemical name** is a precise description of the drug's chemical formula. The **generic name** (*nonproprietary*) in the United States is the name assigned by the U.S. Adopted Names Council to the manufacturer who first develops the drug. When a drug is approved, it is given an *official name,* which may be the same as the nonproprietary name (Lehne, 2006). Drugs with proven therapeutic value are listed by their official name in the USP and NF. Pharmaceutical companies assign a *proprietary name,* also called a **trade (brand) name,** when they market a drug. One generic drug may have several trade names depending on how many companies market the drug. For example, ibuprofen is a generic name; trade names for this drug include Advil, Motrin, Excedrin IB, and Nuprin. *Generic names are not capitalized, but trade names are always capitalized.*

DRUG ACTION

Drug action refers to a drug's ability to combine with a cellular receptor. Depending on the location of cellular receptors affected by a given drug, a drug can have a local effect, a systemic effect, or both. For example, when diphenhydramine hydrochloride (Benadryl) cream is applied to the skin, it has only a local effect; however, when administered

TABLE 25-1 Controlled Substances

Schedule (C-I): Includes substances for which there is a high abuse potential and no current approved medical use (e.g., heroin, marijuana, LSD, other hallucinogens, certain opiates and opium derivatives).
Schedule (C-II): Includes drugs that have a high abuse potential and a high ability to produce physical and/or psychological dependence and for which there is a current approved or acceptable medical use (e.g., narcotics, amphetamines, dronabinol, and some barbiturates).
Schedule (C-III): Includes drugs for which there is less potential for abuse than drugs in Schedule II and for which there is a current approved medical use (e.g., nonbarbiturate sedatives, nonamphetamine stimulants, and limited amounts of certain narcotics). Also, anabolic steroids are classified in Schedule III.
Schedule (C-IV): Includes drugs for which there is a relatively low abuse potential and for which there is a current approved medical use (e.g., sedatives, antianxiety agents, and nonnarcotic analgesics).
Schedule (C-V): Drugs in this category consist mainly of preparations containing limited amounts of certain narcotic drugs (e.g., codeine used as antitussive and antidiarrheals). Federal law provides that limited quantities of these drugs may be bought without a prescription by an individual at least 18 years of age. The product must be purchased from a pharmacist, who must keep appropriate records. However, state laws vary, and in many states such products require a prescription.

From *2010 Delmar Nurse's Drug Handbook* by G. Spratto & A. Woods, 2010, Clifton Park, NY: Delmar Cengage Learning; *Nursing Fundamentals: Caring and Clinical Decision Making* by R. Daniels, R. Grendell, & F. Wilkins, 2010, Clifton Park, NY: Delmar Cengage Learning.

in a tablet or injectable form, it has both a systemic and a local effect.

PHARMACOLOGY

The study of drug effects on living organisms is called pharmacology. This section discusses the pharmacological activities of drug action as related to medication management, drug classification, and routes of administration.

Medication Management

Medication management is to produce the desired drug action by maintaining a constant drug level. Drug action is based on the half-life of a drug. A drug's **half-life** is the time it takes the body to eliminate half of the blood concentration level of the original drug dose. For example, if a drug has a half-life of 8 hours, 50% of the drug's original dose is present in the blood 8 hours after administration, and 25% of the drug is present 16 hours after administration. Because of a drug's half-life, repeated doses are given to maintain a therapeutic drug level over a 24-hour interval. Maintaining a therapeutic drug level ensures antibiotic effectiveness against bacteria within the body, and pain medication provides an effective pain threshold.

Other terms describing drug action include onset, peak plasma level, and plateau. **Onset of action** is the time for the body to respond to a drug after administration. **Peak plasma level** is the highest blood concentration of a single drug dose before the elimination rate equals the rate of absorption. The blood concentration level will decrease steadily once the peak plasma level is reached, unless another dose is given. When a series of scheduled drug doses is administered, the blood concentration level is maintained and is called a **plateau**.

Classification

Drugs are generally classified by the body system with which they interact (e.g., cardiovascular) or by the drug's approved therapeutic usage (e.g., antihypertensive). Drugs with several therapeutic uses are usually classified by their most common use.

Routes

Drugs are prepared in many forms for administration by a specific route (Table 25-2). The route is how the drug is absorbed: oral, buccal, sublingual, parenteral, topical, and respiratory.

Oral Route Most drugs are administered by the oral route because it is the most convenient, least expensive, and safest method, but it acts more slowly than the other routes. Drugs are not given orally to clients with GI intolerance, those on NPO (nothing by mouth) status, or those in a coma.

The buccal or sublingual route is used when small amounts of drugs are required. Buccal and sublingual drugs act quickly because of the oral mucosa's thin epithelium and large vascular system, allowing the drug to be quickly absorbed.

Buccal drugs are placed in the buccal pocket (superior-posterior aspect of the internal cheek next to the molars) for absorption by the mucous membrane. Sublingual medications are made to dissolve quickly when placed under the tongue. For example, nitroglycerin (Nitrostat), an antianginal drug, can be given either sublingually or buccally as prescribed, whereas isoproterenol hydrochloride (Isuprel), a bronchodilator, is given only sublingually, and methyltesterone (Testred), an androgen, is given only buccally.

Parenteral Route **Parenteral** drugs are administered by injection using sterile technique. By definition, parenteral route refers to any route other than the oral-gastrointestinal tract; however, the medical usage of the term excludes topical and respiratory routes. The four routes that nurses use to administer medications parenterally are:

- **Intradermal (ID)**, an injection into the dermis
- **Subcutaneous**, an injection into the subcutaneous tissue
- **Intramuscular (IM)**, an injection into the muscle
- **Intravenous (IV)**, an injection into a vein

Other parenteral routes, such as intrathecal or intraspinal, intrapleural, intracardiac, intra-arterial, and intra-articular, are used by physicians and sometimes by advanced-practice registered nurses.

Topical Route Most topical drugs are given to deliver a drug at or immediately beneath the point of application. Many topical drugs are applied to the skin, but other topical drugs include eye, nose and throat, ear, rectal, and vaginal preparations. Drugs directly applied to the skin are absorbed into the dermis, where they have a local effect or are absorbed into the bloodstream. The vascularity of the skin varies the drug action. Usually several applications over a 24-hour period are required for the desired therapeutic effect.

Transdermal patches are used to deliver medications such as nitroglycerin (Transdermal-NTG), an antianginal, and some supplemental hormone replacements for absorption to produce systemic effects. Some topical drugs, such as eye

SAFETY

Do Not Substitute Drug Forms

Drugs prepared for administration by one route cannot be substituted by the drug prepared for another route. For example, when a client has difficulty swallowing a large tablet or capsule, an oral solution or elixir of the same drug cannot be administered without first consulting the physician. A liquid may be more easily and completely absorbed, producing a higher blood level than a tablet.

PROFESSIONALTIP

Special Considerations for Oral Route

- Chewable tablets are chewed before swallowing; chewing enhances gastric absorption.
- Buccal and sublingual medications must dissolve completely before the client drinks or eats.
- Suspensions and emulsions are administered immediately after shaking and pouring from the bottle.

TABLE 25-2 Types of Drug Preparations

TYPE	DESCRIPTION
Oral Solids	• Tablets: compressed or molded substances, to be swallowed whole, chewed before swallowing, or placed in the buccal pocket or under the tongue (sublingual) • Capsules: substances encased in a hard or a soft soluble cover or gelatin shell that dissolves in the stomach • Caplets: gelatin-coated tablets that dissolve in the stomach • Powders and granules: finely ground substances • Troches, lozenges, and pastilles: designed to dissolve in the mouth • Enteric-coated tablets: coated tablets that dissolve in the intestines • Time-release capsules: encased substances that are further enclosed in smaller casings that deliver a drug dose over an extended period • Sustained-release: compounded substances that release a drug slowly to maintain a steady plasma level
Topicals	• Liniments: substances mixed with an alcohol, oil, or soapy emollient; applied to the skin • Ointments: semisolid substances for topical use • Pastes: semisolid substances, thicker than ointments, absorbed slowly through the skin • Suppositories: gelatin substances designed to dissolve when inserted in the rectum, urethra, or vagina
Inhalants	• Inhalations: drugs or dilutions of drugs administered by the nasal or oral respiratory route for a local or systemic effect
Solutions	• Solutions: contain one or more soluble chemical substances dissolved in water • Enemas: aqueous solutions for rectal instillation • Douches: aqueous solutions that function as a cleansing or antiseptic agent that may be dispensed in the form of a powder with directions for dissolving in a specific quantity of warm water • Suspensions: particles or powder substances that must be mixed with, not dissolved in, a liquid by shaking vigorously before administration • Emulsions: two-phase systems in which one liquid is dispersed in the form of small droplets throughout another liquid • Syrups: substances dissolved in a sugar liquid • Gargles: aqueous solutions • Mouthwashes: aqueous solutions that may contain alcohol, glycerin, and synthetic sweeteners • Nasal solutions: aqueous solutions instilled as drops or sprays • Optic (eye) and otic (ear) solutions: aqueous solutions instilled as drops • Elixirs: solutions that contain water, varying amounts of alcohol, and sweeteners

COURTESY OF DELMAR CENGAGE LEARNING

and nasal drops and vaginal and rectal suppositories, applied directly to the mucous membranes, are absorbed quickly and, depending on the drug's dose (strength and quantity), may cause systemic effects.

Respiratory Route Inhalants such as oxygen and most general anesthetics deliver gaseous or volatile substances that are almost immediately absorbed into systemic circulation. The inhalants, delivered into the alveoli of the lungs, promote fast absorption due to:

- Permeability of the alveolar and vascular epithelium
- Abundant blood flow
- Very large surface area for absorption

Oropharyngeal handheld inhalers deliver topical drugs to the respiratory tract to create local and systemic effects. The three types of inhalers—the metered-dose inhaler, or nebulizer; the turbo-inhaler; and the nasal inhaler—are explained later in this chapter.

PHARMACOKINETICS

Pharmacokinetics is the study of the absorption, distribution, metabolism, and excretion of drugs to determine the relationship between the dose of a drug and the drug's concentration in biological fluids. This knowledge is used by health care providers in medication management.

The physician is concerned mainly with the dose and route that will produce the most therapeutic effects. Pharmacists, physicians, and nurses work together to identify appropriate times for drug administration and to avoid interactions with other substances that might alter the drug's actions. Nurses and physicians monitor the client's response to the drug's action. Drug actions are dependent on four properties: absorption, distribution, metabolism, and excretion.

Absorption

The degree and rate of **absorption**, or movement of a drug from administration site into the bloodstream, depend on several factors: the drug's physicochemical effects, its dosage, its route of administration, its interactions with other substances, and various client characteristics such as age (Blanchard & Loeb, 2006). After ingestion, oral preparations, such as tablets and capsules, disintegrate into smaller particles so that gastric juices can dissolve and prepare the drug for absorption in the small intestines.

Intramuscularly administered drugs are absorbed through the muscle into the bloodstream. Suppositories are absorbed through the mucous membranes into the blood. Intravenous drugs are immediately bioavailable because they are directly injected into the blood.

Distribution

Distribution is the movement of medications from the blood into various body tissues and fluids. Drug distribution in the body is affected by cardiac output, cell membrane permeability, protein-binding capacity of the medication, and body fat. A client's cardiac output can increase or decrease blood flow, and peripheral vascular disease decreases circulation to body tissues. The blood–brain barrier allows only fat-soluble medications through the membrane. A malnourished client or one with liver disease has decreased albumin or protein circulating in the blood, allowing a higher concentration of the medication in the blood. Drug duration is increased in obese clients, resulting in slower drug distribution (Daniels, 2010).

Metabolism

Metabolism is the physical and chemical processing of a drug by the body. Most drugs are metabolized in the liver. The presence of enzymes in the liver that detoxify the drugs determine the rate of metabolism. Some drugs can increase the rate of metabolism.

Excretion

Excretion is the elimination of drugs from the body. This occurs mainly through hepatic metabolism and renal excretion, but the lungs, exocrine glands, skin, and intestinal tract can eliminate some drugs.

Drug Interaction

Drug interaction is the effect one drug can have on another drug. Drug interactions may occur when two drugs are administered at the same time or within a short time interval. Drugs can be purposely combined for a positive effect; for example, hydrochlorothiazide (HydroDIURIL), a potassium-depleting diuretic, and spironolactone (Aldactone), a potassium-sparing diuretic, when combined maintain a normal blood level of potassium. When one drug is purposely given to potentiate the action of another drug, as in preoperative medications, a positive drug interaction occurs.

Not all drug interactions are therapeutic. Some interactions can interfere with the absorption, effect, or excretion of other drugs. For example, calcium products and magnesium-containing antacids can cause inadequate absorption of tetracycline (Tetracyn), an antibiotic, in the digestive tract.

Side Effects and Adverse Reactions

Drug effects other than those therapeutically intended and expected are called *adverse reactions.* A nontherapeutic effect may be mild and predictable (side effect) or unexpected and potentially dangerous (adverse reaction). There are several types of adverse reactions: drug allergy, drug tolerance, toxic effect, and idiosyncratic reactions.

A **drug allergy** (hypersensitivity to a drug) is an antigen–antibody immune reaction occurring when an individual previously exposed to a drug has developed antibodies against the drug. The type of reaction may be mild (skin rash, urticaria, headache, nausea, or vomiting) or severe (anaphylaxis). Drug reactions are often seen on the skin because of its abundant blood supply.

Anaphylaxis is an immediate, life-threatening reaction to a drug, such as penicillin, marked by respiratory distress, sudden severe bronchospasm, and cardiovascular collapse. Anaphylaxis can be fatal if emergency measures are not begun immediately (administration of epinephrine, bronchodilators, and antihistamines).

Drug tolerance occurs when the body is so accustomed to a specific drug that larger doses are needed to produce the desired therapeutic effect. For example, clients with cancer experiencing severe pain may require larger and larger doses of morphine (a narcotic analgesic) to control the pain.

A **toxic effect** occurs when the body cannot metabolize a drug and the drug accumulates in the blood. Digoxin, a cardiac drug, has a narrow margin of safety between an effective therapeutic dose and a toxic dose (Spratto & Woods, 2009).

An **idiosyncratic reaction** is a very unpredictable response that may be an overresponse, an underresponse, or an atypical response. For example, 1 of 40,000 clients will develop aplastic anemia after receiving chloramphenicol (Chloromycetin), an antibiotic (Blanchard & Loeb, 2006).

Food–Drug Interactions

Medication management works to avoid possible food–drug interactions. There are three main types of food–drug interactions:

1. Some drugs interfere with the absorption, excretion, or use in the body of one or more nutrients.
2. Some foods increase or decrease the absorption of a drug into the body.
3. Some foods alter the chemical actions of drugs, preventing the therapeutic effect on the body.

Most interaction problems occur with the use of oral antibiotics, diuretics, anticoagulant, and antihypertensive drugs. Clients on sodium-restricted diets should consult with a pharmacist about the sodium content of prescription and over-the-counter drugs. Some drugs contain almost half the total daily allowance of sodium. Alcohol interacts with many drugs, such as antihistamines, antibiotics, anticoagulants, and sleeping pills. Food–drug interactions vary depending on the dose and the form of the drug taken and the client's age, gender, nutritional status, body weight, and specific medical condition.

Many herbals interact with drugs to change their effect, such as with digoxin, a cardiac drug. Herbal teas such as Woodruff, tonka bean, and melitot contain natural coumarins

LIFE SPAN CONSIDERATIONS

Age-Related Factors Influence Drug Action and Dosing

- Neonates and infants have underdeveloped gastrointestinal systems, muscle mass, and metabolic enzyme systems and inadequate renal function.
- Elderly clients often experience decreased hepatic or renal function and diminished muscle mass.

that can potentiate the effects of Coumadin, an anticoagulant (Spratto & Woods, 2009).

FACTORS INFLUENCING DRUG ACTION

Individual client characteristics such as genetic factors, age, height, weight, and physical and mental conditions can influence drug actions on the body. Genetic factors can interfere with drug metabolism, producing an abnormal sensitivity to certain drugs.

The physician often correlates the client's age, height, and weight to determine the dosage for many drugs. This information must be accurately recorded in the client's medical record. The amount of body fat may also alter drug distribution.

The client's physical condition can also alter the effects of drugs. For example, in an edematous client, the drug must be distributed to a larger volume of body fluids than in a nonedematous client; therefore, the edematous client may require a larger dose to produce the desired action, whereas a dehydrated client may require a smaller dosage. Diseases affecting liver and renal functioning can alter the metabolism and elimination of most drugs.

MEDICATION ORDERS

In health care facilities, medication orders are written on a physician's order form in each client's medical record.

All orders must be written clearly and legibly. A drug order should contain seven parts:

1. Client's name
2. Date and time when the order is written
3. Name of the drug to be administered
4. Dosage
5. Route for administration and special directives about its administration
6. Time of administration and frequency
7. Signature of the person writing the order, such as the physician or advanced-practice registered nurse

Drug prescriptions outside acute care facilities may also specify whether the generic or trade name drug is to be used, the quantity to be given, and how many times the prescription can be refilled.

If, in the nurse's judgment, a drug order is in error, the nurse is responsible and held accountable for questioning that order. The error may be in any part of the drug order, and the nurse should clarify the order with the prescriber. The conversation must be documented in the client's medical record (Smith, 2003). A drug error has serious legal implications if the nurse involved could have been expected, on the basis of experience and knowledge, to have noted the error.

Most agencies have policies relative to medication administration, such as stop dates for certain types of drugs, regularly scheduled times to administer medications as specified in the drug order, and a listing of abbreviations officially accepted for use in the agency. The agency's medical records department maintains the official listing of abbreviations adopted by the medical staff of that agency. Only abbreviations from the official list can be used in any part of the client's medical record at that agency (see appendices).

TYPES OF ORDERS

Medications are prescribed differently, depending on their purpose. Medications can be prescribed as stat, single-dose, scheduled, and prn orders.

Stat Orders

Stat medication orders are those that should be administered immediately, not an hour or two later. Stat orders are often encountered in emergency situations, such as a stat dose of nitroglycerin for a client experiencing chest pain. The client's response to all stat medications must be assessed and documented.

Single-Dose Orders

Single-dose orders are one-time medications. They should be administered either at a time specified by the prescriber or at the earliest convenient time. These orders are often used in preparation for a diagnostic or therapeutic procedure; for example, a laxative may be ordered to prepare a client for a lower GI x-ray.

Scheduled Orders

Scheduled orders are administered as specified until the order is changed or canceled by another order or until the specified number of days has elapsed as set by agency policy. Scheduled orders are used to maintain the desired blood level of the medication.

Agency policy sets the actual times for administering medications over a 24-hour time interval. For example, t.i.d. drugs may be administered at 0800, 1400, and 2000 or at 0900, 1500, and 2100. Medications ordered daily may have a time specified in the order, such as Isophane (NPH) Insulin 10 units subcutaneous daily at 0630, or they will be given at the agency's designated time; for example, Lanoxin 0.25 mg po daily would be given at 0900.

An order specifying the number of days or dosages the client is to receive has an automatic stop date for the drug. For example, an order for tetracycline 250 mg po q6h for 5 days would provide tetracycline 250 mg orally every 6 hours for 5 days, a total of 20 doses. Day 1 begins with the administration of the first dose.

PRN Orders

A prn (as needed) drug is administered when, in the nurse's judgment, the client's condition requires it. This type of order is generally written for laxatives, analgesics, and antiemetics.

For example, a client may have an order for oxycodone hydrochloride (OxyContin), a narcotic analgesic, 5 to 10 mg qid prn. The pain medication is given based on the assessment of the client's pain and as specified in the order.

SYSTEMS OF WEIGHT AND MEASURE

Medication administration requires a knowledge of weight and volume measurement systems. In the United States three different systems of measurement are used in medication management: metric, apothecary, and household.

METRIC SYSTEM

In 1890, the USP adopted the metric system of weights and measures exclusively except for equivalent dosages. In 1944, the Council on Pharmacy and Chemistry of the American Medical Association adopted the metric system exclusively. The metric system is used in every major country of the world except the United States but is used almost exclusively in U.S. health care facilities.

The metric (decimal system) is a simple system based on units of 10. Move the decimal point to the right to change from a larger unit to a smaller unit and move the decimal point to the left to change from a smaller unit to a larger unit. For example:

5 g = 5,000 mg	0.5 mg = 500 mcg
5 mcg = 0.005 mg	1.25 L = 1,250 milliliters (mL)
0.25 g = 250 mg	2.45 kg = 2,450 g

The basic measurement units are the meter (linear), the liter (volume), and the gram (mass, or weight). Important abbreviations and equivalents to remember are:

- Volume (liquid)
  1,000 milliliters = 1 liter (L)
- Weight
  1,000 micrograms (mcg) = 1 milligram (mg)
  1,000 milligrams = 1 gram (g)
  1,000 grams = 1 kilogram (kg)

The metric system uses Latin prefixes to designate subdivisions of the basic units and Greek prefixes to designate multiples of the basic units (Table 25-3).

TABLE 25-3 Metric System Prefixes

PREFIX	EXAMPLE
Latin Prefixes—Subdivisions of the basic unit	deci (1/10, or 0.1) centi (1/100, or 0.01) milli (1/1,000, or 0.001) micro (1/1,000,000 or 0.000001)
Greek Prefixes—Multiples of the basic unit	deka (10) hecto (100) kilo (1,000)

COURTESY OF DELMAR CENGAGE LEARNING

SAFETY

Metric System

A zero is *not* written after a decimal point (1, *not* 1.0), and a zero is always placed in front of the decimal for values less than 1 (0.5) to prevent errors.

APOTHECARY SYSTEM

The apothecary system originated in England and is based on the weight of one grain of wheat. The grain (gr) is the basic unit of weight and the minim (the approximate volume of water that weighs a grain) is the basic unit of volume. Important equivalents and abbreviations are:

- Volume (liquid)
  60 minums (♏) = 1 fluid dram (fl dr, or ʒ)
  8 fluid drams = 1 fluid ounce (fl oz, or ℥)
  16 fluid ounces = 1 pint (pt)
- Weight
  60 grains (gr) = 1 dram (dr, or ʒ)
  8 drams = 1 ounce (oz, or ℥)
  12 ounces = 1 pound (lb)

HOUSEHOLD SYSTEM

The household system of measurement is the least accurate of the three systems. It is not ordinarily used to calculate dosage but only as a reference to help the client. The units of liquid measure are drop (gtt), teaspoon (tsp), tablespoon (Tbsp), ounce (oz), and cup (Figure 25-1). The 16-ounce pound of

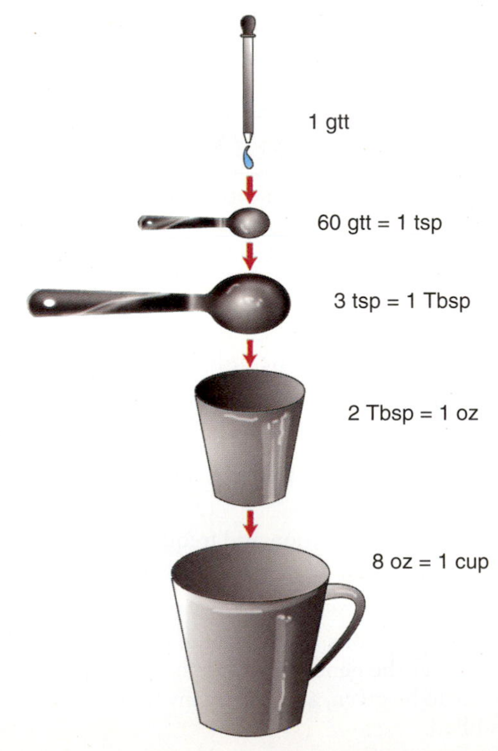

COURTESY OF DELMAR CENGAGE LEARNING

FIGURE 25-1 Relationship Between Household Measures

the household system is used to calculate dosage, with 2.2 lb equal to 1 kg.

The USP recognizes the teaspoon for household medication administration and states that the teaspoon may be regarded as representing 5 mL (American Society of Health-System Pharmacists, 2008). Household spoons are not accurate (varying sizes) for measuring a liquid medication; therefore, the USP recommends using a calibrated oral syringe or dropper for accurate measurement of liquid drug doses.

Household units are generally used in calculating a client's intake and output. Important household equivalents and abbreviations to remember are:

- Volume (liquid)
  - 60 drops (gtt) = 1 teaspoon (tsp)
  - 3 tsp = 1 tablespoon (Tbsp)
  - 2 Tbsp = 1 ounce (oz)
  - 8 oz = 1 cup (c)
  - 2 cups = 1 pint (pt)
  - 2 pints = 1 quart (qt)
- Weight
  - 16 ounces = 1 pound (lb)

APPROXIMATE EQUIVALENTS

The conversion of metric with the apothecary and household systems are *approximate equivalents* (Table 25-4). The approximate equivalents represent quantities usually ordered by physicians using either the metric or apothecary system of weights and volumes for drug doses (American Society of Health-System Pharmacists, 2008). When a dosage is prescribed in the metric system, the pharmacist may dispense the corresponding approximate equivalent in the apothecary system and vice versa. For example, if the physician prescribes magnesium hydroxide (milk of magnesia, MOM) 30 mL, the pharmacist may dispense MOM 1 ounce. The USP and NF reference *exact equivalents* that must be used to calculate quantities in pharmaceutical formularies and prescription compounding.

CONVERTING UNITS OF WEIGHT AND VOLUME

Knowledge of measurement systems and their conversions must be applied when a drug dosage is prescribed in one system and the pharmacy dispenses the equivalent dose in another. The conversions may be accomplished with either a proportion or a ratio. For example:

Proportion

Means (4 and 6)

$$2 : 4 = 6 : 12$$

Extremes (2 and 12)

Ratio

$$\frac{2}{4} = \frac{6}{12}$$

In a proportion, the product (multiplication) of the means equals the product of the extremes. In a ratio, the products of cross-multiplication are equal.

$$4 \times 6 = 24 \qquad 2 \times 12 = 24$$
$$2 \times 12 = 24 \qquad 4 \times 6 = 24$$

If one of the terms is unknown, it can be determined by substituting x for the number. The letter x denotes the unknown or unknown equation. It does not matter if the unknown x is on the right or left when setting up the problem, but when calculating the problem and at the end of the problem, the unknown equation or the unknown x is always put on the left.

$$2{:}x = 6{:}12 \qquad \frac{2}{x} = \frac{6}{12}$$
$$6x = 24 \qquad 6x = 24$$
$$x = 4 \qquad x = 24$$

Proof that the answer is correct can be determined by substituting the answer for the x and multiplying.

Proportion can be used when converting units of weight and volume, conversions within the metric system, conversions between systems, and in drug dosage calculations. When the physician orders morphine gr ¼ and the pharmacist dispenses morphine 15 mg, the nurse is responsible for ensuring the correct dose. The nurse knows that 1 grain equals 60 milligrams;

TABLE 25-4 Approximate Equivalents to the Metric System

METRIC		APOTHECARY		HOUSEHOLD		
Liquid (Volume)						
Liquid	*Weight*	*Liquid*	*Weight*		*Weight*	
0.06 mL	= 60 mg	= 1 ♏	= 1 gr	= 1 gtt	0.4 mg (400 mcg)	= 1/150 gr
1 mL	= 1 g	= 15–16 ♏	= 15 gr	= 15 gtt	1 mg (1,000 mcg)	= 1/60 gr
5 mL	= 5 g	= 1 fl dr	= 1 dr	= 1 tsp	4 mg	= 1/15 gr
15 mL	= 15 g	= 4 fl dr	= 4 dr	= 1 Tbsp	10 mg	= 1/6 gr
30 mL	= 30 g	= 1 fl oz	= 1 oz	= 1 oz	15 mg	= 1/4 gr
240 mL	= 240 g	= 8 fl oz	= 8 oz	= 8 oz	30 mg	= 1/2 gr
380 mL	= 380 g	= 12 fl oz	= 1 lb	= 16 oz	1000 g (1 kg)	= 2.2 lb
500 mL	= 500 g	= 1 pt	= 16 oz	= 1 pt		
1,000 mL	= 1,000 g	= 1 qt	= 32 oz	= 1 qt		

COURTESY OF DELMAR CENGAGE LEARNING

SAFETY

Know What Is Being Calculated

Label all terms (gr, mg, mL, and so on) to avoid errors.

to convert the ordered dose to milligrams, the nurse should use the following calculation:

Proportion	Ratio
1 gr: 60 mg = 1/4 gr: x (the grains cancel out)	$\frac{1\text{ gr}}{4\text{ gr}} \times \frac{x\text{ mg}}{60\text{ mg}}$
$1x = (60\text{ mg})(1/4)$ (divide 60 by 4) $x = 15$ mg	$60 \div 4 = x$ or 15 mg

Conversions Within the Metric System

Dose equivalents within the metric system are computed by either dividing or multiplying. For example, to change milligrams to grams (1,000 mg equals 1 g) or milliliters to liters (1,000 mL equals 1 L), divide the number by 1,000:

250 mg = x g
(move the decimal point three places to the left)
$x = 0.25$ g

or

500 mL = x L
(move the decimal point three places to the left)
$x = 0.5$ L

To convert grams to milligrams or liters to milliliters, multiply the number by 1000:

0.005 g = x mg
(move the decimal point three places to the right)
$x = 5$ mg

or

0.725 L = x mL
(move the decimal point three places to the right)
$x = 725$ mL

Converting the volume of liters and milliliters may be necessary for enemas and irrigating solutions for bladder and wound irrigations. Intravenous solutions are prepackaged, sterile solutions dispensed in volumes as ordered by the physician, such as 50 mL, 100 mL, 250 mL, 500 mL, or 1,000 mL (1 liter).

Conversions between Systems

Converting between systems is necessary when the physician orders nitroglycerin (an antianginal drug) gr 1/150 po for chest pain and the dispensed dose is 0.4 mg:

1 gr: 60 mg = 1/150 gr: x
1 gr x = (60 mg)(1/150 gr)
(the grains cancel out)
$1x = 60/150$ mg
(divide 60 by 150)
$x = 0.4$ mg

COMMUNITY/HOME HEALTH CARE

Converting a Liquid Dose to an Approximate Household Unit

A common error in household units is to equate one drop to one minim. Use a calibrated dropper to administer medications because drops vary in size.

The nurse can use proportion when converting pounds to kilograms (2.2 lb = 1 kg). For example, if the client weighs 154 lb, what is the weight in kilograms?

2.2 lb:1 kg = 154 lb: x
(the pounds cancel out)
$2.2x = 154$
(divide 154 by 2.2)
$x = 70$ kg

Dosage Calculations

Several formulas may be used by the nurse when calculating drug doses. One formula uses ratios based on the *desired dose* and the *dose on hand*. For example, cephalexin hydrochloride (Keftab), an anti-infective cephalosporin, 500 mg po q.i.d. (dose desired) is ordered by the physician; the dose on hand is 250 mg/5 mL. The formula is as follows:

$$\frac{500\text{ mg (desired dose)}}{250\text{ mg (dose on hand)}} \times \frac{x\text{ (quantity desired)}}{5\text{ mL (quantity on hand)}}$$

(cross-multiply)
(milligrams cancel out)
$250x = 500 \times 5$
$250x = 2,500$
(divide 2,500 by 250)
$x = 10$ mL

In another example, the physician orders heparin (an anticoagulant) 10,000 units subcutaneous; the dose on hand is 40,000 units/mL:

$$\frac{10,000\text{ units}}{40,000\text{ units}} \times \frac{x}{1\text{ mL}}$$

(cross-multiply)
(units cancel out)
$40,000x = 10,000$
(zeros cancel out)
$x = 0.25$ mL

Pediatric Dosages

There are several rules to calculate infants' and children's dosages, such as *Young's Rule, Clark's Rule,* and *Fried's Rule.* Another method, body surface area (BSA), is considered to be one of the most accurate methods of calculating medication dosages for infants and children up to 12 years of age (Rice, 2002). No matter which method is used in calculating pediatric drug dosages, the dosages are approximate and, depending on the child's response, may need adjustment.

PROFESSIONALTIP

Reasonable Answer

- *The final step in figuring dosage is to ask whether the answer is reasonable.*
- Seldom are more than 2 or 3 tablets or capsules given of one medication or more than 2 or 3 ounces of a liquid medication.
- Seldom is a parenteral injection, except for IV, given of more than 3 mL.
- If your calculations are outside these parameters, recheck your calculations and have a colleague check the calculations too.

Body surface area refers to the square meter surface area method of relating the surface area of individuals to drug dosage. The BSA based on height and weight gives an approximate dose using the following formula:

$$\frac{\text{Body surface area of child}}{\text{Body surface area of adult}} \times \text{Usual adult dose} = \text{Child's dose}$$

The BSA of an adult is 1.73 square meters (m^2); the 1.73 m^2 is based on an adult weighing 150 pounds.

A nomogram is used to compute the child's BSA (Figure 25-2). Draw a straight line from the child's height in the left column to the child's weight in the right column. The point where this line intersects the body surface area column (designated SA) is the child's BSA. For example: A 3-year-old child is 38 inches tall and weighs 36 pounds. The physician orders meperidine (Demerol) for pain. The average adult dose is 50 mg. How much Demerol should the child receive? From the nomogram the child's BSA is 0.66 m^2.

$$\frac{0.66\ (m^2)}{1.73\ (m^2)} \times 50 \text{ mg}$$

(square meters cancel out)

$$\frac{33}{1.73}$$

(divide 33 by 1.73)

$$= 19.07 \text{ mg} = 19 \text{ mg}$$

Now use the desired dose/dose on hand formula to determine how much to give.

$$\frac{19 \text{ mg}}{50 \text{ mg}} = \frac{x}{1 \text{ mL}}$$

(milligrams cancel out)

(cross-multiply)

$$50x = 19 \text{ mL}$$

$$x = 0.32 \text{ mL}$$

This will have to be given in a tuberculin syringe. Nomograms are used primarily in calculating pediatric drug dosages; however, they are also used when calculating some adult drug dosages such as aminoglycosides and antineoplastic agents.

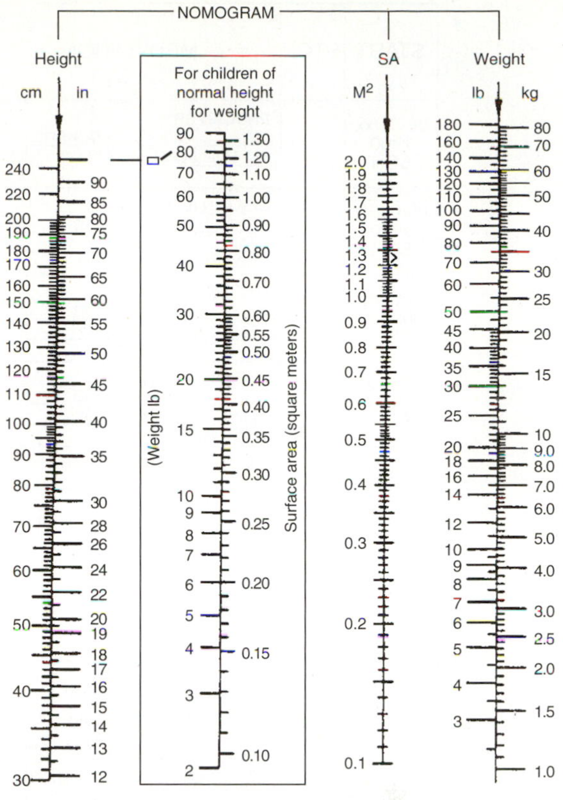

Directions for use: (1) Determine client height. (2) Determine client weight. (3) Draw a straight line to connect the height and weight. Where the line intersects on the SA line is the derived body surface area (M^2).

FIGURE 25-2 **Nomogram for Estimating Body Surface Area** (*From Nelson Textbook of Pediatrics, 17th Edition, by R. E. Behrman, R. Kliegman, & HY.B. Jenson, 2004, Philadelphia: Saunders. Copyright 2000 by Elsevier. Reprinted with permission.*)

DRUG ADMINISTRATION SAFETY

Many drugs must be administered in an efficient and safe manner according to nursing standards of practice and agency policy. Other responsibilities of the nurse include safe storage and maintaining an adequate supply of drugs.

The nurse documents the actual administration of medications on the medication administration record (MAR). The MAR contains the drug's name, dose, route, and frequency of administration. Drug data are entered either by the pharmacist when dispensing the order (computer-generated form; Figure 25-3) or by the nurse when transcribing the order (handwritten onto the form).

GUIDELINES FOR MEDICATION ADMINISTRATION

Nurses use the "seven rights" of drug administration as a guideline to protect clients from medication errors (see Memory Trick on the following page).

1. Right client
2. Right drug
3. Right dose
4. Right route
5. Right time
6. Right documentation
7. Right to refuse

START	STOP	MEDICATION	SCHEDULED TIMES	OK'D BY	0001 HRS. to 1200 HRS.	1201 HRS. to 2400 HRS.
08/31/xx 1800 SCH		PROCAN SR 500 MG TAB-SR 500 MG Q6H PO	0600 1200 1800 2400	WB	0600 LW 1200 LW	1800 GD 2400 WB
09/03/xx 0900 SCH		DIGOXIN (LANOXIN) 0.125 MG TAB 1 TAB QOD PO ODD DAYS-SEPT.	0900	WB	0900 LW	
09/03/xx 0900 SCH		FUROSEMIDE (LASIX) 40 MG TAB 1 TAB QD PO	0900	WB	0900 LW	
09/03/xx 0845 SCH		REGLAN 10 MG TAB 10 MG AC&HS PO GIVE ONE NOW!	0730 1130 1630 2100	WB	0730 LW 1130 LW	1630 GD 2100 GD
09/04/xx 0900 SCH		K-LYTE EFFERVESCENT 25 MEQ TAB 1 EFF. TAB BID PO DISSOLVE AS DIR. START 9-4	0900 1700	WB	0900 LW	1700 GD
09/03/xx 1500 PRN		NITROGLYCERIN 1/50 GR 0.4 MG TAB-SL 1 TABLET PRN* SL PRN CHEST PAIN		WB		
09/03/xx 1700 PRN		DARVOCET-N 100* 1 TAB Q4-6H PO PRN MILD-MODERATE PAIN		WB		
09/03/xx 2100 PRN		MEPERIDINE*(DEMEROL) INJ 50 MG Q4H IM PRN SEVERE PAIN W PHENERGAN		WB		2200 (H) GD
09/03/xx 2100 PRN		PROMETHAZINE (PHENERGAN) INJ 50 MG Q4H IM PRN SEVERE PAIN W DEMEROL		WB		2200 (H) GD

Gluteus	Thigh
A. Right	H. Right
B. Left	I. Left
Ventro Gluteal	
C. Right	J. Right
D. Left	K. Left
E. Abdomen	1 | 2 / 3 | 4

	Nurse's Signature	Initial
7-3	L. White, R.N.	LW
3-11	G. Duncan, R.N.	GD
11-7	W. Baumle, R.N.	WB

Allergies: NKA

Diagnosis: CHF

Patient: Patient, John D.
Patient #: 3-81512-3
Admitted: 08/31/xx
Physician: J. Physician, MD
Room: PCU-14 PCU

COURTESY OF DELMAR CENGAGE LEARNING

FIGURE 25-3 Computerized Medication Administration Record (MAR)

The nurse is legally responsible for knowing the usual dose, the expected action, the side effects, the adverse reactions, and any interactions with other drugs or food of every drug administered. Without this knowledge, the nurse should not administer any medication.

MEMORYTRICK

The seven rights of drug administration are as listed. They can be remembered by memorizing **CDDRTRD**:

- **C** = Right **C**lient
- **D** = Right **D**rug
- **D** = Right **D**ose
- **R** = Right **R**oute
- **T** = Right **T**ime
- **R** = Right to **R**efuse
- **D** = Right **D**ocumentation

Right Client

Never identify a client by calling the person's name because confused clients may answer to any name. Correctly identify the client by checking the client's identification band and by asking the client to state his or her full name. Many institutions ask the nurse to verify the client's name and date of birth (DOB) on the client's name band. Some facilities request nurses to ask the client's birthday, the last four numbers of the Social Security number, or the middle name.

When medications are dispensed with a computer-controlled system, the client is identified by scanning the bar code on the client's wrist band. The unit dose medication bar code is also scanned (Figure 25-4). The two bar codes have to agree before the computer affirms the medication, medication dose, and time.

Right Drug

The medications listed on the electronic medical record, MAR, or, less frequently, medication card are checked against the physician's order before any medication is administered. When procuring a medication, check the label on the container

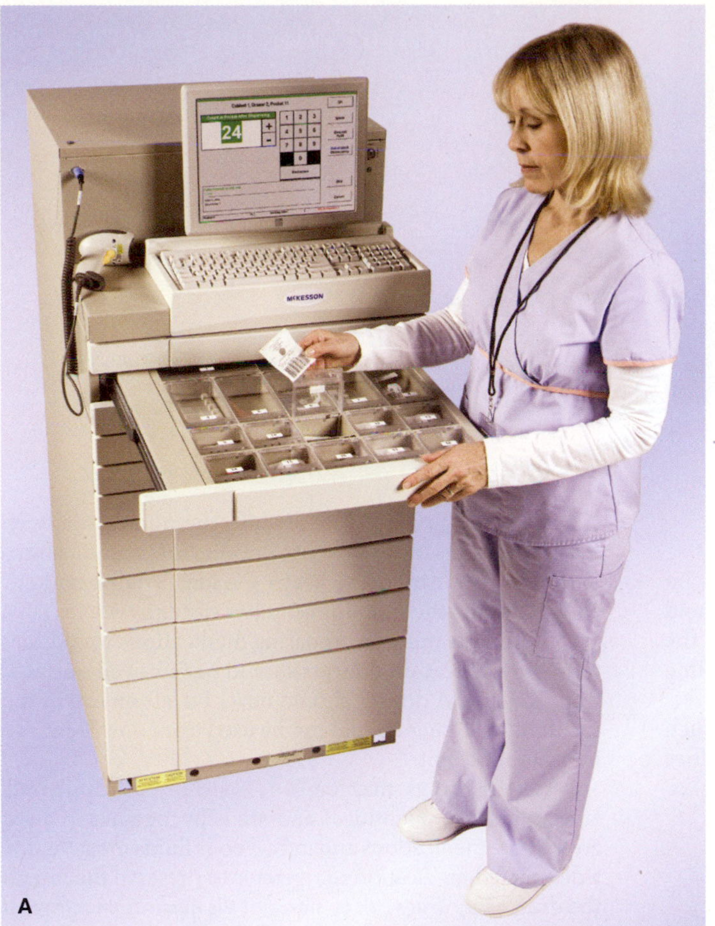

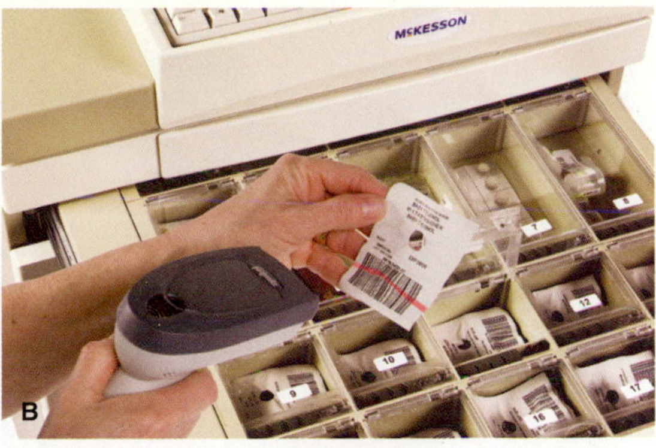

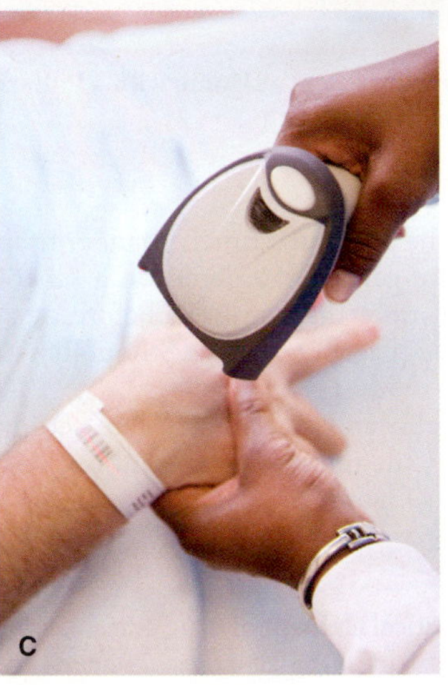

FIGURE 25-4 *A,* **Computer-Controlled Medication Dispensing System;** *B,* **Nurse Scans the Bar Code of a Unit Dose Medication;** *C,* **Nurse Scans the Bar Code on the Client's Wrist Identification Band** (*All images courtesy of McKesson Corporation.*)

against the electronic medical record or MAR at least three times:

1. When removing the drug container from the client's medication drawer
2. When removing the drug from the container
3. Before returning it to the client's medication drawer

Right Dose

Know how to correctly calculate dosages and have them checked before administration. Policy in some facilities requires two nurses to check insulin and heparin dosages to ensure accuracy.

Scored tablets are seldom broken, but if they are, make sure the tablets are broken evenly with tablet scorer. This prevents overdosage or underdosage. After crushing pills with a mortar and pestle, thoroughly cleanse the mortar and pestle to avoid mixing different medications.

Right Route

The route for giving the medication is specified in the written order. If a route is not identified in the order, the route ordered differs from the recommended one, or the route prescribed is questioned, the prescriber should be consulted. For example, the nurse should never substitute an oral medication for an intramuscular medication simply because the oral medication is available.

SAFETY

Medication Administration

- *Never administer medications prepared by another nurse.* You are responsible for a medication error if you administer a medication that was inaccurately prepared by another nurse.
- Listen carefully to the client questioning the addition or deletion of a medication and recheck the order.
- When circumstances prevent giving prescribed medications to the client, the exact reason must be documented in the client's record.
- *Do not leave medications at the client's bedside.*
- Document on the electronic medical record or initial the MAR only for those medications you actually have administered.
- Advise clients not to offer their medications to others and not to take medications belonging to others.

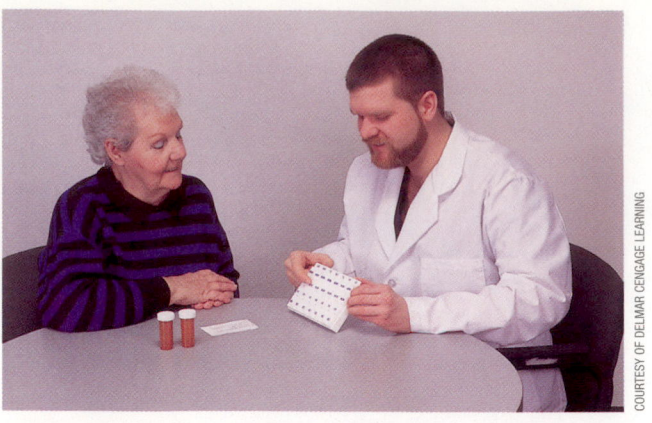
COURTESY OF DELMAR CENGAGE LEARNING

FIGURE 25-5 Assisting Client at Home with a Pillbox Correlated to the Days of the Month

Right Time

Medications have to be given in a timely manner to maintain their effects. They are generally ordered on a schedule and should not be given more than an hour before or after the scheduled time, or as per agency policy, without first checking with the physician.

In the home health and community care settings, such as a retirement home, the nurse has different responsibilities regarding drug safety (Figure 25-5).

Right Documentation

Documentation is a critical element of drug administration. The standard is "*if it was not documented, it was not done.*" Appropriate documentation can prevent many drug errors. The nurse administering a medication must initial the medication on the electronic medical record or MAR for the time the drug was given. Usually space is available for a full signature on the MAR record. Documentation should be done *after* the client has received the drug. Medication times are rescheduled for clients having various diagnostic tests or treatments at the time the medication is to be administered and the change documented.

Right to Refuse

If a client refuses to take a medication, document that a dose was missed, why the dose was missed, and notify the physician. Clients do have the right to refuse a medication, but most will be willing to take it if they understand the actions of the medication.

Drug Supply and Storage

Drugs are dispensed by the pharmacy to nursing units by various methods, accommodating the facility's medication system. After the pharmacy delivers drugs to a nursing unit, the nurse is responsible for their safe storage.

Scheduled drugs are usually dispensed in a unit dose form for each client. **Unit dose** is a system of packaging and labeling each dose of medication by the pharmacy, usually to supply the scheduled drugs for a 24-hour time period. Unit dose drugs are usually stored in a mobile medication dispensing computer system, a medication cart containing individual drawers for each client's medications, or a medication room in separate containers for each client. The unit dose system makes it easy to administer the correct dose, thereby minimizing the number of medication errors.

COMMUNITY/HOME HEALTH CARE

Considerations for Drug Safety

- Encourage and assist the client in removing outdated prescriptions and over-the-counter drugs from medication cabinets.
- Encourage the client or caregivers to maintain drug refills to decrease the risk of missing scheduled medications.
- Use a pillbox or reminder calendar (Figure 25-5) to help the client or caregiver remember to take or administer medications as scheduled.

At the beginning of each shift, the nurse usually checks the medications in each client's drawer. Some medication carts are locked and the nurse keeps the key. The nurse keys in a code to access the mobile computer system.

When the nurse is preparing medications for administration, the medication drawers should be removed one at a time from the cart. A drawer should never be left on top of the cart unattended. Drugs should not be used from one client's supply for another client.

Certain drugs may be **stock supplied** (dispensed and labeled in large quantities) and are kept together in a secured area. Some medications and intravenous fluids must be stored in a designated medication refrigerator to preserve the integrity of the drug. *Only drugs can be stored in the medication refrigerator.*

Narcotics and Controlled Substances

Health care facilities have special forms to record the supply on hand and the administration of narcotics and controlled substances according to federal regulations. These forms usually require the following information for each drug administered:

- Name of the client receiving the drug
- Amount of the drug dispensed
- Time the drug was administered
- Name of the prescribing physician
- Name of the nurse administering the drug

Nurses are required to count the narcotics and controlled substances at specified times, usually at the change of shifts. One nurse going off duty counts the drugs with a nurse coming on duty. Each drug dose must be accounted for on the narcotic record. When the narcotic count does not check, the discrepancy must be reported immediately. Narcotics and controlled substances are kept in a double-locked drawer, box, room, or medication-dispensing cart, such as a computer-controlled dispensing system, as shown in Figure 25-4. The law requires these safety precautions for narcotics and controlled substances.

MEDICATION COMPLIANCE

When clients do not take their prescribed medications consistently or when they adjust the scheduling or dose of the medication, they are *noncompliant.*

Clients may have several reasons why they choose not to take ordered medications. They may not understand the need to take prescribed medications, medications may cost too much for the client on a fixed income, the medication may not provide prompt relief, or the medication may cause undesirable side effects.

Compliance can be enhanced by the nurse teaching the client information on the medications to take at home. Large print or illustrations should be used if the client is elderly. When the nurse teaches the client, include the caregiver. Compliance may be enhanced by giving the client a telephone number to call if questions arise.

LEGAL ASPECTS OF MEDICATION ADMINISTRATION

Remember the "seven rights" for safe administration of medications. Giving the wrong medicine to the client is an error; giving the right medicine but wrong dose or wrong route is an error; giving a medication at the wrong time is an error. The physician must be informed of all errors and needs accurate information to make appropriate decisions. Medications given in error must be documented on the electronic medical record or MAR.

Medication errors must be reported in a timely manner. Incident reports are generally required for medication errors. An incident report, also known as an occurrence or variance report, is documentation of any occurrence or accident that, during the delivery of care, harmed or could have harmed the client. The purpose of an incident report is to provide safety to the client and not to punish the caregiver. Ethically, it is the responsibility of the nurse to complete the incident report so the client's safety is ensured. The report must include the name of the medication, dose given, route, time administered, specific error, time the physician was contacted about the error, what countermeasures were taken, and the clients' response. The nurse includes only accurate and objective facts; no opinions, judgments, assumptions, blame, or incident prevention methods are written in the report. The incident report is not mentioned in the client's medical record. Sometimes nurses discover errors made by other nurses. These must also be reported and documented.

The two purposes of the incident report are to notify the facilities' Risk Management or Continuous Quality Control committee of the incident so that another occurrence of the incident is prevented and to notify the facilities' insurance company of a potential claim and further needed research into the situation. Prompt Risk Management committee review of the incident may prevent litigation. The incident report does not become part of the medical record but may be used if litigation occurs (Daniels, Grendell, & Wilkins, 2010).

Health care institutions should have a national tracking system for medication errors. The USP collects and shares data about actual and potential medication errors. It shares the occurrence of medication errors and methods to prevent the errors with the FDA, the Institute for Safe Medication Practices, and health care professionals (DeLaune & Ladner, 2006). To report medication errors, call 1-800-23-ERROR or go online at http://www.usp.org.

NURSING PROCESS

The nursing process is vital in planning client care and in ensuring safe and accurate medication administration.

ASSESSMENT

The subjective data include medication history and medical history. Objective data include a physical examination and diagnostic and laboratory data.

Medication History

A medication history obtained when a client is admitted to a health care facility should contain information about the client's medication background, including allergies, and use of prescription and over-the-counter drugs.

Allergies Inquire about all medication and food allergies. The nurse asks the client who has had an allergic reaction to a drug to describe the details of the reaction: name of the drug; dosage, route, and number of times the drug was taken before the reaction; onset of the reaction; and evidences of the reaction. Ask about possible contributing factors to the allergic reaction, such as concurrent use of stimulants or depressants (tobacco, alcohol, or illegal drugs) or significant changes in nutritional status.

Allergies to foods should also be discussed because drugs may contain the same substances that cause allergic reactions to some foods. For example, clients who are allergic to shellfish may have a reaction to drugs containing iodine. Vaccines are commonly derived from chick embryos and would be contraindicated for clients with allergies to eggs. If a client has a history of allergies, the nurse may want to obtain an order for an EpiPen® (epinephrine) and oxygen if a new medication is administered.

Prescription Drugs The client should identify all current prescription drugs and describe the following:

- The reason the drug was prescribed and by whom
- The drug's dosage, route, and frequency
- The client's knowledge of the drug's action: side and adverse effects, when to notify the physician, and special administration considerations such as with or without foods

Over-the-Counter Drugs Ask specifically about nonprescription drugs taken by the client. For example, determine if the client takes aspirin, laxatives, or antacids routinely, along with the dosage, route, and frequency of these drugs. Also ask about the use of creams, ointments, patches, or sprays.

Medical History

Gather information about chronic diseases and disorders and correlate these data with the prescription drugs.

Sensory and Cognitive Status Assess for and inquire about sensory deficits such as vision or hearing impairments. Assess the client's cognitive abilities during the history interview by noting if the client is alert and oriented and interacts appropriately.

CRITICAL THINKING

Incorrect Drug

You discover that a similar but incorrect drug (not the drug ordered) is being given IV to a client. What is the first thing you should do? What is your next course of action? How do you feel about the nurse who made the medication error and did not recognize it?

Physical Examination

The client's condition is assessed before administering any drug to establish the client's baseline, or normal, health status. For example, the nurse assesses the client's apical pulse for 1 full minute before administering digoxin (Lanoxin), a cardiac glycoside with positive inotropic effects, to determine that the pulse is above 60 and to assess the heart rhythm. After the client receives the drug, the heart rate is compared with the baseline measurement.

Diagnostic and Laboratory Data

Common laboratory values, such as electrolytes, blood urea nitrogen, creatinine, glucose, complete blood count, and a white blood cell count, are usually monitored over a period to identify trends and to measure the body's response to medications.

Nursing Diagnosis

Once the actual or potential problems are identified, relevant nursing diagnoses can be identified. The North American Nursing Diagnosis Association International (NANDA-I) (2010) nursing diagnoses commonly related to medication administration include:

- *Ineffective **H**ealth Maintenance*
- *Deficient **K**nowledge* (specify)
- *Ineffective **T**herapeutic Regimen Management*
- *Impaired Physical **M**obility*
- *Disturbed **S**ensory Perception*
- *Impaired **S**wallowing*

Planning/Outcome Identification

The care plan and goals are developed based on the nursing diagnoses. For example, the client with a knowledge deficit related to a newly prescribed drug may have the following expected outcomes:

Before discharge the client will:

- Correctly state the actions of the drug in the body
- Prepare the correct dose of the drug
- List the possible side effects of and possible adverse reactions to the drug
- Correctly identify special considerations (i.e., take with food, no alcohol)

Implementation

The main nursing interventions related to medication management are assessment, administration, and teaching. Use the time spent when administering medications to assess the client's knowledge of and response to the drug.

Medication administration requires implementing safety guidelines, following the "seven rights." Medications are administered according to set procedures based on the prescribed route. This section presents information for medication administration by the following routes: oral, including sublingual and buccal; parenteral; site-specific topical applications; and inhalation.

Drug teaching usually takes place in two phases. The first phase is usually a formal teaching session, when the drug's action, route, side and adverse effects, and the specific signs of a drug reaction that require physician notification are explained. Clients may need assistance developing a drug schedule that fits their lifestyle. Teaching the client and/or support person specific procedural techniques, such as subcutaneous injection, may be necessary.

The second phase of client teaching occurs whenever a drug is administered. At each interaction, assess and reinforce the client's knowledge of drugs. When a client is taught self-administration, the teaching plan should identify dates for teaching and a date for achievement of goals.

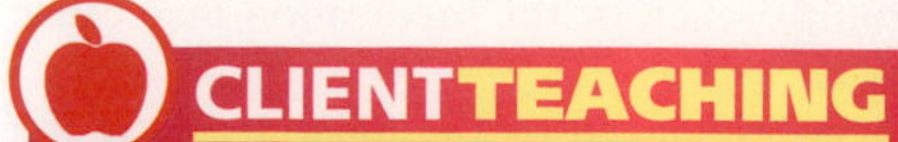

Written Medication Information

Written medication information for clients should be accurate, specific, comprehensive, and presented in a legible and understandable format. It should:

- Include generic and trade names.
- State indications for use, contraindications, precautions, adverse reactions, risks, and storage.
- Provide straightforward instructions.
- Have conspicuous drug warnings.
- Have print size appropriate to client's visual abilities.
- Be appropriate for client literacy level.

Oral Drugs

Oral administration of drugs is the most common route; however, potential risk factors must be considered. Assess the client's ability to take the medication before administering oral drugs by assessing the client's state of consciousness, gag reflex, and presence of nausea and vomiting. These assessments assist in protecting the client from aspiration. **Aspiration** is the inhalation of secretions or fluids into the pulmonary system.

Liquid medications are measured out in a calibrated medicine cup. Doses, smaller than 1 dr, 1 tsp, or 5 mL, are measured in a syringe for accuracy. Solid oral medications are put into a medicine cup or small paper (soufflé) cup, depending on agency policy. Individually wrapped medications should be opened at the bedside.

Remain with the client when administering oral drugs, until all medications have been swallowed. When in doubt that the client has swallowed a pill, don a nonsterile glove and visually inspect the client's mouth using a tongue depressor (Figure 25-6).

Sublingual and Buccal Assess the integrity of the mucous membranes by inspecting under the client's tongue and in the buccal cavity before administering sublingual and buccal drugs. When oral membranes are excoriated or painful, withhold the medication and notify the physician. For buccal drugs that irritate the mucosa, alternate sides of the mouth. Drugs given by these routes are quickly absorbed by the mucosa's abundant blood supply and the thin epithelium.

Enteral **Enteral instillation** is the delivery of drugs through a gastrointestinal tube. Enteral tubes provide a way to directly

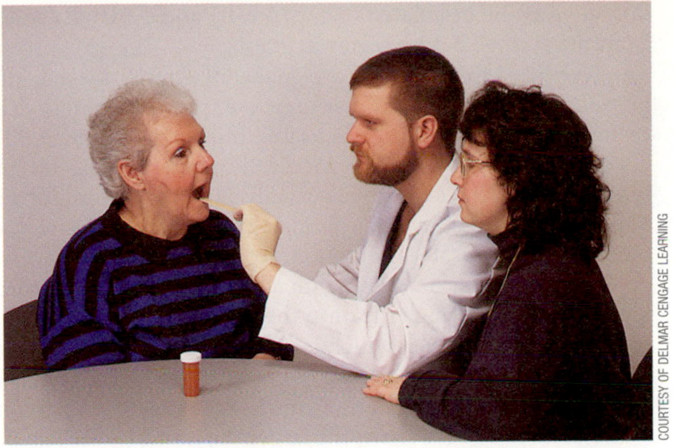

FIGURE 25-6 Check the client's mouth if you are unsure that medications have been swallowed.

instill medications into the gastrointestinal system of clients who cannot take them orally.

There are several types of enteral tubes. A nasogastric tube (NG) is a soft rubber or plastic tube inserted through a nostril and into the stomach. The gastrostomy tube is surgically inserted into the stomach through the abdomen.

Check the tube for **patency** and placement and assess the client for the presence of bowel sounds before administering a medication. Patency is being freely open. When the tube is obstructed or improperly placed, the client is vomiting, or bowel sounds are absent, the instillation of drugs is contraindicated.

Once the patency and placement of the tube are determined, prepare the medication for instillation as prescribed by the physician. When the physician orders a drug in tablet form, crush the tablet into minute particles and dissolve the crushed tablet in 15 to 30 mL of warm water before instillation. Do not dissolve all medications and give at one time. Instead, dissolve each medication in a separate cup in 15 to 30 mL of water and give each medication separately. To clear the tubing, instill 30 mL of water between each medication and at the end of the medication administration. Contact the physician or nurse practitioner to clarify medication administration orders if the client is on a fluid restricted diet. Cold water may cause abdominal cramps when instilled. Open capsules and empty the contents into a liquid.

CLIENT TEACHING

Sublingual and Buccal Drugs

Sublingual Drugs:

- Keep the medication under the tongue until completely dissolved to ensure absorption.
- To prevent accidental swallowing, avoid chewing the tablet or moving it with the tongue.
- Nicotine has a vasoconstrictive effect that slows absorption; therefore, do not smoke until the drug is completely dissolved.

Buccal Drugs:

- Keep the medication in place until completely dissolved to ensure absorption.
- Some tablets take up to an hour to dissolve; therefore, do not drink liquids for an hour.
- Nicotine has a vasoconstriction effect that slows absorption; therefore, do not smoke until the drug is completely dissolved.

PROFESSIONAL TIP

Special Considerations for Enteral Tube Management

- When a client is receiving intermittent tube feedings, schedule medications to prevent the two solutions from being given together.
- An adult client should not receive more than 400 mL of liquid at one time. If feeding and medication administration coincide, give the medication first to ensure that the client receives the prescribed dosage on time; the feeding may not be given in its entirety.
- When the client is receiving a continuous feeding, stop the feeding and aspirate the gastric contents. If the gastric contents are greater than 150 mL, withhold the medication and notify the physician.
- *Never put tablets into tube-feeding bags.*
- For clients who have an NG tube for decompression (removal) of gastric contents, turn off the suction for 20 to 30 minutes after instillation of the medication to allow time for the gastric contents to be emptied into the intestines, where most drugs are absorbed.

Parenteral Drugs

Parenteral medications are given through a route other than the alimentary canal; these routes are intradermal, subcutaneous, intramuscular, or intravenous. The insertion angle of the needle and the depth of penetration indicate the type of injection (Figure 25-7).

Equipment To administer parenteral medications, special equipment such as syringes, needles, ampules, and vials are used.

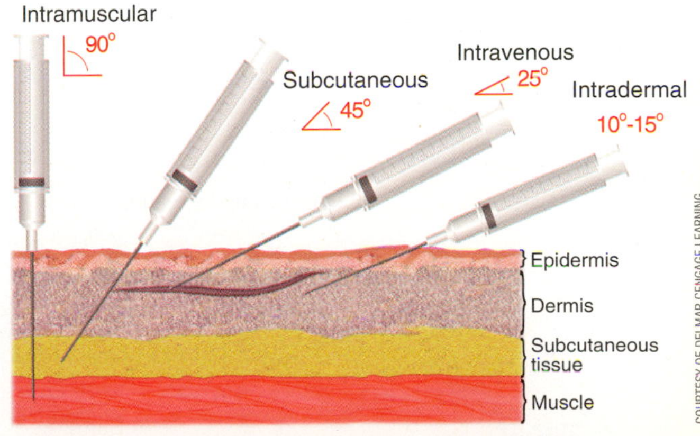

FIGURE 25-7 Angle of Insertion for Parenteral Injections

Syringes A syringe has three basic parts: the hub, which connects with the needle; the barrel, or outside part, which has measurement calibrations; and the plunger, which fits inside the barrel and has a rubber tip (Figure 25-8). The hub, the inside of the barrel, and the shaft and rubber plunger tip must be kept sterile. When handling a syringe, touch only the outside of the barrel and the plunger's handle.

Two designs for syringe hubs are the Luer-Lok tip and the slip tip (see Figure 25-8). The hub of a needle twists into the threaded Luer-Lok tip so that the needle cannot slip off of the syringe. The needle easily slides on and off the slip tip. The choice of syringe type depends on the situation of use and the preference of the user.

Most syringes are disposable, made of plastic, and individually packaged. There are hypodermic, insulin, and tuberculin syringes (Figure 25-9). When a medication is incompatible with plastic, it is usually prefilled into a single-dose glass syringe. Syringes are often packaged with the size and gauge needle commonly used.

The *hypodermic syringe* comes in 2-, 2.5-, and 3-mL sizes. The measurement calibrations are usually in mL, and some syringes have minims. The hypodermic syringe is used most often when a medication is ordered in milliliters. When the order is written in minims, it is safer to use a tuberculin syringe.

The *insulin syringe* is designed especially for use with insulin. For example, if the physician writes the order for 30 units of U-100 insulin, use an insulin syringe calibrated on the 100-unit scale. Always compare the size of the insulin syringe and the strength indicated on the insulin bottle with the physician's order; all three units must be the same. There are three sizes of U-100 insulin syringes: 1 mL, ½ mL, and 3/10 mL (see Figure 25-9). The ½- and 3/10-mL sizes are called low-dose insulin syringes.

The *tuberculin syringe* is a narrow syringe, calibrated in tenths and hundredths of a milliliter (up to 1 mL) on one scale and in sixteenths of a minim (up to 1 minim) on the other scale. This syringe is generally used to administer small or precise doses (i.e., pediatric dosages). The tuberculin syringe should be used for doses 0.5 mL or less.

Prefilled single-dose syringes should not be confused with a unit dose. The prescribed dose must be checked against that in the prefilled syringe and the excess discarded. For example, if the physician orders diazepam (Valium) 5 mg IM as a preoperative sedative and the prefilled single-dose contains 10 mg/2 mL, the dosage must be calculated (5 mg/1 mL) and 1 mL discarded from the syringe before administration.

Needles Most needles are made of stainless steel, disposable, and individually packaged. A prefilled single-dose cartridge is inserted into a reusable injection system holder (Figure 25-10) to give the medication. Depending on the type of holder, the cartridge is usually slid into the holder and tightened in place and the plunger twisted onto the rubber plunger. The reusable holders are called a Tubex are Carpuject, depending on the manufacturer. A needle has three aspects: the hub, which fits onto the syringe hub; the cannula, or shaft; and the bevel, which is the slanted part at the tip of the shaft (Figure 25-11). Needles come in many sizes, from ¼ to 5 inches long, with gauges from 32 to 14. The *gauge* refers to the diameter of the shaft; the larger the number, the smaller the diameter of the shaft. Smaller needles (larger gauge) produce less trauma to the body's tissue; however, the viscosity of a solution must be considered when selecting the gauge.

The *shaft* of the needle indicates its length. The length of the needle is selected based on the client's muscle development and weight and the type of injection, such as intravenous versus intramuscular.

Needles may have a short or a long *bevel*. The bevel length is selected based on the type of injection. Long bevels are sharp and produce less pain when inserted into the subcutaneous or muscle tissues. A short bevel is used for intradermal and intravenous injections to prevent the tissue or blood vessel wall from occluding the bevel.

The hub of the needle should be immediately attached to the hub of the syringe when removed from its sterile wrapper to prevent contamination. The protective cover should remain on the needle until it is ready to be used.

Most syringes come with a protective system to cover needles after giving an injection. Some have an outside shield that slides down over the needle as shown in Figure 25-9A and Figure 25-9D. Another syringe is designed with a plastic hinge as shown in Figure 25-9E. After giving the injection, the nurse slides the plastic hinge over the needle locking it in place. Some syringes automatically retract the needle after the injection is given. Go to the following Web site for an example of this syringe and search for BD Integra retracting syringe: http://www.bd.com.

Used needles must be disposed of in the proper receptacles, such as a sharps container, to prevent needlesticks. All client care areas have sharps containers in most facilities.

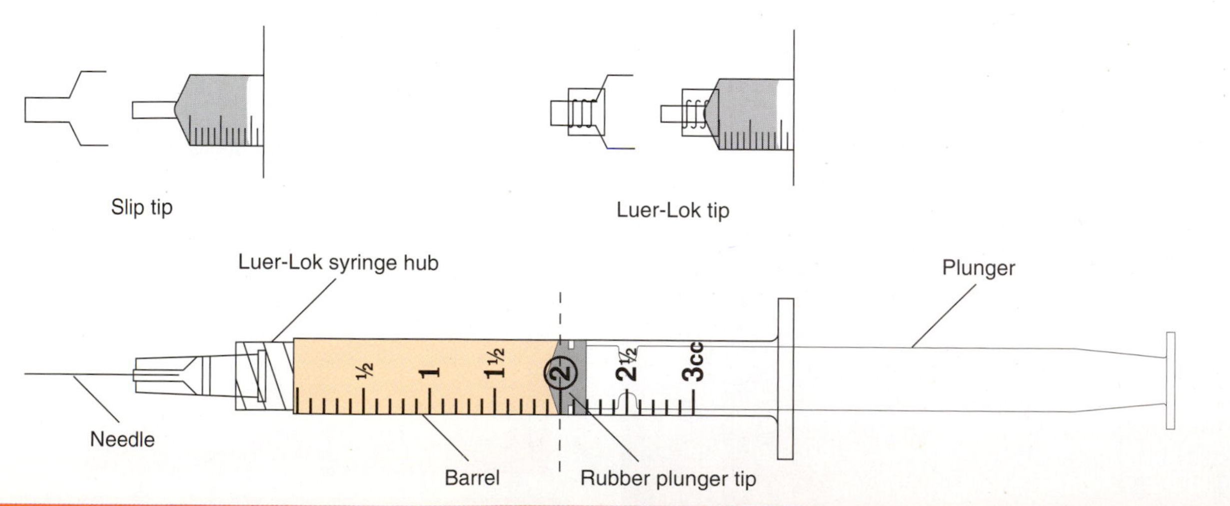

FIGURE 25-8 The Parts of a Syringe with Syringe Tip Options of Slip Tip or Luer-Lok

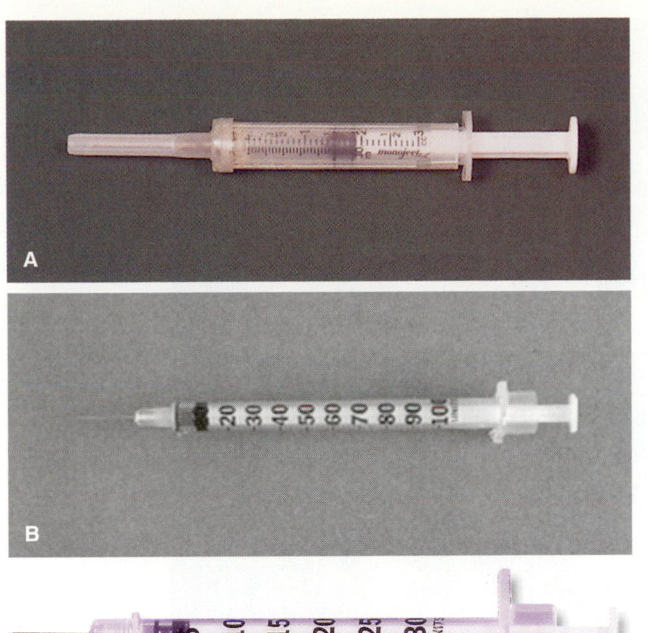

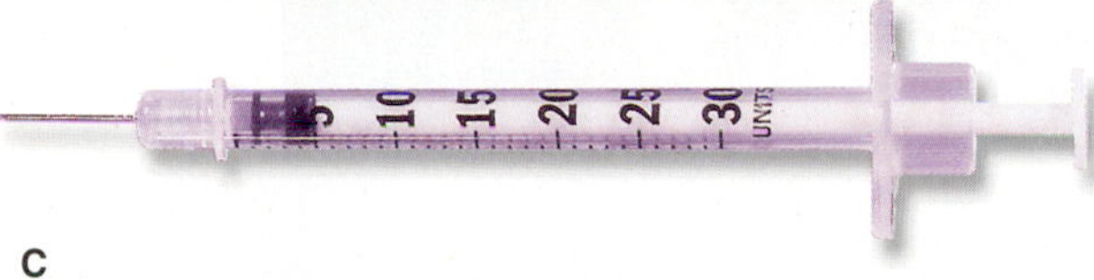

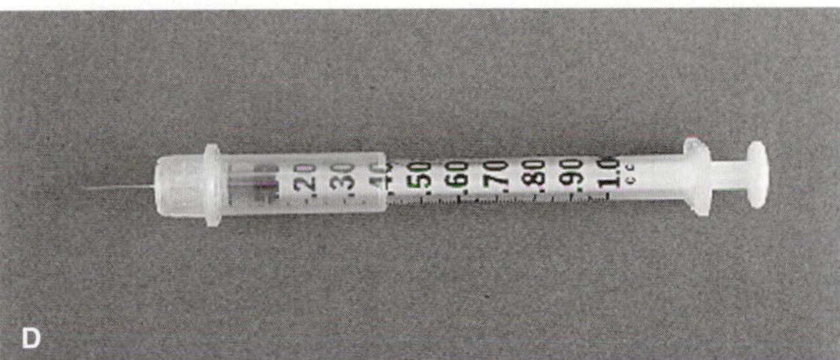

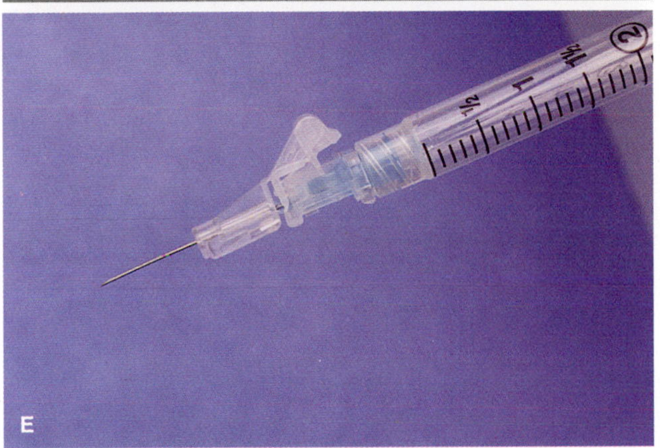

FIGURE 25-9 Types of Syringes; *A,* 3 mL Hypodermic with Plastic Needle Guard; *B,* Standard U-100 Insulin Syringe; *C,* Insulin 3/10 mL; *D,* 1 mL Tuberculin with Plastic Needle Guard; *E,* Syringe with Plastic Hinge that Slides Over the Needle (*Images A, B, C, and D courtesy and copyright Becton, Dickinson and Company. Image E courtesy of Delmar Cengage Learning.*)

Discussion of the needleless system is found under IV therapy later in this chapter.

Ampules and Vials Drugs for parenteral injections must be sterile. Those that deteriorate in solution are dispensed as tablets or powders to be dissolved in a solution immediately before injection. Drugs remaining stable in solution are dispensed in ampules and vials in an aqueous or an oily solution or suspension.

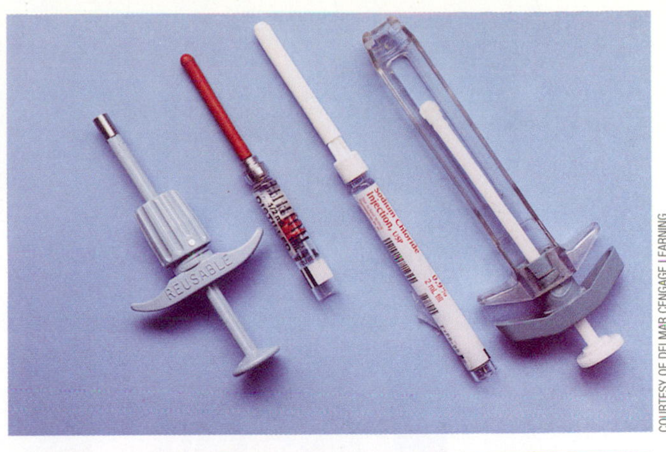

FIGURE 25-10 Prefilled Single-Dose Cartridges with Reusable Injection System Holders

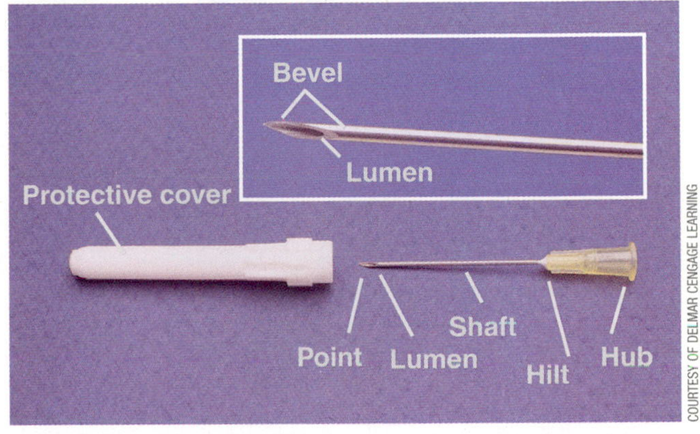

FIGURE 25-11 Parts of a Needle

Ampules are glass containers of single-dose drugs (Figure 25-12A). The glass container has a constriction in the stem to facilitate opening the ampule. When opening an ampule, the nurse slides a plastic shield over the tip to assist in breaking it and to prevent a finger cut (Figure 25-12B). Drugs may be irritating to the subcutaneous tissue, so the needle should be changed after withdrawing a drug from an ampule.

Glass, single- or multiple-dose rubber-capped drug containers are called vials (Figure 25-12D). A vial usually has an easily removed soft metal or plastic cap. The needle should be changed after withdrawing a drug from a vial.

Intradermal Injection Intradermal (ID) or intracutaneous injections are used to administer local anesthetics, identify allergens, and diagnose tuberculosis. An ID injection is administered below the epidermis; drugs are absorbed slowly from this site. Commonly used sites for ID injection are the inner aspect of the forearm, upper back, and upper chest.

The drug's dosage for an ID injection is usually a small amount of solution (0.01 to 0.1 mL). To provide accurate measurement, use a 1-mL tuberculin syringe with a short bevel, 25 to 27 gauge, ⅜- to ½-inch needle. For repeated doses, the sites are rotated. Intradermal injections are administered into the epidermis by angling the needle 10 to 15 degrees to the skin.

Subcutaneous Injection Subcutaneous injections are used to administer insulin and heparin because they are absorbed

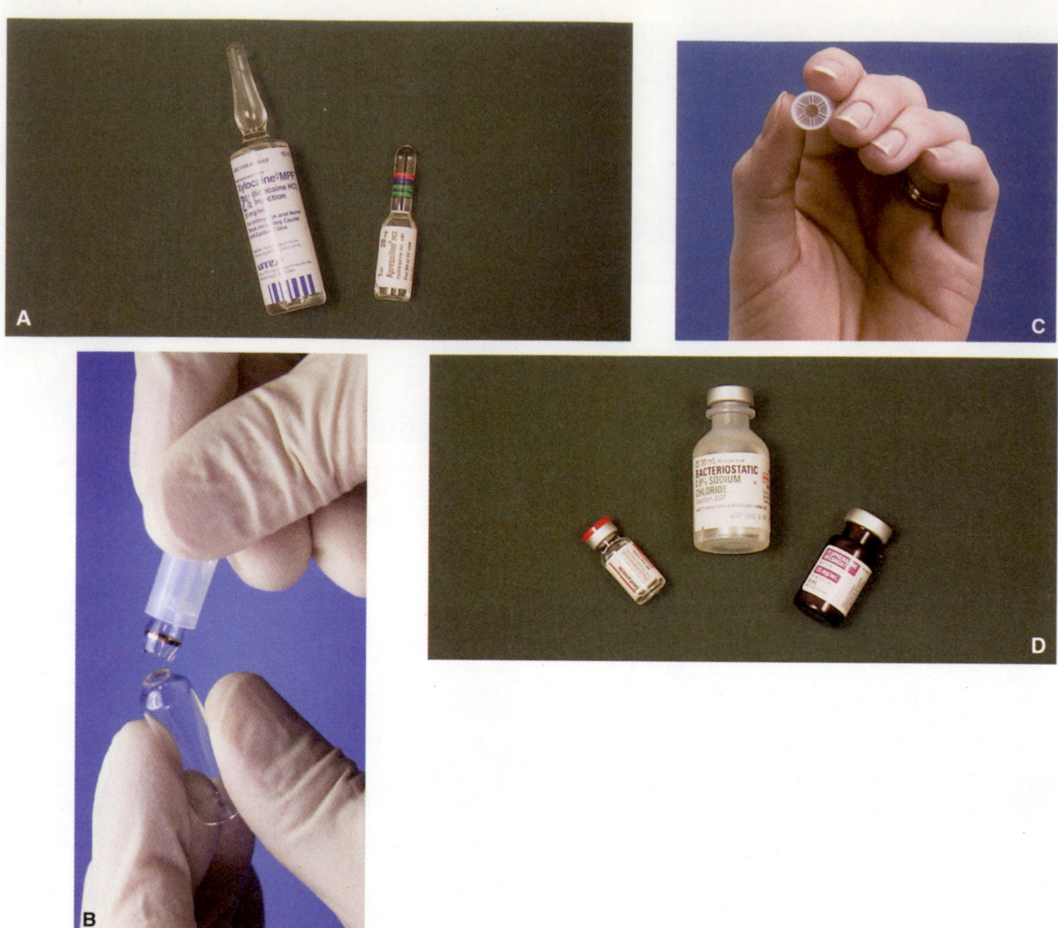

FIGURE 25-12 *A*, Ampules; *B*, Using Safety Cap to Break Ampule; *C*, Safety Cap to Slide Over the Tip of the Ampule When Breaking; *D*, Vials *(Images A and D courtesy of Delmar Cengage Learning. Images B and C courtesy of Sigma-Aldrich.)*

> **PROFESSIONALTIP**
>
> ### Expiration Date
>
> - Laws require manufacturers to put expiration dates on all drugs.
> - To ensure a drug is current, check the expiration date.
> - Return outdated drugs to the pharmacy for proper disposal.

slowly, creating a sustained effect. Subcutaneous injections put the medication between the dermis and the muscle into the subcutaneous tissue. The amount of medication given varies but seldom exceeds 1.5 mL. For repeated doses the site should be rotated.

Common sites for subcutaneous injections include the abdomen, the lateral aspect of the upper arm or the anterior aspect of the upper thigh, the scapular area on the back, and the upper ventrodorsal gluteal area. Select a sterile 0.5- to 3-mL syringe with a 25 to 27 gauge and a ⅜- to ⅝-inch needle. The medication is administered by angling the needle 45 to 90 degrees to the skin.

Intramuscular Injection Intramuscular (IM) injections promote rapid drug absorption and provide another route for drugs that are irritating to subcutaneous tissue. The absorption rate is greater because there are more blood vessels in the muscles than in subcutaneous tissue; however, the client's circulatory status may affect the absorption rate.

> **PROFESSIONALTIP**
>
> ### Heparin Administration
>
> - Heparin is given in the abdomen 2 inches away from the umbilicus and above the iliac crests.
> - When giving heparin subcutaneously, do not aspirate on the plunger; doing so may cause tissue damage and bruising.
> - Do not massage the heparin injection site because it may cause the drug to absorb more quickly.
> - Give heparin at a 90-degree angle with a 3/8-inch needle, unless the client is lean, then give the injection at a 45-degree angle (Berman, Snyder, Kozier, & Erb, 2008).

The four common sites for administering IM injections are the dorsogluteal and ventrogluteal (gluteus maximus muscle), the anterolateral aspect of the thigh (vastus lateralis muscle), and the upper arm (deltoid muscle). These sites are identified by using appropriate anatomic landmarks. An IM injection is administered at a 90-degree angle to the skin, injecting only up to 3 mL into well-developed muscle tissue. See Table 25-5 for amounts of solution to inject in various types of tissue.

Z-Track Injection A Z-track (zigzag) injection is a method for administering IM injections, most commonly in the ventrogluteal and dorsogluteal muscles.

For administration of a Z-track injection, the client is placed in the prone position; the skin is pulled to one side, the needle is inserted at a 90-degree angle, and the medication is administered. After 10 seconds the needle is withdrawn and then the skin is released. Do not massage the site; it may cause tissue irritation. Never inject more than 3 mL in a single site.

IV Therapy The LPN/VN role in IV therapy varies widely from state to state and facility to facility. It is the responsibility of the LPN/VN to know the standards of practice for the state in which one practices. IV therapy requires parenteral fluids (solutions) and special equipment: administration set, IV pole, filter, regulators to control IV flow rate, and an established venous route.

Parenteral Fluids Read the physician's order in the client's medical record to confirm the type and amount of IV solution. Intravenous solutions are sterile and usually packaged in plastic bags. Solutions incompatible with plastic are in glass containers.

Plastic IV solution bags collapse under atmospheric pressure, allowing the solution to enter the infusion set. Plastic solution bags are packaged with an outer plastic bag, which should remain intact until the solution is prepared for administration. The solution bag should be dry when removed from its outer wrapper. If it is wet, the solution should not be used. Moisture on the bag shows that the integrity of the bag has been compromised, and the solution cannot be considered sterile. Return the bag to the department that issued the solution. Glass containers are discussed in the section on equipment.

Parenteral fluids are classified based on their relationship to normal blood plasma. Solutions may be hypotonic, isotonic, or hypertonic. The solution prescribed is based on the client's diagnosis and the goal of therapy. The solution's effect is:

- *Hypotonic fluid.* Lowers osmotic pressure and makes fluid move into the cells. Water intoxication may result if fluid is infused beyond the client's tolerance.
- *Isotonic fluid.* Increases only extracellular fluid volume. Cardiac overload may result if fluid is infused beyond the client's tolerance.
- *Hypertonic fluid.* Increases osmotic pressure and draws fluid from the cells. Cellular dehydration may result if fluid is infused beyond the client's tolerance (Bulechek & McCloskey, 2000).

Common intravenous solutions are shown in Table 25-6.

LIFE SPAN CONSIDERATIONS

Choosing IV Equipment

Neonates, infants, and children are at risk for *Excess Fluid Volume* related to rehydration. A microdrip and special volume-control chamber are used to regulate the fluid amount administered in a specific time.

TABLE 25-5 Summary of Intradermal, Subcutaneous, and Intramuscular Injections

TYPE OF INJECTION	PURPOSE	SITE	NEEDLE SIZE	MAXIMUM DOSE	ANGLE OF INSERTION
Intradermal	Injects medication below the epidermis; drugs are absorbed slowly; typically used for diagnosis of tuberculosis and allergens	Inner aspect of forearm; upper chest; upper back	Syringe with short bevel; 25–27-gauge; 3/8 to 1/2-inch	0.01–0.1 mL	10° to 15°
Subcutaneous	Injects medication between dermis and muscle; absorbed slowly; typically used for insulin and anticoagulants	Abdomen; lateral and anterior aspects of upper arm and thigh; scapular area on back; ventrogluteal area	25-27-gauge, 3/8-5/8-inch needle (varies by size of person)	0.5–1mL	45° to 90°
Intramuscular	Used to promote rapid drug absorption and to provide an alternative route when drug is irritating to subcutaneous tissue	Ventrogluteal; dorsogluteal; anterolateral aspect of thigh (vastus lateralis); upper arm (deltoid)	The gauge and length of needle are selected on the basis of medication volume and viscosity and client's body size	Well-developed adult: 3 mL in a large muscle; infant and small child: 0.5–1 mL; children and elderly: 1–2 mL; deltoid muscle: 0.5–1 mL	90°

COURTESY OF DELMAR CENGAGE LEARNING

TABLE 25-6 Common Intravenous Solutions

TONICITY	SOLUTION	CONTENTS (MEQ/L)	CLINICAL IMPLICATIONS
Hypotonic	Sodium chloride 0.45%	77 Na^+, 77 Cl^-	Daily maintenance of body fluid and establishment of renal function.
Isotonic	Dextrose 2.5% in 0.45% saline	77 Na^+, 77 Cl^-	Promotes renal function and urine output.
	Dextrose 5% in 0.2% saline	77 Na^+, 77 Cl^-	Daily maintenance of body fluids when less Na^+ and Cl^- are required.
	Dextrose 5% in water (D_5W)	38 Na^+, 38 Cl^-	Promotes rehydration and elimination; may cause urinary Na^+ loss; good vehicle for K^+.
	Ringer's lactate	130 Na^+, 4 K^+, Ca^{2+}, 109 Cl^-, 28 lactate	Resembles the normal composition of blood serum and plasma; K^+ level below body's daily requirement.
	Normal saline (NS), 0.9%	154 Na^+, 154 Cl^-	Restores sodium chloride deficit and extracellular fluid volume.
	Dextran 40 10% in NS (0.9%) or D_5W		A colloidal solution used to increase plasma volume of clients in early shock; it should not be given to severely dehydrated clients and clients with renal disease, thrombocytopenia, or active hemorrhaging.
	Dextran 70% in NS		A long-lived (20 hours) plasma volume expander; used to treat shock or impending shock caused by hemorrhage, surgery, or burns. *It can prolong bleeding and coats the RBCs (draw type and cross match before administering).*
Hypertonic	Dextrose 5% in 0.45% saline	77 Na^+, 77 Cl^-	Daily maintenance of body fluid and nutrition; treatment of fluid volume deficit (FVD).
	Dextrose 5% in saline 0.9%	154 Na^+, 154 Cl^-	Fluid replacement of sodium, chloride, and calories (170).
	Dextrose 10% in saline 0.9%	154 Na^+, 154 Cl^-	Fluid replacement of sodium, chloride, and calories (340).
	Dextrose 5% in lactated Ringer's	130 Na^+, 4 K^+, 3 Ca^{2+}, 109 Cl^-, 28 lactate	Resembles the normal composition of blood serum and plasma; K^+ level below body's daily requirement; caloric value 180.
	Hyperosmolar saline 3% and 5% NaCl	856 Na^+, 865 Cl^-	Treatment of hyponatremia; raises the Na osmolarity of the blood, and reduces intracellular fluid excess.
	Ionosol B with dextrose 5%	57 Na^+, 25 K^+, 49 Cl^-, 25 lact., 5 Mg^{2+}, 7 PO^{4-}	Treatment of polyionic parenteral replacement caused by vomiting-induced alkalosis, diabetic acidosis, fluid loss from burns, and postoperative FVD.

From *Fluids and Electrolytes with Clinical Applications: A Programmed Approach* (7th ed.), by J. Kee, B. Paulanka, and C. Polek, 2009, Clifton Park, NY: Delmar Cengage Learning.

LIFE SPAN CONSIDERATIONS

Site for Administering an IM Injection

- For infants and toddlers, use the vastus lateralis site. Select a 22- to 25-gauge needle, ⅝ to 1 inch long. No more than 1 mL is injected into the muscle of a small child and 0.5 mL in an infant (Daniels, Grendell, & Wilkins, 2010). Obtain assistance to hold the infant and child still during an injection.
- For children older than 3 years of age and for adults, the deltoid, dorsogluteal area, or ventrogluteal area may be used. Select a 22 to 25 gauge needle ½ to 1½ inches long (Pope, 2002).
- An older client may have less muscle mass and require a shorter needle (Daniels, Grendell, & Wilkins, 2010).

Equipment Intravenous equipment is disposable, sterile, and prepackaged with user instructions. The user instructions, including a schematic labeling the parts, are usually placed on the outside of the package, which allows the user to read the package before opening. IV equipment requires sterile technique when handling because it is in direct contact with fluids to be infused into the bloodstream.

The administration (infusion) set includes an insertion spike with a protective cap, a drip chamber, tubing with a slide clamp and regulating (roller) clamp, a rubber injection port, and a protective cap over the needle adapter (Figure 25-13). Protective caps keep both ends of the set sterile and are removed only when used. The insertion spike is inserted into the port of the IV solution container.

There are two types of drip chambers: a macrodrip, which releases 10 to 20 drops per milliliter of solution, and a microdrip, which releases 60 drops per milliliter. The drop rate, which varies with the manufacturer, is indicated on the package.

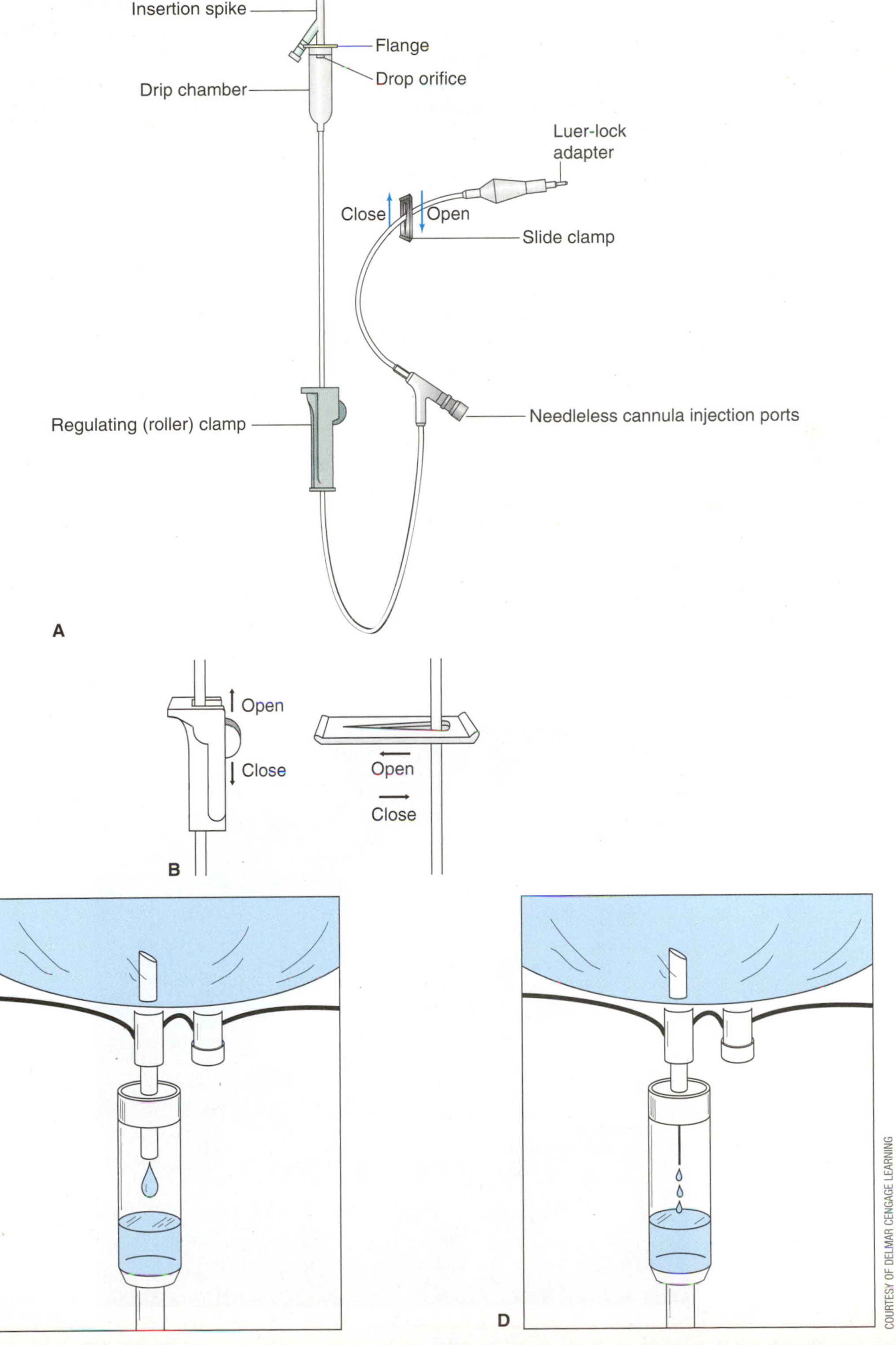

FIGURE 25-13 ***A,*** **Basic IV Administration Set;** ***B,*** **Regulating Roller Clamp and Slide Clamp;** ***C,*** **Macrodrip Chamber;** ***D,*** **Microdrip Chamber**

The roller clamp compresses the plastic tubing to control the flow rate. At the end of the IV tubing is a needle adapter that connects to a sterile injection device inserted into the client's vein. Extension tubing may be used to lengthen the primary tubing or provide additional Y-injection ports for administering additional solutions.

Intravenous Filters Intravenous filters remove particulate matter that may cause irritation and **phlebitis** (inflammation of a vein) from the solution. Intravenous filters come in various sizes. An in-line filter is found in many IV catheters. Then, it is not necessary to add a filter to the tubing.

Needles and Catheters Needles and catheters provide access to the venous system. A variety of devices of different sizes to accommodate the age of the client and the type and duration of therapy are available (Figure 25-14). The larger the number, the smaller the lumen of the needle or catheter; a 20 is larger than a 28.

Butterfly (scalp vein or wing-tipped) **needles** are short, beveled needles with plastic wings attached to the shaft. The wings (which are flexible) are held tightly together to facilitate needle insertion and then are flattened against the skin and taped to prevent dislodgment. These are generally used for short-term or intermittent therapy and for infants and children.

Several types of catheters are used to access peripheral veins. Some of these catheters are threaded over a needle, and others are threaded inside a needle during insertion. **Intracath** refers to a plastic tube inserted into a vein. An **angiocatheter** (angiocath, for short) is a type of intracath with a metal stylet to pierce the skin and vein, then the plastic catheter is threaded into the vein and the metal stylet removed.

Needle-Free System Safety is a concern with IV therapy. Accidental needlestick injuries and puncture wounds with contaminated devices increase the employee's risk for infectious diseases such as AIDS, hepatitis (B and C), and other viral, rickettsial, bacterial, fungal, and parasitic infections. Many health care facilities use totally needle-free IV systems to increase employee safety (Figure 25-15).

Vascular Access Devices Vascular access devices (VADs) include various cannulas, catheters, and infusion ports that allow long-term IV therapy or repeated access to the central venous system. The client's diagnosis and the type and length

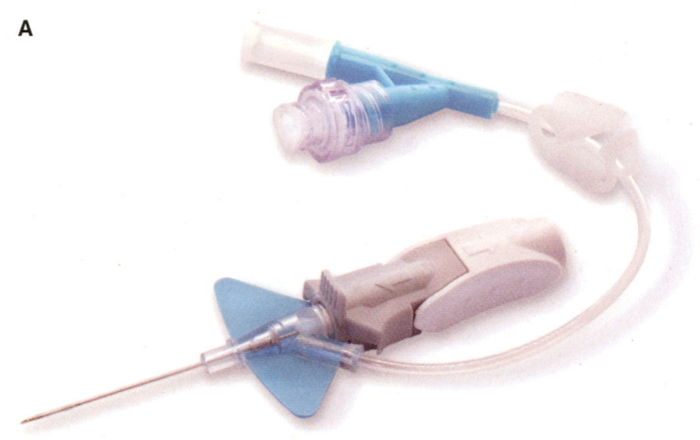

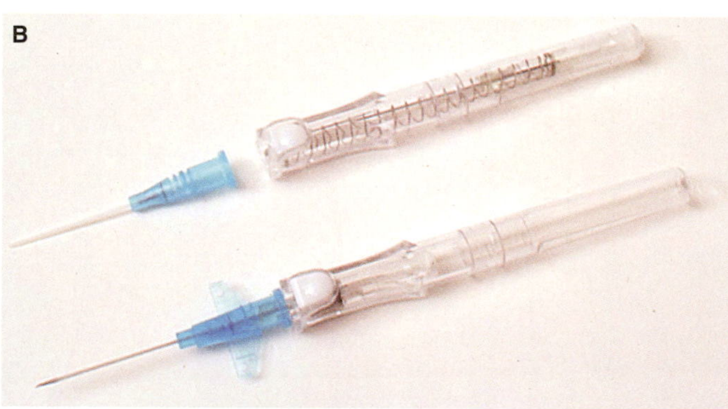

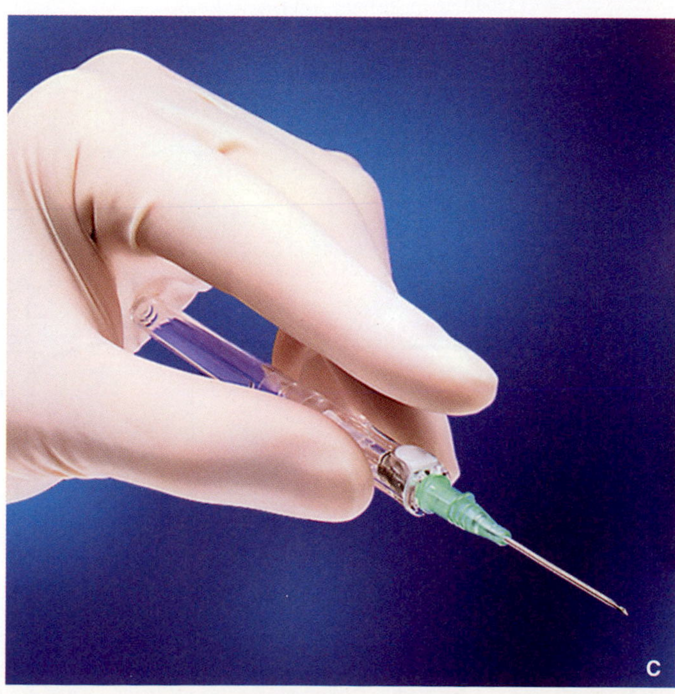

FIGURE 25-14 Peripheral IV Devices; *A*, Butterfly Closed IV catheter system; *B*, Autoguard Shielded IV Catheter; *C*, IV Catheter System Held Between Thumb and Middle Finger for Insertion (*All images courtesy and copyright Becton, Dickinson and Company.*)

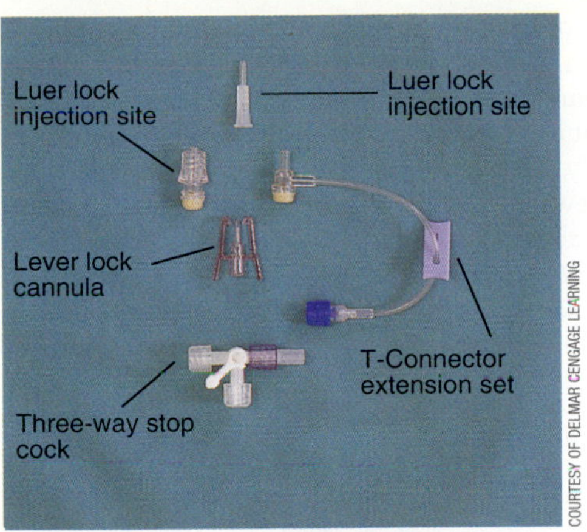

FIGURE 25-15 Needle-Free IV Systems

of treatment determine the kind of VAD used. Central venous catheters (CVCs) are inserted by a physician or an intravenous infusion nurse.

The **implantable port** (a device made of a radiopaque silicone catheter and a plastic or stainless steel injection port with a self-sealing silicone-rubber septum) is another type of VAD. *Only nurses who are specially trained are allowed to access an implanted port because of the risk of infiltration into the tissue if needle placement is incorrect.*

Preparing an Intravenous Solution Before preparing an IV solution, first read the physician's order and the agency's protocol, then gather necessary equipment. Because IV solutions and equipment are sterile, the package expiration date should be checked before use. The IV can be prepared in the client's room or in a nurses' work area.

The IV infusion rate is generally regulated by an infusion pump. Sometimes a time strip is applied to the IV solution bag as a safety check for the infusion pump or to monitor that the infusion rate is the rate prescribed by the physician if an infusion pump is not used (Figure 25-16). Tag the IV tubing

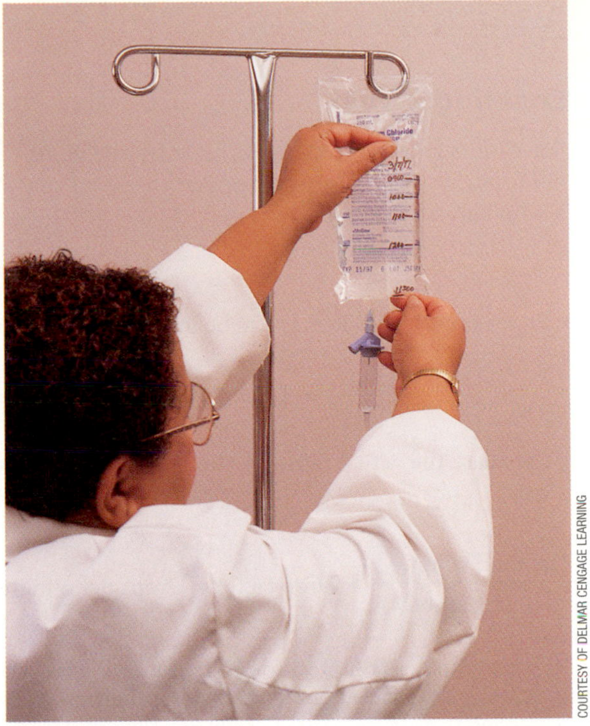

FIGURE 25-16 Applying a Time Strip to the IV Container

with the date and time to notify when the tubing needs to be replaced. Intravenous tubing is changed every 24 to 48 hours according to agency policy. The time strip and the IV tubing tag should be initiated by the nurse.

Initiating IV Therapy Before starting IV therapy, consider the type of fluid to be infused, calculate the flow rate, and assess for a venipuncture site. Altman (2009) suggests that the smallest gauge and shortest needle appropriate be selected (20 to 22 gauge for maintenance fluids and routine antibiotics, 18 to 19 gauge for blood products).

Calculating Flow Rate The physician prescribes the **flow rate**, the volume of fluid to infuse over a set period. For example, 125 mL per hour or 1,000 mL over an 8-hour period. The hourly infusion rate is calculated as follows:

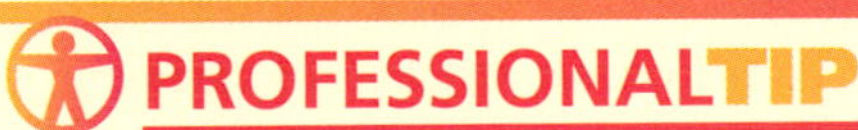

$$\frac{\text{Total volume}}{\text{Number of hours to infuse}} = \text{mL/hour infusion rate}$$

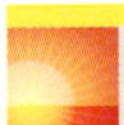

LIFE SPAN CONSIDERATIONS

Selecting Needle Gauge

Consider the client's age and body size and the type of solution to be administered when selecting the gauge of the needle or catheter.

- Infants and small children, 24 gauge
- Preschool through preteen, 24 or 22 gauge
- Teenagers and adults, 22 or 20 gauge
- Elderly, 24 or 22 gauge

PROFESSIONALTIP

Inserting a CVC

When assisting with the insertion of a long-line central catheter, observe the client for symptoms of a pneumothorax:

- sudden shortness of breath or sharp chest pain
- increased anxiety
- a weak, rapid pulse
- hypotension
- pallor or cyanosis

These symptoms indicate accidental puncture of the pleural membrane.

SAFETY

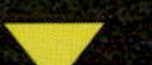

Marking an IV Bag

The ink from a felt-tip pen can leak through the plastic and contaminate the solution. Do not use such a pen.

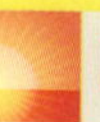

LIFE SPAN CONSIDERATIONS

Locating a Vein

For clients who are elderly or have fragile veins, eliminate the tourniquet or apply it very loosely if a vein can be palpated.

For example, if 1,000 mL is to be infused over 8 hours:

$$\frac{1{,}000}{8} = 125 \text{ mL/hour}$$

Calculate the actual infusion rate (drops per minute) as follows:

$$\frac{\text{Total fluid volume}}{\text{Total time (minutes)}} \times \text{Drop factor} = \text{Drops per minute}$$

For example, if 1,000 mL is to be infused over 8 hours with a tubing drop factor of 10 drops per milliliter:

$$\frac{1{,}000 \text{ mL}}{8(60)\text{min}} \times 10 \text{ drops/mL} = \frac{10{,}000 \text{ drops}}{480 \text{ min}} = \begin{matrix}20.8 \text{ or } 21\\ \text{drops/min}\end{matrix}$$

Another way to calculate the actual infusion rate is to use the hourly infusion rate; for the first example:

$$\frac{125 \text{ mL} \times 10 \text{ drops/mL}}{60 \text{ min}} = 20.8 \text{ or } 21 \text{ drops/min}$$

Consider body size, age, skin condition, clinical status, and impairments when assessing for a potential IV site. Venipuncture site contraindications are as follows:

- Any signs of infection, infiltration, or thrombosis
- Affected arm of a postmastectomy client
- Arm with a functioning arteriovenous fistula (dialysis)
- A paralyzed arm
- Arm with circulatory or neurological impairments

Because venous blood flows upward toward the heart, select a vein for an IV at its most distal end to maintain the integrity of the vein. When a vein is punctured with a needle, fluids can infiltrate (leak from the vein into the tissue at the site of puncture). When IV therapy is discontinued for infiltration, it can only be restarted above the initial puncture site. Generally, it is best to begin with the hand and advance up the arm if new sites are needed. Figure 25-17 illustrates common peripheral sites for initiating IV therapy.

Locating a Vein With the client's arm extended on a firm surface, place a tourniquet on the arm, tight enough to impede venous flow yet loose enough that a radial pulse can still be pal-

PROFESSIONALTIP

Setting Volume to Be Infused

When setting the volume to be infused (e.g., 1,000 mL), set it slightly lower (e.g., 950 mL) so that the alarm goes off before the fluids are completely gone. This practice provides time to have the next bag of fluids ready when all 1,000 mL have been infused. This is especially helpful when having to warm refrigerated fluids. Report to the next shift that the alarm is set to go off early.

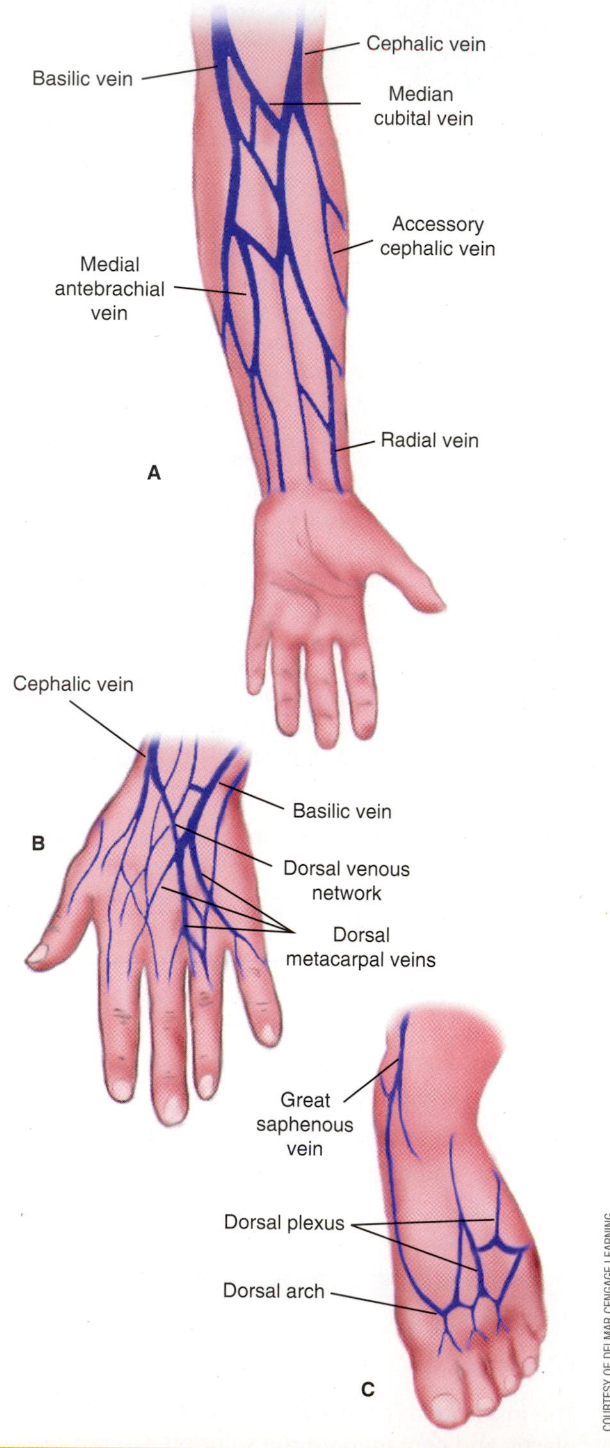

FIGURE 25-17 **Peripheral Veins Used in Intravenous Therapy; *A*, Foreman; *B*, Dorsum of the Hand; *C*, Dorsal Plexus of the Foot**

INFECTION CONTROL

Venipuncture

Standard Precautions must be followed when performing a venipuncture.

pated. Next, the index and middle fingers of the nondominant hand are used to palpate a vein. It should feel soft and resilient and not have a pulse. If no vein can be seen or felt, a warm, moist compress may be applied for 10 to 20 minutes, the area may be massaged toward the heart, or the client may open and close the fist (Berman, Snyder, Kozier, & Erb, 2008; Jensen, 2008a).

Placing the Needle After hand hygiene and gloving is completed, prepare the selected site according to agency policy. Without touching the prepared site, stabilize the vein by placing the thumb of the nondominant hand beside the vein and pulling down, making the skin taut. This technique also makes the needle insertion less painful. Hold the needle at a 10- to 30-degree angle, bevel up to puncture the skin, then lessen the angle to prevent puncturing the back of the vein (Berman et al., 2008; Ellenberger, 1999; Jensen, 2008a). Secure the needle in place according to agency policy.

Administering IV Therapy When the solution has been prepared and the rate calculated, explain the procedure to the client. Administration may be continuous over a 24-hour period, or intermittent, 1,000 mL once in a 24-hour period. Although fluids may be continuous, the type of fluids can change over a 24-hour period. For example, a physician's order might read for the pharmacy to: *Add 40 mEq of KCl to first bag of 1,000 mL of normal saline.*

Intravenous medications may be **piggybacked**, connected to an existing IV to infuse concurrently. Refrigerated solutions and medications should be warmed to room temperature before administration (usually for 30 minutes) for client comfort.

Regulating IV Solution Flow Rate The flow rate for IV solutions can be regulated by calculating the drops per minute and adjusting the drip rate to that number or by the use of volume controllers and pumps (Figure 25-18).

Volume Controllers and Pumps Controllers are devices dependent on gravity to maintain a preselected flow but do not add pressure to overcome resistance (e.g., Dial-a-Flo or Buretrol). Resistance may develop from the use of a large catheter in a small vein, high venous pressure, infusing a viscous solution, or a decrease in the height of the container from the IV site. Resistance causing a decrease in the flow will sound the controller alarm. Volumetric controllers permit flow rates to be set in milliliters per hour.

Pumps maintain a preselected volume delivery by adding pressure when needed. Pumps may be used when large volumes must be delivered in a short period and for viscous fluids. Pumps have maximum pressure limits that sound an alarm when reached. When a drug or solution is administered under high pressure, clients have a greater risk for complications.

Managing IV Therapy Intravenous therapy requires frequent client monitoring to ensure an accurate flow rate. Other nursing actions are to ensure client comfort and position; check the IV solution to ensure that the solution, amount, and timing are correct; monitor expiration dates of the IV system (tubing, venipuncture site, dressing) and change as necessary; and be aware of safety factors.

Client care is coordinated with the maintenance of IV lines. If the facility does not have snaps or Velcro on the gown sleeves, changing the gown and IV tubing when doing site care decreases the number of times the access device is

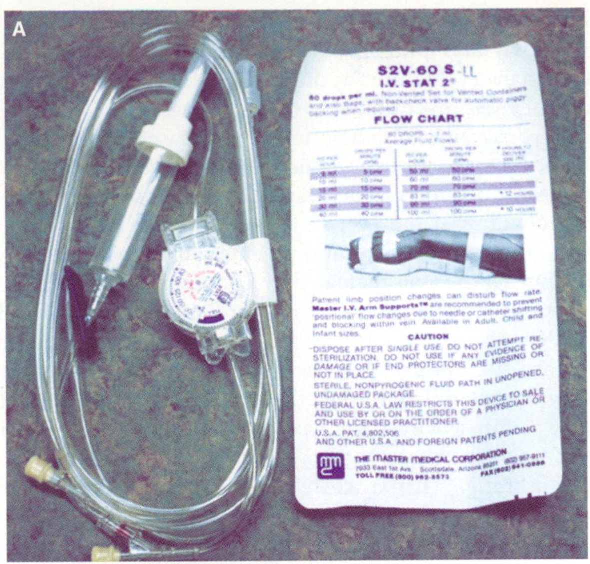

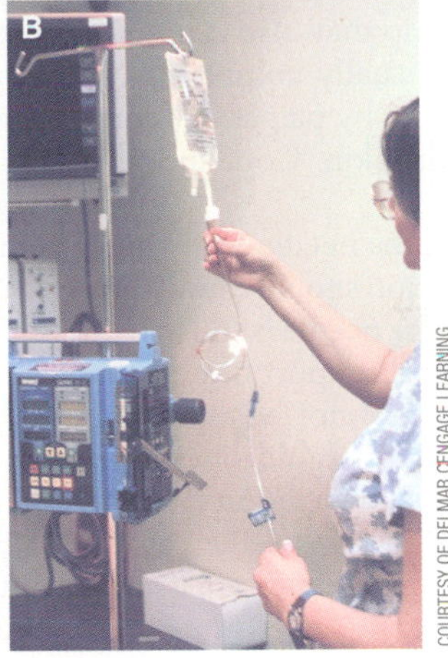

COURTESY OF DELMAR CENGAGE LEARNING

FIGURE 25-18 ***A,*** **Dial-A-Flo In-Line Device to Regulate IV Flow;** ***B,*** **Infusion Pumps Programmed for Specific IV Fluid Volumes and Medication Administration Set Rates**

PROFESSIONALTIP

IV-Related Sepsis

If a client has chills and fever, check how long the IV solution has been hanging and the needle or catheter has been in place. Assess the client's vital signs and for other symptoms of pyrogenic reactions, such as backache, malaise, headache, nausea, and vomiting. If IV-related sepsis occurs, the pulse rate increases, and temperature is usually above 100°F. Stop the infusion, notify the physician, and obtain blood specimens if ordered.

manipulated. This client care action decreases the risk for infiltration and phlebitis. Peripherally inserted devices are changed every 72 hours as directed by the Centers for Disease Control and Prevention (CDC) guidelines.

Hypervolemia **Hypervolemia** (increased circulating fluid volume) may result from rapid IV infusion of solutions, causing cardiac overload, which can lead to pulmonary edema and cardiac failure. If the IV rate is not regulated by a pump, the infusion rate must be monitored hourly to prevent these complications. If the IV is regulated by a pump, check that the rate is flowing correctly on clients at risk for fluid volume overload.

When a solution infuses at a rate greater than prescribed, decrease the rate to *keep vein open* (KVO) and immediately notify the physician. Report the amount and type of solution that was infused over the exact time period and the client's response.

Infiltration **Infiltration** (inadvertent administration of a nonvesicant solution into surrounding tissue) may result from dislodging the device from the vein, inserting the wrong type of device, or using the wrong-gauge needle. Using a high pressure pump may also cause infiltration or vein irritation. The client usually complains of discomfort at the IV site. Inspect the site by palpating for swelling and feeling the temperature of the skin. Cool and pale skin is an indication of infiltration.

Confirm that the needle is still in the vein by pinching the IV tubing. This action should cause **flashback** (blood will rush into the tubing if the needle is still in the vein). If flashback does not occur, the injection port nearest the device is aspirated by an RN. If the port cannot be aspirated, the IV has infiltrated. Follow the institution's guidelines when there is a suspected infiltration, such as notifying an IV nurse or charge nurse. If an infiltration occurred, the needle or catheter is removed from the vein and a sterile dressing applied to the puncture site.

The puncture site may ooze or bleed after the IV has been removed (especially in clients receiving anticoagulants). If oozing or bleeding occurs, apply pressure until it stops and reapply a sterile dressing. Accurately assess and document the degree of edema.

Injury may occur from infiltration. If an IV site is grossly infiltrated, the soft tissue edema may cause nerve compression with permanent loss of function to the extremity. **Extravasation** is the inadvertent administration of a **vesicant** (medication that causes blistering and tissue injury when it escapes from the blood vessel) into surrounding tissue. This may cause significant tissue loss with permanent disfigurement and loss of function (Hadaway, 2002a).

Phlebitis Phlebitis may result from either mechanical or chemical trauma. Inserting a device with too large a gauge, using a vein that is too small or fragile, or leaving the device in place for too long may cause mechanical trauma. Chemical trauma may result from infusing too rapidly or from an acidic solution, hypertonic solution, a solution containing electrolytes (especially potassium and magnesium) or other medications.

Phlebitis may be a precursor of sepsis. Client descriptions of tenderness are usually the first indication of an inflammation. The IV site must be inspected for changes in skin color and temperature (a reddened area or a pink or red stripe along the vein, warmth, and swelling are indications of phlebitis).

If phlebitis is present, the IV infusion must be discontinued. Before removing and discarding the venous device, check the facility's protocol to see whether the tip of the device is to be cultured. If so, it is sent to the laboratory for a culture and sensitivity test. After removing the device, apply a sterile dressing to the site and wet, warm compresses to the affected area. Document the time, symptoms, and nursing interventions.

Intravenous Dressing Change Standard Precautions and aseptic technique are followed for intravenous dressing changes. The frequency of care is determined by institutional protocol and the type of intravenous access device and dressing. Persistent drainage at the IV site may require more frequent dressing changes or may necessitate changing the IV site.

Intravenous Drug Therapy When a rapid drug effect is desired or a medication is irritating to tissue, the IV route is used. Intravenous administration immediately releases medication into the bloodstream; therefore, it can be dangerous. Intravenous medications are administered by one of the following modes:

- Intravenous fluid container
- Volume-control administration set
- Intermittent infusion by piggyback or partial fill
- Intravenous push (IVP or bolus)

Adding Drugs to an Intravenous Fluid Container Before administering IV medications, assess the patency of the infusion system and the condition of the injection site for signs of infiltration and phlebitis. Some IV medications or solutions with high or low pH or high osmolarity are irritating to veins and can cause phlebitis. Also note the client's allergies, drug or solution incompatibilities, the amount and type of diluent needed to mix the medication, and the client's general condition to establish a baseline before administering medication. **Drug incompatibilities** are an undesired chemical or physical reaction between a drug and a solution, between a drug and the container or tubing, or between two drugs. For example, diazepam (Valium) and chlordiazepoxide hydrochloride (Librium) are not compatible with a saline solution; insulin sticks to the inside of the solution bag, so use glass bottles.

Adding Drugs to a Volume-Control Administration Set

A volume-control set is used to administer small volumes of IV solution. They have various names, such as Soluset, Metriset, VoluTrol, or Buretrol. To use this method, do the following:

- Withdraw the prescribed amount of medication into a syringe
- Cleanse the injection port of a partially filled volume-control set with an alcohol swab
- Inject the prepared medication through the port of the volume-control set
- Gently mix the solution in the volume-control chamber
- Check the infusion rate and adjust as necessary

Administering Medications by Intermittent Infusion A common method of administering IV medications is by using a secondary, or partial-fill additive bag, often called IV piggyback (IVPB). The secondary line is a complete IV set (fluid container and tubing with either a microdrip or a macrodrip system) connected to a Y-port of a primary line. The primary line maintains venous access. The IVPB is used for medication administration. When the IVPB medication is incompatible with the primary IV solution, flush the primary IV tubing with normal saline before and after administering the medication. Another method of infusing a medication that is incompatible with the primary line is to disconnect the primary line from the IV catheter, flush the catheter, connect the secondary set IV tubing to the IV catheter and infuse the medication.

Intermittent Infusion Devices When the client requires only IV medications without a quantity of solution, an intermittent infusion device is attached to a peripheral needle or catheter in the client's vein. This device is commonly referred to as a heparin or saline lock, depending on the facility's policy of heparin or saline maintenance. A lock provides continuous venous access, eliminating the need for a continuous IV and increasing the client's mobility.

The device is used to infuse intermittent IVPB or IV push (also called bolus) medications, or it can be converted to a primary IV. An **IV push (bolus)** is the administration of a large dose of medication in a relatively short time, usually 1 to 30 minutes. A saline lock device provides venous access in case of an emergency and is routinely used with cardiac clients.

Administering IV Push Medications An IV push medication can be injected into a saline or a heparin lock (Figure 25-19A) or into a continuous infusion line. When giving an IV push medication into a continuous infusion line, stop the fluids in the primary line by pinching the IV tubing closed while injecting the drug (Figure 25-19B). This technique is safe and prevents having to recalculate the drip rate of the primary infusion line.

Documentation

When IV therapy is begun, the date, time, venipuncture site, number of attempts made, amount and type of fluid, and equipment used must be documented. Each time the insertion site, venipuncture device, or IV tubing is changed, the reason for the change must be documented (e.g., routine, infiltration). The condition of the insertion site and the fluid type, amount, and flow rate are documented each shift and at intervals specified by agency policy. Any complications are precisely documented along with the nurse's actions.

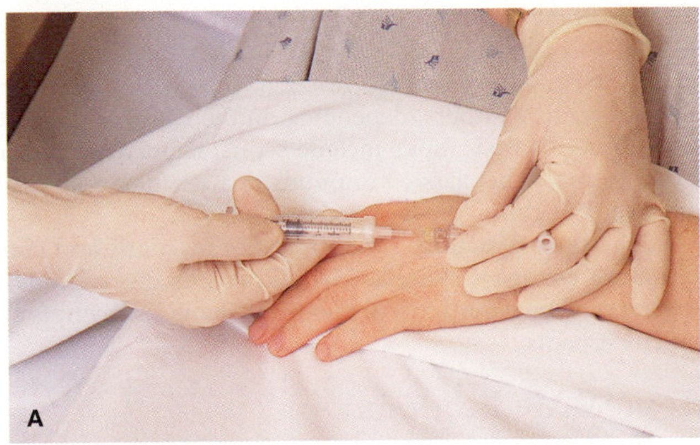

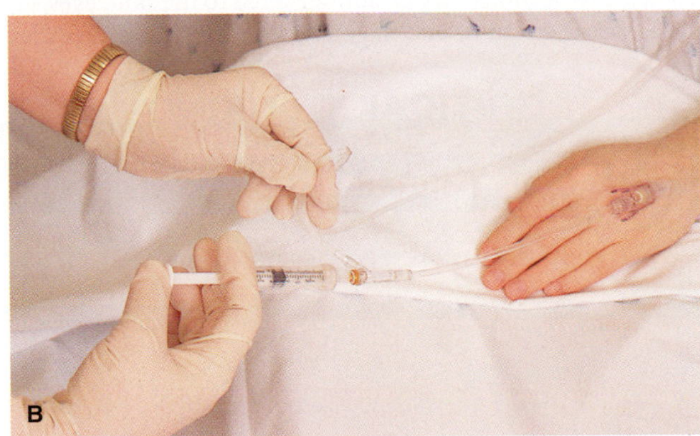

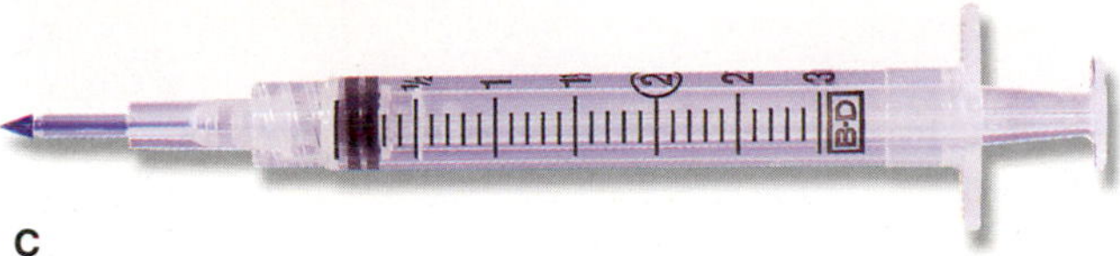

FIGURE 25-19 **Injecting an IV Push (Bolus) Medication; *A*, Into a peripheral saline lock; *B*, Into a primary infusion line. The IV tubing must be pinched closed first; *C*, A needleless syringe to give intravenous medications.** (*Images A and B courtesy of Delmar Cengage Learning. Image C courtesy and copyright Becton, Dickson and Company.*)

PROFESSIONALTIP

New Process for Blood Transfusions

A new process developed by a team of researchers produces an enzyme that strips the A and B antigens from the red blood cell, making the blood useful for all blood types. Commercial production of these enzymes will help make blood transfusion safer by reducing the need for stringent blood typing and matching procedures, eliminating the risk of hemolytic transfusion reactions. The blood supply could be distributed more efficiently and less blood wasted; persons with rare blood types would be able to receive any blood type after the enzyme antigen stripping process (Liu et al., 2007).

Blood Transfusion

A blood transfusion is given to replace blood loss (deficit) with whole blood or blood components. Based on the client's unique needs, the physician determines the type of transfusion, either whole blood or a component of whole blood.

Whole Blood and Blood Products Whole blood contains red blood cells (RBCs) and plasma components of blood. It is used when all the components of blood are needed to restore blood volume and to restore the oxygen-carrying capacity of the blood.

When the physician prescribes whole blood or a blood product, the client's blood is typed and cross matched. If time and the client's condition permit, the family may arrange for donors. The blood is stored in the blood bank after typing and cross matching.

Whole blood has a refrigerated shelf life of 35 days, but platelets must be administered within 3 days after extracted from whole blood. If the RBCs and plasma are frozen, their shelf life is up to 3 years (Kee & Paulanka, 2009).

Initial Assessment and Preparation Perform an initial assessment before administering blood that includes the following:

- Verify that the client has signed a blood administration consent form and that this consent matches what the physician has prescribed.
- Identify the gauge of needle or catheter used if IV in place. The viscosity of whole blood usually requires an 18-gauge needle or catheter to prevent red blood cell damage. If blood is to be infused quickly, a 14- or 15-gauge device must be used.
- Ensure patency of the existing IV site.

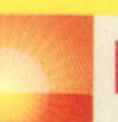

LIFE SPAN CONSIDERATIONS

Initial Assessment

If pediatric, elderly, or clients with congestive heart failure or malnutrition are at risk for circulatory overload, notify the blood bank to divide the 500-mL bag of blood into two 250-mL bags or discuss with the physician other alternatives, such as packed RBCs rather than whole blood.

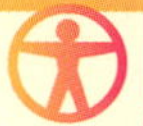

PROFESSIONALTIP

Transfusion Reaction

Transfusion reaction severity is related to the time of onset. Severe reactions usually occur shortly after the blood begins to infuse. At the first sign of a reaction, stop the blood infusion immediately.

- Establish vital signs baseline data, especially temperature, and assess skin for eruptions or rashes.
- Verify label on the whole blood or blood component with the client's blood type before administration, to ensure compatibility. Some facilities require two nurses to verify that the client's name and blood type match the name and blood type on the transfusion bag.
- Assess the client's age and state of nutrition.

Scheduled IV medications should be infused before blood administration to prevent a medication reaction while blood is infusing. If a reaction were to occur, it would not be known whether the medication or the blood was causing the reaction.

Administering Whole Blood or a Blood Component A facility's blood protocol may require that a licensed person sign a release for blood from the blood bank and that two licensed personnel check blood products before infusion. Information that must be on the blood bag label and verified for accuracy includes the client's name and identification number, ABO group and Rh factor, donor number, type of product ordered, and expiration date.

To maintain RBC integrity and decrease the chance of infection, blood administration should begin within 30 minutes after it is received from the bank. Whole blood should not be unrefrigerated for more than 4 hours. Room temperature causes RBC lysis, releasing potassium and causing hyperkalemia.

SAFETY

Blood Transfusion Incompatibilities

Only 0.9% normal saline can be used with a blood product. Blood transfusions are incompatible with dextrose and with Ringer's solution.

Safety Measures Observe the client for the initial 15 minutes for a transfusion reaction. Take vital signs every 15 minutes for the first hour, then every hour while the blood is infusing.

The three basic types of transfusion reactions are allergic, febrile, and hemolytic and may be mild or severe, depending on the cause. Hemolytic reactions may be immediate or delayed up to 96 hours, depending on the cause of the reaction. Other complications include sepsis, hypervolemia, and hypothermia. The classic symptoms of a reaction and sepsis are fever and chills.

The nursing actions for all types of reactions and complications are given in Table 25-7. Table 25-8 gives details of several transfusion reactions, etiologies, signs and symptoms, and treatments.

Topical Medications

Topical medications may be administered to the skin, eyes, ears, nose, throat, rectum, and vagina. The medication provides a

CRITICAL THINKING

Transfusion Reactions

How can transfusion reactions be differentiated?

TABLE 25-7 Nursing Actions for Blood Reactions

IMMEDIATE NURSING ACTION	OTHER MEASURES
• Stop transfusion. • Keep vein open with 0.9% normal saline. • Notify the physician.	• Monitor client's vital signs every 15 minutes for 4 hours or until stable. • Monitor I&O. • Send IV tubing and bag of blood back to the blood bank. • Obtain a blood and urine specimen. • Label specimen "Blood Transfusion Reaction." • Process a transfusion reaction report.

COURTESY OF DELMAR CENGAGE LEARNING

TABLE 25-8 Transfusion Reactions, Etiologies, Signs and Symptoms, and Treatments

REACTION	ETIOLOGY	SIGN AND SYMPTOMS	TREATMENTS
		ACUTE	
Acute hemolytic transfusion reaction (intravascular hemolysis)	Incompatible blood product transfused because of errors during processing the blood products and the type and cross match	Fever, low back pain, pain at IV site, hypotension, tachycardia, abdominal pain, dyspnea, nausea/vomiting, rash/hives, headache, anxiety, renal failure	Stop the transfusion immediately Keep the vein open with a 0.9% normal saline IV Contact physician stat Support vital functions—may require hemodialysis Complete lab tests necessary to determine if blood reaction occurred
Nonhemolytic transfusion reaction	Reaction to donor leukocytes in the blood products	Fever, anemia, increased bilirubin levels	Give premedications to reduce reaction: acetaminophen, diphenydramine, hydrocortisone
Allergic reactions	Recipient antibodies against donor antigens (foreign proteins)	Itching to rashes to anaphylaxis and shock	Stop the transfusion, treat with antihistamines, may resume slowly when symptoms resolved
Transfusion-related acute lung injury (TRALI)	Anti-HLA antibodies and neutrophil antibodies	Acute respiratory insufficiency, chills, fever, cyanosis, hypotension	Support respiratory function, IV steroids
Bacterial contamination of blood product	Endotoxins from gram-negative and gram-positive bacteria	Fever, shock, disseminated intravascular coagulation (DIC), renal failure	High-dose antibiotics, vital organ support, steroids
Circulatory overload	Too rapid a flow rate for client's cardiovascular system	Dyspnea, cough, frothy sputum	Support respiratory system, administer diuretic between units, slower infusion rates for clients with known cardiovascular compromise
Citrate toxicity	Hypocalcemia resulting from citrate binding with calcium in the recipient's bloodstream	Tetany	Monitor for signs and symptoms, monitor calcium level, transfuse extra calcium, if warranted
		DELAYED	
Graft-versus-host disease	Lymphocytes infused with blood product into an immunosuppressed recipient	Fever, hepatitis, bone marrow suppression, overwhelming infection, 90% to 100% mortality rate	Pretransfusion radiation of blood products containing lymphocytes preventing replication of donor lymphocytes and the engrafting process
Disease transmitted with the blood product: bacterial, syphilis, protozoal, viral	Contamination during processing, preexisting donor infection, contamination during donation	Depends on disease transmitted	Careful aseptic technique through all portions of donation and transfusion, careful screening of donors and testing blood products for viruses
Delayed hemolytic reaction	Reaction to donor antibodies	None to fever, mild jaundice and anemia	Conduct additional antibody testing prior to additional blood transfusions
Iron overload	Repeated blood transfusions for chronic anemic conditions, such as sickle cell anemia	Liver failure Cardiac toxicities	Infuse chelation treatment, Desferal®, to bind to iron and remove from system, monitor iron level routinely

COURTESY OF DELMAR CENGAGE LEARNING

local effect but may also have systemic effects. Drugs applied directly to the skin for a local effect include lotions, pastes, creams, ointments, powders, and aerosol sprays. The vascularity of the area determines the rate and degree of the drug's absorption.

Topical drugs provide continuous absorption to produce various effects: to relieve pruritus (itching), to prevent or treat an infection, to provide local anesthesia, to protect the skin, or to create a systemic effect. Topical medications are usually applied two or three times a day to achieve their therapeutic effect.

Before applying a topical preparation, the condition of the skin is assessed for any rashes, open lesions, or areas of erythema and skin breakdown. The nurse checks with the client and the medical record for any known allergies.

Cleanse the area by washing it with soap and warm water, unless contraindicated by a specific order. Allow the skin to thoroughly dry before applying a topical medication. Open wounds require the use of aseptic technique.

When the skin is dry, the medication is applied. To apply a paste, cream, or an ointment, follow Standard Precautions. To prevent cross contamination, use a sterile tongue depressor for removing the medication from the container. Transfer the medication from the tongue blade to a gloved hand for application. Apply the medication in long, smooth strokes in the direction of the hair follicles to prevent the medication from entering the hair follicles. When more medication is removed from the container, a new sterile tongue depressor is used. Assess the area for signs of an allergic reaction 2 to 4 hours after the application.

Eye Medications Eye medications are in the form of drops, ointments, or disks. These drugs are used for diagnostic and therapeutic purposes, to lubricate the eye or socket for a prosthetic eye, and to treat or prevent eye conditions such as glaucoma (elevated pressure within the eye) and infection. Diagnostically, eyedrops are used to dilate the pupil, anesthetize the eye, or stain the cornea to identify abrasions and scars.

Medication disks are inserted at bedtime because they usually cause blurred vision. Follow Standard Precautions when administering eye care and medications; there is a potential for contact with bodily secretions.

Ear Medications Solutions ordered for the ear are often called *otic* (pertaining to the ear) drops or irrigations. Eardrops are instilled to soften ear wax, treat infection or inflammation, produce anesthesia, or facilitate removal of a foreign body.

SAFETY

Prevent Cross Contamination

- Never share a bottle of eyedrops between clients.
- After instillation, discard any solution remaining in the dropper.
- Discard the dropper if the tip is accidentally contaminated (i.e., touching the bottle or any part of the client's eye).

PROFESSIONALTIP

Preventing Systemic Effects of Eyedrops

- Apply pressure to the inner canthus when instilling eyedrops that have potential systemic effects, such as atropine and timolol maleate (Timoptic).
- Gentle pressure over the inner canthus prevents the medication from flowing into the tear duct, thereby decreasing the absorption rate of the drug.

External auditory canal irrigations are usually performed for cleansing purposes.

Inspect the ear for signs of drainage (an indication of a perforated tympanic membrane) before instilling a solution into the ear. Eardrops are usually contraindicated with a perforated tympanic membrane. Aseptic technique must be used if the tympanic membrane is damaged. Otherwise, medical asepsis is used for ear medications.

Nasal Instillations Nasal instillations can be either drops or nebulizers (atomizer or aerosol). Nasal drugs produce one or more of the following effects: shrink swollen mucous membranes, loosen secretions and facilitate drainage, or treat infections of the nasal cavity or sinuses. Because the nose is connected with the sinuses, medical asepsis is used when performing nasal instillations.

COMMUNITY/HOME HEALTH CARE

Considerations for Use of Nasal Inhalers

- The client should have the manufacturer's directions for the specific type of inhaler, such as how to replace a medication cartridge for a nasal aerosol.
- Inhalers are kept at room temperature.
- Aerosols are prepared under pressure, so do not puncture or place in an incinerator.
- No one but the client should use the inhaler.
- Caution that overuse can cause a rebound effect, making the condition worse.
- Ensure that the client knows the expected and adverse effects of the drug. Some of these drugs take several days to 2 weeks of continuous use for the effects to appear.
- Provide the client with a telephone number to call if assistance is needed.

Many of these products are nonprescription drugs, so clients should be taught their correct usage. Nasal decongestants are common over-the-counter drugs to shrink swollen mucous membranes; however, they may have a reverse or rebound effect by increasing nasal congestion when used in excess.

Nebulizers (inhalers) deliver a fine mist containing medication droplets. The client who is discharged with a nasal inhaler must be taught how to store and use the device. Assist clients in the use of atomizers and aerosols:

- Have the client clear the nostrils by blowing the nose.
- Client should be in an upright position with head tilted back slightly.

For atomizers:

- Occlude one nostril to prevent air from entering the nasal cavity and allow the medication to flow freely into the open nostril.
- Insert the atomizer tip into the open nostril and ask the client to inhale, while the atomizer is squeezed once, then ask the client to exhale.

For aerosols:

- Shake the aerosol well before each use.
- Grasp between thumb and index finger and insert the adapter tip into one nostril while occluding the other nostril with a finger, then press the adapter cartridge firmly to release one measured dose of medication.
- Repeat the above steps for the other nostril.
- Have the client keep the head tilted backward for 2 to 3 minutes and breathe through the nose while the medication is being absorbed.

Respiratory Inhalants Respiratory inhalants are delivered by devices that produce fine droplets to be inhaled deep into the respiratory tract. They are absorbed very quickly through the alveolar epithelium into the bloodstream. This section discusses only oropharyngeal handheld inhalers.

Oropharyngeal handheld inhalers deliver medications, such as bronchodilators and mucolytics, that produce both local and systemic effects. Bronchodilators (drugs that dilate the bronchi) improve airway patency and prevent or treat asthma, bronchospasms, and allergic reactions. Mucolytics liquify tenacious (thick) bronchial secretions.

Clients must be able to assemble the turbo-inhaler and form an airtight seal around the inhaling devices. This requirement prevents some clients from using these devices. Bronchodilators are contraindicated for clients with a history of tachycardia.

Rectal Instillations Rectal instillations are in the form of suppositories, ointments, or enemas. Rectal ointments treat local conditions and hemorrhoid symptoms of pain, inflammation, and itching. Rectal suppositories are cone-shaped medications designed to melt at body temperature and be absorbed at a slow and steady rate.

Suppositories are a convenient and safe route for administering drugs that interact poorly with digestive enzymes or have a bad taste or odor. They are used to provide temporary relief for clients who cannot tolerate oral preparations (e.g., to relieve nausea and vomiting). They are also used to reduce fever, relieve pain and local irritation, and stimulate peristalsis and defecation in clients who are constipated.

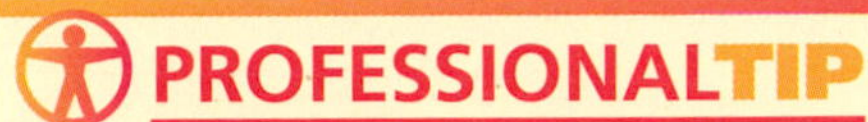

Contraindications for Rectal Suppositories

- Cardiac clients because insertion may stimulate the vagus nerve, causing cardiac dysrhythmias (abnormal heart patterns).
- Clients recovering from rectal or prostate surgery because suppositories may cause pain on insertion and trauma to the tissues.

The rectum should be assessed for irritation or bleeding and sphincter control checked. Some clients may have a problem retaining the suppository. Ask those clients to remain in Sims' position for at least 15 minutes or have the client lie on the abdomen, if allowed, and hold the buttocks closed. When the client is unable to retain a suppository, notify the physician so that another route can be ordered.

Vaginal Instillations Medications inserted into the vagina are suppositories, creams, ointments, gels, foams, or douches. They treat infections, inflammation, and discomfort or as a contraceptive measure.

Vaginal creams, gels, ointments, and foams usually come with a disposable applicator with a plunger to insert the drug. Suppositories are usually inserted with the index finger of a gloved hand; however, small suppositories may come with an applicator. After insertion of these preparations, the client may notice drainage and is told to expect this. To prevent soiling of the underpants, tell the client to wear a perineal pad.

Agency policy usually requires sterile technique when administering a vaginal douche (irrigation). Check that the client does not have an allergy to iodine because many vaginal preparations contain povidone-iodine.

EVALUATION

Administering medications according to the "seven rights" requires the nurse to verify that safe nursing care was provided. Evaluation includes that each client knows the effects, side effects, adverse reactions, special considerations, and when to call the physician for each drug.

A nurse identifying a potential medication risk and initiating actions to prevent client injury is performing another form of evaluation.

Tampon Use

Clients should not use tampons after the insertion of vaginal medications because the tampon can absorb the medication and decrease the drug's effect.

SAMPLE NURSING CARE PLAN

The Client with Deep Vein Thrombosis

M.L., a 45-year-old, was admitted to your floor with a diagnosis of deep vein thrombosis. She noticed swelling of her left leg about a week ago but decided to treat it at home. Four days later the lower leg was very edematous, warm, and painful to move. After an office visit, M.L. was admitted to the hospital. This is her first hospitalization. On examination the left leg is warmer than the right. The left thigh circumference is 3 inches larger than the right. The physician ordered a heparin IV drip after a loading dose bolus was given. The drip contained 10,000 units heparin in 500 mL of D_5W at 10 mL/hour (200 units/hour). The physician anticipates that M.L. will be weaned off the heparin drip and started on subcutaneous heparin within 5 days. At the time of discharge she will be given Coumadin.

NURSING DIAGNOSIS 1 *Ineffective Tissue Perfusion (peripheral)* related to the development of venous thrombi in the deep femoral vein as evidenced by left leg being warmer than right leg and left thigh circumference being 3 inches larger than right thigh circumference

Nursing Outcomes Classification (NOC)
Tissue Perfusion: Peripheral
Tissue Integrity

Nursing Interventions Classification (NIC)
Peripheral Sensation Management
Circulatory Care: Venous Insufficiency

PLANNING/OUTCOMES	NURSING INTERVENTIONS	RATIONALE
M.L. will report an absence of pain.	Maintain on bed rest.	Reduces the possibility of embolus; may decrease the pain and swelling.
	Apply moist heat to the affected extremity.	Provides an analgesic effect; it decreases venospasms and pain.
M.L. will have a decrease of edema.	Elevate the legs above the heart.	Facilitates venous return and decreases the edema.
	Measure the circumference of the left thigh and compare with that of the right thigh.	Provides a quantitative reference point that can be used to evaluate the swelling.
M.L. will experience the same degree of skin temperature in both legs.	Administer the heparin drip at 200 units/hour.	Prevents the conversion of fibrinogen to fibrin and prothrombin to thrombin, thereby limiting the extension of the thrombus.
	Monitor the partial thromboplastin time (PTT).	Monitors heparin therapy because heparin, a short-acting anticoagulant, increases the PTT.

EVALUATION

M.L. is able to ambulate without difficulty or pain. M.L.'s left thigh is only 1/2 inch larger than her right thigh. M.L.'s legs are the same temperature to touch.

SAMPLE NURSING CARE PLAN (Continued)

NURSING DIAGNOSIS 2 *Risk for Injury (bleeding)* related to the administration of an anticoagulant

Nursing Outcomes Classification (NOC)	Nursing Interventions Classification (NIC)
Risk Control	*Health Education*
Safety Behavior: Personal	*Medication Management*

PLANNING/OUTCOMES	NURSING INTERVENTIONS	RATIONALE
M.L. will not demonstrate evidence of bleeding from gums or nose, in urine or stool, or under the skin.	Withhold the medication in the event that bleeding occurs and to notify the physician immediately.	The dose may need to be adjusted.
	Encourage the client to discontinue smoking.	May increase the metabolism of the medication, necessitating an increase in the dose.
M.L. will maintain her prothrombin time (PT) or international normalized ratio (INR) within therapeutic range.	Advise the client to watch food intake.	Foods high in fat and foods rich in vitamin K can interfere with the PT.
	Warn against taking oral contraceptive medication.	Decreases anticoagulant effect.
	Warn against taking aspirin and other over-the-counter medications.	May increase the risk of bleeding; it inhibits platelet formation.

EVALUATION

M.L. has had no bleeding episodes. M.L. still has many questions about taking the oral anticoagulant on discharge. Discharge follow-up will be needed to monitor the client's progress on the oral anticoagulant.

SUMMARY

- The *United States Pharmacopeia* and the *National Formulary* list drug standards for use in the United States.
- The Food and Drug Administration tests all drugs before granting a company the right to market a drug.
- Drugs are usually referred to by their generic name (not capitalized) or by their trade name (always capitalized).
- The safest and least expensive administration route is the oral route, although it is also the slowest to act.
- Parenteral drugs are injected through intradermal (ID), subcutaneous, intramuscular (IM), or intravenous (IV) routes and are typically fast acting.
- The pharmacokinetics of drugs includes absorption, distribution, metabolism, and excretion.
- The "seven rights" of safe drug administration are right client, right drug, right dose, right route, right time, right documentation, and right to refuse.
- Nurses are legally and morally responsible for correct administration of medications.
- Although the physician determines the dose and route of a parenteral drug, the nurse chooses the correct gauge and length of the needle to be used.
- Always monitor client reactions to medications and ensure that clients know the actions, side effects, and contraindications of all medications they take.
- Clients receiving intravenous therapy or blood transfusions require constant monitoring for complications.

REVIEW QUESTIONS

1. A client is unable to swallow the pills ordered by the physician. The best action for the nurse is to:
   1. tell the client to chew the pills.
   2. crush the pills and give them to the client.
   3. call the physician for a change in the orders.
   4. ask the pharmacy to send the medications in liquid form.
2. The client is in the bathroom when the nurse brings the medications. The best action for the nurse is to:
   1. return with the medications when the client is finished in the bathroom.
   2. leave the medications for the client to take when finished in the bathroom.
   3. knock on the bathroom door and give the medications to the client at this time.
   4. ask the nursing assistant to see that the client takes the medications when finished in the bathroom.
3. The best time for the nurse to document medication administration is:
   1. whenever the nurse has time.
   2. before the client receives the medication.
   3. only after the client has received the medication.
   4. toward the end of the shift so all medications can be charted at one time.
4. Standard Precautions are required with: (Select all that apply.)
   1. venipuncture.
   2. IM injections.
   3. oral medications.
   4. nasal instillation.
   5. rectal instillations.
5. A client receiving a blood transfusion tells the nurse, who is taking the first set of 15-minute vital signs, that she is cold (chills) and her chest hurts. The first thing the nurse should do is:
   1. stop the transfusion.
   2. get a warm blanket for the client.
   3. call the blood bank to come and check the blood.
   4. stay with the client and talk quietly to her to help her relax.
6. A 76-year-old client has a peripheral IV infusing in her left arm. The nurse discovers all the following findings in her assessment. To what should the nurse react and treat immediately?
   1. The IV site is bruised without edema.
   2. The patient reports tingling in her hands and muscle cramping.
   3. The patient has a moist cough and distended neck veins.
   4. The patient's urine output was 150 mL for the past 8 hours.
7. The client is complaining of pain at her IV site. The nurse assesses the site and notes that there is a hard cord along the vein, diffuse redness, and slight edema. The nurse opts to remove the IV and does which nursing intervention?
   1. Cleanse the site carefully with chlorhexidine.
   2. Apply warm soaks.
   3. Culture the IV site.
   4. Elevate the extremity.
8. The healthcare provider orders benzylpencillin potassium (Penicillin G Potassium) 2.4 million units IM. The nurse chooses the equipment to administer the medication. The appropriate equipment is a:
   1. 3 mL syringe, a 22 gauge 2 inch long needle, gloves, and an antiseptic cleansing pad.
   2. 3 mL syringe, an 18 gauge 1 inch long needle, gloves, and an antiseptic cleansing pad.
   3. 3 mL syringe, a 22 gauge 5/8 inch long needle, gloves, and an antiseptic cleansing pad.
   4. 3 mL syringe, a 20 gauge short bevel needle, gloves, and an antiseptic cleansing pad.
9. A health care provider orders 2,000 mL D_5W over 24 hours. Drop factor is 10 gtts/mL. The IV should run at how many Run IV at gtts/minute?
   1. 1.4 gtts/min.
   2. 14 gtts/min.
   3. 83 gtts/min.
   4. 833 gtts/min.
10. A nurse gives a client her medications. The client states, "I usually only take 3 pills at 10 AM. Is there a reason I have 4 pills today?" The nurse's best response is:
    1. to state she has the correct number of pills for the client and request she take the pills.
    2. ask the client to wait one moment while she checks the orders again.
    3. to state that orders in the hospital are not always the same as when she is home and request the client take the medication.
    4. to check the orders and, after determining the client is to have 4 pills, explain the reason for the additional pill.

REFERENCES/SUGGESTED READINGS

About BD Integra™ Retracting Syringes. (2008). Retrieved September, 22, 2008, from http://www.bd.com/injection/products/integra

American Society of Health-System Pharmacists. (2008). *AHFS drug information 2008*. Bethesda, MD: Author.

Ampule Breaker/Collar. (2008). Retrieved September, 22, 2008, from http://www.sigmaaldrich.com/catalog/search/ProductDetail/ALDRICH/Z122904

Behrman, R., Kliegman, R., & Jenson, H. (Eds.). (2004). *Nelson textbook of pediatrics* (17th ed.). Philadelphia: W. B. Saunders.

Berman, A., Snyder, S., Kozier, B., & Erb, G. (2008). *Kozier and Erb's fundamental of nursing: Concepts, process, and practice* (8th ed.). Upper Saddle River, NJ: Pearson Prentice Hall.

Blanchard & Loeb. (2006). *Nurse's drug handbook 2006*. Philadelphia: Blanchard & Loeb Publishers, LLC.

Bulechek, G., Butcher, H., McCloskey, J., & Dochterman, J., eds. (2008). *Nursing Interventions Classification (NIC)* (5th ed.). St. Louis, MO: Mosby/Elsevier.

Carroll, P. (2003). Medication errors: The bigger picture. *RN, 66*(1), 52–57.

Charting Tips. (2000a). Documenting IV therapy, part I. *Nursing2000, 30*(2), 73.

Charting Tips. (2000b). Documenting IV therapy, part II. *Nursing2000, 30*(3), 83.

Daniels, R., Grendell, R., & Wilkins, F. (2010). *Nursing fundamentals: Caring and Clinical Decision Making* (2nd ed.). Clifton Park, NY: Delmar Cengage Learning.

Daniels, J., & Smith, L. (1999). *Clinical calculations* (4th ed.). Clifton Park, NY: Delmar Cengage Learning.

DeLaune, S., & Ladner, P. (2006). *Fundamentals of nursing* (3rd ed.). Clifton Park, NY: Delmar Cengage Learning.

Ellenberger, A. (1999). Starting an IV line. *Nursing99, 29*(3), 56–59.

Fitzpatrick, L., & Fitzpatrick, T. (1997). Blood transfusion: Keeping your patient safe. *Nursing97, 27*(8), 34–41

Giving Z-track injections. (2002). *Nursing2002, 32*(9), 81.

Goldy, D. (1998). Circulatory overload secondary to blood transfusion. *American Journal of Nursing, 98*(7), 33.

Hadaway, L. (1999a). Choosing the right vascular access device, part I. *Nursing99, 29*(2), 18.

Hadaway, L. (1999b). Choosing the right vascular access device, part II. *Nursing99, 29*(7), 28–29.

Hadaway, L. (2002a). IV infiltration: Not just a peripheral problem. *Nursing2002, 32*(8), 36–42.

Hadaway, L. (2002b). What you can do to decrease catheter-related infections. *Nursing2002, 32*(9), 46–48.

Hadaway, L. (2003). Infusing without infecting. *Nursing2003, 33*(10), 58–63.

Hrouda, B. (2002). Warming up to IV infusion. *Nursing2002, 32*(3), 54–55.

Jensen, B. (2008a). *Managing peripheral venous access.* Manuscript submitted for publication.

Jensen, B. (2008b). *Transfusing blood and blood products.* Manuscript submitted for publication.

Joint Commission. (2008). Official "do not use" list. Retrieved September 19, 2008, from http://www.jointommission.org/patientsafety/donotuselist

Josephson, D. (1999). *Intravenous infusion therapy for nurses: Principles and practice.* Clifton Park, NY: Delmar Cengage Learning.

Karch, A., & Karch, F. (2002). Double dosing. *American Journal of Nursing, 102*(10), 23.

Karch, A., & Karch, F. (2003). Not so fast. *American Journal of Nursing, 103*(8), 71.

Kee, J., Paulanka, B, & Polek, C. (2009). *Fluids and electrolytes with clinical applications* (7th ed.). Clifton Park, NY: Delmar Cengage Learning.

Larouere, E. (1999). Deaccessing an implanted port. *Nursing99, 29*(6), 60–61.

Lehne, R. (2006). *Pharmacology for nursing care* (6th ed.). St. Louis, MO: Elsevier, Health Sciences Division.

Liu, Q., Sulzenbacher, G., Yuan, H., Bennett, E., Pietz, G., Saunders, K., et al. (2007). Bacterial glycosidases for the production of universal red blood cells. *Nature Biotechnology, 25*(4), 454–464.

Macklin, D. (2000). Removing a PICC. *American Journal of Nursing, 100*(1), 52–54.

Masoorli, S. (2002). How to accurately document IV insertion. *Nursing2002, 32*(6), 65.

Matheny, N., Wehrle, M., Wiersema, L., & Clark, J. (1998). Testing feeding tube placement: Auscultation vs. pH method. *American Journal of Nursing, 98*(5), 37–42.

McConnell, E. (1998). Giving medications through an enteral feeding tube. *Nursing98, 28*(3), 6.

McConnell, E. (1999). Administering a Z-track IM injection. *Nursing99, 29*(1), 26.

McConnell, E. (2001). Instilling ear drops. *Nursing2001, 31*(4), 17.

McConnell, E. (2002). Administering medication through a gastrostomy tube. *Nursing2002, 32*(12), 22.

Metheny, N., & Titler, M. (2001). Assessing placement of feeding tubes, *American Journal of Nursing, 101*(5), 36–45.

Millam, D. (original manuscript), Hadaway, L. (revised manuscript). (2003). On the road to successful I.V. starts. A supplement to *Nursing2003, 33*(5 Suppl.), between pages 64 and 65.

Moorhead, S., Johnson, M., Maas, M., & Swanson, E. (2004). *Nursing Outcomes Classification (NOC)* (3rd ed.). St. Louis, MO: Mosby.

North American Nursing Diagnosis Association International. (2010). *NANDA-I nursing diagnoses: Definitions and classification 2009–2011*. Ames, IA: Wiley-Blackwell.

Obenour, P. (1998). Administering an S.C. medication continuously. *Nursing98, 28*(6), 20.

Pickar, G. (2004). *Dosage calculation* (7th ed.). Clifton Park, NY: Delmar Cengage Learning.

Pope, B. (2002). How to administer subcutaneous and intramuscular injections. *Nursing2002, 32*(1), 50–51.

Przybylek, C. (2002). Two ways to avoid a "sticky" IV situation. *Nursing2002, 32*(11), 47–49.

Rice, J. (2002). *Medications and mathematics for the nurse* (9th ed.). Clifton Park, NY: Delmar Cengage Learning.

Royer, T. (2001). Looking for a vein? Stick with venous ultrasound. *Nursing2001, 31*(11), 72–73.

Saxton, D., & O'Neill, N. (1998). *Math and meds for nurses.* Clifton Park, NY: Delmar Cengage Learning.

Schatzlein, K. (2003). Hold tight: Keeping catheters secure. *Nursing2003, 33*(3), 20–21.

Smetzer, J. (2001). Take 10 giant steps to medication safety. *Nursing2001, 31*(11), 49–53.

Smith, L. (2003). Clarifying a medication order. *Nursing2003, 33*(5), 26.

Spratto, G., & Woods, A. (2010). *Delmar nurse's drug handbook.* Clifton Park, NY: Delmar Cengage Learning.

Togger, D., & Brenner, P. (2001). Metered dose inhalers. *American Journal of Nursing, 101*(10), 26–32.

Trimble, T. (2003a). Peripheral IV starts: Insertion tips. *Nursing2003, 33*(8), 17.

Trimble, T. (2003b). Starting peripheral IVs: Tips for planning ahead. *Nursing2003, 33*(4), 30.

RESOURCES

Infusion Nurses Society, http://www.ins1.org

Institute for Safe Medication Practices, http://www.ismp.org

National Coordinating Council for Medication Error Reporting and Prevention, http://www.nccmerp.org

U.S. Pharmacopeia, http://www.usp.gov

CHAPTER 26
Assessment

MAKING THE CONNECTION

Refer to the following chapters to increase your understanding of health assessment:

Basic Nursing
- ***Communication***
- ***Cultural Considerations***
- ***End-of-Life Care***
- ***Complementary/Alternative Therapies***
- ***Fluid, Electrolyte, and Acid–Base Balance***
- ***Pain Management***

Adult Health Nursing
- ***The Older Adult***

Basic Procedures
- ***Hand Hygiene***
- ***Taking a Temperature***
- ***Taking a Pulse***
- ***Counting Respirations***
- ***Taking Blood Pressure***
- ***Weighing A Client, Mobile and Immobile***

LEARNING OBJECTIVES

Upon completion of this chapter, you should be able to:

- Define key terms.
- Identify the components of functional health patterns.
- Utilize the framework of functional health to facilitate a holistic assessment process.
- Analyze the components of the head-to-toe assessment.
- Incorporate the four assessment techniques within the head-to-toe assessment.
- Utilize the head-to-toe assessment in clinical situations.

KEY TERMS

adventitious breath sounds
affect
auscultation
borborygmi
bradycardia
bradypnea
bronchial sounds
bronchovesicular sounds
crackles
cyanosis
dyspnea
eupnea
health history
hyperventilation
hypoventilation
inspection
orthostatic hypotension
palpation
percussion
pleural friction rub
pulse amplitude

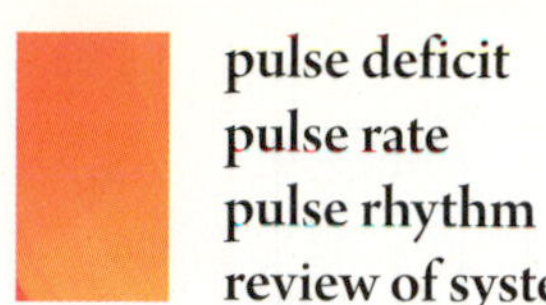

pulse deficit
pulse rate
pulse rhythm
review of systems (ROS)
sibilant wheezes
Snellen chart
sonorous wheeze
stridor
tachycardia
tachypnea
vesicular sounds

INTRODUCTION

Within the scope of the nursing profession, a complete nursing assessment is necessary to analyze each client's needs in a holistic manner. Nursing assessment includes both physical and psychosocial aspects to evaluate a client's condition. Caring, respect, and concern are demonstrated for each client when doing a nursing assessment.

A thorough nursing assessment includes both a health history and a physical examination. For a health history, the client is interviewed to identify how the client adjusts to or lives within the environment. This is subjective data, or information based on client self-report. The physical examination, objective data, includes observations made by the nurse while utilizing the assessment techniques of inspection, palpation, percussion, and auscultation. Other sources of objective data are laboratory tests, x-rays, and measurements of the client's vital signs, height, and weight.

The initial nursing assessment generally occurs within 8 hours of a client's admission to a health care facility and continues throughout the stay. In a physician's office or health care clinic, the nursing assessment would be completed immediately. Most institutions have a standard assessment form (Figure 26-1).

Usually a health history is completed before the physical examination, but in emergency situations or when performing care in a health care facility after the initial admitting assessment, it will be necessary to incorporate history taking into the physical examination. When incorporating a health history into the head-to-toe assessment, the nurse must remember to incorporate questions about the client's habits or usual patterns along with the physical data collected in the head-to-toe assessment. Functional assessment is best done within the framework of the physical assessment because the environment in which each client resides and participates becomes a part of the physical assessment. The functional assessment brings the environment in which the client lives and the physical needs of that client together to establish a holistic picture.

HEALTH HISTORY

A primary focus of the data collection interview is the health history. The **health history** is a review of the client's functional health patterns before the current contact with a health care agency. Whereas the medical history concentrates on symptoms and the progression of disease, the nursing health history focuses on the client's functional health patterns, responses to changes in health status, and alterations in lifestyle. The health history is also used in developing the plan of care.

Demographic Information

Personal data including name, address, date of birth, gender, religion, race/ethnic origin, occupation, and type of health plan/insurance should be included. This information may be useful in understanding a client's perspective.

Reason for Seeking Health Care

The client's reason for seeking health care should be described in the client's own words. For example, the statement "fell off four-foot ladder and landed on right shoulder; unable to move right arm" is the client's actual report of the event that precipitated a need for health care. The client's perspective is important because it explains what is significant about the event from the client's point of view. It is also important to know the time of the onset of symptoms.

Perception of Health Status

Perception of health status refers to the client's opinion of his or her general health. It may be useful to ask clients to rate their health on a scale of 1 to 10 (with 10 being ideal and 1 being poor), along with the client's rationale for the rating score. For example, the nurse may record a statement such as the following to represent the client's perception of health: "Rates health a 7 on a scale of 1 (poor) to 10 (ideal) because he must take medication regularly to maintain mobility, but the medication sometimes upsets his stomach."

Previous Illnesses, Hospitalizations, and Surgeries

The history and timing of any previous experiences with illness, surgery, or hospitalization are helpful in order to assess recurrent conditions and to anticipate responses to illness because prior experiences often affect current responses.

Client/Family Medical History

Ascertain any family history (blood relative) of acute and chronic illnesses that tend to be familial. Health history forms often include checklists of various illnesses that can be used as the basis for questions. It is also helpful to indicate the relative's relationship to the client (e.g., mother, father, sister).

Immunizations/Exposure to Communicable Diseases

A record of current immunizations should be obtained. This is particularly important with children; however, records of immunizations for tetanus, influenza, pneumonia, and hepatitis B are important for adults. A history of childhood or other communicable diseases should be noted. If the client has traveled out of the country, the time frame should be noted in order to determine incubation periods for relevant diseases. Also ask about potential exposure to communicable diseases such as tuberculosis or human immunodeficiency virus (HIV).

DATE:
TIME:

REASON FOR HOSPITALIZATION (E.R. TRIAGE/DIAGNOSIS)

MODE OF ARRIVAL

- Ambulance ☐
- Wheelchair ☐
- Stretcher ☐
- Ambulatory ☐

ONSET OF SYMPTOMS (E.R. TRIAGE)

PAST HISTORY: (Past Surgeries / Hospitalization) (E.R. TRIAGE)

COMMENTS:

VITAL SIGNS		HEALTH HISTORY				PERSON TO NOTIFY IN CASE OF EMERGENCY
TEMP		✓ Only those conditions that patient has history or current condition				
PULSE		GLAUCOMA	☐	GASTRIC ULCERS	☐	NAME
RESP		CANCER	☐	HEPATITIS	☐	
BP		LUNG DISEASE	☐	HIV DISEASE	☐	
HEIGHT	STATED	ASTHMA	☐	DIABETIC # OF YRS ____		RELATIONSHIP
	ACTUAL	KIDNEY DISEASE	☐	ANESTHESIA REACTION	☐	
WEIGHT	STATED	HEART DISEASE	☐	STROKE	☐	
	ACTUAL	PACEMAKER	☐	SEIZURE	☐	HAS POWER OF ATTORNEY FOR HEALTH CARE?
ALLERGIES		HYPERTENSION	☐	TUBERCULOSIS	☐	
FOOD		ALCOHOL	☐	PSYCHIATRIC DX	☐	☐ YES ☐ NO
LATEX ☐		SMOKING	☐	BLOOD TRANSFUSION	☐	TELEPHONE #
OTHER		DRUGS	☐	IN PAST 10 YEARS		

DRUG ALLERGIES	REACTION	DATE
1.		
2.		
3.		
4.		
5.		

MEDICATIONS (E.R. MEDS)

Name	Dose	Freq	Reason	Last Dose

Meds Sent Home: YES ☐ NO ☐ N/A ☐

ORGAN DONATION

Do you want information on organ donation?

YES ☐ NO ☐

Referred to: ☐ Organ Transplant Alliance 887-6189

PATIENT RIGHTS

☐ Received copy of Patient Rights
☐ Verbalizes understanding and ability to implement

SIGNATURES:

Completed by: ____
Entered by: ____

4013

CHRISTUS SPOHN HEALTH SYSTEM

PATIENT ADMISSION
DATA BASE

2705318

NEW: 06/95
REVISED: 02/99.F10

FUNCTIONAL SCREENING (ADULT)

*Physical Therapy:
0 pts = complete independence
1 pt = recent onset of neurological problem
1 pt = recent onset of orthopedic problem
1 pt = recent onset of problem with impaired mobility (ambulation, stair climbing, bed mobility, transferring)
2 pts = open wound or an acute burn
____ TOTAL POINTS
• A Score of 2 or More Points Requires a Physical Therapy Screening.
Physical Therapy Screening Requested
☐ Yes ☐ No

*Occupational Therapy
0 pts = complete independence
1 pt = acute decline in upper extremity function
1 pt = recent onset of a neurological or orthopedic problem
1 pt = recent onset of a problem causing a decrease in ADL function (Bathing, Dressing, Feeding Toileting)
____ TOTAL POINTS
• A Score of 2 or More Points Requires an Occupational Therapy Screen.
Occupational Therapy Screening Requested
☐ Yes ☐ No

*Speech Therapy
0 pts = no identified problems
2 pt = recent onset of swallowing problems
2 pt = recent onset of speech difficulty
1 pt = recent neurological problem affecting ability to follow commands
2 pt = radical ENT surgery
____ TOTAL POINTS
• A Score of 2 or More Points Requires a Speech Therapy Screen.
Speech Therapy Screening Requested
☐ Yes ☐ No

PASTORAL CARE SCREEN

[ ] Would you like a special request sent for a visit from our chaplain?
[ ] Yes [ ] No
[ ] If Yes, Send Request to Pastoral Care

PATIENT INSTRUCTION CHECKLIST

☐ Signal Light	☐ Telephone	☐ Shower	☐ Dentures/Hearing Aid
☐ Bed Controls	☐ Brochure	☐ T.V.	
☐ Light Controls	☐ Visiting Privileges	☐ I.D./Allergy Band On	
☐ Bathroom	☐ Safety Precautions	☐ Pillow Speaker Placement	

PSYCHOSOCIAL/DISCHARGE PLANNING SCREEN

PSYCHOSOCIAL STATUS (circle all that apply)	
History of non-compliance impacting medical treatment	1
History alcohol/chemical abuse needing treatment	1
Suspected neglect/abuse	4
Unsafe home environment (domestic violence/self-neglect)	4
Prolonged confusion/disorientation	1
Illness related anxiety impacting care	1
Ineffective family coping patterns	1
Recent loss of body limb	1
Terminal illness	4
Suicide attempt/Ideation	4
Significant Grief impacting care/treatment	1
Teen Pregnancy (with high risk social factors)	2
Birth Anomalies or retardation	4
Loss of Infant (fetal demise)	4
Adoption	4
Other: ____	

LIVING ARRANGEMENT:

Family Unable to help/no known friends	2
Age > 70 years lives alone	1
Patient admitted from other institution: ___ SNF ___ NH ___ Rehab ___ Other Hospital	1
Patient is disabled	1
Homeless or no address available	3

ADMISSION STATUS:

Readmitted within 1 -30 days	1
Admitted through ER	1

TOTAL OF ALL ____

Low Risk = 0-2
Moderate Risk = 3 pts
High Risk = 4 or > pts
*HIGH RISK requires Social Services consult. Social Services notified ☐ Yes ☐ No

Current Resource Being Utilized:	Yes	No
Home Health	☐	☐
Provider	☐	☐
Private Sitter	☐	☐
Meals on wheels	☐	☐
Hospice	☐	☐
MHMR	☐	☐
Adult Day Program	☐	☐
WIC Program	☐	☐

DME AT HOME
☐ Oxygen ☐ Walker
☐ Wheelchair ☐ Trapeze
☐ Hospital Bed
☐ Bedside commode
Living with ____

VALUABLES BROUGHT WITH PATIENT TO HOSPITAL (SECURITY TAG)

Date: ____

☐ **Cane/Walker**	☐ **Bridgework no. of pieces** ____	☐ **Prothesis type** ____	☐ **Money (purse)**	☐ **Electric Razor**
☐ **Clocks**	☐ **Eyeglasses**	☐ **Hearing Aids L/R**	☐ **Wheelchair**	☐ **Clothing** ____
☐ **Dentures U/L**	☐ **Contact Lens**	☐ **Jewelry**	☐ **Radio**	☐ **Other** ____
☐ **Partial U/L**	☐ **Watches**	☐ **Money (billfold)**	☐ **T.V.**	

I take entire responsibility for keeping in my possession the articles listed above. I am holding nothing in my possession which I have not declared here. I understand and agree that Christus Spohn Health System shall not be liable for the loss or damage to any money, jewelry, eyeglasses, dentures, hearing aids or otther articles of value left in the care, custody and control of the patient or family/significant other.
It is understood and agreed that Christus Spohn Health System maintains a locked safe for money and valuables. The hospital shall not be liable for any of the patient's personal property that is not secured in the valuables storage envelope or in the hospital locked safe.

SIGNATURE OF PATIENT ____
I have fully explained to this patient that Christus Spohn Health System takes no responsibility for articles retained by the patient.
SIGNATURE OF EMPLOYEE RECORDING ARTICLES ____

Valuables given to: ____
VALUABLES STORAGE ENVELOPE: When valuables storage envelope is used, record the following information:
Valuables Storage Envelope Number ____ Date property received ____
Employee taking envelope to cashier ____

2705318-2.F10 02/25/99

FIGURE 26-1 Patient Admission Database (*Courtesy of CHRISTUS Spohn Health System, Corpus Christi, TX.*)

RN ASSESSMENT: DATE: TIME: SIGNATURE:________________________, RN

INSTRUCTION:
1. Complete physical assessment
2. Identify problems/nursing diagnosis for each system as appropriate
3. Prioritize Problems
4. Enter problems for problem list in computer

SYSTEMS	YES	NO	COMMENTS	PROBLEM
NEUROLOGICAL L.O.C. • Alert • Drowsy • Comatose • Disoriented • Cooperative • Agitated				☐ Thought processes, alteration in ☐ Coping, ineffective ☐ Communication, impaired
EYES • Pearl • Vision Normal • Prosthesis				☐ Injury potential ☐ Vision, impaired
MOUTH • Moist • Lesions • Teeth • Other				☐ Sensory, perception ☐ Other
EARS • Responds to normal voice tone • Drainage				
SPEECH • Clear • Slurred • Hoarse / raspy • Aphasic				
RESPIRATORY				
RESPIRATIONS • Rate • Labored				☐ Airway clearance, ineffective ☐ Breathing pattern ineffective
BREATH SOUNDS • Clear • Wheezes • Rales / Rhonchi				☐ Gas exchange; impaired ☐ IF PROBLEM IDENTIFIED SEND RESPIRATORY CONSULT
COUGH • Present • Sputum				☐ Other
MUSCLE / SKELETAL				
EXTREMITIES • Moves all on command WEAKNESS (specify) RA___ LA___ RL___ LL___ • Edema • Normal ambulation • Prosthesis (specify)				☐ Self Care deficit ☐ Mobility impaired, physical ☐ Activity intolerance comfort, alterations in ACUTE ☐ CHRONIC ☐ ☐ Tissue perfusion; alterations in

27053183.F10 02/12/99

SYSTEMS	YES	NO	COMMENTS	PROBLEM
CARDIOVASCULAR Apical Rate [ ] Rhythm (circle one) Regular Irregular On Cardiac Monitor: Yes ☐ No ☐ If Yes: Rhythm ________ Peripheral Pulses: Right / Left Carotid ☐ ☐ Radial ☐ ☐ Popliteal ☐ ☐ Femoral ☐ ☐ Pedal ☐ ☐				☐ Tissue perfusion alterations in ☐ Comfort, alterations in pain: ACUTE ☐ CHRONIC ☐ Post Operative ☐ Other ☐
Pacemaker				
Peripheral Edema				
Chest Pain				
Jugular Vein Distention				
Extremity Discoloration				
Rt. Arm/Hand				
Lt. Arm/Hand				
Rt. Leg/Foot				
Lt. Leg/Foot				
GENITOURINARY				
VOIDING • Normal • Frequency • Burning				☐ Urinary Elimination, alterations in pattern
Decreased Force of urinary stream INCONTINENCE: • Stress • Nocturia				☐ Urinary Retention ☐ Incontinence, Total
UROSTOMY DIALYSIS If Yes: Hemo / Peritoneal Routine schedule Date of last Dialysis Catheter insertion Date Date of last menstrual period				☐ Incontinence, Stress ☐ Comfort, alterations in ACUTE ☐ CHRONIC ☐

GASTROINTESTINAL	YES	NO	COMMENT	PROBLEM
ABDOMEN • Soft • Distended • Tenderness				Bowel elimination alterations in ☐ Diarrhea ☐ Constipation ☐ Incontinence, ☐ Comfort altered pain ACUTE ☐ CHRONIC ☐
ELIMINATION • Bowel Sounds • Diarrhea • Constipation • Incontinence • Ostomy Last B.M. Date:				

SAFETY ASSESSMENT

- ☐ (5) Age greater than 60
- ☐ (5) History of previous falls
- ☐ (3) From nursing home
- ☐ (3) Has had sitter / companion at home

STATUS: MENTAL/PHYSICAL
- ☐ (5) Confused / Judgement Impaired
- ☐ (5) Sensory impairment
- ☐ (5) Combative/Aggressive
- ☐ (5) "Sundowners" Syndrome
- ☐ (5) Noncompliance/uncooperativeness
- ☐ (5) Paralysis / amputee
- ☐ (5) Weakness / debilitation
- ☐ (5) Urgent/frequent elimination needs

________ TOTAL

MEDICATIONS
- ☐ (5) Diuretics
- ☐ (5) Laxatives / G.I. preps
- ☐ (3) Antihypertensives
- ☐ (3) Antiseizures
- ☐ (5) Sedative / hypnotics
- ☐ (3) Analgesics
- ☐ (3) Antipsychotics / antidepressants

- ☐ LEVEL 1 (0-17)
- ☐ LEVEL 2 (18-24)
- ☐ LEVEL 3 (25 or greater)

- ☐ Safety precautions implemented
- ☐ Restraints per protocol
- ☐ Patient/family instructed
- ☐ Color coded band on

INTEGUMENTARY SKIN	YES	NO	COMMENT	PROBLEM
• Color Normal • Warm, dry • Turgor good • Bruises abrasions, lacerations Color, Size, Location			☐ Referral to Social Service (screen for neglect / abuse)	☐ Other: ______ ☐ Tissue perfusion, alterations in ☐ Skin integrity impairment of: actual
• Poor hygiene • Rash, lesions • Scars • Dressing • Pressure points intact • coccyx • heels • elbows • hips • ankles • cast edges • Other______				☐ Skin integrity impairment of: potential ☐ Tissue integrity, comfort, alterations in pain ACUTE ☐ CHRONIC ☐ WOUND CARE ☐
E-Z graph • Vascular access				

Type__________ Insertion Date:__________
Site:__________ Purpose__________

NUTRITIONAL SCREENING

Indicate as appropriate for patient Previous diet ______________
- ☐ (8) TPN/Parental Nutrition
- ☐ (8) Tube Feeding
- ☐ (2) Unplanned weight loss or gain > 20 lbs in 3 months
  - ☐ Referral to S.S. screen for neglect/abuse?
- ☐ (1) Loss of appetite/Eats less than 50% of meal
- ☐ (1) Nausea, vomiting or diarrhea
- ☐ (1) Difficulty chewing
- ☐ (1) Difficulty swallowing

*Diagnosis of:
- ☐ (2) Heart disease, hypertension, CHF, gestational diabetic, hepatic or renal failure, diabetic, anemia, cancer other than ENT, geriatric surgery
- ☐ (5) AIDS, malnutrition, DKA, decubitus ulcer, septic condition requiring ICU, burn patient, ENT cancer
- ☐ (1) modified diet; NPO for 48 hrs.
- ☐ (1) age > 65 years

*LAB VALUES:

Albumin	Glucose	Hgb
☐ (1) 2.5 - 3.0	☐ (1) <60 or > 300	☐ (1) male < 13
☐ (2) < 2.5		☐ (1) female < 11

______ TOTAL SCORE

High Risk - 8 pts or >
Moderate Risk - 5-7 pts
Low Risk - 0-4 pts

☐ SEND NUTRITION SCREEN CONSULT WITH TOTAL SCORE OF 5 OR ABOVE AND IDENTIFY SCORE OF PATIENT IN ORDER

SKIN BREAKDOWN POTENTIAL CHECKLIST

- ______ (1) Fair: Major underlying disease, controlled
- ______ (2) Poor: Uncontrolled underlying disease

MENTAL STATUS
- ______ (1) Lethargic: Listless
- ______ (2) Confused: Inappropriate communication
- ______ (4) Comatose: Unresponsive

MOBILITY / ACTIVITY
- ______ (2) Minor Deficit: Some limitation in movement Needs assistance w / ADL's
- ______ (4) Major Deficit: Movement requires assistance
- ______ (6) Immobile: No voluntary movement

INCONTINENCE
- ______ (1) Mild: Stress incontinence, 1 BM / day
- ______ (4) Frequent: No bladder control, BMs > 2-4 /day
- ______ (6) Total: No bladder control, frequent / continuous BM

NUTRITION
- ______ (2) Fair: Intake < body requirements, eats 75% or less
- ______ (3) Poor: Eats 50% or less, started on TPN or tube feeding
- ______ (4) Compromised: No intake, dehydrated

SKIN INTEGRITY
- ______ (2) Fair: Single stage I or II
- ______ (4) Poor: More than one break in skin integrity

______ TOTAL SCORE OF 8 OR ABOVE, ENTER SKIN INTEGRITY POTENTIAL ON PCP PROBLEM LIST, INITIATE PREVENTATIVE ADL's

PATIENT / SIGNIFICANT OTHER PARTICIPATION IN ADMISSION PROCESS

1. Answered question Yes _____ No _____
2. Volunteered information Yes _____ No _____
3. Family/significant other present Yes _____ No _____
4. Plan of care reviewed with: Patient _____ Family / Significant other_____
5. Comments:

2705318-4.F10

FIGURE 26-1 (Continued)

SAFETY

Assessment for Allergies

It is essential to explore possible allergies before administering any medications. Allergic reactions can be life threatening and can occur with very low dosages of medications. A client's sensitivity to a drug can also change over time, resulting in severe reactions even though the client has successfully taken the drug during prior illnesses or experienced only mild reactions to the drug in the past.

Allergies

Any drug, food, or environmental allergies are noted in the health history, along with the type of reaction to the substance. For example, a client may report that a rash or shortness of breath developed after taking penicillin. This reaction is recorded. Clients may report an "allergy" to a medication because their stomach was upset after ingesting it. This is a side effect that would not preclude administration of the drug in the future.

Current Medications

All medications currently taken, both prescription and over-the-counter, are recorded by name, frequency, and dosage. Ask about birth control pills, laxatives, nonprescription pain relief medications, herbal remedies, and vitamin and mineral supplements. Clients may be hesitant to share herb use with the nurse and medical staff. Ask the client, in an accepting manner, if she is taking any herbal supplements. Sometimes herbal therapies interact with other medications, causing serious side effects.

Developmental Level

Knowledge of developmental level is essential for considering appropriate norms of behavior and for appraising the achievement of relevant developmental tasks. Any recognized theory of growth and development can be applied in order to determine if clients are functioning within the parameters expected for their age-group. For example, if Erikson's stages of psychosocial development are used, validation of an adult client's attainment of the developmental task of generativity versus stagnation can be made by a statement such as "client prefers to spend time with his family; very involved in children's school activities." (Refer to Erickson's Stages of Psychosocial Development in Chapter 10.)

PROFESSIONALTIP

Expired Medications

Remind clients to check all medications for expiration dates before use.

Psychosocial History

Psychosocial history refers to assessment of self-concept and self-esteem as well as usual sources of stress and the client's ability to cope. Sources of support for clients in crisis, such as family, significant others, religion, or support groups, are explored.

Sociocultural History

The client's sociocultural history includes the home environment, family situation, and client's role in the family. For example, the client could be the parent of three children and the sole provider in a single-parent family. The responsibilities of the client are important data through which the impact of changes in health status and the most beneficial care plan for the client are determined. Caffeine and alcohol intake and use of tobacco or recreational drugs also are explored.

Complementary/ Alternative Therapy Use

Alternative therapy and complementary therapy are often used interchangeably but are not the same. Alternative therapy supplants (replaces) traditional medical treatment, and complementary therapy complements or enhances medical practices. Complementary methods are used alongside medical practices to improve the client's health status (Gecsedi & Decker, 2001).

The University of Maryland Medicine (2002) reports that nearly 70% of U.S. citizens have used at least one complementary/alternative therapy in their lifetime. According to a study in a Brooklyn, New York, hospital, one in four clients seen in the emergency department had taken an herbal supplement but did not share their use of herbs with the medical staff (Gulla & Singer, 2000). Herbal use without health care practitioner notification can have serious consequences since some herbs interact with medications and cause serious side effects. The nursing staff can prevent herbal related issues by developing a trusting relationship with clients and asking if they take herbs or do anything to improve their health. As clients share alternative and complementary therapy choices, the nurse enhances a trust relationship by being knowledgeable about the various therapies and genuinely accepting the client's personal choices.

Activities of Daily Living

The activities of daily living (ADLs) is a description of the client's lifestyle and capacity for self-care and is useful both as baseline information and as a source of insight into usual health behaviors. This baseline should include information on nutritional intake and eating habits, elimination patterns, rest/sleep patterns, and activity/exercise.

Review of Systems

The **review of systems (ROS)** is a brief account from the client of any recent signs or symptoms associated with any of the body systems. This can most effectively be obtained as the physical examination is performed. The ROS relies on subjective information provided by the client rather than on the physical examination. When a symptom is encountered, either while eliciting the health history or during the physical examination of the client, as much information as possible about the symptom is obtained. Relevant data include:

- *Location:* The area of the body in which the symptom (such as pain) is felt

- *Character:* The quality of the feeling or sensation (e.g., sharp, dull, stabbing)
- *Intensity:* The severity or quantity of the feeling or sensation and its interference with functional abilities. The sensation can be rated on a scale of 1 (very little) to 10 (very intense)
- *Timing:* The onset, duration, frequency, and precipitating factors of the symptom
- *Aggravating/alleviating factors:* The activities or actions that make the symptom worse or better

PHYSICAL EXAMINATION

A physical examination is performed for all age-groups in all health care settings (home, outpatient facilities, extended care institutions, and acute care facilities) to gather comprehensive, pertinent client data. The physical examination, a picture of the client's physiological functioning, combined with a health and psychosocial assessment, forms a database for decision making. The examination is performed according to the agency's policy, which may vary from one agency to another.

To ensure a thorough assessment of each system, the physical examination is done in a sequential, head-to-toe fashion. This method decreases the number of times the nurse and the client have to change positions and prevents forgetting to examine an area.

The physical or the head-to-toe assessment is performed by using the specific assessment techniques of inspection, palpation, percussion, and auscultation.

INSPECTION

Inspection consists of a thorough visual observation of the client, providing a picture of the body's outward response to its internal functioning. Inspection of the skin, for example, can assist in identifying signs of a fever by the client's flushed face. The skin can also be an indicator of a decreased oxygen supply when **cyanosis**, a bluish or dark purple coloration, is noted in the client's lips, skin, or nail beds. Sharing observations with the client during inspection enhances the holistic data collected. For example, when mentioning the observation of visible scars, the client may discuss previous surgeries or hospitalizations. Instruments such as a penlight and otoscope are often used to enhance visualization.

Effective inspection requires adequate lighting and exposure of the body parts being observed. Show sensitivity to the client's feelings of embarrassment by discussing the technique with the client and using appropriate draping.

PALPATION

Palpation uses the sense of touch to assess texture, temperature, moisture, organ location and size, vibrations, pulsations, swelling, masses, and tenderness. The finger pads are placed flat against the client's skin, exerting slight pressure for light palpation, as seen in Figure 26-2. Assessment of the kidneys, liver, spleen, bowel, and fundal height may be accomplished through deep palpation, in which more pressure is exerted. Pulses are also palpated. The abdomen is palpated for distention, softness, firmness, rigidity, or tenderness.

Palpation requires a calm, gentle approach and is used systematically, with light palpation preceding deep palpation and palpation of tender areas performed last.

SAFETY

Palpation

Deep palpation is a technique requiring significant expertise and beginning nursing students do not perform this procedure without supervision.

PERCUSSION

Percussion uses short, tapping strokes on the surface of the skin to create vibrations of underlying organs. It is used to assess the density of structures or determine the location and size of organs. The fingertips are used to tap the client's body to produce sounds and vibrations. Place the middle finger of the nondominant hand on the client's skin in the area to be percussed, then tap lightly with the middle finger of the dominant hand on the distal phalanx of the middle finger positioned on the body surface (Figure 26-3). Tap twice in

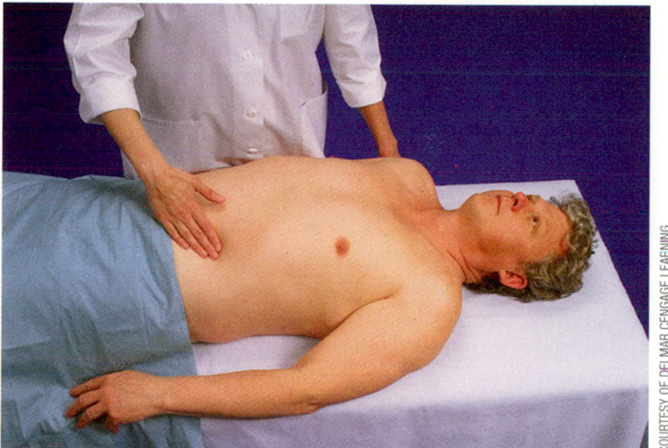
COURTESY OF DELMAR CENGAGE LEARNING

FIGURE 26-2 Light Palpation

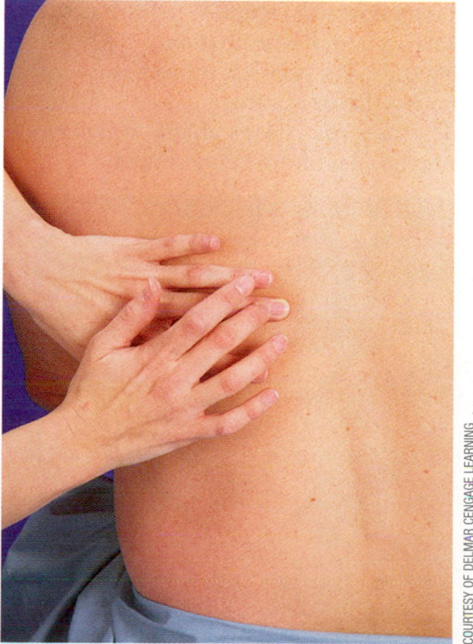
COURTESY OF DELMAR CENGAGE LEARNING

FIGURE 26-3 Percussion

TABLE 26-1 Description of Percussion Tones

TONE	INTENSITY	PITCH	DURATION	QUALITY	NORMAL LOCATION
Dullness	Medium	High	Medium	Thudlike	Liver
Flatness	Soft	High	Short	Extreme dullness	Muscle
Hyperresonance	Very loud	Very low	Long	Booming	Child's lung
Resonance	Loud	Low	Long	Hollow	Peripheral lung
Tympany	Loud	High	Medium	Drumlike	Stomach

COURTESY OF DELMAR CENGAGE LEARNING

one place before moving to a new area. Percussion should not be painful to the client. If it is painful, the percussion should be discontinued and the response documented.

Percussion requires much practice to master, and it is important to be familiar with the sounds produced when percussion is used. Table 26-1 describes the various percussion tones.

AUSCULTATION

Auscultation involves listening to sounds in the body that are created by movement of air or fluid. Areas most often auscultated include the lungs, heart, abdomen, and blood vessels. A stethoscope is used to channel the sound (Figure 26-4).

HEAD-TO-TOE ASSESSMENT

Some important concepts are kept in mind and utilized throughout the examination. The client's privacy is respected by pulling the curtain, closing the door, and providing appropriate draping. When possible, distracting noises such as radio or television and people talking are eliminated. Assessment is performed under natural light because fluorescent light can change the color tones of the skin. All procedures are explained to the client and confidentiality of data acquired during the examination maintained.

The client is positioned to ensure accessibility to the body part being assessed. Figure 26-5 illustrates positions used in conducting a physical examination.

Draping the client prevents unnecessary exposure during the examination. Embarrassment causes tension and restlessness and decreases the client's ability to cooperate. Draping also prevents the client from being chilled.

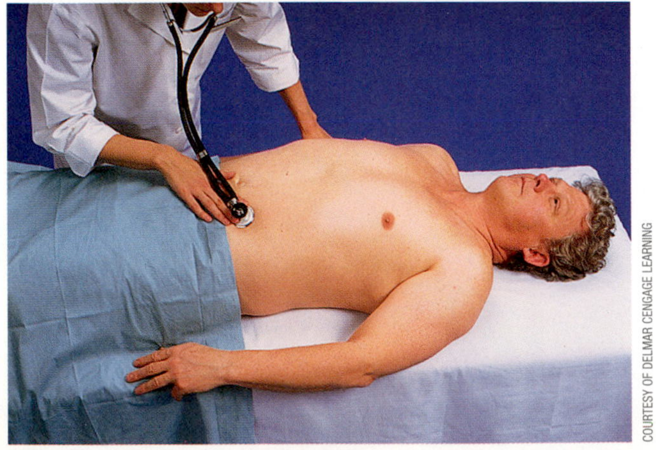

COURTESY OF DELMAR CENGAGE LEARNING

FIGURE 26-4 Auscultation

INFECTION CONTROL

Standard Precautions

Remember to utilize Standard Precautions when in contact with any body fluids by using gloves, gown, or mask as appropriate.

GENERAL SURVEY

During the introductory time, use inspection to make a general assessment of the client. This overview is the first impression of the client and is the beginning point of the head-to-toe assessment. Such aspects as the general state of health and any signs of distress, such as pain or breathing difficulties, the client's awareness of the surroundings, body type and posture, facial expressions, and mood are noted.

Document the general survey data to portray an overall picture of the client. The elderly, disabled, and abused clients will require special consideration during the physical examination.

Elderly

Before assessing elderly clients, it is important to know the normal changes of aging. Aging may reduce the body's tolerance of stress, resistance to illness, and ability to recuperate from illness. Be sure the client understands and can follow instructions and allow extra time for the client having difficulty changing positions.

Disabled Clients

When assessing disabled clients, adapt the process to the client's ability; for example, give a hearing-impaired client

CRITICAL THINKING

Performing a Physical Assessment

Do you feel comfortable performing a complete physical assessment on a client? Identify the areas that are of concern. What could you do to be more confident in performing physical assessments?

Sitting
To examine head, neck, back, posterior thorax and lungs, anterior thorax and lungs, breast, axillae, heart, extremities.

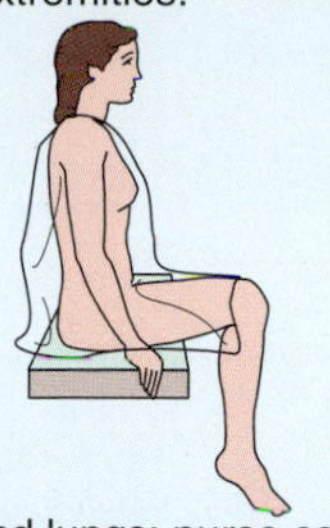

Client can expand lungs; nurse can inspect symmetry. *Institute risk precautions for elderly and debilitated clients.*

Dorsal recumbent
To examine head, neck, anterior thorax and lungs, breast, axillae, heart.

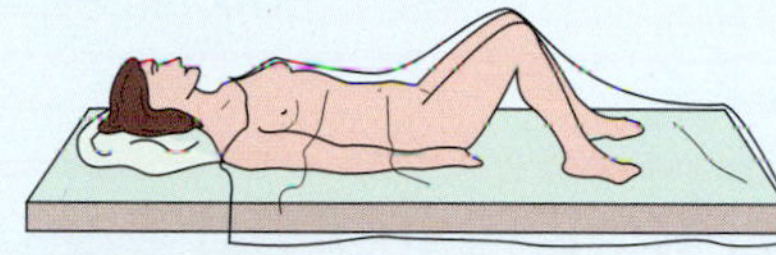

Client comfortable; increases abdominal muscle tension. *Contraindicated in abdominal assessment.*

Prone
To examine posterior thorax and lungs, hip

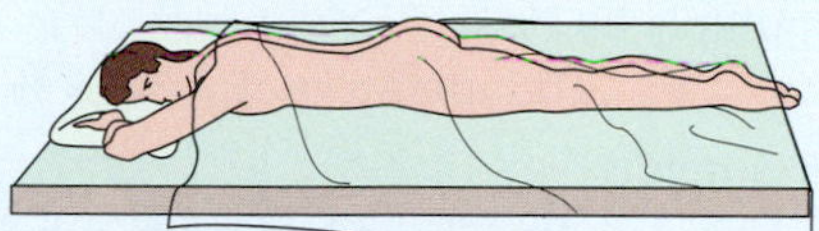

Assessment of hip extension. *Contraindicated in clients with cardiopulmonary alterations.*

Supine
To examine head, neck, anterior thorax and lungs, breasts, axillae, heart, abdomen, extremities.

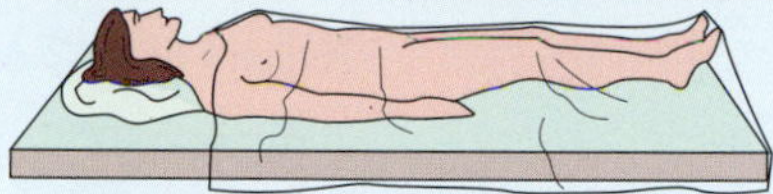

Client relaxed; decreases abdominal muscle tension; nurse can palpate all peripheral pulses. *Contraindicated in clients with cardiopulmonary alterations.*

Sims'
To examine rectum and vagina.

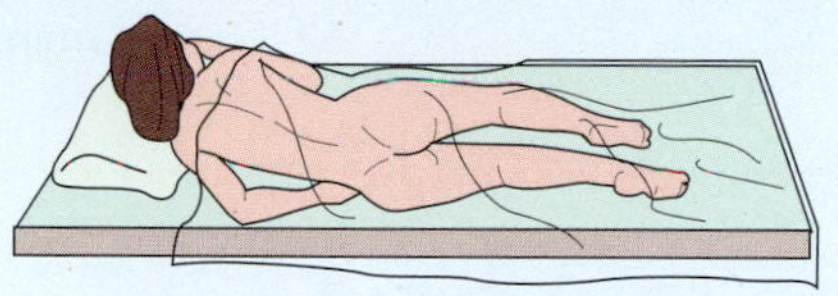

Relaxes rectal muscles. Painful for clients with joint deformities.

Knee-chest
To examine rectum

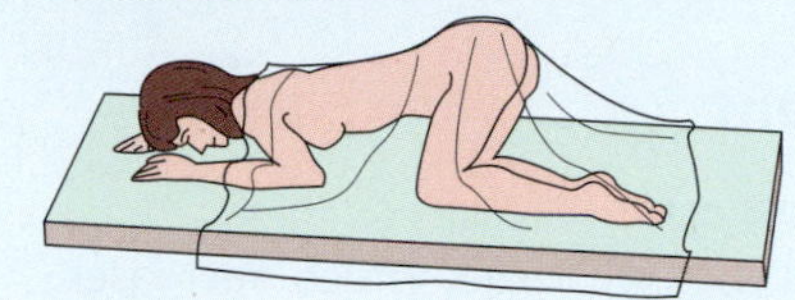

Maximal rectal exposure. *Contraindicated in clients with respiratory alterations.*

Lithotomy
To examine female genitalia, rectum, genital tract.

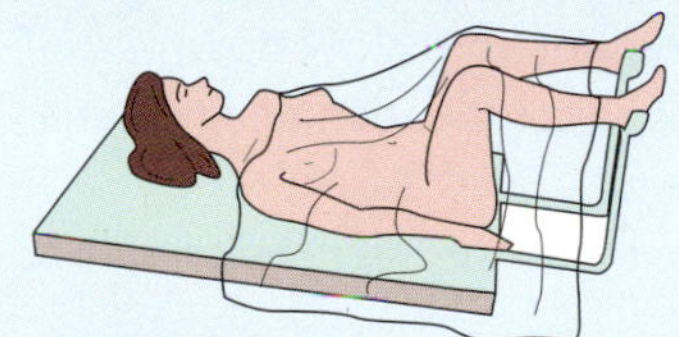

Maximal genitalia exposure; embarrassing and uncomfortable for client. *Contraindicated in clients with joint disorders.*

COURTESY OF DELMAR CENGAGE LEARNING

FIGURE 26-5 Various Positions for Physical Examination

a written questionnaire. Simple, direct sentences and questions or pictures might be required for an intellectually impaired client. It is best to determine the client's ability to participate before conducting the examination. To allay the disabled client's fears and anxiety, encourage a family member to remain with the client during the examination. The client's level of independence and feelings about the disability are noted.

Abused Clients

Observe for signs of abuse, especially in children and the elderly. Symptoms may be psychological as well as physical; for example, refusal to be touched, inability to maintain eye contact, or unwillingness to talk about bruises, burns, or other injuries may indicate abuse. Bruises or lacerations most typically appear on breasts, buttocks, thighs, or genitalia. Inspect for healed scarring or burns and know state laws and agency policies for reporting possible abuse.

Vital Signs

After establishing rapport with the client through introductions, measurement of vital signs is the next step in an assessment. Vital signs are the "signs of life," providing a way of connecting the external inspection with the internal functioning of the client's organs. When checking vital signs, obtain the temperature (T), pulse (P), respirations (R), blood pressure (BP), and pain assessment of the client. See Table 26-2 for normal values and variations.

Temperature

When assessing the client's temperature (T), an electronic, chemical, mercury-free, tympanic, or temporal artery

TABLE 26-2 Vital Signs and Variations

VITAL SIGN	NORMAL READING	VARIATIONS
Temperature	Axillary 36.5°C or 97.6°F Tympanic 37°C or 98.6°F Oral 37°C or 98.6°F Rectal 37.5°C or 99.6°F	<36°C or 96.8°F Hypothermia >38°C or 100.4°F Pyrexia
Pulse	60–100 beats/min.	<60 Bradycardia <100 Tachycardia
Respirations	12–20 resp./min.	<16 Bradypnea >20 Tachypnea
Blood pressure	90/60–140/90	<90/60 Hypotension >140/90 Hypertension

COURTESY OF DELMAR CENGAGE LEARNING

LIFE SPAN CONSIDERATIONS

The Older Client

- All senses are less acute.
- Endorphin level rises with age, which decreases awareness of painful events.
- Temperature normal range is 96°F to 98.9°F.
- Strength and endurance decline.
- Height decreases.
- Digestive and urinary functions slow down.
- Older clients are prone to constipation and nocturia.
- Respirations are slowed.
- Older clients are prone to fatigue, dizziness, and falls.
- Skin is dry.
- Tan to brown irregular macules called "liver spots" or "age spots" appear.
- Genitalia show progressive atrophy. (Andresen, 1998; Scott, 2008; Williams & Keen, 2007)

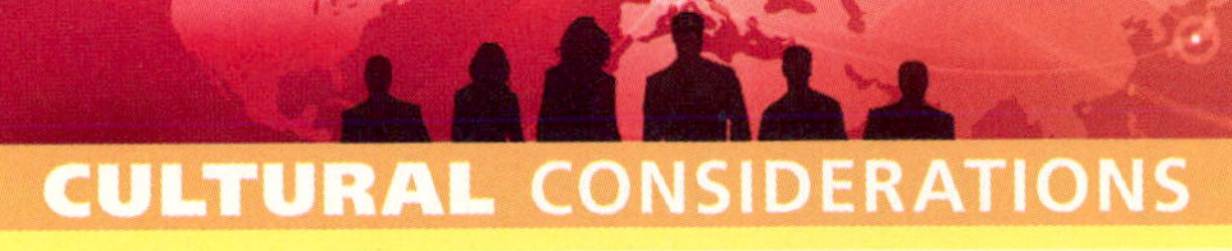

CULTURAL CONSIDERATIONS

Cultural Values and Assessment

Although cleanliness is highly valued by mainstream American society, in some cultures, a daily bath is not believed necessary or desirable. In fact, some cultures do not interpret natural body odors as offensive. Consider the client in the context of cultural beliefs. The terms *dirty*, *unkempt*, or *foul smelling* are value laden and can cloud the assessment process and care provided to a client.

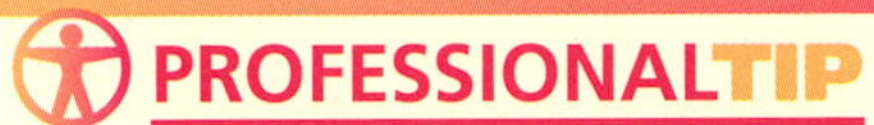

PROFESSIONAL TIP

Temperature Conversion

To convert Fahrenheit to Celsius (centigrade), subtract 32 from the Fahrenheit temperature and multiply by $\frac{5}{9}$:

$$(\text{Temperature } ^\circ\text{F} - 32) \times \tfrac{5}{9} = ^\circ\text{C}$$

Example:

$$98.6^\circ\text{F} - 32 = 66.6 \times \tfrac{5}{9} = 37^\circ\text{C}$$

To convert Celsius to Fahrenheit, multiply the Celsius temperature by $\frac{9}{5}$ and add 32:

$$\tfrac{9}{5} \times \text{temperature}^\circ\text{C} + 32 = ^\circ\text{F}$$

Example:

$$\tfrac{9}{5} \times 40^\circ\text{C} = 72 + 32 = 104^\circ\text{F}$$

thermometer can be used (see Figure 26-6). Body temperature can be taken by five routes: oral, rectal, axillary, skin, or tympanic membrane. The route chosen depends on the client's age and physical condition. Factors such as age, gender, physical activity, and environment affects a person's temperature. Craig, Lancaster, Taylor, Williamson, and Smyth (2002) found ear temperatures in children to be inaccurate. Consumption of hot or cold food or beverage and smoking 15 to 30 minutes before taking an oral temperature can affect the results.

Pulse

Pulse assessment measures a pressure pulsation created when the heart contracts and ejects blood into the aorta. Assessment of pulse characteristics provides clinical data regarding the heart's pumping action and the adequacy of peripheral artery blood flow.

There are many pulse points (Figure 26-7). The most accessible are the radial and carotid sites. The body diverts blood to the brain when a cardiovascular emergency such

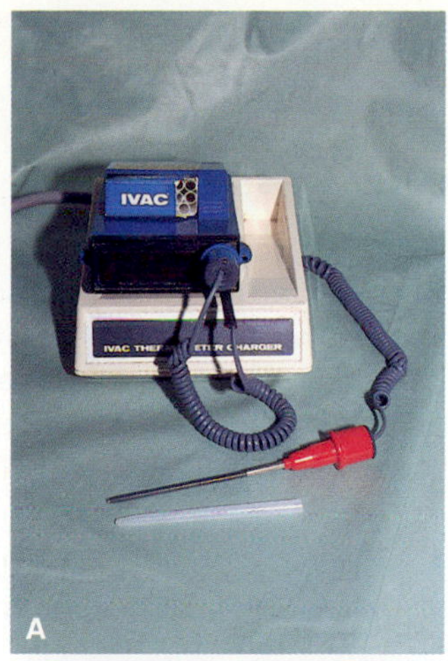

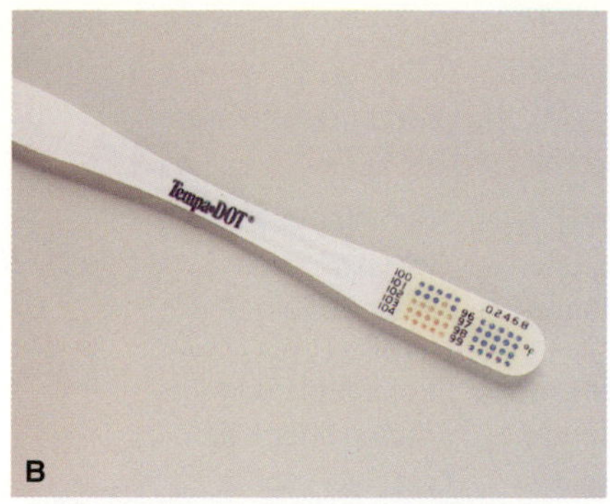

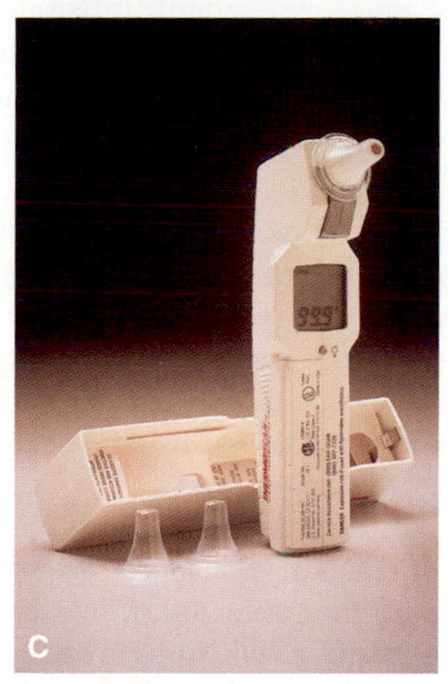

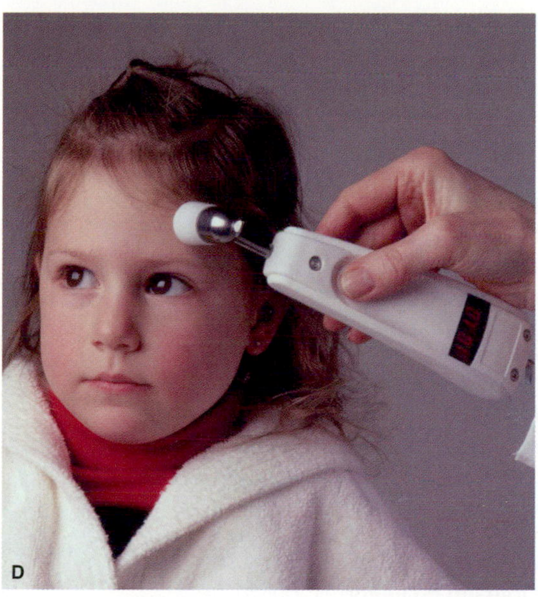

FIGURE 26-6 Different Types of Thermometers for Taking a Client's Temperature: *A*, Electronic Thermometer with a Probe (Red Color Indicates Rectal Thermometer Probe); *B*, Disposable Chemical Thermometer; *C*, Tympanic Thermometer with Disposable Speculums and Infrared-Sensing Electronics; *D*, Temporal Artery Thermometer (*Images A and B courtesy of Delmar Cengage Learning; image C courtesy of The Gilette Company; and image D courtesy of Exergen Corporation, Watertown, MA.*)

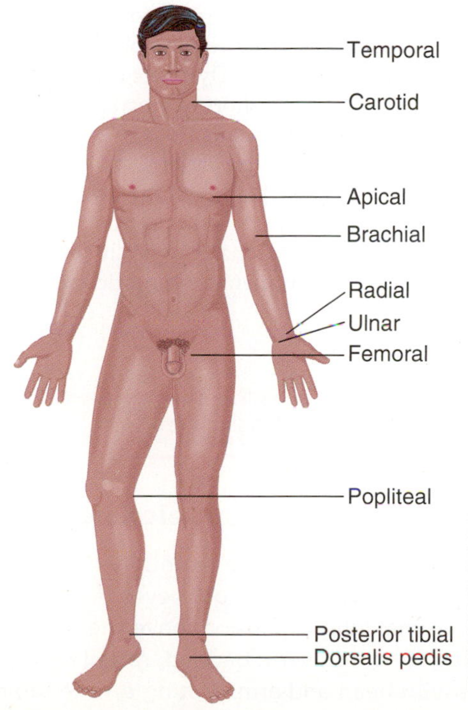

FIGURE 26-7 Pulse Points

as hemorrhage occurs, so in these situations the carotid site should always be used to assess the pulse. Specific pulse sites are shown and pulse point assessments described in Table 26-3.

Pulse rate is an indirect measurement of cardiac output obtained by counting the number of peripheral pulse waves over a pulse point. Assessment of the client's pulse (P) includes the rate, rhythm, and amplitude. A normal pulse rate for adults is between 60 and 100 beats per minute. **Bradycardia** is a heart rate less than 60 beats per minute in an adult. **Tachycardia** is a heart rate greater than 100 beats per minute in an adult.

Pulse rhythm is the regularity of the heartbeat. It indicates how evenly the heart is beating—regular (the beats are evenly spaced) or irregular (the beats are not evenly spaced)—and is also called dysrhythmia.

Pulse amplitude is a measurement of the strength or force exerted by the blood against the arterial wall with each heart contraction. It is described as normal (full, easily palpable), weak (thready and usually rapid), or strong (bounding).

Usual assessment of the radial pulse occurs for 30 seconds, and the number of beats is doubled for documentation. If the pulse rhythm is irregular, the nurse listens to the apical pulse (point of maximum impulse or PMI) for 1 full minute to obtain an accurate pulse rate. In addition, the nurse must assess for a **pulse deficit** (condition in which the apical pulse rate is

TABLE 26-3 Pulse Point Uses

PULSE POINT	USE
Temporal: over temporal bone, lateral and superior to eye	For infants and when radial is inaccessible
Carotid: under lower jaw in neck along medial edge of sternocleidomastoid muscle	For infants and during shock or cardiac arrest when other peripheral pulses are too weak to palpate; also to assess cranial circulation
Apical: left midclavicular line at fourth to fifth intercostal space	To auscultate heart sounds and assess apical-radial deficit
Brachial: between groove of biceps and triceps muscles at antecubital fossa	In cardiac arrest for infants, to assess lower arm circulation, and to auscultate blood pressure
Radial: inner aspect of forearm on thumb side of wrist	To routinely assess pulse
Ulnar: outer aspect of forearm on finger side of wrist	To assess circulation to ulnar side of hand
Femoral: in groin, below inguinal ligament (midpoint between symphysis pubis and anterosuperior iliac spine)	To assess circulation to legs and during cardiac arrest
Popliteal: behind knee, at center in popliteal fossa	To assess circulation to legs and to auscultate leg blood pressure
Posterior tibial: inner aspect of ankle between Achilles tendon and tibia	To assess circulation to feet
Dorsalis pedis: over instep, midway between extension tendons of great and second toe	To assess circulation to feet

COURTESY OF DELMAR CENGAGE LEARNING

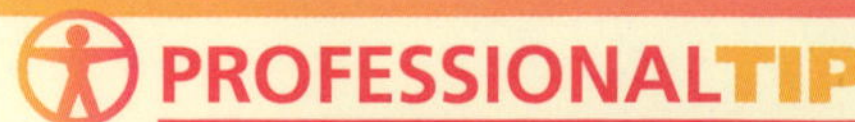

PROFESSIONALTIP

Carotid Pulse Assessment

When assessing a carotid pulse, apply light pressure to only one carotid artery to avoid disruption of cerebral blood flow. Then assess the other one. Only one carotid artery is checked at a time so that the blood supply to the brain is not restricted.

greater than the radial pulse rate). A pulse deficit results from the ejection of a volume of blood that is too small to initiate a peripheral pulse wave.

During the pulse assessment, integrate questions about endurance, fatigue, and any possible episodes of palpitations, "feeling the heart beating," over the chest area.

Respirations

Respiratory assessment measures the breathing pattern. This provides clinical data regarding the pH of arterial blood. Normal breathing is slightly observable, quiet, effortless, regular, and automatic. Assess by observing chest wall expansion and bilateral symmetrical movement of the thorax. Another way to assess breathing is to place the back of the hand next to the client's nose and mouth to feel the expired air.

Assessment of external respirations (R) includes specific characteristics of respirations as well as the use of any type of oxygen equipment, the route, and flow rate. Each respiration includes one complete inhalation (breathing in) and exhalation (breathing out) by the client. When identifying the characteristics of respirations, the rate, depth, and rhythm of each breath is determined.

Eupnea refers to easy respirations with a rate that is age appropriate. **Bradypnea** is a respiratory rate of 10 or fewer breaths per minute. **Tachypnea** is a respiratory rate greater than 24 breaths per minute. **Dyspnea** refers to difficulty breathing as observed by labored or forced respirations by using accessory muscles in the chest and neck. Dyspneic clients are very aware of their respirations and feel short of breath. **Hypoventilation** is characterized by shallow respirations. **Hyperventilation** is characterized by deep, rapid respirations.

Also observe for nasal flaring and the use of accessory muscles for breathing as evidenced by sternal, costal, and subclavicular retractions. Children and males typically utilize abdominal muscles to breathe, but women use thoracic muscles (Fuller &

PROFESSIONALTIP

Positioning for Dyspneic Clients

Dyspneic clients should be maintained in a semi-Fowler's or Fowler's position, never flat in bed. For maximal lung expansion, have the client leaning forward over a padded, raised over-bed table with head and arms resting on the table.

Schaller-Ayers, 2000). During respiration assessment, determine functional ability by asking about any shortness of breath, difficulty in breathing with increased exercise, or problems completing activities of daily living.

Blood Pressure

After checking a client's respirations, assess the client's blood pressure (BP). The most common site for indirect blood pressure measurement is the client's arm over the brachial artery.

When pressure measurements in the upper extremities are not accessible, the popliteal artery, located behind the knee, is the site of choice. Blood pressure can also be assessed in other sites, such as the radial artery in the forearm and the posterior tibial or dorsalis pedis artery in the lower leg. The extremity should be at the level of the heart when blood pressure is measured. Because it is difficult to auscultate sounds over the radial, tibial, and dorsalis pedis arteries, these sites are usually palpated to obtain a systolic reading.

A person's blood pressure is the result of the interaction of cardiac output and peripheral resistance and depends on the speed with which the arterial blood flows, the volume of blood supplied, and the elasticity of the walls of the artery. The force exerted by the blood against the wall of the artery as the heart contracts and relaxes is called the *arterial pressure*. When the ventricles contract and blood is forced into the aorta and pulmonary arteries, the *systolic pressure* is measured. This is the first sound heard. When the heart is in the filling or relaxed stage, the force is described as the *diastolic pressure*. This is when the last sound is heard. The difference between the systolic and diastolic blood pressures is called the *pulse pressure*. A pulse pressure is usually between 30 and 40 mm Hg. Refer to Table 26-4 for normal age-related variations in vital signs.

According to the U.S. Department of Health and Human Services (2003), the client should sit for 5 minutes in a chair rather than on an exam table, with both feet on the floor and the arm supported at heart level. An accurate reading requires the correct width of blood pressure cuff, determined by the circumference of the client's extremity. The cuff bladder encircles 80% of the arm to obtain an accurate blood pressure, and obtaining two measurements ensures accuracy. A falsely elevated reading results if the bladder is too narrow, and a falsely low reading results if it is too wide.

PROFESSIONALTIP

Contraindications for Brachial Artery Blood Pressure Measurement

When the client has any of the following, *do not* measure blood pressure on the involved side:

- Venous access devices, such as an intravenous infusion or arteriovenous fistula for renal dialysis
- Surgery involving the breast, axilla, shoulder, arm, or hand
- Injury or disease to the shoulder, arm, or hand, such as trauma, burns, or application of a cast or bandage

TABLE 26-4 Normal Age-Related Variations in Temperature, Pulse, Respiration, and Blood Pressure

AGE	MEASUREMENT ROUTE	NORMAL RANGE	
		Celsius	Fahrenheit
Newborn	Axillary	35-5–39.5° C	96.0–99.5°F
1 yr	Oral	37.7°C	99.7°F
3 yr	Oral	37.2°C	99.0°F
5 yr	Oral	37.0°C	98.6°F
Adult	Oral	37.0°C	98.6°F
	Axillary	36.4°C	97.6°F
	Rectal	37.6°C	99.6°F
70+ yr	Oral	36.0°C	96.8°F

RESTING PULSE

AGE	NORMAL RANGE	AVERAGE RATE/MIN
Newborn	100–170	140
1 yr	80–170	120
3 yr	80–130	110
6 yr	75–120	100
10 yr	70–110	90
14 yr	60–110	90
Adult	60–100	80

RESTING RESPIRATION

AGE	NORMAL RANGE	AVERAGE RATE/MIN
Newborn	30–50	40
1 yr	20–40	30
3 yr	20–30	25
6 yr	16–22	19
14 yr	14–20	17
Adult	12–20	18

BLOOD PRESSURE

AGE	SYSTOLIC (MM HG)	DIASTOLIC (MM HG)	AVERAGE
Newborn	65–95	30–60	80/60
Infant	65–115	42–80	90/61
3 yr	76–122	46–84	99/65
6 yr	85–115	48–64	100/56
10 yr	93–125	46–68	109/58
14 yr	99–137	51–71	118/61
Adult	100–140	60-90	120/80
Elderly	100–160	60-90	130/80

COURTESY OF DELMAR CENGAGE LEARNING

COMMUNITY/HOME HEALTH CARE

Electronic Sphygmomanometers

Electronic sphygmomanometers are useful for clients who must monitor their own pressure at home. The device electronically inflates and deflates the cuff and displays the systolic and diastolic pressures. They must be recalibrated routinely to ensure an accurate reading.

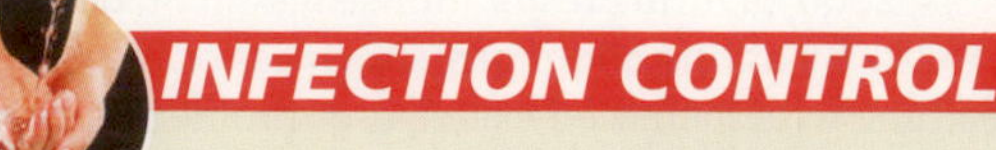

INFECTION CONTROL

Measuring Weight

When standing on a scale, the client wears some type of light foot covering, such as socks or disposable operating room slippers, to prevent the transmission of infection and to enhance comfort.

This is an appropriate time to ask if the client ever becomes light-headed or dizzy when moving from a reclining position to a sitting or standing position. This may occur as a result of an abnormally low blood pressure caused by the inability of the peripheral blood vessels to compensate quickly for the change in position and is referred to as **orthostatic hypotension**.

Pain

According to the Joint Commission standards for ambulatory care, behavioral health care, home care, hospital, health care network, long-term care, and long-term care pharmacy, pain is considered the fifth vital sign. Pain is assessed and recorded along with the client's temperature, pulse, respirations, and blood pressure (JCAHO, 2000a, 2000b; Joint Commission, 2004, 2008). The pain assessment includes pain intensity and quality (character, frequency, location, and duration). Regular assessment and follow-up are according to agency policy. This statement on pain management, "All patients have a right to pain relief," is to be posted in all client care areas (e.g., client rooms, clinic rooms, waiting rooms) (JCAHO, 2000a).

Height and Weight Measurement

Height and weight measurements are as important as the client's vital signs. Routine measurement provides data about growth and development in infants and children. Alterations may indicate illness at any age. Height and weight are routinely taken on visits to physicians' offices, to clinics, on admission to acute care facilities, and in other health care settings.

Height

A height-measuring rod, calibrated in either inches or centimeters, is usually found on a standing weight scale. The client stands erect on the scale's platform and the metal arm, attached to the back of the scale, is extended to gently rest on the top of the client's head. The measurement is read at eye level.

Weight

When a client has an order for "daily weight," the weight should be obtained at the same time of day on the same scale, with the client wearing the same type of clothing. The scale should be balanced before each client is weighed.

Head and Neck Assessment

Assessment of the head and neck determines the client's mental and neurological status and the client's overall **affect** (outward expression of mood or emotion).

Hair and Scalp

The hair and scalp of a client is inspected. Note hair distribution, quantity, texture, and color. The scalp should be smooth and free of any debris or infestations.

Eyes

Examine the eyes to determine if they are symmetrical. Look at the eyebrows and eyelids to see if there is any drooping, which may be a sign of muscle weakness or neurological impairment. Note the color of the sclera and conjunctiva as well as the presence of any drainage.

Assess the pupils to determine their size, shape, and reaction to light. This is accomplished by darkening the room and asking the client to gaze into the distance. Move a light in from the side and notice if the pupil constricts; this is called the *direct light reflex*. Note the pupil size in millimeters both before and after the light response (Figure 26-8). Accommodation is tested by asking the client to focus on an object in the distance; this will dilate the pupils. The client is then asked to move his or her gaze to a near object such as a pen or finger held approximately 3 inches from the nose. The pupils should constrict as they focus on the near object, and the eyes will converge or move in toward midline. This normal response is documented as Pupils Equal, Round, Reactive to Light and Accommodation (PERRLA).

Ask if the client wears glasses and for what reason. Check if any eye problems, such as blurry vision, diplopia (double vision), or difficulty seeing at night, are experienced.

Visual acuity is assessed by a simple, noninvasive procedure using a **Snellen chart** (a chart that contains various-sized letters with standardized numbers at the end of each line of letters). The standardized numbers (called the denominator)

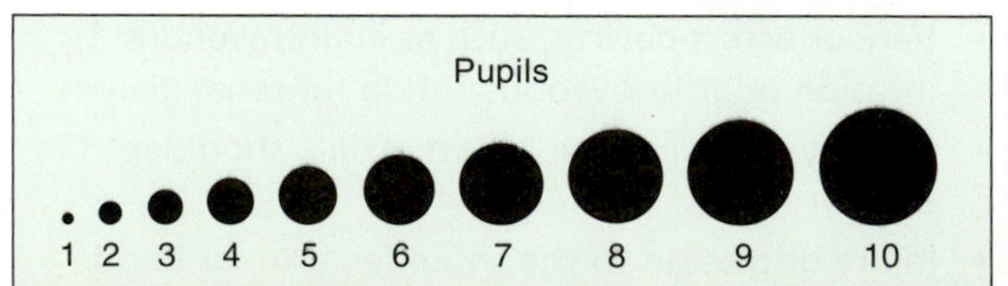

COURTESY OF DELMAR CENGAGE LEARNING

Figure 26-8 Scale Used to Measure Pupil Size in Millimeters

PROFESSIONALTIP

Common Abnormal Breath Odors

- Acetone breath ("fruity" smell) is common in malnourished or diabetic clients with ketoacidosis.
- Musty smell is caused by the breakdown of nitrogen and presence of liver disease.
- Ammonia smell occurs during the end stage of renal failure from a buildup of urea.

indicate the degree of visual acuity when the client is able to read that line of letters at a distance of 20 feet.

Nose

The nose should be symmetrical, midline, and in proportion to other features. Note any deformity, inflammation, or prior trauma. The patency of the nostrils is tested by asking the client to sniff inward while closing off each nostril. Ask the client if the following are ever experienced: nosebleeds, dryness, or decrease in sense of smell.

Lips and Mouth

The lips and mucous membranes of the mouth are observed for color, symmetry, moisture, or lesions. Ask the client with dentures or partial plates to remove them for a more thorough inspection of the mouth. Unusual breath odors are noted. Inspect the oral mucosa by inserting a tongue depressor between the teeth and the cheek. The mucous membranes and gums should be pink, moist, smooth, and free of lesions. Inspection of the tongue assists in determining the client's hydration. The tongue should be pink with a slightly rough texture. During the examination, determine if the client is able to enunciate words appropriately and if there are any voice changes such as hoarseness. Discuss usual dental hygiene practices and obtain the client's history of tobacco usage.

Neck

The neck is assessed for full range of motion. The accessory neck muscles should be symmetrical. As the client moves the head, note any enlargement of the lymph nodes or thyroid gland. Observe for any pulsations in the neck. The carotid pulsation, seen just below the angle of the jaw, normally is the only visible pulsation while the client is in the sitting position.

Mental and Neurological Status and Affect

A head-to-toe assessment incorporates an assessment of the client's mental and neurological status and affect. A client's mental status includes the level of orientation to person, place, and time and the client's responsiveness to the environment. When assessing, observe for responsiveness, the client's ability to follow directions and to respond appropriately to comments and to her name when called.

Neurological assessment of the client focuses on the level of consciousness (LOC), pupil response, hand grasps, and foot pushes. Each of these assessments is discussed in the area of the head-to-toe assessment in which it is observed. The LOC is the client's degree of wakefulness. For example, a client who is alert is fully awake with eyes open and responds to environmental stimuli. The client who is less awake will be drowsy and slow responding to environmental stimuli.

When documenting the client's affect, judgmental words such as *pleasant, happy, cooperative, uncooperative, angry, depressed,* or *hostile* should not be used. Focus specifically on the behaviors exhibited by the client, such as facial expression and verbal and nonverbal behaviors. In doing this, the accuracy of the conversation or the behaviors observed is maintained as well as the legal appropriateness of the assessment.

Skin Assessment

Skin assessment is performed as each area of the body is assessed. Note the color of the skin as well as its moisture or dryness. Inspect and palpate the client's skin, assessing temperature, turgor, edema, and integrity. Palpation of the skin with the dorsal aspect of the hand on the right and left sides of the body provides a comparison of the client's skin temperature. Ask the client if any pain or discomfort in relation to the skin and/or mucous membranes has occurred. Identification of the skin's turgor is best accomplished by gently pinching the skin of the anterior chest and observing the speed of skin return to its previous position. If the skin stays pinched, it may indicate dehydration, and further assessment is needed.

Edema is the visible accumulation of excess interstitial fluid (Daniels, Grendell, & Wilkins, 2010) and is present in overhydration, increased capillary permeability, heart failure, renal failure, cirrhosis of the liver, incompetent lymph system, and varicosities. Vasodilators, calcium antagonists, and nonsteroidal anti-inflammatory drugs (NSAIDS) also cause edema. A client gains 5 to 10 pounds before edema is detected. Assess the weight of clients with congestive heart failure and renal failure on a daily basis. The client is weighed on the same scale, at the same time each day, and with the same amount of clothing so an accurate accounting is made of fluid retention.

Palpate dependent areas (hands, sacrum, legs, ankles, and feet) for edema and assess by firmly applying pressure with a thumb or finger for 5 seconds, noting the amount of indentation (Figure 26-9a). Pitting edema is when an indentation remains after pressure is applied. The degree of edema is based on the depth of indentation and how long it remains. Evaluate pitting edema according to the following rating scale (Assessment Technologies Institute, 2007; Estes, 2010; Gehring, 2002):

+0 no edema

+1 indentation of 2 mm (0–¼ inches), disappears rapidly (trace)

+2 pitting of 4 mm (¼–½ inch), disappears in 10 to 15 seconds (mild)

+3 pitting of 6 mm (½–1 inch), lasts 1 to 2 minutes (moderate)

+4 pitting of 8 mm or more (greater than 1 inch), lasts 2 to 5 minutes (severe) (Figure 26-9b)

Note the location, size, distribution, and appearance of skin lesions throughout the body. Document any breaks or changes in the skin integrity, such as scratches, bruises, skin tears, cuts, and scars from previous injuries or surgeries. Note the general hygiene of the skin and ask the client about usual skin care routines.

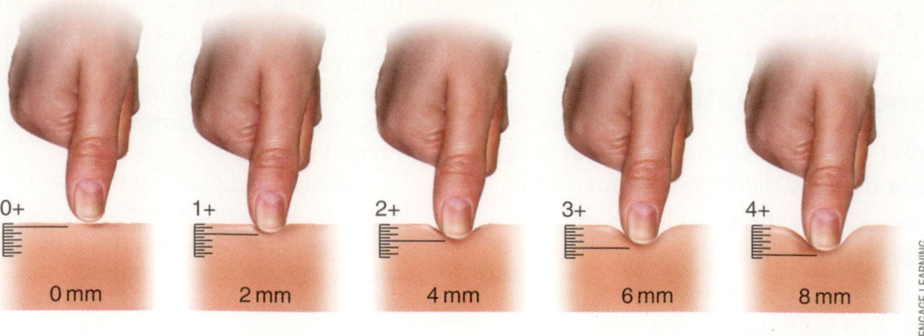
0+
1+
2+
3+
4+
0 mm
2 mm
4 mm
6 mm
8 mm
0+ No pitting edema
1+ Mild pitting edema. 2 mm depression that disappears rapidly.
2+ Moderate pitting edema. 4 mm depression that disappears in 10–15 seconds.
3+ Moderately severe pitting edema. 6 mm depression that may last more than 1 minute.
4+ Severe pitting edema. 8 mm depression that can last more than 2 minutes.
COURTESY OF DELMAR CENGAGE LEARNING

FIGURE 26-9 Assessing edema. Palpate for edema in the lower extremities on the tibia, the dorsal aspect of the foot, and behind the medial malleolus and Assess edema according to the rating scale.

CULTURAL CONSIDERATIONS

Skin, Mouth, and Eye Color

- The darker the client's skin, the more difficult it is to assess changes in color.
- Establish a baseline skin color by observing the least pigmented skin surfaces, which include the volar surfaces of the forearms, the palms of the hands, the soles of the feet, the abdomen, and the buttocks. There should be an underlying red tone in these areas. Absence of this red tone may indicate pallor.
- African American oral mucosa has a bluish hue. Caucasians have pink mucosa (Estes, 2010).
- Oral hyperpigmentation often is found in dark-skinned persons. If the hard palate is not hyperpigmented, it has a yellow discoloration in the presence of jaundice.
- The lips may be used to assess jaundice and cyanosis, and the sclera may be used to assess jaundice if a baseline color has been established for each.
- The conjunctiva reflect color changes of cyanosis or pallor.
- Nail beds are used to note how quickly the color returns after pressure has been released from the free edge of the nail, regardless of the nail bed color.

THORACIC ASSESSMENT

During thoracic assessment, the condition of the client's cardiovascular and respiratory systems along with assessment of the breasts are determined.

Cardiovascular Status

Assessment of the client's cardiovascular status by the LP/VN focuses specifically on listening to the apical pulse, identifying heart tones, and checking the nail beds. The apical pulse (point of maximum impulse or PMI) is determined by using auscultation and palpation. To assess the apical pulse, palpate over the apex of the heart at the fifth left intercostal space at the midclavicular line. A slight, short duration tap against the fingers will be felt, and this is where the apical pulse is auscultated (Figure 26-10). Listening to the apical pulse is the most accurate assessment of the heart rate and should occur for 60 seconds. The apical pulse is assessed first with the diaphragm of the stethoscope for the regularity or irregularity of its rhythm. Second, the bell of the stethoscope is used to differentiate the loudness or tones of the heart. Along with the apical pulse, the other pulse points may be assessed now or when the extremities are assessed.

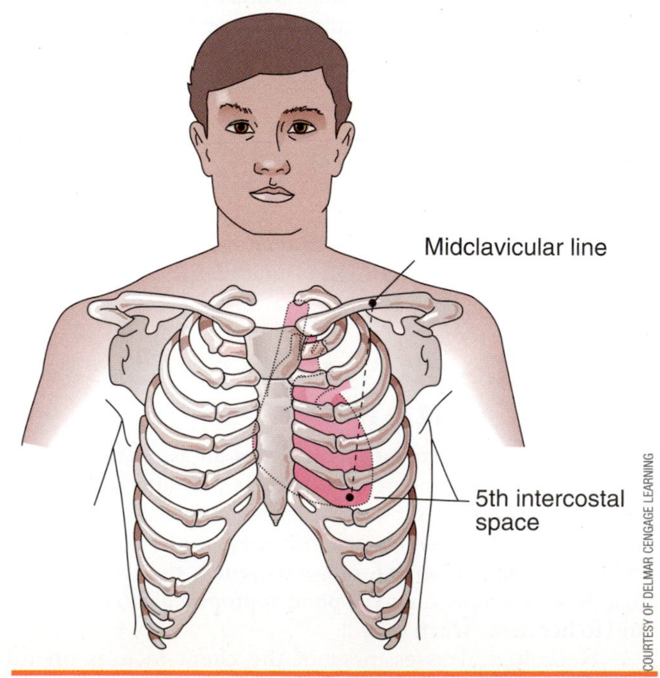
Midclavicular line
5th intercostal space
COURTESY OF DELMAR CENGAGE LEARNING

FIGURE 26-10 Assessing the Apical Pulse

To assess blood perfusion of peripheral vessels and skin, note changes in skin temperature, color, and sensation and changes in the pulses and feel the toes for warmth and color. Because the position of the extremities can affect the skin temperature and appearance, extremities must always be assessed at heart level and at normal room and body temperature. Compare peripheral pulses bilaterally and note changes in strength and quality. The nurse checks the degree to which the tissues are perfused by measuring the SaO_2 with a pulse oximeter. The normal range is 95% to 100% saturation.

The focus of the functional assessment includes personal habits contributing to or preventing cardiovascular disease. Ask about the client's personal exercise habits and elicit information regarding past chest pain or shortness of breath. The client should describe any pain; its location, duration, and precipitating factors; and what is done to alleviate the pain. Also ask if the client has ever fainted or felt dizzy. Any lower leg swelling and its cause should also be noted.

Respiratory Status

Breath sound assessment is performed after assessing the apical pulse rate. The presence of normal and abnormal breath sounds is revealed by respiratory auscultation. Ask the client to breathe only through the mouth during auscultation because mouth breathing decreases air turbulence, which interferes with an accurate assessment.

There are three types of normal breath sounds, each having a unique pitch, quality, intensity, location, and duration in the inspiratory and expiratory phases of respiration:

- **Bronchial sounds**. Loud, high-pitched sounds with a hollow quality heard longer on expiration than inspiration from air moving through the trachea
- **Bronchovesicular sounds**. Medium-pitched, blowing sounds heard equally on inspiration and expiration from air moving through the large airways, posteriorly between the scapula and anteriorly over bronchioles lateral to the sternum at the first and second intercostal spaces
- **Vesicular sounds**. Soft, breezy, low-pitched sounds heard longer on inspiration than expiration resulting from air moving through the smaller airways over the lung's periphery, with the exception of the scapular area

Nonnormal breath sounds are described as either abnormal or **adventitious breath sounds**. Adventitious breath sounds include sibilant wheeze (formerly wheeze), sonorous wheeze (formerly rhonchi), fine and coarse crackle (formerly rales), pleural friction rub, and stridor. **Sibilant wheezes** are high-pitched, whistling sounds heard during inhalation and exhalation. A **sonorous wheeze** is a low-pitched snoring sound that is louder on exhalation. Coughing may alter the sound if caused by mucus. **Crackles** are popping sounds heard on inhalation or exhalation, not cleared by coughing. A **pleural friction rub** is a low-pitched grating sound on inhalation and exhalation. **Stridor** is a high-pitched, harsh sound heard on inspiration when the trachea or larynx is obstructed. Assess breath sounds of the anterior, posterior, and lateral chest wall for normal as well as adventitious breath sounds. Monitor adventitious breath sounds consistently. The lungs are assessed from side to side so the two sides can be compared, as shown in Figure 26-11.

The functional assessment information to be obtained when assessing the respiratory status includes any difficulty breathing or the presence of a cough. Ask the client if the cough is nonproductive or productive and to describe the secretions produced. Terms used to describe secretions expectorated are *thick, thin, yellow, green*. The client's occupational or home environment may affect breathing patterns; exposure to dust, chemicals, vapors, tobacco, smoke, or paint fumes, and irritants such as asbestos are noted.

> **CRITICAL THINKING**
>
> **Assessing Breath Sounds**
>
> When listening to your client's breath sounds, you hear a sound that you think is a pleural friction rub. How do you determine if the sound you heard is really a friction rub?

Wounds, Scars, Drains, Tubes, Dressings

When assessing the thorax, note any type of wounds, scars, drains, tubes, or dressings. Documentation of these include the location, size, and amount of drainage or discharge and, if present, signs of inflammation.

Breasts

Assessment of the breasts is done for both male and female clients. Begin by inspecting the breasts for size and symmetry. It is common to have a slight difference in size of breasts. Note any obvious masses, dimpling (a depression in the surface skin), or inflammation. The skin normally is smooth and even in color. Determine if the nipples and areola are symmetrical in size, shape, and color and note any discharge from the nipples.

Any abnormal area should be palpated for size, consistency, mobility, tenderness, and location of the lesion. Another area to include in breast assessment is the axillary lymph nodes that drain the breasts. Palpate the axilla for enlarged or inflamed lymph nodes, ask if there is any tenderness, and determine if and when the client performs breast self-exams. Note if the client has had a mammogram and when the last one was taken.

> **PROFESSIONALTIP**
>
> **Assessment of the Abdomen**
>
> Although the usual sequence for implementing assessment techniques is inspection, palpation, percussion, and auscultation, assessment of the abdomen entails a different sequence. Because palpation can affect sounds heard on auscultation, the sequence for abdominal assessment is as follows:
>
> - Inspection
> - Auscultation
> - Percussion
> - Palpation

A Anterior
Right midclavicular line
Thyroid cartilage
Trachea
Suprasternal notch
Left upper lobe
Angle of Louis
Right upper lobe
Right middle lobe
Right lower lobe
Left lower lobe
Right anterior axillary line
Midsternal line

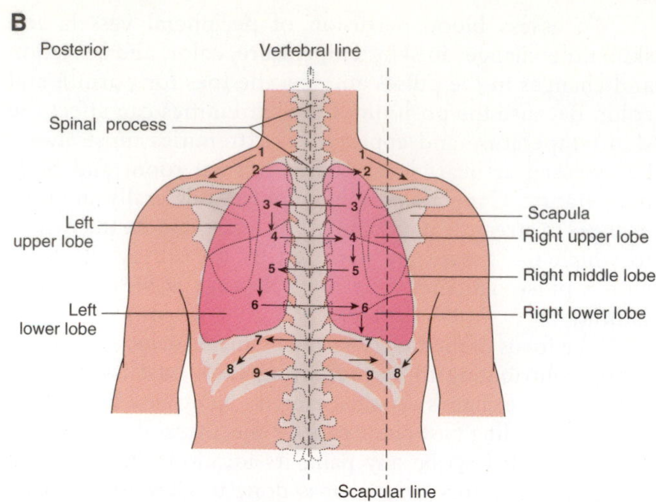

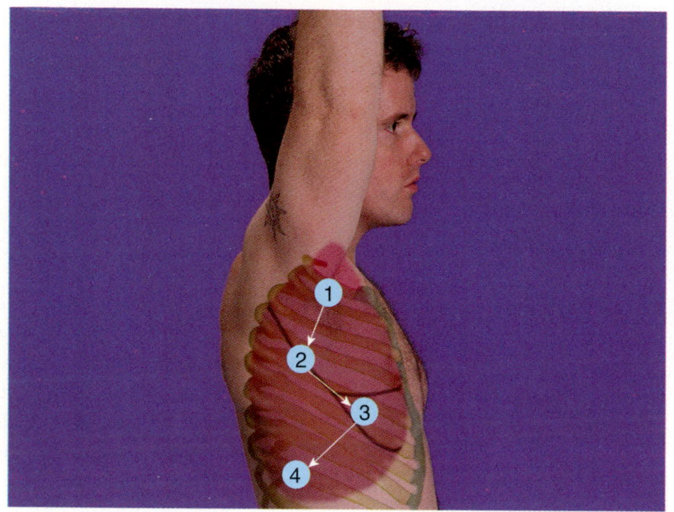

C Right Lateral Thorax

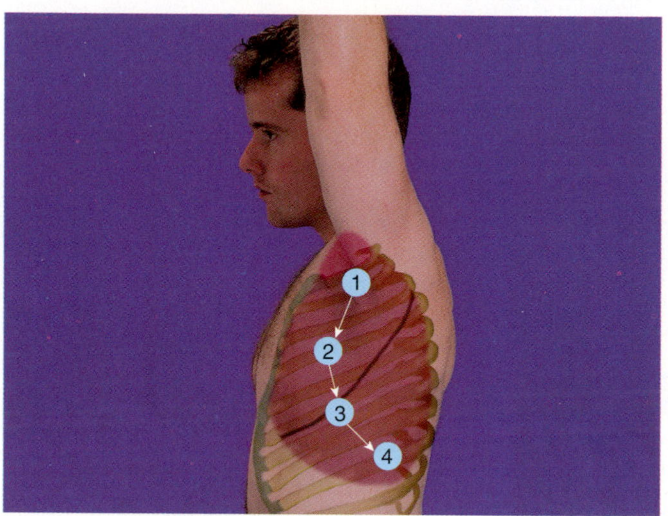

D Left Lateral Throax

COURTESY OF DELMAR CENGAGE LEARNING

FIGURE 26-11 Symmetrical Assessment of Breath Sounds; *A,* Anterior; *B,* Posterior; *C,* Right lateral; *D,* Left lateral. A method of assessing breath sounds is to move the bell of the stethoscope as directed by the arrows in pictures A and B. It is important to find a system that covers all areas of the lungs for thorough lung assessment.

ABDOMINAL ASSESSMENT

Abdominal assessment determines the status of the client's gastrointestinal and genitourinary systems. Note any type of wounds, scars, drains, tubes, dressings, or ostomies. Documentation of these must include the location, size, and amount of drainage or discharge, and if present, signs of inflammation.

Gastrointestinal Status

The abdomen is first inspected for rashes and scars. Assess if the abdomen is flat, rounded, or distended and observe the abdomen for symmetry and visible signs of peristalsis or pulsations. If the abdomen is distended, ask the client questions pertaining to bowel movements and urinary status.

Auscultation is the second component of the abdominal assessment of a client's bowel status. A "bubbly-gurgly" sound, caused by peristalsis and movement of the intestinal contents, can be heard by placing the stethoscope on each quadrant of the abdomen and listening for approximately 1 minute. These sounds should be present in all four quadrants of the abdomen, beginning in the right lower quadrant (RLQ) and moving clockwise around the four quadrants, as shown in Figure 26-12. When approximately 5 to 20 bowel sounds are heard per minute, or one at least every 5 to 15 seconds, the bowel sounds are considered active.

The absence of bowel sounds during 1 minute of auscultation in each quadrant is documented as absent bowel sounds. Bowel sounds of less than five per minute are described as hypoactive, while an excess of 20 or more bowel sounds per minute is defined as hyperactive. High-pitched, loud, rushing sounds heard with or without a stethoscope are termed **borborygmi**. This is caused by the passage of gas through the liquid contents of the intestine.

Percussion of the abdomen is done in all four quadrants. The predominant abdominal percussion sound is tympany caused by percussing over the air-filled stomach and intestines.

Light palpation of the abdomen is done to assess for muscle tone, masses, pulsations, or any signs of tenderness or discomfort. Abdominal muscles may be palpated and should feel relaxed on light palpation, not tightly contracted or

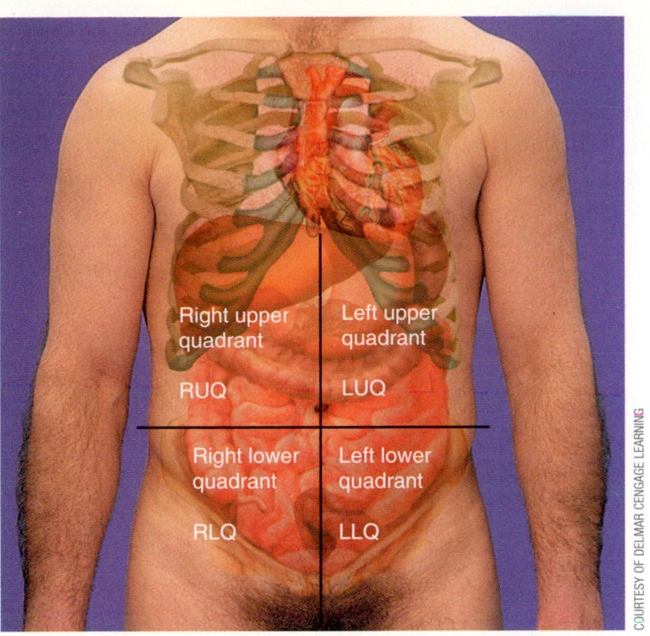

FIGURE 26-12 The Four Quadrants of the Abdomen

spastic. If the client is anxious, muscle contraction may be evident. Palpation of a separation of the rectus abdominis muscle may be felt, especially in clients who are obese or pregnant. The rectus abdominis muscle includes two large, midline muscles that extend from the xiphoid process to the symphysis pubis and can be palpated midline as the client raises his or her head. Rebound tenderness, indicating possible inflammation of the appendix, may be elicited by depressing the abdomen in the right lower quadrant and quickly withdrawing the fingers. This examination is done at the end of the abdominal assessment because of the possibility of increasing the client's level of pain. If any of the abdominal organs can be felt with light palpation, this is abnormal and should be reported to the nursing supervisor. After assessment of bowel sounds, question the client about diet, usual bowel patterns, appetite, weight changes, indigestion, heartburn, nausea, pain, and use of enemas or laxatives.

Genitourinary Status

Assessment of the client's urinary and reproductive status is accomplished mainly by inspection and use of interview skills. Genitourinary assessment includes examination of the abdomen, urinary meatus and genitalia, and assessment of the client's urine.

Inspect the abdomen for any enlargement or fullness. In the normal adult, the abdomen is smooth, flat, and symmetrical. The urinary meatus is inspected for any abnormalities such as inflammation and discharge, which may signal a urethral infection.

In females, observe the appearance of the genitalia (labia, clitoris, vaginal opening). Questions to ask the client that focus on the reproductive history include pregnancies, use of birth control, menstrual cycle history, present sexual activity, use of protection during intercourse, date of the last Pap test, and determination of how any present illness has or will affect sexual activity.

In males, inspect the penis, urethral meatus, foreskin (if uncircumcized), and scrotum. Questions to ask the client that focus on the reproductive history include present sexual activity, use of protection during intercourse, and how the present illness has or will affect sexual activity. Ask if the client performs testicular self-examinations.

Note any lesions or ulcerations that may indicate sexually transmitted disease. The usual voiding pattern and any recent changes should be determined if the client has had any history of urinary tract infections, kidney stones, change in the urinary stream, or painful urination or nocturia.

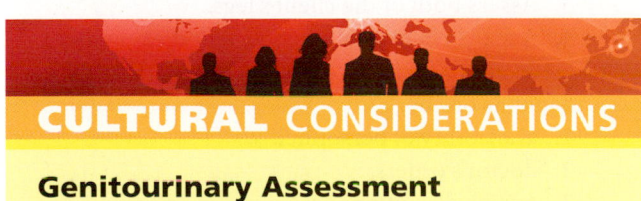

CULTURAL CONSIDERATIONS

Genitourinary Assessment

Middle Eastern women often will remain veiled during this assessment.

MUSCULOSKELETAL AND EXTREMITY ASSESSMENT

Assess symmetry and strength of major muscle groups throughout the head-to-toe assessment. Any time during the assessment when the client is repositioned, observe the range of movement the client utilizes to make that position change. Ask the client to walk across the room and observe the client's movements and posture when sitting up in bed to assess gross motor movement and posture. Assessment of the client's handshake gives an estimate of muscle strength. Palpating muscles lightly identifies swelling, tone, or any specific changes in the shape of the muscles.

Hand grasps and foot pushes assess the strength and equality of the client's extremities. Upper extremity strength is assessed by having the client grasp the nurse's index and middle fingers of each hand. The grasp should be equal in both hands. Foot pushes assess the lower extremities. The nurse's hands are placed on the soles of the client's feet and the client is asked to push both feet against the nurse's hands. The push should be equal in both feet. Ask the client to touch the tip of her nose with a finger and then the tip of the nurse's finger as it is moved to different locations to test the client's coordination skills.

Assess strength and symmetry of some of the major muscle groups by watching gait and postural movements. Note any aids to ambulation. Examine muscles, first in one extremity and then the other; note equality of size, contour, tone, and strength.

Carefully assess the skin of the lower extremities to determine color changes, loss of feeling or hair, change in temperature within the extremity and from one extremity to the other, and presence of varicose veins, ulcers, and edema. Ask if the client experiences any leg pain or cramps or if muscle weakness is experienced or if difficulty or pain when walking or performing routine daily activities occurs. The functional assessment includes asking the client about routine activities such as cooking, shopping, exercise, yard work, and hobbies. Tolerance limitations can be identified by observing for stiffness, crepitus, or fatigue during ambulation. Determine if the client can safely and appropriately perform functions essential for home life and ADLs.

CASE STUDY

K.J., a 17-year-old male, was in a motorcycle accident and sustained fractures of the lower jaw, right humerus, left femur, and right tibia and a dislocated shoulder. His mouth is wired shut, and he has a long arm cast on his right arm, a sling on the left arm, a short leg case on the right lower leg, and skeletal traction on the left leg. He is assigned to you, and you are to complete an assessment on him.

1. You do not have a temporal artery thermometer on your unit. How would you obtain a temperature on K.J.?
2. What would you include when completing the neurological assessment? Why is the neurological assessment so important to this client?
3. When listening to heart tones, you notice a different sound than the usual lubb-dubb. What would you do with this information?
4. Describe how you would listen to breath sounds on K.J. Why is it so important to assess breath sounds on K.J.?
5. Describe how you would assess bowel sounds. Why is it so important to assess bowel sounds on K.J.?
6. K.J. has a catheter inserted. Practice your documentation skills by writing a normal urine finding as if you were charting on K.J.
7. How would you assess for edema? According to the edema rating scale, how would you document pitting edema of 4 mm?
8. Describe how you would assess K.J.'s musculoskeletal system and extremities.

SUMMARY

- Psychosocial needs of clients are identified within the scope of a functional assessment.
- The health history and the physical examination used together present a holistic view of client needs.
- Collection of vital signs is the foundation of each head-to-toe assessment and includes temperature, pulse, respirations, blood pressure, and pain.
- Assessment of a client's mental and neurological status is determined by obtaining information about the client's level of consciousness, pupil response, as well as hand grip and foot push capabilities.
- When describing a client's affect, utilize terms that are descriptive of the specific behavior observed, not a judgment about the behavior.
- Assessing the cardiovascular status of each client includes palpation of specific pulse points.
- Auscultation of lung fields assists in collection of data regarding the breath sounds of the client.
- An abdominal assessment includes use of inspection, auscultation, percussion, and palpation within the four quadrants of the abdomen to establish bowel status and function.
- Through observation of client gait and overall range of movement, some knowledge of the symmetry and strength of muscles is obtained.
- During the assessment of wounds, drains, dressings, and other external devices, maintain accurate documentation of the amount of drainage, color, or other changes.

REVIEW QUESTIONS

1. S.J. is 54 years old. While performing the assessment overview, S.J. states, "I just get so lightheaded when I first get up in the morning." S.J. most likely has:
   1. cyanosis.
   2. hypertension.
   3. orthostatic hypertension.
   4. orthostatic hypotension.

2. During the physical head-to-toe assessment of the client, the nurse checks the pulse and blood pressure. Which of the four assessment techniques did the nurse utilize?
   1. Auscultation, palpation, and inspection.
   2. Auscultation, percussion, and inspection.
   3. Auscultation and palpation.
   4. Palpation and inspection.

3. On admission to your unit, the client verbalizes increased pain in her left leg. What would be the pertinent assessment information to collect about this client?
   1. Listen to the client's bowel sounds.
   2. Check circulation in the right leg.
   3. Assess both of the client's legs.
   4. Ask the client about her current diet.

4. How often a nurse assesses a client's vital signs depends on the:
   1. availability of personnel.
   2. doctor's orders.
   3. nurse's discretion.
   4. client's condition.

5. The nurse checks the radial pulse for 30 seconds and multiplies by 2. She notices an irregularity in the beat. What is the next action the nurse should take?
   1. Check the radial pulse for 60 seconds.
   2. Listen to the apical pulse for 60 seconds.
   3. Listen to the apical for 30 seconds and multiply by 2.
   4. Continue with the rest of the assessment.
6. In what order would a nurse assess a client's abdomen?
   1. Inspection, palpation, percussion, auscultation
   2. Inspection, auscultation, palpation, percussion
   3. Auscultation, palpation, percussion, inspection
   4. Palpation, percussion, inspection, auscultation
7. The best way for a nurse to conduct a physical assessment of the lungs is to: (Select all that apply.)
   1. ask the client to breathe through the nose.
   2. ask the client to breathe through the mouth.
   3. listen to breath sounds on the anterior and posterior chest wall.
   4. listen to breath sounds on the anterior, posterior, and lateral chest wall.
   5. listen to the lung sounds from side to side.
   6. ask the client if the cough is productive or nonproductive.
8. In what position is a client placed in preparation for a rectal exam?
   1. Supine.
   2. Prone.
   3. Sims'.
   4. Right lateral.
9. A 72-year-old woman was recently admitted to a nursing home because of confusion, disorientation, and self-destructive behaviors. She was accompanied by her daughter, who says that she does not have a history of these behaviors. The woman asks the nurse, "Where am I?" The best response for the nurse to make is:
   1. "Don't worry. You're safe here."
   2. "Tell me where you think you are."
   3. "What did your daughter tell you?"
   4. "You're at the community nursing home."
10. The nurse is preparing the client for a physical assessment. The first thing he should do is:
   1. shut the door for privacy.
   2. turn down the sound on the television.
   3. explain the procedure to the client.
   4. listen to lung sounds.

REFERENCES/SUGGESTED READINGS

Andresen, G. (1998). Assessing the older patient. *RN, 61*(3), 46–55.

Assessment Technologies Institute. (2007). *Fundamentals of nursing content mastery series review module*. Stillwell, KS: Author.

Barkauskas, V., Bauman, L., & Darling-Fisher, C. (2002). *Health and physical assessment* (3rd ed.). St. Louis, MO: Mosby.

Bickley, L. S., & Sailagyi, P. (2002). *Bates' guide to physical examination and history taking* (8th ed.). Philadelphia: Lippincott Williams & Wilkins.

Clayton, M. (2006). Communication: An important part of nursing care. *American Journal of Nursing, 106*(11), 70–71.

Craig, J., Lancaster, G., Taylor, S., Williamson, P., & Smyth, R. (2002). Now, hear this: Ear temps in children found to be inaccurate. *Lancet, 360*(9333), 603–609.

Crow, S. (1997). Your guide to gloves. *Nursing97, 27*(3), 26–28.

Daniels, R., Grendell, R., & Wilkins, F. (2010). Nursing fundamentals: Caring and clinical decision making (2nd ed.). Clifton Park, NY: Delmar Cengage Learning.

Estes, M. (2010). *Health assessment and physical examination* (4th ed.). Clifton Park, NY: Delmar Cengage Learning.

Finesilver, C. (2001, April). Perfecting your skills: Respiratory assessment. *RN's Travel Nursing Today*, 16–26.

Fuller, J., & Schaller-Ayers, J. (2000). *Health assessment: A nursing approach*. (3rd ed.). Philadelphia: Lippincott Williams & Wilkins.

Gallauresi, B. (1998). Pulse oximeters. *Nursing98, 28*(9), 31.

Gecsedi, R., & Decker, G. (2001). Incorporating alternative therapies into pain management: More patients are considering complementary approaches. *American Journal of Nursing, 101*(4), 35–39.

Gehring, P. (2002, April). Perfecting your skills: Vascular assessment. *RN's Travel Nursing Today*, 16–24.

Gulla, J., & Singer, A. (2000). Over half of ED patients use alternative therapy. *American Journal of Nursing, 100*(8), 24J.

Heery, K. (2000). Straight talk about the patient interview. *Nursing2000, 30*(6), 66–67.

Hodge, P., & Ullrich, S. (1999). Does your assessment include alternative therapies? *RN, 62*(6), 47–49.

Husain, M., & Coleman, R. (2002). Should you treat a fever? *Nursing2002, 32*(10), 66–70.

Joint Commission. (2004). Nutritional, functional, and pain assessments and screens. Retrieved October 29, 2008, from http://www.jointcommission.org/AccreditationPrograms/Hospitals/Standards/FAWs/Provi

Joint Commission. (2008). Joint Commission urges patients to "speak up" about pain. Retrieved October 29, 2008, from http://www.jointcommission.org/Library/TM_Physicians/tmp_10_08.htm

Joint Commission on Accreditation of Healthcare Organizations. (2000a). Comprehensive accreditation manual for hospitals (CAMH) revised pain management standards. Available: http://www.jcaho.org/standard/pm_hap.html

Joint Commission on Accreditation of Healthcare Organizations. (2000b). Pain assessment and management standards. Available: http://www.jcaho.org/standard/pm_coll.html

Karch, A., & Karch, F. (2000). When a blood pressure isn't routine. *American Journal of Nursing, 100*(3), 23.

Kirton, C. (1997). Assessing bowel sounds. *Nursing97, 27*(3), 64.

Klingman, L. (1999a). Assessing the female reproductive system. *American Journal of Nursing, 99*(8), 37–43.

Klingman, L. (1999b). Assessing the male genitalia. *American Journal of Nursing, 99*(7), 47–50.

Lower, J. (2002). Facing neuro assessment fearlessly. *Nursing2002, 32*(2), 58–64.

Mehta, M. (2003a). Assessing the abdomen. *Nursing2003, 33*(5), 54–55.

Mehta, M. (2003b). Assessing cardiovascular status. *Nursing2003, 33*(2), 56–58.

Mehta, M. (2003c). Assessing respiratory status. *Nursing2003, 33*(2), 54–56.

Murray, R., Zentner, J., & Yakimo, R. (2008). *Health promotion strategies through the lifespan* (8th ed.). Norwalk, CT: Prentice Hall.

O'Hanlon-Nichols, T. (1997). Basic assessment series: The adult cardiovascular system. *American Journal of Nursing, 97*(12), 34–40.

O'Hanlon-Nichols, T. (1998). Basic assessment series: Gastrointestinal system. *American Journal of Nursing, 98*(4), 48–53.

O'Hanlon-Nichols, T. (1998a). Basic assessment series: Musculoskeletal system. *American Journal of Nursing, 98*(6), 48–52.

O'Hanlon-Nichols, T. (1998c). Basic assessment series: The adult pulmonary system. *American Journal of Nursing, 98*(2), 39–45.

O'Hanlon-Nichols, T. (1999). Neurologic assessment. *American Journal of Nursing, 99*(6), 44–50.

Owen, A. (1998). Respiratory assessment revisited. *Nursing98, 28*(4), 48–49.

Pullen, R. (2003). Using an ear thermometer. *Nursing2003, 33*(5), 24.

Rice, K. (1998). Sounding out blood flow with a Doppler device. *Nursing98, 28*(9), 56–57.

Rice, K. (1999). Measuring thigh BP. *Nursing99, 29*(8), 58–59.

Scott, T. (2008). How do I differentiate normal aging of the skin from pathologic conditions? Retrieved October 29, 2008, from http://www.medscape.com/viewarticle/575293_print

Stanley, W. (2003). Nailing a key assessment. *Nursing2003, 33*(8), 50–51.

Thomas, J., & Feliciano, C. (2003). Measuring BP with a Doppler device. *Nursing2003, 33*(7), 52–53.

University of Maryland Medicine. (2002). An introduction to CAM. Available: http://www.umm.edu/altmed/ConsModalities/AnIntroductionToCAMcm.html

U.S. Department of Health and Human Services, National Institutes of Health. (2003). The seventh report of the Joint National Committee on Prevention, Detection, Evaluation, and Treatment of High Blood Pressure JNC 7 Express (NIH Publication No. 03-5233). Washington, DC: Author. Retrieved October 28, 2008, from http://www.nhlbi.nih.gov/guidelines/hypertension/express.pdf

Warner, P., Rowe, T., & Whipple, B. (1999). Shedding light on the sexual history. *American Journal of Nursing, 99*(6), 34–40.

Weber, J., & Kelley, J. (2006). *Health assessment in nursing* (3rd ed.). Philadelphia: Lippincott Williams & Wilkins.

Williams, M., & Keen, P. (2007). Gynecologic assessment of the elderly patient. Retrieved October 28, 2008, from http://www.medscape.com/viewprogram/6881_pnt

CHAPTER 27
Pain Management

MAKING THE CONNECTION

Refer to the following chapters to increase your understanding of pain management:

Basic Nursing

- ***Communication***
- ***Cultural Considerations***
- ***End-of-Life Care***
- ***Complementary/Alternative Therapies***

Intermediate Procedures

- ***Administering Oral, Sublingual, and Buccal Medication***
- ***Withdrawing Medication from an Ampule***
- ***Withdrawing Medication from a Vial***
- ***Administering an Intradermal Injection***
- ***Administering a Subcutaneous Injection***
- ***Administering an Intramuscular Injection***

LEARNING OBJECTIVES

Upon completion of this chapter, you should be able to:

- Define key terms.
- Identify the four components of pain conduction.
- Discuss the gate control theory of pain.
- Describe the types of pain.
- List three guidelines that should be included in a thorough pain assessment.
- Identify three general principles of pain management.
- List the nurse's responsibilities in administration of analgesics.
- Identify site of action of both nonopioid and opioid analgesics.
- Describe three examples of nonpharmacological measures for pain relief.
- List nursing diagnosis for pain.
- Discuss nursing interventions that promote comfort.
- Evaluate client's pain relief.

KEY TERMS

acupuncture
acute pain
adjuvant medications
afferent pain pathway
analgesia
analgesics
ceiling effect
chronic acute pain
chronic nonmalignant pain
chronic pain
colic
cryotherapy
cutaneous pain
distraction
efferent pain pathway
endorphins
epidural analgesia
gate control pain theory
hypnosis
intrathecal analgesia
ischemic pain
mixed agonist-antagonist
modulation
myofascial pain syndromes
neuralgia
nociceptors
noxious stimulus
pain
pain threshold
pain tolerance
patient-controlled analgesia (PCA)
perception
phantom limb pain
progressive muscle relaxation
recurrent acute pain
referred pain
reframing
relaxation techniques
somatic pain
tolerance
transcutaneous electrical nerve stimulation (TENS)
transduction
transmission
visceral pain

INTRODUCTION

Pain is a phenomenon found in all specialties of nursing. No matter the setting, including neonatal intensive care, intraoperative, home care, or clinics, there are challenges in pain management. While other health care team members address pain management with clients, the nurse spends the most time with the client experiencing pain. For example, in an acute care setting, the physician orders the **analgesics** (substances that relieve pain) for the client but may spend only 10 to 15 minutes a day with that client. Nurses are present 24 hours a day, administer the medications, assess the client's response, and report the response to the physician. The nurse's role can be pivotal in relieving the client's pain.

The experience of pain can have a significant impact on a client's health. It is a personal experience affecting all aspects of an individual's health, including physical well-being, mental status, and effectiveness of coping mechanisms. This chapter provides an overview of the complex phenomenon of pain, including pain definitions, pain physiology, and pain assessment. Strategies to control pain are also discussed, including pharmacological, noninvasive, and invasive techniques.

DEFINITIONS OF PAIN

The phenomenon of pain is referenced as far back as the Babylonian clay tablets. Aristotle (4th century B.C.) described pain as an emotion, being the opposite of pleasure. Although emotions certainly play an important role in pain perception, there is much more to the experience than the feelings involved.

In the Middle Ages, pain had religious connotations. Pain was seen as God's punishment for sins or as evidence that an individual was possessed by demons. This definition of pain is still embraced by some clients who might tell the nurse that the suffering is their "cross to bear." Pain relief may not be the goal for those individuals who believe in this definition of pain. Spiritual counseling may need to be implemented before this person is willing to work toward relief.

The most widely accepted definition of **pain** is one developed by the International Association for the Study of Pain (IASP). This organization defines pain as "an unpleasant sensory and emotional experience associated with actual or potential tissue damage or described in terms of such damage" (IASP, 2008). This definition incorporates both the sensory and the emotional components of pain. It also acknowledges that evidence of actual tissue damage is not required in order for the pain to be considered real.

Many pain experts emphasize the subjective nature of pain. Unlike a blood pressure or a blood glucose measurement, the intensity of discomfort the client is feeling cannot be measured with an instrument. McCaffery and Pasero (1999) say it best by defining pain as "whatever the person experiencing it says it is, existing whenever he says it does" (p. 17). All nursing actions are based on what pain means to the client. The first and most important step in assessing a client's pain is to believe the client. The client's description of the pain experience, or self-report, should be the basis of all care decisions. Without it, care will be ineffective (Teeter & Kemper, 2008a).

Because of widespread undertreatment of pain, in 1995 the American Pain Society launched an international campaign to raise awareness about the problem and to promote the routine assessment of pain by health care providers. This quickly led to the incorporation of pain assessment into the daily activities of clinicians as the "fifth vital sign" after the Joint Commission initiated pain management quality standards of care in 2001. However, research conducted by the U.S. Veterans Administration showed no improvement in pain management after adopting this strategy (Mularski et al., 2006). Assessment itself is not enough to ensure adequate pain management for clients. Health care providers must act on the assessment findings (Teeter & Kemper, 2008a).

Although pain has had many definitions throughout history, research in pain physiology shows that pain is a complex phenomenon. Pain is often difficult for clients to describe and nurses to understand, yet it is among the most common complaints leading individuals to seek health care. Until recently, pain was viewed as a symptom that required diagnosis and treatment of the underlying cause. It is now clear that pain itself can be detrimental to the health and healing of clients. Pain control, not just relief from pain once it occurs, must be recognized as a priority in the care of clients in all settings.

NATURE OF PAIN

Pain experience is a signal of tissue damage, as in the pain of cancer and chronic illness. Pain can also be a protective mechanism to prevent further injury, as when a client guards or protects an injured body part. Pain, as a warning of potential tissue damage, may be absent in people with hereditary sensory neuropathies, congenital nerve or spinal cord abnormalities, multiple sclerosis, diabetic neuropathy, alcoholism, leprosy, and nerve or spinal cord injury.

COMMON MYTHS ABOUT PAIN

Pain is often misunderstood and misjudged because it is subjective (depends on the client's perception) and cannot be objectively measured through a laboratory test or diagnostic data. A client's report of the level of pain varies based on cultural and experiential background. The nurse's interpretation of a client's pain is filtered through the nurse's biases and expectations. Some common myths related to pain are discussed in Table 27-1.

TYPES OF PAIN

Pain can be described by its origin or cause and by its nature or description. Pain categorized by its origin is either cutaneous, somatic, or visceral; by its nature, it is either acute or chronic.

Pain Categorized by Origin

Cutaneous pain is caused by stimulating the cutaneous nerve endings in the skin and results in a well-localized "burning" or "prickling" sensation; tangled hair that is pulled during combing causes cutaneous pain. **Somatic pain** is nonlocalized and originates in support structures such as tendons, ligaments, and nerves; twisting an ankle results in somatic pain. **Visceral pain** is discomfort in the internal organs, is less localized, and is more slowly transmitted than cutaneous pain. Pain originating from the abdominal organs is often called **referred pain** because pain is not felt in the organ but instead is perceived at the spot where the organs were located during fetal development, making it difficult to assess (Figure 27-1).

Pain Categorized by Nature

It is important to understand the difference between acute and chronic pain because they each present a different clinical picture.

Acute Pain

Acute pain has a sudden onset, relatively short duration, mild to severe intensity, with a steady decrease in intensity over a period of days to weeks. Once the **noxious stimulus** (underlying pathology) is resolved, the pain usually disappears (Table 27-2). It is usually associated with a specific condition, injury, or tissue damage caused by disease. As healing occurs, acute pain should diminish. Everyone has experienced acute

Table 27-1 Common Myths About Pain

MYTH	FACT
• The nurse is the best judge of a client's pain.	• Pain is a subjective experience; only the client can judge the level and severity of pain.
• If pain is ignored, it will go away.	• Pain is a real experience that is appropriately treated with nursing and medical intervention.
• Clients should not take any measures to relieve their pain until the pain is unbearable.	• Pain control and relief measures are effective in lowering the pain level, which will help clients function more normally and comfortably.
• Most complaints of pain are purely psychological (e.g., "it's all in your head"); only "real" pain manifests in obvious physical signs such as moaning or grimacing.	• Most clients honestly report their perception of pain, both physical and emotional, and need effective intervention and teaching; physical responses vary greatly depending on experience and cultural norms, and visible expressions of pain are not always reliable indicators of its severity.
• Clients taking pain medications will become addicted to the drug.	• Addiction is unlikely when analgesics are carefully administered and closely monitored.
• Clients with severe tissue damage will experience significant pain; those with lesser damage will feel less pain.	• Individuals' perceptions of pain are subjective; the extent of tissue damage is not necessarily proportional to the extent of pain experienced.
• Clients ask for pain medication when they need it.	• Many clients do not ask for medication because they are afraid of side effects, do not want to bother the nurse, have cultural norms and beliefs against it, or believe pain is inevitable and untreatable.

COURTESY OF DELMAR CENGAGE LEARNING

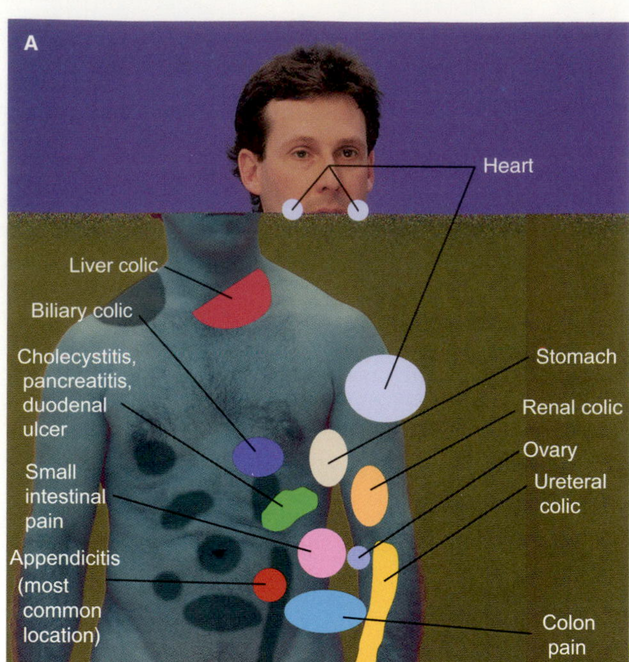

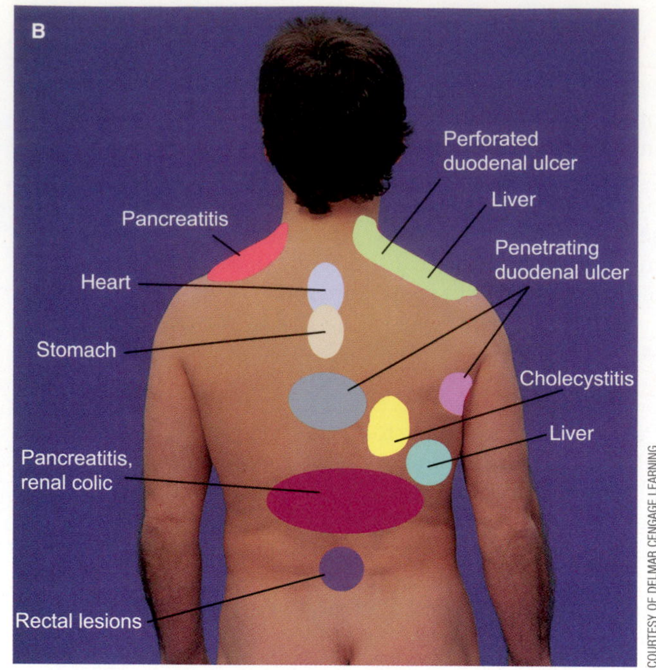

COURTESY OF DELMAR CENGAGE LEARNING

FIGURE 27-1 Areas of Referred Pain; *A,* Anterior View; *B,* Posterior View

pain (e.g., toothaches, headaches, needlesticks, skinned knees, burns, muscle pain, childbirth, postoperative pain, a sprained ankle, and fractures). The client is usually able to pinpoint the hurt. Acute pain is often described as sharp, although deep pain may be described as dull and aching. The client will exhibit elevated heart rate, respiratory rate, and blood pressure and may become diaphoretic and have dilated pupils. These signs resemble those of anxiety, which often accompanies acute pain. Behaviors may include crying and moaning, rubbing the site of pain, guarding, frowning, grimacing, and verbal complaints of the discomfort.

Recurrent acute pain is repetitive painful episodes that recur over a prolonged period or throughout the client's lifetime. Pain-free intervals alternate with painful episodes.

TABLE 27-2 Acute Versus Chronic Pain

	ACUTE	CHRONIC
Time Span	Less than 6 months	More than 6 months
Location	Localized, associated with a specific injury, condition, or disease	Difficult to pinpoint
Characteristics	Often described as sharp, diminishes as healing occurs	Often described as dull, diffuse, and aching
Physiologic Signs	• Elevated heart rate • Elevated BP • Elevated respirations • May be diaphoretic • Dilated pupils	• Normal vital signs • Normal pupils • No diaphoresis • May have loss of weight
Behavioral Signs	• Crying and moaning • Rubbing site • Guarding • Frowning • Grimacing • Complains of pain	• Physical immobility • Hopelessness • Listlessness • Loss of libido • Exhaustion and fatigue • Complains of pain only when asked

COURTESY OF DELMAR CENGAGE LEARNING

Examples of recurrent pain seen in children include recurrent abdominal, chest, limb pain, and headaches. In adults, recurrent pain experience includes migraine headaches, sickle cell crises pain, and angina.

Chronic Pain

Chronic pain is usually defined as long-term (lasting 6 months or longer), persistent, nearly constant, or recurrent pain producing significant negative changes in the client's life. Chronic pain may last long after the pathology is resolved. Although some infants, children, and adolescents experience chronic pain, it is more common in adults. In the United States, one in four individuals lives with chronic pain. Chronic pain is the reason for more than 80% of all physician visits (National Pain Foundation, 2009).

Chronic acute pain occurs almost daily over a long period, months or years, and may never stop. Cancer and severe burns are examples of pathophysiology leading to chronic acute pain. Sometimes the pain ends only at the time of death, as in terminal cancer clients (McCaffery & Pasero, 1999). This type of pain is also called *progressive pain.*

Chronic nonmalignant pain, also called *chronic benign pain,* occurs almost daily and lasts for at least 6 months, ranging from mild to severe intensity. Three critical characteristics of chronic nonmalignant pain are identified by McCaffery and Pasero (1999):

- Caused by non–life-threatening causes
- Not responsive to currently available pain relief methods
- May continue for the rest of the client's life

Examples of pathophysiology leading to chronic nonmalignant pain include the following:

- Many forms of **neuralgia** (paroxysmal pain that extends along the course of one or more nerves)
- Low-back pain
- Rheumatoid arthritis
- Ankylosing spondylitis
- **Phantom limb pain** (a form of neuropathic pain that occurs after amputation with pain sensations referred to an area in the missing portion of the limb)
- **Myofascial pain syndromes** (a group of muscle disorders characterized by pain, muscle spasm, tenderness, stiffness, and limited motion)

When chronic nonmalignant pain is severe enough to disable the client, it is identified as *chronic intractable nonmalignant pain syndrome.*

Signs and Symptoms The signs and symptoms of chronic pain can look very different from those of acute pain. The body cannot tolerate the sympathetic nervous system signs for a long period and, therefore, adapts. Vital signs will often be normal, with no accompanying pupil dilatation or perspiration. Lack of these signs may prompt some health care workers to question the client's description of pain.

The hopelessness, listlessness, and loss of libido (sex drive) and weight of chronic pain are similar to those of depression. The client often describes exhaustion and fatigue. Behaviors include no complaint of pain unless asked and physical inactivity or immobility leading to functional disability. The crying, moaning, guarding, and grimacing that most clinicians associate with pain are absent. Treatment of chronic pain is more complex than that of acute pain. Chronic pain is viewed by pain experts as a disease state rather than a symptom. Management includes identifying the cause of pain, recognizing emotional and environmental factors contributing to the pain, and rehabilitation to improve the client's functional abilities.

PURPOSE OF PAIN

Pain serves as a protective mechanism. If a person touches a hot stove, the pain signal causes the person to pull the hand away immediately. The skin would be seriously burned if this did not happen.

Pain can be a diagnostic tool. The quality and duration of the pain give important clues in determining a client's medical diagnosis. For example, in acute appendicitis, the clinician looks for rebound tenderness (the pain increases after applying firm pressure for several seconds and then quickly releasing the pressure) when palpating the abdomen. This particular type of pain helps confirm the diagnosis of appendicitis rather than other gastrointestinal disorders.

PHYSIOLOGY OF PAIN

When pain occurs, sensory input from injured tissue causes peripheral **nociceptors** (receptive neurons for painful sensations) and central nervous system (CNS) pain pathways to enhance future responses to pain stimuli. Long-lasting changes in cells within the spinal cord **afferent** (ascending) and **efferent** (descending) **pain pathways** may thus occur after a brief noxious stimulus.

Physiological responses (such as elevated blood pressure, respiratory rate, and pulse rate; dilated pupils; perspiration; and pallor) to even a brief acute pain episode will show adaptation within minutes to a few hours. The body cannot sustain the extreme stress response physiologically for more than short periods. The body conserves its resources by physiological adaptation: a return to normal or near normal blood pressure, respiratory rate, and pulse rate; pupil size; and dry skin with little evidence of poor perfusion, *even with continuing pain of the same intensity.*

Stimulation of Pain

The specific action of pain depends on the type of pain. Cutaneous pain rapidly travels through a simple reflex arc from the nerve ending (point of pain) to the spinal cord at approximately 300 feet per second, with a reflex response evoking an almost immediate reaction. This is why, when a hot stove is touched, the person's hand jerks back *before* there is conscious awareness of damage (Figure 27-2). After a hot stove is touched, a sensory nerve ending in the finger skin initiates nerve transmission that travels through the dorsal root ganglion to the dorsal horn in the gray matter of the spinal cord. The impulse then travels though an interneuron that synapses with a motor neuron at the same level in the spinal cord. This motor neuron stimulating the muscle is responsible for the swift movement of the hand away from the hot stove.

In the case of the hot stove, the sensory neuron also synapses with an afferent sensory neuron. The impulse travels up the spinal cord to the thalamus, where a synapse sends the impulse to the brain cortex. Once the impulse is interpreted, the information is consciously available. Then the person is aware of the location, intensity, and quality of pain. Previous experience adds the affective feature to the pain experience.

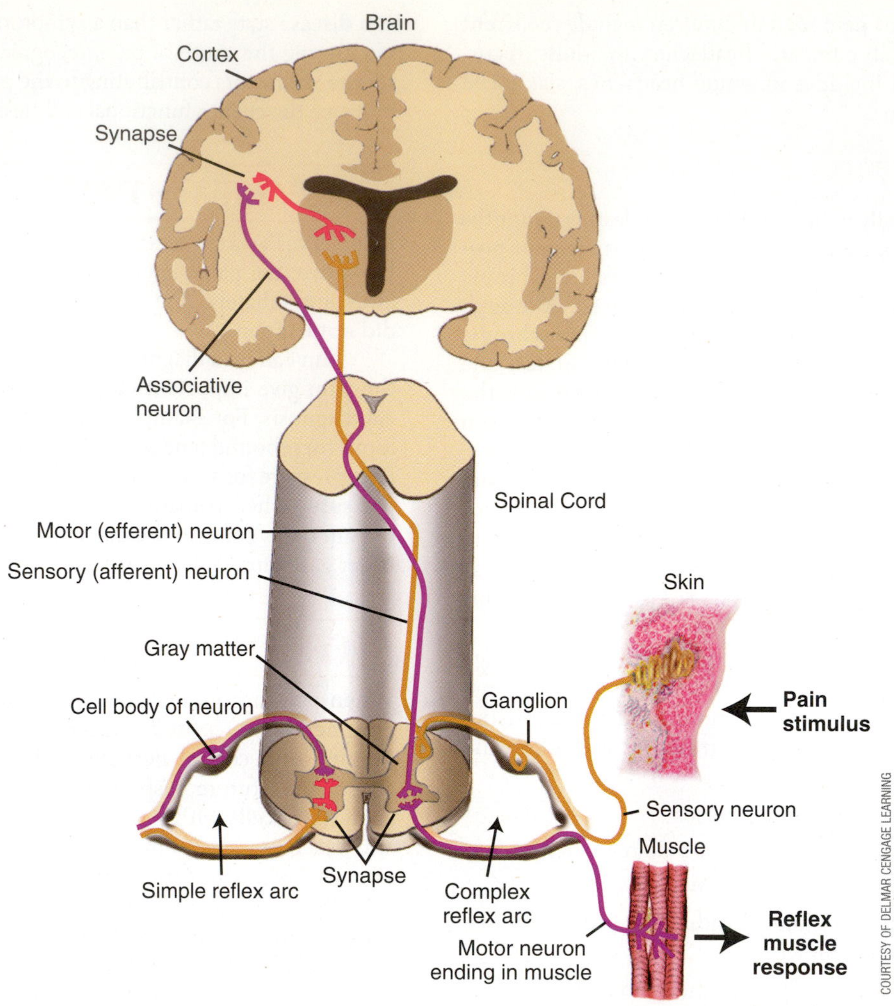

FIGURE 27-2 Reflex Arcs

Descending or efferent motor neuron response moves from the brain through the spinal cord, synapsing with a motor neuron in the spinal cord, and innervates the muscle.

The transmission of visceral pain impulses is slower and less localized than cutaneous pain. Internal organs (including the gastrointestinal tract) have few nociceptors, which is why visceral pain is poorly localized and is felt as a throbbing sensation or dull ache; however, internal organs are very sensitive to distension. The cramping pain of **colic** (acute abdominal pain) results when:

- Constipation or flatus distends the stomach or intestines
- There is hyperperistalsis, as in gastroenteritis
- Something tries to pass through an opening that is too small

The physiology of **ischemic pain**, or pain occurring when the blood supply to an area is restricted or cut off completely, also differs. Blood flow restriction causes inadequate oxygenation of the tissue supplied by those vessels and inadequate removal of metabolic wastes. The onset of ischemic pain is most rapid in an active muscle and much slower in a

PROFESSIONAL TIP

Pain in Americans

According to statistics compiled by the American Pain Foundation in 2007, pain impacts the everyday lives of more Americans than cancer, diabetes, and heart disease *combined*—an estimated 76.5 million Americans per day. Adults between the ages of 45 and 64 were the most likely to report pain; adults over age 65 were least likely. This may reflect age-related changes in pain perception or the underassessment of pain in the elderly.

CRITICAL THINKING

Types of Pain

What are the differences among somatic, cutaneous, visceral, referred, ischemic, acute, chronic, and phantom limb pain?

SAFETY

Ischemic Pain

Administer supplemental oxygen and pain medication quickly to clients with ischemic pain to minimize oxygen deprivation and prevent infarction (tissue death).

passive muscle. Examples of ischemic pain are muscle cramps, myocardial infarction, angina pectoris, and sickle cell crisis. When ischemic pain occurs in a muscle that continues to work, a muscle spasm (cramp) occurs. If the blood supply to the heart is completely cut off or severely restricted and not restored quickly, a myocardial infarction occurs.

Substances released from injured tissue in acute pain episodes lead to stress hormone responses. There is an increase in metabolic rate, enhanced breakdown of body tissue, increased blood clotting, impaired immune function, and water retention. The fight-or-flight reaction is triggered, leading to tachycardia and negative emotions.

THE GATE CONTROL THEORY

Pain transmission and interpretation theories try to describe and explain the pain experience. Early pain theorists focused on the neuroanatomical and neurophysiological mechanisms.

Melzack and Wall (1965) proposed the **gate control pain theory**, which was the first one recognizing that psychological aspects of pain are as important as physiological aspects. The gate control theory combined cognitive, sensory, and emotional components—in addition to the physiological aspects—and proposed that they can act on a gate control system to block the individual's perception of pain. The basic premise is that transmission of potentially painful nerve impulses to the cortex is modulated by a spinal cord gating mechanism and by CNS activity. As a result, the level of conscious awareness of painful sensation is altered.

The theory suggests that nerve fibers that contribute to pain transmission come together at a site in the dorsal horn of the spinal cord. This site is thought to act as a gating mechanism that determines which impulses will be blocked and which will be transmitted to the thalamus. The image of a gate is useful in teaching clients and their families about pain relief measures. If the "gate" is closed, the signal is stopped before it reaches the brain, where awareness of pain occurs. If the gate is open, the signal will continue on through the spinothalamic tract to the cortex, and the client will feel the pain (Figure 27-3). Whether the gate is opened or closed is influenced by impulses from peripheral nerves (the sensory components) and nerve signals that descend from the brain (motivational-affective and cognitive components). For example, stimulation of some types of peripheral nerves by cutaneous stimulation such as massage can close the gate, whereas stimulation of the nociceptors will open the gate.

If a person is anxious, the gate can be opened by signals sent from the brain down to the mechanism in the dorsal horn of the spinal cord. On the other hand, if the person has had

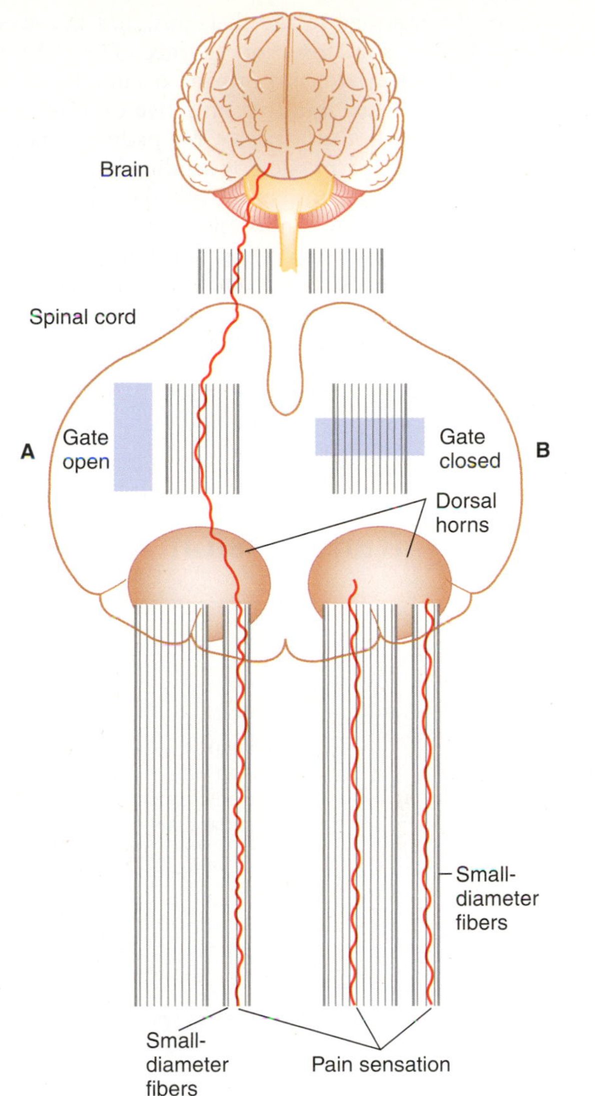

FIGURE 27-3 Gate Control Theory; *A*, An "open gate" allows nerves to transmit pain sensation to the brain; *B*, A "closed gate" stops nerve transmission of pain sensation to the brain.

positive experiences with pain control in the past, the cognitive influence can send signals down to the gating mechanism and close it. The gate theory offered a great benefit by suggesting new approaches to relieving both acute and chronic pain. Pain could be relieved by blocking the transmission of pain impulses to the brain by both physical modalities and by altering the individual's thought processes, emotions, or other behaviors.

CONDUCTION OF PAIN IMPULSES

Conduction of pain impulses refers to the physiologic processes that occur from the initiation of the pain signal to the realization of pain by the individual. Four processes are involved in the conduction of this signal, as illustrated in Figure 27-4. The first, **transduction**, is when a noxious stimulus triggers electrical activity in the endings of afferent nerve fibers (nociceptors). Once the signal is triggered, **transmission** occurs. The impulse travels from the receiving nociceptors to the spinal cord. Projection neurons then carry the message to the thalamus, and the message continues to the somatosensory cortex. Then the third step, **perception** (awareness) of pain, occurs. Here neural messages are converted into the subjective experience. The fourth process, **modulation**, is a CNS pathway that selectively inhibits pain transmission by sending blocking signals back down to the dorsal horn of the spinal cord. Pain modulation is controlled by two endogenous (developing within) analgesic systems (pain killers): endorphins and enkephalins. **Endorphins** (endogenous opiate-like substances) bind to the opioid receptor sites and decrease the perception of pain. Enkephalins also decrease the pain perception in the pain pathway.

FACTORS AFFECTING THE PAIN EXPERIENCE

According to McCaffery and Pasero (1999), the client is the only authority on the existence and nature of his or her pain. Age, previous experience with pain, drug abuse, and cultural norms account for the differences in clients' individual responses to pain.

AGE

Age can greatly influence clients' perception of pain. Individuals may continue pain behaviors learned as children and may

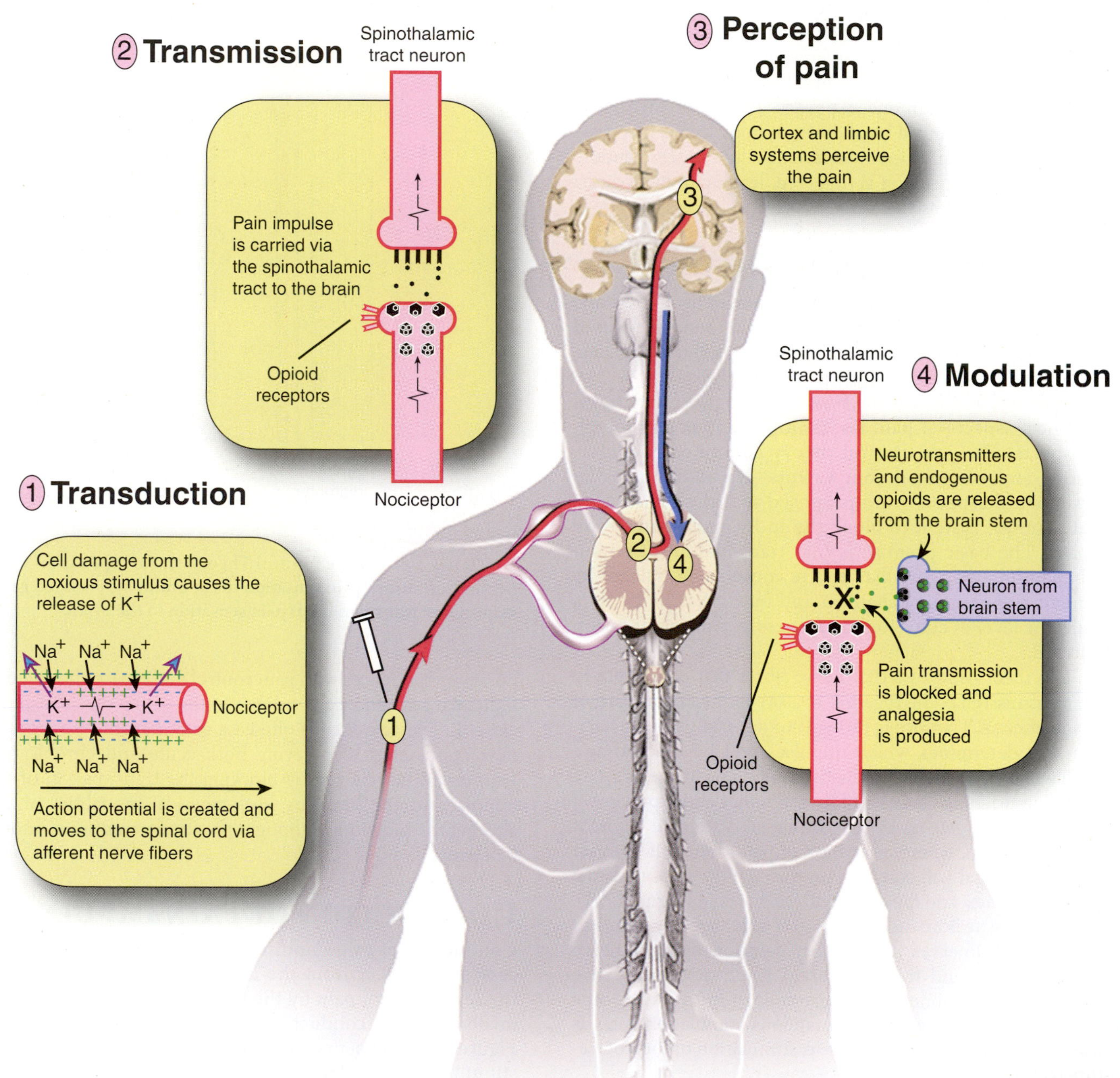

FIGURE 27-4 Conduction of Pain Impulses

LIFE SPAN CONSIDERATIONS

Elders and Pain

Older clients often live with pain, believing that nothing can be done. Pain often is not reported by older clients for fear of being labeled a "bother" or "complainer." Encourage the client to request pain relief as needed.

be reluctant to admit pain or seek medical care because they fear the unknown or fear how treatment may impact their lifestyle. Older adults may ignore their pain, believing it is a consequence of aging. Family and health care members may thoughtlessly support this idea and be less responsive to an older client's complaints of pain.

Previous Pain Experiences

Previous experience with pain often influences clients' reactions. Past coping mechanisms may affect clients' judgments about how pain will affect their lives and which measures they can use to successfully manage the pain on their own. Teaching clients about pain expectations and management methods can often allay their fears and lead to successful pain management.

Drug Abuse

According to Compton (1999), a drug abuser is likely to be *less* tolerant of pain than someone who does not use drugs. Drug abuse may cause changes in the central nervous system, resulting in an exaggerated neurophysiologic response to painful stimuli. To keep a drug abuser comfortable, withdrawal must be prevented.

Cultural Norms

Cultural differences in pain responses can lead to pain management problems. Studies on subjects of various cultures found no significant difference among the groups in the intensity level at which pain becomes perceptible. The same studies showed that the intensity level or duration of pain the client was willing to endure differed significantly. Cultural values guide the expression of pain. Some cultures tolerate pain and "suffering in silence," whereas others fully express pain, including physical and emotional responses. Be careful not to equate the level of pain expression with the level of actual pain experienced but consider cultural and other influences that affect the expression of pain.

JOINT COMMISSION STANDARDS

Each institution should have clearly defined standards for pain management. The Joint Commission Pain Management Standards of Care has made pain management a priority and requires that pain be assessed on admission and throughout the client's stay in an institution. Relating to pain management, the health care organizations are expected to:

- Recognize the right of clients to appropriate assessment and management of their pain
- Assess pain in all clients
- Record the results of the assessment in a way that facilitates regular reassessment and follow-up
- Educate relevant providers in pain assessment and management
- Determine competency in pain assessment and management
- Establish policies and procedures that support appropriate prescription or ordering of pain medications
- Ensure that pain does not interfere with participation in rehabilitation
- Educate clients and their families about the importance of effective pain management
- Include clients' needs for symptom management in the discharge planning process
- Collect data to monitor the appropriateness and effectiveness of pain management (Integrative Pain Center of Arizona, 2003; Joint Commission, 2009; Teeter & Kemper, 2008b)

NURSING PROCESS

The nursing process provides the framework for managing a client's pain.

Assessment

Assessment of the client's pain is a crucial nursing function. During the assessment process, be aware of your own values and expectations about pain behaviors. Just as the client's experience and cultural background help determine how pain is demonstrated, nurses' cultures and experiences help determine which pain behaviors are viewed as acceptable. Be aware of these values and avoid biases when assessing client pain and planning client care. Once a self-assessment about pain has been conducted, the nurse is ready to assess the client.

Pain as the fifth vital sign is assessed and recorded along with the client's temperature, pulse, respiration, and blood pressure. Pain assessment tools are the most effective method to

MEMORYTRICK

Pain Assessment PQRST

P = What Provokes the pain (aggravating factors) and palliative measures (alleviating factors)

Q = Quality of pain (gnawing, pounding, burning, stabbing, pinching, aching, throbbing, and crushing)

R = Region (location) and radiation to other body sites

S = Severity (quantity of pain on 0–10 scale: 0 = no pain and 10 = worst pain experienced) and setting (what causes the pain)

T = Timing (onset, duration, frequency)

(Adapted from Estes, 2010.)

COMPLETE WITH 1ST DOSE OF PAIN MEDICATION	INITIALS	SIGNATURE
1. Onset and frequency (When did it start?) (How often) ______		
2. Provokes (What makes it worse?) ______		
3. Radiates? ______		
4. Severity/Intensity (What is an acceptable level of pain [0–10]) ______		
5. Timing/Duration (How long does it last?) ______		
6. Past & Current analgesic/alternative modalities that make it better. ______		

7. Does your pain affect: sleep__ appetite__ physical activity__ emotions__ social relationships__

COMMENTS:

Source of Information: 1=Patient, 2=Child, 3=Parent, 4=Nurse, 5=Family, 6=Other

Side Effects: 1=Nausa/Vomiting, 2=Resp. Depression, 3=Pruritis, 4=Urinary Retention, 5=Altered Mental Status, 6=None

Safety: 1=Bed low, 2=Call bell in reach, 3=Side rails ×2, 4=Side rails ×4, 5=Bed alert, 6=Family/Sitter

Pediatrics/Noncommunicative Clients (0–10)

A. Verbal/Vocal	B. Body Movements	C. Facial	D. Touching (localizing pain)
0=positive	0=moves easily	0=smiling	0=no touching
1=other complaint, whimper	1=neutral shifting	1=neutral	1=reaching, patting
2=pain, crying	2=tense, flailing arms & legs	2=frown, grimace	2=grabbing
3=screaming		3=clenched teeth	

Nonpharmacological Interventions

1=Cold	7=Massage
2=Distractions	8=Music
3=Environmental Control	9=Positioning
4=Exercises	10=Relaxation
5=Heat	11=TENS
6=Imagery	12=Spiritual Care

Pediatrics

13=Holding
14=Rocking
15=Pacifier
16=Security object

Mode of Administration

PCA	SQ	Rectal (R)
IV	PO	Nasal (N)
IM	SL	
Epidural (EP)		
Transdermal (TD)		

LEVEL OF CONSCIOUSNESS KEY (LOC)*

1. Alert, engages in conversation; puposefully travels with eyes, if mute
2. Lethargic, drowsy, sedate—focuses on personal interchange—but unable to maintain focus
3. Responds only to maximal stimulation (shaking). Response only a grunt or moan—not a clear sentance.
4. Coma—unable to respond at all.

Date/ Time	Location of Pain	Character: Dull, Stabbing, Pressure, Sharp, Throbbing	Severity Rating 0–10	Pharmacologic// (Med Name)/ Nonpharmacologic	Mode of Adminis- tration	Source of Information	B	P	R	LOC / Side Effects	Safety	Time of Evaluation	Evaluation of Interventions/ Frequency Rating 0–10 Response/ Comments	Initails

2006

CHRISTUS SPOHN HEALTH SYSTEM

PAIN MANAGEMENT FLOW SHEET
PATIENT CARE SERVICES

2763751 NEW: 07/99
REVISED: 05/30/2001
FM15

FIGURE 27-5 Pain Assessment and Management (*Courtesy of CHRISTUS Spohn Health System, Corpus Christi, TX.*)

PROFESSIONALTIP

Location of Pain

During intershift report on a postoperative client recovering from abdominal surgery, the nurse reported that the client had stated she had pain and had been medicated with IM Demerol. When greeting her client, the nurse asked the client about the pain she had experienced during the night. The client replied, "Oh, it is fine now, I only had a headache." The night nurse had assumed the client's pain was in her surgical site and chose the medication accordingly. The headache probably could have been relieved with a milder medication. All reports of pain must be thoroughly assessed before implementing any interventions.

identify the presence and intensity of pain in clients. Good nursing practice uses pain assessment tools and accepts the results of the tools (Figure 27-5). Using the "PQRST" mnemonic is an ideal way for a nurse to assess a client's pain. This method is described in the Memory Trick "Pain Assessment PQRST."

Subjective Data

The first step in pain assessment is gathering subjective information regarding the client's pain. A client's pain threshold and pain tolerance level is determined. **Pain threshold** is the intensity level where a person feels pain. It varies with each individual and with each type of pain. **Pain tolerance** is the intensity level or duration of pain the client is able or willing to endure.

The client's description of the pain covers several qualifiers, including its location, onset and duration, quality, intensity, aggravating factors (variables that worsen the pain, such as exercise, certain foods, or stress), alleviating factors (measures the client can take that lessen the effect of the pain, such as lying down, avoiding certain foods, or taking medication), associated manifestations (factors that often accompany the pain, such as nausea, constipation, or dizziness), and what pain means to the client.

Whenever subjective and objective data conflict, the subjective reports of pain are to be considered the primary source.

Location The client can point to the location of the pain on the client's own body or locate it on a body diagram on a pain assessment tool. Ask the client if there is more than one site of pain; if the pain radiates and, if so, to where; and if the pain is deep or superficial.

Onset and Duration Ask the client how long the pain has existed; what, if anything, triggers its onset; and if there are any patterns to the pain (e.g., whether it is worse at certain times of the day or night).

Quality Ask the client what the pain feels like, and record the words used to describe the pain. Clients may use sensory-type words, such as "pricking," "radiating," "burning," or "throbbing." Other clients use words that have an affective connotation, such as "fearful," "sickening," or "punishing." Other words used may be evaluative, such as "miserable" or "unbearable." The quality of pain provides information that may be useful in diagnosing the cause of the pain. For example, pain described as "burning" or "freezing" is usually neuropathic in origin.

Intensity The client may have difficulty in judging the intensity of pain; however, it is important to obtain an estimate of the severity of the pain. This information allows the clinician to evaluate the effectiveness of pain relief measures tried by comparing intensity before and after the interventions.

Pain intensity scales are an effective method for clients to rate the intensity of their pain (Figure 27-6). The simple descriptive pain-intensity scale and the visual analog scale (VAS) are best used by showing the scale to the client and asking the client to point to the spot on the scale that corresponds to the present pain. The pain scale most frequently used with adolescent and adult clients is the verbal 0-to-10 scale. It needs no equipment or supplies and requires only one question: "On a scale of 0 to 10, with 0 being no pain at all and 10 being the worst pain possible, how much do you hurt right now?" If there are multiple painful areas, this question can be asked regarding each area. A study by Twycross et al. (1996) showed that pain ratings of 4 or higher on a 0-to-10 scale interfered with client activities and that scores of 6 and 7 markedly interfered with client quality of life. This study with other studies (Cleeland & Syrjala, 1992) and clinical experience have brought clinicians to believe that a pain level of

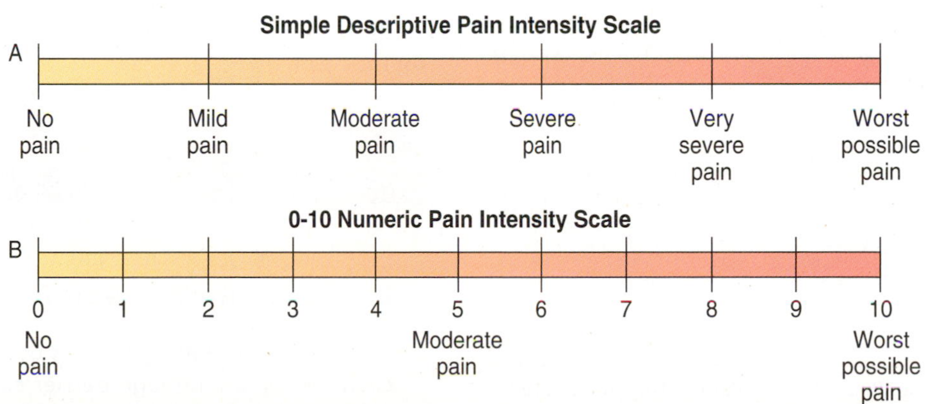

FIGURE 27-6 Pain Intensity Scales; *A*, Simple Descriptive Pain Intensity Scale; *B*, 0-10 Numeric Pain Intensity Scale (*Courtesy of Acute Pain Management: Operative or Medical Procedures and Trauma. Clinical Practice Guideline [AHCPR Publication No. 92-0032].*)

CLIENT TEACHING

Pain at Night

Teach the client that pain is commonly worse at night, when there are fewer distractions. If the client knows this fact, he will not attribute the increased pain to complications.

3 indicates a need to change the pain intervention plan with an increase in analgesics, and/or other medications, or interventions (Office of Quality and Performance, U.S. Department of Veterans Affairs, 2008). Clients must be taught how to correctly use the pain intensity scale.

Although developed for use with children, the FACES Pain Rating Scale (Figure 27-7) can be used effectively with clients when a language barrier exists. A translator is used initially to explain what the faces represent.

Another pain assessment tool is the "Painometer" developed by Dr. Gaston-Johansson (Mattson, 2000). The client positions a pointer between "no pain" and "worst possible pain." Quantifying numbers are on the back. The client also indicates the quality of pain by selecting sensory and affective descriptors from a list.

Aggravating and Alleviating Factors Ask the client about what makes the pain worse and what makes the pain better, including behaviors or activities that influence the pain. This information helps develop the plan of care for the client in pain. If specific activities relieve the pain, incorporate them into the care plan. Being aware of activities that increase the pain can allow for interventions that may prevent the pain. For example, if physical therapy exercises trigger an increase in pain, administer an analgesic according to physician's or nurse practitioner's orders before the treatment.

Associated Manifestations The initial pain assessment includes the impact of pain on the activities of daily living. Pain may cause changes in sleep patterns or the ability to work and carry out the many roles in a client's life. Pain may affect appetite, mood, sexual functioning, or the ability to participate in recreational activities. If pain is interfering with daily life, the client's quality of life is greatly affected.

Pain is fatiguing. It requires a significant amount of energy to deal with pain. The longer a person has pain, the greater the level of fatigue. Although there is no conscious awareness of pain during sleep, there may be dream-state awareness (McCaffery & Pasero, 1999). The stress response (which can be seen even in clients under general anesthesia) continues, and the body physiologically pays the price. Clients also wake up with more pain than they had going to sleep, thereby requiring even more intervention (pharmacologic and nonpharmacologic) to reduce the pain.

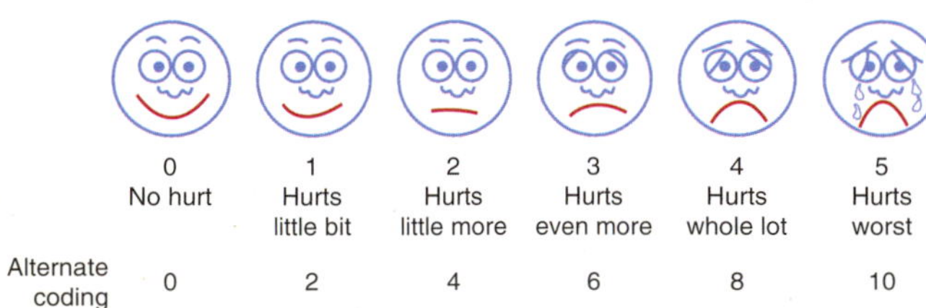

FIGURE 27-7 Wong/Baker FACES Pain Rating Scale (*From Hockenberry, M. J., Wilson, D. Winkelstein, M. L., Wong's Essentials of Pediatric Nursing, ed 7, St. Louis, 2005, p. 1259. Used with permission. Copyright Mosby.*)

LIFE SPAN CONSIDERATIONS

Children and Pain Assessment

Children provide a special challenge in pain assessment. Two useful tools for assessing pain in children are the Wong/Baker FACES Pain Rating Scale and the Oucher scale.

- The Wong/Baker FACES Pain Rating Scale can be used with children as young as 3 years. It helps children express their level of pain by pointing to a cartoon face that most closely resembles how they are feeling (Figure 27-7).
- The Oucher pediatric pain intensity scale (Figure 27-8) consists of two scales: a 0-to-10 numeric scale and a 6-point facial scale. If the child can count from 1 to 10, the numeric scale is used; if not, the facial scale is used. The facial scale has been successfully used in children as young as 3 to 4 years.

Meaning of Pain Because of the motivational-affective components of the pain experience, the meaning of pain can have a great impact on how the client perceives the pain. A frequently cited classic study on this phenomenon was conducted by Beecher (1956), who compared the pain perceived by soldiers wounded in battle to pain perceived by civilians with similar surgical wounds. He found that only 32% of the soldiers required narcotics for pain relief, whereas 85% of the civilians needed the narcotics. This was interpreted that for the soldiers, the wound represented a ticket away from the battlefield; for the civilians, the surgical wound was a depressing event.

Explore with the client what implications the pain may have for the individual. Does it mean that the client's cancer is metastasizing? Or that the client's condition is worsening? All these interpretations may influence the pain experience for the client.

CULTURAL CONSIDERATIONS

Language Barrier and Pain

The FACES Pain Rating Scale is used effectively with clients when a language barrier exists. A translator should be used initially to explain what the faces represent.

OUCHER!™

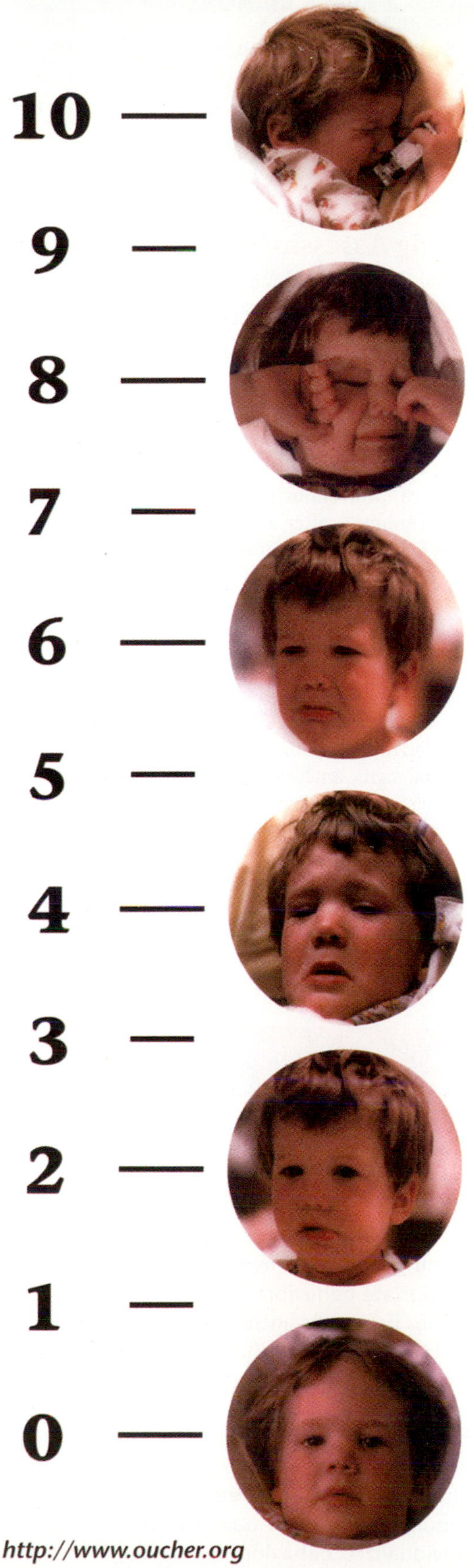

10 —
9 —
8 —
7 —
6 —
5 —
4 —
3 —
2 —
1 —
0 —

http://www.oucher.org

THE OUCHER: A SUMMARY

What is the OUCHER?

The OUCHER is a poster developed for children to help them communicate how much pain or hurt they feel. There are two scales on the OUCHER: A number scale for older children and a picture scale for younger children.

Which scale should be used?

Children who are able to count to 100 by ones or tens and who understand, for example, that 71 is greater than 43, can use the numerical scale. Children who do not understand numbers should use the picture scale. Some children who are able to use the number scale might prefer to use the picture scale. Ask the child which scale he or she would prefer.

How do I use the OUCHER?

Picture scale: The following is an example of how to explain the picture scale to a younger child. The words can be changed when using the picture scale with an older child.

This is a poster called the OUCHER. It helps children tell others how much hurt they have. (For younger children, it might be useful to ask: Do you know what I mean by hurt? If the child is not sure, then an explanation should be provided.) Here's how this works. This picture shows not hurt (point to the bottom picture), this picture shows just a little bit of hurt (point to the 2nd picture), this picture shows a little more hurt (point to the 3rd picture), this picture shows even more hurt (point to the 4th picture), this picture shows a lot of hurt (point to the 5th picture), and this picture shows the biggest hurt you could ever have (point to the 6th picture). Can you point to the picture that shows how much hurt you are having right now?

Once a child selects a picture, their picture selection is changed to a number score from 0-10.

10 – Picture at the top of the scale
8 – Second picture from the top
6 – Third picture from the top
4 – Fourth picture from the top
2 – Fifth picture from the top
0 – Picture at the bottom of the scale

Number scale: The following is an example of how to explain the number scale.

This is a poster called the OUCHER. It helps children tell others how much hurt they have. Here's how it works. 0 means no hurt. Here (point to the lower third of the scale, about 1 to 3), this means you have little hurts; here (point to the middle third of the scale, about 3 to 6) it means you have middle hurts. If your hurt is about here (point to the upper third of the scale, about 6 to 9), it means you have big hurts. But if you point to 10, it means you have the biggest hurt you could ever have. Can you point to the number (or tell me which number) that is like the hurt you are having right now?

The pain score for the number scale is the exact number from 0 to 10 that the child gives you.

What does the score mean? How should it be used?

The person who has pain is the expert or the one who knows best how the pain feels. The OUCHER score gives parents, teachers, nurses, and doctors some idea of how much pain the child is feeling. OUCHER scores can be used as a means to see if certain actions used to relieve pain, such as rest, applying heat or cold, eating or drinking, and medicine make a difference in how much pain the child feels. OUCHER scores can be recorded over a period of hours or days and would be useful information to share with nurses and doctors.

Remember, OUCHER scores only communicate how much pain the child is feeling. Other observations, such as changes in activity, location of the pain, what it feels like, and how long it lasts, are important. If you, as a parent or teacher, are concerned about the child's pain, you should contact your health care provider.

© The Caucasian version of the OUCHER was developed and copyrighted by Judith E. Beyer, PhD, RN, (University of Missouri-Kansas City),1983. The African-American version was developed and copyrighted by Mary J. Denyes, PhD, RN, (Wayne State University), and Antonia M. Villarruel, PhD, RN, (University of Michigan) at Children's Hospital of Michigan, 1990. Cornelia P. Porter, PhD, RN, and Charlotta Marshall, RN, MSN, contributed to the development of the scale. The Hispanic version was developed and copyrighted by Antonia M. Villarruel, PhD, RN, and Mary J. Denyes, PhD, RN, 1990.

For information about the Oucher, write to: Dr. Judith E. Beyer, P.O. Box 411714, Kansas City, MO 64141 or go to the www.OUCHER.com website.

FIGURE 27-8 The Oucher Pain Assessment Tool: For Use with Children 3-12 Years of Age. Caucasian, Hispanic, and African American versions are available. (*The Caucasian version of the Oucher, developed and copyrighted by Judith E. Beyer, RN, PhD, 1983.*)

Objective Data

As discussed when addressing acute versus chronic pain, the objective data often present a different picture depending on the type of pain the client is experiencing.

Physiologic Acute pain activates the sympathetic nervous system, and the client may exhibit elevated heart rate, elevated respiratory rate, elevated blood pressure, diaphoresis, pallor, muscle tension, and dilated pupils. These signs resemble those of anxiety, which often accompanies acute pain. The signs and symptoms of chronic pain show adaptation and, therefore, are different from those of acute pain, with vital signs being normal and no accompanying pupil dilation or perspiration.

Behavioral Acute pain behaviors may include crying and moaning, rubbing the site of pain, restlessness, a distorted posture, clenched fists, guarding the painful area, frowning, and grimacing. The client usually speaks of the discomfort and may be restless or afraid to move.

The client in chronic pain may demonstrate behaviors similar to those of depression, such as hopelessness, listlessness, and loss of libido and weight. Chronic pain often leads to physical inactivity or immobility, which can lead to functional disability. **Distraction** (focusing attention on stimuli other than pain) may also be used by clients. According to McCaffery and Pasero (1999), clients often minimize the pain behaviors they are able to control for several reasons, including:

- To be a "good" client and avoid making demands
- To maintain a positive self-image by not being a "sissy"
- Distraction makes pain more bearable (young children are particularly adept at this)
- Exhaustion

Client pain behaviors include splinting of the painful area, distorted posture, impaired mobility, anxiety, insomnia, attention seeking, and depression. Occasionally, a discrepancy exists between pain behaviors observed by the nurse (objective data) and the client's self-report of pain. Discrepancies between behaviors and the client's self-report can result from good coping skills (e.g., relaxation techniques or distraction), anxiety, stoicism, or cultural differences in pain behaviors. Whenever these discrepancies occur, they should be addressed with the client and the pain management plan renegotiated accordingly.

PROFESSIONALTIP

Assessing the Effect of Pain on Sleep

Questioning clients about the effect pain has on their sleep habits will help clarify the intensity of the pain and its effect on the clients' patterns of daily living. Ask the client whether the pain:

- Prevents the client from falling asleep
- Makes it difficult to find a comfortable sleeping position
- Wakes the client from a sound sleep
- Prevents the client from falling back to sleep
- Leaves the client feeling tired and unrefreshed after sleeping

CRITICAL THINKING

Assessing Pain

A 38-year-old client is unable to rate his pain on a 0-to-10 scale. What actions should the nurse take to perform a pain assessment on this client? (Teeter & Kemper, 2008a)

Ongoing Assessment

The initial assessment obtains a baseline of information about the client's pain, while subsequent assessments provide information regarding the effectiveness of the interventions. Physiologic and behavioral signs and, most important, the client's subjective pain ratings of the intensity all help the health care team determine whether the interventions should be continued or changed. Pain assessments should be performed when the intervention should be providing the most relief. For example, the onset of intravenous morphine is rapid, peaking approximately 20 minutes after administration. If the client has not obtained relief by 20 minutes, the intravenous morphine was ineffective, and the plan of care would need to be changed.

Recording Pain Assessment Findings

Pain assessment is of little value unless the information is recorded in a manner easily understood by the health care team. A flow sheet provides one place to document most of the information used to make pain management decisions, including pain rating, vital signs, analgesic administered, and level of arousal. The client's report of pain must be accepted and recorded, with pain management decisions based on that report.

NURSING DIAGNOSES

The two primary nursing diagnoses used to describe pain are *Acute **Pain*** and *Chronic **Pain***. According to the North American Nursing Diagnosis Association-International (NANDA-I,

CULTURAL CONSIDERATIONS

Perception of Pain

Culture determines the way persons derive meaning from their lives and also determines appropriate behaviors. One's cultural upbringing teaches behaviors, including those that are exhibited when in pain. People from different cultures use different types of words to describe pain (e.g., in sensory or emotional terms). These differences should not be ignored, but be careful not to prejudge a client based on cultural background or ethnicity. Because of the unique experience of pain, the person will exhibit individualized behaviors even though they are influenced by cultural upbringing.

2010), *Acute **P**ain* is defined as "an unpleasant sensory and emotional experience arising from actual or potential tissue damage or described in terms of such damage . . . [with] sudden or slow onset of any intensity from mild to severe, with an anticipated or predictable end and a duration of less than 6 months." *Chronic **P**ain* is defined the same as *Acute **P**ain,* with the last phrase replaced by "constant or recurring without an anticipated or predictable end and a duration of greater than 6 months."

Pain may be the etiology (cause) of other problems (e.g., *Impaired Physical **M**obility,* related to arthritic hip pain). Whether the pain is addressed in the problem statement or the etiology is determined by the client's primary problem. Many diagnoses can be related to the client in pain depending on the effects of the pain:

- ***A**ctivity Intolerance*
- ***A**nxiety*
- ***C**onstipation*
- *Deficient **K**nowledge* (specify)
- *Disturbed **B**ody Image*
- *Disturbed **S**leep Pattern*
- ***F**atigue*
- ***F**ear*
- ***H**opelessness*
- *Impaired **S**ocial Interaction*
- *Ineffective **B**reathing Pattern*
- *Ineffective **C**oping*
- *Ineffective **R**ole Performance*
- *Ineffective **S**elf-Health Management*
- ***P**owerlessness*

Planning/Outcome Identification

When planning care, mutual goal setting with the client experiencing pain is of utmost importance. The nurse and client work together to develop realistic outcomes. Consider both nonpharmacologic and pharmacologic interventions.

Often, several approaches must be combined for adequate relief to be obtained. No matter which type of intervention is being utilized, general principles apply: individualization, prevention, and utilization of a multidisciplinary approach.

Individualize the Approach

A variety of pain relief measures can be tried in many combinations until the goal of pain relief is reached. This often means some trial-and-error of interventions until the right combination is found. It is important to include measures that the client believes will be effective. The cognitive component of pain perception can have a powerful influence on the effectiveness of interventions. This may mean including folk remedies or nonscientific relief measures. It is important to keep an open mind. This comes with the caution to avoid those remedies that may harm the client.

Use a Preventive Approach

Pain is much easier to control if it is treated before it gets severe. Interventions should be implemented when pain is mild or when it is anticipated. For example, medicate a client before a painful dressing change or treatment rather than waiting for the pain to occur.

Use a Multidisciplinary Approach

Pain relief is a complex phenomenon requiring input from various members of the health care team. The nurse's role is pivotal in managing a client's pain. The physician also plays a key role, diagnosing and treating the medical cause of the pain, which includes prescribing appropriate medications. In complex cases, other professionals, such as physical therapists, psychologists, social workers, or chaplains, may be needed. The multidisciplinary team approach is the most successful way to manage chronic pain and improve the quality of a client's life.

Implementation

Pharmacologic and nonpharmacologic interventions can both be effective in caring for clients in pain. Nonpharmacologic techniques may be the primary intervention in some cases of mild pain, with medication available as "backup." Cases of moderate to severe pain may use nonpharmacologic techniques as effective adjunctive, or complementary, treatment.

There are three categories of pain control interventions: pharmacological, noninvasive, and invasive. Each category is discussed separately, but these methods are often used in combination.

Pharmacological Interventions

Caring for a client experiencing pain is a collaborative process. Drug therapy is the mainstay of treatment for pain control. The American Pain Society (APS) provides pain management guidelines that can be used as a framework for providing drug therapy in pain control (APS, 2006; Gordon et al., 2005). These guidelines are based on pain management research and thus are termed *evidence-based.* These guidelines represent concise information that can help nurses, physicians, and other health care workers effectively administer medications for pain relief. The word *action* incorporates these principles of pain management and can be recalled by using the acronym in the "ACTION" Memory Trick (Teeter & Kemper, 2008b).

MEMORYTRICK

Principles of Pain Management

Use the acronym **ACTION** to recall the principles of pain management:

A = Assess clients for pain at regular intervals

C = Choose a variety of interventions for pain

T = Treat pain promptly to avoid escalation of pain

I = Include client-specific cultural, spiritual, and developmental considerations in the pain management plan

O = Optimize the pain management plan through ongoing evaluation

N = Negotiate pain interventions and goals with the client to enhance adherence to the plan

(APS, 2006; Gordon et al., 2005; Teeter and Kemper, 2008b)

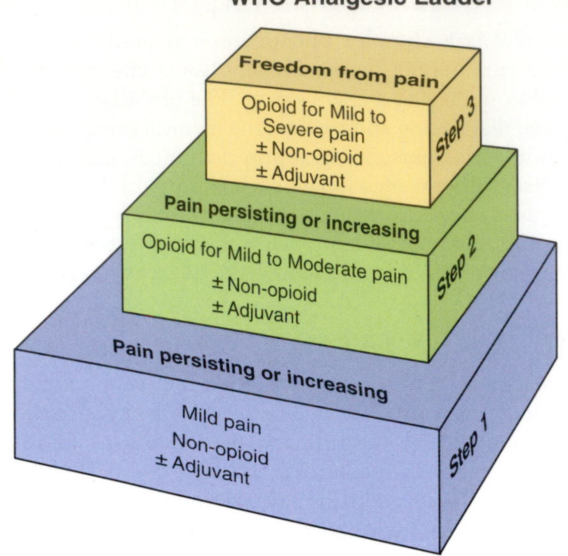

FIGURE 27-9 The WHO analgesic ladder gives guidelines for choosing analgesic therapy for cancer pain based on the level of pain the client is experiencing. (*Courtesy of World Health Organization, 2008, Used with permission.*)

The World Health Organization (WHO, 1990) has made worldwide relief of cancer pain one of its primary goals. In order to help meet this goal, it developed an analgesic ladder to help the clinician determine which analgesic to prescribe (Figure 27-9). Step 1 is for mild pain and includes a nonopioid with or without an adjuvant medication. If pain persists or increases, an opioid for mild to moderate pain can be added (step 2). Step 3, for pain that continues or increases despite step 2 treatments, recommends an opioid for moderate to severe pain with or without a nonopioid or an adjuvant.

All the nonopioids have ceiling doses; that is, if the dose is increased above a certain level, no additional pain relief is provided, only an increase in adverse or toxic effects. This is important to remember for clients who are receiving several medications that contain a nonopioid. For example, a client may be prescribed both acetaminophen for fever and Percocet (a combination drug containing acetaminophen and oxycodone) for pain. Be sure to consider both sources of acetaminophen to ensure that the client does not exceed the 24-hour ceiling dose of 4 grams. Liver necrosis can result from acetaminophen overdose (Lehne, 2004).

Opioids are recommended on step 2 and step 3 of the WHO Pain Relief Ladder. Weak opioids (step 2) include codeine, hydrocodone, and oxycodone. Most often, these drugs are administered orally in combination products containing acetaminophen. As noted previously, dosing of combination products is limited by the ceiling dose of nonopioids. Strong opioids (step 3), such as morphine, hydromorphone, and fentanyl, are given for severe pain (Teeter & Kemper, 2008b). Combining analgesics and the use of adjuvant medication provides effective pharmacologic intervention for clients with pain. **Adjuvant medications** are those drugs used to enhance the analgesic efficacy of opioids, to treat concurrent symptoms that exacerbate pain, and to provide independent analgesia for specific types of pain. The ladder recommends that the analgesic, plus or minus an adjuvant, is chosen based on the level of pain the client is experiencing. This ladder gives health care workers guidelines in determining if the drug regimen is appropriate for the client with cancer pain.

Nurses' Role in Administration of Analgesics The nurse spends the most time with the client in pain and is the team member who most often assesses the effectiveness of pain control interventions. When analgesics are prescribed, the nurse often has choices of drug, route, and interval. For example, the postoperative client may have the following orders:

- Morphine 2.5 to 15 mg IV every 2 to 4 hours prn severe pain
- Vicodin one to two tabs every 3 to 4 hours prn moderate pain

When this client complains of pain, which analgesic should the nurse administer? Which route? Which dose? How frequently? The nurse has a large responsibility in making these decisions but also has autonomy in making these decisions.

McCaffery and Pasero (1999) identify the following as the responsibilities of the nurse in administering analgesics:

- Determine whether to give the analgesic, and if more than one is ordered, which one.
- Assess the client's response to the analgesic, including assessing the effectiveness in pain relief and occurrence of any side effects.
- Report to the physician when a change is needed, including making suggestions for changes based on the nurse's knowledge of the client and pharmacology.
- Teach the client and family regarding the use of analgesics.

Principles of Administering Analgesics "How an analgesic is used is probably more important than which one is used" (McCaffery & Pasero, 1999). Principles should be applied in the administration of analgesics, no matter which one is given.

Establishing and maintaining a therapeutic serum level is important. Peaks and valleys often occur when analgesics are administered in the traditional PRN (as needed) manner. When the dose is administered on an intermittent schedule, a larger dose is often required, causing the client to have a peak serum drug level in the sedation range. The client must wait for the return of pain before requesting the next dose of analgesic. Depending on the length of time it takes to obtain the medication and, once taken, to reestablish an adequate blood level, there could be a period of up to an hour or so without adequate pain control.

Preventive Approach Pain is much easier to control if treated when it is anticipated or at a mild intensity. Once pain becomes severe, the analgesics ordered may not be effective enough to relieve it. Many clinicians still teach their clients to wait to take medication until they are sure they really need it. This practice leads to uncontrolled pain. There are two ways the preventive approach may be implemented:

- ATC (around the clock). When pain is predictable, for example, the first few days following surgery or with

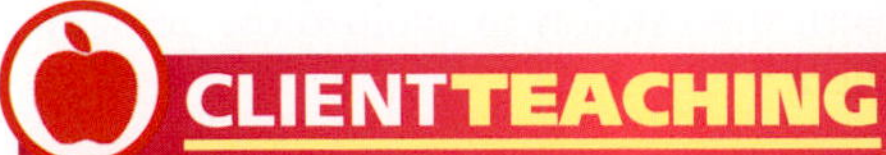

Timed-Release Tablets

Emphasize that the extended-release tablets become immediate release if crushed (e.g., for a client who has difficulty swallowing the tablet).

CLIENT TEACHING

Pain Management

- It is import to take or request pain medication before the pain becomes severe and more difficult to control.
- Numerous nonpharmacologic approaches can be used to augment pharmacologic pain management.
- Pain management is individual. (The client may be taking different medications or dosages than other individuals.)

chronic cancer pain, the medication is administered on a scheduled basis. This prevents the peaks and valleys of serum drug level that can lead to oversedation or toxicity and recurrence of pain, respectively. If the analgesics are ordered by the physician to be given PRN, it can still be a nursing measure to administer the drugs ATC, as long as they are given within the time constraints of the order.

- PRN (Latin for *pro re nata*, which means "as required"). Pain is not always predictable; therefore PRN dosing may be required. For some clients this may be used in addition to scheduled dosing for "breakthrough" pain (pain that surpasses the level of **analgesia**, or pain relief without anesthesia, that the steady level of analgesics is providing). Examples of this include a cancer client on prolonged-release morphine who needs extra analgesics to participate in activities such as shopping or receiving visitors. Another example would be the orthopedic client who is receiving regularly scheduled analgesics for postoperative pain who needs additional pain relief for therapy sessions. In order to implement the preventive approach with PRN dosing, the medications are given as soon as the pain appears, or when it is anticipated to begin.

Titrate to Effect Because of the unique nature of the pain experience, the analgesic regimen needs to be titrated until the desired effect is achieved. This involves adjusting the following:

- *Dosage*. Some clients may require more or less than the standard dose. Many factors may influence the pharmacokinetics in an individual client. The individual's response is assessed, and the dosage of the analgesic is regulated accordingly. In clients with chronic cancer pain, opioid analgesics are increased until pain relief is obtained or unacceptable side effects occur. This may be done because of the lack of a **ceiling effect** (the dosage beyond which no further analgesia occurs) in pure opioids. The lack of a ceiling effect means there is no limit to the dose that can be given. For example, cancer clients have been known to receive more than 1 gram per hour intravenously. Because the dosage is gradually increased, the client develops a **tolerance** (requiring larger and larger doses of an analgesic to achieve the same level of pain relief) to the side effects of the opioid.
- *Interval*. Some clients metabolize the analgesics faster than others. For example, young adults tend to metabolize opioids faster; therefore, they may need more frequent doses. Older clients tend to metabolize them slower, so they require a longer interval between doses.
- *Route*. The appropriate route is chosen depending on how rapidly pain relief is required, the client's ability to take medications orally, the client's diagnosis, and assessment of the client's response to the current route. Intravenous administration provides the most rapid onset of pain relief. All other routes require a lag time for absorption of the analgesic into the circulation. In postoperative pain, IV is the preferred route for opioids when the oral route is not appropriate. If IV access is not available, sublingual, rectal, or transdermal routes are considered.

With cancer pain, the oral route is preferred. If the client is unable to take oral medications, rectal and transdermal routes are preferred because they are less invasive than other routes (Agency for Healthcare Research and Quality, 2007). In addition, tolerance develops at a slower rate with the oral route compared to the more invasive routes.

- *Choice of drug*. If one drug is not providing relief or has unacceptable side effects, another analgesic is tried.

The key to administering an analgesic is to monitor the client's response to it. This includes assessing the effectiveness of pain relief and the occurrence of side effects.

Classes of Analgesics Three classes of drugs are used for pain relief: (a) nonopioid analgesics, (b) opioid analgesics, and (c) analgesic adjuvants already discussed (WHO, 2008).

Nonopioids The medications in this category are useful for a variety of painful conditions, including surgery, trauma, and cancer (APS, 1999). The indications include mild to moderate pain, and they are used in conjunction with opioids. These drugs differ from opioids in several ways in that they:

- Are subject to the ceiling effect.
- Do not produce the effect of tolerance or physical dependence.
- Are antipyretic and should not be given in cases where they may mask an infection.

Ketorolac tromethamine (Toradol) is the only nonsteroidal anti-inflammatory drug (NSAID) available in parenteral form and has proven useful in clients on NPO status who would benefit from a NSAID. Even when administered intramuscularly or intravenously, ketorolac produces significant gastric irritation and the potential for gastric bleeding. The most frequent use of ketorolac is orally or intramuscularly in adults, but some pediatric centers have used it intravenously under strict supervision for a limited course (less than 5 days) in children and adolescents with great success.

Action Action of these drugs is thought to inhibit prostaglandin formation. If prostaglandins are inhibited, the sensory neurons are less likely to receive the pain signal. Thus, this class of analgesics works in the peripheral nervous system.

Opioids The opioid analgesics fall into three classes: pure opioid agonists, partial agonists, and **mixed agonist-antagonists** (a compound that blocks opioid effects on one receptor type while producing opioid effects on a second receptor type). Pure agonists produce a maximal response from cells when they bind to the cells' opioid receptor sites. Morphine (the gold standard against which all other opioids are measured), fentanyl, methadone (Dolophine), hydromorphone hydrochloride (Dilaudid), and codeine are pure agonists. Meperidine (Demerol), although classified as a pure agonist, is not recommended except in clients with a true allergy to all other narcotics because of its neurotoxicity. Meperidine produces clinical analgesia for only 2.5 to 3.5 hours when given intramuscularly in adults.

PROFESSIONALTIP

Ketorolac tromethamine (Toradol)

Ketorolac should not be given to a client with any history of renal dysfunction, gastric irritation, bleeding problems, low platelet count, or allergy to aspirin or other NSAIDs.

Unlike the NSAIDs, pure agonist opioids are not subject to the ceiling effect. As the dosage is increased, pain relief increases.

Action Opioids act in the CNS by binding to opiate receptor sites on afferent neurons. The pain signal is stopped at the spinal cord level and does not reach the cortex where pain is perceived.

Side Effects The only limiting factor in the use of pure agonist opioids is the degree of side effects, particularly respiratory depression and constipation. Other side effects include pruritus and nausea, but the degree to which they are present from each medication varies among individuals. Clients must be instructed regarding these normal responses to opioids and informed that it does not mean that they are allergic to them. A true allergy to opioids would be indicated by a rash or hives that starts after receiving the opioid, a local histamine release at the site of infusion, or anaphylaxis. Clients also need to know that the pruritus and nausea generally subside after 4 to 5 days of opioid therapy. In the meantime, an antihistamine such as diphenhydramine hydrochloride (Benadryl) or hydroxyzine hydrochloride (Atarax, Vistaril) may be used for pruritus, and an antiemetic such as metoclopramide hydrochloride (Clopra) or trimethobenzamide hydrochloride (Tigan) can be used to treat the nausea.

PROFESSIONALTIP

Types of Nonopioid Drugs

- *Salicylates.* These include aspirin and other salicylate salts. Common side effects of aspirin include gastric disturbances and bleeding caused by the antiplatelet effect. Some of the salicylate salts, such as choline magnesium trisalicylate (Trilisate) and salsalate (Salgesic), have fewer gastrointestinal and bleeding effects than aspirin.
- *Acetaminophen*. This nonsalicylate is similar to aspirin in its analgesic action but has no anti-inflammatory effect. Its mechanism of action for pain relief is not known.
- *NSAIDs*. The effectiveness of these drugs varies, with some being close to the effectiveness of aspirin and acetaminophen, whereas others are much stronger. Clients tend to vary in response, so once the maximum recommended dose has been tried with ineffective results, it would be worth trying another NSAID. The drugs in this group inhibit platelet aggregation and are contraindicated in clients with coagulation disorders or on anticoagulation therapy.

LIFE SPAN CONSIDERATIONS

Effects of Meperidine (Demerol)

- In the elderly, most of whom show decreased glomerular filtration rates, there is generally a higher peak and longer duration of action because it takes longer to excrete the opioid as well as its toxic metabolite, normeperidine.
- In pediatric clients receiving intravenous meperidine, analgesia may last for only 1.5 to 2 hours.

Almost all medications used to treat side effects have their own side effect of sedation. Thus, there is the possibility of a cumulative effect of severe sedation. These medications must be used with caution and appropriate monitoring until the client's response is determined. Ondansetron hydrochloride (Zofran) is one antiemetic on the market with little, if any, sedative effect. It received Food and Drug Administration (FDA) approval for use with postoperative nausea and is effective in clients with refractory nausea and vomiting unresponsive to other antiemetics. The current cost per dose, close to $100 in many hospitals, limits its use to the extreme nausea associated with cancer chemotherapy or to clients with refractory nausea and vomiting.

Mixed agonist-antagonist opioids are believed to be subject to the ceiling effect for pain relief, as well as a ceiling effect for respiratory depression. Mixed agonist-antagonist opioids activate one opioid receptor type while simultaneously blocking another type. Butorphanol tartrate (Stadol), pentazocine hydrochloride (Talwin), and nalbuphine hydrochloride (Nubain) are the most frequently used in pain management.

Opioid antagonists include naloxone (Narcan) and naltrexone (Trexal), with the most commonly used being naloxone (Narcan). They work by blocking opioid stimulation of receptor sites. Naloxone effectively reverses opioid side effects of sedation, respiratory depression, and nausea, and *it completely reverses any pain control.*

Alternative Delivery Systems Opioids are administered in more than just the traditional oral, subcutaneous, intramuscular, intravenous, and rectal routes.

Patient-Controlled Analgesia **Patient-controlled analgesia (PCA)** is most often delivered by a device that allows the client to control the delivery of intravenous, epidural, or subcutaneous pain medication in a safe, effective manner through

PROFESSIONALTIP

Constipation and Opioids

Clients who are expected to require opioid analgesics for more than 1 or 2 days should be administered a stool softener as soon as they are taking fluids orally. While they are still NPO, a glycerin or bisacodyl (Dulcolax) suppository should be administered if the client has not had a bowel movement in 1 or 2 days.

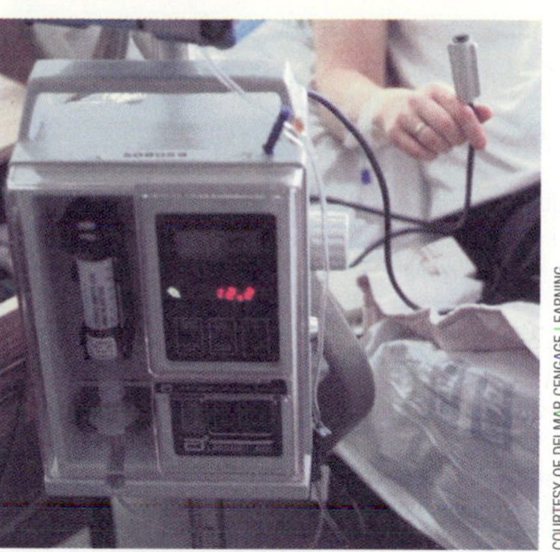

FIGURE 27-10 Client on IV Patient-Controlled Analgesia (PCA)

a programmable pump (Figure 27-10). This system helps eliminate the time required for the nurse to draw up the medication and allows the client control over the pain. The pump has the safety feature of locking out once a maximum dose is reached. This prevents the client from overdosing. The PCA has been successfully used with many types of pain and in many settings, including postoperative, pediatrics, and home health.

Requirements for using a PCA are the cognitive ability to understand how to use the pump and the physical ability to push the button. The nurse teaches the client and family about the PCA pump and pain medication, how to activate the pump, and that the client is the only one to activate the pump. The nurse explains the pain rating scale to the client and continues to regularly monitor the client's pain even when the client is using the pump. Teach the client to "push the button" only when medication for pain is needed. The client or family notifies the nurse if the medication is not controlling the pain so that alternative measures can be taken.

Oral PCA is relatively new in hospitals and is becoming increasingly popular (Rosati et al., 2007). Client teaching is the key for success. The client must understand how pain, pain medication, and pain relief are related and how to maintain a pain-relief diary. A Velcro®-sealed wrist pouch is applied to the client with one or two doses of the prescribed oral analgesic, even controlled substances, in the pouch. The client notifies the nurse when a dose is taken so that it can be replaced. If the client does not comply with the oral PCA policy, it is discontinued.

Medication on demand (MOD®) is another method of oral PCA. The facility pharmacy places eight doses of oral medication in the medication tray, which is then loaded into the device. The cover is closed, locking the medication securely inside. The MOD® locks to an IV pole for easy client access as shown in Figure 27-11A. The client accesses the MOD® with his radio-frequency identification (RFID) wristband, dials in his pain level from 0 to 10 by touching the pad on the front of the device, and receives the prescribed medication. The device is programmed to respond only to a specific client's RFID wristband. Once the client accepts the medication, the device has a lockout interval so the client cannot receive more than the prescribed dose. At the end of the lockout time, a light on the MOD® illuminates, indicating that the client can have medication when needed. Nurses may access the device with a programmed RFID card. The device stores the information for reference, printing, or inclusion in the client's electronic medical record. (Figure 27-11B).

Epidural/Intrathecal Analgesia **Epidural analgesia** refers to administering the opioid via a catheter that terminates in the epidural space, the space outside the dura mater that protects the spinal cord. **Intrathecal analgesia** refers to administering the drug directly into the subarachnoid space. These may be administered as a one-time injection by the anesthesiologist or via a catheter that has been placed. Both of these routes are occasionally referred to as *intraspinal anesthesia.* Because the opioid is delivered close to the site of action, these routes require much lower doses of opioid (usually morphine [Duramorph] or fentanyl [Sublimaze] are used) for pain relief. The incidence of systemic side effects is also much lower with these routes. Duration is longer than systemic routes (e.g., the duration of one dose of intrathecal morphine can last 24 hours).

Transdermal Analgesia Another route of opioid administration is the transdermal patch. The only opioid drug currently available via this route is fentanyl (Duragesic). This medication is on an adhesive patch that attaches to the skin. It is available in 25, 50, 75, and 100 mcg/hour dosages. The fentanyl transdermal patch allows slow infusion of the drug through the skin. The fentanyl patch is indicated for continuous pain with high dosage requirements. The advantage of this route is that it is simple to apply and effective for 72 hours. The disadvantage is that dosage adjustments are difficult to make because of the slow infusion rate. In addition, side effects may not be reversed as rapidly as when opiates are administered via the oral route.

Local Anesthesia Local anesthetics are effective for pain management in a variety of settings. Topical anesthetics are available for teething, sore throats, denture pain, laceration repair, and intravenous catheter insertions. One topical anesthetic, EMLA cream, is a mixture of local anesthetics, combining prilocaine (Citanest) and lidocaine (Xylocaine). It produces complete anesthesia for at least 60 minutes when topically applied on intact skin. Another topical anesthetic, TAC, is available for anesthesia during closure of lacerations. It is a combination of tetracaine hydrochloride (Pontocaine) 0.5%, adrenaline (epinephrine) 1:2000, and cocaine 11.8% in a normal saline solution that can be applied directly to the open wound surface in place of local anesthetic infiltration with a needle. This allows pain-free cleansing of the laceration as well as suturing. Because both adrenaline

LIFE SPAN CONSIDERATIONS

Opioid Analgesia in the Elderly

- Cheyne-Stokes respiratory patterns are not unusual during sleep in the elderly and should not be used as a reason to restrict appropriate opioid pain relief unless accompanied by unacceptable degrees of arterial desaturation (less than 85%).
- The elderly are more sensitive to sedation and respiratory depressant effects and experience a higher peak and longer duration of effect from opioid medications.
- Opioid dose titration must be based on analgesic effects and degree of side effects, such as sedation, urinary retention, constipation, respiratory depression, or exacerbation of Parkinson's disease.

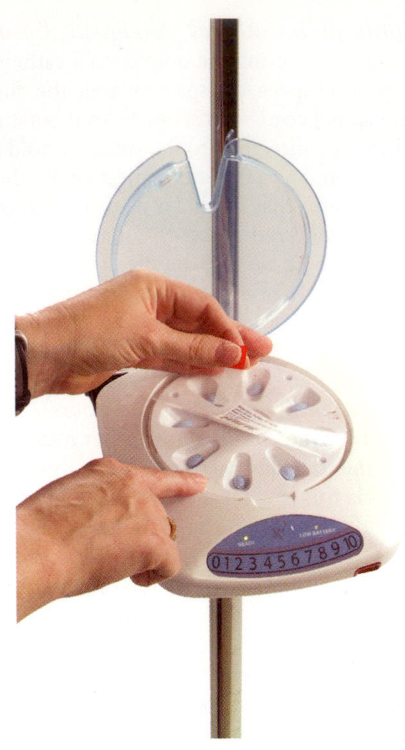

A

After completing a teaching module with hands-on instructions, the client obtains oral pain medication as needed from the MOD®. An illuminated ready light appears indicating to the client that the lockout interval has passed and medication is now available when needed. The client obtains medication as needed without requesting the medication from a nurse. To get the medication, the client:

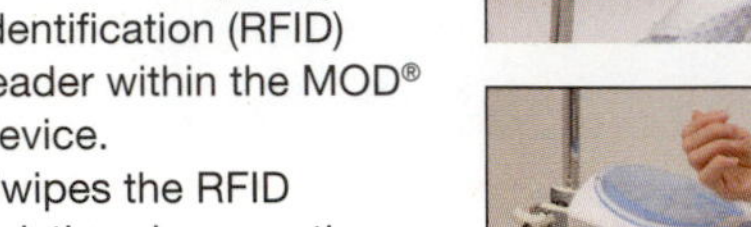

1. Indicates his pain level from 0-10 on the pain scale. This activates the radio frequency identification (RFID) reader within the MOD® device.
2. Swipes the RFID wristband across the MOD®'s faceplate.
3. Removes the prescribed dose of pain medication and self administers the medication.

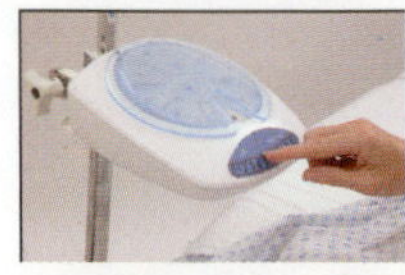

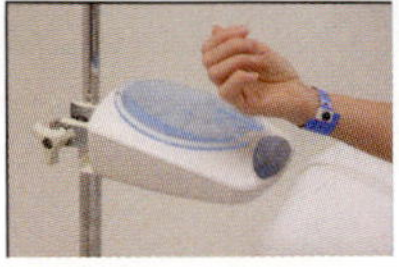

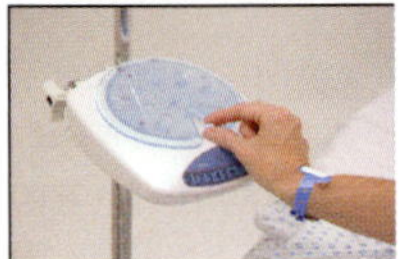

B

FIGURE 27-11 **Oral Patient-Controlled Analgesia Device called Medication on Demand (MOD®); *A*, MOD® is locked to an IV pole for client accessibility. The facility pharmacy places oral medication in the medication tray which is then loaded into the device; *B*, Guidelines for obtaining medication for the MOD®.** ***(Images courtesy of AVANCEN).***

(epinephrine) and cocaine cause vasoconstriction, TAC cannot be used in areas supplied by end-arteriolar blood supply such as a client's digits, ear, or nose. It also is contraindicated on burned or abraded skin because this could lead to increased systemic absorption of cocaine and tetracaine, thus placing the client at risk for seizures.

Noninvasive Interventions

Noninvasive relief measures consist of cognitive-behavioral strategies and physical modalities that use cutaneous stimulation. These treatments can be used to supplement pharmacological therapy and other modalities to control pain. Clients and their families can also be instructed to utilize these treatments at home and in inpatient settings.

Cognitive-Behavioral Interventions The cognitive-behavioral interventions influence the cognitive and the motivational-affective components of pain perception. These methods can not only help influence the level of pain, but also help the client gain a sense of self-control.

Trusting Nurse–Client Relationship Establishing a therapeutic relationship is the foundation for effective nursing care. The clients most likely to be comfortable are those who trust their nurses to be there, to listen, and to act.

Relaxation **Relaxation techniques** (a variety of methods used to decrease anxiety and muscle tension) result in decreased heart rate and respiratory rate and decreased muscle tension. The body's response to pain is almost "tricked" into reversing itself when relaxation exercises are implemented.

Relaxation exercises help reduce pain by decreasing anxiety and decreasing reflex muscular contraction. There are a wide variety of relaxation techniques, including focused breathing, progressive muscle relaxation, and meditation. Simple techniques should be used during episodes of brief pain (e.g., during procedures) or when pain is so severe that the client is unable to concentrate on complicated instructions.

To teach simple relaxation techniques, the nurse can instruct the client to (a) take a deep breath and hold it, (b) exhale slowly and concentrate on going limp; and (c) start yawning (McCaffery & Pasero, 1999). The yawning triggers a conditioned response in the client (i.e., the body associates yawning with relaxation and will relax when the client yawns). The technique can be enhanced if the nurse starts yawning. It is so contagious that even the client compromised by severe pain will usually start yawning with the nurse.

A more complex technique is **progressive muscle relaxation**, a strategy in which muscles are alternately tensed and relaxed. This type of technique is especially useful for clients who do not know what muscle relaxation feels like. By purposely contracting and releasing the muscle groups, the client is able to compare the difference and identify feelings of relaxation. Meditative relaxation techniques are also available, including audiotapes sold in most bookstores.

LIFE SPAN CONSIDERATIONS

Injections and Children

Children lack the cognitive ability to weigh the pain of injection against the pain relief from the medication, so oral and rectal routes are preferred over injections.

PROFESSIONALTIP

Using Distraction

Distraction should never be the *only* pain management intervention used, but it can be very helpful while waiting for other techniques to take effect.

CLIENTTEACHING

Hot or Cold Applications

Teach the client or family that hot or cold applications:

- Must have at least one layer of towel between the heating or cooling device and the skin.
- Should not exceed 20 minutes when placed on the skin (Department of Health, NSW, 2005).
- Should not be applied to tissue that has been exposed to radiation therapy (Agency for Health Care Policy and Research, 1994).

Relaxation is a learned response. The more frequently the client practices these techniques, the more skilled the body will be in learning to relax. Ideally, the best time to teach the client these methods is when pain is controlled or before the pain occurs (e.g., in the preoperative period).

Reframing **Reframing** is a technique that teaches clients to monitor their negative thoughts and replace them with more positive ones. For example, teach a client to replace an expression such as "I can't stand this pain, it's never going away" with one such as "I've had similar pain before, and it's gotten better."

Distraction Distraction focuses one's attention on something other than the pain, therefore placing pain on the periphery of awareness. Successful use of distraction does not eliminate the pain; it makes it less troublesome. The main disadvantage of distraction is that as soon as the distractive stimuli stop, the pain returns in full force. For this reason, the most appropriate use of distraction techniques is for the relief of brief, episodic pain. It can be effective for procedural pain or the period between administration of an analgesic and the onset of the drug. Examples of distraction include the following:

- Active listening to recorded music (have the client tap fingers in rhythm to the beat)
- Reciting a poem or rhyme (children do this well)
- Describe a plot of a novel or movie
- Describe a series of pictures

Guided Imagery Guided imagery uses one's imagination to provide a pleasant substitute for the pain. It incorporates features of both relaxation and distraction. The client imagines a pleasant experience, such as going to the beach or the mountains. The experience should use all five senses to fully involve the client in the image.

The images chosen need to be ones that are pleasant for the client. Describing an ocean cruise would not be appropriate for a person who becomes seasick.

Humor The old saying, "Laughter is the best medicine," carries some truth to it. Although there is nothing very funny about pain, laughing has been shown to provide pain relief. The act of laughing can cause distraction from the pain, induce relaxation by taking deep breaths and releasing tension, release endorphins, and provide a pleasant substitute for pain. Norman Cousins (1991) relates obtaining 2 hours of pain relief from watching episodes of the *Candid Camera* television show and Marx Brothers films. This technique can be implemented by encouraging the client to watch humorous movies, read funny books, or listen to comedy routines. Because different people see humor in different types of situations, be sensitive to what the client views as funny.

Biofeedback Biofeedback is a method that may help the client in pain to relax and relieve tension. Individuals learn to influence their physiological responses to stimuli and thus alter their pain experience.

Cutaneous Stimulation The technique of cutaneous stimulation involves stimulating the skin to control pain. It is theorized that this technique provides relief by stimulating nerve fibers that send signals to the dorsal horn of the spinal cord to "close the gate." The main advantage of these therapies is that many techniques are easy for the nurse to implement and easy to teach the client and family to perform. They are not usually meant to replace analgesic therapy, but to complement it.

Hot and Cold Application In addition to stimulating nerves that can block pain transmission, superficial heat application increases circulation to the area, which promotes oxygenation and nutrient delivery to the injured tissues. It also decreases joint and muscle stiffness. Heat is contraindicated in cases of acute injury because it can increase the initial response of edema. It is also contraindicated in rheumatoid arthritis flare-ups and over topical applications of mentholated ointments. Heat treatments should be limited to 20- to 30-minute intervals because maximum vasodilatation occurs in that time.

Cryotherapy (cold applications) induces local vasoconstriction and numbness, therefore altering the pain sensations. It is contraindicated in any condition where vasoconstriction might increase symptoms (e.g., peripheral vascular disease). For best results, cold therapy should be limited to 20- to 30-minute intervals. Either heat or cold can be used as cutaneous stimulation unless one is specifically contraindicated. Cold often provides faster relief (McCaffery & Pasero, 1999). If the client has used heat or cold before, incorporate the modality that the client believes will be the most effective. Combining the two might provide better relief. An example of this would be to apply a hot pack for 4 minutes, followed by an ice pack for 2 minutes, repeated four times. In a hospital setting, a physician order is required for this therapy.

Acupressure and Massage One of the first responses to pain is to rub the painful part. People seem to instinctively understand the pain-relieving aspects of this intervention. In addition to blocking the pain transmission through nerve stimulation, massage can also promote relaxation. Acupressure is a type of massage that consists of continuous pressure on or the rubbing of acupuncture points. Massage is based on the same principles as acupuncture, but needles are not used. Massage also provides a form of nonverbal communication that can be therapeutic on its own.

Mentholated Rubs Ointments or lotions containing menthol are thought to provide relief by providing a counterirritation to the skin. The menthol gives the client the perception that the temperature of the skin has changed (becoming either warmer or cooler). This alters the sensation of pain or provides a distraction from the pain. Client response varies to mentholated rubs; some gain effective relief, but others have

SAFETY

TENS Contraindications

- No electrodes are placed in the area over or surrounding demand cardiac pacemakers.
- No electrodes are placed over the uterus of a pregnant woman.

poor results. Their use is contraindicated on broken skin, on mucous membranes, or if pain increases.

Transcutaneous Electrical Nerve Stimulation **Transcutaneous electrical nerve stimulation (TENS)** is the process of applying a low-voltage electrical current to the skin through cutaneous electrodes. This modulates pain transmission, as do other cutaneous stimulation methods, but also distracts the client from pain. Research supports the effectiveness of using TENS for the relief of postoperative pain (Agency for Health Care Policy and Research, 1992; Rakel & Frantz, 2003). It has also been used successfully in many pain syndromes (e.g., chronic low-back pain, menstrual cramps, temporomandibular joint [TMJ] syndrome, phantom limb pain, and others). It is administered by specially trained health professionals, usually a physical therapist. Other modalities of pain management should not be abandoned while a trial of TENS occurs.

Exercise Exercise is an important treatment for chronic pain because it helps mobilize joints, strengthens weak muscles, and helps restore balance and coordination. Do not use passive range of motion if it increases discomfort or pain. Immobilization is frequently used to stabilize fractures or for clients with episodes of acute pain. Prolonged immobilization can lead to muscle atrophy and cardiovascular deconditioning.

Psychotherapy Psychotherapy may be beneficial to some clients, particularly those:

- Who are clinically depressed
- Who have a history of psychiatric problems
- Whose pain is difficult to control

Some psychotherapists use **hypnosis** (altered state of consciousness when a person is more receptive to suggestion) to help clients alter pain perception. Hypnosis can be effective but should be used only by specially trained professionals.

Positioning The final noninvasive technique is proper positioning and body alignment. Moving the client with the least possible stress on joints and skin will minimize exposure to painful stimuli. This includes supporting joints appropriately and maintaining wrinkle-free sheets.

Invasive Interventions

Invasive interventions are meant to complement behavioral, physical, and pharmacological therapies in those clients who do not obtain relief from those measures alone. Invasive measures are indicated primarily for chronic cancer pain and in some cases of chronic benign pain. These procedures are usually tried only when noninvasive measures have been attempted first with poor results.

CRITICAL THINKING

Noninvasive Intervention

How would you decide which noninvasive intervention to use with a client?

Nerve Block Neural blockade is the process of injecting a local anesthetic or neurolytic agent into the nerve. An anesthetic agent may be injected to act as a diagnostic tool in order to identify the nerves involved in a pain syndrome. A neurolytic agent is a chemical agent that causes destruction of the nerve and, therefore, creates an interruption in the pain signal.

Neurosurgery Neurosurgical measures for pain control include neurostimulation procedures and destructive or ablative procedures. Neurostimulation procedures involve the implantation of electrical stimulation devices that send impulses to different parts of the nervous system. Some of these devices stimulate areas of the brain; others stimulate the spinal cord. Relief is thought to be provided by blocking the afferent fiber input at the spinal cord level or by stimulating release of endorphins using the body's ability to modulate pain.

Destructive or ablative procedures are used to destroy part of the nervous system that conducts pain. By interrupting the pain signal, it is prevented from reaching the cortex where realization of pain occurs. These procedures are reserved for clients with terminal illness.

Radiation Therapy Radiation can be used as a palliative measure for pain relief in clients with cancer. It can relieve both metastatic pain and pain caused by tumors at the primary cancer site. It enhances other pain management strategies, such as analgesic therapy, because it is aimed specifically at the cause of the client's pain. When administered for pain relief, the smallest dose of radiation is utilized to minimize side effects.

Acupuncture **Acupuncture** is the insertion of small needles into the skin at specific (hoku) sites. The sites are chosen after the practitioner takes a detailed history and uses traditional Asian diagnostic techniques. The needles used for acupuncture have rounded ends that enter the skin without cutting the tissue. The practitioner may twirl or vibrate the needles manually or electrically. It is important that the nurse keep an open mind when the client chooses this therapy, or the client may be reluctant to discuss its use.

EVALUATION

Evaluating pain management interventions is ongoing, focusing primarily on the client's subjective reports. Objective data to evaluate pain management include the following:

- Continuing use of pain assessment tools
- Client's facial expression and posture
- Presence (or absence) of restlessness
- Vital sign monitoring

CASE STUDY

C.S. is a 76-year-old male with arthritis. He and his wife are residents of a nursing home. His wife is bedridden because of a cardiac disorder. Each day, C.S. sits at his wife's bedside and talks to her. Today, C.S. is agitated and short with his wife. He is moving slowly, his knees are edematous, and he winces when he walks.

1. List factors that may indicate that C.S. is experiencing pain.
2. Identify factors that may be impacting C.S.'s pain experience.
3. Describe the nursing actions necessary to perform a comprehensive pain assessment of C.S.

Adapted from *Caring for Clients with Pain*, by M. Teeter and D. Kemper, 2008b, manuscript submitted for publication.

SAMPLE NURSING CARE PLAN

The Client with Chronic Pain

S.J., a 48-year-old woman, injured her back 3 years ago while lifting some boxes of paper at work. Since that time, she has had four epidural steroidal injections for the pain associated with two ruptured discs. Her pain has been intermittent, with some alleviation from the epidural injections. Her last epidural was 3 months ago. She arrives at the clinic stating, "I just don't know how I can go on like this. The pain has been tolerable until last night. I'm hurting so bad!" She is tearful and pacing, saying, "It hurts too much when I sit down." Verbalizes pain is "9" on a 1-to-10 pain intensity scale. Blood pressure is 148/90. Pulse is strong and regular at 92. She has guarded movements.

NURSING DIAGNOSIS 1 *Chronic **Pain***, related to muscle spasm and lower back pain as evidenced by back injury 3 years ago and client statement "I just don't know how I can go on like this. The pain has been tolerable until last night. I'm hurting so bad!"

Nursing Outcomes Classification (NOC)
Comfort Level
Pain Control

Nursing Interventions Classification (NIC)
Pain Management
Medication Management
Coping Enhancement

PLANNING/OUTCOMES	NURSING INTERVENTIONS	RATIONALE
S.J. will verbalize a decrease in pain.	Assess S.J.'s level of pain, determining the intensity at its best and worst.	Determines a baseline for future assessment.
	Listen to S.J. while she discusses the pain; acknowledge the presence of pain.	Decreases anxiety by communicating acceptance and validating her perceptions.
	Discuss reasons why pain may be increased or decreased.	Helps S.J. understand her pain.
S.J. will practice selected noninvasive pain relief measures.	Teach relaxation techniques such as deep breathing, progressive muscle relaxation, and imagery.	Reduces skeletal muscle tension and anxiety, which potentiates the perception of pain.
	Teach S.J. about the use of medication for pain relief. Provide accurate information to reduce fear of addiction.	Lack of knowledge and fear may prohibit S.J. from taking analgesic medications as prescribed.
	Encourage S.J. to rest during the day.	Fatigue increases the perception of pain.

EVALUATION

After practicing relaxation techniques, S.J. rates her pain as a 2 to 3 on the pain intensity scale. S.J. demonstrates the use of deep breathing and progressive muscle relaxation.

(Continues)

SAMPLE NURSING CARE PLAN (Continued)

NURSING DIAGNOSIS 2

Anxiety related to chronic pain as evidenced by pacing and tears

NOC: *Coping; Anxiety Reduction*
NIC: *Anxiety Reduction; Anticipatory Guidance*

CLIENT GOALS

1. S.J. will verbalize an increase in psychological and physiological comfort level.
2. S.J. will demonstrate ability to cope with anxiety as evidenced by normal vital signs and a verbalized reduction in pain intensity.

NURSING INTERVENTIONS

1-1. Assess S.J.'s level of anxiety.

2-1. Encourage S.J. to verbalize angry feelings.

2-1. Speak slowly and calmly.

SCIENTIFIC RATIONALES

1-1. Determines baseline for future assessment.

2-1. Provides an outlet for her anger.

2-2. Avoids escalating S.J.'s anxiety level and increases the likelihood of her comprehension.

EVALUATION

After practicing relaxation techniques, how does S.J. rate her pain on a pain intensity scale?
Is S.J. verbalizing decreased pain intensity?
After a relaxation session, are S.J.'s vital signs within normal ranges?

SUMMARY

- Pain may be defined as "an unpleasant sensory and emotional experience associated with actual or potential tissue damage" (IASP, 2008) and "whatever the client says it is, existing whenever the client says it does" (McCaffery & Pasero, 1999).
- The gate control theory proposes that several processes (sensory, motivational-affective, and cognitive) combine to determine how a person perceives pain.
- Assessment of pain helps establish a baseline of data and helps evaluate the effectiveness of interventions.
- Factors influencing pain perception include age, previous experience with pain, and cultural norms.
- The subjective data to gather include location of pain, onset and duration, quality, intensity (on a scale of 0 to 10), aggravating and relieving factors, and how pain affects the activities of daily living.
- The three general principles to follow with pain relief measures are (a) individualize the approach, (b) use a preventive approach, and (c) use a multidisciplinary approach.

- The nurse carries a great deal of autonomy in administering analgesics, which leads to specific responsibilities for which the nurse is accountable.
- Pharmacologic agents can be therapeutic for clients experiencing pain; however, the medications should not be the only interventions used.
- Noninvasive treatments for pain relief are measures that can supplement pharmacological and invasive treatments for pain relief.
- Invasive techniques are interventions used when the noninvasive and pharmacological measures do not provide adequate relief. Methods include nerve blocks, neurosurgery, radiation therapy, and acupuncture.

REVIEW QUESTIONS

1. According to McCaffery and Pasero, pain may be defined as:
   1. discomfort resulting from identifiable physiologic or iatrogenic sources.
   2. a syndrome of behavioral and physical manifestations that can be objectively identified by the nurse.
   3. whatever the patient says it is, existing whenever and wherever the patient says it does.
   4. a sensory response to noxious stimuli.
2. Which of the following is a useful tool for assessing the intensity of pain that is easy to use?
   1. The gate control scale.
   2. Acute pain monitor.
   3. Numeric pain scale.
   4. Pressure pain monitor.
3. B.L., 45, has experienced chronic low-back pain since a fall 8 years ago. He describes his pain as "a gnawing, constant dull pain" that makes him feel tired. The nurse caring for him recognizes that one of the differences between acute and chronic pain characteristics is:
   1. acute pain is more severe.
   2. chronic pain is often described as dull and is difficult to localize.
   3. chronic back pain is often not real.
   4. acute pain is more diffuse and difficult to describe.
4. N.J., 84 years old, is recuperating from a total hip replacement. Morphine, 8 mg IV q4h PRN, is prescribed for N.J. Her respiratory rate is 18, her pulse rate is 96 beats per minute, and her blood pressure is elevated slightly above her normal level. She is complaining of severe pain, 8 on a scale of 0 to 10. The most appropriate initial nursing intervention is:
   1. question the physician regarding the dosage amount for a client this age.
   2. turn her and then reevaluate her need for opioid analgesia.
   3. administer the medication as ordered.
   4. advise N.J. to cough and breathe deeply since you are unable to give her anything for pain until her respiratory rate is 20.
5. O.R., 55 years old, is hospitalized with an exacerbation of rheumatoid arthritis. She has a favorite television show she watches every afternoon. She reports feeling comfortable during this show and seldom requests pain medication when she is watching it. The nurse's assessment of this phenomenon is that:
   1. the assessment of pain that prompted hospitalization is inaccurate.
   2. O.R. is bored and the boredom usually makes her pain seem worse.
   3. inactivity is the best approach to O.R.'s pain.
   4. distraction is an effective modifier of the pain experience for O.R.
6. Which of the following Joint Commission pain management standards apply to the bedside nurse? (Select all that apply.)
   1. Identify symptoms of pain in the client.
   2. Understand the institutional standards of pain management.
   3. Assess factors impacting the pain experience.
   4. Order the appropriate pain medication for the client.
   5. Implement pain management techniques.
   6. Evaluate the effectiveness of pain management techniques.
7. The client's family expresses concern that the client could overdose with a PCA. The most appropriate response by the nurse is:
   1. "Overdose is not possible with PCA."
   2. "The client receives extensive teaching prior to PCA use, which should prevent overdose."
   3. "The client can stop drug administration but not initiate it, so it is unlikely he will get too much medication."
   4. "The PCA pump is programmed with specific dose limits, reducing the chances of overmedication."
8. A client with terminal cancer is receiving morphine via PCA. The client is grimacing and moaning occasionally but sleeping for short intervals. Respiratory rate is 20, heart rate is 100, and blood pressure is 140/90. What is the most accurate assessment of this client's pain?
   1. The client is able to sleep, so the pain is manageable.
   2. The client is exhibiting respiratory depression and should not receive more medication.
   3. The client may need additional pain medication or an increase in dosage.
   4. The client can be assumed to be comfortable.

9. The nurse is providing preoperative teaching to a client who will most likely receive PCA after surgery. The nurse tells the client that the primary reason for utilizing PCA is that it:
   1. is cost effective.
   2. results in use of less medication.
   3. is convenient for nursing staff.
   4. allows the client control of pain relief.

10. Which factor is most important when determining whether PCA should be used for a client's pain management?
    1. The client's developmental and cognitive abilities.
    2. The client's weight.
    3. The length of the surgical procedure.
    4. The preferences of the surgeon.

REFERENCES/SUGGESTED READING

Acello, B. (2000a). Facing fears about opioid addiction. *Nursing2000, 30*(5), 72.

Acello, B. (2000b). Meeting JCAHO standards for pain control. *Nursing2000, 30*(3), 52–54.

Adler, P., Good, M., Roberts, B., & Snyder, S. (2000). The effects of tai chi on older adults with chronic arthritis pain. *Journal of Nursing Scholarship, 32*(4), 377.

Agency for Health Care Policy and Research. (1992). *Clinical practice guideline: Acute pain management: Operative or medical procedures and trauma* (AHCPR Publication No. 92-0032). Rockville, MD: U.S. Department of Health and Human Services.

Agency for Health Care Policy and Research. (1994). *Clinical practice guideline: Management of cancer pain* (AHCPR Publication No. 94-0592). Rockville, MD: U.S. Department of Health and Human Services.

Agency for Healthcare Research and Quality. (2007). Clinical practice guidelines: Major recommendations. Rockville, MD: Author. Available: http://wwwguideline.gov/summary/summary.aspx?doc_id=3748&nbr=002974&string=p

American Pain Society. (1999). *Principles of analgesic use in the treatment of acute pain and cancer pain* (4th ed.). Glenview, IL: Author.

American Pain Society. (2006). Pain: Current understanding of assessment, management, and treatments. Retrieved July 25, 2006, from http://www.ampainsoc.org/ce/downloads/npc/npc.pdf

American Pain Foundation. (2007). *Pain facts and figures.* Retrieved March 28, 2008, from http://www.painfoundatoin.org/page.asp?file=Newsroom/PainReference.htm.

AVANCEN, LLC. (2008). *A physician introduction to the MOD an oral PCA device for your patients.* Retrieved December 16, 2008, from http://www.avancen.com/news_files/Physician_Information_Flyer.pdf

Beecher, H. (1956). Relationship of significance of wound to pain experienced. *Journal of the American Medical Association, 161,* 1609–1613.

Brand, P., & Yancey, P. (1993). *Pain: The gift nobody wants.* New York: HarperCollins.

Brown, J., Horn, J., Calbert, J., & Nolan-Goslin, K. (1999). A question of pain. *Nursing99, 29*(10), 48–51.

Bulechek, G., Butcher, H., McCloskey, J., & Dochterman, J., eds. (2008). *Nursing Interventions Classification (NIC)* (5th ed.). St. Louis, MO: Mosby/Elsevier.

Chapman, G. (1999). Documenting a pain assessment. *Nursing99, 29*(11), 25.

Choiniere, M. (2001). Burn pain: A unique challenge. *Pain: Clinical Updates, 9*(1). Retrieved January 1, 2009, from http://www.iasp-pain.org/AM/AMTemplate.cfm?Section=Home&CONTENTID=7606&TEMPLATE=/CM/ContentDisplay.cfm

Cleeland, C., & Syrjala, K. (1992). How to assess cancer pain. In D. Turk & R. Melzack (Eds.), *Pain assessment.* New York: Guilford Press.

Collins, P., Auclair, M., Butler, E., Hush, M., Bernstein, B., Aguirre, F., et al. (2000). Educating staff about pain management. *American Journal of Nursing, 100*(1), 59.

Compton, P. (1999). Managing a drug abuser's pain. *Nursing99, 29*(5), 26–28.

Controlling Pain. (2001). Taming pain with TENS. *Nursing2001, 31*(11), 84.

D'Arcy, Y. (2002). How to treat arthritis pain. *Nursing2002, 32*(7), 30–31.

Department of Health, NSW. (2005). Hot or cold packs application (GL2005_015). Retrieved January 30, 2008, from http://www.health.nsw.gov.au/policies/GL/2005/pdf/GL2005_015.pdf

Derby, S. (1999). Opioid conversion guidelines for managing adult cancer pain. *American Journal of Nursing, 99*(10), 62–65.

Dillard, J., & Hirschman, L. (2002). *The chronic pain solution: The comprehensive, step-by-step guide to choosing the best alternative and conventional medicine.* Philadelphia: Bantam Doubleday Dell.

Estes, M. (2010). *Health assessment and physical examination* (4th ed.). Clifton Park, NY: Delmar Cengage Learning.

Faries, J. (1998a). Easing your patient's postoperative pain. *Nursing98, 28*(6), 58–60.

Faries, J. (1998b). Making a smooth switch from IV analgesia. *Nursing98, 28*(7), 26.

Feinberg, S. (2000). Complex regional pain syndrome. *American Journal of Nursing, 100*(12), 23–24.

Flor, H. Birbaumer, N., & Sherman, R. (2000). Phantom limb pain. *Pain: Clinical Updates, 8*(3). Available: http://www.iasp-pain.org/AM/AMTemplate.cfm?Section=Home&TEMPLATE=/CM/ContentDisplay.cfm&CONTENTID=7591

Gordon, D., Dahl, J., Miaskowski, C., McCarberg, B., Todd, K., Paice, J., et al. (2005). American Pain Society recommendations for improving the quality of acute and cancer pain management. *Archives of Internal Medicine, 165,* 1574–1579.

Haddad, A. (2000). Ethics in action: Treating pain in substance abusers. *RN, 63*(1), 21–24.

Hockenberry-Eaton, M., Wilson, D., & Winkelstein, M. L. (2003). *Wong's nursing care of infants and children* (7th ed.). New York: Elsevier Science.

Integrative Pain Center of Arizona. (2003). New JCAHO pain care treatment standards. Retrieved July 20, 2008, from http://www.ipcaz.org/pages/new.html

International Association for the Study of Pain. (2008). IASP pain terminology. Retrieved December 30, 2008, from http://www.iasp-pain.org/AM/Template.cfm?Section=Pain_Definitions&Template=/CM/HTMLDisplay.cfm&ContentID=1728

Joint Commission. (2009). Setting the standard: The Joint Commission and health care safety and quality. Retrieved July 9, 2009, from http://www.jointcommission.org/NR/rdonlyres/6C33FEDB-BB50-4CEE-950B-A6246DA4911E/0/setting_the_standard.pdf

Kedziera, P. (1998). The two faces of pain. *RN, 61*(2), 45–46.

Loeb, J. (1999). Pain management in long-term care. *American Journal of Nursing, 99*(2), 48–52.
Lehne, R. (2004). *Pharmacology for nursing care* (5th ed.). St. Louis, MO: Saunders.
Mattson, J. (2000). The language of pain. *Reflections on Nursing LEADERSHIP, 26*(4), 10–14.
Mayer, D., Torma, L., Byoch, I., & Norris, K. (2001). Speaking the language of pain. *American Journal of Nursing, 101*(2), 44–49.
McCaffery, M. (1979). *Nursing management of the patient with pain* (2nd ed.). Philadelphia: Lippincott Williams & Wilkins.
McCaffery, M. (1999a). Pain control. *American Journal of Nursing, 99*(8), 18.
McCaffery, M. (1999b). Understanding your patient's pain tolerance. *Nursing99, 29*(12), 17.
McCaffery, M. (2001). Using the 0-to-1 pain rating scale. *American Journal of Nursing, 101*(10), 81–82.
McCaffery, M. (2002). Choosing a faces pain scale. *Nursing2002, 32*(5), 68.
McCaffery, M. (2003). Switching from IV to PO: Maintaining pain relief in the transition. *American Journal of Nursing, 103*(5), 62–63.
McCaffery, M. & Ferrell, B. (1999). Opioids and pain management. *Nursing 99, 29*(3), 48–52.
McCaffery, M., & Pasero, C. (1999). *Pain: Clinical manual* (2nd ed.). St. Louis, MO: Mosby.
McCaffery, M., & Robinson, E. (2002). Your patient is in pain: Here's how you respond. *Nursing2002, 32*(10), 36–45.
Melzack, R., & Wall, P. (1965). Pain mechanisms: A new theory. *Science, 150,* 971–979.
Merskey, J., & Bogduk, N. (Eds.). (1994). *Classification of chronic pain* (2nd ed.)., WA: IASP.
Moorhead, S., Johnson, M., Maas, M., & Swanson, E. (2007). *Nursing Outcomes Classification (NOC)* (4th ed). St. Louis, MO: Elsevier, Health Sciences Division.
Morris, D. (2001). Ethnicity and pain. *Pain: Clinical Updates.* Retrieved January 1, 2009, from http://www.iasp-pain.org/AM/AMTemplate.cfm?Section=Home&CONTENTID=7617&TEMPLATE=/CM/ContentDisplay.cfm
Morrison, C. (2000). Fear of addiction: Balancing the facts and concerns about opioid use. *American Journal of Nursing, 100*(7), 81.
Mularski, R. White-Chu, F., Overbay, D., Miller, L., Asch, S. M., & Ganzini, L. (2006). Measuring pain as the 5th vital sign does not improve quality of pain management. *Journal of General Internal Medicine, 21,* 607–612.
National Pain Foundation. (2009). Untying the knot. *National Pain Awareness.* Retrieved January 2, 20009, from http://www.nationalpainfoundation.org/NationalPainAwareness/QA_on_Pain.pdf
North American Nursing Diagnosis Association International. (2010). *NANDA-I nursing diagnoses: Definitions and classification 2009–2011.* Ames, IA: Wiley-Blackwell.
Nichols, R. (2003). Pain management in patients with addictive disease, *American Journal of Nursing, 103*(3), 87–90.
Office of Quality and Performance, U.S. Department of Veterans Affairs. (2008). *Management of postoperative pain—Annotation L: Did the intervention produce adequate and tolerable pain relief?* Retrieved December 15, 2008, from http://www.opq.med.va.gov/cpg/PAIN/pain_cpg/content/algann_1_anno.htm
Pace, J. (2002). Understanding nociceptive pain. *Nursing2002, 32*(3), 74–75.
Panke, J. (2002). Difficulties in managing pain at the end of life. *American Journal of Nursing, 102*(7), 26.
Pasero, C. (1999). Using superficial cooling for pain relief. *American Journal of Nursing, 99*(3), 48–52.
Pasero, C. (2000a). Continuous local anesthetics. *American Journal of Nursing, 100*(8), 22–23.
Pasero, C. (2000b). Oral patient-controlled analgesia. *American Journal of Nursing, 100*(3), 24.
Pasero, C., & McCaffery, M. (2000a). Reversing respiratory depression with naloxone. *American Journal of Nursing, 100*(2), 26.
Pasero, C., & McCaffery, M. (2000b). When patients can't report pain. *American Journal of Nursing, 100*(9), 22–23.
Pasero, C., & McCaffery, M. (2001). The patient's report of pain. *American Journal of Nursing, 101*(12), 73–74.
Pasero, C., & Montgomery, R. (2002). Intravenous fentanyl. *American Journal of Nursing, 102*(4), 73–76.
Perkins, E. (2002). Less morphine, or more? *RN, 65*(11), 51–54.
Portenoy, R., Payne, R., et al. (1999). Oral transmucosal fentanyl citrate (OTFC) for the treatment of breakthrough pain in cancer patients: A controlled dose titration study. *Pain, 79,* 303.
Poulain, P., Langlade, A., & Goldberg, J. (1997). Cancer pain management in the home. *Pain Clinical Updates, 5*(1). Available: http://www.iasp-pain.org/PCU97a.html
Rakel, B., & Frantz, R. (2003). Effectiveness of transcutaneous electrical nerve stimulation on postoperative pain with movement. *Journal of Pain.* 4, 455–464.
Reiff, P., & Niziolek, M. (2001). Troubleshooting TIPS for PCA. *RN, 64*(4), 33–37.
Rosati, J., Gallagher, M., Shook, B., Luwisch, E., Favis, G., Deveras, R., et al. (2007). Evaluation of an oral patient-controlled analgesia device for pain management in oncology inpatients. *Journal of Supportive Oncology, 5*(9), 443–448.
Scholz, M. (2000). Managing constipation that's opioid-induced. *RN, 63*(6), 103.
Slaughter, A., & Pasero, C. (2002). Unacceptable pain levels. *American Journal of Nursing, 102*(5), 75–76.
Smith-Stoner, M. (2003). How Buddhism influences pain control choices. *Nursing2003, 33*(4), 17.
Spratto, G., & Woods, A. (2009). *Delmar's nurses drug handbook.* Clifton Park, NY: Delmar Cengage Learning.
Strevy, S. (1998). Myths and facts about pain. *RN, 61*(2), 42–45.
Teeter, M., & Kemper, D. (2008a). *Assessing pain.* Manuscript submitted for publication.
Teeter, M., & Kemper, D. (2008b). *Caring for clients with pain.* Manuscript submitted for publication.
Thomas, M., & Lundeberg, T. (1996). Does acupuncture work? *Pain Clinical Updates, 4*(3). Available: http://www.iasp-pain. org/PCU96c.html.
Travell, J., & Simons, D. (1983, 1999). *Travell & Simon's myofascial pain and dysfunction: The trigger point manual* (2nd ed., Vols. 1 & 2). Baltimore: Lippincott Williams & Wilkins.
Twycross, R. et al. (1996). A survey of pain in patients with advanced cancer. *Journal of Pain Symptom Management, 12*(5), 273–282.
Vasudevan, S. (1993). *Pain: A four letter word you can live with.* Milwaukee, WI: Montgomery Media.
Victor, K. (2001). Properly assessing pain in the elderly. *RN, 64*(5), 45–49.
Wentz, J. (2003). Understanding neuropathic pain. *Nursing 2003, 33*(1), 22.
Wong, D. (2003). Topical local anesthetics. *American Journal of Nursing, 103*(6), 42–45.
World Health Organization. (1986). *Cancer pain relief.* Geneva: Author.
World Health Organization. (1990). *Cancer pain relief and palliative care* (World Health Organization Technical Report Series, 804). Geneva: Author.
World Health Organization. (2007). *New guide on palliative care services for people living with advanced cancer.* Retrieved December 16, 2008,

from http://www.who.int/mediacentre/news/notes/2007/np31/en

World Health Organization. (2008). *WHO's pain relief ladder.* Retrieved December 16, 2008, from http://www.who.int/cancer/palliative/painladder/en

Young, D., Mentes, J., & Titler, M. (1999). Acute pain management protocol. *Journal of Gerontological Nursing, 26*(5), 10.

RESOURCES

Agency for Healthcare Research and Quality (AHRQ), http://www.ahrq.gov

American Chronic Pain Association, http://www.theacpa.org

American Pain Society (APS), http://www.ampainsoc.org

American Society of Pain Management Nurses, http://www.aspmn.org

City of Hope, http://www.cityofhope.org

International Association for the Study of Pain (IASP), http://www.iasp-pain.org

Joint Commission, http://www.jointcommission.org

National Chronic Pain Outreach Association, http://www.medhelp.org

National Foundation for the Treatment of Pain, http://www.paincare.org

National Guidelines Clearinghouse, http://www.guideline.gov

National Headache Foundation, http://www.headaches.org

National Hospice and Palliative Care Organization, http://www.nhpco.org

National Pain Foundation, http://www.nationalpainfoundation.org

CHAPTER 28
Diagnostic Tests

MAKING THE CONNECTION

Refer to the following chapters to increase your understanding of diagnostic tests:

Basic Nursing
- ***Complementary/Alternative Therapies***
- ***Assessment***
- ***Safety/Hygiene***
- ***Standard Precautions and Isolation***

Basic Procedures
- ***Urine Collection—Closed Drainage System***
- ***Urine Collection—Clean Catch, Female/Male***

Intermediate Procedures
- ***Performing Urinary Catheterization: Female/Male***
- ***Performing a Skin Puncture***

Advanced Procedures
- ***Performing Venipuncture (Blood Drawing)***

LEARNING OBJECTIVES

Upon completion of this chapter, you should be able to:

- Define key terms.
- Discuss the care of the client before, during, and after diagnostic testing.
- Describe the methods of specimen collection.
- Describe common noninvasive and invasive diagnostic procedures.
- Demonstrate the nursing responsibilities for common diagnostic procedures.

KEY TERMS

agglutination
agglutinin
agglutinogen
analyte
aneurysm
angiography
antibody
antigen
arteriography
ascites
aspiration
bacteremia
barium
biopsy
central line
computed tomography
contrast medium
culture
cytology
electrocardiogram
electroencephalogram
electrolyte
endoscopy
enzyme
fluoroscopy
hematuria
invasive
ketone
lipoprotein
lumbar puncture
magnetic resonance imaging (MRI)
necrosis
noninvasive
occult blood
oliguria

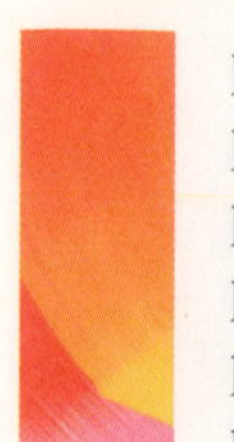

papanicolaou test
paracentesis
phlebotomist
pneumothorax
port-a-cath
procedural sedation
radiography
sensitivity
stable
stress test
thoracentesis
transducer
trocar
type and crossmatch
ultrasound
urobilinogen
venipuncture
void

INTRODUCTION

Information from a thorough history and physical examination determines the need for diagnostic testing. Results of diagnostic procedures are used to formulate a medical diagnosis and to plan a course of treatment. The challenge of cost-effective health care encourages practitioners to rely on basic assessment and to be selective about expensive diagnostic tests. The emphasis on cost containment has changed the nurse's role from doing for the client to teaching clients to do for themselves. The nurse teaches the client, family, and significant others about the diagnostic testing, how to prepare for the specific test(s), and the care required after the test. Although the primary focus is on teaching, the nurse may assist in performing various diagnostic tests. To deliver appropriate care to the client, nurses must know the implications of diagnostic tests and must know anatomy and physiology to understand the nature of diagnostic tests. Nurses can then relate diagnostic tests to specific disease processes and understand the test results.

This chapter discusses common diagnostic tests. The terms *test* and *procedure* are used interchangeably. The term *practitioner* is used to refer to either the physician or an advanced-practice registered nurse. Most state boards of nursing allow advanced-practice registered nurses to order and perform certain diagnostic tests.

DIAGNOSTIC TESTING

Diagnostic tests are either noninvasive or invasive. **Noninvasive** means that the body is not entered with any type of instrument; the skin and other body tissues, organs, and cavities remain intact. **Invasive** means that the body's tissues, organs, or cavities are accessed through some type of instrument.

Client Care

Diagnostic testing is a critical element of assessment. In collaboration with the client, assessment data are used to formulate nursing diagnoses, outcome measures, and a plan of care. Evaluation of the client's expected outcomes requires the incorporation of diagnostic findings.

SAFETY

Diagnostic Testing

To protect your health and safety, as well as that of other health care providers and the client, use Standard Precautions whenever performing invasive or noninvasive procedures.

Preparing the Client for Diagnostic Testing

The nurse plays a key role in scheduling and preparing the client for diagnostic testing. Tests not scheduled correctly inconvenience the client and delay interventions, which may place the client's health at risk. The institution is also at risk to lose money. Table 28-1 outlines a sample protocol of nursing care to prepare a client for diagnostic testing.

Ensure that the client is wearing an identification band and understands those things to be done. Also see that needed consent forms have been signed (Figure 28-1).

Nursing measures to ensure client safety are establish baseline vital signs, identify known allergies, and assess teaching effectiveness. In ambulatory and outpatient centers, there might be only one opportunity to assess and record vital signs. It is important to confirm that the vital signs are normal values for the client. Compare the vital signs taken during and after the procedure to those obtained before as baseline data to accurately assess the client's response to anesthetic agents and the procedure performed.

Advise the client of those things to expect during the procedure. Such teaching can both increase the level of cooperation and decrease the degree of anxiety. The client's family should also be informed of what will happen during the procedure and approximately how long the procedure should last. Know the facility's specific protocols and procedures because these are not standardized.

Care of the Client during Diagnostic Testing

Although client care must be individualized according to the specific procedure, general guidelines for client care during a procedure are outlined in Table 28-2. Protocols are used to assist with client care.

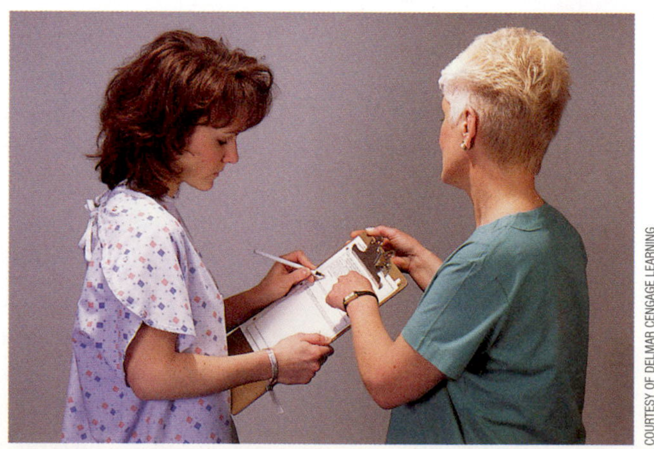

COURTESY OF DELMAR CENGAGE LEARNING

FIGURE 28-1 Preparing a Client for Diagnostic Testing

Table 28-1 Protocol: Preparing the Client for Diagnostic Testing

Purpose	To increase the reliability of the test by providing client teaching on the reason the test is being performed, those things the client can expect during the test, and the outcomes and side effects of the test To decrease the client's anxiety about the test and the associated risks
Supportive Data	Increase the client's knowledge, thereby promoting cooperation and enhancing the quality of the testing Decrease the time required to perform the tests, thereby increasing cost effectiveness Prevent delays by ensuring proper physical preparation
Assessment	Ensure that the client is wearing an identification band Review the medical record for allergies and previous adverse reactions to dyes and other contrast media; a signed consent form; and the recorded findings of diagnostic tests relative to the procedure Assess for the presence, location, and characteristics of physical and communicative limitations or preexisting conditions Monitor the client's knowledge of the reasons for the test and things to expect during and after testing Monitor vital signs, including pain, of the client scheduled for invasive testing, to establish baseline data Assess client outcome measures relative to the practitioner's preferences for preprocedure preparations Monitor level of hydration and weakness for clients who are designated nothing by mouth (NPO)
Report to Practitioner	Notify practitioner of allergy, previous adverse reaction, or suspected adverse reaction following the administration of drugs Notify practitioner of any client or family concerns not alleviated by discussions with nurse
Interventions	Clarify with practitioner whether regularly scheduled medications are to be administered Implement NPO status, as determined by the type of test Administer cathartics or laxatives as noted on the test's protocol; instruct clients who are weak to call for assistance to the bathroom Teach relaxation techniques, such as deep breathing and imagery Establish intravenous (IV) access if necessary for the procedure
Evaluation	Evaluate the client's knowledge of those things to expect Evaluate the client's anxiety level Evaluate the client's level of safety and comfort

Client Teaching	Discuss the following with the client and family, as appropriate to the specific test:
	• The reason for the test and those things to expect
	• An estimate of how long the test will take
	• Specifics of NPO status, including amount of water to drink if oral medication is to be taken
	• Cathartics or laxative: amount, frequency
	• Sputum: cough deeply, do not clear throat
	• Urine: voided, clean-catch specimen; timing of collection
	• Removal of objects (e.g., jewelry or hair clips) that will obscure x-ray film
	• Contrast medium:
	    • Barium: taste, consistency, after-effects (lightly colored stools for 24 to 72 hours; possibly, obstruction/impaction)
	    • Iodine: metallic taste, delayed allergic reaction (itching, rashes, hives, wheezing and breathing difficulties)
	• Positioning during the test
	• Positioning posttest (e.g., immobilize limb after angiography)
	• Posttest (encourage fluid intake if not contraindicated)

Documentation	Record in the client's medical record: • Practitioner notification of allergies or suspected adverse reaction to contrast media • Presence, location, and characteristics of symptoms • Teaching and the client's response to teaching • Responses to interventions (client outcomes)

COURTESY OF DELMAR CENGAGE LEARNING

TABLE 28-2 Protocol: Care of the Client during Diagnostic Testing

Purpose	To increase cooperation and participation by allaying the client's anxiety To provide the maximum level of safety and comfort during a procedure
Supportive Data	Encourage relaxation of the muscles and thus facilitate instrumentation by increasing the client's participation and comfort Ensure efficient use of time during the test and reliable results from the test with proper client preparation
Assessment	Check the client's identification band to ensure the correct client Review the medical record for allergies Assess the client's reaction to the preprocedure sedatives administered prior to the induction of anesthesia during the procedure Assess airway maintenance and gag reflex, if a local anesthetic is sprayed into the client's throat Assess vital signs, including pain, throughout the procedure and compare to baseline data Assess the client's ability to maintain and tolerate the prescribed position Assess the client's comfort level (pain) to ensure the effectiveness of the anesthetic agent Assess for related symptoms indicating complications specific to the procedure (e.g., accidental perforation of an organ)
Report to Practitioner	Notify the practitioner of any client concerns or questions not answered in discussions with the nurse Notify the practitioner of any family members present and their location during the procedure Notify the practitioner when the client is positioned properly and the anesthetic agent has been administered to the client
Interventions	Institute Standard Precautions or appropriate aseptic technique for the specific test Report to all personnel involved in the test any known client allergies Place the client in the correct position, drape, and monitor to ensure that breathing is not compromised Remain with the client during induction and maintenance of anesthesia If the procedure requires the administration of a dye, ensure that the client is not allergic to the dye; if the client has not received the dye before, perform the skin allergy test according to the manufacturer's instructions that accompany the medication Monitor the client's airway and keep resuscitative equipment available Assist the client to relax during insertion of the instrument by telling the client to breathe through the mouth and to concentrate on relaxing the involved muscles Explain what the practitioner is doing so that the client knows what to expect Label and handle the specimen according to the type of materials obtained and the testing to be done Report to the practitioner any symptoms of complications Secure client transport from the diagnostic area Posttest in the diagnostic area: • Assist the client to a comfortable, safe position • Provide oral hygiene and water to clients who were designated NPO for the test, if they are alert and able to swallow • Remain with the client awaiting transport to another area
Evaluation	Evaluate the client's ventilatory status and tolerance to the procedure Evaluate the client's need for assistance Evaluate the client's understanding of what was performed during the procedure Evaluate the client's understanding of findings identified during the procedure Evaluate the client's knowledge of what to expect after the procedure
Client Teaching	Discuss the following with the client and family, as appropriate to the specific test: • Those things that occurred during the procedure • Questions and concerns of the client or family member • Those things to expect during the immediate recovery phase • Those things to report to the nurse during the immediate recovery phase

Table 28-2 Protocol: Care of the Client during Diagnostic Testing (Continued)

Documentation	Record in the client's medical record: • Person who performed the procedure • Reason for the procedure • Type of anesthestic, dye, or other medications administered • Type of specimen obtained and where it was sent • Vital signs and other assessment data such as client's tolerance of the procedure or pain/discomfort level • Any symptoms of complications • Person who transported the client to another area (designate the names of persons who provided transport and the destination)

COURTESY OF DELMAR CENGAGE LEARNING

Standard Precautions are used when possible exposure to body fluids may occur. Protective barriers, such as gown, gloves, and goggles, should be used during invasive procedures.

Label all specimens with the client's name and room number (for hospitalized clients) and the date, time, and specimen source. Some specimens may need to be taken immediately to the laboratory or placed on ice (e.g., arterial blood gases [ABGs]).

Ongoing assessment of the client is required during any procedure. The patency of the client's airway should be continuously assessed because it may be compromised by the client's position, by anesthesia, or by the procedure itself. During an invasive procedure, monitor for signs and symptoms of accidental perforation of an organ (e.g., sudden changes in vital signs).

The nurse has the following additional responsibilities:

- Prepare the procedure room (e.g., ensure adequate lighting)
- Gather and charge for supplies to be used during the procedure
- Test the equipment to ensure it is functional and safe
- Secure proper containers for specimen collection

Practitioners usually have preference cards within the diagnostic testing area that specify the type of equipment to be used, the position in which to place the client, and the type of sedative or anesthetic agent to be used.

Some diagnostic tests are performed with the RN administering IV sedation, also called procedural sedation. **Procedural sedation** is a minimally depressed level of consciousness during which the client retains the ability to maintain a continuously patent airway and respond appropriately to physical stimulation or verbal commands. The nurse managing procedural sedation functions in an expanded role that requires additional education and demonstrated ability beyond the basic education.

Care of the Client after Diagnostic Testing

Postprocedure nursing care is directed toward restoring the client's prediagnostic level of functioning (Table 28-3). Nursing assessment and interventions are based mainly on the nature of the test and whether the client received anesthesia.

The client is closely monitored for signs of respiratory distress and bleeding. Some diagnostic tests require vital signs measurement every 15 minutes for the first hour and then at gradually longer intervals until the client is **stable** (alert and with vital signs within the client's normal range).

Some diagnostic tests use medications that are excreted through the kidneys. The client's intake and output (I&O) is monitored for 24 hours. The client is taught to monitor I&O and to report **hematuria** (presence of blood in the urine).

Clients should receive written instructions when discharged after diagnostic testing. Most agencies have discharge forms on which teaching regarding medications, dietary and activity restrictions, and signs and symptoms to be reported immediately to the practitioner are documented.

LABORATORY TESTS

Common laboratory studies are usually simple measurements to determine the amount or number of **analytes** (i.e., measured substances) present in a specimen. Laboratory tests are ordered by the practitioner to:

- Detect and quantify future disease risk
- Establish or exclude diagnoses
- Assess the disease process severity and formulate a prognosis
- Guide intervention selection
- Monitor the progress of the disorder
- Monitor treatment effectiveness

Specimen Collection

The scheduling and sequencing of laboratory tests are important. All tests requiring **venipuncture** (the use of a needle to puncture a vein to aspirate blood) should be grouped together so the client has only one venipuncture. Fasting laboratory

SAFETY

Radioactive Iodine and Urine Collection

Clients receiving radioactive iodine must have their urine collected and properly discarded in a special container, according to agency policy for handling radioactive medical wastes.

and radiological studies should be scheduled on the same day so that the client is only required to fast for 1 day. The client's comfort level and satisfaction increases with appropriate scheduling.

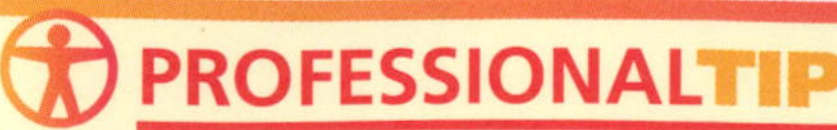

Documentation of Specimen-Collection Difficulties

Document on the laboratory requisition slip and in the nurses' notes any difficulty experienced during collection. Such problems may indicate adverse effects related to the nature of the test and thus must be reported and treated immediately.

Accuracy in laboratory testing requires that:

- The correct requisition form is used
- All requested information is written on the form (e.g., the client's full name and medical number)
- Pertinent data that could influence the test's results, such as medications taken, is included
- Specimen collection from the correct client is confirmed by checking the identification band
- Laboratory results are placed in the correct medical record

VENIPUNCTURE

Various members of the health care team can perform venipuncture. Although laboratories employ **phlebotomists** (individuals who perform venipuncture) to collect blood specimens, nurses must know how to perform venipuncture,

TABLE 28-3 Protocol: Care of the Client after Diagnostic Testing

Purpose	To restore the client's prediagnostic level of functioning by providing care and teaching relative to both those things the client can expect after a test and the outcomes or side effects of the test
Supportive Data	Decrease client anxiety by increasing the client's participation and knowledge of expected outcome measures after a diagnostic test Through proper postprocedure care and client teaching, alert the client to those signs and symptoms that must be reported to the practitioner
Assessment	Check the identification band and call the client by name Assess the client closely for signs of airway distress, adverse reactions to anesthetic or other medications, and other signs that may indicate accidental perforation of an organ Assess for bleeding in those areas where a biopsy was performed Assess the client's vital signs, including pain Assess vascular access lines or other invasive monitoring devices Assess the client's ability to expel air, if air was instilled during a gastrointestinal test Assess the client's knowledge of those things to expect during the recovery phase
Report to Practitioner	Notify the practitioner of any signs of respiratory distress, bleeding, or changes in vital signs; adverse reactions to anesthetic, sedative, or dye; and other signs of complications Notify the practitioner of client or family concerns or questions not answered in discussions with the nurse Notify the practitioner when any results are obtained from the diagnostic test Notify the practitioner when the client is fully alert and recovered (for an order to discharge)
Interventions	Implement the practitioner's orders regarding the postprocedure care of the client Institute Standard Precautions or surgical asepsis as appropriate to the client's care needs Position the client for comfort and accessibility so as to facilitate performance of nursing measures Monitor vital signs according to the frequency required for the specific test Observe the insertion site for hematoma or blood loss; replace pressure dressing, as needed Monitor the client's urinary output and drainage from other devices Enforce activity restrictions appropriate to the test Schedule client appointments as directed by the practitioner
Evaluation	Evaluate the client's respiratory status, especially if an anesthetic agent was used Evaluate the client's tolerance of oral liquids Evaluate the client's understanding of the procedural findings of when the practitioner expects to receive written results Evaluate the client's knowledge of those things to expect after discharge

Table 28-3 Protocol: Care of the Client after Diagnostic Testing (Continued)

Client Teaching	Based on client assessment and evaluation of knowledge, teach the client or family about the following: • Dietary or activity restrictions • Signs and symptoms that should be reported immediately to the practitioner • Medications
Documentation	Record in the client's medical record on the appropriate forms: • Assessment data, nursing interventions, and achievement of expected outcomes • Client or family teaching and demonstrated level of understanding • Written instructions given to the client or family members

COURTESY OF DELMAR CENGAGE LEARNING

because they routinely perform venipuncture in hospital critical care units, the home, and long-term care settings.

Venipuncture can be performed by using either a sterile needle and syringe or a vacuum tube holder with a sterile two-ended needle. Test tubes with different colored stoppers are used to collect blood specimens. The stoppers indicate the type of additive in the test tube. The tubes are universally color coded as follows:

- Red: no additive
- Lavender: ethylenediaminetetraacetic acid (EDTA)
- Light blue: sodium citrate
- Green: sodium heparin
- Gray: potassium oxalate
- Black: sodium oxalate

Arterial Puncture

Arterial blood gases reveal the lung's ability to exchange gases by measuring the partial pressures of oxygen (PaO_2) and carbon dioxide ($PaCO_2$) and evaluates the potential of hydrogen (pH) of arterial blood. Blood gases are ordered to evaluate:

- Oxygenation
- Ventilation and the effectiveness of respiratory therapy
- Acid–base balance in the blood

PROFESSIONALTIP

Arterial Blood Gases

To ensure an accurate determination of the client's actual blood gases, ABGs should not be drawn within 30 minutes after any respiratory treatment.

CLIENTTEACHING

Postarterial Puncture

The client should *immediately* notify the nurse if any pain or numbness occurs in the arm or leg after an arterial puncture. These symptoms indicate impaired circulation.

Arterial blood is drawn from a peripheral artery (e.g., radial or femoral) or from an arterial line. The blood is collected in a 5-mL heparinized syringe. The syringe is then rotated to mix the blood with the heparin to prevent clotting and then placed on ice.

In some agencies, it is within the scope of nursing practice to perform radial artery puncture, but femoral artery puncture is usually performed only by an advanced practitioner because of the associated increased risk of hemorrhage. It is not common practice for student nurses to draw ABG samples, but students often assist with the procedure and care for the client afterward.

The nurse is responsible for assessing the client for symptoms of postpuncture bleeding or occlusion. Apply direct pressure to the puncture site until all bleeding has stopped (a minimum of 5 minutes). Symptoms of impaired circulation include:

- Numbness and tingling
- Bluish color (cyanosis)
- Absence of a peripheral pulse

Capillary Puncture

When small quantities of capillary blood are needed for analysis or when the client has poor veins, a capillary puncture is performed. They are also used for blood glucose analysis. Figure 28-2 illustrates a capillary puncture of a fingertip.

Central Lines

A blood sample can also be collected from a **central line** (a venous catheter inserted into the superior vena cava through the subclavian or internal or external jugular vein). Central lines are used to treat fluid or electrolyte imbalances, such as severe dehydration caused by vomiting. Central lines are inserted when a peripheral route cannot be obtained, can be used for treatment, and to withdraw blood for analysis.

PROFESSIONALTIP

Common Sites for Capillary Puncture

- Inner aspect of a palmar fingertip is the most commonly used site.
- Earlobe is used when the client is in shock or the extremities are edematous.

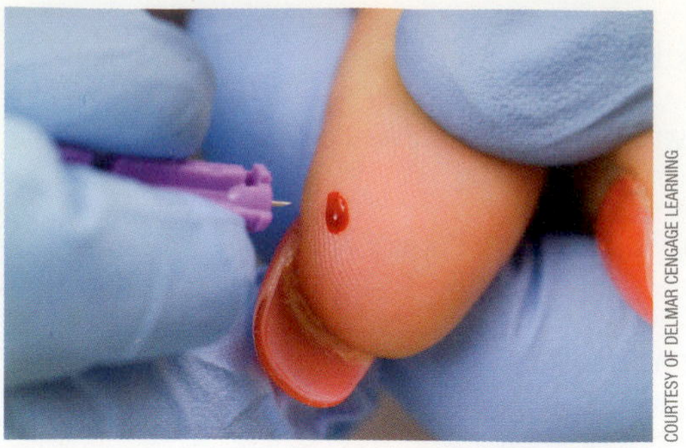
COURTESY OF DELMAR CENGAGE LEARNING

FIGURE 28-2 Capillary Puncture of Fingertip

The first blood sample drawn from a central line cannot be used for diagnostic testing. It must be discarded, with the volume of discard being the same as the dead space (catheter size). Agency protocol should specify the volume to discard relative to the type and size of catheter.

Central line care requires strict sterile technique. The practitioner must write an order for a blood sample to be obtained from a central line.

Peripherally inserted central catheters (PICC) are inserted into one of the major veins in the anticubital fossa or upper extremity and terminate in the superior vena cava. Blood samples can be collected from a PICC line. LPNs are required to successfully complete IV training to manage central lines and PICC lines. LPN nursing care of central lines varies from state to state. LPNs should know and follow the standards of practice for the state of clinical practice.

Implanted Port

Some clients have a **port-a-cath** (a port that has been implanted under the skin) over the third or fourth rib. The port's catheter is inserted into the superior vena cava or right atrium through the subclavian or internal jugular vein.

COMMUNITY/HOME HEALTH CARE

Urine Collection in the Home

Clients in the home should place the urine container in a reclosable ("zipper") plastic bag and refrigerate until delivering to a laboratory. Doing so prevents bacteria growth and promotes accuracy of results.

COMMUNITY/HOME HEALTH CARE

Central Line

Clients receiving prolonged therapy in the home environment usually have a central line in place. Because one of the primary complications of central venous catheter insertion is infection, the nurse must be alert for signs of infection (e.g., fever).

SAFETY

Standard Precautions and Urine Collection

All urine collection requires the use of Standard Precautions to prevent transmission of microorganisms among nurses, clients, and other health care providers. All specimen containers should be sealed in a biohazard bag prior to transport to the laboratory.

This implanted port is used for the same purpose as a central line. Using strict sterile technique, blood can be withdrawn for analysis by accessing the port. This should be performed only by a nurse who has the education to properly do so.

Urine Collection

Urine can be collected for various studies. The type of testing determines the method of collection. The different methods of urine collection are as follows:

- Random collection (routine analysis)
- Timed collection (24-hour urine)
- Collection from a closed urinary drainage system
- Sterile specimen (catheterized)
- Clean-voided specimen

The client's age and the method of collection determine client teaching. The collection method should be written on the laboratory requisition.

Random Collection The practitioner writes the order for a UA (routine urine analysis), also called a random collection. The specimen can be collected at any time using a clean, not sterile, cup. The specimen should be taken immediately to the laboratory to prevent bacterial growth and changes in the urine's analytes.

Timed Collection Timed collection is done over a 24-hour period. The urine is collected in a plastic gallon container that contains preservative(s), some of which are caustic.

For a timed collection, the client is told to **void** (eliminate urine) and discard the specimen at the beginning of the collection. Timing for a 24-hour urine collection begins after the first voiding has been discarded. For example, if the client voids at 1000 hours (24-hour [military] time), that urine should be discarded, but all urine is saved until 1000 hours the following day, when the last urine is saved. The client can void into a clean container and pour the urine into the collection bottle. Toilet tissue should not be dropped into the container used to catch the urine. The collection container should be refrigerated or kept on ice the entire 24 hours to stabilize the analytes and retard bacterial growth.

Collection from a Closed-Drainage System A sterile specimen can be collected from a client with an indwelling Foley catheter and closed-drainage system. A sterile specimen is used for urine culture. The urine specimen should *not* be obtained from the drainage bag because the analytes in the urine drainage bag change, leading to inaccurate results, and bacteria grows quickly in the drainage bag. The closed-drainage tubing has an aspiration port for sterile specimen collection.

Sterile Specimen When a sterile urine specimen is required and the client does not have an indwelling catheter and closed-drainage system, the client is catheterized. A small amount of urine is allowed to run out of the catheter into a basin, then the urine is allowed to flow into a sterile specimen bottle.

Clean-Voided Specimen Clean-voided (clean-catch, or midstream) specimen collection is done to have a specimen uncontaminated by skin flora. The collection technique is different for women and men. The female client is instructed to cleanse from the front to the back and then void into the specimen bottle; the male client is instructed to cleanse from the tip of the penis downward and then void into the specimen bottle.

Stool Collection

The reason for collecting a stool specimen should be explained to the client. The client is then instructed to defecate into a clean bedpan or container and discard used tissue in the toilet. Stools can be collected one time or over 24, 48, or 72 hours. Stools to be collected over a prolonged period must be placed into a container and refrigerated. Once all stools have been collected, the container should be labeled with the client's name, the date and time, and the test to be performed. All stool specimens are placed in a biohazard bag before being transported to the laboratory.

Blood Tests

Many tests can be performed on the blood. Tests specific to the hematologic system are described in Table 28-4.

Type and Crossmatch

A **type and crossmatch** identifies the client's blood type and determines compatibility of blood between a potential donor and recipient (client). There are four basic blood types: A, B, AB, and O. The blood types are determined by the presence or absence of A or B antigens. **Antigens** are substances, usually proteins, that cause the formation of and react specifically with antibodies. **Antibodies** are immunoglobulins produced by the body in response to bacteria, viruses, or other antigenic substances. Type A and type B are antigens that are classified as **agglutinogens**, or substances that cause agglutination (clumping of RBCs). Agglutinins are specific kinds of antibodies whose interaction with antigens manifests as agglutination.

SAFETY

Collecting Stool from a Client with Hepatitis

Write on the requisition form that the client has hepatitis. Doing so alerts laboratory personnel to be especially careful when handling the specimen.

CRITICAL THINKING

Type and Rh

If a client's blood type is AB positive, what are the possible blood types of the client's parents? Can the client receive Rh-negative blood? Explain your answer.

Blood types are also identified as positive or negative, depending on the presence or absence of the Rh factor. The Rh factor is an antigen that may be found on the RBC. The designation *Rh positive* means the antigen is present; *Rh negative* means the antigen is absent. An individual's blood type and Rh are determined genetically.

Crossmatch identifies the compatibility of the donor's blood with that of the recipient. A sample of the recipient's blood is mixed with the blood of a possible donor in the laboratory. If the mixed sample does not agglutinate, it is compatible.

Blood Chemistry

Blood chemistry tests are often grouped together, requiring one requisition and one venous specimen. Tests performed include glucose, electrolytes, enzymes, lipids, creatinine, and protein values. Other tests that may be performed on a blood specimen are listed in Table 28-5.

Blood Glucose Blood for measuring glucose is obtained by either skin puncture or venipuncture and is either fasting (FBS) or nonfasting (usually 2 hours postprandial) blood sugar. If the results of this screening test for diabetes mellitus are abnormal, the practitioner may order a glucose tolerance test, the most accurate test for diagnosing hypoglycemia and hyperglycemia (diabetes mellitus).

Serum Electrolytes An **electrolyte** is a substance that, when in solution, separates into ions and conducts electricity. Some electrolytes act on the cell membrane to allow the transmission of electrochemical impulses in nerve and muscle fibers, whereas others determine the activity of cellular metabolism (Guyton & Hall, 2000).

Cations are ions that have a positive charge, such as sodium (Na^+), potassium (K^+), calcium (Ca^{++}), and magnesium (Mg^{++}). Anions are ions that have a negative charge, including chloride (Cl^-), bicarbonate (HCO_3^-), and phosphate (HPO_4^{--}).

Blood Enzymes Enzymes are globular proteins produced in the body that catalyze chemical reactions within the cells. Enzyme tests are key to diagnosing tissue damage, mainly to the myocardium and, to a lesser degree, to the brain.

Plasma levels of intracellular enzymes elevate in the presence of myocardial **necrosis** (tissue death as the result of disease or injury). Enzymes in the blood are directly proportional to the degree of cellular damage. The enzymes are not used alone in determining a diagnosis but, rather, are reviewed with other diagnostic studies.

Blood Lipids An elevated serum lipid level is one of the controllable contributing risk factors to congestive heart disease (CHD). **Lipoproteins** (blood lipids bound to protein) are measured along with cholesterol.

Text continues on page 626

TABLE 28-4 Tests Specific to the Hematologic System

TEST	EXPLANATION/NORMAL VALUES	NURSING RESPONSIBILITIES
Red blood cells (RBCs)	Number of RBCs per mm^3 of blood. May be low in clients with rheumatoid arthritis. Clients living in high altitudes may have an elevated RBC level. Normal: Male: 4.6–6.2 million/mm^3 Female: 4.2–5.5 million/mm^3	The client is not required to fast for the test.
White blood cells (WBCs)	Number of WBCs per mm^3 of blood. Elevation is associated with infectious processes. Normal: 4,100–10,800 mm^3	The client is not required to fast for the test. Exercise, stress, last month of pregnancy, labor, previous splenectomy, and eating may increase level and alter differential values. Note medications taken that may affect test; aspirin, heparin, and steroids may increase WBC level, whereas antibiotics and diuretics may decrease WBC level.
Differential count	Percentage of types of WBCs in 1 mm of blood.	The client is not required to fast for the test.
Neutrophilis	Increase in bacterial infections and trauma. Normal:	
Segs (mature neutrophils)	Segs: 50%–65%	
Bands (immature neutrophils)	Bands: 0%–5%	
Eosinophils	Increased in allergic reactions or parasitic infestation. Normal: 1%–3%	Corticosteroid therapy causes a decreased level.
Basophils	Increased in allergic reactions and during healing periods. Normal: 0.4%–1.0%	Steroids cause a decreased level.
Lymphocytes	Increased in viral infections and other diseases, such as pertussis and tuberculosis (TB). Decreased in acquired immunodeficiency syndrome (AIDS). Normal: 25%–35%	Steroids cause a decreased level.
Monocytes	Increased in chronic diseases, such as malaria, TB, Rocky Mountain spotted fever. May be low in clients with rheumatoid arthritis. Normal: 4%–6%	
Hemoglobin (Hgb)	Measures the oxygen-carrying compound in RBCs. Normal: Male: 14–18 g/dL Female: 12–16 g/dL Critical value: <5 g/dL	The client is not required to fast for the test. Sample may be drawn from a finger of a child or the heel of an infant.
Hemoglobin electrophoresis	Detects abnormal forms of hemoglobin. Performed after positive sickle cell test. If the hemoglobin electrophoresis is negative, the client has the sickle cell trait. If the hemoglobin electrophoresis is positive, the client has sickle cell anemia. Normal: Hgb S: 0% Hgb F: <2% Hgb Ca: 0%	If the client has had a blood transfusion within the last 12 weeks, the results of the test may be altered.

TABLE 28-4 Tests Specific to the Hematologic System (Continued)

TEST	EXPLANATION/NORMAL VALUES	NURSING RESPONSIBILITIES
Hematocrit (Hct)	Measures the percentage of blood cells in a volume of blood. Clients living in high altitudes may have an increased level. Normal: Male: 40%–54% Female: 38%–47% Critical value: <15% or >60%	The client is not required to fast for the test.
Platelet count	Measures the number of platelets per cubic milliliter of blood. Normal: 150,000–450,000/mm^3 Critical level: <50,000 and >1 million/mm^3	Instruct the client that strenuous exercise and oral contraceptives increase platelet level. Instruct the client that aspirin, acetaminophen, and sulfonamides decrease platelet level. If the client has a low platelet count, maintain digital pressure to the puncture site.
Bleeding time	Measures the length of time for a platelet plug to occlude a small puncture wound. Normal: 1–9 minutes (Ivy method) Critical value: >15 minutes	Notify the laboratory if the client is taking aspirin, anticoagulants, or other medications that may affect the clotting process.
Prothrombin time (PT, protime)	Measures the effectiveness of several blood-clotting factors. Normal: 10–13.4 seconds INR: 2.0–3.0 In the presence of anticoagulant therapy, the values should be 1½–2 times the normal value. Critical value: >20 seconds In the presence of anticoagulant therapy, the critical value should be >3 times the normal critical value.	Ensure that the blood specimen is drawn before the daily dose of warfarin (Coumadin) is administered. Instruct the client that alcohol intake may increase PT and that a diet high in fat may decrease PT. Note those medications taken that may affect results; salicylates, sulfonamides, and methyldopa (Aldomet), as these may increase PT, whereas digitalis and oral contraceptives decrease the level. Instruct the client not to take any medication without notifying the physician, as medications may affect the PT level.
International normalized ratio (INR)	Normal: 0.9–1.1 Clients on anticoagulant drugs should have an INR of 2–3 (2.5–3.5 for the client with a mechanical prosthetic heart valve). The INR is more accurate than PT in monitoring warfarin (Coumadin) therapy.	The daily warfarin (Coumadin) dose should be given after blood has been drawn for the INR.
Partial thromboplastin time (PTT), also called activated partial throboplastin time (APTT)	Normal: PTT: 60–70 sec APTT: 21–35 sec In the presence of anticoagulant therapy, the normal value is 1.5–2.5 times the control value. Critical value: APTT: >70 seconds PTT: >100 seconds	If the client is receiving intermittent heparin doses, schedule the APTT to be drawn 30–60 minutes before the next heparin dose. If heparin is given continuously, the blood specimen can be drawn at any time. If PTT is greater than 100 seconds, the client is at risk for bleeding, and the physician is notified. The antidote for heparin is protamine sulfate. Note whether the client is taking antihistamines, vitamin C, or salicylates, as these prolong PTT time.

(Continues)

Table 28-4 Tests Specific to the Hematologic System (Continued)

TEST	EXPLANATION/NORMAL VALUES	NURSING RESPONSIBILITIES
D dimer test (fragment D dimer, fibrin degradation fragment)	Measures a fibrin split product that is released when a clot breaks. Confirms the diagnosis of disseminated intravascular coagulation (DIC). Screens for deep vein thrombosis (DVT) and pulmonary emboli. Normal: <10 mg/mL	Note whether the client is on thrombolytic therapy, as the results of this test would be increased from negative to positive.

COURTESY OF DELMAR CENGAGE LEARNING

Table 28-5 Additional Tests Performed on Blood Specimen

TEST	EXPLANATION/NORMAL VALUES	NURSING RESPONSIBILITIES
Acid phosphatase	Acid phosphatase is an enzyme found in the prostate gland, seminal fluid, and RBCs. An elevated level is seen in clients with prostatic cancer and hemolytic anemias. If tumors are treated successfully, the level will decrease. A rising level may indicate a poor prognosis. Normal: 0–0.80 U/L	Tell the client that no food or drink restrictions are associated with this test. Apply pressure to the venipuncture site. Observe the site for bleeding. Used in rape investigations.
Adrenocorticotropic hormone (ACTH), corticotropin	Determines the function of the anterior pituitary. Because of diurnal variation, specimens should be drawn in both morning and evening. Normal: 4–22 pmol/L	Emotional or physical stress or recent radioisotope scans can interfere with test results. Drugs that may increase ACTH level include corticosteroids, estrogens, ethanol, and spironolactone. Explain the procedure to the client. This is especially important to decrease the client's stress level. Evaluate the client for increased stress level. Initiate NPO status 12 hours before test. The blood specimen must be drawn with a heparinized syringe, chilled by placing the specimen on ice, and immediately transported to the lab.
ACTH stimulation test, cortisol stimulation test, cosyntropin test	Monitors plasma cortisol level to indicate adrenal gland response to ACTH. Normal: 1 hour: ↑ 20 μg/dL at least above baseline	Note those medications taken that may affect results: cortisone, estrogens, hydrocortisone, and spironolactone may increase plasma cortisol level. Explain the procedure to the client. Initiate NPO status after midnight. For all tests, obtain baseline serum cortisol level. Administer injection of cosyntropin IM or IV. Draw blood specimen 30 to 60 minutes after injection.
Alanine aminotransferase (ALT, formerly serum glutamic pyruvic transaminase [SGPT])	ALT is an enzyme released in response to liver injury. Normal: varies with testing method	Note those medications taken that affect results: many medications may increase level, including antibiotics, narcotics, oral contraceptives, and many others.
Alkaline phosphatase (ALP)	Alkaline phosphatase is an enzyme found primarily in the liver, biliary tract, and bone. Detection is important for determining possible liver and bone disease. Normal: varies widely depending on method	Fasting may be required. Apply pressure to the venipuncture site. Observe the site for bleeding.

TABLE 28-5 Additional Tests Performed on Blood Specimen (Continued)

TEST	EXPLANATION/NORMAL VALUES	NURSING RESPONSIBILITIES
Alpha-fetoprotein (AFP)	Test for tumor marker; elevated in nonseminomatous testicular cancer. Performed between 16 and 18 weeks of pregnancy. A high level is suggestive of neural tube defects. Normal: 0.9 ng/mL 16–18 weeks gestation: 30–43 μg/mL	Apply pressure to site and watch for bleeding or hematoma. Sample must be drawn between 15–20 weeks of gestation.
Amylase (AMS)	Amylase is an enzyme secreted by the pancreas. Elevation indicates pancreatitis. Normal: 25–125 IU/L	Note those medications taken that affect test results; steroids, aspirin, alcohol, some narcotics, some diuretics, and other drugs may increase level, whereas citrate, glucose, and oxalates may decrease level.
Antidiuretic hormone (ADH), vasopressin	Determines the production of ADH by the posterior pituitary. Normal: <1.5 pg/L	Explain the procedure to the client. Note those medications taken that may interfere with test results. Drugs that elevate ADH level include acetaminophen, barbiturates, cholinergic agents, estrogen, nicotine, oral hypoglycemic agents, some diuretics such as thiazides, and tricyclic antidepressants. Drugs that decrease ADH level include alcohol, beta-adrenergic agents, morphine antagonists, and phenytoin (Dilantin). Client should fast for 12 hours before the test. Evaluate the client for high level of physical or emotional stress.
Antinuclear antibodies (ANAs)	ANAs attack cell nuclei. The result is positive in 95% of clients with systemic lupus erythematosus. Levels are low in clients with mononucleosis, rheumatic fever, and liver diseases. Normal: negative at 1:20 dilution	Fasting is not required. Hydralazine (Apresoline) and procainamide (Pronestyl) may increase level. A radioactive scan in the past week may alter results; inform the lab, if applicable.
Antistreptolysin O (ASO)	High titer indicates presence of *beta-hemolytic streptococcus*, which may cause rheumatic fever or acute glomerulonephritis. Upper limit of normal varies with age, season, and geographic area. Normal: Adult: <1:100 12–19 years: <1:200 2–5 years: <1:100	There are no food or fluid restrictions. Antibiotics decrease ASO level. Check urine output if ASO is elevated. Urine output of less than 600 mL/24 h is associated with acute glomerulonephritis.
Antithyroid microsomal antibody, antimicrosomal antibody, microsomal antibody, thyroid autoantibody, thyroid antimicrosomal antibody	Used to detect thyroid microsomal antibodies found in clients with Hashimoto's thyroiditis. Normal: titer <1:100	Explain the procedure to the client.

(*Continues*)

Table 28-5 Additional Tests Performed on Blood Specimen (Continued)

TEST	EXPLANATION/NORMAL VALUES	NURSING RESPONSIBILITIES
Aspartate aminotransferase (AST, formerly serum glutamic oxaloacetic transaminase [SGOT])	AST is an enzyme that indicates inflammation of heart, liver, skeletal muscle, pancreas, or kidneys. Normal: Male: 8–46 U/L Female: 7–31 U/L	Avoid intramuscular (IM) injections; record date and time of any injections. Avoid hemolysis. Withhold medications that affect results, for 12 hours if possible; several medications, such as antihypertensives, cholinergic agents, anticoagulants, digitalis, and others, may increase level, as may exercise.
Arterial blood gases (ABGs)	Direct measurement of the pH, PaO_2, and $PaCO_2$, and calculated measurement of HCO_3^- and SaO_2 from samples of arterial blood. pH = expresses the acidity or alkalinity of the blood. PaO_2 = partial pressure of oxygen in the blood. $PaCO_2$ = partial pressure of carbon dioxide in the blood. SaO_2 = arterial oxygen saturation. HCO_3^- = bicarbonate ion concentration in the blood. The oxygen content of the blood expressed as a percentage of the oxygen carrying capacity of the blood. Normal: / Critical level: pH: 7.35–7.45 / <7.2 or >7.6 PaO_2: 75–100 mm Hg / <40 mm Hg $PaCO_2$: 35–45 mm Hg / <20 or >70 HCO_3^-: 24–28 mEq / <10 or >40 SaO_2: >95% (at sea level) / <60%	Explain that an arterial sample of blood is required. Arterial punctures cause more discomfort than venous. Instruct the client not to move. Assess the adequacy of collateral circulation. The blood sample is drawn in a syringe containing heparin. After the specimen has been obtained, rotate the syringe to mix the blood and heparin. The blood sample is placed on ice and taken immediately to the lab. Apply pressure to the arterial site for 3 to 5 minutes or 15 minutes if client is on an anticoagulant. Assess site for bleeding.
Bilirubin	Measures bilirubin in the blood. Indicates how well the liver is functioning. Normal: Total: 0.1–1.3 mg/dL Direct: 0.0–0.3 mg/dL Indirect: 0.1–1.0 mg/dL	Note those medications taken that affect results; steroids, antibiotics, oral hypoglycemics, narcotics, as well as others may cause increased level, whereas barbiturates, caffeine, penicillins, and salicylates may cause decreased level. Fasting may be required. Do not shake the tube; protect the tube from light.
Blood glucose, fasting blood sugar (FBS)	Measures blood level of glucose (serum values). Results depend on method used by laboratory. Normal fasting glucose: 70–99 mg/dL (3.9–5.5 mmol/L) Impaired fasting glucose (prediabetes): 100–125 mg/dL (5.6–6.9 mmol/L) Diabetes: 126 mg/dL (7.0 mmol/L) and above on more than one testing occasion Critical values: >400 mg/dL <50 mg/dL	Client must fast (except for water) for 12 hours before test. Withhold insulin or oral antidiabetic medications until blood is drawn. Be certain client receives medications and meal after fasting specimen drawn. Cortisone, thiazide, and loop diuretics cause increase.

TABLE 28-5 Additional Tests Performed on Blood Specimen (Continued)

TEST	EXPLANATION/NORMAL VALUES	NURSING RESPONSIBILITIES
2 hour postprandial glucose (2h PPG) or 2 hour postprandial blood sugar (2h PPBS)	Measures blood glucose 2 hours after a meal. Normal: 70–140 mg/dL Diabetic: >140 mg/dL	Instruct the client to eat entire meal and then to not eat anything else until blood is drawn. Notify the laboratory of the time meal was completed.
Blood urea nitrogen (BUN)	Measures urea, end product of protein metabolism. Normal: 5–20 mg/dL	Initiate NPO status 8 hours prior to test, if possible. Note the client's hydration status. Note those medications taken that may affect results, including phenothiazines, nephrotoxic drugs, diuretics (hydrochlorothiazide [Hydro-Diuril], ethacrynic acid [Edecrin], furosemide [Lasix]); antibiotics (bacitracin, gentamicin, kanamycin, methicillin, neomycin); antihypertensives (methyldopa [Aldomet], guanethidine [Ismelin]), sulfonamides, propranolol, morphine, lithium, salicylates.
B-type natriuretic peptide (BNP)	Enables doctors to make the correct diagnosis of heart failure. Secreted from the ventricles of the heart in response to changes in pressure when heart failure develops and worsens. No heart failure: <100 pg/mL Suggests heart failure is present: 100–300 pg/mL Mild heart failure: >300 pg/mL Moderate heart failure: >600 pg/mL Severe heart failure: >900 pg/mL	Explain to client that a blood sample is needed. The test takes about 15 minutes.
CA-15-3	CA-15-3 (cancer antigen) is a tumor marker for monitoring breast cancer. Because benign breast or ovarian disease can also cause elevations, it has limited use in diagnosis. Normal: <22 U/mL	Fasting is not required. Apply pressure to the venipuncture site. Observe the site for bleeding.
CA-19-9	CA-19-9 (cancer antigen) is a tumor marker used primarily in the diagnosis of pancreatic carcinoma. Normal: <37 U/mL	Fasting is not required. Apply pressure to the venipuncture site. Observe the site for bleeding.
CA-125	CA-125 (cancer antigen) is a tumor marker especially helpful in making the diagnosis of ovarian cancer. Normal: 0–35 U/mL	Fasting is not required. Apply pressure to the venipuncture site. Observe the site for bleeding.
Calcitonin, HCT, thyrocalcitonin	Determines thyroid and parathyroid activity. Also used as a tumor marker to detect thyroid cancer and several other cancers. Normal: basal <151 pg/mL	Note those medications taken that may increase calcitonin level, including calcium, cholecystokinin, epinephrine, glucagon, pentagastrin, and oral contraceptives. Explain the procedure to the client. The client should fast 8 hours but may have water.

(*Continues*)

TABLE 28-5 Additional Tests Performed on Blood Specimen (Continued)

TEST	EXPLANATION/NORMAL VALUES	NURSING RESPONSIBILITIES
Carcinoembryonic antigen (CEA)	CEA is found in clients with cancer, especially colorectal cancer. It is especially useful in monitoring treatment response and is occasionally the first sign of tumor recurrence. Normal: <5 ng/mL Smoker <2.5 ng/mL Nonsmoker	Fasting is not required. Apply pressure to the venipuncture site. Observe the site for bleeding. Note whether the client smokes or has a disease that will alter results, such as hepatitis, cirrhosis, or colitis.
Cardiac enzymes Serum AST	Indicates possible tissue damage if elevated. Normal: Male: 7–21 U/L Female: 6–18 U/L	Neither fasting nor NPO status is necessary. Pattern of elevated levels of AST, CPK, and LDH is indicative of myocardial infarction (MI).
Creatine kinase CPK (CK)	Normal: Male: 55–170 U/L Female: 30–135 U/L	CPK is the first enzyme elevated after MI, and peaks within the first 24 hours.
CK isoenzymes	Present in skeletal muscle, brain, lungs, and heart muscle. Normal:	Elevation of an isoenzyme indicates damage to tissue in a specific organ; CK-MB is specific for myocardial cells. Level increases 3–6 hours following MI, peaks in 12–24 hours and returns to normal in 18–24 hours.
CK-MM (muscle)	100%	
CK-BB (brain)	0%	
CK-MB (heart)	0%	
Lactic dehydrogenase (LDH)	Normal: 45–90 U/L Critical level: 300–800 U/L following myocardial infarction	LDH_1 value greater than LDH_2 value is indicative of an acute MI. LDH_5 is elevated with congestive heart failure (CHF).
LDH isoenzymes		
LDH_1 (heart and erythrocytes)	*17.5%–28.3%	
LDH_2 (reticuloendothelial system)	*30.4%–36.4%	
LDH_3 (lungs and other tissues)	*18.8%–26.0%	
LDH_4 (kidney, placenta, pancreas)	*9.2%–16.5%	
LDH_5 (liver and striated muscles)	*5.3%–13.4%	
Cardiac troponin I and T	Proteins found in cardiac muscle. Protein is released when the muscle is injured or dead. Troponin I elevated level in 4–6 hours Normal: <1.5 ng/mL Troponin T elevated level in 4–6 hours Normal: <0.6 ng/mL	Explain to client that blood sample is needed. Test very expensive. Often used in the ED.

*% of total LDH

TABLE 28-5 Additional Tests Performed on Blood Specimen (Continued)

TEST	EXPLANATION/NORMAL VALUES	NURSING RESPONSIBILITIES
CD4 T-cell count	Predictor of HIV progression; baseline taken after positive HIV test. Normal: 500–1,000/mm^3 Critical value: <200/mm^3	Explain the meaning of the test. Provide follow-up explanation of test results.
Cholesterol (lipid profile)	Lipid necessary for steroid, bile, and cell membrane production. Normal: <200 mg/dL (total)	Have client fast 12–14 hours prior to test. No alcohol 24 hours prior to test. Diet intake 2 weeks prior to test will affect results. Note those medications taken that may affect results; steroids, phenytoin, diuretics, and others may elevate level, whereas MAO inhibitors, some antibiotics, lovastatin, and others may decrease level. If elevated, increased risk of coronary artery disease (CAD), hypertension, and MI.
High density lipoprotein (HDL)	Normal: 30–70 mg/dL	
Low density lipoprotein (LDL)	Normal: 60–160 mg/dL	
Very low density lipoprotein (VLDL)	Normal: 25%–50%	
Triglycerides	Normal: 40–150 mg/dL	Elevated level in CAD; level increases when LDL level increases.
Complement assay (total complement, C3 and C4)	Decreased levels in autoimmune diseases due to depletion of complement by antibody–antigen complexes. Normal: C3: Male: 80–180 mg/dL Female: 76–120 mg/dL C4: 15–45 mg/dL	Fasting is not required.
Coombs' test (direct antiglobulin test)	Detects whether immunoglobulins are attached to RBCs. Normal: negative	Note whether the client is taking ampicillin (Unasyn), captopril (Capoten), indomethacin (Indocin), or insulin, as these cause false-positive results.
Cortisol, hydrocortisone	Determines adrenal cortex function. There is normally a diurnal variation, with higher level around 6 to 8 A.M. and lowest levels around midnight. Normal: 8 A.M.: 6–28 μg/dL, or 170–625 nmol/L 4 P.M.: 2–12 μg/dL, or 80–413 nmol/L	Note whether the client has been under physical or emotional stress as either can artificially elevate plasma cortisol level. Likewise, recent use of radioisotopes can interfere with test results. Note those medications taken that may affect results. Drugs that may increase plasma cortisol level include estrogen, oral contraceptives, and spironolactone (Aldactone). Drugs that may decrease plasma cortisol level include androgens and phenytoin (Dilantin). Explain the procedure to the client. Two specimens are drawn—one at 8 A.M. and another at 4 P.M. Assess the client for physical or emotional stress and report to the physician. Indicate times of collection on laboratory requisitions.

(Continues)

TABLE 28-5 Additional Tests Performed on Blood Specimen (Continued)

TEST	EXPLANATION/NORMAL VALUES	NURSING RESPONSIBILITIES
C-reactive protein test (CRP)	An abnormal protein appears in the blood of clients with an acute inflammatory process. Used to monitor the progress of clients with autoimmune disorders such as rheumatoid arthritis. More sensitive than erythrocyte sedimentation rate (ESR). Normal: <6 mg/L	Fast, except for water, for 8 hours. Note those medications that may affect results: nonsteroidal antiinflammatory drugs (NSAIDs), steroids, and salicylates may decrease level; oral contraceptives and intrauterine devices (IUDs) may increase level. Inform laboratory, if applicable.
Culture	Identifies pathogens in blood. Normal: none	There are no food or fluid restrictions. Specimen should be taken immediately to the laboratory. All specimens should be collected prior to initiating antibiotic therapy.
Dexamethasone suppression test (DST), prolonged/rapid DST, cortisol suppression test (ACTH suppression test)	Monitors plasma cortisol level to measure adrenal gland function. Normal: <5 mg/dL	Stress can interfere with test results. Note those medications taken that may affect results, including barbiturates, estrogens, oral contraceptives, phenytoin (Dilantin), spironolactone, steroids, and tetracyclines. Explain the procedure to the client. Weigh the client for baseline weight. Rapid test: Administer dexamethasone 1 mg orally at 11 P.M. with milk or antacid. Administer sedative, if ordered. At 8 A.M., before client rises, draw plasma cortisol level. Overnight 8-mg dexamethasone suppression test: If no cortisol suppression occurs, repeat test using 8 mg dexamethasone. If there is still no cortisol suppression, a prolonged test over 6 days involving six 24-hour urine collections should be done.
Electrolytes	Determines blood electrolyte levels. First four are the most commonly measured.	Sodium and potassium are necessary for cardiac electrical conduction.
Sodium (Na^+)	Measures level of serum sodium. Function in the body: Major electrolyte in extracellular fluid, regulates fluid balance, stimulates conduction of nerve impulses, helps maintain neuromuscular activity. Normal: 135–145 mEq/L	There are no food or fluid restrictions.
Potassium (K^+)	Measures level of serum potassium. Function in the body: Major electrolyte in intracellular fluid, maintains normal nerve and muscle activity, assists in cellular metabolism of carbohydrates and proteins. Normal: 3.5–5.5 mEq/L	There are no food or fluid restrictions. If the client has hypokalemia or hyperkalemia, evaluate the client for cardiac dysrhythmias.

TABLE 28-5 Additional Tests Performed on Blood Specimen (Continued)

TEST	EXPLANATION/NORMAL VALUES	NURSING RESPONSIBILITIES
Electrolytes Continued		
Chloride (Cl^-)	Measures level of serum chloride Function in the body: Major electrolyte in extracellular fluid, functions in combination with sodium to maintain osmotic pressure, assists in maintaining acid–base balance. Normal: 100–110 mEq/L	There are no food or fluid restrictions.
Calcium, total/ionized Ca^{++}	Indicates parathyroid gland function and calcium metabolism. Because ionized calcium is unaffected by serum albumin, it can give more accurate results; however, most laboratories do not have the equipment to perform the test. Normal: Total: 8.5–10.5 mg/dL, or 2.25–2.75 nmol/L Ionized: 4.5–5.6 ng/dL, or 1.05–1.30 nmol/L	Note those medications taken that may affect results. Drugs that may increase serum calcium level include calcium salts, hydralazine, lithium, thiazide diuretics, parathyroid hormone (PTH), thyroid hormone, and vitamin D. Drugs that may decrease serum calcium level include acetazolamide, anticonvulsants, asparaginase, aspirin, calcitonin, cisplatin, corticosteroids, heparin, laxatives, loop diuretics, magnesium salts, and oral contraceptives. Vitamin D and excessive milk ingestion can also interfere with test results. Explain the procedure to the client. Fasting is not required for serum calcium, but might be required if other blood chemistry tests are to be drawn.
Magnesium (Mg^{++})	Measures level of serum magnesium Function in the body: Combines with calcium and phosphorous in intracellular bone tissue, essential for neuromuscular contraction, synthesis of protein, and body temperature regulation. Normal: 1.6–2.6 mEq/L	There are no food or fluid restrictions.
Phosphate (PO_4^{--})	Measures level of serum phosphate Function in the body: An essential intracellular electrolyte, exists in an inverse relationship with calcium. Normal: 3–4.5 mg/dL	Initiate NPO status after midnight. Intravenous fluids containing glucose are sometimes discontinued several hours before the test.
Bicarbonate (HCO_3^-) (total carbon dioxide content or carbon dioxide capacity)	Always in a 20:1 ratio with carbonic acid. Normal: venous 22–29 mEq/L arterial 21–28 mEq/L	There are no food or fluid restrictions. Loss of gastric contents is the most common reason for increased level.
ELISA	Screening test used to indicate the presence of HIV Normal: negative	Inform the client that if the first ELISA test is positive, a second ELISA will be drawn before confirmation is done with Western blot. Provide pretest counseling. Obtain informed consent. Provide or arrange for posttest counseling.

(*Continues*)

TABLE 28-5 Additional Tests Performed on Blood Specimen (Continued)

TEST	EXPLANATION/NORMAL VALUES	NURSING RESPONSIBILITIES
Erythrocyte sedimentation rate (ESR or sed rate test)	Measures, in mm, RBC descent in a normal saline solution after 1 hour. Level is increased in inflammatory, infectious, necrotic, or cancerous conditions, due to increased protein content in plasma. Used to monitor the course of therapy for clients with autoimmune diseases, such as rheumatoid arthritis. Normal: Male: 0–13 mm/h Female: 0–20 mm/h	The test should be performed within 3 hours after the blood is drawn. Menstruation or pregnancy may increase level. Ethanbutal, quinine, aspirin, cortisone, and prednisone may alter results.
Folic acid (Folate level)	Measures folic acid level in the blood. Normal: 5–20 ug/mL, or 14–34 mmol/L	Fasting is not required. Instruct the client not to drink any alcoholic beverages before the test. The test is drawn before folic acid medications are administered. Note whether the client is taking phenytoin (Dilantin), primidone (Mysoline), methotrexate, antimalarial agents, or oral contraceptives, as these cause decreased level.
Follicle-stimulating hormone (FSH)	Determines anterior pituitary function. Usually measured with luteinizing hormone level. Normal: varies with phase of menstrual cycle Follicular: 5–20 mU/mL Midcycle peak: 15–30 mU/mL Luteal: 5–15 mU/mL Postmenopause: 50–100 mU/mL Male: 5–20 mU/mL	Note whether client is taking estrogen or progesterone, as these may decrease FSH level. Recent use of radioisotopes can also interfere with test results. Explain the procedure to the client. Indicate on the laboratory requisition the date of the last menstrual period (LMP) or that the client is postmenopausal. Indicate use of estrogen or progesterone on laboratory requisition. The client should be relaxed and recumbent for 30 minutes before the test.
Gamma-glutamyl transpeptidase (GGT or GGTP)	Enzyme that detects liver cell dysfunction. Normal: 5–38 IU/L	The client must fast for 8 hours prior to test. Note alcohol, Dilantin, and phenobarbital may elevate results, whereas oral contraceptives and clofibrate may decrease results.
Globulin	Key for antibody production. Indicates how well the liver is functioning. Normal: 2.3–3.5 g/dL	Note those medications taken that affect results (see albumin).
Glucose tolerance test (GTT)	Evaluates blood and urine glucose 30 minutes before, and 1, 2, and 3 hours after a standard glucose load. Normal: fasting 70–99 mg/dL 1 hr 160 mg/dL 2 hr 115 mg/dL 3 hr 70–110 mg/dL	The client must fast (except for water) for 6–8 hours prior to the test. Withhold drugs that interfere with results. After administration of glucose load, withhold all food. The client should drink water, however. Collect urine specimens at hourly periods. Administer meal and medications after test is completed.

TABLE 28-5 Additional Tests Performed on Blood Specimen (Continued)

TEST	EXPLANATION/NORMAL VALUES	NURSING RESPONSIBILITIES
Hemoglobin A1c (Hb_{A1c})	Measures the amount of glycated or glycosylated hemoglobin, evaluating average blood glucose level over the past 120 days. Range varies with lab: Normal: <6% Good control: <7% Poor Control: >8%	Fasting is not required. Blood can be drawn at any time.
Hepatitis B surface antigen (HB_sAG)	A positive result indicates presence of hepatitis or that the person is a carrier. Normal: negative	
Human chorionic gonadotropin (hCG)	Test for tumor marker; elevated in germ cell testicular cancer. Normal: negative Female, pregnant: positive, peaks at 8–12 weeks then falls Female, abnormal pregnancy or choriocarcinoma: remains high or increases	Apply pressure to the site and observe for bleeding or hematoma.
Human leukocyte antigen DW4 (HLA-DW4)	Positive (present in 50% of clients with rheumatoid arthritis). Normal: negative	Fasting is not required.
Lead (Pb)	Evaluation or screen for lead toxicity. Especially used in children.	Explain the procedure to the client. Inform client that a blood sample is needed.
Lupus erythematosus test (LE prep)	Positive in 70%–80% of clients with systemic lupus erythematosus. May be positive in clients with rheumatoid arthritis. Used to diagnose and monitor the course of treatment for clients with systemic lupus erythematosus. Normal: negative	Fasting is not required. May be ordered daily for 3 days. Note whether the client is taking Apresoline, Pronestyl, oral contraceptives, quinidine, penicillin, Aldomet, tetracycline, isoniazid, or reserpine, as these may cause false-positive results.
Luteinizing hormone (LH) assay	Determines anterior pituitary function. It can be used to determine whether ovulation has occurred. Can also determine whether gonadal insufficiency is primary or secondary. Normal: Males: 7–24 mU/mL Females: 6–30 mU/mL	Note whether the client is taking estrogen or progesterone, as these may decrease LH level. Recent use of radioisotopes can also interfere with test results. Explain the procedure to the client. Indicate on the laboratory requisition the date of the LMP or that the client is postmenopausal.
Parathyroid hormone (PTH), parathormone	Measures the quantity of PTH to determine hyperparathyroidism or whether hypercalcemia is caused by parathyroid glands. Normal: 10–60 pg/mL	Recent use of radioisotope can interfere with test results. Explain the procedure to the client. Initiate NPO status after midnight, except for water. Obtain morning blood specimen and indicate time of collection.

(*Continues*)

Table 28-5 Additional Tests Performed on Blood Specimen (Continued)

TEST	EXPLANATION/NORMAL VALUES	NURSING RESPONSIBILITIES
Phosphorus	Determines the level of phosphorus in the blood. Normal: 3.0–4.5 mg/dL, or 0.97–1.45 nmol/L	Laxatives or enemas containing sodium phosphate can increase serum phosphorus level. Note those medications taken that may affect results. Drugs that may increase serum phosphorus level include methicillin and excessive vitamin D. Recent carbohydrate ingestion including IV administration causes decreased serum phosphorus level, as do antacids and mannitol. Explain the procedure to the client. Initiate NPO status 12–14 hours before test. Discontinue IV fluids containing glucose for several hours before test, if possible.
Polymerase chain reaction (PCR)	Detects HIV-specific DNA (virus). Normal: negative	Explain the meaning of the test. Provide follow-up explanation of test results.
Progesterone assay	Determines ovulation and function of corpus luteum. Adrenal tumors can elevate level. Normal: Male: <100 ng/dL Female: midcycle: 300–2,400 ng/dL Pregnancy 7–13 weeks 1,500–5,000 ng/dL 14+ weeks 6,500–20,000 ng/dL	Recent use of radioisotopes or hemolysis resulting from rough handling of blood specimen can interfere with test results. Note those medications taken that may interfere with test results, including estrogen and progesterone. Explain the procedure to the client. Indicate the date of LMP on the laboratory requisition.
Prolactin level (PRL)	Determines anterior pituitary secretion. Among the problems indicated by an elevated level are pituitary tumors or primary hypothyroidism. Normal: Female, or male: 0–20 ng/mL Pregnant: 20–400 ng/mL	Note those medications taken that may affect results. Drugs that may increase prolactin level include phenothiazines, oral contraceptives, reserpine, opiates, verapamil, histamine antagonists, monoamine oxidase (MAO) inhibitors, and antihistamines. Drugs that may decrease prolactin level include ergot alkaloid derivatives, clonidine, levodopa, and dopamine. Explain the procedure to the client. The blood specimen should be obtained in the morning and placed on ice if not taken immediately to the laboratory.
Prostate-specific antigen (PSA)	PSA is an antigen detected in all males; level increases with prostatic cancer. It is more sensitive and specific than the acid phosphatase. Normal: <4 ng/mL	Fasting is not required. Apply pressure to the venipuncture site. Observe the site for bleeding.
Protein	Measures total protein in the blood. Normal: 6–8 g/dL	Note those medications taken that may affect results; steroids and hormones such as insulin, and growth hormones may increase level, whereas oral contraceptives and liver toxic drugs may decrease level.

Table 28-5 Additional Tests Performed on Blood Specimen (Continued)

TEST	EXPLANATION/NORMAL VALUES	NURSING RESPONSIBILITIES
Renin assay, plasma renin activity (PRA)	Measures the amount of renin and is used as a screening procedure to detect essential or renal hypertension. When combined with plasma aldosterone level, determines adrenal cortex activity. Normal: Upright position, sodium depleted or restricted diet: 20–39 years: 2.9–24 ng/mL/h >40 years: 2.9–10.8 ng/mL/h Upright position, sodium repleted or normal diet: 20–39 years: 0.1–4.3 ng/mL/h >40 years: 0.1–3.0 ng/mL/h	Pregnancy, salt intake, or licorice ingestion can interfere with test results. Time of day (early in the day), a low-salt diet, or an upright position increases renin value. Note those medications taken that may interfere with test results, including antihypertensives, diuretics, estrogens, oral contraceptives, and vasodilators. Explain the procedure to the client. The client should maintain a normal diet with sodium restricted to 3 grams per day for 3 days before the test. Drugs and licorice should be discontinued for 2 to 4 weeks before the test. The client should stand or sit upright for 2 hours before blood is drawn. Client position, dietary status, time of day, and drugs should be recorded on the laboratory requisition. Blood specimen should be placed in ice and taken immediately to the laboratory. After blood specimen is obtained, the client may resume a normal diet and restart medications.
Rheumatoid factor (RF)	Abnormal protein in serum of approximately 80% of clients with rheumatoid arthritis. Formed as a result of the reaction of IgM to an abnormal IgG. Also elevated in clients with other autoimmune diseases such as systemic lupus erythematosus. Normal: negative	Fasting is preferred.
Sensitivity	Used to identify a pathogen's susceptibility to commonly used antibiotics. Allows the selection of appropriate antibiotic therapy. Normal: none	Specimen should be taken immediately to the laboratory.
Serum acid phosphatase (prostatic) (ACP)	Serum measurement of prostatic acid phosphatase, elevated in malignancy; because it detects cancer in the later stages, no longer commonly used. Normal: 0.0–0.8 U/L	Apply pressure to the site. Observe the site for bleeding or hematoma.
Serum alkaline phosphatase (ALP)	Serum measurement of alkaline phosphates, elevated in malignancy. Normal: 30–120 U/L	Apply pressure to the site. Observe the site for bleeding or hematoma.
Serum creatinine	Specific indicator of renal disease. Normal: 0.4–1.5 mg/dL	Note those medications taken that may affect results, including amphotericin B, cephalosporins (cepfazolin [Ancef]; cephalothin [Keflin]); methicillin; ascorbic acid; barbiturates; lithium carbonate; methyldopa (Aldomet); triamterene (Dyrenium).

(*Continues*)

Table 28-5 Additional Tests Performed on Blood Specimen (Continued)

TEST	EXPLANATION/NORMAL VALUES	NURSING RESPONSIBILITIES
Sickledex (sickle-cell test)	Screening test to determine the presence of Hgb S. Normal: no Hgb S If results are positive, a hemoglobin electrophoresis test is done.	There are no food or fluid restrictions. Note on the laboratory requisition whether the client had a blood transfusion in the past 3 to 4 months.
Thyroid-stimulating hormone (TSH), thyrotropin	Determines thyroid function as well as monitors exogenous thyroid replacement. Normal: 2–10 μU/mL, or 2–10 mU/L	Recent use of radioisotopes may affect test results. Severe illness may decrease TSH level. Drugs that may increase TSH level include antithyroid drugs, lithium, potassium iodide, and TSH injection. Drugs that may decrease TSH level include aspirin, dopamine, heparin, steroids, and T_3. Explain the procedure to the client. The client should be relaxed and recumbent for 30 minutes before the test.
TSH stimulation test	Differentiates between primary and secondary hypothyroidism. Normal: none given	Explain the procedure to the client. Obtain baseline level of radioactive iodine intake or serum T_4. Administer 5–10 units of TSH intramuscularly for 3 days. Repeat radioactive iodine intake or T_4 as indicated for comparison studies.
Thyrotropin-releasing hormone (TRH) test, thyrotropin-releasing factor (TRF) test	Assesses the responsiveness of the anterior pituitary by its secretion of TSH in response to an IV injection of TRH. Also tests the function of the thyroid gland. Normal: undetectable to 15 μU/mL	Pregnancy may increase TSH response to TRH. Note those medications taken that may modify TSH response, including antithyroid drugs, aspirin, corticosteroids, estrogens, levodopa, and T_4. Explain the procedure to the client. Any thyroid preparations should be discontinued for 3–4 weeks before the test.
Thyroxine (T_4) screen	Directly measures the amount of T_4 present. Normal: radioimmunoassay: 5–12 μg/dL, or 65–155 nmol/L	X-ray iodinated contrast studies may increase T_4 levels. Pregnancy will increase T_4 level. Note those medications taken that may affect results. Drugs that may increase T_4 level include clofibrate, estrogens, heroin, methadone, and oral contraceptives. Drugs that may decrease T_4 level include anabolic steroids, androgens, antithyroid drugs, lithium, phenytoin (Dilantin), and propranolol (Inderal). Explain the procedure to the client. Evaluate the client's drug history. If needed, instruct the client to stop exogenous T_4 medications for 1 month prior to test.

TABLE 28-5 Additional Tests Performed on Blood Specimen (Continued)

TEST	EXPLANATION/NORMAL VALUES	NURSING RESPONSIBILITIES
Thyroxine free, FTI, FT_4	Measures the amount of free T_4 that actually enters the cells and is active in metabolism. A true indicator of thyroid activity. Can be used to diagnose thyroid status in pregnant females or clients on drugs that can interfere with results of other tests. Normal: 280–480 pg/dL	Recent radionuclear scans can interfere with test results. Explain the procedure to the client. Blood specimens for T_4 and T_3 uptake must be obtained to calculate T_4.
Total iron-binding capacity (TIBC)	Determines the ability of iron to bind to a protein called transferrin. Normal: 300–360 mg/dL	NPO 12 hours prior to the test. A recent blood transfusion or a diet high in iron may affect test results. Note whether the client is taking oral contraceptives, as these increase TIBC level.
Triglycerides	Form of fat produced in the liver. Normal: 30–150 mg/dL	Client to fast 12–14 hours prior to the test, and have no alcohol for 24 hours before. Diet of prior 2 weeks affects results.
Triiodothyronine (T_3) radioimmunoassay (T_3 by RIA)	Determines thyroid gland function Normal: 110–230 ng/dL, or 1.2–1.5 nmol/L	Radioisotope administration may interfere with test results. Pregnancy increases T_3 results. Note those medications taken that may affect results. Drugs that may increase T_3 level include: estrogen, methadone, and oral contraceptives. Drugs that may decrease T_4 level include anabolic steroids, androgens, phenytoin (Dilantin), propranolol (Inderal), reserpine, and salicylates (high dose). Explain the procedure to the client. Determine whether exogenous T_3 is being taken. With physician's approval, withhold those drugs that would interfere with test results.
Triiodothyronine (T_3) serum free	Measures the amount of free T_3 that actually enters the cells and is active in metabolism. A true indicator of thyroid activity. Can be used to diagnose thyroid status in pregnant females or clients on drugs that can interfere with results of other tests. Normal: 0.2–0.6 ng/dL	Explain the procedure to the client. Blood specimens for T_3 and T_4 uptake must be obtained to calculate T_3.
Troponin I and Troponin T Cardiac-specific (TnI, TnT, cTnI, cTnT)	Used to diagnose a myocardial infarction, to detect and evaluate mild to severe cardiac injury, and to distinguish angina that may be due to other causes. Normal: 0.6 ng/mL	Explain the procedure to the client. Apply pressure to venipuncture site.
Uric acid	Elevated in gout. Normal: Male: 2.1–8.5 mg/dL Female: 2.0–8.0 mg/dL	There are no food or drink restrictions. Note those medications and other substances taken that may affect results, including ascorbic acid, diuretics, levadopa, allopurinol, and Coumadin.

(Continues)

TABLE 28-5 Additional Tests Performed on Blood Specimen (Continued)

TEST	EXPLANATION/NORMAL VALUES	NURSING RESPONSIBILITIES
VDRL (Venereal Disease Research Laboratory), RPR (rapid plasma reagin), FTA-ABS (fluorescent treponemal antibody-absorption test), Reiter test, fluorescent antibody Treponema pallidum immobilization (TPI) test (performed only at Centers for Disease Control and Infection [CDC] in Atlanta, GA)	Blood tests for presence of syphilis. Normal: negative or nonreactive	Explain the test to the client, including amount of blood to be drawn.
Western blot	Confirmatory test for the presence of antibodies to HIV. Normal: negative	Provide pretest counseling. Obtain informed consent. Provide or arrange posttest counseling.

COURTESY OF DELMAR CENGAGE LEARNING

URINE TESTS

Urinalysis assists in the diagnosis of various conditions. Substances not normally found in the urine include RBCs, white blood cells (WBCs), protein, glucose, ketones, and casts. Tests often performed on a urine specimen are found in Table 28-6.

Urine pH

The hydrogen ion concentration in the urine determines the pH. Diabetes mellitus, diarrhea, dehydration, emphysema, and starvation make the urine acidic. Urinary tract infections, chronic renal failure, renal tubular acidosis, and salicylate poisoning make the urine alkaline.

Specific Gravity

Specific gravity measures the number of solutes in a solution. Urea and uric acid, by-products of nitrogen metabolism, are the greatest influence on urine specific gravity.

Specific gravity increases with excess fluid loss from the body. Renal disease decreases specific gravity.

Urine Glucose

Glucose spills into the urine when the blood level of glucose exceeds the renal threshold (180 mg/dL). Measuring urine glucose is not as accurate as measuring the blood glucose level.

PROFESSIONALTIP

Drugs and Laboratory Tests

Note drugs the client is taking when those drugs may influence the results of laboratory tests.

Urine Ketones

Ketones, products of incomplete fat metabolism, are completely metabolized by the liver under normal conditions. The most common cause of ketonuria (excessive ketones in the urine) is diabetes.

Urine Cells and Casts

The urine is normally free of blood cells and casts. In cases of nephritis, renal damage or failure, and urinary stones or infections, the following can occur:

- Bleeding, resulting in RBCs in the urine
- Accumulation of epithelial cells accompanied by cast formation
- WBCs in the urine, indicating infection

STOOL TESTS

Stool specimens are examined for normal substances (such as urobilinogen) and blood, bacteria, and parasites (Table 28-7).

Urobilinogen

Urobilinogen, a colorless derivative of bilirubin, is formed by the normal action of intestinal flora on bilirubin. It increases in situations of severe hemolysis and decreases with most biliary obstructions.

PROFESSIONALTIP

Testing for Blood Lipid Level

To allow for the proper balance between the vascular and extravascular compartment and ensure valid test results, the blood should always be drawn after the client has been sitting quietly for 5 minutes.

TABLE 28-6 Tests Performed on Urine

TEST	EXPLANATION/NORMAL VALUES	NURSING RESPONSIBILITIES
Urinalysis		Explain the procedure and purpose to the client and assist with specimen collection, if needed. Ensure that the specimen is taken to the laboratory in a timely manner.
Color	Clear amber	
Odor	Pleasantly aromatic until left standing; offensive and unpleasant in kidney infection.	
pH	4.6–8.0	
Specific gravity	1.015–1.030	
Glucose	Negative	
Acetone (ketone)	Negative	
Casts	Rare	
Albumin (protein)	Negative	
RBCs	2–3/HPF	
WBCs	4–5/HPF	
Bilirubin	Negative	
Bacteria	Negative	
Leukocyte esterase	Negative	
Nitrites	Negative	
Aldosterone assay	A blood test or 24-hour urine collection to evaluate the adrenal cortex, especially for tumors. The 24-hour urine is more reliable, but the blood specimen is more convenient. Normal, blood: Male: 6–22 ng/dL, or 0.17–0.61 nmol/L Female: 5–30 ng/dL, or 0.14–0.80 nmol/L Normal, urine: 2–80 µg/24 h, or 5.5–72.0 nmol/24 h	Strenuous exercise and stress can increase aldosterone level. Excessive licorice ingestion can decrease aldosterone level. Client should be upright (sitting or standing) for 4 hours before test. Explain the procedure to the client. The client should follow a normal diet with 3 grams of sodium/day and no licorice for at least 2 weeks before the test. Medications should be stopped for at least 2 weeks before the test, if possible. Initiate 24-hour urine collection. Send collection to laboratory immediately upon conclusion.
Bence Jones protein	Bence Jones proteins are immunoglobulins typically found in the urine of clients with multiple myeloma. They may also be associated with tumor metastases to the bone and chronic lymphocytic leukemia. Normal: negative	Instruct the client for a clean-catch or 24-hour urine specimen. Instruct the client not to contaminate specimen with toilet paper or stool.
Creatine clearance	Normal: Male: 95–135 mL/min Female: 85–125 mL/min Minimum: 10 mL/min to maintain life	Instruct the client about the 24-hour urine test. Encourage hourly water intake. Keep urine on ice or in special refrigerator. Cephalosporins and vigorous exercise affect results.
17-hydroxycortico-steriods (17-OHCS)	24-hour urine test that measures adrenal cortex function. Normal: Male: 3–10 mg/24 h Female: 2–6 mg/24 h	Emotional or physical stress or licorice ingestion may increase adrenal activity. Note those medications taken that may affect results. Drugs that may increase 17-OHCS level include acetazolamide, chloral hydrate, ascorbic acid, and erythromycin. Drugs that may decrease 17-OHCS level include estrogens, oral contraceptives, phenothiazines, and reserpine. Explain the procedure to the client. Initiate 24-hour urine collection. Send collection to laboratory immediately upon conclusion.

(Continues)

Table 28-6 Tests Performed on Urine (Continued)

TEST	EXPLANATION/NORMAL VALUES	NURSING RESPONSIBILITIES
17-ketosteroids (17-KS)	24-hour urine test that measures adrenal cortex function. Normal: Male: 5–23 mg/24 h, or 24–88 μmol/24 h Female: 2–15 mg/24 h, or 14–52 μmol/24 h	Stress may increase adrenal activity. Note medications taken that may affect results. Drugs that increase 17-KS level include antibiotics and dexamethasone. Drugs that may decrease 17-KS level include estrogen and oral contraceptives. Explain the procedure to the client. With physician's approval, withhold all drugs for several days before test. Monitor client for stress and report to physician. Initiate 24-hour urine collection. Send collection to laboratory immediately upon conclusion.
Schilling test	Determines vitamin B_{12} absorption by the intestine. Differentiates between pernicious anemia and gastrointestinal malabsorption problems. Normal: 8%–40% of the radioactive vitamin B_{12} is excreted in the urine within 24 hours.	Collect the urine for a 24- to 48-hour period. Laxatives are not given during the test, as they decrease the absorption of vitamin B_{12}.
Urine cortisol, hydrocortisone	24-hour urine test that measures adrenal cortex function. Normal: 22–69 μmol/24 h, or 8–25 mg/24 h	Pregnancy or stress increases cortisol level. Recent radioisotope scans can interfere with test result. Note medications taken that may interfere with test result, including oral contraceptives and spironolactone. Explain the procedure to the client. Assess for stress and report to physician. Initiate 24-hour urine collection. Send collection to laboratory immediately upon conclusion.
Vanillylmandelic acid (VMA) and catecholamines (epinephrine, norepinephrine, metaneprine, normetanephrine, dopamine)	24-hour urine test that diagnoses pheochromocytoma and other adrenal tumors. Normal: VMA: 2–7 mg/24 h, or 10–35 μmol/24 h Epinephrine: 0.5–20.0 μg/24 h, or <275 nmol/24 h Norepinephrine: 15–80 μg/24 h Metanephrine: 24–96 μg/24 h Normetanephrine: 75–375 μg/24 h Dopamine: 65–400 μg/24 h	Certain foods (e.g., tea, coffee, cocoa, vanilla, chocolate), vigorous exercise, stress, or starvation may increase VMA level. Uremia, alkaline urine, or iodinated contrast dyes may falsely decrease VMA level. Note those medications taken that may affect results. Drugs that may increase VMA level include caffeine, epinephrine, levodopa, lithium, and nitroglycerine. Drugs that may decrease VMA level include clonidine, disulfiram (Antabuse), guanethidine, imipramine, MAO inhibitors, phenothiazines, and reserpine. Drugs that may increase catecholamine level include ethyl alcohol, aminophylline, caffeine, chloral hydrate, clonidine (chronic therapy), contrast media (iodine containing), disulfiram (Antabuse), epinephrine, erythromycin, insulin, methenamine, methyldopa, nicotinic acid (large doses), nitroglycerin, quinidine, riboflavin, and tetracyclines. Drugs that may decrease catecholamine level include guanethidine, reserpine, and salicylates.

Table 28-6 Tests Performed on Urine (Continued)

TEST	EXPLANATION/NORMAL VALUES	NURSING RESPONSIBILITIES
Vanillylmandelic acid (VMA) and catecholamines (Continued)		Explain the procedure to the client. The client should be on a VMA-restricted diet for 2–3 days before the test. Items restricted include coffee, tea, bananas, chocolate, cocoa, licorice, citrus fruit, anything with vanilla, and aspirin. Client should not take antihypertensive drugs before the test. Initiate 24-hour urine collection.

COURTESY OF DELMAR CENGAGE LEARNING

Table 28-7 Tests Performed on Stool

TEST	EXPLANATION/NORMAL VALUES	NURSING RESPONSIBILITIES
Stool occult blood (guaiac) Fecal occult blood test (FOBT) Hemoccult	Fecal occult blood screening studies may be utilized as possible indicators of colorectal cancer. Normal: negative for blood	Place a smear of stool on a card. Medications such as anticoagulants, aspirin, iron preparations, NSAIDs, and steroids may cause a false-positive result, whereas vitamin C may cause a false negative. Red meat should not be ingested for 3 days prior to the test. For premenopausal women, wait at least 4 days after menstrual period. Wear gloves when obtaining and handling the specimen.
Clostridium difficile (*C. difficile* toxin)	Evaluation for the etiology of diarrhea, especially postantibiotic diarrhea. Normal: negative	Adhere to standard precautions. Client should be placed in contact isolation.
Fecal fat	Evaluation for malabsorption. Fat in stool is assessed by collecting the client's stool over a 72-hour period. Normal: negative	Instruct client to inform nurse as soon as possible after defecation to collect specimen. Ensure that the client is properly cleaned and dry.
WBC or leukocyte cell count	Evaluation of diarrhea for inflammation and/or infection of the bowel. Evaluates the presence of leukocytes in a single stool specimen. Normal: negative	Explain the procedure to the client. Give client privacy for defecation.
Stool O&P (ova & parasite)	A positive result indicates infection. Normal: negative	Place the stool specimen in a container and take warm to the laboratory. Usually done 3 times.

COURTESY OF DELMAR CENGAGE LEARNING

Occult Blood

Occult blood is invisible blood in the stool that can be detected only by chemical means or with a microscope. The digestive process in the GI tract acts on blood, making it occult. Random sampling for occult blood is done to diagnose gastrointestinal bleeding, ulcers, and malignant tumors (Figure 28-3).

To decrease the possibility of a false-positive result when occult blood is to be used to confirm suspicions of a gastrointestinal disorder, the client is placed on a 3-day diet free of meat, poultry, and fish. Drugs causing a false-positive test for occult blood are salicylate, steroids, and indomethacin.

Parasites

The gastrointestinal tract can harbor parasites and their eggs (ova). Whereas some of these parasites are harmless, others cause clinical symptoms. Most common parasites except pinworms (which can enter the body through both the oral and anal routes) enter the body through the mouth when contaminated water or food is ingested.

Culture and Sensitivity Tests

Culture is the growing of microorganisms to identify the pathogen. Culture and **sensitivity** (C&S) tests are performed

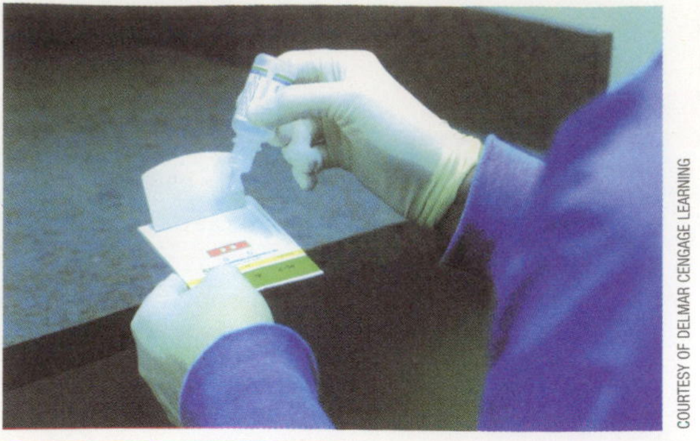

FIGURE 28-3 Applying the Developing Solution to a Stool Sample to Test for Occult Blood

to identify both the pathogen and its susceptibility to commonly used antibiotics. Sensitivity allows the selection of appropriate antibiotic therapy. All C&S specimens should be immediately taken to the laboratory.

Blood Culture

Bacteremia is bacteria in the blood. A blood culture should be procured while the client is having chills and fever. A series of three collections are performed using strict sterile technique. The needle should be changed after the specimen is collected and before injecting the blood sample into the test tube.

Throat (Swab) Culture

The throat normally hosts many organisms. Throat cultures identify such pathogens as beta-hemolytic streptococci, *Staphylococcus aureus*, meningococci, gonococci, *Bordetella pertussis*, and *Corynebacterium diphtheria*. A throat swab is commonly done to identify streptococcal infections, which can cause rheumatic fever or glomerulonephritis if left untreated.

To obtain a throat swab, use a wooden blade to depress the tongue and swab the white patches, exudate, or ulcerations of the throat with a sterile applicator (Figure 28-4). The applicator should not touch any other parts of the mouth. The applicator is then placed in a sterile container.

Sputum Culture

Sputum tests include culture, smear, and cytology. Sputum, created by the mucous glands and goblet cells of the tracheobronchial tree, is sterile until it reaches the throat and mouth, where it comes in contact with normal flora. For a more accurate identification of pulmonary organisms, sputum can be obtained by tracheobronchial suctioning and transtracheal aspiration.

In addition to the organism(s) found in a culture, a sputum smear identifies eosinophils, epithelial cells, and other substances. Smears help diagnose asthma (eosinophils) and fungal infections. The specimen must be refrigerated if it cannot be taken immediately to the laboratory.

Sputum **cytology** (the study of cells) is performed to diagnose cancer of the lungs. The specimen should be collected early in the morning and after a deep cough.

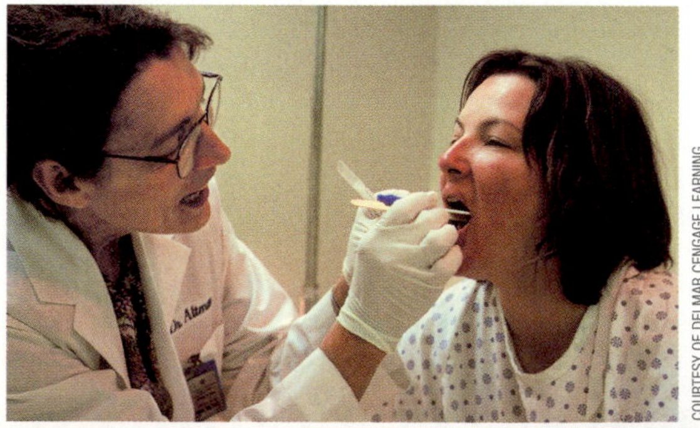

FIGURE 28-4 Swab the sample area using a quick, gentle motion.

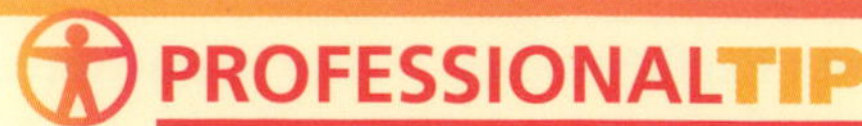

PROFESSIONAL TIP

Cultures

All culture tests should be performed before initiating antibiotic therapy so as to identify the type of pathogen and its sensitivity to specific antibiotics.

CLIENT TEACHING

Pap Smear

Advise female clients to prepare for a Pap smear by:

- Avoiding intercourse, douches, and vaginal creams for 24 hours before the test.
- Informing the practitioners if they are menstruating, as the test will need to be delayed.

Cervical Pap smear testing is recommended every 2 to 3 years after the onset of sexual activity. Annual testing is indicated for those women who:

- Are over 40 years of age.
- Have a family history of cervical cancer.
- Previously had a positive Pap smear.

Urine Culture

Urinary C&S tests are performed whenever a urinary tract infection is suspected.

Stool Culture

Stool C&S is performed to identify bacterial infections. If the client has diarrhea, a rectal swab can be taken and used as a specimen, but fecal material must be visible on the swab for the laboratory to perform the test.

PAPANICOLAOU TEST

The **Papanicolaou test** (a smear method of examining stained exfoliative cells), commonly called a Pap smear, evaluates the metabolic activity, cellular maturity, and morphological variations of cervical tissue. Papanicolaou testing can also be done on specimens from other organs, such as gastric secretions and bronchial aspirations.

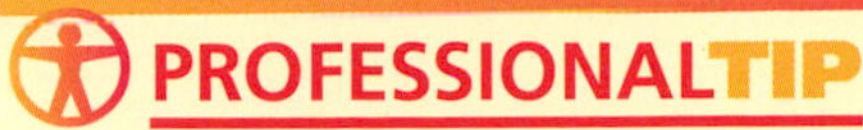

Contrast Media

Carefully monitor those clients scheduled for dye injection studies who have a history of allergies to any foods or drugs because such allergies may predispose them to allergic reactions to contrast media.

RADIOLOGICAL STUDIES

Radiography (the study of film exposed to x-rays or gamma rays through the action of ionizing radiation) is used by the practitioner to study internal organ structure. When used in conjunction with a **contrast medium** (a radiopaque substance that facilitates roentgen imaging of the body's internal structures), **fluoroscopy** (immediate, serial images of the body's structure and function) reveals the motion of organs. X-rays are valuable in formulating a diagnosis and helping to determine if other studies (e.g., a lung lesion requiring biopsy to differentiate between a benign or malignant tumor) are necessary.

Some radiological tests require a contrast medium such as barium and iodine that often interferes with other diagnostic studies. Draw a blood sample for thyroid function before beginning an intravenous pyelogram (IVP), where radioactive iodine dye is administered. If a client needs both an IVP and a barium enema, perform the IVP first because the barium is likely to decrease kidney visualization. Commonly performed radiological studies are described in Table 28-8.

Chest X-Ray

The chest x-ray is the most common radiological study. Chest x-rays are taken from various views (Figure 28-5, p. 636) because multiple views of the chest are needed to assess the entire lung field. To prepare for a chest x-ray, the client should remove all clothing from the waist up and don a gown. The client should also remove all metal objects (jewelry) because metal will appear on the x-ray film, thereby obscuring visualization of parts of the chest. Pregnant women are advised against x-rays; however, if x-ray is absolutely necessary, the woman should be draped with a lead apron to protect the fetus.

SAFETY

X-Rays

- Question the client about the possibility of pregnancy, asthma, and allergic reactions to contrast media (iodine), as well as to other foods and drugs, before scheduling x-rays.
- If the client has not previously received iodine, note this on the requisition to indicate that allergic status is unknown.

Computed Tomography

Computed tomography (CT) is the radiological scanning of the body. X-ray beams and radiation detectors transmit data to a computer that transcribes the data into quantitative measurement and multidimensional images of the internal structures. Figure 28-6 (p. 637) illustrates the sagittal, transverse, and coronal planes used in CT scanning.

The procedure requires the client's informed consent. The client's cooperation is essential during CT scanning because the client will be positioned and asked to remain motionless. Prepare the client by providing an explanation and pictures of what to expect.

Barium Studies

Barium (a chalky white contrast medium) is a preparation that permits roentgenographic visualization of the internal structures of the digestive tract. Barium studies can reveal congenital abnormalities, reflux, spasm, stricture, obstruction, inflammation, ulceration, lesions, varices, and fistula.

Angiography

Angiography allows visualization of vascular structures by using fluoroscopy and a contrast medium. It shows blood flow to the heart, lungs, brain, kidneys, lower extremities, and is useful in diagnosing an **aneurysm** (weakness in the wall of a blood vessel).

TABLE 28-8 Radiologic Studies

TEST	EXPLANATION/NORMAL VALUES	NURSING RESPONSIBILITIES
Radiograph (x-ray)	Most common diagnostic study. Identifies traumatic disorders, i.e., fractures, dislocations, tumors, bone disorders, joint deformities, bone density, and changes in bone relationships. Performed by a technician.	Explain the procedure to the client. Prepare the client as ordered. No specific postprocedure care is required. Administer an analgesic, especially for the arthritic client.
Abdominal x-rays	Determines diaphragm position and gas and fluid distribution in the abdomen.	No preparation is required.

(*Continues*)

TABLE 28-8 Radiologic Studies (Continued)		
TEST	**EXPLANATION/NORMAL VALUES**	**NURSING RESPONSIBILITIES**
Adrenal angiography, Adrenal arteriogram	Study of adrenal glands and arterial system after injection of radiopaque dye to detect benign or malignant tumors or hyperplasia of the adrenal glands. Normal: no growth or enlargement	Assess for allergy to shellfish or iodine, arteriosclerosis, pregnancy, or blood disorders, as they preclude the test. Explain the procedure to the client. Assess for allergies. Informed and written consent must be obtained before the procedure. Note whether client has been taking anticoagulants. Initiate NPO status after midnight. Mark peripheral pulses with a pen before the procedure. Inform the client that a warm flush may be felt when the dye is injected. Observe the puncture site. Monitor vital signs. Monitor peripheral pulses, color, and temperature of extremities. Institute bed rest for 12–24 hours. Apply cold compresses to puncture site, if needed. Force fluids to prevent possible dehydration from the dye.
Adrenal venography	Involves insertion of a catheter through the femoral vein and into the adrenal vein to withdraw a blood specimen to detect the function of each adrenal gland. A contrast dye is injected to visualize size and position of the adrenal glands. Normal: no growth or enlargement	Explain the procedure to the client. Assess for allergies. Obtain informed and written consent. Inform the client that a burning sensation may be experienced when the dye is injected. Although this study involves the venous system, monitor vital signs and injection site as well as pulses, temperature, and color of extremities.
Angiography (cardiac angiogram)	Performed when vessels in a specific organ or vascular area (e.g., heart, kidney) need to be visualized to identify obstruction or abnormality. Involves the insertion of a catheter into a venipuncture site with the injection of a contrast medium, after which angiographic films are taken as the contrast medium enters into the area being studied. Normal: normal vessel	Explain the procedure to the client. Obtain baseline vital signs. Assess for potential allergies to contrast medium.
Arteriography (arteriogram)	Assesses for pathology such as narrowing from atherosclerosis. Normal: normal vessels	Explain the procedure to the client. Assess for potential allergies to contrast medium.
Arthrogram (-graphy)	Visualization of a joint. Radiopaque dye or air is injected into the joint cavity to outline soft tissue, usually on knee/shoulder joints. Local anesthetic and sterile technique are used. Performed by a physician; takes approximately 30 minutes. Normal: absence of lesions, fractures, or tears	Explain the procedure to the client. Obtain informed consent. Client wears an elastic bandage for several days; check for edema. Administer a mild analgesic for pain. Monitor for increased pain. Neither fasting nor sedation is required.
Barium enema	An enema of barium is given while x-rays are taken of the large intestine.	Initiate NPO status the night before. Administer the ordered medication to clean the bowel. Observe the results of the laxatives, and inform the x-ray department if there have been no results. After the test, force oral fluids and administer a cleansing enema, as ordered. Document status of abdomen and stools.

TABLE 28-8 Radiologic Studies (Continued)

TEST	EXPLANATION/NORMAL VALUES	NURSING RESPONSIBILITIES
Barium swallow	The client drinks a glass of barium while x-rays are taken of the esophagus and cardiac sphincter.	Initiate NPO status the evening before. Explain the procedure and the time frame for results. Encourage the client to drink fluids and eat fiber after the test. A laxative is sometimes given after the test. The client should be instructed that bowel movements will be white for 1–2 days. During the test, the client will be tilted on the x-ray table in various positions. There may be repeated pictures taken at half-hour intervals as the barium moves through the bowel. Document the client's tolerance of the procedure and passage of the barium. Because the procedure can be lengthy, encourage the client to take reading material.
Cardiac catheterization (cardiac angiogram, coronary arteriogram)	A catheter is passed into the right and/or left side of the heart to determine oxygen level, cardiac output, and pressure within the heart chambers.	Assess the client for allergy to iodine or shellfish. The client is to fast for 6 hours prior to the test, but medications can be taken with sips of water. Inform the client of the possibility of feeling warm or flushed during the test. After the procedure, assess the peripheral pulses every 15 minutes for 2–4 hours, or according to physician's orders. Assess color, temperature, and pulse in the extremity below the catheter insertion site. Instruct the client to keep the involved extremity straight for 6–8 hours.
Chest x-ray	Provides a two-dimensional image of the lungs without using contrast media. Used to detect the presence of fluid within the interstitial lung tissue or the alveoli; tumors or foreign bodies; and the presence and size of a pneumothorax. The size of the heart can also be determined by chest x-ray.	Explain the test to the client. If appropriate, inquire whether the client may be pregnant, to prevent exposure of the fetus to x-ray. The client is generally required to stand for various views; if the client is unable to stand, views may be obtained with the client in a sitting position, or a portable x-ray may be obtained. Instruct the client to inspire deeply and hold the breath. Instruct the client to remove all metal objects from the chest and neck area and to don a hospital gown that does not have snap closures.
Computed tomography (CT) scan	Provides a three-dimensional cross-sectional view of tissues. Computer-constructed picture interprets densities of various tissues. Most useful for viewing tumors in the chest, abdominal cavity, and brain. There are several different types of CT scans depending on what is being assessed (e.g., brain, cardiac, thoracic, bone, abdomen, pelvic). Angiography or myelography can also be performed via CT scanning.	Explain the procedure to the client. Obtain informed consent. Remove wigs and hairpins and clips for head CT. Initiate NPO status 8 hours prior to scan. Assess for iodine allergy. Observe for signs of anaphylaxis, if dye is used. Check for claustrophobia. Inform the client that the test will take approximately 45 minutes to 1 hour. The client must lie still on a hard, flat table and will be put through a large machine. Because barium will interfere with the test, schedule tests using barium either after or 4 or more days before the scan.

(Continues)

Table 28-8 Radiologic Studies (Continued)

TEST	EXPLANATION/NORMAL VALUES	NURSING RESPONSIBILITIES
Conduitogram	Radiopaque dye is injected through a catheter into either the conduit or a piece of ileum to assess by means of x-ray the length and emptying ability of the conduit as well as the presence of stricture or obstruction.	A conduit is a connection between the bladder or pouch and the outside of the body. Explain the procedure to the client. Assess the client for allergies to iodine-based dye.
Fistula gram	Radiopaque dye or barium is given to drink, and x-rays are taken as the dye or barium passes through the gastrointestinal tract. The dye shows the location of the fistula and how it is connected to the gastrointestinal tract.	Initiate NPO status as ordered. Explain the procedure and the time frame for the results and identify the person who will give the client the results.
Fluoresce in angiography	Following IV injection of sodium fluorescein, rapid-sequence photographs of the fundus are taken with a special camera. Visualization of microvascular structures of the retina and choroid are enhanced, allowing evaluation of the entire retinal vascular bed.	Instill eye drops to dilate the pupils. Start an IV so the sodium fluorescein can be injected. Remove the IV following completion of the test. Inform the client that skin and urine may be yellow for 24–48 hours.
Hysterosalpin-gogram	Radiopaque dye is instilled through the cervix. Used to diagnose uterine cavity and tubal abnormalities. Performed as a part of an infertility workup.	Explain the procedure and prepare the client in the lithotomy position. The test is done in the radiology department. Inquire about allergies to iodine or other dyes. Assist the physician.
Intravenous pyelogram (IVP)	Infusion of radiopaque dye into a vein, allowing visualization of the urinary system. The renal pelvis, ureters, and bladder can be seen. If BUN is over 40 mg/dL, the test may not be performed.	Explain the procedure to the client. Explain that the client will experience a warm feeling during dye injection. Ask the client about allergies. Serve a light supper, then initiate NPO status overnight. Administer a laxative or enema. Schedule test before barium studies. Posttest, observe for untoward reaction to dye. Encourage fluids for 24 hours to eliminate dye.
Kidney-ureter-bladder x-ray (KUB)	Shows abnormalities such as calculi, tumors, or changes in anatomic position.	Explain the procedure to the client. No preparation is required.
Long bone x-rays	Serial x-rays of the long bones to determine bone growth.	Explain the procedure to the client. Instruct the client to keep extremities still while the x-ray is being taken. Shield ovaries, testes, or pregnant uterus. Remove all metallic objects from area being x-rayed.
Lymphangiogram	A contrast dye is injected into the lymph vessels in the hands or feet to examine the lymph vessels and nodes. Used to stage lymphomas and evaluate the effectiveness of chemotherapy and radiation therapy. Normal: normal-sized lymph nodes with no malignant cells	The dye remains in the lymph nodes for 6 months to 1 year, so disease progress can be evaluated with an x-ray. Obtain informed consent. Inform the client that if a blue-colored dye is used, the skin and urine may have a bluish discoloration. Assess the client's breath sounds after the procedure, as lipoid pneumonia is a possible complication if the dye gets into the thoracic duct.

TABLE 28-8 Radiologic Studies (Continued)

TEST	EXPLANATION/NORMAL VALUES	NURSING RESPONSIBILITIES
Mammography	Used to diagnose benign and malignant disorders of the breast.	Explain the procedure to the client. The breast will be compressed, possibly causing discomfort for several seconds. Explain that it is important to have a baseline mammogram done between the ages of 35 and 40 and a breast examination done by a physician or nurse practitioner every 3–4 years. For women ages 40–49, a mammogram should be performed every 1–2 years; for those over 50, an annual mammogram is recommended along with an annual breast examination by physician or nurse practitioner.
Myelogram	X-ray of spinal subarachnoid space following injection of an opaque medium.	Follow nursing responsibilities for lumbar puncture in Table 28-14. Inform the client that the table may be tilted during the procedure. Obtain informed consent according to facility guidelines. Withhold the meal prior to procedure. Administer a light sedative, if ordered. Postprocedure care is determined by the type of medium used; follow physician's orders for activity and fluids.
Orbital CT scan	Allows visualization of abnormalities not readily seen on standard x-rays, delineating size, position, and relationship to adjoining structures. The orbital CT is a series of images reconstructed by a computer and displayed as anatomic slices on an oscilloscope. It identifies space-occupying lesions earlier and more accurately than do other x-ray techniques. It also provides three-dimensional images of orbital structures, especially the ocular muscles and optic nerve. Enhancement with a contrast agent may help define ocular tissue and circulation abnormalities.	Explain the test and the procedure to the client: that the client is positioned on an x-ray table; that the head of the table is moved into the scanner; that the scanner rotates during the test and may make loud, crackling sounds; that if an IV contrast agent is required, the client may feel flushed and warm or experience a transient headache; and that salty taste, nausea, and vomiting may occur following injection of the IV contrast dye. Reassure the client that the reaction is common and that she may signal the technician if she is unable to tolerate the test.
Positron emission tomography (PET) scan	Radioactive tracers are injected intravenously prior to the test. Nuclear imaging is used to confirm tissue that has adequate blood supply and tissue that has become impaired due to a lack of blood.	Instruct the client not to smoke or consume caffeine or alcohol for 24 hours prior to the test. Initiate NPO status from 10 P.M. the evening before the test, except for medications and water. Obtain informed written consent. Encourage the client to drink fluids after the procedure to facilitate faster excretion of the radioactive material.
Pouchogram	Installation of radiopaque dye into the Kock or Indiana pouch. Done with the continent ostomies to determine the state of healing and size of the pouch created.	Assess the client for allergy to iodine. Explain the procedure to the client.

(*Continues*)

TABLE 28-8 Radiologic Studies (Continued)

TEST	EXPLANATION/NORMAL VALUES	NURSING RESPONSIBILITIES
Pulmonary angiography	Assesses the arterial circulation of the lungs. Most often used to detect pulmonary emboli.	Explain the procedure to the client. Assess for allergy to iodine or shellfish. Inform the client that an arterial puncture is required, usually of the femoral artery, and that injection of the dye may cause a flushing or warm sensation due to vasodilation. After the study, assess the arterial puncture site frequently for evidence of bleeding. Assess vital signs and respiratory status. The client may be required to lie flat for up to 6 hours if the femoral artery is used for access. Obtain informed consent per facility policy.
Renal angiography	A catheter is inserted into the femoral artery and threaded into the renal artery. Dye is injected to show blood vessels in the kidney.	Initiate NPO status; administer enema. Assess client for allergy to iodine or shellfish. Check vital signs and peripheral pulses. Institute posttest bed rest, with leg straight. Monitor vital signs, peripheral pulses, urine output, and puncture site.
Voiding cystourethrography	The bladder is filled with dye, and x-rays are taken to observe bladder filling and emptying. Detects structural abnormalities of the bladder and urethra and reflux into the ureters.	Administer enema. Insert a Foley catheter and inject dye into bladder while x-rays are taken. Remove catheter and ask the client to void while more x-rays are taken. Allow the client to express feelings, as this test may be embarrassing.

COURTESY OF DELMAR CENGAGE LEARNING

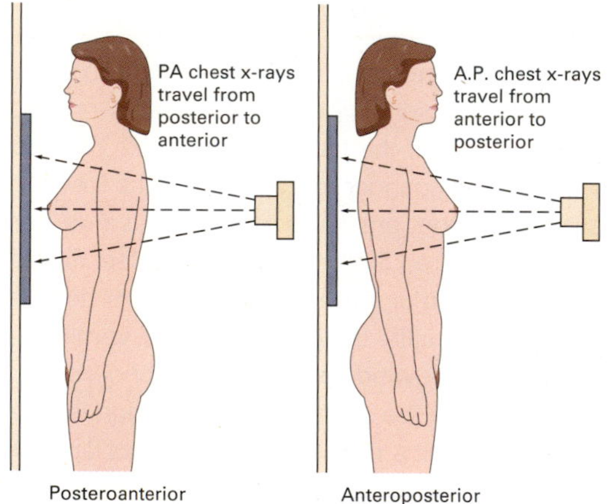

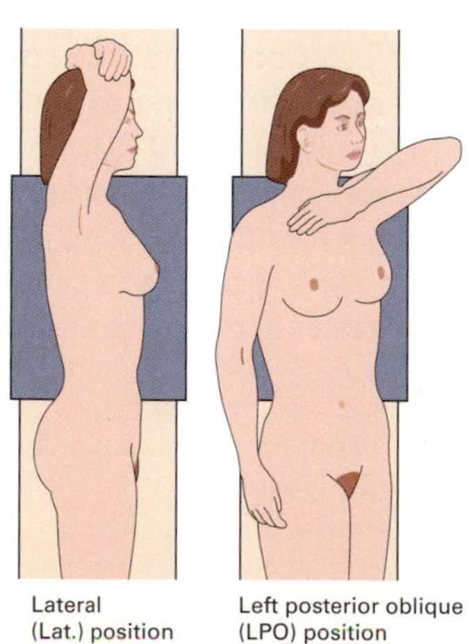

COURTESY OF DELMAR CENGAGE LEARNING

FIGURE 28-5 Radiographic Projection Positions

ARTERIOGRAPHY

Arteriography is the radiographic study of the vascular system after radiopaque dye is injected through a catheter. Using fluoroscopy, the catheter is threaded through a peripheral artery into the area to be studied, such as the aorta or the cerebral, coronary, pulmonary, renal, iliac, femoral, or popliteal artery. With the client on a cardiac monitor, dye is injected through the vascular catheter, and a rapid sequence of films is taken.

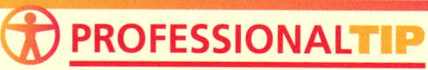

PROFESSIONAL TIP

Computed Tomography

Assess the client's ability to relax, and review imagery relaxation. Sedation can be administered with an order from the practitioner.

SAFETY

Contrast Media

If a contrast medium is used, observe the client for indicators of allergic reaction to the dye, such as respiratory distress, urticaria, hives, nausea, vomiting, decreased production of urine (oliguria), and decreased blood pressure.

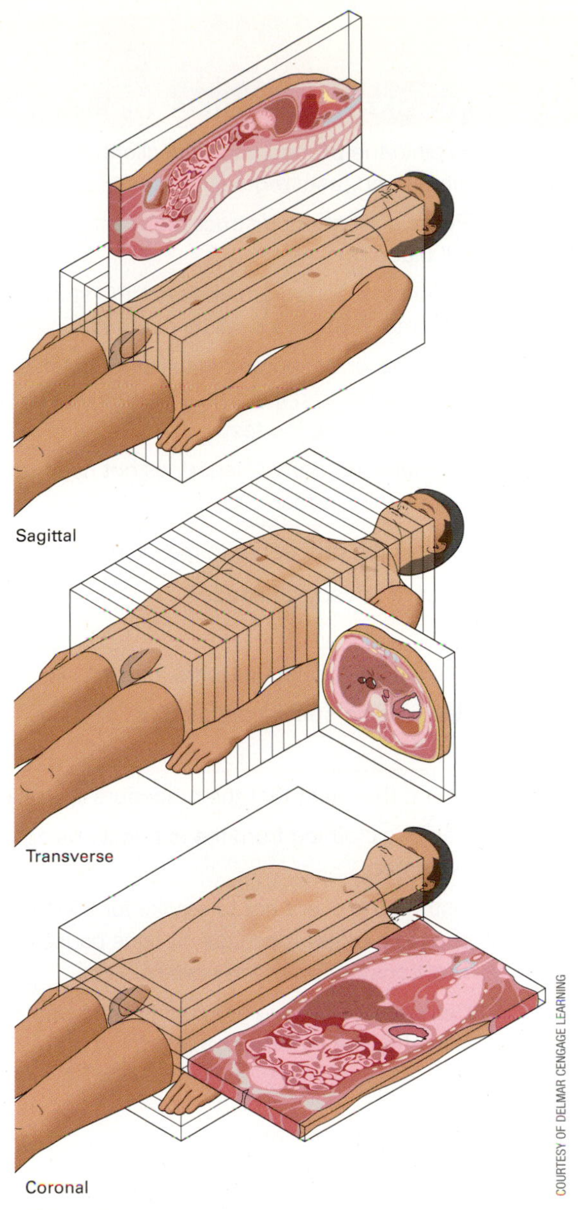

FIGURE 28-6 Computed Tomography

DYE INJECTION STUDIES

Iodine, a common dye used in radiographic studies, might cause the client to experience the following temporary symptoms: shortness of breath, nausea, and a warm to hot flushed sensation. Most dye injection studies are invasive and thus require written informed consent. Assess the client for allergies to iodine and/or the contrast agent prior to administration.

ULTRASONOGRAPHY

An **ultrasound**, also called an echogram or sonogram, is a noninvasive procedure using high-frequency sound waves to visualize deep body structures. To ensure accuracy, this procedure should be scheduled before studies using a contrast medium or air, because the contrast medium would reflect the sound waves differently than body structures do. The client must lie still during the procedure.

Ultrasound is used to evaluate the brain, thyroid gland, heart, abdominal aorta, vascular structures, liver, gallbladder, pancreas, spleen, and pelvis. During pregnancy, an ultrasound is commonly done to evaluate the size of the fetus and placenta. A full bladder is needed to ensure visualization.

To increase the contact between the skin and the **transducer** (instrument that converts electrical energy to sound waves), a coupling agent (lubricant) is placed on the surface of the body area to be studied. The transducer sends sound waves through the body tissue, which are reflected back and recorded. The varying density of body tissues deflects the waves into a differentiated pattern on an oscilloscope. Photographs are taken of the sound wave pattern on the oscilloscope. Table 28-9 describes some ultrasound tests.

MAGNETIC RESONANCE IMAGING

Magnetic resonance imaging (MRI) uses radio waves and a strong magnetic field to make continuous cross-sectional images of the body. During the study, a noniodine IV paramagnetic contrast agent may be used. The study reveals lesions and changes in the body's organs, tissues, and vascular and skeletal structures (Table 28-10).

NUCLEAR SCANS

Radionuclide imaging (nuclear scanning) uses radionuclides (or radiopharmaceuticals) to show morphological and functional changes in the body's structure. A scintigraphic scanner, placed over the area of study, detects emitted radiation and produces a visual image. The results reveal congenital abnormalities, skeletal changes, infections, lesions, and glandular and organ enlargement (Table 28-11). For all nuclear scans, written informed consent is required. The client must remove all jewelry and metal objects.

ELECTRODIAGNOSTIC STUDIES

Electrodiagnostic tests measure electrical activity of the brain, heart, and skeletal muscles. Electrical sensors (electrodes) are placed at certain points to measure the velocity, tone, and direction of the impulses. The impulses are then transmitted to an oscilloscope or printed on graphic paper. Table 28-12 describes the various electrodiagnostic studies.

ELECTROENCEPHALOGRAPHY

An **electroencephalogram (EEG)** is the graphic recording of the brain's electrical activity. During the procedure, electrodes are placed on the client's scalp. The electrodes transmit impulses from the brain to an EEG machine. The machine amplifies the brain's impulses and records the waves on strips of paper. An EEG can reveal not only the presence of a seizure disorder or intracranial lesion but also the type. The absence of the brain's electrical activity is used to confirm death.

ELECTROCARDIOGRAPHY

An **electrocardiogram (EKG or ECG)** is a graphic, noninvasive recording of the heart's electrical activity.

TABLE 28-9 Ultrasound Tests

TEST	EXPLANATION/NORMAL VALUES	NURSING RESPONSIBILITIES
Ultrasound	High-frequency ultrasound waves are sent into the body, and echoes are recorded as they strike tissues of different densities, producing an image or photograph. Useful in distinguishing between cystic and solid masses. Most often used to assess the pelvis, heart, and abdomen. Diagnostic for cysts, tumors, pregnancy, fetal gestational age, and multiple gestation.	Explain the procedure to the client. Most ultrasound tests require no special preparation: Pelvic sonogram: Instruct the client to have a full bladder. Abdominal sonogram: Initiate NPO status at bedtime; prepare bowel as directed. Gallbladder sonogram: Initiate NPO status for 12 hours and institute a fat-free diet the evening before the test. Vaginal sonogram: Client does not need to have a full bladder.
Breast ultrasound	Differentiates between solid and cystic lesions and can be used in conjunction with mammogram findings. Normal: no abnormalities or pathological lesions	Explain the procedure to the client. Provide privacy as needed.
Carotid Doppler	Evaluates carotid arteries in client at high risk or having symptoms of cerebrovascular disease. Normal: no occlusion or stenosis	Explain the procedure to the client. Requires no special preparation.
Doppler ultrasound	Determines patency of veins and arteries in conditions such as arterial occlusive disease, arteriosclerotic disease, or Raynaud's disease. Normal: audible "swishing" sound of the Doppler when placed over vessel A Doppler unit with blood pressure cuffs can measure the pulse volume of arteries and veins. An AB index is obtained by dividing the blood pressure reading in the ankle by the blood pressure reading in the arm (brachial artery). This is known as the ankle-to-brachial arterial blood pressure. There should be a less than 20 mm Hg difference between the pressure in the lower extremity as compared to the pressure in the upper extremity. Normal, AB index: 0.85 or greater	Inform the client that the procedure is painless. Remove clothing from the extremity being evaluated. Instruct the client not to smoke for 30 minutes prior to the test, because nicotine causes vasoconstriction of the vessels. Remove conductive or acoustic gel from the skin after the test is completed.
Echocardiogram	An ultrasound of the heart to determine hypertrophies, cardiomyopathies, or congenital defects. Very helpful in diagnosing valve abnormalities and pericardial effusion. The Doppler technique assesses coronary blood flow and evaluates cardiac valvular disease.	Explain the procedure to the client and assure the client that there is no discomfort during the procedure, although some pressure may be felt on the chest wall from the transducer.
Postvoid bladder ultrasound	Evaluation of urinary bladder for urine retention. Normal: normal size, shape, and position of the bladder; no masses or residual urine	Provide for privacy. Assist client in removing clothing from the waist down.
Thyroid ultrasound	Detects the size, shape, and position of the thyroid gland.	Explain the procedure to the client: that the client will lie supine, with the neck hyperextended; that breathing or swallowing will not be affected by the sound transducer; that a liberal amount of lubricating gel will be placed on the neck for the transducer; and that a series of photos will be taken over a 15-minute period. Assist the client in removing the lubricant.

TABLE 28-9 Ultrasound Tests (Continued)

TEST	EXPLANATION/NORMAL VALUES	NURSING RESPONSIBILITIES
Transrectal bladder ultrasound	Produces an image of the prostate or bladder and surrounding tissue.	Explain the procedure to the client.

COURTESY OF DELMAR CENGAGE LEARNING

TABLE 28-10 Magnetic Resonance Imaging

TEST	EXPLANATION/NORMAL VALUES	NURSING RESPONSIBILITIES
Magnetic resonance imaging (MRI)	Uses magnetic field and radio waves to detect edema, hemorrhage, blood flow, infarcts, tumors, infections, aneurysms, demyelinating disease, muscular disease, skeletal abnormalities, intervertebral disk problems, and causes of spinal cord compression. Can be used in conjunction with a magnetic resonance angiogram (MRA). Provides greater tissue discrimination than do chest x-ray or CT scans. Performed by qualified technologist. Takes approximately 1 hour.	Assess the client for the presence of metal objects within the body (i.e., shrapnel, cochlear implants, pacemakers). Explain the procedure to the client: the client will be required to lie still for up to 20 minutes at a time; the client will be placed within a scanning tunnel; sedation may be required if the client has claustrophobic tendencies; the magnet will make a loud thumping noise as images are obtained (provide earplugs as necessary). As the test may require up to 2 hours to perform, have the client void prior to entering the scanning tunnel. Obtain informed written consent, per facility policy.
Brain MRI	Scans for tumors, pathological lesions and masses, and abnormalities.	Explain the procedure to the client. Evaluate for claustrophobia.
Breast MRI	Delineates and/or differentiates breast disease.	Explain the procedure to the client. Provide privacy as needed. Evaluate for claustrophobia.
Joint MRI	Scans for ligament injuries and abnormalities.	Explain the procedure to the client. Position the client for comfort. Evaluate for claustrophobia.
Soft tissue MRI	Scans for abscesses, masses, tumors, and abnormalities.	Explain the procedure to the client. Evaluate for claustrophobia.
Vertebral MRI	Detects disk disease and used for clarifying x-ray findings.	Explain the procedure to the client and assure that there is no discomfort. Evaluate for claustrophobia.

COURTESY OF DELMAR CENGAGE LEARNING

TABLE 28-11 Nuclear Scans

TEST	EXPLANATION/NORMAL VALUES	NURSING RESPONSIBILITIES
Scan (radioisotope test)	A radioactive substance or isotope is taken up by the part of the body being examined. Sites most frequently studied are the bone, liver, spleen, lungs, heart, urinary tract, thyroid, and brain. The radioactive substance is given orally or intravenously by nuclear medicine personnel.	Explain the procedure to the client: that the client must lie still for 30–60 minutes and that the machine makes clicking noise at times. For liver, spleen, lung, thyroid, and brain scans, no special preparation is required. For a heart scan, initiate NPO status the evening before. For a kidney scan, hydrate as ordered.

(Continues)

TABLE 28-11 Nuclear Scans (Continued)

TEST	EXPLANATION/NORMAL VALUES	NURSING RESPONSIBILITIES
Radioactive iodine uptake (RAIU), iodine uptake, ^{131}I uptake	Uses oral radioactive iodine to determine thyroid function by the thyroid's ability to trap and retain iodine. Normal: 2 hours: 4% to 12% absorbed 6 hours: 6% to 15% absorbed 24 hours: 8% to 30% absorbed	The client who is allergic to iodine or shellfish or is pregnant should not have the test. Client should fast overnight. Drugs that decrease RAIU level include ACTH, antihistamines, saturated solution of potassium iodine, thyroid drugs, antithyroid drugs, and tolbutamide.
Radionuclide angiography (multiplegated radioisotope scan, multigated acquisition scanning, MUGA)	A radioisotope is injected to evaluate the function of the left ventricle. The ejection fraction (a comparison of the volume of blood pumped by the left ventricle to the total volume of blood left in the ventricle) is measured.	
Technetium pyrophosphate scanning	Important in diagnosing acute MIs, with the best accuracy obtained at 48 hours after the client experiences symptoms suggestive of an infarct. A tracer or radioisotope, which is injected intravenously, accumulates in the damaged or infarcted tissue areas, called "hot spots."	Instruct the client not to smoke or consume caffeine or alcohol for 3 hours before the test. Inform the client that the test will take 45–60 minutes.
Ventilation-perfusion scan (lung scan)	Assesses ventilation and perfusion of the lungs. Most often used to detect the presence of pulmonary emboli.	Assess for allergy to iodine and shellfish. Explain the procedure to the client: that a radioactive contrast media will be introduced via an IV access and inhalation of radioactive gas and that the client will be required to hold the breath for short periods as images are obtained.

COURTESY OF DELMAR CENGAGE LEARNING

TABLE 28-12 Electrodiagnostic Studies

TEST	EXPLANATION/NORMAL VALUES	NURSING RESPONSIBILITIES
Cardiac event monitor	Similar to a Holter monitor but worn for an extended period of time (weeks to months) with recording triggered by the client when symptoms occur.	Explain the procedure to the client. Instruct the client to engage in normal daily activities.
Electrocardiogram (EKG or ECG)	Electrodes are placed on the skin to record wave patterns of the electrical conduction of the heart. Detects myocardial damage, rhythmic disturbances, and hyperkalemia.	Explain the procedure to the client. Inform the client that the test is painless.
Electroencephalogram (EEG)	Record of electrical activity generated in the brain and obtained through electrodes applied to the scalp or microelectrodes placed in brain tissue during surgery.	Withhold caffeine due to stimulant effect. Serve meal so that blood sugar will not be altered. Shampoo hair night before test. Explain the procedure to the client: that the test takes approximately 45 minutes to 2 hours; the procedure is painless; the client may be asked to open and close the eyes during the test and that there may be flashing lights or small electrical stimulations.

TABLE 28-12 Electrodiagnostic Studies (Continued)

TEST	EXPLANATION/NORMAL VALUES	NURSING RESPONSIBILITIES
Electromyography (EMG)	Detects primary muscular disorders. A needle electrode is inserted into the muscle being examined. Measures electrical activity of skeletal muscle at rest and during voluntary muscle contraction.	Explain the procedure to the client. Obtain informed written consent. Instruct the client to refrain from consuming caffeine and smoking for 3 hours before the test. Assure client that the needle will not cause electrocution. Inform the client that there will be temporary discomfort when the needle electrode is inserted.
Electromyography (EMG) (Continued)		Observe the site for hematoma or inflammation after the test. The procedure takes approximately 1 hour.
Electroretinogram (ERG)	A record of the changes in the retina's electric potential following stimulation by light. Clinically useful in some clients with retinal disease. Performed by placing a contact lens electrode on the anesthetized cornea. The electrical potential recorded on the cornea is identical to the response that would be obtained if the electrodes were placed directly on the surface of the retina.	Explain the test and procedure to the client.
Esophageal motility studies (manometry)	Evaluates muscle contractions and coordination by using a tube with transducers. Used as a diagnostic tool for disorders of the esophagus and lower esophageal sphincter (LES).	Initiate NPO status 6–8 hours prior to the test.
Holter monitor	A portable EKG monitors and records the electrical conduction of the heart for a period of 24 hours. The heart rhythm is compared to client activities.	Instruct the client to engage in normal daily activities and to keep a journal of symptoms experienced in performing these activities.
Stress test	An EKG taken as the client exercises. Evaluates the effects of exercise on the heart. Often, the client is asked to walk on a treadmill, the incline of which is elevated at various times throughout the test. Used frequently on clients who have CAD.	Explain the procedure to the client. Encourage the client to wear good walking shoes during the test.
Thallium test (myocardial perfusion scan)	A radioactive tracer (Thallium^{201}) is injected and accumulates in myocardial tissue that is well perfused. Accumulation is lessened in areas of myocardial tissue that are not well perfused, areas called "cold spots." The client may be asked to perform exercise, such as riding a bike, during the test to evaluate the perfusion of myocardial tissue during exercise.	Instruct the client to refrain from eating and drinking for 3 hours prior to the test.

COURTESY OF DELMAR CENGAGE LEARNING

Lubricated electrodes are applied to the chest wall and extremities. The client is asked to lie still during the test. The pain-free test can reveal abnormal transmission of impulses and electrical position of the heart's axis.

A portable cardiac monitor (Holter monitor) records the heart's electrical activity, producing a continuous recording over a specified time (e.g., 24 hours) (Figure 28-7). It allows the client to ambulate and perform regular activities. Clients keep a log of activities resulting in the heart beating faster or irregularly. The EKG tracing is reviewed in relation to the client's log to determine if certain activities, such as walking, are associated with abnormal transmission of impulses.

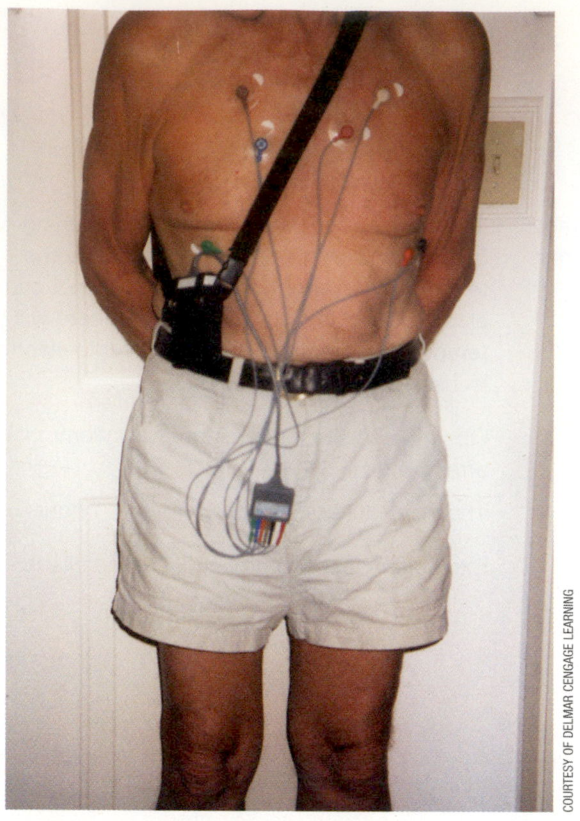

FIGURE 28-7 Holter Monitor

Stress Test

A **stress test** measures the client's cardiovascular fitness. It shows the myocardium's ability to respond to increased oxygen requirements (the result of exercise) by increasing the blood flow to the coronary arteries.

The client walks on a treadmill while connected to an EKG machine. Continuous EKG recordings are made during frequent changes in the treadmill's slope and speed. If the client experiences any symptoms of decreased cardiac output (chest pain, dyspnea, fatigue, or ischemic changes revealed by the EKG monitor), the test is stopped immediately.

Thallium Test

Thallium^{201} is a radioactive isotope that emits gamma rays and closely resembles potassium. Although a radioactive study, the thallium test is discussed here because it is often performed in conjunction with an EKG. Thallium is rapidly absorbed by normal myocardial tissue but is slowly absorbed by areas with poor blood flow and damaged cells. During the test, thallium is administered intravenously, and the scanner detects the radiation and makes a visual image. The light areas on the image represent heavy isotope uptake (normal myocardial tissue), whereas the dark areas represent poor isotope uptake (poor blood flow and damaged cells).

There are two types of thallium test: resting imaging and stress imaging. Resting imaging can detect a myocardial infarction within its first few hours. Stress imaging (thallium stress test) is performed while the client is on a treadmill and being monitored with an EKG. At peak stress, the IV thallium is injected. Scanning is performed in 3 to 5 minutes and again in 2 to 3 hours. The test is stopped immediately if the client becomes symptomatic for ischemia.

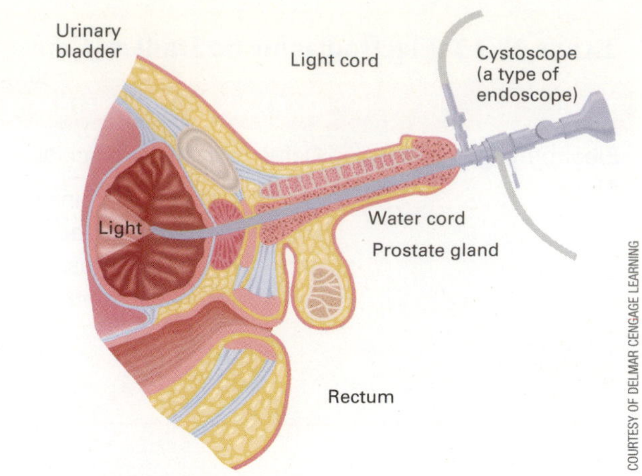

FIGURE 28-8 Cystoscope

ENDOSCOPY

Endoscopy is the visualization of a body organ or cavity through a scope. An endoscope (a metal or fiber-optic tube) is inserted directly into the body structure to be studied (Figure 28-8). A light and, in some studies, a camera at the end of the scope allow the practitioner to assess, via direct visualization or television picture, for lesions and structural problems. The endoscope has an opening at the distant tip that allows the practitioner to administer an anesthetic agent and to lavage, suction, and biopsy tissue. Common endoscopic procedures are listed in Table 28-13.

After the procedure, monitor vital signs, observe for bleeding, and assess for procedural risks (e.g., return of the gag and swallowing reflexes following a bronchoscopy performed under local anesthesia).

ASPIRATION/BIOPSY

Aspiration is performed to withdraw fluid that has abnormally collected or to obtain a specimen. To minimize client discomfort when the skin is pierced by the needle, a local anesthetic is administered in the area to be studied.

A hollow-bore needle with stylet is used to pierce the skin. The stylet is withdrawn once the needle is in place, leaving only the outer needle to aspirate the fluid. A **biopsy** (excision of a small amount of tissue) can be obtained during aspiration or in conjunction with other diagnostic tests (e.g., bronchoscopy). Table 28-14 outlines various aspiration/biopsy procedures.

Bone Marrow Aspiration/Biopsy

The iliac crest and sternum are common sites for bone marrow puncture. A fluid specimen (aspiration) or a core of marrow cells (biopsy) can be obtained. Both tests are often done to obtain the best possible marrow specimen. The test identifies anemias; cancers such as multiple myeloma, leukemia, or Hodgkin's disease; or the client's response to chemotherapy.

Client positioning is determined by the site used: supine for the sternum and side lying for the iliac crest. The site is prepped to decrease the skin's normal flora. Explain to the client that pressure may be experienced as the specimen is withdrawn. The client should hold still because a sudden movement may dislodge the needle.

TABLE 28-13 Endoscopic Procedures

TEST	EXPLANATION/NORMAL VALUES	NURSING RESPONSIBILITIES
Endoscopy	Permits visual examination of internal structures of the body using specially designed instruments. The observation may be done through a natural body opening or through a small incision. A biopsy of suspicious areas may then be done for further study.	Explain the procedure to the client. Initiate NPO status 8–10 hours before test, except for sigmoidoscopy, before which a liquid diet should be followed for several days prior to the examination. Administer a laxative and then a cleansing enema.
Arthroscopy	Endoscopic procedure for direct visualization of a joint. Done in an operating room under sterile conditions and local or general anesthesia.	Perform frequent neurovascular checks. Elevate the client's leg. Apply compression dressing. Administer analgesic for discomfort.
Bronchoscopy	Direct visual examination of the bronchi through a fiber optic scope. Used to remove foreign bodies, for aggressive pulmonary cleansing, and to obtain sputum and tissue specimens.	Obtain written informed consent per facility policy. Explain the procedure to the client: that the client must be NPO for at least 6 hours prior to the test; that, if ordered, preprocedure sedation is administered; that an IV access will be obtained and sedation given during the procedure via this route. Following the procedure, frequently assess vital signs and respiratory status. Assess the client for unusual amounts of bleeding. Inform the client that sputum may be blood tinged initially following the procedure. Maintain the client in a side-lying position until the gag reflex returns. Withhold all food and fluids until the client is fully awake and has a gag reflex.
Colonoscopy	Examination of the rectum, colon, cecum, and ileocecal valve.	Initiate sedation. Cleanse the bowel. Offer only clear liquids after cleansing. Initiate NPO status for 6–8 hours prior to the test. Inform the client that flatulence and cramping will be experienced after the test.
Colposcopy	Direct visualization of the vagina and cervix through a high-powered microscope. Acetic acid is applied to the tissue to dehydrate the cells for improved visualization. Used to diagnose cervical dysplasia or carcinoma in situ of the cervix. Biopsies may be obtained as needed.	Explain the procedure and prepare the client in the dorsal lithotomy position. Assist with the procedure. Prepare biopsy specimens for pathological examination.
Cytoscopy	A cystoscope is passed through the urethra and into the bladder to examine the interior of the bladder for inflammation, stones, tumors, or congenital abnormalities. A biopsy may be performed, and small stones may be removed. Ureteral catheters may be inserted to obtain urine from each kidney. May require topical, spinal or general anaesthesia.	Explain the procedure to the client. Obtain informed written consent. Check vital signs. Instruct in deep breathing, if general anesthesia is to be used. Allow a full liquid diet if topical anesthetic is to be used. Monitor I&O.
Endoscopic retrograde cholangiopan-creatogram (ERCP)	Examination of the common bile duct (CBD) and biliary and pancreatic systems following injection of dye. Sphincterotomy, stone crushing, and stone removal can be done.	Initiate sedation. X-ray is used in conjunction. Initiate NPO status 6–8 hours prior to examination. Inform the client that the test can last up to 2 hours.

(*Continues*)

TABLE 28-13 Endoscopic Procedures (Continued)

TEST	EXPLANATION/NORMAL VALUES	NURSING RESPONSIBILITIES
Esophagogastro-duodenoscopy (EGD)	Examination of the esophagus, stomach, and duodenum. Biopsies can be taken, and dilations done.	Initiate sedation. Initiate NPO status 6–8 hours prior to the examination. Remove dentures and eye wear.
Flexible sigmoidoscopy	Examination of the sigmoid colon and rectum.	Sedation is optional. Administer enemas prior to examination. Inform the client to expect some flatulence and cramping after the examination.
Histeroscopy/ hysteroscopy	Provides a visual evaluation of the endometrium to diagnose or treat a uterine problem, and to perform a procedure such as endometrial ablation.	Explain the procedure to the client. Obtain written informed consent. Client may be asked not to eat or drink for a certain time before the procedure. Some routine lab tests may be done. Client will be asked to empty bladder. Explain to the client that the vaginal area will be cleansed with an antiseptic. The client may feel faint or sick or may have slight vaginal bleeding and cramps for a day or two.
Laparoscopy	Examination of the internal pelvic structures by direct visualization with a laparoscope. Usually performed under general anesthesia. Diagnostic for pelvic disorders and infertility problems.	Explain the procedure to the client. Prepare the client, conduct pre- and postoperative assessment, and institute interventions. Provide discharge instructions on activity and follow-up.
Peg tube placement	Transcutaneous placement of a gastric tube via endoscopy for nutritional (medical) support.	Obtain written informed consent per facility policy. Explain the procedure to the client. Prepare the client, conduct pre- and postoperative assessment, and implement interventions. Assess the site for bleeding after the procedure.

COURTESY OF DELMAR CENGAGE LEARNING

TABLE 28-14 Aspiration/Biopsy Procedures

TEST	EXPLANATION/NORMAL VALUES	NURSING RESPONSIBILITIES
Aspiration procedures		
Arthrocentesis	Procedure to obtain fluid from a joint using strict sterile technique. The knee is anesthetized, the sterile needle is inserted into joint space, and synovial fluid is aspirated. Used to diagnose infections, crystal-induced arthritis, and synovitis, and to inject anti-inflammatory medications. Normal: RBCs, 0; WBCs, 0–150/mm^3, neutrophils, >25%	Explain the procedure to the client. Obtain written informed consent. Assess site for edema, pain. The client should fast if possible. Apply pressure dressing and ice.
Bone marrow aspiration	Evaluates how well the bone marrow is producing RBCs, WBCs, and platelets. Normal: adequate numbers of RBCs, WBCs, and platelets.	Obtain written informed consent. Inform the client that pressure will be felt when the physician aspirates the bone marrow. Assess the site for bleeding after the procedure is completed. Bed rest for 30 minutes.
Gastric acid stimulation	Determines the amount of hydrochloric (HCl) acid in the stomach. If no HCl acid is present, that indicates parietal cells are malfunctioning. Parietal cells secrete the	If the client is having the tube test, initiate NPO status after midnight and instruct the client not to smoke prior to the test. Inform the client that a nasogastric tube is inserted prior to the test so

TABLE 28-14 Aspiration/Biopsy Procedures (Continued)

TEST	EXPLANATION/NORMAL VALUES	NURSING RESPONSIBILITIES
Gastric acid stimulation (Continued)	intrinsic factor that is essential for vitamin B_{12} absorption. Used to diagnose pernicious anemia. Normal tube test: Basal acid output: 2–6 mEq/h Maximal acid output: 16–26 mEq/h Normal, tubeless test: presence of dye in urine (usually blue or blue-green in color)	that gastric contents can be aspirated after the administration of pentagastrin. If the client is having the tubeless test, inform the client of the possibility of a blue or blue-green discoloration of urine. Note any medications taken that affect results; antacids, anticholinergics, and cimetidine (Tagamet) decrease HCl level, whereas adrenergic-blocking agents, cholinergics, steroids, and alcohol elevate HCl level.
Lumbar puncture (LP) (spinal tap)	A needle is inserted into the subarachnoid space to measure cerebrospinal fluid (CSF) pressure and/or to obtain a specimen. Normal pressure: 60–180 mm water pressure Normal specific gravity: 1.007 Normal glucose: 45–100 mg/100 mL Normal complete blood count (CBC): 0 Normal WBC: 0–5 cells/mm^3	Obtain informed written consent. Have the client empty the bowel and bladder prior to procedure. Assist in setting up a sterile field and pouring solutions, if not included in the tray. Assist the client to maintain the position. Postprocedure, deliver the specimen to the lab for testing, keep the client flat in bed for 3–24 hours or as ordered by physician; encourage fluid intake to replace fluids lost; and monitor vital and neurological signs.
Paracentesis	Fluid is withdrawn from the abdominal cavity by inserting a needle into the abdomen. The specimen is analyzed for infection or bleeding.	Have the client empty the bladder prior to the procedure. Prepare the abdomen by scrubbing it with a surgical prep solution and draping it with a sterile drape. Postprocedure, dress the site with a sterile dressing and monitor the site for further drainage. Assess vital signs one time postprocedure.
Pericardiocentesis	Fluid is removed from the pericardial sac for analysis or to relieve pressure.	Obtain written informed consent. Position the client in the semi-Fowler's position during the procedure and attach to an EKG monitor. Postprocedure, take vital signs every 15 minutes and monitor EKG rhythm.
Thoracentesis	Removal of fluid for diagnostic purposes. May also obtain biopsy, instill medications, and remove fluid for client comfort and safety.	Explain the procedure to the client. Obtain written informed consent. Position the client in an upright sitting position, leaning forward. Have client rest the arms on an over-bed table to facilitate this position. Explain to the client that the area will be anesthetized prior to the procedure. Instruct the client to hold as still as possible during the insertion of the thoracentesis needle. Assist the physician during the procedure. Deliver the specimen to the laboratory as soon as possible. Observe the thoracentesis site for bleeding following the procedure. Assess breath sounds before and after the procedure. Report absent breath sounds immediately.
Biopsy procedures	Removal of sample tissue for microscopic study. Tissue may be quickly frozen or placed in formalin before it is chemically stained	Explain the procedure to the client. Follow the physician's orders and/or agency protocol for client preparation.

(Continues)

TABLE 28-14 Aspiration/Biopsy Procedures (Continued)

TEST	EXPLANATION/NORMAL VALUES	NURSING RESPONSIBILITIES
Biopsy procedures (Continued)	and thinly sliced for analysis. Frozen section analysis takes only a few minutes and is often completed while a client is still in surgery. The full biopsy analysis takes 24–48 hours to complete but is the most accurate means of establishing a cancer diagnosis. Tissue biopsy is essential to confirming the type of cancer, the amount of lymph node involvement, and whether the cancer was successfully removed.	Obtain informed written consent.
Breast biopsy	Performed with or without local or general anesthesia and by aspiration, needle biopsy, excision, or incision. Tissue or fluid is obtained and sent to pathology for examination and identification of abnormal cells. Evaluates cystic breast lesions for malignancy. New method of obtaining breast biopsies may be done with the stereotactic mammography studies.	Explain the procedure to the client. Have the client undress down to the waist. Cleanse the biopsy region and shave the area, if needed. Drape the breast and adjacent skin. Provide emotional support prior to, during, and following the procedure. Monitor vital signs. Apply a sterile dressing or bandage. Instruct the client in postbiopsy wound care.
Cardiac biopsy	Done during a cardiac catheterization. The tissue sample is taken from the apex or septum to determine toxicity related to drugs; inflammation; or rejection of a transplanted heart.	Preparation is the same as for cardiac catheterization (see Table 28-8). After the procedure, observe the client for symptoms of a perforation, such as chest pain, decreased blood pressure, or dyspnea.
Endometrial biopsy	Obtained with special biopsy instruments and used to diagnose endometrial tissue abnormalities.	Explain the procedure to the client. Prepare the tissue preservation agent and label and send the sample to pathology. Assist the client in relaxing during the procedure, to offset the discomfort/cramping she may experience.
Liver biopsy	Obtained by inserting a needle into the liver. May be done with ultrasound or CT scan to guide needle placement. Evaluates cirrhosis, cancer, and hepatitis.	Schedule H&H, PT, PTT, and platelet tests prior to the procedure. Instruct the client to refrain from using NSAIDs including aspirin for 1 week prior to the procedure. Prepare the site by scrubbing it with a surgical prep solution and draping with a sterile towel. Monitor for signs of hemorrhage postprocedure by frequently monitoring vital signs and pain. Have the client lie on the right side. Support the biopsy site with a towel or bath blanket for 2 hours. Monitor the site for ecchymosis.
Prostatic biopsy	Removal of a small piece of tissue for microscopic examination.	Monitor for and educate the client about signs and symptoms of hemorrhage, infection, and postprocedure pain.
Testicular biopsy	Determines presence of sperm and rules out vas deferens obstruction.	Monitor for and educate the client about signs and symptoms of infection or hemorrhage.
Thyroid biopsy	Excision of thyroid tissue for histological examination after noninvasive tests prove abnormal or inconclusive. Can be obtained through needle biopsy or open surgical biopsy under general anesthesia.	Explain the procedure to the client. Obtain informed written consent. Assess for allergies. Have coagulation blood studies done. Assess for bleeding and respiratory and swallowing difficulties after the test. To prevent undue strain on the biopsy site, instruct the client to put both hands behind the neck when sitting up. Warn the client that a sore throat is possible after the biopsy.

COURTESY OF DELMAR CENGAGE LEARNING

After the procedure, the client should be kept on bed rest for 1 hour. Monitor vital signs to assess for bleeding (rapid pulse rate, low blood pressure). Instruct the client to report to the practitioner any bleeding or signs of inflammation.

Paracentesis

Paracentesis is the aspiration of fluid from the abdominal cavity. It can be diagnostic, therapeutic, or both. With end-stage liver or renal disease, for instance, **ascites** (an accumulation of fluid in the abdomen) occurs. Pressure from ascites can interfere with breathing and gastrointestinal functioning. In this instance, aspiration is therapeutic. If a specimen for culture is taken, it is also diagnostic.

The client should void and be weighed before the procedure. The client should be placed in a high-Fowler's position in a chair or sitting on the side of the bed. The skin is prepped, anesthetized, and punctured with a **trocar** (a sharply pointed surgical instrument contained in a cannula). The trocar is held perpendicular to the abdominal wall and advanced into the peritoneal cavity. The trocar is removed when fluid appears, leaving the inner catheter in place to drain the fluid. The client is observed for changes resulting from the rapid removal of fluid.

After the procedure, a sterile dressing is applied to the puncture site, and the client is monitored for changes in vital signs and electrolytes. Instruct the client to record the color, amount, and consistency of drainage on the dressing after discharge.

Thoracentesis

Thoracentesis is the aspiration of fluids from the pleural cavity. The pleural cavity normally has a small amount of fluid to lubricate the lining between the lungs and pleura. Inflammation, infection, and trauma may cause increased fluid production, which can impair ventilation.

To facilitate access to the rib cage, position the client with the arms crossed and resting on a bedside table (Figure 28-9). The client should not cough during insertion of the trocar. The practitioner selects, preps, and anesthetizes the puncture site. The trocar is usually inserted into the intercostal space at the place of maximum dullness to percussion. This should be above the seventh rib laterally and above the ninth rib posteriorly.

During the procedure, the client must be carefully monitored for symptoms of a **pneumothorax** (collection of air or gas in the pleural space, causing the lungs to collapse), such as dyspnea, pallor, tachycardia, vertigo, and chest pain. After the procedure, assess for signs of cardiopulmonary changes and a mediastinum shift, as indicated by bloody sputum and changes in vital signs.

Cerebrospinal Fluid Aspiration

Lumbar puncture (LP, "spinal tap") is the aspiration of cerebrospinal fluid (CSF) from the subarachnoid space. The specimen is examined for organisms, blood, and tumor cells. A spinal tap is also performed:

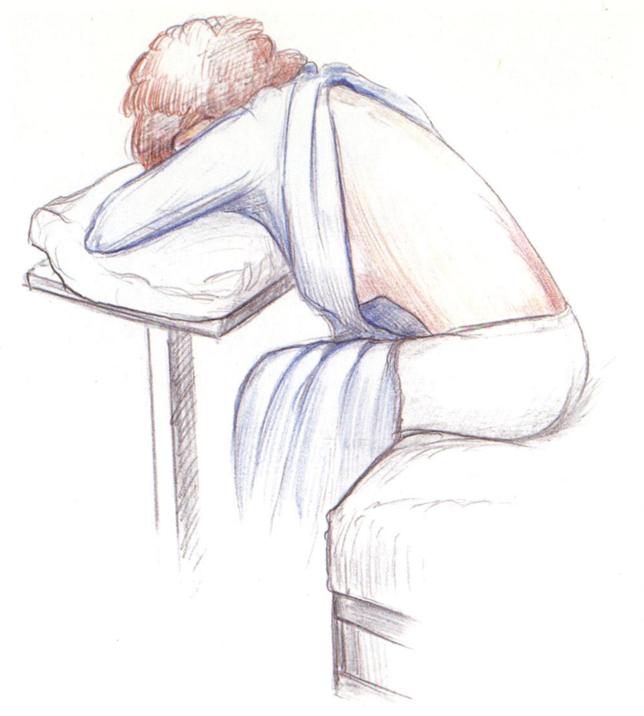

COURTESY OF DELMAR CENGAGE LEARNING

FIGURE 28-9 Client Position for Thoracentesis

- To obtain a pressure measurement when blockage is suspected
- During a myelogram
- To instill medications (anesthetics, antibiotics, or chemotherapeutic agents)

The client assumes a lateral recumbent position, with the craniospinal axis parallel to the floor, the flat of the back perpendicular to the procedure table. The client should assume a flexed knee-chest position to bow the back, thereby separating the vertebrae. Most clients require assistance in maintaining this position throughout the procedure. Face the client and place one hand across the client's shoulder blades and the other hand over the client's buttocks.

The practitioner selects, preps, and anesthetizes the puncture site (usually interspace L3–L4, L4–L5, or L5–S1). The needle and stylet are inserted into the midsagittal space and advanced through the longitudinal subarachnoid space (Figure 28-10).

When positioned, the stylet is removed, leaving the needle in place. An initial CSF pressure reading is taken. If the pressure

CRITICAL THINKING

Thoracentesis

Thoracentesis is an invasive biopsy procedure to remove fluid for diagnostic purposes. What are potential complications associated with a thoracentesis? Why does a physician order a chest x-ray following the procedure?

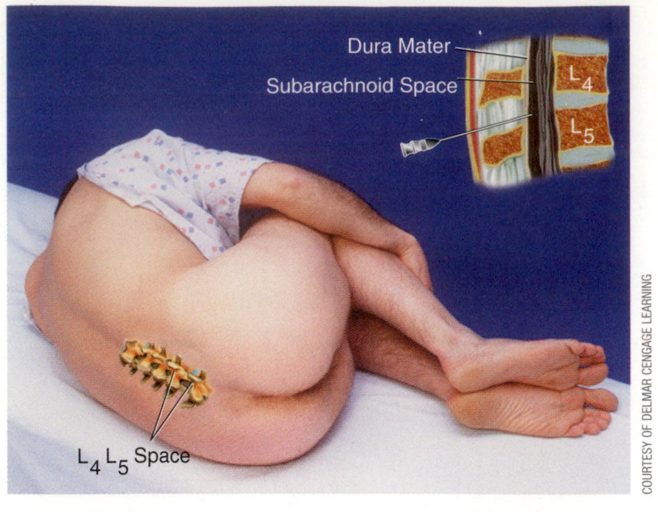

FIGURE 28-10 Lumbar Puncture: Position of client and insertion of the needle into the subarachnoid space are shown.

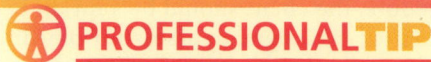

CSF Pressure

The client should be relaxed and quiet during the initial pressure reading because straining increases CSF pressure.

After the procedure, pressure is applied to the puncture site, followed by a sterile bandage to prevent leakage of CSF. The client's neurological and cardiorespiratory statuses are then assessed. A postural headache is the most common complication of a lumbar puncture.

reading is greater than 200 mm H_2O or falls quickly, only 1 or 2 mL of CSF is withdrawn for analysis. If the pressure is less than 200 mm H_2O, an adequate specimen is withdrawn slowly.

After the pressure reading is taken, the stopcock is turned so the CSF slowly flows into a sterile test tube. A sterile cap is placed on the test tube, and the sample is taken to the laboratory. Rapid withdrawal of CSF can cause a transient postural headache. The client's cardiorespiratory status is monitored throughout the procedure.

OTHER TESTS

Other diagnostic tests are described in Table 28-15.

TABLE 28-15 Other Tests

TEST	EXPLANATION/NORMAL VALUES	NURSING RESPONSIBILITIES
Arterial plethysmography (pulse volume recorder)	Determines arteriosclerotic disease in the upper extremities and occlusive disease in the lower extremities. Done by applying three blood pressure cuffs to an extremity. The cuffs are connected to a pulse volume recorder, which records the amplitude of each pulse wave. If there is a decrease in the amplitude of the pulse wave, an occlusion is in the artery proximal to the cuff. A decrease of 20 mm Hg of pressure indicates arterial occlusion. The test is not as reliable as arteriography but also does not have the risks associated with an arteriogram. Normal: normal arterial pulse waves	Explain to the client that the test is painless. Instruct the client to lie still during the test. Instruct the client not to smoke for 30 minutes prior to the test. Instruct the client to remove clothing from the extremity on which the test is to be done.
Audiometric testing	Evaluates both bone and air conduction and determines the degree of hearing loss. The client wears headphones, through which a series of tones is delivered at different frequencies. The client signals to the audiologist when the tones are audible. The results are recorded on an audiogram. The client is kept in a soundproof booth during the test.	Explain the procedure and its purpose to the client. Ensure that the client is not claustrophobic.

Table 28-15 Other Tests (Continued)

TEST	EXPLANATION/NORMAL VALUES	NURSING RESPONSIBILITIES
Brainstem auditory-evoked response (ErA and BAER)	Detects hearing dysfunctions of the central nervous system and cochlear nerve (cranial nerve VII). Valuable for testing comatose clients, clients with neurological damage, and children. An altered appearance of the brainstem waveforms or a delay or loss of a waveform indicates an abnormality including a possible cochlear lesion or acoustic neuroma.	Explain the procedure and its purpose to the client particularly that the client will be in a darkened room and will have both electrodes attached to the head and earphones in place.
Caloric test	Assesses alteration in vestibular function. The client is placed in a supine or Fowler's position and each ear is irrigated with cold and then warm water. Cold water causes rotary nystagmus away from injected ear and back to midline; warm water toward injected ear. Most commonly done on comatose clients. A punctured eardrum or Ménière's disease may contraindicate the test.	Explain the procedure and its purpose to the client. Tell the client that nystagmus, vertigo, nausea, vomiting, and an unsteady gait represent a normal response. Stay with the client and have an emesis basin and tissues available.
Color vision tests	Most common color vision tests use pseudoisochromatic (seemingly the same color) plates comprising patterns of dots of the primary colors superimposed on backgrounds of randomly mixed colors. A client with normal vision can identify the patterns; a client with a color deficiency cannot distinguish between pattern and background.	Explain the test and procedure to the client.
Culture and sensitivity (C&S)	Determines presence of microorganism and identifies the antibiotic that will kill or inhibit growth of microorganism. Drainage from infected lesions is obtained with a sterile swab and is incubated in order to identify the causative organism and to determine antibiotic sensitivity. Normal: negative for microorganism growth.	Ensure that the specimen has been obtained before initiating antibiotic therapy. Specimens should be taken to the laboratory within 30 minutes of being obtained.
Cytology	The study of cells and fluids obtained from various organs by scrapings, brushings, or needle aspiration. Cytologic smears, such as the Pap smear, are routinely done to study cells from the female genital tract. A cytological smear showing evidence of malignancy is followed by a biopsy to facilitate a more comprehensive diagnosis.	Explain the procedure to be used for obtaining cells and fluids for study. Follow agency protocol for client preparation.
Dark field examination of wart scrapings	Microscopic examination to differentiate genital warts from syphilis condylomata.	Take a careful client history. Examine the genital area carefully and provide scalpel and slide, if specimen is to be obtained. Explain the procedure thoroughly to the client.
Dilation and curettage (D&C)	Surgical scraping of the endometrial lining, performed under general, epidural, or paracervical anesthesia and on an outpatient basis. Diagnostic or therapeutic for uterine bleeding disorders.	Explain the procedure to the client. Perform pre- and postoperative assessment and provide care. Provide discharge instructions related to activities and follow-up appointments.

(*Continues*)

TABLE 28-15 Other Tests (Continued)

TEST	EXPLANATION/NORMAL VALUES	NURSING RESPONSIBILITIES
Dynamic infusion cavernosometry and cavernosography (DICC)	Group of diagnostic tests that measure neurovascular events of penile erection.	Perform baseline assessment, monitor during the procedure, and assess for postoperative complications; advise the client of possible discomfort related to the injection. Explain the procedure to the client. Assess for allergies. If preferred by the laboratory, initiate NPO status after midnight. Restrict iodine and thyroid preparations a week before test. Inform the client that radioactive iodine may be given orally or intravenously. Withhold food for 45–60 minutes after the iodine is given. Provide the client with a list of times to report to radiology. Tell the client that he will lie supine for test, which takes about 30 minutes, and that neither isolation nor specific urine precautions are necessary.
Huhner test (postcoital test)	Performed in the office. The couple has intercourse 2 hours before the appointment. A sample of secretions is removed from the vagina and placed on a microscopic slide. The sperm are observed for number and motility in the cervical mucous. Normal: a minimum of 20 sperm per field that demonstrate good motility	Explain the procedure to the client and schedule it near client's normal ovulation. Prepare the client in the lithotomy position. Assist the physician or nurse practitioner with the procedure. Perform microscopic observations as directed.
Nocturnal tumescence penile monitoring	Various devices are attached to the penis at night to monitor swelling (tumescence).	Explain to the client that the test will require application of a device to the penis and that the device is to be worn while sleeping. Show the client the device and explain how to apply it.
Papanicolaou (Pap) smear	Cells are obtained from the external and internal cervical canal. Screening tool for premalignant and malignant cervical changes.	Explain the procedure. Have client empty bladder and undress. Position client in dorsal lithotomy position. Help client relax during procedure. Prepare microscopic slides for pathology. Instruct the client on the importance of having an annual Pap smear.
Past-point testing	Measures the ability or inability to accurately place a finger on some part of the body, usually the client's or examiner's face and fingers. For example, the examiner will instruct the client to close her eyes and touch her nose, then, with eyes open, touch the examiner's nose or the examiner's index finger.	Explain the test and procedure to the client. Explain that it is painless and represents a helpful measure of vestibular function (coordination).
Patch testing	Allergens within occlusive patches are applied to normal skin (usually the upper back) for 48 hours. If the client is allergic to a specific allergen, an erythematous skin reaction will occur.	Clean and dry the skin where the patches are to be applied. Tell the client that the patches must be left in place for the full 48 hours.

Table 28-15 Other Tests (Continued)

TEST	EXPLANATION/NORMAL VALUES	NURSING RESPONSIBILITIES
Pelvic examination (Recommended about 3 years after the beginning of sexual intercourse but no later than age 21 and continue screening through menopause. Screening should be performed every year with the regular Pap test or every 2 years using the newer liquid-based Pap test.)	Performed by a physician or nurse practitioner. The external and internal pelvic structures are visualized, the pelvic organs are palpated via bimanual examination, and the cervix is examined via a speculum. A Pap smear and rectovaginal exam are also performed, and cultures and wet smears may be obtained.	Explain the procedures to the client, prepare the client by having her void and undress, position the client on the examination table in a dorsal lithotomy position, help the client to relax during the examination, prepare slides and culture medium, obtain other supplies, and assist with the procedure.
Postvoid residual (PVR)	Urinary bladder catheterization for the quantification of urine retention.	Explain the procedure to the client. Have the client void prior to the catheterization. Use strict sterile technique during the procedure. Measure and record urine output from the catheterization.
Prostatic smears	Microscopic examination of prostatic secretions obtained via rectal massage performed by a physician.	Explain to the client that to obtain the specimen, the prostate must be massaged via the rectum and that this will cause some discomfort.
Pulmonary function tests (PFTs)	A group of studies used to evaluate ventilatory function. Measurements are obtained directly via spirometer or calculated from the results of spirometer measurements. Bronchodilators may be used during the study. Measurements included are: Tidal volume: the amount of air inhaled and exhaled in one breath: 500 mL at rest. Inspiratory reserve volume: the amount of air inspired at the end of a normal inspiration. Expiratory reserve volume: the amount of air expired following a normal expiration. Residual volume: the amount of air left in lungs after maximal expiration. Vital capacity: the total volume of air that can be expired after maximal inspiration. Total lung capacity: the total volume of air in the lungs when maximally inflated. Inspiratory capacity: the maximum amount of air that can be inspired after normal expiration. Forced vital capacity: the capacity of air exhaled forcefully and rapidly following maximal inspiration. Minute volume: the amount of air breathed per minute.	Explain the procedure to the client. PFTs should not be done within 1–2 hours after a meal. After the test, monitor respiratory status. Advise the client to avoid activity and to rest following the test, as fatigue may result.

(*Continues*)

Table 28-15 Other Tests (Continued)

TEST	EXPLANATION/NORMAL VALUES	NURSING RESPONSIBILITIES
Pulse oximetry	A noninvasive procedure. A transdermal clip is placed on a finger or earlobe to detect the arterial oxygen saturation (SaO_2). Normal: >95% (at sea level)	Explain the procedure to the client. Assess peripheral circulation, as this may alter results. Place the sensor on the earlobe, fingertip, or pinna of the ear. Keep the sensor intact until a consistent reading is obtained. Observe and record readings. Report to the physician measurements below 95%.
Rinne test (tuning fork)	Detects loss of hearing in one or both ears. Tuning fork is struck and placed against the mastoid bone to measure the sound conduction through the bone. The tuning fork is then placed beside and parallel to the ear to test conduction through the air. If the sound is louder when the tines are placed beside the ear, hearing is normal or the hearing loss is sensorineural. If the sound is louder when conducted through the bone, the hearing loss is conductive.	Explain the procedure and its purpose to the client.
Romberg test	Assesses vestibular (balance) function. The client stands with the eyes closed, arms extended in front, and feet together. Normal: slight swaying.	Explain the procedure and its purpose to the client. Stand close and reassure the client that someone will catch him if he begins to fall.
Schiller test	Performed during colposcopy. An iodine solution is applied to the cells of the cervix. Abnormal cells turn white or yellow. Aids in visualization of abnormal tissue and indicates areas for biopsy. Normal: cells turn brown	Explain the reason for the application of the solution. Assist with the biopsy procedure as necessary. Label tissue specimens and send to histology.
Segmented bacteriologic localization cultures	The first 5–10 mL of urine is collected, the next 200 mL is discarded, then 5–10 mL is collected midstream. The prostate is then massaged until prostatic secretions can be collected. Finally, 5–10 mL urine is collected before the bladder is emptied. Four samples are needed in sterile culture tubes.	Ensure that the client is well hydrated and has a full bladder.
Semen analysis	Determines the presence, number, and motility of sperm.	Teach the client about proper collection of sperm.
Skin scrapings	A lesion is scraped with an oiled scalpel blade. The cells are then examined under a microscope. Used to diagnose fungal lesions.	Explain the procedure and its purpose to the client.
Slit-lamp examination	The cornea is examined with the aid of a slit lamp. Provides a visual evaluation and possible treatment of corneal lesions. The exam may reveal disorders such as iritis, corneal abrasions, conjunctivitis, and cataracts.	Explain the procedure and its purpose to the client.
Speech audiometry (Spondee threshold)	Evaluates ability to hear and understand the spoken word. A series of two-syllable words commonly recognized by their vowel sounds (like *toothbrush* and *baseball*) are delivered through earphones. When the client correctly repeats the word, the sound intensity is recorded in decibels. The test is normally conducted in a soundproof booth.	Explain the procedure and its purpose to the client. Ensure that the client is not claustrophobic.

TABLE 28-15 Other Tests (Continued)

TEST	EXPLANATION/NORMAL VALUES	NURSING RESPONSIBILITIES
Sputum analysis	Sputum samples are examined for the presence of bacteria, fungi, molds, yeasts, and malignant cells. Appropriate antibiotic therapy is determined via C&S studies.	Explain the procedure and its purpose to the client. Obtain specimens early in the morning to prevent contamination via ingested food or fluids. Instruct the client to breathe deeply and cough, so as to facilitate collection of a specimen originating from the lower respiratory tract. If necessary, pulmonary suctioning may be used to induce such a specimen. Instruct the client to expectorate sputum into the appropriate container. Deliver specimens to the laboratory as soon as possible.
Tonometry	Used to measure intraocular pressure and to aid in the diagnosis and follow-up evaluation of glaucoma. Two types of tonometric devices are used for assessment: applanation and indentation. An applanation tonometer is the most accurate and commonly used device and measures the force (delineated by the reading on the tension dial on the tonometer) required to flatten a small, standard area of the cornea. An indentation tonometer measures the deformation of the globe in response to a standard weight placed on the cornea. Before use of either apparatus, the eyes are anesthetized with a local ophthalmic solution, such as benoxinate with fluorescein or tetracaine, so that the pressure from the tonometer will not be felt. Normal: 20 mm Hg or lower	Explain the procedure and its purpose to the client. Explain to the client that this test measures the pressure within the eyes and that although the test requires the client's eyes to be anesthetized, the anesthesia will wear off shortly after the examination is complete. Reassure the client that the procedure is painless.
Tympanometry	Measures the movement of the eardrum in response to air pressure in the ear canal. Evaluates the presence of fluid in the middle ear and is commonly used to evaluate otitis media in children or adults.	Explain the procedure and its purpose to the client. Inform the client a small burst of air is introduced through the otoscope, which may produce an uncomfortable sensation.
Tzanck smear	Fluid from the base of a vesicle is applied to a glass slide, stained, and examined under a microscope. Used to diagnose herpes zoster, herpes simplex, varicella, or pemphigus. Normal: negative	Describe to the client how the laboratory technician will obtain the specimen and that although the procedure will likely not be painful, the client must remain still to prevent injury. Provide scalpel blade, glass slide, and stain for collection.
Urethra pressure profile (UPP)	Assesses functional urethral length and general competency of the urethra and sphincter, either at rest or during coughing, straining, or voiding. Functional profile length is the length from bladder outlet to the point in the urethra where urethral pressure equals intravesical pressure. Used to diagnose stress or overflow incontinence or urethral obstruction. Normal: Male: bladder outlet through membranous urethra Female: bladder outlet through mid-urethra	Explain the procedure and its purpose to the client: that it is often performed when the bladder is empty and the client is at rest; that it may be performed simultaneously with CMG; and that the client may be asked to cough or void. Provide privacy, as the test can be embarrassing.

(Continues)

Table 28-15 Other Tests (Continued)

TEST	EXPLANATION/NORMAL VALUES	NURSING RESPONSIBILITIES
Uroflowmetry	Noninvasive assessment of urination. An electronic device connected to a funneled commode calculates the rate of urine flow, volume voided, and time taken to void.	Explain the procedure and its purpose to the client. Instruct the client to void as usual, leaving client alone to do so, if possible.
Weber test (tuning fork)	Detects loss of hearing in one or both ears. Tuning fork is struck and the handle is placed in the middle of the forehead. Clients with normal hearing or bilateral deafness will hear or not hear the sound equally in both ears. Clients with unilateral hearing loss will hear the sound only in the unaffected ear.	Explain the procedure and its purpose to the client.
Wood's light examination	Skin and hair are examined under ultraviolet light (black light) in a darkened room. Used to diagnose fungal infections (tinea) of hair and skin.	Explain the procedure and its purpose to the client. Reassure the client that the rays are not harmful.

COURTESY OF DELMAR CENGAGE LEARNING

CASE STUDY

A 68-year-old male client is admitted to the hospital with a hemoglobin of 9 g/dL and hematocrit of 28%. He is pale, fatigued, complains of muscle weakness, and has a family history of colon cancer. The physician orders a colonoscopy to be performed.

Questions

1. What nursing measures are taken to ensure the client's safety for the colonoscopy?
2. What are the nurse's responsibilities when preparing the client for the colonoscopy?
3. What are the nursing responsibilities when caring for the client during the colonoscopy?
4. What postprocedure nursing care is provided?

SUMMARY

- Most invasive procedures require that the client give written informed consent.
- Prepare clients for diagnostic testing by ensuring client understanding and compliance with preprocedural requirements.
- Clients, families, and significant others must be involved in the testing process; advise them of the estimated procedure time.
- To help offset the discomfort and anxiety experienced during procedures, teach the client how to perform relaxation techniques such as imagery.
- After a diagnostic test, provide care and teach the client those things to expect, including the outcomes or side effects of the test.
- The nurse facilitates the scheduling of diagnostic tests, performs client teaching, performs or assists with procedures, and assesses clients for adverse responses.
- Schedule diagnostic procedures to promote client comfort and cost containment.
- Standard Precautions are used when obtaining a specimen or assisting with an invasive procedure.
- Before a procedure, obtain baseline vital signs and assess the client's preparation for testing.
- After a procedure, assess the client for secondary procedural complications and perform any necessary nursing interventions.

REVIEW QUESTIONS

1. After the client voided, he reports feeling lower abdominal pressure, fullness, and a need to void again. When the client tries to urinate, no urine is voided. Which diagnostic test will the physician order?
   1. Uric acid.
   2. 17-ketosteroids (17-KS).
   3. Postvoid residual.
   4. Urine cortisol.
2. When preparing a client for diagnostic testing, nursing measures to ensure client safety include: (Select all that apply.)
   1. establishing baseline vital signs.
   2. identifying known allergies.
   3. assessing teaching effectiveness.
   4. checking the identification band.
   5. evaluating the client's respiratory status.
   6. obtaining written informed consent for invasive procedures.
3. The nurse is preparing a client for a bronchoscopy. Which statement made by the client indicates the need for further teaching?
   1. "The procedure is invasive and requires a signed consent."
   2. "The nurse will start an IV in my hand or arm."
   3. "The nurse will check my vital signs frequently."
   4. "I will be able to drink water again as soon as the procedure is over."
4. When scheduling a series of tests, the nurse knows to schedule:
   1. a barium enema before an upper GI.
   2. an ultrasound after all other tests.
   3. an upper GI before a gallbladder x-ray.
   4. a gallbladder x-ray before any barium studies.
5. A test that combines a radioactive scan with an electrodiagnostic study is a:
   1. MUGA.
   2. brain scan.
   3. thallium stress test.
   4. radioactive iodine uptake test.
6. Place the nursing actions in the correct order when providing care for a client undergoing diagnostic testing:
   A. Correctly label specimen(s)
   B. Obtain baseline vital signs
   C. Provide written discharge instructions
   D. Ensure client is wearing identification band
   E. Monitor for signs of complications
   1. C, B, D, A, E
   2. D, B, A, E, C
   3. B, D, C, A, E
   4. B, D, E, C, A
7. A newly diagnosed diabetic client asks the nurse, "What is a hemoglobin A1C test?" The best response by the nurse is:
   1. "The procedure is ordered once a year and requires a 12-hour fasting prior to the blood draw."
   2. "The urine test evaluates the amount of glucose in the bloodstream."
   3. "The blood test evaluates the average blood glucose over 120 days."
   4. "The test requires a finger stick blood sample that evaluates the average blood glucose over 180 days."
8. Nursing responsibilities for common diagnostic testing procedures include: (Select all that apply.)
   1. remaining with the client during induction of anesthesia.
   2. placing the client in the correct position for the procedure.
   3. assessing the client's allergies to dye and contrast agents.
   4. referring the client's medical questions and concerns to family.
   5. creating an individualized care plan for the client's procedure.
   6. assessing the client's comfort level (pain).
9. The physician has ordered an occult blood stool test to confirm suspicions of a GI disorder. Which of the following does not cause a false-positive test result?
   1. Steroids.
   2. Grapefruit.
   3. Salicylate.
   4. Meat.
10. Nursing responsibilities when caring for a client that is scheduled for a chest x-ray include:
    1. instructing the client to inspire deeply and hold the breath.
    2. inquiring whether the client may be pregnant.
    3. instructing the client to remove all metal objects from the chest and neck area.
    4. all of the above.

REFERENCES/SUGGESTED READING

Ahmed, D. (2000). Hidden factors in occult blood testing. *American Journal of Nursing, 100*(12), 25.

Beattie, S. (2007). Bone marrow aspiration and biopsy. *RN, 70*(2), 41–43.

Bourg, M. (2007). Screening for microalbuminuria. *Nursing2007, 37*(2), 70.

Carr, M., & Grey, M. (2002). Magnetic resonance imaging. *American Journal of Nursing, 102*(12), 26–33.

Clinical Rounds. (2002). Quick blood test identifies heart failure. *Nursing2002, 32*(6), 34.

Connolly, M. (2001). Chest X-rays: Completing the picture. *RN, 64*(6), 56–62.

Daniels, R. (2010). Delmar's guide to laboratory and diagnostic tests 2nd edition. Clifton Park, NY: Delmar Cenage Learning.

Darty, S., Thomas, M., Neagle, C., Link, H., Wesley-Farrington, D., & Hundley, G. (2002). Cardiovascular magnetic resonance imaging. *American Journal of Nursing, 102*(12), 34–38.

Deatcher, J. (2008). Diabetes under control: Prediabetes. Are you or your patients at risk for type 2 diabetes? *American Journal of Nursing, 108*(7), 77–79.

Ernst, D. (1999). Collecting blood culture specimens. *Nursing99, 29*(7), 56–58.

Gallauresi, B. (1998). Pulse oximeters. *Nursing98, 28*(9), 31.

Guyton, A., & Hall, J., (2000). *Textbook of medical physiology* (10th ed.). Philadelphia: W. B. Saunders.

Hill, J., & Newton, J. (1998). Contrast echo: Your role at the bedside. *RN, 61*(10), 32–35.

Josephson, D. (2004). *Intravenous infusion therapy for nurses: Principles and practice.* Clifton Park, NY: Delmar Cengage Learning.

Kayyali, A., Singh Joy, S., & Cutugno, C. (2008). Informing practice: "Point-of-care" glucometers. *American Journal of Nursing, 108*(9), 72cc.

Kee, J. (2006). *Laboratory and diagnostic tests with nursing implications* (7th ed.). Upper Saddle River, NJ: Prentice Hall.

Lawrence, B., & Tasota, F. (2003). Detecting neuromuscular problems with electromyography. *Nursing2003, 33*(4), 82.

Lewis, K. (2000). *Sensible analysis of the 12-lead ECG.* Clifton Park, NY: Delmar Cengage Learning.

McEnroe-Ayers, D. (2002a). EBCT: Beaming in on coronary artery disease. *Nursing2002, 32*(4), 81.

McEnroe-Ayers, D. (2002b). Preparing a patient for cardiac catheterization. *Nursing2002, 32*(9), 82.

Montes, P. (1997). Managing outpatient cardiac catheterization. *American Journal of Nursing, 97*(8), 34–37.

Neighbors, M., & Tannehill-Jones, R. (2006). *Human disease* (2nd ed.). Clifton Park, NY: Delmar Cengage Learning.

Nursing2002. (2002). Teaching your patient about cardiovascular tests. *Nursing2002, 32*(1), 62–64.

Prue-Owens, K. (2006). Use of peripheral venous access devices for obtaining blood samples for measurement of activated partial thromboplastin time. *Critical Care Nurse, 26*(1), 30–38.

Rushing, J. (2007). Obtaining a throat culture. *Nursing2007, 37*(3), 20.

Ryan, D. (2000). Is it an MI? A lab primer. *RN, 63*(2), 26–30.

Tasota, F. (2002). Full-body scans: Screening for problems. *Nursing2002, 32*(7), 22.

Tasota, F., & Tate, J. (2001a). Assessing thyroid function with serum tests. *Nursing2001, 31*(1), 22.

Tasota, F., & Tate, J. (2001b). Diagnosing pulmonary embolism with spiral CT. *Nursing2001, 31*(5), 75.

Tasota, F., & Tate, J. (2001c). Digital mammography: Enhanced imaging in real time. *Nursing2001, 31*(4), 70.

Tasota, F., & Tate, J. (2001d). Interpreting the highs and lows of platelet counts. *Nursing2001, 31*(2), 25.

Tasota, F., & Tate, J. (2001e). Teaching patients about lipid levels. *Nursing2001, 31*(3), 68.

Tasota, F., & Tate, J. (2001f). Using PET to detect abnormalities. *Nursing2001, 31*(11), 24.

White, L., & Duncan, G. (2002). *Medical-surgical nursing: An integrated approach* (2nd ed.). Clifton Park, NY: Delmar Cengage Learning.

Wong, F. (1999). A new approach to ABG interpretation. *American Journal of Nursing, 99*(8), 34–36.

RESOURCES

Harvard Health Publications, Harvard Medical School, http://www.health.harvard.edu/diagnostic-tests

National Library of Medicine, http://www.nlm.nih.gov

The Cleveland Clinic, http://my.clevelandclinic.org

UNIT 8 Nursing Procedures

CHAPTER 29
Basic Procedures

PROCEDURE 29-1 Hand Hygiene

OVERVIEW

Hand hygiene is a general term that includes *hand washing* (using plain soap and water), *antiseptic hand wash* (using antimicrobial substances and water), *antiseptic hand rub* (using alcohol-based hand rub), and *surgical hand antisepsis* (using antiseptic hand wash or antiseptic hand rub preoperatively by surgical personnel to eliminate transient and reduce resident hand flora) (Centers for Disease Control and Prevention [CDC], 2007). *When hands are visibly dirty, wash hands with soap (plain or antimicrobial) and water. If hands are not visibly soiled, an alcohol-based hand rub may be used* (Siegel, Rhinehart, Jackson, & Chiarello, 2007).

Hand washing is the rubbing together of all surfaces and crevices of the hands using a soap or chemical and water. Hand washing is a component of all types of isolation precautions and is the most basic and effective infection-control measure to prevent and control the transmission of infectious agents.

The three essential elements of hand washing are soap or chemical, water, and friction. Soaps that contain antimicrobial agents are frequently used in high-risk areas such as emergency departments and nurseries. Friction is the most important element of the trio because it physically removes soil and transient flora.

Hand washing is performed after arriving at work, before leaving work, between client contacts, after removing gloves, when hands are visibly soiled, before eating, after excretion of body waste (urination and defecation), after contact with body fluids, before and after performing invasive procedures, and after handling contaminated equipment. The exact duration of time required for hand washing depends on the circumstances. A washing time of 10 to 15 seconds is recommended to remove transient flora from the hands. High-risk areas, such as nurseries, usually require about a minimum 2-minute hand wash. Soiled hands usually require more time (CDC, 2007). According to the CDC Standard Precautions (Siegel, Rhinehart, Jackson, & Chiarello, 2007), artificial fingernails or extenders are not recommended when having direct contact with clients at risk for infection or with potential adverse outcomes, that is, clients in intensive care or surgery. The CDC recommends following agency policy regarding wearing nonnatural nails when caring for clients other than those previously mentioned.

ASSESSMENT

1. Assess the environment **to establish if facilities are adequate for washing the hands.** Is the water clean? Is soap available? Is there a clean towel to dry hands?
2. Assess your hands **to determine if they have open cuts, hangnails, broken skin, or heavily soiled areas.**
3. Maintain short natural nails. **Short nails harbor fewer microorganisms and do not harm clients when providing care.**

POSSIBLE NURSING DIAGNOSIS

Risk for Infection

PLANNING

Expected Outcomes

1. The caregiver's hands are washed adequately to remove microorganisms, transient flora, and soiling from the skin.

Equipment Needed

- Soap
- Paper or cloth towels
- Sink
- Running water

delegation tips

All hospital personnel are expected to maintain proper hand hygiene technique and routinely practice Standard Precautions.

PROCEDURE 29-1 Hand Hygiene (Continued)

IMPLEMENTATION—ACTION/RATIONALE

ACTION	RATIONALE
Handwashing	
1. Remove jewelry. Wristwatch may be pushed up above the wrist (mid-forearm). Push sleeves of uniform or shirt up above the wrist at mid-forearm level.	1. Provides access to skin surfaces for cleaning. Facilitates cleaning of fingers, hands, and forearms.
2. Assess hands for hangnails, cuts, or breaks in the skin, and areas that are heavily soiled.	2. Intact skin acts as a barrier to microorganisms. Breaks in skin integrity facilitate development of infection and should receive extra attention during cleaning.
3. Turn on the water. Adjust the flow and temperature. Temperature of the water should be warm.	3. Running water removes microorganisms. Warm water removes less of the natural skin oils.
4. Wet hands and lower forearms thoroughly by holding under running water. Keep hands and forearms in the down position with elbows straight. Avoid splashing water and touching the sides of the sink or faucet.	4. Water should flow from the least contaminated to the most contaminated areas of the skin. Hands are considered more contaminated than arms. Splashing of water facilitates transfer of micro-organisms. Touching of any surface during cleaning contaminates the skin.
5. Apply about 5 mL (1 teaspoon) of liquid soap. Lather thoroughly.	5. Lather facilitates removal of microorganisms. Liquid soap harbors less bacteria than bar soap.
6. Thoroughly rub hands together for about 10 to 15 seconds. Interlace fingers and thumbs and move back and forth to wash between digits. Wash palms, back of hands, and wrists with firm rubbing and circular motions (Figure 29-1-1). Special attention should be provided to areas such as the knuckles and fingernails, which are known to harbor organisms (Figure 29-1-2).	6. Friction mechanically removes microorganisms from the skin surface. Friction loosens dirt from soiled areas.
7. Rinse with hands in the down position, elbows straight. Rinse in the direction of forearm to wrist to fingers.	7. Flow of water rinses away dirt and microorganisms.
8. Blot hands and forearms to dry thoroughly. Dry in the direction of fingers to wrist and forearms. Discard the paper towels in the proper receptacle.	8. Blotting reduces chapping of skin. Drying from cleanest (hand) to least clean area (forearms) prevents transfer of microorganisms to cleanest area.
9. Turn off the water faucet with a clean, dry paper towel (Figure 29-1-3).	9. Prevents contamination of clean hands by a less clean faucet.

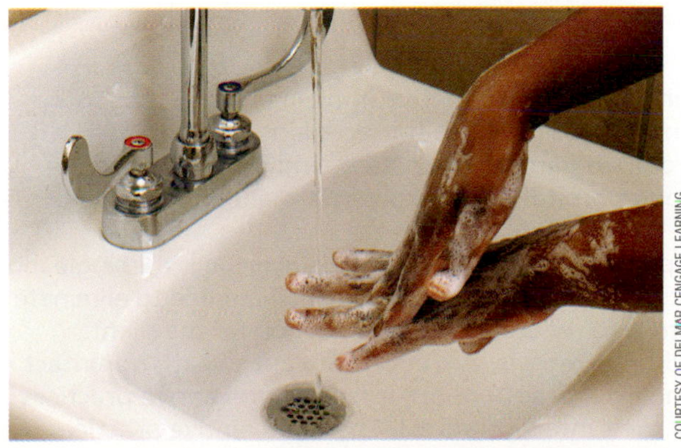

FIGURE 29-1-1 Lather thoroughly and rub hands together.

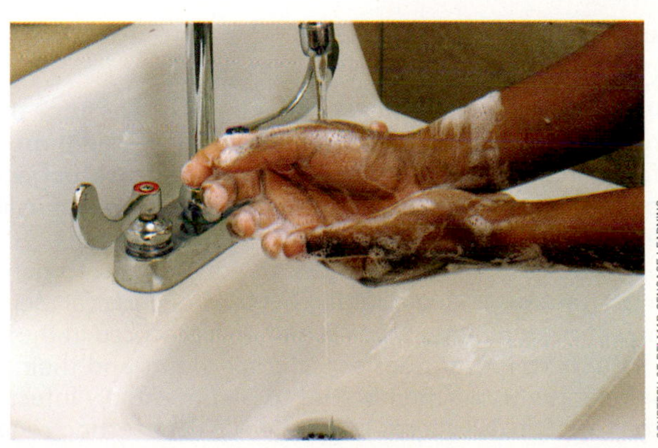

FIGURE 29-1-2 Give special attention to fingernails and knuckles.

(Continues)

PROCEDURE 29-1 Hand Hygiene (Continued)

ACTION	RATIONALE

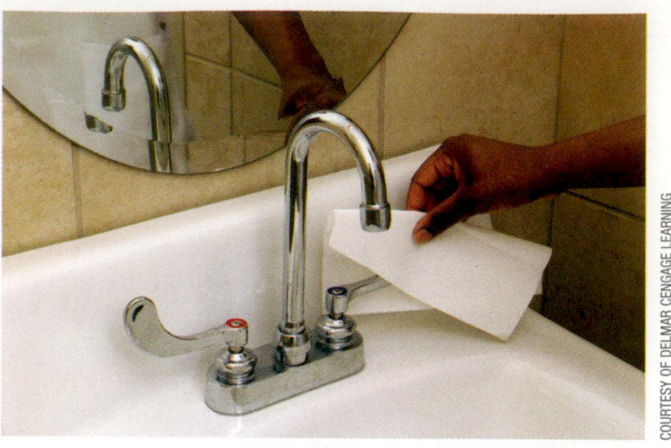

FIGURE 29-1-3 Turn off faucet with a clean, dry paper towel.

Alcohol-Based Hand Rub

ACTION	RATIONALE
10. Apply the manufacturer's recommended amount of product to one hand.	10. Amount of rub required varies by product.
11. Rub hands together, covering hands and fingers on all sides.	11. Spreads rub to cover all aspects of hands and fingers.
12. Continue rubbing until hands are dry.	12. Allows the alcohol-based hand rub to remove or destroy transient microorganisms and reduce resident flora.

EVALUATION

- The hand hygiene was adequate to control topical flora and infectious agents on the hands.
- The hands were not recontaminated during or shortly after the hand hygiene.

DOCUMENTATION

No documentation is needed for routine hand hygiene by the nurse.

PROCEDURE 29-2 Use of Protective Equipment

OVERVIEW

Infection control is an essential area of concern for the nurse in any setting. Effective implementation prevents or reduces the incidence of health care associated (nosocomial) infections. The hospitalized client is at increased risk for infection because of added exposure to pathogens, compromised immunologic state, and potential invasive procedures. Development of infection can delay healing, prolong hospital stay, or cause permanent disability or even loss of life.

Medical asepsis is the process of reducing microorganisms and preventing their spread. Hand hygiene is the single most important technique for infection control. Surgical asepsis takes this further with procedures implemented to eliminate any microorganisms. Medical asepsis is practiced in the surgical arena to reduce the risk of infection for the client.

Standard Precautions consider all clients and their bodily fluids, secretions, excretions (except sweat), nonintact skin, and mucous membranes to be potentially infectious. Standard Precautions are infection preventive practices that apply to all clients in any health care setting regardless of their infection status. These preventive practices include hand hygiene; wearing gloves, gown, masks, and eye protection or face shield; and injection safety.

(Continues)

PROCEDURE 29-2 Use of Protective Equipment (Continued)

Appropriate protective items are worn according to the interaction with the client (Siegel, Rhinehart, Jackson, & Chiarello, 2007):

- Gloves are required when hand contact with any body fluids is anticipated. This includes touching mucous membranes and nonintact skin. Latex-free and powder-free gloves are recommended. Hands are washed after the gloves are removed.
- Impervious gowns must be worn by health care workers to prevent soiling of clothing by splashes of blood or body fluids, and masks, along with eye protection, are mandated if splashes toward the face are anticipated.
- Masks are worn when caring for clients on airborne and/or droplet precautions and immunocompromised clients.
- Hair is covered by a cap when in the semirestricted and restricted areas of the surgical suite and in areas of the hospital where special procedures are done (i.e., bone marrow transplant).
- Eye protection (goggles) or face shields are worn during care activities that may be associated with splashes or sprays of blood or body fluids.
- Soiled protective items are removed promptly after use and disposed of as appropriate.

ASSESSMENT

1. Assess if Standard Precautions are followed or if specific isolation precautions are needed for the client's condition. **The type of microorganism and mode of transmission determine the degree of precautions.**
2. Assess the client's laboratory results **to learn which organism the client is infected with and the client's immune responses.**
3. Assess what nursing measures are required before entering the room **to have all the necessary equipment ready.**
4. Assess the client's knowledge for the need to wear a cap, gown, and mask during care **to direct client teaching.**
5. Assess whether the isolation is airborne, droplet, or contact and which isolation attire is necessary.

POSSIBLE NURSING DIAGNOSIS

Ineffective Protection
Social Isolation
Situational Low Self-Esteem

PLANNING

Expected Outcomes

1. The client and staff will remain free of health care associated infection.
2. The health care provider will be protected from infection when caring for the client.
3. The staff will avoid transmitting microorganisms to others.
4. The client will interact on a social level with nurse, family members, and other visitors.

Equipment Needed

- Gloves, clean—sterile if necessary
- Gown, sterile or clean
- Cap
- Mask
- Goggles
- Face mask

delegation tips

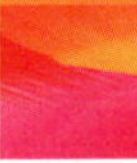

Donning and removing gloves, caps, and masks is a skill that is required of all personnel, including ancillary personnel. Proper technique should be monitored by the nursing staff.

IMPLEMENTATION—ACTION/RATIONALE

ACTION	RATIONALE
* Check client's identification band * Explain procedure before beginning *	
1. Wash hands.	1. Reduces the transmission of microorganisms.
2. First put on the cap or surgical hat/hood. Hair should be tucked in a manner so that all hair is covered (Figure 29-2-1).	2. Because hair acts as a filter when left uncovered, it collects bacteria in proportion to its length, curliness, and oiliness. Loose hair may fall in the surgical area. Shedding hair may lead to surgical wound infection.

(Continues)

PROCEDURE 29-2 Use of Protective Equipment (Continued)

ACTION	RATIONALE

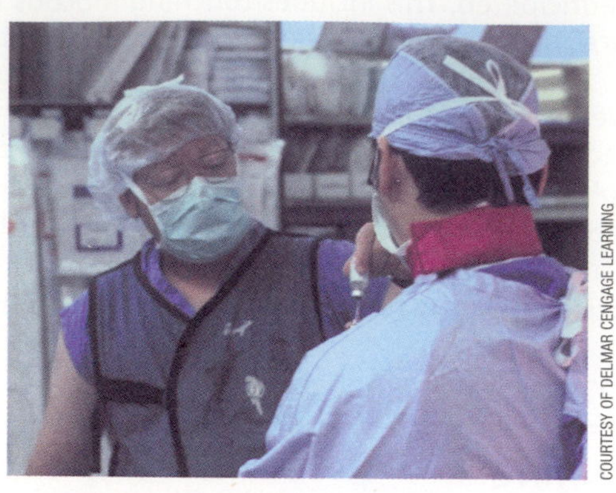

FIGURE 29-2-1 Caps and surgical caps cover the head, and hair is tucked in.

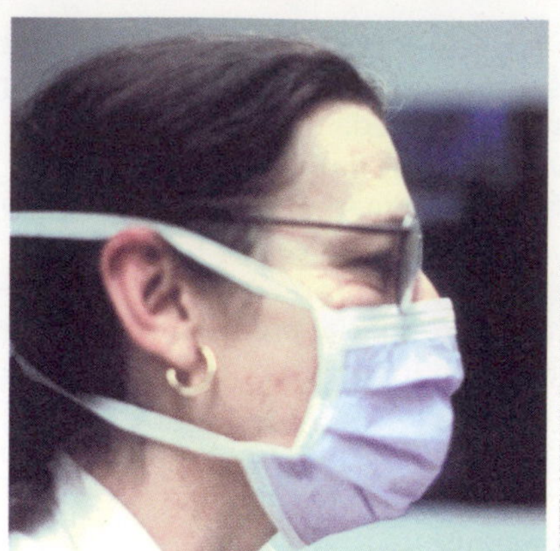

FIGURE 29-2-2 Bottom of the mask fits snugly under the chin.

3. Apply a mask around mouth and nose and secure in a manner that prevents venting. For masks with strings:
   a. Hold mask by top and pinch center (metal strip) over bridge of nose.
   b. Pull top two strings over ears and secure at top, back of head.
   c. Tie two lower ties around back or nape of neck so bottom of mask fits snugly under chin (Figure 29-2-2).

   Rationale: 3. Masks are worn to contain and filter droplets of microorganisms that are expelled when talking, sneezing, or coughing. Masks prevent the transmission of oral and nasopharyngeal organisms between the nurse and client.

4. Open gown, slip arms into sleeves, and secure at neck and waist (Figure 29-2-3 A and B).

   Rationale: 4. Gowns act as a protective barrier and should be worn to reduce exposure to blood, body fluid, or other potentially infectious liquids.

5. Protective eyewear is worn whenever health care provider or client are at risk for splash and contamination. These are applied as goggles/glasses or face shields that have elastic ties for around the ears.

   Rationale: 5. Protective eyewear reduces the incidence of contamination to the eyes. If eyewear or face shields become contaminated, they should be discarded immediately and replaced with a clean barrier.

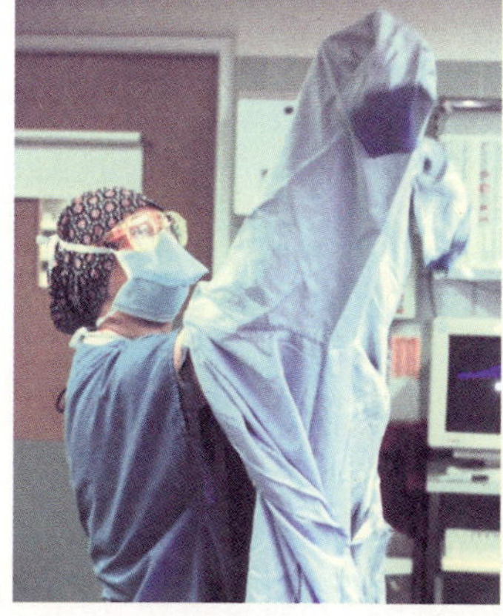
A

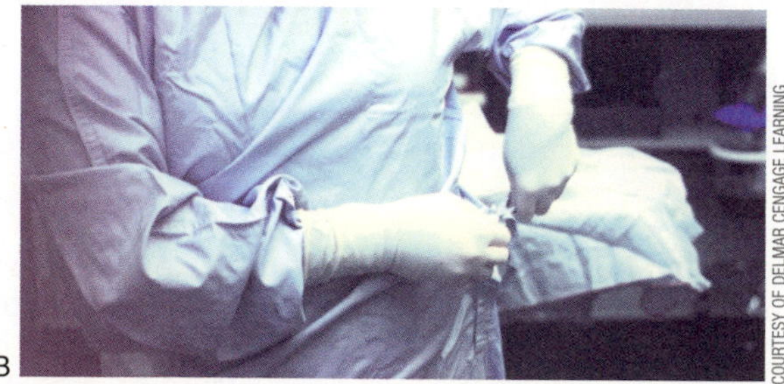
B

FIGURE 29-2-3 *A,* The gown is put on before the gloves. *B,* Tie the gown at the neck and waist.

(Continues)

PROCEDURE 29-2 Use of Protective Equipment (Continued)

ACTION	RATIONALE
6. Don clean gloves. If sterile gloves are required for a procedure, use open or closed method.	6. Gloves are worn to prevent gross contamination of the hands. They should be changed between clients and hands washed. The open method is used when performing procedures that require sterile technique but do not require donning a sterile gown or when both gloves need to be changed without assistance during a surgical procedure (Procedure 30-2). The closed method is used by scrubbed personnel in the operating room.
7. The open glove technique: a. Slide the hands into the gown all the way through the cuffs on the gown. b. Pick up the cuff of the left glove using the thumb and index finger of the right hand. c. Pull the glove onto the left hand, leaving the cuff of the glove turned down. d. Take the gloved left hand and slide the fingers under the cuff of the right glove, keeping the gloved fingers under the folded cuff. e. Pull the glove onto the right hand. f. Rotate the arm as the cuff of the glove is pulled over the gown.	7. The open glove method is commonly used for sterile procedures or when both gloves need to be changed without assistance during a surgical procedure.
8. The closed glove technique: a. Slide the hands into the gown all the way through the cuffs on the gown. b. Use right hand to pick up left glove. c. Place the glove on the upward-turned left hand—palm side down thumb to thumb with the fingers extending along the forearm pointing toward the elbow. d. Hold the glove cuff and sleeve cuff together with the thumb of the left hand. e. The right hand stretches the cuff of the left glove over the opened end of the sleeve. f. Work the fingers into the glove as the cuff is pulled onto the wrist. g. The right glove is done in the same manner.	8. The closed glove technique is used by the scrubbed personnel in the operating room. This is preferred because the possibility of the glove touching the skin is eliminated.
9. Enter the client's room and explain the rationale for wearing the attire.	9. Minimizes anxiety and feelings of isolation.
10. After performing necessary tasks, remove gown, gloves, mask, and cap before leaving the room.	10. Reduces transmission of organisms.
11. Removal of gown: Untie gown and remove from shoulders. Fold and roll gown down in front into a ball, so contaminated area is rolled onto center of gown. Dispose in approved receptacle.	11. Reduces transmission of organisms.
12. Removal of gloves:	12.
a. Grasp outside cuff of one glove and pull off, turning inside out. Hold it with the remaining gloved hand (Figures 29-2-4 and 29-2-5).	a. Reduces risk of contamination.
b. Pull the second glove off without touching the outside of the second glove (Figure 29-2-6). Turn the second glove over the first glove as it is removed (Figure 29-2-7). Dispose into receptacle with first glove (Figure 29-2-8).	b. Reduces risk of contamination.
13. Removal of mask: Untie bottom strings of mask first, then top strings, and lift off face. Hold mask by strings and discard.	13. Prevents contaminated surface of mask from contacting uniform.

(Continues)

PROCEDURE 29-2 Use of Protective Equipment (Continued)

ACTION	RATIONALE

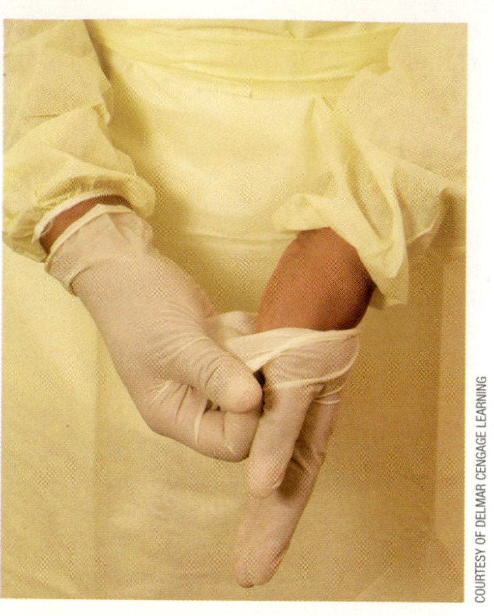

FIGURE 29-2-4 Grasp the outside cuff to remove the gown.

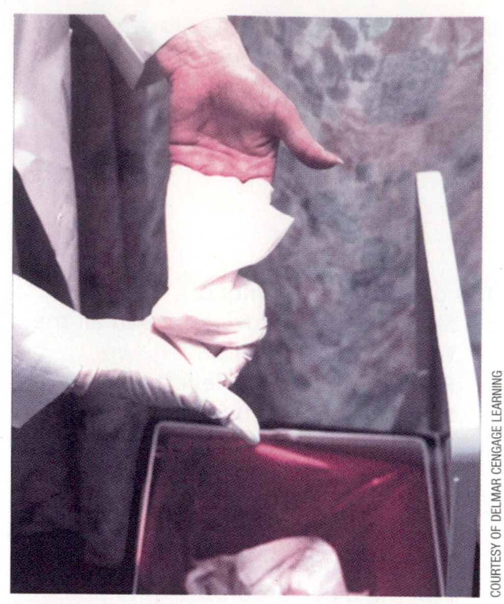

FIGURE 29-2-5 As the glove is removed, turn the glove inside out.

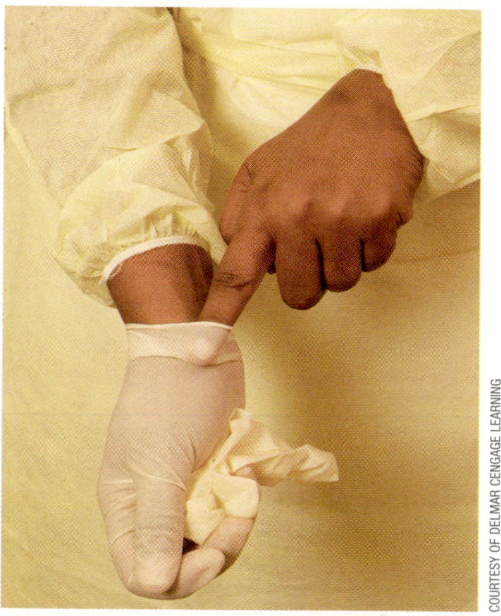

FIGURE 29-2-6 As the first glove is removed, place it inside the palm of the second glove. To remove the second glove, place a finger inside the glove and slide the glove down the hand.

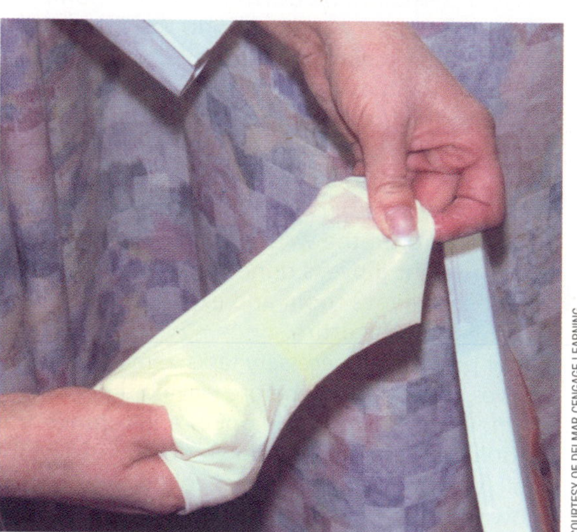

FIGURE 29-2-7 The second glove covers the first glove so that only the clean side of the glove is exposed.

ACTION	RATIONALE
14. Removal of cap: Grasp top surface of cap and lift from head.	14. Minimizes contact of hands to hair.
15. Wash hands.	15 Reduces transmission of microorganisms.

(Continues)

PROCEDURE 29-2 Use of Protective Equipment (Continued)

ACTION	RATIONALE

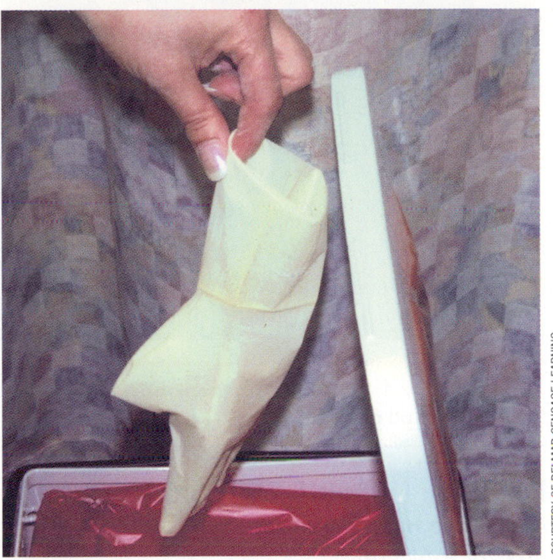

FIGURE 29-2-8 Place the contaminated gloves in the trash.

EVALUATION

- The client remains free of any health care associated infection.
- The health care provider and staff are protected from infection and microorganisms are contained without cross contamination.
- The client interacts on a social level with nurse, family members, and other visitors.

DOCUMENTATION

Nurses' Notes

- Type of protective barriers used and any breaks in isolation technique
- Client's compliance with and verbalization of understanding and adjustment to isolation
- Family members' compliance of isolation procedures

PROCEDURE 29-3 Taking a Temperature

OVERVIEW

Vital signs are generally taken with automatic measurement devices or a Dinamap with the results displayed on an electronic panel (Figure 29-3-1). The same basic procedural steps are used when obtaining the vital signs manually, such as with a BP cuff and stethoscope or thermometer. With the Dinamap, the temperature (T), pulse (P), blood pressure (BP), and pulse oximetry are automatically taken by applying a BP cuff and pulse oximetry sensor and correctly placing a thermometer probe. The electronic device promptly provides vital information to the nurse. Automated measurement devices simplify taking vital signs, but the nurse learns to manually take vital signs correctly and accurately in case of a malfunction of the electronic device or if one is not available. Therefore, the manual methods of obtaining vital signs are explained in Procedures 29-3 to 29-7. Specific vital signs are defined in the separate procedures. Refer to Chapter 26, Assessment"; Chapter 35, "Respiratory System"; and Chapter 36, "Cardiovascular System" for more detailed information on vital sign assessment.

Monitoring body temperature is a basic skill necessary in nursing and medical decision making. When heat production exceeds heat loss and body temperature rises above the normal range, pyrexia (fever) occurs. Pyrexia can accompany any inflammatory response, loss of body fluid, or prolonged exposure to high temperatures. When

(Continues)

PROCEDURE 29-3 Taking a Temperature (Continued)

the body is exposed to temperatures lower than normal for a prolonged length of time, hypothermia occurs. Hospitalized clients are at particular risk for infection and accompanying fever. Clients are stressed by their presenting conditions, and their bodies are further stressed by the hospital environment; thus, they are more susceptible to the infectious agents found there. Hypothermia generally occurs in response to prolonged exposure to cold weather or as a result of being immersed in cold water. Accurate monitoring and recording of a client's temperature is essential for diagnosis, treatment, and monitoring of the client.

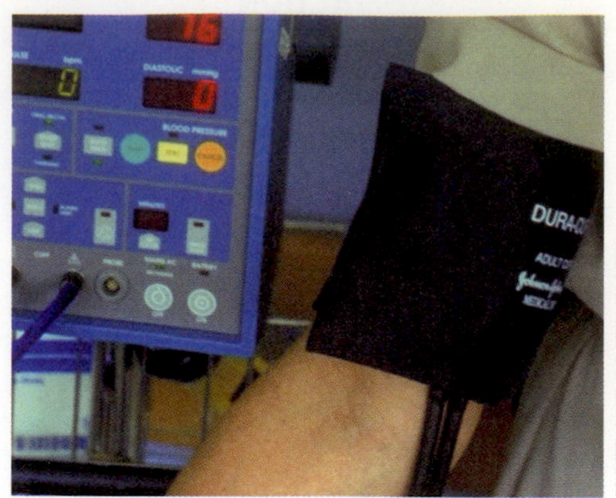

FIGURE 29-3-1 Health care personnel automatically take the T, P, BP, and pulse oximetry with the Dinamap.

ASSESSMENT

1. Assess body temperature for changes when exposed to pyrogens (endogenous or exogenous substances that cause fever) or to extreme hot or cold external environments **because such environments may indicate the cause of an infection.**
2. Assess the client for the most appropriate site to check temperature **to obtain an accurate reading.**
3. Confirm that the client has not consumed hot or cold food or beverage nor smoked for 15 to 30 minutes before the measurement **because these activities may alter the oral reading.**
4. Assess for mouth breathing and tachypnea **because both can cause an inaccurate oral reading.**
5. Assess for oral lesion, especially herpetic lesions, **because herpes viruses are extremely contagious and require implementation of Standard Precautions of the Centers for Disease Control and Prevention. Clients with herpetic lesions should have their own glass thermometer or disposable thermometer to prevent transmission to others.**

POSSIBLE NURSING DIAGNOSES

*Ineffective **H**ealth Maintenance*
*Risk for **I**nfection*
***H**ypothermia*
***H**yperthermia*
*Ineffective **T**hermoregulation*
*Deficient **F**luid Volume*
*Risk for Imbalanced **B**ody Temperature*

PLANNING

Expected Outcomes

1. An accurate temperature reading will be obtained.
2. The client will verbalize understanding of the reason for the procedure.

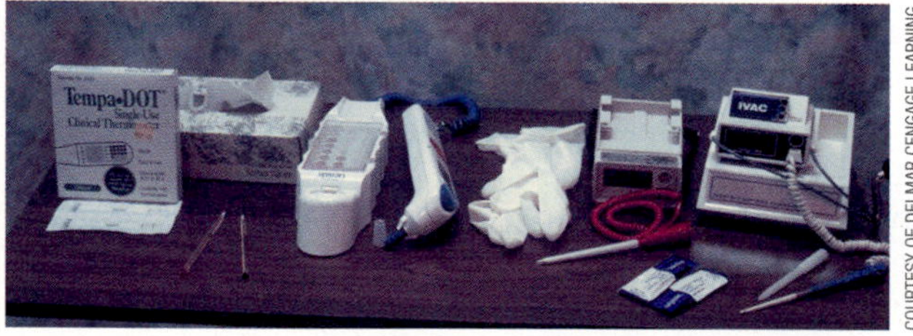

FIGURE 29-3-2 Various types of thermometers are used to take a client's temperature.

Equipment Needed (Figure 29-3-2)

- Vital signs automatic measurement device (Dinamap) or manual thermometer (one of the following)
  - — Electronic thermometer with disposable protective sheath
  - — Tympanic membrane thermometer with probe cover
  - — Disposable, single-use chemical strip thermometer
  - — Glass (mercury free): oral or rectal at client's bedside, usually color coded to avoid cross use
- Lubricant for rectal and glass thermometer
- Two pairs of nonsterile gloves
- Tissues

(Continues)

PROCEDURE 29-3 Taking a Temperature (Continued)

delegation tips

The skill of temperature measurement is often delegated to ancillary personnel; however, the nurse retains responsibility for knowledge of the client's temperature and appropriate actions. The expectation is that ancillary personnel will have documented instruction and competency validation of their ability to:

- *Select the correct route for measurement of the temperature.*
- *Correctly position the client for measurement.*
- *Correctly perform the measurement according to established guidelines and record on the appropriate flow sheet (clinical record).*
- *Recognize and report abnormal findings to the nurse.*

IMPLEMENTATION—ACTION/RATIONALE

* Check client's identification band * Explain procedure before beginning *

ACTION	RATIONALE
1. Review medical record for baseline data and factors that influence vital signs.	1. Establishes baseline, provides direction in device selection, and helps determine site to use for measurement. Vital signs are measured in the order of temperature, pulse, and respiration (TPR); blood pressure (BP); and pulse oximetry, usually without interruptions, to provide the nurse with an objective clinical database to direct decision making.
2. Explain to the client that vital signs will be assessed. Encourage the client to remain still and refrain from drinking, eating, and smoking, and to avoid mouth breathing, if possible. Do not take vital signs within 30 minutes of the client drinking, eating, or smoking, as these activities give false readings.	2. Encourages participation, allays anxiety, and ensures accurate measurements. Cold or hot liquids and smoking alter circulation and body temperature. Mouth breathing can alter temperature.
3. Assess client's toileting needs and proceed as appropriate.	3. Prevents interruptions during measurements, communicates caring, and promotes client comfort.
4. Gather equipment.	4. Facilitates organization and establishes client trust when the health care worker is prepared and does not have to leave the room for supplies multiple times.
5. Provide for privacy.	5. Decreases embarrassment.
6. Wash hands and apply gloves when appropriate.	6. Hands are washed before and after every contact with a client to reduce the transmission of microorganisms. Gloves are worn to avoid contact with bodily secretions and to reduce transmission of microorganisms.
Oral Temperature—Electronic Thermometer	
7. Repeat Actions 1 to 6.	7. See Rationales 1 to 6.
8. Place disposable protective sheath over probe.	8. Reduces transmission of microorganisms.
9. Grasp top of the probe's stem. Avoid placing pressure on the ejection button (Figure 29-3-3).	9. Pressure on the ejection button releases the sheath from the probe.
10. Place tip of thermometer under the client's tongue and along the gumline to the posterior sublingual pocket lateral to center of lower jaw (Figure 29-3-4).	10. Sublingual pocket contains superficial blood vessels.
11. Instruct client to keep mouth closed around thermometer.	11. Maintains thermometer in proper place and decreases amount of time required for an accurate reading.
12. Thermometer will signal (beep) when a constant temperature registers (Figure 29-3-5).	12. Signal indicates final temperature reading.

(Continues)

PROCEDURE 29-3 Taking a Temperature (Continued)

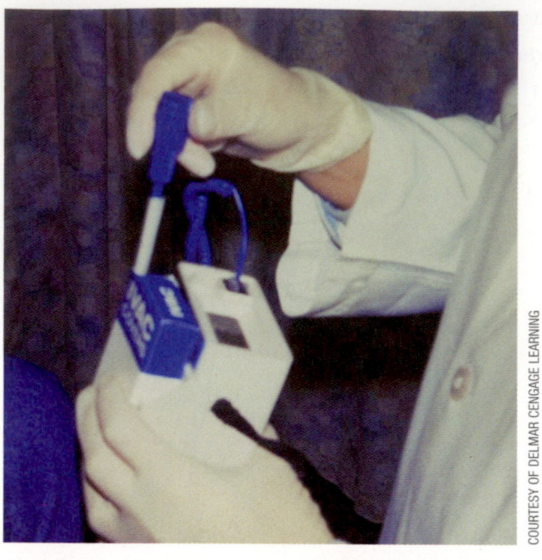

FIGURE 29-3-3 Place disposable protective sheath over probe.

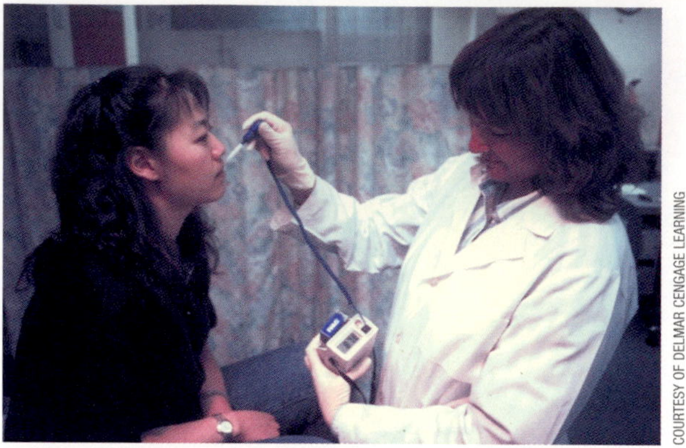

FIGURE 29-3-4 Place probe tip in the posterior sublingual pocket.

ACTION	RATIONALE
13. Read measurement on digital display of electronic thermometer. Push ejection button to discard disposable sheath into receptacle and return probe to storage well.	13. Reduces transmission of microorganisms. Ensures that the electronic system is ready for next use.
14. Inform client of temperature reading.	14. Promotes client's participation in care.
15. Remove gloves and wash hands.	15. Reduces transmission of microorganisms.
16. Record reading according to institution policies.	16. Accurate documentation by site allows for comparison of data.
17. Return electronic thermometer unit to charging base, checking that it is plugged in.	17. Ensures charging base is plugged into electrical outlet and thermometer is ready for next use.
18. Wash hands.	18. Reduces transmission of microorganisms.
Tympanic Temperature: Infrared Thermometer	
19. Repeat Actions 1 to 6.	19. See Rationales 1 to 6.
20. Position client in Sims' or sitting position.	20. Promotes access to ear.
21. Remove probe from container and attach probe cover to tympanic thermometer unit (Figure 29-3-6).	21. Prevents contamination.

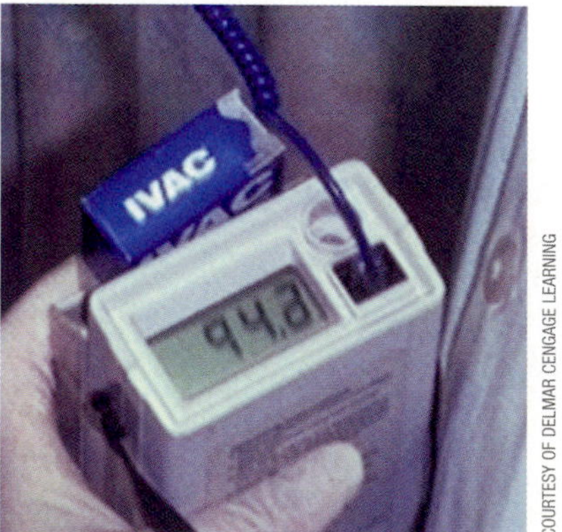

FIGURE 29-3-5 Listen for audible beep signal when temperature registers.

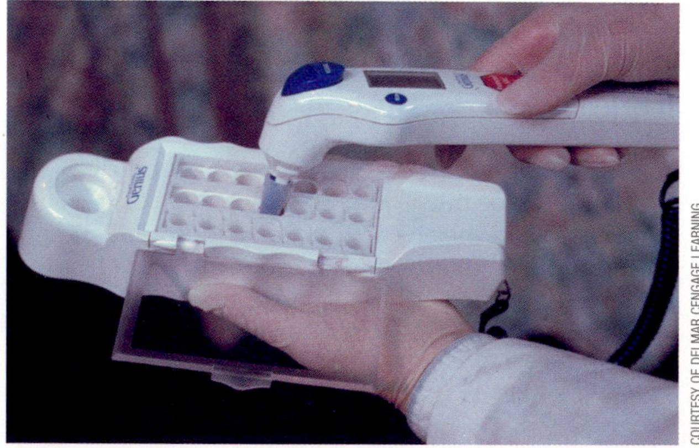

FIGURE 29-3-6 Attach disposable probe cover to unit.

(Continues)

PROCEDURE 29-3 Taking a Temperature (Continued)

ACTION	RATIONALE
22. Turn client's head to one side. For an adult, pull pinna upward and back; for a child, pull down and back. Gently insert probe with firm pressure into ear canal (Figure 29-3-7).	22. Provides access to ear canal. Gentle insertion prevents trauma to external canal. Firm pressure is needed to ensure probe will record an accurate temperature.
23. Remove probe after the reading is displayed on digital unit (usually 2 seconds).	23. Reading is displayed within seconds.
24. Discard probe cover into receptacle and replace probe in storage container.	24. Reduces transmission of microorganisms. Protects reusable probe from damage.
25. Return tympanic thermometer to storage unit.	25. Recharges batteries of unit for future use.
26. Record reading according to institution policy.	26. Promotes accurate documentation for data comparison.
27. Wash hands.	27. Reduces transmission of microorganisms.
Using a "Tempa-Dot"	
28. Repeat Actions 1 to 6.	28. See Rationales 1 to 6.
29. Position the client in a sitting or lying position.	29. Promotes client's comfort, and promotes site access for temperature measurement.
30. Prepare Tempa-Dot according to directions (Figure 29-3-8). • Oral measurement: Place Tempa-Dot under tongue as far back as possible. Have client press tongue down on thermometer and keep mouth closed for 60 seconds. Remove thermometer; read the last blue dot; ignore any skipped dot. • Axillary measurement: Place thermometer high in the armpit, vertical to the body, with dots against the torso. Lower client's arm to hold thermometer in place. Remove thermometer after 3 minutes.	30. Promotes accurate measurement and client safety.
31. Record temperature, indicate the method, and discard the thermometer.	31. Nursing documentation, practice clean technique.
32. Wash hands.	32. Reduces transmission of microorganisms.

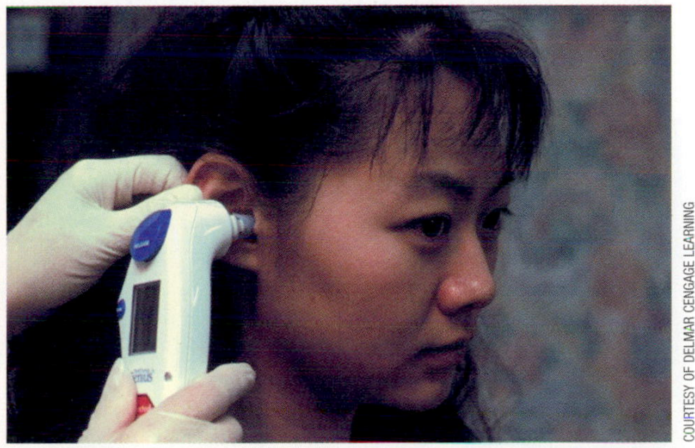

COURTESY OF DELMAR CENGAGE LEARNING

FIGURE 29-3-7 Insert temperature probe into ear canal.

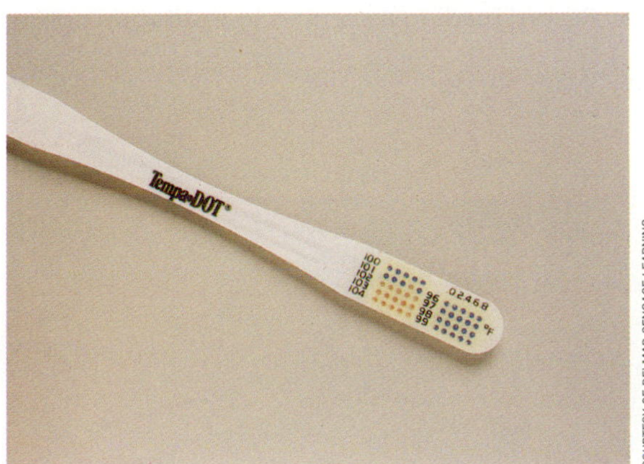

COURTESY OF DELMAR CENGAGE LEARNING

FIGURE 29-3-8 "Tempa-Dot" Single-Use Disposable Thermometer

(Continues)

PROCEDURE 29-3 Taking a Temperature (Continued)

ACTION	RATIONALE
Oral Temperature: Plastic Thermometer	
A glass thermometer is not generally used. Mercury glass thermometers are no longer recommended for use (National Institutes of Health, 2008).	
33. Repeat Actions 1 to 6.	33. See Rationales 1 to 6.
34. Select correct color tip of thermometer from client's bedside container (Figure 29-3-9).	34. Identifies correct device; a blue tip usually denotes an oral thermometer.
35. Remove thermometer from storage container, hold at end away from bulb and rinse under cool water.	35. Cleansing removes disinfectant, which can irritate oral mucosa. Cool water prevents expansion of the colored solution. Touching the bulb will heat the solution and cause an inaccurate reading.
36. Use a tissue to dry thermometer from bulb's end toward fingertips.	36. Wipe from area of least contamination to most contaminated area.
37. Read thermometer by locating colored solution level. It should read 35.5°C (96°F).	37. Thermometer must be below normal body temperature to ensure an accurate reading.
38. If thermometer is not below normal body temperature reading, grasp thermometer with thumb and forefinger and shake vigorously by snapping the wrist in a downward motion to move colored solution to a level below normal.	38. Shaking briskly lowers level of colored solution in column. Because glass thermometers break easily, make sure that nothing in the environment comes in contact with the thermometer when shaking it.
39. Place thermometer in client's mouth under the tongue and along the gumline to the posterior sublingual pocket. Instruct client to hold lips closed (Figure 29-3-10).	39. Ensures contact with large blood vessels under the tongue. Prevents environmental air from coming in contact with the bulb.
40. Leave in place as specified by institution policy, usually 3 to 5 minutes.	40. Thermometer must stay in place long enough to ensure an accurate reading.
41. Remove thermometer and wipe with a tissue away from fingers toward the bulb's end (Figure 29-3-11).	41. Mucus on thermometer may interfere with the effectiveness of the disinfectant solution. Wipe from area of least contamination to most contaminated area.
42. Read at eye level and rotate slowly until colored solution level is visualized.	42. Ensures an accurate reading.
43. Shake thermometer down, cleanse glass thermometer with soapy water, rinse under cold water, and return to storage container.	43. Mechanical cleansing removes secretions that promote growth of microorganisms. Hot water may cause coagulation of secretions and cause expansion of colored solution in the thermometer.
44. Remove and dispose of gloves in receptacle. Wash hands.	44. Reduces transmission of microorganisms.
45. Record reading according to institution policy.	45. Accurate documentation by site allows for comparison of data.
46. Wash hands.	46. Reduces transmission of microorganisms.

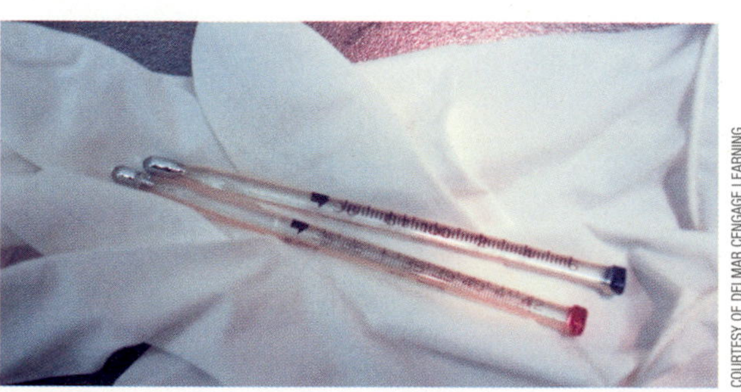

COURTESY OF DELMAR CENGAGE LEARNING

FIGURE 29-3-9 Oral (blue tip) and Rectal (red tip) Glass Thermometer

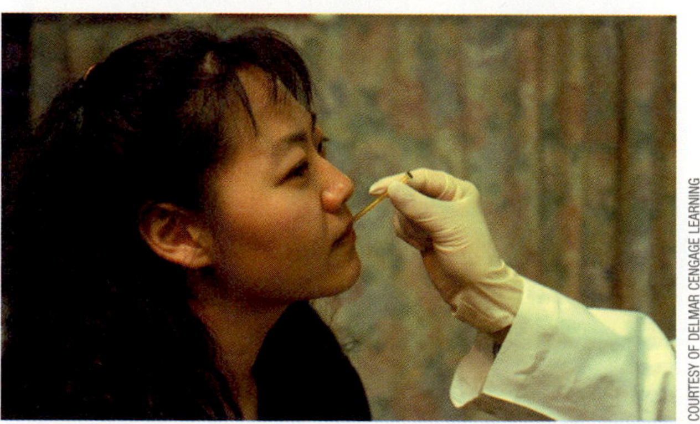

COURTESY OF DELMAR CENGAGE LEARNING

FIGURE 29-3-10 Place bulb of thermometer in the posterior sublingual pocket. Have client close lips around thermometer.

(Continues)

PROCEDURE 29-3 Taking a Temperature (Continued)

ACTION	RATIONALE
Rectal Temperature	
47. Repeat Actions 1 to 6.	47. See Rationales 1 to 6.
48. Place client in the Sims' position with upper knee flexed. Adjust sheet to expose only anal area.	48. Proper positioning ensures visualization of anus. Flexing knee relaxes muscles for ease of insertion.
49. Place tissues in easy reach. Apply gloves.	49. Tissue is needed to wipe anus after device is removed.
50. Prepare the thermometer.	50. Ensures a smooth procedure and an accurate reading.
51. Lubricate sheath or probe covering tip of rectal thermometer. (A rectal thermometer usually has a red tip or cap.)	51. Promotes ease of insertion of thermometer or probe.
52. With dominant hand, grasp thermometer. With other hand, separate buttocks to expose anus (Figure 29-3-12).	52. Aids in visualization of anus.
53. Instruct the client to take a deep breath. Insert the thermometer or probe gently into anus: infant, 1.2 cm (0.5 inches); adult, 3.5 cm (1.5 inches). If resistance is felt, do not force insertion.	53. Relaxes anal sphincter. Gentle insertion decreases discomfort to client and prevents trauma to mucous membranes.
54. Hold plastic thermometer in place for 3 to 5 minutes. If taking the rectal temperature with an electronic probe, remove it after the reading is displayed on digital unit (usually 2 seconds).	54. Prevents trauma to mucosa and breakage of glass thermometer.
55. Wipe off secretions on the glass thermometer with a tissue. Dispose of tissue in a receptacle.	55. Removes secretions and fecal material for visualization of mercury level. Prevents transmission of microorganisms.
56. Read measurement and inform the client of the temperature reading.	56. Promotes client's participation in care.
57. While holding glass thermometer in one hand, use other hand to wipe anal area with tissue to remove lubricant or feces. Dispose of soiled tissue. Cover client.	57. Prevents contamination of clean objects with soiled thermometer, decreases skin irritation, and promotes client comfort. Prevents embarrassment.
58. Wash thermometer.	58. Reduces transmission of microorganisms.
59. Remove and dispose of gloves in receptacle. Wash hands.	59. Reduces transmission of microorganisms.
60. Record reading according to institution policy.	60. Accurate documentation by site allows for comparison of data.

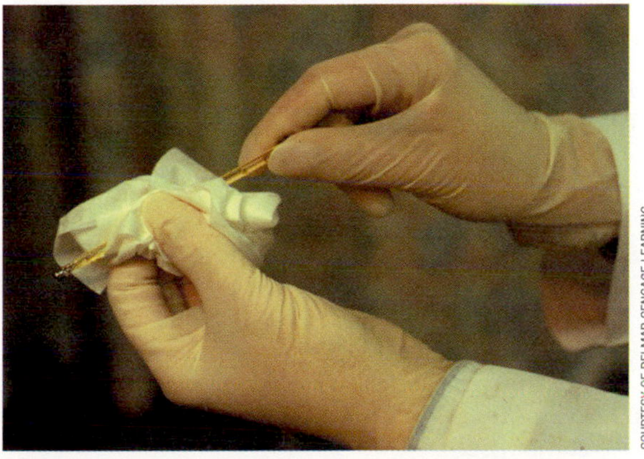

COURTESY OF DELMAR CENGAGE LEARNING

FIGURE 29-3-11 Wipe the thermometer with a tissue from fingertips to bulb end.

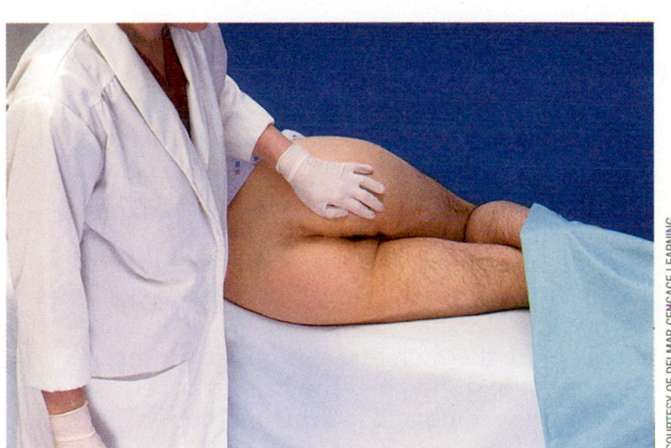

COURTESY OF DELMAR CENGAGE LEARNING

FIGURE 29-3-12 Preparation for the insertion of a rectal thermometer.

(Continues)

PROCEDURE 29-3 Taking a Temperature (Continued)

ACTION	RATIONALE
Axillary Temperature	
61. Repeat Actions 1 to 6.	61. See Rationales 1 to 6.
62. Remove client's arm and shoulder from one sleeve of gown. Avoid exposing chest.	62. Exposes axillary area.
63. Make sure axillary skin is dry; if necessary, pat dry.	63. Removes moisture and prevents a false low reading.
64. Prepare thermometer.	64. Ensures accurate use of thermometer.
65. Place thermometer or probe into center of axilla. Fold the client's upper arm straight down, and place arm across the client's chest. On a thin client, make sure flesh rather than a hollow armpit surrounds the thermometer or probe.	65. Puts device in contact with axillary blood supply. Maintains the device in proper position.
66. Leave glass thermometer in place as specified by institution policy (usually 6 to 8 minutes). Leave an electronic thermometer in place until signal is heard.	66. Device must stay in place long enough to ensure an accurate reading. Signal indicates final temperature reading.
67. Remove and read thermometer.	67. Allows accurate reading of temperature.
68. Inform client of temperature reading.	68. Promotes client's participation in care.
69. If using a thermometer, shake down the solution. Wash glass thermometer with soapy water, rinse under cold water, and return to storage container. If using an electronic thermometer, push ejection button to discard disposable sheath into receptacle and return probe to storage well.	69. Prevents breakage of glass thermometer and transmission of microorganisms. Removing the disposable sheath reduces transmission of microorganisms and ensures that the electronic system is ready for next use.
70. Assist the client with replacing the gown.	70. Promotes comfort.
71. Record reading according to institution policy.	71. Promotes accurate documentation for data comparison.
72. Wash hands.	72. Reduces transmission of microorganisms.
Disposable (Chemical Strip) Thermometer	
73. Repeat Actions 1 to 6.	73. See Rationales 1 to 6.
74. Apply tape to appropriate skin area, usually forehead.	74. Tape must be in direct contact with the client's skin.
75. Observe tape for color changes.	75. Color indicates temperature reading (refer to the manufacturer's instructions).
76. Record reading and indicate method.	76. Promotes accurate documentation for data comparison.
77. Wash hands.	77. Reduces transmission of microorganisms.
Noninvasive Temporal Artery Scan Thermometer (Temporal Scanner)	
78. Repeat Actions 1 to 6.	78. See Rationales 1 to 6.
79. Locate the client's exposed temporal artery.	79. The temporal artery has an accurate arterial temperature because the vessel has little vasomotor control and a reliable rate of perfusion (Exergen Corporation, 2009).
80. Place the thermometer sensor head in the center of the forehead halfway between the eyebrows and the hairline.	80. The scanner crosses the temporal artery by scanning across half of the forehead.
81. Slide the thermometer straight across the forehead, stopping at the hairline.	81. Maintain direct contact with the skin for an accurate reading.
82. Record reading and indicate method.	82. Promotes accurate documentation for data comparison.
83. Wash hands.	83. Reduces transmission of microorganisms.

(Continues)

PROCEDURE 29-3 Taking a Temperature (Continued)

ACTION	RATIONALE

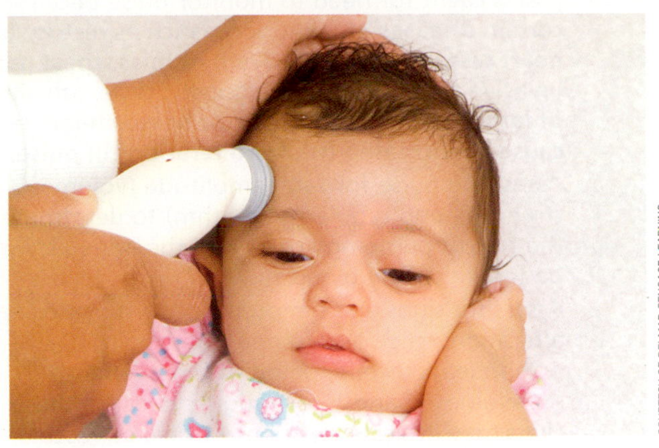

FIGURE 29-3-13 The child's temperature is taken with a temporal artery thermometer.

EVALUATION

- Establish client's baseline temperature.
- Compare temperature with the client's baseline temperature.
- Evaluate the client's condition for trauma caused by the instrument.

DOCUMENTATION

Vital Signs Flow Sheet or Electronic Medical Record

- Temperature measurement and site
- If using a paper flow sheet, plot the temperature on a graph to identify patterns, or sudden elevations and drops (a condition known as spiking). If the facility uses electronic medical records, enter the vital signs in the computer.

Medication Administration Record

- Antipyretic (fever-reducing) medications and temperature reading

Nurses' Notes

- Response to antipyretic medications

PROCEDURE 29-4 Taking a Pulse

OVERVIEW

A pulse is the number of heart beats in 1 minute. Pulse assessment is the measurement of a pressure pulsation created when the heart contracts and ejects blood into the aorta. Assessment of pulse characteristics provides clinical data regarding the heart's pumping action and the adequacy of peripheral artery blood flow. The radial pulse is most often used for basic assessment; however, other site areas are used in total assessment and when determining circulation to specific areas. Pulse rate is an indirect measurement of cardiac output obtained by counting the number of peripheral pulse waves over a pulse point. A normal pulse rate for adults is between 60 and 100 beats per minute. Pulse rhythm is the regularity of the heartbeat. It indicates how evenly the heart is beating. Pulse amplitude (also called pulse strength or volume) is a measurement of the strength or force exerted by the blood against the arterial wall with each heart contraction. It is described as normal (full, easily palpable), weak (thready and usually rapid), or strong (bounding).

PULSE-TAKING TECHNIQUES

Palpation

- Palpation of a pulse involves the index and middle fingers of one hand. Start with gentle pressure to locate the strongest pulsation and then use firmer palpation for the counting. When counting, also assess the rhythm and quality of the pulse. Measure the pulse for 30 and 60 seconds and then multiply the counts if need be to obtain the 1-minute reading.

(Continues)

PROCEDURE 29-4 Taking a Pulse (Continued)

Auscultation

- Auscultation is usually used to assess the apical pulse. The apical pulse is the most accurate pulse, especially when the peripheral pulse is difficult to locate. Auscultation requires the stethoscope. The stethoscope is equipped with a bell and a diaphragm. The diaphragm side is normally used for low-pitch sound, such as normal heart sound, bowel sound, or breath sound; the bell side is used for high-pitch sound, such as murmur and abnormal heart sound.

Doppler

- An ultrasonic Doppler device is used when the pulse cannot be detected by palpation. The Doppler detects the peripheral pulses in situations such as cardiopulmonary collapse in obese clients, infants with small arms, or clients with edema or peripheral vascular disease in which palpation of the pulse is difficult.
- A vendor-recommended conductive gel be applied to the skin as a coupling medium for ultrasound transmission. The transmitting device (probe) is then placed over the artery assessed. The Doppler usually is equipped with both high- and low-frequency probes. A high-frequency (8 to 10 Hz) probe is usually used on the surface vessel sites. A low-frequency (2 to 3 Hz) probe often is used for deeper sites, such as obstetric assessment.
- The sounds are amplified and heard through an earpiece or speaker attached to the device, assessing with low volume initially. Tilt the back of the probe toward the hand at an angle of about 45 degrees. Search the area of the assessed artery and tilt the probe for best Doppler sounds. Adjust the sound volume control to a comfort level for counting.

ASSESSMENT

1. Assess client for need to monitor pulse **because certain diseases or conditions, such as history of heart disease or cardiac dysrhythmias, chest pain, invasive cardiovascular diagnostic tests, infusion of large volume of IV fluids, or hemorrhage, can cause an increased risk for alterations in pulse.**
2. Assess the pulse for rate, amplitude (volume, strength), and regularity (rhythm) to determine the heart's pumping action and the adequacy of peripheral artery blood flow.
3. Assess for signs and symptoms of cardiovascular alterations, such as dyspnea, chest pain, orthopnea, syncope, palpitations, edema of extremities, cyanosis, or fatigue, **because these signs may indicate deficient cardiac or vascular function.**
4. Assess client for factors that may affect the character of the pulse, such as age, medications, exercise, change in position, or fever. **This enables the nurse to accurately assess for the significance of an alteration in pulse.**
5. Assess for the appropriate site for measuring pulse **so the pulse will be accurate.**
6. Assess the baseline heart rate and rhythm in the client's chart **to compare it with the current measurement.**
7. Assess circulatory status by using appropriate site (Table 29-4-1) **because pulses may be affected by surgery, medical condition, arterial blood draws, or poor circulation.**

POSSIBLE NURSING DIAGNOSES

Decreased Cardiac Output
Ineffective Peripheral Tissue Perfusion

TABLE 29-4-1 Pulse Point Assessment

PULSE POINT	LOCATION	ASSESSMENT CRITERIA
1. Temporal	Over the temporal bone, lateral to the eye, upper to the ear	Accessible; used routinely for infants and when radial is inaccessible
2. Carotid	Bilateral, under the lower jaw, beneath the sternomastoid muscles. Carotid pulse best represents the aortic pulse for its close location to the central circulation. Palpation of the carotid artery on the neck may cause stimulation of the carotid sinus and result in decrease of the pulse rate	Accessible; used routinely for infants and during shock or cardiac arrest when other peripheral pulses are too weak to palpate; also used to assess cranial circulation Take a carotid pulse on only one side of the neck at a time (Figure 29-4-1)
3 Apical	Left ventricle, fourth to fifth intercostal space, on the midclavicular line	Used to auscultate heart sounds and assess apical-radial deficit

(Continues)

PROCEDURE 29-4 Taking a Pulse (Continued)

TABLE 29-4-1 Pulse Point Assessment (Continued)

PULSE POINT	LOCATION	ASSESSMENT CRITERIA
4. Brachial	Inner side between the groove of bicep and tricep muscles at the antecubital fossa	Used in cardiac arrest for infants, to assess lower arm circulation, and to auscultate blood pressure
5. Radial	On the thumb side, inner aspect of the wrist	Accessible; used routinely in adults to assess character of peripheral pulse
6. Ulnar	On the little finger side, outer aspect of the wrist	Used to assess circulation to ulnar side of hand and to perform the Allen test
7. Femoral	Below the inguinal ligament, in the anterior medial aspect of the thigh, midway to the anterior-superior iliac spine and symphysis pubis	Used to assess circulation to legs and during cardiac arrest
8. Popliteal	Behind the knee. Medial or lateral to the popliteal fossa	Used to assess circulation to legs and to auscultate leg blood pressure
9. Posterior Tibial	Inner side of the ankle, between the Achilles tendon and tibia	Used to assess circulation to feet
10. Pedal/Dorsal Pedal	Lateral to the extension tendon, from the great toe toward the ankle or between the first and second metatarsal bones on the dorsum (upper) part of the foot (General Practice Notebook, 2009)	Used to assess circulation to feet

COURTESY OF DELMAR CENGAGE LEARNING

PLANNING

Expected Outcomes

1. Pulse rate, quality, rhythm, and volume will be within normal range for the client's age group.
2. The client will be comfortable with the procedure and demonstrate an understanding regarding its importance.

Equipment Needed

- Vital signs automatic measurement device (Dinamap) or watch with a second hand or digital display
- Stethoscope
- Alcohol swab
- Gloves

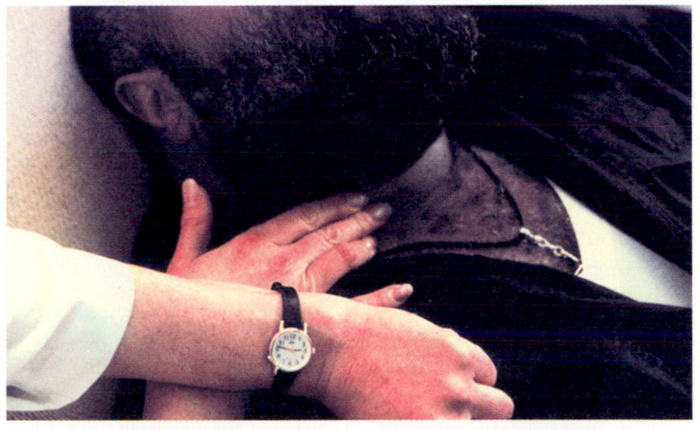

COURTESY OF DELMAR CENGAGE LEARNING

FIGURE 29-4-1 Take a carotid pulse on only one side of the neck at a time.

delegation tips

The radial pulse assessment is often delegated to trained ancillary personnel; however, the nurse is responsible for knowing the results. Assessment of the apical pulse may be delegated to specially prepared staff. The assessment of peripheral circulation is delegated after proper training in the monitoring of peripheral sites for the presence of abnormal color, motion, or sensation in the extremity. The absence of pulses is immediately reported for further assessment by the nurse, and the nurse is responsible for reviewing the data collected in a timely manner and revalidating the results, if indicated. The institution's policy should clearly indicate the training and validation requirements before the nurse delegates the monitoring of apical pulses and peripheral vascular assessments on stable clients. These tasks should not be delegated if the client is unstable.

(Continues)

PROCEDURE 29-4 Taking a Pulse (Continued)

IMPLEMENTATION—ACTION/RATIONALE

ACTION	RATIONALE
* Check client's identification band * Explain procedure before beginning *	
Taking a Radial (Wrist) Pulse	
1. Wash hands.	1. Reduces transmission of microorganisms.
2. Inform client of the site(s) at which you will measure pulse.	2. Encourages participation and allays anxiety.
3. Flex client's elbow and place lower part of arm across chest.	3. Maintains wrist in full extension and exposes artery for palpation. Placing client's hand over chest will facilitate later respiratory assessment without undue attention to your action. (It is difficult for any person to maintain a normal breathing pattern when someone is observing and measuring.)
4. Support client's wrist by grasping outer aspect with thumb.	4. Stabilizes wrist and allows for pressure to be exerted.
5. Place your index and middle fingers on inner aspect of client's wrist over the radial artery and apply light but firm pressure until pulse is palpated (Figure 29-4-2).	5. Fingertips are sensitive, facilitating palpation of pulsating pulse. The nurse may feel his or her own pulse if palpating with thumb. Applying light pressure prevents occlusion of blood flow and pulsation.
6. Identify pulse rhythm or regularity.	6. Palpate pulse until rhythm is determined. Describe as regular or irregular.
7. Determine pulse volume or amplitude.	7. Quality of pulse strength is an indication of stroke volume. Describe as normal, weak, strong, or bounding.
8. Count pulse rate by using second hand on watch. For a regular rhythm, count number of beats for 30 seconds and multiply by 2. For an irregular rhythm, count number of beats for a full minute, noting number of irregular beats.	8. An irregular rhythm requires a full minute of assessment to identify the number of inefficient cardiac contractions that fail to transmit a pulsation, referred to as a "skipped" or irregular beat.
Taking an Apical Pulse	
9. Wash hands.	9. Reduces transmission of microorganisms.
10. Raise client's gown to expose sternum and left side of chest.	10. Allows access to client's chest for proper placement of stethoscope.
11. Cleanse earpiece and diaphragm of stethoscope with an alcohol swab.	11. Decreases transmission of microorganisms from one health care practitioner to another (earpiece) and from one client to another (diaphragm).

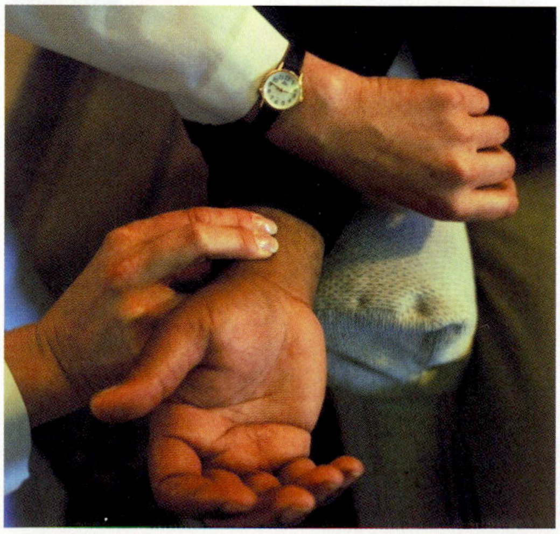

COURTESY OF DELMAR CENGAGE LEARNING

FIGURE 29-4-2 Place index and middle finger over radial artery and apply light but firm pressure until pulse is palpated.

(Continues)

PROCEDURE 29-4 Taking a Pulse (Continued)

ACTION	RATIONALE

TABLE 29-4-2 3-Point And 4-Point Scales for Measuring Pulse Volume

3-POINT SCALE		4-POINT SCALE	
SCALE	DESCRIPTION OF PULSE	SCALE	DESCRIPTION OF PULSE
0	Absent	0	Absent
1+	Thready/weak	1+	Thready/weak
2+	Normal	2+	Normal
3+	Bounding	3+	Increased
		4+	Bounding

COURTESY OF DELMAR CENGAGE LEARNING

12. Put stethoscope around your neck.

12. Ensures stethoscope is nearby for frequent use.

13. Locate apex of heart:
    - With client lying on left side, palpate and locate suprasternal notch.
    - Then, move to the left of the sternum and palpate for the second intercostal space. Palpate second intercostal space to left of sternum.
    - Place index finger in intercostal space, counting downward until fifth intercostal space is located.
    - Move index finger along fourth intercostal space left of the sternal border and to the fifth intercostal space, on the midclavicular line to palpate the apical impulse, called the point of maximal impulse (PMI) by some practitioners (Figure 29-4-3).
    - Keep index finger of nondominant hand on the apical impulse.

13. Identification of landmarks facilitates correct placement of the stethoscope at the fifth intercostal space in order to hear apical impulse.
    - Ensures correct placement of stethoscope.

14. Inform client that you are going to listen to his or her heart. Instruct client to remain silent.

14. Elicits client support. Stethoscope amplifies noise.

15. With dominant hand, put earpiece of the stethoscope in your ears and grasp diaphragm of the stethoscope in palm of your hand for 5 to 10 seconds.

15. Dominant hand facilitates psychomotor dexterity for placement of earpiece with one hand. Heat warms metal or plastic diaphragm and prevents startling client.

16. Place diaphragm of stethoscope over the apical impulse and auscultate for sounds S1 and S2 to hear lub-dub sound (Figure 29-4-4).

16. Movement of blood through the heart valves creates S1 and S2 sounds. Listen for a regular rhythm (heartbeats are evenly spaced) before counting.

17. Note regularity of rhythm.

17. Establishment of a rhythmic pattern determines length of time to count the heartbeats to ensure accurate measurement.

18. Start to count while looking at second hand or digital display of watch. Count lub-dub sound as one beat:
    - For a regular rhythm, count rate for 30 seconds and multiply by 2.
    - For an irregular rhythm, count rate for a full minute, noting number of irregular beats.

18. Ensures sufficient time to count irregular beats.

19. Share your findings with client.

19. Promotes client participation in care.

(Continues)

PROCEDURE 29-4 Taking a Pulse (Continued)

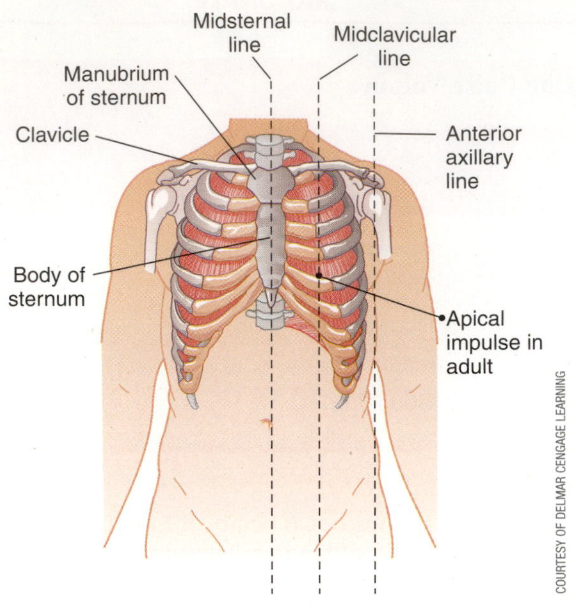

FIGURE 29-4-3 The apical impulse (still called PMI by some practitioners) is located along the fourth intercostal space left of the sternal border and to the fifth intercostal space on the midclavicular line.

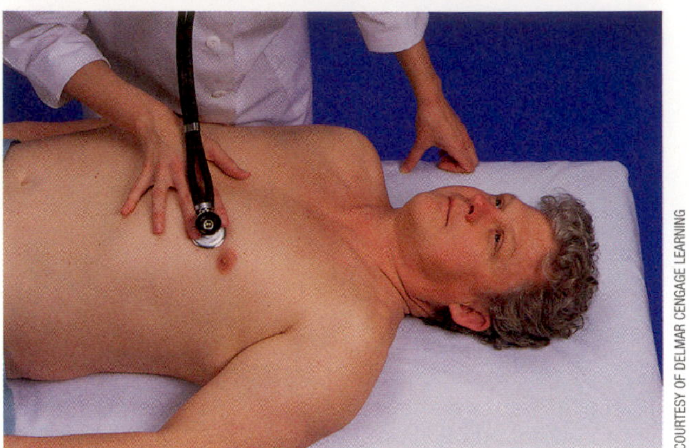

FIGURE 29-4-4 Place diaphragm of stethoscope over the apical impulse to hear the heart rate.

20. Record by site the rate, rhythm, and, if applicable, number of irregular beats.
21. Wash hands.

20. Record rate and characteristics at bedside to ensure accurate documentation.
21. Reduces transmission of microorganisms

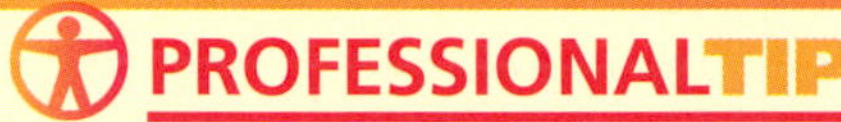

PMI versus Apical Impulse

The term *point of maximal impulse* (PMI) is not used as frequently because a cardiac abnormality can cause a stronger impulse in a different area. Therefore, the mitral landmark is now called the apical impulse (Estes, 2010).

EVALUATION

- Compare client's pulse with baseline rate, amplitude (volume, strength), and rhythm (regularity) to detect any changes.
- If pulse is irregular or abnormal, ask another nurse to check the pulse and then report to health care provider.
- Evaluate pulse site as required by client's condition and compare bilateral pulses. Example: For clients with poor peripheral circulation in the lower extremities, compare both pedal/dorsal or both posterior tibial pulses.

DOCUMENTATION

Nurses' Notes and/or Flow Sheet or Electronic Medical Record

- Pulse rate
- Observations regarding regularity, volume, or rate
- New irregularities in pulse reported to the client's health care provider

PROCEDURE 29-5 Counting Respirations

OVERVIEW

Respiratory assessment is the measurement of the breathing pattern. Assessment of respirations provides clinical data regarding the pH of arterial blood.

Normal breathing is slightly observable, effortless, quiet, automatic, and regular. It can be assessed by observing chest wall expansion and bilateral symmetric movement of the thorax or by placing the back of the hand next to the client's nose and mouth to feel the expired air.

When assessing respiration, ascertain the rate, depth, and rhythm of ventilatory movement. Assess the rate by counting the number of breaths taken per minute. Note the depth and rhythm of ventilatory movements by observing for the normal thoracic and abdominal movements and symmetry in chest wall movement. Normal respirations are characterized by a rate ranging from 12 to 20 breaths per minute.

One inspiration and expiration cycle is counted as one breath. The nurse can observe the rise and fall of the chest wall and count the rate by placing the hand lightly on the chest to feel it rise and fall (Figure 29-5-1). Count the number of respirations for a 30-second interval and multiply by 2 if respirations are regular and even. If the client is experiencing any respiratory difficulty, count the rate for a full minute.

Also observe alterations in the movement of the chest wall: Costal (thoracic) breathing occurs when the external intercostal muscles and the other accessory muscles are used to move the chest upward and outward; diaphragmatic (abdominal) breathing occurs when the diaphragm contracts and relaxes as observed by movement of the abdomen. Dyspnea refers to difficulty in breathing as observed by labored or forced respirations through the use of accessory muscles in the chest and neck to breathe. Dyspneic clients are acutely aware of their respirations and complain of shortness of breath.

Respiratory alterations may cause changes in skin color as observed by a bluish appearance of the nail beds, lips, and skin. The bluish color (cyanosis) results from reduced oxygen level in the arterial blood. Changes in the level of consciousness (restlessness, anxiety, and dyspnea) may also occur with decreased oxygen level. Clients assume a forward-leaning position or may have to stand to increase the expansion capacity of the lungs.

Metabolic alterations such as diabetic ketoacidosis can cause Kussmaul's respirations, which are abnormally deep but regular.

Apnea is the cessation of breathing for several seconds. Persistent apnea is called respiratory arrest. Irregular rhythm with alternating periods of apnea and hyperventilation is called Cheyne-Stokes respirations. The cycle begins with slow, shallow breaths that gradually increase to abnormally deep and rapid respirations, which then gradually slow and return to shallow breathing followed by apnea. This is common in clients who are dying.

ASSESSMENT

1. Assess the movement of client's chest wall **to see if it is equal bilaterally, if the movement is labored, or if the client is using accessory muscles to breathe.**
2. Assess the rate of respirations **to identify slow, rapid, or irregular respirations or even periods of apnea.**
3. Assess the depth of the client's breaths **to monitor shallow, deep, or uneven respirations. Think if there might be something influencing the client's respirations. Is the client in pain, frightened, talking, or smoking?**
4. Assess for risk factors such as fever, pain, anxiety, diseases, or trauma to the chest wall **that may alter the respirations because certain conditions may cause increased risk of alterations in respirations.**
5. Assess for factors that normally influence respirations such as age, exercise, anxiety, pain, smoking, medications, or postural changes **so that an accurate assessment can be made.**

POSSIBLE NURSING DIAGNOSES

*Impaired **G**as Exchange*
*Impaired Spontaneous **V**entilation*
*Ineffective **A**irway Clearance*
*Ineffective **B**reathing Pattern*

PLANNING

Expected Outcomes

1. An accurate evaluation of a client's respiratory rate and character is obtained.
2. The respiratory rate and character is normal.

Equipment Needed

- Watch with a second hand or digital display
- Stethoscope if needed

delegation tips

The skill of respiratory rate measurement is often delegated to properly trained ancillary personnel; however, the nurse is responsible for this information and appropriate action. Respiration counts over 30 (adult) or 60 (child) should be immediately reported to the nurse for further assessment.

(Continues)

PROCEDURE 29-5 Counting Respirations (Continued)

IMPLEMENTATION—ACTION/RATIONALE

ACTION	RATIONALE
* Check client's identification band * Explain procedure before beginning *	
1. Wash hands.	1. Reduces transmission of microorganisms.
2. Be sure chest movement is visible. Client may need to remove heavy clothing.	2. Facilitates observation of chest wall and abdominal movements.
3. Observe one complete respiratory cycle. If it is easier, place the client's hand across the abdomen and your hand over the client's wrist.	3. Helps determine what constitutes a breath. Helps to determine what to count. Hand rises and falls with inspiration and expiration.
4. Start counting with first inspiration while looking at the second hand of a watch (Figure 29-5-1). • Infants and children: Count a full minute. • Adults: Count for 30 seconds and multiply by 2. If an irregular rate or rhythm is present, count for 1 full minute.	4. Respiratory rate is one complete cycle (inspiration and expiration). • Infants and children usually have an irregular rate.
5. Observe character of respirations: • Depth of respirations by degree of chest wall movement (shallow, normal, or deep) • Rhythm of cycle (regular or interrupted)	5. Reveals volume of air movement into and out of the lungs.
6. Observe skin color and level of consciousness	6. Reveals reduced oxygen level in arterial blood.
7. Replace client's gown if needed.	7. Prevents embarrassment and chilling.
8. Record rate and character of respirations.	8. Record rate and characteristics at bedside to ensure accurate documentation.
9. Wash hands.	9. Reduces transmission of microorganisms.

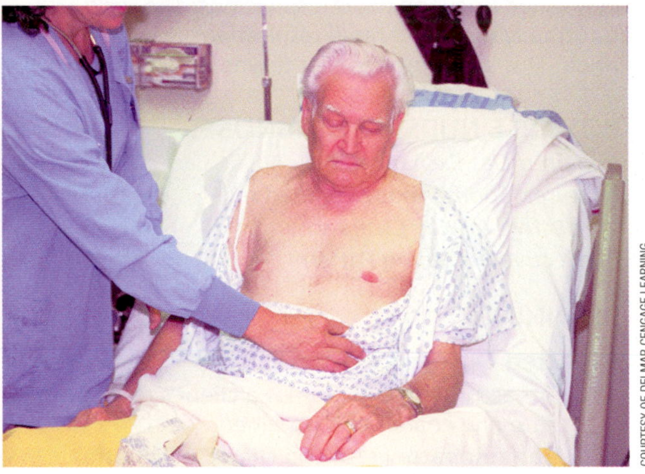

COURTESY OF DELMAR CENGAGE LEARNING

FIGURE 29-5-1 Observe the depth of respirations and rhythm of cycle. Placing the client's hand across the abdomen and your hand over the client's wrist may make counting respirations easier.

EVALUATION

- Evaluate client's respirations as a baseline value.
- Compare respirations with baseline to detect any alterations.

DOCUMENTATION

Vital Signs Flow Sheet or Electronic Medical Record

- Respiratory rate

Nurses' Notes

- Depth, rhythm, and character of respirations
- Respiratory rate outside the normal age range, an irregular rhythm, inadequate depth, or any abnormal characteristics such as dyspnea

PROCEDURE 29-6 Taking Blood Pressure

OVERVIEW

Blood pressure is the pressure exerted on the walls of blood vessels because of cardiac output and volume of circulating blood. Blood pressure measurement is performed during a physical examination, at initial assessment, and as part of routine vital signs assessment. Depending on the client's condition, the blood pressure is measured by either a direct or indirect technique.

The indirect method requires use of the sphygmomanometer and stethoscope for auscultation and palpation as needed. The most common site for indirect blood pressure measurement is the client's arm over the brachial artery. When the client's condition prevents auscultation of the brachial artery, assess the blood pressure in the forearm or leg sites. When pressure measurements in the upper extremities are not accessible, the popliteal artery, located behind the knee, is the site of choice. See Figure 29-6-1 for the location of the artery sites. Blood pressure can also be assessed in other sites, such as the radial artery in the forearm and the posterior tibial or dorsalis pedis artery in the lower leg. Because it is difficult to auscultate sounds over the radial, tibial, and dorsalis pedis arteries, these sites are usually palpated to obtain a systolic reading.

The direct method requires an invasive procedure in which an intravenous catheter with an electronic sensor is inserted into an artery and the artery-transmitted pressure on an electronic display unit is read.

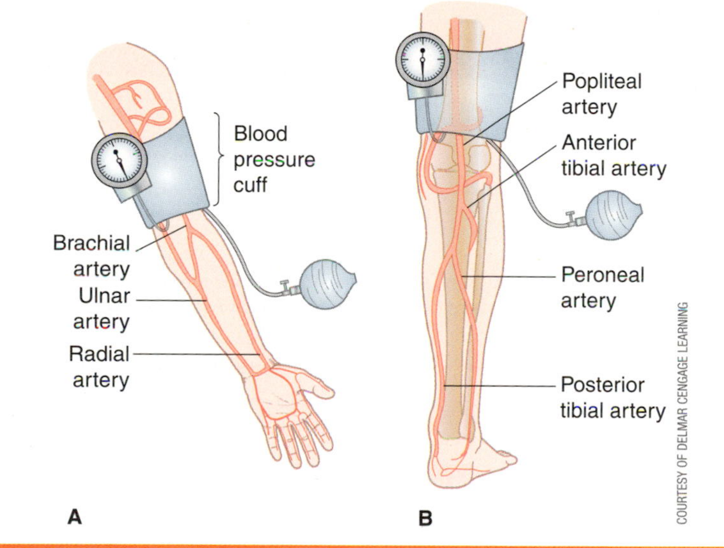

FIGURE 29-6-1A & B: Alternative blood pressure artery sites.

ASSESSMENT

1. Assess the condition of the potential blood pressure (BP) site **so that a site with an injury or surgery proximal to the site can be avoided.**
2. Assess the artery for any compromise to it **so that compressing the artery briefly will not cause decrease in circulation.**
3. Assess the distal pulse **to check if it is intact and palpable.**
4. Assess the circumference of the extremity for the right size cuff **so an accurate reading can be obtained.**
5. Assess for factors that affect blood pressure, such as age, anxiety, fear, medications, smoking, eating, or exercising within 30 minutes before BP assessment, and postural changes **so an accurate reading can be obtained.**
6. Determine client's baseline blood pressure by reading the medical record **so a comparison can be made with each BP reading.**

(Continues)

PROCEDURE 29-6 Taking Blood Pressure (Continued)

POSSIBLE NURSING DIAGNOSES

Ineffective Peripheral Tissue Perfusion
Decreased Cardiac Output
Deficient Knowledge (blood pressure control)

PLANNING

Expected Outcomes

1. An accurate estimate of the arterial pressure at diastole and systole is obtained.
2. Blood pressure is within the expected range for the client.
3. Client understands why the blood pressure is taken and what it means.

Equipment Needed

- Vital signs automatic measurement device (Dinamap) or stethoscope and sphygmomanometer/bladder with aneroid dial
- Gloves, if required
- Alcohol swabs

delegation tips

The measurement of blood pressure is often delegated to ancillary personnel who have been properly educated to use both manual and electronic equipment; however, the nurse is responsible for carefully monitoring this information for significant changes and taking appropriate action. The delegation of blood pressure measurement would be reserved for a client in stable physical condition and measured at sites without intravenous solutions infusing, dialysis shunt or fistula, painful extremity, or recent mastectomy.

TABLE 29-6-1 Classification of Hypertension and Prehypertension from the Joint National Committee on Prevention, Detection, Evaluation, and Treatment of High Blood Pressure

CLASSIFICATION BY BP CATEGORY	SYSTOLIC BP (mm Hg)	DIASTOLIC BP (mm Hg)
Normal	<120	<80
Prehypertension	120–139	80–89
Stage 1 hypertension	140–159	90–99
Stage 2 hypertension	≥160	≥100

BP, Blood Pressure

Pickering, T.G., Hall, J.E., Appel, L.J., Falkner, B.E., Grares, J., Hill, M.N., et al. (2005). Part I: Blood pressure measurement in humans: A statement for professionals from the subcommittee of professional and public education of the American Heart Association Council on high blood pressure research. Hypertension, 45, 142–161.

IMPLEMENTATION—ACTION/RATIONALE

ACTION	RATIONALE
* Check client's identification band * Explain procedure before beginning *	
Asculation Method Using Brachal Artery	
1. Wash hands.	1. Reduces transmission of microorganisms.
2. Determine which extremity is most appropriate for reading. Do not take a pressure reading on an injured or painful extremity or one in which an intravenous line is running.	2. Cuff inflation can temporarily interrupt blood flow and compromise circulation in an extremity already impaired or a vein receiving intravenous fluid.
3. Select a cuff size appropriate for the client. Estimate by inspection, or measure with a tape, the circumference of the bare upper arm at the midpoint between the shoulder (acromion) and the elbow (olecranon process) (Figure 29-6-2).	3. The bladder inside the cuff should encircle 80% of the arm in adults and 100% of the arm of children less than 13 years old. If in doubt, use a larger cuff to ensure equalization of pressure on the artery and accurate measurement.

(Continues)

PROCEDURE 29-6 Taking Blood Pressure (Continued)

ACTION	RATIONALE

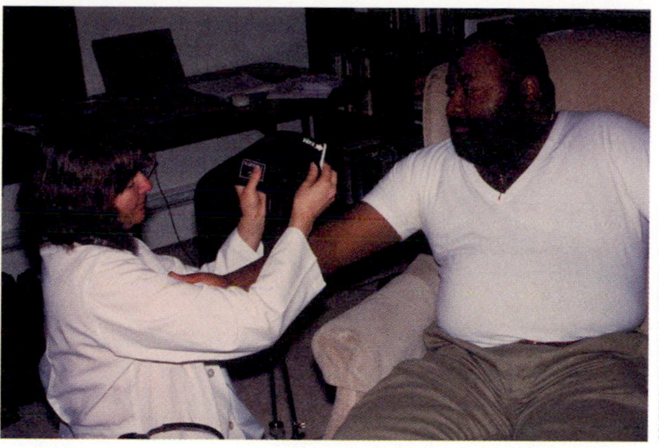

FIGURE 29-6-2 Select a cuff size appropriate for the client.

ACTION	RATIONALE
4. Have the client's bared arm resting on a support so the midpoint of the upper arm is at the level of the heart. Extend the elbow with palm turned upward.	4. Blood pressure increases when the arm is below the level of the heart and decreases when the arm is above the level of the heart.
5. Make sure the bladder cuff is fully deflated and the pump valve moves freely. Place the manometer so the center of the aneroid dial is at eye level and easily visible to the observer.	5. Equipment must be visible and function properly to obtain an accurate reading.
6. Palpate the brachial artery, in the antecubital space, and place the cuff so that the midline of the bladder is over the arterial pulsation. Next, wrap and secure the cuff snugly around the client's bare upper arm. The lower edge of the cuff should be 1 inch (2 cm) above the antecubital fossa (bend of the elbow) (Figures 29-6-3 and 29-6-4).	6. Ensures even pressure distribution over the brachial artery. Rolling up the sleeve may form a tourniquet around the upper arm. Always use a bare arm.

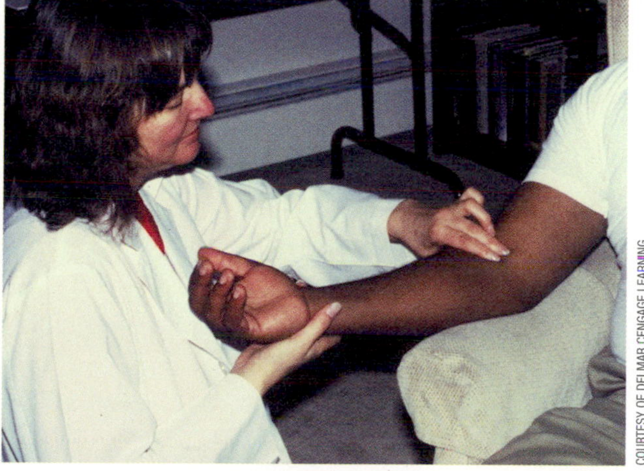

FIGURE 29-6-3 Palpate the brachial artery to determine placement of the stethoscope.

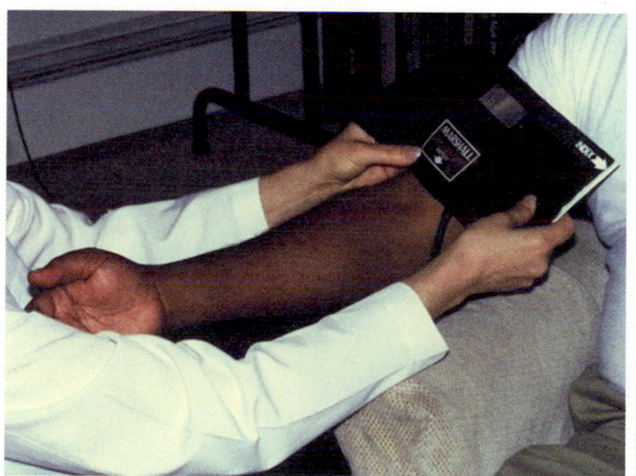

FIGURE 29-6-4 Center the blood pressure cuff over the brachial artery.

(Continues)

PROCEDURE 29-6 Taking Blood Pressure (Continued)

ACTION	RATIONALE
7. Inflate the cuff rapidly to 70 mm Hg and increase by 10-mm increments while palpating the radial pulse. Note the level of pressure at which the pulse disappears and subsequently reappears during deflation. Let all the air out of the cuff in preparation for reinflating the cuff to take the BP reading. Let the arm rest 1 minute before reinflating the cuff. This is called the two-step method of obtaining a BP by obtaining a baseline prior to obtaining the BP reading.	7. The palpatory method provides the necessary preliminary approximation of systolic blood pressure to ensure an accurate reading. When frequent measurements are required, such as every 15 minutes, the palpatory method is generally not incorporated with each pressure check.
8. Insert the earpieces of the stethoscope into the ear canals with a forward tilt to fit snugly.	8. The bell, the low-frequency position of the stethoscope, enhances sound transmission from chest piece to ears.
9. Relocate the brachial artery with your nondominant hand, and place the bell of the stethoscope over the brachial artery pulsation. The bell is held firmly in place, ensuring that the head is in direct contact with the skin and not touching the cuff (Figure 29-6-5).	9. Sound is heard best directly over the artery. Wedging the head of the stethoscope under the edge of the cuff results in considerable extraneous noise and may cause an inaccurate reading.
10. With the dominant hand, turn the valve clockwise to close. Compress the pump to inflate the cuff rapidly and steadily until the manometer registers 20 to 30 mm Hg above the level previously determined by the palpation.	10. Prevents air leaks during inflation. Ensures the cuff is inflated to a pressure greater than the client's systolic pressure.
11. Partially unscrew (open) the valve counterclockwise to deflate the bladder at 2 mm/sec while listening for the appearance of the five phases of the Korotkoff sounds. Note the manometer reading for these sounds. 1. A faint, clear tapping sound that increases in intensity 2. Swishing sound 3. Intense sound 4. Abrupt, distinctive muffled sound 5. No sound	11. Maintains constant release of pressure to ensure hearing first systolic sound. Identify manometer readings for each of the five phases. • Identify two consecutive tapping sounds to confirm systolic reading. • The American Heart Association (2002) recommends using Phase 4 as the diastolic level in children less than 13 years old. Even though 5 phases of Korotkoff sounds have been identified, most clients have only 2 clearly distinct sounds (Phases 1 and 5), identified as the systolic and diastolic sounds.

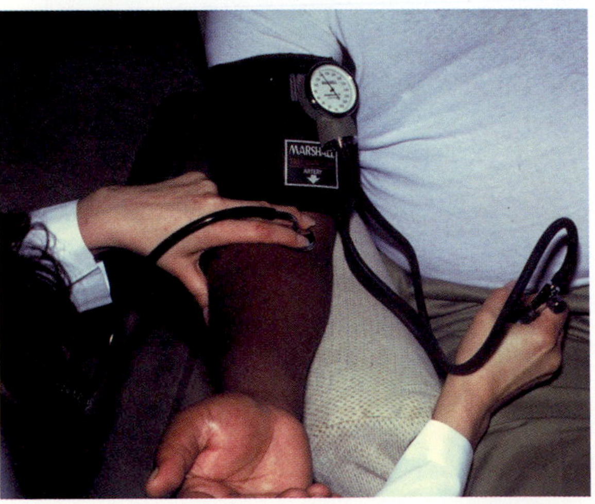

COURTESY OF DELMAR CENGAGE LEARNING

FIGURE 29-6-5 The stethoscope diaphragm should not touch the blood pressure cuff.

(Continues)

PROCEDURE 29-6 Taking Blood Pressure (Continued)

ACTION	RATIONALE
12. After the last Korotkoff sound is heard, deflate the cuff slowly for at least another 10 mm Hg to ensure that no other sounds are audible; then, deflate rapidly and completely.	12. Prevents arterial occlusion and client discomfort from numbness or tingling.
13. Allow the client to rest for at least 30 seconds and remove cuff. (A measurement should be repeated after 30 seconds and the two readings averaged. It may be done in the same or opposite arm) (American Heart Association, 2005).	13. Releases trapped blood in the vessels. Ensures accurate measurement.
14. Inform the client of the reading.	14. Promotes client's participation in health care.
15. The systolic (Phase 1) and diastolic (Phase 5) pressure should be immediately recorded, rounded off (upward) to the nearest 2 mm Hg. (In children and when sounds are heard nearly to the level of 0 mm Hg, the Phase 4 pressure should also be recorded, e.g., 136/104/96).	15. Ensures accuracy.
16. If appropriate, lower bed and place call light in easy reach.	16. Promotes client's safety.
17. Put all equipment in proper place.	17. Fosters maintenance of equipment.
18. Wash hands.	18. Reduces transmission of microorganisms.

EVALUATION

- Evaluate the blood pressure reading for accuracy by comparing with the medical record.
- Evaluate the client's blood pressure for being within the normal range.
- Identify variations in the client's blood pressure of more than 5 to 10 mm Hg from one arm to the other.
- Evaluate if the client's blood pressure changes significantly when he or she stands up.
- Report abnormal measurements to charge nurse or health care provider.

DOCUMENTATION

Vital Signs Flow Sheet or Electronic Medical Record

- Blood pressure measurement
- Site where recording was done
- Method of obtaining the pressure—auscultation or palpation

PROCEDURE 29-7 Performing Pulse Oximetry

OVERVIEW

Pulse oximetry is a quick, easy, noninvasive method to assess the arterial blood oxygen saturation of a client by using an external sensor. There are several types of sensors; however, the most common for adult use is a finger sensor. The finger is placed between a clip mechanism. On one side of the clip are light-emitting diodes (a red and an infrared); a photon detector is on the other side. The beam of light goes through the tissue and blood vessels, and the photon detector receives the light and measures the amount of light absorbed by oxygenated and unoxygenated hemoglobin. Unoxygenated hemoglobin absorbs more red light and oxygenated hemoglobin absorbs more infrared light. The amount of each light and, hence, the arterial blood oxygen saturation (SaO_2) is determined by the spectrum of light. Other types of sensors, using the same principle of spectrometry, are used on the toes, nose, ear, forehead, or around the hand or foot. Special sensors are available for the neonatal hand and pediatric toe.

(Continues)

PROCEDURE 29-7 Performing Pulse Oximetry (Continued)

ASSESSMENT

1. Assess the client's hemoglobin level. **Because pulse oximetry measures the percent of SaO_2, the results of the oxygenation status are affected. The results appear normal if the hemoglobin level is low because all hemoglobin available to carry O_2 is completely saturated; therefore, it is important to know the hemoglobin level.**
2. Assess the client's color. **If the client has vasoconstriction of the extremities, an inaccurate recording may be obtained.**
3. Assess the client's mental status **as this assists in general evaluation of oxygen delivery to the brain and indicates a high level of CO_2.**
4. Assess the client's pulse rate. The pulse oximeter measures pulse rate. **Manually assessing the pulse is a cross-reference to indicate functioning of the oximeter.**
5. Assess the area where the sensors are placed **to determine whether it is an area with adequate circulation (no scars or thickened nails).**
6. Remove nail polish and/or acrylic nails, **which interfere with sensor measurements.**

POSSIBLE NURSING DIAGNOSES

*Impaired **G**as Exchange*
*Ineffective **T**issue Perfusion*
*Risk for Impaired **S**kin Integrity*

PLANNING

Expected Outcomes

1. The SaO_2 will be in a normal range for the client (95%– 100% in the absence of chronic respiratory disease).
2. The client will be alert and oriented.
3. The client's color will remain normal.
4. The client will tolerate the placement of sensors.
5. There will not be any skin irritation or pressure from sensors.

Equipment Needed

- Vital signs automatic measurement device (Dinamap) with pulse oximetry or hand-held pulse oximeter
- Proper sensor
- Alcohol wipe or soap and water
- Nail polish remover if necessary

delegation tips

Ancillary personnel routinely perform pulse oximetry. They should be instructed on acceptable parameters and to report any abnormal findings to the nurse.

IMPLEMENTATION—ACTION/RATIONALE

ACTION	RATIONALE
* Check client's identification band * Explain procedure before beginning *	
1. Wash hands.	1. Reduces transmission of microorganisms.
2. Select an appropriate sensor. Sensors are commonly used for the fingertips. (See Figure 29-7-1.)	2. The sensor is selected based on the size of the person and the site to be used.
3. Select an appropriate site for the sensor. Fingers are most commonly used; however, toes (Figure 29-7-2), earlobes, nose, forehead (Figure 29-7-3), hands, and feet are used. Assess for capillary refill and proximal pulse. If the client has poor circulation, use an earlobe, forehead, or nasal sensor instead. In children, sensors are used on the hand, foot, or trunk. If elderly clients have thickened nails, pick another site.	3. Decreased circulation alters the O_2 saturation measurement.
4. Clean the site with an alcohol wipe. Remove artificial nails or nail polish if present or select another site. Clean any tape adhesive. Use soap and water if necessary to clean the site.	4. Polish and artificial fingernails alter the results.

(Continues)

PROCEDURE 29-7 Performing Pulse Oximetry (Continued)

ACTION	RATIONALE

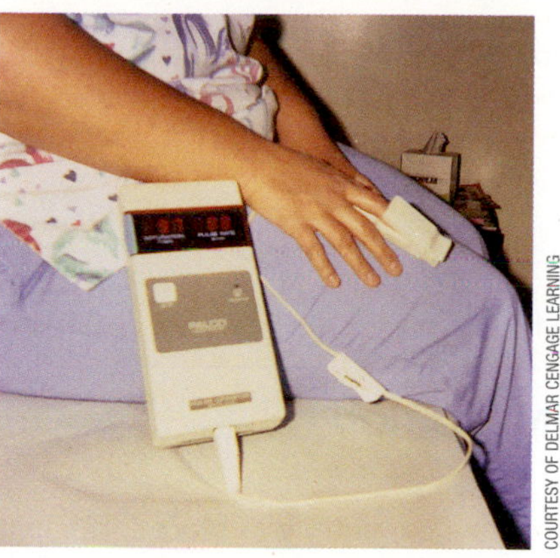

COURTESY OF DELMAR CENGAGE LEARNING

FIGURE 29-7-1 A pulse oximeter determines a client's O_2 saturation.

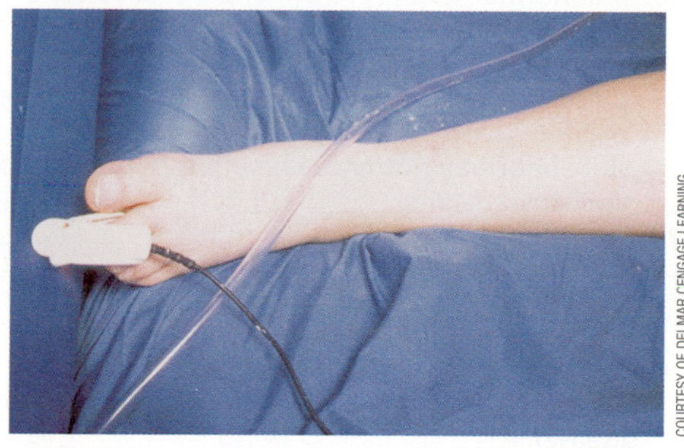

COURTESY OF DELMAR CENGAGE LEARNING

FIGURE 29-7-2 A pulse oximeter sensor may be place on a toe.

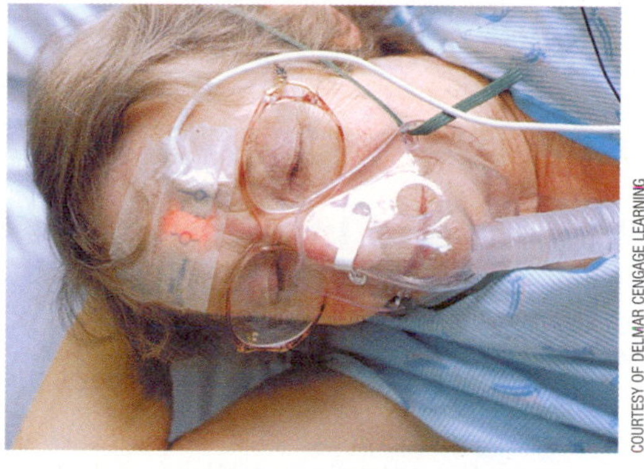

COURTESY OF DELMAR CENGAGE LEARNING

FIGURE 29-7-3 A pulse oximeter sensor may also be placed on the forehead.

ACTION	RATIONALE
5. Apply the sensor. Make sure the photon detectors are aligned on opposite sides of the selected site.	5. Proper application is necessary for accurate results.
6. Connect the sensor to the oximeter with a sensor cable. Turn on the machine. Initially a tone is heard, followed by an arterial wave-form fluctuation with each arterial pulse. In most oximeters if the battery is low, a low-battery light illuminates when 15 minutes of battery life are remaining. Plug in oximeters even when not in use.	6. The tone and wave-form fluctuation indicate the machine is detecting blood flow with each arterial pulsation.
7. Adjust the alarm limits for high and low O_2 saturation levels according to the manufacturer's directions. Pulse rate limits usually are also set. Adjust volume.	7. The alarms indicate that the saturation levels or pulse rates are outside the designated levels and alert the nurse of abnormal O_2 saturation levels and pulse rates.
8. If taking a reading, note the results. If the oximeter is being used for constant monitoring, move the site of spring sensors every 2 hours and adhesive sensors every 4 hours.	8. Prevents skin breakdown from pressure and skin irritation from the adhesive.
9. Cover the sensor with a sheet or towel to protect it from exposure to bright light.	9. Ambient light sources such as sunlight or warming lights may interfere with the sensor and alter the SaO_2 results.

(Continues)

PROCEDURE 29-7 Performing Pulse Oximetry (Continued)

ACTION	RATIONALE
10. If abnormal results are obtained, first assess the client. Are the client's hands cold? Is the sensor correctly placed on the client's finger? Is the pulse oximetry device broken? Obtain the pulse oximetry with another device. If the results are still abnormal, notify the health care provider of abnormal results.	10. A low SaO_2 level requires medical attention because permanent tissue damage may result from low oxygen saturation.
11. Wash hands.	11. Reduces transmission of microorganisms.

EVALUATION

- The SaO_2 is in the normal range for the client (95%– 100% in the absence of chronic respiratory disease).
- The client is alert and oriented.
- The client's color is normal.
- The client tolerates the placement of sensors.
- There is no skin irritation or pressure from sensors.

DOCUMENTATION

Nurses' Notes

- Time pulse oximetry was placed, the location of the sensor, baseline readings, and hemoglobin level

Flow Sheet

- Pulse, oxygen, flow rate, and saturation readings

PROCEDURE 29-8 Weighing a Client, Mobile and Immobile

OVERVIEW

A client's weight is essential data used in monitoring his or her response to a variety of therapies. Changes in a client's weight could necessitate an alteration in the assessment and intervention plans. Weigh a client on the same scale, the same time of day, and wearing the same amount of clothing. An accurate weight is important to ensure appropriate care.

ASSESSMENT

1. Assess the client's ability to stand independently and safely on a scale. **Consider factors requiring the use of a sling scale: The client is somnolent or comatose; paralyzed; too weak to stand; or unsteady when standing.**
2. Determine if clothing is similar to that worn during previous weight measurement **to help determine accuracy of the new weight.**

POSSIBLE NURSING DIAGNOSES

*Imbalanced **N**utrition: More Than Body Requirements*
*Imbalanced **N**utrition: Less Than Body Requirements*
*Excess **F**luid Volume*
*Deficient **F**luid Volume*

PLANNING

Expected Outcomes

1. Health care provider obtains accurate weight.
2. Client incurs no injuries.
3. Client maintains privacy.

Equipment Needed

- Scale: standing electronic or balance scale (see Figure 29-8-1), wheelchair scale, sling scale (Figure 29-8-2), or bed scale.
- Recommended disinfectant
- 1 to 3 other staff members to assist when using sling scale
- Plastic cover for sling scale
- Gloves (when applicable)

(Continues)

PROCEDURE 29-8 Weighing a Client, Mobile and Immobile (Continued)

delegation tips

The skill of weighing the mobile and immobile client is routinely delegated to trained ancillary personnel. The personnel should be instructed to do the following:

- *Select the correct scale for measurement.*
- *Properly and safely position the client for measurement.*
- *Correctly and safely perform the measurement according to established guidelines and record on the appropriate flow sheet (clinical record).*
- *Recognize and report abnormal findings promptly to the nurse.*

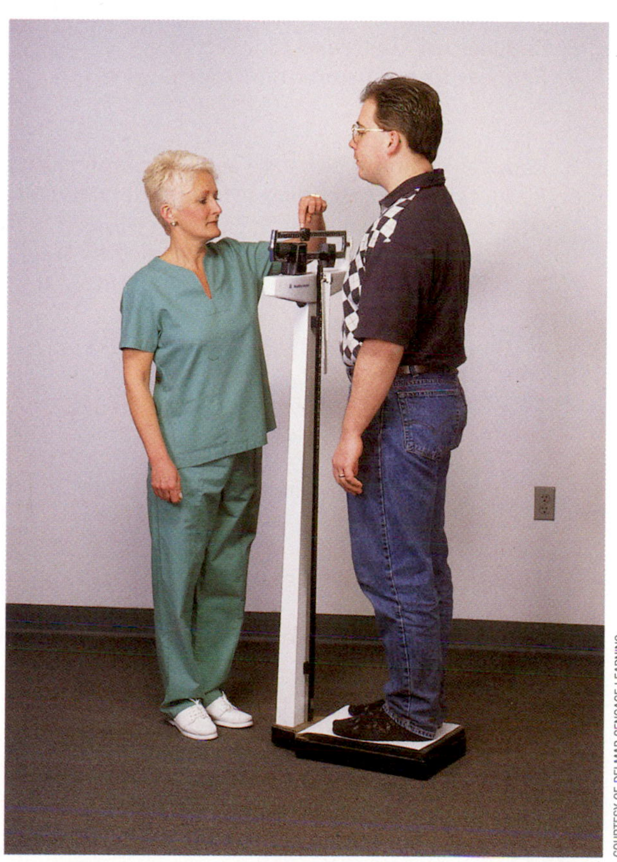
A
COURTESY OF DELMAR CENGAGE LEARNING

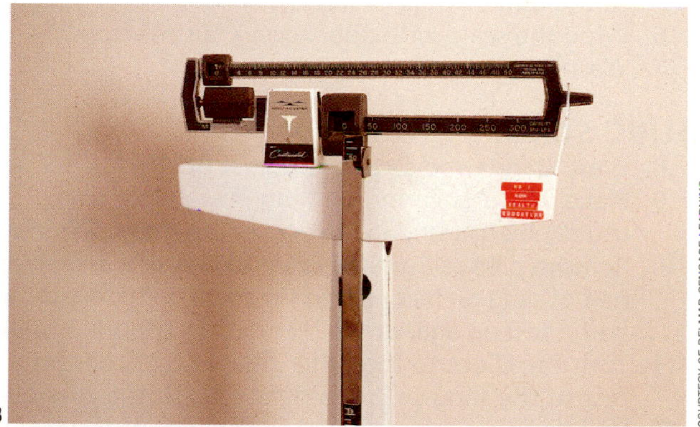
B
COURTESY OF DELMAR CENGAGE LEARNING

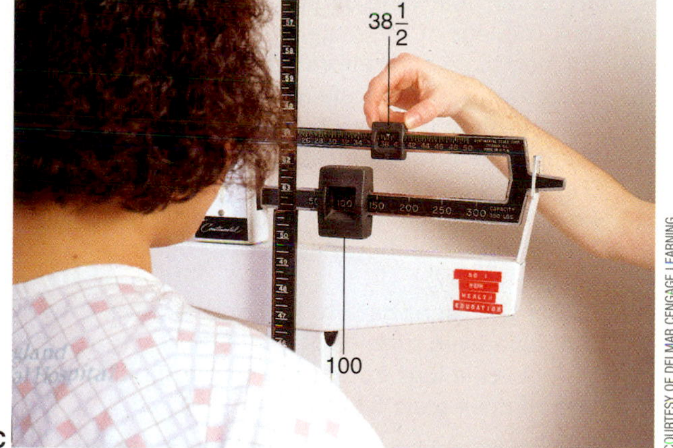

C
COURTESY OF DELMAR CENGAGE LEARNING

FIGURE 29-8-1 ***A,*** **The standing balance or digital scale weighs ambulatory clients.** ***B,*** **Prior to weighing the client, set both weight indicators to zero and make sure the tip of the balance beam is balanced in the middle of the mark.** ***C,*** **Move the both weight indicators on the balance beam until the tip of the beam is balanced in the middle of the mark. In the photo, the lower weight indicator is on 100, and the top one is on 38½, indicating the client weighs 138½ pounds.**

IMPLEMENTATION—ACTION/RATIONALE

ACTION	RATIONALE
* Check client's identification band * Explain procedure before beginning *	
STANDING SCALE	
1. Wash hands.	1. Reduces transmission of microorganisms.
2. Place the scale near the client.	2. Reduces risk of fall or injury.
3. Turn on the electronic scale and calibrate it to zero.	3. Ensures accurate reading.

(Continues)

PROCEDURE 29-8 Weighing a Client, Mobile and Immobile (Continued)

ACTION	RATIONALE
4. Ask client to remove shoes if necessary, step up on the scale, and stand still.	4. Obtains weight.
Electronic scale: Read weight after digital numbers have stopped fluctuating.	Reading is not accurate when the numbers are still fluctuating.
Balance scale: Slide the larger weight into the notch most closely approximating the client's weight. Slide the smaller weight into the notch so the balance rests in the middle. Add the two numbers for the client's weight.	Weights on scale must be balanced to obtain accurate reading.
5. Ask the client to step down. Assist the client back to the bed or chair, if necessary.	5. Reduces risk of injury if client needs assistance.
6. Wipe the scale with appropriate disinfectant.	6. Reduces risk of spread of infection.
7. Wash hands.	7. Reduces transmission of microorganisms.
SLING SCALE	
8. Wash hands and put on gloves if needed.	8. Reduces risk of health care associated infection.
9. Place plastic covering on sling if available (can usually be ordered in bulk from the manufacturer).	9. Reduces risk of spreading infection between clients.
10. Remove pillows. Turn the client to one side and place half of sling on bed next to the client, with remaining half rolled up against the client's back (Figure 29-8-3).	10. Most accurate weight will be obtained by leaving no other bedding between the client and sling.
11. Turn the client to the other side, and unroll the rest of the sling so it lays flat beneath the client.	11. Turning in this manner maximizes client comfort.
12. Roll the scale over the bed so the legs of the scale are underneath the bed (Figure 29-8-4). Open and lock the legs of the scale.	12. Ensures equipment is being used safely to reduce risk of injury.
13. Turn on scale and calibrate to zero.	13. Ensures accurate reading.
14. Lower arms of the scale and slip hooks through holes in sling (Figure 29-8-5).	14. Attaches sling to scale to obtain weight.
15. Pump scale until sling rests completely off the bed (Figure 29-8-6).	15. Ensures accurate weight.
16. Remind the client to remain still. Read weight after digital numbers have stopped fluctuating (Figure 29-8-7).	16. Reading is not accurate when the numbers are still fluctuating.
17. Lower the client back to bed and remove arms of the scale from sling (Figure 29-8-8).	17. Prepares for removal of sling.
18. Unlock scale legs, return to their original position, and remove scale from bed.	18. Allows for removal of equipment that obstructs proximity to the client, thereby facilitating removal of the sling.

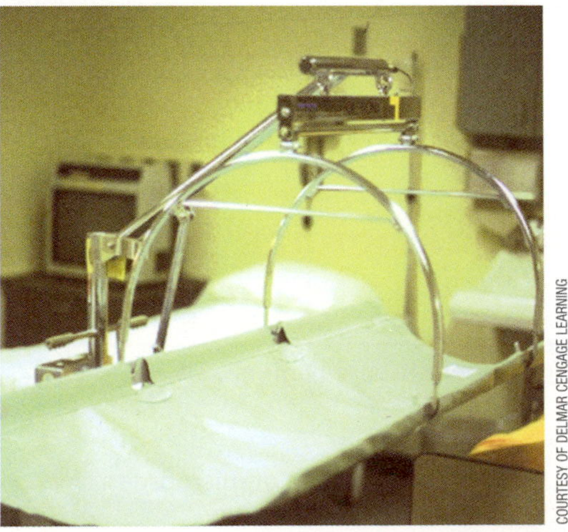

COURTESY OF DELMAR CENGAGE LEARNING

FIGURE 29-8-2 The sling scale weighs clients in bed.

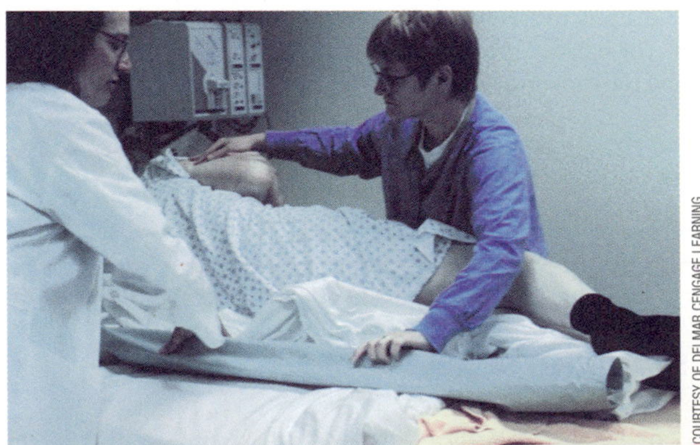

COURTESY OF DELMAR CENGAGE LEARNING

FIGURE 29-8-3 Turn client on one side and place sling on the bed.

(Continues)

PROCEDURE 29-8 Weighing a Client, Mobile and Immobile (Continued)

ACTION	RATIONALE

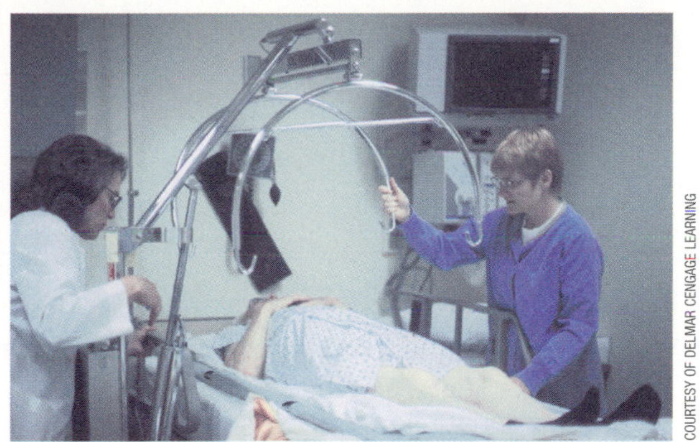

FIGURE 29-8-4 After unrolling the rest of the sling under the client, move the scale into position over the bed.

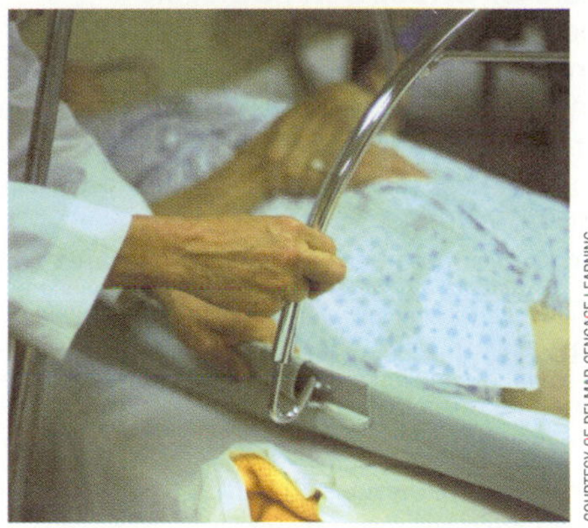

FIGURE 29-8-5 Attach the hooks through the holes in the sling.

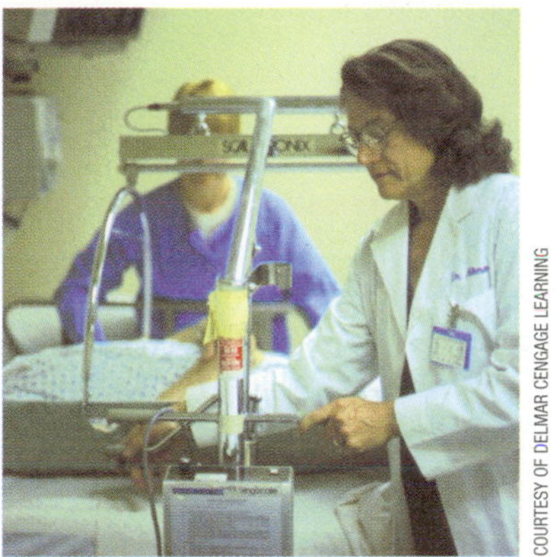

FIGURE 29-8-6 Pump the scale until the sling lifts completely off the bed.

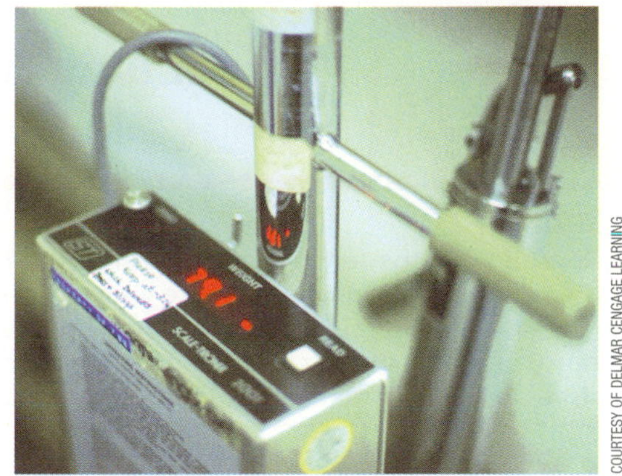

FIGURE 29-8-7 Read the weight after the numbers have stopped fluctuating.

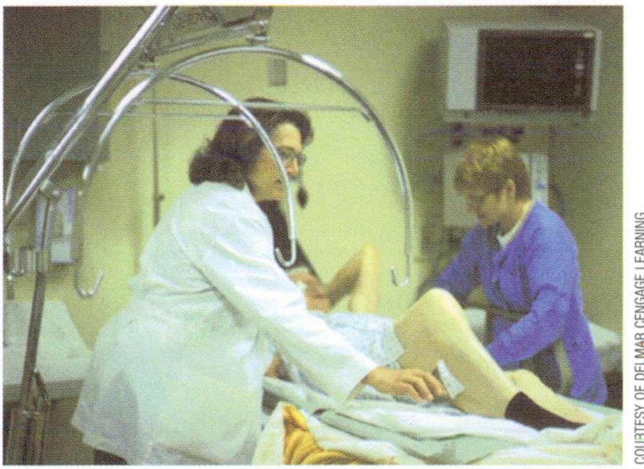

FIGURE 29-8-8 Lower the client back to the bed and remove the sling.

ACTION	RATIONALE
19. Turn the client on his or her side, roll up sling, turn client to the other side.	19. Facilitates removal of the sling.
20. Realign the client with pillows and covers.	20. Ensures comfort and privacy.
21. Remove plastic covering from the sling and discard as per hospital policy.	21. Reduces risk of spread of infection and health care associated infection.
22. Remove gloves and wash hands.	22 Reduces transmission of microorganisms.

(Continues)

PROCEDURE 29-8 Weighing a Client, Mobile and Immobile (Continued)

ACTION	RATIONALE
Bed Scale or Under-Bed Pod Scale Some beds have scales built into the bed that electronically weigh the client. Other beds weigh clients after rolling the bed onto four pods that are connected to a digital monitor.	
23. Place the same amount of bedding on the bed and clothing on the client.	23. Ensures accurate client weight.
24. Turn on electronic weight monitor and weigh client.	24. Obtain an accurate digital weight.

EVALUATION

- Compare weight obtained to previously recorded weight. Repeat weight if large discrepancy is noted.
- If large discrepancy still remains, notify appropriate health care team members.

DOCUMENTATION

Vital Signs Flow Sheet or Electronic Medical Record

- Date, time of day, and the weight of the client on the appropriate flow sheet

PROCEDURE 29-9 Proper Body Mechanics

OVERVIEW

Body mechanics is the term used when referring to lifting techniques and involves proper body alignment, balance, and synchronized movements that are vital when lifting and ambulating clients (Daniels, 2010). Proper use of body mechanics maximizes the power and energy of the musculoskeletal and neurological systems and prevents strains and injury to muscles, joints, and tendons. Correct body mechanics decreases work-related musculoskeletal injuries, diminishes excessive strain and fatigue, and minimizes the potential for injury (Figure 29-9-1). It is imperative that

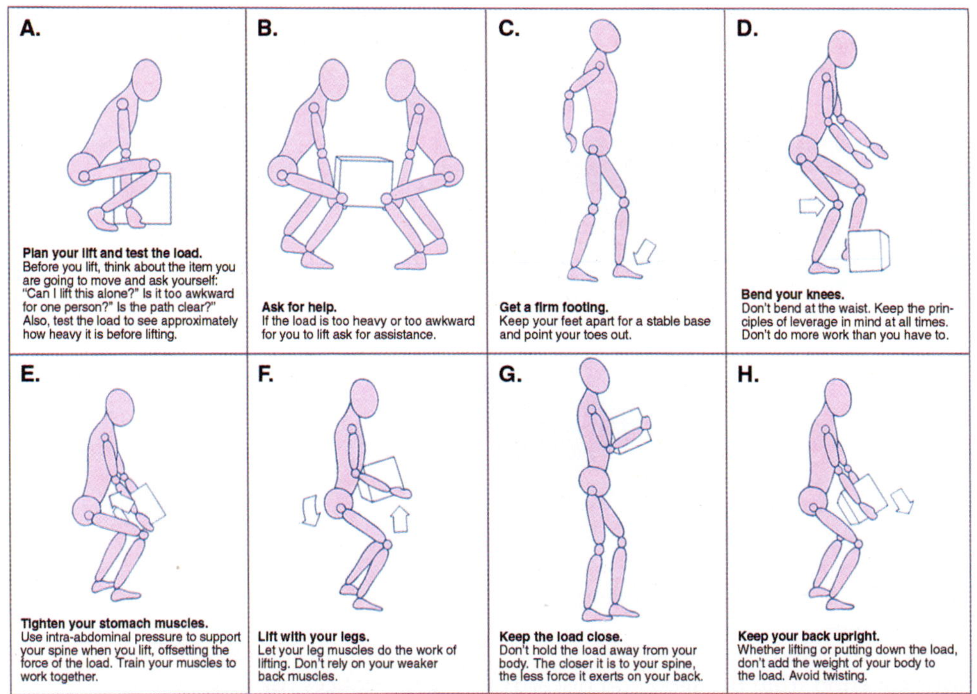

FIGURE 29-9-1 Always follow these eight rules for lifting. *(Reprinted with permission from Ergodyne Corporation, St. Paul, MN.)*

(Continues)

PROCEDURE 29-9 Proper Body Mechanics (Continued)

nurses know and use proper lifting techniques and seek assistance as needed to avoid injury to self and clients. Knowledge of various client transfer techniques, specialized lifting skills of transfer from bed to stretcher and from bed to chair or wheelchair, and the use of the bed transfer board and a hydraulic lift are reviewed in the following procedure. Specific tips for client and staff safety are highlighted.

ASSESSMENT

1. Assess the need and degree to which the client requires assistance to achieve physical movement. **Identifies client's ability to attain maximum level of self-help before initiating intervention.**
2. Identify the type of physical movement required **to ensure the use of proper body mechanics such as pushing, pulling, or lifting.**
3. Identify the potential need for assistive equipment to accomplish the goal of safe lifting **to minimize the risk of client/nurse injury.**
4. Identify any unusual risks to safe lifting, such as an extra-heavy client or a home care setting. **Allows nurse to plan modifications to ensure good body mechanics and reduce the risk of injury.**
5. Assess the situation for obstacles, heavy clients, poor handholds, or equipment or objects in the way. Reduce or remove safety hazards prior to lifting the client or object.
6. Assess the situation for slippery surfaces, including wet floors; slippery shoes on client, helper, or nurse; and towels, linen, or paper on the floor. Resolve the slippery surface before lifting the client or object.
7. Assess the situation for hidden risks, including client confusion, combativeness, orthostatic hypotension, drug effects, pain, or fear.
8. Assess the client's vital signs, pain status, and need for pain medications before ambulating. Assess incisional areas and/or areas of injury.
9. Check equipment to ensure that it is in working order to facilitate a safe and uninterrupted transfer. Especially check locks on wheelchair.
10. Identify all equipment and tubes connected to the client and take appropriate preventive measures. Frequently, clients that require lifting or transfer have intravenous tubing, other tubing, and/or orthopedic equipment.
11. Assess the client's understanding of the steps required to achieve the goal of a safe transfer and the ability to assist. **Explanation of the steps in a clear, concise fashion will decrease anxiety, secure cooperation, and ease physical requirements for both the client and the nurse/caregiver.**

POSSIBLE NURSING DIAGNOSES

*Risk for **I**njury*
*Impaired Physical **M**obility*

PLANNING

Expected Outcomes

1. Clients will be safely lifted/transferred by staff utilizing appropriate equipment and correct body mechanics.
2. Accidents during lifting of clients will be avoided by using proper body alignment and mechanics.
3. Heavy lifting will be facilitated by mechanical devices and a team effort.
4. Clients and families will be taught safe lifting/transfer techniques to facilitate this process in home and extended-care environments.
5. The nurse will practice safe lifting and proper body mechanics when performing nursing care that requires bending or lifting.
6. Staff and clients are not injured by using correct body mechanics and utilizing appropriate equipment.

Equipment Needed

- Transfer or gait belts
- Wheelchair equipped with working locks
- Transfer board
- Draw or lift sheet
- Nonslip shoes or slippers
- Safety or gait belt
- Stretcher equipped with working locks
- Hydraulic lift

delegation tips

Delegation to ancillary personnel of the moving, transferring, and lifting of clients is an expectation of their role after proper instruction and/or certification. Ancillary personnel are routinely expected to place the bed at proper height, use a wide base of support, properly position the client, and safely use assistive devices. After repositioning the client, ancillary personnel are expected to evaluate the client's level of comfort. The client who requires complex turning or lifting devices needs the supervision of the professional nurse.

(Continues)

PROCEDURE 29-9 Proper Body Mechanics (Continued)

IMPLEMENTATION—ACTION/RATIONALE

ACTION	RATIONALE
* Check client's identification band * Explain procedure before beginning *	
1. Wash hands.	1. Reduces the transmission of microorganisms.
2. Assess the client situation as stated in previous **Assessment** section.	2. Allows the nurse to anticipate and plan for unexpected events.
3. Maintain low center of gravity by bending at the hips and knees, not the waist. Squat down rather than bend over to lift and lower (Figure 29-9-2).	3. Provides for the equal distribution of body weight and assists in maintaining safe balance.
4. Establish a wide support base with feet spread apart (Figure 29-9-3).	4. Provides stability and lowers the center of gravity.
5. Use feet to move, not a twisting or bending motion from the waist.	5. Assists in maintaining correct body alignment, which increases strength to lift, push, pull, and carry.
6. When pushing or pulling, stand near the object and stagger one foot partially ahead of the other.	6. Provides a safety net for avoiding potential back injuries.
7. When pushing a client or an object, lean into the client or object and apply continuous light pressure. When pulling a client or an object, lean away and grasp with light pressure. Never jerk or twist your body to force a weight to move.	7. Firm pressure will provide continuous movement of the object and will avoid abrupt movements that require the expenditure of increased energy.
8. When stooping to move an object, maintain a wide base of support with feet, flex knees to lower body, and maintain straight upper body.	8. Provides the appropriate mechanics for the strength and endurance to achieve the task and to stand up straight upon completion.
9. When lifting or carrying an object, squat in front of the object, take a firm hold, and assume a standing position by using the leg muscles and keeping the back straight.	9. This stance will avoid the use of the back, diminish the potential for spinal twisting, and provide the lifter with a firm center of gravity and strength to lift the required weight.
10. When rising up from a squatting position, arch your back slightly. Keep the buttocks and abdomen tucked in and rise up with your head first.	10. Keeps the back from bowing and increasing the strain on the back muscles.
11. When lifting or carrying heavy objects, keep the weight as close to your center of gravity as possible.	11. Reduces the strain on arm, leg, and back muscles.
12. When reaching for a client or an object, keep the back straight. If the client or object is heavy, do not try to lift the client or object without repositioning yourself closer to the weight (Figure 29-9-4).	12. Avoids straining the back and arm muscles.

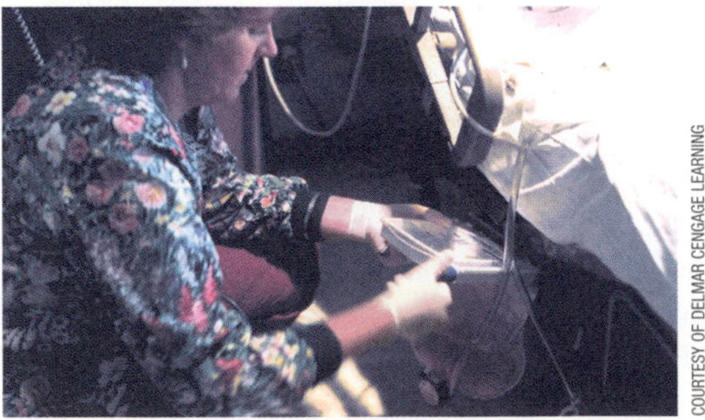
COURTESY OF DELMAR CENGAGE LEARNING

FIGURE 29-9-2 Squat rather than bend to maintain good posture.

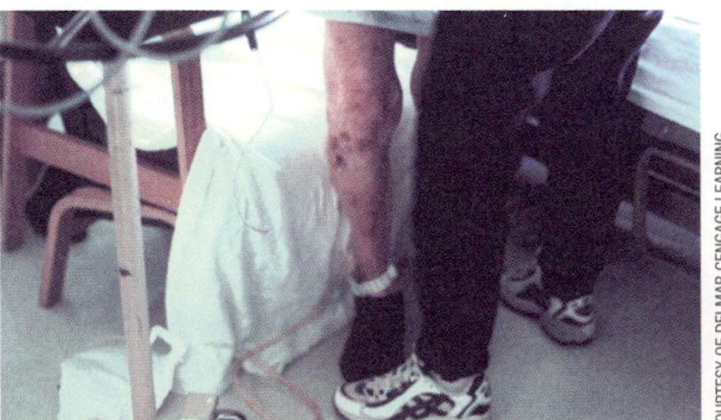
COURTESY OF DELMAR CENGAGE LEARNING

FIGURE 29-9-3 Spread feet apart to establish a wide base of support.

(Continues)

PROCEDURE 29-9 Proper Body Mechanics (Continued)

ACTION	RATIONALE
13. Use safety aids and equipment. Use gait belts (Figure 29-9-5), lifts (Figure 29-9-6), draw sheets, and other transfer assistance devices (Figure 29-9-7). Encourage clients to use handrails and grab bars (Figure 29-9-8). Wheelchair, cart, and stretcher wheels are locked when they are not actually being moved.	13. Reduces the strain on the nurse and improves the safety for the client.

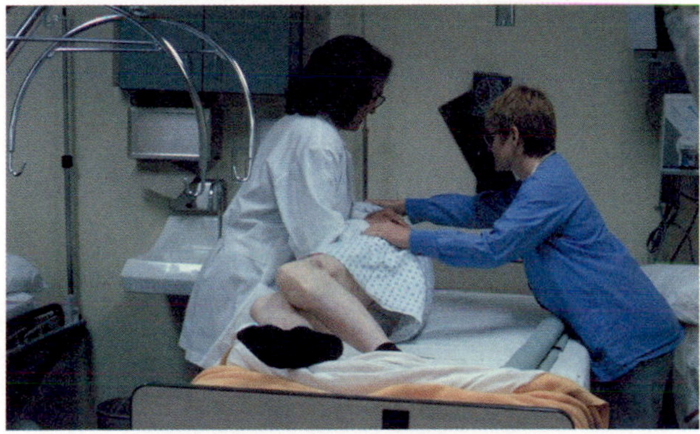
COURTESY OF DELMAR CENGAGE LEARNING

FIGURE 29-9-4 Keep your back straight when reaching.

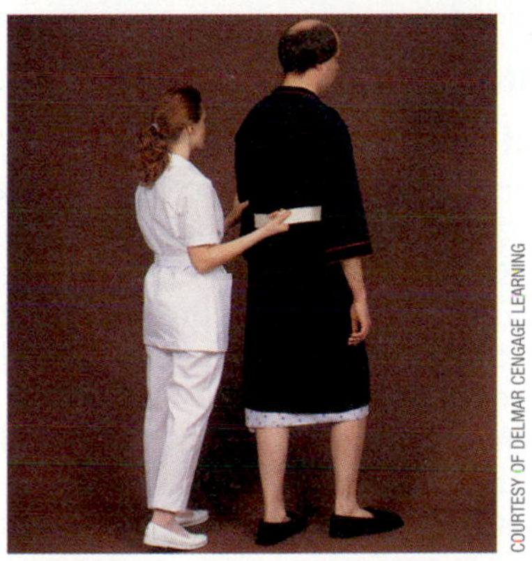
COURTESY OF DELMAR CENGAGE LEARNING

FIGURE 29-9-5 Use gait belts for better grip and control.

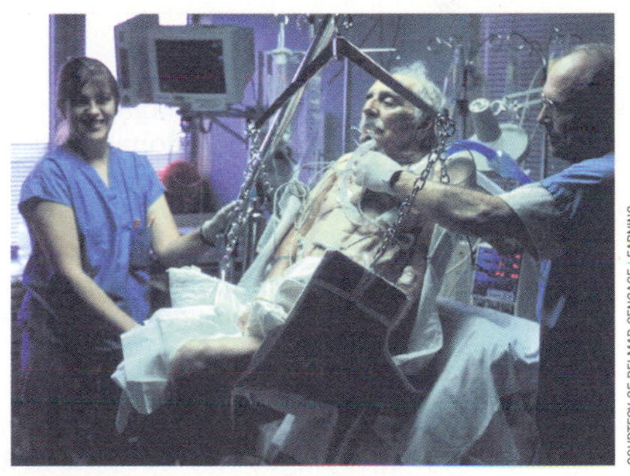
COURTESY OF DELMAR CENGAGE LEARNING

FIGURE 29-9-6 Use lifts to carry the weight of the client. Monitor equipment, lines, tubes, and drains and adjust as needed to prevent them from being dislodged.

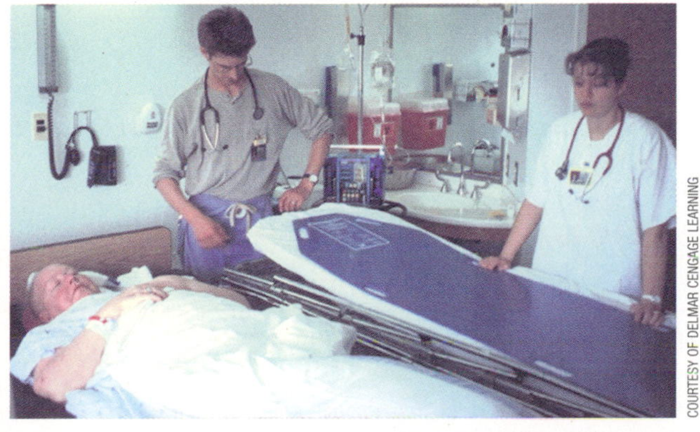
COURTESY OF DELMAR CENGAGE LEARNING

FIGURE 29-9-7 Use a transfer board to reduce shearing forces and to reduce effort needed to slide the client.

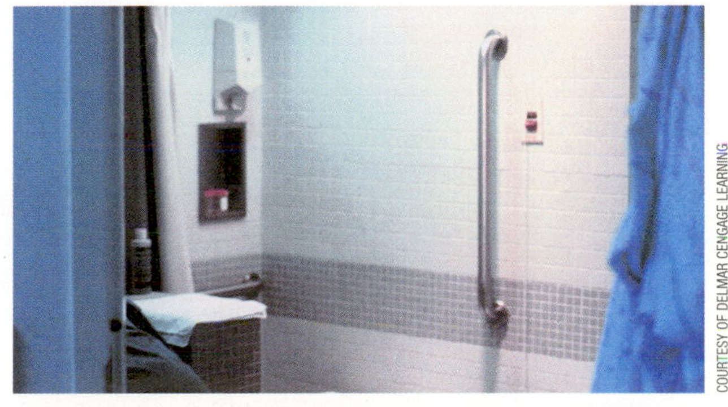
COURTESY OF DELMAR CENGAGE LEARNING

FIGURE 29-9-8 Encourage clients to use handrails and grab bars.

(Continues)

PROCEDURE 29-9 Proper Body Mechanics (Continued)

EVALUATION

- The client or object is lifted and/or moved without sustaining injury or damage.
- The nurse who is lifting and moving clients or objects is not injured.

DOCUMENTATION

Nurses' Notes

- Type of lift or transfer in the progress notes
- Client's tolerance of the lift or move

PROCEDURE 29-10 Performing Range-of-Motion (ROM) Exercises

OVERVIEW

Range of motion (ROM) is the natural range of movement of muscles and joints. When an individual is capable of moving the muscles and joints through their full range of movements in daily activities, he is performing active ROM exercises.

Clients recovering from a stroke or any client with limited movement may need health care personnel to do passive ROM and move the muscles and joints through the natural ROM for the joint. Passive ROM (PROM) exercises seek to maintain or improve the current level of functional mobility of a client's extremities. The nurse provides, assists with, and teaches the client functional movements in all available planes and directions of involved joints. ROM exercises prevent contractures and shortening of muscles and tendons, increase circulation to extremities, decrease vascular complications of immobility, and facilitate comfort for the client.

ASSESSMENT

1. Be aware of the client's medical diagnosis. **Understand the expected functional limits of a client with this diagnosis.**
2. Familiarize yourself with the client's current range of motion. Note any joint pain, stiffness, or inflammation that might limit the client's motion. **Understanding the client's current ROM will help you assess the functional limits of movement of each joint.**
3. Assess client consciousness and cognitive function. **Client is encouraged to participate in ROM as actively as possible.**

POSSIBLE NURSING DIAGNOSES

Impaired Physical Mobility
Risk for Activity Intolerance

PLANNING

Expected Outcomes

1. Client will maintain or improve current functional mobility in all involved joints and extremities.
2. Client will regain or improve strength and/or voluntary movement in involved joints and extremities.
3. Client will avoid complications of immobility, including pressure ulcers, contractures, decreased peristalsis, constipation, fecal impaction, orthostatic hypotension, pulmonary embolism, and thrombophlebitis.

Equipment Needed

- No special equipment is needed, except gloves when contact with body fluids is possible.

delegation tips

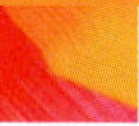

Administering passive ROM exercises may be delegated to properly trained ancillary personnel. Outcomes must be reported to the nurse.

IMPLEMENTATION—ACTION/RATIONALE

ACTION	RATIONALE
* Check client's identification band * Explain procedure before beginning *	
1. Wash hands, wear gloves if contact with body fluids is possible.	1. Reduces the transmission of microorganisms.
2. Provide for privacy, including exposing only the extremity to be exercised.	2. Decreases physical exposure and embarrassment.

(Continues)

PROCEDURE 29-10 Performing Range-of-Motion (ROM) Exercises (Continued)

ACTION	RATIONALE
3. Adjust bed to comfortable height for performing ROM.	3. Prevents muscle strain and discomfort for nurse.
4. Lower bed rail only on the side you are working.	4. Prevents falls.
5. Describe the passive ROM exercises you are performing, or verbally cue client to perform ROM exercises with your assistance.	5. Exercises all joint areas.
6. Start at the client's head and perform ROM exercises down each side of the body.	6. Provides a systematic method to ensure that all body parts are exercised.
7. Repeat each ROM exercise three to five times as the client tolerates, with five times as maximum. Perform each motion in a slow, firm manner. Encourage full joint movement, but do not go beyond the point of pain, resistance, or fatigue.	7. Provides exercise to the client's tolerance or to a level that will maintain the joint function.
8. Perform the movements listed in Table 29-10-1. Figures 29-1 through 29-4 give examples to follow.	8. The ROM exercises optimize the performance of the movements, to preserve muscle tone and joint flexibility.

TABLE 29-10-1 Defining Joint Range of Motion

JOINT MOVEMENT	RANGE	MUSCLE GROUP(S)
1. Temporomandibular Joint (TMJ) (Synovial Joint)		
a. Open mouth.	1–2.5 in.	Masseter, temporalis
b. Close mouth.	Complete closure	
c. *Protrusion:* Push out lower jaw.	0.5 in.	Pterygoideus lateralis
d. *Retrusion*: Tuck in lower jaw.	0.5 in.	
e. *Lateral motion*: Slide jaw from side to side.	0.5 in.	Pterygoideus lateralis, pterygoideus medialis
2. Cervical Spine (Pivot Joint)		
a. *Flexion*: Rest chin on chest.	45° each side	Sternocleisdomastoid
b. *Extension*: Return head to midline.	45°	Trapezius
c. *Hyperextension*: Tilt head back.	10°	Trapezius
d. *Lateral flexion*: Move head to touch ear to shoulder.	40° each side	Sternocleidomastoid
e. *Rotation*: Turn head to look to side.	90° each side	Sternocleidomastoid, trapezius

(Continues)

PROCEDURE 29-10 Performing Range-of-Motion (ROM) Exercises (Continued)

Table 29-10-1 Defining Joint Range of Motion (Continued)

JOINT MOVEMENT	RANGE	MUSCLE GROUP(S)
3. Shoulder (Ball-and-Socket Joint)		
a. *Flexion*: Raise straight arm forward to a position above the head.	180°	Pectoralis major, coracobrachialis, deltoid, biceps brachii
b. *Extension*: Return straight arm forward and down to side of body.	180°	Latissimus dorsi, deltoid, triceps brachii, teres major
c. *Hypertension*: Move straight arm behind body.	50°	Latissimus dorsi, deltoid, teres major
d. *Abduction*: Move straight arm laterally from side to a position above the head, palm facing away from head.	180°	Deltoid, supraspinatus
e. *Adduction*: Move straight arm download laterally and across front of body as far as possible.	230°	Pectoralis major, teres major
f. *Circumduction*: Move straight arm in a full circle.	360°	Deltoid, coracobrachialis, latissimus dorsi, teres major
g. *External rotation*: Bent arm lateral, parallel to floor, palm down, rotate shoulder so fingers point up.	90°	Infraspinatus, teres minor, deltoid
h. *Internal rotation*: Bent arm lateral, parallel to floor, rotate shoulder so fingers point down.	90°	Subscapularis, pectoralis major, latismus dorsi, teres major
4. Elbow (Hinge Joint)		
a. *Flexion*: Bend elbow, move lower arm toward shoulder, palm facing shoulder.	150°	Biceps brachii, brachialis, brachioradialis
b. *Extension*: Straighten lower arm forward and downward.	150°	Triceps brachii
c. *Rotation for supination*: Elbow bent, turn hand and forearm so palm is facing upward.	70°–90°	Biceps brachii, supinator
c. *Rotation for pronation*: Elbow bent, turn hand and forearm so palm is facing downward.	70°–90°	Pronator teres, pronator quadratus

PROCEDURE 29-10 Performing Range-of-Motion (ROM) Exercises (Continued)

TABLE 29-10-1 Defining Joint Range of Motion (Continued)

JOINT MOVEMENT	RANGE	MUSCLE GROUP(S)
5. Wrist (Condyloid Joint)		
a. *Flexion*: Bend wrist so fingers move toward inner aspect of forearm.	80°–90°	Flexor carpi radialis, flexor carpi ulnaris
b. *Extension*: Straighten hand to same plane as arm.	80°–90°	Extensor carpi radialis longus, extensor carpi radialis brevis, extensor carpi ulnaris
c. *Hypertension*: Bend wrist so fingers move back as far as possible.	80°–90°	Extensor carpi radialis longus, extensor carpi radialis brevis, extensor carpi ulnaris
d. *Radial flexion*: abduction—Bend wrist laterally toward thumb.	Up to 20°	Extensor carpi radialis longus, extensor carpi radialis brevis, flexor carpi radialis
e. *Ulnar flexion*: adduction—Bend wrist laterally away from thumb.	30°–50°	Extensor carpi ulnaris, flexor-carpi ulnaris
6. Hand and Fingers (Condyloid and Hinge Joints)		
a. *Flexion*: Make a fist.	90°	Interosseus dorsales manus, flexor digitorum superficialis
b. *Extension*: Straighten fingers.	90°	Extensor indicis, extensor digiti minimi
c. *Hyperextension*: Bend fingers back as far as possible.	30°–50°	Extensor indicis, extensor digiti minimi
d. *Abduction*: Spread fingers apart.	25°	Interosseus dorsales manus
e. *Adduction*: Bring fingers together.	25°	Interosseus palmares
7. Thumb (Saddle Joint)		
a. *Flexion*: Move thumb across palmar surface of hand.	90°	Felxor pollicis brevis, opponens pollicis
b. *Extension*: Move thumb away from hand.	90°	Extensor Pollicis brevis, extensor pollicis longus
c. *Abduction*: Move thumb laterally.	30°	Abductor pollicis brevis, abductor pollicis longus
d. *Adduction*: Move thumb back to hand.	30°	Adductor pollicis transversus, adductor pollicis obliquus

(Continues)

PROCEDURE 29-10 Performing Range-of-Motion (ROM) Exercises (Continued)

TABLE 29-10-1 Defining Joint Range of Motion (Continued)

JOINT MOVEMENT	RANGE	MUSCLE GROUP(S)
e. *Opposition*: Touch thumb to tip of each finger of same hand.	Touching	Opponens pollicis, flexor pollicis brevis 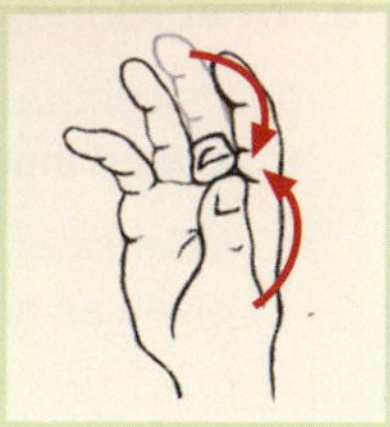
8. Hip (Ball-and-Socket Joint) 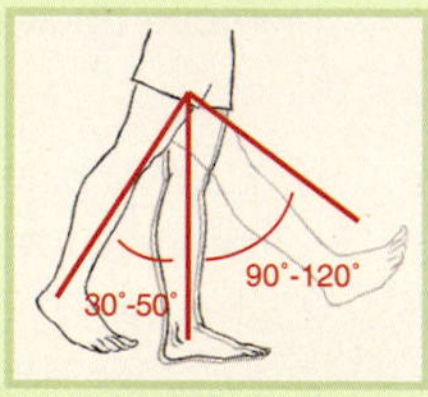		
a. *Flexion*: Move straight leg forward and upward.	90°–120°	Psoas major, iliacus, iliopsoas
b. *Extension*: Move leg back beside the other leg.	90°–120°	Gluteus maximus, adductor magnus, semitendinosus, semimembranosus
c. *Hyperextension*: Move leg behind body.	30°–50°	Gluteus maximus, semitendinosus, semimembranosus
d. *Abduction*: Move leg laterally from midline.	40°–50°	Gluteus medius, gluteus minimus 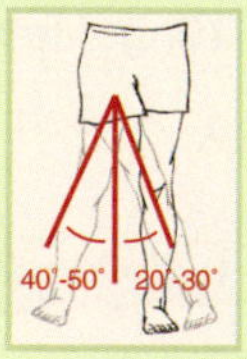
e. *Adduction*: Move leg toward and past midline.	20°–30° past midline	Adductor magnus, adductor brevis, adductor longus
f. *Circumduction*: Move leg backward in a circle.	360°	Psoas major, gluteus maximus, gluteus medius, adductor magnus 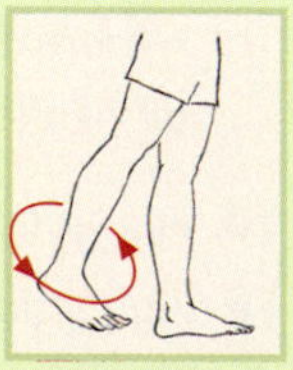
g. *Internal rotation*: Turn foot and leg inward, pointing toes toward other leg.	90°	Gluteus minimus, gluteus medius, tensor fasciae latae 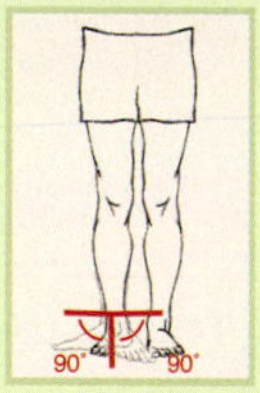
h. *External rotation*: Turn foot and leg outward, pointing toes away from other leg.	90°	Obturator externus, obturator internus, quadratus femoris
9. Knee (Hinge Joint) 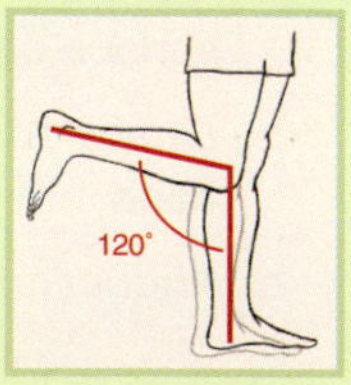		
a. *Flexion*: Bend knee to bring heel back toward thigh.	120°–130°	Biceps femoris, semitendinosus, semimembranosus
b. *Extension*: Straighten each leg, place foot beside other foot.	120°–130°	Rectus femoris, vastus lateralis, vastus medialis, vastus intermedius
10. Ankle (Hinge Joint) 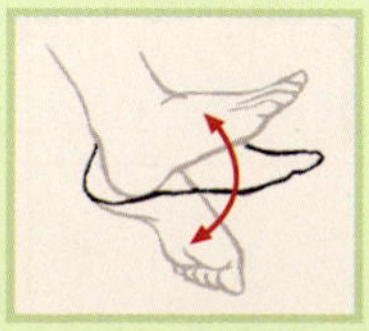		
a. *Plantar flexion*: Point toes downward.	45°–50°	Gastrocnemius, soleus
b. *Dorsiflexion*: Point toes upward.	20°	Peroneus, tertius, tibialis anterior

PROCEDURE 29-10 Performing Range-of-Motion (ROM) Exercises (Continued)

TABLE 29-10-1 Defining Joint Range of Motion (Continued)

JOINT MOVEMENT	RANGE	MUSCLE GROUP(S)
11. Foot (Gliding Joint)		
a. *Eversion*: Turn sole of foot laterally.	5°	Peroueus longus, peroneus brevis
b. *Inversion*: Turn sole of foot medially.	5°	Tibialis posterior, tibialis anterior
12. Toes (Condyloid)		
a. *Flexion*: Curve toes downward.	35°–60°	Flexor hallucis brevis, lumbricales pedis, flexor digitorum brevis
b. *Extension*: Straighten toes.	35°–60°	Extensor digitorum longus, extensor digitorum brevis, extensor hallucis longus
c. *Abduction*: Spread toes apart.	Up to 15°	Interosseus dorsales pedis, abductor hallucis
d. *Adduction*: Bring toes together.	Up to 15°	Adductor hallucis, interosseus plantares

ACTION | **RATIONALE**

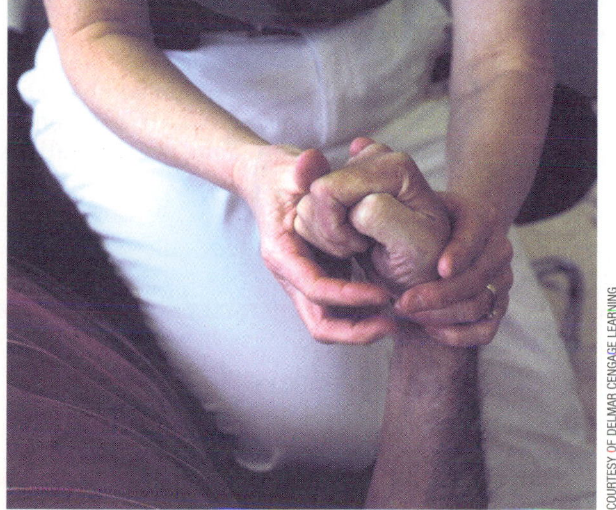

COURTESY OF DELMAR CENGAGE LEARNING

FIGURE 29-10-1 Flex and extend the wrist.

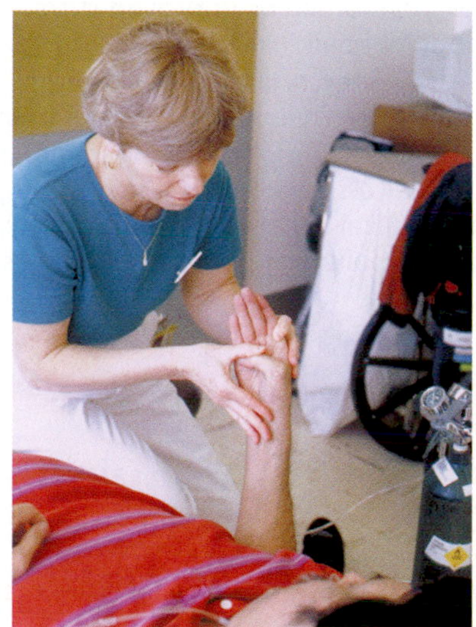

COURTESY OF DELMAR CENGAGE LEARNING

FIGURE 29-10-2 Flex and extend the fingers.

ACTION	RATIONALE
9. Observe client's joints and face for signs of exertion, pain, or fatigue during movement.	9. Alerts nurse to discontinue exercise.
10. Replace covers and position client in proper body alignment.	10. Promotes comfort.
11. Place side rails in original position.	11. Prevents falls.
12. Place call light within reach.	12. Facilitates communication.
13. Wash hands.	13. Reduces the transmission of microorganisms.

(Continues)

PROCEDURE 29-10 Performing Range-of-Motion (ROM) Exercises (Continued)

ACTION | **RATIONALE**

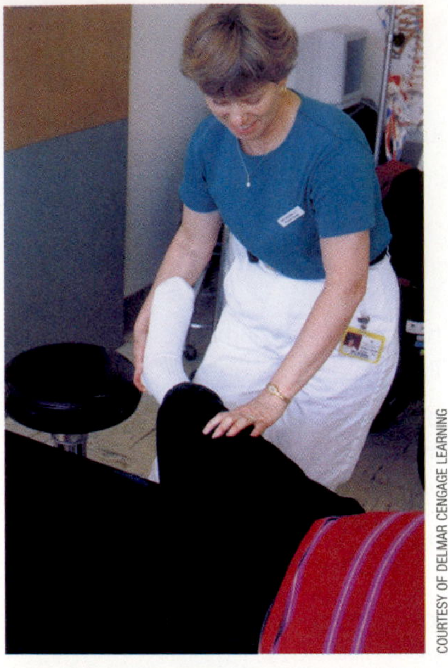

FIGURE 29-10-3 Slide the leg away from the client's midline, then return.

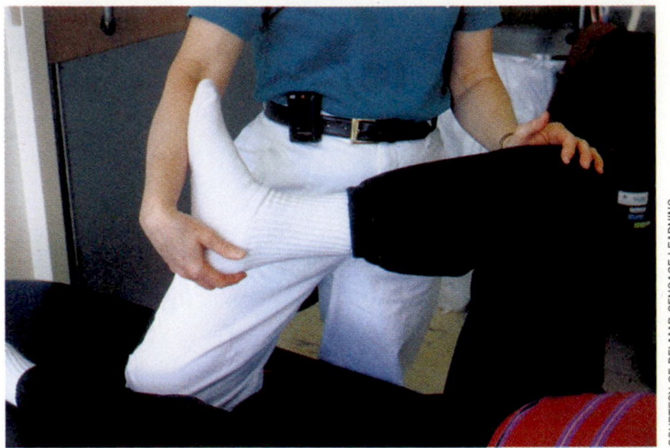

FIGURE 29-10-4 Flex and extend the knee.

EVALUATION

- Client has maintained or improved current functional mobility in all involved joints and extremities.
- Client has regained or improved strength and/or voluntary movement in involved joints and extremities.
- Client has avoided complications of immobility, including pressure ulcers, contractures, decreased peristalsis, constipation, fecal impaction, orthostatic hypotension, pulmonary embolism, and thrombophlebitis.

DOCUMENTATION

Nurses' Notes

- Performance of ROM exercises. Include joints and extremities on which ROM was performed, the types and degrees of limitation observed, the extent of the client's active involvement in exercises, any reports of pain or discomfort, and any observations of intolerance to exercise.
- Unusual findings

PROCEDURE 29-11 Ambulation Safety and Assisting from Bed to Walking

OVERVIEW

Client ambulation (assisted or unassisted walking) is encouraged soon after the onset of illness or surgery to prevent the complications of immobility. First, assess the strength, endurance, mobility, and orientation of the client. Assist with client ambulation, especially if equipment (IV infusions, urinary catheters, closed chest drainage systems, drainage tubes) is present. Evaluate client ambulation to plan the progression of activity.

Clients at high risk for falls include those with prolonged hospitalization, those taking sedatives or tranquilizers, confused clients, or those with a history of physical restraint use. A great majority of falls:

- Occur in the evening
- Occur in the client's room
- Involve wheelchairs
- Involve confused clients
- Involve unattended clients
- Involve clients with poor footwear

(Continues)

PROCEDURE 29-11 Ambulation Safety and Assisting from Bed to Walking (Continued)

- Occur with poor lighting
- Involve clients with poor vision
- Occur with clients experiencing neuromuscular impairment

Awareness of risk factors for falls allows many client injuries to be prevented. When the client is comfortably able to tolerate sitting on the side of the bed and then standing at the side of the bed, progressive ambulation activities are initiated. Disturbances in balance, coordination, proprioception (spatial position), as well as weakness, low endurance, and deconditioning often occur as consequences of medical/surgical procedures. These clients need assistance with ambulation. Gait belts provide client safety when ambulating.

Continually evaluate the client's strength and endurance during the entire ambulation process.

ASSESSMENT

1. Determine the client's most recent activity level and tolerance **to evaluate the client's current ambulatory ability.**
2. Assess the client's current status, including vital signs, fatigue, pain, and medications **to identify conditions that might adversely affect ambulation.**
3. **To evaluate the client's environment for safety:** Check for handrails to help the client stand and to hold onto while walking. Check that the floor is level, clean, and not slippery or wet. Make sure there is adequate lighting so the client can see where he or she is going.
4. Assess the client's ambulation equipment, including the use of a walker, cane, or other assistive device **to determine whether the equipment is in safe condition.**
5. Check the client's clothing **to determine that the client's shoes or slippers are safe to walk in and that he or she has adequate covering for warmth and privacy.**
6. While the client is ambulating, assess his or her gait and bearing. **Determines how well he or she is tolerating the activity and allows detection of hypotension, diaphoresis, breathlessness, or weakness.**
7. After ambulation, assess the client's ability to recover from the activity, including exhaustion, energy, and recovery times. **Determine if modifications need to be made in the distance, type of assistance, or length of time the client is ambulating.**

POSSIBLE NURSING DIAGNOSES

*Risk for **I**njury*
*Impaired **P**hysical Mobility*
***A**ctivity Intolerance*

PLANNING

Expected Outcomes

1. The client will be able to walk a predetermined distance, with assistance as needed, and return to the starting point.
2. While walking, the client will not suffer any injury.
3. The client will be able to increase the distance he or she can walk and/or will require less assistance to accomplish the distance on a regular basis.

Equipment Needed

- Gait belt (transfer) as needed (PRN)
- Assistive devices
- Shoes or nonslip footwear

delegation tips

The ambulation and safe movement of clients is routinely delegated after proper instruction regarding planning the move, arranging for adequate help, if necessary, and positioning oneself close to the client to prevent injury.

IMPLEMENTATION—ACTION/RATIONALE

ACTION	RATIONALE
* Wash hands * Check client's identification band * Explain procedure before beginning *	
Ambulation Safety	
1. When assisting a client with an intravenous (IV) infusion, place the IV pole with wheels at the head of the bed before having the client dangle the legs, so there is room to swing the legs from the bed to the floor. If orders allow, place a saline lock on the IV.	1. Prevents the client's legs from becoming tangled in the IV pole or tubing, causing a fall or causing the tubing to become dislodged. Provides more freedom of movement.
2. If the facility does not maintain IVs on IV poles, transfer the IV infusion from the bed IV pole to the portable IV pole. The client or the nurse can guide the portable IV pole ahead during ambulation (Figure 29-11-1).	2. Supports the IV while the client ambulates.

(Continues)

PROCEDURE 29-11 Ambulation Safety and Assisting from Bed to Walking (Continued)

ACTION

RATIONALE

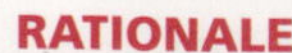

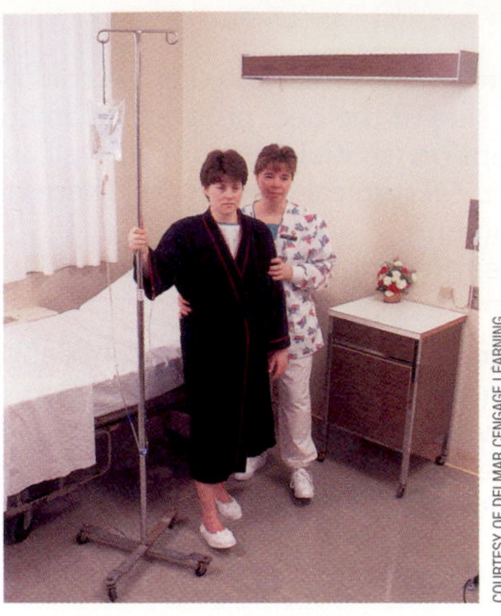

FIGURE 29-11-1 Ambulating client with an IV.

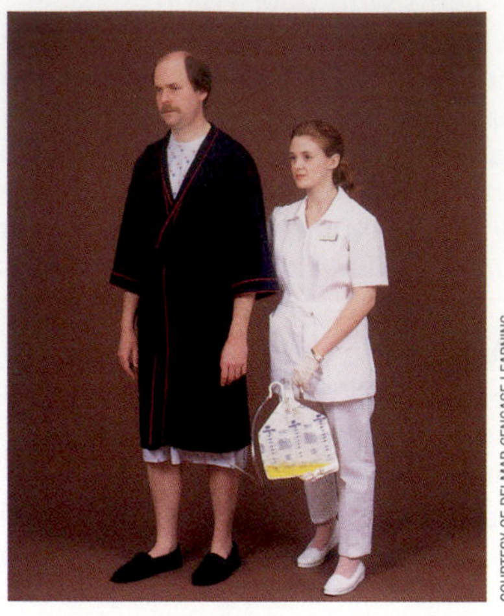

FIGURE 29-11-2 Ambulating client with a urinary drainage bag.

3. When assisting the client with a urinary drainage bag, empty the drainage bag before ambulation. Have the client sit on the side of the bed with legs dangling.
   Remove the urinary drainage bag from the bed. The nurse or client can hold the urinary drainage bag during ambulation. Make sure the drainage bag remains below the level of the bladder (Figure 29-11-2).

   Rationale: 3. Emptying the bag reduces the weight of the bag. An empty bag kept below the level of the bladder reduces the risk of urine flowing back into the bladder, and, hence, reduces risk of contamination.
   Having the nurse hold the drainage bag allows the client to concentrate on safe ambulation.

4. When the client has a drainage tube such as a T-tube, Hemo Vac, or Jackson–Pratt drainage system, be sure to secure the drainage tube and bag before ambulation. Place a rubber band around the drainage tube near the drainage bag. Secure the drainage tube and bag with a safety pin through the rubber band. Allow slack. The safety pin is secured to the client's gown or robe (Figure 29-11-3). Make sure the safety pin is unfastened after the walk so that the tubing is not accidentally pulled when removing the gown.

   Rationale: 4. Prevents the tubing from becoming dislodged or tangled in clothing or other tubes.

5. Ambulating the client with a closed chest tube drainage system often requires two nurses, one assisting the client and one nurse managing the closed chest tube drainage system. While the client is sitting on the edge of the bed with feet

   Rationale: 5. Two nurses allow one to focus on the client's safety and ambulation while the other focuses on maintaining the chest drainage system and keeping tubes from becoming dislodged.

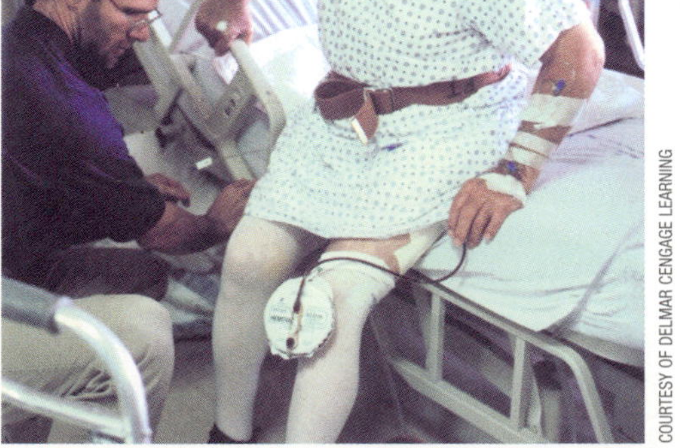

FIGURE 29-11-3 Secure tubes and drainage bags prior to ambulation so that they do not become dislodged.

(Continues)

PROCEDURE 29-11 Ambulation Safety and Assisting from Bed to Walking (Continued)

ACTION	RATIONALE
dangling, remove the hangers from the drainage system. Hold the closed chest tube drainage system upright at all times. Handle all IVs, tubes and chest tubes gently so as not to dislodge any drains.	
6. Use a transfer belt or gait belt when ambulating a client who is weak. For additional safety, a wheelchair can be pushed along behind the client for ready access if the client feels weak, tired, or faint.	6. The transfer belt is a 2-inch-wide webbed belt worn by the client for stabilization during transfers and ambulation. It provides more support for the client by having the nurse hold the back of the belt.
7. If a client feels faint or dizzy during dangling, return the client to a supine position in bed and lower the head of the bed. Monitor the client's blood pressure and pulse.	7. Keeps the client from falling from the bed. Lowering the head of the bed allows gravity to support blood flow to the brain in the hypotensive client.
8. If the client feels faint or dizzy during ambulation, allow the client to sit in a chair. Stay with the client for safety. Request another nurse to secure a wheelchair if not already available to return the client to bed.	8. May stop the client from progressing to full syncope.
9. If the client feels faint or dizzy during ambulation and starts to fall, ease the client to the floor while supporting and protecting the client's head. Position yourself next to and slightly behind the ambulating client, thus being able to step behind the client and safely ease the client to the floor. Ask other personnel to assist you in returning the client to bed. Assess orthostatic blood pressures.	9. Easing the client to the floor prevents injury to the client.
10. Encourage the client to void before ambulating, especially with elderly clients.	10. Prevents need to interrupt ambulation. Restroom may not be readily available.
Bed to Walking	
11. Inform client of the purposes and distance of the walking exercise.	11. Reduces client anxiety and increases cooperation.
12. Elevate the head of the bed and wait several minutes.	12. Prevents orthostatic hypotension.
13. Lower the bed height.	13. Reduces distance client has to step down, thus decreasing risk of injury.
14. Encourage client to actively move legs, or this may be done passively.	14. Stimulates flow of blood, especially elevation of systolic blood pressure to prevent possible orthostatic hypotension.
15. With one arm on the client's back and one arm under the client's upper legs, move the client into the dangling position.	15. Provides client support and reduces risk of falling.
16. Encourage client to dangle at side of bed for several minutes.	16. Prevents orthostatic hypotension. Allows for assessing tolerance for the sitting position.
17. Place gait belt around client's waist; secure the buckle in front. Place ambulation device such as a walker within reach of the client, if necessary. Assist client into standing position (Figure 29-11-4). Make sure bed is locked and floor is not slippery. Client shoes should have nonslip soles.	17. Provides handholds for the caregiver to support the client. Provides for client and caregiver safety.
18. Stand in front of client with your knees touching client's knees.	18. Prevents client from sliding forward if dizziness or faintness occurs.
19. Place arms under client's axilla.	19. Supports client's trunk.
20. Assist client to a standing position, allowing client time to balance.	20. Reduces risk of fall.
21. If client is able to proceed with ambulating, assume a position beside the client and assist the client as necessary using the gait belt. Place yourself in a guarding position so as to assist client quickly and safely, if necessary. Use additional assistance, as necessary.	21. Provides for client and caregiver safety.

(Continues)

PROCEDURE 29-11 Ambulation Safety and Assisting from Bed to Walking (Continued)

ACTION	RATIONALE

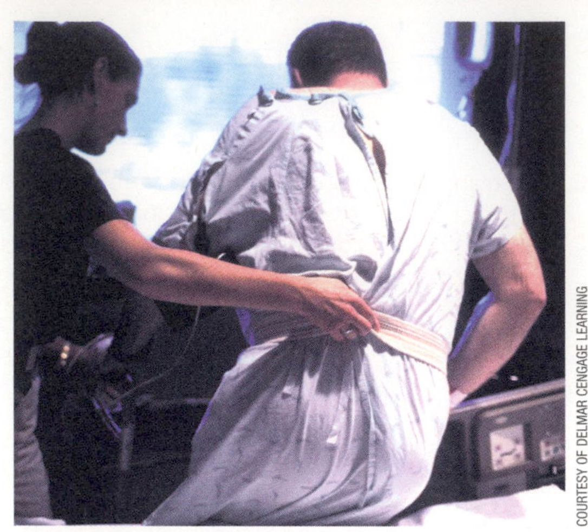

FIGURE 29-11-4 Assist the client to stand.

ACTION	RATIONALE
22. Following ambulation, return client to bed, remove gait belt, and monitor vital signs, as necessary. Make the client comfortable, and make sure all lines and tubes are secure.	22. Promotes safety and comfort.
23. Place the call light within reach of the client.	23. Provides for client safety.
24. Move the bedside table close to the bed and place items of frequent use within reach of the client.	24. Provides for client safety.
25. Wash hands.	25. Reduces the transmission of microorganisms.

EVALUATION

- The client was able to walk a predetermined distance, with assistance as needed, and return to the starting point.
- While walking, the client did not suffer any injury.
- The client was able to increase the distance walked and/or required less assistance to accomplish the distance on a regular basis.

DOCUMENTATION

Nurses' Notes

- Distance the client was able to ambulate and how the client tolerated the ambulation
- Assistive devices the client required and teaching done regarding using the device
- Special concerns or unusual findings observed while ambulating the client

PROCEDURE 29-12 Assisting with Crutches, Cane, or Walker

OVERVIEW

Mobility is an important part of everyone's life. Being able to move about in the environment can mean the difference between living at home and living in a health care facility. Being able to move independently improves a client's emotional, mental, and physical well-being.

Clients who cannot safely walk unassisted can use devices designed to aid them in walking independently. The three most common devices used are crutches, canes, and walkers.

The appropriate device for each client is determined by the client's health care provider, physical therapist, or nurse. These caregivers often work together to determine which device is best for the client. This decision is based on the client's ability to bear weight on the legs, upper arm strength, stamina, and the presence or absence of unilateral weakness.

(Continues)

PROCEDURE 29-12 Assisting with Crutches, Cane, or Walker (Continued)

Crutches are used by clients who cannot bear any weight on one leg, who can only bear partial weight on one leg, and who have full weight-bearing ability on both legs. Several types of crutches are available, depending on the length of time the client requires the assistance and the client's upper-body strength.

A cane is used by clients who can bear weight on both legs but one leg or hip is weaker or impaired. There are several types of canes as well. The standard, straight cane is used most often. There are also canes with three or four legs on the end, called quad canes, to increase a client's stability when walking.

Walkers are used by clients who require more support than a cane provides. Walkers are available with or without wheels. Walkers without wheels provide the most stability, but they must be lifted with each step. Walkers with wheels are somewhat less stable, but a client who does not have the upper-body strength to lift the walker repeatedly can push it along while walking.

ASSESSMENT

1. Assess the reason the client requires an assistive device. Is it a long-term need or a short-term need? **Helps determine which device to use.**
2. Assess the client's physical limitations. How much weight is the client able to bear? Can the client bear weight on both legs or just one? Is the upper body strength good? Does the client tire easily? **Assesses safety and comfort.**
3. Assess the client's physical environment. Is the client at home or in a medical facility? Is the environment suited to assistive needs and the assistive device the client will be using? Are the hallways wide enough? Well lit? Are the doorways wide enough? Are there stairs used frequently, and if so, how many? Do the doors swing open far enough? **Assesses safety and comfort.**
4. Assess the client's ability to understand and follow directions regarding use of an assistive device. Can the client understand the instructions? Can he or she remember them? Has the client used this device in the past? Is there a language barrier that might limit understanding? **Assesses safety, educational, comfort, and effectiveness.**

POSSIBLE NURSING DIAGNOSES

Impaired Physical Mobility
Risk for Trauma
Deficient Knowledge (assistive devices for mobility)

PLANNING

Expected Outcomes

1. The client will be able to demonstrate safe and independent ambulation with the assistance of crutches, a cane, or a walker.
2. The client will feel confident and safe while using the assistive device.

Equipment Needed

- Gait belt
- Assistive device: crutches, cane, or walker
- Tape measure
- Nonslip footwear

delegation tips

Ambulation of clients with assistive devices is frequently delegated to ancillary personnel. The initial teaching of and ongoing assessment of the proper use of the device is not delegated. The nurse or physical or occupational therapist is responsible to observe the client's technique, reteach if necessary, and document the client's proficiency.

IMPLEMENTATION—ACTION/RATIONALE

* Check client's identification band * Explain procedure before beginning *

ACTION	RATIONALE
1. Assess client for strength, mobility, range of motion, visual acuity, perceptual difficulties, and balance. *Note:* The nurse and physical therapist often work together on assessment and choosing the correct assistive equipment of ambulation.	1. Helps determine the client's capabilities and amount of assistance required.
2. Measure client for size of crutches and adjust crutches to fit. While client is supine, measure client from heel to axilla. When client is standing, the crutch pad should fit 1.5 to 2 inches below axilla (Figure 29-12-1). Adjust hand grip so elbow is at 30-degree flexion.	2. Increases client safety and comfort. Space between crutch pad and axilla prevents pressure on radial nerves. Elbow flexion allows for space between crutch pad and axilla.

(Continues)

PROCEDURE 29-12 Assisting with Crutches, Cane, or Walker (Continued)

ACTION	RATIONALE

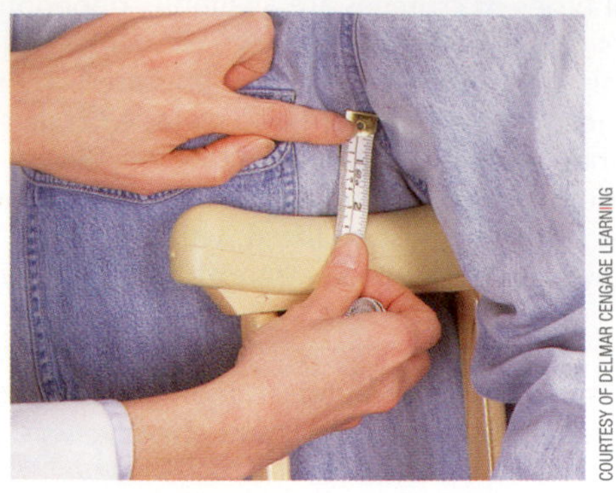

COURTESY OF DELMAR CENGAGE LEARNING

FIGURE 29-12-1 Adjusting the crutches to fit the client will increase comfort and stability.

ACTION	RATIONALE
3. Provide a robe or other covering as well as nonslip foot coverings or shoes.	3. Provides for privacy and safety.
4. Lower the height of the bed.	4. Allows client to sit with feet on the floor and increases safety.
5. Dangle the client at the side of the bed for several minutes. Assess for vertigo or nausea.	5. Allows for stabilization of blood pressure, thus preventing orthostatic hypotension.
6. Apply gait belt around the client's waist if balance and stability are unknown or unreliable. It is good practice to use a gait belt the first time the client is out of bed.	6. Provides support and promotes safety.
7. Demonstrate to client the method of holding crutches while he or she remains seated. This should be with elbows bent 30 degrees while hands are on the hand grips and pads 1.5 to 2 inches below the axilla. Instruct client to position crutches 4 to 5 inches laterally and 4 to 6 inches in front of feet. With weight on hands, not axilla.	7. Increases comprehension and cooperation, decreases anxiety.
8. Assist the client to a standing position by having client place both crutches in nondominant hand. Then, using the dominant hand, push off from the bed while using the crutches for balance. Once erect, the extra crutch can be moved into the dominant hand.	8. Allows for stability while promoting independence.
9. Instruct the client to remain still for a few seconds while assessing for vertigo or nausea. Stand close to the client to support as needed. While client remains standing, check for correct fit of the crutches.	9. Promotes client comfort, support, and safety. If the client becomes dizzy, sit client back down and wait before trying again.
Two-Point Gait (Figure 29-12-2A)	
10. Move the left crutch and right leg forward 4 to 6 inches. Move the right crutch and left leg forward 4 to 6 inches. Repeat the two-point gait.	10. The two-point gait (used for partial weight-bearing) provides a strong base of support. The client must be able to bear weight on both legs. This gait is faster than the four-point gait.
Three-Point Gait (Figure 29-12-2B)	
11. Advance both crutches and the weaker leg forward together 4 to 6 inches. Move the stronger leg forward, even with the crutches. Repeat the three-point gait.	11. The three-point gait (used for partial or non-weight-bearing) provides a strong base of support. This gait can be used if the client has a weak or non-weight-bearing leg.

(Continues)

PROCEDURE 29-12 Assisting with Crutches, Cane, or Walker (Continued)

ACTION	RATIONALE
Four-Point Gait (Figure 29-12-2C)	
12. Position the crutches 4.5 to 6 inches to the side and in front of each foot. Move the right crutch forward 4 to 6 inches and move the left foot forward, even with the left crutch. Move the left crutch forward 4 to 6 inches and move the right foot forward, even with the right crutch. Repeat the four-point gait.	12. The four-point gait (used for partial or full weight-bearing) provides greater stability. Weight bearing is on three points (two crutches and one foot or two feet and one crutch) at all times. The client must be able to bear weight with both legs.
Swing-Through Gait (Figure 29-12-2D)	
13. Move both crutches forward 4 to 6 inches. Move both legs forward in a swinging motion past the crutches. Repeat the swing-through gait.	13. The swing-through gait permits a faster pace. This gait requires greater balance, strength, and more practice.

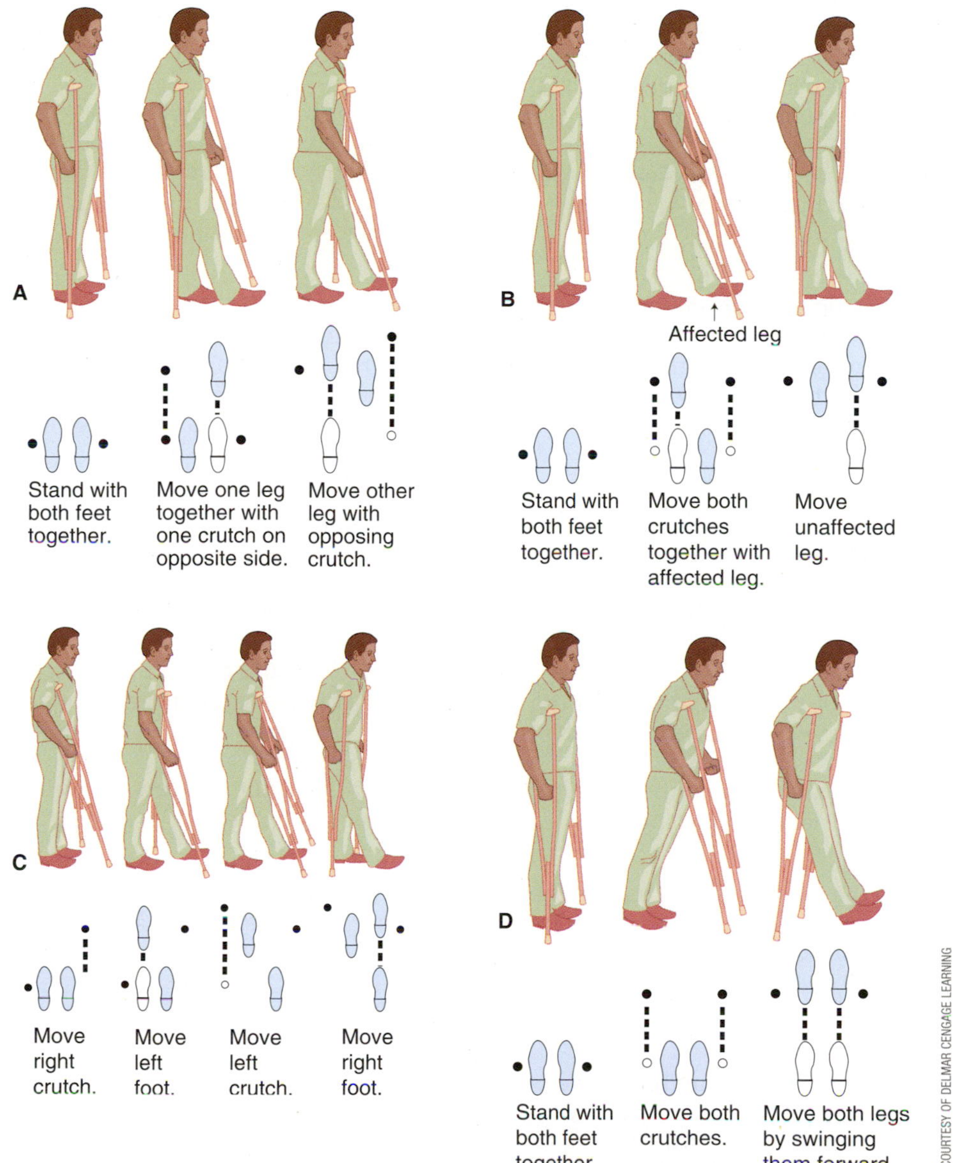
A
Stand with both feet together.
Move one leg together with one crutch on opposite side.
Move other leg with opposing crutch.
B
Affected leg
Stand with both feet together.
Move both crutches together with affected leg.
Move unaffected leg.
C
Move right crutch.
Move left foot.
Move left crutch.
Move right foot.
D
Stand with both feet together.
Move both crutches.
Move both legs by swinging them forward.
COURTESY OF DELMAR CENGAGE LEARNING

FIGURE 29-12-2 Various Crutch Gaits; *A*, Two-Point Gait (partial weight bearing); *B*, Three-Point Gait (partial or non–weight bearing); *C*, Four-Point Gait (partial or full weight bearing); *D*, Swing through Gait (non-weight-bearing)

(Continues)

PROCEDURE 29-12 Assisting with Crutches, Cane, or Walker (Continued)

ACTION	RATIONALE
Walking Upstairs	
14. Stand beside and slightly behind client. Instruct client to position the crutches as if walking. Place body weight on hands. Place the strong leg on the first step. Pull the weak leg up and move the crutches up to the first step. Repeat for all steps.	14. Prevents weight bearing on the weaker leg. When ascending stairs, crutches should follow the legs, thereby allowing stability if the client's weight shifts down the stairs while moving. This allows the client to catch him or herself instead of falling backward.
Walking Downstairs	
15. Position the crutches as if walking. Place weight on the strong leg. Move the crutches down to the next lower step. Place partial weight on hands and crutches. Move the weak leg down to the step with the crutches. Put total weight on arms and crutches. Move strong leg to same step as weak leg and crutches. Repeat for all steps. A second caregiver standing behind the client holding on to the gait belt will further decrease the risk of falling.	15. Prevents weight bearing on the weaker leg. Crutches in front of the legs while descending stairs allow the client more forward stability if his or her weight shifts down the stairs while client is moving. This allows client to catch self before falling forward.
16. Set realistic goals and opportunities for progressive ambulation using crutches.	16. Crutch walking takes up to 10 times the energy required for unassisted ambulation.
17. Consult with a physical therapist for clients learning to walk with crutches.	17. The physical therapist is the expert on the health care team for crutch-walking techniques.
18. Wash hands.	18. Reduces transmission of microorganisms.
Sitting with Crutches	
19. Instruct client to back up to chair until it is felt with the back of the legs.	19. Allows for less turning, better stability, and increased safety.
20. Place both crutches in the nondominant hand and use the dominant hand to reach back to the chair.	20. Increases safety by giving the client an idea of how far away he or she is from the seat.
21. Instruct client to lower slowly into the chair.	21. Decreases pain and possible injuries.
Walking with a Cane	
22. Repeat Actions 1 to 6.	22. See Rationales 1 to 6.
23. Have the client push up from the sitting position while pushing down on the bed with arms.	23. Promotes autonomy as well as increases upper body strength.
24. Have the client stand at the bedside for a few moments with cane in hand opposite the affected leg.	24. Allows the client to gain balance. Allows more control of cane.
25. Assess the height of the cane. With the cane placed 6 inches ahead of the client's body, the top of the cane should be at wrist level with the arm bent 25% to 30% at the elbow.	25. A 25% to 30% bend at the elbow provides for better muscle strength and support than if the arm is straight.
26. Walk to the side and slightly behind the client, holding the gait belt if needed for stability.	26. Allows the nurse to provide stability or assistance if the client needs it.
Cane Gait	
27. Move the cane and the weaker leg forward at the same time for the same distance (Figure 29-12-3). Place weight on the weaker leg and the cane. Move the strong leg forward. Place weight on the strong leg.	27. The cane helps provide a wide base of support for the body when the weight is on the weaker leg.
Sitting with a Cane	
28. Have client turn around and back up to the chair. Have client grasp the arm of the chair with the free hand and lower self into the chair. Be sure to place the cane out of the way but within reach.	28. The cane provides additional support as client lowers self into the chair.
29. Consult with a physical therapist for clients learning to walk with a cane.	29. The physical therapist is the expert on the health care team for cane-walking techniques.
30. Wash hands.	30. Reduces transmission of microorganisms.

(Continues)

PROCEDURE 29-12 Assisting with Crutches, Cane, or Walker (Continued)

ACTION	RATIONALE

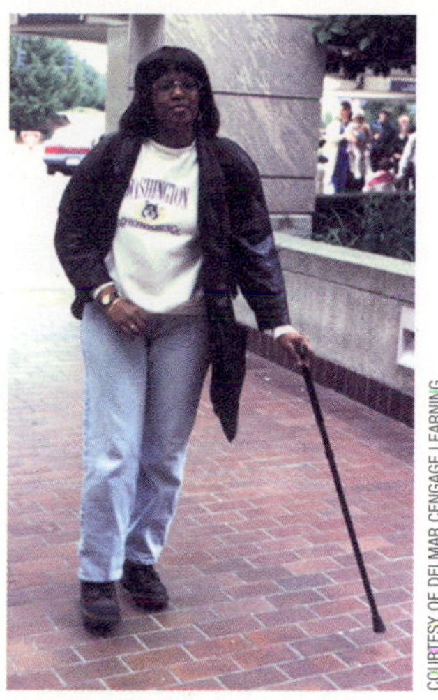

FIGURE 29-12-3 Move the cane and the weaker leg forward. Cane should be in alignment with client.

Walking with a Walker

ACTION	RATIONALE
31. Repeat Actions 1 to 6.	31. See Rationales 1 to 6.
32. Place the walker in front of the client.	32. Positions the walker for use and provides stability when the client is standing.
33. Have the client put the nondominant hand on the front bar of the walker or on the hand grip for that hand, whichever is more comfortable. Then, using the dominant hand to push off from the bed and the nondominant hand for stabilization, help the client to an erect position.	33. Uses upper body strength and encourages independence.
34. Have the client transfer hand to the walker handgrips.	34. Allows the client to maintain balance while transferring weight.
35. Be sure the walker is adjusted so the handgrips are just below waist level and the client's arms are slightly bent at the elbow.	35. Provides maximum support from the arms while ambulating.
36. Walk to the side and slightly behind the client, holding the gait belt if needed for stability.	36. Provides stability or assistance if the client needs it.

Walker Gait

ACTION	RATIONALE
37. Move the walker and the weaker leg forward at the same time (Figure 29-12-4). Place as much weight as possible or as allowed on the weaker leg, using the arms for supporting the rest of the weight. Move the strong leg forward and shift the weight to the strong leg (Figure 29-12-5).	37. Provides support for a weak or non–weight-bearing leg by using arm and upper body strength.

Sitting with a Walker

ACTION	RATIONALE
38. Have the client turn around in front of the chair and back up until the back of the legs touch the chair. Have client place hands on the chair armrests, one hand at a time, then lower self into the chair using the armrests for support.	38. Using the armrests of the chair is a more stable support than using the walker.
39. Consult with a physical therapist for clients learning to walk with a walker.	39. The physical therapist is the expert on the health care team for walker techniques.
40. Wash hands.	40. Reduces transmission of microorganisms.

(Continues)

PROCEDURE 29-12 Assisting with Crutches, Cane, or Walker (Continued)

ACTION **RATIONALE**

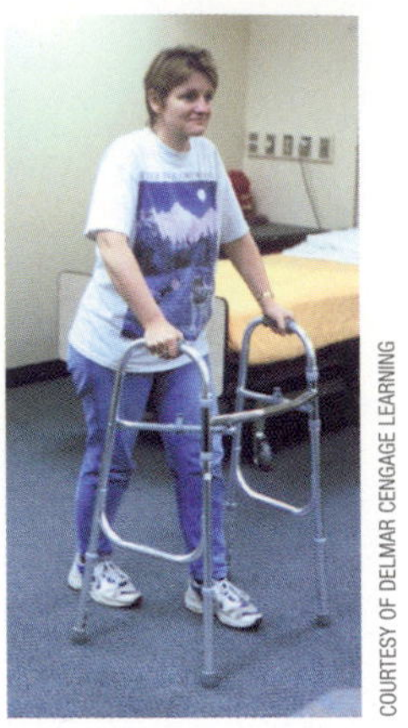

FIGURE 29-12-4 **Move the walker and the weaker leg forward.**

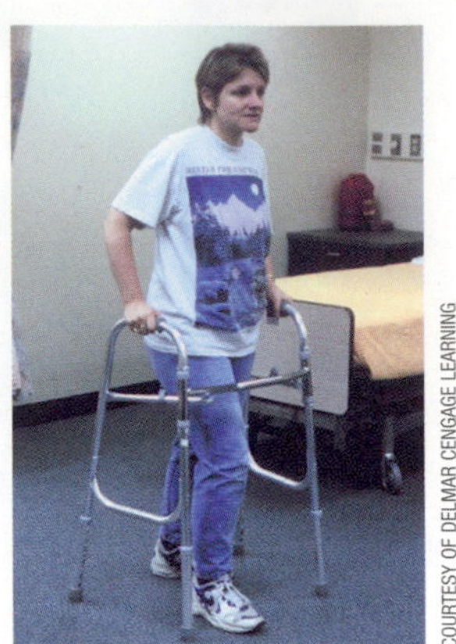

FIGURE 29-12-5 **Use the arms to support the rest of the weight and move strong leg forward.**

EVALUATION

- The client is able to demonstrate safe and independent ambulation with the assistance of crutches, a cane, or a walker.
- The client feels confident and safe while using the assistive device.

DOCUMENTATION

Nurses' Notes

- Type of device the client is using, the level of understanding regarding the use of the device, how far the client is able to walk using the device, and the client's response to the activity

Kardex

- Information that is pertinent to nurses or therapists regarding type of device or a particular client's needs

PROCEDURE 29-13 Turning and Positioning a Client

OVERVIEW

Clients are not always able to independently move and position themselves in bed. Proper turning and positioning allows the health care provider to make clients as comfortable as possible, prevent contractures and pressure sores, make portions of the client's body available for treatment or procedures, and allows clients greater access to their environment. There are three key concepts to remember when positioning a client: pressure, friction, and skin shear.

Any area that contacts the surface the client is lying on is a pressure site. Because of circulatory compromise, the pressure sites over bony prominences are at the highest risk of skin breakdown and ulceration. Always assess the blood flow to skin and tissue areas put under increased pressure when placing a client in a given position. When repositioning a client, be sure the sheets under the client are smooth. This helps prevent areas of increased pressure that could contribute to pressure sores.

Skin shear is caused when the skin is dragged across a hard surface. The deep layers of skin are torn by the resistance of being dragged. This damage to the skin can lead to skin breakdown and ulceration. To prevent skin shear, or friction burn from the sheets, do not drag a client across the bed. Lift the client into proper position or use a turning sheet.

(Continues)

PROCEDURE 29-13 Turning and Positioning a Client (Continued)

Friction is caused when the skin is dragged across a rough surface, thereby causing heat and damaging the skin's surface. Any damage to the skin's integrity can lead to infection and skin breakdown.

Clients who cannot reposition themselves must be repositioned at least every two hours and more frequently if they are uncomfortable, incontinent, or have poor circulation, fragile skin, decreased cognition, decreased sensation, or poor nutritional status. When repositioning a client, assess the skin for redness and integrity. Areas of redness should be resolved before the client is repositioned on that area. Areas of redness that do not resolve within 30 minutes after pressure relief should be documented. A plan to reposition the client more frequently may need to be instituted. Areas of prolonged redness are more likely to sustain tissue damage, as are tissue areas covering bony prominences. Hip, back, neck, or head conditions may require that a client be turned keeping the body in alignment, turning as one unit, as a log. This is called log rolling. Remember that proper body mechanics are essential to protect the caregiver's back and to ensure client safety.

ASSESSMENT

1. Assess the client's ability to move independently. **Determine if the client can assist with turning and repositioning.**
2. Assess the client's flexibility. **If clients have contractures or other flexibility limitations, their positions may need to be modified to allow for the restrictions.**
3. Assess the client's age, medical diagnosis, cognitive status, skin integrity, nutritional status, continence, altered sensation, as well as the overall condition of the musculoskeletal system. **Helps determine the client's potential for pressure sore development.**
4. Assess the physician's or qualified practitioner's orders for specific restrictions regarding client positioning **to ensure the correct positioning is implemented.**

POSSIBLE NURSING DIAGNOSES

Risk for Impaired Skin Integrity
Impaired Physical Mobility
Activity Intolerance
Acute Pain

PLANNING

Expected Outcomes

1. The client will maintain skin integrity without skin burns, pressure areas, or pressure ulcers.
2. The client will be comfortable as evident by verbal and nonverbal cues.

Equipment Needed

- Pillows
- Rolled blankets or towels
- Footboard
- Heel protectors
- Hand rolls
- Gloves (if chance of exposure to body fluids)

delegation tips

Turning and positioning are routinely delegated to ancillary personnel who have received the appropriate training. The caregiver must protect him or herself and the client from injury and report the client's response to the activity to the nurse.

IMPLEMENTATION—ACTION/RATIONALE

ACTION	RATIONALE
* Check client's identification band * Explain procedure before beginning *	
1. Wash hands.	1. Reduces the transmission of microorganisms.
2. Gather all necessary equipment. Provide for client privacy.	2. Ensures client dignity and allows for a smooth procedure.
3. Secure adequate assistance to safely complete task.	3. Prevents caregiver back and muscle strain as well as provides for client safety.
4. Adjust bed to comfortable working height. Lower side rail on side of bed from which you are assisting client.	4. Prevents caregiver back and muscle strain.
5. Follow proper body mechanics guidelines: When moving a client in bed, position the bed so that your legs are slightly bent at the knees and hips. Maintain the natural curves in your back while lifting. Position one foot slightly in front of	5. Prevents caregiver back injury and muscle strain and promotes client safety. Spreading feet to create a wide base helps prevent loss of balance.

(Continues)

PROCEDURE 29-13 Turning and Positioning a Client (Continued)

ACTION	RATIONALE
the other and spread feet apart to create a wide base for balance. When your arms are placed under the client, slowly lean backward onto your back leg using your body weight to help you lift the client to one side of the bed. Do not extend or rotate your back to move a client in bed. If you cannot move the client easily, always ask for and obtain assistance for both your and the client's safety (Figure 29-13-1). Be sure the floor is not slippery and that the bed is locked. Always use a turning sheet when rolling a client because this gives you better support and control of the client (Figure 29-13-2).	
6. Position drains, tubes, and IVs to accommodate for new client position.	6. Prevents accidental dislodgment and/or discomfort from movement by reduced mechanical tension.
7. Place or assist client into appropriate starting position. Monitor client status, and provide adequate rest breaks or support as necessary.	7. Prevents client injury.
Moving from Supine to Side-Lying Position	
8. Slide your hands underneath the client. Move the client to one side of the bed by lifting the client's body toward you in stages—first the upper trunk, then the lower trunk, and finally the legs. Lift the client's body; do not drag the client across the sheets. Move to other side of bed. Roll the client to side-lying position by placing the client's inside arm next to the client's body with the palm of the hand against the hip. Cross the client's outside arm and leg toward midline and log roll the client toward you using the client's outside shoulder and hip for leverage while maintaining stability and control of top arm and leg.	8. Prevents shearing of skin tissue. Maintains client body alignment. Protects caregiver's back and prevents muscle strain. Prevents client injury and shearing of skin tissue.
Maintaining Side-Lying Position	
9. Repeat Actions 1 to 8.	9. See Rationales 1 to 8.
10. Pillows may be placed to support the client's head and arms (Figure 29-13-3). An additional pillow	10. Provides support and comfort.

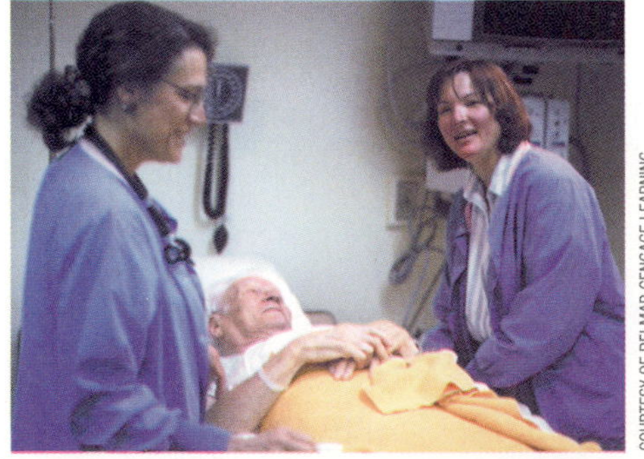

FIGURE 29-13-1 If the client is heavy or hard to move, always obtain assistance for both the client's and your safety.

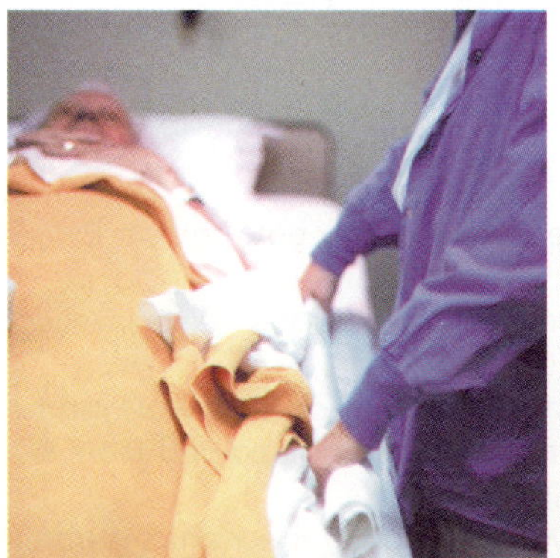

FIGURE 29-13-2 When rolling a client, use a turning sheet for better support and control.

(Continues)

PROCEDURE 29-13 Turning and Positioning a Client (Continued)

ACTION	RATIONALE

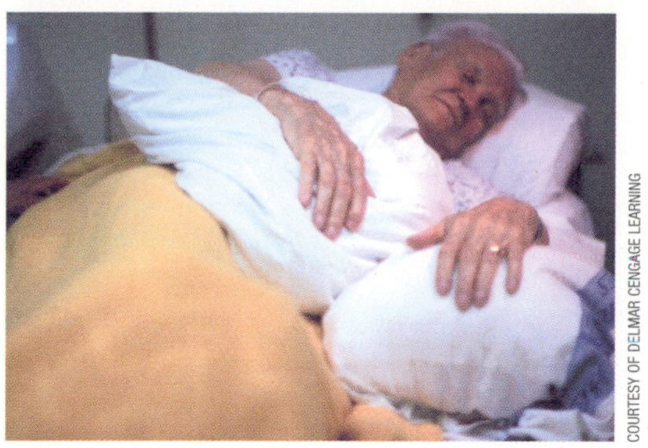

FIGURE 29-13-3 Place pillows to support the head and arms.

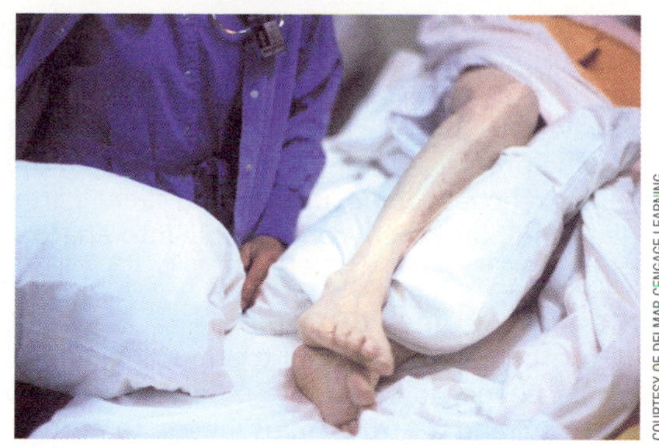

FIGURE 29-13-4 Place pillows to support the leg, ankle, and foot.

may be used to support the topside leg, and fully and equally support the thigh, knee, ankle, and foot (Figure 29-13-4). Move the lower arm forward slightly at the shoulder and bend the elbow for comfort. If the client is unstable, a pillow placed against the back will provide additional support and keep the client from rolling supine.

Moving from Side-Lying to Prone Position

ACTION	RATIONALE
11. Repeat Actions 1 to 8.	11. See Rationales 1 to 8.
12. Remove positioning towels, pillows, or other support devices. Assess whether the client's position in bed needs to be adjusted to accommodate the continued movement into prone. Move the client's inside arm next to the client's body with palm against hip. Roll the client onto the stomach using the shoulder and hip as key points of control. The head must be placed in a comfortable position to one side without excessive pressure to sensitive areas. Pillows under the trunk are placed as needed to relieve pressure and increase comfort. The client's arms are placed comfortably at the client's side and the legs are uncrossed with the feet approximately a foot apart.	12. Ensures comfort and safety in movement.

Maintaining Prone Position

ACTION	RATIONALE
13. A shallow pillow or a folded towel may be used to support the client's head comfortably as well as a pillow placed under the abdomen to support the back. An additional pillow may be placed under the lower leg to reduce the pressure of the toes and forefoot against the bed.	13. Provides support and comfort.

Moving from Prone to Supine Position

ACTION	RATIONALE
14. Repeat Actions 1 to 8.	14. See Rationales 1 to 8.
15. Remove positioning towels, pillows, or other supporting devices. Slide your hands underneath the client. Move the client segmentally to one side of the bed to accommodate the new position. Position the inside arm next to the client's body with the client's palm next to the hip. Roll the	15. Provides support and comfort.

(Continues)

PROCEDURE 29-13 Turning and Positioning a Client (Continued)

ACTION	RATIONALE
client to supine by log rolling the client toward you using the client's outside shoulder and hip for leverage. Have the client's face positioned away from the direction of the roll to prevent undue pressure to the face or neck. When the client reaches supine, uncross the client's arms and legs and place them comfortably into anatomic positions.	
Maintaining Supine Position	
16. A footboard may be used to support the foot as well as heel protectors or a pillow placed between the heel and gastrocnemius muscle to reduce the pressure on the heels. Assess and compare warmth, sensation, color, and movement of feet. To prevent excessive external rotation of the lower extremity, a trochanter roll is used. For comfort, additional pillows are used to support the client's head, arms, or lower back.	16. Provides support and comfort. Heel protectors and routine assessment of the feet help to prevent pressure sores. Trochanter rolls and pillows help to prevent displacement of the acetabulum (hip joint).
Log Rolling	
17. Repeat Actions 1 to 8.	17. See Rationales 1 to 8.
18. Use three nurses. Place a turning/draw sheet under client's head, back, and buttocks (if not already present).	18. Provides for client safety. Reduces shearing force.
19. Place pillow between client's legs.	19. Keeps legs in alignment with body.
20. Have client fold arms across chest.	20. Prevents getting the client's arms trapped or injured.
21. Roll up draw sheet on the far side until it is next to the client.	21. Provides support under the heavy parts of the client and places the nurses' hands close to the weight to be turned.
22. One nurse places hands under the client's far leg, another holds rolled draw sheet at client's buttocks, and third nurse holds rolled draw sheet at chest and shoulder level.	22. Ensures client is turned like a log, as a unit.
23. Nurse nearest the client's head gives the signal to turn: 1-2-3 turn.	23. Ensures a smooth, coordinated turn.
24. Tuck pillows at client's back and abdomen.	24. Helps maintain side-lying position.
25. Assess the client for comfort and proper alignment.	25. Comfort is subjective. Ensures alignment.
26. Procedure can be reversed to reposition client on back or opposite side.	26. Reduces pressure ulcer development.
27. Be sure to replace side rails to upright position as well as to lower bed to beginning position.	27. Provides for client safety.
28. Place call light within reach of the client.	28. Provides for client safety.
29. Move bedside table close to bed and place items of frequent use within reach of the client.	29. Provides for client safety.
30. Wash hands.	30. Reduces the transmission of microorganisms.

EVALUATION

- Safe and proper body alignment and movement were achieved for both client and caregiver.
- The client is comfortable in the new position as evident by verbal and nonverbal cues.
- The client's skin and underlying organs and tissues were protected from pressure, friction, and shear.

DOCUMENTATION

Nurses' Notes

- Client's new position and time of the position change
- Report or observation of pain, discomfort, or dyspnea
- Integumentary assessment, including color and integrity of skin and length of time redness persists over bony prominences

PROCEDURE 29-14 Moving a Client in Bed

OVERVIEW

Prolonged immobility is uncomfortable and presents an increased risk of many complications. Muscle wasting, clot formation, and skin breakdown are the most common risks associated with immobility. Clients who are unable to move themselves in bed or are only able to assist with moving in bed are at risk for discomfort and complications related to immobility. Often, clients' restlessness in bed will cause them to slide down toward the foot of the bed. This is especially true in beds where the head raises up to a Fowler's or semi-Fowler's position. If the client slides down toward the foot of the bed while the head is elevated, it leads to reduced respiratory effort, reduced lung capacity, and skin breakdown, thus impairing the client's recovery.

The nurse often moves a client to a more comfortable position. Repositioning a client is sometimes done by a single staff member, but often it requires two or more people to do this procedure safely.

ASSESSMENT

1. Assess the client's ability to assist with repositioning. Determine if the client can move with the aid of an overhead trapeze or the side rail. Judge how much assistance will be needed. **Determines safety for the client and the nurse and good body mechanics for the nurse.**
2. Assess the client's ability to understand and follow directions and assist and cooperate with the move. **Affects how the procedure is completed and client teaching.**
3. Assess the client's environment and bed for cleanliness. Has the client been restless, sweaty, or incontinent? Check to see if the sheets are turned or twisted. Tubes, lines, wires, traction, casts, or splints are moved carefully. **Affects how the procedure is completed. Affects what additional procedures are performed. Prepares the caregivers to keep tubes and equipment from becoming dislodged, tipped, or pulled.**

POSSIBLE NURSING DIAGNOSES

Impaired Physical Mobility
Activity Intolerance
Risk for Impaired Skin Integrity

PLANNING

Expected Outcomes

1. The client will be moved in bed without injury to self.
2. The client will be moved in bed without injury to the staff.
3. The client will report an increase in comfort following the move.
4. All tubes, lines, and drains will remain patent and intact.

Equipment Needed

- Hospital bed with side rails
- Trapeze if required
- Turn sheet or draw sheet

delegation tips

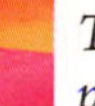

Turning and positioning is routinely delegated to ancillary personnel who have received appropriate training. The caregiver protects himself and the client from injury and reports the client's activity response to the nurse.

IMPLEMENTATION—ACTION/RATIONALE

ACTION	RATIONALE
* Check client's identification band * Explain procedure before beginning *	
Moving a Client Up in Bed with One Nurse	
1. Wash hands.	1. Reduces the transmission of microorganisms.
2. Elevate bed to just below waist height. Lower head of bed if tolerated by client. Lower side rails on the side where you are standing.	2. Lessens strain on nurse's back muscles.
3. Remove the pillow and place it against the headboard.	3. Prevents having to move against the pillow. Provides padding of the headboard if the client should be moved too high in the bed.
4. Have client hold on to the overhead trapeze, if available (Figure 29-14-1).	4. Promotes client autonomy by allowing the client to assist with the move.

(Continues)

PROCEDURE 29-14 Moving a Client in Bed (Continued)

ACTION	RATIONALE

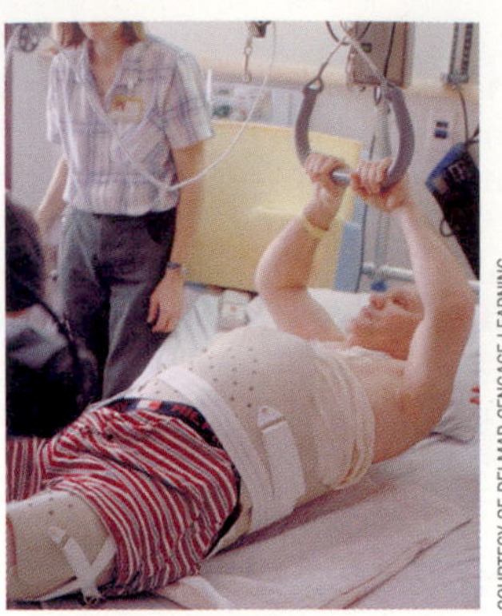

FIGURE 29-14-1 Have client hold onto the overhead trapeze, if one is available, to assist in the move.

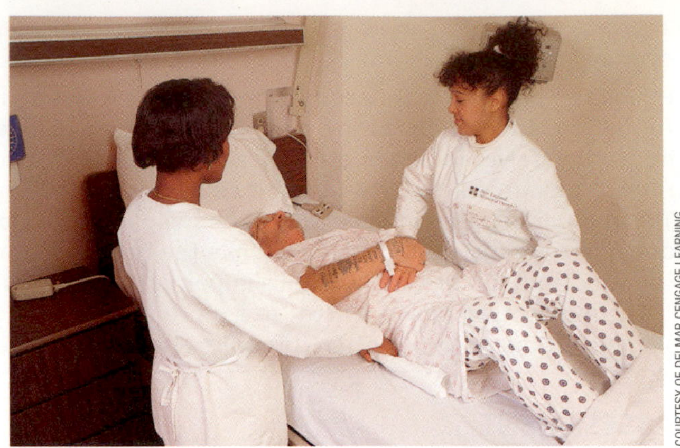

FIGURE 29-14-2 Have the client bend the knees and place feet on the bed.

ACTION	RATIONALE
5. Have the client bend the knees and place the feet flat on the bed if able (Figure 29-14-2).	5. Allows the client to assist in the move; promotes client autonomy.
6. Stand at an angle to the head of the bed, feet apart, knees bent, feet toward the head of the bed.	6. Promotes good body mechanics.
7. Slide one hand and arm under the client's shoulder, the other under the client's thigh.	7. Distributes the client's weight more evenly. Promotes good lifting technique.
8. Rock forward toward the head of the bed, lifting the client with you. Simultaneously have the client push with the legs.	8. Allows a smooth motion to lift the client. Client assistance lessens strain on nurse's back muscles; promotes client autonomy.
9. If the client has a trapeze, have the client pull up holding onto the trapeze as you move the client upward in bed.	9. Client assistance lessens strain on nurse's back muscles; promotes client autonomy.
10. Repeat these steps until the client is moved up high enough in bed.	10. Large or very immobile clients are often not moved far enough in one step.
11. Return the client's pillow under the head.	11. Promotes client comfort.
12. Elevate head of bed, if tolerated by client.	12. Promotes comfort; facilitates eating and drinking; facilitates communication.
13. Assess client for comfort.	13. Comfort is subjective.
14. Adjust the client's bedclothes as needed for comfort.	14. Promotes comfort.
15. Lower bed and elevate side rails.	15. Promotes client safety.
16. Wash hands.	16. Reduces the transmission of microorganisms.

Moving a Client Up in Bed with Two or More Nurses

ACTION	RATIONALE
17. Wash hands and apply gloves if needed.	17. Reduces the transmission of microorganisms.
18. Elevate bed to just below waist height. Lower head of bed if tolerated by client. Lower side rails.	18. Lessens strain on nurses' back muscles.
19. With two nurses, place turn/draw sheet under client's back and head.	19. Reduces shearing force, which can precipitate skin breakdown.
20. Roll up the draw sheet on each side until it is next to the client (refer to Figure 29-14-3).	20. Provides support under the heavy parts of the body and places the nurse's hands close to the weight to be moved.
21. Follow previous Actions 3 to 5.	21. See Rationales 3 to 5.
22. The nurses stand on either side of the bed, at an angle to the head of the bed, with knees flexed, feet apart in a wide stance.	22. Promotes good body mechanics.

(Continues)

PROCEDURE 29-14 Moving a Client in Bed (Continued)

ACTION	RATIONALE

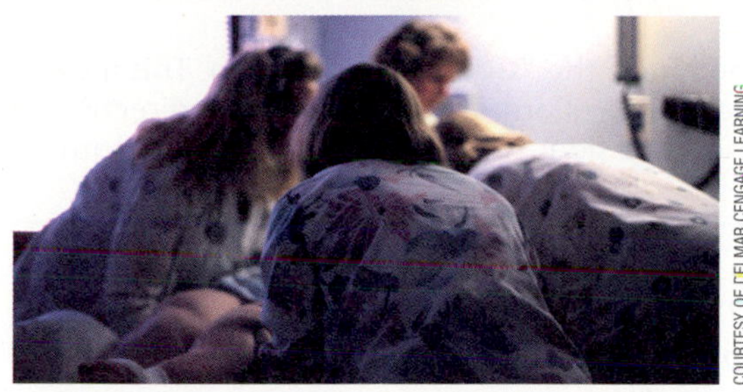

FIGURE 29-14-3 At the signal from the lead nurse, lift and pull in one smooth motion. A gentle, smooth, coordinated motion does not jar or injure the client.

ACTION	RATIONALE
23. The nurses hold their elbows as close as possible to their bodies.	23. Allows the muscles of the torso to assist the arm muscles in bearing and moving the weight of the client.
24. The lead nurse gives the signal to move: 1-2-3 go. The nurses lift the turn/draw sheet off the bed and toward the head of the bed in one smooth motion. Simultaneously, the client pushes with the legs or pulls using the trapeze. Nurses take care to move the client with a gentle, smooth, coordinated motion so as not to jar or injure the client.	24. Allows a smooth motion to lift the client. Client assistance lessens strain on the nurses' back muscles; promotes client autonomy.
25. Repeat previous Actions 10 to 16.	25. See previous Rationales 10 to 16.

EVALUATION

- The client was moved without injury to self or staff.
- The client reported an increase in comfort following the move.
- All tubes, lines, and drains remained intact.

DOCUMENTATION

Nurses' Notes

- Time and position the client was moved
- Unusual findings

PROCEDURE 29-15 Transferring from Bed to Wheelchair, Commode, or Chair

OVERVIEW

Client activity is an important part of the healing process. Activity improves muscle tone, increases venous return to the heart, and stimulates peristalsis. Moving a client from the bed to a chair is an important part of client activity.

Moving a client from the bed to a chair, wheelchair, commode, or stretcher is called a transfer. Transferring a client requires good planning to avoid injury to the client and the nurse. When transferring a client, consider the client's ability to assist with the transfer. If the client is unable to provide any assistance or is large, one or more staff members are needed to help perform the transfer safely.

The most frequent complication in transferring a client is falling during the transfer. Gait belts provide client safety during a transfer. If a client starts to fall during the transfer, lower him or her gently to the floor, making sure the head does not strike anything. If a client does fall, obtain assistance and perform a thorough assessment of the client before moving him or her.

Another possible hazard in client transfers is pulling on or dislodging indwelling tubes or catheters. Think ahead about ways tubes will move with the transfer and try to avoid snagging them. Take care to appropriately anchor all tubes and catheters before transferring a client.

Clients are also at risk of damage to their skin during a transfer. Sliding across the sheets, side rails, and wheelchair armrest can bruise or injure the client. Use a transfer board or pad any sharp exposed areas to help prevent injury to the client.

(Continues)

PROCEDURE 29-15 Transferring from Bed to Wheelchair, Commode, or Chair (Continued)

Be sure the client is wearing shoes or slippers with firm, nonslip soles when transferring a client. Even if the client is standing only briefly, the feet need protecting from potential injury and contamination from the floor and the client from slipping.

When transferring a client with weakness on one side of the body, use the "Good to go" maxim. This means that the client needs to lead off with the "good" or strong side of the body. Perform the transfer in the direction of the good side, so the client pivots and supports the weight on the good side. This allows maximum strength and stability on the client's part.

ASSESSMENT

1. Assess the client's current level of mobility. Determine how much the client is able to assist with the transfer. Assess for pain or confusion, which might impair ability to assist. Check for a "weak" side. **Affects how the procedure is completed.**
2. Assess for any impediments to mobility, including casts, drainage tubes, catheters, IVs, or intubation. **Affects how the procedure will be carried out. Prepares caregivers to keep tubes and equipment from becoming dislodged, tipping, or pulling.**
3. Assess the client's level of understanding and anxiety regarding the procedure. **Affects how the procedure is completed and client teaching.**
4. Assess the client's environment. Assess the available space for maneuvering the wheelchair to the bed. **Affects how the procedure is completed and safety and good body mechanics for caregivers.**
5. Assess the equipment. Check the bed and chair height. See whether they are adjustable. Check for chair footings and wheelchair brakes. **Affects safety for client and caregivers.**

POSSIBLE NURSING DIAGNOSES

*Impaired Physical **M**obility*
***A**ctivity **I**ntolerance*
*Risk for **I**njury*

PLANNING

Expected Outcomes

1. The client will be transferred from the bed to the wheelchair, commode, or chair without pain or injury.
2. Drainage tubes, IVs, or other devices will be intact.
3. The client's skin will be intact and undamaged.

Equipment Needed

- Bed
- Wheelchair, chair, or commode
- Any splints, braces, or supportive equipment specific to the client
- Shoes or slippers with nonskid soles
- Gait belt
- Transfer board (if necessary)

delegation tips

Assisting a client from a bed to a wheelchair, commode, or chair is a skill routinely delegated to properly trained ancillary personnel.

IMPLEMENTATION—ACTION/RATIONALE

* Check client's identification band * Explain procedure before beginning *

ACTION	RATIONALE
1. Wash hands.	1. Reduces transmission of microorganisms.
2. Assess client for ability to assist with the transfer and for presence of cognitive or sensory deficits.	2. Allows planning regarding the amount of assistance and cooperation to expect from the client.
3. Lock the bed in position.	3. Prevents the bed from rolling during the procedure.
4. Place any splints, braces, or other devices on the client.	4. Provides support and prevents injury to the client.
5. Place the client's shoes or slippers on the client's feet.	5. Provides a nonslip surface for stability.
6. Lower the height of the bed to lowest possible position.	6. Reduces distance client has to step down, thus decreasing risk of injury.

(Continues)

PROCEDURE 29-15 Transferring from Bed to Wheelchair, Commode, or Chair (Continued)

ACTION	RATIONALE
7. Slowly raise the head of the bed if this is not contraindicated by the client's condition.	7. Minimizes lifting.
8. Place one arm under the client's legs and one arm behind the client's back. Slowly pivot the client so the client's legs are dangling over the edge of the bed and the client is in a sitting position on the edge of the bed (Figure 29-15-1).	8. Supports the client while sitting him or her upright.
9. Allow client to dangle for 2 to 5 minutes. Help support client if necessary (Figure 29-15-2).	9. Allows time for assessing client's response to sitting; reduces possibility of orthostatic hypotension.
10. Bring the chair or wheelchair close to the side of the bed. Place it at a 45-degree angle to the bed. If the client has a weaker side, place the chair or wheelchair on the client's strong side.	10. Minimizes transfer distance. Allows the client to pivot on the stronger leg.
11. Lock wheelchair brakes and elevate the foot pedals. For chairs, lock brakes if available.	11. Provides stability.
12. If using a gait belt to assist the client, place it around the client's waist.	12. Provides a secure handhold for the nurse during the transfer.
13. Assist client to side of bed until feet are firmly on the floor and slightly apart.	13. Moves client into proper position for transfer. Provides stable footing for client.
14. Grasp the sides of the gait belt or place your hands just below the client's axilla. Using a wide stance, bend your knees and assist the client to a standing position.	14. Wide stance increases nurse stability and minimizes strain on the back. Avoids putting pressure directly on the axilla, and risking nerve damage or shoulder subluxation.
15. Standing close to the client, pivot until the client's back is toward the chair.	15. Moves client into proper position to be seated.
16. Instruct the client to place hands on the arm supports, or place the client's hands on the arm supports of the chair.	16. Allows client to gain balance and judge distance to seat.
17. Bend at the knees and ease the client into a sitting position.	17. Increases stability and minimizes strain on back.
18. Assist client to maintain proper posture. Support weak side with pillow if needed.	18. Increases client comfort.
19. Secure the safety belt, place client's feet on feet pedals, and release brakes if you will be moving the client immediately. Make sure tubes and lines, arms, and hands are not pinched or caught between the client and the chair (Figure 29-15-3).	19. Ensures client safety; prepares client for movement.

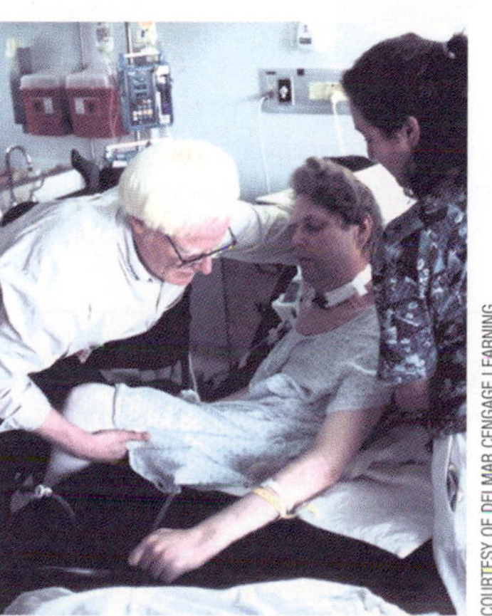

COURTESY OF DELMAR CENGAGE LEARNING

FIGURE 29-15-1 Pivot the client to a sitting position on the edge of the bed.

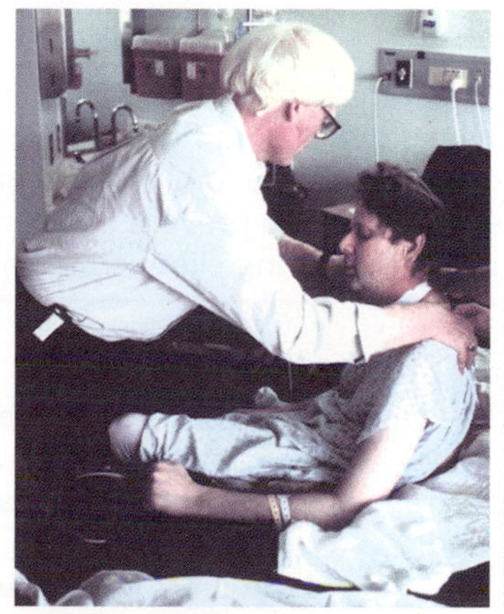

COURTESY OF DELMAR CENGAGE LEARNING

FIGURE 29-15-2 Support the client, if needed, while the client adjusts to the sitting position.

(Continues)

PROCEDURE 29-15 Transferring from Bed to Wheelchair, Commode, or Chair (Continued)

ACTION	RATIONALE
If a client is sitting in a wheelchair, position the footrests in a position of client comfort (Figure 26-15-4); if in a chair, offer a footstool if available.	
20. Wash hands.	20. Reduces the transmission of microorganisms.

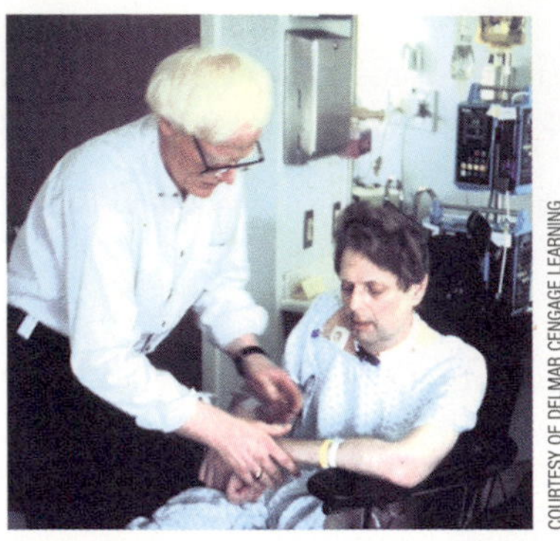

FIGURE 29-15-3 **Once the client is moved, make sure skin, tubing, or equipment is not pinched between the client and the chair.**

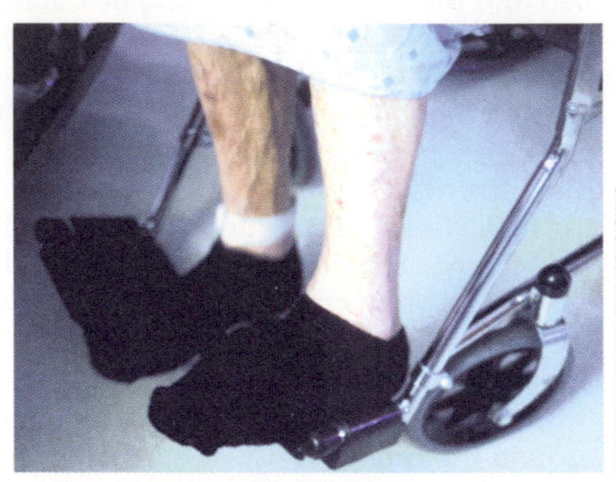

FIGURE 29-15-4 **Position the wheelchair footrests or use a footstool if the client is sitting in a chair.**

EVALUATION

- Client was transferred from the bed to the wheelchair without pain or injury.
- Drainage tubes, IVs, or other devices remain intact.
- Client's skin is intact and undamaged.

DOCUMENTATION

Nurses' Notes

- Client's tolerance of the activity, any aids that were required, how much assistance was required, and the client's ability to assist
- Unusual events during the transfer

PROCEDURE 29-16 Transferring from Bed to Stretcher

OVERVIEW

Some clients are not strong enough to sit erect in a wheelchair or have some injury that prevents them from sitting, so they are moved while lying flat. The most commonly used equipment for transferring a client is a stretcher (gurney). A stretcher is a narrow, cartlike bed that rolls on wheels. For client safety, stretchers are equipped with side rails or safety straps to prevent accidental falls during transport. The wheels on a stretcher lock to prevent accidental movement during client transfers.

ASSESSMENT

1. Assess the client's current level of mobility. **Knowing whether a client is able to assist with the transfer affects how the transfer is performed.**
2. Assess for injury. **Caregivers keep the client in the same alignment as much as possible.**
3. Assess for any impediments to mobility such as a cast, drainage tubes, IVs, or intubation. **This affects how the transfer is performed.**
4. Assess the client's level of understanding of the procedure. **This affects client comfort, anxiety, and cooperation.**
5. Assess the client's environment. Assess how close the stretcher will move to the bed and the height of the bed. **This allows for a safe transfer. Plan for good body mechanics.**

(Continues)

PROCEDURE 29-16 Transferring from Bed to Stretcher (Continued)

6. Make sure the stretcher is safe to use. Check for working brakes, side rails, safety straps that are intact and usable, and an IV pole attachment if needed. **This allows for a safe transfer. Plan for good body mechanics.**

POSSIBLE NURSING DIAGNOSES

Impaired Physical Mobility
Activity Intolerance

PLANNING

Expected Outcomes

1. The client will be transferred from the bed to the stretcher without pain or injury.
2. Drainage tubes, IVs, or other devices will remain intact.
3. The client's skin will be intact and undamaged.

Equipment Needed

Transferring a Client with Minimum Assistance

- Bed
- Stretcher

Transferring a Client with Maximum Assistance

- Bed
- Stretcher
- Pillows
- Transfer/slider boards
- Lift sheet
- Other qualified personnel to assist

delegation tips

Assisting a client from a bed to a stretcher is a skill routinely delegated to properly trained ancillary personnel.

IMPLEMENTATION—ACTION/RATIONALE

ACTION	RATIONALE
* Check client's identification band * Explain procedure before beginning *	
Minimum Assistance	
1. Wash hands.	1. Reduces the transmission of microorganisms.
2. Raise the height of bed to 1 inch higher than the stretcher and lock brakes of bed.	2. Reduces distance nurse must bend, thus preventing back strain; prevents bed from moving.
3. Instruct client to move to side of bed close to stretcher. Lower side rails of bed and stretcher. Leave side rails on opposite side up.	3. Decreases risk of client falling.
4. Stand at outer side of stretcher and push it toward bed.	4. Diminishes the gap between bed and stretcher; secures the stretcher position.
5. Instruct client to move onto stretcher with assistance as needed.	5. Promotes client independence.
6. Cover client with sheet or bath blanket.	6. Promotes comfort; protects privacy.
7. Elevate side rails on stretcher and secure safety belts about client. Release brakes of stretcher.	7. Prevents falls.
8. Stand at head of stretcher to guide it when pushing.	8. Pushing, not pulling, ensures proper body mechanics.
9. Wash hands.	9. Reduces the transmission of microorganisms.
Maximum Assistance	
10. Repeat Actions 1 and 2.	10. See Rationales 1 and 2.
11. Assess amount of assistance required for transfer. Usually 2 to 4 staff members are required for the maximum-assisted transfer.	11. Promotes client independence; ensures that enough staff are present before beginning transfer.
12. Lock wheels of bed and stretcher.	12. Prevents falls.
13. Have one nurse stand close to client's head.	13. Supports client's head during the move.
14. Log roll the client (keep in straight alignment) and place a lift sheet under the client's back, trunk, and upper legs. The lift sheet can extend under the head if client lacks head control abilities.	14. Prevents flexion and rotation of client's hips and spine; maintains correct body alignment.

(Continues)

29-16 Transferring from Bed to Stretcher (Continued)

ACTION	RATIONALE
15. Empty all drainage bags (e.g., T-tube, Hemovac, Jackson–Pratt). Record amounts. Secure drainage system to client's gown before transfer.	15. Decreases possibility of spills; prevents dislodging of tubes.
16. Move client to edge of bed near stretcher. Lift up and over to avoid dragging.	16. Prevents dragging, which causes shearing force.
17. Because the client is now on the side of the bed, without the side rail up, the nurse on nonstretcher side of bed holds the stretcher side of the lift sheet up (by reaching across the client's chest) to prevent the client from falling onto the stretcher or off the bed.	17. Protects the client from falling.
18. Place pillow and slider board overlapping the bed and stretcher (Figure 29-16-1).	18. Protects head from injury. Slider board eases movement of the client.
19. Have staff members grasp edges of lift sheet. Be sure to use good body mechanics (Figure 29-16-2).	19. Provides surface for client to slide on. Prevents dragging and shearing.
20. On the count of three, have staff members pull lift sheet and the client onto the stretcher.	20. Working in unison makes the overall job easier and prevents staff injury.
21. Position client on stretcher, place pillow under head, and cover with a sheet or bath blanket.	21. Promotes comfort and provides for privacy.
22. Secure safety belts and elevate side rails of stretcher.	22. Prevents falls.
23. If IV is present, move it from bed IV pole to stretcher IV pole after client transfer.	23. Prevents tubing from being pulled and IV from being dislodged.
24. Wash hands.	24. Reduces the transmission of microorganisms.

EVALUATION

- The client was transferred from the bed to the stretcher without pain or injury.
- All drainage tubes, IVs, or other devices remain intact.
- Assess whether the client's skin is intact and undamaged.

DOCUMENTATION

Kardex

- Amount of assistance the transfer required and amount the client was able to assist

Nurses' Notes

- Time, date, reason for transfer, type of transfer, and how the client tolerated the activity

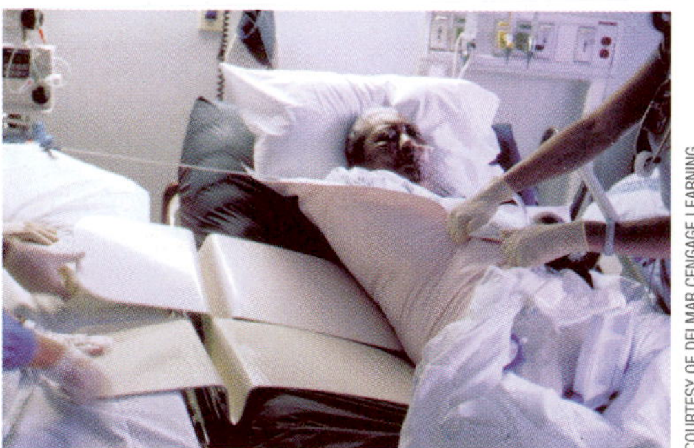

COURTESY OF DELMAR CENGAGE LEARNING

FIGURE 29-16-1 Place pillow and slider board overlapping the bed and stretcher.

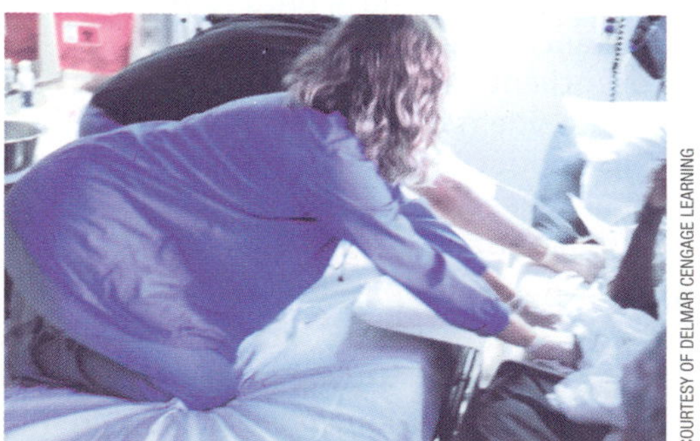

COURTESY OF DELMAR CENGAGE LEARNING

FIGURE 29-16-2 Firmly grasp edges of lift sheet.

PROCEDURE 29-17 Bed Making: Unoccupied Bed

OVERVIEW

After the client takes a bath, clean linens are placed on the bed to promote comfort and decrease transmission of microorganisms. If the client is able to get out of bed, assist the client to a chair and proceed with making the bed. After surgery, the client is returned to a clean bed with the linens folded to the foot of the bed to promote easy client transfer.

ASSESSMENT

1. Assess your equipment. Check for all linens necessary to change the bed. Check for a dirty linen hamper. **Facilitates a smooth procedure.**
2. Assess whether the bed needs cleaning before placing clean sheets on it. **Reduces the transmission of microorganisms.**
3. Assess the client's needs in the bed. Check for profuse drainage, incontinence, or special needs for comfort or skin integrity. **Determines how the procedure is performed.**
4. Assess the client's ability to be out of bed in a safe place while changing linens. **Assures client safety.**

POSSIBLE NURSING DIAGNOSIS

Risk for Impaired Skin Integrity

PLANNING

Expected Outcomes

1. The client will have clean linens on the bed.
2. The clean linens will be appropriate to the client's needs and condition.

Equipment Needed

- Bottom sheet (fitted, if available)
- Top sheet
- Protective disposable pad
- Draw sheet (regular top sheet may be used)
- Blanket
- Spread
- Pillowcase (each pillow on the bed)
- Mattress pad (optional)
- Antiseptic solution, washcloth, and towel
- Laundry bag
- Nonsterile gloves

delegation tips

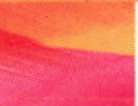

Bed making is usually delegated to ancillary personnel. Their instruction should include safety precautions for themselves and the client, and understanding the appropriate use of Standard Precautions.

IMPLEMENTATION—ACTION/RATIONALE

* Wash hands * Check client's identification band * Explain procedure before beginning *

ACTION	RATIONALE
1. Place hamper by client's door if linen bags are not available. Assess condition of blanket and/or bedspread.	1. Provides for proper disposal of soiled linens. Allows for organization of supplies.
2. Gather linens and gloves. Place linens on a clean, dry surface in reverse order of usage at the client's bedside (pillowcases, top sheet, draw sheet, bottom sheet).	2. Provides easy access to items.
3. Inquire about the client's toileting needs and attend as necessary.	3. Provides for client comfort and prevents interruptions during bed making.
4. Assist client to a safe, comfortable chair.	4. Increases client's comfort and decreases risk of falls.
5. Apply gloves.	5. Reduces risk of infection from soiled, contaminated linens.
6. Position bed: flat, side rails down, adjust height to waist level.	6. Promotes good body mechanics and decreases back strain.
7. Remove and fold blanket and/or bedspread. If clean and reusable, place on clean work area.	7. Keeps reusable bed linens clean.

(Continues)

PROCEDURE 29-17 Bed Making: Unoccupied Bed (Continued)

ACTION	RATIONALE
8. Remove soiled pillowcases by grasping the closed end with one hand and slipping the pillow out with the other. Place the soiled cases on top of the soiled sheet, and place the pillows on clean work area.	8. Allows easy removal of the pillowcases without contamination of uniform by soiled linens and keeps pillows clean.
9. Remove soiled linens: Start on the side of the bed closest to you; free the bottom sheet and mattress pad (if used) by lifting the mattress and rolling soiled linens to the middle of the bed. Go to the other side of the bed, repeat action.	9. Prevents tearing and fanning of linens. Linens are folded from cleanest area to most soiled to prevent contamination.
10. Fold (do not fan or flap) soiled linens: head of bed to middle, foot of bed to middle. Place in linen bag, keeping soiled linens away from uniform.	10. Fanning or flapping linens increases the number of microorganisms in the air. Folding linens reduces the risk of transmission of infection to others.
11. Check mattress. If the mattress is soiled, clean it with an antiseptic solution and dry it thoroughly.	11. Reduces the transmission of microorganisms.
12. Remove gloves, wash hands, and apply a second pair of clean gloves (when appropriate).	12. Reduces the transmission of microorganisms to clean linens.
13. Open the clean mattress pad lengthwise onto the bed. Unfold half the pad's width to the center crease and smooth the pad flat. If there are elastic bands to hold the pad in place, slide them under the corners of the mattress.	13. Facilitates making bed in an organized, time-saving manner by not having to go from one side of the bed to the other.
14. Proceed with placing the bottom sheet onto the mattress. Linens differ from facility to facility. Bottom sheets may be fitted or they may be flat. Proceed to the appropriate action for the linen available.	14. Use linen available at the facility.
Fitted Bottom Sheet	
15. Position yourself diagonally toward the head of the bed.	15. Ensures good body mechanics and efficient procedure.
16. Start at the head with seamed side of the fitted sheet toward the mattress.	16. Placement of seamed side toward mattress prevents irritation to the client's skin.
17. Lift the mattress corner with your hand closest to the bed; with your other hand, pull and tuck the fitted sheet over the mattress corner; secure at the head of the bed.	17. Prevents straining of back muscles; decreases the chance that the sheet will pull out from under the mattress.
18. Pull and tuck the fitted sheet over the mattress corners at the foot of the bed.	18. Prevents straining of back muscles; decreases the chance that the sheet will pull out from under the mattress.
Flat Regular Sheet	
19. Unfold the bottom sheet with the seamed side toward the mattress. Align the bottom edge of the sheet with the edge of the mattress at the foot of the bed.	19. Placement of the seamed side toward the mattress prevents irritation to the client's skin. Ensure proper placement of the sheet so that it can be tightly secured at the top and on both sides of the bed.
20. Allow the sheet to hang 10 inches (25 cm) over the mattress on the side and at the top of the bed.	20. Proper placement of linens ensures adequate sheeting for all sides of the bed.
21. Position yourself diagonally toward the head of the bed. Lift the top of the mattress corner with the hand closest to the bed and smoothly tuck the sheet under the mattress.	21. Prevents straining of back muscles; decreases the chance that the sheet will pull out from under the mattress.
22. Miter the corner at the head of the bed using the following technique (Figure 29-17-1).	22. Secures sheet tightly to the mattress, with the triangular fold providing a smooth tuck to keep the linen in place.
23. Face the side of bed and lift and lay the edge of the sheet onto the bed to form a triangular fold.	23. Forms the base for the tuck.

(Continues)

PROCEDURE 29-17 Bed Making: Unoccupied Bed (Continued)

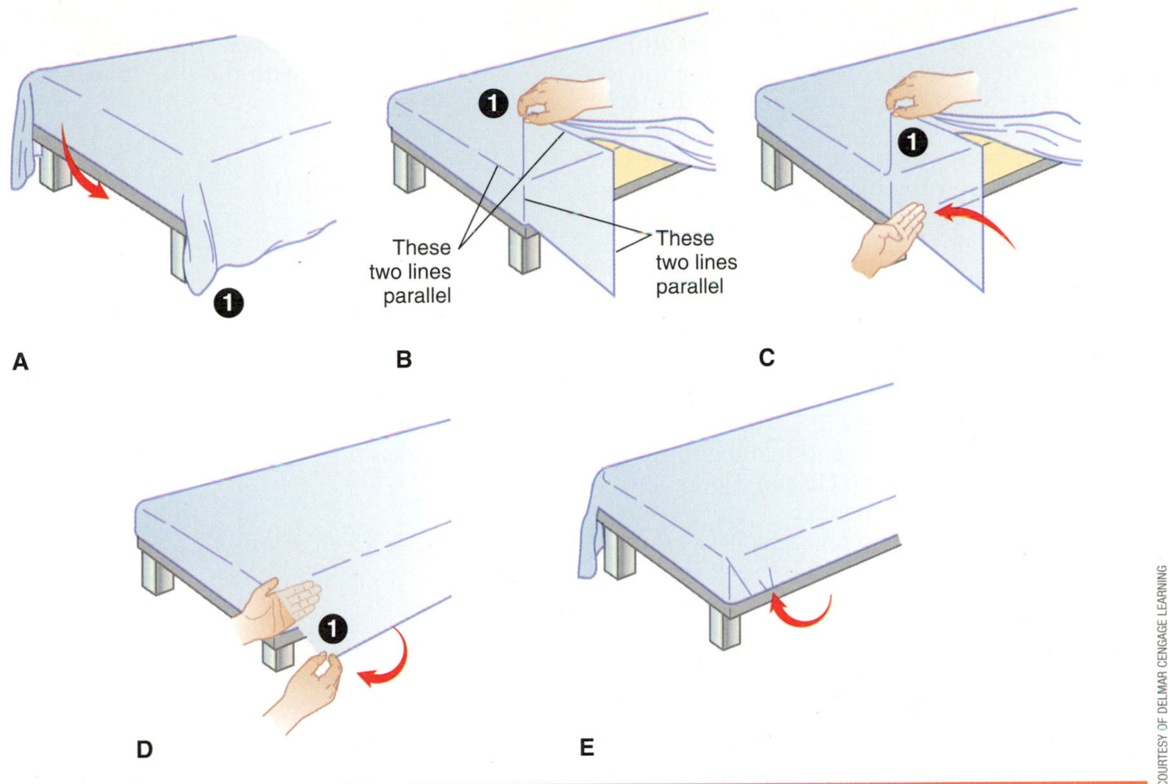

FIGURE 29-17-1 Steps in making a mitered corner; *A*, Tuck the lower edge of the sheet under the mattress; *B*, Grasp the triangular point of the sheet and raise it parallel to the edge of the mattress; *C*, Tuck the sheet that hangs below the mattress under the mattress; *D*, Bring the triangular point down alongside the bed; E, Tuck the sheet under the mattress with palms down.

ACTION	RATIONALE
24. With your palms down, tuck the lower edge of sheet (hanging free at the side of the mattress) under the mattress.	24. Forms the first half of the tuck.
25. Grasp the triangular fold; bring it down over the side of the mattress. Allow the sheet to hang free at the side of the mattress.	25. Will form the final portion of the mitered corner when tucked in.
26. Place the draw sheet on the bottom sheet and unfold it to the middle crease (Figure 29-17-2).	26. Provides a sheet to lift and move the client in bed without having to use the bottom sheet and remake the bed. Helps to keep the bottom sheet clean.
27. Face the side of the bed, palms of hands down. Tuck both the bottom and draw sheets under the mattress. Ensure that the bottom sheet is tucked smoothly under the mattress all the way to the foot of the bed.	27. Keeps sheet taut, in place, and wrinkle-free, thereby decreasing the risk of skin irritation.
28. Go to the other side of the bed, unfold the bottom sheet, and repeat the actions used to apply the mattress pad and bottom sheet.	28. Unfolding decreases air current; air currents can spread microorganisms.
29. Unfold the draw sheet, if used, and grasp the free-hanging sides of both the bottom and draw sheets. Pull toward you, keeping your back straight, and with a firm grasp (sheets taut) tuck both sheets under the mattress. Use your arms and open palms to extend the linen under the mattress. Place the protective pad on the bottom sheet.	29. Uses your body's weight in pulling the sheet taut and prevents strain on your back muscles.

(Continues)

PROCEDURE 29-17 Bed Making: Unoccupied Bed (Continued)

ACTION	RATIONALE
30. Place the top sheet on the bed and unfold lengthwise, placing the center crease (width) of the sheet in the middle of the bed. Place the top edge of the sheet (seam up) even with the top of the mattress at the head of the bed. Pull the remaining length toward the bottom of the bed.	30. Saves time and movement, making one side of the bed at a time. Seam will be folded down to prevent contact with the client's skin, which can result in irritation.
31. Unfold and apply the blanket or spread. Follow the same technique as used in applying the top sheet (Figure 29-17-3).	31. Provides warmth.
32. Miter the bottom corners. With your palms down, tuck the lower edge of the sheet under the mattress. Grasp the triangular fold and bring it down over the side of the mattress. Allow the sheet to hang free at the side of the mattress (Figures 29-17-4 and 29-17-5).	32. Secures linen at the foot of the bed.
33. Face the head of the bed and fold the top sheet and blanket over 6 inches (15 cm) (Figure 29-17-6). Fanfold the sheet and blanket	33. Allows the client easy access to the bed.
34. Apply a clean pillowcase on each pillow (Figure 29-15-7). With one hand, grasp the closed end of the pillowcase. Gather the pillowcase and turn it	34. Keeps clean pillowcase away from your uniform.

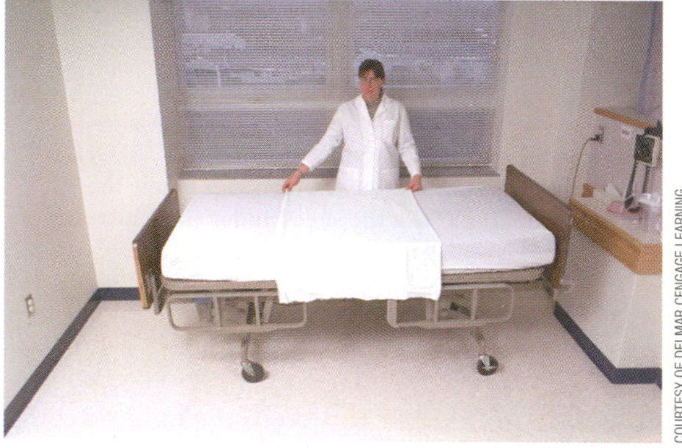

FIGURE 29-17-2 The draw sheet is placed on top of the bottom sheet and may be used as a turning sheet.

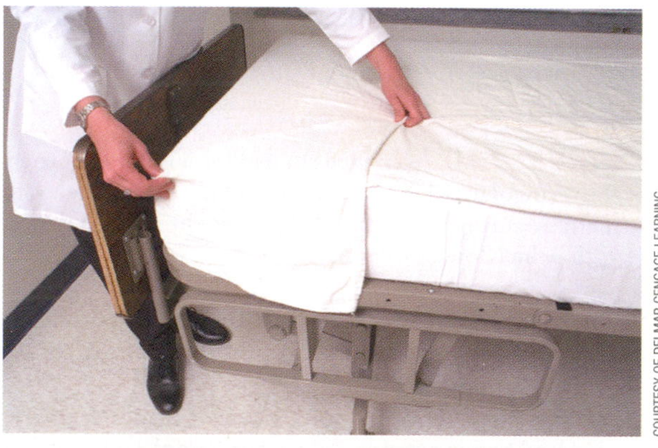

FIGURE 29-17-4 Lift and lay the edge of the sheet and blanket on the bed to form a triangular fold.

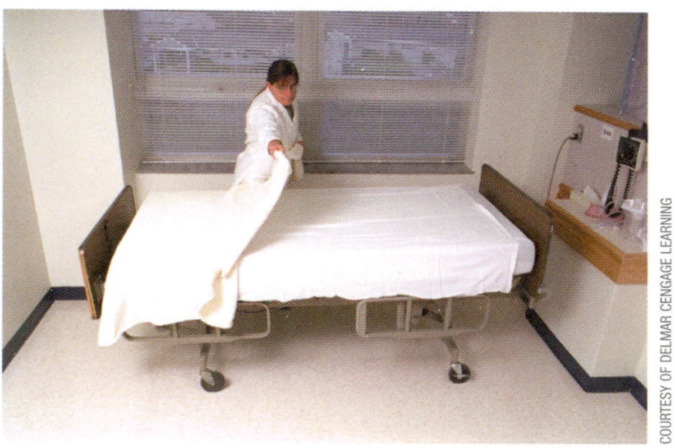

FIGURE 29-17-3 Place the blanket or spread over the top sheet.

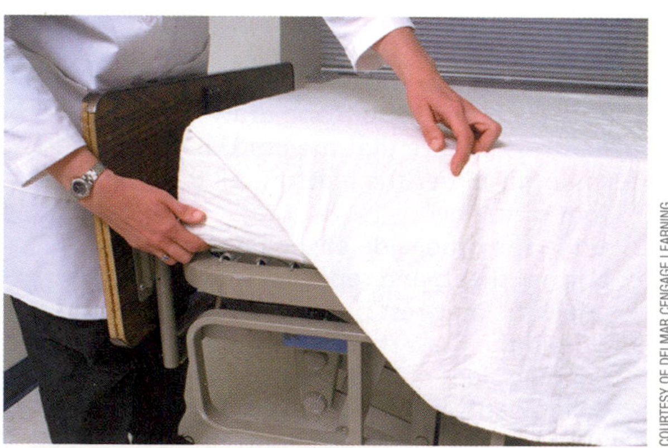

FIGURE 29-17-5 Bring the triangular fold down and let it hang freely at the side of the mattress.

(Continues)

PROCEDURE 29-17 Bed Making: Unoccupied Bed (Continued)

ACTION	RATIONALE

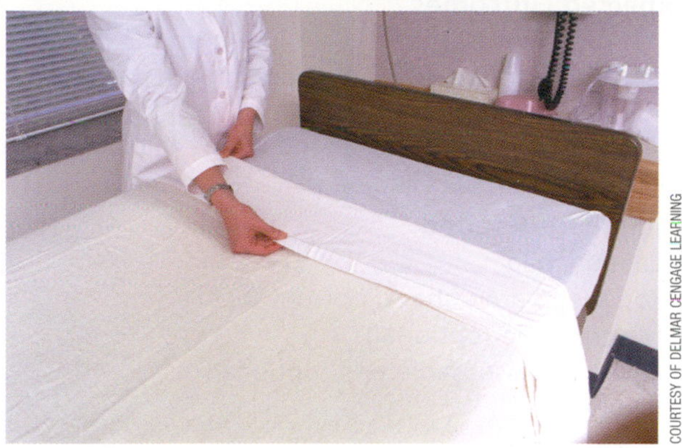

FIGURE 29-17-6 Fold a cuff with the top sheet and blanket.

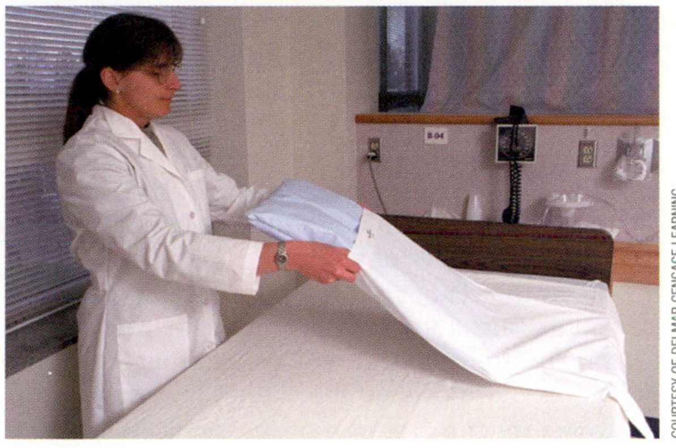

FIGURE 29-17-7 A quick method of applying a clean pillowcase on a pillow.

ACTION	RATIONALE
inside out over hand. With same hand, grasp the middle of one end of the pillow. With the other hand, pull the case over the length of the pillow. The corners of the pillow should fit snugly into the corners of the case.	
35. Return the bed to the lowest position and elevate the head of the bed 30 to 45 degrees. Put side rails up on side, farthest from client.	35. Provides for client safety.
36. Inquire about toileting needs of the client; assist as necessary.	36. Saves client energy and provides time to care for the client's needs.
37. Assist the client back into the bed and pull up the side rails; place call light in reach; take vital signs.	37. Promotes client safety and a means to call for assistance. Sitting up in a chair and movement may cause changes in the client's vital signs.
38. Remove gloves and wash hands.	38. Reduces the transmission of microorganisms.

EVALUATION

- Confirm that fresh linens were placed on the bed in a manner appropriate to the client's needs.

DOCUMENTATION

Nurses' Notes

- Client's tolerance to being out of bed. (Linen changes are not generally documented.)

PROCEDURE 29-18 Bed Making: Occupied Bed

OVERVIEW

After the client takes a bath, clean linens are placed on the bed to promote comfort and decrease the transmission of microorganisms. If the client is unable to get out of bed, change the linens around the client. Assistance is needed if the client is in traction or cannot be turned. Care is taken to avoid disturbing the traction weights. If the client cannot be turned, change the linens from head to toe. Place a waterproof draw sheet on the beds of clients who are incontinent or have profuse drainage. The type and amount of linens placed on the bed will vary based on the type of bed the client is using. Air beds and Clinitron beds, for example, use only minimal linens under the client.

(Continues)

PROCEDURE 29-18 Bed Making: Occupied Bed (Continued)

ASSESSMENT

1. Assess your equipment. **Facilitates a smooth procedure.**
2. Assess whether the bed needs cleaning before placing clean sheets on it. **Reduces the transmission of microorganisms.**
3. Assess the client's needs in the bed. Check for profuse drainage, incontinence, or special needs for comfort or skin integrity. **Determines how the procedure is performed.**
4. Assess the client's ability to assist with the procedure, including mobility, mental status, and muscle strength. **Determines whether assistance is needed to change the client's linens.**
5. Assess for the presence of dressings, IV lines, tubes, or any equipment that may be attached to the client. **Provides for client safety.**

POSSIBLE NURSING DIAGNOSIS

Risk for Impaired Skin Integrity

PLANNING

Expected Outcomes

1. The client will have clean linens on the bed.
2. The clean linens will be appropriate to the client's needs and condition.
3. The linens will be changed with a minimum of trauma to the client.

Equipment Needed

- Laundry bag
- Top sheet, draw sheet, bottom sheet
- Mattress pad (optional)
- Protective disposable pad (optional)
- Pillowcase
- Blanket
- Bath blanket
- Antiseptic solution, washcloth, and towel
- Nonsterile gloves (if needed)

delegation tips

Bed making is usually delegated to ancillary personnel. Their instruction should include the appropriate use of Standard Precautions and safety precautions for themselves and the client, such as the proper movement of the client in bed, how to manage drains and dressings, and the use of proper body mechanics. In certain situations where the client is in critical condition and multiple tubes, especially chest tubes, are present, the nurse assists.

IMPLEMENTATION—ACTION/RATIONALE

* Wash hands * Check client's identification band *

ACTION	RATIONALE
1. Explain procedure to client.	1. Promotes client cooperation.
2. Bring equipment to the bedside.	2. Facilitates procedure organization.
3. Cover client with a bath blanket (Figure 29-18-1). Remove top sheet and blanket. Loosen bottom sheet at foot and sides of bed. Lower side rail nearest the nurse, if necessary for access.	3. Bath blanket prevents exposure and chills. Facilitates easy removal of linens. Lowering only side rail close to nurse reduces client's risk of falls.
4. Position client on side, facing away from you. Reposition pillow under head.	4. Provides space to place clean linens.
5. Fanfold or roll bottom linens close to client toward the center of the bed (Figure 29-18-2).	5. Keeps soiled linen together. Promotes comfort when client later rolls to other side.
6. Place clean bottom linens with the center fold nearest the client. Fanfold or roll clean bottom linens nearest client and tuck under soiled linen (Figure 29-18-3). If fitted sheets are not available, maintain an adequate amount of sheet at head of bed for tucking. Have sheet even with bottom of mattress.	6. Provides for maximum fit of sheets and decreases chance of wrinkles.
7. If fitted sheets are not available, miter bottom sheet at head of bed. To miter, lift the mattress and tuck the sheet over the edge of the mattress, lift edge of sheet that is hanging to form a triangle, and lay upper part of sheet back onto bed; tuck the lower hanging section under the mattress. Repeat for each corner. Tuck the sides of the sheet under the mattress.	7. Holds linens firmly in place.

(Continues)

PROCEDURE 29-18 Bed Making: Occupied Bed (Continued)

ACTION	RATIONALE

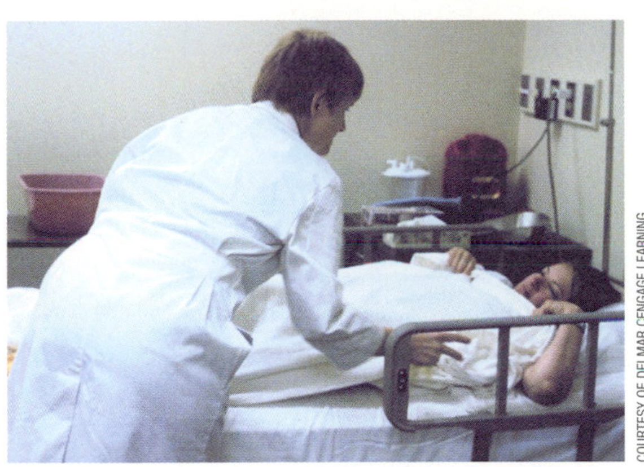

COURTESY OF DELMAR CENGAGE LEARNING

FIGURE 29-18-1 Cover the client with a bath blanket for warmth and modesty while top sheet and blanket are removed.

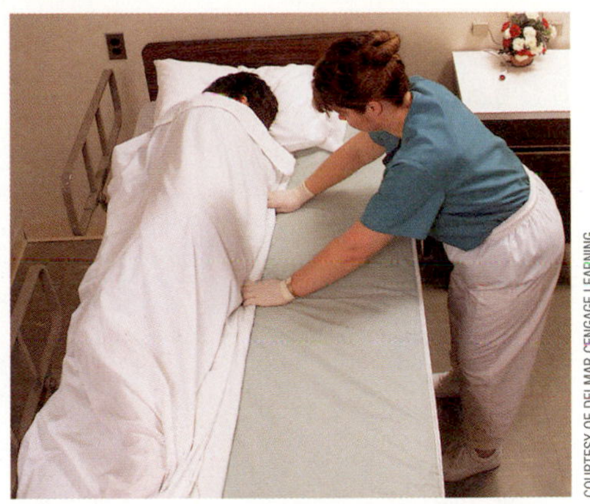

COURTESY OF DELMAR CENGAGE LEARNING

FIGURE 29-18-2 When changing an occupied bed, fanfold the bottom linens toward the center of the bed close to the client. Change gloves, if soiled, before handling clean linen.

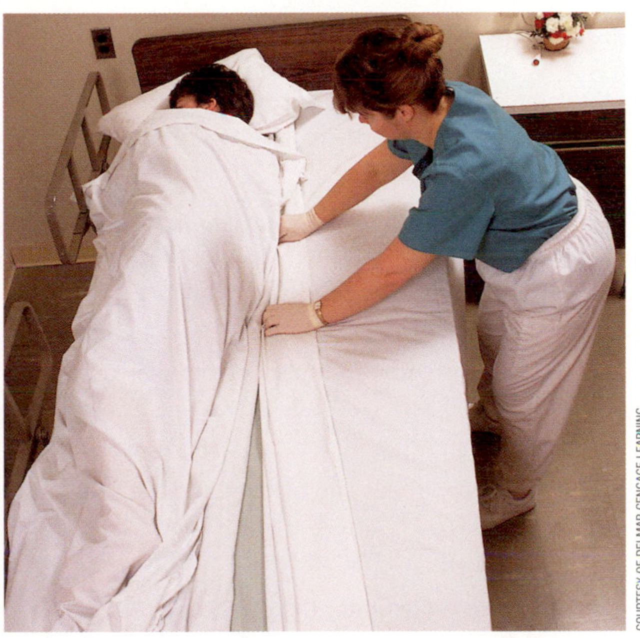

COURTESY OF DELMAR CENGAGE LEARNING

FIGURE 29-18-3 Fanfold or roll clean bottom sheet on the bed and tuck under soiled linen.

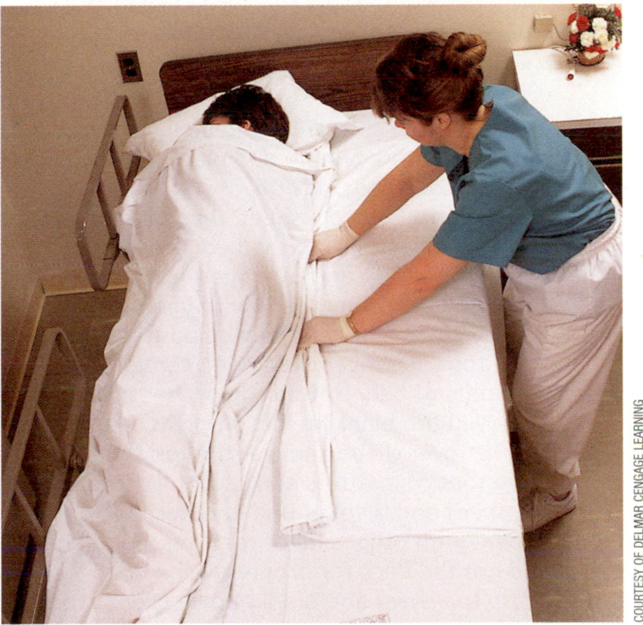

COURTESY OF DELMAR CENGAGE LEARNING

FIGURE 29-18-4 Fanfold or roll draw sheet on the bed and tuck under soiled linen.

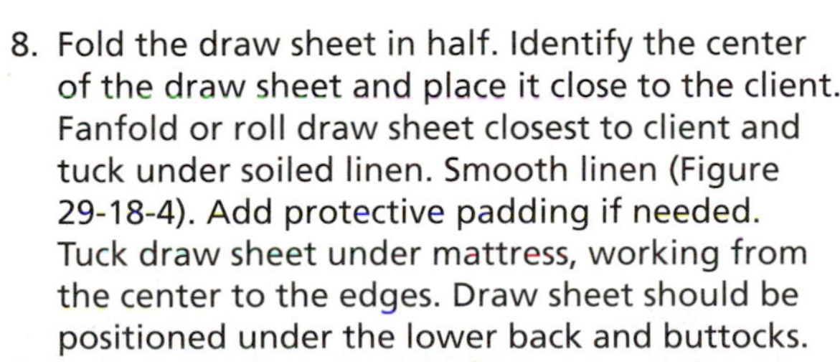

ACTION	RATIONALE
8. Fold the draw sheet in half. Identify the center of the draw sheet and place it close to the client. Fanfold or roll draw sheet closest to client and tuck under soiled linen. Smooth linen (Figure 29-18-4). Add protective padding if needed. Tuck draw sheet under mattress, working from the center to the edges. Draw sheet should be positioned under the lower back and buttocks.	8. Draw sheet facilitates moving and lifting clients while in bed.
9. Roll client over onto side facing you. Raise side rail.	9. Positions client off soiled linen. Protects client from falling.

(Continues)

PROCEDURE 29-18 Bed Making: Occupied Bed (Continued)

ACTION	RATIONALE

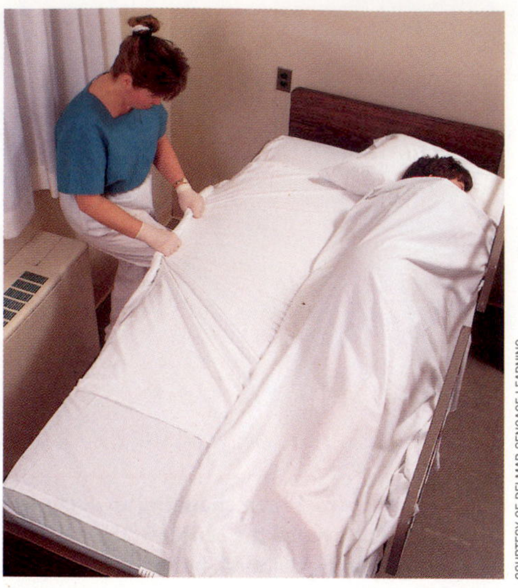

FIGURE 29-18-5 Unfold/unroll the bottom sheet and draw sheet. Grasp each sheet with knuckles up and over the sheet and pull tightly while leaning back with your body weight.

ACTION	RATIONALE
10. Move to other side of bed. Remove soiled linens by rolling into a bundle and place in linen bag without touching uniform.	10. Prevents cross contamination.
11. Unfold/unroll bottom sheet, then draw sheet. Look for objects left in the bed. Grasp each sheet with knuckles up and over the sheet and pull tightly while leaning back with your body weight (Figure 29-18-5). Client may be positioned supine.	11. Tight sheets keep linens wrinkle free and decrease the risk of skin irritation. Leaning back uses body weight for good body mechanics.
12. Place top sheet over client with center of sheet in middle of bed. Unfold top of sheet over client. Remove bath blankets left on client. Place top blanket over client, same as the top sheet.	12. Provides client with top sheet and blanket to prevent chilling.
13. Raise foot of mattress and tuck the corner of the top sheet and blanket under. Miter the corner. Repeat with other side of mattress. Bend knees and not the back for proper mechanics.	13. Secures top sheet and blanket in place.
14. Grasp top sheet and blanket over client's toes and pull upward, then make a small fanfold in the sheet.	14. Provides room under the tight top sheet and blanket for client to move feet. Prevents toe decubitus and sheet burns from pressure.
15. Remove soiled pillowcase. Grasp center of clean pillowcase and invert pillowcase over hand/arm. Maintain grasp of pillowcase while grasping center of pillow. Use other hand to pull pillowcase down over pillow. Place pillow under client's head.	15. Provides clean pillowcase without shaking pillow or pillowcase. Promotes comfort.
16. Wash hands.	16. Reduces the transmission of microorganisms.

EVALUATION

- The client has clean, unwrinkled linen.
- The linen placed on the bed is suitable for the client's special needs.
- The linen was changed with a minimum of pain and trauma to the client.

DOCUMENTATION

Nurses' Notes

- How the client tolerated the bed change, and any unusual findings. (Bed change is not generally documented.)

(Continues)

PROCEDURE 29-19 Bathing a Client in Bed

OVERVIEW

Bathing clients is an essential component of nursing care and a critical time to assess the client. Whether the nurse performs the bath or delegates the activity to another health care provider, the nurse is responsible for ensuring that the hygienic needs of the client are met. Cleansing baths are provided as routine client care for personal hygiene. Following are the five types of cleansing baths:

1. Shower
2. Tub
3. Self-help, or assisted bed bath
4. Complete bed bath
5. Partial bath

There are several variations of bed bath depending on the client's ability to assist with care. The complete bed bath is provided to dependent clients confined to bed. The nurse washes the client's entire body during a complete bed bath. A partial bed bath and a self-help bed bath are variations of the complete bed bath.

After washing a client's hair, cover the head with a towel even if still washing the rest of the body. Most heat is lost from the head, and older clients chill very quickly and have difficulty regulating their temperature.

ASSESSMENT

1. Assess the client's level of ability to assist with the bath. **Determine if the client is able to follow directions. Check the client's ability to assist with cleaning any portion of the body.**
2. Assess the client's level of comfort with the procedure. Check into potential cultural, sexual, or generational issues. **Determine whether the client is uncomfortable, tense, or nervous about being bathed by someone else.**
3. Assess the environment. Verify that the equipment needed is available. Assess if the client has skin intact or dressings, IV lines, or drainage tubes in place. Check whether clean, warm water is available. **Determine whether the need for modesty and privacy can be met. The environment should be conducive to a clean, safe, and comfortable procedure.**

POSSIBLE NURSING DIAGNOSES

Risk for Impaired Skin Integrity
Bathing/Hygiene Self-Care Deficit

PLANNING

Expected Outcomes

1. Clients will be cleaned without damage to their skin.
2. Clients' privacy will be maintained throughout the procedure.
3. Clients will participate in their own hygiene as much as possible.
4. Clients will not become overly tired or experience increased pain, cold, or discomfort as a result of the bath.

Equipment Needed

Some facilities provide packs of microwaveable pre-moistened cloths for baths. For the traditional bed bath, these items are needed:

- Bath towels
- Washcloths
- Bath blanket
- Washbasin
- Soap
- Soap dish
- Lotion
- Deodorant
- Clean gown
- Clean linen
- Disposable, latex-free gloves

delegation tips

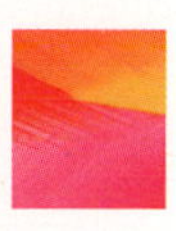

This skill is routinely delegated to ancillary personnel who should allow the client to perform as much of the bath as possible or permitted. The caregiver employs Standard Precautions, properly positions the client, and observes and reports the client's skin condition and color to the nurse. The nurse retains the responsibility to assess the client.

(Continues)

PROCEDURE 29-19 Bathing a Client in Bed (Continued)

IMPLEMENTATION—ACTION/RATIONALE

ACTION	RATIONALE
* Check client's identification band * Explain procedure before beginning *	
1. Assess the client's preferences about bathing.	1. Provides client opportunity to participate in care.
2. Prepare environment. Close doors and windows, adjust temperature, provide time for elimination needs, and provide privacy.	2. Protects from chills during bath and increases sense of privacy.
3. Wash hands. Apply gloves. Gloves should be changed when emptying water basin.	3. Reduces the transmission of microorganisms.
4. Lower side rail on the side close to you. Position client in a comfortable position close to the side near you.	4. Prevents unnecessary reaching. Facilitates use of good body mechanics.
5. If bath blankets are available, place bath blanket over top sheet. Remove top sheet from under bath blanket. Remove client's gown. Bath blanket should be folded to expose only the area being cleaned at that time. Towels may also be used for bath blankets. Top sheets are not used as bath blankets because they are not absorbent and do not prevent chilling.	5. Prevents exposure of client. Promotes privacy. Protects from chills.
6. Fill washbasin two-thirds full. Permit client to test temperature of water with hand. Water should be changed when a soap film develops or water becomes soiled.	6. Prevents accidental burns or chills.
7. Wet the washcloth and wring it out.	7. Prevents unnecessarily wetting of client.
8. Make a bath mitten with the washcloth. To make a mitten, grasp the edge of the washcloth with the thumb; fold a third over the palm of the hand; wrap remainder of cloth around hand and across palm, and grasp the second edge under the thumb; fold the extended end of the washcloth onto the palm and tuck under the palmar surface of the cloth.	8. Prevents ends of washcloth from dragging across skin. Promotes friction during bath.
9. Wash the face (Figure 29-19-1). Ask the client about preference for using soap on the face. Use a separate corner of the washcloth for each eye, wiping from inner to outer canthus. Wash neck and ears. Rinse and dry well. Male clients may want to shave at this time. Provide assistance with shaving as needed.	9. Some clients may not use soap on the face. Using separate corners of washcloth reduces risk of transmitting microorganisms from one eye to the other eye. Patting dry reduces skin irritation and drying.
10. Wash arms, forearms, and hands. Wash forearms and arms using long, firm strokes in the direction of distal to proximal. Arm may need to be supported while being washed. Wash axilla. Rinse and dry well. Apply deodorant or powder if desired. Immerse client's hand into basin of water. Allow hand to soak about 3 to 5 minutes. Wash hands, interdigit area, fingers, and fingernails. Rinse and dry well.	10. Long strokes promote circulation. Soaking hands softens nails and loosens soil from skin and nails. Strokes directed distal to proximal promote venous return.
11. Wash chest and abdomen. Place bath towel lengthwise over chest and abdomen, then fold bath blanket to waist. Lift bath towel and wash	11. Promotes privacy and prevents chills. Long strokes promote circulation. Perspiration and soil collect within skin folds.

(Continues)

PROCEDURE 29-19 Bathing a Client in Bed (Continued)

ACTION	RATIONALE

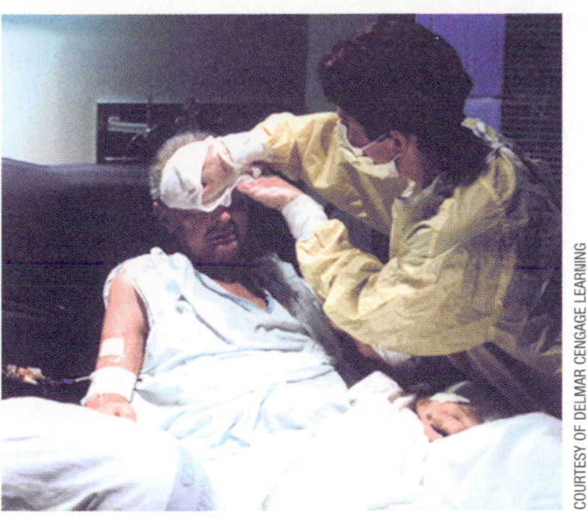

FIGURE 29-19-1 **Wash the client's face first.**

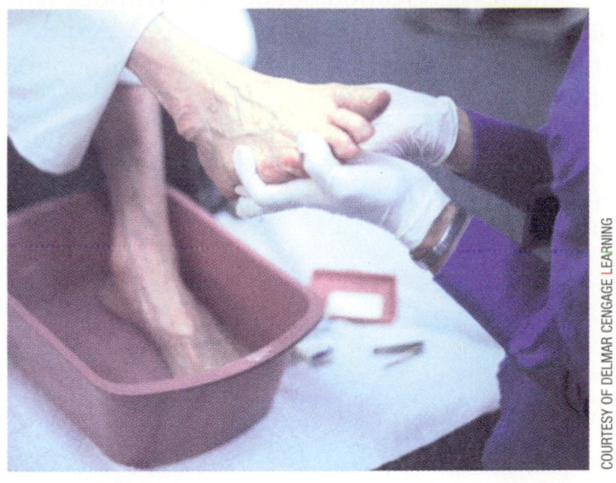

FIGURE 29-19-2 **Place feet in basin. Clean interdigits and soles of feet.**

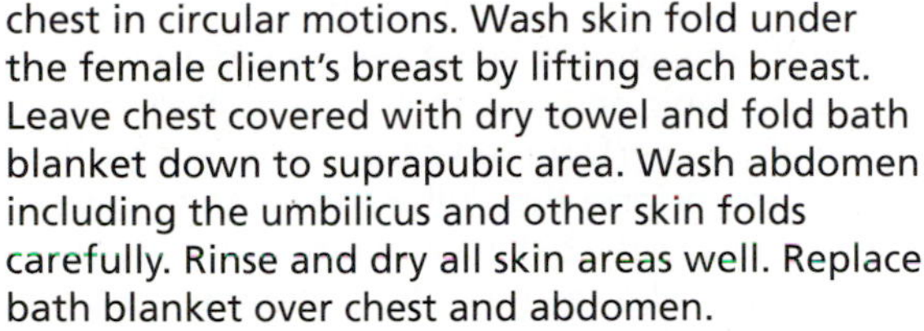

chest in circular motions. Wash skin fold under the female client's breast by lifting each breast. Leave chest covered with dry towel and fold bath blanket down to suprapubic area. Wash abdomen including the umbilicus and other skin folds carefully. Rinse and dry all skin areas well. Replace bath blanket over chest and abdomen.

12. Wash legs and feet. Expose leg farthest from you by folding bath blanket to midline. Bend the leg at the knee. Grasp the heel, elevate the leg from the bed, and cover bed with bath towel. Place washbasin on towel. Place client's foot into washbasin (Figure 29-19-2). Allow foot to soak while washing the leg with long, firm strokes in the direction of distal to proximal Gently wash the legs of clients with deep vein thrombosis (DVT) or other coagulation issues; do not use firm strokes. Rinse leg and dry well. Clean soles, interdigits, and toes. Carefully examine the foot and between the digits of a diabetic for pressure sores or ulcerations. Rinse foot and dry well. Apply lotion to legs and feet if they are dry but do not massage legs, as an embolus may occur. Perform the same procedure with the other leg and foot.

    12. Supports joints to prevent strain and fatigue. Soaking foot loosens dirt, softens nails, and promotes comfort.

13. Wash back. Assist client into prone or side-lying position facing away from you. Wash the back and buttocks using long, firm strokes. Rinse and dry well. Give back rub and apply lotion.

    13. Exposes back and buttocks for washing. Back rub promotes relaxation and circulation.

14. Perineal care: Assist client to supine position. Perform perineal care (see Procedure 29-20).

    14. Removes genital secretions and soil.

15. Apply lotion as desired or needed. Apply clean gown.

    15. Lotion lubricates skin.

16. Wash hands.

    16. Reduces the transmission of microorganisms.

(Continues)

PROCEDURE 29-19 Bathing a Client in Bed (Continued)

EVALUATION

- The client was cleaned adequately without skin damage.
- The client's modesty was maintained throughout the procedure.
- The client participated in the procedure as much as possible.
- The client remained comfortable during the procedure.

DOCUMENTATION

Nurses' Notes

- Client was bathed. Indicate how much of the bath the client assisted with and how well the client tolerated the activity.
- Unusual findings including rashes, open sores, poor turgor, and so on.

PROCEDURE 29-20 Perineal Care

OVERVIEW

The perineum is the external structure of the pelvic floor. It is composed of the skin and muscle surrounding the genitalia; it is the area between the scrotum and anus in the male and between the vulva and anus in the female. Care of the perineum and genitalia is directed toward maintaining a hygienic perineal environment. Perineal and genital care is usually self-care; however, alterations in the client's ability to perform self-care or alterations in the perineum and genitalia are reasons for nurses or other care providers to perform this skill. Perineal and genital care is an emotionally and culturally difficult subject. Many cultures have specific beliefs and taboos regarding the perineal/genital area. Many people are embarrassed by the idea of anyone else seeing or touching their genitals, particularly a stranger. Be aware of these possibilities when approaching genital/perineal care. In general, a professional, nonjudgmental approach will put the client more at ease with the procedure. Ask the client or the client's caregiver, if possible, about any preferences the client may have in this area.

ASSESSMENT

1. Evaluate client status: level of consciousness, ability to ambulate, ability to perform self-care, frequency of urination and defecation, skin condition. **This allows the nurse to decide who, where, how, and when to perform perineal care.**
2. Identify cultural preferences for perineal care. **Perineal care is strongly associated with cultural practices, for example, who may touch the perineal area and how, and the proper way to "wipe." To the extent possible, these preferences are identified and incorporated into the client's care.**
3. Assess the client's perineal health. Ask the male client if he has any perineal/genital itching or discomfort. Ask the female client if she has any urethral, vaginal, or anal discharge. **Determines the presence of signs and symptoms that may need additional assessment and intervention.**
4. Determine if the client is incontinent of urine or stool. **Affects how the procedure is done and what additional procedures may be necessary.**
5. Assess whether the client has recently had perineal/genital surgery. **Affects how the procedure is done and what additional procedures may be necessary.**

POSSIBLE NURSING DIAGNOSES

Risk for Impaired Skin Integrity
Bathing/Hygiene Self-Care Deficit

PLANNING

Expected Outcomes

1. Perineum and genitalia will be dry, clean, and free of secretions and unpleasant odors.
2. The client will report feeling comfortable and clean in the perineal area.
3. The client will not experience discomfort or undue embarrassment during the procedure.
4. The perineum will be free of skin breakdown or irritation.

Equipment Needed

- Personal protective equipment (gloves, gown)
- Toilet paper/washcloths
- Waterproof pads

(Continues)

PROCEDURE 29-20 Perineal Care (Continued)

- Cleansing solution, if needed
- Perineal wash bottle (fill with plain, warm water).
- Water receptacle (bedpan or toilet if client is ambulatory)
- Dry towels
- Perineal treatment (i.e., ointment or lotions) if necessary
- Linen receptacle
- Room deodorizer

delegation tips

This skill is routinely delegated to ancillary personnel who should be trained in Standard Precautions and proper client positioning, and to report color, odor, and amount of any discharge, if present, to the nurse.

IMPLEMENTATION—ACTION/RATIONALE

* Check client's identification band * Explain procedure before beginning *

ACTION	RATIONALE
1. Wash hands and wear gloves. If appropriate and splashing is likely, wear gown, mask, and goggles.	1. Reduces the transmission of microorganisms.
2. Close privacy curtain or door.	2. Provides privacy.
3. Position client.	3. If client is ambulatory, perineal care may be done either with client on or standing at the toilet. If perineal care is to be performed in the bed, place the client on the side or over a deep bedpan.
4. Place waterproof pads under the client in the bed or under bedpan if used.	4. Protects bed linen.
5. Remove fecal debris with toilet paper and dispose in toilet.	5. May require several attempts. If performing at the bedside, may collect paper in disposable pad or linens until end of procedure.
6. Spray perineum with washing solution if indicated. Alternatively, plain water may be used.	6. Several perineal solutions are available, which may or may not require rinsing. Carefully evaluate this requirement. Solutions that require rinsing may cause skin breakdown if left on the skin.
7. Wash perineum with wet washcloths (front to back on females), changing to clean area on washcloth with each wipe (Figure 29-20-1). Wash the penis on the male (Figure 29-20-2).	7. Maximizes cleaning; prevents spread of rectal flora to vagina and meatus.
8. Carefully examine gluteal folds and scrotal folds for debris. Gently visualize vulva for debris.	8. Fecal material causes irritation and skin breakdown rapidly when left in contact with skin.
9. If soap is used, spray area with clean water from the peri-bottle.	9. Rinses soap, which can irritate the skin, from the area.
10. Change gloves.	10. Reduces the transmission of microorganisms.
11. Dry perineum carefully with towel.	11. Residual moisture provides an ideal environment for the growth of microorganisms.
12. If indicated, apply barrier lotion or ointment.	12. Barrier ointments may be used if client is incontinent or skin folds tend to harbor moisture.
13. Reposition or dress client as appropriate.	13. Promotes client comfort.
14. Dispose of linens and garbage according to hospital policy.	14. Prevents spread of disease or bacteria.
15. Wash hands.	15. Reduces the transmission of microorganisms.
16. Deodorize room if appropriate.	16. Promotes client comfort. This may also be done at the beginning of the procedure.

(Continues)

PROCEDURE 29-20 Perineal Care (Continued)

ACTION	RATIONALE

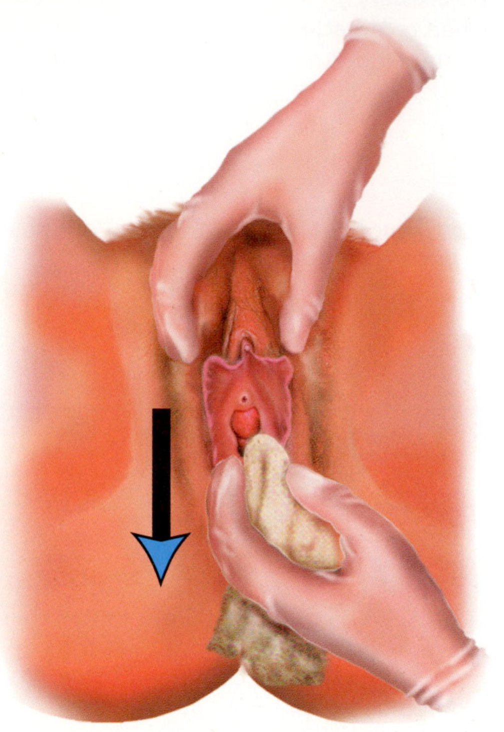

FIGURE 29-20-1 Wash the female perineum from front to back.

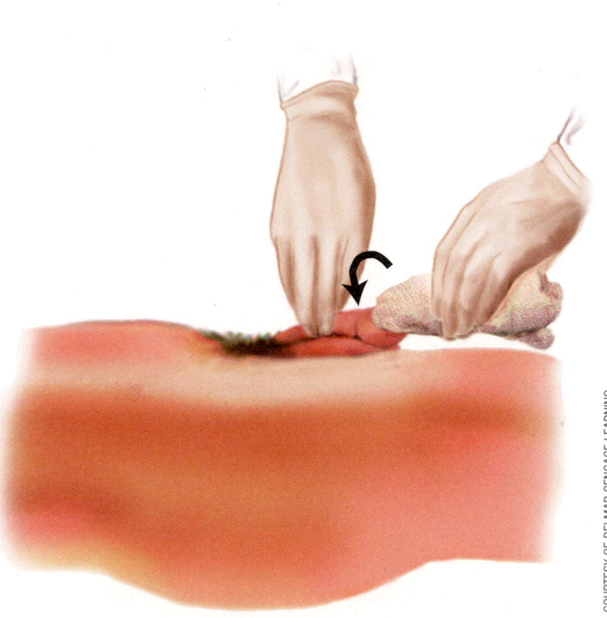

FIGURE 29-20-2 Wash the penis with a warm, wet washcloth in circular motions.

EVALUATION

- The perineum and genitalia are dry, clean, and free of secretions and unpleasant odors.
- The client reports feeling comfortable and clean in the perineal area.
- The client did not experience discomfort or undue embarrassment during the procedure.

DOCUMENTATION

Nurses' Notes

- Time and type of perineal care provided
- Unusual findings such as skin breakdown, infection, or unusual drainage
- Client special preferences or cultural considerations

Kardex

- Special preferences or cultural considerations

PROCEDURE 29-21 Routine Catheter Care

OVERVIEW

An indwelling catheter is used to provide continuous drainage of urine from the bladder. The catheter, which is attached to a drainage bag, may be used for episodic or long-term urinary drainage. Because the catheter is in the bladder through the urethra, bacteria may enter the urinary system; therefore, care must be taken to ensure that the surrounding area is clean to decrease contamination of the catheter by bacterial flora. Clients may be embarrassed or frightened by the catheter and related care and, therefore, require emotional support.

(Continues)

PROCEDURE 29-21 Routine Catheter Care (Continued)

ASSESSMENT

1. Assess catheter patency and urine color, consistency, and amount while performing the care **to determine if catheter and drainage system are functioning correctly.**
2. Determine the condition of the urinary meatus and perineal area **to monitor for redness, swelling, or drainage, stool, or vaginal discharge, as indicators of infection. External infections may migrate up the catheter and lead to urinary tract infection.**
3. Determine the client's emotional reaction and feelings related to the catheter. **This may prevent untoward reactions to the care and allow the nurse to help the client deal with some deeper emotional issues.**

POSSIBLE NURSING DIAGNOSES

Risk for Infection
Risk for Impaired Skin Integrity

PLANNING

Expected Outcomes

1. The client will be free of signs and symptoms of urinary tract infection.
2. The client will understand the reason for the catheter and related cares.
3. The meatus and surrounding area will be clean and free of drainage.

Equipment Needed

- Clean latex-free gloves
- Washcloth, soap, and water
- Waterproof pad
- Antiseptic solution
- Sterile swabs

delegation tips

Routine catheter care is a procedure ancillary personnel are able to perform after proper instruction and supervision. Instruction should include notifying the nurse regarding the appearance of catheter drainage and any problems with catheter tubing, such as leaks.

IMPLEMENTATION—ACTION/RATIONALE

* Check client's identification band * Explain procedure before beginning *

ACTION	RATIONALE
1. Wash hands.	1. Reduces the transmission of microorganisms.
2. Check institutional protocol or care plan.	2. Ensures proper procedure.
3. Provide privacy.	3. Protects client dignity.
4. Place client in supine position and expose perineal area and catheter.	4. Allows for visualization of field. If unable to visualize the perineal area with the client supine, try placing the client in a side-lying position.
5. Place waterproof pad under client.	5. Protects bed linens.
6. Put on clean gloves.	6. Reduces transmission of microorganisms.
7. After performing perineal care (Procedure 29-20), cleanse meatus if there is excessive purulent drainage with nonirritating antiseptic solutions on cotton balls.	7. Moving from the most clean area out decreases risk of recontamination.
8. Wash catheter from meatus out to end of catheter, taking care not to pull on catheter.	8. Moving from most clean area out does not transmit bacteria to meatal area predisposing the client to a urethral or bladder infection.
9. Be sure to repeat catheter care any time it becomes soiled with stool or other drainage.	9. Reduces chance of infection.
10. Place linen or cotton balls in proper receptacle for laundry or disposal.	10. Reduces transmission of infection to other clients.
11. Wash hands.	11. Reduces transmission of microorganisms.

(Continues)

PROCEDURE 29-21 Routine Catheter Care (Continued)

EVALUATION

- The client is free of signs and symptoms of urinary tract infection.
- The client understands the reason for the catheter and related care.
- The meatus and surrounding area are clean, intact, and free of drainage.

DOCUMENTATION

Nurses' Notes

- Time the procedure was performed and condition of area surrounding the catheter

PROCEDURE 29-22 Oral Care

OVERVIEW

The oral cavity functions in mastication, secretion of mucus to moisten and lubricate the digestive system, secretion of digestive enzymes, and absorption of essential nutrients. Common problems occurring in the oral cavity include the following:

- Bad breath (halitosis)
- Dental cavities (caries)
- Plaque
- Periodontal disease
- Inflammation of the gums (gingivitis)
- Inflammation of the oral mucosa (stomatitis)

Poor oral hygiene and loss of teeth may affect a client's social interaction and body image as well as nutritional intake. Daily oral care is essential to maintain the integrity of the mucous membranes, teeth, gums, and lips. Through preventive measures, the oral cavity and teeth can be preserved. Preventive oral care consists of fluoride rinsing, flossing, and brushing.

Fluoride

Researchers determined that fluoride can prevent dental caries. Fluoride is a common component of many mouthwashes and toothpastes; however, people with excessive dryness or irritated mucous membranes should avoid commercial mouthwashes because of the alcohol content, which causes drying of mucous membranes. Educate clients about fluoride being an excellent preventive measure against dental caries, but excessive fluoride exposure can affect the color of tooth enamel.

Flossing

Floss daily in conjunction with brushing of teeth. Flossing prevents the formation of plaque, removes plaque between the teeth, and removes food debris. Cavities and periodontal disease are prevented by regular flossing. Many floss holders are available to facilitate flossing.

Brushing

Teeth should be brushed after each meal. Brushing is performed using a dentifrice (toothpaste) that contains fluoride to aid in preventing dental caries. An effective homemade dentifrice is the combination of two parts salt with one part baking soda. Brushing removes plaque and food debris and promotes blood circulation of the gums. Dentures are brushed using the same brushing motion as that used for brushing teeth.

ASSESSMENT

1. Assess whether the client is able to assist with oral care and to what extent. **Promotes independence where possible.**
2. Evaluate whether the client has an understanding of proper oral hygiene. **Promotes self-care and teaching.**
3. Check whether the client has dentures. **Determines how oral care is performed.**

(Continues)

PROCEDURE 29-22 Oral Care (Continued)

4. Assess the condition of the client's mouth. **Determines how oral care is performed.**
5. Assess whether inflammation, bleeding, infection, or ulceration is present. **Determines how oral care is performed. Determines the need for additional assessment and intervention.**
6. Assess what cultural practices to consider. **Determines how oral care is performed.**
7. Assess whether there are any appliances or devices present in the client's mouth such as braces, endotracheal tube, or bridgework. **Determines how oral care is performed.**
8. Check that the proper equipment is available to perform oral care. **Ensures a smooth procedure.**

POSSIBLE NURSING DIAGNOSES

Risk for Infection
Impaired Oral Mucous Membrane
Bathing/Hygiene Self-Care Deficit
Deficient Knowledge-Oral Hygiene

PLANNING

Expected Outcomes

1. Client's mouth, teeth, gums, and lips will be clean and free of food particles.
2. Any inflammation, bleeding, infection, or ulceration present will be noted and treated.
3. The oral mucosa will be clean, intact, and well hydrated.

Equipment Needed

Brushing and Flossing

- Toothbrush
- Toothpaste with fluoride
- Emesis basin
- Towel
- Cup of water
- Nonsterile gloves
- Dental floss, floss holder
- Mirror
- Lip moisturizer

Denture Care

- Denture brush
- Denture cleaner
- Emesis basin
- Towel
- Cup of water
- Nonsterile gloves
- Tissue
- Denture cup

Special Care Items for Clients with Impaired Physical Mobility or Who Are Unconscious (comatose)

- Soft toothbrush or toothette
- Tongue blade
- 3 × 3 gauze sponges
- Cotton-tip applicators
- Prescribed solution
- Plastic Asepto syringe
- Suction machine and catheter

delegation tips

Oral care is routinely delegated to ancillary personnel, who allow the client to perform as much of the oral care as possible or permitted. The caregiver is educated to employ Standard Precautions, to properly position the client, and to observe and report the client's mucous membrane condition and color to the nurse.

IMPLEMENTATION—ACTION/RATIONALE

ACTION	RATIONALE
* Check client's identification band * Explain procedure before beginning *	
Self-Care Client: Flossing and Brushing	
1. Assemble articles for flossing and brushing.	1. Promotes efficiency.
2. Provide privacy.	2. Relaxes the client.
3. Place client in a high Fowler's position.	3. Decreases risk of aspiration.
4. Wash hands and apply gloves.	4. Reduces the transmission of microorganisms.
5. Arrange articles within client's reach.	5. Facilitates self-care.

(Continues)

PROCEDURE 29-22 Oral Care (Continued)

ACTION	RATIONALE
6. Assist client with flossing and brushing as necessary. Position mirror, emesis basin, water with straw near the client, and a towel across the chest (Figure 29-22-1).	6. Flossing and brushing decrease microorganism growth in the mouth. Use of mirror permits cleaning back and sides of teeth.
7. Assist client with rinsing mouth.	7. Removes toothpaste and oral secretions.
8. Reposition client, raise side rails, and place call button within reach.	8. Promotes comfort, safety, and communication.
9. Rinse, dry, and return articles to proper place.	9. Promotes a clean environment.
10. Remove gloves, wash hands, and document care.	10. Reduces the transmission of microorganisms and documents nursing care.
Self-Care Client: Denture Care	
11. Assemble articles for denture cleaning (Figure 29-22-2).	11. Promotes efficiency.
12. Provide privacy.	12. Relaxes the client.
13. Assist client to a high Fowler's position.	13. Facilitates removal of dentures.
14. Wash hands and apply gloves.	14. Reduces the transmission of microorganisms and exposure to body fluids.
15. Assist client with denture removal: a. Top denture: • With gauze, grasp the denture with thumb and forefinger and pull downward. • Place in denture cup. b. Bottom denture: • Place thumbs on the gums and release the denture. Grasp denture with thumb and forefinger and pull upward. • Place in denture cup.	15. Breaks seal created with dentures without causing pressure and injury to oral membranes. Prevents breaking of dentures.
16. Apply toothpaste to brush, and brush dentures either with cool water in the emesis basin or under running water in the sink. Pad sink with towel to protect dentures in case they are dropped. Some clients prefer to clean dentures by soaking them in a cup with water and an effervescent denture cleaning tablet.	16. Facilitates removal of microorganisms.
17. Rinse thoroughly.	17. Removes toothpaste.
18. Assist client with rinsing mouth and replacing dentures.	18. Freshens mouth and facilitates intake of solid food.

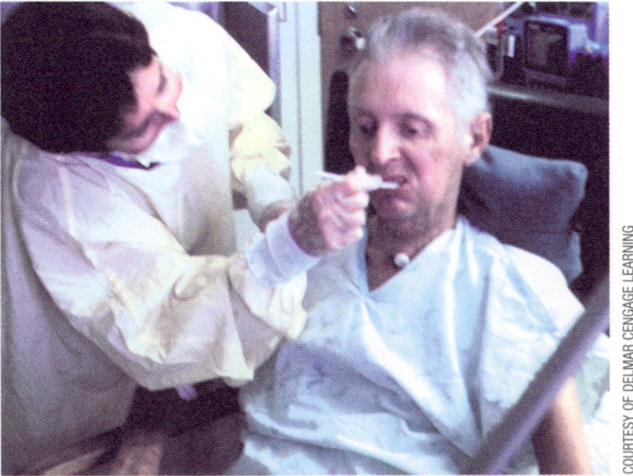

COURTESY OF DELMAR CENGAGE LEARNING

FIGURE 29-22-1 Promote independence but assist with flossing or brushing as necessary.

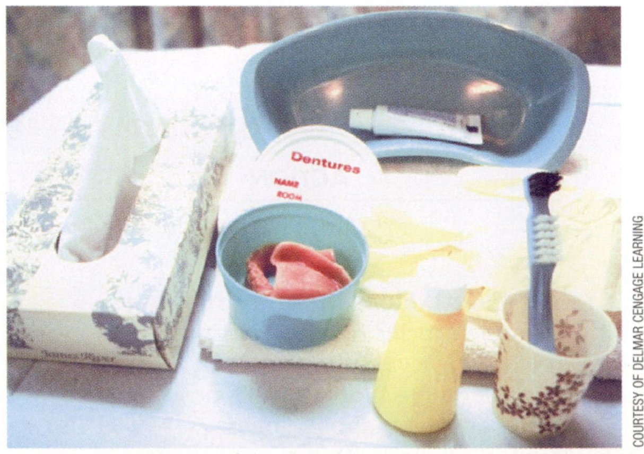

COURTESY OF DELMAR CENGAGE LEARNING

FIGURE 29-22-2 Assemble articles for denture care.

(Continues)

PROCEDURE 29-22 Oral Care (Continued)

ACTION	RATIONALE
19. Reposition client, with side rails up and call button within reach.	19. Promotes comfort, safety, and communication.
20. Rinse, dry, and return articles to proper place.	20. Maintains a clean environment.
21. Remove gloves and wash hands.	21. Reduces the transmission of microorganisms.
Full-Care Client: Brushing and Flossing	
22. Assemble articles for flossing and brushing.	22. Promotes efficiency.
23. Provide privacy.	23. Relaxes client.
24. Wash hands and apply gloves.	24. Reduces the transmission of microorganisms and exposure to body fluids.
25. Position client as condition allows: high Fowler's, semi-Fowler's, or lateral position, head turned toward side (Figure 29-22-3).	25. Decreases risk of aspiration.
26. Place towel across client's chest or under face and mouth if head is turned to one side.	26. Catches secretions.
27. Moisten toothbrush or toothette, apply small amount of toothpaste, and brush teeth and gums.	27. Moistens mouth and facilitates plaque removal.
28. Grasp the dental floss in both hands or use a floss holder and floss between all teeth; hold floss against tooth while moving floss up and down sides of teeth.	28. Removes plaque and prevents gum disease.
29. Assist the client in rinsing mouth.	29. Removes toothpaste and oral secretions.
30. Reapply toothpaste and brush the teeth and gums using friction in a circular motion. On inner and outer surfaces of teeth, hold brush at 45-degree angle against teeth and brush from sulcus to crowns of teeth. On biting surfaces, move brush back and forth in short strokes. All surfaces of teeth should be brushed from every angle.	30. Permits cleaning of back and sides of teeth and decreases microorganism growth in mouth.
31. Assist the client in rinsing and drying mouth.	31. Removes toothpaste and oral secretions.
32. Apply lip moisturizer, if appropriate.	32. Maintains skin integrity of lips.
33. Reposition client, raise side rails, and place call button within reach.	33. Promotes comfort, safety, and communication.
34. Rinse, dry, and return articles to proper place.	34. Provides an orderly environment.
35. Remove gloves and wash hands.	35. Reduces the transmission of microorganisms.

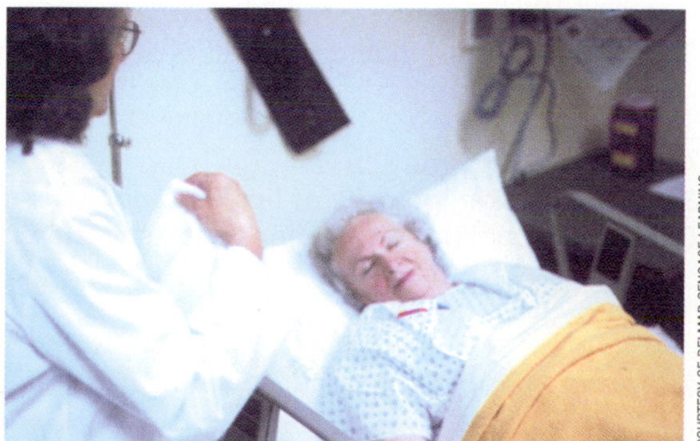

COURTESY OF DELMAR CENGAGE LEARNING

FIGURE 29-22-3 If client is unable to sit up, turn head to the side.

(Continues)

PROCEDURE 29-22 Oral Care (Continued)

ACTION	RATIONALE
Clients at Risk for or with an Alteration of the Oral Cavity	
36. Follow Actions 22 to 24.	36. See Rationales 22 to 24.
37. Bleeding:	37.
a. Assess oral cavity with a padded tongue blade and flashlight for signs of bleeding.	a. Determines whether bleeding is present, amount, and specific areas.
b. Proceed with the actions for oral care for a full-care client except:	b.
• Do not floss.	• Decreases risk of bleeding and trauma to gums.
• Use a soft toothbrush, toothette, or a tongue blade padded with 3 × 3 gauze sponges to gently swab teeth and gums.	• Decreases risk of bleeding and trauma to gums.
• Dispose of padded tongue blade into a biohazard bag according to institutional policy.	• Promotes proper disposal of contaminated waste.
• Rinse with tepid water.	• Cleanses mouth.
38. Infection or ulceration:	38.
a. Assess oral cavity with a tongue blade and flashlight for signs of infection.	a. Determines appearance, integrity, and general condition.
b. Culture lesions as ordered.	b. Identifies growth of specific microorganisms.
c. Proceed with the actions for oral care for a full-care client except:	c.
• Do not floss.	• Prevents irritation, pain, and bleeding.
• Use prescribed antiseptic solution.	• Antiseptic solutions decrease growth of microorganisms.
• Use a tongue blade padded with 3 × 3 gauze sponges to gently swab the teeth and gums.	
• Dispose of padded tongue blade into a biohazard bag according to institutional policy.	• Promotes proper disposal of contaminated materials.
• Rinse mouth with tepid water.	• Cleanses mouth.
• Apply additional solution as prescribed.	• Provides a coating that promotes healing of the tissue.
Unconscious (Comatose) Client	
39. Follow Actions 22–24.	39. See Rationales 22 to 24.
40. Place the client in a lateral position, with the head turned toward the side.	40. Prevents aspiration.
41. Use a floss holder and floss between all teeth.	41. Prevents transfer of microorganisms from a client bite.
42. Moisten toothbrush or toothette, and brush the teeth and gums using friction in a circular motion. Do not use toothpaste. Brush teeth as described in Action 30.	42. Permits cleaning of back and sides of teeth and decreases microorganism growth in mouth. Toothpaste may foam and cause aspiration.
43. After flossing and brushing, rinse mouth with an Asepto syringe (do not force water into the mouth) and perform oral suction.	43. Promotes cleansing and removal of secretions and prevents aspiration.
44. Dry the client's mouth.	44. Prevents skin irritation.
45. Apply lip moisturizer.	45. Maintains skin integrity of lips.
46. Leave the client in a lateral position with head turned toward side for 30 to 60 minutes after oral hygiene care. Suction one more time. Remove the towel from under the client's mouth and face.	46. Prevents pooling of secretions and aspiration.
47. Dispose of any contaminated items in a biohazard bag and clean, dry, and return all articles to the appropriate place.	47. Promotes proper disposal of contaminated materials.
48. Remove gloves and wash hands.	48. Reduces the transmission of microorganisms.

(Continues)

PROCEDURE 29-22 Oral Care (Continued)

EVALUATION

- The client's mouth, teeth, gums, and lips are clean and free of food particles.
- Inflammation, bleeding, infection, or ulceration are noted and cared for.
- The oral mucosa is clean, intact, and well hydrated.
- The oral care was performed with a minimum of trauma to the client.

DOCUMENTATION

Nurses' Notes

- Unusual findings

PROCEDURE 29-23 Eye Care

OVERVIEW

Eyes need little daily care and are continually cleansed by the production of tears and movement of eyelids over the eyes. Some clients, however, do have special eye care needs.

Contact Lenses

Self-care is the best method of care for a client with contact lenses; however, accidents or illness may render a client unable to remove or care for the lenses. Some lenses may be left on the cornea for up to a week without damage. Most must be removed daily for cleaning and to prevent hypoxia of the cornea. It is a nursing responsibility to determine whether the client is wearing contact lenses and to properly care for the lenses and the client's eyes. In acute care situations, encourage the client to wear glasses if possible and send the contact lenses home with a family member.

Prosthetic Eyes

Some clients have an artificial eye (ocular prosthesis) in place. Artificial eyes are created to look identical to the client's biologic eye. They are generally made from glass or plastic. Some artificial eyes are permanently implanted in the eye socket, but others must be removed daily for cleaning. The eye socket should also be gently cleansed to remove crusts and mucus, and the prosthesis replaced in the eye socket.

ASSESSMENT

1. Determine if the client is wearing contact lenses or has an ocular prosthesis. If the client is unable to answer questions, you will need to find out another way. Does it indicate in the client's chart if the client wears contact lenses or has a prosthesis? Are there family members present to ask? **This affects the eye care given.**
2. Are the eye care supplies needed available? If the client can tell you what kind of eye care products he or she normally uses, ask or have a family member bring these products from home. **This affects eye care given.**
3. Assess whether the client can do his or her own eye care. If not, evaluate what kind of assistance the client needs. **This promotes maximum independence in the client.**

POSSIBLE NURSING DIAGNOSES

Ineffective Health Maintenance
Bathing/Hygiene Self-Care Deficit
Disturbed Sensory Perception (Visual)

PLANNING

Expected Outcomes

1. The client's contact lenses will be safely removed and stored.
2. The client's ocular prosthesis will be safely removed, cleaned, and either stored or returned to the client's eye socket.
3. The client's contacts or prosthesis will be cared for with a minimum of trauma to the client's eyes.
4. The client's eyes will be free of crusts and exudate.

Equipment Needed

Artificial Eye

- Storage container
- Mild soap
- 3 × 3 gauze sponges
- Cotton balls
- Towel
- Emesis basins

(Continues)

PROCEDURE 29-23 Eye Care (Continued)

- Eye irrigation syringe (optional)
- Running water
- Sterile gloves
- Biohazard bag
- Saline solution
- Protector pad

Contact Lenses

- Lens container
- Soaking solution—type used by client
- Towel
- Suction cup (optional)
- Scotch tape (optional)
- Nonsterile gloves

delegation tips

Eye care requires the assessment and intervention of the nurse and delegation to ancillary personnel is inappropriate.

IMPLEMENTATION—ACTION/RATIONALE

ACTION	RATIONALE
* Check client's identification band * Explain procedure before beginning *	
Artificial Eye Removal	
1. Inquire about client's care regimen and gather equipment accordingly.	1. Promotes continuity of care.
2. Provide privacy.	2. Relaxes the client.
3. Wash hands; apply gloves.	3. Reduces the transmission of microorganisms.
4. Place client in a semi-Fowler's position.	4. Facilitates procedure and client participation.
5. Place the cotton balls in an emesis basin filled halfway with warm tap water.	5. Dry cotton balls could cause irritation.
6. Place 3 × 3 gauze sponges in bottom of second emesis basin and fill halfway with mild soap and tepid water.	6. Gauze serves as padding to prevent breakage of the prosthesis.
7. Grasp and squeeze excess water from a cotton ball. Wash the eyelid with the moistened cotton ball, starting at the inner canthus and moving outward toward the outer canthus. After each use, dispose of cotton ball in biohazard bag. Repeat procedure until eyelid is clean (without dried secretions).	7. Eliminating the excess water prevents water from running down the client's face. Cleansing the eyelid prevents contamination of the lacrimal system (inner canthus area). Disposal of cotton balls reduces transmission of microorganisms to other health care workers.
8. Remove the artificial eye:	8. Cleanses the artificial eye.
a. Using dominant hand, raise the client's upper eyelid with index finger and depress the lower eyelid with thumb.	a. Promotes removal of artificial eye.
b. Cup nondominant hand under the client's lower eyelid.	b. Cupping reduces dropping and possible breaking of the eye.
c. Apply slight pressure with index finger between the brow and the artificial eye and remove it. Place it in an emesis basin filled with warm, soapy water.	c. Applying pressure will help the prosthesis to slip out.
9. Grasp a moistened cotton ball and cleanse around the edge of the eye socket. Dispose of the soiled cotton ball into biohazard bag.	9. Cleanses the eye socket. Disposal of cotton ball reduces transmission of microorganisms to other health care workers.
10. Inspect the eye socket for any signs of irritation, drainage, or crusting. Note: If the client's usual care regimen or physician order requires irrigation of the socket, proceed with Action 11; otherwise, go to Action 12.	10. Indicates an infection.

(Continues)

PROCEDURE 29-23 Eye Care (Continued)

ACTION	RATIONALE
11. Eye socket irrigation:	11. Cleanses the eye socket and removes secretions.
a. Lower the head of the bed and place the client in a supine position. Place protector pad on bed; turn head toward socket side and slightly extend neck.	a. Positioning of client facilitates ease in performing the procedure and client comfort.
b. Fill the irrigation syringe with the prescribed amount and type of irrigating solution (warm tap water or normal saline).	b. Ensures compliance with client's regimen or prescribed orders.
c. With nondominant hand, separate the eyelids with your forefinger and thumb while resting fingers on the brow and cheekbone.	c. Keeps the eyelid open and the socket visible.
d. Hold the irrigating syringe in dominant hand several inches above the inner canthus; with thumb, gently apply pressure on the plunger, directing the flow of solution from the inner canthus along the conjunctival sac.	d. Prevents injury to the client.
e. Irrigate until the prescribed amount of solution has been used.	e. Ensures compliance with client's regimen of prescribed orders.
f. Wipe the eyelids with a moistened cotton ball after irrigating. Dispose of soiled cotton ball in biohazard bag.	f. Reduces the transmission of microorganisms to prosthesis.
g. Pat the skin dry with the towel.	g. Prevents maceration of the skin.
h. Return the client to a semi-Fowler's position.	h. Promotes client comfort.
i. Remove gloves, wash hands, and apply clean gloves.	i. Reduces the transmission of microorganisms.
12. Rub the artificial eye between index finger and thumb in the basin of warm, soapy water.	12. Creates cleaning with friction and prevents breakage of the prosthesis.
13. Rinse the prosthesis under running water or place in the clean basin of tepid water. Do not dry the prosthesis. *Note:* Either reinsert the prosthesis (Action 14) or store in a container (Action 15).	13. Removes soap and secretions. Keeping the artificial eye wet prevents irritation from lint or other particles that might adhere to it and facilitates reinsertion.
14. Reinsert the prosthesis:	14. Allows for client comfort.
a. With the thumb of the nondominant hand, raise and hold the upper eyelid open.	a. Facilitates reinsertion of the prosthesis without discomfort to the client.
b. With the dominant hand, grasp the artificial eye so that the indented part is facing toward the client's nose and slide it under the upper eyelid as far as possible.	b. Positions the prosthesis for insertion.
c. Depress the lower lid.	c. Allows the prosthesis to slide into place.
d. Pull the lower lid forward to cover the edge of the prosthesis.	d. Holds the prosthesis in place.
15. Place the cleaned artificial eye in a labeled container with saline or tap water solution.	15. Protects the prosthesis from scratches and keeps it clean.
16. Grasp a moistened cotton ball and squeeze out excessive moisture. Wipe the eyelid from the inner to the outer canthus. Dispose of the soiled cotton ball in a biohazard bag.	16. Squeezing the cotton ball removes moisture. Cleansing the eyelid prevents contamination of lacrimal system. Disposal of cotton ball reduces the transmission of microorganisms to other health care workers.
17. Clean, dry, and replace equipment.	17. Promotes a clean environment.
18. Reposition the client, raise side rails, and place call light in reach.	18. Promotes client's comfort, safety, and communication.
19. Dispose of biohazard bag according to institutional policy.	19. Reduces the transmission of microorganisms to other health care workers.
20. Remove gloves and wash hands.	20. Same as Rationale 19.

(Continues)

PROCEDURE 29-23 Eye Care (Continued)

ACTION	RATIONALE
Contact Lens Removal	
21. Assess level of assistance needed and provide privacy.	21. Level of assistance determines level of intervention. Privacy reduces anxiety.
22. Wash hands.	22. Reduces the transmission of microorganisms.
23. Assist the client to a semi-Fowler's position if needed.	23. Facilitates removal of lens.
24. Drape a clean towel over the client's chest.	24. Provides a clean surface and facilitates the location of a lens if it falls during removal.
25. Prepare the lens storage case with the prescribed solution.	25. Hard lenses can be stored dry or in a special soaking solution. Soft lenses are stored in sterile normal saline without a preservative.
26. Instruct the client to look straight ahead. Assess the location of the lens. If it is not on the cornea, either you or the client should gently move the lens toward the cornea with pad of index finger (Figure 29-23-1).	26. Client's position promotes easy removal of lens. Positioning lens on the cornea aids removal. Use of the finger pad of the index finger prevents damage to cornea and lens.
27. Remove the lens.	27. Provides for cleaning and storage of the lens.
a. Hard lens:	a.
• Cup nondominant hand under the eye.	• Cupping the hand under eye helps catch the lens and prevent breakage.
• Gently place index finger on the outside corner of the eye and pull toward the temple and ask client to blink. Catch the lens in your nondominant hand.	• Pulling the corner of the eye tightens the eyelid against the eyeball. Pressure on the upper edge of lens causes the lens to tip forward.
b. Soft lens:	b.
• With nondominant hand, separate the eyelid with your thumb and middle finger.	• Separating the eyelid exposes the lower edge of lens.
• With the index finger of the dominant hand gently placed on the lower edge of the lens, slide the lens downward onto the sclera and gently squeeze the lens.	• Positions lens for easy grasping with the pad of the index finger, which prevents injury to the cornea and lens. Squeezing the lens allows air to enter and release the suction.
• Release the top eyelid (continue holding the lower lid down) and remove the lens with your index finger and thumb.	• Ensures control of the lens.
Note: If Action 27 is unsuccessful, secure a suction cup to remove the contact lens. If you are unable to remove the lens, notify the physician or qualified practitioner.	• Suction cup is used to remove a lens from an unconscious or dependent client.

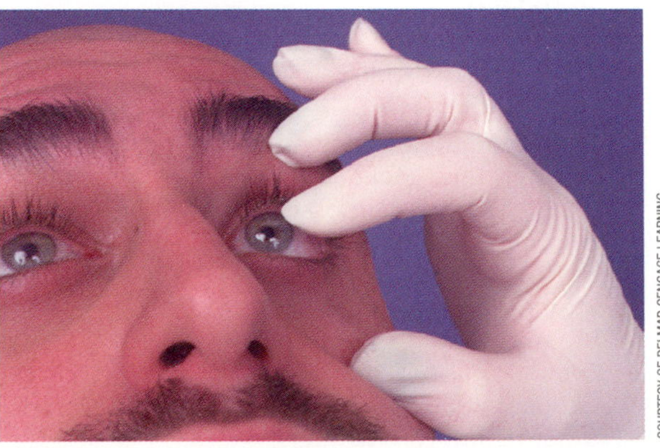
COURTESY OF DELMAR CENGAGE LEARNING

FIGURE 29-23-1 If the lens is not on the cornea, gently move it toward the cornea with the pad of the index finger.

(Continues)

PROCEDURE 29-23 Eye Care (Continued)

ACTION	RATIONALE
28. Store the lens in the correct compartment of the case ("right" or "left"). Label with the client's name. Note: Some soft lenses are thrown away after a timed usage. Check with client before disposing of contact lens.	28. Storage prevents damage to the lenses and ensures that each lens will be reinserted into the correct eye.
29. Remove and store the other lens by repeating Actions 27 and 28.	29. Refer to Rationales 27 and 28.
30. Assess eyes for irritation or redness.	30. Signs of corneal irritation.
31. Store the lens case in a safe place.	31. Prevents damage or loss.
32. Dispose of soiled articles and clean and return reusable articles to proper location.	32. Reduces the transmission of infection.
33. Reposition the client, raise side rails, and place call light in reach.	33. Promotes client comfort, safety, and communication.
34. Remove gloves and wash hands.	34. Reduces the transmission of infection.

EVALUATION

- The client's contact lenses were safely removed and stored.
- The client's ocular prosthesis was safely removed, cleaned, and either stored or returned to the client's eye socket.
- The client's contacts or prosthesis were cared for with a minimum of trauma to the client's eyes.
- The client's eyes are free of crusts and exudate.
- The client is comfortable.

DOCUMENTATION

Nurses' Notes

- Whether the client wears contact lenses
- Location and condition of the lenses
- Whether the client requires assistance to place and remove the contact lenses
- Whether the client has an ocular prosthesis and which eye
- Condition of the prosthesis and the condition of the eye socket
- Care performed on the prosthesis and the socket and how the client tolerated the activity
- Client teaching

Kardex

- Whether the client wears contact lenses or glasses or has an ocular prosthesis
- Special care requirements

PROCEDURE 29-24 Giving a Back Rub

OVERVIEW

Giving a back rub is a basic nursing skill. Back massage is an effective means of building a sense of trust and increased rapport between the nurse and client. Clients are often touch-deprived in the busy health care industry of today. The small amount of time that it takes to do a simple back massage can often soothe and relax a "difficult" client and increase the effectiveness of the nurse–client relationship.

Massage is performed in many different ways, from light strokes to heavy kneading. Various forms include effleurage, deep or gentle stroking, and petrissage, a kneading performed with the tips of the fingers and thumbs or palm of the hand. Massage stimulates circulation and promotes lymphatic drainage, thereby helping to rid the body of metabolic wastes, speed healing, and provide gentle relaxation. However, do not massage over areas of skin that are red or white and remain that color for over a minute. Massaging over these areas may damage the tissue. Do not massage over open skin areas or boney prominences that do not have fatty tissue. Massage can open lines of communication and improve the therapeutic relationship between a nurse and client.

(Continues)

PROCEDURE 29-24 Giving a Back Rub (Continued)

ASSESSMENT

1. Assess the client's willingness to have a massage. **The client may not want a massage or may not enjoy the tactile experience of a massage.**
2. Assess the client for contraindications of a back rub. Conditions include open sores or lesions, vertebral fractures, burns, and signs of pressure ulcers. **To prevent injuring the client.**
3. Assess any limitations the client has in positioning **to determine if the client has any conditions that prohibit a side-lying or prone position.**
4. Assess the client for fatigue, stiffness, or soreness in the back and shoulders. **Knowing areas of particular concern allows you to focus your energies toward "trouble areas."**
5. Assess the client for anxiety or emotional disturbances. **Massage can help reduce anxiety and calm people in distress.**
6. If possible, have the client quantify the degree of discomfort using a 1 to 10 rating scale. **Quantifying the results can provide more validity to the intervention.**

POSSIBLE NURSING DIAGNOSES

Anxiety (mild)

*Impaired Physical **M**obility*

PLANNING

Expected Outcomes

1. The client will experience a reduction in tension, anxiety, pain, and fatigue.
2. The client's circulation to the back is improved.
3. The nurse will establish a better rapport with the client.

Equipment Needed

- Quiet environment, free of interruptions, with a comfortable room temperature
- Comfortable bed or massage table that allows a client to lie in a side-lying or prone position
- Bath blanket
- Bath towel, to absorb excess moisture, oils
- Lotion, baby powder, or massage oil
- Gloves if necessary

delegation tips

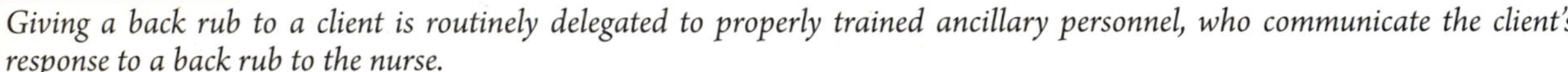

Giving a back rub to a client is routinely delegated to properly trained ancillary personnel, who communicate the client's response to a back rub to the nurse.

IMPLEMENTATION—ACTION/RATIONALE

ACTION	RATIONALE
* Check client's identification band * Explain procedure before beginning *	
1. Wash your hands and apply gloves if necessary.	1. Reduces the transmission of microorganisms.
2. Help client to a prone or side-lying position.	2. Allows exposure of back and shoulder area.
3. Drape the bath blanket and undo the client's gown, exposing the back, shoulder, and sacral area but keeping the remainder of the body covered.	3. Prevents chilling and excess exposure.
4. Pour a small amount of lotion in your hand and warm between your palms for a few moments. The lotion bottle can also be submerged in a bowl of warm water for a few minutes to warm the lotion. Baby powder may be substituted for oils or lotions.	4. Prevents the shock of cold lotion being applied to the body. Some clients may be sensitive to oils or lotions.
5. Begin in the sacral area with smooth, circular strokes, moving upward toward the shoulders. Gradually lengthen the strokes to the upper back, scapulae, and upper arms. Apply firm, continuous pressure without breaking contact with the client (Figures 29-24-1).	5. Applying firm, continuous pressure increases circulation and relaxation.
6. Assess client's back as you are massaging for areas of redness and signs of decreased circulation.	6. Monitors for signs of early skin breakdown.
7. Provide a firm, kneading massage to areas of increased tension if desired, in areas such as the shoulders and gluteal muscles.	7. Firm, kneading strokes can decrease muscle tension, reducing pain and increasing relaxation.

(Continues)

PROCEDURE 29-24 Giving a Back Rub (Continued)

ACTION	RATIONALE

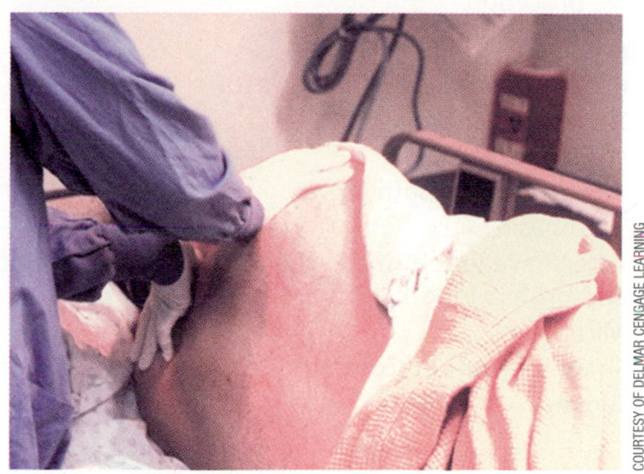

FIGURE 29-24-1 Apply firm, continuous pressure without breaking contact between your hands and the client's skin.

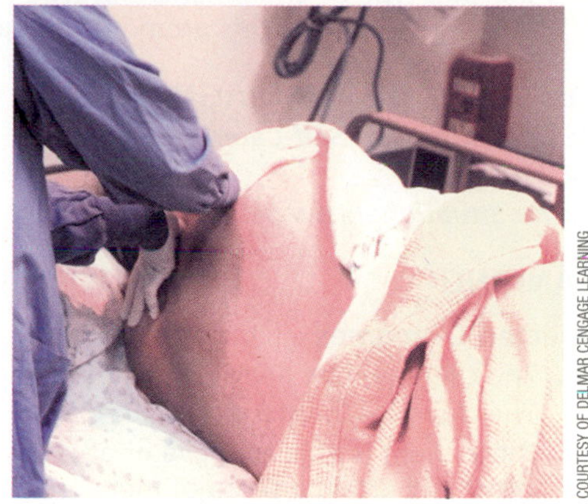

FIGURE 29-24-2 Finish the massage with light brushstrokes, using the fingertips.

ACTION	RATIONALE
8. Complete the massage with long, very light brushstrokes, using the tips of the fingers (Figure 29-24-2).	8. This is a very relaxing stroke and signals an end to the massage.
9. Gently pat or wipe excess lubricant off the client and cover the client.	9. Prevents soiling of the bed with excess lotions and keeps the client warm.
10. Wash hands.	10. Reduces the transmission of microorganisms.

EVALUATION

- The client experienced a reduction in tension, anxiety, pain, and fatigue.
- The nurse established better rapport with the client.

DOCUMENTATION

Nurses' Notes

- Time and date the back rub was performed
- Client's response to the back rub
- Complaints of pain or tension the client reported
- Unusual findings

PROCEDURE 29-25 Shaving a Client

OVERVIEW

Shaving is usually done after a bath or shower and as often as required to remove unwanted facial hair. Most men shave every day, although the facial hair of older clients does not grow as rapidly. If a beard or mustache is present, it is groomed daily and trimmed as appropriate. Do not shave off beards or mustaches without the client's permission. Some clients on anticoagulants may prefer to shave with an electric shaver instead of a safety razor.

ASSESSMENT

1. Assess whether the client is able to perform self-care. **Promote independence when possible.**
2. Assess the client's skin for areas of redness, skin breakdown, moles, or skin lesions. **Shaving could irritate the skin further.**
3. Assess whether the client has a bleeding tendency or is on anticoagulants. **If there is an increased risk of bleeding, an electric razor is used.**
4. If the client prefers to shave himself, assess the client's ability to manipulate the razor. **The client must be able to shave safely.**

(Continues)

PROCEDURE 29-25 Shaving a Client (Continued)

5. Assess the client's preference for the type of shaving, type of equipment, and type of lotion (if there are options). **This promotes independence.**

POSSIBLE NURSING DIAGNOSES

Dressing/Grooming Self-Care Deficit
Risk for Injury
Risk for Situational Low Self-Esteem

PLANNING

Expected Outcomes

1. The client will be neat and well groomed.
2. The client's skin integrity will remain intact.
3. If the client is able to shave or able to assist, the client will attain a sense of independence.
4. The client will be comfortable following the procedure.

Equipment Needed

- Electric razor or disposable razor
- Shaving cream or soap
- Warm water
- Washcloth and bath towel
- Washbasin
- Aftershave lotion (if the client has no skin irritation and prefers lotion)
- Mirror
- Sharp scissors and comb if mustache care required
- Gloves

delegation tips

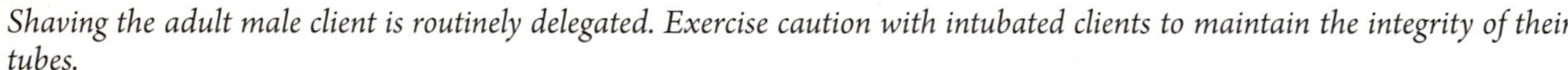

Shaving the adult male client is routinely delegated. Exercise caution with intubated clients to maintain the integrity of their tubes.

IMPLEMENTATION—ACTION/RATIONALE

* Check client's identification band * Explain procedure before beginning *

ACTION	RATIONALE
1. Wash hands and apply gloves.	1. Reduces transmission of microorganisms.
2. Assist the client to a comfortable position. If the client can shave himself, set up the equipment and supplies, including warm water, and watch the client for safety. Adjust lighting as needed.	2. Facilitates comfort and ease of shaving. Encourages sense of self-control and independence.
3. Place a towel over the client's chest and shoulder.	3. Protects the client and gown from soil.
4. Raise the bed to a comfortable height.	4. Facilitates comfort of staff.
5. Fill a washbasin with water at approximately 44°C (110°F). Check temperature for comfort.	5. Warm water helps soften the skin and beard.
6. Place the washcloth in the basin and wring out thoroughly. Apply the cloth over the client's entire face.	6. Warm water helps soften the skin and beard. Warmth can be relaxing.
7. Apply shaving cream.	7. Helps soften the whiskers.
8. Take the razor in the dominant hand and hold it at a 45-degree angle to the client's skin. Start shaving across one side of the client's face. Use the nondominant hand to gently pull the skin taut while shaving. Use short, firm strokes in the direction hair grows (Figure 29-25-1). Use short, downward strokes over the upper lip area.	8. Holding the skin taut prevents razor cuts and discomfort during shaving.
9. Rinse the razor in water as cream accumulates.	9. Keeps the cutting edge of the razor clean.
10. Check the face to see if all the facial hair is removed.	10. Ensures a neat appearance.
11. After all the facial hair is removed, rinse the face thoroughly with a moistened washcloth.	11. Promotes comfort and cleanliness.
12. Dry the face thoroughly and apply aftershave lotion if desired.	12. Stimulates and lubricates the skin.
13. Assist the client to a comfortable position and allow him to inspect the results of the shave.	13. Facilitates comfort and a sense of control.

(Continues)

PROCEDURE 29-25 Shaving a Client (Continued)

ACTION	RATIONALE

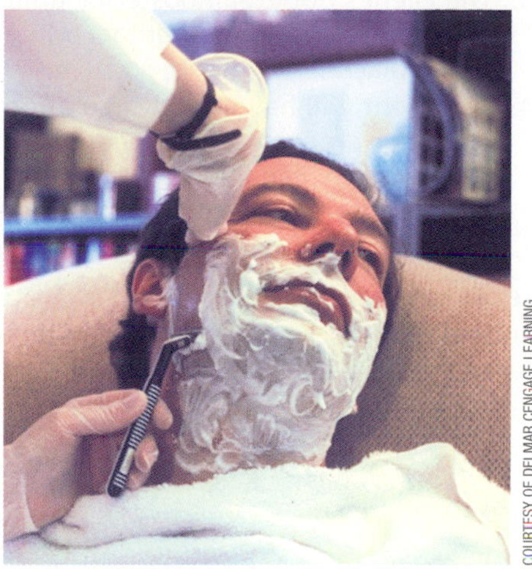

COURTESY OF DELMAR CENGAGE LEARNING

FIGURE 29-25-1 Shave with short, firm strokes in the direction the hair grows.

ACTION	RATIONALE
14. Dispose of equipment in proper receptacle.	14. Equipment should not be shared between clients in accordance with Standard Precautions because disruption of skin and bleeding may occur. The client may, however, keep his own razor. Clean and store it at the bedside.
15. Wash hands.	15. Reduces the transmission of microorganisms.

EVALUATION

- The client is neat and well groomed.
- The client's skin integrity remained intact.
- If the client was able to shave or able to assist, the client attained a sense of independence.
- The client is comfortable following the procedure.

DOCUMENTATION

Nurses' Notes

- Procedure, if the client was able to assist, and how the client tolerated the activity
- Unusual findings or injury that may have occurred

PROCEDURE 29-26 Applying Antiembolic Stockings

OVERVIEW

Antiembolic stockings also called TED® hose or elastic stockings, are used to promote circulation by compression and are useful to prevent thrombophlebitis. They are used on the legs of a client after surgery, on clients who are immobile, and on clients who have vascular disorders such as thrombophlebitis, varicose veins, and other conditions of impaired circulation of the lower extremities.

ASSESSMENT

1. Assess the condition of the client's lower extremities, noting edema, color, temperature, intact skin, ulcers, or infections. **Establishes a baseline for comparison.**
2. Assess the quality and equality of peripheral pulses in the legs (either dorsalis pedis or posterior tibial pulses) **to determine circulatory status.**
3. Assess the client's understanding of the reasons for, and the use of, the antiembolic stockings **to determine the amount of client teaching required.**

(Continues)

PROCEDURE 29-26 Applying Antiembolic Stockings (Continued)

4. Assess the client for signs and symptoms of deep vein thrombosis, such as increased calf size or color change, **to determine the appropriateness of the TED® hose placement.**

POSSIBLE NURSING DIAGNOSES

Risk for Impaired Skin Integrity
Decreased Cardiac Output
Ineffective Tissue Perfusion

PLANNING

Expected Outcomes

1. The client will experience no signs or symptoms of deep venous thrombosis or thrombophlebitis.
2. The client's venous return will be improved.
3. The client's popliteal, posterior tibial, and dorsalis pedis pulses will remain intact while stockings are in place.
4. The client will have good circulation while stockings are in place, as evident by warm skin temperature, capillary return within normal limits, sensation present, and no edema present in both extremities.

Equipment Needed

- Antiembolic stockings and package directions (latex-free, if necessary)
- Tape measure

delegation tips

Ancillary personnel routinely remove and reapply antiembolic stockings. Instruction is given to staff to apply stockings while client is supine in bed and to inspect and report any skin breakdown, impaired circulation, or excessive edema to the nurse.

IMPLEMENTATION—ACTION/RATIONALE

ACTION	RATIONALE
* Check client's identification band * Explain procedure before beginning *	
1. Wash hands.	1. Reduces transmission of microorganisms.
2. Review the orders with the client, including the reason for the stockings and the type of stockings ordered (e.g., knee or thigh high).	2. Facilitates compliance.
3. With the client in a supine position in bed, measure the client's leg for the correct size: • Thigh-high stockings: from Achilles tendon to the gluteal fold, circumference of the midthigh • Below-the-knee stockings: from the Achilles tendon to the popliteal fold, circumference of the midcalf	3. Supine position encourages venous return and decreases swelling, thereby allowing accurate measurement for size of stockings.
4. Compare the obtained measurements with the package insert to ascertain proper size.	4. Correct size is essential for stockings to apply the appropriate pressure for adequate venous return without compromise to circulation.
5. Apply stockings. The best time to apply stockings is early in the morning, before the client gets out of bed or immediately after surgery. Keep client in supine position until stockings are applied.	5. Feet are less swollen in the morning because the feet have been in a nondependent position during the night and most venous return has occurred. This, of course, is not the case in a client who has been up frequently during the night.
6. Open the package and turn stockings inside out over hand and arm. Place hand deep enough inside a stocking to grasp the stocking toe.	6. Because stockings contain strong elastic, application can be difficult if not initiated from the bottom up and if stockings are not turned inside out. Wrinkles in stockings can also occur if a systematic approach is not used for application.
7. Using the hand inside the stocking, hold onto the client's toes. Invert the stocking with the other hand and pull it over the hand and the client's toes. Release toes.	7. See Rationale 6.

(Continues)

PROCEDURE 29-26 Applying Antiembolic Stockings (Continued)

ACTION	RATIONALE
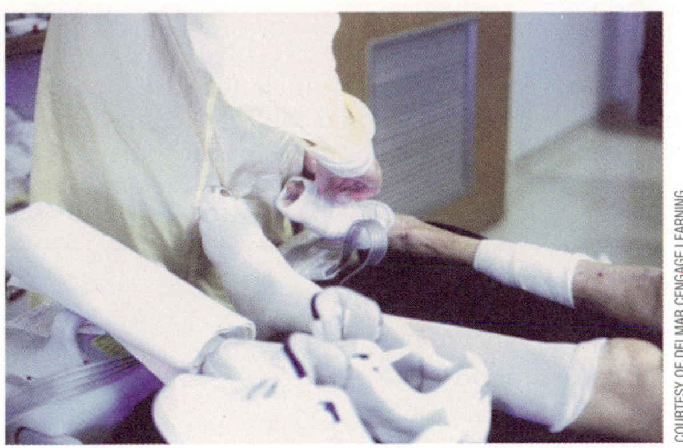 COURTESY OF DELMAR CENGAGE LEARNING FIGURE 29-26-1 **Place the stocking over the client's toes and foot.**	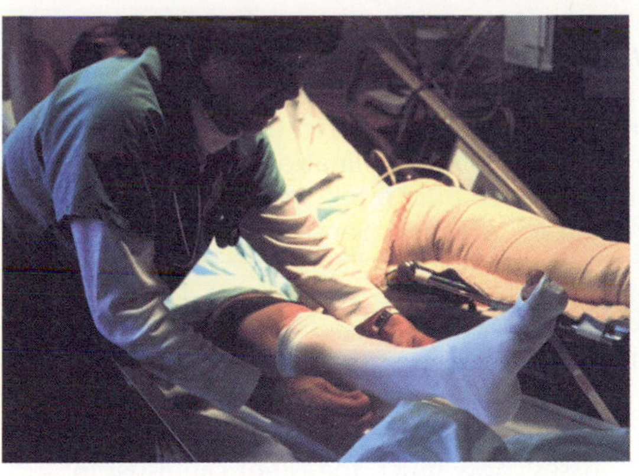 COURTESY OF DELMAR CENGAGE LEARNING FIGURE 29-26-2 **Pull the stocking smoothly and evenly up the client's leg.**
8. Hold each side of the stocking and pull it from the client's toes to the heel in one motion (Figure 29-26-1).	8. See Rationale 6.
9. Continuing to hold each side of the stockings, firmly pull the stocking up by using the thumbs to guide the stockings upward over the ankles and up the client's leg (Figure 29-26-2).	9. See Rationale 6.
10. Repeat with the other leg, if necessary.	10. See Rationale 6.
11. Smooth and remove any wrinkles in the stockings.	11. Wrinkles can create skin breakdown and can cause a tourniquet effect on the leg.
12. Assess circulatory and neurostatus of feet. (CMS: circulatory, movement, sensation)	12. Establishes baseline assessment.
13. Wash hands.	13. Reduces transmission of microorganisms.

EVALUATION

- The client has not experienced any signs or symptoms of deep venous thrombosis or thrombophlebitis.
- The client's venous return is improved.
- The client's popliteal, posterior tibial, and dorsalis pedis pulses remain intact while stockings are in place.
- The client has good circulation while stockings are in place, as evident by warm skin temperature, capillary return within normal limits, sensation within normal limits, and no edema in either extremities.

DOCUMENTATION

Nurses' Notes

- Use of stockings
- Skin integrity, any presence of venous problems, and circulatory status of extremities
- Equality of pedal pulses
- Size and length of stockings

PROCEDURE 29-27 Assisting with a Bedpan or Urinal

OVERVIEW

Voiding and bowel elimination for the client confined to bed require a bedpan and/or a urinal. Reduced mobility, pain, privacy issues, the need for assistance, delays in getting assistance when needed, and the fear of interruption can all alter normal elimination patterns. Fear of creating embarrassing noises, sights, or odors may compel the client to reduce fluid intake or avoid the urge to eliminate while in the hospital. This can lead to an increased risk of urinary tract infection. Sensitivity and proper technique by caregivers support the client on bed rest.

ASSESSMENT

1. Assess your equipment. Do you have the necessary items within reach? **Prevents having to stop the procedure and leave the client's bedside.**
2. Assess how much the client can assist in positioning and removing the bedpan. **Determines how the procedure is done and whether assistance is required.**
3. Check whether the client is confused, combative, in traction, or immobile. **Determines how the procedure is done and whether assistance is required.**
4. Check for casts, braces, or dressings that need protecting from accidental contamination with waste products. **Determines how much preparation is needed before toileting.**
5. Check for privacy and unexpected interruptions. **Determines if extra steps are needed to ensure privacy before toileting.**
6. Assess if client has orders to record intake and output. **Determines need to take steps for measurement and may require containers with measurement markings.**

POSSIBLE NURSING DIAGNOSES

Constipation
Bowel Incontinence
Stress Urinary Incontinence
Urge Urinary Incontinence
Urinary Retention
Toileting Self-Care Deficit
Situational Low Self-Esteem
Powerlessness

PLANNING

Expected Outcomes

1. Clients will be able to void and defecate when necessary.
2. Clients will have as much privacy and comfort as allowable, given their physical condition.
3. Intake and output will be accurately measured as needed.
4. The urinal or bedpan will be placed without skin damage.
5. The bedpan will be removed and emptied without spillage.

Equipment Needed

- Bedpan (regular or fracture) or urinal
- Disposable gloves
- Bedpan cover
- Toilet paper
- Washcloth and towel

delegation tips

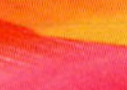

This skill is routinely delegated to ancillary personnel educated in Standard Precautions and proper body positioning, and to report color, odor, and amount of output to the nurse.

IMPLEMENTATION—ACTION/RATIONALE

ACTION	RATIONALE
* Check client's identification band * Explain procedure before beginning *	
Positioning a Bedpan	
1. Close curtain or door.	1. Provides for privacy.
2. Wash hands; apply gloves.	2. Reduces transmission of microorganisms.
3. Lower head of bed so client is in supine position.	3. The supine position will increase ability of client to move to side-lying position.
4. Elevate bed.	4. Ensures proper body mechanics.
5. Assist client to side-lying position using side rail for support.	5. Provides for best position for proper placement of bedpan.

(Continues)

PROCEDURE 29-27 Assisting with a Bedpan or Urinal (Continued)

ACTION	RATIONALE
6. Powder edge of bedpan if necessary.	6. For comfort; prevents bedpan from sticking to the skin.
7. While holding the bedpan with one hand, help the client roll onto his or her back, while pushing against the bedpan (toward the center of the bed) to hold it in place (Figure 29-27-1A).	7. Prevents dislocation or alignment of bedpan.
8. Alternate: Help the client raise the hips using the over-bed trapeze, and slide the pan in place (Figure 29-27-1B). Alternate: If the client is unable to turn or raise hips, use a fracture pan instead of a bedpan (Figure 29-27-2A&B). With a fracture pan, the flat side is placed toward the client's head.	8. Provides an alternate way to position the pan. Fracture pan reduces the amount of movement and lift required to place the pan.
9. Check placement of bedpan by looking between client's legs.	9. May prevent spillage from misalignment of bedpan.
10. If indicated, elevate head of bed to 45-degree angle or higher for comfort.	10. Check order of physician or qualified practitioner; bed remains flat if client has a spinal cord injury or spinal surgery. Elevating the head of bed creates a more normal elimination position.
11. Place call light within reach of client; place side rails in upright position, lower bed, and provide privacy.	11. Privacy allows for a more comfortable elimination environment; elevated side rails provide for safety.
12. Remove gloves; wash hands.	12. Reduces transmission of microorganisms.
Positioning a Urinal	
13. Repeat Actions 1 and 2.	13. See Rationales 1 and 2.
14. Lift the covers and place the urinal (Figure 29-27-2C) so the client may grasp the handle and position it. If the client cannot do this, you must position the urinal and place the penis into the opening (Figure 29-27-3).	14. Ensures proper placement of the urinal and reduces the risk of spillage.
15. Remove gloves; wash hands.	15. Reduces transmission of microorganisms.

A

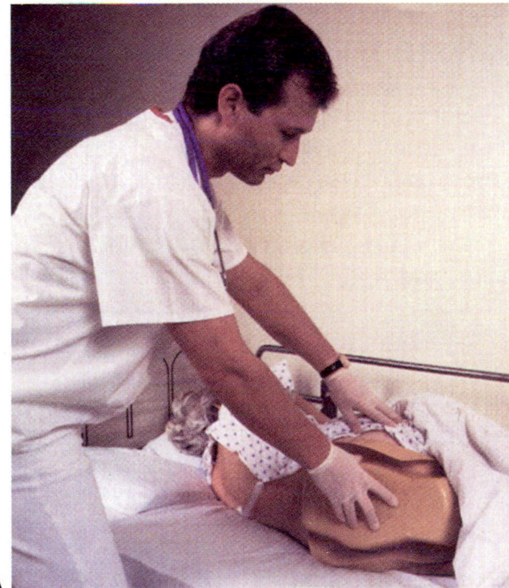

B

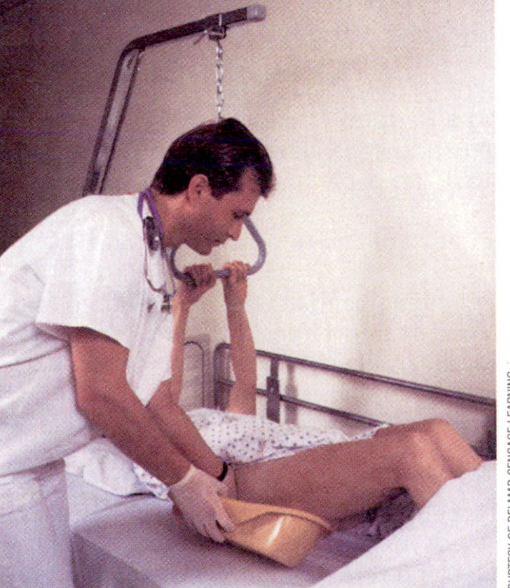

COURTESY OF DELMAR CENGAGE LEARNING

FIGURE 29-27-1 Positioning a bedpan: *A*, Hold the bedpan in place with one hand and have the client roll onto the pan. *B*, A client uses the trapeze bar to raise hips when given a bed pan.

(Continues)

PROCEDURE 29-27 Assisting with a Bedpan or Urinal (Continued)

ACTION | **RATIONALE**

A
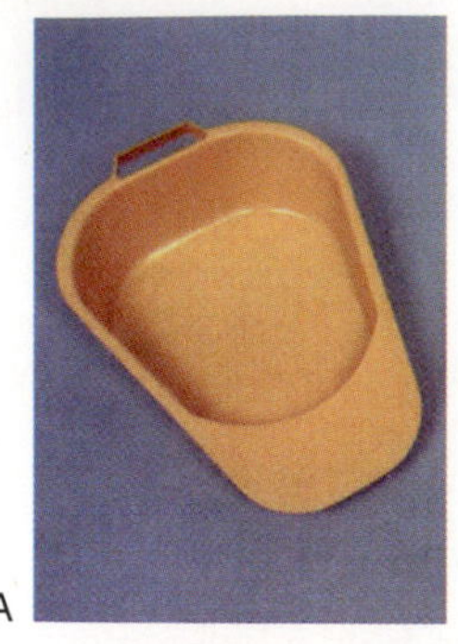
B
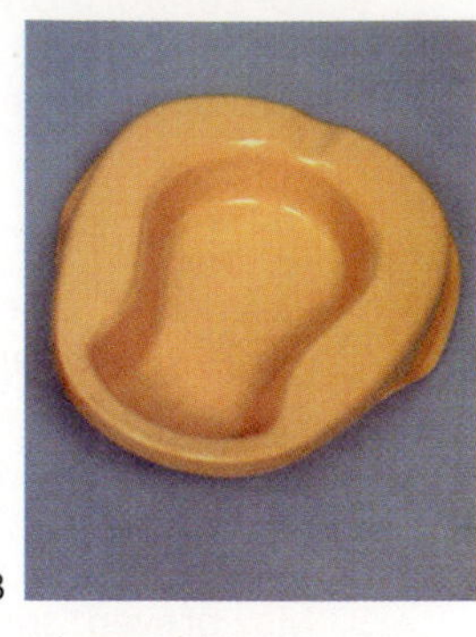
C
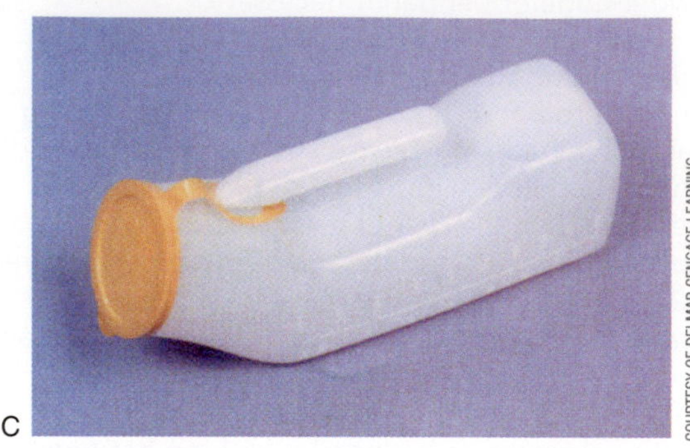
COURTESY OF DELMAR CENGAGE LEARNING

FIGURE 29-27-2 Bedpans and urinals are used when clients are on bed rest; *A*, A fracture pan is used when the client is unable to turn or raise hips; *B*, A bedpan is offered to clients who do not have mobility problems; *C*, A urinal is used by a male when on bed rest.

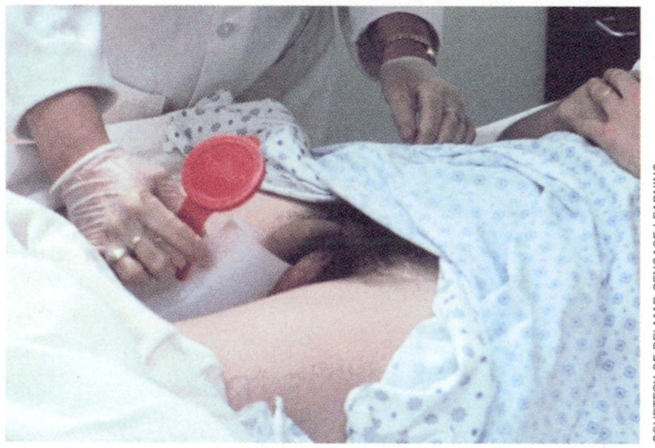
COURTESY OF DELMAR CENGAGE LEARNING

FIGURE 29-27-3 If the client is unable to assist, place the penis into the opening of the urinal.

Removing a Bedpan

ACTION	RATIONALE
16. Wash hands; apply gloves.	16. Reduces transmission of microorganisms.
17. Gather toilet paper and washing supplies.	17. Having supplies at the bedside allows smooth and safe completion of the procedure.
18. Lower head of bed to supine position.	18. Increases client's ability to move to side-lying position.
19. While holding bedpan with one hand, roll client to side and remove the pan, being careful not to pull or shear skin sticking to the pan and being careful not to spill contents.	19. Prevents possible spillage of bedpan contents.
20. Assist with cleaning or wiping; always wipe from front to back.	20. Client may not be able to clean self; wiping from front to back decreases chances of cross contamination from anus to urethra.
21. Empty bedpan (observe and measure urine output and check for occult blood if ordered), clean bedpan, and store it in proper place.	21. Promotes privacy and decreases the chance of spilling contents. Assess for constipation and diarrhea.
22. Remove soiled gloves. Wash hands.	22. Reduces transmission of microorganisms.

(Continues)

PROCEDURE 29-27 Assisting with a Bedpan or Urinal (Continued)

ACTION	RATIONALE
23. Allow client to wash hands.	23. Provides for physical hygiene and comfort.
24. Place call light within reach; recheck that side rails are in the upright position.	24. Ensures client safety and comfort.
25. Wash hands.	25. Reduces transmission of microorganisms.
Removing a Urinal	
26. Wash hands and apply gloves.	26. Reduces transmission of microorganisms.
27. Empty the urinal, measuring urine output if ordered; rinse the urinal; and replace it within the client's reach. Observe odor and color of urine before discarding.	27. Provides a way to measure the client's output. Keeping the urinal within reach promotes client autonomy. Helps evaluate for concentrated urine, infection, and renal problems.
28. Remove soiled gloves. Wash hands.	28. Reduces transmission of microorganisms.
29. Allow client to wash hands.	29. Provides for physical hygiene and comfort.
30. Place call light within reach; recheck that side rails are in the upright position.	30. Ensures client safety and comfort.
31. Wash hands.	31. Reduces transmission of microorganisms.

EVALUATION

- The client was able to void or defecate as needed.
- The client's request for assistance was answered promptly.
- The bedpan or urinal was removed and emptied without spillage.
- Ordered tests were performed and samples were collected.
- The client's skin integrity was maintained without skin shear or tearing.
- The client was provided with as much privacy and comfort as possible.

DOCUMENTATION

Nurses' Notes

- Elimination and voiding; include color, odor, consistency, and any unusual findings such as blood or mucus
- Client complaints such as constipation or burning with urination
- Condition of the client's skin

Intake and Output Record

- Time the client voided and the amount of urine voided

PROCEDURE 29-28 Applying a Condom Catheter

OVERVIEW

The condom catheter is an external drainage system that collects urine from male clients with incontinence. It is less invasive than a retention catheter and allows less contact of the skin with urine than a disposable brief or protective disposable underpad. Condom catheters require an order from an appropriate health care provider.

ASSESSMENT

1. Assess skin integrity around the penis and perineal area **to look for signs of irritation and skin breakdown.**
2. Assess the client for ability to cooperate with the application and retention of the condom catheter **to determine what type of teaching is necessary.**

(Continues)

PROCEDURE 29-28 Applying a Condom Catheter (Continued)

3. Assess the amount and pattern of urinary incontinence **to determine if the condom catheter is the best continence method for the client.**
4. Assess for latex allergy.

POSSIBLE NURSING DIAGNOSES

*Impaired **U**rinary Elimination*
*Risk for Impaired **S**kin Integrity*
*Toileting **S**elf-Care Deficit*

PLANNING

Expected Outcomes

1. The client will have a condom catheter in place without leakage or discomfort.
2. The client will have no skin irritation from the condom catheter.
3. The client will understand the reason for, and cooperate with, the placement and retention of the condom catheter.

Equipment Needed

- Condom catheter kit with adhesive strip
- Urinary drainage bag
- Clean gloves
- Basin with warm water and soap
- Towel and washcloth

delegation tips

Application of a condom catheter may be delegated to properly trained ancillary personnel. The need for condom drainage and the ongoing assessment of the client's skin condition is followed up by the nurse.

IMPLEMENTATION—ACTION/RATIONALE

ACTION	RATIONALE
* Check client's identification band * Explain procedure before beginning *	
1. Wash hands.	1. Reduces transmission of microorganisms.
2. Protect the client's privacy by closing the door and pulling curtains around the bed.	2. Allows privacy for the client.
3. Position the client in a comfortable position, preferably a supine position, if tolerated by the client. Raise the bed to a comfortable height for the nurse.	3. Facilitates the cleaning and application of the catheter. Raising the bed to a comfortable height promotes good body mechanics.
4. Apply nonsterile latex-free gloves.	4. Prevents possible transmission of microorganisms.
5. Fold the client's gown across the abdomen and the sheet just below pubic area.	5. Provides minimal exposure of the client, thereby reducing the client's embarrassment.
6. Assess the client's penis for any signs of redness, irritation, or skin breakdown.	6. A significant amount of skin breakdown may require an indwelling catheter. Provides baseline data for comparison with future assessments.
7. Clean the client's penis with warm soapy water. Retract the foreskin on the uncircumcised male and clean thoroughly in folds.	7. Removes microorganisms that could enter the urinary meatus and cause a urinary tract infection. Avoids trapping microorganisms in folds around the meatus.
8. Return the client's foreskin to its normal position.	8. Failure to return the foreskin to a normal position can lead to swelling of the penis and possible vascular constriction.
9. Shave any excess hair around the base of the penis if required by institutional policy.	9. Prevents discomfort from the adhesive strip when the condom catheter is removed.
10. Rinse and dry the area.	10. Moist warm environment can lead to the growth of microorganisms.
11. If a condom kit is used, open the package containing the skin preparation. Wipe and apply skin preparation solution to the shaft of the penis. If the client has an erection, wait for termination of erection before applying the catheter.	11. Preparation solution protects the client's skin from irritation. An erection may occur from manipulation of the penis while cleaning the area. This is a normal reaction and will terminate in a few minutes.
12. Apply the double-sided adhesive strip around the base of the client's penis in a spiral	12. Applying the adhesive in a spiral fashion does not compromise circulation of the penis. Encircling the

(Continues)

PROCEDURE 29-28 Applying a Condom Catheter (Continued)

ACTION	RATIONALE

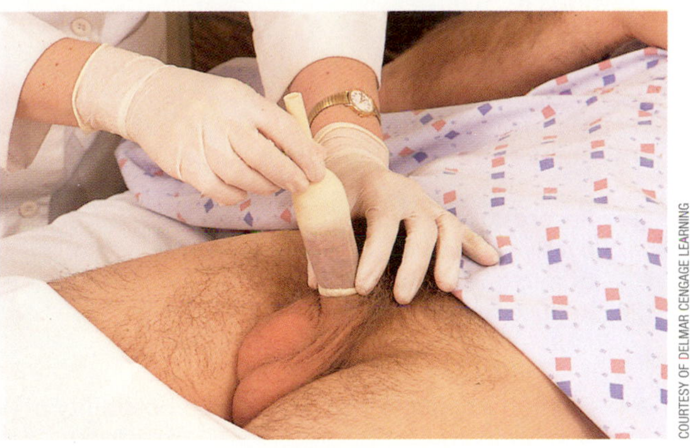

COURTESY OF DELMAR CENGAGE LEARNING

FIGURE 29-28-1 Unroll the condom from the distal portion of the penis upward to the base. Leave 1 to 2 inches between the tip of the penis and the end of the condom.

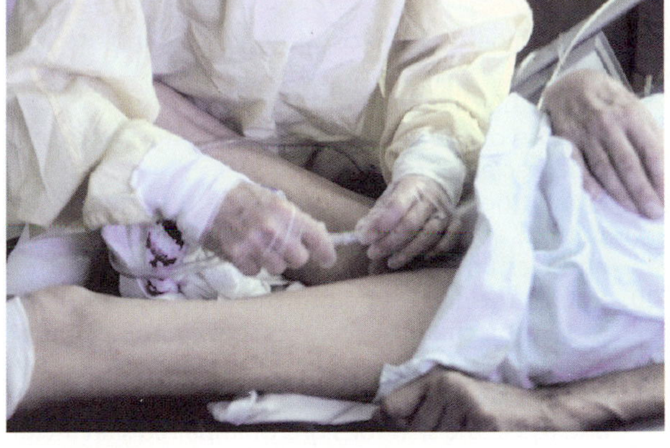

COURTESY OF DELMAR CENGAGE LEARNING

FIGURE 29-28-2 Attach the drainage bag tubing to the condom tubing.

ACTION	RATIONALE
fashion. The strip is applied 1 inch from the proximal end of the penis. Do not completely encircle the penis or tightly encompass penis.	penis can constrict the penis, impair circulation, and cause edema.
13. Position the rolled condom at the distal portion of the penis and unroll it, covering the penis and the double-sided strip of adhesive. Leave a 1- to 2-inch space between the tip of the penis and the end of the condom (Figure 29-28-1).	13. The condom sticks to the adhesive and remains in place. The extra spacing prevents pressure and erosion of the tip of the penis.
14. Gently press the condom to the adhesive strip.	14. Enables the condom to adhere evenly to the adhesive strip.
15. Attach the drainage bag tubing to the catheter tubing (Figure 29-28-2). Make sure the tubing lays over the client's legs, not under (Figure 29-28-3). Secure the drainage bag to the side of the bed below the level of the client's bladder or to the drainage bag attached to the leg.	15. Promotes urine flow away from the client. Constant exposure to urine and moisture can irritate the penis. Prevents reflux of the urine onto the penis and microorganisms from entering the penis.

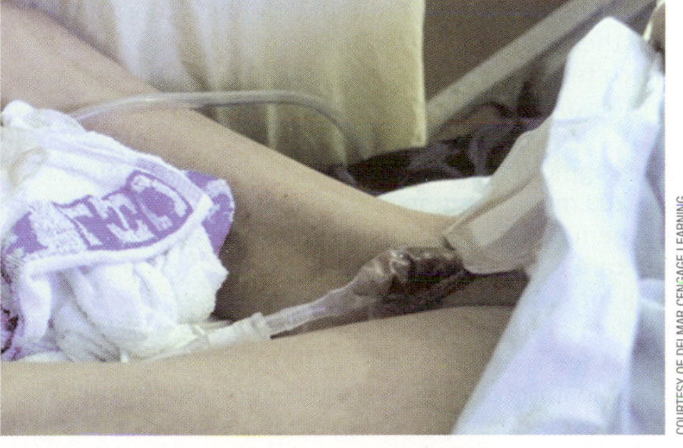

COURTESY OF DELMAR CENGAGE LEARNING

FIGURE 29-28-3 Make sure the drainage bag tubing lies over the client's leg.

(Continues)

PROCEDURE 29-28 Applying a Condom Catheter (Continued)

ACTION	RATIONALE
16. Determine that the condom and tubing are not twisted.	16. If the condom or tubing is twisted, the urine cannot flow out and the condom will leak or fall off.
17. Cover the client.	17. Maintains privacy of the client.
18. Dispose of the used equipment in appropriate receptacle.	18. Reduces transmission of microorganisms.
19. Empty the bag, measure the client's urinary output, and record every 4 hours. Remove gloves and wash hands after procedure.	19. Records output and prevents bag from becoming overly full and/or too heavy. Reduces transmission of microorganisms.
20. Return the client's bed to the lowest position and reposition client to comfortable or appropriate position.	20. Reduces potential injury from falls.
21. Remove the condom once a day to clean the area and assess the skin for signs of impaired skin integrity.	21. Promotes hygiene and reduces the possibility of skin breakdown.

EVALUATION

- The client's condom catheter is in place without leakage or discomfort.
- The client does not have any skin irritation from the condom catheter.
- The client understands the reason for, and cooperates with, the placement and retention of the condom catheter.

DOCUMENTATION

Nurses' Notes

- Time the procedure was performed
- Condition of the client's skin, recording any irritation, rashes, or open areas
- Client teaching performed

Intake and Output Record

- Amount of urine emptied from the urine drainage bag

PROCEDURE 29-29 Administering an Enema

OVERVIEW

An enema is a solution inserted into the rectum and sigmoid colon to remove feces and/or flatus. Enemas can also be used to instill medications. A cleansing enema is probably the most common type of enema. This type of enema stimulates peristalsis via irritation of the colon/rectum and by causing intestinal distention with fluid. There are two general types of cleansing enemas: the large-volume enema and the small-volume enema.

A large-volume enema is designed to clean the colon of as much feces as possible. In a large-volume enema, between 500 and 1,000 mL of fluid are instilled into the rectum/colon, and the client is asked to retain the fluid as long as possible.

Small-volume enemas are designed to clear the rectum and the sigmoid colon of fecal matter. Small-volume enemas are delivered with the traditional enema kit using 50 to 200 mL of solution, but most frequently they are administered using a prepackaged disposable kit. Prepackaged enemas are easily administered and available over-the-counter in most drugstores. This makes them ideal for home care use.

An oil retention enema is a small-volume enema that instills oil into the rectum, retained for up to an hour to soften very hard stool. It is often followed by a large-volume cleansing enema. A small-volume enema can deliver a medicated solution directly to the rectal mucosa. This method is useful when the rectum is the area to be medicated, if the client is unable to take oral medications, or if rapid absorption of the medication is required. The return-flow enema, used to remove flatus and stimulate peristalsis, is frequently given following abdominal surgery to reduce intestinal distention and to stimulate the resumption of bowel function.

Many different solutions are used for enemas, including tap water, normal saline, hypertonic solutions, soap solutions, oil, and carminative solutions. Tap water is a hypotonic solution. Because it is a less concentrated solution

(Continues)

PROCEDURE 29-29 Administering an Enema (Continued)

than the body's cells, it is drawn into the body and may cause water toxicity, electrolyte imbalance, or circulatory overload. Normal saline is an isotonic solution. It is the same concentration as the body's own fluids and is considered a safe enema solution. It is important that children and infants be given only normal saline enemas because their small size predisposes them to fluid imbalances. Prepackaged small-volume enemas use hypertonic solutions to draw fluid from the body to lubricate the stool and distend the rectum. Hypertonic solutions are contraindicated in dehydrated clients and small children. Carminative solutions are used to prevent gas from forming.

Enemas are contraindicated in clients with bowel obstruction, inflammation, or infection of the abdomen or if the client has had recent rectal or anal surgery. If there is any question regarding the advisability of administering an enema, consult the client's health care provider.

ASSESSMENT

1. Identify the type of enema ordered as well as the rationale for the enema. **Allows the nurse to verify the appropriateness of the type of enema ordered.**
2. Assess the physical condition of the client. Determine if the client has bowel sounds. Assess for a history of constipation, hemorrhoids, or diverticulitis. Determine if the client is able to hold a side-lying position or to retain the enema solution. **Allows the nurse to plan the procedure with the client's limitations in mind.**
3. Assess the client's mental state, including ability to understand and cooperate with the procedure, the client's knowledge level regarding the procedure, and any preexisting fears the client may have regarding the procedure. Knowing if the client can comprehend and cooperate with the procedure helps the nurse plan ahead. **Many clients have preexisting fears and beliefs regarding enemas and their administration.**

POSSIBLE NURSING DIAGNOSES

Constipation
Risk for Deficient Fluid Volume
Risk for Situational Low Self-Esteem

PLANNING

Expected Outcomes

1. The client's rectum will be free of feces and flatus.
2. The client will experience a minimum of trauma and embarrassment from the procedure.

Equipment Needed

Large-Volume Cleansing Enema

- Absorbent pad for the bed
- Disposable gloves
- Bedside commode or bedpan if client will not be able to ambulate to bathroom
- Lubricant
- Enema container
- Tubing with clamp and nozzle
- Toilet tissue
- Washcloth, towel, and basin

Small-Volume Prepackaged Enema

- Prescribed prepackaged enema
- Lubricant if the tip is not prelubricated
- Toilet tissue
- Bedpan or commode if the client cannot use the bathroom
- Absorbent pad for bed
- Gloves

Return-Flow Enema

- Absorbent pad for the bed
- Disposable gloves
- Bedside commode or bedpan if client will not be able to ambulate to bathroom
- Prescribed solution
- Lubricant
- Enema container
- Tubing with clamp and nozzle
- Toilet tissue

delegation tips

Administering an enema is a procedure that ancillary personnel perform after proper instruction and supervision. Instruct ancillary personnel to notify the nurse if any difficulty in administering or negative reactions such as severe cramping or inability to retain the enema occur. Results are documented and reported to the nurse.

(Continues)

PROCEDURE 29-29 Administering an Enema (Continued)

IMPLEMENTATION—ACTION/RATIONALE

* Check client's identification band * Explain procedure before beginning *

ACTION	RATIONALE
Administering an Enema	
1. Wash hands.	1. Reduces transmission of microorganisms.
2. Assess client's understanding of procedure and provide privacy.	2. Prepares client for procedure.
3. Apply gloves.	3. Prevents contact with feces.
4. Prepare equipment.	4. Ensures a smooth procedure.
5. Place absorbent pad on bed under client. Assist client in attaining left lateral position with right leg flexed as sharply as possible. If there is a question regarding the client's ability to hold the solution, place a bedpan on the bed nearby (Figure 29-29-1).	5. Facilitates flow of solution into the rectum and colon. The flexed leg provides the best exposure of the anus.
6. Steps 6 to 12 are specific instructions for administering a large-volume cleansing enema. Enemas administered to adults are usually given at 105° to 110°F (40.5° to 43°C), and those administered to children are usually administered at 100°F (37.7°C). Solution should be at least body temperature to prevent cramping and discomfort.	6. Enemas work best when solution is warm. If enemas are too hot, damage can be done to the bowel mucosa. If enemas are too cold, spasms may occur.
7. Pour solution into the bag or bucket; add water if needed. Open clamp and allow solution to prime tubing. Clamp tubing when primed.	7. Expels air from the tubing, which could cause intestinal distention and discomfort.
8. Lubricate 5 cm (2 inches) of the rectal tube unless the tube is part of a prelubricated enema set (Figure 29-29-2).	8. Minimizes trauma to the anal sphincter during insertion of the rectal tube.
9. Hold the enema container level with the rectum. Ask the client to take a deep breath. Simultaneously, slowly and smoothly insert rectal tube into rectum approximately 7 to 10 cm (3 to 4 inches) in an adult. The rectum of an adult is usually 10 to 20 cm (4 to 6 inches). The tube	9. A deep breath helps relax the sphincter. Insertion of rectal tube toward the umbilicus guides tube along rectum.

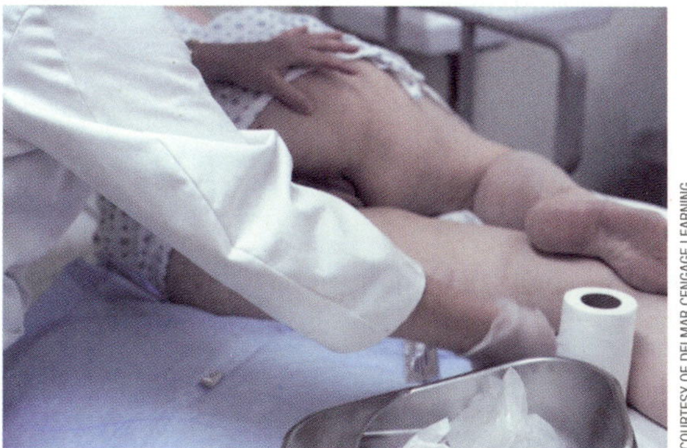

COURTESY OF DELMAR CENGAGE LEARNING

FIGURE 29-29-1 Position the client in the left lateral position with the right leg flexed.

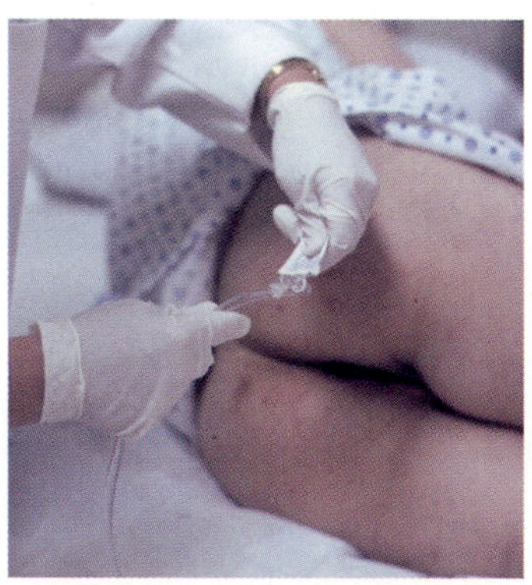

COURTESY OF DELMAR CENGAGE LEARNING

FIGURE 29-29-2 Lubricate 2 inches of the rectal tube with lubricant.

(Continues)

PROCEDURE 29-29 Administering an Enema (Continued)

ACTION	RATIONALE
should be inserted beyond the internal sphincter. Aim the rectal tube toward the client's umbilicus (Figure 29-29-3).	
10. Raise the solution container and open clamp. (If using an enema set, gently squeeze the container holding solution). The solution should be 30 to 45 cm (12 to 18 inches) (Figure 29-29-4) above the rectum for an adult and 7.5 cm (3 inches) above the rectum for an infant.	10. Solution should be at a height above rectum that allows gravity flow of solution into the rectum, but does not cause damage to the rectal lining because of a too-rapid increase in rectal pressure.
11. Slowly administer the fluid.	11. Decreases the incidence of intestinal spasms and cramps.
12. When solution has been completely administered or when the client cannot hold any more fluid, clamp the tubing, remove the rectal tube, and dispose of it properly. Steps 13 to 15 are specific instructions for administering a small-volume prepackaged enema.	12. The urge to defecate indicates that a sufficient amount of fluid has been administered.
13. Remove prepackaged enema from packaging. Be familiar with any special instructions included with the enema. The packaged enema may be stood in a basin of warm water to warm the fluid before use.	13. Prepare the enema.
14. Remove the protective cap from the nozzle and inspect the nozzle for lubrication. If the lubrication is not adequate, add more.	14. Prevents trauma to the rectal mucosa.
15. Squeeze the container gently to remove any air and prime the nozzle (Figure 29-29-5).	15. Reduces introduction of air into the rectum.
16. Have the client take a deep breath. Simultaneously, gently insert the enema nozzle into the anus, pointing the nozzle toward the umbilicus.	16. Relaxes the rectal sphincter. Pointing the nozzle toward the umbilicus positions the nozzle away from the rectal walls.
17. Squeeze the container until all the solution is instilled and remove the nozzle from the anus (Figure 29-29-6).	17. Allows the client to get the full benefit of the solution.

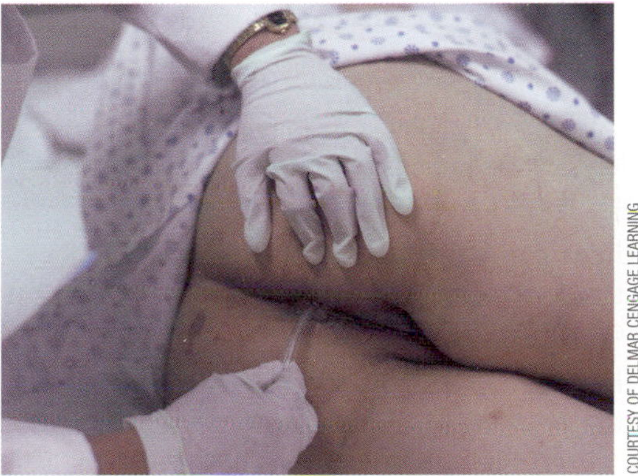

COURTESY OF DELMAR CENGAGE LEARNING

FIGURE 29-29-3 Gently and smoothly insert the rectal rube into the rectum.

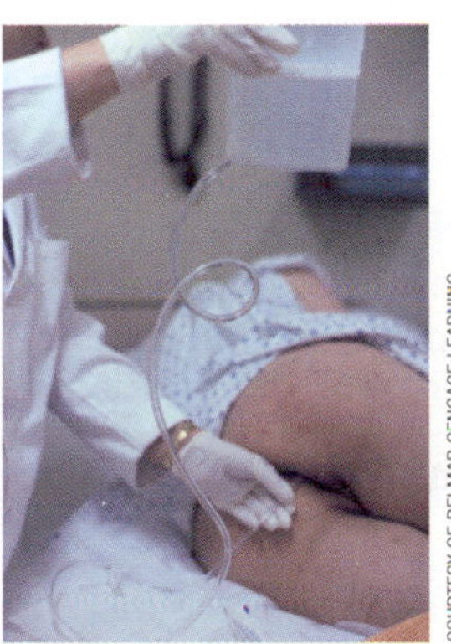

COURTESY OF DELMAR CENGAGE LEARNING

FIGURE 29-29-4 Raise the container 12 to 18 inches above the rectum and instill the solution.

(Continues)

PROCEDURE 29-29 Administering an Enema (Continued)

ACTION | 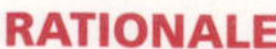 **RATIONALE**

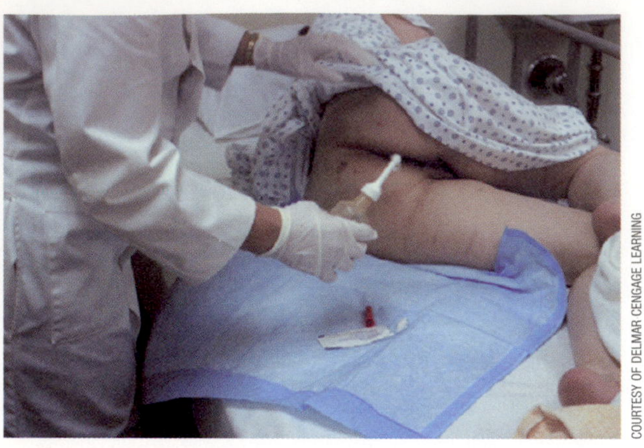

FIGURE 29-29-5 Squeeze the prepackaged enema container gently to remove any air and prime the nozzle.

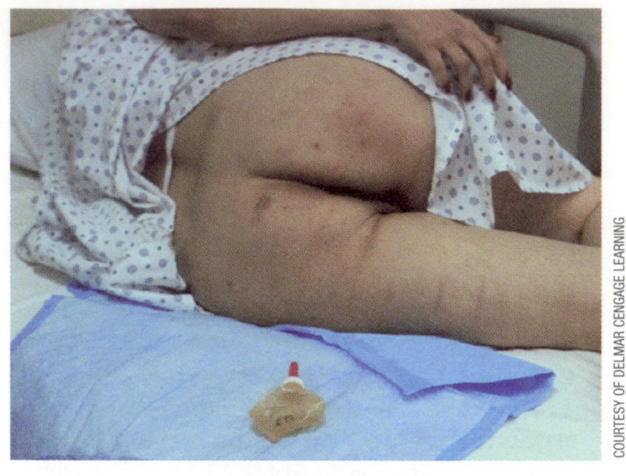

FIGURE 29-29-6 Squeeze the container until all the solution is instilled and remove the nozzle from the anus.

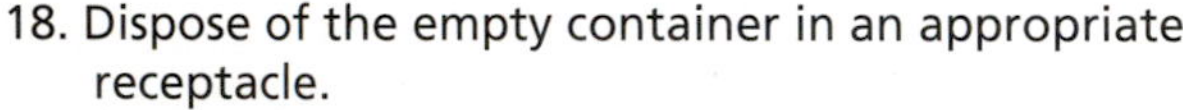

18. Dispose of the empty container in an appropriate receptacle.
    - Rationale: 18. Prevents the spread of microorganisms.
19. Clean lubricant, any solution, and any feces from the anus with toilet tissue.
    - Rationale: 19. Minimizes skin irritation.
20. Have the client continue to lie on the left side for the prescribed length of time. A client may need to expel a large-volume cleansing enema soon after administration. Usually, a client can hold a small-volume prepackaged enema the recommended minutes stated on the package.
    - Rationale: 20. Certain types of enemas are more effective when retained for a specified amount of time. It is easier for the client to retain the enema in a lying position, where gravity can be resisted.
21. When the client has retained the enema for the prescribed amount of time, assist to the bedside commode or toilet or onto the bedpan. If the client is using the bathroom, instruct not to flush the toilet when finished.
    - Rationale: 21. Client will be prepared to expel fluid and feces. Caregiver can see results of the enema.
22. When the client is finished expelling the enema, assist to clean the perineal area if needed.
    - Rationale: 22. Prevents skin breakdown and excoriation.
23. Return the client to a comfortable position. Place a clean, dry protective pad under the client to catch any solution or feces that may continue to be expelled.
    - Rationale: 23. Provides comfort for the client and protects the linen from potential soiling.
24. Remove gloves and wash hands.
    - Rationale: 24. Reduces transmission of microorganisms.

EVALUATION

- The client's rectum is free of feces or flatus.
- The client experienced a minimum of trauma and embarrassment from the procedure.

DOCUMENTATION

Nurses' Notes

- Time and date of the procedure
- Type of enema given, amount of fluid infused and returned, and amount and description of the feces expelled
- Client's tolerance for the procedure and any complaints or unusual findings

Medication Administration Record (MAR)

- If this is a medicated enema, be sure to note it on the MAR.

Intake and Output Record (I/O)

- If the amount of fluid returned is significantly less than the amount infused, note this on the I&O record.

PROCEDURE 29-30 Measuring Intake and Output

OVERVIEW

One of the most basic methods of monitoring a client's health is measuring intake and output, commonly called "I&O." By monitoring the amount of fluids a client takes in and comparing this to the amount of fluid a client puts out, the health care team gains valuable insights into the client's general health as well as monitors specific disease conditions.

To maintain good health, fluid intake approximately equals fluid output. Intake that exceeds output can indicate medical conditions ranging from renal failure to congestive heart failure. Output that exceeds intake can be caused by things as serious as life-threatening diarrhea or as benign as diuretic medications. An accurate record of a client's fluid balance is an important nursing function.

I&O monitoring is often ordered by the health care provider but can also be initiated by the nurse. Ideally, I&O is monitored over several days to obtain an accurate record of the client's status. In critical situations, the client's I&O is monitored and reported on an hourly basis. A urine output of less than 30 mL per hour is reported.

A daily weight is often done in conjunction with I&O because it indicates fluid retention or loss. One gallon of water weighs 8 pounds. An 8-pound weight gain over a 24- to 48-hour period indicates a life-threatening condition for the client. A significant change in a client's weight or a significant difference in a client's total I&O is reported to the client's health care provider.

Intake is any fluid consumed or infused. Generally, liquid intake is anything that is liquid at room temperature and includes water, juice, coffee, milk, ice cream, soup broth, gelatin, and popsicles. However, some facilities are including other items as liquid intake, such as oatmeal, cream of wheat, and soups. Follow the health care facility's policy when documenting. Ice is documented as one-half the total amount of mL within a container. Be sure to calculate the amount of water the client has consumed from the bedside water pitcher. Any fluids infused through IV lines, central lines, feeding tubes, or irrigant that is not returned is considered intake. Blood and blood products as well as the saline used to flush IV lines before and after the transfusion are also included in this count. IV piggybacks, fluids used to measure cardiac output, central line flushes, and TKO (to keep open) fluids are also considered in the intake total.

Urine is the largest component of output fluid volume, but diarrhea, diaphoresis, wound drainage, gastric or other fluids removed by suction, and bleeding are all fluid losses as well. These losses are measured or estimated and recorded in the total output.

Clients who are able to understand and cooperate with the I&O measurement may keep track of their fluid balance. Particularly in clients who are on a fluid restriction, client understanding and participation can greatly increase cooperation.

ASSESSMENT

1. Assess the client's risk factors for fluid overload, such as congestive heart failure, renal failure, or ascites **because edema results from excess volume in extracellular fluid spaces and transferring of fluid into tissues.**
2. Determine if the client is receiving fluids or medications that predispose to fluid overload, such as large amounts of IV fluids or steroid therapy **because steroids cause sodium and water retention and excretion of potassium.**
3. Assess the client's risk factors for fluid loss, such as diaphoresis, rapid respirations, diarrhea, gastric suction, blood loss, or wound drainage **because dehydration results from reduction of fluid within the tissues and circulatory system.**
4. Determine if the client's urine output is in excess of fluid intake **because the kidneys excrete excess fluid during periods of overhydration and conserve body water during periods of dehydration.**
5. Assess the client's ability to understand and cooperate with intake and output measurement **because cooperation in these measurements will help ensure accuracy.**

POSSIBLE NURSING DIAGNOSES

Excess Fluid Volume
Deficient Fluid Volume
Risk for Deficient Fluid Volume

PLANNING

Expected Outcomes

1. The client's fluid intake and output will be accurately measured and recorded.
2. The client will participate in the recording of fluid intake and output if possible.

Equipment Needed

- I&O form at bedside
- I&O graphic record in chart or electronic medical record
- Glass or cup
- Bedpan, urinal, or bedside commode
- Graduated container for output
- Nonsterile gloves
- Sign at bedside stating client is on I&O

(Continues)

PROCEDURE 29-30 Measuring Intake and Output (Continued)

delegation tips

Intake and output measurement may be delegated to ancillary personnel, who should be knowledgeable regarding the following:

- *Obtaining accurate measurements and reporting incontinence*
- *Observing the amount, color, and any odor from the output*
- *Protecting themselves from contamination from a body fluid and storing collection containers in designated areas*
- *Recording measurements on proper clinical records*

IMPLEMENTATION—ACTION/RATIONALE

ACTION	RATIONALE
* Check client's identification band * Explain procedure before beginning *	
1. Wash hands.	1. Reduces transmission of microorganisms.
2. Explain the rules of I&O record. All fluids taken orally are recorded on the client's intake and output form (sometimes called a fluid balance flow sheet).	2. Elicits client support.
• Client must void into bedpan, urinal, or "hat" in toilet for collecting urine, not into toilet.	• Fluid voided into the toilet cannot be measured.
• Toilet tissue is disposed of in plastic-lined container, not in bedpan.	• Liquids absorbed into toilet tissue cannot be measured by volume.
Intake	
3. Measure all oral fluids in accord with agency policy (e.g., cup =150 mL, glass = 240 mL). Record all IV fluids as they are infused.	3. Provides for consistency of measurement.
4. Record time and amount of all fluid intake in the designated space on bedside form (e.g., oral, tube feedings, IV fluids).	4. Documents fluids.
5. Transfer 8-hour total fluid intake from bedside I&O record to graphic sheet or 24-hour I&O record on client's chart or client's electronic medical record.	5. Provides for data analysis of the client's fluid status.
6. Record all fluid intake in the appropriate column of the 24-hour record or enter intake appropriately into the electronic medical record.	6. Documents intake by type and amount.
7. Complete 24-hour intake record by adding all 8-hour totals or checking that the computer has calculated data appropriately.	7. Provides consistent data for analysis of the client's fluid status over a 24-hour period.
Output	
8. Wash hands and apply nonsterile gloves.	8. Reduces potential for transmission of pathogens.
9. Empty urinal, bedpan, or Foley drainage bag (Figure 29-30-1) into graduated container or commode "hat" (Figure 29-30-2).	9. Provides accurate measurement of urine.
10. Remove gloves and wash hands.	10. Prevents cross contamination.
11. Record time and amount of output (e.g., urine, drainage from nasogastric tube, drainage tube) on I&O record.	11. Documents output.
12. Transfer 8-hour output totals to graphic sheet or 24-hour I&O record on the client's chart or client's electronic medical record.	12. Provides for data analysis of the client's fluid status.
13. Complete 24-hour output record by totaling all 8-hour totals or checking that the computer has calculated data appropriately.	13. Provides consistent data for analysis of the client's fluid status over a 24-hour period.
14. Wash hands.	14. Reduces transmission of microorganisms.

(Continues)

PROCEDURE 29-30 Measuring Intake and Output (Continued)

ACTION | RATIONALE

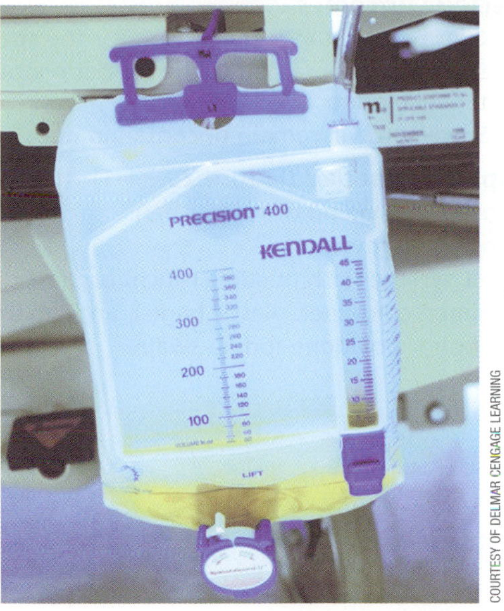

COURTESY OF DELMAR CENGAGE LEARNING

FIGURE 29-30-1 Urine in the Foley drainage bag must be measured.

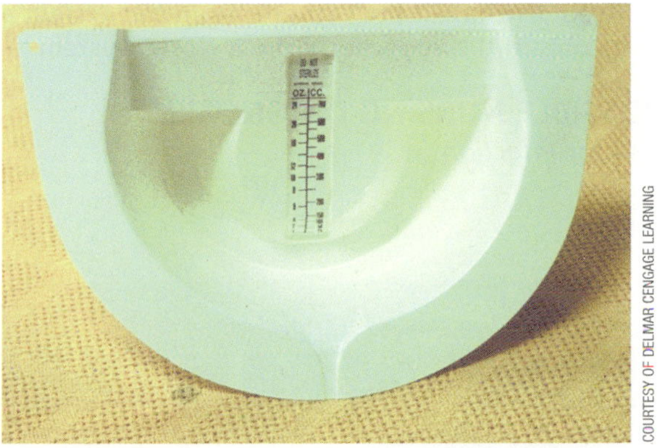

COURTESY OF DELMAR CENGAGE LEARNING

FIGURE 29-30-2 Measure urine, drainage, or other output in graduated specimen containers.

EVALUATION

- The client's fluid intake and output was accurately measured and recorded.
- Note if the client was able to participate in the recording of fluid intake and output to the best of his ability.
- Note and report any abnormal findings to the client's health care provider.

DOCUMENTATION

Intake and Output Record

- All fluid I&O
- Totals at the end of every shift
- Totals for 24 hours

Nurses' Notes

- Unusual findings, excessive intake, excessive output, or serious imbalance of intake and output and report to the client's health care provider

PROCEDURE 29-31 Urine Collection—Closed Drainage System

OVERVIEW

Indwelling catheters are used frequently in acute care settings for episodic or continuous drainage of urine. Specimens may be required to evaluate urine content, such as electrolytes, dilution, hormones, glucose, or renal function. Bacteria can be identified in urine specimens to determine if the catheter needs to be removed or if antibiotic therapy is indicated. Catheter tubing is generally designed to allow for easy access to obtain specimens without disconnecting the catheter from the tubing. Careful technique prevents contamination of the system and risk for infection.

(Continues)

PROCEDURE 29-31 Urine Collection—Closed Drainage System (Continued)

ASSESSMENT

1. Identify the purpose of the urine test **to determine the amount of urine needed and the proper container for collection.**
2. Assess the client's understanding of the test **to determine the amount of instruction needed.**
3. Identify the type of collecting tubing attached to the indwelling catheter **to determine if you need to disconnect the catheter from the system or obtain the specimen from a closed system.**

POSSIBLE NURSING DIAGNOSIS

Risk for Infection

PLANNING

Expected Outcomes

1. Client understands the reason for the specimen.
2. Specimen is obtained in the proper container in a timely manner.
3. Specimen will remain uncontaminated.

Equipment Needed (Figure 29-31-1)

- Nonserrated clamp or rubber band
- Nonsterile gloves
- 10-mL syringe with needle (1-inch) or plastic cannula
- Specimen container, plastic bag(s), and labels
- Alcohol or povidone-iodine swabs

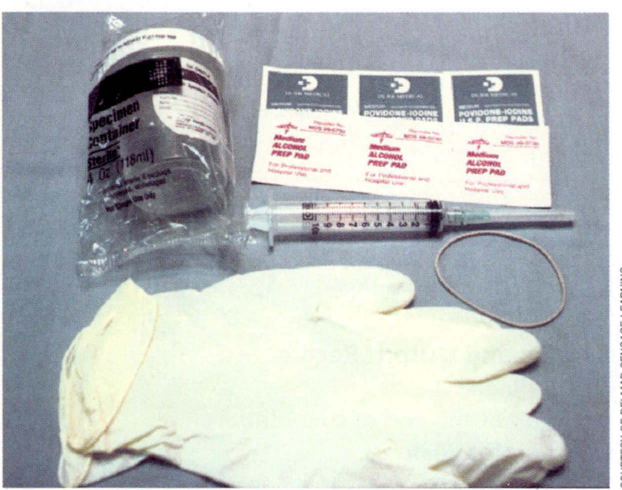

COURTESY OF DELMAR CENGAGE LEARNING

FIGURE 29-31-1 Assemble equipment to collect urine from a catheter drainage system.

delegation tips

Obtaining a urine specimen from an indwelling catheter requires the skill and problem-solving ability of a nurse. This task cannot be delegated to ancillary personnel.

IMPLEMENTATION—ACTION/RATIONALE

ACTION	RATIONALE
* Check client's identification band * Explain procedure before beginning *	
1. Wash hands.	1. Reduces transmission of microorganisms.
2. Check health care provider's order.	2. Determines test and container needed for the specimen.
3. Provide privacy.	3. Maintains client dignity.
4. Check for urine in the tubing.	4. Determines if there is sufficient urine in the collecting tubing for a specimen. *Urine from the collection bag should not be used for sterile specimens.*
5. If more urine is needed, clamp the tubing using a nonserrated clamp or a rubber band for 10 to 15 minutes (Figure 29-31-2).	5. Collects 10 mL of urine, which is needed for most urinalyses.

(Continues)

PROCEDURE 29-31 Urine Collection—Closed Drainage System (Continued)

ACTION	RATIONALE
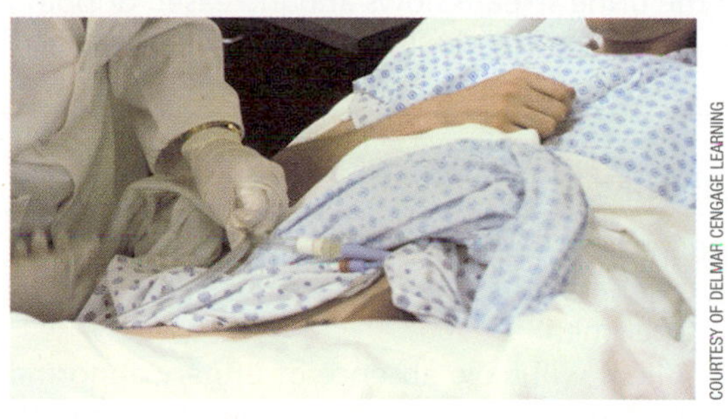 **Figure 29-31-2** Clamp the tubing by folding it over and securing it with a rubber band to collect an adequate sample.	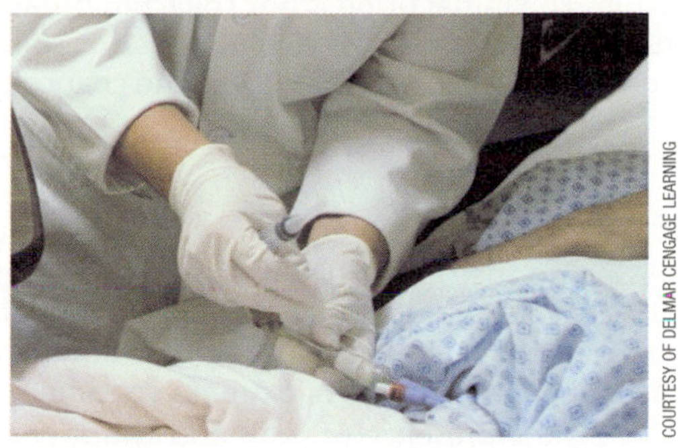 **Figure 29-31-3** Cleanse the sample port and insert a sterile needle or sterile plastic cannula and syringe into the sample port.
6. Put on clean gloves.	6. Practices Standard Precautions.
7. Clean sample port with an alcohol or povidone-iodine swab.	7. Prevents entrance of microorganisms into the system.
8. Insert sterile needle or sterile plastic cannula of syringe into the sample port of catheter at a 45-degree angle and withdraw 10 mL of urine (Figure 29-31-3).	8. Obtains specimen with sufficient volume for most urine tests.
9. Put urine into sterile container and close tightly, taking care not to contaminate the lid of the container.	9. Prevents contamination of specimen and spill of urine.
10. Place needle and syringe into sharps container; never recap a contaminated needle.	10. Prevents accidental needlesticks.
11. Remove clamp and rearrange tubing avoiding dependent loops.	11. Reestablishes urine flow and drainage into the system.
12. Label specimen container, put it in doubled plastic bags, and send to the laboratory.	12. Ensures right test and controls transfer of pathogens.
13. Wash hands.	13. Reduces transmission of microorganisms.

EVALUATION

- Client understands the reason for the specimen.
- Specimen was obtained in the proper container in a timely manner.
- Specimen remained uncontaminated.

DOCUMENTATION

Nurses' Notes

- Date and time the specimen was sent to the laboratory
- Date, time, client name and room number, and test(s) ordered

Intake and Output Record

- Amount of urine collected for the specimen

PROCEDURE 29-32 Urine Collection—Clean Catch, Female/Male

OVERVIEW

A clean urine specimen for culture and sensitivity is collected without using an invasive method such as catheterization. This procedure is referred to as a clean-voided, clean-catch, or midstream urine specimen in that it is not a sterile procedure such as catheterization but, rather, a method of obtaining a clean specimen. This procedure is best accomplished with the client on the toilet because the use of a urinal or bedpan increases the risk of contamination. The client is asked to clean him or herself and initiate urination. After the client starts voiding,

(Continues)

PROCEDURE 29-32 Urine Collection—Clean Catch, Female/Male (Continued)

a sterile collection cup is placed under the stream of urine and a specimen collected. Hence, it is called midstream collection. The initial urine is not collected because this portion of the stream flushes the urethral opening and meatus of any bacteria. The end urine is not collected because as the urine stream slows and increased dripping and contact with the meatus occurs, the chance of contamination increases. The clean-catch specimen is sent to a laboratory for analysis.

ASSESSMENT

1. Evaluate the client's ability to obtain a clean-catch specimen **to determine if the client is able to clean himself appropriately and understands the need to obtain a midstream specimen.**
2. Assess the presence of signs and symptoms of urinary tract infections or other abnormalities **because burning or the inability to control urination may hamper the client's ability to obtain a clean specimen.**

POSSIBLE NURSING DIAGNOSES

*Impaired **U**rinary Elimination*

*Acute **P**ain*

*Deficient **K**nowledge* (collecting clean-catch urine specimen)

PLANNING

Expected Outcomes

1. Client will be able to obtain a clean, midstream specimen.
2. Client will have absence of urinary abnormalities, such as burning, tingling, pain upon urination, or inability to control stream.
3. Client will understand procedure.

Equipment Needed

- Sterile collection container with lid and label
- Sterile midstream kit, antiseptic towelettes, or cotton balls with antiseptic solution
- Toilet paper
- Nonsterile latex-free gloves

delegation tips

Collection of a clean-catch specimen may be delegated to ancillary personnel properly trained in the technique of cleaning the client and obtaining the voided specimen.

IMPLEMENTATION—ACTION/RATIONALE

ACTION	RATIONALE
* Check client's identification band * Explain procedure before beginning *	
1. Check orders and assess need for the procedure.	1. Provides understanding of the purpose of the procedure.
2. Gather equipment.	2. Provides for organization.
3. Assess the client's ability to complete the procedure, including understanding, mobility, and balance.	3. Improves compliance and likelihood of obtaining clean specimen.
4. If the nurse is to perform the procedure: Wash hands and apply gloves. If the client performs the procedure, instruct the client to wash hands before and after the procedure. If the client wishes, provide a pair of gloves.	4. Decreases transmission of microorganisms.
5. Provide privacy.	5. Decreases embarrassment.
6. Using sterile procedure, open kit or towelettes. Open sterile container, placing the lid with sterile side up on a firm surface (Figure 29-32-1).	6. Prevents contamination of the specimen.
7. Female client: Sit with legs separated on the toilet. Use the thumb and forefinger to separate the labia, or have the client separate the labia with fingers (Figure 29-32-2). With the labia separated, use a downward stroke (from the top of the labia down toward the rectal area), and cleanse one side of the labia with the towelette (Figure 29-32-3).	7. Provides access for cleaning the labia. Cleanses area and prevents contamination of clean area. Prevents contamination by feces. Keeping labia separated avoids contamination and decreases microorganisms in specimen.

(Continues)

PROCEDURE 29-32 Urine Collection—Clean Catch, Female/Male (Continued)

ACTION	RATIONALE
 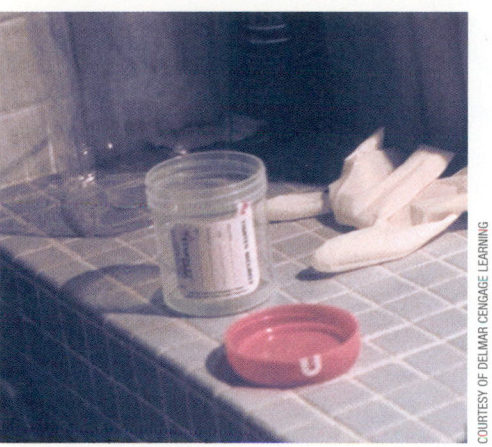	FIGURE 29-32-1 Place the lid on a firm surface, sterile side up. Do not touch the inside of the lid.
Discard the towelette and repeat the procedure on the other side with another towelette, keeping the labia separated at all times. With a third towelette, use a downward stroke from the top of the urethral opening to the bottom. Discard the towelette.	
8. Male client: Stand in front of toilet. Pull back the foreskin (if present in uncircumcised male) and clean with a single stroke around meatus and glans. Use a circular motion, starting with the head of the penis at the urethral opening, moving down the glans shaft. Discard the towelette and repeat the procedure with another towelette, keeping the foreskin retracted. Wipe the head of the penis three times using a circular motion. Use a new towelette each time.	8. Prevents contamination of microorganisms from foreskin. Single strokes and moving away from opening prevents contamination of the urethral opening.
9. Ask the client to begin to urinate into the toilet. After the stream starts with good flow, place the collection cup under the stream of urine (Figure 29-32-4). Avoid touching the skin with the container. Fill the container with 30 to 60 mL of urine and remove the container before urination ceases. Wipe with toilet paper.	9. The specimen is collected midstream to avoid contamination of urine that touches the labia. The initial urine flushes bacteria from the orifice and the end urine may have contact with the meatus or labia and, hence, be contaminated.

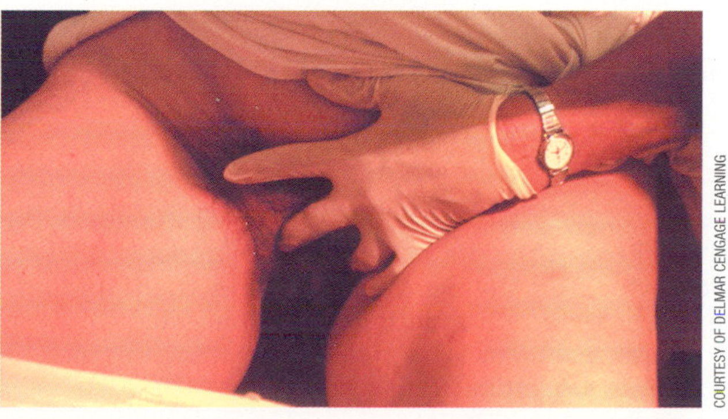

FIGURE 29-32-2 Separate the labia with the fingers of the nondominant hand.

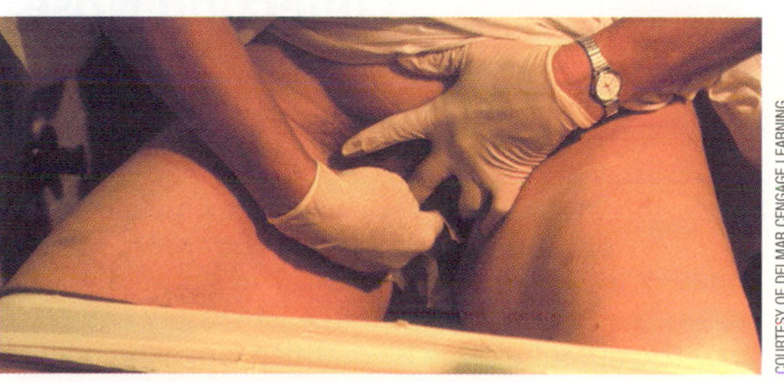

FIGURE 29-32-3 Cleanse each side and down the middle using a single downward stroke for each towelette. Keep the labia separated.

(Continues)

PROCEDURE 29-32 Urine Collection—Clean Catch, Female/Male (Continued)

ACTION	RATIONALE

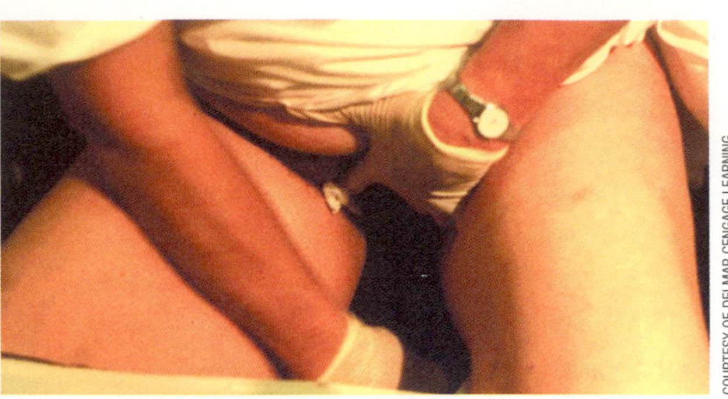

FIGURE 29-32-4 **Ask the client to begin to urinate into the toilet. After the stream starts with good flow, place the collection cup under the stream of urine. Remove the cup before urination ceases.**

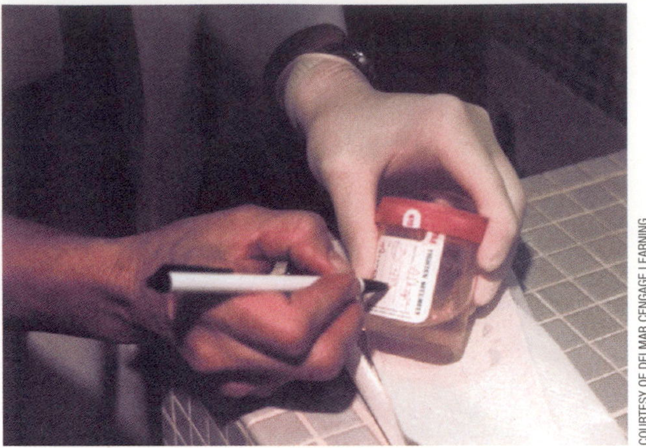

FIGURE 29-32-5 **Label the container with the client's name, the date, and time specimen collected.**

ACTION	RATIONALE
10. Place the sterile lid back onto the container and close tightly. Clean and dry the outside of the container with a towelette. Wash hands. Label and enclose in a double-bagged plastic biohazard bag, and follow facility policy for transporting specimen to the laboratory (Figure 29-32-5).	10. Prevents contamination of clean specimen, prevents spillage, and ensures accuracy.
11. Remove and dispose of gloves and wash hands	11. Decreases transmission of microorganisms.

EVALUATION

- Clean midstream specimen obtained.
- Client understood procedure.
- Client had no statement of burning, pain, or inability to initiate urination.

DOCUMENTATION

Nurses' Notes

- Procedure
- Date and time specimen was collected
- Characteristics of urine
- Client's signs and symptoms associated with urination
- Time urine specimen sent to lab

PROCEDURE 29-33 Collecting Nose, Throat, and Sputum Specimens

OVERVIEW

A nose, throat, or sputum specimen is a simple diagnostic tool for clients with signs or symptoms of upper respiratory or sinus infections. Nose and throat specimens are collected from the client using a sterile swab. Sputum specimens are collected in a sterile cup. Sputum specimens are also obtained via a specimen trap connected to suction. Specimens are sent to the laboratory and placed in a culture medium to allow pathogenic organisms to grow. The organism type is identified, enabling diagnosis and appropriate antimicrobial therapy.

(Continues)

PROCEDURE 29-33 Collecting Nose, Throat, and Sputum Specimens (Continued)

ASSESSMENT

1. Assess the client's understanding of the purpose of the procedure **so the client cooperates.**
2. Assess the type of nasal or sinus drainage **to determine what kind of collection equipment is needed.**
3. Review the health care provider's orders for the cultures requested **so repeat cultures are not done.**
4. Assess the client for postnasal drip, sinus headache or tenderness, nasal congestion, or sore throat **to know the purpose of the procedure.**
5. Identify whether the client has received recent antimicrobials and obtain a specimen before treatment, if possible.

POSSIBLE NURSING DIAGNOSES

Risk for Infection
Anxiety
Risk for Injury
Deficient Knowledge (regarding the procedure)

PLANNING

Expected Outcomes

1. An adequate specimen will be obtained and sent to the laboratory.
2. The procedure will be performed with a minimum of trauma to the client.

Equipment Needed

- Two sterile swabs in sterile culture tubes or a flexible wire sterile swab with cotton tip for nose or throat cultures
- Tongue blades
- Penlight
- Facial tissues
- Clean, disposable latex-free gloves
- Nasal speculum (optional)
- Emesis basin or clean container
- Sterile specimen cup, or sputum specimen collector

delegation tips

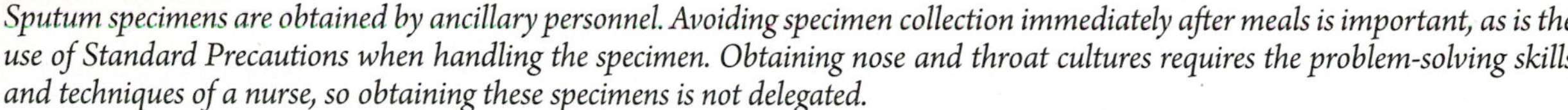

Sputum specimens are obtained by ancillary personnel. Avoiding specimen collection immediately after meals is important, as is the use of Standard Precautions when handling the specimen. Obtaining nose and throat cultures requires the problem-solving skills and techniques of a nurse, so obtaining these specimens is not delegated.

IMPLEMENTATION—ACTION/RATIONALE

* Check client's identification band * Explain procedure before beginning *

ACTION	RATIONALE
1. Wash hands and put on clean gloves.	1. Reduces transmission of microorganisms.
2. Ask the client to sit erect in the bed or on a chair facing the nurse.	2. Provides easy access to the nose or throat.
3. Prepare a sterile swab for use by loosening the top of the container.	3. Prevents contamination of the swab.
Collecting Throat Culture	
4. Ask the client to tilt the head backward, open the mouth, and say "ah."	4. Promotes visualization of the pharynx, relaxes the throat muscles, and minimizes the gag reflex.
5. Depress the lateral anterior one-third of the tongue with a tongue blade for better visualization.	5. Promotes visualization of the pharynx. Depressing the lateral aspect rather than the middle of the tongue decreases stimulation of the gag reflex.
6. Insert the swab without touching the cheek, lips, teeth, or tongue.	6. Prevents contamination of the specimen with oral flora.
7. Swab the tonsillar area from side to side in a quick, gentle motion (Figure 29-33-1).	7. Ensures collection of microorganisms. Retains microorganisms in the culture tube and ensures the life of bacteria for testing.
8. Withdraw the swab without touching adjacent structures and place in the culture tube. Crush ampule at bottom of tube and push swab into liquid medium (Figure 29-33-2).	8. Prevents contamination from outside microorganisms and erroneous culture results.

(Continues)

PROCEDURE 29-33 Collecting Nose, Throat, and Sputum Specimens (Continued)

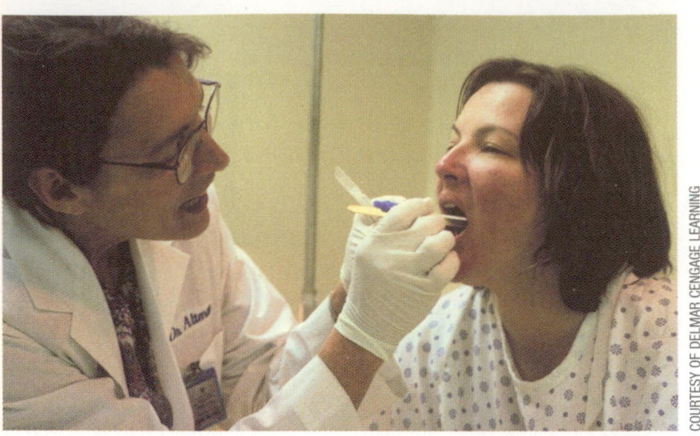
COURTESY OF DELMAR CENGAGE LEARNING

FIGURE 29-33-1 **Swab the sample area using a quick, gentle motion.**

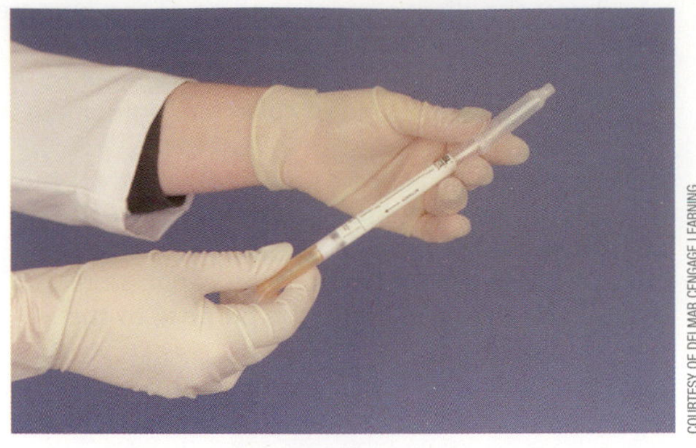
COURTESY OF DELMAR CENGAGE LEARNING

FIGURE 29-33-2 **Crush ampule to release the culture medium.**

ACTION	RATIONALE
9. Secure the top to the culture tube and label with the client's name.	9. Prevents identification mistakes.
10. Discard the tongue depressor. Remove gloves and discard. Wash hands.	10. Reduces transmission of microorganisms.
Collecting Nose Culture	
11. Instruct the client to blow nose and check nostrils for patency with penlight.	11. Clears nasal passages of mucus containing resident bacteria.
12. Ask the client to occlude one nostril, then the other, and exhale.	12. Determines the optimal nasal passage from which to obtain the specimen.
13. Ask the client to tilt the head back.	13. Promotes visualization of the sinuses.
14. Insert the swab into the nostril until it reaches the inflamed mucosa and rotate the swab.	14. Ensures the swab will be covered with the appropriate exudate.
15. Withdraw the swab without touching adjacent structures and place in culture tube. Crush ampule at bottom of tube and push swab into liquid medium.	15. Prevents contamination from normal nasal flora and erroneous culture results.
16. Secure the top to the culture tube and label with the client's name.	16. Prevents identification mistakes.
17. Remove gloves and discard. Wash hands.	17. Reduces transmission of microorganisms.
Collecting of Nasopharyngeal Culture	
18. Follow Actions 11 to 17, except use a swab on a flexible wire that can reach the nasopharynx via the nose.	18. Allows for access to the nasopharyngeal area.
Collecting a Sputum Culture	
19. Explain to the client that the specimen must be sputum, coughed up from the lungs.	19. Promotes client cooperation.
20. Have a sterile specimen cup ready for the sample and some tissues at hand.	20. The specimen must be collected in a sterile cup to prevent contamination.
21. Have the client take several deep breaths and then cough deeply.	21. Helps loosen secretions so the client will be able to provide a specimen.
22. Have the client expectorate the sputum into the sterile cup without touching the inside of the cup.	22. Prevents contamination of the specimen.
23. Place the lid on the specimen container without touching the inside of the lid or the container.	23. Prevents contamination of the specimen.
24. Provide the client with tissues and make him comfortable.	24. Promotes client comfort.

(Continues)

PROCEDURE 29-33 Collecting Nose, Throat, and Sputum Specimens (Continued)

ACTION	RATIONALE

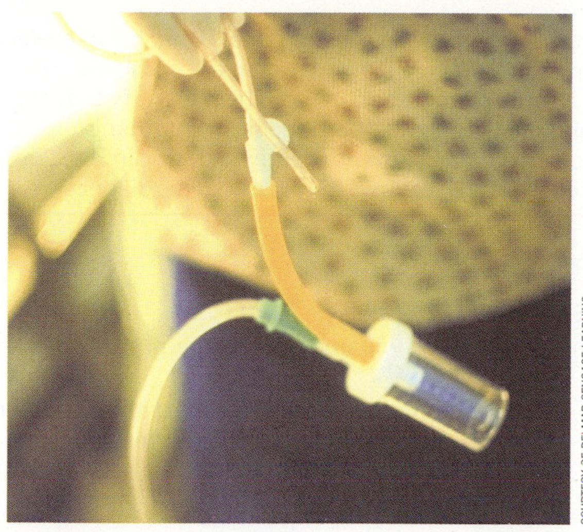

FIGURE 29-33-3 Sputum collector for use with suction.

Alternative Sputum Collection Method

* Generally used if the client is unable to expectorate an adequate sample.*

ACTION	RATIONALE
25. Obtain a sterile suction catheter and an in-line sputum collection container.	25. Prevents contamination of the specimen.
26. Provide the client with warm humidified air for about 20 minutes if it is not contraindicated by the client's condition.	26. Helps loosen secretions in the lungs.
27. Hook up the sputum collector to the suction tubing and a suction device (Figure 29-33-3). Hook up the suction catheter to the sputum collector.	27. Prepare the equipment before having the client cough.
28. If the client is able to cooperate, have him take several deep breaths and cough.	28. Loosens the secretions and brings them up to the back of the throat.
29. As the client is coughing up sputum, carefully insert the catheter either orally or nasopharyngeally into the back of the throat and suction the sputum into the specimen container.	29. Obtains a sterile specimen that is not contaminated with saliva.
30. Safely dispose of the suction catheter.	30. Prevents spread of microorganisms.
31. Close the specimen container.	31. Prevents contamination of the specimen.
32. Provide tissues or other measures for client comfort.	32. Promotes client comfort.
33. Wash hands.	33. Reduces transmission of microorganisms.
34. Label each specimen with the client's name and send to the laboratory.	34. Promotes the correct diagnosis for the client.

EVALUATION

- An adequate specimen was obtained.
- The procedure was performed with a minimum of trauma to the client.

DOCUMENTATION

Nurses' Notes

- Date, time, and site from which the specimen was obtained
- Bleeding or obvious trauma as a result of the procedure
- Description and time the specimen was collected and if the specimen is the first morning specimen, not pooled secretions

PROCEDURE 29-34 Collecting a Stool Specimen

OVERVIEW

Stool specimens are not collected as frequently as urine or blood specimens, but they are extremely valuable in evaluating and diagnosing a variety of gastrointestinal diseases. The most common tests on a stool specimen are occult blood, culture, fecal fat, fecal leukocyte, and OVA and parasite (parasite screen). A stool specimen can help identify GI bleeding; screen for carcinomas, polyps, diverticulitis, and colitis; diagnose and monitor various pathogenic microorganisms; diagnose inflammatory bowel disorders, pancreatitis, and malabsorption syndrome; and identify parasitic infestations. A single specimen is often not diagnostic, and at least three stool cultures are required for a pathogenic diagnosis.

ASSESSMENT

1. Assess the client's or family member's understanding of the need for the test **so the nurse can provide needed teaching.**
2. Assess the client's ability to cooperate with the procedure to collect the specimen **to maintain privacy while a sample is obtained.**
3. Assess the client's medical history for bleeding or GI disorders. **The nurse can initiate screening tests.**
4. Assess any medications the client receives that can cause GI bleeding, such as anticoagulants, steroids, or acetylsalicylic acid, **to help determine the need for testing and/or the possible source of bleeding.**

POSSIBLE NURSING DIAGNOSES

Constipation
Diarrhea
Deficient Knowledge (need and test procedure)

PLANNING

Expected Outcomes

1. The client will understand the purpose of the test.
2. The client will be able to collect the specimen, or allow the specimen to be collected.
3. The test will be conducted properly and results recorded.

Equipment Needed

- Paper towel
- Disposable gloves
- Wooden applicator
- Specimen container
- Gloves
- Clean, dry bedpan, bedside commode, or toilet "hat"

delegation tips

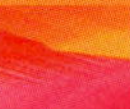

The collection of stool is delegated. Ancillary personnel are instructed to report the presence of red blood in the stool immediately to the nurse.

IMPLEMENTATION—ACTION/RATIONALE

* Check client's identification band * Explain procedure before beginning *

ACTION	RATIONALE
1. Wash hands and apply clean gloves.	1. Reduces transmission of microorganisms from fecal specimen to nurse.
2. Depending on agency policy, assist client as needed to bedside commode or toilet. Have client void before moving bowels. Then, prepare for specimen collection. If client is not ambulatory, use a bedpan. For the toilet, use "hat" (Figure 29-34-1). Place the "hat" in the back section of the toilet to collect a stool specimen and the front section to collect a urine specimen.	2. Allows client privacy and the ability to move bowels in a more normal physiological position.
3. Instruct the client not to contaminate the specimen with urine, vaginal discharge, or toilet paper.	3. Minimizes risk of skewed laboratory results.
4. Ask the client to notify you as soon as the specimen is available.	4. Reduces the risk of contamination of specimen, allows the nurse to collect a fresh specimen, and reduces embarrassment to client.

(Continues)

PROCEDURE 29-34 Collecting a Stool Specimen (Continued)

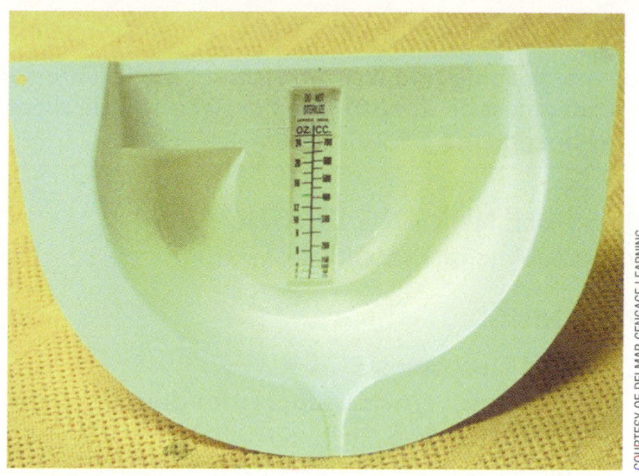

COURTESY OF DELMAR CENGAGE LEARNING

FIGURE 29-34-1 Place the commode "hat" in the back of the toilet to collect a stool specimen.

ACTION	RATIONALE
5. Assist the client with hygiene, help the client back to bed (as required), and ensure client comfort before turning attention to specimen.	5. Promotes client cleanliness and dignity.
6. Apply gloves and wear gown if client is on isolation or at risk for infectious stool, such as *vancomycin-resistant enterococcus* (VRE) or *clostridium difficile* (C. difficile or c diff).	6. Reduces the risk of transmission of microorganisms.
7. Assess the stool for color, consistency, and odor, and presence or absence of visible blood or mucus.	7. Facilitates comprehensive client assessment.
8. Using one or two tongue blades (depending on how much specimen is needed and for which test), transfer a representative sample of stool to the specimen card (Figure 29-32-2) or container, taking care not to contaminate the outside of the container (or the inside of a sterile specimen cup). If using a culture swab, swab in a representative area of stool, particularly if any purulent material is visible. Check with laboratory regarding the volume of stool needed for a particular test.	8. Provides a high-quality sample for optimal results.
9. Close the card, place the lid on the container, or place the swab in the culture tube (according to agency policy) as soon as specimen is collected.	9. Reduces the risk of spread of microorganisms and reduces odor.
10. Place the specimen container in a plastic biohazard bag for transport to the lab after proper labeling is done according to agency policy. Be careful not to contaminate the outside of bag. Provide requisition for test according to agency policy.	10. Properly identifies specimen to client; makes transport of specimen to lab more aesthetic for personnel. Provides client privacy. Reduces spread of microorganisms.
11. Dispose of rest of stool according to agency policy.	11. Reduces spread of microorganisms.
12. Remove gloves and wash hands.	12. Reduces spread of microorganisms.
13. Send specimen to laboratory immediately.	13. Maximizes quality of specimen for testing.

EVALUATION

- Note presence or absence of color change in the guaiac paper.
- Note color, character, and consistency of stool.
- Ask the client to explain the rationale and procedure for the stool test.

DOCUMENTATION

Nurses' Notes

- Date and time the collection was obtained
- Color, character, and consistency of the stool
- When the results of the test were reported to the health care provider

PROCEDURE 29-35 Applying Velcro Abdominal Binders

OVERVIEW

Abdominal Velcro binders support the abdomen and hold abdominal dressings in place. Stretch net binders are not designed for support but simply to hold dressings in place. The binder must be smooth, the right size for the client, and not interfere with circulation or put too much pressure on the bound area.

ASSESSMENT

1. Assess the reason the binder is needed **to determine the correct binder and correct placement.**
2. Assess the client's skin condition for rashes, inflammation, open areas, or dressings **to provide a baseline for future assessments.**
3. Assess and measure the client **to determine what size binder is needed.**
4. Assess for any special circumstances that may affect the placement of the binder, such as dressings, tubing, catheters or IV lines **to determine a plan for binder placement.**
5. Assess the client's understanding of the reasons for the binder and the method of placing the binder **to determine what types of client teaching is needed.**

POSSIBLE NURSING DIAGNOSES

*Impaired Physical **M**obility*

PLANNING

Expected Outcomes

1. Binder will provide support for dressings or soft tissue.
2. Binder will not be too tight or compress the skin.
3. Client will assist in placement of the binder as much as possible.

Equipment Needed

- Correct binder (latex free if indicated)

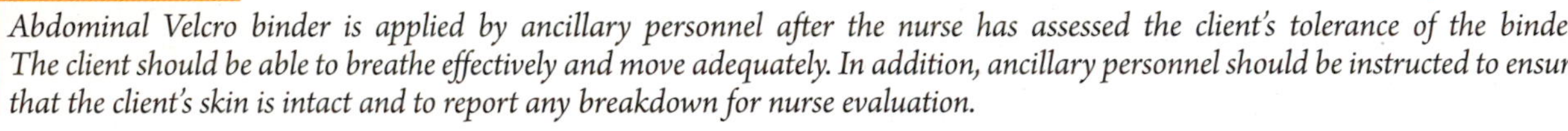

delegation tips

Abdominal Velcro binder is applied by ancillary personnel after the nurse has assessed the client's tolerance of the binder. The client should be able to breathe effectively and move adequately. In addition, ancillary personnel should be instructed to ensure that the client's skin is intact and to report any breakdown for nurse evaluation.

IMPLEMENTATION—ACTION/RATIONALE

* Check client's identification band * Explain procedure before beginning *

Abdominal Binders

ACTION	RATIONALE
1. Wash hands.	1. Reduces transmission of microorganisms.
2. Choose correct-size binder.	2. The correct size will make the binder most effective.
3. Help the client into the proper position to place the binder. • For abdominal Velcro binders, the client should lie supine and lift the hips, or, alternatively, position the client on one side, and roll the client onto the binder.	3. Applying binders can be awkward if the client is not positioned correctly. If binders are too high, they interfere with breathing.
4. Secure binder with Velcro. Check for snug fit.	4. Velcro closure will keep binder in place.
5. Adjust if necessary. Be sure that binders are not restricting breathing or circulation. Be sure that sterile dressings are in place between the binder and any wound.	5. Binders that are too tight may make breathing difficult and may contribute to skin irritation or breakdown. Binders are generally not sterile.
6. Wash hands.	6. Reduces transmission of microorganisms.

(Continues)

PROCEDURE 29-35 Applying Velcro Abdominal Binders (Continued)

ACTION | **RATIONALE**

EVALUATION

- Binder provides support for dressings or soft tissue.
- Binder is not too tight and does not compress the skin.
- Client assists in placement of the binder as much as possible.

DOCUMENTATION

Nurses' Notes

- Time, date, and type of binder
- Difficulty the client experienced with the procedure

PROCEDURE 29-36 Application of Restraints

OVERVIEW

A restraint is a physical or mechanical method of involuntarily restricting movement and physical activity so that the confused, agitated, or disoriented client is protected from causing harm to self and/or to others. Restraints may be used to prevent movement during a procedure. If a client is restless or confused, a restraint may be used to prevent the client from damaging therapeutic equipment.

According to the Centers for Medicare and Medicaid Service's Final Rule for Patient Rights, effective January 8, 2007, a physician or licensed independent practitioner is required to evaluate the client within 1 hour of the initiation of restraints or seclusion within a hospital accredited for Medicare-deemed status. Registered nurses or physician assistants may evaluate the client within 1 hour of the application of restraints or seclusion if they are trained and have consulted with the attending physician or licensed independent practitioner as soon as possible after the evaluation (American Academy of Physician Assistants, 2009). Nurses or caregivers may not restrain or confine clients without documented necessity; however, the nurse or caregiver is liable if a confused client sustains injury without appropriate protection, which may include restraints. Interpretation of the Acute Medical and Surgical (Nonpsychiatric) Care restraint standards Section PC.03.03.23 requires client assessment within 15 minutes of the initiation of restraints or seclusion. After the first 15 minutes, the nurse uses clinical judgment or health care practitioner orders to establish a routine for assessing the client needs. The nurse has a legal and ethical duty to keep clients safe. The decision to restrain a client and how much are delicate balancing acts of nursing judgment.

Restraints range from a simple arm board to prevent movement of a wrist or elbow to the more commonly used soft restraints of mesh or soft canvas. They are designed to gently restrain the client without damaging the skin. According to the Joint Commission, the nature of a device does not determine if the device is a restraint but, rather, the intended device use (physical restriction), involuntary application, and/or client need that determines if the device is a restraint. If a full bed-side rail (a bed rail extending the full length of the bed) prevents a client from getting out of bed, the side rail is considered a restraint. However, if a client uses the side rail to assist in leaving the bed, it is not considered a restraint (Joint Commission, 2008).

ASSESSMENT

1. Assess the client's level of consciousness. **This helps determine the client's ability to protect himself from potential harm.**
2. Assess the client's degree of orientation. **A client who is confused regarding time, place, or person is more likely to be at risk of injuring himself. A client who is agitated or angry may be at risk of injuring others.**
3. Assess the client's physical condition. **A client who has weakness, paralysis, or impaired balance or mobility is at increased risk of injury. Impaired vision or hearing also increases the client's risk of injury.**
4. Assess the client's history for falls, accidents, confusion, agitation, or self-inflicted injury. **A client who has a history of this type is at increased risk for injury.**
5. Assess the client's intent. **A client who is verbalizing threats to harm self or others is at increased risk of injury.**
6. Assess the need for restraints. Determine if the client's treatment plan requires and allows restraints, if orders are in place, and hospital policies and laws are specified. **This will prevent**

(Continues)

PROCEDURE 29-36 Application of Restraints (Continued)

Table 29-36-1 The Joint Commision Restraint/Seclusion Standards for Nonpsychiatric Clients

To protect a client from injuring himself or others, it may be necessary to place him in seclusion or in restraints. This can be done in the absence of a licenced independent practitioner (LIP) in a crisis situation. Each organization must determine who is competent to make this decision when an LIP is not available. The Joint Commission provides the following time frames related to restraint and seclusion.

Time Frames for Restraint or Seclusion for an Adult Client	
Adult client in restrain/seclusion	Order must be obtained from LIP within 1 hour of start of restrains/seclusion.
Adult client evaluated in person by LIP	1. LIP evaluation to be completed within 1 hour of initiation of restraint/ seclusion. 2. If client is released prior to expiration of original order, an LIP in-person evaluation must be conducted within 24 hours of initiation of restraints.
LIP reorders restrain after evaluation by qualified staff	Every 4 hours until adult client is released from restrain/seclusion.
In-person evaluation by LIP	Every 8 hours until adult client is released from restrain/seclusion.
Time Frames for Restraint or Seclusion for Children and Youth Clients	
Child or youth is put into restraint/ seclusion	Order must be ordered from LIP within 1 hour of initiation.
Evaluation of child or youth by LIP in person	1. LIP must perform an in-person evaluation within the first 2 hours for youth 9-17 or for children under 9. 2. LIP in-person evaluation must be done within 24 hours of initiation of restraints if youth or child is released prior to expiration of original order.
Restraint and evaluation reordered by LIP by performed by qualified staff	This occurs every 2 hours for youth (9-17) and every 1 hour for children (under 9) until child is released.
Evaluation in-person by LIP	Every 4 hours for children and youth (17 or younger) until child or youth is released.

Adapted from The Joint Commission. (2005). Restraint and Seclusion, Retrieved August 3, 2008, from http://www.jointcommission.org/Accreditation-programs/BehavioralHealthCare/Standards/FAQs/Provision+of+Care+Treatment+and+Services/Restraint+and+Seclusion/Restraint_Seclusion.htm.

the inappropriate use of restraints and is necessary for legal protection in the event of an injury.

7. Assess client and family knowledge regarding the use of and rationale for restraints or protective devices. **The more the client and family understand regarding the reason for restraints, the more cooperative and understanding they will be.**

POSSIBLE NURSING DIAGNOSES

Risk for Injury
Powerlessness
Deficient Knowledge (need for restraints)
Impaired Physical Mobility

PLANNING

Expected Outcomes

1. The client will remain uninjured.
2. The client will not suffer injury or impairment from the restraints.
3. The client's therapeutic equipment will remain intact and functional.
4. Others will not be harmed by the client.
5. The client will be restrained just enough to prevent injury.

Equipment Needed

- Restraints appropriate to the client's condition and type of restraint required
- Cotton batting or foam padding

(Continues)

PROCEDURE 29-36 Application of Restraints (Continued)

delegation tips

Delegation of the application of restraints to ancillary personnel is acceptable if appropriate orders are in place and proper training has occurred. The assessment of the need for and the type of restraints required and their proper application and maintenance requires the professional nurse's observation and documentation. A physician or health care practitioner must evaluate the client within 1 hour of the application of the restraint and write an order for the restraint as deemed necessary.

IMPLEMENTATION—ACTION/RATIONALE

ACTION	RATIONALE
* Wash hands * Check client's identification band *	
Chest Restraint	
1. Explain that the client will be wearing a jacket attached to the bed. Explain that this is for safety.	1. Promotes client cooperation.
2. Place the restraint over the client's hospital gown or clothing.	2. Provides for client privacy and prevents the restraint from rubbing the client's skin.
3. Place the restraint on the client with the opening in the front.	3. Allows movement but restricts freedom.
4. Overlap the front pieces, threading the ties through the slot/loop on the front of the vest (Figure 29-36-1A).	4. Secures the restraint.
5. If the client is in bed, secure the ties to the movable part of the mattress frame with a half-knot or quick-release knot (Figures 29-36-2 and 29-36-3). Refer to Figure 29-36-4 for guidance in tying the half knot or quick-release knot.	5. Allows the restraint to move with the bed if the head of the bed is raised or lowered.
6. If the client is in a chair, cross the straps behind the back of the chair and secure the straps to the chair's lower legs, out of the client's reach (Figure 29-36-1B). If it is a wheelchair, be sure the straps will not get caught in the wheels.	6. Provides support for the client to sit up while restricting freedom.
7. Step back and assess the client's overall safety. Be sure the restraint is loose enough not to be a hazard to the client but tight enough to restrict the client from getting up and harming him or herself.	7. Looking at the overall picture allows one to see possible missed dangers.
8. Wash hands.	8. Prevents spread of microorganisms.

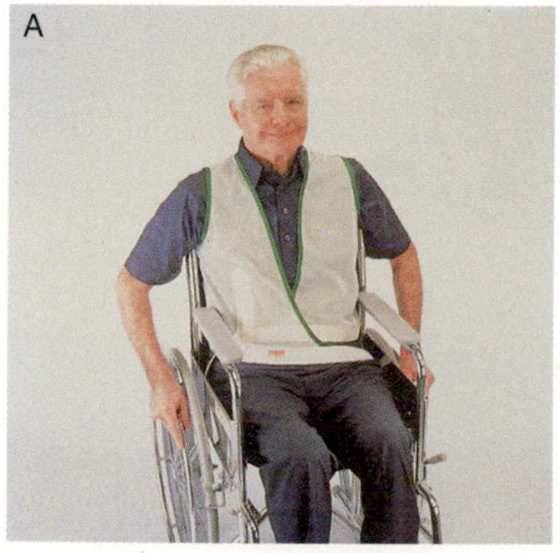

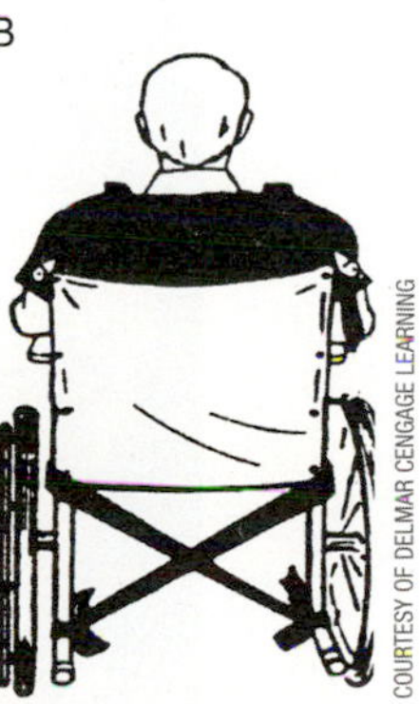

FIGURE 29-36-1 Vest restraint; *A,* Place the restraint on the client with the opening in the front, overlapping the front pieces, and threading the ties through the slot/loop on the front of the vest. *B,* Secure the straps with a slip (easy-release) knot on the opposite side of the wheelchair kick spur.

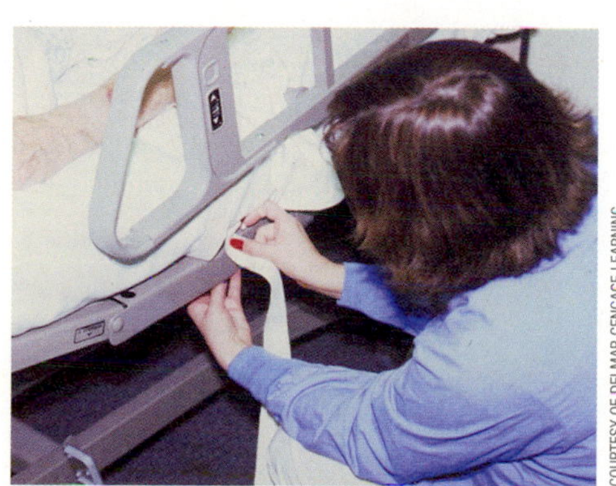

FIGURE 29-36-2 Secure ties to the movable part of the frame with a half-knot or quick-release knot.

(Continues)

PROCEDURE 29-36 Application of Restraints (Continued)

ACTION	RATIONALE

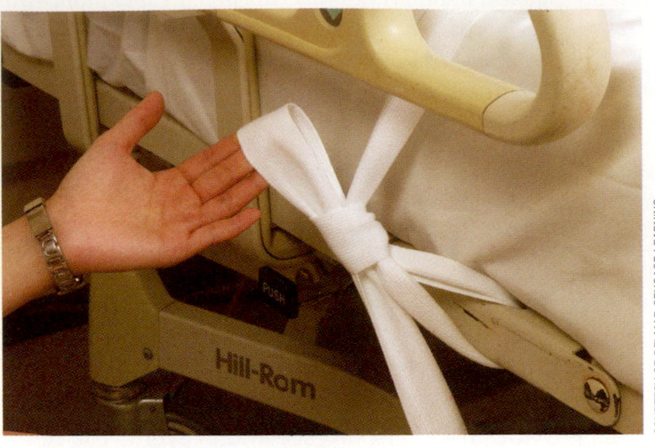

COURTESY OF DELMAR CENGAGE LEARNING

FIGURE 29-36-3 A half-knot or quick-release knot.

Applying Wrist or Ankle Restraints

ACTION	RATIONALE
9. Explain to the client that you are placing a wrist or ankle band that will restrict movement.	9. Promotes client cooperation.
10. Wrap the restraint around the client's wrist/ankle and fasten with Velcro grips.	10. Secures the restraint, and prevents the restraint from overtightening at the wrist.
11. Secure the restraint to the movable portion of the mattress frame with a half-knot or quick-release knot.	11. When the head or foot of the client's bed is moved, the restraint will move with it.
12. Slip two fingers under the restraint to check for tightness (Figure 29-36-5). Be sure the restraint is tight enough that the client cannot slip it off but loose enough that the neurovascular status of the client's extremity is not impaired.	12. If the restraint is too tight, the client's neurovascular status may be impaired, causing injury to the client.

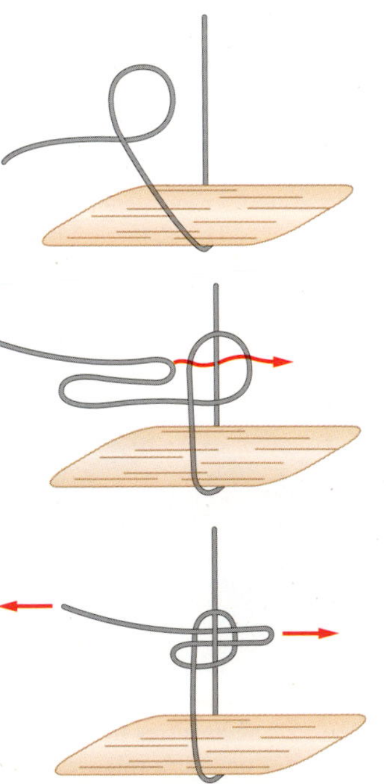

COURTESY OF DELMAR CENGAGE LEARNING

FIGURE 29-36-4 Steps for a half-knot or quick release knot.

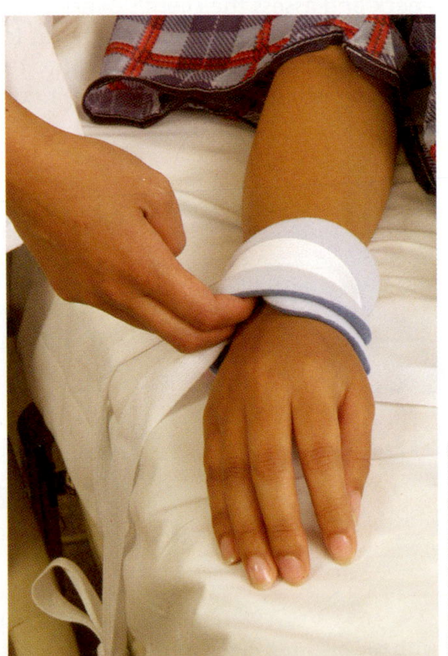

COURTESY OF DELMAR CENGAGE LEARNING

FIGURE 29-36-5 Slip two fingers under the restraint to check for tightness.

(Continues)

PROCEDURE 29-36 Application of Restraints (Continued)

ACTION	RATIONALE
13. Step back and assess the client's overall safety. Be sure the restraint is loose enough not to be a hazard to the client but tight enough to restrict the client from getting up and harming himself.	13. Looking at the overall picture can allow you to see dangers you might have missed.
14. Place the call light within the client's reach.	14. Allows the client to contact the nurse to have any needs met. Provides the client with an increased sense of safety.
15. Assess the client 15 minutes after the initiation of restraints or seclusion with special attention to the client's emotional status, safety of the restraint placement, and the client's neurovascular status. After the first 15 minutes, the nurse uses clinical judgment or health care practitioner orders to establish a routine for assessing the client needs. A physician or health care practitioner must evaluate the client within 1 hour of the application of the restraint and write an order for the restraint as deemed necessary.	15. Assures that the client remains safe. Clients may try to escape from restraint and injure themselves in the attempt. States, institutions, Centers for Medicare and Medicaid Services, and the Joint Commission have regulations outlining the frequency of client checks if the client is in restraints. Be aware of regulations that apply.
16. Wash hands.	16. Prevents spread of microorganisms.

EVALUATION

- The client remains uninjured.
- The client has not suffered injury or impairment from the restraints.
- The client's therapeutic equipment has remained intact and functional.
- Others have not been harmed by the client.
- The client is restrained just enough to prevent injury.

DOCUMENTATION

Nurses' Notes

- Use of restraints including reason the client was restrained, type of restraint placed, time the restraints were placed, condition of the client's skin at the site of restraint at the time of placement, and any unusual findings at the time the client was restrained.
- Nurses' notes should be made at least every 2 hours even if a flow sheet is used.
- Ongoing need for restraints
- If the client's status changes, restraints may no longer be necessary.

Flow Sheet

- Some institutions have flow sheets that are used when a client is restrained. These flow sheets document the frequency of client checks, the client's condition, and how often the restraints are released.

PROCEDURE 29-37 Performing the Heimlich Maneuver

OVERVIEW

Foreign body obstruction of the breathing passages has consistently ranked as one of the top 10 causes of accidental deaths in the United States. Complete or partial airway obstruction by a foreign body can occur in numerous settings. In adults, large, poorly chewed pieces of food are most frequently the cause of airway obstruction. Pediatric clients are at risk for choking, especially the infant and young child, and in this population, food (e.g., grapes, hot dogs, raisins, and peanuts) as well as foreign bodies (e.g., coins, beads, marbles, thumbtacks, and paper clips) often cause airway obstruction. A health care provider successfully treats a client's airway obstruction with the Heimlich maneuver or subdiaphragmatic abdominal thrusts. It is important in the pediatric population to differentiate airway obstruction as a result of infection (e.g., epiglottitis) versus a foreign body aspiration.

(Continues)

PROCEDURE 29-37 Performing the Heimlich Maneuver (Continued)

Health professionals frequently teach the Heimlich maneuver to the general public because most food/foreign body obstructions occur outside the hospital/clinic settings. It is important to have a good comfort level with this skill as well as the ability to disseminate this information in an easily understood manner to the public.

ASSESSMENT

1. Assess air exchange. A foreign body obstruction is complete or partial. Partial airway obstruction has some air exchange. If the client can cough, this should be encouraged, and do not interfere with the client's efforts. In the event of partial airway obstruction, the client will usually cough but may wheeze between coughs. **If the client has complete airway obstruction as indicated by a weak, ineffective cough, high-pitched inspiratory noises (stridor), and signs of respiratory distress (cyanosis, loss of consciousness), intervention is necessary.**
2. Establish airway obstruction. The universal sign of airway obstruction is clutching the neck with hands (Figure 29-37-1). In addition, the inability to talk or breathe as well as cyanosis and the progression to an unconscious state indicate airway obstruction. **Determine the problem.**
3. In the pediatric client, differentiate between infection and airway obstruction. Fevers, gradually increasing respiratory distress, retractions, stridor, and drooling are all signs of infection. **With an infection airway obstruction, it is important to maintain an upright position, keep the child as calm as possible, and seek immediate medical attention.** The Heimlich maneuver is not appropriate for an infection airway obstruction.

POSSIBLE NURSING DIAGNOSES

*Impaired **G**as Exchange*
*Ineffective **A**irway Clearance*
*Ineffective **B**reathing Pattern*
*Risk for **S**uffocation*
*Risk for **A**spiration*
***F**ear*

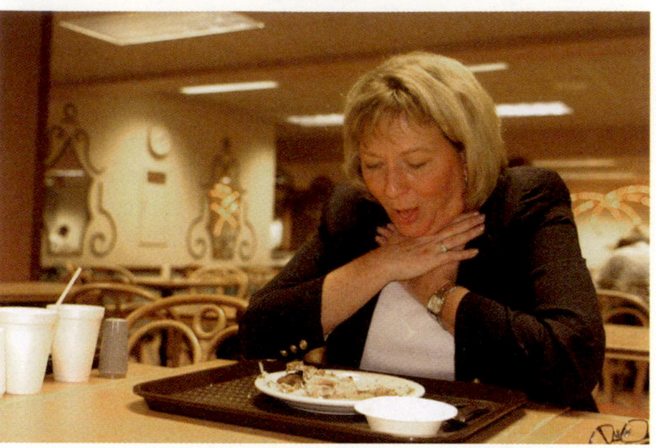

COURTESY OF DELMAR CENGAGE LEARNING

FIGURE 29-37-1 The universal sign of airway obstruction is clutching the neck with hands.

PLANNING

Expected Outcomes

1. The client will demonstrate improved clinical status as evident by airway clearance or establishment of a patent airway.
2. The client will demonstrate improved gas exchange as evident by absence of signs and symptoms of partial or complete airway obstruction (e.g., cough, wheezing, stridor, loss of consciousness, cyanosis).
3. The client will experience minimal discomfort during the Heimlich maneuver or other method of airway clearance.
4. The client will not experience complications related to airway obstruction/hypoxia.

Equipment Needed

- An individual with the training to perform this procedure

delegation tips

The Heimlich maneuver is performed by any trained individual. A technique adjustment of chest thrusts rather than subdiaphragmatic abdominal thrusts are given to choking clients with obesity and late term pregnancy (American College of Emergency Physicians Foundation, 2009).

PROCEDURE 29-37 Performing the Heimlich Maneuver (Continued)

IMPLEMENTATION—ACTION/RATIONALE

ACTION	RATIONALE
* Check client's identification band * Explain procedure before beginning *	
Foreign Body Obstruction—All Clients	
1. Assess airway for complete or partial blockage.	1. If there is good air exchange and the client is able to forcefully cough, do not intervene or interfere with the client's attempts to expel the foreign body.
2. Encourage attempts to cough and breathe.	2. Attempts to cough will provide a more forceful effort. If complete airway obstruction is apparent, the Heimlich maneuver or alternative method of subdiaphragmatic thrust is performed immediately.
3. Activate emergency response assistance if respiratory distress or complete blockage; for example, ask bystander to call 911.	3. Provides follow-up care by professionally trained personnel.
Conscious Adult Client—Sitting or Standing (Heimlich Maneuver)	
4. Stand behind the client and wrap your arms around the client's waist (Figure 29-37-2).	4. Proper positioning provides an effective subdiaphragmatic thrust.
5. Make a fist with one hand and grasp the fist with your other hand, placing the thumb side of the fist against the client's abdomen. The fist is placed midline, below the xiphoid process and lower margins of the rib cage and above the navel (Figure 29-37-3).	5. Correct hand placement is important to prevent internal organ damage.
6. Perform a quick upward thrust into the client's abdomen; each thrust is separate and distinct.	6. This subdiaphragmatic thrust produces an artificial cough by forcing air from the lungs.
7. Repeat this process 6 to 10 times until the client either expels the foreign body or loses consciousness.	7. Attempts to dislodge food or a foreign body to relieve airway obstruction is continued as long as necessary because of the serious consequences of hypoxia.

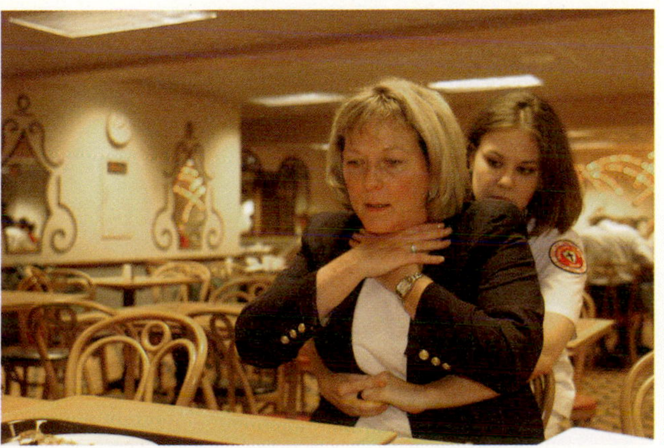
COURTESY OF DELMAR CENGAGE LEARNING

FIGURE 29-37-2 Stand behind the client and wrap your arms around the client's waist.

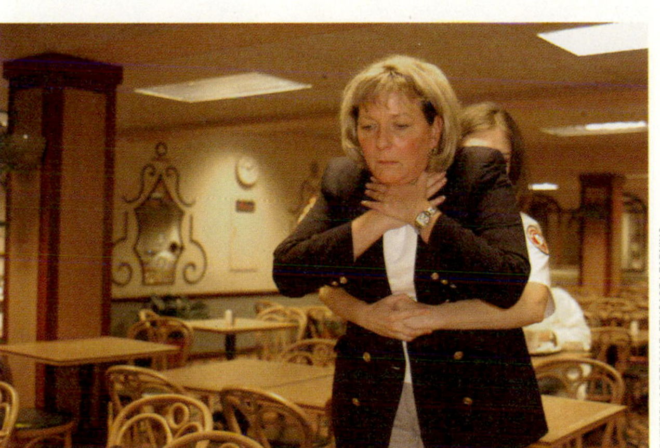
COURTESY OF DELMAR CENGAGE LEARNING

FIGURE 29-37-3 The fist is placed midline, below the xiphoid process and lower margins of the rib cage and above the navel.

(Continues)

PROCEDURE 29-37 Performing the Heimlich Maneuver (Continued)

ACTION	RATIONALE
Unconscious Adult Client or Adult Client Who Becomes Unconscious	
8. Repeat Actions 1 to 3.	8. Determines the need for intervention and summons essential help.
9. Position the client supine; kneel astride the client's abdomen.	9. Proper positioning provides an effective subdiaphragmatic thrust.
10. Place the heel of one hand midline, below the xiphoid process and lower margin of the rib cage and above the navel. Place the second hand directly on top of the first hand.	10. Proper positioning provides an effective subdiaphragmatic thrust.
11. Perform a quick upward thrust into the diaphragm, repeating 6 to 10 times.	11. A client who becomes unconscious may become more relaxed so that the previously unsuccessful Heimlich maneuver may be successful.
12. Perform a finger sweep:	12. Should only be used on the unconscious client, who will not fight the action.
a. Use one hand to grasp the lower jaw and tongue between your thumb and fingers and lift. This will open the mouth and pull the tongue away from the back of the throat.	a. Draw the tongue away from any foreign body lodged in the back of the throat.
b. Using the index finger of the other hand, do a finger sweep to remove any foreign body that can be easily seen and removed, as shown in Figure 29-37-4 (ACEP Foundation, 2009a).	
Caution must be used to prevent pushing the foreign body farther down into the airway.	
13. Open the client's airway and attempt ventilation.	13. The brain can suffer irreversible damage if it is without oxygen for more than 4 to 6 minutes.
14. Continue sequence of Heimlich maneuver, finger sweep, and rescue breathing as long as necessary.	14. Lifesaving efforts must continue until they are successful, or until the rescuer becomes exhausted and cannot go on.
Airway Obstruction—Infants and Small Children	
15. Differentiate between infection and airway obstruction.	15. Infectious complications that lead to airway obstruction require immediate medical attention, establishment of a patent airway (intubation or emergency tracheotomy), and treatment of the underlying infection. Food/foreign body airway obstruction also needs immediate attention; however, airway management differs for each scenario.

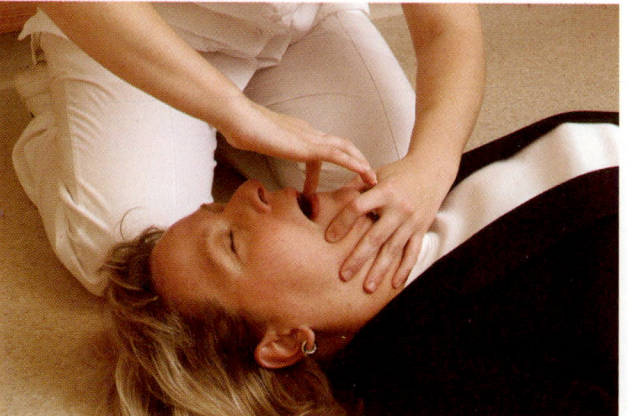

COURTESY OF DELMAR CENGAGE LEARNING

FIGURE 29-37-4 Use a sweeping motion with the index finger to remove any foreign body that can be easily seen and removed.

(Continues)

PROCEDURE 29-37 Performing the Heimlich Maneuver (Continued)

ACTION	RATIONALE
Infant Airway Obstruction	
16. Straddle infant over your forearm in the prone position with the head lower than the trunk. Support the infant's head, positioning a hand around the jaws and chest.	16. Proper positioning is essential for success of the maneuver and prevention of other organ damage.
17. Deliver five back blows between the infant's shoulder blades (Figure 29-37-5).	17. Provides correct technique for dislodging the obstruction.
18. Keeping the infant's head down, place the free hand on the infant's back and turn the infant over, supporting the back of the child with your hand and thigh.	18. Safely rotates the infant's position to continue lifesaving procedures.
19. With your free hand, deliver five thrusts in the same manner as infant external cardiac compressions (Figure 29-37-6).	19. Technique for dislodging the obstruction.
20. Assess for a foreign body in the mouth of an unconscious infant and utilize the finger sweep only if a foreign body is visualized.	20. A blind finger sweep is avoided in infants and children because a foreign object can be pushed back farther into the airway, increasing obstruction.
21. Open airway and assess for respiration. If respirations are absent, attempt rescue breathing. Assess for the rise and fall of the chest; if not seen, reposition infant and attempt rescue breathing again.	21. Many times some air can get around the foreign body causing the airway obstruction. This allows for some oxygenation of the client. Without oxygen, irreversible brain damage can occur within 4 to 6 minutes.
22. Repeat the entire sequence again: five back blows, five chest thrusts, assessment for foreign body in oral cavity, and rescue breathing as long as necessary.	22. Lifesaving efforts must continue until they are successful or until the rescuer becomes exhausted and cannot go on.
Small Child—Airway Obstruction (Conscious, Standing or Sitting)	
23. Assess air exchange and encourage coughing and breathing. Provide reassurance to the child that you are there to help.	23. Inability to breathe is a distressing event for anyone, especially a small child who may not fully understand the circumstance. Reassurance is important to gain the child's trust and cooperation with the maneuvers necessary to help him or her, especially if the child is conscious.

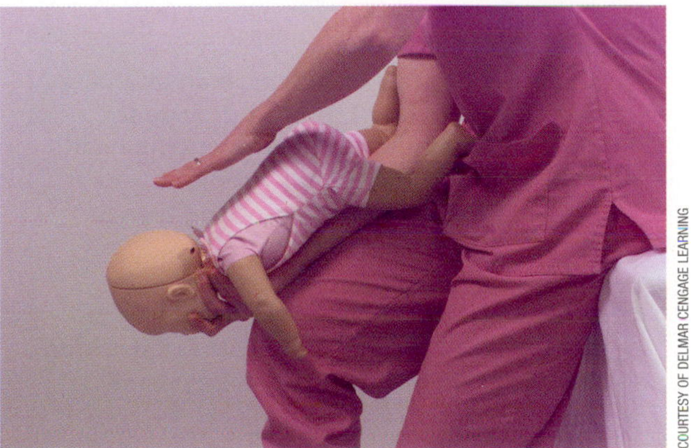
COURTESY OF DELMAR CENGAGE LEARNING

FIGURE 29-37-5 Place the infant in prone position, supporting the head with a hand around the jaws and chest, then deliver five blows between the infant's shoulder blades.

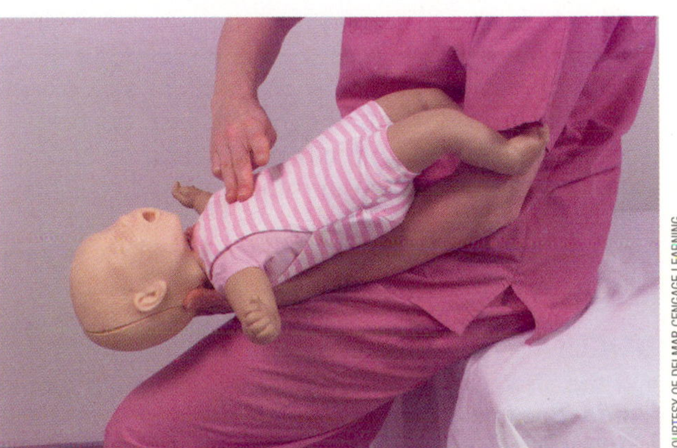
COURTESY OF DELMAR CENGAGE LEARNING

FIGURE 29-37-6 Turn the infant face up, supporting the back of the child with hand and thigh. Deliver five chest thrusts with fingers place just below the nipple line.

(Continues)

PROCEDURE 29-37 Performing the Heimlich Maneuver (Continued)

ACTION	RATIONALE
24. Ask the child if he or she is choking. If the response is affirmative, follow the steps outlined below. In addition, if the child has poor air exchange (and infection has been ruled out), initiate the following steps:	24. Many small children are capable of responding to simple questions such as "Are you choking?"
a. Stand behind the child with your arms wrapped around his or her waist and quickly administer 6 to 10 subdiaphragmatic abdominal thrusts.	a. Proper positioning is essential for success of the maneuver and prevention of other organ damage.
b. Continue until foreign object is expelled or the child becomes unconscious.	b. Lifesaving efforts must continue until they are successful or until the rescuer becomes exhausted and cannot go on.
Small Child—Airway Obstruction (Unconscious)	
25. Position the child supine and kneel at the child's feet and gently deliver five subdiaphragmatic abdominal thrusts in the same manner as for an adult but more gently.	25. This is the recommended position for small children; the astride position may be used for larger children. Proper positioning is essential for success of the maneuver and prevention of other organ damage.
26. Open airway by lifting the lower jaw and tongue forward. Perform a finger sweep only if a foreign body is visualized.	26. Opens the airway and allows visualization of the oral cavity. A blind finger sweep can cause increased obstruction by pushing a foreign object farther back into the airway.
27. If breathing is absent, begin rescue breathing. If the chest does not rise, reposition the child and attempt rescue breathing again.	27. Many times some air can get around the foreign body causing the airway obstruction. This allows for some oxygenation of the client. Without oxygen, irreversible brain damage can occur within 4 to 6 minutes.
28. Repeat this sequence as long as necessary.	28. Lifesaving efforts must continue until they are successful or until the rescuer becomes exhausted and cannot go on.
29. Wash hands.	29. Reduces transmission of microorganisms.

EVALUATION

- The client demonstrates improved clinical status as evident by airway clearance or establishment of a patent airway.
- The client demonstrates improved gas exchange as evident by absence of signs and symptoms of partial or complete airway obstruction (e.g., cough, wheezing, stridor, loss of consciousness, cyanosis).
- The client experienced minimal discomfort during the Heimlich maneuver or other method of airway clearance.
- The client did not experience complications related to airway obstruction/hypoxia.

DOCUMENTATION

- If the airway obstruction occurs in the health care setting, document the following in the narrative notes and in the emergency procedure notes if needed:
  - — Time and date of onset of symptoms
  - — Presentation, including onset and type of symptoms
  - — Type (complete or partial) and cause of obstruction, if known
  - — Interventions utilized to alleviate obstruction
  - — Results of interventions
  - — Other emergency support needed (e.g., emergency tracheotomy)
- If the airway obstruction occurs in an alternate setting (e.g., restaurant, home), provide the following information to the responding health care providers for documentation:
  - — Presentation, including onset and type of symptoms
  - — Type (complete or partial) and cause of obstruction, if known
  - — Interventions utilized to alleviate obstruction
  - — Length of time with airway obstruction
  - — Results of interventions

PROCEDURE 29-38 Performing Cardiopulmonary Resuscitation (CPR)

OVERVIEW

Cardiac or respiratory arrest can occur at any time to individuals of all ages. It is a crisis event that can be the result of an accident (e.g., foreign body aspiration, motor vehicle accident, drowning) or a disease process (e.g., cardiac arrhythmia, epiglottitis). Cardiopulmonary resuscitation (CPR) is the basic lifesaving skill utilized in the event of cardiac, respiratory, or cardiopulmonary arrest to maintain tissue oxygenation by providing external cardiac compressions and/or artificial respiration.

This lifesaving skill is initiated in the event that an individual is found with or develops the absence of a pulse or respiration or both. The basic goals of CPR, which are often referred to as the ABCD of emergency resuscitation, are as follows:

A: Establish **A**irway
B: Initiate **B**reathing
C: Maintain **C**irculation
D: **D**efibrillate

Cardiopulmonary resuscitation must be initiated immediately once it is determined that a cardiac or pulmonary arrest has occurred. Lack of oxygen to the tissues can result in permanent cardiac and brain damage within 4 to 6 minutes.

Cardiopulmonary resuscitation is a basic lifesaving skill that nurses are expected to perform not only in the hospital and other clinical settings but in the outside environments as well. It is expected that nurses maintain certification in the administration of CPR to individuals of all ages and participate in annual review or recertification courses. In addition, this skill is frequently taught to the lay public and caregivers of medically fragile individuals.

ASSESSMENT

1. Assess responsiveness and level of consciousness by gently shaking or tapping the client while shouting, "Are you OK?" **It is important to differentiate an unconscious individual from someone who is intoxicated, hypoglycemic, sleeping, or in shock. In addition, it is important to touch clients in case they are hearing impaired.**
2. Assess the amount and abilities of any available assistance. **CPR cannot be performed indefinitely by a single individual. If in the hospital or a clinical setting, activate the appropriate "code" to signify there is an emergency situation. If outside the hospital, call for help to activate emergency assistance (e.g., call 911 or the local emergency medical service).**
3. Assess the client's position. **Proper positioning, in a supine position (flat) on a hard surface, is essential to assess respiratory and cardiac status and to adequately perform cardiopulmonary resuscitation. Care must be taken when positioning the client with a suspected neck injury.**
4. Assess respiratory status by looking for chest rise and fall, listening for air exchange, and feeling for the presence of air movement. **Presence of respirations contraindicates the initiation of artificial respiration. In addition, assessment of the respiratory status will uncover complicating factors, including foreign body obstruction and vomit or other excessive airway secretions. These complicating factors need to be resolved in order to open the airway before the initiation of artificial respirations.**
5. Assess circulatory status by using the carotid or brachial pulse points. **Presence of pulse contraindicates the initiation of external chest compressions.**

POSSIBLE NURSING DIAGNOSES

Ineffective Airway Clearance
Ineffective Breathing Pattern
Impaired Gas Exchange
Impaired Spontaneous Ventilation
Decreased Cardiac Output

PLANNING

Expected Outcomes

1. Client will experience improved clinical status, as evident by:
   - Patent airway with spontaneous respirations
   - Return of cardiac circulation
2. Client does not experience negative sequela related to hypoxic event.
3. Client does not have damage inflicted by incorrect positioning for CPR (e.g., paralysis from manipulation of neck injury, cracked ribs or sternum).
4. Cardiopulmonary resuscitation will be terminated only in the following situations:
   - Cardiopulmonary resuscitation was successful in reestablishing respirations and circulation.
   - The client is placed on advanced life support (e.g., intubated and transferred to the intensive care unit).
   - The rescuer is unassisted, fatigued, and unable to continue.

(Continues)

PROCEDURE 29-38 Performing Cardiopulmonary Resuscitation (CPR) (Continued)

- The physician or qualified practitioner pronounces the client dead and orders CPR to be discontinued.

Equipment Needed

Hospital or Clinical Setting

- Hard, flat surface (e.g., chest compression board)
- Body substance isolation items
  - — Gloves
  - — Face shield
  - — Mask/CPR oral barrier device
- Ambu®-bag
- Oral airway
- Emergency resuscitation cart (including defibrillator)
- Documentation forms

Outside: Public Environment

- Hard, flat surface (e.g., floor)
- Body substance isolation items, if available
  - — Gloves
  - — Face shield
  - — Mask/CPR oral barrier device

delegation tips

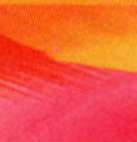

The administration of CPR to adults and children is a skill delegated to ancillary personnel and caregivers after proper instruction and CPR certification.

IMPLEMENTATION—ACTION/RATIONALE

ACTION	RATIONALE
CPR: One Rescuer—Adult, Adolescent	
1. Assess responsiveness by tapping or gently shaking client while shouting, "Are you OK?"	1. Prevents injury to a client who is not experiencing cardiac or respiratory arrest. Also assists in assessing level of consciousness and possible etiology of crisis.
2. Activate emergency medical system (EMS). In the hospital or clinical setting, follow institutional protocol. In the community or home environment, activate the local emergency response system (e.g., 911).	2. Activates assistance from personnel trained in advanced life support. Note: According to the CPR guidelines (American Heart Association [AHA], 2005), rescuers should notify the EMS or phone 911 for unresponsive adults before beginning CPR.
3. Position client in a supine position on a hard, flat surface (e.g., floor or cardiac board). Use caution when positioning a client with a possible head or neck injury.	3. Proper positioning facilitates assessment of the cardiac and respiratory status and successful external cardiac massage. Prevents further damage to a potential head or neck injury.
4. Apply appropriate body substance isolation items (e.g., gloves, face shield) if available (Figure 29-38-1).	4. Prevents transmission of disease.

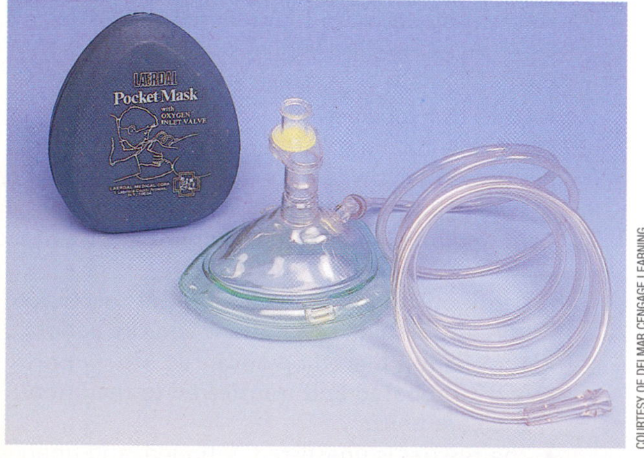

COURTESY OF DELMAR CENGAGE LEARNING

FIGURE 29-38-1 Facemask for artificial resuscitation.

(Continues)

PROCEDURE 29-38 Performing Cardiopulmonary Resuscitation (CPR) (Continued)

ACTION	RATIONALE
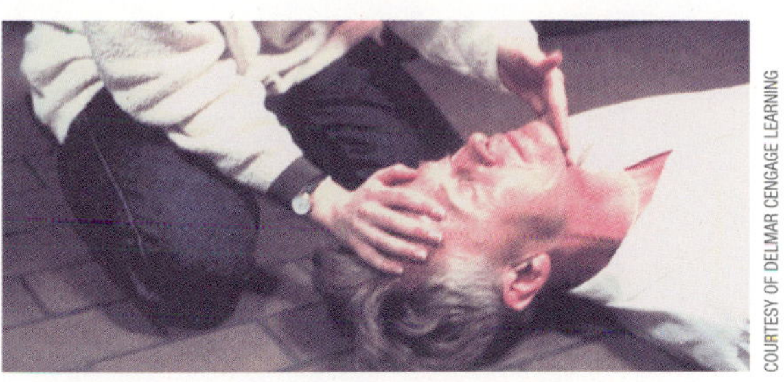 COURTESY OF DELMAR CENGAGE LEARNING **FIGURE 29-38-2 Use the head-tilt/chin-lift method to open airway.**	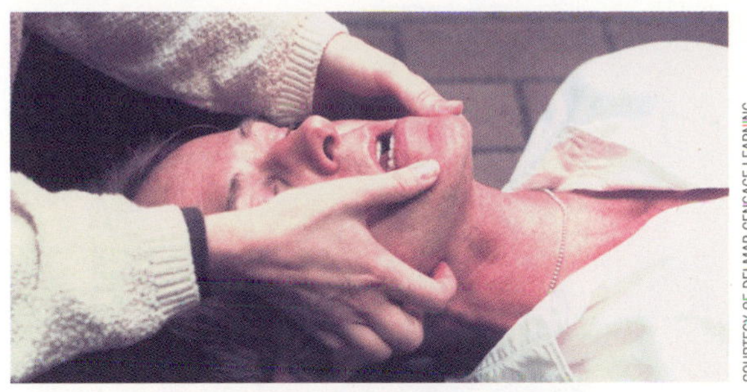 COURTESY OF DELMAR CENGAGE LEARNING **FIGURE 29-38-3 The jaw-thrust method is used to open the airway if a neck injury is suspected.**
5. Position self. Face the client on your knees parallel to the client, next to the head, to begin to assess the airway and breathing status.	5. Proper positioning prevents rescuer fatigue and facilitates CPR by allowing the rescuer to move from chest compressions to artificial breathing with minimal movement.
6. Open airway. The most commonly used method is the head-tilt/chin-lift method. This is accomplished by placing one hand on the client's forehead and applying a steady backward pressure to tilt the head back while placing the fingers of the other hand below the jaw at the location of the chin and lifting the chin (Figure 29-38-2). In the event of a suspected head or neck injury, this lift is modified and the jaw thrust is used without head extension. To perform the jaw thrust, place hands at the angles of the lower jaw and lift, displacing the mandible forward (Figure 29-38-3). Additionally, if available, insert oral airway.	6. A patent airway is essential for successful artificial respirations. The head-tilt/chin-lift assists in preventing the tongue from obstructing the airway. The jaw thrust is used when a head or neck injury is suspected because it prevents extension of the neck and decreases the potential of further injury.
7. Assess for respirations. Look, listen, and feel for air movement (3 to 5 seconds).	7. Cardiopulmonary resuscitation should not be administered to a client with spontaneous respirations or pulse because of the potential risk of injury.
8. If respirations are absent: • Occlude nostrils with the thumb and index finger of the hand on the forehead that is tilting the head back (Figure 29-38-4). • Form a seal over the client's face mask using either your mouth or the appropriate respiratory assist device (e.g., Ambu®-bag and mask) and give two full breaths of 1 second per breath (AHA, 2005), allowing time for both inspiration and expiration (Figure 29-38-5). The volume of each rescue breath should provide visible chest rise (AHA, 2005–2006). • In the event of a serious mouth or jaw injury that prevents mouth-to-mouth ventilation, mouth-to-nose ventilation may be used by tilting the head as described earlier with one hand and using the other hand to lift the jaw and close the mouth.	8. Occluding the nostrils and forming a seal over the client's mouth will prevent air leakage and provide full inflation of the lungs. Excessive air volume and rapid inspiratory flow rates can create pharyngeal pressures that are greater than esophageal opening pressures. This will allow air into the stomach, resulting in gastric distention and increased risk of vomiting.
9. Assess for the rise and fall of the chest: • If the chest rises and falls, continue to Action 10. • If the chest does not move, assess for excessive oral secretions, vomit, airway obstruction, or improper positioning.	9. Visual assessment of chest movement helps confirm an open airway. A volume of 800 to 1,200 mL is usually sufficient to make the chest rise in most adults.

(Continues)

PROCEDURE 29-38 Performing Cardiopulmonary Resuscitation (CPR) (Continued)

ACTION | **RATIONALE**

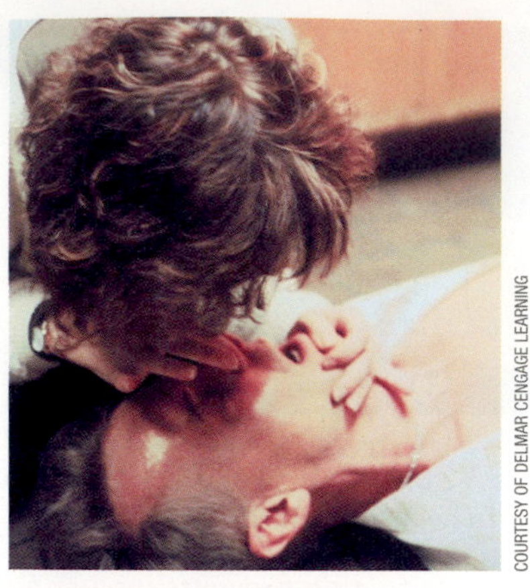

FIGURE 29-38-4 Occlude both nostrils with fingers.

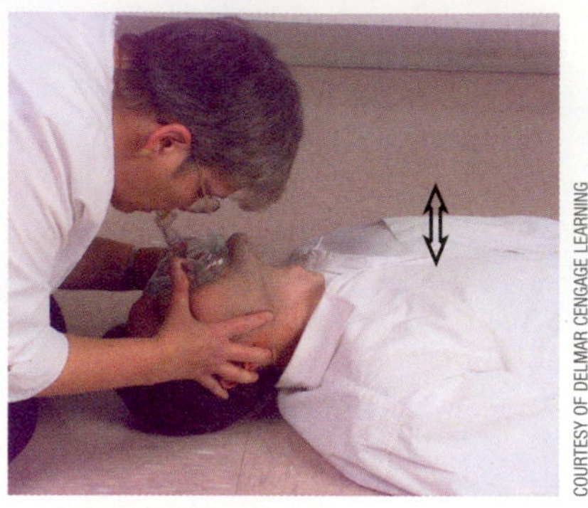

FIGURE 29-38-5 Give two full breaths.

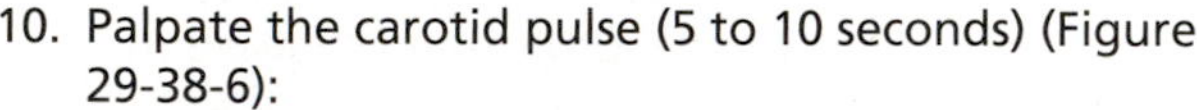

10. Palpate the carotid pulse (5 to 10 seconds) (Figure 29-38-6):
    - If present, continue rescue breathing, at the rate of 12 breaths per minute.
    - If absent, begin external cardiac compressions.

10. Performing chest compressions on an individual with a pulse could result in injury. Additionally, the carotid pulse may persist when peripheral pulses are no longer palpable. Hyperventilation assists in maintaining blood oxygen levels. Additionally, a pulse may be present for approximately 6 minutes after respirations have ceased.

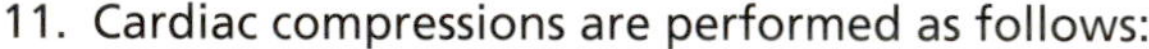

11. Cardiac compressions are performed as follows:
    - Maintain a position on knees parallel to sternum.
    - Position the hands for compressions:
    a. Using the hand nearest to the legs, use the index finger to locate the lower rib margin and quickly move the fingers up to the location where the ribs connect to the sternum.
    b. Place the middle finger of this hand on the notch where the ribs meet the sternum and the index finger next to it.
    c. Place the heel of the opposite hand next to the index finger on the sternum (Figure 29-38-7).

11. Irreversible brain and tissue damage can occur if a client is hypoxic for more than 4 to 6 minutes. Proper positioning is essential for the following reasons:
    - Allows for maximum compression of the heart between the sternum and vertebrae.
    - Compressions over the xiphoid process can lacerate the liver.
    - Keeping fingers off the chest during compressions reduces the risk of rib fracture.

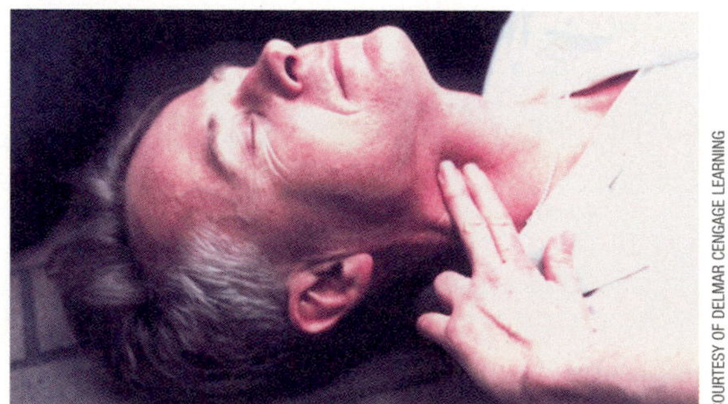

FIGURE 29-38-6 Palpate for a carotid pulse.

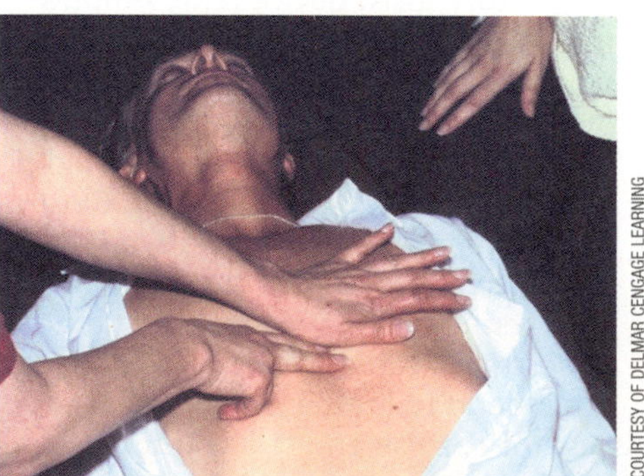

FIGURE 29-38-7 Place the heel of one hand next to the index finger on the client's sternum.

(Continues)

PROCEDURE 29-38 Performing Cardiopulmonary Resuscitation (CPR) (Continued)

ACTION	RATIONALE
d. Remove the first hand from the notch and place it on top of the hand that is on the sternum so they are on top of each other. e. Extend or interlace fingers and do not allow them to touch the chest (Figure 29-38-8). f. Keep arms straight with shoulders directly over hands on sternum and lock elbows (Figure 29-38-9). g. Compress the adult chest 3.8–5.0 cm (11/2–2 inches) at the rate of approximately 100 compressions per minute. h. The heel of the hand must completely release the pressure between compressions, but it should remain in constant contact with the client's skin. i. Use the mnemonic "one and, two and, three and . . . " to keep rhythm and timing. j. Ventilate client as described in Action 8.	
12. Maintain the compression rate for approximately 100 times per minute, interjecting 2 ventilations after every 30 compressions. (compression:ventilation rate at 30:2)	12. Faster rate increases blood flow to key organ tissues.
13. Reassess the client after four cycles.	13. Determines return of spontaneous pulse and respirations and need to continue CPR.
CPR: Two Rescuers—Adult, Adolescent 14. Follow the steps above with the following changes: • One rescuer is positioned facing the client parallel to the head while the other rescuer is positioned on the opposite side facing the client parallel to the sternum next to the trunk (Figure 29-38-10). • The rescuer positioned at the client's trunk is responsible for performing cardiac compressions	14. Proper positioning allows one rescuer to perform artificial respirations while the other administers chest compressions without getting in each other's way. In addition, this facilitates ease in changing positions when one of the rescuers becomes fatigued. Palpating the carotid pulse with each chest compression during the first full minute

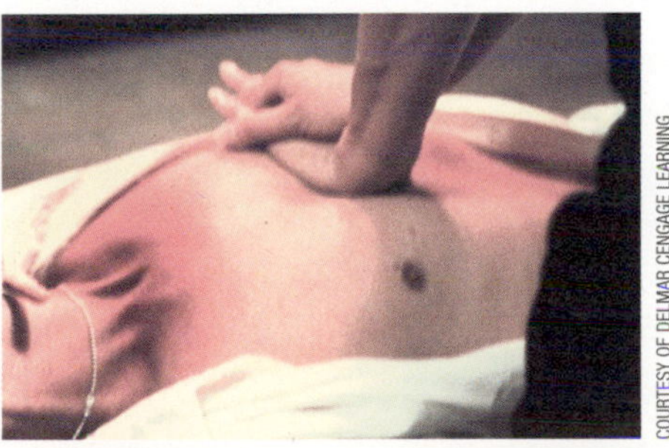

FIGURE 29-38-8 Extend or interlace the fingers.

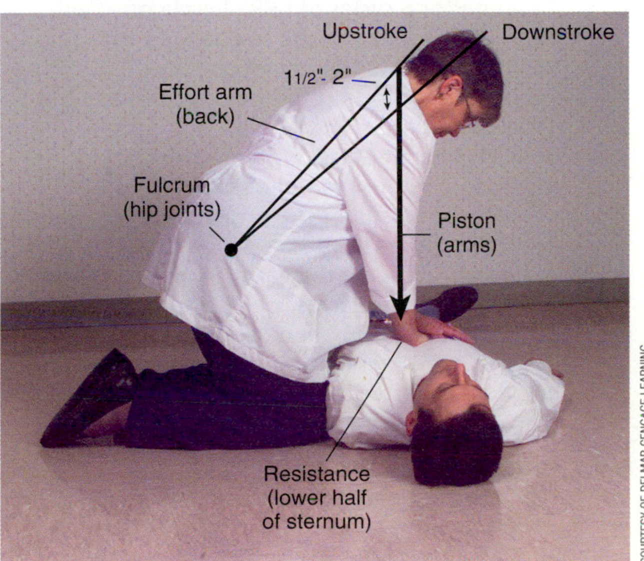

FIGURE 29-38-9 Proper position of rescuer. Keep arms straight and lock elbos.

(Continues)

PROCEDURE 29-38 Performing Cardiopulmonary Resuscitation (CPR) (Continued)

ACTION	RATIONALE

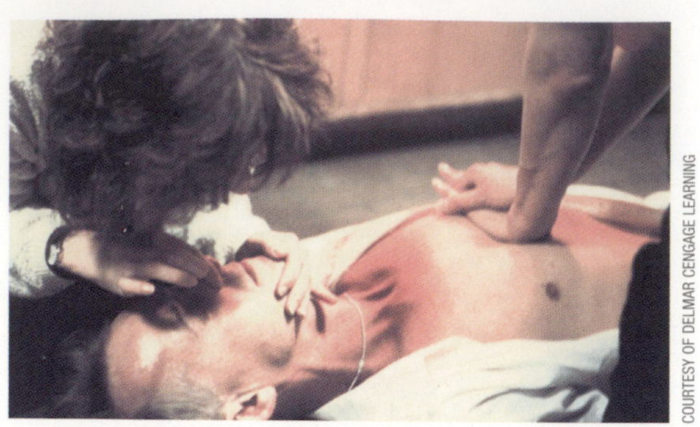

FIGURE 29-38-10 **Two-rescuer positioning. One person kneels on each side of the client.**

and maintaining the verbal mnemonic count. This is rescuer 1. According to the 2005 CPR guidelines, the rescuer is to make the chest compressions hard and fast and allow the chest to recoil after each compression.

Rationale: assures that adequate stroke volume is delivered with each compression.

- The rescuer positioned at the client's head is responsible for monitoring respirations, assessing the carotid pulse, establishing an open airway, and performing rescue breathing at the rate of 10 to 12 breaths per minute. This is rescuer 2.

Rationale: Two rescuers are needed because one person cannot maintain CPR indefinitely. According to studies, the chest compression rescuer fatigues in as little as 1 to 2 minutes (AHA, 2005–2006). When a rescuer becomes fatigued, chest compressions can become ineffective, decreasing the volume of oxygenated blood circulated to key organs and tissue.

- Maintain the compression rate for approximately 100 times per minute, interjecting two ventilations after every 15 compressions. (compression:ventilation rate at 15:2)
- Rescuer 2 palpates the carotid pulse with each chest compression during the first full minute.
- Rescuer 2 is responsible for calling for a change. Rescuers should change every 2 minutes or 5 cycles of CPR (1 cycle of CPR = 30 compressions: 2 rescue breaths). Rescuer 2 follows this protocol:
- Rescuer 1 calls for a change and completes the 15 chest compressions.
- Rescuer 2 administers two breaths and then moves to a position parallel to the client's sternum and assumes the proper hand position.
- Rescuer 1 moves to the rescue breathing position and checks the carotid pulse for 5 seconds. If cardiac arrest persists, rescuer 1 says, "continue CPR" and delivers one breath. Rescuer 2 resumes cardiac compressions immediately after the breath.

CPR: One Rescuer—Child (1 to onset of adolescence/puberty)

15. Assess responsiveness, position the child, apply appropriate body substance isolation, position self, open airway, and assess for respirations as described in Actions 1, 3–7. Remember respiratory arrest is more common in the pediatric population.

Rationale: 15. See Rationales 1 and 3 to 7.

(Continues)

PROCEDURE 29-38 Performing Cardiopulmonary Resuscitation (CPR) (Continued)

ACTION	RATIONALE
16. If respirations are absent, begin rescue breathing: • Give two slow breaths (1–1 ½ sec/breath), pausing to take a breath in between. • Use only the amount of air needed to make the chest rise. When you see the chest rise and fall, you are using the right volume of air.	16. Hypoxia can cause irreversible brain and tissue damage after 4 to 6 minutes. • The volume of air in a small child's lungs is less than an adult's. Excessive air volume and rapid inspiratory rates can increase pharyngeal pressures that exceed esophageal opening pressures. This allows air to enter the stomach, causing gastric distention, increasing the risk of vomiting, and further compromising the client's respiratory status.
17. Palpate the carotid pulse (5 to 10 seconds). If present, ventilate at a rate of once every 3 to 5 seconds or 12 to 20 breaths per minute. If absent, begin cardiac compressions.	17. Performing chest compressions on a child with a pulse could result in injury. Additionally, the carotid pulse may persist when peripheral pulses are no longer palpable. Hyperventilation assists in maintaining blood oxygen levels. Additionally, a pulse may be present for approximately 6 minutes after respirations have ceased.
18. Cardiac compressions (child 1–7 years): • Maintain a position on knees parallel to child's sternum. • Position the hands for compressions: a. Locate the lower margin of the rib cage using the hand closest to the feet and find the notch where the ribs and sternum meet. b. Place the middle finger of this hand on the notch and then place the index finger next to the middle finger. c. Place the heel of the other hand next to the index finger of the first hand on the sternum with the heel parallel to the sternum (1 cm above the xiphoid process). d. Keeping the elbows locked and the shoulders over the child, compress the sternum one-third to one-half the depth of the chest at the approximate rate of 100 times per minute. e. At the end of every 30th compression, administer 2 ventilations (1 second).	18. Irreversible brain and tissue damage can occur if a client is hypoxic for more than 4 to 6 minutes. Proper positioning is essential for the following reasons: • Allows for maximum compression of the heart between the sternum and vertebrae. • The backward tilt of the head lifts the back of small children. • Compressions over the xiphoid process can lacerate the liver. • Keeping fingers off the chest during compressions reduces the risk of rib fracture. • Keeping one hand on the child's forehead helps maintain an open airway.
f. Reevaluate the child after 20 cycles. If respirations are still absent, call 911.	f. Guidelines published by the AHA (2005) recommend that a 1-minute CPR be performed for infants and children up to the onset of adolescence/puberty before calling 911. In institutions, follow hospital protocol.
CPR: One Rescuer—Infant (1–12 months)	
19. Assess responsiveness, activate emergency medical system, position the child, apply appropriate body substance isolation, position self, open airway, and assess for respirations as described in Actions 1, 3–7. Remember, respiratory arrest is more common in the pediatric population.	19. See Rationales 1 and 3 to 7.
20. If respirations are absent, begin rescue breathing:	20. Irreversible brain and tissue damage can occur if a client is hypoxic for more than 4 to 6 minutes. Proper positioning is essential for the following reasons:
• Avoid overextension of the infant's neck.	• It is believed that overextension of an infant's head can cause a closing or narrowing of the airway.

(Continues)

PROCEDURE 29-38 Performing Cardiopulmonary Resuscitation (CPR) (Continued)

ACTION	RATIONALE
• Place a small towel or diaper under the infant's shoulders or use a hand to support the neck.	• Proper positioning with support allows maximum compression of the heart between the sternum and vertebrae.
• Make a tight seal over both the infant's nose and mouth and gently administer artificial respirations.	• Making a complete seal over the infant's mouth and nose prevents air leakage.
• Give two slow breaths (1 second per breath), pausing to take a breath in between. • Use only the amount of air needed to make the chest rise.	• The volume of air in a small child's lungs is less than an adult's. Excessive air volume and rapid inspiratory rates can increase pharyngeal pressures that exceed esophageal opening pressures. This allows air to enter the stomach, causing gastric distention, increasing the risk of vomiting, and further compromising the client's respiratory status.
21. Assess circulatory status using the brachial pulse: • Locate the brachial pulse on the inside of the upper arm between the elbow and shoulder by placing your thumb on the outside of the arm and palpating the proximal side of the arm with the index finger and middle fingers. • If a pulse is palpated, continue rescue breathing 12 to 20 times per minute or once every 3 to 5 seconds. • If a pulse is absent, begin cardiac compressions.	21. The carotid pulse is often difficult to locate in the infant; therefore the brachial artery is the recommended site.
22. Cardiac compressions (infant 1–12 months): • Maintain a position parallel to the infant. Infants can easily be placed on a table or other hard surface. • Place a small towel or other support under the infant's shoulders/neck. • Position the hands for compressions: a. Using the hand closest to the infant's feet, locate the intermammary line where it intersects the sternum. b. Place the index finger 1 cm below this location on the sternum and place the middle finger next to the index finger. c. Using these two fingers, compress in a downward motion one-third to one-half the depth of the chest at the rate of 100 times per minute. d. Keep the other hand on the infant's forehead. e. At the end of every thirtieth compression, administer two ventilations (30 compressions: 2 ventilations) (1 second per breath).	22. Irreversible brain and tissue damage can occur if a client is hypoxic for more than 4 to 6 minutes. Proper positioning is essential for the following reasons: • Allows for maximum compression of the heart between the sternum and vertebrae. • A small towel, diaper roll, or some other type of support is necessary for effective cardiac compressions. • Compressions over the xiphoid process can lacerate the liver. • Keeping other fingers and hands off the chest during compressions reduces risk of rib fracture. • Keeping one hand on the infant's forehead helps maintain an open airway.
f. Reevaluate infant after 20 cycles. If respirations are still absent, call 911.	f. Guidelines published by the AHA (2005) recommend that about 5 cycles of CPR be performed for unresponsive infants and children up to the onset of adolescence/puberty before calling 911. In institutions, follow hospital protocol.
CPR: Two Rescuers—Child (1 to onset of adolescence/puberty) and Infant (1–12 months)	
23. Follow Action 14 for two-rescuer CPR for adults with the following changes: • Utilize the child or infant procedure for chest compressions. • Change the ratio of compressions to ventilation to 15:2 (15 chest compressions to 2 ventilations). • Deliver the ventilation on the upstroke of the third compression.	23. Improper hand placement can cause internal organ damage or other medical complications in infants or children. Delivering ventilation during the upstroke phase allows for full lung expansion during inspiration.

(Continues)

PROCEDURE 29-38 Performing Cardiopulmonary Resuscitation (CPR) (Continued)

ACTION	RATIONALE
CPR—Neonate or Premature Infant	
24. Follow the infant guidelines with the following changes for chest compressions: • Encircle the chest with both hands. • Position thumbs over the midsternum. • Compress the midsternum with both thumbs. • Compress one-third to one-half the depth of the chest at a rate of 100 to 120 times per minute.	24. Improper hand placement can cause internal organ damage or other medical complications in infants or children.
25. If properly trained use an automated external defibrillator (AED). Use adult defibrillation pads for adults. Use the pediatric system for children 1 to 8 years of age, if available. Use AED after 5 cycles of CPR on children age 1 to the onset of adolescence/puberty. In hospital setting, use defibrillator as specified by institution protocol. Defibrillator should be placed only by properly trained personnel.	25. The use of an AED can increase the client's chances for survival by restoring rhythm and circulation. Protocol in hospital setting include the use of defibrillator with codes and can increase survival. Injury to self, staff, or the client may occur with untrained personnel.

EVALUATION

- There should be a constant evaluation for the return of spontaneous pulse and respirations.
- Successful intervention with CPR is illustrated as follows:
  - — An open airway is maintained, as evident by the visible chest rise and fall.
  - — The resistance and compliance of the client's lungs is felt.
  - — Airway movement during expiration is felt and heard.
  - — Circulation indicators, such as color, improve.
  - — The client has return of spontaneous pulse and respirations, as evidenced by a palpable carotid or brachial pulse and the presence of respiratory effort.
- Assist with transfer to hospital/advanced life-support unit.
- If CPR was unsuccessful, assist in notifying next of kin and providing psychosocial support.

DOCUMENTATION

Nurses' Notes/Code Record

- Time and condition in which the client was found
- Interventions that were implemented, including accurate times, results of the implementations, orders received from the physicians, vital signs of the client, timing of the incident, and status of the client afterward

Medication Administration Record

- Medications the client received, including time and route, during the procedure
- If the incident occurs in a noninstitutional setting, report findings and interventions to aid personnel when they arrive

PROCEDURE 29-39 Admitting a Client

OVERVIEW

The procedure for admitting a client to a health care facility is extremely important. First impressions of the facility and caregivers are lasting ones. A calm, caring approach instills confidence in the client and the belief that the client's needs are important. Orienting the client to the room, nursing unit, and facility will help the client to be comfortable in the health care environment.

ASSESSMENT

1. Assess the client's comfort level about being in a health care facility. **Identifies needed nurse–client interactions.**
2. Assess client's physical and mental state. **Provides basis for nursing care. Shows caring and concern for the client.**

(Continues)

PROCEDURE 29-39 Admitting a Client (Continued)

3. Assess client's knowledge of reason for admission. **Provides basis for nurse–client interaction and client teaching.**

POSSIBLE NURSING DIAGNOSES

Fear
Anxiety
Deficient Knowledge (health care facility)

PLANNING

Expected Outcomes

1. Client will be comfortable in health care facility.
2. Client will understand how to use call bell system, bed controls, television, and telephone.
3. The client will adjust to facility routine.

Equipment Needed

- Admission kit: wash basin, emesis basin, pitcher, glass, etc.
- Client orientation materials
- Valuables envelope (if needed)
- Belongings checklist
- Admission Nursing Assessment form
- Sphygmomanometer, stethoscope, thermometer

delegation tips

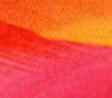

Admitting a client may be delegated to ancillary personnel after proper instruction. The nursing assessment must be performed by the nurse and may not be delegated.

IMPLEMENTATION—ACTION/RATIONALE

ACTION	RATIONALE
* Wash hands *	
1. Welcome client to unit. Introduce yourself by name and title. Ask client to state his or her name.	1. Verifies identification.
2. Orient client to room and nursing unit. Describe items such as nurse call bell system, location of bathroom, place for clothing, bed controls, television, telephone, visiting hours, meal times, Standard Precautions, and review items in client education materials such as client rights and other written information about the facility.	2. Reduces client anxiety; allows fuller participation in care.
3. Provide privacy for client to change into pajamas or hospital gown, if not already done.	3. Respects client privacy.
4. Show client ID bracelet to double-check proper identification. Attach bracelet to wrist. (This may have been done in Admitting Department.) Review drug allergies and attach allergy bracelet to same wrist, according to agency policy.	4. Confirms client identification; promotes client safety.
5. Document and store client's belongings and valuables according to agency policy.	5. Reduces the risk of loss.
6. Begin nursing assessment, according to agency policy.	6. Starts development of client database.
7. Perform any other actions, as directed by agency policy.	7. Different facilities have different needs, regulations, and guidelines for client admission.

EVALUATION

- The client is comfortable in the health care facility.
- The client uses call bell system, bed controls, television, and telephone.
- The client has adjusted to facility routing.

DOCUMENTATION

- Complete admitting nursing assessment record
- Time and condition of client on admission
- All valuables sent to the safe
- Client's belongings
- Client's comfort level

PROCEDURE 29-40 Transferring a Client

OVERVIEW

Transferring a client to a different unit in a health care facility can be very stressful to the client. It may mean that the client's condition has deteriorated (transferring to ICU) or improved (transferring to a rehabilitation unit after a hip replacement), thus requiring different treatments.

However short the stay before a transfer, the client has a sense of knowing the environment and the health care personnel on that unit. Explaining the reason for transfer to the client and family, as well as gathering all equipment, medications, and assisting in collecting client's personal belongings, help ease the stress of a transfer.

Introducing the client and family to health care personnel working on the new unit and sharing some of the client's personal preferences in the client's presence (i.e., prefers one pillow and an extra blanket) shows caring and concern for the client and helps ensure continuity of care.

ASSESSMENT

1. Assess client's knowledge and feelings about the transfer. **Allows for explanations and discussion about the situation.**
2. Assess which equipment is to be transferred with the client and that those medications and client's personal belongings are ready to move. **Provides organization to the transfer and encourages completeness.**
3. Assess readiness of new unit to accept client. **Allows transfer to proceed smoothly with no waiting.**

POSSIBLE NURSING DIAGNOSES

Anxiety
Fear
Hopelessness

PLANNING

Expected Outcomes

1. Client will understand reason for transfer.
2. Client will be safely moved with needed equipment and medications and all personal belongings.
3. Client's move will be communicated to appropriate department for continuity of care (i.e., Dietary, Pharmacy).

Equipment Needed

- Client's medical record (if not electronic)
- Client's imprint card
- Client's medications
- Stretcher or wheelchair
- Cart to carry client's belongings

delegation tips

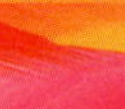

Ancillary personnel may assist with transferring a client. The nurse is responsible for transferring the client's medical record and medications and for giving a thorough report to the accepting nurse on the new unit.

IMPLEMENTATION—ACTION/RATIONALE

ACTION	RATIONALE
* Wash hands * Check client's identification band *	
1. Check to see if order is needed to initiate transfer according to agency policy.	1. Policies differ among facilities.
2. Call nursing unit of new location to see if bed is ready and to give report.	2. Provides continuity of care.
3. Explain the transfer to the client (and family, if appropriate). Answer any questions. Allay anxieties about moving.	3. Keeps client informed and promotes cooperation.
4. Review the valuables and belongings checklist completed on admission. Compare with belongings.	4. Ensures all of client's belongings are transferred with the client. Prevents loss.
5. Gather records and any other equipment that is transferred with the client, according to agency policy, such as eyedrops, other medications, IV pump, and respiratory therapy equipment.	5. Helps make transfer more efficient and reduces multiple trips to new area.

(Continues)

PROCEDURE 29-40 Transferring a Client (Continued)

ACTION	RATIONALE
6. Transfer client by appropriate vehicle (wheelchair, stretcher). Accompany client to new unit. Transfer care to another staff member in person. Ensure that call bell is within reach or staff member is in room before leaving client.	6. Enhances continuity of care. Promotes safety.
7. Document time of transfer and any other information required by agency policy.	7. Promotes communication among members of the health care team.
8. Upon return to unit, notify appropriate personnel according to agency policy that client has left the unit. Arrange for personnel to clean the bed and surroundings the client left.	8. Prepares bed for new admission. Reduces transfer of microorganisms.

EVALUATION

- The client understands the reason for transferring to a new unit.
- The client is safely moved with needed equipment and medications and all personal belongings.
- The client's move was communicated to appropriate departments for continuity of care.

DOCUMENTATION

- Client's condition when leaving unit
- Equipment and medications transferred with the client
- Personal belongings sent with client.
- Report on client given to receiving nurse
- Departments notified of client's transfer

PROCEDURE 29-41 Discharging a Client

OVERVIEW

A client may be discharged from a health care facility to another facility or to home. This can be a frightening experience depending on the level of recuperation the client has achieved, the amount and type of medications prescribed, dietary needs or restrictions, and other treatments to be conducted. Being transferred from one facility to another is seen either as improvement or as a lack of progress in recovery.

Discuss with the client and family the discharge process. Complete all paperwork and all discharge teaching. Collect the client's belongings and valuables (as documented on admission) so they accompany the client. These things make the discharge process pleasant and effective.

ASSESSMENT

1. Assess client's feelings about being discharged. **Opens communication about the discharge.**
2. Assess that family and home or the other facility is prepared to receive the client. **Provides a smooth process with less stress for the client.**
3. Assess client's or family's knowledge of care at home. **Ensures continuity of care.**

POSSIBLE NURSING DIAGNOSES

Anxiety

PLANNING

Expected Outcomes

1. Client will complete discharge to another facility with no problems.
2. Client will feel confident about care at home.

Equipment Needed

- Required facility paperwork
- Stretcher or wheelchair
- Cart for client's belongings

For Discharge to Home

- Prescriptions
- Instructions—care, diet, medications, follow-up appointment

(Continues)

PROCEDURE 29-41 Discharging a Client (Continued)

delegation tips

Ancillary personnel assist with the physical movements of discharging a client. The nurse reviews with the client prescriptions and instructions on care, diet, medications, and making a follow-up appointment.

IMPLEMENTATION—ACTION/RATIONALE

ACTION	RATIONALE
* Wash hands * Check client's identification band *	
1. Check order for discharge.	1. Most agency policies require order for discharge.
Discharge to Another Facility	
2. Explain discharge to client, and family, if appropriate.	2. Includes client in care. Promotes cooperation.
3. Complete intra-agency transfer form, according to policy. Be sure to note last time of medication doses. Complete nursing discharge summary. Prepare transfer paperwork, according to policy.	3. Facilitates continuity of care. Promotes client safety.
4. Notify receiving agency of impending transfer. Provide report and confirm ability to receive client.	4. Facilitates continuity of care. Ensures that new facility will accept client before client leaves current facility.
5. Arrange for transportation to new facility. Call transportation company according to agency policy.	5. Reduces waiting time; facilitates continuity of care.
6. Review the valuables and belongings checklist completed on admission. Compare with belongings.	6. Ensures all of client's belongings leave with the client. Prevents loss.
7. When personnel from transportation company arrive, assist client transfer to stretcher or wheelchair. Provide transportation personnel with required information, such as client's DNR status, for transfer. See that client's belongings accompany client, along with any required paperwork or equipment.	7. Provides continuity of care.
Discharge to Home	
8. Discuss discharge with client, and family, if appropriate. Confirm that discharge teaching has been done. Ask client if there are any questions about self-care at home. If so, follow up with appropriate personnel (typically, RN).	8. Promotes client cooperation. Allays anxiety.
9. LP/VN or RN (according to agency policy) reviews with client: prescriptions to be filled, including telling client when next dose is due based on medications administered in the facility; food and drug interactions and any other essential medication information; care of incision or dressings, if indicated; dietary needs or restrictions or other pertinent information; and when client should make appointment for follow-up with private physician.	9. Promotes continuity of care.
10. Have client/family provide return demonstration of skills required for self-care at home.	10. Demonstrates that learning has occurred.
11. Check that transportation to home is available. Check client room area for any personal belongings.	11. Reduces waiting time.

(Continues)

PROCEDURE 29-41 Discharging a Client (Continued)

ACTION	RATIONALE
12. Complete any paperwork with client, as required by agency policy.	12. Meets regulatory requirements.
13. Escort client to transportation vehicle.	13. Promotes client safety.
For Any Discharge	
14. Notify appropriate personnel according to agency policy that client left the unit. Arrange for personnel to clean the bed and surroundings the client left.	14. Prepares bed for new admission. Reduces transfer of microorganisms.

EVALUATION

- The client encountered no problems in discharge to another facility.
- The client, with the assistance of family, is confident about care at home.

DOCUMENTATION

- Date and time of discharge
- Belongings and valuables with client

Discharge to Another Facility

- Person receiving report on client
- Company transporting client

Discharge to Home

- Mode of taking client to transportation vehicle
- Person taking client home
- Prescriptions and instructions given to client

PROCEDURE 29-42 Initiating Strict Isolation Precautions

OVERVIEW

Occasionally, a client is placed in isolation to prevent the spread of an infectious process. Barrier protective equipment is put on outside the room before providing any client care. All linens and trash are double-bagged, according to agency policy, before he is removed from an isolation room. Meals are served on disposable dishes.

Visitors may be limited because everyone entering the room must wear barrier protective equipment. Some clients feel the isolation very profoundly. Paperback books (to be discarded later), TV, and other diversional activities help the client pass the time.

ASSESSMENT

1. Review physician's orders for isolation to ensure proper setup.
2. Assess client's and family's understanding of client's condition and reason for isolation to identify required teaching needed.

POSSIBLE NURSING DIAGNOSES

Social Isolation
Impaired Social Interaction
Deficient Knowledge (disease process, isolation)
Risk for Powerlessness
Risk for Loneliness

PLANNING

Expected Outcomes

1. The room will be set up for the appropriate type of isolation.
2. The client and family will understand the client's condition and the reason for isolation.

Equipment Needed

- Isolation sign
- Disposable gowns
- Gloves (nonsterile and sterile)
- Goggles or face shield
- Disposable masks
- Impermeable bags (for linen and trash)
- Tape or bag ties and labels
- Disposable vital signs equipment (single-use thermometers, stethoscope, and sphygmomanometer) if available
- Disposable water pitcher and cups
- Linen
- Room with sink and running water
- Other supplies relative to client's condition

(Continues)

PROCEDURE 29-42 Initiating Strict Isolation Precautions (Continued)

delegation tips

Initiating strict isolation precautions is a nursing responsibility. Properly trained ancillary personnel may provide some client care according to agency policy.

IMPLEMENTATION—ACTION/RATIONALE

ACTION	RATIONALE
* Check client's identification band * Explain procedure before beginning * * Note: Barrier protection must be on before checking client's ID *	
1. Review physician orders and agency protocols relative to the type of isolation precautions: a. Implement protocol related to the type of disinfectants needed to eliminate specific microorganisms. b. Alert housekeeping regarding the room number and type of isolation supplies needed in the room. c. Make sure the room has proper ventilation (the door remains closed at all times) and that the bed and other electrical equipment are functioning properly.	1. Ensures compliance without unnecessary stress being placed on the client and family. Allows housekeeping to have the necessary supplies on their cleaning carts. Provides for client comfort and decreases the spread of microorganisms. Limits the number of personnel coming into the client's room and the client's exposure to microorganisms.
2. Place appropriate isolation supplies outside the client's room and place isolation sign on the door.	2. Ensures staff follows isolation protocol and alerts visitors to check with the nurses' station before entering the room.
3. Gather appropriate supplies to take in the room: a. Linen b. Impermeable bags c. Disposable vital signs equipment, if available d. Wound care supplies, if appropriate	3. Provides for organized care, hand hygiene, proper isolation, and client care materials. Decreases the spread of microorganisms and the number of times caregivers go into and out of the room.
4. Remove jewelry, lab coat, and other items not necessary for providing client care.	4. Decreases the spread of resident and transient microorganisms.
5. Wash hands and don disposable clothing: a. Apply mask by placing the top of the mask over the bridge of your nose (top part of mask has a lightweight metal strip) and pinch the metal strip to fit snugly against your skin. b. Apply cap to cover hair and ears completely, if policy requires cap. c. Apply gown to cover outer garments completely: Hold gown in front of body and place arms through sleeves (Figure 29-42-1A). Pull sleeves down to wrist. Tie gown securely at neck and waist (Figure 29-42-1B, C). d. Don nonsterile gloves and pull gloves to cover gown's cuff. e. Don goggles or face shield.	5. Disposable garments act as a barrier protecting from contact with pathogens. e. Eyeglasses do not offer adequate protection.
6. Enter client's room with all gathered supplies; if client is to receive medications, bring them at this time.	6. Prevents trips into and out of client room and keeps supplies clean.
7. Assess client and family knowledge relative to client's diagnosis and isolation: a. Reason isolation initiated b. Type of isolation c. Duration of isolation d. How to apply barrier protection	7. Client's and family's understanding of isolation procedures will increase their participation in care.

(Continues)

PROCEDURE 29-42 Initiating Strict Isolation Precautions (Continued)

ACTION	RATIONALE

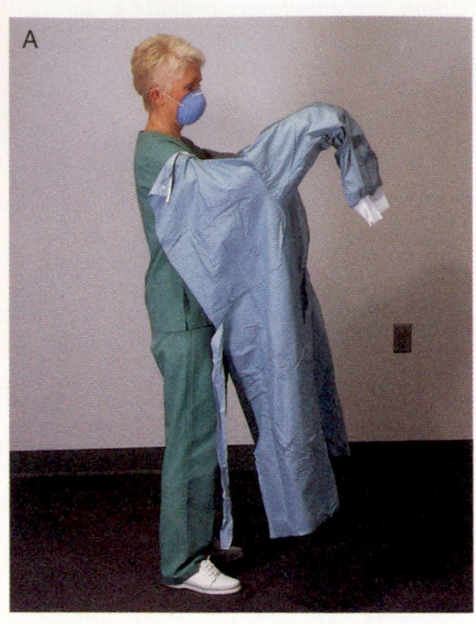

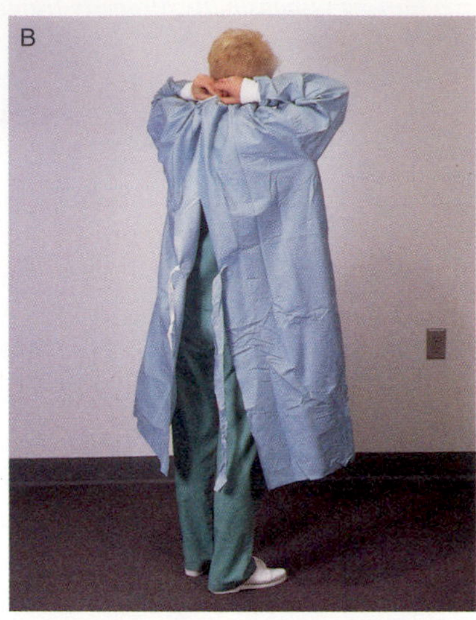

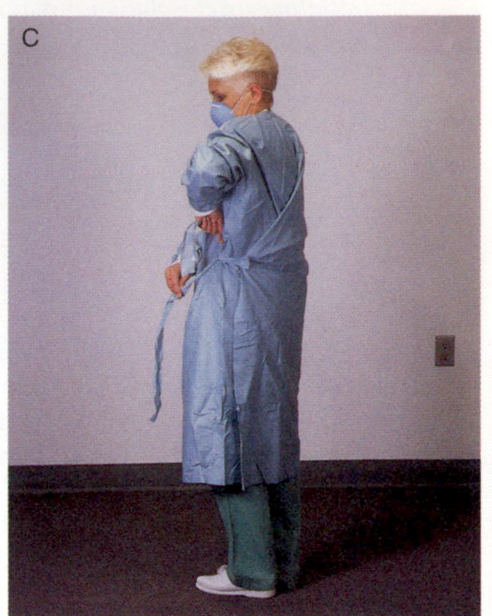

COURTESY OF DELMAR CENGAGE LEARNING

FIGURE 29-42-1 Donning disposable gowns; *A*, Hold gown in front of the body and place arms through the sleeves. *B*, Fasten neck ties. *C*, Fasten waist ties.

ACTION	RATIONALE
8. Assess vital signs, administer medications if appropriate, and perform other functions of nursing care to meet client needs. Record assessment data on a piece of paper, avoiding contact with any articles in the client's room.	8. Allows for data collection and the performance of client care measures.
9. Dispose of soiled articles in the impermeable bags, which should be labeled correctly according to contents. If soiled reusable equipment is removed from the room, label bag accordingly.	9. Impermeable bags prevent the leakage of contaminated materials, thereby preventing the spread of infection. Labeling is a warning to other personnel that the contents are infectious.
10. Double-bag soiled linen according to agency policy in an impermeable bag or in plastic linen bag.	10. Double-bagging allows the washing of soiled linen without human contact. When linen is double-bagged, the first bag is removed before washing and the second bag goes into the machine with the dirty linen and dissolves.
11. Replenish supplies before leaving the client's room by having another staff member bring the clean supplies and transfer at the door. Ask client if anything is needed (e.g., juice or personal care items).	11. Decreases the number of times staff members go in and out of the room.
12. Before leaving, let the client know when you will return and make sure call light is accessible.	12. Decreases a feeling of abandonment; provides client with a means of communication.
13. Exiting the isolation room: a. Untie gown at waist. b. Remove one glove by grasping the glove's cuff and pulling down so that the glove turns inside out (glove on glove) and dispose of it. With your ungloved hand, slip your fingers inside the cuff of the other glove, pull it off, inside out, and dispose of it.	13. Gloves are removed inside out to avoid contact with skin. The gown is removed and folded with hands touching only the inside of the garment. Only the ties and the inside of the cap are touched with your hands. All articles are disposed of as soon as they are removed.
c. Grasp and release the ties of the mask, and dispose of it.	c. If a client has an airborne-spread disease, the mask may be removed last.
d. Release neck ties of the gown and allow the gown to fall forward. Place fingers of dominant	

(Continues)

PROCEDURE 29-42 Initiating Strict Isolation Precautions (Continued)

ACTION	RATIONALE

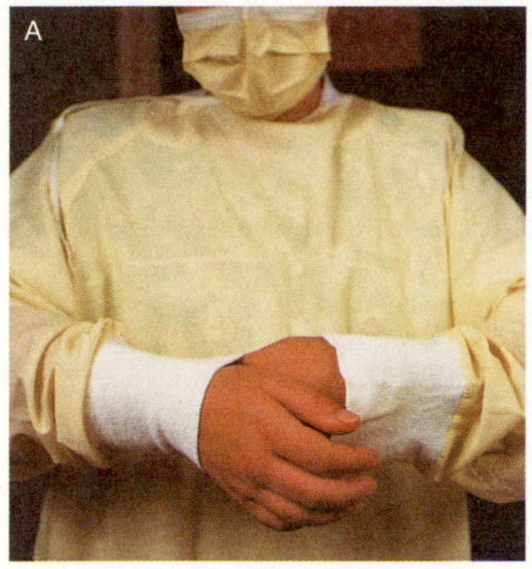

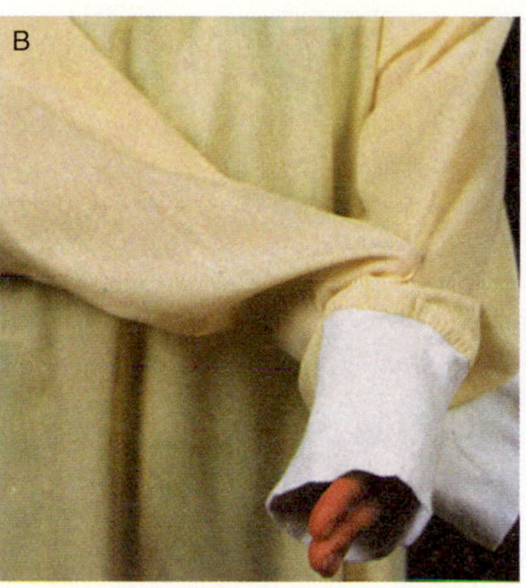

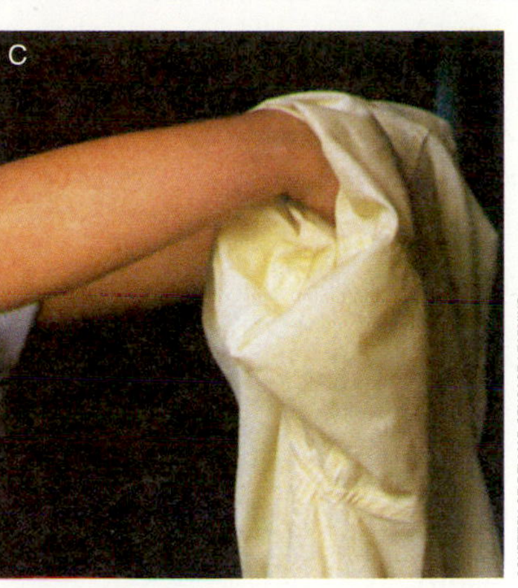

FIGURE 29-42-2 Removing disposable gown: *A*, Place fingers of dominant hand inside the cuff of the other hand and pull gown down over other hand; *B*, With the gown-covered hand, pull gown down over the dominant hand. *C*, As the gown is removed, fold the outside of the gown together and dispose of it.

ACTION	RATIONALE
hand inside cuff of other hand and pull down over other hand (Figure 29-42-2A). With gown-covered hand, pull gown over the dominant hand (Figure 29-42-2B). While gown is still on arm, fold outside of gown together, remove, and dispose of it (Figure 29-42-2C). e. Remove cap by slipping your finger under the cap and removing from the front to back and dispose of it.	
14. Wash hands. Don nonsterile gloves and remove bags from the client's room. Exit room and close door. Dispose of bags according to agency protocol. Remove gloves and wash hands.	14. Reduces transmission of microorganisms.

EVALUATION

- The appropriate type of isolation was instituted.
- The client and family express understanding of the client's condition and the reason for isolation.

DOCUMENTATION

Nurses' Notes

- Date, time, and type of isolation instituted
- Client response to isolation
- Client and family teaching regarding isolation
- Document on appropriate electronic medical record or flow sheet

REFERENCES/SUGGESTED READING

American Academy of Physician Assistants (AAPA). (2009). Joint Commission Standards-restraint and seclusion. Retrieved March 15, 2009 from http://www.aapa.org/gandp/joint-commission-restraint.html

American College of Emergency Physicians Foundation. (2009a). What to do in a medical emergency. Retrieved March 15, 2009, from http://www.emergencycareforyou.org/EmergencyManual/WhatToDoInMedical Emergency

American College of Emergency Physicians Foundation. (2009b). How to perform CPR. Retrieved March 15, 2009, from http://www.emergencycareforyou.org/EmergencyManual/HowToPerformCPR/Default/aspx

American Heart Association. (2005). 2005 American Heart Association guidelines for cardiopulmonary resuscitation and emergency cardiovascular care (Part 3: Overview of CPR). *Circulation, 112,* IV-12–IV-18. Retrieved March 15, 2009, from http://circ.ahajournals.org/cgi/content/full/112/24_suppl/IV-12

American Heart Association. (2005–2006). Highlights of the American Heart Association guidelines for cardiopulmonary resuscitation and emergency cardiovascular care. *Currents in Emergency Cardiovascular Care, 16*(4). Retrieved March 15, 2009, from http://www.americanheart.org/presenter.jhtml?identifier+3012268

Centers for Disease Control and Prevention. (2007). Guideline for hand hygiene in health-care settings. Available: http://www.cdc.gov/mmwr/preview/mmwrhtml/ rr5116a1.htm

Daniels, R. (2010). *Delmar's guide to laboratory and diagnostic tests, 2nd edition.* Clifton Park, NY: Delmar Cengage Learning.

Exergen Corporation. (2009). *Exergen temporal artery thermometry: Changing the way the world take temperature.* Retrieved March 8, 2009 from http://exergencorporations.web.officelive.com/Thermal.aspx

General Practice Notebook. (2009). Dorsalis pedis pulse. Retrieved on March 4, 2009, from http://www.gpnotebook.co.uk/simplepage.cfm?ID=-1818623972

Infection Control. (2002). "Hand hygiene" news. *Nursing2002, 32*(5), 32hn6.

Joint Commission. (2008). Provision of care, treatment, and services. Retrieved March 9, 2009 from HYPERLINK "http://www.jointcommission.org/AccreditationPrograms/BehavioralHealthCare/Standards/O" http://www.jointcommission.org/AccreditationPrograms/BehavioralHealthCare/Standards/09_FAQs/PC/Restraint+_Seclusion.htm

Martin, P. (2003). CPR when the patient's pregnant. *RN, 66*(8), 34–39.

National Institutes of Health. (2008). NIH policy manual (OD/OM/ORFDO/DEP 301-496-3537). Retrieved March 3, 2009, from http://www1.od.nih.gov/oma/manualchapters/intramural/3033/main.html

Nelson, A., Owen, B., Lloyd, J., Fragala, G., Matz, M., Amato, M., et al. (2003). Safe patient handling and movement. *American Journal of Nursing, 103*(3), 32–43.

NANDA International. (2009). *NANDA-I nursing diagnoses: Definitions and classification 2009–2011.* Ames, IA: Wiley-Blackwell.

Parini, S., & Myers, F. (2003). Keeping up with hand hygiene recommendations. *Nursing2003, 33*(2), 17.

Pullen, R. (2003). Caring for a patient on pulse oximetry. *Nursing2003, 33*(9), 30.

Ramponi, D. (2001). Eye on contact lens removal. *Nursing2001, 31*(8), 56–57.

Siegel, J., Rhinehart, E., Jackson, M., & Chiarello, L. (2007). Guideline for isolation precations: Preventing transmission of infectious agents in healthcare settings. Retrieved December 5, 2009 from http://www.cdc.gov/ncidod/dhqp/pdf/guidelines/Isolation2007.pdf

CHAPTER 30
Intermediate Procedures

PROCEDURE 30-1 Surgical Asepsis: Preparing and Maintaining a Sterile Field

OVERVIEW
Preparing and maintaining a sterile field is basic to many nursing procedures, such as inserting a urinary catheter and changing surgical dressings. It takes practice to develop a "sterile conscience," a consistent awareness of what is sterile, and to maintain the sterility.

ASSESSMENT
1. Assess all packages to determine that they are dry and intact. **Assesses the sterility of packages.**
2. Assess the local environment for a dry, horizontal, stable area. **A dry, flat workspace is best for a sterile field.**

POSSIBLE NURSING DIAGNOSIS
Risk for Infection

PLANNING
Expected Outcomes
1. Sterility of the field and all packages, while being opened, will be maintained.
2. Sterility of the procedure will be maintained.

Equipment Needed
- Sterile kit as needed for procedure
- Sterile gloves (if not in kit)
- Sterile drape (if needed)
- Sterile solution (if needed)
- Other sterile items as required

delegation tips

Only nurses should prepare and maintain a sterile field, with the exception of surgical technicians in the OR.

IMPLEMENTATION—ACTION/RATIONALE

ACTION	RATIONALE
* Wash hands * Check client's identification band*	
1. Gather equipment for the type of procedure: a. Select only clean, dry packages marked sterile, and read listing of contents. b. Check the package for integrity and expiration date.	1. Prevents break in technique during procedure. If the package is moist or outdated, it is considered contaminated and cannot be used.
2. Select a clean area in the client's environment to establish the sterile field.	2. Promotes access to the sterile field during the procedure.
3. Explain procedure to the client; provide specific instructions if client assistance is required during the procedure.	3. Gains client's understanding and cooperation during the procedure.

(Continues)

PROCEDURE 30-1 Surgical Asepsis: Preparing and Maintaining a Sterile Field (Continued)

ACTION	RATIONALE
4. Inquire about and attend to the client's toileting needs.	4. Prevents break in technique during the procedure.
5. Hospital environment: If the procedure is to be performed at the client's bedside, the client should be in a private room or moved to a clean treatment room if available.	5. Minimizes microorganisms in the environment.
6. Home environment: Secure privacy and remove pets from the room.	6. Puts the client at ease and promotes a clean environment.
7. Position client and attend to comfort measures; the client's position should provide easy access to the area and facilitate good body mechanics during the procedure.	7. Helps the client relax and prevents movement during the procedure; prevents reaching, decreasing the risk of contamination and back strain.
8. Wash hands.	8. Reduces transmission of microorganisms.
9. Place sterile package (drape or tray) in the center of the clean, dry work area.	9. Prevents reaching over exposed sterile items when wrapper is removed.
Drape	
10. Open the wrapper, pulling away from the body first.	10. Prevents contamination.
11. Grasp the top edge of the drape with fingertips of one hand.	11. Edges are considered unsterile.
12. Remove the drape by lifting up and away from all objects while it unfolds; discard the outer wrapper with other hand.	12. If the drape touches an unsterile object, it is contaminated and must be discarded.
13. With free hand, grasp the other drape corner, keeping it away from all objects.	13. Avoids contamination.
14. Lay the drape on the surface, with the drape bottom first touching the surface farthest from you; step back and allow the drape to cover the surface.	14. Prevents you from reaching over the sterile field; stepping back decreases risk that drape will touch your uniform.
Tray	
15. Remove outer wrapping and place the tray on the work surface so that the top flap of the sterile wrapper opens away from you.	15. Prevents reaching over the sterile items.
16. Reach around the tray, not over it. With thumb and index fingertips grasping the wrapper's top flap, gently pull up, then down to open over the surface.	16. Only the edges of the field can be contaminated, pulling up frees the top folded flap.
17. Repeat the same steps to open the side flaps.	17. Keeps the arm from reaching over the sterile field.
18. Grasp the corner of the bottom flap with fingertips, step back, and pull flap down (Figure 30-1-1).	18. Creates a sterile work surface.

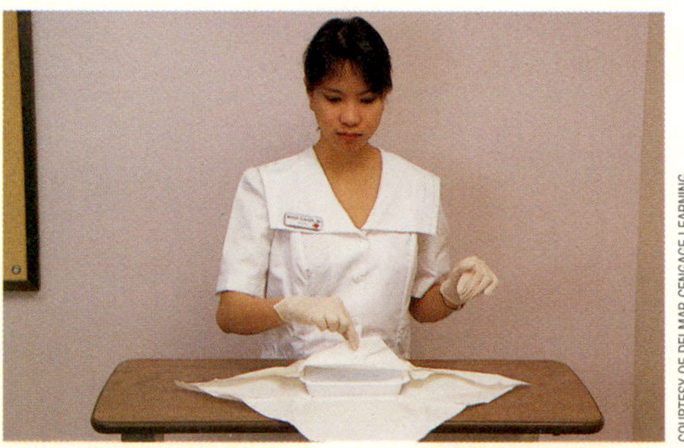
COURTESY OF DELMAR CENGAGE LEARNING

FIGURE 30-1-1 Grasp the corner of the bottom flap with fingertips, step back, and pull flap down (gloves not required for this procedure).

(Continues)

PROCEDURE 30-1 Surgical Asepsis: Preparing and Maintaining a Sterile Field (Continued)

ACTION	RATIONALE
Adding Additional Sterile Items to Sterile Field	
19. While facing the sterile field, step back, remove the outer wrapper, and grasp the item in your nondominant hand so that the top flap will open away from you.	19. Keeps your dominant hand free, item remains sterile.
20. With your dominant hand, open the flaps as previously described.	20. Prevents reaching over the sterile item.
21. With your dominant hand, pull the wrapper back and away from the sterile field (toward your nondominant arm holding the item) and place the item onto the field.	21. Prevents the wrapper from touching the sterile field.
22. When adding additional gauze or dressings to the sterile field, open the package as directed, grasp the top flaps of the wrapper and pull downward (Figure 30-1-2), then drop the contents onto the center of the field (Figure 30-1-3).	22. Prevents contamination of item and sterile field.

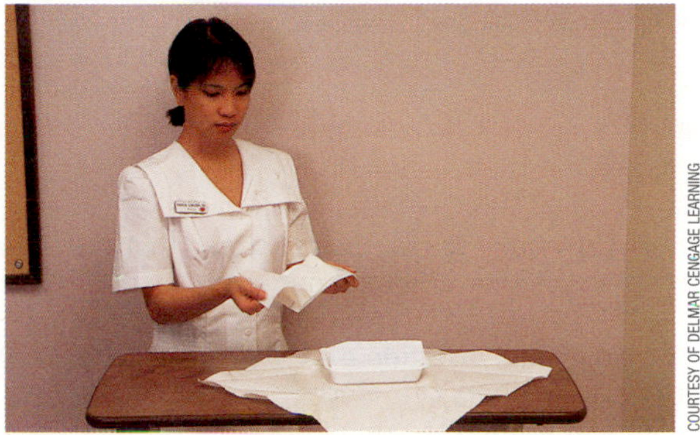

FIGURE 30-1-2 Grasp the flaps of the wrapped supply and pull downward.

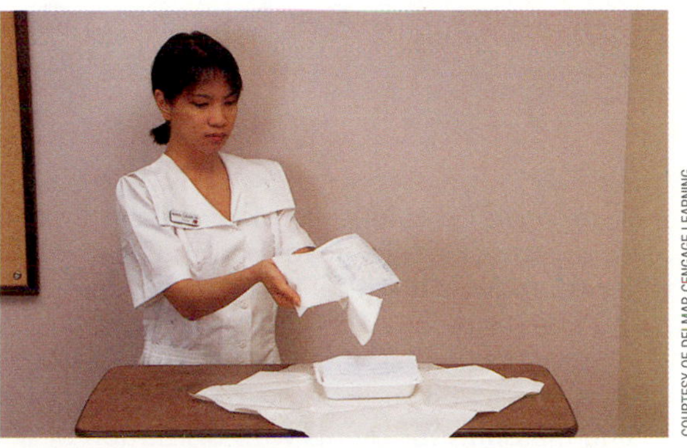

FIGURE 30-1-3 Add contents to the sterile field by holding the package 6 inches (15 cm) above the field and allowing the contents to drop onto the field.

ACTION	RATIONALE
Adding Solutions to Sterile Field	
23. Read the labels and strengths of all solutions three times before pouring.	23. Ensures proper solution and strength.
24. Remove the lid from the bottle of solution and invert the lid onto a clean surface.	24. Inverting the lid prevents contamination of the inner surface.
25. Hold the bottle, label facing ceiling, 4 to 6 inches (10 to 15 cm) over the container on the sterile field; slowly pour the solution into the container to avoid splashing. Pour from the side of the sterile field. Do not reach over it.	25. Prevents the label from getting wet. If the solution splashes onto the label, the field is contaminated because moisture conducts microorganisms from the nonsterile surface. Prevents contamination. If the solution splashes out of the container and the drape becomes wet, the field is contaminated.
26. Replace the lid on the container, label the container with the date and time, and initial the container.	26. Sterility of the solution will be lost if exposed to air for an extended period.
Using Sterile Gloves	
27. Wash hands and perform open gloving (see Procedure 30-2).	27. Prevents transmission of microorganisms.
28. Continue with procedure, keeping gloved hands above waist level at all times, touching only items on the sterile field.	28. Decreases chance of contamination.
29. If using a solution to cleanse a site, use the sterile forceps to prevent contamination of gloves; dispose of forceps after use or process instruments according to agency policy.	29. Prevents field contamination.

(Continues)

PROCEDURE 30-1 Surgical Asepsis: Preparing and Maintaining a Sterile Field (Continued)

ACTION	RATIONALE
30. Postprocedure, dispose of all contaminated items in appropriate receptacle.	30. Decreases risk of transmission of microorganisms to all health care workers.
31. Remove gloves as shown in Procedure 30-2.	31. Minimizes risk of contact with infectious wastes on the gloves.
32. Reposition the client.	32. Promotes client comfort.
33. Clean the environment; wash hands.	33. Prevents transmission of microorganisms.

EVALUATION

- Sterility of field was maintained.
- Sterility of procedure was maintained.

DOCUMENTATION

- Procedure completed following sterile technique.

PROCEDURE 30-2 Performing Open Gloving

OVERVIEW

Asepsis, or sterile technique, consists of those practices that eliminate all microorganisms and spores from an object or area. The use of sterile gloves is at the heart of aseptic technique. The ability to manipulate sterile items without contaminating them is critical to many diagnostic and therapeutic interventions. Common nursing procedures that require sterile technique are:

- All invasive procedures, either intentional perforation of the skin (injection, insertion of IV needles or catheters) or entry into a body orifice (tracheobronchial suctioning, insertion of a urinary catheter)
- Nursing measures for clients with disruption of skin surfaces (changing a surgical wound or IV site dressing) or destruction of skin layers (trauma and burns)

There are two methods for applying sterile gloves: open and closed. The open method is used most frequently when performing procedures that require the sterile technique, such as dressing changes, but that do not require donning a sterile gown.

ASSESSMENT

1. Assess the glove package. Is it intact? Is it wet or otherwise contaminated? **Assesses the sterility of the glove.**
2. Assess the local environment. Is there an area suitable for opening the package and applying the gloves? Is it dry? Is it reasonably stable and horizontal? Are there obvious airborne contaminants? **A flat, clear workspace is necessary to successfully carry out the procedure.**
3. Assess the correct glove size for proper fit. **Gloves come in many sizes, and proper fit is conducive to maintaining asepsis.**

POSSIBLE NURSING DIAGNOSIS

Risk for Infection

PLANNING

Expected Outcomes

1. Sterility of the gloves will be maintained while they are being applied.
2. Sterility of the procedure will be maintained.

Equipment Needed (Figure 30-2-1)

- Package of proper-sized sterile gloves

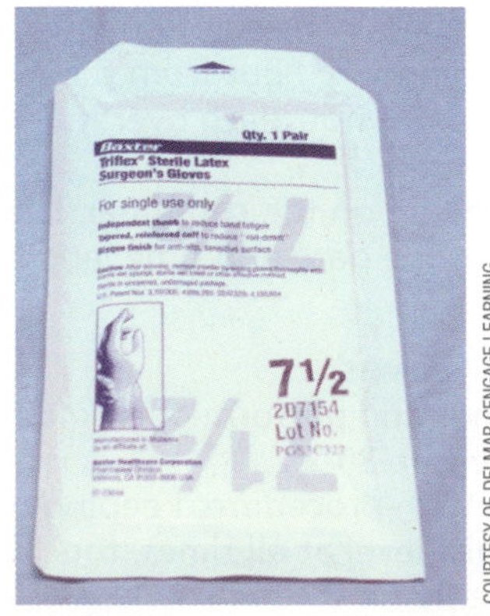

COURTESY OF DELMAR CENGAGE LEARNING

FIGURE 30-2-1 Sterile Gloves

(Continues)

PROCEDURE 30-2 Performing Open Gloving (Continued)

delegation tips

Sterile gloving is only delegated if the personnel are specifically trained, such as in a surgical suite or a testing laboratory setting.

IMPLEMENTATION—ACTION/RATIONALE

ACTION	RATIONALE
1. Wash hands.	1. Reduces transmission of microorganisms.
2. Read the manufacturer's instructions on the package of sterile gloves; proceed as directed in removing the outer wrapper from the package (Figure 30-2-2), placing the inner wrapper onto a clean, dry surface (Figure 30-2-3). Open inner wrapper to expose gloves (Figure 30-2-4).	2. Different manufacturers package gloves differently; the instructions will tell you how to open properly to avoid contamination of the inner wrapper; any moisture on the surface will contaminate the gloves.

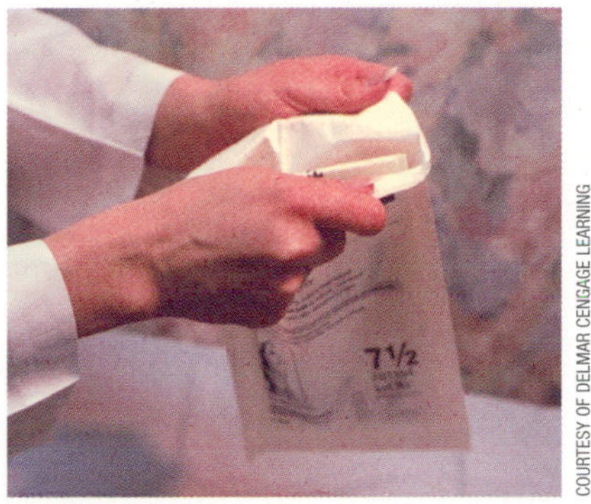

COURTESY OF DELMAR CENGAGE LEARNING

FIGURE 30-2-2 Remove the outer wrapper of the sterile glove package.

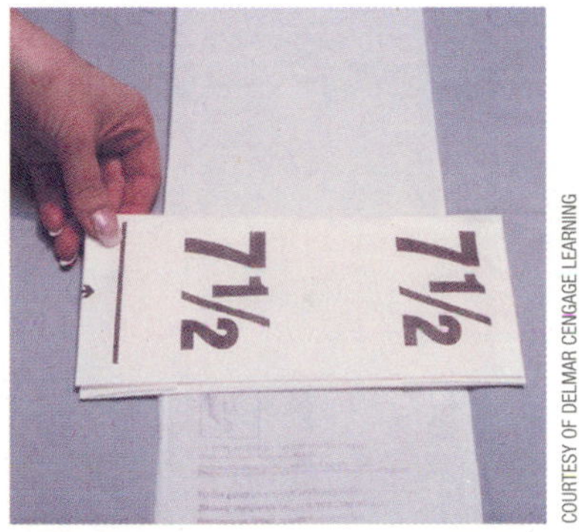

COURTESY OF DELMAR CENGAGE LEARNING

FIGURE 30-2-3 Place the gloves in the inner wrapper on a clean dry surface.

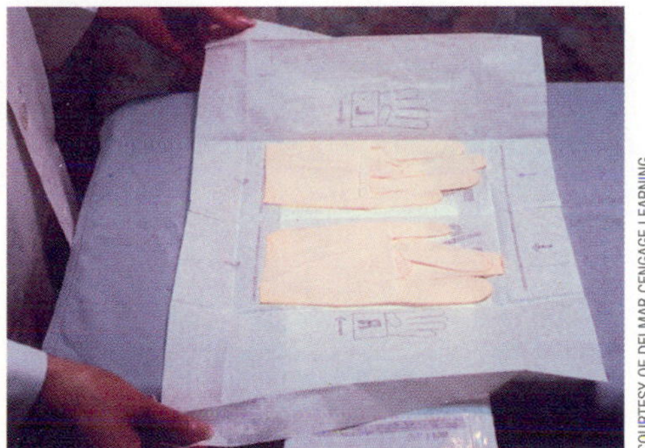
COURTESY OF DELMAR CENGAGE LEARNING

FIGURE 30-2-4 Open the inner wrapper to expose the gloves.

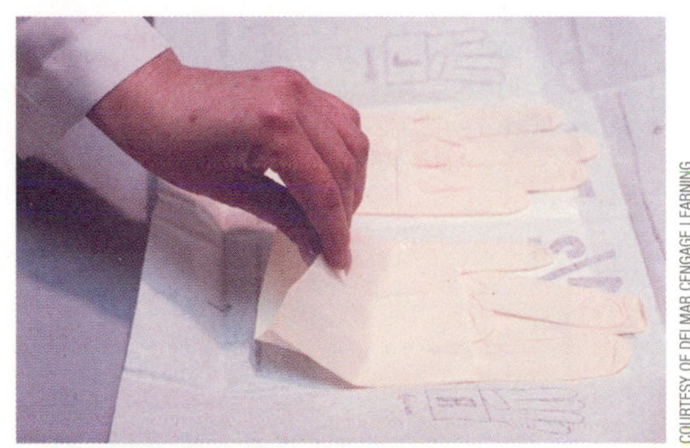
COURTESY OF DELMAR CENGAGE LEARNING

FIGURE 30-2-5 Grasp first cuff with the nondominant hand.

ACTION	RATIONALE
3. Identify right and left hand; glove dominant hand first.	3. Dominant hand should facilitate motor dexterity during gloving.
4. Grasp the 2-inch (5-cm) wide cuff with the thumb and first two fingers of the nondominant hand, touching only the inside of the cuff (Figure 30-2-5).	4. Maintains sterility of the outer surfaces of the sterile glove.
5. Gently pull the glove over the dominant hand, making sure the thumb and fingers fit into the proper spaces of the glove (Figure 30-2-6).	5. Prevents tearing the glove material; guiding the fingers into proper places facilitates gloving.

(Continues)

PROCEDURE 30-2 Performing Open Gloving (Continued)

ACTION	RATIONALE

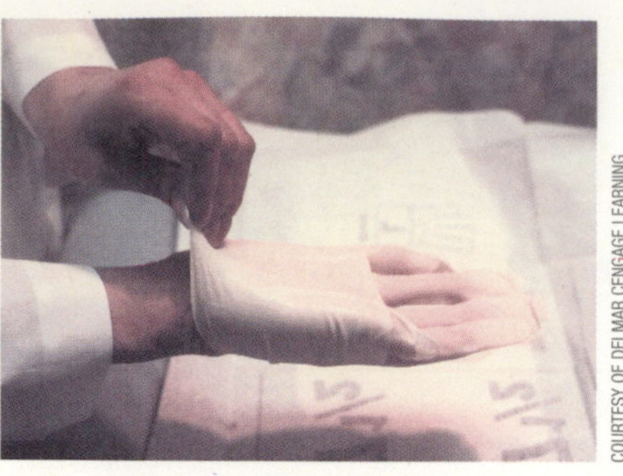

FIGURE 30-2-6 Pull the glove over the dominant hand.

6. With the gloved dominant hand, slip your fingers under the cuff of the other glove, gloved thumb abducted, making sure it does not touch any part on your nondominant hand (Figure 30-2-7).

   6. Cuff protects gloved fingers, maintaining sterility.

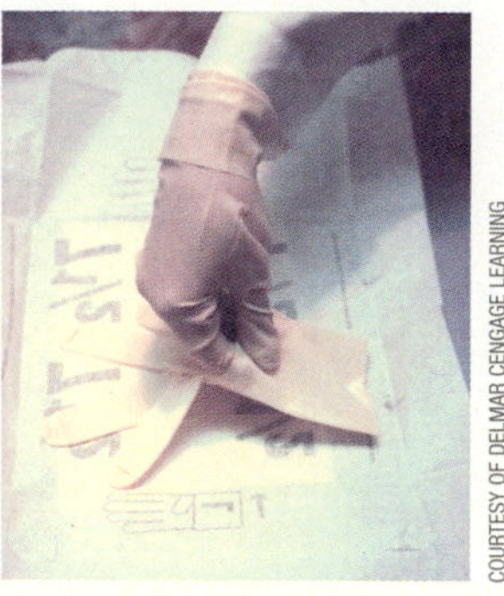

FIGURE 30-2-7 Slip fingers under the cuff of the second glove.

7. Gently slip the glove onto your nondominant hand, making sure the fingers slip into the proper spaces (Figures 30-2-8 and 30-2-9).

   7. Contact is made with two sterile gloves.

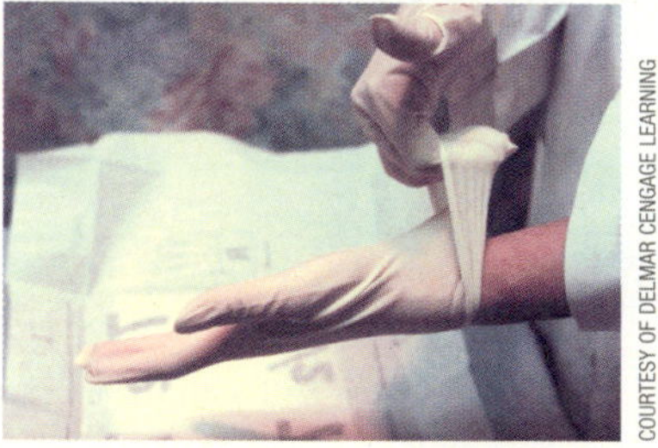

FIGURE 30-2-8 Pull on the second glove.

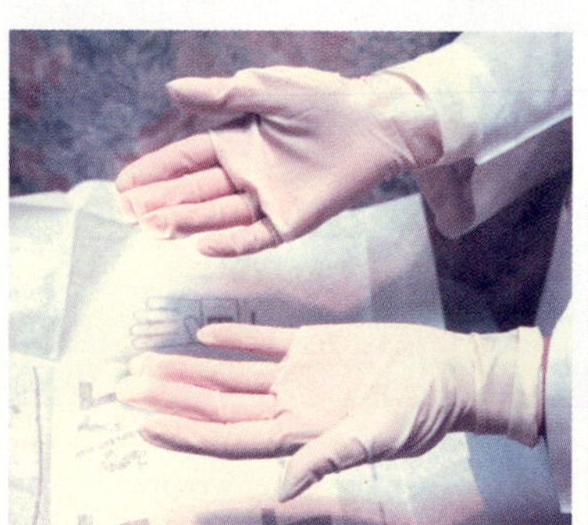

FIGURE 30-2-9 Make sure all fingers are in the proper spaces.

8. With gloved hands, interlock fingers to fit the gloves onto each finger. If the gloves are soiled, remove by turning inside out as follows:

   8. Promotes proper fit over the fingers.

(Continues)

PROCEDURE 30-2 Performing Open Gloving (Continued)

ACTION	RATIONALE
Removing Gloves If the gloves are soiled, remove them by turning inside out as follows:	
9. With your dominant hand, grasp the other glove at the wrist. Avoid touching the skin of your wrist with the fingers of the glove. Pull the glove off, turning it inside out. (Figure 30-2-10).	9. Prevents the transfer of microorganisms.
10. Place removed glove in palm of gloved hand.	10. Prevents the transmission of microorganisms.
11. Place thumb of ungloved hand inside the cuff of the gloved hand touching only the inside of the glove (Figure 30-2-11).	11. Reduces the transmission of microorganisms.

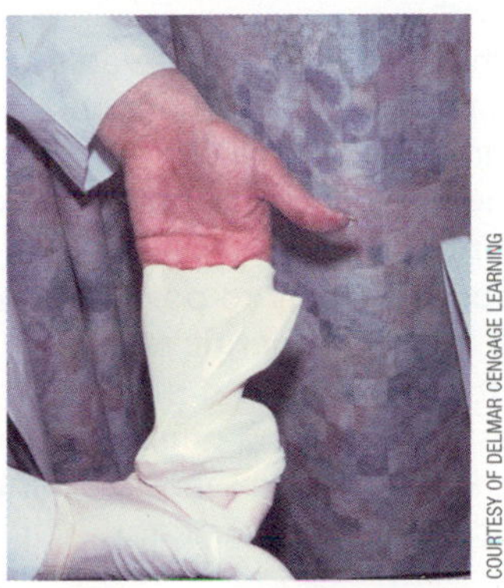

COURTESY OF DELMAR CENGAGE LEARNING

FIGURE 30-2-10 Pull glove off, turning it inside out.

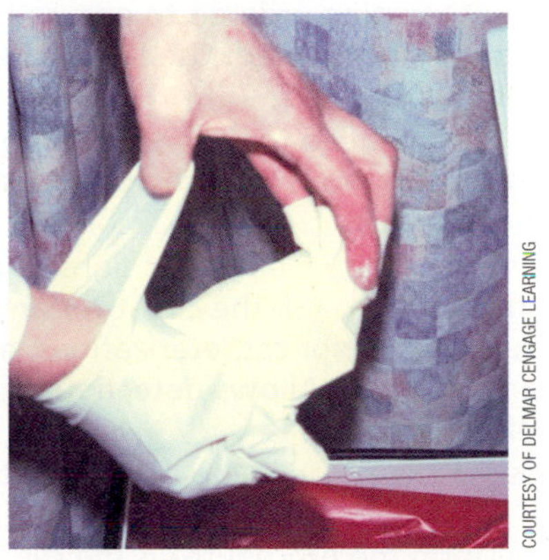

COURTESY OF DELMAR CENGAGE LEARNING

FIGURE 30-2-11 Slip uncovered thumb into the opposite glove.

ACTION	RATIONALE
12. Pull glove off, turning it inside out and over the other glove (Figure 30-2-12).	12. Reduces the transmission of microorganisms.
13. Dispose of soiled gloves according to institutional policy and wash hands (Figure 30-2-13).	13. Prevents the transfer of microorganisms.

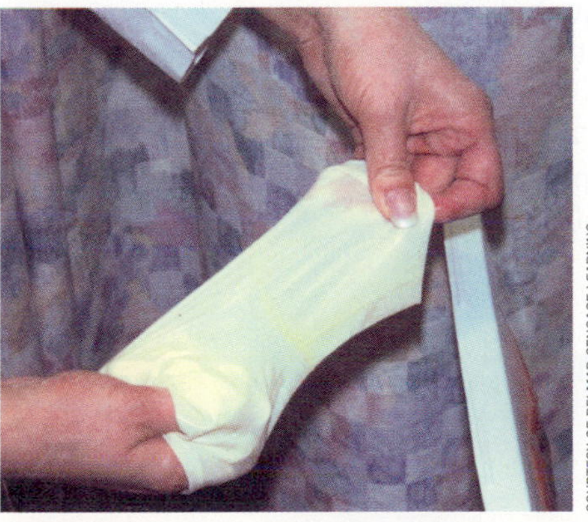

COURTESY OF DELMAR CENGAGE LEARNING

FIGURE 30-2-12 When soiled gloves are removed correctly, only the inside, clean surface of one glove is exposed.

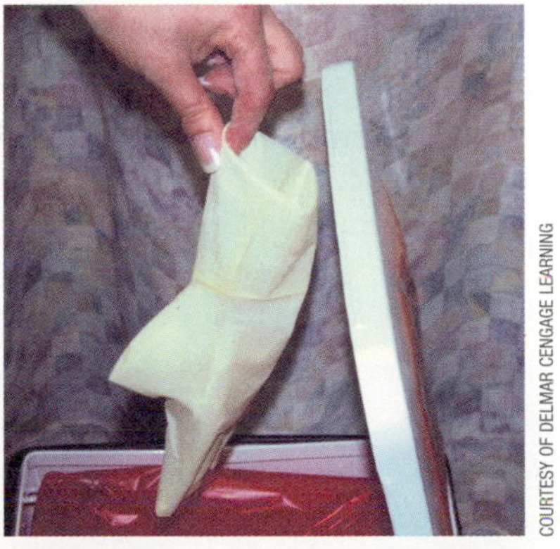

COURTESY OF DELMAR CENGAGE LEARNING

FIGURE 30-2-13 Dispose of gloves in appropriate receptacle.

EVALUATION

- Sterility of the gloves, sterile field, and procedure was maintained without breaks.

DOCUMENTATION

Nurses' Notes

- Procedure was performed using sterile technique.
- Document on appropriate electronic medical record or flow sheet.

PROCEDURE 30-3

Performing Urinary Catheterization: Female/Male

OVERVIEW

Catheterization involves passing a rubber or plastic tube into the bladder via the urethra to drain urine from the bladder or to obtain a urine specimen. Intermittent catheterization may be used to obtain a sample or to relieve bladder distention. Indwelling catheters may be used short-term to keep the bladder empty, prevent urinary retention, or allow precise measurement of urine. Long-term indwelling, or retention, catheters are used to control incontinence, prevent retention, or prevent the leakage of urine. Catheterization is a sterile procedure.

ASSESSMENT

1. Assess the need for catheterization and the type of catheterization ordered **to ensure the proper procedure is performed.** Use latex-free catheter if client has latex allergy.
2. Assess for the need for perineal care before catheterization **to reduce the transmission of microorganisms.**
3. Assess the urinary meatus for signs of infection or inflammation. Ask the client for any history of difficulty with prior catheterizations, anxiety, or urinary strictures. **Allows detection of potential complications.**
4. Assess the client's ability to assist with the procedure. Can she maintain the proper position while you perform the procedure? Is the client agitated, and could she contaminate the sterile field? Will you need assistance to hold her legs in position? **Determines how the procedure is to be carried out.**
5. Assess the light. Will you be able to see well enough to place the catheter, or do you need a secondary light source? **Determines what preparation needs to be done to ensure a successful procedure.**
6. Assess for an allergy to povidone-iodine and/or latex **to avoid an allergic reaction.**
7. Watch for indications of distress or embarrassment, especially if the nurse is of the opposite gender, **to determine what teaching and support are needed.** Explore further if indicated.

POSSIBLE NURSING DIAGNOSES

*Impaired **U**rinary Elimination*
Urinary Retention
*Risk for **I**nfection*
*Risk for **I**mpaired Skin Integrity*
*Deficient **K**nowledge* (insertion of a catheter)

PLANNING

Expected Outcomes

1. A catheter will be inserted without pain, trauma, or injury to the client.
2. The client's bladder will be emptied without complication.
3. The nurse will maintain the sterility of the catheter during insertion.

Equipment Needed

- Straight or indwelling catheter with drainage system (Figure 30-3-1)
- Sterile catheterization kit (Figure 30-3-2)
- Adequate lighting source
- Nonsterile latex-free gloves
- Blanket or drape
- Soap and washcloth
- Warm water
- Towel

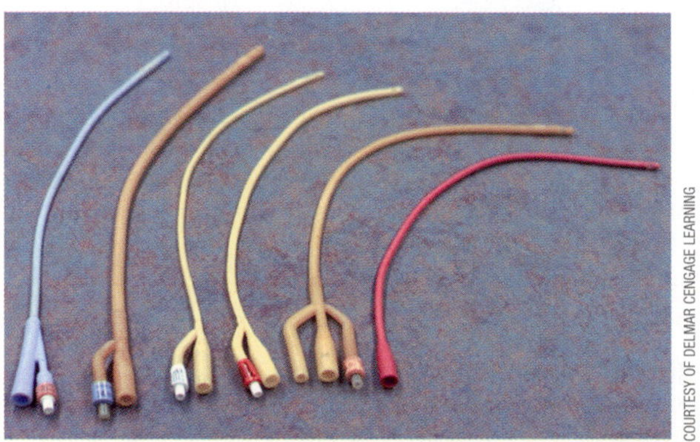

FIGURE 30-3-1 Indwelling and Straight Catheters

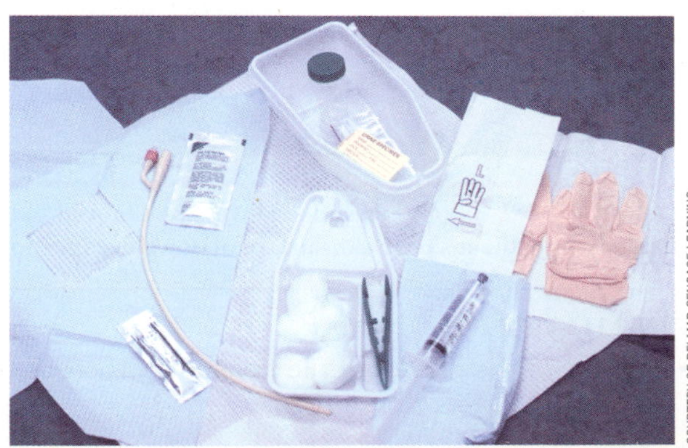

FIGURE 30-3-2 Catheterization Kit

(Continues)

PROCEDURE 30-3 Performing Urinary Catheterization: Female/Male (Continued)

delegation tips

Insertion of an indwelling catheter in a female client is generally not delegated to ancillary personnel. The delegation of this skill depends on institution policy and the availability of licensed staff versus properly trained ancillary personnel. Male urinary catheterization may be delegated to properly trained ancillary personnel depending on institution policies. The nurse is responsible to evaluate the client for contraindications to delegating this procedure, such as the risk for a difficult or traumatic insertion. The nurse may then decide to perform the procedure or to defer to the health care practitioner.

IMPLEMENTATION—ACTION/RATIONALE

ACTION	RATIONALE
* Check client's identification band * Explain procedure before beginning *	
Performing Female Urinary Catheterization	
1. Gather the equipment needed. Read the label on the catheterization kit. Note if the catheter is included in the kit and, if so, what type it is. Gather any supplies you will need that are not in the prepackaged kit.	1. Promotes efficiency in the procedure. Kits from various manufacturers come with different equipment. The catheter may or may not be packaged in the kit. Sterile gloves and the urine drainage bag may also need to be gathered separately.
2. Identify client by reading arm band assessing two client identifiers.	2. Verifies correct client.
3. Provide for privacy. Assess for allergy to povidone-iodine.	3. Promotes client dignity. Prevents known allergic reactions.
4. Set the bed to a comfortable height to work, and raise the side rail on the side opposite to you.	4. Promotes proper body mechanics and ensures client safety.
5. Assist the client to a supine position with legs spread and feet together (Figure 30-3-3).	5. Relaxes muscles and allows visualization of the area to facilitate insertion of the catheter.
6. Drape the client's abdomen and thighs for warmth if needed.	6. Promotes client comfort and warmth.
7. Ensure adequate lighting of the perineal area.	7. Facilitates proper execution of technique.
8. Wash hands and apply nonsterile latex-free gloves.	8. Reduces transfer of microorganisms.
9. Wash perineal area.	9. Reduces transfer of microorganisms.
10. Remove gloves and wash hands.	10. Reduces transfer of microorganisms.
11. Remove plastic wrap from catheterization kit. Place catheterization kit between client's legs and open the catheterization kit, using aseptic technique (Figure 30-3-4).	11. Provides an area for the sterile equipment to be laid out and assembled. Establish the sterile field close to the client. If the client is able to cooperate, the sterile field can sometimes be established in the open area between the client's legs. Plastic wrap may be used as receptacle for contaminated supplies.

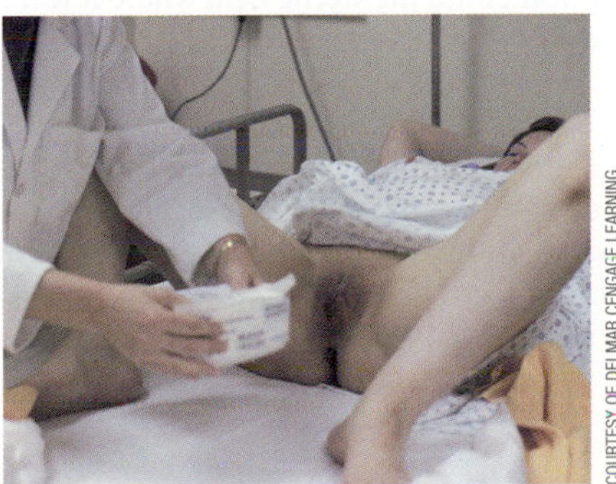
COURTESY OF DELMAR CENGAGE LEARNING

FIGURE 30-3-3 Position the client supine with legs spread.

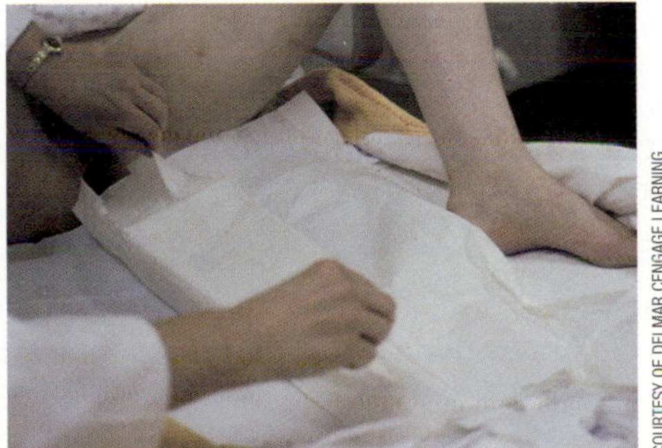
COURTESY OF DELMAR CENGAGE LEARNING

FIGURE 30-3-4 Open the catheterization kit, using the wrapper to establish a sterile field between the client's legs.

(Continues)

PROCEDURE 30-3 Performing Urinary Catheterization: Female/Male (Continued)

ACTION	RATIONALE
a. Open the top flap away from your body by grasping the corner of the outer surface between your thumb and finger only.	a. Outer surface is considered contaminated.
b. Grasp the outer surface of the left and right flaps and open.	b. Maintains sterile technique.
c. Grasp the proximal (closest) flap and open towards you. Avoid touching the inside of the flap or package with your hands or clothing.	c. Opening the proximal flap last prevents reaching over the sterile field.
12. If the catheter is not included in the kit, drop the sterile catheter onto the field using aseptic technique. Add any other items needed.	12. Prevents contamination of the sterile equipment and the sterile field.
13. Apply sterile gloves. These may be included in the kit.	13. Prevents contamination of the sterile equipment and the sterile field.
14. Place the sterile drape from the catheterization kit between the client's thighs, close to the perineum, and be careful not to touch nonsterile areas with sterile gloves.	14. Provides a sterile field at the procedural site.
15. If inserting a retention catheter, attach the syringe filled with sterile water to the Luerlock tail of the catheter. Inflate and deflate the retention balloon. Keep water-filled syringe attached to the port. (Figure 30-3-5).	15. Tests the patency of the retention balloon. A new catheter must be obtained if the balloon leaks or does not inflate.

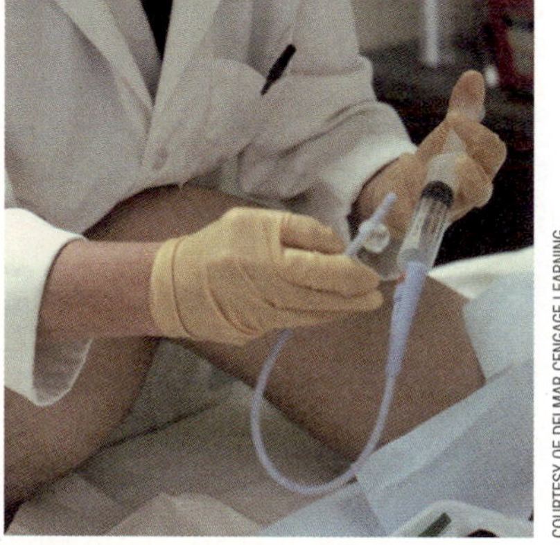
COURTESY OF DELMAR CENGAGE LEARNING

FIGURE 30-3-5 Inflate and deflate the retention balloon to test its patency.

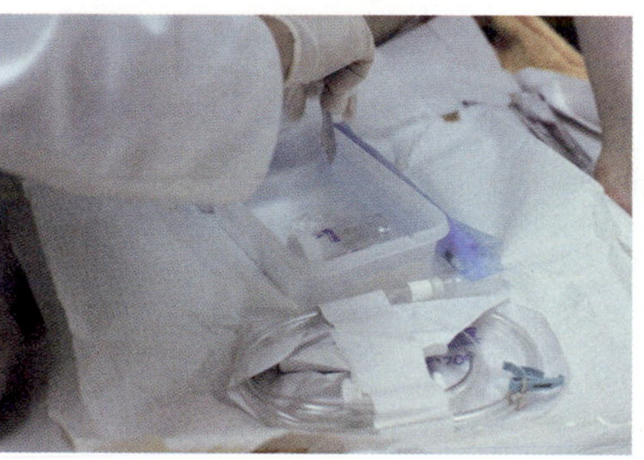
COURTESY OF DELMAR CENGAGE LEARNING

FIGURE 30-3-6 Open the lubrication package and squeeze lubricant onto the sterile field where it will be used to lubricate the catheter.

ACTION	RATIONALE
16. Attach the catheter to the urine drainage bag if it is not preconnected.	16. The catheter and drainage system may be preconnected; otherwise, connect it before catheterization to avoid exposing the client to ascending infection from an open-ended catheter.
17. Open supplies: a. Open povidone-iodine or other antimicrobial solution and pour over cotton balls. b. Squeeze lubrication package onto sterile field.	17. Maintains sterile technique and facilitates execution of the procedure.
18. Generously coat the distal portion of the catheter with water-soluble, sterile lubricant and place it nearby on the sterile field (Figure 30-3-6).	18. Facilitates catheter insertion.

(Continues)

PROCEDURE 30-3 Performing Urinary Catheterization: Female/Male (Continued)

ACTION	RATIONALE
19. Place the fenestrated drape from the catheterization kit over the client's perineal area with the labia visible through the opening.	19. Provides a sterile field at the procedural site. Prevents accidental contamination from adjacent areas.
20. Gently spread the labia minora with the fingers of your nondominant hand and visualize the urinary meatus (Figure 30-3-7).	20. Helps locate the meatus, so the catheter can be placed in the correct spot.
21. Holding the labia apart with your nondominant hand, use the forceps to pick up a cotton ball soaked in povidone-iodine, and cleanse the periurethral mucosa. Use one downward stroke for each cotton ball and dispose. Keep the labia separated with your nondominant hand until you insert the catheter (Figure 30-3-8).	21. Cleans the area and minimizes the risk of urinary tract infection by removing surface pathogens.

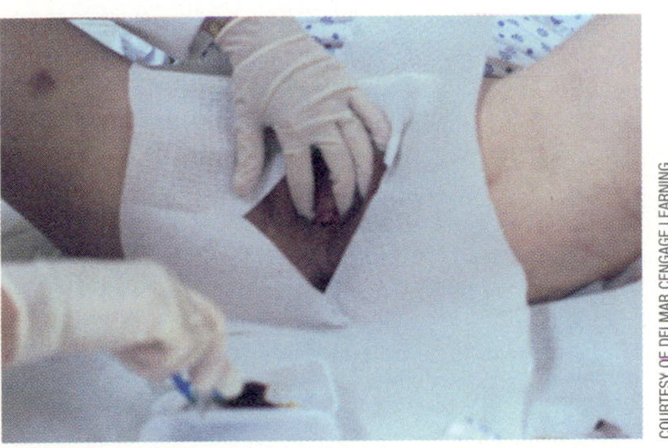

COURTESY OF DELMAR CENGAGE LEARNING

FIGURE 30-3-7 Spread the labia minora and visualize the urinary meatus.

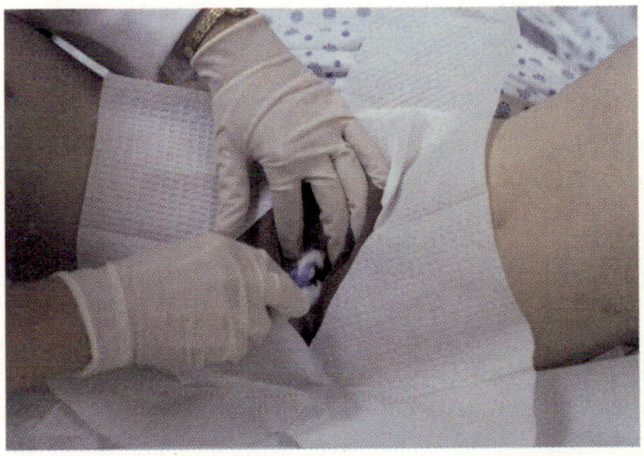

COURTESY OF DELMAR CENGAGE LEARNING

FIGURE 30-3-8 Using forceps, pick up a cotton ball soaked in povidone-iodine. Cleanse the periurethral mucosa.

ACTION	RATIONALE
22. Holding the catheter in the dominant hand, steadily insert the catheter into the meatus until urine is noted in the drainage bag or tubing (Figure 30-3-9).	22. Provides a visual confirmation that the catheter tip is in the bladder.

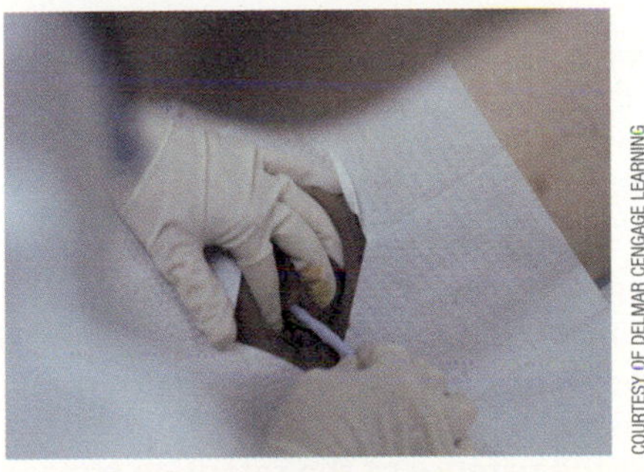

COURTESY OF DELMAR CENGAGE LEARNING

FIGURE 30-3-9 Steadily insert the catheter into the meatus.

ACTION	RATIONALE
23. If the catheter will be removed as soon as the client's bladder is empty, insert the catheter another inch and hold the catheter in place as the bladder drains.	23. The catheter needs to be inserted far enough to allow complete bladder drainage, but not so far as to possibly irritate the bladder, causing spasms.
24. If the catheter will be indwelling with a retention balloon, continue inserting another 1 to 3 inches.	24. Ensures adequate catheter insertion before retention balloon is inflated.

(Continues)

PROCEDURE 30-3 Performing Urinary Catheterization: Female/Male (Continued)

ACTION	RATIONALE
25. Inflate the retention balloon using the manufacturer's recommendations or according to the health care provider's instructions.	25. Ensures retention of the balloon. Retention catheters are available with a variety of balloon sizes. Use a catheter with the appropriate-size balloon.
26. Instruct the client to immediately report discomfort or pressure during balloon inflation; if pain occurs, discontinue the procedure, deflate the balloon, and insert the catheter farther into the urethra. If the client continues to complain of pain with balloon inflation, remove the catheter and notify the client's health care provider.	26. Pain or pressure indicates inflation of the balloon in the urethra; further insertion will prevent misplacement and further pain or bleeding.
27. Once the balloon has been inflated, gently pull the catheter until the retention balloon is resting snugly against the bladder neck (resistance will be felt when the balloon is properly seated).	27. Maximizes continuous bladder drainage and prevents urine leakage around the catheter.
28. Secure the catheter according to institutional policy. Securing the catheter to the client's thigh is usually acceptable; be sure to leave enough slack so that it does not pull on the bladder (Figure 30-3-10).	28. Prevents excessive traction from the balloon rubbing against the bladder neck, inadvertent catheter removal, or urethral erosion.

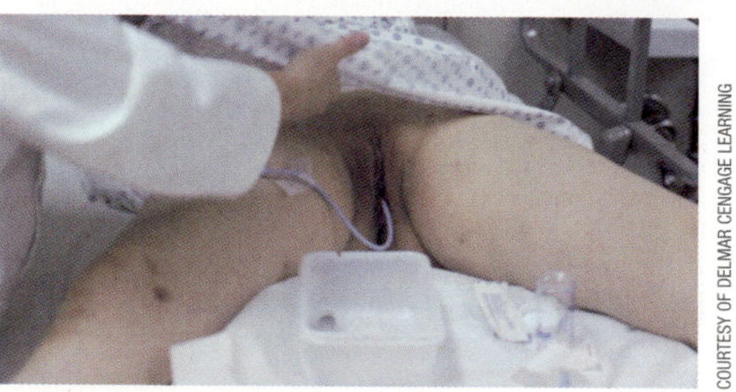

COURTESY OF DELMAR CENGAGE LEARNING

FIGURE 30-3-10 Tape the catheter to the client's thigh.

ACTION	RATIONALE
29. Place the drainage bag below the level of the bladder. Do not let it rest on the floor. Make sure the tubing lies over, not under, the leg.	29. Maximizes continuous drainage of urine from the bladder (drainage is prevented when the drainage bag is placed above the abdomen).
30. Wash the perineal area with soap and water.	30. Removes antiseptic solution to prevent skin irritation.
31. Dispose of equipment, remove gloves, and wash hands.	31. Prevents transfer of microorganisms
32. Assist client to a comfortable position and lower the bed.	32. Promotes client comfort and safety.
33. Assess the color, odor, quality, and amount of urine.	33. Monitors urinary status.
34. Wash hands.	34. Reduces transmission of microorganisms.
Performing Male Urinary Catheterization	
35. Repeat Actions 1 to 14.	35. See Rationales 1 to 14.
36. Place the fenestrated drape from the catheterization kit over the client's perineal area with the penis extending through the opening.	36. Provides a sterile field at the procedural site. Prevents accidental contamination from adjacent areas.
37. If inserting a retention catheter, attach the syringe filled with sterile water to the Luerlock tail of the catheter. Inflate and deflate the retention balloon. Keep water-filled syringe attached to the port.	37. Tests the patency of the retention balloon. A new catheter must be obtained if the balloon leaks or does not inflate.
38. Attach the catheter to the urine drainage bag if it is not preconnected.	38. The catheter and drainage system may be preconnected; otherwise it is connected before catheterization to avoid exposing the client to ascending infection from an open-ended catheter.
39. Open povidone-iodine or other antimicrobial solution and pour over cotton balls. Remove the cap from the water-soluble lubricant syringe.	39. Maintains sterile technique.

(Continues)

PROCEDURE 30-3 Performing Urinary Catheterization: Female/Male (Continued)

ACTION	RATIONALE
40. With your nondominant hand, gently grasp the penis and retract the foreskin (if present). With your dominant hand, use the forceps to pick up a saturated cotton ball. Place the cotton ball on the meatus. Using a circular motion and cleanse from the meatus to the base of the penis. Discard cotton ball. Cleanse the meatus three times using a new saturated cotton ball each time (Figure 30-3-11).	40. Removes microorganisms and minimizes the risk of urinary tract infection.

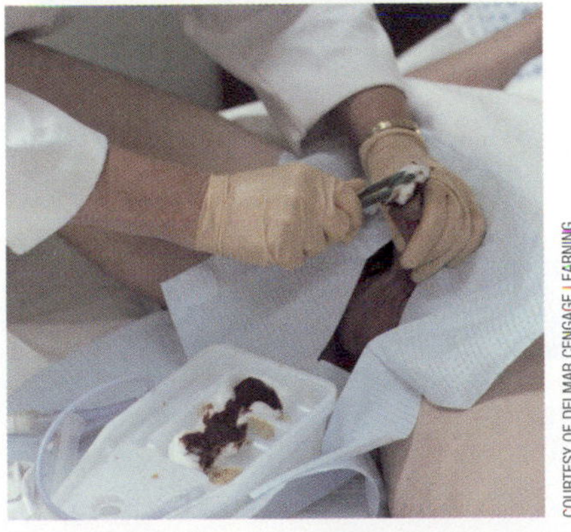

FIGURE 30-3-11 Cleanse the glans penis with a povidone-iodine solution.

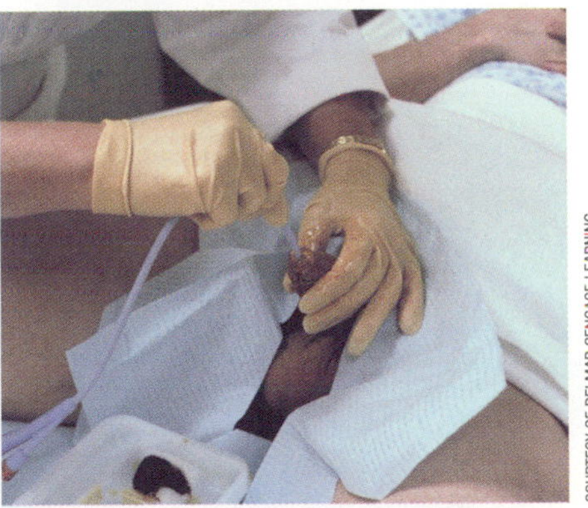

FIGURE 30-3-12 Steadily insert the catheter.

ACTION	RATIONALE
41. Hold the penis perpendicular to the body and pull up gently.	41. Facilitates catheter insertion by straightening urethra.
42. Inject 10 mL sterile, water-soluble lubricant (use a 2% Xylocaine lubricant whenever feasible) into the urethra.	42. Avoids urethral trauma and discomfort during catheter insertion and facilitates insertion.
43. Holding the catheter in the dominant hand, steadily insert the catheter about 8 inches until urine is noted in the drainage bag or tubing (Figure 30-3-12).	43. Provides a visual confirmation that the catheter tip is in the bladder.
44. If the catheter will be removed as soon as the client's bladder is empty, insert the catheter another inch, place the penis in a comfortable position, and hold the catheter in place as the bladder drains.	44. The catheter needs to be inserted far enough to allow complete bladder drainage, but not so far as to possibly irritate the bladder, causing spasms.
45. If the catheter will be indwelling with a retention balloon, continue inserting until the hub of the catheter (bifurcation between drainage port and retention balloon arm) is met.	45. Ensures adequate catheter insertion before retention balloon is inflated.
46. Inflate the retention balloon with sterile water per manufacturer's recommendations or according to the health care provider's orders (Figure 30-3-13).	46. Ensures retention of the balloon. Retention catheters are available with a variety of balloon sizes. Use a catheter with the appropriate size balloon.
47. Instruct the client to immediately report discomfort or pressure during balloon inflation; if pain occurs, discontinue the procedure, deflate the balloon, and insert the catheter farther into the bladder. If the client continues to complain of pain with balloon inflation, remove the catheter and notify the client's health care provider.	47. Pain or pressure indicates inflation of the balloon in the urethra; further insertion will prevent misplacement and further pain or bleeding.
48. Once the balloon has been inflated, gently pull the catheter until the retention balloon is resting snugly against the bladder neck (resistance will be felt when the balloon is properly seated).	48. Maximizes continuous bladder drainage and prevents urine leakage around the catheter.

(Continues)

PROCEDURE 30-3 Performing Urinary Catheterization: Female/Male (Continued)

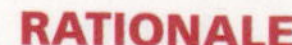

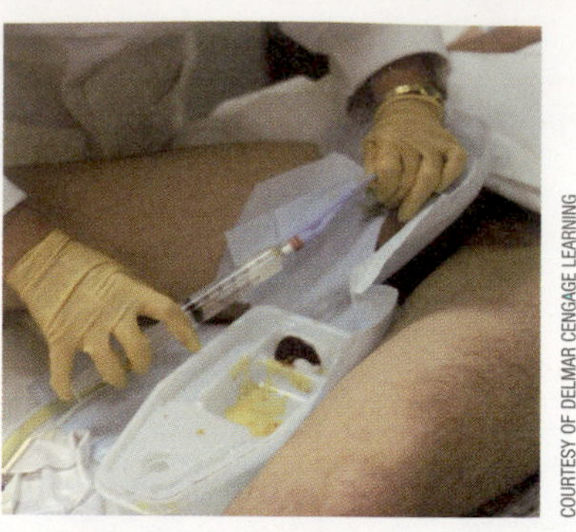

COURTESY OF DELMAR CENGAGE LEARNING

FIGURE 30-3-13 Inflate the retention balloon.

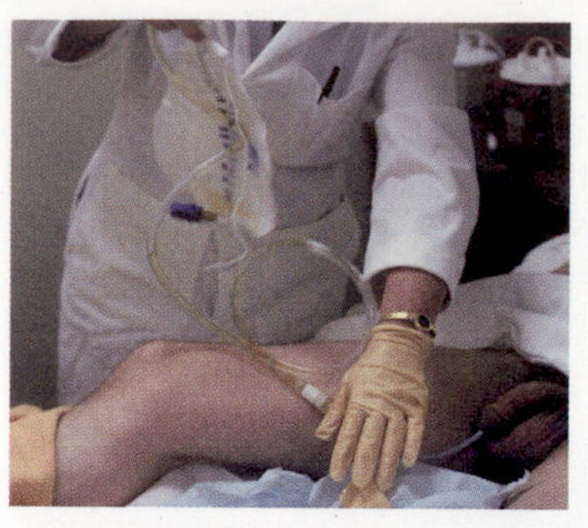

COURTESY OF DELMAR CENGAGE LEARNING

FIGURE 30-3-14 Place the drainage bag tubing over the leg.

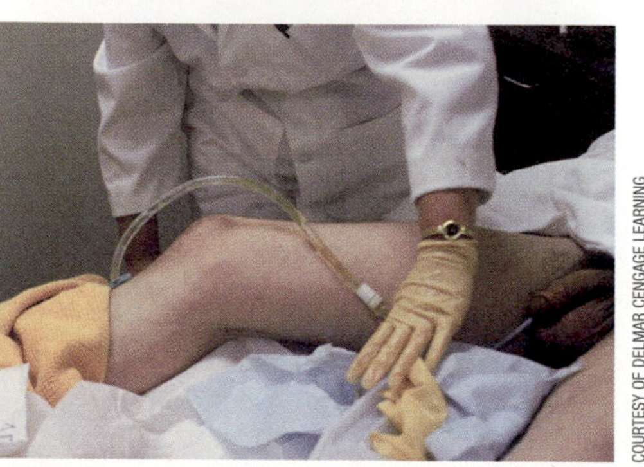

COURTESY OF DELMAR CENGAGE LEARNING

FIGURE 30-3-15 Place the drainage bag below the level of the bladder, but do not rest it on the floor.

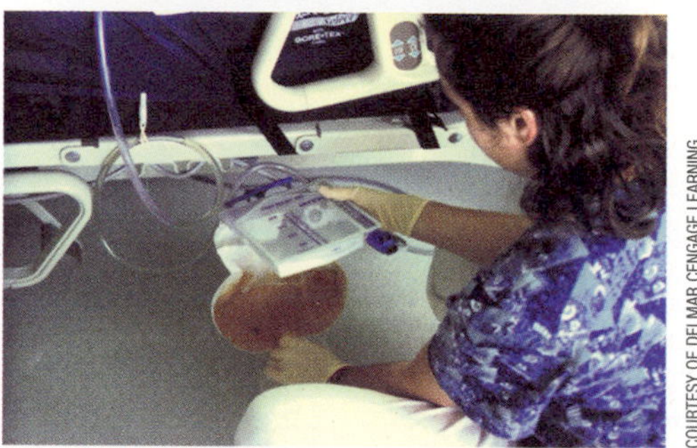

COURTESY OF DELMAR CENGAGE LEARNING

FIGURE 30-3-16 Monitor the urinary status. Assess and document the amount, color, and quality of urine.

ACTION	RATIONALE
49. Secure the catheter to the client's thigh according to institutional policy. Allow enough slack in the catheter so that it will not pull on the bladder when the client moves.	49. Prevents excessive traction from the balloon rubbing against the bladder neck, inadvertent catheter removal, or urethral erosion.
50. Place the drainage bag below the level of the bladder. Do not let it rest on the floor. Make sure the tubing lies over, not under, the leg (Figures 30-3-14 and 30-3-15).	50. Maximizes continuous drainage of urine from the bladder (drainage is prevented when the drainage bag is placed above the abdomen).
51. Clean perineal area with soap and water, and dry the area.	51. Removes antiseptic solution to prevent skin irritation.
52. Dispose of equipment, remove gloves, and wash hands.	52. Prevents transfer of microorganisms.
53. Assist client to a comfortable position. Lower the bed.	53. Promotes client comfort and safety.
54. Assess and document the amount, color, odor, and quality of urine (Figure 30-3-16).	54. Monitors urinary status.
55. Wash hands.	55. Reduces transmission of microorganisms.

EVALUATION

- The catheter was inserted without pain, trauma, or injury to the client.
- The client's bladder was emptied without complication.
- The nurse maintained the sterility of the catheter during insertion.

DOCUMENTATION

Nurses' Notes

- Time and date the catheter was inserted
- Size and type of catheter used, including the size of the retention balloon and the amount of sterile water used to inflate the balloon
- Client's response to the procedure and the amount, color, and quality of urine returned
- Document on appropriate electronic medical record or flow sheet.

Intake and Output Record

- Amount of urine returned

PROCEDURE 30-4 Irrigating a Urinary Catheter

OVERVIEW

Open intermittent irrigation of a urinary catheter is generally done for one of two reasons: either to instill medication into the bladder or to irrigate the catheter itself, which may be blocked by either blood clots or urinary sediment. This irrigation is referred to as "open" because the closed bladder drainage system is opened where the drainage tubing inserts into the urinary catheter; the catheter is generally indwelling. Maintaining sterility of the system is paramount in this type of irrigation.

ASSESSMENT

1. Identify the following items in the health care provider's orders: type of irrigation (bladder or catheter); purpose of the irrigation; type and amount of solution to irrigate with; any premedication ordered; and any other details of the order. **Allows the nurse to anticipate responses to the procedure and assess pertinent features of the client's condition.**
2. Assess the condition of the client as it relates to the procedure: patency of the catheter, characteristics of urinary drainage, and total intake and output status of the client. **Establishes a baseline of the client's condition as it relates to elimination and in the case of PRN catheterization, which may indicate whether there is a need for the procedure.**
3. Assess for current pain or bladder spasms. **Even when medication is not specifically ordered, medicating for pain before the procedure can increase client comfort, and if irrigation does not relieve spasms, the client may need medication afterward.**
4. Assess client's knowledge about the procedure **to determine need for education and reduce anxiety about the procedure.**
5. If this is a repeat of the procedure, read the charting from previous times. **Provides a history of how this client tolerates the procedure and of any teaching done.**

POSSIBLE NURSING DIAGNOSES

Risk for Infection
Impaired Urinary Elimination
Acute Pain
Urinary Retention

PLANNING

Expected Outcomes

1. Urinary catheter will be patent.
2. Sediment/blood clots will be passed through the catheter.
3. Bladder will be free of sources of local irritation.
4. Urinary pH will be lowered to a more acidic state.

Equipment Needed

- Sterile gloves
- Nonsterile latex-free gloves
- Sterile cover for the end of the drainage tubing
- Disposable, water-resistant drape or towel
- Sterile Asepto or Toomey syringe with container for irrigant
- Sterile antiseptic swabs
- Sterile irrigating solution (labeled with date and time of opening, if opened)

delegation tips

The procedure of irrigating a urinary catheter cannot be delegated because it requires the skills and problem-solving abilities of a nurse.

IMPLEMENTATION—ACTION/RATIONALE

ACTION	RATIONALE
* Check client's identification band * Explain procedure before beginning *	
1. Verify the need for bladder or catheter irrigation.	1. Ensures that procedure is being applied correctly, to reduce unnecessary opening of the system and risk of infection.
2. For prn catheter irrigation, palpate for full bladder and check current output against previous totals.	2. If irrigation is on an as-needed basis, it may not be needed at this time.

(Continues)

PROCEDURE 30-4 Irrigating a Urinary Catheter (Continued)

ACTION	RATIONALE
3. Check health care provider's orders for type of irrigation, irrigant, and the amount.	3. Ensures procedural accuracy.
4. If this is a repeat procedure, read previous documentation in the record.	4. Establishes prior client response to procedure.
5. Assemble all supplies.	5. Having all supplies in room enables the nurse to maintain sterility of supplies once they are opened and laid out.
6. Premedicate client if ordered or needed.	6. Increases comfort for the procedure.
7. Educate client as needed based on what the client already knows.	7. Knowledge will increase client compliance and decrease anxiety.
8. Provide for client privacy with a closed door or curtain.	8. Decreases client anxiety.
9. Assist the client to a dorsal recumbent position.	9. Facilitates the flow of irrigant into the bladder.
10. Wash hands.	10. Decreases transmission of microorganisms.
11. Apply nonsterile latex-free gloves and empty the collection bag of urine.	11. Starting with an empty collection bag makes it easier to identify clots or sediment passed as a result of irrigation.
12. Remove gloves and wash hands.	12. Reduces transmission of microorganisms.
13. Expose the indwelling catheter and place the water-resistant drape underneath it.	13. Protects the bedclothes and client from urine and body fluids.
14. Open the sterile syringe and container. Stand it up carefully in or on the wrapper and add 100 to 200 mL sterile diluent without touching or contaminating the tip of the syringe or the inside of the receptacle.	14. Enables nurse to maintain sterility of gloves once they are applied.
15. Open the end of the antiseptic swab package, exposing the swab sticks, and the sterile cover for drainage tube.	15. Enables nurse to maintain sterility of gloves once they are applied.
16. Apply the sterile gloves.	16. Maintains sterility of the procedure.
17. Using the antiseptic swab sticks, disinfect the connection between the catheter and the drainage tubing.	17. Minimizes risk of contaminating the system.
18. After the disinfectant dries, loosen the ends of the connection.	18. Enables the nurse to open the connection without accidentally contaminating either end.
19. Grasp the catheter and tubing 1 to 2 inches from their ends, with catheter in the nondominant hand.	19. Maintains sterility of the procedure and allows the nurse to be positioned to use the dominant hand for the syringe.
20. Fold the catheter to pinch it closed between the palm and last three fingers; use the thumb and first finger to hold the sterile cap for the drainage tube.	20. Allows for one nurse to handle all equipment simultaneously, thus maintaining sterility.
21. Separate the catheter and tube, covering the tube tightly with the sterile cap.	21. Maintains sterility of equipment.
22. Fill the syringe with 30 mL for catheter irrigation, 60 mL for bladder irrigation. Insert the tip of the syringe into the catheter and gently instill the solution into the catheter (Figures 30-4-1 and 30-4-2).	22. Catheter can be irrigated with 30 mL of solution, minimizing bladder discomfort, while irrigating a bladder takes 60 mL.
23. Clamp catheter if ordered (medicated solution). If not clamped, irrigant may be released into a collection container or aspirated back into the syringe (Figure 30-4-3).	23. Fine sediment or clear irrigant with medication can run freely; material with more solids (sediment or clots) may need gentle aspiration.
24. If the bladder or catheter is being irrigated to clear solid material, repeat irrigation until return is clear.	24. Clearing the catheter completely in this irrigation means a lower total number of irrigations and less opening of the system, thus decreasing the risk of infection.

(Continues)

PROCEDURE 30-4 Irrigating a Urinary Catheter (Continued)

ACTION	RATIONALE

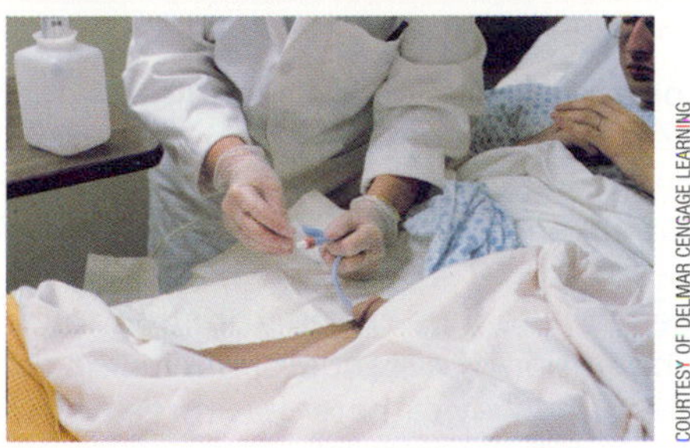

FIGURE 30-4-1 Separate the catheter and tube.

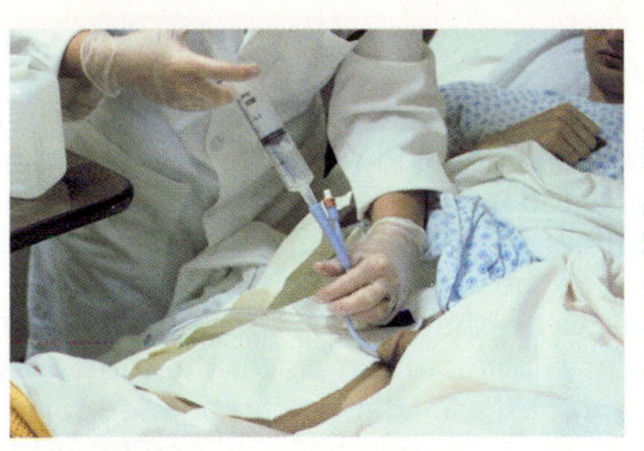

FIGURE 30-4-2 Insert the tip of the syringe into the catheter and gently instill the solution.

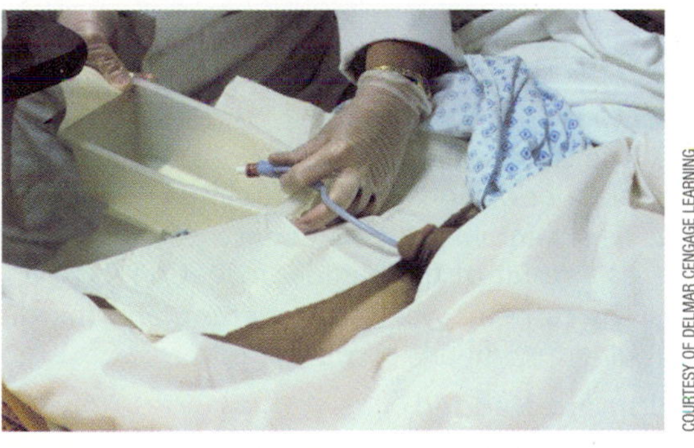

FIGURE 30-4-3 Irrigant is released into a collection container.

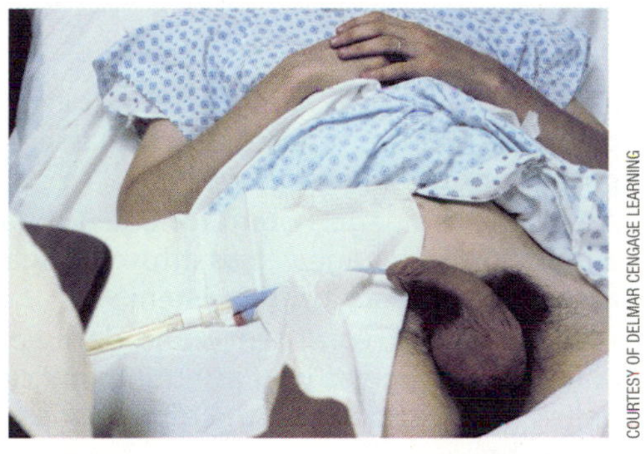

FIGURE 30-4-4 Reconnect the tubing to the catheter.

ACTION	RATIONALE
25. Reconnect system and remove sterile gloves. Wash your hands (Figure 30-4-4).	25. Maintains sterility of system and reduces transmission of microorganisms.
26. Record the type of irrigation, total amount of irrigant used, and the color and quality of return.	26. Evaluation of the urinary tract status and catheter.
27. Monitor client for pain, urine color and clarity, any solid material passed, and total intake and output.	27. Monitoring output after irrigation evaluates the efficacy of the treatment.
28. Wash hands.	28. Reduces transmission of microorganisms.

EVALUATION

- Urinary catheter remains patent.
- Any sediment/blood clots were passed through the catheter.
- Bladder is free of local irritation.
- Urinary pH was more acidic.

DOCUMENTATION

Nurses' Notes

- Assessment indicating need for irrigation, such as decreased output, increased sediment, clots, bladder spasms/pain, or palpation of a full bladder
- Type of irrigant and amount in each instillation
- Amount and quality of returns (returns often include urine trapped in the bladder)
- Medication given before or after the procedure and response to same
- Urine output, color, and clarity and any solids passed 30 to 60 minutes after procedure
- Client response, especially changes in pain, spasms, or discomfort
- Document on appropriate electronic medical record or flow sheet.

Medication Administration Record

Record:

- Type of irrigant, if medicated, and amount in each instillation
- Any medication given before or after the procedure

Intake and Output Record

Document:

- Amount of urine emptied from the drainage bag prior to and following the procedure
- Amount of irrigant instilled

PROCEDURE 30-5 Irrigating the Bladder Using a Closed-System Catheter

OVERVIEW

Surgical procedures such as prostate resections and bladder surgery or traumatic injury may require frequent or continuous bladder irrigation. To prevent the potential introduction of infectious organisms, and as a practical matter, open bladder irrigation is not used in these cases. A closed bladder irrigation system is preferable under these circumstances. Closed bladder irrigation may be used to instill medication, encourage hemostasis, or flush clots and debris out of the catheter and bladder.

A three-way catheter is used for closed bladder irrigation. If the client will require closed irrigation following surgery, the surgeon often places the three-way catheter during the operation. If a standard indwelling catheter has been placed, a Y adapter can be used for intermittent irrigation. A three-way catheter has three ports: one for inflation of the retention balloon, one for urine drainage, and one for instilling irrigant.

As with open bladder irrigation, closed bladder irrigation is a sterile procedure. The irrigant, tubing, and drainage systems must be maintained as a closed sterile system to decrease the risk of infection. Because of the risk of blockage from clots and debris, the system must also be monitored closely for equal amounts of irrigant instilled and irrigant returned.

ASSESSMENT

1. Assess the client for bladder distention or complaints of fullness or discomfort **to assess the patency of the drainage system.**
2. Assess the drainage system for equal or larger amounts of drainage versus infused irrigant **to assess the patency of the system.**
3. Assess the color, consistency, and clarity of the bladder drainage as well as noting any clots or debris present **to assess the effectiveness of the irrigation.**

POSSIBLE NURSING DIAGNOSES

*Risk for **I**nfection*
*Impaired **U**rinary Elimination*
***U**rinary Retention*
*Acute **P**ain*

PLANNING

Expected Outcomes

1. The client will not exhibit signs or symptoms of bladder or urinary tract infection.
2. The client will not experience pain or discomfort as a result of the bladder irrigation.
3. The catheter will remain patent, and the client's bladder will not be distended.

Equipment Needed

- Three-way indwelling catheter or Y adapter
- IV pole
- Ordered irrigation solution
- Sterile gloves
- Closed-irrigation tubing
- Large urine collection bag
- Antiseptic swabs

delegation tips

This procedure cannot be delegated. Bladder irrigation using a closed-system catheter requires the skills of a nurse.

IMPLEMENTATION—ACTION/RATIONALE

ACTION	RATIONALE
* Check client's identification band * Explain procedure before beginning *	
Intermittent Bladder Irrigation Using a Standard Indwelling Catheter and a Y Adapter	
1. Wash hands.	1. Prevents spread of microorganisms.
2. Close privacy curtain or door.	2. Provides privacy.
3. Hang the prescribed irrigation solution from an IV pole.	3. Different solutions may be ordered depending on the results the health care provider desires. Bladder irrigant is generally packaged in 2,000- to 4,000-mL bottles.
4. Insert the clamped irrigation tubing into the bottle of irrigant and prime the tubing with fluid, expel all air and reclamp the tube (Figure 30-5-1).	4. Prevents introduction of air into the bladder.

(Continues)

PROCEDURE 30-5 Irrigating the Bladder Using a Closed-System Catheter (Continued)

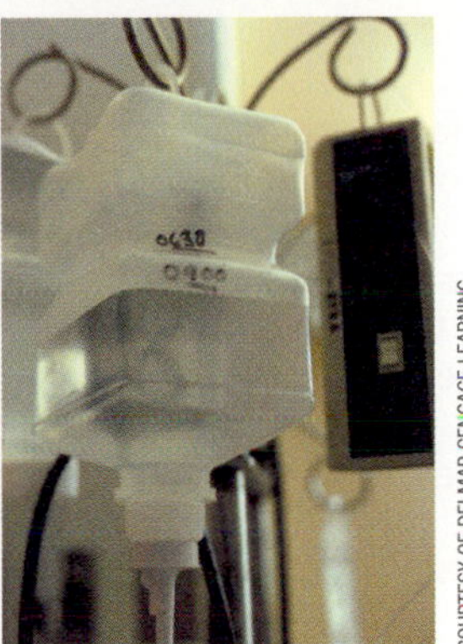

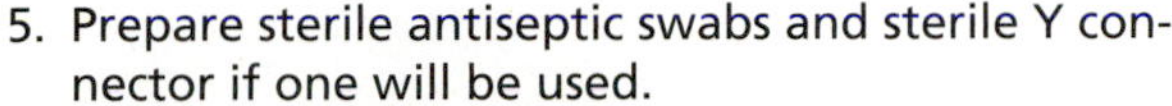

FIGURE 30-5-1 Insert the clamped irrigation tubing into the bottle of irrigant.

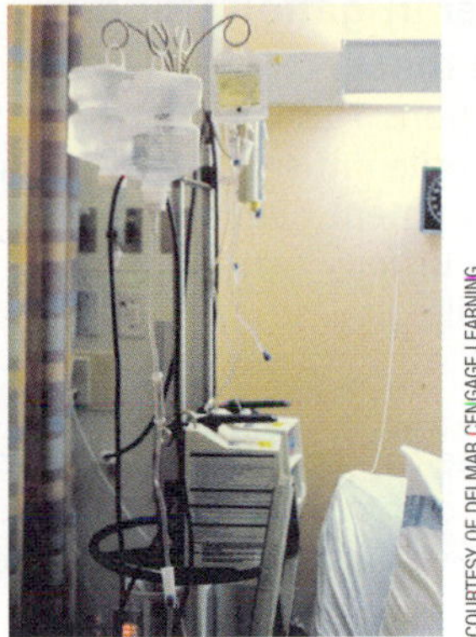

FIGURE 30-5-2 Clamp the irrigant tubing.

ACTION	RATIONALE
5. Prepare sterile antiseptic swabs and sterile Y connector if one will be used.	5. Prevents contamination of sterile gloves and field.
6. Clamp the urinary catheter.	6. Prevents urine leakage onto the bed linens.
7. Apply sterile gloves.	7. Minimizes the client's risk of infection.
8. Unhook the drainage bag from the indwelling catheter.	8. Allows the Y adapter to be inserted into the system.
9. While holding the drainage tubing and the drainage port of the catheter in your nondominant hand, cleanse both the tubing and the port with antiseptic swabs.	9. Reduces risk of contamination and infection.
10. Connect one port of the Y connector to the drainage port of the catheter.	10. Provides a bifurcation for irrigant to instill as well as urine to drain.
11. Connect another port of the Y adapter to the drainage tubing.	11. Collects the urine and drained irrigant. This may be the established urine collection bag or a new, sterile bag that is large enough to hold the increased volume of drainage.
12. Attach the third port of the Y adapter to the irrigant tubing.	12. Instills the irrigant into the closed system.
13. Unclamp the urinary catheter and establish that urine is draining through the catheter into the drainage bag.	13. If the urine does not flow freely after unclamping, the catheter may have become clogged with a clot or debris. Notify the client's health care provider of the lack of urine drainage.
14. To irrigate the catheter and bladder, clamp the drainage tubing distal to the Y adapter.	14. Prevents the irrigant from bypassing the bladder and flowing directly into the drainage bag.
15. Unclamp irrigation tubing and instill the prescribed amount of irrigant.	15. The bladder normally feels full when it contains approximately 300 mL of urine. If a prescribed amount of irrigant was not ordered, do not instill more than 150 mL of irrigant. If the client has undergone bladder surgery, do not instill irrigant without knowing the specific amount ordered.
16. Clamp the irrigant tubing (Figure 30-5-2).	16. Prevents further instillation of irrigant.
17. If the health care provider has ordered the irrigant to remain in the bladder for a measured length of time, wait the prescribed length of time.	17. Some irrigation solutions contain medication and are meant to remain in contact with the bladder wall for a prescribed length of time.
18. Unclamp the drainage tubing and monitor the drainage as it flows into the drainage bag.	18. Assess the drainage for volume, color, clarity, and the presence of any clots or debris.

(Continues)

PROCEDURE 30-5 Irrigating the Bladder Using a Closed-System Catheter (Continued)

ACTION	RATIONALE
Closed Bladder Irrigation Using a Three-Way Catheter	
19. Follow Actions 1 to 4.	19. See Rationales 1 to 4.
20. Prepare sterile antiseptic swabs and any other sterile equipment needed.	20. Prevents contamination of sterile gloves and field.
21. Clamp the urinary catheter.	21. Prevents leakage of urine onto the bedclothes.
22. Apply sterile gloves.	22. Minimizes the client's risk of infection when connecting the irrigant to the catheter and drainage system.
23. Remove the cap from the irrigation port of the three-way catheter (Figure 30-5-3).	23. Allows access for the irrigant tubing.
24. Cleanse the irrigation port with the sterile antiseptic swabs.	24. Minimizes the risk of infection.
25. Attach the irrigation tubing to the irrigation port of the three-way catheter.	25. Connects irrigant to the system.
26. Remove the clamp from the catheter and observe for urine drainage (Figure 30-5-4).	26. Ensures catheter remains patent after being clamped. Some surgical procedures can cause bleeding and clotting of the catheter.
If intermittent irrigation has been ordered:	
27. Follow Actions 15 to 16.	27. See Rationales 15 to 16.
28. If the health care provider has ordered the irrigant to remain in the bladder for a measured length of time, clamp the drainage tube before instilling the irrigant and wait the prescribed length of time.	28. Some irrigation solutions contain medication and are meant to remain in contact with the bladder wall for a prescribed length of time.
29. Monitor the drainage as it flows into the drainage bag.	29. Assesses the drainage for volume, color, clarity, and the presence of any clots or debris.
If continuous bladder irrigation has been ordered:	
30. Adjust the clamp on the irrigation tubing to allow the prescribed rate of irrigant to flow into the catheter and bladder.	30. Regulates the amount of irrigant flowing in and out of the bladder to prevent distention or damage to any surgical site.
31. Monitor the drainage for color, clarity, debris, and volume as it flows back into the drainage bag.	31. Assesses for bleeding, clotting, and blockage of urine drainage or other complications.
32. Tape the catheter securely to the thigh (Figure 30-5-5).	32. Prevents the catheter from becoming dislodged.
33. Remove gloves and wash hands.	33. Reduces transmission of microorganisms.

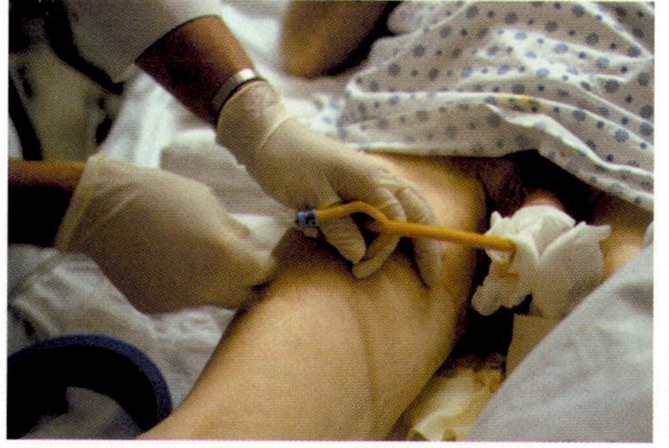

COURTESY OF DELMAR CENGAGE LEARNING

FIGURE 30-5-3 Remove the cap from the irrigation port of the three-way catheter.

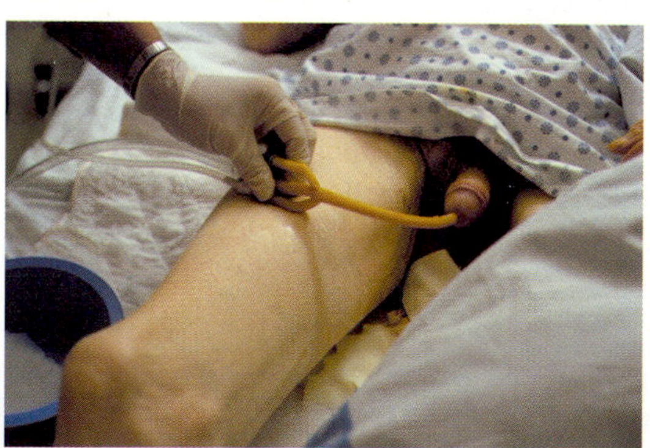

COURTESY OF DELMAR CENGAGE LEARNING

FIGURE 30-5-4 Attach the irrigation tubing, remove the clamp from the catheter, and observe for urine drainage. Carefully observe the drainage for color, clarity, and the presence of debris.

(Continues)

PROCEDURE 30-5 Irrigating the Bladder Using a Closed-System Catheter (Continued)

ACTION	RATIONALE

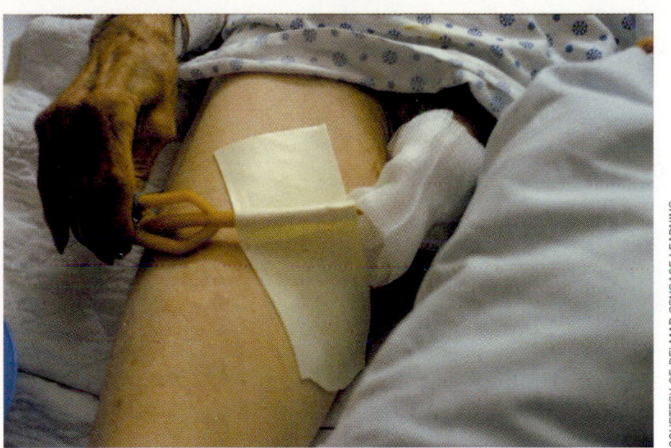

COURTESY OF DELMAR CENGAGE LEARNING

FIGURE 30-5-5 Securely tape the catheter to the thigh to prevent it from becoming dislodged.

EVALUATION

- The client does not exhibit signs or symptoms of bladder or urinary tract infection.
- The client has not experienced pain or discomfort as a result of the bladder irrigation.
- The catheter remains patent, and the client's bladder is not distended.

DOCUMENTATION

Intake and Output Record

- Amount of irrigant instilled and amount of drainage measured. Subtracting the used irrigant from the drainage total will leave the amount of the client's urine output.

Nurses' Notes

- Client's tolerance for the procedure
- Color, clarity, volume, and debris in the drainage
- Document on appropriate electronic medical record or flow sheet.

PROCEDURE 30-6 Changing a Bowel Diversion Ostomy Appliance: Pouching a Stoma

OVERVIEW

A colostomy is an opening surgically created from the ascending, transverse, or descending colon to the abdominal wall. An ileostomy is an opening from the ileum to the abdominal wall. Colostomies and ileostomies function to discharge waste (liquids, solids, and gases) to the outside of the body. Pouching a fecal diversion ensures that the client's peristomal skin remains intact and provides the client with artificial continence.

The purpose of creating ileostomies and colostomies is to improve survival and the quality of life. Anger, grief, body image disturbances, socialization disturbances, depression, and helplessness often accompany these procedures.

ASSESSMENT

1. Inspect the stoma for color and texture. **Allows the nurse to determine the viability and turgor of the stoma.**
2. Inspect the condition of the skin surrounding the stoma. **Alterations in skin integrity prohibit a closed drainage system from adhering to the skin.**
3. Measure the dimensions of the stoma before obtaining an ostomy appliance system from central supply. **Alleviates the problem of obtaining the wrong size equipment.**

(Continues)

PROCEDURE 30-6 Changing a Bowel Diversion Ostomy Appliance: Pouching a Stoma (Continued)

POSSIBLE NURSING DIAGNOSES

*Risk for Impaired **S**kin Integrity*
*Impaired **S**kin Integrity*
*Disturbed **B**ody Image*
*Deficient **K**nowledge*
*Risk for Deficient **F**luid Volume*

PLANNING

Expected Outcomes

1. Peristomal skin integrity will remain intact.
2. Irritated or denuded peristomal skin will heal.
3. Client will acknowledge the change in body image.
4. Client will express positive feelings about self.
5. Client will maintain fluid balance.

Equipment Needed

- Clean washcloth or 4 × 4 gauze pads
- Warm tap water
- Appropriate drainable ostomy appliance (Figures 30-6-1 and 30-6-2)
- Scissors
- Pen or pencil
- Nonsterile latex-free gloves

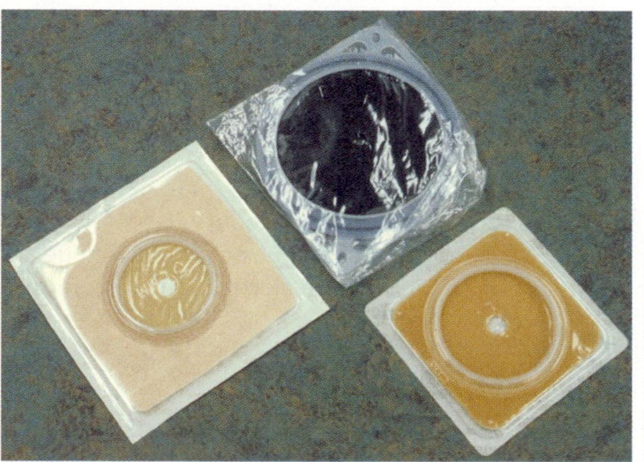
COURTESY OF DELMAR CENGAGE LEARNING

FIGURE 30-6-1 Ostomy Skin Barriers (Also Called Wafers)

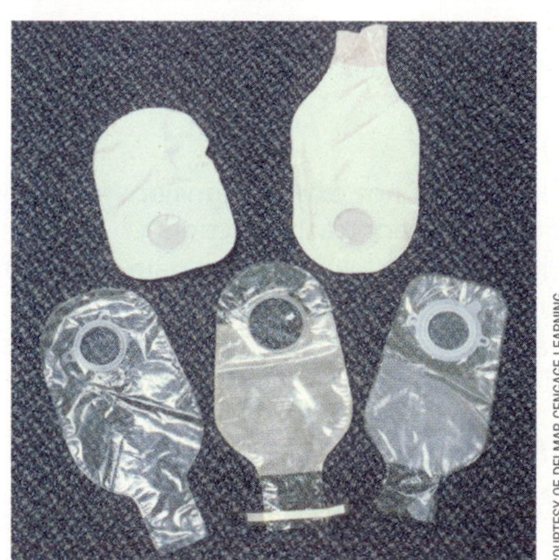
COURTESY OF DELMAR CENGAGE LEARNING

FIGURE 30-6-2 Ostomy Drainage Bags

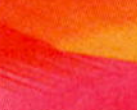

delegation tips

This procedure cannot be delegated to ancillary personnel. Changing an ostomy appliance requires the skills and problem-solving ability of a nurse.

IMPLEMENTATION—ACTION/RATIONALE

* Check client's identification band * Explain procedure before beginning *

ACTION	RATIONALE
1. Wash hands.	1. Prevents spread of microorganisms.
2. Assemble drainable pouch and wafer.	2. Ensures that all equipment is ready to use.
3. Apply nonsterile latex-free gloves.	3. Practices clean technique.
4. Remove current ostomy appliance after emptying pouch of stool, if present.	4. Prevents contamination of surrounding environment if stool accidentally leaks from appliance when removed from client's skin.
5. Dispose of appliance in appropriate waste container.	5. Practices infection control.
6. Remove gloves and wash hands.	6. Prevents spread of microorganisms.

(Continues)

PROCEDURE 30-6 Changing a Bowel Diversion Ostomy Appliance: Pouching a Stoma (Continued)

ACTION	RATIONALE
7. Apply nonsterile latex-free gloves.	7. Follows Standard Precautions.
8. Cleanse stoma and skin with warm tap water. Pat dry (Figure 30-6-3).	8. Gentle care of the stoma prevents injury to the mucosa, which has no nerve endings and is very friable.
9. Measure stoma using a measuring guide for appropriate length and width of stoma at base (where skin meets stoma) (Figure 30-6-4).	9. Correct measurement of the stoma's dimensions ensures a good fit of the ostomy appliance without excess skin at the base of the stoma exposed to stool.
10. Place gauze pad over orifice of stoma to wick stool while you are preparing the wafer and pouch for application.	10. Ensures a good seal of the wafer to the client's skin.
11. Trace pattern onto paper backing of wafer.	11. Inaccurate pattern size results in either laceration of the stoma by the wafer or maceration of peristomal skin from constant contact with stool.
12. Cut wafer as traced.	12. Ensures a snug fit.
13. Attach clean pouch to wafer. Make sure port closure is closed (Figure 30-6-5).	13. Preattaching the pouch to the wafer saves time and prevents stool from leaking underneath the wafer during application process.
14. Remove gauze pad from orifice of stoma.	14. It is easier to visualize the stoma.
15. Remove paper backing from wafer and place on skin with stoma centered in cutout opening of wafer (Figure 30-6-6).	15. Paper backing needs to be removed from wafer in order for wafer to adhere to skin.

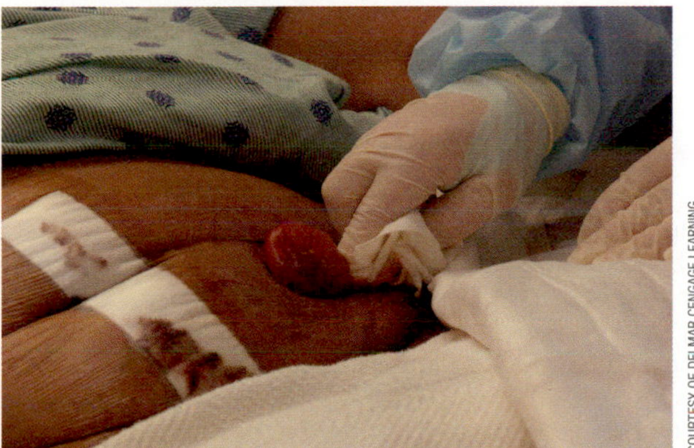

COURTESY OF DELMAR CENGAGE LEARNING

FIGURE 30-6-3 Cleanse the stoma and surrounding skin with warm water.

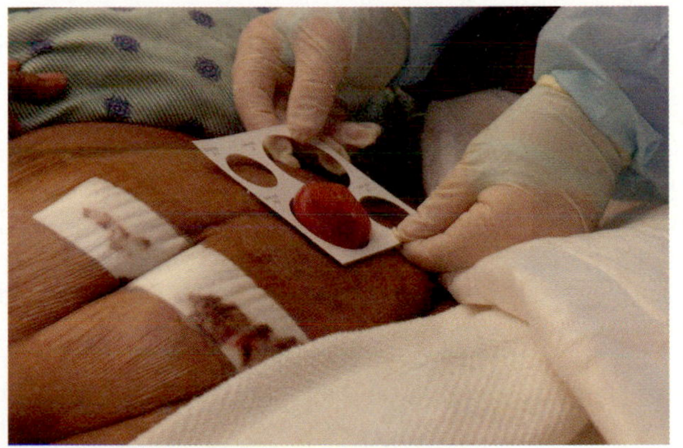

COURTESY OF DELMAR CENGAGE LEARNING

FIGURE 30-6-4 Measure the stoma using a measuring guide.

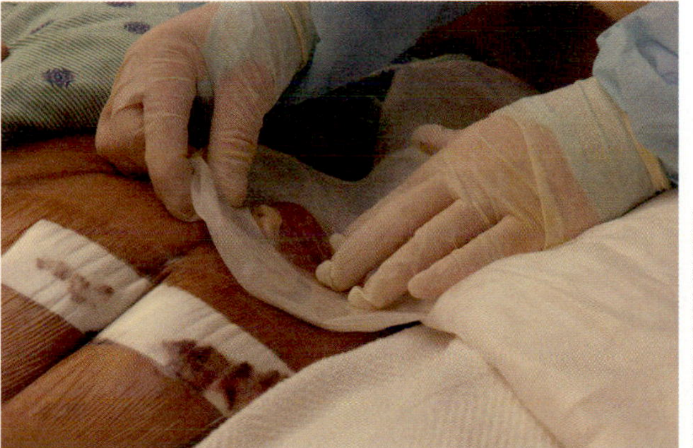

COURTESY OF DELMAR CENGAGE LEARNING

FIGURE 30-6-5 Place the wafer and pouch with the stoma centered in the cutout opening of the wafer.

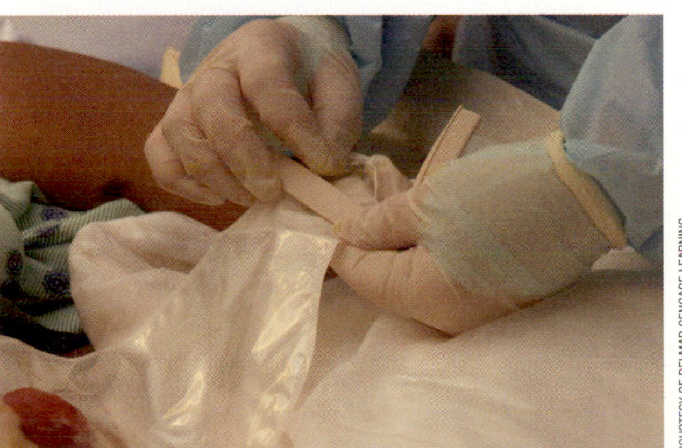

COURTESY OF DELMAR CENGAGE LEARNING

FIGURE 30-6-6 Apply closure clamp to pouch.

(Continues)

PROCEDURE 30-6 Changing a Bowel Diversion Ostomy Appliance: Pouching a Stoma (Continued)

ACTION	RATIONALE
16. Tape the wafer edges down with hypoallergenic tape (optional).	16. Ensures that the edges of the wafer will not adhere to client's clothing.
17. Dispose of used materials, remove gloves, and wash hands.	17. Reduces transmission of microorganisms.

EVALUATION

- Peristomal skin integrity remains intact.
- Irritated or denuded peristomal skin integrity is healed.
- Client acknowledges the change in body image.
- Client expresses positive feelings about self.
- Client maintains fluid balance.

DOCUMENTATION

Nurses' Notes

- Assessment of peristomal skin
- Assessment of stoma
- Stoma measurements (length, width, height)
- Color and amount of drainage
- Peristomal skin care if alteration in skin integrity was noted
- Type of ostomy pouch applied
- Document on appropriate electronic medical record or flow sheet.

PROCEDURE 30-7 Application of Heat and Cold

OVERVIEW

Heat application is used to promote vasodilatation, increase capillary permeability, decrease blood viscosity, increase tissue metabolism, and reduce muscle tension. Moist heat can be in the form of immersion of a body part in a warmed solution or water. It can also be accomplished by wrapping body parts in dressings that are saturated with warmed solution.

Dry heat can be used to enhance circulation, promote healing, reduce swelling and inflammation, reduce pain, reduce muscle spasms, and increase systemic temperature.

Cold therapy is used to decrease blood flow to an area by promoting vasoconstriction and increased blood viscosity. These changes facilitate clotting and control bleeding. Cold decreases tissue metabolism, reduces oxygen consumption, and decreases inflammation and edema formation. Cold therapy has a local anesthetic effect by raising the threshold of pain receptors. It causes a decrease in muscle tension. Cold is used to reduce fever.

ASSESSMENT

1. Assess the area to receive heat or cold treatment for circulation. **Heat increases circulation; adequate vasculature must be present to be effective. Cold decreases circulation; adequate circulation must be present to prevent further tissue damage.**
2. Assess the skin sensation and integrity around the area to be treated. **Heat treatment cannot be used over areas of blisters, burns, or redness indicative of burning.**
3. Assess for open wounds that may be affected by the treatment. **Moist heat provides an ideal climate for the growth of microorganisms. Moist heat should be applied to open wounds only with orders from a physician or qualified practitioner.**
4. Check the client's systemic temperature. **If large areas are exposed to heat or cold, the total body temperature may be increased or decreased.**
5. Assess age. **Tolerance to heat and cold varies with individuals and is related to age, thinner layers of skin, or general sensitivity to heat and cold.**

POSSIBLE NURSING DIAGNOSES

*Ineffective **T**issue Perfusion*
*Acute **P**ain*
*Risk for Impaired **S**kin Integrity*
*Risk for Imbalanced **B**ody Temperature*
*Ineffective **T**hermoregulation*
*Risk for **I**njury*

(Continues)

PROCEDURE 30-7 Application of Heat and Cold (Continued)

PLANNING

Expected Outcomes

1. The client will derive the intended benefits of the heat or cold treatment.
2. The client will not experience any injury to skin integrity.

Equipment Needed

- Aquathermia pad
- Commercial heat or cold pack
- Solution for heat or cold treatment
- 4 × 4 gauze and waterproof pads
- Nonsterile latex-free gloves
- Sterile gloves if open wounds
- Towels
- Heat cradle
- Portable sitz bath
- Peri-care equipment
- Timer or clock

delegation tips

These procedures are routinely delegated to properly trained ancillary personnel. Reassessment of the client after application to maintain proper temperature and to evaluate the client response is essential.

IMPLEMENTATION—ACTION/RATIONALE

* Check client's identification band * Explain procedure before beginning *

Moist Heat

ACTION	RATIONALE
1. Check the physician's order and the reason for warm compress.	1. A physician's or nurse practitioner's order is generally required.
2. Wash hands.	2. Reduces transmission of microorganisms.
3. Assess the client's skin for areas of redness, breakdown, or scar tissue. If open wounds are involved, carefully assess the open wounds. Explain to client the reason for the compress.	3. Provides baseline information for comparison assessments. Because scar tissue may be heat sensitive or insensitive, this area should be avoided, if possible, when the compress is applied. Any open wounds should be avoided unless the treatment is specific for these areas. Client understanding of reason for compress may improve compliance.
4. Review the client's condition, medical diagnosis, and any history of diabetes mellitus or impairments in sensation.	4. Sensation is often impaired in peripheral vascular disease, diabetes, and especially in peripheral neuropathy. People with impairments in sensation may not be able to identify when the compresses are too hot. The risk of burns is greater with moist heat than with dry heat. The client's history and medical diagnosis may alert you to other problems.
5. Warm the container of sterile saline or tap water by placing it in a bath basin filled with hot tap water. Sterile saline should be warmed to 105°–113°F. If you are using a commercial compress, follow the manufacturer's directions for heating the compress.	5. Sterile saline is used to prevent any contamination of the wound. A temperature above 113°F will cause further injury.
6. Place a waterproof pad under the body area that needs the warm compress (Figure 30-7-1).	6. Protects the client's bed and clothing.
7. Pour the sterile saline into the sterile basin. Soak an appropriate-size piece of gauze or a towel, wring out the excess saline, and place it on the affected area (Figure 30-7-2). Wear gloves if there is any drainage of the client's body fluids. Wear sterile gloves if there is an open wound.	7. A sterile basin is used to prevent further contamination. Excess saline may increase the chance of burns.

(Continues)

PROCEDURE 30-7 Application of Heat and Cold (Continued)

ACTION	RATIONALE

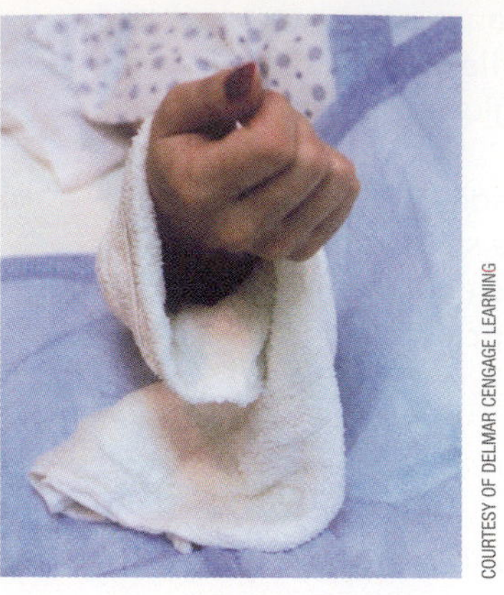

FIGURE 30-7-1 Place a waterproof pad under the body area to protect the client's bed and clothing.

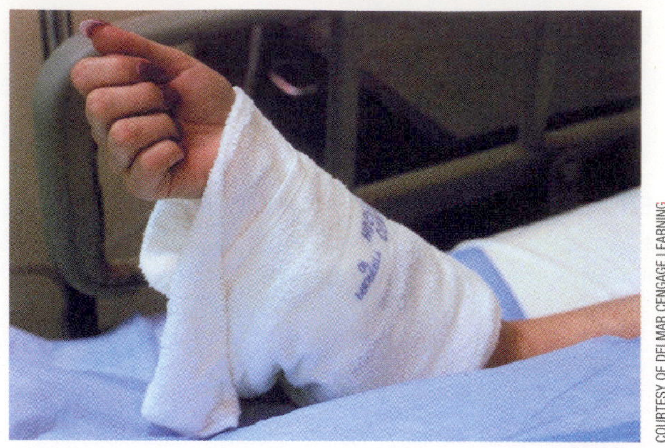

FIGURE 30-7-2 Place the moist towel on the area being treated.

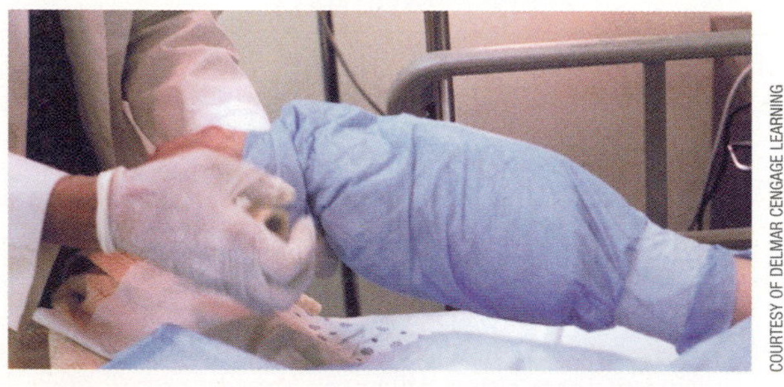

FIGURE 30-7-3 Wrap the hot, moist towel with a waterproof pad and secure the pad.

ACTION	RATIONALE
8. Wrap the area with a waterproof pad or apply a disposable heat or Aquathermia pad (Figure 30-7-3).	8. Maintains or holds in the heat.
9. Check the client's skin periodically for signs of heat intolerance. Tell the client to report any signs of discomfort immediately.	9. Signs of intolerance may include redness or further swelling.
10. If it is tolerated, leave the compress in place for approximately 20 minutes and then remove it.	10. Application of moist heat for a longer period of time may damage the client's skin and predispose the client to edema formation from circulatory congestion.
11. Dry the affected area with sterile towels if there is an open wound and with clean towels if there is no open wound.	11. The client may feel chilled when the warm compress is removed. Dry the area completely to prevent chilling.
12. Properly dispose of all single-use equipment according to hospital protocol.	12. Proper disposal of all other equipment reduces transmission of microorganisms.
13. Remove gloves, if they were worn, and wash hands.	13. Reduces transmission of microorganisms.
14. Reassess the condition of the client's skin.	14. The condition of the client's skin and any signs of heat sensitivity should be assessed and documented.

(Continues)

PROCEDURE 30-7 Application of Heat and Cold (Continued)

ACTION	RATIONALE
15. Record the procedure: condition of the client's skin and length of time of moist heat application. Report any abnormal findings to the physician.	15. Communicates procedure and findings to other members of the health care team and legally documents the care provided.
Sitz Bath	
16. Wash hands and assemble equipment (Figure 30-7-4).	16. Reduces transmission of microorganisms and organizes time.
17. Run tap water to preferred temperature (between 100°F and 110°F). Have client test the temperature on the dorsal surface of the wrist.	17. Prevents burn injury.
18. For toilet insert model, raise the seat of the toilet. Set the basin on the rim of the toilet bowel. Fill water bag and prime tubing. Close the clamp. Hang the water bag above the toilet. Thread the tubing through the front of the basin. Secure the tubing in the notch in the bottom of the basin.	18. Basin will rest on the bowl. Water bag will create a gentle swirling of water. The higher the bag, the more forceful the flow and the faster the water will run out.
19. For stand-alone model, fill basin with water (Figure 30-7-5).	19. Allows client to sit in the water.
20. Pad the seat with a towel (Figure 30-7-6).	20. Provides client comfort.
21. Always use Standard Precautions when assisting with perineal care treatments. Have client remove and dispose of peri-pad in a biohazard receptacle.	21. Prevents infection. Dressings that contain blood are disposed of in a biohazard container to prevent the spread of microorganisms.

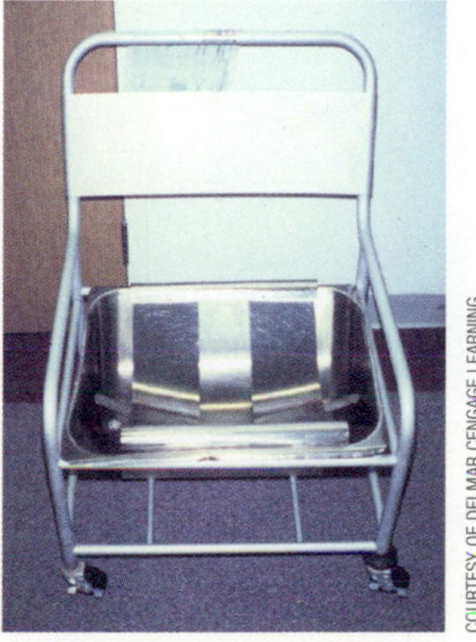
COURTESY OF DELMAR CENGAGE LEARNING

FIGURE 30-7-4 Portable Sitz Bath

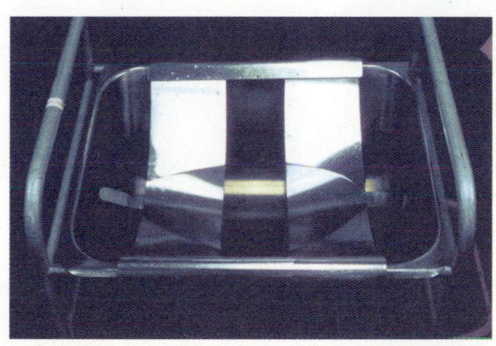
COURTESY OF DELMAR CENGAGE LEARNING

FIGURE 30-7-5 Fill the sitz bath basin with warm water.

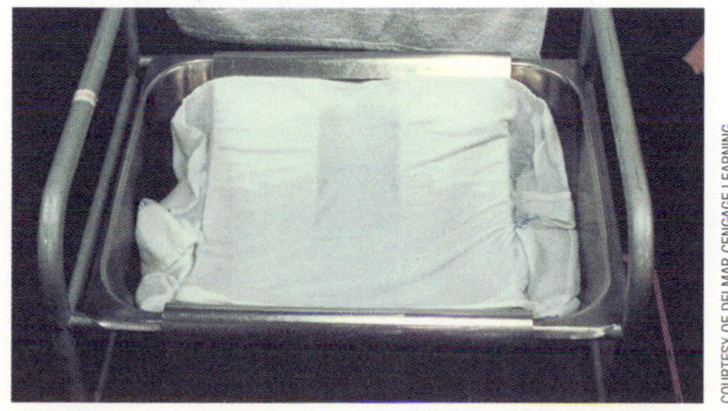
COURTESY OF DELMAR CENGAGE LEARNING

FIGURE 30-7-6 Pad the seat of the sitz bath with a towel for comfort.

(Continues)

PROCEDURE 30-7 Application of Heat and Cold (Continued)

ACTION	RATIONALE
22. Ensure that the floor is dry. Assist client to the bathroom if necessary.	22. Prevents injury from falling.
23. Have client sit in the basin (Figure 30-7-7). For toilet insert model, demonstrate how to unclamp the tubing to start the water flow.	23. Water flow is soothing and helps cleanse the area.
24. Cover client's lap for warmth and modesty (Figure 30-7-8).	24. Provides client comfort and privacy.
25. Ensure that the client can reach the call button. Instruct the client to call before standing up.	25. Water may splash over the floor, creating a slipping hazard.
26. After 20 minutes (or sooner if client is finished), help the client dry the area by gently patting with clean towels.	26. Warm soaks should last no longer than 20 minutes to prevent rebound vasoconstriction.
27. Assist client to bed. Encourage client to lie flat or elevate hips for 20 minutes.	27. Prevents congestion and decreases swelling.
28. For toilet insert model, empty remaining water into toilet. Rinse basin and bag. Clean according to institutional policy. For stand-alone model, empty water from drain trap into basin (Figure 30-7-9). Clean according to institutional policy.	28. Prepares equipment for the next use.

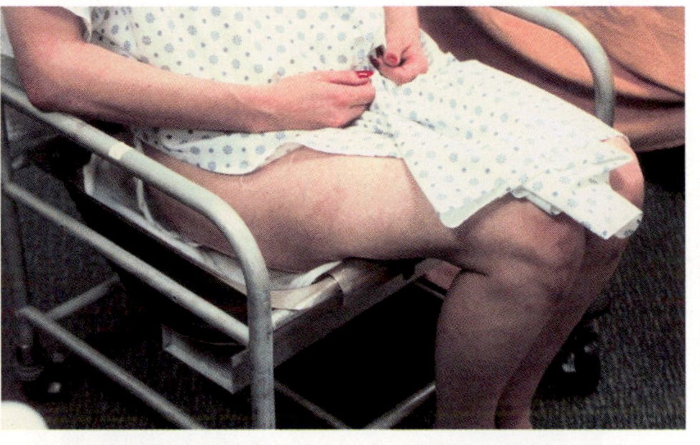
COURTESY OF DELMAR CENGAGE LEARNING

FIGURE 30-7-7 Have the client sit in the basin.

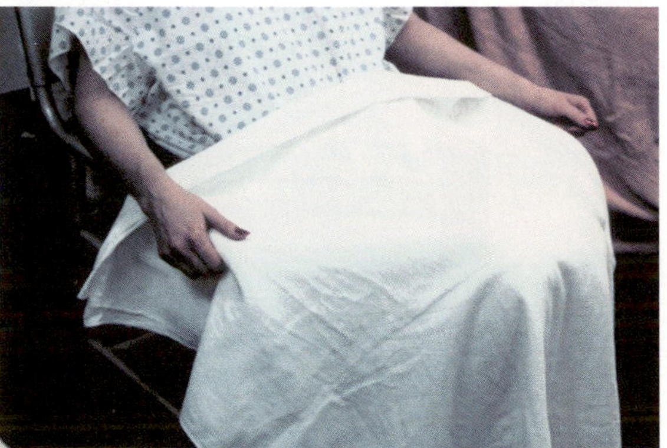
COURTESY OF DELMAR CENGAGE LEARNING

FIGURE 30-7-8 Cover the client's lap with a blanket or towel for modesty.

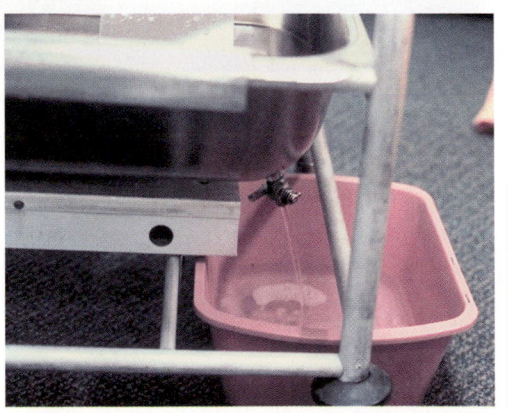
COURTESY OF DELMAR CENGAGE LEARNING

FIGURE 30-7-9 Empty water from drain tap into a basin for disposal.

Dry Heat

ACTION	RATIONALE
29. Check the physician's or qualified practitioner's order and the purpose of the heat treatment.	29. An order is required. Because there are many purposes of heat treatment, it is helpful to know what outcomes are expected and the site/sites to be treated.

(Continues)

PROCEDURE 30-7 Application of Heat and Cold (Continued)

ACTION	RATIONALE
30. Determine if there are any underlying problems that may affect the use of heat treatment, such as decreased sensation; decreased mentation; or a history of diabetes mellitus, bleeding disorders, peripheral vascular disease, or peripheral neuropathy. Heat should not be used over areas of scarring.	30. If the client has decreased sensation or mental status, heat treatment should be used only if the client can be observed closely. Heat should not be applied over areas where the client cannot alert the nurse about the sensation of burning.
31. Wash hands.	31. Reduces transmission of microorganisms.
32. Check the skin for lotions or ointments and remove if present.	32. Lotions and ointments retain heat and can lead to an increased risk of burning.
33. Gather equipment and complete as follows: *For a disposable heat pack:*	33.
• Activate the pack according to the manufacturer's directions. Some packs must be heated in boiling water, others can be heated by microwave, and some require bending and chemical activation (Figure 30-7-10).	• Manufacturer's directions should be followed because activation differs. If a microwave is used to heat a pack that should be heated in boiling water, the bag might break.
• Wrap the pack in a towel or protective covering (some manufacturers include cover). Do not use pins. Use tape if needed to secure the towel.	• A barrier between the client's skin and the heat source is necessary to avoid burns.
• Discard after use.	• Chemically activated packs will not reactivate once activated. In medical facilities, gel packs cannot be reheated in common areas without causing the transmission of microorganisms. In the home setting, packs activated by boiling or the microwave can be used on the same client again.
For an Aquathermia pad: • Follow manufacturer's directions.	• There are various brands of Aquathermia pads and each one may have slight differences in operating instructions.
• Fill the control unit with distilled water or as indicated by manufacturer's directions.	• Distilled water prevents the accumulation of mineral deposits that will damage equipment.
• Check the control unit and tubing for leaks. Turn on the unit and check the temperature of the water with a thermometer after several minutes. The proper temperature of the water is 105°F. Some units require that the control unit is level with the pad to function because overcoming gravity can put undue strain on the motor (Figure 30-7-11).	• This will ensure that the control unit is properly functioning. If there is a leak in the tubing, another pad should be obtained because this presents an electrical danger to the client and the staff.
34. Wash hands.	34. Reduces transmission of microorganisms.

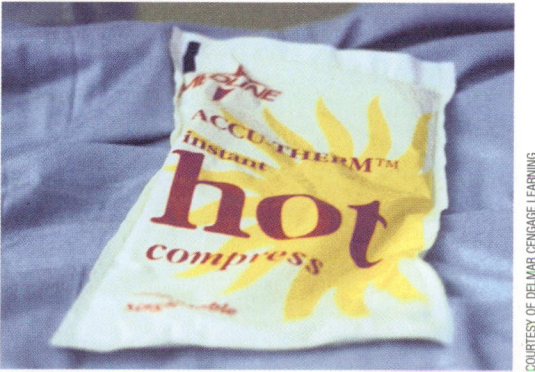

COURTESY OF DELMAR CENGAGE LEARNING

FIGURE 30-7-10 Disposable Hot Pack

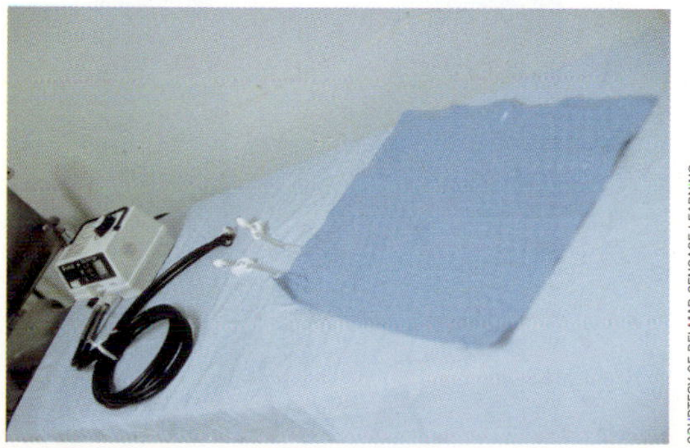
COURTESY OF DELMAR CENGAGE LEARNING

FIGURE 30-7-11 Aquathermia Pad

(Continues)

PROCEDURE 30-7 Application of Heat and Cold (Continued)

ACTION	RATIONALE
Application of Cold	
35. Wash hands.	35. Reduces transmission of microorganisms.
36. Assess the client's sensation and skin color at the site of planned application. Determine if any tissue damage is present. Assess for bleeding or wound drainage (Figure 30-7-12).	36. Provides baseline data for post-treatment comparison.
37. Identify whether the client has a history of circulatory impairment or neuropathy (Figure 30-7-13).	37. Cold causes vasoconstriction and decreased metabolism and can cause tissue damage in people with impaired circulation and sensation.
38. Check the physician's or qualified practitioner's order and the reason for the application of cold.	38. A physician's or qualified practitioner's order is needed in most situations of cold treatment. The reason for application of cold should be taught to the client.
39. If using an ice bag with moist gauze or towels, fill the bag three-fourths full with ice and remove the remaining air from the bag. Close the bag. Check for leaks. Wrap the bag in a towel or protective cover and place it on the affected area. If cold soaks are being applied, use the appropriate-size basin for the body part to be soaked.	39. If air is removed from the bag, the bag will be easier to mold to the client's body. The bag is wrapped to prevent injury to the client's skin or exposed tissue because direct cold can cause damage.
40. If an ice collar is used, fill the collar three-fourths full with ice and remove the remaining air from the collar before closing the collar. Check for leaks. Place the collar in a protective cover and around the client's neck.	40. Easier to mold to the client's body. The collar is wrapped to prevent injury to the client's skin.

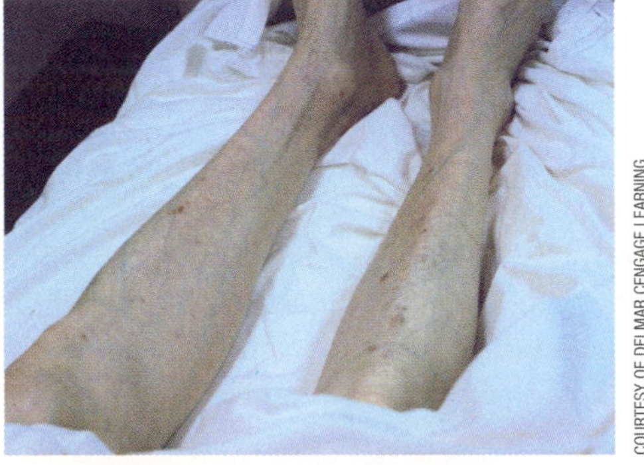
COURTESY OF DELMAR CENGAGE LEARNING

FIGURE 30-7-12 Assess the skin at the site of planned cold application for color, sensation, wounds, or skin irritation.

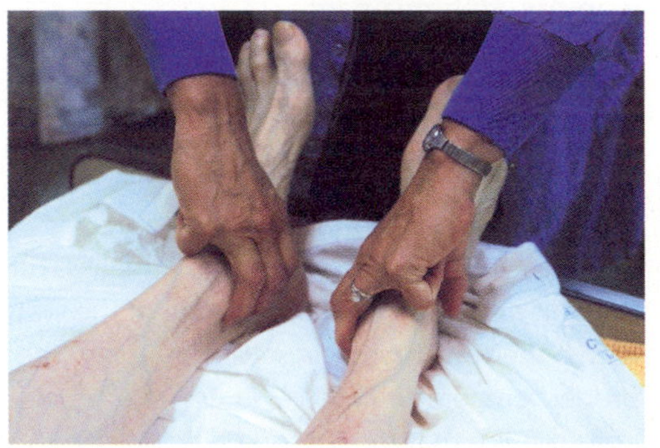
COURTESY OF DELMAR CENGAGE LEARNING

FIGURE 30-7-13 Assess for circulatory or neuropathy before beginning the procedure.

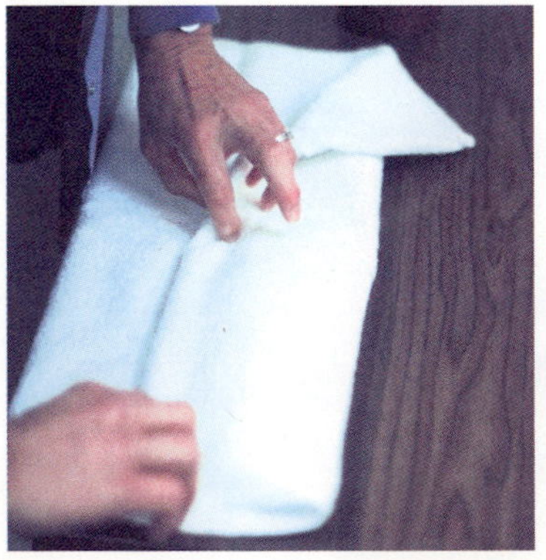
COURTESY OF DELMAR CENGAGE LEARNING

FIGURE 30-7-14 Wrap the cold pack in a towel.

(Continues)

PROCEDURE 30-7 Application of Heat and Cold (Continued)

ACTION	RATIONALE
41. If a disposable cold pack is used, activate the pack according to the manufacturer's directions, wrap the pack in a towel (Figure 30-7-14), and place it on the affected area (Figure 30-7-15). Some packs come with covers. Secure the pack in place with tape, elastic wrap, or bandage (Figures 30-7-16, 30-7-17, and 30-7-18). Dispose of the pack after the treatment.	41. When the pack is squeezed or kneaded, an alcohol-based solution is released, creating the cold temperature. The pack cannot be used again.
42. Assess the client's skin periodically for signs of cold intolerance or tissue damage.	42. Signs of intolerance to cold are pallor, blanching, mottling, or numbness of the skin.
43. If the client can tolerate the cold, leave the cold application in place for approximately 20 minutes at approximately 15°C (59°F).	43. Longer application can cause tissue damage, especially because the client's pain sensation is decreased in the presence of cold. A reflex vasodilation occurs after 20 minutes, thereby negating the therapeutic effect of the cold treatment.
44. Dispose of equipment according to agency policy.	44. Reduces transmission of microorganisms.
45. Reassess the condition of the client's skin or exposed tissue.	45. The client's skin should be assessed, and any signs of cold changes and intolerance should be documented.
46. Wash hands.	46. Reduces transmission of microorganisms.

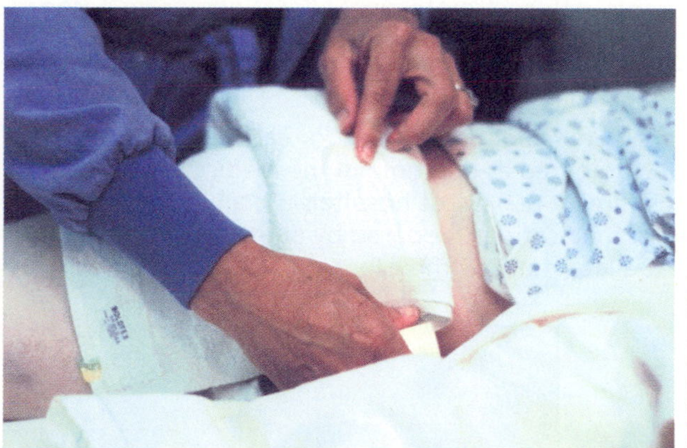
COURTESY OF DELMAR CENGAGE LEARNING

FIGURE 30-7-15 Place the cold pack on the affected body area.

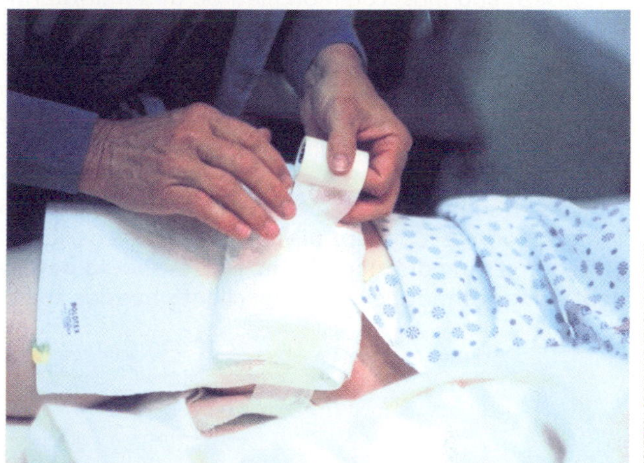
COURTESY OF DELMAR CENGAGE LEARNING

FIGURE 30-7-16 Secure the cold pack to the area with tape.

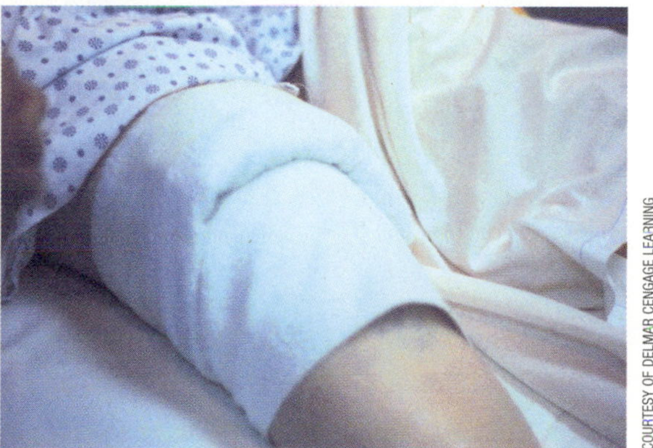
COURTESY OF DELMAR CENGAGE LEARNING

FIGURE 30-7-17 Cold pack properly wrapped in a towel and secured with tape.

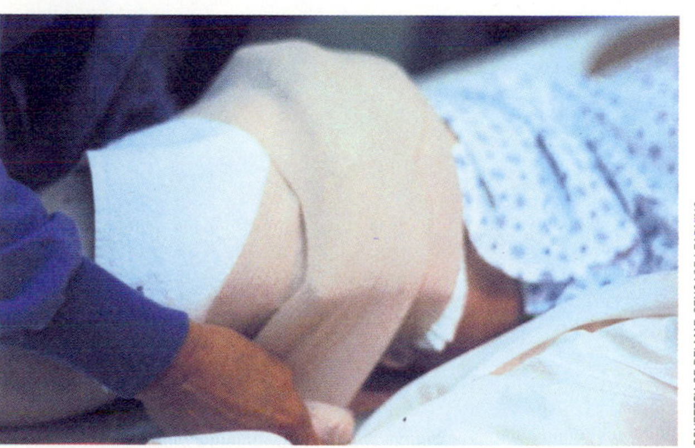
COURTESY OF DELMAR CENGAGE LEARNING

FIGURE 30-7-18 Elastic wrap may be used to hold bulky cold wraps in place.

(Continues)

PROCEDURE 30-7 Application of Heat and Cold (Continued)

EVALUATION

- The client derived the intended benefits of the heat or cold treatment.
- The client had no injury to skin integrity.

DOCUMENTATION

Nurses' Notes

- Document the procedure and the client's response to the procedure
- Record the equipment used
- Record the length of time of application
- Record the client's skin condition after the procedure

PROCEDURE 30-8 Administering Oral, Sublingual, and Buccal Medications

OVERVIEW

The easiest and most common method of administering a medication is usually by mouth (Figure 30-8-1). Clients may be taught to administer the medication by themselves at home, or a nurse can prepare the medications and dispense to clients. Oral medications are contraindicated for clients with gastrointestinal alterations, using nasogastric tube or gastrostomy tube, or who have a poor gag reflex. Clients with an inability to swallow because of neuromuscular disorder, esophageal stricture, or lesion of the mouth or those who are unresponsive or comatose are also ineligible to receive oral administration of medication.

Nurses need to know the action, normal dosage, side effects, and nursing implications for each drug they administer. In some settings, medications for several clients may be prepared at one time in the medication room or medication cart by carefully identifying each client's doses (Figure 30-8-2). Most hospitals use a computerized, limited-access medication system. Nurses should never administer medications prepared by another individual, and medications cannot be left at the client's bedside to be taken at a later time by the client.

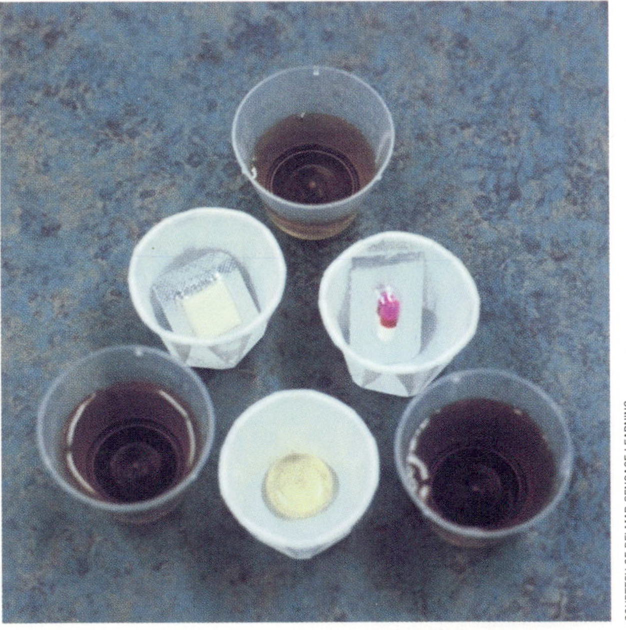

COURTESY OF DELMAR CENGAGE LEARNING

FIGURE 30-8-1 Oral, Sublingual, and Buccal Medications

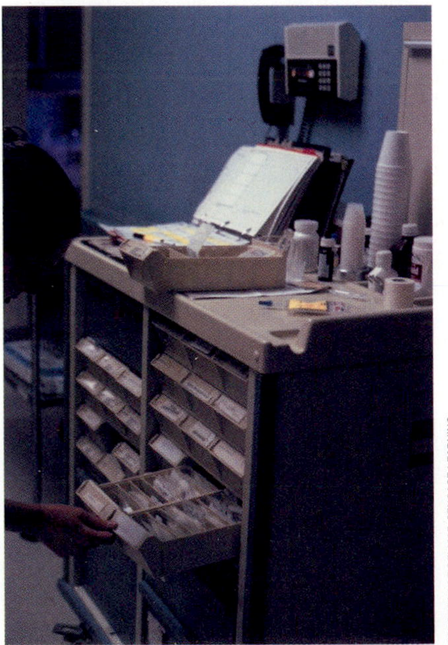

COURTESY OF DELMAR CENGAGE LEARNING

FIGURE 30-8-2 In some settings, medications for several clients are prepared at the medication cart at the same time.

(Continues)

PROCEDURE 30-8 Administering Oral, Sublingual, and Buccal Medications (Continued)

ASSESSMENT

1. Assess the seven rights: right client, right medication, right route, right dose, right time, right to refuse, and right documentation. **Prevents errors in medication administration.**
2. Review the action, purpose, normal dosage and route, common side effects, time of onset and peak action, and nursing implications of each drug **so the client's response to the medication may be monitored.**
3. Assess the client's condition to be sure the order of the health care provider is appropriate **because the client's condition may have changed since the order was written.**
4. Assess the client's ability to swallow food and fluid **because an alternate route for medication may be needed if unable to swallow a pill.**
5. Assess for any contraindications for administering an oral medication such as nausea and vomiting, gastric suction, or gastric surgery resulting in decreased peristalsis **because alterations in gastrointestinal function may interfere with drug absorption and excretion.**
6. Assess the client's medical record for a history of allergies to food or medications **so these medications can be avoided.**
7. Assess the client's knowledge about the use of medications **so client teaching can be tailored to client's needs. This may also assess compliance for taking the drugs at home or reveal drug dependence or abuse.**
8. Assess the client's age **because pediatric or geriatric clients may have special needs according to their ability to swallow a pill.**
9. Assess the client's need for fluids **because swallowing a pill is usually easier with fluid and promotes fluid intake; however, fluid restrictions are sometimes necessary.**
10. Assess the client's ability to sit or turn to the side. **The client must be able to swallow the pill without aspiration.**

POSSIBLE NURSING DIAGNOSES

Noncompliance
Impaired Swallowing
Deficient Knowledge (medication regimen)

PLANNING

Expected Outcomes

1. The client will swallow the prescribed medication.
2. The client will be able to explain the purpose and schedule for taking the medication.
3. The client will have no gastrointestinal discomfort or alterations in function.
4. The client will show the desired response to the medication such as pain relief, regular heart rate, or stable blood pressure.
5. The client will not have an allergic reaction.

Equipment Needed

- Health care provider's order for the medication
- Medication administration record (MAR)
- Medication cart or dispensing computer
- Medication tray
- Disposable medication cups
- Glass of water, juice, or other liquid
- Drinking straw
- Mortar and pestle, if needed
- Pill-cutting device, if needed
- Paper towels

delegation tips

The procedure of medication administration and assessment of effects is not delegated to ancillary personnel in acute care settings. This may vary in state or federal institutions. Ancillary personnel are generally informed about the medications the client is receiving if adverse effects are anticipated or are being monitored.

IMPLEMENTATION—ACTION/RATIONALE

ACTION	RATIONALE
1. Wash hands.	1. Reduces the number of microorganisms.
2. Arrange the medication tray and cups in the medication room or on the medication cart outside the client's room. Most hospitals use a computerized limited-access medication cart. Follow institutional protocol.	2. Organizing medications and equipment saves time and reduces the possibility of error.

(Continues)

PROCEDURE 30-8 Administering Oral, Sublingual, and Buccal Medications (Continued)

ACTION	RATIONALE

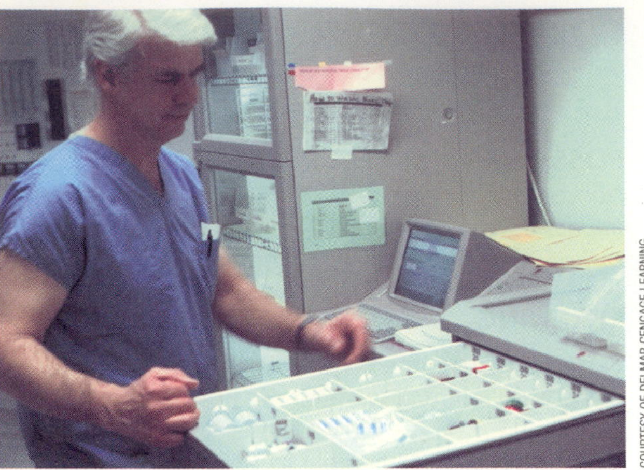

COURTESY OF DELMAR CENGAGE LEARNING

FIGURE 30-8-3 Prepare oral medication following the five rights: right client, time, medication, dose, and route.

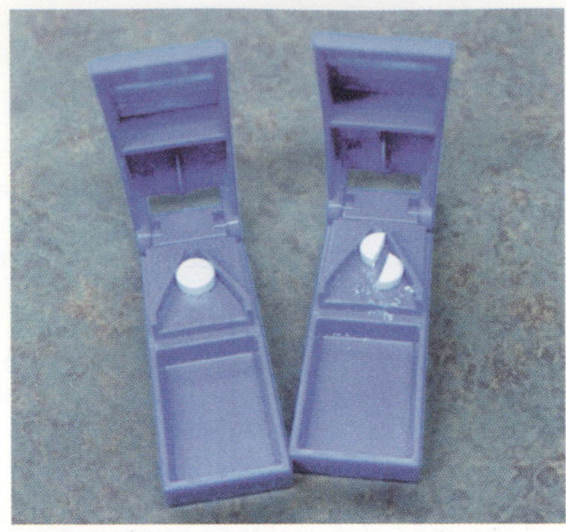

COURTESY OF DELMAR CENGAGE LEARNING

FIGURE 30-8-4 Scored tablets may be broken, if necessary.

ACTION	RATIONALE
3. Unlock the medication cart or log on to the computer.	3. Medications need to be safeguarded.
4. Prepare the medication for one client at a time following the first five rights. Select the correct drug from the medication drawer according to the MAR (Figure 30-8-3). Calculate the drug dosage if needed.	4. The first five rights are right client, right time, right medication, right dose, and right route. Comparing the MAR with the label reduces error. Double-checking reduces error in calculation.
5. To prepare a tablet or capsule: Pour the required number of tablets or capsules into the bottle cap and transfer the medication to a medication cup without touching them.	5. Avoids wasting expensive medications and avoids contamination of medication.
• Scored tablets may be broken, if necessary, using gloved hands or with a pill-cutting device (Figure 30-8-4).	• Tablets that are not scored are not meant to be broken. The medication's effectiveness would be diminished if the tablet were broken or crushed.
• A unit-dose tablet should be placed directly into the medicine cup *without* opening it until it is administered to the client.	• The wrapper maintains cleanliness and identification until it is administered.
• For clients with difficulty in swallowing, some tablets may be crushed into a powder using a mortar and pestle or by being placed between two paper medication cups and ground with a blunt object, then mixed in a small amount of applesauce. *Time-released or specially coated medications must not be crushed.* Check with the pharmacy if you are uncertain (Figure 30-8-5).	• A large tablet is usually easier to swallow if it is ground and mixed with soft food.
6. To prepare a liquid medication: Remove the bottle cap from the container and place cap upside down on the cart. Hold the bottle with the label up and place the medication cup at eye level on a level surface while pouring (Figure 30-8-6). Fill the cup to the desired level using the surface or base of the meniscus as the scale, not the edge of the liquid on the cup. Wipe lip of bottle with paper towel.	6. Placing the bottle cap upside down on the cart prevents contamination of the inside of the container. Holding the bottle with the label up keeps spilled liquid from obliterating the label. Holding the medication cup at eye level ensures an accurate dose. Wiping the lip of the bottle prevents the bottle cap from sticking.

(Continues)

PROCEDURE 30-8 Administering Oral, Sublingual, and Buccal Medications (Continued)

ACTION	RATIONALE
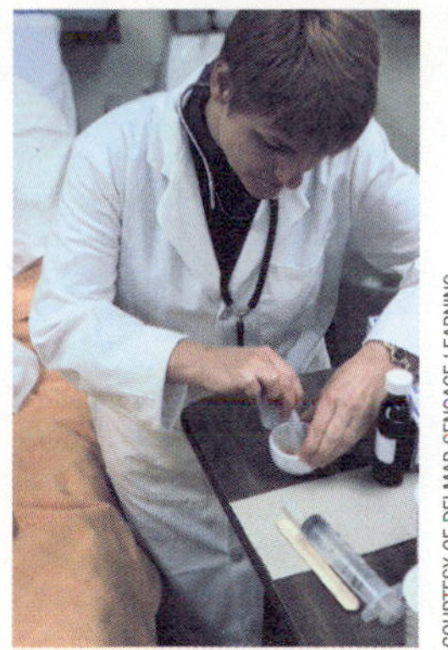 **FIGURE 30-8-5** Some medications may be crushed and mixed with a soft food, such as applesauce, for clients who have difficulty in swallowing.	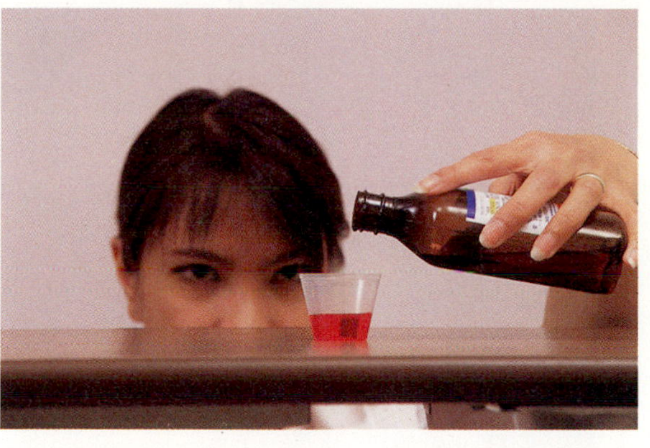 **FIGURE 30-8-6** Measure liquid medications at eye level on a level surface.
7. To prepare a narcotic, obtain the key to the narcotic drawer and check the narcotic record for the drug count when signing out the dose. If the drug count does not agree with records, report to charge nurse immediately.	7. Controlled substance laws require records of each dose dispensed. Early identification of errors assists in corrective action. Facility may require an incident report be filed.
8. Check expiration date on all medications.	8. Expired medications may lose their effectiveness.
• Double-check the MAR with the prepared drugs.	• Reduces risk of error.
• Return stock medications to their shelf or drawer.	• Ensures safety of stock medications.
• Place MARs with the client's medications.	• Ensures identification of medications.
• Do not leave drugs unattended.	• Drugs are safeguarded by nurse.
9. Administer medications to client: Observe the correct time to give the medication.	9. Ensures the therapeutic effect of the drug when given within 30 minutes of the prescribed time. (*Right time.*)
• Identify the client using two identifiers by reading the client's name bracelet, repeating the name, and/or asking the client to state his or her name (Figure 30-8-7). Additionally, check the hospital number if name alert or client is not reliable.	• Identification bracelets made at the time of admission are the most reliable source of identification even if the client is unable to state his or her name. (*Right client.*)
• Check the drug packaging if it is present to ensure the medication type and dosage.	• Prevents giving the wrong medication or wrong dose. (*Right medication, right dose.*)
• Assess the client's condition and the form of the medication.	• Allows you to assess the route of the medication and if this route is appropriate. (*Right route.*)
• Perform any assessment required for specific medications such as a pulse or blood pressure.	• Determines whether the medication should be given at that time or not.
• Explain the purpose of the drug and ask if the client has any questions, assessing the client's sixth right to refuse the medications.	• Improves compliance with drug therapy.
• Assist the client to a sitting or lateral position.	• Prevents aspiration during swallowing.
• Allow client to hold the tablet or medication cup.	• Client becomes familiar with medications.
• Give a glass of water or other liquid, and straw if needed, to help the client swallow the medication (Figure 30-8-8).	• Promotes client comfort in swallowing and can improve fluid intake.
• For *sublingual* medications, instruct client to place medication under the tongue and allow it to dissolve completely.	• Drug is absorbed through the mucous membranes into the blood vessels. If swallowed, the drug may be destroyed by gastric juices or detoxified in the liver too quickly so that its intended effects will not occur.

(Continues)

PROCEDURE 30-8 Administering Oral, Sublingual, and Buccal Medications (Continued)

ACTION | RATIONALE

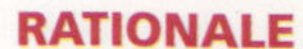

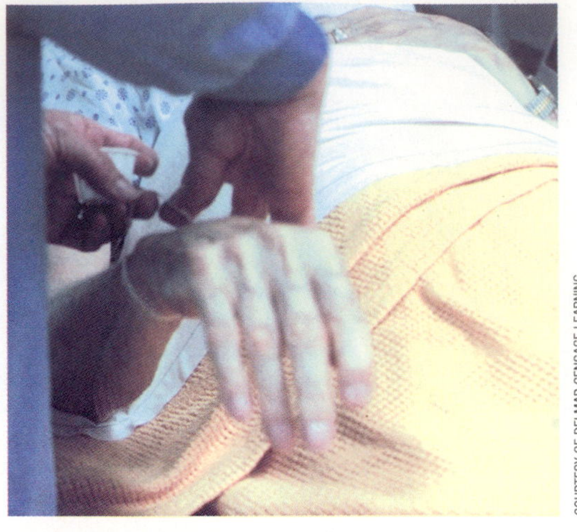

COURTESY OF DELMAR CENGAGE LEARNING

FIGURE 30-8-7 Identify the client using two identifiers by reading the client's name bracelet and asking his or her name before administering medication.

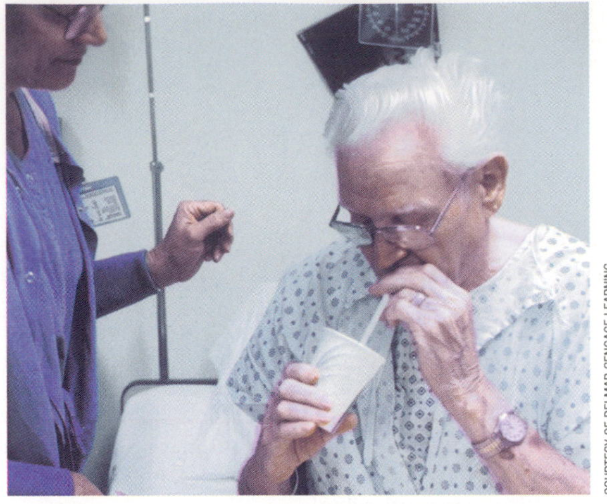

COURTESY OF DELMAR CENGAGE LEARNING

FIGURE 30-8-8 Allow the client to hold the tablet, and give water or juice to help him swallow the medication.

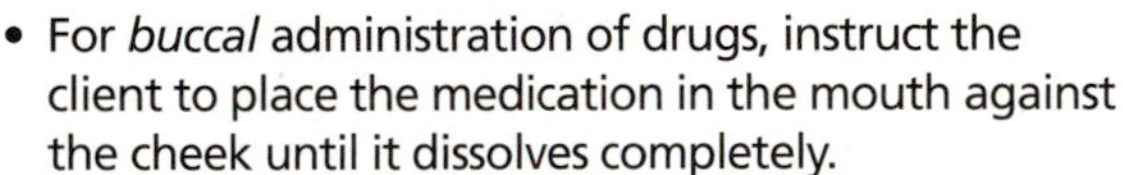

ACTION	RATIONALE
• For *buccal* administration of drugs, instruct the client to place the medication in the mouth against the cheek until it dissolves completely.	• Promotes local activity on mucous membranes.
• For oral medications given through a *nasogastric tube*, crush tablets or open capsules and dissolve powder with 20 to 30 mL of warm water in a cup. Be sure medication will still be properly absorbed if crushed and dissolved. Check placement of the feeding tube or nasogastric tube before instilling anything but air into the tube.	• Allows medication administration via nasogastric or feeding tube. Ensures that the medication is absorbed and utilized correctly.
• Remain with the client until each medication has been swallowed or dissolved.	• Ensures that the client receives the dose and does not save it or discard it.
• Assist the client into a comfortable position.	• Maintains client's comfort.
10. Dispose of soiled supplies and wash hands.	10. Reduces transmission of microorganisms.
11. Document (seventh right) the time and route of medication administration on the MAR and return it to the client's file.	11. Prevents administration error.
12. Return the cart to the medicine room; restock the supplies as needed. Clean the work area.	12. Assists other staff in completing duties efficiently.

EVALUATION

- Evaluate the client's response to the drug within 30 minutes of administration or sooner if an allergic reaction is anticipated.
- Ask client or caregiver to discuss the purpose, action, dosage schedule, and side effects of the drug.

DOCUMENTATION

Medication Administration Record

- Date and time each drug was administered, including initials and signature
- If drug is withheld, circle the time the drug was scheduled on the MAR.
- Document on appropriate electronic medical record or flow sheet.

Nurses' Notes

Document:

- Date, time, and reason a drug was withheld
- Response to drug administered

PROCEDURE 30-9 Withdrawing Medication from an Ampule

OVERVIEW

Ampules are containers that hold a single dose of medication. The ampules are made of clear glass and have a distinctive shape with a constricted neck. The head of the ampule is broken off at the neck, and the medication is withdrawn with a filter needle and syringe (Figure 30-9-1).

The neck of the ampule is often colored and usually scored. This scoring allows the neck to be broken off easily from the body to obtain the medication. Place a sterile piece of gauze around the neck of the ampule and break the neck in an outward motion. The gauze protects the nurse's fingers from the glass.

Medication can become trapped in the uppermost portion of the ampule. Before opening the ampule, flick the upper portion of the ampule with a fingernail to drop the medication from the upper segment down into the body of the ampule. This step may need to be repeated several times.

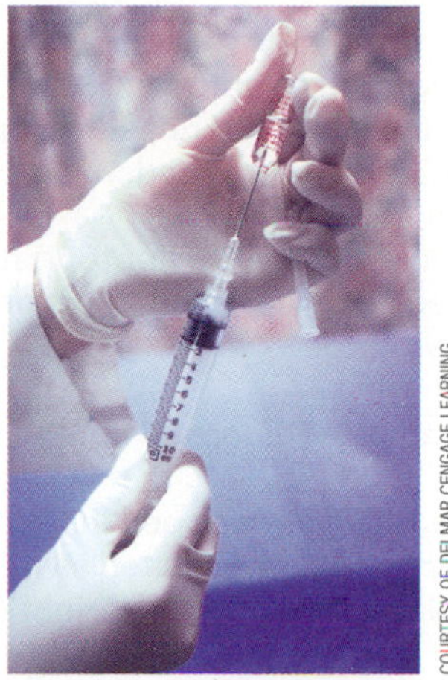

FIGURE 30-9-1 Withdrawing medication from an ampule.

ASSESSMENT

1. Identify the correct ampule, including medication, dosage strength, dosage volume, dosage route, and expiration date **to avoid medication errors.**
2. Assess the syringe, filter needle, and injection needle for expiration date and package intactness **to evaluate the sterility of the equipment.**
3. Assess the fluid in the ampule for cloudiness, particulate matter, or color changes **to evaluate for usability of the medication.**
4. Identify the medication's intended action, purpose, normal dosage range, time of action, common side effects, and nursing implications **to avoid medication errors.**

POSSIBLE NURSING DIAGNOSES

Risk for Impaired Skin Integrity
Risk for Infection

PLANNING

Expected Outcomes

1. The correct medication ampule will be selected.
2. The medication will be drawn into an appropriate syringe.
3. Microorganisms will not be introduced into the sterile system.
4. Foreign objects will not be introduced into the sterile system.

Equipment Needed (Figure 30-9-2)

- Medication ampule
- Sterile gauze pad or alcohol pad
- Syringe with filter needle
- Replacement needle
- Clean work space
- Medication administration record (MAR)

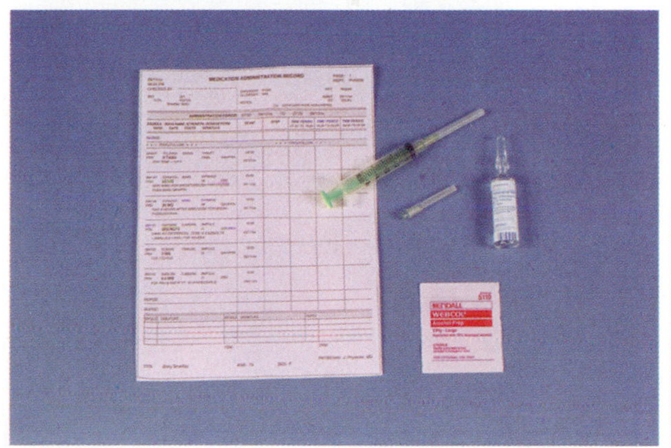

FIGURE 30-9-2 Syringes, needles, medication ampules, and alcohol wipes are used to withdraw medication from an ampule.

delegation tips

The procedure of medication administration is not delegated to ancillary personnel in acute care settings. This may vary in state or federal institutions. Ancillary personnel are generally informed about the medications the client is receiving if adverse effects are anticipated or are being monitored.

(Continues)

PROCEDURE 30-9 Withdrawing Medication from an Ampule (Continued)

IMPLEMENTATION—ACTION/RATIONALE

ACTION	RATIONALE
1. Wash hands.	1. Decreases transmission of microorganisms.
2. Select appropriate ampule (Figure 30-9-3).	2. Ensures client receives correct medication.
3. Select syringe with filter needle (Figure 30-9-4).	3. Filter needle entraps any glass fragments.
4. Obtain a sterile gauze pad.	4. Using a gauze pad prevents cuts on the jagged edge of the broken ampule.
5. Select and set aside the appropriate length of safety needle for planned injection.	5. Accurate needle length ensures the medication is administered where it is intended.
6. Clear a work space.	6. Prevents contamination with microdroplets that may spill when the ampule is broken.
7. Observe ampule for location of the medication.	7. The medication frequently becomes trapped in the top of the ampule.
8. If the medication is trapped in the top, flick the neck of the ampule repeatedly with your fingernail while holding the ampule upright (Figure 30-9-5).	8. Flicking the neck and top of the ampule moves the medication into the body of the ampule.

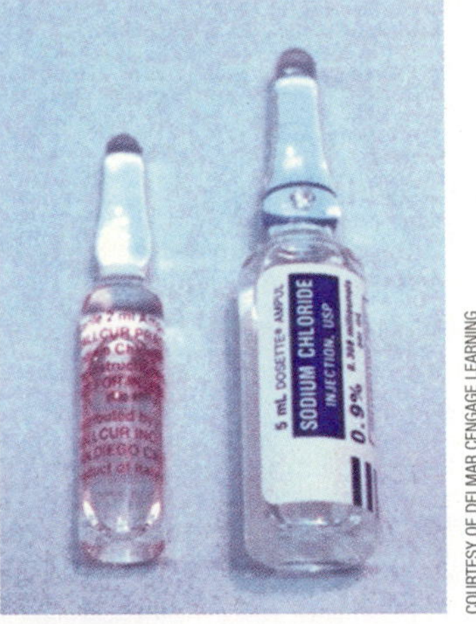

COURTESY OF DELMAR CENGAGE LEARNING

FIGURE 30-9-3 Medication Ampules

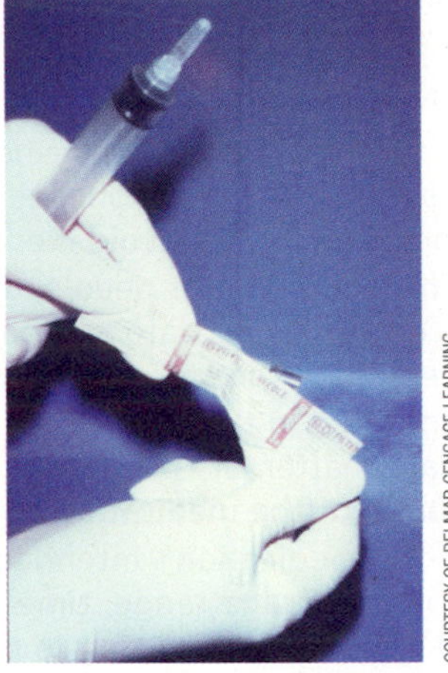

COURTESY OF DELMAR CENGAGE LEARNING

FIGURE 30-9-4 Select a syringe and filter needle.

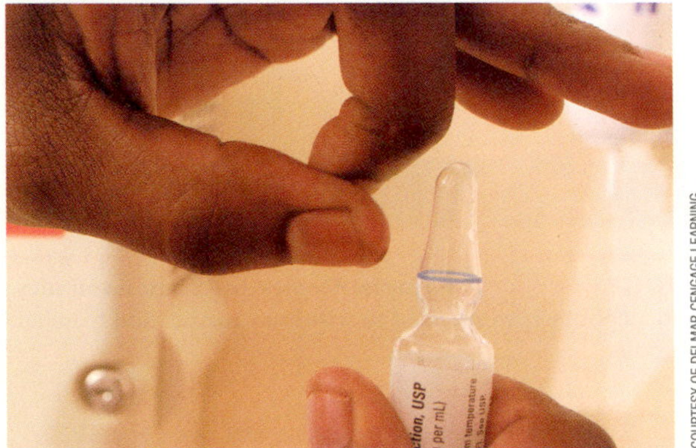

COURTESY OF DELMAR CENGAGE LEARNING

FIGURE 30-9-5 Flick the neck of the upright ampule to dislodge medication from the top of the vial.

(Continues)

PROCEDURE 30-9 Withdrawing Medication from an Ampule (Continued)

ACTION	RATIONALE
9. Wrap the sterile gauze pad around the neck and snap off the top in an outward motion directed away from self (Figures 30-9-6 and 30-9-7).	9. The gauze prevents the nurse from being cut by the jagged edge of the broken ampule. The outward motion provides added safety for the nurse.
10. Invert ampule and place the filter needle into the liquid. Gently withdraw medication into the syringe (Figure 30-9-8).	10. Inverting the ampule allows all of the medication to be withdrawn into the syringe. Surface tension will hold the medication in the ampule until the negative pressure of the syringe barrel draws it into the syringe.
11. Alternately, place the ampule on the counter, hold and tilt slightly with the nondominant hand. Insert the needle below the level of liquid and gently draw liquid into the syringe, tilting the ampule as needed to reach all the liquid.	11. While it is more difficult to read the syringe calibrations, it is easier to hold the ampule steady. Choose the method most comfortable for you.
12. Remove the filter needle and replace with the safety injection needle.	12. The filter needle is designed to trap glass particles and must not be used for client injections.
13. Dispose of filter needle and glass ampule (including lid) in appropriate sharps container.	13. Needles or sharp glass objects must always be disposed of in puncture and leak-proof containers to provide safety for clients and health care workers.
14. Label the syringe with drug, dose, date, and time.	14. Prevents medication errors from taking place.
15. Wash hands.	15. Decreases transmission of microorganisms.

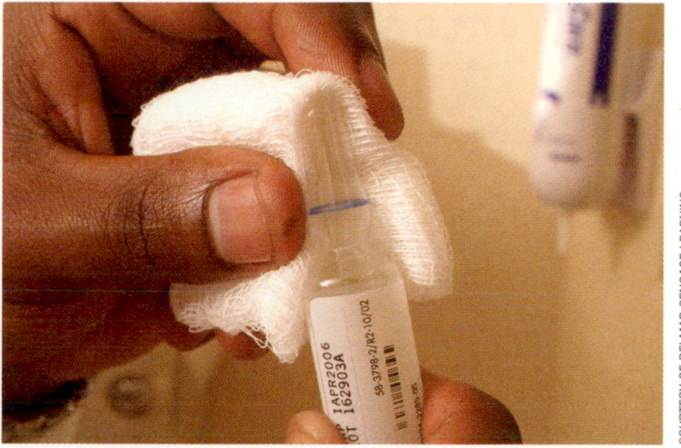

COURTESY OF DELMAR CENGAGE LEARNING

FIGURE 30-9-6 Wrap gauze or alcohol pad around the neck to protect fingers.

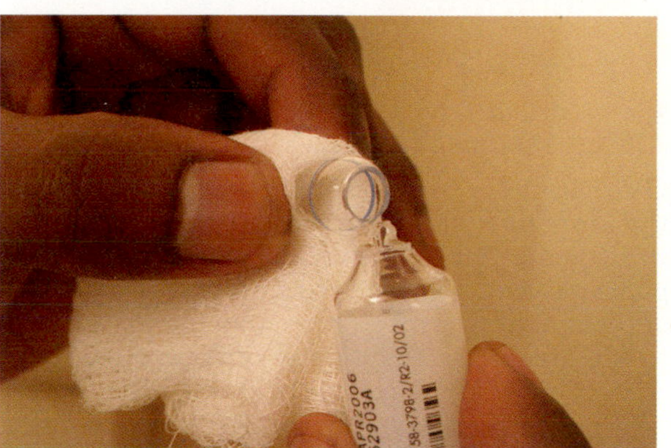

COURTESY OF DELMAR CENGAGE LEARNING

FIGURE 30-9-7 Snap the top of the ampule off in an outward motion away from self.

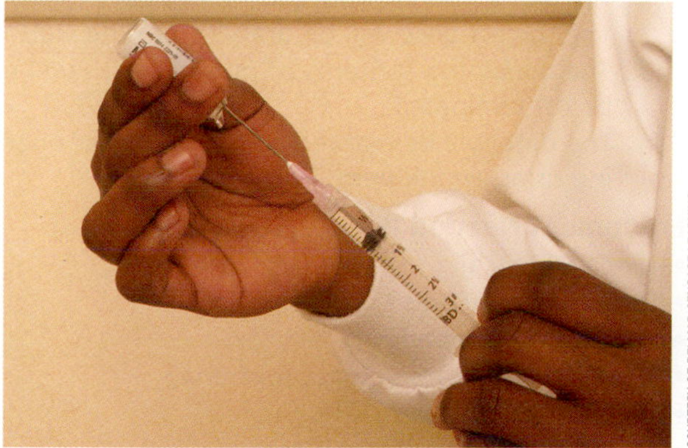

COURTESY OF DELMAR CENGAGE LEARNING

FIGURE 30-9-8 Invert ampule and gently draw the liquid into the syringe. Remove the filter and replace with the injection needle.

(Continues)

PROCEDURE 30-9 Withdrawing Medication from an Ampule (Continued)

EVALUATION
- The correct medication ampule was selected.
- The medication was drawn into an appropriate syringe.
- Microorganisms were not introduced into the sterile system.
- Foreign objects were not introduced into the sterile system.

DOCUMENTATION
Medication Administration Record

Document:
- Name of the medication
- Dosage drawn up
- Date and time the medication was drawn up

If the medication drawn up is a controlled substance, document in the Controlled Substances Record Book:
- Name of the medication
- Dosage drawn up
- Date and time the medication was drawn up
- Any controlled substance that was wasted
- Name of nurse drawing up the controlled substance

Controlled substances must be documented at the time they are removed from the locked cabinet. Documentation on the MAR is done after the medication is administered.

PROCEDURE 30-10 Withdrawing Medication from a Vial

OVERVIEW
Vials are often used to package multidose or single-dose parenteral medication. A vial is a small glass or plastic bottle with a rubber seal at the top. Vials come with a protective plastic or metal cap that prevents the rubber from being punctured before use. The rubber top must be cleaned with 70% alcohol with every usage of the medication. In order to aspirate the medication from the vial, an equal amount of air must be injected into the vial before attempting to withdraw any medication. In order to draw the medication out of the vial, the entire vial should be turned upside down. The syringe should be held at eye level to ensure an accurate amount of medication is drawn into the syringe.

ASSESSMENT
1. Assess the expiration date on the vial to be sure it is current **to avoid administering outdated medications.**
2. Assess the contents of the medication vial you are about to use for the correct medication in the correct dosage strength **to avoid medication error.**
3. Assess the contents of the vial for color, consistency, and debris **to avoid administering contaminated medication.**
4. Assess the integrity of the vial and its stopper **to avoid using a vial that may be contaminated.**
5. Assess the integrity of the syringe and needle that will be used to withdraw the medication **to avoid using equipment that may be contaminated.**

POSSIBLE NURSING DIAGNOSES
Risk for Infection

Risk for Injury

PLANNING
Expected Outcomes
1. The correct medication will be drawn from the vial using sterile technique.
2. The correct dose will be drawn from the vial.
3. The remaining contents of multiuse vials will not be contaminated.
4. The date will be marked on the vial after opening using an ink pen.

Equipment Needed (Figure 30-10-1)
- Medication vial
- Syringe with needle
- Alcohol sponge pad
- Nonsterile latex-free gloves (optional)
- Clean work space
- Medication administration record (MAR)

(Continues)

PROCEDURE 30-10 Withdrawing Medication from a Vial (Continued)

ACTION	RATIONALE

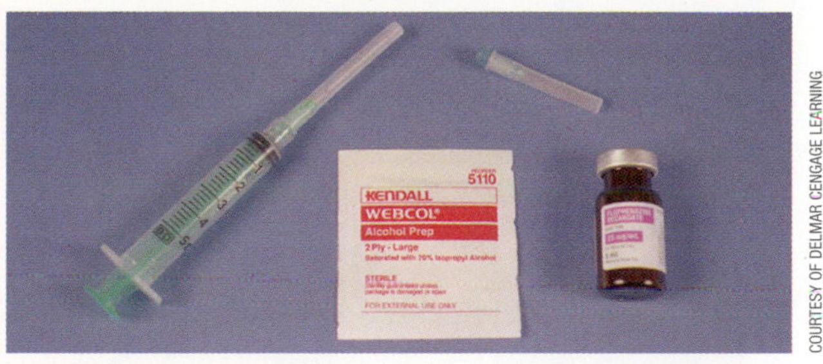

COURTESY OF DELMAR CENGAGE LEARNING

FIGURE 30-10-1 Syringe, needle, vial of medication, and alcohol wipes are used to withdraw medication from a vial.

delegation tips

The procedure of medication administration is not delegated to ancillary personnel in acute care settings. This may vary in state or federal institutions. Ancillary personnel are generally informed about the medications the client is receiving if adverse effects are anticipated or are being monitored.

IMPLEMENTATION—ACTION/RATIONALE

ACTION	RATIONALE
1. Wash hands. Apply nonsterile latex-free gloves (optional).	1. Decreases transmission of microorganisms.
2. Select the appropriate vial (Figure 30-10-2).	2. Prevents medication errors.
3. Verify health care provider's orders.	3. Prevents medication errors.
4. Check expiration date on vial.	4. Avoids giving expired medication, which may have altered potency.
5. Determine the route of medication delivery and select the appropriate size syringe and needle.	5. The route of medication delivery is essential to selecting the appropriate size syringe and needle.
6. While holding the syringe at eye level, withdraw the plunger to the desired volume of medication.	6. Holding the syringe at eye level makes it easier to read the syringe calibrations and increases accuracy.
7. Clean the rubber top of the vial with a 70% alcohol pad. Use a circular motion starting at the center and working out (Figure 30-10-3).	7. Ensures that the center of the rubber top is the cleanest area for needle entry. Reduces potential contamination with microorganisms.
8. Using sterile technique, uncap the needle and lay the needle cap on a clean surface.	8. Prevents spread of microorganisms.

COURTESY OF DELMAR CENGAGE LEARNING

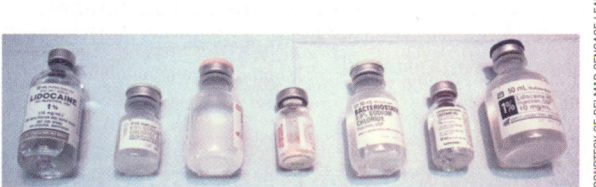

FIGURE 30-10-2 Carefully select the ordered medication.

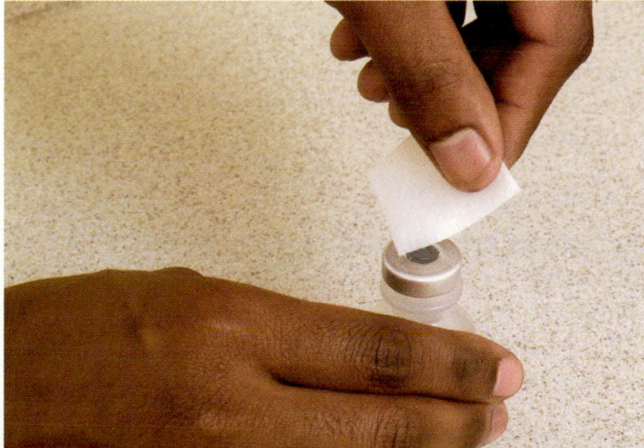

COURTESY OF DELMAR CENGAGE LEARNING

FIGURE 30-10-3 Clean the rubber top of the vial with a 70% alcohol pad.

(Continues)

PROCEDURE 30-10 Withdrawing Medication from a Vial (Continued)

ACTION	RATIONALE

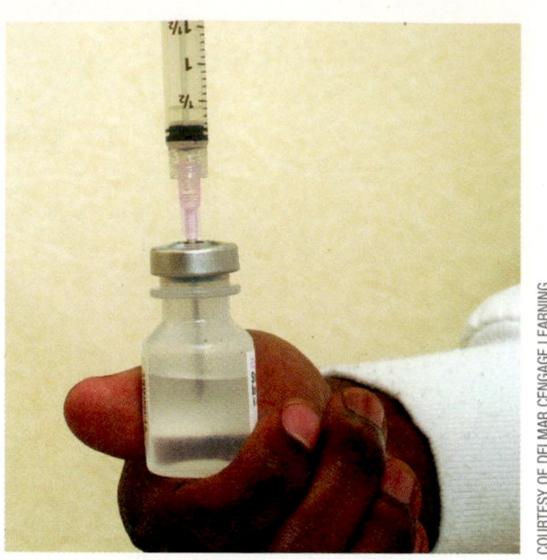

FIGURE 30-10-4 Place the needle into the vial through the center of the rubber top.

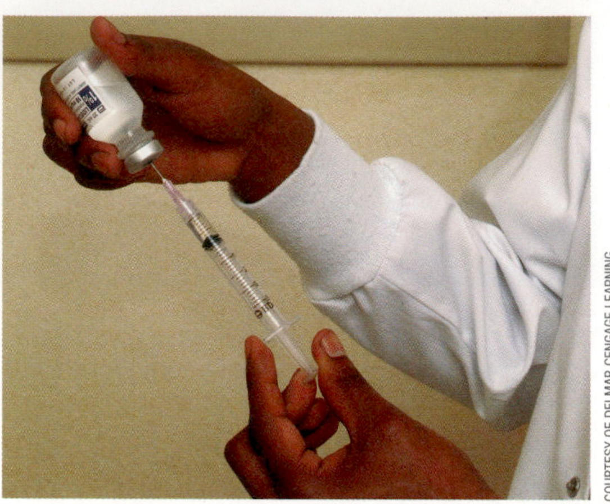

FIGURE 30-10-5 Invert the vial and slowly withdraw the medication until the appropriate dosage has been reached.

ACTION	RATIONALE
9. Placing the needle in the center of the vial, inject the air slowly. Do not cause turbulence (Figure 30-10-4).	9. Adding air prevents the buildup of negative pressure in the vial. Turbulence, which can result in air bubbles forming within the vial, can affect the accuracy of the volume of liquid being withdrawn.
10. Invert the vial and slowly, using gentle negative pressure, withdraw the medication. Keep the needle tip in the liquid (Figure 30-10-5).	10. Decreases the number of air bubbles that tend to form with unsteady, fast, jerky motions. Keeping the needle tip in the liquid prevents drawing in air.
11. With the syringe at eye level, determine that the appropriate dose has been reached by volume.	11. Ensures client receives the ordered dose of medication.
12. Slowly withdraw the needle from the vial. Follow the institution's policy regarding recapping and changing needles.	12. Avoids splatter of medication and potential contamination of nearby supplies. Keeps the needle sterile.
13. Using ink, mark the current date and time and initials on the vial.	13. Prevents using a medication that has been opened too long per institutional protocol.
14. Label the syringe with drug, dose, date, and time.	14. Prevents medication errors.
15. Wash hands.	15. Decreases transmission of microorganisms.

EVALUATION

- The vial was current and the rubber seal intact.
- The correct amount of medication was withdrawn.
- The needle did not become contaminated or damaged.

DOCUMENTATION

Medication Administration Record

Document:

- Name of the medication
- Dosage drawn up
- Date and time the medication was drawn up

If the medication drawn up is a controlled substance, document in the Controlled Substances Record Book:

- Name of the medication
- Dosage drawn up
- Date and time the medication was drawn up
- Any controlled substance that was wasted
- Name of nurse drawing up the controlled substance

Controlled substances must be documented at the time they are removed from the locked cabinet. Documentation on the MAR is done after the medication is administered.

PROCEDURE 30-11 Administering an Intradermal Injection

OVERVIEW

An intradermal injection is a method used to administer medications just below the skin. Potent medications that should be absorbed slowly are given intradermally because of the less richly supplied blood vessels of this layer; however, the client may respond rapidly and should be monitored for allergic reactions.

The most common reason for an intradermal injection is skin testing such as tuberculin screening or allergy testing. Only small amounts (0.01 to 0.10 mL) of fluid are given intradermally.

The most common sites for injections are forearms, upper chest, and upper back. The site should be lightly pigmented, free of lesions, and hairless. Because these areas are easily accessible, the nurse can monitor the reaction (Figure 30-11-1).

A tuberculin or small hypodermic syringe is used with a short (¼ to ½ inch), fine (26 to 27) gauge needle.

As of April 2001, a Federal Needle Stick Safety and Prevention Law requires safe medical devices. The position of the Occupational and Safety Health Act (OSHA) provides that whenever exposure to blood-borne pathogens is anticipated, controls to eliminate employee exposure should be used, hence, safe devices. Examples of such devices are needle-protected or needleless systems. In the case of intradermal injections, safety syringes or needles should be used. These can be safety-glide needles or safety-retraction or slide syringes. Instruction should be provided appropriate to manufacturers' specifications.

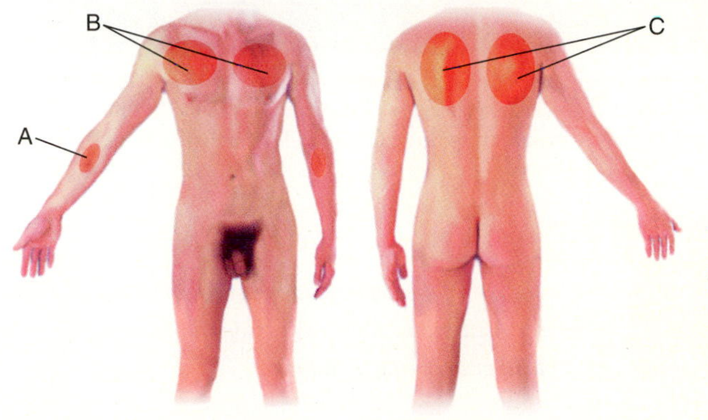

FIGURE 30-11-1 Common Intradermal Injection Sites: *A*, Inner Aspect of the Forearm; *B*, Upper Chest; *C*, Upper Back

ASSESSMENT

1. Assess the seven rights: right client, right medication, right route, right dose, right time, right to refuse, and right documentation. **Prevents errors in medication administration.**
2. Review health care provider's order **so the drug is administered safely and correctly.**
3. Review information regarding the expected reaction to the allergen **to anticipate the type of reaction a client may have.**
4. Assess for the indications for intradermal injection, including the client's allergy history, **so the nurse will not administer a substance to which the client is known to be sensitive.**
5. Check the expiration date of the medication vial **because the drug loses its potency over time.**
6. Assess client's knowledge regarding the medication to be received **so client education may be tailored according to need.**
7. Assess the client's response to discussion about an injection **because some clients may express anticipatory anxiety, which may increase pain.**

POSSIBLE NURSING DIAGNOSES

Risk for Infection
Impaired Skin Integrity
Deficient Knowledge (procedure)
Anxiety
Fear

PLANNING

Expected Outcomes

1. The client will experience only minimal pain or burning at the injection site.
2. The client will experience no allergic reaction or other side effects from the injection.
3. The client will be able to explain the significance of the presence or absence of a skin reaction.
4. The client will keep follow-up appointments within the recommended time frame to have responses to the medication evaluated.

(Continues)

PROCEDURE 30-11 Administering an Intradermal Injection (Continued)

Equipment Needed

- Tuberculin syringe, 1 mL (Figure 30-11-2)
- Needle (25- to 27-gauge, ¼- to ⅝-inch)
- Antiseptic or alcohol swabs
- Medication ampule or vial
- Medication card or medication administration record
- Nonsterile latex-free gloves

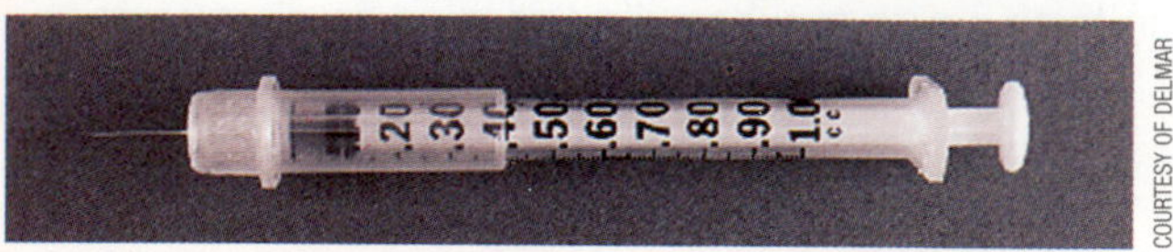

COURTESY OF DELMAR CENGAGE LEARNING

FIGURE 30-11-2 Syringes come in many sizes. Select a 1-mL tuberculin safety-syringe for intradermal injections.

delegation tips

The procedure of medication administration is not delegated to ancillary personnel in acute care settings. This may vary in state or federal institutions. Ancillary personnel are generally informed about the medications the client is receiving if adverse effects are anticipated or are being monitored.

IMPLEMENTATION—ACTION/RATIONALE

ACTION	RATIONALE
* Check client's identification band * Explain procedure before beginning *	
1. Wash hands and put on nonsterile latex-free gloves.	1. Reduces transmission of microorganisms.
2. In the inpatient setting, close door or curtains around bed and keep gown or sheet draped over body. In the outpatient setting, close door to exam or treatment room. Identify client and assess right to refuse (sixth right).	2. Provides privacy. Ensures that medication is given to right client.
3. Select injection site (Figure 30-10-1). • Inspect skin for bruises, inflammation, edema, masses, tenderness, and sites of previous injections. • Forearm site should be 3 to 4 finger widths below antecubital space and one hand width above wrists on inner aspect of forearm.	3. Injection site should be free of lesions. Repeated daily injections should be rotated. Ensures a clear site for interpreting results.
4. Select 1 mL tuberculin syringe and ¼- to ⅝-inch 25- to 27-gauge needle.	4. Ensures that needle will be inserted into the dermis.
5. Assist client into a comfortable position. Forearm site: Relax the arm with elbow and forearm extended on a flat surface. Distract client by talking about an interesting subject.	5. Relaxation minimizes discomfort. Distraction reduces anxiety.
6. Use alcohol pad or antiseptic swab in a circular motion to clean skin at site.	6. Circular motion and mechanical action of swab remove secretions containing microorganisms.

(Continues)

PROCEDURE 30-11 Administering an Intradermal Injection (Continued)

ACTION	RATIONALE
7. While holding the swab between fingers of nondominant hand, pull the cap from needle.	7. Swab remains accessible during procedure. Prevents contamination of needle.
8. Administer injection:	8.
• With nondominant hand, stretch skin over site with forefinger and thumb.	• Needle penetrates tight skin easier than loose skin.
• Insert needle slowly at a 5- to 15-degree angle, bevel up, until resistance is felt; then advance to no more than ⅛ inch below the skin. The needle tip should be seen through the skin.	• Ensures needle tip is in the dermis.
• Slowly inject the medication. Resistance will be felt.	• Dermal layer is tight and does not expand easily when fluid is injected.
• Note a small bleb, like a mosquito bite, forming under the skin surface (Figure 30-11-3).	• Indicates the medication was deposited in the dermis.
9. Withdraw the needle while applying gentle pressure with the antiseptic swab.	9. Supporting tissue around injection site minimizes discomfort.
10. Do not massage the site.	10. Prevents medication from being dispersed into the tissue and altering test results.
11. Assist the client to a comfortable position.	11. Promotes comfort.
12. Discard the uncapped needle and syringe in a sharps container.	12. Decreases risk of needlestick.
13. Remove gloves and wash hands.	13. Reduces transmission of microorganisms.
14. Document (seventh right).	14. Maintains legal record and prevents medication errors.

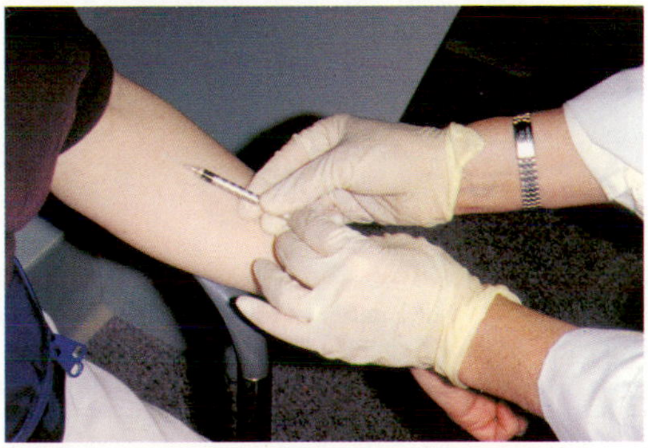

COURTESY OF DELMAR CENGAGE LEARNING

FIGURE 30-11-3 Note a small bleb, like a mosquito bite, forming under the skin surface as the medication is injected.

EVALUATION

- The client experienced only minimal pain or burning at the injection site.
- The client experienced no allergic reaction or other side effects from the injection.
- The client was able to explain the significance of the presence or absence of a skin reaction.
- The client kept all follow-up appointments within the recommended time frame to have responses to the medication evaluated.

DOCUMENTATION

Medication Administration Record

- Date, time, medication, dose, route, site, and signature or initials.

Nurses' Notes

Document:

- Date and time of skin reaction
- Date and time of any systemic side effects of the medication. Report to health care provider.

PROCEDURE 30-12 Administering a Subcutaneous Injection

OVERVIEW

A subcutaneous injection is a method used to administer medications into the loose connective tissues just below the dermis of the skin. Medications that do not need to be absorbed as quickly as those given intramuscularly are given subcutaneously because of the less richly supplied blood vessels in the subcutaneous tissue; however, the client may respond more rapidly to a subcutaneous injection than to oral medication and should be monitored for potential side effects, allergic reactions, the risk of infection, or bleeding.

Only small (0.5- to 1-mL) doses of isotonic, nonirritating, nonviscous, and water-soluble medications should be given subcutaneously, such as anticoagulants, insulin, tetanus toxoid, allergy medications, epinephrine, and vitamin B_{12}. If larger volumes of medications remain in these sensitive tissues, a sterile abscess could form, causing a hard, painful lump.

The most common sites for subcutaneous injections are the vascular areas around the outer aspect of the upper arms, the abdomen, and the anterior aspect of the thighs (Figure 30-12-1). Because these areas are easily accessible, the client may learn how to self-administer medications. Rotation of sites of injections should be observed so that no site is used more often than every 6 to 7 weeks.

For a subcutaneous injection, a 2- to 3-mL syringe or a 1-mL syringe is recommended. U-100 insulin syringes in 30-, 50-, and 100-unit sizes are used for subcutaneous insulin injections. The most commonly used needle for a subcutaneous injection is a ⅝-inch 25-gauge needle. Adjustments need to be made for pediatric, obese, or cachectic clients.

As of April 2001, a Federal Needle Stick Safety and Prevention Law requires safe medical devices. The position of the Occupational and Safety Health Act (OSHA) provides that whenever exposure to blood-borne pathogens is anticipated, controls to eliminate employee exposure should be used, hence, safe devices. Failure to comply with using safe devices and safe disposal can result in fines. Examples of safe devices are needle-protected or needleless systems with proper disposal in clearly marked sharps containers. In the case of subcutaneous injections, safety syringes or needles should be used. These can be safety-glide or retraction needles or slide syringes. Instruction should be provided appropriate to manufacturers' specifications.

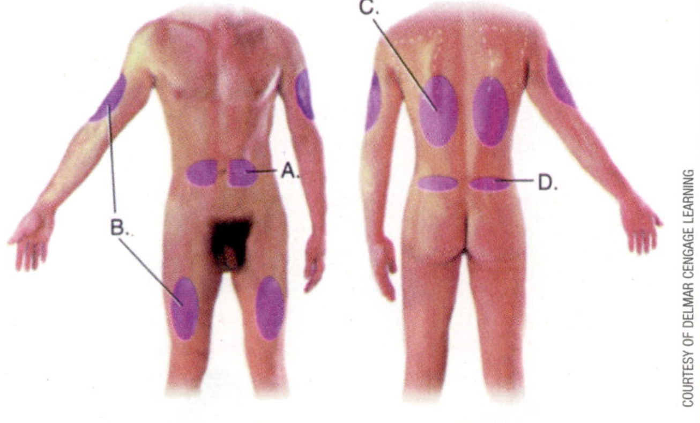

FIGURE 30-12-1 Subcutaneous Injection Sites: *A*, Abdomen; *B*, Lateral and Anterior Aspects of Upper Arm and Thigh; *C*, Scapular Area of Back; *D*, Upper Ventrodorsal Gluteal Area

ASSESSMENT

1. Assess the seven rights: right client, right medication, right route, right dose, right time, right to refuse, and right documentation. **Prevents errors in medication administration.**
2. Review health care provider's order **so the drug is administered safely and correctly.**
3. Review information regarding the drug ordered, such as action, purpose, time of onset and peak action, normal dosage, common side effects, and nursing implications **to anticipate the drug's effects and anticipate a reaction.**
4. Assess client for factors that may influence an injection such as circulatory shock or reduced local tissue perfusion **because reduced tissue perfusion will interfere with the absorption and distribution of the drug.**
5. Assess for previous subcutaneous injections **in order to rotate sites and avoid repeating a dose in the same site.**
6. Assess for the indications for subcutaneous injection **because an injection is preferred for clients who are confused or unconscious, are unable to swallow a tablet, or have a gastrointestinal disturbance, including the use of nasogastric suction.**
7. Assess the client's age **because older clients or pediatric clients have special needs based on their physiologic status.**
8. Assess client's knowledge regarding the medication to be received **so client education may be tailored according to need.**
9. Assess the client's response to discussion about an injection **because some clients may express anticipatory anxiety, which may increase pain.**
10. Check the client's drug allergy, history **as an allergic reaction could occur.**

(Continues)

PROCEDURE 30-12 Administering a Subcutaneous Injection (Continued)

POSSIBLE NURSING DIAGNOSES

Risk for Infection
Impaired Skin Integrity
Anxiety
Deficient Knowledge (procedure)
Fear

PLANNING

Expected Outcomes

1. The client will experience only minimal pain or burning at the injection site.
2. The client will experience no allergic reaction or other side effects from the injection.
3. The client will be able to explain the action, side effects, dosage and schedule of the medication, and rationale for rotation of sites.

Equipment Needed (Figures 30-12-2 and 30-12-3)

- Syringe appropriate for the medication being given
- Needle (25- to 27-gauge, ⅜- to ⅝-inch)
- Antiseptic or alcohol swabs
- Medication ampule or vial
- Medication record
- Nonsterile latex-free gloves

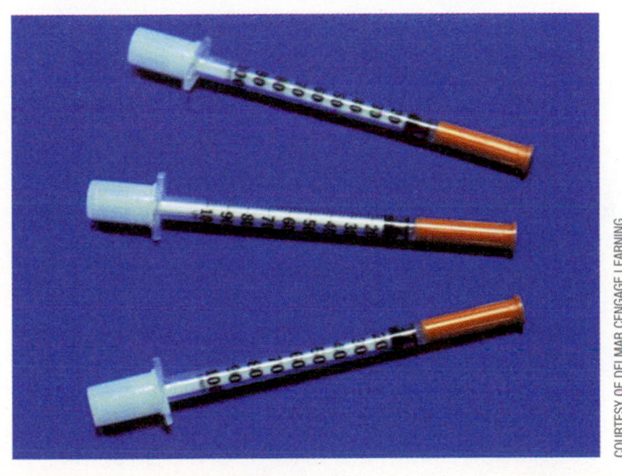

COURTESY OF DELMAR CENGAGE LEARNING

FIGURE 30-12-2 100-unit insulin syringes are used to administer insulin subcutaneously.

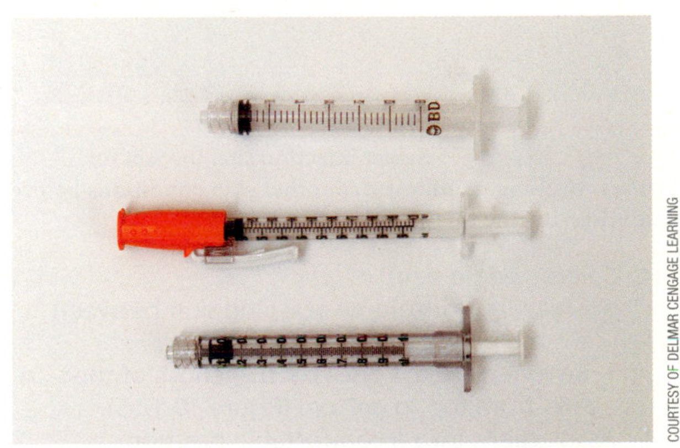

COURTESY OF DELMAR CENGAGE LEARNING

FIGURE 30-12-3 Syringes that are used for a subcutaneous injection include a 3-mL syringe, and insulin syringe, and a tuberculin syringe.

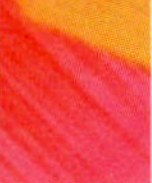

delegation tips

The procedure of medication administration is not delegated to ancillary personnel in acute care settings. This may vary in state or federal institutions. Ancillary personnel are generally informed about the medications the client is receiving if adverse effects are anticipated or are being monitored.

IMPLEMENTATION—ACTION/RATIONALE

* Check client's identification band * Explain procedure before beginning *

ACTION	RATIONALE
1. Wash hands and put on nonsterile latex-free gloves.	1. Reduces the number of microorganisms.
2. Close door or curtains around bed and keep gown or sheet draped over client. Identify client using two different identifiers.	2. Provides privacy. Ensures that medication is given to the right client.
3. Select injection site (Figure 30-12-1).	3. Injection site should be free of lesions.
• Inspect skin for bruises, inflammation, edema, masses, tenderness, and sites of previous injections and avoid these areas (Figure 30-12-4).	• Repeated daily injections should be rotated.
• Use subcutaneous tissue around the abdomen, lateral aspects of upper arm or thigh, or scapular area.	• Avoids injury to underlying nerves, bone, or blood vessels.

(Continues)

PROCEDURE 30-12 Administering a Subcutaneous Injection (Continued)

ACTION	RATIONALE

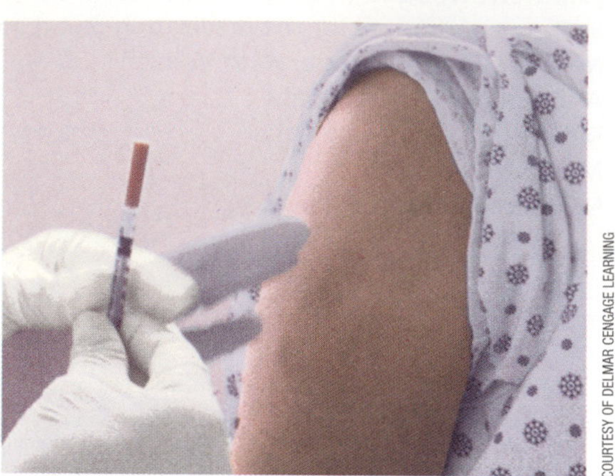

FIGURE 30-12-4 Select injection site. Inspect for bruises, swelling, tenderness, or other skin conditions before administering the injection.

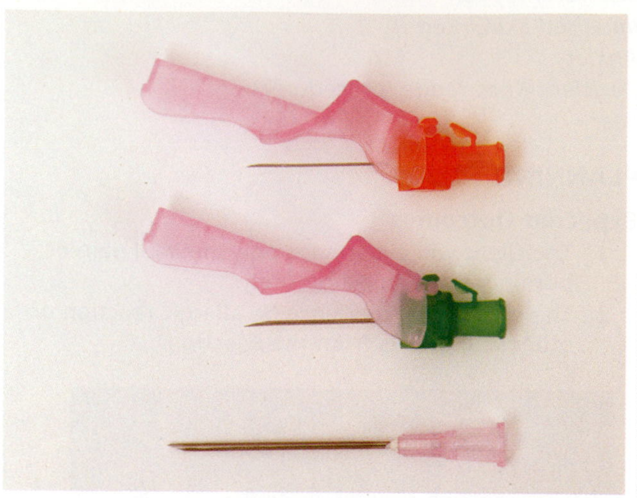

FIGURE 30-12-5 Shown are different types of needles used for an injection that have safety shields to protect against accidental needle sticks after the injection is given.

ACTION	RATIONALE
4. Select needle size: • Measure skinfold by grasping skin between thumb and forefinger. • Be sure needle is one-half the length of the skinfold from top to bottom (Figure 30-12-5).	4. Ensures that needle will be inserted into subcutaneous tissue.
5. Assist client into a comfortable position: • Relax the arm, leg, or abdomen. • Distract client by talking about an interesting subject or explaining what you are doing step by step.	5. Relaxation minimizes discomfort. Distraction reduces anxiety.
6. Use alcohol swab or antiseptic swab to clean skin at site.	6. Circular motion and mechanical action of swab remove microorganisms.
7. While holding swab between fingers of nondominant hand, pull cap from needle.	7. Swab remains accessible during procedure. Prevents contamination of needle.
8. Administer injection:	8.
• Hold syringe between thumb and forefinger of dominant hand like a dart.	• Quick, smooth injection is easier with proper position of syringe.
• Pinch skin with nondominant hand (Figure 30-12-6).	• Needle penetrates tight skin easier than loose skin. Pinching skin elevates subcutaneous tissue.
• Inject needle quickly and firmly (like a dart) at a 45- to 90-degree angle (Figure 30-12-7).	• Quick, firm injection minimizes discomfort. Angle depends on amount of subcutaneous tissue present and the site used.
• Release the skin.	
• Grasp the lower end of the syringe with nondominant hand and position dominant hand to the end of the plunger. Do not move the syringe.	• Injection requires smooth manipulation of syringe parts. Movement of syringe may cause discomfort.
• Pull back on the plunger to ascertain that the needle is not in a vein. If no blood appears, slowly inject the medication. (Aspiration is contraindicated with some medications; check with the pharmacy if you are unclear.)	• Aspiration of blood indicates intravenous placement of needle so procedure may have to be abandoned.

(Continues)

PROCEDURE 30-12 Administering a Subcutaneous Injection (Continued)

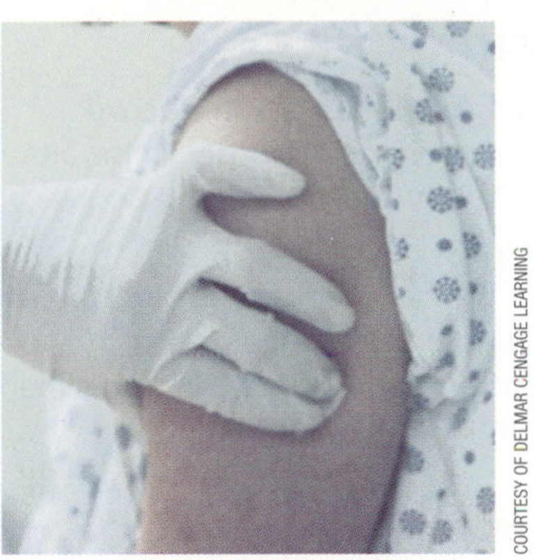
COURTESY OF DELMAR CENGAGE LEARNING

FIGURE 30-12-6 Pinch the skin with the nondominant hand.

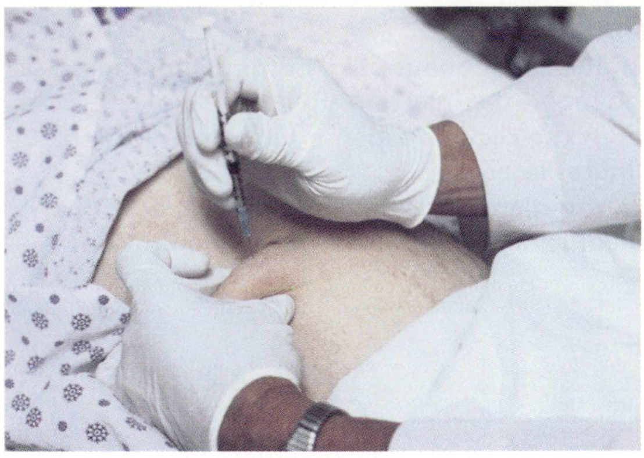
COURTESY OF DELMAR CENGAGE LEARNING

FIGURE 30-12-7 When injecting at a 90° angle, hold the syringe like a dart and pierce the skin quickly and firmly.

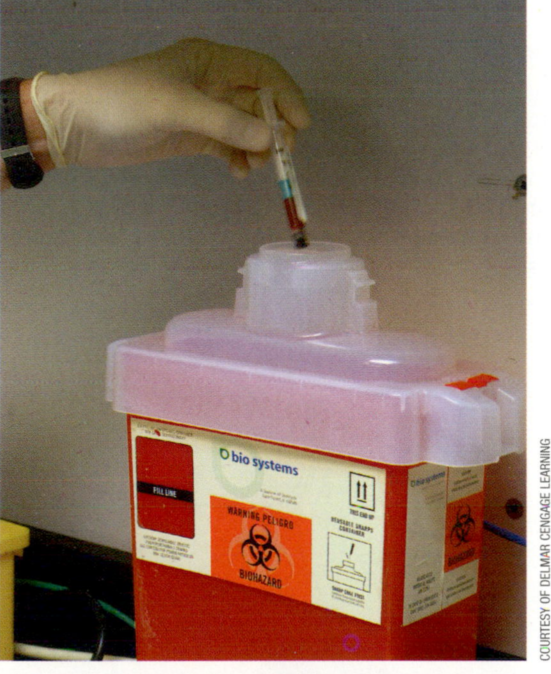

COURTESY OF DELMAR CENGAGE LEARNING

FIGURE 30-12-8 Dispose the uncapped needle in a specified biohazard sharps container.

ACTION	RATIONALE
9. Remove hand from injection site and quickly withdraw the needle. Apply pressure with the antiseptic swab. Do not push down on the needle with the swab while withdrawing it, because this will cause more pain.	9. Supporting tissue around injection site minimizes discomfort. Removing hand before withdrawing needle reduces chance of needlestick.
10. Apply pressure. Some medications should not be massaged. Ask the pharmacy if you are unclear.	10. Stimulates circulation and improves drug distribution and absorption.
11. Discard the uncapped needle and syringe in a disposable needle receptacle (Figure 30-12-8).	11. Decreases risk of needlestick.
12. Assist the client to a comfortable position.	12. Promotes comfort and encourages client to remain still.
13. Remove gloves and wash hands.	13. Reduces transmission of microorganisms.

(Continues)

PROCEDURE 30-12 Administering a Subcutaneous Injection (Continued)

ACTION	RATIONALE

EVALUATION
- Ask the client about pain, burning, numbness, or tingling at the injection site.
- Assess the client's response to the medication 30 minutes later.
- Ask the client to discuss the purpose, action, schedule, and side effects of the medication.

DOCUMENTATION
Medication Administration Record
- Date, time, medication, dose, route, site of injection, and signature or initials

Nurses' Notes
- Date and time of response to the medication
- Date and time of any side effects of the medication
- Document on appropriate electronic medical record or flow sheet (seventh right).

PROCEDURE 30-13 Administering an Intramuscular Injection

OVERVIEW
An intramuscular injection is a method used to administer medications into the deep muscle tissue. Medications will be absorbed quickly because of the richly supplied blood vessels in the muscle. Most aqueous medications are absorbed in 10 to 30 minutes. Average-sized adults can tolerate up to 3 mL of medication injected into a large muscle because muscle is less sensitive to irritating and viscous drugs than subcutaneous tissue.

The most common sites for intramuscular injections are the vastus lateralis, the ventrogluteal, the dorsogluteal, and the deltoid muscles (Figure 30-13-1). The *vastus lateralis* muscle is located on the anterior lateral aspect of the

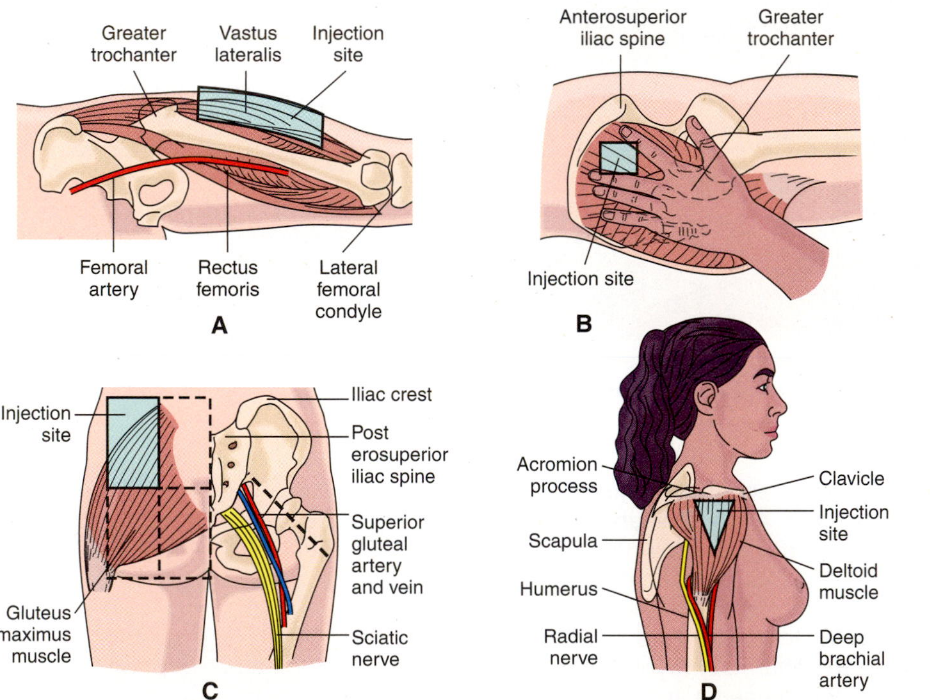

FIGURE 30-13-1 Intramuscular injection sites. *A,* Vastus lateralis: Identify greater trochanter; place hand at lateral femoral condyle; injection site is middle third of anterior lateral aspect. *B,* Ventrogluteal: Place palm of left hand on right greater trochanter so that index finger points toward anterosuperior iliac spine; spread first and middle fingers to form a V; injection site is the middle of the V angle. *C,* Dorsogluteal: Place hand on iliac crest and locate the posterosuperior iliac spine. Draw an imaginary line between the trochanter and the iliac spine; the injection site is the outer quadrant. *D,* Deltoid: Locate the lateral side of the humerus from two to three finger widths below the acromion process in adults or one finger width below the acromion process in children.

(Continues)

PROCEDURE 30-13 Administering an Intramuscular Injection (Continued)

ACTION	RATIONALE

thigh. This easily accessible site is the preferred site for clients of all ages because it has no major blood vessels or nerves nearby. The *ventrogluteal* site is the preferred site in adults because it is located deep and away from major blood vessels and nerves. It is preferred over the dorsogluteal for the following reasons: There is less risk of damage to the sciatic nerve and blood vessels; this site is less painful because the muscle is most often not tense even in an anxious client. The *dorsogluteal* muscle in the upper outer quadrant of the buttock poses greater risk of damage to the sciatic nerve, major blood vessels, and the greater trochanter bone. It should not be used in children younger than 5 years of age because this muscle is not developed. The *deltoid* muscle is found on the upper arm about 1 to 2 inches below the acromion process. Major nerves and blood vessels are beneath this site, and only small volumes of medication should be injected.

Originally the Z-track method of intramuscular injections was used as a special procedure for only certain medications. Medications such as iron dextran and hydralazine hydrochloride can be irritating to the tissues and stain the skin. Using the Z-track method prevents potentially irritating medications from being tracked up through the tissues by interrupting the injection tract. This method can help reduce pain also with nonstaining or irritating substances.

There are many different types and sizes of syringes. Prefilled syringes that consist of a prefilled barrel and needle assembly placed in a reusable plunger are often used (Figure 30-13-2). For an intramuscular injection, a 2- to 3-mL syringe is recommended with a 1¼- to 1½-inch, 19- to 23-gauge needle. Adjustments need to be made for pediatric, obese, or cachectic clients.

As of April 2001, a Federal Needle Stick Safety and Prevention Law requires safe medical devices. The position of the Occupational and Safety Health Act (OSHA) provides that whenever exposure to blood-borne pathogens is anticipated, controls to eliminate employee exposure should be used, hence, safe devices. Failure to comply with using safe devices and safe disposal can result in fines. Examples of safe devices are needle-protected or needleless systems with proper disposal in sharps containers clearly marked. With intramuscular injections, safety syringes or needles should be used. These can be safety-glide or retraction needles or slide syringes. Instruction should be provided appropriate to manufacturers' specifications.

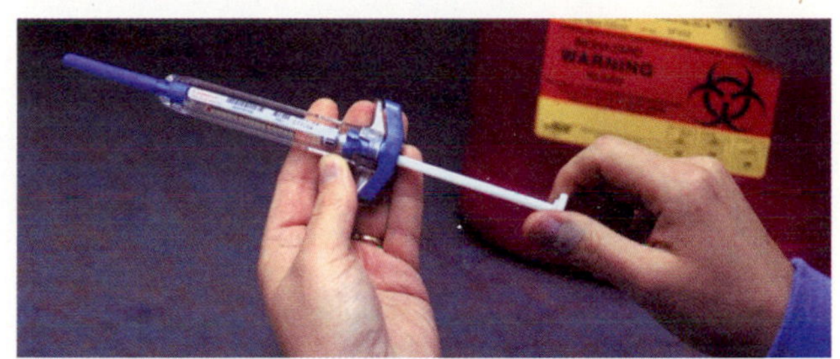

COURTESY OF DELMAR CENGAGE LEARNING

FIGURE 30-13-2 A prefilled syringe consists of a prefilled barrel and needle assembly placed in a reusable plunger.

ASSESSMENT

1. Assess the seven rights: right client, right medication, right route, right dose, right time, right to refuse, and right documentation. **Prevents errors in medication administration.**
2. Review health care provider's order **so the drug is administered safely and correctly.**
3. Review information regarding the drug ordered, such as action, purpose, time of onset and peak action, normal dosage, common side effects, and nursing implications **to anticipate the drug's effects and anticipate a reaction.**
4. Assess client for factors that may influence an injection, such as circulatory shock, reduced local tissue perfusion, or muscle atrophy **because reduced tissue perfusion will interfere with the absorption and distribution of the drug.**
5. Assess for previous intramuscular injections **to rotate sites and avoid repeating a dose in the same site.**
6. Assess for the indications for intramuscular injection **because an injection is preferred for clients who require the fast action of the medication, are confused or unconscious, are unable to swallow a tablet, or have a gastrointestinal disturbance, including the use of nasogastric suction.**
7. Assess the client's age **because older clients or pediatric clients have special needs based on their physiologic status.**
8. Assess client's knowledge regarding the medication to be received **so client education may be tailored according to need.**
9. Assess the client's response to discussion about an injection **because some clients may express anticipatory anxiety, which may increase pain.**
10. Assess the client's size and muscle development. **Assists in identification of appropriate site, needle size, angle to be used, and amount of medication that can be administered in the site.**
11. Check the client's allergy history, **as an allergic reaction could occur.**

(Continues)

PROCEDURE 30-13 Administering an Intramuscular Injection (Continued)

POSSIBLE NURSING DIAGNOSES

Risk for Infection
Impaired Skin Integrity
Anxiety
Deficient Knowledge (injection)
Fear

PLANNING

Expected Outcomes

1. The correct client will receive the correct medication.
2. The client will experience only minimal pain or burning at the injection site.
3. The client will experience no allergic reaction or other side effects from the injection.
4. The client will be able to explain the action, side effects, dosage, and schedule of the medication.
5. The client will obtain the expected benefit from the medication.
6. The client will not experience pain or skin staining secondary to the medication when Z-track injection is given.

Equipment Needed (Figures 30-13-3 and 30-13-4)

- Safety-syringe (1- to 3-mL)
- Safety-needle (19- to 23-gauge, 1¼ to 1½ inches)
- Antiseptic or alcohol swabs
- Medication ampule or vial
- Medication record
- Nonsterile latex-free gloves

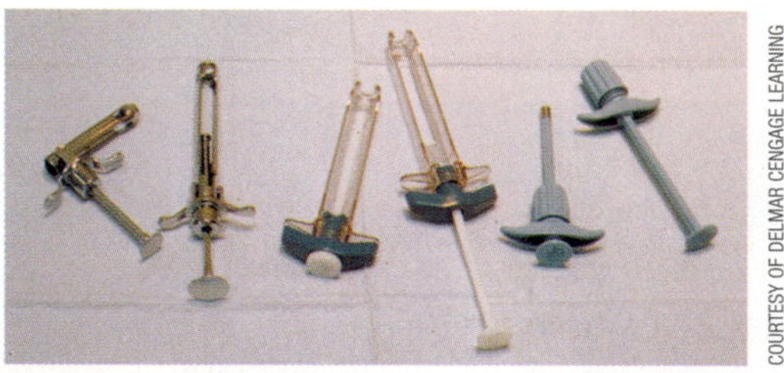

FIGURE 30-13-3 Shown are various types of prefilled syringe plungers.

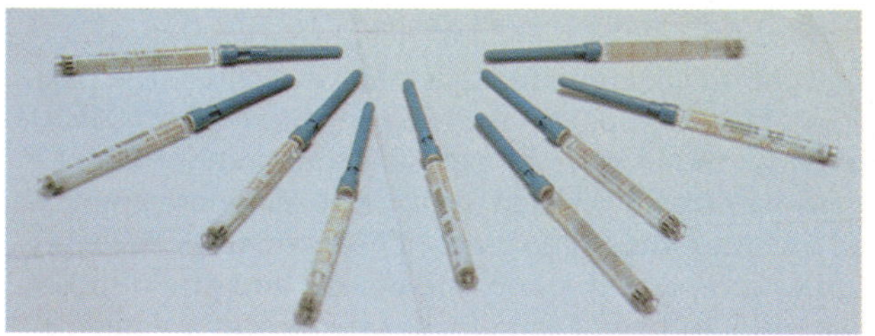

FIGURE 30-13-4 Prefilled Barrel and Needle Cartridges

delegation tips

The procedure of medication administration is not delegated to ancillary personnel in acute care settings. This may vary in state or federal institutions. Ancillary personnel are generally informed about the medications the client is receiving if adverse affects are anticipated or are being monitored.

IMPLEMENTATION—ACTION/RATIONALE

ACTION	RATIONALE
* Check client's identification band * Explain procedure before beginning *	
1. Wash hands and put on nonsterile latex-free gloves.	1. Reduces the number of microorganisms.
2. Close door or curtains around bed and keep gown or sheet draped over client. Identify client using two different identifiers.	2. Provides privacy. Ensures that medication is given to the right client.
3. Select injection site (Figure 30-13-1). • Inspect skin for bruises, inflammation, edema, masses, tenderness, and sites of previous injections.	3. Injection site should be free of lesions. • Repeated daily injections should be rotated.

(Continues)

PROCEDURE 30-13 Administering an Intramuscular Injection (Continued)

- Use anatomic landmarks.
  - Avoids injury to underlying nerves, bone, or blood vessels. Site should be selected based on muscle development, type, and amount of medication, and comfortable access to site.

4. Select needle size: Assess size and weight of client and site to be used.

   4. Ensures that needle will be inserted into the muscle.

5. Assist client into a comfortable position:
   - For vastus lateralis, lying flat or supine with knee slightly flexed.
   - For ventrogluteal, lying on side or back with knee and hip slightly flexed.
   - For dorsogluteal, lying prone with feet turned inward or on side with upper knee and hip flexed and placed in front of lower leg.
   - For deltoid, standing with arm relaxed at side or sitting with lower arm relaxed on lap or lying flat with lower arm relaxed across abdomen (Figure 30-13-5).
   - Distract client by talking about an interesting subject.

   5. Relaxation minimizes discomfort. Distraction reduces anxiety.

6. Use antiseptic swab or alcohol swab to clean skin at site.

   6. Circular motion and mechanical action of swab remove secretions containing microorganisms.

7. While holding swab between fingers of nondominant hand, pull cap from needle.

   7. Swab remains accessible during procedure. Prevents contamination of needle.

8. Administer injection:
   - Hold syringe between thumb and forefinger of dominant hand like a dart.
     - Quick, smooth injection is easier with proper position of syringe.
   - Spread skin tightly or pinch a generous section of tissue firmly—for cachectic clients.
     - Needle penetrates tight skin more easily than loose skin.
   - Inject needle quickly and firmly (like a dart) at a 90-degree angle (Figure 30-13-6).
     - Quick, firm injection minimizes discomfort.
   - Release the skin.
     - Injection requires smooth manipulation of syringe parts. Movement of syringe may cause discomfort.

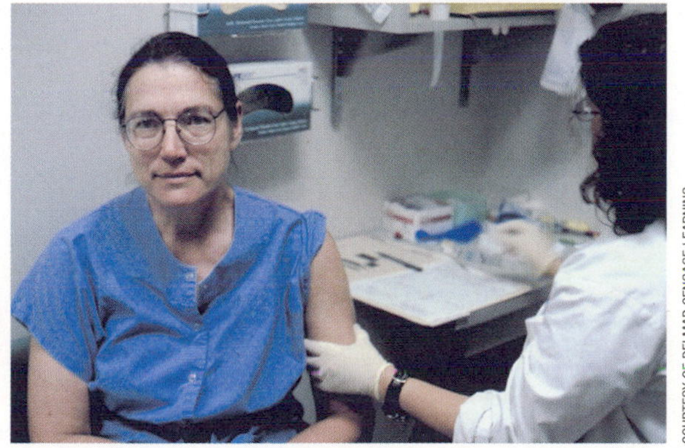

COURTESY OF DELMAR CENGAGE LEARNING

FIGURE 30-13-5 Have the client stand or sit with arm relaxed at side.

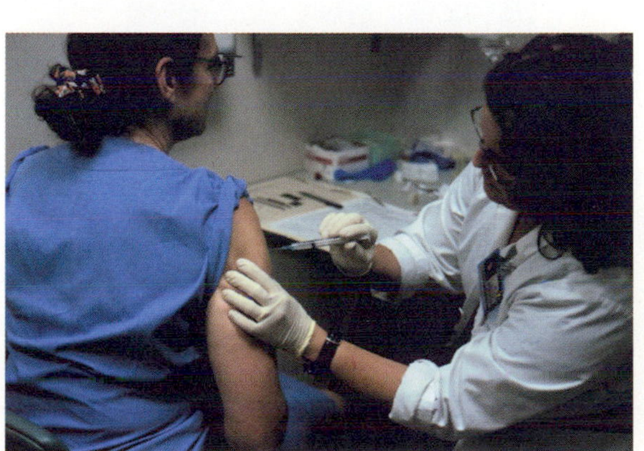

COURTESY OF DELMAR CENGAGE LEARNING

FIGURE 30-13-6 Inject needle quickly and firmly at a 90° angle.

(Continues)

PROCEDURE 30-13 Administering an Intramuscular Injection (Continued)

ACTION	RATIONALE
• Grasp the lower end of the syringe with non-dominant hand and position dominant hand to the end of the plunger. Do not move the syringe. • Pull back on the plunger and aspirate to ascertain if needle is in a vein. If no blood appears, slowly inject the medication.	• Aspiration of blood indicates intravenous placement of needle so procedure may have to be abandoned.
9. Remove nondominant hand and quickly withdraw the needle. Apply pressure with the antiseptic swab.	9. Supporting tissue around injection site minimizes discomfort. Removing hand before withdrawing needle prevents needlestick.
10. Apply pressure. Certain protocols suggest gentle massage action.	10. Pressure prevents medication from leaking out of site. Gentle massage stimulates circulation and improves drug distribution and absorption.
11. Discard the uncapped needle and syringe in a specified biohazard sharps container.	11. Decreases risk of needle stick.
12. Assist the client to a comfortable position.	12. Promotes comfort.
13. Remove gloves and wash hands.	13. Reduces transmission of microorganisms.
Z-track Injection	
14. Wash hands and put on gloves.	14. Reduces the number of microorganisms.
15. Use antiseptic swab or alcohol swab to clean skin at site.	15. Circular motion and mechanical action of swab remove secretions containing microorganisms.
16. Create an air lock. Add 0.1 to 0.2 mL of air to the dose in the syringe (Figure 30-13-7). The air will push the medication out of the needle when the last of the medication has been injected (Figure 30-13-8).	16. The injected medication is followed by air to clear the medication from the needle.
17. Using your nondominant hand, pull the skin and subcutaneous tissue to the side or downward	17. Pulling the tissue to the side or downward prior to the injection will break the injection track after removing the needle and not allow the

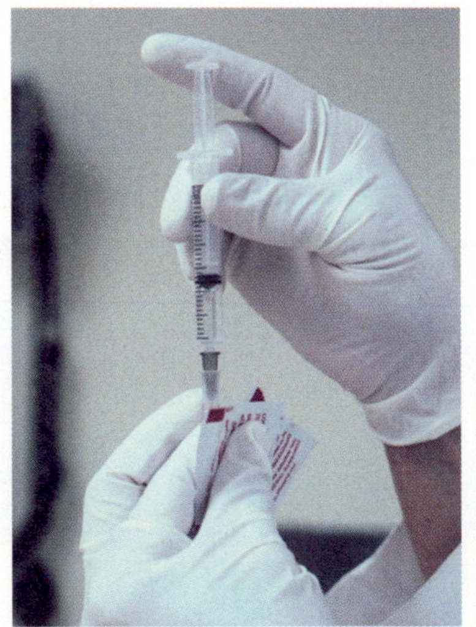

FIGURE 30-13-7 Add 0.1 to 0.2 mL of air to the medication in the syringe.

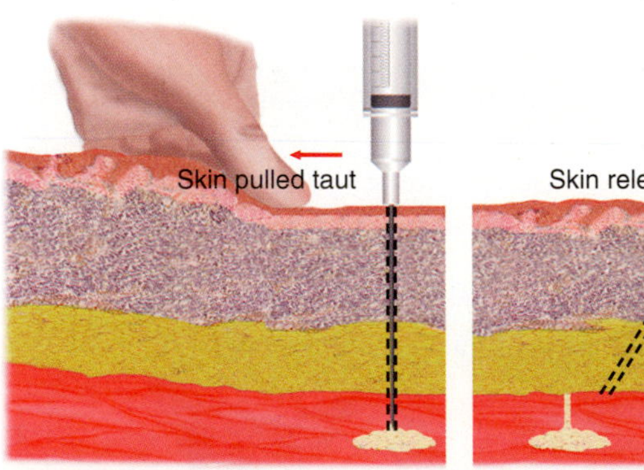

FIGURE 30-13-8 Administering intramuscular injection using Z-track technique.

(Continues)

PROCEDURE 30-13 Administering an Intramuscular Injection (Continued)

ACTION	RATIONALE
about an inch, out of alignment with the underlying muscle (Figure 30-13-5). (Do not use this technique in the deltoid; dorsogluteal is the preferred site).	medication to track back up to the surface of the skin. Also, by pulling the tissue tight, the skin becomes firm and facilitates entry of the needle(Figure 30-13-8).
18. Using sterile technique, remove the needle guard using your nondominant hand.	18. Ensures the needle is not contaminated with microorganisms.
19. While maintaining traction on the skin, using your dominant hand, dart the needle into the skin at a 90-degree angle.	19. Darting the needle is more comfortable for the client. A 90-degree angle will ensure the needle reaches muscle tissue and is not trapped in the subcutaneous or adipose tissue.
20. Aspirate for a minimum of 5 seconds. Observe for a blood return.	20. Blood from small vessels can take up to 5 seconds to appear in the syringe.
21. If no blood return is present, slowly (at a rate of 1 mL/10 seconds) inject the medication.	21. Allows the medication to diffuse, causing less stretch on the muscle fibers and thus is better tolerated by the client.
22. Allow the needle to stay in place for 10 seconds after the medication is injected.	22. Allows the medication to diffuse before the needle is removed, which decreases the chance that any medication will be tracked back up through the skin.
23. While still maintaining traction on the skin with the nondominant hand, smoothly remove the needle and allow the skin to return to its normal position.	23. Holding traction on the tissue prevents any irritation caused by the needle being removed. Allowing the tissue to slide over the track seals the track.
24. Do not rub or wipe the skin after removal of the needle.	24. This can cause seepage of the medication back to the surface and result in irritation.
25. Discard the uncapped needle and syringe in a specified biohazard sharps container.	25. Decreases risk of needlestick.
26. Assist the client to a comfortable position.	26. Promotes comfort.
27. Remove gloves and wash hands.	27. Reduces transmission of microorganisms.

EVALUATION

- The correct client received the correct medication.
- Ask the client about any pain, burning, numbness, or tingling at the injection site.
- Assess the client's response to the medication 10 to 30 minutes later.
- Ask the client to explain the purpose, action, schedule, and side effects of the medication.
- The client obtains the expected benefit.

DOCUMENTATION

Medication Administration Record

- Name of medication
- Dosage
- Route of administration
- Location of injection
- Time administered
- Initials and signature of nurse administering medication

Nurses' Notes

- Time and type of client complaint
- Medication administered
- Outcome of treatment (client response)
- Nurse's signature
- Document on appropriate electronic medical record or flow sheet (seventh right).

(Continues)

PROCEDURE 30-14 Administering Eye and Ear Medications

OVERVIEW

Eye Medications

Eye medications refer to drops, ointment, and disks. These drugs are used for diagnostic and therapeutic purposes—to lubricate the eye or socket for a prosthetic eye and to prevent or treat eye conditions such as glaucoma (elevated pressure within the eye) and infection. Diagnostically, eyedrops can be used to anesthetize the eye, dilate the pupil, and stain the cornea to identify abrasions and scars.

Review the abbreviations used in medication orders to ensure that the medication is instilled in the correct eye. Cross contamination is a potential problem with eyedrops. Adhere to the following safety measures to prevent cross contamination:

- Each client should have his or her own bottle of eyedrops.
- Discard any solution remaining in the dropper after instillation.
- Discard the dropper if the tip is accidentally contaminated by touching the bottle or any part of the client's eye.

Ear Medications

Solutions ordered to treat the ear are often referred to as otic (pertaining to the ear) drops or irrigation. Eardrops may be instilled to soften ear wax, to produce anesthesia, to treat infection or inflammation, or to facilitate removal of a foreign body, such as an insect. External auditory canal irrigations are usually performed for cleaning purposes and less frequently for applying heat and antiseptic solutions.

Before instilling a solution into the ear, inspect the ear for signs of drainage, which is an indication of a perforated tympanic membrane. Eardrops are usually contraindicated when the tympanic membrane is perforated. If the tympanic membrane is damaged, all procedures must be performed using sterile technique; otherwise, medical asepsis is used when instilling medication into the ear.

Certain conditions have contraindications for specific drugs (e.g., hydrocortisone eardrops are contraindicated in clients with a fungal infection or a viral infection such as herpes).

ASSESSMENT

1. Assess the seven rights: right client, right medication, right route, right dose, right time, right to refuse, and right documentation. **Prevents errors in medication administration.**
2. Assess the condition of the client's eyes and/or ears. Are there any contraindications to administering this medication present? Is there drainage from the ear indicating a possible tympanic rupture? If so, the medication administration must be done using sterile technique. **Reassessing the client before every medication dose prevents possibly injuring the client.**
3. Assess the medication order. Is the medication for only one eye/ear or both? With eye medications be sure to understand the abbreviations used for right eye (OD), left eye (OS), and both eyes (OU). **Prevents errors in medication administration.**

POSSIBLE NURSING DIAGNOSES

Risk for Injury
Deficient Knowledge (medication regime)
Disturbed Sensory Perception (visual or auditory)

PLANNING

Expected Outcomes

1. The right client will receive the right dose of the right medication via the right route at the right time.
2. The client will encounter minimum discomfort during the medication administration procedure.
3. The client will receive maximum benefit from the medication.

Equipment Needed (Figure 30-14-1)

Eye Medication

- Medication administration record (MAR)
- Eye medication
- Tissue or cotton ball
- Nonsterile latex-free gloves (if needed)

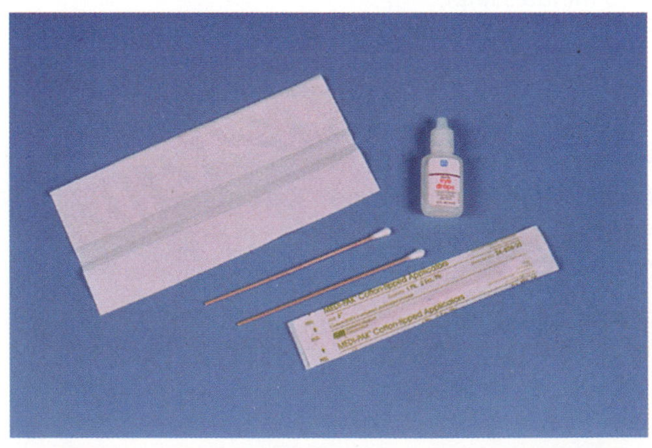

COURTESY OF DELMAR CENGAGE LEARNING

FIGURE 30-14-1 Supplies needed for administering eye and ear drops.

(Continues)

PROCEDURE 30-14 Administering Eye and Ear Medications (Continued)

Ear Medication
- Medication administration record (MAR)
- Medication
- Nonsterile latex-free gloves
- Cotton-tipped applicator
- Tissue

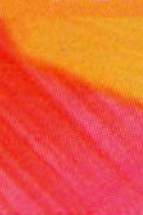

delegation tips

The procedure of medication administration is not delegated to ancillary personnel in acute care settings. This may vary in state or federal institutions. Ancillary personnel are generally informed about the medications the client is receiving if adverse effects are anticipated or are being monitored.

IMPLEMENTATION—ACTION/RATIONALE

ACTION	RATIONALE
* Check client's identification band * Explain procedure before beginning *	
Eye Medication	
1. Check with the client and the chart for any known allergies or medical conditions that would contraindicate use of the drug.	1. Prevents occurrence of adverse reactions.
2. Gather the necessary equipment.	2. Promotes efficiency.
3. Follow the seven rights of drug administration.	3. Promotes safety.
4. Take the medication to the client's room and place on a clean surface.	4. Decreases risk of contamination of bottle cap.
5. Identify client using two different identifiers.	5. Accurately identifies the client.
6. Inquire if the client wants to instill medication. If so, assess the client's ability to do so.	6. Some clients are used to instilling their own medication.
7. Wash hands, and don nonsterile latex-free gloves if needed.	7. Reduces transmission of microorganisms. Decreases contact with bodily fluids.
8. Place client in a supine position with the head slightly hyperextended.	8. Minimizes drainage of medication through the tear duct.
Instilling Eyedrops	
9. Remove cap from eye bottle and place cap on its side.	9. Prevents contamination of the bottle cap.
10. Place a tissue below the lower lid.	10. Absorbs the medication that flows from the eye.
11. With dominant hand, hold eyedropper ½–¾ inch above the eyeball; rest hand on client's forehead to stabilize.	11. Reduces risk of dropper touching eye structure, and prevents injury to the eye.
12. Place hand on cheekbone and expose lower conjunctival sac by pulling down on cheek.	12. Stabilizes hand and prevents systemic absorption of eye medication.
13. Instruct the client to look up and drop prescribed number of drops into center of conjunctival sac (Figure 30-14-2).	13. Reduces stimulation of the blink reflex; prevents injury to the cornea.
14. Instruct client to gently close eyes and move eyes. Briefly place fingers on either side of the client's nose to close the tear ducts and prevent the medication from draining out of the eye (Figure 30-14-3).	14. Distributes solution over conjunctival surface and anterior eyeball.
15. Remove gloves; wash hands.	15. Reduces transmission of microorganisms.
16. Document (seventh right) on the MAR the route, site (which eye), and the time administered.	16. Provides documentation that the medication was given.

(Continues)

PROCEDURE 30-14 Administering Eye and Ear Medications (Continued)

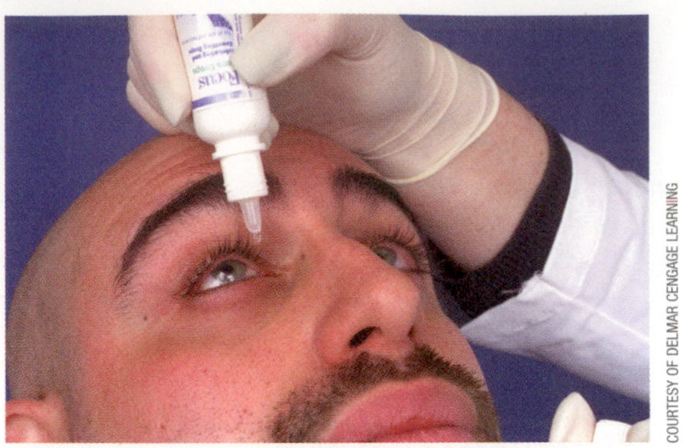
COURTESY OF DELMAR CENGAGE LEARNING

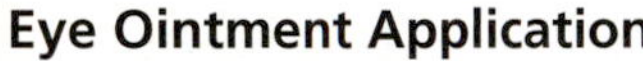

FIGURE 30-14-2 Have the client look upward while instilling drops into the lower conjunctival sac.

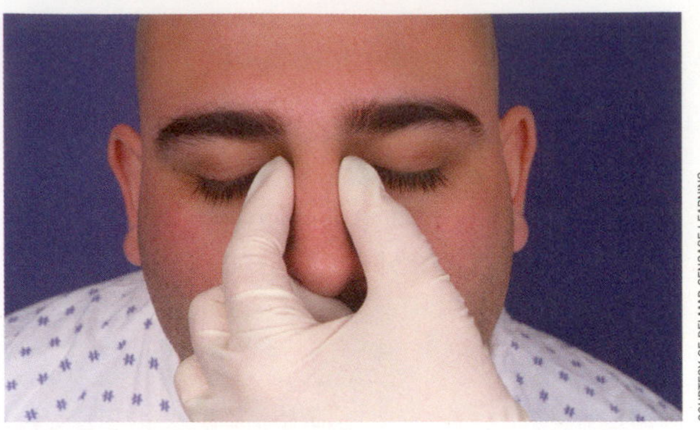
COURTESY OF DELMAR CENGAGE LEARNING

FIGURE 30-14-3 Placing the fingers on the sides of the client's nose closes the tear ducts and prevents the medication from draining out of the eye.

ACTION	RATIONALE
Eye Ointment Application	
17. Repeat Actions 1 to 8.	17. See Rationales 1 to 8.
18. Lower lid:	18.
• With nondominant hand, gently separate client's eyelids with thumb and finger and grasp lower lid near margin immediately below the lashes; exert pressure downward over the bony prominence of the cheek.	• Provides access to the lower lid.
• Instruct the client to look up.	• Reduces stimulation of the blink reflex and keeps cornea out of the way of the medication.
• Apply eye ointment along inside edge of the entire lower eyelid, from inner to outer canthus.	• Ensures drug is applied to entire lid
19. Upper lid:	19.
• Instruct client to look down.	• Keeps cornea out of the way of the medication.
• With nondominant hand, gently grasp client's lashes near center of upper lid with thumb and index finger, and draw lid up and away from eyeball.	
• Squeeze ointment along upper lid starting at inner canthus.	• Ensures that medication is applied to entire length of lid.
20. Repeat actions 15 to 16.	20. See Rationales 15 to 16.
Medication Disk	
21. Repeat Actions 1 to 8.	21. See Rationales 1 to 8.
22. Open sterile package and press dominant, sterile gloved finger against the oval disk so that it lies lengthwise across fingertip.	22. Promotes sticking of disk to fingertip.
23. Instruct the client to look up.	23. Reduces stimulation of the blink reflex and keeps cornea out of the way of the medication.
24. With nondominant hand, gently pull the client's lower eyelid down and place the disk horizontally in the conjunctival sac.	24. Allows the disk to automatically adhere to the eye.
• Then pull the lower eyelid out, up, and over the disk.	• Secures the disk in the conjunctival sac.
• Instruct the client to blink several times.	• Allows the disk to settle into place.
• If disk is still visible, repeat steps.	• Ensures correct placement of the disk.

(Continues)

PROCEDURE 30-14 Administering Eye and Ear Medications (Continued)

ACTION	RATIONALE
• Once the disk is in place, instruct the client to gently press the fingers against the closed lids; do not rub eyes or move the disk across the cornea.	• Secures disk placement. Prevents corneal scratches.
• If the disk falls out, pick it up, rinse under cool water, and reinsert.	• Preserves medication. This is not a sterile procedure. Health care provider must wear gloves to pick up disk.
25. If the disk is prescribed for both eyes (OU), repeat Actions 22 to 24.	25. Ensures both eyes are treated at the same time.
26. Repeat Actions 14 to 16.	26. See Rationales 14 to 16.
Removing an Eye Medication Disk	
27. Repeat Actions 3 and 5 to 8.	27. See Rationales 3 and 5 to 8.
28. Remove the disk:	28.
• With nondominant hand, invert the lower eyelid and identify the disk.	• Exposes the disk for removal.
• If the disk is located in the upper eye, instruct the client to close the eye, and place your finger on the closed eyelid. Apply gentle, long, circular strokes; instruct client to open the eye. Disk should be located in corner of eye. With your fingertip, slide the disk to the lower lid, then proceed.	• Safely moves the disk to the lower conjunctival sac.
• With dominant hand, use the forefinger to slide the disk onto the lid and out of the client's eye.	• Safely removes the disk without scratching the cornea.
29. Remove gloves; wash hands.	29. Reduces transmission of microorganisms.
30. Record on the MAR the removal of the disk.	30. Provides documentation that the disk was removed.
Ear Medication	
31. Check with client and chart for any known allergies.	31. Prevents the occurrence of hypersensitivity reactions.
32. Check the MAR against the health care provider's written orders.	32. Ensures accuracy in identification of the medication.
33. Wash hands.	33. Reduces transfer of microorganisms.
34. Place the client in a side-lying position with the affected ear facing up.	34. Facilitates the administration of the medication.
35. Straighten the ear canal by pulling the pinna down and back for children less than 3 years of age or upward and outward in adults and older children.	35. Opens the canal and facilitates introduction of the medication.
36. Instill the drops into the ear canal by holding the dropper at least ½ inch above the ear canal (Figure 30-14-4).	36. Prevents injury to the ear canal.
37. Ask the client to maintain the position for 2 to 3 minutes.	37. Allows for distribution of the medication.
38. Place a cotton ball on the outermost part of the canal, if approved by the health care prescriber.	38. Prevents the medication from escaping when the client changes to a sitting or standing position.
39. Wash hands.	39. Reduces the transmission of microorganisms.

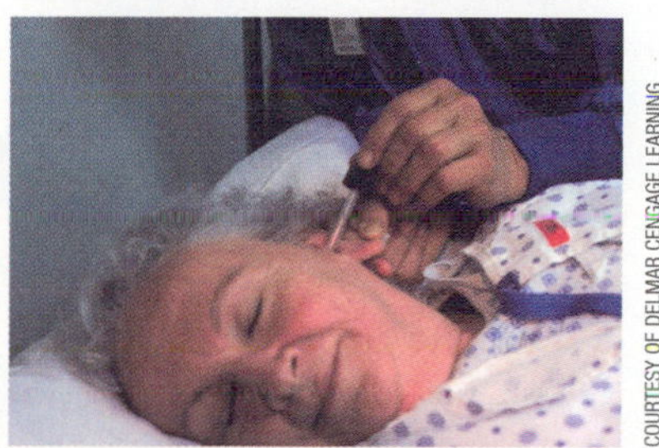

COURTESY OF DELMAR CENGAGE LEARNING

FIGURE 30-14-4 Slowly instill the drops, holding the dropper at least ½ inch above the ear canal.

(Continues)

PROCEDURE 30-14 Administering Eye and Ear Medications (Continued)

EVALUATION

- The right client received the right dose of the right medication via the right route at the right time.
- The procedure was performed with minimum trauma and/or discomfort to the client.
- The client received maximum benefit from the medication.
- All the prescribed medication went into the eye or ear, and none was spilled.

DOCUMENTATION

Medication Administration Record (MAR)

- Date, time, medication, location, and dosage administered
- If an ordered medication was not given, note this, usually by circling the time of the missed medication.

NURSES' NOTES

- If an ordered medication was not given, record the reason.
- If an as-needed medication was given, note the reason for giving the medication and the client's response.
- Document on appropriate electronic medical record or flow sheet (seventh right).

PROCEDURE 30-15 Administering Skin/Topical Medications

OVERVIEW

Topical medications are applied directly to the skin or mucous membranes. These types of medications are used for their local effect or to produce systemic effects by absorption from percutaneous routes. Topical medications include creams, ointments, and lotions. Topical medications applied to the skin are commonly used to relieve itching, prevent local infections, moisten the skin, or for vasodilation. Most topical medications are used for local effects; however, certain medications can be absorbed percutaneously to provide systemic effects, such as topical nitroglycerin, nicotine patches, or certain estrogen products.

ASSESSMENT

1. Assess the seven rights: right client, right medication, right route, right dose, right time, right to refuse, and right documentation. **Prevents errors in medication administration.**
2. Assess the area where treatment will be applied **to establish a baseline condition of the skin for future comparison.**
3. If drug is being used for systemic effect, assess for area free of scars, moles, or other skin aberrations **to facilitate selection of a site with no barriers to absorption.**
4. Check the client's allergy history, **as an allergic reaction could occur.**

POSSIBLE NURSING DIAGNOSIS

Risk for Impaired Skin Integrity

PLANNING

Expected Outcomes

1. Good skin integrity
2. Relief of itching, irritation, or pain
3. Improved circulation

Equipment Needed (Figure 30-15-1)

- Correct medication
- Correct applicator (cotton balls, sterile gauze pad, tongue blades, or cotton applicator)
- Nonsterile latex-free gloves (sterile gloves if broken skin integrity)
- Basin with warm water
- Mild soap (if appropriate and not contraindicated by skin condition or interaction with medication)
- Washcloth and towel
- Gauze dressing, tape as indicated
- Disposable waterproof pad
- Chart or medication sheet for medication verification
- Nonsterile latex-free gloves

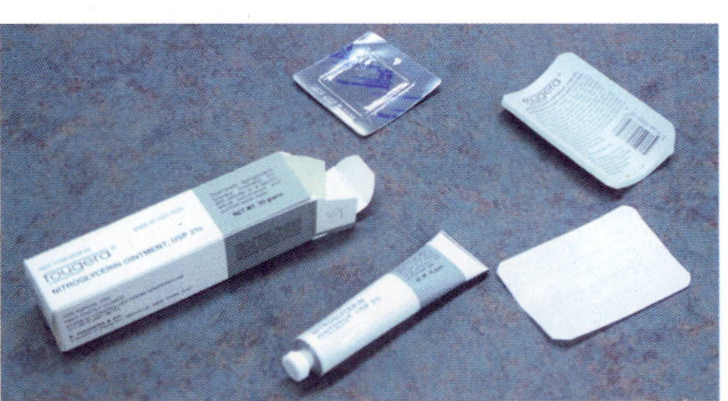

COURTESY OF DELMAR CENGAGE LEARNING

FIGURE 30-15-1 Lotions, creams, ointments, and patches are used to dispense topical medications.

(Continues)

PROCEDURE 30-15 Administering Skin/Topical Medications (Continued)

delegation tips

The application of some creams, lotions, and ointments may be delegated to properly trained ancillary personnel, but these are generally over-the-counter preparations and not prescription medications.

IMPLEMENTATION—ACTION/RATIONALE

ACTION	RATIONALE
* Check client's identification band * Explain procedure before beginning *	
1. Wash hands.	1. Reduces transmission of microorganisms.
2. Obtain order for medication from health care provider.	2. Prevents inappropriate medication administration. An order is needed for any medication.
3. Ascertain client's allergic status.	3. Avoids allergic reactions. Nurses are responsible for medication errors including reactions. Charts may not always be current regarding allergies or an oversight might have occurred.
4. If unfamiliar with medication, read label and insert or seek appropriate information.	4. Prevents inappropriate medication administration and errors. Medications should never be administered without knowledge about the medication.
5. Select medication and verify medication with orders (**first medication verification**).	5. Prevents medication errors.
6. Check medication expiration date.	6. Outdated medications may not be effective.
7. Read medication label again before leaving medication room or cart as available in facilities (**second medication verification**).	7. Avoids medication errors.
8. Take the medication to the client's room and introduce yourself to the client. In some facilities, topical medications used for skin irritations are kept in the client's room, so verification must be done at the bedside.	8. Identifies appropriate medication with right client.
9. Ask the client if he or she has had the medication before and to describe its effect. Ascertain client's allergy status.	9. Provides another verification for the medication. Prevents allergic reaction.
10. Explain the purpose of the medication.	10. Helps to inform and involve the client in his or her care and promotes learning more about condition.
11. Read the label for the third time (**third medication verification**) and check the client's identification band.	11. Avoids medication errors.
12. Position the client appropriately for administration of medication. Keep client draped for privacy.	12. Keeps the client in a comfortable position for medication administration. Protects privacy.
13. Put on gloves. If dressing is over area to be treated, remove, discard, and change gloves.	13. Decreases contact with microorganisms.
14. If an open wound, clean area to be treated with mild soap (if no allergies or reactions to soap) and water. If skin is irritated, use only warm water. If administering a systemically absorbed topical medication, clean the skin surface thoroughly and pat skin dry, leaving no residues of soap. Do not rub vigorously because absorption can be altered (Figure 30-15-2).	14. Soap can irritate an open wound. If skin is already irritated, soap may cause more irritation. Systemically absorbed medication can be effected by residue on the skin or rubbing, which causes vasodilation.
15. Assess the client's skin condition, making notation of circulation, drainage, color, temperature, or any altered skin integrity.	15. Information can be compared with future assessment and effect of medication.

(Continues)

PROCEDURE 30-15 Administering Skin/Topical Medications (Continued)

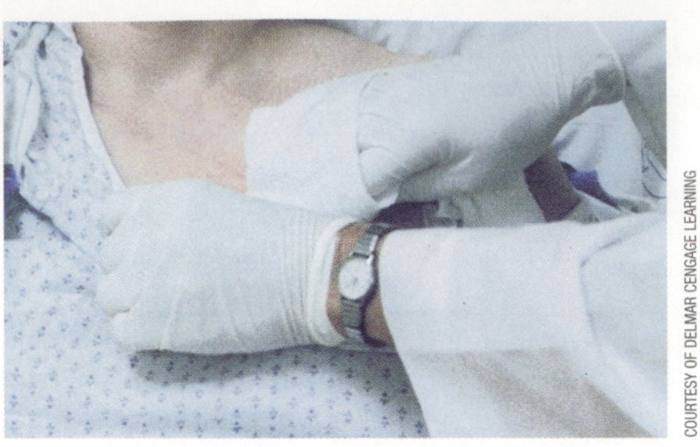

FIGURE 30-15-2 Cleanse the skin before applying topical medication.

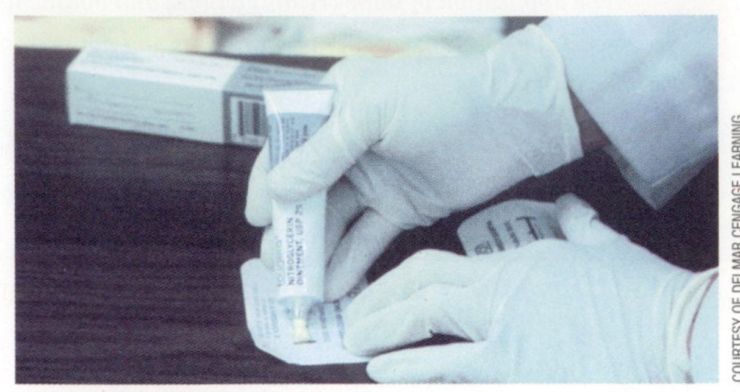

FIGURE 30-15-3 Squeeze the correct dose out onto the enclosed medication measuring strip.

ACTION	RATIONALE
16. Change gloves.	16. Prevents spread of microorganisms and avoids absorption of medication by caregivers. (This is especially important with systemically absorbed medication.)
17. Apply medication according to label. If lotion or ointment, apply a thin layer and smooth into skin as indicated.	17. Medication dosages have been studied and are recommended according to certain standards.
18. If an aerosol spray is used, shake the container and administer according to direction. Spray evenly over affected area and avoid spraying close to client's or caregiver's face.	18. Aerosol may need to be mixed to be effective. Avoid inhalation because it may have adverse effects on the mucous membranes and lungs.
19. If gels or pastes are used, applicators may be needed. Apply evenly. If applying over an area with hair growth, follow direction of hair.	19. Apply evenly to affected areas. Excess gel or paste will be wasted because absorption can only occur at skin level. The client will experience less discomfort if hair growth pattern is followed.
20. If powders are used, dust lightly and avoid inhalation by client and caregiver.	20. Excess powder will be wasted because absorption can only occur at skin level. Inhalation can cause untoward effects on the lungs and mucous membranes.
21. If nitroglycerin ointment or paste are used, follow instructions and orders carefully to administer correct dosage.	21. Nitroglycerin is systemically absorbed and accurate dosing is essential. If thick lines of ointment are applied, the dose will be different; therefore, the manufacturer's suggestions must be followed carefully for safe use of this drug.
• Remove the old ointment strip and clean the old site thoroughly. New ointment will be applied in a different area.	• If areas of ointment from previous doses are not removed, the client will be receiving more than one dose at a time.
• Cleanse the new site with the appropriate cleaner.	• Ensures proper absorption of the medication.
• Squeeze the dose out onto the enclosed medication measuring strip (Figure 30-15-3). Nitroglycerin paste dosages are measured in inches and applied to the paper measuring strip before being applied to the client.	• Use care not to over- or undermedicate by squeezing out a line of ointment that is too thick or too thin.
• Flatten the roll of nitroglycerin so the ointment will be spread over a wider area when applied to the client.	• The wider area of contact and thinner coating of ointment increases absorption.

(Continues)

PROCEDURE 30-15 Administering Skin/Topical Medications (Continued)

ACTION	RATIONALE
• Apply the measuring paper, ointment side down, to a portion of the client's body without hair.	• Using a nonhairy area increases the absorption of the medication.
• Tape the paper in place.	• Keeps the medication in place.
22. If a transdermal patch is used, follow the manufacturer's directions and apply the patch to a smooth, cleaned skin surface.	22. Patches offer a more reliable means of controlling dosage; however, patches are generally more expensive than ointments.
• Remove the old patch and wash the site of the old patch.	• Prevents overdose.
• Wash and prepare the skin at a new site.	• Allows for maximal medication absorption.
• Remove the protective covering over the transdermal portion of the patch and apply the new patch (Figure 30-15-4).	• Removing the protective covering allows the medication to be absorbed.
• Write the date and time on the patch.	• Alerts caregivers of when the patch was applied.
23. Remove gloves; wash hands.	23. Reduces transmission of microorganisms.
24. Document (seventh right) the medication given, the site it was applied to, and the client's response to the medication.	24. Proper documentation is essential for safe client care.

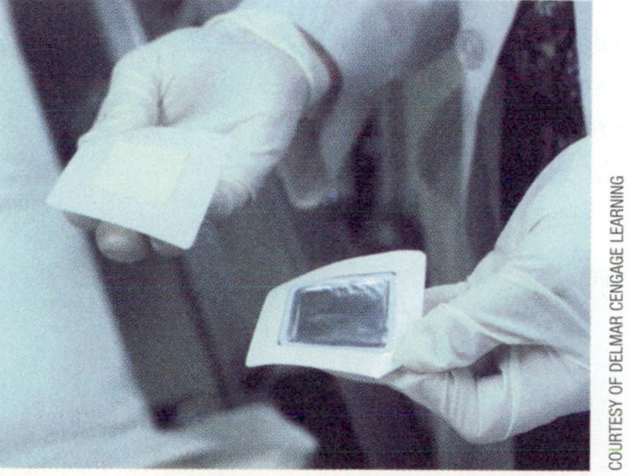
COURTESY OF DELMAR CENGAGE LEARNING

FIGURE 30-15-4 When applying a transdermal patch, remove the protective covering and apply the patch.

EVALUATION

- The client's skin integrity was maintained.
- The client experienced relief of itching, irritation, or pain if this was the intent of the medication.
- The client experienced maximum effect from the topical medication.
- The client experienced no allergic reaction.

DOCUMENTATION

Medication Administration Record

- Date, time, and site of application of the topical medication.

Nurses' Notes

- Changes in the client's skin integrity, coloration, or sensation
- If medication was for irritation, itching, or rash, document any improvement or change
- Unusual findings or client complaints
- Document on appropriate electronic medical record or flow sheet.

PROCEDURE 30-16 Administering Nasal Medications

OVERVIEW

Nasal medications may be administered by drops or sprays. Sprays may be packaged as pump sprays, sprays in aerosolized containers (pressurized containers, sometimes called nasal nebulizers), or powdered turbo inhalers. Prescribed medications are generally available in pump sprays or aerosolized sprays, whereby sprays and nasal drops are available in over-the-counter medications. Nasal medications may be used to achieve local effects on the nasal mucosa, indirect effects on the sinuses, or a systemic effect. Examples of medications that have systemic effects and are available in nasal sprays are insulin, agents to suppress nicotine use, and agents to treat migraine headaches. The four groups of sinuses (frontal, ethmoid, sphenoid, and maxillary) communicate with the nasal fossae and are lined with mucous membranes similar to those that line the nose. Even though it is unlikely that nasal medications penetrate the sinuses, positioning may aid in decreasing inflammation and congestion in the mucous membranes adjacent to the sinuses, thereby indirectly decreasing pressure in the sinuses. To medicate the mucous membranes adjacent to the frontal sinuses, the client will assume a supine position with the head turned to the affected side to be treated. To medicate the mucous membranes adjacent to the ethmoid sinuses, the client will lie supine with his or her head leaning back over the side of the bed with the client's head supported by the nurse's hand to avoid muscle strain on the client's neck. Although the nose is not considered a clean or sterile cavity, because of its connection with the sinuses, employ medical asepsis when performing nasal instillation.

ASSESSMENT

1. Assess the seven rights: right client, right medication, right route, right dose, right time, right to refuse, and right documentation. **Prevents errors in medication administration.**
2. Assess the client's nasal congestion and nasal obstruction **to determine if the medicine can be inhaled to reach the nasal mucosa and to determine the effectiveness of the medication.**
3. Assess the color, quantity, and odor of the client's discharge and the color and moistness of the nasal mucosa **to check for signs and symptoms of infection, to discern tissue damage, and to establish a baseline for future assessments.**
4. Assess the client's pain and/or discomfort level in the areas of sinuses **because this is another symptom of infection. May determine if the client can use the inhaler or drops.**
5. Assess the client for systemic conditions that may be adversely affected by nasal medications (see manufacturer's information). **Clients with cardiovascular conditions and hypertension may need to use caution with medications containing sympathomimetic** ingredients.

POSSIBLE NURSING DIAGNOSES

*Impaired **O**ral Mucous Membrane*
*Impaired **T**issue Integrity*

PLANNING

Expected Outcomes

1. The client will be free of nasal congestion.
2. The client will be free of nasal discharge and odor.
3. The client will breathe freely through the nasal passages.
4. The client will be free of sinus pain and nasal pain.
5. The client's nasal passages will be moist and pink.

Equipment Needed (Figure 30-16-1)

- Medication in spray, drops, or aerosolized form
- Nonsterile latex-free gloves
- Tissue as needed
- Dropper as needed

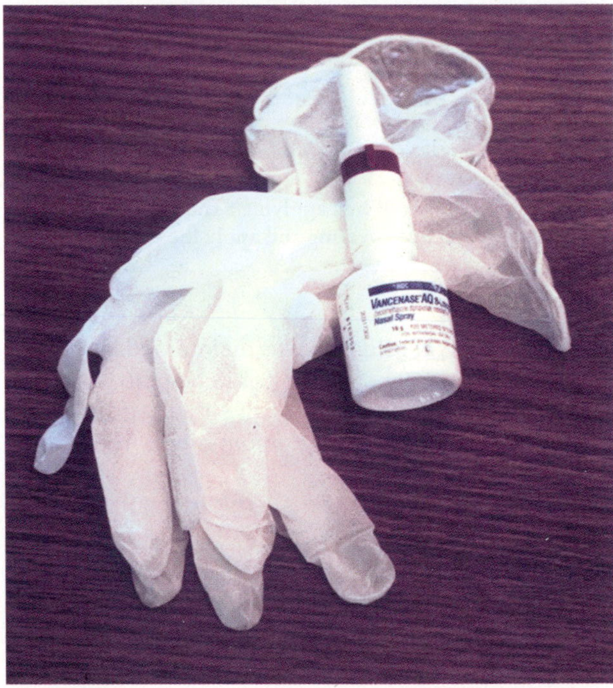

COURTESY OF DELMAR CENGAGE LEARNING

FIGURE 30-16-1 Nasal medication spray and latex-free gloves are needed when administering nasal medication to a client.

(Continues)

PROCEDURE 30-16 Administering Nasal Medications (Continued)

delegation tips

The procedure of medication administration is not delegated to ancillary personnel in acute care settings. This may vary in state or federal institutions. Ancillary personnel are generally informed about the medications the client is receiving if adverse effects are anticipated or are being monitored.

IMPLEMENTATION—ACTION/RATIONALE

ACTION	RATIONALE
* Check client's identification band * Explain procedure before beginning *	
1. Wash hands. Wear a mask if the client is coughing or sneezing. Don nonsterile latex-free gloves.	1. Reduces transmission of microorganisms. Respiratory-related microorganisms are easily transferred by the hands and air droplets. Gloves prevent absorption of medication through the skin of health care worker.
2. Explain the purpose of the medication and the position desired for the client.	2. Ensures nose drops will reach the area of treatment by gravity with the client assuming a dependent position.
3. Explain to the client the sensation of the local effects of the medications, such as burning, tingling, and effect on taste buds. If drops are used, explain to the client that a sensation of medications may be felt in the posterior oral pharynx.	3. Some nasal medications cause undesirable tastes. If this occurs, the health care provider may order other medications or encourage mouthwashes after treatment. Prepares the client for sensation that may be felt.
4. Have the client clear the nostrils by blowing the nose.	4. Removes discharge that would prevent medication from contacting the mucous membrane.
Nose Drops	
5. Follow the seven rights and three checks of safe medication administration.	5. Prevents medication error.
6. Ask client to lie supine and hyperextend the neck (Figure 30-16-2). Turn head to the appropriate position described in the Overview.	6. Allows the nose drops to reach the appropriate area.
7. Squeeze some medication into dropper.	7. Makes medication ready to administer.
8. Have client exhale and occlude one nostril with a finger.	8. Readies client to inhale as medication is administered.
9. Insert dropper about 3⁄8 inch into the nostril, keeping it away from the sides of the nostril. Ask client to inhale as prescribed dosage of medication is administered.	9. Prevents getting microorganisms back into medication bottle. Medication is distributed better during inhalation.
10. Discard any unused medication remaining in the dropper.	10. Prevents contamination of medication.
11. Client may blot excess drainage but may not blow the nose and should remain in position for 5 minutes.	11. Removes discomfort of drainage on face. Allows time for medication to be absorbed.
12. Repeat on other nostril if ordered.	12. Generally, both nostrils are treated.
Nasal Inhalers	
13. Repeat Actions 1 to 5.	13. See Rationales 1 to 5.
14. Explain the manufacturer's directions and how inhalers work.	14. Clients will be more compliant if they understand the use of the inhalers and that a fine cold mist will be released into the nasal passage via a pressurized container.
15. Have the client assume an upright position. Squeeze nose drops into dropper.	15. The client should be as comfortable as possible. Makes medication ready to administer.
16. Have the client exhale and occlude one nostril with a finger.	16. Readies the client to inhale as medication is administered.

(Continues)

PROCEDURE 30-16 Administering Nasal Medications (Continued)

ACTION	RATIONALE

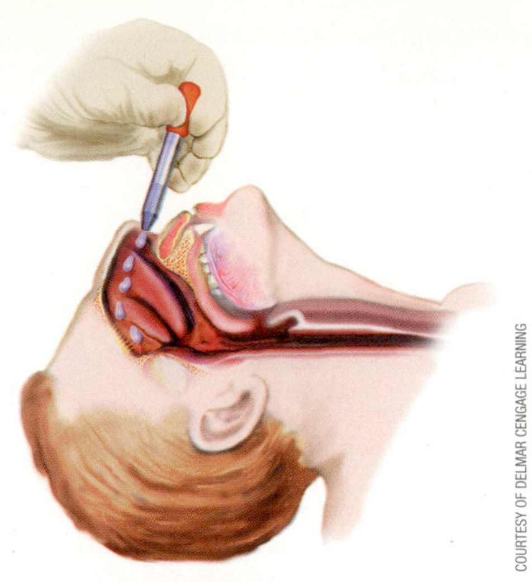

FIGURE 30-16-2 Positioning a client for nose drop instillation.

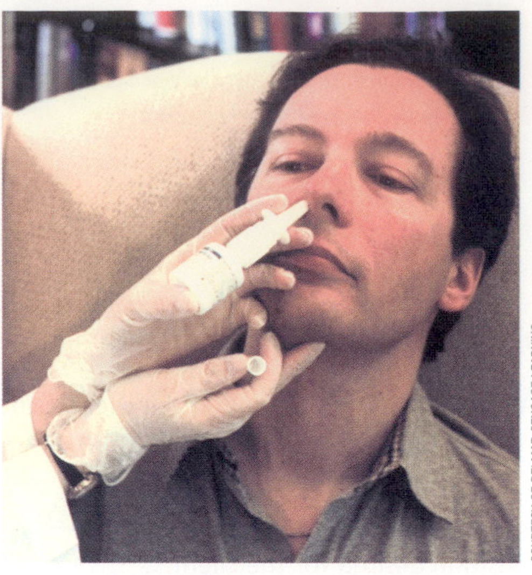

FIGURE 30-16-3 Ask the client to inhale while the spray is administered.

ACTION	RATIONALE
17. Ask the client to inhale while the spray is administered (Figure 30-16-3).	17. Nasal medications are more effective if instilled during inhalation.
18. Repeat the procedure on the other nostril.	18. Most often, both nostrils are treated.
19. Remove all soiled supplies and dispose of them according to Standard Precautions. Remove gloves. Wash hands carefully.	19. Decreases the chance of transmission of microorganisms. Respiratory diseases are especially easily transmitted.
20. Evaluate the effect of the medication in 15 to 20 minutes.	20. Identifies if the medication is effective without adverse side effects.

EVALUATION

- The client is free of nasal congestion.
- The client is free of nasal discharge and odor.
- The client breathes freely through the nasal passages.
- The client is free of sinus pain and nasal pain.
- The client's nasal passages are moist and pink.
- The client is free of adverse side effects secondary to the nasal medication.

DOCUMENTATION

Medication Administration Record

- Time and date medication was given, amount (number of drops may be necessary), and nostril medicated.

Nurses' Notes

- Results of the treatment
- Adverse or unpleasant side effects
- Document (seventh right) on appropriate electronic medical record or flow sheet

PROCEDURE 30-17 Administering Rectal Medications

OVERVIEW

The administration of rectal medications is an important responsibility for nurses in numerous health care settings. Rectal suppositories include medications that produce both local and systemic effects. Suppositories that produce a local effect include laxatives, which promote defecation. Medications to help relieve nausea, fever, or bladder spasms can also be administered via rectal suppository but produce a systemic effect.

(Continues)

PROCEDURE 30-17 Administering Rectal Medications (Continued)

ASSESSMENT

1. Assess the seven rights: right client, right medication, right route, right dose, right time, right to refuse, and right documentation. **Prevents errors in medication administration.**
2. Review the health care provider's order and identify the medication to be delivered, verifying dosage, route, time, and correct client. **This ensures safe and correct administration of medications.**
3. Assess the client's need and appropriateness for rectal medication administration and review the client's history for contraindications. **A history of rectal surgery or bleeding may contraindicate use of a suppository.**
4. Consider any adjustments that may need to be taken in delivery of medications resulting from the age of the client. **This allows the nurse to deliver the medication in a correct manner if the client is an infant, child, or adult.**
5. Observe the client for the desired therapeutic effects or any adverse reactions, and document this response appropriately **to determine the effectiveness of the treatment.**
6. Assess the client's knowledge and understanding of the procedure. **Explaining the procedure will decrease client fear and anxiety and will promote understanding and cooperation. If physically able, the client may wish to self-administer the medication.**
7. Assess the client's rectal area to determine condition of skin, mucosa, and presence of hemorrhoids or other rectal conditions. **Preventive action can be taken to protect injured skin and ensure client comfort.**

POSSIBLE NURSING DIAGNOSES

Dysfunctional Gastrointestinal Motility
Constipation
Nausea
Chronic Pain

PLANNING

Expected Outcomes

1. The medication will be delivered appropriately and safely following the seven rights of medication administration.
2. The desired outcome will be verbalized by the client and documented appropriately by the nurse.
3. The treatment will be completed as quickly and efficiently as possible to decrease discomfort and anxiety.
4. Client will state relief of complaint after medication administration.

Equipment Needed (Figure 30-17-1)

- Medication (suppository or medicated enema)
- Water-soluble lubricant
- Nonsterile latex-free gloves
- Tissue or washcloth
- Bedpan if client physically immobile
- Medication administration record
- Towels or pads (such as disposable "Blue pads")

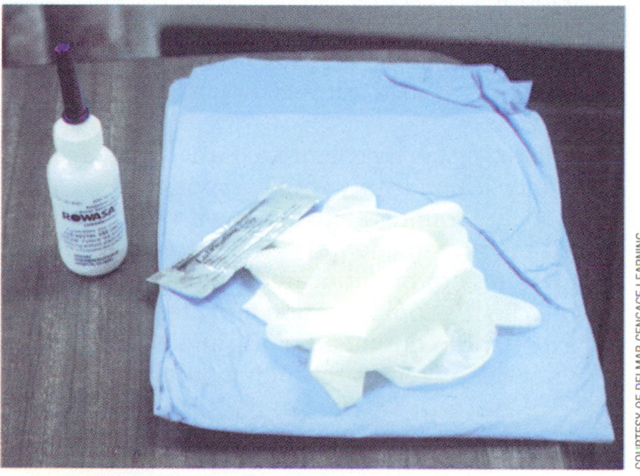

COURTESY OF DELMAR CENGAGE LEARNING

FIGURE 30-17-1 Latex-Free Gloves, Protective Pad, Water Based Lubricant, and Rectal Medication

delegation tips

The procedure of medication administration is not delegated to ancillary personnel in acute care settings. This may vary in state or federal institutions. Ancillary personnel are generally informed about the medications the client is receiving if adverse effects are anticipated or are being monitored.

(Continues)

PROCEDURE 30-17 Administering Rectal Medications (Continued)

IMPLEMENTATION—ACTION/RATIONALE

* Check client's identification band * Explain procedure before beginning *

ACTION	RATIONALE
1. Assess the client's need for the medication.	1. Allows the nurse to determine the need and effectiveness of the medication.
2. Check the health care provider's written order.	2. Ensures safe and accurate administration of medication.
3. Check the medication administration record against the written order to verify the correct client, medication, route, time, and dosage.	3. Decreases the chance of a medication error and ensures accuracy (right dosage, right route, right time, right client, right medication, right to refuse, and right documentation).
4. Assess client for any drug allergies.	4. Decreases the risk for an allergic reaction.
5. Review the client's history for any previous surgeries or bleeding.	5. Contraindications for rectal administration may be discovered.
6. Gather the equipment needed for the procedure before entering the client's room.	6. Prevents numerous trips to gather supplies and helps the procedure flow smoothly.
7. Provide privacy for client.	7. Maintains dignity and self-image.
8. Wash hands.	8. Reduces transmission of microorganisms.
9. Ask the client to state his or her full name and check his or her identification band.	9. Ensures correct client (right client).
10. Apply nonsterile latex-free gloves (Figure 30-17-2).	10. Prevents contact with fecal material.
11. Assist client into Sims' (left) position with upper leg drawn up toward chest. Provide protection under client such as towel or pad.	11. The descending colon is on the left side; this is a more anatomically correct position. Exposes the anus to identify placement. Provides comfort to client who may fear soiling linen.
12. Visually assess the client's external anus.	12. Determines presence of any active bleeding.
13. Remove suppository from wrapper and lubricate rounded end along with insertion finger. If a medicated enema is used, lubricate the enema tip if it is not prelubricated (Figure 30-17-3).	13. Lubrication decreases friction and decreases discomfort.
14. Tell client a cool sensation and pressure will be experienced during administration. Encourage slow, deep breaths through mouth.	14. Prepares the client for administration. Relaxes the rectal sphincter.

COURTESY OF DELMAR CENGAGE LEARNING

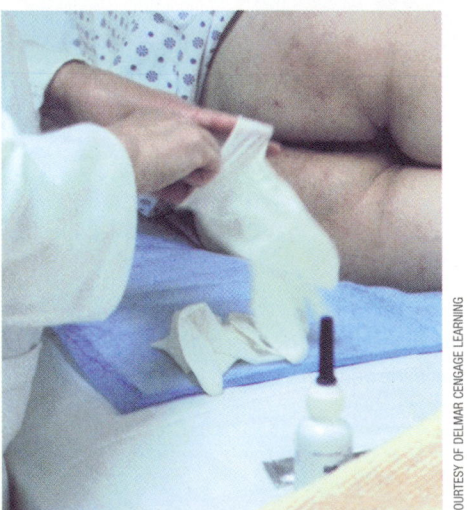

FIGURE 30-17-2 Apply latex-free gloves before administering rectal medications.

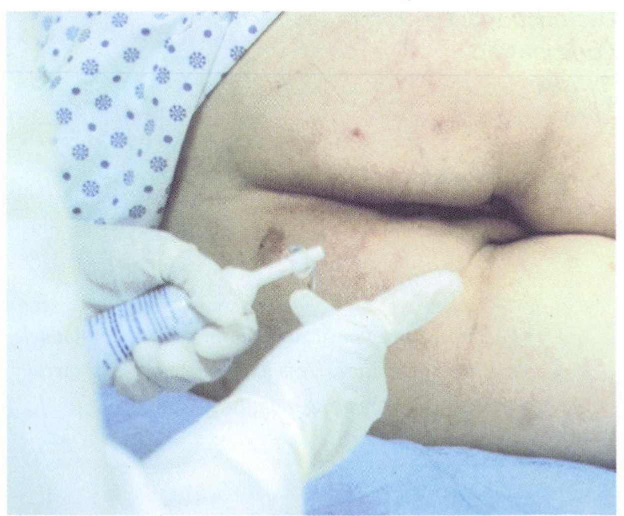

FIGURE 30-17-3 The enema needs to be lubricated with water soluble lubricant.

(Continues)

PROCEDURE 30-17 Administering Rectal Medications (Continued)

ACTION	RATIONALE
15. Retract buttocks with nondominant hand, visualizing the anus (Figure 30-17-4). Using the dominant index finger, slowly and gently insert the suppository through the anus, past the internal sphincter, and against the rectal wall (Figure 30-17-5). Depth of insertion will differ if client is a child or infant. If instilling a medicated enema, gently insert the enema tip past the internal sphincter and instill the contents by slowly squeezing (Figure 30-17-6).	15. Slow insertion minimizes pain. Correct placement ensures adequate absorption and less chance for expulsion of medication.
16. Remove finger or enema tip and wipe client's anal area with a washcloth or tissue.	16. Removes lubricant externally. Promotes cleanliness and comfort.
17. Remove and discard gloves.	17. Reduces transfer of microorganisms.
18. Wash hands.	18. Reduces transfer of microorganisms.
19. Have client remain in position for 10 to 15 minutes.	19. Keeps suppository or medicated fluid in place for better absorption.
20. Place call light in client's reach.	20. Gives client control over situation.
21. Document administration of medication (seventh right).	21. Provides documentation of medication administration.
22. Document effectiveness or any side effects on nursing notes.	22. Communicates effectiveness of treatment with other caregivers.

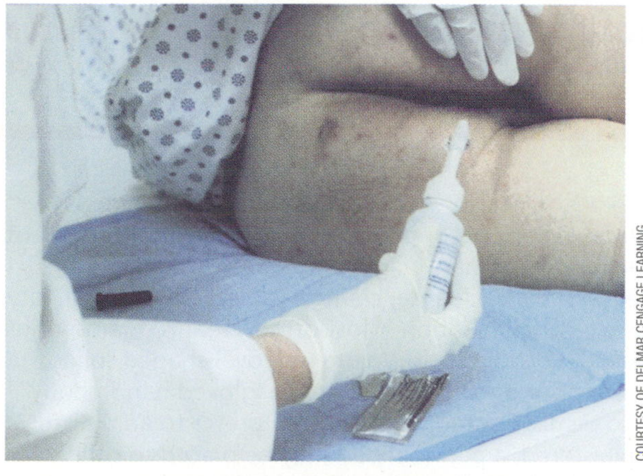

FIGURE 30-17-4 Retract the buttocks and visualize the anus.

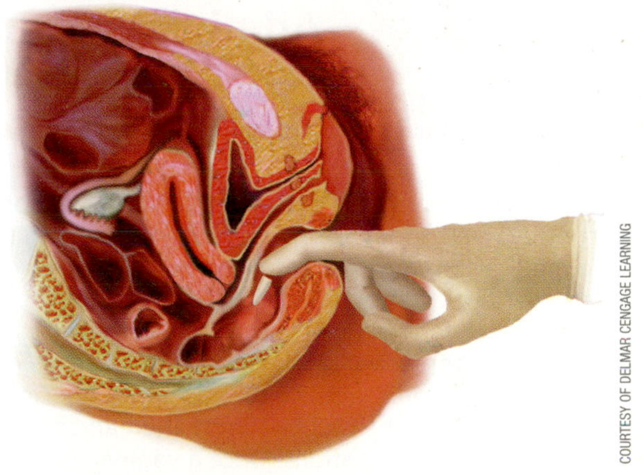

FIGURE 30-17-5 Inserting a Rectal Suppository

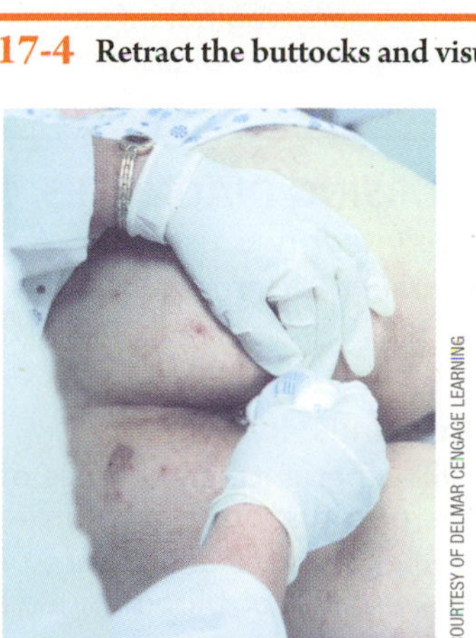

FIGURE 30-17-6 When administering an enema, gently insert the enema tip and instill the contents by slowly squeezing the bottle.

(Continues)

PROCEDURE 30-17 Administering Rectal Medications (Continued)

EVALUATION

- The medication was delivered appropriately and safely, following the seven rights of medication administration.
- The desired outcome was verbalized by the client and documented appropriately by the nurse.
- The treatment was completed as quickly and efficiently as possible to decrease discomfort and anxiety.
- Client stated relief of complaint after medication administration.

DOCUMENTATION

Medication Administration Record

- Name of medication
- Dosage
- Route of administration
- Time administered
- Initials and signature of nurse administering medication

Nurses' Notes

- Time and type of client complaint
- Medication administered
- Outcome of treatment (client response)
- Health care provider notified, if needed
- Nurse's signature
- Document on appropriate electronic medical record or flow sheet.

PROCEDURE 30-18 Administering Vaginal Medications

OVERVIEW

Vaginal medications come in the form of creams, suppositories, foams, jellies, or irrigations (commonly known as douches). Vaginal medications are generally used to treat infections, irritations, or pruritis requiring topical treatment. These medications may be prescribed by a physician or nurse practitioner, or many vaginal medications can be purchased over-the-counter (OTC). Irrigations or douches can be used to soothe, cleanse, change vaginal acidity/alkalinity, or disinfect the vagina; however, if used excessively, they can cause vaginal irritation. Most often, creams, foams, or jellies are administered with an applicator or inserter. Suppositories are individually foil-wrapped, oval-shaped solids that require refrigeration. Once the suppository is inserted by an applicator or directly with a finger (gloved hand), body temperature causes the suppository to melt and the medication to be distributed. Clients often prefer to administer their own vaginal medications. Once a vaginal medication is administered, a perineal pad may be placed to collect any drainage and discharge. Pericare and personal hygiene are essential because many vaginal infections cause foul-smelling discharge and irritation. Assess the client's level of pain, pruritis, burning, or general discomfort to establish a baseline for future assessment.

ASSESSMENT

1. Assess the client's comfort level. Evaluate the level of burning, irritation, pruritis, pain, and odor **to establish a baseline for assessment of treatment.**
2. Assess the client's knowledge of the purpose of the medication and treatment. **Enables client to understand and monitor effects of medication.**
3. If the client prefers to self-administer the medication, assess the client's ability to do so, such as ability to manipulate the applicator or insert a suppository the appropriate distance. **Clients may prefer to self-administer vaginal medications for privacy, but if medication is not properly inserted, it will not be effective.**

POSSIBLE NURSING DIAGNOSES

*Impaired **T**issue Integrity*
*Ineffective **S**exuality Patterns*

PLANNING

Expected Outcomes

1. Client will experience an absence of vaginal infection, pruritus, burning, or irritation.
2. Client will experience an absence of foul-smelling, curdlike, or blood-tinged discharge.
3. Client will understand the importance of continued treatment until infection is absent.
4. Client will understand the importance of personal hygiene in combination with medication.

(Continues)

PROCEDURE 30-18 Administering Vaginal Medications (Continued)

5. Client will understand the need to properly clean and store equipment.

Equipment Needed (Figure 30-18-1)

- Vaginal medication: cream, foam, jelly, or suppository
- Applicator (if needed)
- Water-soluble lubricating jelly (for suppository)
- Nonsterile latex-free gloves
- Perineal pad
- Paper towel, toilet tissue, or tissue paper
- Washcloth and warm water (optional)

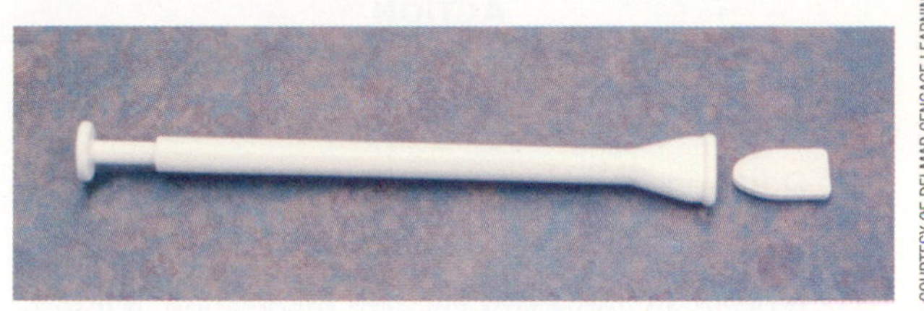

COURTESY OF DELMAR CENGAGE LEARNING

FIGURE 30-18-1 Vaginal Medication and Applicator

delegation tips

The procedure of medication administration is not delegated to ancillary personnel in acute care settings. This may vary in state or federal institutions. Ancillary personnel are generally informed about the medications the client is receiving if adverse effects are anticipated or are being monitored.

IMPLEMENTATION—ACTION/RATIONALE

ACTION	RATIONALE
* Check client's identification band * Explain procedure before beginning *	
1. Check the medication administration record against the health care provider's orders to verify the correct client, medication, route, time, and dosage.	1. Decreases the chance of a medication error and ensures accuracy (right dosage, right route, right time, right client, and the right medication).
2. Assess the client for any drug allergies.	2. Decreases the risk for an allergic reaction.
3. Ask the client to void.	3. Provides for client comfort during the procedure.
4. Wash hands.	4. Reduces transmission of microorganisms.
5. Arrange equipment at client's bedside.	5. Promotes organization.
6. Provide privacy by closing door and curtains.	6. Protects the client's privacy.
7. Assist the client into a dorsal-recumbent or Sims' position (Figure 30-18-2).	7. Allows for administration and for medication to remain in vagina.
8. Drape the client as appropriate, such as over the client's abdomen and lower extremities. Provide towel or protective pad on bed.	8. Provides privacy. Prevents linen from becoming soiled.

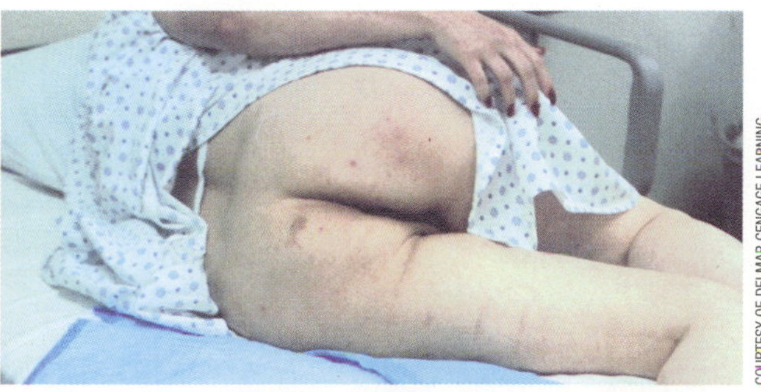

COURTESY OF DELMAR CENGAGE LEARNING

FIGURE 30-18-2 The client is placed in Sim's position for administering vaginal medication.

(Continues)

PROCEDURE 30-18 Administering Vaginal Medications (Continued)

ACTION	RATIONALE
9. Position lighting to illuminate vaginal orifice.	9. Assists in visualization of vagina and proper administration of medication.
10. Don nonsterile latex-free gloves and assess the perineal area for redness, inflammation, discharge, or foul odor.	10. Decreases transmission of microorganisms and risk of reaction to latex. Provides baseline data.
11. If using an applicator, fill with medication. If inserting a suppository, remove the suppository from the foil and position in the applicator (applicator is optional) (Figure 30-18-3). An applicator may be used for suppositories, or a gloved finger may be used. The foil is discarded. Apply water-soluble lubricant to suppository or applicator (optional for applicator).	11. Prepares medication for insertion. Lubricant provides comfort and ease of insertion.
12. For suppository, with nondominant hand, retract the labia (Figure 30-18-4).	12. Allows visualization of the vaginal orifice and eases insertion of medication.
13. With dominant hand, insert the applicator 2 to 3 inches into the vagina, sliding the applicator posteriorly (Figure 30-18-5). Push the plunger to administer the medication (Figure 30-18-6). With a suppository, insert the tapered end first with the index finger or applicator along the posterior wall of the vagina (approximately 3 inches) (Figure 30-18-7).	13. Medication must be inserted completely to provide coverage of the entire vagina. When medication is deposited at the posterior end of the vagina, gravity will allow medication to move toward the orifice.

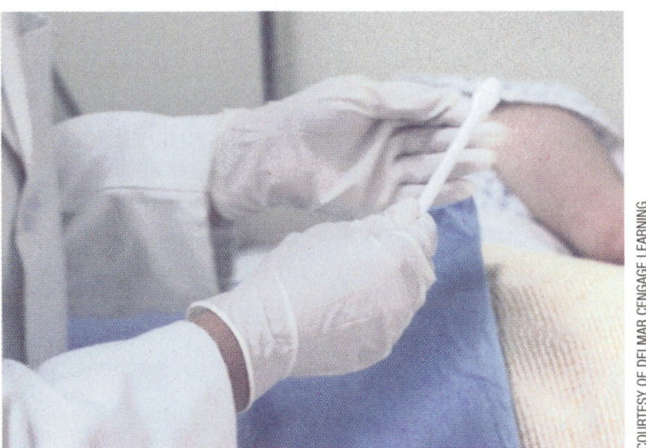

FIGURE 30-18-3 Place the vaginal suppository in the applicator.

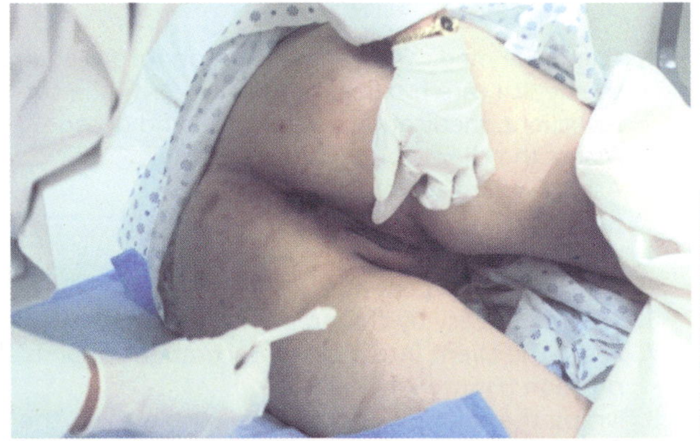

FIGURE 30-18-4 Retract the labia with the nondominant hand.

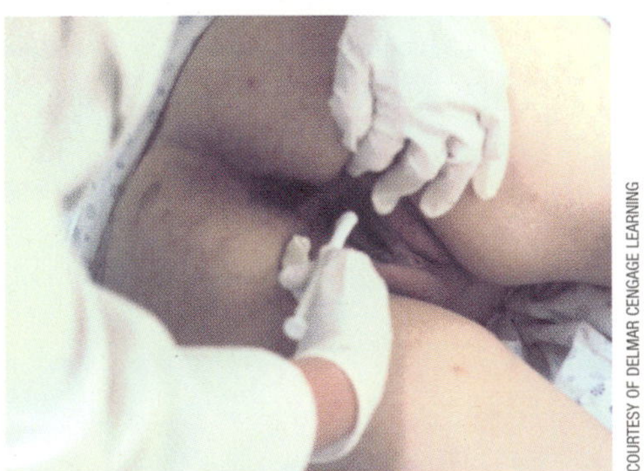

FIGURE 30-18-5 Slide the applicator 2 to 3 inches into the vagina.

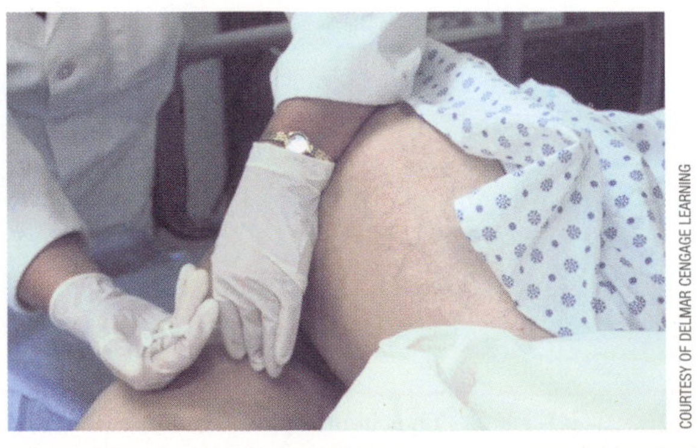

FIGURE 30-18-6 Push the plunger to administer the medication.

(Continues)

PROCEDURE 30-18 Administering Vaginal Medications (Continued)

ACTION	RATIONALE
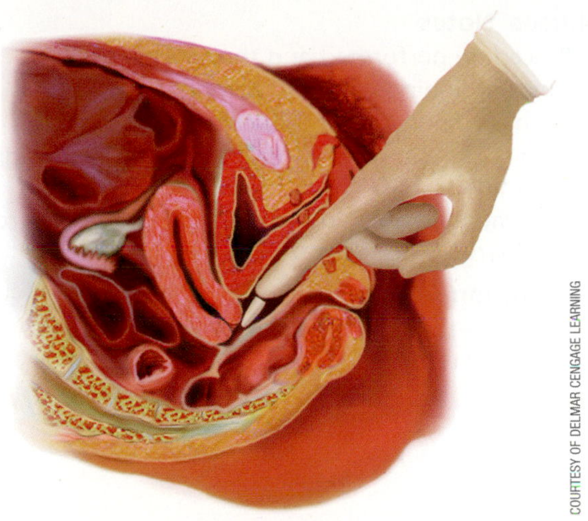 FIGURE 30-18-7 Inserting a vaginal suppository along the posterior wall of the vagina.	
14. Withdraw the applicator and place on a towel.	14. Reduces transmission of microorganisms.
15. If administering a douche or irrigation:	15.
• Warm solution to slightly above body temperature (105° to 110°F). Check using the back of the hand or the wrist.	• Avoids burning the client. The mucous membranes of the vagina are sensitive.
• Position the client in a semirecumbent position on a bedpan, on a toilet seat, or in a tub.	• Provides comfort during procedure and allows for appropriate drainage of irrigation solution.
• Apply lubricant to the irrigation nozzle and insert approximately 3 inches into the vagina.	• Provides comfort.
• Hang the irrigant container approximately 2 feet above the client's vaginal area.	• Height is necessary for drainage by gravity. If the container is too high, the flow will be too forceful and uncomfortable.
• Open the clamp and allow a small amount of solution to flow into the vagina.	• Allows the client to evaluate the temperature.
• Move the nozzle and rotate around the entire vaginal area. If the labia are inflamed, allow the solution to flow over the labia as well. If the client is on the toilet seat, alternate between closing off the labia and allowing solution to be expelled.	• Rotation allows for irrigation throughout vagina. Closing off labia allows medication to stay in and flush total vagina.
16. Wipe and clean the client's perineal area, including the labia, from the front to the back with toilet tissue. Some clients may prefer that the perineal area is also cleaned with a washcloth and warm water.	16. Provides comfort for client and avoids spread of infective agents to perineal area.
17. Apply a perineal pad.	17. Protects client from discomfort of drainage and spread of infection or irritation to perineal area.
18. Wash the applicator (if reusable) with soap and warm water and store in appropriate container in client's room.	18. Applicator can only be used for individual clients; however, some applicators and inducers are reusable and must be appropriately cleaned and stored to prevent reinsertion of infective agents.
19. Remove gloves and wash hands.	19. Reduces transmission of microorganisms.
20. Instruct the client to remain flat for at least 30 minutes.	20. Allows maximum contact between the medication and the vaginal mucous membranes.
21. Raise side rails and place the call light in reach.	21. Provides for client comfort and safety.

(Continues)

PROCEDURE 30-18 Administering Vaginal Medications (Continued)

EVALUATION

- Client experiences an absence of vaginal infection, pruritus, burning, or irritation.
- Client experiences an absence of foul-smelling, curd-like, or blood-tinged discharge.
- Client understands the importance of continued treatment until infection is absent.
- Client understands the importance of personal hygiene in combination with medication.
- Client understands the need to properly clean and store equipment.

DOCUMENTATION

Nurses' Notes

- Procedure performed and the results
- Unusual findings or client complaints
- Client's response to treatment
- Client's signs and symptoms associated with vaginal condition
- Document (seventh right) on appropriate electronic medial record or flow sheet.

Medication Administration Record

- Date and time the medication/treatment was administered

PROCEDURE 31-19 Administering Nebulized Medications

OVERVIEW

A nebulizer is a device that is used to aerosolize medications into a mist for delivery directly into the lungs. Medication that is inhaled in the form of small droplets is absorbed immediately into the mucosa and bloodstream and is available to the body within minutes. This method of medication delivery is one of the fastest noninvasive methods of medication delivery. Many medications can be delivered by inhalation, but currently this delivery method is used primarily for medications designed to ease respiratory distress symptoms such as those seen with asthma.

There are two types of nebulizers: the single-dose nebulizer, which is driven by an air compressor, wall air, or wall oxygen, and the portable metered-dose inhaler. The single-dose, compressor-driven nebulizer delivers smaller droplets, allowing faster, more complete assimilation of the medication. The single-dose nebulizer can be filled with any type of medication that is ordered and can be used by clients who cannot coordinate use of the metered-dose inhaler. The primary drawback of the single-dose nebulizer is its lack of portability. The nebulizer must also be loaded with medication for each use, thus delaying the client's relief.

The metered-dose inhaler has the benefit of being small and portable. It can be carried in the client's pocket. Because the meter dispenses measured doses of the preloaded medication, no special training is needed to prime the inhaler. The primary drawback of a metered-dose inhaler is the need to coordinate dispensing the dose and inhalation. A spacer or extender chamber may be attached to the mouthpiece of the inhaler to hold the medication in suspension and provide the client an opportunity to inhale all the medication so that the dose is not lost during exhalation.

ASSESSMENT

1. Assess the seven rights: right client, right medication, right route, right dose, right time, right to refuse, and right documentation. **Prevents errors in medication administration.**
2. Assess the client's respiratory status. Note if the client is using accessory muscles for respiration or if there is flaring of the nares. Auscultate the client's chest for wheezes and crackles. **Respiratory distress is the primary reason to administer nebulized medications.**
3. Evaluate the history of this episode of the client's distress. Take a complete history from the client or a reliable informant about the symptoms and length of time the client has had them. Respiratory distress can have many causes. Asthma, bronchitis, a foreign object in the airways, and chronic obstructive pulmonary disease can all cause respiratory distress. **Assessing the client's current symptoms provides more accurate diagnosis and care. The client's history of asthma does not mean that this episode of distress is asthma.**

(Continues)

PROCEDURE 30-19 Administering Nebulized Medications (Continued)

4. Assess the client's ability to use the nebulizer or metered-dose inhaler. Determine the client's ability to understand and follow the directions, to hold and manipulate the equipment, and to coordinate the release of the medication with inhalation. **Determines the type of equipment used for the client. Very young children may need a mask instead of a mouthpiece on the nebulizer. The elderly may need specialized dispensers for their metered-dose inhalers.**
5. Assess the medication(s) currently ordered by the health care provider: action, purpose, common side effects, time of onset, and peak of action. **Permits the nurse to anticipate what to observe from the client.**
6. Assess the medications the client is currently taking, including over-the-counter drugs. **Some medications can interact. Beta-blockers (propranolol, atenolol, and betalol) can antagonize the beta agonists and cause or increase asthma symptoms.**
7. Assess the client's knowledge regarding the medications and use of the nebulizer or metered-dose inhaler. **Allows the nurse to determine the need for client education to promote compliance.**
8. Verify the client's drug allergy history, **as an allergic reaction could occur.**

POSSIBLE NURSING DIAGNOSES

*Impaired **G**as Exchange*
*Ineffective **B**reathing Pattern*
*Deficient **K**nowledge* (proper use of the nebulizer or metered-dose inhaler)
***A**nxiety*
***F**ear*

PLANNING

Expected Outcomes

1. The client will experience improved gas exchange.
2. The client's breathing pattern will become effective.
3. The client will demonstrate understanding of the need for the medication and use of the nebulizer or metered-dose inhaler.
4. The client will not experience any adverse effects secondary to medication interactions.
5. The client's anxiety level will decrease following treatment.

Equipment Needed (Figures 30-19-1 and 30-19-2)

Handheld Nebulizer
- Medication administration record
- Nebulizer set (cup, tubing, cap, T-shaped tube, mouthpiece, or mask) or prepackaged nebulizer and applicator
- Medication(s)
- Saline
- Air compressor, wall air, or wall oxygen

Metered-Dose Inhaler
- Metered-dose inhaler
- AeroChamber, if appropriate

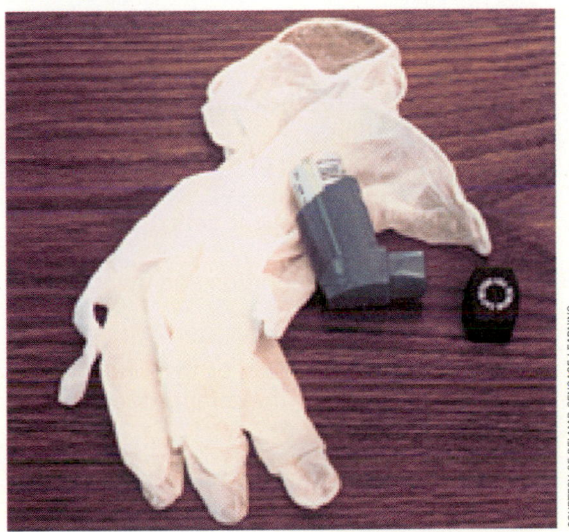
COURTESY OF DELMAR CENGAGE LEARNING

FIGURE 30-19-1 Handheld Metered-Dose Inhaler

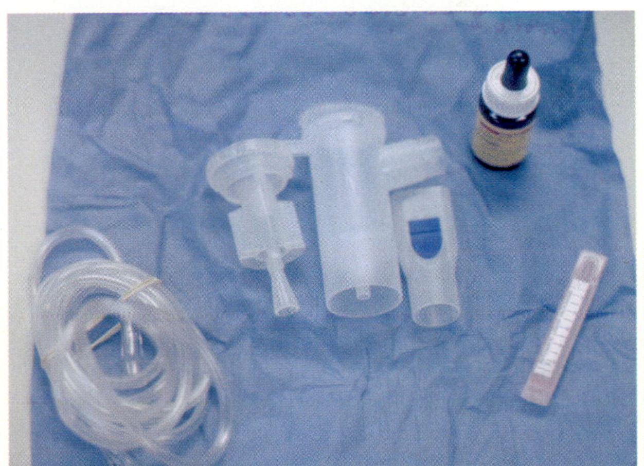
COURTESY OF DELMAR CENGAGE LEARNING

FIGURE 30-19-2 Nebulizer Cup, Tubing, Cap, T-Shaped Tube, Mouthpiece, and Medication

(Continues)

PROCEDURE 30-19 Administering Nebulized Medications (Continued)

delegation tips

The procedure of medication administration is not delegated to ancillary personnel in acute care settings. This may vary in state or federal institutions. Ancillary personnel are generally informed about the medications the client is receiving if adverse effects are anticipated or are being monitored.

IMPLEMENTATION—ACTION/RATIONALE

* Check client's identification band * Explain procedure before beginning *

ACTION	RATIONALE
Single-Dose Handheld Nebulizer	
1. Assess the client's ability to use the nebulizer.	1. Ensures client compliance and accurate use of the nebulizer.
2. Check the medication administration record against the health care provider's written order to verify the correct client, medication, route, time, and dosage.	2. Decreases the chance of a medication error and ensures accuracy (right dosage, right route, right time, right client, and the right medication).
3. Assess the client for any drug allergies.	3. Decreases the risk for an allergic reaction.
4. Wash hands.	4. Reduces transmission of microorganisms
5. Set up and prepare the medication(s) for one client at a time.	5. Ensures the client receives the right medication(s).
6. Look at the medication at eye level if using a dropper to dispense the solution into the nebulizer.	6. Ensures accuracy.
7. Carefully pour the entire amount of the drug(s) into the nebulizer cup.	7. Determines the correct amount of medicine and ensures accurate dosage.
• Avoid touching the drug while pouring into the nebulizer cup.	• Reduces the transmission of microorganisms.
8. Cover the cup with the cap and fasten.	8. Prevents spillage of the medication.
9. Fasten the T-piece to the top of the cap.	9. Provides a connector for the mouthpiece.
10. Fasten a short length of tubing to one end of the T-piece.	10. Provides dead space to prevent room air from entering the system and medicated aerosol from escaping.
11. Fasten the mouthpiece or mask to the other end of the T-piece.	11. Provides a portal for the client to inhale the aerosolized medication.
• Avoid touching the nebulizer mouthpiece or the interior part of the mask.	• Reduces transmission of microorganisms.
12. Identify the client prior to the administration of the medication(s).	12. Ensures that the right client gets the medication.
13. Identify the medication(s) to the client and clearly explain the therapeutic purpose(s) of the medication.	13. Promotes client's cooperation and awareness of the medication's effects.
14. Advise the client to sit in an upright position.	14. Promotes better expansion of the lungs.
15. Attach tubing to the bottom of the nebulizer cup and attach the other end to the air compressor or wall air.	15. Provides a conduit for the compressed air.
• Before turning it on, adjust the wall oxygen valve to 6 liters/min (or less per health care provider's orders).	• Drives the medication into a mist or wet aerosol form.
• Leave the air on for about 6 to 7 minutes until the medications are used up.	• Allows the client to receive the entire dose of medication.

(Continues)

PROCEDURE 30-19 Administering Nebulized Medications (Continued)

ACTION	RATIONALE
16. Instruct the client to breathe in and out slowly and deeply through the mouthpiece/mask.	16. Promotes better deposition and efficacy of the medication in the airways.
• The client's lips should be sealed tightly around the mouthpiece.	
17. Remain with the client long enough to observe the proper inhalation-exhalation technique.	17. Ensures the correct use of the nebulizer to get the full effects from the medications administered.
18. Wash hands.	18. Reduces transmission of microorganisms.
19. When the nebulizer cup is empty, turn off the compressor or wall air.	19. Stops the aerosolization.
• Detach the tubing from the compressor and the nebulizer cup.	• Prepares components for cleaning or disposal.
• If the nebulizer is disposable, dispose of the nebulizer in the appropriate container.	• Prevents transmission of microorganisms.
• If the nebulizer is to be reused for this client, carefully wash, rinse, and dry the nebulizer components.	• Prevents transmission of microorganisms.
20. Assess the client immediately following the treatment for results or adverse effects from the treatment.	20. Determines the effectiveness of the treatment.
21. Reassess the client 5 to 10 minutes following the treatment.	21. Some effects may be delayed.
22. Wash hands.	22. Reduces transmission of microorganisms.
Metered-Dose Nebulizer	
23. Assess the client for ability to use the metered-dose nebulizer.	23. Ensures client compliance.
24. Check the medication administration record against the health care provider's order to verify the correct client, medication, route, time, and dosage.	24. Decreases the chance of a medication error and ensures accuracy (right dosage, right route, right time, right client, and the right medication).
25. Assess the client for any drug allergies.	25. Decreases the risk for an allergic reaction.
26. Wash hands.	26. Decreases transmission of microorganisms.
27. Shake the prepackaged nebulizer.	27. Thoroughly mixes the medication.
28. Place the nebulizer into the applicator.	28. Allows for proper administration of the medication.
29. Place the AeroChamber onto the nebulizer if needed (Figure 30-19-3).	29. The AeroChamber provides dead space for the medicated mist while the client inhales.

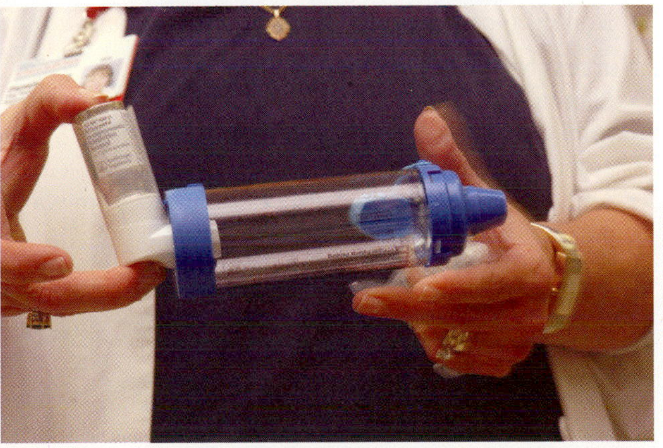

COURTESY OF DELMAR CENGAGE LEARNING

FIGURE 30-19-3 Preparing a Metered-Dose Inhaler and Medication

(Continues)

PROCEDURE 30-19 Administering Nebulized Medications (Continued)

ACTION	RATIONALE

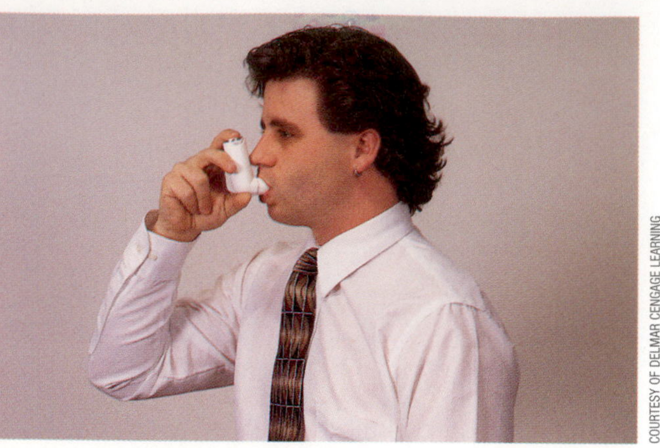
COURTESY OF DELMAR CENGAGE LEARNING

FIGURE 30-19-4 Self-Administration with a Metered-Dose Inhaler

ACTION	RATIONALE
30. Have the client exhale and place the mouthpiece in his or her mouth (Figure 30-19-4).	30. Prepares for delivery of the medication to the lungs.
31. Have the client press down on the prepackaged dispenser and simultaneously inhale slowly until lungs feel full. Hold breath for 10 seconds and exhale slowly.	31. Draws medication into the lungs. Allows medication to reach alveoli.
32. If there is an AeroChamber attached to the nebulizer, have the client inhale slowly and deeply.	32. Allows for proper delivery of the medication.
33. Observe the client for several minutes to assess for possible adverse effects from the medication.	33. Reactions can occur right away.
34. Have the client rinse his or her mouth.	34. The medication may leave a metallic taste.
35. Wash hands.	35. Prevents transmission of microorganisms.
36. Document the medication administration (seventh right).	36. Provides a record of medication administration.

EVALUATION

- The client experienced improved gas exchange.
- The client's breathing pattern became effective.
- The client demonstrates understanding of the need for the medication and the use of the nebulizer or metered-dose inhaler.
- The client did not experience any adverse effects secondary to medication interactions.
- The client's anxiety level decreased following treatment.

DOCUMENTATION

Medication Administration Record

- Name of medication(s)
- Dosage
- Route
- Site
- Time of administration
- Initials of the nurse who administered the medication(s)
- Signature of the nurse identifying the initials

Nurses' Notes

- Client's assessment parameters
- Name of medication, dosage, route, and time of administration
- Amount of oxygen delivered per minute from wall oxygen or air compressor machine
- Signature and initials of the nurse
- Client's response
- Document on appropriate electronic medical record or flow sheet.

PROCEDURE 30-20

Applying a Dry Dressing

OVERVIEW

A closed surgical wound can be described as a wound that was caused, revised, or debrided by a surgical intervention. Closed wounds are generally categorized as clean. They may be closed with sutures, staples, or tapes. The general purpose of the closed wound dressing is to cover and protect as well as absorb the minimal drainage that may occur with this type of wound. Dressing care may vary according to the surgeon's preference and institutional policy. General guidelines for the closed surgical wound dressing is covered in this procedure.

There are different approaches to wound care. Cleaning solutions can dry the wound and interfere with wound healing at the cellular level. Furthermore, clients may be allergic or sensitive to these solutions. Although they reduce the risk of infection, frequent application may not be necessary. In many cases, sterile normal saline, sterile water, or pH-neutral solutions will be adequate to cleanse the wound. It is standard for the surgeon to do the first postoperative dressing change. The initial dressing is maintained for 24 to 48 hours postoperatively, unless conditions of the dressing call for contacting the health care provider for a dressing change order. Until the removal of the initial dressing, reinforce the dressing as needed.

The frequency of the dressing change depends on the needs of the wound and the preference of the health care provider. This will usually be specified in the orders. It is important to follow agency guidelines and observe the preferences of the health care provider.

ASSESSMENT

1. Assess the client's comfort level postoperatively upon arrival from the operating room, before wound care, and as needed throughout the postoperative course. **Surgical wounds are painful. If clients are made comfortable with appropriate pain medications and positioning, there will be better tissue gas exchange from deep breathing, coughing, and early ambulation, thereby promoting healing of tissues. Clients will be more cooperative and less anxious during dressing changes if they are comfortable.**
2. Assess the external appearance of the initial postoperative dressing and subsequent dressings. **The initial dressing may need to be reinforced. Excess saturation with drainage, blood, or other bodily fluids, dislodgement, or anything unusual about the dressing should be brought to the attention of the health care provider. The appearance of the external portion of the dressing provides information about needed supplies.**
3. Assess the appearance of the wound and drains once the dressing is removed. **Inspection of the wound is important for assessment of the skin and tissues and for determining dressing supply needs. Assessment includes noting signs of infection as evident by redness, swelling, foul odor, amount of drainage, color of wound exudate (yellow and viscous would indicate purulent), or unusual pain or tenderness; signs of tissue trauma as evident by swelling or ecchymosis; evidence of bleeding or leakage of tissue fluids from the site; and the position of indwelling catheters, drainage tubes, and the sutures or stabilizing devices closing the wound and supporting the drains.**
4. Assess the client's understanding about the postoperative care of the surgical wound site. **It is important to take into consideration the client's ability to understand verbal and written instructions and the cultural and social variations that may affect the delivery of health care and client/family education.**
5. If solutions are to be used on the wound, assess the client's allergy status and test a drop of solution on the skin. **This prevents an adverse reaction.**

POSSIBLE NURSING DIAGNOSES

*Impaired **S**kin Integrity*
*Impaired **T**issue Integrity*
*Risk for **I**nfection*

PLANNING

Expected Outcomes

1. The site will be inspected for signs of infection, drainage, drainage tubes, and position of sutures or staples.
2. The initial postoperative dressing will be reinforced until changed by the health care provider.
3. The site will have the appropriate dressing applied.
4. The client/family will verbalize and/or demonstrate understanding and the ability, if indicated, to perform the dressing change and associated wound care of the surgical wound site.

Equipment Needed (Figure 30-20-1)

- Nonsterile latex-free gloves
- Container for proper disposal of soiled dressing
- Sterile 4 × 4 gauze pads
- Washcloth (optional)
- ABD pads (optional)
- 2-inch tape (foam or paper)
- Cleaning solution (if ordered)

(Continues)

PROCEDURE 30-20 Applying a Dry Dressing (Continued)

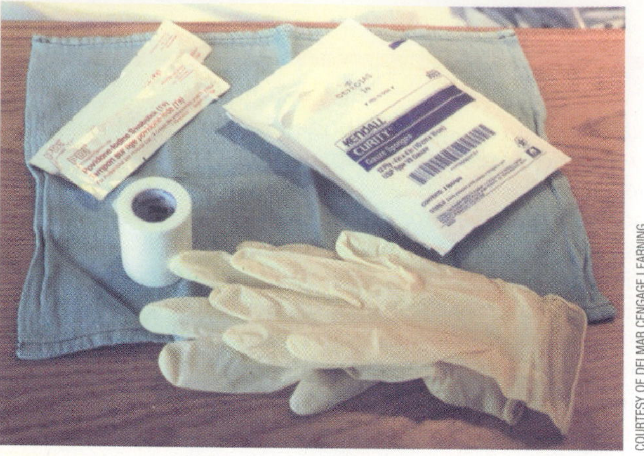

COURTESY OF DELMAR CENGAGE LEARNING

FIGURE 30-20-1 Clean gloves, gauze sponges, tape, and antiseptic solution are used to change a dry dressing.

delegation tips

The application of bandages is not delegated to ancillary personnel. Family members may be taught this before the client's discharge. Occasionally, ancillary personnel will be delegated the task of applying a clean dry gauze as skin protection, but the nurse is responsible for assessing the integrity of the client's skin.

IMPLEMENTATION—ACTION/RATIONALE

ACTION	RATIONALE
* Check client's identification band * Explain procedure before beginning *	
1. Gather supplies.	1. Promotes a smooth work flow.
2. Provide privacy; draw curtains; close door.	2. Maintains client comfort and privacy while body is exposed during procedure.
3. Wash hands.	3. Reduces transmission of microorganisms.
4. Apply nonsterile latex-free gloves.	4. Promotes infection control and protection from body fluids.
5. Remove dressing and place in appropriate receptacle. Remove soiled gloves with contaminated surfaces inward and discard in appropriate receptacle; apply nonsterile latex-free gloves.	5. Dressings and gloves soiled with body fluids are considered contaminated and subject to biohazard disposal in the correct manner per institution protocol.
6. Assess the undressed wound for signs of redness, foul odor, swelling, irritation, drainage, dehiscence, bleeding, or skin breakdown.	6. These may be signs of infection or inadequate wound healing.
7. Remove used exam gloves.	7. Exam gloves that are used to remove the old dressing are considered contaminated and should be removed and discarded appropriately.
8. Wash hands.	8. Reduces transmission of microorganisms.
9. Set up supplies. Open 4 × 4 gauze packages. • If incision requires cleaning, pour cleaning solution on 4 × 4 gauze pads (consult health care provider's orders and institution policy regarding cleaning incisions).	9. Following the removal of the dressing, you will have a better idea of what supplies are needed.
10. Apply a new pair of clean gloves.	10. This is considered to be a clean procedure after the initial dressing is removed if the skin margins are approximated with the skin closures.

(Continues)

PROCEDURE 30-20 Applying a Dry Dressing (Continued)

ACTION	RATIONALE

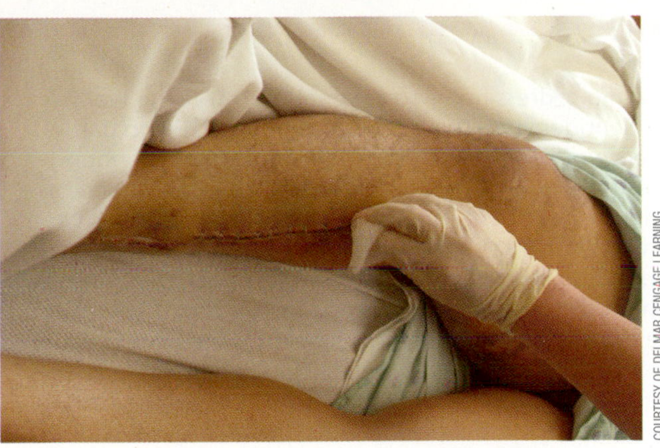

FIGURE 30-20-2 Clean the suture lines gently.

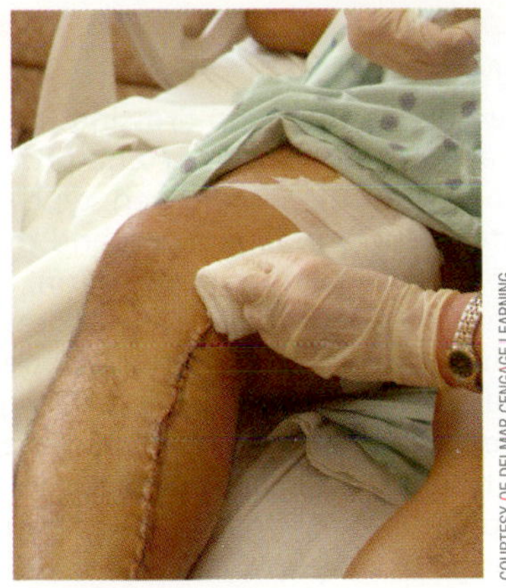

FIGURE 30-20-3 Apply 4 × 4 gauze pads, folded in half. Tape the gauze in place.

ACTION	RATIONALE
11. Cleanse wound if indicated. Grasp the edges of the gauze that contains cleaning solution. • **Incision:** Moving from top to bottom, clean the incision line first (Figure 30-20-2). Clean each side of incision using a new gauze for each swipe. • **Drain:** Using a circular motion, begin at the drain site and move outward. If additional cleaning is required, obtain a new gauze and clean from drain site outward.	11. Wounds are cleansed from least contaminated to most contaminated.
12. Remove gloves and wash hands.	12. Reduces transmission of microorganisms.
13. Apply nonsterile latex-free gloves.	13. Promotes infection control.
14. Apply a new dressing using 4 × 4 gauze pads folded in half to the 2 × 4 size. Place the folded gauze pad lengthwise on wound and tape lightly or apply tubular mesh for those with sensitive skin (Figure 30-20-3). Initial the dressing, citing date and time it was changed. • **Optional:** An ABD pad may be applied on top of the dressing for added protection over sutures or for client comfort.	14. A light dressing of 4 × 4 pads may be the only dressing that is needed to protect the incision from clothing or to collect a small amount of tissue drainage. This maintains a record of the dressing change for the next nurse.
15. Dispose of dressings appropriately, remove gloves, and then wash hands.	15. Reduces transmission of microorganisms.
16. Conduct client/family education about the dressing, which may include teaching the dressing technique to the client/family.	16. Educates the client/family and prepares for discharge.

EVALUATION

- Assess client comfort level during dressing change procedure.
- Determine whether the client's privacy was protected during the dressing change.
- Assess whether the correct supplies were brought in for the dressing change and whether any modifications need to be made to the dressing change.
- Determine the effectiveness of client/family education by having the client/family return-demonstrate the dressing or verbally review the steps of the dressing.

DOCUMENTATION

Nurses' Notes

- Date and time dressing done
- Brief description of the wound site
- Brief description of the site care done and dressing applied
- Client comfort before and after dressing change
- Client/family education done and evaluation of the teaching
- Document on appropriate electronic medical record or flow sheet.

(Continues)

PROCEDURE 30-21 Applying a Wet to Damp Dressing

OVERVIEW

The purpose of a wet to damp dressing (also known as wet to moist dressing) is to cover and protect the wound, collect exudate, promote healing, and promote light surface debridement. The decision to apply a wet to damp dressing depends on the wound bed, type of tissue and presence of eschar, amount of exudate, stage of wound healing, state of surrounding tissue, and the presence of infection.

Wound healing is promoted by a warm, moist environment; however, it is imperative to avoid moisture on the surface of the dressing. A wet external dressing can act as a wick with the external environment and draw contamination into the wound. Gentle debridement of a red wound is accomplished with a wet to damp dressing. One must be careful not to apply a dressing so wet that it ends up macerating the surrounding good tissue. Wet dressings are contraindicated in black eschar wounds, where the eschar represents full-thickness tissue destruction, because bacteria will multiply under such a dressing.

The wet to damp dressing consists of gauze, applied wet and allowed to become "near dry" before the next dressing change. Specifics of the wet to damp dressings vary according to the preferences of the surgeon and wound specialist, institutional policy, and outcome measurement standards used to evaluate the effectiveness of the dressing. General guidelines for a simple wet to damp dressing are covered.

ASSESSMENT

1. Assess the client's comfort level **to assess the need for medication before the dressing change**. Clients will be more cooperative and less anxious during dressing changes if they are comfortable.
2. Assess the external appearance of the dressing **to evaluate dressing adequacy as well as needed supplies**.
3. Assess the appearance of the wound and drains once the dressing is removed, noting redness, swelling, purulent drainage, or ecchymosis **to determine the condition of the wound and the effectiveness of the wet to damp dressing**.
4. Assess the client's understanding regarding the dressing changes and wound care **to determine any client teaching needed**.
5. Assess the client's healing response to previous treatments. The effectiveness of the wet to moist application should be routinely reassessed and the treatment modified if healing is not occurring.

POSSIBLE NURSING DIAGNOSES

*Impaired **S**kin Integrity*
*Impaired **T**issue Integrity*
*Risk for **I**nfection*
*Acute **P**ain*

PLANNING

Expected Outcomes

1. The site will be inspected for healing, signs of infection, and drainage.
2. The site will have the appropriate dressing applied.
3. The client/family will verbalize and/or demonstrate understanding and the ability, if indicated, to perform the dressing change and associated wound care of the surgical wound site.
4. The client will experience minimal discomfort during the procedure.

Equipment Needed (see Figure 30-21-1)

- Nonsterile latex-free gloves
- Container for proper disposal of soiled dressing
- Sterile gloves
- Moisture-proof gown (optional)
- Sterile towel
- Normal saline or ordered solution
- Sterile bowl
- Sterile 4 × 4 gauze pads, multiple
- Cover sponges or fluffs (optional)
- ABD dressing pads
- 2-inch tape (foam or paper)
- Tubular mesh (optional)
- Montgomery straps (optional)

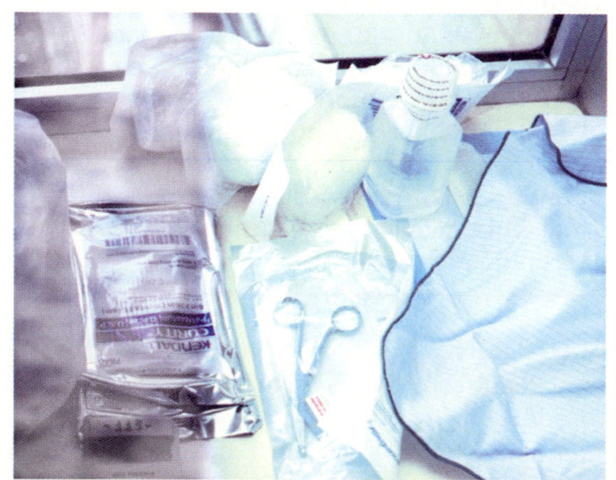

FIGURE 30-21-1 Sterile bandages, sterile saline, sterile scissors, and a sterile field are necessary to create a wet-to-damp dressing.

(Continues)

PROCEDURE 30-21 Applying a Wet to Damp Dressing (Continued)

delegation tips

Applying a wet to damp dressing requires sterile technique and professional assessment skills and cannot be delegated to ancillary personnel.

IMPLEMENTATION—ACTION/RATIONALE

* Check client's identification band * Explain procedure before beginning *

ACTION	RATIONALE
1. Review order of health care provider for wound care and gather supplies.	1. Promotes a smooth work flow.
2. Provide privacy; draw curtains; close door.	2. Maintains client comfort and privacy while body is exposed during procedure.
3. Assess need for pain medication. Pain is rated on a scale from 0 (lowest) to 10 (greatest). Assess need based on quality, pain pattern, location, and last pain medication received.	3. Removal of a wet to damp or moist dressing may be painful to the client, so careful assessment of pain medication needs before the dressing change is important.
4. Wash hands.	4. Reduces transmission of microorganisms.
5. Apply nonsterile latex-free gloves. If there is copious drainage or the wound is infected, wear a gown, a mask, and eye protection.	5. Provides infection control and protection from body fluids.
6. Remove dressing, noting number of gauze pads used and place them in appropriate receptacle (Figure 30-21-2). If it is found that the dressing is extremely dry and removal will result in injury, a small amount of saline to loosen that portion of the dressing is indicated (Figure 30-21-3).	6. To counteract the problem of an extremely dry dressing, increase the wetness of the dressing or increase the frequency of dressing changes. Provides number of gauze pads needed to replace the dressing.
7. Observe the undressed wound for healing (granulation and approximation of edges), signs of infection (inflammation, edema, warmth, pain), and drainage.	7. Allows for evaluation of effectiveness of treatment.
8. Cleanse the skin around the incision if necessary with a clean, warm, wet washcloth.	8. Dried blood or drainage on the surrounding skin can be an irritant and a medium for microbes.

COURTESY OF DELMAR CENGAGE LEARNING

FIGURE 30-21-2 Carefully remove the old dressing, allowing the old dressing to debride the wound as you pull it away.

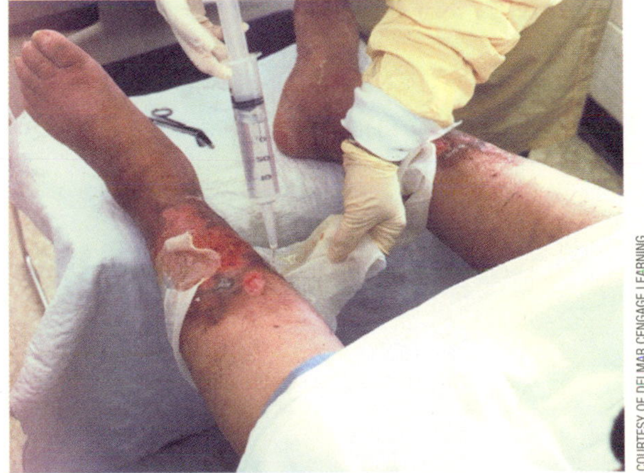

COURTESY OF DELMAR CENGAGE LEARNING

FIGURE 30-21-3 If the dressing is too dry and removing it will cause injury, use a small amount of saline to loosen the portion of the dressing that adheres too tightly to the wound.

(Continues)

PROCEDURE 30-21 Applying a Wet to Damp Dressing (Continued)

ACTION	RATIONALE
9. Remove gloves and wash hands.	9. Reduces transmission of microorganisms.
10. Set up supplies in a sterile field, including pouring ordered solutions into appropriate containers if indicated for the dressing.	10. Maintains sterility.
11. Apply sterile gloves.	11. This is a sterile dressing change.
12. Place gauze or packing material in the bowl with the normal saline or specified solution.	12. Wets gauze or packing material for dressing.
• Wring excess solution from gauze or packing. Avoid overwringing the dressing to prevent excessive drying.	• If too wet, wound bed can get soupy, increasing chance of bacterial growth.
• Gently place wet gauze over the area (Figure 30-21-4).	• Dresses the wound.
13. Apply external dressing of dry 4 3 4 gauze pads, cover sponges, fluffs, or ABD pads (Figure 30-21-5).	13. Prevents excess drying and protects wound.
• Secure dressing in place with tape, Montgomery straps, or tubular mesh (Figure 30-21-6).	• Tape for short-term dressings in clients who are not sensitive to adhesives. For long-term dressings or for those who are sensitive to tape, use Montgomery straps or tubular mesh to prevent skin irritation.
14. Remove gloves and wash hands.	14. Reduces transmission of microorganisms.
15. Mark the dressing with the date and time it was changed. Initial the dressing.	15. Maintains a record of the dressing change and provides for continuity of care.
16. Conduct client/family education about the dressing, which may include teaching the dressing technique to the client/family.	16. Educates the client/family and prepares for discharge.

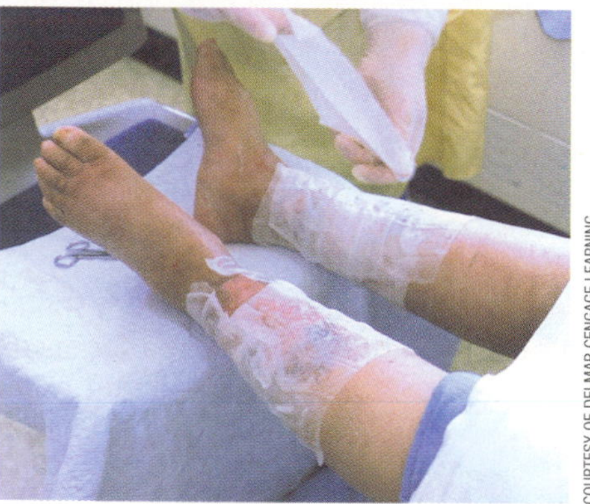
COURTESY OF DELMAR CENGAGE LEARNING

FIGURE 30-21-4 Place the gauze on the wound.

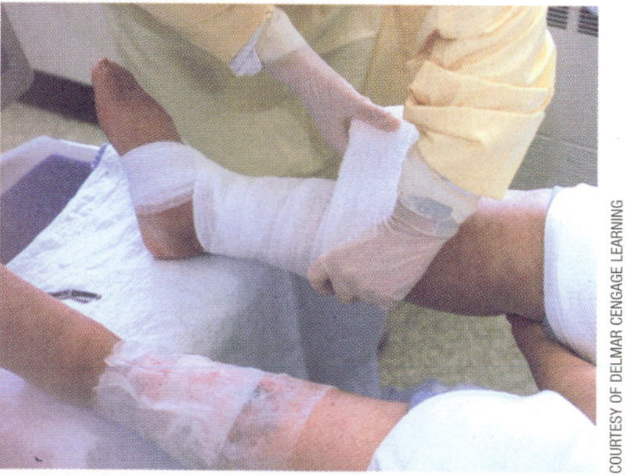
COURTESY OF DELMAR CENGAGE LEARNING

FIGURE 30-21-5 Wrap the wet gauze with an external dressing of dry gauze bandages.

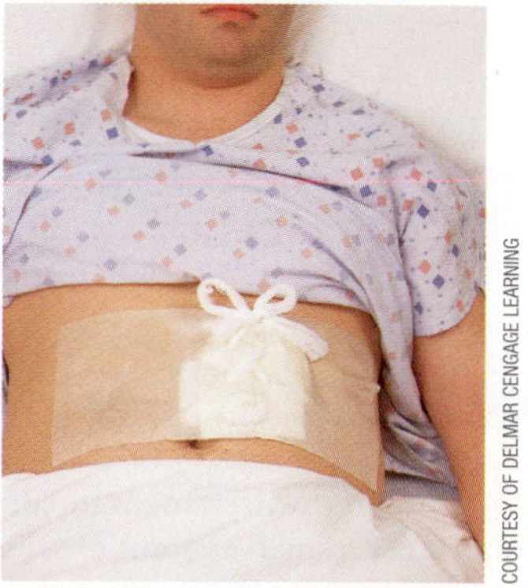
COURTESY OF DELMAR CENGAGE LEARNING

FIGURE 30-21-6 Montgomery Straps

(Continues)

PROCEDURE 30-21 Applying a Wet to Damp Dressing (Continued)

EVALUATION

- The site was inspected for healing, signs of infection, and drainage.
- The site had the appropriate dressing applied.
- The client/family verbalized or demonstrated understanding and the ability, if necessary, to perform the dressing change and associated wound care of the surgical wound site.
- The procedure was performed with minimal discomfort to the client.

DOCUMENTATION

Nurses' Notes

- Administration of pain medication before dressing change
- Date and time dressing done
- Brief description of the wound site
- Brief description of the site care done and dressing applied
- Client comfort before and after dressing change
- Client/family education done and evaluation of the teaching
- Document on appropriate electronic medical record or flow sheet.

PROCEDURE 30-22 Culturing a Wound

OVERVIEW

Bacterial wound contamination is one of the most common causes of altered wound healing. A surgical wound can become infected preoperatively, intraoperatively, or postoperatively. Nicks or abrasions created during preoperative shaving may be a source of pathogens. The risk for intraoperative exposure to pathogens increases when the respiratory, gastrointestinal, genitourinary, and oropharyngeal tracts are opened. Nonsurgical wounds from trauma, pressure ulcers, or disease can become infected as well.

If the amount of bacteria in the wound is sufficient or the client's immune defenses are compromised, clinical infection may become apparent 2 to 11 days postoperatively. Infection slows healing by prolonging the inflammatory phase of healing, competing for nutrients, and producing chemicals and enzymes that are damaging to the tissues. Identifying the infectious agent in a wound is an important step in wound healing.

ASSESSMENT

1. Assess the wound and the surrounding tissues for signs of infection. Check for heat, redness, inflammation, and drainage. Check the color and consistency of the drainage. Check the smell and color of the wound. **Allows for intervention to detect and treat infection.**
2. Assess the client's overall status, including vital signs, for signs of infection such as fever, chills, or elevated white blood cell count (WBC). **Allows for intervention to detect and treat infection.**

POSSIBLE NURSING DIAGNOSES

Risk for Infection
Impaired Skin Integrity
Disturbed Body Image

PLANNING

Expected Outcomes

1. The wound culture will be collected with a minimum of pain and trauma to the client.
2. The wound culture will be representative of the flora present in the wound, without contamination by flora outside the wound.

Equipment Needed (see Figure 30-22-1)

- Nonsterile latex-free gloves
- Sterile gloves and dressing supplies
- Normal saline and irrigation tray
- Culture tube and swab
- Moisture-proof container or bag

(Continues)

PROCEDURE 30-22 Culturing a Wound (Continued)

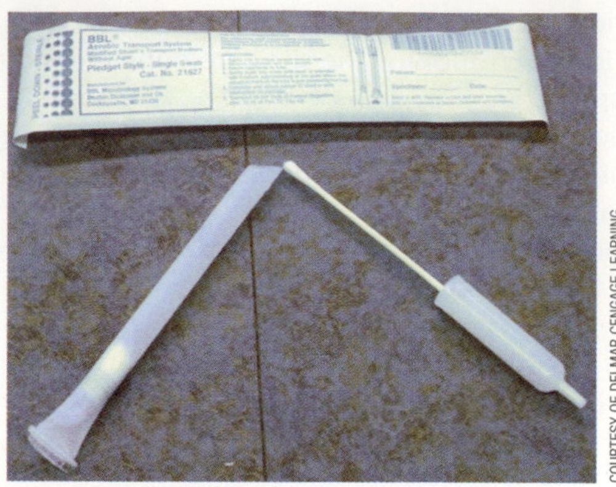
COURTESY OF DELMAR CENGAGE LEARNING

FIGURE 30-22-1 Sterile Culture Tube and Swab

delegation tips

Obtaining a wound culture requires nursing assessment and aseptic technique, and is potentially an invasive procedure; therefore, delegation to ancillary personnel is not appropriate.

IMPLEMENTATION—ACTION/RATIONALE

* Check client's identification band * Explain procedure before beginning *

ACTION	RATIONALE
1. Wash hands, apply nonsterile latex-free gloves, and remove old dressing. Place old dressing in moisture-proof container and remove and discard gloves. Wash hands again.	1. Reduces transmission of microorganisms. Makes the wound accessible for obtaining the culture.
2. Open the dressing supplies using sterile technique and apply sterile gloves.	2. Maintains sterile environment.
3. Assess the wound's appearance; note quality, quantity, color, and odor of discharge.	3. Provides assessment of the amount and character of the wound's drainage before irrigation. Reddened areas and heavy drainage suggest infection.
4. Irrigate the wound with normal saline before culturing the wound; do not irrigate with antiseptic.	4. Decreases the risk of culturing normal flora and other exudates such as protein; an antiseptic may destroy the bacteria.
5. Using a sterile gauze pad, absorb the excess saline, then discard the pad.	5. Prevents maceration of tissue caused by excess moisture.
6. Remove the culture tube from the packaging (Figure 30-22-2). Remove the culture swab from the culture tube and gently roll the swab over the granulation tissue. Avoid eschar and wound edges (Figure 30-22-3).	6. Decreases the chance of collecting superficial skin microorganisms.
7. Replace the swab into the culture tube, being careful not to touch the swab to the outside of the tube. Recap the tube. Crush the ampule of medium located in the bottom or cap of the tube (Figure 30-22-4).	7. Avoids contamination with microorganisms. Releases the medium to surround the swab.
8. Remove gloves, wash hands, and apply sterile gloves. Dress the wound with sterile dressing.	8. Reduces transmission of microorganisms. Prevents contamination of the wound.

(Continues)

PROCEDURE 30-22 Culturing a Wound (Continued)

ACTION	RATIONALE

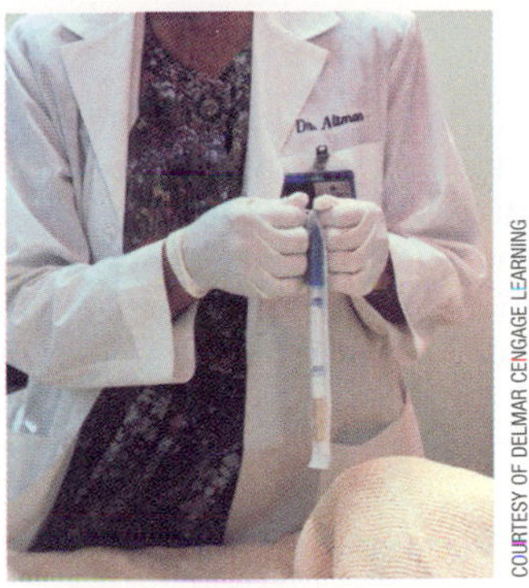

COURTESY OF DELMAR CENGAGE LEARNING

FIGURE 30-22-2 Remove the culture tube from the packaging.

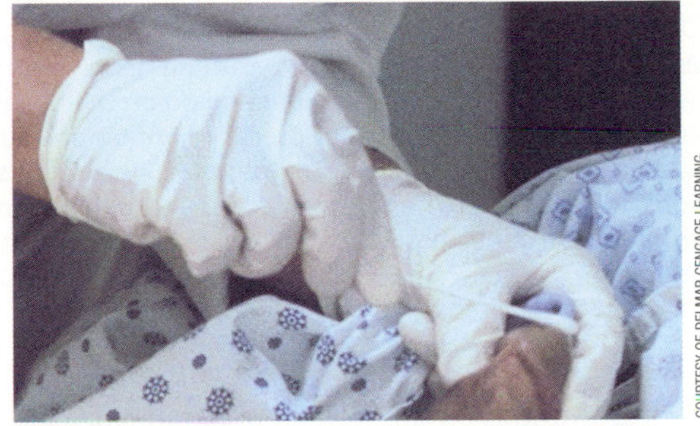

COURTESY OF DELMAR CENGAGE LEARNING

FIGURE 30-22-3 Roll the swab over the area to be cultured.

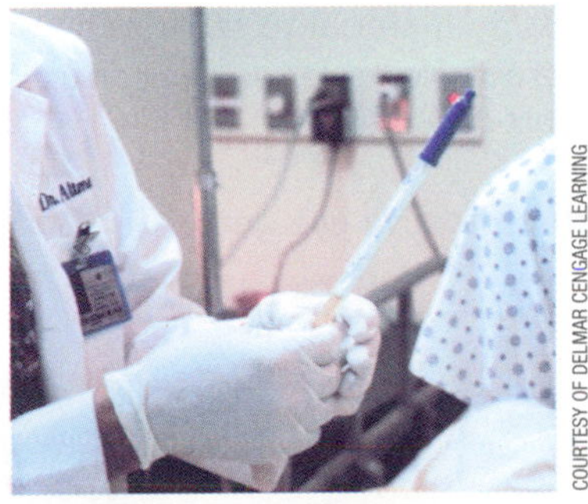

COURTESY OF DELMAR CENGAGE LEARNING

FIGURE 30-22-4 Crush the ampule to release the medium inside the culture tube.

ACTION	RATIONALE
9. Label the specimen, place in biohazard transport bag, and arrange to transport the specimen to the laboratory according to institutional policy.	9. Ensures proper handling of specimen.
10. Remove gloves and wash hands.	10. Reduces transmission of microorganisms.
11. Document assessment findings, actions taken, and that specimen was obtained.	11. Promotes continuity of care and records information for evaluation.

EVALUATION

- Assess whether the wound culture was collected with a minimum of pain and trauma to the client.
- Determine whether the wound culture is representative of the flora present in the wound, without contamination by other bacteria.

DOCUMENTATION

Nurses' Notes

- Time and method of collection of the culture, and what was done with the specimen
- Fill out the lab requisition form with the client's information as well as time and date specimen was collected, location of the culture, and requested tests. Often there are duplicate numbered or coded labels on the lab slips. One copy is placed in the chart.
- Document on appropriate electronic medical record or flow sheet.

(Continues)

PROCEDURE 30-23 Irrigating a Wound

OVERVIEW

Wound irrigation is the process of washing debris, drainage, or exudate out of the wound to promote healing. The fluid used to irrigate a wound varies depending on the health care provider's orders. Fluids commonly used include normal saline, acetic acid, and specially prepared antibiotic solutions. If cytotoxic solutions are used, then the area must be flushed/irrigated afterward with normal saline. Wounds that require irrigation also vary. They may be simple open lacerations; tunneled pressure ulcers; or complex, open abdominal wounds extending down to the abdominal fascia. Wound irrigation is a sterile procedure. Take care not to contaminate the wound and not to become contaminated with wound drainage.

ASSESSMENT

1. Assess the current dressing **to determine what equipment will be needed to replace it with a clean dressing and whether the dressing has been adequate to protect the wound and contain any drainage or exudate.**
2. Assess the client to determine if able **to understand the need for the wound irrigation and cooperate with the procedure.**
3. Assess whether the client has concerns about pain or body image regarding this wound and the irrigation **to determine what client teaching and support will be most effective.**
4. Assess the client's environment **to plan if the necessary equipment and supplies are available, including irrigant, hand hygiene facilities, and an adequate work area to lay out supplies and establish a sterile field.**

POSSIBLE NURSING DIAGNOSES

*Impaired **S**kin Integrity*
*Risk for **I**nfection*
*Acute **P**ain*

PLANNING

Expected Outcomes

1. The wound will be free of exudate, drainage, and debris.
2. The wound will be free of signs and symptoms of infection.
3. The procedure will be performed with a minimum of trauma and pain to the client.

Equipment Needed (see Figure 30-23-1)

- Sterile latex-free gloves
- Nonsterile latex-free gloves
- Sterile irrigation kit (basin, piston irrigation syringe, solution container)
- Irrigation solution (per health care provider's order)
- Waterproof pad
- Sterile dressing material to redress the wound
- Moisture-proof container or bag for use after the irrigation procedure
- Gown
- Mask with protective eye gear

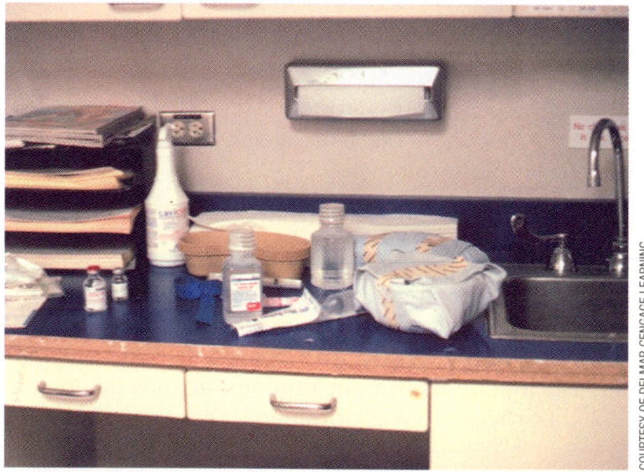

COURTESY OF DELMAR CENGAGE LEARNING

FIGURE 30-23-1 Sterile solution, sterile syringes, and a sterile basin are used to irrigate a wound.

delegation tips

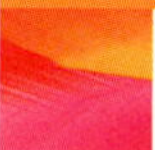

Wound irrigation requires nursing assessment, aseptic technique, and monitoring of wound healing. This procedure is not delegated to ancillary personnel.

(Continues)

PROCEDURE 30-23 Irrigating a Wound (Continued)

IMPLEMENTATION—ACTION/RATIONALE

ACTION	RATIONALE
* Check client's identification band * Explain procedure before beginning *	
1. Confirm the health care provider's order for wound irrigation and note the type and strength of the ordered irrigation solution.	1. Wound irrigation is a dependent nursing action that requires a medical order stating the type of solution to be used.
2. Assess the client's pain level and medicate if needed with analgesic 60 minutes before procedure if the medication is to be given orally (PO) or intramuscularly (IM).	2. Allows time for medication to be absorbed to increase the analgesic effect.
3. Place a waterproof pad on the bed. Assist the client onto the pad. Then assist the client into a position that will allow the irrigant to flow through the wound and into the basin from the cleanest to dirtiest area of the wound.	3. Positioning of the client and placement of a waterproof pad will decrease contamination of bed linen.
4. Wash hands and apply nonsterile latex-free gloves, gown, and mask with protective eye gear if splashes from wound fluid or blood are anticipated. Remove and discard old dressing in appropriate receptacle.	4. Reduces transmission of microorganisms.
5. Assess the wound's appearance and note quality, quantity, color, and odor of drainage.	5. Provides assessment of wound status.
6. Remove gloves and wash hands.	6. Reduces transmission of microorganisms.
7. Prepare the sterile irrigation tray and dressing supplies. Pour the room-temperature irrigation solution into the solution container.	7. Prevents introduction of microorganisms into the wound. Reduces client discomfort.
8. Apply sterile gloves (new gown and goggles if needed).	8. Promotes sterile environment. Follows Standard Precautions.
9. Position the sterile basin below the wound so the irrigant will flow from the cleanest area to the dirtiest area and into the basin.	9. Decreases possibility of wound contamination.
10. Fill the piston or bulb syringe with irrigant and gently flush the wound. Hold the syringe approximately 1 inch above the wound bed to irrigate. Refill the syringe and continue to flush the wound until the solution returns clear and no exudate is noted or until the prescribed amount of fluid has been used (Figures 30-23-2 and 30-23-3).	10. Decreases trauma to granulation tissue, yet provides the ideal pressure for cleansing and removal of debris.

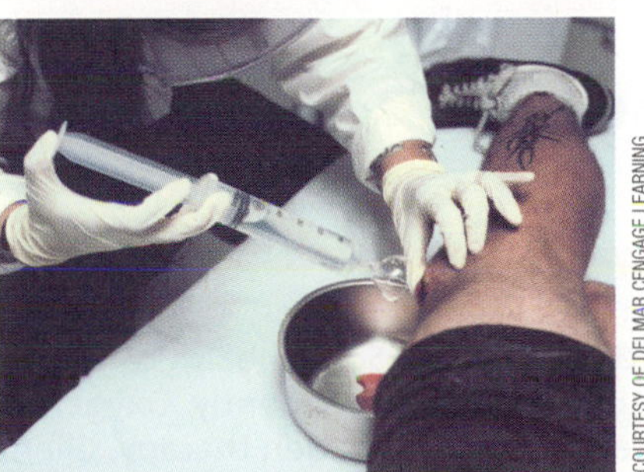

COURTESY OF DELMAR CENGAGE LEARNING

FIGURE 30-23-2 Gently flush the wound.

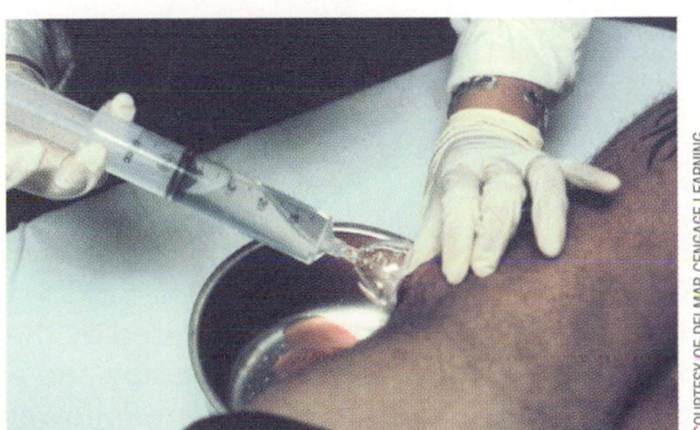

COURTESY OF DELMAR CENGAGE LEARNING

FIGURE 30-23-3 Hold the syringe close to the wound, but be careful not to touch the wound with the syringe.

(Continues)

PROCEDURE 30-23 Irrigating a Wound (Continued)

ACTION	RATIONALE

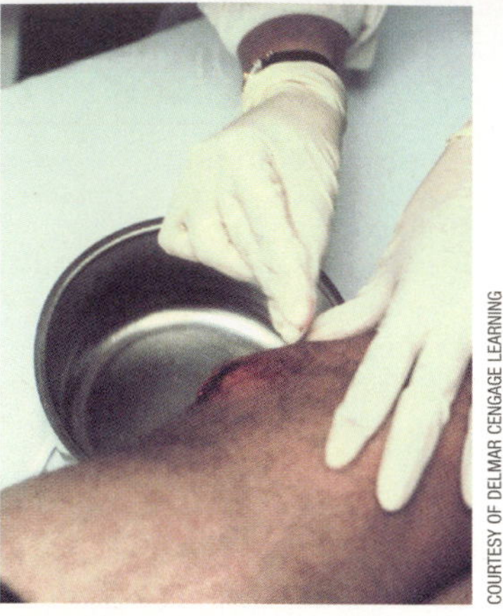

FIGURE 30-23-4 Dry the edges of the wound with sterile gauze.

ACTION	RATIONALE
11. Dry the edges of the wound with sterile gauze (Figure 30-23-4).	11. Prevents maceration of tissues caused by excess moisture.
12. Assess the wound's appearance and drainage.	12. Provides indication of change in wound status.
13. Apply a sterile dressing.	13. Protects the wound from microorganisms.
14. Dispose of dressings and equipment. Remove gown, mask with protective eye gear, and gloves. Wash hands.	14. Reduces transmission of microorganisms.
15. Document all assessment findings and actions taken.	15. Records information for evaluation.

EVALUATION

- Assess whether the wound is free of exudate, drainage, and debris.
- Assess whether the wound is free of signs and symptoms of infection.
- Evaluate whether the procedure was performed with a minimum of trauma and pain to the client.

DOCUMENTATION

Nurses' Notes

- Wound's appearance and quality, quantity, color, and odor of drainage
- Client's tolerance of the procedure and any observations regarding the client's body image
- Document on appropriate electronic medical record or flow sheet.

Kardex

- Special equipment or techniques required with the client to provide the information to other staff members

PROCEDURE 30-24 Administering Oxygen Therapy

OVERVIEW

Administration of oxygen must be ordered by the physician or qualified practitioner. Some health care facilities will have protocols that govern oxygen therapy and allow the nurse to begin therapy independently. Oxygen is a drug, so medication administration criteria are followed in addition to the steps unique to oxygen therapy. Clients unable to maintain adequate PO_2 and O_2 saturation levels on room air are candidates for oxygen therapy. An adequate airway is essential to effectiveness of the treatment. It is best to treat the hypoxia with the lowest oxygen dose possible. Some clients with a normal oxygen level are also given oxygen if they are at risk for complications related to hypoxia; for example, the myocardial infarction client often receives oxygen therapy to prevent dysrhythmias.

(Continues)

PROCEDURE 30-24 Administering Oxygen Therapy (Continued)

The health care provider orders the oxygen delivery system and flow rate, and the nurse monitors client response to the therapy. The dosage of oxygen may be ordered as an FIO_2 (fraction of inspired oxygen), which is expressed as a percentage or as liters per minute (L/min). Respiratory therapists may be available to assist in the administration of oxygen therapy and client assessment.

ASSESSMENT

1. Determine client history and acute and chronic health problems. **Clients with carbon dioxide retaining chronic obstructive pulmonary disease (COPD) will need lower amounts of oxygen so as not to obliterate their hypoxic respiratory drive. They may already be on oxygen and need long-term continuous therapy.**
2. Assess the client's baseline respiratory signs, including airway, respiratory pattern, rate, depth, and rhythm, noting indications of increased work of breathing. **Helps determine the client's need for oxygen as well as response to the therapy.**
3. Check the extremities and mucous membranes closely for color. **Gives some indication of oxygenation, although problems with circulation and tissue perfusion can also alter these factors.**
4. Review arterial blood gas (ABG) and pulse oximetry results. **These are the most important determinants of the effectiveness of the pulmonary system and determine the need for therapy as well as changes in therapy.**
5. Note lung sounds for wheezes/crackles. **Secretions will interfere with airway patency and diffusion of oxygen and carbon dioxide across the alveolar-capillary bed.**
6. Assess the nares, behind the earlobes, cheek, tracheostomy site, or other places where oxygen tubing or equipment is in constant contact with the skin **to look for signs of skin irritation or breakdown.**

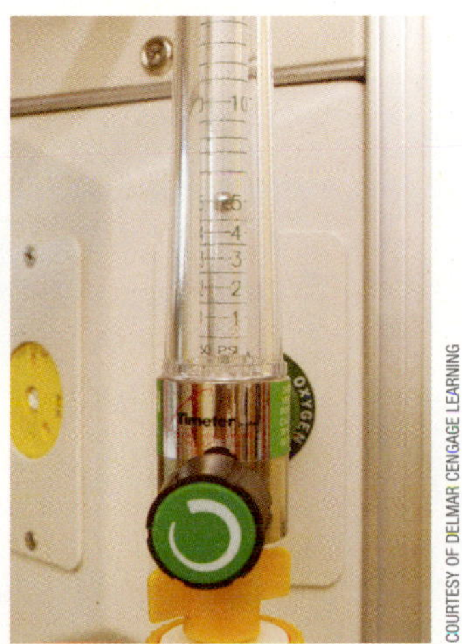

FIGURE 30-24-1 In-Line Oxygen and Flow Meter

POSSIBLE NURSING DIAGNOSES

*Impaired **G**as Exchange*
*Ineffective **B**reathing Pattern*
*Risk for **I**njury*
*Ineffective **A**irway Clearance*
*Risk for Impaired **S**kin Integrity*
***A**ctivity Intolerance*

PLANNING

Expected Outcomes

1. Oxygen level will return to normal in blood and tissues as evident by oxygen saturation greater than or equal to 92%, skin color normal.
2. Respiratory rate, pattern, and depth will be within the normal range for client.
3. The client will not develop any skin or tissue irritation or breakdown.
4. The client will demonstrate methods to clear secretions and maintain optimal oxygenation.
5. Breathing efficiency and activity tolerance will be increased.
6. The client will understand the rationale for the therapy.

Equipment Needed (see Figures 30-24-1 and 30-24-2)

- Stethoscope
- Oxygen source—portable or in-line
- Oxygen flow meter
- Oxygen delivery device: nasal cannula, mask, tent, or T-tube with adapter for artificial airway
- Oxygen tubing
- Pulse oximeter
- Humidifier and distilled or sterile water (not needed with low flow rates per nasal cannula)

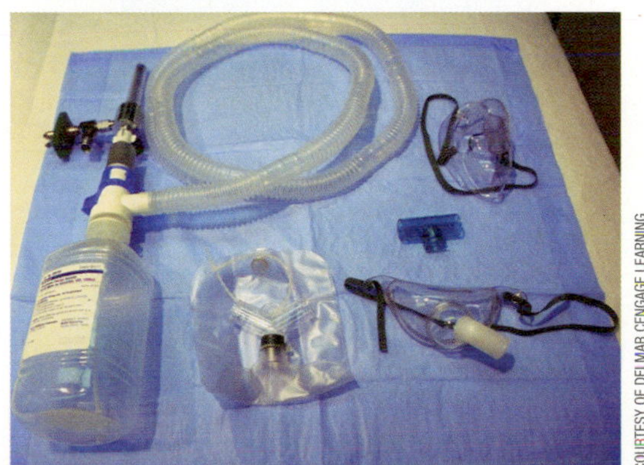

FIGURE 30-24-2 Humidifier, reservoir bag, tracheostomy mask, T-tube, and a simple face mask are used when administering oxygen therapy.

(Continues)

PROCEDURE 30-24 Administering Oxygen Therapy (Continued)

delegation tips

The initiation of oxygen therapy requires assessment by a nurse or respiratory care practitioner. All personnel are responsible to maintain fire/safety precautions when oxygen is in use. Ancillary personnel should be instructed to report dyspnea, tachycardia, any changes in the client's activity tolerance, a respiratory rate less than 12 or greater than 20 breaths per minute in the adult client, or changes in mental status. Ancillary personnel should be instructed how to properly reapply respiratory therapy equipment, how to initiate assistance with activities of daily living for the client requiring oxygen therapy, and to report any abnormal client responses.

IMPLEMENTATION—ACTION/RATIONALE

ACTION	RATIONALE
* Check client's identification band * Explain procedure before beginning *	
Nasal Cannula (see Figure 30-24-3)	
1. Wash hands.	1. Reduces transmission of microorganisms.
2. Verify the health care provider's order.	2. Ensures correct dosage and route.
3. Remind clients who smoke of the reasons for not smoking while O_2 is in use.	3. Increases compliance with procedures. Oxygen supports combustion.
4. If using humidity, fill humidifier to fill line with distilled water and close container.	4. Prevents drying of the client's airway and thins any secretions.
5. Attach humidifier to oxygen flow meter.	5. Allows the oxygen to pass through the water and become humidified.
6. Insert humidifier and flow meter into oxygen source in wall or portable unit.	6. Gives access to oxygen. Reduces possibility of inserting into wrong outlet. Many institutions also have compressed air available from outlets very similar in appearance to oxygen outlets. Green always stands for oxygen. Be sure to plug the flow meter into the green outlet.
7. Attach the oxygen tubing and nasal cannula to the flow meter and turn it on to the prescribed flow rate (1 to 5 L/min). Use extension tubing for ambulatory clients so they can get up to go to the bathroom.	7. Rates above 6 L/min are not efficacious and can dry the nasal mucosa.
8. Check for bubbling in the humidifier.	8. Ensures proper functioning.
9. Place the nasal prongs in the client's nostrils (Figure 30-24-4). Secure the cannula in place by adjusting the tubing around the client's ears and using the slip ring to stabilize it under the client's chin (Figure 30-24-5).	9. Keeps delivery system in place so client receives the amount of oxygen ordered.

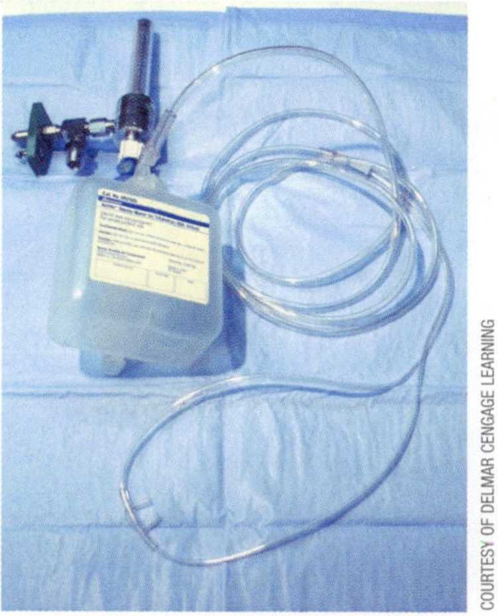

COURTESY OF DELMAR CENGAGE LEARNING

FIGURE 30-24-3 Nasal cannula and oxygen attached to a humidifier.

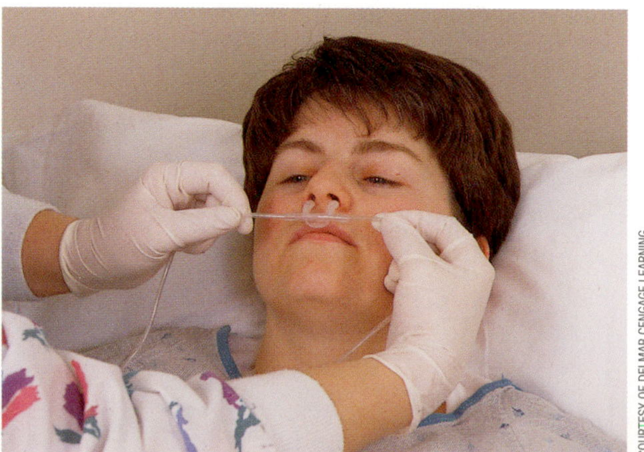

COURTESY OF DELMAR CENGAGE LEARNING

FIGURE 30-24-4 Insert cannula prong into nostrils (gloves are optional).

(Continues)

PROCEDURE 30-24 Administering Oxygen Therapy (Continued)

ACTION	RATIONALE
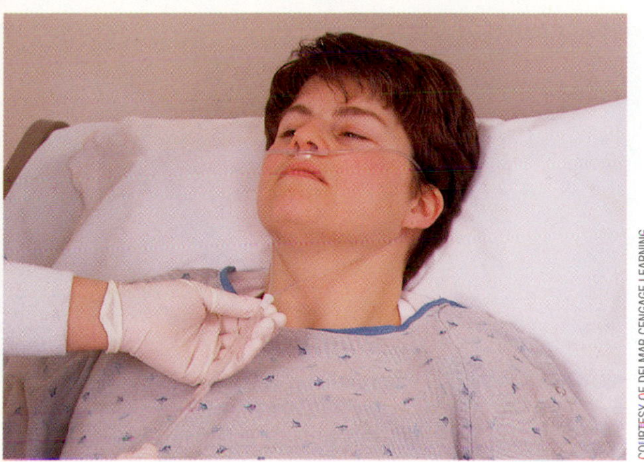 COURTESY OF DELMAR CENGAGE LEARNING **FIGURE 30-24-5** Adjust Tubing	
10. Check for proper flow rate every 4 hours and when the client returns from procedures.	10. Ensures that client receives proper dose. The nasal cannula is a low-flow system because it administers oxygen while the client also inspires room air. The actual dose of oxygen received by the client will vary depending on the client's respiratory pattern.
11. Assess client's nostrils every 8 hours. If the client complains of dryness or has signs of irritation, use sterile lubricant to keep mucous membranes moist. Add humidifier if not already in place.	11. Dry membranes are more prone to breakdown by friction or pressure from nasal cannula.
12. Monitor vital signs, oxygen saturation, and client condition every 4 to 8 hours (or as indicated or ordered) for signs and symptoms of hypoxia.	12. Detects any untoward effects from therapy.
13. Wean client from oxygen as soon as possible using standard protocols.	13. Oxygen is not without side effects and should be used only as long as needed. Problems with reimbursement may develop if criteria for therapy are not met.
Mask: Venturi (high-flow device), simple mask (low flow), partial rebreather mask, nonrebreather mask, and face tent	
14. Repeat Actions 1 to 6.	14. See Rationales 1 to 6.
15. Attach appropriately sized mask (Figure 30-24-6 and Figure 30-24-7) or face tent to oxygen tubing and turn on flow meter to prescribed flow rate. The Venturi mask will have color-coded inserts that list the flow rate necessary to obtain the desired percentage of oxygen. Allow the reservoir bag of the nonrebreathing or partial rebreathing mask to fill completely.	15. Ensures proper fit; size needed is based on the client's size. Checks the oxygen source and primes the tubing and mask or tent.
16. Check for bubbling in the humidifier.	16. Ensures proper functioning.
17. Place the mask or tent on the client's face, fasten the elastic band around the client's ears, and tighten until the mask fits snugly.	17. Prevents loss of oxygen from the sides of the mask.
18. Check for proper flow rate every 4 hours.	18. Ensures that client is receiving the proper dose.

(Continues)

PROCEDURE 30-24 Administering Oxygen Therapy (Continued)

ACTION	RATIONALE

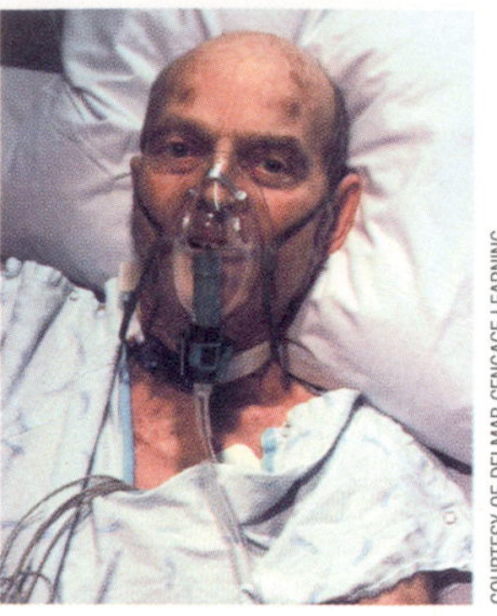

FIGURE 30-24-6 Make sure that the mask is the appropriate size for the client.

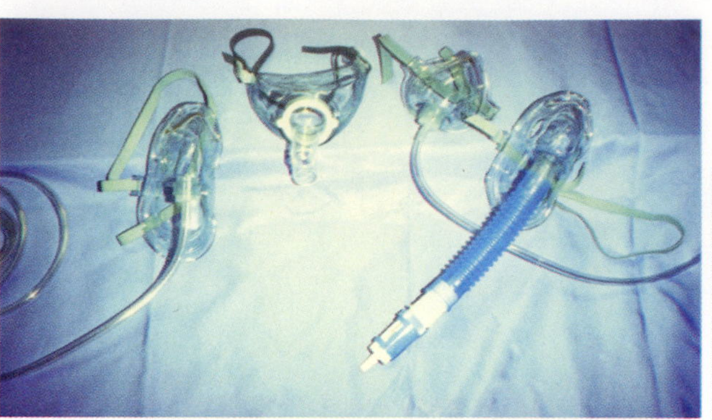

FIGURE 30-24-7 Simple oxygen mask, tracheostomy mask, pediatric mask, and Venturi mask are different types of oxygen masks.

ACTION	RATIONALE
19. Ensure that the ports of the Venturi mask are not under covers or impeded by any other source.	19. Air must be entrained to mix room air and oxygen coming from source to ensure proper oxygen percentage (FIO_2).
20. Assess client's face and ears for pressure from the mask and use padding as needed.	20. Provides client comfort and prevents skin breakdown.
21. Wean client to nasal cannula and then wean off oxygen per protocol.	21. Oxygen is not without side effects and should be used only as long as needed. The nasal cannula provides a lower FIO_2 than the mask. Problems with reimbursement may develop if criteria for therapy are not met.

EVALUATION

- Oxygen level returned to normal in blood and tissues as evident by oxygen saturation ≥92%; skin color normal for client.
- Respiratory rate, pattern, and depth are within the normal range.
- The client did not develop any skin or tissue irritation or breakdown.
- Breathing efficiency and activity tolerance are increased.
- The client understands the rationale for the therapy.

DOCUMENTATION

Nurses' Notes

- O_2 saturation and respiratory status
- Method of oxygen delivery and rate
- Client's assessment parameters and response to treatment
- Changes in mental status
- Document on appropriate electronic medical record or flow sheet.

PROCEDURE 30-25 Performing Nasopharyngeal and Oropharyngeal Suctioning

OVERVIEW

Suctioning secretions is necessary to maintain a patent airway for a client who is unable to effectively clear secretions by coughing. It is considered a sterile procedure, thereby preventing the introduction of microorganisms into the client's airway and lungs.

Suctioning is performed as often as necessary to remove excess secretions, depending on the amount of secretions the client is generating and the client's ability to clear the airway. The client's airway and oxygenation are evaluated to determine the need for suctioning.

(Continues)

PROCEDURE 30-25 Performing Nasopharyngeal and Oropharyngeal Suctioning (Continued)

Wall suction should be set at 100 to 120 mm Hg for adults, 50 to 100 mm Hg for children, and 40 to 60 mm Hg for infants. Portable suction should be set at 8 to 15 mm Hg for adults, 5 to 8 mm Hg for children, and 3 to 5 mm Hg for infants.

ASSESSMENT

1. Assess respirations for rate, rhythm, depth, and bubbling or gurgling noises **to evaluate airway.**
2. Auscultate lung fields **to evaluate airway and determine need for suctioning.**
3. Monitor arterial blood gases and/or pulse oximetry values **to determine oxygen level and adequate air exchange.**
4. Assess for anxiety and restlessness, **which may be signs of airway distress and/or hypoxia.**
5. Assess the client's understanding of the suctioning procedure **to decrease the client's anxiety.**

POSSIBLE NURSING DIAGNOSES

*Ineffective **A**irway Clearance*
*Impaired **G**as Exchange*
***A**nxiety*

PLANNING

Expected Outcomes

1. The client will have no coarse bubbling or gurgling noises with respirations.
2. The client will report breathing comfortably.
3. The client will have no apparent anxiety or restlessness.
4. The client will have arterial blood gases and pulse oximetry values within normal limits.
5. The client will express understanding of the suctioning process.

Equipment Needed

- Suction source (wall or portable with collection bottle)
- Sterile suction kit
- Sterile gloves (if not in kit)
- Sterile water-soluble lubricant
- Small bottle of sterile water or normal saline (if not in kit)
- Tubing connected to suction source
- Personal protective equipment: gown, mask, and goggles or face shield

delegation tips

Nasopharyngeal and oropharyngeal suctioning is generally performed by the nurse. Properly trained ancillary personnel may perform oropharyngeal suctioning in some situations.

IMPLEMENTATION—ACTION/RATIONALE

ACTION	RATIONALE
* Check client's identification band * Explain procedure before beginning *	
1. Choose the most appropriate route (nasopharyngeal or oropharyngeal) for your client. If nasopharyngeal approach is considered, inspect the nares with a penlight to determine patency. Alternately, you may assess patency by occluding each nare in turn with finger pressure while asking the client to breathe through the remaining nare.	1. The oropharyngeal approach is easier but requires that the client cooperate; it may also produce gagging more readily. The nasopharyngeal route is more effective for reaching the posterior oropharynx but is contraindicated in clients with a deviated nasal septum, nasal polyps, or any tendency toward excessive bleeding (low platelet count, use of anticoagulants, recent history of epistaxis or nasal trauma).
2. Advise the client that suctioning may cause coughing or gagging but emphasize the importance of clearing the airway.	2. Promotes cooperation and reduces anxiety.
3. Wash hands.	3. Reduces transmission of microorganisms.
4. Position the client in a high Fowler's or semi-Fowler's position.	4. Maximizes lung expansion and effective coughing.

(Continues)

PROCEDURE 30-25 Performing Nasopharyngeal and Oropharyngeal Suctioning (Continued)

ACTION	RATIONALE
5. If the client is unconscious or otherwise unable to protect his or her airway, place in a side-lying position.	5. Protects the client from aspiration in the event of vomiting.
6. Connect extension tubing to suction device if not already in place, and adjust suction control to between 100 and 120 mm Hg for adult.	6. Excessive negative pressure can cause tissue trauma, whereas insufficient pressure will be ineffective.
7. Put on gown and mask and goggles or face shield.	7. Protects nurse from splattering of body fluids.
8. Using sterile technique, open the suction kit. Consider the inside wrapper of the kit to be sterile, and spread the wrapper out carefully to create a small sterile field.	8. Produces an area in which to place sterile items without contaminating them.
9. Open a packet of sterile water-soluble lubricant and squeeze out the contents of the packet onto the sterile field.	9. Lubricant will be used to further lubricate the catheter tip if the nasopharyngeal route is used.
10. If sterile solution (water or saline) is not included in the kit, pour about 100 mL of solution into the sterile container provided in the kit.	10. Will be used to lubricate the catheter and to rinse the inside of the catheter to clear secretions.
11. If gloves are wrapped, carefully lift the wrapped gloves from the kit without touching the inside of the kit or the gloves themselves. Lay the wrapped gloves next to the suction kit, and open the wrapper. Put on the gloves using sterile gloving technique (Procedure 30-2).	11. Keeps gloves sterile for handling the sterile suction catheter to avoid introducing pathogens into the client's airway.
12. If a cup of sterile solution is included in the suction kit, open it.	12. Will be used to lubricate the catheter and to rinse the inside of the catheter to clear secretions.
13. Designate one hand as *sterile* (able to touch only sterile items) and the other as clean (able to touch only unsterile items).	13. Usually, the dominant hand is the sterile hand, while the nondominant hand is clean. This prevents contamination of sterile supplies while allowing unsterile items to be handled.
14. *Using your sterile hand*, pick up the suction catheter. Grasp the plastic connector end between your thumb and forefinger and coil the tip around your remaining fingers.	14. Prevents accidental contamination of the catheter tip.
15. Pick up the extension tubing *with your clean hand*. Connect the suction catheter to the extension tubing, taking care not to contaminate the catheter (Figure 30-25-1).	15. The extension tubing is not sterile.
16. Position your clean hand with the thumb over the catheter's suction port.	16. Suction is activated by occluding this port with the thumb. Releasing the port deactivates the suction.
17. Dip the catheter tip into the sterile solution, and activate the suction. Observe as the solution is drawn into the catheter.	17. Tests the suction device as well as lubricates the interior of the catheter to enhance clearance of secretions.

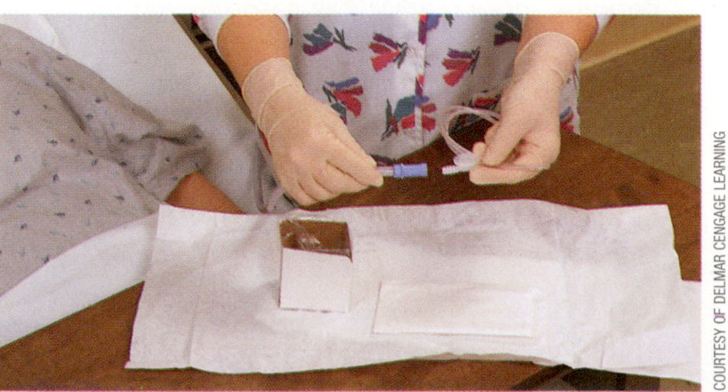
COURTESY OF DELMAR CENGAGE LEARNING

FIGURE 30-25-1 Attach catheter to tubing.

(Continues)

PROCEDURE 30-25 Performing Nasopharyngeal and Oropharyngeal Suctioning (Continued)

ACTION	RATIONALE
18. For oropharyngeal suctioning, ask the client to open his or her mouth. Without activating the suction, use sterile hand to gently insert the catheter and advance it until you reach the pool of secretions or until the client coughs. Do not poke catheter in oropharynx.	18. To minimize trauma, do not apply suction while the catheter is being advanced.
19. For nasopharyngeal suctioning, estimate the distance from the tip of the client's nose to the earlobe and grasp the catheter between your thumb and forefinger at a point equal to this distance from the catheter's tip.	19. Ensures placement of the catheter tip in the oropharynx and not in the trachea.
20. Dip the tip of the suction catheter into the water-soluble lubricant to coat catheter tip liberally.	20. Promotes the client's comfort and minimizes trauma to nasal mucosa.
21. Use *sterile* hand to insert the catheter tip into the nostril with the suction control port uncovered. Advance the catheter gently with a slight downward slant. Slight rotation of the catheter may be used to ease insertion (Figure 30-25-2). Advance the catheter to the point marked by your thumb and forefinger.	21. Guides the catheter toward the posterior oropharynx along the floor of the nasal cavity.
22. If resistance is met, *do not force the catheter*. Withdraw it and attempt insertion via the opposite nostril.	22. Forceful insertion may cause tissue damage and bleeding.
23. With *clean* hand, apply suction by occluding the suction control port with your thumb; at the same time, slowly rotate the catheter by rolling it between your thumb and fingers while slowly withdrawing it. Apply suction for no longer than 15 seconds at a time.	23. Prolonged suction applied to a single area of tissue can cause tissue damage.
24. Repeat step 23 until secretions have been cleared, allowing for brief rest periods between suctioning episodes.	24. Promotes complete clearance of the airway.
25. Withdraw the catheter by looping it around your fingers as you pull it out.	25. Allows you to maintain control over the catheter tip as it is withdrawn.
26. Dip the catheter tip into the sterile solution and apply suction.	26. Clears the extension tubing of secretions that would promote bacterial growth and could block tubing.

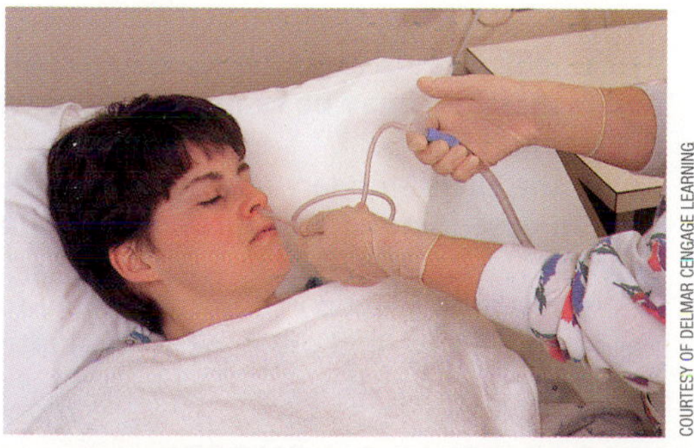

FIGURE 30-25-2 Insert catheter into nostril. (This nurse is left-handed.)

(Continues)

PROCEDURE 30-25 Performing Nasopharyngeal and Oropharyngeal Suctioning (Continued)

ACTION	RATIONALE
27. Disconnect the catheter from the extension tubing. Holding the coiled catheter in your gloved hand, remove the glove by pulling it over the catheter. Discard catheter and gloves in an a ppropriate container.	27. Contains the catheter and secretions in the glove for disposal.
28. Discard remaining supplies in the appropriate container and wash your hands.	28. Prevents transmission of microorganisms. Suctioning and coughing may produce an unpleasant taste.
29. Provide the client with oral hygiene if indicated or desired.	29. Suctioning and coughing may produce an unpleasant taste.

EVALUATION

- Check breath sounds for a patent airway.
- Ask client if breathing is easier.
- Assess client for signs of dyspnea.
- Review arterial blood gases and/or pulse oximetry results.
- Assess consistency, color, amount, and odor of secretions.

DOCUMENTATION

Nurses' Notes

- Date and time of suctioning procedure
- Client's tolerance of the procedure
- Amount, consistency, color, and odor or secretions
- Arterial blood gases and/or pulse oximetry results
- Document on appropriate electronic medical record or flow sheet.

PROCEDURE 30-26 Performing Tracheostomy Care

OVERVIEW

A tracheotomy is an incision made into the trachea with insertion of a cannula for airway management. Tracheostomy is the creation of an opening into the trachea through the neck. The two terms can be used interchangeably. A tracheostomy is performed for the client with potential or present airway obstruction, for ventilatory assistance, to provide pulmonary hygiene, to decrease the anatomic dead space in the client with chronic obstructive pulmonary disease, to avoid prolonged endotracheal intubation, and to provide an airway for clients with severe obstructive sleep apnea syndrome. The tracheostomy is performed below the level of the vocal cords and allows air to enter and exit the tracheostomy rather than through the upper airway. The tracheostomy tube can have a single or double cannula. The determination of the tube design used is based on the needs of the client. The double cannula tube allows for the tube to be cleaned to prevent obstruction caused by dried secretions. During the acute phase after a tracheostomy has been performed, all care must be performed using sterile technique. Once care of the tracheostomy tube becomes a client procedure, a clean technique is used.

ASSESSMENT

1. Assess respirations for rate, rhythm, and depth **to evaluate the airway.**
2. Assess the client's lung sounds **to determine the need for suctioning.**
3. Assess the client's arterial blood gases and/or pulse oximetry values **to evaluate air exchange and blood oxygen levels.**
4. Assess the movement of air through the tracheostomy tube **to evaluate the air exchange through the tube and determine whether there is any obstruction.**
5. Assess the amount and color of tracheal secretions **to evaluate for bleeding, infection, and the need for suctioning.**
6. Assess for anxiety, restlessness, and fear. **Anxiety and restlessness may be symptoms of airway distress and hypoxia.**
7. Assess the client's understanding of the procedure **to determine client education and support needed.**
8. Assess the area around the tracheostomy for redness, swelling, and drainage **to evaluate skin integrity.**

POSSIBLE NURSING DIAGNOSES

Ineffective Airway Clearance
Risk for Infection
Risk for Suffocation
Impaired Skin Integrity

(Continues)

PROCEDURE 30-26 Performing Tracheostomy Care (Continued)

Impaired Verbal Communication
Deficient Knowledge (Tracheostomy Care)
Anxiety
Impaired Gas Exchange

PLANNING

Expected Outcomes

1. The client's airway will be free of obstruction.
2. The procedure will be performed with a minimum of client anxiety.
3. The client's skin will remain intact and free of redness and excoriation.
4. The client will remain free of signs and symptoms of infection.
5. The client will have cannulas free of secretions and clean, secure ties.

Equipment Needed

Cleaning the Inner Cannula

- Sterile latex-free gloves
- Nonsterile latex-free gloves
- Disposable inner cannula (if available)
- Tracheostomy care kit: 2 basins, tracheostomy brush, tracheostomy ties (twill tape, commercially available Velcro ties)
- Hydrogen peroxide
- Sterile water or sterile saline
- Cotton-tip applicators
- Tracheostomy dressing (4 × 4 gauze without cotton lining)

delegation tips

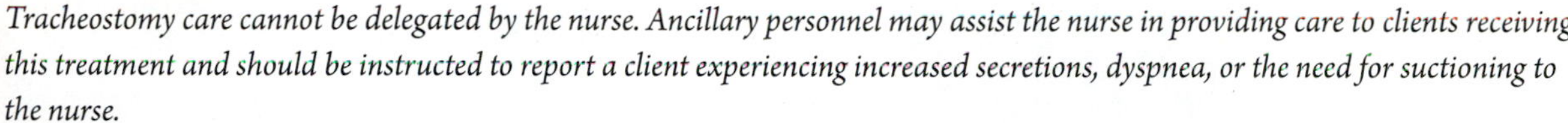

Tracheostomy care cannot be delegated by the nurse. Ancillary personnel may assist the nurse in providing care to clients receiving this treatment and should be instructed to report a client experiencing increased secretions, dyspnea, or the need for suctioning to the nurse.

IMPLEMENTATION—ACTION/RATIONALE

ACTION	RATIONALE
* Check client's identification band * Explain procedure before beginning *	
1. Wash hands and apply nonsterile latex-free gloves.	1. Reduces transmission of microorganisms.
2. Remove soiled dressing and discard. Remove gloves and discard. Wash hands.	2. Prevents contamination of other areas.
Conventional/Reusable Inner Cannula	
3. Open tracheostomy care set (Figure 30-26-1).	3. Provides sterile equipment for use in the procedure.
4. Place hydrogen peroxide solution in one basin and sterile water or saline in a second basin.	4. Prepare solutions prior to applying gloves.
5. Apply sterile gloves.	5. Uses aseptic technique.
6. Dip the applicator in the basin of hydrogen peroxide.	6. Prevents contamination of the applicator.
7. Remove inner cannula.	7. Allows for cleaning.
8. Place inner cannula in basin of hydrogen peroxide.	8. Loosens secretions.
9. Clean the area under the neck plate of the tracheostomy tube using a cotton applicator moistened with hydrogen peroxide (Figure 30-26-2).	9. Decreases microorganisms and removes crusting.
10. Rinse area under neck plate with cotton applicator moistened with sterile water or saline.	10. Removes hydrogen peroxide from the skin.
11. Dry skin under neck plate with cotton-tip applicator.	11. Prevents skin excoriation from moisture.

(Continues)

PROCEDURE 30-26 Performing Tracheostomy Care (Continued)

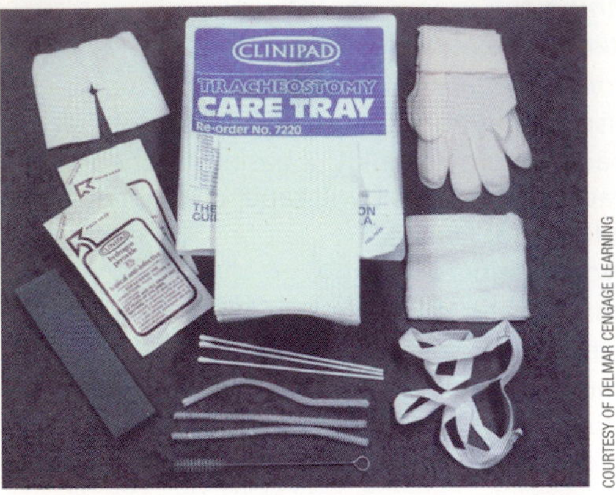

COURTESY OF DELMAR CENGAGE LEARNING

FIGURE 30-26-1 Tracheostomy Care Kit and Supplies

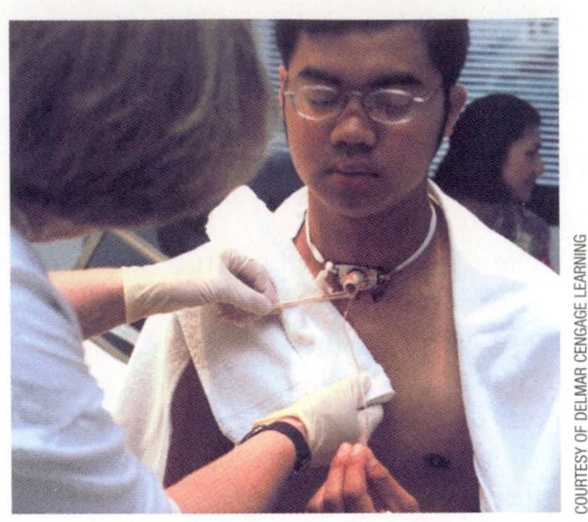
COURTESY OF DELMAR CENGAGE LEARNING

FIGURE 30-26-2 Clean the area under the neck plate with a cotton applicator moistened with hydrogen peroxide.

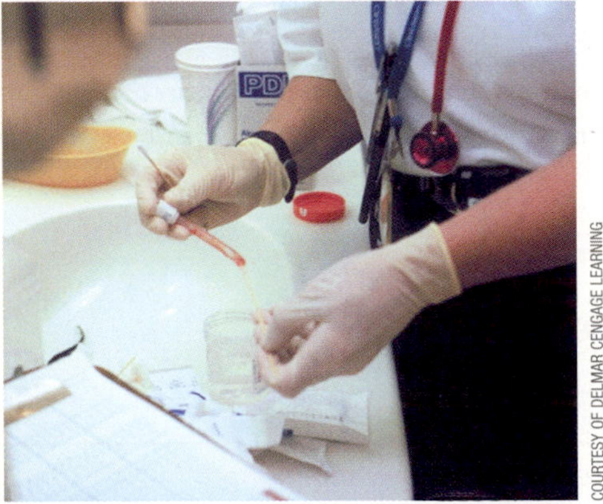
COURTESY OF DELMAR CENGAGE LEARNING

FIGURE 30-26-3 Use a sterile cotton-tipped applicator to clean the inner cannula area and remove crusted secretions.

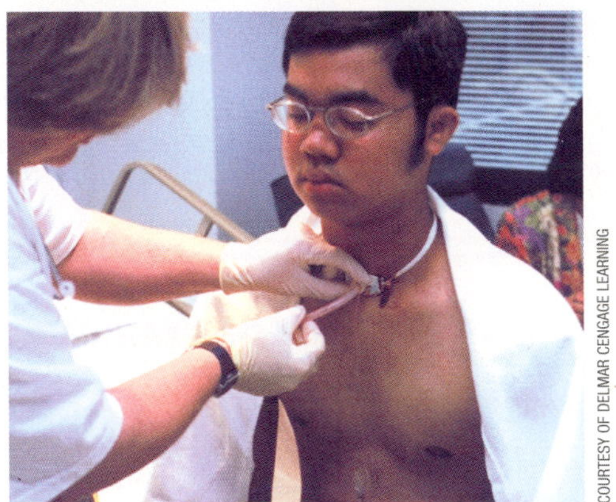
COURTESY OF DELMAR CENGAGE LEARNING

FIGURE 30-26-4 Carefully reinsert inner cannula and lock into place.

ACTION	RATIONALE
12. Apply tracheostomy gauze under neck plate of tube. Note: if using tracheostomy gauze under neck plate of tube, change gauze frequently to prevent infection and skin breakdown.	12. Prevents rubbing and irritation of the skin.
13. Use a tracheostomy brush or sterile cotton-tip applicator to clean inner cannula (Figure 30-26-3).	13. Removes crusted secretions.
14. Rinse inner cannula with sterile water or sterile saline.	14. Removes hydrogen peroxide from inner cannula.
15. Dry inner cannula.	15. Prevents introduction of solutions into the trachea.
16. Reinsert inner cannula and lock it into place (Figure 30-26-4).	16. Prevents accidental removal of the inner cannula during coughing.
17. Remove gloves and wash hands.	17. Reduces transmission of microorganisms.
Disposable Inner Cannula	
18. Wash hands. Open disposable cannula container without touching cannula.	18. Reduces transmission of microorganisms.

(Continues)

PROCEDURE 30-26 Performing Tracheostomy Care (Continued)

ACTION	RATIONALE
19. Apply sterile gloves.	19. Uses aseptic technique.
20. Remove inner cannula and discard.	20. Disposable inner cannulas are not to be reused.
21. Replace inner cannula with new disposable cannula.	21. Provides a clean open cannula.
22. Remove gloves and wash hands.	22. Prevents transmission of microorganisms.
Two-Person Technique of Changing Tracheostomy Ties	
23. Cut two pieces of twill tape about 12 to 14 inches in length.	23. Prepares equipment before beginning procedure.
24. Make a fold about 1 inch below the end of each piece of twill tape and cut a half-inch slit lengthwise in the center of the fold.	24. Prepares tape for insertion.
25. Have a second person gently hold the tracheostomy tube in place with fingers on both sides of the neck plate.	25. Prevents accidental movement of the tracheostomy tube resulting in coughing and accidental decannulation.
26. Untie old tracheostomy ties and discard.	26. Removes tracheostomy ties.
27. Insert the split end of the tracheostomy tape through the opening on one side of the tracheostomy tube neck plate. Pull the distal end of the tracheostomy tie through the cut end and pull tightly.	27. Secures tracheostomy tie within neck plate.
28. Repeat procedure with second piece of twill tape.	28. Secures tracheostomy tube.
29. Tie tracheostomy tapes with a double knot at the side of the neck.	29. Secures tracheostomy tube.
30. Insert one finger under tracheostomy tapes.	30. Ensures that tube has been tied securely.
31. Insert tracheostomy gauze under neck plate of tube.	31. Prevents irritation of skin from secretions and rubbing of tracheostomy tube.
32. Discard all used materials and wash hands.	32. Reduces transmission of microorganisms.
One-Person Technique of Changing Tracheostomy Ties	
33. Follow Actions 23 to 24 and 27 to 29.	33. See Rationales 23 to 24 and 27 to 29.
34. Hold the neck plate firmly with one hand; untie and remove old tracheostomy tapes and discard.	34. Prevents dislodgment while untying and removing old tracheostomy tapes.
35. Place one finger under tracheostomy ties.	35. Checks for tightness and security.
36. Discard all used materials and wash hands.	36. Reduces transmission of microorganisms.

EVALUATION

- Airway is free of obstruction.
- Client anxiety was minimal during procedure.
- There is no evidence of infection.
- Airway is patent.
- Cannulas free of secretions, and clean, secured ties.
- Client's skin intact and free of redness and excoriation.

DOCUMENTATION

Nurses' Notes

- Date, time, procedure performed, and client's tolerance of the procedure
- Size and type of tracheostomy tube in place
- Amount and consistency of any secretions
- Condition of the client's skin
- Client teaching and participation
- Document on appropriate electronic medical record or flow sheet.

PROCEDURE 30-27 Performing Tracheostomy Suctioning

OVERVIEW

Suctioning secretions is necessary to maintain the airway of a client who is unable to clear his or her own secretions by coughing. Some clients may be able to cough but not effectively enough to expel the secretions. Suctioning the client's airway is considered a sterile procedure. Using sterile technique prevents the introduction of contagion into the client's airway and lungs.

Suctioning is performed as often as necessary to remove excess secretions. The procedure may be performed as often as every 5 minutes or as infrequently as every few hours, depending on the amount of secretions the client is generating and the client's ability to clear his or her own airway. Evaluate the client's airway and oxygenation to determine the need for suctioning. Wall suction should be set at 100 to 120 mm Hg for adults, 50 to 100 mm Hg for children, and 40 to 60 mm Hg for infants. Portable suction set at 8 to 15 mm Hg for adults, 5 to 8 mm Hg for children, and 3 to 5 mm Hg for infants.

ASSESSMENT

1. Assess respirations for rate, rhythm, and depth **to evaluate airway.**
2. Auscultate lung fields **to evaluate airway and determine need for suctioning.**
3. Monitor arterial blood gases and/or pulse oximetry values **to determine oxygen levels and adequate air exchange.**
4. Assess passage of air through the tracheostomy tube **to determine air exchange and obstruction of the tube.**
5. Monitor tracheal secretions for amount, color, consistency, and odor **to assess for evidence of bleeding or signs of infection and need for suctioning.**
6. Assess for anxiety and restlessness, **which may be signs of airway distress and/or hypoxia.**
7. Assess the client's understanding of the suctioning procedure **to decrease the client's anxiety.**

POSSIBLE NURSING DIAGNOSES

Impaired Gas Exchange
Anxiety
Ineffective Airway Clearance
Risk for Infection

PLANNING

Expected Outcomes

1. The client will have no crackles or wheezes in large airways and the absence of cyanosis.
2. The client will report breathing comfortably and will have no apparent anxiety or restlessness.
3. The client will have minimal amount of thin, normal-colored secretions.
4. The client will maintain a patent airway.
5. The client will maintain adequate pulse oximetry.

Equipment Needed

- Sterile latex-free gloves
- Mask, eye protection, and gown if appropriate
- Source of negative pressure (suction machine or wall suction)
- Sterile suction catheter
- Oxygen or Ambu-bag
- Equipment for tracheostomy care or tracheostomy care tray

delegation tips

Suctioning a tracheostomy is not delegated by the nurse. Ancillary personnel may assist the nurse in providing care to clients receiving this treatment and should be instructed to report a client experiencing increased secretions, dyspnea, or the need for suctioning to the nurse.

IMPLEMENTATION—ACTION/RATIONALE

ACTION	RATIONALE
* Check client's identification band * Explain procedure before beginning *	
1. Assess depth and rate of respirations; auscultate breath sounds.	1. Determines need for suctioning.
2. Assemble supplies on bedside table.	2. Organizes work.
3. Wash hands.	3. Reduces transmission of microorganisms.

(Continues)

PROCEDURE 30-27 Performing Tracheostomy Suctioning (Continued)

ACTION	RATIONALE
4. Position the client in a high Fowler's or semi-Fowler's position.	4. Maximizes lung expansion and effective coughing.
5. Connect extension tubing to suction device, if not already in place, and adjust suction control to between 100 and 120 mm Hg.	5. Excessive negative pressure can cause tissue trauma, hypoxemia, and atelectasis, whereas insufficient pressure will be ineffective.
6. Put on gown and mask and goggles or face shield.	6. Protects from splattering body fluids.
7. Using sterile technique, open tracheostomy care kit. Consider the inside wrapper of the kit to be sterile, and spread the wrapper out carefully to create a small sterile field. Add sterile suction catheter if not in kit.	7. Produces an area in which to place sterile items without contaminating them.
8. If gloves are wrapped, carefully lift the wrapped gloves from the kit without touching the inside of the kit or the gloves themselves. Lay the wrapped gloves down and open the wrapper. Put on the gloves using sterile gloving technique.	8. Reduces introduction of pathogens into the client's airway.
9. Pour hydrogen peroxide in one basin and sterile water or saline in the other.	9. Provides solution to clean inner cannula and to lubricate the catheter and rinse the inside of the catheter to clear secretions.
10. Designate one hand as *sterile* (able to touch only sterile items), usually the dominant hand, and the other as *clean* (able to touch only nonsterile items), the nondominant hand.	10. Prevents contamination of sterile supplies while allowing you to handle unsterile items.
11. *Using your sterile hand*, pick up the suction catheter. Grasp the plastic connector end between your thumb and forefinger and coil the tip around your remaining fingers.	11. Prevents accidental contamination of the catheter tip.
12. Pick up the extension tubing *with your clean hand*. Connect the suction catheter to the extension tubing, taking care not to contaminate the catheter.	12. The extension tubing is not sterile.
13. If client is not receiving oxygen, administer oxygen or use Ambu-bag with *clean* hand before beginning procedure.	13. Hyperoxygenates client and prevents hypoxia during suctioning.
14. Remove inner cannula and place in basin of hydrogen peroxide to loosen secretions, if reusable, or set aside if disposable. Do not dispose of disposable cannula until new inner cannula is securely in place.	14. Allows easier passage of the suction catheter. Retain old cannula until you are sure the new cannula fits correctly.
15. Position your clean hand with the thumb over the catheter's suction port, dip the catheter tip into the sterile solution, and activate the suction. Observe as the solution is drawn into the catheter.	15. Tests the suction device as well as lubricating the interior of the catheter to enhance clearance of secretions.
16. Remove thumb from suction port.	16. Deactivates the suction.
17. Using your *clean* hand, remove the oxygen delivery device from the tracheostomy tube and place it on a clean surface.	17. Permits access to the tracheostomy tube. Placing the oxygen device on a clean surface reduces contamination (the sterile glove wrapper may be used for this purpose).
18. Without occluding the suction control port, insert the catheter tip into the tracheostomy tube and advance it until the client coughs or resistance is met (Figure 30-27-1) and withdraw slightly.	18. Minimizes trauma when suction not applied while the catheter is being advanced.
19. Apply suction by occluding the suction control port with your thumb, while slowly rotating the	19. Prolonged suction can cause tissue damage, atelectasis, and hypoxemia.

(Continues)

PROCEDURE 30-27 Performing Tracheostomy Suctioning (Continued)

ACTION	RATIONALE
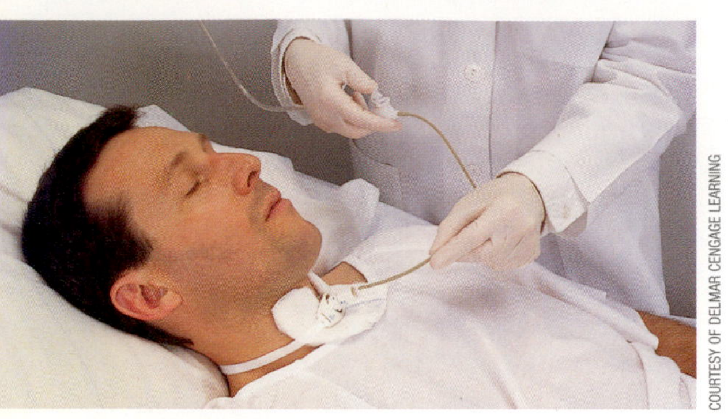 FIGURE 30-27-1 Suction Tracheostomy	
catheter between your thumb and finger and slowly withdrawing it. Apply suction for no longer than 15 seconds at a time.	
20. Repeat step 19 until all secretions have been cleared, allowing brief rest periods between suctioning episodes. Encourage client to breathe deeply between suctioning episodes. Provide oxygen between passes of the suction catheter.	20. Promotes complete clearance of the airway.
21. Withdraw the catheter and dip it into the cup of sterile saline, applying suction.	21. Cleans suction catheter of secretions.
22. Clean inner cannula using tracheostomy brush and rinse well in sterile water or sterile saline. Dry (or open new disposable inner cannula).	22. Removes secretions and maintains patent inner cannula.
23. Reinsert inner cannula and lock into place.	23. Prevents secretions from obstructing outer cannula.
24. Reapply oxygen delivery device.	24. Reoxygenates the client and restores supplemental oxygen and humidification.
25. Dip the catheter tip into the sterile solution and apply suction.	25. Clears the extension tubing of secretions, which would promote bacterial growth.
26. Disconnect the catheter from the extension tubing. Holding the coiled catheter in your gloved hand, remove the glove by pulling it over the catheter. Discard catheter and gloves in an appropriate container.	26. Contains the catheter and secretions in the glove for disposal.
27. Discard remaining supplies in the appropriate container.	27. Follow institutional policy regarding disposal of client care supplies.
28. Wash hands.	28. Reduces transmission of pathogens.
29. Provide the client with oral hygiene if indicated/desired.	29. Suctioning and coughing may produce an unpleasant taste.

EVALUATION

- Ask client whether breathing is easier.
- Auscultate breath sounds for a patent airway.
- Review arterial blood gases and/or pulse oximetry values.
- Assess client for signs of dyspnea.
- Evaluate consistency, color, amount, and odor of secretions.

DOCUMENTATION

Nurses' Notes

- Date and time of suctioning procedure
- Client's tolerance of the suctioning procedure
- Amount, consistency, color, and odor of secretions
- Arterial blood gases and/or pulse oximetry values
- Document on appropriate electronic medical record or flow sheet.

PROCEDURE 30-28

Postoperative Exercise Instruction

OVERVIEW

Preoperative teaching of postoperative exercises prepares the client physically and emotionally for the impending surgery. The goal of instruction is to have the client demonstrate the performance of exercises while verbalizing why the exercises are used during the postoperative phase.

Several postoperative exercises help speed recovery from surgery. Turning, deep breathing, and coughing facilitate removal of accumulated pulmonary secretions. Clients may experience their worst postoperative pain while doing these exercises. Inhaled gases and oxygen have a drying effect on the respiratory mucosa, which increases the viscosity of secretions, making them difficult to raise with coughing.

To prevent respiratory complications, teach clients to breathe deeply to achieve sustained maximum inspiration (SMI). SMI promotes the reinflation of the alveoli and the removal of mucus secretions.

Several devices help encourage clients to perform SMI exercises. The breathing devices, called incentive spirometers, measure the client's ventilatory volume and provide the user with a tangible reward for generating an adequate respiratory flow. When the client takes a deep breath, the ball moves upward and the amount of air is measured, thereby making the results visible to the client.

Turning, deep breathing, coughing, and using spirometry prevent respiratory complications by doing the following:

- Promoting pulmonary circulation
- Promoting the exchange of gases by increasing lung compliance
- Facilitating the removal of mucus secretions from the tracheobronchial tree

Postoperatively the client is encouraged to move in bed and perform leg exercises. These exercises assist in preventing circulatory complications that can arise from anesthetic agents that depress the metabolic and heart rates. Early ambulation also increases respiratory function and the return of peristalsis.

ASSESSMENT

1. Assess the client's current understanding of postoperative procedures. **Establishes baseline for teaching.**
2. Assess the client's ability to understand the postoperative exercise instructions. **Establishes baseline for teaching. Affects how the teaching and procedures will be performed.**
3. Assess any preoperative limitations the client may have that would prevent or impair the ability to perform the postoperative exercises accordingly. **Establishes baseline for teaching. Affects how the teaching and procedures will be performed. Allows modification of the exercises.**

POSSIBLE NURSING DIAGNOSES

*Acute **P**ain*

*Impaired Physical **M**obility*

*Impaired **G**as Exchange*

*Risk for Impaired **S**kin Integrity*

PLANNING

Expected Outcomes

1. The client will be able to successfully demonstrate postoperative exercises, deep breathing, coughing, pillow splinting, turning and proper body alignment, leg and foot exercises, and out-of-bed transfers.
2. The client will be able to successfully demonstrate proper use of the incentive spirometer.

Equipment Needed (see Figure 30-28-1)

- Educational materials
- Pillow
- Tissue
- Nonsterile latex-free gloves
- Disposable, volume-oriented incentive spirometer

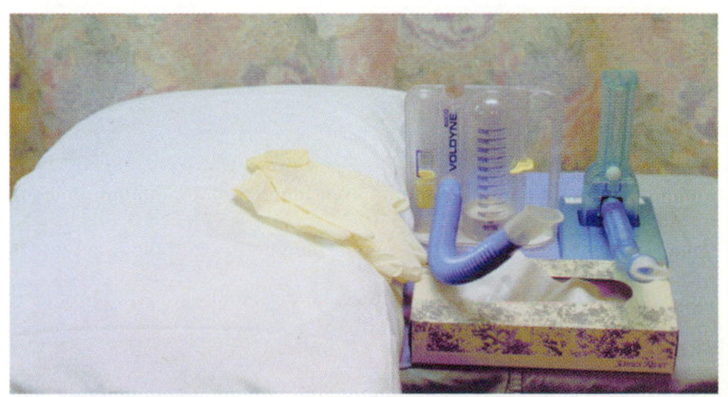

COURTESY OF DELMAR CENGAGE LEARNING

FIGURE 30-28-1 Incentive spirometers encourage deep breathing. A pillow may be used to splint the incision site. Tissues are used to cover the mouth when coughing.

(Continues)

PROCEDURE 30-28 Postoperative Exercise Instruction (Continued)

delegation tips

Postoperative instruction requires the assessment and intervention of a nurse. Ancillary staff may reinforce the information and directions taught to the client.

IMPLEMENTATION—ACTION/RATIONALE

ACTION	RATIONALE
* Check client's identification band * Explain procedure before beginning *	
1. Wash hands and organize equipment.	1. Reduces the transmission of microorganisms and promotes efficiency.
2. Apply nonsterile latex-free gloves.	2. Reduces the transmission of microorganisms.
3. Place client in a sitting position.	3. Promotes full chest expansion.
4. Demonstrate deep breathing exercises.	4. Shows the client how to breathe deeply.
• Place one hand on abdomen (umbilical area) during inhalation.	• Exerts counterpressure during inhalation.
• Expand the abdomen and rib cage on inspiration.	• Promotes maximum chest expansion.
• Inhale slowly and evenly through your nose until you achieve maximum chest expansion.	• Maintains full expansion of the alveoli.
• Hold breath for 2 to 3 seconds.	• Increases the pressure, thereby preventing immediate collapse of the alveoli.
• Slowly exhale through your mouth until maximum chest contraction has been achieved.	• Promotes maximum chest contraction.
5. Have the client return-demonstrate deep breathing and repeat 3 to 4 times.	5. Reinforces learning. Promotes increased air exchange.
6. Instruct the client on the use of an incentive spirometer (Figure 30-28-2).	6. Reinflates the alveoli and removes mucus secretions.
• Hold the volume-oriented spirometer upright.	• Promotes proper functioning of the device.
• Take a normal breath and exhale, then seal lips tightly around the mouthpiece; take a slow, deep breath to elevate the balls in the plastic tube, hold the inspiration for at least 3 seconds.	• Allows for greater lung expansion; holding the inspiration increases the pressure, preventing the immediate collapse of the alveoli.
• The client simultaneously measures the amount of inspired air volume on the calibrated plastic tube.	• Encourages the client to do respiratory exercises.
• Remove the mouthpiece, exhale normally.	• Allows normal expiration.
• Take several normal breaths.	• Provides the client the opportunity to relax.
7. Have the client repeat the procedure 4 to 5 times.	7. Encourages sustained maximal inspiration and loosens secretions.

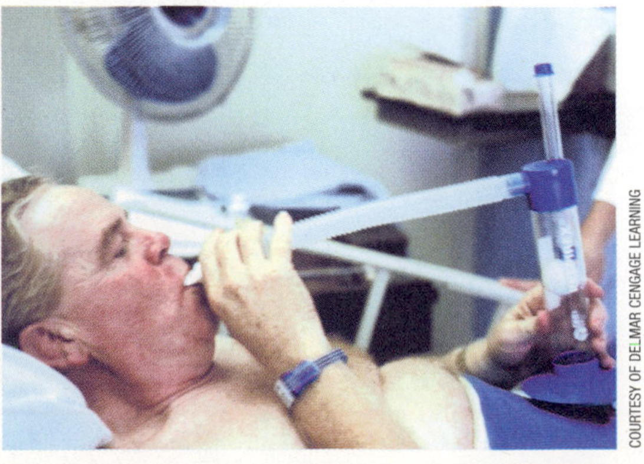
COURTESY OF DELMAR CENGAGE LEARNING

FIGURE 30-28-2 Instruct the client to take a slow, deep breath to elevate the ball in the tube.

(Continues)

PROCEDURE 30-28 Postoperative Exercise Instruction (Continued)

ACTION	RATIONALE
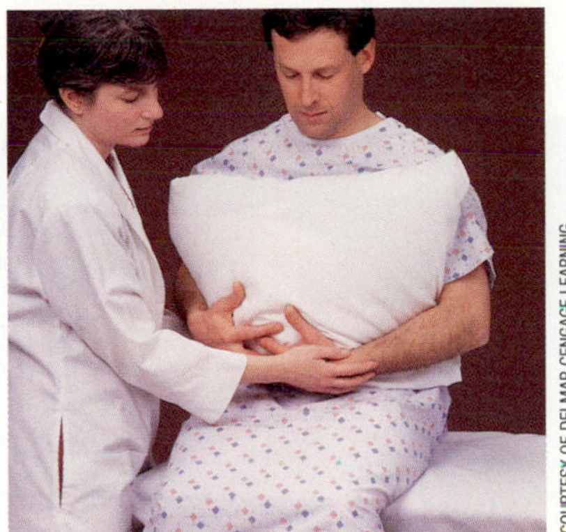 COURTESY OF DELMAR CENGAGE LEARNING **FIGURE 30-28-3** Use a pillow to support the abdominal muscles when coughing.	
8. Have the client cough after the incentive effort. See the following section.	8. Facilitates the removal of secretions.
9. Demonstrate splinting and coughing.	9. Shows the client how to raise mucus secretions from the tracheobronchial tree.
• Have the client slowly raise head and sniff the air.	• Increases the amount of air and helps aerate the base of the lungs.
• Have the client slowly bend forward and exhale slowly through pursed lips.	• Dries the tracheal mucosa as air flows over it. There is a slight increase in carbon dioxide level, which stimulates deeper breathing.
• Repeat breathing 2 to 3 times.	• Loosens mucus plugs and moves secretions to the main bronchus.
• When the client is ready to cough, have client place a folded pillow against the abdomen with clasped hands (Figure 30-28-3).	• Elevates the diaphragm and expels air in a more forceful cough; supports the abdominal muscles and reduces pain while coughing, if the client has an abdominal incision.
• Have client take a deep breath and begin coughing immediately after inspiration is completed by bending forward slightly and producing a series of soft, staccato coughs.	• Removes secretions from the main bronchus.
• Have a tissue ready.	• Preparation for sputum disposal.
10. Have the client return-demonstrate splinting and coughing.	10. Fosters learning.
11. Wash the incentive spirometer mouthpiece under running water and store in a clean container. Disposable mouthpieces should be changed every 24 hours.	11. Reduces transmission of microorganisms.
12. Teach the client leg and foot exercises (Figure 30-28-4).	12. To improve venous blood return from the legs.
• Have the client, with heels on bed, push the toes of both feet toward the foot of the bed until the calf muscles tighten, then relax feet. Pull the toes toward the chin, until calf muscles tighten; then relax feet (Figure 30-28-4A).	• Causes contraction and relaxation of the calf muscles.
• With heels on bed, lift and circle each ankle, first to the right and then to the left; repeat three times, relax (Figure 30-28-4B).	• Causes contraction and relaxation of the quadriceps muscles.
• Flex and extend each knee alternately, sliding foot up along the bed; relax (Figure 30-28-4C).	• Causes contraction and relaxation of the quadriceps muscles.
13. Have the client return-demonstrate the leg and foot exercises.	13. Fosters learning of how to improve venous blood return.

(Continues)

PROCEDURE 30-28 Postoperative Exercise Instruction (Continued)

ACTION | **RATIONALE**

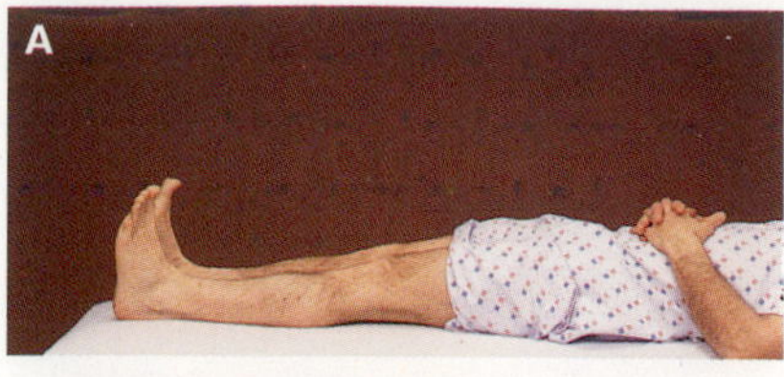

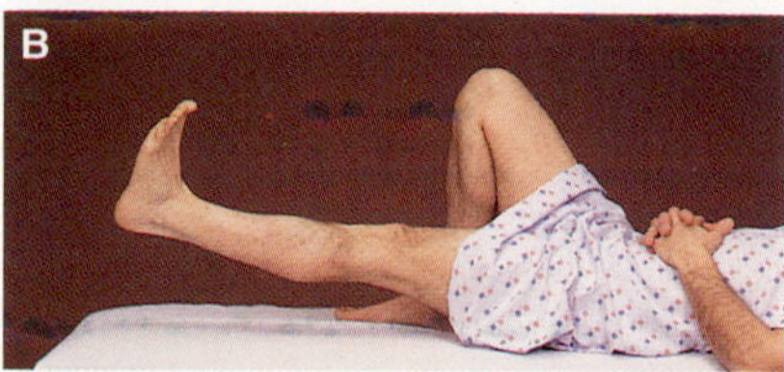

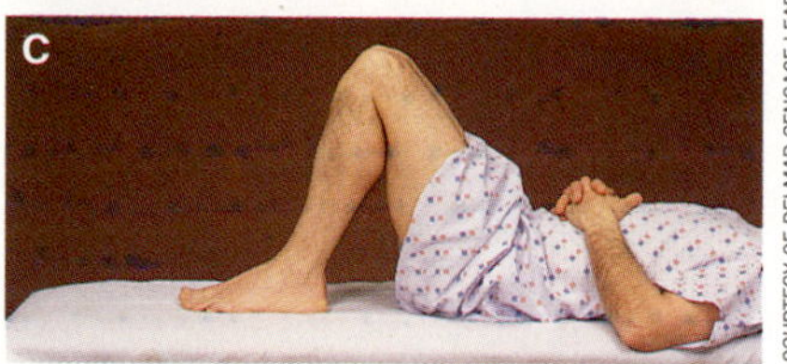

FIGURE 30-28-4 Leg exercises improve venous blood return. *A,* Flex foot forward; *B,* Lift leg up and flex foot forward; *C,* Bend the knee.

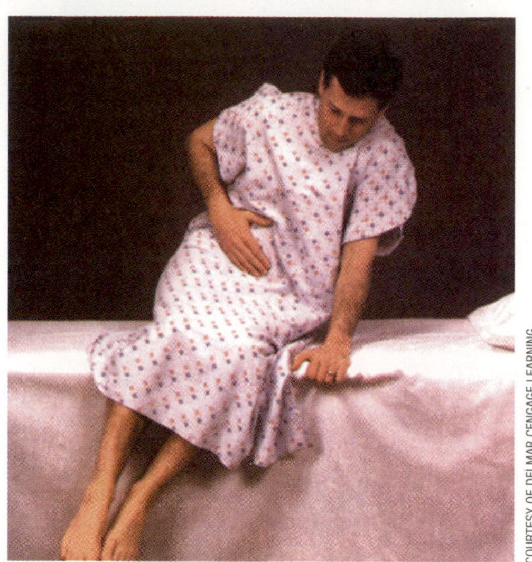

FIGURE 30-28-5 Using the hand to splint the incision site when sitting up in bed will reduce the pain and pressure at the incision site.

14. Explain how to turn in bed and get out of bed.
    - *Rationale:* Elicits client cooperation.
15. Instruct the client who has a left-sided abdominal or chest incision to turn to the right side of bed and sit up as follows:
    - Flex the knees.
    - With the right hand, splint the incision with hand or small pillow.
    - Turn toward right side by pushing with the left foot and grasping the shoulder of the nurse or partial side rail of the bed with the left hand.
    - Rise up to a sitting position on the side of the bed by using the left arm and hand to push down against the mattress or side rail.
    - *Rationale:* Fosters learning how to turn and get out of bed without putting pressure on the incision line.
16. Reverse instructions (use left side instead of right) for the client with a right-sided incision according to Action 15 (Figure 30-28-5).
    - *Rationale:* Same as Rationale 15.
17. Instruct clients with orthopedic surgery (e.g., hip surgery) how to use a trapeze bar.
    - *Rationale:* Facilitates movement in bed without putting pressure on a leg or hip joint.
18. Wash hands.
    - *Rationale:* Reduces transmission of microorganisms.

EVALUATION

- The client is able to successfully demonstrate postoperative exercises, deep breathing, coughing, pillow splinting, turning and proper body alignment, leg and foot exercises, and out-of-bed transfers.
- The client is able to successfully demonstrate proper use of the incentive spirometer.

DOCUMENTATION

Nurses' Notes

- Document teaching the client postoperative exercises.
- Note the client's level of understanding and cooperation with the teaching.
- Document on appropriate electronic medical record or flow sheet.

Preoperative Checklist

- Initial the check-off area for documentation of preoperative teaching.

PROCEDURE 30-29 Performing a Skin Puncture

OVERVIEW

Skin punctures are performed when small quantities of capillary blood are needed for analysis or when the client has poor veins. Capillary puncture is also commonly performed for blood-glucose analysis. The common sites for capillary punctures are:

- Heel—most common site for neonates and infants
- Fingertip—the inner aspect of palmar fingertip used most commonly in children and adults
- Earlobe—used when the client is in shock or the extremities are edematous

ASSESSMENT

1. Assess the condition of the client's skin at the potential puncture site **to determine whether it is intact, free of bruising, and can be used without causing undue trauma to the site.**
2. Assess the circulation at the potential puncture site **to determine whether it is a good site to obtain a sample, and to determine if healing at the site might be compromised.**
3. Assess the client's comfort level regarding the procedure **to determine client education and support needed.**
4. Assess the cleanliness of the client's skin **to determine how much cleansing is needed before the skin puncture.**

POSSIBLE NURSING DIAGNOSES

Risk for Impaired Skin Integrity
Acute Pain
Anxiety

PLANNING

Expected Outcomes

1. An adequate blood specimen will be obtained.
2. The client will suffer minimal trauma during the specimen collection.
3. The specimen will be collected and stored in a manner compatible with the ordered tests.

Equipment Needed

- Antiseptic 70% isopropanol or povidone-iodine
- Microhematocrit tubes or micropipette (collection tubes)
- Sterile 2×2 gauze
- Sterile lancet
- Nonsterile latex-free gloves
- Hand towel or absorbent pad

delegation tips

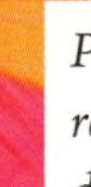

Properly trained ancillary personnel may perform skin puncture. Agency policy usually dictates certification and recertification requirements for this skill. Proper client and specimen identification are of the utmost importance and must be consistently demonstrated by the ancillary personnel.

IMPLEMENTATION—ACTION/RATIONALE

ACTION	RATIONALE
* Check client's identification band * Explain procedure before beginning *	
1. Wash hands.	1. Reduces transmission of microorganisms.
2. Check the client's identification band if appropriate.	2. Ensures the correct client.
3. Explain the procedure to the client.	3. Allays anxiety and encourages cooperation.
4. Prepare supplies: • Open sterile packages. • Label specimen collection tubes. • Place in easy reach.	4. Ensures efficiency.
5. Apply nonsterile latex-free gloves.	5. Follows Standard Precautions.

(Continues)

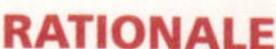

PROCEDURE 30-29 Performing a Skin Puncture (Continued)

ACTION	RATIONALE

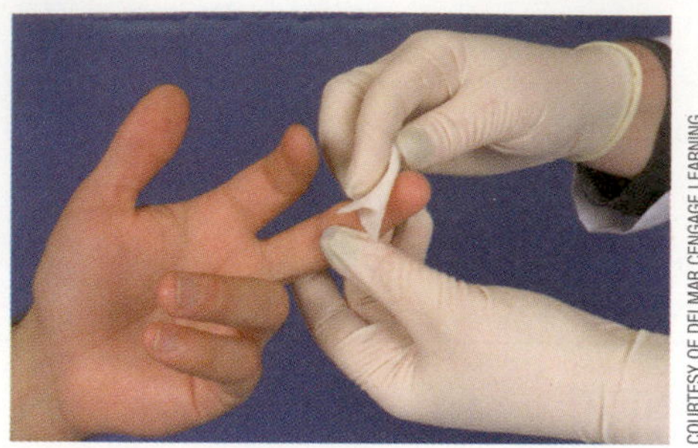
COURTESY OF DELMAR CENGAGE LEARNING

FIGURE 30-29-1 Cleanse the puncture site and allow it to dry.

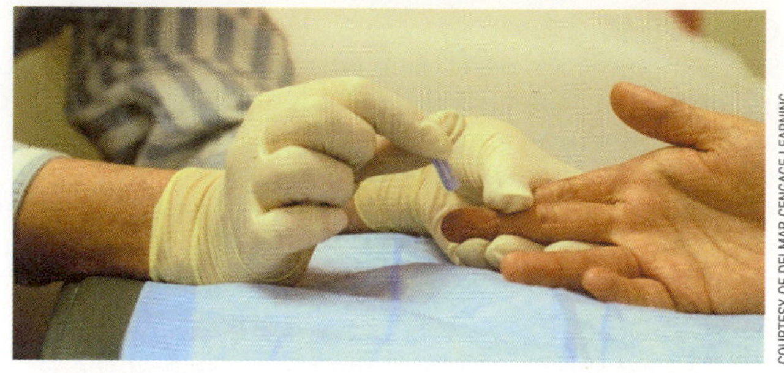
COURTESY OF DELMAR CENGAGE LEARNING

FIGURE 30-29-2 Use a quick stab to puncture the skin.

ACTION	RATIONALE
6. Select site: lateral aspect of the fingertips in adults/children; heel for neonates and infants.	6. Avoids damage to nerve endings and calloused areas of the skin.
7. Place the hand or heel in a dependent position; apply warm compresses if fingers or heel are cool to touch.	7. Increases the blood supply to the puncture site.
8. Place hand towel or absorbent pad under the extremity.	8. Prevents soiling the bed linen.
9. Cleanse puncture site with an antiseptic and allow it to dry. Use 70% isopropanol if the client is allergic to iodine (Figure 30-29-1).	9. Reduces skin surface bacteria; povidone-iodine must dry to be effective.
10. With nondominant hand, apply gentle milking pressure above or around the puncture site. Do not touch the puncture site.	10. Increases blood to puncture site and maintains asepsis.
11. Read directions carefully before using the lancet. • With the sterile lancet at a 90-degree angle to the skin, use a quick stab to puncture the skin (about 2 mm deep) (Figure 30-29-2). • With the automatic unistik, push the lancet into the body of unistik until it clicks. Hold the body of the unistik and twist off the lancet cap. Place the end of the unistik tightly against the client's finger and press the lever. The needle automatically retracts after use.	11. Provides a blood sample with minimal discomfort to the client.
12. Wipe off the first drop of blood with sterile 2 × 2 gauze; allow the blood to flow freely (Figure 30-29-3).	12. The first drop may contain a large amount of serous fluid, which could affect the results. Pressure at the puncture site can cause hemolysis.
13. Collect the blood into the tube(s). If blood for a platelet count is to be collected, obtain this specimen first (Figure 30-29-4).	13. Allows blood collection; avoids aggregation of platelets at the puncture site.
14. Apply pressure to the puncture site with a sterile 2 × 2 gauze.	14. Controls bleeding.
15. Place contaminated articles into a sharps container.	15. Reduces the risk of needlestick.
16. Remove gloves; wash hands.	16. Reduces transmission of microorganisms.
17. Position client for comfort with call light in reach.	17. Provides for comfort and communication.
18. Wash hands.	18. Reduces transmission of microorganisms.

(Continues)

PROCEDURE 30-29 Performing a Skin Puncture (Continued)

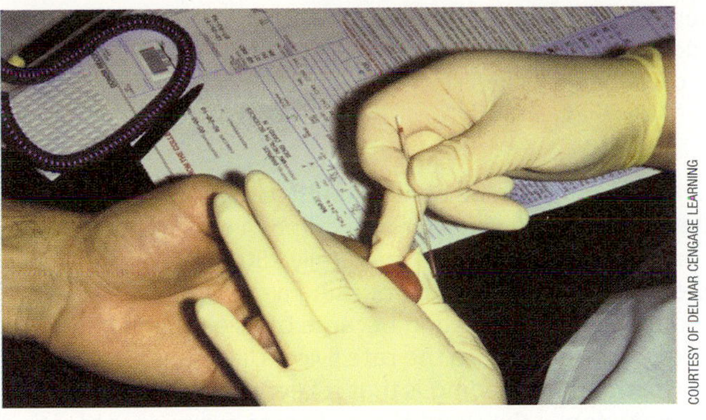

FIGURE 30-29-3 Allow the blood to flow from the puncture site to ensure that an adequate amount can be obtained.

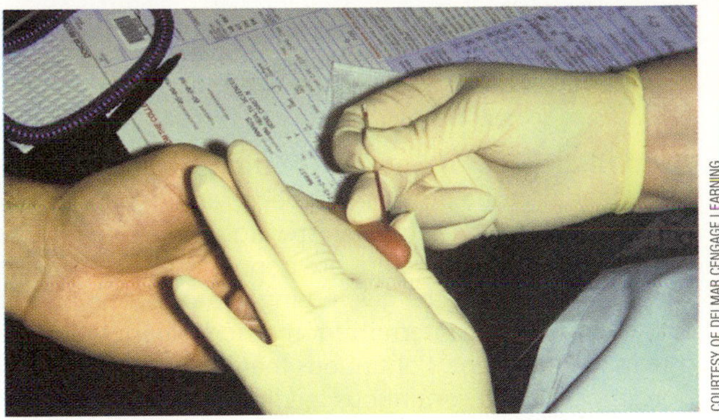

FIGURE 30-29-4 Collect a small sample of blood.

EVALUATION

- Specimen is adequate.
- No trauma to client.

DOCUMENTATION

Nurses' Notes

- Puncture site and the reason for the puncture.
- Report test results if the testing is performed at the time of the puncture.

PROCEDURE 30-30 Feeding and Medicating via Enteral Tube

OVERVIEW

Enteral nutrition is a procedure whereby liquid food (formula) is instilled directly into the stomach or small intestines using a tube. Other names for this procedure are tube feedings and gastric gavage. Candidates for tube feedings are clients who have a functional gastrointestinal (GI) tract and will not, should not, or cannot eat. Tube feedings are used for clients who are (or may become) malnourished and in whom oral feedings are insufficient to maintain adequate nutritional status.

Enteral tube feedings maintain the structural and functional integrity of the GI tract, enhance the utilization of nutrients, and provide a safe and economic method of feeding.

Enteral tube feedings are contraindicated in clients with the following:

- Diffused peritonitis
- Intestinal obstruction that prohibits normal bowel functioning
- Intractable vomiting; paralytic ileus
- Severe diarrhea

Enteral tube feedings are used with caution in clients with the following:

- Severe pancreatitis
- GI ischemia
- Enterocutaneous fistula

Feeding Tubes

Most feeding tubes are made of silicone or polyurethane, which are durable and biocompatible with formulas. They vary in diameter (8–12 French) and length in accord with the route and formula. The health care provider selects the route and type of feeding tube on the basis of the anticipated duration of feeding, the condition of the GI tract, and the potential for aspiration.

A nasogastric, small-bore feeding tube is generally used when the anticipated duration of use is short.

The gastrostomy tube is placed through an opening in the abdominal wall into the intestines. This is done via an enterostomy, the surgical creation of an artificial fistula into the intestines. Tube enterostomies can be placed at various points along the GI tract and are performed when long-term tube feeding is anticipated or when obstruction makes nasoenteral tube feeding impossible.

(Continues)

PROCEDURE 30-30 Feeding and Medicating via Enteral Tube (Continued)

Percutaneous endoscopic gastrostomy (PEG) tube placement is performed by the health care provider at the bedside or in the endoscopy room; insertion of a PEG tube does not require general anesthesia surgery. This method of enteral feeding is more common than conventional enterostomies; it is less risky because surgery is not required, and it is more economic.

Administration of Enteral Feedings

Once feeding tube position has been radiographically verified, the formula can be administered as prescribed. There are two typical methods of administering tube feedings. Intermittent feeding is given four to six times a day in the form of a bolus. Intermittent feedings are generally given through a large-bore tube. The bolus (generally 250–400 mL of formula for adult clients) can be given using a large syringe fit into the end of the feeding tube or using a gravity drip over 20 to 30 minutes. The intermittent method is generally practiced in the home care setting because of its ease and need for minimal equipment. Continuous feeding delivers formula with a pump to regulate the rate. Most clients with a small-bore tube receive continuous feeding. One of the advantages of continuous feeding is that it keeps gastric volume small, minimizing residual volume and reducing the risk of aspiration pneumonia; the client is less likely to experience bloating, nausea, abdominal distention, and diarrhea. Continuous feeding is recommended for the seriously ill or comatose client.

Safety Considerations

Clients receiving enteral nutrition through a tube feeding are at risk for aspiration. Auscultate for bowel sounds to determine gastric motility. If the bowel sounds are hypoactive or absent, stop or withhold additional feeding and notify the health care provider.

Always assess placement of the feeding tube before administering any liquids. Clients who are receiving continuous gastric feeding should be assessed every 4 hours for tube placement and residual gastric contents. Aspirate gastric contents with a syringe. Observe and check the pH of the aspirate. If less than 100 mL, replace stomach contents after checking the residual to prevent fluid and electrolyte imbalance.

Client safety and comfort require daily cleansing of the feeding tube exit site. Cleanse the skin with a clean washcloth, soap, and water. Enterostomy tubes require surgical asepsis of the exit site until the incision heals; rotate the tubes within the stoma to promote healing. Report any observations of redness, irritation, or gastric leakage at the site. Between feedings, a prosthetic device may be used to cover the ostomy opening.

The PEG tubes require daily rotation to relieve pressure on the skin. Notify the health care provider if unable to rotate the PEG; it may be an indication of internal embedding of the tube into the gastric wall. When the tube is internally embedded, it can cause gastric acid reflux, which results in skin breakdown, sepsis, and cellulitis. Care must be taken to avoid dislodgment of the tube. Keep it secured to the client's abdomen with tape, being careful not to use excessive tension. The PEG tubes require frequent flushing to prevent clogging. These tubes have small lumens. If a tube becomes clogged, flush it with 60 mL of lukewarm tap water.

ASSESSMENT

1. Assess the client for signs of gastric distress, such as nausea, vomiting, and cramping, **to determine the client's tolerance for the tube feeding.**
2. Assess the feeding tube placement every 4 hours **to confirm tube placement in the intestines.**
3. Assess the client's respiratory status **to evaluate for pulmonary aspiration of gastric contents.**
4. Assess the client's ongoing nutritional status **to evaluate the effectiveness of the tube feeding.**
5. Assess the client's intake and output **to evaluate for fluid deficit or excess**.

POSSIBLE NURSING DIAGNOSES

Risk for Imbalanced Nutrition: Less Than Body Requirements
Risk for Deficient Fluid Volume
Risk for Aspiration
Risk for Impaired Skin Integrity
Impaired Oral Mucous Membrane

PLANNING

Expected Outcomes

1. The client will receive the correct feeding formula and the correct volume of formula over the correct time period.
2. The client will not experience any undesirable effects: aspiration, nausea, vomiting, abdominal distention, cramping, diarrhea, or constipation.
3. The client's weight and nutritional status will remain stable or improve.
4. The client will not experience any adverse skin or gastrointestinal effects from the gastrostomy or PEG tube.

Equipment Needed

- Asepto syringe or 20- to 50-mL syringe
- Emesis basin
- Clean towel
- Disposable gavage bag and tubing
- Formula
- Infusion pump for feeding tube (if needed)
- Water to follow feeding
- Nonsterile latex-free gloves

(Continues)

PROCEDURE 30-30 Feeding and Medicating via Enteral Tube (Continued)

delegation tips

Feedings via gastrostomy tubes may be given by properly trained ancillary personnel if the facility and the state permit. The ancillary personnel must be properly trained in assessing tube placement, proper positioning of the client, and in the administration of the correct type and rate of feeding. All medications must be administered by a nurse.

IMPLEMENTATION—ACTION/RATIONALE

ACTION	RATIONALE
* Check client's identification band * Explain procedure before beginning *	
1. Review client's medical record for formula, amount, and time.	1. Verifies health care provider's prescription for appropriate formula and amount.
2. Wash hands and gather equipment and formula.	2. Reduces transmission of microorganisms and promotes efficiency during procedure.
3. Identify client by checking armband.	3. Verifies correct client.
4. Explain procedure to client.	4. Increases client compliance and reduces anxiety.
5. Assemble equipment. Add color to formula per institutional policy. If using a bag, fill with prescribed amount of formula (Figure 30-30-1).	5. Ensures efficiency when initiating feeding. Color will distinguish formula aspirate.
6. Place client on right side in high Fowler's position.	6. Reduces risk of pulmonary aspiration in the event client vomits or regurgitates formula.
7. Provide for privacy.	7. Places client at ease.
8. Wash hands and don nonsterile latex-free gloves.	8. Reduces transmission of pathogens.
9. Observe for abdominal distention; auscultate for bowel sounds.	9. Assesses for delayed gastric emptying; indicates presence of peristalsis and ability of GI tract to digest nutrients.
10. Check feeding residuals (Figure 30-30-2). Insert syringe into adapter port, aspirate stomach contents, and determine amount of gastric residual. If residual is greater than 50 to 100 mL (or in accordance with agency protocol), hold feeding until residual diminishes. Instill aspirated contents back into feeding tube.	10. Indicates whether gastric emptying is delayed. Reduces risk of regurgitation and pulmonary aspiration related to gastric distention. Prevents electrolyte imbalance.
11. Administer tube feeding.	11. Provides nutrients as prescribed.

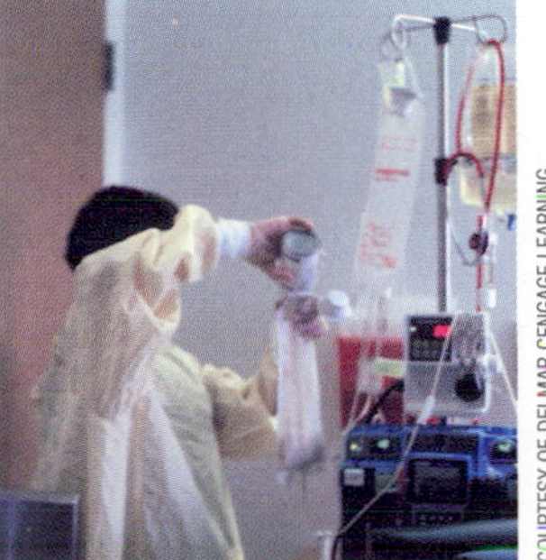
COURTESY OF DELMAR CENGAGE LEARNING

FIGURE 30-30-1 Fill the bag with the prescribed amount of formula.

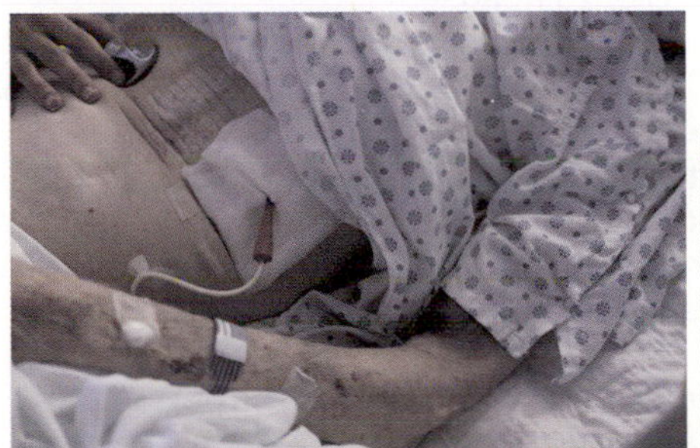
COURTESY OF DELMAR CENGAGE LEARNING

FIGURE 30-30-2 Check that the feeding tube is intact and in place, auscultate for bowel sounds, and look for abdominal distention.

(Continues)

PROCEDURE 30-30 Feeding and Medicating via Enteral Tube (Continued)

ACTION	RATIONALE
Intermittent Bolus	
12. Pinch the tubing.	12. Prevents air from entering tubing.
13. Remove plunger from barrel of syringe and attach to adapter.	13. Provides system to delivery feeding.
14. Fill syringe with formula (Figure 30-30-3).	14. Allows gravity to control flow rate, reducing risk of diarrhea from bolus feeding.
15. Allow formula to infuse slowly; continue adding formula to syringe until prescribed amount has been administered.	15. Prevents air from entering stomach. Decreases risk of diarrhea.
16. Flush tubing with 30 to 60 mL or prescribed amount of water.	16. Ensures that remaining formula in tubing is administered and maintains patency of tube; prevents air from entering the stomach.
17. Remove syringe and replace cap into adaptor port	17. Prevents airs from entering the stomach and prevents gastric contents from leaving the stomach.

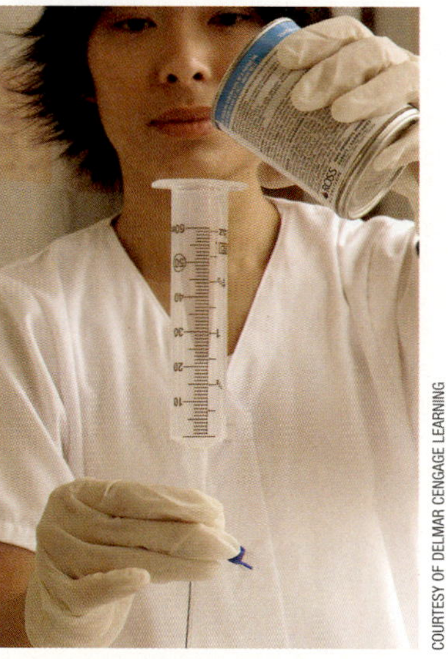

FIGURE 30-30-3 Fill syringe with formula.

ACTION	RATIONALE
Intermittent Gavage Feeding	
18. Hang bag on IV pole so that it is 18 inches above the client's head.	18. Allows gravity to promote infusion of formula.
19. Fill bag with ordered amount of feeding. Remove air from tubing by opening clamp on tubing and allow feeding to flow through tubing.	19. Prevents air from entering stomach. Decreases risk of diarrhea.
20. Attach distal end of tubing to feeding tube adapter and adjust drip to infuse over prescribed time.	20. Allows gravity to control flow rate, reducing risk of diarrhea from bolus feeding.
21. When bag empties of formula, add 30 to 60 mL or prescribed amount of water; close clamp.	21. Prevents air from entering stomach and reduces risk for gas accumulation. Maintains patency of feeding tube.
22. Remove tubing from adaptor port and cap adaptor port.	22. Prevents air from entering stomach and prevents gastric contents from leaving the stomach.
23. Change bags every 24 hours.	23. Decreases risk of microorganism multiplication in bag and tubing.

(Continues)

PROCEDURE 30-30 Feeding and Medicating via Enteral Tube (Continued)

ACTION	RATIONALE
Continuous Gavage	
24. Check tube placement at least every 4 hours.	24. Ensures that feeding tube remains in stomach.
25. Check residual at least every 4 hours.	25. Indicates ability of GI tract to digest and absorb nutrients.
26. If residual is above 100 mL, stop feeding.	26. Reduces risk of regurgitation and pulmonary aspiration related to gastric distention.
27. Add prescribed amount of formula to bag for a 4-hour period; dilute with water if prescribed.	27. Provides client with prescribed nutrients and prevents bacterial growth (formula is easily contaminated).
28. Hang gavage bag on IV pole. Prime tubing.	28. Removes air from tubing.
29. Thread tubing through feeding pump and attach distal end of tubing to feeding tube adapter; keep tubing straight between bag and pump.	29. Provides for controlled flow rate; prevents loops in tubing.
30. Program rate.	30. Infuses formula over prescribed time.
31. Monitor infusion rate and signs of respiratory distress or diarrhea.	31. Prevents complications associated with continuous gavage.
32. Flush tube with water every 4 hours as prescribed or following administration of medications.	32. Maintains patency of tube.
33. Replace disposable feeding bag at least every 24 hours, in accord with institution protocol.	33. Decreases transmission of microorganisms.
34. Elevate head of bed at least 30 degrees at all times and turn client every 2 hours.	34. Prevents aspiration and promotes digestion and reduces skin breakdown.
35. Provide oral hygiene every 2 to 4 hours.	35. Provides comfort and maintains the integrity of buccal cavity.
36. Administer water as prescribed with and between feedings.	36. Ensures adequate hydration.
37. Remove gloves and wash hands.	37. Reduces transmission of microorganisms.
Instilling Medications into Enteral Tubes	
38. Wash hands and don nonsterile gloves.	38. Reduces spread of microorganisms.
39. Assist the client to high or semi-Fowler's position.	39. Gravity assists to keep medications down.
40. Place linen saver over bed linens.	40. Prevents soiling during procedure.
41. Verify nasogastric (NG) tube placement.	41. Ensures tube placement is correct.
42. Attach syringe to tube and pour 30 mL of prepared medication into syringe.	42. Readies medication to be given.
43. Open clamp on tube.	43. Allows medication into tube.
44. Hold syringe at a slight angle; add more medication before syringe empties.	44. Allows medication to flow at a slow, steady rate.
45. For two or more medications, give each separately, with 5-mL water rinse between medications.	45. Ensures each medication is given.
46. As syringe empties with the last of the medication, slowly add 30 to 50 mL water.	46. Clears medication from the sides and distal end of tube to prevent clogging.
47. Before tube empties of water, clamp the tube, detach and dispose of the syringe.	47. Prevents air from getting into the stomach. Disposes of used equipment.
48. Place clients with an NG tube on the right side with head slightly elevated for 30 minutes.	48. Prevents regurgitation.
49. Remove gloves and wash hands.	49. Reduces spread of microorganisms.

EVALUATION

- The client received the correct feeding formula and the correct volume of formula over the correct time period.
- Client did not experience any undesirable effects such as aspiration, nausea, vomiting, abdominal distention, cramping, diarrhea, or constipation.
- Client's weight and nutritional status remained stable or improved.

(Continues)

PROCEDURE 30-30 Feeding and Medicating via Enteral Tube (Continued)

- Client did not experience any adverse skin or gastrointestinal effects from the gastrostomy or PEG tube.

DOCUMENTATION

Nurses' Notes

- Time, date, formula, and amount of feeding, and client's response
- Amount of residual aspirated before the feeding
- Tube placement checked and method used
- If the dressing at the tube insertion site was changed and the condition of the client's skin
- If the tube was rotated or adjusted
- Any client complaints or adverse effects such as bloating, nausea, vomiting, diarrhea, or constipation
- Document on appropriate electronic medical record or flow sheet.

Medication Administration Record

- Date and time the feeding was instilled (per institution specifications)

Intake and Output Record

- Amount of tube feeding instilled and the amount of water used to flush the feeding tube

REFERENCES/SUGGESTED READINGS

Altman, G. (2010). *Fundamental and advanced nursing skills 3rd edition.* Clifton Park, New York: Delmar, Cengage Learning.

Gray, M. (2008). Securing the indwelling catheter. *AJN*, 108(12), 44–50.

Lord, L. (2001). How to insert a large-bore nasogastric tube. *Nursing2001, 31*(9), 46–48.

Metheny, N., & Titler, M. (2001). Assessing placement of feeding tubes, *AJN, 101*(5), 36–45.

Metules, T. (2007). Hands-on help hot and cold packs. *RN*, 70(1), 45–48.

North American Nursing Diagnosis Association International. (2010). *NANDA-I nursing diagnoses: Definitions and classification 2009–2011.* Ames, IA: Wiley-Blackwell.

Raymond, M. (2008). Piercing ears to test glucose. *RN*, 71(12), 23.

CHAPTER 31
Advanced Procedures

PROCEDURE 31-1 Inserting and Maintaining a Nasogastric Tube

OVERVIEW

Nasogastric (NG) tubes are used for several purposes, including feeding for nutrition when the client is comatose, semiconscious, or unable to consume sufficient nutrition orally. Nasogastric suction tubes are used for decompression of gastric content after gastrointestinal surgery and to obtain gastric specimens for diagnosis of peptic ulcer. Tubes are used for irrigation to clean and flush the stomach after oral ingestion of poisonous substances. Finally, NG tubes are used to document the presence of blood in the stomach, monitor the amount of bleeding from the stomach, and identify the recurrence of bleeding in the stomach.

The two most commonly used NG tubes are the single-lumen Levin's tube and the double-lumen Salem sump tube.

The gastrointestinal tract is considered to be a clean area rather than a sterile one. The procedure to place an NG tube is performed using clean technique unless it is performed in conjunction with gastrointestinal surgery.

ASSESSMENT

1. Assess client's consciousness level **to determine the ability of the client to cooperate during the procedure.**
2. Check the client's chart for any previous medical history of nostril surgery or injury or unusual nostril bleeding. **Reduces risk of injury from the tube.**
3. Use a penlight to assess nostrils for a deviated septum. **Facilitates choice of nostril and size of tube.**
4. Ask the client to breathe through each nostril, occluding the other with a finger. **Facilitates choice of nostril and decreases chance that tube will interfere with respirations.**
5. Assess for latex allergy. **Prevents reaction to latex and determines need to use latex-free tubes and gloves.**

POSSIBLE NURSING DIAGNOSES

Imbalanced Nutrition: Less Than Body Requirement
Impaired Swallowing
Risk for Aspiration
Risk for Diarrhea
Impaired Oral Mucous Membrane
Risk for Deficient Fluid Volume
Acute Pain
Impaired Skin Integrity

PLANNING

Expected Outcomes

1. Client's nutritional status will improve, as indicated by increased body weight, physical strength, and mental status.
2. Client's nutritional needs will be met with the assistance of tube feeding.
3. Client will maintain a patent airway, as evident by absence of coughing, no shortness of breath, and no aspiration.
4. Client will not have diarrhea caused by nasogastric feeding.
5. Mouth mucous membranes will remain moist and intact.
6. Client will maintain a normal fluid volume, as evident by good skin texture, muscle tone, and blood volume.
7. Client's comfort level will increase.
8. Skin around the tube will remain intact, with no redness or blisters.

Equipment Needed

- Nasogastric tube: adult, 14 to 18 French; child/infant, 5 to 10 French; single-lumen (Levin's tube): feeding; double-lumen (Salem sump tube): feeding, suction, irrigation
- Water-soluble lubricant
- Syringe with catheter tip or adapter, 50 mL

PROCEDURE 31-1 Inserting and Maintaining a Nasogastric Tube (Continued)

- Glass of tap water with straw, or ice
- Towel or tissue
- Emesis basin with ice chips
- Tongue blade
- pH chemstrip
- Stethoscope
- Hypoallergenic tape, rubber band, and safety pin
- Personal protective equipment: gown; disposable, nonsterile latex-free gloves; face shield or goggles; and mask
- Penlight or flashlight
- Disposable irrigation set (if needed)
- Wall mount or portable suction equipment (if needed)
- Administration set with pump or controller for feeding tube

delegation tips

Inserting and maintaining a nasogastric tube is the responsibility of a nurse. Oral hygiene for the client may be delegated.

IMPLEMENTATION—ACTION/RATIONALE

* Check client's identification band * Explain procedure before beginning *

ACTION	RATIONALE
1. Review client's medical history for conditions that have resulted in a loss of the gag reflex.	1. To assess for any nostril surgery and abnormal bleeding. A client without a gag reflex is at risk for aspiration.
2. Identify client by checking armband. Assess client's consciousness and ability to understand. Develop a hand signal.	2. Verifies correct client. Decreases anxiety and promotes cooperation.
3. Provide privacy. Prepare the equipment, putting tissues, a cup of water, and an emesis basin nearby.	3. Provides privacy. Facilitates an efficient procedure.
4. Prepare the environment; raise the bed and place it in a high Fowler's position (45 to 60 degrees). Cover the chest with a towel.	4. Prevents back strain and facilitates insertion.
5. Wash hands and then put on gloves and personal protective equipment.	5. Reduces transmission of microorganisms. Protects from body fluids.
6. Assess client's nostrils with penlight and have the client blow nose one nostril at a time.	6. Decreases discomfort and unnecessary trauma by choosing the more patent nostril for insertion.
7. Using the NG tube, measure the distance from the tip of the nose to the earlobe and then to the xiphoid process of the sternum and mark this distance on the tube with a piece of tape (Figure 31-1-1).	7. Determines the approximate amount of tube needed to reach the stomach.
8. Lubricate first 4 inches of the tube with water-soluble lubricant.	8. Facilitates passage into the naris.
9. Ask the client to slightly flex the neck backward.	9. Makes insertion easier.
10. Gently insert the tube into a naris (Figure 31-1-2).	10. Promotes passage of tube with minimal trauma to mucosa.
11. Ask the client to tip the head forward once the tube reaches the nasopharynx—this is usually where the client starts to gag. If the client continues to gag, stop for a moment.	11. Tipping the head forward facilitates passage of the tube into the esophagus instead of the trachea. Tube may stimulate gag reflex. Allows the client to rest, reduces anxiety, and prevents vomiting.
12. Advance the tube several inches at a time as the client swallows. If gag reflex is present, have the client swallow water or ice chips as tube is advanced.	12. Assists in advancing the tube past the oropharynx. The action of swallowing facilitates the insertion process. With each swallow, the tracheal opening is closed to prevent inspiration. Clients who do not have a gag reflex are at risk for aspiration.

(Continues)

PROCEDURE 31-1 Inserting and Maintaining a Nasogastric Tube (Continued)

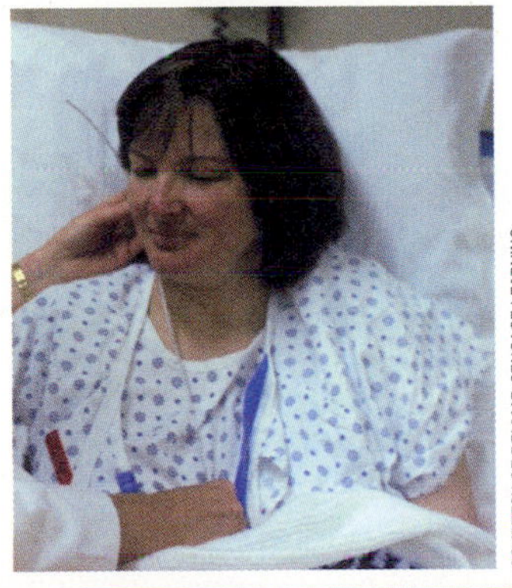

FIGURE 31-1-1 Measure the distance from the nose to earlobe to the xiphoid process to determine how much tube will need to be inserted to reach the stomach.

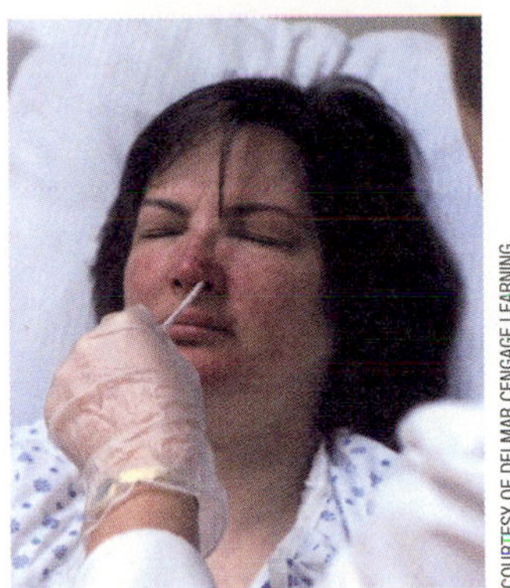

FIGURE 31-1-2 Gently insert the tube into the naris.

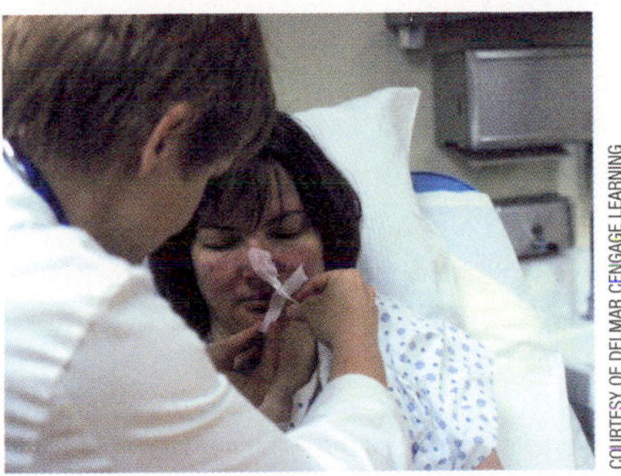
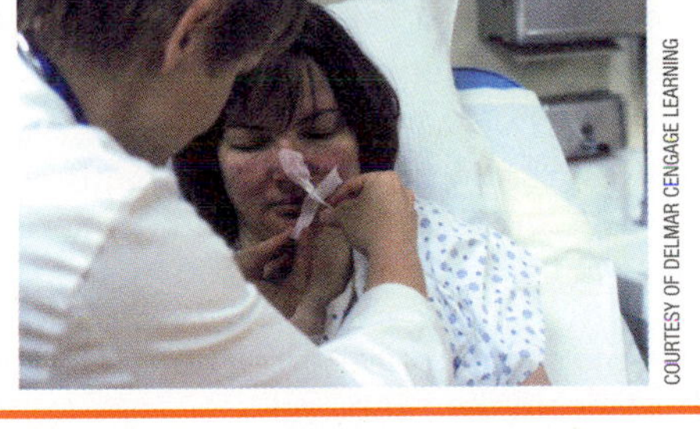

FIGURE 31-1-3 Secure the tube to the nose.

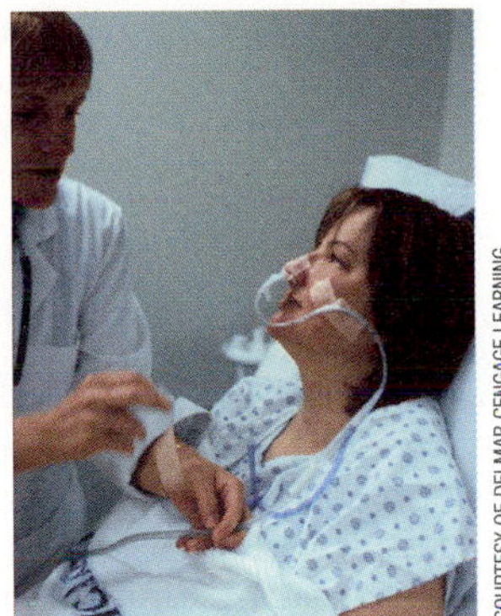

FIGURE 31-1-4 Tape the tube to the cheek as well, if desired, to provide extra support.

ACTION	RATIONALE
13. Withdraw the tube immediately if there are signs of respiratory distress.	13. Prevents trauma to bronchus or lung.
14. Advance the tube until the taped mark is reached.	14. Enables the tube to reach the stomach.
15. Wipe or wash body oils off tip of nose and allow to dry. Split a 4-inch strip of tape lengthwise 2 inches. Secure the tube with the tape by placing the wide portion of the tape on the bridge of the nose and wrapping the split ends around the tube (Figure 31-1-3). Tape to cheek as well if desired (Figure 31-1-4).	15. Prevents tube displacement.
16. Check the placement of the tube: • Aspirate for gastric content, assess the color and quality of the content. If required, measure with pH indicator strip (Figure 31-1-5). Follow protocol regarding reinsertion of contents versus discarding. • Prepare the client for x-ray checkup, if prescribed.	16. Ensures correct placement. A pH below 5 indicates the tube is in the stomach.
17. Connect the distal end of the tube to suction, draining bag, or adapter according to the purpose of this nursing intervention.	17. Establishes an appropriate pathway for intervention.
18. Secure the tube with tape, or with rubber band and safety pin, to client's gown.	18. Enhances the level of comfort and secures the tubing system.

(Continues)

PROCEDURE 31-1 Inserting and Maintaining a Nasogastric Tube (Continued)

ACTION	RATIONALE
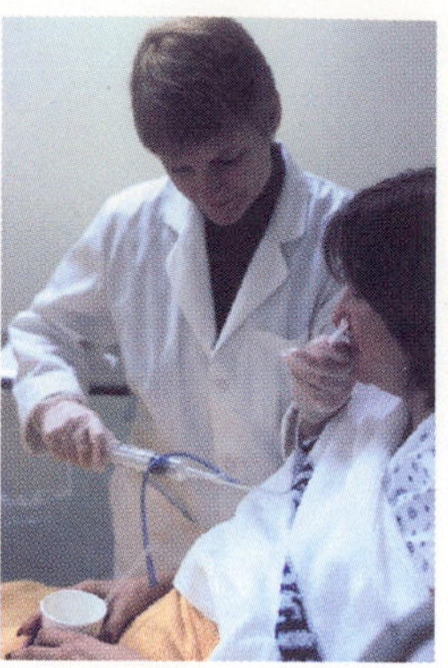 FIGURE 31-1-5 Aspirate a sample of gastric content to check for pH.	
19. Remove protective equipment, dispose of contaminated materials in proper container, and wash hands.	19. Implements Standard Precautions.
20. Position client comfortably and place the call light in easy reach.	20. Decreases client's anxiety and provides access to help if needed.
21. Document procedure.	21. Records implementation of intervention and promotes continuity of care.
Maintaining a Nasogastric Tube	
22. Wash hands and apply gloves.	22. Reduces transmission of microorganisms.
23. Follow the steps in Action 16 to check the proper tubing position before instilling anything per NG tube or at least every 8 hours.	23. Prevents complications from dislocation of the tube.
24. Assess for signs that the tube has become blocked, including epigastric pain and vomiting, and/or the inability to pass medications or feedings through the tube.	24. Prevents complications from the loss of beneficial effects from the tube.
25. Remember never to irrigate or rotate a tube that has been placed by the health care provider during gastric or esophageal surgery.	25. Rotation or irrigation may disturb incisions.
26. Provide oral hygiene and assist client to clean nares daily.	26. Enhances client's comfort and the integrity of skin and nose mucosa.
27. Remove gloves, dispose of contaminated materials in proper container, and wash hands.	27. Reduces transmission of microorganisms.

EVALUATION

- Client's nutritional status improves, as indicated by increased body weight, physical strength, and mental status.
- Client's nutritional needs are met with the assistance of tube feeding.
- Client maintains a patent airway, as evident by absence of coughing, no shortness of breath, and no aspiration.
- Client does not have diarrhea caused by nasogastric feeding.
- Mouth mucous membranes remain moist and intact.
- Client maintains a normal fluid volume, as evident by good skin texture, muscle tone, and blood volume.
- Client's stomach decompressed and comfort level increases.
- Skin around the tube remains intact, with no redness or blisters.

DOCUMENTATION

Nurses' Notes

- Type of NG tube inserted, the naris used, how the client tolerated the procedure, and the methods used to verify placement
- Care provided to the client to increase comfort of the NG insertion naris
- Any unusual findings

(Continues)

PROCEDURE 31-1 Inserting and Maintaining a Nasogastric Tube (Continued)

- Document on appropriate electronic medical record or flow sheet

Intake and Output Record

- Amount of fluid the client drank to aid insertion of the NG tube
- Amount of gastric contents removed for testing
- Amount of gastric suctioning

PROCEDURE 31-2 Performing Venipuncture (Blood Drawing)

OVERVIEW

Obtaining a sample of blood through venipuncture is a commonly used procedure for many diagnostic tests. Blood test results are a source of valuable information to screen for disease, to evaluate the progress of therapy, and to monitor the well-being of the client. The nurse is often required to obtain a variety of specimens. Because some specimens require special handling, it is important to be familiar with the particular test that is ordered.

There are three primary methods of obtaining blood specimens: venipuncture, skin puncture, and arterial stick. Venipuncture is the most common method and involves inserting a large-bore needle into a vein. The nurse attaches either a syringe or a vacutainer tube for the collection of the blood specimen. Skin puncture is the easiest way to obtain a small specimen from the finger, toe, or heel. A lancet is used for the puncture, and a drop of blood is collected through a capillary tube. An arterial stick is the most complicated and requires special assessment skills and techniques.

As with any procedure, it is important to review the employer's policies and procedures as well as their state's nurse practice act.

ASSESSMENT

1. Determine which test(s) is ordered and be familiar with any special conditions associated with the timing of the collection or the handling of the specimen. Many specimens may be collected at very specific times (i.e., before or after administration of a drug, while the client is NPO, or after fasting). Other specimens may require special handling (i.e., ice is used to transport for ammonia level; heparinized collection containers are needed for platelet count; and so on). A blood specimen drawn at the incorrect time or put into an incorrect collection container cannot be used. Test results will be delayed and the client has to be stuck again.
2. Assess the integrity of the veins that may be used in the procedure. Identify any conditions that may contraindicate venipuncture. Avoid veins injured by infiltration or phlebitis or compromised by surgery (i.e., modified radical mastectomy). **Using a damaged vein may cause further injury to the vein. A compromised site may not provide an adequate amount of blood for the specimen and may lead to another venipuncture for the client. In addition, drawing samples from sites near IV infusion solutions may alter the composition of the blood sample.**
3. Review the client's medical history to determine if there are any expected complications from the venipuncture. **Clients with a history of abnormal clotting disorders, low platelets, or related disorders (hemophilia) may be at risk for increased bleeding at the site or hematoma formation.**
4. Determine the client's ability to cooperate with the procedure. **Many clients are fearful of needles—especially children—and additional help may be needed. Very young children may need to have the extremity restrained during the procedure.**
5. Review the physician's or qualified practitioner's order. Check for appropriateness of the test as well as the frequency of the test. Critically ill clients may require frequent blood tests and venipuncture. **Combining tests and carefully evaluating frequency may reduce unnecessary blood loss for the client.**

POSSIBLE NURSING DIAGNOSES

Deficient Knowledge (purpose of blood sample and procedure)
Risk for Infection
Impaired Tissue Integrity
Anxiety
Fear
Risk for Injury

(Continues)

PROCEDURE 31-2 Performing Venipuncture (Blood Drawing) (Continued)

PLANNING

Expected Outcomes

1. Venipuncture site will show no evidence of continued bleeding or hematoma.
2. The venipuncture site will show no evidence of signs and symptoms of infection.
3. The laboratory test will be properly acquired and appropriately handled after collection.
4. The client will be able to discuss the purpose of the test and describe the procedure.
5. The client will report minimal anxiety associated with the procedure.

Equipment Needed

- Disposable gloves
- Alcohol swabs
- Rubber tourniquet
- Sterile 2 × 2 gauze pads
- Band-Aid or adhesive tape (precut)Assessment
- Band-Aid or adhesive tape (precut)
- Appropriate blood collection tubes
- Labels for each collection tube with the appropriate client information included
- Completed laboratory requisition forms
- Needle/equipment disposal container
- Small pillow or folded towel to support the extremity if needed
- Syringe method: sterile needles: 20- to 21-gauge for adults, 23- to 25-gauge butterfly for older adults, 23- to 25-gauge butterfly for children
- Vacutainer method: Vacutainer tube with needle holder; sterile double needles (20- to 21-gauge for adults, 23- to 25-gauge for children)

delegation tips

The procedure of performing a venipuncture for the purposes of blood drawing is frequently delegated to properly trained ancillary personnel. Documentation of their competency and skill should be available to the nurse, and periodic reevaluation should occur according to agency and state policy. The ancillary personnel should be reminded to not obtain blood specimens from an extremity above the site of infusing fluids and to report to the nurse any complications or concerns the client might express postprocedure.

IMPLEMENTATION—ACTION/RATIONALE

* Check client's identification band * Explain procedure before beginning *

ACTION	RATIONALE
1. Validate client's identification.	1. Verifies correct client.
2. Wash hands.	2. Reduces transmission of microorganisms.
3. Bring equipment to bedside or exam room. Transfer client to the exam room, especially small children.	3. Provides an organized approach to the procedure. Keeps their hospital room a "safe haven."
4. Close curtain or door.	4. Provides privacy.
5. Raise or lower bed/table to comfortable working height.	5. Maintains good body mechanics during the procedure.
6. Before selecting an appropriate site for the venipuncture, assess the extremities for the presence of an arteriovenous shunt used for dialysis or history of a mastectomy.	6. Extremities with a shunt or on the same side of the body as a mastectomy should not be used.
7. Position client's arm; extend arm to form a straight line from shoulder to wrist. Place pillow or towel under upper arm to enhance extension. Client should be in a supine or semi-Fowler's position.	7. Helps stabilize the arm. The bed should support the client's body (when possible) in case the client feels faint during the procedure.
8. Apply disposable gloves.	8. Reduces the risk of infection to both the client and the nurse (Standard Precautions).
9. Apply the tourniquet 3 to 4 inches above the venipuncture site. Most often, the antecubital fossa site is used. The tourniquet should be able to be removed by pulling the end with a single motion.	9. Provides improved visibility of the veins as they dilate in response to decreased venous return of blood flow from the extremity to the heart.

(Continues)

PROCEDURE 31-2 Performing Venipuncture (Blood Drawing) (Continued)

ACTION	RATIONALE
10. Check for the distal pulse. If there is no pulse felt, then the tourniquet is applied too tightly and must be reapplied more loosely.	10. Impedes arterial flow, preventing venous filling.
11. Have client open and close fist several times, leaving fist clenched before venipuncture.	11. Increases the venous distension and enhances visibility of the vein.
12. Maintain tourniquet for only 1 to 2 minutes.	12. Prolonged time may increase client discomfort and alter some laboratory results (falsely elevated serum potassium).
13. Identify the best venipuncture site through palpation; the ideal site is a straight, prominent vein that feels firm and slightly rebounds when palpated. Palpate potential site.	13. Straight, intact veins are easier to puncture. A thrombosed vein is rigid, or rolls easily, and is difficult to stick.
14. Select the vein for venipuncture. (If the tourniquet has been on too long, release it and let the client rest for 1 to 2 minutes before reapplying the tourniquet.)	14. Increases client comfort and ensures accurate laboratory results.
15. Prepare to obtain the blood sample. Technique varies depending on equipment used:	15.
• *Syringe method:* Have syringe with appropriate needle attached.	• A needle with a very small bore can damage the red cells as the blood is drawn and lead to inaccurate test results.
• *Vacutainer method:* Attach double-ended needle to vacutainer tube and have the proper blood specimen tube resting inside the vacutainer. Do not puncture the rubber stopper yet.	• The long end of the needle is used to puncture the vein, and the short end enters the blood tube.
16. Cleanse the venipuncture site according to agency policy using a circular method at the site and extending 2 inches beyond the site. Allow to dry.	16. Cleans the skin surface of bacteria that may cause infection at the site. Allowing the alcohol to dry reduces stinging. Povidone-iodine must dry to be effective.
17. Remove the needle cover and warn that client will feel the needlestick.	17. Clients will be better able to control their reaction if they know what to expect.
18. Place the thumb or forefinger of the nondominant hand 1 inch below the site and pull the skin taut.	18. Helps stabilize the vein during insertion.
19. Hold syringe needle or vacutainer at a 15- to 30-degree angle from the skin with the bevel up.	19. This angle reduces the chance of penetrating through the vein during insertion. The needle causes less trauma to the skin and vein when the bevel is up during insertion.
20. Slowly insert needle/vacutainer.	20. Prevents puncture through the other side of the vein.
21. Technique varies depending on equipment used:	21.
• *Syringe method:* Gently pull back on syringe plunger and look for blood return. Obtain desired amount of blood into the syringe.	• If blood does not appear, the needle is not in the vein.
• *Vacutainer method:* Hold vacutainer securely and advance specimen tube into needle of holder. Be careful not to advance the needle into the vein. The blood should flow into the collection tube. After the collection tube is full, grasp the vacutainer firmly, remove the tube, and insert additional specimen collection tubes as indicated (Figure 31-2-1).	• Pushing the needle through the stopper breaks the vacuum and causes the flow of blood into the collection tube. Failure of blood to appear in the collection tube indicates the vacuum in the tube has been lost or the needle is not in the vein.
22. After the specimen collection is completed, release the tourniquet.	22. Reduces bleeding from pressure when the needle is removed.
23. Apply 2 × 2 gauze over the puncture site without applying pressure and quickly withdraw the needle from the vein.	23. Helps prevent the skin from pulling with the needle removal.

(Continues)

PROCEDURE 31-2 Performing Venipuncture (Blood Drawing) (Continued)

ACTION	RATIONALE

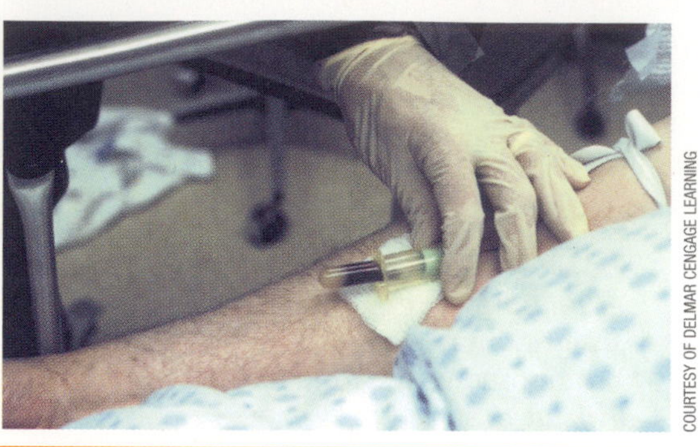

COURTESY OF DELMAR CENGAGE LEARNING

FIGURE 31-2-1 Allow the tube to fill with blood. When it is full, remove the tube and insert additional tubes if needed.

ACTION	RATIONALE
24. Immediately apply pressure over the venipuncture site with the gauze for 2 to 3 minutes or until the bleeding has stopped. Tape the gauze dressing over the site (or apply the Band-Aid).	24. Direct pressure stops the bleeding and minimizes formation of a hematoma. You may avoid using tape or a Band-Aid if, after applying pressure, no bleeding is present. Many clients are sensitive to tape, and its removal can be painful.
25. Syringe method: • Using one hand, insert the syringe needle into the appropriate collection tube and allow vacuum to fill. You may also remove the stopper from each vacutainer collection tube, remove the needle from the syringe, fill the tube, and replace the stopper.	25. Using a one-handed method to fill the syringe helps reduce the chance of needlestick injury. • This alternative method allows you to control the speed and amount of fill in the collection tubes.
26. If any of the blood tubes contain additives, gently rotate back and forth 8 to 10 times.	26. Ensures that the additive is properly mixed throughout the specimen.
27. Inspect the client's puncture site for bleeding. Reapply clean gauze and tape, if necessary.	27. Keeps site clean and dry.
28. Assist client into a comfortable position. Return bed to low position with side rails up, if appropriate.	28. Provides comfort and safety for the client.
29. Check tubes for any external blood and decontaminate with alcohol as appropriate.	29. Prevents contamination to other equipment and personnel.
30. Check tubes for proper labeling. Place tubes into appropriate bags/containers for transport to the laboratory.	30. Ensure the specimens are properly identified. Follows Standard Precautions.
31. Dispose of needles, syringes, and soiled equipment into proper container.	31. Prevents spread of disease and needlestick injury.
32. Remove and dispose of gloves.	32. Reduces transmission of microorganisms.
33. Wash hands.	33. Reduces transmission of microorganisms.
34. Send specimens to the laboratory.	34. Facilitates timely handling of specimens and accurate results.

EVALUATION

- Venipuncture site shows no evidence of continued bleeding or hematoma.
- Venipuncture site shows no signs or symptoms of infection.
- The blood specimen is properly acquired and appropriately handled after collection.
- The client is able to discuss the purpose of the test and describe the procedure.
- The client reports minimal anxiety associated with the procedure.

DOCUMENTATION

Nurses' Notes

- Date and time of the venipuncture, the site used for the procedure, any complications, the tests to be run, and the disposition of the specimens
- Client's reaction to the procedure and the condition in which the client was left (i.e., bed lowered with side rails up)
- Document on appropriate electronic medical record or flow sheet

PROCEDURE 31-3 Preparing an IV Solution and Starting an IV

OVERVIEW

An intravenous solution is a method of correcting or preventing a fluid and electrolyte disturbance. Clients who are acutely ill, are NPO after surgery, or have severe burns are examples of those who require IV therapy.

The solution in an IV bag is ordered by the health care provider according to the client's needs and is changed at least every 24 hours, or per the institution's policy, to decrease the risk of infection. Tubing is used to connect the solution in the IV bag with the client's IV catheter or needle. Use needleless systems if available. OSHA requires safe devices.

Performing venipuncture in order to establish venous access is a priority for clients with fluid and electrolyte disturbances, clients who are critically ill, clients who are NPO after surgery, or clients who, for other reasons, are not able to take fluids or food by mouth. Venous access can be used for infusions of IV fluids, emergency medications, parenteral nutrition, blood products, and routine IV medications.

There are a variety of IV needles and catheters. They vary in gauge from small bore to large bore. A 20- to 22-gauge flexible catheter is used for adults, and a 22- to 24-gauge catheter is used for pediatric clients. If large volumes of fluid or blood products are anticipated to be given, a larger bore (18- or 19-gauge) is recommended.

A commonly used angiocatheter has an over-the-needle catheter (ONC) made of plastic, Teflon, or other materials. These flexible catheters have a metal stylet that is used to pierce the skin and vein and a plastic catheter that is threaded into the vein and attached to the IV tubing after the stylet has been removed.

The other type of IV needle is a straight steel needle that is inserted into the vein and secured after being attached to an IV tubing. With an increased emphasis on safety, many health care facilities use a safety-shielded intravenous catheter or retractable needle system when placing a peripheral IV line. This consists of a traditional metal stylet used for the skin puncture covered by the plastic or Teflon angiocatheter. Once the IV line is successfully placed, the person initiating the IV pushes a button and the stylet retracts completely into a protective casing, thereby reducing the risk of needlestick injury.

The Centers for Disease Control and Prevention (CDC) guidelines must be followed to decrease the risk of infection for the client by changing the IV solution every 24 hours, changing the IV site and catheter every 48 to 72 hours, and changing the IV tubing every 72 hours. Occupational Safety and Health Administration (OSHA) standards are necessary to prevent exposure to blood-borne pathogens through the use of gloves, sharps containers, and special training for health care workers.

ASSESSMENT

1. Check the health care provider's order for the IV solution to be infused and rate of flow **to determine the optimal needle size and type to use and ensure accurate administration.**
2. Review information regarding the solution and insertion of the IV and nursing implications **in order to insert the catheter and administer the solution safely.**
3. Know the agency's policy regarding who may start an IV **because many agencies require that nurses have special training before they can perform this procedure.**
4. Check all additives in the solution and other medications **so that there will be no incompatibilities of additives with the solution.**
5. Assess the client's veins to **optimize planning of the IV site.**
6. Check the client's fluid, electrolyte, and nutritional status **to provide baseline data for comparison with the client's response to IV therapy.**
7. Assess the client's understanding of the purpose of the procedure **so that client teaching can be used to decrease anxiety.**

POSSIBLE NURSING DIAGNOSES

Deficient Knowledge (need for IV)
Risk for Infection
Excess Fluid Volume
Deficient Fluid Volume
Impaired Skin Integrity
Risk for Injury

PLANNING

Expected Outcomes

1. The appropriate fluids at the ordered dosages will be available for IV infusion.
2. The IV infusion will be sterile, without precipitate or contamination.
3. The IV will be inserted into the vein without complications and will remain patent.
4. Fluid and electrolyte balance will be restored.
5. Nutrition will be restored or maintained.
6. The IV site will remain free of swelling and inflammation.

(Continues)

PROCEDURE 31-3 Preparing an IV Solution and Starting an IV (Continued)

Equipment Needed

- Appropriate safety needle or catheter for venipuncture
- Tourniquet
- Povidone-iodine swabs (3) or chlorhexidine alcohol (chloroprep)
- Alcohol swab sticks (3) (not needed if using chlorhexidine alcohol)
- Disposable gloves
- Arm board, if needed
- Towel or absorbent drape
- Povidone-iodine ointment (not used in all institutions)
- Gauze dressing
- Tape
- Scissors
- IV solution and tubing

delegation tips

Initiating IV therapy via venipuncture involves assessment and the use of medical asepsis. It is an invasive procedure not delegated by the nurse unless other licensed personnel have been trained and certified to perform the procedure. Ancillary personnel who will be caring for the client need to be instructed to handle the extremity with the IV gently and to report any complaints of pain or swelling in the affected extremity to the nurse.

IMPLEMENTATION—ACTION/RATIONALE

* Check client's identification band * Explain procedure before beginning *

ACTION	RATIONALE
1. Check health care provider's order for an IV and the solution. Identify client.	1. Ensures accurate insertion of catheter and administration of the solution to the correct client.
2. Wash hands.	2. Reduces transmission of microorganisms.
3. Prepare solution bag by removing protective cover from bag.	3. Allows for access to the solution container.
4. Inspect the bag for leaks, tears, or cracks. Inspect the fluid for clarity, particulate matter, and color. Check expiration date.	4. Prevents infusing contaminated or outdated solution.
5. Prepare a label for the IV bag: • On the label, note date, time, and your initials. • Attach the label to the bag. Keep in mind that the bag will be inverted when it is hanging. Make sure the label can be read when the IV is hanging.	5. • Communicates when the bag was opened. • Labeling the bag upside-down makes identification easier when the bag is hanging.
6. Open new infusion set. Unroll tubing and close roller clamp.	6. Prevents fluid from leaking after IV bag is spiked.
7. Grasp the port of the IV bag with your nondominant hand, remove the plastic tab covering the port (Figure 31-3-1), and insert the full length of the spike into the bag's port (Figure 31-3-2).	7. Promotes rapid flow of solution through new tubing without air bubbles.
8. Compress drip chamber to fill halfway.	8. Allows the chamber to provide a clear measurement of drip rate when the IV is flowing.
9. Loosen protective cap from the end of the IV tubing, open roller clamp, and flush tubing with solution (Figure 31-3-3 A and B).	9. Removes air from tubing.
10. Close roller clamp and replace cap protector.	10. Prevents fluid from leaking and maintains sterility.
11. Take prepared fluid and needed equipment to bedside.	11. Ensures smooth procedure without accidents or contamination.
12. Check client's identification band and explain procedure.	12. Ensures correct client and decreases anxiety.
13. Wash hands and put on mask and gown if needed.	13. Reduces transmission of microorganisms.

(Continues)

PROCEDURE 31-3 Preparing an IV Solution and Starting an IV (Continued)

ACTION	RATIONALE

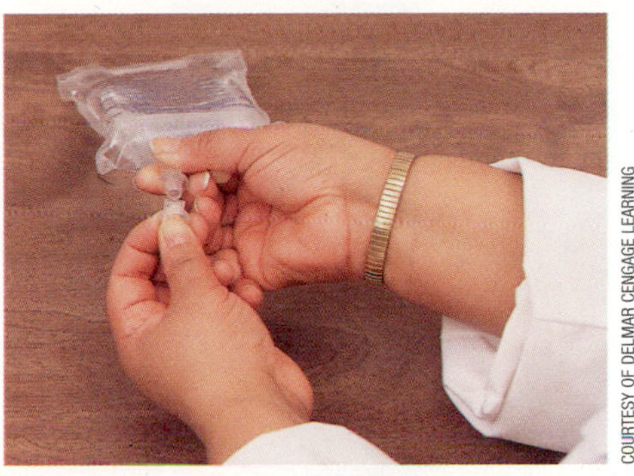

FIGURE 31-3-1 Open the IV plastic bag and pull down the plastic tab covering the port with one hand while pinching the port with the other hand.

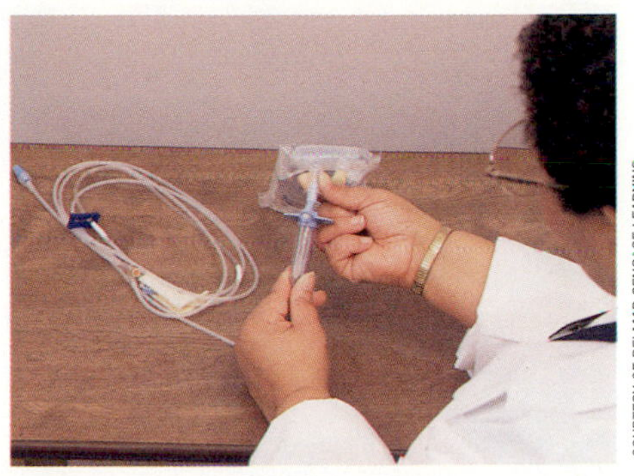

FIGURE 31-3-2 Remove the cap from the spike and spike the IV port.

A

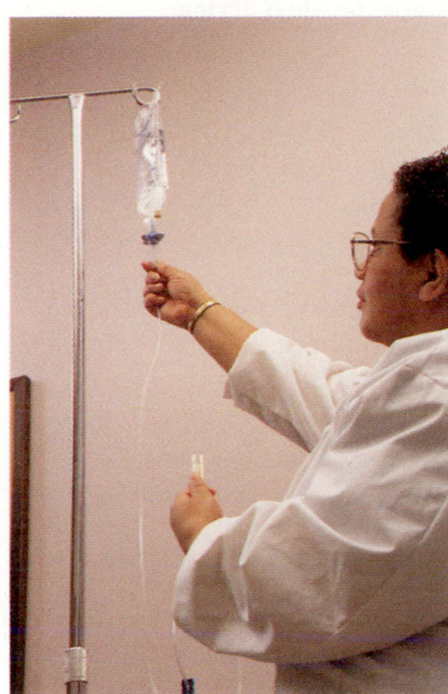

B

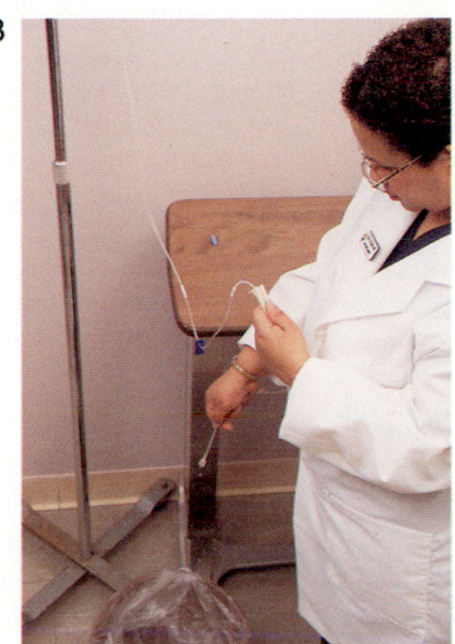

FIGURE 31-3-3 Priming the IV tubing. Open the roller clamp on the tubing to allow the fluid to enter the tube and expel the air.

ACTION	RATIONALE
14. Assess the extremities for the presence of an arteriovenous shunt used for dialysis or history of mastectomy before selecting an appropriate site for the IV.	14. Extremities with a shunt or on the same side as the mastectomy should not be used for an IV site.
15. Inspect potential veins to be used:	15. Promotes ease of placement of catheter.
• Place a tourniquet around the upper arm, close to the axilla.	• Distends vein to allow visual and tactile examination.
• Examine the veins as they dilate.	• Evaluates viability of the veins.
• Palpate the vein to test for firmness (Figure 31-3-4).	• Determines best site for venipuncture and IV placement.
• Release the tourniquet.	• Prevents engorgement of vein.
16. Select vein for venipuncture:	16.
• Use most distal part of the vein first.	• If the vein is later damaged, the proximal part can be used.
• Avoid bony prominences.	• Increases client comfort.
• Avoid client's wrist or hand.	• Bending increases risk of infiltration or phlebitis.
• Avoid client's dominant hand and arm.	• Allows freedom of movement.
• Avoid an extremity with decreased sensation.	• Promotes earlier detection of infiltration.
• Avoid an area of skin affected by a rash or infection.	• Decreases risk of infection.

(Continues)

PROCEDURE 31-3 Preparing an IV Solution and Starting an IV (Continued)

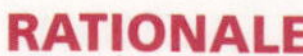

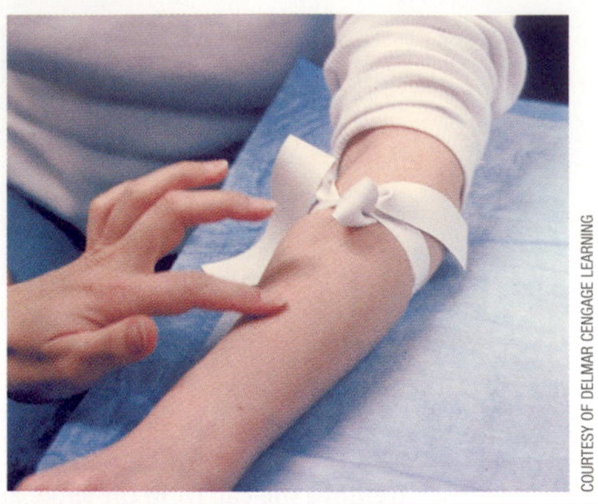

COURTESY OF DELMAR CENGAGE LEARNING

FIGURE 31-3-4 Inspect the site for potential veins to use, and palpate to further locate a vein and test for firmness.

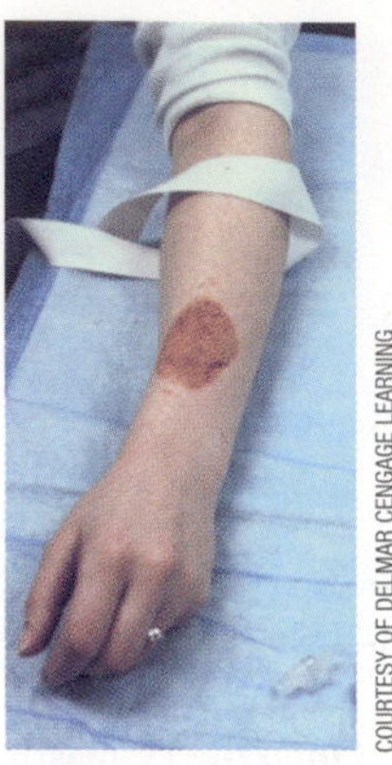

COURTESY OF DELMAR CENGAGE LEARNING

FIGURE 31-3-5 After scrubbing the insertion site with alcohol and povidone-iodine, allow it to dry. *Note:* The tourniquet is released while the site is drying.

ACTION	RATIONALE
17. Select safety shield or angiocatheter that is appropriate for ordered IV fluid. Select the correct size (gauge and length) of catheter.	17. Particular intravenous therapies require specific sizes of intravenous access. Age and quality or location of veins can affect choice of size.
18. Prepare supplies: • Place towel or drape on table for supplies. • Place supplies on towel. • Open needle adapter end of IV tubing set.	18. Provides a clean working surface for an efficiently performed procedure.
19. Shave hair on skin at site if necessary.	19. Ensures adherence of dressing and a less painful removal. Avoid shaving because it causes small abrasions that increase the risk of infection.
20. Ask client to rest arm in a dependent position, if possible.	20. Allows better venous dilation and visibility.
21. Put on disposable gloves.	21. Reduces transmission of microorganisms.
22. Prepare insertion site (Figure 31-3-5):	22.
• Place absorbent drape under the arm.	• Reduces transmission of microorganisms.
• Scrub the insertion site with 3 alcohol swabs then 3 povidone-iodine swabs. • Follow institution protocol. Some facilities use chlorhexidine alcohol instead of iodine. • Use separate swab and start in the middle of the site and work outward.	• Alcohol removes fat on the skin and vigorous scrubbing in circular motion with povidone-iodine removes bacteria. Prevents bacteria from being reintroduced to the site.
• Allow the antiseptic solution to air dry.	• Povidone-iodine or chlorhexidine alcohol must be dry to be effective.
23. Apply tourniquet 5 to 6 inches above the insertion site.	23. Allows the vein to engorge for easier venipuncture.
• Secure it tightly enough to occlude venous flow, not arterial flow.	• Decreased arterial flow prevents venous filling.
• Check presence of distal pulse.	• Ensures arterial flow is present.
24. Perform the venipuncture:	24.
• Anchor the vein by placing thumb over vein and stretching the skin against the direction of insertion 2 to 3 inches distal to the site.	• Stabilizes the vein for ease of venipuncture.
• Insert the stylet needle at a 10- to 30-degree angle with the bevel up (Figure 31-3-6).	• Prevents puncture of posterior wall of vein.
• Watch for a quick blood return through the flashback chamber of the ONC.	• Venous pressure from tourniquet causes backflow of blood into catheter or tubing.
• Verify needle placement in a vein, not an artery.	• Some veins are close to an artery. Arterial blood is bright red and pulses.
• Advance ONC ¼ inch into the vein while it is parallel to the skin.	• Ensures the catheter is in the vein.

(Continues)

PROCEDURE 31-3 Preparing an IV Solution and Starting an IV (Continued)

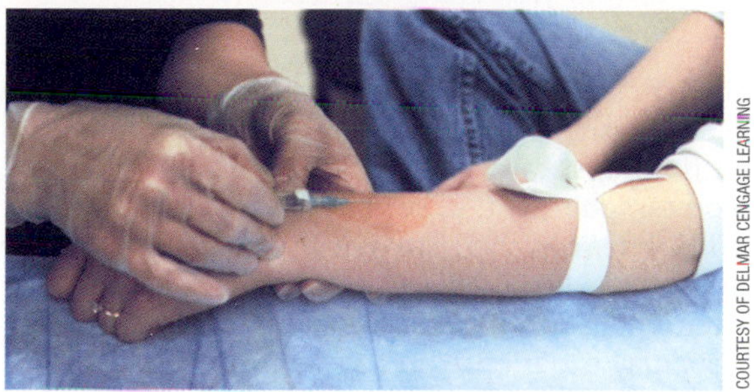

FIGURE 31-3-6 Insert the needle with the beveled side up. Keep the angle low, 10 to 30°.

FIGURE 31-3-7 Loosen the stylet and advance the catheter into the vein until the hub rests on the skin at the venipuncture site.

ACTION	RATIONALE
• Loosen stylet and advance catheter into vein until hub rests at venipuncture site (Figure 31-3-7).	• Ensures proper placement of the catheter.
• Do not reinsert stylet.	• Prevents the catheter from being punctured by the stylet.
• Hold thumb over vein above catheter tip.	• Prevents blood from leaking out of vein until IV tubing is connected.
• Release the tourniquet.	• Reestablishes venous blood flow.
25. Attach IV tubing to ONC.	25.
• Stabilize the catheter with one hand.	• Maintains catheter placement.
• Remove the stylet from ONC or, if using a safety catheter, push the button on the protective casing and stylet will fully retract into the casing.	• Provides entry portal for IV fluids. Reduces risk of inadvertent needlestick injury.
• Quickly release pressure over vein and quickly connect needle adapter of IV set to hub of ONC.	• Reduces blood loss.
• Begin infusion at slow rate to keep vein open.	• Prompt initiation of infusion maintains patency of IV.
26. Secure catheter in place:	26.
• Place tape over the hub of the catheter.	• Ensures catheter's safe position.
• Place transparent dressing over the site and secure.	• Controls bleeding and prevents infection. Allows visualization of site through transparent dressing.
• Secure tubing in loop fashion with tape.	• Prevents dislodgement of IV if tubing is pulled.
27. Regulate flow or, if applicable, attach tubing to infusion device or rate controller if used. Turn on pump and set flow rate (see Procedure 31-4, Setting the IV Flow Rate).	27. Sets flow rate at prescribed rate.
28. Remove gloves and dispose with all used materials.	28. Reduces transmission of microorganisms.
29. Place label with date and time of insertion and size and gauge of catheter on the dressing. Follow protocol for scheduled dressing change.	29. Provides information to schedule next dressing change.
30. Wash hands.	30. Reduces transmission of microorganisms.

EVALUATION

- The appropriate fluids at the ordered dosages were available for IV infusion.
- The IV infusion was sterile, without precipitate or contamination.
- The IV was inserted into the vein without complications and remains patent.
- Fluid and electrolyte balance were restored.
- Nutrition was restored or maintained.
- The IV site remains free of swelling and inflammation.

DOCUMENTATION

Nurses' Notes

- Date and time the IV was inserted
- Type and gauge of catheter
- Date of dressing placement
- Fluid to be infused or if a saline or heparin lock
- Client's reaction to the procedure
- Document on appropriate electronic medical record or flow sheet

PROCEDURE 31-4

Setting the IV Flow Rate

OVERVIEW

Setting the rate of an IV infusion according to the health care provider's order is a nursing responsibility. The flow rate can be controlled by the roller clamp on the IV tubing or by an infusion pump. It is important for the rate to be accurate to prevent complications in fluid balance. A rate that is too fast can result in fluid overload, which is potentially serious in clients with cardiovascular, renal, or neurologic impairment, as well as in very young or very old clients. If an infusion is set too slow, the vein may clot or the more serious complication of circulatory collapse in a dehydrated or severely injured client who required large volumes of fluid could develop.

Sudden changes in the rate of infusion may be accidental or positional. A confused client may loosen the roller clamp or get tangled in the IV tubing. A client who gets up to walk may experience an increase in the IV rate. Changes in flow rate can occur with tubing and a roller clamp or infusion devices.

An infusion pump is an electronic device used to deliver a prescribed amount of fluid over a period of time in milliliters per hour. Pumps may have a drop sensor that counts each drop of fluid and sounds an alarm if the flow rate differs from what is programmed. An alarm sounds when the bag is empty or when pressure increases in the system, as in the case of an infiltrated IV.

An IV controller delivers fluid by gravity, so the bag must be at least 36 inches above the IV site. The number of drops per minute, as well as the IV tubing size and viscosity of the fluid, are necessary to calculate the actual volume delivered per hour. The controller cannot force fluid into the vein like a pump, so infiltrations are detected more quickly; however, the sensitivity of the pump system increases the number of alarms caused by client movement.

A volume-control device is a calibrated chamber placed between the IV bag and the drip chamber so that a small volume of IV fluid (<200 mL) can flow into the chamber and then infuse without the danger that the whole bag will be infused into the client.

ASSESSMENT

1. Check the health care provider's order for the IV to be infused and rate of flow **to ensure accurate administration.**
2. Review information regarding the solution and nursing implications **in order to administer the solution safely.**
3. Assess the patency of the IV **to ensure that the solution will enter the vein and not the surrounding tissue.**
4. Assess the skin at the IV site **so that the solution will not be administered into an inflamed or edematous site, which could cause injury to the tissue.**
5. Assess the client's understanding of the purpose of the IV infusion **so that client teaching can be tailored to his needs.**

POSSIBLE NURSING DIAGNOSES

*Excess **F**luid Volume*
*Risk for Deficient **F**luid Volume*
*Deficient **K**nowledge (IV infusion)*

PLANNING

Expected Outcomes

1. The fluid will be infused into the vein without complications.
2. The IV catheter will remain patent.
3. The fluid and electrolyte balance will return to normal.
4. The client will be able to discuss the purpose of the IV therapy.

Equipment Needed

- Watch with a second hand
- IV solution in a bag
- IV tubing
- IV infusion pump (optional)
- Volume control device (optional)
- Paper and pencil

delegation tips

Setting the rate of the IV after establishing the infusion is the responsibility of the nurse. This procedure is not delegated unless other licensed personnel have been trained and certified to perform the procedure. Ancillary personnel may be instructed to report an infusion that is dripping too fast or an IV bag that is almost empty. It is the nurse's responsibility to monitor the infusion, but ancillary personnel may also be instructed to report observations such as swelling, leaking, or client concerns about pain, numbness, or tingling at the site or in the extremity used for the infusion.

PROCEDURE 31-4 Setting the IV Flow Rate (Continued)

IMPLEMENTATION—ACTION/RATIONALE

ACTION	RATIONALE
* Check client's identification band * Explain procedure before beginning *	
1. Check health care provider's order for the IV solution and rate of infusion. Check client's identification armband.	1. Ensures accurate administration of the solution to the correct client.
2. Wash hands.	2. Reduces transmission of microorganisms.
3. Prepare to set flow rate:	3.
• Have paper and pencil ready to calculate flow rate.	• A nurse unfamiliar with IV fluid rates should calculate the rate at first.
• Review calibration in drops per milliliter (gtt/mL) of each infusion set.	• Drops per milliliter vary with manufacturer and tubing type. Macrodrip tubing varies from 10 to 15 gtt/mL. Microdrip tubing generally delivers 60 gtt/mL.
4. Determine hourly rate by dividing total volume by total hours. *Example 1:* The order reads 1000 mL D_5W with 20 mEq KCl over 8 hours: $\frac{1000\text{ mL}}{8\text{ hr}} = 125\text{ mL/hr}$ *Example 2:* Three liters are ordered for 24 hours: $\frac{3000\text{ mL}}{24\text{ hr}} = 125\text{ mL/hr}$	4. Provides a prescribed hourly rate.
5. Mark a length of tape placed on the IV bag with the hourly time periods according to the rate.	5. Provides a visual check of the fluid infused to be sure the rate is correct.
6. Calculate the minute rate based on the drop factor of the infusion set: $\frac{\text{mL/ hr}}{60\text{ min}} = \text{mL/min}$ $\text{Drop factor} \times \text{mL/min} = \text{gtt/min}$ $\frac{\text{mL hr} \times \text{drop factor}}{60\text{ min}} = \text{gtt/min}$ $\frac{\text{hourly rate} \times \text{drop factor}}{60\text{ min}} = \text{gtt/min}$ • Microdrip example: $\frac{125\text{ mL} \times 60\text{ gtt/mL}}{60\text{ min}} = \frac{7500\text{ gtt}}{60\text{ min}} = 125\text{ gtt/min}$ • Macrodrip example: $\frac{125\text{ mL} \times 15\text{ gtt/mL}}{60\text{ min}} = 31\text{ gtt/min}$	6. Formulas calculate how many drops per minute to be infused.
7. Set flow rate:	7.
• *For regular tubing without a device:* Count drops in drip chamber for 1 minute while watching second hand of watch and adjust the roller clamp as necessary (Figure 31-4-1).	• Ensures that infusion is administered as ordered.
• *For an infusion pump:* Insert the tubing into the flow control chamber, select the desired rate (generally calibrated in milliliters per minute), open the roller clamp, and push start button.	• Pumps the solution through the tubing at the rate set.
• *For a controller:* Place IV bag 36 inches above the IV site, select the desired drops per minute, open the roller clamp, and count drops for 1 minute to verify rate.	• The controller works by gravity.

(Continues)

PROCEDURE 31-4 Setting the IV Flow Rate (Continued)

ACTION	RATIONALE

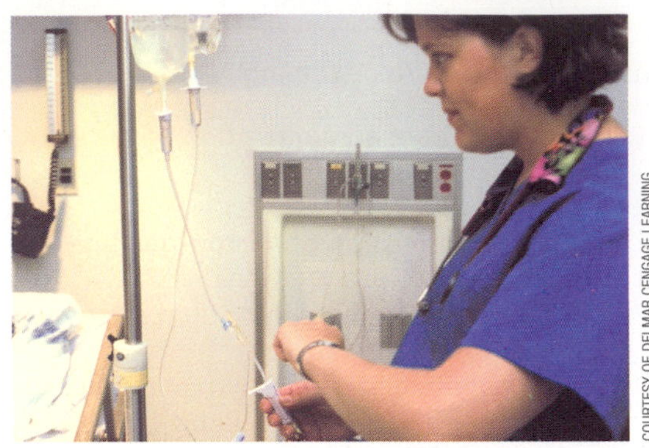

FIGURE 31-4-1 Count the drips in the drip chamber for 1 minute.

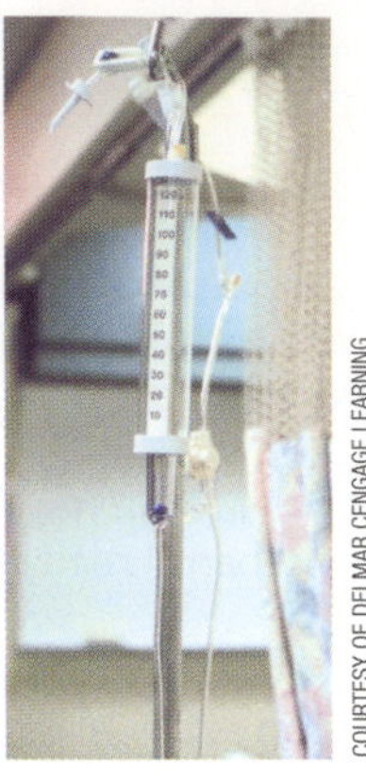

FIGURE 31-4-2 The volume-control device is placed between the IV bag and the client. It is filled with 1 to 2 hours worth of IV fluid.

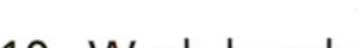

ACTION	RATIONALE
• *For volume-control device:* Place device between IV bag and insertion spike of IV tubing, fill with 1 to 2 hours amount of IV fluid, and count drops for 1 minute (Figure 31-4-2).	• The amount of fluid in the volume control chamber depends on the amount of fluid to be infused per hour: 50 mL/hour = 50 to 100 mL of fluid 100 mL/hour = 100 to 200 mL of fluid
8. Monitor infusion rate and IV site for infiltration.	8. Infusion devices may fail.
9. Assess infusion when alarm sounds.	9. Sounds when a drip has not been sensed. It can be caused by an empty IV bag, a kink in the tubing, a clotted needle, an infiltrated IV, or another malfunction of the device.
10. Wash hands.	10. Reduces transmission of microorganisms.

EVALUATION

- The fluid is infusing into the vein without complications.
- The IV catheter remains patent.
- The fluid and electrolyte balance returned to normal.
- The client is able to discuss the purpose of IV therapy.
- The client receives the correct amount of IV fluid.

DOCUMENTATION

Flow Sheet

- Date and time IV solution was started
- Rate of infusion in drops per minute and milliliters per hour
- Any changes in the IV rate

Nurses' Notes

- Client's response to the IV therapy
- Changes in condition caused by a complication in the IV infusion
- Document on appropriate electronic medical record or flow sheet

PROCEDURE 31-5 Administering Medications via Secondary Administration Sets (Piggyback)

OVERVIEW

A medication is given intravenously when a rapid response to a drug is required or when several medications need to be given IV on a regular schedule. This is best accomplished by using an existing IV as the basic infusion and adding medications by "piggyback" when they are ordered. It also carries the highest risk of side effects because of the immediate response of the medication and the inability to correct a medication administration error.

(Continues)

PROCEDURE 31-5 Administering Medications via Secondary Administration Sets (Piggyback) (Continued)

The drug is diluted and mixed with a small volume (50 to 100 mL) of compatible solution and then joined to the primary IV line for infusion. The bag is connected to the upper Y-port of the primary infusion line and hung higher than the primary IV bag, thus the name piggyback. The piggyback infusion works because of the backflow valve. When the piggyback infusion starts flowing, the valve stops the flow of the primary infusion. After the piggyback infusion is complete and the solution within the tubing falls below the level of the primary infusion drip chamber, the valve opens and the primary infusion flows.

It is important to note that some medications can be irritating to the lining of blood vessels. Other medications, when injected into a vein that is beginning to infiltrate, will injure the tissue to such an extent that tissue could slough, become abscessed, or become necrotic. No IV medication should be administered through IV sites that are suspected to be inflamed or infiltrated. Use needleless systems if available. Safety needles and syringes are required by OSHA standards.

ASSESSMENT

1. Check the health care provider's order or the medication administration record (MAR) for the medication, dosage, and time and route of administration **to ensure accurate administration.**
2. Review information regarding the drug, including action, purpose, side effects, normal dose, peak onset, and nursing implications, **in order to administer the drug safely.**
3. Determine additives in the solution of an existing IV line **so that the medication will be compatible with the solution.**
4. Assess the placement of the IV catheter in the vein **to ensure that the medication will enter the vein and not the surrounding tissue.**
5. Assess the skin at the IV site **so that the medication will not be administered into an inflamed or edematous site, which could cause injury to the tissue.**
6. Check the client's drug allergy history, **because an allergic reaction could occur rapidly and be fatal.**
7. Assess the client's understanding of the purpose of the medication **so that client teaching can be tailored to needs.**
8. Assess the compatibility of the piggyback IV medication with the primary IV solution **to avoid an adverse reaction such as the formation of precipitate in the IV tubing.**

POSSIBLE NURSING DIAGNOSES

Risk for Infection
Risk for Injury
Impaired Skin Integrity
Deficient Knowledge (medication)

PLANNING

Expected Outcomes

1. The drug is infused into the vein without complications.
2. The IV site remains free of swelling and inflammation.
3. The client will be able to discuss the purpose of the drug.
4. The client is free from allergic reaction.

Equipment Needed

- Disposable gloves
- Medication prepared in a labeled infusion bag
- Short microdrip or macrodrip tubing set for piggyback (needleless system preferred)
- Safety sterile needles, 21- or 23-gauge, if needleless system is not available
- Antiseptic swab
- Adhesive tape
- IV pole
- Medication administration record (MAR)

delegation tips

The skill of medication administration is not delegated to ancillary personnel in acute care settings. This may vary in state or federal institutions. Ancillary personnel are generally informed about the medications the client is receiving if adverse effects are anticipated or are being monitored.

IMPLEMENTATION—ACTION/RATIONALE

ACTION	RATIONALE
* Check client's identification band * Explain procedure before beginning *	
1. Check health care provider's order.	1. Ensures accurate administration of medication.
2. Wash hands. *Gloves are not necessary if you are adding fluids to an existing infusion line.*	2. Reduces transmission of microorganisms.
3. Check client's identification armband.	3. Ensures medication is given to the correct client.

(Continues)

PROCEDURE 31-5 Administering Medications via Secondary Administration Sets (Piggyback) (Continued)

ACTION	RATIONALE
4. Prepare medication bag:	4.
• Close clamp on tubing of infusion set.	• Prevents leakage of solution.
• Spike medication bag with infusion tubing.	• Provides a method of infusing the medication into the system.
• Open clamp.	• Allows the solution to fill the tubing.
• Allow tubing to be filled with solution to evacuate air from tubing.	• Prevents air embolus.
5. Hang piggyback medication bag above level of primary IV bag. Use extender found in the piggyback tubing package to lower the primary bag (Figure 31-5-1).	5. Relationship between height of the bags affects the flow rate to the client.
6. Connect piggyback tubing to primary tubing at Y-port:	6. Ensures medication in piggyback bag is infused.
• For needleless system, remove cap on port and connect tubing (Figure 31-5-2).	• A needleless system is preferred to prevent accidental needlesticks.
• If a needle is used, clean port with antiseptic swab and insert small-gauge needle into center of port.	• A small-gauge needle does less damage to the rubber stopper on the port.
• Secure tubing with adhesive tape.	• Prevents accidental removal of tubing.
7. Administer the medication:	7.
• Check the prescribed length of time for the infusion.	• Each medication has a recommended rate for IV piggyback administration.
• Regulate flow rate of piggyback by adjusting regulator clamp (Figure 31-5-3).	• Medication infuses through primary line.
• Observe whether backflow valve on piggyback has stopped flow of primary infusion during drug administration (Figure 31-5-4).	• Prevents backup of medication into primary infusion line.
8. Check primary infusion line when medication is finished:	8.
• Regulate primary infusion rate.	• Reestablishes primary infusion.
• Leave secondary bag and tubing in place for next drug administration.	• Reduces risk for entry of microorganisms by repeated changes of tubing.

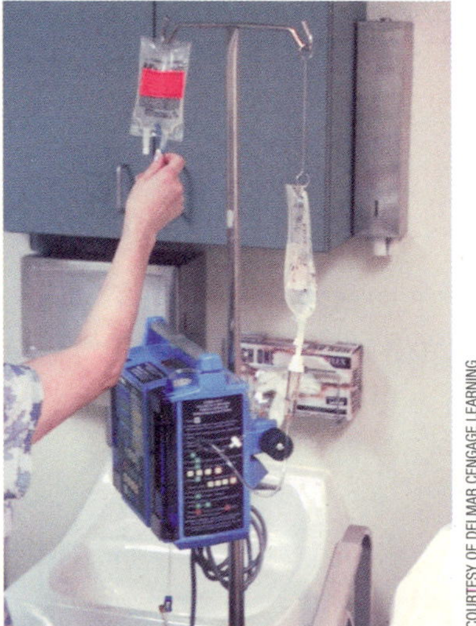
COURTESY OF DELMAR CENGAGE LEARNING

FIGURE 31-5-1 Hang the piggyback bag higher than the primary IV bag.

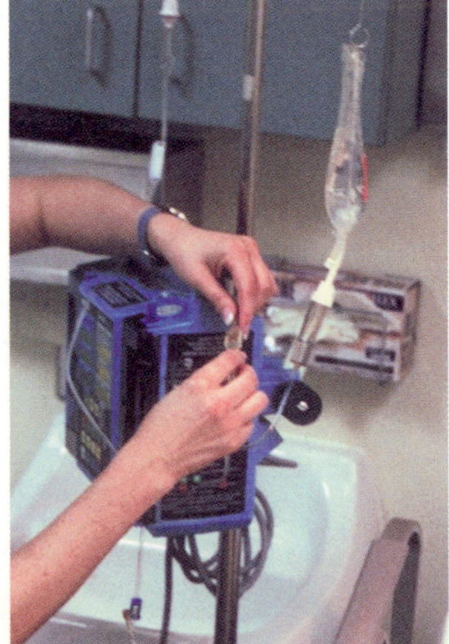
COURTESY OF DELMAR CENGAGE LEARNING

FIGURE 31-5-2 Connect the needleless system tubing.

(Continues)

PROCEDURE 31-5 Administering Medications via Secondary Administration Sets (Piggyback) (Continued)

ACTION	RATIONALE

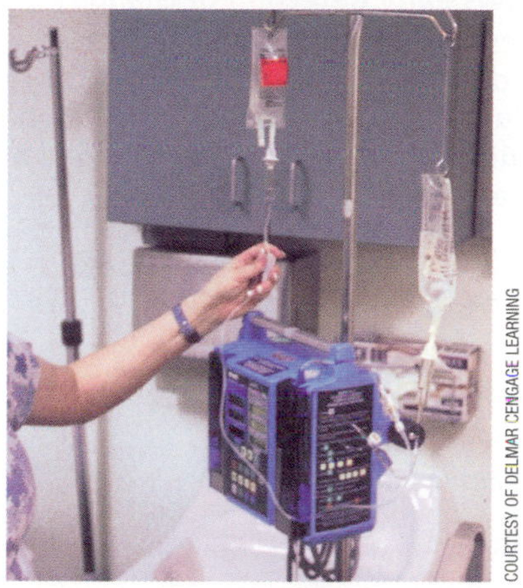

FIGURE 31-5-3 Regulate the flow rate of the piggyback by adjusting the regulator clamp.

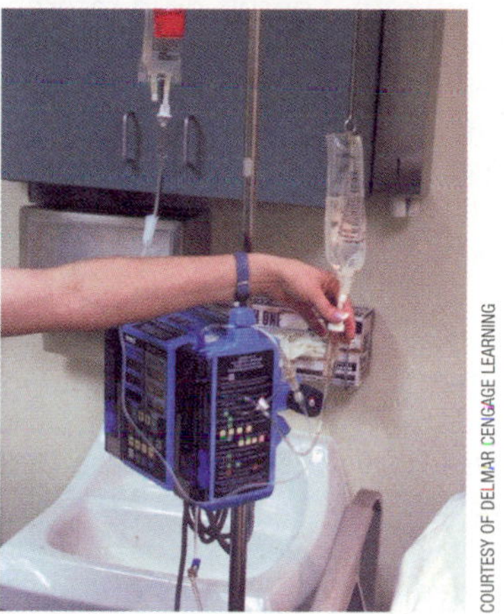

FIGURE 31-5-4 Double-check that the primary infusion has stopped flowing.

ACTION	RATIONALE
9. Dispose of all used materials and place needles in needle biohazard sharps container.	9. Reduces transmission of microorganisms.
10. Wash hands.	10. Reduces transmission of microorganisms.

EVALUATION

- The drug was infused into the vein without complications.
- The IV site remained free of swelling and inflammation.
- The client was able to discuss the purpose of the drug.

DOCUMENTATION

Medication Administration Record

- Date, time, dose, and route of medication

Flow Sheet

- Date, time, and volume of fluid infused IV piggyback

Nurses' Notes

- Client's response to the medication
- Any serious side effects and report them to the health care provider immediately
- Document on appropriate electronic medical record or flow sheet

Intake and Output Record

- Amount of fluid infused

PROCEDURE 31-6 Assessing and Maintaining an IV Insertion Site

OVERVIEW

Assessing an established IV site requires knowledge about the length of time since the insertion, the condition of the dressing, and the site itself. The site should be without redness, swelling, pain, or discharge. When palpating the vein, it should have the characteristics of a healthy vein without signs of infection or phlebitis. Knowledge of both the IV solution and medications to be given and their potential side effects on the veins should be included in the assessment. Intravenous solutions with electrolytes and medications can have irritant properties that would require more frequent IV monitoring.

PROCEDURE 31-6 Assessing and Maintaining an IV Insertion Site (Continued)

ASSESSMENT

1. Review the order for IV therapy: Identify potential side effects from medication actions, and fluid rate. Consult drug reference books or pharmacists for information. **Decreases the risk of medication errors.**
2. Identify potential risk factors for your client's condition that might indicate fluid and electrolyte imbalances. **Allows targeted assessment and monitoring.**
3. Assess for dehydration: sunken eyes, dry skin, mucous membranes, flattened neck veins, vital sign changes, inelastic skin turgor, decreased urine output, behavior changes, and confusion. **Allows intervention to increase fluids and reduce dehydration.**
4. Assess for fluid overload: periorbital edema, distended neck veins, auscultation of crackles or wheezes in lungs, changes in vital signs, and level of consciousness. **Allows intervention to decrease fluids.**
5. Determine the client's risk for developing complications from IV therapy: very young or very old, heart or renal failure. **Allows the procedure to be modified if needed, and promotes targeted assessment to look for signs of risk-related problems.**
6. Observe IV site for complications, that is, signs of infection, phlebitis, or infiltration: redness, swelling, pallor, or warmth at the IV site and surrounding tissue, and bleeding or drainage. **Allows interventions to reduce further damage.**
7. Observe IV site for patency by briefly compressing the IV cannulated vein above the site. Note slowing or momentary cessation of IV rate with a positive blood return. **Provides ongoing assessment of current patency status. Allows early detection of changes.**
8. Assess the client's knowledge regarding the need for the IV therapy. **Allows for teaching, including information and education regarding medications, fluid needs, and signs of IV site irritation or phlebitis.**

POSSIBLE NURSING DIAGNOSES

*Impaired **T**issue Integrity*
*Risk for Impaired **S**kin Integrity*
*Risk for **I**nfection*
*Excess **F**luid Volume*
*Deficient **F**luid Volume*

PLANNING

Expected Outcomes

1. The client will have a patent IV, without signs of infection or inflammation.
2. The client's fluid and electrolyte imbalance will return to normal and will be maintained.
3. The client will be able to report signs of inflammation or infiltration.
4. The client's IV rate will be administered and maintained per order.
5. The client's IV dressing will remain intact, clean, and dry.

Equipment Needed

- Clean gloves
- Gauze dressing
- Tape

delegation tips

Assessing and maintaining the IV after establishing the infusion is the responsibility of the nurse. This procedure is not delegated unless other licensed personnel have been trained and certified to perform the procedure. Ancillary personnel may be instructed to report an infusion that is dripping too fast or an IV bag that is almost empty. It is the nurse's responsibility to monitor the infusion, but ancillary personnel may also be instructed to report any observations, such as swelling, leaking, client concerns about pain, numbness, or tingling at the site or in the extremity used for the infusion. Ancillary personnel may also be involved in monitoring the client's daily weight, if ordered, along with intake and output. Ancillary personnel should be instructed not to obtain vital signs on an extremity with solutions infusing.

IMPLEMENTATION—ACTION/RATIONALE

ACTION	RATIONALE
* Check client's identification band * Explain procedure before beginning *	
1. Review health care provider's order for IV therapy.	1. Ensures accuracy in the administration of IV therapy.
2. Review client's history for medical conditions or allergies.	2. Decreases risk of fluid overload and allergic reactions.
3. Review client's IV site record and intake and output record.	3. Assesses for potential problems with fragile IV sites and fluid balance.

(Continues)

PROCEDURE 31-6 Assessing and Maintaining an IV Insertion Site (Continued)

ACTION	RATIONALE

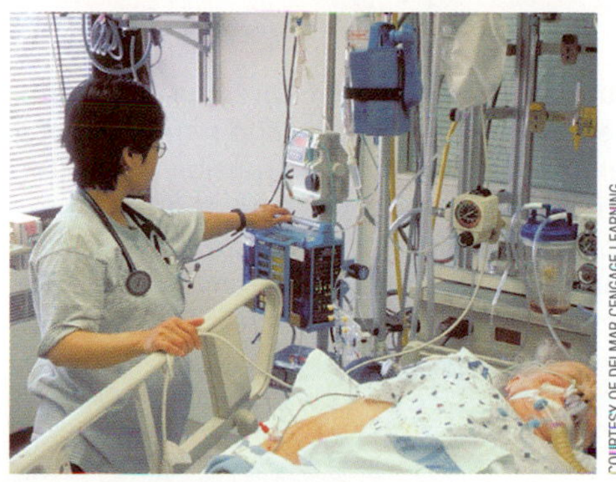

FIGURE 31-6-1 Check the IV fluid rate, volume, tubing, and additives at the beginning of the shift.

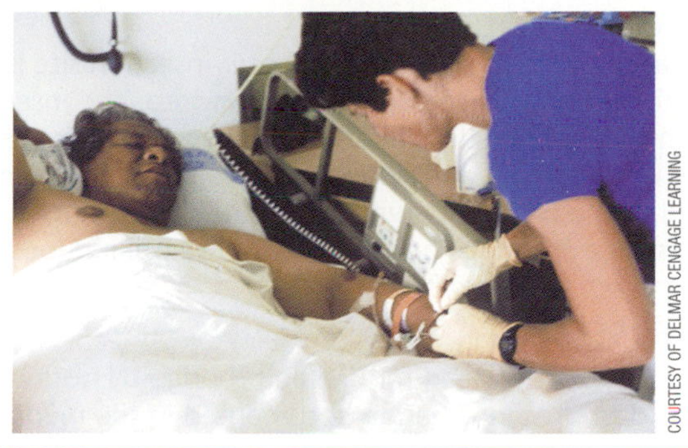

FIGURE 31-6-2 Check the IV dressing site every hour.

ACTION	RATIONALE
4. Wash hands.	4. Decreases transmission of microorganisms.
5. Obtain client's vital signs.	5. Assesses for changes in cardiovascular system.
6. Check IV fluid for correct fluid, additives, rate, and volume at the beginning of your shift (Figure 31-6-1).	6. Ensures client is receiving correct therapy.
7. Check IV tubing for tight connections every 4 hours.	7. Ensures that no fluid leaks from tubing and connections.
8. Check gauze IV dressing hourly to be sure it is dry and intact (Figure 31-6-2).	8. Ensures there is no sign of infiltration or infection at IV insertion site.
9. If the gauze is not dry and intact, remove the dressing and observe site for redness, swelling, or drainage.	9. Ensures there is no sign of inflammation or infection at IV site.
10. Replace with new dry sterile gauze dressing if site is okay.	10. Protects IV insertion site.
11. If an occlusive dressing is used, do not remove the dressing when assessing the site.	11. Ensures there is no sign of inflammation or infection at IV site.
12. Observe vein track for redness, swelling, warmth, or pain hourly.	12. These are early signs of phlebitis or infiltration.
13. Document IV site findings on appropriate electronic medical record or IV flow sheet.	13. Provides documentation of frequent IV site observation.
14. Wash hands.	14. Decreases transmission of microorganisms.

EVALUATION

- IV site observed on an hourly basis to avoid complications of phlebitis and infiltration.
- Client reported no signs or symptoms of redness, swelling, and pain.

DOCUMENTATION

Flow Sheet

- Name of IV solution with additives
- Hourly rate of fluids
- IV site condition
- Time checked
- Initials/signature of nurse

PROCEDURE 31-7 Changing the Central Venous Dressing

OVERVIEW

Because the central venous catheter insertion site is a direct route to the circulatory system, care must be taken to keep the insertion site clean and infection-free. The insertion site is inspected frequently for signs and symptoms of infection, such as inflammation, heat, or drainage. Regular, aseptic dressing changes help decrease the possibility of infection at the insertion site and systemically. Policies vary from institution to institution regarding the type of dressing to apply as well as the frequency with which they are changed. Be aware of the policy at your institution and the rationale for it. Dressings that have become wet or are pulling loose from the insertion site must be changed immediately.

ASSESSMENT

1. Assess the need for dressing change by noting the last dressing change documented in the medical record and standard of care recommended by the manufacturer and the institution. **This decreases the risk of infection by following the standard of care.**
2. Assess the timing of the dressing change as it relates to medication, IV fluid and transfusion schedules, and as well as the time of the client's daily shower or bath. **This allows the nurse to avoid simultaneous administration of medication and the need for two dressing changes in one day.**
3. Assess the type of central venous access in place **in order to obtain the appropriate supplies.**
4. Assess the integrity of the skin at the site **for signs of infection or bleeding.**
5. Assess the client and caregiver's knowledge of the purpose and care of the catheter **so a teaching plan can be developed.**

POSSIBLE NURSING DIAGNOSES

Risk for Infection
Impaired Skin Integrity
Deficient Knowledge

PLANNING

Expected Outcomes

1. Skin is intact at catheter site, has normal color, is not edematous, and has no drainage.
2. Client has no signs of systemic infection such as fever, malaise, or chills.

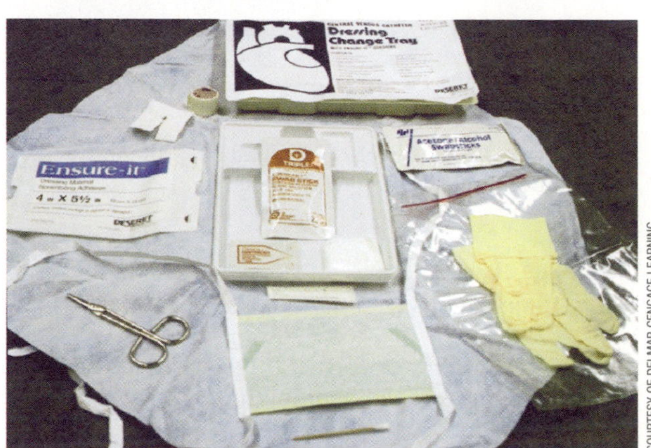

COURTESY OF DELMAR CENGAGE LEARNING

FIGURE 31-7-1 Central venous catheter dressing change supplies.

3. Catheter and tubing are intact.
4. Client and caregiver are able to perform skin care and dressing change.

Equipment Needed: (see Figure 31-7-1)

- Povidone-iodine swabs, chlorhexidine or agency-approved antiseptic solution
- Povidone-iodine ointment
- Sterile gauze, tape, or moisture transparent dressing
- Label with date and time of dressing change
- Latex-free clean gloves
- Mask
- Latex-free sterile gloves

delegation tips

Changing the central venous catheter dressing is a skill involving assessment and the use of sterile technique. It is a procedure not delegated by the nurse unless other licensed personnel have been trained and certified to assist with the procedure. Ancillary personnel who will be caring for the client need to be instructed to report any disruption of the closed dressing, along with complaints of pain, redness, or swelling at the insertion site.

(Continues)

PROCEDURE 31-7 Changing the Central Venous Dressing (Continued)

IMPLEMENTATION—ACTION/RATIONALE

ACTION	RATIONALE
* Check client's identification band * Explain procedure before beginning *	
1. Wash hands and put on latex-free clean gloves.	1. Reduces the number of microorganisms.
2. Put on mask.	2. Reduces the number of microorganisms.
3. Remove old dressing carefully (see Figures 31-7-2 and 31-7-3), being careful not to dislodge the central catheter.	3. Skin integrity may be impaired.
4. Note drainage on dressing for color, odor, consistency, and amount.	4. Potential for bleeding or infectious material.
5. Inspect skin at insertion site for redness, tenderness, or swelling (see Figure 31-7-4).	5. Assesses for infection.
6. Palpate tunneled catheter for presence of Dacron cuff, using care not to palpate close to the exit site.	6. Documents proper placement of catheter.
7. Visually inspect catheter from hub to skin.	7. Checks whether catheter has a crack or is split or cut.
8. Remove gloves and put on latex-free sterile gloves.	8. Prevents transmission of microorganisms from skin to exit site.
9. Clean exit site according to institution protocol. Most use alcohol wipes first, then povidone-iodine swab beginning at the catheter and moving out in a circular manner for 3 cm to maintain aseptic technique (see Figure 31-7-5).	9. Eliminates microorganisms by chemical and mechanical means.
10. Some institutions use povidone-iodine ointment to exit site (check agency policy).	10. Reduces growth of bacteria at exit site.
11. Apply transparent dressing (see Figures 31-7-6, 31-7-7, and 31-7-8). Some institutions prefer to omit the gauze dressing to allow visualization of the site; in this case, only apply the transparent dressing.	11. Prevents bacteria from entering exit site.
12. Label with date and time of dressing change (see Figure 31-7-9).	12. Documents time to plan for next change.
13. Secure tubing to client's clothing.	13. Prevents accidental displacement.
14. Remove gloves and dispose of all used materials according to agency policy.	14. Reduces transmission of microorganisms.
15. Wash hands.	15. Reduces transmission of microorganisms.

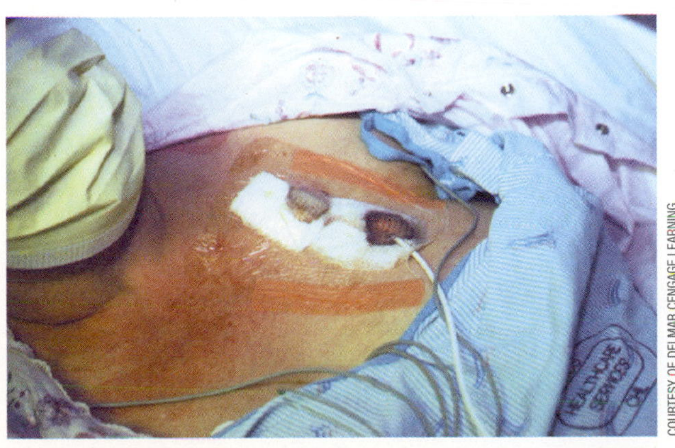

COURTESY OF DELMAR CENGAGE LEARNING

FIGURE 31-7-2 Inspect the dressing.

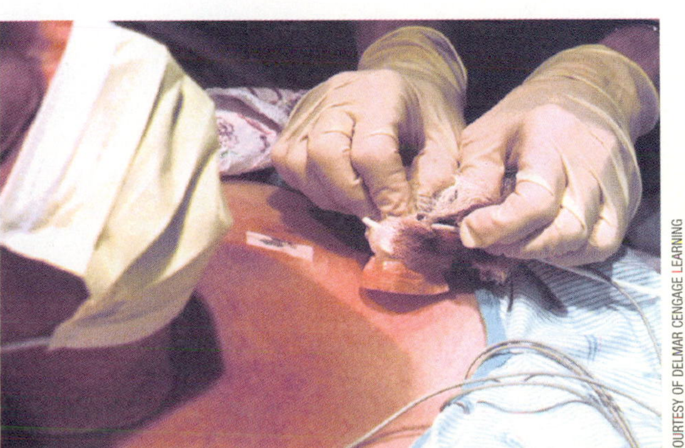

COURTESY OF DELMAR CENGAGE LEARNING

FIGURE 31-7-3 Be careful not to dislodge the catheter when removing the old dressing.

(Continues)

PROCEDURE 31-7 Changing the Central Venous Dressing (Continued)

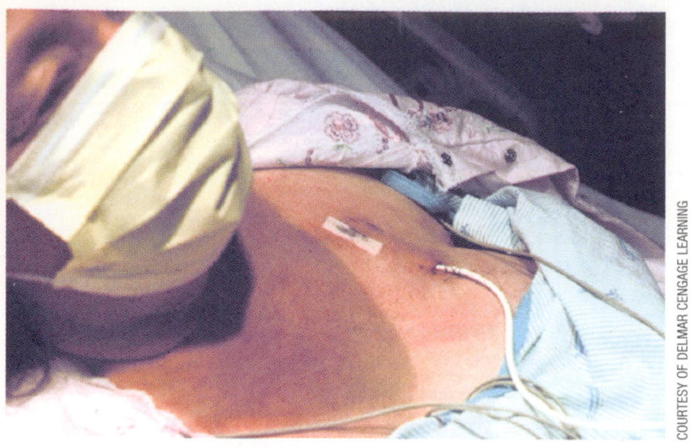

FIGURE 31-7-4 Inspect the site for redness, tenderness, and swelling.

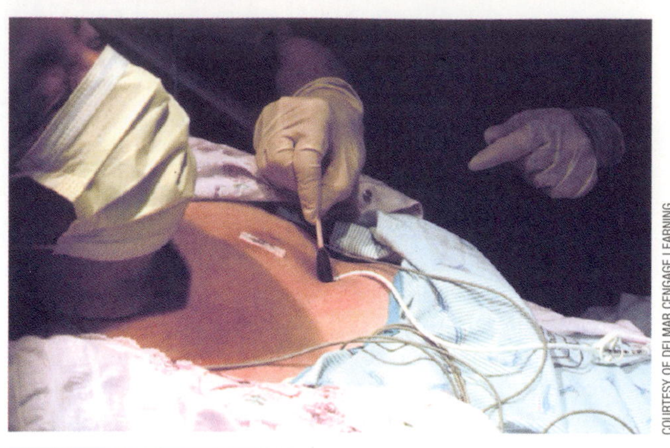

FIGURE 31-7-5 Clean the site with povidone-iodine swab.

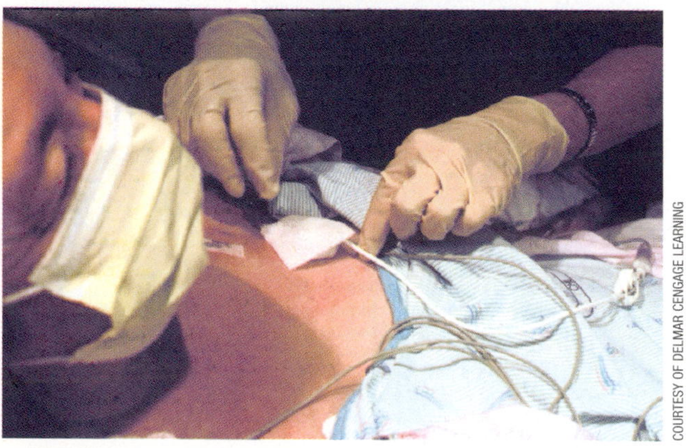

FIGURE 31-7-6 Slide the first piece of gauze directly over and under the catheter.

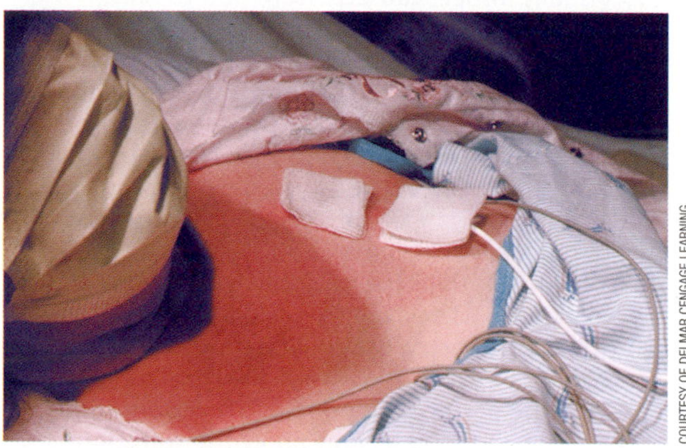

FIGURE 31-7-7 Place the next piece of gauze directly over the insertion site.

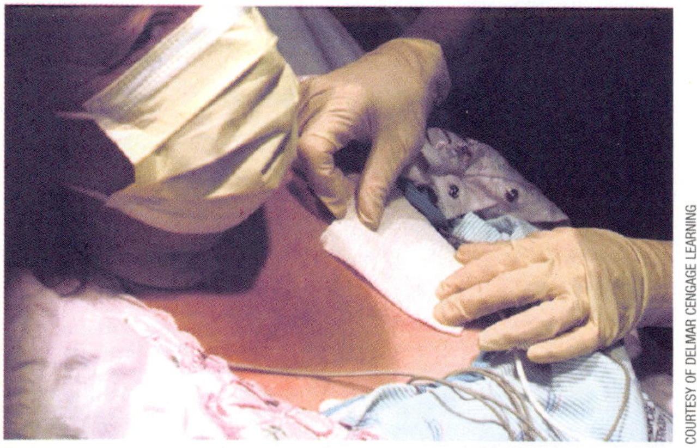

FIGURE 31-7-8 Place a larger piece of gauze over the area and secure with tape or transparent dressing.

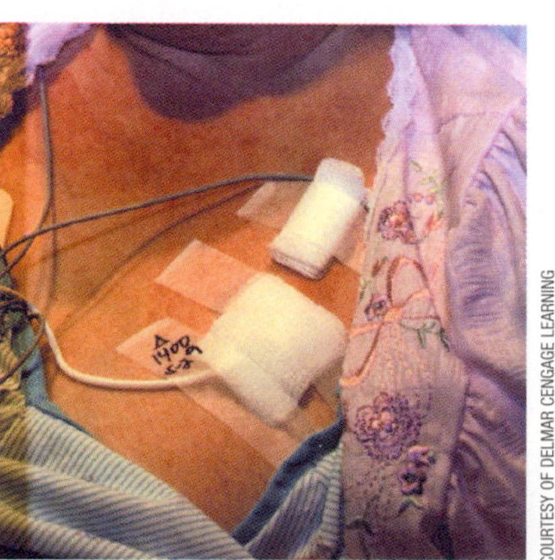

FIGURE 31-7-9 Write the date and time of the dressing change on the dressing.

(Continues)

PROCEDURE 31-7 Changing the Central Venous Dressing (Continued)

EVALUATION

- The client's skin is intact at catheter site, has normal color, and is not edematous.
- The client has no signs of systemic infection such as fever or malaise.
- The central venous catheter and tubing are intact.
- Client and caregiver are able to perform skin care and dressing change.

DOCUMENTATION

Nurses' Notes

- The date and time the dressing was changed
- The type of ointment and dressing applied
- The condition of the skin at the site
- The presence of any exudate or bleeding at the site
- The client or caregiver's ability to perform the dressing change
- Document on appropriate flow sheet or electronic medical record (EMR)

PROCEDURE 31-8 Removing Skin Sutures and Staples

OVERVIEW

Sutures and staples are a surgical means of closing a wound by sewing, wiring, or stapling the edges of the wound together. Most wounds are sutured in layers to maintain alignment of the tissues and reduce scarring. Sutures are generally removed 7 to 10 days after surgery, depending on where the wound is located and how well it is healing. Suture removal requires a health care provider's orders. Timing is important because sutures left in too long can increase the risk of infection and irritation from a foreign substance.

Sutures placed deep within the tissue layers are made of absorbable materials. Surface sutures are made of wire, nylon, or cotton. Continuous sutures are made with one thread, tied at the beginning and end of the suture line. Interrupted sutures are tied individually. Staples are used for large incision areas where the risk of dehiscence is greater, such as in sterneotomies, in clients with increased adipose tissue, abdominal areas, and wounds that fail to heal or adhere.

ASSESSMENT

1. Assess the wound **to determine whether the edges are approximate and healing.** In deep wounds, palpate around the suture site for edema or any evidence of failure of tissue to adhere below the skin's surface.
2. Assess **for any signs of infection**, such as increased warmth, redness, exudate or drainage, and pain.
3. Assess for any conditions **that impede the healing process**, such as age, immunosuppression, diabetes, obesity, smoking, radiation, poor cellular nutrition, infection, and deep wounds.

POSSIBLE NURSING DIAGNOSES

Impaired Skin Integrity
Risk for Infection
Acute Pain
Deficient Knowledge (fear of dehiscence)
Impaired Physical Mobility

PLANNING

Expected Outcomes

1. The wound is healing, with the edges of the wound well-approximated.
2. There is no redness or signs of infection.
3. The procedure is performed with a minimum of pain and trauma to the client.

Equipment Needed

- Suture removal kit or sterile forceps with sterile suture removal scissors
- Gauze size as appropriate for wound area to be covered
- Biohazard bag or appropriate waterproof disposable bag
- Sterile saline, prepackaged antiseptic swabs, or gauze for cleaning if appropriate
- Examination gloves
- Sterile gloves if dressings are to be applied

(Continues)

PROCEDURE 31-8 Removing Skin Sutures and Staples (Continued)

- Adhesive strips or butterfly adhesive tape as needed
- Sterile gauze to wipe stitches or sutures from forceps and scissors
- Tincture of benzoin as indicated

delegation tips

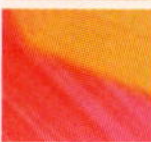

Suture removal is a skill requiring aseptic technique and wound assessment by a nurse and, therefore, is not delegated to ancillary personnel.

IMPLEMENTATION—ACTION/RATIONALE

* Check client's identification band * Explain procedure before beginning *

ACTION	RATIONALE
1. Wash hands.	1. Reduces transmission of microorganisms.
2. Assess the wound to determine whether the edges of the wound are well-approximated and healing has occurred.	2. Health care providers often have standing orders for sutures to be removed at a specified date. If the wound is not well-healed, sutures should be left in place longer and the health care provider notified.
3. Close the door and curtains around the client's bed.	3. Provides for privacy.
4. Raise the bed to a comfortable level.	4. Provides for proper body mechanics.
5. Position the client for comfort with easy access and visibility of the suture line.	5. Facilitates removal of the sutures and allows for careful observation of suture line.
6. Drape the client so that only the suture area is exposed.	6. Provides for privacy.
7. Open the suture removal kit on a clean surface and assemble any supplies needed within easy access.	7. Facilitates removal of sutures.
8. Apply clean gloves to remove the old dressing and place it in a disposable bag.	8. Follows Standard Precautions protocol.
9. Remove gloves and wash hands.	9. Reduces transmission of microorganisms.
10. If dressings are to be used, assemble equipment and supplies on sterile field.	10. Protects client from microorganisms.
11. Apply sterile gloves according to institutional policy. Clean the incision with saline-soaked gauze pads, antiseptic swabs, or per institutional policy.	11. Protects the incision from microorganisms on the nurse's hands. Protects the nurse from possible contact with bodily fluids. Various opinions exist regarding use of cleansing solutions for wound care.
12. When removing an interrupted suture, hold forceps in your nondominant hand and grasp the suture near the knot (Figure 31-8-1).	12. Pulls the suture up and away from the client's skin.
13. Place the curved edge of the scissors under the suture or near the knot (Figure 31-8-2).	13. Facilitates clipping of the suture.
14. Cut the suture close to the skin where the suture emerges from the skin (not in the middle). Pull the long end and remove it in one piece.	14. Facilitates suture removal. Avoids pulling large amounts of contaminated suture through tissue.
15. If the client has a continuous suture, cut both the first and second suture before removing them.	15. Facilitates suture removal without traumatizing the incision line.
16. Some policies require the removal of every other suture, with the remaining sutures removed at a later time. Assess the suture line to ensure that the edges remain approximated.	16. Any dehiscence should be detected early, and every other suture can be left in place.
17. Discard the sutures onto the gauze squares as they are removed and place the gauze squares in the disposable bag when all the sutures have been removed.	17. Decreases transmission of microorganisms and follows Standard Precaution protocol.
18. Assess the suture line to ensure that the edges remain approximated and that all sutures have been removed.	18. Detects early signs of dehiscence. Ensures that sutures do not remain in the skin when they are no longer needed.

(Continues)

PROCEDURE 31-8 Removing Skin Sutures and Staples (Continued)

ACTION	RATIONALE
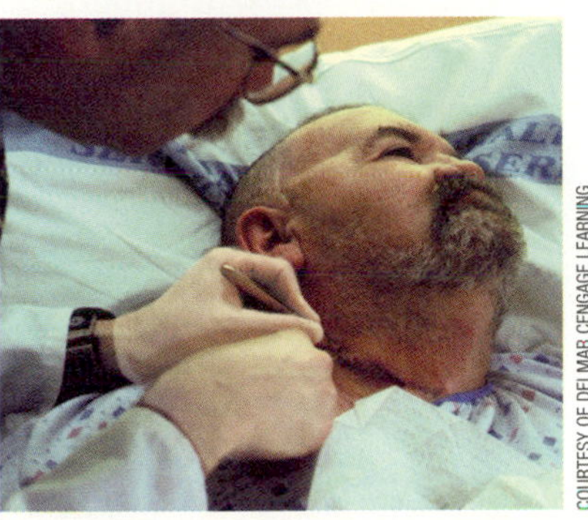 **FIGURE 31-8-1 Hold forceps in your nondominant hand and grasp the suture near the knot.**	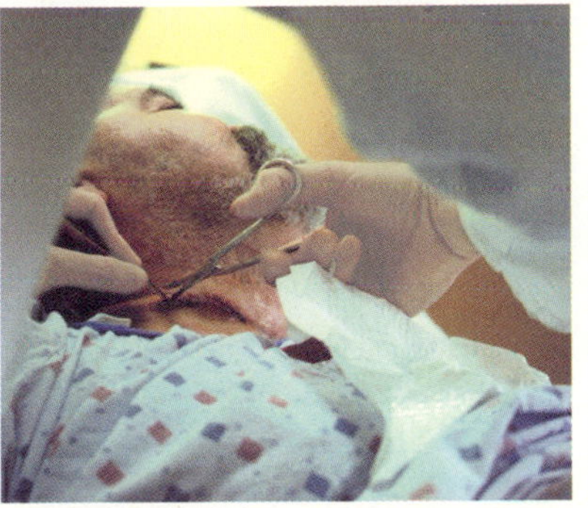 **FIGURE 31-8-2 Hold the scissors in your dominant hand. Place the curved edge of the scissors under the suture.**
19. Apply adhesive strips or butterfly tape adhesive strips across the suture line to secure the edges. The amount of reinforcement varies depending on the adherence of the suture line and the length of the suture line. Adhesive skin closures may be placed 1 inch apart or closer together. Tincture of benzoin may be applied to skin adjacent to the incision.	19. If the suture line pulls apart a little after the sutures are removed, adhesive skin closures can be used to reinforce the suture line. Helps adhesive adhere to skin.
20. Dispose of the soiled equipment.	20. Reduces odors in the client's room and reduces transmission of microorganisms.
21. Remove gloves and wash hands.	21. Reduces transmission of microorganisms.
22. If removing staples:	22.
• Repeat Actions 2–11.	• Prepares for staple removal.
• Use a staple extractor to remove every other staple. Place the lower tip of staple remover under the staple and squeeze the handles together. The ends of the staple will extract from the skin. Move the staple away from the skin surface and release the staple into a disposal container. Assess the wound for adherence. Move on to the next staple if the skin has adhered well.	• When removing staples, it is best to remove every other staple and assess wound adherence before removing all staples. A staple extractor is designed to remove the staple with a minimum of discomfort and trauma to the surrounding skin and tissue.
• Repeat Actions 19 to 21.	• See Rationales 19 to 21.

EVALUATION

- The wound is intact, edges are adhered, and there are no signs of infection or drainage.
- Sutures/staples removed with a minimum of pain and trauma to the client.

DOCUMENTATION

Nurses' Notes

- Procedure and findings at wound site, such as redness, pain, or drainage
- Time sutures/staples were removed
- Follow-up instructions and client teaching provided
- Document on appropriate electronic medical record or flow sheet

REFERENCE/SUGGESTED READING

Altman, G. (2010). *Fundamental and advanced nursing skills.* (3rd ed.). Clifton Park, NY: Delmar Cengage Learning.

SECTION II
Adult Health Nursing

UNIT 9 Essential Concepts

CHAPTER 32
Anesthesia

MAKING THE CONNECTION

Refer to the following chapters to increase your understanding of anesthesia:

Basic Nursing
- ***Legal and Ethical Responsibilities***
- ***Fluid, Electrolyte, and Acid–Base Balance***
- ***Pain Management***

Adult Health Nursing
- ***Surgery***

LEARNING OBJECTIVES

Upon completion of this chapter, you should be able to:

- Define key terms.
- Describe the difference between regional and general anesthesia.
- Identify the purposes of sedation.
- Describe the effects of sedation or general anesthesia on memory and cognitive function.
- Discuss the types of monitoring necessary to ensure client safety during sedation.
- Describe the signs and symptoms and risks of oversedation.
- Discuss the dangers involved in aspiration of gastric contents and how gastric aspiration is prevented during anesthesia.
- List the medications that are typically given on the day of surgery.
- List and describe the different types of regional anesthesia.
- Describe the risks involved with regional and general anesthesia.
- Discuss the residual effects of anesthesia on the client.
- List three methods of postoperative pain management and explain briefly how each is administered.

KEY TERMS

amnesia
analgesia
anesthesia
anesthesiologist
anesthetist
capnography
general anesthesia
orthostatic hypotension
regional anesthesia
sedation
synergism

INTRODUCTION

Anesthesia refers to the absence of normal sensation. **Analgesia** refers to pain relief without producing anesthesia. The delivery of general anesthesia to prevent pain during surgery began in the United States in the 1800s. When surgeons began using anesthesia routinely, they soon realized the need for someone trained in its administration and turned to the nurses with whom they worked daily. Early nurse anesthetists were trained on the job by the surgeons with whom they worked.

Anesthesia is now a specialty of both nursing and medicine. Experienced registered nurses (RNs) with a baccalaureate degree can become certified registered nurse anesthetists (CRNAs) after completing two or more years of graduate education in nurse anesthesia. In November 2001, the Centers for Medicare and Medicaid Services (CMS) published an anesthesia care rule stating a governor could notify CMS of the desire to opt out of the federal physician supervision requirement for nurse anesthetists administering anesthesia to Medicare clients (AANA, 2000). Since then, 13 states have opted out of the supervision rule (AANA, 2005).

Today there are more than 37,000 CRNAs who administer more than 30 million anesthetics in the United States each year and are the only anesthesia providers in two-thirds of all the U.S. rural hospitals (AANA, 2009). CRNAs often work in groups with anesthesiologists.

An **anesthesiologist** is a licensed physician educated and skilled in the delivery of anesthesia who also adds to the knowledge of anesthesia through research or other scholarly pursuits. An **anesthetist** is a qualified RN, dentist, or physician who administers anesthetics.

Before administering an anesthetic, the anesthesia provider assesses the client's health status, discusses the risks and benefits of anesthesia with the client, and plans an anesthetic appropriate for the client and the surgical procedure. Surgical nurses prepare clients to talk with their anesthesia providers by encouraging them to ask any questions they have about anesthesia and the care they will receive.

The use of anesthesia is essential to the health and well-being of clients undergoing surgery. Although anesthesia prevents any sensation of pain, it also temporarily eliminates or diminishes the client's ability to control many essential physiologic functions such as respiration, heart rate, and temperature regulation. In addition to ensuring adequate levels of anesthesia throughout a surgical procedure, the anesthesia provider monitors and, when necessary, controls physiologic functions such as respiratory rate and blood pressure. Before the end of the surgery, the anesthesia provider administers appropriate medications to ensure that the client is comfortable when emerging from the anesthetic. Pain may be relieved with local anesthetic infiltration, opioid analgesics, or nonopioid analgesics.

PREANESTHETIC PREPARATION

Preparing a client for anesthesia and surgery is a cooperative effort involving the surgeon, the anesthesia provider, and the

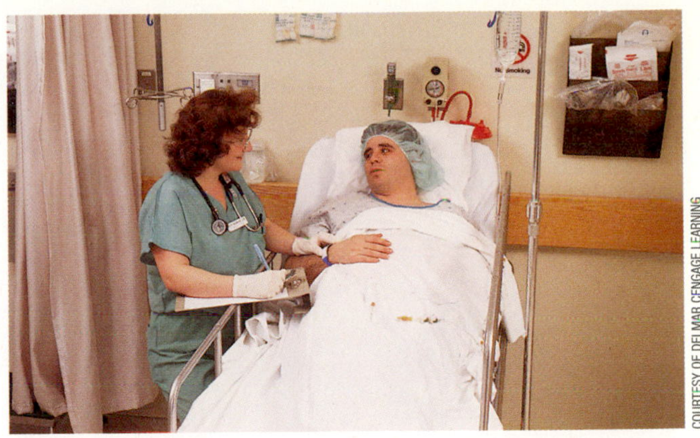

COURTESY OF DELMAR CENGAGE LEARNING

FIGURE 32-1 A nurse prepares a client for anesthesia and surgery.

nursing staff who cares for the client both before and after surgery (Figure 32-1). The client may undergo general (total body) anesthesia, where the control of body functions is temporarily lost; regional anesthesia, where a region of the body is made insensible to pain; or local anesthesia, where only a small area of the body is made insensible to pain.

ORAL INTAKE

Normally, only air should enter the trachea and lungs. The body prevents foreign material from entering the trachea by coughing forcefully when something other than air enters or by tightly closing the vocal cords to prevent entry of the foreign substance. Anyone who has ever drank something and had it go down the trachea knows how uncomfortable it is and how hard the body works to cough up the foreign substance.

General anesthesia removes a person's ability to guard the airway by coughing or closing the vocal cords. Passive regurgitation of stomach contents into the back of the throat can occur at any time during the delivery of general anesthesia. Aspiration of gastric contents into the lungs can cause significant illness or death. An important step in preventing aspiration of gastric contents is ensuring that the stomach is as empty as possible. In the past, adults have been instructed not to eat or drink anything for at least 8 hours before surgery and usually nothing past midnight the night before surgery. More recent information, however, strongly indicates that adults need not go without clear liquids for 8 or more hours before surgery; 2 hours are sufficient (ASA, 1999; ASA, 2007). In fact, the amount of liquid in a person's stomach at the time of surgery may actually be decreased if water is taken a couple of hours

CRITICAL THINKING

Physical Assessment and Anesthesia

What is the relevance of physical assessment and anesthesia?

LIFE SPAN CONSIDERATIONS

Anesthesia for Pediatric Clients

- Have a parent present when the anesthesiologist examines the child and performs the preoperative assessment.
- Explain the procedure at the child's level of understanding, such as "This mask will help you go to sleep for a while."
- Allow the child to play with a mask.

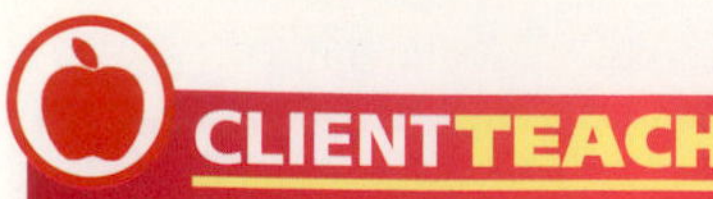

CLIENT TEACHING

Oral Intake Before Surgery

- Clearly explain to clients those things that they will or will not be allowed to eat or drink before surgery.
- Emphasize the need to exactly follow the instructions related to the time at which eating or drinking must cease before surgery.
- Discuss taking usual medications with doctor before surgery.

before surgery. Some anesthesia providers still prefer that their clients not have anything to eat or drink for at least 8 hours before surgery; others may allow water up to 2 hours before.

PREOPERATIVE MEDICATION

Most scheduled medications that a person receives while in the hospital or takes at home every day are continued until the time of surgery. Give oral medications with just enough water to swallow them, even when a client is having surgery first thing in the morning. The anesthesia provider usually writes orders specifying how the morning medication should be managed. Diabetic drugs and cardiovascular medications such as antihypertensives and heart medications are especially important for the client to receive.

Exceptions to the practice of continuing scheduled medications before surgery include administration of drugs such as insulin and oral antihyperglycemics, nonsteroidal anti-inflammatory drugs (NSAIDs) such as aspirin, and anticoagulants such as heparin or warfarin (Coumadin). Because food is withheld, giving insulin or oral antihyperglycemic drugs is likely to result in a dangerously low blood sugar level. The way insulin and glucose administration is handled depends on the severity of the client's disease and the preference of the physician and anesthesia provider. Anticoagulants and NSAIDs affect clotting. With some types of surgery, the bleeding caused by aspirin-like drugs or low-dose heparin is more likely. In some cases, no NSAIDs are allowed for 10 days to 2 weeks before surgery. In other circumstances, they are taken right up until surgery. Low-dose heparin or heparinoids may be given preoperatively to prevent postoperative thromboembolism, but higher doses of heparin and any dose of Coumadin is stopped before surgery to allow coagulation times to return to within normal ranges. Coumadin is usually stopped a week to 10 days before surgery and heparin within a few hours of surgery. Health care providers may order laboratory work the morning of surgery if the client takes anticoagulants to check the INR or PT for Coumadin and APTT or PTT levels for heparin.

Additional medications may be ordered to prepare the client for surgery or anesthesia. Surgeons often order prophylactic antibiotics. The anesthesia provider may order a sedative to help the client sleep the night before surgery or to ease the client's anxiety while waiting for surgery. Opioids like morphine or meperidine (Demerol) also are used for pain relief or to ease the induction of anesthesia. Atropine may be given to decrease oral secretions and prevent aspiration. Some anesthesia providers prefer to give preoperative medications in the operating room to precisely control the medication's effect on the client. This is especially true for very sick clients.

LIFE SPAN CONSIDERATIONS

Fasting: Infants and Small Children

Infants and small children have a high metabolic need and tolerate only short periods of fasting, 4 hours or less.

PROFESSIONAL TIP

Preanesthetic Care

- Health care providers explain the risks and benefits of anesthesia and the surgical procedure and have the client sign consent forms before they administer any preoperative medications. The client must be alert to sign consent forms.
- Complete the preoperative checklist.
- Make sure all preoperative orders are executed, especially those for blood tests, preoperative medications, and blood from the blood bank.
- Check, verify, and document the presence or absence of drug allergies for each client.
- Administer regular daily oral medications with a small sip of water as ordered.
- Remind the client of the importance of following instructions regarding any eating or drinking restrictions.
- Administer preoperative medications at the ordered time. Timing can be crucial to achieving the desired effect at the correct time.
- If the client responds abnormally to the preoperative medication, notify the anesthesia department immediately.
- Be sure the client's chart is complete when it goes to the operating room with the client. Recent diagnostic test results are especially important to include; otherwise, surgery may be delayed while these results are sought.
- Make sure the client's consents are in order and included in the chart when the client is transported to surgery.

CONSENT

Consent for anesthesia is usually obtained on the same form as is surgical consent, or a separate anesthesia consent form may be used instead of or in addition to the combined consent. In either case, for informed consent to be obtained, the anesthetic must be discussed with the client by someone with expert knowledge of anesthesia, usually an anesthesia provider or the surgeon.

SEDATION

Sedation refers to a reduction of stress, excitement, or irritability and involves some degree of central nervous system (CNS) depression. Sedation is used to decrease awareness of events, relieve anxiety, control the physiologic changes that often accompany anxiety, and ease the induction of general anesthesia. This is welcome news to many clients who fear local or regional anesthesia because they do not want to be awake and see and hear anything during surgery or a diagnostic procedure.

Different sedatives given in combination have a greater effect on the client than does any one of the sedatives given alone. This phenomenon is called **synergism**. The synergistic effect that occurs when different sedative drugs are administered together makes respiratory depression and unconsciousness more likely. In general, benzodiazepines (diazepam [Valium] and midazolam hydrochloride [Versed]) are better sedatives than are opioids (morphine and fentanyl citrate [Sublimaze]). If a client's anxiety is caused by pain, an opioid is a better choice of sedative because the opioid relieves the pain that caused the anxiety.

Sedative medications are administered based on the client's physical condition, weight, mental state, and the procedure being performed, with close observation of the effects of the drugs on the client.

The amount of sedation required by a client for comfort is always balanced with the amount of stimulation experienced as a result of pain or anxiety. Sedation and general anesthesia both involve CNS depression; thus sedation and anesthesia exist on a continuum. As sedation becomes deeper and deeper, it eventually becomes general anesthesia. Sometimes, the line between sedation and general anesthesia is very difficult to distinguish. When sedation becomes general anesthesia, all of the risks of general anesthesia are present, including airway obstruction, respiratory arrest, and aspiration of gastric contents. For this reason, all but the lightest sedation should be administered by an anesthetist or another provider skilled and experienced in airway assessment, protection, and management, as well as assessment of oxygenation and ventilation.

Sedation and Monitoring

Sedation is often used to alleviate client anxiety and discomfort during procedures performed under local anesthesia. Properly administered, local anesthetic injection blocks the painful stimulus of small incisions and minor surgical procedures; however, local anesthetic administration can cause significant discomfort because of edema and tissue irritation caused by the acidity of the local anesthetic solution. Most clients are uncomfortable knowing they are undergoing surgery and prefer to be less alert during the procedure. Procedural sedation (also known as moderate sedation and conscious sedation), decreases the client's perception of these physical and mental discomforts.

During local anesthesia and sedation, the client must remain conscious and in control of his own airway and breathing reflexes. Oversedation is likely to result in airway obstruction and places the client at risk for aspiration of gastric contents. Because sedatives are CNS depressants and, thus, respiratory depressants, give supplemental oxygen to clients during sedation. Monitoring during sedation is done through observation by an individual knowledgeable and experienced in the assessment of respiratory volume and airway patency.

The Joint Commission standards for monitoring clients undergoing procedural sedation require that the BP be measured at frequent and regular intervals and the heart rate and oxygenation be continually monitored by pulse oximetry. They also require the continual monitoring of respiratory rate and pulmonary ventilation. Cardiac rhythm for clients with significant cardiovascular disease or predisposition to dysrhythmias is monitored with an EKG (Joint Commission, 2009).

One method of monitoring pulmonary ventilation is **capnography** that measures a client's carbon dioxide concentration. The capnogram displays the CO_2 level as a waveform (Srinivasa & Kodali, 2008). The individual monitoring the client's breathing and vital signs is devoted to that task to the exclusion of any other duties.

Residual Effects of Sedation

Sedation usually persists beyond the duration of the surgical procedure. The length of time it takes to recover from sedation depends on the health of the client, the properties of the drugs used, other drugs the client may be taking, and the amount of sedative drugs administered.

Amnesia (the inability to remember things) produced by sedatives is commonly found even in clients who appear to be completely recovered. Such clients will probably not remember any instructions given to them during or soon after the procedure. Given that minor procedures and surgery are commonly performed on an outpatient basis, some clients may be discharged before regaining the ability to remember verbal instructions. All instructions should thus be given in writing and explained to the person responsible for taking the client home. Some facilities put the discharge instructions on a CD-ROM, DVD, or video for the client to take home and review.

If heavy sedation was used or the procedure ends suddenly, the client may remain significantly sedated after the procedure is over because the CNS stimulation ended while the CNS depressant effect of the sedative remains. The client is closely monitored until the effects of the sedative medications wear off enough for the client to wake and become oriented.

REGIONAL ANESTHESIA

In **regional anesthesia** a region of the body is temporarily rendered insensible to pain by injection of a local anesthetic. Local anesthetics are a class of drugs that temporarily block the transmission of small electrical impulses through nerves (Table 32-1). The duration of anesthesia produced by a local anesthetic depends on the drug used, the amount injected, and into which part of the body the drug is injected. The amount of insulation surrounding a nerve fiber, the anatomic location of the fiber, and the diameter of the fiber all influence the ease with which nerve impulses are blocked by local anesthetics.

Types of Regional Anesthesia

There are three types of regional anesthesia: local anesthesia, nerve blocks, and spinal and epidural blocks.

Local Anesthesia

Clinically, the use of local anesthetics to block nerves is identified by different names depending on the amount of local anesthetic used and where it is injected. When a small amount of local anesthetic drug is injected either into the

Table 32-1 Drugs Used For Sedation And Anesthesia

Local anesthetics	chloroprocaine (Nesacaine) procaine (Novocain) tetracaine (Pontocaine) bupivacaine (Marcaine) dibucaine (Nupercaine, Nupercainal) lidocaine (Xylocaine) prilocaine (Citanest)
General anesthetics	enflurane (Ethrane) halothane (Fluothane) isoflurane (Forane)
Intravenous anesthetics	methohexital sodium (Brevital) thiopental sodium (Pentothal) diazepam (Valium) midazolam hydrochloride (Versed) fentanyl citrate (Sublimaze)
Adjuncts to anesthesia	succinylcholine chloride (Anectine, Quelicin, Sucostrin) tubocurarine chloride (Tubocurarin)

Adapted from *Pharmacology for Nurses: A Pathophysiologic Approach*, by M. Adams, L. Holland, and P. Bostwick, 2008, Upper Saddle River, NJ: Pearson Prentice Hall.

skin and subcutaneous tissues around a cut or at the site of a needle puncture for a central line placement, it is called local anesthesia. The anesthetic is not aimed at a specific nerve; rather it anesthetizes all small superficial nerves in the target area. Local anesthesia is most commonly performed using lidocaine (Xylocaine) and lasts approximately 1 hour. Serious side effects of lidocaine (Xylocaine) are convulsions, respiratory depression, and dysrhythmias leading to cardiac arrest. Lidocaine with preservatives or epinephrine are used only for local anesthesia and never given for dysrhythmias (Adams, Holland, & Bostwick, 2008). Occasionally, for some types of plastic surgery, this type of anesthesia is used over a large area of the body. In this case, longer-acting local anesthetics are used. Because very small amounts of local anesthetics are generally used, the risk of local anesthetic toxicity is also small.

SAFETY

Preventing Choking and Aspiration

To prevent choking and aspiration after the use of an oral anesthetic solution (e.g., viscous lidocaine) or spray, fluids and foods must be withheld until the gag reflex returns.

Topical anesthesia, achieved with direct application of a local anesthetic to tissue, is desired in some situations (e.g., before insertion of an IV). The anesthetic takes the form of an ointment, lotion, solution, or spray.

Nerve Blocks

When a local anesthetic is injected more deeply into the body and/or is directed at a specific nerve or nerves, it is called a *nerve block*. Nerve blocks are often called by the name of the specific nerve or nerves they block. Examples include an ulnar nerve block in the arm or a brachial plexus block of all the nerves in the arm. Nerve blocks are often performed using lidocaine (Xylocaine), mepivacaine (Carbocaine), or bupivacaine (Marcaine) and may last from 1 to 12 hours.

Spinal and Epidural Blocks

Blocks also are identified according to where the local anesthetic is injected. One example is an *epidural block*, for which local anesthetic is injected into the epidural space near the spinal cord to anesthetize several spinal nerves at once. With spinal blocks (also called subarachnoid blocks), the local anesthetic is injected into the cerebrospinal fluid (CSF), where it can bathe uninsulated spinal nerves as they exit the spinal cord to the periphery of the body (Figure 32-2).

Spinal and epidural blocks are generally used to anesthetize a significant area of the body. They are capable of safely

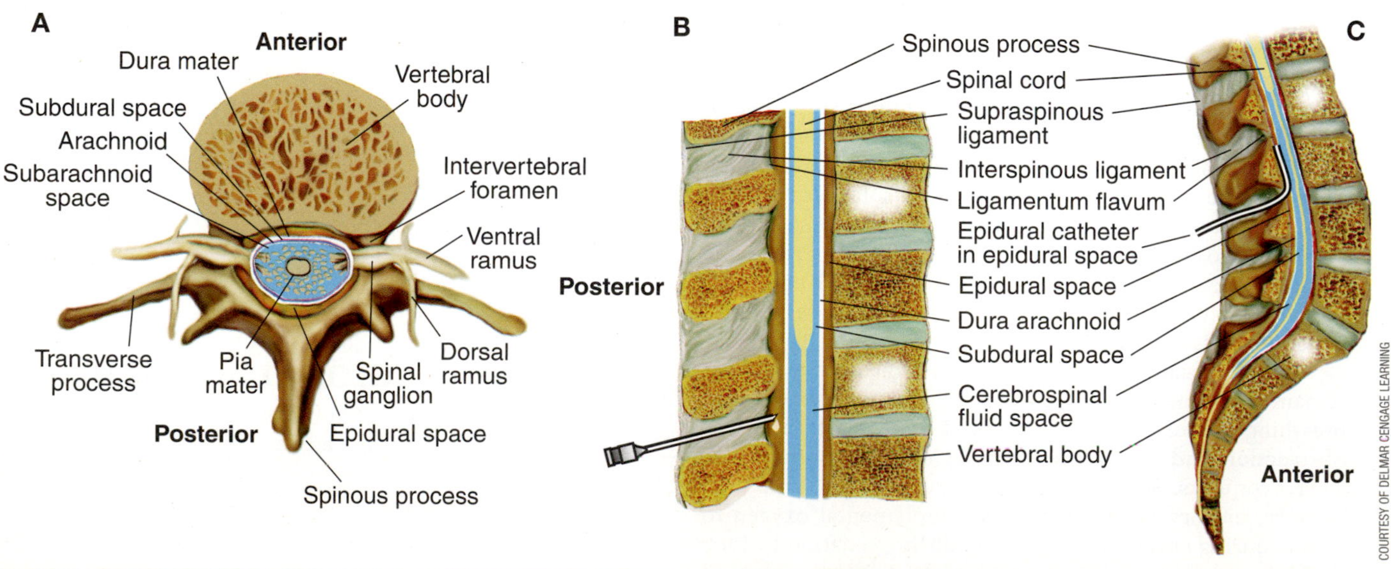

Figure 32-2 *A*, Cross-Sectional Anatomy of the Spine; *B*, Side View of Spinal Anatomy with the Tip of an Epidural Needle Placed in the Epidural Space; *C*, Side View of Spinal Anatomy with the Tip of an Epidural Catheter Placed in the Epidural Space

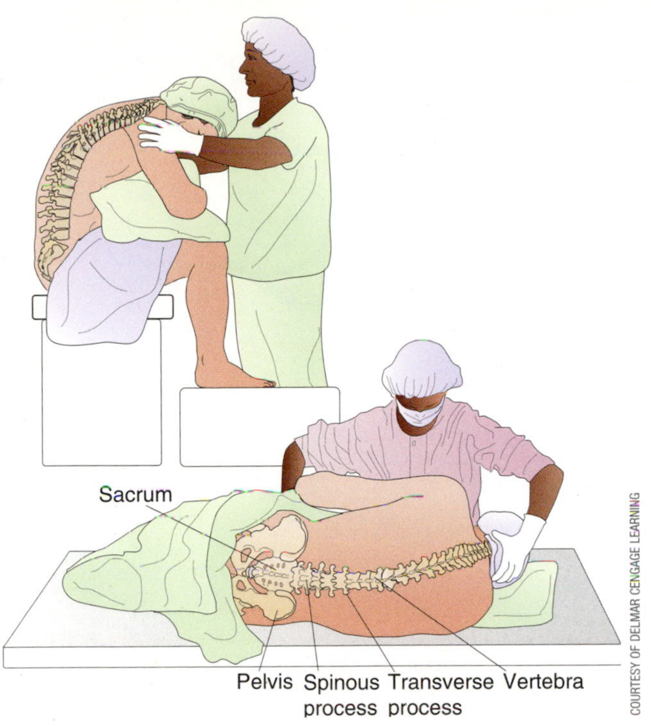

FIGURE 32-3 Correct positions for performing a spinal block or inserting an epidural catheter into the lumbar area. The assistance of trained personnel is crucial to the proper positioning, reassurance, and safety of the client.

producing anesthesia sufficient for surgery in the abdomen, pelvis, perineum, or lower extremities. When an epidural block is performed, a catheter is usually inserted into the epidural space, making it possible to inject additional doses of drug. The client must either be sitting in a bent-over position or lying on the side with head and knees as close together as possible (Figure 32-3). Either position separates the vertebra, making insertion of the needle or catheter possible. Epidural blocks have an added advantage in that by varying the way the anesthetic is used, the block can produce analgesia (pain relief without producing anesthesia), complete anesthesia, and even profound muscular relaxation (needed for some types of surgery). This allows epidural anesthesia to be used not only for surgical procedures, but also for analgesia during labor and for postoperative pain relief.

Spinal blocks are most often performed using lidocaine (Xylocaine) or bupivacaine (Marcaine) and last from 1 to 3 hours. Epidural blocks are most commonly performed using bupivacaine (Marcaine), and the block can be continued as long as local anesthetic is injected through the catheter into the epidural space.

Opioids such as morphine and fentanyl citrate (Sublimaze) may be added to the local anesthetic in either of these blocks to intensify the analgesic or anesthetic effect, or to provide postoperative pain relief after the block has worn off.

One type of complication is peculiar to spinal and epidural regional anesthetics. When CSF leaks out through a hole made in the dural membrane during performance of a subarachnoid block or an accidental dural puncture during the attempted performance of an epidural block, a postdural puncture headache (PDPH) may result. The headache is caused by the loss of CSF from around the brain. The headache is relieved by lying down and returns when the individual sits up or stands. Pain commonly occurs in both the front and the back of the head and is sometimes accompanied by neck and shoulder stiffness. Photophobia or double vision may be present with severe headache. The onset of the headache is usually not immediate and may take 1 to 2 days to become bothersome. Treatment involves adequate hydration to allow the normal production of CSF; analgesics; and bed rest in a supine position. One treatment for significant or persistent PDPH is a procedure called an epidural blood patch, which involves injecting 15 to 20 mL of the client's own blood into the epidural space. Once the blood clots, it plugs the hole in the dural membrane. Another treatment involves connecting an IV infusion to the epidural catheter to replace the lost CSF and treat the headache.

RESIDUAL EFFECTS OF REGIONAL ANESTHESIA

All anesthetics wear off as the drug responsible for causing the anesthesia is removed, metabolized, and eliminated. Some effects wear off faster than others. The client may be wide awake and able to carry on a conversation but have residual effects that are not detected by casual observation. Motor, sensory and sympathetic residual block effects are common.

Residual Motor Block

A motor block is a temporary condition caused when local anesthetic blocks nerves that carry instructions to skeletal muscles telling them to contract. Motor block results in the inability to move a body part and is usually the last effect to develop and the first to wear off. It results only when the regional block is very dense and complete.

A complete motor block results in a temporary paralysis, with the client being incapable of moving the blocked part despite tremendous effort. With a complete motor block, there is usually no function in any other type of nerve in the same area. A client with a complete motor block of any part of the body would not likely be released from the recovery area. Clients experiencing residual (incomplete) motor block may be released from recovery. A client who has had any type of block involving the legs is not allowed to get out of bed without assistance until it is demonstrated that a complete recovery of motor strength in the legs is regained. Even a small amount of residual motor block greatly increases the possibility that a client will fall.

As a regional block begins to wear off, motor function begins to return first, sensation begins to return next, and sympathetic nervous function returns last. Motor function and sensation is detected easily by asking the client to move the blocked part or by touching the skin and asking the client whether it feels normal. The return of sympathetic function is more difficult to detect. Orthostatic hypotension may occur even after motor and sensory functions have completely returned and the regional block appears to have worn off. To prevent fainting, the nurse assists the client in getting out of bed until she is able to do so without any dizziness or significant decrease in blood pressure.

Residual Sensory Block

Normal sensation may not have returned completely upon client discharge from the recovery area. As the regional block wears off, sensation returns gradually. As sensation begins to return, the client experiences a "pins-and-needles" feeling in an arm or leg that has been blocked and may feel touch or pressure before recovering complete sensation. Until complete recovery of normal sensation, any blocked areas are frequently checked and carefully protected, as the client may be unaware that a finger or hand, for example, is being pinched or denied blood supply.

Residual Sympathetic Block

The last nerve fibers to recover as a local anesthetic wears off are those responsible for carrying instructions to the muscles that surround blood vessels. When these sympathetic nerves are blocked, veins and arteries dilate, lowering the blood pressure. The venous system has a large capacity, and venous dilation results in the pooling of a large amount of blood. This decreases the amount of blood that returns to the heart, and the blood pressure falls. The amount of blood that pools is greatest in parts of the body that are farthest below the level of the heart. Even in a client who has had a spinal or epidural block and is lying supine, a significant amount of venous pooling occurs, resulting in lower-than-normal blood pressure. If the same client is allowed to sit up, even more venous pooling will occur, less blood will return to the heart, and blood pressure will fall substantially. This phenomenon of having a large drop in blood pressure when sitting up or standing is called **orthostatic hypotension**. *Orthostatic* signifies that it involves body position, and hypotension means low blood pressure. Clients who have had a spinal or epidural block are more likely to have orthostatic hypotension the higher in the spinal column the level of their block.

GENERAL ANESTHESIA

General anesthesia involves unconsciousness, complete insensibility to pain, amnesia, motionlessness, and muscle relaxation. With general anesthesia, the body also loses the ability to control many important functions, including the abilities to maintain an airway, control vital functions such as breathing and heart rate, and regulate temperature. These functions are controlled by the anesthesia provider during administration of general anesthesia.

General anesthesia involves four overlapping stages: induction (going to sleep), maintenance, emergence (waking up), and recovery.

Induction and Airway Management

The induction of general anesthesia is a short but critical period during which the client is rendered unconscious, vital functions are controlled, and enough anesthetic drug is introduced into the body to keep the client asleep during surgery. In adults, drugs are usually injected into an IV line to quickly produce unconsciousness, and additional anesthetic is then inhaled (Table 32-1).

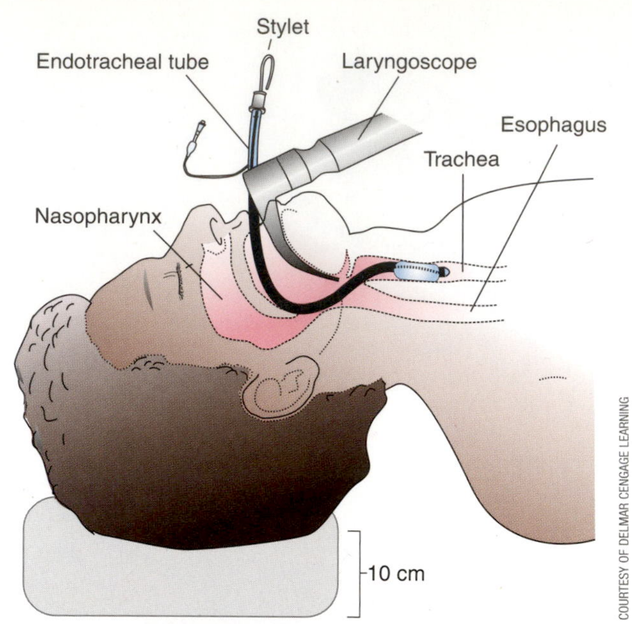

FIGURE 32-4 Placing an Endotracheal Tube in the Trachea with Direct Visualization by Laryngoscopy

Immediately after the induction of general anesthesia, the anesthesia provider secures the airway using a cuffed endotracheal tube (ETT) (Figure 32-4). An ETT provides a breathing passage from outside the client to within the client's trachea.

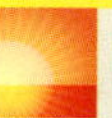

LIFE SPAN CONSIDERATIONS

Induction of Anesthesia in Small Children

Inhalation of an anesthetic vapor is used first, then an IV line is started and additional IV drugs are administered.

Maintenance

General anesthesia is maintained with some combination of IV and inhaled drugs. Figure 32-5 shows a client connected to an anesthesia machine by a breathing circuit.

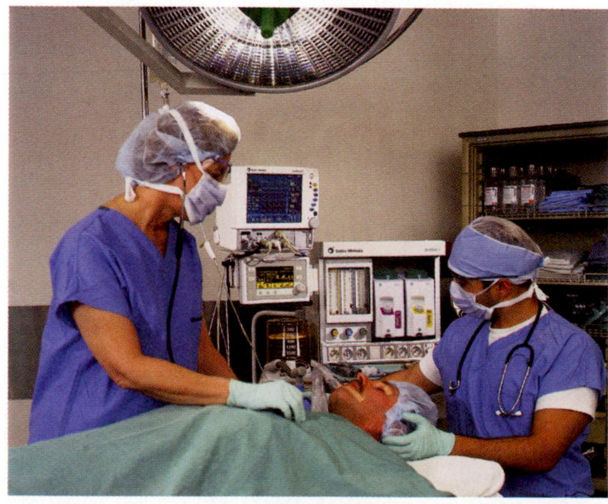

FIGURE 32-5 A typical anesthesia machine is a complex equipment set. This machine has anesthetic vaporizers and flowmeters to deliver oxygen, nitrous oxide, and air. It also supports a ventilator and equipment to monitor ventilation, oxygen content of inspired gas, client oxygen saturation, blood pressure, heart rate, and respiration. (Pictured above is the Datex-Ohmeda Aestiva/5 Anesthesia Delivery System equipped with a Cardiocap/5 Monitor.) (*Reprinted with permission of Datex-Ohmeda, Inc.*)

Skeletal Muscle Relaxation

Some types of surgery require complete relaxation of skeletal muscles. In these cases, the anesthesia provider administers a skeletal muscle relaxant such as pancuronium bromide (Pavulon) or vecuronium bromide (Norcuron) to completely paralyze the client. These types of drugs prevent clients from breathing on their own, requiring the anesthesia provider to ventilate clients during surgery. Paralysis is eliminated before emergence from anesthesia so the client can breathe independently again.

Inadequate reversal of paralysis presents as anything from total skeletal muscle paralysis to the inability of the client to cough and clear the airway. If the client is having difficulty breathing, basic life support is provided until the arrival of an anesthesia provider.

EMERGENCE

Emergence from general anesthesia occurs when anesthetic drugs are allowed to wear off. The anesthesia provider carefully controls the timing and amount of anesthetic drug given in order for the client to emerge from general anesthesia at the desired time. The initial phase of emergence is usually quite quick, allowing the client to awaken enough to respond to verbal directions and maintain an airway. After this time, the client's breathing tube usually is removed, and the client is taken to the postanesthesia care unit (recovery room). If, for some reason, the client is left on a ventilator and with a breathing tube in place, the anesthesia provider takes the client to an intensive care unit asleep instead of waking the client up from the anesthetic.

RECOVERY

Recovery from general anesthesia is not complete simply because the client has regained consciousness. The client may not remember what has happened for minutes or even hours after receiving an anesthetic. The ability to think clearly often takes longer to return, with some residual thinking difficulty persisting for several days or even weeks. Inhalation anesthetics are eliminated from the body through the lungs, and very small amounts of anesthetic are still being exhaled for several weeks. Many anesthetic drugs are stored in body fat and released back into the bloodstream very slowly after anesthetic administration has ended. The speed of this release depends on the amount of anesthetic given during the surgery, the length of the surgery, and how deeply the client is breathing.

> **LIFE SPAN CONSIDERATIONS**
>
> **Oxygenation and Ventilation in the Elderly Client**
>
> - Impaired mobility allows secretions to pool in the lungs. Therefore, elderly clients must be monitored more closely, and secretions suctioned.
> - Most anesthetic agents cause decreased respiratory rate and decreased tidal volume, putting elderly clients at greater risk for hypoventilation.

Oxygenation and Ventilation

Almost all anesthetics are respiratory depressants. Benzodiazepines, opioids, and inhalation anesthetic agents have significant respiratory depressant effects. Any one of these drugs may be used in a dose that causes apnea, or lack of respirations for more than 10 seconds, during a general anesthesia. When used in combination their effect on respiration is at least additive. When the rate or depth of respirations decrease, the elimination of carbon dioxide is retarded, and carbon dioxide builds up in the blood and in the lungs. Oxygen saturation is monitored by pulse oximetry. Even small amounts of supplemental oxygen given to a client whose rate or depth of breathing is decreased adds significantly to the amount of oxygen in the bloodstream. This is the most important reason that oxygen is given to even healthy clients when they are recovering from general anesthesia.

Heart Rate and Blood Pressure

Few direct effects on heart rate (HR) and blood pressure (BP) regulation are seen during recovery from general anesthesia. Some anesthetic techniques that are heavily based on opioids, such as fentanyl citrate (Sublimaze) or sufentanil citrate (Sufenta), can cause a slow HR, but as long as BP is maintained, no specific treatment is necessary. Although most general anesthetics are myocardial depressants, the depressive effects of current agents are mild, especially after anesthetic administration is ended.

Most HR and BP changes seen during recovery result from factors related indirectly to the anesthetic. Both HR and BP increase as a result of sympathetic stimulation. Pain, hypoxia, and fear can all result in sympathetic stimulation with an increase in HR and BP. Discovering and addressing the source of the client's fear often reduces the anxiety. When the causes of sympathetic stimulation are addressed, HR and BP should normalize.

Temperature Regulation and Shivering

With general anesthesia, the body loses its natural ability to regulate temperature. General anesthetic agents dilate the blood vessels close to the surface of the body, exposing the client's warm blood to the cool exterior. During anesthetization, the client is mostly uncovered in a cold operating room, and the body's surgical area is cleaned with cold solutions. After this is done, the client's insulating covering (skin and subcutaneous fat) is cut open to expose the warm interior of the body and allow its heat to escape. Room temperature intravenous (IV) fluids are infused into the veins, and the client breathes cool gases. Surgical clients lose a great amount of heat at a time when the body is least able to respond to warm the tissues. Hypothermia adds to the CNS depression resulting from any residual anesthetics. Surface warming with a forced-air warming blanket is an effective way to increase the temperature of a client intraoperatively and when recovering from general anesthesia; warm cloth blankets also maintain body warmth. Figure 32-6 shows use of a forced-air warming blanket.

All potent inhalation agents are associated with shivering during emergence from general anesthesia when the blood level of the anesthetic agent is very low. The cause of the shivering is not clear but does not appear to be related to the client's body temperature. (Of course, postoperative clients

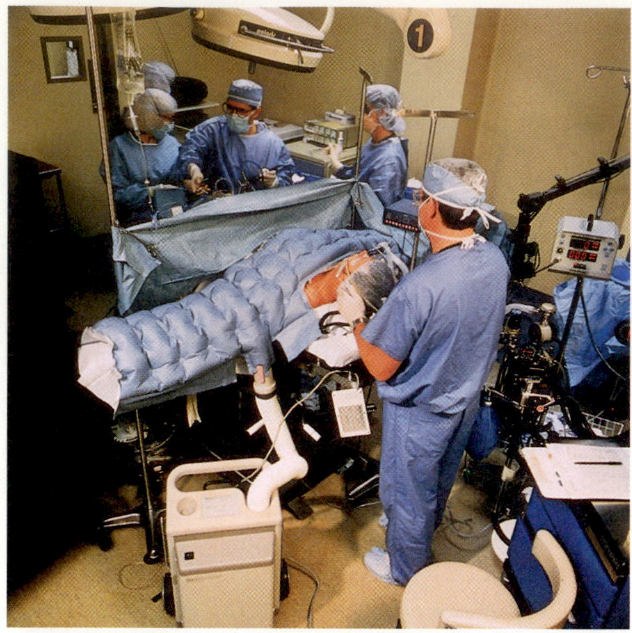

FIGURE 32-6 **A forced-air warming blanket applied to the upper abdomen, chest, and arms or lower torso of a client during surgery. The unit on the floor to the left of the anesthesia provider (foreground) is the heating unit, which contains a fan that pushes warm air through the hose and into the blanket, much like a furnace pushes warm air through heating ducts and into a house. Warm air exits hundreds of pinholes on the surface of the blanket and next to the client. (*Courtesy of Mallinckrodt Medical, Inc.*)**

also shiver when they are cold.) The key to eliminating shivering postoperatively is to ensure client warmth and encourage deep breathing so that the anesthetic is eliminated as quickly as possible.

Fluid Balance

Surgical procedures and the injuries that necessitate them have major effects on the body's distribution of fluid. Appropriate care during anesthesia sometimes necessitates the delivery of a large volume of IV fluid. This IV fluid does not stay in the vascular system long, moving out of the vascular space to replace losses from the interstitial and intracellular spaces.

Trauma, whether caused by an accidental injury or a surgical incision, results in fluid losses or shifts in three general areas as follows: direct blood loss, evaporation through the surgical wound, and fluid shifts. Large volumes of fluid are lost to the air through the surgical wound, especially during abdominal procedures. A major abdominal procedure, for example, can result in the loss of up to 10 mL/kg/hour of fluid by evaporation.

CRITICAL THINKING

Client Monitoring After Anesthesia

Why must clients be monitored very closely after receiving an anesthetic?

POSTOPERATIVE PAIN MANAGEMENT

Pain has many causes. Postoperative pain results from tissue injury, release of local and hormonal substances, inflammation, mental outlook, and, perhaps, neural hyperexcitability related to excessive noxious input. As such, baseline postoperative pain, pain from pressure placed on an incision, and pain from client movement each respond best to different pain-relieving strategies.

The amount of medication needed to relieve pain depends on the intensity and type of pain, the size of the client, and the client's age. The opioid dose for an elderly client is started at 25–50% of the usual adult dose and then slowly increased by 25–50% increments until the client reports a mild pain level (McDonald, 2006). The opioid of choice for elderly is morphine with hydromorphone hydrochloride (Dilaudid) as the second choice (McDonald, 2006). Monitor the elderly closely for opioid toxicity on a pain scale they understand.

PATIENT-CONTROLLED ANALGESIA

Patient-controlled analgesia (PCA) allows clients to self-administer pain medication by pushing a button when they experience pain. After an IV catheter is in place, a client-controlled analgesia pump is connected "piggyback" to the IV line. The pump is programmed to deliver a predetermined dose of morphine, hydromorphone hydrochloride (Dilaudid), or fentanyl citrate (Sublimaze) when the client pushes a button. It will not, however, deliver unlimited amounts. A set time must pass between each successive dose, and when the total dose of opioid delivered in any hour reaches a preset limit, the pump will not deliver any more medicine until the next hour. This is referred to as lockout.

Properly programmed, PCA allows the client a great deal of control over when pain medicine is received, which is likely to help decrease anxiety. Patient-controlled analgesia also results in a shorter interval between the need for pain medicine and its administration, better pain relief than that obtained with intermittent IM injections, and a reduction in nursing time necessary for the delivery of pain medicine. It does not, however, decrease the need for client assessment of pain while the PCA machine is in use.

REGIONAL ANALGESIA

Regional analgesia and anesthesia have many applications in the relief of postoperative pain. Regional anesthetics do not cease working when the surgery ends and provide pain relief for a variable period of time afterward. The duration of postoperative pain relief can be extended by continuing the infusion of pain medication into the epidural space or by adding opioids to either epidural or spinal anesthetics.

Local Anesthetics

Local anesthetics, either alone or in combination with opioids, are administered into the epidural space at low concentrations that do not cause complete anesthesia. This type of pain relief is most commonly used for women in labor who receive epidural analgesia. Local anesthetic in low concentrations is

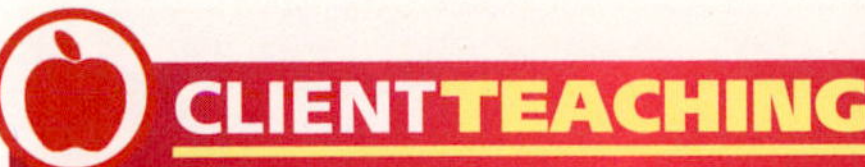

Patient-Controlled Analgesia (PCA)

- Only the client should push the button to administer more analgesic.
- The client should not ask visitors to push the button.

a powerful analgesic. If local anesthetic is administered in a way to relieve pain in the lower extremities, clients are usually confined to bed, because even dilute concentrations of local anesthetic may affect the strength of leg muscles enough to increase the risk of falling. Clients receiving analgesia via an epidural block are watched carefully to ensure that they do not develop pressure necrosis in the blocked areas.

Opioids

The spinal cord has receptors for opioids, and when opioids are added to a spinal or epidural anesthetic, they provide pain relief even after the anesthetic block has worn off. Morphine added to a spinal or epidural anesthetic provides hours of postoperative pain relief, often enough so that no other pain medication is needed; it may even provide better pain relief than do IM injections or intravenous PCA. Opioids are added to spinal or epidural anesthetics as a single dose or be infused into the epidural space postoperatively. Although spinal and epidural morphine provide excellent pain relief, they may also produce significant respiratory depression. Fortunately, the respiratory depression after spinal or epidural morphine administration is rarely rapid in onset. Respiratory depression is very rare with properly dosed epidural or spinal fentanyl citrate (Sublimaze). With current client selection and dosing protocols, life-threatening respiratory depression is a rare event. When it does occur, it can be detected long before it causes harm, by observing the client frequently, noting respiratory rate and depth, and periodically measuring oxygen saturation by pulse oximetry.

PROFESSIONAL TIP

Postanesthetic Care

- Immediately report to the anesthesia provider or surgeon any client breathing difficulty or a respiratory rate of 12 breaths per minute or less.
- Immediately report to the surgeon or the anesthesia department a fall in the client's BP or increase in HR.
- Verify client's ability to stand or walk with normal motor strength and coordination and without any dizziness before allowing the client to get up without assistance.
- Do not allow clients to rub their eyes. Clients who are still drowsy may try to rub out protective eye moisturizer and, in the process, cause painful corneal abrasions.
- Observe clients immediately and hourly for bladder distention. Both regional and general anesthesia can sometimes cause temporary urinary retention.
- If clients have an epidural catheter for postoperative pain management, ensure that they change positions from time to time to prevent pressure necrosis. Do not allow the lateral aspect of the leg to rest on the side rails.
- Report to the anesthesia department as soon as possible any headache that gets worse when the client sits up or stands.
- Before giving discharge instructions, verify that the client's ability to remember instructions has returned. Always share discharge instructions with the individual responsible for taking the client home and provide the client with a written copy of the instructions.

CASE STUDY

C.P. is in the recovery room after outpatient surgery. She received a general anesthetic and is now awake, breathing deeply, and talking to the staff. She has received morphine sulfate intravenously and is quite comfortable. Before being discharged home from the surgery center, C.P. rests in an easy chair in the transitional recovery area. The nurse taking care of her notices that she asks questions about things that have already been discussed and has even asked one question three times.

The following questions will guide your development of a nursing care plan for the case study.

1. After making these observations, what nursing diagnoses and goals might the nurse identify for C.P.?
2. List nursing interventions in caring for C.P.
3. Identify teaching approaches.

SUMMARY

- In addition to ensuring an adequate level of anesthesia throughout a surgical procedure, the anesthesia provider monitors and controls physiologic functions.
- Some anesthesia providers prefer that clients not have anything to eat or drink for at least 8 hours before surgery. Others allow water up to 2 hours before surgery.
- Most scheduled medications that a client takes every day are continued up to and including the morning of surgery.
- Sedation depresses brain activity, decreasing awareness, reducing anxiety, and easing the induction of general anesthesia.
- Oversedation results in respiratory depression, which can cause airway obstruction, and places the client at risk for aspiration of gastric contents.
- Regional anesthesia by the injection of a local anesthetic temporarily renders a "region" of the body insensible to pain.
- General anesthesia produces unconsciousness, complete insensibility to pain, amnesia, motionlessness, and muscle relaxation.
- A person is unlikely to remember what has happened for minutes to hours after sedation or a general anesthetic.
- Intravenous patient-controlled analgesia (PCA) allows clients to self-administer pain medication by pushing a button on the PCA machine. Limits are programmed into the machine to prevent overdose.
- Local anesthetics, alone or in combination with opioids, can be injected into the epidural space at low concentrations to provide postoperative analgesia.
- Spinal and epidural morphine can produce dangerous respiratory depression. This can be detected by frequent observations of the client's respiratory rate and depth and by periodic measurement of oxygen saturation via pulse oximetry.

REVIEW QUESTIONS

1. Clients are at risk for aspiration of gastric contents into the lungs when receiving a general anesthetic because:
   1. general anesthesia causes stomach distention.
   2. general anesthesia eliminates protective airway reflexes.
   3. gastric peristalsis is reversed during general anesthesia.
   4. vomiting normally occurs during general anesthesia.

2. The most dangerous result of oversedation is:
   1. lack of response to verbal directions.
   2. longer recovery time and resultant delayed discharge.
   3. prolonged amnesia.
   4. inability to breathe adequately.

3. What is a sign that a client has a postdural puncture headache following a spinal or epidural regional block?
   1. The headache subsides after intake of plenty of liquids.
   2. The headache begins after the surgical procedure.
   3. The headache worsens when the client sits up or stands.
   4. The client is confused in addition to having a headache.

4. After cessation of a general anesthetic, how long might it be before the client can think as clearly as before the client received the anesthetic?
   1. Before being discharged from the recovery room.
   2. Within 2 hours.
   3. Six hours.
   4. Several days.

5. What effect might a spinal or epidural anesthetic block still have after normal sensation and motor function have returned?
   1. Decrease in pulse rate when the client is lying in bed.
   2. Decrease in blood pressure when the client stands up.
   3. Inhibition of protective airway reflexes.
   4. Sore muscles.

6. A client returned from surgery and has a PCA for pain. The main purpose of the PCA is:
   1. the client controls pain medication administration.
   2. so the nurse does not have to stop caring for another client to administer medication to the client in pain.
   3. better pain relief for the client than intermittent IM injections.
   4. less time needed to assess the client's pain level.

7. A client is given fentanyl citrate (Sublimaze) with a spinal anesthetic for pain relief. To adequately assess the client for respiratory depression the nurse: (Select all that apply.)
   1. notes respiratory rate and depth.
   2. observes the color the mucous membranes.
   3. measures oxygen saturation with a pulse oximeter on a regular basis.
   4. monitors the client's ventilation by capnography.
   5. checks apical and peripheral pulses.
   6. observes symmetry of chest wall movements and use of accessory muscles.

8. A client had a regional anesthesia. During postoperative care, the nurse assesses for residual effects of the anesthesia by: (Select all that apply.)
   1. asking the client questions and listening to his responses.

2. asking the client to move an area blocked by the anesthesia.
3. touching the client's legs and asking if the touch feels normal.
4. assisting the client to a sitting position and asking if she is dizzy.
5. assessing the client's mental alertness.
6. assessing the motor strength in her legs.

9. A client has a nonunion fracture of the fifth phalange and is having a nerve block as the anesthesia. What client statement indicates to the nurse that more teaching is needed about the anesthesia and scheduled procedure?
   1. I may be awake but sleepy throughout the surgery.
   2. I will not be able to move my lower arm during surgery.
   3. I will not have any painful feeling in my lower arm or hand during surgery.
   4. I will be unconscious and put to sleep prior to and during the surgery.
10. The main priority of the anesthesia provider during a general anesthetic is monitoring the:
   1. blood pressure at frequent intervals.
   2. oxygenation by pulse oximetry.
   3. respiratory rate and pulmonary ventilation.
   4. cardiac rhythm by an EKG.

REFERENCES/SUGGESTED READINGS

Adams, M., Holland, L., & Bostwick, P. (2008). *Pharmacology for nurses: A pathophysiologic approach.* Upper Saddle River, N.J.: Pearson Prentice Hall.

American Association of Nurse Anesthetists (AANA). (2001). Administration puts politics before patients; Implements cumbersome anesthesia care rule. Retrieved on April 2, 2009 at http://www.aana.com/Advocacy.aspx?ucNavMenu_TSMenuTargetID=49&ucNavMenu_TSMenuTargetType=4&ucNavMenu_TSMenuID=6&id=2575&terms=administration+puts+politics+before+patients%3a+implements+cumbersome+anesthesia+care+rule

American Association of Nurse Anesthetists (AANA). (2002). New Hampshire becomes fifth state to opt out of federal anesthesia requirement. Retrieved on April 2, 2009 at http://www.aana.com/news.aspx?ucNavMenu_TSMenuTargetID=171&ucNavMenu_TSMenuTargetType=4&ucNavMenu_TSMenuID=6&id=690&terms=opt+out

American Association of Nurse Anesthetists (AANA). (2005). *Governor Rounds removes physician supervision for South Dakota CRNAs.* Retrieved on March 31, 2009 at http://www.aana.com/news.aspx?ucNavMenu_TSMenuTargetID=62&ucNavMenu_TSMenuTargetType=4&ucNavMenu_TSMenuID=6&id=854&terms=opt+out

American Association of Nurse Anesthetists (AANA). (2008). Education of nurse anesthetists in the United States–At a glance. Retrieved on March 31, 2009 at http://www.aana.com/BecomingCRNA.aspx?ucNavMenu_TSMenuTargetID=18&ucNavMenu_TSMenuTargetType=4&ucNavMenu_TSMenuID=6&id=1018

American Association of Nurse Anesthetists (AANA). (2009). Qualifications and capabilities of the certified registered nurse anesthetist. Retrieved on March 31, 2009 at http://www.aana.com/BecomingCRNA.aspx?ucNavMenu_TSMenuTargetID=102&ucNavMenu_TSMenuTargetType=4&ucNavMenu_TSMenuID=6&id=112

American Society of Anesthesiologists (ASA). (1999). 1998 House of delegates passes two new practice guidelines. Retrieved on March 31, 2009 at http://www.asahq.org/Newsletters/1999/02_99/1998_0299.html

American Society of Anesthesiologists (ASA). (2007). Revised guidelines issued for anesthesia, pain relief during labor and delivery. Retrieved on March 31, 2009 at http://www.asahq.org/news/asanews040207.htm

Berkowitz, C. (1997). Epidural pain control—Your job, too. *RN,* 60(8), 22–27.

Carroll, P. (2002). Procedural sedation: Capnography's heightened role. *RN,* 65(10), 54–62.

Clinical News. (1999). "NPO after midnight" outdated? *AJN,* 99(2), 18.

Connolly, M. (1999). Postdural puncture headache. *AJN,* 99(11), 48–49.

Crenshaw, J. (1999). New guidelines for preoperative fasting. *AJN,* 99(4), 49.

Joint Commission. (2009). Standards for operative or other high-risk procedures and/or the administration of moderate or deep sedation or anesthesia. Retrieved on April 1, 2009 at http://www.jointcommission.org/NR/rdonlyres/6530941D-98AD-4AC7-8944-9DDE1116E503/0/OBS_Standards_Sampler_2007_final.pdf

Joint Commission Resources. Joint Commission on Accreditation of Healthcare Organizations. (2000). New definitions, revised standards address the continuum of sedation and anesthesia. *Joint Commission Perspectives,* 20(4), 10.

Kodali, B. (2008). Capnograms during procedural sedation. Retrieved on April 1, 2009 at http://www.capnography.com/new/index.php?option=com_contetn&view=article&id+245&

Kost, M. (1999). Conscious sedation: Guarding your patient against complications. *Nursing99,* 29(4), 34–39.

Kreger, C. (2001). Spinal anesthesia and analgesia. *Nursing2001,* 31(6), 36–41.

McDonald, D. (2006). Postoperative pain management for the aging patient. *Geriatrics Aging,* 9(6), 395-398.

Messinger, J., Hoffman, L., O'Donnell, J., & Dunworth, B. (1999). Getting conscious sedation right. *AJN, 99*(12), 44–49.

O'Donnell, T., Bragg, K., & Sell, S. (2003). Procedural sedation: Safely navigating the twilight zone. *Nursing2003,* 33(4), 36–41, 44.

Pasero, C., & McCaffery, M. (1999). Providing epidural analgesia. *Nursing99, 29*(8), 34–39.

Scott, J., & Stanski, D. (1987). Decreased fentanyl and alfentanil dose requirements with age: A simultaneous pharmacokinetic and pharmacodynamic evaluation. *Journal of Pharmacology and Experimental Therapeutics,* 240, 159–166.

Srinivasa, V., & Kodali, B. (2008). Applications of capnography. Retrieved on November 6, 2009 at http://www.capnography.com/outside/sedation.htm

Wong, D. (2003). Topical local anesthetics. *AJN,* 103(6), 42–45.

Woomer, J., & Berkheimer, D. (2003). Using capnography to monitor ventilation. *Nursing2003,* 33(4), 42–43.

RESOURCES

American Association of Nurse Anesthetists, http://www.aana.com

American Society of Anesthesiologists, http://www.asahq.org

American Society of Peri Anesthesia Nurses, http://www.aspan.org

American Society of Regional Anesthesia and Pain Medicine, http://www.asra.com

Anesthesia Patient Safety Foundation, http://www.gasnet.org/societies/apsf/

Foundation for Anesthesia Education and Research, http://www.faer.org

Society for Education in Anesthesia, http://www.seahq.org

CHAPTER 33
Surgery

MAKING THE CONNECTION

Refer to the following chapters to increase your understanding of perioperative nursing:

Basic Nursing

- ***Legal and Ethical Responsibilities***
- ***Communication***
- ***Cultural Considerations***
- ***Fluid, Electrolyte, and Acid–Base Balance***
- ***Assessment***
- ***Pain Management***

Adult Health Nursing

- ***Anesthesia***
- ***Respiratory System***
- ***Cardiovascular System***
- ***Musculoskeletal System***
- ***Integumentary System***

Basic Procedures

- ***Hand Hygiene***
- ***Transferring from Bed to Stretcher***
- ***Applying Antiembolic Stockings***

Intermediate Procedures

- ***Postoperative Exercise Instruction***

Advanced Procedures

- ***Removing Skin Sutures and Staples***

LEARNING OBJECTIVES

Upon completion of this chapter, you should be able to:

- Define key terms.
- List risk factors in a preoperative nursing assessment.
- List information in a general teaching plan for a preoperative client.
- Identify common nursing care for the preoperative, intraoperative, and postoperative phases.
- Describe the principles of asepsis and their application to nursing practice.
- Discuss nursing interventions to prevent or treat postoperative complications.
- Identify information needed by the postoperative client before discharge.
- Discuss the physiologic changes of aging that affect the elderly client's response to surgery.
- Plan care for a postoperative client.

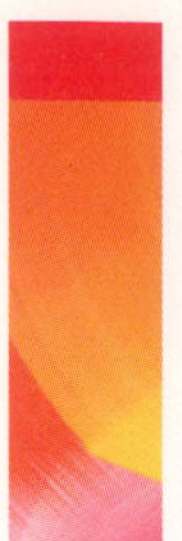

KEY TERMS

Aldrete Score
ambulatory surgery
asepsis
aseptic technique
circulating nurse
dehiscence
evisceration
first assistant
informed consent
intraoperative phase
perioperative
postoperative phase
preoperative phase
scrub nurse
sterile
sterile conscience
sterile field
surgery

INTRODUCTION

Surgery refers to the treatment of injury, disease, or deformity through invasive operative methods. Surgery is a unique experience, with no two clients responding alike to similar operations. Even the same client may respond differently to two separate surgical situations or to the same surgery performed at a later time. Surgery is a major stressor for every client. To a client, there is no such thing as minor surgery; anxiety and fear are normal. Surgery, even when planned well in advance, is a stressor that produces both psychological (anxiety, fear) and physiologic (neuroendocrine) stress reactions. Surgery is a stressful experience because it involves entry into the human body.

Surgeries are classified as minor (presenting little risk to life) or major (possibly involving risk to life) and are performed for a variety of reasons. Table 33-1 lists indications for surgery.

The term **perioperative** encompasses the preoperative (before surgery), intraoperative (during surgery), and postoperative (after surgery) phases of surgery. Each phase refers to a particular time during the surgical experience, and each requires a wide range of specific nursing behaviors and functions. Perioperative nursing has one continuous goal: to provide a standard of excellence in the care of the client before, during, and after surgery. Nursing activities are geared to meet the client's psychosocial needs as well as immediate physical needs.

Individuals face surgery with their own values. Each client has specific expectations of the surgical experience and distinct hopes for the outcome of the surgery. The nurse takes an active part in the entire perioperative process to ensure quality and continuity of client care.

PREOPERATIVE PHASE

The **preoperative phase** is that time during the surgical experience that begins with the client's decision to have surgery and ends with the transfer of the client to the operating table.

The outcome of surgical treatment is tremendously enhanced by accurate preoperative nursing assessment and careful preoperative preparation. The client must be assessed by the nurse both physiologically and psychologically. Assessment of the client involves the integration of factors relating to the client's illness, physical condition, related medical conditions, and current surgical diagnosis. Regardless of how minor the surgical procedure, a thorough health history is essential and available to the perioperative team throughout the client's surgical experience.

The psychological well-being of the client has an impact on the surgical outcome. The surgical client is at risk for anxiety related to the surgical experience and the outcome of surgery. Fear and anxiety are normal responses to the stress of surgery and affect the client's ability to cope with the proposed plan of care. Because individuals differ in their perceptions of the meaning of surgery, the degree of anxiety and fear experienced varies. If fear and anxiety become excessive, however, these emotions interfere with recovery by magnifying the normal physiologic stress response. By assessing and being aware of the fears and anxieties of the surgical client, the nurse provides support and information so that stress does not become overwhelming. The most common fears related to surgery are:

- Fear of the unknown
- Fear of pain and discomfort

TABLE 33-1 Indications for Surgery

TYPE OF SURGERY	PURPOSE	EXAMPLE
Diagnostic	Determine cause of symptoms	Biopsy Exploratory laparotomy
Curative	Remove a diseased body part or replace a body part to restore function	Cholecystectomy Total knee arthroplasty
Palliative	Relieve symptoms without curing disease	Tumor resection associated with cancer
Restorative	Strengthen a weakened area	Herniorrhaphy
Cosmetic	Improve appearance Change shape	Face lift Mammoplasty

COURTESY OF DELMAR CENGAGE LEARNING

- Fear of mutilation and disfigurement
- Fear of anesthesia
- Fear of disruption of life patterns
  — Separation from family/significant others
  — Sexuality
  — Financial
  — Permanent/temporary limitations
- Fear of death/not waking up
- Fear of not being in control

Fear of the unknown is the most prevalent fear before surgery and is the fear the nurse can most easily allay through client education and preoperative teaching.

Preoperative Physiologic Assessment

Physiologic assessment includes a physical examination and a review of the client's laboratory values and diagnostic studies. Laboratory and diagnostic studies are divided into those that are routine and those that are performed specifically to evaluate the client's primary disease process or coexisting condition. The common preoperative laboratory tests include:

- Hemoglobin and hematocrit (Hgb and Hct)
- White blood cell (WBC) count
- Blood typing and cross matching (screening)
- Serum electrolytes
- Prothrombin time (PT), International Normalized Ratio (INR), and partial thromboplastin time (PTT)
- Bilirubin
- Liver enzymes: alanine aminotransferase (ALT) and aspartate aminotransferase (AST)
- Urinalysis
- Blood urea nitrogen (BUN) and creatinine

Although it is common practice to obtain a chest x-ray for many clients admitted to the hospital, this study is increasingly omitted for healthy children and healthy adults younger than age 40 years in whom the physical examination is normal and there is no reason to suspect pulmonary or cardiac disease. Additional radiographic or fluoroscopic examinations, sonograms, radioisotopic scans, magnetic resonance imaging, and computerized tomography scans provide useful information about the nature of the disease process and its anatomic location and extent. Any organ that is undergoing major surgery is adequately evaluated with these techniques before the operation.

Electrocardiograms (ECGs) are routinely performed in middle-age and elderly clients undergoing surgery because of the prevalence of ischemic heart disease in these age groups. It is also of value to have a baseline study for comparison in case subsequent ECGs are needed.

Preoperative testing is completed several days before the date of surgery. The type and amount of screening depends on the age and condition of the client, the nature of the surgery, and the surgeon's preference. Surgeons (doctors who perform surgery) are coming under increasing economic pressure to minimize routine testing procedures. The current trend is based on cost versus benefits, moving away from extensive testing in the absence of indicative/warranting data from the health history and physical examination.

The nurse's role in preoperative testing is to ensure that the ordered tests are performed, that the results are placed in the client's chart, and that abnormal results are reported to the physician immediately.

The physiologic nursing assessment is completed before surgery. Preoperative assessment takes place in the surgeon's office, in the hospital during hospitalization, or in the hospital or ambulatory surgery unit on the day of surgery. The nurse collects client health data by interviewing the client, the family, significant others, and health-care providers. Data collection also is accomplished through review of the client's records, assessment, and/or consultation. Assessment is essential to establishing nursing diagnoses and predicting outcomes (Association of periOperative Registered Nurses [AORN], 2002b). When performing the nursing assessment, the nurse screens the client for risks that may contribute to complications in the perioperative period. The nurse's role in the preoperative phase ensures client safety, understanding, and compliance with health care treatment. The variables affecting surgical status are age, medications, nutrition, fluid and electrolytes, and various body systems.

Age

Surgery is performed on individuals of any age, although persons at both extremes of age (infants and elders) are at greater risk for complications. Infants easily become dehydrated or fluid overloaded with resultant electrolyte imbalances. Because their metabolic rate is two to three times that of adults, infants can receive formula up to 6 hours before surgery, and breastfed infants can be nursed up to 4 hours before surgery. Infants may then have clear liquids for up to 2 hours before surgery.

Body temperature regulation and the renal, immune, and respiratory systems are different in infants than in adults. Renal function in the infant is comparatively less efficient because of a lower glomerular filtration rate and less efficient renal tubular function (Phillips, 2007). This leads to retention of anesthesia and medications and to fluid overload. Because of a comparatively larger ratio of body surface area to body mass, infants are also more prone to hypothermia when placed in a cool environment or when large areas of their body surface is exposed. Furthermore, an immature immune system renders the infant more susceptible to infections. Because of a smaller and less developed anatomic structure and enlarged tongue and lymphoid tissue, the infant is also more prone to respiratory obstruction. The nursing process and nursing care is tailored to meet the unique needs of the infant client.

Elderly clients experience many physiologic changes associated with aging and are more likely to have degenerative disease in many organs. Elders are more likely to become

LIFE SPAN CONSIDERATIONS

Surgery in the Elderly Client

Morbidity and mortality rates for surgical clients older than age 90 years are much higher than for those age 70 to 75 years (Hogstel, 2001). Elderly clients do not tolerate emergency or long, complicated surgery as well as do younger clients because of a lesser ability to adapt to physical and psychological stress.

dehydrated and are thus less able to adapt to fluid loss during surgery. The elderly client is also more sensitive to central nervous system depressants used during the perioperative period; however, even elderly clients favorably tolerate extensive surgery when carefully assessed and managed.

Nutritional Status

Nutritional assessment includes evaluation of individual deficiencies or excesses that place the client at greater risk for complications during surgery. Surgery increases the body's need for nutrients necessary for tissue healing and resistance to infection.

Nutritional deficiencies place the client at greater risk for fluid and electrolyte imbalance, delayed wound healing, and wound infections. The malnourished individual has diminished stores of carbohydrates and fats; in such instances, proteins are used for energy instead of tissue building and restoration. In addition to carbohydrates and fats, vitamins B complex and C are also significant because these vitamins are essential to healing. Poor nutritional status also adversely affects liver and kidney function, leaving the client with a poor tolerance for anesthetic agents and a tendency for bleeding.

Nutritional excesses or obesity increase the risk for respiratory, cardiovascular, and gastrointestinal complications. Obesity makes access to the surgical site more difficult, which prolongs surgical time and increases the amount of anesthetic agents required. Because inhalation anesthetics are absorbed by and stored in adipose tissue and released postoperatively, recovery time from anesthesia is slower in the overweight client. Adipose tissue is less vascular and more difficult to suture, which predisposes the client to wound infection, delayed wound healing, and increased incidence of wound complications, including postoperative incisional hernias. Failure to exercise and ambulate increases the chances of decreased respiratory function, accompanied by atelectasis and pneumonia, and also leads to decreased wound healing and an increased risk of thrombus formation. Often, obese clients also have other chronic conditions, such as hypertension or diabetes mellitus that increase the likelihood of surgical complications. In some surgical situations, such as joint replacement, surgery is delayed until nutritional status improves and the client loses weight.

Fluid and Electrolyte Status

Dehydration and hypovolemia, with correlating electrolyte disturbances, predispose a client to complications during and after surgery. Both are caused by diarrhea, excessive nasogastric suctioning, inadequate oral intake, vomiting, and/or bleeding. The complications of fluid and electrolyte imbalance are numerous and varied. Changes in fluid and electrolyte balance affect cellular metabolism, renal function, and oxygen concentration in the circulation. Nursing care focuses on administering parenteral fluids or blood products as prescribed, keeping a detailed intake and output record, and evaluating results of laboratory studies.

Respiratory Status

Respiratory assessment includes detection of acute and chronic problems. Because acute respiratory infections may lead to bronchospasms or laryngospasms, surgery for clients with these conditions is delayed or contraindicated. Chronic respiratory problems, such as asthma and chronic obstructive pulmonary disease, impair the client's gas exchange and increase the risk associated with inhalation anesthetic agents. Clients with chronic respiratory problems are more likely to develop atelectasis and pneumonia.

Respiratory assessment as performed by the nurse includes assessing breath sounds, color of the skin and mucous membranes, and for shortness of breath (dyspnea) and coughing. All clients, and especially those clients who smoke and have chronic lung disease, are taught deep breathing, use of incentive spirometry, coughing, and preoperative turning.

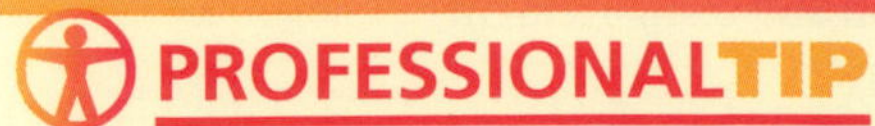

Client's Psychological Condition

The client "who fears dying while under anesthesia runs a greater risk of cardiac arrest on the operating table than [do] clients with known cardiac disease" (Phillips, 2007).

- The psychological condition of the client can have a stronger influence than does the physical condition.
- Encourage clients to express their feelings and fears about receiving anesthetic and having surgery.
- Observe the client for nonverbal clues indicating anxiety.
- To reduce client anxiety, explain what happens throughout the surgical experience.

Cardiovascular Status

Cardiovascular assessment focuses on such diseases as angina, recent myocardial infarction or cardiac surgery, hemophilia, hypertension, and congestive heart failure. Clients with a history of cardiac disease are prone to developing complications such as dysrhythmias, hypotension, myocardial infarction, congestive heart failure, cardiac arrest, stroke, shock, deep vein thrombosis, thrombophlebitis, or pulmonary embolism.

Also assess for anxiety; elevated blood pressure; slow, rapid, or irregular pulse; chest pain; edema; coolness or cyanosis/discoloration of extremities; weakness; and shortness of breath (dyspnea). All clients are taught postoperative leg exercises to prevent thrombophlebitis. The goal of nursing care is to improve the client's cardiovascular condition to the highest degree possible by promoting rest alternated with activity; encouraging a low-sodium and low-cholesterol diet; administering heart medications; and judiciously administering parenteral fluids and recording intake and output.

Renal and Hepatic Status

Because many medications and anesthetic agents are detoxified by the liver and excreted by the kidneys, renal and hepatic sufficiency constitute a major concern. Renal disease affects fluid and electrolyte balance and protein equilibrium. Liver disease causes bleeding tendencies and carbohydrate, fat, and amino acid imbalances that impair wound healing and increase the risk of infection. Assess for symptoms of urinary frequency, dysuria, and anuria and record the color and amount of the urine. Also assess for a history of bleeding tendencies, easy

CLIENT TEACHING

Postoperative Leg Exercises

Activity	Instructions
Leg lifts	1. While lying on back or in a semi-sitting position, raise the leg off the bed. 2. Hold for count of five. 3. Lower leg to the bed. 4. Repeat five times then proceed to other leg. Perform every hour.
Dorsiflexion and hyper-extension of ankles	1. Flex ankles and raise toes toward head, stretching posterior calf. 2. Hold for a count of two. 3. Relax. 4. Repeat five times, then proceed to other foot. Perform every hour.
Foot circles	1. Point the toe and raise the leg slightly off the bed. 2. Use the great toe to trace a circle in the air, first to the right and then to the left. 3. Repeat five times, then proceed to the other foot. Perform every hour.

bruising, nosebleeds, and use of anticoagulants. The most commonly ordered preoperative tests to assess renal function are urinalysis, blood urea nitrogen (BUN), and creatinine. The most common liver tests are prothrombin time (PT), partial thromboplastin time (PTT), bilirubin, and the liver enzymes alanine aminotransferase (ALT) and aspartate aminotransferase (AST). Nursing care focuses on administering fluids and adequate nutrition, monitoring fluid intake and output, and evaluating results of laboratory tests.

Neurological, Musculoskeletal, and Integumentary Status

Assess the client's overall mental status, including level of consciousness; orientation to person, place, and time; and the ability to understand and follow instructions. Note skin condition, including turgor and any rashes, bruises, lesions, or previous incisions. Assess client mobility and sensation through observation of both range of motion and ability to ambulate and through client statements. Note any abnormalities, injuries, or previous surgery and assess the risk for falls. The presence of internal or external prostheses or implants such as pacemakers, heart valves, or joint prosthesis is also noted, because the presence of these may necessitate preoperative antibiotics.

Thin clients, clients undergoing long surgical procedures or vascular procedures, and elderly clients are the most vulnerable to neurological, musculoskeletal, or integumentary injuries. Some underlying disease processes, such as edema, infection, cancer, osteoporosis, arthritic joints, or neck or back problems, also place a client at greater risk for injury. Clients who are malnourished, anemic, obese, hypovolemic, paralyzed, or diabetic are also prone to skin breakdown. Information gathered about the neurological, musculoskeletal, and integumentary systems is used to prepare the surgical site, for surgical positioning, and as a comparative basis for postoperative assessments and complication screening.

Endocrine and Immunological Status

Clients with diabetes are scheduled as early in the morning as possible, and a fasting glucose drawn immediately before surgery. Surgery is a stressor, and stress raises the serum glucose level in the client with diabetes. Thus the morning dose of insulin usually is adjusted.

When anesthetized during surgery, the diabetic client exhibits very few symptoms of glucose imbalance. Serum glucose must therefore be checked frequently during surgery, usually by the anesthesia provider. Stability is attained by the administration of insulin, glucose, or both. Besides hyperglycemia and hypoglycemia, a diabetic client is more prone to fluid and electrolyte imbalances, infection including respiratory and urinary tract infections, neurogenic bladder, impaired wound healing, ketoacidosis, deep vein thrombosis, thrombophlebitis, and pulmonary embolism.

Because the immunological system protects the client from infections, the immunocompromised surgical client is very prone to infection. Clients receiving steroids or chemotherapy, or who have systemic lupus erythematosus, Addison's disease, or acquired immunodeficiency syndrome (AIDS) are considered immunocompromised. The immune response in these clients is weakened or deficient, resulting in an increased incidence of infection. Because surgery breaks the integrity of the skin and the normal inflammatory response is suppressed, wound healing may be impaired. Strict adherence to aseptic technique (covered later in this chapter) is thus even more imperative. Prevention of infection is crucial in these clients. The role of the nurse is to communicate the presence of potential immunosuppression to other health care team members involved in the client's care and to prevent infection by practicing aseptic technique.

Medications

Knowledge of the client's use of drugs for recreational or therapeutic purposes is essential to preoperative assessment. The history of medication usage by the client should include type and frequency of use for over-the-counter, prescription, and street drugs. The use of certain drugs affects the client's reaction to anesthetic agents and surgery. Some drugs increase surgical risks; these medications usually are temporarily discontinued before surgery. Other medications, such as heart or hypoglycemic medications, may still be given even though the client is to undergo surgery; the surgeon or anesthesia provider writes specific orders in such instances. Dosages of medications may also be adjusted during the perioperative period.

Chronic alcohol use increases surgical risk because it is often accompanied by impaired nutrition and liver disease. Postoperatively, the client may exhibit delirium tremens or acute withdrawal syndrome. Furthermore, pain medication may be less effective.

PROFESSIONALTIP

Questions to Assess Psychosocial Status

- Why are you having surgery?
- When did this problem start?
- What do you think caused this problem?
- Has this caused any problems in your relationships with others?
- Has your problem prevented you from working?
- Are you able to take care of your own needs?
- Are you experiencing any discomfort or pain?
- What are you expecting from this surgery?
- Is there anything that you do not understand regarding your surgery?
- Are you worried about anything?
- Will someone be available to assist you when you return home?

CULTURAL CONSIDERATIONS

Impending Surgery

- Some clients desire special religious rites before surgery.
- Some clients may not want to receive blood transfusions or other treatments.
- All client beliefs are respected.

Psychosocial Health Assessment

The psychosocial health status of the client is also assessed. The nurse elicits the client's perceptions of surgery and the expected outcome. The nurse also ascertains the client's coping mechanisms and the client's knowledge level and ability to understand. The data collected are incorporated into nursing care throughout the perioperative experience.

Cultural beliefs can influence a client's perception of surgery. For example, some cultures believe that surgery is a "final effort" performed only when all other possible treatments have been of no avail. Furthermore, surgeries that cause changes in the appearance of the body can alter body image and self-esteem; the client may worry about being sexually attractive or active after surgery.

The nurse provides an opportunity for the client to express his spiritual values and beliefs. Many clients wish to see a member of the clergy before having surgery.

Surgical Consent

An **informed consent** is a legal form signed by the client and witnessed by another person that grants permission to the client's physician to perform the procedure described by the physician. An informed consent is needed whenever these situations occur:

- Anesthesia is used.
- The procedure is considered invasive.
- The procedure is nonsurgical but has more than a slight risk of complications (such as with an arteriogram).
- Radiation or cobalt therapy is used.

Informed consent protects both the client (against unauthorized procedures) and the physician and the health care facility and its employees (against claims that an unauthorized procedure was performed). Although the ultimate responsibility for obtaining the informed consent lies with the physician, the nurse often obtains and witnesses the client's signature and ensures that the client signs the consent form voluntarily and is alert and comprehending of the action.

Most hospitals use a standard preprinted form. The information written by the health care personnel is specific to the individual client. The client's signature on the consent form indicates the information has been read and is correct. The client has the right to refuse treatment even after signing the consent. When this occurs, the nurse informs the physician immediately of the client's decision.

Preoperative Teaching

The client about to have surgery is at risk for knowledge deficit related to preoperative procedures and protocols and postoperative expectations. The potential benefits of preoperative teaching include reduced anxiety and more rapid recovery with fewer complications and shorter hospitalization. Reduction in anxiety has a secondary benefit: The client usually requires less medication for pain. The purposes of preoperative teaching are to (1) answer questions and concerns about surgery, (2) ascertain the client's knowledge of the intended surgery, (3) ascertain the need or desire for additional information, and (4) provide information in a manner most conducive to learning.

One-on-one sessions constitute the most personal method of instruction, but try to include the family or significant other when possible. The level of learning increases when more than one teaching medium is used. For example, using materials such as videotapes, charts, tours, anatomic models, pictures, and brochures reinforces both visual and auditory learning. Demonstration followed by return demonstration is helpful. Written instructions serve as a reference for later use. Make instructions simple, using terms the client can understand. Any unfamiliar words or concepts are thoroughly explained.

Clients are often interested in any information that describes the sights, sounds, tastes, feelings, odors, and temperature of what they are about to experience. For example, the feeling of relaxation from preoperative medications; the sounds of instruments or equipment in the operating room (OR); the pressure from the automatic blood pressure cuff; the warmth or coolness of skin-preparation solutions; or the brightness of the OR lights are all sensations the client may experience. Analogies or stories of real or fictitious situations of sensory experiences help the client understand. The teaching methods used strongly influence the client's learning and retention of information.

Preoperative teaching begins as soon as surgery is agreed upon. Instructions given over the phone and/or mailed to the client during the time leading up to surgery are beneficial.

Just before surgery, a brief review with additional information tailored to the needs of the client are given. Give the client an opportunity to ask questions.

Information always is targeted to the client's needs and according to the client's level of knowledge and anxiety. Mild-to-moderate anxiety actually heightens a person's alertness and motivates learning. Mildly anxious clients receive the most complete instructions. Moderately anxious clients receive less information but more attention to specific areas of concern. Severely anxious clients receive only basic information but are encouraged to verbalize their concerns. Clients in a state of panic are unable to learn; in such cases, no instruction is given, and the surgeon is notified.

CLIENT TEACHING

Preoperative Teaching

- Introduce self
  - Identify role in client's care
- Determine client's knowledge level and need or desire for addition information
- Explain the routine for the day of surgery
  - Restricted food or fluid intake
  - Intravenous fluids
  - Premedication
  - Time of surgery
  - Anticipated length of surgery
  - Transportation to the OR
  - Special skin preparations
  - Type of surgical incision (Figure 33-1)
- Familiarize client with the OR environment
  - Operating room lights and table
  - Accessory equipment
  - Monitoring equipment
  - Anesthesia induction
- Include significant others
  - Time to arrive at the hospital
  - Location of the surgical waiting area
  - What to expect when the client returns to the unit
- Explain postanesthesia care unit (PACU)
  - Location of recovery room
  - Purpose of recovery room
  - Routine of postanesthesia care
- Identify anticipated dressings, drains, catheters, casts, etc.
- Demonstrate and evaluate client's proficiency with:
  - Coughing and deep breathing exercises
  - Turning
  - Incentive spirometry
  - Extremity exercises
  - Any special transfer procedures or aids required after surgery
- Describe pain management strategies appropriate for the specific surgical procedure

PHYSICAL PREPARATION

Extremely close attention is given to identifying the proper client both verbally and by reading the identification name band and to verifying the operative procedure. This is completed through client statements, surgeon verification, and the signed surgical consent form. *Particular attention is given to differentiating between right and left operative sites.*

Special care is given to the preparation of the operative site to lessen the chance of infection. The operative site is thoroughly cleansed with an antiseptic soap such as povidone-iodine to reduce the number of microorganisms on the skin. Typically, the operative site is not shaved, but if shaving is to be performed, it is done in the OR immediately before surgery. To reduce the number of bacteria in the gastrointestinal tract for gastrointestinal, peritoneal, perianal, or pelvic surgery, an enema is ordered. Enemas prevent contamination of the peritoneal area by fecal content passed during surgery. The reduction in colon size related to the loss of bulk also helps prevent colon injury and increases visualization of the operative site. Enemas are usually given the night before surgery. If the enema is done at home, give the client detailed instructions. Many types of surgery require special preparations. The specific protocol for each surgical procedure is available from the health care facility or the physician.

Check the client's vital signs, including blood pressure, temperature, pulse, and respirations. Some changes in vital signs are normal as a result of anxiety. If marked differences exist from the baseline data, however, the surgeon is notified.

Assist the client in putting on a hospital gown, hair cap and, if ordered, antiembolic hose sized according to client size. Institutional policy usually requires the removal of all jewelry, including body jewelry. Hairpins, wigs, and prostheses also are removed. The nurse is responsible for recording the disposition of any personal items removed for surgery.

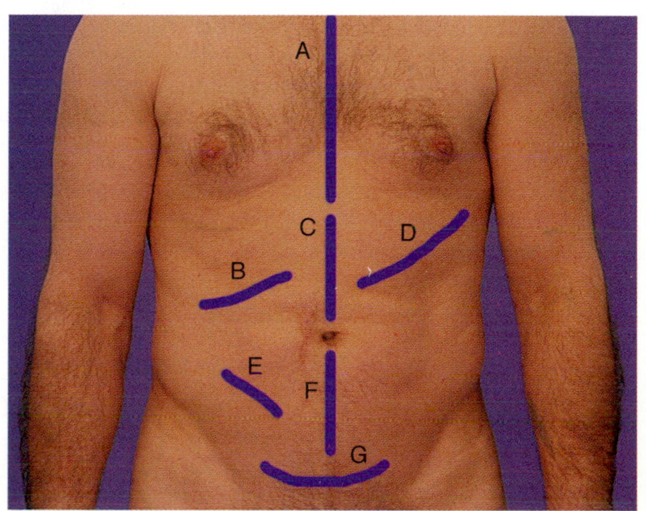

FIGURE 33-1 Common Surgical Incisions; *A*, Sternal Split; *B*, Oblique Subcostal; *C*, Upper Vertical Midline; *D*, Thoracoabdominal; *E*, McBurney; *F*, Lower Vertical Midline; *G*, Pfannenstiel

SAFETY

Iodine Allergy, Latex Allergy

- Each client is asked about allergy to iodine and latex.
- If a client is allergic to either, document the allergy on the client's record and inform the surgeon and OR personnel so that an iodine-free solution and latex-free equipment is used.

If policy requires, nail polish (from at least one nail, if dark polish) is removed to read oxygen saturation via pulse oximetry. Makeup is also removed so that skin color is observed.

Allergies to medication, food, and chemicals (including contrast agents) are verified, as are previous blood reactions. The nurse differentiates between a medication intolerance and a true allergic reaction. With an intolerance to certain medications, the client may experience side effects that are unpleasant. For example, many clients experience nausea when given morphine; although unpleasant, this is not a drug allergy. A true allergy produces a skin reaction or anaphylactic reaction, where the client experiences cardiorespiratory reactions that may be life threatening, such as hypotension and pulmonary edema. A client with multiple food allergies is also prone to hypersensitivities to medications. When allergies are identified, the client's chart is marked accordingly, and an allergy wrist band is put on the client. By being aware of and alerting other team members to the client's allergies, client safety and comfort are maintained.

Verify the NPO (nothing by mouth) status of the client for the time specified by the surgeon's order. Restricting oral intake reduces the possibility of aspiration. If surgery takes place in the afternoon, the client has a clear liquid breakfast if ordered by the surgeon. Careful client instruction is required because surgery may need to be postponed if the client eats or drinks.

In addition to the previously outlined preparations, remove dentures and bridgework to prevent loss, damage, and possible dislodgement and airway obstruction during the surgery. Ensure that the client has an empty bladder by allowing time for the client to void before transfer to surgery.

Identify any sensory deficits of the client and communicate this information to other health-care team members.

PROFESSIONALTIP

Implementing NPO Status

- Explain reasons for NPO status to the client.
- Remove any food and water from the client's overbed table and nightstand.
- Mark the client's door and bed with an NPO sign.
- Mark the client's Kardex, electronic medical records, and other nursing information sources.
- Notify the dietary department.

LIFE SPAN CONSIDERATIONS

Preparation for Surgery

For pediatric clients:

- Provide physical and psychological preparation at the child's level of understanding.
- Listen carefully to the child to promote understanding.
- Ask the child to point to the operative site on self or doll.
- Be honest and truthful.

The elder client may have:

- Increased risk of complications including infection.
- Increased incidence of coexisting conditions.
- Unpredictable response to medications and anesthetics.
- Greater need for support from family and significant other.
- Increased skin and bone fragility.
- Nutritional and financial deficiencies.
- Impaired vision and hearing.
- Impaired or slowed thought processes and cognitive abilities.
- Fear of death, loss of independence, and change in lifestyle.

Glasses, contact lenses, and hearing aids are usually removed to prevent loss or damage; if policy allows, however, it is best to leave these items in place so the client is better able to see and hear. Then the nurse is responsible for communicating the presence of these aids to the surgical team members.

The surgeon or anesthesiologist (a doctor trained in providing anesthesia) may order preoperative medication. The nurse gives the medication by the prescribed route (intramuscular, intravenous, or oral) at the specified time (typically 1 hour before surgery). Preoperative medications may be ordered "on call," which means that the nurse is notified by a member of the surgical team when the preoperative medication is to be given. Before administering the medication, ask the client to void. After administering the preoperative medication, raise the side rails of the gurney or bed, put the bed in the lowest position, and instruct the client not to get up without assistance.

When the surgical team is ready, the client is transported on a gurney by a member of the OR team, typically an orderly. The client is always transported feet first and with the side rails up to ensure safety and minimize the likelihood of dizziness and nausea. The client may be taken to a preoperative holding area first (Figure 33-2 on following page). The nurse instructs the family or significant others where to wait.

The information collected as part of preoperative preparation is documented in the client record, usually on a preoperative checklist. Figure 33-3 (p. 976) illustrates a typical preoperative checklist. This checklist is completed before the client leaves the clinical unit or upon the client's admission to ambulatory surgery.

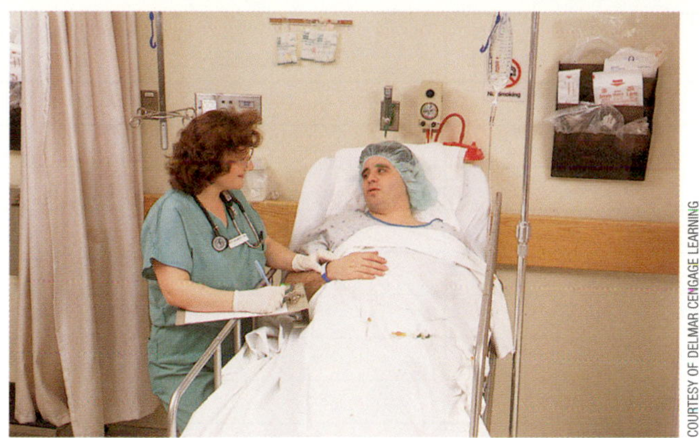
COURTESY OF DELMAR CENGAGE LEARNING

FIGURE 33-2 **The holding area is used for clients who are waiting to have surgery.**

The nurse also verbally communicates to other health-care members any necessary information collected.

INTRAOPERATIVE PHASE

The **intraoperative phase** is the time during the surgical experience that begins when the client is transferred to the OR table and ends when the client is admitted to the postanesthesia care unit (PACU).

PHYSICAL DESCRIPTION OF THE OPERATING ROOM ENVIRONMENT

For the purposes of preventing wound infections, the surgical suite is environmentally controlled. Personnel restriction and geographic isolation from other areas of the hospital or clinic are part of this control. Constant filtered airflow and positive air pressure in the OR also aid in environmental control. Clean areas and contaminated areas are separated within the suite. Equipment and supplies needed for each client are in the surgical suite so members of the surgical team do not have to leave the area.

ORs vary in size depending on the amount of equipment needed for each particular type of operation. Supplies and furniture are limited to prevent dust collection and are usually made of stainless steel to withstand corrosive disinfectants. Furniture and equipment are easily movable on wheels. In addition to general illumination from ceiling lights, the operative site is illuminated by overhead operating lights. Figure 33-4 shows a typical OR. The temperature of the room can be adjusted but usually is maintained at a cool 66°F to 68°F. This provides comfort for the surgical team (the members of which wear gowns, gloves, and masks under hot lights). This temperature also is an unfavorable environment for bacterial incubation and growth.

The client entering the OR is confronted with an environment that is most likely unfamiliar. The OR is cold. The surgical team members dress in surgical scrubs and have their hair covered by caps and their faces covered by surgical masks, making them appear impersonal and distant. The sounds of equipment being prepared can be unfamiliar and alarming. The terminology used in conversations among OR personnel may be foreign. These elements combined with the sight of ominous overhead lights and the feel of the hard OR table may increase the client's fear, anxiety, and feelings of powerlessness.

MEMBERS OF THE SURGICAL TEAM

The surgical team is a group of hospital personnel assigned to see a client successfully through an operative procedure. At no other time during hospitalization will the ratio of personnel to client be greater than when the client is undergoing surgery. The surgical team includes **sterile dressed** (without microorganisms) team members: the surgeon, the **first assistant** (a physician or RN who assists the surgeon in performing hemostasis, tissue retraction, and wound closure), and the **scrub nurse** (an LP/VN, RN, or surgical technologist who, under the direction of the circulating nurse, prepares and maintains the integrity, safety, and efficiency of the **sterile field** throughout the operation). These team members scrub their arms and hands, don sterile gowns and gloves, and then perform their duties in the sterile field. The sterile field is that area surrounding the client and the surgical site that is free from all microorganisms. It is created by using sterile drapes to drape the work area and the client. Other team members, dressed in nonsterile attire, include the anesthesia provider (an anesthesiologist or anesthetist) and **circulating nurse** (an RN responsible for management of personnel, equipment, supplies, environment, and communication throughout a surgical procedure). These team members perform their duties outside of the sterile field. Each team member has a clearly defined role and duties. Clear communication among team members and coordination of their activities improve the most favorable outcome for the client.

ASEPSIS

Prevention of infection is the responsibility of the entire surgical team. The environment of the surgical client contains both pathogenic (disease-producing) and nonpathogenic microorganisms. When the skin, a prime barrier to infection, is broken, as during surgery, susceptibility to a bacterial invasion increases. Bacteria carried by dust or nose and throat droplets are easily transported by air currents.

Asepsis is the absence of pathogenic microorganisms. **Aseptic technique** is a collection of principles used to control and/or prevent the transfer of pathogenic microorganisms from sources within (endogenous) and outside (exogenous) the client. For example, scrubbed persons wear sterile gowns and gloves; sterile drapes are used to create a sterile field; items used in a sterile field are sterilized; and those working within a sterile field maintain the integrity of the sterile field. Aseptic technique is applicable to other nursing functions such as changing dressings, inserting a Foley catheter, or preparing for an obstetrical delivery. Thus, the practice of aseptic technique is not confined to the OR, but applies to other clinical nursing units and other procedures as well.

The practice of aseptic technique requires the development of **sterile conscience**, an individual's personal sense of honesty and integrity with regard to adherence to the principles of aseptic technique. Aseptic technique must be strictly followed. Doing so requires constant assessment and monitoring of self and others. It is sometimes easier or less expensive to overlook an infraction of aseptic technique rather than to correct that infraction. This must never be allowed. Compromising the principles of aseptic technique may increase the likelihood of infection and, thus, harm to the client.

	CK (✓)	COMMENTS	NURSE CK (✓)
COMPLETE NIGHT BEFORE SURGERY			
List allergies			
Procedure scheduled			
Surgical permit signed/witnessed			
History/physical on chart and/or dictated			
Preanesthetic evaluation done			
Able to state type and purpose			
Demonstrates ability to perform: Deep breathing, turning and coughing exercises			
Leg exercises			
P.M. care with shower or bath given			
Nail polish removed and makeup removed			
Old chart requested and obtained			
Type and crossmatch for ______ units of blood			
Blood consent signed and witnessed			
Labor work a. CBC ______ b. UA ______			
Tonsillectomy and adenoidectomy patients: a. ___PTT b. ___PT c. ___Platelets			
If ordered by MD: a. ECG ___ b. Chest X-ray ___			
Add other lab work ordered (specify)			
Notify surgeon of abnormal lab work			
New progress note and physician order sheet on chart			
Weight			
NPO after midnight (if applicable)			
Signature of Nurse ______________________________		Date ____________	
COMPLETE DAY OF SURGERY			
Jewelry removed and secured with responsible party			
Dental prosthesis and contact lenses removed			
Voided on call to surgery			
Indwelling catheter ordered and inserted			
Tampon removed			
Identiband and/or bloodband on/checked for accuracy			
Time _______ Pulse _______ Resp _______ B/P _______ Temp. _______			
Pre-op medicine given medication ________________ Time _______ AM PM			
Siderails up and bed to lowest level			
Patient instructed not to get out of bed without nursing assistance			
Addressograph plate/MARs on chart			
VS 30 minutes after pre-op (if remains on unit)			
BP _______ P _______ R _______ T _______			
Old chart sent to surgery per request			
Surgical prep done and checked			
To surgery Time _______ Via _______			

Signature of Nurse ______________________________ Date ____________

Holding Room Nurse Signature ______________________________ Date ____________

COURTESY OF DELMAR CENGAGE LEARNING

FIGURE 33-3 Sample Preoperative Checklist

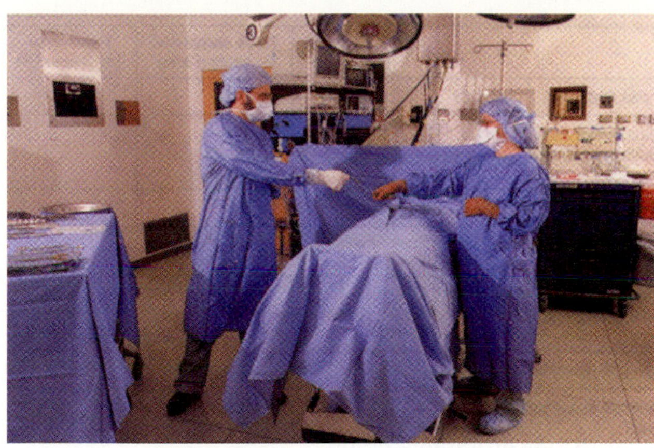

FIGURE 33-4 Typical Operating Room and Proper Surgical Attire (*Photo courtesy of the U.S. Army.*)

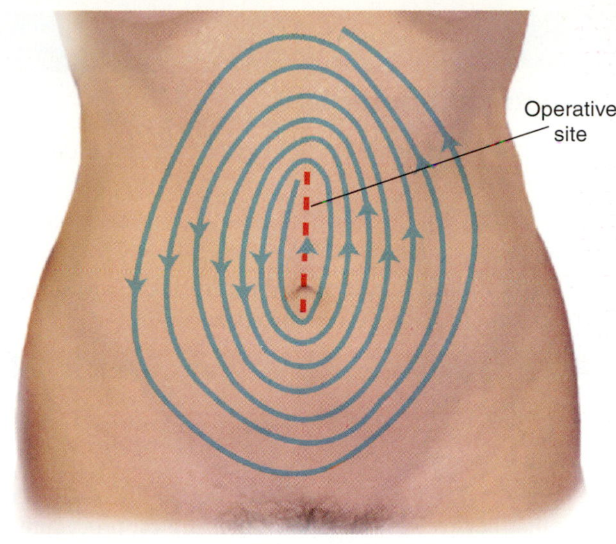

FIGURE 33-5 Skin Preparation at Operative Site

CRITICAL THINKING

Sterile Conscience

How can you use a sterile conscience when providing nursing care?

SURGICAL HAND SCRUB

An item is considered sterile when all microorganisms are removed. The skin, however, cannot be sterilized. For this reason, the sterile team members wear gloves as barriers between the sterile field and the skin. Because accidental tearing or puncturing of the surgical glove and resultant introduction of microorganisms into the surgical wound are possible, the sterile team members must take measures to lower the number of microorganisms on their hands and arms. The surgical hand scrub, performed before gowning and gloving, removes soil and transient (not always present and easily removed) microorganisms from the hands and forearms. The antimicrobial soap used lowers the count of resident (almost always present and not easily removed) microorganisms and continues to prevent sudden bacterial rebound or regrowth after the scrub is completed. The surgical scrub thus reduces the possibility of transmission of microorganisms from the surgical team to the client.

Watches, rings, and bracelets are removed before the surgical hand scrub. Fingernails must be short, clean, and healthy. Artificial nails cannot be worn (AORN, 2002a), although unchipped fingernail polish that has been applied within the last 4 days may be allowed (AORN, 2002b). The hands and forearms should be free of breaks in skin integrity.

SURGICAL SKIN PREPARATION

Like the skin of the surgical team members, the skin surface at the client's incision site also cannot be sterilized. As with the surgical hand scrub, the goal of surgical skin preparation at the client's incision site is to lower the number of microorganisms on and near the incision site.

Typically, the client is asked to shower or to wash the operative site either before arriving at the surgical facility or immediately before surgery. The client is then transferred to the OR. After general anesthesia induction or regional block completion or before local infiltration of the operative site, the circulating nurse performs the surgical skin preparation. Using aseptic technique, the circulating nurse scrubs the area with an antimicrobial soap. Typically the soap used is povidone-iodine (containing iodine) or chlorhexidine, thus potential allergies to iodine must be verified. The circulating nurse scrubs a generous area surrounding the operative site to allow for extension of the surgical incision if the need arises. The scrub is completed in an ever-widening circular motion from the incision site, which is considered clean, to the periphery, which is considered dirty (Figure 33-5). Once the periphery is reached, the sponge is discarded, never brought back toward the center of the area. The concept of cleansing from the center (incision site) to the periphery also applies to skin preparation for other procedures such as intravenous (IV) insertion, chest tube insertion, thoracentesis, or subclavian catheter placement. Surgical skin preparation lasts 5 to 10 minutes. After the scrub is completed, the area is blotted dry with sterile towels. An antiseptic solution, often also iodine based, is then applied in the same manner.

INTRAOPERATIVE NURSING CARE

The success of nursing care in the OR is measured by client outcomes. The AORN has established client outcome standards for evaluating perioperative clients upon completion of surgery. These outcomes state that the client is to be free from infection and injury related to positioning, foreign objects, or chemical, physical, and electrical hazards. In addition, skin integrity and fluid and electrolyte balance are to be maintained. Consequently, nursing care in the OR strives to provide these standards to all clients undergoing surgery.

Although the responsibilities of the circulating nurse and scrub nurse may seem to be a series of tasks or duties, these same tasks and duties provide quality nursing care to the client. The nurse planning for surgery is involved in selection of equipment and supplies, room preparation, and formation of the sterile field before the delivery of actual nursing care.

After completion of surgery, the circulating nurse applies and secures the dressing. When the anesthesia provider is ready, the client is transferred to a stretcher or a gurney. The unconscious or semiconscious client is placed in a side-lying or semiprone position unless contraindicated by the surgical procedure. If the client is supine, the client's head is turned to the side in case the client vomits. The client is then taken to the PACU, accompanied by the anesthesia provider and another surgical team member.

SAFETY

Electrical Equipment

- Electrical equipment is plugged into grounded outlets.
- Electrical equipment is regularly checked by a bioelectronic technician.
- A grounding pad is placed under the client and in direct contact with the client's skin.

POSTOPERATIVE PHASE

The **postoperative phase** is the time during the surgical experience that begins with the end of the surgical procedure and lasts until the client is discharged not just from the hospital or institution, but from medical care by the surgeon. Upon transfer from the OR, the client usually goes to the PACU (Figure 33-6). All clients who receive general anesthesia, spinal anesthesia, or regional anesthesia are admitted to the PACU. Occasionally, clients who have undergone surgery with local anesthesia or no anesthesia or who have received only IV sedation are placed in the PACU for a short period to be monitored closely until their conditions stabilize. The PACU is usually located next to the OR. Typically, it is one large room with individual units for clients along the perimeter of the room. Each of these units has an oxygen delivery system, suction, various other supplies, and cardiac, respiratory, and blood pressure monitoring devices. Curtains are pulled to provide privacy if needed, but an open view allows continual assessment of all clients.

Postoperative Nursing Care

The postanesthesia care nurse is an RN specially trained in caring for immediate postoperative clients. The goal of postanesthesia nursing care is to promote recovery from anesthesia and the immediate effects of surgery. The postanesthesia nurse has knowledge and skill in recognizing and treating anesthetic and surgical complications very quickly. The postanesthesia nurse is empathetic and is able to assess and manage pain for the client who is not able to express himself.

Upon the client's arrival in the PACU, the anesthesia provider verbally reviews the client's anesthesia and operative procedure with the postanesthesia nurse. The postanesthesia nurse begins the following nursing assessment and care in the immediate postoperative period:

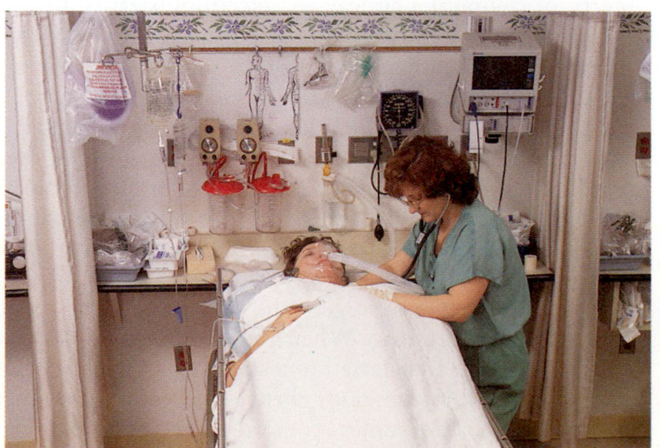

Figure 33-6 Postanesthesia Care Unit (PACU)

- Time of arrival in recovery room
- Patency of airway
- Respirations
- Presence of artificial airway devices
  - Oral airway
  - Nasopharyngeal airway
  - Endotracheal airway
- Oxygen saturation
- Need for supplemental oxygen
  - Mode of administration
  - Flow rate
- Breath sounds
- Color of skin, nail beds, and lips
- Presence of cardiac dysrhythmias
- Other vital signs
  - Blood pressure, pulse
- Skin condition (moist or dry, warm or cool) and skin temperature
- Initiate Aldrete Score
- Intravenous infusion
  - Type of solution
  - Amount in bottle or bag
  - Flow rate
  - Appearance and location of IV site
- Dressings
  - Amount and character of drainage
- Drains and tubes
  - Intactness and function
  - Connection to drainage and/or suction
  - Amount and character of drainage
- Level of consciousness
- Activity level
- Other assessments according to surgical procedure
- Pain

The postanesthesia nurse notes the client's arrival time to the unit and immediately begins to assess the patency of the airway by placing a hand above the client's nose and mouth to feel exhalation. The quality and quantity of respirations are then immediately observed, as is the presence of an artificial airway. The client is attached to a pulse oximeter (Figure 33-7), and breath sounds are auscultated. The color and condition of the skin are noted as part of the respiratory assessment. The lips are checked for circumoral pallor. Peripheral cyanosis may be an indication of hypothermia rather than respiratory distress. Thus, correlating with the "ABCs" of airway, breathing, and circulation, the respiratory system is assessed first.

Because most clients admitted are unconscious and have received muscle relaxants during surgery, respiratory exchange is often affected. Snoring, stridor, labored chest movement, sternal retractions, cyanosis, and apnea are all signs of respiratory distress. Respiratory distress is the gravest of all complications because respiratory crisis and subsequent death occurs in a matter of minutes if distress is not observed and treated quickly. In

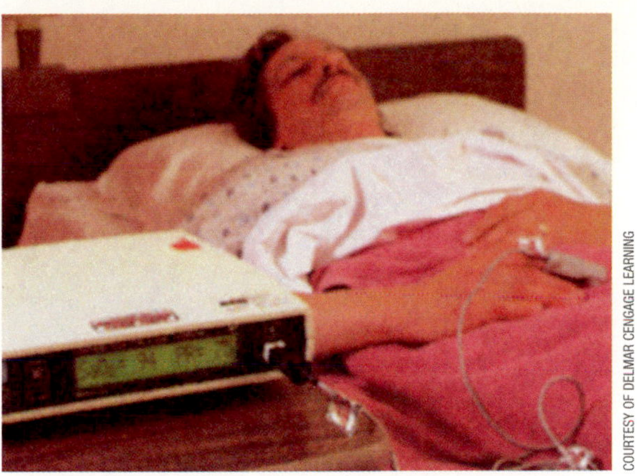
COURTESY OF DELMAR CENGAGE LEARNING

FIGURE 33-7 Client with Pulse Oximeter on Finger

the event of any signs of respiratory distress, the postanesthesia nurse must be alert to the possibility of respiratory arrest and be ready to initiate cardiopulmonary resuscitation.

The **Aldrete Score**, also known as the Postanesthetic Recovery Score, is used in PACUs to objectively assess the physical status of clients recovering from anesthesia and serves as a basis for discharge from the PACU (Table 33-2). The Aldrete Score was adapted to also assess the readiness of clients for discharge from ambulatory surgery. The first five items are used for discharge from the PACU. Clients are assessed at the time of admission to the PACU and every 15 minutes until discharge. The first five items include assessing activity, respiration, consciousness, circulation, and color (oxygen saturation). Each of the five items is scored from 0 to 2, according to the degree of functional disturbance. The score is expressed as a total score, with 10 being the maximum. Typically, a minimum score of 8 is required for discharge from the PACU.

Fluid intake and output are assessed. The amounts and types of IV solutions hanging are identified, as are any added medications. The IV fluids are infused according to the surgeon's order and are run at a specified rate. The IV site is assessed for patency, redness, and swelling. The client is restrained as necessary to maintain patency of the IV site. All other infusions and irrigations are also assessed.

Dressings and/or peripads are checked for any evidence of bloody drainage and the amount noted so that any subsequent appearance of blood may be accurately evaluated. All drainage tubes are then connected, and the type of drain and the drainage amount are recorded according to physicians' orders. Table 33-3 outlines common types of drains placed in surgery. Urinary output is also monitored. Scanty urinary drainage (<50 mL/hour or as ordered) is reported to the surgeon.

TABLE 33-2 Aldrete Score/Postanesthetic Recovery Score

Activity	Able to move 4 extremities voluntarily or on command	2
	Able to move 2 extremities voluntarily or on command	1
	Able to move 0 extremities voluntarily or on command	0
Respiration	Able to breathe deeply and cough freely	2
	Dyspnea or limited breathing	1
	Apneic	0
Consciousness	Fully awake	2
	Arousable on calling	1
	Not responding	0
Circulation	B/P ± 20% of preanesthetic level	2
	B/P ± 20% to 50% of preanesthetic level	1
	B/P ± 50% of preanesthetic level	0
Color	Normal	2
	Pale, dusky, blotchy, jaundiced, other	1
	Cyanotic	0
Additional Assessments: Aldrete Score/ Postanesthetic Recovery Score for Clients Having Anesthesia on an Ambulatory Basis		
Dressing	Dry and clean	2
	Wet but stationary or marked	1
	Growing area of wetness	0
Pain	Pain free	2
	Mild pain handled by oral medication	1
	Severe pain requiring parenteral medication	0
Ambulation	Able to stand up and walk straight	2
	Vertigo when erect	1
	Dizziness when supine	0
Fasting/ Feeding	Able to drink fluids	2
	Nauseated	1
	Nausea and vomiting	0
Urine Output	Has voided	2
	Unable to void but comfortable	1
	Unable to void and uncomfortable	0

Courtesy of J. Antonio Aldrete, M.D., M.S., Defuniak Springs, FL.

Surgical drains are placed so the wound can drain freely of blood clots, body fluids, pus, and necrotic material that otherwise would collect in the wound and provide a rich medium for bacterial growth. Figure 33-8 illustrates common drainage devices. All drains are inserted at the operative site and exit through the incision or a separate stab wound adjacent to the incision. The type of drain is chosen according to the location of wound, size of wound, and type of drainage anticipated. The use of drains decreases pain and infection and aids wound healing; however, if the wound is draining, the skin is not closed, and a pathway exists for the entrance of microorganisms. Drain sites can thus also be a source of infection. Potential complications of drains include hemorrhage, sepsis, drain loss, and bowel herniation. Nursing care for drains includes assessing the color, character, and odor of drainage; ensuring the patency of the drain (making sure there are no kinks in the tubing); and ensuring that the drain does not accidentally become

Table 33-3 Description, Uses, and Nursing Care of Common Drainage Devices Placed During Surgery

TYPE	EXAMPLE	DESCRIPTION	USES	NURSING CARE
Passive	Penrose	A single-lumen, soft latex tube that works with gravity directly from the surgical incision	To remove drainage when more than a minimal amount of drainage is expected	• Inspect dressing • Check underneath client to ensure drainage has not leaked from the side of the dressing • Always keep a dressing over drain • Check safety pin through end of drain
Active	Hemovac Jackson-Pratt J-Vac Relia Vac Surgivac	Closed wound drainage system with drain and reservoir having self-suction when reservoir is compressed	Used after multiple types of procedures; provides continuous gentle suction of the operative site to increase drainage of serosanguinous fluid and collapse tissue to facilitate healing	• Assess the drainage system as appropriate to client's condition for: 1. Continued drainage 2. Maintained decompression 3. Air-tight tubings 4. Need for emptying • To reactivate suction, wash hands and wear gloves and eye/face protection • Empty reservoirs every 8 hours, when drainage nears the full line, or as ordered by the physician
Passive or active	Davol Sump Axiom Sump	Large, multilumen tube with a larger main port for drainage and/or suction and with smaller side port(s) for irrigation and/or air venting to help prevent tissue from being suctioned against catheter and damaged	To drain intra-abdominal fluids from abscesses, cysts, or hematomas	• Use one of the smaller or sump ports for continuous irrigation • Calculate intake and output carefully with irrigations • Place impervious pads underneath client • Change dressings frequently when saturated • Attach to catheter drainage bag if not attached to suction; do not plug sump ports
	Chest tube ThoraKlex Pleure Vac	Large single-lumen drain attached to closed water-seal drainage system	To drain fluid or air from pleural cavity	• Assess breath sounds and respirations, including depth, rate, symmetry of chest expansion, color of mucous membranes, and presence of crepitus with suction off or tubing clamped • If present, assess amount and type of suction • Ensure that connections are tight and sealed with tape • Keep chest tube drainage reservoir lower than client's chest • Observe for air leaks in air leak indicator or drainage chamber of drainage reservoir • Place petroleum jelly gauze nearby for quick access should the tube become dislodged • Measure drainage at least every 8 hours (more frequently if in a critical care unit or client's condition warrants it) • Clamp or milk the chest tube only if ordered by surgeon • Notify surgeon if drainage is greater than 100 mL/hour • Change drainage system when 2/3 full

COURTESY OF DELMAR CENGAGE LEARNING

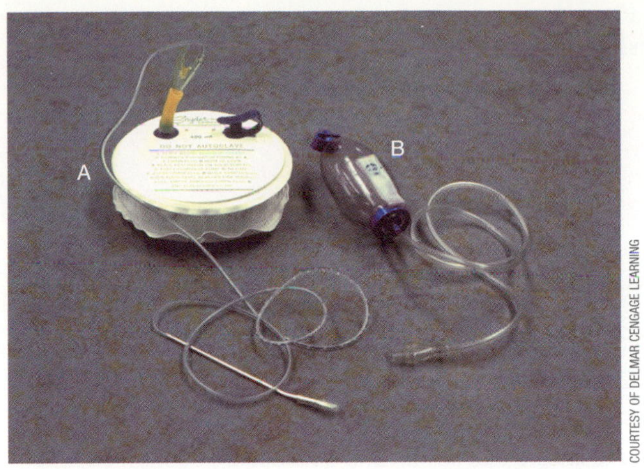

FIGURE 33-8 Common Drainage Devices; *A*, Hemovac; *B*, Jackson-Pratt

dislodged. Table 33-4 lists additional nursing care according to surgical procedure.

Part of the neurological assessment involves assessing the activity level or the ability to move extremities voluntarily. The ability to move extremities on command indicates voluntary movement. Hearing is the first sensation to return to the client after having been anesthetized. Clients in the PACU are asked to squeeze the postanesthesia nurse's hands and to plantarflex and dorsiflex the feet.

CONTINUING NURSING CARE IN THE PACU

After the client has been admitted and assessed in PACU, the postanesthesia nurse checks the surgeon's and the anesthesia provider's orders and initiates any therapy designated for the PACU.

The postanesthesia nurse charts on a separate nursing record for the PACU. Anything unusual must be adequately documented. If vital signs are in the normal range, the postanesthesia nurse checks them every 15 minutes. If vital signs are unstable, they are checked every 5 minutes or as often as necessary until stable. If vital signs fail to stabilize, the surgeon and anesthesia provider are notified. The surgical site is checked at least every 30 minutes. If any initial bleeding has not subsided, the surgeon is notified. Routine checks are continued until the client is discharged from the PACU.

The postanesthesia nurse determines whether the client meets the criteria for discharge from the PACU. Typically, the client's vital signs are stable and within the client's normal limits. The Aldrete Score is 8 to 10. If the score is 7 or less, a surgeon's or anesthesia provider's order is required for discharge. Also before client discharge, the dressing is checked, changed, or reinforced according to orders. All other parameters are reassessed and charted. Institutional protocol dictates minimum stay in the PACU. Adults are typically kept in the PACU for a minimum of 1 hour, except outpatients, who go to the ambulatory surgery unit when they are awake and when postmedication time is fulfilled. Children are typically kept in the PACU until they are awake, stable, and have an Aldrete Score of 8 to 10. When criteria for discharge are met, the postanesthesia nurse calls the clinical unit or ambulatory surgery unit and reports the client's name, vitals, surgery, and any other pertinent information. The client is then transferred to the appropriate unit.

LATER POSTOPERATIVE NURSING CARE

Before the client's arrival in the clinical unit, the nurse prepares for the client. The linen is changed, the bed linen folded down, and the room cleared of clutter. Special required equipment, as directed by the postanesthesia nurse, is gathered. An emesis basin and tissue are available. The nurse is ready to assess the client in an organized manner, focusing on the body system affected by surgery.

Upon the client's arrival in the clinical unit, the nurse assists in transferring the client to the bed. Nursing assessment and care of the client upon admission to the clinical unit includes the following:

- Time of arrival in unit
- Transfer from cart to bed
  - — Place bed in lowest, locked position, with side rails up
  - — Place client in position of comfort, or as ordered
- Vital signs including airway assessment and breath sounds
- Color of skin, nail beds, and lips
- Skin condition (moist or dry, warm or cool)
- Level of consciousness
- Activity level
- Intravenous infusion
  - — Type of solution
  - — Amount in bottle or bag
  - — Flow rate
  - — Appearance and location of IV site
- Dressings
  - — Amount and character of drainage
- Drains and tubes
  - — Intactness and function
  - — Connection to drainage and/or suction
  - — Amount and character of drainage
- Urinary output
  - — Need to void or time of voiding
  - — Presence of patency and catheter; output/hour
- Pain
  - — Last dose of analgesia
  - — Current pain location, intensity, quality
- Compare assessment with PACU report
- Call light within reach
  - — Reorient client to usage
- Location of family or significant others
- Postoperative orders

A brief assessment, including vital signs, is completed every 15 minutes for 1 hour; every 30 minutes for 2 hours; and every hour for 4 hours, or as prescribed by the physician. The possibilities of postanesthetic complications continue, but as time passes, different postsurgical complications may develop; the nurse is responsible for managing these.

1. The client is at risk for *Ineffective **Airway** Clearance* caused by atelectasis and hypostatic pneumonia. Respiratory

TABLE 33-4 Additional Nursing Care According to Classification or Type of Surgical Procedure

CLASSIFICATION OR TYPE OF SURGICAL PROCEDURE	NURSING CARE	
Orthopedic	• Expose wet casts to the air. • Check surgeon's orders for positioning of client; operated extremities typically are elevated. • Check for digital warmth, color, mobility, circulation (pulses), and sensation in affected extremity.	
Urologic	• Attach all catheters to drainage. • Closely monitor continuous irrigation to ensure that flow in and flow out are equal; if obstructed, the bladder could rupture. • Increase or decrease irrigation flow rate according to amount of bleeding. • Assess for chills or elevated pulse, possibly indicative of hemolysis or bacterial infection. • Assess abdomen for signs of distension and rigidity and report, especially if client complains.	
Oral	• Suction frequently and carefully around sutures. • Observe breathing; ensure that drainage or packing does not obstruct airway. • Apply ice bag, when ordered. • Remove dental packs as ordered and assess every 15 minutes for further bleeding.	
Eye, ears, nose, and throat (EENT)	*Eye surgery*	• Assess for facial paralysis. • Minimize head movement, coughing, vomiting, and restlessness.
	Ear surgery	• Assess edema and tracheal patency (listening for stridor and observing for restlessness).
	Nose surgery	• Maintain open airway; suction orally; and apply ice.
	Tonsillectomy	• Place on side to facilitate drainage: elevate head of bed; have suction available; and observe closely for bleeding, vomiting, and obstruction.
Neurologic	• Assess level of consciousness; be alert to drowsiness, slurred speech, disorientation, or irritability that differs from that exhibited in the preoperative state. • Observe for pupil changes: inequality, constriction, and nonreactivity to light. • Assess for respiratory changes such as snoring, retraction of cheeks and trachea, shallowness, and slowed rate. • Monitor blood pressure and pulse; an elevated blood pressure coupled with a lowered pulse leads to shock. • Observe extremity movement for weakness, paralysis, and rigidity; observe for unilateral drooping of facial features. • Use caution when medicating.	
	Laminectomy or discectomy	• Move only as ordered. • Assess sensation, circulation, and motion of extremities distal to incision.
	Craniotomy	• Position as ordered. • Complete a neurological check. • Use Trendelenburg position only with permission of the surgeon.

Table 33-4 Additional Nursing Care According to Classification or Type of Surgical Procedure (Continued)

CLASSIFICATION OR TYPE OF SURGICAL PROCEDURE	NURSING CARE
Vascular (all grafts, carotid endarterectomy, femoral-popliteal bypass)	• Assess color, sensation, warmth, and mobility of extremity. • Observe presence and strength of pedal and post-tibial pulses. • Complete a neurological check for carotid endarterectomy. • Frequently check all dressings and the area directly beneath the client. • Drainage can roll around a curved body part leaving the dressing appearing dry. However, check the area directly under curved body structures for bleeding.
Thoracic	• Closely observe chest tube for patency, amount of bleeding, and air leaks. Tape all connections. Mark drainage container upon client's admission and discharge. Assess fluctuation of drainage in tubing. Attach suction as ordered. • Observe respirations closely with regard to color change, restlessness, apprehension, dyspnea, or mediastinal shift. • Elevate head of bed 30°, unless contraindicated. • Encourage coughing and deep breathing. • Use caution in administering narcotics, especially morphine sulfate, as client cannot afford respiratory depression.
	Pneumonectomy: • Do not turn on nonoperative side. Alternately turn from back to operated side.
	Lobectomy and resection: • May turn client to either side.
Gynecologic	• Assess vaginal drainage.

COURTESY OF DELMAR CENGAGE LEARNING

complications can still occur with any anesthetized client. As in the PACU, the postoperative client is at risk for ineffective airway clearance, ineffective breathing patterns, and aspir.ation. Now, however, nursing measures are directed toward preventing ineffective airway clearance caused by atelectasis and hypostatic pneumonia, both of which usually occur within the first 48 hours postoperatively. In postoperative atelectasis, the bronchioles of the lungs become plugged with mucus so that air cannot reach the alveoli. The alveoli then collapse. The client develops dyspnea, fever, tachypnea, tachycardia, and cyanosis. In postoperative hypostatic pneumonia, stagnant mucus promotes the growth of bacteria, and atelectasis then develops into a secondary infection. To prevent these complications, actively encourage the client to cough, deep breathe (with and without incentive spirometry), and turn as instructed preoperatively. Encourage the client to sit up and ambulate as soon and as often as ordered. Ensure adequate pain relief measures so that mobility is well tolerated.

2. The client is at risk for ***Peripheral Neurovascular Dysfunction, Excess/Deficient Fluid Volume, and Activity Intolerance***. The client continues to be at risk for decreased cardiac output and fluid volume deficit. Implement measures to prevent deep vein thrombosis, thrombophlebitis, pulmonary embolism, complications of fluid overload, fluid deficit, hypokalemia, and syncope.

The stress response to surgery, inactivity, pressure related to body position, obesity, and injury to pelvic veins during surgery contributes to the formation of deep vein thrombosis, thrombophlebitis, or pulmonary embolism. These complications may appear immediately after surgery or 1 to 2 weeks later. Routinely assess for a positive Homans' sign and for warm, tender, reddened, hardened areas in the calves. To assess for Homans' sign, ask the client to forcefully dorsiflex the foot. If pain is felt in the calf of the leg, it is considered a positive Homans' sign; if no pain is felt, it is considered a negative finding. A positive Homans' sign may indicate thrombophlebitis and is reported to the surgeon. Deep vein thrombosis and thrombophlebitis may lead to a pulmonary embolus, although there is no warning of pulmonary embolism. When pulmonary embolism occurs, the client experiences dyspnea, chest pain, cyanosis, cough, hemoptysis, tachycardia, and fever coupled with an elevated white blood cell count. If the embolism is large enough, shock develops rapidly. Pulmonary embolism may be fatal.

To prevent the formation of deep vein thrombosis, thrombophlebitis, and pulmonary embolism, encourage the client to ambulate to the extent the client is able. When in bed, encourage the client to perform postoperative leg exercises each hour. Antiembolism stockings are ordered, or a sequential compression device, which is a boot applied to the legs to simulate walking by alternate inflation. Remove the boots and antiembolism stockings every day to cleanse the skin. Antiembolism stockings and the sequential compression device are not substitutes for leg exercises. Encourage the client to perform leg exercises.

When ordered, low-molecular-weight heparin, enoxaparin (Lovenox), is administered to hemostatically stable clients who have undergone pelvic, abdominal, or thoracic surgery. It is given subcutaneously every 12 hours or daily as ordered until discharge. If preoperative INR levels were within normal range, no laboratory test is necessary to determine the drug's effect. The regimen is ordered at the surgeon's discretion.

Measure intake and output and monitor laboratory findings (e.g., electrolytes, hematocrit, hemoglobin, and serum osmolality) and signs and symptoms of hemorrhage by assessing vital signs, skin color and condition, dressings, drains, and tubes, as in the PACU.

Clients often experience syncope when changing from a lying position to a sitting or standing position. Assist the client to change positions slowly, proceed in steps, and allow time for the client's internal equilibrium to adjust. Check the radial pulse frequently and ask the client if he is dizzy or nauseated. If syncope occurs during ambulation, ask for assistance in obtaining a wheelchair for the client, use a nearby chair, or lower the client to the floor until the client recovers. Although frightening for the client, syncope is not physiologically threatening unless the client is injured in a fall.

3. The client may be at risk for *Imbalanced **N**utrition: Less than Body Requirements* related to nausea and vomiting, hiccups, abdominal distension, constipation, and NPO status. Gastrointestinal complications become more prevalent after immediate postoperative recovery. The client may also experience pain related to hiccups and slowed gastrointestinal function.

   Anesthetic agents, narcotics, hypotension, and the manipulation of the bowel during surgery cause nausea and vomiting. Handling of the bowel during pelvic and abdominal surgery causes peristalsis to stop or severely slow. Bowel function normally returns 2 to 5 days after surgery. If bowel inactivity persists, a paralytic ileus develops. As bowel function resumes, continue to assess the client for bowel sounds and, if a nasogastric tube is present, a reduction in drainage. As peristalsis returns in a discontinuous fashion, the client experiences distention along with flatulence and gas pains. After bowel sounds resume in all quadrants, the client is removed from NPO status according to the surgeon's orders. Provide good oral hygiene when the client is NPO and administer antiemetics as needed for nausea and vomiting.

   Hiccups are caused by irritation of the phrenic nerve. Impulses then cause the diaphragm to contract rhythmically and violently. Abdominal distention, gastric distention, and the presence of a nasogastric tube are common causes, but electrolyte and acid–base disturbances, intestinal obstruction, and intra-abdominal bleeding also initiate hiccups. Notify the surgeon when hiccups are prolonged.

   Gas pains and signs and symptoms of abdominal distention are minimized by early and frequent ambulation and resumption of oral intake. Frequently repositioning the client encourages movement of air through the intestines, relieving gas pains. As air rises and peristalsis moves from right to left, the client is moved from lying on the left side (where air will rise on the right), to lying supine, to lying on the right side (where air will rise on the left). If the client can tolerate it and there are no contraindications, lying prone with the head turned to the side places pressure on the abdomen, forcing air to rise and move out through the rectum. Other nursing care measures to relieve abdominal distention might include irrigation of the nasogastric tube, if present. Irrigating the nasogastric tube may also relieve hiccups.

   Constipation is a major source of discomfort for the client. Analgesics combined with decreased activity and NPO status are very constipating. Oral fluids and activity are encouraged. If ordered, the medical regimen of stool softeners and suppositories are indicated.

4. The client is at risk for developing ***U**rinary Retention* related to anesthesia, immobility, and pain. The client is also at *Risk for **I**nfection* related to Foley catheter placement. The quantity and quality of urine are more directly related to cardiac output and the perfusion of the kidneys than to anesthesia, immobility, and pain; although a stress response following surgery causes the body to retain fluids for 24 to 48 hours after surgery. Urine output should be at least 30 mL per hour if a catheter is in place. The catheter is assessed for patency. If not catheterized, the client should void at least 200 mL at the first postoperative voiding. Most clients void within 6 to 8 hours after surgery; however, urinary retention occurs frequently in the postoperative period, especially following abdominal or pelvic surgery. Anesthesia depresses the urge to void. Narcotics, vagolytic agents (anticholinergics), and spinal anesthesia also interfere with the ability to initiate voiding. Facilitate voiding by encouraging fluid intake and assisting the client to void in an anatomically correct position depending on the client's condition. Privacy, running water, indirect bladder pressure (placing a firm hand over the bladder), and warm water over the perineum may also encourage voiding.

   If the client has not voided, use a noninvasive bladder ultrasound instrument to measure the bladder volume. If the facility does not have a bladder scanner, palpate, inspect, and percuss the bladder to check for distention. The surgeon orders a Foley catheter inserted if the client has a distended bladder or has not voided after 8-10 hours.

5. The client may become at risk for *Disturbed **S**ensory Perception* related to anesthesia, narcotics, change of environment, fluid and electrolyte imbalances, sleep deprivation, hypoxia, and sensory deprivation or overload. The client may also experience *Acute **P**ain* related to the surgical incision; ***H**ypothermia* related to anesthesia and surgical environment; and ***H**yperthermia* related to infection. Alterations in neurological function vary and manifest as pain, fever, or delirium. Assessing the level of consciousness is a priority. A change in level of consciousness may be the first indication of a stroke and/or increased intracranial pressure. Determining the level of consciousness is difficult, especially in the elderly client or at night, when clients are groggy from being awakened. Often, thoughts will clear if the client is given the opportunity to thoroughly awaken. Encouraging the presence of loved ones, offering explanations, and listening to the client decreases sensory perceptual alterations. Encouraging previous sleep patterns,

providing uninterrupted sleep, and alternating rest and activity also is beneficial.

Assess and record subjective data regarding pain location, intensity on a scale of 0 to 10, quality, and duration as well as factors contributing to pain. Objective data such as grimacing and crying are also recorded. Analgesics are usually ordered for administration via patient-controlled analgesia (PCA) or epidural analgesia or intravenously, intramuscularly, or orally, all on a PRN (as needed) basis. Encourage the client to ask for medication before the pain becomes severe. Offer medication before activity or painful procedures such as wound irrigation. Attend to analgesic requests promptly. Ensuring comfort encourages the client's full participation in coughing, deep breathing, turning, and ambulation.

Hypothermia is common in the first few hours following surgery. Offer blankets as needed. Because of the normal inflammatory response, temperature may later elevate to a low-grade fever. If temperature rises higher than 101°F, notify the surgeon. Atelectasis and dehydration cause elevated temperature (higher than 101°F) in the first 24 to 48 hours after surgery. After 48 hours, temperature higher than 101°F indicates a wound, respiratory, or urinary tract infection; thrombophlebitis; or pulmonary embolism.

The nurse's primary role is to prevent infection by using aseptic technique. Once a fever has occurred, follow orders to ascertain the cause of the elevation by taking urine, wound, blood, or sputum cultures. Administer antipyretics as ordered. Providing light covers and clothing, performing frequent linen changes, offering cool washcloths, and ensuring a cool environment are measures that may increase comfort.

6. The surgical client is at *Risk for Impaired **S**kin Integrity and Risk for **I**nfection* related to surgical incision. The nurse generally does not remove the primary dressing without an order to do so. Bleeding is monitored by circling the drainage on the dressing and then reassessing later to ascertain whether the drainage area has increased in size. The dressing also is reinforced with additional absorbent dressings as needed. In some institutions, the dressing is changed as necessary after the first dressing change. Some surgeons prefer no dressing if there is no drainage or drains.

Drainage on dressings and in drains typically changes from sanguinous to serosanguinous to serous over several hours to several days, depending on the type of surgery. The amount also decreases over the same time period. Purulent, odorous drainage is a sign of infection. A sudden increase in drainage is a sign of impending wound separation. Always notify the surgeon of any excessive or abnormal drainage.

All wounds heal by primary, secondary, or tertiary intention. In primary intention, the wound layers are sutured together and have no gaping edges. The wound generally heals in 8 to 10 days but may take up to 3 months. There is minimal scar formation. Most surgical wounds are of this type.

In secondary intention, the wound heals by filling in with granulation tissue and by contracting where the skin edges are not approximated. This method is used for ulcers when there is not enough tissue to approximate the edges or for infected wounds when drainage is desirable. Wounds healing by secondary intention are assessed according to the presence of granulation tissue having a red, granular appearance. Wound healing is slow, possibly taking many months or years. Thus wound healing by primary intention is preferable.

In tertiary intention, the approximation of tissue edges is delayed. This allows an infection to drain or an area of extensive tissue removal to begin healing. The edges of the wound are closed 4 to 6 days later. Because areas of granulation tissue are brought together at this time, the scar is usually much wider (Figure 33-9).

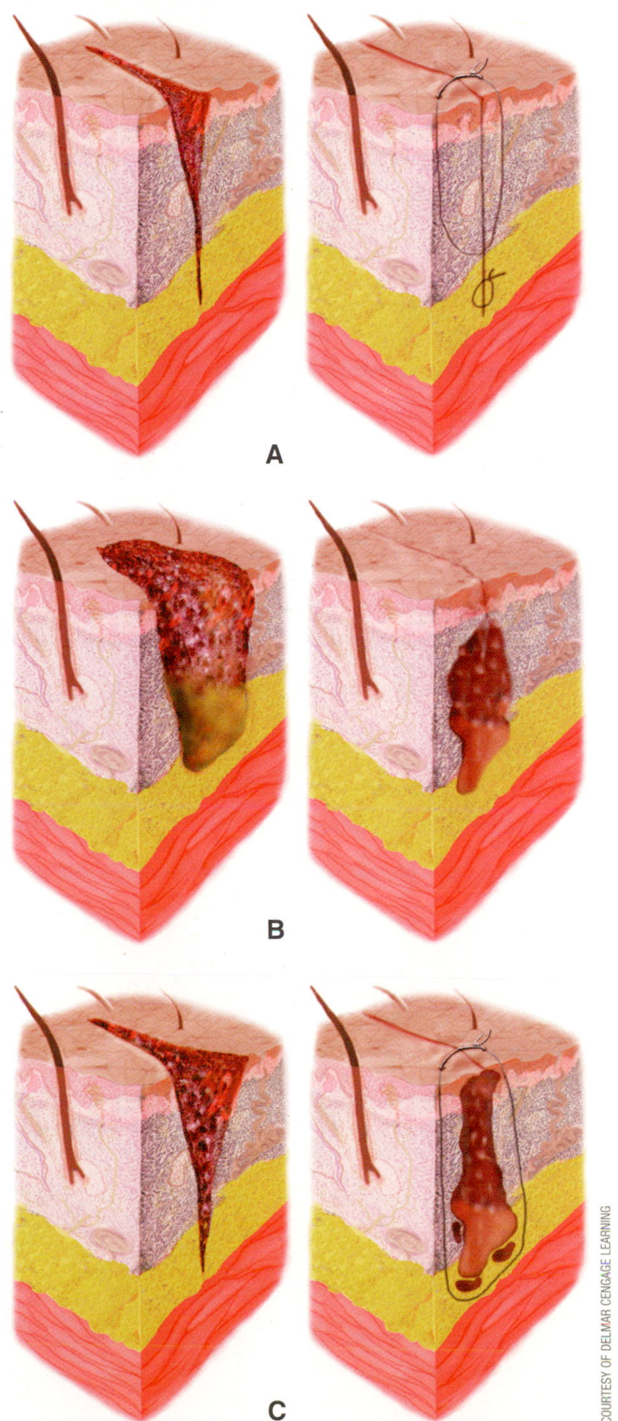

COURTESY OF DELMAR CENGAGE LEARNING

FIGURE 33-9 Wound Healing; *A*, Primary Intention; *B*, Secondary Intention; and *C*, Tertiary Intention

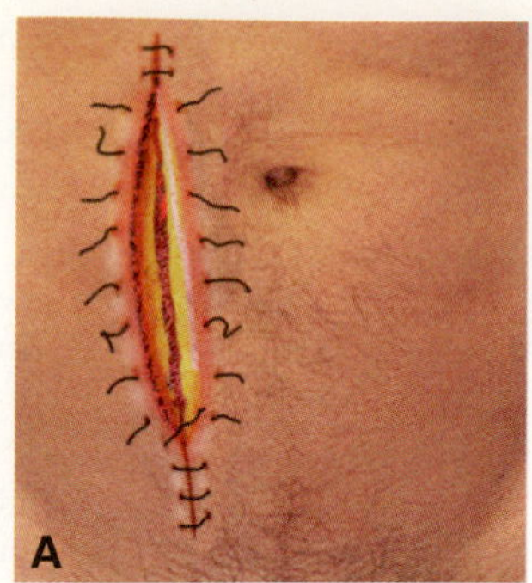

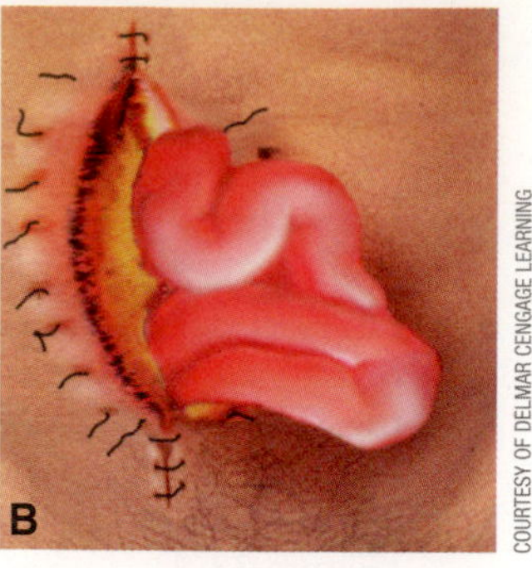

COURTESY OF DELMAR CENGAGE LEARNING

FIGURE 33-10 *A*, Dehiscence; *B*, Evisceration

Wound dehiscence and evisceration are serious complications of wound healing. **Dehiscence** occurs when the wound edges separate. **Evisceration** occurs when the wound separates completely and the viscera protrude from the wound (Figure 33-10). Both are more likely to occur 7 to 10 days after surgery and are preceded by a sudden spillage of serosanguinous drainage. Dehiscence and evisceration are more likely to occur in the very elderly client, the malnourished client, the client with an infection, or the client with abdominal distention who is straining severely. If evisceration occurs, the viscera is immediately covered with sterile saline dressings and the surgeon notified of the wound disruption.

When dressings are changed, the surgical incision is cleansed to remove debris and bacteria from the incision. The choice of cleansing agent depends on the physician's prescription as well as institutional protocol. It is recommended that isotonic solutions such as normal saline or lactated ringers be used.

The major principles to keep in mind when cleansing a surgical incision are:

- Use Standard Precautions at all times.
- Use a sterile swab or gauze and work from the clean area out toward the dirtier area. Begin over the incision line and swab downward from top to bottom. Change the swab and proceed again on either side of the incision, using a new swab each time (Figure 33-11).

The surface closures (staples or sutures) are removed as the incision heals. Continuous sutures are made with one thread and tied at the beginning and end of the suture line. Intermittent sutures are each tied individually. In blanket continuous sutures, the single thread is grounded again in the last suture exit (Figure 33-12). Some surgical wounds are closed with dissolvable sutures and special tape strips and others with special adhesive glue. The dissolvable sutures are not removed and the glue wears off. Sometimes no bandage is applied when the wound is closed with glue.

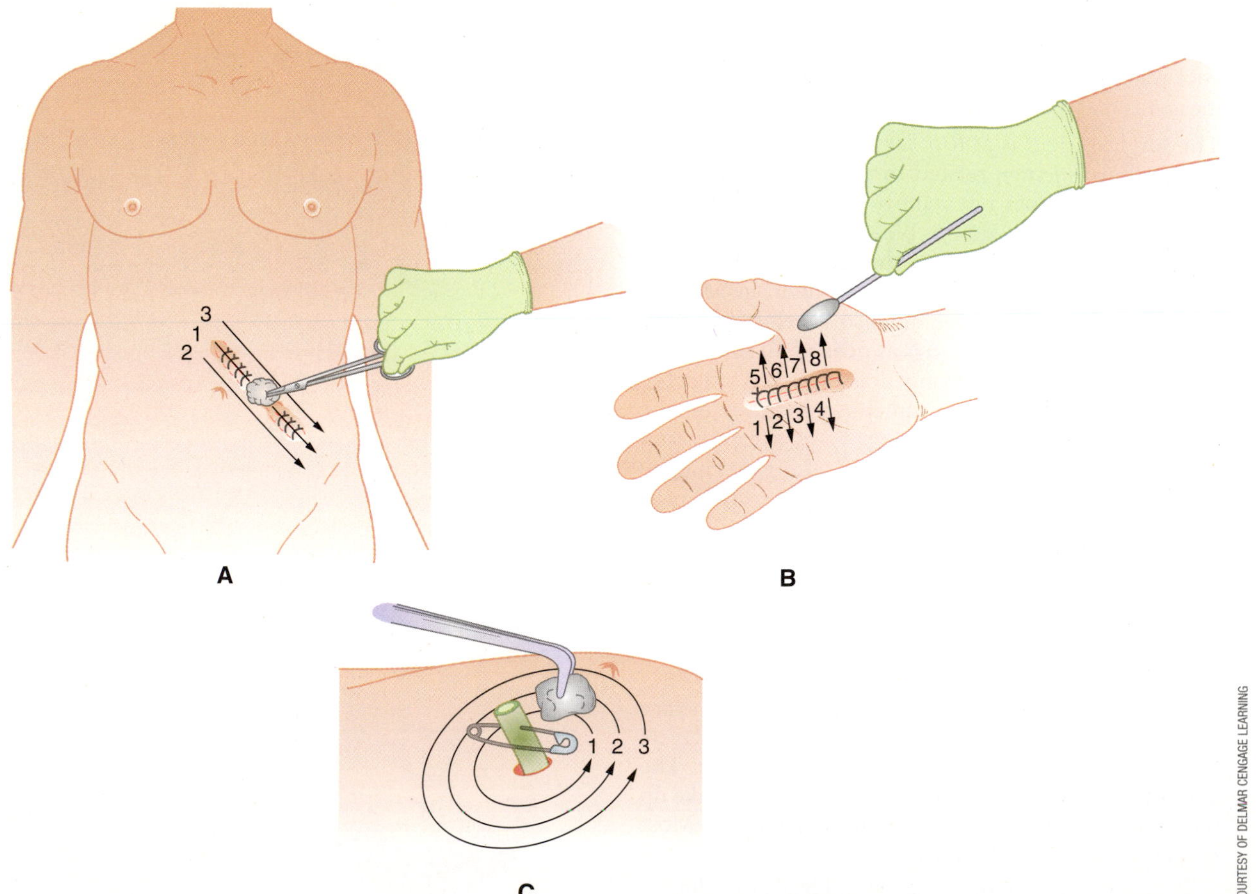

COURTESY OF DELMAR CENGAGE LEARNING

FIGURE 33-11 Use a clean, sterile swab for each stroke when cleansing a surgical incision. *A*, Gently clean the incision, then each side alternately; *B*, Gently wipe swab outward, away from the incision; *C*, Clean around a drain site in a circular motion.

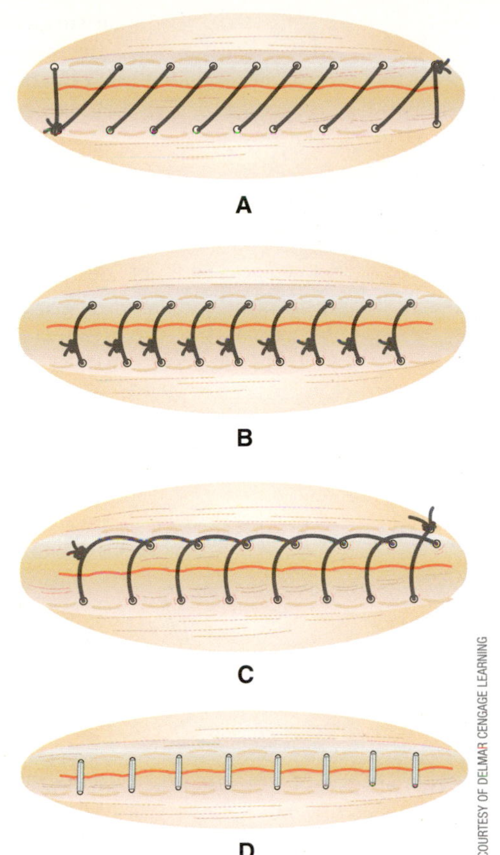

FIGURE 33-12 Skin Closure Methods; *A*, Continuous; *B*, Intermittent; *C*, Blanket Continuous; *D*, Staples

The incisional dressing keeps the incision clean and protects it from physical trauma and bacterial invasion. Generally, the same kind of dressing is put on as was taken off. As the incision heals and drainage lessens, a small, thinner dressing usually is applied.

COMMUNITY/HOME HEALTH CARE

Dressing Wounds

- Because of early discharge, clients are often sent home with incisions that need dressing changes.
- Ascertain the client's support system, including caregivers, the home environment, and available resources.
- Teach the client and/or home caregiver the correct method of changing the dressing.
- Have the client and/or home caregiver change the dressing before the client is discharged.
- Provide a list of signs and symptoms of complications of wound healing.
- At times, a referral for home care nursing is necessary.

COMMUNITY/HOME HEALTH CARE

Postoperative Care

For proper home care, the client and family must be given information about the following topics:

- Medication regimen
- Diet
- Activity restrictions
- Follow-up appointments
- Wound care
- Special instructions

The specifics for each topic will vary with each client and will depend on the surgical procedure and the client's age and physical condition.

Bandages and binders are applied over the incision dressing to secure, immobilize, or support a body part; to hold the dressing in place; or to prevent or minimize swelling of a body part. Bandages are long rolls of material, such as gauze, webbing, or muslin, designed for wrapping around body parts. Figure 33-13 illustrates several different methods of bandaging. Binders are bandages made for specific body parts, usually the abdomen or arm (sling) (Figure 33-14). Abdominal binders support the abdomen of an obese client following abdominal surgery. A sling is a cloth support with adjustable straps that wrap around the back to provide support for an injured arm; it maintains the arm in a set position.

During dressing changes and after the dressing has been removed, the surgical wound is assessed for skin edge approximation, edema, and bleeding. The skin edges may be slightly reddened and swollen from the normal inflammatory response. Possible signs of a wound infection include increased suture tension, warmth, erythema, drainage, odor, pain, and induration around the incision site. Wound healing is enhanced by promoting nutrition, discouraging smoking, and performing proper wound cleansing. The practice of aseptic technique cannot be emphasized enough in preventing nosocomial infections in a surgical incision.

7. Clients are at risk for *Anxiety or Ineffective Coping* related to disturbance in body image, change in lifestyle, financial strain, or a poor prognosis. Many clients undergo a psychological adjustment to surgery. Taking time to listen to the client as well as offering simple explanations and reassurances supports the client needs to combat anxiety.

As the client recovers and is ready for discharge from the hospital, the client is at risk for *Deficient Knowledge* related to home care. Ideally, the client receives home care instructions from the moment of admission. Adequate teaching about home care results in a quicker recovery, fewer complications, and greater independence.

Minimally invasive surgery (MIS) is replacing much of the traditional types of surgery. MIS is

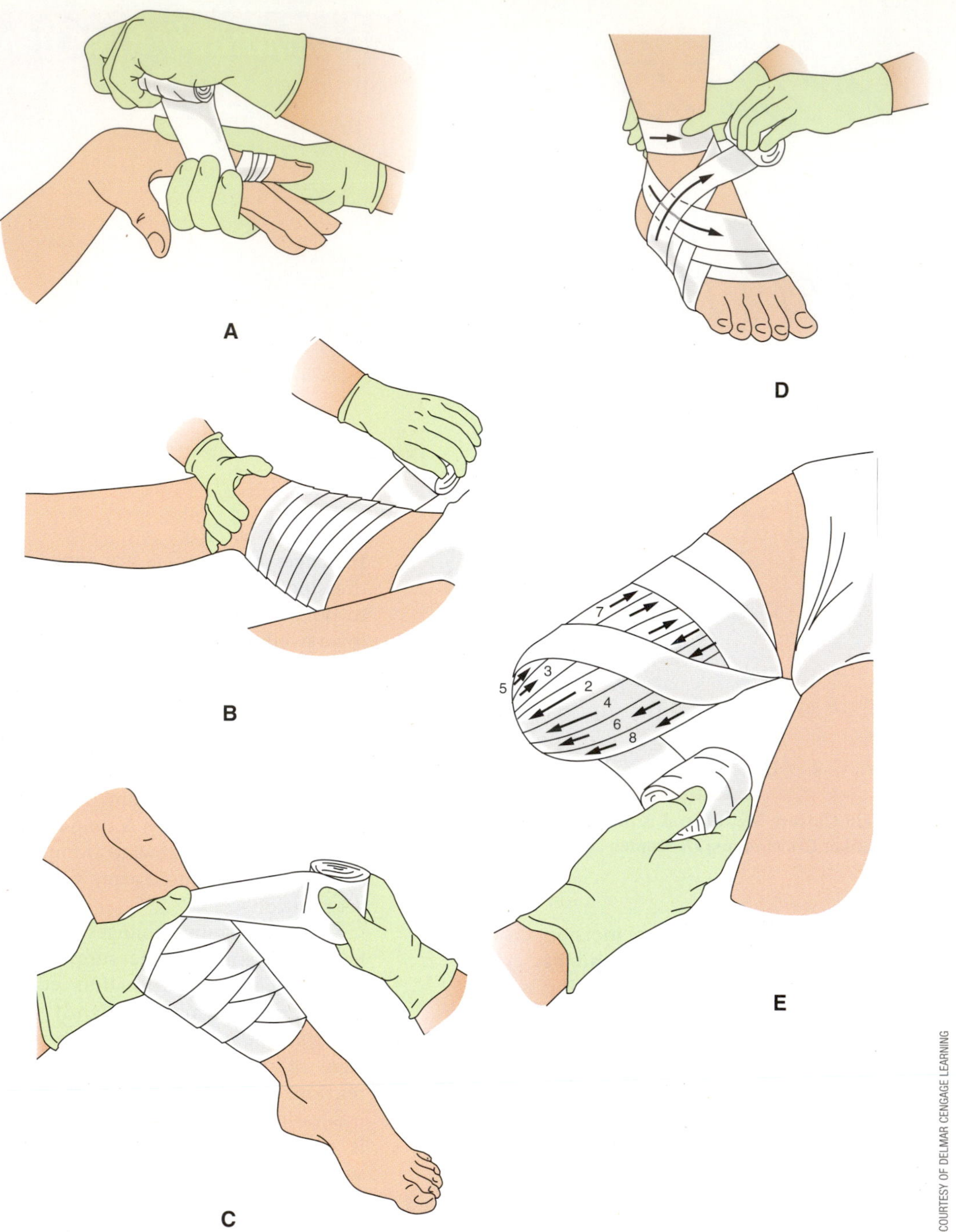

FIGURE 33-13 Common Bandaging Methods; *A,* Circular turns are wrapped around a body part several times to anchor the bandage or supply support. *B,* Spiral turns begin with a circular turn and then proceed up the body part, with each turn covering two-thirds the width of the preceding turn. *C,* Spiral reverse turns begin with a circular turn. The bandage is then reversed or twisted, once each turn, to accommodate a limb that gets larger as the bandaging progresses. *D,* Figure-eight turns crisscross in the shape of a figure eight and are used on a joint that requires movement. *E,* Recurrent turns are anchored with circular turns, follow a back-and-forth motion, and are completed with circular turns; they are used to cover a fingertip, head, or residual limb.

completed with three to five small incisions in which a videoscope and specialized instruments are inserted into the small incisions to complete the surgery (see Figure 33-15). The same traditional type of surgery would require a much longer incision through larger areas of tissue and muscle. The layout of the surgical room is different than the usual surgery suite. See Figure 33-16 for a layout of the surgical room and surgical system of a console, patient cart, and vision cart. Abdominal, thoracic, pelvic, and spine surgeries are performed by MIS. The advantages of MIS are less postoperative pain, decreased hospital stay, less risk of infection, prompt return to normal activities and work, and less overall postoperative complications. Specific MIS surgery is discussed throughout the various system chapters (Ohio State University Medical Center, 2009; George Washington University Hospital, 2009).

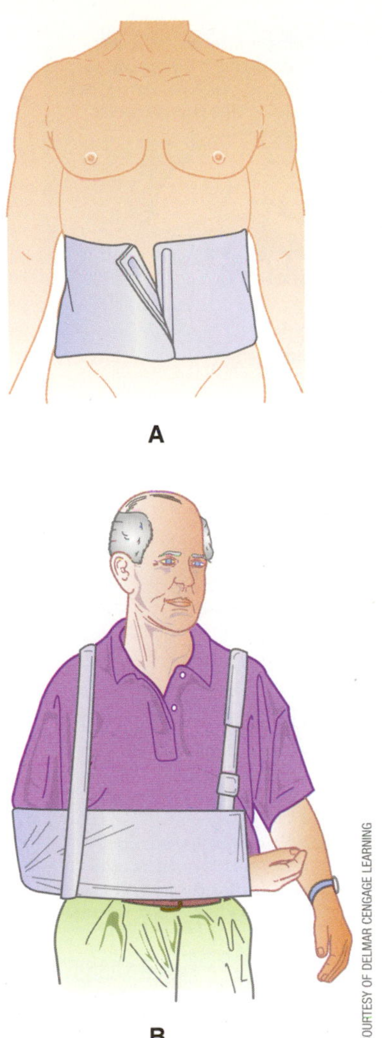

FIGURE 33-14 Common Binders: *A*, Abdominal; *B*, Arm Sling

AMBULATORY SURGERY

Ambulatory surgery is defined as surgical care performed under general, regional, or local anesthesia involving less than 24 hours of hospitalization. Other names for ambulatory surgery include same-day, one-day, outpatient, in and out, or short-stay surgery.

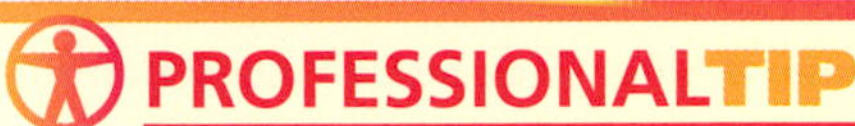

PROFESSIONALTIP

Ambulatory Surgery

- Precertification documents are approved before the preadmission visit.
- Preadmission diagnostic tests, preoperative nursing assessment, and initial teaching are usually performed the day before the scheduled surgery.
- On the day of surgery, care is focused on the immediate needs of the client.

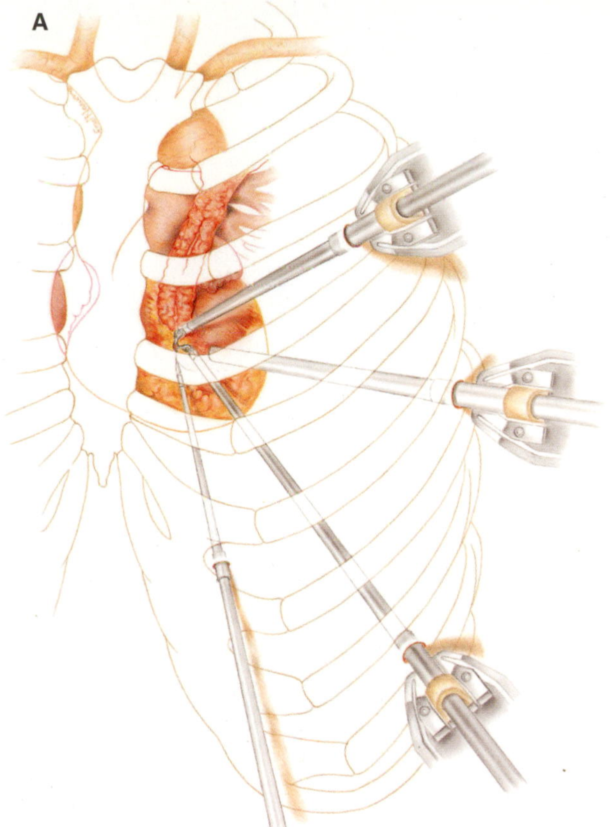

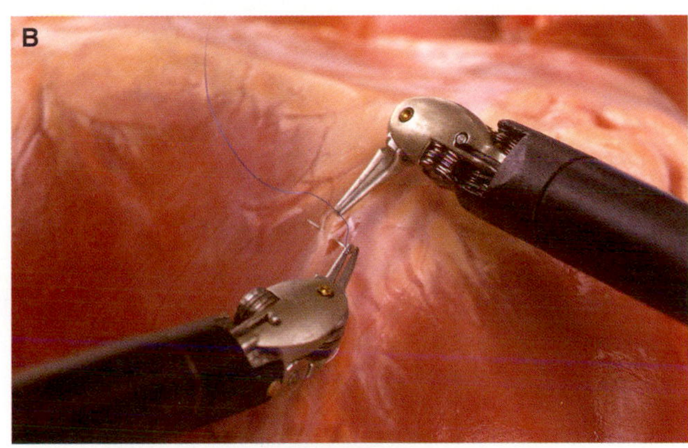

FIGURE 33-15 Minimally invasive surgery (MIS); *A*, Surgeons, using small incisions, introduce specialized instruments into the body to perform surgery. *B*, Special instruments are manipulated by the surgeons to perform surgery. (*© 2009 Intuitive Surgical, Inc.*)

The trend in health care is to promote wellness. Clients are encouraged to accept more personal responsibility for their state of health. In the past, the message sent to clients was that the client is sick, and the medical community will provide all care. Today, ambulatory surgery clients are sent an entirely different message: that the postoperative client is not sick and, except for a few minor limitations, can often resume normal daily activities soon after undergoing anesthesia and surgery.

Ambulatory surgery provides the longest period of time for the client to receive skilled postoperative care or monitoring without formal admission to the hospital. The practice of ambulatory surgery attempts to overcome the risk of premature dismissal while meeting fiscal requirements. The emphasis

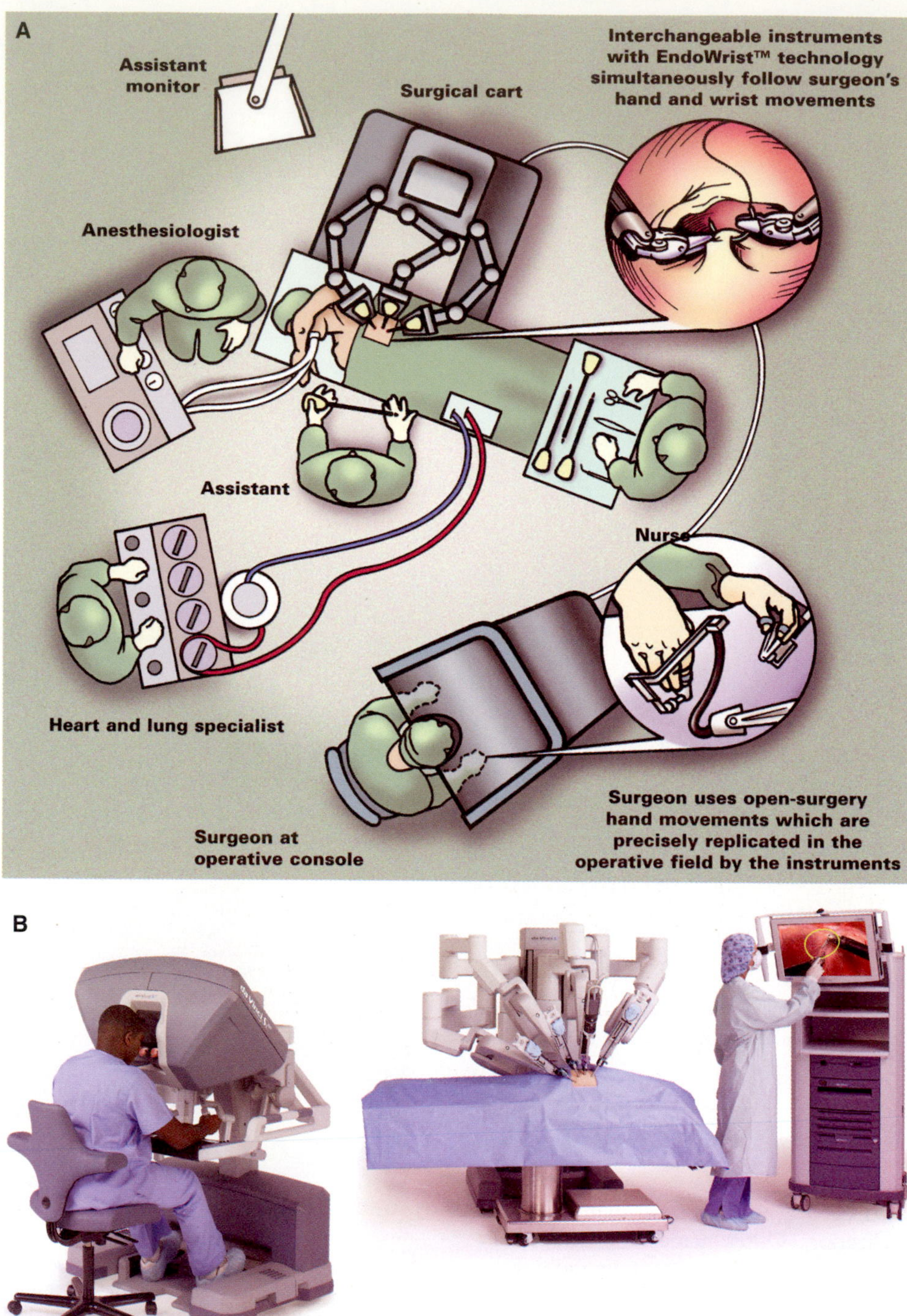

FIGURE 33-16 Minimally Invasive Surgical Suite; *A*, Typical Layout of a MIS Surgical Suite; *B*, Surgeon at the Da Vinci Si Console with Patient Cart and Surgical Nurse at the Vision Cart (*© 2009 Intuitive Surgical, Inc.*)

on cost containment coupled with government reductions in Medicare and Medicaid payments has further promoted the concept of ambulatory surgery.

To further reduce health care costs, few clients are admitted to the hospital before the day of surgery. Most surgical clients are processed through the ambulatory surgery unit. These clients are called "day of surgery" or "A.M. admit" clients. Necessary laboratory work, radiology tests, or other examinations are completed on an outpatient basis before the day of surgery. Even clients undergoing extensive surgeries such as open-heart surgery (a coronary artery bypass), craniotomy, or total joint replacement are admitted the day of surgery. Then, after discharge from the perioperative suite, the client either is admitted to the hospital as an inpatient or is sent home from the ambulatory surgery unit.

In addition to fiscal considerations, the growth of ambulatory surgery can also be traced to technological advances. Clients now require shorter recovery periods as a result of new procedural technology, such as laparoscopic cholecystectomy. The introduction of shorter-acting anesthetic agents also decreases the immediate postoperative recovery time, facilitating the client's ability to function independently upon discharge from the ambulatory surgery setting.

The benefits of ambulatory surgery are many. Ambulatory surgery decreases cost to the client, institution, insurance carriers, and governmental agencies. The risk of acquiring a nosocomial infection is also decreased. The client experiences less disruption to personal life and less psychological distress related to hospitalization. With ambulatory surgery, the client especially benefits from early postoperative ambulation.

Ambulatory surgery is performed in several different settings. Hospital-based integrated facilities are formal ambulatory surgery programs incorporated into existing inpatient surgery programs. Clients are cared for preoperatively and postoperatively in the ambulatory surgery unit but are mixed with inpatients on the OR schedule. This type of facility also allows preoperative processing of day-of-surgery clients. Hospital-affiliated facilities consist of a separate department with designated preoperative, intraoperative, and postoperative areas. Such a facility is located within the hospital, adjacent to the hospital, or at a satellite location. Freestanding facilities are independently owned and operated and are not affiliated with a hospital or medical center. In the past, physicians generally owned such facilities, but today the trend is for health care corporations to own these facilities. Some doctors' offices also have facilities for performing minor ambulatory surgery.

The Aldrete Score has been modified for use with clients having anesthesia on an ambulatory basis. Five assessments were added to the Aldrete Score for this purpose (Table 33-2). Attainment of these criteria indicates that clients can care for themselves at home and accomplish activities of daily living independently and safely. The points are totaled at regular intervals (usually every half hour), and clients are discharged home when their total score is 18 or higher.

ELDERLY CLIENTS HAVING SURGERY

Elderly clients (older than 65 years of age) are at risk for developing complications from surgery or anesthesia. Unfortunately, because an increased incidence of disease correlates with increasing age, more elderly clients require surgery than does any other age group. As the percentage of elderly persons in the whole population rises, the number of surgeries on elders is increasing. Because of the complex needs of the elderly client undergoing surgery, knowledge in promoting health and rehabilitation in the elderly client is necessary.

Surgery is a stressor. Because of depleted energy sources, the elderly client may not have sufficient resilience to react defensively to this stressor. The risk of complications from surgery further increases in elderly clients who have one or more chronic diseases. In these clients, surgery then can be the source of a downward spiraling effect toward debilitation or possibly death.

Elderly clients vary in their abilities to respond to the stress of surgery. Physiologic changes related to the aging process inhibit the elderly client from readily coping with surgery. The number of physiologic changes in the very elderly client (older than 80 years of age) is markedly greater than that in those in their sixties and seventies. Breathing capacity, renal blood flow, cardiac output, and conduction velocity of the nervous system all diminish. Table 33-5 lists the physiologic changes in the elderly client along with correlating nursing interventions for postoperative care. Aging affects all body systems, and the nurse's

TABLE 33-5 Physiologic Changes of Aging and Related Postoperative Nursing Interventions

BODY SYSTEM	CHANGES	NURSING INTERVENTIONS
Cardiovascular	• Decreased elasticity of the vascular system • Decreased cardiac output • Decreased peripheral circulation	• Closely monitor vital signs and peripheral pulses • Encourage early ambulation • Use antiembolism stockings • Monitor intake and output, including blood loss • Monitor preoperative response to activity and compare to postoperative response
Respiratory	• Decreased vital capacity • Decreased alveolar volume • Decreased movement of cilia	• Closely monitor respirations • Auscultate breath sounds frequently • Encourage coughing and deep breathing • Turn frequently • Monitor oxygen saturation

(Continues)

Table 33-5 Physiologic Changes of Aging and Related Postoperative Nursing Interventions (Continued)

BODY SYSTEM	CHANGES	NURSING INTERVENTIONS
Urinary	• Decreased glomerular filtration rate • Decreased bladder muscle tone • Weakened perineal muscles	• Monitor intake and output every 1 to 2 hours • Assist frequently with toileting • Monitor fluid and electrolyte status
Gastrointestinal	• Decreased gastric and intestinal motility • Altered digestion and absorption • Decreased food consumption	• Assess for obesity and malnutrition • Encourage fluids and activity • Encourage high-protein foods and supplements • Assist with meals as needed • Provide companionship during mealtime
Immunological	• Decreased level of gamma globulin • Decreased plasma proteins	• Follow strict aseptic technique • Monitor temperature • Assess incision site
Neurological	• Decreased conduction velocity • Decreased visual acuity • Loss of hearing • Decreased sensation	• Allow use of glasses and hearing aids • Orient to environment • Provide for safe environment • Repeat information as needed • Use medications sparingly • Provide written instructions • Allow for extra education time
Integumentary	• Lack of elasticity • Loss of collagen • Decreased subcutaneous fat	• To prevent shearing forces on skin when positioning client, lift rather than slide client • Pad bony prominences • Use tape that is easy to remove • Use warm prepping solutions, irrigating solutions, and IV solutions intraoperatively • Provide extra blankets • Ensure warm room temperature • Turn frequently • Encourage early ambulation

COURTESY OF DELMAR CENGAGE LEARNING

knowledge of these changes and the interventions geared toward each assist in preventing and detecting complications of surgery.

The elderly client has a lifetime of experiences that affects the response to surgery. A lifetime of watching family and friends experience surgery, illness, and death particularly influences personal reactions to impending surgery. Because of the variation in such experiences, each client reacts differently to similar situations. Simply talking with the client to provide information or listening to the client's fears helps prepare the client for upcoming surgery.

Third-party reimbursement policies often require elderly clients to undergo surgical procedures on an outpatient basis. Because many elderly clients have neurological deficits and other chronic disease processes, the elderly outpatient poses a particular challenge. Additional postoperative self-care deficits may result from the surgical procedure and the effects of anesthesia. Elderly clients often live alone and lack the support systems necessary for home care. In order to provide realistic discharge planning, the nurse assesses the ability of the client, family, and friends to provide care at home.

CASE STUDY

G.S., a 74-year-old retired school teacher who is married and the father of four and the grandfather of sixteen, weighs 275 lbs. He has undergone a right hemicolectomy, wherein the right side of his colon was removed because of cancer. He has a history of smoking but has no other health problems. The surgery was uncomplicated, and he is in the PACU. He has a midline incision with a Penrose drain and a stab wound with a Jackson-Pratt drain adjacent to the incision. He also has a nasogastric tube attached to low intermittent suction. He is alert and oriented and moves all four extremities freely. His blood pressure is normal for him in comparison to his preoperative levels. He is breathing regularly and easily at a rate of 16 breaths per minute, and his skin color is normal. His oxygen saturation, however, is 86% with additional oxygen given via mask.

The following questions will guide your development of a nursing care plan for the case study.

1. What risk factors for developing postoperative complications can you identify for G.S.?
2. What is his Aldrete Score at this point?
3. What nursing measures can you institute to promote oxygenation?
4. What type of drainage is expected from the incision and the drains during the first 1 to 2 days?
5. What nursing observations can be made and reported to indicate to the surgeon that the nasogastric tube can be removed?
6. What nursing measures can be implemented to prevent deep vein thrombosis, thrombophlebitis, and pulmonary embolism?
7. Write and prioritize three individualized nursing diagnoses and goals for G.S.
8. What information will G.S. need before discharge?

SUMMARY

- Surgery is a major stressor for all clients. Anxiety and fear are normal. Fear of the unknown is both the most prevalent fear before surgery and the fear easiest for the nurse to help the client overcome.
- The outcome of surgical treatment is tremendously enhanced by accurate preoperative nursing assessment and careful preoperative preparation. Information gathered through preoperative assessment and risk screening is later used to prepare the surgical site, for surgical positioning, and as a comparative basis for postoperative assessments and complication screening.
- The teaching methods that the nurse uses strongly influence the degree of learning and the retention of information.
- Aseptic technique is a collection of principles used to control and/or prevent the transfer of microorganisms from sources within (endogenous) and outside (exogenous) the client. All clinical nursing units practice these principles. The sterile conscience governs personal behavior with regard to adherence to aseptic technique.
- Nursing care in the OR focuses on the safety and protection of the client.
- Postoperative nursing assessments are completed in an organized manner, focusing first on the priorities of airway, breathing, and circulation, and then on the body system affected by surgery.
- The nurse prevents the formation of deep vein thrombosis, thrombophlebitis, and pulmonary embolism through encouraging early ambulation and postoperative leg exercises and by providing antiembolism stockings and/or sequential stockings, if ordered.
- Ambulatory surgery is defined as surgical care performed under general, regional, or local anesthesia and involving fewer than 24 hours of hospitalization. Cost containment, governmental changes, and technological advances promote the concept of ambulatory surgery.
- Because of the physiologic changes and complex needs of the elderly client undergoing surgery, the nurse's knowledge assists in promoting health and rehabilitation in the elderly surgical client.

REVIEW QUESTIONS

1. Client education is:
    1. completed when time allows.
    2. started when discharge is scheduled.
    3. always more beneficial when completed in a structured group setting.
    4. directed toward the client's family when the client is unable to learn.
2. A client is scheduled for surgery. The role of the nurse in obtaining consent includes:
    1. judging the quality of the explanation and ascertaining the client's understanding of the consent form.
    2. acting as a witness to the signature of the client.

3. administering the preoperative medication before the client signs the consent.
4. ensuring that coercion was used to obtain the client's signature on the consent.

3. Upon the client's admission to the PACU, the nurse knows to first:
   1. take the client's blood pressure.
   2. assess the airway.
   3. assess the client's level of consciousness.
   4. check the incision site.

4. The nurse is making a preoperative assessment on a client. Of the following findings, the most important item to know for a client who is having general anesthesia is:
   1. hearing impaired.
   2. a right-leg amputee.
   3. color blind.
   4. a smoker.

5. The nursing intervention that has the greatest impact on reducing overall surgical risk is:
   1. encouraging activity and early ambulation.
   2. assessing blood pressure.
   3. ensuring adequate nutrition.
   4. monitoring intake and output.

6. An elderly client is returning to the unit from surgery. The nursing interventions specifically geared toward elderly care are: (Select all that apply.)
   1. carefully monitoring vital signs and peripheral pulses.
   2. lifting the client rather than sliding client when repositioning.
   3. encouraging early ambulation.
   4. repeating information as needed.
   5. following strict aseptic technique.
   6. using tape that is easily removed.

7. The surgical client's most common fear is of the unknown. The nurse can ease the client's fears by:
   1. listening to the client's concerns about surgery.
   2. taking time from busy schedule and sitting beside the client for a few minutes.
   3. asking the client's family to stay with the client.
   4. teaching the client about the surgical process and answer questions.

8. A 73-year-old client is scheduled for prostate surgery. His vital signs are T 98.2, P 74, R 14, and BP160/92. He drinks heavily and smokes a pack of cigarettes a day. What is the client's risk factors pending his upcoming surgery? (Select all that apply.)
   1. Hepatic status.
   2. Fluid and electrolyte status.
   3. Age.
   4. Cardiovascular status.
   5. Respiratory status.
   6. Musculoskeletal system.

9. The PACU nurse asks a new surgical client if he has the ability to wiggle his toes and move his feet. She is assessing his: (Select all that apply.)
   1. hearing since that is the first sensation to return after anesthesia.
   2. ability to pull his drain from the wound.
   3. likeliness of becoming combative after surgery.
   4. ability to voluntarily move his extremity.
   5. Homans' sign in both lower extremities.
   6. circulation to the extremities.

10. A client returns to the PACU following a craniotomy. After assessing the airway, the first priority of the nurse is to:
    1. attach all tubes to drainage.
    2. place the client in Trendelenburg position.
    3. check abdomen for bowel sounds.
    4. assess level of consciousness and extremity movement.

REFERENCES/SUGGESTED READINGS

Aldrete, J. (1995). The post-anesthesia recovery score revisited. *Journal of Clinical Anesthesiology*, 7(1), 89–91.

Association of periOperative Registered Nurses (AORN). (2002a). Artificial nails. AORN Online Journal. [Online]. Available: www.aorn.org/journal/2002/juneci.htm

Association of periOperative Registered Nurses (2002b). Standards, recommended practices, and guidelines, Denver, CO: Author.

Brenner, Z. (1999). Preventing postoperative complications. *Nursing99*, 29(10), 34-39.

Bryant, R., & Nix, D. (2006). *Acute and chronic wounds: Current management concepts* (3rd ed.). St. Louis, MO: Mosby

Burden, N., Defazio-Quinn, D., & O'Brien, D. (2000). *Ambulatory surgical nursing*. Philadelphia: W. B. Saunders.

Cizzell, J. (1994). Back to basics: Test your wound assessment skills. *AJN*, 94(6), 34–35.

Crenshaw, J., & Winslow, E. (2002). Preoperative fasting: Old habits die hard. *AJN*, 102(5), 36–44.

Erwin-Toth, P., & Hocevar, B. (1995). Wound care: Selecting the right dressing. *AJN*, 95(2), 46–51.

Fort, C. (2002). Get pumped to prevent DVT. *Nursing2002*, 32(9), 50–52.

George Washington University Hospital. (2009). Thinking big about small incisions. *George Washington University Hospital Health News*. Retrieved on April 25, 2009 at http://gwashington.uhspublications.com/spring2009/story1.html

Gilchrist, B. (1990). Washing and dressings after surgery. *Journal of the Wound Care Society*, 86(50), 71.

Grogan, T. (1999). Bringing bloodless surgery into the mainstream. *Nursing99*, 29(11), 58–61.

Hogstel, M. (2001). *Gerontology: Nursing care of the older adult*. Clifton Park, NY: Delmar Cengage Learning.

Lewis, S., Collier, I., & Heitkemper, M. (2002). *Medical–surgical nursing: Assessment and management of clinical problems* (5th ed.). St. Louis, MO: Mosby.

Monahan, F., Sands, J., Neighbors, M., Marek, J., & Green-Nigro, C. (2006). *Phipps' medical-surgical nursing: Health and illness perspectives* (8th ed.). St. Louis, MO: Mosby.

Motta, G. (1993). How moisture retentive dressings promote healing. Nursing 93, 23(12), 26–33.

Ohio State Universtity Medical Center. (2009). What is minimally invasive surgery? Retrieved on April 25, 2009 at http://cmis.osu.edu/8880.cfm

Phillips, J. (1998). Wound dehiscence. *Nursing98*, 28(3), 33.

Phillips, N. (2007). *Berry and Kohn's operating room technique* (11th ed.). St. Louis, MO: C.V. Mosby Co.

Smeltzer, S., Bare, B. Hinkle, S., & Cheever, K. (2008). *Brunner and Suddarth's textbook of medical-surgical nursing* (11th ed.). Philadelphia: Lippincott Williams & Wilkins.

Surgical Associates at Virginia Hospital Center. (2009). Surgical wound care: Frequently asked questions. Retrieved on April 25, 2009 at http://www.SurgicalAssociatesVHC.com

Talabiska, D. (1995). *Malnutrition in the elderly. Newlines in Multi-Vitamin Infusion*, 4(2), 1, 2, 6.

Vernon, S., & Molnar-Pfeifer, G. (1997). Are you ready for bloodless surgery? *AJN*, 97(9), 40–47.

Winslow, E., & Jacobson, A. (2001). The case against artificial nails. *Nursing2001*, 31(10), 30.

RESOURCES

Association of periOperative Registered Nurses (AORN), http://www.aorn.org

Intuitive Surgical, Inc., http://www.intuitivesurgical.com

CHAPTER 34
Oncology

MAKING THE CONNECTION

Refer to the following chapters to increase your understanding of oncology nursing:

Basic Nursing
- ***Legal and Ethical Responsibilities***
- ***End-of-Life Care***
- ***Pain Management***
- ***Diagnostic Tests***

Adult Health Nursing
- ***Surgery***
- ***Hematologic and Lymphatic Systems***
- ***Gastrointestinal System***
- ***Neurological System***
- ***Endocrine System***
- ***Reproductive System***
- ***Integumentary System***
- ***Immune System***
- ***The Older Adult***

LEARNING OBJECTIVES

Upon completion of this chapter, you should be able to:

- Define key terms.
- Explain how the behavior of cancer cells differs from that of normal cells.
- Describe the role of the nurse in cancer detection.
- Discuss three medical treatments for cancer.
- Describe four complications that can occur in advanced cancer.
- Discuss ways the licensed practical/vocational nurse can aid the client in coping with cancer.

KEY TERMS

alopecia
anorexia
antineoplastic
benign
biologic response modifier (BRM)
bone marrow transplantation (BMT)
cachexia
cancer
carcinogen
carcinoma
chemotherapy
curative surgery
differentiation
extravasation
leukemia
lymphoma
malignant
metastasis
neoplasm
oncology
palliative surgery
photodynamic therapy (PDT)
radiotherapy
reconstructive surgery
sarcoma
stomatitis
tumor marker
vesicant

INTRODUCTION

Cancer is a disease resulting from the uncontrolled growth of abnormal cells, which causes malignant cellular tumors. One in three Americans will develop some type of cancer during their lifetime. Cancer is the second-leading cause of death in the United States and can develop in individuals of any race, gender, age, socioeconomic status, or culture. It is not a single disease but, rather, a group of more than 200 different diseases that can attack any tissue or organ of the body.

According to the American Cancer Society (ACS), in the 1930s fewer than one in five cancer clients survived 5 years after diagnosis. In the 1940s, one in four survived 5 years. Today, 66% of people diagnosed with cancer will be alive in 5 years (ACS, 2003; ACS, 2008). Survival rates are influenced by the type of cancer, the progression of the disease at diagnosis, and the client's response to the treatment.

INCIDENCE

In the United States, men have a one in two lifetime risk of developing cancer, whereas women have a risk of one in three (ACS, 2008). Incidence and mortality rates are usually greater for African Americans than for Anglo Americans. The incidence of cancer is greater in the elderly population than in any other age group. In men, the most common cancers are prostate, lung, colorectal, and urinary bladder; in women, they are breast, lung, colorectal, and uterine cancer (Figure 34-1).

The ACS estimates that 1,437,180 new cancer cases were diagnosed in the United States in 2008. Not included in this estimate are basal- and squamous-cell skin cancers and noninvasive cancers except for urinary bladder cancer. More than 1 million cases of highly curable basal- and squamous-cell skin cancers were estimated to be diagnosed in 2008 (ACS, 2008).

In 2008, approximately 170,000 cancer deaths were estimated to be caused by tobacco. About one-third of the 565,650 cancer deaths estimated for 2008 are related to nutrition, physical inactivity, obesity, and other lifestyle factors and could be prevented (ACS, 2008).

PATHOPHYSIOLOGY

Cancer is a disease characterized by neoplasia, an uncontrolled growth of abnormal cells. Unlike normal cells, which reproduce in an orderly manner and grow for a purpose, cancer cells develop rapidly and undiscriminatingly, and they serve no useful function because they grow at the expense of healthy tissue. Neoplasms, any abnormal growth of new tissue, can be found in any body tissue. Neoplasms may be benign (not progressive and, thus, favorable for recovery) or malignant (becoming progressively worse and often resulting in death).

Benign neoplasms are not cancerous and are usually harmless. They grow slowly, are encapsulated and well-defined, and do not spread to neighboring tissues. Unless their location interferes with vital functions, benign neoplasms are associated with a favorable prognosis.

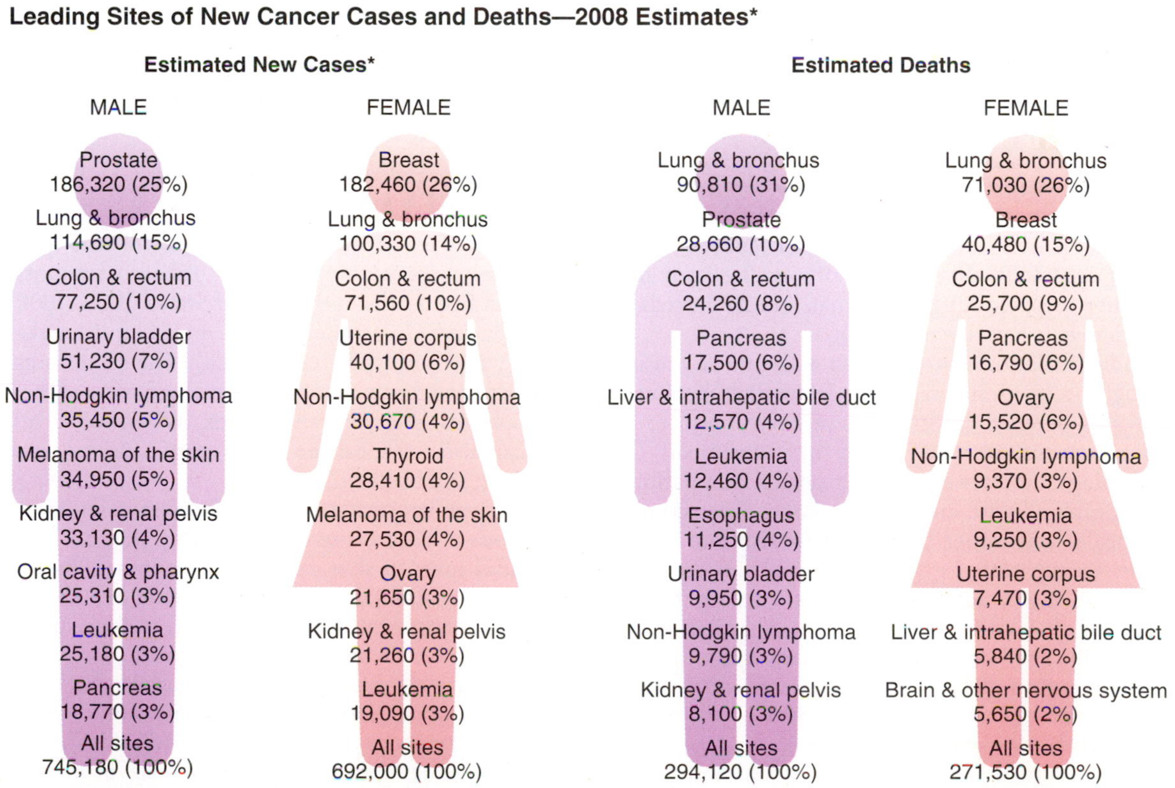

Leading Sites of New Cancer Cases and Deaths—2008 Estimates*

Estimated New Cases*		Estimated Deaths	
MALE	FEMALE	MALE	FEMALE
Prostate 186,320 (25%)	Breast 182,460 (26%)	Lung & bronchus 90,810 (31%)	Lung & bronchus 71,030 (26%)
Lung & bronchus 114,690 (15%)	Lung & bronchus 100,330 (14%)	Prostate 28,660 (10%)	Breast 40,480 (15%)
Colon & rectum 77,250 (10%)	Colon & rectum 71,560 (10%)	Colon & rectum 24,260 (8%)	Colon & rectum 25,700 (9%)
Urinary bladder 51,230 (7%)	Uterine corpus 40,100 (6%)	Pancreas 17,500 (6%)	Pancreas 16,790 (6%)
Non-Hodgkin lymphoma 35,450 (5%)	Non-Hodgkin lymphoma 30,670 (4%)	Liver & intrahepatic bile duct 12,570 (4%)	Ovary 15,520 (6%)
Melanoma of the skin 34,950 (5%)	Thyroid 28,410 (4%)	Leukemia 12,460 (4%)	Non-Hodgkin lymphoma 9,370 (3%)
Kidney & renal pelvis 33,130 (4%)	Melanoma of the skin 27,530 (4%)	Esophagus 11,250 (4%)	Leukemia 9,250 (3%)
Oral cavity & pharynx 25,310 (3%)	Ovary 21,650 (3%)	Urinary bladder 9,950 (3%)	Uterine corpus 7,470 (3%)
Leukemia 25,180 (3%)	Kidney & renal pelvis 21,260 (3%)	Non-Hodgkin lymphoma 9,790 (3%)	Liver & intrahepatic bile duct 5,840 (2%)
Pancreas 18,770 (3%)	Leukemia 19,090 (3%)	Kidney & renal pelvis 8,100 (3%)	Brain & other nervous system 5,650 (2%)
All sites 745,180 (100%)	All sites 692,000 (100%)	All sites 294,120 (100%)	All sites 271,530 (100%)

*Excluding basal and squamous cell skin cancer and *in situ* carcinomas except urinary bladder.
Percentages may not total 100% due to rounding.

FIGURE 34-1 Leading Sites of New Cancer Cases and Deaths—2008 Estimates (*American Cancer Society Cancer Facts and Figures, 2008. Reprinted with Permission.*)

Malignant neoplasms form irregularly shaped masses with fingerlike projections. They usually multiply quickly and spread to distant body parts through the bloodstream or the lymph system. This process is called metastasis. Patterns of metastasis will differ depending on the type of cancer.

Cancers are usually named according to the site of the primary tumor or to the type of tissue involved. There are four main classifications of cancer according to tissue type:

- **Lymphomas** (cancers occurring in infection-fighting organs, such as lymphatic tissue)
- **Leukemias** (cancers occurring in blood-forming organs, such as the spleen, and in bone marrow)
- **Sarcomas** (cancers occurring in connective tissue, such as bone)
- **Carcinomas** (cancers occurring in epithelial tissue, such as the skin)

The exact mechanism that causes cancer is unknown, but most authorities believe that cancer develops from a combination of factors rather than from a single factor. Environmental, genetic, and viral factors have been implicated in the development of cancer. Chemical substances that initiate or promote the development of cancer are known as carcinogens. These agents are thought to alter the DNA in the cell nucleus.

CLIENT TEACHING

Dietary Guidelines to Reduce the Risk of Cancer

- Choose most foods from plant sources.
  - Eat five or more servings of fruits and vegetables each day, especially green and dark-yellow vegetables and those in the cabbage family.
  - Consume other foods from plant sources including breads, cereals, pastas, beans (legumes), and soy products.
- Limit intake of high-fat foods, particularly from animal sources.
  - Choose foods low in fat.
  - Limit consumption of meats, especially red meats and high-fat meats.
- Be physically active and achieve and maintain a healthy weight.
  - Physical activity can help by balancing caloric intake with energy expenditures or by other mechanisms.
- Limit or eliminate consumption of alcoholic beverages.

(ACS, 2002; ACS, 2008)

RISK FACTORS

Many risk factors, such as environmental, lifestyle, genetic, and viral, may increase an individual's chances of developing cancer.

Environmental Factors

The first environmental carcinogen was discovered in 1760, when Percival Pott noted that chimney sweeps had a very high rate of what is now known to be scrotal cancer because they were exposed to cancer-causing oils in the soot that was rubbed into their clothing. Since that time, hundreds of chemical carcinogens have been identified.

Many individuals come into contact with cancer-causing agents through occupational exposure. Industrial chemicals, such as asbestos or vinyl chlorides, have been found to be carcinogenic. For workers who handle these chemicals, the risk of developing cancers is greatly increased if occupational exposure is combined with cigarette smoking. Tobacco may act synergistically with other substances to promote cancer development. Occupational exposure to coal tar, creosote, arsenic compounds, or radium constitutes a risk factor for development of skin cancer. The effects of carcinogenic agents are usually dose dependent. The larger the dose or the longer the duration of exposure, the greater is the risk of cancer development. It is estimated that 80% of all cancers are associated with environmental exposures and might be prevented if exposure is avoided. Occupational Safety and Health Administration (OSHA) established safety standards and levels of exposure for those likely to be exposed to chemical carcinogens at work.

In 1993, the U.S. Environmental Protection Agency (EPA) declared secondhand smoke a human carcinogen. Approximately 3,000 nonsmoking adults die each year of lung cancer from breathing secondhand smoke (ACS, 2008).

Lifestyle Factors

Lifestyle factors include the use of tobacco, sun exposure, alcohol consumption, and diet. Tobacco accounts for nearly one in five deaths in the United States (ACS, 2008). Tobacco use includes cigarettes, cigars, pipes, and smokeless forms (e.g., snuff and chewing tobacco). The same carcinogens are found in all forms of tobacco, causing cancer of the oral cavity, esophagus, pharynx, and larynx. When tobacco is smoked, it can also cause cancer of the lung, pancreas, uterus, cervix, kidney, and bladder.

Overexposure to the sun's ultraviolet rays over long periods of time is the cause of many skin cancers. The most serious form of skin cancer is melanoma. The ACS (2008) estimates 62,480 newly diagnosed cases of melanoma in 2008. Other factors predisposing a person to skin cancer are family history, multiple nevi, and atypical nevi.

Heavy alcohol consumption has also been implicated in mouth, throat, esophageal, and liver cancers. Alcohol is hypothesized to cause 5% of cancer deaths. Alcohol and tobacco used together greatly increase the risk of oral and esophageal cancers. The combined effect of alcohol and tobacco is greater than the sum of their individual effects (ACS, 2008). Despite the epidemiological evidence linking alcohol to cancer, the exact carcinogen in alcohol is yet to be determined. Table 34-1 lists some risk factors for cancer.

Table 34-1 Risk Factors for Cancer

Breast Cancer

- Family history (immediate female relatives)
- High-fat diet
- Obesity after menopause
- Early menarche, late menopause
- Alcohol consumption
- Postmenopausal estrogen and progestin
- First child after age 30

Cervical Cancer

- Multiple sexual partners
- Having sex at early age
- Exposure to human papillomavirus
- Smoking

Colorectal Cancer

- Family history (immediate relatives)
- Low-fiber diet
- History of rectal polyps

Esophageal Cancer

- Heavy alcohol consumption
- Smoking

Lung Cancer

- Cigarette smoking
- Asbestos, arsenic, and radon exposure
- Secondhand smoke
- Tuberculosis

Skin Cancer

- Excessive exposure to ultraviolet radiation (sun)
- Fair complexion
- Work with coal, tar, pitch, or creosote
- Multiple or atypical nevi (males)

Stomach Cancer

- Family history
- Diet heavy in smoked, pickled, or salted foods

Testicular Cancer

- Undescended testicles
- Consumption of hormones by mother during pregnancy

Prostate Cancer

- Increasing age
- Family history
- Diet high in animal fat

COURTESY OF DELMAR CENGAGE LEARNING

Research suggests that an increase in dietary fiber may help prevent colon cancer. Some studies have suggested that obesity is a significant risk factor for breast, colon, endometrial, and prostate cancers. Studies have also shown that diets high in salt-cured, smoked, and nitrite-cured foods increase an individual's risk for cancer of the stomach and esophagus. Food substances that may reduce cancer risk include cruciferous vegetables (cabbage, broccoli, cauliflower, brussels sprouts, kohlrabi); possibly vitamins A, E, and C; and selenium. Some foods have been found to contain carcinogens in the forms of additives or as by-products of storage. On the basis of current knowledge, the ACS has offered dietary guidelines to reduce cancer risk.

GENETIC FACTORS

Some families have a high incidence of certain types of cancer. Women whose mothers, grandmothers, or sisters have had breast cancer have twice the risk of developing cancer as those whose first-degree relatives have not had the disease (ACS, 2008). Leukemia and cancers of the colon, stomach, prostate, lung, and ovary may also run in families. Therefore, relatives of persons with these cancers should be carefully monitored.

VIRAL FACTORS

Although viruses have been linked to several cancers, their exact role is unclear. It has been theorized that they incorporate themselves into the genetic structure of the cell. Herpes simplex II virus and some of the human papillomaviruses that are transmitted sexually are known to predispose women to cervical cancer. Reducing the number of sexual partners can reduce the risk of contracting these viruses.

CLIENT TEACHING

Lifestyle Guidelines to Reduce the Risk of Cancer

- Do not smoke or use tobacco in any form.
- Avoid overexposure to the sun and indoor tanning.
- Eat a healthy diet.
- Get plenty of exercise.
- Have a physical examination on a routine basis, including a mammogram, Pap smear, testicular, and colon examinations.
- Get plenty of sleep (6 to 8 hours per night).
- Keep weight within normal limits.
- Practice regular self-examinations and see your physician if any changes are noted.
- Know and follow health and safety rules at the workplace.
- Avoid unprotected sexual behaviors.

DETECTION

When cancer develops, the earlier it is detected the more likely it is to be controlled. In some cases, a diagnosis is made before symptoms become apparent. Cancer is usually found by the affected individual, who notices a warning sign, or by a health-care provider during a checkup. A cancer checkup is recommended every 3 years for persons ages 20 to 39 years and annually for those ages 40 years and older. Risk assessment is the first step in cancer prevention. The cancer examination includes both a medical history of exposures to environmental agents and a comprehensive family history.

If cancer is suspected, various diagnostic studies are performed depending on the suspected primary or metastatic site of the cancer. They include laboratory studies or blood tests, radiologic studies, endoscopy, cytology, and biopsy. Nurses educate clients about such tests as well as assist in client preparation.

Although no one blood test can confirm a cancer diagnosis, some malignancies do alter the chemical composition of the blood. Specialized laboratory tests have been developed to detect **tumor markers**, substances such as specific proteins, antigens, genes, hormones, or enzymes that are found in the serum and indicate the possible presence of malignancy. Tumor markers are not 100% accurate because benign processes can also cause elevations; they are, however, useful in monitoring response to treatment or detecting a relapse. (See Table 34-2 for cancer-screening guidelines.)

CRITICAL THINKING

Cancer Detection

Which diagnostic tests should a person have as part of a routine physical to detect cancer?

CLIENT TEACHING

Warning Signs of Cancer

The professional nurse educates individuals about the warning signs of cancer. The seven warning signs can be easily remembered through an acronym, CAUTION.

C: Change in bladder or bowel habits, such as absence of urination or bowel movement or excessive urination or stool.

A: A sore that does not heal within a realistic period of time.

U: Unusual bleeding or discharge from any body orifice, such as the vagina, the nipple, or the penis. The unusual discharge can be bloody, purulent, clear, or viscous. The keywords are *unusual* and *any body orifice*.

T: Thickening or the presence of a lump of the breast, testicle, or any part of the body.

I: Indigestion or difficulty swallowing for a prolonged period of time.

O: Obvious change in a wart or mole, such as color, size, texture.

N: Nagging cough or hoarseness that is prolonged.

If any of these warning signs are observed, encourage client to see a health-care provider.

Courtesy of Daniels, R, Nosek, L., & Nicoll, L. (2010). Contemporary medical-surgical nursing. Clifton Park, NY: Delmar, Cengage Learning.

COMMON DIAGNOSTIC TESTS

Commonly used diagnostic tests for clients who present with symptoms of cancer are listed in Table 34-3. See Basic Nursing Diagnostic Tests, for explanation/normal values and nursing responsibilities related to each test.

STAGING OF TUMORS

Staging determines the extent of the spread of cancer. The TNM classification proposed by the American Joint Commission on Cancer is one of the most frequently used systems. The T refers to the anatomical size of the primary tumor; N, the extent of lymph node involvement; and M, the presence or absence of metastasis (Table 34-4). Use of this internationally recognized staging system for tumors ensures a reliable comparison of clients in many different hospitals. Staging is important because it influences decisions about treatment modalities and helps predict overall prognosis.

GRADING OF TUMORS

Normal body cells have individual characteristics that allow them to perform different body functions. This process is called **differentiation**. Tumor cells that retain many of the identifiable tissue characteristics of the original cell are termed *well differentiated*. Tumor cells having little similarity to the tissue of origin are termed *undifferentiated*. Tumor grading is based primarily on the degree of differentiation of malignant cells. Grading evaluates tumor cells in comparison with normal cells. Pathologists indicate tumor cell grades by using the Roman numerals I through IV; the higher the grade, the higher the number and the worse the prognosis. Thus, a grade I tumor is the most differentiated, and a grade IV tumor is the most undifferentiated (or least differentiated). Tumors containing poorly differentiated cells are more aggressive in growth and may display uncharacteristic behaviors, leading to a poorer prognosis. Grading criteria vary for different neoplasms.

Table 34-2 Screening Guidelines

SITE	AGE TO BEGIN	RECOMMENDATIONS	PREFERRED/ALTERNATIVE
Colorectal	50	One of the following initially: fecal occult blood or fecal immunochemical test annually; flexible sigmoidoscopy every 5 years; barium enema every 5 years; colonoscopy every 10 years.	Combination testing rather than a single diagnostic test.
Prostate	50	Protein-specific antigen (PSA) test and digital rectal exam (DRE) to men who have a life expectancy of at least 10 years.	Begin at age 45 for African-American men and men with a strong family history.
Breast	20	Beginning at age 20, breast self-exams monthly and clinical breast exams every 3 years. Beginning at age 40, add annual mammograms and clinical breast exams.	Women at greater risk may begin mammograms at earlier age, or have additional tests performed (MRI, ultrasound, etc.).
Cervical	21, or 3 years after beginning vaginal intercourse	Pap test annually. After total hysterectomy with cervix removal screening is not necessary unless the surgery was performed as treatment for cervical cancer.	Pap test may be every 2 years, with a liquid-based test. A woman 30 or older with three normal test results in a row may be screened every 2–3 years. As an alternative HPV DNA testing and cytology could be done every 3 years. High-risk women may get screened more often. Women older than 70 years of age with three or more consecutive normal Pap tests in past 10 years may choose to stop screening.
Endometrium	35	Annual screening with biopsy for women with or at risk for HNPCC (hereditary nonpolyposis colon cancer).	All women at menopause should be educated about risks and symptoms and be encouraged to report any unexpected spotting or bleeding.

From *Cancer facts & figures*, by ACS Recommendations, 2006, Atlanta, GA: American Cancer Society; *Understanding Neoplasms*, by R. Teasley, in press.

TREATMENT MODALITIES

After cancer is diagnosed, staged, and graded, a medical treatment plan is developed. The most common treatment methods used are surgery, radiation therapy, and **chemotherapy** (use of drugs to treat illness); biotherapy/immunotherapy, hormone therapy, targeted therapy, photodynamic therapy, and bone marrow transplantation also are used. These methods may be used alone or in combination.

SURGERY

Surgery is the oldest form of cancer treatment and remains the most common method of treatment today. Surgery is classified as curative, palliative, or reconstructive.

The goal of **curative surgery** is to heal or restore to health; this involves excising all of the tumor, the involved surrounding tissue, and the regional lymph nodes. Surgery most often has curative results when performed in the early stages of cervical, breast, or skin cancer.

CRITICAL THINKING

Teaching Risk Factors for Cancer

A neighbor, a 45-year-old female, asks you if there is anything she can do to "cancer-proof" her lifestyle. She tells you that there have been several incidences of cancer diagnosed in family members, although none have been in her immediate family. What is the best answer you can give her?

Table 34-3 Common Diagnostic Tests for Cancer Detection

Laboratory Tests

- Acid phosphatase (elevated)
- Alkaline phosphatase (elevated)
- Bence Jones protein
- CA-15-3
- CA-19-9
- CA-125
- CEA (carcinoembryonic antigen)
- Fecal occult blood test (FOBT) or fecal immunochemical test (FIT)
- PSA (prostate-specific antigen)
- Stool for occult blood (Guaiac)
- Serum calcitonin

Radiologic Studies

- X-ray studies
- Computerized axial tomography (CT scan or CAT scan)
- Magnetic resonance imaging (MRI)
- Scans (radioisotope test)
- Ultrasound
- Mammograms

Invasive Diagnostic Techniques

- Endoscopy
- Cytology
- Biopsy

COURTESY OF DELMAR CENGAGE LEARNING

Because 70% of clients show evidence of metastasis at diagnosis, cure is not always possible, and **palliative surgery** may be necessary. This surgery is effective in relieving symptoms in more advanced stages of cancer, although it does not alter the course of the disease. It is usually performed in an attempt to relieve complications such as obstructions or to surgically interrupt nerve pathways for intractable pain. It may also be used to insert special access devices or to place tubes for enteral nutrition.

Reconstructive surgery is performed to reestablish function or rebuild for a better cosmetic effect. Reconstructive surgery to areas such as the head, neck, breast, and extremities minimizes deformity. The surgery is completed all at once or done in stages.

Radiation Therapy

Radiation therapy is the second most common method of treating cancer. Radiation therapy, or **radiotherapy,** uses high-energy ionizing radiation to kill cancer. Ionizing radiation penetrates tissue cells and deposits energy within them. This intense energy causes breakage in chromosomes within the cell, thus preventing the ability of the cell to replicate. Cell death occurs hours, days, or even years after treatment, depending on the rate of mitosis.

The goal of radiation therapy is to eradicate malignant cells without causing harm to healthy tissues. Some cells are more sensitive to radiation than others. Better vascularized, better oxygenated cells and those that divide rapidly are the most sensitive.

It is used alone or as an adjunct to other therapies. As a single treatment modality, it is most often used when the disease is localized. Preoperative radiation is frequently used to reduce the tumor mass before surgery. Postoperative radiation therapy is frequently used to decrease the risk of local recurrence after surgery. Some chemotherapeutic drugs increase the sensitivity of cancer cells to radiation and thus are used together with radiation. Radiation therapy is classified as curative or palliative. It is frequently used to alleviate symptoms of metastasis, such as pain.

There are two types of radiation therapy: external radiation and internal radiation.

External Radiation

External radiation, or teletherapy, is performed with special equipment that can deliver high-energy radiation. Treatments are usually administered on an outpatient basis, divided over many days or weeks. Customized shielding blocks are created to protect healthy tissues, and immobilization devices are used to maintain the exact position for each treatment. Dyes or tattoos may be used to designate reference points on the skin.

Nursing care is directed toward client teaching, safety, and performing interventions that provide relief from side effects. Undesirable side effects that are most likely to occur include varying degrees of skin reactions and gastrointestinal discomfort, such as abdominal cramping, diarrhea, loss of appetite, and fatigue. Treatments have a cumulative effect and may thus produce symptoms after the therapy has been completed.

Internal Radiation

Internal radiation delivers radioactive isotopes directly within the body. Clients treated with internal sources of radiation are a source of radioactivity. Isotopes are introduced into the body by sealed or unsealed sources.

With sealed sources, radioactive elements are encapsulated in special containers such as tubes, wires, needles, seeds, or capsules. These containers are implanted close to the cancer cells to deliver a highly concentrated dose of radiation to the cancer cells. Radioactive implants are used in the treatment of

CLIENT TEACHING

External Radiation

- Do not wash off the skin markings used to designate reference points for treatment.
- Client is alone in the room during treatment.
- Client must lie absolutely still.
- Treatment typically lasts 1 to 3 minutes.
- Treatment is usually painless.

Table 34-4 Staging of Tumors: TNM Classification

STAGE	TUMOR	LYMPH NODE	METASTASIS
I	<2 cm diameter Mobile Often superficial Confined to organ of origin	No involvement	No evidence
II	2 to 5 cm diameter No as mobile Extension into adjacent tissue	Palpable, mobile >2 to 3 cm diameter Firmer than normal	No evidence
III a	>5 cm diameter Not mobile Regional involvement	No involvement	No evidence
III b	<2 to >5 cm diameter Mobile or not mobile Localized or extended	>2 to 3 cm diameter Firmer than normal	No evidence
IV a	>10 cm diameter Extension into another organ; major arteries, veins, or nerves; or bone	No involvement or >2 to 3 cm diameter Firmer than normal	No evidence
IV b	No evidence to >10 cm diameter	3 to 5 cm diameter Partially mobile Firm to hard; or >5 cam diameter Extended and fixed to bone, large blood vessels, skin, or nerves	No evidence
IV c	No evidence to >10 cm diameter	No evidence to >10 cm diameter Fixed and destructive Extension to second or distant stations	Solitary or multiple

COURTESY OF DELMAR CENGAGE LEARNING

SAFETY

Internal Radiation

Client care is modified based on the three factors related to the degree of exposure to sealed-source radiation by:

- Preparing everything outside of the room so that as little time as possible is spent close to the client.
- Having several nurses assigned to care for the client so that the time of exposure for each nurse is lessened.
- Wearing a lead apron or other shielding device, as provided.

cancers of the tongue, lip, breast, vagina, cervix, endometrium, rectum, bladder, and brain.

Because sources are sealed, body fluids are not radioactive. Personnel caring for clients who have sealed sources must still be familiar with the hazards of radiation, however. Generally, the degree of exposure is dependent on three factors:

- The distance between the individual and the source (Figure 34-2)
- The amount of time an individual is exposed
- The type of shielding provided

Radioactive isotopes also are placed in suspensions or solutions as unsealed sources of radiation. They are given orally or parenterally or instilled into intrapleural or peritoneal spaces.

Some radioactive elements used in unsealed radiation sources are eliminated in body secretions, including urine and stool; thus health care workers must take special

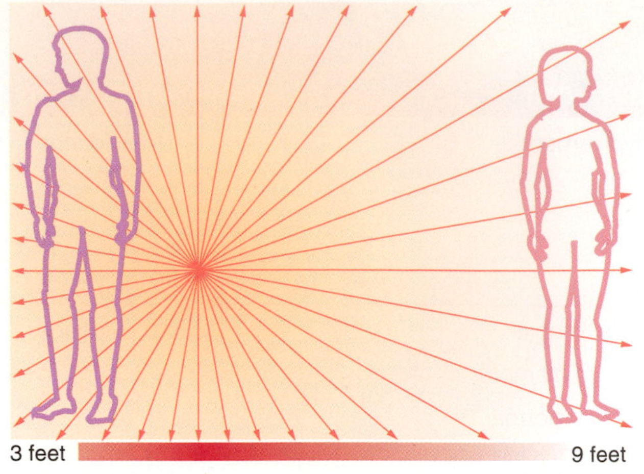

FIGURE 34-2 Radiation dose decreases with distance. (*Courtesy of the U.S. Nuclear Regulatory Commission.*)

precautions to avoid exposure. Agency policies and procedures as well as Standard Precautions are followed closely. Unsealed sources are not usually radioactive as long as the sealed sources.

CHEMOTHERAPY

Chemotherapy is used to cure, prevent, or relieve cancer symptoms. Drugs used in chemotherapy are called **antineoplastics** because they inhibit the growth and reproduction of malignant cells. To understand how anticancer drugs work, one must have a basic understanding of the cell cycle.

Almost all anticancer drugs kill cancer cells by affecting DNA synthesis or function, but they vary in how they exert their activity within the cell cycle. Most chemotherapeutic drugs are classified as cell-cycle specific (CCS) or cell-cycle nonspecific (CCNS).

CCS drugs attack cancer cells when the cells enter a certain phase of reproduction. These agents are most effective against rapidly growing tumors. Many of the drugs are "schedule dependent" because they produce a greater cell kill when given in multiple, repeated doses.

CCNS drugs can destroy cancer cells in any phase of the cell cycle and are used for large tumors that have fewer actively dividing cells. These drugs are not schedule dependent but, rather, dose dependent. This means that the number of cells destroyed is determined by the amount of drug given.

Anticancer agents are cytotoxic (toxic to cells) and destroy both normal and abnormal cells. They are most effective against cells that reproduce rapidly, such as those in bone marrow, gastrointestinal lining, hair follicles, and the ova and sperm. Because cells multiply at their most rapid rate at the beginning of the disease, the drugs work best against cancer in its earliest stages.

Many of these drugs are given in combination with or after radiation or surgery to achieve maximum effect. They are usually given intermittently over an extended period. Drug resistance can occur.

The most common routes of administration are oral and intravenous. A few drugs are given topically, subcutaneously, or intramuscularly. Recently, other methods have been introduced to increase the local concentration of the drug at the tumor site, including intrathecal injection and intracavity instillation. Table 34-5 lists some commonly used drugs.

Careful attention is given to intravenous administration. Leakage of fluid from the vein into the surrounding tissues during infusion is called **extravasation**. Because most chemotherapeutic drugs are irritating to the tissues, extravasation is a potentially serious problem, especially if the drugs administered are **vesicants**. These agents are so irritating that they can cause blistering and even necrosis. All sites must be monitored carefully. Pain, swelling, redness, and the presence of vesicles are all signs of extravasation. Additional signs include the following:

PROFESSIONAL TIP

Chemotherapy and Protective Equipment

- Because many chemotherapy drugs are carcinogenic, the nurse preparing and administering the chemotherapy wears protective equipment.
- All personnel involved in any aspect of handling chemotherapeutic agents receive instructions about the known risks of the drugs, the proper use of protective equipment, the applicable skill procedures, and the policies regarding pregnant personnel.

COMMUNITY/HOME HEALTH CARE

Home Care After Chemotherapy

Teach clients receiving chemotherapy to monitor the side effects of therapy at home.

- Inspect the skin daily for any signs of rash or dermatitis, which indicates hypersensitivity to a drug.
- Report taste loss and tingling in the face, fingers, or toes, which may signal peripheral neuropathy.
- Report signs of dizziness, headache, confusion, slurred speech, or convulsions, which are signs of central nervous system (CNS) toxicity.
- Report signs of unusual bleeding or bruising; fever; sore throat; or mouth sores, which may signal developing myelosuppression.
- Report signs of jaundice; yellowing of the eyes; clay-colored stools; or dark urine, which signals developing hepatic dysfunction.
- Report a continued cough or shortness of breath, which indicates developing pulmonary fibrosis.

Table 34-5 Drugs Commonly Used in Chemotherapy

Antimetabolites (CC5)	**Antibiotics (CCNS)**	**Antihormonal Agents (CCNS)**
cytarabine (Cytosar)	dactinomycin (Cosmegan)*	flutamide (Eulexin)
fluorouracil (Adrucil 5-FU)	daunorubicin (Cerubidine)*	goserelln acetate (Zoladex)
methotrexate (Mexate, Folex)	doxorubicin hydrochloride (Adriamycin)*	tamoxifen (Nolvadex)
6-mercaptopurine (Purinethol)	mitomycin (Mutamycin)*	
	mithramycin (Mithracin)	
	bleomycin (Blenoxane)	
Vinca Plant Alkaloids (CCS)	**Hormones (CCNS)**	**Nitrosureas (CCNS)**
vinblastine sulfate (Velban)*	diethylstilbestrol (DES)	carmustine (BiCNU)
vincristine sulfate (Oncovin)*	megestrol acetate (Megace)	lomustine (CeeNU)
	medroxyprogesterone acetate (Depo-Provera)	
	testosterone (Histerone, Testoderm)	
	tamoxifen citrate (Nolvadex)	
Alkylating Agents (CCNS)	**Corticosteroids**	**Miscellaneous Agents**
busulfan (Myleran)	dexamethasone (Decadron)	etoposide (VePesid)
chlorambucil (Leukeran)	hydrocortisone sodium succinate (Solu-Cortef)	L-asparaginase (Elspar)
cisplatin (Platinol)	prednisone (Deltasone)	procarbazine hydrochloride (Matulane)
cyclophosphamide (Cytoxan)		
mechlorethamine hydrochloride (Mustargen)*		
melphalan (Alkeran)		
thiotepa (Thiotepa)		

Frequently Used Combinations

CAF	cyclophosphamide, doxorubicin, and fluorourcil (5-FU)
CHOP	cyclophosphamide, doxorubicin, vincristine (Oncovin), and prednisolone
C-VAMP	cyclophosphamide, vincristine, doxorubicin, and methyl-prednisolone
CVP	cyclophosphamide, vincristine, and prednisone
ECF	epirubicin, cisplatin, and fluorourcil
FEC	fluorourcil, epirubicin, and cyclophosphamide
MMM	mitomycin, methotrexate, and mitoxantrone
MOPP	mechlorethamine hydrochloride (Mustargen), vincristine, procarbazine, and prednisone
MVP	mitomycin, vinblastine, and cisplatin

*= vesicant drug

COURTESY OF DELMAR CENGAGE LEARNING

- Pain or burning at the site or along the vein
- Absent or sluggish blood return
- Redness 6 to 12 hours later
- Swelling
- Diffuse hardening

If extravasation occurs, the drug is stopped immediately and protocols for treatment initiated.

Improved infusion techniques, control of symptoms such as nausea and vomiting, and cost-containment restrictions have reduced the length of hospitalizations for clients undergoing chemotherapy. Teaching clients and family members to monitor side effects in the home setting is thus an essential function of the **oncology** (study of tumors) nurse.

Clients also are advised that their lifestyle may need adjustment to accommodate the side effects of chemotherapy. Clients are instructed to pace themselves according to their energy level and allow time for rest throughout the day. It is also important to inform clients that even between treatments they may not have the same amount of energy as before treatment initiation. Many clients do not experience any adverse effects, but some experience life-threatening toxicity. Nursing care of the client receiving chemotherapy requires not only a thorough understanding of the drugs used to destroy the cancer, but also skills in helping clients and families cope with the side effects of the therapy.

Biotherapy

Biotherapy/immunotherapy is performed with **biologic response modifiers (BRMs)**, agents that stimulate the body's natural immune system to control and destroy malignant cells. Some BRMs are being evaluated in trial studies. Biotherapy is used after surgery, radiation, and chemotherapy have removed the bulk of the tumor. Some agents currently used include interferons, monoclonal antibodies, interleukin-2, tumor necrosis factor, *bacillus Calmette-Guérin (BCG),* and colony-stimulating factors. Side effects are usually less severe than those seen in chemotherapy and include fever, malaise, myalgia, and headache. Because an anaphylactic reaction can occur, the client must be closely monitored.

Photodynamic Therapy

Photodynamic therapy (PDT) has a 90% effective rate when used for esophageal cancer and early-stage lung cancer (Cancer Treatment Centers of America, 2009b). PDT is also used as an investigation therapy for obstructive lung cancer, Barrett's esophagus, and head, neck and skin cancer. The client is injected with a light-activated drug (Photofrin) that targets cancerous cells. Twenty-four to 48 hours after injecting the drug, a low-power laser light is directed by a fiberoptic guide to the cancerous tissue area through an endoscope. The light stimulates the drug to destroy the cancerous cells, but the surrounding healthy tissue is not harmed. An advantage of PDT is the client has the procedure performed on an outpatient basis with slight sedation and is relatively pain free. There is less risk than with a surgical procedure, and there are fewer side effects. The side effects of PDT are discomfort from local swelling, nausea, fever, and constipation. The client experiences sunburn, redness, and swelling if the skin and eyes are exposed to a bright light or sunlight.

SAFETY

Chemotherapy and Contamination

- Any personnel handling blood, vomitus, or excreta from clients who have received chemotherapy within the previous 48 hours wears disposable latex gloves and a disposable gown.
- Place contaminated linen in specially marked laundry bags according to agency procedures.

Hormone Therapy

Some cancerous cells need estrogen, progesterone, or testosterone to grow. The goal of hormone therapy is to deprive the cancerous cells of these hormones. Clients may have the ovaries (**oophorectomy**) or testicles (**orchiectomy**) removed. Another method of depriving the cells of hormonal stimulation is to give women with early-stage breast cancer tamoxifen citrate (Nolvadex) and to give men luteinizing hormone-releasing hormone (LHRH). LHRH prevents the testes from producing testosterone. Tamoxifen is a systemic treatment and increases the chances for endometrial cancer. Hormone therapy is effective for a time in men, but eventually prostate cancer grows without hormone stimulation. The hormone therapy is no longer effective when this occurs (Cancer Treatment Centers of America, 2009c).

Targeted Cancer Therapy

Most targeted cancer therapies are in preclinical testing (animal research) and clinical trial (human research). Some drugs have been approved by the U.S. Food and Drug Administration (FDA). The goal of targeted cancer therapy is to stop the growth and spread of cancer cells by preventing normal cells from changing into cancerous cells at the molecular or cellular level. This therapy is more effective than present treatments and causes less harm to healthy cells. An example of targeted therapy is STI-571, or imatinib mesylate (Gleevac®), which is a small-molecule drug used to treat gastrointestinal stromal tumor and chronic myeloid leukemia (National Cancer Institute, 2006).

Bone Marrow Transplantation

Bone marrow transplantation (BMT) is used for cancers that respond to high doses of chemotherapy or radiation therapy. Treatment involves aspirating and storing a fraction of bone marrow, exposing the client to high-dose drug therapy or total-body irradiation, and then reinfusing the bone marrow after the treatment is complete.

The bone marrow used in transplantation can be the client's own marrow (autologous), marrow taken from an identical twin (syngeneic), or marrow taken from a histocompatibly matched donor, preferably a sibling (allogeneic).

Client expenses for BMT are high, ranging from $50,000 to $100,000 for an autologous transplant, and $100,000 to $200,000 for an allogeneic transplant unless covered or partially covered by insurance (NBMTLink, 2009). The average length of hospital stay is 35 to 40 days. Complications can be life-threatening and include infection, bleeding, gastrointestinal effects, renal insufficiency, veno-occlusive disease (deposits of fibrin obstruct venules of liver), and graft-versus-host disease (new bone marrow cells recognize environment as foreign and try to destroy the host). Clients who undergo autologous BMT do not experience graft-versus-host disease.

SYMPTOM MANAGEMENT

Cancer clients undergoing treatment experience a variety of secondary problems. One of the most important responsibilities of the oncology nurse is to formulate nursing interventions to manage these problems.

Bone Marrow Dysfunction

Cancer treatments kill both malignant cells and normal cells in bone marrow. Blood counts are monitored carefully during and after treatment.

A low white-cell count increases the risk of infection. A decreased neutrophil count (<500 mm^3) is an indicator that special infection prevention measures should be initiated. Scrupulous hand hygiene is the most effective method of controlling bacterial infection. Personnel maintain strict asepsis when changing dressings or performing invasive procedures. Clients avoid contact with anyone who is ill. Antimicrobial soaps are used for bathing clients. The skin and mucous membranes are inspected daily for signs of infection. Vital signs are taken every 4 hours and the client observed for fever and chilling.

Clients with a platelet count of <50,000 mm^3 are monitored for bleeding. Their skin is inspected daily for bruises or petechiae. Shaving is undertaken with an electric razor to minimize the chance of cutting the skin. Stool and urine are monitored for occult blood. Observe the client for bleeding from the vagina, rectum, nose, mouth, and venipuncture sites. If bleeding occurs, pressure is applied to the site for 5 minutes. Any bleeding that does not stop in 5 minutes is reported. A soft toothbrush is recommended for oral care. Aspirin or any medication containing acetylsalicylic acid is not given.

Nutritional Alterations

Cytokines are substances secreted by the tumor in an attempt to cannibalize the body and by the immune system to fight the tumor. Cytokines make the body digest muscle for energy instead of using stored fat for this purpose. This state of malnutrition and protein (muscle) wasting is called **cachexia**. It occurs in conjunction with lung, pancreatic, stomach, bowel, and prostate cancers but rarely with breast cancer.

In some cases, untreated cachexia, rather than the cancer itself, is the cause of death. Untreated cachexia also decreases the effectiveness of cancer treatments and increases the side effects of these treatments. Treating cachexia with drugs has met with little success.

A registered dietitian understands cancer cachexia and can identify appetizing foods that are nutrient and calorie dense. Foods that appeal to the client are eaten anytime. The use of liquid nutritional supplements and a multivitamin is often recommended (Wilkes, 2000).

Hallmarks of malnutrition are a weight loss of 10% or more or a serum albumin level <3.4 g/dL. Clients unable to maintain sufficient oral intake for long periods are given enteral or total parenteral nutrition (TPN). Nutritional problems associated with cachexia include anorexia, nausea and vomiting, altered taste sensation, mucosal inflammation, and dysphagia.

Anorexia

Anorexia, or the loss of appetite, is a common concern among individuals with cancer. It is generally best for these clients to eat small, frequent, high-calorie (carbohydrate and fat-rich) meals. Try to ascertain the client's likes and dislikes. Highly seasoned foods help increase taste. Clients are encouraged to eat when they are feeling best. Weight is monitored weekly.

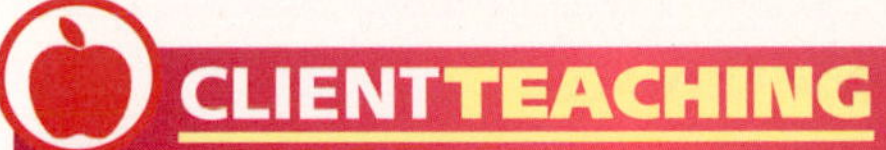

Increasing Nutritional Intake

- Drink 4 ounces of a nutritional supplement before breakfast.
- Eat breakfast (if desired), and then take a walk. Doing so will help build muscle and increase appetite.
- Drink another 4 ounces of nutritional supplement 1 hour before having a lunch consisting of whatever foods are appealing.
- Have another 4 ounces of nutritional supplement at midafternoon and at bedtime.
- If not hungry for dinner, take another walk.

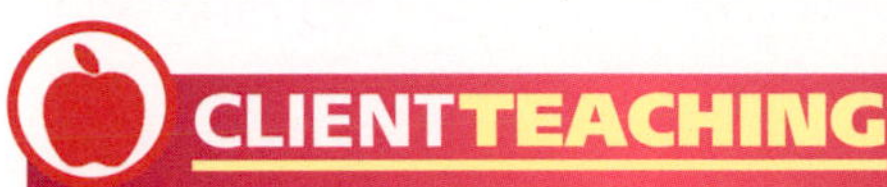

Enhancing Taste Sensation

- Tart food usually enhances taste sensation.
- Many foods taste better if they are cold or at room temperature.
- Using plastic utensils reduces metallic taste.

Nausea and Vomiting

Nausea and vomiting usually occur within 3 to 4 hours after chemotherapy is administered and may last up to 72 hours. Antiemetics are given before chemotherapy and continued afterward as needed (Table 34-6). Small, frequent feedings of complex carbohydrates may be beneficial. Liquids are given 30 to 60 minutes before meals. Although highly seasoned foods may increase taste, they often also increase nausea and vomiting. Cool, bland foods are more easily tolerated. Avoid foods with strong odors. Frequent mouth care helps remove the taste of chemotherapy and increase the likelihood of the client's wanting to eat. The client should be monitored for dehydration and electrolyte imbalances.

Table 34-6 Commonly Used Antiemetics
prochlorperazine (Compazine)
metoclopramide (Reglan)
ondansetron hydrochloride (Zofron)
lorazepam (Ativan)
dolasetron (Anzemet)

COURTESY OF DELMAR CENGAGE LEARNING

PROFESSIONALTIP

Mucosal Inflammation

- The condition of the client's mouth provides a clue to the appearance and integrity of other areas of the gastrointestinal tract because mucosal inflammation caused by cancer treatments affects all mucosa.
- Mucositis (inflammation of the mucous membrane) in the esophagus, also called esophagitis, causes painful swallowing.
- In female clients, mucosal inflammation is found in the vagina, causing pain, itching, and discharge.

Altered Taste Sensation

Taste sensation is altered because cancer cells release substances that stimulate bitter taste buds, causing a bitter or metallic taste in the mouths of some clients. Some find they no longer enjoy the taste of red meat, and others say they have an aversion to sweets.

Mucosal Inflammation

Stomatitis, or inflammation of the mucous membrane of the oral cavity, occurs in one-half of cancer clients receiving treatment. It usually occurs 7 to 14 days after chemotherapy administration and lasts 2 to 3 weeks. To minimize stomatitis, assess for early signs and symptoms such as edema, ulceration, erythema, excessive saliva, and infection. If the client is receiving a chemotherapy drug that is known to cause stomatitis (e.g., methotrexate) oral care is administered at least four times a day.

Avoid rough, chewy foods and acidic foods. Straws are beneficial because food is taken in the back of the mouth and swallowed. Popsicles and frozen fruit bars sometimes help numb and lessen pain. Avoid commercial mouthwashes containing alcohol. A saline rinse may be helpful after meals. If the client has dentures, remove them at night. Viscous Xylocaine rinses are ordered for pain. Lemon and glycerine swabs are not used because lemon is irritating to mouth lesions.

Dysphagia

Dysphagia, difficulty in swallowing, often occurs in clients with esophageal cancers, or in those receiving radiotherapy.

Artificial saliva is ordered for severe dryness. A softer diet along with nutritional supplements is prescribed. Dry foods such as toast can scratch the delicate tissues of the throat. Food puréed in a blender is easier to tolerate. Encourage clients to take plenty of time to chew and swallow.

Pain

Approximately 60% to 90% of all individuals with progressive malignancy experience pain. The pain may be acute, but it is more likely to be chronic (>3 months in duration).

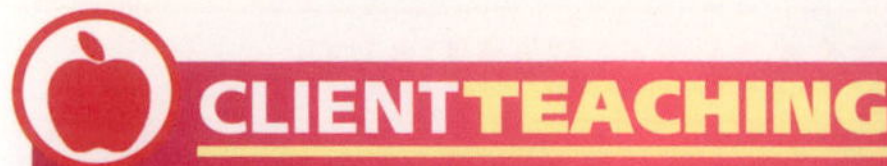

CLIENTTEACHING

Stomatitis

- Use soft bristle toothbrush.
- Avoid flossing if bleeding or discomfort occurs.
- Avoid tobacco products and alcohol because of their drying effects.

Pain usually does not occur until the advanced stages of the disease. The most common causes of pain are metastatic bone disease, venous or lymphatic obstruction, or nerve compression.

Pain causes anxiety, depression, and feelings of helplessness in addition to physical discomfort. It can affect the client's sleeping habits, eating patterns, work, family, and social relationships. Ultimately, pain can affect the client's quality of life.

Noninvasive pain-relief techniques are useful in pain management. They include cutaneous stimulation (heat, cold, massage); transcutaneous electrical nerve stimulation (TENS); relaxation techniques; imagery; and hypnosis. Most of these techniques are inexpensive and easy to perform. They have few side effects and can usually be done in any environment. They also give the client some control over the treatment of pain. Although not every client responds successfully to these measures, it is worthwhile to attempt them before using invasive techniques.

The Agency for Health Care Policy and Research (AHCPR, 1994) developed Cancer Pain Guidelines for clients, family members, and health care professionals. Some points emphasized by the guidelines include:

- Cancer pain can be managed effectively through relatively simple means in up to 90% of cancer clients in the United States. Skin patches, slow-release tablets, and client-controlled pumps are now available to complement standard drugs.
- The mainstay of pain assessment is the client self-report. Because there is no standard test for pain, the nurse must respect the client's report of pain and regard it as the single most reliable indicator.
- The simplest dosage schedules and least invasive pain management modalities are used first. Nonopioids are the first step in the analgesic ladder. They are tried first for mild to moderate pain.

PROFESSIONALTIP

Inadequate Pain Control in the Cancer Client

A major reason given for inadequate pain control in the cancer client is the fear of inducing respiratory depression. This, however, is a rare occurrence in the cancer client.

- Morphine is the most commonly used opioid for moderate to severe pain because it is available in a wide variety of dosage forms, it has well-characterized pharmacokinetics and pharmacodynamics, and it is relatively low in cost. Morphine can be given orally, subcutaneously, intramuscularly, intravenously, rectally, and intraspinally. It can also be given in sustained-release preparations.
- Health-care providers work to prevent pain rather than try to treat pain after it has occurred. Analgesics work better when given regularly around the clock before pain becomes severe. A major nursing responsibility is to teach the client to request pain medication before the pain becomes severe. When medication is ordered around the clock, the nurse does not hesitate to wake the client to administer analgesics.

If pain control is not achieved with noninvasive techniques or medications, neurosurgical procedures such as nerve blocks are an option.

Fatigue

Fatigue occurs as a direct result of cancer treatment or because of anemia, chronic pain, stress, depression, insufficient rest, or inadequate nutritional intake. Although the etiology is not well understood, fatigue is often related to the effects of the tumor itself (Greifzu, 1998). Fatigue contributes to client noncompliance with the treatment regimen.

Frequent rest periods are provided for the client. Assess for the presence and pattern of fatigue. Proper planning allows the client to be active when energy level is higher, which in turn restore a greater sense of control. Evaluate factors that increase or decrease fatigue, such as nutritional intake. Blood count is monitored for anemia.

Alopecia

Alopecia, the thinning or loss of hair, is induced by chemotherapy or radiation treatments. The extent of hair loss depends on the dose and duration of the therapy. Scalp hair is most commonly affected, but pubic, axillary, and facial hair, even eyebrows and eyelashes, also are affected. The treatments cause hair loss by interfering with the growth processes in the hair follicle. This results in weakening of the hair shaft, thereby causing the hair to break off at the surface of the scalp. Hair loss usually begins 2 to 3 weeks after the initial treatment. Drug-induced alopecia is not permanent. Hair usually begins to grow back within 8 weeks after treatment is completed. The color and consistency of the hair may change.

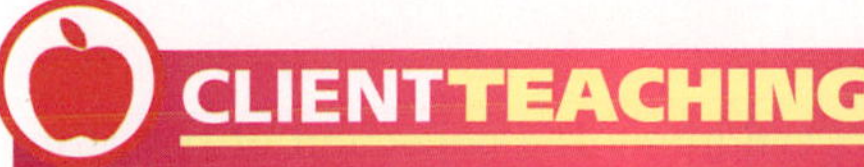

Alopecia, Threat to Body Image

Encourage client to:

- Buy a wig or hairpiece before treatment actually begins so that it will match the client's normal hair.
- Wear hats, scarves, or bandanas to cope with the change in body image caused by hair loss.
- Focus on other positive aspects rather than on just physical appearance.

Odors

Unpleasant odors emanating from the cancer client are a source of embarrassment. These odors are usually associated with drainage, exudates, or incontinence. Fortunately, meticulous nursing care can eliminate most offending odors. Change soiled linens, drainage pads, and dressings immediately. Wash the client's skin gently with soap and warm water. Protective creams are used if the areas are not receiving radiation. Room deodorizers are helpful but should be used cautiously because many clients experience nausea when exposed to the odors from room fresheners. Placing a drop of oil of wintergreen or oil of cloves on a cotton ball near the ventilation system can sometimes lend a light freshness to the environment.

Dyspnea

One-half of all clients with terminal cancer experience dyspnea, or difficulty in breathing. Possible causes include fluid accumulation in the chest, infection such as pneumonia, fibrosis caused by radiation, and anemia. Lungs are auscultated every 4 hours. Oxygen is ordered. Fluid is drained by an invasive procedure called a thoracentesis. High-Fowler positioning maximizes ventilation. Plan care to keep activity to a minimum to balance oxygen requirements and oxygen supply. Oxygen status is monitored with a pulse oximeter. Report a sustained reading of less than 90%. Avoid pulling the privacy curtain or shutting the client's door unless absolutely necessary because either of these actions reduces air flow and creates more anxiety.

Bowel Dysfunctions

Cancer clients frequently exhibit changes in bowel patterns. Constipation, diarrhea and subsequent perineal skin breakdown, and bowel obstructions are common elimination disorders.

Constipation results from decreased motility of the colon. It is frequently caused by chemotherapy, opioid analgesic, or inactivity. Monitor and record the frequency of the client's bowel movements. Constipation is an early sign of vincristine toxicity. Fluid consumption is encouraged and a stool softener is given daily. Clients at risk for constipation are started on a high-fiber diet, with increased intake of bran and prune juice.

Common causes of diarrhea include radiation therapy, chemotherapy, antibiotics, tube feedings, hyperosmolar dietary supplements, stress, and fecal impactions. Clients develop fluid and electrolyte imbalances from constant diarrhea. If the client is receiving a chemotherapy drug known to cause diarrhea (such as fluorouracil [Adrucil] or doxorubicin hydrochloride [Adriamycin]), a low-residue and lactose-free diet is encouraged. Instruct the client to avoid foods that stimulate the gastrointestinal tract, such as warm liquids and coffee.

Bananas (which are high in potassium) and sports drinks (which contain sodium and potassium) help replace lost fluids and electrolytes without irritating the gastrointestinal tract.

The perineum is kept clean and dry after each loose stool. Note signs of fluid and electrolyte imbalances, such as thirst, dry mucous membranes, and decreased skin turgor. The potassium level is monitored. Measure and record the amount, frequency, and characteristics of all client bowel movements.

Antidiarrheal medications such as Lomotil or Imodium are given for every loose stool. Sitz baths help soothe sore or broken-down tissues.

Bowel obstructions occur more commonly in conjunction with advanced abdominal malignancies and are suspected if the client has received radiation or has adhesions from previous surgeries. Symptoms include nausea, vomiting, and abdominal pain. Surgery is required to relieve the obstruction.

Pathological Fractures

Pathological fractures are a major problem in cancers that metastasize to bone. These cancers weaken the bone to the point that normal activities cause painful breaks. Thus, limbs are supported and handled gently, and extreme care is taken when moving clients. Special devices such as splints are used for extra protection. Weight-bearing restrictions are ordered.

Ascites

Abdominal cancers cause ascites, or fluid accumulation in the abdomen. Clients experience abdominal swelling and difficult breathing. Symptoms are treated temporarily with an invasive procedure called a paracentesis, wherein a small, plastic tube is advanced through the abdominal wall and excess fluid is withdrawn. Chemotherapy drugs sometimes are instilled in an attempt to prevent the fluid from returning. Visually assess the abdomen. A protruding abdomen indicates ascites as well as intestinal distention and enlarged organs. Measure abdominal girth at the umbilicus daily with a tape measure to monitor changes, then auscultate the abdomen in all four quadrants. Gurgling bowel sounds heard every 5 to 15 seconds indicate normal peristalsis. Decreased or absent bowel sounds indicate peritonitis or paralytic ileus. Fluid accumulation is confirmed by percussing for shifting dullness. When a large amount of fluid is present, fluid waves are seen. Gentle palpation is used to detect pain and tenderness as well as abdominal masses. The nurse carefully documents any abnormal findings.

Weigh the client daily to monitor weight gain. Fluid consumption is restricted. Good skin care, especially to the abdomen, is essential. Fowler positioning maximizes ventilation. Clients are observed closely for electrolyte imbalance if large amounts of fluids are withdrawn via paracentesis.

Sexual Alterations

Many chemotherapy drugs interfere with sexual functioning and reproduction. Premenopausal women may become infertile. Those younger than 35 years of age may regain their fertility after therapy is completed. Men may experience impotence, decreased libido, interrupted sperm production, and ejaculation problems. Women experience vaginal dryness.

Encourage clients and their partners to express their feelings and concerns to each other and to explore other avenues of sexual expression, such as cuddling, kissing, and stroking. Birth control is practiced during therapy and for 1 or 2 years after therapy (depending on physician recommendation) to ensure that all chemotherapy drugs are eliminated and will have no ill effects on a pregnancy. Eggs and sperm may be saved before treatment.

MEDICAL EMERGENCIES

Medical emergencies occur in approximately 20% of clients with advanced-stage cancer. Early recognition and treatment can prevent irreversible complications and improve the quality of life. Four complications with which to be familiar are hypercalcemia, spinal cord compression, superior vena cava syndrome, and cardiac tamponade.

HYPERCALCEMIA

Hypercalcemia occurs commonly and can be a potentially fatal complication if not detected early. It is found most often in clients with malignant tumors that have metastasized to bone, such as breast cancer. The condition occurs when the serum calcium level rises >10.5 mg/dL.

Early symptoms of hypercalcemia, such as nausea, vomiting, constipation, and weakness, may be overlooked because these are common side effects of many cancer therapies. Later symptoms such as dehydration, renal failure, coma, and cardiac arrest develop swiftly.

Hypercalcemia is treated aggressively with intravenous normal saline and furosemide (Lasix), which increase calcium excretion. Clients also are given drugs to decrease bone reabsorption. Monitor the serum calcium level when Lasix is administered. Teach clients early symptoms of hypercalcemia so they recognize a recurrence. These clients are also at increased risk for pathological fractures because calcium has been released from the bones, leaving them very fragile.

SPINAL CORD COMPRESSION

Spinal cord compression can result in permanent paralysis if not treated promptly. Cancers of the lung, breast, and prostate carry the greatest risk of metastasizing to the spinal cord. The chief symptom of metastasis to the spinal cord is back pain. The discomfort is aggravated by lying down, coughing, or moving, and may be relieved by sitting upright.

Treatment is aimed at reducing tumor size to decrease pressure on the spinal cord. Radiation, surgery, and steroid therapy are used. Pain medications are given frequently, and clients are supported carefully during transfers.

SUPERIOR VENA CAVA SYNDROME

Superior vena cava syndrome is a collection of symptoms caused by an obstruction of the superior vena cava. It occurs more frequently in conjunction with lung cancer and lymphomas. Typically, clients experience dyspnea and swelling of the face and neck. Edema in the upper extremities, chest pain, and coughing may also occur. Central nervous system symptoms such as headache, visual disturbances, and alteration in consciousness rarely occur.

The goal of treatment is to reduce tumor size. Radiation along with diuretics is usually ordered. Administer oxygen as ordered and provide a calm, restful environment. Encourage the client to limit activities and lie in Fowler's position. Carefully monitor respirations. Lower extremities should not be elevated, as doing so will increase venous return to an already engorged area.

CARDIAC TAMPONADE

Cardiac tamponade is caused by the formation of pericardial fluid, which reduces cardiac output by compressing the heart. Tumor metastasis to the pericardium is associated with lung cancer, breast cancer, Hodgkin's disease, lymphoma, melanoma, gastrointestinal tumors, and sarcoma. Common symptoms of cardiac tamponade include a rapid, weak pulse; distended neck veins during inspiration; ankle or sacral edema; pleural effusion; ascites; enlarged spleen; lethargy; and altered consciousness.

Treatment is aimed at aspirating the fluid constricting the heart (pericardiocentesis). Reassure the client, explain the procedure, and administer medication for pain.

PSYCHOSOCIAL ALTERATIONS

Perhaps of all the problems that clients with cancer experience, none is more challenging than the associated psychosocial alterations. The mere diagnosis of cancer invokes fear and misunderstanding. A myriad of emotions may surface initially. These may range from deep depression to denial and total refusal of treatment. Anxiety, sadness, and withdrawal are common. Some clients feel that the disease is a punishment for some misguided deed. Each client responds differently to the diagnosis, depending on individual coping mechanisms and support systems.

Research has identified effective and ineffective coping mechanisms. Clients who seek information or share feelings tend to cope more effectively than do those who submit to treatment and procedures without asking questions or who use small talk to avoid discussing threatening issues.

Cancer affects not only the client, but the client's family as well. Responses of family members to the disease have a significant impact on the client's coping. The client and family face issues such as loss of control, changes in body image, and financial burdens, which can be a huge problem.

The nurse has several roles in this context. The client needs time and space to adjust to the diagnosis. Be available to offer support and reassurance. Answer questions, but do not bombard the client with information. Interpret information given by the physician and help the client formulate questions to ask the physician. Encourage the client to express feelings and fears about the illness.

The initial treatment is very frightening for most cancer clients. Allay anxiety by giving information about the treatment's purpose, adverse reactions, and signs and symptoms to report to the physician. Explaining procedures and answering questions in simple language help the client and family regain a feeling of some control. Treatment modalities cause many discomforts, but if the client knows what to expect, the distress can generally be handled. Symptom management is critical in preventing lifestyle disruptions.

Families and clients facing the terminal phase of cancer are confronted with a complex set of problems. The client and family face separation and impending death. Some families demand that extraordinary measures be taken to keep the client alive. Some search for meaning in life and experience a genuine closeness. Give the client and family privacy and time to share feelings. Sometimes, the only psychosocial support the client needs is to have someone sitting by the bedside. Touch, especially at times when words are hard to find, can often be the most comforting intervention.

As the client's condition deteriorates, physical needs become more pronounced. Focus on keeping the client comfortable and free of pain. Hospice care is designed to provide spiritual, emotional, and physical support during the final days of illness. The goal of hospice is to keep the client as comfortable as possible. Pain relief and symptom management are stressed. The focus is shifted from cure to care. Care is given in an institution, but most hospice care is given in the home. Hospice care is medically managed and nurse coordinated. Members of the hospice team typically include a chaplain, physician, nurse, social worker, physical therapist, and home health aide, as well as various volunteers. The team functions to ensure that the client's plan of care is carried out and that family members receive adequate support. The family is instructed in ways to provide care. Bereavement counseling is offered to help family members deal with their loss.

COMMUNITY/HOME HEALTH CARE

Psychosocial Aspects of Cancer

- Clients may see themselves as burdens to their families.
- Family caregivers may be angry that their own needs must go unmet.
- Family caregivers may feel inadequate with regard to caring for the client.
- Medical equipment such as a hospital bed, commode chair, or wheelchair may need to be brought into the home. These may have an impact on family member state of mind and disposition with regard to the family member with cancer.

NURSING PROCESS

ASSESSMENT

Subjective Data

The client interview serves as a forum for ascertaining the client's perception of the illness, treatment, and prognosis; health practices; and health concerns. The client's significant other also is interviewed to ascertain support systems.

Objective Data

Vital signs are measured, and a head-to-toe assessment is performed. Past hospital records are reviewed along with the current record. Laboratory reports, biopsy results, treatment modalities, and comments from other health care professionals are studied.

CRITICAL THINKING

Nursing Intervention Rationale

What is the rationale for each nursing intervention given for the possible nursing diagnoses identified in this chapter?

Nursing diagnoses for a client with cancer includes the following:

NURSING DIAGNOSES	PLANNING/OUTCOMES	NURSING INTERVENTIONS
Fear related to cancer diagnosis	The client will express anxieties and fears to family and/or health care providers.	Review the client's previous experience with cancer to ascertain any current misconceptions based on past beliefs. Encourage the client to share feelings regarding the diagnosis to facilitate identification of coping strategies. Explain hospital routines and focus on the recommended treatment, including its purpose and potential side effects. Accurate descriptions that convey what the client can expect eases fears associated with the unknown. A calm, reassuring environment also enhances coping abilities.
Anticipatory Grieving related to potential loss of body function	The client will express grief to family and/or health care providers.	Open, honest discussions help the client cope with the situation. Be aware that mood swings, hostility, and other negative behaviors often occur. Discuss the loss of body function with the client. Ask what the loss of body function means to the client. Encourage the client to seek help and support from close family members.
Imbalanced Nutrition: Less than Body Requirements related to side effects of chemotherapy	The client will maintain body weight.	Encourage the client to eat a high-calorie, nutrient-rich diet. Supplements are useful. Some clients benefit from frequent, small meals and snacks. Foods high in protein, such as cheese, fish, and poultry, are also recommended. Provide oral hygiene before and after meals. Administer antiemetics approximately 30 minutes before meals. Mints, hard candies, and saltine crackers may help if the client complains of metallic taste. Nondietary interventions include varying the surroundings, using small plates, eating at a table with friends, and minimizing food odors. Monitor intake and output along with daily weight.
Risk for Impaired Skin Integrity related to chemotherapy and radiation	The client will maintain skin integrity.	Assess skin frequently for side effects of cancer therapy. (A reddening or tanning effect develops with radiation. Skin reactions such as rashes, pruritus, and alopecia develop with chemotherapy.) Use lukewarm water and soap to gently wash the client's skin. Skin often becomes sensitive during radiation treatments.
Risk for Infection related to side effects of chemotherapy	The client will remain free of infection.	Monitor vital signs at least every shift. White blood count is monitored and protective isolation is instituted if the count falls <500 mm^3. Educate the client, staff, and visitors in all aspects of infection prophylaxis. Thorough hand hygiene is the most important means of preventing and controlling the transmission of organisms. Fresh flowers and raw fruits and vegetables transmit microbes and therefore are eliminated. The client should not be exposed to anyone who has an infection or who has been recently vaccinated against or exposed to a communicable disease. Visitors are limited.

Nursing diagnoses for a client with cancer includes the following: (Continued)

NURSING DIAGNOSES	PLANNING/OUTCOMES	NURSING INTERVENTIONS
Risk for Injury related to altered clotting factors secondary to side effects of chemotherapy	The client will remain free of injury related to bleeding.	Every shift, assess the client for signs of bleeding (petechiae, ecchymoses, hematomas, bleeding gums, epistaxis, tarry stools, hematuria, frank or prolonged bleeding from puncture sites) because transfusions may be indicated. Monitor platelet count, which is an indicator of clotting ability. Institute special precautions if the count falls <50,000 mm^3. Apply pressure to all puncture sites for 3 to 5 minutes. Doing so prevents prolonged bleeding, which causes damage to underlying tissues such as nerves. Instruct the client to use a soft toothbrush or sponge for oral hygiene to prevent damage to oral mucosa, which is particularly susceptible to bleeding. Instruct the client to use an electric razor when shaving.
Fatigue related to analgesics, anemia, stress, increased metabolism, and chemotherapy	The client will experience less fatigue.	Plan frequent rest periods for the client to restore energy, and schedule activities when the client has the most energy. Monitor nutritional intake, as adequate nutrients are necessary to meet energy needs. Recognize that weakness places the client at increased risk for injury. Because fatigue may make activities of daily living difficult to complete, assistance may need to be provided.

Evaluation: Evaluate each outcome to determine how it has been met by the client.

SAMPLE NURSING CARE PLAN

The Client with Lung Cancer

H.S. is a 54-year-old carpenter. He is admitted with pain over his left scapula and radiating to his left arm. He describes having dyspnea and a productive cough. He denies any recent weight loss but does acknowledge experiencing extreme fatigue for the last 2 months. H.S. has been a chronic smoker for 20 years. A chest x-ray reveals an area of density in the left lung. A needle biopsy confirms small-cell lung cancer. A computed tomography (CT) scan confirms extrathoracic involvement. His physician referred H.S. to an oncologist for palliative chemotherapy. H.S. is to receive his first treatment of cisplatin (Platinol) and etoposide (VePesid). H.S. states that he is not sure about this treatment because it will not cure him and he does not know how he will keep breathing. He has never before been hospitalized.

NURSING DIAGNOSIS 1 *Death Anxiety* related to unfamiliar surroundings and uncertainty regarding change in health status as evidenced by H.S.'s statement that he does not know how he will keep breathing and the fact that he has never before been hospitalized

Nursing Outcomes Classification (NOC)
Anxiety Control
Acceptance: Health Status
Fear Control

Nursing Interventions Classification (NIC)
Anxiety Reduction
Coping Enhancement
Emotional Support

(Continues)

SAMPLE NURSING CARE PLAN (Continued)

PLANNING/OUTCOMES	NURSING INTERVENTIONS	RATIONALE
H.S. will share his feelings regarding his dyspnea.	Ascertain what the physician has told H.S. and what conclusions H.S. has reached. Encourage H.S. to share his feelings concerning cancer.	Helps decrease fear of the unknown. Identifies the source of any misconception that is increasing anxiety.
H.S. will express less anxiety about being in the hospital.	Maintain frequent contact with H.S. Explain the hospital routine and care H.S. will receive.	Reassures H.S. that he is not alone. An unfamiliar environment increases anxiety.

EVALUATION

H.S. shares his feelings about his diagnosis and treatment regimen. H.S. exhibits less anxiety about the change in his health status and hospitalization.

NURSING DIAGNOSIS 2 *Impaired **G**as Exchange* related to decreased lung capacity and increased secretions as evidenced by dyspnea, productive cough, and dense area in left lung

Nursing Outcomes Classification (NOC)
Respiratory Status: Gas Exchange
Respiratory Status: Ventilation
Tissue Perfusion: Pulmonary

Nursing Interventions Classification (NIC)
Airway Management
Respiratory Monitoring
Oxygen Therapy

PLANNING/OUTCOMES	NURSING INTERVENTIONS	RATIONALE
H.S. will report less dyspnea with oxygen saturation >90%.	Monitor pulmonary status by auscultating breath sounds; checking rate, depth, and pattern of respirations; evaluating skin color for cyanosis; and monitoring pulse oximetry.	Provides information regarding pulmonary status changes indicating either improvement or onset of complications.
	Position H.S. in Fowler's position.	Promotes expansion of lungs and respiratory muscles.
	Administer oxygen at prescribed level.	Corrects hypoxemia and provides oxygen for metabolic needs.
	Administer opioids with caution.	Opioids can depress the respiratory center.
	Monitor amount, color, and consistency of sputum.	Changes in sputum suggest infection or change in pulmonary status.
	Plan care and treatments within H.S.'s tolerance.	Oxygen demands increase with activity.

EVALUATION

Adequate ventilation with oxygen saturation >90% is maintained.

SAMPLE NURSING CARE PLAN (Continued)

NURSING DIAGNOSIS 3 *Acute **P**ain* related to tumor growth and tissue destruction as evidenced by verbal report of pain over left scapula radiating to left arm

Nursing Outcomes Classification (NOC)
Pain Control
Comfort Level

Nursing Interventions Classification (NIC)
Pain Management
Medication Management
Emotional Support

PLANNING/OUTCOMES	INTERVENTIONS	RATIONALE
H.S. will report less pain after pain-relief measures.	Provide routine comfort measures such as repositioning and backrub.	Noninvasive pain-relief techniques are helpful in pain management.
	Teach H.S. to request pain medication before onset of pain.	Keeps pain under control.
	Have H.S. rate pain on a scale of 0 to 10 (0 = no pain and 10 = worst pain).	Provides a method of evaluating the subjective experience of pain.
	Teach H.S. relaxation techniques.	Decreases the perception of pain.
	Document H.S.'s response to the pain-control regimen and adjust as needed.	Identifies effectiveness of pain-relief techniques.

EVALUATION

H.S. reports less pain; <2 on a scale of 0 to 10.

NURSING DIAGNOSIS 4 *Fatigue* related to chronic pain and dyspnea as evidenced by client's description of dyspnea and extreme fatigue for 2 months

Nursing Outcomes Classification (NOC)
Activity Tolerance
Energy Conservation

Nursing Interventions Classification (NIC)
Activity Therapy
Energy Management

PLANNING/OUTCOMES	INTERVENTIONS	RATIONALE
H.S. will report feeling less fatigued.	Plan care to allow for rest periods.	Helps conserve energy.
	Assess for related factors such as nutritional imbalances, lack of sleep, and causes of stress.	Reduces fatigue.
	Have H.S. rate fatigue on a scale of 0 to 10 (0 = not tired, 10 = total exhaustion) for a 24-hour period.	Identifies peak energy and exhaustion times.
	Teach energy-conservation strategies such as planning ahead, setting priorities, scheduling rest periods, and resting before a difficult task.	Decreases physical and psychological stress.

EVALUATION

H.S. exhibits less fatigue in light of having frequent rest periods daily.

NURSING DIAGNOSIS

Anticipatory Grieving related to loss of body function as evidenced by H.S.'s statement that he does not know how he will keep breathing

NOC: *Coping, Grief Resolution*
NIC: *Anticipatory Guidance, Coping Enhancement, Grief Work Facilitation*

NURSING GOAL

H.S. will verbalize his loss and develop coping skills as he acknowledges his illness as terminal.

NURSING INTERVENTIONS

1. Provide opportunities for H.S. to express his feelings.
2. Answer all of H.S.'s questions honestly.
3. Encourage H.S.'s participation in his care.
4. Encourage family support and visits from friends.
5. Utilize appropriate referrals to professionals, such as clergy, as needed.

SCIENTIFIC RATIONALES

1. Helps identify H.S.'s coping strategies.
2. Helps H.S. cope.
3. Gives H.S. a greater sense of control.
4. Assures H.S. that he is not alone and provides time to discuss concerns openly.
5. Facilitates the grief process and spiritual care.

EVALUATION

Has H.S. come to terms with the reality of his diagnosis and prognosis?

CONCEPT CARE MAP 34-1

CASE STUDY

J.D. is a 70-year-old man with a history of prostate cancer, which was treated with palliative hormones and radiation. His admitting diagnosis is adenocarcinoma of the prostate with widespread bone metastasis. J.D. is married and has one grown daughter, who often helps with his care. His chief concern is severe back pain. The physician has ordered intrathecal morphine sulfate and aspirin 10 g for pain relief.

The following questions will guide your development of a nursing care plan for the case study.

1. List symptoms typically seen in clients diagnosed with prostate cancer.
2. Identify the population most at risk for developing prostate cancer.
3. List three possible risk factors for prostate cancer.
4. Discuss the rationale for the physician's orders including aspirin along with morphine sulfate.
5. Discuss the rationale for benzodiazepines not being used for pain relief.
6. List the subjective and objective data the nurse would want to obtain.
7. When you walk into J.D.'s room, he greets you with a smile and continues talking and joking with his daughter. While assessing him, you note that his vital signs are normal. You ask him to rate his pain on a scale of 0 to 10. He pauses to think about it, then rates the pain at 8. In the chart, you must record your nursing assessment by circling the appropriate number on the scale. Which number do you think you should circle?
8. Write three individualized nursing diagnoses and goals for J.D.
9. Discuss which oncological emergency J.D. is most likely to develop.

SUMMARY

- Cancer is the second most common cause of death in the United States.
- Most cancers are curable if treated early.
- Benign neoplasms are localized and encapsulated and do not spread.
- Malignant neoplasms spread to neighboring tissues via blood and lymph.
- Biopsy is the most accurate diagnostic test for cancer.
- The most common medical treatments for cancer are surgery, radiation, and chemotherapy. They may be used alone or in combination.
- Surgery is the treatment of choice for early cancers.
- Chemotherapy is the treatment of choice for metastatic cancers. It is also the treatment most responsible for increasing cancer cure rates in recent years.
- Lung cancer is the leading cause of cancer death among men and women. Eighty percent of all cases are related to smoking.
- Quality of life, not quantity of life, is the ultimate goal for clients living with cancer.

REVIEW QUESTIONS

1. The nurse carefully monitors the client's intravenous chemotherapy. An early indicator that extravasation may be occurring is when:
   1. the fluid stops infusing.
   2. edema is noted at the site.
   3. blood returns when the bottle is lowered.
   4. burning occurs at the site.
2. A breast cancer client states that the doctor says he is going to prescribe hormone therapy. Which of the following hormones would probably be ordered?
   1. Thyroxin.
   2. Parathormone.
   3. Progesterone.
   4. Testosterone.
3. A cancer client develops a low white-cell count. She is placed on neutropenic precautions. Which of the following menu selections would be best?
   1. Meat loaf, mashed potatoes, green beans, and fruit gelatin.
   2. Meat loaf, mashed potatoes, marinated carrots, and a garden salad.
   3. Meat loaf, mashed potatoes, chef salad, and tapioca.
   4. Meat loaf, mashed potatoes, green beans, fruit salad, and a cookie.
4. When stomatitis develops, it is best to encourage the client to:
   1. drink plenty of orange juice.
   2. use lemon and glycerine swabs frequently.
   3. brush teeth before and after eating.
   4. rinse with commercial mouthwash as needed.
5. Clients receiving radiation are encouraged to:
   1. wash and dry the skin carefully and apply lotion.
   2. not bathe.
   3. not apply deodorants or lotions.
   4. wash the skin with soap and apply baby powder.
6. The client asks the nurse to explain the implications of the TNM system. His physician told him "the news is not good; your tumor is classified as $T_2 N_2 M_1$." The nurse's response is based on the knowledge that:
   1. this is a local classification system used by the physicians at this particular hospital.
   2. this is an international system used by oncologists as a standardized method of defining a tumor and tumor activity.
   3. the numbers used are indicative of tumor growth and spread, with the smaller numbers meaning more aggressive growth.
   4. only the physician can interpret any findings to the client.
7. A difference between normal cells and cancer cells is that cancer cells:
   1. adhere to their area of origin.
   2. are well differentiated.
   3. multiply at will.
   4. cannot move freely around the body.
8. Choose risk factors for cancer: (Select all that apply.)
   1. use of oral birth control pills.
   2. consumption of a high fiber diet.
   3. heavy alcohol consumption.
   4. use of smokeless tobacco instead of smoking cigarettes.
   5. consumption of five servings of fruits and vegetables daily.
   6. multiple sexual partners with unprotected sex.
9. A nurse is caring for a client with advanced cancer. The first priority of nursing intervention is:
   1. support limbs and gently turn client to prevent a pathological fracture.
   2. monitor ascites by measuring abdominal girth at the umbilicus.
   3. listen to the client share her concerns about losing her hair.
   4. administer oral morphine sulfate for break through pain.

10. The nurse meets the psychosocial needs of the client with cancer and his family's needs by:
    1. conversing on a superficial level so she does not always have to think about her condition.
    2. allowing the client personal time to adjust to diagnosis but answer questions and provide support as needed.
    3. allaying anxiety by not giving any information about treatment options or adverse reactions.
    4. providing all the physical care for the client so the family is not involved with these needs.

REFERENCES/SUGGESTED READINGS

Agency for Health Care Policy and Research. (1994). *Clinical practice guidelines: Management of cancer pain* (AHCPR Publication No. 94-0592). Rockville, MD: U.S. Department of Health & Human Services.

American Cancer Society (ACS). (2000). Cancer Facts & Figures 2000. [Online]. Retrieved on May 2, 2009 from http://www.cancer.org/docroot/STT/stt_0_2000.asp?sitearea=STT&level=1

American Cancer Society (ACS). (2002). Cancer news roundup. *Nursing*2002, 32(10), 32hn6–32hn7.

American Cancer Society (ACS). (2003). Cancer Facts & Figures 2003. [Online]. Retrieved on May 2, 2009 from http://www.cancer.org/docroot/STT/stt_0_2003.asp?sitearea=STT&level=1

American Cancer Society (ACS). (2006). *Cancer facts & figures 2006*. Atlanta: American Cancer Society.

American Cancer Society (ACS). (2007). Global Cancer: Facts & Figures 2007. Retrieved on May 2, 2009 from http://www.cancer.org/downloads/STT/Global_Cancer_Facts_and_Figures_2007_rev.pdf

American Cancer Society (ACS). (2008). Cancer Facts & Figures 2008. Retrieved on May 2, 2009 from http://www.cancer.org/docroot/STT/stt_0_2008.asp?sitearea=STT&level=1

American Pain Society. (1992). *Principles of analgesic use in the treatment of acute and chronic cancer pain* (3rd ed.). Skokie, IL: Author.

Baird, S., Donehower, M., Stalsbroten, V., & Ades, T. (Eds.) (1997). *A cancer source book for nurses* (7th ed.). Atlanta, GA: American Cancer Society.

Belcher, A. (1992). *Cancer nursing*. St. Louis, MO: Mosby.

Blackburn, G. (1998). Wasting away: Cancer cachexia. *Health News*, 4(4), 4. Waltham, MA: Massachusetts Medical Society.

Bral, E. (1998). Caring for adults with chronic cancer pain. *AJN*, 4(98), 27–32.

Bulechek, G., Butcher, H., McCloskey, J., & Dochterman, J., eds. (2008). *Nursing Interventions Classification (NIC)* (5th ed.). St. Louis, MO: Mosby/Elsevier.

Cancerbackup. (2009). Combination chemotherapy regimen. Macmillan Cancer Support. Retrieved on May 5, 2009 from http://www.cancerbackup.org.uk/Treatments/Chemotherapy/Combinationregimen

Cancer Treatment Centers of America. (2009a). Biotherapy/Immunotherapy. Retrieved on May 1, 2009 from http://www.cancercneter.com/conventional-cancer-treatment/biotherapy-immunotherapy.cfm

Cancer Treatment Centers of America. (2009b). Photodynamic therapy. Retrieved on May 1, 2009 from http://www.cancercneter.com/conventional-cancer-treatment/photodynamic-therapy.cfm

Cancer Treatment Centers of America. (2009c). Hormone Therapy. Retrieved on May 1, 2009 from http://www.cancercneter.com/conventional-cancer-treatment/hormone-therapy.cfm

Chapman, D., & Goodman, M. (2000). *Cancer nursing principles* (5th ed.). Boston, MA: Jones & Bartlett.

Chiramannil, A. (1998). Lung cancer. *AJN*, 4(98), 46–47.

Dell, D. (2001). Regaining range of motion after breast surgery. *Nursing2001*, 31(10), 50–52.

Erickson, J. (1994, November). Update on Hodgkin's Disease. *Nurse Practitioner*, 63–67.

Estes, M. (2010). *Health assessment & physical examination* (4th ed.). Clifton Park, NY: Delmar Cengage Learning.

Fieler, B. (1997). Side effects and quality of life in patients receiving high-dose rate brachytherapy. *Oncology Nursing Forum*, 24(3), 545.

Galvan, T. (2001). Dysphagia: Going down and staying down. *AJN*, 101(1), 37–42.

Greifzu, S. (1998). Fighting cancer fatigue. *RN*, 61(8), 41–43.

Harris, L. (2002). Ovarian cancer: Screening for early detection. *AJN*, 102(10), 46–52.

Held-Warmkessel, J. (1998). Chemotherapy complications: Helping your patient cope with adverse reactions. *Nursing98* 4(28), 41–45.

Kediziera, P. (1998). The two faces of pain. *RN*, 61(2), 45–46.

Kohr, J. (1995). Measuring your patient's pain. *RN*, 58(4), 39–40.

Langhorne, M., Fulton, J., & Otto, S. (2007). *Oncology nursing* (5th ed.). St. Louis: Mosby.

Lewis, S., Heitkemper, M., & Dirksen, S. (2007). *Medical–surgical nursing: Assessment and management of clinical problems* (7th ed.). St. Louis, MO: Mosby.

Machia, J. (2001). Breast cancer: Risk, prevention & Tamoxifen. *AJN*, 101(4), 26–35.

McCaffery, M., & Ferrell, B. (1994, July). How to use the new AHCPR cancer pain guidelines. *AJN*, 42–47.

McCarron, E. (1995, June). Supporting the families of cancer patients. *Nursing95*, 48–51.

McConnell, E. (2001). Myth & Facts about dysphagia. *Nursing2001*, 31(7), 29.

Moorhead, S., Johnson, M., Maas, M., & Swanson, E. (2007). *Nursing Outcomes Classification (NOC)* (4th ed). St. Louis, MO: Elsevier—Health Sciences Division.

Monahan, F., Sands, J., Neighbors, M., & Marek, J. (2006). *Phipps' medical-surgical nursing: Health and illness perspectives* (8th ed.). St. Louis, MO: Mosby Elsevier.

Myers, J. (2000). Chemotherapy-induced hypersensitivity reaction. *AJN*, 100(4), 53–54.

National Bone Marrow Transplant Link (NBMTLink). (2009). Resource guide for bone marrow/stem cell transplant. Retrieved on April 30, 2009 from http://www.nbmtlink.org/resources_support/rg/rg_costs.htm

National Cancer Institute. (2006). Targeted cancer therapies: Questions and answers. National Cancer Institute Fact Sheet. Retrieved on May 4, 2009 from http://www.cancer.gov/cacncertopics/factsheet/Therapy/targeted/print?page=&keyword

Otto, S. (2001). *Oncology nursing* (4th ed.). St. Louis, MO: Mosby.

Porth, C., & Matfin, G. (2008). *Pathophysiology: Concepts of Altered Health States* (8th ed.). Philadelphia: Lippincott Williams & Wilkins.

Researchers say new drug may boost effects of cancer radiation. (1998, May 12). *Corpus Christi Caller Times*.

Resnick, B., & Belcher, A. (2002). Breast reconstruction. *AJN*, 102(4), 26–33.

Sargent, C., & Murphy, D. (2003). What you need to know about colorectal cancer. *Nursing2003*, 33(2), 36–41.

Schweid, L., & Werner-McCullough, M. (1994, September). Will you recognize these oncological crises? *RN*, 23–27.

Smeltzer, S., Bare, B., Hinkle, J., & Cheever, K. (2008). *Brunner & Suddarth's Textbook of Medical Surgical Nursing, North American Edition* (11th ed.) Philadelphia: Lippincott Williams & Wilkins

Tamoxifen for breast cancer prevention. (1998, December 15). *Healthnews*, 4(15).

Teasley, R. (in press). *Understanding Neoplasms.*

Thaler-DeMers, D. (2000). The cancer survival toolbox. *AJN*, 100(4), 52.

Timby, B., Smith, N., & Scherer, J. (2002) *Introductory Medical-Surgical Nursing* (8th ed.) Philadelphia: Lippincott Williams & Wilkins.

U.S. Preventive Services Task Force. (2002). Screening for colorectal cancer: Recommendations and rationale. *AJN*, 102(9), 107–114.

Watson, A., & Coyne, P. (2003). Recognizing the faces of cancer pain. *Nursing2003*, 33(4), 32hn1–32hn8.

Weber, M. (1995). Clinical snapshot: Chemotherapy-induced nausea and vomiting. *AJN*, 95(4).

White, L., & Spitz, M. (1994). Cancer risk and early detection assessment. *Capsules and Comments in Oncology Nursing*, 2(1), 2–3.

Wilkes, G. (2000). Nutrition: The forgotten ingredient in cancer care. *AJN*, 100(4), 46–51.

Woodward, W., & Thobaben, M. (1994). Special home health care nursing challenges: Patients with cancer. *Home Health Care Nurse*, 12(3), 33–37.

Zuckerman, D. (2002). The breast cancer information gap. *RN*, 65(2), 39–41.

RESOURCES

American Cancer Society (ACS), http://www.cancer.org

American Pain Society, http://www.ampainsoc.org/

Breast Cancer Network of Strength, http://www.networkofstrength.org/

National Cancer Institute, http://www.cancer.gov

National Coalition for Cancer Survivorship (NCCS), http://www.canceradvocacy.org

UNIT 10 Nursing Care of the Client: Oxygenation and Perfusion

CHAPTER 35
Respiratory System

MAKING THE CONNECTION

Refer to the following chapters to increase your understanding of the respiratory system:

Basic Nursing
- ***Assessment***
- ***Diagnostic Tests***

Adult Health Nursing
- ***Oncology***
- ***Cardiovascular System***
- ***Hematologic and Lymphatic Systems***

Basic Procedures
- ***Performing the Heimlich Maneuver***

Intermediate Procedures
- ***Administering Oxygen Therapy***
- ***Performing Nasopharyngeal and Oropharyngeal Suctioning***
- ***Performing Tracheostomy Care***

Delmar's Heart & Lung Sounds on StudyWare CD™: Lung Sounds

LEARNING OBJECTIVES

Upon completion of this chapter, you should be able to:

- Define key terms.
- Describe components of a complete respiratory assessment.
- Identify normal parameters for common respiratory diagnostic studies.
- Discuss the etiology, medical–surgical management, and nursing care for clients with respiratory disorders.
- Prepare a nursing care plan for a client with a respiratory disorder.

KEY TERMS

adventitious breath sound
asthma
atelectasis
audible wheeze
bronchial sound
bronchiectasis
bronchitis
bronchovesicular sound
caseation
cavitation
chemoreceptor
coarse crackle
diffusion
emphysema
empyema
epistaxis
external respiration
fine crackle
hemopneumothorax
hemothorax
internal respiration
liquefaction necrosis
lung stretch receptor
perfusion
pleural effusion
pleural friction rub
pleurisy
pneumonia
pneumothorax
primary tubercle
respiration
sibilant wheeze
sonorous wheeze
status asthmaticus
stridor
surfactant
ventilation
vesicular sound

INTRODUCTION

Respiratory disorders account for millions of the dollars spent in the U.S. health care arena. From loss of time on the job because of the common cold to care for those with chronic respiratory disorders, the cost of respiratory disease is staggering. This chapter explores the various respiratory disorders, with a focus on the nursing process.

ANATOMY AND PHYSIOLOGY REVIEW

The primary function of the respiratory system is delivery of oxygen to the lungs and removal of carbon dioxide from the lungs.

Thoracic Cavity

The chest cage is a closed compartment bounded on the top by the neck muscles and at the bottom by the diaphragm. The walls of the chest cage are formed by the ribs and intercostal muscles laterally, the thoracic vertebrae posteriorly, and the sternum anteriorly. The inside of the chest cage is called the *thoracic cavity*. Contained within the thoracic cavity are the lungs. The lungs are cone-shaped, porous organs separated from the other chest organs by the mediastinum. The lungs lie free, except for their attachment to the heart and trachea, and are encased in the pleura, a thin, transparent double-layered serous membrane lining the thoracic cavity. The layers of the pleura are the *parietal pleura*, which lie adjacent to the chest wall and produce pleural fluid, and the *visceral pleura*, which adhere to the surface of the lungs and absorb pleural fluid. The area between the two pleura is known as the *pleural space* or pleural cavity.

The pleural space contains 5 to 20 mL of fluid, which allows the layers of the pleura to slide on each other yet hold together. The pressure within the pleural space is less than that of outside air. This difference in pressure creates a suction that prevents the lungs from collapsing on exhalation.

The right lung is larger than the left and is divided into three sections, or lobes: upper, middle, and lower. The left lung is divided into two lobes: upper and lower (Figure 35-1). The upper portion of the lung is referred to as the apex (plural, apices). The lower portion is called the base. The lungs possess a dual blood supply: bronchial circulation and pulmonary circulation. Bronchial circulation begins with the bronchial artery, which provides the passageways of the lungs with blood to meet nutritional needs and ends when the venous blood enters the pulmonary veins. Pulmonary circulation is the route by which blood is delivered to the alveoli for gas exchange (Figure 35-2).

Conducting Airways

The conducting airways are tube-like structures that provide a passageway for air as it travels to the lungs. These are the nasal passages, mouth, pharynx, larynx, trachea, bronchi, and bronchioles (Figure 35-1). The conducting airways are lined with

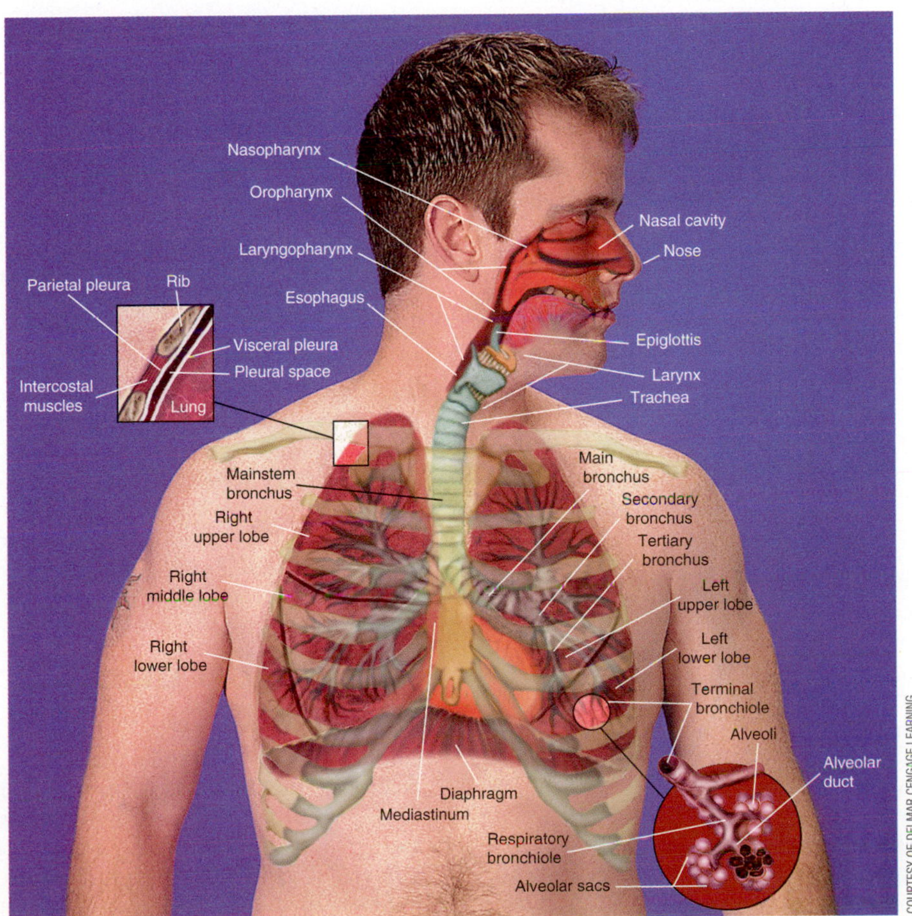

Figure 35-1 Structures of the Respiratory Tract

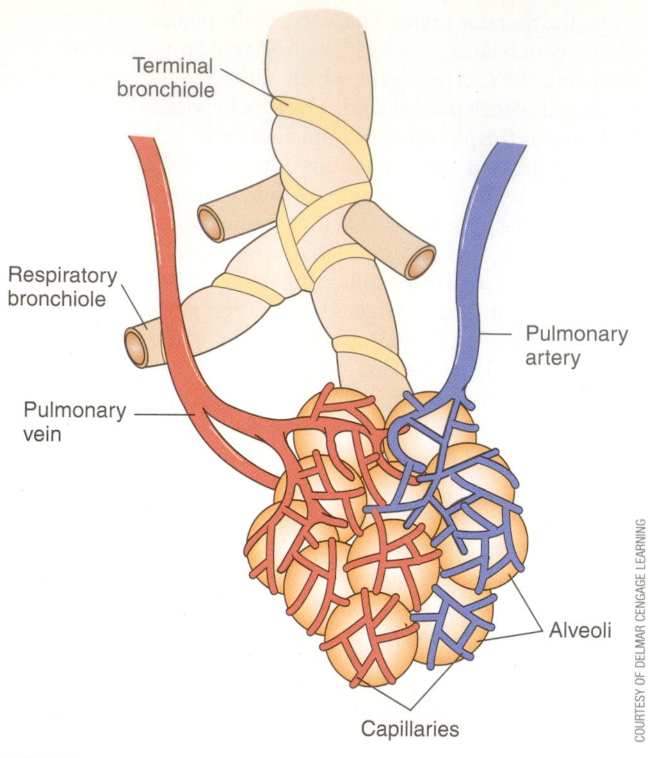

FIGURE 35-2 **Gas exchange occurs at the alveolar capillary membrane.**

epithelial tissue containing serous glands, mucus-secreting Goblet cells, and hair-like projections called *cilia*. The mucus of the Goblet cells together with the cilia form a mucociliary blanket that protects the respiratory system from foreign particles. The constant upward motion of the cilia propels the mucociliary blanket toward the pharynx, where foreign matter is expectorated or swallowed.

The nasal passages are the preferred route for air to enter the respiratory tract. In addition to the function of filtering inspired air, the nasal passages are richly supplied with blood vessels that warm and moisten the air. Because the mouth lacks cilia and abundant blood supply, breathing through the mouth reduces the ability to filter, warm, and moisten inspired air.

Connecting the nasal passages and mouth to the lower parts of the respiratory tract is the *pharynx*. Located behind the oral cavity, the pharynx serves as a passageway for both inspired air into the larynx and ingested food passing into the digestive system. At the distal portion of the pharynx is the larynx, also known as the voice box.

The *larynx* contains the vocal cords and is the passageway for air entering and leaving the trachea. The larynx is composed of four structures: the uppermost thyroid cartilage (Adam's apple), the cricoid cartilage (which lies at the lower edge of the larynx), the epiglottis (a leaf-shaped structure that covers the larynx during swallowing), and the glottis (the triangular space between relaxed vocal cords).

The *trachea*, commonly known as the windpipe, is a tube composed of connective tissue mucosa and smooth muscle supported by C-shaped rings of cartilage that extends into the bronchi. The trachea is 2.0 to 2.5 cm wide (approximately 1 inch) and 10 to 12 cm long (approximately 4 to 6 inches). The trachea terminates by branching into two tubes: the right and left primary bronchi. The *bronchi* are somewhat smaller in diameter than the trachea, and each passes into its respective lung.

The right bronchus is wider and more vertically positioned than the left. This difference in positioning allows foreign matter to enter the right bronchus more easily than the left. Within the lungs, the bronchi branch off into increasingly smaller diameter tubes until they become the terminal *bronchioles*. These branch further, forming alveolar ducts that end in numerous saclike, thin-walled structures called the *alveoli*. Collectively, the alveoli and the alveolar ducts resemble a cluster of grapes. The branching makes this portion of the respiratory tract resemble an inverted tree, giving rise to the term *bronchial tree* (Figure 35-1).

Respiratory Tissues

The respiratory tissues perform the function of gas exchange. The alveoli constitute the primary site of gas exchange. The alveolar ducts are smooth, muscular tubes containing abundant alveolar macrophages that remove foreign particles (e.g., bacteria). The alveoli, into which the alveolar ducts terminate, consist of interconnected spaces with thin walls, or septa, occupied by a network of capillaries called the *alveolar capillary membrane*.

The alveoli contain two specialized types of cells. Type I alveolar cells are flat, squamous, epithelial cells across which gas exchange occurs. Type II alveolar cells produce a phospholipid substance called **surfactant**. Surfactant coats the inner surfaces of the alveoli, reduces the surface tension of pulmonary fluids, allows gas exchange, and prevents the collapse of the airways. Each lung contains approximately 300 million alveoli.

Respiration

Respiration is a process of gas exchange. This process is necessary to supply cells with oxygen for metabolism and to remove the waste by-product carbon dioxide. There are two types of respiration: external respiration and internal respiration. **External respiration** is the exchange of gases between the inhaled air, now in the alveoli, and the blood in the pulmonary capillaries. **Internal respiration** is the exchange of gases at the cellular level between tissue cells and blood in systemic capillaries (Figure 35-3). These functions depend on the adequacy of ventilation, perfusion, and diffusion. **Ventilation** is the movement of gases into and out of the lung. **Perfusion** is the flow of blood through the vessels of a specific organ or body part. Pertaining to the respiratory system, **diffusion** is the movement of gases across the alveolar capillary membrane from areas of high concentration to areas of lower concentration. Factors that affect ventilation, perfusion, and diffusion affect respiration (Table 35-1).

Neuromuscular Control of Respiration

Unlike the heart muscle, the respiratory muscles must receive continuous neural stimuli to function. Regulation of respiration is integrated by neurons located in the pons and medulla of the brain. The control of respiration is influenced by involuntary (automatic) and voluntary components. Involuntary components include chemoreceptors, lung stretch receptors, and impulses from other sources. **Chemoreceptors** monitor the levels of carbon dioxide and

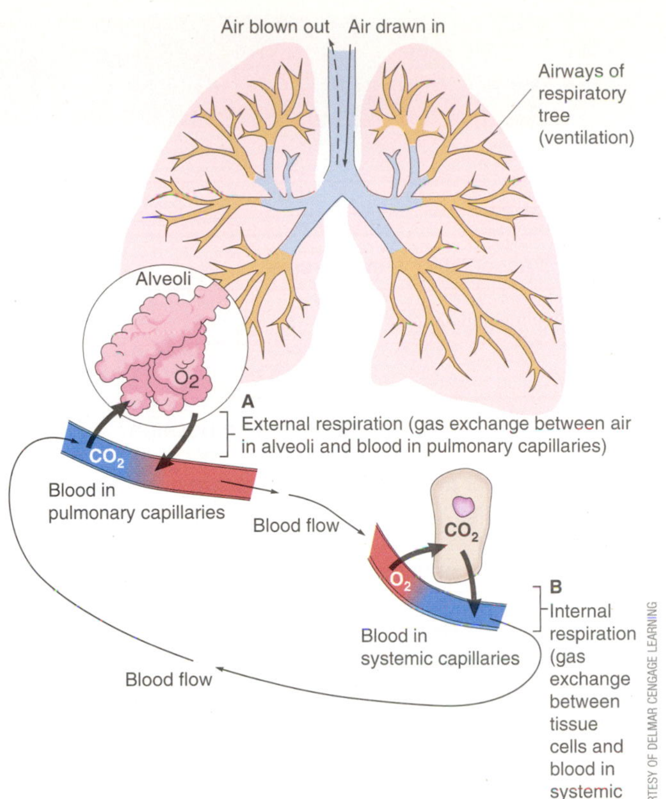

FIGURE 35-3 *A*, External Respiration; *B*, Internal Respiration

oxygen and the acidity/alkalinity (pH) of the blood. Normally, chemoreceptors initiate respiration in response to an increase of carbon dioxide in the blood. With certain chronic pulmonary disorders, such as emphysema, chemoreceptors become more responsive to a low level of oxygen. This becomes significant when administering oxygen to persons whose drive to breathe depends on a low level of oxygen in the blood. **Lung stretch receptors** monitor the pattern of breathing and prevent overexpansion of the tissues. Many other sources involuntarily send impulses to the respiratory center. For example, if a person becomes frightened or angry, the respiratory rate increases in response to stimuli from the autonomic nervous system. Voluntary components of respiratory control integrate breathing with acts such as talking and speaking.

The diaphragm acts as the primary muscle of respiration. During inspiration, the diaphragm contracts and flattens out in response to stimuli from the respiratory center, increasing the length of the thoracic cavity. At the same time, the intercostal muscles contract, elevating the ribs and increasing the diameter of the thoracic cavity. The total thoracic space increases, reducing the pressure within the thoracic cavity. The pressure within the thoracic cavity then becomes negative in relation to that of atmospheric pressure, and air moves into the thoracic cavity. Upon expiration, the respiratory center signals the diaphragm and intercostal muscles to relax. The thoracic cavity returns to its original size. Aided by the elastic recoil of the lungs, the decrease in size of the thoracic cavity increases pressure, and air moves out of the lungs.

TABLE 35-1 Factors Affecting Ventilation, Perfusion, and Diffusion

Ventilation	Position: Dependent areas receive majority of air. Lung volume: Low volume results in shunting air to lung apices. Disease: Bronchial constriction and airway collapse decrease ventilation.
Perfusion	Position: Dependent areas receive majority of blood. Hypoxia: Results in vasoconstriction and decreased perfusion. Blockage: Results in decreased or absent perfusion to distal areas.
Diffusion	Alveolar capillary membrane: Alterations may occur in thickness and permeability of membrane.

COURTESY OF DELMAR CENGAGE LEARNING

GAS EXCHANGE

Gas exchange occurs at the alveolar capillary membrane (Figure 35-2). Venous blood from the right ventricle is pumped into the pulmonary arteries and travels to the alveolar capillary network, where it is exposed to the inhaled air. Because of the higher concentration of oxygen in the alveoli, oxygen diffuses into the blood within the alveolar capillary network. The majority of oxygen binds to the iron atoms of the hemoglobin molecule in the red blood cells. Approximately 1% to 3% of oxygen dissolves into the blood plasma.

The exchange of carbon dioxide also occurs within the alveoli. Within the alveolar capillary network, the carbon dioxide detaches from hemoglobin and diffuses into the alveolar space. Carbon dioxide is removed from the alveolar space when exhalation occurs. The blood within the pulmonary capillary network is now oxygenated and travels to the heart via the pulmonary veins. Oxygenated blood is sent to the body via the aorta and the arterial network (Figure 35-3).

ASSESSMENT

To understand the assessment of the respiratory system, the student must be familiar with related terminology (Table 35-2).

HEALTH HISTORY

Nursing assessment begins with a complete history. The client is questioned regarding allergies, occupation, lifestyle, and health habits such as smoking or alcohol use (Box 35-1). Ask about other health problems that affect the respiratory system, such as pneumonia or cardiac problems. Symptoms such as dyspnea, decreased exercise tolerance, and cough are explored

Table 35-2 Respiratory Terms

TERM	DEFINITION
Eupnea	Normal breathing
Apnea	Cessation of breathing, possibly temporary in nature
Dyspnea	Labored or difficult breathing, possibly normal if associated with exercise
Bradypnea	Abnormally slow breathing
Tachypnea	Abnormally rapid breathing
Orthopnea	Discomfort or difficulty with breathing in any but an upright sitting or standing position
Kussmaul's respirations	Abnormal respiratory pattern characterized by irregular periods of increased rate and depth of respiration; most often seen with diabetic ketoacidosis
Biot's respirations	Abnormal respiratory pattern characterized by irregular periods of apnea alternating with short periods of respiration of equal depth; most commonly seen with increased intracranial pressure
Cheyne-Stokes respirations	Abnormal respiratory pattern characterized by initially slow, shallow respirations that increase in rapidity and depth and then gradually decrease until respiration stops for 10 to 60 seconds; pattern then repeats itself in the same manner
Anoxia	Without oxygen
Hypoxia	Lack of adequate oxygen in inspired air such as occurs at high altitude
Hypoxemia	Insufficient amount of oxygen in the blood possibly due to respiratory, cardiovascular, or anemia-related disorders
Cyanosis	Bluish, grayish, or purplish discoloration of the skin caused by abnormal amounts of reduced (oxygen-poor) hemoglobin in the blood; not always a reliable indicator of hypoxia
Acrocyanosis	Cyanosis of the fingertips and toes; often caused by vasomotor disturbances associated with vasoconstriction
Circumoral cyanosis	Bluish discoloration encircling the mouth
Oxygen saturation	Amount of oxygen combined with hemoglobin

COURTESY OF DELMAR CENGAGE LEARNING

in depth. Following a complete history, the nurse completes a physical assessment of the client.

Inspection

Physical assessment of the respiratory system starts with inspection. Note the client's color, level of consciousness, and emotional state. Respirations are observed for their rate, depth, quality, rhythm, and breathing pattern. Symmetry of chest wall movement is also noted. The nurse observes for use of accessory muscles to aid breathing. The position the client assumes provides information on respiratory status because individuals having trouble breathing often lean forward.

Palpation and Percussion

The next steps in the respiratory assessment are palpation and percussion. These are normally done by the registered nurse or physician. Through the use of palpation and percussion, areas of varying densities in the lung can be detected. The density of lung tissues changes with disease states such as pneumonia, pneumothorax, and pleural effusion.

Auscultation

The client should breathe slowly through the mouth while the listener assesses breath sounds at each location for the length of a complete inspiration and expiration. Breath sounds are assessed for duration, pitch, and intensity. Figure 35-4 illustrates the recommended stethoscope location for each auscultation.

Normal Breath Sounds

Under normal circumstances, **bronchial sounds** are heard over the sternum (Figure 35-5). These loud, high-pitched tubular, hollow-like sounds last longer during expiration than during inspiration. When heard in areas other than the sternum, bronchial sounds indicate fluid, exudate, or lung tissue

BOX 35-1 QUESTIONS TO ASK AND OBSERVATIONS TO MAKE WHEN COLLECTING DATA

Subjective Data

- Do you have seasonal or environmental allergies?
- Have you been coughing? If so, are you coughing up any mucous? What does it look like?
- Do you get frequent upper respiratory infections?
- Have you ever had pneumonia? If so, when and how often?
- Have you had the pneumonia vaccine?
- Do you get a flu shot annually?
- Do you have any chronic lung conditions such as asthma or emphysema?
- Are you experiencing any difficulty breathing?
- Have you experienced any shortness of breath with exertion or activity?
- Is your nose feeling stuffy and congested?
- Does your throat hurt or feel sore?
- Have you experienced changes in your voice?
- Do you currently or have you ever smoked?
- If you no longer smoke, when did you quit?
- If you smoke, how long have you smoked? What do you smoke? And, how much do you smoke each day?
- Does your chest feel tight when you breathe?
- Are you experiencing any chest pain or discomfort when breathing?

Objective Data

- Check vital signs.
- Check pulse oximetry levels.
- Observe respiratory effort.
- Observe use of accessory muscles.
- Assess color of mucous membranes and nail beds.
- Assess for sputum production.
- Record the quality, color, and odor of the sputum.
- Observe client's activity tolerance.
- Assess supplemental oxygen requirements.
- Auscultate lung sounds.
- Report chest x-ray results or other diagnostic test results.
- Record the quality, color, and odor of the sputum.

compression. **Bronchovesicular sounds** are heard over the anterior one-third of the chest near the sternum and also around the scapula posteriorly (Figure 35-5). Bronchovesicular sounds have a medium pitch and intensity with inspiration and expiration being equal in duration. They may be heard in the periphery of the lung when consolidation and fluid are present.

Vesicular sounds are heard over the majority of the lungs (Figure 35-5). These soft, low-pitched sounds are best heard during inspiration and may be inaudible during expiration.

Adventitious Breath Sounds

Abnormal breath sounds are called **adventitious breath sounds** and include **fine crackles** (rales), **coarse crackles** (rales), **sonorous wheezes** (rhonchi), **sibilant wheezes**, **pleural friction rub**, and **stridor**. Table 35-3 describes the general characteristics of these adventitious breath sounds.

COMMON DIAGNOSTIC TESTS

Commonly used diagnostic tests for clients with respiratory disorders are listed in Table 35-4. Table 35-5 lists normal values for arterial blood gases.

INFECTIOUS/INFLAMMATORY DISORDERS

Infectious/inflammatory disorders of the upper respiratory tract, pneumonia, tuberculosis, and pleurisy/pleural effusion are discussed in the following sections.

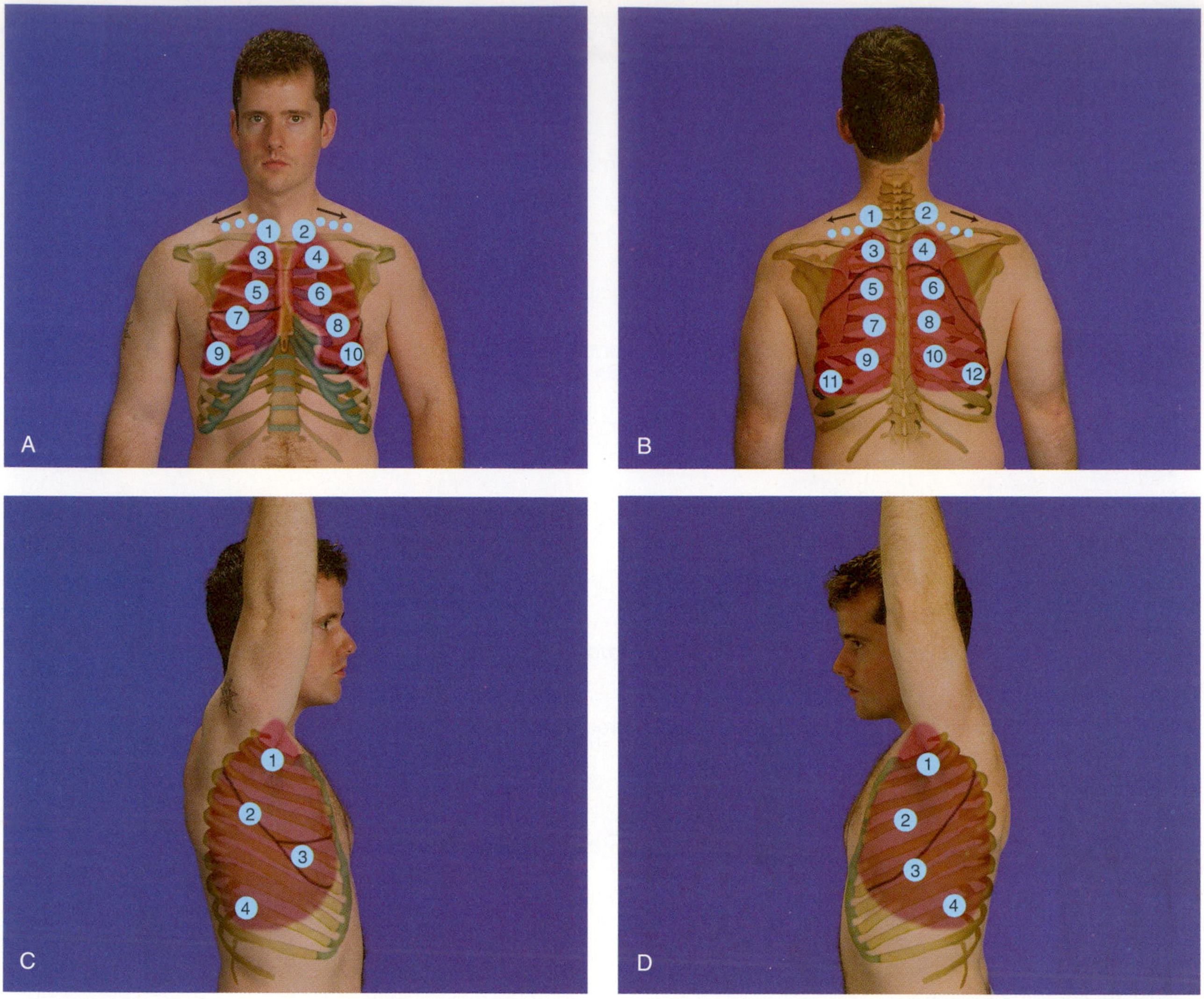

COURTESY OF DELMAR CENGAGE LEARNING

FIGURE 35-4 Stethoscope Locations for Each Auscultation; *A,* Anterior Thorax; *B,* Posterior Thorax; *C,* Right Lateral Thorax; *D,* Left Lateral Thorax

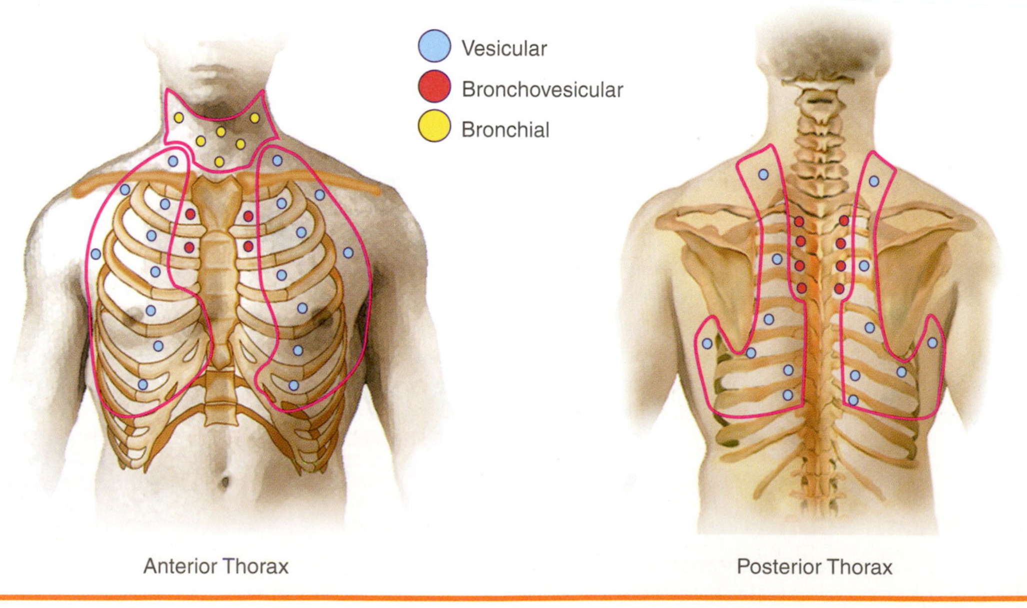

COURTESY OF DELMAR CENGAGE LEARNING

FIGURE 35-5 Location of Breath Sounds

TABLE 35-3 Characteristics of Adventitious Breath Sounds

BREATH SOUND	RESPIRATORY PHASE	TIMING	DESCRIPTION	CLEAR WITH COUGH	ETIOLOGY	CONDITIONS
Fine crackle (rale)	Predominantly inspiration	Discontinuous	Dry, high-pitched crackling, popping, short duration; roll hair near ears between your fingers to simulate this sound	No	Air passing through moisture in small airways that suddenly reinflate	COPD, congestive heart failure (CHF), pneumonia, pulmonary fibrosis, atelectasis
Coarse crackle (coarse rale)	Predominantly inspiration	Discontinuous	Moist, low-pitched crackling, gurgling; long duration	Possibly	Air passing through moisture in large airways that suddenly reinflate	Pneumonia, pulmonary edema, bronchitis, atelectasis
Sonorous wheeze (rhonchi)	Predominantly expiration	Continuous	Low pitched; snoring	Possibly	Narrowing of large airways or obstruction of bronchus	Asthma, bronchitis, airway edema, tumor, bronchiolar spasm, foreign body obstruction
Sibilant wheeze	Predominantly expiration	Continuous	High pitched; musical	Possibly	Narrowing of large airways or obstruction of bronchus	Asthma, chronic bronchitis, emphysema, tumor, foreign body obstruction
Pleural friction rub	Inspiration and expiration	Continuous	Creaking, grating	No	Inflamed parietal and visceral pleura; can occasionally be felt on thoracic wall as two pieces of dry leather rubbing against each other	Pleurisy, tuberculosis, pulmonary infarction, pneumonia, lung abscess
Stridor	Predominantly inspiration	Continuous	Crowing	No	Partial obstruction of the larynx, trachea	Croup, foreign body obstruction, large airway tumor

COURTESY OF DELMAR CENGAGE LEARNING

TABLE 35-4 Common Diagnostic Tests for Respiratory Disorders

Laboratory Tests

- Hemoglobin
- Arterial blood gases (ABGs)
- Pulmonary function tests (PFTs)
- Sputum analysis

Radiologic Studies

- Chest x-ray
- Ventilation-perfusion scan (V/Q scan)
- Computerized axial tomography (CAT scan)
- Pulmonary angiography

Other

- Pulse oximetry
- Bronchoscopy
- Thoracentesis
- Magnetic resonance imaging (MRI)

COURTESY OF DELMAR CENGAGE LEARNING

TABLE 35-5 Arterial Blood Gases: Normal Values

MEASUREMENT IN BLOOD	NORMAL VALUE
Acidity or alkalinity (pH)	7.35 to 7.45
Partial pressure of oxygen (PaO_2)	80 to 100 mm Hg
Partial pressure of carbon dioxide ($PaCO_2$)	35 to 45 mm Hg
Bicarbonate ion (HCO_3)	24 to 28 mm Hg
Arterial oxygen saturation (SaO_2)	95% to 100%

COURTESY OF DELMAR CENGAGE LEARNING

INFECTIOUS/INFLAMMATORY DISORDERS OF THE UPPER RESPIRATORY TRACT

Infectious and inflammatory disorders of the upper respiratory tract are common and usually self-limiting. Among the causal factors of infectious and inflammatory disorders are various viruses (rhino viruses, influenza viruses) and bacteria *(streptococci and pneumococci)*. Group A *beta-hemolytic streptococci* infections of the upper respiratory system are associated with serious sequelae such as rheumatic fever. Allergic reactions frequently play a role in the development of sinusitis and pharyngitis. Laryngitis is associated with factors such as pollution, smoking, and excessive use of the voice. Breathing cold air decreases local immune responses of the respiratory tract. This fact coupled with closer and prolonged contact with others indoors during the colder months leads to an increased incidence of acute upper respiratory tract inflammatory disorders.

The signs and symptoms that occur with acute upper respiratory tract infection or inflammation are a result of the inflammatory process. Early signs and symptoms include general malaise, low-grade fever, localized redness, and edema of affected tissues. Joint pain is common with viral disorders. The client may complain of nasal or sinus congestion and headache. Drying of the mucous membranes coupled with edema cause local discomfort such as sore throat. Cough and nasal or sinus discharge may occur. Nasal secretions that are thick and purulent indicate bacterial infection.

PROFESSIONALTIP

Influenza

Influenza (the flu) is a contagious respiratory illness caused by influenza viruses that lead to mild to severe illness and, at times, death. Influenza viruses are spread from person to person in respiratory droplets of coughs and sneezes. The Centers for Disease Control and Prevention (2009) estimates that 5% to 20% of Americans get the flu, more than 200,000 people are hospitalized from flu complications, and about 36,000 people die from influenza during each flu season, from November to March. The best way to prevent the flu is to get a flu vaccination each year. There are two types of influenza vaccines available: the "flu shot" and the nasal-spray flu vaccine. Currently there are four antiviral medications approved for treatment of influenza in the United States. Oseltamivir (Tamiflu) and zanamivir (Relenza) are recommended by the CDC due to the emerging influenza A resistance to the other two medications, amantadine (Symmetrel) and rimantadine (Flumadine) (National Institute of Allergy and Infectious Diseases, 2009). For more information on influenza, visit http://www.cdc.gov/flu/ or http://www3.niaid.nih.gov/topics/Flu/

MEDICAL–SURGICAL MANAGEMENT

Medical

Most clients with acute upper respiratory tract infections or inflammatory disorders are treated in a clinic or office setting. Unless the disorder becomes chronic or bacterial infection occurs, treatment is symptomatic. When infection is suspected, specimens for culture and sensitivity are obtained, and appropriate antibiotic therapy is initiated.

Surgical

Disorders that develop into chronic conditions (e.g., tonsillitis and sinusitis) may require surgical intervention to remove or drain affected tissues.

Pharmacological

Nonprescription antipyretic, analgesic, anti-inflammatory medications are used to reduce discomfort, fever, and inflammation. Antitussives are used to suppress cough and allow for rest. To aid in removal of secretions, expectorants are used. Bacterial infections are treated with various antibiotics according to culture and sensitivity studies. Comfort measures such as saline gargles may be useful.

Diet

Fluids are advocated to liquefy secretions and hydrate dry mucous membranes. Nausea may occur if secretions are swallowed as opposed to expectorated. The client should cover cough to prevent spread and be encouraged to cough up all secretions and dispose of them in a tissue. With severe coughing, emesis may occur. The client is encouraged to rest before meals and may require an antitussive to reduce coughing.

Activity

Normally, activity does not need to be restricted, but energy level may decrease. The client who is infectious is encouraged to avoid contact with others. Strenuous activity should be avoided to reduce oxygen requirements and coughing.

Nursing Management

Client teaching about signs and symptoms of a respiratory infection, avoiding items causing an allergic response, and taking all prescribed antibiotics is the main nursing responsibility. Hand washing is vital in preventing the spread of infection.

NURSING PROCESS

Assessment

Subjective Data

Subjective data include information about present signs and symptoms, onset of symptoms, exposure to allergens or infected individuals, and frequency of the disorder. Common symptoms include sore throat, nasal congestion, dyspnea, and headache.

Objective Data

Objective data include fever and inflammation, redness, edema, and drying of the mucous membranes of the oropharynx. Secretions are evaluated for their color, viscosity, amount, and odor, which will help in identifying the specific illness. The client may have hoarseness and a cough. Culture and sensitivity studies may reveal a causative organism and, thus, guide antibiotic therapy. If infection with group A *beta-hemolytic streptococci* is suspected, an antistreptolysin O (ASO) titer is done to reveal the presence of antibodies formed in reaction to this bacteria. Nonspecific diagnostic studies include elevated white blood cell count and erythrocyte sedimentation rate.

Nursing diagnoses for a client with an upper respiratory infection or inflammatory disorder include the following:

NURSING DIAGNOSES	PLANNING/OUTCOMES	NURSING INTERVENTIONS
*Deficient **K**nowledge* related to signs and symptoms of respiratory bacterial infection, potential allergens, and antibiotic therapy	The client will be able to state the signs and symptoms of bacterial infection.	Educate client regarding signs and symptoms indicating a respiratory bacterial infection, such as purulent or green secretions, fever.
	The client will be able to identify individual potential allergens.	Assist physician in allergy testing. Teach client to avoid those things that precipitate an allergic response.
	The client will complete entire course of antibiotic therapy.	Instruct client to complete the entire course of antibiotics.
*Ineffective **A**irway Clearance* related to nasal secretions	The client will verbalize a decrease or absence of nasal congestion.	Encourage client to blow the nose and not "snuffle" secretions back up into nose.

Evaluation: Evaluate each outcome to determine how it has been met by the client.

PNEUMONIA

Pneumonia is inflammation of the bronchioles and alveoli accompanied by consolidation, or solidification of exudate, in the lungs. It can result from bacteria, viruses, mycoplasms, fungi, chemical exposures, or parasite invasions. Pneumonia can also be caused by aspiration, oversedation, or inadequate ventilation. Pneumonia remains a common cause of hospitalization and is often a cause of death, particularly among the elderly. Under normal circumstances, the alveolar macrophages are able to remove foreign matter. When confronted with overwhelming numbers of virulent microorganisms, however, this protective mechanism fails. The invading organism irritates the walls of the alveoli. In response to this irritation, the alveolar walls secrete exudate (an accumulation of fluid in the pulmonary passageways). Eventually, the alveoli fill with the exudate, resulting in consolidation. The exudate within the alveoli interferes with gas exchange.

Risk factors for the development of pneumonia include immobility, depressed cough reflex (caused by anesthesia or cerebrovascular accident [CVA]), alterations in respiratory function (e.g., chronic obstructive pulmonary disease [COPD]), advanced age, and numerous other chronic debilitating conditions (e.g., congestive heart failure [CHF], diabetes mellitus). Common bacterial causes of pneumonia are *Streptococcus pneumoniae, Pneumococcus, Staphylococcus aureus, Klebsiella pneumoniae,* and *Pseudomonas aeruginosa.* A common, serious viral source of pneumonia is the *Cytomegalovirus,* which affects clients with compromised immune status, such as those taking immunosuppressant medications or those infected with human immunodeficiency virus (HIV).

CLIENT TEACHING

Pneumonia

- Discuss pertinent information about medications being taken.
- Instruct in measures to prevent spread of infection (covering the mouth and nose with a tissue when coughing or sneezing).
- Encourage disposal of tissues in a closed paper sack.
- Outline individual's specific risk factors (age, chronic respiratory condition, cardiac condition).
- Instruct in methods to prevent future infection (avoiding crowds and obtaining vaccine).
- Encourage increase in oral fluid intake, if appropriate for client.

Pneumocystis carinii pneumonia can also occur in the immunosuppressed client. The invading organism associated with *Pneumocystis carinii* pneumonia is thought to be a protozoan. The infecting microorganisms that cause pneumonia are spread by airborne droplets or direct contact with infected individuals or carriers.

Chemical pneumonia is caused by entry of irritating substances into the pulmonary passageways. A common source of chemical pneumonia is the aspiration of gastric contents. Inhalation of irritating substances can also result in a chemical pneumonia. Pneumonia is now classified according to the causative factor rather than the area of the lung affected (e.g., aspiration pneumonia). The right middle and lower lobes are affected by pneumonia more frequently than the right upper and left lobes because of the anatomy of the right bronchus and the effects of gravity.

A high fever of sudden onset is often the presenting complaint of the client. The elderly client, however, may be seriously ill and have only a low-grade fever. A productive cough yielding abnormally thick and discolored sputum may be present. Associated respiratory symptoms include dyspnea, coarse crackles, and diminished breath sounds. Most clients complain of pleuritic chest pain, which is stabbing in nature and increases on inspiration. Pain occurs as a result of irritation of the pleura lying adjacent to the affected alveoli.

In the case of bacterial pneumonia, white blood cell count increases and may go as high as 40,000/mm^3. Pneumonia caused by viruses or mycoplasms may produce a normal or a lowered white blood cell count. Chest x-ray reveals consolidation in the affected areas. Bacterial pneumonia is likely to produce isolated areas of consolidation on a chest x-ray, whereas viral and chemical pneumonia appear as more diffuse areas of consolidation. Arterial blood gases (ABGs) may reveal a decrease in PaO_2 or oxygen saturation caused by interference with gas exchange. Pulmonary function tests (PFTs) are usually within normal limits unless the client has an underlying pulmonary disorder such as emphysema.

MEDICAL–SURGICAL MANAGEMENT

Medical

Clearing the airways of exudate and maintaining adequate oxygenation are the goals of treatment for clients with pneumonia. Postural drainage and percussion may be ordered to aid the client in mobilizing secretions. Aerosol or nebulization treatments may also be utilized, often with added medications. The client is encouraged to cough and deep breathe, particularly following respiratory treatments. Incentive spirometry, which measures the amount of air inspired in one inhalation, is ordered to aid the client when coughing and deep breathing are inadequate (e.g., after surgery) (Figure 35-6). If the client is unable to mobilize secretions, suctioning of the respiratory tract is indicated. When secretions are overwhelming, the physician may perform a bronchoscopy in order to remove them. Intravenous fluids are utilized to maintain adequate hydration, especially in the presence of fever. Adequate hydration promotes liquefaction of respiratory secretions and thus aids in their removal. Pulse oximetry or ABGs are done to assess the level of oxygenation. Supplemental oxygen is used when oxygenation is inadequate.

Pharmacological

The treatment of choice for bacterial pneumonia is specific based on a sputum specimen for culture and sensitivity. It should be obtained before initiating antibiotic therapy. After a specimen has been obtained, the physician may start therapy with a broad-spectrum antibiotic. If laboratory data indicate

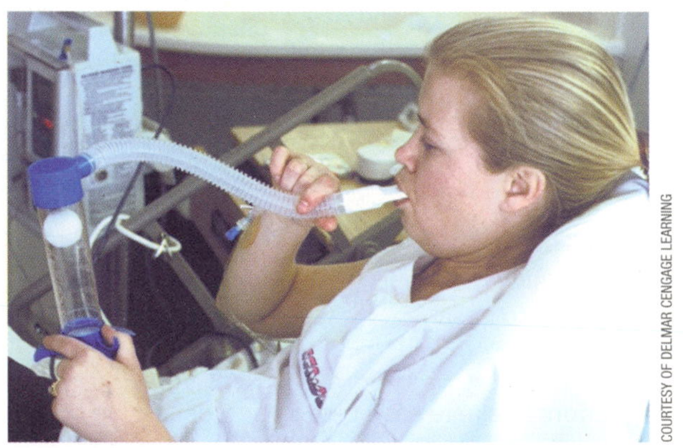
COURTESY OF DELMAR CENGAGE LEARNING

FIGURE 35-6 An Incentive Spirometer

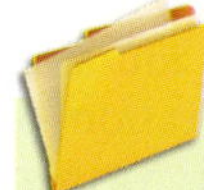

COLLABORATIVE CARE

Postural Drainage, Medications

Respiratory therapists work together with nurses in providing postural drainage for clients with pneumonia or other respiratory problems when exudate drainage from the lungs is desired. They also collaborate on administering aerosol or nebulized medications.

LIFE SPAN CONSIDERATIONS

Respiratory Status in the Older Client

- Respiratory effort increases because muscles atrophy, the diaphragm flattens out, costochondral cartilage calcifies, ligaments and joints stiffen, and intervertebral discs degenerate.
- Alveolar gas exchange diminishes because of a decrease in the lung's elastic recoil, which causes air to be trapped, especially in the lower lobes, for a portion of the respiratory cycle.
- The medulla becomes less sensitive to changes in carbon dioxide and oxygen levels, thereby rendering the respiration triggering mechanism less active.
- Ciliary activity diminishes, thereby increasing susceptibility to infection.
- Cough reflex decreases.
- Aspiration risk increases because of the decrease in the cough reflex.

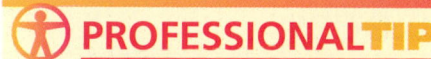

Assessment and Respiratory Assistive Devices

When caring for clients with respiratory assistive devices in place, assess the following:

- Oxygen
  - Mode of delivery (e.g., nasal cannula, face mask)
  - Percentage of oxygen that is being delivered (e.g., 25%, 40%)
  - Flow rate of the oxygen (e.g., 2 L/min, 4 L/min)
  - Humidification provided and oxygen warmed
- Incentive spirometer
  - Frequency of use
  - Volume achieved
  - Number of times client reaches goal with each use

resistant microorganisms, a specific antibiotic will be started. Antiviral agents, such as acyclovir sodium (Zovirax), are utilized for clients with chronic respiratory problems related to viral pneumonia. Prophylactic antibiotic therapy is often utilized for viral pneumonia to prevent a secondary bacterial infection. To promote opening and clearing of the airways, bronchodilators, and mucolytic agents are administered via aerosol or nebulization by the respiratory therapist or nurse. Expectorants may be given orally. Cough suppressants and pain relievers, especially those containing narcotics such as codeine sulfate, are administered only with discretion, because they may further inhibit the client's ability to clear the airways.

Diet

The client with pneumonia is encouraged to drink fluids to aid in the liquefaction of respiratory secretions. Small, frequent, nutritionally balanced meals are preferred. Respiratory treatments that promote coughing should be avoided immediately before and after meals to prevent nausea and vomiting associated with vigorous coughing.

LIFE SPAN CONSIDERATIONS

Oxygen Therapy in Children

- Any child receiving oxygen therapy should not play with friction toys or use a nylon or wool blanket.
- Oxygen concentration must be measured near the child's head with an oxygen analyzer. Prolonged exposure to a high concentration can be toxic to certain tissues (retina in preterm babies and lungs in all children), especially in children with asthma or cystic fibrosis.

Activity

Bed rest or limited activity promotes optimal tissue oxygenation; however, range-of-motion exercises and progressive ambulation prevent immobility complications.

Health Promotion

Pneumococcal vaccine (Pneumovax 23), a vaccine that prevents infection caused by *Streptococcus pneumonia*, should be given to clients at risk of developing pneumonia, such as those with chronic respiratory or cardiac conditions, and the older adult. Usually only one dose of vaccine is needed, but under certain circumstances a second dose may be given. A second dose is recommended for clients who have: a damaged or removed spleen, sickle-cell disease, HIV infection or AIDS, cancer, leukemia, lymphoma, multiple myeloma, nephrotic syndrome, organ or bone transplant, or are taking medication that lowers immunity (chemotherapy, long-term steroids). When a second dose is given, it should be given five years after the first dose. Medicare pays for this vaccine (ALA, 2009).

Nursing Management

Auscultation of lungs for breath sounds, assessment of vital signs, and monitoring pulse oximetry and/or ABGs are nursing responsibilities. Encourage deep breathing, use of incentive spirometer, and the intake of fluids. Reposition clients who are on bed rest at least every 2 hours. Assist with range-of-motion exercises and ambulation when able.

NURSING PROCESS

Assessment

Subjective Data

Data gathered in the history include the onset, duration, and severity of cough; the color, amount, and odor of sputum if present; the onset and duration of elevated temperature; and the presence or absence of night sweats.

Objective Data

The client's level of consciousness should be noted. Evidence of dyspnea, orthopnea, tachypnea, and cyanosis may be present. On auscultation of the lung fields, moist crackles or diminished breath sounds may be heard. In the event of obstruction of the airways, sibilant wheezes occur. All vital signs are taken before and after drug therapy to provide information regarding the severity of the illness and the efficacy of treatment. The color, amount, viscosity, and odor of sputum are noted.

Nursing diagnoses for a client with pneumonia include the following:

NURSING DIAGNOSES	PLANNING/OUTCOMES	NURSING INTERVENTIONS
*Ineffective **A**irway Clearance* related to inability to remove airway secretions	The client will have clear breath sounds upon auscultation.	Encourage client to breathe deeply and cough a minimum of every 2 hours. Teach use of the incentive spirometer to encourage lung expansion. Administer aerosol and nebulizer treatments as ordered. Assess breath sounds and respiratory rate prior to and following respiratory procedures to evaluate their effectiveness. Encourage fluids to liquefy thickened secretions. For clients who are able, assist in sitting up or ambulating three to four times daily; those on bed rest, turn every 2 hours. Administer medications as ordered. Provide oral care several times a day.
*Impaired **G**as Exchange* related to inflammatory changes in alveolar capillary membrane	The client will have an oxygen saturation of 92% or greater.	Monitor pulse oximetry and/or ABGs. Administer supplemental oxygen as ordered.
***A**ctivity Intolerance* related to hypoxia secondary to pneumonia	The client will be able to complete activities of daily living (ADL) and activity as ordered and without complaints of fatigue.	Encourage client to complete ADL according to ability and the physician's orders. To prevent client fatigue, alternate periods of activity and care with periods of rest.

Evaluation: Evaluate each outcome to determine how it has been met by the client.

TUBERCULOSIS

Pulmonary tuberculosis (TB) is an infection of the lung tissue by *Mycobacterium tuberculosis*. Infection by tubercle bacilli can occur in other parts of the body, but with less frequency. In pulmonary tuberculosis, the tubercle bacilli are inhaled into the lungs. Whether infection occurs depends on the host's susceptibility, the virulence of the tubercle bacilli, and the number of bacilli inhaled. Tuberculosis is not as highly contagious as once thought. Prolonged exposure to the bacilli is required to produce infection. In addition, persons with uncompromised immune systems are able to combat the bacilli and do not develop the disease. Those at risk for tuberculosis include persons suffering from malnutrition, those living in crowded conditions, persons with compromised immune status, and health care workers providing care to high-risk individuals.

Once inhaled in sufficient numbers, the tubercle bacilli cause an inflammatory response within the alveoli of the lung. A small nodule called a **primary tubercle,** containing tubercle bacilli, forms in the lung tissue. In an attempt to isolate the primary tubercles, the body forms a fibrous outer coating around each tubercle. This fibrous surface interferes with the blood and nutritional supplies to the tubercle. In time, the interior of the tubercle becomes soft and cheese-like as a result of decreased perfusion, a process known as

caseation. Then the tubercle may become calcified and is called a Ghon's tubercle.

Liquefaction necrosis, where the tissue dies and changes to a liquid or semi-liquid state, may occur; this fluid may then be coughed up. A cavity is formed at the site where the primary tubercle liquefied and ruptured. This is called **cavitation.**

Following the advent of antitubercular medications in the 1950s, the incidence of TB decreased dramatically until 1985. From 1985 to 1992, TB cases increased 20%, but from 1992 have decreased 39%. In 2007, the total number of cases of TB (13,293 persons) in the United States was the lowest it has been since the study started in 1953 (ALA, 2009). New forms of TB, resistant to conventional drug therapy, have surfaced. Some of the factors that may be responsible for the increase in TB cases are increased numbers of persons with compromised immune systems (e.g., many AIDS clients also have TB); increased mobility of the world's population (persons from areas of high TB incidence moving to areas of low incidence); widespread IV drug abuse; increased numbers of those with poor access to health care; and increased numbers of those living in impoverished conditions. Direct health care costs for TB are $703.1 million each year (ALA, 2008a).

Symptoms of TB develop gradually following infection and include the following: low-grade fever that recurs in a specific pattern, persistent cough, hemoptysis, hoarseness, dyspnea on exertion, night sweats, fatigue, weight loss, and enlarged lymph nodes.

The Mantoux skin test is the preferred screening method for TB. Purified protein derivative (PPD) of killed tubercle bacilli 0.1 mL is injected intradermally in the inner forearm. The test is evaluated by measuring the area of induration (palpable swelling) that occurs 48 and 72 hours following injection. A reddened area with no induration is not considered positive. A positive skin test, however, indicates only that the client has been infected with and developed antibodies against the tubercle bacillus (Table 35-6). It is important for clients to know that the test will thereafter always be positive throughout the individual's lifetime. The Food and Drug Administration recently approved a new TB blood test called QuantoFERON-TB that is used for detecting TB and latent TB infection. The client receives the results from this test in less than 24 hours (ALA, 2008a).

The bacteria can remain alive but inactive in the body, often for a lifetime, so a client is given prophylactic treatment, usually isoniazid (INH), for 6 to 12 months. Other medications used against tuberculosis are outlined in Table 35-7. If INH has not been given and the person later in life is under physical or emotional stress, which weakens the immune system, the bacteria may become active and cause TB disease.

A negative reaction does not rule out the possibility of TB exposure. Individuals at high risk, such as those who are infected with HIV or who have compromised immune status, may have a negative reaction because they are unable to develop antibodies. Immediately following exposure to TB, a skin test may reveal a false-negative result because it can take up to 10 weeks for an infected individual to develop the antibodies. An additional skin test may be done in 10 to 12 weeks. If the second TB test is positive, the client's history is reviewed for the presence of symptoms suggesting TB, and further evaluation is indicated.

Chest x-ray and sputum specimens are utilized to confirm a diagnosis of TB. Inpatient clients are placed in airborne respiratory isolation until cultures are completed with results. Sputum is tested for the presence of acid-fast bacilli (AFB). The sputum specimen is collected when the client arises in the morning to prevent specimen contamination with ingested food and liquids. In most instances, three specimens collected on consecutive days and testing positive for AFB indicate a positive diagnosis of TB. The TB diagnosis is confirmed if the TB bacilli grow in a culture. Individuals who are unable

TABLE 35-6 Classification of the Tuberculin Reaction

CLASSIFIED AS POSITIVE	POPULATION
Induration of 5 mm or more	• HIV-positive persons • Recent contacts of TB case • Persons with chest x-rays consistent with old, healed TB • Clients with organ transplants or other immunosuppressed persons
Induration of 10 mm or more	• Injection drug users • Recent arrivals (<5 years) from high-prevalence countries • Residents and employees of high-risk congregate settings (prisons, nursing homes, mental institutions, residential facilities for AIDS patients, and homeless shelters) • Persons with medical conditions that have been shown to increase the risk of TB, such as silicosis; persons who are 10% or more below ideal body weight; and persons with some hematologic disorders (leukemias and lymphomas) and other malignancies • Mycobacteriology laboratory personnel • Children < 4 years of age, or children and adolescents exposed to adults in high-risk categories
Induration of 15 mm or more	*Persons with no risk factors for TB*

COURTESY OF DELMAR CENGAGE LEARNING

Table 35-7 Tuberculosis Medications

DRUG	MEDICATION PRECAUTIONS AND INFORMATION
First-Line Drugs	
ethambutol hydrochloride (Myambutol)	Monthly vision checks are important for acuity and distinction of red and green colors. Take medication with food.
isoniazid (INH) (Laniazid)	Alcohol ingestion interferes with metabolism and may cause hepatitis. Check baseline and monthly hepatic enzymes. Report signs of neuropathy and hepatitis. Have client take pyridoxine (vitamin B_6) to decrease side effects.
pyrazinamide (PMS Pyrazinamide)	Take medication with food and drink 2 liters of liquids daily. Check baseline and monthly uric acid and liver enzymes.
Rifamate	A combination of isoniazid and rifampin.
rifampin (Rifadin)	Body secretions (urine, sweat, tears) turn orange while taking the medication.
rifapentine (Priftin)	As effective as rifampin but taken less frequently. Body secretions (urine, sweat, tears) turn orange. Drug must be given with at least one other tuberculosis drug.
Rifater	A combination of isoniazid, rifampin, and pyrazinamide.
streptomycin sulfate	Have monthly audiograms to check auditory function. Check baseline and monthly renal function.
Second-Line Drugs	
cycloserine (Seromycin)	Observe for mental alertness. While taking the medication, monitor renal and liver function, drink 2 to 3 liters of fluid daily, and avoid alcohol.
ethionamide (Trecator-SC)	Given with other antitubercular drugs to prevent resistant organisms from developing.
kanamycin sulfate (Kantrex)	Drug may cause steatorrhea and electrolyte imbalance.
para-amino-salicylate (Sodium P.A.S.)	Must be taken with other antitubercular drugs; taken with meals.

COURTESY OF DELMAR CENGAGE LEARNING

to produce sputum, including children and older adults, may have stomach contents aspirated for AFB testing. Chest x-ray may reveal the presence of primary tubercles, calcified lesions, and cavitation in the lung.

Medical–Surgical Management

Medical

Most clients are treated briefly in the hospital, with long-term treatment continuing at home. In the hospital, follow Airborne Precautions in addition to Standard Precautions. The precautions include placing the client in an isolation room with negative air pressure (air inflow is controlled through one vent and air outflow is exhausted through another vent directly to the outside and is not recirculated to other rooms.). The doors and windows of the client's room must be kept closed to maintain control of air flow. Caregivers should wear N95 particulate respirator masks because standard isolation masks do not prevent *Mycobacterium tuberculosis* from passing through (Figure 35-7). The Centers for Disease Control and Prevention recommend periodic TB skin testing for health care personnel.

Surgical

In the past, surgical intervention involving the removal of affected lung tissues was common. With the advent of effective chemotherapy (treatment with drugs), however, surgical intervention is now rarely utilized.

Pharmacological

Multidrug-resistant TB (MDR TB) can develop when a client does not complete the full therapy or is inadequately treated. A new strain of TB called extensively-drug resistant tuberculosis (XDR TB) is a strain with extensive resistance to second-line drugs. XDR TB is a public threat worldwide and is raising concerns of a future epidemic of TB that is virtually untreatable (ALA, 2008b). Active TB is treated with a combination of medications. Three medications—isoniazid (Laniazid, which is most effective), rifampin (Rifadin), and pyrazinamide (PMS Pyrazinamide)—are

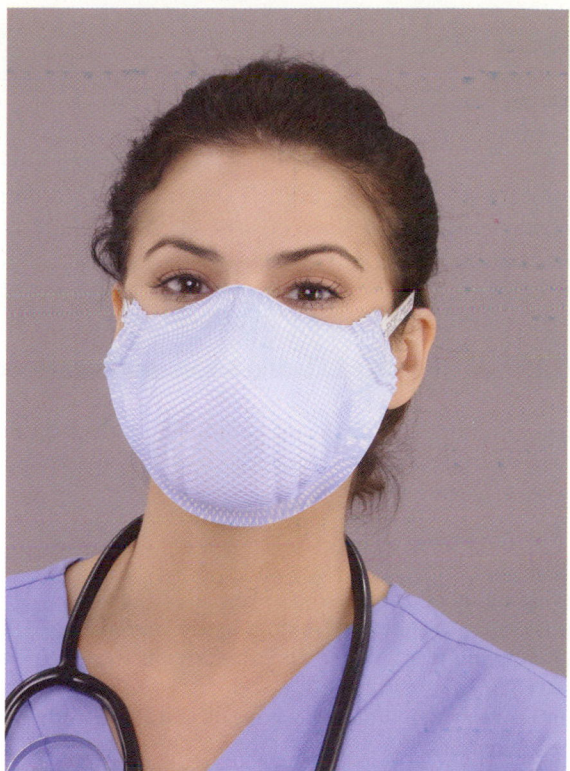

FIGURE 35-7 A particulate respirator fits tightly around the nose and face. (*Photo courtesy of Moldex Metric Inc; www.moldex.smugmug.com*)

given for several months. This is followed by a regimen of rifampin and isoniazid for an additional time. The combination of three drugs is given initially to rapidly decrease the number of active bacilli in the body and to prevent the development of MDR TB. Long-term therapy is required because TB bacilli have long periods of metabolic inactivity. Those clients with bone and joint infections, meningitis, or resistant forms of TB are treated for longer periods. Clients who are HIV positive require a longer regimen of isoniazid and pyrazinamide; prophylactic treatment with isoniazid is indicated from then on. Ethambutol hydrochloride (Myambutol) and streptomycin sulfate are added to the treatment regimen if the infecting organism is resistant to one of the three normally used medications. Infection with MDR TB requires the use of kanamycin sulfate (Kantrex), capreomycin sulfate (Capastat Sulfate), and cycloserine

SAFETY

Caregivers in Health Care Institutions

- Be aware of risks when caring for a client with TB.
- Follow Standard Precautions and Airborne Precautions.
- Use face and/or eye shield in addition to particulate mask when performing sputum-induction procedure.
- Plan care to limit prolonged exposure to client.
- Wash hands frequently and thoroughly.

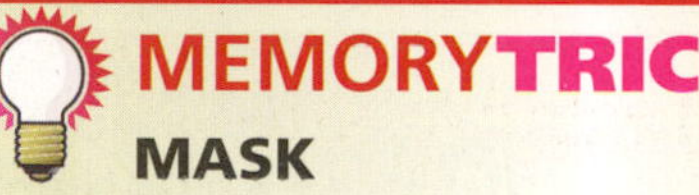

MEMORY TRICK

MASK

A memory trick for the nurse to use to remember how to correctly wear and use an N95 particulate respirator mask when providing care for a TB client is the term **MASK**:

M = Make sure you are using the correct size mask.

A = Always wear an N95 particulate respirator mask (NOT a surgical mask).

S = Seal between face and respirator must be tightly fitted and intact.

K = Keep N95 particulate respirator mask on until after you leave the client's room.

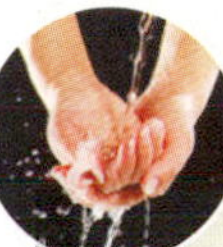

INFECTION CONTROL

Use of a Particulate Respirator

- Follow facility's procedure for fit-testing.
- Use the correct size mask.
- Put on respirator before entering client's room and remove after leaving client's room.
- Ensure that the respirator is free of holes.
- Check that the seal between face and respirator is intact.
- Discard soiled or damaged respirators.
- Have client wear N95 respirator when leaving the room.

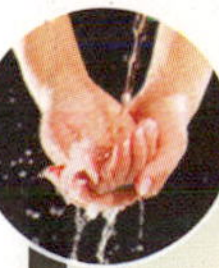

INFECTION CONTROL

Tuberculosis

- Instruct client to cover mouth and nose when coughing or sneezing.
- Double-bag secretions and dispose of them as infectious waste.
- Use disposable items for care when possible.
- Thoroughly clean and disinfect nondisposable items.

CLIENT TEACHING

Side Effects of Rifampin

- Urine, saliva, or tears may turn orange.
- May permanently discolor contact lenses.
- Birth control pills and implants become less effective. Use alternative methods of birth control.

CRITICAL THINKING

Tuberculosis Precautions

A nurse is working in a medical clinic when a client comes to the desk and informs her that one of his friends has TB, and that he was told to come to the clinic to get checked. The client is coughing continuously. The nurse knows that it will be 45 minutes before she can get him in to see the physician. What should the nurse do?

(Seromycin). The client is considered noninfectious following three negative AFB sputum specimens. At that point, the client may return to work and other normal activities. Prophylactic treatment of high-risk individuals is recommended to reduce their chances of developing the disease following their exposure.

Taking multiple drugs can be confusing and lead to noncompliance. The development of two new drugs has been valuable. These drugs are Rifater, a combination of isoniazid, rifampin, and pyrazinamide, and Rifamate, a combination of isoniazid and rifampin.

Diet

The client with TB often has nutritional deficits. Correcting these deficits assists the client in overcoming the disease process. Dietary management is based on the type of deficiency present. A well-balanced diet is encouraged for all clients with TB. Fluids are encouraged to aid in the liquefaction of respiratory secretions.

Activity

Activity is restricted based on the client's tolerance. The client who is severely compromised from a respiratory standpoint may be placed on bed rest. If the client's condition allows, activity is encouraged because it promotes lung expansion and aids in the removal of static secretions. The client in isolation whose condition permits it may ambulate in the hallways, as long as a particulate respirator mask is worn by the client while outside of the room.

COMMUNITY/HOME HEALTH CARE

The Client with Tuberculosis

Advise the client of the following:

- Keep all clinic appointments.
- Take all medications exactly as directed for duration of treatment.
- Until tested and noninfectious:
  - Put used tissues in a closed paper sack and throw away.
  - Avoid close contact with anyone; wear a mask.
  - Sleep alone in bedroom.
  - Air out bedroom often, using a fan in the window to blow air outside.
  - Thoroughly clean articles such as eating utensils.

Health Promotion

Prevention of TB is preferred to treatment. In areas where the disease remains endemic (seldom in the United States), a vaccine containing attenuated tubercle bacilli, *bacillus Calmette-Guérin* (BCG), may be given, but its effectiveness has not been proven. Individuals receiving it will test positive to the tuberculin skin test.

Any person who has had close contact with a client with TB without practicing appropriate protective measures should be tested. Other measures that decrease the likelihood of TB include adequate nutrition, housing, and health care access, and treatment of individuals who have or are at risk for developing TB.

Nursing Management

Assess client for low-grade fever, night sweats, and persistent cough. Teach client and family about the disease process and stress the importance of absolute compliance with the treatment plan.

NURSING PROCESS

Assessment

Subjective Data

The history includes questions about the presence of signs and symptoms of TB, such as night sweats, dyspnea on exertion or at rest in late disease, anorexia, loss of muscle strength, and fatigue. Pleuritic pain occurs when the pleura is involved.

Objective Data

Objective data include weight loss; persistent, low-grade fever; and persistent cough. The cough may be nonproductive early in the disease. Later, the cough is productive and yields thick, purulent sputum. Eventually, hemoptysis (blood spitting) occurs. Auscultation of breath sounds reveals coarse crackles. In the presence of cavitary disease, breath sounds are diminished or absent in the affected areas. Sputum is observed as to amount, color, odor, and consistency.

Nursing diagnoses for a client with TB include the following:

NURSING DIAGNOSES	PLANNING/OUTCOMES	NURSING INTERVENTIONS
*Ineffective **B**reathing Pattern* related to pulmonary infectious process	The client will have color and respiratory rate within normal limits and will not complain of dyspnea.	Assess client's color, respiratory rate, and respiratory effort and auscultate the breath sounds. Plan care activities to allow client uninterrupted periods of rest. Assist client in assuming the position that most aids respiratory effort. Administer medications as ordered. Encourage fluids if not otherwise contraindicated.
*Deficient **K**nowledge* related to disease process and its treatment	The client will verbalize an understanding of the disease process and its treatment.	Teach client and family about the basic pathophysiology of TB, how the infection is contracted, who is at risk of developing an infection, the signs and symptoms of TB infection, and complications that may arise. Present information regarding the actions, side effects, and untoward effects of the drugs being administered. Teach client signs and symptoms of adverse drug reactions to report to the physician. Emphasize the necessity of long-term therapy to cure TB. Inform client and family that symptoms decrease and are often gone long before the organism is eliminated from the body.
*Ineffective **T**herapeutic Regimen Management* related to client value system	The client will continue medication regimen for the prescribed length of time.	Include client and family in making decisions about care, when appropriate. Allow client to be an active participant in care decisions, to increase personal responsibility and accountability. Visits from public health or home care nurses may be necessary to monitor client for compliance. Explore reasons for noncompliance with client and family, and identify strategies to increase compliance. Refer client who is unable to afford the cost of medications to agencies such as the local health department for assistance. Begin directly observed therapy if the client continues to be noncompliant. Directly observed therapy involves sending the nurse or another health care worker to the client to administer the medications and verify that they are taken.

Evaluation: Evaluate each outcome to determine how it has been met by the client.

SAMPLE NURSING CARE PLAN

The Client with TB

R.D. is an 87-year-old man who is admitted to the hospital with a chief complaint of productive cough and fatigue. Four months ago, R.D. was placed in a long-term care facility because of his inability to care for himself at home after his wife's death 1 year previously. Since admission to the long-term care facility,

(*Continues*)

SAMPLE NURSING CARE PLAN (Continued)

R.D. has lost 15 pounds. The nurses at the facility report that R.D. has experienced progressive fatigue, dyspnea on exertion, cough, night sweats, and anorexia. Initially, his cough was nonproductive, but it is now productive of moderate amounts of thick, purulent sputum that is occasionally streaked with blood. Vital signs are temperature 99.8°F, pulse 108 beats/min, respirations 26 breaths/min, and blood pressure 138/86 mm Hg. A TB skin test done at the long-term care facility 1 week ago was evaluated as negative at 6 mm. Sputum specimens for AFB reveal the presence of active tubercle bacilli, and chest x-ray is positive for TB. Auscultation of breath sounds reveals crackles in the right lower half of the lung. R.D. says, "I don't understand why I can't breathe good and what all this fuss is about."

NURSING DIAGNOSIS 1 *Ineffective Breathing Pattern* related to infectious pulmonary process as evidenced by dyspnea on exertion and productive cough

Nursing Outcomes Classification (NOC)	Nursing Interventions Classification (NIC)
Respiratory Status: Airway Patency	*Airway Management*
Respiratory Status: Ventilation	*Ventilation Assistance*
Energy Conservation	*Energy Management*

PLANNING/OUTCOMES	NURSING INTERVENTIONS	RATIONALE
R.D. will have respiratory rate, oxygen saturation, and color within desired ranges and will not complain of dyspnea.	Initially and periodically assess R.D.'s respiratory status, including color, respiratory rate, respiratory effort, oxygen saturation, breath sounds, level of consciousness, cough, and sputum.	Provides a database from which the plan of care can be formulated and against which the effectiveness of treatment is evaluated. Subsequent assessments evaluate the effectiveness of interventions and may modify the care plan.
	Assist R.D. in assuming a position that most aids respiratory effort.	Allows for greater ease of respiration and lung expansion.
	Alternate care activities with periods of rest.	Allows R.D. to compensate for the increased oxygen demand required by activity.
	Encourage activity within R.D.'s tolerance.	Promotes expansion of the lungs.
	Encourage fluids.	Promotes liquefaction of respiratory secretions.
	Administer medications for fever as ordered.	Persistent fever leads to dehydration, which hinders the removal of respiratory secretions.
	Administer oxygen as ordered to maintain an SaO_2 of 95% or greater.	Necessary for optimal cellular function.
	Administer antitubercular drugs as ordered.	Decreases the number of viable tubercle bacilli.

EVALUATION

R.D. verbalizes a decrease in dyspnea and cough. R.D.'s color, respiratory rate, and oxygen saturation are within normal limits.

SAMPLE NURSING CARE PLAN (Continued)

NURSING DIAGNOSIS 2 *Risk for Infection* spread related to viable bacilli in secretions as evidenced by AFB in sputum

Nursing Outcomes Classification (NOC)
Knowledge: Infection Control

Nursing Interventions Classification (NIC)
Health Education

PLANNING/OUTCOMES	NURSING INTERVENTIONS	RATIONALE
R.D. will verbalize both those situations that allow for the transmission of the tubercle bacilli and the means to prevent their transmission.	Place R.D. in a negative air pressure, private room; keep door closed at all times. On the door, place Airborne Precaution signs indicating that R.D. has an infectious process and asking visitors to see nursing personnel before visiting. Instruct visitors to wear N95 respirators when in R.D.'s room, to limit the length of their visits, to avoid intimate contact, and to wash their hands when leaving the room.	Prevents transmission of the tubercle bacilli in air that has been circulated into and out of R.D.'s room. Prevents inadvertent contact and exposure. The nature of the infection is not revealed publicly to maintain client confidentiality. Visitors are informed of precautions to take to prevent exposure.
	Instruct R.D. to cover his mouth and nose when coughing and sneezing.	Aids in the containment of the tubercle bacilli.
	Instruct R.D. to cough up secretions in tissues and to place the tissues in a plastic bag. Dispose of contained secretions as infectious waste.	Aids in preventing the spread of the tubercle bacilli.
	Inform the long-term care facility and family/significant others of the positive results of the AFB studies. Instruct those persons who have been exposed to R.D. to have a TB skin test.	Known exposure to active tubercle bacilli necessitates testing to identify individuals who may have become infected.
	Observe Standard Precautions and Airborne Precautions.	Decreases the likelihood of transmitting the tubercle bacilli (and other infectious diseases) to staff and other clients.
	Wear a fitted N95 respirator when in R.D.'s room.	Prevents the inhalation of tubercle bacilli, which are able to pass through a simple surgical mask.

EVALUATION

Persons exposed to R.D. have been tested for TB. Those with TB are being treated.

(*Continues*)

SAMPLE NURSING CARE PLAN (Continued)

NURSING DIAGNOSIS 3 *Deficient Knowledge* related to disease process and its treatment as evidenced by client statement: "I don't understand why I can't breathe good and what all this fuss is about."

Nursing Outcomes Classification (NOC)	Nursing Interventions Classification (NIC)
Knowledge: Disease Process	*Teaching: Disease Process*
Knowledge: Treatment Regimen	*Teaching: Individual*

PLANNING/OUTCOMES	NURSING INTERVENTIONS	RATIONALE
R.D. will verbalize an understanding of the disease process and the required medication regimen.	Assess R.D.'s present level of knowledge regarding TB and its treatment.	Provides a database regarding R.D.'s present level of knowledge regarding TB and its treatment. Client education can then be individualized to build and expand on that knowledge base. Misinformation can also be corrected.
	Provide information in small amounts and use a variety of approaches (e.g., verbal, written, video).	Increases the likelihood of learning and stimulates the various senses.
	Encourage and allow time for R.D. to ask questions.	Provides a means to clarify information and for the nurse to evaluate learning and correct misconceptions.
	Have R.D. verbalize signs and symptoms of adverse medication effects to report to the staff.	Provides a means to clarify information and for the nurse to evaluate learning and correct misconceptions.

EVALUATION

R.D. verbalizes individual treatment regimen and its purpose. R.D. reports adverse effects of medication to health care personnel to allow for early intervention.

PLEURISY/PLEURAL EFFUSION

Pleurisy is a painful condition that arises from inflammation of the pleura, or sac that encases the lung. This pleuritic pain is sharp and stabbing in nature. Pain increases on inspiration as the irritated pleura rub over each other. Inflammation of the pleura occurs with many disorders, such as viral infections, cancer of the lung, trauma, tuberculosis, congestive heart failure, and pulmonary embolism. The inflamed pleura secrete increased amounts of pleural fluid into the pleural cavity, creating a **pleural effusion**. As fluid accumulates within the pleural space (cavity), it compresses the lung tissue (Figure 35-8). Collapse, or **atelectasis**, results if the effusion is left untreated. Those areas of collapsed lung tissue are unable to take part in gas exchange, thereby decreasing oxygenation. **Empyema** is the term to describe infected pleural exudate.

The primary manifestation of pleurisy is pain on inspiration. Signs and symptoms of pleural effusion depend on the amount of lung tissue compressed and the source of the effusion. With large pleural effusions, the mediastinum (heart, great vessels, and trachea) shifts toward the unaffected side; this can be detected by inspection, and heart sounds will move toward the unaffected side. Magnetic resonance imaging (MRI) or computerized tomography (CT) studies are useful in detecting pleural effusions, particularly small ones. A chest x-ray will show pleural effusions of 250 mL of fluid or more. If empyema is suspected, culture and sensitivity studies will identify the presence and type of infection. The client with empyema will also have an elevated temperature and white blood cell count.

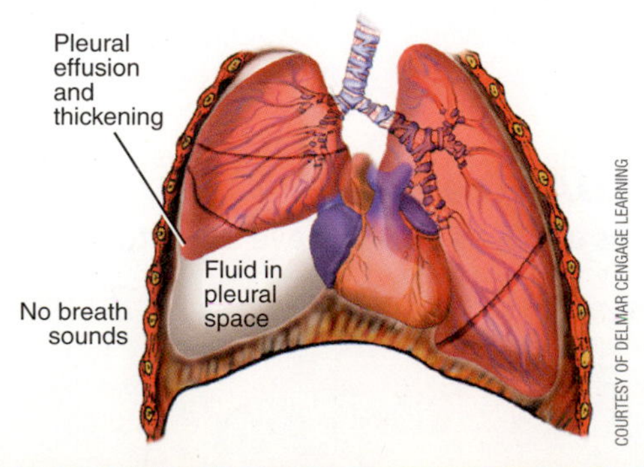

FIGURE 35-8 Pleural Effusion

PROFESSIONALTIP

Assessment of Client with a Chest Tube

- Obtain vital signs as ordered.
- Be alert for dyspnea.
- Record and describe amount of drainage.
- Look for loops of tubing containing drainage.
- Monitor water level in the water seal. Fluctuation (called tidaling) should occur with respirations and will stop when lung is reexpanded, tubing is kinked, connections are not tight, or chest tube becomes dislodged.
- Keep chest drainage system below the level of the client's chest.
- Every 2 hours, monitor client's response to coughing and deep breathing.
- If the chest tube is accidentally dislodged, cover opening with petrolatum gauze and tape only three sides of the dressing to create a one-way valve in which air can exit the pleural space on exhalation to prevent a tension pneumothorax from occurring (Daniels, Nosek, Nicoll, 2007).
- Assess for pain and discomfort.
- Ensure chest tube patency.
- Auscultate breath sounds in each lung lobe.
- Assess chest tube insertion site for signs of infection.
- Assess and palpate skin at chest tube insertion site for puffiness and crepitus (crackling).
- Observe for signs of subcutaneous emphysema.

MEDICAL–SURGICAL MANAGEMENT

Medical

Treatment is aimed at eliminating the underlying cause, maintaining adequate oxygenation to the tissues, and preventing complications such as atelectasis and pneumonia. Oxygenation is evaluated by ABGs and/or pulse oximetry. Supplemental oxygen is given to maintain an oxygen saturation of 95% or greater. Respiratory treatments to aid lung expansion such as incentive spirometry are used.

Surgical

Larger pleural effusions require that a thoracentesis be performed by the physician to remove accumulated fluid. After the overlying tissues are anesthetized, a large-bore needle is placed into the pleural space. Fluid is removed (no more than 1500 mL) and may be sent to the laboratory for diagnostic purposes (e.g., culture, cytology). If fluid accumulation continues, a thoracotomy tube is placed into the pleural space to drain fluid continuously. Following administration of local anesthetics, the physician places a large-bore catheter into the pleural space. This catheter is attached to an underwater seal chest tube drainage device (Figure 35-9). It prevents the negative pressure within the pleural space from pulling air into the pleural space, and allows for the drainage of accumulated fluid or air. Most chest tube devices have a chamber to which suction may be applied to assist in the removal of fluid or air from the pleural space. It can also be sealed with a Heimlich (one-way) valve. A chest x-ray is done to evaluate the chest tube's placement and effectiveness.

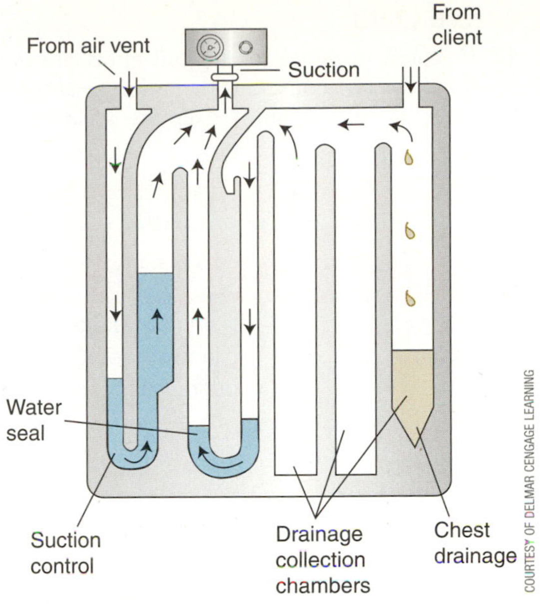

FIGURE 35-9 Underwater Seal Chest Drainage Device

Pharmacological

If a pleural effusion is small and does not interfere greatly with respiratory function, diuretics are used to promote removal of fluid from the pleural space. Furosemide (Lasix) and bumetanide (Bumex) may be given for this purpose. If empyema is present, specific therapy is used once the causative agent is identified. Pain relief is a high priority. Analgesia that also decreases inflammation is preferred. Ketorolac tromethamine (Toradol) or other nonsteroidal anti-inflammatory drugs are often used. Severe pain may require narcotics. For extensive inflammation, corticosteroids may be utilized.

Activity

The client's activity is limited to prevent fatigue. High Fowler's position assists respirations.

NURSING MANAGEMENT

Assess the client's color, respiratory rate and effort, and level of consciousness. Monitor vital signs and breath sounds. If a chest tube is in place, watch that all tubes are in place and the drainage device is working properly. A variety of closed-drainage chest tube systems are available. Empty drainage per agency policy. Encourage the client to use the incentive spirometer.

NURSING PROCESS

ASSESSMENT

Subjective Data

A nursing history is obtained from the client regarding onset, duration, and severity of symptoms. The client usually describes both chest pain that increases with each inspiration and difficulty breathing.

Objective Data

The client's color, respiratory rate, and effort are evaluated along with the level of consciousness. Abnormalities in vital signs are noted. Breath sounds over the areas of involvement are diminished or absent. A pleural friction rub may be audible. Dyspnea, cyanosis, and hypoxia occur in proportion to the severity of the condition. If a chest tube is in place, the amount and color of drainage are assessed.

Nursing diagnoses for a client with a pleural effusion include the following:

NURSING DIAGNOSES	PLANNING/OUTCOMES	NURSING INTERVENTIONS
*Acute **P**ain* related to inflammation of the pleura	Using a scale of 0 to 10, the client will verbalize a decrease in the level of pain.	Administer pain medications as ordered. Assist the client in attaining the position that allows for greatest comfort. Elevate the head of the bed. Provide diversional activities.
*Impaired **G**as Exchange* related to compressed lung	The client will maintain an oxygen saturation of 95% or greater and a respiratory rate of 14 to 22 bpm and will have clear breath sounds.	Monitor vital signs and pulse oximetry. Provide supplemental oxygen as ordered. Encourage client to breathe deeply or use the incentive spirometer as ordered. Administer diuretics and anti-inflammatory medications as ordered. Assist physician with the thoracentesis or the placement of a thoracotomy tube. Collect specimen for culture and sensitivity and other studies as ordered.
*Risk for **A**ctivity Intolerance* related to hypoxia secondary to pleural effusion	The client will increase activity without complaining of fatigue.	Stagger periods of activity with periods of rest. To prevent fatigue, plan activities around therapies.
*Bathing/Hygiene **S**elf-care Deficit* related to mobility restriction	The client will increase self-care activities as mobility increases.	Assist client with hygiene and self-care needs, but encourage participation in self-care activities within the limits of the physician's orders.

Evaluation: Evaluate each outcome to determine how it has been met by the client.

SEVERE ACUTE RESPIRATORY SYNDROME

Severe acute respiratory syndrome (SARS) is a viral respiratory illness with flu-like symptoms that is caused by the SARS associated coronovirus (SARS-CoV). It was identified in China in late 2002, and first reported in Asia in February 2003 (CDC, 2008). A total of 8,098 people became sick with SARS, and 773 died worldwide during the outbreak (CDC, 2005a). SARS spread worldwide over several months before the outbreak ended (National Institutes of Health, 2009c).

It appears that SARS spreads by close personal contact or contact with infectious material (respiratory secretions). This happens when a client with SARS coughs or sneezes droplets onto themselves, others, or nearby surfaces.

The incubation period is generally 2 to 7 days. Then an elevated temperature of > 100.4°F (>38°C) occurs and may be associated with chills, headache, malaise, body aches, respiratory symptoms, pneumonia, and even respiratory failure. After 2 to 7 days, clients may develop a dry, nonproductive cough and dyspnea.

There is no specific treatment for SARS. Support treatment is provided based on the symptoms.

Nursing Management

Follow Standard Precautions (hand hygiene and eye protection), Contact Precautions (gown and gloves), and Airborne Precautions (isolation room with negative pressure and use of N-95 respirators). Monitor client's vital signs. Assess breath sounds. Provide routine care with uninterrupted rest periods.

ACUTE RESPIRATORY TRACT DISORDERS

Acute respiratory tract disorders include atelectasis, pulmonary embolism, pulmonary edema, acute respiratory distress syndrome, and acute respiratory failure.

ATELECTASIS

Atelectasis refers to the collapse of a lung or a portion of a lung. The most common cause of atelectasis is airway obstruction. A bronchiole becomes blocked with secretions, and the alveoli distal to it collapse (Figure 35-10). Airway obstruction of this nature is common after surgery and with immobility problems. Anesthesia, pain, narcotics, and immobility can cause hypoventilation and retention of secretions.

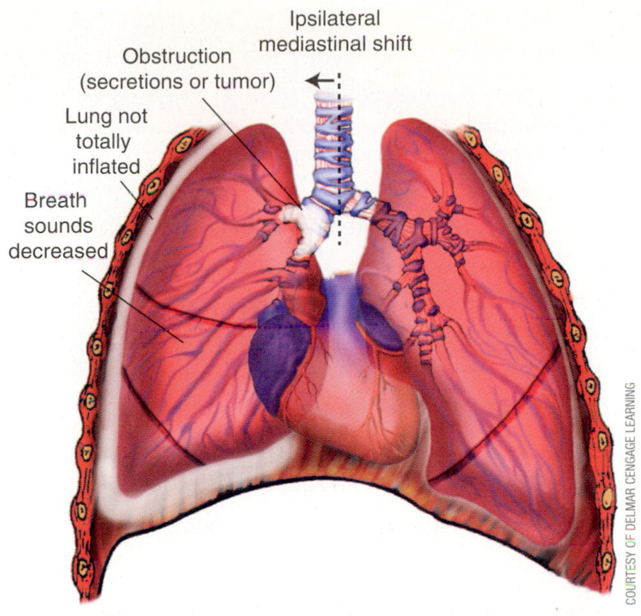

FIGURE 35-10 Atelectasis (Collapsed Lung)

Hypoventilation can cause atelectasis, which increases hypoventilation. Atelectasis can occur with compression of lung tissue, as in pleural effusion or pneumothorax. Insufficient surfactant results in increased recoil properties of the lungs, leading to atelectasis.

Signs of respiratory distress are proportional to the amount of lung tissue involved. When large areas of the lung are involved, orthopnea or cyanosis may develop. Breath sounds are diminished or absent over collapsed areas. Chest wall movement may decrease on the affected side. Oxygenation decreases as shown by ABGs or pulse oximetry. Pulse and respiratory rate increase as the heart and lungs work harder to meet the body's oxygen needs. Trapped secretions are a growth medium for microorganisms. An elevated temperature indicates secondary infection (pneumonia). Chest x-ray shows the areas of collapse. Bronchoscopy (insertion of a bronchoscope into the trachea) is used to directly visualize the area of obstruction and obtain a specimen for diagnostic purposes.

MEDICAL–SURGICAL MANAGEMENT

Medical

The physician orders incentive spirometry and deep breathing and coughing exercises to promote expansion of the lungs. Postural drainage and percussion aids in the removal of any static secretions. If the client is unable to cough up secretions, suctioning of the respiratory tract is performed. Bronchoscopy may be done to remove secretions and obtain specimens. Arterial blood gases and pulse oximetry are utilized to evaluate the need for supplemental oxygen. Oxygen is administered to maintain an oxygen saturation of 95% or greater.

Surgical

Clients with pneumothorax or pleural effusion as the underlying cause of atelectasis require removal of trapped air or fluid via thoracentesis or placement of a thoracotomy tube (refer to the sections on pleural effusion and pneumothorax). Atelectasis resulting from the growth of a tumor requires removal of the tumor.

Pharmacological

Adequate pain control aids the client, particularly the surgical client, to breathe deeply and cough. Client-controlled analgesia or a routine schedule of pain medication may be used to provide effective pain management. Bronchodilators may be used to open the airways. Mucolytic agents are used to liquefy secretions. Bronchodilators, such as albuterol sulfate (Ventolin), and mucolytics, such as acetylcysteine (Mucomyst), may also be administered via updraft or nebulizer treatments. The client with an infection requires treatment with an appropriate antibiotic.

Diet

Unless otherwise contraindicated, fluids are encouraged to promote liquefaction of trapped respiratory secretions.

Activity

Activity promotes lung expansion. Immobile clients are turned a minimum of every 2 hours and assisted to do range-of-motion exercises. Surgical clients may do leg exercises as well as deep breathing and coughing. Ambulation is recommended if the client's condition allows. If the client is unable to walk, sitting up in a chair is encouraged. To prevent fatigue, rest periods are planned between activities.

NURSING MANAGEMENT

Monitor for pain, shortness of breath, fatigue, dyspnea, cyanosis, anxiety, and level of consciousness. Assess for Homans' sign. Teach client how to cough, deep breathe, and use the incentive spirometer. Encourage ambulation as client's condition allows. Turn immobile clients at least every 2 hours.

NURSING PROCESS

ASSESSMENT

Subjective Data

Clients who smoke, those who are immunocompromised, and those who have known chronic respiratory or cardiovascular diseases are at increased risk of developing atelectasis. The client is asked about the onset, duration, and severity of symptoms such as pain, cough, and dyspnea. The client may complain or show signs of air hunger, shortness of breath, fatigue, and anxiety.

Objective Data

Assess the client for changes in level of consciousness, an early sign of decreased oxygenation. Periodically evaluate for dyspnea, tachypnea, cyanosis, and restlessness. Measure vital signs frequently, with particular attention to respiratory rate and effort. Auscultation reveals diminished or absent breath sounds over the areas of atelectasis. Crackles (rales) or sonorous wheezes may be heard if pneumonia develops. Note objective indicators of pain such as facial grimacing, and validate by subjective questioning. Assess the effectiveness of the client's cough. A productive cough is evaluated for amount, color, consistency, and odor of secretions.

Nursing diagnoses for a client with atelectasis include the following:

NURSING DIAGNOSES	PLANNING/OUTCOMES	NURSING INTERVENTIONS
*Impaired **G**as Exchange* related to decreased alveolar–capillary surface	The client will have an oxygen saturation of 95% or greater, a respiratory rate of 14 to 22 bpm, and clear breath sounds.	Establish a schedule for coughing and deep breathing. Encourage client to ambulate and/or sit up in a chair three to four times daily. Turn the immobile client every 2 hours or more frequently. Assess client's vital signs and breath sounds every 4 hours or more frequently as situation warrants. Encourage fluids if client's condition allows. Administer respiratory treatments and medications as ordered. Assess secretions (sputum) for color, amount, consistency, and odor.
*Risk for **A**ctivity Intolerance* related to hypoxia secondary to atelectasis	The client will complete activity without complaints of shortness of breath, dyspnea, or fatigue.	Encourage some activity, such as walking, to promote lung expansion, and alternate with periods of rest to avoid client fatigue. Provide assistance with ADL as client's condition requires. Place client in a high or semi-Fowler's position to aid lung expansion. Position client on the unaffected side.
*Deficient **K**nowledge* related to the complications of surgery and/or immobility	The client will verbalize the purpose of deep breathing, coughing, and activity following surgery, and will demonstrate deep breathing and coughing.	Teach all preoperative and immobile clients to cough and breathe deeply at least every 2 hours and have the client demonstrate to ensure that learning has occurred. Teach the surgical client to splint the surgical incision to minimize discomfort that might occur with coughing and deep breathing. Instruct clients at risk for developing atelectasis in the use of incentive spirometry. Emphasize the importance of early ambulation and activity to promote lung expansion.

Evaluation: Evaluate each outcome to determine how it has been met by the client.

PULMONARY EMBOLISM

Pulmonary embolism (PE) develops when a bloodborne substance lodges in a branch of a pulmonary artery and obstructs flow. A common source of PE is deep vein thrombosis. Other sources are air from intravenous infusions; fat from long-bone fractures; and amniotic fluid. The size and location of the emboli determine the severity and outcome of the condition.

Pulmonary emboli rarely develop before adulthood. As age increases, the risk for pulmonary embolism becomes greater because of the development of arteriosclerosis and other vascular changes associated with aging. Other factors increasing the risk for PE are heredity, smoking, peripheral vascular disease, diabetes mellitus, and oral contraceptive use.

Emboli interfere with gas exchange to the pulmonary circulation distal to the emboli, resulting in hypoxemia. The client describes breathlessness and dyspnea. Pulse oximetry or ABGs will show the degree to which oxygenation has been affected. Obstruction of a main branch of a pulmonary artery can result in lung infarction, necrosis, and may even lead to death.

All clients at risk for PE are observed for signs and symptoms of deep vein thrombosis, such as localized calf tenderness or swelling. Measures to prevent thrombus formation are taken for these individuals. Any signs of thrombophlebitis are immediately reported to the physician.

Signs and symptoms of PE are abrupt in onset. The client becomes anxious and restless. Sudden, sharp chest pains or back pain of a pleuritic nature (worse on inspiration) develop. Dyspnea and cough, along with hemoptysis, occur. Venous return is diminished, resulting in jugular venous distention. The client becomes diaphoretic. A low-grade fever develops in response to inflammation. A high temperature indicates lung infarction. Diagnosis of PE is often done by a ventilation/perfusion lung scan, but the gold standard is pulmonary angiography. Arterial blood gases show hypoxia and respiratory alkalosis. A spiral CT scan of the lungs may be ordered, and can be performed within a few seconds.

MEDICAL–SURGICAL MANAGEMENT

Medical

Preventive measures are instituted for the client at risk of developing deep vein thrombosis. Following surgery, antiembolism stockings, sequential compression devices (SCDs), intermittent pneumatic compression devices (e.g., PlexiPulse), and early ambulation are indicated. When hypoxia occurs, supplemental oxygen is given to increase oxygenation. The underlying cause of the PE is treated when identified.

Surgical

In severe cases, the physician may remove the clot via an embolectomy. This procedure is usually done at the time of angiography. Clients who experience successive episodes of PE may require a venacaval plication or filter. This surgical procedure involves placing a sieve-like device in the inferior vena cava to catch emboli before they enter pulmonary circulation (National Heart Lung and Blood Institute, 2009b).

Pharmacological

The client at risk of developing deep vein thrombosis and/or PE may be treated with enoxaparin (Lovenox). Lovenox is often used in the postoperative client to prevent clot formation. After PE has developed, anticoagulation is ordered to prevent the formation of further clots. Heparin sodium is initially used to establish anticoagulation and is administered parenterally by either the intravenous or subcutaneous route. After adequate anticoagulation is established, warfarin sodium (Coumadin) therapy is initiated and may be given concurrently with heparin while the client is hospitalized until Coumadin level is therapeutic. Coumadin alone is given orally when the client is discharged. If the clot is large or lies in a branch of a main pulmonary artery, fibrinolytic therapy may be used. Fibrinolytics lyse, or dissolve, the clot versus inhibiting the formation of new clots. Examples of fibrinolytic agents are alteplase recombinant (Activase) and streptokinase (Streptase). These agents may be administered intra-arterially at the site of the clot or intravenously to achieve a systemic effect. Narcotic analgesics such as morphine are used to control pain.

CLIENT TEACHING

Anticoagulant Therapy (Coumadin)

Stress the importance of:

- Follow-up laboratory testing
- Using a soft toothbrush to prevent trauma to the gums (bleeding)
- Inspecting the skin for bruises or petechiae
- Using an electric razor to avoid scratching skin
- Reporting nosebleeds, tarry stool, hematuria, or hematemesis to the physician
- Eating a consistent amount of green, leafy vegetables daily (differing amounts alter anticoagulant effects)
- Avoiding other medications including aspirin (it has an anticoagulant effect) without approval from physician
- In the female client, monitor menstrual flow for excessive amount

LIFE SPAN CONSIDERATIONS

Older Adults at Risk for Pulmonary Embolism

The risk of developing a pulmonary embolism increases with age. For each 10 years after age 60, the risk of developing a pulmonary embolism doubles (NHLBI, 2009c).

Diet

Fluids are encouraged to prevent hemoconcentration leading to clot formation. Unless contraindicated, fluids are encouraged for the client at risk of developing PE.

Activity

To prevent the formation of clots, activity is encouraged. After a clot has formed, however, the client's activity is restricted to prevent the clot from moving and becoming an embolus. Activities such as sitting, crossing the knees, or prolonged bending at the hips are to be avoided because they promote venous stasis.

NURSING MANAGEMENT

Assess the abrupt onset of pleuritic chest pain for location, duration, severity, and character. Assess lung sounds, monitor pulse oximetry, vital signs, jugular veins for distension, peripheral pulses, and capillary refill. Encourage deep breathing and provide supplemental oxygen as ordered. Monitor results of

APTT, INR, PT, hemoglobin, and hematocrit. Do not massage site if deep vein thrombosis (DVT) has occurred.

NURSING PROCESS

ASSESSMENT

Subjective Data

The client's history is obtained to identify potential risk factors for the development of PE. Ask the client about the onset, duration, and severity of symptoms. Shortness of breath, dyspnea, and severe pleuritic chest pain are abrupt in onset. Pain is evaluated as to onset, location, duration, severity, and character.

Objective Data

Pulse oximetry measurements are monitored. The client's respirations are rapid and shallow. Pallor progressing to cyanosis develops as oxygenation decreases. The client becomes diaphoretic. Increased anxiety or a change in level of consciousness may be the first indication of PE. The pulse increases in response to anxiety and in an attempt to supply oxygen to the body's cells. Blood pressure may increase or decrease in response to hypoxia, anxiety, and pain. Temperature may elevate in response to inflammation and tissue necrosis. On auscultation, breath sounds may or may not be decreased. The jugular veins may be distended.

Nursing diagnoses for a client with pulmonary embolism include the following:

NURSING DIAGNOSES	PLANNING/OUTCOMES	NURSING INTERVENTIONS
Impaired ***G****as Exchange* related to alteration in pulmonary circulation	The client will maintain an oxygen saturation of 95% or greater, have a respiratory rate of 14 to 22 bpm, and have color within normal limits.	Assess client for indications of decreasing oxygenation. Auscultate breath sounds every 4 hours or more often. Assess peripheral pulses and capillary refill. Encourage deep breathing and coughing. Provide supplemental oxygen to maintain oxygen saturation at greater than 95% or as ordered. Administer anticoagulants (Heparin, Lovenox, Coumadin) as ordered. Encourage fluids, unless contraindicated, to prevent hemoconcentration.
Acute ***P****ain* related to decreased perfusion of lung tissue	Using a scale of 0 to 10, the client will indicate decreased pain.	Administer pain medication as ordered and monitor for relief. Assist client in assuming a position of comfort. If possible, place client in a high Fowler's position to aid respiratory effort.
Risk for ***I****njury* related to anticoagulation/fibrinolytic therapy	The client will be free of abnormal bleeding and maintain hemoglobin and hematocrit within normal limits.	Assess for evidence of bleeding. Monitor lab reports for activated partial thromboplastin time (APTT), international normalized ratio (INR), prothrombin time (PT), decrease in platelet count, and hemoglobin and hematocrit levels. Evaluate blood pressure and pulse for signs of bleeding (i.e., rapid pulse and low blood pressure). Check stool for occult blood. Assess gums for bleeding.

Evaluation: Evaluate each outcome to determine how it has been met by the client.

PULMONARY EDEMA

Acute pulmonary edema is a life-threatening condition characterized by a rapid shift of fluid from plasma into the pulmonary interstitial tissue and the alveoli (Figure 35-11). As a result, gas exchange is markedly impaired. Pulmonary edema generally has a cardiac cause such as left ventricular failure or myocardial infarction, or a noncardiac cause such as fluid overload, inhalation of noxious gases, opiate overdose, aspiration, sepsis, or radiation injury.

The hallmark of acute pulmonary edema is a cough producing a copious amount of frothy, blood-tinged sputum (hemoptysis), often appearing pinkish. The client rapidly becomes dyspneic, orthopneic, and cyanotic. Anxiety ranging from restlessness to panic occurs. Heart and respiratory rate increase. Progressive crackles (rales) are heard in the lung fields on auscultation. Initially, fine crackles (rales) are present in the posterior bases of the lung. As pulmonary edema progresses, the crackles (rales) become increasingly coarser, louder, and more diffuse. Wheezes are heard in the presence of significant

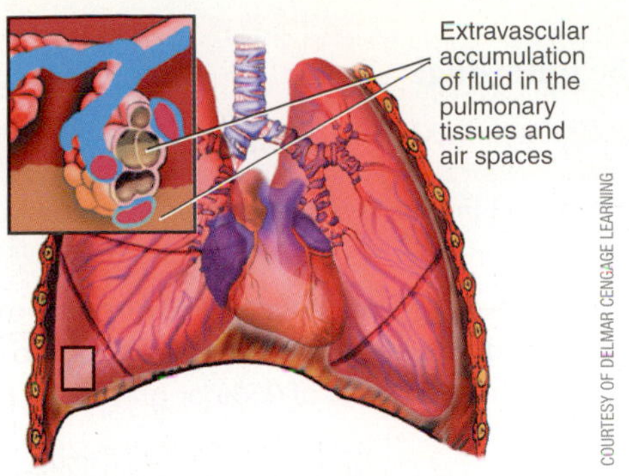

FIGURE 35-11 Pulmonary Edema

airway obstruction by fluid. Left untreated, the client deteriorates rapidly as oxygenation decreases. The client's history is crucial to identify the cause. Noncardiogenic pulmonary edema can quickly become respiratory failure.

MEDICAL–SURGICAL MANAGEMENT

Medical

The goals of medical management are to remove fluid from the alveoli and pulmonary interstitial space, prevent further influx of fluid, improve oxygenation, and decrease workload of left ventricle. Arterial blood gases and pulse oximetry values are used to assess oxygenation. Oxygen is administered per physician's order when hypoxia is present. Noncardiogenic pulmonary edema often requires ventilation support and treatment of the cause.

Pharmacological

A diuretic such as furosemide (Lasix) is the primary treatment for cardiogenic pulmonary edema. When the pumping force of the left ventricle is impaired, a digitalis preparation is given to improve the contractile force of the myocardium. To prevent further influx of fluid into the lungs, venous pooling is enhanced. This also decreases the workload on the heart by limiting venous return. Morphine is used to promote vasodilation and, thus, venous pooling and to relieve anxiety. Bronchodilators are administered to dilate airways obstructed with fluid.

Diet

A sodium-restricted diet may be ordered to prevent fluid retention. Intake and output as well as daily weight are measured to monitor fluid balance.

Activity

Bed rest reduces the workload on the heart and lungs. High Fowler's position aids respiratory effort and enhances venous pooling. Activities are increased slowly according to the physician's orders and the client's ability to tolerate activity.

NURSING MANAGEMENT

Monitor ABGs and pulse oximetry and administer oxygen as ordered. Assess breath sounds, vital signs, and level of consciousness. Keep client in high Fowler's position. Keep an accurate intake and output record. Monitor client's weight daily.

NURSING PROCESS

ASSESSMENT

Subjective Data

The nurse must be aware of the conditions that predispose the client to pulmonary edema. The client may describe feeling anxious, breathless, and fatigued.

Objective Data

Breath sounds are auscultated for the presence of crackles (rales). Report increasingly coarse and diffuse crackles (rales) to the physician. Assess the client's level of consciousness, respiratory rate and effort, and color. Dyspnea, tachypnea, cyanosis and/or pallor may be present. Assess oxygenation via pulse oximetry or ABGs. A productive cough may be present, as may symptoms of CHF, such as rapid weight gain and peripheral edema. Pulse may be rapid and weak. Blood pressure may increase in response to anxiety and decreased oxygenation.

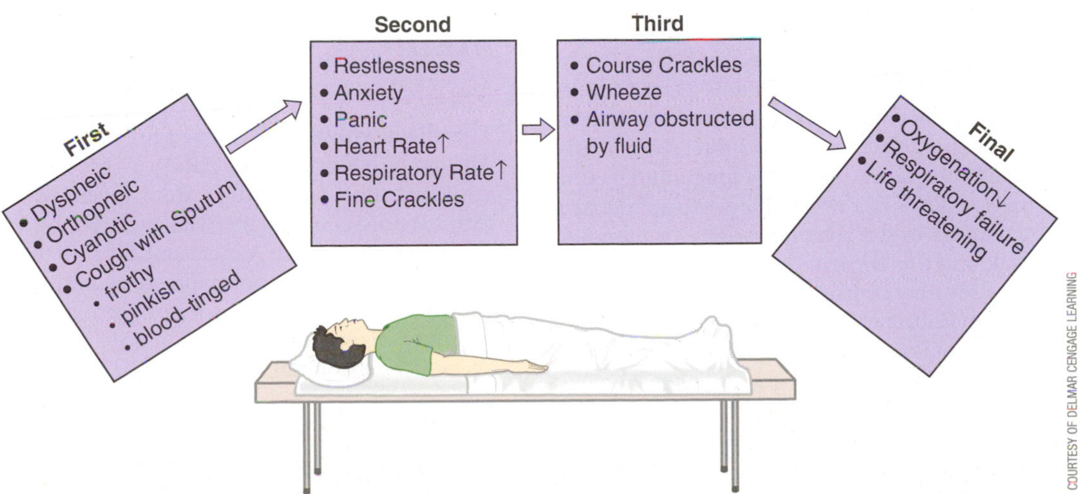

CONCEPT MAP 35-1 Progression of Pulmonary Edema

Nursing diagnoses for a client with pulmonary edema include the following:

NURSING DIAGNOSES	PLANNING/OUTCOMES	NURSING INTERVENTIONS
*Impaired **G**as Exchange* related to fluid in the lung tissue	The client will maintain an oxygen saturation of 95% or greater and will have respiratory rate, color, and blood gases within normal limits and clear breath sounds.	Place client in high Fowler's or orthopneic position (sitting upright leaning forward). Continually assess oxygenation with ABG or pulse oximetry measurements and provide supplemental oxygen to maintain an oxygen saturation of 95% or greater or per physician's order. Frequently assess respiratory rate, breath sounds, apical heart rate, and blood pressure. Administer respiratory treatments as ordered. Assist client with activities to reduce the workload on the heart and lungs, and alternate periods of activity with periods of rest to prevent client fatigue. Administer medications as ordered and evaluate the effectiveness of each. Monitor lab reports for electrolyte values.
*Excess **F**luid Volume* related to altered tissue permeability	The client's weight will return to normal.	Weigh client daily. Monitor I&O. Frequently assess the client for peripheral edema. Provide client with a low-sodium diet as ordered. Administer diuretics per order and evaluate their effectiveness. Monitor lab reports for electrolyte values. Monitor the rate at which intravenous fluids are given. Teach client and family symptoms of fluid excess, medication information, and dietary modifications.

Evaluation: Evaluate each outcome to determine how it has been met by the client.

ACUTE RESPIRATORY DISTRESS SYNDROME

Acute respiratory distress syndrome (ARDS; formerly called adult respiratory distress syndrome) is a life-threatening condition characterized by severe dyspnea, hypoxemia, and diffuse pulmonary edema. The condition usually follows a major assault on multiple body systems or severe lung trauma. Underlying causes include trauma, sepsis, coronary artery bypass surgery, major thoracic or vascular surgery, renal failure, severe pulmonary infections, inhalation lung injuries, and acute drug poisoning. ARDS is a noncardiogenic pulmonary edema, caused by damage to the alveolocapillary membranes allowing fluid to leak into the lungs under normal pressure.

Gas exchange is severely impaired by the damage to the pulmonary capillary membrane and the presence of fluid in the alveoli. The surfactant is rendered inactive, resulting in the collapse of the alveoli, further reducing gas exchange. Hypoxemia, resistant to conventional oxygen therapy, develops.

The client with ARDS is critically ill, as reflected by severe dyspnea, tachypnea, and cyanosis. Arterial blood gases will show $PaO_2 < 70$ mm Hg, $PaCO_2 > 35$ mm Hg, bicarbonate ion < 22 mEq/L, and initially elevated then steadily decreasing pH. The ABGs and pulse oximetry reveal severe hypoxemia and progressive respiratory and metabolic acidosis. On auscultation, the lung fields are filled with diffuse coarse crackles (rales) and sonorous wheezes. The client will have a productive cough yielding blood-tinged sputum. Chest x-ray shows widely scattered infiltrates, often referred to as a "white out."

MEDICAL–SURGICAL MANAGEMENT

Medical

The client with ARDS is cared for in the intensive care unit. The underlying cause of ARDS is ascertained and treated; until that time, supportive care is given. Mechanical ventilatory support is necessary, with multiple other systems often also being supported. A mechanical ventilator allows the oxygen percentage, pulmonary pressure, and lung volume to be controlled. Oxygenation is monitored with ABGs and pulse oximetry. Respiratory secretions are removed by frequent bronchial suctioning.

Pharmacological

Pharmacological therapy includes high doses of corticosteroids such as hydrocortisone sodium succinate (Solu-Cortef) or methylprednisolone sodium succinate (Solu-Medrol). Furosemide (Lasix) and other diuretics are given to remove fluids and increase urinary output. Aminophylline (Aminophyllin) is administered to open the bronchi. While the client is on the mechanical ventilator, pancuronium bromide (Pavulon) is given to suppress the client's own respiratory effort. Blood pressure can fall dangerously low, and vasopressors such as dopamine hydrochloride (Intropin) may be required to maintain the blood pressure within an acceptable range.

Diet

Total parenteral nutrition (TPN) may be given to the client, especially during the acute phase of the illness. When possible, enteral feedings are preferred.

Activity

The client with ARDS will be on bed rest. Special beds that provide movement and pressure adjustment prevent the complications associated with immobility. According to the ARDS Support Center (2009a), prone positioning improves oxygenation and may prevent further lung damage.

Nursing Management

Monitor client's level of consciousness, response to stimuli, vital signs, ABGs, pulse oximetry, and breath sounds. Suction excess secretions. Provide frequent oral care. Plan for uninterrupted rest periods. Assess for restlessness and anxiety.

NURSING PROCESS

Assessment

Subjective Data

The client history is typically gathered from family members or significant others because the client is usually too ill to communicate.

Objective Data

The client's level of consciousness and response to stimuli are assessed, and the client is observed for restlessness and anxiety. Vital signs are measured every 15 minutes or more often. Heart rate is increased, and arrhythmias may be present. Blood pressure is usually low. Respiratory rate, rhythm, and effort are assessed for signs of dyspnea, nasal flaring, cyanosis, tachypnea, and other indications of respiratory distress. Arterial blood gases and pulse oximetry values are assessed to evaluate oxygenation and acid–base balance. Diffuse, coarse crackles (rales) and wheezes are heard throughout the lung fields.

Nursing diagnoses for a client with ARDS include the following:

NURSING DIAGNOSES	PLANNING/OUTCOMES	NURSING INTERVENTIONS
*Impaired **G**as Exchange* related to pulmonary capillary membrane damage	The client will have an oxygen saturation of 95% or greater, ABGs within normal limits, and respiratory rate and effort within normal limits.	Provide adequate oxygenation and ventilation as ordered. Monitor ABGs and pulse oximetry to evaluate oxygenation and acid–base balance. Assess the client's respiratory rate and effort and auscultate the lungs frequently. Suction the respiratory tract as necessary to remove excess secretions, and provide oral care frequently.
***A**nxiety* related to difficulty breathing and mechanical ventilation	The client, if able, will verbalize a decrease in anxiety or will exhibit fewer objective signs of anxiety, such as restlessness and facial grimacing.	Describe care and purposes to the client. Allow rest periods between periods of activity to avoid overwhelming the client with stimuli. Plan care to allow for uninterrupted rest. Allow family and significant others to visit and participate in care, as appropriate. Assess client for signs of sensory overload/deprivation.

Evaluation: Evaluate each outcome to determine how it has been met by the client.

ACUTE RESPIRATORY FAILURE

Acute respiratory failure is not a disease entity in and of itself; rather, the term is used to refer to conditions wherein there is a failure of the respiratory system as a whole. This condition occurs as a result of the client literally becoming too tired to continue the "work" of breathing. Mechanical ventilatory support is required during the acute phase. Clients with preexisting pulmonary conditions coupled with acute respiratory tract infections are at risk for developing acute respiratory failure.

CHRONIC RESPIRATORY TRACT DISORDERS

Asthma, chronic obstructive pulmonary disease (COPD), chronic bronchitis, emphysema, and bronchiectasis are discussed following.

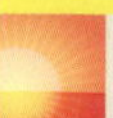

LIFE SPAN CONSIDERATIONS

Asthma and Age

In children:

- Asthma attacks often become less severe and less frequent as the child ages.
- Asthma attacks are usually associated with definite allergens.
- Oral bronchodilators should be taken 30 to 60 minutes before exercise, inhaled bronchodilators 15 to 20 minutes before exercise.

In adults:

- Asthma attacks usually become more severe and more frequent as the individual ages.
- Asthma attacks are usually not associated with definite allergens.

ASTHMA

Asthma is a condition characterized by intermittent airway obstruction in response to a variety of stimuli. The epithelial lining of the airways responds by becoming inflamed and edematous. Bronchospasm occurs in the smooth muscles of the bronchi and bronchioles. Secretions increase in viscosity. Elastic recoil decreases. All of these changes result in a reduction of the diameter of the airways, making breathing more difficult. Some clients who develop asthma in childhood experience spontaneous recovery.

Asthma is classified as extrinsic or intrinsic. Extrinsic asthma is caused by substances outside the body that precipitate the asthma response, such as pollen, house dust, or food additives. Intrinsic asthma is diagnosed when no extrinsic factor can be identified and the asthma is the result of internal factors such as emotional stress, exercise, or fatigue. An asthma attack that does not respond to treatment and persists is known as **status asthmaticus**.

The hallmark of an asthma attack is sudden onset of wheezing, increasing dyspnea, and chest tightness. Mild asthma usually is controlled by routine medication. Severe asthma attacks usually occur at night and require extra medication. With severe attacks, wheezing may be audible to the unaided ear. Expiratory wheezes are common as air attempts to escape through the narrowed airways. Both inspiratory and expiratory wheezes may be heard. *Absence of wheezing could indicate complete closure of the airway*. The respiratory rate rises initially, but as the client tires, the rate may decrease. Nasal flaring and costal and sternal retractions may be present, particularly in the young client. The client uses accessory muscles to assist respiratory effort. Cough occurs as the respiratory secretions become thick and block the airways. Cyanosis and a decrease in oxygen saturation occur. Heart rate elevates, as may blood pressure. The client becomes anxious and may complain of a sense of impending doom. These responses are thought to be caused by a release of catecholamines. Values of ABGs indicate hypoxia and respiratory acidosis. Chest x-ray shows hyperinflation of the lungs. Pulmonary function tests reveal an abnormal flow rate and lung volume. With a severe asthma attack, apnea and sudden death can occur in minutes.

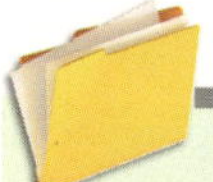

COLLABORATIVE CARE

Assessment and Teaching for Asthma

Respiratory therapists and nurses work together in assessing breath sounds and respiratory effort. Teaching the client how to use a nebulizer or inhalers and aerosol treatment is a collaborative effort of nurses and respiratory therapists.

MEDICAL–SURGICAL MANAGEMENT

Medical

The client with allergies should avoid specific antigens that might bring on an attack. Some clients with asthma are aided by controlling psychological stressors. Routine physical exercise is beneficial in treating exercise-induced asthma. The client with asthma should avoid other respiratory irritants such as cigarette smoke and air pollution. Clients who develop asthma later in life show more symptoms as they age.

Pharmacological

The primary treatment for an acute asthma attack is pharmacological. A combination of medications is used to open the narrowed airways. Medications used to dilate the bronchi include bronchodilators such as aminophylline (Aminophyllin) and terbutaline sulfate (Brethine, Bricanyl); beta agonists such as epinephrine (Primatene Mist) and albuterol sulfate (Ventolin); and anticholinergics such as atropine sulfate and ipratropium bromide (Atrovent). Corticosteroids such as prednisone (Delatsone) are utilized to decrease inflammation. Mucolytic agents such as acetylcysteine (Mucomyst) aid in liquefying secretions. Supplemental oxygen is given when indicated.

Diet

Adequate fluid intake is maintained to promote liquefaction of secretions. Foods, such as dairy products, which contribute to mucous production, should be avoided during or immediately following an asthma attack.

Activity

Incorporate several rest periods for the client. Use relaxation techniques to manage anxiety. The client should not overexert to the point of dyspnea, wheezing, or fatigue. If overexertion occurs, the client should sit down and sip warm water. This promotes slower, regular breathing; bronchodilation; and loosens secretions.

NURSING MANAGEMENT

Obtain history about previous asthma attacks. Evaluate wheezes for location, duration, and phase of respiration when they occur. Monitor pulse oximetry and ABGs for oxygenation and acid–base balance.

COMMUNITY/HOME HEALTH CARE

Asthma

- Prohibit smoking in the home, especially if a child has asthma.
- Use a humidifier, especially in the bedroom of the person with asthma.
- Use fans to circulate air.

NURSING PROCESS

ASSESSMENT

Subjective Data

A detailed history is taken regarding exposure to triggering stimuli before past asthma attacks. Also, the onset, duration, and severity of symptoms such as dyspnea are noted.

Objective Data

Note the effectiveness of ventilation. Wheezes are evaluated as to their duration, location, and the phase of respiration during which they occur (e.g., inspiration). Wheezes heard without the aid of a stethoscope are called **audible wheezes**. Respiratory rate, depth, rhythm and effort; position assumed; and client color are evaluated. Monitor pulse oximetry or lab reports of ABG values to determine oxygenation and acid–base balance. If sputum is produced, note its color, amount, viscosity, and odor.

Nursing diagnoses for a client with asthma include the following:

NURSING DIAGNOSES	PLANNING/OUTCOMES	NURSING INTERVENTIONS
*Inefficient **B**reathing Pattern* related to narrowed airways	The client will have respiratory rate and color within normal limits, clear breath sounds on auscultation, and ABG or pulse oximetry values within normal limits.	Assist client in assuming a position that facilitates ventilation. Administer medication as ordered. Assist client in the use of inhalers and aerosol treatments. Assess oxygenation by ABG or pulse oximetry values and administer supplemental oxygen, as ordered. Frequently assess respiratory rate and effort as well as color as client's condition dictates and auscultate the lung fields for presence of wheezes. If sputum is produced, note its color, amount, viscosity, and odor. Frequently assess vital signs as client's condition dictates. Unless otherwise contraindicated, encourage fluid intake to promote liquefaction of respiratory secretions.
*Deficient **K**nowledge* related to asthma, asthma treatment, and individual triggers for asthma attacks	The client will verbalize an understanding of both the pathophysiology and treatment of asthma, including the medications taken and their purposes and side effects. The client will also identify individual triggers and means of avoiding these triggers.	Teach client and family about the disease process; the purpose, effect, adverse effects, side effects, and use of all prescribed medications, especially inhalers and respiratory aerosol equipment. Assist client in establishing a medication schedule that will facilitate regular and timely taking of medications. Instruct client to use the inhaler prior to meals to aid in breathing while eating. If client is taking steroids, teach to rinse mouth after using the inhaler so as to prevent fungal infection. Encourage exercise because it increases respiratory reserve and improves overall physical condition. Assist client in identifying triggering stimuli and ways to avoid them. Teach client and family signs and symptoms of asthma attacks and respiratory tract infections. Teach client to avoid crowded areas and close contact with persons with infections.
***A**nxiety* related to perceived threat of dying	The client will verbalize a decrease in anxiety.	Provide client with explanations for all care. Provide care in a calm, unhurried manner. Plan care to allow client uninterrupted periods of rest. Allow client to make decisions regarding care, if possible. Provide client with opportunities to discuss anxiety with staff, family, or significant others.

Evaluation: Evaluate each outcome to determine how it has been met by the client.

CHRONIC OBSTRUCTIVE PULMONARY DISEASE

Chronic obstructive pulmonary disease (COPD), also called chronic obstructive lung disease (COLD), is a term used for two closely related respiratory diseases: chronic bronchitis and emphysema. These two diseases often occur together. Most clients have a long history of heavy cigarette smoking (NHLBI, 2009a). First signs are chronic cough, sputum production, or shortness of breath. It gradually gets worse over time. There is no known cure. In the United States, about 12 million adults have COPD. It is the fourth leading cause of death. In 2007, the national cost for COPD was approximately $42.6 billion (ALA, 2007a).

CHRONIC BRONCHITIS

Bronchitis is an inflammation of the bronchial tree accompanied by hypersecretion of mucus. The condition becomes chronic if cough and sputum are present on most days for 3 months a year for 2 consecutive years or for 6 months in 1 year (NHLBI, 2001b). Constant irritation of the bronchi results in hypertrophy of the mucus-secreting glands. The bronchioles fill with exudate, and subsequent infections are common. There may be narrowing of large and small airways. Environmental factors, especially cigarette smoke, play an important role in the development of chronic bronchitis.

The client usually has a history of recurrent respiratory infections, dyspnea, cyanosis, and chronic or recurrent cough yielding copious amounts of sputum. Often, the sputum is purulent or green in color. Over the course of time, the chest wall configuration becomes slightly distended. Coarse crackles (rales) are present throughout the lung fields. Breath sounds may be diminished or absent over the periphery of the lung fields. Elevation of pulmonary artery pressure results in increased workload for the right ventricle and in signs and symptoms of right-sided congestive heart failure (CHF), such as peripheral edema and fatigue. Arterial blood gases reveal increased $PaCO_2$ and decreased PaO_2. The red blood cell count elevates, as do hemoglobin and hematocrit. The increases in the amounts of red blood cells and hemoglobin represent an attempt by the body to compensate for the lower oxygen level. Chest x-ray shows hyperexpansion of the lungs. When CHF occurs, the chest x-ray also shows an enlarged heart.

MEDICAL–SURGICAL MANAGEMENT

Medical

The goals of medical treatment are to decrease symptoms of airway irritation, decrease airway obstruction related to secretions and inflammation, prevent infection, maintain oxygenation, and increase the client's exercise tolerance. Respiratory therapy includes the use of updraft (nebulizer) and aerosol treatments, along with percussion and postural drainage. Humidification of inspired air helps liquefy secretions. Supplemental oxygen is administered based on ABG or pulse oximetry values. The neurological stimulus to breathe becomes altered in some clients with chronic bronchitis so that breathing is initiated when the blood level of oxygen falls instead of when the level of carbon dioxide rises. Consequently, when the level of oxygen in the blood is relatively high in relation to the level of carbon dioxide, the stimulus to breathe is reduced and further depresses the CNS. When supplemental oxygen is necessary, it is maintained at the lowest possible flow rate to maintain oxygenation and prevent depression of the client's respiratory drive. Evaluate the client with chronic bronchitis and CHF for signs of fluid overload. Daily weight, intake, and output are monitored.

Pharmacological

Current medications used include beta-adrenergic agonists, cholinergic antagonists, methylxanthines, corticosteroids, cromolyn sodium/nedocromil, and leukotriene modifiers. Bronchodilators such as theophylline (Theo-dur) given orally, and ipratropium bromide (Atrovent) given as an inhalation aerosol (metered dose inhaler [MDI]) or inhalation solution (nebulizer) are used to open airways. Tiotropium bromide (Spiriva) is a once-daily inhalation powder administered using a HandiHaler device. Salmeterol (Serevent), given by a dry powder inhaler (DPI) is a long-acting $beta_2$-selective agonist used for chronic maintenance therapy. Inhalation aerosol (MDI) or inhalation solution (nebulizer) treatments with bronchodilators such as albuterol (Proventil, Ventolin) or metaproterenol sulfate (Alupent) are often used in conjunction with oral medications. Prednisone (Meticorten), a corticosteroid, is given as short-term therapy for acute exacerbations. If steroids are required on a long-term basis, they may be given by inhalation to prevent some adverse systemic effects. Mucolytic medications such as acetylcysteine (Mucomyst) are given to reduce the viscosity of purulent and nonpurulent pulmonary secretions. Guaifenesin (Robitussin, Naldecon Senior EX, Mucinex) are expectorants given to loosen phlegm and thin bronchial secretions. If infection occurs, broad-spectrum antibiotics are given. Immunization against influenza viruses and *Streptococcus pneumoniae* is recommended.

The client with chronic bronchitis who also has CHF will receive medications to aid the function of the weakened heart. Digoxin (Lanoxin) strengthens the force of the contraction of the heart muscle. Diuretics such as furosemide (Lasix) are given to remove fluid by increasing urinary output. Supplemental potassium chloride (K-Dur, Kay-Ciel elixir) is given if the client's potassium level decreases from effect of the diuretic.

Diet

Encourage the client to eat a well-balanced diet. If the client also has CHF, sodium intake is restricted. Unless contraindicated, fluids are encouraged. Offer small, frequent meals to clients experiencing shortness of breath.

Activity

Activity is restricted to decrease the workload on the heart and lungs. With acute exacerbations, the client is placed on bed rest. The level of activity is then slowly increased based on the client's tolerance.

Programs of breathing exercises and graded (easy to difficult) exercise regimes assist the client to achieve the maximum level of activity tolerance. Breath-retaining exercises such as coughing techniques, pursed-lip breathing, and diaphragmatic or abdominal breathing are taught. The client is monitored from a respiratory standpoint while exercising. The goal is to increase the client's capacity for all ADLs.

NURSING MANAGEMENT

Obtain history of onset, duration, and severity of symptoms. Note changes in level of consciousness, mental status, respiratory rate and effort, color, and use of accessory muscles. Obtain sputum specimen for culture and sensitivity. Monitor vital signs. Assess for weight gain, peripheral edema, and neck vein distention.

NURSING PROCESS

ASSESSMENT

Subjective Data

A thorough past medical history is obtained, including information about the onset, duration, and severity of symptoms. The client may describe fatigue and difficult breathing.

Objective Data

Note changes in level of consciousness or mental status, color, respiratory rate and effort, the position the client assumes to aid respiratory effort, and the use of accessory muscles. Review ABGs or pulse oximetry values. Auscultate lung fields for crackles (rales) and diminished breath sounds. Note color, amount, viscosity, and odor of sputum. Obtain specimens for culture and sensitivity, if indicated. Frequently measure vital signs. The pulse may be elevated and irregular. Blood pressure may be elevated or low. An elevated temperature may indicate infection. Assess for peripheral edema, neck vein distention, and rapid weight gain.

Nursing diagnoses for a client with chronic bronchitis include the following:

NURSING DIAGNOSES	PLANNING/OUTCOMES	NURSING INTERVENTIONS
*Ineffective **A**irway Clearance* related to thicker and increased amounts of respiratory secretions	The client's color, respiratory rate, and ABG values will be within normal limits.	Frequently assess level of consciousness, mental status, vital signs, respiratory effort, and color, and auscultate breath sounds at least every 4 hours. Obtain sputum specimens as ordered, and assess sputum for amount, viscosity, color, and odor. Assist client in assuming the position that most aids respiratory effort, usually an upright position. Administer oxygen and respiratory treatments as ordered and assess their effectiveness. Evaluate results of diagnostic and laboratory tests (ABGs) and notify the physician of abnormalities. Alternate care with periods of uninterrupted rest. Administer antibiotics and bronchodilators as ordered and evaluate their effectiveness. Provide client with a well-balanced diet and, unless otherwise contraindicated, encourage fluids. Assess client for signs and symptoms of CHF (i.e., fine crackles heard on auscultation, peripheral edema, weight gain, and fatigue). Report any signs and symptoms of CHF to the physician.
*Deficient **K**nowledge* related to chronic bronchitis and its treatment and prevention	The client will verbalize signs and symptoms to report to the physician, safety precautions to take with medication and equipment, medication and respiratory treatment regimen, and techniques for facilitating breathing.	Teach client to avoid respiratory infections, maintain adequate nutrition, increase fluid intake, and obtain adequate rest; the purpose, expected effects, and side effects of medications; and to administer respiratory treatments and medications prior to eating to aid in breathing. Instruct client to rinse mouth following use of inhaler. Teach client to self-administer oxygen. Provide information regarding both the use of equipment and safety measures for the equipment. Refer client to an established respiratory rehabilitation program. If such a program is not available, instruct client in breathing techniques. Encourage regular exercise within the client's limitations. Encourage client to obtain immunization against influenza viruses and *Streptococcus pneumoniae*.

Evaluation: Evaluate each outcome to determine how it has been met by the client.

EMPHYSEMA

Emphysema is a complex and destructive lung disease wherein air accumulates in the tissues of the lungs. The airways lose their elasticity and the walls thicken, resulting in narrower lumens. Airflow is impeded as it leaves the lungs (i.e., during expiration). The alveoli distal to these airways become overdistended with trapped air (Figure 35-12). Rupture of the alveolar wall may occur. The alveolar capillary membrane is destroyed, resulting in a loss of available area for gas exchange. Cigarette smoking is the most common cause of emphysema. Deficiency in alpha-1-antitrypsin is a familial disorder that leads to the development of emphysema. Alpha-1-antitrypsin is an enzyme that inhibits the activity of the enzyme elactase, which breaks down lung tissue.

Emphysema develops slowly over a period of years. The earliest symptom is a daily morning cough with clear sputum. Later, the client notes increasing dyspnea in response to activity. The degree of dyspnea corresponds to the degree of hypoxia, which is usually mild at rest but becomes increasingly severe in response to activity. In advanced stages of the disease, hypoxia is evident even at rest. With infection, a cough yielding purulent sputum occurs. The client's complexion appears ruddy, or reddish in color. The chest becomes barrel shaped (Figure 35-13) as the chest cage enlarges to accommodate distended lung tissues. The respiratory rate elevates. The expiratory phase of respiration becomes increasingly difficult. Accessory muscles are used to aid respiratory effort. Because of destruction of the alveoli, bronchial breath sounds are heard in the periphery of the lungs. As the disease progresses, breath sounds diminish and eventually disappear over the periphery of the lungs. Arterial blood gases reveal the degree of hypoxia depending on the severity of the disease. Hypercapnia, or retention of carbon dioxide, is not as likely as with chronic bronchitis. The extra effort required to breathe increases metabolic need, resulting in weight loss. Chest x-ray reveals hyperinflated lung tissue and a flattened diaphragm, which has been displaced by distended lung tissues. Pulmonary function studies reveal a decrease in expiratory volume. Polycythemia and elevation of hemoglobin and hematocrit occur in response to prolonged hypoxia.

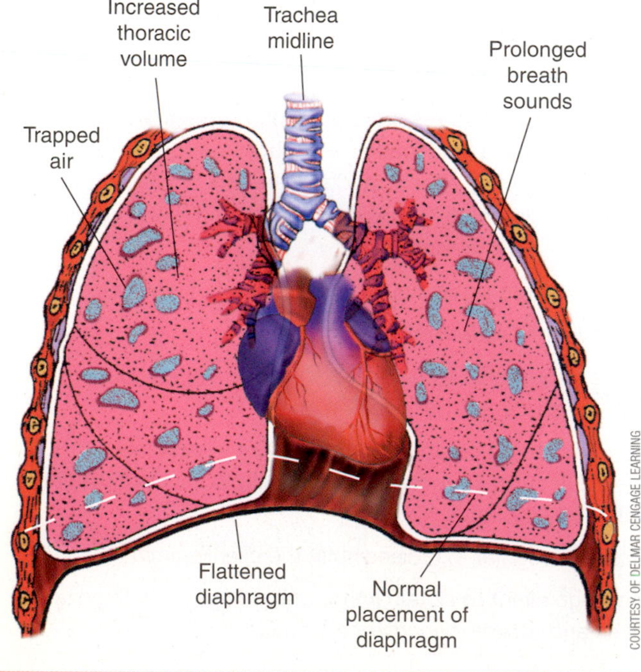

FIGURE 35-12 **Emphysema**

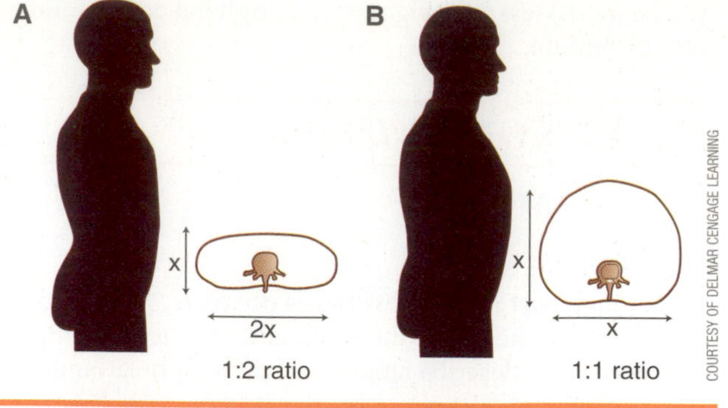

FIGURE 35-13 **Changes in Chest Configuration and Posture; *A,* The normal ratio of the anterior posterior diameter to the lateral diameter is 1:2; *B,* With a barrel chest, the ratio between the diameters is 1:1.**

MEDICAL–SURGICAL MANAGEMENT

Medical

The goals of treatment are to prevent further damage to the lung tissues, maintain adequate oxygenation, prevent infection, and improve the client's activity tolerance. The client who smokes should stop or, at least, decrease the number of cigarettes smoked daily. Supplemental oxygen is given to maintain oxygenation. The client with advanced emphysema and severe, chronic hypoxia may be maintained at PaO_2 of 55 to 59 mm Hg and/or oxygen saturation of 90% or greater. As with chronic bronchitis, the client with emphysema is given supplemental oxygen at the lowest possible flow rate, usually 2 to 3 L/min, to prevent respiratory and CNS depression.

Pharmacological

The client with emphysema receives many of the same medications used to treat chronic bronchitis. To open airways that have become fibrotic, theophylline and similar preparations are used. Steroids may be required for exacerbations. The client with emphysema usually does not need mucolytic agents, unless infection is present. Antibiotics are used to treat and prevent respiratory tract infections. The client should receive immunizations against influenza and *Streptococcus pneumoniae.* The client who smokes may use nicotine gum or transdermal patches to aid in smoking cessation.

Diet

The client with emphysema requires a diet high in carbohydrates to supply the energy necessary for breathing. If a negative nitrogen balance exists because of the client's using muscle tissue to provide energy, a diet high in protein is ordered. Dietary supplements such as Ensure may be needed to supply the necessary calories and nutrients. Unless contraindicated, fluids and small, frequent meals are encouraged.

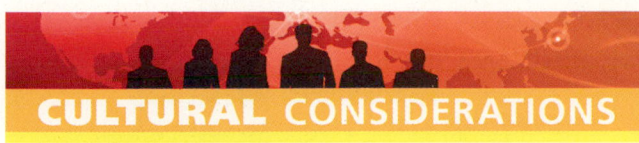

CULTURAL CONSIDERATIONS

Skin Color/Cyanosis

- For a client with highly pigmented skin, establish a baseline skin color.
- Observe skin surfaces that have the least amount of pigmentation, such as the palms, the soles of the feet, the abdomen, mucous membranes, or the inner aspect of forearms.

Activity

The client is placed on bed rest. Level of activity is increased based on the client's oxygenation. Oxygen saturation is evaluated periodically as the activity level is increased to determine the effect of activity on oxygenation.

Health Promotion

The client with emphysema benefits from a respiratory rehabilitation program. The client is taught breathing exercises similar to those taught to the client with chronic bronchitis. A graded exercise program is also used for the client with emphysema. Group programs that aid in smoking cessation are useful for the client who smokes.

Nursing Management

Review factors that increase client's dyspnea and those that relieve dyspnea. Evaluate client's nutritional status, vital signs, ABGs, pulse oximetry, color, and level of consciousness. Assist with ADL. Plan for uninterrupted periods of rest.

NURSING PROCESS

Assessment

Subjective Data

Included in the history is information regarding the timing of dyspnea, those factors that exacerbate dyspnea, and those factors that relieve dyspnea.

Objective Data

Assess sputum for color, amount, viscosity, odor, and vital signs. An elevated pulse may indicate hypoxia and/or infection. Auscultation of the lungs will reveal the presence of adventitious, diminished, or absent breath sounds. Note the client's position to aid respiratory effort, color, respiratory rate and effort, and use of accessory muscles to aid breathing. Evaluate the client's nutritional status by weighing the client and measuring nutrient and caloric intake. Review results of laboratory and diagnostic tests.

Nursing diagnoses for a client with emphysema include the following:

NURSING DIAGNOSES	PLANNING/OUTCOMES	NURSING INTERVENTIONS
*Impaired **G**as Exchange* related to destruction of the alveoli	The client's respiratory rate, color, and ABG values will be within normal limits.	Assess the client's level of consciousness and mental status. Frequently evaluate client's respiratory rate, respiratory effort, color, and oxygenation with ABG and/or pulse oximetry. Assess the effect of activity on oxygenation, particularly when activity is being increased and provide supplemental oxygen as ordered. Auscultate the lungs and report abnormalities to the physician. Assess client's vital signs: heart rate and temperature elevations may indicate infection, an elevated pulse may indicate hypoxia. Review results of diagnostic and laboratory tests and report abnormalities. Administer medications and respiratory treatments as ordered. Assist client in assuming the position that offers the most comfort and most aids respiratory effort. Instruct client in breathing techniques, such as pursed-lip breathing.
*Risk for **A**ctivity Intolerance* related to hypoxia	The client will complete activity without experiencing fatigue or dyspnea.	Assist client with ADL and hygiene needs. Plan care and treatments to allow client uninterrupted periods of rest. Allow rest before and after meals. As activity increases, assess the effects on oxygenation.

(*Continues*)

Nursing diagnoses for a client with emphysema include the following: (Continued)

NURSING DIAGNOSES	PLANNING/OUTCOMES	NURSING INTERVENTIONS
*Imbalanced **N**utrition: Less than Body Requirements* related to increased energy requirements to maintain respiration	The client will achieve or maintain a weight within normal limits for height.	Assess client's weight and evaluate in relation to the client's height. Evaluate client's diet for nutritional adequacy and review client's food likes and dislikes. Provide a well-balanced diet based on client's likes and dislikes. Provide nutritional supplements as ordered. Avoid activities or procedures prior to meals that might reduce appetite (e.g., enemas). Administer medications and respiratory treatments prior to meals to aid in breathing.

Evaluation: Evaluate each outcome to determine how it has been met by the client.

BRONCHIECTASIS

Bronchiectasis is chronic dilation of the bronchi. The main causes of this disorder are pulmonary TB infection, chronic upper respiratory tract infections, and complications of other respiratory disorders of childhood, particularly cystic fibrosis. The bronchi become distended and eventually lose their elastic recoil property. The mucociliary blanket's function is impaired, and secretions thicken. Secretions accumulate in the bronchi, resulting in a medium for infection. Airflow is hindered, reducing gas exchange.

The client with bronchiectasis describes a frequent or chronic productive cough, dyspnea, weight loss, and fatigue. Sputum is thick and sometimes purulent when infection is present. Crackles, which clear on coughing, are heard scattered throughout the lungs and are more prominent early in the morning. Accessory muscles are used to aid respiration. Over a period of time, right-sided CHF and peripheral edema develop. Arterial blood gases reveal elevated $PaCO_2$, decreased PaO_2, and respiratory acidosis. Polycythemia and elevated hemoglobin and hematocrit levels are present. Chest x-ray shows slight hyperinflation of lung tissue and, in the presence of CHF, cardiomegaly. Respiratory flow rate decreases, and lung volume increases, as demonstrated by pulmonary function studies. Table 35-8 compares asthma, chronic bronchitis, emphysema, and bronchiectasis.

MEDICAL–SURGICAL MANAGEMENT

Medical

Medical treatment is aimed at removing respiratory secretions, preventing or eliminating infection, and maintaining adequate oxygenation. Percussion and postural drainage are used to aid in the removal of secretions. Aerosol and updraft respiratory treatments may be ordered before percussion and drainage. If the client is unable to expectorate secretions, bronchial suctioning is performed. The physician performs a bronchoscopy to remove especially tenacious and copious secretions. Arterial blood gases and/or pulse oximetry values are evaluated to assess the need for supplemental oxygen. Daily weight and I&O are performed to detect signs of CHF. Pulmonary function studies evaluate the severity of lung damage.

CRITICAL THINKING

COPD Disorders

What are the differences and the similarities of the two disorders classified as COPD?

Pharmacological

Mucolytic agents are given to promote liquefaction of respiratory secretions. Antibiotics are ordered to treat and prevent infection. The client is immunized against influenza and against *Streptococcus pneumoniae* with the pneumococcal vaccine (Pneumovax 23). Bronchodilators are indicated to open the fibrotic airways. Inflammation is treated with oral steroids such as prednisone (Meticorten) and/or by inhalation with beclomethasone dipropionate (Beclovent). The client with cystic fibrosis is required to take pancreatic enzymes, pancrelipase (Pancrease capsules, Cotazym capsules), to replace those that are missing with this disorder. If CHF occurs, the client is treated with digoxin (Lanoxin), furosemide (Lasix), and potassium supplements, as indicated.

Diet

To provide energy for breathing, the diet should be high in carbohydrates and calories. Protein is supplemented if necessary. Dietary supplements such as Ensure may be needed. Fluids are encouraged, unless otherwise contraindicated. Sodium is restricted in the diet of the client with CHF to prevent fluid retention. The diet for the client with cystic fibrosis is restricted in fats because fats are not properly absorbed.

Activity

During acute exacerbations or in the presence of serious infection, activity is limited. The client is placed on bed rest. Activity is progressively increased depending on the client's

TABLE 35-8 Signs and Symptoms of Asthma, Chronic Bronchitis, Emphysema, and Bronchiectasis

	ASTHMA	CHRONIC BRONCHITIS	EMPHYSEMA	BRONCHIECTASIS
History	Intermittent attacks of dyspnea and wheezing	Recurrent respiratory infections, chronic cough	Insidious onset, dyspnea on exertion to dyspnea at rest	Cystic fibrosis, recurrent respiratory infections, TB
Cough	Present during attack	Chronic or recurrent productive cough	Present with infections	Frequent or chronic productive cough
Sputum	Thick	Copious, purulent, green	Scanty mucoid, unless infection present	Thick, tenacious, sometimes purulent secretions
Weight	No weight loss	Slight or no weight loss	Weight loss common	Commonly, weight loss or failure to gain
Appearance	Flushed then cyanotic	Commonly cyanosis ("blue bloater")	Ruddy complexion ("pink puffer")	Clubbing of fingernails
Chest Configuration	Slight overdistention	Slight overdistention	Overdistention prominent ("barrel chest")	Slight overdistention
Breath Sounds	Audible wheezing Prolonged expiration	Coarse crackles (rales)	Bronchial breath sounds in peripheral lung fields Diminished or absent in late disease	Crackles
Edema	Infrequent	Peripheral edema common, especially in ankles	Infrequent	Peripheral edema in late disease
Right-sided CHF (Cor Pulmonale)	Infrequent	Frequent	Infrequent	Frequent late in disease
CO Retention (Hypercapnia)	Sometimes	Common	Unlikely	Common in late disease
Hypoxemia	Depends on severity of attack	Possibly severe	Usually mild, especially at rest	Possibly severe in late disease and with infection
Dyspnea	Increases during attack	Progressive	Dyspnea on exertion to dyspnea at rest usually presenting symptom	With respiratory infection and late disease
Accessory Muscles Used for Respiration	Yes	Yes	Yes	Yes
Poly cythemia	Uncommon	Late in disease	Yes	In late disease
Respiratory Failure	Possible	Common	Possible	Common

COURTESY OF DELMAR CENGAGE LEARNING

tolerance. Respiratory rehabilitation and graded exercise programs are useful in the treatment of bronchiectasis. Regular exercise is encouraged, particularly for the pediatric client with cystic fibrosis.

NURSING MANAGEMENT

Review client's history for recent and past respiratory infections, TB, and cystic fibrosis. Monitor vital signs. An increased heart rate may indicate hypoxia and/or infection, and an

PROFESSIONALTIP

Cystic Fibrosis

Cystic fibrosis (CF) is an inherited life-threatening disorder that causes severe lung damage and nutritional deficiencies. Improvements in the treatment of CF have increased the life expectancy of a client with CF from 10 years of age in 1962 to 37 years of age in 2009 (National Institutes of Health, 2009a). Treatment for CF is aimed at relieving symptoms and complications. New antibiotics such as inhaled tobramycin sulfate (TOBI) are more effective in treating infections, and other drugs, such as dornase alfa recombinant (Pulmozyme) and azithromycin (Zithromax, Zmax) slow the progression of the lung disease. Mechanical chest physical therapy devices used daily, such as electric chest clappers and inflatable vibrating vests help loosen and remove thick mucus from the lungs. Lung transplantation may be an option for clients with severe lung damage. Respiratory failure is the most dangerous consequence of CF (Mayo Clinic, 2009). For more information about CF visit the Cystic Fibrosis Foundation at http://www.cff.org

elevated temperature may indicate infection. Note weight loss and muscle wasting. Monitor breath sounds and suction mucous as necessary.

CHEST TRAUMA

Pneumothorax/hemothorax is discussed following.

PNEUMOTHORAX/ HEMOTHORAX

Normally, the pleural space between the visceral and parietal pleura contains pleural fluid and is held together by surface tension. The pleural space is a closed compartment with a negative pressure compared to the lungs or the atmosphere. When the integrity of the pleura is interrupted, air from the atmosphere or from the lungs moves between the pleura, creating a space. This air in the pleural space is known as a **pneumothorax** (Figure 35-14). The lung tissue underlying the pneumothorax is compressed and unable to fully expand. If the pneumothorax is large enough, the entire lung may collapse from the compression.

A pneumothorax may be referred to as traumatic (closed or open), spontaneous, tension, or a hemopneumothorax. A closed pneumothorax occurs when there is no communication between the pleura and the external environment. An example of a closed pneumothorax is when blunt trauma to the chest causes a broken rib that pierces the pleura and lung, allowing air to enter between the pleura. An open pneumothorax exists when there is direct communication between the external environment and the pleural space as in a gunshot wound. A spontaneous pneumothorax occurs without an obvious underlying cause. A tension pneumothorax is a life-threatening condition wherein air enters the pleural space on inspiration but is unable to exit on expiration. The air thus continues to accumulate in the pleural space, compressing the underlying structures. If left untreated, a tension pneumothorax collapses the lung and encroaches on the structures on the opposite side. The structures of the mediastinum shift to the unaffected side as more and more air accumulates in the pleural space. Without intervention, tension pneumothorax will result in cardiopulmonary arrest. Tension pneumothorax is often associated with mechanical ventilation. The pressure exerted by the ventilator on compromised lung tissue interrupts the integrity of the pleura. Air continues to enter the pleural space but is unable to exit as mechanical ventilation continues. In the case of a pneumothorax associated with trauma or surgery, bleeding of adjacent vessels into the pleural cavity often occurs. Blood within the pleural space is referred to as a **hemothorax**. When accompanied by air, the condition is called a **hemopneumothorax**.

The severity of injury and the amount of lung tissue affected determine the signs and symptoms the client exhibits. The client with a small pneumothorax may be asymptomatic or may complain of minor dyspnea, whereas the client with a significant pneumothorax may exhibit signs of severe respiratory distress. Dyspnea, tachypnea, orthopnea, and cyanosis may be present. Oxygenation is impaired. Pleuritic pain is common. Breath sounds are absent in the area of the pneumothorax. The client with an accompanying hemothorax exhibits signs and symptoms of shock associated with blood loss.

MEDICAL–SURGICAL MANAGEMENT

Medical

For the affected lung to reexpand, the air and/or blood must be removed from the pleural space. When the blood loss

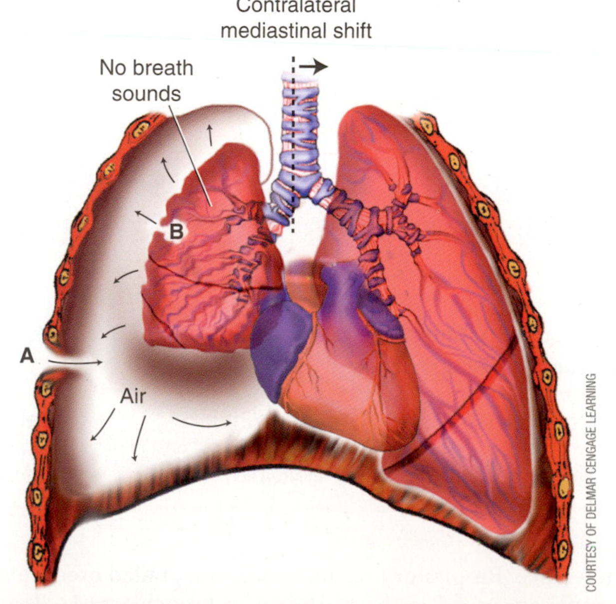

FIGURE 35-14 Pneumothorax; *A*, Penetrating Wound; *B*, Ruptured Bleb on the Lung

associated with a hemothorax is significant, fluid and blood replacement may be necessary.

Surgical

A thoracotomy tube, or chest tube, is inserted by the physician into the pleural space to drain fluid and air and allow the lung to reexpand. The tube is placed in the midaxillary line at approximately the fifth intercostal space. To drain air alone, the tube is placed in the anterior chest at the midclavicular line and the fourth intercostal space. The thoracotomy tube is connected to an underwater seal drainage device (refer back to Figure 35-9). The underlying cause of the hemopneumothorax then must be treated.

A recurrent spontaneous pneumothorax may require a pleural cortication to prevent further episodes. This involves roughing the adjacent surfaces of the visceral and parietal pleura so the resulting scar tissue will improve adhesion between the two surfaces. Emergency treatment for a tension pneumothorax that is severely compromising the function of the heart and lungs is placing a large-bore needle into the anterior chest at the fourth intercostal space. A thoracotomy tube is then inserted until the lung(s) are fully reexpanded and to prevent a recurrence.

Pharmacological

To control pleuritic pain, narcotic analgesics such as morphine sulfate or meperidine (Demerol) are prescribed. Analgesics may be given orally or parenterally depending on the severity of the pain. Before insertion of a thoracotomy tube, intravenous narcotics may be given prophylactically. Tissues adjacent to the area of the pneumothorax are injected with local anesthetics before insertion of a thoracotomy tube.

Diet

A well-balanced diet with sufficient amounts of protein is encouraged for healing. The client with other injuries and conditions may require TPN or enteral feedings.

Activity

If hypoxia is present, activity restrictions are necessary. The presence of other injuries or conditions may also necessitate activity restrictions. After the client is adequately oxygenated and stable, activity is encouraged to promote expansion of the lungs.

Nursing Management

Gather information about recent chest injuries or falls. Assess level of consciousness, mental status, color, respiratory effort, and chest wall movement. Monitor vital signs. Auscultate for breath sounds. When a chest tube is in place, assess function, patency, and amount and character of drainage.

NURSING PROCESS

Assessment

Subjective Data

Gather information about the source of the pneumothorax. Ask the client about previous pneumothoraces, recent chest injury, falls, and severe coughing. The client often describes being very anxious.

Objective Data

Assess the client's level of consciousness and mental status and the client's color, respiratory effort, and chest wall movement. Chest wall movement is decreased on the affected side. When a large pneumothorax is present, the trachea shifts toward the unaffected side. Dyspnea and cyanosis may occur. The cough is forceful and nonproductive. Respiratory rate and heart rate are elevated. Blood pressure may be elevated because of the presence of pain and anxiety or may be low because of blood loss. Breath sounds are diminished or absent over the affected areas. Note the location, duration, and severity of pain. When a chest tube is inflated, assess for function, patency, and amount and character of drainage.

Nursing diagnoses for a client with a pneumothorax include the following:

NURSING DIAGNOSES	PLANNING/OUTCOMES	NURSING INTERVENTIONS
*Ineffective **B**reathing Pattern* related to decreased lung expansion	The client's respiratory rate and color will be within normal limits, and the client will have clear breath sounds in affected area.	Monitor the amount and character of drainage from the chest tube and note chest tube drainage as output. Observe fluctuations (tidaling) in the water seal chamber, which indicates that the tube is in the pleural space. Investigate the absence of tidaling because this may indicate that the lung is fully reexpanded or that the tube is occluded or kinked. Observe for bubbling in the water seal chamber, which indicates an air leak. Assess the connections and chest tube to determine if leaks are present. If no air leaks are present, notify the physician because the air leak may be within the client's lungs. Encourage client to cough and deep breathe to prevent further respiratory complications.

(*Continues*)

Nursing diagnoses for a client with a pneumothorax include the following: (Continued)

NURSING DIAGNOSES	PLANNING/OUTCOMES	NURSING INTERVENTIONS
*Acute **Pain** related to pleural space irritation*	The client will verbalize a decrease in pain on a scale of 0 to 10.	Assist client in assuming the position that most aids respiration. Most clients find this to be the orthopneic position.
		Assess vital signs and respiratory status.
		Administer pain medications as ordered. Remember that respiratory depression is possible with narcotic medications.
		Provide diversional activities.

Evaluation: Evaluate each outcome to determine how it has been met by the client.

NEOPLASMS OF THE RESPIRATORY TRACT

Neoplasms discussed following include benign neoplasms, lung cancer, and laryngeal cancer.

BENIGN NEOPLASMS

A benign tumor or cyst in the lung has sharply defined edges, as revealed on an x-ray. Peripheral tumors usually have no symptoms. Bronchial tumors may cause obstruction, infection, or atelectasis.

LUNG CANCER

Malignant tumors (carcinomas) of the lung may originate within the lung or may result from metastasis from other tumor sites (e.g., breast, colon, or kidney). Men, especially those older than 40 years of age, are more likely to have lung cancer than are women. The number of deaths is still rising among women, but has reached a plateau for men (ALA, 2007c). Cigarette smoking is the most important risk factor for lung cancer. Air pollution and exposure to carcinogens such as asbestos are also risk factors, especially among smokers, for developing lung cancer. Exposure to radiation or radon is also known to cause lung cancer. Prognosis depends on the size of the tumor when diagnosed and the specific cell type (Figure 35-15).

Symptoms develop late in the course of lung cancers. Peripheral lesions generally have few symptoms. Initially, the client may complain of a chronic cough or wheezing. Central lesions cause obstruction and erosion of the bronchi. As the tumor grows and occludes the air passages, the client may experience shortness of breath, dyspnea, and blood-tinged sputum. Pain occurs relatively late in the course of the disease and indicates that the tumor has grown to a significant size to put pressure on adjacent nerves and other structures. Although some tumors can be seen on chest x-ray, many cannot. Low-dose helical CT scans and MRI scans are more reliable studies when assessing soft-tissue structures. To confirm a diagnosis, cytology studies are performed on specimens collected via bronchoscopy, needle biopsy, or mediastinoscopy. Lung scans are occasionally useful for diagnosis. Before initiating treatment, the client is evaluated for metastatic disease using bone and total body scans.

Family members and significant others often need assistance in coping with their feelings.

MEDICAL–SURGICAL MANAGEMENT

Medical

Treatment of lung cancer depends on the type and stage of the cancer.

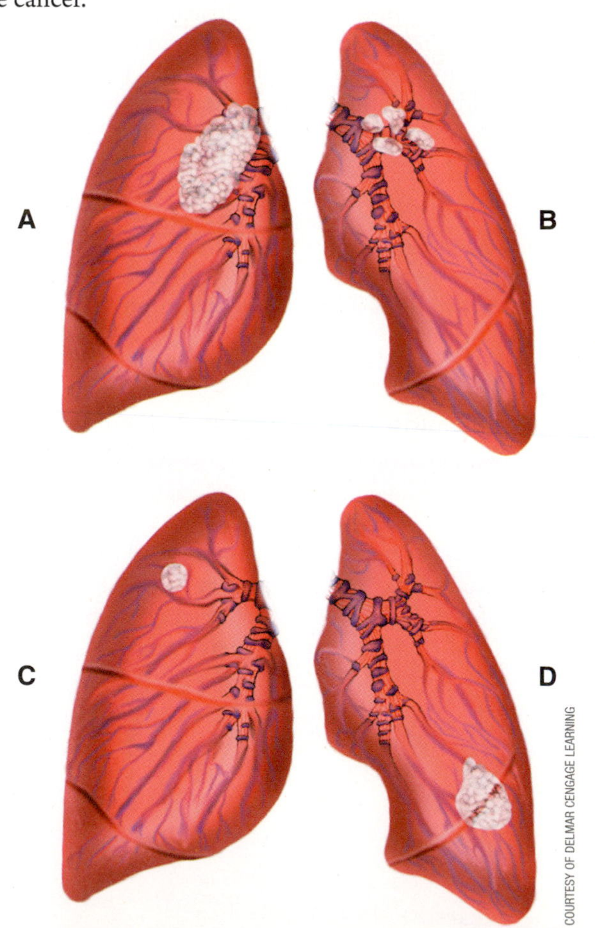

FIGURE 35-15 Lung Cancers; *A*, Small-Cell Carcinoma; *B*, Epidermoid (Squamous-Cell) Carcinoma; *C*, Adenocarcinoma; *D*, Large Cell (Undifferentiated) Carcinoma

COMMUNITY/HOME HEALTH CARE

Client with Laryngeal Stoma

- Humidify home, especially in winter.
- The client and family must know how to suction the respiratory tract and care for the respiratory equipment.
- Use warm water to clean around the stoma.
- Do not use tissues, linty cotton, or soap for cleansing.
- Wear a bib or dressing over the stoma to filter and warm incoming air.
- Do not swim or splash water in the stoma when showering or bathing.
- Notify the physician if any signs of respiratory infection develop, such as fever, cough, yellow or green mucus, or redness around the stoma.
- Keep follow-up appointments with physician.

Surgical

Surgical intervention involves the removal of the tumor and adjacent lung tissue. Pneumonectomy is the removal of an entire lung. Lobectomy is the removal of a lobe of a lung. Segmental resection is the removal of a segment of a lung. The client will have a thoracotomy tube on the operative side. Radiation and chemotherapy are often used in conjunction with surgery. The incidence of lung tumor recurrence following surgery is high. Surgery is often indicated for early non–small-cell carcinomas.

Pharmacological

The specific type of chemotherapy used depends on the cell type and the extent of tumor growth.

Health Promotion

The foremost method of preventing lung cancer is to avoid smoking or to cease smoking. Avoid the secondhand smoke of others.

Nursing Management

Review client's history for smoking, exposure to carcinogens, and other risk factors. Gather information about onset and severity of symptoms. Assess for pain. Monitor breath sounds, vital signs, and drainage from chest tube. Assist to semi-Fowler's position or lying on the affected side. Monitor ABGs and provide oxygen as indicated. When pain medication is given, monitor for respiratory depression. Aid client to express feelings of grief about diagnosis.

NURSING PROCESS

Assessment

Subjective Data

Review the client's history for smoking, exposure to carcinogens, and other risk factors. Gather information regarding the onset, duration, and severity of symptoms. The client may report hoarseness, chronic cough, pain, and shortness of breath. Assess pain for location, character, duration, and severity.

Objective Data

Note the color, amount, consistency, and odor of sputum. Before surgery, wheezing or decreased breath sounds may be heard on the affected side. Following surgery, breath sounds are diminished or absent on the affected side. Monitor the amount and color of drainage from the thoracotomy tube. Assess the wound for hemorrhage and infection. Respiratory rate and effort may be increased. Pulse rate may be elevated as a result of a variety of factors including decreased oxygenation, hemorrhage, and infection. Hypotension occurs with significant blood loss. High blood pressure may indicate pain, anxiety, or other underlying pathology such as essential hypertension.

Nursing diagnoses for a client with lung cancer include the following:

NURSING DIAGNOSES	PLANNING/OUTCOMES	NURSING INTERVENTIONS
Ineffective Breathing Pattern related to disease process	The client's respiratory rate and color will be within normal limits.	Frequently monitor client's level of consciousness, vital signs, color, and respiratory effort. Auscultate breath sounds.
		Assess oxygenation and provide supplemental oxygen as indicated.
		Stagger activities with periods of rest to prevent overtaxing client's reserves.
		Assist client in assuming the position that maximizes respiratory effort by positioning client in semi-Fowler's position or lying on the affected side.
		Monitor lab reports for blood gas levels.

(*Continues*)

Nursing diagnoses for a client with lung cancer include the following: (Continued)

NURSING DIAGNOSES	PLANNING/OUTCOMES	NURSING INTERVENTIONS
Chronic ***Pain*** related to Lung cancer	The client will state pain is decreased on a scale of 0 to 10.	Administer pain medication and monitor for respiratory depression. Provide diversional activities. Assist client in assuming a position of comfort.
Anticipatory ***Grieving*** related to prognosis and perceived separation from significant others	The client will be able to express to significant others and/or staff feelings related to diagnosis and prognosis.	Aid the client in expressing feelings of grief related to the diagnosis. Hope should not be eliminated, but false hope should not be encouraged. Allow the client and family time to express their feelings.

Evaluation: Evaluate each outcome to determine how it has been met by the client.

LARYNGEAL CANCER

The American Cancer Society (2007) estimated that in 2008 approximately 12,250 Americans would be diagnosed with laryngeal cancer, and about 3,670 persons would die from it. Risk factors for cancer of the larynx include smoking, chronic alcohol abuse, chronic laryngitis, and overuse of the voice. Laryngeal cancer is relatively asymptomatic. The client may experience hoarseness or difficulty speaking above a whisper. If either persists for more than 2 weeks, medical care should be sought. Difficulty swallowing is sometimes present. Laryngeal pain radiating to the ear or a lump in the throat are often signs of metastasis.

MEDICAL–SURGICAL MANAGEMENT

Treatment is determined by the extent of tumor growth.

Surgical

Surgical removal of the larynx, a laryngectomy, is used to treat laryngeal cancer. A radical or modified radical neck dissection may be performed if the cancer has spread to surrounding tissues and lymph nodes. Radical neck dissection operations have been performed for almost 100 years and include the removal of lateral neck lymph nodes and tissues, the submandibular gland, the sternocleidomastoid muscle, the jugular vein and the spinal accessory nerve (Georgetown University Hospital, 2009). A modified radical neck dissection removes all the lymph nodes in one or both sides of the neck without removing neck muscles. The jugular vein and spinal accessory nerve may be removed (National Cancer Institute, 2009). Radiation may be used as an adjunct to surgery or as primary treatment if the tumor is detected in the early stages. Following surgery, a permanent tracheostomy is necessary to allow air to enter the respiratory tract. A small incision is made into the trachea and below the Adam's apple, and a plastic tracheostomy tube is inserted.

NURSING MANAGEMENT

Monitor respiratory status. Suction secretions and provide tracheostomy care. Teach client stoma protection. Keep head of bed elevated and provide extra humidity. Refer client to the American Cancer Society for support at www.cancer.org.

NURSING PROCESS

ASSESSMENT

Subjective Data

Obtain a history of the onset, duration, and severity of symptoms, such as hoarseness or laryngitis and alcohol and tobacco use. The client may describe ear pain and difficulty breathing and swallowing.

Objective Data

Evaluate the client's respiratory status for other respiratory problems that may accompany laryngeal cancer, such as COPD. Examine sputum for the presence of blood.

Nursing diagnoses for a client with laryngeal cancer include the following:

NURSING DIAGNOSES	PLANNING/OUTCOMES	NURSING INTERVENTIONS
Ineffective ***Airway*** *Clearance* related to tracheostomy tube	The client's respiratory rate and color will be within desired ranges, and the client will have clear breath sounds to auscultation.	Suction frequently following surgery to remove static secretions and provide routine tracheostomy care. Provide small, frequent feedings of liquid or pureed food to prevent choking. Assist client to turn, cough, and deep breathe two to four times an hour.

Nursing diagnoses for a client with laryngeal cancer include the following: (Continued)

NURSING DIAGNOSES	PLANNING/OUTCOMES	NURSING INTERVENTIONS
		Teach client stoma protection. Assess respirations two to four times an hour, if secretions are copious. Auscultate lung sounds. Keep head of bed elevated. Provide extra humidity.
*Impaired Verbal **C**ommunication* related to removal of the larynx	The client will be able to communicate needs.	Before surgery, establish a means of communication to be used afterward. If available, a manual or computer word/picture board works well. Keep call light by client's bed. Avoid mouthing communications, as this is frustrating to the client and is time consuming. As possible, ask questions that require only a "yes" or "no" answer. Refer client to the local support group (Lost Chord Club) or the American Cancer Society. Provide written information and materials.
*Deficient **K**nowledge* related to tracheostomy care	The client will verbalize precautions and safety measures for a tracheostomy; how to use equipment; how to suction the respiratory tract; how to change a tracheostomy tube; and actions to take in an emergency.	Teach client and family how to suction the respiratory tract, care for the tracheostomy, and use respiratory equipment. Instruct client and family in what to do in case of an emergency, such as secretions clogging the tracheostomy tube. Advise client not to swim and to avoid aspirating water when showering or bathing. Advise client to avoid extremely cold temperatures. Cover tracheostomy site for warming or cosmetic purposes with a porous material without frayed or loose threads.

Evaluation: Evaluate each outcome to determine how it has been met by the client.

DISORDERS OF THE NOSE

The most common disorder of the nose is epistaxis, or nose bleed.

EPISTAXIS

Epistaxis is hemorrhage of the nares or nostrils. It is either unilateral, which is most common, or bilateral. Epistaxis may be primary in nature, stemming from drying of the nasal mucosa, local irritation, or trauma, or may occur secondary to uncontrolled hypertension or coagulopathies (e.g., thrombocytopenia, anticoagulant therapy). The diffuse vascularity and proximity of blood vessels to the surface of the nasal mucosa make the nares a susceptible avenue for hemorrhage. Blood loss can be minimal to severe. With significant blood loss, hypovolemic shock occurs.

MEDICAL–SURGICAL MANAGEMENT

Medical

The client with epistaxis usually arrives at an urgent care facility or emergency room after unsuccessful attempts to stop the bleeding. Signs of airway obstruction or aspiration require immediate attention. The goals of treatment are to maintain airway, stop bleeding, identify the cause, and prevent recurrence. Nosebleeds are usually responsive to compression of the nares. Maintain firm pressure for 5 minutes. If bleeding persists, the client should blow the nose and clear the nasal passages. Resume pressure for a full 10 minutes. Epistaxis that continues following these measures requires more aggressive treatment. Bleeding sites that cannot be visualized require a sterile nasal packing inserted after application of a local anesthetic. In severe cases, a nasostat is inserted. This device resembles a Foley catheter and provides direct compression to the site of bleeding via

INFECTION CONTROL

Epistaxis

Wear gloves, goggles or a face mask, and a gown when caring for a client with epistaxis. A cough or sneeze can splatter blood.

a balloon. Clients with severe nosebleeds may require fluid and blood replacement to prevent hypovolemic shock. Persistent or recurrent epistaxis may require surgical ligation of the artery supplying the area.

Pharmacological

Sites of bleeding that can be visualized are cauterized by the physician using silver nitrate sticks. Hemostasis also is accomplished by packing the affected nostril with epinephrine 1:1000 on cotton packing.

Nursing Management

Evaluate overt blood flow and visually examine the posterior oropharynx for hidden bleeding. Monitor vital signs. Have client sit up with head bent slightly forward, breathe through the mouth, and allow blood to run freely from the nose into a container. Avoid tipping the head back as blood will flow down the esophagus causing nausea and vomiting. Then, wearing gloves, compress the nares for 5 minutes. Suction through the mouth to prevent aspiration. Monitor for nausea and vomiting caused by swallowed blood.

NURSING PROCESS

Assessment

Subjective Data

Ask about the onset, precipitating events, duration, and frequency of epistaxis, as well as associated symptoms such as nausea, vomiting, headache, and lightheadedness. The client with an occult bleeding in the back of the throat may complain of needing to swallow frequently.

Objective Data

Evaluate blood flow for amount, consistency, color, and rate (or severity). Overt bleeding from the nose may be present. This bleeding can vary in flow, from a continuous drip to a pulsating stream of blood. Visually examine the posterior oropharynx of the client with an occult epistaxis to assess blood flow. Vomiting may be present. Lowered blood pressure and rapid heart rate are signs of hypovolemic shock. Conversely, the client with uncontrolled hypertension has an abnormally high systolic blood pressure. Prothrombin time (PT), APTT, INR, and other clotting studies will be abnormal with underlying coagulopathies. Decreased red blood cell count, hemoglobin, and hematocrit are evidence of significant bleeding.

Nursing diagnoses for a client with epistaxis include the following:

NURSING DIAGNOSES	PLANNING/OUTCOMES	NURSING INTERVENTIONS
*Impaired **G**as Exchange* related to airway obstruction	The client's respiratory rate, color, and blood gases will be within normal limits.	Place client in a high Fowler's position, with the head bent slightly forward. Instruct client to breathe through the mouth and allow the blood to escape freely from the nose and into a container. This aids in preventing obstruction of the airway and swallowing of blood. Monitor client for signs and symptoms of airway obstruction. Assess client's color, respiratory rate and effort, and breath sounds. Monitor pulse oximetry and lab reports of ABGs and administer supplemental oxygen as indicated.
*Risk for **A**spiration* related to epistaxis	The client will develop no complications related to aspiration.	Place client in the position previously described to aid in preventing aspiration of blood. Assess client for signs of aspiration, such as choking, coarse crackles (rales) on auscultation, or elevated temperature. Suction the respiratory tract through the mouth to remove secretions and blood.
*Deficient Fluid **V**olume* related to blood loss	The client will maintain adequate fluid volume.	With a gloved hand, compress the nares for 5 minutes. If bleeding persists, have client blow nose to clear passages, then compress nares for 10 minutes. If bleeding continues following compression attempts, prepare to assist the physician with procedures such as cautery or insertion of nasal packing.

Nursing diagnoses for a client with epistaxis include the following: (Continued)

NURSING DIAGNOSES	PLANNING/OUTCOMES	NURSING INTERVENTIONS
		Administer medications to control blood pressure, as ordered. After hemostasis has been established, the clots formed should not be removed or dislodged, as this will lead to recurrence of bleeding. Every 30 minutes, evaluate the blood pressure and pulse of the client who shows signs of volume depletion. Assess for orthostatic hypotension as a means of measuring volume depletion. A decrease in systolic blood pressure of greater than 10 mm Hg when the position is changed from lying to sitting or standing indicates hypovolemia. Administer intravenous fluids, as ordered.

Evaluation: Evaluate each outcome to determine how it has been met by the client.

CASE STUDY

P.W. is a 77-year-old woman with a history of smoking two to three packs of cigarettes per day for the past 60 years. P.W. has been diagnosed with COPD for the past 4 years. She has required supplemental oxygen at 2 L/min for the last 18 months. Three days ago, P.W. was admitted with chief complaints of increasing dyspnea on exertion and a productive cough yielding thick, green-yellow sputum. She states that she does "not know why she is coughing up this awful stuff."

Physical examination of P.W. this morning revealed vital signs of T = 101.5°F, P = 124 beats/min, R = 38 breaths/min, BP = 168/74 mm Hg, and sonorous and sibilant wheezes on expiration and in the posterior lung fields, with superimposed coarse crackles heard in the right posterior lower lung field. She is unable to ambulate to the bathroom or complete other ADL because of the dyspnea. Chest x-ray showed a large area of consolidation in the right lower lobe. Sputum culture is still pending.

The following questions will guide your development of a nursing care plan for the case study.

1. List the clinical manifestations that indicate P.W. is experiencing an infection concomitant with her COPD.
2. Explain why COPD predisposes a client to respiratory infection.
3. Explain why the physician will increase P.W.'s oxygen flow to 3 to 4 L/min.
4. List the subjective and objective data the nurse should obtain during the nursing assessment.
5. Identify three nursing diagnoses and client goals that would be pertinent to P.W.'s care.
6. List the above diagnoses in order of priority, with number one being the highest.
7. Describe client outcomes indicating that P.W.'s treatment and nursing care regimen have been successful.

SUMMARY

- The primary function of the respiratory system is delivery of oxygen to the lungs and removal of carbon dioxide from the lungs.
- Pneumonia is a lung infection wherein infectious secretions accumulate in the air passages and interfere with gas exchange. Clients with chronic pulmonary disorders or problems of immobility are at increased risk of developing pneumonia.
- Pulmonary TB is an infection of the lung tissue caused by the *Mycobacterium tuberculosis*. Treatment of TB requires the long-term administration of pharmacological agents.

- A common respiratory tract disorder associated with immobility and the administration of anesthetic agents is atelectasis. Clients at risk are encouraged to cough and breathe deeply to aid in preventing atelectasis.
- Obstruction of a pulmonary artery by a bloodborne substance is known as pulmonary embolism. Deep vein thrombosis is a common cause of pulmonary emboli.
- Chronic obstructive pulmonary disease is a collective term used to refer to chronic bronchitis and emphysema, which often occur together.
- Traumatic disorders of the respiratory tract include pneumothorax and hemothorax, wherein the underlying lung tissue is compressed and eventually collapses.
- Cigarette smoking is indicated as a major causative factor in the development of respiratory disorders, such as lung cancer, cancer of the larynx, emphysema, and chronic bronchitis.

REVIEW QUESTIONS

1. The physician orders 2 to 3 L/min of oxygen to be delivered to the client with COPD because:
   1. no client ever requires more than 2 to 3 L/min of oxygen.
   2. the client requests it.
   3. a higher flow rate may suppress the client's drive to breathe.
   4. 2 to 3 L/min is the maximum flow that a nasal cannula can effectively deliver.
2. A particulate respirator mask is used by the nurse caring for a client with TB because:
   1. regular masks allow the tubercle bacilli to pass through.
   2. this mask is more comfortable for long-term use.
   3. this type of mask allows the nurse to be in close contact with the client for prolonged periods of time.
   4. there is no need for this type of mask when caring for clients with TB.
3. The nurse is teaching a client about lung cancer. Which statement best demonstrates the client correctly understands the risk factors for lung cancer?
   1. "I work with asbestos everyday and it is safe now."
   2. "Having asthma does not make me more at risk for getting lung cancer."
   3. "I should stop chewing tobacco and drinking alcohol."
   4. "My wife smokes and I do not, so I do not have to worry."
4. A client with severe epistaxis arrives at an urgent care clinic. When assessing this client, the nurse's initial action should be to:
   1. identify the cause of the bleeding.
   2. stop the bleeding.
   3. assess for a patent airway.
   4. teach the client how to prevent recurrence.
5. The nurse's assessment of a client with pulmonary edema indicates the following: thick frothy sputum, cough, and dyspnea. On the basis of these findings, the most appropriate nursing diagnosis is:
   1. ineffective airway clearance.
   2. Activity Intolerance.
   3. altered tissue perfusion.
   4. acute pain.
6. A client needs to be tested for tuberculosis when the nurse takes a medical history that includes complaints of:
   1. cough, night sweats, hemoptysis.
   2. weight gain, diarrhea, vomiting.
   3. fever > 102°F, fatigue, dry mouth.
   4. weight loss, stridor, chills.
7. The health care provider has prescribed furosemide (Lasix) for a client with a pleural effusion as part of the treatment plan. Which of the following statements made by the client regarding furosemide (Lasix) indicates that further teaching is needed by the nurse?
   1. "I will probably need to urinate more frequently."
   2. "This medication will help remove fluid from my pleural space."
   3. "The nurse will monitor my intake and output each shift."
   4. "I should take this medication at bedtime."
8. Parents of a newly diagnosed 14-year-old asthmatic client ask the nurse what medications will be prescribed for their child. The nurse informs the parents that common medications for asthma include: (Select all that apply.)
   1. bronchodilators.
   2. antibiotics.
   3. Corticosteroids.
   4. diuretics.
   5. mucolytic agents.
   6. beta agonists.
9. A client with a pneumothorax is brought to the emergency department. Which of the following assessments will the nurse be able to make?
   1. Decreased respirations, low blood pressure, constricted pupils.
   2. Cyanosis, dyspnea, tracheal shift, and tachycardia.
   3. Clammy skin, dilated pupils, slow pulse, and low blood pressure.
   4. Dyspnea, agitation, visual hallucinations, and elevated blood pressure.

10. A client informs the nurse that she is not sure how to use her incentive spirometer. The most appropriate response from the nurse would be:
    1. "The incentive spirometer measures the amount of air inspired in one inhalation."
    2. "The incentive spirometer is a device that a client will use after surgery."
    3. "Would this be a good time for me to teach you and demonstrate?"
    4. "Did someone from the respiratory department teach you?"

REFERENCES/SUGGESTED READINGS

American Cancer Society (ACS). (2003). *Cancer facts and figures 2003.* Atlanta, GA: Author.

American Cancer Society (ACS). (2007). Overview: laryngeal and hypopharyngeal cancer. How many people get laryngeal and hypopharyngeal cancers? Retrieved April 1, 2009 from http://www.cancer.org/docroot/CRI/content/CRI_2_2_1X_How_many_people_get_these_cancers_23.asp?sitearea=

American Cancer Society (ACS). (2009). Lung cancer. Retrieved April 11, 2009 from http://www.cancer.org/docroot/PRO/content/PRO_1_1x_Lung_Cancer.pdf.asp?sitearea=PRO

American Lung Association (ALA). (2007a). Chronic obstructive pulmonary disease fact sheet. Retrieved April 11, 2009 from http://www.lungusa.org/site/apps/nlnet/content3.aspx?c=dvLUK9O0E&b=2058829&content_id={EE451F66-996B-4C23-874D-BF66586196FF}¬oc=1

American Lung Association (ALA). (2007b). HIV and tuberculosis fact sheet. Retrieved April 10, 2009 from http://www.lungusa.org/site/apps/nlnet/content3.aspx?c=dvLUK9O0E&b=2060731&content_id={A3132347-3F7C-4ED7-AB4C-34FBEE5B0D4C}¬oc=1

American Lung Association (ALA). (2007c). Lung cancer fact sheet. Retrieved April 11, 2009 from http://www.lungusa.org/site/apps/nlnet/content3.aspx?c=dvLUK9O0E&b=4294229&ct=3232839

American Lung Association (ALA). (2008a). Trends in tuberculosis morbidity and mortality. Retrieved April 10, 2009 from http://www.lungusa.org/atf/cf/{7a8d42c2-fcca-4604-8ade-7f5d5e762256}/TB_TRENDS_AUG_2008.PDF

American Lung Association (ALA). (2008b). Tuberculosis fact sheet. Retrieved April 10, 2009 from http://www.lungusa.org/site/apps/nlnet/content3.aspx?c=dvLUK9O0E&b=4294229&ct=3052619

American Lung Association (ALA). (2009). Influenza and pneumonia. Retrieved April 10, 2009 from http://www.lungusa.org/site/pp.asp?c=dvLUK9O0E&b=4074717

Andrews, C., & Kearney, K. (2002). Preventing air embolism. *AJN, 102*(1), 34–36.

ARDS Support Center. (2009a). Frequently asked questions about ARDS. Retrieved April 11, 2009 from http://www.ards.org/learnaboutards/whatisards/faq/

ARDS Support Center. (2009b). Learn about ARDS. Retrieved April 11, 2009 from http://ards.org/learnaboutards/

Avalos-Bock, S. (2001). The hard truth about the PPD skin test. *Nursing2001, 31*(6), 56–57.

Bulechek, G., Butcher, H., McCloskey, J., & Dochterman, J., eds. (2008). *Nursing Interventions Classification (NIC)* (5th ed.). St. Louis, MO: Mosby/Elsevier.

Carroll, P. (2001). How to intervene before asthma turns deadly. *RN, 64*(5), 52–58.

Centers for Disease Control and Prevention (CDC). (2005a). Basic information about SARS. Retrieved April 11, 2009 from http://www.cdc.gov/ncidod/sars/factsheet.htm

Centers for Disease Control and Prevention (CDC). (2005b). Current SARS situation. Retrieved April 11, 2009 from http://www.cdc.gov/ncidod/sars/situation.htm

Centers for Disease Control and Prevention (CDC). (2008). NIOSH topic area: Severe acute respiratory syndrome (SARS). Retrieved July 17, 2009 from http://www.cdc.gov/niosh/topics/SARS/

Centers for Disease Control and Prevention(CDC). (2009). Influenza: The disease. Retrieved July 20, 2009 from http://www.cdc.gov/flu/about/disease/index.htm

Chan, S., & Goldrick, B. (2003). Emerging infections. *AJN, 103*(6), 60–62.

Daniels, R., Nosek, L., & Nicoll, L. (2007). *Contemporary medical-surgical nursing.* Clifton Park, NY: Delmar Cengage Learning.

Davies, P. (2002). Guarding your patient against ARDS. *Nursing2002, 32*(3), 36–41.

Diehl-Oplinger, L., & Kaminski, M. F. (2002). Flash pulmonary edema. *Nursing2002,* 32(7), 96.

Dirkes, S., & Winklerprins, A. (2002). Help for ARDS patients. *RN, 65*(8), 52–58.

Dunn, N. (2001). Keeping COPD patients out of the ED. *RN, 64(2),* 33–37.

Eckler, J. (2002). Keeping pulmonary tuberculosis at bay. *Nursing2002, 32*(12), 70.

Ellmers, K., & Criddle, L. (2002). Cystic fibrosis. *RN, 65*(9), 60–66.

Estes, M. E. Z. (2010). *Health assessment & physical examination* (4th ed.). Clifton Park, NY: Delmar Cengage Learning.

Finesilver, C. (2001). Perfecting your skills: Respiratory assessment. *Travel Nurse Today supplement to RN* (April) 16–26.

Georgetown University Hospital. (2009). Neck dissection patient information. Retrieved July 17, 2009 from http://www.georgetownuniversityhospital.org/body.cfm?id=1016#3

Goodfellow, L., & Jones, M. (2002). Bronchial hygiene therapy. *AJN, 102*(1), 37–43.

Hayes, D. (2001). Stemming the tide of pleural effusions. *Nursing2001, 31*(5), 49–52.

Lazzara, D. (2001). Respiratory distress. *Nursing2001, 31*(6), 58–63.

Lazzara, D. (2002). Eliminate the air of mystery from chest tubes. *Nursing2002, 32*(6), 36–43.

Lindell, K., & Jacobs, S. (2003). Idiopathic pulmonary fibrosis. *AJN, 103*(4), 32–41.

Little, C. (2002). Chronic bronchitis. *Nursing2001, 32*(9), 52–55.

Marion, B. (2001). A turn for the better: "Prone positioning" of patients with ARDS. *AJN, 101*(5), 26–33.

Marthaler, M., Keresztes, P., & Tazbir, J. (2003). SARS: What have we learned? *RN, 66*(8), 58–66.

Mayo Clinic. (2009). Cystic fibrosis. Retrieved July 20, 2009 from http://www.mayoclinic.com/health/cystic-fibrosis/DS00287

McConnell, E. (2002). Providing tracheostomy care. *Nursing2002, 32*(1), 17.

Miracle, V. (2002). Asthma attack. *Nursing2002, 32*(11), 104.

Moorhead, S., Johnson, M., Maas, M., & Swanson, E. (2007). *Nursing Outcomes Classification (NOC)* (4th ed.). St. Louis, MO: Mosby.

National Cancer Institute. (2009). Metastatic squamous neck cancer with occult primary treatment (PDQ). Retrieved July 17, 2009 from http://www.cancer.gov/cancertopics/pdq/treatment/metastatic-squamous-neck/Patient/page4

National Heart Lung and Blood Institute (NHLBI). (2009a). COPD: what causes COPD? Retrieved April 11, 2009 from http://www.nhlbi.nih.gov/health/dci/Diseases/Copd/Copd_Causes.html

National Heart Lung and Blood Institute (NHLBI). (2009b). How is pulmonary embolism treated? Retrieved April 11, 2009 from http://www.nhlbi.nih.gov/health/dci/Diseases/pe/pe_treatments.html

National Heart Lung and Blood Institute (NHLBI). (2009c). Who is at risk for pulmonary embolism? Retrieved April 11, 2009 from http://www.nhlbi.nih.gov/health/dci/Diseases/pe/pe_risk.html

National Institute of Allergy and Infectious Diseases. (2009). Flu (influenza). Retrieved July 20, 2009 from http://www3.niaid.nih.gov/topics/Flu/understandingFlu/DefinitionsOverview.htm

National Institutes of Health(NIH). (2009a). Fact sheet: Cystic fibrosis. Retrieved July 20, 2009 from http://www.nih.gov/about/researchresultsforthepublic/CysticFibrosis.pdf

National Institutes of Health (NIH). (2009b). Pleural disorders. Retrieved April 11, 2009 from http://www.nlm.nih.gov/medlineplus/pleuraldisorders.html

National Institutes of Health (NIH). (2009c). Severe acute respiratory syndrome. Retrieved April 11, 2009 from http://www.nlm.nih.gov/medlineplus/severeacuterespiratorysyndrome.html

Perkins, L., & Shortall, S. (2000). Ventilation without intubation. *RN, 63*(1), 34–38.

Phipps, W., Monahan, P., Sands, J., Marek, J., & Neighbors, M. (2003). *Medical–surgical nursing: Health and illness perspectives* (7th ed.). St. Louis, MO: Mosby.

Pope, B. (2002). Asthma. *Nursing2002, 32*(5), 44–45.

Pullen, R. (2003). Teaching bedside incentive spirometry. *Nursing2003, 33*(8), 24.

Schultz, T. (2002). Community-acquired pneumonia. *Nursing2002, 32*(1), 46–49.

Shortall, S., & Perkins, L. (1999). Interpreting the ins and outs of pulmonary function tests. *Nursing99, 29*(12), 41–47.

Spratto, G., & Woods, A. (2010). *2010 Delmar nurse's drug handbook.* Clifton Park, NY: Delmar Cengage Learning.

Tasota, F., & Davies, P. (2001). Diagnosing pulmonary embolism with spiral CT. *Nursing2001, 31*(5), 75.

Togger, D., & Brenner, P. (2001). Metered dose inhalers. *AJN, 101*(10), 26–32.

Wisniewski, A. (2003). Chronic bronchitis and emphysema: Clearing the air. *Nursing2003, 33*(5), 46–49.

Woods, A. (2002). Pneumonia. *Nursing2002, 32*(11), 56–57.

World Health Organization (WHO). (2009). Severe acute respiratory Syndrome. Retrieved April 11, 2009 from www.who.int/csr/sars/travel/en/index.html

Zorb, S. (2002). Transplantation offers hope. *RN, 65(9)*, 66–68.

RESOURCES

American Cancer Society (ACS),
http://www.cancer.org

American Lung Association,
http://www.lungusa.org

American Thoracic Society,
http://www.thoracic.org

Centers for Disease Control and Prevention (CDC),
http://www.cdc.gov

Cystic Fibrosis Foundation,
http://www.cff.org

International Association of Laryngectomees,
http://www.theial.com/ial/

CHAPTER 36
Cardiovascular System

MAKING THE CONNECTION

Refer to the following chapters to increase your understanding of the cardiovascular system:

Basic Nursing
- ***Wellness Concepts***
- ***Fluid, Electrolyte, and Acid–Base Balance***
- ***Assessment***
- ***Pain Management***
- ***Diagnostic Tests***

Adult Health Nursing
- ***Respiratory System***
- ***Hematologic and Lymphatic Systems***
- ***Endocrine System***

Basic Procedures
- ***Hand Hygiene***
- ***Use of Protective Equipment***
- ***Taking a Pulse***
- ***Taking Blood Pressure***
- ***Weighing a Client, Mobile and Immobile***
- ***Ambulation Safety and Assisting from Bed to Walking***
- ***Applying Antiembolic Stockings***

Delmar's Heart & Lung Sounds on StudyWare™: Heart Sounds

LEARNING OBJECTIVES

Upon completion of this chapter, you should be able to:

- Define key terms.
- Describe the anatomy and physiology of the cardiovascular system.
- Relate laboratory results to each disorder.
- Describe basic heart dysrhythmias.
- Explain the pathophysiology of each disorder.
- Describe nursing interventions in caring for clients with cardiovascular conditions.

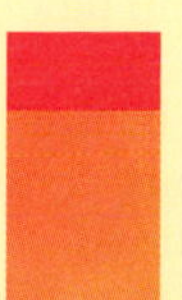

KEY TERMS

aneurysm
angina pectoris
annulus
arteriosclerosis
ascites
atherosclerosis
baseline level
bradycardia
cardiac cycle

cardiac output (CO)
cardiac tamponade
depolarization
dyspnea
dysrhythmia
embolus
heart sound
hemolysis
Homans' sign
hypertrophy
implantable cardioverter-defibrillator (ICD)
myocardial infarction
myocarditis
necrosis
orthopnea
palpitation
paroxysmal nocturnal dyspnea
pericardial friction rub
pericardiocentesis
pericarditis
peripheral resistance
phlebitis
phlebothrombosis
primary hypertension
repolarization
sclerotherapy
secondary hypertension
stasis dermatitis
stent
stroke volume (SV)
tachycardia
thrombectomy
thrombophlebitis
thrombosis
thrombus
transesophageal echocardiography (TEE)
varicosities
vasoconstrict
vasodilate
vein ligation
vein stripping
Virchow's triad

INTRODUCTION

Since 1900, heart disease has been the leading cause of death in the United States every year except in 1918 during the flu epidemic (AHA, 2007a). In 2003, 911,163 deaths were attributed to cardiovascular disease (CVD) compared to 869,724 deaths in 2007 (AHA, 2007a). The death rate for cardiovascular disease is declining because of public education in modifying and decreasing risk factors such as smoking, high-fat diets, and minimal exercise.

This chapter reviews the anatomy and physiology of the cardiovascular system. Pathophysiology, medical management, and nursing interventions related to cardiovascular conditions are discussed with an emphasis on decreasing risk factors and improving lifestyles.

ANATOMY AND PHYSIOLOGY REVIEW

The cardiovascular system consists of the heart and its vasculature and the peripheral vascular system. The heart is located in the lower anterior area of the mediastinum with the apex near the diaphragm. The heart apex tips forward and to the left of the client's chest cavity. In an average lifetime, the heart will pump 80 million gallons of blood.

The peripheral vascular system consists of arteries, arterioles, capillaries, venules, and veins. The arteries carry oxygenated blood away from the left side of the heart to the body tissues, and the veins carry deoxygenated blood back to the right side of the heart. The capillaries connect the arterioles to the venules. The venules and veins contain 60% to 70% of the body's total blood volume.

The cardiovascular system provides oxygen, nutrients, and hormones to the cells and removes carbon dioxide and waste products of cellular metabolism from body cells. Body temperature is maintained by the distribution of heat throughout the body produced by the metabolic activity of muscles and other body organs.

STRUCTURE OF THE HEART

The heart is encapsulated by a protective sac called the pericardium and consists of three layers: endocardium, myocardium, and epicardium. The endocardium is made of endothelium cells that line the inside of the heart, the four heart valves, and is continuous with the endothelial lining of the arteries, capillaries, and veins making the circulatory system a closed system. Therefore, if a person has a systemic blood infection the heart lining and valves are also affected. The myocardium consists of striated muscle and varies in thickness depending on the heart chamber. The left ventricle pumps blood to the body and is, therefore, the thickest chamber. The outside of the heart is surrounded by the epicardium. The pericardium consists of two layers: the parietal pericardium and visceral pericardium. The parietal layer (outer layer) is a fibrous loose sac that surrounds the heart and the visceral layer lines the great vessels and is also called the epicardium when it lines the heart. The pericardial space is between the two pericardium layers and is filled with fluid (see figure 36-1).

The heart is a hollow muscular organ containing four chambers that fill and empty of blood with each contraction (**depolarization**) and recovery phase (**repolarization**) of the cardiac muscle. The upper chambers are the atria and the lower chambers are the ventricles (Figure 36-1). When the atria contract, blood is forced into the ventricles. Contraction of the right ventricle pumps blood into the pulmonary arteries and on to the lungs (pulmonary circulatory system). Contraction of the left ventricle pumps blood into the aorta and out to the entire body (systemic circulatory system). The myocardium of the left ventricle is thicker than the right ventricle because more force is needed to pump blood throughout the body.

There are four valves in the heart: tricuspid, bicuspid (mitral), pulmonic, and aortic. One end of fibrous cords called *chordae tendineae* is attached to the cusps of the tricuspid and mitral valves, and the other end is attached to papillary muscles on the ventricular walls. The chordae tendineae keep the valves from inverting when the ventricles contract, thus preventing blood from flowing back into the atrium.

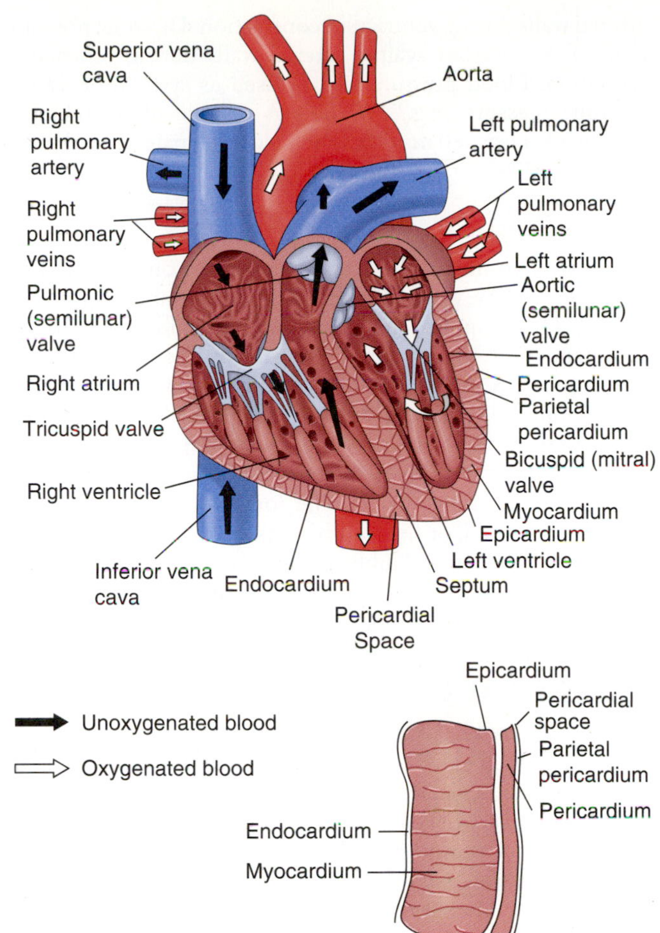

FIGURE 36-1 Internal View of the Heart with Aorta, Vena Cava, and Pulmonary Arteries and Veins

The pulmonic and aortic valves prevent blood from flowing back into the ventricles from the pulmonary artery and aorta during repolarization.

CIRCULATION OF BLOOD

Blood enters the heart through veins and leaves the heart through arteries. With the contraction of the right ventricle, blood is forced through the pulmonic valve into the pulmonary artery. Blood circulates through the pulmonary circulatory system, where carbon dioxide is exchanged for oxygen in the lungs. The blood then returns to the left atrium through the pulmonary veins, providing oxygenated blood for systemic circulation. When the left ventricle contracts, blood is forced through the aortic valve into the aorta, beginning systemic circulation. Blood is then distributed throughout the body and returns to the right atrium of the heart through the inferior and superior vena cava.

STROKE VOLUME AND CARDIAC OUTPUT

Heart rate (HR) is the number of ventricular contractions per minute as determined by auscultation of the heart or palpation of a pulse. Each time the heart beats, the ventricle pumps 60 to 80 mL of blood. The volume of blood ejected from the left ventricle with each contraction or systole is known as the **stroke volume (SV)**. Normal stroke volume is approximately 70 mL. The amount of blood ejected in 1 minute is known as the **cardiac output (CO)**. Therefore, CO is determined by multiplying HR for 1 minute by the stroke volume (CO = HR × SV) (Bender, 2008). If the heart has a strong ventricular contraction, more blood is pumped by the heart into the systemic circulatory system. Therefore, CO has a direct effect on the circulating volume of arterial blood.

CORONARY ARTERIES

Coronary arteries supply nutrients and oxygen to the muscle tissue of the heart. The two coronary arteries, which branch off the aorta, are the right coronary artery and the left coronary artery (Figure 36-2). The right coronary artery divides into the posterior descending artery (interventricular artery) and the marginal artery and supplies blood to the anterior area of the right and left ventricles, the posterior area of the right ventricle, the AV node, and the posterior section of the interventricular septum. The left coronary artery divides into the anterior descending artery and the circumflex artery. The left anterior descending (LAD) artery supplies blood to the anterior section of the interventricular septum, anterior area of the left ventricle, and the lateral aspect of the left ventricle. The circumflex artery nourishes the left atrium and ventricle.

CONDUCTION SYSTEM

The specialized cardiac muscle cells are capable of conducting electrical impulses from one part of the heart to another. For the heart to beat regularly in a rhythmic sequence, electrical impulses follow a set pattern through the conduction system of the heart. The conduction system, consisting of the sinoatrial node (SA node), atrioventricular node (AV node), bundle of His, bundle branches, and Purkinje fibers, controls the heartbeat (Figure 36-3).

The SA node located in the superior aspect of the right atrium initiates electrical impulses that cause the heart

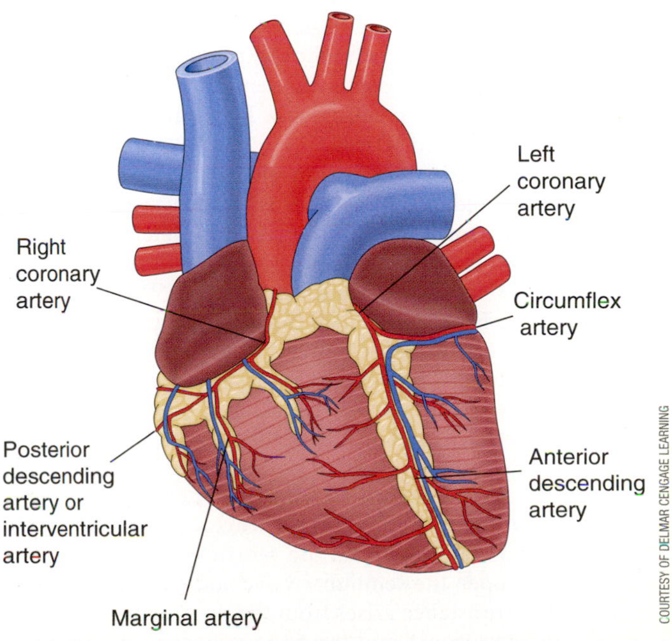

FIGURE 36-2 Coronary Arteries that Supply Blood to the Heart Tissue

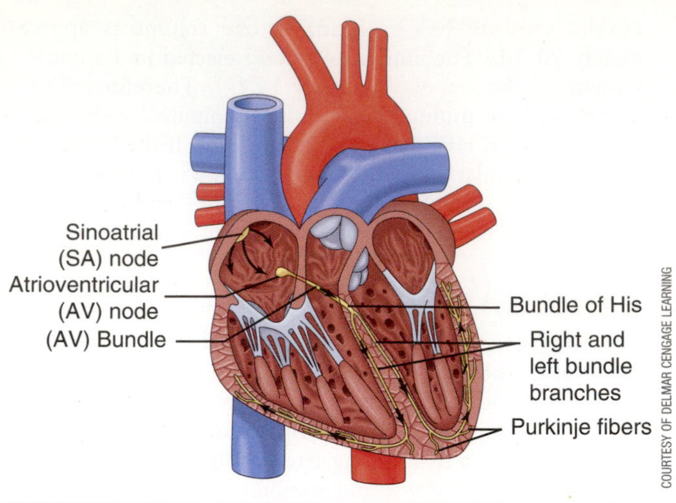

FIGURE 36-3 Conduction System of the Heart

to beat. It is called the pacemaker of the heart. Electrical impulses from the SA node pass through the muscle fibers of the right and left atria, causing the atria to contract almost simultaneously. Atrial impulses are transmitted to the AV node located in the lower part of the right atrium. There is a short delay in the impulse at the AV node that allows the atria to complete their contraction and empty the blood into the ventricles. The electrical impulse is transmitted from the AV node into a group of specialized conduction fibers called the AV bundle or the bundle of His. Once the impulse leaves the AV node, it travels down the fibers of the bundle of His into the interventricular septum. The fibers separate into right and left bundle branches dividing into smaller and smaller branches, called Purkinje fibers. These terminate in the ventricular muscle, causing the ventricles to contract. When an impulse has completely gone through the conduction system of the heart and the ventricles have contracted, a **cardiac cycle** is completed.

The end-diastolic volume (EDV) is the amount of blood in the ventricles after the ventricular rest and filling phase of the cardiac cycle. In the healthy heart, the EDV is usually around 120 mL. The end-systolic volume (ESV) is the amount of blood in the ventricles after the ventricular contraction and ejection phase of the cardiac cycle. In the healthy heart, the ESV is usually around 50 mL.

Ejection fraction (EF) is an indicator of ventricle functioning and is reduced in patients with myocardial infarction and diagnostic for heart failure (HF). To determine the EF, stroke volume is divided by end-diastolic volume (EF = SV/EDV). In healthy hearts, the EF is between 50% and 70% of the EDV. The EF is determined through echocardiography.

Four factors influence stroke volume and CO: preload, afterload, contractility, and HR. **Preload** refers to the amount of pressure within the ventricles. This is determined by the amount of stretch or tension derived from the ventricular filling and the pressure exerted by fluid volume on the myocardium at the end of diastole (ventricular end-diastolic pressure), or just before contraction. **Afterload** is the force that resists ejection of blood from the ventricles, or the force that is needed to open the semilunar valve and eject blood during systole. This resistance arises from the pulmonary circulation for the right ventricle, and from the systemic circulation for the left ventricle. **Contractility** refers to the strength of cardiac contraction. Systolic pressure is the force exerted against arterial walls during ventricular contraction. Diastolic pressure is the force exerted against arterial walls during ventricular relaxation. Blood pressure is expressed as systolic pressure/diastolic pressure (e.g., 120/80). A systolic blood pressure reading of at least 80 mm Hg is needed to palpate a radial pulse (Bender, 2008).

Heart Sounds

There are two normal **heart sounds** heard on auscultation; S_1 and S_2. They yield a sound like "lubb-dubb." S_1, or the "lubb," is the sound of the mitral and tricuspid valves closing simultaneously. The S_1 sound is heard on the left fifth intercostal space. S_2, or the "dubb," is the simultaneous closing of the pulmonic and aortic valves, heard on the right second intercostal space. There is a slight pause after the "lubb-dubb" is heard. Clients with congestive heart failure (CHF) may have a third sound known as S_3. The low-pitched sound occurs after the S_2 sound, or the "dubb," making the heart sound like the word "Kentucky" ("lubb-dubb-by"). The S_3 sound also is described as a gallop because of the similarity in sound to a horse's gallop.

ARTERIOLES AND ARTERIES

The arteries are thick-walled tubes consisting of three layers or tunics (Figure 36-4). The inner layer is called the *tunica intima* and consists of a single layer of smooth endothelial cells. The middle layer is the *tunica media* and is composed of smooth muscle cells. The smooth muscle layer of the artery receives nerve stimulation from the sympathetic nervous system. The suppleness of the smooth muscle allows the vessel to **vasoconstrict** (decrease in diameter) and **vasodilate** (increase in diameter). The outer layer, the *tunica adventitia* or *tunica externa*, consists of a connective tissue sheath with some of its collagen fibers fusing with those of the surrounding tissue to hold the vessels in place. The elastic connective tissue allows the artery to expand and recoil with each contraction of the ventricle as an increased volume of blood is pumped through the vessel. The arteries have thick walls, so they can withstand the increased pressure from the left ventricle pumping blood through the body.

The arteries divide and branch into smaller vessels called *arterioles*. The same three layers are present in the walls, but as the arterioles approach the capillaries their walls become

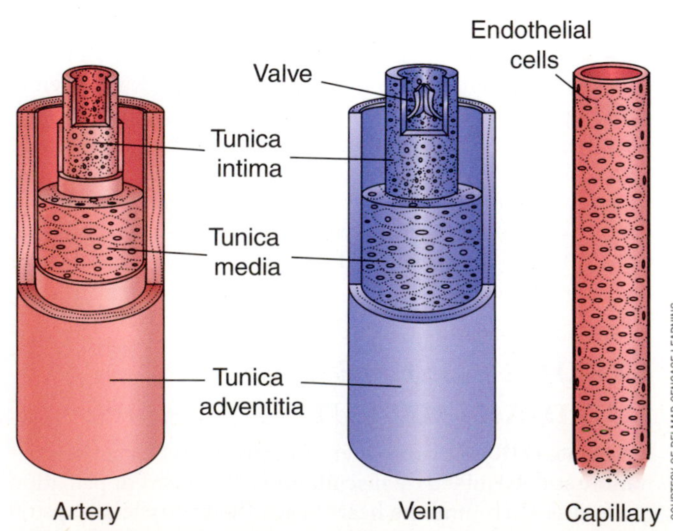

FIGURE 36-4 Tunic Layers of Each Type of Vessel

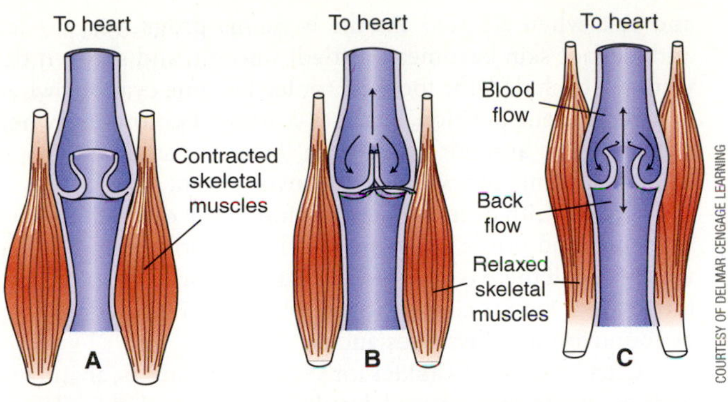

FIGURE 36-5 Valves in the veins hold the blood at a certain level in the vein. *A*, Contracted skeletal muscles apply pressure to veins and assist with the circulation of blood. *B*, Valves prevent the backflow of blood. *C*, Incompetent valves allow a backflow of blood.

thinner. The outer layer is reduced to a very thin layer of connective tissue.

CAPILLARIES

Capillaries are very tiny thin vessels that connect the smallest arterioles with the smallest venules. They have only one layer of endothelial cells whose cell membranes are the semipermeable membrane that allows the exchange of oxygen, nutrients, carbon dioxide, and waste products between the tissues of the body and the blood.

VENULES AND VEINS

Venules are small vessels that emerge from the capillaries and gradually increase in size to eventually form veins. Veins have three layers or tunics like the arteries, but the middle layer of a vein is thinner with less smooth muscle and elastic tissue. The elasticity of the smooth muscles allow the walls of the veins to dilate more easily. Endothelial flaps, called *valves*, are on the inside lining of veins. The valves open and close with each contraction of the surrounding skeletal muscles. The valves assist the blood in returning to the heart. Blood is held by the valves until skeletal muscle contractions move the blood toward the heart against gravity (Figure 36-5).

HEALTH HISTORY

There are three goals when obtaining a health history from a client: (1) identify present and potential health problems, (2) identify possible familial and lifestyle risk factors, and (3) involve the client in planning long-term health care.

Ascertain the onset of the symptoms, the predisposing factors that cause the symptoms, and the client's treatment of the symptoms. Ask about the client's activity level or limitations in activity. Determine if appetite has increased or decreased. Evaluate the client's ability to sleep, the need for the trunk of the body to be supported with pillows when sleeping, or the need to sleep in a chair.

Major risk factors associated with cardiovascular diseases are age, gender, heredity (including race), smoking, dyslipidemia (presence of increased total serum cholesterol and low-density lipoprotein [LDL]), high blood pressure, physical inactivity, overweight, obesity, and diabetes mellitus. An individual's response to stress may be a contributing factor. Additional contributing factors for women include menopause, use of birth control pills, and high triglyceride level.

Advancing age, male gender, diabetes, heredity, and family history of chest pain or myocardial infarctions are risk factors that cannot be altered. Alterable risk factors are physical inactivity, smoking, contraceptive method, dyslipidemia, overweight, obesity, and triglyceride level. A change in diet may alter the last four factors.

There are two objectives in assisting the client toward a healthier lifestyle: (1) to educate the client about the risk factors; and (2) to determine what risk factors the client would like to modify. Once this is determined, assist the client to establish goals and determine actions to achieve the goals.

ASSESSMENT

Assessment includes clients' self-report of symptoms as well as physical findings and confirming lab data.

SUBJECTIVE DATA

The typical concerns expressed by a client with a cardiac disorder are chest pain, **dyspnea** (difficulty breathing), edema, fainting, palpitations, diaphoresis, and fatigue. When a client talks about having chest pain, ascertain the time of onset, situation occurring at the onset of pain, location and radiation of pain, severity of chest pain, duration, past episodes of chest pain, and methods used to alleviate pain. Using the Memory Trick: Pain Assessment PQRST is an ideal way for a nurse to assess a client's pain. This method is described in the Memory Trick: Pain Assessment PQRST. Women are more likely to experience shortness of breath, fatigue, back or jaw pain, and atypical discomfort such as a feeling of indigestion or nausea and vomiting (Nagle & Nee, 2002; AHA, 2007b).

The client may be experiencing several types of dyspnea. Exertional dyspnea occurs when a person participates in moderate activity and becomes short of breath. This occurs in the early stages of HF and indicates that the heart is not able to meet the demands of the body during moderate activity. **Orthopnea** is when a client has difficulty breathing while lying down and must sit upright or stand to relieve the

MEMORYTRICK

Pain Assessment PQRST

P = Provoker of pain (aggravating factors) and palliative measures (alleviating factors)

Q = Quality of pain (gnawing, pounding, burning, stabbing, pinching, aching, throbbing, and crushing)

R = Region (location) and radiation to other body sites

S = Severity (quantity of pain on 0–10 scale, 0 = no pain and 10 = worst pain experienced) and setting (what causes the pain)

T = Timing (onset, duration, and frequency)

(Adapted from Estes, 2010)

dyspnea. This occurs in a more advanced stage of HF. **Paroxysmal nocturnal dyspnea** usually occurs 2 to 5 hours after an individual falls asleep. The person suddenly awakens, is sweating, and has difficulty breathing.

A client has fainting spells for various physical and psychological reasons. Cardiac clients faint because of decreased CO causing decreased blood flow to the brain.

A client may describe a "fluttering" or "pounding" sensation in the chest. This is known as **palpitations**. If these sensations occur during exercise, it is a sign that the heart has to work harder to meet the demands of the body. Palpitations may also be caused by anxiety, ingestion of a large meal, lack of adequate rest, or a large intake of caffeine.

A cardiac client will usually experience fatigue increasing throughout the day because the heart is not able to keep up with the demands of the body. Frequent rest periods will help alleviate some of the fatigue.

The typical concerns expressed by the client with a peripheral vascular disorder are pain, paresthesia (decreased sensation in an area), and/or paralysis in the hands, thigh, calf, ankles, foot, abdomen, or lower back. The quality of pain (aching, cramping, sharp, or throbbing) and any numbness or tingling is noted.

OBJECTIVE DATA

In a head-to-toe assessment on a cardiac client, the skin, neck veins, respirations, heart sounds, abdomen, and extremities are carefully assessed. Observe the skin for cyanosis in the earlobes, lips, mucous membranes, and finger-and toenails. Assessment of skin turgor may indicate fluid volume. If the skin is dry and has poor turgor, the client may be dehydrated from diuretics. If a client has distended internal and external jugular veins when the head of the bed is gradually elevated to a 45-degree angle or higher, there may be right-sided HF. Assess the quality of respirations for rate and ease of breathing, signs of dyspnea, and coughing. Heart sounds are assessed for the normal S_1 and S_2 sounds. If the typical lubb-dubb is heard, the valves are closing properly.

While listening to the heart, the radial pulse should be palpated to account for every heartbeat. If a heartbeat is heard through the stethoscope but not felt in the radial pulse, the heart has decreased CO to the extremities. If the abdomen is distended, the client may have **ascites**, which is excess fluid in the abdomen. After assessing the heart and lung sounds, check the peripheral pulses. Pulses on both sides of the body should be checked at the same time to determine adequate bilateral perfusion. It is important to check pedal pulses in both feet to determine blood flow to each foot. Pulse amplitude can be described as absent, diminished, normal, increased, and bounding (Gehring, 2002).

If the hands and feet are cold or have mottling, this indicates decreased CO. Capillary refill should be less than 3 seconds in the fingers and toes.

Note if the feet, ankles, or legs are edematous (Figure 36-6). A client may gain 10 pounds before edema is detected. Weigh cardiac clients with edema daily. The weight must be taken on the same scale, at the same time of day, with the client wearing the same amount of clothing.

Decreased circulation to an area results in coolness in the ischemic area, pallor, paresthesia, and paralysis. Paresthesia and paralysis result from a lack of oxygenated blood and nourishment to the nerves. Symptoms of paresthesia are numbness and tingling.

If an artery in the leg is occluded, the foot and/or leg become reddish in color when the leg is in a dependent position, and pale when elevated. As the ischemia progresses, the leg and/or foot skin becomes mottled, smooth, and shiny. If the veins are occluded, the foot and/or leg become cyanotic when in a dependent position, and has a normal coloration when elevated. The anterior area of the lower leg and ankle has a brown pigmentation with venous involvement.

Clients with decreased circulation to the extremities have hardened and brittle nails and less hair distribution. The leg will be cool if there is an arterial circulatory problem but warm if there is a venous circulatory problem. Skin ulcerations may be found around the ankles and toes.

Check the client's ankles for **stasis dermatitis**, an inflammation of the skin caused by decreased circulation. Waste products that normally are carried away by the circulatory system remain in the tissues, causing pruritus and irritation of the skin. At first, the ankle area is reddened and edematous, then vesicles form and start oozing. The skin becomes crusted, thickened, and brown.

A positive **Homans' sign** is present in some cases of deep vein thrombosis (DVT). To test for Homans' sign, dorsiflex the client's foot. If there is pain in the calf of the leg or behind the knee, the Homans' sign is positive and may indicate the presence of a venous clot. Do not do a Homans' sign if there is a diagnosis of a thrombus, because the clot may be dislodged with the procedure.

Refer to Box 36-1, "Questions to Ask and Observations to Make When Collecting Data" for guidance in completing client cardiac assessments.

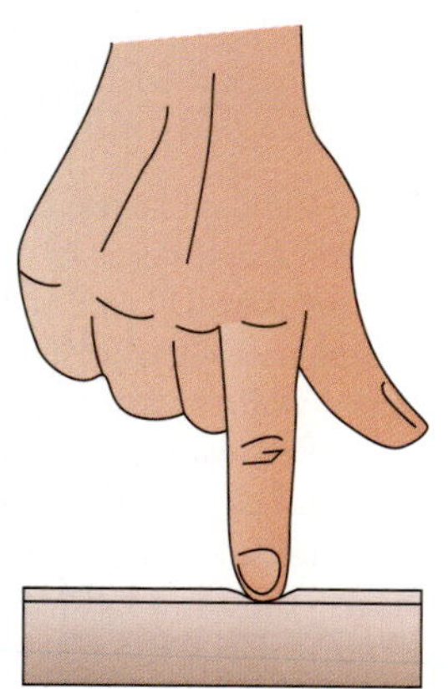

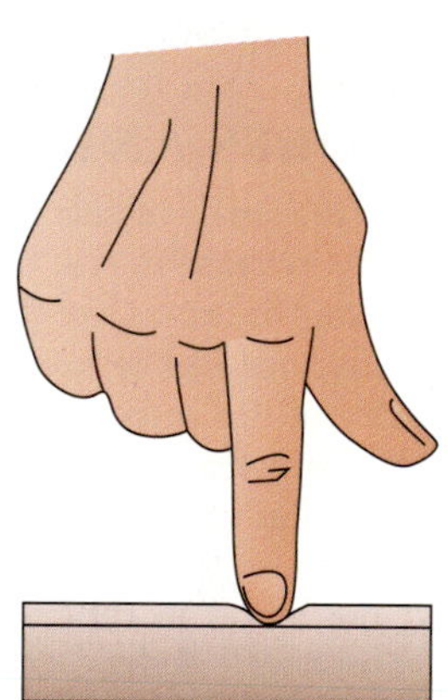

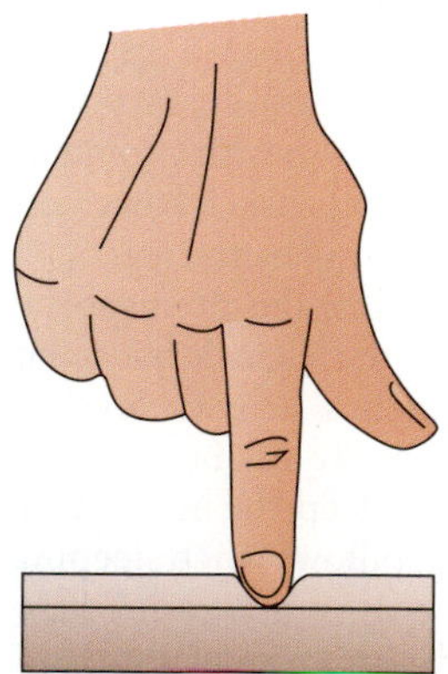

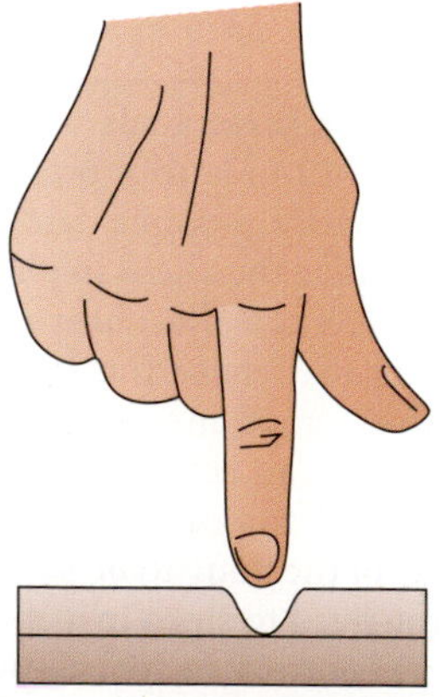

COURTESY OF DELMAR CENGAGE LEARNING

FIGURE 36-6 Edema Rating Scale: Press down for 5 seconds, then time how long indentation remains.

BOX 36-1 QUESTIONS TO ASK AND OBSERVATIONS TO MAKE WHEN COLLECTING DATA

SUBJECTIVE DATA

Have you experienced chest pain? Radiating pain? Nausea? Indigestion? Fatigue?

What activities cause chest pain?

Have you felt palpitations or your heart flutter?

Do you ever feel dizzy or lightheaded?

Tell me about your memory.

On how many pillows do you sleep?

Do you awaken short of breath?

List prescription and over the counter medications you are taking.

Do you use any herbal supplements?

Describe your daily exercise habits.

Are you on any specific type of diet?

Do you weigh yourself at regular intervals? Have you noticed a weight gain of 5 pounds or more from one day to the next?

How often do you urinate during the daytime? During the night?

Are you sexually active? Have there been any changes in the last year?

Do you experience swelling in your feet or ankles?

Can you climb a flight of stairs without becoming short of breath?

Can you walk a block without feeling cramps in your legs?

How do you cope with stress?

How do you relax?

OBJECTIVE DATA

Take vital signs; temperature, pulse, respirations, and pulse oximetry.

Check pupils.

Check capillary refill.

Check the skin, lips, fingers, and feet for cyanosis.

Listen to the apical pulse and palpate the radial pulse at the same time.

Listen to breath sounds on anterior and posterior aspects of chest

Listen to bowel sounds.

Palpate abdomen for edema or tautness.

Examine legs, ankles, and feet for swelling.

Examine legs for hair distribution.

Check for areas for decreased sensation.

Check peripheral pulses noting the quality, rhythm, and amplitude.

Check extremities for areas of brownish discoloration, ulcerations, and bruising.

Complete a Homans' sign.

COMMON DIAGNOSTIC TESTS

Commonly used diagnostic tests for clients with symptoms of cardiovascular system disorders are listed in Table 36-1. Cardiac biomarkers that diagnose, evaluate, and monitor clients with possible acute coronary syndrome (ACS) are troponin I, troponin T, CK, CK-MB, and myoglobin. AST and LDH are not specific for heart damage and are not recommended for clients suspected with ACS (American Association for Clinical Chemistry, 2008). Troponins are replacing CK and CK-MB in some settings because they are more specific for heart injury (versus skeletal muscle injury) and are elevated for a longer period of time. Troponins elevate within 3–4 hours after injury and may remain elevated for 10–14 days (see Table 36-2 for elevation times of biomarkers). The greater the tissue damage the greater the elevation. Muscular injection, strenuous exercise and drugs that affect muscles do not elevate troponin levels as they do with CK (Bender, 2008). Other general tests ordered with cardiac biomarkers are ABGs, comprehensive metabolic panel, basic metabolic panel, electrolytes, and CBC.

A newer cardiac biomarker test used with troponin and an ECG to identify clients at a greater risk of an MI is ischemia modified albumin (IMA). If IMA is not present in a client who has experienced chest pain for a few minutes to a few hours, it is not likely that the client has ischemia. IMA is not as valuable with a client who has experienced chest pain for several hours because the IMA level may have risen and returned to normal within that time frame.

CARDIAC RHYTHM/ DYSRHYTHMIA

As a basis for understanding cardiac dysrhythmias, the normal sinus rhythm must first be understood.

NORMAL SINUS RHYTHM

The electrical conduction of the heart begins with the SA (refer to Figure 36-7) node located in the superior section of the right atrium. From the SA node, the electrical impulse spreads in wave fashion through the atria similar to the ripples from a pebble dropped in water. The firing of the SA node and the electrical impulse spreading across both atria yields a P wave on the ECG. The P wave represents the electrical activity causing the contraction of both atria.

After the atria contract, the electrical impulse reaches the AV node, where it pauses for approximately one-tenth of a second, allowing blood to enter both ventricles. The electrical impulse then starts down the AV bundle that divides into right and left bundle branches in the interventricular septum. The electrical impulse continues from the right and the left bundle branches to the Purkinje fibers that transmit the electrical impulse to the myocardial cells resulting in depolarization or contraction of the ventricles. On an ECG the QRS complex represents the electrical impulse as it travels through the AV node, AV bundle, bundle branches, Purkinje fibers, and myocardial cells, ending with the

TABLE 36-1 Common Diagnostic Tests for Cardiovascular System Disorders

Laboratory Tests
- Arterial blood gasses (ABGs)
- Basic metabolic panel (BMP)
- Cardiac biomarkers
  - Creatine kinase (CK)
  - CK-MB (CK_2)
  - High-sensitivity C-reactive protein (hs-CRP)
  - B-type natriuretic peptide (BNP)
  - N-terminal pro BNP (NT-pro-BNP)
  - Troponin
  - Myoglobin
  - Ischemia-Modified Albumin (IMA)
- Complete blood count (CBC)
- Comprehensive metabolic panel (CMP)
- Cystatin C
- Platelet count
- Hemoglobin (Hgb)
- Hematocrit (Hct)
- Electrolytes
- Erythrocyte sedimentation rate (ESR)
- Glomerular filtration rate (GFR)
- Glucose
- Glycosylated hemoglobin (HbA_1c)
- Liver function
- Prothrombin time (PT)
- Partial thromboplastin time (PTT)
- International normalized ratio (INR)
- Serum lipids (lipid profile)
  - Cholesterol
  - High-density lipoprotein (HDL)
  - Low-density lipoprotein (LDL)
  - Very low-density lipoprotein (VLDL)
  - Triglycerides
- Thyroid stimulating hormone (TSH)
- Urinalysis (UA)

Radiologic Tests
- Chest x-ray
- Cardiac positron emission tomography scan
- Radionuclide angiography (multiplegated radioisotope scan, multigated acquisition scanning, MUGA)
- Technetium pyrophosphate scanning
- Thalium scan

Other Diagnostic Tests
- Cardiac biopsy
- Cardiac catheterization
- Echocardiogram
- Electrocardiogram (ECG)
- Holter monitor
- Magnetic resonance imaging (MRI)
- Pericardiocentesis
- Pulse oximetry
- Stress test
- Arterial plethysmography (pulse volume recorder)
- Venous plethysmography (cuff pressure test)

COURTESY OF DELMAR CENGAGE LEARNING

TABLE 36-2 Cardiac Biomarkers Elevation Times

CARDIAC BIOMARKER	ONSET OF ELEVATION	DURATION OF ELEVATION AFTER INJURY
Troponin I	4–6 hours	4–7 days
Troponin T	4–6 hours	10–14 days
Creatine kinase-MB (CK-MB)	4–6 hours	48–72 hours
Myoglobin	Less than 3 hours (Myoglobin is not specific to the heart. However, it is the first biomarker to elevate.)	
Ischemia modified albumin (IMA)	Few minutes to a few hours	IMA is not as valuable with a client who has experienced chest pain for several hours because the IMA level may have risen and returned to normal within that time frame.

COURTESY OF DELMAR CENGAGE LEARNING

ventricles contracting. The Q wave is not always present on the ECG strip.

The pause after the QRS complex is called the ST segment. This represents the period between the contraction and the beginning of the recovery or repolarization of the ventricular muscles. The T wave represents the repolarization of the ventricles.

After the repolarization of the ventricles, the entire cycle begins again at the SA node. In this way the P wave, QRS complex, and T waves are repeated with each

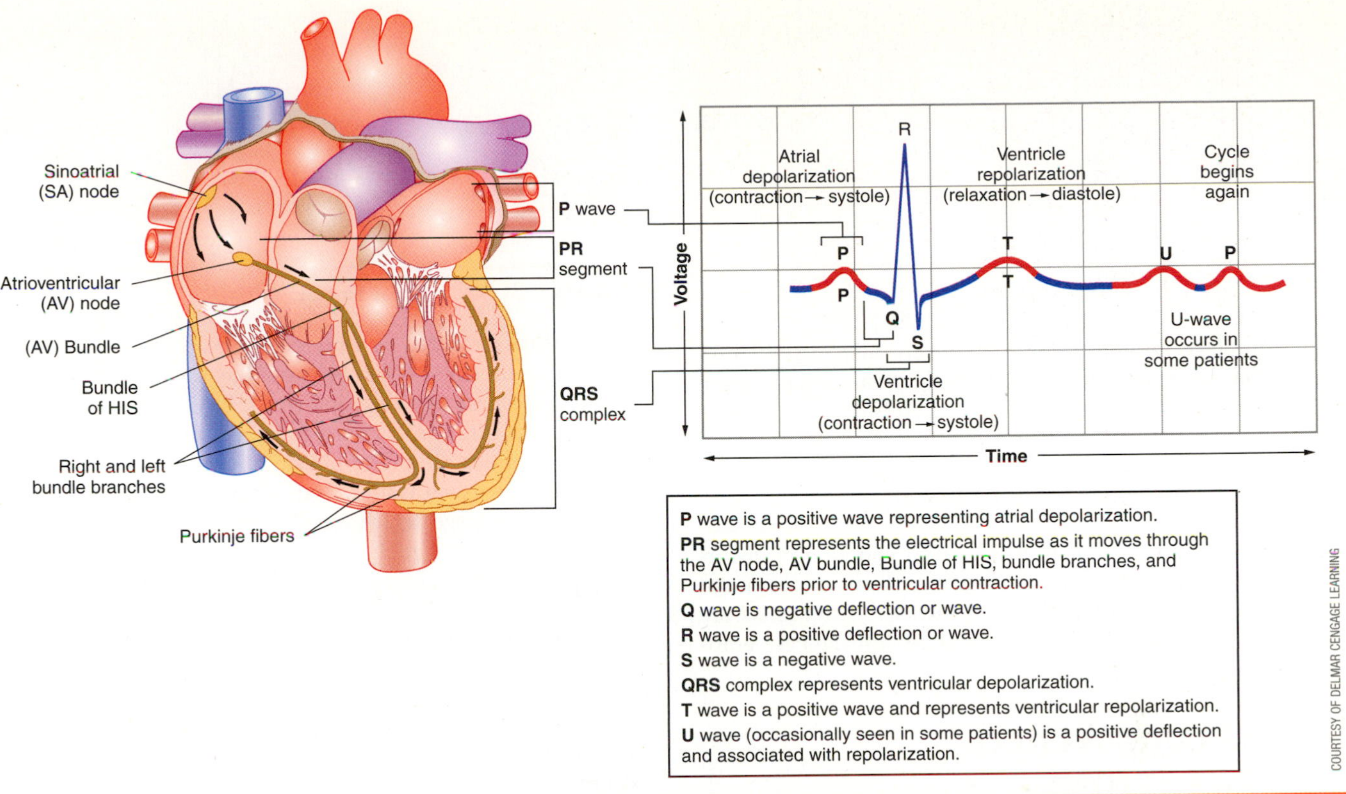
Sinoatrial (SA) node
Atrioventricular (AV) node
(AV) Bundle
Bundle of HIS
Right and left bundle branches
Purkinje fibers
P wave
PR segment
QRS complex
Voltage
Time
Atrial depolarization (contraction → systole)
Ventricle repolarization (relaxation → diastole)
Cycle begins again
Ventricle depolarization (contraction → systole)
U-wave occurs in some patients
R
P
Q
S
T
U
P wave is a positive wave representing atrial depolarization.
PR segment represents the electrical impulse as it moves through the AV node, AV bundle, Bundle of HIS, bundle branches, and Purkinje fibers prior to ventricular contraction.
Q wave is negative deflection or wave.
R wave is a positive deflection or wave.
S wave is a negative wave.
QRS complex represents ventricular depolarization.
T wave is a positive wave and represents ventricular repolarization.
U wave (occasionally seen in some patients) is a positive deflection and associated with repolarization.
COURTESY OF DELMAR CENGAGE LEARNING

FIGURE 36-7 Relationship of the Conduction System to an ECG Strip

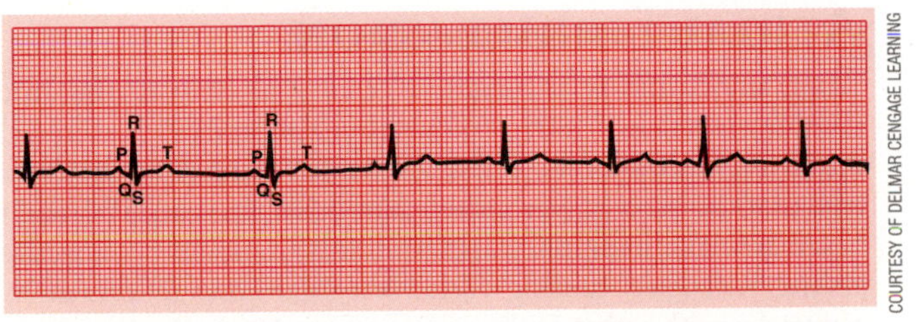
R
P
T
Q
S
COURTESY OF DELMAR CENGAGE LEARNING

FIGURE 36-8 An ECG Strip Showing a Normal Sinus Rhythm with the P Wave, QRS Complex, and T Wave Identified

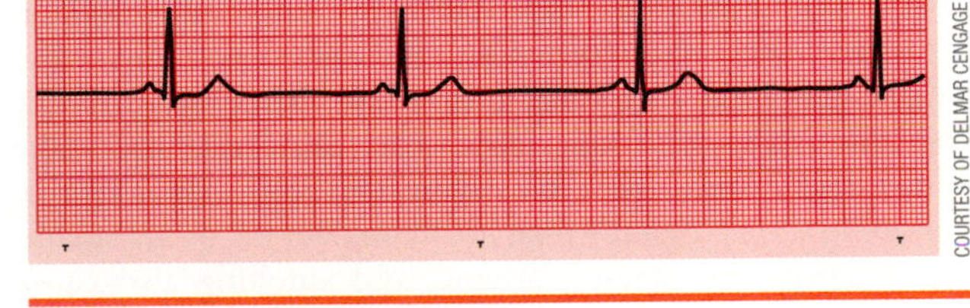
COURTESY OF DELMAR CENGAGE LEARNING

FIGURE 36-9 Sinus Bradycardia

heartbeat. Figure 36-8 shows an ECG strip of normal sinus rhythm.

DYSRHYTHMIAS

A **dysrhythmia** is an irregularity in the rate, rhythm, or conduction of the electrical system of the heart. Dysrhythmia can occur in the atria, ventricles, or any part of the conduction system. Specialized cells in the heart muscle have the ability to generate an electrical impulse. Under certain conditions these cells start sending impulses to other cells in the heart, causing irregular beats called *ectopic beats*. The most common causes of dysrhythmias are coronary artery disease (CAD), CHF, and myocardial infarction (MI). Other causes of dysrhythmias are electrolyte imbalances and drug toxicity.

Symptoms of a client experiencing a dysrhythmia vary from asymptomatic to cardiac arrest. The client experiences fainting, seizures, fatigue, decreased energy level, exertional dyspnea, chest pain, and palpitations.

BRADYCARDIA

Sinus bradycardia is a HR of 60 beats per minute or less (Figure 36-9). Causes of sinus bradycardia are myocardial ischemia, electrolyte imbalances, vagal stimulation, beta blockers, heart block, drug toxicity, intracranial tumors, sleep, and vomiting. The treatment for bradycardia is the administration of atropine. Some clients with bradycardia may require a permanent pacemaker. Asymptomatic bradycardia related to physical fitness is usually not treated.

TACHYCARDIA

Tachycardia is a sinus rhythm with a HR ranging from 100 to 150 beats per minute (Figure 36-10, following page). Causes of tachycardia are exercise, emotional stress, fever, medications, pain, anemia, thyrotoxicosis, pericarditis, HF, excessive caffeine intake, and tobacco use. When the heart is beating at this rate, there is limited time for the ventricles to fill with

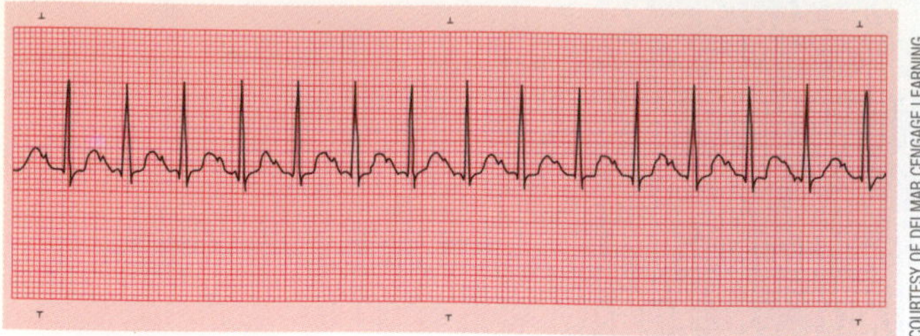

COURTESY OF DELMAR CENGAGE LEARNING

FIGURE 36-10 Sinus Tachycardia

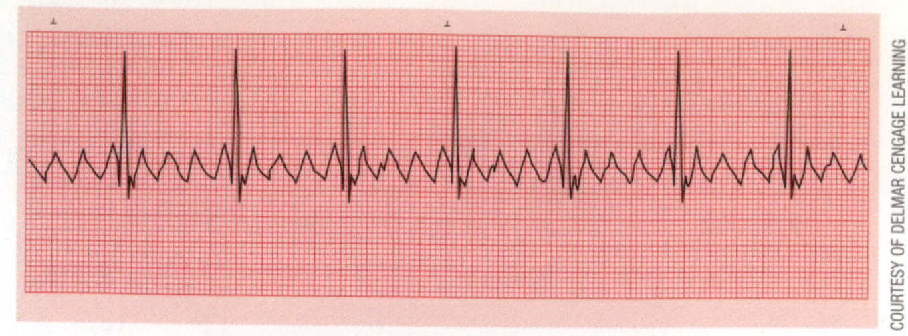

COURTESY OF DELMAR CENGAGE LEARNING

FIGURE 36-11 Atrial Flutter

blood, and less blood is pumped to the coronary arteries and throughout the body. The client may experience anginal pain. The treatment for sinus tachycardia depends on the cause.

ATRIAL DYSRHYTHMIAS

Atrial dysrhythmias occur from electrical conduction disturbances in the atria, resulting in premature beats or abnormal atrial rhythms. Common causes for atrial dysrhythmias are myocardial infarction, CHF, electrolyte imbalances, emotional stress, and drugs.

PREMATURE ATRIAL CONTRACTIONS

A premature atrial contraction (PAC) is an ectopic impulse not originating in the sinoatrial node, but in the atrial tissue. This causes an atrial depolarization to occur earlier in the cycle than expected, thus the term *premature atrial contraction.*

PACs do not cause physical symptoms depending on how often they occur. Generally they are benign and occur several times a day in healthy individuals. If their occurrence causes an increase or decrease in the pulse rate, they should be evaluated. PACs can be a symptom of myocardial ischemia, developing CHF, digitalis toxicity, hypokalemia, or an inflammatory condition. Stress, caffeine, and smoking also cause PACs. PACs can be the first indication that more serious atrial dysrhythmias could occur if not treated properly.

ATRIAL TACHYCARDIA

Atrial tachycardia is an ectopic impulse that causes the atria to contract at the rate of 140 to 250 beats per minute. This is sometimes referred to as a *supraventricular dysrhythmia*, meaning the impulse causing the dysrhythmia is occurring above the ventricles. This dysrhythmia occurs as a continuous rhythm or as short, sudden eruptions that start and end spontaneously.

Atrial tachycardia occurs with hypokalemia, digitalis toxicity, and ischemia. Potassium supplements are given for hypokalemia. If an increased level of serum digitalis is the cause, digitalis is withheld until the level returns to normal. An artificial pacemaker may be surgically inserted to regulate the atrial tachycardia.

PAROXYSMAL SUPRAVENTRICULAR TACHYCARDIA

Paroxysmal supraventricular tachycardia (PSVT) was previously called paroxysmal atrial tachycardia (PAT). PSVT is a rapid atrial beat accompanied by an abnormal conduction in the AV node. The dysrhythmia occurs suddenly (paroxysmally) and is usually initiated by a premature beat. PSVT can stop as abruptly as it begins. It can be caused by myocarditis, caffeine, alcohol ingestion, smoking, and stress. PSVT may also be present in clients with coronary artery disease, mitral valve prolapse, and acute pericarditis. The physician performs vagal stimulation procedures such as the Valsalva maneuver and carotid sinus pressure or massage, which usually stops the dysrhythmia.

ATRIAL FLUTTER

Atrial flutter, a rapid contraction of the atria, yields a HR of 250 to 350 beats per minute (Figure 36-11). The ECG displays a sawtooth wave pattern. The AV node attempts to block some of the atrial impulses, but usually the ventricles are also contracting at a rate of 300 beats per minute. This causes a decreased blood supply to the body because the atria and ventricles are unable to fill with blood when they are contracting at such a fast rate. This requires immediate intervention.

ATRIAL FIBRILLATION

Atrial fibrillation is an erratic electrical activity of the atria, resulting in a rate of 350 to 600 beats per minute (Figure 36-12). Atrial depolarization is so uncoordinated during the dysrhythmia that the atria quiver rather than contract. The AV node is bombarded with impulses and randomly transmits the impulses to the ventricles, causing varied irregular contractions of the ventricles with a ventricular rate of 100 to 180 beats per minute. The underlying cause is mitral valve disease or dysfunction,

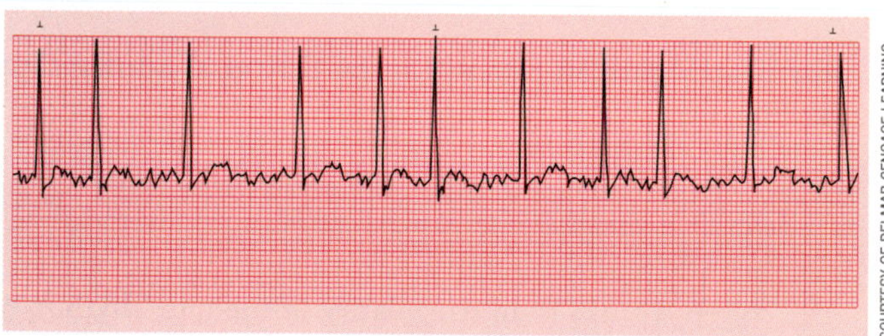

COURTESY OF DELMAR CENGAGE LEARNING

FIGURE 36-12 Atrial Fibrillation

LIFE SPAN CONSIDERATIONS

Antidysrhythmic Medications

Antidysrhythmic medication doses are reduced in the elderly if they have hepatic or renal impairment.

CAD, acute MI, hypertensive heart disease, HF, cardiomyopathy, or hyperthyroidism. Because the atria are not contracting properly, blood pools in the atria, predisposing the person to thrombi forming on the walls of the atria. The clots can dislodge and travel to the brain, lungs, and other parts of the body. Most cardiac clients take a low dose (81 mg) of aspirin daily to prevent clot formation. Once the underlying condition is treated, atrial fibrillation may stop. If the dysrhythmia cannot be controlled with medication, cardioversion may be necessary.

VENTRICULAR DYSRHYTHMIAS

Ventricular dysrhythmias originate in the ventricles. They are more life threatening than atrial dysrhythmias because the ventricles supply blood to the lungs and body. These dysrhythmias must be treated promptly.

PREMATURE VENTRICULAR CONTRACTIONS

Premature ventricular contractions (PVCs) arise from ectopic beats in the ventricles and are the most common ectopic beats (Figure 36-13). PVCs can easily be identified on the ECG because of the wide, bizarre QRS complexes. No P waves precede the QRS complex.

Coronary artery disease is the most common cause of PVCs. Other causes of PVCs are myocardial ischemia, CHF, electrolyte imbalances, digitalis toxicity, anxiety, exercise, hypoxia, caffeine, and excessive alcohol consumption.

If PVCs occur without the presence of other cardiac conditions, there is no treatment other than removing the precipitating cause, such as stress or caffeine. Potassium supplements are given for hypokalemia induced PVCs. Administering oxygen may increase the oxygen perfusion to the myocardial tissue and decrease the frequency of premature beats.

PROFESSIONAL TIP

Six authors from Stanford reported a 7-year study on 1,847 heart failure-free clients in the Archives of Internal Medicine in 2008. Forty-six percent of the clients developed PVCs during exercise and 34% developed PVCs while recovering from the exercise period. Nine percent of these clients died in 5 years. The study conclusion was that clients experiencing PVCs in the recovery or rest period after exercise had an almost "doubled propensity-adjusted mortality rate" (Lundberg, 2008, p. 93).

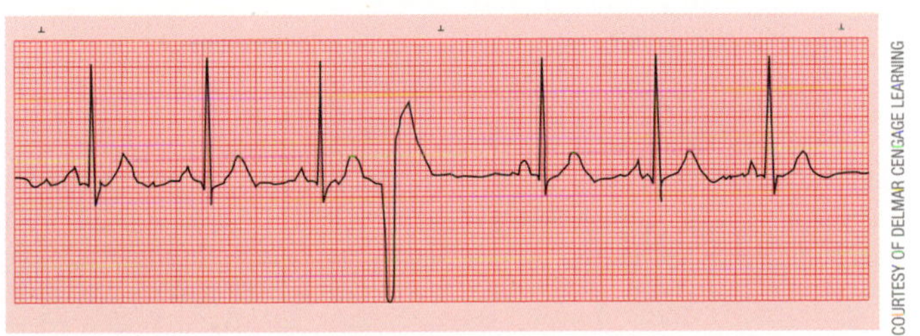

COURTESY OF DELMAR CENGAGE LEARNING

FIGURE 36-13 Premature Ventricular Contraction

VENTRICULAR TACHYCARDIA

Ventricular tachycardia (VT) is the occurrence of three or more consecutive PVCs. The ventricular rate may go as high as 140 to 240 beats per minute. Underlying conditions in which VT occurs are cardiomyopathy, hypoxemia, digitalis toxicity, and electrolyte imbalance.

During VT, the client has a low blood pressure, weak or absent peripheral pulses, body weakness, and may become unconscious. The ventricle is beating so rapidly that it is unable to fill with blood or eject blood properly. This causes blood to back up in the pulmonary circulation, leading to pulmonary congestion.

It is important that VT be treated promptly because a ventricular tachycardia rhythm may lead into ventricular fibrillation, a life-threatening dysrhythmia. The client is given oxygen, and an intravenous line is inserted if one is not already in place. The drug of choice is amiodarone (Cardarone) given intravenously. Lidocaine hydrochloride (Xylocaine HCL), sotalol (Betapace), and magnesium sulfate (Magnesium) may also be given. If the VT is not controlled with medications, the client is cardioverted if peripheral pulses are present, or defibrillated if peripheral pulses are absent.

Cardioversion

Cardioversion is the delivery of a synchronized electrical shock to change a dysrhythmia to a rhythm that circulates more blood to the body tissues and improve oxygenation of the tissues. The electrical shock is delivered on the R wave because a shock during ventricular depolarization may cause ventricular fibrillation. Cardioversion is done as an elective or emergency treatment. Electrodes are placed to the right of the sternum below the clavicle and at the apex of the heart. The electrodes are lubricated with a special gel or placed on gel pads or defibrillator pads. The electrical current delivered through the electrodes depolarizes the myocardium and allows the heart's pacemaker to reestablish a sinus rhythm.

The client is NPO for 8 hours before an elective cardioversion. Diuretics and digitalis preparations are withheld 24 to 72 hours before the cardioversion because they make myocardium cells less responsive to conversion to a normal rhythm or may cause a serious dysrhythmia after the cardioversion. Anticoagulants and oral antidysrhythmics are still given before cardioversion. Anticoagulants are given so a thrombus is not released into the system. A sedative such as diazepam (Valium) or midazolam hydrochloride (Versed) is given intravenously before the procedure. Monitor the client's vital signs and ECG strip closely for the first hour afterward and then as ordered by the physician.

Defibrillation

Defibrillation is the delivery of an unsynchronized, high-energy electrical shock during an emergency situation, such as a cardiac arrest or pulseless VT, to convert the life-threatening dysrhythmia or arrhythmia to a sinus rhythm. Defibrillation is done by a physician or a nurse who has had special education to handle emergency situations. Paddles are lubricated with a special gel, or gel pads or defibrillator pads are applied to the skin where the paddles will be placed. The paddles are placed to the right of the sternum below the clavicle and at the apex of the heart. When the electrical shock is delivered to the client, everyone stands clear of the bed to prevent them from also receiving the electrical shock. More than one

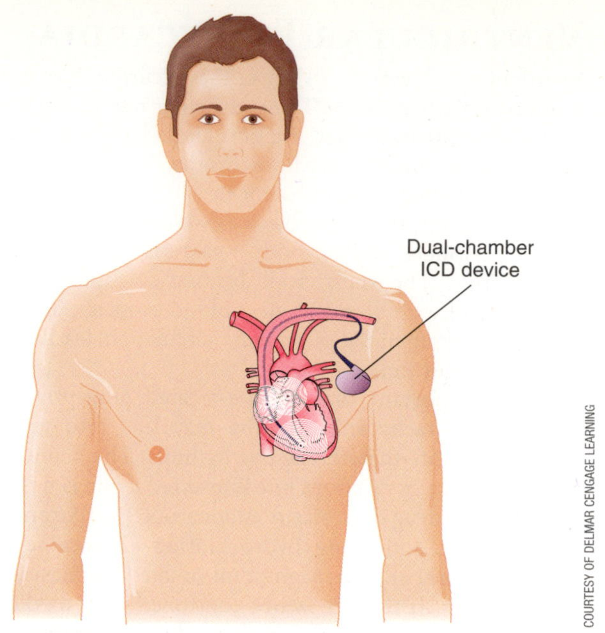

FIGURE 36-14 **An Implantable Cardiovert-Defibrillator: A dual-chamber ICD device with a pulse generator is implanted below the collarbone and endocardial leads positioned in the heart through a vein.**

electrical shock may be delivered in an attempt to convert the rhythm.

If conservative measures do not control the VT and the client has periodic episodes of VT, an **implantable cardioverter-defibrillator (ICD)** is implanted in the client (Figure 36-14). This device senses the dysrhythmia and automatically sends an electrical shock directly to the heart to defibrillate it.

Most ICDs have 1–3 endocardial leads that are guided through a vein into the right side of the heart where they become embedded into the heart tissue. The pulse generator is placed under the skin below the collarbone. The ICD detects VT and ventricular fibrillation (VF) through the leads attached to the heart muscle. Once VT or VF is detected, an electrical shock is sent from the pulse generator. The ICD is capable of delivering three more shocks to the heart muscle if the heart does not return to normal sinus rhythm (NSR). Usually, clients are converted to NSR with the first shock. Some ICDs also deliver cardiac resynchronization therapy (CRT) for clients with advanced HF. These devices have three leads; one lead is placed in the right atrium and one lead is placed in each of the ventricles. When this device functions as an ICD, it senses abnormal heart beats and delivers a shock to the heart to initiate a normal rhythm. When functioning as a CRT, it coordinates the beating of the ventricles so they effectively work together and pump blood throughout the body (FDA, 2002). Some ICDs also function as a pacemaker and an ICD; delivering shocks as needed to correct abnormal rhythms but also initiating heartbeats when the heartbeat is too slow. Another ICD, called antitachycardia pacing (ATP), sends a fast impulse to correct the rhythm after an ICD shock and detects and treats rapid atrial heartbeats (Stanford Hospital and Clinics, 2009; FDA, 2002). ICDs store the client's dysrhythmic activity and allow the health care practitioner to test the electrophysiologic activity noninvasively (AHA, 2007).

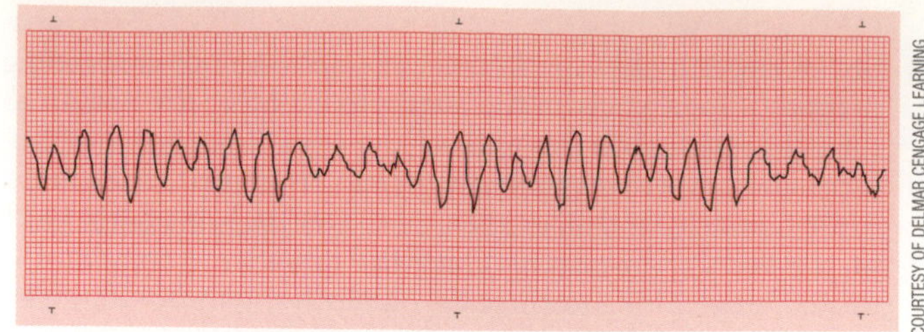

FIGURE 36-15 **Ventricular Fibrillation (VF)**

Complications after the insertion of an ICD are atelectasis, pneumonia, pneumothorax, thrombus, and a seroma at the generator site (a swelling from serum collecting around the device that initiates the shock). According to Shaffer (2002), anger and depression are common, expected side effects.

VENTRICULAR FIBRILLATION

The most common cause for VF is CAD. VF is a disorganized, chaotic quivering of the ventricles. The ventricles are unable to contract, and no blood is ejected into the circulatory system. The ECG reading is a series of jagged, unidentifiable waves (Figure 36-15). The client will not have a pulse, blood pressure, or respirations. This dysrhythmia is serious. Aggressive measures must be taken to initiate CPR and defibrillate the client immediately.

VENTRICULAR ASYSTOLE

Ventricular asystole is represented by a P wave or a straight line on the ECG (Figure 36-16). The ventricles are not contracting, and the client is in cardiac arrest. The client loses consciousness and has no pulse or respirations. Aggressive treatment should be initiated within 1 minute to prevent chemical changes within the body that jeopardize recovery. CPR is started, and the client is defibrillated. Atropine sulfate and epinephrine are given intravenously.

ATRIOVENTRICULAR BLOCKS

In atrioventricular blocks, the electrical conduction is interrupted to some degree between the atria and ventricles at the AV node. The extent of interruption is classified as first degree, second degree, or third degree.

FIRST-DEGREE AV BLOCK

In first-degree block, the impulse is delayed in traveling through the AV node. The impulse eventually reaches the

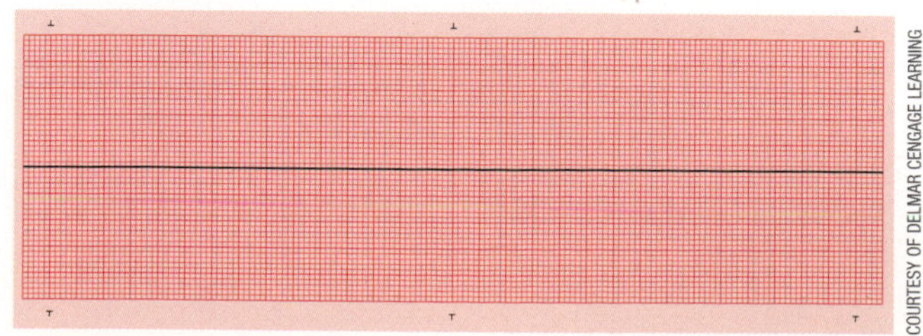

FIGURE 36-16 **Asystole**

ventricles but is delayed. There are no physical symptoms or treatment for first-degree block.

Second-Degree AV Block

In second-degree block, some of the impulses pass through the AV node to the ventricles and others are blocked. Symptoms include irregular pulse, vertigo, and weakness. A temporary pacemaker may be inserted until the conduction pattern is stabilized. If the dysrhythmia persists, a permanent pacemaker may be implanted. When the impulse is blocked, the ECG reveals an extended PR interval that is not followed by a QRS complex.

Third-Degree AV Block

Third-degree heart block is when no impulses are able to pass from the atria through the AV node to the ventricles. The atria and ventricles beat independently of each other. The causes of third-degree block are myocardial ischemia, drug toxicity, and electrolyte imbalances. Atropine sulfate may be given to improve conduction through the AV node. A permanent pacemaker is usually required to control the dysrhythmia.

A pacemaker is an electronic device that stimulates the heart to beat when the heartbeat is slow or drops below a set HR. It consists of one or two lead wires that are attached to the endocardium of the right atrium, right ventricle, or both, and a pulse generator that is "the 'brain' of the pacemaker" (Stanford Hospital and Clinics, 2009). The electrodes sense the heart's electrical activity and relay the information to the pulse generator. The purpose of the pacemaker is to regulate the HR and increase CO. When the heart beats slower than the programmed rate, an electrical impulse is sent to the lead that causes the heart to beat faster. Pacemakers are used for bradycardia, tachycardia, myocardial infarction, and heart block.

Some pacemakers have leads in the atrium, ventricle, or both to sense electrical activity and set the beating pace of one or both chambers. Sometimes in CHF the ventricles do not pump effectively together, decreasing the amount of blood pumped throughout the body. A biventricular pacemaker paces the ventricles together increasing the pumping effectiveness of the ventricles. The pacing of a biventricular pacemaker is called *cardiac resynchronization therapy* because it puts the ventricles back in synch.

A pacemaker is used either temporarily or permanently. A temporary pacemaker is used until a client's condition improves or until a permanent pacemaker is inserted. With a temporary pacemaker, the pulse generator remains outside of the body. The permanent pacemaker has a lead wire threaded through a vein to the heart and the pulse generator is implanted subcutaneously under the collarbone. An ECG of a client with a pacemaker shows the impulse from the pulse generator by a pacemaker spike, a vertical line before each QRS on the ECG strip.

Before discharge, teach clients to take accurate apical and radial pulses. Inform clients to report dizziness, fainting, or fever. Clients are taught to have regular pacemaker checks or transtelephonic monitoring in which an ECG strip is sent by phone to a designated hospital or physician's office.

SAFETY

Pacemaker and ICD

Encourage the client to carry an ID card and wear a medical identification tag indicating the presence of a pacemaker or ICD.

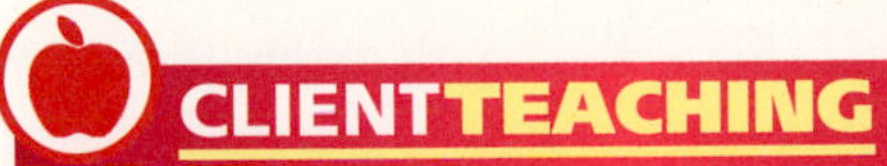

Pacemaker

- High-tension wires, high-voltage electrical generators, or MRIs may cause pacemaker malfunction.
- Avoid contact sports.
- Pacemakers may activate airport security alarms.

Medical–Surgical Management

Pharmacological

Dysrhythmias originating in the atria are treated with amiodarone (Cardarone), diltiazem hydrochloride (Cardizem, Dilacor, Tiazac), and digitalis (Digoxin). Dysrhythmias originating in the ventricles are treated with amiodarone (Cardarone), lidocaine hydrochloride (Xylocaine HCL), and magnesium sulfate.

Diet

The client is usually placed on a low-fat, low-cholesterol diet. Caffeine consumption is restricted.

Nursing Management

Monitor vital signs including apical pulse. Provide rest periods throughout the day. Explain all procedures and treatments. Encourage client to verbalize concerns about condition and potential complications. Teach relaxation methods.

NURSING PROCESS

Assessment

Subjective Data

Inquire if the client has experienced palpitations, lightheadedness, nausea, dyspnea, anxiety, fatigue, or chest discomfort.

Objective Data

If a client is experiencing dysrhythmias, check the HR, blood pressure, and respirations. While listening to the apical pulse and respirations, note abnormal heart sounds and monitor breath sounds for crackles. Crackles indicate the lungs are filling with fluid. Observe the skin for pallor and cyanosis, especially during and after activity/exercise. Urine output may decrease.

Nursing diagnoses for a client with dysrhythmias include the following:

NURSING DIAGNOSES	PLANNING/OUTCOMES	NURSING INTERVENTIONS
*Decreased **C**ardiac **O**utput* related to inadequate electrical conduction	The client will have increased CO.	Apply electrodes for telemetry monitoring. Balance activity with rest periods, and monitor vital signs during activity and at rest. Listen to the apical pulse, especially noting rate and rhythm. Elevate the extremities so they are not in a dependent position.
***A**nxiety* related to fear of potential diagnosis, treatment regimen, and death	The client will relate fears of potential cardiac problems.	Care for the client in a calm, confident, and efficient manner. Remain with the client and explain procedures and treatments. Encourage client input regarding the care. Encourage the client to verbalize concerns about the dysrhythmia and potential future complications. Teach the client relaxation activities.
*Deficient **K**nowledge* related to electrical conduction of the heart and treatment methods	The client will describe electrical disorder and treatment methods.	Explain medication administration times, action, side effects, and symptoms that need reporting. Provide written instructions to the client and family. Explain symptoms of dysrhythmias such as fatigue, edema, palpitations, lightheadedness, nausea, dyspnea, and anxiety. If a pacemaker is needed, explain to client and family the purpose, insertion procedures, and home care.

Evaluation: Evaluate each outcome to determine how it has been met by the client.

INFLAMMATORY DISORDERS

Inflammatory disorders include rheumatic heart disease, infective endocarditis, myocarditis, pericarditis, and valvular heart disease.

RHEUMATIC HEART DISEASE

Rheumatic heart disease is a complication of rheumatic fever and is also linked to group A streptococcus after an upper respiratory infection. Rheumatic fever is a systemic inflammatory disease that occurs 2 to 3 weeks after an inadequately treated pharyngitis caused by group *A beta-hemolytic streptococcus*. Symptoms of rheumatic fever are a mild fever, polyarthritis, carditis, chorea, and a rash. The endocardium, myocardium, and epicardium can become inflamed, with the most damage occurring to the mitral valve. The mitral valve becomes incompetent because of thickening and stenosis of the valve leaflets. Mitral prolapse (valve leaflets flip back into the left atrium during systole) may result.

A person who had rheumatic fever is more likely to have a recurrence. It is treated with intravenous antibiotics, anti-inflammatory agents, corticosteroids, and strict bed rest. The main goal is to treat the inflammation, prevent cardiac complications, and prevent the recurrence of the disease. These clients are placed on prophylactic antibiotic therapy before dental procedures or invasive surgery. Antibiotic therapy reduced the mortality from 15,000 in 1950 to 3,676 in 1999 (AHA, 2001c).

INFECTIVE ENDOCARDITIS

Infective endocarditis is an inflammation or infection of the inside lining of the heart, particularly the heart valves. The etiology of inflammatory endocarditis is a collagen-vascular disease or rheumatic fever. Infective endocarditis is caused by bacteria, fungi, or virus. As the microorganisms invade the valves, they form fibrinous substances called *vegetations*. The vegetations cause scar tissue on the valves resulting in hard, brittle valves that do not close properly and allow blood to flow back into the previous chamber. The valve is said to be insufficient. Sometimes the vegetations cause the valve flaps to grow together, resulting in a narrowing of the opening. This is called a *valvular stenosis*. The mitral valve is more frequently affected than any other. When the mitral valve is affected, it is termed *mitral insufficiency* or *mitral stenosis*.

Historically, rheumatic fever was the common cause of endocarditis. Clients at risk for endocarditis are individuals that use IV drugs, are immunosuppressed, have dental caries and abscesses, and a history of valvular heart disease. Goldrick (2003) reports that endocarditis is associated with body piercing.

There are two forms of endocarditis: acute and subacute. Symptoms of acute endocarditis are tachycardia, pallor, diaphoresis, and symptoms of a systemic infection, such as temperature of 103°F and shaking chills. Clients with subacute endocarditis have low-grade fever, malaise, weight loss, and anemia. Clients with both types may have murmurs and symptoms of CHF, such as dyspnea, peripheral edema, and pulmonary congestion.

Endocarditis is diagnosed by the client's history and symptoms. **Transesophageal echocardiography (TEE)** can confirm the diagnosis by ultrasonic imaging of the cardiac structures through the esophagus. The erythrocyte sedimentation rate (ESR) and WBC are elevated. A blood culture and sensitivity is done to determine the causative organism and the most effective antibiotic.

Medical–Surgical Management

Surgical

Surgical repair or replacement of a valve is done in severe cases.

Pharmacological

Clients are treated with antimicrobial drugs (endocarditis) and intravenous antibiotics. The antibiotics are usually continued for 2 to 6 weeks. The most commonly used antibiotics are penicillin V potassium (V-Cillin K), vancomycin hydrochloride (Vancocin), and gentamicin sulfate (Garamycin).

Diet

Provide the client with a well-balanced nutritious diet, with between-meal snacks.

Activity

The client is on bed rest to decrease the workload of the heart. Provide a calm, quiet environment.

Health Promotion

Clients who previously had endocarditis or have a mitral valve prolapse are more prone to develop endocarditis. They should take antibiotics prophylactically before having dental work and genitourinary or gastrointestinal invasive procedures. Amoxicillin trihydrate (Amoxil) 1 hour before the procedure and again after the procedure is the usual order.

Nursing Management

Administer oxygen as needed, and measure blood pressure and pulse before and after activity to monitor toleration. Note apical pulse rate and rhythm and assess breath sounds for adventitious sounds. Balance activity with rest periods. Monitor BUN and creatinine levels if a client is on vancomycin hydrochloride (Vancocin) or gentamicin sulfate (Garamycin) because both of these drugs are nephrotoxic.

MYOCARDITIS

Myocarditis is an inflammation of the myocardium of the heart. Lymphocytes and leukocytes invade the muscle fibers of the heart, causing the chambers to enlarge and the muscle to weaken. This can lead to CHF. Myocarditis is caused by bacteria, viruses, fungi, or parasites. It can also be an autoimmune reaction such as with rheumatic fever or lupus erythematosus. Usually the cause is a virus. Myocarditis is more prevalent in clients with AIDS.

Acute myocarditis presents with flulike symptoms of fever, pharyngitis, myalgias, and gastrointestinal complications. The client will also have chest pain and should be monitored for signs of CHF. A **pericardial friction rub** is often heard if the pericardium becomes involved. The friction rub is a "squeaky" sound heard through the stethoscope when the two inflamed pericardial surfaces rub together with the contraction of the heart.

Myocarditis diagnostic symptoms are nonspecific. They include elevated ESR and elevated LDH, CK, and SGOT levels. The diagnosis of myocarditis can be confirmed with an endomyocardial biopsy.

Medical–Surgical Management

Pharmacological

Digitalis preparations are given to try to prevent CHF. Broad-spectrum antibiotics are also given to treat the infection. Anti-inflammatory agents may be given to reduce the inflammation. Oxygen is administered as needed.

Activity

The client is placed on bed rest to decrease the workload of the heart.

Nursing Management

Monitor the client for symptoms of CHF or pericarditis. Place the client in a semi-Fowler's position to assist with breathing. Provide a quiet environment and frequent rest periods. Apply a pulse oximeter to monitor oxygen saturation.

PERICARDITIS

When the membranous sac surrounding the heart becomes inflamed, the condition is called **pericarditis**. Causative organisms are viral, bacterial, fungal, or parasitic. Inflammation can also occur from rheumatic or collagen-vascular conditions such as systemic lupus erythematosus. The most common cause of pericarditis is idiopathic, meaning no known cause. Symptoms of pericarditis are severe precordial pain (pain on the anterior surface of the chest over the heart) and a pericardial friction rub. The pain may radiate to the neck, back, or abdomen and become worse when the client coughs or lies on the left side. If the client sits erect and leans forward, the pain is relieved. Pericardial effusion (excess fluid in pericardial space) may develop. **Cardiac tamponade** will result if the fluid rapidly increases and hinders the functioning of the ventricle. The S_1 and S_2 sounds are often muffled and hard to hear because of fluid accumulation.

With inflammation, scar tissue develops in the pericardial sac. Heart movement is limited by the scar tissue and cardiac failure results.

Medical–Surgical Management

Medical

The physician performs a **pericardiocentesis** to aspirate the excess fluid from the pericardial sac. A needle is inserted through the chest wall into the pericardial space.

Surgical

If fibrotic scar tissue in the pericardium hinders heart performance, a pericardiectomy or pericardial window is done. Pericardiectomy is removal of the pericardium. When a pericardial window is done, a section of the parietal pericardium is cut and tacked back onto itself, allowing fluid to escape from the pericardial sac.

Pharmacological

Clients are given antipyretics, analgesics, and anti-inflammatory agents. The infection is combated with antibiotics. A digitalis preparation and diuretic are given to improve the pumping action of the heart and decrease fluid retention.

Nursing Management

Assess the client's apical pulse and blood pressure and monitor the ECG for dysrhythmias. Assess for signs of cardiac tamponade such as decreased pulse and blood pressure, muffled heart sounds, increased respirations, restlessness, and oliguria. Administer oxygen as needed, and assist the client to a position of comfort. Administer analgesics, antibiotics, and anti-inflammatory agents as ordered and monitor the client's responses. Encourage the client to verbalize concerns and fears.

VALVULAR HEART DISEASES

Valvular heart disease occurs when the valves do not open and close properly. When the valve does not close completely, blood leaks back into the chamber from which it was pumped. This is called regurgitation. The client with valvular heart disease often has a history of rheumatic fever.

STENOSIS AND INSUFFICIENCY

The definitions, symptoms, diagnostic findings, medical–surgical management, and nursing interventions for mitral and aortic valve conditions are covered in Table 36-3.

MITRAL VALVE PROLAPSE

Mitral insufficiency can lead to mitral valve prolapse in which the valve leaflets, chordae tendineae, and papillary muscle become damaged. The valve leaflets flip back into the left atrium when the left ventricle contracts. This condition affects more women than men. Often the client remains asymptomatic. The symptoms that a client may experience depend on how seriously the mitral valve is affected. Sometimes clients experience palpitations and fatigue caused by decreased CO. They also may experience angina, dizziness, and syncope. Some clients have panic attacks. Often a click or murmur is heard.

Medical–Surgical Management

Medical

Clients with valvular heart disease are to take antibiotics prophylactically before any dental procedures and genitourinary or gastrointestinal invasive procedures.

Table 36-3 Mitral and Aortic Valve Stenosis and Insufficiency

VALVE CONDITION	DEFINITION	SYMPTOMS	DIAGNOSTIC FINDINGS	MEDICAL-SURGICAL MANAGEMENT	NURSING INTERVENTIONS
Mitral stenosis	The diseased valve becomes narrowed and the leaflets thickened, preventing blood from freely flowing from the left atrium into the left ventricle.	Gradual onset of symptoms: exertional dyspnea, fatigue, orthopnea, paroxysmal nocturnal dyspnea, murmur. **Later symptoms:** peripheral edema, atrial fibrillation, jugular venous distention, hepatomegaly, abdominal distention, hypotension, thrombus from blood pooling in the left atrium.	**Chest x-ray:** hypertrophy and enlargement of left atrium and right ventricle. **ECG:** atrial fibrillation. **Echocardiogram:** fusion of valve leaflets, enlarged left atrium, decreased blood flow through valve.	**Medical management:** diuretics, digitalis, anticoagulants, antidysrhythmics, prophylactic antibiotics for invasive procedures, low-sodium diet, semi-Fowler's position, activity restrictions as needed. **Surgical management:** commissurotomy, percutaneous balloon mitral valvuloplasty, mitral valve replacement.	Encourage rest periods, administer oxygen, elevate head of bed, reposition frequently to decrease pressure points, elevate legs, low-sodium diet, monitor for signs of right and left-sided HF, teach stress reduction techniques, daily weight.

TABLE 36-3 Mitral and Aortic Valve Stenosis and Insufficiency (Continued)

VALVE CONDITION	DEFINITION	SYMPTOMS	DIAGNOSTIC FINDINGS	MEDICAL-SURGICAL MANAGEMENT	NURSING INTERVENTIONS
Mitral insufficiency	The valve leaflets become hard and do not close completely. Blood backs up in both the left atria and ventricle, causing both chambers to hypertrophy.	Gradual onset of symptoms: exertional dyspnea, palpitations, fatigue, atrial fibrillation, loud murmur and gallop.	**Chest x-ray:** hypertrophy and enlargement of left atrium and left ventricle. **ECG:** atrial fibrillation.	**Medical management:** same as mitral stenosis. **Surgical management:** valvuloplasty, mitral valve replacement.	Same as mitral stenosis, teach exercise modification.
Aortic stenosis	The valve cusps become hard and calcify due to rheumatic fever, syphilis, a congenital anomaly, or the aging process.	Syncope, exertional dyspnea, arrhythmias, angina, murmur, and gallop; sudden death may occur. **Later symptoms as the disease progresses:** paroxysmal atrial tachycardia, orthopnea.	**Chest x-ray:** enlargement of left ventricle, calcification of aortic valve. **ECG:** hypertrophy of left ventricle inverted T wave echocardiogram fusion of valve leaflets, regurgitation.	**Medical management:** same as mitral stenosis. **Surgical management:** percutaneous balloon aortic valvuloplasty, aortic valve replacement.	Same as mitral stenosis.
Aortic insufficiency	The valve cusps become so hardened they do not close completely. The blood no longer flows through the aorta but backs up into the left ventricle.	Palpitations, chest pain, exertional dyspnea, nocturnal angina, dizziness, fatigue, decreased activity, intolerance, paroxysmal nocturnal dyspnea, visible pulsation of the neck veins, murmur, lung congestion.	**Chest x-ray:** hypertrophy and enlargement of left ventricle.	**Medical management:** same as mitral stenosis. **Surgical management:** aortic valve replacement.	Same as mitral stenosis, teach exercise modification.

COURTESY OF DELMAR CENGAGE LEARNING

Surgical

When the activities of a client with valvular heart disease become curtailed because of decreased CO and the symptoms can no longer be controlled by medical means, surgery is performed. The type of surgery performed will depend on the client's overall condition and on the involved valve.

For the mitral valve, surgery alleviates the symptoms, but it does not cure the condition. Surgeries frequently have to be repeated. A commissurotomy is done for mitral stenosis, which surgically separates the valve leaflets. For mitral regurgitation or insufficiency, a valvuloplasty is becoming the treatment of choice. A percutaneous mitral valvuloplasty is a repair of perforated cusps or torn chordae tendineae. The risk of a thrombus is less with valvuloplasty than with grafts or prosthetic valves. An annuloplasty, a repair of an **annulus** or valvular ring, can also be done (see Figure 36-17A). The annulus is tightened with a purse-string suture or an annular ring. The mitral valve is replaced when other repair measures are not feasible.

The aortic valve is not repaired, only replaced, if the symptoms cannot be controlled by medical means. The preferred treatment for a client with an aortic stenosis is percutaneous aortic valvuloplasty. This treatment is often used in elderly or high risk surgical clients. A catheter is advanced to the affected valve and a balloon is inflated in the stenosed valve. The narrowed valvular space is expanded by the balloon, leaving a wider opening. Later, large balloons may be used to expand the opening as needed.

Mitral and tricuspid valves are now repaired or replaced with robotically-assisted closed-chest heart surgery. Cardiac surgeons perform these minimally invasive valve surgeries with a robot. Some valves are still repaired and replaced with the open chest method, but there are several advantages to robotically assisted surgery. They require smaller incisions with minimal scarring. The client experiences less trauma,

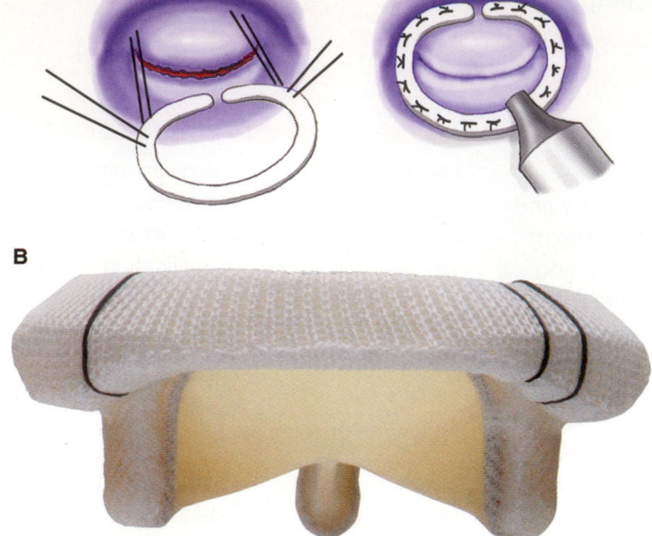

FIGURE 36-17 *A,* **Annuloplasty** *B,* **Carpentier-Edwards Perimount Mitral Pericardial Bioprosthesis** (*Image A courtesy of Delmar Cengage Learning; image B courtesy of Edwards LifeScience.*)

pain, and bleeding. Clients have a decreased need for pain medication and a decreased risk of infection. The hospital stay is shorter than open heart surgery and the recovery is quicker, with a prompt return to daily activities.

There are two types of replacement valves: mechanical and biological. The mechanical valve is the caged-ball valve (Figure 36-17B). There is a greater risk of a thromboembolism with a caged-ball valve. Clients remain on anticoagulant therapy with both types of valves. The biological valves come from calves, pigs, or humans. The disadvantage of the biological valves is tissue degeneration and calcification of the valve. Carpentier-Edwards produced the first biomechanical valve that consists of a mechanical device and natural tissue.

NURSING MANAGEMENT

Assess for dyspnea, fatigue, palpitations, lightheadedness, cough, and numbness and tingling in the extremities. Provide rest periods during the day. Encourage smokers to stop. Refer client and family to dietitian for information on low-sodium diets. Encourage client's input regarding care decisions.

NURSING PROCESS

ASSESSMENT

Subjective Data

Review past medical history for conditions such as rheumatic fever or streptococcal infections. Document if the client has experienced any dyspnea, palpitations, fatigue, cough, lightheadedness, or numbness and tingling in the extremities.

Objective Data

Take the vital signs and listen to the apical pulse for rate, rhythm, murmurs, and S_3 sound. Auscultate breath sounds for adventitious sounds. Note edema, jugular distention, cyanosis, and equality of peripheral pulses. Test for Homans' sign because dysrhythmias may produce clots.

Nursing diagnoses for a client with cardiac valvular disorders include the following:

NURSING DIAGNOSES	PLANNING/OUTCOMES	NURSING INTERVENTIONS
*Decreased **C**ardiac Output* related to structural changes in valves	The client will have increased CO.	Administer oxygen as needed. Help the client balance activities with rest periods. The pulse should return to the baseline within 10 minutes of activity; if not, activity has been excessive. Discourage smoking and refer clients to support groups to assist them to stop smoking.
*Excess **F**luid Volume* related to decreased CO	The client will have a decrease in edema.	Administer diuretics as needed. Support extremities so they are not in a dependent position. Encourage the client to maintain a low-sodium diet.
***A**nxiety* related to threat to or change in health status	The client will list ways to cope with stressors.	Calmly explain the procedures before doing them. Encourage the client's input to decisions regarding care. Assist the client and the client's family in identifying ways to cope with stressors. Teach relaxation techniques.

Nursing diagnoses for a client with cardiac valvular disorders include the following: (Continued)

NURSING DIAGNOSES	PLANNING/OUTCOMES	NURSING INTERVENTIONS
Deficient Knowledge related to disease process and treatment	The client will relate the disease process and needed self-care management.	Explain the valvular disease process, medication actions, dosage times, and medication side effects to report. Refer the client and family members to the dietitian for low-sodium diet instructions. Encourage the client to begin an appropriate exercise program.

Evaluation: Evaluate each outcome to determine how it has been met by the client.

OCCLUSIVE DISORDERS

Occlusive disorders include arteriosclerosis, angina pectoris, and myocardial infarction.

ARTERIOSCLEROSIS

Arteriosclerosis is a narrowing and hardening of arteries. A buildup of lipids, collagen, and smooth muscle cells narrows the lumen of the vessel. Decreased blood flow through the vessel causes decreased perfusion to cells beyond the narrowed or hardened area.

There are three types of arteriosclerosis: atherosclerosis, calcific sclerosis, and arteriolar sclerosis. **Atherosclerosis** is fatty deposits on the inner lining of vessel walls. The fat deposit is called *plaque*. In calcific sclerosis, calcium deposits are on the middle layer of the wall of the arteries. Hypertension causes a thickening of the arterioles and is called *arteriolar sclerosis*. With these conditions, vessels lose their elasticity, resulting in various conditions, such as arteriosclerotic heart disease, angina, myocardial infarction, stroke, and peripheral vascular disease.

ANGINA PECTORIS

When coronary arteries lose elasticity or become narrow as a result of plaque collection, the heart muscle receives less blood and oxygen. Physical exertion, emotional stress, smoking, exposure to extreme cold, heavy meals, or an arterial spasm may cause a temporary inadequate blood and oxygen supply to the heart. Myocardial ischemia and angina pectoris result. Myocardial ischemia is a temporary inadequate blood and oxygen supply to the myocardial tissues. When this temporary condition occurs, the person experiences chest pain or **angina pectoris.**

At first, the person may experience a squeezing pain under the sternum, which radiates to the left shoulder. For some, the pain may radiate to the right shoulder, jaw, or ear. The discomfort may vary from mild discomfort to immobilizing pain. Anginal attacks usually increase in frequency and severity over time. The severity of the condition depends on the development of collateral circulation.

Collateral circulation develops as larger vessels gradually narrow or harden. Blood that normally passes through the larger vessels is shunted into surrounding smaller vessels. These vessels enlarge in an attempt to supply blood to the affected area. Collateral circulation increases the blood supply to tissues with an inadequate blood supply.

Many people experiencing ischemic attacks do not experience angina. This is called silent myocardial infarct or ischemia. Symptoms are chest pressure or heaviness, restlessness, shortness of breath with increased respiratory rate, a sensation of epigastric fullness with noisy belching, numbness or tingling in both arms or shoulders, physical or mental fatigue, and dizziness. The person may also experience a change in sleep patterns and mental alertness. The person states that he or she "feels funny." Clients that are more likely to experience a silent myocardial infarction are women, older adults, and individuals with diabetes or a history of HF (Overbaugh, 2009).

Two other types of angina are unstable angina and Prinzmetal's angina. Unstable angina occurs at rest or with minimal exertion and is not relieved with nitroglycerin. The client is more susceptible to myocardial infarction and sudden death. Prinzmetal's angina is caused by a coronary artery spasm and occurs at rest.

There is a high incidence of angina pectoris in clients with hypertension and diabetes mellitus. The diagnosis of angina is made after reviewing the client's history, lifestyle, laboratory tests, and stress test. A lipid profile (cholesterol, HDL, LDL, and triglycerides), hs-CRP, and lipoprotein A [Lp(a)] are evaluated. Angina pectoris is diagnosed by a stress test, thallium scan, or a coronary arteriogram.

MEDICAL–SURGICAL MANAGEMENT

Medical

Treatment for angina includes measures to increase the blood supply to the affected area. Clients are administered 162 to 325 mg of chewed or crushed aspirin by mouth because it prevents platelet aggregation and vasoconstriction. Oxygen is given at 2 to 4 L/min per nasal cannula to maintain the SaO_2 >90%. Nitroglycerin tablets 0.3 to 0.4 mg are given sublingually every 5 minutes up to 3 doses because it is a vasodilator and increases the oxygen supply to the myocardium. If the pain is not relieved with the nitroglycerin, morphine sulfate 2 to 4 mg IV push is administered because it is a vasodilator and analgesic. The morphine dose can be repeated every 5 to 15 minutes until the pain is under control. The nurse should closely monitor the BP, respirations, and SaO_2 because the side effects

MEMORY TRICK

MONA for Anginal Pain

M = Morphine sulfate 2 to 4 mg IV push

O = Oxygen 2 to 4 L/min per nasal cannula to maintain SaO_2 above 90%

N = Nitroglycerin tablets 0.3 to 0.4 mg sublingually every 5 minutes up to 3 doses

A = Aspirin 162 to 325 mg by mouth (chewed or crushed)

(Overbaugh, 2009)

of morphine are hypotension and respiratory depression. A mnemonic to recall the treatment of angina is MONA (see Memory Trick: MONA). Even though the letters are not in the order of administration, it helps the nurse recall the treatment for angina (Overbaugh, 2009).

Silent ischemia is treated in the same way symptomatic ischemia is treated. The client needs to be educated about cardiac risk factors, the importance of following the prescribed medical regimen, and maintaining regular physical checkups.

Surgical

A percutaneous transluminal coronary angioplasty (PTCA) may be done if only one coronary artery is involved and if the atherosclerotic material is small and has not hardened. When a PTCA is done, atherosclerotic matter is pressed against the walls of the coronary vessels to improve circulation to myocardial tissue supplied by that coronary artery (Figure 36-18). A guidewire is inserted to the stenosed area, and a special balloon-tipped catheter is placed in the narrowed sclerotic area. When the balloon is inflated, the atherosclerotic material is pressed against the wall of the vessel. The vessel, now open, allows more blood to flow to the myocardial tissue. During this procedure, a piece of the atherosclerotic material may break off and occlude the vessel. If this occurs, the client would have to undergo immediate coronary artery bypass graft (CABG) surgery. Other complications of the procedure are occlusion of the vessel because of a vascular spasm.

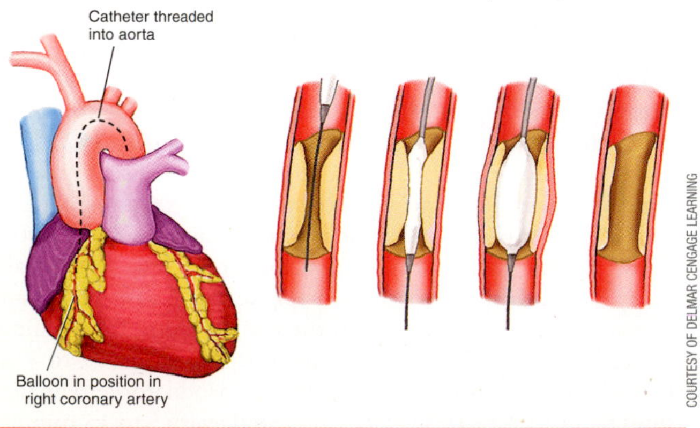

FIGURE 36-18 Demonstration of the Function of a Balloon-Tipped Catheter During a PTCA Procedure

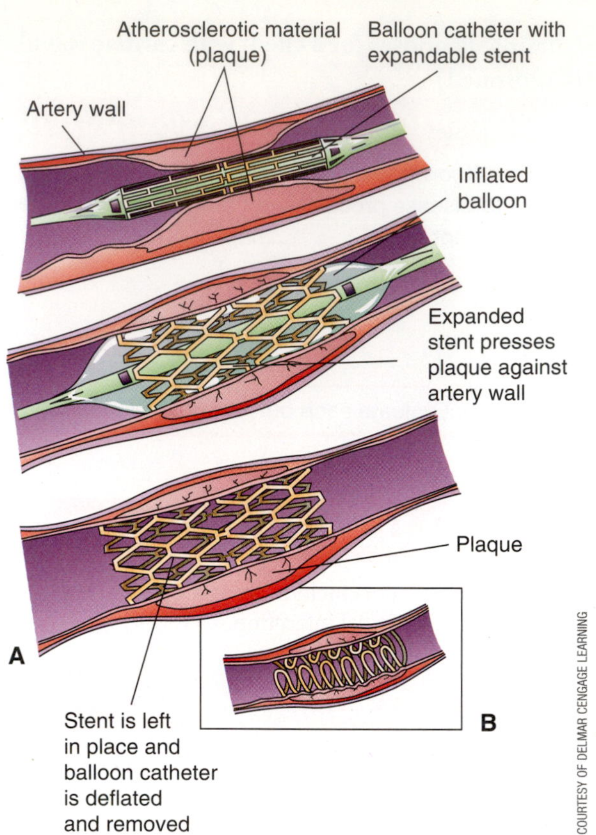

FIGURE 36-19 Placement of a Stent in a Coronary Artery; *A*, Palmaz-Schatz Stent; *B*, Gianturco-Roubin Ex-Stent

An intracoronary **stent** may be implanted into a stenosed vessel to prevent the vessel from collapsing and to keep the atherosclerotic plaque pressed against the vessel wall. A stent is a tiny metal tube with holes in it (Figure 36-19). The procedure is sometimes done when a vessel collapses after a PTCA or in place of a PTCA. The stent is tightly wrapped around a balloon catheter. When the balloon catheter has been threaded through a vessel to the stenosed area, the balloon is inflated and the stent expands and presses the plaque against the vessel wall. The stent remains in the vessel and the catheter is withdrawn.

If a CABG is performed, the internal mammary artery, the saphenous vein, or an accordion type of synthetic graft material is used. The vein or synthetic material is grafted to the aorta and passed beyond the obstruction in the coronary vessel (Figure 36-20). The graft provides an increased blood supply to the affected myocardium. The client then has less angina and an increased tolerance for activities.

A minimally invasive direct coronary artery bypass graft (MID CABG) surgery is now an option for clients whose surgeons use a left internal mammary artery to bypass an occlusion in the left anterior descending artery (see Figure 36-20B). With a MID CABG the client is not connected to a heart bypass machine and only small incisions (2–3 inches) are needed for the procedure. There is decreased risk of infection and the client experiences less bleeding and pain. The average recovery time is 2 to 4 weeks compared with 6 to 8 weeks with the traditional heart surgery.

Another recent advance in CABG surgery is Cardica's C-Port Flex-A System that completes the vessel anastomosis by arranging tiny, stainless steel staples attaching the bypass

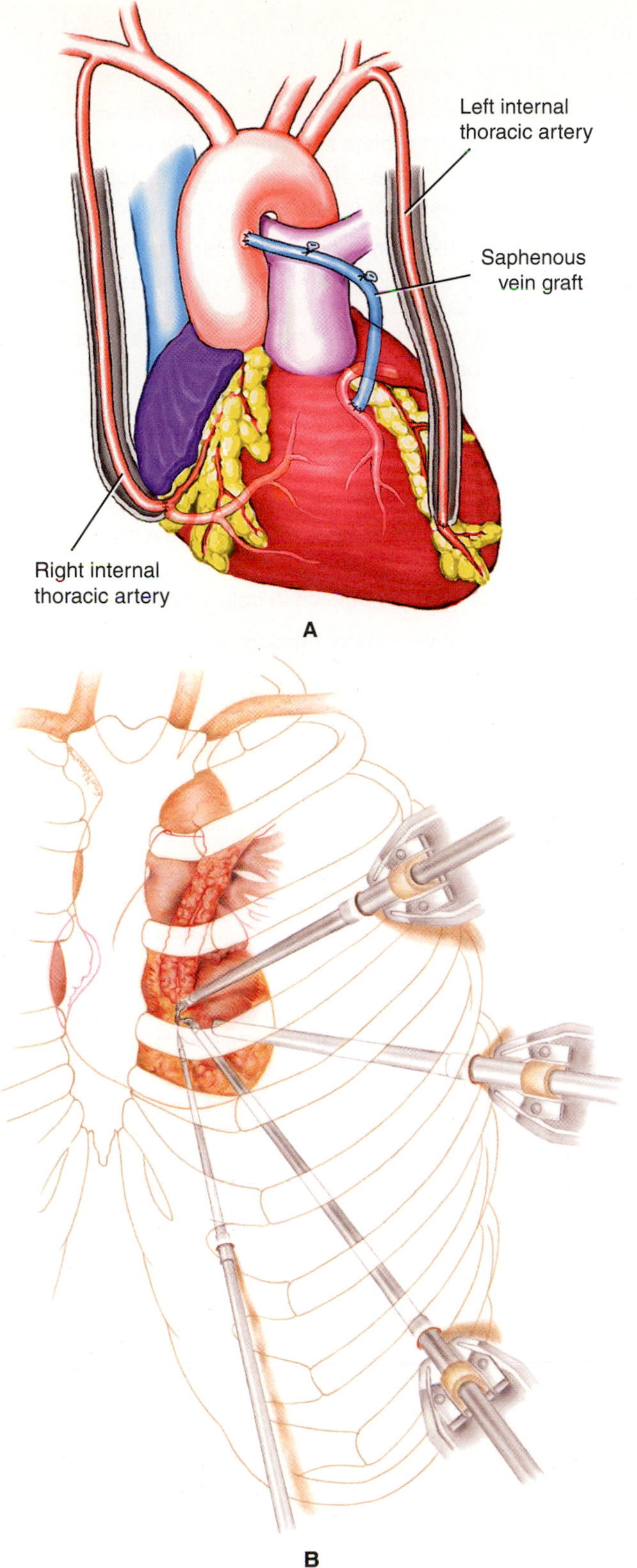

FIGURE 36-20 ***A*, Coronary Artery Bypass Graft (CABG) with the Saphenous Vein and Intern Mammary Vein; *B*, Robotic-assisted Surgery Completing a CABG (*Image A courtesy of Delmar Cengage Learning; image B courtesy of Intuitive Surgical, Inc. ©2005.*)**

vessel to the coronary artery. (To view the Cardica C-Port Flex-A System used in a robotic CABG or an animation of the C-Port Flex-A System, go to http://www.cardica.com.) The anastomosis is completed with robotic arms in a minimally invasive surgery while the heart is still beating. There is no need for a heart bypass machine or a sternotomy. This surgery has all the advantages of a minimally invasive surgery (Broadcast Newsroom, 2009).

Pharmacological

Vasodilators, such as nitroglycerin tablets, cause the blood vessels to dilate, providing an increased blood supply to tissues. The client may not need as much analgesic medication if beta blockers are given. Beta-adrenergic blockers and calcium channel blockers slow the HR and decrease the oxygen demand of the heart. Calcium channel blockers also dilate vessels and decrease spasms of the coronary vessels. All of these measures provide an increased blood supply to the myocardium.

Diet

The client is placed on a low-fat, low-cholesterol, sodium-restricted diet. Sodium restriction may vary from no salt to 4 grams daily depending on the ability of the client's kidneys to excrete excess sodium. An increase of fruits and vegetables is recommended in the diet.

Activity

Activity should be slower and for shorter periods of time with more rest periods.

Health Promotion

To prevent coronary artery disease from resulting in angina, it is recommended that a person limit fat intake to 30 grams or less per day and exercise 5 times per week for at least 30 minutes. Simple activities such as parking a car farther from an entrance to increase walking distance and taking stairs instead of an elevator improve circulation and help decrease cholesterol levels. Activities such as gardening or housework are also good.

Nursing Management

Assess pain and medicate client as ordered. Monitor vital signs. Emphasize taking rest periods. Encourage client to always carry nitroglycerin and to get regular exercise as recommended by the physician. Answer questions about the low-fat, low-cholesterol, sodium-restricted diet that is prescribed.

NURSING PROCESS

Assessment

Subjective Data

Ask the client to describe the pain regarding type, radiation, onset, duration, and precipitating factors.

Objective Data

Observe and document the client's actions during the anginal attack. Take vital signs and attach the client to an ECG monitor and observe for any dysrhythmias.

Nursing diagnoses for a client with angina include the following:

NURSING DIAGNOSES	PLANNING/OUTCOMES	NURSING INTERVENTIONS
*Acute **P**ain* related to decreased oxygen supply to the myocardium	The client will experience decreased episodes of angina.	Administer nitroglycerin tablets sublingually. The pain should be relieved within 1 to 2 minutes. If the pain has not stopped after 3 doses 5 minutes apart, notify the emergency personnel. Administer other medication such as beta blockers or calcium channel blockers as ordered and monitor client's response.
***A**nxiety* related to perceived threat of death or change in lifestyle	The client will relate concerns and practice stress reduction techniques.	Assist the client in learning to decrease personal expectations and to live within personal activity limitations. Emphasize the importance of getting adequate rest and stopping before becoming too exhausted.
*Deficient **K**nowledge* related to disease process, medications, and treatment regimen	The client will explain the disease process, medication actions, dosage times and side effects, and self-care practices.	Explain the cause of angina. Teach the client to avoid stressful situations that may produce angina. Other ways to prevent angina are to sleep in a warm room, eat smaller proportions at mealtimes, and not exercise outside in cold weather. Inform the client to always carry nitroglycerin in a tightly closed container. Nitroglycerin may cause orthostatic hypotension, so inform the client to sit after taking it and to change position slowly after taking the medication. Encourage the client to start and maintain a regular exercise program as recommended by the physician.

Evaluation: Evaluate each outcome to determine how it has been met by the client.

MYOCARDIAL INFARCTION

In 2002, an estimated 1.1 million persons in the United States had an acute myocardial infarction (MI), and about 45% died. Half of those who died did so before arriving at a hospital (Nagle & Nee, 2002). The most common cause for myocardial infarction is atherosclerosis.

A **myocardial infarction** is caused by an obstruction in a coronary artery, resulting in necrosis (death) to the tissues supplied by the artery. The obstruction is usually caused by atherosclerotic plaque, a thrombus, or an embolism. The area most commonly affected is the left ventricle.

Obstruction of a large coronary artery damages the myocardial tissue and affects the pumping efficiency of the heart. A client's prognosis is better if a small coronary artery or arteriole is obstructed and there is good collateral circulation to the heart. If a large vessel is obstructed and the client does not have sufficient collateral circulation, the client may die immediately.

The typical symptoms of men experiencing an MI are feelings of chest heaviness or tightness that progresses to a severe gripping pain in the lower sternal area. Pain also occurs in the arm, neck, back, or epigastric area and may or may not radiate to these areas. The pain is not relieved by rest or nitroglycerin, and the client becomes short of breath (dyspneic), diaphoretic, and anxious. The client frequently becomes nauseated and vomits. The pulse may be irregular, rapid, and weak, and the blood pressure is low. The skin is pale and then turns cyanotic. Even though a person may not experience the typical MI symptoms, the condition can still be serious or fatal. Complications such as HF and stroke may also occur.

Women experiencing an MI present with atypical symptoms that often delay an accurate diagnosis. Women are more likely to have upper abdominal pain, heartburn, nausea, dyspnea, fatigue, lethargy, dull pain, anxiety, as well as chest pain (Cheek & Cesan, 2003; Joy, 2006). Women have pain in the back or left side of the chest rather than substernally and report the symptoms as a numb, tingling, burning, or stabbing sensation (Overbaugh, 2009).

A myocardial infarction is diagnosed by client symptoms, ECG tracings, cardiac biomarker values, and a radioactive isotope scan; however, in women the ECG stress test has less diagnostic value than in men. An exercise echocardiography is more reliable for women (Cheek & Cesan, 2003). When an

PROFESSIONALTIP

Risk Factors for Myocardial Infarction

- Overweight
- Cigarette smoking
- Hypertension
- Diabetes
- Family history of heart disease
- High cholesterol level
- High LDL

(Lab Tests Online, 2009)

MI is evolving in men, the ECG has an elevated ST segment, which eventually changes into an inverted T wave.

A CK-MB fraction that measures an isoenzyme specific to the cardiac muscle increases within 3 to 6 hours of the onset of a myocardial infarct, peaks in 18 to 24 hours, and returns to normal in 72 hours. CK studies are performed as soon as the client is admitted and then every 8 hours until four samples have been obtained. A CK-MB fraction >5% indicates myocardial damage.

Two other important lab values for diagnosing an MI are cardiac troponin I and myoglobin. Cardiac troponin I is a protein found in cardiac cells. When cardiac cells are damaged, the protein is released, resulting in an elevated level (normal level is <0.6 ng/mL) for 7 days. Within an hour of an MI, the myoglobin blood level increases, peaks in 4 to 12 hours, and returns to normal in 18 hours. If an MI is suspected, the lab value must be obtained quickly.

During the first 3 days after the infarction, the client may have a low-grade fever and an increased white cell count. The infarcted heart tissue is soft and necrotic and incapable of responding to electrical stimuli. Life-threatening dysrhythmias are most likely to occur at this time. Four to seven days after the infarction, the infarcted tissue is the softest and weakest. An aneurysm, or ballooning effect, can occur in the infarcted area with the potential of rupturing. There is a possibility of the ventricle rupturing from the time of the infarct to 2 weeks after the infarct. Collateral circulation begins forming around the edges of the infarct, but it will be 2 to 3 weeks before the collateral circulation functions effectively. Two to three months will pass before the heart muscle regains maximum strength.

Medical–Surgical Management

Medical

Medical–surgical management focuses on reducing oxygen demands, increasing oxygen supply to the myocardium, relieving pain, improving tissue perfusion, and preventing complications and further tissue damage. Immediately after an MI, a client is admitted into a coronary care unit. The client's heart is constantly monitored for dysrhythmias, and vital signs are monitored for any changes.

Three dysrhythmias that may occur after an MI are ventricular fibrillation, bradycardias, and tachycardias. Ventricular fibrillation is treated by defibrillation. Atropine and, if needed, a temporary pacer is inserted for bradycardias. Two tachycardias that may occur are atrial fibrillation and ventricular tachycardia. Atrial fibrillation is treated with digoxin (Lanoxin) diltiazem hydrochloride (Cardizem), or amiodarone hydrochloride (Cordarone). Ventricular tachycardia is treated with Cordarone, lidocaine hydrochloride (Xylocaine), or cardioversion. If dysrhythmias continue, magnesium may be given.

Medical complications that can occur following an MI are acute left ventricular failure, cardiogenic shock, pericarditis, embolism and/or thrombosis, and cardiac rupture. The health care team must closely monitor the client for signs of these complications. Women have a worse prognosis and die more often than men after a heart attack or bypass surgery (Cheek & Cesan, 2003).

Surgical

Primary treatment may be PTCA instead of thrombolytic therapy. Along with balloon compression, a stent(s) may be inserted. Clients with multiple vessels occluded, or for whom thrombolytic therapy and PTCA have not been effective, have the CABG procedure performed.

Pharmacological

Oxygen is given by a Venturi mask or nasal cannula. Morphine sulfate is given intravenously for pain. Medications include nitrates (IV or sublingually) to relieve pain and dilate coronary arteries, sedatives to calm and relax the client, and a stool softener to prevent rectal straining.

Thrombolytic therapy is sometimes used within 3 to 6 hours of the myocardial infarction to dissolve a clot blocking an artery and reperfuse the area. Medications such as streptokinase (Streptase), anistreplase (Eminase), and alteplase recombinant (Activase) are used. A possible complication from thrombolytic therapy is bleeding. Be alert for symptoms of hemorrhaging in the gastrointestinal tract (hematemesis and tarry stools), retroperitoneum (low back pain and numbness in lower extremities), or cerebrum (headache, vomiting, and confusion). Heparin therapy inhibits further clotting. Aspirin and/or clopidogrel (Plavix) is given to prevent vasoconstriction and platelet aggregation.

Diet

Until the client is stabilized, a diet is withheld in case a PTCA or CABG procedure is required. Fluids may be offered during the acute stage. A liquid diet is progressed to a regular low-fat, low-cholesterol, low-sodium diet. The client tolerates small frequent feedings better than three large meals. Avoid caffeine and extremely hot and cold foods.

Activity

It is vital that the client receive physical, mental, and emotional rest. Less stimuli places less demand on the heart. Explain procedures so the client understands the care provided.

The client is usually limited to bed rest during the first 24 hours and progressed to sitting in a chair by the second day. If pain returns or other complications occur, the client is back to bed rest. Early ambulation is encouraged to prevent thrombosis. During and after each activity, assess the client's tolerance by monitoring the HR for an increase of 20 beats per minute, checking for a decrease in systolic blood pressure, and observing for dyspnea and dysrhythmias. Document verbal and nonverbal statements of fatigue and chest pain.

Before discharge, low-intensity tests are performed to determine the types of activities in which the client may engage at home. When the client is able to climb two flights of stairs, sexual activity is resumed.

Health Promotion

A diet of less than 30 grams of fat per day reduces the progression of atherosclerosis, but there is no documented evidence that diet will prevent the disease in clients with hereditary hyperlipidemia. Regular exercise, 30 minutes at least 5 days per week, and smoking cessation help prevent an MI.

Participation in a cardiac rehabilitation program provides the client with monitored exercise sessions as well as education and counseling about reducing the risk of future heart problems and coping with a new lifestyle. Because women have a worse prognosis than men, it is critical for women to participate in a cardiac rehabilitation program.

Nursing Management

Assess for pain. Observe for verbal and nonverbal signs of pain. Have client describe symptoms. Monitor vital signs, breath sounds, pedal pulses, and ECG strips. Maintain client on bed rest with call light and other items within reach. Accurately record I&O. Provide a quiet, calm environment. Balance activity with rest periods.

NURSING PROCESS

Assessment

Subjective Data

Note the medications the client has taken, including over-the-counter medications, anticoagulants, and thrombolytic medications. Assess pain regarding onset, duration, intensity, location, radiation, and precipitating factors; ask the client to describe the symptoms. Not all persons having angina or an MI will experience or state having pain. Some may describe feelings of chest heaviness, indigestion, or "something not right." Explore these statements with the client so the client can explain them in more detail. Dizziness, weakness, and shortness of breath may be expressed. Ask how the client tried to relieve pain.

Objective Data

Assess vital signs, skin changes, breath sounds, and ECG rhythm strips. Monitor vital signs for an irregular or increased pulse, hypotension, or slight temperature elevation. The client may have pallor, cyanosis, diaphoresis, vomiting, cool clammy skin, or confusion. Assess breath sounds for lung congestion, and monitor the ECG for dysrhythmias. Note any client clenching of hands or clutching at the chest.

Nursing diagnoses for a client with myocardial infarction include the following:

NURSING DIAGNOSES	PLANNING/OUTCOMES	NURSING INTERVENTIONS
*Decreased **C**ardiac Output* related to damaged heart tissue	The client will have increased CO.	Maintain bed rest with head of bed elevated 30° until the condition is stabilized. Auscultate breath sounds and palpate pedal pulses every 4 hours. Administer oxygen per mask or nasal cannula at 2 to 4 L/min. Start an IV so medications such as morphine and antidysrhythmics can be administered. If beta blockers are administered, monitor closely for a drop in HR and blood pressure. Constantly monitor the client for dysrhythmias. Place a rhythm strip on the chart at least once per shift. Monitor I&O. Administer medications as prescribed by the physician.
*Acute **P**ain* related to decreased oxygenation of myocardial tissue	The client will verbalize decrease in frequency and intensity of chest pain.	Maintain client on bed rest and observe for verbal and nonverbal signs of pain such as grimacing, diaphoresis, or increased HR. Ask the client to rate the pain on a scale of 0 to 10, 0 being no pain and 10 extreme pain. Administer analgesic, usually morphine and oxygen, as ordered.
*Risk for **A**ctivity Intolerance* related to decreased circulation to body tissues	The client will increase activities with decreased symptoms of angina, dyspnea, cyanosis, and dysrhythmia.	Place objects within reach of the client. Balance activity with rest periods. Assist the client and partner to discuss their fears and feelings candidly about resuming sexual activity.
*Death **A**nxiety* related to change in health status and threat of death	The client will verbalize situations that are causing stress.	Encourage the family and client to verbalize their feelings. Provide a quiet, calm environment to relax the client and family. Administer sedatives to help the client relax and provide periods of uninterrupted rest. Since the myocardial client may be in denial, be aware of denial symptoms such as attempting to conduct business over the phone while hospitalized or statements that the pain is really nothing.

Evaluation: Evaluate each outcome to determine how it has been met by the client.

HEART FAILURE

HF is often the final stage of many other heart conditions. A weakened muscle wall from a myocardial infarction or a heart that has been stressed over a period of time to meet metabolic needs of the body can cause HF. HF develops when the heart is no longer capable of meeting the oxygen needs of the body. The muscles of the left ventricle **hypertrophy** (increases in muscle mass), and often the ventricular chamber enlarges in an attempt to meet the oxygen needs of the body.

Both the right and left ventricles act as pumps for the heart. Each of these pumps can fail separately, resulting in two types of HF: right-sided HF and left-sided HF. HF usually begins on the left side. Some of the causes of right-sided failure are untreated left ventricular failure, right ventricular myocardial infarction, chronic obstructive coronary disease, cor pulmonale, and pulmonic valve stenosis. Left-sided failure is caused by left ventricular myocardial infarction, aortic valve stenosis, prolapsed valve complications, and hypertension. Notice that right- and left-sided failure are caused by a defect of the ventricle or an increased resistance in the path of the blood pumped by the ventricles. This causes an increased workload for the involved ventricle.

When left-sided HF occurs, the left ventricle is not able to completely empty of blood or effectively pump blood out through the aorta to the body systems. Usually the right ventricle continues to pump adequate quantities of blood. This causes blood to back up in the left ventricle, left atrium, and pulmonary veins. The lungs become congested with fluid as fluid leaks through the capillaries and fills air spaces in the lungs. The client becomes cyanotic, dyspneic, restless, and coughs up blood-tinged sputum. The breath sounds have moist crackles. Often the client has tachycardia with low blood pressure because the heart is not able to pump sufficient blood to meet the body's demands. The client may have decreased urinary output because enough blood is not pumped through the kidneys. As the blood oxygen level decreases, the client becomes confused.

As the right side of the heart fails, blood becomes congested in the inferior vena cava, causing edema first in the extremities and then in the trunk of the body. As the condition progresses, the client experiences edema of the ankles, lower legs, thighs, and finally in the abdomen. The excess abdominal fluid causes the client to be anorectic. Hepatomegaly (enlargement of the liver) and splenomegaly (enlargement of the spleen) develop. The jugular veins in the neck become distended when the client is sitting or standing, and pitting edema occurs in the lower extremities. Refer to Figure 36-6. Oliguria occurs as decreased amounts of blood are pumped through the kidneys.

In the early stages of HF, the client experiences fatigue, dyspnea with slight exertion, pedal edema, and a slight cough with a small amount of expectoration. The client may also have paroxysmal nocturnal dyspnea.

CRITICAL THINKING

Lifestyle Changes for MI

What would you teach a client to assist him in decreasing risk factors for an MI?

What lifestyle changes could you take to decrease the risk factors for an MI?

Medical–Surgical Management

Medical

Goals for treating HF are to improve circulation to the coronary arteries and decrease the workload of the left ventricle. To meet these goals, cardiac efficiency is increased with medication; oxygen requirements of the body are decreased by bed rest with the head elevated 45 degrees; edema and pulmonary congestion are treated with medications, diet, and restricted fluid intake; and fluid retention is monitored by weighing the client daily. A chest x-ray directly visualizes the ventricles and evidence of lung congestion. An ECG is done and arterial blood gases are evaluated. The client's oxygen saturation level is monitored by pulse oximetry. Depending on the seriousness of the client's condition, a pulmonary artery catheter (Swan-Ganz catheter) may be inserted to determine left ventricular function.

In right-sided failure, the symptoms of edema, hepatomegaly, and neck vein distention are significant diagnostic evidence.

Surgical

Two mechanical devices are available: an intra-aortic balloon pump and a ventricular assist device (VAD). An intra-aortic balloon is threaded through the femoral artery to the descending aorta (Figure 36-21). The pump is synchronized with the contractions of the left ventricle so the balloon inflates during diastole and deflates during systole. Inflation of the balloon increases the blood flow to the coronary arteries, thus increasing oxygenation of the myocardium. Deflation of the balloon allows the left ventricle to pump blood to the body tissues with less peripheral resistance.

The ventricular assist device (VAD) does not replace the heart, but it assists a weakened heart to pump sufficient blood throughout the body. It is referred to as "a bridge to transplant" because a client uses the VAD while waiting for a heart transplant. Some clients who are not transplant candidates may use the VAD until death. A left VAD takes blood from the left ventricle and delivers it to the aorta (see Figure 36-22); a right VAD takes blood from the right ventricle and delivers it to the pulmonary artery. Potential complications are bleeding, blood clots, respiratory failure, renal failure, infection, stroke, and device failure.

Pharmacological

Medications to reduce the heart's workload in moderate HF are angiotensin converting enzymes (ACE) inhibitors, angiotensin receptor blockers, vasodilators, nitrates, beta blockers, diuretics, digitalis, and aspirin (Table 36-4). The client with HF will receive diuretics such as furosemide (Lasix) to decrease fluid retention. ACE inhibitors, such as captopril (Capoten) or enalopril (Vasotec), are given to reduce blood pressure and peripheral arterial resistance and improve CO. Beta blockers carvedilol (Coreg) and metoprolol succinate (Toprol XL), the only beta-blockers approved for HF in the United States, are then added (Ammon, 2001). A digitalis preparation may be required to increase the strength and contractility of the heart muscle. Vasodilators such as nitroglycerin (Cardabid) are given to dilate the veins so the blood will stay in the peripheral vessels and decrease blood return to the right side of the heart, thereby decreasing the workload on the heart. Clients in severe HF who are already taking an ACE inhibitor may be given spironolactone (Aldactone) (Ahmed, 2008). Morphine sulfate is given in the acute phase to control pain and decrease anxiety.

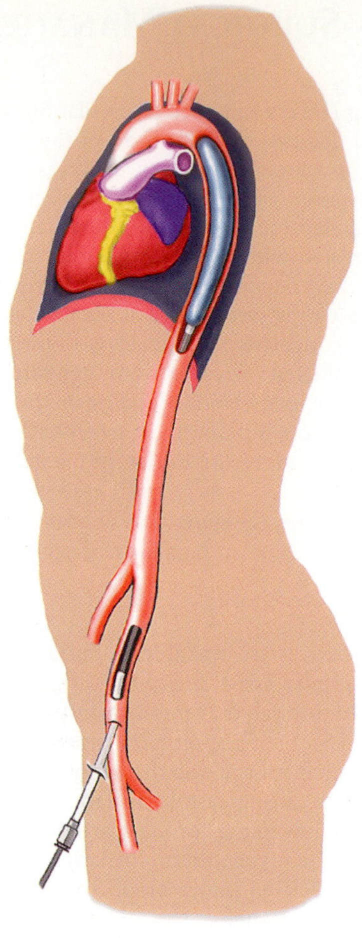

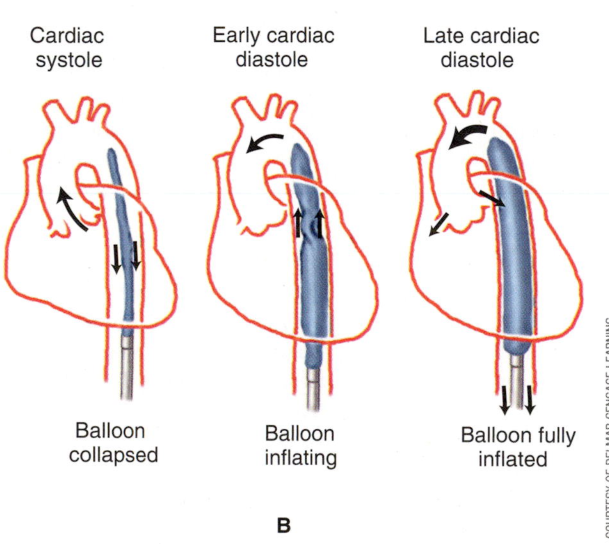

FIGURE 36-21 An intra-aortic balloon pump increases circulation to the coronary arteries and decreases the workload of the left ventricle.

Diet

A daily weight and strict intake and output are necessary to assess fluid retention. Sometimes fluid intake is limited. The client is generally on a low-sodium diet.

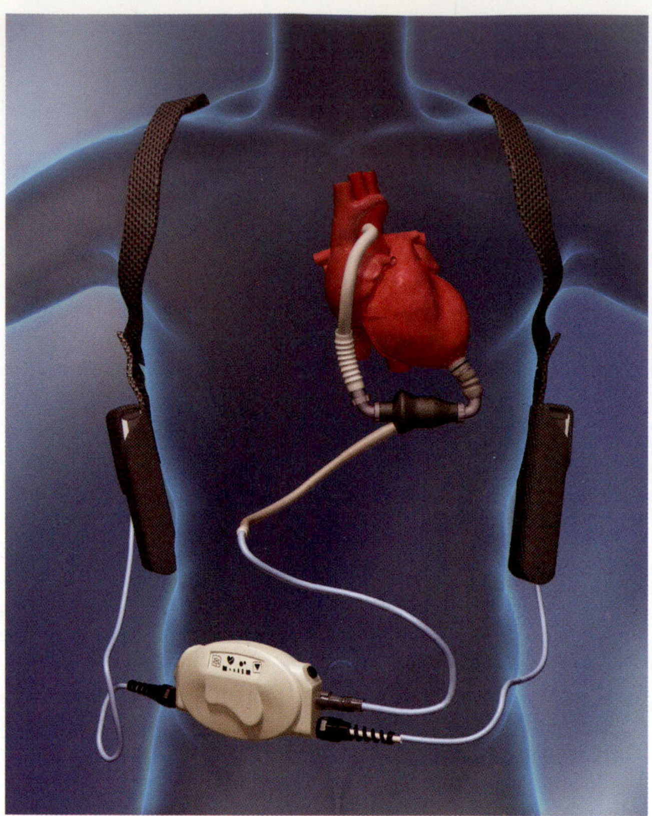

FIGURE 36-22 The cannula of the ventricular assist device (VAD) takes blood from the left atrium to the aorta, bypassing the ineffective left ventricle. (*Reprinted with permission from Thoratec Corporation.*)

PROFESSIONALTIP

Digoxin in Older Adults

HF is the leading cause of hospitalization in adults 65 years of age and older. New data indicates that a low dose (0.125 mg/day or lower) of digoxin decreases hospitalization due to HF and may also reduce mortality. Lower doses also decrease the risk of digoxin toxicity and the need for frequent serum digoxin levels. Digoxin in low doses is recommended for older adults with chronic HF (Ahmed, 2008).

Activity

Activity orders will depend on the client's activity tolerance. The client's activity may vary from strict bed rest to ambulation depending on the severity of the condition. When in bed, the head of the bed is elevated 45 degrees. Visitation privileges are monitored to provide rest periods.

Health Promotion

The most common cause of HF is left ventricular failure after a myocardial infarction. To prevent HF following coronary artery disease, a diet low in fat, high in fiber, and balanced in caloric intake to maintain optimum weight is recommended. Stress reduction and a regular exercise program will also decrease the risk of developing HF. Clients with congenital heart defects may not be able to prevent HF, but following the prescribed medical regimen may prevent the early development of HF.

TABLE 36-4 Recommended and Contraindicated Medications in Heart Failure

RECOMMENDED MEDICATIONS FOR HEART FAILURE THERAPY	CONTRAINDICATED MEDICATIONS FOR HEART FAILURE PATIENTS
• Loop diuretics for volume overload • ACE inhibitors (titrate upward to optimal dose) • Beta blockers (titrate upward to optimal dose with support and monitoring) • Digitalis • Spironolactone for advanced heart failure (with optimal doses of ACE inhibitors and beta blockers. Monitor for complications such as hyperkalemia) • ARBs if ACE inhibitors are not tolerated	• Alcohol • Cocaine • Antiarrhythmic agents except amiodarone • Calcium channel blockers except amlodipine • NSAIDs (associated with development of CHF and interact with ACE inhibitors) • Thiazolidinediones (may cause fluid retention) • Metformin

From State of the Science for Care of Older Adults with Heart Disease, by C. Deaton, J. Bennett, & B. Riegel, (2004). In *Nursing Clinics of North America, 39*(3), 495–528; Polypharmacy and Comorbidity in Heart Failure, by F. Masoudi & H. Krumholz, (2003), in *British Journal of Medicine, 327*(7414), 513–514.

NURSING MANAGEMENT

Monitor client's level of consciousness, skin color and turgor, and jugular veins for distension. Assess breath, heart, and bowel sounds. Check capillary refill and peripheral and abdominal edema. Weigh client daily at same time, on same scale, in same type of clothes. Monitor electrolytes and vital signs. Keep bed in semi-Fowler's position. Maintain accurate intake and output. Provide frequent rest periods and minimal interruptions at night. Teach about disease process, medications, and diet.

NURSING PROCESS

ASSESSMENT

Subjective Data

Ask the client about dyspnea, orthopnea, fatigue, anxiety, weight gain, edema, pain, or difficulty in performing activities of daily living.

Objective Data

Assess the client's level of consciousness to determine circulation of blood to the brain. Check skin color for pallor or cyanosis. Assess skin turgor to help determine the level of hydration. Jugular distention indicates right ventricle functioning. Assess breath sounds for adventitious sounds and heart sounds for gallop or murmurs. Bowel sounds may be hypoactive depending on the amount of fluid retention in the abdomen. Check peripheral pulses and capillary refill to assess the level of circulation to the extremities. Assess edema in the extremities and abdomen according to the edema rating scale. Monitor the client's weight daily for possible increase from fluid retention. The physician should be notified if there is a gain of more than 2 pounds in one day. Monitor I&O and assess for oliguria.

Nursing diagnoses for a client with HF include the following:

NURSING DIAGNOSES	PLANNING/OUTCOMES	NURSING INTERVENTIONS
Decreased **C***ardiac Output* related to mechanical failure of heart muscle	The client's vital signs will remain stable. The client will have decreased adventitious breath sounds.	Take an apical pulse on all cardiac clients, especially checking the rate and rhythm. Monitor the client's HR and rhythm by telemetry. Auscultate breath sounds every 4 hours. Administer diuretics, digitalis, and vasodilators as prescribed. Closely monitor the electrolytes, especially the potassium level, as diuretics can deplete the potassium level. Administer potassium supplements as ordered. Take the apical pulse before giving a digitalis preparation. If the HR is below 60, withhold the medication and notify the physician. In some institutions the HR can drop to 50 before the physician is notified if the client is taking a calcium channel blocker or beta-blocker along with digitalis.

(*Continues*)

Nursing diagnoses for a client with HF include the following: (Continued)

NURSING DIAGNOSES	PLANNING/OUTCOMES	NURSING INTERVENTIONS
*Impaired **G**as Exchange* related to decreased CO and pulmonary edema	The client will have increased gas exchange.	Provide oxygen by mask or nasal cannula at 2 to 6 L/min. Apply a pulse oximeter and monitor the oxygenation status. If the pulse oximeter is ≤90%, notify the physician. Elevate the head of the bed to a semi-Fowler's or Fowler's position to relieve pressure on the diaphragm.
*Excess **F**luid Volume* related to decreased cardiac output and decreased renal output	The client will have less edema of the extremities.	Encourage elevation of the client's legs, not letting them hang in a dependent position. Maintain an accurate intake and output. Weigh daily at the same time each day, on the same scales, and with the client wearing the same type of clothing. If the client is on a fluid-restricted diet, offer hard candies to quench the thirst.
*Risk for **A**ctivity Intolerance* related to edema, dyspnea, and fatigue	The client will have an increased tolerance for activity.	Schedule nursing care so the client is given frequent rest periods with minimal interruptions at night. Teach the client to take frequent rest periods and to stop activities before becoming tired. Monitor the client's vital signs for an increase or decrease in HR or blood pressure, especially after periods of activity. Have an occupational therapist assist the client in energy saving methods. Instruct the client to call the physician if there is more dyspneic, fatigue, less activity tolerance, or weight gain or loss when at home.

Evaluation: Evaluate each outcome to determine how it has been met by the client.

COR PULMONALE

In this condition, the heart is affected because of a lung condition that interferes with the exchange of carbon dioxide and oxygen in the alveoli. The carbon dioxide level increases in the blood. For some unknown reason, the pulmonary arteries vasoconstrict, causing pulmonary hypertension. The right ventricle is forced to pump against increased pulmonary pressure. The right ventricle enlarges and finally weakens in the attempt to pump blood into the lungs. The symptoms the client experiences and medical and nursing care are the same as for right-sided HF.

CARDIAC TRANSPLANTATION

Cardiac transplantations are done for cardiomyopathy, end-stage coronary artery disease, and valvular disease. Recipients are evaluated for emotional stability, minimal disease involvement, and a good support system. The heart donor and the recipient's tissues are matched.

The transplant is performed by removing the recipient's heart except for posterior sections of the atria. The posterior sections of the atria are removed from the donor's heart, and then the heart is sutured to the recipient's posterior atria.

The recipient must remain on an immunosuppressant medication for the remainder of life so the donor heart is not rejected. Some immunosuppressant medications are azathioprine (Imuran), cyclosporine (Sandimmune), antithymocytic globulin, ATG (Atgam), antilymphocytic globulin (ALG), rapamycin, and FK 506 (Prograf).

PERIPHERAL VASCULAR DISORDERS

Disorders in this category include aneurysm, hypertension, venous thrombosis/thrombophlebitis, varicose veins, Buerger's disease, and Raynaud's disease.

ANEURYSM

An **aneurysm** is a localized dilation occurring in a weakened section of an artery's medial layer. The main cause for aneurysms is atherosclerosis (Mayo Clinic, 2002). Some aneurysms occur because of congenital conditions such as Marfan's syndrome or because of trauma to the vessel wall. Two other possible causes of an aneurysm are an increased turbulence in a section of the vessel and a slower production of smooth muscle cells. Clients have a higher tendency to develop an aneurysm if they smoke cigarettes and have hypertension.

Aneurysms can occur in any artery but occur most often in the abdominal aorta. Abdominal aneurysms occur more frequently in men over the age of 55 (Mayo Clinic, 2002). Other involved vessels are the ascending, transverse, and descending aorta, thoracic aorta, popliteal arteries, and femoral arteries.

Deposits of atherosclerotic plaque on the tunica intima cause a hardening of the vessel, and the media layer of the vessel loses elasticity. Atherosclerosis and a lack of elastin in the vessel wall predisposes the vessel to a weakened area, which develops into an aneurysm.

Symptoms of an aneurysm depend on its location. Aneurysms are often asymptomatic until they start leaking or pressing on other structures. A thoracic aneurysm may press on surrounding structures, causing dull upper back pain or deep, scattered chest pain. Pressure on the trachea and bronchus may cause dyspnea, coughing, wheezing,and hoarseness. Pressure on the esophagus causes dysphagia.

The most common location of an abdominal aortic aneurysm is between the renal and iliac arteries. There may be no symptoms, but as it enlarges and presses on other vessels, organs, and nerves, the client may experience abdominal, back, or flank pain. The client may feel a pulse in the abdomen when in a supine position. A tender pulsating mass may be palpated slightly left of the umbilicus. Popliteal and femoral aneurysms may cause decreased pedal pulses. Rupture of an aneurysm is an emergency situation. Signs of rupture may include hypotension, tachycardia, pallor, cool and clammy skin, and intense abdominal, back, or groin pain. An aneurysm is usually diagnosed when a client has an x-ray or ultrasound done for other conditions/symptoms.

Medical–Surgical Management

Medical

If the client has hypertension, control of the hypertension is the focus of care. Aneurysms are monitored for enlargement. Thrombi formation and ischemia may also result.

Surgical

Before elective surgery, the status of the client's carotid arteries and peripheral vessels are checked with a Doppler ultrasound. Cardiac status is usually evaluated by a stress test or cardiac catheterization before surgery is scheduled. The surgeon often orders an angiogram, ultrasound, or CT scan of the affected vessel before surgery to assess the blood supply to the area surrounding the aneurysm. Before surgery, 4 to 8 units of blood are placed on hold because hemorrhage is a possibility. The surgeon clamps the aorta, removes the section of the vessel involving the aneurysm, and replaces it with a section of the client's saphenous vein or a synthetic graft (Figure 36-23). Complications that can occur from clamping the aorta are myocardial infarctions, strokes, and renal damage. Vessels below the repaired aneurysm may become occluded because of decreased blood flow during surgery or from plaque that has broken off from the wall of the vessel. A nasogastric tube may be inserted to decrease pressure on the aneurysm repair site and incision. After surgery, the client may be in the ICU with mechanical ventilator assistance in breathing.

Pharmacological

Clients with aortic aneurysms may be given propranolol hydrochloride (Inderal) to decrease the pressure of the blood coming from the heart. Clients with hypertension are given antihypertensive medications and diuretics. Analgesics are given to control pain.

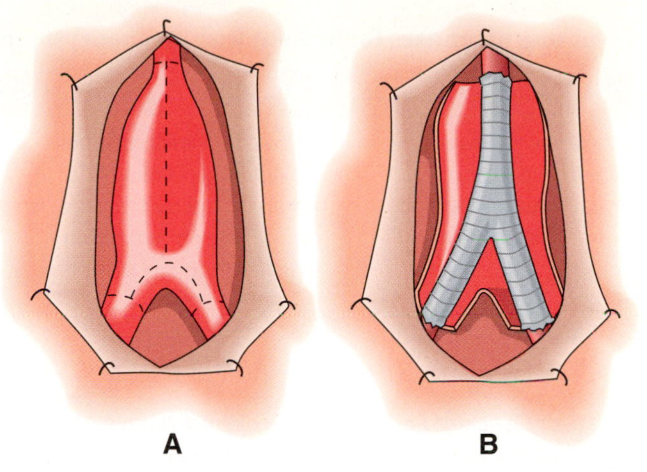

FIGURE 36-23 *A*, **Aortoiliac Aneurysm;** *B*, **Bifurcated Synthetic Graft**

Activity

Any activity that increases blood pressure, especially exercise and lifting, can increase pressure in the arteries and should be avoided.

Health Promotion

Clients are encouraged not to smoke. Education for the hypertensive client includes the importance of closely monitoring the blood pressure and taking antihypertensive medication as prescribed.

Nursing Management

Preoperatively, monitor vital signs and peripheral pulses. Assess capillary refill, feet for mottling, and for edema. Postoperatively, add checking operative site frequently. Check function and drainage of NG tube. Measure abdomen for increasing size indicating internal hemorrhage. Measure output hourly for at least 25 to 30 mL of urine.

NURSING PROCESS

Assessment

Subjective Data

Preoperatively, the client may be concerned about an abdominal pulsation when reclining. The client may have chest, back, abdominal, or flank pain depending on the aneurysm location. Postoperatively, listen for statements of pain and assess the level of pain according to a scale of 1 to 10 or the facility-approved scale.

Objective Data

Palpate the abdomen for a pulsating mass, and check vital signs. Immediate intervention is needed if symptoms of bleeding or a rupturing aneurysm occur. Check the peripheral pulses before surgery. Pulses can then be compared preoperatively and postoperatively. Postoperatively, assess the extremities for color, warmth, peripheral pulses, and sensation.

Nursing diagnoses for a client with an aneurysm include the following:

NURSING DIAGNOSES	PLANNING/OUTCOMES	NURSING INTERVENTIONS
*Ineffective **Tissue** Perfusion (Peripheral)* related to decreased arterial blood flow	The client will have well-oxygenated tissues as manifested by strong pulses and the skin remaining baseline color and warm.	Monitor for symptoms of an occluded vessel (pain, paleness, cyanosis, and coldness). Monitor the temperature, color, and fullness of the peripheral pulses in both extremities and compare them to the preoperative pulses. Assess capillary refill and client's feet for mottling and darkened areas on the toes and soles of the feet. Notify physician immediately if any of these symptoms occur.
*Risk for Deficient **Fluid** Volume* related to hemorrhage	The client will have adequate fluid volume.	Monitor vital signs closely for signs of hemorrhage. Check the operative site frequently to make sure the dressing is dry. Turn the client to make sure blood is not pooling under the client's body. Monitor for other signs of hemorrhaging. Measure the abdomen for increasing abdominal girth indicating internal bleeding. If the client has low back pain, there may be hemorrhaging in the retroperitoneal space. Other symptoms of hemorrhage are lightheadedness, dizziness, and tachycardia. Check for adequate functioning and drainage of the NG tube to decrease pressure on the aneurysm repair site and incision.
*Ineffective **Tissue** Perfusion (Renal)* related to interruption of blood flow during surgery	The client will have a urine output above 25 mL/hour.	Measure hourly output to make sure the client has at least 25 to 30 mL of urine per hour. Assess for edema which could indicate fluid overload or a vessel occlusion. Provide fluids as ordered.

Evaluation: Evaluate each outcome to determine how it has been met by the client.

HYPERTENSION

Hypertension (HTN), also known as high blood pressure, is defined as an elevated arterial blood pressure. A systolic blood pressure at or above 140 or a diastolic blood pressure at or above 90 indicates hypertension. Fifty million adults in the United States have hypertension (NIH, 2002).

Before age 55, more men than women have hypertension, but after age 55, more women have hypertension (CDC, 2002). Unalterable risk factors include African-American race, male gender, aging, postmenopausal women, and family history of hypertension. Modifiable risk factors include smoking, lack of exercise, obesity, stress, low socioeconomic status, diet high in sodium and fat, alcohol intake, and oral contraceptives.

When the cause of hypertension is unknown, it is called **primary hypertension** or "essential hypertension." Eighty to ninety-five percent of clients with hypertension have primary hypertension (Klabunde, 2007). In 5% to 10% of the cases, the cause of hypertension is another condition within the body such as renal artery stenosis, chronic renal disease, primary hyperaldosteronism, sleep apnea, hyper- or hypothyroidism, pheochromocytoma, preeclampsia, or aortic coarctation (Klabunde, 2007); this is known as **secondary hypertension.** Arteriosclerosis, atherosclerosis, hypernatremia (increased sodium in the blood) or prolonged stress may also cause hypertension.

Malignant hypertension is a rapidly progressing, severe elevation of BP (diastolic 120 mm Hg). It damages small arterioles in the major organs. Arteriole inflammation in the eyes is the primary distinguishing finding. It is most common in black males younger than 40 years of age.

Renal diseases that interfere with blood flow to the kidneys cause them to release an enzyme called renin. The released renin interacts with plasma proteins, forming a vasopressor called *angiotensin*. Vasoconstriction caused by angiotensin increases blood pressure when more force is required to push the blood through the vessel. Vasodilation decreases vascular or **peripheral resistance** (pressure within a vessel that resists the flow of blood such as plaque buildup or vasoconstriction). Figure 36-24 depicts how renal disease causes hypertension.

Arteriosclerosis causes the vessel walls to have less elasticity, decreasing their ability to expand and recoil. Because the vessel is not able to expand, more pressure is needed to force the blood through the vessel. The plaque buildup causes resistance to blood flow through the vessel, and more pressure is needed to get the blood through the vessel. Hypernatremia (increased blood sodium) causes vasocongestion, and the heart must pump with more force, increasing the pressure in the arteries, thus causing HTN.

Stress stimulates the sympathetic nervous system, which supplies nerves to the smooth muscles of the arteries, arterioles, veins, and venules. Stimulation of these smooth muscles

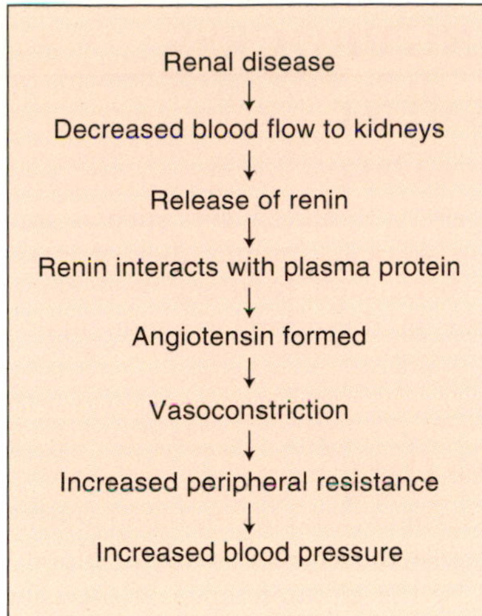

COURTESY OF DELMAR CENGAGE LEARNING

FIGURE 36-24 Pathophysiology of Renal Diseases and Hypertension

causes the vessels to constrict, leading to elevated blood pressure.

Some complications of HTN are cerebral vascular accident (stroke), myocardial infarction, HF, and renal failure. Table 36-5 lists the recognized classification of blood pressure.

TABLE 36-5 Classification of Blood Pressure

CATEGORY	SYSTOLIC (MM HG)		DIASTOLIC (MM HG)
Normal	<120	and	<80
Prehypertension	120–139	or	80–89
Hypertension			
Stage 1	140–159	or	90–99
Stage 2	≥160	or	≥ 100

From *The Seventh Report of the Joint National Committee on Prevention, Detection, Evaluation, and Treatment of High Blood Pressure*, 2003, Bethesda, MD: National Institutes of Health.

MEDICAL–SURGICAL MANAGEMENT

Medical

The main goal for a client with HTN is keeping the blood pressure within normal limits. The regimen is referred to as a stepped-care approach. The first step is to encourage the client to try some diet and lifestyle changes, including losing weight if >15% over optimum weight; limiting sodium, saturated fat, cholesterol, and alcohol intake; exercising on a regular basis; stopping the use of nicotine; and maintaining an adequate intake of calcium, magnesium, and potassium. This step is tried for 3 to 6 months, and if the BP then is < 140/90 mm Hg, these steps are continued. If the BP still remains high, the second step is the addition of a diuretic or a beta-blocker to the client's care regimen. The client is again evaluated for a period of time, usually 2 months. If the BP still is not <140/90 mm Hg, the third step of increasing the drug dosage, trying another drug, or adding a second antihypertensive drug from another class of drugs is implemented. If the BP is maintained at <140/90 mm Hg, the regimen is continued. If the BP is still high, the last step is implemented by adding a second or third antihypertensive drug.

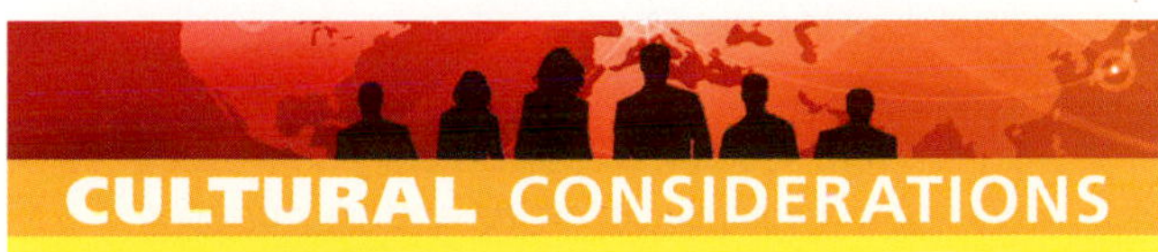

Hypertension

African-American clients develop hypertension earlier in life, and it is more severe at any decade of life, than other ethnic groups.

Pharmacological

Diuretics are usually the first pharmacological step in treating HTN. Diuretics increase the renal excretion of sodium and water from the body, decreasing the total fluid volume. When less fluid is in the body, less pressure or force is needed to pump the blood through the body.

Beta-adrenergic blocking agents are given to block the epinephrine and norepinephrine receptor sites. With these receptor sites blocked, the vessels do not constrict and the blood has less resistance flowing through the vessel. Diuretics and antihypertensive medications may cause impotence.

Diet

A low-fat, low-cholesterol, and low-sodium diet is encouraged. Restricting sodium intake to 2.3 grams of sodium or 6 grams of sodium chloride per day assists in decreasing blood pressure. Avoiding processed foods, carbonated drinks, and most cereals helps decrease sodium intake. Encourage the client to have an adequate intake of potassium, magnesium, and calcium. These minerals are obtained by eating fresh oranges, bananas, broccoli, and collards. Fresh foods are better sources for minerals than frozen foods. Yogurt is a good calcium supplement. The National Committee on Prevention, Detection, Evaluation, and Treatment of High Blood Pressure recommends that clients with hypertension not consume more than 2 ounces of alcohol at a time and no more than twice a week.

Activity

A regular aerobic exercise regimen assists in lowering blood pressure. The client is to gradually increase the exercise period to

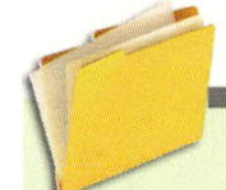

COLLABORATIVE CARE

Hypertension

Assisting a client to eliminate hypertension is a multidisciplinary task. Members of the care team most often include physician, nurses, dietitian, fitness center therapist, smoking cessation counselor, and stress management advisor.

CRITICAL THINKING

Lifestyle Changes for Hypertension

How can you best teach the hypertensive client ways to modify the present lifestyle?

30 to 45 minutes 3 to 5 times per week with a pulse rate at 75% of the target HR (target HR = 220 – age × 0.75). Walking, swimming, and jogging are excellent aerobic exercises.

Health Promotion

Measures to prevent hypertension are exercising regularly; reducing sodium in the diet; maintaining an optimum weight; reducing and managing stress; maintaining intake of potassium, calcium, and magnesium; decreasing alcohol consumption; and ceasing smoking.

NURSING MANAGEMENT

Monitor BP. Make referrals to assist in lifestyle changes. Explain pathophysiology, risk factors, suggested lifestyle changes, and complications.

NURSING PROCESS

ASSESSMENT

Subjective Data

Ask about general lifestyle habits such as smoking, alcohol consumption, exercise routine, dietary intake, and family history of hypertension. Note any dizziness, blurred vision, and headache in the occipital region upon rising in the morning.

Objective Data

The basic assessment is taking the blood pressure. An accurate reading requires the correct width of blood pressure cuff, determined by the circumference of the client's extremity. The cuff bladder should encircle 80% of the arm to obtain an accurate blood pressure (JNC 7 Express, 2003). The blood pressure is taken in both arms in supine and sitting positions. Before taking the blood pressure, the client should rest quietly in a chair, rather than on an exam table, for 5 minutes with both feet on the floor and the arm supported at heart level. If the client has an elevated BP, a repeat blood pressure is taken 15 minutes later and compared to previous readings. Measure client height and weight, heart sounds, and peripheral pulses.

Nursing diagnoses for a client with hypertension include the following:

NURSING DIAGNOSES	PLANNING/OUTCOMES	NURSING INTERVENTIONS
*Ineffective **H**ealth Maintenance* related to lack of knowledge about lifestyle habits contributing to hypertension	The client will relate needed changes in lifestyle habits to decrease blood pressure.	Make referrals to the appropriate personnel to teach the client lifestyle changes. These may include a dietitian, smoking cessation clinic, fitness center, or stress management seminars. Explain the pathophysiology, risk factors, lifestyle changes, medication actions and side effects, and complications of hypertension.
***N**oncompliance* related to individual's value system (lack of physical symptoms and expense of medication)	The client will keep appointments for regular check-ups and take medications as prescribed.	Regularly inquire about the client's satisfaction in regard to the prescribed regimen of diet, exercise, and prescribed medication(s). If the client cannot afford needed medications, refer the client to financial assistance programs. Encourage the client to become an active participant in the treatment because this will give the client a sense of control over the condition. Encourage the client to record BP readings, weekly weight, exercise activities, and dietary intake as a way of giving a sense of control and encouraging compliance.
*Imbalanced **N**utrition: More than Body Requirements* related to excess caloric intake and excess sodium intake	The client will maintain weight at no more than 15% over optimum weight and have no more than 2.3 grams of sodium per day.	Give basic dietary instructions as stated under medical management or make a referral to a dietitian. Weigh the client at scheduled appointments.

Nursing diagnoses for a client with hypertension include the following: (Continued)

NURSING DIAGNOSES	PLANNING/OUTCOMES	NURSING INTERVENTIONS
*Sexual **D**ysfunction* related to altered body structure or function and side effects of antihypertensive medications	The client will state satisfaction with sexual function while taking antihypertensive medications.	Because diuretics and antihypertensive medications may cause impotence, discuss this effect in an open and candid manner, so the client and spouse will be feel comfortable discussing sexual difficulties.

Evaluation: Evaluate each outcome to determine how it has been met by the client.

SAMPLE NURSING CARE PLAN

The Client with Hypertension

T.L., a 28-year-old African-American client, is in his last year of law school and is clerking for a prestigious law firm. He and his fiancé plan to marry as soon as he graduates. During the last week he has had four dizzy spells and a headache at the base of his skull upon awakening for the last 2 days. His father has a history of hypertension, so T.L. is aware that his symptoms may indicate high blood pressure. T.L. stops by the clinic on his way home from work and asks the nurse to check his blood pressure. The nursing assessment has the following data.

Subjective data: States he has had four dizzy spells and has awakened with a headache in the occipital lobe the last two mornings. T.L. has 1 glass of wine at lunch and 2–3 beers in the evening to relax from the tension of school and work. Most of his meals are at fast-food establishments and have a high fat content. T.L. does not smoke. He used to jog 4 mornings a week but quit when he started clerking. He has had nocturia for the last 3 weeks. He is not taking any medication. T.L. states he is concerned about having hypertension because he does not want to take medication.

Objective data: T 98.6°F, AP 78 beats/min, R 16 breaths/min, BP 142/92 mm Hg, Wt 190 lbs (optimum weight 160). No edema noted in hands, feet, or legs.

NURSING DIAGNOSIS 1 *Ineffective **H**ealth Maintenance* related to ineffective individual coping as evidenced by high-fat diet, lack of exercise, stressful job, and alcohol intake

Nursing Outcomes Classification (NOC)
Health-Promoting Behavior
Knowledge: Health Promotion

Nursing Interventions Classification (NIC)
Health Education
Self-Responsibility Facilitation
Risk Identification

PLANNING/OUTCOMES	NURSING INTERVENTIONS	RATIONALE
T.L. will change lifestyle habits by engaging in aerobic exercises at least 3 times a week for 30 to 45 minutes, stating three ways to reduce stress, and limiting alcohol consumption to 2 ounces twice a week.	Refer T.L. to a dietitian to learn ways to cut fat and sodium in his diet.	Knowledge encourages compliance.
	Discuss ways T.L. can exercise and still meet responsibilities of work, school, and personal and social life.	Encourages exercise if he sees ways that he can still meet responsibilities of life.
	Explain alcohol content in various beverages.	Encourages compliance.

EVALUATION

T.L. begins exercising with his fiancé 3 times a week. T.L. uses breathing techniques and a hot shower to reduce daily stress. T.L. limits alcohol consumption to 1 beer a day.

NURSING DIAGNOSIS 2 *Imbalanced **N**utrition:* More than Body Requirements, related to excessive caloric intake as evidenced by 30 pounds overweight and high-fat diet

(Continues)

SAMPLE NURSING CARE PLAN (Continued)

Nursing Outcomes Classification (NOC)	Nursing Interventions Classification (NIC)
Nutritional Status	*Nutrition Management*
Teaching: Nutrition	*Nutrition Monitoring*

PLANNING/OUTCOMES	NURSING INTERVENTIONS	RATIONALE
T.L. will lose 30 pounds and maintain a low-fat, low-sodium diet.	Refer T.L. to a weight support group.	It is easier to lose weight with support of others.
	Encourage T.L. to record a weekly weight and daily intake of fat.	Promotes self-care.

EVALUATION

T.L. is maintaining a diet low in sodium and no more than 30 grams of fat per day. T.L. keeps a weekly record of his weight.

NURSING DIAGNOSIS 3 *Anxiety* related to threat to or change in health status and stress as evidenced by alcohol consumption to relax and statement of not wanting to take medications

Nursing Outcomes Classification (NOC)	Nursing Interventions Classification (NIC)
Anxiety Reduction	*Anxiety Reduction*
Coping	*Anticipatory Guidance*

PLANNING/OUTCOMES	INTERVENTIONS	RATIONALE
T.L. states preventive measures to reduce blood pressure.	Have T.L. identify stress factors in life.	Action to cope with stressors can be taken only if stressors are identified.
	Discuss stress reduction techniques with T.L.	Knowledge promotes compliance.
	Discuss risk factors of hypertension and ways to reduce it.	Promotes identification of risk factors in personal life.
	Explain to T.L. and his fiancé that hypertension is a chronic condition, possibly without symptoms, but with some potentially serious complications.	Knowledge promotes compliance.

EVALUATION

T.L. states four ways to reduce blood pressure.

VENOUS THROMBOSIS/ THROMBOPHLEBITIS

The terms *phlebitis, thrombosis, phlebothrombosis,* and *thrombophlebitis* are often used interchangeably even though each word has a separate meaning and etiology. **Phlebitis** is an inflammation in the wall of a vein without clot formation. The formation of a clot in a vessel is a **thrombosis**, and a formed clot that remains at the site where it formed is a **thrombus**. If the thrombus moves, it becomes an **embolus**, a mass such as a blood clot or an air bubble that circulates in the bloodstream. **Phlebothrombosis** is the formation of a clot because of blood pooling in the vessel, trauma to the vessel's endothelial lining, or a coagulation problem with little or no inflammation in the vessel. **Thrombophlebitis** is the formation of a clot caused by an inflammation in the wall of the vessel.

In 1846, Virchow listed three factors leading to the formation of a clot: pooling of blood, vessel trauma, and a coagulation problem. These are known as **Virchow's triad**. Risk factors for thrombi formation are prolonged bed rest, leg trauma, oral contraceptives, obesity, varicose veins, hip fractures, and total hip and knee replacement.

There are two types of thrombi: a superficial thrombus and a deep vein thrombus (DVT). A superficial vein thrombus forms in a superficial vein such as the saphenous vein in the leg.

A DVT forms in the deep veins of the arms, pelvic area, or legs, but the legs are the most common site. Leg veins in which clots form are the femoral, popliteal, iliac, and deep veins of the calf.

Phlebitis can either form spontaneously or as a result of IV catheters or cannulas, IV medications such as potassium or antibiotics, or direct trauma to a vein. A clot may then form as red blood cells pass over the damaged area, rupture, and start the clotting process.

Phlebitis manifests as a reddened streak over a vein. If a clot is in a superficial vein, the site becomes reddened, warm, tender, and swollen. A hardening is palpated in a section of the vein. There are no symptoms with a deep vein thrombus, or there may be warmth and tenderness at the site, unilateral edema of the affected extremity, positive Homans' sign, dilation of superficial veins, and cyanosis of the foot. The client may say the leg feels "tight" or "heavy." If the clot is in the calf of the leg, the calf may feel tender. If the swelling restricts the arterial blood flow, the leg may be cool and pale. If there are obvious clinical signs of a thrombosis, Homans' sign should not be assessed because the clot may be dislodged and become an embolus.

A complication of a DVT is a pulmonary embolus that may result in death. Symptoms of a pulmonary embolus are sudden and severe chest pain, dyspnea, and tachypnea. Emboli may travel and block other vessels in the heart, brain, or peripheral vessels.

Medical–Surgical Management

Medical

A superficial phlebitis or thrombus may need no treatment, or warm soaks may be applied to the affected area. Acetaminophen or an NSAID is given for pain. Elevating the extremity decreases swelling and improves venous return. Some doctors recommend the application of elastic support hose. If a DVT is diagnosed, the client is placed on bed rest. Once the client improves and becomes ambulatory, below-the-knee compression stockings are recommended.

Surgical

If a clot has formed in a large vein and all conservative methods have failed, the clot may be removed surgically. This procedure is called a **thrombectomy** and is performed only if the tissue in the area becomes ischemic or gangrenous or if the client has a history of thromboemboli.

Another surgical procedure is a vena cava interruption surgery (venacaval plication) in which a Greenfield vena cava filter or umbrella filter is placed in the inferior vena cava to prevent thromboemboli from traveling from the lower extremities to the lungs, heart, or brain. Figure 36-25 shows these filters and their placement in the vena cava. The procedure is done on clients with a history of pulmonary emboli.

Pharmacological

If a client is at risk for a thrombus or phlebitis, anticoagulant therapy is initiated. A prophylactic heparin dose is given. Enoxaparin injection (Lovenox), a low-molecular-weight heparin, is used prophylactically after hip replacement surgery. It should be used cautiously with clients on oral anticoagulants.

If a clot forms, the client is immediately started on heparin as an IV bolus and then followed with a continuous IV drip of heparin. Before heparin is started, a partial thromboplastin time (PTT) or activated partial thromboplastin time (APTT) and a platelet count are drawn by the laboratory to establish a baseline level. The heparin dose is regulated by the PTT or the APTT. For effective heparin therapy, the client's PTT or APTT level should be 2.5 times the baseline. A **baseline level** is a value at a particular time that serves as a reference point for future value levels.

Clients are usually discharged on Coumadin. Because of rapid hospital discharges, clients are often started on Coumadin the next day after heparin has been initiated. Once the Coumadin dose is regulated, heparin is stopped.

CLIENT TEACHING

Thrombophlebitis

- Drink 2 to 3 quarts of water per day.
- Do not sit with legs crossed.
- Elevate both legs when sitting.
- Avoid sitting or standing for extended periods.
- Wear support hose.
- When standing, shift weight frequently and occasionally stand on tiptoes to stimulate the calf muscle to pump blood.
- Notify the physician immediately if leg pain, tenderness or swelling, difficulty breathing, or chest pain is experienced.

A

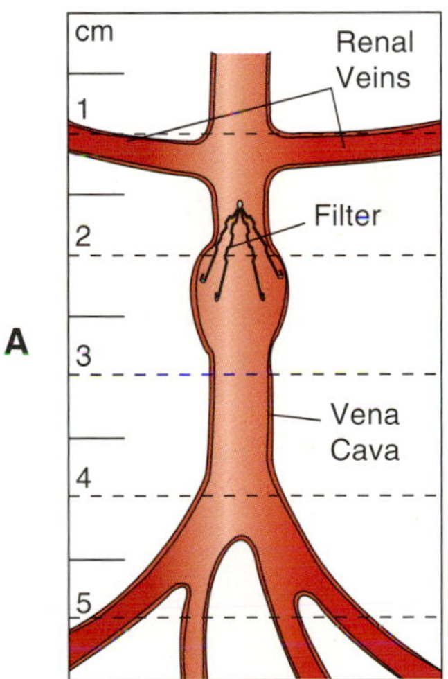

B

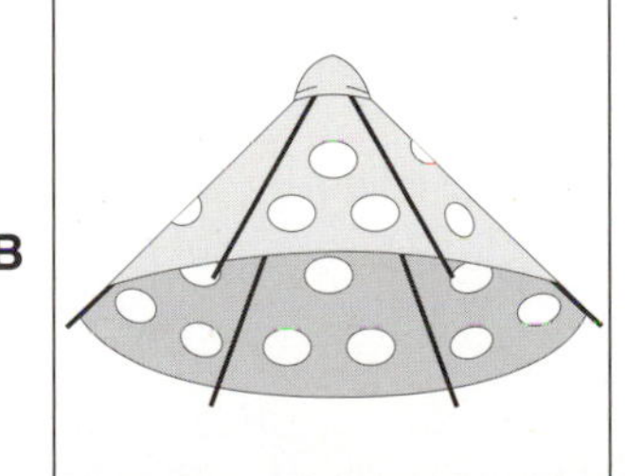

COURTESY OF DELMAR CENGAGE LEARNING

Figure 36-25 Filter in the Vena Cava Prevents an Embolus from Traveling to the Heart, Lungs, or Brain; *A*, Greenfield Filter in Place; *B*, Umbrella Filter

After the initial Coumadin dose, the daily Coumadin dose is regulated by the prothrombin time (PT) or the International Normalized Ratio (INR). The client generally remains on Coumadin for 3 to 6 months.

Thrombolytic drugs, urokinase (Abbokinase), streptokinase (Streptase), and tissue plasminogen activator, t-PA (Alteplase), are used locally and systemically if there is a massive DVT. Streptokinase should only be used on the same client once every 6 months. If the client has had a recent streptococcal infection, streptokinase may not be effective (Spratto & Woods, 2010). The main complication in a client receiving thrombolytic drugs is bleeding. Heparin and Coumadin are given after the thrombolytic drugs to prevent thrombi formation.

Diet

Adequate hydration is important for clients at risk for thrombi. This is accomplished orally or intravenously.

Activity

During the acute stage, the client is placed on bed rest to prevent the clot from dislodging and embolizing. Later, the leg is elevated periodically to improve venous return and decrease swelling. The client's leg should never be massaged because a clot could be dislodged and become an embolus.

Health Promotion

Prevention is the best way to treat a DVT. Early ambulation, adequate hydration, alternating pneumatic compression devices, prophylactic anticoagulants, elevation of legs, leg exercises, and deep breathing exercises all contribute to the prevention of thrombi.

Nursing Management

Monitor vital signs for changes and IV sites for redness and warmth. Do not do a Homans' sign if there is a diagnosis of a thrombus. Measure the circumference of the affected leg. Assess peripheral pulses and capillary refill. If on anticoagulant drugs, assess for signs of bleeding. When on bed rest, elevate the entire affected leg. Remove elastic support or pneumatic compression stockings daily for hygiene.

NURSING PROCESS

Assessment

Subjective Data

Ask the client if there was any recent injury to the extremity, if the affected area is tender to the touch, or if there have been clots previously. Note any chest pain, dyspnea, tachycardia, or hemoptysis.

Objective Data

Check IV sites at least once per shift to see if a phlebitis or reddened area is developing at the insertion site. If a positive Homans' sign is detected during an assessment, notify the physician and do not perform another Homans' sign until a clot has been ruled out. Assess the skin for redness, tenderness, hardness, or warmth, and measure both legs to determine baseline measurements. Measure the circumference of the affected leg every shift to determine an increase or decrease in swelling. Assess peripheral pulses every 4 hours and more frequently if the client experiences increased pain in the leg, cyanosis of the foot or extremity, or increased swelling. These are signs of an occlusion.

Nursing diagnoses for a client with a venous thrombosis include the following:

NURSING DIAGNOSES	PLANNING/OUTCOMES	NURSING INTERVENTIONS
*Ineffective **T**issue Perfusion (Peripheral)* related to decreased venous blood flow and/or clot formation	The client will have adequate tissue perfusion.	Elevate the client's entire affected leg when on bed rest to improve venous return. When elevated, the leg should be slightly flexed at the knee with a pillow under the thigh and calf. Apply elastic support or intermittent pneumatic compression stockings on the client. Use intermittent pneumatic compression stockings only if a clot is not present. If the client has received thrombolytic or anticoagulant drugs, assess for signs of bleeding, which include hematuria, bruising, bleeding from the gums, and blood in the stool. Monitor pedal pulses and capillary refill and measure thigh or calf circumference daily.
*Acute **P**ain* related to inflammatory process	The client will state absence of pain.	If the client has phlebitis, apply warm moist soaks to the affected area as ordered. Administer acetaminophen or a nonsteroidal anti-inflammatory as ordered for discomfort.
***A**nxiety* related to possibility of the clot becoming an embolus	The client will express anxiety about possible embolus.	Encourage client to discuss the possibility of embolus formation.

Evaluation: Evaluate each outcome to determine how it has been met by the client.

VARICOSE VEINS

Varicose veins, also called **varicosities**, are visibly prominent, dilated, and twisted veins, usually in the lower extremities, but the veins in the esophagus (esophageal varices) and anus (hemorrhoids) can also be affected. Usually, the saphenous vein is affected in the leg. Women are more prone to varicose veins than men. Risk factors for developing varicose veins are a familial tendency, congenital abnormalities, pregnancy, obesity, constrictive clothing, and occupations that require prolonged standing. Pregnancy and obesity cause more pressure in the veins of the legs.

The causes of varicose veins are incompetent valves and veins that have lost their elasticity. The wall of the vessel is weakened from a lack of elastin or collagen and is unable to support the normal pressure of the blood in the vessel. The vein dilates as the blood in it flows backward. As the walls of the vein dilate, the valves become incapable of holding the blood and allow blood to leak backward through the space between the valves. Refer to Figure 36-5C. The client has pain in the feet and ankles, swelling, and ulcers on the skin. Trendelenburg's test is used for diagnosis.

MEDICAL–SURGICAL MANAGEMENT

Medical

Varicose veins are usually treated conservatively with elastic support hose, elevation of the legs when sitting, not crossing legs, and ankle and leg exercises.

Sclerotherapy involves injecting a chemical into the vein, causing the vein to become sclerosed (hardened) so blood no longer flows through it. A compression bandage or elastic stocking is applied to the extremity for 4 to 5 days. The client wears support hose for 5 more weeks. Complications of the procedure are **necrosis** (tissue death) at the injection site, vasospasm, allergic responses, and **hemolysis** (destruction of red blood cells).

Surgical

In more severe cases, varicose veins can be ligated (tied off) or stripped. **Vein stripping** involves introducing a wire into a vein. The wire has collapsible claws on the end. As the wire is withdrawn, the claws expand and strip the walls of the vein. This measure is used when there is a threat of thrombus or leg ulcers. **Vein ligation** is tying off an involved section of a vein with suture. Endovenous laser ablation is another method of treating varicose veins.

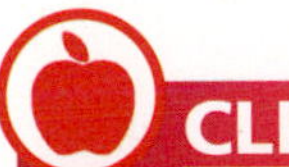

CLIENT TEACHING

Varicose Veins

Apply support hose after the legs have been elevated for an extended time, 10 to 15 minutes, so the venous blood drains from the legs. Application before getting out of bed in the morning is ideal. Do not fold or roll hose down from the top because this would act like a tourniquet, causing pooling of blood. Smooth the hose on the legs because wrinkles or creases may cause extra pressure, leading to stasis or pooling of blood or pressure ulcers. Remove hose daily so the leg can be washed and dried before reapplication.

Pharmacological

Analgesics are given for leg discomfort. Anticoagulants may be given to prevent clot formation.

Activity

The client is encouraged to exercise regularly. Walking is a very good exercise to improve circulation because the blood circulates faster in response to an increased heartbeat. Muscles in the legs apply pressure to the veins, forcing the blood toward the heart. Ankle exercises such as rotating the ankle in circular motions also improves circulation.

Health Promotion

Encourage clients with a familial tendency for varicose veins to elevate their legs 6 to 10 inches on a small stool when sitting in a chair. Frequent position changes and not standing in one spot for extended times also improve circulation.

NURSING MANAGEMENT

Assist the client in elevating the legs above the heart when in bed or elevating the feet 6 to 10 inches on a pillow or stool when sitting in a chair.

After sclerotherapy, the affected area may be tender and discolored. Most discoloration will disappear in a few weeks, but a darkened pigmentation may last for 6 to 8 months. Repeated sclerotherapy may be needed. Encourage the client to maintain a walking exercise program to improve circulation to the legs.

After a vein stripping, the client is on bed rest for the first 24 hours. Elastic hose are worn continuously for 5 days to compress the blood into the deeper veins and for 5 weeks after the surgery. Administer pain medication 30 minutes before the client ambulates until walking is tolerated without discomfort. Encourage walking and leg exercises.

BUERGER'S DISEASE (THROMBOANGIITIS OBLITERANS)

Buerger's disease is an inflammatory disease of small and medium arteries and veins that leads to vascular obstruction. Inflammation occurs in the adventitia and media layers of the vessels and may affect only a portion of the vessel or the entire vessel. Hands and feet are mainly involved, but the wrists and lower extremities may also be affected. The distal tips of the hands and feet are pale, but as the disease progresses, the hands and feet become reddened when held in a dependent position. At first, pain in the palm of the hand and arch of the foot is the main symptom. Pain becomes more severe with disease progression, and as ischemia affects the nerves, the client may experience numbness, burning, pain when at rest, and decreased sensation in the hands and lower extremities. The dorsalis pedis, posterior tibia, and ulnar and radial pulses are weak or absent. Skin color changes, cold sensitivity, ulcers, and gangrene occur in the later stages.

Buerger's disease occurs primarily in men between the ages of 20 and 40 of Israeli, Indian, and Asian descent. There is a correlation between smoking and Buerger's disease. Tests for diagnosis include arteriography and Doppler ultrasound.

MEDICAL–SURGICAL MANAGEMENT

Medical

The client is encouraged to stop smoking and is referred to a smoking clinic or seminar. Buerger-Allen exercises are recommended and explained. Buerger-Allen exercises consist of elevating the legs until they blanch and supporting them at that angle for 2 to 3 minutes. The legs are then lowered to a dependent position until they become red and supported at that level for 5 to 10 minutes. The legs are then placed flat on the bed with the client in a supine position for 10 minutes. The exercises are repeated as tolerated by the client.

Surgical

A sympathectomy (excision of a nerve, plexus, or ganglion of the sympathetic portion of the autonomic nervous system) is done to relieve pain and prevent vasospasm in the affected area. Digits and toes are amputated if gangrene occurs.

 Pharmacological

Analgesics are given to control pain. Vasodilators are given to increase circulation to the affected area.

NURSING MANAGEMENT

Nursing diagnoses and interventions are the same as for other obstructive vascular conditions and are described under Raynaud's disease.

RAYNAUD'S DISEASE/ PHENOMENON

Raynaud's disease or primary Raynaud's is an intermittent spasm of the digital arteries and arterioles resulting in decreased circulation to the fingers and toes. Sometimes the tip of the nose and ears are also affected. The cause of the condition is unknown but seems to be related to vasospastic disorders, a disturbance with the innervation of the sympathetic nervous system, and angiography complications.

MEMORYTRICK

Peripheral Vascular Disorders Assessment

The nurse remembers 5 **P**s when assessing clients with peripheral vascular disorders:

P = Pain
P = Pulse
P = Pallor
P = Paresthesia
P = Paralysis

During a spasm that lasts approximately 15 minutes, the fingers become pale and then cyanotic. As the circulation returns to the fingers, the fingertips become reddened and the person experiences a tingling or throbbing pain in the fingers. Some people experience only pallor and cyanosis. The episode may last 1 to 2 hours. Symptoms usually occur when the person is exposed to cold or experiences emotional stress. Gangrene is not common but can occur in the fingertips. Ulcerations can also occur and are difficult to heal because of decreased circulation in the fingers.

When associated with a connective tissue or collagen vascular disease, medications, or occupational trauma, the condition is called Raynaud's phenomenon or secondary Raynaud's. Raynaud symptoms may occur 10 years before the related disease is diagnosed. A 2-year history of signs and symptoms with no evidence of underlying disease, especially an autoimmune disease, is necessary for a diagnosis of Raynaud's disease.

Raynaud's is more prevalent in cold climates. Women are nine times more likely to be affected than men (Raynauds Association, 2008). Primary Raynaud's begins between the ages of 15 and 25 (NIAMS, 2006). Secondary Raynaud's begins later in life, between the ages of 35 to 40 (NIAMS, 2006). Persons who use vibrating hand tools such as air hammers or grinding wheels or who perform repetitive movements such as typing or playing the piano are at risk.

Diagnostic examinations include a complete blood count, digital blood pressure measurement, digital plethysmography waveforms, and a cold-challenge test. A digital blood pressure of 30 mm Hg below the brachial pressure indicates a digital artery obstruction. A sedimentation rate, antinuclear antibody, and rheumatoid factor determine the presence of autoimmune diseases. During a cold-challenge test, thermistors are placed on the fingers and a baseline temperature is taken. The hands are submerged into ice water for 20 seconds and then removed. The temperature of the hands is then taken every 5 minutes until it returns to the baseline level. Hand x-rays determine the presence of subcutaneous calcium deposits and narrowing of bone in the digits. The diagnostic tests distinguish between Raynaud's phenomenon and Raynaud's disease. If a client has unilateral or single-digit Raynaud's, an obstruction or emboli is suspected.

MEDICAL–SURGICAL MANAGEMENT

Medical

Raynaud's phenomenon is treated conservatively. The client is assessed regularly for symptoms of autoimmune diseases. If the symptoms of Raynaud's are caused by a vasospastic disease, relief is best achieved with medications. Alternative therapies such as relaxation techniques and biofeedback may be beneficial.

Surgical

A sympathectomy is sometimes done to alleviate the client's symptoms; however, it usually provides temporary relief and is not a routine treatment.

 Pharmacological

Calcium channel blockers, such as nifedipine (Adalat, Procardia), amlodipine (Norvasc), and diltiazem hydrochloride (Cardizem), improve symptoms in severe Raynaud's phenomenon by vasodilating small vessels in the hands and feet and decreasing the frequency and intensity of attacks (Mayo Clinic, 2008). Clients may be given nifedipine (Adalat, Procardia) at night for severe cases of Raynaud's phenomenon. Clients may also take the medication 1 to 2 hours before engaging in an outdoor activity during cold weather. They may not need to take the medication during warmer months. Alpha blockers, such as prazosin hydrochloride (Minipress) and doxazosin mesylate (Cardura), interfere with the effects of norepinephrine, a hormone causing vasoconstriction. Some clients benefit from topical nitroglycerin. Other drugs in Raynaud's research trials are losartan potassium (Cozaar), sildenafil citrate (Viagra), fluoxetine hydrochloride (Prozac), and prostaglandins (Mayo Clinic, 2008).

Beta blockers, birth control pills, cold medications, and diet pills cause some clients to have Raynaud's phenomenon. Chemotherapy drugs such as bleomycin sulfate (Blenoxane) and cisplatin, CDDP (Platinol), also cause secondary Raynaud's.

Health Promotion

Encourage the client to avoid decongestants, caffeine, exposure to cold, repetitive hand movements, and stressful situations. Also encourage the client to quit smoking and avoid secondary smoke because nicotine is a potent vasoconstrictor. Stress management techniques (e.g., biofeedback and tai chi) may assist in alleviating some distress from the condition. Wearing mittens in cold weather or when handling cold foods keeps fingers warmer than wearing gloves. Keeping the entire body warm is helpful.

Nursing Management

Assess digits for pallor, blanching, cyanosis, rubor, coldness, and texture. Encourage client to keep indoor temperature at a comfortable level. Teach relaxation exercises to enhance circulation. Encourage the use of mitts when pushing shopping carts and the wearing of wear mittens and socks to bed. Apply lotion regularly to prevent dry, chapped skin.

NURSING PROCESS

Assessment

Subjective Data

Ask the client how frequently the vasospastic episodes occur, what symptoms are experienced, what triggers the episodes, which digits are affected during an episode, and how long the incident lasts. Inquire about daily activities the client finds difficult, such as tying shoes, washing dishes, or handling frozen foods. Obtain a history of occupational activities.

Objective Data

Assess the digits for pallor, blanching, cyanosis, rubor, coldness, and texture. If the disease is longstanding, the digits may be tapered and the skin shiny in appearance. There may be ulcerated or gangrenous areas on the fingertips.

Nursing diagnoses for a client with Raynaud's disease include the following:

NURSING DIAGNOSES	PLANNING/OUTCOMES	NURSING INTERVENTIONS
*Ineffective **Tissue** Perfusion (Peripheral)* related to vasospasm of peripheral arteries	The client will have fewer vasospastic episodes and increased circulation in digits.	Encourage the client to use caution when engaging in activities that may cause a cut or scratch because healing may be impaired because of decreased circulation. If a client has ulcers, wash the areas with soap and water and administer prescribed medications such as ciprofloxacin (Cipro) and intravenous iloprost.
*Acute **Pain*** related to decreased circulation in digits	The client will experience decreased pain as vasospasms are controlled.	Teach client to keep the indoor temperature at a comfortable level to avoid ischemic attacks. Encourage client to avoid dramatic changes in environmental temperatures (e.g., entering a cold air-conditioned room during hot summer months). Encourage the client to wear woolen or wind-proof gloves or mittens and layered clothes when exposed to colder temperatures. Mittens may be better than gloves so the fingers can obtain warmth from each other. Chemical warming devices may be used inside gloves and shoes. Encourage the client to stop smoking and make a referral to a smoking cessation clinic. Teach the client relaxation exercises that may decrease the number of ischemic attacks.
*Situational Low **Self-esteem*** related to inability of hands to perform activities of daily living	The client will learn ways to handle activities of daily living.	Encourage client to use mitts or potholders when removing items from the freezer or handling cold food to decrease the risk of a Raynaud's episode. Clients can wear mittens or

(*Continues*)

Nursing diagnoses for a client with Raynaud's disease include the following: (Continued)

NURSING DIAGNOSES	PLANNING/OUTCOMES	NURSING INTERVENTIONS
		socks to bed. Use of insulated mugs, foam rubber holders, or stemware glasses may reduce ischemic attacks. Instruct client to wash vegetables under tepid water instead of cold, to bathe in lukewarm water, and to apply lotion regularly to prevent dry and chapped skin. Encourage client to use gloves when pushing shopping carts or operating some vibrating machines because this may decrease the cold sensation and soften the vibration.

Evaluation: Evaluate each outcome to determine how it has been met by the client.

CASE STUDY

L.J., a 55-year-old truck driver, is admitted to the emergency room with a feeling of heavy squeezing pressure in his sternal area. The pain is radiating to his left shoulder. He is diaphoretic, short of breath, and nauseated. He states the sternal pain came on suddenly while watching a football game. He had been mowing his yard and decided to rest. The emergency physician gives L.J. a nitroglycerin tablet and connects him to an ECG monitor. Cardiac biomarkers (CK-MB, troponin, and myoglobin) with an IMA and a chest x-ray are requested STAT. Morphine sulfate 2 mg is given intravenously. Oxygen is given by mask at 4 liters/minute. L.J.'s apical pulse is 102 beats/min and his blood pressure is 130/88 mm Hg. A cardiac catheterization with fluoroscopy is ordered to determine the patency of the coronary blood vessels and functioning of the heart muscle.

Three hours after admission, crackles are heard in the lungs.

The following questions will guide your development of a nursing care plan for the case study.

1. List symptoms/clinical manifestations, other than L.J.'s, that a client may experience when having a myocardial infarction.
2. List two reasons morphine sulfate was given to L.J.
3. List two other diagnostic tests that may have been ordered for L.J.
4. List subjective and objective data a nurse would want to obtain about L.J.
5. Write three individualized nursing diagnoses and goals for L.J.
6. L.J. is moved from the critical care unit. List pertinent nursing actions a nurse would do in caring for L.J. related to:

   oxygenation — activity
   cardiac output — medications
   comfort/rest — teaching

7. List teaching that L.J. will need before his discharge.
8. List at least three successful client outcomes for L.J.
9. How might the MI symptoms for a woman differ from L.J.'s symptoms?

SUMMARY

- The function of the heart is to pump blood through the vascular system. Blood is the medium by which oxygen and nutrients are provided to the body cells and carbon dioxide and waste products are removed from the body cells.
- The coronary arteries supply blood to the heart. If the blood flow through these vessels becomes diminished or occluded, ischemia to the heart tissue occurs, resulting in angina or a myocardial infarction.
- Typical symptoms experienced by a person with cardiac problems include chest pain, dyspnea, edema, fainting, palpitations, diaphoresis, and fatigue.
- A lipid profile and cardiac biomarkers provide diagnostic information about the risk of heart disease and the occurrence of a myocardial infarction.
- A dysrhythmia is an irregularity in the rate, rhythm, or conduction of the electrical system of the heart.

- Inflammatory or infectious conditions of the heart include endocarditis, myocarditis, and pericarditis. Endocarditis may cause valvular heart disease with the possibility of the valve needing to be surgically repaired (valvuloplasty) or replaced with a mechanical (caged-ball valve or tilting-disk valve) or biological valve from a calf, pig, or human.
- Atherosclerosis causes a narrowing and occluding of vessels and is a primary cause of angina and myocardial infarction.
- Surgical treatment for angina includes a PTCA, intracoronary stent, transcatheter ablation, or a coronary artery bypass graft.
- Heart failure is often the final stage of many other heart conditions in which the heart is no longer able to fulfill the demands of the body.
- To assess the peripheral vascular system, the nurse assesses pain, pulse, pallor, paresthesia, and paralysis.
- Three factors leading to the formation of a clot—pooling of blood, vessel trauma, and a coagulation problem—are called Virchow's triad.
- A client with a DVT may be asymptomatic or may have warmth and tenderness at the site, edema of the extremity, a positive Homans' sign, cyanosis of the foot, and a sensation of heaviness or tightness in the extremity.
- It is important for the nurse to measure the leg circumference every shift and check peripheral pulses for the client with a thrombus.
- The cause of varicose veins is incompetent valves and veins that have lost their elasticity.
- Primary Raynaud's disease is an intermittent spasm of the digital arteries and arterioles, resulting in decreased circulation to the digits.
- Symptoms of an aneurysm depend on the location of the aneurysm in the body. Aneurysms are often asymptomatic until they start leaking or pressing on other structures.

REVIEW QUESTIONS

1. To assess a client with right-sided heart failure, the nurse would:
    1. listen for a pericardial friction rub.
    2. listen for a muffled S_1 and S_2 heart sound.
    3. check for distended neck veins with the bed at a 45-degree angle.
    4. assess for radiation of the squeezing sensation under the sternum.
2. It is important to teach a client with angina to:
    1. take antibiotics before having dental work.
    2. carry nitroglycerin tablets at all times.
    3. perform the Valsalva maneuver daily.
    4. massage the carotid sinuses in the neck.
3. A nursing intervention to improve cardiac output is:
    1. encouraging the client to verbalize fears.
    2. teaching the side effects of new medications.
    3. a referral to a dietitian for low-sodium diet instructions.
    4. administer oxygen per physician orders.
4. Instructions to a client on anticoagulant therapy include:
    1. taking Coumadin twice a day.
    2. watching for symptoms of bleeding.
    3. taking over-the-counter medications as needed.
    4. no dietary or activity limitations.
5. The first step of the stepped-care approach in treating hypertension is:
    1. lifestyle changes.
    2. diuretics.
    3. beta blockers.
    4. adding a second or third antihypertensive.
6. A client is admitted to the emergency room with chest pain. The first nursing intervention is:
    1. attach the client to an ECG monitor.
    2. administer oxygen.
    3. listen to the heart sounds.
    4. order cardio biomarkers.
7. A client is diagnosed with coronary artery disease and his physicians recommended a coronary bypass giving the client the option of a robotic CABG. The client and his wife ask the advantages of a robotic CABG as compared to a traditional CABG. The nurse states the advantages of robotic CABG as: (Select all that apply.)
    1. The client has less bleeding.
    2. The client's recovery is 6 to 8 weeks.
    3. The client will require less medication.
    4. The surgeon will do a complete sternotomy.
    5. The client has a risk of increased infection.
    6. The client's hospital stay is shorter.
8. What ECG wave represents ventricular repolarization?
    1. P wave.
    2. QRS complex.
    3. ST segment.
    4. T wave.
9. A client is admitted to the floor from an intensive care unit and has a pacemaker pulse generator lying beside his body. The client asks whether he will have to live the rest of his life with the pulse generator hanging from his body. The nurse's best response is:
    1. No, this is a temporary pacemaker. Your heart has maintained a regular rhythm for 2 days. As your heartbeat continues to stabilize, it will be removed.
    2. No, this is a temporary pacemaker. If you would need a permanent pacemaker, the energy source would be placed in a belt you will wear around your waist.

3. Yes. The pacemaker wires will be connected to an energy source and placed in a belt you will wear around your waist.
4. No, this pacemaker will be changed to an ICD that will regulate your heart with intermittent electrical shocks. It will also regulate the rhythm of your heart.

10. A client was admitted to the unit from the postoperative recovery room. He has a history of venous thrombus. Nursing measures to prevent the formation of a clot are to: (Select all that apply.)

1. ambulate the client as soon as ordered.
2. encourage the client to exercise his legs, such as making circular movements with his feet to increase circulation.
3. encourage the client to rest in bed when he is dismissed.
4. request an order for a pneumatic compression device if the client does not have one.
5. check Homans' sign every shift.
6. limit his fluid intake to 200 mL per shift.

REFERENCES/SUGGESTED READINGS

Ahmed, A. (2008). An update on the role of digoxin in older adults with chronic heart failure. *Geriatrics Aging, 11*(1), 37–41.

American Association for Clinical Chemistry. (2006). IMA. Retrieved on January 14, 2009 from http://labtestsonline.org/understanding/analytes/ima/multiprint.html

American Association for Clinical Chemistry. (2008). Cardiac biomarkers. Retrieved on January 14, 2009 from http://labtestsonline.org/understanding/analytes/a1c/glance.htmardiac_biomarkers/glance-2.html

American Association for Clinical Chemistry. (2009). Cardiac risk assessment. Retrieved on 1/19/09 from http://labtestsonline.org/understanding/analytes/cardiac_risk/glance.html

American Heart Association (AHA). (2001a). Rheumatic heart disease statistics. Retrieved from http://216. 185.112.5/presenter.jhtml?identifier=4712

American Heart Association (AHA). (2001b). Women, heart disease and stroke statistics. Retrieved from http://216. 185.112.5/presenter.jhtml?identifier=4787

American Heart Association (AHA). (2007). Implantable cardioverter defibrillator. Retrieved on January 16, 2009 at http://www.americanheart.org/presenter.jhtml?identifier=11227

American Heart Association (AHA). (2007a). Cardiovascular disease death rates decline, but risk factors still exact heavy toll. *AHA News*. Retrieved January 12, 2009 from http://www.americanheart.org/print_presenter.jhtml?identifier=3052670

American Heart Association (AHA). (2007b). Heart attack symptoms and warning signs. *AHA News*. Retrieved January 12, 2009 from http://www.americanheart.org/print_presneter.jhtml?identifier=4595

Ammon, S. (2001). Managing patients with heart failure. *AJN, 101*(12), 34–40.

Baker, S., & Graziano, J. (2003). A new device for heart failure. *RN, 66*(3), 32–35.

Beattie, S. (1999). Cut the risks for cardio cath patients. *RN, 62*(1), 50–54.

Beattie, S. (2002). New biomarkers may predict CAD. *RN, 65*(9), 47–54.

Bender, R. (in press). *Assessing the Cardiovascular System.*

Bither, C., & Apple, S. (2001). Home management of the failing heart. *AJN, 101*(12), 41–45.

Bond, E., Nelson, K., Germany, C., & Smart, A. (2003). The left ventricular assist device. *AJN, 103*(1), 32–39.

Breen, P. (2000). DVT: What every nurse should know. *RN, 63*(4), 58–62.

Broadcast Newsroom. (2009). Reminder: Cardica announces webcast of internationally renowned cardiothoracic surgeon, Dt. Sudhir Srivastava, performing robotic cardiac bypass surgery using revolutionary anastomosis device. Retrieved on January 19, 2009 from http://www.broadcastnewsroom.com/articles/viewarticle.jsp?id=622186

Bubien, R. (2000). A new beat on an old rhythm. *AJN, 100*(1), 42–50.

Bulechek, G., Butcher, H., McCloskey, J., & Dochterman, J., eds. (2008). *Nursing Interventions Classification (NIC)* (5th ed.). St. Louis, MO: Mosby/Elsevier.

Carelock, J., & Clark, A. (2001). Heart failure: Pathophysiologic mechanisms. *AJN, 101*(12), 26–33.

Centers for Disease Control and Prevention (CDC). (2002). Health, United States 2002. Retrieved from www.cdc. gov/nchs/data/hus/tables/2002/02hus068.pdf

Chase, S. (2000). Hypertensive crisis. *RN, 63*(6), 62–67.

Chavez, J., & Brewer, C. (2002). Stopping the shock slide. *RN, 65*(9), 30–34. Delmar Cengage Learning.

Cheek, D., & Cesan, A. (2003). What's different about heart disease in women? *Nursing2003, 33*(8), 36–42.

Cleveland Clinic. (2009a). Robotically assisted heart surgery. Retrieved on January 19, 2009 from http://my.clevelandclinic.org/heart/services/surgery/roboticallyassisted.aspx

Cleveland Clinic. (2009b). What is minimally invasive heart surgery. Retrieved on January 19, 2009 from http://my.clevelandclinic.org/heart/disorders/mini_invasivehs.aspx

Corona, G. (1999). Pacemakers: Keeping the beat today. *RN, 62*(12), 50–55.

Crumlish, C., Bracken, J., Hand, M., Keenan, K., Ruggiero, H., & Simmons, D. (2000). When time is muscle. *AJN, 100*(1), 26–35.

Dakin, C. (2008). New approaches to heart failure in the ED. *American Journal of Nursing, 108*(3), 68–71.

Daniels, R. (2010). Delmar's guide to laboratory and diagnostic tests, (2nd ed.). Clifton Park, NY: Delmar Cengage Learning.

Darty, S., Thomas, M., Neagle, C., Link, H., Wesley-Farrington, D., and Hundley, G. (2002). Cardiovascular magnetic resonance imaging. *AJN, 102*(12), 34–37.

Davis, S. (2002). How the heart failure picture has changed. *Nursing2002, 32*(11), 36–44.

Day, M. (2003). Recognizing and managing DVT. *Nursing 2003, 33*(5), 36–41.

deSouza, I. and Ward, C. (2008). *Ventricular tachycardia.* Retrieved January 16, 2009 from http://emedicine.medscape.com/article/760963-print

Fort, C. (2002). Get pumped to prevent DVT. *Nursing 2002, 32*(9), 50–52.

Freeman, J., & Hedges, C. (2003). Cardiac arrest: The effect on the brain. *AJN, 103*(6), 50–54.

Gehring, P. (April 2002). Perfecting your skills: Vascular assessment. *Travel Nursing Today (supplement to RN)* 16–24.

George, E., & Tasota, F. (2003). Predicting heart disease with C-reactive protein. *Nursing2003, 33*(5), 70–71.

Goldrick, B. (2003). Endocarditis associated with body piercing. *AJN, 103*(1), 26–27.

Goodreau, L. (2003). Coronary stenting—with a twist. *RN, 66*(1), 32–36.

Granger, B., & Miller, C. (2001). Acute coronary syndrome. *Nursing2001, 31*(11), 36–43.

Halm, M., & Penque, S. (1999). Heart disease in women. *AJN, 99*(4), 26–31.

Hays, D. (2003). Picturing reciprocal changes in an MI. *Nursing 2003, 33*(5), 53.

Hiller, G. (1999). Atrial fibrillation. *Nursing99, 29*(2), 27–31.

Hurley, M. (2003). The latest hypertension guidelines. *RN, 66*(8), 43–45.

Joint National Committee on Prevention, Detection, Evaluation, and Treatment of High Blood Pressure. (2003). The Seventh Report of the Joint National Committee on Prevention, Detection, Evaluation, and Treatment of High Blood Pressure. Retrieved from www.nhlbi.nih.gov/guidelines/ hypertension/index.htm

Joy, S. (2006). Women may delay treatment for acute myocardial infarction. *American Journal of Nursing, 107*(7), 16.

Klabunde, R. (2007). Cardiovascular physiology concepts. Retrieved on January 20, 2009 from http://www.cvphysiology.com/Blood%20Pressure/BP023.htm

Kowalczyk, T. (2002). A low-tech approach to venous congestion. *RN, 65*(10), 26–30.

Lab Tests Online. (2009). Cardiac Risk Assessment. Retrieved January 19, 2009 from http://labtestonline.org/understanding/analytes/cardiac_risk/glance.html

Lazzara, D. (1999). Shocking facts about semiautomatic defibrillation. *Nursing99, 29*(4), 55–57.

Lewis, A. (1999). Cardiovascular emergency. *Nursing99, 29*(6), 49–51.

Lewis, S., Heitkemper, M., & Dirksen, S. (2004). *Medical–surgical nursing: Assessment and management of clinical problems* (6th ed.). St. Louis, MO: Mosby.

Linton, A., Matteson, M., & Maebius, N. (2000). Introductory nursing care of adults (2nd ed.). Philadelphia: W. B. Saunders.

Lundberg, G. (2008). The Medscape medical minute: Recovery PVCs during treadmill testing tied to heart disease. *Medscape Journal of Medicine, 10*(4), 93. Retrieved on January 16, 2009 from http://www.medscape.com/viewarticle/571891_print

Macklin, D. (2003). Phlebitis. *AJN, 103*(2), 55–60.

Malacaria, B., & Feloney, C. (2003). Going with the flow of anticoagulant therapy. *Nursing2003, 33*(3), 36–42.

Mancini, M., & Kaye, W. (1999). AEDs: Changing the way you respond to cardiac arrest. *AJN, 99*(5), 26–30.

Marcolongo, E. (2003). Isolated systolic hypertension—not your usual silent killer. *Nursing2003,* 33(1), 32hn1–32hn3.

Martin, T. (2002). How heart failure complicates care. *Nursing2002, 32*(7), 32hn1–32hn5.

Mayo Clinic (2002). Aneurysms. Retrieved from www. mayoclinic.com/findinformation./invoke.cfm?objectid=FE3FE459-7DIE-405F-95E9339CD2E974B

Mayo Clinic. (2008). Raynaud's disease. Retrieved on January 21, 2009 from http://www.mayoclinic.com/health/raynauds-disease/DS00433/DSECTION=treatments-an

McAvoy, J. (2000). Cardiac pain: Discovering the unexpected. *Nursing2000, 30*(3), 34–39.

McConnell, E. (2002a). Applying antiembolism stockings. *Nursing2002, 32*(4), 17.

McConnell, E. (2002b). Using an automated external defibrillator. *Nursing2002, 32*(10), 18.

McCormick, J., & Deeg, M. (2000). Pharmacologic treatment of dyslipidemia. *AJN, 100*(2), 55–60.

McGrath, A. (1997). Clinical snapshot: Raynaud's syndrome. *AJN, 97*(1), 34–35.

McKinney, B. (1999). Solving the puzzle of heart failure. *Nursing99, 29*(5), 33–39.

Metules, T. (1999). Cardiac tamponade. *RN, 62*(12), 26–31.

Metules, T. (2003). IABP therapy: Getting patients treatment fast. *RN, 66*(5), 56–62.

Miracle, V. (2001a). Act fast during a hypertensive crisis. *Nursing 2001, 31*(9), 50–51.

Miracle, V. (2001b). Putting the brakes on pericarditis. *Nursing2001, 31*(4), 44–45.

Moorhead, S., Johnson, M., Maas, M., & Swanson, E. (2007). *Nursing Outcomes Classification (NOC)* (4th ed). St. Louis, MO: Elsevier–Health Sciences Division.

Mosley, M., Oenning, V., & Melinik, G. (1999). Methemoglobinemia. *AJN, 99*(5), 47.

Nagle, B., & Nee, C. (2002). Acute myocardial infarction. *Nursing2002, 32*(10), 50–54.

National Institute of Arthritis and Musculoskeletal and Skin Diseases (NIAMS). (2006). *Raynaud's Phenomenon* (NIH Publication No.06-4911). Retrieved on January 21, 2009 from http://www.niams.nih.gov/Health_Info/Raynauds_Phenomenon/default.asp

National Institutes of Health (NIH). (2002). New recommendations to prevent high blood pressure issues. Retrieved from http://www.nhlbi.nih.gov/news/press/02-10-15.htm

North American Nursing Diagnosis Association International. (2010). *NANDA-I nursing diagnoses: Definitions and classification 2009–2011*. Ames, IA: Wiley-Blackwell.

Oliver-McNeil, S. (2001). Treating hypertrophic cardiomyopathy without surgery. *Nursing2001, 31*(2), 32cc1–32cc4.

Overbaugh, K. (2009). Acute coronary syndrome. *American Journal of Nursing, 109*(5), 42–60.

Palatnik, A. (2001). How cardiac drugs do what they do. *Nursing2001, 31*(5), 54–60.

Pope, B. (2002). Heart failure. *Nursing2002, 32*(8), 50–51.

Pope, W. (2002). Angioplasty & stenting in the carotid? *RN, 65*(6), 54–59.

Raynaud's Association, Inc. (2008). What is Raynaud's? Retrieved on January 21, 2009 from http://www.raynauds.org/raynauds/index.cfm

Reger, T., & Vargas, G. (1999). The return of the radial artery in CABG. *AJN, 99*(9), 26–30.

Ross, G., & DeJong, M. (1999). Pericardial tamponade. *AJN, 99*(2), 35.

Ryan, D. (2000). Is it an MI? A lab primer. *RN, 63*(1), 26–30.

Shaffer, R. (2002). ICD therapy: The patient's perspective. *AJN, 102*(2), 46–49.

Sims, J., & Miracle, V. (2001). Getting the lowdown on hypotension. *Nursing2001, 31*(10), 56–57.

Siomko, A. (2000). Demystifying cardiac markers. *AJN, 100*(1), 36–40.

Spratto, G., & Woods, A. (2010). 2010 Delmar's Nurses Drug Handbook. Clifton Park, NY: Delmar Cengage Learning.

Stanford Hospital and Clinics. (2009). Pacemaker/implantable cardioverter defibrillator (ICD) insertion. Stanford University Medical Center. Retrieved January 16, 2009 from http://www.stanfordhospital.com/healthLib/greystone/heartCenter/heartProcedures/cemakerImplantableCardioverterDefibrillatorICDInsertion

U.S. Food and Drug Administration (FDA). (2002). Medtronic In Sync ICD model 7272dual chamber implantable cardioverter defibrillator system with cardiac resynchronization therapy—P010031. Retrieved on January 16, 2009 from http://www.fda.gov/cdrh/mda/docs/p010031.html

U.S. Food and Drug Administration (FDA). (2004). Ventricular assist device (VAD). Retrieved on January, 19, 2009 from http://www.fda.gov/heartheatlh/treatments/medialdevices/vad.html

Willis, K. (2001). Gaining perspective on peripheral vascular disease. *Nursing2001, 31*(2), 32hn1–32hn4.

Woods, A. (1999). Managing hypertension. *Nursing99, 29*(3), 41–46.

Woods, A. (2001). Improving the odds against hypertension. *Nursing2001, 31*(8), 36–41.

Woods, A. (2002). High blood pressure (hypertension). *Nursing2002, 32*(4), 54–55.

Zangerm, D., Solomon, A., & Gersh, B. (2000). Contemporary management of angina: Part II. Medical management of chronic stable angina. *American Family Physician, 61*(1), 129–138.

RESOURCES

American Heart Association, http://www.americanheart.org

National Heart, Lung, and Blood Institute, http://www.nhlbi.nih.gov

President's Council on Physical Fitness and Sports, http://www.fitness.gov

Raynaud's Association, Inc., http://www.raynauds.org

The Mended Hearts, Inc., http://www.mendedhearts.org

U.S. Food and Drug Administration, http://www.fda.gov

FDA heart health online illustration: Prosthetic heart valve, http://www.fda.gov/hearthealth/flash/fda_26.html

FDA heart health online illustration: Ventricular assist device, http://www.fda.gov/hearthealth/flash/fda_25.html

CHAPTER 37
Hematologic and Lymphatic Systems

MAKING THE CONNECTION

Refer to the following chapters to increase your understanding of the hematologic and lymphatic systems:

Basic Nursing
- ***Fluid, Electrolyte, and Acid–Base Balance***
- ***Assessment***
- ***Pain Management***

Adult Health Nursing
- ***Oncology***
- ***Respiratory System***
- ***Cardiovascular System***
- ***Endocrine System***
- ***Immune System***

Basic Procedures
- ***Hand Hygiene***
- ***Initiating Strict Isolation Precautions***

Intermediate Procedure
- ***Administering an Intramuscular Injection (Z-track technique)***

LEARNING OBJECTIVES

Upon completion of this chapter, you should be able to:

- Define key terms.
- Relate anatomy and physiology of the blood and lymph systems to disease processes.
- Relate diagnostic test results to the blood and lymph disorders.
- Describe nursing interventions in caring for clients with blood and lymph disorders.
- Assist in developing a nursing care plan for clients with blood and lymph disorders.

KEY TERMS

agranulocytosis
apheresis
autologous
bands
blastic phase
erythrocytapheresis
fibrinolysis
hemarthrosis
hematocrit
hematopoiesis
hemolysis
hyperuricemia
idiopathic
leukocytosis
leukopenia
lymphoma
phlebotomy
purpura
reticulocyte
sickle
thrombocytopenia

INTRODUCTION

The hematologic system of the body consists of blood and blood-forming organs. Blood consists of formed elements (red blood cells, white blood cells, and platelets) and plasma. As blood is pumped through the body, it carries essential substances to the tissues and removes waste products from the tissues. Disorders of the hematologic system usually result from abnormal production or functioning of the cells. Some of these disorders are the result of genetics, environment, or pathogenic organisms.

The lymph system consists of lymph vessels, nodes, and organs. Lymph vessels collect and return lymph fluid to the blood vessels through the right and left lymphatic ducts at the right and left subclavian veins. The functions of the lymph system are assisting with immunity, controlling edema, and absorbing digested fats.

Medical management, nursing diagnoses, goals, and interventions are given for each blood and lymph disorder. A thorough understanding of the blood and lymph disorders equips the nurse to provide quality client care.

ANATOMY AND PHYSIOLOGY REVIEW

The anatomy and physiology of the blood and lymphatic systems are discussed in the following section.

Blood

The heart pumps 5 to 6 liters of blood per minute through the circulatory system of an adult. Blood is an aqueous mixture consisting of plasma and cells (Figure 37-1).

Plasma

Plasma is a straw-colored liquid consisting of approximately 90% water and 10% proteins. The water component assists in transporting body nutrients, hormones, antibodies, electrolytes, and waste; regulating blood volume; and controlling body temperature. The proteins are albumin, globulins, and fibrinogen. Albumin controls the volume of the blood and blood pressure by osmotic pressure that pulls tissue fluid into the capillary system. There are three types of globulins: alpha, beta, and gamma. Alpha and beta globulins are secreted by the liver and are carrier molecules for substances. Gamma globulins are antibodies important in the immune response of the body. Fibrinogen changes into fibrin, a solid that controls bleeding in the blood-clotting mechanism of the body. The formed elements in plasma are red blood cells (RBCs), white blood cells (WBCs), and platelets.

Red Blood Cells

Red blood cells, also called erythrocytes, are the most numerous blood cells in the body, generally 4.5 to 6.1 million/mm^3 in an adult. RBCs are biconcave disks that do not have a nucleus. They are about the size of the smallest capillary but are flexible and capable of changing shape so they can squeeze through the capillaries.

RBCs, in conjunction with the respiratory and circulatory systems, oxygenate body tissues. In the capillary bed of the alveoli, blood receives oxygen (O_2), and carbon dioxide (CO_2) is eliminated. The O_2-enriched RBCs (oxyhemoglobin) carry O_2 to systemic capillaries, where O_2 is exchanged for carbon dioxide (CO_2). The CO_2-laden blood then returns the CO_2 to the alveoli in the lungs, where it is again exchanged for oxygen. The CO_2 is exhaled from the body with each breath. Hemoglobin is a protein in the RBC that carries O_2 and is responsible for the exchange of O_2 and CO_2.

The average life span for an RBC is 120 days. Blood cells originate from a single stem cell that proliferates and differentiates into lymphoid stem cells or blood stem cells (Figure 37-2). The lymphoid stem cells further divide and differentiate into T cells and B cells. The blood stem cells divide and differentiate

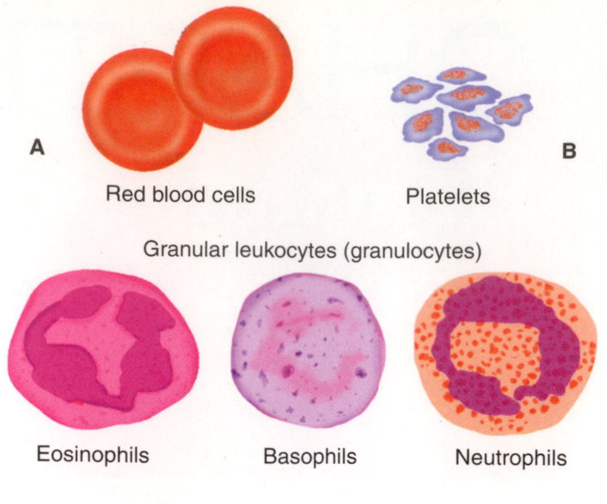

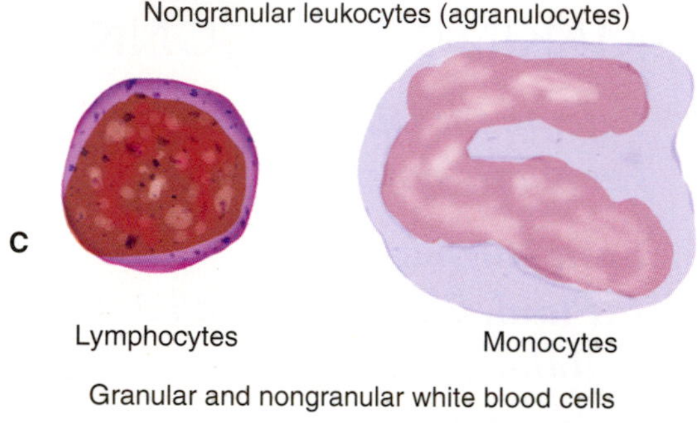

FIGURE 37-1 The Cells in Blood; *A*, Red Blood Cells (erythrocytes); *B*, Platelets (thrombocytes); *C*, White Blood Cells (leukocytes)

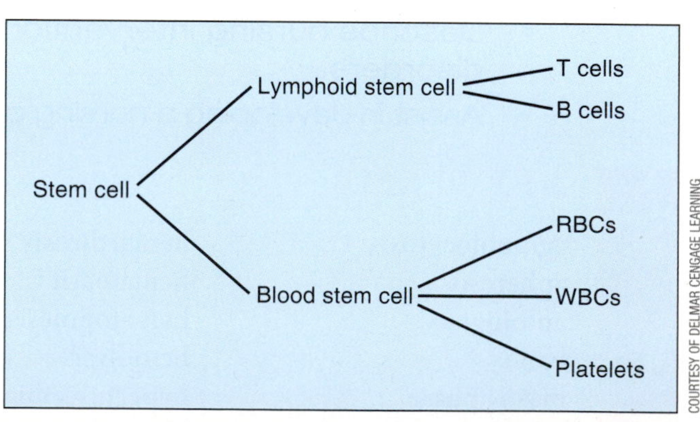

FIGURE 37-2 Origin of T Cells, B Cells, RBCs, WBCs, and Platelets

into RBCs, WBCs, and platelets. The process of blood cell production and development is called **hematopoiesis**. RBCs are produced daily by the bone marrow according to the demand of the body. When the partial pressure of O_2 decreases, a renal hormone, erythropoietin, stimulates the bone marrow to produce more immature RBCs (**reticulocytes**), which are released into the bloodstream. These reticulocytes develop into mature red blood cells. The number of circulating reticulocytes is used as a diagnostic tool for RBC disorders.

As RBCs age, their outer membrane deteriorates and they are destroyed by large macrophages in the liver and are filtered out of the body by the spleen. The iron from heme in the old RBCs is used in the production of new RBCs.

Hematocrit is the percentage of blood cells in a volume of blood. A normal hematocrit for a woman is 38% to 47% and, for a man, 40% to 54% (Daniels, 2009).

White Blood Cells

White blood cells (WBCs), also called leukocytes, fight infection and assist with immunity. The life span of a WBC varies, depending on the type of WBC. Neutrophils, basophils, and eosinophils live from a few hours to days, whereas lymphocytes and monocytes live from days to years. The normal WBC count is 4,100 to 10,800/mm^3 of blood (Daniels, 2009). An increased number of WBCs (**leukocytosis**) may signify the presence of an infection, inflammation, tissue necrosis, or leukemia. A decreased number of WBCs (**leukopenia**) may indicate bone marrow failure, a massive infection, dietary deficiencies, drug toxicity, or an autoimmune disease.

WBCs are classified as granulocytes or polymorphonuclear leukocytes (PMNs, or polys) and agranulocytes. The granulocytes have granules (grainy substances) in their cytoplasm, and the agranulocytes do not. Granulocytes are divided into three types: the neutrophils, eosinophils, and basophils. Agranulocytes are classified into two groups: monocytes and lymphocytes. Neutrophils are the most numerous, comprising approximately 60% of the total number of WBCs. The main function of neutrophils is to digest and kill microorganisms. If a client has an acute infection, the bone marrow is stimulated to produce more neutrophils, resulting in an increased circulation of immature neutrophils called **bands**. An increased production of neutrophils indicates the presence of an acute infection. An increased number of basophils and especially of eosinophils indicates an allergic response.

Monocytes become macrophages, cells that destroy dead and injured cells and bacteria. There are two types of lymphocytes, T cells and B cells, which are involved in the body's immune response.

Platelets

Platelets (thrombocytes) are not typical cells but non-nucleated, granular ovoid, or spindle-shaped cell fragments. The normal life span of a platelet is approximately 10 days. Platelets are active in the clotting mechanism of the body. When platelets flow over a rough or damaged area in a vessel, they adhere to the area and release thromboplastin and clotting factors that start the blood-clotting process. They also secrete prostaglandins and serotonin, which cause the vessel to constrict, thereby decreasing the blood flow through the area. Prothrombin, thromboplastin, and calcium ions form thrombin, which joins with fibrinogen to form fibrin. The fibrin strands seal the opening or area, and a clot is formed (Figure 37-3).

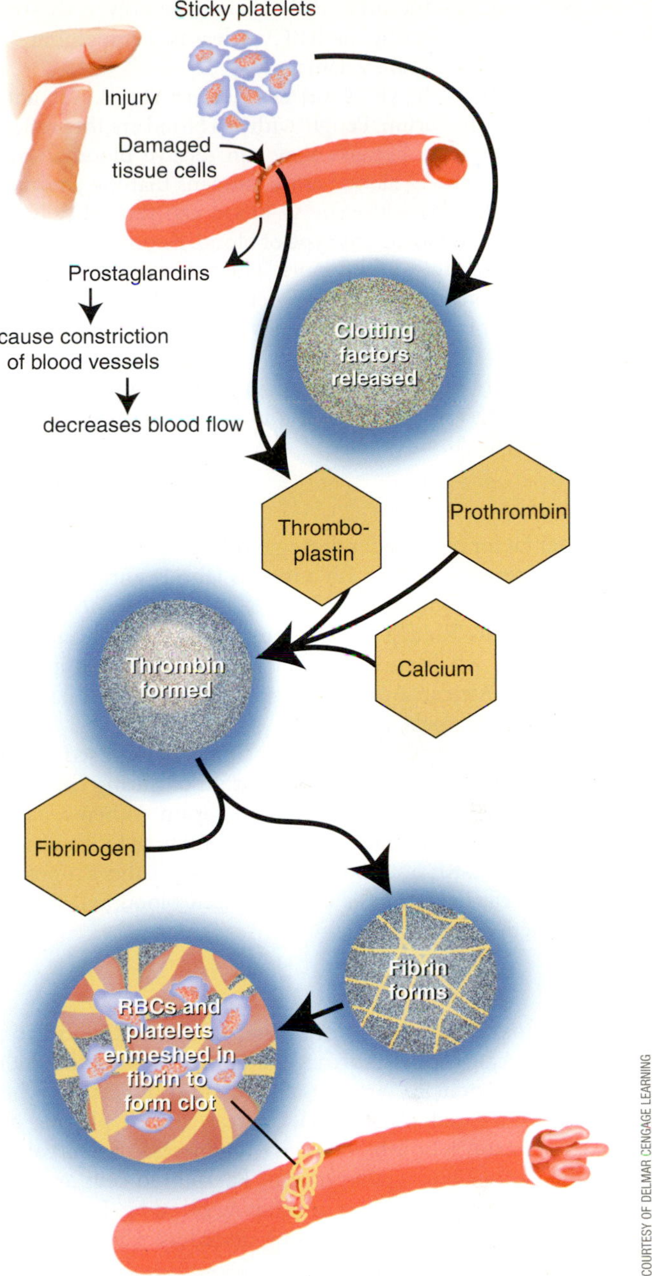

FIGURE 37-3 The Process of Clot Formation

Blood Types

Genetically determined antigens called agglutinogens are located on the surface of RBC membranes. The A and B antigens constitute the ABO blood group. If the A antigen is on the RBC membrane, the client has type A blood. If the B antigen is on the RBC membrane, the client has type B blood. If both an A and a B antigen are present, the client has type AB blood, and if no antigen is present, the client has type O blood.

Type A blood has anti-B antibodies in the serum, and type B blood has anti-A antibodies. If a person with type A blood receives type B blood during a transfusion, the anti-B antibodies attack the infused RBCs and hemolyze (destroy) them. The hemolyzing of RBCs releases hemoglobin that potentially causes kidney damage.

A person with AB blood has neither anti-A nor anti-B antibodies in the serum. People with AB blood are theoretically universal recipients because they can receive blood from all blood types. Type O blood has no antigens that the antibodies can attack. Persons with type O blood can theoretically give blood to persons having any type of blood. Persons with type O blood are called universal donors. The terms *universal recipient* and *universal donor* are only theoretical because during blood transfusions, blood incompatibilities can occur because of other types of antigens.

There are 14 different blood groups and more than 100 different antigens. The different blood groups vary in number with different ethnic groups.

Rh Factor

Another factor to consider during blood transfusions is the Rh factor. Persons who have Rh antigens (the D antigen) are Rh positive. Those who do not have Rh antigens on their RBC membranes are Rh negative. Approximately 85% of Caucasian people have Rh-positive blood and 15% have Rh-negative blood. The African-American population has 93% and 7%, respectively (Daniels, 2009).

If a person with Rh-negative blood is exposed to Rh-positive blood during a blood transfusion or during childbirth, anti-Rh antibodies form in the blood serum. When a person with Rh-negative blood is exposed a second time to Rh-positive blood, the anti-Rh antibodies will react with the Rh-positive blood and cause hemolysis of the infused blood and a severe blood reaction.

Blood Transfusions

Blood transfusions are given to replace needed blood components because of hemorrhage, anemia, clotting disorders, or blood deficiencies. Transfusable blood products are whole blood, packed red cells, platelets, fresh frozen plasma, and cryoprecipitate. Whole blood is given to increase blood volume and the various blood components. Packed red cells are given for anemia. Platelets assist in controlling bleeding. Fresh frozen plasma is administered for clotting disorders. Cryoprecipitate corrects fibrinogen deficiencies.

Before blood products are given, the lab does a type and crossmatch to check compatibility between the donor's blood type and Rh factor and the client's blood type and Rh factor. The lab also checks all blood products for HIV and hepatitis B and C viruses. When administering a blood transfusion, handle blood gently so the cells are not damaged. Administer blood within 30 minutes of obtaining it from the laboratory refrigerator. Take baseline vital signs—temperature, pulse, and blood pressure—before administering the blood product. Once the transfusion is started, temperature and pulse are measured after 15 minutes, 30 minutes, and then hourly; blood pressure is measured hourly during the transfusion. Blood is generally administered through a peripheral vein using an 18- or 19-gauge cannula. A large cannula is used so the blood cells do not break when passing through the cannula.

Before the transfusion, two nurses check the compatibility of the blood product with the client's blood. The first 50 mL is given within 5 to 10 minutes. The client is observed closely for a hemolytic blood reaction during this time. If a client experiences any symptoms of a reaction, the infusion is stopped immediately and the physician notified. Follow institutional protocol.

A blood transfusion should be completed within 4 hours of the start of administration. No medications are given at the blood administration site during infusion. Blood is administered with 0.9% sodium chloride solution since other solutions cause the blood to clot.

Autologous Transfusion If time and the client's condition permit, **autologous** ("from self") blood as opposed to homologous ("from a donor") blood is collected and saved for the client. This may be used for elective surgeries. An alternate procedure is to recover the blood lost during surgery and transfuse it back into the client. The use of autologous blood eliminates the possibility of a transfusion reaction and prevents the transmission of disease.

> **CULTURAL CONSIDERATIONS**
>
> **Jehovah's Witnesses and Blood**
>
> - Many Jehovah's Witnesses agree to autologous blood transfusions.
> - Some Jehovah's Witnesses allow the use of certain blood volume expanders and carry a card identifying the desired expanders.

LYMPHATIC SYSTEM

The lymphatic, or lymph, system is a separate vessel system. The two main functions of the lymph system are to transport excess fluid from the interstitial spaces to the circulatory system and to protect the body against infectious organisms.

Lymph Fluid and Vessels

Lymph fluid is pale yellow. Fluid and substances move from the plasma through the capillary walls and become interstitial fluid (Figure 37-4). As fluid accumulates in the interstitial space, pressure within the interstitial space increases. The interstitial fluid then diffuses through the lymphatic vessel wall into the lymph vessel.

Semilunar valves in the lymphatic vessels assist the lymph system in returning the interstitial fluid, which is now called lymph, to the venous system. When the valves do not work properly or the vessels become obstructed, edema occurs. The pumping action or contractions of the skeletal muscles and the rhythmic action of the respiratory muscles assist in the movement of the lymph toward the subclavian veins. The right lymphatic duct drains lymph from the right side of the head, neck, thorax, and arm into the right subclavian vein. The lymph from the rest of the body drains into the left subclavian vein through the thoracic duct.

Lymph Nodes

Lymph nodes are scattered throughout the body along the lymph vessels (Figure 37-5) and contain dense patches of lymphocytes and macrophages. Lymphocytes act against such foreign particles as viruses and bacteria. Macrophages ingest and destroy foreign

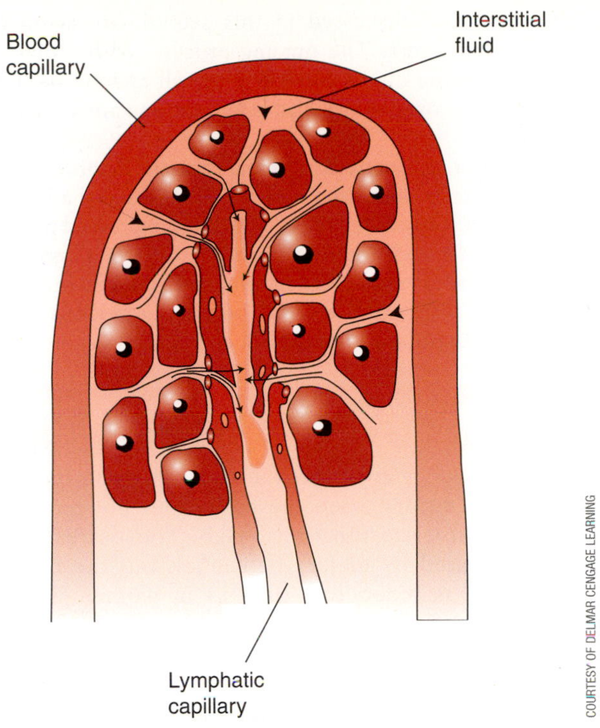

FIGURE 37-4 Flow of Fluid from the Blood into the Lymphatic System

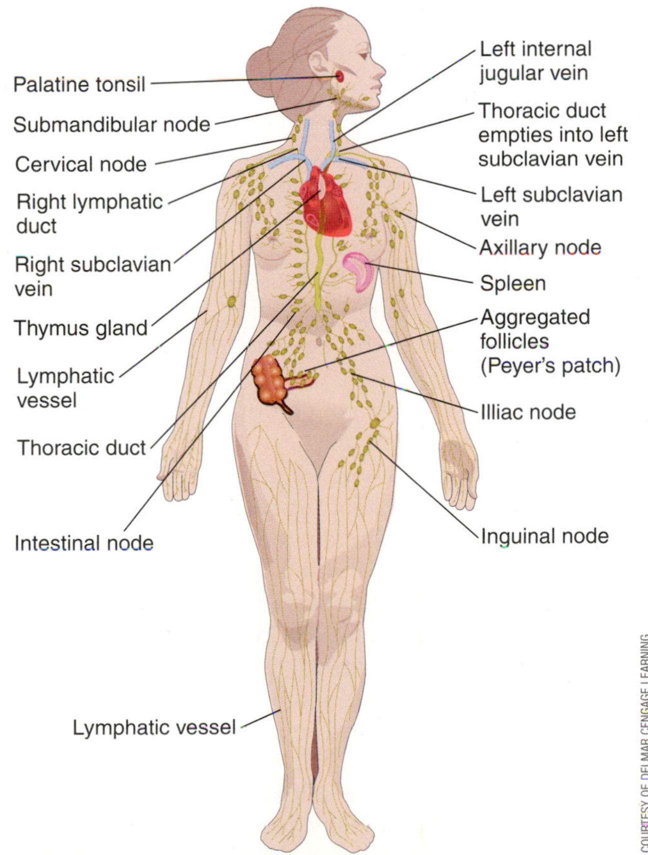

FIGURE 37-5 The Lymphatic System

substances, damaged cells, and cellular debris. The superficial lymph nodes in the neck, axilla, and groin can be palpated, especially when infected and swollen. The tonsils in the pharynx and Peyer's patch in the mucosal lining of the ileum are located deeper within the body and cannot be palpated.

As lymph is collected from body tissues, cancer cells enter the lymphatic system and escape into the circulation or to other body tissues, such as the lungs. Wherever the cancer cells collect, more cancer cells are produced. This is the way cancer spreads to other body parts. Lymph nodes are biopsied to check for the spread of cancer.

Lymph Organs

The spleen and thymus are lymph organs. The spleen removes old RBCs, platelets, and microorganisms from the blood. Approximately 350 mL of blood are stored in the spleen and approximately 200 mL can be pumped out within a minute into the body as needed (Thibodeau & Patton, 2009). During an infection, the spleen enlarges to produce and release monocytes and lymphocytes. Lymphocytes in the lymph tissue differentiate into T lymphocytes (T cells) and B lymphocytes (B cells).

In infancy and childhood, the thymus gland is large but decreases in size with age. In advanced age, it is replaced with fat and connective tissue. The thymus performs an important role in the special processing and proper functioning of the thymus-derived T lymphocytes (T cells). The T cells are actively involved in immunity.

ASSESSMENT

Information is based on client report, physical examination, and diagnostic tests.

Subjective Data

Biological and demographic data, including age, sex, ethnic background, and race, are important for many hematologic problems. Inquire about the client's occupation and hobbies because of possible exposure to radiation or chemicals. Past military experience is also important because some military personnel have been exposed to toxic chemicals. Obtain a medication history, including prescription and over-the-counter medications. Note recent or recurring infections, night sweats, palpitations, bleeding problems, previous blood transfusions, and any complications.

Assess neurological functioning by asking if the client has experienced any cognitive or mental difficulties or numbness and tingling of the extremities. A headache may indicate a low erythrocyte count or intracranial bleeding. Note hearing or vision difficulties.

Ask about past surgeries and any complications from surgeries; if the client has had a duodenal, gastric, or ileal resection, the absorption of iron and vitamin B12 may be affected. Alcohol use affects vitamin intake and is caustic to the gastrointestinal (GI) tract. Ask about the presence of blood in the stool or urine and any anorexia, nausea, vomiting, oral discomfort, or problems with taste perception. A diet history is helpful when reviewing the erythrocyte level. Inquire if the client has difficulty accomplishing ADLs because of decreased energy.

Objective Data

Begin by obtaining the client's height, weight, and vital signs. An elevated temperature is an indication of an infection. Note recent weight gains or losses.

Laboratory tests are very important when assessing the hematologic and lymphatic systems. The nurse compares past and present laboratory results.

Palpate the lymph nodes in the neck, axillae, and groin; normal findings include small (0.5–1.0 cm) nodes that are freely movable, firm, and nontender. Tender nodes indicate inflammation. Hard, fixed nodes may be malignant. See Table 37-2 for the general "Rules of Thumb" regarding abnormal lymph findings.

Next, inspect the skin and extremities for petechiae, bruises, lesions, and brittle nails. Check urine and stool for blood. Note dyspnea, an enlarged abdomen, or swollen joints. Refer to Box 37-1, Questions to Ask and Observations to Make When Collecting Data, for guidance in completing the client's hematology and lymphatic assessment.

COMMON DIAGNOSTIC TESTS

Commonly used diagnostic tests for clients with symptoms of blood and lymph system disorders are listed in Table 37-3.

RBC DISORDERS

Reduced production of RBCs results in anemia, of WBCs results in infections, and of platelets results in bleeding. RBC disorders discussed in this section are anemias and polycythemia vera. The nursing process for anemias is presented after the discussion of sickle cell anemia because the nursing diagnoses, goals, and interventions are similar for all anemias.

Anemia is a common hematopoietic disorder in which the client has a decreased number of RBCs and a low hemoglobin level. The causes for anemia are a decreased production of RBCs, an increased destruction of RBCs, or a loss of blood. Anemias discussed in this section are iron deficiency anemia, hypoplastic (aplastic) anemia, pernicious anemia, acquired hemolytic anemia, and sickle cell anemia.

IRON DEFICIENCY ANEMIA

Iron deficiency anemia is the most common type of anemia and occurs when the body does not have enough iron to synthesize functional Hgb. The decrease in iron may be caused by dietary deficiency, but the most common cause is blood loss such as in women with heavy menstrual periods or slow, chronic blood loss from a peptic ulcer, kidney or bladder tumor, colon polyp, or colorectal cancer (Mayo Clinic, 2009). Decreased iron absorption, menstruating women, or an increased need for iron such as

BOX 37-1 QUESTIONS TO ASK AND OBSERVATIONS TO MAKE WHEN COLLECTING DATA

Subjective Data

Do you smoke?
Have you gained or lost weight in the last six months?
Do you feel fatigued?
Have you noticed a decrease in your energy levels?
Do you get frequent colds or infections?
Do you ever have dizzy spells?
Do your teeth or gums bleed?
Have you experienced any changes in skin color or sensation? (See Table 37-1.)
Have you noticed any change in the sensation in your fingers and toes?
Do you experience numbness in your hands or feet?
Do you notice excessive bruising?
Do you have any swollen "glands"? If so, is the swelling always there or does it come and go? When is the swelling the worst? Is there any associated heat?
Do you have any sores that do not heal? Where are they?
Do you bruise easily?
Do you experience joint pain?
To your knowledge, have you been exposed to HIV?

Objective Data

Observe for apparent lymph nodes in the neck.
Inspect skin for lesions
Palpate the supraclavicular lymph bilaterally in the indentation just superior to the outer one third of the clavicle.
Inspect shoulder, elbow, wrist, and finger joints for edema, bruising, and deformity.
Examine the axillae bilaterally for redness and visible swelling.
Inspect and palpate lymph nodes.
Inspect for size and symmetry of extremities. If one extremity is asymmetrical and increased in size, it may be indicative of lymph drainage obstruction on that side.
Note and document any wounds or ulcerations, bruising or changes in vascular patterns.
While your patient is lying supine, palpate the liver and spleen for tenderness, nodules, or enlargement.
Inspect hip, knee, ankle, and toe joints for edema, bruising, and deformity.
Observe the backs of the legs for changes in vascular pattern.
Inspect joints for edema or deformity and symmetry in size and shape bilaterally.
Using the pads of the second, third, and fourth fingers, lightly palpate for superficial lymph nodes.
Use a gentle circular motion in each lymph node area moving the overlying skin with your fingers.
Note any enlargement or palpable nodes. Observe your client's face during palpation for any signs of discomfort with the exam. All lymph nodes should normally be nonpalpable and nontender. Lymph nodes do not have a pulse, so if one is palpated, it is definitely not lymph.
For lymph nodes that are palpable, be careful to note size, shape, mobility, temperature, and consistency.
Palpate the tissues around any enlarged nodes for changes adjacent to them.

TABLE 37-1 Common Skin Findings in the Presence of Blood Disorders

Pallor	Pale color of the skin. Lack of circulating oxygen to tissues. May indicate abnormal destruction of or lack of production of RBCs.
Purpura	Purplish discoloration greater than 0.5 cm in diameter resulting from bleeding under the skin. May be caused by intravascular defects, platelet disorders, or infection (Seidel, Ball, Dains, & Benedict, 2006).
Petechiae	Reddish discoloration less than 0.5 cm in diameter. Also caused by platelet disorders, infection, and vasculitis.
Ecchymosis	Red-purple bruising caused by tissue injury and bleeding underneath the skin.
Spider angioma	Small red center with red "spider leg" projections. May be caused by liver disease and vitamin B deficiency (Seidel, Ball, Dains, & Benedict, 2006).

COURTESY OF DELMAR CENGAGE LEARNING

during growth periods or pregnancy are also causes. Iron deficiency anemia is more frequently found in premature or low-birthweight infants, adolescent girls, alcoholic clients, and the elderly. The symptoms are fatigue, palpitations, tachycardia, exertional dyspnea, weakness, and pallor. Clients with chronic anemia have pica, stomatitis, glossitis, and brittle hair. Diagnostic tests reveal decreased RBCs, a low Hgb level, a low Hct, a low serum iron, and a high total iron-binding capacity (TIBC).

MEDICAL–SURGICAL MANAGEMENT

Pharmacological

An oral iron preparation, usually ferrous sulfate (Feosol) is ordered. These preparations are not given with food or milk because they interfere with iron absorption. The administration of iron with orange juice or vitamin C–rich drinks increases iron absorption. Iron dextran (InFeD), an intramuscular iron preparation, is given only in the upper, outer quadrant of the buttocks, deep IM with Z-track method.

CRITICAL THINKING

Iron Deficiency Anemia

How are the symptoms of iron deficiency anemia related to a decreased red blood cell count and decreased hemoglobin?

TABLE 37-2 General "Rules of Thumb" Regarding Abnormal Lymph Findings

Inflamed Lymph Nodes	Malignant Lymph Nodes
Enlarged	Small
Soft	Hard
Mobile	Attached to over- or underlying surfaces
Tender	Nontender

COURTESY OF DELMAR CENGAGE LEARNING

Diet

A diet high in iron is encouraged. Foods rich in iron are red meats, fish, raisins, apricots, dried fruits, dark green vegetables, dried beans, eggs, and iron-enriched whole-grain breads. An increase of vitamin C in the diet assists in the absorption of iron. If the client has a loss of appetite, small frequent snacks are tolerated better than three large meals.

Activity

Space daily activities to provide rest periods between times of exercise.

APLASTIC ANEMIA

The bone marrow decreases or stops functioning in a client with aplastic anemia. The client with aplastic anemia has pancytopenia, a decrease in the number of RBCs, WBCs, and platelets. In most cases the cause is unknown, but genetic factors are suspected. Secondary aplastic anemia is caused by exposure to viruses, chemicals (benzene or airplane glue), radiation, or medications. Some medications that cause aplastic anemia are chloramphenicol (Chloromycetin), mephenytoin (Mesantoin), trimethadione (Tridione), mechlorethamine or nitrogen mustard (Mustargen), methotrexate (Folex PFS), 6-mercaptopurine or 6-MP (Purinethol), and phenylbutazone (Butazolidin). Symptoms include fatigue, weakness, palpitvations, headaches, fever, mouth ulcers, petechiae, gingival bleeding, and epistaxis. These clients are extremely ill. Diagnosis is confirmed by a bone marrow aspiration.

TABLE 37-3 Common Diagnostic Tests for Blood and Lymphatic System Disorders

Partial thromboplastin time (PTT)
Activated partial thromboplastin time (APTT)
Bleeding time
Blood culture and sensitivity
Coombs' test (direct antiglobulin test)
D-dimer test (fragment D-dimer, fibrin degradation fragment)
Erythrocyte sedimentation rate (sed rate, ESR)
Folic acid (folate level)
Hematocrit (Hct)
Hemoglobin (Hgb)
Hemoglobin electrophoresis
International normalized ratio (INR)
Platelet count
Protein electrophoresis (immunofixation electrophoresis)
Prothrombin time (PT, protime)
Red blood cells (RBCs)
Serum ferritin
Sickledex (Sickle cell test)
Total iron binding capacity (TIBC)
White blood cells (WBCs)
Differential count
Granulocytes
Basophils
Eosinophils
Neutrophils
Bands
Agranulocytes
Lymphocytes
Monocytes
Bone marrow aspiration
Radiologic lymphangiogram

COURTESY OF DELMAR CENGAGE LEARNING

MEDICAL–SURGICAL MANAGEMENT

Medical

The cause of aplastic anemia is removed if possible. Immunosuppressive therapy with antithymocyte globulin or ATG (Atgam) and cyclosporine is given to suppress the reaction causing the aplastic anemia and to allow the client's bone marrow to recover. A client who has a good response will improve in 3 to 6 months. The response rate is 70% to 80% (Aplastic Anemia & MDS International Foundation, 2006). Transfusions of packed red cells and platelets are given as needed.

Surgical

A bone marrow transplant is performed if the client's bone marrow fails to respond to treatment. Cyclosporine (Sandimmune), an immunosuppressant, is given for a bone marrow transplant to decrease the graft rejection. The best response occurs in a young client who has not previously had a transfusion because transfusions increase bone marrow graft rejection. Bone marrow transplants from a human leukocyte antigen- (HLA-) matched sibling donor are the treatment of choice for clients younger than 30 years of age. The treatment of choice for an older adult or a client who does not have an HLA-matched sibling donor is immunosuppression with ATG and cyclosporine. (Bone marrow transplants are discussed in the section on acute myelocytic leukemia.)

Pharmacological

Infections are treated with antibiotics. Steroids and androgens are sometimes used to stimulate the bone marrow.

PERNICIOUS ANEMIA

The parietal cells of the gastric mucosa secrete a protein intrinsic factor that is essential for the proper absorption of vitamin B_{12}. Pernicious anemia is an autoimmune disease in which the parietal cells are destroyed and the gastric mucosa atrophies. Without the secretion of the intrinsic factor, vitamin B_{12} cannot be absorbed in the distal portion of the ileum.

The onset of the disease occurs around the age of 60. Pernicious anemia occurs most frequently in women of Northern European descent and some African Americans. Pernicious anemia occurs in clients who have had a gastrectomy with the section of the stomach removed that secretes the intrinsic factor. High levels of serum homocysteine and methylmalonic acid (MMA) are confirming diagnostic tests (NIH, 2009).

Pernicious anemia has an insidious onset because the body can store 3 to 5 years' worth of vitamin B_{12} in the liver. Neurologic changes, paresthesia, and numbness occur before lab tests identify vitamin B_{12} deficiency (Holcomb, 2001). Symptoms include extreme weakness, a sore tongue, edema of the legs, ataxia, dizziness, dyspnea, headache, fever, blurred vision, tinnitus, jaundice with pallor, poor memory, irritability, and loss of bladder and bowel control. The client has decreased sensitivity to heat and pain because of neurological involvement. Clients with pernicious anemia are highly susceptible to gastric carcinoma and are monitored closely for symptoms.

MEDICAL–SURGICAL MANAGEMENT

Pharmacological

Topical anesthetics are given to relieve oral discomfort during the acute phase of the disease. Vitamin B_{12}, cyanocobalamin crystalline (Rubesol-1000) is given IM until the Hct returns to normal. Then it is given monthly for the rest of the client's life. The frequency of administration depends on the client's

PROFESSIONALTIP

Vitamin B_{12} Deficiency

Strict vegetarians are at risk for vitamin B_{12} deficiency. A dietary supplement of vitamin B_{12} is the treatment.

symptoms and response to the medication. Oral administration of vitamin B_{12} is not effective because vitamin B_{12} cannot be absorbed without the intrinsic factor. Folic acid or folate (Folvite) is prescribed. Encourage the client to increase folic acid in the diet by eating green leafy vegetables, meat, fish, legumes, and whole grains. Iron is usually not prescribed because once the condition is corrected with regular administration of cyanocobalamin, erythrocytes are produced and the Hgb and Hct return to normal.

ACQUIRED HEMOLYTIC ANEMIA

In hemolytic anemias, **hemolysis**, or destruction of RBCs, occurs, and iron and hemoglobin are released. Several causes for acquired hemolytic anemia are an autoimmune reaction, radiation, blood transfusion, chemicals, arsenic, lead, or medications. Sulfisoxazole (Gantrisin), penicillin, and methyldopa (Aldomet) are medications that cause hemolysis. A substance produced by the bacterium *Clostridium perfringens* also causes hemolysis. Clients may not notice symptoms or experience a severe reaction. Symptoms are mild fatigue and pallor. More severe symptoms include jaundice, palpitations, hypotension, dyspnea, and back and joint pain. Diagnostic tests reveal a low Hgb and Hct and an increased level of lactate dehydrogenase (LDH). LDH is an enzyme in the heart, liver, kidneys, skeletal muscle, brain, RBCs, and lungs. As these tissues are damaged, LDH is released into the bloodstream, causing an elevated LDH.

MEDICAL–SURGICAL MANAGEMENT

Medical

Treatment is aimed at removing the cause, if possible. Clients are given blood transfusions or **erythrocytapheresis** (a procedure that removes abnormal RBCs and replaces them with healthy RBCs).

Surgical

The spleen destroys RBCs. In severe cases of hemolytic anemia, a splenectomy is performed in an attempt to stop the destruction of RBCs.

Pharmacological

Corticosteroids are administered to decrease the autoimmune response. Folic acid is given to increase the production of RBCs.

SICKLE CELL ANEMIA (INHERITED HEMOLYTIC ANEMIA)

Sickle cell anemia is also known as inherited hemolytic anemia or sickle cell disease. This genetic disorder has abnormal hemoglobin S rather than hemoglobin A in the RBCs. Sickle cell anemia is caused by a recessive gene or genes that are passed through the generations (Figure 37-6). The client with one s gene has sickle cell trait (Hb sA) and is asymptomatic but is a carrier of the disease. The client with sickle cell anemia has two s genes (Hb ss) and manifests symptoms.

The condition occurs most frequently in African-American clients, with an estimated 1,000 infants born with sickle cell disease each year in the United States (SCDAA, 2005). It also occurs in persons from Asia Minor, India, and the Mediterranean and Caribbean areas.

Sickle cell tests are done on infants to diagnose sickle cell trait or disease. A screening test to detect the presence of Hb S is Sickledex or sickle cell test. If Hb S is present, a hemoglobin electrophoresis is done to distinguish between sickle cell trait and sickle cell disease. If the hemoglobin electrophoresis test is negative, the client has the sickle cell trait and not sickle cell disease.

Situations that precipitate sickle cell crisis are dehydration, deoxygenation, acidosis, and temperature changes (Platt, Beasley, Miller, & Eckman, 2002). In these situations crystallization of hemoglobin is promoted, which forces the RBCs to **sickle**, i.e., become crescent-shaped and elongated

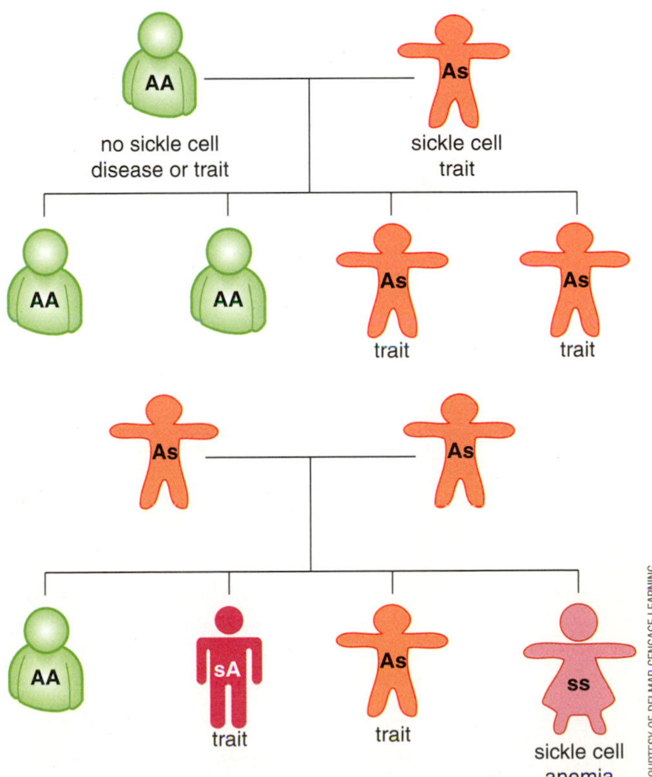

FIGURE 37-6 Inheritance of the Sickle Cell Trait and Sickle Cell Anemia

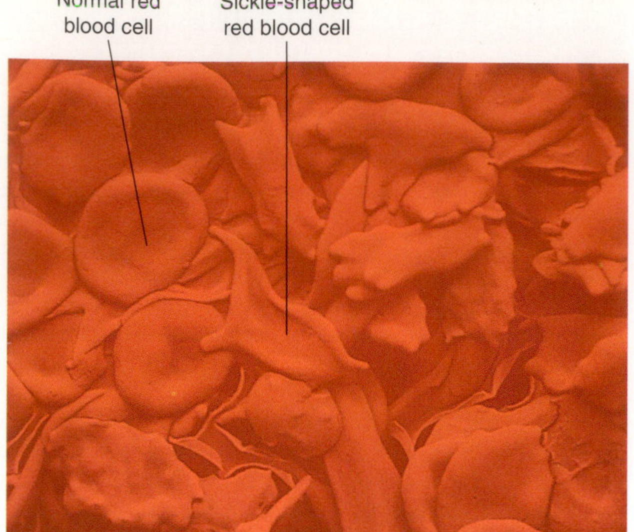

FIGURE 37-7 Blood Cells Magnified through a Scanning Electron Microscope Show Normal and Sickle-Shaped Red Blood Cells (*Courtesy of Phillips Electronic Instruments Company.*)

and obstruct vessels, especially capillaries (Figure 37-7) (Platt et al., 2002). The area normally supplied by these obstructed blood vessels becomes infarcted and ischemic. The destruction of sickled RBCs in 12 to 15 days causes chronic anemia; the heart enlarges in an attempt to circulate more blood for adequate oxygenation of body tissues. Other symptoms include fatigue, jaundice, chronic leg ulcers, tachypnea, dyspnea, and arrhythmias. When the client experiences a sickle cell crisis, there is fever, severe pain, and loss of blood supply to various organs because of obstructed vessels. Areas most frequently affected are the joints, bone, brain, lungs, liver, kidneys, and penis. Joints become painful, swollen, and immobile. Clients experience cerebrovascular accidents, renal failure, pulmonary infarction, shock, and priapism (a continuous, painful erection).

Assess extremity circulation frequently by doing capillary refill, peripheral pulses, and temperature. Application of warm compresses to painful areas relieves pain. Encourage the client to avoid restrictive clothing and anything that may restrict circulation. Teach clients to avoid high altitudes and have adequate fluid intake.

CLIENT TEACHING
Sickle Cell Anemia

- Encourage client to avoid high altitudes and nonpressurized airplanes.
- Encourage adequate fluid intake because dehydration causes a sickle cell crisis.
- Treat all infections promptly.
- Encourage client to tight-fitting, restrictive clothing, and strenuous exercise, smoking, and cold temperatures.
- Encourage client to receive yearly flu vaccine and pneumococcal vaccine.

MEDICAL–SURGICAL MANAGEMENT

Medical

Infections are treated promptly with antibiotics. Large amounts of oral and intravenous fluids (3–5 L/day) are given to remove the by-products of broken RBCs. Oxygen is administered based on pulse oximetry and ABGs to combat deoxygenation. Skin grafting is necessary for chronic leg ulcers.

Genetic counseling is recommended for clients with sickle cell trait and sickle cell anemia. There may be more openness to counseling if the counselor is from the same community as the client.

Pharmacological

Hydroxyurea (Droxia) reduces the frequency of painful crisis and the need for blood transfusions in adults (Spratto & Woods, 2004). Folic acid or folate (Folvite) is administered daily to assist in the production of RBCs. Pentoxifylline (Trental) reduces blood viscosity and increases RBC flexibility. Blood transfusions are given during a crisis.

Patient-controlled analgesia (PCA) with morphine is effective during a crisis. The client is progressed from narcotics to nonnarcotic analgesics as indicated.

CRITICAL THINKING
Anemias

Use the table and compare the etiologies, diagnostic tests, symptoms, treatments, and nursing interventions of the listed anemias.

	Iron deficiency anemia	Aplastic anemia	Pernicious anemia	Acquired hemolytic anemia	Sickle cell anemia
Etiology					
Diagnostic tests					
Symptoms					
Treatments					
Nursing interventions					

Nursing Management

Assess weight, vital signs, apical and peripheral pulses, breath sounds, color, abdominal tenderness, and signs of bruising or jaundice. Review client's history for possible familial illnesses. Encourage client to follow treatment regimen. Monitor laboratory test results. Administer blood products as ordered and monitor for a possible reaction.

NURSING PROCESS

Assessment

Subjective Data

Obtain a history of the client's medical problems, including a history of familial hematopoietic illnesses. Some anemias may be caused by drugs and environmental conditions, so information about medications taken and about environmental situations at work and in recreational settings is important. The client is asked about fatigue, dyspnea with exertion, palpitations, dizziness, pain, petechiae, tingling and numbness in the extremities, blurred vision, and oral discomfort.

Objective Data

The client's weight and vital signs; apical pulse and peripheral pulses; breath sounds; sensation and movement in the extremities; abdominal tenderness; and edema, pallor, and signs of bruising or jaundice are assessed. A thorough assessment of the cardiac system is completed because severe anemia causes cardiac enlargement and arrhythmias.

Nursing diagnoses for a client with decreased erythrocytes and hemoglobin may include the following:

NURSING DIAGNOSES	PLANNING/OUTCOMES	NURSING INTERVENTIONS
Deficient Knowledge related to prescribed treatment regimen	The client will relate the prescribed treatment regimen.	Teach the cause of the particular type of anemia and, if possible, ways to avoid the occurrence of that anemia in the future. For iron deficiency anemia, teach the importance of taking and increasing iron in the diet. Instruct clients with pernicious anemia to obtain a vitamin B_{12} injection at regularly scheduled times. Teach clients with hemolytic anemias the significance of following the prescribed regimens.
Activity intolerance related to imbalance between oxygen supply and demand	The client will increasingly tolerate activity.	Assist the client as needed with activities of daily living. Teach the client to alternate periods of rest with activity.
Ineffective Tissue Perfusion (Peripheral) related to a decreased hemoglobin concentration in the blood	The client will have increased tissue perfusion.	Administer oxygen as needed to relieve symptoms of dyspnea. Monitor Hgb, Hct, RBCs, pulse oximetry, electrolytes, vital signs, and mental alertness. Monitor for symptoms of obstructed vessels such as pain, leg ulcerations, abdominal tenderness, dyspnea, confusion, and blurred vision. Administer blood products as ordered and monitor the client closely after blood transfusions for possible reactions such as chills, fever, dyspnea, pruritus, wheezing, and pain in the lumbar region.

Evaluation: Evaluate each outcome to determine how it has been met by the client.

SAMPLE NURSING CARE PLAN

The Client with Sickle Cell Anemia

R.T., a 19-year-old African-American client, was diagnosed with sickle cell anemia 5 years ago. R.T. works for a computer company and has been working 12-hour days to get a system installed. He felt fatigued lately and decided to relax by playing golf on a warm Saturday morning. After the seventh hole, R.T. experienced dyspnea and tingling and numbness in his legs. After the next hole, he experienced severe pain in his ankles and knees. He was taken to the local medical center, where he was admitted. The physician ordered oxygen by nasal cannula, IV fluids, and a PCA pump with morphine sulfate.

NURSING DIAGNOSIS 1 *Acute **P**ain* related to occlusion of small vessels by sickled cells as evidenced by severe pain in the knees and ankles

Nursing Outcomes Classification (NOC)
Comfort Level
Pain Control

Nursing Interventions Classification (NIC)
Pain Management
Emotional Support
Heat/Cold Application

PLANNING/OUTCOMES	NURSING INTERVENTIONS	RATIONALE
R.T. will state pain has been relieved.	Assess pain type, location, and intensity.	Identifies where vessels may be occluded.
	Monitor analgesic administration by PCA pump.	Assesses relief from pain.
	Support joints and lower extremities with pillows.	Relieves joint pain.
	Keep bed linens off knees and ankles with a bed cradle.	Keeps linen from putting pressure on painful areas.

EVALUATION

The morphine in the PCA pump relieved R.T.'s pain, and oral analgesics were ordered.

NURSING DIAGNOSIS 2 *Ineffective **T**issue Perfusion (Cardiopulmonary and Peripheral)* related to a decreased number of RBCs and decreased oxygenation as evidenced by dyspnea and tingling and numbness in his ankles and knees

Nursing Outcomes Classification (NOC)
Tissue Perfusion: Peripheral
Circulation Status

Nursing Interventions Classification (NIC)
Oxygen Therapy
Intravenous Therapy

PLANNING/OUTCOMES	NURSING INTERVENTIONS	RATIONALE
R.T. will experience improved circulation in his extremities.	Elevate the head of the bed.	Allows lungs to expand more fully.
	Administer oxygen as needed.	Oxygen increases blood oxygen level.
	Administer IV fluids as ordered.	Decreases the possibility of RBCs' sickling.
	Encourage R.T. to drink 8 to 10 glasses of water daily.	Prevents RBCs from sickling.
	Monitor for symptoms of obstructed vessels such as pain, leg ulcerations, abdominal tenderness, dyspnea, confusion, and blurred vision.	Vessels supplying blood to other vital organs can become obstructed.
	Administer blood products as ordered.	Improves the blood oxygen concentration.
	Closely monitor for possible blood transfusion reactions such as chills, fever, dyspnea, pruritus, wheezing, and pain in the lumbar region.	Administration of blood products may cause adverse reactions.

SAMPLE NURSING CARE PLAN (Continued)

EVALUATION

Circulation in lower extremities has improved as manifested by prompt capillary refill and strong pedal and popliteal pulses. Extremities are warm to touch.

NURSING DIAGNOSIS 3 *Deficient Knowledge* related to prescribed treatment regimen as evidenced by a lack of rest and working long hours

Nursing Outcomes Classification (NOC)
Knowledge: Energy Conservation
Knowledge: Treatment Regimen

Nursing Interventions Classification (NIC)
Self-Modification Assistance
Teaching: Individual

PLANNING/OUTCOMES	NURSING INTERVENTIONS	RATIONALE
R.T. will relate the prescribed treatment regimen before discharge.	Teach R.T. the pathophysiology related to sickle cell disease.	Improves compliance with the medical regimen.
	Encourage R.T. to take medications as ordered.	Improves circulation and postpones sickle cell crisis situations.
	Explain the importance of avoiding stressful situations and the symptoms of infection.	These situations increase oxygen demands.
	Explain the importance of adequate rest on a routine basis.	Allows adequate oxygenation and reduces stress.

EVALUATION

R.T. states his RBCs have Hgb S rather than Hgb A, and a lack of oxygen causes his RBCs to sickle. Sickling is caused by fatigue, lack of oral fluids, emotional and physical stress, infection, exposure to cold and anesthesia. He knows the purpose and side effects of each medication and the times he is to take them. R.T. states he is to avoid high altitudes. R.T. states that he will try to routinely have enough rest.

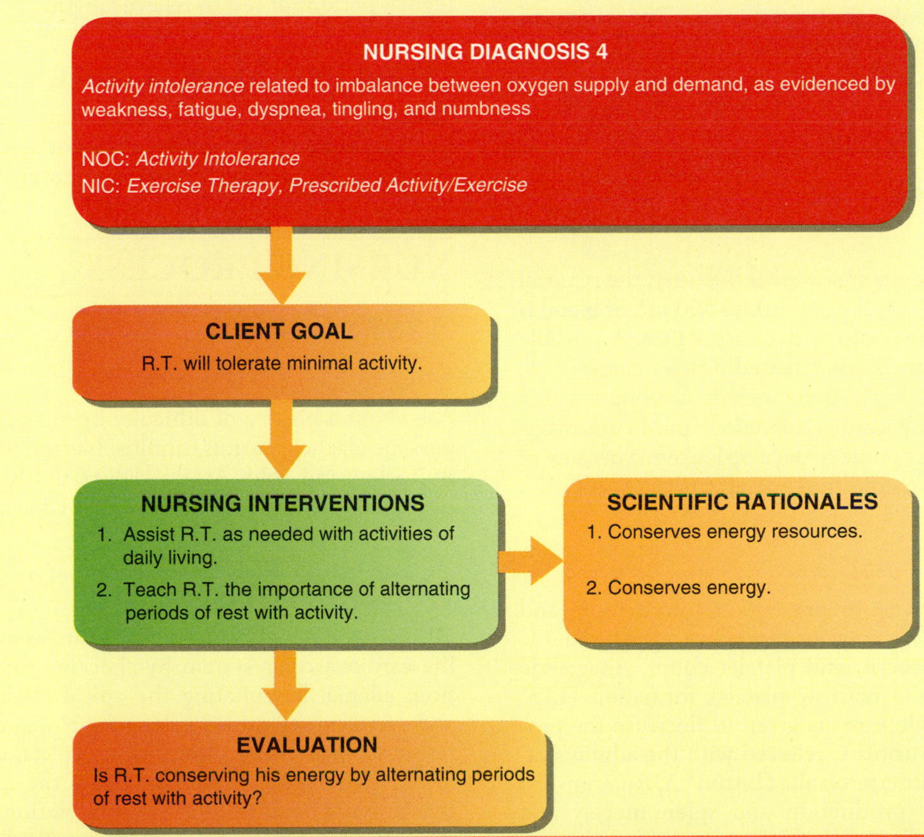

NURSING DIAGNOSIS 4
Activity intolerance related to imbalance between oxygen supply and demand, as evidenced by weakness, fatigue, dyspnea, tingling, and numbness
NOC: Activity Intolerance
NIC: Exercise Therapy, Prescribed Activity/Exercise
CLIENT GOAL
R.T. will tolerate minimal activity.
NURSING INTERVENTIONS
1. Assist R.T. as needed with activities of daily living.
2. Teach R.T. the importance of alternating periods of rest with activity.
SCIENTIFIC RATIONALES
1. Conserves energy resources.
2. Conserves energy.
EVALUATION
Is R.T. conserving his energy by alternating periods of rest with activity?

CONCEPT CARE MAP 37-1

POLYCYTHEMIA

Polycythemia is a disease in which there is an increased production of red blood cells. Usually the numbers of WBCs and platelets are also increased. The increase in RBCs increases the blood volume and viscosity and decreases the ability of the blood to circulate freely. There are two types of polycythemia: polycythemia vera (PV) (primary polycythemia) and secondary polycythemia. The average age for a diagnosis of polycythemia vera is between the ages of 60 and 65. It is more prevalent in Jewish men of Eastern European ancestry (The Leukemia and Lymphoma Society, 2007). Clients with PV have a mutation of the JAK2 (Janus kinase 2) gene, but the exact role of the mutated gene in the cause is not known. A DNA abnormality occurs in an early marrow cell that produces all of the blood cells in the individual. Secondary polycythemia is a compensatory mechanism as the body makes more red blood cells in response to low oxygenation caused by long-term hypoxia, as in chronic obstructive pulmonary disease, chronic heart failure, smoking, or living in a high altitude.

Symptoms of the two types are the same. As the blood viscosity and volume increase, the client experiences headaches, dizziness, tinnitus, blurred vision, fatigue, weakness, pruritus, exertional dyspnea, angina, and increased blood pressure and pulse. The client's complexion becomes ruddy (reddish), and the palms, earlobes, and cheeks are flushed. Some clients experience a burning sensation in the feet. The client is susceptible to thrombi formation because of the increased viscosity of the blood and increase in platelets. Even though there are more RBCs produced in polycythemia, the RBCs have a shorter life span than normal. When RBCs die, uric acid is released, causing **hyperuricemia** (increased uric acid blood level). The elevated uric acid levels cause or aggravate gout symptoms. The Hgb and Hct increase in the same proportion as the RBCs (Leukemia & Lymphoma Society, 2007).

MEDICAL–SURGICAL MANAGEMENT

Medical

The treatment for polycythemia is **phlebotomy**, the removal of blood from a vein. Generally 350 mL to 500 mL of blood is withdrawn at regular intervals to decrease RBCs. A possible side effect of phlebotomy is an increased platelet count (LLS, 2007). Polycythemia complications include cerebral vascular accident, thrombosis, myocardial infarction, and hemorrhage. Clients with PV are more prone to develop leukemia because of the disease process and medication side effects (LLS, 2007).

Pharmacological

Low-dose aspirin is given to prevent clot formation, and hydroxyurea (Hydrea®), a myelosuppressive agent, reduces the hemoglobin, hematocrit, and platelet count. Anagrelide (Agrylin®) reduces bone marrow platelet formation (LLS, 2007). Allopurinol (Zyloprim) is given to decrease the production of uric acid. Pruritus is relieved with the administration of antihistamines. Interferon alfa (Intron® A, Roferon-A®) reduces bone marrow production and splenomegaly and relieves pruritus. Interferon alfa is an option for younger clients with splenomegaly. However, interferon alfa is not used as often because of the expense and the side effects of the drugs (Stuart & Viera, 2004). Alkylating agents are not used as frequently because of the incidence of leukemia in clients using these drugs (Stuart & Viera, 2004). Radioactive phosphorus (32p) decreases the production of blood cells in the bone marrow and is used along with phlebotomy.

> **CLIENT TEACHING**
>
> **Polycythemia**
>
> - Drink at least 3 L of water daily.
> - Elevate feet when resting.
> - Avoid tight or restrictive clothing.
> - Wear support hose.
> - Take medications as ordered.
> - Report chest pain, joint pain, fever, or activity intolerance to physician.
> - Keep appointments for laboratory testing and physician checks.

Diet

The client is placed on a diet that has increased calories and protein. A diet low in sodium decreases fluid volume. Iron-containing foods are avoided.

Activity

Activities of daily living are adjusted so the client can have regular periods of rest to relieve fatigue.

NURSING MANAGEMENT

Monitor vital signs, nutritional status, and oxygenation. Keep accurate I&O. Initiate passive or active leg exercises or encourage ambulation. Encourage compliance with regimen.

NURSING PROCESS

ASSESSMENT

Subjective Data

Ask about a history of difficulty breathing, chest pain, dizziness, headache, pruritus, tinnitis, blurred vision, and sensitivity to hot and cold. Assess client's nutritional status for an inadequate dietary intake because of GI symptoms of fullness and dyspepsia.

Objective Data

Observe the skin for bruises and changes in skin color. Assess the cardiovascular system by checking for neck vein distention, edema, auscultating the apical pulse, palpating radial and pedal pulses, and checking for Homans' sign. Assess the respiratory system by observing for epistaxis and dyspnea and listening to the breath sounds. Check the central nervous system through pupil response, disorientation, and the presence of numbness or tingling.

Nursing diagnoses for a client with polycythemia include the following:

NURSING DIAGNOSES	PLANNING/OUTCOMES	NURSING INTERVENTIONS
*Deficient **K**nowledge* related to disease process and treatment	The client will relate disease process and treatment.	Explain the cause of the disease, possible symptoms, side effects of medications, and possible future complications to report. Teach client to report headache, chest pain, dyspnea, or redness, swelling, or tenderness in the arms or legs to the physician or nurse practitioner immediately.
*Ineffective **T**issue Perfusion (Peripheral)* related to decreased blood circulation	The client will have 2+ peripheral pulses.	Administer oxygen as needed for dyspnea. Check vital signs frequently and assess Homans' sign and signs of thrombi formation. Explain phlebotomy process.
*Risk for **I**njury* related to dizziness	The client will relate measures to avoid injury.	Encourage the client to change positions slowly to prevent dizziness. Encourage activities of daily living when the client is feeling well. Teach client to avoid activities that cause bruising or trauma.

Evaluation: Evaluate each outcome to determine how it has been met by the client.

WBC DISORDERS

WBC disorders include leukemia and agranulocytosis.

LEUKEMIA

Leukemia is a malignancy of blood-forming tissues in which the bone marrow produces increased numbers of immature white blood cells that are incapable of protecting the body from infections. The increased number of WBCs crowds out the other cells in the bone marrow, causing a decreased production of RBCs and platelets. Anemia and bleeding result from the decreased number of RBCs and platelets.

Leukemia is divided into 4 categories: acute myelogenous leukemia (AML), acute lymphocytic leukemia (ALL), chronic myelogenous leukemia (CML), and chronic lymphocytic leukemia (CLL). An estimated 44,790 new cases of leukemia were diagnosed in 2009 (ACS, 2009a).

Because of the increased production of immature WBCs, clients with acute leukemia generally are fighting persistent infections and have fever and chills. The decreased number of RBCs causes symptoms of anemia such as fatigue, pallor, malaise, tachycardia, and tachypnea. The decreased platelet production causes bleeding tendencies, and the client experiences petechiae, bruising, epistaxis, melena, gingival bleeding, and increased menstrual bleeding. The client also experiences weight loss, night sweats, and swollen lymph nodes. As the malignant cells invade the central nervous system, the client experiences headaches, seizures, vomiting, blurred vision, and difficulty maintaining balance (ACS, 2007a). Some clients experience bone pain because the rapid production of WBCs crowds the cells in the bone marrow.

ACUTE LEUKEMIA

Acute leukemias have a rapid onset and must be treated quickly for a good prognosis. ALL has a more rapid onset than AML. ALL is the more common type of leukemia in childhood with most cases occurring between the ages of 2 and 4 years of age (LLS, ACS, 2009c). The 5-year survival rate for a child with ALL is more than 80%. (ACS, 2009c).

AML and CLL are more common in adults (LLS, 2009). AML in childhood occurs more frequently during the first 2 years of life and in teenage years. However, AML is more common in older people with the average age for a diagnosis at 67 years-of-age. The 5-year survival rate of a child with AML is more than 50%; more adults die from AML (ACS, 2009b).

Medical–Surgical Management

Medical

Diagnosis of acute leukemia is confirmed with a CBC and a bone marrow biopsy. A lumbar puncture determines the presence of malignant cells in the central nervous system. An x-ray, MRI, CT scan, or Gallium scan and bone scan of the chest and skeleton determine the presence of infection and bone marrow tissue involvement.

Bone marrow transplantation is used with relapsed ALL clients and AML clients. High doses of chemotherapy and radiation therapy are given to the client to destroy the bone marrow. Leukemic white blood cells and healthy bone marrow cells are both destroyed, placing the client at a high risk for infection and death. Identical human leukocyte antigen (HLA) bone marrow from a sibling, the client, or an antigen-matched donor is given intravenously in a manner similar to a blood transfusion. The transfused bone marrow finds its way to the client's bone marrow and starts producing WBCs, RBCs, and platelets. The bone marrow is matched in a process very similar to the process of crossmatching blood. If the client's own bone marrow is used, it is removed from the client, treated with chemotherapy, and then reinfused into the client.

Maningo (2002) describes a fast-emerging alternative to bone marrow transplantation, peripheral blood stem cell transplantation. The stem cell donor (client or HLA-matched donor) is given growth factors such as granulocyte colony-stimulating factor (filgrastim [Neupogen]) and granulocyte macrophage–colony-stimulating factor (sargramostim [Leukine]) to increase the number of circulating blood stem cells. The peripheral stem cells, collected with a large-bore central vascular access device, are separated out of the whole blood. The RBCs, platelets, WBCs, and plasma are returned to the donor. The stem cells are then infused. Engraftment occurs in 2 to 4 weeks.

Pharmacological

Initial doses of chemotherapy are called **induction doses**. Small doses of chemotherapy given every 3 to 4 weeks to maintain remission are called **maintenance therapy**.

Leukemic cells lie dormant in the brain and spinal area because the chemotherapeutic drugs are unable to pass through the blood–brain barrier. Intrathecal (within the spinal canal) administration of methotrexate has decreased recurrences of ALL. Methotrexate is given by a lumbar puncture into the cerebrospinal fluid or through a subcutaneous cerebrospinal reservoir. Sometimes radiation therapy is also used on the brain and spinal area.

AML is treated with chemotherapeutic agents, blood products, and antibiotics. Chemotherapeutic agents used in treating acute leukemia are listed in Table 37-4.

Table 37-4 Chemotherapeutic Agents to Treat Leukemia

LEUKEMIA	CHEMOTHERAPEUTIC AGENTS
Acute lymphocytic leukemia (ALL)	vincristine (Oncovin) daunorubicin or daunomycin (Cerubidine) doxorubicin (Adriamycin) cytarabine (Cytosar) etoposide (VePesid) dexamethasone (Decadron) prednisone (Deltasone) 6-mercapotopurine or 6-MP (Purinethol) methotrexate (Methotrexate)
Acute myelogenous leukemia (AML)	daunorubicin HCl (Cerubidine) cytarabine or ara-C (Cytosar-U) 6-thioguanine or 6-TG (Thioguanine) vincristine (Oncovin) etoposide (VePesid)
Chronic myelogenous leukemia (CLL)	fludaravine (Fludara) pentostatine (Nipent) cladrivine (2-CdA, Leustatin) chlorambucil (Leukeran) COP (Cytoxan, Oncovin, and prednisone)
Chronic lymphocytic leukemia (CML)	Tyrosine kinase inhibitors are more effective than chemotherapy. hydroxyurea (Hydrea)

COURTESY OF DELMAR CENGAGE LEARNING

Diet

Avoid extremely hot or cold foods and drinks as well as alcohol. A bland, high-protein, high-carbohydrate diet is usually ordered.

Activity

Encourage clients to alternate periods of rest with activity and keep frequently used items nearby to conserve energy.

CHRONIC LEUKEMIA

Chronic leukemia generally occurs in adults with a gradual increase in the white cell count over months or years. The prognosis depends on the severity of the disease at the time of diagnosis.

CLL clients have increased abnormal B lymphocytes, with a WBC count between 20,000 and 100,000. CLL develops with advanced age and has a higher incident rate in men than in women (ACS, 2007e). There are two types of CLL. One type of CLL grows slowly, rarely needs treatment with a survival average of 15 years. The other type grows faster with a survival average of 8 years. The CLL cells have a protein called ZAP-70 and a substance called CD38. Clients with cells with lower levels of ZAP-70 and CD38 have a better survival rate (ACS, 2007f).

CML is characterized by the Philadelphia chromosome, indicating a possible genetic link. Treatment for CML has improved over the last few years and clients are surviving at least 5 years after diagnosis (ACS, 2008b). The WBC count ranges from 15,000 to 500,000. Most clients feel good and maintain a relatively normal life until later in the disease process, when the chronic recessed phase changes into an intensified stage that resembles an acute phase of leukemia. This acute phase is called a **blastic phase**, in which there is an increased production of WBCs. When this occurs, the general condition spirals downhill and the client soon dies. The most common cause of death in the leukemic client is viral and fungal pneumonia.

Medical–Surgical Management

Medical

Diagnosis of chronic leukemia is confirmed with a CBC and a bone marrow biopsy.

In the CML chronic phase, the HLA-identical allogenic bone marrow is given, and the client's own treated bone marrow is given in the blastic phase. Autologous or allogenic peripheral blood stem cell transplantation is used.

Pharmacological

Refer to Table 37-4 for chemotherapeutic agents used in treating CLL and CML. Chemotherapy does not extend the length of life but seems to give a better quality of life by prolonging the chronic phase. Fludarabine (Fludara), a purine analog, is the most effective single drug used to treat CLL. Purine analogs have significant side effects and cause increase susceptibility to infections. Alkylating agents, such as chlorambucil (Leukeran), and cyclophosphamide (Cytoxan) are used in treating CLL clients who cannot tolerate aggressive treatment. Monoclonal antibodies are medications that boost the client's immune system to respond and kill cancer cells. These medications attach to specific targeted substances on the surface of the cancer cells. Alemtuxumab (Campath) attaches to the CD52 antigen on the B and T lymphocytes. Campath is used when the client is no longer responding to chemotherapy. It is given subcutaneously or intravenously. Since it increases the risk for infections, it is given with antibiotics and antiviral medications (ACS, 2007b). Rituximab (Rituxan), a monoclonal antibody, targets the CD20 antigen on the surface of B lymphocytes. It is used along with chemotherapy for CLL and is given intravenously once a week (ACS, 2007b).

Chemotherapy is no longer the main treatment for CML. Imatinib mesylate (Gleevec) is one of the main drugs to treat CML. Chemotherapy is used in treating CML after the tyrosine kinase inhibitors are no longer effective. Hydroxyurea (Hydrea) is an oral pill taken to decrease very high WBC counts and to decrease spleen enlargement.

Diet

The client is on a diet high in protein, carbohydrates, and vitamins. A bland, nonirritating diet prevents oral mucosal irritation. Alcohol is avoided.

Activity

It is important for the client to learn methods to conserve energy, such as placing frequently used items nearby.

Nursing Management

Assess for pain. Monitor for symptoms of infection and bleeding. Check platelet count results. Follow proper hand hygiene procedure and teach it to all visitors. Provide frequent oral care with soft toothbrush or cotton swabs. Assist with or provide daily personal hygiene with antimicrobial soap. Monitor vital signs and report any temperature over 100°F. Encourage client to use an electric razor. Administer antiemetics, stool softener, and vitamins as ordered. Encourage client to talk about concerns and fears.

NURSING PROCESS

Assessment

Subjective Data

Ask the client or family about chromosomal abnormalities, exposure to chemicals, viral infections, and previous chemotherapy or radiation therapy. Ask the client to describe the location, type, and duration of pain, especially in bones or joints. Note symptoms of infection such as the presence of a cough or pain or burning on urination. Document a history of bleeding such as epistaxis, gingival bleeding, melena, or hematuria. Fatigue, malaise, and irritability are often described.

Objective Data

Note signs of infection, bleeding, and chemotherapy complications. Common sites for infection include the mouth, pharynx, lungs, skin, bladder, and perianal area. During chemotherapy, the reduced white cell count may stop the formation of pus, so infection may manifest as redness, swelling, and pain.

Assess for bleeding by monitoring the platelet count because bleeding occurs easily if the platelet count falls below 50,000. Clients bleed from any orifice, so inspect all body discharge. Occult blood is present in the urine and stool.

Chemotherapy complications are nausea, vomiting, and stomatitis. Alopecia occurs 1 to 2 weeks after treatments are initiated.

Nursing diagnoses for a client with leukemia include the following:

NURSING DIAGNOSES	PLANNING/OUTCOMES	NURSING INTERVENTIONS
*Deficient **K**nowledge* related to disease process and treatment	The client will relate treatment methods and possible complications of chemotherapy.	Teach the client to observe for signs of infection and bleeding. Review side effects of chemotherapy and radiation with the client, family members, and significant others.
*Risk for **I**nfection* related to increased production of immature white blood cells	The client will describe ways to prevent infection.	Follow good hand hygiene techniques. Teach proper hand hygiene to the family and friends who come into contact with the leukemic client. Use antimicrobial soaps for the client's daily bath. Provide frequent oral care with a soft toothbrush and nonirritating mouthwash to prevent open sores and stomatitis. Wash the perianal area after each bowel movement to decrease bacterial contamination and prevent rectal fissures.

(*Continues*)

Nursing diagnoses for a client with leukemia include the following: (Continued)

NURSING DIAGNOSES	PLANNING/OUTCOMES	NURSING INTERVENTIONS
		Avoid taking a rectal temperature and giving suppositories. Monitor the temperature every 4 hours for signs of infection. Report any temperature over 100°F to the physician. Administer antibiotics and antifungals as ordered. Closely monitor respiratory rate and breath sounds.
*Risk for **Injury*** related to decreased production of platelets	The client will identify ways to avoid injury and prevent bleeding.	Frequently observe the client for signs of bleeding such as epistaxis, gingival bleeding, petechiae, ecchymoses, hematemesis, enlarged abdomen, hematuria, melena, and confusion, which occur from intracranial hemorrhage. Administer stool softeners frequently to prevent anal irritation from hard stools. Use cotton swabs instead of a toothbrush for oral care. Encourage the client to use an electric razor. Avoid giving injections as much as possible. If a catheter is needed, lubricate it well to avoid trauma to the mucosal lining of the urethra.
*Imbalanced **Nutrition**: Less than Body Requirements* related to effects of disease process and chemotherapy on gastrointestinal tract	The client will choose nonirritating, high-protein, high-carbohydrate meals and snacks.	Administer antiemetics as ordered to relieve nausea and vomiting. Suggest that the client may tolerate small frequent feedings better than three large meals. Provide the client with a high-protein, high-carbohydrate diet to prevent infection and provide needed energy. Administer vitamin supplements as ordered. Teach the client to avoid raw fruits and vegetables as these foods contain more bacteria than cooked foods.
*Ineffective **Coping*** related to uncertainty about treatment of disease and prognosis	The client will identify ways to cope with concerns about disease process.	Inform the client of the possibility of alopecia from therapy treatments. Suggest client purchase a wig prior to initiation of chemotherapy treatments. Encourage the client to voice concerns and fears. Teach the client, family members, and significant others to monitor and report signs of infection and bleeding. Refer to support groups, social workers, and clergy as needed.

Evaluation: Evaluate each outcome to determine how it has been met by the client.

AGRANULOCYTOSIS

A severely reduced number of granulocytes (basophils, eosinophils, and neutrophils) is called **agranulocytosis** (see Memory Trick). The primary cause is an adverse reaction to medication or medication toxicity, especially with administration of phenylbutazone (Butazolidin), chloramphenical (Chloromycetin), penicillin derivatives, cephalosporins, phenytoin (Dilantin), antihistamines, vincristine (Oncovin), propythiouracil, diuretics, chlorpromazine hydrochloride (Thorazine), fluphenazene (Prolixin), promazene hydrochloride (Sparine), and sulfonamides and their derivatives. Other causes of agranulocytosis are neoplastic disease, chemotherapy, radiation therapy, and bacterial and viral infection. The causative agent suppresses the bone marrow, reducing the production of leukocytes.

The client exhibits the symptoms of infection: headache, fever, chills, and fatigue as well as mucous membrane ulcerations of the nose, mouth, pharynx, vagina, and rectum. The white blood count and neutrophils are low.

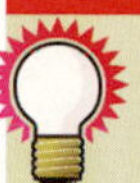

MEMORYTRICK

Granulocytes

There are three types of granulocytes: basophils, eosinophils, and neutrophils. A way to remember the granulocyte cells is to recall **G-BEN**:

G = Granulocytes
B = Basophils
E = Eosinophils
N = Neutrophils

Medical–Surgical Management

Medical

The main goals of treatment are to remove the cause of the bone marrow suppression and either prevent or treat any infection. When the client's temperature is elevated, blood cultures are performed. Mucosal ulcerations are cultured. Blood transfusions are given to provide mature leukocytes. Filgrastim (Neupogen), a human granulocyte colony-stimulating factor, is given. Protective isolation is instituted.

Pharmacological

Antibiotics specific for cultured microorganisms are given.

Diet

A soft, bland diet high in calories, protein, and vitamins is ordered.

Activity

Periods of activity must be balanced with periods of rest to prevent weakness and fatigue.

INFECTION CONTROL

The Client with Agranulocytosis

- Perform hand hygiene frequently and follow aseptic technique when caring for the client.
- Keep client's environment very clean.
- The client should avoid crowds.
- Screen guests so no one with a cold or any type of infection visits the client.
- Teach client to avoid hot or cold environments.
- Ensure that the client reports any signs or symptoms of infection.

Nursing Management

Assess vital signs and monitor for temperature over 100.6°F. Auscultate lungs for crackles and wheezes. Balance periods of activity with periods of rest. Use strict asepsis for all procedures. Perform thorough hand hygiene before caring for client. Screen everyone coming into contact with the client for signs of infection. Encourage intake of adequate fluids. Monitor WBC count.

NURSING PROCESS

Assessment

Subjective Data

The client may describe having extreme fatigue, weakness, headache, chills, and fever. Inquire about all medications taken, including over-the-counter and prescription drugs.

Objective Data

Assess vital signs especially for a temperature over 100.6°F. Mucosal ulcerations may be reddened. Auscultate the lungs for crackles and wheezes.

A nursing diagnosis for a client with agranulocytosis includes the following:

NURSING DIAGNOSES	PLANNING/OUTCOME	NURSING INTERVENTIONS
Risk for Infection related to decreased leukocyte production	The client will not have signs and symptoms of infection.	Thoroughly cleanse hands before caring for the client. Screen all persons for signs of infection before allowing them near the client. Monitor vital signs for signs of infection. Use strict asepsis for all procedures. Encourage the client to drink an adequate amount of fluids. Monitor WBC count. Provide personal hygiene to prevent infection. Provide client with periods of rest between activities.

Evaluation: Evaluate each outcome to determine how it has been met by the client.

COAGULATION DISORDERS

Coagulation disorders include disseminated intravascular coagulation, hemophilia, and thrombocytopenia.

DISSEMINATED INTRAVASCULAR COAGULATION

Disseminated intravascular coagulation (DIC) is not a disease in itself but a syndrome that occurs because of a primary disease process or condition. A few of the conditions in which DIC may occur are burns, acute leukemia, metastatic cancer, polycythemia vera, pheochromocytoma, shock, acute infections, septic abortion, abruptio placenta, blood transfusion reactions, and trauma.

DIC is a condition of alternating clotting and hemorrhaging. The primary disease stimulates the clotting mechanism, causing many microthrombi (very small clots) to form and block the circulation in the arterioles and capillaries. With the formation of the numerous small clots, the body's fibrinolytic process responds in an attempt to stop the clot formation, thus causing hemorrhaging (Figure 37-8). This can be a very serious and potentially fatal condition.

The occlusion of blood vessels with the clots causes infarcts and necrosis of organs and tissues. The kidneys are the most commonly affected organ.

If a client with a predisposing condition develops **purpura** (reddish purple patches on the skin indicative of hemorrhage), bleeding tendencies, or renal impairment, the nurse assesses for DIC. Symptoms of DIC present as oozing from a venipuncture, mucus membrane, or surgical wound. The oozing progresses rapidly into a hemorrhage within a few hours to a day. The client has decreased urine output from decreased blood flow or renal infarction.

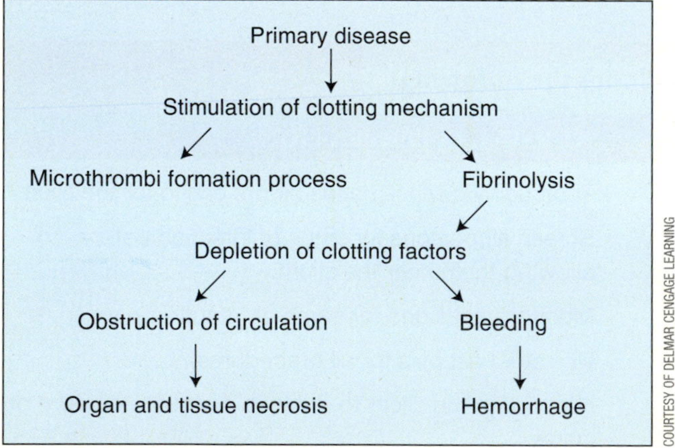

FIGURE 37-8 Pathophysiology of DIC

MEDICAL–SURGICAL MANAGEMENT

Medical

DIC is diagnosed by the client's symptoms and laboratory tests. With DIC there is an increased prothrombin time, partial thromboplastin time, thrombin time, and a decreased fibrinogen and platelet count. A laboratory test that confirms the diagnosis is the D dimer, which measures a fibrin split product that is released when a clot breaks.

The primary disease or condition must be treated. For example, if the primary disease is an infection, an antibiotic is given. If cancer is the primary disease, chemotherapy is given.

DIC is treated by administering whole blood or blood products to normalize the clotting factor level. Platelets and packed red cells are given to replace those lost during hemorrhage. Cryoprecipitate or fresh-frozen plasma is given to normalize clotting factor levels.

Pharmacological

Heparin has no effect on the thrombi that are already formed but is given to prevent the formation of more microthrombi. The administration of heparin is controversial because of the risk of hemorrhage. After thrombi formation is controlled with heparin, aminocaproic acid (Amicar) is given to stop the bleeding because it stops the fibrinolytic process. **Fibrinolysis** is the process of breaking fibrin apart.

NURSING MANAGEMENT

Be aware of precipitating conditions. Monitor I&O closely. Watch for purpura on the chest and abdomen, a common first sign. Monitor vital signs, peripheral pulses, and neurological checks. Avoid giving injections and venipunctures when possible.

NURSING PROCESS

ASSESSMENT

Subjective Data

Ask the client about previous conditions such as infectious processes, trauma, or cancer. Client statements of joint pain indicate bleeding into the joint. Document recent visual changes.

Objective Data

Observe and record the amount of bleeding from any wound or body orifice. Monitor I&O closely. Purpura on the chest and abdomen is a common first sign. Abdominal tenderness is often present. Note presence of pulmonary edema, hypotension, tachycardia, absence of peripheral pulses, confusion, restlessness, convulsions, and coma.

A nursing diagnosis for a client with DIC includes the following:

NURSING DIAGNOSES	PLANNING/OUTCOME	NURSING INTERVENTIONS
Risk for Injury related to altered clotting factors	The client will experience a minimal amount of injury.	Monitor vital signs, peripheral pulses, neurological checks, and urine output.
		Check urine and stool for the presence of blood.
		Assess for abdominal bleeding by checking for abdominal firmness or rigidity.
		If abdominal bleeding is suspected, measure the abdominal girth every 4 hours.
		Assess surgical wounds and all body orifices for bleeding and apply pressure to any oozing site.
		Assess color, warmth, sensation, and movement of extremities.
		Observe for changes in mental status.
		Avoid giving injections and venipunctures as much as possible.
		Observe for signs of orthostatic hypotension.

Evaluation: Evaluate each outcome to determine how it has been met by the client.

HEMOPHILIA

Hemophilia is an inherited bleeding disorder in which there is a lack of clotting factors. Approximately 18,000 persons in the United States have hemophilia (CDC, 2005). There are two types of hemophilia: hemophilia A is lacking clotting factor VIII, and hemophilia B (Christmas disease) is lacking clotting factor IX, along with an absence of a plasma protein, which results in nonformation of thromboplastin. The hemophilia trait is carried on the recessive X chromosome, so a mother is asymptomatic but can pass the trait to the son, who then manifests the symptoms of hemophilia (Figure 37-9). In the male population, hemophilia A occurs at the rate of 1:5,000 and hemophilia B occurs at the rate of 1:10,000 (NHF, 2006). Genetic counseling is often advantageous for clients who are carriers or who have hemophilia. There is no family history of hemophilia B in 33% of those with the disorder. These cases result from a new or spontaneous gene mutation (NHF, 2006). It is rare for a female to have hemophilia, but it can happen if the father has the disease and the mother is a carrier (NHF, 2002a).

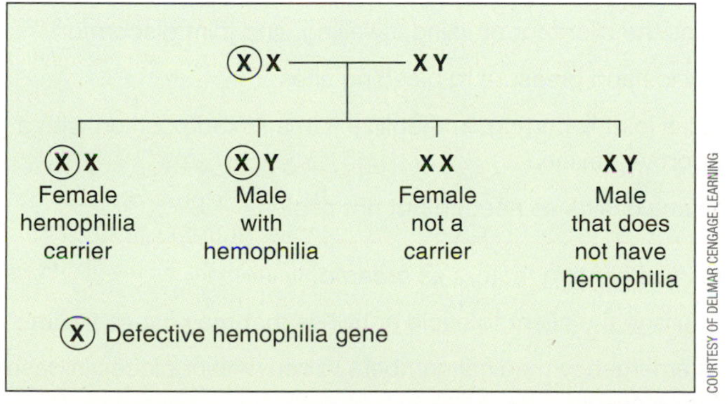

FIGURE 37-9 Hemophilia Inheritance Pattern between a Female Hemophilia Carrier and a Male without Hemophilia

There are three classifications of hemophilia: severe (factor level less than 1% of normal), moderate (factor level 1% to 5% of normal), and mild (factor level 40% of normal). The main symptom of hemophilia is bleeding. The client with severe hemophilia bleeds with minor trauma to an area but can also bleed spontaneously. **Hemarthrosis** (bleeding into the joints) occurs most frequently, causing pain, swelling, redness, and fever. Spontaneous ecchymoses and bleeding from the mouth and gastrointestinal and urinary tracts may occur. The most common cause of death is intracranial hemorrhage. Clients with mild hemophilia will not have spontaneous muscle and joint bleeding but will bleed after minor or major surgery. This condition could prove fatal if the diagnosis is not determined promptly.

Medical–Surgical Management

Medical

Hemophilia is diagnosed by a deficient or absent blood level of factors VIII or IX. The prothrombin time (PT), thrombin time, platelet count, and bleeding time are normal, but the partial thromboplastin time (PTT) is usually prolonged.

The National Hemophilia Foundation's Medical and Scientific Advisory Council (MASAC) recommend that hemophilia A be treated with Recombinant (genetically engineered) factor VIII. Cryoprecipitate is not recommended because of the risk of hepatitis and HIV infections (NHF, 2002a). For hemophilia B, the MASAC recommends Recombinant factor IX concentrates. Plasma-derived factor VIII concentrates still has the possibility of transmitting HIV-1, HIV-2, or hepatitis B or C, even with the use of improved viral–depleting processes (NHF, 2009). About

COMMUNITY/HOME HEALTH CARE

Hemophilia

It is important for the client and family to understand the disease process, learn how to recognize signs and symptoms of bleeding, and be able to administer treatments at home. The client should:

- Obtain medical care for trauma, cuts, edema, or pain in muscles and joints.
- Wear a Medic-Alert tag.
- Not take aspirin.
- Use a soft-bristled toothbrush and carefully perform oral hygiene.
- Prevent injuries by wearing gloves and long-sleeved clothing when doing household chores and participating in noncontact sports and activities.

90% of hemophilia clients treated with plasma concentrates in the early 1980s were infected with HIV; more than 50% of these client have died (NHF, 2006).

Pharmacological

Desmopressin acetate is available in a parenteral form (DDAVP Injection) and a highly concentrated intranasal spray (Stimate Nasal Spray) in clients with mild hemophilia A. Desmopressin is not used in children under 2 years of age, pregnant women, or in hemophilia A clients who do not receive adequate Factor VIII levels with the medication (NHF, 2009).

NURSING MANAGEMENT

Assess for signs of bleeding: petechiae, ecchymoses, hematemesis, melena, epistaxis, hematuria, hemarthrosis, and abdominal rigidity. Note edematous or immobile joints. Encourage client to wear Medic-Alert bracelet and avoid activities that cause trauma. Advise not to take aspirin, and to use an electric razor and a soft toothbrush.

NURSING PROCESS

ASSESSMENT

Subjective Data

Assess the client for pain and ask what measures were used in the past to relieve pain and bleeding.

Objective Data

Assess the client for bleeding by checking for petechiae, ecchymoses, hematuria, hematemesis, melena, epistaxis, hemarthrosis, abdominal firmness and rigidity, and frank bleeding. Note edematous or immobile joints.

Nursing diagnoses for a client with hemophilia include the following:

NURSING DIAGNOSES	PLANNING/OUTCOMES	NURSING INTERVENTIONS
*Deficient **Knowledge*** related to disease process	The client will relate symptoms to report and treatment methods if bleeding occurs.	Discuss ways to improve the safety of the client's home environment. Advise client not to take aspirin and encourage the client to use an electric razor and soft-bristled toothbrush. Teach family members or significant others administration of clotting factors for prophylactic purposes and if injury occurs. Encourage client to wear Medic-Alert bracelet. Refer for genetic counseling. Refer client and family to a hemophilia treatment center.
*Acute **Pain*** related to bleeding into tissues and joints	The client will have minimal pain.	Assess the client for bruising, swelling, and joint discomfort. Apply ice and pressure to bleeding sites. When a joint is hurting, immobilize it in a flexed position with a supportive device. Give analgesics as needed but not aspirin.
*Risk for **Injury*** related to altered clotting factors	The client will take precautions to avoid injury.	Transfuse clotting factors as ordered. Encourage the client to avoid activities that may cause trauma. Post emergency medical numbers in convenient places in case of future need.

Evaluation: Evaluate each outcome to determine how it has been met by the client.

THROMBOCYTOPENIA

Thrombocytopenia is a decrease in the number of platelets in the blood. The decrease may be related to:

- Decreased platelet production as in aplastic anemia, tumors, leukemia, and chemotherapy
- Decreased platelet survival as in infection or viral illnesses
- Increased platelet destruction as in DIC or thrombocytopenic purpura that is either drug induced or **idiopathic** (occurring without a known cause)

Withdrawal of the causative drug usually allows the platelet count to return to normal in 1 to 2 weeks. The acute form of idiopathic thrombocytopenic purpura (ITP) is an autoimmune process caused by an autoantibody-destroying platelet antigen.

Petechiae, ecchymoses, and bleeding from mucous membranes are observed. Bleeding may occur in internal organs. The platelet count is very low; the bleeding time is prolonged; Hgb and Hct is low; and bone marrow aspiration shows mostly immature platelets.

Medical–Surgical Management

Medical

Transfusions of platelet concentrates are given, or **apheresis** (removal of unwanted components) is performed on the client's blood to remove the autoantibodies.

Surgical

A splenectomy is performed because the spleen is the primary site of platelet destruction. This treatment is usually reserved until all other treatments have been unsuccessful.

Pharmacological

Corticosteroids are given to prolong platelet life and strengthen the capillaries. Immunosuppressive drugs, gamma globulin, and vitamin K are given.

Diet

A high-fiber diet is eaten to prevent constipation and the need to strain when having a bowel movement.

Activity

Activity is undertaken thoughtfully and carefully to prevent any trauma.

Nursing Management

Monitor for signs of bleeding (ecchymoses, petechiae, and rigid abdomen). Check laboratory reports for low platelet count, Hgb, and Hct, and prolonged bleeding time. Encourage a high-fiber diet to prevent constipation. Assess pain and administer analgesics as ordered. Monitor vital signs and mental status.

NURSING PROCESS

Assessment

Subjective Data

Ask the client about medications being taken and any recent infection.

Objective Data

Observe for petechiae, ecchymoses, and any signs of blood or internal bleeding.

Nursing diagnoses for a client with thrombocytopenia include the following:

NURSING DIAGNOSES	PLANNING/OUTCOMES	NURSING INTERVENTIONS
*Acute **Pain*** related to hemorrhage	The client will verbalize having less pain.	Assess client's pain on 0 (least) to 10 (most) pain scale and client's ability to cope with pain. Administer analgesic as ordered, and note client's response.
*Risk for **Injury*** related to thrombocytopenia	The client will have minimal injury.	Monitor client's vital signs and neurological and mental status. Assess client's skin and excretions for signs of bleeding. Handle client very carefully when turning, assisting out of bed, and in all other care situations.

Evaluation: Evaluate each outcome to determine how it has been met by the client.

LYMPH DISORDERS

A **lymphoma** is a tumor of the lymphatic system. Two malignant lymphomas discussed in this chapter are Hodgkin's disease and non-Hodgkin's lymphoma (NHL). The overview and medical management of each disease are presented separately. The nursing process for both diseases is presented together because the nursing diagnoses, goals, and interventions are the same.

HODGKIN'S DISEASE

Hodgkin's disease (Hodgkin's lymphoma) is a rare lymphoma that usually arises as a painless swelling in a lymph node. The diagnosis is confirmed when Reed-Sternberg cells (Hodgkin cells) are biopsied from the swollen lymph node. There are two types of Hodgkin's disease (HD), the classical Hodgkin's disease and the nodular lymphocyte predominance Hodgkin disease (NLPHD). HD has an abnormal B lymphocyte that is larger than normal lymphocytes. The abnormal B lymphocytes are known as Reed-Sternberg cells (Hodgkin cells) and confirm the diagnosis when biopsied from a swollen lymph node. NLPHD is confined to lymph nodes in the neck and under the arm (ACS, 2009d). HD affects children and adults, but occurs most frequently in early adulthood between the ages of 15–40 and in adults after 55 years of age (ACS, 2009d).

Risk factors are mostly unknown, but reduced immune function and certain infectious agents are involved. There is a slightly higher risk for HD in clients who had mono (infectious mononucleosis) caused by the Epstein-Barr virus (ACS, 2009d).

Clients with Hodgkin's disease most commonly have painless enlarged lymph nodes in the neck, in the area above the clavicles, and in the groin. Lymph nodes in the mediastinum may also be enlarged but are not usually diagnosed until the nodes enlarge and press on the mediastinal structures, causing dyspnea and a cough. A chest x-ray or a computed tomography (CT) scan confirms the involvement of the mediastinal lymph nodes. Other symptoms are weight loss, fatigue, pruritus, recurrent high fever, night sweats, anemia, thrombocytopenia, and lowered resistance to infections.

If a client has painless, enlarged lymph nodes and the symptoms of an elevated temperature of 100°F without any known cause other than HD, drenching night sweats, and weight loss of more than 10% of the body weight in a 6-month period, more intense treatment is recommended. Hodgkin's lymphoma spreads throughout the body in a predictable pattern. From the site of the original swollen gland, the disease spreads to nearby lymph nodes and then to other lymphatic tissue in the body such as the liver, spleen, and bone marrow. The invasion of other nodes and lymphatic tissue determines the prognosis of the disease. See Table 37-5 for the Ann Arbor Staging System for HD.

TABLE 37-5 Ann Arbor Staging System For Hodgkin's Disease with 5-Year Relative Survival Rate

STAGE	NODE AND ORGAN INVOLVEMENT	DESCRIPTION OF ANN ARBOR STAGING CLASSIFICATION	5-YEAR RELATIVE SURVIVAL RATE
I	Cervical nodes Stage I	Enlargement of single lymph node region (I) or of a single extralymphatic organ (IE)	90% to 95%
II	Mediastinal nodes Stage II	Involvement of two or more lymph node regions on the same side of the diaphragm (II) or involvement of extralymphatic organ and one or more lymph node region on the same side of the diaphragm (IIE)	90% to 95%
III	Splenic hilar nodes; Periaortic nodes; Iliac nodes; Mesenteric nodes; Inguinal nodes; Spleen; Splenic hilar nodes; Portahepatic nodes; Celiac nodes Stage III	Involvement of lymph node region on both sides of the diaphragm (III) plus involvement of the spleen (IIIS) or with involvement of extralymphatic organ (IIIE) or both (IIISE)	80% to 85%
IV	Pulmonary infiltrates; Axillary nodes; Liver; Splenic hilar nodes; Small intestine; Bone Stage IV	Scattered involvement of one or more extralymphatic organs with or without involving lymph nodes (IV)	Approximately 60% to 70%

Table 37-5 Ann Arbor Staging System for Hodgkin's Disease with 5-Year Relative Survival Rate (Continued)

STAGE	NODE AND ORGAN INVOLVEMENT	DESCRIPTION OF ANN ARBOR STAGING CLASSIFICATION	5-YEAR RELATIVE SURVIVAL RATE
If an organ outside of the lymph system but next to involved lymph nodes is affected, the letter "E" is added to the stage number, i.e., IE.			
If the spleen is involved, the letter "S" is added to the stage number, i.e., IIS.			
If the client has lost more than 10% of body weight in a 6-month time frame, has a temperature above 100°F without any known cause other than HD, and drenching night sweats, the letter "B" is added to the stage number, i.e., IIIB.			
If a client has tumors that are 1/3 as wide as the chest or 4 inches across, the letter "X" is added to the stage number, i.e., IIX.			

Adapted from Overview: Hodgkin's disease. By American Cancer Society (ACS), 2009d, retrieved May 13, 2009, from http://www.cancer.org/docroot/CRI/content/CRI_2_2_1X_What_is_Hodgkins_disease_20.asp?sitearea=CRI; Ann Arbor Staging Classification for Hodgkin Disease. By CureSearch, 2001, retrieved May 13, 2009, from http://www.curesearch.org/articleprint.aspx?ArticleId=3325

COURTESY OF DELMAR CENGAGE LEARNING

PROFESSIONALTIP

Serious HD Factors

If a client is male, older than 45 years of age, has tumors that are one-third as wide as the chest or tumors 4 inches across, a WBC >15,000, Hgb <10.5, lymphocyte count <600, and a low blood albumin level, the prognosis is worse, and more intense treatment is recommended.

Medical–Surgical Management

Medical

Diagnostic tests include CBC, platelet count, bone marrow aspiration, chest x-ray, abdominal CT scan, lymphangiogram, and lymph node biopsy.

Localized Hodgkin's disease stages I and II are treated with radiation therapy. Clients with massive mediastinal involvement and those who have relapsed after radiation therapy alone are treated with radiation therapy and chemotherapy.

During radiation therapy, the client may experience weight loss, nausea and vomiting, skin reactions, esophagitis, fatigue, and bone marrow suppression. The client's blood count is monitored closely during therapy to check for infection and bleeding tendencies. If the WBC level drops too low, the client will be more susceptible to infections. A decrease in RBCs and platelets causes a bleeding tendency. Long-term complications from radiation therapy include hypothyroidism, radiation pneumonitis, immune system impairment, herpes zoster, and the development of a second cancer.

Generalized Hodgkin's disease stages III and IV are treated with combination chemotherapy, which is administering a series of combined drugs over a set period. Serious late complications of chemotherapy are infertility and a secondary malignancy or cancer.

Surgical

Sometimes a laparotomy is done to see if the liver and spleen are involved. The rationale of performing the procedure is being questioned since the overall treatment plan is not altered.

Pharmacological

During radiation therapy, antiemetics, such as ondansetron HCl (Zofran), are given for nausea and vomiting. Analgesics are given for esophagitis discomfort.

Chemotherapy drugs are often given in combinations. The main chemotherapy treatment for HD is ABVD, a combination of 4 drugs: adriamycin (Doxorubicin), bleomycin, vinblastine (Velban), and dacarbazine (DTIC). When the disease does not respond to other treatments, MOPP (nitrogen mustard (Mustargen), vincristine sulfate (Oncovin), procarbazine HCl (Matulane), and prednisone (Deltasone) is used. Sometimes MOPP alternating with ABVD or ABV (adriamycin, bleomycin, and vinblastine) are used. Zofran or Kytril are given for nausea and Zantac for an upset stomach with MOPP. These drugs are usually administered intravenously or through an implanted venous port. Allopurinol (Zyloprim) is given to prevent uric acid renal stones caused by the rapid destruction of cells during therapy.

If the disease process does not respond well to chemotherapy, an option for the client is a bone marrow or peripheral blood stem cell transplant with high-dose chemotherapy. Rituximab (Rituxan), a monoclonal antibody, is presently in trial for use with HD.

Diet

During therapy, the client is on a high-calorie, high-protein diet. Encourage an intake of 2,500 mL of fluid per day to prevent the formation of renal stones.

Activity

Extra rest periods may be necessary to cope with fatigue that occurs with Hodgkin's disease.

NON-HODGKIN'S LYMPHOMA

Non-Hodgkin's lymphoma (NHL) is more common than Hodgkin's disease and is the fifth most-common cancer in the United States. The incidence rate for NHL has almost doubled since the 1970s. Approximately 66,120 new cases are estimated for 2008. The 5-year relative survival rate is 63% and the 10-year rate is 51% (ACS, 2007g).

NHL originates from the B lymphocytes and the T lymphocytes. NHL arising from the B lymphocytes occurs in the older adult population; NHL arising from the T lymphocytes manifests in malignant skin diseases such as mycosis fungoides or Sezary syndrome. More men are affected than women. NHL does not have the Reed-Sternberg cell present.

Symptoms of NHL are enlarged painless lymph nodes in the neck, axillary, abdominal, and inguinal areas. Other symptoms include fever, night sweats, excessive tiredness, indigestion, abdominal pain, loss of appetite, and bone pain.

MEDICAL–SURGICAL MANAGEMENT

Medical

The diagnosis of NHL is confirmed by a lymph node biopsy. Physicians use the same staging system as for Hodgkin's disease.

Pharmacological

There are two different chemotherapy regimens, CHOP and CVP: CHOP combines cyclophosphamide (Cytoxan), doxorubicin HCl (Adriamycin), vincristine sulfate (Oncovin), and prednisone (Deltasone); CVP combines cyclophosphamide (Cytoxan), vincristine sulfate (Oncovin), and prednisone (Deltasone). Other chemotherapy drugs used are chlorambucil (Leukeran), fludaravine (Fludara), and etoposide (VePesid). Bone marrow or peripheral blood stem cell transplantation is used for HD clients who have a relapse.

NURSING MANAGEMENT

Assess for enlarged, painless lymph nodes. Monitor vital signs, weight, and voice changes. Review blood test results. Encourage deep breathing and adequate fluid intake. Provide a high-calorie, high-protein diet in small, frequent meals.

NURSING PROCESS

ASSESSMENT

Subjective Data

Ask if the client is experiencing pruritus, night sweats, weight loss, decreased appetite, fever, fatigue, weakness, or chest pain.

Objective Data

Assess weight, vital signs, and for skin infections; dyspnea; cough; voice changes; enlarged lymph nodes in the neck, axilla, and groin; and edema in the extremities. Bone scan shows fractures and tumor infiltration. Review blood tests for hypercalcemia if bone lesions are present, and a CBC often indicates anemia. When the client is having radiation or chemotherapy treatments, the assessment includes observing for dysphagia, nausea and vomiting, skin rashes, and alopecia.

Nursing diagnoses for a client with Hodgkin's disease or non-Hodgkin's lymphoma include the following:

NURSING DIAGNOSES	PLANNING/OUTCOMES	NURSING INTERVENTIONS
*Ineffective **B**reathing Pattern* related to tracheobronchial obstruction from enlarged mediastinal nodes	The client will complete activities of daily living without dyspnea.	Elevate the head of the bed to assist the client's breathing. Encourage the client to take frequent deep breaths to expand the lungs and prevent infection; assess the client's breathing pattern every shift and as needed for dyspnea.
*Risk for **I**nfection* related to radiation/chemotherapy treatments, decreased WBCs and pruritus	The client will remain free of infection.	Monitor the lab results for lowered WBCs. Teach the client the importance of avoiding situations where there is exposure to infections. Provide cool sponge baths or oral medication to relieve pruritus. Assess the radiated skin areas for redness or breaks in the skin. Encourage the client to report symptoms of dyspnea, sore throat, and burning or frequency of urination.
*Imbalanced **N**utrition: Less than Body Requirements* related to decreased appetite	The client will consume an adequate amount of a nutritional diet.	Serve attractive high-calorie, high-protein meals in a pleasant environment. Offer six to eight smaller meals throughout the day to decrease a feeling of fullness. A soft, bland diet is more palatable during radiation or chemotherapy treatments. Avoid hot, spicy foods that are caustic to mucous membranes and lead to infection. Encourage an adequate intake of fluids to prevent constipation and renal stones. Weigh the client biweekly or more frequently if needed.

Nursing diagnoses for a client with Hodgkin's disease or non-Hodgkin's lymphoma include the following: (Continued)

NURSING DIAGNOSES	PLANNING/OUTCOMES	NURSING INTERVENTIONS
Anxiety related to disease and therapy treatments	The client will cope effectively with disease process and therapy treatments.	Listen to the concerns of the client regarding the effect of the disease on lifestyle, family, and finances. Encourage the family to express their concerns and discuss effective ways to deal with the diagnosis and treatment. Refer the client and family to clergy and social agencies when appropriate.

Evaluation: Evaluate each outcome to determine how it has been met by the client.

PLASMA CELL DISORDER

The main plasma cell disorder is myeloma.

MULTIPLE MYELOMA

There were an estimated 19,920 new cases of multiple myeloma diagnosed in 2008, and an estimated 10,690 persons died from it (ACS, 2009e). More cases occur in men older than age 65 (ACS, 2009e).

The plasma cells, mainly in bone marrow, become malignant, crowd out normal cell production, destroy normal bone tissue, and thereby cause pain. The normal production of antibodies is changed, making the client susceptible to infections. The first sign of myeloma is often bone pain, especially in the ribs, spine, and pelvis. The long bones ache; joints are swollen and tender; and a low-grade fever and general malaise are present. The client tires easily and has weakness from anemia. The weakened bones fracture easily. The cause of myeloma is not known.

Diagnosis is made with bone marrow biopsy showing large numbers of immature plasma cells and x-rays showing demineralization and osteoporosis. Bence Jones protein is found in the urine of many clients with myeloma. The client will also have hypercalcemia, hyperuricemia, anemia, and hypercalciuria.

MEDICAL–SURGICAL MANAGEMENT

Medical

Multiple myeloma is not curable, so treatment is symptomatic. Intensive chemotherapy followed by autologous peripheral blood stem cell transplantation may restore normal blood cell production.

Surgical

A laminectomy is required if any vertebrae collapse. If the client gets kidney stones from the large amount of calcium in the blood and urine, surgery may be required.

Pharmacological

Steroids such as prednisone and dexamethasone (Decadron) along with antineoplastic drugs such as cyclophosphamide (Cytoxan), meophalan (Alkeran), vincristine sulfate (Oncovin), and doxorubicin HCl (Adriamycin) are given. Some drugs are used in combination, such as VAD (vincristine, doxorubicin, and dexamethasone). Pamidronate (Aredia) and zoledronic acid (Zometa), bisphosphonates, are given intravenously for bone problems. Radiation therapy is used to treat bone pain or bone that is not responding to chemotherapy. Interferon is given when the client is in remission because it seems to extend the remission (ACS, 2009e).

> **CLIENT TEACHING**
>
> **Myeloma**
>
> - Drink 3 to 4 L of fluids per day.
> - Exercise to decrease bone demineralization.
> - Monitor for symptoms of hypercalcemia and notify physician if symptoms occur.

If the serum calcium level increases above 10 mg/dL, the physician orders an IV of normal saline infused at a high rate followed by diuretics.

Diet

Six small meals per day are often tolerated better than the usual three meals per day; nutritious meals based on the client's food preferences are recommended. A fluid intake of 3 to 4 L per day is essential to minimize the complications of excessive calcium in the blood and urine.

Activity

It is important to keep the client as mobile as possible. Walking stimulates calcium resorption and decreases demineralization. When the client is in bed, it is important to reposition the client frequently using a lift sheet to decrease the risk of pathological fractures.

NURSING MANAGEMENT

Assess for bone pain. Monitor laboratory test results for hypercalcemia. Provide six small meals each day of client's preferred foods. Encourage fluid intake to 3 to 4 L per day. Encourage ambulation. Monitor vital signs.

NURSING PROCESS

ASSESSMENT

Subjective Data

The client describes constant pain that increases with movement. The pain is usually in the back, ribs, or pelvis. Achiness in the long bones and joints and general malaise also is described.

Objective Data

Assess pain using a 0 (none) to 10 (most) pain scale. Temperature is elevated. The client's ability to perform activities of daily living is decreased. Monitor the level of blood calcium.

Nursing diagnoses for a client with multiple myeloma include the following:

NURSING DIAGNOSES	PLANNING/OUTCOMES	NURSING INTERVENTIONS
*Chronic **Pain*** related to disease process	The client will express a decrease in pain level.	Assess the client's pain level with pain scale. Administer analgesic as ordered and monitor the client's response.
*Risk for **Injury*** related to bone demineralization	The client will have minimal injuries.	Handle client gently and reposition the client using a lift sheet. Keep the client's personal items within easy reach.
*Risk for **Infection*** related to disease process and pharmaceutical agents	The client will have few infections.	Thoroughly cleanse hands before caring for the client. Teach the client and family proper hand hygiene. Assist the client with personal hygiene as needed. Screen visitors for signs of infections before allowing them to visit the client.

Evaluation: Evaluate each outcome to determine how it has been met by the client.

CASE STUDY

J.J., 46, owns a hobby shop. He has had a cold for 3 weeks that has recently settled in his chest. He has been tired lately and takes naps each evening before the evening meal. His wife noticed several bruises on his arms and legs, but J.J. could not recall any particular injury. J.J. has gradually lost 10 pounds during the last 3 months but has not been concerned about it. When J.J. went to the clinic for some antibiotics for his cold, the nurse practitioner completed a physical assessment and ordered a chest x-ray and CBC. The nurse practitioner noticed the WBCs were 250,000/mm^3; RBCs, 4.2 million/mm^3; and platelets, 100,000/mm^3. After several other tests were performed during the next few days, a diagnosis of chronic myelogenous leukemia (CML) was confirmed.

The following questions will guide your development of a nursing care plan for the case study.

1. List the symptoms occurring in J.J. that are typical of CML.
2. List five other typical symptoms of CML that were not stated in the case study.
3. List other diagnostic tests that could be done to confirm the diagnosis of CML.
4. List subjective and objective data the nurse would obtain about J.J.
5. Write three individualized nursing diagnoses and goals for J.J.
6. List nursing interventions for J.J.
7. List community resources specific to locale that could assist J.J. and his family during his illness with CML.
8. List discharge teaching the nurse would give to J.J. and his family.
9. List successful client outcomes for J.J.
10. List chemotherapeutic agents and side effects of the agents that may be prescribed for J.J.
11. List other medical treatments that may be ordered for J.J.
12. What measures could the nurse take to meet the emotional needs of J.J. and his family?

SUMMARY

- The main formed components of the blood are red blood cells, white blood cells, and platelets.
- The lymphatic system is composed of lymph vessels that drain lymph into the venous system; lymph nodes that filter microorganisms in the body; and lymph organs, the spleen and thymus.
- Sickledex and hemoglobin electrophoresis are diagnostic tests for sickle cell anemia.
- Some of the symptoms of anemia are fatigue, pallor, exertional dyspnea, and tachycardia.
- Symptoms of polycythemia vera are headache, epistaxis, dizziness, tinnitus, blurred vision, fatigue, weakness, pruritus, exertional dyspnea, angina, and increased blood pressure and pulse.
- Polycythemia vera is treated with chemotherapeutic agents.
- DIC is not a disease but a complication of a disease or condition that causes the client to alternate between forming many small clots and hemorrhaging.
- Hemophilia is a recessive X chromosome inherited bleeding disorder in which the client is lacking clotting

factors. The main symptom is spontaneous bleeding or bleeding caused by trauma.

- The two types of malignant lymphomas are Hodgkin's disease and non-Hodgkin's lymphoma. Clients with both types of lymphoma have enlarged lymph nodes.
- Hodgkin's disease is diagnosed by the presence of the Reed-Sternberg cell in the swollen lymph nodes. Non-Hodgkin's lymphoma arises from the B lymphocytes and T lymphocytes and does not have the Reed-Sternberg cell in the lymph system.

REVIEW QUESTIONS

1. A client has iron deficiency anemia. To improve iron absorption, the nurse serves Feosol with:
  1. milk.
  2. an orange.
  3. water.
  4. processed cheese.

2. A thorough assessment of the cardiac system on a client with sickle cell anemia is important because:
  1. the heart enlarges in an attempt to provide the oxygen needs to the body tissues.
  2. cells sickle more easily in the heart chambers.
  3. more cardiac force is needed to pump RBCs with Hbg S.
  4. people with sickle cell anemia are prone to bradycardia.

3. Clients with leukemia are prone to infections because:
  1. there are too many WBCs.
  2. the bone marrow is not producing WBCs.
  3. the bone marrow is producing too many cells.
  4. the WBCs are incapable of fighting infections.

4. Symptoms that alert a nurse that a client may have DIC are:
  1. tinnitus and numbness and tingling in the extremities.
  2. jaundice, palpitations, and dyspnea.
  3. purpura, bruising, and decreased urine output.
  4. ruddy complexion, epistaxis, and tinnitus.

5. A nurse teaches a client with non-Hodgkin's lymphoma about his disease condition. He knows that the teaching is successful when the client says:
  1. "I will use an electric razor."
  2. "I will take folic acid as prescribed."
  3. "I will apply ice and pressure to bleeding sites."
  4. "I will avoid exposure to infections."

6. A client had the axillary lymph nodes removed. Which one of the following activities is avoided in the affected arm?
  1. Using fingernail polish.
  2. Wearing rings.
  3. Blood pressure checks.
  4. Pulse checks.

7. A nurse examines a client's skin and notes multiple purplish areas randomly distributed over the abdomen. The areas measure more than 0.5 cm in diameter. The nurse records these areas as:
  1. purpura.
  2. petechiae.
  3. spider angioma.
  4. liver disease.

8. A Maine lobsterman was admitted to the unit with an infection in his right hand that he acquired while handling lobster bait. The nurse would most likely find palpable, tender lymph nodes in the:
  1. inguinal region.
  2. supraclavicular region.
  3. periaortic region.
  4. axillary region.

9. A client is at risk of developing a deep vein thrombosis. The nurse anticipates receiving an order for: (Select all that apply.)
  1. compression stockings.
  2. a sequential compression device.
  3. low molecular weight heparin.
  4. bed rest.
  5. a leg massage.
  6. a vitamin K injection.

10. What laboratory value confirms to the nurse that his client has DIC?
  1. Elevated white blood count.
  2. Elevated platelet count.
  3. Presence of fibrin degradation products.
  4. Elevated hematocrit.

REFERENCES/SUGGESTED READINGS

American Cancer Society (ACS). (2003). Cancer Facts & Figures 2003. [Online]. http://search.cancer.org/search?q=cancer+facts+and+figures+&start=30&num=10&access=p&entqr=0&restrict=cancer&output=xml_no_dtd&sort=date%3AD%3AL%3Ad1&ie=UTF-8&client=amcancer&ud=1&site=amcancer&oe=UTF-8&proxystylesheet=amcancer&ip=71.97.143.207

American Cancer Society (ACS). (2007a). How is acute lymphocytic leukemia diagnosed? Retrieved on May 12, 2009 at http://www.cancer.org/docroot/CRI/content/CRI_2_4_3X_How_Is_Acute_Lymphocytic_Leukemia_Diagnosed.asp?sitearea=

American Cancer Society (ACS). (2007b). Detailed Guide: Leukemia-Chronic lymphocytic (CLL) Monoclonal antibodies. Retrieved on

May 12, 2009 at http://www.cancer.org/docroot/CRI/content/CRI_2_4_4X_Monoclonal_Antibodies_62.asp?sitearea=

American Cancer Society (ACS). (2007c). Detailed Guide: Leukemia-Acute myeloid (AML) Chemotherapy (AML). Retrieved on May 12, 2009 at http://www.cancer.org/docroot/CRI/content/CRI_2_4_4x_Chemotherapy_AML.asp?sitearea=

American Cancer Society (ACS). (2007d). Detailed Guide: Leukemia-Acute lymphocytic (ALL) Chemotherapy (AML). Retrieved on May 12, 2009 at http://www.cancer.org/docroot/CRI/content/CRI_2_4_4X_Chemotherapy_57.asp?sitearea=

American Cancer Society (ACS). (2007e). Detailed Guide: Leukemia-Chronic lymphocytic (CLL). What are the key statistics about chronic lymphocytic leukemia? Retrieved on May 12, 2009 at http://www.cancer.org/docroot/CRI/content/CRI_2_4_1X_What_Are_the_Key_Statistics_About_Chronic_Lymphocytic_Leukemia.asp?sitearea=

American Cancer Society (ACS). (2007f). Detailed Guide: Leukemia-Chronic lymphocytic (CLL). What is chronic lymphocytic leukemia? Retrieved on May 12, 2009 at http://www.cancer.org/docroot/CRI/content/CRI_2_4_1X_What_Is_Chronic_Lymphocytic_Leukemia.asp?sitearea=

American Cancer Society (ACS). (2007g). Detailed Guide: Lymphoma, non-Hodgkin type. Retrieved on May 12, 2009 at http://www.cancer.org/docroot/CRI/content/CRI_2_4_1X_What_Is_Non_Hodgkins_Lymphoma_32.asp?sitearea=CRI

American Cancer Society (ACS). (2008a). Detailed Guide: Leukemia-Chronic myeloid (CML). Chemotherapy. Retrieved on May 12, 2009 at http://www.cancer.org/docroot/CRI/content/CRI_2_4_4x_Chemotherapy_CML.asp?sitearea=

American Cancer Society (ACS). (2008b). Detailed Guide: Leukemia-Chronic myeloid (CML). What are the key statistics about chronic myeloid leukemia (CML)? Retrieved on May 12, 2009 at http://www.cancer.org/docroot/CRI/content/CRI_2_4_1x_What_Are_the_Key_Statistics_About_Chronic_Myeloid_Leukemia_CML.asp?sitearea=

American Cancer Society (ACS). (2009a). Cancer Facts and Figures 2009. Retrieved on May 12, 2009 at http://www.cancer.org/downloads/STT/500809web.pdf

American Cancer Society (ACS). (2009b). Detailed Guide: Leukemia – Acute Myeloid (AML). What are the key statistics about acute myeloid leukemia (AML)? Retrieved on May 12, 2009 at http://www.cancer.org/docroot/CRI/content/CRI_2_4_1x_What_Are_the_Key_Statistics_About_Acute_Myeloid_Leukemia_AML.asp?sitearea=

American Cancer Society (ACS). (2009c). Detailed Guide: Leukemia-Acute myeloid (AML). What are the key statistics about childhood leukemia. Retrieved on May 12, 2009 at http://www.cancer.org/docroot/CRI/content/CRI_2_4_1X_What_are_the_key_statistics_about_childhood_leukemia_24.asp?rnav=cri

American Cancer Society (ACS). (2009d). Overview: Hodgkin's disease. Retrieved on May 13, 2009 at http://www.cancer.org/docroot/CRI/content/CRI_2_2_1X_What_is_Hodgkins_disease_20.asp?sitearea=CRI

American Cancer Society (ACS). (2009e). Detailed Guide: Multiple myeloma. Retrieved on May 12, 2009 at http://www.cancer.org/docroot/CRI/content/CRI_2_4_2X_What_are_the_risk_factors_for_multiple_myeloma_30.asp?rnav=cri

Aplastic Anemia & MDS International Foundation. (2006). Aplastic anemia. http://www.aamds.org/aplastic/disease_information/about_the_diseases/aplastic_anemia.php

Atassi, K., & Harris, M. (2001). Disseminated intravascular coagulation. *Nursing2001*, 31(3), 64.

Barry, D., & Schaefer, J. (2003). Hemophilia forces parents to make a tough decision: A nurse's child requires a venous access device implant. *AJN*, 103(1), 64A–64C.

Bulechek, G., Butcher, H., McCloskey, J., & Dochterman, J., eds. (2008). *Nursing Interventions Classification (NIC)* (5th ed.). St. Louis, MO: Mosby/Elsevier.

Centers for Disease Control and Prevention (CDC). (2005). Bleeding disorders. Retrieved on May 12, 2009 at http://www.cdc.gov/ncbddd/hbd/hemophilia.htm

Daniels, R. (2009). *Delmar's guide to laboratory and diagnostic tests* (2nd ed.). Clifton Park, NY: Delmar Cengage Learning.

Day, M. (2001). Sickle cell crisis. *Nursing2001*, 31(5), 88.

Gioia, K., Kleinert, D., & Hannon, M. (1999). What's wrong with this patient? *RN*, 62(2), 43–45.

Gorman, K. (1999). Sickle cell disease. *AJN*, 99(3), 38–43.

Hoffman, K. (2008). *Assessing the hematologic and lymphatic systems.* Manuscript submitted for publication.

Holcomb, S. (2001). Anemia: Pointing the way to a deeper problem. *Nursing2001*, 31(7), 36–42.

Leukemia & Lymphoma Society. (2007). Polycythemia Vera. Retrieved on May 14, 2009 at http://www.leukemia-lymphoma.org/attachments/National/br_1178803767.pdf

Leukemia & Lymphoma Society (LLS). (2009). Leukemia. Retrieved on May 11, 2009 at http://www.leukemia-lymphoma.org/all_page?item_id=7026&viewmode=print

LymphomaInfo. (2009). Hodgkin's chemotherapy – MOPP. 2009 Deep Dive Media, LLC. Retrieved on May 15, 2009 at http://www.lymphomainfo.net/therapy/chemotherapy/mopp.html

LymphomaInfo. (2009). Adult Hodgkin's lymphoma: Chemotherapy. 2009 Deep Dive Media, LLC. Retrieved on May 15, 2009 at http://www.lymphomainfo.net/hodgkins/chemo.html

Maningo, J. (2002). Peripheral blood stem cell transplant. *Nursing2002*, 32(12), 52–55.

Mayo Clinic. (2009). Iron deficiency anemia. Retrieved on May 9, 2009 at http://www.mayoclinic.com/health/iron-deficiency-anemia/DS00323/METHOD=print&DS

McBrien, N. (1997). Clinical snapshot: Thrombocytopenic purpura. *AJN*, 97(2), 28–29.

Mitchell, R. (1999). Sickle cell anemia. *AJN*, 99(5), 36–37.

Moorhead, S., Johnson, M., Maas, M., & Swanson, E. (2007). *Nursing outcomes classification (NOC)* (4th ed). St. Louis, MO: Elsevier – Health Sciences Division.

National Hemophilia Foundation (NHF). (2002a). Bleeding disorders information center/hemophilia A. Retrieved on May 14, 2009 at http://www.hemophilia.org/NHFWeb/MainPgs/MainNHF.aspx?menuid=180&contentid=45&rptname=bleeding

National Hemophilia Foundation (NHF). (2002b). Bleeding disorders information center/hemophilia B. Retrieved on May 14, 2009 at http://www.hemophilia.org/NHFWeb/MainPgs/MainNHF.aspx?menuid=181&contentid=46&rptname=bleeding

National Hemophilia Foundation (NHF). (2007). Fast facts. Retrieved on May 12, 2009 at http://www.hemophilia.org/NHFWeb/MainPgs/MainNHF.aspx?menuid=259&contentid=476

National Hemophilia Foundation (NHF). (2009). MASAC recommendations concerning products licensed for the treatment of hemophilia and other bleeding disorders (MASAC Document #190). Retrieved November 9, 2009 at www.hemophilia.org

National Institutes of Health (NIH). (2009). How is pernicious anemia diagnosed? Retrieved on May 10, 2009 at http://www.nhlbi.nih.gov/health/dci/Diseases/prnanmia/prnamia_diagnosis.html

North American Nursing Diagnosis Association International. (2010). *NANDA-I nursing diagnoses: Definitions and classification 2009–2011.* Ames, IA: Wiley-Blackwell.

Platt, A., Beasley, J., Miller, G., & Eckman, J. (2002). Managing sickle cell pain . . . and all that goes with it. *Nursing2002*, 32(12), 32hn1–32hn7.

Sickle Cell Disease Association of America, Inc. (SCDAA). (2005). Who is affected? Retrieved on May 10, 2009 at http://www.sicklecelldisease.org/about_scd/affected1.phtml

Sidel, H., Ball, J., Dains, J., & Benedict, G. (2006). *Mosby's guide to physical examination* (6th ed.). St. Louis, MO: Mosby Elsevier

Spratto, G., & Woods, A. (2008). *2009 edition Delmar's nurses drug handbook*. Clifton Park, NY: Delmar Cengage Learning.

Stuart, B., & Viera, A. (2004). Polycythemia vera. American Family Physician. Retrieved on May 11, 2009 at http://www.aafp.org/afp/AFPprinter/20040501/2139.html?print=yes

Thibodeau, G., & Patton, K. (2009). *Anatomy and physiology* (7th ed.) St. Louis, MO: Mosby.

Voshall, B. (2008). *Caring for clients with coagulation and lymphatic disorders*. Manuscript submitted for publication.

RESOURCES

American Cancer Society (ACS), http://www.cancer.org

Aplastic Anemia & MDS International Foundation, Inc., http://www.aamds.org

Blood and Marrow Transplant Information Network, http://www.bmtinfonet.org

Cancer Information Service (CIS), http://cis.nci.nih.gov/

Center for Sickle Cell Disease, http://www.sicklecell.howard.edu/

Cooley's Anemia Foundation, http://www.thalassemia.org/

Information for Sickle Cell and Thalassemic Disorders, http://sickle.bwh.harvard.edu/

National Cancer Institute, http://www.cancer.gov/

National Heart, Lung, and Blood Institute, http://www.nhlbi.nih.gov/

National Hemophilia Foundation, http://www.hemophilia.org

National Marrow Donor Program, http://www.marrow.org

Sickle Cell Disease Association of America, Inc., http://www.sicklecelldisease.org

The Leukemia & Lymphoma Society, http://www.leukemia_lymphoma.org

The Lymphoma Foundation, http://www.lymphomafoundation.org/

UNIT 11 Nursing Care of the Client: Digestion and Elimination

CHAPTER 38
Gastrointestinal System

MAKING THE CONNECTION

Refer to the following chapters to increase your understanding of the gastrointestinal system:

Basic Nursing
- ***End-of-Life Care***
- ***Wellness Concepts***
- ***Fluid, Electrolyte, and Acid–Base Balance***
- ***Assessment***
- ***Pain Management***
- ***Diagnostic Tests***

Adult Health Nursing
- ***Oncology***
- ***Endocrine System***
- ***Immune System***
- ***Mental Illness***
- ***The Older Adult***

Basic Procedures
- ***Collecting a Stool Specimen***
- ***Applying Velcro Abdominal Binders***

Intermediate Procedures
- ***Changing a Bowel Diversion Ostomy Appliance: Pouching a Stoma***
- ***Irrigating a Wound***
- ***Feeding and Medicating via Enteral Tube***

Advanced Procedures
- ***Inserting and Maintaining a Nasogastric Tube***

LEARNING OBJECTIVES

Upon completion of this chapter, you should be able to:

- Define key terms.
- Discuss diagnostic tests associated with the digestive system.
- Discuss components necessary for a complete assessment of the digestive system.
- List medical and surgical management for clients with digestive disorders.
- Describe nursing interventions for clients with digestive disorders.
- Assist with the formulation of nursing care plans for clients with digestive disorders.

KEY TERMS

adhesion
appendicitis
ascites
calculi
cholecystitis
cholelithiasis
cirrhosis
colostomy
constipation
diverticula
diverticulitis
diverticulosis
effluent
gastric ulcer
gastritis
glycogenesis
glycogenolysis
hematemesis
hemorrhoid
hepatitis
ileostomy
intussusception
jaundice
ligation
melena
occult blood test (guaiac)
pancreatitis
peptic ulcer
peristalsis
peritonitis
polyp
postprandial
steatorrhea
stoma
stomatitis
volvulus

INTRODUCTION

Disorders and diseases of the gastrointestinal system and accessory organs can affect not only the digestive process and nutrient absorption but the lifestyle of the individual as well.

ANATOMY AND PHYSIOLOGY REVIEW

The digestive system, also known as the *gastrointestinal (GI) tract or the alimentary system,* is responsible for breaking down complex food into simple nutrients the body can absorb and convert into energy (Figure 38-1). This process is known as digestion.

Mouth/Esophagus

Digestion begins in the mouth, where the teeth mechanically break food down into smaller pieces by chewing and mixing it with saliva. The chemical breakdown of cooked starches is begun in the mouth by the enzyme ptyalin, a salivary amylase. The food is then swallowed as a small ball or bolus and transported down the esophagus, a hollow, muscular tube approximately 10 inches long. **Peristalsis**, coordinated rhythmic contractions of the muscles, pushes the bolus through the esophagus. The cardiac sphincter, also called the *lower esophageal sphincter (LES),* located at the distal end of the esophagus, relaxes and allows the food to pass into the stomach.

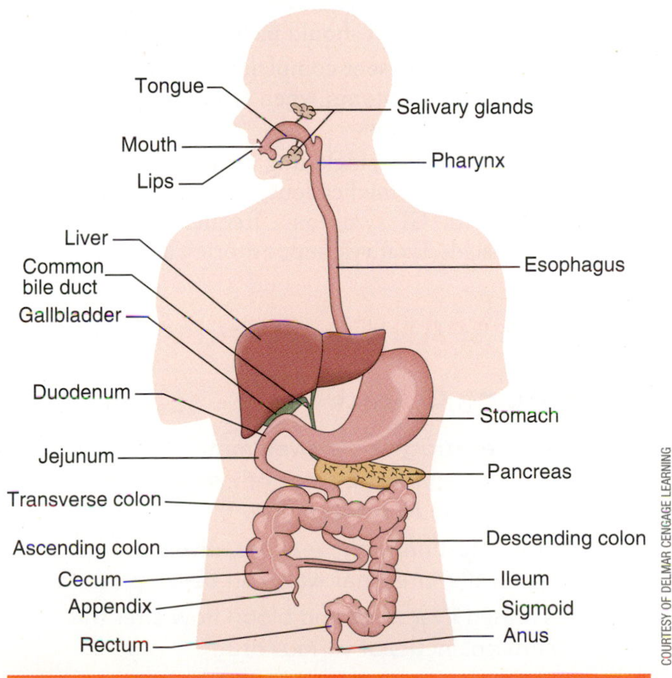

FIGURE 38-1 The Digestive System

Stomach

Further mechanical and chemical breakdown of the food occurs in the stomach, a J-shaped muscular organ located beneath the diaphragm. The stomach secretes gastric juices that contain hydrochloric acid (HCl) and pepsinogen, a nonactive form of the enzyme pepsin. HCl and pepsin are responsible for beginning the breakdown of protein and continuing the breakdown of starches. Starch digestion in the stomach gradually stops because of the acidic environment. Mucus is secreted to protect the lining of the stomach. The stomach also secretes an intrinsic factor necessary for vitamin B_{12} absorption and gastrin to stimulate HCl release.

The peristaltic movement of the stomach mixes the partially digested food and digestive enzymes into a semiliquid mass called **chyme**. The chyme will not pass into the small intestine until it is the proper consistency and particles are 1 millimeter or less. On average, the stomach empties in 3 to 4 hours. Carbohydrates are digested most readily, followed by proteins, with fats taking the longest to pass from the stomach. When the chyme has reached the proper consistency, the pyloric sphincter relaxes, releasing a portion at a time of the chyme into the small intestine.

Small Intestine

The small intestine is approximately 20 to 25 feet long and is responsible for absorbing nutrients from the chyme. The small intestine also secretes digestive enzymes, mucus to protect the mucosa, and hormones to aid in the absorption of nutrients.

The chyme enters the duodenum, the first 10 to 12 inches of the small intestine. The duodenum is responsible for absorbing calcium and iron as well as neutralizing the acids in the chyme. Enzymes from the pancreas and bile from the liver enter the duodenum from the common bile duct by way of the ampulla of vater; it is here that fats are digested.

The jejunum, the middle 8 to 10 feet of the small intestine, is responsible for absorption of fats, proteins, and carbohydrates. Vitamin B_{12} and bile salts are absorbed in the ileum, the distal 12 feet of the small bowel.

Large Intestine

The chyme enters the large intestine, also known as the *colon,* through the ileocecal valve into the cecum, a small pouch to which the appendix is attached. The colon is approximately 4 to 5 feet long and consists of the ascending or right colon, the transverse colon, the descending or left colon, and the sigmoid colon, an S-shaped segment before the rectum. The colon absorbs water, electrolytes, and bile salts.

The last 5 inches of the large intestine comprise the rectum. The distal end of the rectum forms the anal canal composed of muscles that control defecation. The opening to the anal canal is called the anus.

Accessory Organs

The digestive system also has accessory organs that aid in the digestion of food. The accessory organs include the pancreas, liver, and gallbladder (Figure 38-2).

Pancreas

The pancreas is a fish-shaped glandular organ 6 to 8 inches long extending from the duodenum across the abdomen behind the stomach. The pancreas has both endocrine and exocrine functions. The endocrine functions, which include the production of glucagon and insulin to regulate the blood sugar level, are presented in the endocrine system chapter.

The pancreas produces three main groups of enzymes in pancreatic juice for its exocrine function. The enzymes are:

amylase—converts carbohydrates into glucose
lipase—aids in fat digestion
protease—breaks down protein

Liver

The liver is the largest glandular organ of the body. It is located in the right upper quadrant of the abdomen. The liver is one of the most vascular organs, filtering 1,500 mL of blood per minute. Some of the many functions of the liver are to:

- Produce and secrete bile, which emulsifies fats
- Convert glucose into glycogen for storage (**glycogenesis**)
- Convert glycogen to glucose when blood sugar level drops (**glycogenolysis**)
- Metabolize hormones
- Break down nitrogenous wastes to urea
- Incorporate amino acids into proteins
- Filter blood and destroy bacteria
- Produce prothrombin and fibrinogen, which are necessary for blood clotting
- Manufacture cholesterol
- Produce heparin
- Store vitamin B_{12} and fat-soluble vitamins A, D, E, and K
- Detoxify poisonous substances

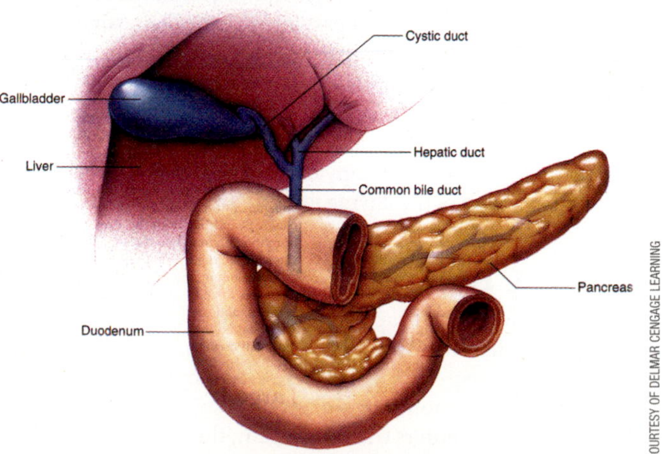

Figure 38-2 Accessory organs. Bile travels from the liver to the gallbladder via the hepatic and cystic ducts. The bile is released into the duodenum via the common bile duct. The pancreas releases its digestive juice into the duodenum.

Gallbladder

The gallbladder is a pear-shaped sac attached to the undersurface of the liver. The liver produces bile and transports the bile to the gallbladder through the hepatic and cystic ducts. The gallbladder stores and concentrates the bile until it is needed in the small intestine. When fats enter the small intestine, the gallbladder releases the bile through the cystic duct into the common bile duct and finally into the small intestine. The cystic duct, hepatic duct, and pancreatic duct combine to form the common bile duct.

Effects of Aging

As the body ages, several changes occur in the digestive system (Table 38-1). It is important to educate clients about these changes and ways they can adapt their lifestyles.

ASSESSMENT

A thorough assessment is necessary to collect data on which to make an accurate nursing diagnosis. For clients describing GI symptoms, the assessment should include the following:

1. History of the present complaint, including length and frequency of symptoms, when symptoms occur, as well as aggravating factors
2. Medication history, including prescribed and over-the-counter (OTC) medications, and their effectiveness. Clients with GI symptoms frequently self-medicate with antacids, laxatives, suppositories, and enemas.

LIFE SPAN CONSIDERATIONS

The Aging GI Tract

- Loss of elasticity and slowed motility of the GI tract, accompanied by lack of exercise, make the elderly prone to constipation.
- As the intestinal wall weakens, diverticuli, or scars on the intestinal wall, can develop.
- Decreased liver mass and blood flow alter the pharmacokinetics of various drugs.

TABLE 38-1 Changes in the Digestive System with Aging

COMMON CHANGES	RESULT	IMPLICATIONS FOR NURSES
Decrease in peristalsis	Food moves more slowly through digestive system. Bowel movements are more infrequent. Increase in constipation. Feeling full and bloated and may eat less.	Increase fiber and fluid intake. Encourage smaller, frequent meals. Offer fiber supplements.
Oral changes	Dentures are common. Chewing is more difficult. Eating and drinking time may be prolonged. Number of taste buds decreases.	Make sure dentures fit. Cut food into small bites. Teach that softer foods may be better tolerated. Some clients may start using more salt and seasonings to compensate for less flavor; monitor salt usage.
Decrease in enzyme secretion	Food is harder to digest. Increase in indigestion. Intolerance to some food and seasonings.	Encourage water between meals. Avoid foods that are not tolerated while ensuring adequate nutrient intake.
Decrease in saliva	Food is more difficult to chew. Swallowing becomes difficult.	Encourage fluid intake with meals. Have clients chew food well and do two swallows with each bite of food. Have clients sit up to eat.

COURTESY OF DELMAR CENGAGE LEARNING

3. A complete nutritional history; a note should be made of any foods that increase or decrease symptoms. Also, assess if meals aggravate symptoms or if symptoms occur within a specific time period after a meal. Note the fiber and fat content of the diet as well as the amount of fluids typically consumed.
4. Psychosocial factors, including compliance and noncompliance with health status. Meal patterns should be evaluated: note whether the client eats alone, eats large meals at regular intervals, or snacks all day.
5. Physical examination, including inspection, auscultation, percussion, and palpation of the abdomen. An evaluation of the client's ability to chew and swallow is also important.
6. Bowel elimination patterns, including frequency, consistency, and amounts of bowel movements.
7. Evaluation of diagnostic data, including laboratory analysis and radiologic and endoscopic examinations.

Refer to Box 38-1, Questions to Ask and Observations to Make When Collecting Data, for guidance in completing client gastrointestinal assessments.

COMMON DIAGNOSTIC TESTS

Commonly used diagnostic tests for clients with digestive disorders are listed in Table 38-2.

DISORDERS OF THE GASTROINTESTINAL TRACT

Disorders of the gastrointestinal tract include stomatitis, esophageal varices, gastroesophageal reflux disease, gastritis, ulcers, appendicitis, diverticulosis and diverticulitis, inflammatory bowel disease, irritable bowel syndrome, intestinal obstruction, hernias, peritonitis, hemorrhoids, and constipation.

STOMATITIS

Stomatitis is a painful condition characterized by inflammation and ulcerations in the mouth. Stomatitis can be caused by infections, damage to the mucous membranes by irritants, or chemotherapy.

MEDICAL–SURGICAL MANAGEMENT

Medical

Cultures may be done to determine whether an infectious process is present.

Pharmacological

Because the client's mouth can be sore, topical anesthetics such as xylocaine may be used. Analgesics may also be ordered. If an infection is present, the appropriate medication is ordered.

Diet

Dietary restrictions are based on what the client is able to tolerate. Bland, soft foods or liquids are usually tolerated best. As the sores heal, the diet may be advanced as tolerated. It is important to monitor dietary intake because caloric and fluid intake may be poor as a result of discomfort.

NURSING MANAGEMENT

Monitor caloric and fluid intake for adequacy. Encourage the client to eat soft, bland foods and liquids. Assess for mouth discomfort and check mouth for inflammation and ulcerations. Provide oral care and administer medications as ordered.

TABLE 38-2 Common Diagnostic Tests for Gastrointestinal Disorders

Laboratory Tests
- Complete blood count (CBC)
- Prothrombin time (PT)
- Partial thromboplastin time (PTT)
- Bilirubin
- Albumin
- Globulin
- Total protein
- Alkaline phosphatase
- Lactate hydrogenase (LDH-5)
- Gamma-glutamyl transpeptidase (GGT or GGTP)
- Aspartate aminotransferase (AST/SGOT)
- Alanine aminotransferase (ALT/SGPT)
- Cholesterol
- Triglycerides
- Amylase
- Carcinoembryonic antigen (CEA)
- HAA, now called hepatitis B surface antigen (HBsAG)
- Stool O & P
- Stool occult blood (guaiac)
- Fecal occult blood test (FOBT)
- Hemocult

Radiologic Studies
- Barium swallow
- Upper gastrointestinal tract (UGI) with small bowel follow-through
- Abdominal x-rays
- CT scans
- Ultrasound
- Barium enema
- Gallbladder series

Other
- Flexible sigmoidoscopy
- Esophagogastroduodenoscopy (EGD)
- Endoscopic retrograde cholangiopancreatogram (ERCP)
- Colonoscopy
- Esophageal motility studies (manometry)
- Gastric secretion analysis
- Liver biopsy
- Peritoneal aspiration

COURTESY OF DELMAR CENGAGE LEARNING

NURSING PROCESS

ASSESSMENT

Subjective Data

Clients usually describe pain in the mouth and difficulty swallowing.

Objective Data

Observations include inflamed mucosa of the mouth with ulcerations frequently present.

Nursing diagnoses for a client with stomatitis include the following:

NURSING DIAGNOSES	PLANNING/OUTCOMES	NURSING INTERVENTIONS
*Acute **P**ain* related to Stomatitis	The client will verbalize increase in comfort within 1 hour of initiation of treatment.	Assess the client frequently for discomfort. Administer medications such as topical xylocaine and analgesics as ordered. Allow for rest periods as indicated.
*Imbalanced **N**utrition: Less than Body Requirements* related to inadequate caloric and fluid intake	The client will maintain caloric intake of 1,500 calories per day within 48 hours of treatment initiation. The client will maintain a fluid intake of 2,000 mL per day within 48 hours of treatment initiation.	Monitor daily caloric intake and consult with the dietitian to assist with food selection. Administer IV fluids as ordered and monitor I&O.
*Impaired **O**ral Mucous Membranes* related to stomatitis	The client will have less inflammation and a decrease in the size of the ulcers by 36 hours after treatment initiation.	Monitor the stomatitis every shift to assess status of condition. Provide oral care every 4 hours. Administer medications as ordered to combat the infection.

Evaluation: Evaluate each outcome to determine how it has been met by the client.

BOX 38-1 QUESTIONS TO ASK AND OBSERVATIONS TO MAKE WHEN COLLECTING DATA

Subjective Data

Do you wear dentures? If yes, do they fit properly?
Do you consume alcohol?
Obtain a history of alcohol use/abuse.
How much alcohol do you consume in a week?
Do you smoke cigarettes, cigars, or a pipe?
Do you chew tobacco?
Do you smoke, inhale, or ingest illicit drugs?
Do you have pain or discomfort in your mouth?
Do you have difficulty swallowing?
What kind of foods and liquids do you consume?
Do you consume acidic foods?
What is your ideal weight? Do you have unexplained weight loss? Weight gain?
Have you ever vomited bloody stomach contents?
Have you vomited stomach contents that look like coffee grounds?
Are you easily fatigued?
Describe your energy level now compared to 6 months ago.
Do you have a history of liver disease?
Do your bowel movements appear black and tarry?
Are your bowel movements constipated, watery?
Do you have diarrhea? Persistent or occasional?
Have you passed blood clots in your stool?
Have you ever experienced bloody diarrhea alternating with normal bowel movements?
Do you experience heartburn? How often do you have heartburn?
Do you take any OTC medications to treat the heartburn? Do you get relief from these medications?
Do you have heartburn, acid regurgitation into the throat or mouth, or increased salivation after bending over to tie your shoes or retrieve something from the floor?
Do you have increased difficulty swallowing when lying down, bending over, or straining?
Have you experienced a burning sensation in the chest, throat, or behind the sternum?
Do you belch frequently?
Do you have a burning or squeezing pain when swallowing?
Have you experienced the sensation of food being caught in your throat or like you are choking?
Have others mentioned that you frequently have bad breath?
Do you have frequent chest pain? Describe the chest pain. How long does it last?
Is the chest pain related to any particular activity? Does it seem to occur after a heavy meal?
Are you hoarse in the morning?
Do you have difficulty breathing in the morning?
Do you cough in the morning? During the night?
Do any foods irritate your stomach, cause indigestion, belching, or bloating? Do you take any medications to relieve stomach discomfort, pain, or indigestion?
Do you take NSAIDs?
What do you think causes the discomfort, pain, or indigestion?
What relieves the discomfort, pain, or indigestion?
Do you notice more discomfort or pain at one time more than another?
Have you missed work because of stomach discomfort, pain, or indigestion?

Objective Data

Inspect the oral mucosa for ulcers or lesions.
Assess the mucous membranes for dryness, cracked lips, erythema, bleeding, and presence and appearance of saliva.
Assess the surface of the tongue.
Inspect the gingiva for redness and swelling.
Assess the teeth for caries and firmness within the gums.
Assess vital signs.
Guaiac all stools for occult blood.
Observe for hematemesis and melena.
Assess and measure amount of blood vomited.
Assess lab data for H & H, liver profiles, albumin, pre-albumin, bilirubin, WBCs, and neutrophils.
Assess the skin and sclera for presence of jaundice.
Weigh the client every day and evaluate BMI.
Assess for recent weight loss and/or weight gain.
Assess eating habits for types of food/beverages consumed, and time and frequency of meals.
Assess breath odor for halitosis.
Assess voice for hoarseness.
Assess for frequent belching.
Assess breath sounds for cough and wheezing.
Inspect the abdomen for distention.
Assess for presence of bowel sounds.
Assess for presence and location of abdominal pain.
Assess for rebound abdominal tenderness.
Keep client NPO as ordered.
Monitor I&O.
Maintain IV fluids for hydration.

ESOPHAGEAL VARICES

A varix is an enlarged, tortuous vein or, occasionally, an artery. Although varices can occur in any part of the digestive system, they occur most frequently in the distal veins of the esophagus. The varices are often associated with cirrhosis of the liver or any other condition that causes chronic obstruction of drainage from the esophageal veins into the portal veins. Swelling of the veins causes the walls to weaken, making them prone to ulceration and bleeding. Anything that causes increased abdominal venous pressure, such as sneezing, coughing, vomiting, the Valsalva maneuver, swallowing large, poorly chewed pieces of food, and the erosion of vessel walls by gastric acid, can cause the varices to rupture.

Varices have no symptoms, so clients may not be aware of them until they start bleeding. Death may ensue rapidly if the hemorrhaging varix is not treated immediately.

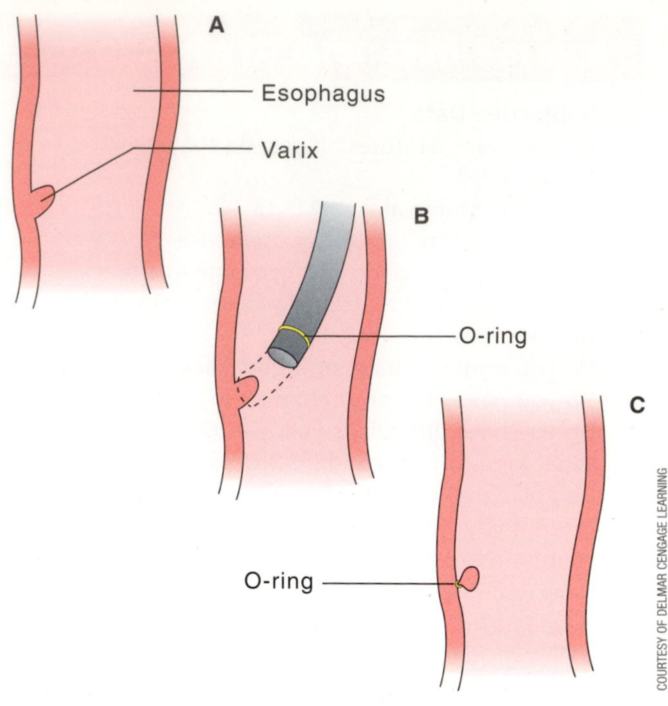

FIGURE 38-3 Banding of an Esophageal Varix; *A*, Varix; *B*, Insertion of Tube with O-Ring; *C*, O-Ring is Placed around the Varix

MEDICAL–SURGICAL MANAGEMENT

Medical

The varices may be treated with sclerotherapy, ligation, or balloon tamponade. Sclerotherapy is a procedure in which a caustic substance is injected into the varix. An esophagogastroduodenoscopy (EGD) is performed and a sclerosing agent is injected through a special needle. Several treatments are necessary to cause formation of scar tissue and to stop the bleeding. After the bleeding has stopped and the client has stabilized, the remaining treatments may be done on an outpatient basis.

Complications to sclerotherapy include mediastinal inflammation secondary to extra esophageal injection, perforation, ulceration, stricture secondary to scar formation, and rebleeding.

Esophageal **ligation**, also called banding, involves placing a rubber band, tie, or O-ring on the varix (Figure 38-3). An EGD is performed to guide the placement of the bands. The complications include rebleeding and stricture formation.

In a case where varices are actively bleeding, a three- or four-lumen balloon tamponade, known as a Minnesota or Sengstaken-Blakemore tube, is passed into the esophagus. The balloon is then inflated in the esophagus to put direct pressure onto the bleeding varices. The balloon is periodically deflated to prevent necrosis of the esophageal tissue. Isotonic saline lavages also are administered through the tube. During the procedure, the client must be kept NPO with the head of the bed elevated 30 to 45 degrees. Complications include perforation of the esophagus from the balloon pressure and necrosis of the surrounding tissue.

Surgical

A portosystemic shunt is performed to relieve the pressure on the esophageal veins by redirecting blood from the portal vein to the inferior mesenteric vein. Some of the blood bypasses the liver and reenters the circulatory system (Figure 38-4).

A nonsurgical but invasive procedure, transjugular intrahepatic portosystemic shunt (TIPS), may also be performed. With this procedure, the right internal jugular vein is used to place a cannula into the hepatic and portal veins. A connection is made through the liver tissue between the hepatic and portal veins. A stent is placed in the connection. This allows some of the blood to bypass the liver and relieve pressure in the portal vein. This procedure is done in x-ray and is used with clients who are too unstable for surgery (also refer to Figure 38-9).

Pharmacological

Octreotide (Sandostatin) is given by IV to help control the bleeding by decreasing blood flow to the gut, thus lowering pressure in the portal system. Analgesics may be necessary following sclerotherapy if clients have chest discomfort. Clients should avoid NSAIDs, aspirin, and all anticoagulants. Sucralfate (Carafate) liquid may be given to coat the esophagus, protecting it from erosion by gastric acid. IV rehydration as well as blood transfusions may be necessary for clients with active bleeding.

Activity

If varices are bleeding or have recently bled, the client should remain on bed rest. If no active bleeding is present, the client may be ambulatory but should avoid strenuous exercise.

NURSING MANAGEMENT

Monitor vital signs. Explain tests and procedures. Allow time for client to express fears and concerns about the varices. Check laboratory test results for changes. Explain reasons to avoid strenuous activity. Assess for nausea and dizziness.

NURSING PROCESS

ASSESSMENT

Subjective Data

Assessment includes history of liver disease or alcohol abuse and nausea. With esophageal varices there is no abdominal pain. The symptom of abdominal pain helps distinguish esophageal

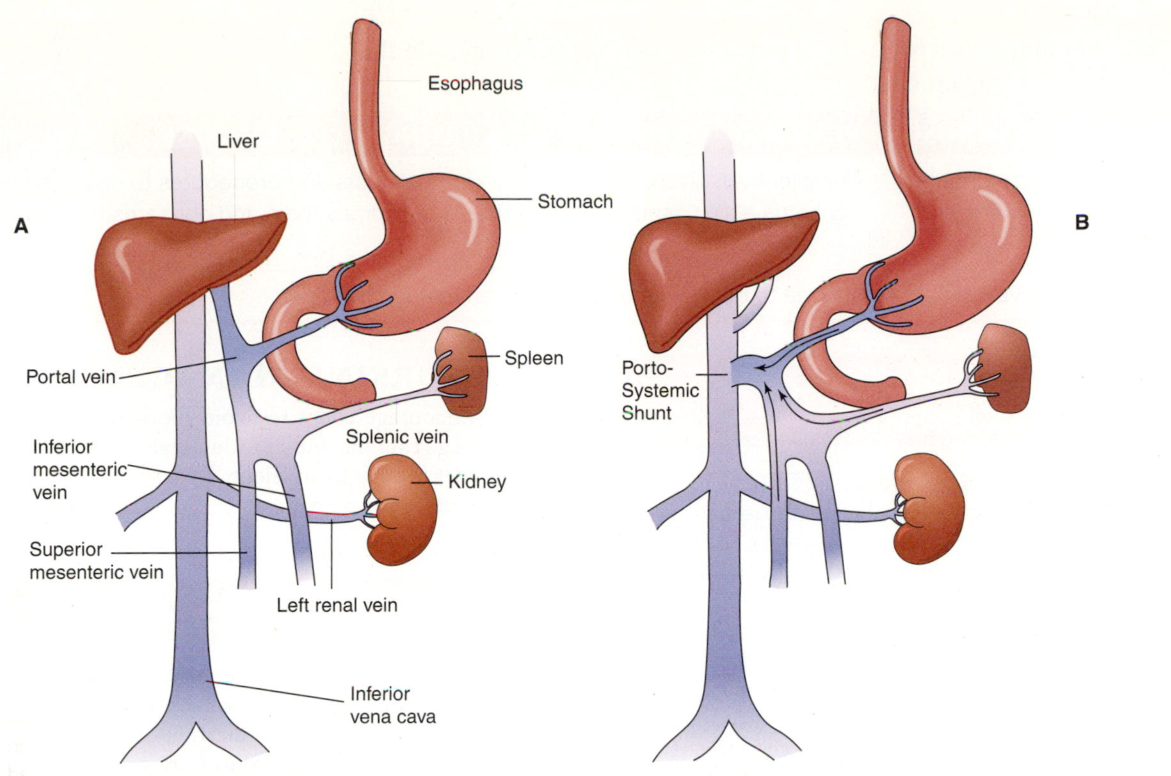

FIGURE 38-4 *A*, **Normal Circulation of Abdominal Organs;** *B*, **An Example of a Portosystemic Shunt (May be Performed in Clients with Elevated Portal Vein Pressure That Is Resistant to Medical Management)**

varices from bleeding gastric ulcers, which generally do cause pain that worsens after eating (Movius, 2006).

Objective Data

Assessment includes testing stools for **occult blood (guaiac)** and **melena** (black, sticky, tar-like stools containing partially broken-down blood), and assessing for **hematemesis**, or vomiting blood. Review hemoglobin and hematocrit (H & H) to evaluate anemia and liver profile for elevated bilirubin and globulin levels and a decrease in albumin.

If cirrhosis of the liver is present, **jaundice**, a yellowing of the skin, mucous membranes, and sclerae of the eyes, is present. Jaundice results when the liver is unable to fully remove bilirubin from the blood. Nutritional status may be poor if the client abuses alcohol.

Nursing diagnoses for a client with esophageal varices include the following:

NURSING DIAGNOSES	PLANNING/OUTCOMES	NURSING INTERVENTIONS
*Risk for Deficient **Fluid** Volume* related to bleeding esophageal varices (if the varices are not actively bleeding)	The client will maintain adequate fluid volume.	Monitor vital signs every 4 hours including orthostatic blood pressures. Orthostatic blood pressure is obtained by taking the blood pressure when the client is lying down and then when standing. A 20 mm Hg difference in blood pressures from lying to standing would indicate a change in fluid volume, possibly indicating varix bleeding. Monitor for nausea and dizziness. Monitor H & H every 4 to 8 hours as ordered. A decrease in H & H values would indicate bleeding.
*Deficient **Fluid** Volume* related to bleeding esophageal varices and gastric loss from vomiting	The client will maintain an H & H within normal limits. The client's blood pressure will be within 20 mm Hg of baseline with no orthostatic changes.	Monitor H & H. Frequently monitor vital signs. Administer IV fluids, electrolyte replacement, and blood transfusions as ordered.

(*Continues*)

Nursing diagnoses for a client with esophageal varices include the following: (Continued)

NURSING DIAGNOSES	PLANNING/OUTCOMES	NURSING INTERVENTIONS
Anxiety related to change in health status, threat of death	The client will discuss concerns about health status.	Explain all tests and procedures to decrease anxiety. Allow client to express fears and concerns regarding condition.

Evaluation: Evaluate each outcome to determine how it has been met by the client.

GASTROESOPHAGEAL REFLUX DISEASE

In gastroesophageal reflux disease (GERD), gastric secretions flow upward into the esophagus, damaging the tissues. An inability of the lower esophageal sphincter (LES) to fully close contributes to this condition. Environmental and physical factors contribute to decreased pressure in the LES. Fatty foods, caffeine, nicotine, calcium channel blockers, and NSAIDs decrease the tightness of the sphincter. Symptoms include belching, dysphagia, esophagitis, epigastric pain, heartburn, flatulence, melena, and bleeding. Diagnosis is made by symptoms, a 24-hour pH monitoring, and an esophageal motility test. An endoscopy determines the extent of esophagitis and rules out a malignancy.

Medical–Surgical Management

Medical

GERD is generally treated conservatively with diet and medications. Clients are encouraged to lose weight if they are overweight.

Surgical

A fundoplication is done to alleviate symptoms. A fundoplication is a laparoscopic procedure in which the LES is tightened by wrapping and suturing the fundus of the stomach around the esophagus.

Pharmacological

GERD is treated conservatively with antacids, H_2 receptor antagonists, proton pump inhibitors, cytoprotective agents, and gastrointestinal motility agents.

Diet

A low-fat, high-protein diet is recommended. The client is encouraged to avoid caffeine, milk products, alcohol, peppermint, licorice, and spicy foods.

CLIENT TEACHING

GERD

- Lose weight as needed.
- Avoid fatty foods, alcohol, nicotine, caffeine, and spicy foods.
- Take medications as instructed.
- Elevate head of the bed 2 to 4 inches on blocks.
- Avoid wearing constrictive clothing.

Nursing Management

Encourage client to avoid foods that increase the symptoms (e.g., caffeine, milk products, alcohol, and fatty foods). Obtain diet history from client. Observe for melena and signs of discomfort or pain.

GASTRITIS

Gastritis is an inflammation of the stomach mucosa occurring when the stomach has been exposed to irritating substances such as medications, smoke, food allergens, or toxic chemicals. Another contributing factor to gastritis is impaired mucosal defenses, which occur when the epithelial cells of the stomach are not able to secrete an adequate quantity or quality of mucus to protect the stomach. The presence of the bacteria *Helicobactor pylori* (*H. pylori*) has also been associated with gastritis.

Medical–Surgical Management

Medical

Diagnosis of gastritis is based on history and symptoms. An UGI or EGD is done to help diagnose the condition. If *H. pylori* is suspected, a biopsy is obtained during an EGD and a culture is performed.

Pharmacological

Treatment for gastritis is primarily pharmacological involving antacids and histamine (H_2) receptor antagonists (also call H_2 blockers). A proton pump inhibitor such as omeprazole (Prilosec) or prostaglandins is used. If *H. pylori* is present, bismuth preparations are used to inhibit *H. pylori* growth and antibiotics to eliminate the bacteria (Table 38-3).

NSAIDs such as ibuprofen (Motrin) and indomethacin (Indocin) have been shown to compromise mucosal defenses and increase acid secretion. Clients who are on NSAIDs chronically, such as clients with arthritis, need to be evaluated to determine whether other analgesics would be effective or if a prostaglandin should be taken with the NSAIDs.

Diet

Although studies have shown that dietary modifications have little impact on the rate of gastritis healing, some modifications are indicated. Any foods that aggravate symptoms are eliminated. Also, foods that increase acid secretions, such as milk, coffee, decaffeinated coffee, tea, colas, and chocolate, should be consumed only in small amounts or eliminated if possible. Eating before bedtime is avoided because it increases nocturnal acid secretions.

Table 38-3 Medications Used for Ulcers and Gastritis

MEDICATION	PURPOSE	NURSING IMPLICATIONS
Antacids • aluminum hydroxide (Amphogel) • aluminum hydroxide and magnesium hydroxide (Maalox) • dihydroxyaluminum sodium carbonate (Rolaids)	Seal impaired mucosa. Neutralize acids.	Antacids containing aluminum hydroxide may cause constipation. Antacids containing magnesium hydroxide may cause diarrhea; monitor serum electrolytes; do not give with other meds.
H_2 Receptor Antagonists • ranitadine HCl (Zantac) • cimetidine (Tagamet)	Decrease gastric acid secretion.	Do not give within 1 hour of antacids.
Proton Pump Inhibitor • omeprazole (Prilosec)	Stop gastric acid secretion.	Give with food. Suspend granules in an acid liquid. Takes 4 days to achieve blood level.
Prostaglandins • misoprostol (Cytotec)	Decrease gastric acid secretion. Enhance mucosal defenses.	Give when NSAIDs need to be continued.
Bismuth Compounds • bismuth subsalicylate (Pepto-Bismol)	Enhance mucosal barriers. Inhibit *H. pylori* growth.	Do not give within 1 hour of H_2 blockers.
Antibiotics • ampicillin (Omnipen) • metronidazole (Flagyl)	Eliminate *H. pylori*.	Some antibiotics will cause N/V if taken with alcohol. Do not give with antacids or meals with the exception of Flagyl, which must be taken with food. Clients are usually placed on two different antibiotics simultaneously.

COURTESY OF DELMAR CENGAGE LEARNING

Health Promotion

Smoking and alcohol aggravate the mucosal lining of the stomach and significantly impair gastritis healing. Smoking and alcohol consumption are minimized or eliminated if possible.

Nursing Management

Encourage client to minimize or eliminate smoking and alcohol consumption (if applicable) and any foods that aggravate symptoms. Teach client about medications.

NURSING PROCESS

Assessment

Subjective Data

Clients with gastritis may have no symptoms or may describe epigastric pain or burning, or nausea. They may also state that certain foods aggravate symptoms.

Objective Data

Stools may test positive for blood.

Nursing diagnoses for a client with gastritis include the following:

NURSING DIAGNOSES	PLANNING/OUTCOMES	NURSING INTERVENTIONS
*Acute **P**ain* related to gastric acid on inflammation	The client will experience less pain within 24 hours of onset of treatment as identified by pain scale.	Administer medications and provide diet as ordered. Assess client for improvement of symptoms. Implement education about lifestyle changes.
*Deficient **K**nowledge* related to condition, therapy, and symptoms of potential complications	The client will verbalize understanding of condition and symptoms of complications and will comply with treatment regimen.	Educate regarding medication regimen and lifestyle changes. If the client smokes or drinks alcohol, provide information on smoking and drinking cessation. Discuss dietary modifications.

Evaluation: Evaluate each outcome to determine how it has been met by the client.

ULCERS

Peptic ulcers are erosions that form in the esophagus, stomach, or duodenum resulting from an acid/pepsin imbalance. **Gastric ulcers** refer to erosions in the stomach and are correlated to exposure to irritants such as NSAIDs, smoking, alcohol, food allergens, toxic chemicals, *H. pylori* infections, and impaired mucosal defenses. Impaired mucosal defenses occur when the epithelial cells of the stomach are not able to secrete an adequate quantity or quality of mucus to protect the stomach.

Clients with gastric ulcers frequently complain of pain 1 to 2 hours after eating. Eating may not relieve pain or may even increase pain. Weight loss is common. Risk factors include alcohol use, stress, and NSAID use.

Stress ulcers are a type of gastric ulcer that form when gastritis becomes erosive and starts bleeding. As the name implies, stress ulcers occur in clients whose bodies are experiencing stress, such as clients who have experienced major surgery, trauma, burns, chemotherapy, or radiation therapy. Clients with chronic respiratory disorders also experience stress ulcers because hypoxia can lead to impaired mucosa. Bleeding may be massive resulting in significant blood loss or can be slow and insidious. Because of the multiple sites of bleeding, stress ulcers are difficult to manage.

Duodenal ulcers refer to ulcers in the duodenum. Incidents of duodenal ulcers have been correlated to a high secretion of HCl. Clients with duodenal ulcers frequently complain of pain 2 to 4 hours after eating. Nocturnal pain may be present, occurring between midnight and 3:00 a.m. Eating frequently relieves symptoms. Weight gain is common. Risk factors include a history of pulmonary disease, cirrhosis, chronic pancreatitis, and/or chronic renal failure.

If an ulcer erodes through a blood vessel, the client may experience a life-threatening hemorrhage. A perforation occurs if the ulcer erodes through the wall of the stomach or small intestine resulting in gastric or intestinal contents entering the abdominal cavity and causing peritonitis.

Diagnosis of ulcers is based on symptoms, history, and an UGI or EGD performed to visualize the ulcer. If an *H. pylori* infection is suspected, a biopsy is obtained during an EGD and a culture is performed.

MEDICAL–SURGICAL MANAGEMENT

Medical

If an ulcer bleeds, an EGD may be performed, and the ulcer is either injected with epinephrine to cause vasoconstriction or a special electrical probe is used to cauterize or burn the tissue that is bleeding. A nasogastric (NG) tube is inserted to remove gastric contents and blood, and iced isotonic saline is instilled to help cause vasoconstriction and stop the bleeding.

Surgical

The most commonly performed surgery for peptic ulcers is a vagotomy, in which a section of the vagus nerve is cut removing vagal innervation to the fundus of the stomach. This eliminates the production of hydrochloric acid, decreases function of the gastrin hormone, and slows motility of the stomach. A vagotomy eliminates the complications of the more aggressive surgeries, such as gastrectomies.

If the ulcer continues to bleed or if the ulcer has perforated, the client is taken to surgery and a gastrectomy is performed. The portion of the stomach or duodenum that is perforated is removed and the bowel is reconnected with an anastomosis.

Complications from gastrectomies include gastric dumping in which the stomach experiences **postprandial** (after eating) rapid gastric emptying. Clients experience abdominal pain, nausea, vomiting, explosive diarrhea, weakness, and dizziness. Clients with gastric dumping have malabsorption of nutrients because the food passes too quickly to permit absorption, thus leading to malnutrition. In addition, many clients with significant symptoms limit dietary intake to avoid symptoms, compounding the malnutrition and weight loss issues.

Management of gastric dumping includes small, frequent meals of high fiber and high protein and avoidance of simple carbohydrates.

Pharmacological

Treatment of ulcers is primarily pharmacological involving antacids, histamine (H_2) receptor antagonists (also called H_2 blockers), proton pump inhibitors, or prostaglandins. If *H. pylori* is present, bismuth preparations are generally used to inhibit its growth and antibiotics to eliminate the bacteria (refer to Table 38-3).

NSAIDs such as ibuprofen (Motrin) and indomethacin (Indocin) have been shown to compromise mucosal defenses and increase acid secretion. For clients who are on NSAIDs chronically, such as clients with arthritis, one needs to evaluate whether other analgesics would be effective or whether a prostaglandin should be taken with the NSAIDs.

Diet

Although studies have shown that dietary modifications have little impact on the rate of ulcer healing, some modifications are indicated. Foods that aggravate symptoms are eliminated. Also, foods that increase acid secretions, such as milk, coffee, decaffeinated coffee, tea, colas, and chocolate, should be consumed only in small amounts or eliminated if possible. Eating close to bedtime is avoided because it increases nocturnal acid secretions.

Health Promotion

Smoking and alcohol aggravate the mucosal lining of the stomach and duodenum and significantly impair ulcer healing. Smokers also experience a higher ulcer recurrence rate. Stress has been shown to increase the rate of peptic ulcers. Although the type or severity of stress may not be significant, the client's interpretation of the events as stressful is. Clients need to develop mechanisms for reducing stress such as exercise, biofeedback, and relaxation.

NURSING MANAGEMENT

Encourage lifestyle changes when necessary regarding smoking, alcohol, and stress. Teach relaxation techniques. Monitor weight and laboratory test results. Discourage having a bedtime snack to prevent acid secretions at night. Assess pain including relationship to eating a meal.

NURSING PROCESS

Assessment

Subjective Data

Clients with gastric ulcers are often asymptomatic or may describe epigastric pain or burning 1 to 2 hours after eating, and nausea or bloating. Clients may experience an increase of symptoms when they eat and therefore may decrease dietary intake. When questioned about lifestyle, NSAID usage, stress, smoking, and alcohol use may be discovered.

Clients with duodenal ulcers may exhibit no symptoms or may complain of pain 2 to 4 hours after eating. Eating will frequently decrease symptoms, so clients will often eat more frequently. When questioned about lifestyle, stress, smoking, and alcohol consumption may be discovered. The client may also have a history of pulmonary disease, cirrhosis, chronic pancreatitis, and/or chronic renal failure.

A client who is actively bleeding from an ulcer will experience an acute onset of epigastric pain, shortness of breath, and nausea.

Objective Data

Clients with gastric ulcers may show a weight loss and stools may test positive for blood. An H & H may show anemia.

Clients with duodenal ulcers may show a weight gain and stools may test positive for blood. An H & H may show anemia.

The client who is actively bleeding from an ulcer will show signs of shock: pale clammy skin, an elevated pulse rate, and a drop in blood pressure. The client may also have hematemesis. Laboratory tests show a low H & H and stools test positive for blood.

Nursing diagnoses for a client with ulcers include the following:

NURSING DIAGNOSES	PLANNING/OUTCOMES	NURSING INTERVENTIONS
*Acute **Pain*** related to gastric acid on ulcerated mucosa	The client will experience less pain within 24 hours of onset of treatment as identified on pain scale.	Assess clients for decrease of pain. Administer medications as ordered. Assess for elevated BP.
*Deficient **Knowledge*** related to condition, therapy, and symptoms of complications	The client will verbalize understanding of factors related to condition and symptoms of complications. Client will comply with treatment regimen.	Identify client's learning style and provide information in a manner compatible with the learning style. Educate regarding medication regimen, lifestyle changes, and signs and symptoms of possible complications. If indicated, provide client with smoking cessation information and stress reduction techniques such as exercise and biofeedback.
*Deficient Fluid **Volume*** related to bleeding ulcer	The client will exhibit normal fluid volume as evidenced by stable H & H and blood pressure within 20 mm Hg of baseline.	Check vital signs every 4 hours and PRN including orthostatic blood pressure. Monitor for dizziness and nausea. Check stool for blood. Administer IV fluids, electrolyte replacement, and blood transfusions as ordered.

Evaluation: Evaluate each outcome to determine how it has been met by the client.

APPENDICITIS

Appendicitis is the inflammation of the vermiform appendix, a 10-cm small, slender tube attached to the cecum. The appendix may be inflamed, gangrenous, or ruptured. If the opening to the appendix becomes blocked with feces, the *E. coli* multiply in the appendix and infection develops with pus formation. If it ruptures, fecal content spills into the abdominal cavity causing peritonitis, which may be fatal. It is most common in young adults, but can occur at any age (Atassi, 2002a). A barium enema or an ultrasound is ordered to confirm inflammation in the appendiceal area.

Medical–Surgical Management

Early diagnosis and treatment are necessary for the best client outcome. A white blood count and differential will usually show a WBC >10,000/mm^3 and neutrophils >75%. An elevated temperature indicates infection. Rebound tenderness in the right lower quadrant (RLQ) of the abdomen (at McBurney's point) is a positive diagnostic finding. An appendectomy is performed along with other abdominal surgeries as a preventive measure.

Surgical

A surgical procedure called an appendectomy is necessary before the appendix ruptures. Appendectomies are the most common emergency surgery and require a hospital stay of a few days if the appendix has ruptured. If no rupture has occurred, a laparoscopic appendectomy, in which the appendix is removed through a scope, may be done. This requires only a small incision and allows the client to be discharged 24 hours after the surgery.

Pharmacological

Preoperatively, no analgesics are administered so that symptoms will not be masked by the medication. Fluids and electrolytes may need to be replaced before surgery. Antibiotics are usually given preoperatively. Postoperatively, analgesics are administered for relief of incisional discomfort. Antibiotics are usually given postoperatively, especially if a perforation is present.

Diet

Preoperatively and initially postoperatively, the client is NPO. If a perforation with peritonitis occurred, the client is kept NPO longer, and an NG tube is inserted until bowel sounds return. Clear liquids and then full liquids and finally a regular diet is given as normal bowel function returns.

Activity

Initially postoperatively, the client is encouraged to turn, cough, and deep breathe every 2 hours. Next, the client is encouraged to increase ambulation gradually. Activity restrictions depend on the severity of the appendicitis. Driving, exercise, and lifting will be limited for a few weeks to allow for incisional healing.

NURSING MANAGEMENT

Assess pain. Keep client NPO. Monitor vital signs, especially temperature. Assess bowel sounds. Monitor the results of the CBC, especially WBC and neutrophils. Postoperatively, encourage client to turn, cough, and deep breathe every 2 hours. Encourage ambulation. Advance diet from liquid to regular as bowel function returns.

NURSING PROCESS

ASSESSMENT

Subjective Data

Clients with appendicitis describe abdominal pain, typically located in the RLQ around McBurney's point (halfway between the umbilicus and the right iliac crest). Clients also complain of anorexia (a loss of appetite) and nausea.

Objective Data

Clients may have vomiting and fever. Bowel sounds may be diminished or absent. Rebound tenderness, pain that occurs when fingers are pressed into the RLQ and then released suddenly, may be present. A CBC will show WBCs elevated $> 10{,}000/mm^3$ with neutrophils $> 75\%$.

Nursing diagnoses for a client with appendicitis include the following:

NURSING DIAGNOSES	PLANNING/OUTCOMES	NURSING INTERVENTIONS
*Acute **P**ain* related to appendicitis/appendectomy	The client will experience a decrease in pain as evidenced by improved mobility and as identified on pain scale.	Preoperatively, monitor client's pain and check abdomen for rigidity. Provide an ice pack to help relieve pain as ordered; never use heat. Postoperatively, give analgesics as ordered and medicate prior to activities such as ambulation. Teach client to use a pillow to splint the incision when coughing. If client is having difficulty passing flatus, administer enemas or a rectal tube as ordered, and encourage ambulation.
*Impaired **S**kin Integrity* related to the abdominal incision	The client will verbalize signs and symptoms of infection and factors that enhance wound healing, by discharge.	Administer antibiotics as ordered. Educate the client that incision may be left open to the air after 24 hours; that showers may be taken, per physician instruction; and signs and symptoms of infection and activity restrictions. If adhesive strips are present, leave in place until they no longer cover the incision (approximately 10 days to 2 weeks).

Evaluation: Evaluate each outcome to determine how it has been met by the client.

DIVERTICULOSIS AND DIVERTICULITIS

Diverticula are saclike protrusions of the intestinal wall. **Diverticulosis** refers to a condition of the colon in which multiple diverticula are present (Figure 38-5). The exact cause of diverticulosis is not known; however, a diet low in fiber is believed to contribute to the formation of the pouches. Diverticulosis affects >50% of the elderly population (Marrs, 2006). It is asymptomatic unless perforation or hemorrhage occur.

Diverticulitis refers to the inflammation of one or more diverticula generally in the sigmoid colon. It is a complication of diverticulosis and is thought to be caused by stool impacted in the diverticula.

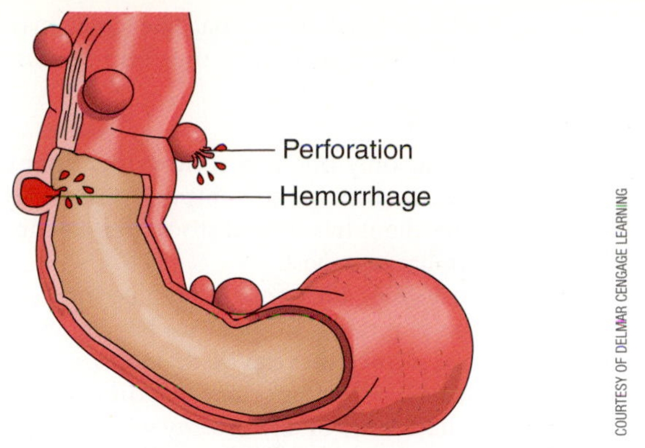

FIGURE 38-5 Diverticula in the sigmoid colon. Diverticulosis is almost always located in the descending or sigmoid colon.

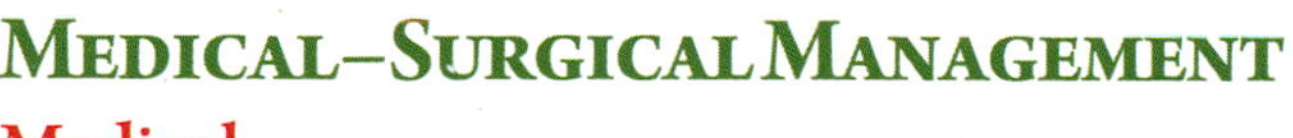

MEDICAL–SURGICAL MANAGEMENT

Medical

Diverticulosis is typically asymptomatic and needs no intervention. Most cases of diverticulitis are treated with analgesics, antibiotics, bed rest, NPO to rest the bowel, and IV fluid hydration.

A barium enema or abdominal ultrasound is usually ordered when diverticulitis is suspected. A flexible sigmoidoscopy is also performed.

Surgical

If bleeding or perforation of the diverticula occurs, or if an abscess forms, surgery is required to remove the affected portion of the bowel. A colon resection is performed. A **colostomy** may be required. A colostomy is a surgically created opening from the colon through the abdominal wall to relieve either a disease or functional problem in the large intestine.

Stool consistency depends on the placement of the **stoma** (surgical opening between a cavity and the surface of the body) in the colon. A colostomy is named for the part of the colon where it is located. An ascending colostomy takes its name from the ascending colon and would be on the right side of the abdomen. It has a liquid output. A transverse colostomy would be more toward the midline of the abdomen and has a pasty liquid output. A descending colostomy or sigmoid colostomy has a more solid output. Figure 38-6 shows the different colostomy sites.

If a large amount of inflammation is present, a temporary colostomy is performed to allow the colon to heal. The colon is reconnected at a later time. Sometimes a permanent colostomy needs to be performed.

Pharmacological

Clients who have been identified as having diverticulosis are usually placed on fiber supplements or stool softeners. Clients with diverticulitis are treated with sulfa antibiotics and other antimicrobial agents. Analgesics also are ordered for discomfort.

Diet

A high-fiber diet is believed to help reduce the occurrence of diverticulosis and diverticulitis. Clients experiencing diverticulitis will be NPO to rest the bowel. Once the diverticulitis begins healing, the client is placed on clear liquids and then advanced to a bland, low-residue diet while the diverticulitis heals.

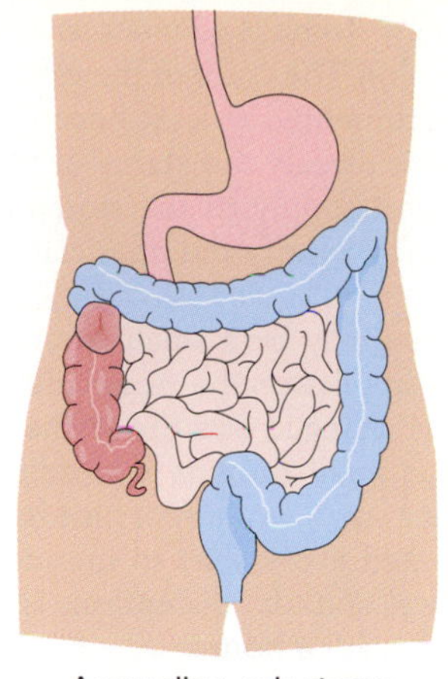
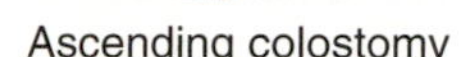

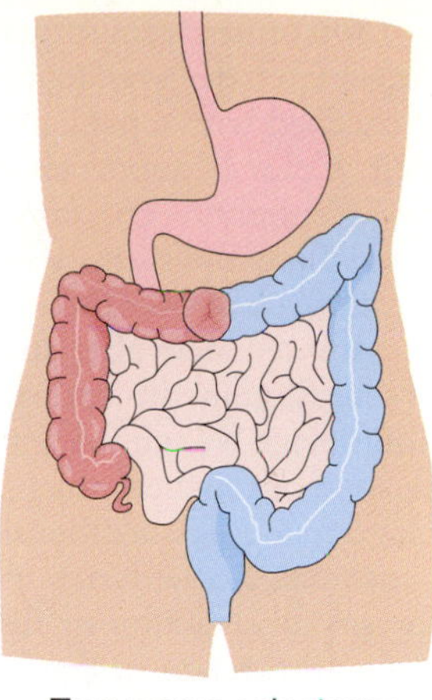

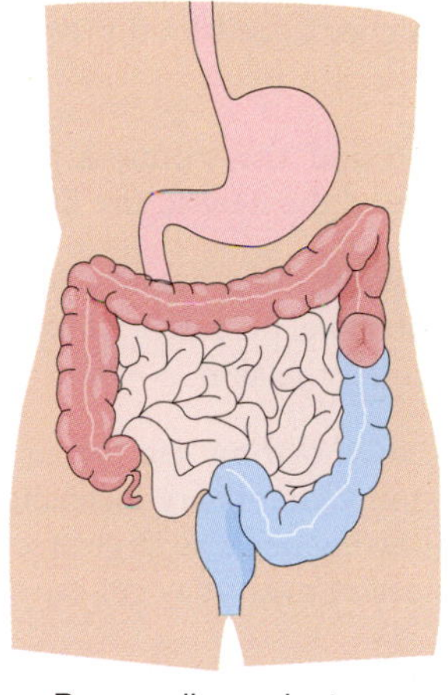

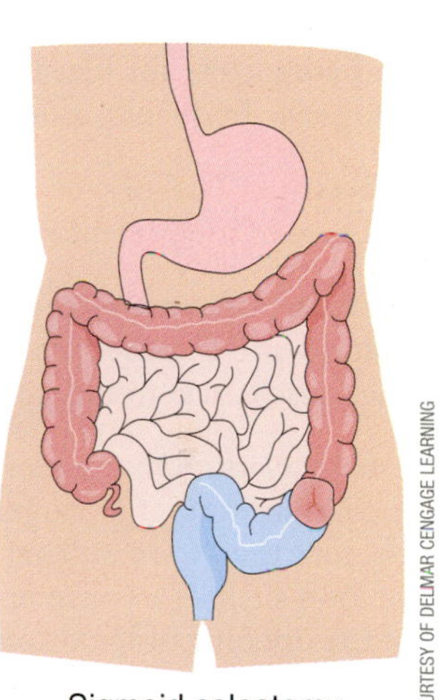

FIGURE 38-6 Colostomy Sites (Blue Area Is Colon Removed)

If surgery is performed, the client is NPO until bowel sounds return. The client is then started on clear liquids, advanced to full liquids as more bowel function returns, and then finally advanced to a regular diet. A high-fiber diet is encouraged for clients once the diverticulitis episode has resolved.

Activity

For clients experiencing diverticulitis, bed rest and decreased mobility are encouraged to allow the bowel to rest. In clients who have had a bowel resection, activity will gradually be progressed postoperatively.

STOMA/OSTOMY MANAGEMENT

Assessment

Provide the client with an opportunity to ask questions and begin coping with a possible altered body image. Before ostomy surgery, the surgeon and the enterostomal (ET) nurse talk with the client and explain the reason for the surgery and the possibilities of ostomy surgery. Choosing the site or placement of the stoma depends on the type of ostomy being created, the lifestyle of the client, and the contours of the client's abdomen.

On return from surgery, the new stoma is edematous and ranges from deep red to dusky in color. The color of the stoma is checked with a penlight and documented at least once per shift. Color is important because it reveals the status of the blood supply to the stoma. If blood supply to the stoma is inadequate, the stoma will turn black. Notify the physician if the stoma becomes black.

Immediately after surgery there may be a small amount of serosanguineous drainage in the appliance, the stool-collection device. When the appliance is changed and the stoma is cleaned or touched when swollen, a small amount of bleeding may occur. Reassure the client that a small amount of bleeding is normal. Bowel function is checked every shift to monitor for any obstruction or ileus. Bowel sounds, distention, and abdominal tenderness are checked every 4 hours.

Complications

Hemorrhage Bleeding or hemorrhage may occur at the incision site or stoma site. It is important to check the incision and stoma site for bleeding and to check the blood pressure and pulse frequently after surgery.

Infection The risk of infection around the stoma is great because of the presence of stool around the new suture line.

Hernia A hernia is the most frequent complication of an ostomy and is caused when a loop of bowel pushes up through the muscle next to the stoma and under the skin.

Obstruction Obstruction of the bowel ostomy may occur as a complication after surgery. Ileostomy clients are instructed to chew their food well before swallowing because large pieces of food such as an olive or large piece of meat may get caught at the opening of the ostomy.

Prolapse The bowel may sometimes telescope out through the stoma, resembling an elephant's trunk. If the bowel continues to work, this is not an emergency. The physician or ET nurse may be able to replace the bowel back into the abdomen; if not, the mucosa of the bowel may become injured, so the prolapse is corrected surgically. Prolapse can be frightening for the client, and its possibility is discussed in postoperative teaching.

Electrolyte Imbalance An ileostomy with a high output of effluent can cause electrolyte imbalances by loss of large amounts of potassium and protein. The client may have difficulty learning to cope with an appliance that is always filling and the need to take in enough fluid, protein, and potassium to replace the lost nutrients.

Skin Excoriation The skin around a high-output ostomy may become excoriated if an appliance that protects the skin cannot be found. Ileostomy effluent contains digestive juices that, if left on the skin, will start to digest the skin, resulting in red, open areas. To prevent this problem, correct appliance fitting that will stay in place is important for these clients.

Discharge Teaching for the Ostomy Client

Assessment

As the client prepares to go home, it is important to assess the client's or the family's ability to handle ostomy care at home. The client may still be dealing with an altered body image and not want to look at or touch the stoma. The family may have to help with care and be supportive until the client can assume the care.

Appliances

If the client has only one bowel movement per day, a closed appliance that is taken off and emptied once a day is all that is needed. If the client has several stools per day, an open-ended drainable appliance is best.

For ileostomies, the one- or two-piece open-end appliance offers ease in emptying. Effluent usually varies from liquid to pasty, so an appliance that can be drained several times per day without taking it off is important. A skin barrier is also necessary for the ileostomy or any ostomy with liquid output.

Irrigation

Irrigation is a means of regulating some colostomies. Descending or sigmoid colostomies are irrigated daily or every other day for control of evacuation. After irrigation, the client may wear a small security appliance or a gauze pad over the stoma the rest of the day. The disadvantage of irrigation is that it takes about an hour or more to perform. The decision to irrigate is made by the client, with the consent of the surgeon, after healing has taken place. To irrigate a colostomy, a cone tip is needed on the end of the irrigation catheter. Using the cone on the tip of the tubing prevents the end of the tube from poking into the side of the bowel and injuring the bowel and helps hold the fluid in the bowel. The cone needs to be lubricated liberally with water-soluble lubricating jelly.

Support Person

Upon discharge, the client and family receive the telephone number of the hospital and unit where treatment was received so they may call if questions arise. Seeing the ET nurse again in 4 to 6 weeks is sometimes recommended to check how the client is doing with ostomy care. If there is a local stoma support group, a person from the group may call or visit the client at home and invite the client and family to come to the group sessions.

Having ostomy surgery is no reason to stop any life activity. People with ostomies live full, active, productive lives.

Nursing Management

Assess bowel sounds frequently. Monitor severity of symptoms such as pain, diarrhea, constipation, abdominal distention, anorexia, nausea, vomiting, and fever. Check CBC reports for increased WBC and low H & H. Explain all tests and treatments and answer questions.

NURSING PROCESS

Assessment

Diverticulosis often has no symptoms, and therefore, clients may not be aware they have it.

Subjective Data

Clients with diverticulitis frequently describe left lower abdominal pain, constipation or diarrhea, bloating, anorexia, and nausea.

Objective Data

Assessment shows abdominal distention with tenderness on palpation, decreased bowel sounds, fever, vomiting, and stools that test positive for blood. A CBC will show an increased WBC and, if bleeding is present, a low H & H.

Nursing diagnoses for a client with diverticulosis or diverticulitis include the following:

NURSING DIAGNOSES	PLANNING/OUTCOMES	NURSING INTERVENTIONS
*Acute **Pain*** related to diverticulitis	The client will verbalize a decrease in pain within 24 hours after intervention as measured by the pain scale.	Encourage bed rest to allow healing. Maintain client as NPO. Administer analgesics and antibiotics as ordered.
*Risk for **Infection*** related to abscess formation or perforation	The client will verbalize understanding of signs and symptoms of possible complications.	Monitor vital signs and pain level every 4 hours and assess abdomen every 4 hours for increased tenderness and distention. Educate the client to notify staff of chills, shortness of breath, or increasing pain.
***A**nxiety* related to possible surgery	The client will verbalize fears related to surgery and exhibit decreased anxiety regarding the procedure and follow-up treatment.	Explain all tests and treatments to decrease the client's anxiety level. Answer all concerns and questions. Allow the client to verbalize fears and concerns. If a colostomy is planned, arrange a consult with an enterostomal therapist to help answer concerns.

Evaluation: Evaluate each outcome to determine how it has been met by the client.

SAMPLE NURSING CARE PLAN

The Client with Diverticulitis

W.D. is a 67-year-old man admitted to the hospital with abdominal pain that started 2 days ago. The pain has been increasing in intensity and is now accompanied by nausea and anorexia. Physical assessment reveals temperature 101.7°F, pulse 96, respirations 24, and blood pressure of 162/90. W.D.'s abdomen is tender on palpation. He is in obvious discomfort and is unable to lie on his back. W.D. states he has not been eating any food or drinking adequate fluids for 24 hours. Skin turgor is poor. An abdominal ultrasound is ordered and identifies diverticulitis. An IV of D5 1/2 NS with 20 mEq KCl, droperidol (Inapsine) IV for nausea, meperidine (Demerol) IM for pain, and IV antibiotics are ordered. W.D. is placed on I&O, bed rest with bathroom privileges, and is made NPO. W.D. states that he does not understand why all this is being done. His first two voidings are 50 mL each and very concentrated (dark-gold colored).

NURSING DIAGNOSIS 1 *Deficient **K**nowledge* related to diagnosis and treatment regimen, as evidenced by W.D.'s statement that he does not understand why all this is being done

Nursing Outcomes Classification (NOC)
Knowledge: Disease Process
Knowledge: Treatment Regimen

Nursing Interventions Classification (NIC)
Teaching: Disease Process
Teaching: Individual

PLANNING/OUTCOMES	NURSING INTERVENTIONS	RATIONALE
W.D. will verbalize understanding of treatment plan.	Assess W.D.'s knowledge level of diverticulosis/diverticulitis.	Helps client relate new information and integrate it into his behavior.
	Assess W.D.'s learning style and present information in a compatible manner.	Increases understanding and retention.
	Monitor for signs of pain and fatigue.	They impair learning.
	Answer questions and reinforce information.	Reinforces the new information learned.

(*Continues*)

SAMPLE NURSING CARE PLAN (Continued)

EVALUATION

W.D. verbalizes understanding of the disease process and treatment regimen.

NURSING DIAGNOSIS 2 *Acute **P**ain* related to diverticulitis as evidenced by tender abdomen

Nursing Outcomes Classification (NOC)
Comfort Control
Pain Control

Nursing Interventions Classification (NIC)
Pain Management
Medication Management

PLANNING/OUTCOMES	NURSING INTERVENTIONS	RATIONALE
W.D. will verbalize a decrease in pain within 24 hours of pain intervention.	Assess pain by the use of a scale of 1 (no pain) to 10 (extreme pain).	Provides objective measure of the client's perceived discomfort and effectiveness of analgesics.
	Medicate with analgesics as ordered.	Provides pain relief.
	Encourage W.D. to request analgesics before pain becomes intense.	Provides better control of pain.
	Monitor effectiveness of the pain medication by reassessing the pain 45 minutes after the analgesic is given.	Provides a measure of analgesic effectiveness.

EVALUATION

W.D. demonstrates adequate pain relief as demonstrated by a decrease in pain scale.

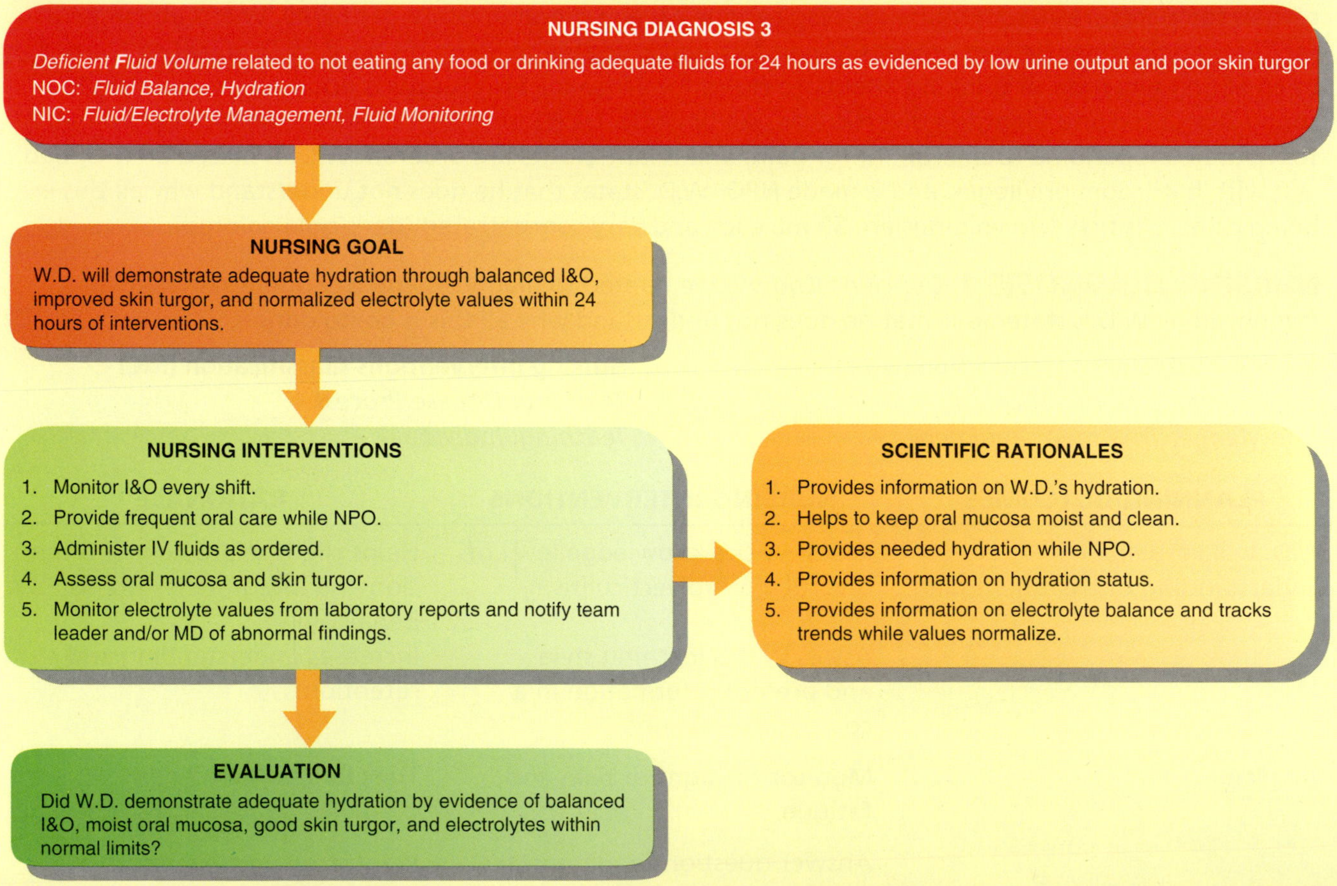

NURSING DIAGNOSIS 3

*Deficient **F**luid Volume* related to not eating any food or drinking adequate fluids for 24 hours as evidenced by low urine output and poor skin turgor
NOC: *Fluid Balance, Hydration*
NIC: *Fluid/Electrolyte Management, Fluid Monitoring*

NURSING GOAL

W.D. will demonstrate adequate hydration through balanced I&O, improved skin turgor, and normalized electrolyte values within 24 hours of interventions.

NURSING INTERVENTIONS

1. Monitor I&O every shift.
2. Provide frequent oral care while NPO.
3. Administer IV fluids as ordered.
4. Assess oral mucosa and skin turgor.
5. Monitor electrolyte values from laboratory reports and notify team leader and/or MD of abnormal findings.

SCIENTIFIC RATIONALES

1. Provides information on W.D.'s hydration.
2. Helps to keep oral mucosa moist and clean.
3. Provides needed hydration while NPO.
4. Provides information on hydration status.
5. Provides information on electrolyte balance and tracks trends while values normalize.

EVALUATION

Did W.D. demonstrate adequate hydration by evidence of balanced I&O, moist oral mucosa, good skin turgor, and electrolytes within normal limits?

CONCEPT CARE MAP 38-1

INFLAMMATORY BOWEL DISEASE

Inflammatory bowel disease (IBD) is the term used to describe Crohn's disease and ulcerative colitis (UC), which are diseases characterized by inflammation and ulcerations of the bowel (Table 38-4). The symptoms of IBD are not confined to the bowel but can affect many of the body's systems, such as uveitis and inflammatory process in the eye (Cox, Evans, Withers, and Titmuss, 2008). Potential extraintestinal manifestations may be found in other internal organs, eyes, blood, skin, and musculoskeletal system. Thirty percent of IBD clients have at least one extraintestinal manifestation (Rayhorn & Rayhorn, 2002).

Crohn's disease is characterized by lesions that affect the entire thickness of the bowel and can occur anywhere throughout the colon and small intestine. Symptoms include abdominal pain, diarrhea that usually does not contain blood, fever, anorexia, weight loss, and **steatorrhea** (fatty stools). Electrolyte imbalance, iron-deficiency anemia, and amino acid malabsorption occur when the disease involves the jejunum and the ileum. Long-term complications of Crohn's disease include bowel obstructions, fistulas, abscesses, and perforation. The risk for colorectal cancer, although not as high as in UC, is still increased. There is malabsorption of fat and fat-soluble vitamins.

UC is characterized by mucosal lesions occurring typically in the rectal area and sigmoid colon and progressing throughout the colon. Symptoms include fever, anorexia, weight loss, cramping, spasms, abdominal pain, and bloody diarrhea. Long-term complications include fissures, abscesses, and an increased risk for colorectal cancer.

The gold standard for diagnosing IBD is an endoscopic examination with a biopsy.

MEDICAL–SURGICAL MANAGEMENT

Medical

Treatment for Crohn's disease and UC is similar. Crohn's disease, however, is more debilitating because it involves more of the GI tract. UC is more limited but can still produce significant symptoms.

An endoscopy done on a UC client reveals continuous mucosal inflammation and ulceration, loss of mucosal vascularity, diffuse erythema, and often purulent exudate. Any granuloma found in the biopsy confirms Crohn's disease (Rayhorn & Rayhorn, 2002). The goals of treatment are to control inflammation, relieve symptoms, maintain fluid and electrolyte balance, provide adequate nutrition, and prevent complications.

Surgical

In severe cases of UC resistant to medical management, the colon is removed and an ileostomy is performed, curing the disease. An **ileostomy** is an opening created in the small intestine (ileum). The output from an ileostomy is a thin liquid, usually of a yellowish-green color. This thin output is called **effluent**. It generally has no odor, and it may get thicker in time as the body adapts to the need to retain moisture. Many ileostomies have almost constant effluent output. The Kock continent ileostomy has a pouch made inside the abdomen to hold the effluent until the client is ready to empty the pouch. Figure 38-7 illustrates a Kock continent ileostomy.

Most clients with Crohn's disease need surgery at some point to repair the structural damage caused by scarring. Intestinal obstructions and perforations may also occur in Crohn's disease, necessitating further surgery. Surgical intervention, however, does not cure the disease.

TABLE 38-4 Comparison of Crohn's Disease and Ulcerative Colitis

PARAMETER	CROHN'S DISEASE	ULCERATIVE COLITIS (UC)
Involvement	Patchy areas. Can involve small and large intestine.	Starts in lower colon and spreads progressively throughout colon. Affects only the colon.
Tissue affected	Affects entire thickness of bowel.	Affects mucosal lining of bowel.
Long-term complications	Intestinal obstruction, fistulas, abscesses, perforations; cancer risk increases with age.	Fissures, abscesses, increased risk for colorectal cancer.
Surgical intervention	Usually needed at some point to repair structural damage. Does not cure or limit the progress of the disease.	Ileostomy performed in approximately 20% of cases to remove the colon. Cures the disease.
Cause	Unknown: possibly altered immune state.	Unknown: possibly enteric bacterium *E. coli.*
Stools	3 to 4 semisoft/day; rarely bloody; steatorrhea and mucus present.	15 to 20 liquid/day; blood present; no steatorrhea.

COURTESY OF DELMAR CENGAGE LEARNING

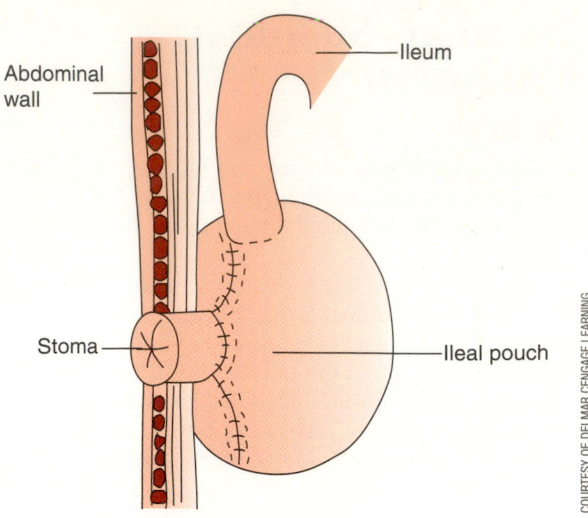

FIGURE 38-7 Kock Continent Ileostomy

Pharmacological

Treatment for both UC and Crohn's disease includes 5-ASA compounds such as sulfasalazine (Azulfidine) or salicylates such as mesalamine (Rowasa) or olsalazine sodium (Dipentum). If inflammation is severe, corticosteroids also are administered. In cases resistant to the 5-ASA compounds and corticosteroids, immunosuppressors are used. If an infection is present, antibiotics are administered. According to Rayhorn and Rayhorn (2002), clients are seldom given antidiarrheal medications because they may predispose the client to toxic megacolon.

Clients need IV fluid and electrolyte replacement during severe flare-ups. In the most severe cases, clients are placed on total parenteral nutrition (TPN) to allow for complete bowel rest and to improve nutritional status.

Diet

Protein and calorie malnutrition is a concern in clients with IBD. Because of the severe cramping, pain, and diarrhea brought on by foods, these clients typically put themselves on a very restrictive diet that is not nutritionally balanced. Clients with Crohn's disease may also have malabsorption of iron and vitamin B_{12}.

Nutritional support includes modifying the diet to eliminate foods that exacerbate symptoms while maintaining a balanced diet. A high-calorie, low-residue, high-protein, low-fat diet is recommended (Rayhorn & Rayhorn, 2002).

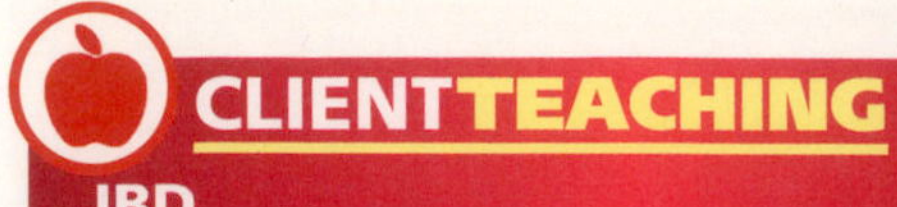

CLIENT TEACHING

IBD

- Schedule a colon cancer screening regularly.
- When taking oral corticosteroids, strictly adhere to the prescribed schedule.

Health Promotion

Although stress has not been shown to exacerbate the symptoms of Crohn's disease or UC, the impact on the client's lifestyle can be significant, especially with Crohn's disease. Support groups can be beneficial. Encourage clients to develop mechanisms to help them cope with the disease process. Exercise, meditation, and biofeedback may be helpful.

NURSING MANAGEMENT

Assess the abdomen for tenderness, distention, and bowel sounds. Monitor weight, vital signs, and stools. Maintain an accurate I&O and calorie count. Provide high-calorie, high-protein small, frequent meals and snacks. Encourage verbalization of feelings.

NURSING PROCESS

ASSESSMENT

Subjective Data

Clients describe mild abdominal spasms and cramping, which may increase to severe abdominal pain, nausea, and anorexia. Clients with UC have an urge to defecate with the cramping.

Objective Data

Clients have abdominal tenderness on palpation, guarding, distention, weight loss, diarrhea, an elevated WBC count, and fever. In clients with Crohn's disease, steatorrhea and iron-deficiency anemia may be present. In clients with UC, stools may be positive for blood and the H & H may be low. The serum potassium, magnesium, and albumin levels are usually low. Because Crohn's disease is so debilitating, clients may become depressed.

Nursing diagnoses for a client with Crohn's disease or UC include the following:

NURSING DIAGNOSES	PLANNING/OUTCOMES	NURSING INTERVENTIONS
*Imbalanced **N**utrition: Less than Body Requirements* related to postprandial pain, bowel hypermobility, and decreased absorption	The client will demonstrate adequate nutritional status as exhibited by maintaining weight within range for height and body type.	Monitor I&O every shift; caloric count and weight daily. Administer IV fluid and electrolyte replacement as ordered. Provide high-calorie, high-protein supplements as ordered along with small, frequent meals. Administer TPN, a high-calorie and nutrient-dense IV solution, as ordered. Closely monitor lab reports for electrolytes and glucose level.

Nursing diagnoses for a client with Crohn's disease or UC include the following: (Continued)

NURSING DIAGNOSES	PLANNING/OUTCOMES	NURSING INTERVENTIONS
*Risk for Deficient **Fluid** Volume* related to diarrhea and altered intake	The client will exhibit adequate hydration as evidenced by electrolytes within normal range, moist mucous membranes, and I&O nearly equal within 48 hours of intervention. The frequency and amount of diarrhea will decrease within 48 hours of intervention.	Administer 5-ASA compounds, corticosteroids, and immunosuppressors as ordered. Monitor I&O every shift. Administer IV fluid and electrolyte rehydration as ordered.
***P**owerlessness* related to impairment in lifestyle secondary to disease process	The client will verbalize a plan to seek support, by discharge.	Provide client with information on national organizations and local support groups. Arrange social work consult if needed. Allow client to verbalize feelings.
Evaluation: Evaluate each outcome to determine how it has been met by the client.		

IRRITABLE BOWEL SYNDROME

Irritable bowel syndrome (IBS) refers to a group of symptoms—cramping, abdominal pain, bloating, constipation, or diarrhea. Some clients have both constipation and diarrhea which alternate in appearance. There is no organic cause, but the movement of feces and gas through the colon and the absorption of fluids are affected. When feces stay in the colon too long and too much water is absorbed, constipation results. When feces is pushed through the colon too fast by spasms, little water is absorbed and diarrhea results. Spasms also temporarily trap gas or feces, preventing them from moving forward, and therefore causing pain.

The colon seems to be more sensitive and reactive especially to certain foods and stress. Since the colon is partly controlled by the autonomic nervous system, it responds to stress. It may contract too much or too little, and too much water or too little water may be absorbed.

In the United States, one in five persons has IBS, making it one of the most common gastrointestinal disorders. Only a small proportion of people seek medical treatment, while most will treat the symptoms themselves. IBS occurs more frequently in women than in men, and usually begins around age 20 (NIDDK, 2009b).

There is no diagnostic test for IBS, but clients presenting with the aforementioned symptoms often undergo testing to rule out other disorders. Criteria for a diagnosis of IBS include:

1. Abdominal pain or discomfort for at least 12 weeks (not necessarily consecutive) out of the previous 12 months.
2. At least two of the following three features must be present:
    - Abdominal pain or discomfort is relieved by having a bowel movement.
    - When abdominal pain or discomfort begins, there is a change in how often the client has a bowel movement.
    - When abdominal pain or discomfort begins, there is a change in the form of the stool or the way it looks.

MEDICAL-SURGICAL MANAGEMENT

Medical

The goal of treatment is to relieve the symptoms. Foods that make the symptoms worse are eliminated from the diet. Increasing dietary fiber is often helpful. Anxiety-reducing measures often relieve symptoms. If the client has severe anxiety or depression, counseling may be required.

Pharmacological

Anticholinergic medications are administered before meals. Clients with constipation may be given tegaserod maleate (Zelnorm), usually for 4 weeks. Bulk-forming psyllium hydrophilic muciloid (Metamucil) may also be used.

Clients who primarily have diarrhea and have not responded to other therapies may be given alosetron hydrochloride (Lotronex). It should be used with caution because it can have serious side effects, such as severe constipation or decreased blood flow to the colon.

Diet

The client is instructed to eliminate from the diet those foods that aggravate the symptoms and discomfort. Foods often associated with making IBS symptoms worse include wheat, rye, barley, chocolate, milk products, alcohol, and caffeinated drinks. Foods high in fiber such as bran, cereal, beans, fruits, and vegetables may reduce symptoms. Large meals cause cramping and diarrhea.

Activity

Regular exercise may help relieve symptoms. Seldom is weight loss a problem.

Nursing Management

Encourage the client to write down what is eaten, what symptoms are present and when they occur, and which foods always make the client feel bad. Then eliminate those foods causing symptoms or making the client feel bad. Suggest that the client eat five or six small meals instead of three large meals each day. Encourage the client to exercise regularly and practice stress-relieving measures such as progressive relaxation or guided imagery.

NURSING PROCESS

Assessment

Subjective Data

Some clients describe cramping, abdominal pain, and diarrhea during or soon after a meal, others complain of constipation, and still others report alternating diarrhea and constipation. Abdominal fullness, gas, and bloating also often occur.

Objective Data

The client's stools will be either very loose (diarrhea) or very hard and difficult to pass (constipation). Mucus may be passed with the bowel movement. ***No** weight loss, bleeding, or fever is associated with IBS.*

Nursing diagnoses for a client with irritable bowel syndrome include the following:

NURSING DIAGNOSES	PLANNING/OUTCOMES	NURSING INTERVENTIONS
Diarrhea related to rapid movement of feces through the colon with too little fluid being absorbed	The client will have normally formed stools.	Encourage frequent meals. Add high-fiber foods gradually to meals. Teach client to eliminate gas-forming foods and other foods causing symptoms from the diet. Teach stress-reducing measures.
Constipation related to delayed movement of feces through the colon with too much fluid being absorbed	The client will have regularly passed, soft, formed stools.	Encourage increased fluid intake unless contraindicated, and increase consumption of high-fiber foods. Encourage regular exercise such as walking. Administer medications as prescribed. Teach stress-reducing measures.

Evaluation: Evaluate each outcome to determine how it has been met by the client.

INTESTINAL OBSTRUCTION

An intestinal obstruction occurs when the contents cannot pass through the intestine. Obstructions occur in the large or the small intestine, with most occurring in the ileum. Obstructions may be mechanical, neurogenic, or vascular in origin.

A mechanical obstruction may be a partial or complete obstruction caused by a tumor; fecal impaction; hernia; **volvulus**, a twisting of the bowel on itself; **intussusception**, a telescoping of the bowel where the bowel slides inside itself (Figure 38-8); or **adhesions**, scar tissue in the abdomen from previous surgeries or disease process such as Crohn's disease.

A neurogenic obstruction, known as a *paralytic ileus,* occurs when nerve transmission to the bowel is interrupted by trauma, infection, or medications, resulting in a portion of the bowel being paralyzed.

A vascular obstruction occurs when blood flow to a portion of the bowel is interrupted, as in atherosclerosis, and that portion of the bowel becomes necrotic.

When the small intestine becomes obstructed, large amounts of fluid, bacteria, and swallowed air build up in the bowel proximal to the obstruction. The normal process of

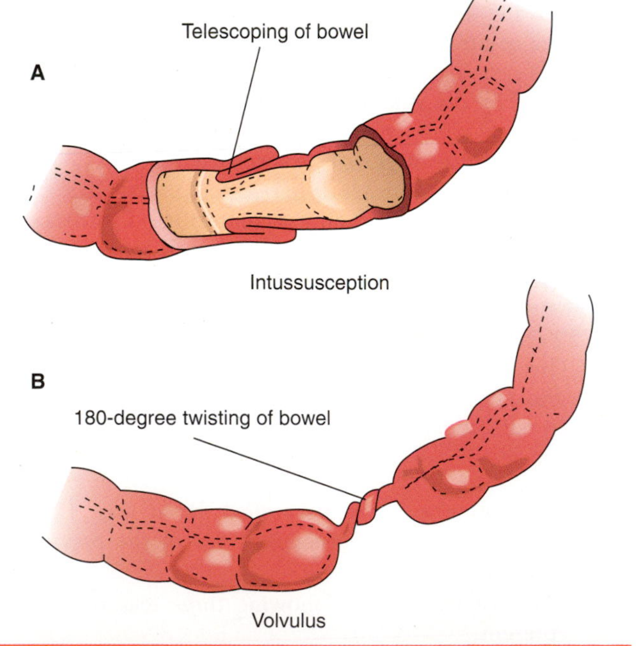

FIGURE 38-8 Bowel obstructions can be caused by *A,* an intussusception; or *B,* a volvulus.

secretion and absorption of the electrolyte-rich fluid is interrupted. Distention and poor absorption occur when water and salts move from the circulatory system to the lumen of the intestine.

An abdominal x-ray and a barium enema or UGI with small bowel follow-through are ordered when a bowel obstruction is suspected.

Medical–Surgical Management

Medical

Treatment of the obstruction depends on the cause and location. Some can be treated medically by inserting an NG tube for decompression, providing IV fluids for rehydration, and treating the cause, such as the use of enemas for fecal impaction.

Surgical

Most bowel obstructions require surgery. A bowel resection is performed to remove the portion of the bowel affected by the obstruction.

Pharmacological

Nonnarcotic analgesics are used to avoid the intestinal motility decrease caused by opioids. Antibiotics also are ordered.

Diet

Clients are kept NPO until the obstruction is cleared and then slowly progressed from a clear liquid diet to a regular diet as more bowel function returns.

Activity

In cases of paralytic ileus, ambulation is encouraged to help bowel function return. Encourage clients who have had a bowel resection to turn, cough, and deep breathe every 2 hours initially postoperatively. Activity is progressed the next day.

Nursing Management

Assess abdomen for tenderness, distention, and bowel sounds. Monitor vomiting for fecal material. Assess weight daily. Accurately record I&O and limit ice chips when NPO. Check laboratory reports for low sodium and potassium and elevated BUN, amylase, and H & H.

NURSING PROCESS

Assessment

Subjective Data

Clients report symptoms of colicky abdominal pain, nausea, constipation, and bloating.

Objective Data

Objective assessment includes abdominal distention and tenderness on palpation. Vomiting temporarily relieves the abdominal pain. Vomitus may include fecal material, which is a poor prognostic sign (Lynch and Sarazine, 2006).

Laboratory analysis demonstrates decreased levels of sodium and potassium, elevated BUN, elevated amylase, and elevated H & H caused by hemoconcentration.

Nursing diagnoses for a client with intestinal obstruction include the following:

NURSING DIAGNOSES	PLANNING/OUTCOMES	NURSING INTERVENTIONS
*Deficient **Fluid** Volume* related to vomiting, shift in fluids, and NPO status	The client will exhibit adequate hydration within 48 hours of initiation of treatment as evidenced by moist mucous membranes, electrolytes within normal limits, and I&O approximately equal.	Monitor I&O every shift. Administer IV fluid and electrolyte replacements as ordered. Allow limited ice chips to prevent further electrolyte imbalance in clients with NG tubes. Assess weight daily.
*Acute **Pain*** related to distention, edema, or ischemia	The client will verbalize increased comfort within 1 hour of analgesic administration as measured on pain scale.	Administer nonnarcotic analgesics as ordered. In clients with a paralytic ileus, encourage ambulation to encourage return of bowel function. Maintain and monitor NG tube as ordered for abdominal decompression. Check bowel sounds every 4 hours or PRN.
*Deficient **Knowledge*** related to disease process, treatment regimen, and possible surgery	The client will verbalize treatment course, possible complications, and possible need for surgery.	Identify client's learning style and present information in a manner compatible with learning style. Include intestinal decompression, need for ambulation, need for good oral care due to fecal drainage, and surgery.

Evaluation: Evaluate each outcome to determine how it has been met by the client.

HERNIAS

A hernia occurs when the wall of a muscle weakens and the intestine protrudes through the muscle wall. Hernias that do not return to the abdominal cavity with rest or manipulation and cause complete bowel obstruction are said to be *incarcerated*. If the blood supply to the hernia is cut off, the hernia is said to be *strangulated*. Immediate surgery is required to restore blood flow. If not done, gangrene develops, which may be fatal.

Several types of hernias exist. In an umbilical hernia, a portion of the bowel protrudes through the umbilicus. In children, these generally resolve on their own once the child begins to walk. Umbilical hernias most commonly occur in multiparous women or in adults with cirrhosis and **ascites** (abnormal accumulation of fluid in the peritoneal cavity). Because of a high risk for strangulation in adults with umbilical hernias, surgery is usually performed.

Abdominal hernias occur in the midline of the abdomen between the umbilicus and the xyphoid process. Most are asymptomatic, with a few causing pain on exertion that resolves with reclining and rest. Inguinal hernias, the most common hernia, occur in the groin area. Inguinal hernias frequently occur after activities, such as lifting, that increase intraabdominal pressure; they subside with relaxation. Pain is located lower than in the abdominal hernia. Femoral hernias occur when the intestine pushes into the passageway carrying blood vessels and nerves to the legs and are more common in women than in men. A hiatal hernia occurs when a portion of the stomach protrudes into the mediastinal cavity through the diaphragm. Symptoms of hiatal hernias include indigestion and heartburn, especially after eating a large meal.

Upon evaluation and recommendation of a physician, some hernias can be reduced or pushed back into place. This can be accomplished by having the client recline, applying direct pressure to the hernia, and, in some cases, having the client exhale to decrease intraabdominal pressure. The nurse should never try to reduce a hernia.

MEDICAL–SURGICAL MANAGEMENT

Medical

Some hernias have no symptoms or minimal symptoms, so clients may not be aware they have one or may learn to live with it by reducing it when needed. Clients who are a poor surgical risk may use a truss, a device that applies pressure to the hernia, thus keeping the intestine in the abdominal cavity.

Surgical

Hernias are repaired with surgery called herniorrhaphy. The surgery is typically performed on an outpatient basis, with clients going home the same day. If the surgery is more complicated because the hernia is incarcerated, the client may stay overnight. If the hernia is strangulated, a bowel resection may be required.

Surgical repair of a hiatal hernia involves reinforcing the esophagus with a portion of the stomach. The surgery is performed laparoscopically, with the client remaining in the hospital 3 to 5 days postoperatively. Initially, the client will have an NG tube. The NG tube is removed 24 to 48 hours later and the diet gradually progressed to a soft diet.

Diet

Clients with hiatal hernias modify their dietary patterns by eating small frequent meals. Clients are encouraged not to eat after the evening meal, lie down for 2 hours after eating, or consume aggravating foods.

NURSING MANAGEMENT

Assess abdomen for bowel sounds and bulge in abdominal wall. Encourage client with hernia to eat small, frequent meals and avoid lying down for 2 hours after eating.

NURSING PROCESS

ASSESSMENT

Subjective Data

Clients may describe pain at the site of the hernia.

Objective Data

Assessment may show a bulge through the abdominal wall. If the hernia is strangulated, the client will have the symptoms of a bowel obstruction.

Nursing diagnoses for a client with a hernia include the following:

NURSING DIAGNOSES	PLANNING/OUTCOMES	NURSING INTERVENTIONS
*Acute **Pain*** related to tissue edema	The client will experience less pain within 1 hour of intervention as measured on the pain scale.	Administer analgesics as ordered. Evaluate aggravating activities (e.g., straining to have a bowel movement) and provide information on modification if indicated. Educate regarding signs of complications and when to notify staff of symptoms.
*Ineffective **Tissue Perfusion** (Gastrointestinal)* related to strangulation	The client will have minimal tissue necrosis.	Assess abdomen for bowel sounds every 4 hours. Insert NG tube to decrease abdominal distention as ordered. Administer IV hydration as ordered. Prepare client for surgery as ordered. Keep client NPO.

Evaluation: Evaluate each outcome to determine how it has been met by the client.

PERITONITIS

Peritonitis is the inflammation of the peritoneum, the membranous covering of the abdomen. Peritonitis is caused by irritating substances such as feces, gastric acids, bacteria, or blood in the abdominal cavity. A ruptured portion of the digestive system (such as the appendix), a ruptured tubal pregnancy, or invasion of tumors through the gastric wall can lead to peritonitis. Peritonitis is a serious, life-threatening condition. Complications of peritonitis include adhesions (scar tissue), paralytic ileus, and pneumonia.

MEDICAL–SURGICAL MANAGEMENT

Surgical

Treatment is primarily surgical with repair of the cause and irrigation of the abdominal cavity with saline and antibiotic solutions. Drains are left in the abdomen for several days postoperatively to allow any remaining fluid to drain. Because bowel function usually stops as a result of the irritating substances, an NG tube is placed to decompress the abdomen and relieve nausea.

Pharmacological

Analgesics are ordered postoperatively for discomfort. If an ileus develops, nonnarcotic analgesics are ordered. Antibiotics are ordered preoperatively and postoperatively.

Diet

Clients are NPO preoperatively and postoperatively until bowel sounds return. Clients are then placed on a clear liquid diet and slowly progressed to a regular diet as more bowel function returns.

Activity

Preoperatively, clients are placed on bed rest and encouraged to turn, cough, and deep breathe. Because clients tend to breathe shallowly with peritoneal inflammation, pulmonary hygiene is important. Activity is increased postoperatively, as soon as tolerated, to increase lung expansion and to encourage bowel function return. Exercise, lifting, and driving are restricted until the incision heals.

NURSING MANAGEMENT

Assess vital signs and administer antipyretics as ordered. Monitor I&O, signs of dehydration, and fluid and electrolyte replacement. Provide comfort measures (cool cloth, oral hygiene, back rub). Maintain patency of NG tube. Encourage coughing and deep breathing and teach incision splinting. Keep client in semi-Fowler's position to help localize purulent exudate. Follow surgical asepsis for wound care. Empty drainage devices as required. If drainage does not flow into a device, change dressings frequently to keep drainage off the skin. If the wound is still draining when the client is discharged, teach client/family aseptic technique for changing dressings.

NURSING PROCESS

ASSESSMENT

Subjective Data

Clients describe abdominal pain, nausea, and constipation.

Objective Data

Assessment reveals vomiting, absent bowel sounds, a tense or distended abdomen with tenderness on palpation, shallow and rapid respirations, weak and rapid pulse, dry mucous membranes, low urine output, fever, and limited mobility because of pain. Laboratory analysis will show an increased WBC. If the client is bleeding, the H & H will be low. Sodium, potassium, and chloride may be low.

Nursing diagnoses for a client with peritonitis include the following:

NURSING DIAGNOSES	PLANNING/OUTCOMES	NURSING INTERVENTIONS
*Deficient **F**luid Volume* related to gastric losses and restricted intake	The client will maintain hydration as indicated by an I&O that is nearly equal and electrolytes within normal limits.	Monitor I&O every shift. Monitor for signs of dehydration: dry mucous membranes, poor skin turgor, and low urine output. Monitor electrolytes as ordered. Administer IV rehydration and electrolyte replacement as ordered.
***H**yperthermia* related to inflammatory process and dehydration	The client will maintain temperature within normal limits.	Assess VS including temperature every 4 hours. Administer antipyretics as ordered; probably rectal suppositories due to NPO status. Monitor for dehydration: decrease in urine output, dry mucous membranes, and poor skin turgor. Provide comfort measures: cool cloth to the head or neck, assistance to turn, and a back rub with cooling lotion.

(*Continues*)

Nursing diagnoses for a client with peritonitis include the following: (Continued)

NURSING DIAGNOSES	PLANNING/OUTCOMES	NURSING INTERVENTIONS
*Acute **Pain*** related to abdominal distention	The client will have less pain and improved mobility within 1 hour of receiving analgesics as measured on the pain scale.	Administer analgesics as ordered. Encourage activity such as coughing and deep breathing after analgesics. Teach splinting of incision for cough and deep breathing. Monitor NG tube to decompress abdomen. Maintain patency of NG tube.

Evaluation: Evaluate each outcome to determine how it has been met by the client.

HEMORRHOIDS

Hemorrhoids are swollen vascular tissues in the rectal area. They may be internal or external. Hemorrhoids may be caused by straining with constipation or sitting on the toilet (reading) for an extended time. Hemorrhoids frequently occur with pregnancy. Hemorrhoids can cause burning, pruritis, and pain with defecation. At times, they can bleed, leading to anemia.

MEDICAL–SURGICAL MANAGEMENT

Medical

Sitz baths or warm compresses on the rectal area for 20 minutes, 4 times a day, often helps decrease swelling.

Surgical

If bleeding continues despite medical intervention, or if discomfort is significant, hemorrhoids can be surgically removed by a hemorrhoidectomy. For external hemorrhoids, surgery is performed on an outpatient basis by placing a band around the hemorrhoid as for esophageal varices, allowing it to necrose and fall off. For internal hemorrhoids, sclerotherapy, cryotherapy, or laser is performed. This usually requires that the patient stay overnight in the hospital. Hemorrhoids can recur after surgical removal if the cause is not eliminated.

Pharmacological

Treatment includes the administration of creams and suppositories to decrease inflammation, some with cortisone to decrease swelling. Fiber supplements and stool softeners are ordered to keep bowel movements soft.

Diet

Bowel movements are kept soft with a high-fiber diet of 20 to 30 grams of fiber per day and at least 2,500 mL of fluid intake daily.

NURSING MANAGEMENT

Teach client to modify bowel habits (sit on toilet only for short periods), increase fiber in diet to 20 or 30 grams per day, and increase fluid intake to 2,500 mL per day. Provide sitz baths several times a day or teach client how to do it.

NURSING PROCESS

ASSESSMENT

Subjective Data

Clients describe rectal burning, pain, and pruritis with bowel movements; constipation; and, occasionally, bright red bleeding. A dietary history is obtained to determine fiber and fluid intake.

Objective Data

If hemorrhoids are external, they can be visualized during a physical examination. If chronic bleeding is present, laboratory analysis may show a low H & H.

Nursing diagnoses for a client with hemorrhoids include the following:

NURSING DIAGNOSES	PLANNING/OUTCOMES	NURSING INTERVENTIONS
*Acute **Pain*** related to edema and inflammation of swollen vascular tissues	The client will verbalize a decrease in discomfort within 48 hours of initiation of treatment.	Provide sitz baths or warm compresses for 20 minutes, 4 times a day. Administer creams and suppositories as ordered. Increase fiber and fluids in diet to keep stools soft to avoid straining.
*Deficient **Knowledge*** related to diet, causes of condition, treatment, and potential complications	The client will be able to verbalize treatment regimen and long-term management of hemorrhoids.	Determine client's learning style and present information in a manner compatible with learning style. Educate client about increasing fiber in diet to 20 to 30 grams per day, increasing fluid intake to 2,500 mL per day, causes of hemorrhoids, possible complications such as anemia, and modification of bowel habits (such as not sitting on the toilet for long periods).

Evaluation: Evaluate each outcome to determine how it has been met by the client.

CONSTIPATION

Constipation is characterized by hard, infrequent stools that are difficult and/or painful to pass. Constipation can be caused by tumors, low-fiber diet, inactivity, some diseases that interfere with the mechanical functioning of the bowel (such as multiple sclerosis), or some medications (such as narcotics, antidepressants, or anti-Parkinson drugs).

MEDICAL–SURGICAL MANAGEMENT

Pharmacological

Fiber supplements and stool softeners are ordered. Laxatives and enemas may be ordered, but long-term use is avoided because they interrupt normal bowel function. If constipation is caused by medications the client is taking, the client should discuss other options with the physician, such as modifying the dosage or changing medications.

Diet

Fiber is increased to 20 to 30 grams per day. Fluid intake is increased to 2,500 mL per day.

Activity

Increase activity level if possible because exercise, such as walking, increases motility in the colon.

> **LIFE SPAN CONSIDERATIONS**
>
> **Constipation in the Older Client**
>
> The slowing of peristalsis, which is part of the aging process, leads to constipation in the older client. An increase in dietary fiber and fluid intake (water) helps to prevent constipation. A regular schedule for bowel evacuation also helps.

NURSING MANAGEMENT

Assess dietary intake of fiber and fluids and activity/exercise level. Review medications client is taking for any causing constipation. Encourage regular schedule for bowel evacuation.

NURSING PROCESS

ASSESSMENT

Subjective Data

Clients describe infrequent, difficult to pass stools. Dietary assessment of fiber and fluids usually reveals inadequate intake. Ask client to describe activity/exercise level.

Objective Data

Bowel movements are hard-formed.

Nursing diagnoses for a client with constipation include the following:

NURSING DIAGNOSES	PLANNING/OUTCOMES	NURSING INTERVENTIONS
Constipation related to inadequate intake of fiber and fluids	The client will have soft stools every other day by one week from intervention.	Encourage client to increase fiber in the diet to 20 to 30 grams a day and fluid intake to 2,500 mL a day. Administer fiber supplements and stool softeners as ordered. Determine fluid preferences of client and always have fluids at client's bedside within reach. Help the client establish a regular schedule for bowel movements, usually 30 minutes after a meal.
Deficient Knowledge related to dietary sources of fiber and the importance of adequate fluid intake and exercise	The client will be able to select a menu high in fiber and fluids utilizing nutrients from the food pyramid within 48 hours and verbalize the need for adequate exercise.	Assess client's learning style and present information in a manner compatible with learning style. Teach client about foods that are high in fiber (fruits, vegetables, whole grains) as well as importance of fluid intake. Discuss with client the importance of exercise in maintaining bowel function.

Evaluation: Evaluate each outcome to determine how it has been met by the client.

DISORDERS OF THE ACCESSORY ORGANS

Disorders of the accessory organs include cirrhosis, hepatitis, pancreatitis, and cholecystitis/cholelithiasis.

CIRRHOSIS

Cirrhosis refers to the chronic, degenerative changes in the liver cells and thickening of surrounding tissue that result from the liver repairing itself after chronic inflammation.

Causes of cirrhosis include chronic hepatitis, repeated exposure to toxic substances, disease processes (such as sclerosing cholangitis and hemochromatosis), cancer, and chronic alcohol abuse. Alcohol abuse accounts for most cases of cirrhosis.

Because the liver is responsible for so many functions, complications of cirrhosis can be significant and include malnutrition, hypoglycemia, clotting disorders, jaundice, portal hypertension, ascites, hepatic encephalopathy, and hepatorenal syndrome.

Liver dysfunction causes several organ-related complications. Malnutrition results from the liver's inability to absorb fat and fat-soluble vitamins and leads to muscle wasting, weight loss, and fatigue. Hypoglycemia occurs when the liver is unable to perform glycogenolysis efficiently. When the liver is not able to produce sufficient amounts of prothrombin and fibrinogen, clotting disorders arise.

Portal hypertension results when blood flow through the cirrhotic liver is inhibited, resulting in blood backflowing in the portal vein. Portal hypertension leads to distention of the esophageal veins, resulting in esophageal varices; distention of rectal veins, resulting in hemorrhoids; and distention of the splenic vein, resulting in splenomegaly.

Because the liver is responsible for metabolizing medications, clients frequently become intolerant to some medications. Jaundice, a yellow discoloration of the skin, is usually present. Jaundice occurs when the liver is unable to convert bilirubin, an end product of red blood cell breakdown, into a water-soluble form that can be excreted in the bile. The extra bilirubin collects in areas that contain elastin, such as the sclera of the eyes, the skin, and the nail beds.

Fluid accumulates in the pleural cavity in the form of pleural effusions. Fluid may also accumulate in the peritoneal cavity. This condition is called ascites. The cause of ascites is the congestion of blood in the portal system.

Hepatic encephalopathy is a condition in which ammonia accumulates in the brain. Fluid is pulled into the extracellular compartment, accelerating brain stem herniation. Confusion, lethargy, and/or coma may occur. Symptoms of impending hepatic encephalopathy are disorientation and *asterixis* (liver flap), a flapping tremor of the hands. When the client extends the arms and hands in front of the body, the hands rapidly flex and extend.

Hepatorenal syndrome is a complication of cirrhosis in which the client goes into renal failure. Symptoms include oliguria (diminished production of urine), azotemia (excess nitrogen in the blood), anorexia, fatigue, and weakness.

Cirrhosis is a form of end-stage liver disease for which there is no cure. The process of cirrhosis can be slowed by removing the cause (i.e., abstaining from alcohol), but the damage cannot be reversed. Clients in end-stage liver disease are evaluated to determine whether they qualify for a liver transplant.

MEDICAL–SURGICAL MANAGEMENT

Medical

The physician performs a paracentesis to remove the fluid from the abdomen and relieve pressure on the diaphragm and lungs. A small incision is made and a trochar inserted into the abdomen to drain the fluid. Albumin may be infused at the same time to pull excess fluid back into the vascular system.

Surgical

If the client continues to develop ascites after medical treatment, a LeVeen or Denver peritoneal venous shunt is used. The pressure-regulated shunt is implanted in the peritoneal cavity and threaded through the subcutaneous tissue into the superior vena cava, returning the fluid back to the vascular system. As fluid pressure builds in the peritoneal cavity, a valve opens and drains the fluid into the superior vena cava.

If esophageal varices are present, an EGD with sclerotherapy or banding is done to prevent hemorrhage (refer to Figure 38-3).

If portal hypertension cannot be controlled with medications, a portosystemic shunt or a transjugular intrahepatic portosystemic shunt (TIPS) may be performed. The shunt redirects the blood flow, thereby relieving the portal hypertension, and decreases the risk of rupturing distended veins in the esophagus (Figure 38-9).

Pharmacological

A potassium-sparing diuretic, such as spironolactone (Aldactone), decreases ascites and pleural effusion. Lactulose (Cholac) moves ammonia from the blood into the bowel. The lactulose acts as a laxative and causes the body to excrete the stool containing ammonia. Tap water enemas may also be ordered to help the body eliminate the ammonia.

Propranolol hydrochloride (Inderal), an antihypertensive medication, is ordered to lower portal hypertension. All unnecessary medications are avoided because the liver cannot metabolize them.

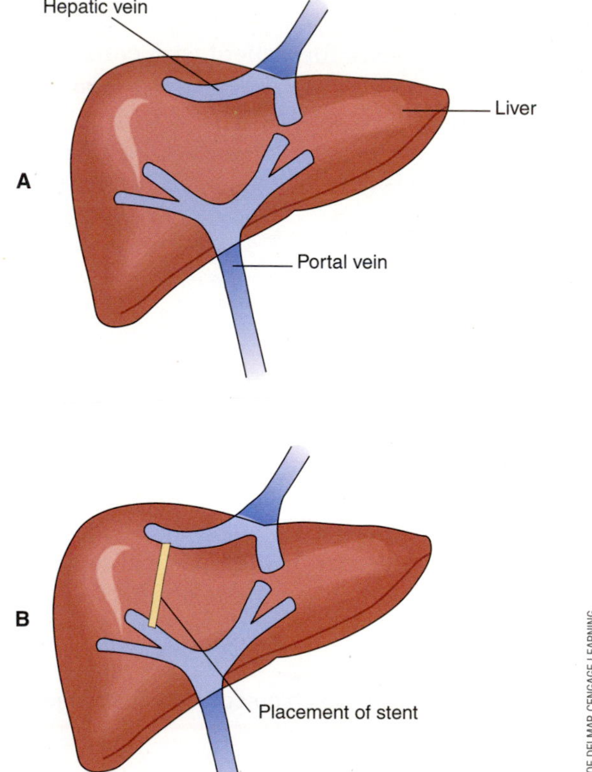

FIGURE 38-9 *A,* **Blood Flow before TIPS;** *B,* **TIPS is performed in radiology on clients deemed too unstable for the surgery necessary for a portosystemic shunt. A stent is placed to redirect the blood flow.**

Diet

Clients with cirrhosis are placed on a low-protein diet, usually 40 grams per day. If ascites is present, sodium will also be restricted to 2 grams or less per day to decrease the amount of fluid retained by the body. Fluids also are restricted to 1,000 mL to 2,000 mL per day depending on the severity of fluid accumulation.

Activity

Because fatigue is such a common symptom of cirrhosis, the client's tolerance for activity will be diminished. Plan rest periods during the day, and schedule activities between rests.

SAFETY

Cirrhosis

If hepatic encephalopathy is present, precautions are taken to ensure the client's safety, such as elevating bedrails and allowing the client to ambulate only with assistance, especially if the client's gait is unsteady.

Nursing Management

Monitor vital signs and mental status. Restrict fluid intake as ordered. Accurately record I&O. Weigh client daily and measure abdominal girth. Provide low-sodium, low-protein diet. Turn client every 2 hours and monitor for redness and skin breakdown. Assist with or provide frequent oral hygiene.

NURSING PROCESS

Assessment

Subjective Data

Clients describe fatigue, nausea, anorexia, weakness, and indigestion.

Objective Data

Assessment shows ascites, jaundice, enlarged liver and spleen, petechiae (small bruises on the skin), vomiting, weight loss, fever, epistaxis, and decreased breath sounds. Lethargy, confusion, or coma is present if encephalopathy has occurred.

Laboratory analysis includes a CBC, which will demonstrate low WBCs, RBCs, Hgb, and platelets. A liver panel will show an elevated bilirubin, alkaline phosphatase, GGT, ALT, and AST. Albumin will be low. PT, PTT, and clotting times will be delayed.

Nursing diagnoses for a client with cirrhosis include the following:

NURSING DIAGNOSES	PLANNING/OUTCOMES	NURSING INTERVENTIONS
*Disturbed **Thought** Processes* related to elevated serum ammonia level and hepatic coma	The client will experience an improved level of orientation within 48 hours of initiation of treatment.	Administer tap water enemas and lactulose as ordered to eliminate ammonia-rich stools. An NG tube may be placed to give lactulose if the client is comatose. Monitor ammonia level. Elevate bedrails to prevent injury. As coma lessens, reorient client frequently.
*Excess **Fluid** Volume* related to ascites	The client will have less ascites by discharge.	Weigh daily. Educate client to notify physician of weight gain of 1½ lbs or more in 1 week. Measure abdominal girth daily. Restrict fluid to 1,000 to 2,000 mL per day depending on the severity of the ascites. Provide low-sodium diet of 500 to 2,000 mg a day depending on severity of the ascites. Teach client how to measure fluids and calculate sodium in diet. If a paracentesis is done, check vital signs every 15 minutes during the procedure and after the procedure until the vitals are stable. The amount of fluid removed from the abdomen is measured and sent to the laboratory.
*Risk for Impaired **Skin** Integrity* related to accumulation of bile salts in skin, poor skin turgor, ascites, and edema	The client will not experience skin breakdown while hospitalized.	Provide egg crate mattress. Turn client every 2 hours. Monitor skin closely for redness and skin breakdown. Apply lotion to skin frequently, especially to pressure areas. Assist with ADLs to promote good hygiene and conserve client's energy.

(*Continues*)

Nursing diagnoses for a client with cirrhosis include the following: (Continued)

NURSING DIAGNOSES	PLANNING/OUTCOMES	NURSING INTERVENTIONS
Imbalanced Nutrition: Less than Body Requirements related to inadequate diet, anorexia, or vomiting	The client will eat a balanced diet of 1,500 calories a day.	Offer small, high-calorie meals frequently. Offer high-nutrient supplements if client is unable to maintain adequate caloric intake. Assist and encourage client to eat. Provide frequent oral hygiene. Observe for changes in mental status that would interfere with caloric intake (e.g., increased lethargy).

Evaluation: Evaluate each outcome to determine how it has been met by the client.

HEPATITIS

Hepatitis is a chronic or acute inflammation of the liver caused by a virus, bacteria, drugs, alcohol abuse, or other toxic substances. There is a diffuse inflammatory reaction with liver cells degenerating and dying. The functions of the liver slow down. Because viral infections are the most common cause of hepatitis, emphasis will be placed on viral hepatitis within the chapter.

Researchers are still learning about the viruses that cause hepatitis. Seven viruses are known to cause hepatitis: A, B, C, D, E, F, and G.

Dustia (2005) describes hepatitis F as similar to hepatitis A and E and hepatitis G usually as a coinfection with hepatitis C. Hepatitis F has no serologic test and is diagnosed by seeing the virus with an electron microscope. Hepatitis G is transmitted by blood. Most clients have no symptoms, and 90% to 100% develop chronic infection. The viruses are similar and have almost identical signs and symptoms. Incubation period, mode of transmission, treatment and prognosis vary. See Table 38-5 for a summary of hepatitis viruses A–E.

MEDICAL–SURGICAL MANAGEMENT

Treatment is focused on resting the liver and early detection of complications. The liver is rested by modifying the diet so that less bile is needed to digest the food. Treatment is related to the signs and symptoms present and the prevention of transmission.

Pharmacological

Antiemetics such as hydroxyzine hydrochloride (Atarax, also Vistaril) or trimethobenzamide hydrochloride (Tigan) are given before meals for nausea. IV hydration with vitamin C for healing may be ordered. A vitamin B complex also is ordered to help clients absorb fat-soluble vitamins. Vitamin K may be ordered if clotting time is prolonged. All unnecessary medications, especially sedatives, are avoided.

Those exposed to hepatitis B by needle puncture or sexual contact should have hepatitis B immunoglobin (HBIG). Vaccines for hepatitis A (HAV) and hepatitis B (HBV) are available. HAV vaccine is recommended for persons 2 years of age and older at risk for exposure to hepatitis A such as homosexuals, IV drug users, travelers to countries with poor sanitation conditions, and laboratory workers who handle live hepatitis A virus (CDC, 2009). HBV vaccine is recommended as a routine vaccination for all 0 to 18 years olds and for those in high-risk groups (CDC, 2009). The Food and Drug Administration approved a combined hepatitis A and B vaccine in September 2001. It is recommended for persons younger than age 18 years and those in a high-risk group.

Diet

Diet modifications include decreasing fat intake to decrease the amount of bile needed in the digestive tract. A low-protein diet is needed if the client's liver is no longer able to metabolize the protein. Anorexia is a common symptom that can be treated with small, frequent, high-calorie meals. Fluids are restricted if the client retains fluids. No alcoholic beverages are recommended for at least 1 year or longer.

Activity

Bed rest is usually recommended for the first several weeks, generally at home unless the serum bilirubin is greater than 10 mg/dL or the PT is prolonged. If either occurs, hospitalization is usually recommended. Once bed rest is no longer necessary, activity is increased gradually because fatigue will be present for up to several months. Rest periods are included throughout the day.

NURSING MANAGEMENT

Follow Standard Precautions with all clients and Enteric Precautions for hepatitis A and E. Teach clients to always follow proper hand hygiene. For hepatitis A and E, be careful about consuming contaminated food and/or water. Hepatitis B spreads through blood and body fluids. Health care workers are at risk for hepatitis B and C. Most clients with hepatitis have flu-like symptoms, weight loss, hepatomegaly, jaundice, dark yellow urine, and light stools. Monitor laboratory test results for increased levels of bilirubin, GGT, AST, ALT, LDH, and alkaline phosphatase. Clotting time and PT are prolonged. Encourage low-fat, low-protein, high-calorie frequent small meals and fluid intake of 2,500 to 3,000 mL daily. Bed rest is important for the first several weeks and then a gradual increase in activity with rest periods several times a day.

Table 38-5 Comparison of Different Types of Viral Hepatitis

	A	B	C	D	E
Etiologic Agent	Hepatitis A virus (HAV)	Hepatitis B virus (HBV)	Hepatitis C virus (HCV)	Hepatitis D virus (HDV)	Hepatitis E virus (HEV)
Transmission	Fecal-oral; contaminated water or food; person to person	Blood or body fluids from infected person	Blood	Only persons with hepatitis B can get hepatitis D; blood and blood products; needlesticks; seldom sexual; rarely perinatal	Oral-fecal route; contaminated water; person to person uncommon
Risk Groups	Household/sexual contact with infected person; international travelers	Intravenous drug users; sexual/ household contact with infected person; infants born to infected mothers; health care workers; multiple sex partners	Blood transfusions or organ transplants prior to 1992; sharing needles; exposure to blood and blood products	Needle sharing; needlesticks	Mainly travel to countries where endemic
Incubation Period	15–50 days	45–160 days	14–180 days	15–60 days	15–60 days
Infectious Period	Usually less than 2 months	Before symptoms appear; lifetime if chronic	Before symptoms appear; lifetime if chronic	Not determined	Not determined
Diagnostic Tests	IgM anti-HAV	HBsAg	EIA-3; RIBA serum ALT increased 10x; HCVRNA-PCR	IgG anti-HDV and/ or Igm anti-HDV	None available
Symptoms	Flu-like; jaundice; dark yellow urine; light colored stools	Flu-like; may have jaundice; dark yellow urine; light colored stools	80% have no symptoms; flu-like	Flu-like; may have jaundice; dark yellow urine; light colored stools	Abdominal pain; anorexia; dark yellow urine; jaundice; fever
Prevention	Standard Precautions; Enteric Precautions; hepatitis A vaccine (entire series); immune globulin (for short term)	Standard Precautions; reduce risk behaviors; hepatitis B vaccine (entire series); immune globulin (for short term)	Standard Precautions; reduce risk behaviors; no vaccine	Standard Precautions; reduce risk behaviors; hepatitis B vaccine; if client already has hepatitis B, no prevention for hepatitis D	Standard Precautions; be sure water safe when traveling; no vaccine
Treatment	Immune globulin within 2 weeks of exposure	Immune globulin (HBIg); alpha interferon; lamivudine (Epivir-HBV); adefovirdipivoxil (Hepsera)	Peginterferon alfa-2a (Pegasys); ribavirin (Virazole)	Alpha interferon	None given

(*Continues*)

Table 38-5 Comparison of Different Types of Viral Hepatitis (Continued)

	A	B	C	D	E
Prognosis	Rarely fatal; no chronicity; resolves on its own in several weeks	No cure; may become chronic	75% to 85% have chronic infection; 70% develop chronic liver disease	Low risk of chronicity	No evidence of chronicity

Data from Viral Hepatitis A. By Centers for Disease Control and Prevention (CDC), 2009a, retrieved from www.cdc.gov/ncidod/diseases/hepatitis/a/fact.htm; Viral Hepatitis B. By CDC, 2009b, retrieved from www.cdc.gov/ncidod/diseases/hepatitis/b/fact.htm; Viral Hepatitis C. By CDC, 2009c, retrieved from www.cdc.gov/ncidod/diseases/hepatitis/c/fact.htm; Viral Hepatitis D. By CDC, 2009d, retrieved from www.cdc.gov/ncidod/diseases/hepatitis/slideset/hep-d.htm; Viral Hepatitis E. By CDC, 2009e, retreived from www.cdc.gov/ncidod/diseases/hepatitis/slideset/hep-e.htm; Peginterferon alfa-2a plus ribavirin for chronic hepatitis C virus infection, by M. W. Fried, M. L. Shiffman, et al., 2002e, *New England Journal of Medicine, 347*(13), 975; Resolution of chronic delta hepatitis after 12 years of interferon alpha therapy. By D. T. Lau, D. E. Kleiner, Y. Park, A. M. DiBisceglie, & J. H. Hoofnagle, 1999, *Gastroenterology, 117*(5), 1229-33; What I need to know about hepatitis C. By NIDDK, 2006, retrieved from www.niddk.nih.gov/health/digest/pubs/hep/hepc/hepc.htm; Viral hepatitis A to E and Beyond. By National Institute of Diabetes and Digestive and Kidney Diseases (NIDDK) 2008a, retrieved from www.niddk.nih.gov/health/digest/pubs/hep/hepa-e/hepa-e.htm; What I need to know about hepatitis A. By NIDDK, 2008b, retrieved from www.niddk.nih.gov/health/digest/pubs/hep/hepa/hepa.htm; What I need to know about hepatitis B. By NIDDK, 2008c, retrieved from www.niddk.nih.gov/health/digest/ pubs/hep/hepb/hepb.htm; Speaking out about the silent epidemic, by S. Parini, 2001, *Nursing 2001*, 31(3), 36–42; FDA approves new treatment for chronic hepatitis B. By U.S. Food and Drug Administration, 2002, retrieved from www.fda.gov/bbs/topics/ANSWERS/2002/ANS01163.html.

NURSING PROCESS

Assessment

Subjective Data

Symptoms include fatigue, anorexia, photophobia, nausea, headaches, abdominal pain, generalized muscle aches, chills, pruritis, and bloating.

Objective Data

The client may have weight loss, hepatomegaly, fever, jaundice, dark amber urine, and clay-colored stools.

Laboratory analysis shows an increased level of bilirubin, GGT, AST, ALT, LDH, and alkaline phosphatase. Clotting time and PT are prolonged. Specific hepatitis test is elevated (refer to Table 38-5).

CRITICAL THINKING

Hepatitis and Lifestyle

What lifestyle changes are necessary with a diagnosis of hepatitis A, B, C, or D?

Nursing diagnoses for a client with hepatitis include the following:

NURSING DIAGNOSES	PLANNING/OUTCOMES	NURSING INTERVENTIONS
*Deficient **K**nowledge* related to disease process, treatment regimen, and mode of transmission	The client will be able to explain disease process, incubation period, and mode of transmission, by discharge. The client will practice precautions to prevent spread of disease. The client will be able to select a menu using foods from the food guide pyramid and maintain a low-fat, low-protein diet.	Assess client's learning style and present information in a manner compatible with learning style. Educate about disease process and incubation period. Teach proper hand hygiene technique and emphasize importance of washing hands after using the bathroom. Emphasize that client cannot donate blood. Emphasize importance of follow-up laboratory analysis. Instruct in selection of low-fat, low-protein diet. For clients with hepatitis A, teach client to disinfect articles contaminated with feces (such as the toilet), not to prepare food for others, and not to share articles such as eating utensils or toothbrushes. For clients with hepatitis B, teach to avoid sexual contact until they test negative for HBsAg or their partners are immunized with the HBV vaccine.

Nursing diagnoses for a client with hepatitis include the following: (Continued)

NURSING DIAGNOSES	PLANNING/OUTCOMES	NURSING INTERVENTIONS
		For clients with hepatitis C, teach that it is unknown whether it can be transmitted through sexual contact, so precautions are recommended until more is known.
*Imbalanced **N**utrition: Less than Body Requirements* related to inadequate caloric intake, fat intolerance, nausea, and vomiting	The client will maintain a caloric intake of 2,000 calories/day.	Monitor I&O every shift. Weigh daily. Offer small, frequent, high-calorie, low-fat meals. Encourage low-protein diet of 40 gm of protein. Monitor daily calorie count. Offer largest meal in morning, as food tends to be tolerated better in the morning. Encourage fluid intake of 2,500 to 3,000 mL daily. Note color and consistency of stools and color of urine. Administer antiemetic 30 minutes before meals as ordered.
***F**atigue* related to decreased energy production and altered body chemistry	The client will verbalize plan to modify activity, by discharge.	Educate client regarding reasons for fatigue and that fatigue may be present for several months. Encourage client to maintain bed rest for several weeks. Advise client that when resuming normal activity, rest periods should be included until stamina returns.

Evaluation: Evaluate each outcome to determine how it has been met by the client.

PANCREATITIS

Pancreatitis is an acute or chronic inflammation of the pancreas caused when pancreatic enzymes digest the lining of the pancreas. Pancreatitis occurs when obstruction of the pancreatic duct occurs as a result of gallstones, tumors, exposure to chemicals or alcohol, or injury to the pancreas. In severe cases, the pancreas can hemorrhage, resulting in a life-threatening condition.

Medical–Surgical Management

Medical

Treatment depends on the cause of the pancreatitis. If the pancreatitis results from exposure to chemical or alcohol abuse, treatment is primarily medical. An NG tube is inserted to rest the bowel and relieve abdominal distention.

Surgical

If the pancreatitis is caused by structural changes such as gallstones, an endoscopic retrograde cholangiopancreatogram (ERCP) with stone removal is performed. Surgery to relieve the pancreatic duct obstruction is necessary in cases where tumors or injury are the causes of the pancreatitis.

Pharmacological

Insulin is administered if the client's pancreas is unable to secrete enough to maintain normal blood sugar level. If nausea and vomiting are present, antiemetics are ordered. Meperidine (Demerol) is ordered for analgesia because morphine sulfate may cause spasms of the sphincter of Oddi. Atropine sulfate or propantheline bromide (Pro-Banthine) is ordered to decrease pancreatic activity. Antacids or an H_2 receptor antagonist is ordered to prevent stress ulcers.

Diet

Clients are kept NPO while the serum amylase level is elevated to decrease the demand for digestive enzymes in the bowel. An NG tube is inserted to decrease pancreatic activity and to prevent nausea, vomiting, and abdominal distention. As the serum amylase level begins to decrease, clients are started on clear liquids and slowly advanced to a bland, low-fat, high-protein, high-carbohydrate diet. No coffee or alcohol is allowed.

IV rehydration is necessary while the client is NPO. If the pancreatitis is severe and the client must be NPO for a prolonged period, TPN, a high-calorie, high-nutrient IV solution, is administered.

Activity

Clients are generally placed on bed rest to decrease metabolic rate. Activity is increased as the serum amylase decreases.

Nursing Management

Monitor and maintain NG tube. Weigh client daily and maintain client on bed rest. Assess pain and administer an analgesic. Monitor vital signs. Provide personal hygiene. Assess and maintain IV hydration and TPN if ordered. Accurately record

I&O. Monitor laboratory results, especially serum amylase, bilirubin, electrolytes, and H & H.

NURSING PROCESS

Assessment

Subjective Data

Clients describe excruciating epigastric pain that radiates to the back. Pain may decrease by leaning forward or lying in a fetal position. Nausea and anorexia are also present.

Objective Data

Assessment includes steatorrhea, vomiting, low-grade fever, tachycardia, and jaundice. Laboratory analysis shows an elevated serum amylase followed by an elevated urine amylase and serum lipase, leukocytosis, and an increased Hct. Glucose, alkaline phosphatase, and bilirubin may also be elevated.

Nursing diagnoses for a client with pancreatitis include the following:

NURSING DIAGNOSES	PLANNING/OUTCOMES	NURSING INTERVENTIONS
*Acute **Pain*** related to inflammation and edema of the pancreas	The client will verbalize a decrease in pain as evidenced by pain scale by 1 hour after initiation of interventions.	Monitor NG tube to decompress the abdomen. Position client in most comfortable position. Assess pain for increasing severity that would indicate worsening pancreatitis. Administer analgesics as ordered and monitor for relief. Monitor serum amylase, WBCs, and H & H for signs of increasing severity of pancreatitis or hemorrhage.
*Imbalanced **Nutrition**: Less than Body Requirements* related to NPO status, nausea, vomiting, and altered ability to digest nutrients	The client will experience no further weight loss during hospitalization.	Monitor I&O every shift. Administer IV rehydration or TPN as ordered. Weigh client daily. Maintain bed rest to decrease the metabolic rate. Insert NG tube to decompress the abdomen as ordered.
*Risk for Deficient **Fluid** Volume* related to vomiting, NG tube, or hemorrhage	The client will maintain adequate hydration as evidenced by I&O that is nearly equal, electrolytes within normal limits, and moist mucous membranes.	Monitor I&O every shift. Administer IV hydration or TPN as ordered. Monitor electrolyte levels and H & H as ordered.

Evaluation: Evaluate each outcome to determine how it has been met by the client.

CHOLECYSTITIS AND CHOLELITHIASIS

Cholecystitis is an inflammation of the gallbladder. In >90% of the cases, gallstones are present. **Cholelithiasis** is the presence of gallstones or **calculi** (concentration of mineral salts) in the gallbladder. Not all gallstones cause cholecystitis. Some gallstones pass out of the gallbladder and into the duodenum with the client unaware of the stones. Sometimes gallstones migrate into the cystic or common bile duct causing an obstruction that, in turn, leads to cholecystitis. The exact cause of the formation of these stones is not known.

These two diseases are more common in multiparous women, age 45 and older; obese people; those who use birth control pills or control cholesterol with gemfibrozil (Lopid); and people with a history of a disease of the small intestine such as Crohn's disease. Also, clients on sudden weight reduction diets that are low in fat will cause the bile to pool in the gallbladder, increasing the risk for gallstone formation.

Ultrasound of the gallbladder is ordered if gallstones are suspected.

Medical–Surgical Management

In asymptomatic clients, no intervention is necessary.

Medical

If stones are lodged in the common bile duct, an ERCP is performed.

Surgical

A sphincterotomy, an incision in the ampulla of vater, is performed to enlarge the opening of the common bile duct. Stones are then removed or crushed. If the stones are too large or in the case of clients with repeated episodes of cholelithiasis, a cholecystectomy, the surgical removal of the gallbladder, is performed. The cholecystectomy is performed laparoscopically or by making a large abdominal incision.

Laparoscopic cholecystectomies have become the surgery of choice for cholelithiasis and cholecystitis. The gallbladder is removed by making four small incisions and extracting the gallbladder through an endoscope. If the cholecystectomy is performed laparoscopically, it is more difficult to perform an exploration of the common bile duct, especially in clients with cholecystitis. An ERCP may need to be performed if stones remain in the common bile duct (CBD). Clients are ready for discharge 24 hours after the surgery.

The cholecystectomy can also be performed by making a large abdominal incision. A cholangiogram can be performed easily, and therefore this type of procedure is more common in clients with much inflammation of the gallbladder. If damage has occurred to the CBD from severe inflammation or a stone, a T-tube will be left in place to allow the bile to drain into a collection bag. This allows the CBD to heal. Clients are typically ready for discharge 3 to 7 days after surgery.

Pharmacological

In acute cholecystitis, analgesics are ordered to relieve discomfort. Meperidine (Demerol) is preferred because morphine sulfate is believed to increase sphincter spasms. IV hydration is ordered if the client is unable to maintain hydration. Antiemetics are ordered for nausea and vomiting. In clients who have surgery, analgesics are ordered after surgery to control discomfort.

Diet

In clients with mild or moderate symptoms, a clear liquid diet to rest the bowel, followed by small frequent meals low in fat, may resolve the symptoms.

If clients are to have surgery, they will be NPO before surgery and initially after surgery until bowel sounds return. They are started on clear liquids first and then advanced, as tolerated, to a regular diet.

Activity

In acute cases of cholecystitis, bed rest is recommended to decrease metabolic rate. If surgery is performed, the client is encouraged to turn, cough, and deep breathe every 2 hours initially after surgery. On the day after surgery, the client is assisted out of bed and encouraged to gradually increase activity. Clients who have a laparoscopic cholecystectomy are ambulated within hours of returning from the recovery room. Clients usually leave the hospital later on the day of surgery, but may stay overnight depending on their overall condition (University of Michigan Health System, 2009). Clients return to normal activities within 4-5 days and typically return to previous activity level 2 weeks after surgery. Clients who have an incision restrict lifting, driving, and exercise until incisional healing is complete, usually 4 to 6 weeks.

Nursing Management

Monitor vital signs and bowel sounds. Assess pain, nausea, and vomiting and administer analgesic and/or antiemetic. Prepare for surgery by teaching deep breathing, coughing, splinting incision, incentive spirometry use, and leg exercises. Monitor and maintain NG tube if used. Accurately record I&O.

NURSING PROCESS

Assessment

Subjective Data

Clients describe pain in the right upper quadrant radiating to the right scapular area that occurs 2 to 4 hours after a meal containing significant amounts of fat, nausea, flatulence, and indigestion.

Objective Data

Assessment shows vomiting, occasionally a fever, jaundice, steatorrhea, clay-colored stools, and dark amber urine. Laboratory analysis shows increased alkaline phosphatase, GGT, WBCs, and bilirubin.

Nursing diagnoses for a client with cholecystitis and cholelithiasis include the following:

NURSING DIAGNOSES	PLANNING/OUTCOMES	NURSING INTERVENTIONS
*Acute **Pain*** related to inflammation or blocked bile duct	The client will experience less pain as evidenced by pain scale within 1 hour of initiation of treatment.	Keep client NPO or on a clear liquid diet as ordered. Administer analgesics as ordered. Monitor NG tube to decompress the abdomen as ordered. Observe for jaundice and bile flow obstruction.
*Ineffective **Breathing** Pattern* related to decreased lung expansion because of pain	The client will demonstrate appropriate breathing pattern and will not have respiratory complications while hospitalized.	Assist client to cough and breathe deeply every 2 hours. Teach use of incentive spirometer. Teach splinting techniques for comfort and to facilitate breathing. Turn client every 2 hours and ambulate as soon as indicated.
*Risk for Deficient **Fluid** Volume* related to nausea, NG tube, NPO, or bile drainage	The client will maintain adequate hydration as evidenced by I&O that is nearly equal and moist mucous membranes.	Monitor I&O every shift including NG drainage and T-tube drainage if present. Administer IV hydration as ordered. Maintain patency of NG tube.

Evaluation: Evaluate each outcome to determine how it has been met by the client.

NEOPLASMS OF THE GASTROINTESTINAL SYSTEM

Neoplasms of the gastrointestinal system may occur anyplace in the GI system. Signs, symptoms, and treatment vary according to where the cancer occurs. Oral cancer, colorectal cancer, and liver cancer are discussed following.

ORAL CANCER

Oral cancer refers to cancers of the lips, tongue, oral cavity, and pharynx. According to the American Cancer Society (ACS, 2009), 35,720 new cases are expected that year. Risk factors are tobacco use and excessive consumption of alcohol. Symptoms include a mouth sore that bleeds easily and does not heal, a lump, or difficulty chewing, swallowing, or moving tongue or jaw. On the lips, the cancer may be a growth.

MEDICAL–SURGICAL MANAGEMENT

Surgical

Treatment is primarily surgical and involves removal of the cancer with excision of tissue and lymph nodes surrounding the cancer. In cases of cancer involving the pharynx, a radical neck dissection is performed, which requires reconstruction of the pharynx. Clients undergoing radical neck dissection frequently have a tracheostomy.

Pharmacological

Chemotherapy is not effective against most oral cancers and is, therefore, used only in the most severe cases with metastases. Medications ordered are based on the client's symptoms. If the client is experiencing side effects from the radiation such as nausea, antiemetics are ordered.

If a client has surgery, analgesics are ordered postoperatively. Analgesics are also ordered if the cancer has progressed and is causing discomfort.

Diet

Because the surgery is in the oral area, it may be difficult to maintain adequate nutrition. Depending on the extent of the surgery, clients require a soft diet or, in some cases, nutritional supplements to allow the surgical area to heal. Tube feedings, either by a feeding tube or by a gastrostomy tube (a special tube inserted through the abdomen into the stomach), are frequently needed in clients who have undergone a radical neck dissection.

Activity

If the surgery is minor, no activity restrictions are necessary. If surgery is extensive, postoperatively, the client will need to turn, cough, and deep breathe. Activity is increased postoperatively. Clients receiving radiation treatments frequently experience fatigue and need scheduled rest periods.

Other Therapies

In cases where the lesion cannot be surgically removed, radiation and/or radium implants is/are used. High-energy radiation is used to destroy cancer cells. Clients may experience irritated skin, swallowing difficulties, dry mouth, nausea, diarrhea, hair loss, or fatigue. Radiation is usually administered daily for a specified period. If radium implants are used, a radioactive capsule is implanted into the area.

NURSING MANAGEMENT

Encourage all clients to refrain from tobacco use and excessive alcohol consumption. Maintain feeding tube and administer tube feedings as ordered. Preoperatively, teach client to turn, cough, and deep breathe, and encourage client to practice postoperatively. Weigh client daily and accurately record I&O.

NURSING PROCESS

ASSESSMENT

Subjective Data

Clients describe a sore throat, difficulty swallowing, or a painful area in the mouth.

Objective Data

Assessment reveals a sore or lesion of the lips or in the oral cavity, and hoarseness.

Nursing diagnoses for a client with oral cancer include the following:

NURSING DIAGNOSES	PLANNING/OUTCOMES	NURSING INTERVENTIONS
Fear related to diagnosis and long-term prognosis	The client will verbalize fear and express plan to cope with diagnosis.	Allow client time alone and with significant others and client and family to express fears and concerns. Answer questions. Encourage contact with support system (e.g., clergy). Discuss past experiences with stress and individual responses to those situations.

Nursing diagnoses for a client with oral cancer include the following: (Continued)

NURSING DIAGNOSES	PLANNING/OUTCOMES	NURSING INTERVENTIONS
*Imbalanced **N**utrition: Less than Body Requirements* related to oral surgery or radical neck dissection	The client will maintain weight while hospitalized.	Monitor I&O every shift. Weigh client daily. Administer tube feedings and IV rehydration as ordered and introduce fluids, when indicated. Monitor for aspiration.
*Disturbed **B**ody Image* related to disfiguring surgery	The client will verbalize feelings regarding surgery and altered body image.	Allow client time to verbalize feelings. Answer questions. Discuss options (e.g., plastic surgery or makeup). Provide information on support groups.

Evaluation: Evaluate each outcome to determine how it has been met by the client.

COLORECTAL CANCER

Colorectal cancer is the third most common site of new cancers and deaths in the United States (ACS, 2009). Almost all colorectal cancers arise from **polyps**, an abnormal growth of tissue that protrudes into the colon. Risk factors for colorectal cancer include age 50 or older, history of polyps, family history of polyps and/or colorectal cancer, a history of ulcerative colitis, and a diet high in fat and low in fiber.

Prognosis is very good if the cancer is caught in the early stages. Recommended routine screenings for early detection include fecal occult blood testing and colonoscopy depending on personal and family history.

A colonoscopy or barium enema may demonstrate the disease. A CBC may show anemia if the cancer is bleeding. A CEA may be effective in detecting recurrent cancer but is not a valid screening test. Signs and symptoms include a change in bowel habits, guaiac-positive stools, and abdominal pain.

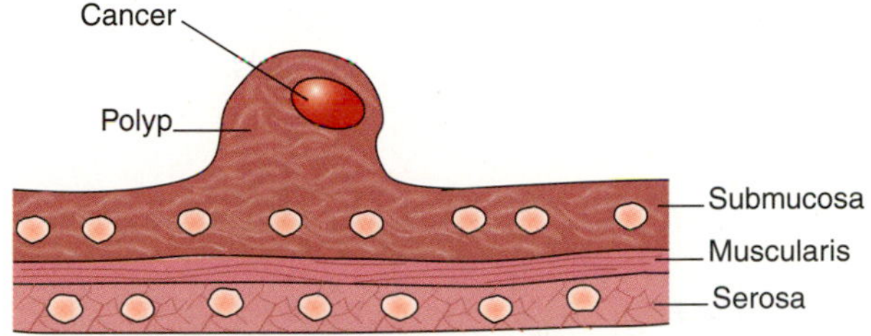

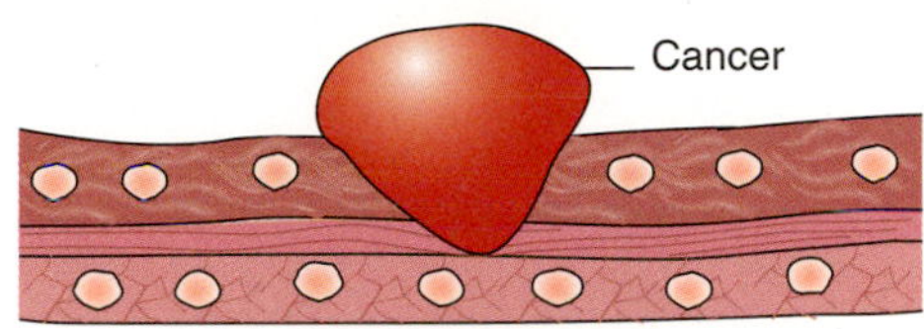

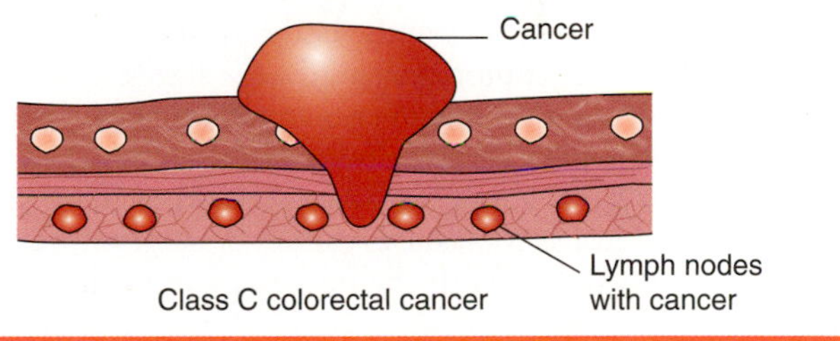

COURTESY OF DELMAR CENGAGE LEARNING

FIGURE 38-10 Classes of Colorectal Cancer

MEDICAL–SURGICAL MANAGEMENT

Surgical

Treatment is surgical to remove the cancer. In class A tumors, a colonoscopy is performed with a polypectomy, the removal of the polyp. In class B or C tumors, a colon resection is done (Figure 38-10). In some cases, a colostomy, either temporary or permanent, is performed. In class D tumors, surgery is done only to relieve symptoms (e.g., bowel obstruction). Follow-up colonoscopies must be performed throughout the client's life to monitor for recurrence of the disease.

Pharmacological

In cases of class B, C, and D tumors, chemotherapy is given after the surgery. Side effects of chemotherapy include nausea, vomiting, weight loss, hair loss, fatigue, and dry skin. Medications to combat some side effects of the chemotherapy are ordered. Immunotherapy as an adjunct therapy for class C and D tumors is ordered to boost the immune system.

Diet

Preoperatively, the client is NPO. Postoperatively, the client is NPO and an NG tube is in place until bowel sounds return. The client is then started on a clear liquid diet and progressed to a high-fiber, low-fat diet.

Activity

Postoperatively, the client is encouraged to turn, cough, and deep breathe every 2 hours. The client is ambulated the next day and activity is progressed.

Other Therapies

No significant benefits have been found with the use of radiation on colorectal cancer; however, radiation may be used on metastatic sites in class D tumors.

Nursing Management

Encourage all clients to have recommended routine screenings, fecal occult blood test, and colonoscopy, based on their personal and family history. Prepare client for side effects (hair loss, fatigue, nausea, and dry skin) when chemotherapy is used. Postoperatively, maintain the NG tube. Assess bowel sounds. Encourage turning, coughing, deep breathing, use of incentive spirometer, leg exercises, and ambulation.

NURSING PROCESS

Assessment

Subjective Data

Clients describe a change in bowel habits and possibly abdominal pain.

Objective Data

Stools may be guaiac positive for blood. An H & H may show anemia.

Nursing diagnoses for a client with colorectal cancer include the following:

NURSING DIAGNOSES	PLANNING/OUTCOMES	NURSING INTERVENTIONS
Fear related to diagnosis and long-term prognosis	The client will verbalize fear and express plan to cope with diagnosis.	Allow client time alone and with significant others and allow client and family to express fears and concerns. Answer questions and encourage contact with support system (e.g., clergy). Discuss past experiences with stress and identify individual responses to those situations.
*Deficient **Knowledge*** related to disease process, treatment options, and follow-up	The client will be able to explain disease process, treatment, and follow-up care.	Determine client's learning style and present information in a manner compatible with the learning style. Educate client regarding disease process and discuss treatment options. Recognize that information may need to be presented more than once.

Evaluation: Evaluate each outcome to determine how it has been met by the client.

LIVER CANCER

Primary liver cancer is rare. Most liver tumors are metastatic from other sites in the body. Most cases of primary liver cancer are asymptomatic until later stages. Risk factors for primary liver cancer include a history of cirrhosis, hepatitis B, and exposure to toxic chemicals.

A primary liver tumor can be removed surgically if the disease is not extensive. Metastases cannot be surgically removed and are usually treated with chemotherapy and radiation.

Obesity

According to the National Heart Lung and Blood Institute (NHLBI), the body mass index (BMI) measures body fat in relation to an individual's height and weight. The BMI determines an individual's weight according to categories of underweight, normal weight, overweight, or obese. According to the World Health Organization, an individual is overweight with a BMI of 30 or greater and morbidly obese with a BMI of 40 or greater. The NHLBI website provides a formula to automatically calculate an individual's BMI: http://www.nhlbisupport.com/bmi/

The National Center for Health Statistics (2007) reported that more than one third of adult Americans (>72 million people) were obese in 2005 to 2006 (Ogden, Carrol, McDowell, & Flegal, 2007). Between 2000 and 2005, the number of obese cases rose 24% and morbidly obese cases with a BMI of >40 and 50 increased 50% and 75%, respectively.

A 1990 study by Blumberg and Mellis reported that 78% of preoperative bariatric clients felt health care professionals "always" or "usually" treated them with disrespect. Another study 12 years later in 2002 by Kaminsky and Gadaleta revealed very similar results. Kaminsky and Gadaleta concluded their results were because health care providers do not understand the disease of obesity, its causes, or the medical consequences if not treated. Little data suggest that health care providers' attitudes affected their delivery of care. In other words, the medical/nursing care was provided but the "caring" attitude was not perceived. Clients having bariatric surgery deserve respect for privacy and deserve kind, compassionate care. To provide clients with compassionate, quality care, health care providers may desire to analyze personal attitudes toward obesity and take appropriate steps to care for each individual as a valued person of worth.

The obese client presents challenges to the health care provider. The extra soft tissue makes it difficult to assess heart and lung sounds, and significant abnormalities can be missed. A nurse needs the appropriate equipment to assess and care for the obese client, such as an extra large blood pressure cuff to obtain an accurate reading. A blood pressure cuff that is too small gives an elevated reading. An echocardiograph may be more accurate than an EKG. Fatigue and lethargy along with nausea and

SAFETY

Weight Limitations with Equipment

When caring for an obese client, consider the weight limits on equipment such as stretchers, toilets, and bedside commodes. If these weight limitations are not considered, staff and clients are at risk for injury (Wolf, 2008).

vomiting are possible symptoms of a cardiac or glycemic emergency (Wolf, 2008). Obese clients have more difficulty breathing and present issues with intubation. A guided ultrasonography assists with IV insertion, and an extra long needle is used for central venous catheter placement. Obese clients are at risk for rapid skin breakdown, hypercoagulopathy leading to venous thromboembolism, and pulmonary emboli after surgery. Pneumonia is a risk because of immobility, difficulty taking deep breaths, and extra soft tissue on the chest (Wolf, 2008). Signs of hypoxia are lethargy, mental status changes, and restlessness. Regular-size stretchers are not safe because the client makes the stretcher top-heavy and causes it to tip over. Skin pressure sores also may occur from the side rails. Therefore, bariatric stretchers and beds provide stability and client safety.

Medical-Surgical Management

Health care professionals are reluctant to discuss weight loss with clients. In a national study of adults with a BMI of ≥30 only 42% reported that a health care provider discussed the need for weight loss (Calonge, 2004). The health care provider could suggest a monitored weight-loss program with nutritional counseling and exercise to assist the overweight client. If these interventions do not work and the client desires to lose weight, the health care provider makes a referral to a bariatrician (a specialist in the treatment of obesity and obese diseases).

Bariatric surgery may be a client option and includes a restrictive or malabsorptive surgery. The laparoscopic adjustable gastric band is a restrictive surgery. A band is placed laproscopically around the proximal stomach distal to the gastroesophagel junction as shown in Figure 38-11A. A tube is connected to the band and threaded through the abdomen to the abdominal wall, where it is connected to an access port. The access port is anchored to the fascia. Throughout the next year, the physician injects saline into the access port to restrict the stomach size so the client loses weight.

The Roux-en-Y gastric bypass is a malabsorptive surgery. A section of the stomach close to the gastroesophageal junction is divided from the remaining stomach by stapling along the dividing line as shown in Figure 38-11B. A section of the jejunum is anastomosed to the stomach pouch. The remaining stomach, duodenum, and proximal jejunum are anastomosed distally on the jejunum. Weight loss occurs for 2 reasons: the restricted stomach area cannot hold as much food and the bypassed bowel section cannot absorb as many calories and nutrients from ingested food. Thus, it is called a malabsorptive surgery. This surgery bypasses the part of the small intestine that absorbs calcium, iron, and other nutrients placing the client at risk for chronic nutritional deficits and vitamin B_{12} anemias. After the surgery, the client is placed on multivitamin and mineral supplements.

Nursing Management

Postoperatively the nurse maintains the client's oxygen saturation at 92% by administering 2 to 4 L of oxygen by nasal cannula or, if client tolerates it, room air. Encourage the client to use the incentive spirometer every 2 hours. The head of the bed is elevated to 45° to enhance breathing. If the client uses a continuous positive airway pressure device (CPAP),

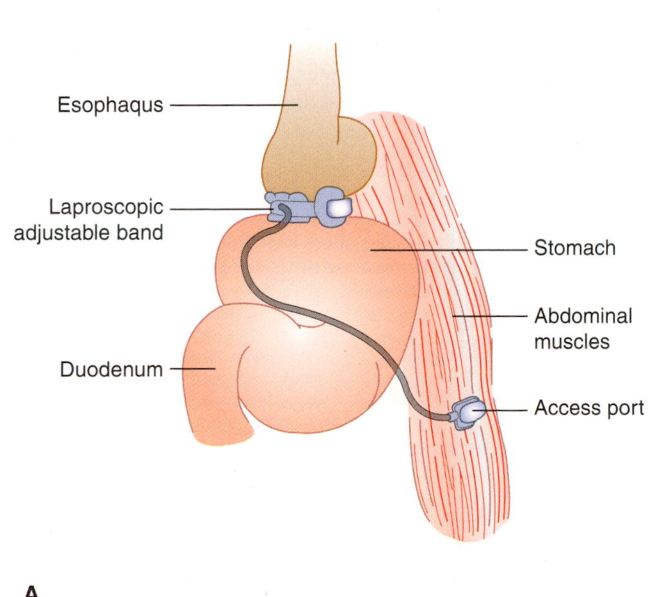

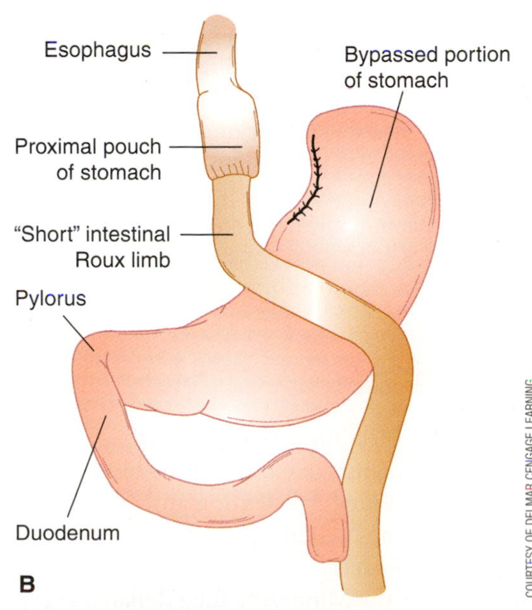

Figure 38-11 Types of Bariatric Surgery; *A*, Laparoscopic Adjustable Gastric Banding; *B*, Roux-en-Y Gastric Bypass

continue using it in the hospital. The nurse assesses pain regularly, monitors PCA use, and obtains appropriate orders to manage pain (Sammons, 2002). If an NG tube is in place, the nurse does not reposition the NG tube as the movement may damage the suture line. The client takes sips of water and, if tolerated, slowly progresses to eating very small portions of pureed food or juices. The nurse teaches diet modifications and exercise to assist the client in controlling weight. Weight loss is a lifetime challenge.

Postoperative complications are nausea and dumping syndrome. The nurse assesses for abdominal distension, diarrhea, cramping, hypotension, flushing, and tachycardia indicating symptoms of dumping syndrome that last 20 to 30 minutes. Dumping syndrome is a common side effect caused by eating simple sugars. It is a benign problem that possibly can be modified by decreasing the ingestion of simple sugar.

CASE STUDY

R.J. is a 52-year-old woman admitted to the hospital with acute abdominal pain. R.J. complains of right upper quadrant pain radiating to the back. She has had previous episodes, usually occurring about 2 hours after eating. This episode, however, is not resolving. R.J. also complains of nausea. Her vital signs are BP 152/88 mmHg, pulse 92 beats/min, and respirations 24 breaths/min and shallow. R.J. is a slightly obese female who states she has recently been dieting to lose weight. Laboratory analysis includes a CBC with slightly elevated WBCs, elevated bilirubin, and elevated alkaline phosphatase. An IV is started, and R.J. is given meperidine (Demerol) IM for pain. R.J. has been made NPO. An ultrasound of the gallbladder is ordered.

The following questions will guide your development of a nursing care plan for this case study.

1. List subjective and objective data a nurse would want to obtain about R.J.
2. List risk factors other than those R.J. has that would put a client at risk for developing cholecystitis.
3. List two nursing diagnoses and goals for R.J.
4. The ERCP is successful in removing the CBD stone. The decision is made to perform a laparoscopic cholecystectomy. What teaching will R.J. need?
5. Why is meperidine (Demerol) the medication of choice for pain control?
6. List at least three successful outcomes for R.J.

SUMMARY

- The gastrointestinal system is a complex system composed of the digestive tract as well as accessory organs.
- Disorders of the GI tract affect the breakdown and absorption of nutrients, breakdown of wastes and by-products, and the lifestyle of the individual.
- Because the liver is responsible for so many functions in the body, disorders of the liver can affect other systems significantly.
- Peptic ulcers may be either gastric or duodenal. *H. pylori* is a common cause of ulcers and can be treated with antibiotics.
- Diverticulosis is a commonly occurring disorder in the United States and is believed to be caused by a low-fiber diet.
- Inflammatory bowel disease includes both Crohn's disease and ulcerative colitis. IBD can lead to nutritional imbalances, bowel obstructions, alterations in the structure of the intestine, and affected lifestyle.
- Bowel obstructions have multiple causes and can lead to electrolyte imbalances, dehydration, and possibly sepsis.
- Viral hepatitis is a concern for health care professionals at risk for exposure. Standard precautions must be used to prevent the transmission of the virus.
- Colorectal cancer is one of the most preventable forms of cancer if routine screenings are performed.

REVIEW QUESTIONS

1. A client with a bleeding esophageal varix:
   1. should be encouraged to vomit the blood to decrease abdominal distention and pressure.
   2. should have an NG tube placed to suction blood from the stomach.
   3. should have the Minnesota tube deflated every 4 hours.
   4. will not need follow-up once the bleeding has stopped.

2. A client with a perforated duodenal ulcer:
   1. requires an EGD to repair the perforation.
   2. may need diet modification after surgery.
   3. will have a vagotomy performed.
   4. may experience an increased risk for cholecystitis.

3. Clients with hepatitis C:
   1. should be instructed that all the mechanisms of transmission are not known.
   2. will have a negative HCV if they are a carrier.
   3. should be instructed that recombinant interferon alpha-2b will cure the hepatitis C.
   4. are not contagious until symptoms develop.
4. Crohn's disease:
   1. can be cured by removing the colon.
   2. usually causes clients to gain weight from the slower metabolism of nutrients.
   3. can be a debilitating disease leading to depression.
   4. is cured as long as the clients remain on 5-ASA compounds.
5. Hernias are a protrusion through the muscle wall and:
   1. can be easily reduced by the nurse applying gentle pressure.
   2. are benign occurrences that do not need any intervention.
   3. can lead to bowel obstructions.
   4. are caused by a lack of exercise.
6. Postoperative care of clients who have undergone gastric bypass surgery includes:
   1. immobilization of abdominal wound to stabilize the incision areas.
   2. keeping the head of the bed flat to avoid stressing the incision.
   3. allowing only sips of fluids and small amounts of food in soft consistency.
   4. bed rest to prevent complications from surgery in obese patients.
7. An excessively overweight client expressing a desire to lose weight must be advised initially to:
   1. decrease caloric intake.
   2. follow a weight loss diet and increase activity level.
   3. consider a referral for surgical intervention.
   4. participate in vigorous exercise.
8. A nurse gave dietary instructions to a client recently diagnosed with ulcerative colitis. What dietary choice indicates the client understands the appropriate foods to eat? (Select all that apply.)
   1. Apple.
   2. Lettuce salad.
   3. Refined pasta.
   4. Chunky peanut butter.
   5. Cream of asparagus soup.
   6. Cottage cheese.
9. A client is returning to the unit with a bowel resection from an intestinal obstruction. What is the nurse's first action when the client returns to the room?
   1. Encourage ambulation to stimulate the return of bowel function.
   2. Connect NG tube to suction to decompress the abdomen.
   3. Identify client's learning style and teach information in a manner compatible with learning style.
   4. Assess for pain and administer an analgesic as ordered.
10. A client is admitted to the unit with the diagnosis of a peptic ulcer. When assessing the client, the nurse would most likely find:
    1. epigastric pain that increases when the stomach is empty.
    2. stools that are fatty and foul smelling.
    3. alternating episodes of diarrhea and constipation.
    4. pain in the upper quadrant radiating to the right scapular area that occurs 2–4 hours after eating fatty foods.

REFERENCES/SUGGESTED READINGS

Ables, A., Simon, I., & Melton, E. (2007). Update on Helicobacter pylori treatment. *American Family Physician, 75*(3), 351–358.

American Cancer Society. (2007). What are the risk factors for stomach cancer? Retrieved March 28, 2008 from http://www.cancer.org/docroot/cri/content/cri

American Cancer Society. (2009a). Cancer facts & figures 2009. Retrieved from http://www.cancer.org/docroot/home/index.asp

American Cancer Society. (2009b). Colorectal cancer: Statistics and incidences. Retrieved from http://www.cancer.org/docroot/CRI/CRI_2_3x.asp?dt=10

Atassi, K. (2002a). Appendicitis. *Nursing2002, 32*(8), 96.

Atassi, K. (2002b). Bleeding esophageal varices. *Nursing2002, 32*(4), 96.

Barba, K., Fitzgerald, P., & Wood, S. (2007). Managing peptic ulcer disease: Learn how it develops and how to help your patient heal. *Nursing2007*, July, 1–4.

Bazensky, I., Shoobridge-Moran, C., & Yoder, L. (2007). Colorectal cancer: An overview of the epidemiology, risk factors, symptoms, and screening guidelines. *MedSurg Nursing, The Journal of Adult Health, 16*(1), 46–51.

Beattie, S. (2007). Bedside emergency: Hemorrhage. *RN, 70*(8), 30–35.

Blumberg, P., & Mellis, L. (1985). Medical students' attitudes toward the obese and the morbidly obese. *International Journal of Eating Disorders, 4*(2), 169–175.

Boekhold, K. (2000). Who's afraid of hepatitis C? *AJN, 100*(5), 26–31.

Bulechek, G., Butcher, H., McCloskey, J., & Dochterman, J., eds. (2008). *Nursing Interventions Classification (NIC)* (5th ed.). St. Louis, MO: Mosby/Elsevier.

Bunting, T. (2001). Putting the lid on gastroesophageal reflux. *Nursing2001, 31*(6), 46–49.

Calonge, N. (2004). Screening for obesity in adults: Recommendations and rationale. *American Journal of Nursing, 104*(5), 94–105.

Cameron, C., & Sawatzky, J. (2008). Postoperative pain management: The challenges of the patient with Crohn's disease. *MedSurg Nursing, The Journal of Adult Health, 17*(2), 85–91.

Cameron, J. (1998). *Current surgical therapy* (6th ed.). St. Louis, MO: Mosby.

Centers for Disease Control and Prevention (CDC). (2001). FDA approval for a combined hepatitis A and B vaccine. *MMWR, 50*(37), 806–807. Retrieved May 28, 2009 from www.cdc.gov/mmwr/preview/mmwrhtml/mm5037a4.htm

Centers for Disease Control and Prevention (CDC). (2009a). Viral hepatitis A. Retrieved May 28, 2009 from www.cdc.gov/ncidod/diseases/hepatitis/a/fact.htm

Centers for Disease Control and Prevention (CDC). (2009b). Viral hepatitis B. Retrieved May 28, 2009 from www.cdc.gov/ncidod/diseases/hepatitis/b/fact.htm

Centers for Disease Control and Prevention (CDC). (2009c). Viral hepatitis C. Retrieved May 28, 2009 from www.cdc.gov/ncidod/diseases/hepatitis/c/fact.htm

Centers for Disease Control and Prevention (CDC). (2009d). Viral hepatitis D. Retrieved May 28, 2009 from www.cdc.gov/ncidod/diseases/hepatitis/slideset/hep-d.htm

Centers for Disease Control and Prevention (CDC). (2009e). Viral hepatitis E. Retrieved May 28, 2009 from www.cdc.gov/ncidod/diseases/hepatitis/slideset/hep-e/htm

Chene, B., & Decker, A. (2001). Battling hepatitis C. *RN, 64*(4), 54–58.

Clinical Rounds. (2003). Acetaminophen linked to most liver failure cases. *Nursing2003, 33*(3), 34.

Cole, L. (2001). Unraveling the mystery of acute pancreatitis. *Nursing2001, 31*(12), 58–63.

Cox, C., Evans, P., Withers, T., & Titmuss, K. (2008). The importance of gastrointestinal nurses being HLA-B27 aware. *Gastrointestinal Nursing, 6*(9), 32–40.

Daniels, R. (2009). *Delmar's guide to laboratory and diagnostic tests* (2nd ed.). Clifton Park, NY: Delmar Cengage Learning.

Day, M. (2008). Fight back against inflammatory bowel disease. *Nursing2008, 38*(11), 34–42.

Durston, S. (2005). What you need to know about viral hepatitis. *Nursing2005, 35*(8), 36–42.

Edmondson, D. (2008). Esophageal cancer—A tough pill to swallow. *Nursing2008*, April, 44–51. http://www.nursingcenter.com/ce/nursing

Erwin-Toth, P. (2001). Caring for a stoma. *Nursing2001, 31*(5), 36–40.

Estes, M. (2010). *Health assessment & physical examination* (4th ed.). Clifton Park, NY: Delmar Cengage Learning.

Farrar, J. (2001). Acute cholycystitis. *AJN, 101*(1), 35–36.

Framp, A. (2006). Diffuse gastric cancer. Retrieved from http://gateway.ut.ovid.com/gw1/ovidweb.cgi

Frazzoni, M., DeMicheli, E., Zentilin, P., & Savarino, V. (2004). Pathophysiological characteristics of patients with non-erosive reflux disease differ from those of patients with functional heartburn. *Alimentary Pharmacological Therapy, 20*, 81–88.

Fried, M., Shiffman, M., et al. (2002). Peginterferon alfa-2a plus ribavirin for chronic hepatitis C virus infection. *New England Journal of Medicine, 347*(13), 975.

Galvan, T. (2001). Dysphagia: Going down and staying down. *AJN, 101*(1), 37–42.

Hairon, N. (2008). New IBS guidance focuses on improving diagnosis and care. *Nursing Times, 104*(9), 23–24.

Harris, T. (2009). Does cigarette smoking increase the risk of developing ulcerative colitis or Crohn's disease? *Internet Journal of Academic Physician Assistants, 6*(2).

Heitkemper, M., & Jarrett, M. (2001). It's not all in your head: Irritable bowel syndrome. *AJN, 101*(1), 26–33.

Kaminsky, J., & Gadaleta, D. (2002). A study of discrimination within the medical community as viewed by obese patients. *Obese Surgery Journal, 12*(1), 14–18.

Klonowski, E., & Masoodi, J. (1999). The patient with Crohn's disease. *RN, 62*(3), 32–37.

Krumberger, J. (2002). When the liver fails. *RN, 65*(2), 26–29.

Krupp, K., & Heximer, B. (1998). Going with the flow: How to prevent feeding tubes from clogging. *Nursing98, 28*(4), 54–55.

Lau, D., Kleiner, D., Park, Y., DiBisceglie, A., & Hoofnagle, J. (1999). Resolution of chronic delta hepatitis after 12 years of interferon alpha therapy. *Gastroenterology, 117*(5), 1229–33.

Lee, C., Kelly, J., & Wassef, W. (2007). Complications of bariatric surgery. *Current Opinion in Gastroenterology, 23*(6), 636–643. Retrieved July 15, 2009 from http://www.medscape.com/viewarticle/565072_print

Lee, L., & Grap, M. (2008). Care and management of the patient with ascites. *MedSurg Nursing, The Journal of Adult Health, 17*(6), 376–381.

Lord, L. (2001). How to insert a large-bore nasogastric tube. *Nursing2001, 31*(9), 46–48.

Lynch, B., & Sarazine, J. (2006). A guide to understanding malignant bowel obstruction. *International Journal of Palliative Nursing, 12*(4), 164–171.

McConnell, E. (2001a). Administering total parenteral nutrition. *Nursing2001, 31*(11), 17.

McConnell, E. (2001b). Myths & facts . . . about dysphagia. *Nursing2001, 31*(7), 29.

McConnell, E. (2001c). What's behind intestinal obstruction? *Nursing2001, 31*(10), 58–63.

Marrs, J. (2006). Abdominal complaints: Diverticular disease. *Clinical Journal of Oncology Nursing, 10*(2), 155–157.

Mehta, M. (2003). Assessing the abdomen. *Nursing2003, 33*(5), 54–55.

Metheny, N., & Titler, M. (2001). Assessing placement of feeding tubes. *AJN, 101*(5), 36–45.

Moorhead, S., Johnson, M., Maas, M., & Swanson, E. (2007). *Nursing Outcomes Classification (NOC)* (4th ed). St. Louis, MO: Elsevier – Health Sciences Division.

Movius, M. (2006). What's causing that gut pain? Appendicitis? Diverticulitis? Constipation? MI? *RN, 69*(7), 25–29.

National Cancer Institute. (2008a). *U.S. National Institutes of Health: Esophageal cancer.* Retrieved July 14, 2008 from http://www.cancer.gov/cancertopics/types/esophageal/

National Cancer Institute. (2008b). *U.S. National Institutes of Health: Stomach (gastric) cancer screening.* Retrieved July 26, 2008 from http://www.cancer.gov/cancertopics/types/stomach

National Heart Lung and Blood Institute (NHLBI). (2009). *Calculate your body mass index.* Retrieved July 15, 2009 from http://www.nhlbisupport.com/bmi/

National Institute of Diabetes and Digestive and Kidney Diseases. (2006). Chronic hepatitis C: Current disease management. Retrieved July 14, 2008 from www.niddk.nih.gov/health/digest/pubs/chrnhepc/chrnhepc.htm

National Institute of Diabetes and Digestive and Kidney Diseases. (2008a). Viral hepatitis A to E and beyond. Retrieved May 29, 2009 from www.niddk.nih.gov/health/digest/pubs/hep/ hepa-e/hepa-e.htm

National Institute of Diabetes and Digestive and Kidney Diseases. (2008b). What I need to know about hepatitis A. Retrieved May 29, 2009 from http://digestive.niddk.nih.gov/ddiseases/pubs/viralhepatitis/index.htm

National Institute of Diabetes and Digestive and Kidney Diseases. (2008c). What I need to know about hepatitis B. Retrieved May 29, 2009 from http://digestive.niddk.nih.gov/ddiseases/pubs/viralhepatitis/index.htm

National Institute of Diabetes and Digestive and Kidney Diseases. (2009a). What I need to know about hepatitis C. Retrieved July 14, 2008 from www.niddk.nih.gov/health/digest/pubs/hep/hepc/hepc.htm

National Institute of Diabetes and Digestive and Kidney Diseases. (2009b). NIDDK recent advances and emerging opportunities: Digestive diseases and nutrition. Retrieved July 14, 2009 from www2.niddk.nih.gov/NR/rdonlyres/B36A7E82-C94A-4599-A749-7D2609F8A09E/0/DDN_508compliant.pdf

North American Nursing Diagnosis Association International. (2010). *NANDA-I nursing diagnoses: Definitions and classification 2009–2011*. Ames, IA: Wiley-Blackwell.

Ogden, C., Carrol, M., McDowell, M., & Flegal, K. (2007). Obesity among adults in the United States–No statistically significant change since 2003–2004. Centers for Disease Control and Prevention National Center for Health Statistics. Retrieved July 15, 2005 from http://www.cdc.gov/nchs/data/databriefs/db01.pdf

Parini, S. (2001). Hepatitis C: Speaking out about the silent epidemic. *Nursing2001, 31*(3), 36–42.

Parini, S. (2003). Hepatitis C: Update your knowledge of this silent stalker. *Nursing2003, 33*(4), 57–63.

Perry, J., Jagger, J., & Parker, G. (2003). Statistically, your risk of HCV infection has dropped. *Nursing2003, 33*(6), 82.

Rayhorn, N., & Rayhorn, D. (2002). An in-depth look at inflammatory bowel disease. *Nursing2002, 32*(7), 36–42.

Sammons, D. (2002). Roux-en-Y gastric bypass. *American Journal of Nursing, 102*(10), 24A–24D.

Sargent, C., & Murphy, D. (2003). What you need to know about colorectal cancer. *Nursing2003, 33*(2), 36–41.

Schlapman, N. (2001). Spotting acute pancreatitis. *RN, 64*(11), 54–58.

Snyder, D. (2005). Evidence-based recommendations for older adults with Helicobacter pylori or those using nonsteroidal anti-inflammatory drugs. *Gastroenterology Nursing, 28*(4), 309–314.

Spratto, G., & Woods, A. (2009). *2009 PDR nurse's drug handbook*. Clifton Park, NY: Thomson Learning Center.

University of Michigan Health System. (2009). Laproscopic cholecystectomy. Retrieved November 30, 2009 from http://www.med.umich.edu/1libr/aha/aha_llapch_crs.htm

U.S. Food and Drug Administration. (2002). FDA approves new treatment for chronic hepatitis B. Retrieved from www. fda.gov/bbs/topics/ANSWERS/2002/ANS01163.html

Wolf, L. (2008). The obese patient in the ED. *American Journal of Nursing, 108*(12), 77–80.

RESOURCES

American Liver Foundation, http://go.liverfoundation.org/

Crohn and Colitis Foundation of America, Inc., www.ccfa.org

Hepatitis Foundation International (HFI), www.hepfi.org

National Digestive Diseases Information Clearinghouse (NDDIC), http://digestive.niddk.nih.gov/

National Institute of Diabetes and Digestive and Kidney Diseases, http://www2.niddk.nih.gov/

United Ostomy Associations of America — Ostomy, Colostomy, http://www.uoaa.org/

CHAPTER 39
Urinary System

MAKING THE CONNECTION

Refer to the following chapters to increase your understanding of the urinary system:

Basic Nursing
- ***Arenas of Care***
- ***Wellness Concepts***
- ***Assessment***
- ***Diagnostic Tests***

Adult Health Nursing
- ***Cardiovascular System***
- ***Reproductive System***
- ***The Older Adult***

Basic Procedures
- ***Hand Hygiene***
- ***Use of Protective Equipment***
- ***Perineal Care***
- ***Routine Catheter Care***
- ***Measuring Intake and Output***
- ***Urine Collection: Closed Drainage System***
- ***Urine Collection—Clean Catch, Female/Male***

Intermediate Procedures
- ***Performing Urinary Catheterization: Female/Male***
- ***Irrigating a Urinary Catheter***
- ***Irrigating the Bladder Using a Closed-System Catheter***

LEARNING OBJECTIVES

Upon completion of this chapter, you should be able to:

- Define key terms.
- Describe the anatomy and physiology of the urinary system.
- Relate diagnostic test results to urinary disorders.
- Discuss the pros and cons of peritoneal dialysis/hemodialysis and kidney transplantation, including lifestyle changes for the client receiving dialysis.
- List four drug classifications and two examples of each used in the treatment of urinary disorders.
- State two changes in the urinary system related to the normal aging process.
- Compare and contrast acute and chronic renal failure, including nursing care.
- Assist in formulating a nursing care plan for clients with urinary disorders.

KEY TERMS

anasarca
azotemia
cachectic
calculus
cystitis
dialysate
dialysis
dysuria
erythropoiesis
fulguration
glomerular filtration rate (GFR)
hematuria
ileal conduit
intravesical
litholapaxy
lithotripsy
micturition
nephrotoxic
nocturia
nocturnal enuresis
oliguria
overflow incontinence
polyuria
pyelonephritis
pyuria
renal colic
residual urine
retroperitoneal
stress incontinence
urge incontinence
urgency
urinary incontinence (UI)
urinary retention
urolithiasis

INTRODUCTION

Urology is the study of disorders of the urinary system. The National Kidney Foundation estimates that more than 26 million Americans have chronic kidney disease and more than 26 million more are at increased risk (National Kidney Foundation [NKF], 2008). Disorders of the urinary system may seriously affect an individual's health and, thereby, affect the lives of family members. Clients are treated by a urologist, specialist in urinary tract disorders, or a nephrologist, specialist in structure, function, and diseases of the kidney.

According to the National Kidney Foundation (2009b), the warning signs of kidney disease are:

- Burning or difficulty during urination
- Increase in the frequency of urination, especially at night (**nocturia**)
- Passage of bloody appearing urine
- Puffiness around the eyes, or swelling of the hands and feet, especially in children
- Pain in the small of the back just below the ribs (not aggravated by movement)
- High blood pressure

ANATOMY AND PHYSIOLOGY REVIEW

The urinary system consists of two kidneys, two ureters (upper urinary tract), a urinary bladder, and a urethra (lower urinary tract) (Figure 39-1). The kidneys manufacture urine (Figure 39-2). Urine normally consists of 95% water; the nitrogenous waste products of protein, which are urea, uric acid, and creatinine; the excessive electrolytes sodium,

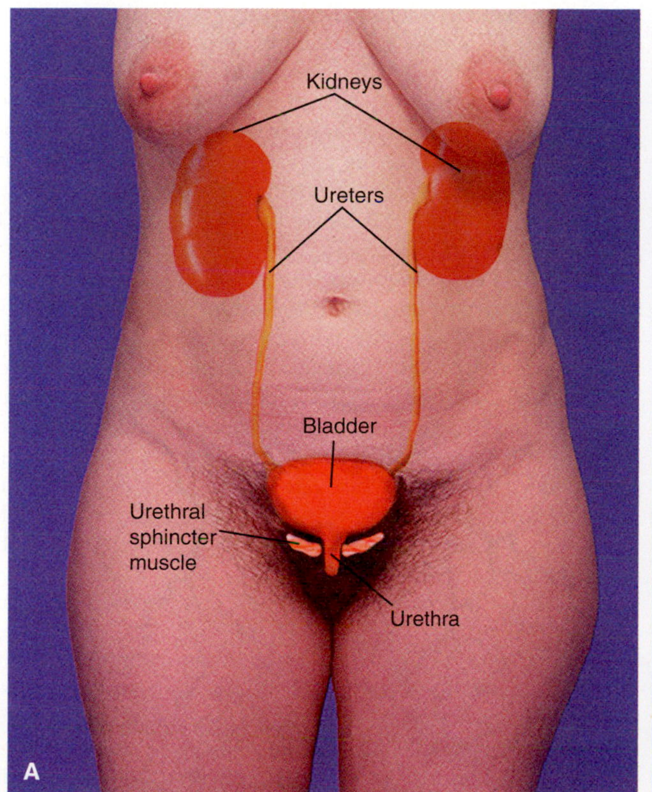

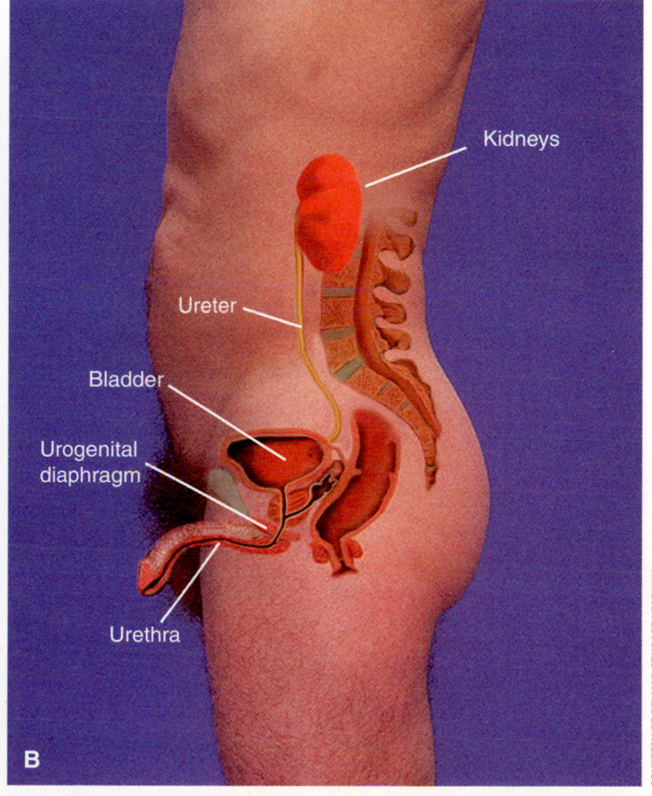

COURTESY OF DELMAR CENGAGE LEARNING

FIGURE 39-1 Urinary Tract; *A*, Female; *B*, Male

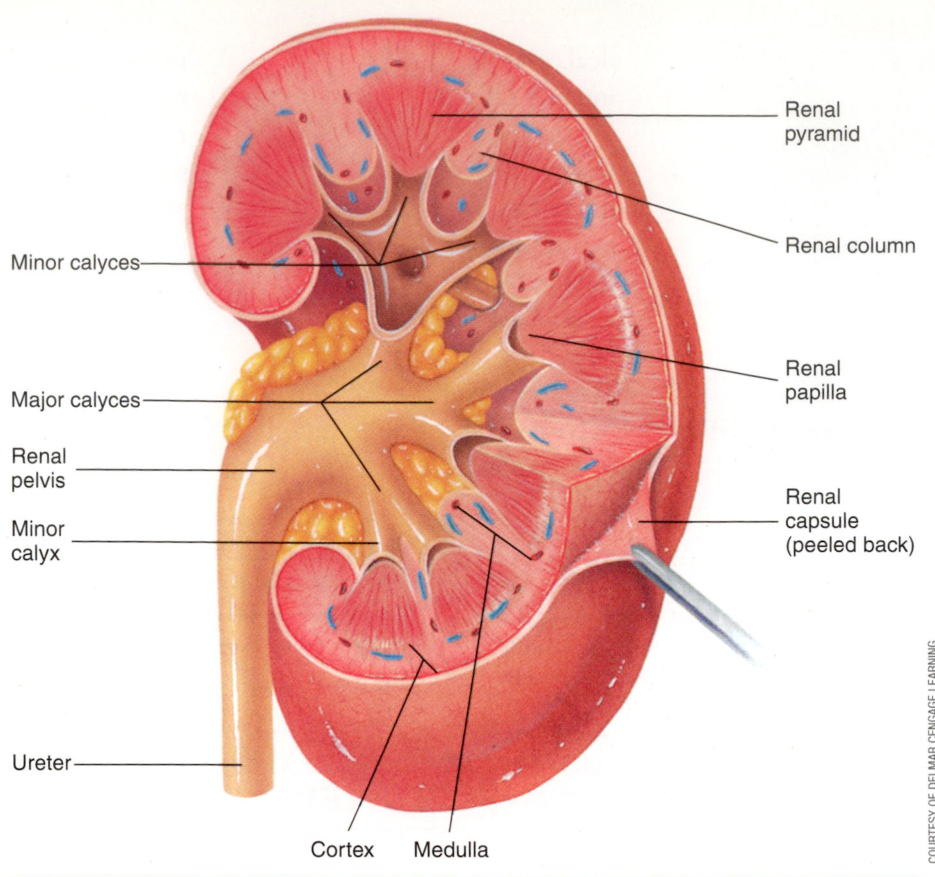

FIGURE 39-2 The Internal Anatomy of the Kidney

calcium, potassium, and phosphates; bile pigments; hormones; and metabolized drugs and toxins. Urine moves steadily by peristalsis through the ureters into the urinary bladder (Figure 39-3). The urine remains in the urinary bladder until capacity has been reached (about 500 mL) or until the body feels the **urgency** or desire to urinate

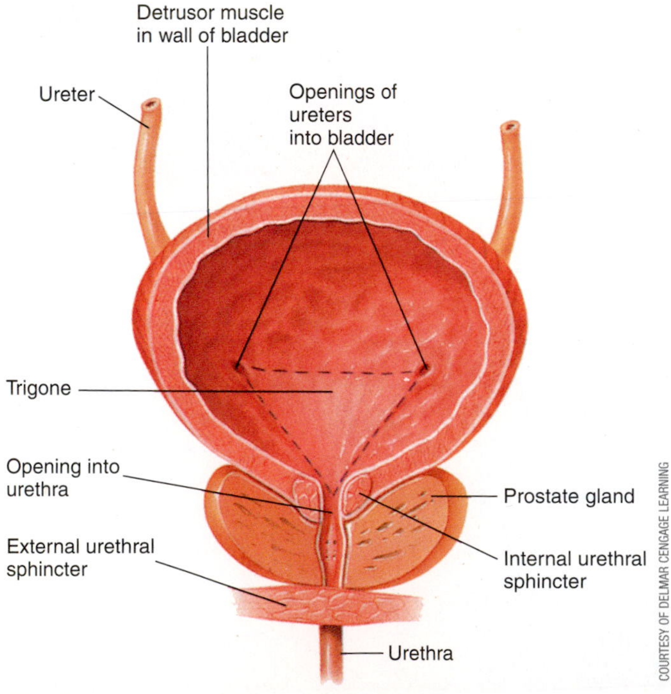

FIGURE 39-3 The Anatomy of the Urinary Bladder

(about 250 mL). The urine is then expelled from the bladder through the urethra, which is shorter in females than in males. **Micturition**, the process of expelling urine from the urinary bladder, is also called urination or voiding.

The kidneys are located beneath the false ribs, in the **retroperitoneal** space (behind the peritoneum outside the peritoneal cavity) of the abdominal cavity. The kidneys also assist in acid–base balance, raise blood pressure by secreting the enzyme renin, and produce the hormone erythropoietin, which is responsible for **erythropoiesis** (the production of red blood cells and their release by the red bone marrow).

Within the kidneys are microscopic units called nephrons, which are responsible for urine formation (Figure 39-4). The nephron winds into the cortex and medulla of the kidney. Each nephron includes a renal corpuscle, which consists of a glomerulus, a ball-like network of capillaries formed from an arteriole and held within a cuplike Bowman's capsule. The Bowman's capsule is attached to a long, intricate, ultrathin looped and coiled tubular structure called the renal tubule. Continuing on from the glomerulus is an arteriole that forms a capillary network around the tubule. Blood flowing through this system is collected by venioles.

Most of the contents of the blood, except for large molecules and blood cells, are forced out of the blood from the capillaries of the glomerulus and into the Bowman's capsule (glomerulofiltration). This occurs because of the high capillary blood pressure within the glomerulus. The glomerular basement membrane assists with the process of filtration. The **glomerular filtration rate (GFR)** is the amount of fluid filtered from the blood into the capsule per minute and an accurate measure of the functioning status of the kidneys. The material filtered from the blood

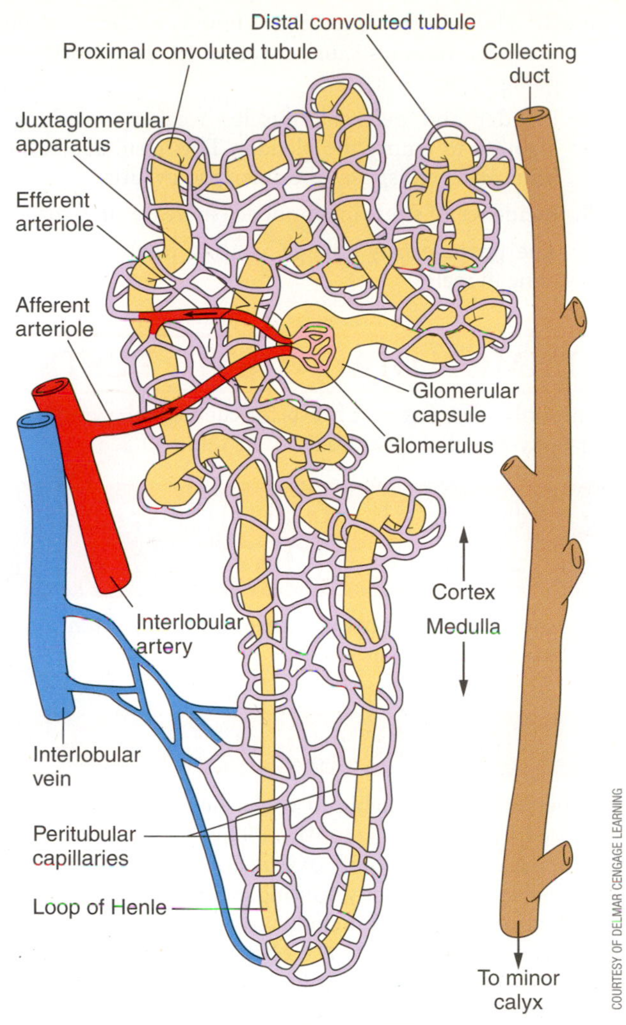

FIGURE 39-4 The Anatomy of a Nephron

is called glomerular filtrate, which contains water, electrolytes, glucose, various toxic substances, waste products (urea and creatinine), and just about everything else in the blood except large protein molecules and blood cells. As the filtrate passes through the first parts of the tubular structure, various substances such as necessary amounts of electrolytes, glucose, and water are reabsorbed (tubular reabsorption) back into the circulatory system through the capillaries or into the interstitial fluid. Tubular secretion then removes certain ions, nitrogen waste products, and drugs from the blood in the capillaries and adds it to the filtrate. The remaining filtrate—water, urea, excess electrolytes, toxic substances, and wastes, all of which constitute urine—continues through the tubules into the collecting duct, which collects urine from many nephrons. The urine passes from the collecting duct into the pelvis of the kidney, then through the ureter into the bladder and out of the body through the urethra. The kidneys process about 200 quarts of blood a day to eliminate 2 quarts of waste products and extra water as urine (NIDDK, 2006).

ASSESSMENT

Assessment of the urinary system is included in the baseline data for all clients. The client may be reluctant to discuss urinary problems. Assist the individual to relax by asking open-ended questions, using familiar terms, and making sure the client understands the medical terms (Table 39-1).

TABLE 39-1 Urinary Terms

TERMS	DEFINITION
Anuria	Cessation of urine production or urine output <100 mL/day
Dysuria	Painful or difficult urination
Hematuria	Blood in the urine
Nocturia	Excessive urination at night
Oliguria	Diminished capacity to form and excrete urine (<500 mL/day)
Polyuria	Excreting an abnormally large quantity of urine
Urgency	Feeling the need to urinate immediately

COURTESY OF DELMAR CENGAGE LEARNING

A more in-depth assessment is performed when clients are at high risk for renal disease because of exposure to nephrotoxins; an altered health state such as diabetes mellitus, pregnancy, or hypertension; trauma, dehydration, or fluid retention, which can compromise renal function; and those with suspected or active renal disease.

SUBJECTIVE DATA

Ask the client to describe how the symptoms developed and progressed. Is there pain? Is it sharp or a dull ache? Constant or intermittent? Does it radiate to the groin, genital area, or leg? Is the pain associated with urination? Have headaches been experienced?

Next, the client can describe the urine and urination pattern. Is there difficulty starting the stream? Is there urgency, frequency, incontinence, or hematuria? Does the bladder feel empty after voiding? Does the client have pruritis or dry skin?

OBJECTIVE DATA

If edema is present, ask the client if it is always present or if it disappears during the night. Monitor I&O and vital signs, and palpate the client's bladder for retention. Weigh the client. Assess mucous membranes for moisture and the skin for dryness and uremic frost. Evaluate urine for color, clarity, and odor. Review diagnostic tests.

CRITICAL THINKING

Clinical Setting Activity: Urinalysis Results

Research and evaluate the urinalysis results of a client in the clinical setting. Were abnormal results detected? If so, what course of treatment was ordered for the client? What nursing interventions should be implemented?

Box 39-1 QUESTIONS TO ASK AND OBSERVATIONS TO MAKE WHEN COLLECTING DATA

Subjective Data

Do you have any urinary health problems?

Do you have any family members with any urinary health problems?

How do you view your overall urinary health?

What was different today than any other day that brought you here?

How often do you urinate in the day and at night?

Are you urinating as much as you are drinking?

How many glasses of water do you drink a day?

Does it ever hurt or burn when you urinate?

Do you leak urine when you cough or exercise?

Do you have trouble starting your urine stream?

Does your urine have a strong odor or appear dark yellow?

Do you ever see blood in your urine?

Are you experiencing sleep disturbances?

Do you experience shortness of breath on exertion?

Objective Data

Check vital signs

Inspect color, odor, and consistency of the urine

Observe client for signs of anorexia

Observe client's activity tolerance and for signs of fatigue

Assess client for nausea and/or metallic taste in the mouth

Assess skin condition for pruritus

Measure and record intake and output

Weigh client daily

Monitor client for impaired cognition

Report diagnostic test results

CHANGES WITH AGING

The following changes are found in the urinary system as a result of aging:

1. Nephrons decrease, resulting in decreased filtration and gradual decrease in excretory and reabsorptive functions of renal tubules.
2. Glomerular filtration rate decreases, resulting in decreased renal clearance of drugs.
3. Blood urea nitrogen (BUN) increases 20% by age 70. The creatinine clearance test is a better index than the BUN of renal function in the elderly.
4. Sodium-conserving ability is diminished.
5. Bladder capacity decreases, causing increased frequency of urination and nocturia.
6. Renal function increases when the client is lying down, sometimes causing a need to void shortly after going to bed.
7. Bladder and perineal muscles weaken, resulting in inability to empty the bladder. This results in residual urine and predisposes the elderly to cystitis.
8. Incidence of stress incontinence increases in females.
9. The prostate may enlarge, causing frequency or dribbling in males.

COMMON DIAGNOSTIC TESTS

Commonly used diagnostic tests for clients with symptoms of urinary system disorders are listed in Table 39-2.

IMPAIRED URINARY ELIMINATION

Disorders in this category include urinary retention and urinary incontinence.

URINARY RETENTION

A person who is unable to void when there is an urge to void has **urinary retention**. This creates urinary stasis and increases the possibility of infection. The urine may overflow the bladder's capacity, causing incontinence.

A variety of causes include a response to stress; benign prostatic hypertrophy (BPH), obstruction of the urethra by **calculi** (concentration of mineral salts, known as stones), tumor, or infection; interference with the sphincter muscles during surgery; or as a side effect of medications or perineal trauma.

The client may experience discomfort and anxiety from urinary retention. Frequency of urination and voiding small amounts may also occur. A distended bladder can be palpated above the symphysis.

Treatment may include urinary analgesics and antispasmodics to help the client relax. Cholinergic medications such as bethanechol chloride (Urecholine) may be ordered to promote detrusor muscle contraction and bladder emptying. A urinary catheter may be used to empty the bladder, or surgery may be performed to remove any obstruction.

When a client is unable to void, check for residual urine. Immediately after the client voids, use a bladder scan or insert an intermittent straight catheter, if ordered, and measure the urine output. The bladder scan is preferred because it reduces the risk of urinary tract infection (UTI). The urine left in the bladder, **residual urine**, should be less than 50 mL.

URINARY INCONTINENCE

Urinary incontinence (UI) is the involuntary loss of urine from the bladder. UI may be a complication of urinary tract problems or neurologic disorders and may be permanent or temporary. Medications such as sedatives, hypnotics, diuretics, anticholinergics, antipsychotics, and alpha antagonists may be associated with UI.

More than 25 million men and women in the United States experience UI, with women twice as often as men

Table 39-2 Common Diagnostic Tests for Urinary System Disorders

URINALYSIS	
Urinalysis	
Color	Bilirubin
Odor	Glucose
Albumin (protein)	Specific gravity
Acetone (ketone)	Bacteria
RBCs	Casts
WBCs	pH
Culture and sensitivity (C & S)	
Creatinine clearance	
Residual urine (postvoiding residual urine)	
BLOOD TESTS	
Blood urea nitrogen (BUN)	
Serum creatinine	
Antistreptolysin O titer (ASO titer)	
Serum electrolytes	
Sodium	Calcium
Potassium	Phosphorus
Chloride	Uric acid
URINE TESTS	
Voiding cystourethrography	
Kidney-ureter-bladder (KUB) x-ray	
Computed tomography (CT; spiral CT)	
Magnetic resonance imaging (MRI)	
Intravenous pyelogram (IVP)	
Renal angiography	
Renal scan	
Ultrasound	
Portable ultrasonic bladder scan	
Retrograde pyelogram	
URODYNAMIC TESTS	
Uroflowmetry	
Cystometrogram (CMG)	
Urethra pressure profile (UPP)	
ENDOSCOPIC EXAMS	
Cystoscopy	
Biopsy	
Renal biopsy	

COURTESY OF DELMAR CENGAGE LEARNING

(National Association for Continence, 2008). This is not just a physiological problem but also affects the client's emotional, psychological, and social well-being. UI can occur in clients of any age but is more common in older adults. All types of incontinence can be treated at any age. Keeping the perineal area dry and intact is a goal for all clients. UI is classified as stress, urge, overflow, total, or nocturnal enuresis.

Stress Incontinence

Stress incontinence is the most common type of incontinence. It is not a disease or a natural, inevitable effect of aging. Anyone can be affected; however, women are more likely to have this condition than men. In stress incontinence there is leakage of urine when a person does anything that strains the pelvic floor, such as coughing, laughing, jogging, dancing, sneezing, lifting, making a quick movement, or even walking. Medical management depends on the underlying cause. Treatment may include bladder retraining, medicines such as conjugated estrogens (Premarin Vaginal Cream), or surgery. Surgery may be necessary to restore the support of the pelvic floor muscles or to reconstruct the sphincter but is used after other treatments are unsuccessful. Another possible treatment is having collagen injected into the tissues surrounding the urethra thus causing the urethra to close enough to prevent urine from leaking out. The procedure is done in a nonsurgical outpatient setting. Surgical procedures include internal mesh support of the urethra, formation of a urethral sling to elevate and compress the urethra, and implantation of an artificial sphincter. Several support prostheses and external barriers are available.

The client can be taught pelvic floor exercises (Kegel exercises) to strengthen the muscles, thereby preventing or minimizing stress incontinence. Kegel exercises involve having the client tighten the pelvic floor muscles to stop the flow of urine when urinating, and then releasing the muscles to start the flow of urine again. Once the client can do this, the exercise may be done anytime, anyplace. Practicing the exercise 10 times, 7 or 8 times a day strengthens the pelvic floor muscles.

CLIENT TEACHING

Performing Pelvic Muscle Exercises (Kegel Exercises)

The nurse instructs the client to do the following when learning Kegel exercises:

- To learn how to control the pelvic floor muscles, tighten the pelvic floor muscles to stop the flow of urine when urinating.
- Then, release the pelvic floor muscles to start the flow of urine again.
- Now, practice (without urinating) tightening and holding the pelvic floor muscles for a count of 3 to 5 seconds and then release the muscles.
- Perform each contraction 10 times, three times daily.
- This exercise can be done anytime, anyplace.
- Develop a schedule or routine to remember to do daily Kegel exercises (e.g., when drinking morning coffee, working at the kitchen sink, waiting at a stoplight).

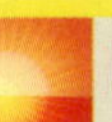

LIFE SPAN CONSIDERATIONS

Elderly Clients and UTIs

- Elderly clients are more prone to UTIs because of incomplete emptying of the bladder, fecal incontinence with perineal soiling, and a decrease in urine acidity.
- Incomplete emptying of the bladder in women is caused by bladder or uterine prolapse or loss of pelvic muscle tone; in men it is caused by an enlarged prostate gland.
- In elderly clients, sometimes the only sign of a UTI or urosepsis is new onset of mental changes or confusion (National Institutes of Health, 2006).

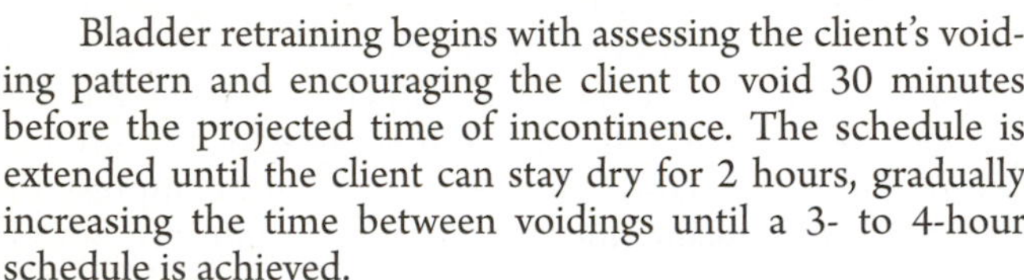

Bladder retraining begins with assessing the client's voiding pattern and encouraging the client to void 30 minutes before the projected time of incontinence. The schedule is extended until the client can stay dry for 2 hours, gradually increasing the time between voidings until a 3- to 4-hour schedule is achieved.

URGE INCONTINENCE

Urge incontinence occurs when a person is unable to suppress the sudden urge or need to urinate. Sometimes urine may leak without any warning. An irritated bladder is often the cause. Infection or very concentrated urine may irritate the bladder.

Treatment includes clearing up an infection, if present, and encouraging the client to have a fluid intake of 3,000 mL per day. This prevents the urine from becoming concentrated. Less fluid does not prevent incontinence but may promote infection.

OVERFLOW INCONTINENCE

When the bladder becomes so full and distended that urine leaks out, it is called **overflow incontinence**. This occurs when a blocked urethra or bladder weakness prevents normal emptying. The blockage may be an enlarged prostate. The distended bladder cannot contract with enough force to expel a stream of urine. Bladder weakness occurs most often in persons who have diabetes, drink a large quantity of alcohol, and have decreased nerve function. Bladder retraining may alleviate the situation.

TOTAL INCONTINENCE

When no urine can be retained in the bladder, it is termed total incontinence. The client may be able to manage with an indwelling catheter. A neurologic problem is usually the cause. Surgery to make a temporary or permanent urinary diversion may be required. Kobayashi, Nomura, Yamada, Fujimoto, and Matsumoto (2005) surgically performed the Mitrofanoff procedure, which creates a catheterizable channel between an abdominal stoma and the bladder. Clients can then empty their bladder with a catheter.

MEMORYTRICK

DRIP

There are several causes of incontinence that can be reversed or corrected. A memory trick to easily identify the reversible causes of incontinence is **DRIP:**

D = Delirium (a new onset of delirium)
R = Restriction (restricted mobility)
I = Infection (a new infection)
P = Polyuria (increase in urination as seen in diabetes)

NOCTURNAL ENURESIS

Incontinence that occurs during sleep is called **nocturnal enuresis**. Limiting fluid intake after 6 p.m. helps the client remain continent during the night. The total fluid intake for 24 hours, however, should remain the same. The bladder should be emptied immediately before going to bed.

NURSING MANAGEMENT

Identify impaired urinary elimination based on subjective and objective data. Assess vital signs. Encourage adequate fluid intake. Teach Kegel exercises. Initiate bladder retraining.

INFECTIOUS DISORDERS

Infectious disorders of the urinary system are called urinary tract infections (UTIs). There are two types: lower UTIs affect the bladder (cystitis) and urethra, and upper UTIs affect the kidneys (pyelonephritis, and acute and chronic glomerulonephritis) and ureters.

CYSTITIS

Cystitis is an inflammation of the urinary bladder. It is more common in females because their short urethra allows bacteria to ascend through the urethra from the vagina or rectum to the urinary bladder. Also, bacteria from an infected kidney can descend through the ureter into the urinary bladder. Most urinary tract infections are caused by *Escherichia coli*, but some are caused by *Candida albicans*. Other common causes of cystitis are coitus, prostatitis, and diabetes mellitus.

As women age, pelvic floor muscles relax, leading to a decreased ability to empty the bladder completely. This contributes to stasis of urine and promotion of bacterial growth, as in pregnancy or benign prostatic hypertrophy. In men, cystitis usually occurs secondary to another infection such as epididymitis or prostatitis.

Once bacteria enter the bladder, they multiply, causing redness and swelling of the wall of the bladder. These changes result in urinary frequency, dysuria, pyuria, hematuria, and sometimes burning and urgency with urination. These symptoms increase as the bladder distends with even a small volume of urine.

A clean-catch midstream urinalysis showing a bacteria count greater than 100,000 organisms/mL confirms the diagnosis. Microscopic examination of the urine also shows **hematuria** (blood in the urine) and pus.

Medical–Surgical Management

Medical

Treatment of cystitis includes medication and fluids. Recurrence of a UTI usually occurs when it is not effectively treated. Obtaining and sending a urine specimen for C & S before the administration of any urinary antimicrobial is necessary to determine the most effective medication. A repeat urinalysis after 2 or 3 days on medication confirms its effectiveness. Chronic lower urinary tract infections are often a factor in the development of pyelonephritis.

Diet

Encourage fluid intake. Clients are usually asked to drink between 3 and 4 liters of noncaffeinated fluid per day. The intake of meats and whole grains makes the urine more acidic and may discourage the growth of bacteria in the urinary bladder. Drinking cranberry juice has been advised for years, but how it worked was not understood. Research suggests that condensed tannins in the juice prevent E. coli from sticking to the urinary tract (Lynch, 2004).

Pharmacological

Cystitis treatment entails the use of antimicrobial medication in conjunction with urinary tract analgesics. Cystitis is generally treated with trimethoprim-sulfamethoxazole (TMP-SMZ, Bactrim), ciprofloxacin (Cipro), cephalexin (Keflex), nitrofurantoin (Macrobid, Macrodantin), Amoxicillin (Amoxil), doxycycline calcium (Vibramycin), and Augmentin. Determine whether the client is allergic to sulfonamides or penicillins before administering the medication. The antimicrobial ordered is determined by the results of the urine culture and sensitivity. The length of treatment is related to the type of cystitis, acute or chronic. Some physicians may order a single dose or short course (3 or 4 days) of antimicrobial therapy rather than the traditional 7- to 10-day course. **Dysuria** (difficult or painful urination) related to a burning sensation when voiding can be alleviated with the use of the urinary tract analgesic phenazopyridine hydrochloride (Pyridium), which causes red-orange urine and stains clothing and toilets.

Activity

Because cystitis causes frequency of urination, call lights must be answered promptly for clients on bed rest or those in need of assistance to the bathroom. Clients on bed rest are generally not able to empty their bladder completely when using a bedpan. Encourage orders for bathroom privileges or using a commode chair. Help allay the client's fears of being incontinent with properly timed bladder management.

Nursing Management

Monitor vital signs. Accurately record intake and output. Encourage fluid intake, especially water and cranberry juice. Encourage the client to void more frequently and women to void after intercourse. Teach clients that when taking Pyridium the urine will be red-orange and will stain clothing. Encourage cotton-crotch undergarments. Teach those who wear an incontinence control product to change it frequently.

NURSING PROCESS

Assessment

Subjective Data

The client will usually describe having frequency or urgency of urination or nocturia. This is annoying and embarrassing, regardless of age or sex. Burning and pain when voiding are common reasons clients seek medical care. Even clients with an indwelling catheter may complain of dysuria, burning, and frequency. Clients often feel body discomfort and malaise.

Objective Data

Perineal irritation may be noticed when the client with a catheter pulls on it in hopes of alleviating the bladder pain. The urine will smell foul and appear cloudy. Hematuria may be present (Figure 39-5). The elderly population in particular may become anorexic and develop a low-grade fever. The urinalysis will indicate the presence of bacteria, and the C & S will identify the specific microorganism causing the UTI and the medication to which the pathogen is most sensitive.

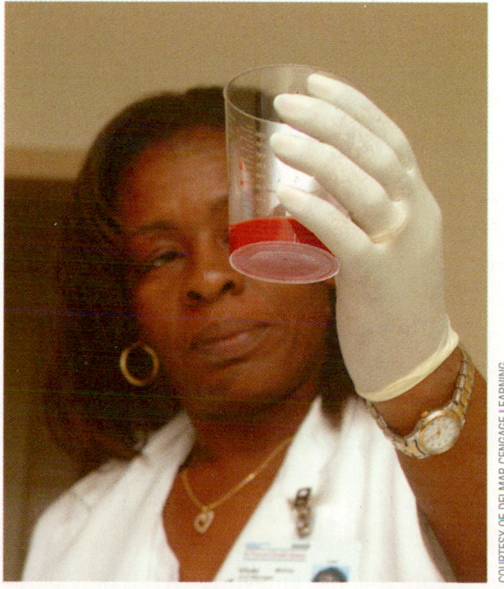
COURTESY OF DELMAR CENGAGE LEARNING

FIGURE 39-5 Nurse Examining and Measuring Hematuria Sample from Client with a UTI

Nursing diagnoses for a client with cystitis include the following:

NURSING DIAGNOSES	PLANNING/OUTCOMES	NURSING INTERVENTIONS
*Impaired **U**rinary Elimination* related to UTI	The client will return to usual pattern of urinary elimination.	Encourage a large amount of fluid intake, at least 3,000 mL each day, especially water and cranberry juice twice a day. Administer urinary tract analgesics and antimicrobial medications as ordered. Alert the client, if Pyridium is being taken, that the urine will be red-orange and will stain clothing.
*Deficient **K**nowledge* related to treatment regimen and prevention of recurrence	The client will comply with treatment regimen and practice preventive habits.	Discuss the importance of taking all medication ordered even after the symptoms are relieved. Teach or reinforce the following preventive measures. Clean the perineum from front to back. If nylon undergarments are worn, they should have a cotton crotch. Wearing tight-fitting jeans and thongs, and taking long bike rides may be irritating to the perineum. Perfumed perineal products such as menstrual products, douches, powder, or bubble bath may also be contributing factors to bladder infections. Spermicidal contraceptive products can be irritating, thus contributing to a lower UTI. Advise the client to void more frequently and not retain urine in the bladder. Advise women to void after sexual intercourse. Teach the elderly client who uses incontinence control products, to change the product frequently to prevent cystitis. When this client is hospitalized, plan time for frequent ambulation to the bathroom or commode chair.

Evaluation: Evaluate each outcome to determine how it has been met by the client.

CRITICAL THINKING

Assessment Scenario

A 24-year-old female client comes into the emergency department complaining of frequency and dysuria on urination.

1. What assessment should the nurse perform?
2. What tests might be ordered?
3. What instructions should the nurse teach the client?

PYELONEPHRITIS

Pyelonephritis, also known as pyelitis or nephropyelitis, is a bacterial infection of the renal pelvis, tubules, and interstitial tissue of one or both kidneys. Bacteria generally ascend from the urinary bladder through the ureter and enter the kidney in the renal pelvis. Bacteria can also enter from the blood and lymph. Pyelonephritis can be secondary to ureterovesicular reflux (backflow of urine from the bladder into the ureters) or when urine cannot drain from the pelvis of the kidney because of an obstruction blocking the kidney or ureter. Pyelonephritis may occur during pregnancy, with prostatitis, when bacteria are introduced during a cystoscopy or catheterization, or from trauma to the urinary tract. Pyelonephritis can be an acute illness or a chronic condition leading to the development of high blood pressure and/or chronic renal failure.

Escherichia coli is the microorganism most often cultured. The inflamed kidney becomes edematous and the renal blood vessels become congested. Sometimes abscesses form in the kidney. The urine is usually cloudy, containing mucus, blood, and pus.

Medical–Surgical Management

Medical

Diagnostic tests that may be ordered include a CT scan, an ultrasound (when CT scan is contraindicated), a urinalysis with a C&S, complete blood count [CBC], BUN, and serum creatinine.

Collect urine specimens before the administration of any antimicrobial medication. Medical treatment and care are focused on preventing pyelonephritis from becoming chronic. Follow-up care and treatment may be necessary for up to 6 months.

Pharmacological

Pyelonephritis is generally treated with sulfonamides, such as trimethoprim-sulfamethoxazole (TMP-SMZ, Bactrim) or the antimicrobial ciprofloxacin hydrochloride (Cipro). Cipro may not be indicated if the client has renal damage. Antipyretics are used to reduce fever and analgesics to manage pain.

Diet

As with infections in general, the individual's diet should be light during the febrile stage. Fluids must be increased to 3,000 mL per day by mouth and supplemented intravenously when indicated.

Activity

Because the disease process causes fatigue, bed rest is maintained during the acute phase of pyelonephritis. Diversionary activities are important while on bed rest. When the client is allowed to ambulate, dizziness related to the analgesic medication taken for pain may be a problem.

Nursing Management

Encourage client to verbalize concerns and fears. Answer questions honestly. Monitor I&O and observe output. Encourage fluid intake to 3,000 mL per day and cranberry juice twice a day. Cleanse perineum from front to back. Encourage client to empty bladder frequently. Promote rest periods during the day. Weigh client daily. Monitor adequate pain management. Monitor and record diagnostic test results.

NURSING PROCESS

Assessment

Subjective Data

In acute pyelonephritis the client is acutely ill with malaise, urgency in urination, and pain during voiding and in the flank area. **Renal colic**, severe pain in the kidney that radiates to the groin, may occur, impairing urination. The client may describe being hot, with or without chills. In chronic pyelonephritis, only a general symptom of nausea may be present. The client may be very anxious that this kidney infection will cause permanent kidney damage.

Objective Data

Assessment may find the client tender on one or both sides of the lower back. Temperature, pulse, and respiratory rate may all be elevated. The urine is foul smelling, cloudy, and often hematuria is noted. The urinalysis results show bacteria and **pyuria** (pus in the urine), and the CBC indicates leukocytosis. The client with chronic disease will have the systemic signs of vomiting, diarrhea, and elevated blood pressure. Some clients with pyelonephritis may be asymptomatic.

Nursing diagnoses for a client with pyelonephritis include the following:

NURSING DIAGNOSES	PLANNING/OUTCOMES	NURSING INTERVENTIONS
Anxiety related to unknown prognosis	The client will verbalize fears and concerns to family and health care team.	Encourage the client to verbalize fears and concerns. Use active listening and observe for behavioral signs of anxiety. Answer questions honestly.
Impaired Urinary Elimination related to UTI	The client will regain normal urinary pattern.	Encourage drinking cranberry juice in the morning and evening. Encourage fluid intake to 3,000 mL per day, especially water. Monitor intake and output. Evaluate kidney function by measuring and observing urine output and monitoring the results of blood and urine tests.
Deficient Knowledge related to disease process, treatment regimen, and prevention	The client will verbalize understanding of disease process, treatment regimen, and preventive measures.	Teach or reinforce the hygiene measure of cleansing the perineum from front to back and practice this when doing perineal care on any client. Instruct the client on the importance of taking all the antimicrobial medication as prescribed in order to eliminate the bacteria. Teach the client to refrain from using perfumed perineal products such as menstrual pads, tampons, or douches, and avoid bubble baths and hot tubs because they can be irritating to the tissues of the genital area.

(*Continues*)

Nursing diagnoses for a client with pyelonephritis include the following: (Continued)

NURSING DIAGNOSES	PLANNING/OUTCOMES	NURSING INTERVENTIONS
		Encourage the client to empty the bladder frequently to avoid distention. Promote rest periods, which aid the healing process. Inform the client to call the physician immediately if there is a decrease in urine output or signs of infection (elevated temperature, chills, flank pain, urgency, fatigue, nausea, and vomiting). Teach client to weigh daily and report sudden weight gain (2 pounds/week) to the physician. Emphasize the importance of keeping all appointments with the physician for follow-up care and when signs of infection appear. Teach the client the importance of long-term treatment and monitoring for chronic pyelonephritis.

Evaluation: Evaluate each outcome to determine how it has been met by the client.

ACUTE GLOMERULONEPHRITIS

Glomerulonephritis is a condition that can affect one or both kidneys. In both acute and chronic disease, the glomerulus within the nephron unit becomes inflamed. It is predominantly a disease of children and young adults when the cause is bacterial. The viral form can affect all ages. The prognosis for most clients is a full recovery; however, some may develop chronic glomerulonephritis. Acute glomerulonephritis during childhood is known as Bright's disease.

Clients may develop symptoms 1 to 3 weeks after an upper respiratory infection (tonsillitis or pharyngitis with fever) or skin infection caused most commonly by group A *β-hemolytic streptococcus*. The infection triggers an autoimmune response and the glomeruli are attacked by antibodies at the site of the glomerular basement membrane, resulting in inflammation. Some clients are asymptomatic. A nephrotoxic drug or systemic disease such as diabetes or lupus may also be a cause (NIDDK, 2006).

Immunologic effects on the body are not completely understood. Direct effects on the glomeruli result in the reduced ability of the glomeruli to function. The glomeruli become more permeable, resulting in the loss of red blood cells and protein from the blood. These substances escape from the body in the urine. The inflammatory process causes thickening of the membrane of the glomeruli and potential scarring.

Diagnostic tests on blood and urine as well as KUB x-rays will be performed. BUN, serum creatinine, potassium, erythrocyte sedimentation rate (ESR), and antistreptolysin O titer (ASO titer) will be elevated. Urinalysis will show proteinuria and red blood cells. A CBC and electrolytes are ordered. Cultures of the throat and skin may be ordered to rule out *Streptococcus*.

Medical–Surgical Management

Medical

Prevention of renal complications and complications to cardiac and cerebral functioning is the focus of care. Medical treatment must start as soon as the client is diagnosed to restore kidney function. Management includes drug therapy, diet, and rest. Treatment is correlated with the blood pressure and the results of urine testing for red blood cells and protein. The client is not considered to be free from the disease until the urine tests negative for protein and red blood cells for 6 months.

Plasmapheresis may be indicated if there is no response from other treatments and if the client also has Goodpasture's syndrome. Between 150 and 400 mL of blood is removed from the client and put in a cell separator. Here the blood is divided into plasma and formed elements which are mixed with a plasma replacement and returned to the client through a vein. Another technique filters the client's own plasma to remove a specific disease mediator (antibody) and then returns the plasma to the client.

Pharmacological

Prophylactic antimicrobial therapy may be administered. The drug of choice is penicillin. If the client is allergic to penicillin, erythromycin is ordered. Diuretic and antihypertensive medication furosemide (Lasix) may be ordered. Corticosteroids, chemotherapeutic drugs such as cyclophosphamide (Cytoxan), and/or immunosuppressive agents such as azathioprine (Imuran) may be ordered to control the inflammatory response. Corticosteroids and immunosuppressive drugs may be prescribed to treat the underlying causes of glomerulonephritis, such as lupus or vasculitis (Mayo Clinic, 2009).

Diet

Fluid retention often requires fluid restriction. The restriction is adjusted according to the client's I&O record and daily weight. Protein in the client's diet will be regulated according to the BUN and the creatinine blood levels. The kidneys need to rest; however, particularly in children, it may not be necessary to restrict protein. Potassium will need to be replaced if the diuretic promotes its excretion. Sodium may be restricted to prevent fluid retention. Strict intake and output are necessary to monitor kidney function.

COMMUNITY/HOME HEALTH CARE

Sodium Restriction

When water at home is naturally high in sodium or if water is chemically softened, teach the client to use low-sodium bottled water in cooking and for the drinking allowance.

Activity

Physical and emotional rest are essential. Compliance with bed rest may be difficult, especially for a child or the client who feels well. Bed rest is indicated until the inflammation subsides, urinary flow increases, and as long as the client has hematuria or proteinuria. During this time a strict turning schedule needs to be followed because skin breakdown is more likely in the presence of edema. When ambulation is allowed, the client may feel weak from the effects of anemia and inactivity.

Nursing Management

Monitor vital signs and I&O. Blood pressure should be monitored closely. Assess for headache, flank pain, and edema. Weigh client daily. Assess heart and lung sounds. Monitor results of diagnostic tests. If fluids are restricted, work with client on fluid intake schedule. Encourage client to follow schedule. Assist with or provide oral hygiene several times a day. Refer for dietary consultation if protein and sodium are restricted.

NURSING PROCESS

Assessment

Subjective Data

The health history will likely reveal a recent sore throat, skin infection, flulike symptoms, and a headache. The client describes flank pain as the kidneys become congested. Other symptoms the client may describe are headache, malaise, anorexia, cola-colored "smokey" urine, and a marked decrease in the amount of urine (**oliguria**). Facial edema may be the first sign noticed, may impair vision, and may cause the client to have negative feelings about body image.

Objective Data

Vital signs will generally show an increase in body temperature and blood pressure. Facial (periorbital) edema is present. The edema will progress to dependent areas such as the sacral area and the legs. Monitor daily the location and degree of edema. Ascites may also develop. Assess the general condition of the skin and skin integrity. Weigh the client to establish a baseline weight. Assess heart and lung sounds for signs of heart failure and pulmonary edema (unusual heart sounds and crackles in the lungs). Neck veins may be distended. Dyspnea on exertion or when recumbent, and shortness of breath, may both be noted. Urine output is decreased and cola colored to red colored urine is present.

Monitor results of diagnostic tests: urine for red blood cells and protein (albumin) and blood for BUN, serum creatinine, potassium, ESR, ASO titer, and specific gravity, all of which will be elevated.

Nursing diagnoses for a client with acute glomerulonephritis include the following:

NURSING DIAGNOSES	PLANNING/OUTCOMES	NURSING INTERVENTIONS
Fear related to potential permanent damage to the kidneys	The client will communicate fears of kidney damage to the family and the health care personnel.	Provide client and family with support and understanding. Encourage client to discuss fears. Explain the importance of protecting the client from other infections. Allow no one with an upper respiratory infection to visit the client. Discuss the importance of compliance with medications, bed rest, and diet to prevent permanent damage to kidneys. Emphasize the importance of keeping the follow-up visits to the laboratory for tests and to the physician's office. Arrange consultation with social services to assist the client in arranging time off from work and to help the client and family with their financial needs.
Excess Fluid Volume related to compromised regulatory mechanism secondary to renal dysfunction	The client will have decreased edema and adequate urinary output.	Fluids will be restricted with specific amounts designated throughout the day. For example, 900 mL of fluids for a day might be divided in the following manner: 7 a.m. to 3 p.m. 600 mL; 3 p.m. to 11 p.m. 200 mL; 11 p.m. to 7 a.m. 100 mL. Encourage compliance to the fluid amounts. Maintain accurate intake and output records hourly.

(*Continues*)

Nursing diagnoses for a client with acute glomerulonephritis include the following: (Continued)

NURSING DIAGNOSES	PLANNING/OUTCOMES	NURSING INTERVENTIONS
		Provide oral hygiene several times a day. Advise that thirst may be relieved by sucking on hard candy or, if allowed, a few ice chips. Provide eye care with normal saline to promote comfort from the periorbital edema.
*Impaired **S**ocial Interaction* related to changes in body image	The client will resume social interaction.	Encourage client to keep in contact with friends and relatives by telephone. Encourage keeping appointments with the physician and laboratory.
*Imbalanced **N**utrition: More than Body Requirements* related to the disease process	The client will comply with nutritional restrictions.	Once the client's condition warrants solid foods, arrange a dietary consultation to incorporate food preferences and religious and/or cultural needs. Finances may be an issue if the family has to incorporate foods that are not usually part of its budget. Teach client to plan menus and to read food labels in order to comply with the dietary restrictions. Before discharge, teach client and family about diet, fluids, and activity restrictions and measuring fluid intake and urine output. Provide client with guidelines listing reasons to call the physician.

Evaluation: Evaluate each outcome to determine how it has been met by the client.

CHRONIC GLOMERULONEPHRITIS

The prognosis for acute glomerulonephritis is often good when treatment is begun early; however, chronic glomerulonephritis generally leads to permanent kidney damage. Those who develop chronic glomerulonephritis may have neither symptoms nor a recent history of an infection. Chronic diseases, such as diabetes mellitus or systemic lupus erythematosus, often mask renal symptoms and the client does not seek medical care until kidney function is impaired. It may take up to 30 years for the signs of renal insufficiency to develop.

Chronic glomerulonephritis is a slowly progressive, destructive process affecting the glomeruli, causing loss of kidney function. The kidney decreases in size as glomeruli are destroyed. If end-stage renal disease (ESRD) develops, the client may die quickly.

Nephrons lose their ability to filter nitrogenous wastes from the blood. Protein (albumin) and red blood cells escape into the urine and are present on a urinalysis. Nitrogenous waste remains in the blood, and the BUN level increases. As glomeruli are destroyed, the serum level of creatinine also increases. BUN and serum creatinine are checked on a regular basis to monitor renal function. Serum electrolyte levels are also monitored. Anemia is evaluated with a CBC.

MEDICAL–SURGICAL MANAGEMENT

Medical

Prevention of further renal damage as well as heart or cerebral complications is the focus of care. Management includes drug therapy, diet, and bed rest. Exposure of the client to infection of any kind must be avoided. Blood transfusion may be required for severe anemia. The client may be transferred to a facility where dialysis and/or kidney transplantation can be performed.

Pharmacological

Diuretic and antihypertensive medications are ordered. Antimicrobial therapy is generally given prophylactically. Monitor for side effects from all medications and report to the physician immediately.

Diet

Fluid intake is adjusted according to urinary output. Protein allowed in the diet will be regulated according to the BUN and the creatinine blood levels. As these levels increase, protein will be restricted to decrease the nitrogenous wastes. Sodium and potassium restrictions will be determined by the serum electrolyte levels. Carbohydrates are usually increased in the diet to provide adequate energy.

Activity

Bed rest is indicated when the client has hematuria or albuminuria.

NURSING MANAGEMENT

Assist client with ADLs and encourage bed rest with diversional activities. Monitor vital signs and I&O. Measure urine hourly or as ordered. Assess color and consistency of urine. Assess lung sounds, edema, speech, and mental functioning. Assist client to reposition frequently and assess skin. Weigh client daily. Monitor laboratory reports.

NURSING PROCESS

ASSESSMENT

Subjective Data

Clients may describe a morning headache, pruritis, a decreased ability to concentrate, fatigue, and dyspnea making it difficult to perform ADLs. Facial edema and/or blurring of vision caused by retinal edema may also be reported by clients.

Objective Data

As chronic glomerulonephritis develops, fluid retention becomes evident, leading to shortness of breath, especially at night. Monitor vital signs; hypertension is usually present. Assess lung sounds every shift for crackles, a sign of fluid retention. Monitor weight daily, and note the degree of edema, its location, and if it is pitting or nonpitting. **Anasarca** is generalized edema that appears as the client's condition deteriorates. Assess skin for color, presence of ecchymosis or rash, dryness, and evidence of scratching. Note mental functioning, irritability, tremors, ataxia, or slurred speech.

As nephrons lose their ability to concentrate urine, the urine becomes pale and dilute. Closely monitor I&O because initially, polyuria develops, giving the client a false sense that recovery will be soon. Monitor results of blood and urine tests.

Nursing diagnoses for a client with chronic glomerulonephritis include the following:

NURSING DIAGNOSES	PLANNING/OUTCOMES	NURSING INTERVENTIONS
*Impaired **U**rinary Elimination* related to the failing kidney function	The client will have adequate urine output.	Measure urine output hourly, or every 4 or 8 hours as ordered. Parameters will be set by the physician for immediate notification. Assess and document the color and consistency of the urine. Measure intake to determine compliance with the amount of fluids permitted. Weigh client daily at the same time each day, on the same scale and with the same clothes.
*Excess **F**luid Volume* related to compromised regulatory mechanism	The client will have decreased edema.	Assess and describe the location of the edema. Administer medications as ordered for treatment of the edema. Monitor electrolyte values. Maintain fluid intake at restricted amount. Document I&O.
***A**nxiety* related to threat to or change in health status (potential dialysis treatment)	The client will communicate less anxiety about possible treatment with dialysis.	Assist client to express concerns about possible treatment with dialysis. Arrange for a dialysis nurse to visit client. Provide written information about dialysis.
*Risk for Impaired **S**kin Integrity* related to immobility and edema	The client will maintain skin integrity.	Assess skin every time the client is repositioned. Cleanse the skin frequently, especially when crystals of urea form on the skin, causing itching and dryness.

Evaluation: Evaluate each outcome to determine how it has been met by the client.

OBSTRUCTIVE DISORDERS

Disorders of this type include urolithiasis, urinary bladder tumors, renal tumors, and polycystic kidney.

URINARY CALCULI

Approximately 1 million Americans each year have kidney stones (NKF, 2009c). **Urolithiasis** is a calculus,

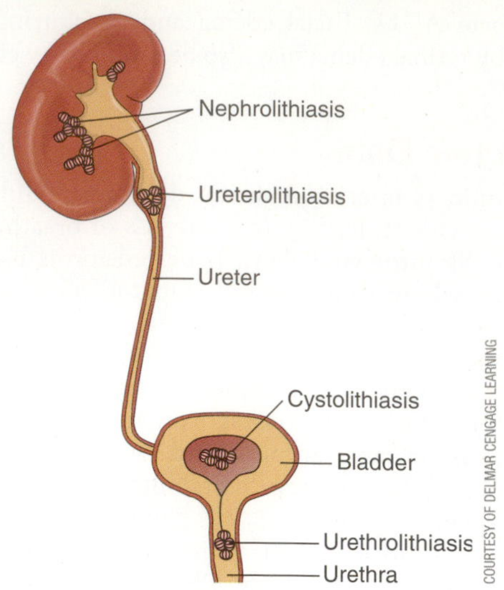

FIGURE 39-6 Common Locations of Urinary Calculi Formation

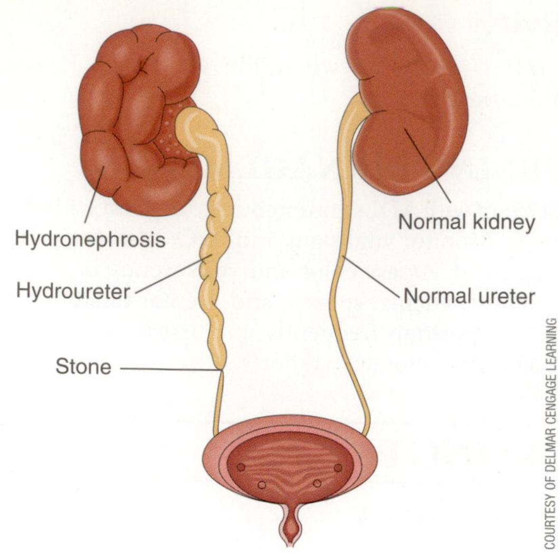

FIGURE 39-7 Hydronephrosis and Hydroureter Resulting from a Stone in the Ureter

or stone, formed in the urinary tract. A **calculus** (plural—calculi) is a solid mass of mineral salts occurring within a hollow organ such as the renal pelvis, ureters, bladder, or urethra (Figure 39-6). A urinary calculus can range in size from microscopic to 10 to 20 mm in diameter.

Calculi are formed when minerals precipitate out of solution and collect within hollow areas. The reason stones form has not yet been identified, but individuals who are immobile, hyperparathyroid, or have recurrent UTIs are predisposed. When a person is immobile for long periods, calcium is pulled from the bones into the blood. The nephrons filter the excess calcium out of the blood into the urine. Calculi can also lodge in and obstruct an indwelling catheter. The size and location of the stone within the urinary system greatly affects the degree of pain and other symptoms present. When the stone is in the kidney, the pain is dull and constant mainly in the back just below the ribs near the spine. Stones in the ureter often cause ureteral colic, an excruciating, intermittent pain that begins in the flank and radiates into the groin, inner thigh, or genitalia. It is caused by spasm of the ureter as the calculus moves down the ureter. The client often has nausea and vomiting.

If a calculus becomes lodged anyplace along the ureter and urine cannot pass, a condition called hydronephrosis and/or hydroureter occurs. The kidney and/or ureter become enlarged with the accumulated urine (Figure 39-7).

Tests to confirm the diagnosis and determine the size and location of the stone include spiral CT scan, KUB, IVP, cystoscopy, and ultrasound. A BUN and serum creatinine indicate whether the calculus has damaged kidney function. A urinalysis with a culture and a CBC may be ordered to determine whether an infection is present. A 24-hour urine may be sent to the laboratory to determine whether there is abnormal excretion of calcium oxalate, phosphorus, and uric acid.

MEDICAL–SURGICAL MANAGEMENT

Medical

All urine is strained whether voided or from an indwelling catheter drainage bag. Urine from a catheter drainage bag is drained and strained every 2 to 4 hours. All strained particles are saved for the physician or sent to the laboratory.

A very small calculus may be flushed out by peristalsis and fluids. The client is encouraged to drink at least 4,000 mL of fluid per day, unless contraindicated by other health problems. The urologist may insert a small, pliable catheter stent into the ureter or urethra to allow temporary drainage of urine around the calculus.

PROFESSIONALTIP

Risk Factors for Kidney Stone Development

The following factors may increase a client's risk of developing kidney stones:

- Diet: high protein, high sodium, foods containing oxalate
- Lack of fluids: causes a higher concentration of substances that can form stones
- Family/personal history
- Age/sex: common between 20 to 70 years of age, men more likely to develop
- Limited activity: on bed rest or sedentary for long periods of time
- Hypertension: doubles the risk of forming stones
- Obesity: higher body mass index (particularly in women)
- Gastric bypass surgery, inflammatory bowel disease, or chronic diarrhea: changes in digestive process that affect absorption of calcium increase the level of substances in urine that form stones

Adapted from Mayo Clinic, 2009, Kidney Stones Risk Factors, from http://www.mayoclinic.com/health/kidney-stones/DS00282/DSECTION=risk-factors

Extracorporeal shock wave **lithotripsy** (ESWL) is a noninvasive method of crushing a calculus in the urinary system with ultrasonic waves to shatter or pulverize the stones into tiny pieces that are small enough to be passed in the urine. Sedation or light anesthesia is used to maintain comfort during the procedure due to the pain caused by the shock waves. The procedure requires 30 minutes to 2 hours to complete. The client is placed in a warm-water bath, and ultrasonic waves aimed at the stone break the stone into small pieces. An alternate method is to appropriately place a fluid-filled bag on the client's body and aim the ultrasonic waves at the stone through the bag, or the client is placed on a soft cushion. There is some discomfort and the client may be bruised where the ultrasonic waves hit the body. The urine will be slightly bloody for 24 to 48 hours and must be strained. The client should drink large amounts of fluids (3,000 mL to 4,000 mL per day) unless contraindicated. Clients should avoid taking aspirin and other drugs that affect blood clotting for several weeks before the procedure (NIDDK, 2007a).

Ureteroscopy is used for mid- and lower-ureter stones. The small fiber-optic ureteroscope is passed through the urethra and bladder into the ureter. The stone is either removed in a cage-like device or shattered with a shock wave and the pieces removed (NIDDK, 2007b).

Surgical

The surgeon may choose from several surgical procedures, depending on the location and size of the calculus. These include nephroscopic removal, pyelolithotomy, or nephrolithotomy (Figure 39-8).

Percutaneous nephrolithotomy is an endoscopic procedure in which a small incision is made in the fleshy area on the client's side between the ribs and the hip. A catheter is inserted and an ultrasonic probe is inserted through the catheter. Ultrasound waves directed at the stone break it into small pieces that can be withdrawn through the catheter. The catheter is left in place until the edema subsides, usually 1 or 2 days.

A bladder calculus may be crushed with special surgical instruments and the fragments washed out through a catheter. This is called a **litholapaxy**.

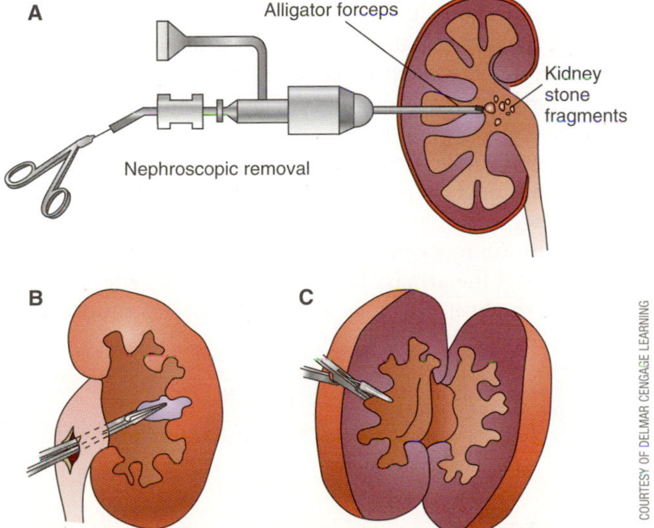

FIGURE 39-8 Methods of Removing Urinary Stones; *A*, Nephroscopic Removal (percutaneous nephrolithotomy); *B*, Pyelolithotomy, Removal Through the Renal Pelvis; *C*, Nephrolithotomy, Removal Through Incision into the Kidney

Pharmacological

Narcotic analgesics are generally prescribed for the severe pain often called renal colic. Antispasmodics such as propantheline bromide (Pro-Banthine) or belladonna preparations may be ordered to relieve ureteral spasms. Antibiotics may be ordered prophylactically.

Drug therapy is specific to stone composition. Allopurinol (Zyloprim) reduces the serum urate level, preventing calcium oxalate stones. Diuretics, such as hydrochlorothiazide (Esidrex, Ezide, Hydro-Par), are prescribed to decrease the amount of calcium released by the kidneys in the urine. Tiopronin (Thiola) and penicillamine (Cuprimine) are given to prevent the formation of cystine stones by reducing the amount of cystine in the urine. Aluminum hydroxide gel (Amphojel) binds with excess phosphates in the gastrointestinal tract. The phosphates are then excreted. Rarely, clients with hypercalciuria are given sodium cellulose phosphate (Calcibind) to bind with calcium in the intestines and facilitate excretion of calcium and prevent it from leaking into the urine.

Diet

In the past, clients who formed calcium stones were told to avoid foods high in calcium. It was believed that foods high in calcium, including dairy products, may contribute to the formation of calcium stones. Recent studies have shown that eating foods high in calcium may help prevent calcium stones, but taking calcium in pill form may increase the risk of developing stones (NIDDK, 2007a). When the stones contain uric acid, purine-rich foods (meat, fish, and poultry) are restricted, and organ meats, anchovies, and sardines avoided. Foods rich in oxalic acid (broccoli, asparagus, chocolate, tea, rhubarb, and spinach) are restricted when oxalate stones form. A deficiency of pyridoxine, thiamin, and magnesium may also contribute to the formation of oxalate stones.

Sometimes an effort is made to change the pH of the urine and thus prevent the formation of calculi. Acid-ash or alkaline-ash diets are used. Acid-ash foods are meats, fish, poultry, eggs, cereals, cranberries, and plums. Alkaline-ash foods are vegetables and all other fruits. These diets are often difficult for the client to maintain.

Drinking large amounts of fluid, at least half of it water, dilutes the urine and helps move any microscopic calculi through the system. Up to 4,000 mL per day of fluid is indicated for a client with renal calculi, unless contraindicated by another health problem such as heart failure.

Activity

Exercising regularly helps reduce the formation of calculi and keeps calculi moving through the urinary tract. Clients on bed rest should perform active range-of-motion (ROM) exercises daily in addition to frequent turning and positioning.

Nursing Management

Strain all urine. Monitor I&O. Encourage 4,000 mL per day of fluid intake unless contraindicated. Refer to dietitian for special acid-ash or alkaline-ash diet. Encourage active ROM exercises for clients on bed rest. Assess for pain and administer analgesic as ordered.

NURSING PROCESS

Assessment

Subjective Data

Many individuals are asymptomatic until the calculus begins to move or becomes too large. When the stone moves, the client usually describes intractable pain (pain not relieved by ordinary measures). The pain is often described as beginning in the flank and radiating down to the groin and inner thigh. Nonverbal client behaviors may indicate pain by tossing and turning when in bed or the inability to sit still when out of bed. If the calculus is not moving, the client may describe symptoms of infection such as lethargy, frequency of urination, persistent urge to urinate, dysuria, burning on urination, or feeling very warm. Nausea and vomiting are often reported. The client may express feelings of frustration related to the inability to complete daily tasks.

Objective Data

Assess hematuria, vomiting, intake and output, and vital signs. Elevated pulse and blood pressure may indicate pain. Check urine for stones when it is strained. Assess for cloudy, foul smelling urine and fever and chills if infection is present.

Nursing diagnoses for a client with urolithiasis include the following:

NURSING DIAGNOSES	PLANNING/OUTCOMES	NURSING INTERVENTIONS
*Acute **Pain** related to irritation of the urinary tract and the mobility of calculi*	The client will verbalize a reduction in pain.	Develop a pain management plan. Inquire about intensity, location, duration, and alleviating factors of pain. Observe for nonverbal signs of pain. Provide comfort measures and diversionary activities and administer analgesics and antispasmodics as ordered.
*Impaired **Urinary** Elimination* related to blockage of urine flow by the calculi	The client will return to normal urine elimination.	Encourage fluids to dilute the urine and flush out the calculi. Monitor urine for color and amount. Assist client to ambulate, if able. Accurately monitor intake and output. If a ureteral catheter is in place, measure and record the urine output from it separately from the urine output from the bladder.

Evaluation: Evaluate each outcome to determine how it has been met by the client.

URINARY BLADDER TUMORS

The American Cancer Society estimates approximately 70,980 new cases of urinary bladder cancer in 2009 (ACS, 2009b). Men are affected four times more often than women. Bladder cancer occurs most frequently after the age of 50. The only early warning signs are increased urinary frequency and painless, intermittent hematuria. As the disease progresses, the client may present with a UTI, painful urination, back pain, and abdominal pain. The main risk factor is cigarette smoking. Those individuals who smoke nicotine products have twice the risk of developing bladder cancer as do nonsmokers. Other risk factors are working with dyes, rubber, leather, or paint products; arsenic in drinking water; genetics; bladder birth defects; low fluid consumption; chemotherapy and radiation therapy; and chronic bladder inflammation (ACS, 2009d).

Benign papillomas are the most common urinary bladder tumor. Although papillomas are quite small, they should be treated aggressively because they are considered to be premalignant. Cancer cells develop mainly in the area where the ureters enter the urinary bladder. The primary sites for metastasis are the liver, lungs, or bones. Symptoms resulting from

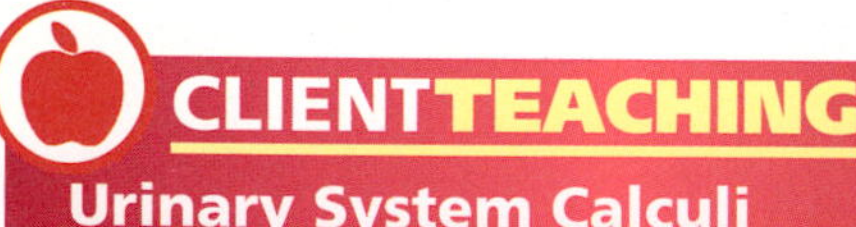

Urinary System Calculi

A person with a family history of stones or who has had more than one stone is at risk to develop another stone. Instruct these clients to:

- Drink plenty of fluids—water is best—to prevent stone formation.
- Avoid immobility.
- Take medications and modify diet as prescribed.
- Keep a record of intake and output.
- Learn how to strain urine.

CULTURAL CONSIDERATIONS

Bladder Cancer

Caucasians are almost 2 times as likely to have bladder cancer as African Americans (ACS, 2009).

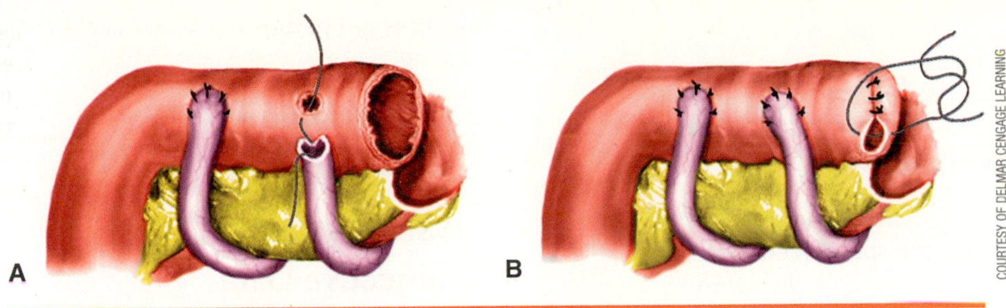

FIGURE 39-9 Ileal Conduit; *A*, Ureters Implanted into Ileal Segment; *B*, Closure of Proximal End of Ileal Conduit

obstruction of the ureters are often the reason the client seeks medical care. Diagnostic studies usually include a urinalysis, a cystoscopic visualization and biopsy of the lesions, an IVP, CT scan, urine cytology and culture, tumor marker studies, retrograde pyelography, chest x-ray, MRI, ultrasound, bone scan, and PET scan.

MEDICAL–SURGICAL MANAGEMENT

Surgical

For superficial or early stage bladder cancer, a transurethral resection (TUR) is most commonly performed. The urologist places a resectoscope into the bladder through the urethra to remove the tumor. The tumor tissue is sent to pathology for examination. Surgical removal of small tumors is generally done by **fulguration** (a procedure to destroy tissue with long, high-frequency electric sparks) to burn the lesions off the internal bladder wall. Other surgical procedures used are laser surgery or snaring of the lesion. These procedures are usually performed with cystoscopic visualization. Several times a year, the client who has had bladder lesions should be monitored for recurrence of the lesions. A cytologic examination is done on any lesion(s) noted during a cystoscopic examination.

A cystoscopic examination is performed with either local anesthesia and sedation or general anesthesia. After the procedure, the client's legs may be sore from the lithotomy position used. Analgesics will be prescribed for use as needed. After a cystoscopic procedure, the client may experience urinary frequency, burning on urination, and the presence of pink-tinged urine.

When the pathology of tissue specimens indicates a need for more extensive surgery, either a partial or total cystectomy may be performed. The surgery may be done in conjunction with radiation therapy or chemotherapy.

When the urinary bladder is completely removed, a urinary diversion is necessary. Consideration is made for age, extent of the disease, and the prognosis. One option is a bilateral cutaneous ureterostomy, in which the ureters are implanted directly into the abdominal wall. Another option is for the ureters to be implanted into a piece of the ileum, which is then attached to the abdominal wall as a stoma. This is known as an **ileal** ("wet") **conduit** (Figure 39-9).

Other methods of urinary diversion are the implantation of the ureters into the sigmoid colon (ureterosigmoidostomy) and the creation of a continent stoma with a pouch of bowel. This urinary diversion is known either as a Kock (Figure 39-10) or Mainz pouch or a Gilchrist ileocecal reservoir, depending on which surgical procedure was used. A newer method is to create a neobladder, a urinary reservoir composed of a piece of ileum, to route the urine back into the urethra, restoring close-to-normal urination (ACS, 2009a).

Pharmacological

One chemotherapy treatment is the instillation of an antineoplastic drug within the urinary bladder (**intravesical**). The most common and most effective intravesical therapy used for treating low-stage bladder cancer is Bacillus Calmette-Guerin (BCG). BCG causes the client's immune system to attack the bladder cancer. Systemic chemotherapy may also be used. Medications to relieve symptoms such as pain and nausea are important for the client's well-being.

Diet

If proctitis (inflammation of the rectum and anus) or diarrhea occurs, a low-residue diet is ordered to facilitate normal bowel elimination.

Activity

When the client is on bed rest, turning and positioning are important to maintain skin integrity because the client may be emaciated as a result of significant weight loss. Activity should be encouraged as the client's condition warrants. During the intravesical instillation of an antineoplastic drug, the client will have to change positions every 15 minutes, for a period of several hours, to evenly distribute the chemotherapeutic drug around the urinary bladder.

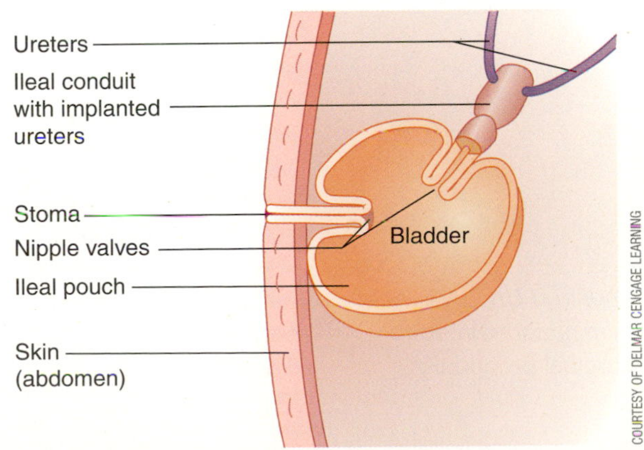

FIGURE 39-10 Urinary Diversion—Koch Pouch

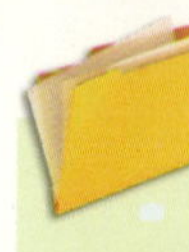

COLLABORATIVE CARE

Urinary Diversions

Nurses work together with the enterostomal therapist to provide the specialized care and teaching required for a urinary diversion.

Nursing Management

Encourage clients to reduce or eliminate the use of nicotine products and report urinary frequency and painless hematuria to their physician. After a cystoscopic examination, administer analgesic as needed for sore legs from lithotomy position. Encourage client to have adequate fluid intake and to express fears and concerns, especially if a urinary diversion is performed. Refer client to local ostomy support group.

NURSING PROCESS

Assessment

Subjective Data

The client will describe having painless, intermittent hematuria and changes in voiding patterns. Fatigue may also be mentioned. As the cancer progresses, the client may experience abdominal and back pain.

Objective Data

Weakness will be noted if the client has become anemic from the hematuria. Check urine specimen with a reagent strip for blood, review results of diagnostic tests, and assess the client's understanding of current health situation.

Nursing diagnoses for a client with urinary bladder tumors include the following:

NURSING DIAGNOSES	PLANNING/OUTCOMES	NURSING INTERVENTIONS
*Deficient **K**nowledge* related to surgery and treatment regimen	The client will describe surgical changes and treatment regimen.	If surgical removal of bladder lesions is done as an outpatient procedure, teach the client to observe for pink-tinged urine and to notify the physician if bright red urine is seen. Discuss the use of analgesics as ordered for pain of bladder spasms. Encourage adequate fluid intake. For urinary diversions: Refer the client with a stoma to the enterostomal therapist for specialized care and teaching. The therapist will assist the client with the appliance and skin care protocol. Monitor the color and integrity of the stoma daily to ensure that the tissue is receiving adequate circulation. The stoma is normally red and edematous for a time postoperatively. The stoma will remain red in color but will shrink in size during the healing process. If the stoma color changes, notify the physician. Refer to a local ostomy group for ongoing support and assistance or to the United Ostomy Association, which provides support and literature. Teach the signs and symptoms related to potential problems that should be reported to the physician. Encourage the intake of fluids, up to 3,000 mL per day, unless contraindicated. Teach about the medications to be taken at home. Encourage the client to attend all scheduled follow-up visits. Assist the client to plan the gradual return to the routines of driving, lifting, sexual activities, and work.
*Impaired **U**rinary Elimination* related to surgical procedure	The client will maintain adequate urinary elimination.	Accurately monitor urine output because this is the major postoperative concern. Assist client to discuss feelings about the altered urinary elimination method.

Nursing diagnoses for a client with urinary bladder tumors include the following: (Continued)

NURSING DIAGNOSES	PLANNING/OUTCOMES	NURSING INTERVENTIONS
		Assist the client with a bilateral cutaneous ureterostomy to use leg bags for easier ambulation. Change the leg bag tubing back to straight bag drainage to promote uninterrupted sleep. Teach the client how to use both a leg bag and a straight bag drainage system.

Evaluation: Evaluate each outcome to determine how it has been met by the client.

RENAL TUMORS

The American Cancer Society estimates that there will be approximately 57,760 new cases of kidney cancer in 2009 (ACS, 2009c). A unilateral renal cell adenocarcinoma is the most common tumor and is seen more often in men between the ages of 50 and 70. Risk factors include smoking, obesity, familial incidence, preexisting renal disorders, hypertension, and workplace exposure to asbestos, cadmium, some herbicides, benzene, and organic solvents, particularly trichloroethylene.

Intermittent, painless hematuria is often ignored by the client, and medical attention is not sought until the malignancy is quite advanced. By this time, the client usually has experienced weight loss, dull flank pain, gross hematuria, and a mass that may be palpable in the flank area. Lymph nodes in the area of the kidney, the renal vessels, and/or the inferior vena cava may become involved. The primary sites for metastases are the lungs, liver, brain, and bone. A pathological fracture may be the reason for admission of the client, resulting in the diagnosis of kidney cancer.

A helical (spiral) CT scan or standard CT scan are commonly used to provide detailed images of the kidney. Other diagnostic studies used to evaluate the kidney or the status of other body systems possibly involved are MRI, IVP, angiography, ultrasound, urinalysis, CBC, biopsy, PET, and bone scan.

CULTURAL CONSIDERATIONS

Renal-Cell Carcinoma

Those most at risk are:

- African-American clients, who have a slightly greater rate
- People with a strong family history of renal cell cancer
- Siblings (brothers or sisters) of those affected
- Those exposed to asbestos, cadmium, some herbicides, benzene, and organic solvents, particularly trichloroethylene, at their job (ACS, 2009e)

MEDICAL–SURGICAL MANAGEMENT

Medical

The physician may insert a nephrostomy tube into the renal pelvis of each kidney to evaluate their function. Treatment options may include immunotherapy, targeted therapy, chemotherapy, radiation therapy, or a combination of these depending on the stage of the cancer and the client's overall health. Chemotherapy and/or radiation therapy have proved to be of minimal benefit.

Surgical

Usually a laparoscopic nephrectomy, the preferred method, or an open radical nephrectomy is performed if the other kidney is healthy and the disease is localized. The surgeon may enter the thoracic as well as the abdominal cavity during this procedure. If the chest is opened, the client will have a closed-chest drainage system postoperatively. A nasogastric drainage tube may be in place and attached to suction. Hemorrhage and compromised respiratory effort are the postoperative problems for which to observe.

Pharmacological

If the client is receiving radiation therapy treatments, antiemetics or antispasmodics may be ordered. Analgesics are ordered to control pain and facilitate respirations and client activity. An antiemetic will usually be ordered to promote comfort and to encourage eating.

Diet

The client having a nephrectomy will have intravenous fluids until food can be tolerated. A well-balanced diet is then ordered. Fluid intake of at least 2,000 mL per day is needed to maintain adequate hydration. The use of alcohol should be avoided. If the client is **cachectic** (in a state of malnutrition and wasting) because of the cancer's pathology, parenteral nutrition may be indicated.

Activity

Encourage ambulation during the client's recovery. Frequent rest periods are necessary even after discharge.

Nursing Management

Encourage client to express feelings and concerns about diagnosis. Observe for signs of grieving. Answer questions honestly. Assess neurologic status, lung sounds, peripheral pulses, and vital signs. Accurately record I&O. Provide preoperative teaching.

NURSING PROCESS

Assessment

Subjective Data

The client will describe having a dull pain in the flank area and noticing blood in the urine intermittently; however, the client often comments that there is no difficulty in urinating. Fatigue and weight loss are also described.

Objective Data

Observe client for weight changes. Monitor vital signs and diagnostic test results. Assess the client's lung sounds for possible respiratory distress resulting from metastases. Hematuria may be present. A mass may be palpated in the client's flank area.

Nursing diagnoses for a client with renal tumors include the following:

NURSING DIAGNOSES	PLANNING/OUTCOMES	NURSING INTERVENTIONS
***F**atigue* related to disease process and treatment	The client will understand reason for fatigue and not feel guilty for taking rest periods.	Discuss with client that fatigue is a result of blood loss in the urine and growth of the tumor. Because there is increased fatigue following any surgery, plan nursing care so the client will have several periods of uninterrupted rest each day.
*Anticipatory **G**rieving* related to diagnosis, treatment, and prognosis	The client will maintain open communications with family and health care members.	Actively listen to what the client says. Encourage the client to express feelings about the diagnosis and treatment. Observe for signs of grieving such as crying, denial, anger, or withdrawal. Answer questions honestly. Assist client in identifying strengths and coping skills. Make referrals to other professionals as needed.
*Deficient **K**nowledge* related to limited information of disease process and treatment regimen	The client will verbalize understanding of information taught.	Inform client of the assessments to be done: neurological status, lung sounds, the incision, Homans' sign, peripheral pulses, vital signs, and serum electrolyte values. Teach the importance of accurate intake and output records. Provide routine preoperative teaching. Encourage client to eat a well-balanced diet to enhance healing. Instruct client not to wash off the skin markings if radiation therapy is being used. Teach the name, purpose, dosage, schedule, and side effects of all medications and the importance of drinking plenty of fluids and ambulating as tolerated. Inform client and family of community resources and support groups. Point out the importance of following the instructions for care when discharged and keeping physician appointments.

Evaluation: Evaluate each outcome to determine how it has been met by the client.

POLYCYSTIC KIDNEY

Approximately 600,000 Americans have polycystic kidney disease (PKD), which is the fourth leading cause of kidney failure (NIDDK, 2007c). Two major inherited forms of PKD include autosomal-dominant PKD, about 90 % of all cases, and autosomal recessive PKD, a rare form. Acquired cystic kidney disease (ACKD) is associated with kidney failure and dialysis. Approximately 90% of clients on dialysis for 5 years develop ACKD (NKF, 2009d). In PKD, multiple grape-like clusters of fluid-filled cysts develop in and greatly enlarge both kidneys. They compress and eventually replace functioning kidney tissue. PKD has an insidious onset that becomes obvious between 30 and 50 years of age.

Early symptoms include hypertension, polyuria, and urinary tract infections. Flank pain and headache are common. Recurrent hematuria and proteinuria develop. Diagnosis is made by x-ray or sonogram showing the cysts. BUN and creatinine are used to monitor kidney function.

The goal of medical management is to preserve kidney function, prevent infections, and relieve pain. Hypertension is carefully managed with antihypertensive medications, diuretics, and fluid and dietary modifications. Eventually, dialysis or renal transplantation may be needed.

RENAL FAILURE

According to the NIDDK (2006), any acute or chronic loss of kidney function is called renal failure and is the term used when some kidney function remains. Total, or nearly total, and permanent kidney failure is called ESRD. It may take only a few days or weeks to lose renal function or it may deteriorate slowly over decades. Disorders of renal failure are either acute or chronic.

ACUTE RENAL FAILURE

The rapid deterioration of renal function with rising blood levels of urea and other nitrogenous wastes (**azotemia**) is termed acute renal failure (ARF). The nephrons are unable to regulate the fluid and electrolyte or the acid–base balance of the blood. Predisposing factors include acute glomerular disease; severe, acute kidney infection; decreased cardiac output; trauma; or hemorrhage.

There are three major forms depending on the location of the cause: postrenal ARF (disrupted urine flow), prerenal ARF (disrupted blood flow to the kidney), and intrarenal ARF (renal tissue damage). Both postrenal ARF and prerenal ARF are reversible situations if they are identified early and treatment is begun. Undiagnosed postrenal ARF and prerenal ARF lead to intrarenal ARF. Diagnostic testing to identify the cause of ARF includes an ultrasound, CT scan, MRI, and, on occasion, a kidney tissue biopsy.

POSTRENAL ARF

Postrenal ARF is caused by an obstruction. It should be checked out first when a client has an unexplained decrease in urine output or has anuria. Kidney function can be easily restored by removing the obstruction. Urine volume will vary depending on the location and degree of obstruction. Catheterization, ultrasound, and retrograde pyelogram are used to diagnose an obstruction. An obstruction may be caused by renal calculi, blood clots, edema, tumors, urethral strictures, benign prostatic hypertrophy (BPH), pregnancy, or a nerve disorder. Postrenal failure can be ruled out if there is no obstruction. If an obstruction is confirmed, relief of the obstruction is imperative to minimize renal damage and resolve azotemia. When postrenal failure is prolonged, both blood creatinine and BUN will rise.

PRERENAL ARF

Any abnormal decline in kidney perfusion that reduces glomerular perfusion can cause prerenal failure. Common causes include extremely low blood pressure from severe bleeding, infection, shock, congestive heart failure, myocardial infarction, or severe dehydration. Fluid volume status does not indicate perfusion. Effective arterial blood volume (EABV) is the amount of fluid in the vascular space that effectively perfuses the kidneys. Even in fluid volume excess situations, such as low cardiac output caused by heart failure, the EABV falls, causing prerenal failure. The kidney interprets a fall in EABV as fluid volume deficit.

The glomeruli are then unable to filter waste from the blood. The renal tubules are structurally intact, and the kidneys can resume normal functioning if perfusion is restored fairly quickly. Ischemia results from prolonged inadequate perfusion, which can cause acute tubular necrosis (ATN).

The client generally has pale, cool skin; orthostatic hypotension; and oliguria. The BUN-to-creatinine ratio increases from 10:1 to more than 20:1. This increase occurs because of greater reabsorption of urea when fluids flow slowly through the tubules. A urinalysis shows a low sodium level (<20 mEq/L), high osmolality (>500 mOsm/L), and high specific gravity (>1.020). This results because the kidneys are retaining sodium and water in an attempt to correct the perceived fluid volume deficit.

When the client truly has a fluid volume deficit, treatment consists of intravenous fluids and albumin, plasma, or blood to restore the EABV. When the cause is inadequate cardiac output, inotropic agents such as dobutamine hydrochloride (Dobutrex) or amrinone lactate (Inocor) are used.

INTRARENAL ARF

Tissue damage of the glomeruli and/or tubules causes a loss of renal function known as intrarenal ARF. Glomerulonephritis and ATN are the main reasons for renal tissue damage. The antigen/antibody complexes formed in glomerulonephritis become trapped in the basement membrane, where they cause inflammation. The glomeruli then become more permeable, so red blood cells and protein are allowed to enter the filtrate and ultimately the urine.

Most intrarenal failure cases are caused by ATN and are the most common cause of nosocomial acute renal failure. ATN is the result of ischemia or toxic insult to the renal tubules. Ischemia may result from untreated prerenal failure or severe hypoxemia. Radiographic contrast dye, pigments (myoglobin and hemoglobin), aminoglycoside and cephalosporin antibiotics, and NSAIDs are all **nephrotoxic** (substances that causes kidney tissue damage) and can cause acute tubular necrosis.

The BUN-to-creatinine ratio in acute tubular necrosis is usually normal between 10:1 and 15:1; however, both the BUN and creatinine are greatly elevated. For example, the BUN may be 70 mg/dL and the creatinine 7 mg/dL. Urine sodium is more than 40 mEq/L, urine osmolality less than

CLIENT TEACHING

Acute Renal Failure

Teach clients at risk for ARF (older clients; diabetic clients; and clients with renal, heart, or liver disease) to:

- Immediately report to health care provider signs of fluid retention, pain on urination, and changes in urine output (amount or appearance).
- Avoid chronic use of and high doses of NSAIDs.
- Follow sodium and fluid restrictions as prescribed.
- Advise all health care providers of condition.

300 mOsm/L, and specific gravity less than 1.010. There are three phases to the clinical course of ATN: oliguric/nonoliguric, diuretic, and recovery. The first phase is either oliguric or nonoliguric depending on the causative factor.

Oliguric/Nonoliguric Phase

A nonoliguric phase is usually seen when nephrotoxic agents are the causative factor. When adequate urine output is maintained, dialysis is needed less often, and the morbidity and mortality rates are lower.

An oliguric phase, which may last 1 to 2 weeks, is seen more often when ischemia is the causative factor. Oliguria, voiding less than 400 mL/24 hours, can cause fluid volume overload; electrolyte imbalance, specifically high potassium and phosphorus, and low sodium and calcium; metabolic acidosis; and uremia.

Diuretic Phase

The diuretic phase is seldom seen because early dialysis keeps extracellular fluid volume at a fairly normal level. If it were seen, there would be a tremendous increase in urine output.

Recovery Phase

As renal function begins to improve, the client's urine output returns to normal and serum and urine laboratory test values move closer to normal. There is usually a short period of rapid improvement and then a period (may be several months) of slower improvement. Some clients will have residual renal insufficiency and a few will require long-term dialysis.

Medical–Surgical Management

Medical

Acute renal failure is often reversible, and complications can be prevented with early diagnosis and treatment. The goal is to have kidney function stabilized and returned to normal. Problems to be alert for are fluid volume overload, electrolyte imbalances, metabolic acidosis, high rate of catabolism, uremia, hemotologic abnormalities, and infection.

Dialysis is now an early treatment in ATN. Homeostasis is maintained while the cause of ATN is determined and treated. Permanent kidney damage may thus be averted. See the section on dialysis later in this chapter.

Surgical

The obstructions causing postrenal failure are often removed surgically. The exact procedure will depend on what type of obstruction is present and its location.

Pharmacological

Drugs used to treat acute renal failure include antihypertensives, diuretics, cardiotonics (inotropics), phosphate-binding antacids, potassium-lowering agents, and electrolyte replacement. It is important to ensure that drugs used are not nephrotoxic. See Table 39-3 for drugs used in acute renal failure.

TABLE 39-3 Drugs Used in Acute Renal Failure

DRUGS	NURSING RESPONSIBILITIES
Antihypertensives methyldopa (Aldomet) minoxidil (Loniten) clonidine HCl (Catapres) hydralazine HCl (Apresoline)	Monitor BP and pulse, weigh daily, monitor for postural hypotension and K, Na, Cl, and CO_2 levels, I&O.
Diuretics furosemide (Lasix) hydrochlorothiazide (HydroDiuril)	Monitor output, maintain fluid restrictions, weigh client daily.
Cardiotonics/inotropics digoxin (Lanoxin) amrinone lactate (Inocor)	Assess apical pulse before giving, report blood level of digoxin, monitor BP and P, monitor blood level of potassium.
Phosphate-binding antacids aluminum hydroxide gel (Amphojel)	Monitor serum potassium, assess BP and P, and for constipation.
Potassium exchange sodium polystyrene sulfonate (Kayexalate)	Monitor serum potassium, assess BP and P, and for constipation.
Electrolyte replacement calcitrol (Rocaltrol) calcifediol (Calderol)	Monitor blood calcium and phosphate levels, report metallic taste.

COURTESY OF DELMAR CENGAGE LEARNING

Diet

Restrictions generally include sodium, potassium, phosphorus, protein, and fluids. The amounts allowed are based on the laboratory tests results. Carbohydrates and fats are increased to be sure energy needs are met and protein will be spared as a source of energy. Clients with a high rate of catabolism often require total parenteral nutrition (TPN) to provide adequate nutrition.

Activity

Because the client is often weak and may also be confused, activity is restricted during the initial phase of acute renal failure. As recovery becomes evident, ambulation is begun.

Nursing Management

Accurately record I&O (often hourly). Monitor vital signs, BUN, creatinine, and serum electrolytes and protein. Weigh client daily. Assess skin turgor, lung sounds, and jugular vein distention. Provide fluids within prescribed limits. Ask dietitian to discuss dietary restrictions with client. Provide or assist with oral hygiene before meals. Listen to client's concerns.

NURSING PROCESS

Assessment

Subjective Data

The client may describe diarrhea; nausea, possibly with vomiting; swelling; loss of appetite; headache; increasing fatigue; and/or a change in mental alertness. Anxiety and fear related to not knowing what is happening is often expressed.

CRITICAL THINKING

Assessment Scenario

A 52-year-old male client has been admitted to the hospital for chest pain. After a couple of days in the hospital, the nurse notices the client has a total urinary output of 325 mL in 24 hours and has edema in both ankles. The lab results for this client are: sodium 130 mEq/L, BUN 28, and serum creatinine 2.5.

1. What might be going on with the client at this time?
2. What is significant about the client's lab results?
3. What type of diet may this client need to be on? Why?

Objective Data

Physical findings will depend on how far the disease process has progressed. Assess for hypertension, GI bleeding and/or bruising, reduction in urine output, anasarca, poor skin turgor, and dry mucous membranes because vomiting or diarrhea can cause dehydration. In a severe stage, the client may be drowsy and have muscle twitching and convulsions.

The BUN and serum creatinine will be elevated, as are the serum electrolytes potassium and phosphorus. The serum electrolyte calcium will be low. Blood level of red blood cells will decrease as the production of erythropoietin decreases. Leukocyte level will increase in the presence of an infection.

Nursing diagnoses for a client with acute renal failure include the following:

NURSING DIAGNOSES	PLANNING/OUTCOMES	NURSING INTERVENTIONS
Excess Fluid Volume related to sodium and water retention	The client will maintain a stable fluid volume.	Monitor BUN, creatinine, and serum electrolyte and protein levels. Accurately measure urine output, often on an hourly basis. Parameters are often set for notification of the physician. Weigh daily to identify weight gain related to fluid retention. One pound of weight gain is equivalent to 500 mL of retained fluid. Assess skin turgor, edema, BP, lung sounds, jugular vein distention, pulse and respiratory rate and quality. Provide fluids within the prescribed limits. Teach client about importance of fluid restrictions.
Impaired Nutrition: Less than Body Requirements related to anorexia, dietary restrictions, and increased catabolism	The client will have stabilized weight within normal limits.	Arrange for a dietary consultation to provide food in keeping with the prescribed restrictions and client preferences, including cultural and religious factors. Suggest 6 small meals throughout the day. Offer antinausea medications before meals. Provide or assist with oral hygiene prior to meals. Monitor weight and serum albumin level weekly.

(*Continues*)

Nursing diagnoses for a client with acute renal failure include the following: (Continued)

NURSING DIAGNOSES	PLANNING/OUTCOMES	NURSING INTERVENTIONS
Anxiety related to the disease process	The client will verbalize anxieties with the family and health care workers.	Establish rapport with the client. Listen to the client's concerns. Maintain open communications to foster expression of anxieties.

Evaluation: Evaluate each outcome to determine how it has been met by the client.

SAMPLE NURSING CARE PLAN

The Client with Acute Renal Failure

R.H., age 65, has had a history of heart trouble for several years. He is admitted because he has urinated very little for 2 days, he gets dizzy when he gets up from lying down, and he cannot get his shoes on because his feet are "fat." He states that he does not know what is happening to him. Results of laboratory tests are BUN 90 mg/dL, creatinine 4 mg/dL, urine sodium 15 mEq/L, and urine specific gravity 1.030.

NURSING DIAGNOSIS 1 *Excess Fluid Volume* related to sodium and water retention as evidenced by "fat feet," urine sodium 15 mEq/L, and urine specific gravity 1.030

Nursing Outcomes Classification (NOC)
Fluid Balance
Electrolyte & Acid–Base Balance

Nursing Interventions Classification (NIC)
Electrolyte Management
Fluid Management

PLANNING/OUTCOMES	INTERVENTION	RATIONALE
R.H. will have reduced fluid volume excess.	Accurately measure and record intake and output.	Provides information about retention of intake.
	Weigh R.H. daily—same time, scale, clothes.	Allows weight comparisons.
	Assess skin turgor, edema, BP, lung sounds for crackles.	Provides information about fluid in tissue, lungs, or vascular system.
	Monitor BUN, creatinine, and serum electrolyte and protein levels.	Gives insight to kidney functioning.
	Administer inotropics or cardiotonic medications as ordered.	Strengthens heartbeat, which will give better perfusion to kidneys.
	Provide fluids within prescribed limits.	Prevents fluid excess.

EVALUATION

R.H.'s feet are no longer "fat." His urine sodium is 18 mEq/L and urine specific gravity is 1.027.

NURSING DIAGNOSIS 2 *Impaired urinary Elimination* related to decreased perfusion as evidenced by his urinating very little for 2 days and BUN–creatinine ratio of 22.5:1

Nursing Outcomes Classification (NOC)
Urinary Elimination
Knowledge: Disease Process

Nursing Interventions Classification (NIC)
Urinary Elimination Management
Teaching: Disease Process

SAMPLE NURSING CARE PLAN (Continued)

PLANNING/OUTCOMES	NURSING INTERVENTIONS	RATIONALE
R.H. will increase amount of urination to 1,200 mL/day.	Administer diuretics as ordered.	Increases water elimination by enhancing sodium excretion by the kidneys.
	Accurately measure and record intake and output.	Provides information about fluid movement through the body.

EVALUATION

R.H. is urinating 1,000 mL/day. His BUN is 50 mg/dL and creatinine is 3 mg/dL.

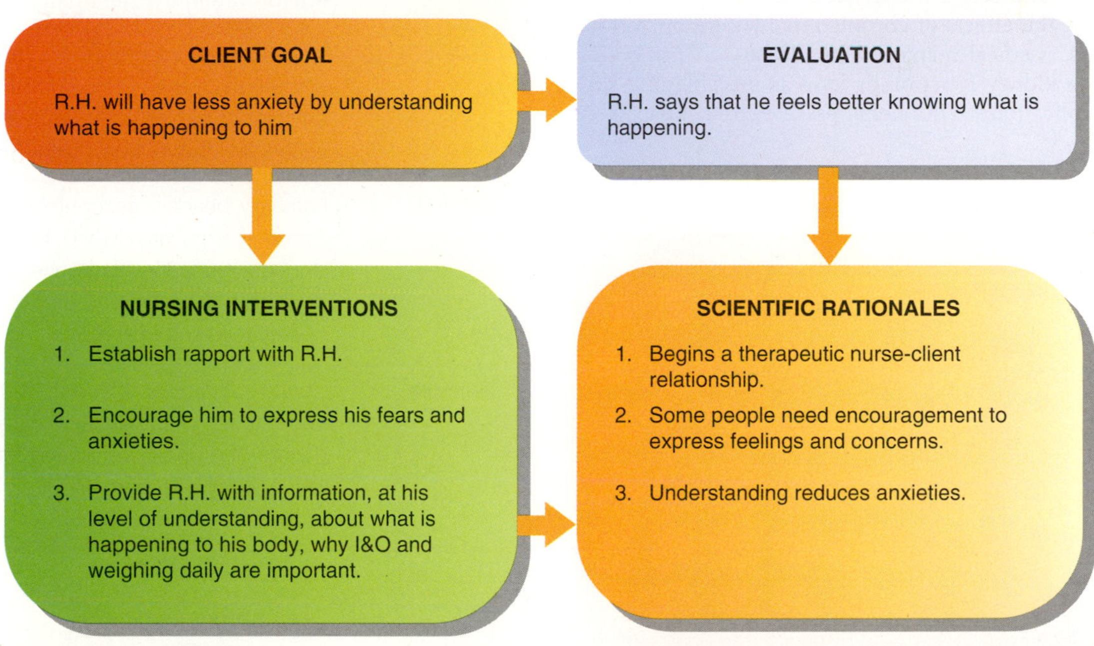

NURSING DIAGNOSIS
Anxiety related to the disease process as evidenced by his statement that he does not know what is happening to him
Nursing Outcomes Classification (NOC): *Acceptance: Health Status*
Nursing Interventions Classification (NIC): *Teaching: Individual*
CLIENT GOAL
R.H. will have less anxiety by understanding what is happening to him
EVALUATION
R.H. says that he feels better knowing what is happening.
NURSING INTERVENTIONS
1. Establish rapport with R.H.
2. Encourage him to express his fears and anxieties.
3. Provide R.H. with information, at his level of understanding, about what is happening to his body, why I&O and weighing daily are important.
SCIENTIFIC RATIONALES
1. Begins a therapeutic nurse-client relationship.
2. Some people need encouragement to express feelings and concerns.
3. Understanding reduces anxieties.

CONCEPT CARE MAP 39-1

CHRONIC RENAL FAILURE/ END-STAGE RENAL DISEASE

Chronic renal failure is a slow, progressive condition in which the kidney's ability to function ultimately deteriorates. This condition is not reversible. The kidneys have an amazing capability to perform effectively, even though most of the nephrons are destroyed.

Renal erythropoietin decreases, causing anemia. Hypertension, acidosis, and glucose intolerance usually are also present. Urea in the blood is extremely elevated. As the disease progresses, uremia develops.

There are three stages of chronic renal failure: reduced renal reserve, renal insufficiency, and end-stage renal disease (ESRD). Symptoms of reduced renal reserve are not apparent until more than 40% of the nephrons fail. A prolonged urine concentration test or a decline in GFR may be the only evidence of reduced renal reserve. When 75% of the nephrons stop functioning, renal insufficiency occurs. BUN and creatinine are above normal, and the client may have nocturia and polyuria. The onset of ESRD occurs when at least 90% of the nephrons fail: BUN and creatinine levels rise, polyuria changes to oliguria, and severe fluid and electrolyte imbalances are evident.

When the kidneys become unable to filter blood, an alternate method for filtration is necessary. Lifetime dialysis becomes inevitable unless kidney transplantation is performed and is successful. Life expectancy varies with the initial cause of chronic renal failure and the person's overall health at the time of diagnosis.

According to the National Kidney Foundation (2008), 485,000 Americans have ESRD. There are numerous causes of chronic renal failure. The four leading causes are diabetes mellitus 45%, hypertension 27%, glomerulonephritis 8.2%, and polycystic kidney 2.2% (NKF, 2008). Nephrotoxic drugs, including some over-the-counter drugs, aggravate the situation.

The diagnosis is confirmed when the BUN is at least 50 mg/dL and the serum creatinine level is greater than 5 mg/dL.

Medical–Surgical Management

Medical

Chronic renal failure is a multisystem disease process. See Table 39-4 for the effects of chronic renal failure on various body systems. Medical management focuses on preserving the remaining kidney function as long as possible and preventing complications. This helps preserve the integrity of

Table 39-4 Effects of Chronic Renal Failure by Body System

SYSTEM	EFFECT
Urinary	Oliguria from renal insufficiency Azotemia
Blood	Anemia from decreased red blood cell production Decreased platelet activity, causing bleeding tendency
Cardiovascular	Hypervolemia and tachycardia Hypertension and dysrhythmias from hyperkalemia
Respiratory	Dyspnea, pulmonary edema Hyperventilation from metabolic acidosis Eventually Kussmaul respirations
Gastrointestinal	Urea in the blood is converted to ammonia by the mouth, causing uremic halitosis Hiccups, anorexia, and nausea from edema within the gastrointestinal tract
Skin	Dry skin with pruritis from uremic frost (excretion of urea through the skin with an odor of urine); pallor with anemia, yellowish-brown skin color
Nervous	Lethargy, headaches, confusion, impaired concentration with disorientation, depression, decreased level of consciousness, sleep disturbances, and uremic encephalopathy resulting in seizures and coma
Sensory	Peripheral neuropathy with numbness and tingling of extremities with complaints of a prickly, crawling feeling in the feet and legs, especially at night, sleep problems
Reproductive	Decrease in libido Decreased sperm count Amenorrhea Impotence Delayed puberty
Musculoskeletal	Joint pain and muscle cramping/twitching Bone demineralization from Hypocalcemia
Immune	Greater chance of infections from immunosuppression Decrease in antibody production

COURTESY OF DELMAR CENGAGE LEARNING

CLIENT TEACHING

Herbal Facts for Renal Clients

Use of herbal supplements may be unsafe for renal clients because their bodies are unable to clear waste products effectively. Listed below are facts about herbs that every renal client should know (NKF, 2009e):

- The government does not regulate herbal supplements, so the exact contents and affects are unknown.
- Many herbs can interact with prescription drugs.
- Check with the physician, dietitian, or pharmacist regarding safety, dosage, duration of use, interaction with prescription drugs, etc. for all herbal products.
- Any interaction between herbs and medications could potentially put a transplant client at risk for rejection or losing the kidney.
- Herbs that may be toxic to the kidneys are artemisia absinthium (wormwood plant), periwinkle, autumn crocus, tung shueh, chuifong tuokuwan (Black Pearl), vandelia cordifolia, and horse chestnut.

the person's life. Fluid retention increases the risk of complications such as edema (ascites), hypertension, and heart failure. Electrolytes are monitored and regulated.

Pharmacological

Antihypertensives such as methyldopa (Aldomet) and propranolol hydrochloride (Inderal) are used to control hypertension. Diuretics such as furosemide (Lasix) are used to treat fluid retention; anticonvulsants, phenytoin (Dilantin) to control seizures; antiemetics, prochlorperazine (Compazine) to control vomiting; and antipruritics, cyproheptadine hydrochloride (Periactin) to control itching. Calcium acetate (Phos-Lo) is used to lower the phosphate level in the blood; however, it can be constipating. A low renal erythropoietin level causing anemia is often treated with epoetin alpha (Epogen). An iron supplement is used to decrease the anemia-related symptoms. Multivitamins with folic acid are used because dialysis promotes the loss of water-soluble vitamins.

Diet

Diet restrictions are similar to those in acute renal failure. Sodium, potassium, phosphorus, and protein are restricted. Fluids are also limited. Modifications are made as kidney function deteriorates. With consistent compliance, symptoms decrease, resulting in fewer complications. Resources are available for clients to obtain assistance with dietary restrictions. Meal ideas are published in newsletters such as *NephroNotes*. Long-term dietary compliance is a challenge, and daily activities as well as special events during the year are a continual reminder of the client's dietary restrictions. As with other chronic diseases, those with renal failure need to have all family members and friends encouraging them to adapt to their restrictions. Dietitians can assist the family to incorporate religious and cultural dietary practices. The person with chronic renal failure may also have to incorporate dietary guidelines for additional diagnoses such as diabetes mellitus and/or coronary artery disease.

With the progression of chronic renal disease, dialysis becomes necessary. Fluid restrictions must be followed, and the amount allowed divided throughout the day. The greatest amount of fluid should be allowed during the day, incorporating enough fluids with oral medications. Some fluids should be planned for the evening meal, with a small amount to be allowed during the night; for example, days—500 mL, evenings—200 mL, and nights—100 mL. Protein restriction is closely monitored and regulated with the blood albumin level. The development of hyperkalemia will lead to a diet restricted in potassium. Foods high in potassium include dried fruits or dried beans and peas, peanuts, bananas, sweet potatoes, spinach, products with tomatoes, oranges, chocolate, artichokes, avocados, pumpkins, and mushrooms.

Activity

The client is encouraged to participate in activities of daily living. Safety becomes a significant factor during periods when the client has weakness, fatigue, or mental confusion. Confusion is seen in clients who have uremic encephalopathy. When bed rest is required, turning, ROM exercises, and skin care are important. As symptoms continue to become more severe, the client will need total assistance for all ADLs.

Nursing Management

Monitor daily weight, skin turgor, vital signs, and lung sounds. Provide prescribed amount of fluids and accurately record intake and output (sometimes hourly). Assist with or provide oral hygiene before meals and as needed. Administer an antiemetic 30 minutes before meals. Arrange for a dietitian to plan meals with the client. Assist with or provide bathing frequently, followed by applying lotion on the skin. Encourage repositioning at least every 2 hours, ROM exercises, and use of an egg-crate mattress or Clinitron bed. Monitor for mental confusion. Refer client and family to the National Kidney Foundation website at www.kidney.org for more information.

NURSING PROCESS

Assessment

Subjective Data

Inquire about the client's past medical history including treatments for maintenance of renal disease. Take a complete medication history, including the use of over-the-counter drugs. Description of fatigue, joint pain, severe headaches, nausea, anorexia, some chest pain, intractable singultus (hiccups), decreased libido, menstrual irregularities, and impaired concentration is given by the client. The client may feel uncomfortable talking directly to the nurse if uremic halitosis is a problem.

Objective Data

Note changes in the client's neurological status such as reduced alertness and awareness. Kussmaul respirations appear as coma develops. Halitosis with a urine odor and "uremic frost," a white powder on the skin, result from the accumulation of urates. Observe for dark-colored urine and bloody or tarry stools, which could indicate bleeding in the intestinal tract.

Nursing diagnoses for a client with ESRD include the following:

NURSING DIAGNOSES	PLANNING/OUTCOMES	NURSING INTERVENTIONS
*Excess **Fluid** Volume* related to compromised renal mechanism	The client will understand the importance of prescribed (restricted) fluid amounts.	Monitor daily weight, intake and output (maybe hourly), skin turgor, edema, blood pressure, respirations, and lung sounds. Provide prescribed amounts of fluids. Teach client to plan nutritional and fluid intake within the prescribed amounts. Monitor laboratory reports for serum albumin level and serum electrolyte levels.

(*Continues*)

Nursing diagnoses for a client with ESRD include the following: (Continued)

NURSING DIAGNOSES	PLANNING/OUTCOMES	NURSING INTERVENTIONS
*Imbalanced **N**utrition: Less than Body Requirements* related to dietary restrictions, GI distress, anorexia	The client will stabilize weight within normal limits and participate in dietary plan.	Provide or assist with complete mouth care before meals because uremic halitosis leaves a metallic taste in the client's mouth. Provide a clean, quiet, odor-free environment for meals. Suggest 6 small meals throughout the day. Encourage self-feeding. Arrange a consultation with the dietitian to plan alternate ways to prepare foods allowed on the diet. Ask the family to bring favorite foods, within the dietary restrictions, from home. Administer antiemetics 30 minutes before meals to control nausea.
*Risk for Impaired **S**kin Integrity* related to altered metabolic state leading to pruritis from "uremic frost"	The client will maintain skin integrity.	Bathe skin frequently to remove "uremic frost." Encourage the use of emollients and lotions on the skin. Administer antihistamines, as ordered, for the temporary relief of itching. Assist the client to change position every 2 hours. Provide an egg-crate mattress or Clinitron bed.
*Ineffective **C**oping* related to uncertainty of long-term compliance of the treatment regimen	The client will verbalize feelings and intention to comply with treatment.	Encourage the client to discuss feelings about long-term lifestyle changes. Refer client to the National Kidney Foundation website at www.kidney.org for information about client services and treatments for diseases of the kidney. Include the client and family in rehabilitation and discharge planning to ensure compliance. Topics for these sessions include diet, rest, medications, fluid restrictions, intake and output, activities, dialysis, required lab tests, and frequent visits to the physician. Incorporate into the discharge planning and teaching the client's socioeconomic needs, cultural background, role in the family unit, accessibility to medical care, and anticipated follow-up care. Complete referrals before discharge to lessen client anxiety.
		Consider future needs of a newly diagnosed client with end-stage renal disease and include the availability of dialysis, vocational rehabilitation, home health care, financial assistance with medical needs, and psychological therapy for the client and family.

Evaluation: Evaluate each outcome to determine how it has been met by the client.

DIALYSIS

As the kidneys continue to deteriorate, nitrogenous waste products accumulate in the circulatory system. These waste products need to be removed artificially with **dialysis**, a mechanical means of removing nitrogenous waste from the blood by imitating the function of the nephrons. It involves filtration and diffusion of wastes, drugs, and excess electrolytes and/or osmosis of water across a semipermeable membrane into a dialysate solution. The **dialysate** is a solution designed to approximate the normal electrolyte structure of plasma and extracellular fluid.

There are two types of dialysis: hemodialysis and peritoneal dialysis. These treatments can be obtained throughout the country at dialysis centers or at hospital dialysis units.

Hemodialysis

Hemodialysis is performed by a machine with an artificial semipermeable membrane used to filter the blood. This machine is often referred to as an artificial kidney. A graft or fistula is surgically prepared to access the client's circulatory system. Figure 39-11 illustrates several ways this can be done. With each hemodialysis treatment, a catheter is inserted into the graft or fistula. The client's blood is circulated through the semipermeable membrane (Figures 39-12 and 39-13). Excess fluids are removed by osmosis, and by-products of protein metabolism, especially urea and uric acid, as well as creatinine, drugs, and excess electrolytes, are removed from the blood by diffusion or filtration. In return, the client receives fluids, electrolytes, and blood products, as necessary. The solution (dialysate) is especially prescribed to meet the client's metabolic needs.

For the entire process, Standard Precautions must be followed and strict asepsis maintained. The client is weighed before and after each dialysis session to determine if fluid is being retained. It is important to keep the client comfortable and provide diversionary activities during the treatment. Hemodialysis is usually performed 3 times a week and takes 3 to 4 hours each time.

The graft or fistula site requires strict aseptic care and must be assessed daily for signs of infection: redness, swelling, or drainage. Assess circulation through the site by palpation or feeling the area and/or listening with a (Doppler) stethoscope. A thrill should be felt and/or a bruit should be heard. Lack of these signs may indicate a blood clot, which requires immediate surgical attention. Patency must be documented. Assess pulses peripheral to the graft site.

Blood pressure and blood draws are never done on the extremity where the graft or fistula is placed. Also, restraints or intravenous solutions are never applied to or inserted into that extremity. All health care personnel should know the location of the hemodialysis access site. These sites should not be used for any other purpose than dialysis.

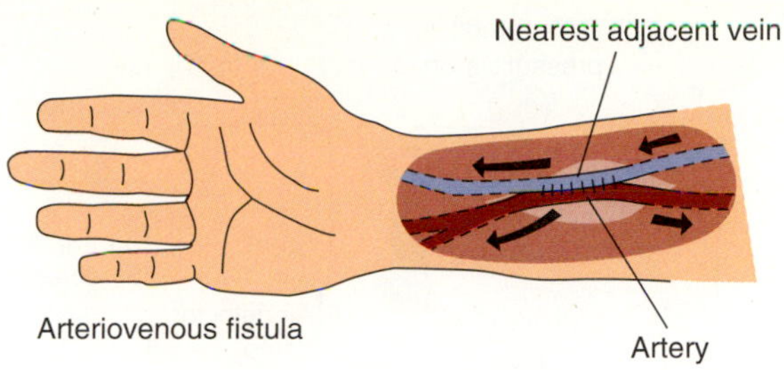

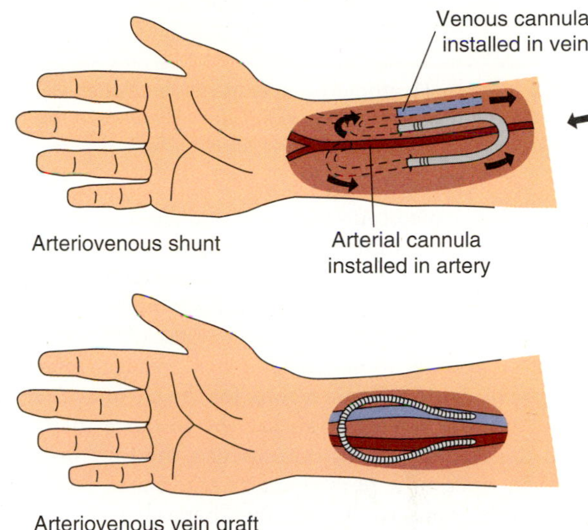

Figure 39-11 Types of Hemodialysis Access Sites

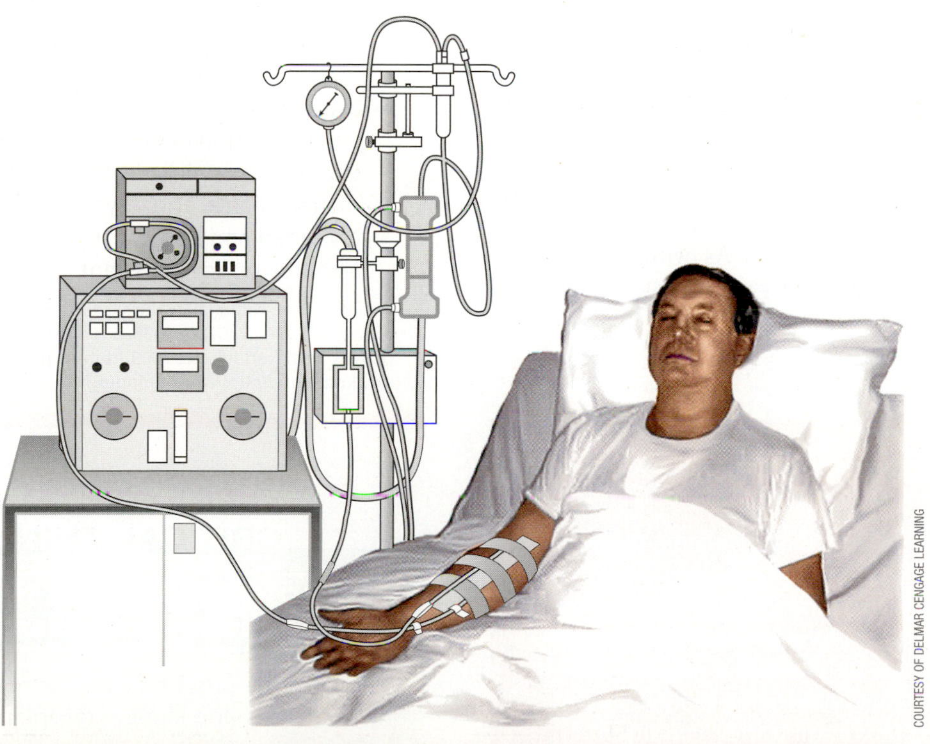

Figure 39-12 Client Receiving Hemodialysis

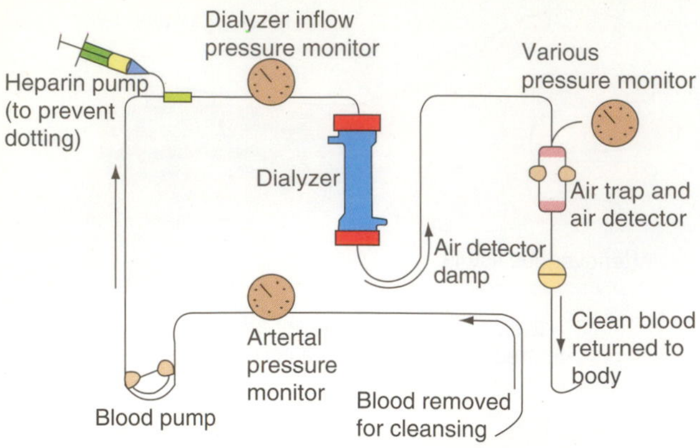

FIGURE 39-13 Hemodialysis (*Adapted from National Institute of Diabetes and Digestive and Kidney Diseases 2006, Treatment Methods for Kidney Failure: Hemodialysis.*)

Because most medications are removed during dialysis, they are generally not administered until after the dialysis session. Vancomycin hydrochloride (Vancocin) is not removed during dialysis and so is often used. If the client is hypertensive before dialysis, nifedipine (Procardia) is given because of its fast action.

Possible complications include hemorrhage, infection, and emboli formation. Some factors for the client and family to consider about hemodialysis are the distance they must travel to the dialysis center, the expense, the time involved, and the presence of a permanent arteriovenous (AV) line. Clients can be taught to do their own hemodialysis at a center. Portable units are being developed to make hemodialysis more usable in the client's home. This is a growing trend with home health care.

Continuous renal replacement therapy (CRRT), a slow, gentle form of dialysis, is available.

PERITONEAL DIALYSIS

Peritoneal dialysis uses the peritoneal lining of the abdominal cavity as the membrane through which diffusion and osmosis occur instead of the artificial kidney machine. It is usually performed 4 times a day or overnight 7 days a week. A Tenc khoff or a flanged-collar catheter is placed by the physician, under aseptic conditions, into the client's peritoneal space. The client must void just before catheter insertion to prevent accidental puncture of the bladder. As with hemodialysis, weigh the client before and after each dialysis session. Also auscultate bowel sounds.

CLIENT TEACHING

Dialysis

Clients who are receiving dialysis need a significant amount of teaching. All clients should have the process thoroughly explained. Other teaching topics are the importance of physician and laboratory visits, and observations for which the physician needs to be notified. Clients undergoing dialysis should wear Medic Alert tags stating their condition.

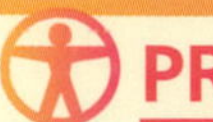

PROFESSIONAL TIP

Nutrition for Dialysis Clients

Dialysis clients need to follow strict dietary and fluid guidelines. Listed below is information and discussion of several of these guidelines.

- Refer the client to a dietitian. A dietitian with special training in care for kidney health is called a renal dietitian.
- Monitor and record how much fluid the client drinks and ensure that fluid restrictions are followed as ordered by the physician.
- Teach client to limit or avoid sodium and to eat fresh foods that are naturally low in sodium.
- Potassium levels can rise between dialysis sessions and affect the client's heartbeat. Evaluate serum potassium levels and assess client for cardiac arrhythmias.
- Educate client that foods high in potassium must be avoided or limited as ordered (refer to Chapter 24 for a listing of foods high in potassium). Potassium can be reduced from potatoes and other vegetables by peeling and soaking them in a large container of water for several hours, then dicing or shredding, and cooking in fresh water (Figure 39-14).
- Teach client that foods high in phosphorus should be avoided. The client will probably need to take a phosphate binder such as Renagel, PhosLo, Tums, or calcium carbonate with food to control the serum phosphorus level between dialysis sessions.
- Clients on dialysis are encouraged to eat high-quality protein.
- Instruct client to not take over-the-counter vitamin supplements as they may contain vitamins and minerals that are harmful to dialysis clients. The physician may prescribe a vitamin and mineral supplement such as Nephrocaps for the client.

Adapted from National Institute of Diabetes and Digestive and Kidney Diseases (NIDDK), 2008, Eat right to feel right on hemodialysis, retrieved July 26, 2009 from http://kidney.niddk.nih.gov/kudiseases/pubs/eatright/index.htm

CRITICAL THINKING

Peritoneal Dialysis, Hemodialysis, and Kidney Transplantation

What are the pros and cons for peritoneal dialysis, hemodialysis, and kidney transplantation?

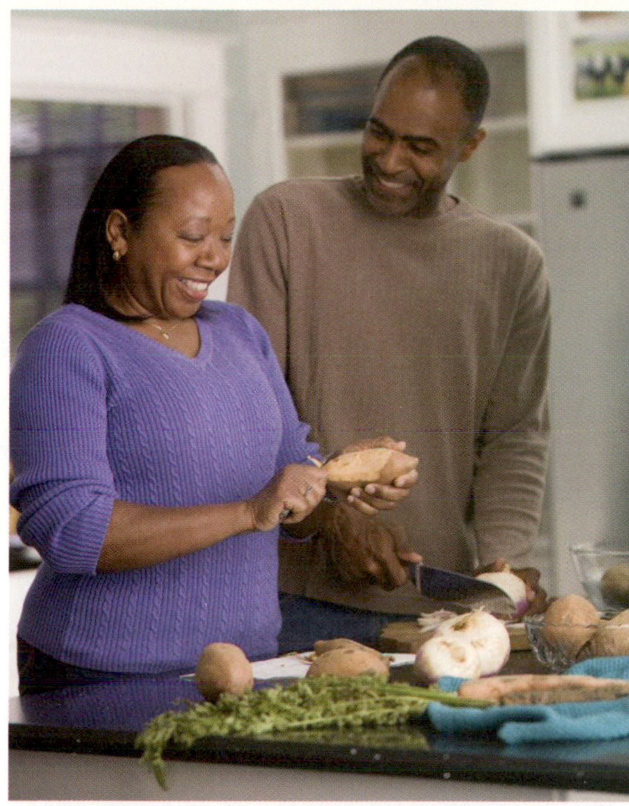

FIGURE 39-14 **Hemodialysis clients need to follow strict dietary guidelines.** (*Courtesy of Centers for Disease Control and Prevention/photo by Cade Martin.*)

The dialysate, held within a sterile soft container similar to an IV bag, is instilled aseptically through the catheter into the abdominal cavity. *To decrease client discomfort, the dialysate should be at body temperature and not instilled too rapidly.* Severe pain should not be experienced. The container, still connected to the catheter, is then rolled up and the dialysate remains in the abdominal cavity for a specified length of time. The client is free to ambulate during this time. The container is then unrolled and lowered below the abdominal cavity to allow the dialysate to drain, by gravity, back into the container. The dialysate now contains excess fluids, nitrogenous waste, and other impurities. The outflow of dialysate is inspected for color, sediments, and amount. The fluid should be light yellow and clear enough to read the printing on the bag when placed on a white towel. Usually 2 liters of dialysate are exchanged each time. If the outflow does not at least equal the inflow, the client is asked to turn from side to side to increase the outflow.

Peritoneal dialysis may be performed manually by the nurse, client, or family member as just described; by a cycler machine; or by continuous ambulatory peritoneal dialysis (CAPD). The cycler machine automatically completes dialysis after sterile setup and connection; CAPD is performed by the client. After the dialysate is aseptically installed, the empty bag is rolled up under the clothing, and the client can go about normal activities. Every 6 to 8 hours, the solution is drained into the bag, which is then discarded following standard precaution guidelines. A new bag of dialysate is attached and instilled. This provides continuous dialysis 24 hours per day, 7 days per week. The client's lifestyle is only minimally disrupted. Peritoneal dialysis is less expensive, easier to perform, less stressful for the client, and almost as effective as hemodialysis.

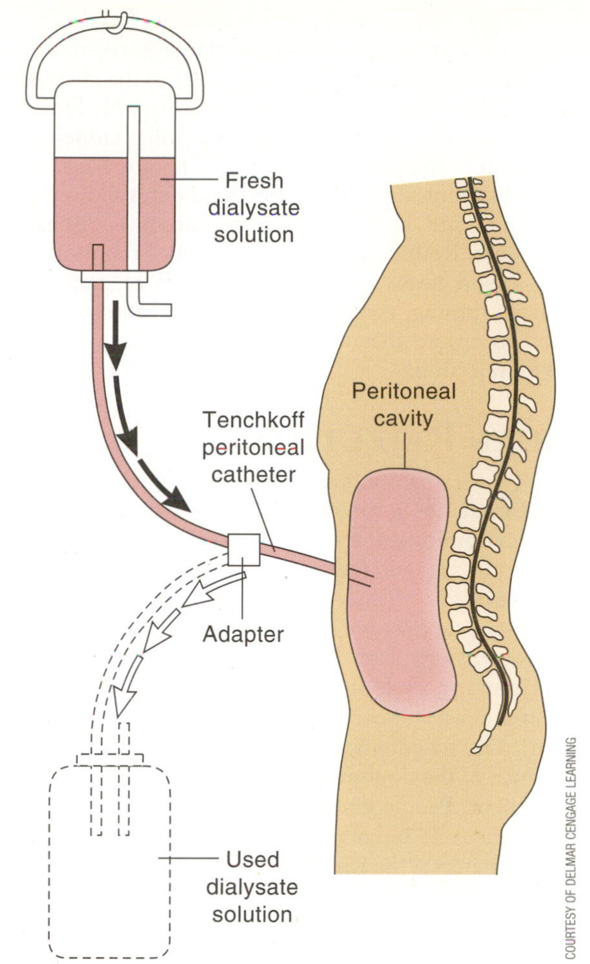

FIGURE 39-15 **Peritoneal Dialysis Setup**

The main complication of peritoneal dialysis is infection. Strict aseptic care of the catheter site is necessary. Standard Precautions are essential in caring for the dialysis client. Figure 39-15 shows a peritoneal dialysis setup.

KIDNEY TRANSPLANTATION

According to the Open Procurement and Transplantation Network (OPTN, 2006), 16,000 kidney transplants will be performed in 2006. Transplants are either from a live donor (usually a relative) or a cadaver. There are approximately 76,000 persons on the waiting list for a kidney transplant (United Network for Organ Sharing, 2008).

Before being placed on the nationwide donor waiting list, the client with ESRD must be tissue- and blood-typed to determine a compatible donor. Insurance coverage varies for this procedure. Lack of funds does not exclude anyone from needed care. Since 1973, an amendment to the Social Security Act allows Medicare to pay 80% of the cost for treating ESRD clients, regardless of age, including dialysis and kidney transplantation.

When a donor kidney becomes available, the client is transported to the transplant medical center. The donor kidney can be preserved for 36 hours in solution or up to 72 hours if it is attached to an irrigating pump with perfusion maintained while en route to the recipient. Through a lower abdominal incision, the surgeon attaches the donor kidney to the client's blood supply. The donor kidney is usually placed in the iliac fossa anterior to the iliac crest. The donor ureter is anastomosed (surgical connection of tubular structure) to the client's ureter or surgically implanted into the client's urinary bladder (Figure 39-16). Generally, the client's nonfunctioning kidney is left in place to reduce the postoperative risk of hemorrhage.

After a couple days of bed rest, the client is allowed increasing activities and, if no complications occur, is discharged in 1 to 3 weeks. Routine nursing care includes monitoring urine output, blood tests, vital signs, and level of consciousness. Encourage turning, coughing, and deep breathing. Assess the incision to ensure that wound closure is intact. In addition, assess for rejection.

Organ Rejection

Signs of rejection include generalized edema, tenderness over the graft site, fever, decreased urine output, hematuria, edema (extremities or eyes), weight gain, oliguria or anuria, and/or an increase in feeling tired. The BUN and creatinine will be elevated.

Immunosuppressive drug therapy is begun to decrease the chance of organ rejection. These drugs include azathioprine (Imuran), cyclophosphamide (Cytoxan), cyclosporine (Sandimmune), and corticosteroids such as prednisone (Meticorten). The scheduling and dosage of these drugs vary with acceptance of the donor kidney and the side effects exhibited by the client. People continue to survive many years with a kidney transplant and maintain a quality life.

Researchers at the University of Cincinnati have discovered a new therapy for transplant clients. The cancer drug, bortezomib, used for cancer of plasma cells, is effective in treating and/or reversing rejection episodes that do not respond to standard therapies (American Association of Kidney Patients, 2009).

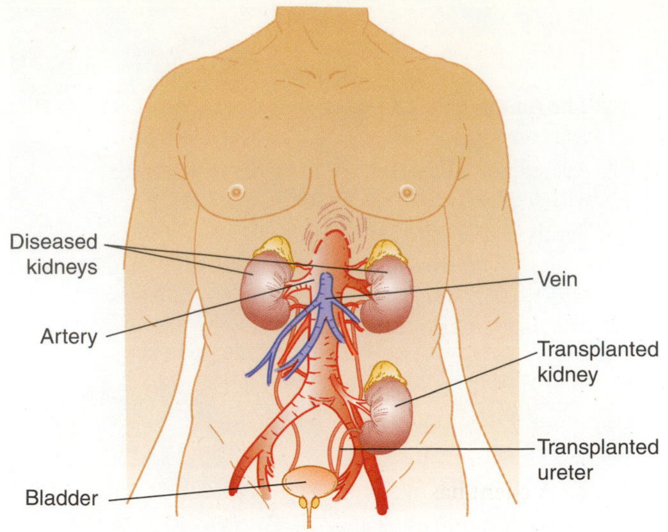

Figure 39-16 Kidney Transplantation (*Adapted from National Institute of Diabetes and Digestive and Kidney Diseases, 2006, Treatment Methods for Kidney Failure: Transplantation.*)

Complications

The greatest complication in renal transplantation is infection. The immunosuppressive therapy to prevent rejection of the kidney increases the risk and masks the usual signs of infection. The client and family must learn how to recognize these signs of infection. There will be only a slight increase in temperature, development of a cough, low back pain, cloudy urine, or wound drainage. The client must always monitor urine output.

CASE STUDY

A.R., 56, is a client in the extended care facility. She has amyotrophic lateral sclerosis (ALS) with muscle weakness that has progressed and involves her legs and arms. A hydraulic lift is used to transfer her out of bed. A student nurse and a classmate enter with the lift to assist A.R. OOB, when she asks to use the bedpan. As they help her onto the bedpan, they recall that the staff nurse gave A.R. the bedpan about a half hour ago. Returning in a few minutes, they help A.R. off the bedpan and notice the urine is cloudy with a foul odor. A.R. is not on I&O; however, they notice that there is a very small amount of urine. She tells them that she does not know why she is going to the bathroom so often and why her urine smells bad.

The following questions will guide your development of a nursing care plan for the case study.

1. What subjective data should be gathered? What objective data should be gathered?
2. List diagnostic tests that may be ordered.
3. Write two nursing diagnoses for A.R., related to her cystitis/UTI.
4. Write a goal related to each of A.R.'s nursing diagnoses.
5. List pertinent nursing actions for the care of A.R. for each of the following areas as they relate to the cystitis/UTI:
    - elimination—bladder
    - diet and fluids
    - safety, comfort, and rest
    - teaching (client and nursing staff)
6. List two classifications of medications used for the treatment of an UTI.
7. List two successful client outcomes for A.R.

SUMMARY

- The functions of the urinary system are reflected in their relationship with nearly all of the systems in the body.
- Accurate intake and output is imperative for every client with a urinary system disorder.
- Teach proper perineal care, especially to female clients of all ages, about cleansing from front to back.
- Diet management is important for clients with renal calculi, glomerulonephritis, renal failure, and dialysis.
- Encourage an adequate intake of fluids for clients unless fluids are restricted.
- Monitor laboratory test results for BUN, creatinine, and electrolytes.
- Level of consciousness, vital signs, lung sounds, edema, and urine characteristics are important to monitor.
- Strict aseptic care is mandatory for dialysis clients.

REVIEW QUESTIONS

1. A client has been admitted for chronic pyelonephritis. She is jittery and states she is concerned. Which of the following signs would indicate potential kidney damage?
   1. Urine output is 100 mL on your shift.
   2. Blood pressure is decreased with a rapid pulse.
   3. Blood pressure is elevated with a decreased pulse.
   4. BUN and creatinine clearance are within normal limits.

2. A male client, age 64, has had hematuria for several years. He is admitted to your same-day surgical unit scheduled for cystoscopic fulguration. Postoperatively, which of the following would you anticipate?
   1. Blood in the urine.
   2. An elevated temperature.
   3. Hypotension.
   4. Smoky urine.

3. A male client, age 29, had impetigo 2 weeks before his noting a decrease in urine output and urine that "did not look right." His admission diagnosis is acute glomerulonephritis. He is on intake and output with fluid restriction. Which of the following comments indicates knowledge of his nursing care?
   1. "I had my wife empty my urinal."
   2. "My urine still looks pretty bad."
   3. "I put my call light on so you can empty my urinal."
   4. "My wife helped me out of bed, so I urinated in the bathroom."

4. A client with chronic glomerulonephritis is discharged home with home health care. As the LP/VN assigned to her case, you are planning her a.m. care. While preparing the bath supplies, she says, "Please do not use any soap. My skin is so dry and flaky." The rationale for this would be:
   1. kidney failure leads to uremia.
   2. the bladder does not concentrate urine.
   3. her blood sugar is elevated.
   4. confusion leads to comments of this nature.

5. A client is attending classes to be able to do his own peritoneal dialysis. He states he feels well and is eager to continue to learn. He asks if washing his hands before the procedure is important. The best response is:
   1. "Yes, only if you have not done so today."
   2. "Yes, as you want to keep the procedure as clean as possible."
   3. "No, since you just went to the bathroom."
   4. "No, because all the equipment is sterile."

6. A client has been diagnosed with renal carcinoma. The client states, "My husband will leave me if I lose my hair from chemotherapy." What would be the most appropriate answer for this client?
   1. "You seem to be concerned that your relationship with your husband might change."
   2. "You should focus on your disease and not your hair."
   3. "Why don't you wait and see if your husband leaves you before you get too upset."
   4. "Everything is going to be fine. Don't worry about your hair loss."

7. A client has an order for a throat and skin culture; what might the physician be testing for?
   1. Nephrolithiasis.
   2. Glomerulonephritis.
   3. Nephrotic syndrome.
   4. Chronic renal failure.

8. The nurse is teaching a new hemodialysis client about dietary restrictions. Which of the following client statements indicates that further teaching is needed?
   1. "Peeling, dicing up, and boiling potatoes in fresh water when cooking helps to lower the amount of potassium."
   2. "I need to eat high quality protein in my diet."
   3. "Drinking several glasses of orange juice each day will keep me healthy."
   4. "I should only take vitamin supplements prescribed by my physician."

9. A client is scheduled for hemodialysis today and has called to see if she should take her blood pressure pills prior to coming in for the procedure. The nurse should inform the client:
   1. "Take your pills after your procedure is completed."
   2. "It is ok to take your pills prior to coming in for your procedure."

3. "No, do not take your blood pressure pills at all, today."
4. "You can take your blood pressure pills after we get your treatment started. I want to check your blood pressure first."

10. A women presents to the urgent care center with dysuria and hematuria, and states that she has a history of cystitis. The nurse assesses for which of the following symptoms that are indicative of cystitis?
    1. Frequency and urgency of urination, flank pain, nausea, and vomiting.
    2. Chills and flank pain.
    3. Fever, nausea, vomiting and flank pain.
    4. Frequency and urgency of urination, suprapubic pain, and foul smelling urine.

REFERENCES/SUGGESTED READINGS

American Association of Kidney Patients. (2009). Cancer drug may treat rejection. Retrieved April 18, 2009 from http://www.aakp.org/newsletters/Kidney-Transplant/January-2009/Drug-May-Treat-Rejection/

American Cancer Society. (2008). Cancer facts and figures 2008. Retrieved April 18, 2009 from http://www.cancer.org/downloads/STT/2008CAFFfinalsecured.pdf

American Cancer Society. (2009a). Detailed guide: Bladder cancer surgery. Retrieved July 25, 2009 from http://www.cancer.org/docroot/CRI/content/CRI_2_4_4X_Surgery_44.asp?rnav=cri

American Cancer Society. (2009b). What are the key statistics for bladder cancer? Retrieved July 25, 2009 from http://www.cancer.org/docroot/CRI/content/CRI_2_4_1X_What_are_the_key_statistics_for_bladder_cancer_44.asp?sitearea=

American Cancer Society. (2009c) What are the key statistics for kidney cancer? Retrieved July 25, 2009 from http://www.cancer.org/docroot/CRI/content/CRI_2_4_1X_What_are_the_key_statistics_for_kidney_cancer_22.asp?sitearea=

American Cancer Society. (2009d). What are the risk factors for bladder cancer? Retrieved July 25, 2009 from http://www.cancer.org/docroot/CRI/content/CRI_2_4_2X_What_are_the_risk_factors_for_bladder_cancer_44.asp?rnav=cri

American Cancer Society. (2009e). What are the risk factors for kidney cancer? Retrieved July 25, 2009 from http://www.cancer.org/docroot/CRI/content/CRI_2_4_2X_What_are_the_risk_factors_for_kidney_cancer_22.asp?rnav=cri

Arbique, J. (2003). Stop UTIs in their tracts. *Nursing2003, 33*(6), 32hn1–32hn4.

Bulechek, G., Butcher, H., McCloskey, J., & Dochterman, J., eds. (2008). *Nursing Interventions Classification (NIC)* (5th ed.). St. Louis, MO: Mosby/Elsevier.

Campbell, D. (2003). How acute renal failure puts the brakes on kidney function. *Nursing2003, 33*(1), 59–63.

Castner, D., & Douglas, C. (2005). Now onstage: Chronic kidney disease. *Nursing2005, 35*(12), 58–63.

Castina, S., Boyington, A., & Dougherty, M. (2002). Urinary incontinence. *AJN, 102*(8), 85–87.

Dowling-Castronovo, A., & Specht, J. (2009). Assessment of transient urinary incontinence in older adults. *American Journal of Nursing, 109*(2), 62–71.

Gray, M., Ratliff, C., & Donovan, A. (2002). Tender mercies: Providing skin care for an incontinent patient. *Nursing2002, 32*(7), 51–54.

Growe, S. (2009). Manuscript submitted for publication. Henderson, NV.

Hayes, D. (2003). Performing peritoneal dialysis. *Nursing2003, 33*(3), 17.

Kaplow, R., & Barry, R. (2002). Continuous renal replacement therapies. *AJN, 102*(11), 26–33.

Kobayashi, M., Nomura, M., Yamada, Y., Fujimoto, N., & Matsumoto, T. (2005). Bladder-sparing surgery and continent urinary diversion using the appendix (Mitrofanoff procedure) for urethral cancer. *International Journal of Urology, 12*(6), 581–584.

Lynch, D. (2004). Cranberry for preventions of urinary tract infections. *American Family Physician, 70*, 2175–2177.

Martchev, D. (2008). Improving quality of life for patients with kidney failure. *RN 71*(4), 31–36.

Martin, C. (2009). Unpublished manuscript. Denver, PA.

Mason, D., Newman, D., & Palmer, M. (2003). Changing UI practice: People have the right to be continent. *AJN, 103*(3), 129.

Mayo Clinic. (2009). Glomerulonephritis treatments and drugs. Retrieved July 24, 2009 from http://www.mayoclinic.com/health/glomerulonephritis/DS00503/DSECTION=treatments-and-drugs

McConnell, E. (2002). Protecting a hemodialysis fistula. *Nursing2002, 32*(11), 18.

Moorhead, S., Johnson, M., Maas, M., & Swanson, E. (2007). *Nursing Outcomes Classification (NOC)* (4th ed.). St. Louis, MO: Mosby.

National Association for Continence (NAFC). (2008). Prevalence. Retrieved from http://www.nafc.org/media/statistics/prevalence-2/

National Institute of Diabetes and Digestive and Kidney Diseases (NIDDK). (2006a). Glomerular Diseases. Retrieved April 18, 2009 from http://kidney.niddk.nih.gov/kudiseases/pubs/glomerular/index.htm

National Institute of Diabetes and Digestive and Kidney Diseases (NIDDK). (2006b). Treatment methods for kidney failure: hemodialysis. Retrieved July 26, 2009 from http://kidney.niddk.nih.gov/kudiseases/pubs/hemodialysis/index.htm

National Institute of Diabetes and Digestive and Kidney Diseases (NIDDK). (2006c). Treatment methods for kidney failure: transplantation. Retrieved July 26, 2009 from http://kidney.niddk.nih.gov/kudiseases/pubs/transplant/index.htm

National Institute of Diabetes and Digestive and Kidney Diseases (NIDDK). (2007a). Kidney stones in adults. Retrieved April 18, 2009, from http://kidney.niddk.nih.gov/kudiseases/pubs/stonesadults/index.htm

National Institute of Diabetes and Digestive and Kidney Diseases (NIDDK). (2007b). Kidney stones: what you need to know. Retrieved April 18, 2009 from http://kidney.niddk.nih.gov/kudiseases/pubs/stones_ES/index.htm

National Institute of Diabetes and Digestive and Kidney Diseases (NIDDK). (2007c). Polycystic kidney disease. Retrieved April 18, 2009 from http://kidney.niddk.nih.gov/kudiseases/pubs/polycystic/index.htm

National Institute of Diabetes and Digestive and Kidney Diseases (NIDDK). (2008). Eat right to feel right on hemodialysis. Retrieved July 26, 2009 from http://kidney.niddk.nih.gov/kudiseases/pubs/eatright/index.htm

National Institutes of Health (NIH). (2006). Kidney infection (pyelonephritis). Retrieved April 18, 2009 from http://www.nlm.nih.gov/medlineplus/ency/article/000522.htm

National Kidney Foundation (NKF). (2003). About kidney disease. Retrieved from www.kidney.org/general/aboutdisease/index.cfm

National Kidney Foundation (NKF). (2008). The problem of kidney and urologic disease. Retrieved April 18, 2009 from www.kidney.org/news/newsroom/fs_new/prblmkd&urologd.cfm

National Kidney Foundation (NKF). (2009a). Diet and kidney stones. Retrieved April 18, 2009 from http://www.kidney.org/atoz/atozItem.cfm?id=41

National Kidney Foundation (NKF). (2009b). How your kidneys work. Retrieved April 18, 2009 from http://www.kidney.org/kidneydisease/howkidneyswrk.cfm#whatare

National Kidney Foundation (NKF). (2009c). Kidney stones. Retrieved April 18, 2009 from http://www.kidney.org/atoz/atozItem.cfm?id=84

National Kidney Foundation (NKF). (2009d). Polycystic kidney disease. Retrieved April 18, 2009 from http://www.kidney.org/atoz/atozItem.cfm?id=102

National Kidney Foundation (NKF). (2009e). Use of herbal supplements in chronic kidney disease. Retrieved April 18, 2009 from http://www.kidney.org/news/newsroom/fs_new/herbalsuppckd.cfm

Newman, D. (2003). Stress urinary incontinence in women. *AJN, 103*(8), 46–55.

Newman, D., & Giovannini, D. (2002). The overactive bladder: A nursing perspective. *AJN, 102*(6), 36–45.

North American Nursing Diagnosis Association International. (2010). *NANDA-I nursing diagnoses: Definitions and classification 2009–2011*. Ames, IA: Wiley-Blackwell.

Organ Procurement and Transplantation Network (OPTN). (2006). Scientific registry of transplant recipients annual report. Retrieved April 19, 2009 from www.ustransplant.org/annual_reports/current/107_dh.htm

Paton, M. (2003). Continuous renal replacement therapy. *Nursing2003, 33*(6), 48–50.

Patraca, K. (2005). Measure bladder volume without catheterization. *Nursing 2005, 35*(4), 46–47.

Polt, C. (2006). Taking the pressure off for women with stress incontinence. *Nursing2006, 36*(2), 49–51.

Rice, J. (2002). *Medications and mathematics for the nurse* (9th ed.). Clifton Park, NY: Delmar Cengage Learning.

Roth, R., & Townsend, C. (2002). *Nutrition and diet therapy* (8th ed.). Clifton Park, NY: Delmar Cengage Learning.

Scherer, J., & Timby, B. (2002). *Introductory medical-surgical nursing* (8th ed.). Philadelphia: Lippincott Williams & Wilkins.

Schofield, C. (2002). Patient may have a UTI—What next? *Nursing2002, 32*(10), 17.

Schultz, J. (2002). Urinary incontinence: Solving a secret problem. *Nursing2002, 32*(11), 53–55.

Smith, D. (1999). Gauging bladder volume without a catheter. *Nursing99, 29*(12), 52–53.

Stockert, P. (1999). Getting UTI patients back on track. *RN, 62*(3), 49–52.

Stothers, L. (2002). A randomized trial to evaluate effectiveness and cost effectiveness of naturopathic cranberry products as prophylaxis against urinary tract infection in women. *Canadian Journal of Urology,* (9), 1558–1562.

United Network for Organ Sharing (UNOS). (2008). U.S. transplant waiting list passes 100,000. Retrieved April 18, 2009 from http://www.unos.org/news/newsDetail.asp?id=1165

Van Snell, S., & Miller-Anderson, M. (2007). Stress incontinence: It's no laughing matter. *RN, 70*(4), 25–29.

Wetherbee, S. (2006). New weapons to snuff out kidney cancer. *Nursing2006 36*(12), 58–63.

Williams, L., & Hopper, P. (2003). *Understanding medical surgical nursing*. (2nd ed.). Philadelphia: F. A. Davis.

Zabat, E. (2003). When your patient needs peritoneal dialysis. *Nursing2003, 33*(8), 52–54.

RESOURCES

American Association of Kidney Patients, http://www.aakp.org

American Foundation for Urologic Disease, http://www.afud.org

American Society of Nephrology, http://www.asn-online.org

Bard, C.R. Bard, Inc., http://www.crbard.com

Interstitial Cystitis Association, http://www.ichelp.org

Medic Alert® Foundation, http://www.medicalert.org

National Association for Continence (NAFC), http://www.nafc.org

National Kidney and Urologic Diseases Information Clearinghouse, http://www.kidney.niddk.nih.gov

National Kidney Foundation, http://www.kidney.org

Polycystic Kidney Disease Foundation, http://www.pkdcure.org

The Simon Foundation for Continence, http://www.simonfoundation.org

UNIT 12 Nursing Care of the Client: Mobility, Coordination, and Regulation

CHAPTER 40
Musculoskeletal System

MAKING THE CONNECTION

Refer to the following chapters to increase your understanding of the musculoskeletal system:

Basic Nursing
- ***Wellness Concepts***
- ***Assessment***
- ***Pain Management***
- ***Diagnostic Tests***

Adult Health Nursing
- ***Oncology***
- ***Cardiovascular System***
- ***Immune System***
- ***The Older Adult***

Basic Procedures
- ***Performing Passive Range-of-Motion (ROM) Exercises***
- ***Ambulation Safety and Assisting from Bed to Walking***
- ***Assisting with Crutches, Cane, or Walker***
- ***Turning and Positioning a Client***
- ***Moving a Client in Bed***
- ***Transferring from Bed to Wheelchair, Commode, or Chair***
- ***Transferring from Bed to Stretcher***

LEARNING OBJECTIVES

Upon completion of this chapter, you should be able to:

- Define key terms.
- List the diagnostic tests used in the evaluation of orthopedic disorders and diseases.
- Describe preventive nursing care of the orthopedic client (e.g., positioning, mobility).
- Identify the various types of casts used in the treatment of orthopedic disorders.
- Describe nursing care of clients with orthopedic devices.
- List four types of fractures and their related treatment.
- Discuss the nursing care of the client undergoing a total hip replacement.
- Utilize the nursing process to plan nursing care including physical and emotional needs of the orthopedic client.

KEY TERMS

amphiarthrosis
amputation
arthroplasty
bruxism
closed reduction
contracture
crepitus
diarthrosis
dislocation
fracture
Heberden's nodes
internal fixation
kyphosis
locomotor
lordosis
open reduction
orthopedics
osteoporosis
paresthesia
phantom limb pain
scoliosis
sprain
strain
subluxation
synarthrosis
tophi
windowing

INTRODUCTION

Orthopedics, also spelled orthopaedics, is the branch of medicine that deals with the prevention or correction of the disorders and diseases of the musculoskeletal system. It involves the muscles, skeleton, joints, and supporting structures such as ligaments and tendons.

The prime concern of the nurse caring for a client with **locomotor** (pertaining to movement or the ability to move) disorders is the prevention of **contractures** (permanent shortening of a muscle) or deformities. The objective of all caregivers is to maintain good body alignment, preserve muscle tone, prevent disuse, and continue joint motion for the client with acute or long-term therapeutic or rehabilitative needs. Caring for orthopedic clients also requires an understanding of basic principles that apply to all clients whether they are in traction, casts, or recovering from surgery.

ANATOMY AND PHYSIOLOGY REVIEW

The musculoskeletal system consists of bones, muscles, tendons, ligaments, cartilage, and joints. When it is functioning properly, the musculoskeletal system allows an individual to stand erect and ambulate. Figure 40-1 identifies the bones of the skeleton.

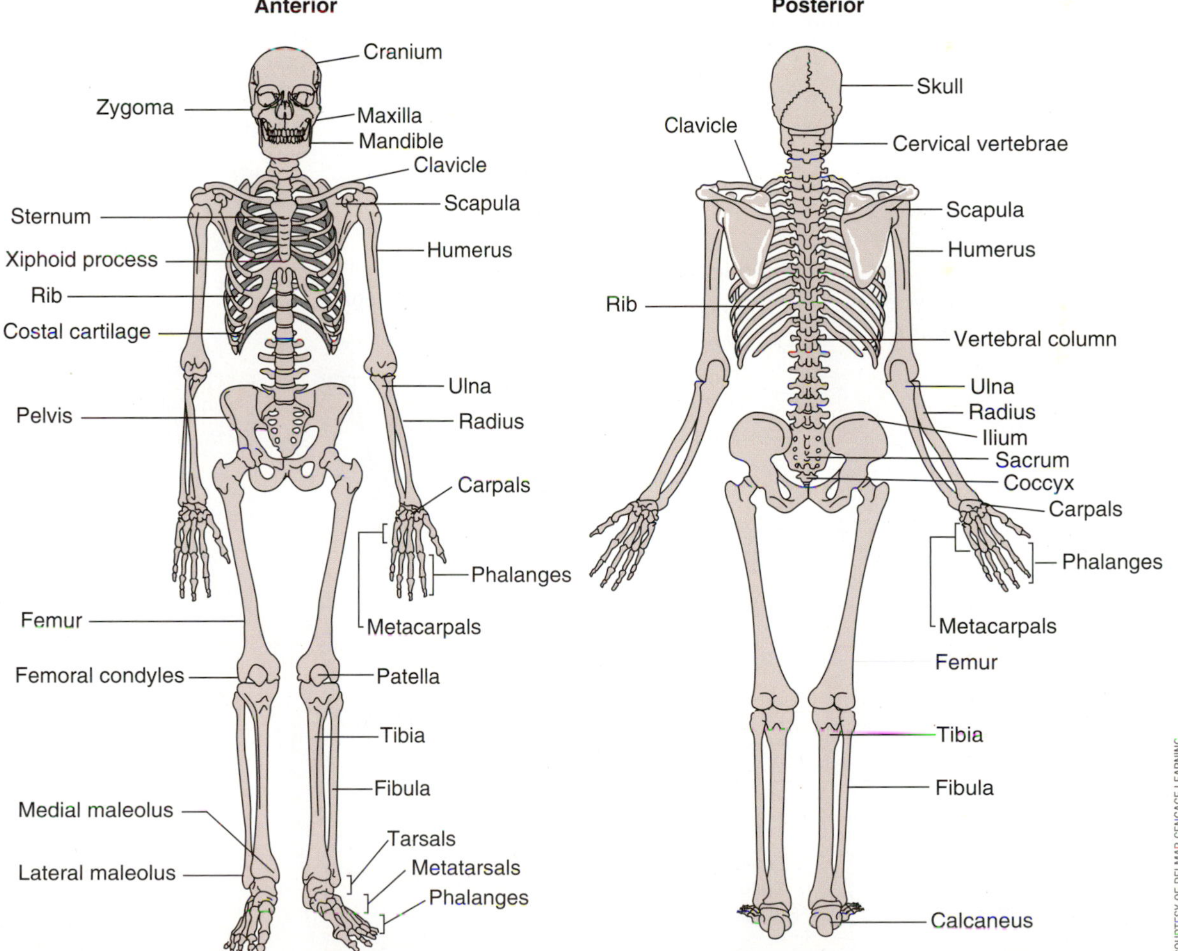

FIGURE 40-1 Anterior and Posterior Views of the Adult Human Skeleton

The skeletal system consists of bones attached to each other by cartilage and strong ligaments. The functions of the skeleton are to:

- Provide the body with structural framework
- Act as a protective casing for internal organs such as the brain, heart, and lungs
- Allow movement by muscles attached to the skeleton
- Store calcium, phosphorus and magnesium and release these minerals when the body requires them
- Manufacture blood cells in the red bone marrow

Bones in the skeletal system are classified as long, short, flat, or irregular. Examples include the humerus, a long bone; the phalanges of the finger, short bone; occiput, flat bone; and the vertebrae, irregular bone. Figure 40-2 illustrates these bones.

There are two types of bone. One type of bone is *cancellous,* which resembles a sponge with spaces and is found in the epiphysis or end of the long bones as well as in all other bones. The other type is *cortical* bone, which is compact bone and is found in the diaphysis or shaft of the long bones. Short bones consist of cancellous bone covered by a layer of compact bone. Flat bones are made of cancellous bone layered between compact bone. Generally, the makeup of irregular bones is similar to that of flat bones.

The muscular system is composed of muscle fibers and tendons innervated by nerves (Figure 40-3). The muscle fibers vary in size and shape and are arranged according to a muscle's function. The muscles act as motors controlled by nerve impulses from the cerebral cortex. The muscles and the skeleton work together to permit body movement. Muscles are attached to bones by tendons.

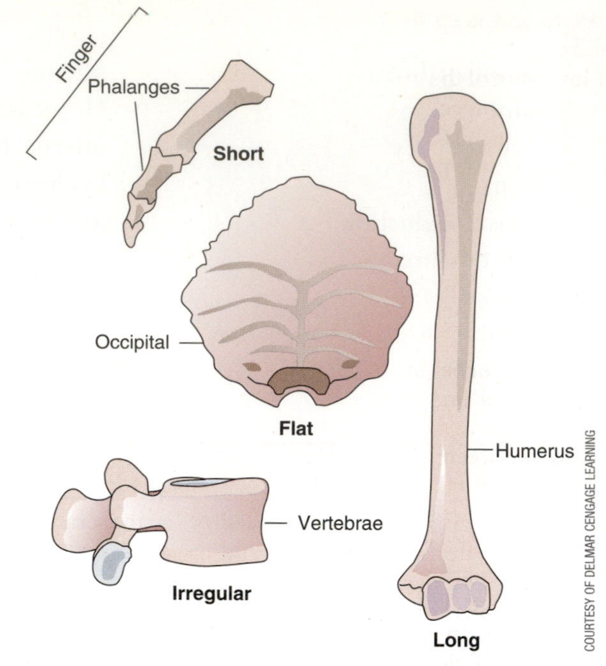

FIGURE 40-2 Bone Shape Classification

The action of muscles is to contract or shorten. Muscles are arranged within the body as opposing pairs to act as antagonists to each other. For example, the biceps flex the forearm and the triceps extend it.

Muscles are surrounded and divided by fibrous envelopes called fascia. In the extremities, the muscles surround and give support to main blood vessels and nerves. Muscles also give

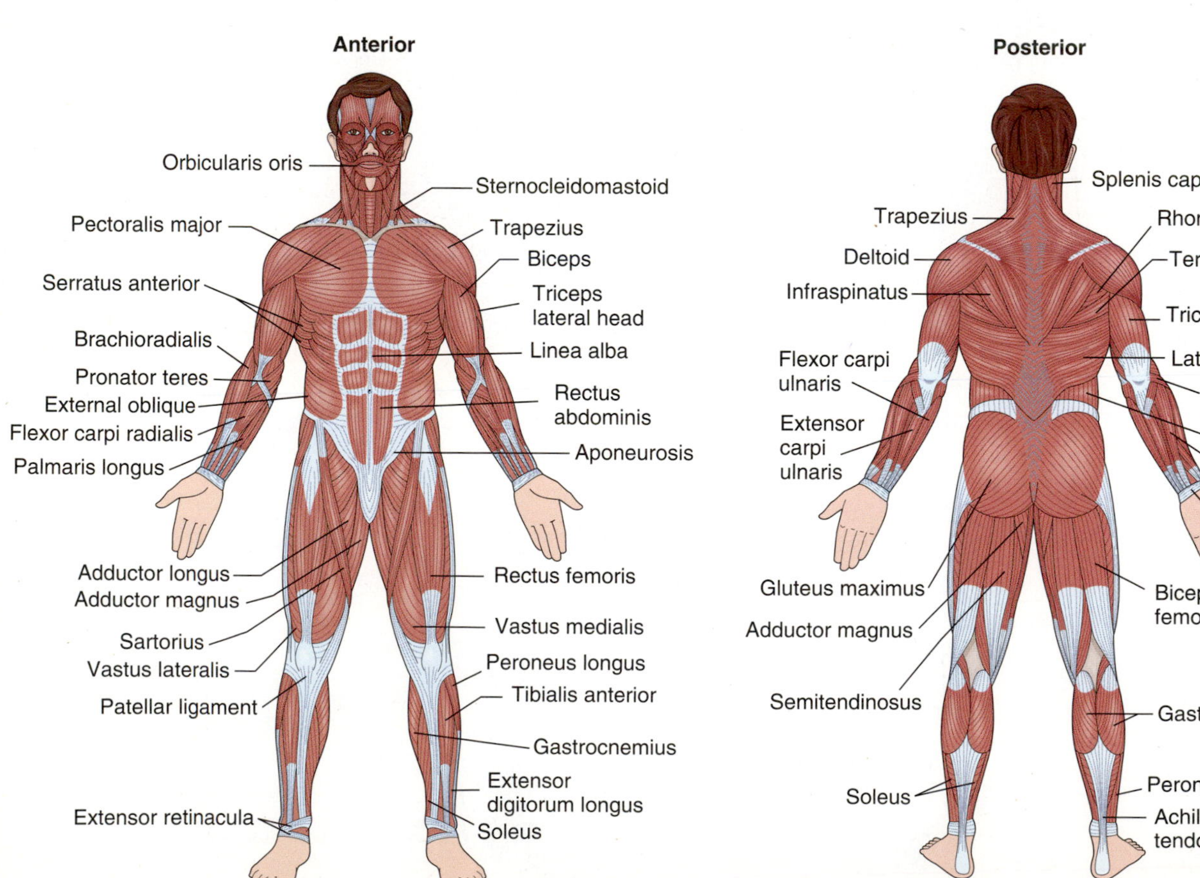

FIGURE 40-3 Muscular System: Anterior and Posterior Views

support to and keep the body erect as well as give shape to the body.

Movement of the muscles may be either voluntary or involuntary. Muscles attached to bone can function at the will of the person (voluntary). Involuntary muscles, found within body organs, regulate the physical activity of the organs so the organs can perform their functions. These actions are not under the person's control. Involuntary muscles are located in the intestinal tract, the pupil of the eye, and in the heart and blood vessels.

A joint is a junction of two or more bones. There are three types of joints: diarthrosis, synarthrosis, and amphiarthrosis. **Diarthrosis** joints are freely movable, such as the hinge (elbow, knee), ball and socket (hip and shoulder), pivot (skull and first vertebrae), gliding (wrist), and saddle (thumb). **Synarthrosis** joints are immovable, such as the suture line between the temporal and occipital bones of the skull. **Amphiarthrosis** joints are slightly movable, such as the vertebrae and pelvic bones separated by fibrous cartilage. Figure 40-4 illustrates types of joints.

The ends of articulating joints are covered with a smooth articular cartilage. The joint capsule is composed of an outer fibrous layer and an inner synovial layer that secretes synovial fluid. This clear fluid acts as a lubricating fluid for the joints.

Other structures related to the musculoskeletal system include bursa, fascia, tendons, and ligaments. Bursae are sacs filled with fluid that facilitate joint movement by making it possible for muscles and tendons to move or glide over ligaments or bones. Fascia is connective tissue that covers a muscle. Tendons are strong fibrous tissue attaching muscle to bones, providing mobility. Ligaments grow out of the periosteum and lash bones together more firmly.

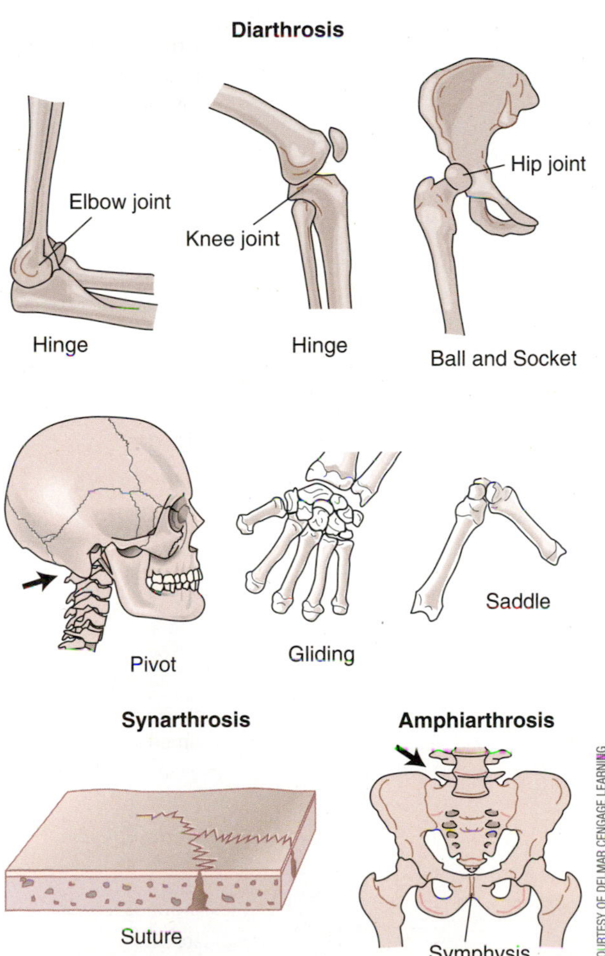

FIGURE 40-4 Joints Classified by the Degree of Movement Permitted

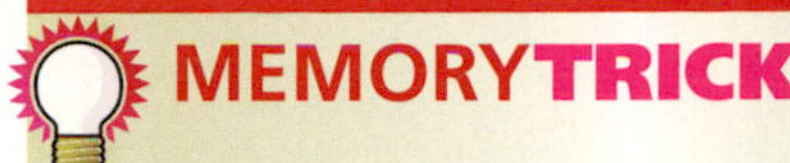

Tendons **tend** to bind muscles to bones, and ligaments bind bone to bone.

ASSESSMENT

Assessment of the musculoskeletal system ranges from a basic assessment of functional abilities done by the nurse to a complete physical exam by the physician for diagnosis of specific muscle and joint disorders. The extent of the physical exam depends on the client's symptoms, health history, and any other physical signs.

Inspect and palpate to evaluate bone integrity, posture, joint function, muscle strength, and gait. Also assess the client's ability to perform basic activities of daily living.

The medical history includes information on any past medical or surgical disorders and any symptoms relative to onset, duration, or location of discomfort or pain. Ask if activity makes symptoms better or worse. A family medical history should also be obtained.

Assessment of the bony skeleton includes notation of deformities, body alignment, abnormal growths, shortened extremities, amputations, abnormal angulation other than at the joints, and **crepitus**, a grating or crackling sensation or sound.

Assessment of the spine necessitates exposure of the client's back, buttocks, and legs for adequate visualization. Note differences in the height of the shoulders or iliac crests. Gluteal folds should appear symmetrical. The vertebral column should be straight and perpendicular to the floor, with the spine convex through the thoracic portion and concave through the cervical/lumbar portion.

Three common spinal curvatures are scoliosis, kyphosis, and lordosis. A lateral curving deviation is known as **scoliosis**. Scoliosis is seen most frequently in school-age children and adolescents. **Kyphosis** (hump back) is seen as an increased roundness of the thoracic spinal curve. This condition is frequently seen in older persons with osteoporosis. **Lordosis** (sway back) is an exaggeration of the lumbar spine curvature as seen in pregnancy as a woman's body adjusts its center of gravity. These three curvatures are illustrated in Figure 40-5.

Assessment of the articular system includes range of motion (limited, active, and passive), stability of joints, deformities and any nodular formation, and pulses in the extremities. Normal ranges of motion (ROM) are shown in Figure 40-6. Assess for the angle of the joint movement; presence of pain, tenderness, and crepitus; and client's ability to move joint by self through full range of motion (active), with limited movement (limited), or with assistance only (passive) (Estes, 2006). When assessing passive ROM, remember to keep the motion steady and avoid causing any pain.

ROM includes assessment of the client's ability to change position, muscle strength and coordination, and the size of

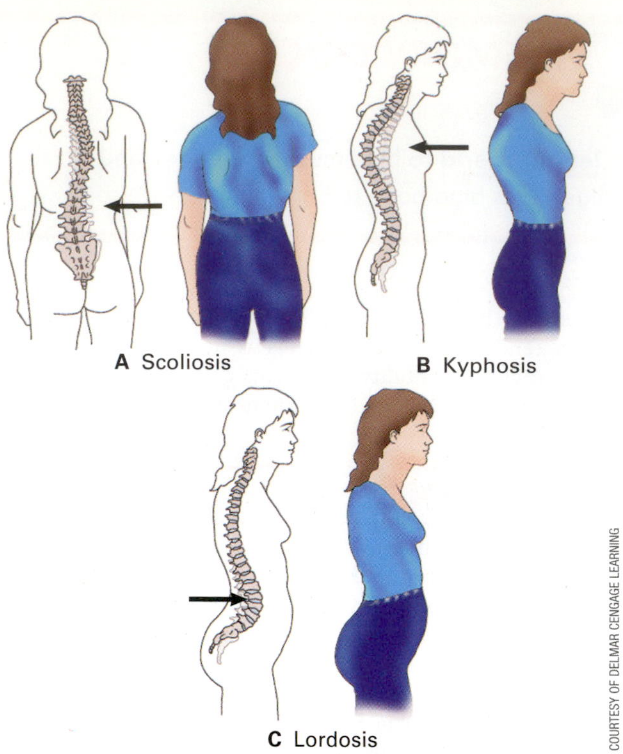

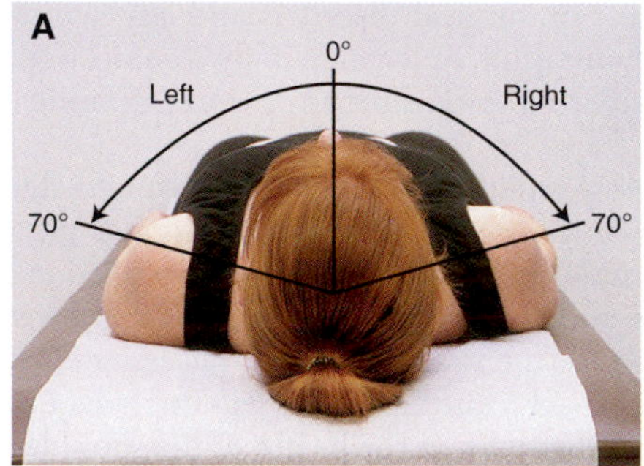

FIGURE 40-5 Curvatures of the Spine

individual muscles. Assess muscle groups for strength and equality with the client using the movements of ROM. Compare the right and left muscles in strength and size. Normal muscle strength is equal bilaterally. Assess if the client has voluntary movement against gravity and resistance. Table 40-1 describes two grading scales used in assessing muscle strength; grading scale of 0-5 and the Lovett scale. Figure 40-7 shows assessment of muscle strength and resistance. Assess for involuntary movements (Estes, 2006).

Joints are examined for excessive fluid. The knee is the most common site for fluid accumulation. Edema and an elevated temperature may be signs of active inflammation in the joint. Normal joint movement is stable and smooth. If there is a snap or crack sound when a joint is passively moved, it may indicate a ligament slipping over a bony prominence.

Deformities are caused by several factors, including contractures, dislocations, and **subluxation** (a partial separation of an articular [joint] surface). Nodular formations are produced by musculoskeletal diseases such as gout, rheumatoid arthritis, and osteoarthritis.

Pulse points in the extremities are palpated to assess for weak or absent pulses. The strength of the pulse in affected extremities is compared with that of nonaffected extremities. Note skin color and temperature and check capillary refill by pressing down on the client's fingernail or toenail for a few seconds, then release and note the time it takes for the client's nail

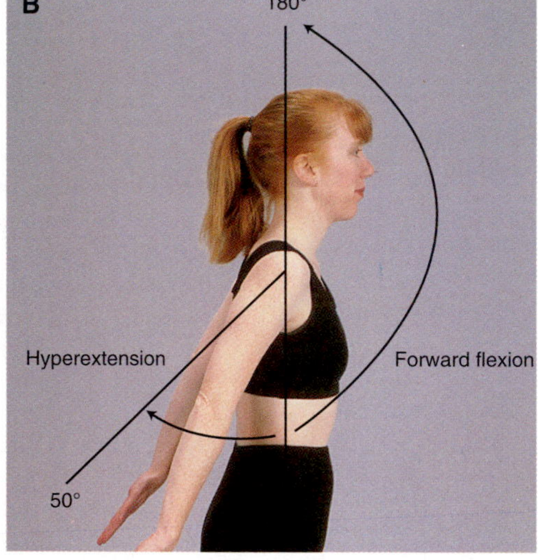

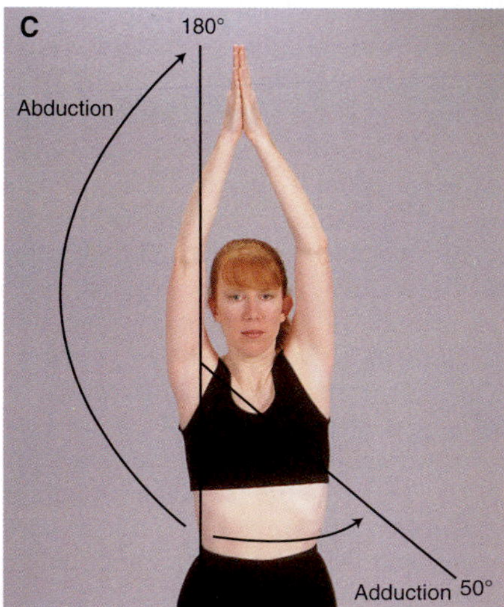

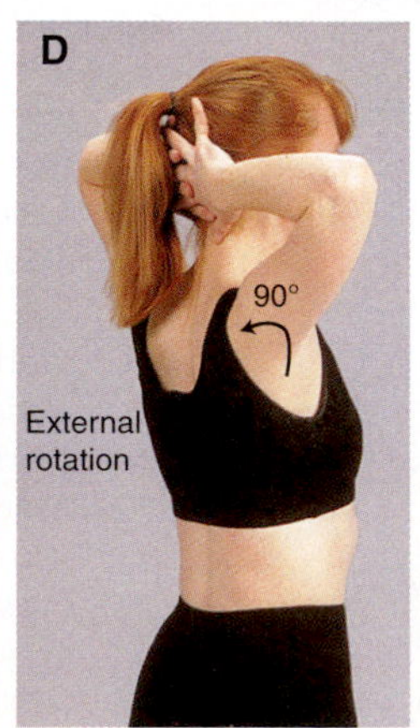

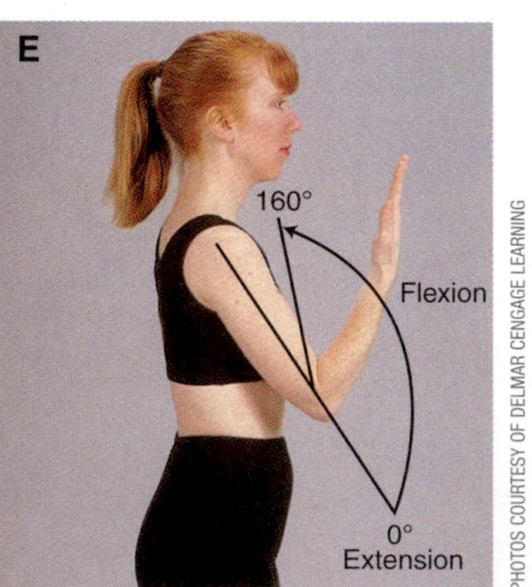

FIGURE 40-6 Range of Joint Motion; *A*, Cervical Spine Rotation; *B*, Shoulder Flexion and Hyperextension; *C*, Shoulder Abduction and Adduction; *D*, Shoulder Rotation; *E*, Elbow Flexion and Extension (*Continues*)

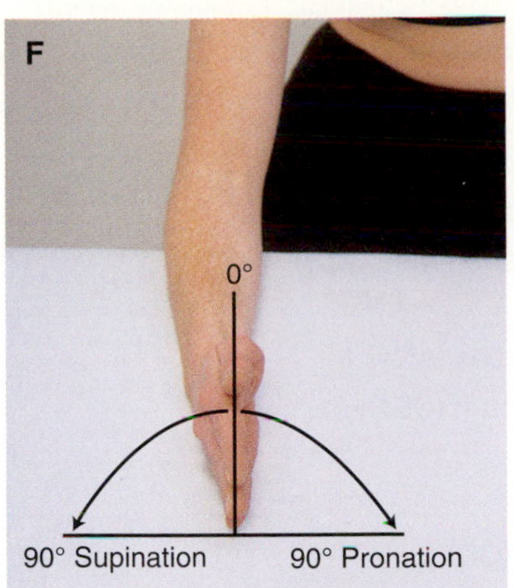

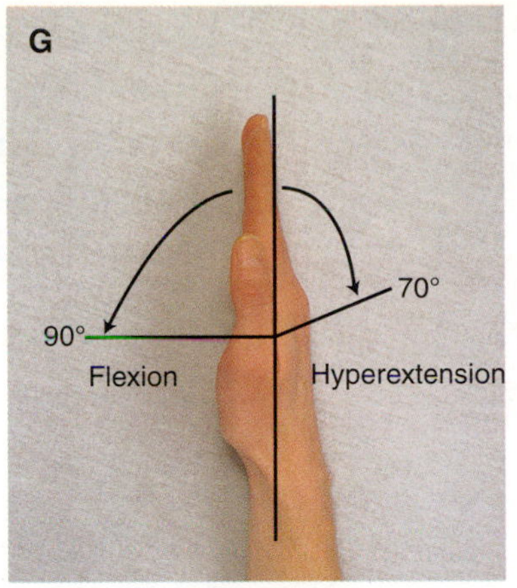

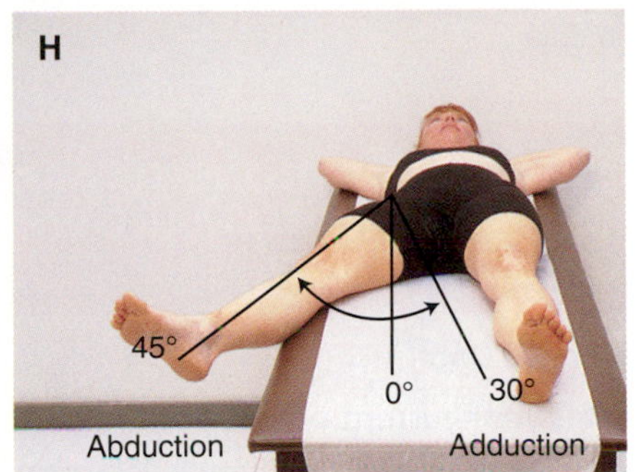

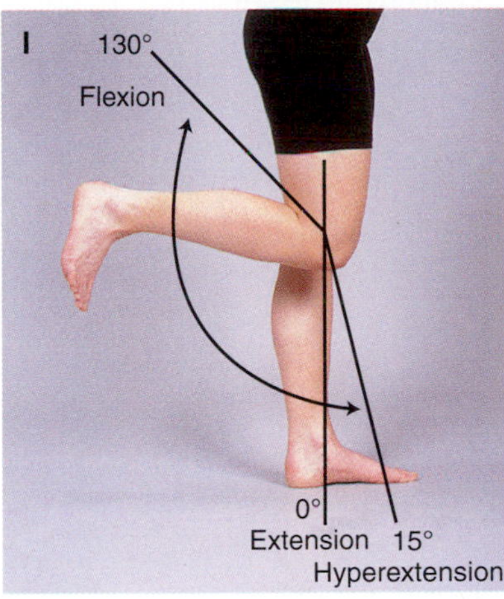

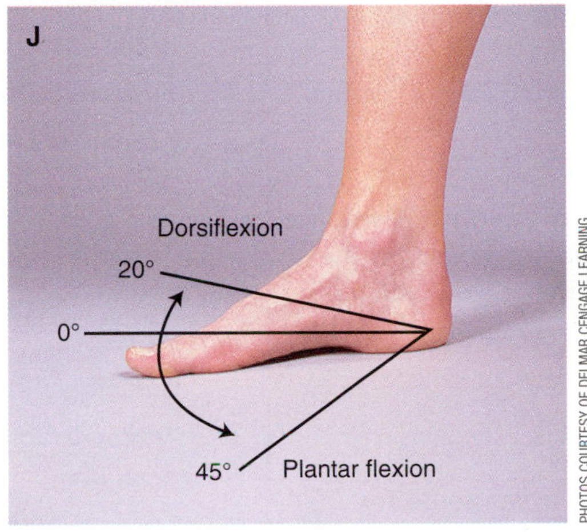

PHOTOS COURTESY OF DELMAR CENGAGE LEARNING

FIGURE 40-6 (Continued) *F,* Elbow Supination and Pronation; *G,* Wrist Flexion and Hyperextension; *H,* Hip Abduction and Adduction; *I,* Knee Flexion, Extension, and Hyperextension; *J,* Dorsiflexion and Plantar Flexion

TABLE 40-1 Assessing Muscle Strength

GRADING	DESCRIPTION	LOVETT SCALE
0	No contraction	Zero (0)
1	Slight contraction	Trace (T)
2	Full ROM with gravity eliminated (passive motion)	Poor (P)
3	Full ROM with gravity	Fair (F)
4	Full ROM against gravity, some resistance	Good (G)
5	Full ROM against gravity, full resistance	Normal (N)

Adapted from *Assessing the Musculoskeletal System,* by S. Wise, in press, and *Caring and Clinical Decision Making* (2nd ed.). Clifton Park, NY: Delmar Cengage Learning.

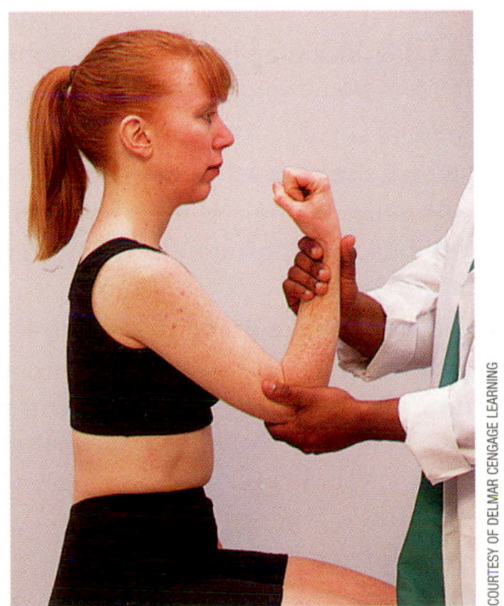

COURTESY OF DELMAR CENGAGE LEARNING

FIGURE 40-7 Assessment of Muscle Strength

to return to normal color. The color should return immediately (less than 2 seconds); if a client has an arterial disorder, the color will take longer than 2 seconds to return to normal. Refer to Box 40-1 for guidance in completing client musculoskeletal assessments.

BOX 40-1 QUESTIONS TO ASK AND OBSERVATIONS TO MAKE WHEN COLLECTING DATA

Subjective Data

What is your current occupation?

Describe your current activity level, sport participation, and lifestyle.

What leisure or recreation activities or exercise regimen do you enjoy?

Have you gained or lost any weight over the last few months?

Describe a typical 3-day diet.

Do you need assistance to care for yourself? Assistance to the bathroom? Assistance cleaning house? If the answer is yes, ask: Who is available to assist you with mobility or self-care activities?

Do you have any pain?

Do you take any medication for pain?

Have you ever broken any bones?

Have you gone to a chiropractor or masseuse for treatment?

Does muscle or joint pain or discomfort have an adverse impact on your ability to sleep and rest?

Tell me how you feel about yourself.

Do you feel in control of your life?

Tell me about your relationship with your spouse and family

Objective Data

Obtain vital signs, including height and weight. Compare to ideal body weight chart.

Assess the volume (1+, 2+, 3+, 4+) of peripheral pulses.

Observe the gait, use of assistive devices, and range of motion. Is the ability to transfer or ambulate limited?

Observe body build and posture. Visually scan the body for deformities.

Assess muscle strength according to grading scale.

Visually scan the body for symmetry, contour, and size of muscles, and muscle atrophy. Clients must be assessed bilaterally to compare one extremity or muscle group with the other side.

Assess for crepitus.

Assess for swelling and tenderness.

Assess for pain on a scale of 1–10, with 0 being no pain and 10 being the worst pain ever felt.

Assess ROM of joints.

Adapted from Wise (2008).

TABLE 40-2 Common Diagnostic Tests for Clients with Musculoskeletal Disorders

Laboratory Tests

Alkaline phosphatase (ALP)

Aspartate aminotransferase (AST)

Aldolase (ALD)

Antinuclear antibodies (ANA)

Complete blood count (CBC)

- WBC
- Hg

C-reactive protein (CRP)

Creatine kinase (CK-MM)

Erythrocyte sedimentation rate (ESR)

Lactate dehydrogenase (LDH)

Rheumatoid factor (RF)

Serum calcium

Serum phosphorus

Uric acid

- serum
- urine

Radiologic Studies

Arthrogram/graphy

Bone scan

Computed tomography (CT scan)

Dual energy x-ray absorptiometry scan (DEXA)

Electromyography (EMG)

Indium (white blood cell) scan

Magnetic resonance imaging (MRI)

Myelogram

Radiography (x-ray)

Other Tests

Arthrocentesis

Arthroscopy

Joint aspiration

Somatosensory evoked potentials (Evoked potentials)

COURTESY OF DELMAR CENGAGE LEARNING

COMMON DIAGNOSTIC TESTS

Commonly used diagnostic tests for clients with symptoms of musculoskeletal system disorders are listed in Table 40-2.

MUSCULOSKELETAL TRAUMA

Trauma to the musculoskeletal system causes a variety of injuries to clients of all ages. Such injuries include strains, sprains, dislocations, fractures, and compartment syndrome.

CRITICAL THINKING

Client Assessment

After reading the anatomy and physiology and assessment sections of the text, examine the accompanying photo of a client.

1. Identify the anatomical abnormality.
2. List the variations from the norm that you identify.

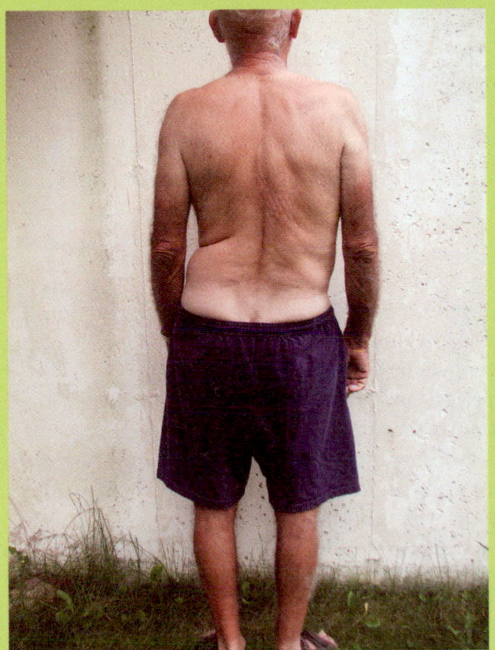

(Courtesy of Dick Hill. Photo by Susan Hill.)

STRAIN

A **strain** is an injury to a muscle or tendon caused by overuse or overstretching. A strain may be either acute or chronic. An acute strain may be caused when an individual performs unaccustomed exercises vigorously. A chronic strain may develop after repeated overuse of certain muscles. Individuals with acute strains experience sudden severe pain, whereas the onset is gradual in chronic strains, with the affected part feeling only stiff and sore.

Chronic strains require no specific treatment, but acute strains require rest and possibly immobilization. Immediately after injury, apply cold packs for 20- to 30-minute periods, and then remove for 1 hour during a 24-hour period to reduce any edema. Then apply heat for the client's comfort. In the case of a severe strain when the muscle may be completely ruptured, surgical repair may be necessary.

SPRAIN

A **sprain** is an injury to ligaments surrounding a joint caused by a sudden twist, wrench, or fall. Symptoms include pain, edema, loss of motion, and ecchymosis. X-ray will reveal soft tissue edema but no evidence of joint or bone injury. Immediate treatment is RICE (rest, ice, compression, and elevation). The client rests and ice is applied to the injured area. The part may then be immobilized with an elastic compression bandage or a brace and elevated. After the edema has decreased significantly, a cast may be applied.

DISLOCATION

Dislocation occurs when articular surfaces of a joint are no longer in contact. The bones are literally "out of joint." The displaced bone may hinder the blood supply, damage nerves, tear ligaments, or rupture muscle attachments. Traumatic dislocations are considered orthopedic emergencies. Congenital dislocations are present at birth, whereas spontaneous or pathologic dislocations are caused by diseases affecting joints.

Symptoms of a dislocation include localized joint pain, loss of function of the joint, and a change in the length of the extremity and contour of the joint. Diagnosis is based on the symptoms, physical exam, and x-rays. X-rays reveal either a complete or partial separation of the articulating surfaces.

FRACTURE

A **fracture** is a break in the continuity of a bone. Fractures occur when the forces from outside the body are greater than the strength of the bone, causing the bone to break. Fractures usually involve soft tissue (edema and bleeding), damaged nerves, and tendons. Most fractures are caused by accidents. These may be the result of direct force, torsion or twisting, or violent contractions of highly developed muscles. Other fractures may be the result of a disease process that weakens the bone. This type of fracture is known as *pathologic* or *spontaneous*. Individuals considered at high risk for fractures include those who have predisposing bone conditions such as metastatic or primary bone tumors or osteoporosis, poor coordination, diminished vision, dizzy spells, or general weakness.

There are more than 90 different classifications of fractures. Some of the more common types include greenstick or incomplete, simple or closed, compound or open, impacted or telescoped, spiral, comminuted, compression, and stress or fatigue.

In a *greenstick* fracture, the continuity of the bone is not completely disrupted but has splintering on one side and bending on the other. This fracture is seen most frequently in children. An uncomplicated (clean) fracture in which the skin remains intact is called a *closed or simple* fracture; the fractured surfaces are not contaminated by outside air. In a *compound or open* fracture, the bone is broken and the skin is also broken, allowing the bone to protrude and be susceptible to a greater chance for infection. An *impacted* fracture is also called a telescoped fracture; one portion of a bone fragment is forcibly driven into another. A *spiral* fracture twists around the shaft of the bone. This type of fracture may occur from a twisting force. In a *comminuted* fracture, the bone is splintered into many unaligned fragments. A *compression* fracture usually occurs when a bone, such as a vertebra, becomes weakened from osteoporosis. A fall or lifting excess weight causes a compression or crushing of the vertebral body (Zdeblick, 2009). *Stress or fatigue* fractures occur from repetitive overuse of a bone and are one of the five most common injuries of runners (Reeser, 2007). Various types of fractures are shown in Figure 40-8.

Healing time for fractures is affected by the age of the client and the type of injury or any underlying disease process, and may take weeks, months, or even years before healing is complete. The average healing time for an uncomplicated fracture is

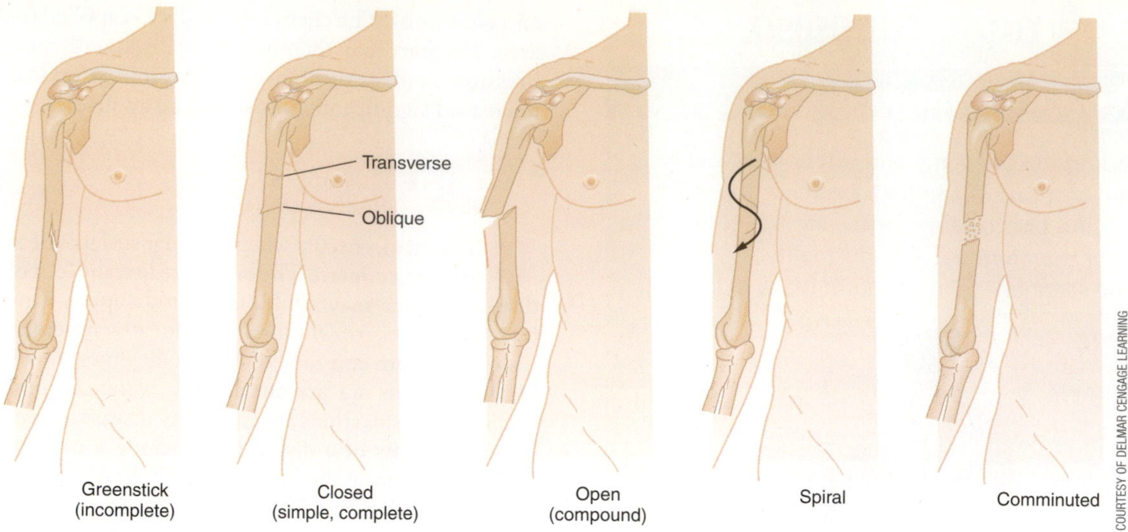

FIGURE 40-8 Classifications of Common Bone Fractures

6 to 8 weeks. The sequence of healing takes place beginning with the formation of a hematoma, then granulation tissue formation, callus formation, callus ossification, and ultimately remodeling.

Hematoma formation begins with the formation of a clot that serves as a fibrin network. Bleeding comes from ruptured vessels within the bone as well as from tears in the periosteum and adjacent tissues. The hematoma is not absorbed but develops into granulation tissue. Granulation tissue forms a soft tissue callus that surrounds the fracture site and serves as a temporary splint. Callus ossification is the result of deposits of calcium salts in the callus forming rigid bone in excess as a protective measure. The formation of bone binds the bone ends together. Remodeling is completed by osteoclastic activity, whereby excess bone is gradually reduced and removed by absorption until the original shape and outline of the fractured bone is reestablished. Figure 40-9 outlines the healing sequence.

Complications of a fracture include infection, fat embolism syndrome, and compartment syndrome. Complications may delay healing or be life threatening.

Infections may result from an open fracture in which the bone extends through the skin, allowing contamination from the outside. They may also occur following surgical repair of a fracture using an internal fixation device. Any infection may lead to a delayed union of the bone.

Fat embolism syndrome is usually associated with fractures of the long bones, multiple fractures, or crushing injuries. An embolus usually occurs within 24 to 72 hours following a fracture but may occur up to a week after injury. Much is still unclear about how a fat embolism occurs (Walls, 2002). When a small area of the lungs is involved, the symptoms are pain, tachycardia, and dyspnea. Larger areas of lung involvement produce more pronounced symptoms, including severe pain, dyspnea,

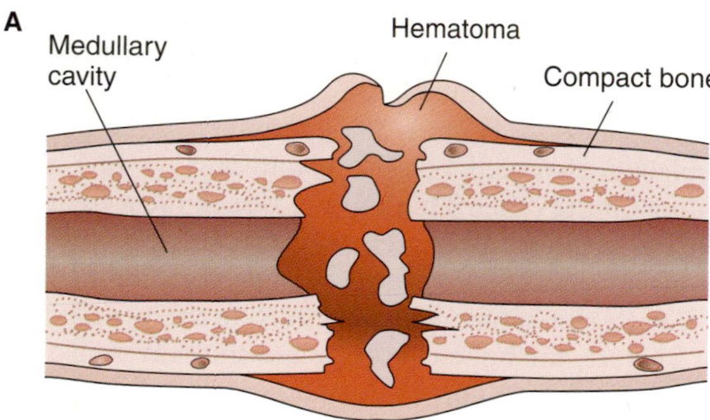

Medullary cavity

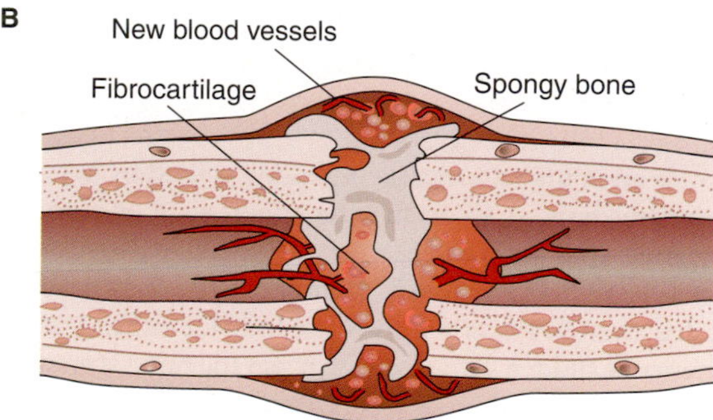

Fibrocartilage
Spongy bone
Spongy bone forms close to developing blood vessels; fibrocartilage forms away from new blood vessels.

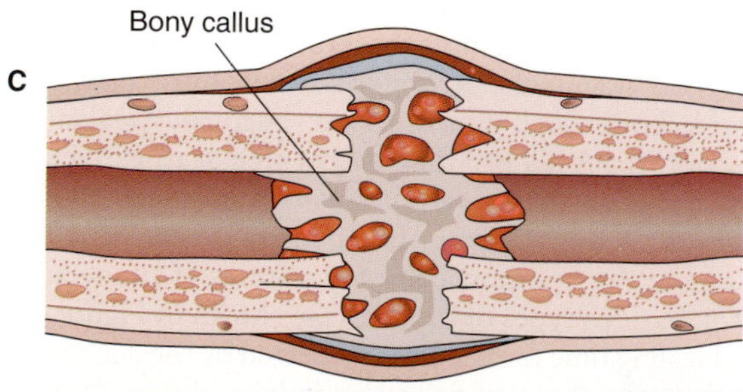

Bony callus

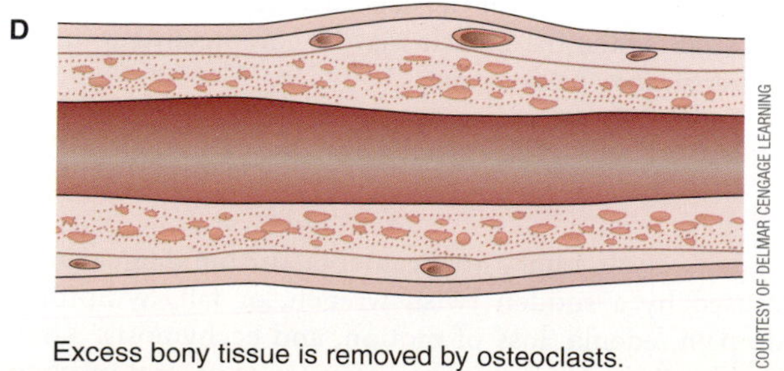

Bony callus replaces fibrocartilage.

D
Excess bony tissue is removed by osteoclasts.
Closed (simple, complete)
COURTESY OF DELMAR CENGAGE LEARNING

FIGURE 40-9 Steps of Bone Repair

cyanosis, restlessness, and shock. Petechiae may appear over the neck, upper arms, chest, or abdomen. Treatment consists of bed rest, respiratory support, oxygen, and IV fluids.

MEDICAL–SURGICAL MANAGEMENT

Medical

The treatment of a fracture requires immediate attention. The most important objectives are to (1) realign the fracture, (2) maintain the alignment, (3) regain the function of the injured part, and (4) prevent complications. The method of treatment depends on the first aid given; the site, severity, and type of the fracture; and the age and condition of the client.

Closed Reduction Repair of a fracture accomplished without surgical intervention is called **closed reduction**. External manipulation is used to correct bone position. This manipulation requires three maneuvers: traction and countertraction, angulation, and rotation. Following the reduction, x-rays are taken to visualize the fracture alignment. The part is then immobilized by using a cast, bandage, or traction. Local or general anesthesia may be used to make the reduction easier and less painful to the client.

Casts Casts are made either from plaster bandages or synthetic materials such as fiberglass. The cast should include the joint above and below the affected part. The major purposes of casts are immobilization, support and protection of the affected part, prevention of deformities resulting from conditions such as arthritis, and the correction of deformities such as scoliosis.

A fiberglass cast weighs less, wears longer, breathes better, and is more penetrable to x-rays than plaster casts (AAOS, 2007a). A dry cast should be odorless, shiny in appearance, resonant (produces vibrating sound on percussion) when percussed, and have a temperature similar to the room air. Moisture occurring from any underlying drainage gives the cast a musty smell, dullness on percussion, a lusterless color, and cool temperature.

Numerous types of casts exist. Long and short arm casts allow the fingers to be visible; long and short leg casts allow the toes to be visible. A spica cast is used for hip, shoulder, and thumb dislocations or injuries. The hip spica has an abduction bar that keeps the cast in the correct position. A walking cast with a cast shoe facilitates client ambulation. Body casts are used to immobilize the spine following surgical spinal fusions, unstable spinal injuries, or for degenerative disorders. Figure 40-10 shows different types of casts.

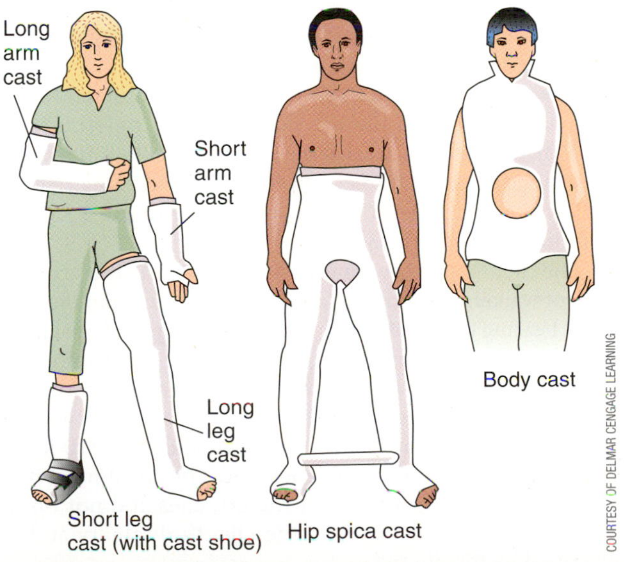

FIGURE 40-10 Casts Used to Correct Musculoskeletal Disorders

CLIENT TEACHING

Casts

Because plaster casts dry from the inside out, they should not be covered or dried with a hairdryer or heat lamp. Allow moisture and heat from the drying cast to evaporate naturally. Inform clients that the heat they feel during the application, drying, and setting process is normal and should subside in 10 to 15 minutes. To avoid indentation, a drying cast is placed on pillows and not on a hard surface. For the same reason, when handling the cast, only the palms of the hands are used. Plaster casts cause clients to feel cold when they are drying. Apply blankets only to body areas that are not covered with the cast. Synthetic casts dry in minutes to a couple of hours. Teach the client not to insert any objects such as rulers or hangers into the cast to relieve itching as the skin is soft and can be damaged. After the cast has dried, use a hairdryer to blow cool air inside the cast to alleviate itching.

Keep the plaster cast dry because the cast weakens if it gets wet. Sometimes a waterproof cast is applied so the client can shower or possibly swim. Obtain physician approval for swimming with a cast.

After the application and drying of a cast, the doctor may order a cast cut to allow visualization of a body area or to relieve pressure. This procedure is known as **windowing**. A cast is also split in half or bivalved to relieve pressure.

When a cast is removed, the client becomes conscious of aches and discomforts caused by the constricted joint structures and immobilized muscles. Minimize the client's discomfort by supporting the joint and maintaining the part in the same position as it was in the cast. The skin is cool and pale with mottling and edema present. A yellow exudate, which is part dead skin and part secretions from oil sacs, is on the skin. This exudate is not rubbed or forced off.

Traction The principle of traction is to have two forces pulling in opposite directions. Traction consists of weights and counterweights. Countertraction forces are provided by the weight of the client's body or other weight such as elevating the foot of the bed. Traction is used to reduce a fracture, immobilize an extremity, lessen muscle spasms, or correct or prevent a deformity.

Types of traction are skeletal, skin, and manual. Skeletal traction requires the surgical insertion of pins (Steinmann) or wires (Kirschner) through the bones. Skeletal traction is

LIFE SPAN DEVELOPMENT

Cast Removal

Children often are afraid when a cast is removed. Letting the child feel and see the cast cutter before starting to remove the cast alleviates fear.

continuous and is used most frequently for fractures of the femur, tibia, and cervical spine. Head tongs (e.g., Gardner-Wells tongs) are fixed in the skull to apply traction that immobilizes cervical fractures. An external fixation (fixator) is applied outside of the body to stabilize a break. Two or more pins are placed on either side of the fracture and attached to the fixator. The pins or screws remain in place with the fixator for 6 weeks or until the fracture heals, which may take up to a year or longer if complicated (The Ohio State University Medical Center, 2008). Figure 40-11 shows examples of traction devices.

Skin traction is a nonsurgical method of providing necessary pull for shorter periods, such as Buck's traction (Figure 40-11).

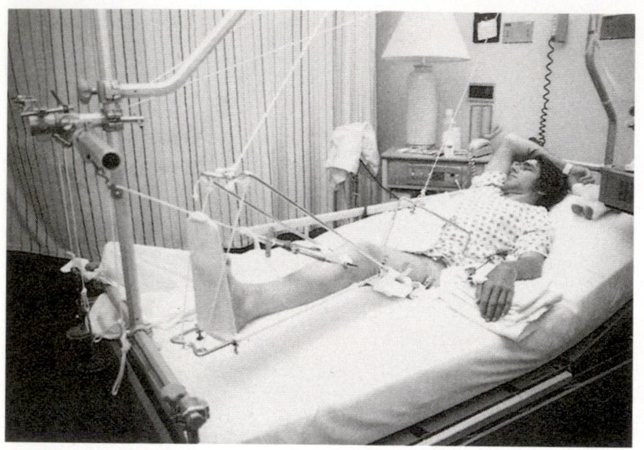

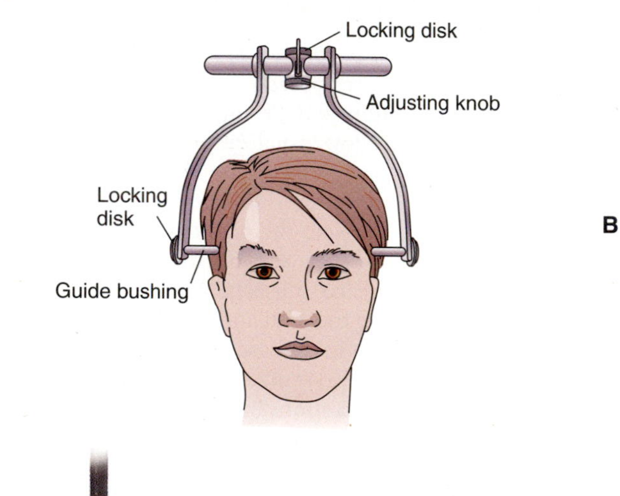

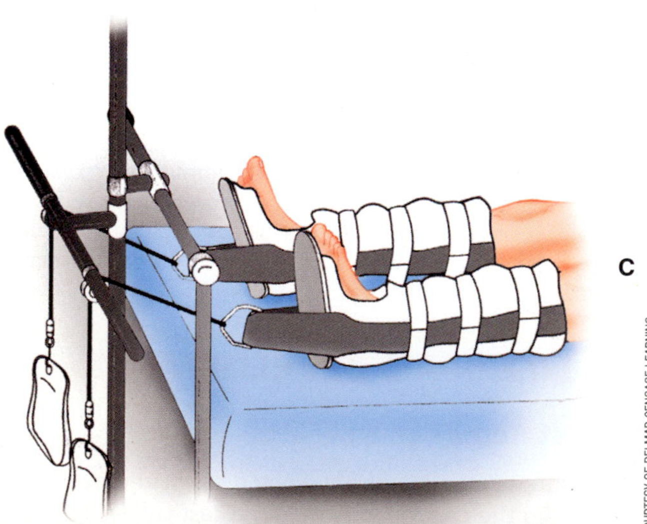

FIGURE 40-11 **Types of Traction Devices; *A*, Skeletal Traction; *B*, Head Tongs; *C*, Buck's Traction, a Type of Skin Traction**

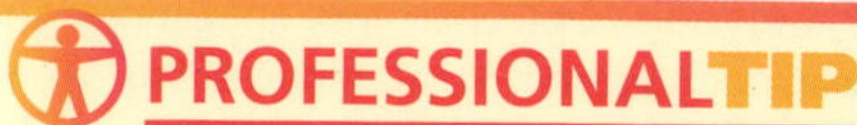

PROFESSIONALTIP

Pin Care

Pin care varies with health-care providers' orders and hospital protocol, therefore, basic guidelines are provided.

- Keep the pin site clean and dry.
- Cleanse the pin site with prescribed solution and a gauze pad using sterile technique.
- Use a new gauze pad for each pin.
- Remove any crust from the pin site.
- Remove all drainage from the pin site.
- Notify the health care provider if there is redness, swelling, purulent drainage, or pain at the pin site or if the pin becomes loose.
- Notify the health care provider if the client develops a fever of 101.5°F.

(The Ohio State University Medical Center, 2008)

Materials used include tapes, traction strips, cervical halters, pelvic belts, and lower extremity boots. Skin traction is frequently used to temporarily immobilize a part or stabilize a fracture. The disadvantage of skin traction for adult use is that it does not adequately control rotation and cannot be maintained for the length of time necessary for adult healing. Tapes and bandages are applied smoothly to prevent any pressure areas.

A nurse caring for a client in traction knows the purpose of the traction, how it accomplishes its purpose, and any complications associated with the use of the traction. It is also important to know the extent of the injury and the movements and positions allowed. Care of the client includes maintenance of the injured part, general body alignment, the alignment of the traction apparatus, and range of motion in as many joints as possible.

Rehabilitation The physician determines when the bone has healed sufficiently for rehabilitation. Healing is monitored by periodic x-rays and physical examinations. The major objective of rehabilitation is to assist the client to return to the former level of functioning. Rehabilitation programs vary depending on the injury and the client.

The nurse has a major role in client education reinforcing the directions of both the physician and the physical therapist. Patience and encouragement are extremely important in assisting the client to feel comfortable in learning self-care techniques. Teach the client to report any unusual signs or symptoms to the physician.

The client learns proper use of equipment such as crutches, canes, or walkers. Crutches allow ambulation with limited or no weight bearing on the affected extremity. Walkers allow limited weight bearing and provide stability when the client ambulates. Canes allow the client to walk with balance and support.

The tripod position is the basic stance for crutch walking. Tips of the crutches are placed approximately 8 to 10 inches in front of and lateral to the client's feet. The client must place his weight on the handpiece of the crutches and not on the axilla. Crutch gaits depend on the client's disability and are prescribed by the physician.

Canes are held in the hand *opposite* the affected extremity. In normal walking, the opposite arm and leg move together.

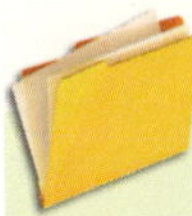

COLLABORATIVECARE

Use of Crutches, Canes, and Walkers

Nurses collaborate with physical therapists to assist clients in the use of crutches, canes, and walkers. Clients generally go to physical therapy to learn how to use the walking aid, and nurses reinforce the teaching when they see clients using their walking aid.

This same action is done when walking with a cane. Walkers provide more support than canes or crutches. They are especially useful for clients who have poor balance. The client places the walker 12 to 18 inches in front and walks toward the walker holding onto the hand grips.

Surgical

Open reduction is a surgical procedure that enables the surgeon to reduce (repair) the fracture under direct visualization. When an open reduction/**internal fixation** (ORIF) is done, orthopedic devices are used to maintain the reduction. Some of the devices used include pins, screws, nails, plates, wires, and rods. These internal fixation devices are inserted through bone fragments or fixed to the sides of the bones.

The major disadvantage of the open reduction is the possibility of introducing infection into the bone. Possible complications include impaired circulation and accidental injury to major nerves, blood vessels, and bone caused by the fixation devices. X-rays are taken during and after the open reduction to evaluate the alignment of the fracture.

Pharmacological

Analgesics are given to relieve pain. Muscle relaxants, such as cyclobenzaprine hydrochloride (Flexeril), also are prescribed for muscle spasms. Severe or continued pain indicates complications and is given immediate attention. Stool softeners, such as docusate sodium (Colace), are given to prevent constipation in the immobilized client.

Diet

The client is encouraged to eat regular meals with foods that provide fiber, protein, calcium, phosphorus, and fluids. For the client whose dietary intake is inadequate, vitamin and mineral supplements, especially calcium and phosphorus, are included. Consultation with a dietitian regarding client food preferences may be necessary.

Activity

Client activity and exercise are important in maintaining muscle strength and tone and minimizing cardiovascular problems. Joints that are not immobilized are exercised either actively or passively to maintain function. *Isometric* (maintaining constant resistive force) exercises help maintain muscle strength of immobilized muscles.

Nursing Management

Frequent and accurate assessment of the musculoskeletal trauma area includes circulation (color), movement, and sensation (CMS). CMS is very important. Provide comfort measures and administer analgesia as ordered. An important nursing responsibility is the prevention of constipation, skin breakdown, urinary calculi, and respiratory complications from immobility.

NURSING PROCESS

Assessment

Subjective Data

The neurovascular assessment of a client with a fracture may reveal subjective data of pain, especially on movement; muscle spasms; and paresthesia.

Objective Data

Assess for edema, shortening and deformity of the affected limb, hematoma, and pallor. Check pulses in the affected and unaffected extremity and compare with each other. Take the client's vital signs routinely, and note the client's general physical and mental condition. Check the skin, especially over bony prominences, for color and temperature.

When the client has a cast applied, check all cast edges for smoothness. Also check the cast for spots indicating wound drainage, including the color and amount. Mark the size of the drainage spot on the cast with a ballpoint pen and indicate the date and time. Then an increase in the size of the drainage spot can easily be identified. Assess extremities including fingers, toes, hands, and feet for changes in skin color, pulse, or temperature. Check all traction wires, pulleys, and weights. Weights should hang free and are not removed unless a health-care provider writes specific orders for removal. When providing pin care, nurses use sterile technique according to health-care facility guidelines. Observe for drainage and infection at the pin sites.

PROFESSIONALTIP

Neurovascular Assessment

- CMS assessments are performed on clients following musculoskeletal trauma; after surgery, if nerve or blood vessel damage is possible; and following casting, splinting, and bandaging.
- The CMS assessment is performed every 15 to 30 minutes for several hours, and then every 3 to 4 hours.
- All findings are documented.
- Tingling and numbness are relieved by flexing fingers or toes or repositioning extremity.
- Remember 6 Ps when performing a CMS assessment:
    1. Paresthesia (unrelieved tingling or numbness)
    2. Pain
    3. Pallor (Assessment may reveal a slow capillary return. Normal capillary refill is 2 to 4 seconds.)
    4. Paralysis
    5. Puffiness (edema)
    6. Pulselessness

Nursing diagnoses for a client with musculoskeletal trauma include the following:

NURSING DIAGNOSES	PLANNING/OUTCOMES	NURSING INTERVENTIONS
*Acute **P**ain* related to fracture	The client will have relief of pain with medication.	Assess for pain and swelling. Provide comfort measures. Administer medications for pain as ordered.
*Risk for Impaired **S**kin Integrity* related to immobility	The client's skin remains intact.	Change client position, if allowed, maintaining correct body alignment. Check bony prominences and keep the client's skin clean and dry. For the client in a cast, check the edges of the cast for roughness, keep the exposed skin next to the cast clean and dry. Inspect all body pressure points including the head, ears, and heels; turn the client as orders direct; and check for friction rubs. Instruct clients not to place anything inside the cast or use objects to scratch, causing skin breakdown or infections. Avoid getting the cast wet.
*Impaired Physical **M**obility* related to loss of integrity of bone structures	The client will perform range-of-motion exercises in unaffected joints. The client will demonstrate use of adaptive devices to improve mobility.	If the client in a cast is allowed to turn, use an overhead trapeze. Assist client in performing ROM exercises. Assist client in use of adaptive devices.

Evaluation: Evaluate each outcome to determine how it has been met by the client.

RHABDOMYOLYSIS

Crushing injuries most commonly cause rhabdomyolysis, the release of myoglobulin (muscle protein) from damaged muscle cells (MedlinePlus®, 2007). Myoglobin, creatine kinase (CK), and other inflammatory mediators escape from the injured muscle tissue into the circulation. The circulating myoglobin, filtered by the kidneys, can precipitate, causing renal tubular obstruction. About 15% of rhabdomyolysis cases will have acute renal failure (Walls, 2002). Two other major problems are respiratory distress from muscle weakness and fluid and electrolyte imbalance. Standard treatment includes IV fluids to maintain circulating blood volume and renal perfusion so the myoglobin is flushed from the kidneys.

COMPARTMENT SYNDROME

Compartment syndrome is a form of neurovascular impairment that may lead to permanent injury of an affected limb caused by progressive constriction of blood vessels and nerves. It occurs with any orthopedic injury as a result of bleeding into the tissue, tissue edema, or prolonged external pressure (cast or tight dressing). If untreated, in 4 to 6 hours it leads to irreversible damage to nerves and muscles, and within 24 to 48 hours permanent loss of normal limb function. Accurate, regular assessments and early detection are the best ways to avoid permanent disability. A neurovascular assessment that reveals throbbing pain not relieved by narcotic analgesics or greater in comparison with the injury, greater pain with passive motion than active, diminished capillary refill, weak or unequal pulses, **paresthesia** (numbness or tingling), and paralysis indicates this orthopedic emergency. Treatment consists of relieving pressure by removing the cast or dressing or by performing a fasciotomy. A surgical fasciotomy is an incision into the fascia to relieve pressure on the nerves and blood vessels.

CRITICAL THINKING

Immobility Complications

Prepare a teaching plan for an immobile client to prevent constipation, skin breakdown, urinary calculi, and respiratory complications.

INFLAMMATORY DISORDERS

Inflammatory disorders involve inflammation of the joints and include conditions such as rheumatoid arthritis, bursitis, and osteomyelitis.

RHEUMATOID ARTHRITIS

Rheumatoid arthritis is an autoimmune disease of unknown etiology, with recurring inflammation involving the synovium or lining of the joints. It can also affect the lungs, heart, blood vessels, muscles, eyes, and skin. Rheumatoid arthritis is a potentially destructive and disabling disease. The course is variable with either slow or rapid progress and/or periods of remissions. Women are affected more often than men. Rheumatoid arthritis occurs at any age; however, it most commonly affects young adults. In children, it occurs in a form known as juvenile rheumatoid arthritis (Still's disease). See the immune system chapter for more information on rheumatoid arthritis.

BURSITIS

Bursitis is inflammation of the bursa, a sac filled with synovial fluid that facilitates joint movement. Major bursae are found in the shoulder, knee, hip, and elbow. The inflammation is usually the result of trauma or repetitive movements. The client experiences painful joint movement. Diagnosis is made from the client's symptoms and x-ray, which shows a calcified bursa. Treatment includes rest of the joint and the administration of anti-inflammatory drugs including salicylates and nonsteroidal anti-inflammatory drugs (NSAIDs). For some clients, corticosteroids may be injected into the bursa.

OSTEOMYELITIS

Osteomyelitis is the inflammation of the bone and bone marrow. The most common cause of osteomyelitis is the introduction of pathogenic bacteria into a penetrating injury such as an open fracture. Bone infections may also result from the spread of infection from another site such as infected teeth, tonsils, or an upper respiratory infection. The most common pathogen causing osteomyelitis is *Staphylococcus aureus*. Other organisms found in osteomyelitis are *Pseudomonas* and *Escherichia coli*. Osteomyelitis may become a chronic disabling problem affecting the quality of life. The affected bone may have spontaneous fractures.

Local symptoms of an acute infection are sudden pain and tenderness of the affected bone, warmth, redness, edema, and pain on movement. General symptoms with acute severe bone infections include chills, elevated temperature, rapid pulse, and marked leukocytosis.

MEDICAL–SURGICAL MANAGEMENT

Medical

The client is placed on bed rest, and the infected bone is kept at rest with the use of sandbags or casts. Antibiotics are given IV as soon as osteomyelitis is suspected. Unless the infective process is controlled early, a bone abscess forms (Figure 40-12). Cultures of the abscess may indicate a need for change in the antibiotic therapy. The abscess may drain naturally; however, it usually requires an incision, allowing it to drain. The abscess cavity of dead bone tissue does not liquefy easily, drain, and heal as in soft tissue abscesses. A bone sheath forms around the sequestrum (dead bone), giving the appearance of healing; however, chronically infected sequestrum has the tendency to produce recurrent abscesses throughout the life of the individual.

Surgical

A sequestrectomy to remove the dead bone tissue may need to be performed. Strict aseptic technique is maintained when changing any dressings. Because infected bone is extremely painful, unnecessary movement is avoided and the affected extremity handled very gently.

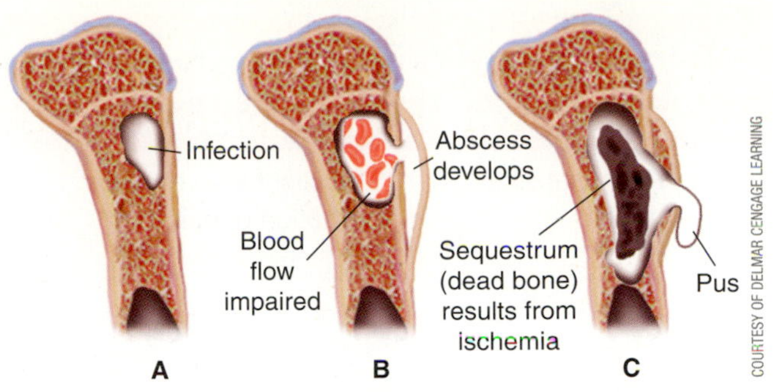

FIGURE 40-12 *A,* Osteomyelitis; *B,* Without early treatment, an abscess forms; *C,* Bone dies (sequestrum) and pus forms.

Pharmacological

Osteomyelitis is treated with vigorous antibiotic therapy and analgesics. Wound irrigations with antiseptics or antibiotics are often prescribed by the physician. Specific drugs given are determined by the causative organism.

Diet

A high-calorie, high-protein diet is generally ordered for the client with osteomyelitis. Dietary supplements of vitamins and calcium are also given. Fluids are increased as tolerated, and a high-fiber diet is encouraged due to analgesic use and immobilization.

Activity

Absolute rest of the affected extremity is needed. Avoid excessive handling of the extremity because it is very painful. The extremity is handled in a smooth, unhurried manner, supporting the joints above and below the affected area.

NURSING MANAGEMENT

Maintain the client on bed rest and the infected bone at absolute rest. Avoid excessive handling of the affected extremity. Administer IV antibiotics, analgesics, and dietary supplements (vitamins and calcium) as ordered. Maintain strict asepsis if wound irrigations are ordered. Encourage the client to drink more fluids and to eat the high-calorie, high-protein diet ordered. Provide for diversional activities.

NURSING PROCESS

ASSESSMENT

Subjective Data

Inquire about pain, muscle spasms, and tenderness in the bone. Ask about any traumas, surgeries, and other diseases.

Objective Data

Observe the client for signs of infection, including chills, elevated temperature, pain, redness, and edema of the affected extremity. The client may also experience headaches, restlessness, and irritability.

Nursing diagnoses for a client with osteomyelitis include the following:

NURSING DIAGNOSES	PLANNING/OUTCOMES	NURSING INTERVENTIONS
*Acute **Pain** related to* inflammation	The client will verbalize reduction of pain.	Protect client from jerky movements and falls. Assess wound appearance and new sites of pain. Provide diet high in protein and vitamin C. Administer pain medications as ordered.
*Impaired Physical **Mobility*** related to pain	The client will maintain movement of unaffected extremities.	Encourage and assist client to maintain active ROM or perform passive ROM to unaffected extremities.
*Risk for Impaired **Skin** Integrity* related to immobility	The client will maintain skin integrity.	Handle the affected extremity gently, protect it from injury, keep it in good body alignment and level with the body. Irrigate wound as ordered. Use aseptic technique when irrigating the affected area and when changing the dressing. Assess skin and bony prominences for reddened areas. Encourage adequate fluid intake.

Evaluation: Evaluate each outcome to determine how it has been met by the client.

DEGENERATIVE DISORDERS

Degenerative disorders include osteoporosis, degenerative joint disease, and total joint arthroplasty.

OSTEOPOROSIS

Osteoporosis is an increase in the porosity of bone. It is a common disorder in bone metabolism in which both mineral and protein matrix components are diminished and the bone becomes brittle and fragile. There is an increased susceptibility to fractures of the hip, spine, and wrist.

Ten million individuals in the United States have osteoporosis, and another 34 million have low bone mineral density, which places them at risk for osteoporosis (NOF, 2008d). Of those affected by osteoporosis, 80% are women (NOF, 2008d). In 2005, more than 2 million osteoporosis related fractures occured, including 297,000 hip fractures, 547,000 vertebral fractures, 397,000 wrist fractures, 135,000 pelvic fractures, and 675,000 fractures of other types (NOF, 2008d).

Osteoporosis has been called the "silent disease" because there are no symptoms of bone loss. As the bone tissue loses density, fractures and kyphosis occur. Very slight trauma fractures the brittle bones. With multiple vertebral fractures, the individual experiences a loss of height.

The only way to determine whether an individual has osteoporosis is to measure bone mineral density (BMD). The recommended type of BMD test is the dual-energy x-ray absorptiometry (DXA or DEXA) that identifies low bone density prior to a fracture and predicts the chances of a person having a fracture in the future (NOF, 2008a, 2008c, 2008d). The test measures the bone density of the spine, hip, or total body and is painless, noninvasive, and safe.

MEDICAL–SURGICAL MANAGEMENT

There is no cure for osteoporosis. Prevention through diet, regular exercise, eliminating tobacco and alcohol use, having BMD testing, and taking medication is possible for most people (NOF, 2002e).

PROFESSIONALTIP

Absolute Fracture Risk

A DXA machine is in development that reports an *absolute fracture risk*. The report uses a client's bone mineral density results, age, risk factors for osteoporosis, and fractures to determine the client's risk of a fracture in the next 10 years. The information enables health care providers to determine appropriate osteoporosis treatment (NOF, 2008d).

PROFESSIONALTIP

Osteoporosis

Risk factors for osteoporosis include being female, having thin or small bones, history of fractures, advanced age, family history of osteoporosis, postmenopause without estrogen replacement therapy, amenorrhea, eating disorders, low calcium intake, inactive lifestyle, smoking, excessive alcohol intake, use of corticosteroids or anticonvulsant medications, and low testosterone level in men.

Pharmacological

Several medications are approved for the prevention and treatment of osteoporosis. Alendronate sodium (Fosamax) and alendronate plus vitamin D3 (Fosamax plus D™), risedronate (Actonel®) and risedronate with calcium (Actonel® with calcium), and zoledronic acid (Reclast®) are used for prevention and treatment of osteoporosis in postmenopausal men and women. Ibandronate (Boniva®) is used for prevention and treatment of postmenopausal women only. Calcitonin (Forical® and Miacalcin®) is used in treatment of osteoporosis in women at least 5 years beyond menopause. Raloxifen (Evista®), an estrogen agonists/antagonists or selective estrogen receptor modulators (SERMs), is used for the prevention and treatment of osteroporosis in postmenopausal women. Estrogen is used both for prevention and treatment, but according to the FDA, other medications should be used first (NOF, 2008c). Estrogen is used both for prevention and treatment, but according to the FDA, other medications should be used first (NOF, 2008c). Teriparatide (Forteo®), a parathyroid hormone, is used in the treatment of postmenopausal men and women with very low BMD and at risk of a fracture. The FDA recommends the client take teriparatide for no more than 2 years (NOF, 2008c).

Testosterone-replacement therapy may be used for men with low testosterone levels.

Nonnarcotic analgesics are prescribed for relief of pain. The client also is advised to take supplemental vitamin D with calcium.

Diet

Encourage the client to maintain an adequate balanced diet rich in calcium and vitamin D. A reduction in the consumption of caffeine, alcohol, excess protein, and smoking cessation is recommended.

Activity

Encourage the client to practice good body mechanics and posture and to walk, preferably outdoors for the benefits of sunshine (vitamin D). This is effective in preventing further bone loss and stimulating new bone formation.

Nursing Management

Encourage clients to prevent osteoporosis through a diet adequate in calcium and vitamin D, regular exercise, and eliminating tobacco and alcohol use. Teach correct body mechanics and encourage good posture.

CULTURAL CONSIDERATIONS

Osteoporosis

- Significant risk has been reported in persons of all ethnic backgrounds.
- White women older than age 65 have twice as many fractures as African American women (NOF, 2002c).
- White men are at greater risk for osteoporosis, but osteoporosis is found in men from all ethnic groups (NOF, 2002d).

COMMUNITY/HOME HEALTH CARE

Osteoporosis

- Maintain physical activity—walking, isometric exercises.
- Remove potential hazards, such as throw rugs.
- Eat a diet high in calcium and vitamin D.
- Be out in the sun 10 to 15 minutes a day.
- Move items down from top shelves of cupboards because it is difficult to see or reach the items as a result of curvature changes in the spine.
- Wear sturdy shoes.

NURSING PROCESS

Assessment

Subjective Data

This includes the client's gender, age, and family health history. Note any symptoms the client expresses regarding altered body image or back or neck pain that worsens when coughing, sneezing, straining, or standing. Take a nutritional history. Note lifestyle patterns such as smoking, inactivity, or immobilization. A medical history regarding any medications is also important.

Objective Data

Kyphosis, gait impairment, and poor posture are noted.

Nursing diagnoses for a client with osteoporosis include the following:

NURSING DIAGNOSES	PLANNING/OUTCOMES	NURSING INTERVENTIONS
*Chronic **Pain*** related to disease process	The client will express minimal discomfort.	Administer analgesics as ordered; teach client about the medications. Handle client carefully; instruct client to avoid any twisting movements. The bed should have a firm mattress or bed board for support.

(*Continues*)

Nursing diagnoses for a client with osteoporosis include the following: (Continued)

NURSING DIAGNOSES	PLANNING/OUTCOMES	NURSING INTERVENTIONS
*Risk for **I**njury* related to disease process	The client will practice correct body mechanics.	Teach client correct body mechanics.
*Impaired Physical **M**obility* related to disease process	The client will maintain physical activity.	Teach client about types of exercises and physical activities that help maintain bone mass and isometric exercises to strengthen muscles. Encourage ambulation with the client using a walker or cane if necessary.

Evaluation: Evaluate each outcome to determine how it has been met by the client.

OSTEOARTHRITIS (DEGENERATIVE JOINT DISEASE)

Osteoarthritis (OA) is considered a "wear-and-tear" disease and is characterized by slow and steady progressive breakdown of cartilage. It is a nonsystemic, noninflammatory disorder causing bones and joints to degenerate. It is the most common type of arthritis. The etiology is unknown, but predisposing factors include increased age, obesity, an injury to a joint, poor posture, or occupations that put strain on joints. Genetics plays a role in OA, especially in the hands (Arthritis Foundation, 2002b). The weight-bearing joints of the lower extremities as well as the hands and cervical and lumbar vertebrae are the joints most frequently affected. The cartilage covering the bone becomes thin and then wears off. The synovial membrane thickens and fibrous tissue around the joint ossifies. The effects of degenerative changes on the knee joint are shown in Figure 40-13.

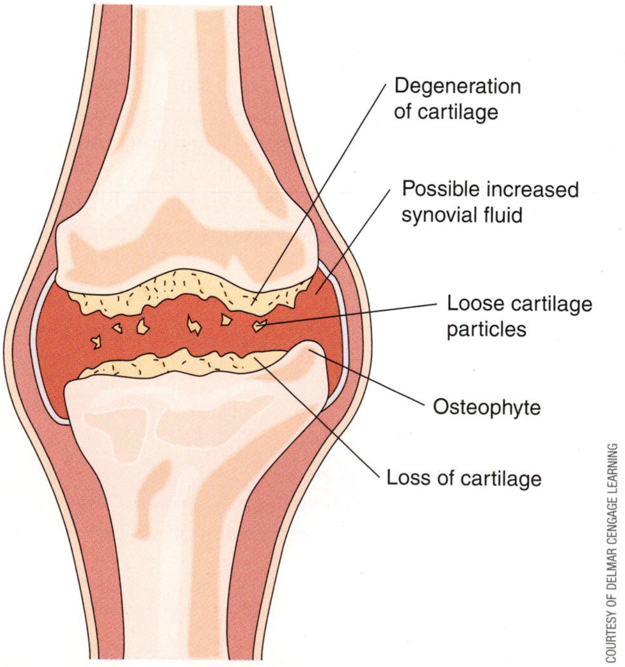

Degeneration of cartilage

Possible increased synovial fluid

Loose cartilage particles

Osteophyte

Loss of cartilage

COURTESY OF DELMAR CENGAGE LEARNING

FIGURE 40-13 Degenerative Changes in the Cartilage of the Knee Due to Osteoarthritis

The onset of osteoarthritis begins during middle age, and by age 65 most people have some degeneration. Symptoms include early morning stiffness and pain after physical activity. There is joint enlargement and characteristic hypertrophic spurs, called **Heberden's nodes**, in the terminal interphalangeal finger joints. More women are affected with OA, especially in the hands. The hips are more affected in men.

Diagnosis is made from the client's symptoms and examination of the joints that are enlarged and tender. X-ray shows a narrowing of joint spaces and gross irregularities of joint structure. A CT scan or MRI shows vertebral joint involvement.

MEDICAL–SURGICAL MANAGEMENT

Medical

No treatment exists to stop the degenerative process; therefore, treatment focuses on relief of the client's discomfort. Medical management includes local heat and rest for the affected joint, weight reduction for obese clients to relieve strain on affected joints, and orthotic devices (braces, canes, crutches) to support the joints. Physical therapy can provide exercises to strengthen muscles and keep joints flexible and teach self-management skills.

Surgical

Surgical procedures such as total hip or knee replacement may be recommended for clients with severe osteoarthritis. Osteotomy may help correct malalignment situations. Refer to the section on total joint arthroplasty in this chapter.

Pharmacological

Pharmacological treatment includes the use of aspirin or NSAIDs. Narcotics are avoided because of the chronic nature of the disease. Steroids may be used and are sometimes injected into a joint to provide immediate relief of pain and to stop the degenerative process temporarily. If the client has vertebral involvement with muscle spasms, cyclobenzaprine hydrochloride (Flexeril) may be given to relax the muscles.

CLIENT TEACHING

Osteoarthritis

- Set priorities each day, and do the most important activities first.
- Do not plan too many activities for one day.
- Plan rest periods during the day between activities.
- Prevent rushing and stressful situations by planning ahead.
- Lose weight, if necessary.
- When knees or hips are affected, avoid climbing stairs, bending, stooping, or squatting.

Nursing Management

Encourage clients to maintain a proper weight for height and to practice good posture. Provide rest and heat for the affected joint. Collaborate with physical therapy for muscle-strengthening exercises and self-management skills.

NURSING PROCESS

Assessment

Subjective Data

The client describes nonspecific symptoms such as general musculoskeletal pain, joint stiffness especially on rising, and joint pain or tenderness. Note weight gain, occupation, and any conditions or situations that exacerbate the client's joint pain. Some of these situations include cold weather, overexercising, or extreme fatigue. Assess the client's understanding of the disease and its effect on lifestyle and ability to perform activities of daily and social living.

Objective Data

This includes edema and tenderness around the joints and bony enlargements of distal interphalangeal joints (Heberden's nodes).

Nursing diagnoses for a client with osteoarthritis include the following:

NURSING DIAGNOSES	PLANNING/OUTCOMES	NURSING INTERVENTIONS
*Chronic **Pain*** related to joint tenderness and edema	The client will express minimal discomfort.	Handle the affected extremity gently and apply heat as ordered. Administer prescribed analgesic and evaluate its effectiveness.
*Impaired Physical **Mobility*** related to joint deterioration	The client will maintain mobility within the parameters of the disease process.	Coordinate with physical therapy and assist in a planned exercise program as ordered. Advise client to plan rest periods during the day.

Evaluation: Evaluate each outcome to determine how it has been met by the client.

TOTAL JOINT ARTHROPLASTY

Joint replacement or **arthroplasty** is the replacement of both articular surfaces within a joint capsule. The hip, knee, shoulder, and fingers are the joints most frequently replaced. Replacements consist of metal and polyethylene and may be cemented in the prepared bone with methyl methacrylate, which has properties similar to bone. See Figure 40-14 for knee- and hip-replacement components.

Newer techniques use porous-coated cementless artificial joint components. These allow bone to grow into the joint component and securely fix the prosthesis. This reduces the incidence of prosthesis failure. Joint replacement is usually an elective procedure, and clients may wish to have autologous blood transfusions whereby they predonate their own blood in case a blood transfusion is needed.

Total Hip Replacement

Total hip replacement is the replacement of a damaged hip with an artificial joint. The hip is replaced with a traditional procedure or a minimally invasive procedure. The minimally invasive method has less pain, less muscle injury, shorter hospitalization, and a faster rehabilitation. The incisions are 2 to 3 inches or less, whereas the traditional method has a 10- to 12-inch incision on the side of the hip and possibly with a portable suction device in place (AAOS, 2007c). The traditional method has more drainage and the drain is removed when the drainage is 30 mL or less. The hip prosthesis by either method can be cemented in place or be coated with a special textured metal or bone-like substance that is not cemented into the joint. A cemented ball and a noncemented socket are sometimes used (AAOS, 2007d).

Surgical complications are venous thrombosis, bleeding, respiratory problems, and, after several years, the hip prosthesis may loosen or need replacing. Potential problems with the hip replacement include dislocation of the prosthesis, excessive wound drainage, and infection. To prevent venous thrombosis, antiembolism stockings are worn. They are removed twice daily to inspect the skin.

After a total hip replacement, the client's hip and leg are kept in a position of abduction and extension. The knees are kept apart by using a foam V-wedge, several pillows, or an abductor pillow. When the client turns from the back to a side-lying position, the entire leg is supported with pillows to keep the hip abducted. The client usually prefers to lie on the unaffected side. Instruct the client to avoid acute hip flexion of greater than 90 degrees. The legs should not

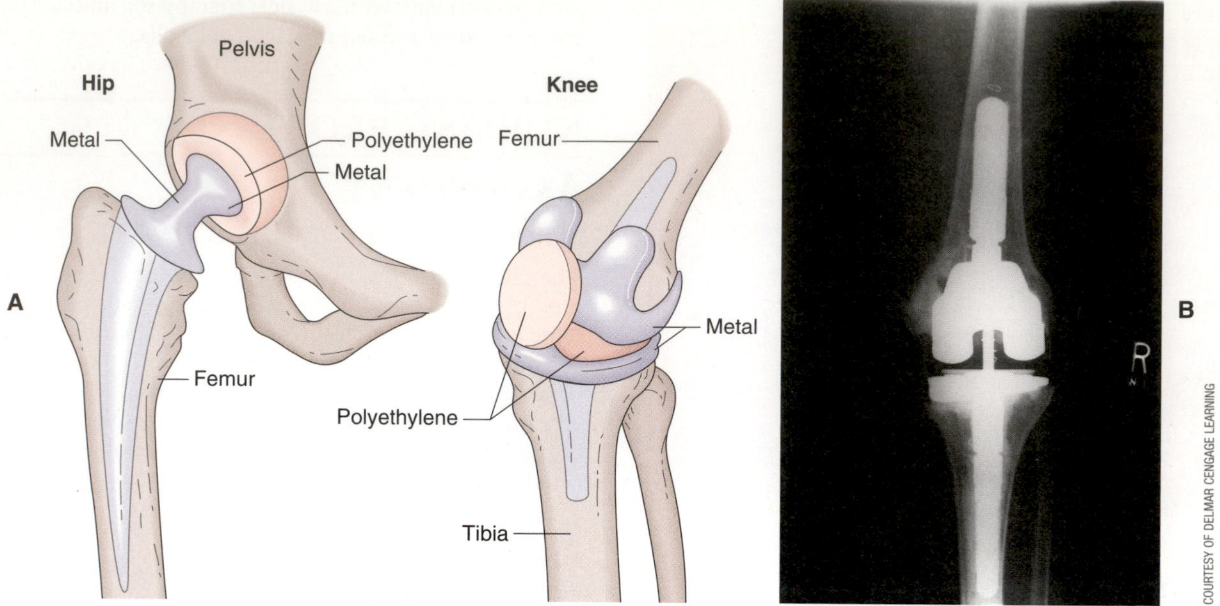

FIGURE 40-14 *A,* **Total Hip and Knee Replacement;** *B,* **Radiograph of a Total Knee Replacement (Anterior-Posterior View). The patella is plastic, and, therefore, it is not visible here.**

be crossed nor the hips flexed to pull up a blanket or sheet. A fracture bedpan is used until the client can ambulate to the bathroom. Use a raised toilet seat in the bathroom or a bedside commode. Any specific client turning, movement, and positioning are ordered by the physician. Vital signs and CMS checks are performed routinely. Encourage the client to cough and deep breathe or use an incentive spirometer after surgery to prevent respiratory problems. Inspect the dressings frequently.

The goal for clients who have total hip or knee joint replacement is to ambulate independently. Ambulatory activity progresses rapidly for clients with joint replacement. Clients who have total hip replacement are usually out of bed the night of surgery or early the next day. Physical therapy teaches exercises to strengthen the hip muscles. Gait training begins with the use of a walker and progresses to the use of crutches or a cane. The client avoids hip flexion of more than 90 degrees and stair climbing for at least 3 months.

TOTAL KNEE REPLACEMENT

Total knee replacement, like hip replacement, is considered for clients experiencing severe pain and functional disability related to joint destruction. The prosthesis chosen for the replacement provides the client with a painless, stable, and functional joint.

Immediately after surgery a firm compression dressing is applied to the operative site. The physician may order a special ice machine applied to circulate ice water around the knee. The cold water decreases pain and swelling. After the dressing is removed, a CPM machine helps increase circulation to the operative area and promotes flexibility within the knee joint. The surgeon orders the frequency of use and the amount of tension, flexion, and extension produced by the machine. A sequential compression device (SCD) is used or antiembolism stockings worn to minimize the development of thrombophlebitis. After the arthroplasty, the client wears an adjustable soft knee immobilizer to stabilize the leg when walking. The client may transfer out of bed to a wheelchair with the immobilizer in place. No weight bearing is allowed on the knee until it is prescribed by the surgeon.

The most common complication after total knee replacement is blood clots in the leg veins. The orthopedic surgeon may order periodic elevation of legs, leg exercises to improve circulation, support hose, and an anticoagulant (AAOS, 2007e).

NURSING MANAGEMENT

Perform neurovascular assessment of the affected extremity as well as incision assessment, vital signs, lung sounds, pedal pulses, and I&O. Maintain the client's hip in a position of abduction and extension for 6 to 10 days as ordered. Keep client's skin and bed dry and clean. Encourage the client to cough and deep breathe and to use the trapeze to raise hips off the bed for bedpan use.

NURSING PROCESS

ASSESSMENT

Subjective Data

Assess for irritability, restlessness, orientation, and neurovascular assessment of the affected extremity for pain, numbness, tingling, and paresthesia.

Objective Data

Assess the incision for approximation, redness, and drainage and the skin over all bony prominences. Assess for tachypnea, dyspnea, hypoxemia, and crackles and wheezes in the lungs (signs of fat embolism). Vital signs, pedal pulses, and I&O are also assessed.

The client with a total hip replacement is assessed for position of the affected hip. The hip should be maintained in a position of abduction and extension. The most prominent symptom of a dislocation is a clicking, popping sound. Other symptoms are a sudden sharp pain that is unrelieved by narcotic analgesics, loss of leg motion, and edema of the affected hip. The client is not moved, and the physician is notified immediately.

Assessment of the client with a total knee replacement includes the neurovascular status of the leg and the dressing and drainage device. Vital signs, intake and output, and the color and temperature of the extremity are also assessed. The knee is elevated and the nurse monitors the ice machine and CPM machine.

Nursing diagnoses for a client undergoing arthroplasty surgery include the following:

NURSING DIAGNOSES	PLANNING/OUTCOMES	NURSING INTERVENTIONS
*Impaired **S**kin Integrity* related to immobility and surgical incision	The client's skin will remain free from redness or any other signs of breakdown.	Maintain a clean and dry dressing. If a drainage device is used, assess functioning. Keep client's skin and bed clean and dry. Assess bony prominences for redness. Provide high-protein diet with dairy products and vitamin C.
*Impaired Physical **M**obility* related to surgery	The client will ambulate following physician's direction.	Keep hip in a position of abduction. Use an abductor pillow or wedge to maintain the position when turning the client. Encourage client to use the trapeze to raise hips off the bed to use the bedpan. Assist client in accomplishing activities of daily living.
*Ineffective Peripheral **T**issue Perfusion* related to surgery and immobility	The client will have adequate circulation of extremity.	Encourage client to cough and deep breathe. Monitor vital signs until stable. Assess pedal pulses and capillary refill in both extremities.

Evaluation: Evaluate each outcome to determine how it has been met by the client.

MUSCULOSKELETAL DISORDERS

Musculoskeletal disorders discussed include amputations, temporomandibular joint disease/disorder, and carpal tunnel syndrome.

AMPUTATIONS

An **amputation** is the removal of all or part of an extremity. Amputations are done in response to injuries resulting in extensive laceration of arteries or nerves, or diseases such as malignant tumors, infections, and peripheral vascular disorders. Other disease conditions that may require amputation include extensive osteomyelitis or congenital disorders. In severe trauma situations, an amputation may be done to save the client's life.

Recent advances in microsurgical techniques have allowed replantation (limb reattachment) in some injuries. These procedures involve the use of microscopes and highly specialized instruments to reconnect severed nerves and blood vessels. Amputations involving the hand or wrist are more likely considered for replantation rather than an injury involving a large muscle mass because of extensive tissue, bone, and muscle damage. Any amputation creates a major physical and psychological adjustment for the client.

MEDICAL–SURGICAL MANAGEMENT

Medical

Rehabilitation for the client with an amputation requires the effort of the entire rehabilitation team. The client's physical and psychological responses to the amputation are monitored by all members of the team. If appropriate, counseling and job training will enable many clients to return to their jobs.

Surgical

Before surgery, the surgeon evaluates the client and makes several decisions. These decisions include necessity of an amputation, type of amputation (open or closed), level of amputation, potential for rehabilitation, and type of prosthesis and rehabilitation program.

The surgeon attempts to save as much of the limb as possible. A closed amputation is done by using skin flaps to cover the bone end of the extremity. This type of amputation is done when there is no evidence of infection. Sometimes a Guillotine (open) amputation is necessary. This amputation requires a straight cut and allows for free drainage of infectious material. Tissue, bone, and vessels are severed at the same level without skin flaps. The major indication for doing an open amputation is infection.

The level of an amputation is determined by the vascular supply and is never higher than absolutely necessary. If the blood flow at the site of the incision is normal, the amputation is performed at that level. If the bleeding is scant, a higher level

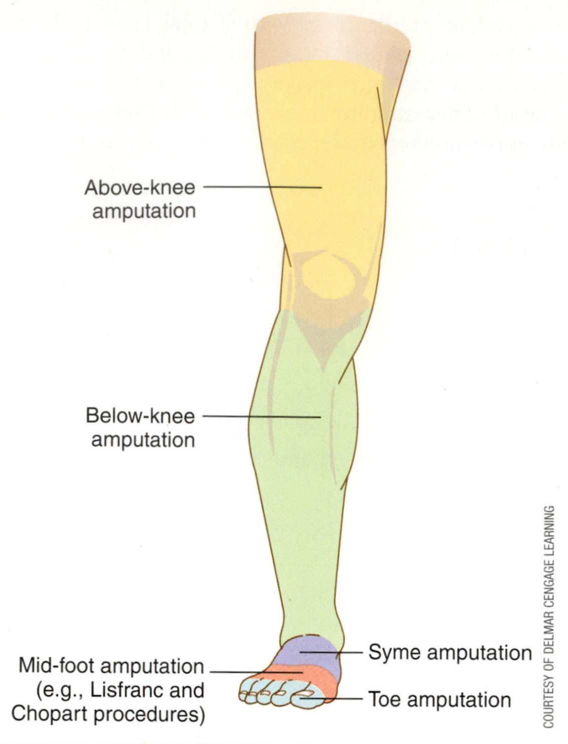

FIGURE 40-15 Different Amputation Levels

of amputation is performed to ensure adequate postoperative healing. See Figure 40-15 for different lower-extremity amputation levels.

Pharmacological

Narcotic analgesics are required immediately after surgery. After several days, pain is controlled with nonnarcotic analgesics. If infection exists, appropriate antibiotic therapy is ordered.

Diet

A balanced diet with adequate vitamins and protein is essential for adequate wound healing. Many elderly clients are poorly nourished or require special diets. Nutritional care plans are discussed with the physician and a dietitian.

Activity

The surgeon determines postoperative positioning of the stump. The stump is alternately placed in an extended position or elevated on pillows for short periods. Encourage the client to spend some time in the prone position. This position helps stretch the flexor muscles and prevents contractions of the hip. Physical therapy starts exercises to prevent contractures and increase muscle strength and assists with ambulation as soon after surgery as possible.

CRITICAL THINKING

Phantom Limb Pain

How would you explain phantom limb pain to a client?

NURSING MANAGEMENT

Perform routine postoperative care by encouraging deep breathing, coughing, and turning; assessing pain on a 1 to 10 scale; and administering analgesics as ordered. The residual limb is shaped for prosthesis by using a figure-8 wrapping of wide elastic bandages. Some physicians prefer a two-way elastic compression shrinker that forms the residual limb to the prosthesis. Other more rigid dressings are also used.

Encourage client to eat a balanced diet with extra protein for wound healing. Collaborate with physical therapy regarding bed exercises, transfer techniques, and later ambulation.

NURSING PROCESS

ASSESSMENT

Subjective Data

Subjective assessment data include pain, sensations felt on the extremity to be amputated, and the emotional status of the client. If a client has experienced chronic pain before the amputation, pain may seem mild following the surgery. Severe pain may indicate a hematoma or excessive pressure from a cast or elastic bandage on a bony prominence. Sometimes the client confuses **phantom limb pain** with the incisional pain. Phantom limb pain is the sensation that there is pain, soreness, tingling, burning, and stiffness in the amputated limb. The sensory sensations of the missing limb remain in the brain causing the feelings of phantom pain. Phantom pain decreases as inflammation subsides at the incisional site.

Objective Data

Objective assessment data include the color and temperature of the skin, pulse, and responses to limb movement. The unaffected extremity also is assessed for function and circulation.

PROFESSIONALTIP

Robotic Ankle

Hugh Herr developed a robotic ankle that simulates the action of the human ankle-foot. The prosthesis is made with springs and an electric motor so it propels the person with each step, giving the person a natural appearing gait. The robotic ankle makes one less tired when walking and improves balance (MIT, 2007).

Nursing diagnoses for a client who has an amputation include the following:

NURSING DIAGNOSES	PLANNING/OUTCOMES	NURSING INTERVENTIONS
*Impaired **S**kin Integrity* related to amputation	The client will remain free from infection.	Inspect the incision for any inflammation, excessive drainage, edema, increased pain, and hypersensitivity to touch. Use aseptic technique for all dressing changes. Monitor vital signs.
*Disturbed **B**ody Image* related to loss of limb	The client will participate in the care of the residual limb.	Handle the residual limb gently and treat it as though a prosthesis will be worn. Encourage client to watch dressing change and eventually assist with and do the dressing changes. Encourage client to express feelings and concerns about the amputation.
*Impaired Physical **M**obility* related to loss of limb	The client will demonstrate improved physical mobility.	Encourage client to participate in physical therapy and to perform ROM exercises. Assist client when ambulating with assistive devices.

Evaluation: Evaluate each outcome to determine how it has been met by the client.

SAMPLE NURSING CARE PLAN

The Client with a Below-the-Knee Amputation

R.S. is a 76-year-old resident in a retirement home. She has remained active since her retirement from the secretarial job she held for 20 years. Her health history indicates she has had circulatory problems with inadequate peripheral circulation resulting from atherosclerosis. Her physician hospitalized her for a planned below-the-knee amputation on the left leg and has ordered an arteriogram to assist in determining the site for the amputation. The arteriogram determines the point of adequate circulatory status to promote wound healing after the limb is amputated.

The nurse's assessment of R.S.'s vital signs are blood pressure 120/68 mm Hg, pulse 72 beats/minute, and respirations 18 breaths/minute. Femoral pulses are present in both extremities; however, the pedal pulse in her left foot is barely palpable, and the skin is cool and pale. She stated that lately her left foot is always cold and is a bluish-black color. R.S. expresses concern about her ability to take care of herself after she loses her foot.

NURSING DIAGNOSIS 1 *Disturbed **B**ody Image* related to scheduled amputation as evidenced by statement of concern over losing foot

Nursing Outcomes Classification (NOC)
Psychosocial Adjustment: Life Change
Grief Resolution

Nursing Interventions Classification (NIC)
Body Image Enhancement
Grief Work Facilitation

PLANNING/OUTCOMES	NURSING INTERVENTIONS	RATIONALE
R.S. will communicate her concerns and feelings about the changes in her body image.	Involve R.S. in participating in her daily care.	Gives sense of independence.
	Encourage R.S. to voice her concerns.	Helps resolve concerns.

(*Continues*)

SAMPLE NURSING CARE PLAN (Continued)

PLANNING/OUTCOMES	NURSING INTERVENTIONS	RATIONALE
	Provide positive reinforcement when R.S. attempts to adapt to body changes.	Encourages client to continue adapting.

EVALUATION

R.S. has demonstrated beginning acceptance of body changes by taking an active interest in her appearance.

NURSING DIAGNOSIS 2 *Situational Low **S**elf-Esteem* related to loss of body part as evidenced by expression of concern about ability to care for self

Nursing Outcomes Classification (NOC)
Psychosocial Adjustment: Life Change
Decision Making

Nursing Interventions Classification (NIC)
Coping Enhancement
Support Group
Cognitive Restructuring

PLANNING/OUTCOMES	NURSING INTERVENTIONS	RATIONALE
R.S. will identify at least two positive qualities about herself.	Encourage R.S. to express her feelings about herself.	Helps identify positive qualities.
	Involve R.S. in decision making regarding her care.	Helps maintain a sense of control over her life.
	Provide R.S. with positive feedback.	Gives a feeling of acceptance and approval.

EVALUATION

R.S. has voiced two positive qualities about herself.

NURSING DIAGNOSIS 3 *Deficient **K**nowledge* related to postoperative care and activity as evidenced by concern about ability to care for self

Nursing Outcomes Classification (NOC)
Knowledge: Treatment Regimen

Nursing Interventions Classification (NIC)
Teaching: Procedure/Treatment

PLANNING/OUTCOMES	NURSING INTERVENTIONS	RATIONALE
R.S. swill perform stump wrapping correctly.	Encourage R.S. to participate in the care of the residual limb.	Helps client adjust to body changes.
	Demonstrate how to wrap her stump, then allow her to do it several times.	Helps client to know how to care for self.

EVALUATION

R.S. demonstrated the ability to care for the residual limb by wrapping the stump correctly.

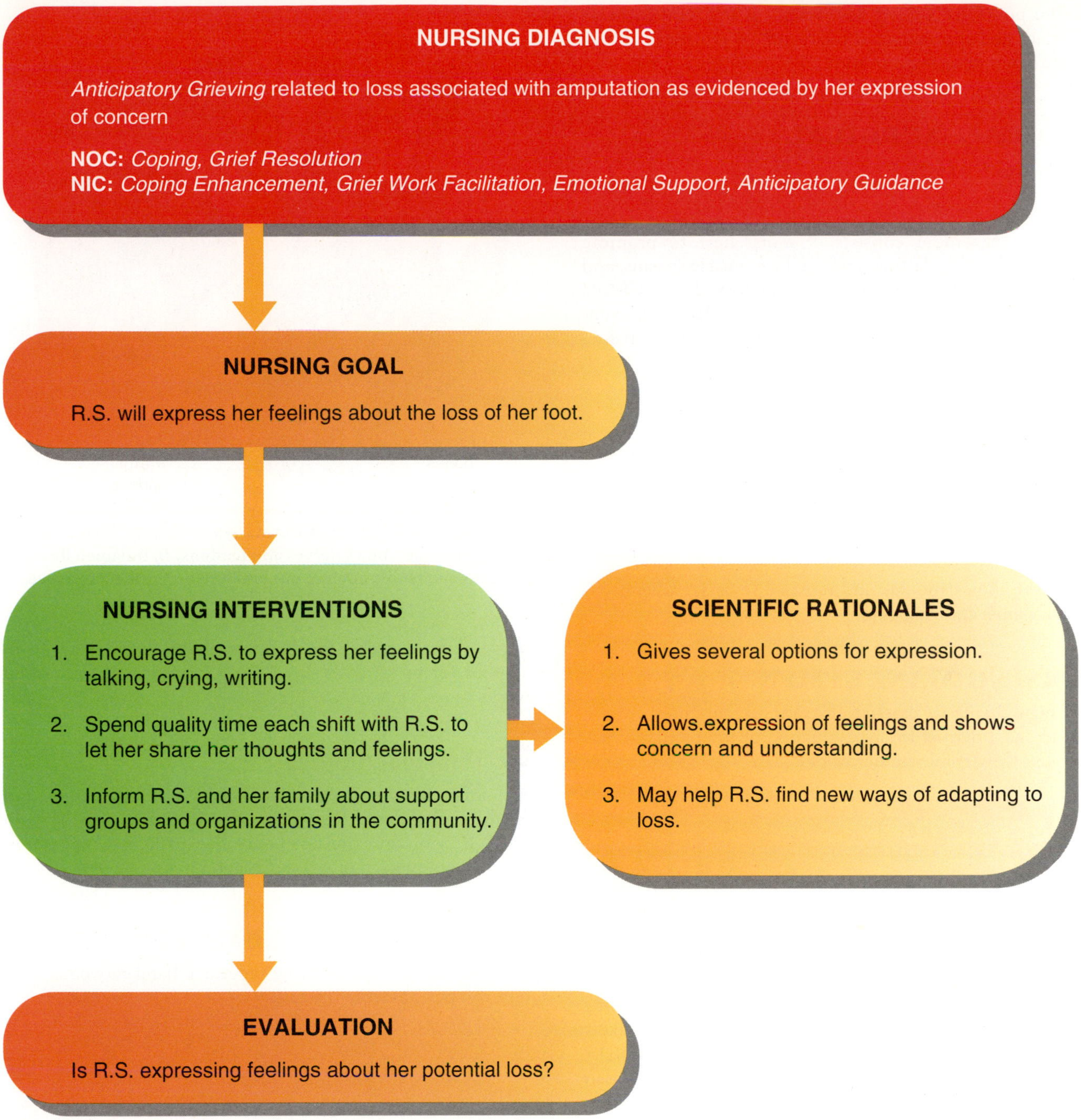

NURSING DIAGNOSIS

Anticipatory Grieving related to loss associated with amputation as evidenced by her expression of concern

NOC: *Coping, Grief Resolution*
NIC: *Coping Enhancement, Grief Work Facilitation, Emotional Support, Anticipatory Guidance*

NURSING GOAL

R.S. will express her feelings about the loss of her foot.

NURSING INTERVENTIONS

1. Encourage R.S. to express her feelings by talking, crying, writing.
2. Spend quality time each shift with R.S. to let her share her thoughts and feelings.
3. Inform R.S. and her family about support groups and organizations in the community.

SCIENTIFIC RATIONALES

1. Gives several options for expression.
2. Allows.expression of feelings and shows concern and understanding.
3. May help R.S. find new ways of adapting to loss.

EVALUATION

Is R.S. expressing feelings about her potential loss?

CONCEPT CARE MAP 40-1

TEMPOROMANDIBULAR JOINT DISEASE/DISORDER

Temporomandibular joint disease/disorder (TMD) is commonly referred to as TMJ. It is a collection of conditions affecting the temporomandibular joint and/or the muscles of mastication. More than 10 million people in the United States have TMD. It affects both males and females, but 90% of those seeking treatment are females between puberty and menopause (The TMJ Association, 2002).

The temporomandibular joint is the articular surface between the mandible and temporal bone of the skull. It is a combined hinge and gliding joint. Normally, the mandible moves smoothly, appears symmetrical, and is without deformity. Causes for TMD include trauma, stress, teeth clenching, or grinding (**bruxism**), and joint diseases such as rheumatoid arthritis or osteoarthritis. Common symptoms of TMD include limited jaw movement, clicking or crepitus when the jaw moves, popping when chewing or talking, and radiating pain in the face, neck, or shoulders. The clicking is caused by displaced cartilage. The jaw may lock as a result of muscle spasms.

Diagnosis of TMD may include an x-ray to evaluate the bony structure, a CT scan to evaluate any degenerative changes, an MRI or arthrography, and an evaluation of the teeth and jaw in a bite position. Nursing assessment of the joint includes movement and appearance. If the mandible protrudes, it may indicate a mandibular dislocation.

Medical–Surgical Management

Medical

Medical management consists of moist heat to promote muscle relaxation, cold therapy to reduce muscle spasms, and analgesics or nonsteroidal anti-inflammatory drugs. Clients may be fitted with a dental retainer or bite plate to prevent teeth clenching or grinding, or splints to help realign malocclusions.

Surgical

Procedures such as arthroscopy or surgery to reshape the joint may be done in some cases that do not respond to medical treatment.

Diet

A soft diet allows the jaw and muscles to relax. Clients are advised against chewing gum.

Nursing Management

Encourage clients to practice relaxation techniques. Advise client to see a dentist for an evaluation of the teeth and jaw and to use the dental retainer or bite plate if given one.

CARPAL TUNNEL SYNDROME

Carpal tunnel syndrome occurs when the median nerve in the wrist is compressed by inflamed, edematous flexor tendons and tenosynovium (Figure 40-16). Symptoms include pain, paresthesia, and weakness of the thumb, index, middle and part of ring fingers, but never the little finger. Persons performing assembly line work or extensive keyboarding are especially at risk. Assemblers are three times more likely to have carpal tunnel than data-entry personnel (NINDS, 2002). Arthritis or fractures may also be a cause. Diagnosis is based on a physical examination and the subjective symptoms of the client and may be confirmed by motor nerve velocity studies.

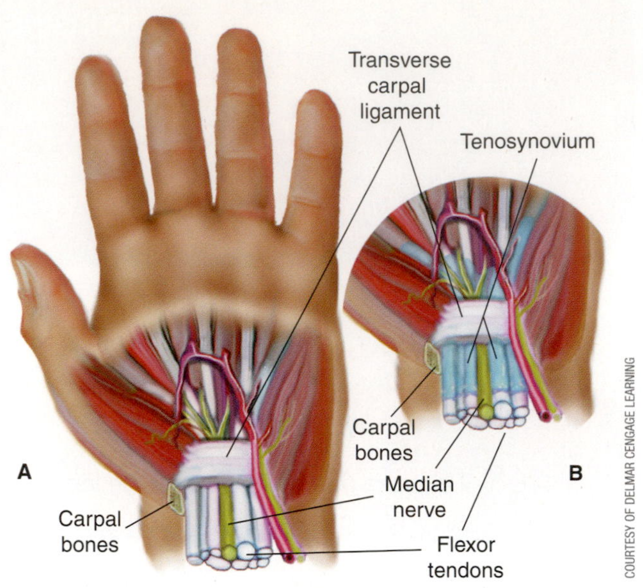

Figure 40-16 Carpal Tunnel Syndrome; *A*, Cross-section of carpal tunnel shows nerves and tendons; *B*, Inflamed flexor tendons and tenosynovium put pressure on the median nerve.

Medical–Surgical Management

Medical

Treatment consists of rest for the hands. Splints to immobilize the hand and wrist also are used to help relieve some of the discomfort.

Surgical

If conservative treatment does not control the symptoms, surgery is necessary to relieve the pressure on the median nerve. After surgery, the hand is elevated and may be in a splint for up to 2 weeks. Lifting is restricted for several weeks.

Pharmacological

Anti-inflammatory drugs may decrease inflammation and edema and reduce symptoms. NSAIDs may provide pain relief. If symptoms are not controlled with these measures, cortisone is injected into the carpal tunnel.

Nursing Management

Encourage clients performing repetitive hand movements to take rest periods from the task.

NURSING PROCESS

Assessment

Subjective Data

Subjective assessment data consist of the client's description of tingling in the hands and numbness in the thumb, index, middle and part of the ring fingers. The client may also state that there is a feeling of "puffiness" in the affected hand and that the client is unable to grasp or hold small objects. Waking in the middle of the night with pain and a feeling that the entire hand is asleep is very common.

Objective Data

Objective assessment data include atrophy of the padded area at the base of the thumb.

Nursing diagnoses for a client with carpal tunnel syndrome include the following:

NURSING DIAGNOSES	PLANNING/OUTCOMES	NURSING INTERVENTIONS
*Acute **P**ain* related to inflammation and swelling causing pressure on the median nerve	The client will have less discomfort.	Administer analgesics as ordered and teach client about use, side effects, and dosage. Encourage client to wear wrist brace. Encourage client to refrain from repetitive hand movements.
*Risk for **D**isuse Syndrome* related to tingling and numbness of hand and wrist	The client will use fingers and hand.	Teach client to do ROM exercises, and to prevent twisting and turning of wrist.

Evaluation: Evaluate each outcome to determine how it has been met by the client.

SYSTEMIC DISORDERS WITH MUSCULOSKELETAL MANIFESTATIONS

Systemic disorders that result in musculoskeletal symptoms include gout and Lyme disease.

GOUT

Gout is a metabolic disease of ineffective purine metabolism resulting in deposits of needlelike crystals of uric acid in connective tissue, joint spaces, or both. Middle-aged men are most commonly affected, but it may occur in women after menopause. Gout may be primary (an inherited problem with purine metabolism), secondary (complication from another disease or from use of certain drugs), or idiopathic (unknown cause). Up to 18% of clients with gout have a family history of the disease (NIAMS, 2002b). The excessive use of alcohol interferes with uric acid removal from the body and may contribute to or exacerbate symptoms.

The acute gout attack begins abruptly with severe constant pain. The joint becomes swollen, red, and tender. The great toe is the joint most frequently involved; however, any joint may be affected. The course of gout is variable, with one to two attacks being severe. If the disease is untreated, the attacks may occur with increasing frequency. Clients with symptoms of gout develop **tophi**, which are subcutaneous nodular deposits of sodium urate crystals appearing in various parts of the body, including the rim of the ears, the knuckles, and great toe. Diagnosis is made from the client's health history and an examination of the affected joint. Aspiration of the joint synovial fluid may show urate crystals. The client should be instructed to avoid foods high in purine, such as liver, sardines, sweetbreads, anchovies, gravies, and asparagus. Avoid excessive use of alcohol. Oral fluid intake is increased to 3,000 mL per day to reduce the possibility of urate stone formation in the kidneys.

To reduce inflammation, NSAIDs are given, especially indomethacin (Indocin) and ibuprofen (Motrin). Colchicine (Colsalide) is added in acute cases. When tophi develop, medicine to reduce hyperuricemia is used, such as allopurinol (Zyloprim) and probenecid (Benemid).

LYME DISEASE

Lyme disease is caused by a spirochete, *Borrelia burgdorferi*, carried by deer ticks. In the United States, it has been reported in nearly all states, but Lyme disease is endemic in Connecticut, Delaware, Maryland, Massachusetts, Minnesota, New Jersey, New York, Pennsylvania, Rhode Island, and Wisconsin. The onset of the disease is most prevalent in May (7%), June (25%), July (29%), and August (13%) (MMWR, 2005).

These ticks should be removed by using a tweezers. Early manifestations occur from spring through late fall. People living in states with a high incidence of Lyme disease should wear protective clothing and check for ticks frequently. Insect repellent containing 20% to 30% DEET is applied to exposed parts of the body and to clothing (CDC, 2008). For preventive protection, household pets wear a flea and tick collar, are given monthly preventive medication, and also are checked frequently for ticks.

For most individuals, the first symptom is a red rash called erythema migrans. It starts as a red spot at the site of the tick bite and expands, resembling a bull's eye. Other symptoms are headache, neck stiffness, fever, swelling in the knees and other large joints, and muscle pain. For those individuals untreated with antibiotics, arthritis (joint swelling and pain), fatigue, and neurological abnormalities such as facial palsy, meningitis, and encephalitis become evident. The antibody test ELISA is used to identify antibodies to *B. burgdorferi* in blood or spinal fluid specimens. Antibiotics such as doxycycline (Vibramycin), cefuroxime exetil (Ceftin), or amoxicillin (Amoxil) speed healing of the rash and may prevent arthritis and neurologic symptoms.

CASE STUDY

G.E., a 40-year-old truck driver, was getting ready to help unload his cargo. He was climbing into the truck when he lost his balance and fell to the ground, twisting his left leg. He stated he was in severe pain and was unable to stand. His coworkers called the emergency ambulance service to transport him to the hospital. Upon arrival in the emergency department, the nurse immediately took G.E.'s vital signs, which were temperature 98.6°F, pulse 92 beats/minute, respirations 24 breaths/minute, and blood pressure 158/90 mm Hg. The nurse also noted that G.E.'s face was flushed and his left leg was shorter than his right.

The following questions will guide your development of a nursing care plan for the case study.

1. List five types of fractures.
2. Based on the action of the fall, what type of fracture do you think G.E. sustained?
3. What diagnostic measures will determine whether or not G.E. has a fracture of his left leg?
4. What would be the best immediate care for G.E.?
5. List four nursing interventions for clients in traction.
6. What possible treatment options are best for G.E.'s injury?
7. What objective and subjective data are important for the nurse to obtain regarding G.E.'s injury?

SUMMARY

- When assessing the client with a musculoskeletal disorder, the nurse evaluates any changes in appearance, including alignment, loss of motion, and any signs of circulatory impairment.
- Treatment of a fracture includes any one or more of the following methods: closed reduction, open reduction that may include internal fixation, casts, and traction.
- Compartment syndrome is a serious form of neurovascular impairment. Symptoms include severe pain that is not relieved with narcotic analgesics, sluggish capillary refill, weak pulses, numbness, and paralysis.
- When a client is in traction, it is important to remember to preserve body alignment, maintain continuous pull and countertraction, keep the ropes moving freely through the pulleys, use the prescribed amount of weights, and keep the weights hanging freely.
- Osteoarthritis is characterized by slow progressive degeneration of joint articular cartilage.
- Hips, knees, and fingers are the joints most frequently considered for replacement.
- After total hip replacement, the hip is kept in a position of abduction and extension.
- After total knee replacement surgery, some clients use a CPM machine that promotes knee joint flexibility and increased circulation to the operative area.
- Individuals at greatest risk for developing osteoporosis are postmenopausal women and older adults who are generally inactive.

REVIEW QUESTIONS

1. A client is admitted to the hospital and expresses concerns for his job. This information will become what part of his nursing care plan?
   1. Nursing diagnosis.
   2. Goal.
   3. Validating data.
   4. Evaluation.

2. A client returned from surgery with an internal fixation of the right femur. The nursing primary treatment goal of the repaired fracture is:
   1. aid in the formation of osteoclasts.
   2. establish a callus between the broken ends of bone.
   3. aid in the formation of granulation tissue.
   4. prevent further injury to the fractured limb.

3. A nurse enters the room and notices a client in skeletal traction is lying with poor positioning and alignment. The nurse repositions the client in good alignment to prevent the possible deformity of:
   1. scoliosis.
   2. lordosis.
   3. contracture.
   4. muscle atony.

4. A client is admitted to the hospital with osteoarthritis (degenerative joint disease). Upon assessing the client, the nurse expects to find: (Select all that apply.)
   1. nausea after each meal.
   2. joint stiffness especially on arising.
   3. an increased appetite.
   4. muscle spasms after exercising.
   5. Heberden's nodes.
   6. pain after physical exercise.

5. A 48-year-old man has suffered low-back pain and sciatica for over 2 years. He is admitted to the hospital for evaluation and treatment of this problem. A thorough assessment of his level of discomfort from low-back pain is important primarily because:

1. this will provide a baseline for later comparison.
2. this is a method for identifying clients with "low back neurosis."
3. clients who have pain localized to the back and radiating to one extremity are probably not candidates for surgery.
4. surgery is contraindicated for clients who have had pain for less than 2 years.

6. In preparing a teaching plan for an adult who has had an arthroscopy, what following information will the nurse include?
1. Client should check extremity for color, mobility, and sensation at least every 2 hours after the procedure.
2. Client may return to regular activities immediately after procedure.
3. Remove compression dressing 6 to 8 hours after procedure.
4. Keep extremity in flexion for 24 hours after procedure.

7. A client just returned from surgery for the repair of a right fractured tibia and fibula and has a cast applied to the extremity. The nurse first:
1. listens to the breath sounds for respiratory complications.
2. listens to the abdomen for bowel sounds.
3. covers the client with a warm blanket.
4. checks the right toes for circulation, sensation, and movement.

8. A client was admitted to the hospital following a motorcycle accident with multiple fractures to the left leg. A long leg cast was applied and 6 hours after surgery the client is expressing extreme pain in his left leg after receiving medication by a PCA. The nurse suspects compartment syndrome. If the nurse is correct, what other symptoms would the client have? (Select all that apply.)
1. Sluggish capillary refill.
2. Pain from the lower spine down the back of the leg.
3. Numbness or tingling in the leg.
4. Weak pulse in the left toes and strong pulse in the right toes.
5. Increased length of the right leg.
6. Foul odor from the cast.

9. An appropriate nursing diagnosis for a client with a recent amputation is:
1. *Ineffective Peripheral **T**issue Perfusion.*
2. *Risk for **I**njury.*
3. ***N**ausea.*
4. *Disturbed **B**ody Image.*

10. A client was admitted to the hospital with a fracture after a skiing accident. One of the most common fractures from this type of accident is:
1. comminuted.
2. greenstick.
3. spiral.
4. impacted.

REFERENCES/SUGGESTED READINGS

American Academy of Orthopaedic Surgeons (AAOS). (2007a). Care of casts and splints. Retrieved April 8, 2009, from http://orthoinfo.aaos.org/topic.cfm?topic=a00204

American Academy of Orthopaedic Surgeons (AAOS). (2007b). Compartment syndrome. Retrieved April 8, 2009, from http://orthoinfo.aaos.org/topic.cfm?topic=a00204

American Academy of Orthopaedic Surgeons (AAOS). (2007c). Minimally invasive total hip replacement. Retrieved April 8, 2009, from http://orthoinfo.aaos.org/topic.cfm?topic=A00404

American Academy of Orthopaedic Surgeons (AAOS). (2007d). Total hip replacement. Retrieved April 8, 2009, from http://orthoinfo.aaos.org/topic.cfm?topic=A00377

American Academy of Orthopaedic Surgeons (AAOS). (2007e). Total knee replacement. Retrieved April 8, 2009, from http://orthoinfo.aaos.org/topic.cfm?topic=A00389

Arthritis Foundation. (2002a). Gout. Retrieved April 9, 2009, from http://ww2.arthritis.org/conditions/diseaseCenter/gout.asp

Arthritis Foundation. (2002b). Osteoarthritis. Retrieved April 9, 2009, from http://ww2.arthritis.org/conditions/DiseaseCenter/oa.asp

Bailey J. (2003). Getting a fix on orthopedic care. *Nursing2003, 33*(6), 58–63.

Bryant, G. (2001). Stump care. *AJN, 101*(2), 67–71.

Bulechek, G., Butcher, H., McCloskey, J., & Dochterman, J., eds. (2008). *Nursing Interventions Classification (NIC)* (5th ed.). St. Louis, MO: Mosby/Elsevier.

Burke, S. (2001). Boning up on osteoporosis. *Nursing2001, 31*(10), 36–42.

Centers for Disease Control (CDC). (2008). Lyme disease. Retrieved April 9, 2009, from http://www.cdc.gov/ncidid.dvbid/lyme?prevention/ld_Prevention_Avoid.htm

Curry, L., & Hogstel, M. (2002). Osteoporosis. *AJN, 102*(1), 26–32.

D'Arcy, Y. (2002). How to treat arthritis pain. *Nursing2002, 32*(7), 30–31.

Daniels, R. (2009). *Delmar's guide to laboratory and diagnostic tests.* Clifton Park, NY: Delmar Cengage Learning.

Daniels, R., Grendell, R., & Wilkins, F. (2010). *Nursing fundamentals: Caring & clinical decision making* (2nd ed.). Clifton Park, NY: Delmar Cengage Learning.

Estes, M. (2010). *Health assessment & physical examination* (4th ed.). Clifton Park, NY: Delmar Cengage Learning.

Fort, C. (2002). Getting a fix on long-bone fracture. *Nursing2002, 32*(6), 32hn1–32hn6.

Fort, C. (2003). How to combat 3 deadly trauma complications. *Nursing2003, 33*(5), 58–63.

Hayes, D. (2003a). How to wrap an above-the-knee amputation stump. *Nursing2003, 33*(1), 70.

Hayes, D. (2003b). How to wrap a below-the-knee amputation stump. *Nursing2003, 33*(2), 28.

Ignatavicius, D. (2002). Catching compartment syndrome early. *Nursing2002, 32*(11), 10.

Infectious Disease Society of America (IDSA). (2007). Updated guidelines on diagnosis, treatment of Lyme disease. Retrieved April 9, 2009, from http://www.idsociety.org/Content.aspx?id=3744

Ingham Regional Orthopedic Hospital, A McLaren Health Service. (2004). Regaining an active lifestyle: A helpful guide for patient undergoing knee replacement surgery. Retrieved April 10, 2009, from http://www.irmc.org/documents/Health%20Articles/KNEE%20REPLACEMENT%20BROCHURE.pdf

Lawrence, B., & Tasota, F. (2003). Detecting neuromuscular problems with electromyography. *Nursing2003, 33*(4), 82.

Leslie, M. (2000). When the ache is not arthritis. *RN, 63*(3), 38–40.

Lewis, A. (1999). Orthopedic and vascular emergencies. *Nursing99, 29*(12), 54–56.

Lindgren, V. (2003). When to suspect this bone disorder. *RN, 66*(6), 32–36.

Maher, A. (2002). Assessment of the musculoskeletal system. In A. B. Maher, S. W. Salmond, & T. A. Pellino (eds.), Orthopaedic nursing (3rd ed., pp. 189–210). Philadelphia: W. B. Saunders Company.

McClung, B. (2001). Reducing your risk of osteoporosis. A Guide to Women's Health (supplement to *Nursing2001)*, April, 4–8.

McConnell, E. (2001). Myth & facts . . . about gout. *Nursing2001, 31*(5), 73.

McConnell, E. (2002a). Assessing neurovascular status in a casted limb. *Nursing2002, 32*(9), 20.

McConnell, E. (2002b). Myths & facts . . . about compartment syndrome. *Nursing2002, 32*(2), 92.

MedlinePlus®. (2007). Rhabdomyolysis. Retrieved April 7, 2009, from http://www.nlm.nih.gov/medlineplus/ency/article/000473.htm

MedlinePlus®. (2009). Lyme disease. Retrieved April 7, 2009, from http://www.nlm.nih.gov/medlineplus/print/lymedisease.html

MMWR Weekly. (June 15, 2005). Lyme disease—United States, 2003–2005. Retrieved April 7, 2009, from http://www.cd.gov/mmwr/preview/mmwrhtml/mm5623al.htm

Moorhead, S., Johnson, M., Maas, M., & Swanson, E. (2007). *Nursing Outcomes Classification (NOC)* (4th ed). St. Louis, MO: Elsevier–Health Sciences Division.

National Institute of Allergies and Infectious Diseases (NIAID). (2008). Lyme disease. Retrieved April 9, 2009, from http://www3.niaid.nih.gov/topics/lymeDisease/

National Institute of Arthritis and Musculoskeletal and Skin Diseases (NIAMS). (2006a). Osteoarthritis. Retrieved April 9, 2009, from http://www.niams.nih.gov/Health_Info/Osteoarthritis/default.asp

National Institute of Arthritis and Musculoskeletal and Skin Diseases (NIAMS). (2006b). Questions and answers about gout. Retrieved April 9, 2009, from http://www.niams.nih.gov/Health_Info/Gout/default.asp

National Institute of Neurological Disorders and Stroke (NINDS). (2008). Carpal tunnel syndrome fact sheet. Retrieved April 9, 2009, from http://www.ninds.nih.gov/disorders/carpal_tunnel/detail_carpal_tunnel.htm

National Osteoporosis Foundation (NOF). (2008a). Osteoporosis bone density. Retrieved April 9, 2009, from http://www.nof.org/osteoporosis/bonemass.htm

National Osteoporosis Foundation (NOF). (2008b). Osteoporosis: men. Retrieved April 9, 2009, from http://www.nof.org/men/index.htm

National Osteoporosis Foundation (NOF). (2008c). Prevention: Five steps to prevention. Retrieved April 9, 2009, from http://www.nof.org/prevention/index.htm

National Osteoporosis Foundation (NOF). (2008d). Fast facts on osteoporosis. Retrieved April 8, 2009, from http://www.nof.org/osteoporosis/diseasefacts.htm

North American Nursing Diagnosis Association International. (2010). *NANDA-I nursing diagnoses: Definitions and classification 2009–2011*. Ames, IA: Wiley-Blackwell.

O'Hanlon-Nichols, T. (1998). Basic assessment series: Musculoskeletal system. *AJN, 98*(6), 48–52.

Overdorf, J., Pachuki-Hyde, L., Kressenick, C., McClung, B., & Lucasey, C. (2001). Osteoporosis: There's so much we can do. *RN, 64*(12), 30–34.

Pauldine, E. (2003). Taking a bite out of Lyme disease. *Nursing2003, 33*(4), 49–52.

Preboth, M. (2001). Lyme disease: New guidelines. *American Family Physician, 63*(10), 2065–2067.

Queensland Government. (2009). Introduction to stump care. Retrieved April 8, 2009, from http://www.health.qld.gov.au/qals/docs/stump_care.pdf

Reeser, J. (2007). Stress fractures. Retrieved April 7, 2009, from http://emedicine.medscape.com/article/309106-overview

Rogers, D. (2003). New meaning for safe sex. *RN, 66*(1), 38–41.

Rupert, S. (2002). Pathogenesis and treatment of rhabdomyolysis. *Journal of the American Academy of Nurse Practitioners, 14*(2), 82.

Sauret, J. M., Marinides, G., & Wang, G. K. (2002). Rhabdomyolysis. *American Family Physician, 65*(1), 907.

Spratto, G., & Woods, A. (2009). *2009 PDR nurse's drug handbook*. Clifton Park, NY: Delmar Cengage Learning.

Sullivan, M., & Sharts-Hopko, N. (2000). Preventing the downward spiral. *AJN, 100*(8), 26–31.

The Ohio State University Medical Center. (2008). External fixator. Retrieved July 27, 2009 from http://medicalcenter.osu.edu/PatientEd/Materials/PDFDocs/surgery/ortho/externalfixation.pdf

The TMJ Association. (2009). Changing the face of TMJ. Retrieved April 9, 2009, from http://www.tmj.org/

University of Iowa Health Care. (2008). Cast care. Retrieved April 8, 2009, from http://www.uihealthcare.com/topics/bonesjointsmuscles/bone3418.html

Wade, C. (2000). Keeping lyme disease at bay. *AJN, 100*(7), 26–31.

Walls, M. (2002). Orthopedic trauma. *RN, 65*(7), 52–56.

Wise, S. (in press). Assessing the musculoskeletal system.

Yarnold, B. (1999). Hip fracture. *AJN, 99*(2), 36–40.

Zdeblick, T. (2009) Compression and wedge fractures. Retrieved April 7, 2009, from http://www.spineuniverse.com/displayarticle.php/article1441.html

RESOURCES

American Occupational Therapy Association, Inc., http://www.aota.org

American Physical Therapy Association, http://www.apta.org

Arthritis Foundation, http://www.arthritis.org

National Amputation Foundation, http://www.nationalamputation.org

National Institute of Arthritis and Musculoskeletal and Skin Diseases (NIAMS), http://www.niams.nih.gov

National Osteoporosis Foundation, http://www.nof.org

OrthoIllustrated Orthopaedic Surgery Patient Education, http://www.orthoillustrated.com

Osteoporosis and Related Bone Diseases, http://www.osteo.org

The TMJ Association, Ltd., http://www.tmj.org

CHAPTER 41
Neurological System

MAKING THE CONNECTION

Refer to the following chapters to increase your understanding of the neurological system:

Basic Nursing
- ***Assessment***
- ***Diagnostic Tests***

Adult Health Nursing
- ***Oncology***
- ***Cardiovascular System***
- ***Musculoskeletal System***
- ***Endocrine System***
- ***The Older Adult***

Basic Procedures
- ***Performing Passive Range-of-Motion (ROM) Exercises***
- ***Ambulation Safety and Assisting from Bed to Walking***
- ***Turning and Positioning a Client***
- ***Transferring from Bed to Wheelchair, Commode, or Chair***

LEARNING OBJECTIVES

Upon completion of this chapter, you should be able to:
- Define key terms.
- Identify basic functional areas of the human neurological system.
- Perform a neurological screening and a basic neurological examination.
- Prepare a client for common neurological diagnostic examinations.
- Derive a Glasgow Coma Scale score for a client.
- Recognize common symptoms of neurological disorders.
- Plan interventions for a client with a neurological disorder.

KEY TERMS

affect
agnosia
anosognosia
aphasia
areflexia
ataxia
aura
automatism
autonomic nervous system (ANS)
awareness
bradykinesia
central nervous system (CNS)
cephalalgia
chorea
coprolalia
decerebration
dysarthria
dysphagia
emotional lability
encephalitis

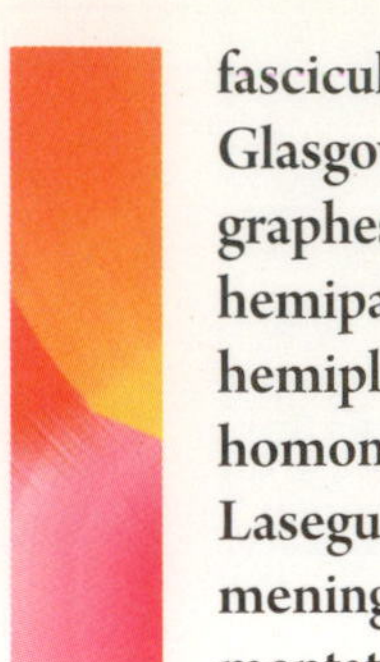

fasciculation
Glasgow Coma Scale
graphesthesia
hemiparesis
hemiplegia
homonymous hemianopia
Lasegue's sign
meningitis
mentation
neuralgia
neurogenic shock
neurotransmitter
nuchal rigidity
nystagmus
orientation
paraplegia
peripheral nervous system (PNS)
postictal
quadriplegia
sclerotic
somatic nervous system (SNS)
spinal shock
status epilepticus
stereognosis
tetraplegia
unilateral neglect
vertigo

INTRODUCTION

The human neurological system (called nervous system) is highly complex, controlling and integrating all other body systems. This system controls motor, sensory, and autonomic functions of the body. This is accomplished by coordination and initiation of cellular activity through the transmission of electrical impulses and various hormones.

ANATOMY AND PHYSIOLOGY REVIEW

The nervous system is divided into the **central nervous system (CNS)**, consisting of the brain and spinal cord; the **peripheral nervous system (PNS)**, which consists of the cranial nerves and spinal nerves; and the **autonomic nervous system (ANS)**, which is part of the peripheral nervous system and consists of the sympathetic and parasympathetic systems.

Central Nervous System

The CNS comprises the brain and the spinal cord (Figure 41-1).

The Brain

The brain, composed of gray matter and white matter, controls, initiates, and integrates body functions through the use of electrical impulses and complex molecules. The gray matter, on the outer part of the brain, contains billions of neurons. Neurons, the basic cells of the nervous system, have three major components: the cell body, the axon, and the dendrites (Figure 41-2). The axon carries impulses away from the cell body, and the dendrites carry impulses toward the cell body. The cell body controls the function of the neuron. Functions include the conduction of impulses and the release of neurotransmitters. **Neurotransmitters** are chemical substances that excite, inhibit, or modify the response of another neuron (Hickey, 2008). Neuroglial cells are in the central and peripheral nervous systems and are not neurons. They protect, support, and nourish the neurons.

The white matter of the inner structures of the brain contains association and projection pathways that transmit nerve impulses to communicate information to the different areas of the brain. These communication pathways are necessary for integration of brain activity (Hickey, 2008).

The brain is contained within the skull, or cranium, which is a bony, rigid box that protects the brain tissue. There are three coverings of the brain, called meninges. They are the *dura mater, arachnoid mater,* and *pia mater* (Figure 41-1A). These coverings provide protection, support, and small amounts of nourishment.

The brain is divided into two hemispheres. The right side of the brain receives information from and controls the left side of the body. The left hemisphere receives information from and controls the right side of the body. Both hemispheres of the brain communicate through nerve fibers in the corpus callosum. A predominate hemisphere exists for special tasks so that confusion does not occur. The right side specializes in the perception of physical environment, art, nonverbal communication, music, and spiritual aspects. The left hemisphere generally specializes in analysis, calculation, problem solving, verbal communication, interpretation, language, reading, and writing.

The Spinal Cord

The spinal cord is a continuation of the brainstem. It exits the skull through the *foramen magnum*, an opening in the base of the skull. The spinal cord is approximately 45 centimeters, or 18 inches, in length and is the thickness of one finger. The cord is divided into right and left halves and has a shallow groove, called the posterior median sulcus, on the dorsal side and a deep groove, called the anterior median fissure, on the ventral side (Figure 41-3A). The cord tapers to a thin tip, called the conus medullaris, at the first lumbar vertebrae, and terminates as a thin cord of connective tissue, called the filum terminale, which continues as far as the second sacral vertebrae (Figure 41-3A and B). The vertebral column provides vertical support for the cord. The meninges cover the spinal cord, providing protection. Reflex activity is initiated within the spinal cord.

There are 31 pairs of spinal nerves originating from the spinal cord. Each pair contains a dorsal, or posterior, nerve root and a ventral, or anterior, nerve root (Figure 41-3C). The dorsal nerve roots carry sensory impulses from the body to the brain; the ventral nerve roots carry motor impulses from the spinal cord to the body. The spinal cord has an H-shaped appearance of gray matter within the white matter (Figure 41-3D). The horns forming the H shape are referred to as the anterior (ventral) horns, the posterior (dorsal) horns, and the lateral horns. These horns contain the cell bodies of neurons that innervate the skeletal muscles.

Cerebrospinal Fluid

Cerebrospinal fluid (CSF) is produced primarily in the choroid plexus. Five hundred milliliters of CSF are produced daily, with excess being reabsorbed by the arachnoid villi in the subarachnoid space. The circulation of CSF is from the lateral ventricles to the third and fourth ventricles. From there, it enters the subarachnoid space to flow around the spinal cord and the brain.

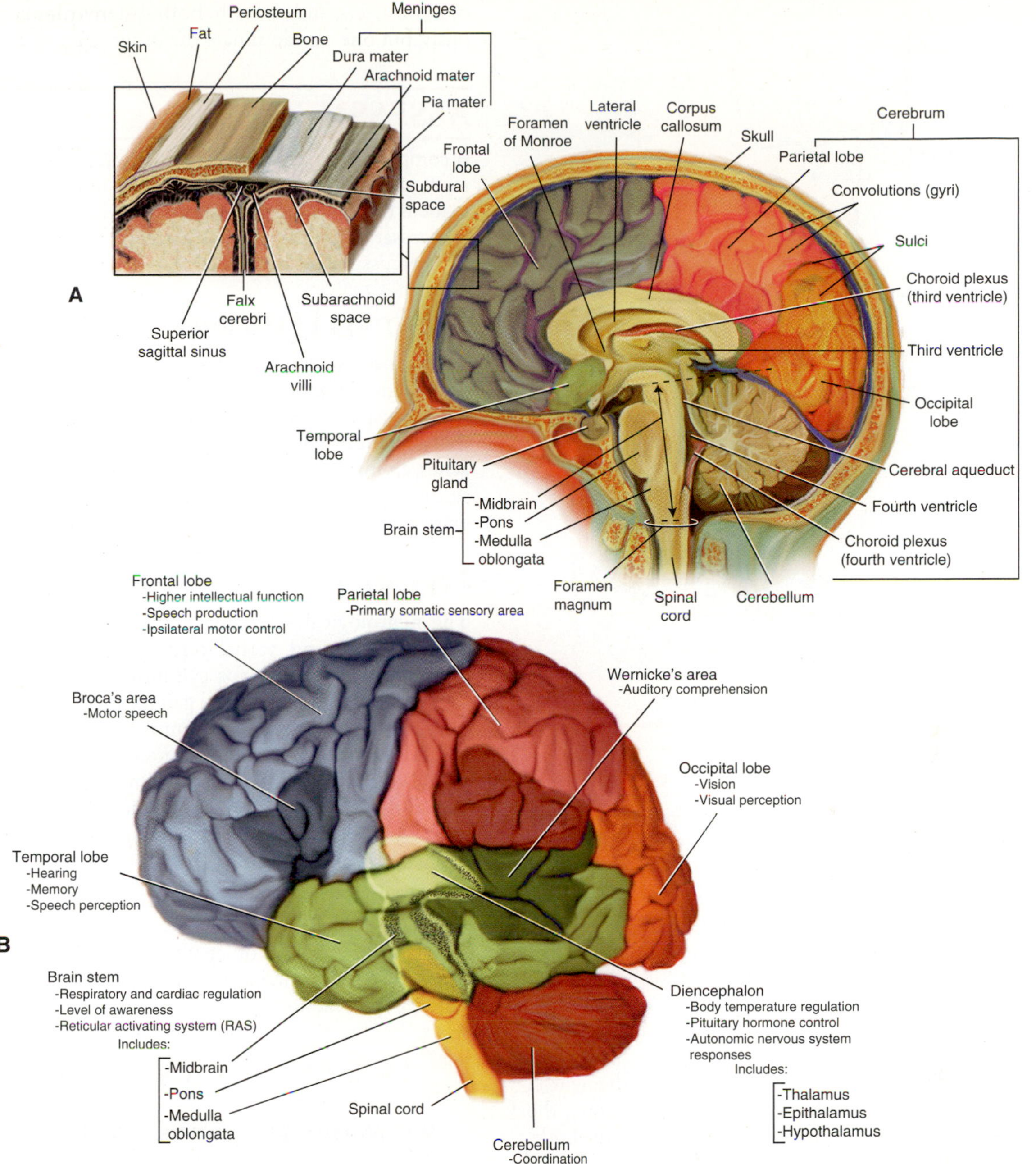

FIGURE 41-1 The central nervous system includes the brain, spinal cord, and meninges. *A*, Structures of the Brain; *B*, Functional Area of the Brain.

Cerebrospinal fluid absorbs shock and bathes the brain and spinal cord. It contains glucose, protein, urea, and salts. These nutritive substances are delivered to the CNS cells, and the waste and toxic substances are removed.

Peripheral Nervous System

All of the nerve tissue outside of the CNS is part of the peripheral nervous system (PNS). The PNS consists of the cranial nerves and the spinal nerves and has both sensory and motor components. The PNS can be divided into the **somatic nervous system** and the ANS. The somatic portion connects the CNS to the skin and skeletal muscles. It is involved in conscious activities, such as walking. The autonomic portion connects the CNS to visceral organs such as the heart, stomach, intestines, and various glands. It is involved in unconscious activities, such as breathing.

Cranial Nerves

The 12 pairs of cranial nerves have sensory, motor, or mixed functions. Table 41-1 lists functions and describes assessment of cranial nerves. The cranial nerves originate from the brain or brainstem, with most originating from the brainstem. Although always identified by Roman numerals, the cranial nerves also have names.

Spinal Nerves

Thirty-one pairs of spinal nerves exit from the spinal cord through the vertebral column: cervical, 8 pairs; thoracic, 12 pairs;

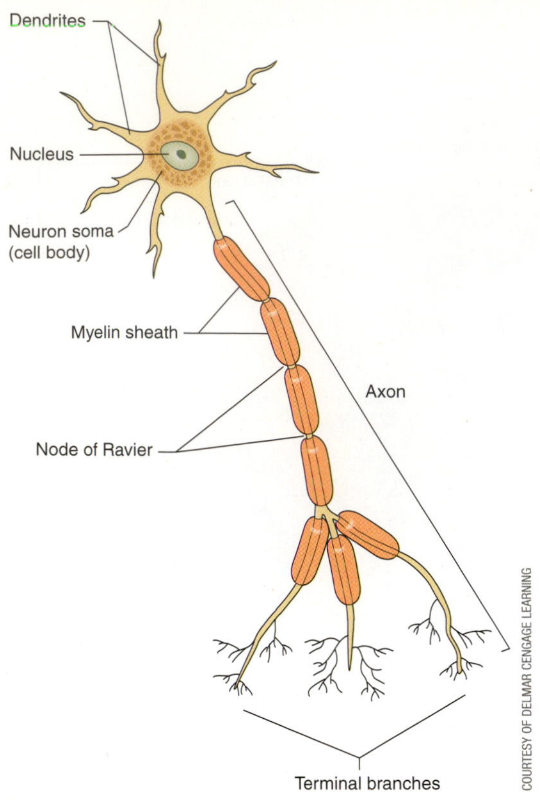

FIGURE 41-2 Neuron (Nerve Cell) Structure

lumbar, 5 pairs; sacral, 5 pairs; and coccyx, 1 pair. The dorsal, or posterior, nerve roots carry sensory impulses to the brain. The ventral, or anterior, nerve roots carry motor impulses from the spinal cord and brain to the muscles. Motor and sensory impulses are transmitted from the body and internal organs.

Reflex activity is a stereotypical response to a stimulus that is initiated by the nervous system (Hickey, 2008). The three classifications of reflexes are muscle stretch, or deep tendon; superficial, or cutaneous; and pathological (see section on assessment of reflexes). Reflex activity requires the function of five areas in the nervous system: the sensory fibers, the neuron relaying the impulse, the association center in the brain, the neuron relaying the motor impulse from the brain to the body, and the specific organ involved. Disease processes at any of these areas can cause an abnormal reflex response.

Autonomic Nervous System

The main function of the ANS is to maintain internal homeostasis. There are two subdivisions of the ANS: the sympathetic system and the parasympathetic system. The sympathetic system, activated by stress, prepares the body for the "fight-or-flight" response. The sympathetic system causes increased heart rate, increased blood pressure, vasoconstriction, decreased peristalsis, dilated pupils, increased secretions of epinephrine and sweat, and decreased secretions of digestive juices and saliva (Table 41-2).

The parasympathetic system conserves, restores, and maintains vital body functions, slowing heart rate, increasing gastrointestinal activity, and activating bowel and bladder evacuation.

The sympathetic and parasympathetic systems work antagonistically to regulate the smooth muscles, the heart, and the glands of the body. When one system increases an action, the other system decreases the action. Thus, when one stimulates, the other inhibits; when one dilates, the other one constricts, and so forth. Both systems function simultaneously, but one can dominate the other as needed.

ASSESSMENT

A complete health history and a neurological screening assessment allow the nurse to identify areas of dysfunction in order to focus the neurological assessment. Observation (inspection) is necessary for most of the assessment; palpation, auscultation, and percussion are also used.

Health History

A baseline assessment is essential to ascertaining changes in neurological functioning. Any change from the baseline assessment must be identified and early intervention initiated. A thorough health history includes asking the client about headaches, clumsiness, loss of or change in function of an extremity, seizure activity, numbness or tingling, change in vision, pain, extreme fatigue, personality changes, and mood swings.

Neurological Assessment

The neurological screening involves assessment of level of consciousness and verbal responses to specific questions; selected cranial nerves for eye movement and visual acuity; muscle strength; movement; gait for motor function; and tactile and pain sensation of extremities for sensory screening.

A complete nursing assessment of neurological function includes assessment of the following areas: cerebral function, cranial nerve function, motor function, sensory function, and reflexes. Neurological nursing assessment is discussed in more detail in the next section.

Cerebral Function

Areas of assessment of cerebral function include level of consciousness, mental status, intellectual function, emotional status, pupil reaction, and communication.

LIFE SPAN CONSIDERATIONS

Neurological Changes with Aging

Remember the following with regard to the elderly client:

- Nerve impulse transmission slows.
- Cardiovascular system changes that lead to a decreased oxygen supply to the brain affect mental acuity, sensory interpretation, and motor ability.
- The amount of neurotransmitters produced diminishes, and the enzyme activity that degrades neurotransmitters increases.
- Changes in neurotransmitters affect sleep, temperature control, and mood.
- The brain tends to atrophy, leaving the cortical bridging veins, which connect the brain to the meninges, vulnerable to trauma and bleeding.

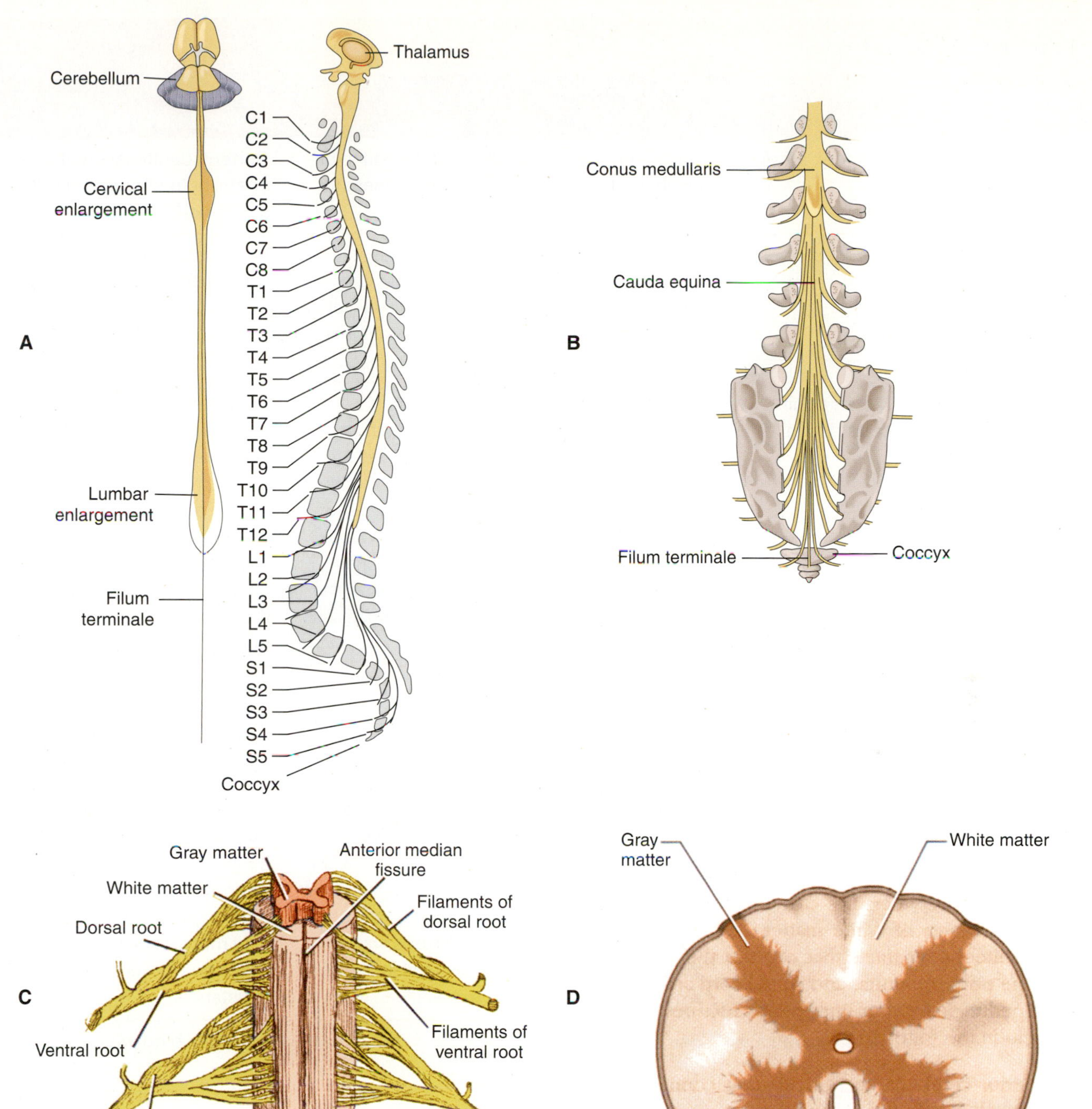

FIGURE 41-3 *A*, **Spinal Cord and Spinal Nerves;** *B*, **Conus Medullaris and Filum Terminale;** *C*, **Anterior View of Spinal Cord;** *D*, **H-Shaped Appearance of Gray Matter and White Matter in the Spinal Cord**

Level of Consciousness Level of consciousness is assessed by determining the client's awareness and orientation and is the most important indicator of change in neurological status. **Awareness** is the person's ability to perceive environmental stimuli and body reactions and then respond with thought and action. The client's awareness is assessed through four components: orientation, memory, calculation, and fund of knowledge (Lower, 2002).

A more objective assessment is made using the **Glasgow Coma Scale**, an objective tool for assessing consciousness in clients, most frequently in clients with head injuries. With the Glasgow Coma Scale, eye opening, verbal response, and motor response are scored using measurable criteria (Table 41-3). The totaled scores indicate coma severity. A score of 15 indicates a fully oriented person. A score of 3 is the lowest possible score, indicating deep coma. A score of 7 or less is considered a state of coma.

Changes in the Glasgow Coma Scale indicate changes in client condition. To prevent further damage to the brain in instances of decreasing scores, the nurse acts quickly. The physician must be notified immediately and measures taken to decrease intracranial pressure (see section on increased intracranial pressure).

TABLE 41-1 Cranial Nerves

CRANIAL NERVE	FUNCTION	ASSESSMENT	EXPECTED FINDINGS
Olfactory (I)	Sensory: smell	Have client identify smells such as coffee or alcohol with one nostril occluded; repeat for opposite nostril.	Correct identification of smell or ability to choose smell from a list of choices.
Optic (II)	Sensory: vision	Ask client to read printed material, identify number of fingers held in front of client, or read from Snellen eye chart. Test visual fields by having client identify when the examiner's finger enters visual field.	Vision intact or correctable with lenses; visual field intact.
Oculomotor (III)	Motor: pupil constriction	Cranial nerves III, IV, and VI are tested together. Inspect for ptosis, or drooping of eyelid. Assess extraocular eye muscles by having client follow the examiner's finger to each quadrant of the visual field. Assess for accommodation by asking the client to look at the examiner's finger held 4 to 6 inches from the client's nose, and then to follow the finger to 18 inches from the client's nose. Ask client about double vision.	Pupils are equal and round and react equally to light. No ptosis or double vision. Eyes move smoothly and consensually inward and downward. As the examiner's finger moves away from the client, the pupil will accommodate by dilating; as the finger moves closer; the pupil will normally constrict.
Trochlear (IV)	Motor: upper eyelid elevation, extraocular eye movement	See oculomotor (III).	Eyes should move smoothly and consensually upward and outward without nystagmus or diplopia.
Trigeminal (V)	Sensory: cornea, nose, and oral mucosa Motor: mastication	Test corneal reflex by lightly touching cornea with a small piece of cotton. Check sensation of face by touching lightly with a cotton ball while the client's eyes are closed and asking the client whether sensation is present. Check motor function by having client clench jaws shut while the examiner palpates the contraction of the temporalis and masseter muscles.	Corneal reflex as evidenced by rapid blinking when cotton swept across cornea. Feeling cotton ball on face indicates that facial sensation is intact. Jaw movement symmetrical and able to overcome resistance.
Abducens (VI)	Motor: extraocular eye movement	See oculomotor (III).	Eyes move outward.
Facial (VII)	Motor: facial muscles; Sensory: taste (anterior two-thirds of tongue)	Ask client to smile, show teeth, wrinkle forehead, or whistle. Have client close eyes lightly and keep them closed against the examiner's trying to open them. Have client identify salt and sugar when dabbed on tongue.	Facial movement symmetrical, sense of taste intact.
Acoustic (VIII)	Sensory: hearing, equilibrium	Assess ability to hear ticking watch or whispered voice. Observe gait for swaying. Perform Romberg test (refer to assessment of motor function).	Sense of hearing intact; no swaying or loss of balance.
Glossopharyngeal (IX)	Sensory: sensation to throat and taste (posterior one-third of tongue) Motor: swallowing	Have client identify taste of salt and sugar on back of tongue. Have client say "ah" and assess for symmetrical position of uvula. Test gag reflex by touching back of pharynx with tongue depressor. Observe swallowing ability and speech patterns.	Taste sensation intact; uvula raises symmetrically; gag reflex intact; swallowing and speech intact.

TABLE 41-1 Cranial Nerves (Continued)

CRANIAL NERVE	FUNCTION	ASSESSMENT	EXPECTED FINDINGS
Vagus (X)	Motor and sensory	Test along with glossopharyngeal nerve.	
Spinal accessory (XI)	Motor: movement of uvula, soft palate, sternocleidomastoid muscle, trapezius muscle	Place examiner's hand on side of client's face and ask client to turn head against resistance; have client shrug shoulders against resistance of the examiner's hand.	Ability to move shoulder and head against resistance.
Hypoglossal (XII)	Motor: tongue movement	Ask client to stick out tongue and observe for symmetry, deviation to side; have client push tongue against tongue depressor and move tongue from side to side.	Tongue should be centrally aligned, able to push against resistance of tongue depressor; no fasciculations (involuntary twitching of muscle fibers) should be present.

COURTESY OF DELMAR CENGAGE LEARNING

TABLE 41-2 Sympathetic and Parasympathetic Responses

SYSTEM	SYMPATHETIC RESPONSE	PARASYMPATHETIC RESPONSE
Neurological	Pupils dilated Heightened awareness	Pupils normal size
Cardiovascular	Increased heart rate Increased myocardial contractility Increased blood pressure	Decreased heart rate Decreased myocardial contractility Vasodilation
Respiratory	Increased respiratory rate Increased respiratory depth Bronchial constriction	Bronchial relaxation
Gastrointestinal	Decreased gastric motility Decreased gastric secretions Increased glycogenolysis Decreased insulin production Sphincter contraction	Increased gastric motility Increased gastric secretions Sphincter dilatation
Genitourinary	Decreased urine output Decreased renal blood flow	Normal urine output

COURTESY OF DELMAR CENGAGE LEARNING

Orientation is the person's awareness of self in relation to person, place, and time. Using open-ended communication techniques, instruct the client to "tell me your first and last name and age," "tell me the month, day, year, and day of the week," "tell me where you are (city, state, hospital)," in order to ascertain the client's level of orientation. The client also is asked to open and close his eyes or open and close his fist.

Mental Status Assessment of mental status requires observation of the client's appearance, behavior, posture, mood, gestures, movements, and facial expressions. The nurse compares these behaviors to expected behaviors based on the client's age, health status, educational level, and social position. Mood is assessed by observation and asking the client about moods and feelings.

Intellectual Function Intellectual function is the ability of the brain to perform thought processes. Ability to concentrate, memory function (both long-term and short-term), recall, calculation activities, and fund of knowledge are all aspects of intellectual function.

Nursing assessment of intellectual function involves asking individuals to perform certain tasks, such as the following:

- Repeating a series of numbers, such as 1, 3, 7, 1
- Telling what the individual ate for breakfast

TABLE 41-3 Glasgow Coma Scale

BEHAVIOR	RESPONSE	SCORE
Eye opening response	Spontaneous	4
	To verbal command	3
	To pain	2
	No response	1
Best verbal response	Oriented, conversing	5
	Disoriented, conversing	4
	Use of inappropriate words	3
	Incomprehensible sounds	2
	No response	1
Best motor response	Obeys verbal commands	6
	Moves to localized pain	5
	Flexion withdrawal to pain	4
	Abnormal posturing—decorticate	3
	Abnormal posturing—decerebrate	2
	No response	1
Total		3 to 15

COURTESY OF DELMAR CENGAGE LEARNING

A

B

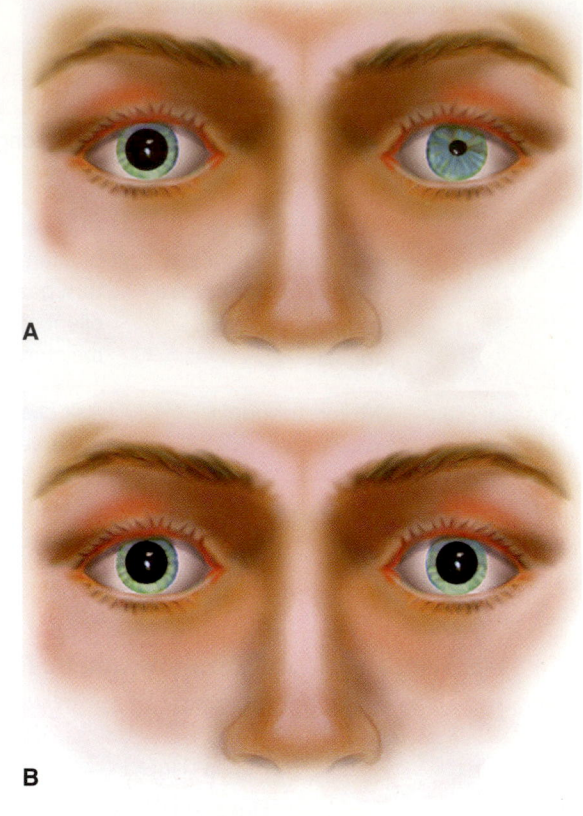

FIGURE 41-4 ***A*, Unequal Pupils; *B*, Dilated, Fixed Pupils** (*Images courtesy of Delmar Cengage Learning.*)

- Adding two numbers, for example, 2 + 6
- Reporting what is on the national news

The nurse determines the client's ability to process thoughts by evaluating the responses to questions such as these. For purposes of comparison, the client's ability to perform these tasks before assessment should be ascertained by asking the family. For example, if the client was math illiterate before the nursing assessment, the client will still not be able to add or subtract.

Emotional Status Emotional status is assessed by observation of the client's **affect** (emotional response or mood). Is affect appropriate for the situation? Is affect labile (prone to rapid change)? Is affect consistent with verbal communication?

Pupil Reaction Size, equality, and roundness of pupils are assessed (Figure 41-4). Size is measured in millimeters. Pupils are evaluated for symmetry of size and for reaction to light. The nurse briefly shines a penlight into the client's eye by passing the light from the outer edge of the eye toward the center of the eye (Figure 41-5). Reaction is assessed as being brisk, sluggish, or nonreactive; consensual reaction (the opposite pupil responding at the same time) is also noted. Accommodation is assessed as described in Table 41-1 under cranial nerve III.

The abbreviation PERRLA is used for documenting pupils that are equal, round, and reactive to light and that demonstrate accommodation. This abbreviation is used only when pupil reaction is normal. If any part of the assessment is abnormal in one or both eyes, the assessment findings are written out for clarity.

CULTURAL CONSIDERATIONS

Neurological Assessment

- Consider language and cultural norms when performing the mental status assessment.
- An interpreter may be required to ensure that the client understands the questions or directions.

Communication Both written and oral communication are assessed. Various specialized areas of the nervous system are involved in communication. The inability to communicate verbally, termed **aphasia**, is caused by the inability to form words or the inability to understand written or spoken words. To assess communication function, various approaches are necessary. Ask the client to follow a simple command such as "Close your eyes." Also use a written card instructing the client to complete a simple task such as "Touch your nose." Note the ability to form words; appropriate use of words; speech patterns, clarity, rate, and flow; and voice modulation. During the health history, ask the client about health care expectations to evaluate the client's ability for verbal expression. Have the client write his name and address on paper to evaluate the ability to write.

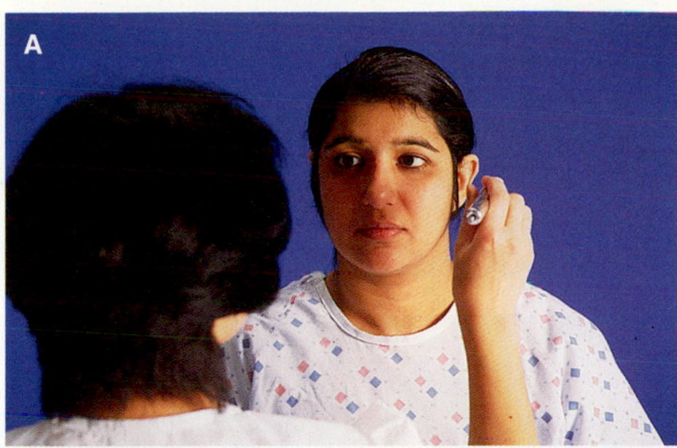

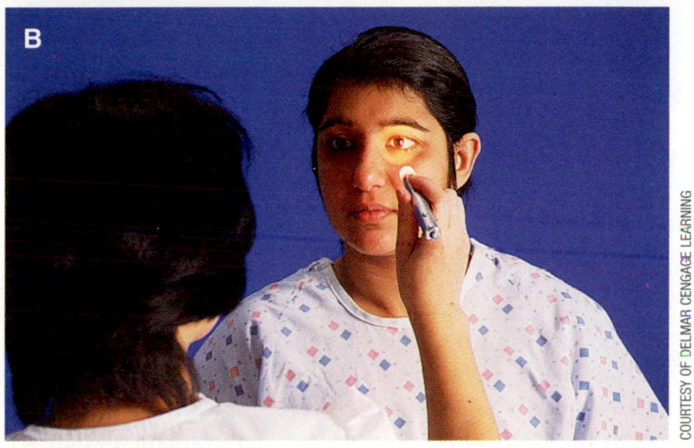

COURTESY OF DELMAR CENGAGE LEARNING

FIGURE 41-5 Pupil Assessment; *A*, Starting Position, with Penlight to Side of Pupil; *B*, Moving Penlight Directly in Front of Pupil

Cranial Nerve Function

Cranial nerve function essentially reflects brainstem activity. A complete cranial nerve examination, if required, is usually performed by the physician or advanced-practice nurse.

Motor Function

The neurological screening includes assessment of muscle strength, arm and leg movement, and gait. A complete motor function assessment is performed if a deficit is identified. A complete motor function assessment includes evaluating muscle size, symmetry, tone, and strength; coordination; balance; and posturing.

Muscle Size and Symmetry Muscle size and symmetry are assessed by palpating major muscle groups of the arms and legs and then comparing them to the muscle groups of the opposite side of the body. Unilateral atrophy indicates a nervous system problem.

PROFESSIONALTIP

Assessment of Pupils

To ensure accuracy in assessing direct light reflex and consensual light reflex, the beginning examiner focuses the beam of light a total of four times, twice in each eye.

Muscle Tone Muscle tone is assessed during palpation of major muscle groups for size and symmetry, while at rest and during passive movement. Muscle tone is described as normal, flaccid, spastic, or rigid. Flaccid muscles are hypotonic, or soft and flabby. Spastic muscles are at first resistant to passive movement, but then release resistance. Rigid muscles may have tremors but are constantly rigid. Rigidity is a more constant state of spasticity, with fewer periods of release of resistance.

Muscle Strength To assess muscle strength, each extremity is placed through passive movement. The client is then asked to move the extremity, first against gravity, by lifting the extremity off the bed, then against resistance, by lifting against slight resistance exerted by the nurse's hand pushing on the extremity. Strength is graded on a scale of 0 to 5 (Table 41-4).

Coordination Coordination, a function of the cerebellum, is assessed by asking the client to perform repetitious movement. The client should close her eyes and repeatedly, rapidly touch her own nose with alternate index fingers (Figure 41-6). Lower extremity coordination is assessed by asking the client to run the heel of one foot down the opposite shin, and then repeat with the other heel (Figure 41-7). Inability to perform these movements is termed **ataxia**, incoordination of voluntary muscle action.

Balance Balance is evaluated by using the Romberg test. The client stands with the feet together, arms extended in front, and eyes closed. Balance is observed; a slight swaying is normal.

Posturing Abnormal posturing occurs with injury to the motor tract. Two types for which to observe are flexion

TABLE 41-4 Muscle Strength

SCORE	DEFINITION
5/5	Full power of contraction
4/5	Fair or moderate power of contraction
3/5	Just able to overcome force of gravity
2/5	Can move, but cannot overcome power of gravity
1/5	Minimal contractile power
0/5	No movement

COURTESY OF DELMAR CENGAGE LEARNING

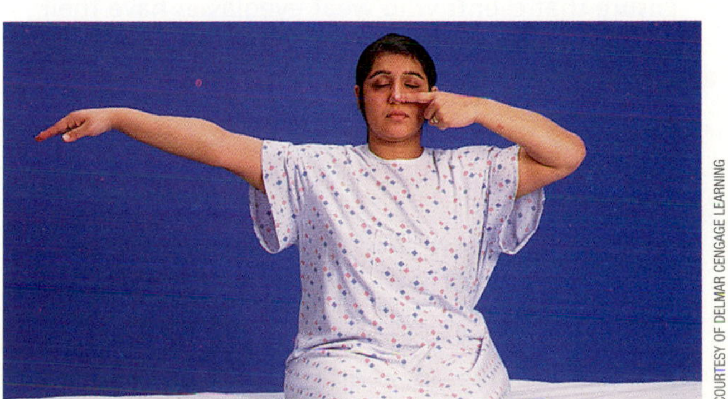

COURTESY OF DELMAR CENGAGE LEARNING

FIGURE 41-6 Assessment of Coordination: Fingertip-to-Nose Touch

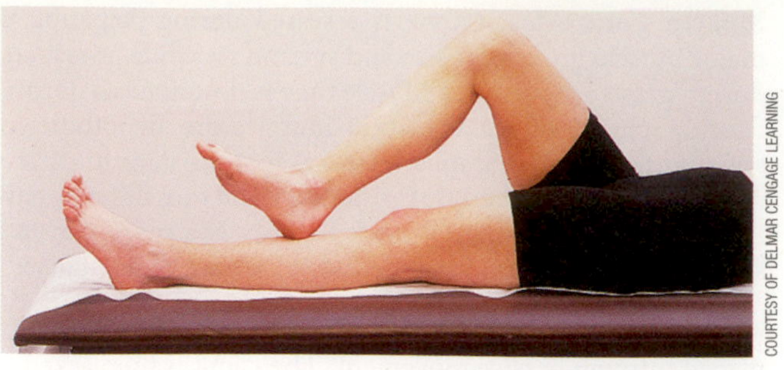

FIGURE 41-7 Assessment of Coordination: Heel Slide

(formerly decorticate) and extension (formerly decerebrate) posturing (Lower, 2002). Flexion posturing is characterized by flexion of the arms, adduction of the upper extremities, and extension of the lower extremities. Lesions of the cerebral hemispheres or internal structures of the brain cause flexion posturing. Extension posturing is caused by brainstem injury and is characterized by an arcing of the back, backward flexion of the head, adduction and hyperpronation of the arms, and extension of the feet (Figure 41-8).

Abnormal posturing may be present either at all times or in response to stimuli such as loud noises, bright lights, or painful stimuli. The nurse notes whether bilateral or unilateral posturing is present, and, if intermittent, the cause of the posturing. The presence of either type of posturing is reported at once, because either represents an ominous sign of cerebral dysfunction. Extension posturing represents greater dysfunction than does flexion posturing, and any change from flexion to extension posturing indicates a worsening of condition.

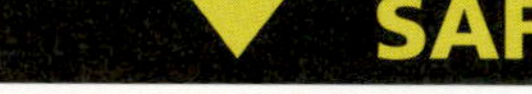

Romberg Test

Always stand in front of the client during the Romberg test, anticipating that the client might fall.

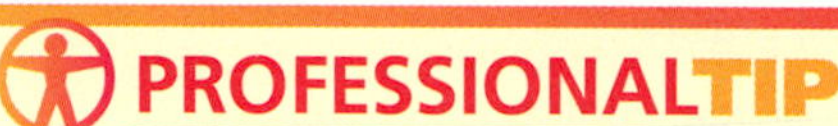

Assessing Coordination

Ensure that clients who wear eyeglasses have their glasses on before the assessment is performed.

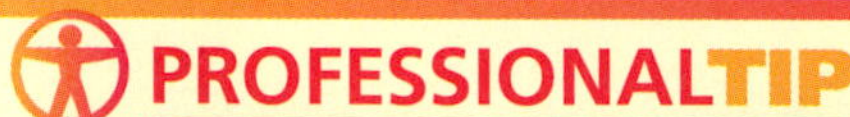

Assessing Pain and Temperature Sensory Function

- Test upper and lower extremities
- Begin with the upper arms, moving down to the hands; then work from thighs to feet (proximodistal)

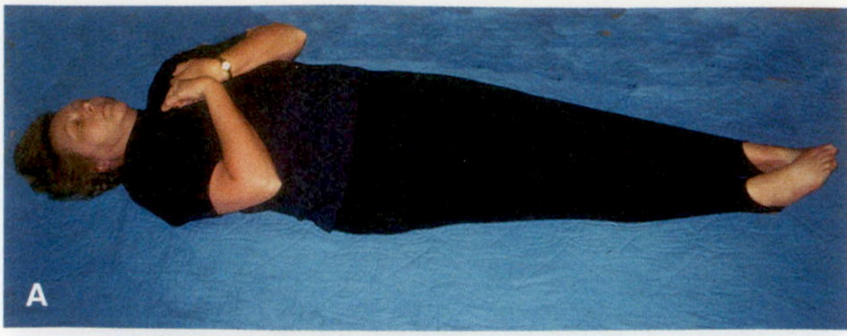

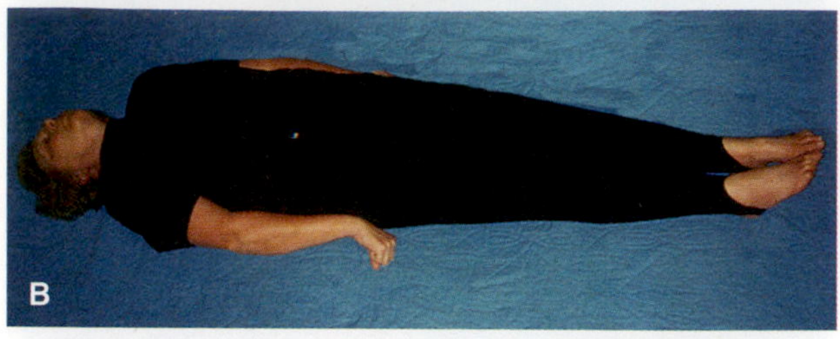

FIGURE 41-8 Abnormal Posturing; *A*, Flexion Posturing; *B*, Extension Posturing (*Photos courtesy of John White, Corpus Christi, TX.*)

Sensory Function

A subjective examination of sensory function, performed with the client's eyes closed, is generally done only when a dysfunction is suspected. Different pathways are used to transmit different sensory impulses. To evaluate all pathways, the examiner must test tactile sensation, pain and temperature, vibration, proprioception, stereognosis, graphesthesia, and integration of sensations.

Tactile Sensation Tactile sensation is tested by using a cotton ball to lightly touch the client's arms, hands, upper legs, and feet. Comparison is done side to side. The client, with eyes closed, indicates whether the cotton ball is felt.

Pain and Temperature Sensations of pain and temperature are transmitted along the same pathways and are evaluated using a sharp and dull touch. A paper clip or cotton-tipped applicator is used.

Touch the client with the rounded end of a paper clip or cotton-tipped applicator to test for dull sensation, and the pointed end of a paper clip or uncovered end of the applicator to test for sharp sensation. The client's ability to distinguish sharp and dull is noted, again comparing both sides of the body.

Vibration Vibration is tested using a tuning fork. Strike the tuning fork on the palm, holding only the handle, then place the end of the handle first on the client's wrists and then on the ankles and ask whether vibrations are felt (Figure 41-9). The client's eyes should be closed during the test.

SAFETY

Sensation

Do not use a safety pin to test pain because skin integrity may be compromised.

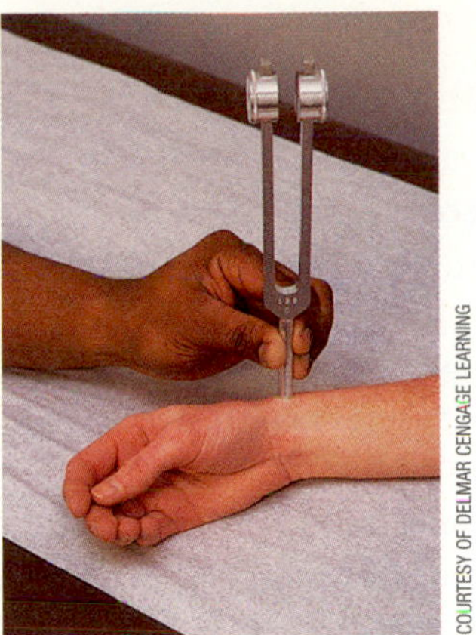

FIGURE 41-9 Assessment of Vibration

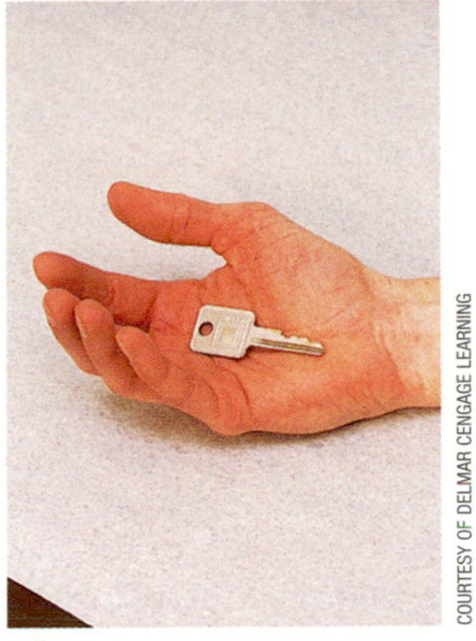

FIGURE 41-10 Assessment of Stereognosis

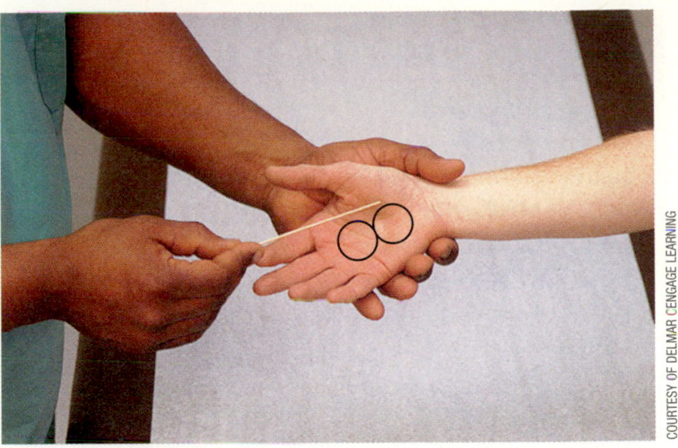

FIGURE 41-11 Assessment of Graphesthesia

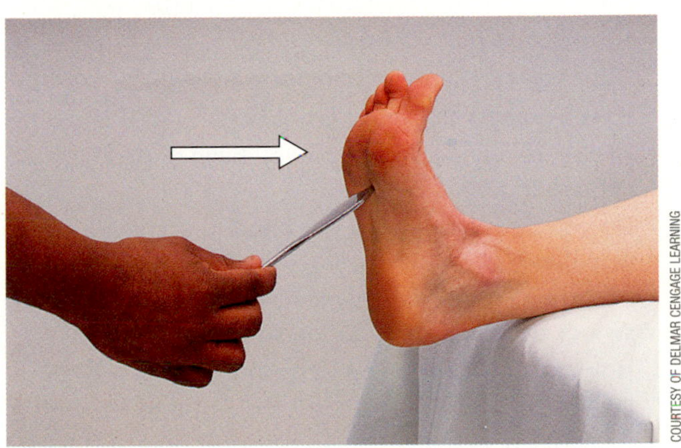

FIGURE 41-12 Pathologic Reflex: Babinski

Proprioception Proprioception is the sense of joint position in space. With the client's eyes remaining closed, move a joint of the client's finger or extremity up or down in space and ask the client to distinguish the direction of movement of the digit or extremity as being either up or down.

Stereognosis **Stereognosis** is the ability to recognize an object by feel. Place a familiar object such as a coin or key in the client's hand and ask what the object is. The sensation is a function of the brain, not of the spinal pathways (Figure 41-10).

Graphesthesia **Graphesthesia** is the ability to identify letters, numbers, or shapes drawn on the skin. Hold the client's hand and, with the stick end of a cotton-tipped applicator or a closed pen, trace an outline on the open palm, ensuring that the letter, number, or shape is right side up for the client (Figure 41-11).

Integration of Sensation Integration of sensation is a higher cortical function. A two-point discrimination test is performed by touching the client simultaneously on opposite sides of the body with a sharp object and asking the client to ascertain the number of objects felt. The normal response is two. If only one is felt, the brain function of integration is abnormal.

Reflexes

Both deep tendon reflexes and superficial reflexes are assessed. Deep tendon reflexes are involuntary contractions of muscles or muscle groups responding to brisk stretching near the insertion site of the muscle (Smeltzer & Bare, 2008). Testing these reflexes is generally the responsibility of the physician or registered nurse, although the LP/VN should be familiar with these assessments, as abnormal reflex responses are an early indicator of motor or sensory dysfunction.

Superficial, or cutaneous, reflexes are elicited by irritating the skin on the area assessed. They are diminished or absent with dysfunction of the reflex arc.

The superficial reflex generally assessed is the plantar. To assess the plantar reflex, the handle of the reflex hammer is used to stroke the outer aspect of the sole of the foot from the heel and across the ball of the foot to just below the big toe. Plantar flexion, or curling under of the toes, should occur.

Abnormal Reflexes The absence of deep tendon reflexes in clients is considered an abnormal finding. A fanning of the toes and dorsiflexion of the big toe in response to the assessment of the plantar reflex is called a positive Babinksi's reflex (Figure 41-12). This abnormal response indicates corticospinal disease and is the most important abnormal superficial reflex.

Refer to Box 41-1, "Questions to Ask and Observations to Make When Collecting Data," for guidance in completing client neurological assessments.

BOX 41-1 QUESTIONS TO ASK AND OBSERVATIONS TO MAKE WHEN COLLECTING DATA

Subjective Data

Do you have headaches? On a scale of 0 to 10, with 0 being no pain and 10 being the most pain you have experienced, rate your headaches. How long have you had these headaches?

Describe the headache to me. What makes the headache feel better? What make the headache feel worse?

Point to the area of your head where you have headaches.

Have you had a seizure?

If you have seizures, do you have an aura?

What precipitates (causes) your seizures?

Have you had any numbness or tingling?

Have you fallen recently?

Describe your sense of balance.

Have you had any vision problems?

Are there any activities that you have difficulty completing?

Do you have the energy you need to accomplish daily activities?

Have you or your family members noticed any mood swings or changes in your personality?

How many hours do you sleep at night?

Do you have back pain? On a scale of 0 to 10, with 0 being no pain and 10 being the most pain you have experienced, rate your back pain. How long have you had the back pain?

Describe the pain to me. What makes the back pain feel better? What make the back pain feel worse?

Have you had any difficulty with any of your extremities? Weakness? Lack of function?

How does the condition affect your life?

Has this condition affected your sexual relationships?

What do you do to cope with your condition?

Does the client answer questions appropriately?

During the subjective data assessment, determine if the client answers questions appropriately.

Objective Data

Assess client's orientation to person, place, and time.

Assess level of consciousness.

Is the client clean and neatly groomed?

Assess client's intellectual function by asking the client to:

Repeat a series of numbers, such as 6, 3, 7, 9.

Tell me what you had for breakfast.

Add 8 + 9.

Tell me a recent news event.

Assess appropriateness of verbal responses to questions.

Does the client have the expected behaviors based on the client's age, health status, educational level, and social position?

Have the client write a complete sentence.

Ask the client to complete a verbal request, such as "Cross your arms."

Check coordination by asking the client to touch his own nose with alternate index fingers.

Ask the client to close his eyes, then place a common object in the client's hand and ask him to identify the object.

Draw a number in the clients palm, and ask him to identify the number.

Asses the client's visual field. As the examiner's finger moves away from the client, does the pupil accommodate by dilating? Constrict as the finger moves closer to the client? Do the eyes move smoothly and consensually upward, downward, inward and outward? As the client's eyes follow your finger as you move it up, down, back, and forth in the path of the client's visual field, does the client see the finger at all times? Check the size, roundness, equality, reaction, and accommodation of the client's pupils.

Assess the client's sense of smell by introducing nonoffensive odors to the client.

Do the client's facial expressions match the conversation?

Check trigeminal nerve by swiping a piece of cotton over the client's check area.

Can the client smile? Frown?

Observe the client's posture. Does the client slump or sit erect?

Note the client's gait and ability to balance. Is the gait symmetrical, and how does the client approach you?

Assess muscle strength in all extremities. Do all extremities have full range of motion?

Assess superficial reflexes.

Does the client have a gag reflex?

Can the client stick out his tongue?

Complete the Glasgow Coma Scale.

COMMON DIAGNOSTIC TESTS

Commonly used diagnostic tests for clients with symptoms of nervous system disorders are listed in Table 41-5.

HEAD INJURY

Head injuries involve trauma to the scalp, skull, or brain.

SCALP

Scalp injuries bleed profusely because of the abundance of blood vessels in the scalp. As with any break in skin integrity, infection is of major concern. The wound is cleansed and irrigated to remove foreign matter before closing the wound with sutures or butterfly dressings.

SKULL

Skull injuries and fractures of the skull may occur with or without brain injury. A fracture is usually caused by extreme force. Skull fractures are considered closed if the dura mater is intact and open if the dura mater is torn. The clinical manifestation of skull fracture is localized pain. If the brain is injured, other symptoms occur.

Types of skull fractures are linear fracture, comminuted fracture, depressed fracture, and basilar fracture. Linear fractures are nondisplaced cracks in the bone. Comminuted fractures occur when the bone is broken into fragments. Depressed fractures have bone fragments pressing into the intracranial cavity. Basilar skull fractures are of the bones in the base of the skull.

Basilar fractures are of particular concern because of the proximity of the fragile sinus bones and the adhesion of the dura mater to this area. The dura mater can easily tear, and CSF can leak from the ears or nose. Two tests determine if the drainage is CSF; a dextrostick dipped in the liquid and the halo test. Because CSF has a high glucose level, a dextrostick is placed in the liquid. If the dextrostick reveals the presence of glucose, the liquid is CSF. The drainage can also be checked, by placing a drop on a white sheet. When the liquid dries, a yellow halo appears around the edges of the pink or bloody drainage if it is CSF (halo test). The internal carotid artery and cranial nerves can also be damaged easily with a basilar skull fracture.

TABLE 41-5 Common Diagnostic Tests for Nervous System Disorders

- Lumbar puncture (LP)
- Electroencephalogram (EEG)
- Electromyogram (EMG)
- Imaging procedures: computerized tomography (CT), positron emission tomography (PET), single-photon emission computed tomography (SPECT), magnetic resonance imaging (MRI)
- Cerebral angiography
- Brain scan
- Myelogram

COURTESY OF DELMAR CENGAGE LEARNING

LIFE SPAN CONSIDERATIONS

Reflexes

The absence of the Achilles reflex in the elderly client is not considered abnormal.

BRAIN

Brain injuries are caused by primary injuries of acceleration–deceleration force, rotational force, or penetrating missile. Acceleration injuries are caused by moving objects striking the head, such as a baseball bat. Deceleration injuries result when the head is moving and strikes a solid object such as a car dashboard. Rotational injuries are hyperextension, hyperflexion, or lateral flexion of the head, which cause twisting of the cerebrum on the brainstem, such as a whiplash injury. Penetrating missile injuries are a direct penetration of an object, such as a bullet, into brain tissue (Urden, Stacy, & Lough, 2009).

OPEN INJURY

Skull fractures and penetrating injuries are referred to as open head injuries. Hemorrhaging from the nose, pharynx, or ears; ecchymosis over the mastoid area (Battle's sign); or blood in the conjunctiva may occur in conjunction with open head injuries. Raccoon eyes (ecchymosis around both eyes) indicates a basilar skull fracture. Cerebrospinal fluid may leak from the ears or nose. A computed tomography (CT) scan or magnetic resonance imaging (MRI) determines the extent of injury. Neurological deficits depend on the extent and area of injury.

CLOSED INJURY

Closed head injuries are caused by blunt force to the head. Coup injuries are caused by the impact of the head against an object. Contrecoup injuries are caused by the impact of the brain against the opposite side of the skull (Figure 41-13).

Types of closed head injuries are concussion, contusion, and laceration. Concussions are transient neurological deficits caused by shaking the brain. Clinical manifestations may include immediate loss of consciousness lasting from minutes to hours, momentary loss of reflexes, respiratory arrest for several seconds, and amnesia for the period immediately before and after the event. Headaches, drowsiness, confusion, dizziness, irritability, visual disturbances, and unsteady gait may also occur (Hickey, 2008).

Post-concussion syndrome may develop after the injury, as manifested by headache and dizziness. Nervousness, irritability, emotional lability, fatigue, insomnia, loss of **mentation** (ability to concentrate, remember, or think abstractly), and sometimes other neurological deficits occur. This syndrome may last from several weeks up to a year (Hickey, 2008).

Contusions are surface bruises of the brain. Symptoms depend on the area of injury. Frequently, the client is unconscious for a longer period than with a concussion. The client becomes conscious only to drift back into unconsciousness. Pulse, blood pressure, and respirations are below normal. Skin is cool and pale. Cerebral edema occurs with widespread injury (see section on cerebral edema).

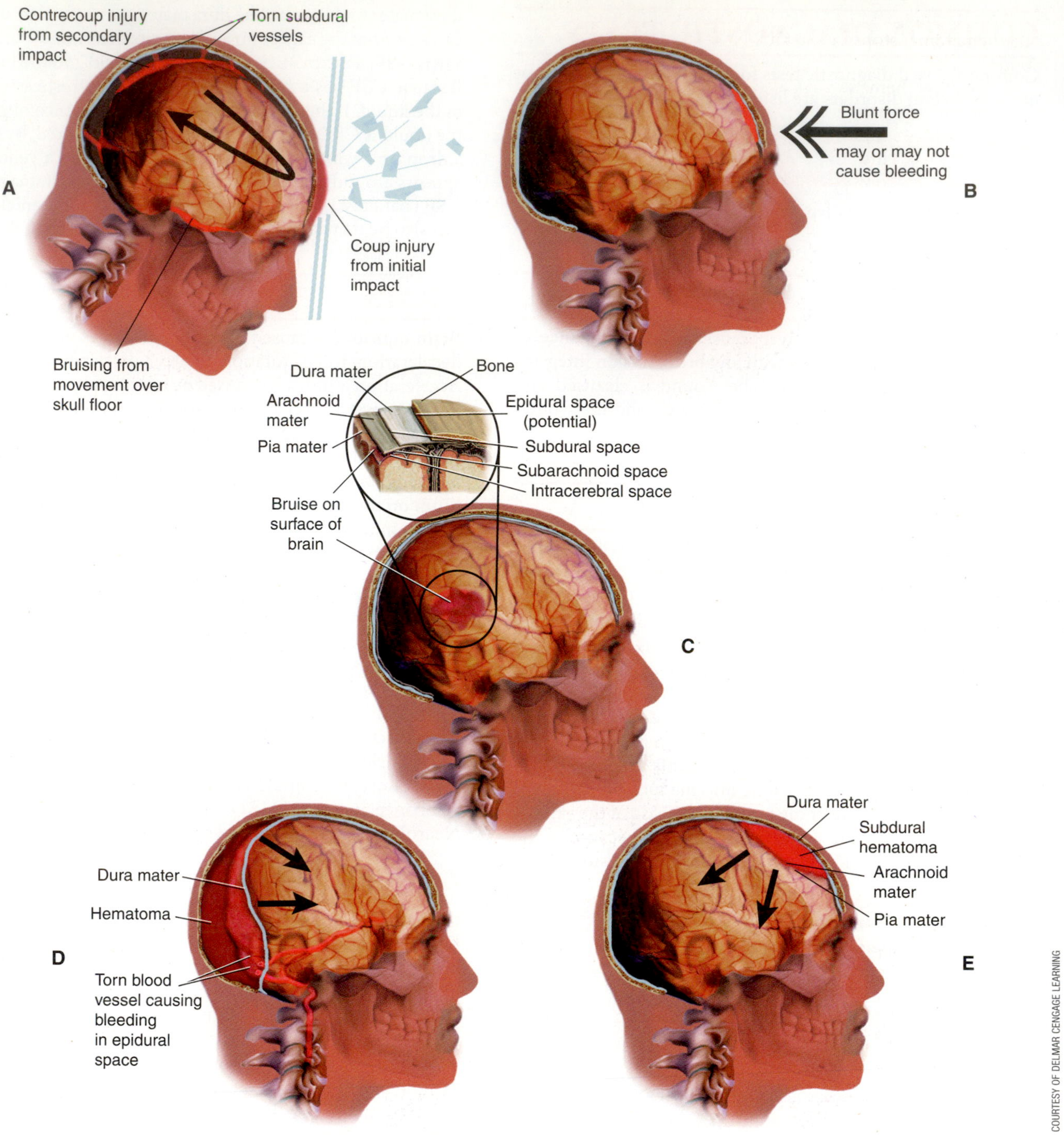

FIGURE 41-13 Brain Injuries; *A*, Coup/Contrecoup; *B*, Concussion; *C*, Contusion; *D*, Epidural Hematoma; *E*, Subdural Hematoma

Return of consciousness may be followed by cerebral irritability to stimuli. Headache and dizziness may be present for an indefinite period. Permanent damage causes either changes in mental function or seizure disorders. Prognosis ranges from full recovery to death.

Cerebral laceration is the tearing of cortical tissue. Symptoms of brainstem injury include deep coma from time of impact, extension posturing, autonomic dysfunction, nonreactive pupils, and respiratory difficulty. The ability to relay nerve impulses from high levels in the brain is lost. Diffuse axonal injury (DAI) usually occurs in conjunction with brainstem injuries. This widespread damage to nerve cells in the white matter of the brain causes immediate coma, extension posturing, and increased intracranial pressure (ICP).

Hemorrhage

Intracranial hemorrhage, usually due to an arterial bleed, is a common complication of any head injury. Bleeding occurs in the epidural space, subdural space, subarachnoid space, ventricles, or intracerebrally. Neurological change is caused by pressure on the brain resulting from the space-occupying hemorrhage. With epidural hematoma (bleeding in the epidural space), momentary unconsciousness is followed by a conscious state of a few hours within that day, depending on the rapidity of the bleeding. As the bleeding continues, neurological status begins to deteriorate, with decreasing level of consciousness; headache; seizures; hemiparesis; **decerebration** (severing spinal cord); and dilated, fixed pupils. This is a medical emergency, and the treatment is surgery to evacuate the hematoma, stop the bleeding, and relieve pressure on the brain.

Subdural hematomas (bleeding in the subdural space) cause immediate pressure on the brain. Subdural hematomas are acute (within 48 hours of injury), subacute (from 2 to 14 days after injury), or chronic (from 2 weeks to months after injury). Common symptoms are headache, drowsiness, slow mentation, and confusion. The symptoms slowly progress as the size of the subdural clot increases, causing increased pressure on the brain. Small hematomas are usually reabsorbed. Large hematomas require surgical removal.

Subarachnoid (below the arachnoid) and intraventricular (within the ventricles of the brain) hemorrhages are common in severe head injury. The symptoms include those listed for hematoma, as well as **nuchal rigidity**, stiffness or inability to bend the neck. Blood in the subarachnoid space interferes with the reabsorption of CSF, further increasing intracranial pressure.

Intracranial hematomas from contusions usually occur in the temporal or frontal lobes; from shearing forces, they usually occur deep in the brain. The hematoma usually expands rapidly. The injury usually causes immediate unconsciousness. Headache, deteriorating level of consciousness, hemiplegia, and dilated pupils are initial signs of an internal hematoma. As intracranial pressure increases, herniation of the brainstem occurs, causing changes in pupils, respirations, and vital signs. Craniotomy along with evacuation and control of bleeding may be performed depending on the condition of the client, extent of cerebral contusion, and accessibility of the bleeding site.

Signs and symptoms of increased intracranial pressure include deterioration in level of consciousness; confusion; difficulty in rousing; and, initially, restlessness. Other signs and symptoms are changes in pupil size or reaction to light. The pupil gradually dilates and becomes less responsive to light. Muscle weakness progressing to **hemiplegia** (paralysis of one side of the body) or **paraplegia** (paralysis of lower extremities), and abnormal posturing occurs. Headache and vomiting are experienced by some clients. Vital sign changes generally do not occur until the increased intracranial pressure has progressed to the point of involving the brainstem. An increase in systolic blood pressure and a widening pulse pressure accompanied by a slowing pulse are the effects of pressure on the brainstem.

Cerebral Edema and Increased Intracranial Pressure

The brain is contained in a rigid container, the skull. The only normal opening to the adult skull is the foramen magnum at the base of the skull. Intracranial pressure is a result of the pressure exerted by the contents of the skull, which are the brain, blood, and CSF.

Regulatory mechanisms maintain intracranial pressure between 0 and 15 mm Hg. The Monroe-Kellie hypothesis states that when one component of the cranial contents increases in volume, the volumes of the other components decrease in order to compensate and maintain intracranial pressure between 0 and 15 mm Hg. As long as this ability to compensate remains effective, no neurological changes occur.

In decompensation, the volume increase is so excessive that intracranial pressure cannot be maintained below 15 mm Hg by decreasing the volume of the remaining components. Neurological changes are exhibited because of cellular hypoxia and displacement of the brain, which compresses neurons, especially in the brainstem. These changes include deteriorating level of consciousness; decreased motor response to commands; fixed, dilated pupils; and vital sign changes known as Cushing's triad or reflex. Cushing's triad refers to bradycardia, widening pulse pressure along with increasing systolic pressure, and respiratory irregularities. Respiratory changes include periods of apnea, decreased respiratory rate and depth, and irregular respirations.

Causes of increased intracranial pressure are increased blood volume resulting from vascular vasodilation; increased volume of brain tissue resulting from edema, infection, tumor, or hemorrhage; or increased volume of CSF resulting from overproduction, decreased reabsorption, or interruption of CSF circulation. If intracranial pressure continues to increase, brain herniation will occur at the tentorial notch or through the foramen magnum, resulting in death.

Medical–Surgical Management

Management of head injury is focused on early recognition and treatment of increasing intracranial pressure and maintenance of normal body functions.

Medical

Intracranial pressure is monitored with an ICP device that has a small tube placed in the ventricles of the brain. CSF is drained through a ventricular drain (ventriculostomy) if the intracranial pressure increases (Daniels, 2007). Suctioning may be necessary but is *never* done through the nose on a head injury client because of the possibility of CSF leakage. Oxygen is given to maintain cerebral perfusion. Pulse oximetry and arterial blood gases (ABGs) are checked.

If the client has an endotracheal tube in place, the $PaCO_2$ level can drop below normal. This decrease causes a slightly alkaline pH, which decreases vasodilation and, thus, intracranial pressure.

Surgical

Decompression is performed surgically by placing burr holes in the skull to allow room for the expansion of the brain. A space-occupying lesion such as a tumor, hematoma, or abscess is surgically removed. Excess CSF is drained from the ventricles.

Pharmacological

Corticosteroids, such as dexamethasone (Decadron), are given to reduce cerebral edema. Antacids, such as Mylanta or

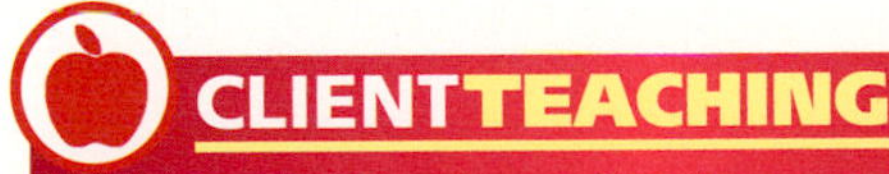

Surgery for Head Injury

Inform the client of the following:

- The head is shaved in the area of the incision.
- Edema of the head and face are present after surgery but will gradually disappear.
- A mechanical ventilator is used for a day or two after surgery.

Maalox, or histamine receptor antagonists, such as ranitidine (Zantac), are given to decrease both the side effects of corticosteroids and stress-induced gastric acidity. Osmotic diuretics, such as mannitol (Osmitrol), are administered to rapidly reduce fluid in the brain tissue; muscle relaxants, sedatives, barbiturates, or muscle-paralyzing agents are administered to decrease activity and reduce the oxygen need of the brain.

Antipyretic drugs are used to decrease body temperature and the metabolic needs of the brain, thereby reducing the volume of blood sent to the brain to supply oxygen and glucose. Anticonvulsants are given to prevent or treat seizure activity.

Activity

Activity is limited to keep the metabolic needs of the brain to a minimum. Increased metabolic needs require more oxygen and glucose supplied by increases in blood volume in the cranium, which further increases intracranial pressure.

Nursing Management

Frequently monitor level of consciousness, eye movements, pupil changes, vital signs, I&O, pulse oximetry and Glasgow Coma Scale score. Monitor the ICP if a device is in place. Maintain airway patency and administer oxygen as ordered. Keep head of bed at 30 to 40 degrees and client's head positioned at midline. Watch for signs of arm/leg muscle weakness, muscle twitching, nausea or vomiting, and visual or hearing disturbance. Fluids often are restricted.

NURSING PROCESS

Assessment

Nursing assessment for any head injury is focused on neurological status. At the nursing shift change, nurses may complete a neurologic assessment together for consistency in assessing the neuropathy.

Subjective Data

Subjective data includes a history of what happened, including type of trauma (acceleration, deceleration, or missile), site of blow, and any loss of consciousness, including timing, length, and ability to be roused.

Objective Data

A neurological screening is done to obtain a baseline neurological status; then, a more in-depth neurological exam is performed to identify any early signs of increasing intracranial pressure.

Frequent assessment of neurological status, including level of consciousness, motor function, eye movement, pupil size and reaction, protective reflexes, and vital signs, allows for early recognition of and intervention for increasing intracranial pressure. Nursing observation also includes assessing for double vision, headache, nausea, and bleeding from any orifice. Ipsilateral pupil reaction (reaction of the pupil on the same side as the injury or lesion) occurs as a result of pressure on the oculomotor nerve caused by increased intracranial pressure or cerebral edema. Assess for factors that cause increased intracranial pressure.

If a client is undergoing intracranial surgery, assess the teaching needs of the client and family. Also assess the emotional and psychosocial needs and support systems.

Longer-term care involves assessment of bowel elimination status to prevent the need for straining, skin assessment to prevent skin breakdown, and assessment for complications of immobility.

Nursing diagnoses for a client with a head injury include the following:

NURSING DIAGNOSES	PLANNING/OUTCOMES	NURSING INTERVENTIONS
*Ineffective **T**issue/ Perfusion (Cerebral)* related to disruption in cerebral blood flow	The client will demonstrate improvement or maintenance on Glasgow Coma Scale.	Assess neurological status of client every 15 to 60 minutes. Note findings on Glasgow Coma Scale. Compare findings to previous assessments to uncover changes in condition. Administer oxygen as ordered to supply a high concentration of oxygen to the brain. Position client with head of the bed at 30 to 40 degrees and client's head at midline to promote venous drainage from the head. Minimize physical activity to prevent increasing metabolic demands.
*Ineffective **B**reathing Pattern* related to neurological impairment of respiratory status or mechanical ventilation	The client will have an effective breathing pattern.	Assess respiratory status every 15 to 60 minutes. Administer oxygen as ordered to maintain blood oxygen concentration. Provide mechanical ventilation if necessary. Continually assess ABG levels or pulse oximeter readings to identify need for assisting respirations to prevent vasodilation in the brain and increasing intracranial pressure.

Nursing diagnoses for a client with a head injury include the following: (Continued)

NURSING DIAGNOSES	PLANNING/OUTCOMES	NURSING INTERVENTIONS
*Interrupted **Family** Processes* related to sudden crisis	The client and/or family will demonstrate effective coping mechanisms.	Assess family's coping mechanisms. Involve the family in client care as appropriate. Provide information about the client in an ongoing fashion. Provide teaching about the injury and pathophysiology involved. Prepare family for possible outcomes of the injury, such as paralysis or death. Collaborate with clergy, social services, mental health counselors, and support groups. Teach the family to report increased drowsiness, arm/leg weakness, muscle twitching, nausea or vomiting, visual or hearing disturbances, and so on. Inform the family that the client is not aware of the symptoms and that signs and symptoms of the head injury are not immediately apparent.

Evaluation: Evaluate each outcome to determine how it has been met by the client.

BRAIN TUMOR

Brain tumors are space-occupying intracranial lesions, either benign or malignant. Brain tumors are classified by location or tissue type. Intracranial lesions are primary lesions, which develop initially in brain tissue; extensions of tumors of the meninges, cranial nerves, or pituitary gland; or metastatic lesions from tumors originating in other body systems.

The etiology of primary lesions is unknown. Clinical manifestations differ according to the area of the lesion and the rate of growth. Intracranial pressure increases as compensatory mechanisms are no longer able to balance tumor growth. Clinical manifestations commonly include alteration in consciousness, decreased mental functioning, headaches, seizures, or vomiting (sometimes sudden and projectile). Other signs and symptoms are relative to the functions of areas involved, such as visual problems resulting from occipital lobe tumors.

Diagnostic evaluation is by CT scan, MRI, or electroencephalogram (EEG). Total body scans, chest x-rays, and needle biopsies of the tumor are performed to identify the type of tumor and, thus, serve as a basis for medical treatment.

MEDICAL–SURGICAL MANAGEMENT

Medical

Medical management is based on tumor type, growth rate, and assessment of the client. Radiation therapy is used for specific tumor types or for inoperable tumors. The goal is to destroy the tumor cells that are more susceptible to radiation than are normal cells. Radiation is used with surgery and chemotherapy.

Surgical

Surgical intervention removes tumors (benign or malignant) to decrease the space occupied by the lesion or obtains tissue for biopsy. Some CSF is removed to relieve increased pressure.

Pharmacological

Dexamethasone (Decadron) is given to decrease cerebral edema. Phenytoin (Dilantin) is given to prevent seizure activity. Antacids and H_2 blockers, such as cimetidine (Tagamet) or ranitidine (Zantac), are given to prevent gastric irritation. Analgesics, nonsteroidal anti-inflammatory drugs (NSAIDs), or codeine are used for headaches, and stool softeners are administered to prevent straining. A protective mechanism called the blood–brain barrier prevents many potentially harmful substances from reaching the brain tissue or CSF. It prevents chemotherapeutic agents from reaching the brain except in very large doses that are not well tolerated by other body systems. Antineoplastic agents are administered on the basis of tumor type and whether the client meets the requirements for receiving the drug. Antineoplastic alkylating agents (carmustine [BICNU, Gliadel], lomustine [CCNU], and semustube [Methyl-CCNU]) inhibit cell division in rapidly replicating cells. Temozolomide (Temodar) crosses the blood–brain barrier and is used for clients with gliaoblastoma multiforme.

Another alternative way of administering chemotherapeutics is to use the intrathecal (directly into the spinal canal) route. Sometimes chemotherapy disk-shaped wafers are left in the cavity after tumor removal. The wafers release the chemotherapy drug over the next few days (Mayo Clinic, 2008). The surgical insertion of an Ommaya reservoir under the scalp can also allow direct insertion of chemotherapy into the CNS.

NURSING MANAGEMENT

Prepare client and family for surgery in a caring, compassionate manner. Explain procedures, including shaving the head. The client generally will stay in the ICU for several days.

NURSING PROCESS

ASSESSMENT

Subjective Data

Ask the client about fatigue, pain, headache, weakness, and ability to perform daily activities. Note sensory/perceptual alterations such as hearing, visual, tactile, kinesthetic, or olfactory changes. Assess the client's pain and evaluate effectiveness of interventions. A thorough psychosocial assessment, including changes in personality or judgment, serves as the basis for providing emotional support.

Objective Data

Assess functional ability, mobility, and mental status, including motor strength, gait, ability to perform activities of daily living (ADLs), and level of consciousness. Note signs of neurological changes, deficits, or increased intracranial pressure, such as restlessness, changes in logic, changes in vital signs, pupil responses, speech abnormalities, seizure activity, or changes in respiratory patterns.

Nursing diagnoses for a client with a brain tumor include the following:

NURSING DIAGNOSES	PLANNING/OUTCOMES	NURSING INTERVENTIONS
***A**nxiety* related to fear of unknown and treatment plans	The client will demonstrate effective use of coping mechanisms.	Allow client to verbalize feeling of anxiety and discuss coping patterns previously used. Observe for verbal and nonverbal cues of anxiety. Provide emotional support by listening and guiding client to explore feelings of helplessness, fear of the unknown, and potential impending death. Maintain a calm demeanor. Teach client and family about diagnostic tests, treatments, and expected outcomes. Collaborate with pastoral care, physician, social services, and family to provide emotional support. Teach relaxation exercises and techniques such as slow, deep breathing and progressive muscle relaxation. Administer tranquilizers and sedatives as ordered.
*Disturbed **S**ensory Perception* (visual, auditory, kinesthetic, tactile) related to displacement/compression of brain tissue	The client will maintain sensory perceptions.	Maintain communication. Provide a safe environment. Provide orientation and appropriate stimuli. Encourage some social interaction.
*Imbalanced **N**utrition: Less than Body Requirements* related to side effects of treatment and disease process	The client will maintain weight within 5 pounds of initial weight.	Assess client's weight every other day. Provide frequent small feedings of high-calorie and high-protein foods. Offer foods of client's choice. Use nutritional supplements to maintain weight. Offer fluids frequently.

Evaluation: Evaluate each outcome to determine how it has been met by the client.

CEREBROVASCULAR ACCIDENT/TRANSIENT ISCHEMIC ATTACKS

Cerebrovascular accident (CVA), or stroke, is a "brain attack." It happens in the brain rather than the heart and causes a sudden loss of brain function accompanied by neurological deficit. It is a medical emergency and immediate treatment is crucial for the best outcome just as it is for a heart attack (NSA, 2002c). Stroke is the third leading cause of death in the United States, with nearly 144,000 deaths each year (NSA, 2009a). Approximately 795,000 strokes will occur in 2009 (NSA, 2009a). Refer to Figure 41-14 and complete the Stroke Risk Scorecard to evaluate your stroke risk (NSA, 2009b).

Strokes are caused by ischemia (oxygen deprivation) resulting from a thrombus, embolus, severe vasospasm, or cerebral hemorrhage. Blood supply to the brain is interrupted, causing neurological deficits of sensation, movement, thought, memory, or speech. The loss of function can be temporary or permanent.

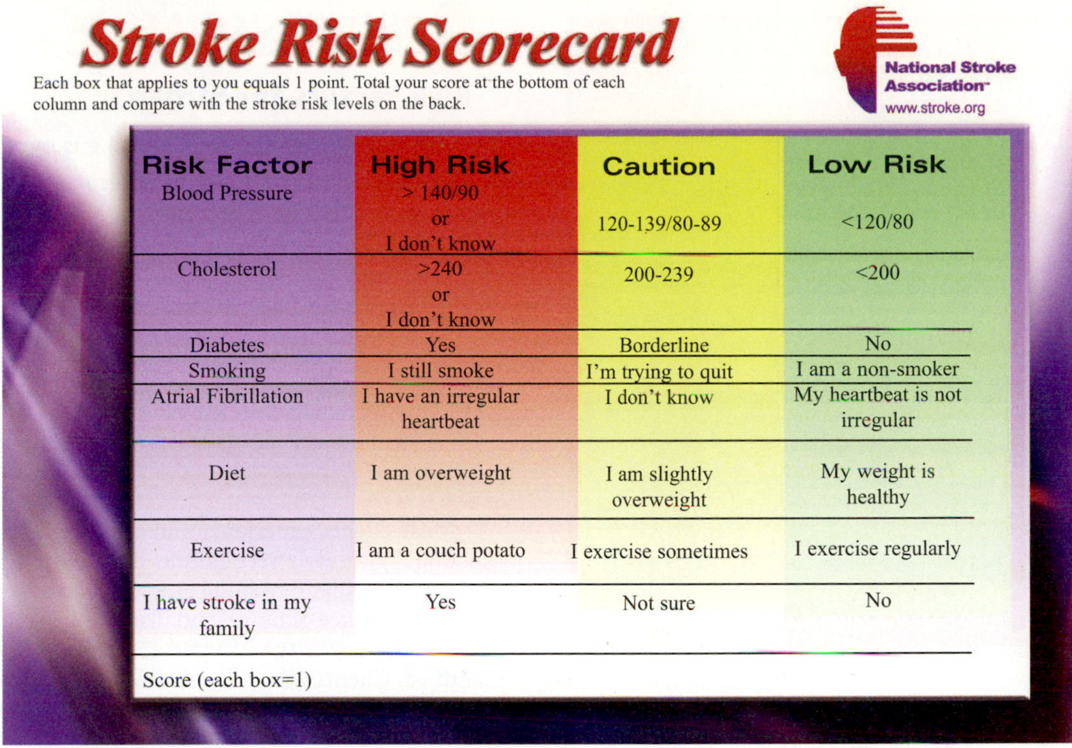

Stroke Risk Scorecard

Each box that applies to you equals 1 point. Total your score at the bottom of each column and compare with the stroke risk levels on the back.

National Stroke Association
www.stroke.org

Risk Factor	High Risk	Caution	Low Risk
Blood Pressure	> 140/90 or I don't know	120-139/80-89	<120/80
Cholesterol	>240 or I don't know	200-239	<200
Diabetes	Yes	Borderline	No
Smoking	I still smoke	I'm trying to quit	I am a non-smoker
Atrial Fibrillation	I have an irregular heartbeat	I don't know	My heartbeat is not irregular
Diet	I am overweight	I am slightly overweight	My weight is healthy
Exercise	I am a couch potato	I exercise sometimes	I exercise regularly
I have stroke in my family	Yes	Not sure	No
Score (each box=1)			

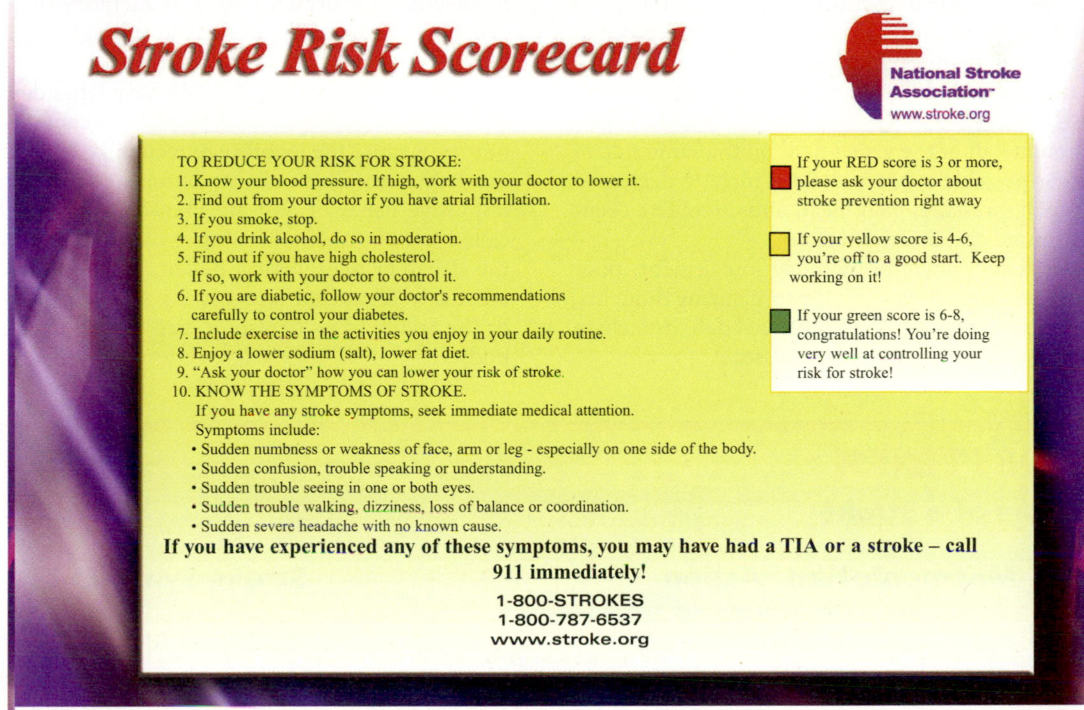

Stroke Risk Scorecard

National Stroke Association
www.stroke.org

TO REDUCE YOUR RISK FOR STROKE:

1. Know your blood pressure. If high, work with your doctor to lower it.
2. Find out from your doctor if you have atrial fibrillation.
3. If you smoke, stop.
4. If you drink alcohol, do so in moderation.
5. Find out if you have high cholesterol. If so, work with your doctor to control it.
6. If you are diabetic, follow your doctor's recommendations carefully to control your diabetes.
7. Include exercise in the activities you enjoy in your daily routine.
8. Enjoy a lower sodium (salt), lower fat diet.
9. "Ask your doctor" how you can lower your risk of stroke.
10. KNOW THE SYMPTOMS OF STROKE.
    If you have any stroke symptoms, seek immediate medical attention.
    Symptoms include:
    - Sudden numbness or weakness of face, arm or leg - especially on one side of the body.
    - Sudden confusion, trouble speaking or understanding.
    - Sudden trouble seeing in one or both eyes.
    - Sudden trouble walking, dizziness, loss of balance or coordination.
    - Sudden severe headache with no known cause.

If your RED score is 3 or more, please ask your doctor about stroke prevention right away

If your yellow score is 4-6, you're off to a good start. Keep working on it!

If your green score is 6-8, congratulations! You're doing very well at controlling your risk for stroke!

If you have experienced any of these symptoms, you may have had a TIA or a stroke – call 911 immediately!

1-800-STROKES
1-800-787-6537
www.stroke.org

FIGURE 41-14 Stroke Risk Scorecard (*© 2009 National Stroke Association. National Stroke Association holds copyright to all of its educational publications and materials. In addition, National Stroke Association is the sole distributor of those publications and materials.*)

Transient ischemic attacks (TIAs) are mini-strokes and frequently precede a stroke. A TIA is a temporary or transient episode of neurological dysfunction caused by temporary impairment of blood flow to the brain. The loss of motor or sensory function may last from a few seconds to minutes to 24 hours. The classic symptoms are sudden blurring of vision or blindness, loss of balance or coordination, difficulty speaking or understanding simple statements, and weakness/numbness/paralysis in the face, arm, or leg (NSA, 2002b, 2008).

Clinical manifestations of TIA or CVA vary according to the location of interrupted blood supply in the brain. As with head injury, the specific functions of the involved area of the brain are interrupted, causing the symptoms. Common neurological deficits are motor deficits of hemiplegia (paralysis of one side of the body on the side opposite of the brain lesion), **hemiparesis** (weakness of one side of the body), **dysarthria** (impairment of speech caused by muscle dysfunction), and dysphagia (impairment of swallowing muscles). **Emotional**

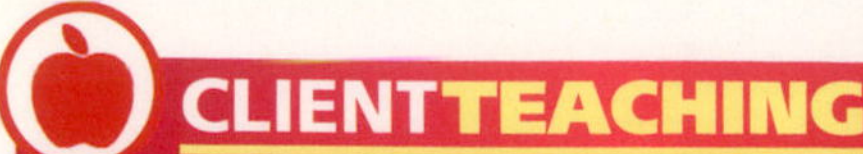

CLIENT TEACHING

Stroke-Prevention Guidelines

- Have an annual blood pressure check.
- Be aware of cholesterol level.
- Consume lesser amounts of sodium (salt) and fat.
- Exercise daily.
- Do not smoke.
- If you drink alcohol, do so in moderation.
- Check with a doctor for symptoms of atrial fibrillation.
- Check cholesterol level.
- Control diabetes.
- Check with a doctor for circulation problems.
- See a doctor immediately with any stroke-like symptoms.

(National Stroke Association, 2009)

PROFESSIONAL TIP

Risk Factors for Stroke

- The major risk factor for stroke is hypertension.
- Other risk factors are diabetes mellitus, atherosclerosis, aneurysm, cardiac disease, high blood cholesterol, obesity, sedentary lifestyle, smoking, stress, drug abuse (especially of cocaine), and use of oral contraceptives. Clients with more than one risk factor are at even greater risk.
- One in twenty people who have a TIA will have a stroke within 2 days (NSA, 2009b)

lability (loss of emotional control), inability to control behavior, and inability to process multiple pieces of information are also common manifestations of a stroke.

Sensory deficits include visual deficits of double vision, decreased visual acuity, and **homonymous hemianopia**, the loss of vision in half of the visual field on the same side of both eyes. Other possible sensory deficits include decreased sensation to touch, pressure, pain, heat, and cold. The client also may be confused and disoriented.

Intellectual deficits include memory impairment, poor judgment, short attention span, difficulty organizing thoughts, and inability to reason or calculate. Emotional deficits include depression and decreased tolerance to stressors.

Most clients experience initial bowel and bladder dysfunction. With early recognition of the problem and use of bowel and bladder retraining programs, however, most clients regain continence of bowel and bladder.

Differences in the affected side of the brain have been identified. Clients with left-side CVA tend to have communication deficits of aphasia, or inability to communicate. These clients tend to be slow and cautious in behavior and have intellectual impairments such as memory deficits or loss of problem-solving skills. Defects in the right visual field occur, and hemiplegia occurs on the right side.

Clients with right-side CVA have left-sided paralysis and defects in the left visual field. Spatial–perceptual defects, called **agnosia**, cause the inability to recognize familiar objects such as a hairbrush. These clients demonstrate poor judgment and impulsive behavior and are unaware of the deficits. This is called **anosognosia**, which is gross or unconscious denial of the stroke or neurological deficit. Furthermore, these clients are easily distracted and usually show **unilateral neglect**, or the failure to recognize or care for the affected side of the body.

MEMORY TRICK

Indicators of a Stroke

Mnemonic	Mnemonic Hint	Action	Stroke Symptom
S	Smile	Ask the client to smile.	One side of the face may droop.
T	Talk or speak	Ask the client to say a simple sentence, e.g., The grass is green.	The speech is slurred or garbled.
R	Raise both arms	Ask the client to raise both arms.	One arm is weak and falls downward.
T	Tongue	Ask the client to stick his tongue out.	Tongue moves to one side.
T	Time	If any of these signs are present in a nonhospitalized client, call 911 to transport the client to an acute facility	

Adapted from National Stroke Association (NSA). (2009a). Stroke 101. Retrieved on June 3, 2009 at http://www.stroke.org/site/DocServer/STROKE_101_Fact_Sheet.pdf?docID=454; and Santa Rosa County Citizen Service Center. (2009) Blood Clots/Stroke – They now have a fourth indicator, the tongue. Retrieved on June 3, 2009 at http://www.santarosa.fl.gov/hr/documents/identiyastroke.pdf

PROFESSIONALTIP

Medication and Cerebrovascular Accident

Calcium channel blockers should not be used for the client with CVA because they dilate blood vessels and increase cerebral perfusion.

Cerebral edema and increased intracranial pressure may further complicate neurological status. Cerebral edema maximizes in 3 to 5 days following CVA. Neurological deficits begin to resolve within 2 days as cerebral edema decreases. Gradual progression in the return of various functions from proximal to distal can occur for 1 to 2 years.

Medical–Surgical Management

Medical

Medical management of the client with CVA is directed toward airway maintenance and supportive therapy during the first 24 to 48 hours. Early diagnosis of the cause and type of stroke is necessary to determine the appropriate treatment. Maintaining adequate cerebral perfusion and preventing cerebral edema reduce neurological deficit. Respiratory failure is treated with mechanical ventilation; temperature is regulated, with the help of a hypothermia blanket if necessary. (See the section on increased intracranial pressure for information on prevention and treatment.)

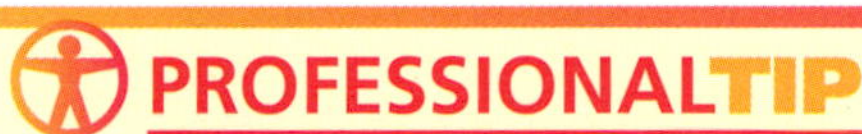

Caregivers for Client with CVA

- Give the CVA client ample time to process and then answer the question before proceeding with more conversation.
- To provide consistency in understanding the needs of a client with a CVA, assign the same caregiver to the client whenever possible.

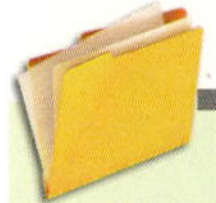

COLLABORATIVECARE

Post-CVA Care

Depending on the location of the CVA and the extent of neurologic deficit, collaboration with physical, occupational, and speech therapists is necessary for the client to reach the optimal functional level of recovery.

COMMUNITY/HOME HEALTH CARE

Post-CVA Care

- Consult with the family to evaluate the home for safety and use of wheelchair or walker, if needed.
- Evaluate the client's ability to perform self-care so that assistive devices or personal assistance is obtained.
- Determine whether a hospital bed or other medical equipment will need to be rented.

To prevent further loss of function, a focus on rehabilitation begins on admission. After a stroke, all effort is made to maintain self-care and mobility.

Surgical

Surgical removal of the thrombus (thrombolectomy) or embolus (embolectomy) may be necessary to relieve pressure on the brain.

Pharmacological

Antihypertensive agents are used to control blood pressure. Anticoagulants, aspirin, heparin, or Coumadin are used to prevent further clot formation in cases of stroke caused by thrombi. To dissolve the clot, thrombolytic agents such as alteplase (Activase), anistreplase (Eminase), streptokinase (Streptase), or urokinase (Abbokinase) are given within 3 hours of the stroke. A stroke caused by bleeding would not be treated with thrombolytic agents. Dexamethasone (Decadron) is be used to reduce intracranial pressure. Anticonvulsants such as phenytoin (Dilantin) is used if convulsions are present.

Diet

Fluid is restricted for a few days after a CVA. The client will, however, be given intravenous fluids or tube feedings. The gag reflex is assessed to identify choking risk and food restrictions implemented accordingly.

Activity

In cases of an embolic or thrombolic stroke, the client's bed is kept flat with the head midline to increase cerebral perfusion. In the event of a hemorrhagic stroke, the head of the bed is elevated to decrease cerebral perfusion. The type of CVA and the physician's judgment determines the length of time the client stays in bed.

Nursing Management

Maintain a patent airway and fluid and electrolyte balance. Administer oxygen and medications as ordered. Monitor vital signs, neurologic status, I&O, pulse oximetry, and ABGs. Ensure adequate nutrition. Provide careful mouth and eye care. Keep client's body in correct alignment, using a footboard to prevent foot drop and contractures. Turn client at least every 2 hours to prevent pneumonia. Perform and assist client to perform range of motion (ROM) exercises using the unaffected side to exercise the affected side. Communicate with the client; often an unresponsive client can hear. Set realistic short-term goals. Involve the client's family in client care when possible.

NURSING PROCESS

ASSESSMENT

Subjective Data

Subjective data include client statements regarding how the client is feeling, frustration level with limitations, reports of pain, numbness, tingling, and sensory deficits of vision or hearing.

Objective Data

Give specific attention to the objective assessment findings of level of consciousness, respiratory status, hemiparesis, hemiplegia, mobility, and cognitive perceptual functioning, including the inability to think clearly and the ability to understand the condition.

Nursing diagnoses for a client with a CVA include the following:

NURSING DIAGNOSES	PLANNING/OUTCOMES	NURSING INTERVENTIONS
*Deficient **K**nowledge* related to home care	The client and/or family will verbalize or demonstrate home health care management.	Assess client's and family's needs for discharge teaching and knowledge level about necessary home care. Develop a multidisciplinary plan for client and family teaching. Provide education in verbal, written, and picture forms to accommodate the varying possible impairments from the stroke. Teach small segments of information at a time and reinforce teaching, then, to ascertain effectiveness of teaching, have client and family return demonstrate or verbalize knowledge. Primary areas of teaching are medication administration; dosages, actions, and side effects to report to the physician; mobility needs; self-care needs; safety factors; communication; swallowing; elimination; and skin care.
*Impaired Verbal **C**ommunication* related to neuromuscular impairment	The client will communicate needs to the caregiver.	Assess communication deficits and consult a speech therapist to determine a method of communication, if deficits are apparent. Allow time for the client to attempt to communicate needs; anticipate needs to prevent client frustration in trying to communicate. Use gestures, pictures, and closed questions (those requiring only a "yes" or "no" answer). Provide paper and pencil if dominant side is unaffected.
*Unilateral **N**eglect* related to neuromuscular impairment	The client will move paralyzed extremities with assistance from functioning extremities.	Adapt environment to prevent injury of the client with unilateral neglect by positioning water and personal items on the unaffected or unneglected side. Approach the client from the unneglected side. Gradually cue client to remind to tend to the neglected side. Remind client of safety factors such as arm trailing over edge of wheelchair or close proximity of a wall on the neglected side. Teach client and family to place small bites of food on unaffected side and to check for food in the cheek on the affected side after meals. Instruct client to scan environment for safety factors at all times. Teach client how to dress and tend to neglected side. Place arm either in a sling if client is ambulatory, or on a wheelchair tray if client is in a wheelchair.

Evaluation: Evaluate each outcome to determine how it has been met by the client.

EPILEPSY/SEIZURE DISORDER

Epilepsy is a disorder of cerebral function in which the client experiences sudden attacks of altered consciousness, motor activity, or sensory phenomenon. Convulsive seizures are the most common type. Most recurrent seizure patterns are caused by epilepsy. Most clinicians and authors use the term "seizure disorder" for epilepsy or seizures (Hickey, 2008).

A seizure is initiated by an electrical disturbance in the neurons, which, in turn, causes an aberrant discharge of electrical activity from any part of the cerebral cortex and possibly from other areas of the brain (Samuels, 2004). This electrical discharge may cause involuntary episodes of loss of consciousness, excessive muscular movement or loss of muscle tone, and changes in behavior, mood, sensation, and/or perception (Smeltzer, Bare, Hinkle, & Cheever, 2008).

The etiology of the electrical disturbance may be birth trauma, hypoxia, infection, tumor, alcohol toxicity, drugs, drug withdrawal, carbon monoxide or lead poisoning, vascular abnormalities such as CVA, hypoglycemia electrolyte imbalance, or fever. Often, the cause is idiopathic, or unknown.

Seizures are classified as generalized or partial. In generalized seizures, the entire brain is affected simultaneously, causing bilateral, symmetrical reactions. Generalized seizures are classified as tonic and/or clonic (grand mal), absence (petit mal), or myoclonic.

Tonic–clonic seizures involve rigid tonic contractions of muscles and loss of postural control followed by a clonic stage of intermittent contraction and relaxation. Incontinence of stool or urine is common. Absence seizures involve loss of conscious activity without the muscular involvement of tonic–clonic seizures. Myoclonic seizures are very mild, sudden, involuntary contractions of a muscle group or rapid, forceful movements. They usually occur in the trunk or extremities and involve no loss of consciousness.

Partial seizures initiate in a focal point in the brain and involve the function of those specific neurons. Partial seizures are either simple or complex. In simple partial seizures, the area affected may be a hand, a finger, the ability to talk, or a sense such as smell. Consciousness is not lost.

Complex partial seizures generally involve loss of consciousness and produce cognitive, affective, psychosensory, or psychomotor symptoms. The client performs inappropriate purposive behaviors, called **automatisms**, or mechanical, repetitive motor behaviors performed unconsciously, such as lip-smacking. **Auras**, peculiar sensations that precede a seizure, may take the form of a taste, smell, sight, or sound; dizziness; or a "funny" feeling. After the seizure, the client typically cannot remember the episode.

Diagnostic testing to determine the type of seizure activity includes an EEG to identify abnormal electrical activity and/or the focal point of the seizure. Sleep and video EEGs document changes in electrical activity of the brain. CT scans identify or rule out lesions, degenerative changes, or vascular abnormalities.

MEDICAL–SURGICAL MANAGEMENT

Surgical

Surgical intervention is indicated for a very small percentage of clients; those for whom pharmacological treatment has not been effective and when the focal points are identified. Microsurgery is used to irradiate focal points of abnormal electrical discharge caused by tumor, vascular abnormality, or abscess.

Pharmacological

The primary method of controlling seizure activity is pharmacological. Seizure activity is controlled with an anticonvulsant agent or a combination of anticonvulsants in 75% of clients (Hickey, 2008). Phenytoin (Dilantin), phenobarbital (Phenobarbital), carbamazepine (Tegretol), valproic acid (Depakene), and primidone (Mysoline) are often used. Anticonvulsant agents are started one at a time in gradually increasing doses. The client's blood level is monitored for therapeutic range, and the client is assessed for side effects of the drug and signs of drug toxicity, such as drowsiness, dizziness, gastric distress, rash, blood dyscrasias, and ataxia.

The goal is to obtain seizure control with minimal side effects. Any anticonvulsant is gradually discontinued. Abrupt

SAFETY

Precautions During a Seizure

If the client is in bed:

- Be sure the side rails are up.
- Put padding (blankets) on the side rails to prevent injury.

If the client is out of bed:

- Carefully ease the client to the floor.
- Move nearby objects so that the client will not be injured.
- Place a soft item beneath the client's head.

Whether the client is in or out of bed:

- Never leave the client alone.
- Do not restrain the client.
- Do not attempt to put anything in the client's mouth after the seizure has begun.
- Loosen any restrictive clothing around the client's neck.
- Turn the client's head to the side.
- Monitor seizure activity carefully, noting the exact time that the seizure began and ended.

After the seizure:

- Call the client by name and ask to perform a simple command.
- Test the client's memory by asking to remember two words.
- Ask the client whether an aura was experienced before the seizure.
- Check the oral cavity—especially the tongue—for injury.
- Offer comfort and reassurance, as the client is frightened and embarrassed.
- Document everything observed.
- Keep the client in a side-lying position if the client remains lethargic.

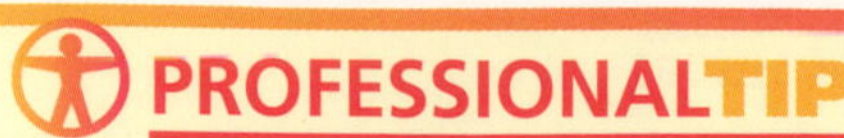

Long-Term Use of Dilantin

The client on Dilantin requires good oral hygiene because of hyperplasia of the gums, which become edematous and enlarged.

withdrawal can cause **status epilepticus**, an acute prolonged episode of seizure activity lasting at least 30 minutes with or without loss of consciousness (Smeltzer, Bare, Hinkle, & Cheever, 2008). Status epilepticus is a medical emergency that results in respiratory arrest and irreversible brain damage.

Diet

Nutritionally balanced meals are required. The client should not consume alcohol.

Activity

Adequate rest is required. Driving, operating machinery, and swimming are not allowed until seizures are controlled.

Nursing Management

Monitor for toxic signs of anticonvulsant medications. Stress importance for compliance with prescribed medication schedule. Encourage scrupulous oral hygiene. Warn client not to drink alcoholic beverages. Encourage client to have anticonvulsant medication blood level checked regularly.

NURSING PROCESS

Assessment

Subjective Data

Include client statements of experiences before the seizure and activity the client was performing when the seizure occurred. Determine whether an aura was experienced and the sensations that were manifested, and ascertain if the client has a prior history of seizure disorder.

Objective Data

Assessment of the nature of the seizure and sequencing of events is important in determining cause and management of seizure activity. During the seizure, assess the client's respiratory status and observe for muscular stiffness or flaccidity, the position of the eyes and head, the size and equality of the pupils, automatism, any cry or sounds made, and incontinence of urine or stool. Note the duration of the phases of the seizure, total duration, and whether unconsciousness occurred. Note if the onset of seizure activity was observed, along with what the client was doing when the seizure began.

After the seizure, assess airway and observe the client for **postictal** (after a seizure) signs of paralysis of arms or legs, inability to speak, sleep following seizure, difficulty in awakening from sleep, confusion, or general dazed affect (Smeltzer, Bare, Hinkle, & Cheever, 2008; Hickey, 2008). The postictal phase lasts from several minutes to hours. Assess the client for signs of injury and vital signs. Clients on anticonvulsant therapy are assessed thoroughly because of the wide variety of side effects involving multiple body systems.

Nursing diagnoses for a client with a seizure include the following:

NURSING DIAGNOSES	PLANNING/OUTCOMES	NURSING INTERVENTIONS
Ineffective Airway Clearance related to mucus accumulation during the seizure and uncontrollable tonic–clonic muscle contractions involving the respiratory muscles	The client will maintain an effective airway during seizure activity.	Following tonic–clonic activity, turn client to the side to allow secretions to drain from the airway. Prepare to suction oropharynx if necessary to clear airway. Assess skin color and respiratory rate and depth during and following seizure. Administer oxygen as needed. Insert oral airway or epistick if client's jaw is not clenched. Never insert an object if the jaw is already clenched. Do not place fingers between client's teeth. Loosen restrictive clothing.
Risk for Injury related to seizure activity	The client will be free of injury related to seizure activity.	During seizures in bed, use blankets or protective pads to pad side rails. If client is standing or sitting, ease client to the floor when seizure activity begins. Place client in a supine position, but do not physically restrain client. Remove objects from around client so that he will not hit them. After the seizure, assess airway and turn client to the side to allow secretions to drain from the mouth. Observe client for injuries (e.g., tongue lacerations; broken bones; body lacerations or bruising). Maintain a low-stimulus environment to prevent further seizure activity.

Nursing diagnoses for a client with a seizure include the following: (Continued)

NURSING DIAGNOSES	PLANNING/OUTCOMES	NURSING INTERVENTIONS
		Teach client about ways of maintaining a safe environment, including driving restrictions; lying down in a safe area if an aura is experienced; showering instead of tub bathing; either avoiding swimming or swimming with a partner if the physician allows; and wearing a medical identification tag.
*Ineffective **Coping*** related to anxiety secondary to seizure disorder and altered self-concept	The client will verbalize fears and concerns about seizure activity; and will use effective coping methods.	Allow client to verbalize fears and concerns. Explore coping mechanisms with client. Collaborate with mental health counselor or clergy to assist client in development of coping mechanisms.

Evaluation: Evaluate each outcome to determine how it has been met by the client.

HERNIATED INTERVERTEBRAL DISK

Herniated intervertebral disks are a major cause of chronic back pain. Most clients with herniated disks are 30 to 50 years of age. Most herniated disks occur in the lumbar or cervical spine because of the flexibility of these regions (Hickey, 2008). This can occur either suddenly from trauma, lifting, or twisting or gradually from aging, osteoporosis, or degenerative changes. Most herniated disks are caused by trauma, such as falls, accidents, or repeated lifting. Degenerative changes related to arthritis, aging, or repeated minor injuries predispose the client to herniated intervertebral disks.

The intervertebral disk is a cartilaginous cushion between vertebral bodies (Figure 41-15). In herniation, or rupture of the disk, the nucleus pulposus protrudes into the fibrous ring, the annulus fibrosus. This protrusion presses on the spinal cord and nerve roots, causing pain, motor changes, sensory changes, and alterations in reflexes.

The nerve root affected and the degree of compression leads to specific symptoms. Ninety percent to 95% of lumbar herniations occur at the L-4 to L-5 and S-1 levels (Hickey, 2008). Low-back pain that radiates across the buttock and down the leg along the path of the sciatic nerve is the most common symptom. The affected leg tingles and is numb. Sneezing, straining, stooping, standing, sitting, blowing the nose, and jarring movements aggravate the pain. Positions of comfort are lying on the back, with knees flexed and a small pillow under the head, or lying on the unaffected side, with the affected knee flexed.

Motor weakness is experienced. Paresthesia and numbness of the leg and foot occur. Knee and ankle reflexes are diminished or absent. **Lasegue's sign**, pain experienced upon gentle raising of the fully extended leg of the supine-positioned client to 20 to 60 degrees, stems from stretching of the inflamed sciatic nerve. With a low-back herniated disk, however, the client is unable to extend the knee because of severe pain radiating down the hip and leg. Symptoms vary with the area and degree of nerve root compression.

Cervical herniation commonly occurs at levels C-5 to C-6 or C-6 to C-7. Symptoms of lateral herniation include pain and paresthesia in the neck, arms, and shoulders. Loss of muscle strength and reflexes also occur, as does muscle atrophy.

Because of anatomic position, cervical disks herniate centrally more frequently than do lumbar disks, thereby compressing the spinal cord. Symptoms are weakness of the lower extremities and unsteady gait. Spasticity and hyperactive reflexes develop in the lower extremities. Difficulty in voiding and sexual dysfunction occur.

Degenerative spinal cord disease can follow compression from a herniated disk. Spinal cord tumors and herniated lumbar disk are differential diagnoses that are ruled out through the use of MRI or CT scans.

MEDICAL–SURGICAL MANAGEMENT

Medical

Conservative medical treatment, i.e., providing rest, stress reduction and immobility of the spine, and pain relief, often is tried for several weeks. Physical therapy is ordered, with exercises to strengthen back muscles and possibly ultrasound treatments.

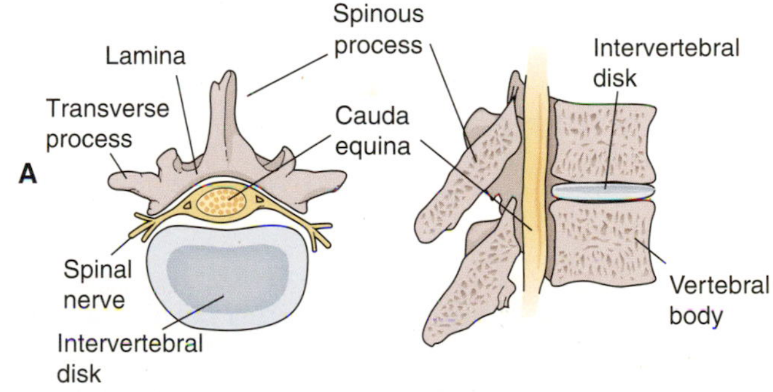

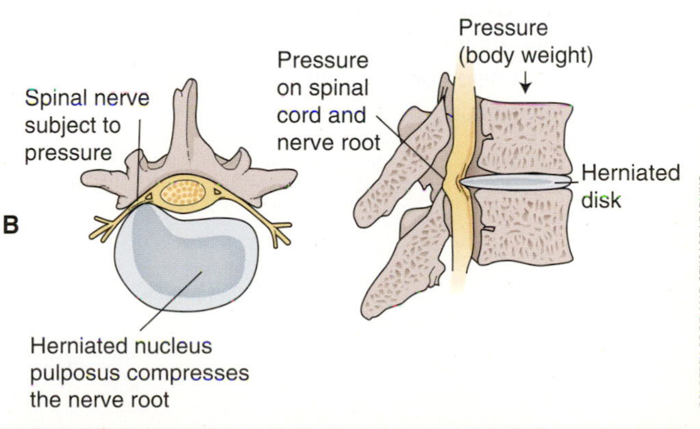

FIGURE 41-15 ***A*, Normal Intravertebral Disk; *B*, Herniated Disk**

A transcutaneous electrical nerve stimulation (TNS) unit may also be used to decrease pain.

Surgical

Surgery to remove the herniated disk is performed when neurological deficit or pain are not responsive to conservative treatment or when symptoms require immediate surgical intervention.

 Pharmacological

Narcotic analgesics, such as hydrocodone bitartrate with acetaminophen (Vicodin), and nonnarcotic analgesics, such as tramadol hydrochloride (Ultram), are ordered for pain control. Antiinflammatory drugs, steroids, or NSAIDs, such as ibuprofen (Motrin) or naproxen (Anaprox), are prescribed to reduce the inflammatory response. Clients in chronic pain sometimes benefit from an antiepileptic drug, e.g., gabapentin (Neurontin), because it treats neuropathic pain. Muscle relaxants, such as methocarbamol (Robaxin), are given to reduce spasms of surrounding muscles, which decreases the pain. Antianxiety medications, such as diazepam (Valium), are given to decrease muscle tension and promote rest. Short-term oral corticosteroids may be ordered, or local or epidural corticosteroid injections may be used

Diet

To decrease the workload on the involved muscles, weight reduction is advocated if the client is overweight. A high-protein diet with calcium, vitamin D, and phosphorus is necessary for bone repair and prevention of osteoporosis. Fiber is necessary for bowel function because constipation is a common side effect of analgesics.

Activity

Bed rest, a support garment (back brace) or cervical collar, a firm mattress, and traction are used to decrease stress on the affected vertebrae. Postoperatively, log-roll turning prevents injury to the vertebrae and spine.

The client may not lift or carry more than 5 pounds for at least 8 weeks. Twisting movements are avoided. The client cannot drive a car until the surgeon permits. Sitting is limited during the early postoperative period; the client either stands or lies down. Physical therapy is focused on muscle strengthening and client comfort. Heat therapy, ultrasound, and exercises promote comfort and healing.

Nursing Management

Preoperatively, monitor neurological status and vital signs. Encourage client to cough, deep breathe, use incentive spirometer, and move legs as allowed. Provide adequate fluids to prevent renal stasis and constipation.

Postoperatively, monitor vital signs, neurovascular status of legs, and check dressing for any bleeding. If drain is in place (e.g., Hemovac or Jackson-Pratt drain), check frequently and empty at end of shift and record on I&O sheet. Use the log-rolling technique for turning the client.

NURSING PROCESS

Assessment

Subjective Data

Assessment includes eliciting client statements about motor and sensory function, pain, and effectiveness of comfort measures.

Objective Data

Assessment entails a neurological evaluation of motor and sensory function of the extremities innervated below the herniated area. Reflex testing is a part of the nursing assessment in some facilities. Assess range of motion (ROM) of the affected extremity. Assess the client's knowledge about the disease process, the planned treatment including pain management and surgery, and the postsurgical care. Assess bowel and bladder elimination for potential nerve involvement or effects of immobility. Note gait alteration and bending limitations.

Nursing diagnoses for a client with a herniated intervertebral disk include the following:

NURSING DIAGNOSES	PLANNING/OUTCOMES	NURSING INTERVENTIONS
*Chronic **Pain*** related to nerve compression or surgical intervention	The client will experience increased comfort.	Assess pain intensity and location, as well as activities or position when pain began. Have the client rate pain on a scale of 1 to 10.
		Maintain activity level as ordered by physician. Provide diversional activities.
		Place client in position of comfort, usually on back, with knees slightly flexed and a small pillow beneath head, or on unaffected side, with affected extremity flexed and a pillow between the legs.
		Maintain immobility of vertebrae with corset, brace, or traction.
		Apply moist heat as prescribed and administer medications to relieve pain, relax muscles, and relieve inflammation and anxiety, as ordered. Document effectiveness.

Nursing diagnoses for a client with a herniated intervertebral disk include the following: (Continued)

NURSING DIAGNOSES	PLANNING/OUTCOMES	NURSING INTERVENTIONS
Impaired Physical Mobility related to nerve compression or surgical intervention	The client will have no complications of immobility.	Assess for complications of immobility. Turn client every 1 to 2 hours. The client tends to limit position to one of comfort. Assist the client to log roll, that is, move the body as a unit without twisting the back. Ambulate as ordered by the physician.

Evaluation: Evaluate each outcome to determine how it has been met by the client.

SPINAL CORD INJURY

Spinal cord injury (SCI) occurs from trauma to the spinal cord or from compression of the spinal cord caused by injury to the supporting structures. Each year, almost 12,000 new spinal cord injuries occur. Most of the victims are males between the ages of 16 and 30 years. Leading causes of injury in the order of prevalence are motor vehicle accidents; falls; acts of violence; and sporting accidents (Spinal Cord Injury Information Network, 2009).

Numerous classification systems exist for SCIs. Spinal cord injuries are classified by level of injury, mechanism of injury, or neurological or functional level (Figure 41-16). The injury may be considered complete or incomplete. When injury is complete, no impulses are carried below the level of injury. There is complete disruption of the spinal cord functions, including motor (voluntary) movement, sensation, and reflexes to areas innervated by the spinal nerves at and below the level of the injury. In an incomplete injury, some of the spinal cord tracts are affected while others are able to carry impulses normally.

The mechanism of injury is usually an acceleration–deceleration event that causes hyperflexion, hyperextension, axial loading, or excessive rotation injury (Hickey, 2008). Hyperflexion is the extreme forward movement of the head, which causes compression of the vertebral bodies and damage to the posterior ligaments and intervertebral disks, as shown in Figure 41-17A. Hyperextension is the extreme backward movement of the head, causing injury to the posterior vertebral structures and the anterior ligaments, as shown in Figure 41-17B. Axial loading or compression occurs when extreme pressure is placed on the spinal column, such as in diving accidents or falls landed on feet or buttocks (Figure 41-17C). Compression of the vertebrae shatters the vertebral body. Compression fractures and posterior ligament injury can also be caused by excessive rotation, or turning the head beyond the normal range.

Classification of injury by cause includes concussion, contusion, laceration, transection, hemorrhage, or damage to blood vessels supplying the spinal cord. Immediately after injury to the spinal cord, an autodestructive process begins, with chemical and vascular changes that lead to ischemia and necrosis of the spinal cord.

Spinal shock (cessation of motor, sensory, autonomic, and reflex impulses) and **areflexia** (the absence of reflexes) occur immediately upon transection of the spinal cord or upon injury to the spinal cord. Flaccid paralysis of all skeletal muscles, loss of spinal reflexes, loss of sensation, and absence of autonomic function below the level of injury also occur. The diaphragm is innervated at levels C3 through C5. Injuries in this area cause partial or complete disruption of respiratory function. The client does not perspire below the level of the injury. Bowel and bladder function is lost either for a few days to months, or permanently, although this loss generally lasts from 1 to 6 weeks.

As spinal shock resolves, reflex activity returns below the level of injury. The client with a lower motor neuron injury continues to experience flaccid paralysis, areflexia, hypotonic bowel and bladder function, and sexual dysfunction. Lower motor neuron injury causes paraplegia, or paralysis of lower extremities.

Neurogenic shock, a hypotensive situation resulting from the loss of sympathetic control of vital functions from the brain, may occur during spinal shock. This happens in clients with injury above the sixth thoracic vertebra. The client develops orthostatic hypotension, bradycardia, decreased cardiac output, loss of ability to sweat below the level of injury, and poikilothermia (body temperature adjusts to room temperature).

Upper motor neuron injury results in spastic paralysis, loss of voluntary skeletal muscle movement, and reflexive bowel, bladder, and sexual responses. Complete upper motor neuron injury results in **quadriplegia (tetraplegia)**, or dysfunction or paralysis of both arms, both legs, bowel, and bladder. Injuries above C5 affect respiratory function because of innervation of the diaphragm and accessory respiratory muscles. Mechanical ventilation is required to keep the client alive. Fractures below the cervical vertebrae result in diaphragmatic breathing, if the phrenic nerve is functioning.

Once spinal shock has passed, the client with an injury above the sixth thoracic vertebra is at risk for developing *autonomic dysreflexia* or *autonomic hyperreflexia*. Autonomic dysreflexia is an emergency situation resulting in a hypertensive crisis (elevated systolic pressures of 260 to 300 mm Hg), bradycardia, severe headache, and possibly stroke or seizure activity. The cause is noxious stimuli such as a full bladder, a fecal impaction, a wrinkle in clothing, menstrual cramps, an erection, an ingrown toenail, a bladder infection, or sitting on catheter tubing. Autonomic reflexes below the level of the injury cause vasoconstriction in this area. The controlling impulses from the higher cortical levels do not transmit past the level of injury but cause bradycardia and vasodilation above the level of injury. Skin above the level of injury is warm and moist, but skin below the level of injury is cold, with goose flesh (Beare & Meyers, 1998; Hickey, 2008).

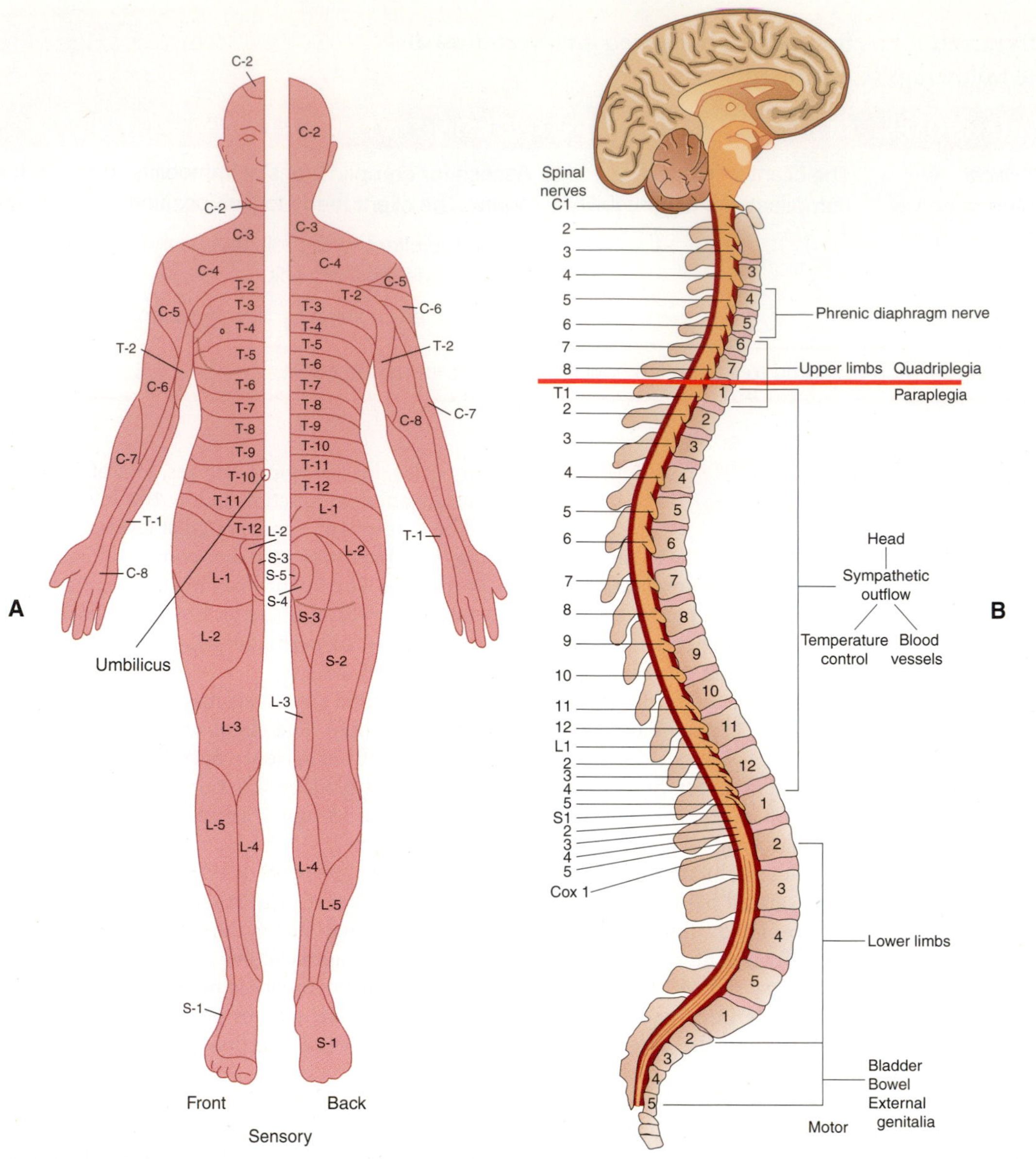

FIGURE 41-16 Spinal Cord—Levels of Injury; *A*, Areas of Sensory Function (Dermatomes); *B*, Areas of Motor Function

The noxious stimuli must be removed, if possible, and the client placed in a sitting position immediately. Assess blood pressure immediately and monitor every few minutes until within normal limits (Huston & Boelman, 1995). The drug of choice, nitroprusside sodium (Nipride), is given if the conservative measure does not work. Nifedipine (Procardia) is also used. Prevent autonomic dysreflexia when possible, recognize when it develops, and treat immediately. Once autonomic dysreflexia is relieved, the client may develop hypotension from the decreased sympathetic response and the residual effects of medication and positioning changes. A pattern of individual response to stimuli and of sympathetic response is soon identified for the client; however, the client with an upper motor neuron injury above T-6 is always at risk for developing autonomic dysreflexia. Some clients experience the first episode years after the injury.

The extent of permanent injury cannot be determined immediately because of necrosis, edema, and spinal shock. Functional loss depends on the level, degree, and type of injury.

MEDICAL–SURGICAL MANAGEMENT

Medical

Medical management of the client with spinal cord injury begins before reaching the hospital. Further damage to the spinal cord is prevented by immobilizing the head, neck, and vertebral column with devices such as rigid cervical collars and splinting backboards. All trauma clients are treated as potential spinal cord injuries. When the client reaches the emergency room, x-rays of the spine are taken before removing the immobilizing devices.

Respiratory function is continuously assessed, and ventilatory support is provided as necessary. The client may have multiple injuries, necessitating astute diagnostic skills by the emergency room physician. Assessment of the trauma client involves evaluating for internal hemorrhaging, cardiac contusion, head injury, hemorrhagic shock, and spinal shock resulting from the spinal cord injury. A thorough assessment is done to specifically evaluate the degree of deficit and to establish the level or degree of injury.

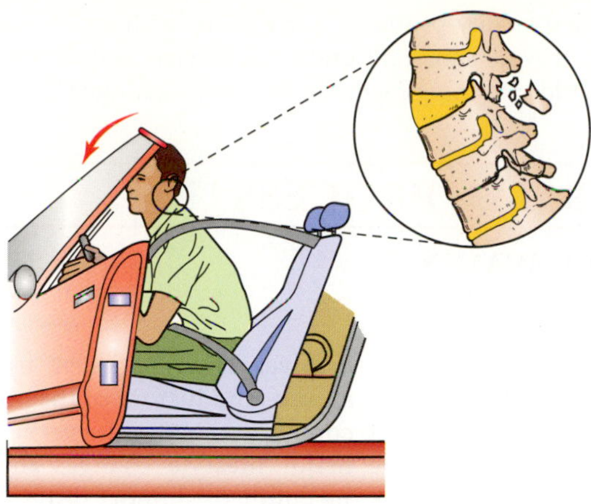

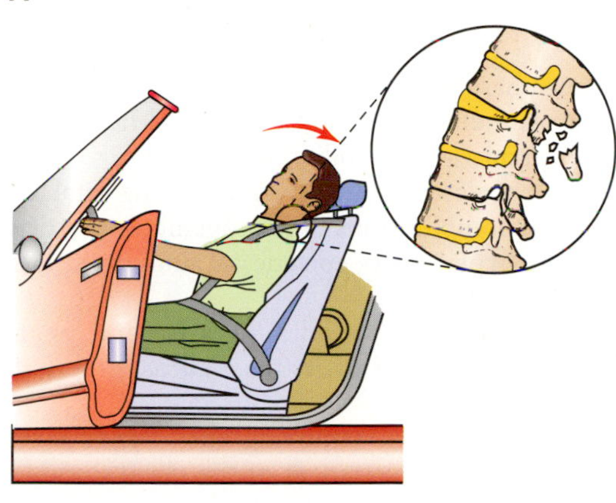

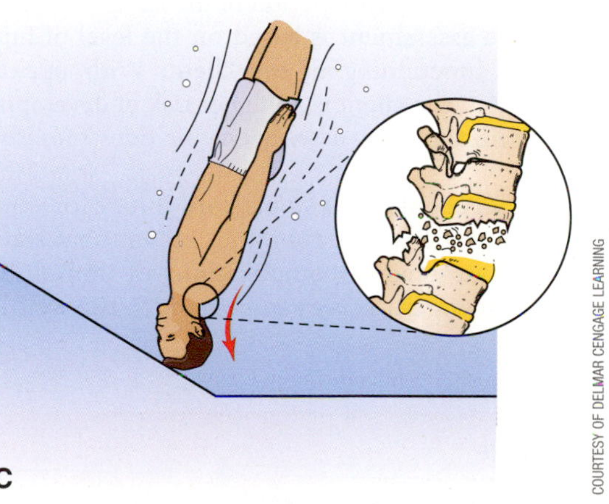

FIGURE 41-17 Acceleration/Deceleration Injuries; ***A*, Hyperflexion: The extreme forward movement of the head causes compression of the vertebral bodies and damage to the posterior ligaments and intervertebral disks; *B*, Hyperextension: Extreme backward movement of the head causes injury to the posterior vertebral structures and the anterior ligaments; *C*, Axial loading or compression: Extreme pressure is placed on the spinal column, such as in diving accidents or falls landing on feet or buttocks**

Blood pressure monitoring is crucial. A systolic BP below 90 mm Hg should be avoided or corrected as soon as possible because one episode can send the client into shock and cause permanent damage (Baker & Saulino, 2002).

Immobilization of the spinal cord continues to be the focus of care during early medical management of the client. Traction is used to maintain alignment of the spinal column. Cervical tongs and halo devices are used to apply traction and to immobilize the cervical spine (Figure 41-18). Under local anesthesia, cervical tongs and halo rings are applied with spring-loaded pins that are embedded into the scalp. Antiseptic solution is used to cleanse the scalp, and a local anesthetic is injected into the insertion sites. Traction weights are applied to the cervical tongs or halo rings after the insertion pins are firmly embedded. Body casts, jackets, vests, or braces are used to immobilize thoracic and lumbar fractures.

Surgical

Surgical interventions are performed for decompression, realignment, and stabilization of the vertebral column, depending on the nature of the injury. A laminectomy is performed to decompress the spinal cord with fusion or placement of Harrington rods to stabilize the vertebral column. Realignment is maintained by surgical manipulation of the vertebral column.

If the client has respiratory involvement, an endotracheal tube is put in place to provide mechanical ventilatory support. Following urgent treatment, a tracheostomy is performed to continue ventilation.

Pharmacological

Nitroprusside sodium (Nipride) and nifedipine (Prodardia) are ordered to reduce blood pressure in cases of autonomic dysreflexia.

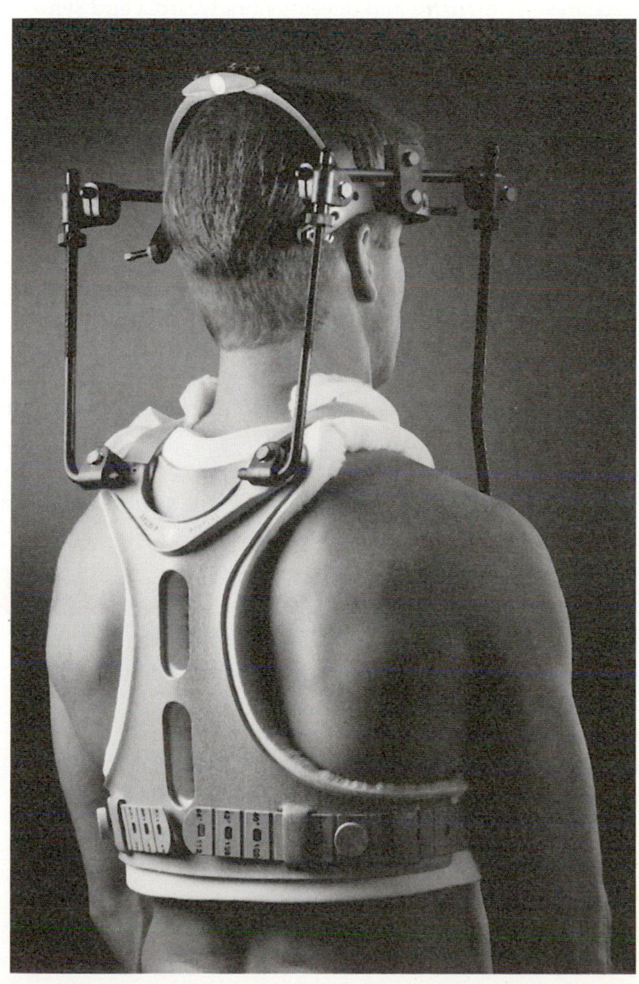

FIGURE 41-18 Halo Vest (*Courtesy of DePuy AcroMed.*)

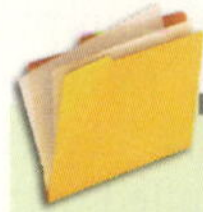

COLLABORATIVECARE

After a Spinal Cord Injury

The interdisciplinary team works together to optimize the functional capabilities of the client. The physical therapist works on activity level, the occupational therapist on ADLs, the speech therapist on swallowing and communication, and nursing coordinates the team and reinforces what the client has been taught. The focus is to prevent disabilities and maximize and strengthen functional ability.

Activity

Initially, immobilization of the spinal column is necessary. In the acute phase, ROM for all joints is performed to prevent mobility loss and muscle contracture. As the spine is stabilized, the client's activity progresses to sitting up in a chair, performing strengthening exercises, and increasing endurance. The nurse observes for the complication of orthostatic hypotension.

Orthostatic hypotension is caused by the venous pooling of blood in the lower body and extremities resulting from impairment of the sympathetic nervous system. The client becomes hypotensive and develops bradycardia and syncope. Asystole may even occur. Prevention of orthostatic hypotension also requires the application of full leg support stockings and pneumatic boots and the gradual lowering of the lower extremities. Monitor the client's vital signs throughout the mobilization process to ascertain tolerance to the procedure. After spinal shock has subsided, active rehabilitation begins.

Nursing Management

After stabilization, turn client frequently to prevent embolism, pneumonia, and skin breakdown. Use log-rolling technique. Keep call light within client's reach. Provide passive and active ROM exercises as allowed. Maintain adequate nutrition and fluid intake. If client has a halo device, perform pin-site care following facility protocol. For a client with a vest, jacket, or brace, provide skin care under the device. Implement bowel and bladder training regimen. Monitor vital signs.

NURSING PROCESS

Assessment

Subjective Data

Subjective assessment involves eliciting input from the client regarding sensation, pain, and history of the accident. Note how the client is coping with the injury, the resulting disability, and the major lifestyle changes that have occurred. Evaluate how the family or support system is coping with the changes.

Objective Data

In the acute phase of care of the client with a spinal cord injury, nursing assessment focuses on the critical factors of airway, breathing, circulation, disability, and exposure.

Assess circulatory status by monitoring vital signs and observing for complications of neurogenic shock; orthostatic hypotension; hypertensive episodes of autonomic dysreflexia; and hemorrhaging.

Assess disability by performing a baseline neurological assessment (as described under the Neurological Assessment section in this chapter).

Exposure refers to removing the client's clothing to perform a thorough assessment of the client's body for skin condition and for entrance and exit wounds. Monitor body temperature because of the neurological deficit in temperature regulation caused by dysfunction of the ANS.

Subacute assessment is based on the level of injury and neurological functioning of the client. With upper motor neuron injuries, the client is at higher risk of developing autonomic dysreflexia; thus, assessment includes monitoring for these signs.

Assess all clients with spinal cord injury for skin condition, bowel and bladder function, respiratory status, and signs and symptoms of complications of immobility. Psychosocial assessment is very important to the well-being of the client.

Nursing diagnoses for a client with a spinal cord injury in the subacute phase of care include the following:

NURSING DIAGNOSES	PLANNING/OUTCOMES	NURSING INTERVENTIONS
Risk for Injury related to motor and sensory deficits secondary to spinal fractures	The client will not experience additional injury.	Assess the client's risk factors for additional injury. Monitor skin condition for pressure areas or shearing injuries from sliding across sheets or the mats in physical therapy. Turn client frequently to prevent pressure areas. Use enough personnel to turn client correctly to maintain alignment of client's spinal column. Provide a call light that the client can operate; teach to call nurse for assistance as necessary. Reinforce wheelchair safety factors and observe client for use of wheelchair.

Nursing diagnoses for a client with a spinal cord injury in the subacute phase of care include the following: (Continued)

NURSING DIAGNOSES	PLANNING/OUTCOMES	NURSING INTERVENTIONS
		Prevent falls when transferring client to wheelchair. Prevent foot drop. Provide passive and active ROM exercises. Maintain adequate fluid intake and nutrition. Provide routine care for halo device by opening vest on one side to cleanse skin under vest at least daily and to assess for skin breakdown. Repeat procedure on the other side. Monitor pin sites of halo device every shift for placement. Perform pin site care using facility protocol.
Powerlessness related to changes in motor and sensory function and in lifestyle	The client will make decisions regarding care, treatment, and future.	Explain all procedures and care options. Allow client to participate in care decisions. Establish an open, trusting relationship with client to foster therapeutic communication. Allow time for client to express concerns, anger, and fears. Foster a positive environment for client to explore feelings and accept disability. Assess for signs and symptoms of depression. Collaborate with mental health professional to provide assistance in coping with lifestyle changes. Collaborate with family and support people to include them in the plan of care.
Autonomic Dysreflexia related to noxious stimulation secondary to overstimulation of ANS	The client will state factors that cause autonomic dysreflexia, describe treatment, and notify the nurse if experiencing symptoms of dysreflexia.	Teach client causes and symptoms of autonomic dysreflexia: increased blood pressure, sudden throbbing headache, chills, pallor, goose flesh, nausea, and/or metallic taste in mouth. Prevent bladder distention and fecal impaction by implementing a bowel and bladder training program. Observe for bradycardia, vasodilatation, flushing, and diaphoresis above the level of spinal cord injury. If these symptoms occur, immediately notify the physician and administer medications as ordered to decrease blood pressure. Raise head of bed and lower legs to reduce blood pressure. Then, remove the noxious stimuli, which may include constrictive clothing, shoes, splints, or linens. Assess client for a distended bladder and empty the bladder if distended. Observe urine for signs of infection and obtain a urine specimen for culture, if needed to identify the cause of the reaction. Check for fecal impaction using xylocaine viscous per physician's order to decrease stimulation. Monitor blood pressure every few minutes.

Evaluation: Evaluate each outcome to determine how it has been met by the client.

PARKINSON'S DISEASE

Parkinson's disease (PD) is a chronic, progressive, degenerative disease affecting the area of the brain controlling movement. The cause is unknown in most cases, but toxicity, hypoxia, or encephalitis may precede the onset of PD. Vascular and genetic factors have been implicated. Drugs such as cocaine, haloperidol (Haldol), and chlorpromazine (Thorazine) may cause a parkinsonian syndrome. The theory is that these drugs interfere with the synthesis or storage of dopamine.

Typical signs and symptoms of PD are muscular rigidity, **bradykinesia** (slowness of voluntary movement and speech), resting tremors, muscular weakness, and loss of postural reflexes. Muscular rigidity along with bradykinesia impairs the person's ability to perform daily activities and speech.

Rigidity is noted along with increased muscle tone when the client is at rest. Stiffness of the trunk, head, and shoulders is present. The rigidity causes loss of arm swing when walking. A cogwheel phenomenon results from the muscle contractions breaking through the muscular rigidity. The alternating rigidity and rhythmic contractions causes a jerking-like movement. Motor impairment progressively affects facial expressions, eye blink, and voice, causing a typical presentation of a mask-like face and a monotone voice.

Resting tremors, usually in the upper extremities, are present when the hand is motionless. The hand moves in a "pill-rolling" motion. When the client is moving or sleeping, the tremors are usually absent. Tremors also occur in other areas, including the feet, lips, tongue, or jaw. The tremors usually begin unilaterally in one area and progress to other areas and then to the opposite side of the body. Anxiety and concentration tend to increase the degree of tremors.

The posture and gait of people with PD is characterized by bowed head, forward-bent trunk, drooped shoulders, and flexed arms. The gait is characterized by shuffling movement and small steps. Balance is affected, resulting in a tendency to fall forward. Figure 41-19 shows the classic posture of a client with PD.

Autonomic dysfunction includes drooling, **dysphagia** (difficulty swallowing), excessive sweating, hyperactivity of oil glands, and constipation. Orthostatic hypotension may occur from loss of the peripheral autonomic response. Urinary incontinence and frequency occur.

Mental changes may also occur. Intelligence is not impaired, but problems with judgment and emotional stability may occur. Dementia, depression, cognitive, perceptual, or memory deficits may occur. The major cause of death is from the complications of immobility or injury. Fatigue increases all signs and symptoms. There is no definitive diagnostic procedure for PD. The diagnosis is based on history, physical, and the client's response to anti-Parkinson's medications. Imaging studies and EEG are performed to rule out other neurological diseases. Position emission tomography (PET) scanning is performed as a way of researching information about the degeneration of the neurons that make dopamine (National Institute Neurological Disorders and Stroke, 2006c). In cases of early onset, it is important to differentiate from Wilson's disease, an increased absorption of copper, for which testing is available.

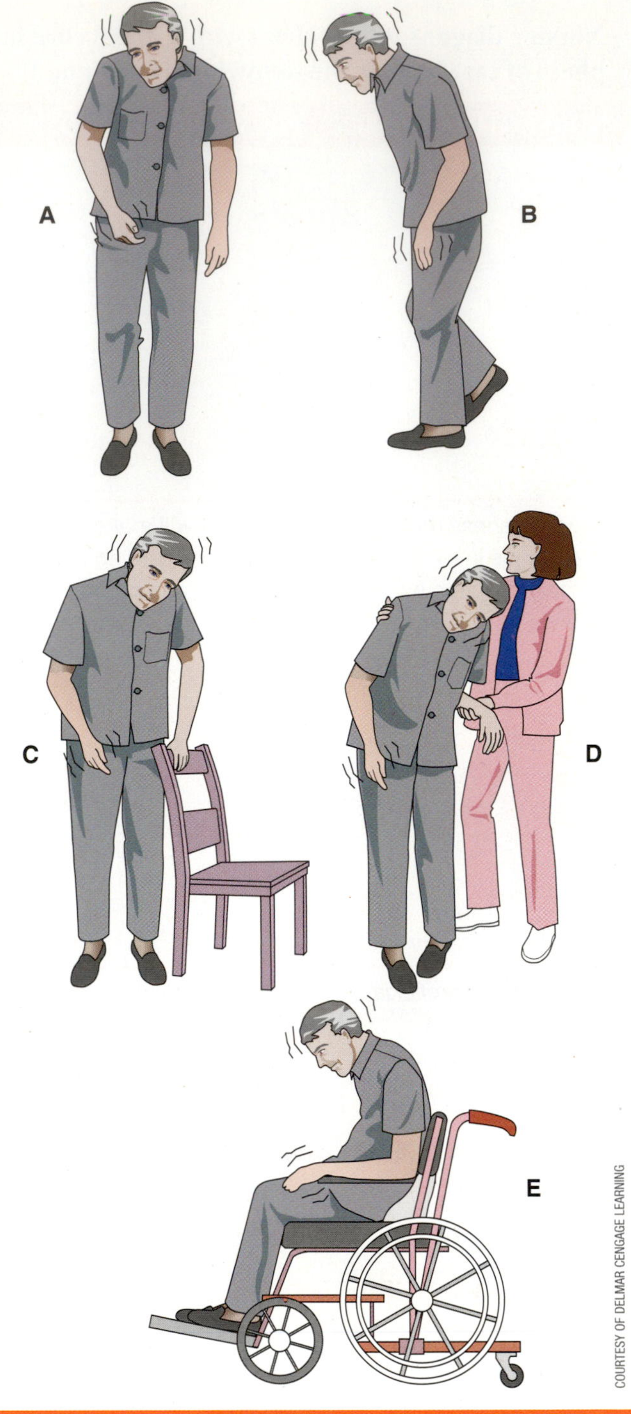

FIGURE 41-19 **Progression of Parkinson's Disease; *A*, Flexion of Affected Arm; *B*, Shuffling Gait; *C*, Need for Sources of Support to Prevent Falling; *D*, Progression of Weakness to Point of Needing Assistance for Ambulation; *E*, Profound Weakness**

Medical–Surgical Management

Medical

The goals of medical management are to control the symptoms, provide supportive therapy and maintenance, maintain function via physiotherapy, and provide psychotherapy as necessary.

Surgical

Surgical procedures are usually only used in clients who are unresponsive to drug therapy. Ablation procedures (thalamotomy, pallidotomy, and subthalamic nucleotomy) destroy areas of the brain to control intractable tremors or akinesia. The risk of causing permanent neurological deficits is high. Deep brain stimulation has been approved by the U.S. Food and Drug Administration to reduce the severity of symptoms (National Institute of Neurological Disorders and Stroke, 2006c). In deep brain stimulation, an electrode is placed in the thalamus, globus pallidus, or subthalamic nucleus to deliver a specific current to the targeted brain location. These jolts of electricity counter balance the hyperactivity of these parts of the brain in clients with PD. Surgical interventions are believed to be most effective in relatively young clients with unilateral tremor. Still in the experimental stages are neural tissue transplants, gene therapy, and stem cell transplantation.

Pharmacological

Drug therapy is used to control the symptoms of PD. Levodopa (L-Dopa) is converted into dopamine in the basal ganglia to replace the deficit of dopamine. Dopamine is not given orally because it is metabolized before reaching the brain. L-Dopa, a precursor to dopamine, is given orally and reaches the brain to be converted into dopamine.

Dopadecarboxylase inhibitors such as carbidopa-levodopa (Sinemet) prevent the conversion of levodopa (L-Dopa) to dopamine in peripheral tissue. Dopamine in the peripheral tissue causes numerous side effects as well as decreases the amount of L-dopa available to the brain. Dopadecarboxylase inhibitors that do not cross the blood–brain barrier are used to inhibit the enzyme that changes L-dopa to dopamine so that the conversion in the brain is not inhibited.

Anticholinergic drugs, such as trihexyphenidyl hydrochloride (Artane), cycrimine hydrochloride (Pagitane hydrochloride), and benztropine mesylate (Cogentin), are administered to control tremors and rigidity. Anticholinergics are used alone for mild symptoms or if levodopa is contraindicated. In other instances, they may be administered in conjunction with levodopa.

PROFESSIONALTIP

Pallidotomy

Pallidotomy, an operation of the 1950s for PD, is being used again. Improved surgical equipment and clients who no longer benefit from medications are causing a resurgence in the use of pallidotomy.

Using MRI and stereotactic equipment, the physician can pinpoint the area of the brain that is causing the unwanted symptoms. A probe is then inserted into the brain through a small hole in the client's head. A small lesion is made deep in the brain to interrupt the electrical pathways that cause the rigidity and tremors. The surgery relieves symptoms but does not cure PD. Furthermore, associated risks such as paralysis and bleeding must be considered (PDF, 2002).

COMMUNITY/HOME HEALTH CARE

Adaptations for the Client with Parkinson's Disease

- Arrange for bathroom facilities and bedroom on first floor.
- Remove crepe- or rubber-soled shoes from the client because they may drag on the floor, especially on carpeting.
- Remove throw rugs or other obstacles over which the client may trip.
- Install handrails at steps, hallways, and bathroom.
- Have no highly waxed floors.
- Provide assistance to client as needed.

CLIENTTEACHING

Parkinson's Disease

Advise caregivers to:

- Encourage the client to be as independent as possible.
- Protect the client from injury and unnecessary stress and fatigue.

Advise the client to:

- Use adaptive devices (e.g., cane, walker, feeding utensils).
- Take medications at scheduled times to maintain level in the body.
- Avoid taking multivitamins, foods high in vitamin B_6, and high-protein foods when taking levodopa.
- Prevent constipation by drinking plenty of water and, possibly, using a stool softener.
- Have intraocular pressure measured frequently if client has glaucoma.

Amantadine hydrochloride (Symmetrel), an antiviral agent, is effective in treating parkinsonian symptoms. The mechanism by which the drug works is not known, but the theory is that it either releases dopamine storage areas or delays the reuptake of dopamine.

Ethopropazine hydrochloride (Parsidol), a phenothiazine derivative, is used in combination with other anti-Parkinson drugs to alleviate symptoms. Dopamine agonist-ergot derivatives, such as pergolide mesylate (Permax), directly stimulate the dopamine receptors to improve the use of available dopamine. The monoamine oxidase inhibitor (MAOI), selegiline hydrochloride (Eldepryl), inhibits dopamine breakdown. The tricyclic antidepressants, amitriptyline hydrochloride (Elavil) and imipramine hydrochloride (Tofranil), alleviate depression as well as other symptoms.

Diet

Puréed foods or tube feedings are required because of dysphagia. Maintenance of weight may require high- or low-calorie diets. In the early stages of PD, a diet high in antioxidants may alleviate some symptoms. Free-radicals are attracted to cells that produce dopamine. Antioxidants are chemicals that destroy free radicals, thus allowing the release of dopamine. A diet that discourages the formation of free radicals is high in complex carbohydrates (such as those found in whole-grain breads and lentils), low in fat, and high in vitamins A and E. See Box 41-2 for foods high in antioxidants. Large doses of supplemental vitamins A and E are also given. A high-fiber diet helps prevent constipation.

SAFETY

Mealtime

The client with PD must be monitored for choking while eating because of dysphagia.

BOX 41-2 FOOD HIGH IN ANTIOXIDANTS

Dark-colored fruits and vegetables:
Leafy green vegetables
Broccoli
Tomatoes
Carrots
Garlic
Red kidney beans
Pinto beans
Blueberries
Cranberries
Strawberries
Plums
Apples

Teas:
Green tea
Black tea

Activity

Ambulation with assistance is necessary to maintain joint mobility and prevent injury. Ambulate at the client's pace because the bradykinesia becomes worse when the client attempts to hurry.

Other Therapies

Physical therapy is directed toward maintaining joint mobility, posture, and gait. Occupational therapy focuses on maintaining optimal functioning in achieving ADL. Speech therapy is used to promote communication and maintain swallowing function. Psychotherapy addresses the implications of living with a chronic disease, depression, and the possible psychiatric side effects of the medication regimen.

Nursing Management

Encourage independence. Fatigue may cause more dependence. Assist to establish a regular bowel routine by encouraging the client to drink at least 2,000 mL of liquids daily and eat high-fiber foods. Provide an elevated toilet seat. Assist client and family to express feelings and frustrations.

NURSING PROCESS

Assessment

Subjective Data

Nursing assessment focuses on functional ability and activities. It includes eliciting client statements about symptom control and emotional status. Ascertain bowel and bladder elimination patterns.

Objective Data

Objective assessment involves evaluation of tremors, muscular rigidity, movement, posture, and gait for degree of impairment. Assessment of swallowing ability is necessary to maintain adequate nutrition and prevent aspiration. Evaluate mental/emotional status for signs and symptoms of depression or dementia.

Assess skin for diaphoresis, or excessive oil production; skin integrity; and signs of injury from falls. Obtain supine, sitting, and standing blood pressures to assess for orthostatic hypotension.

Nursing diagnoses for a client with Parkinson's disease include the following:

NURSING DIAGNOSES	PLANNING/OUTCOMES	NURSING INTERVENTIONS
*Impaired **P**hysical Mobility* related to muscle rigidity, gait disturbance, and bradykinesia	The client will maintain optimal mobility.	Assess degree of muscle involvement by testing ROM, muscular rigidity, tremors, and gait. Perform passive and active ROM exercises to maintain function. Administer medications within the time window that provides a constant therapeutic level for symptom control. Ambulate, as client is able to tolerate. Frequently turn client when in bed.
*Bathing/Hygiene and Dressing/Grooming **S**elf-care Deficit* related to immobility, tremors, and bradykinesia	The client will maintain optimal independence in self-care.	Assess client's ability to perform self-care. Encourage client to perform as much self-care as possible. Consult with occupational therapy for methods to increase the ability to perform self-care. Assist with daily care that the client is unable to perform alone.
*Impaired **S**wallowing* related to neuromuscular Impairment	The client will swallow with minimal choking and coughing and no aspiration.	Position client sitting upright when eating with client's head slightly forward and never extended to facilitate swallowing. Encourage client to take small bites. Provide small bites of food or pureed foods to prevent client from choking. Have suction equipment available during meals.

Evaluation: Evaluate each outcome to determine how it has been met by the client.

MULTIPLE SCLEROSIS

Multiple sclerosis (MS) is a chronic, progressive, degenerative disease of the CNS characterized by a loss of myelin in the brain, spinal cord, or both and by the occurrence of **sclerotic** (hardened) patches (Figure 41-20). The disease interferes with the conduction of impulses. The neurological deficit that occurs depends on which nerve cells are affected. The cause of MS is unclear, but research suggests that it is an abnormal response to the body's immune system. The disease is more prevalent among people of Northern European ancestry (NMSS, 2003). Diagnosis is usually made between the ages of 20 and 50 years. Women are affected two to three times more often than are men (NMSS, 2003).

The white matter of the brain and spinal cord consists of axons covered by a white, lipid substance called myelin. This myelin sheath is an insulator that is involved in the conduction of impulses.

As sclerotic tissue replaces the myelin, neurological function returns. Nerve fibers begin to degenerate as periods of exacerbation become more frequent. Degeneration of the nerve fibers leads to permanent neurological deficits.

Signs and symptoms of MS vary according to the areas of demyelination. The client may have one symptom or a combination of symptoms. Periods of exacerbation and remission also make diagnosis difficult. Symptoms may vary from hour-to-hour or day-to-day. Medical diagnosis is generally based on history and on elimination of other possible diagnoses. Magnetic resonance imaging and CT scan can be used to identify lesions of sclerotic tissue as the disease progresses. Cerebrospinal fluid reveals increased white blood cells, protein, and immunoglobulin (IgG), a diagnostic indicator.

Client symptoms may be sensory, motor, or other disturbances. Sensory symptoms include visual disturbances, numbness, paresthesia (burning, prickling, tingling), pain, and decreased sense of temperature. Motor symptoms include decreased muscle strength, spasticity, paralysis, or bowel and bladder incontinence or retention.

Ataxia (loss of balance or coordination), **nystagmus** (constant, involuntary eye movements in any direction), speech disturbances, tremors, and **vertigo** (dizziness) occur. Other possible symptoms are sexual dysfunction and mood changes ranging from depression to euphoria. Profound fatigue is common.

Exacerbations are frequently precipitated by periods of emotional or physical stress, such as infections, pregnancy, trauma, or fatigue. Hot baths or strenuous exercise may aggravate motor symptoms. Periods of exacerbation last hours to months. Commonly, the periods of exacerbation become more frequent as the disease progresses. Complications such as urinary tract infection, pneumonia, pressure ulcers, contractures, and depression frequently occur. As the disease progresses and permanent neurological deficits occur, the client becomes bedridden, has difficulty speaking and handling oral secretions, and/or develops emotional and intellectual disturbances.

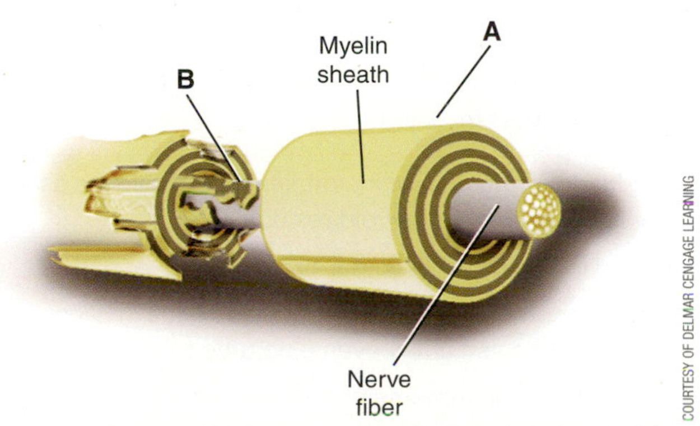

FIGURE 41-20 *A*, Normal Nerve Fiber and Myelin Sheath; *B*, Multiple Sclerosis Destruction of Myelin Sheath

CLIENT TEACHING

Temperature Sensation

Because the client with MS has a decreased sense of temperature, advise to:

- Be careful when cooking or otherwise around the kitchen stove.
- Use a bath thermometer to test bath or shower water so as to prevent burning.
- Use only the low setting on a heating pad.

MEDICAL–SURGICAL MANAGEMENT

There is no cure or specific treatment for MS. Treatment goals are to limit exacerbations, prevent complications, and maintain functional level.

Pharmacological

The treatment of choice for relapsing–remitting MS is interferon beta (Avonex, Betaseron). For 2 or 3 months, clients usually experience flu-like symptoms after each injection. For clients who cannot take either of these two drugs, glatiramer acetate (Copaxone) is an option. The steroids adrenocorticotropic hormone (ACTH) or prednisone (Delasone) are used to decrease periods of exacerbation. Muscle relaxants such as dantrolene sodium (Dantrium) or baclofen (Lioresal) are used for muscle spasticity.

The immunosuppressive agents azathioprine (Imuran), cyclophosphamide (Cytoxan), or cyclosporine (Sandimmune) are administered to decrease immune response. Propantheline bromide (ProBanthine) is often used for urinary frequency and urgency. Bethanechol chloride (Urecholine) may be helpful for the client with a neurogenic bladder. Trimethoprim sulfamethoxazole (Bactrim or Septra) or nitrofurantoin macrocrystals (Macrodantin) is given prophylactically when urinary tract infections are a problem.

CRITICAL THINKING

Multiple Sclerosis

What are the most important things to teach a client with multiple sclerosis?

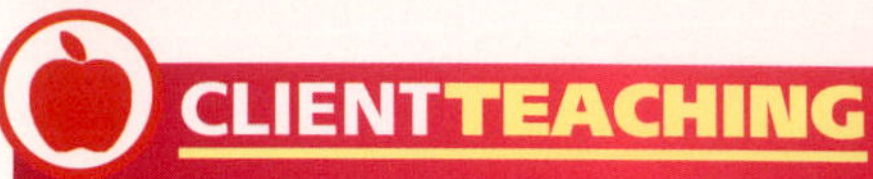

COMMUNITY/HOME HEALTH CARE

Adaptive Devices

To assist the client with MS in self-care:

- Purchase a raised toilet seat.
- Use a long-handled comb and shoe horn.
- Modify clothing so that the client can dress self.

CLIENT TEACHING

Risk of Falling

Advise the client with MS to:

- Use assistive devices such as a walker or cane.
- Wear high-topped (above the ankles) shoes, with laces.
- Watch feet when walking to know where they are stepping.

Diet

A well-balanced diet complete with roughage is necessary to promote bowel elimination. Plenty of fluids are also necessary. If the client is obese, a dietitian should be consulted for meal planning to help the client lose weight while maintaining adequate nutrition.

Activity

The goal of maintaining the highest possible functional level must be individualized to each client. Daily exercise is necessary for clients with limited motor involvement. Physical therapy may be necessary to prevent contractures, maintain muscle strength, or prevent loss of function from spasticity, or for gait training. Passive/active ROM exercises should be done several times per day. Occupational therapy may be used to maintain or attain self-care. Daily skills of cooking, doing laundry, or maintaining a job may also be encouraged.

NURSING MANAGEMENT

Emphasize avoiding stress, infections, and fatigue. Encourage independence and individualized ways of performing daily activities. Stress the importance of a well-balanced diet, high in fiber to prevent constipation. Encourage adequate fluid intake and regular urination.

NURSING PROCESS

ASSESSMENT

Subjective Data

Subjective assessment includes eliciting client statements of symptoms and an historical accounting of exacerbations and remissions. Subjective data should include incidence of visual disturbances, hazy vision, loss of central vision, or diplopia (double vision). Note symptoms of weakness, numbness, fatigue, bowel or bladder problems, sexual dysfunction, emotional instability, vertigo, changes in gait, urinary incontinence or retention, constipation, or difficulty swallowing. Pain is not common.

Objective Data

Objective assessment includes observation of gait for spastic or ataxic gait and a complete neurological examination.

Nursing diagnoses for a client with MS include the following:

NURSING DIAGNOSES	PLANNING/OUTCOMES	NURSING INTERVENTIONS
*Impaired **P**hysical Mobility* related to muscle weakness, ataxia, spasticity, or perceptual impairment	The client will maintain optimal mobility within physical limitations.	Assess motor status every 4 to 24 hours. Provide active and passive ROM every 8 hours. Ambulate client four times daily with use of assistive devices as necessary. Turn bedridden clients every 2 hours. Use pillows, splints, high-topped (above the ankles) shoes with laces to maintain proper body alignment. Encourage client to perform daily activities as able given the limitations of the disease.
*Impaired **U**rinary Elimination* related to changes in innervation of the bladder	The client will have adequate bladder elimination with minimal postvoid residual, urinary tract infections, and episodes of incontinence.	Assess for bladder retention or incontinence. Catheterize as necessary for retention or postvoid residual. Maintain fluid intake of 1,000 cc per day. Develop bladder program to meet individual needs of client. Toilet client at scheduled times even if no urge to go. Assess for signs and symptoms of urinary tract infection, such as elevated temperature and burning on urination.

Nursing diagnoses for a client with MS include the following: (Continued)

NURSING DIAGNOSES	PLANNING/OUTCOMES	NURSING INTERVENTIONS
*Situational Low **S**elf-esteem* related to neuromuscular and perceptual impairment	The client will verbalize positive statements of self-esteem.	Assess client's concept of self in relation to changes brought about by the disease process. Teach client about the disease process. Allow client to verbalize feelings. Assist client in methods of adapting to change. Collaborate with other health care providers, such as mental health counselors and physicians. Refer client to local support groups (see Resources).
***S**exual Dysfunction* related to changes in sensation, genitalia, and musculature, and psychological response to diagnosis	The client will seek counseling concerning sexual dysfunction.	Allow client to verbalize concerns. Suggest adaptations (planning time for sexual contact so as to conserve energy; alternatives to sexual intercourse, such as touching or holding). Refer client to appropriate health care providers.

Evaluation: Evaluate each outcome to determine how it has been met by the client.

SAMPLE NURSING CARE PLAN

The Client with MS

D.B., a 37-year-old wife and the mother of two children, ages 3 years and 5 years, was diagnosed with MS 2 days ago. She presents with decreased sensation (paresthesia) in the lower extremities and muscle weakness of the right lower extremity. She has also experienced episodes of loss of central vision. Fatigue has affected her ability to care for her children and perform household tasks. She states, "I do not know what is going to happen to me." She is crying and states, "I do not know about MS or how I am going to take care of my children," and "I cannot get my housework done, and my children need more from me than I can give right now."

Her employer is concerned about her ability to perform her teaching responsibilities, but because he values her excellence as a teacher, he is willing to give her a few weeks off. She has bruises on her thigh, face, and arm from a fall that she experienced several days ago. The client presents in an outpatient clinic for follow-up care.

NURSING DIAGNOSIS 1 *Deficient **K**nowledge* related to disease process and lifestyle changes as evidenced by client statements, "I do not know what is going to happen to me, I do not know about multiple sclerosis or how I am going to take care of my children."

Nursing Outcomes Classification (NOC)
Knowledge: Disease Process

Nursing Interventions Classification (NIC)
Teaching: Disease Process

PLANNING/OUTCOMES	NURSING INTERVENTIONS	RATIONALE
D.B. will verbalize knowledge of the disease process, pathophysiology,	Assess D.B.'s knowledge of diagnosis, treatment regimen, and lifestyle changes. Ask specific questions.	Provides a frame of reference for D.B., helping her to relate new information and integrate it into her behavior.

(Continues)

SAMPLE NURSING CARE PLAN (Continued)

PLANNING/OUTCOMES	NURSING INTERVENTIONS	RATIONALE
prognosis, and treatment, including the need to reduce stressors in her life, eat a balanced diet, drink adequate fluids, and get adequate rest.	Begin teaching information about the pathophysiology and signs and symptoms of MS.	Assists understanding about the disease.
	Discuss needed lifestyle changes, such as planning rest periods, avoiding stressors, eating a balanced diet, and drinking plenty of fluids.	Helps understanding of necessary changes in life.
	Emphasize the importance of keeping a diary of symptoms, activities, and feelings to identify stressors that exacerbate symptoms.	Helps identify activities that exacerbate the symptoms.
	Provide information about the Multiple Sclerosis Society and offer available pamphlets.	Provides resources to strengthen D.B.'s knowledge base.
	Provide the name and telephone number of a contact from the local MS support group or of another client who is willing to share.	Provides a great deal of emotional support as well as practical solutions to problems.

EVALUATION

D.B. verbalizes accurate information regarding the disease process, prognosis, and treatment. She states that by reducing stressors, maintaining a balanced diet, taking in adequate fluids, and obtaining plenty of rest, she can prevent exacerbations of MS.

NURSING DIAGNOSIS 2 *Impaired **H**ome Maintenance* related to fatigue, neuromuscular impairment, and difficulty in performing child care and household tasks as evidenced by client statements, "I cannot keep my housework done, my children need more from me than I can give right now" and by objective data including decreased sensation in lower extremities, muscle weakness, and fatigue.

Nursing Outcomes Classification (NOC)
Family Functioning

Nursing Interventions Classification (NIC)
Home Maintenance Assistance

PLANNING/OUTCOMES	NURSING INTERVENTIONS	RATIONALE
By the next appointment, D.B. will identify concerns and solutions to accomplishing home maintenance management.	Allow D.B. to verbalize concerns about home maintenance management.	Gives D.B. time to plan and organize tasks and responsibilities within her ability to perform home maintenance management.
	Assist D.B. in identifying areas of concern, items that can be delegated, and possible solutions.	Can then investigate methods of solving her home maintenance problems.
	Assess the extended family's ability to assist with home maintenance management.	May uncover opportunities that she had not considered.

SAMPLE NURSING CARE PLAN (Continued)

PLANNING/OUTCOMES	NURSING INTERVENTIONS	RATIONALE
	Ask D.B. to start identifying ways to decrease workload and to set priorities for expending energy.	Helps focus on needed changes.
	Collaborate with social services to identify social agencies that can be of assistance.	Gives other possible solutions to achieving home maintenance management.
	Plan activities around rest periods.	Conserves strength and prevents fatigue.
	Identify peak energy times and plan activities with peak energy in mind.	Allows more to be accomplished.

EVALUATION

D.B. identifies that she is able to care for her children with the assistance of her husband and her mother, but that she does not have the strength to maintain the housekeeping responsibilities. Following further discussion of family commitments and availability of social supports, D.B. agrees to request weekly assistance from the women's group at her church.

NURSING DIAGNOSIS 3

Risk for Injury related to muscle weakness, decreased sensory perception (vision, tactile, kinesthetic), and fatigue as evidenced by recent falls

NOC: *Risk Control, Falls Occurrence, Safety Behavior: Home Physical Environment, Safety Behavior: Personal*

NIC: *Fall Prevention, Environmental Management: Safety, Surveillance: Risk Identification*

CLIENT GOAL

D.B. will remain free of injury.

NURSING INTERVENTIONS	SCIENTIFIC RATIONALES
1. Teach D.B. to identify risk-factors in the environment.	1. Avoids injury.
2. Teach D.B. to identify risk factors of the disease process.	2. Reduces her risk of injury.
3. Teach D.B. to avoid hot baths, hot tubs, and saunas because muscle weakness and paresthesia is exacerbated by the heat.	3. Prevents exacerbation of weakness and decreased sensation, thereby reducing her risk of injury.
4. Teach safety factors of wearing well-fitting, oxford-style shoes.	4. Decreases the risk of falling by providing support for feet.

EVALUATION

Have injuries been prevented by increasing D.B.'s awareness of the risks involved with the disease process?

AMYOTROPHIC LATERAL SCLEROSIS (LOU GEHRIG'S DISEASE)

Amyotrophic lateral sclerosis (ALS) is a progressive, fatal disease characterized by the degeneration of motor neurons in the cortex, medulla, and spinal cord. The cause of the disease is not known, but a viral immune response or genetic defect are suggested by current research. Age at onset is 40 to 70 years; men are affected two to three times more often than are women. Average time from onset to death is 3 years, but some clients with ALS have remained active 10 to 20 years after diagnosis.

The upper and lower motor neurons degenerate and deteriorate, causing atrophy of the muscles innervated by those neurons. The involved motor neurons are in the anterior horns of the spinal cord and lower brainstem. The muscles of the hands, forearms, and legs usually atrophy first. As the disease progresses, most body muscles are affected. Muscle spasticity and reduced muscle strength result when upper motor neurons are involved. Lower motor neuron involvement causes muscle flaccidity, paralysis, and muscle atrophy. Sensory and intellectual function are not affected. Respiratory function, ability to communicate, and emotional lability are affected as the disease progresses. Drooling, inability to handle oral secretions, and impaired swallowing occur.

MEDICAL–SURGICAL MANAGEMENT

There is no known cure for ALS. The focus of medical management is to treat the symptoms and to promote independence for as long as possible.

Pharmacological

Muscle relaxants including diazepam (Valium), baclofen (Lioresal), and dantrolene sodium (Dantrium) are used to reduce spasticity. Quinidine is prescribed for muscle cramping. Increased salivation is treated with trihexyphenidyl hydrochloride (Artane), clonidine hydrochloride (Catapres), or amitriptyline hydrochloride (Elavil).

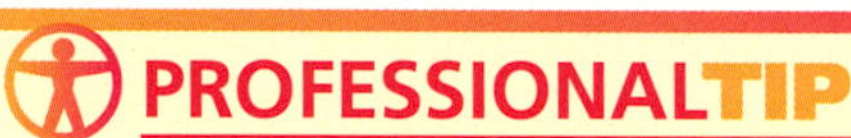

Advance Directives

Before the client with ALS becomes unable to communicate, suggest some advantages of drawing up a living will or giving someone power of attorney for health care.

Riluzole (Rilutek) is the only drug currently approved for use in ALS treatment. Riluzole is believed to reduce damage to motor neurons by decreasing the release of glutamate. Clinical trials with ALS clients showed that riluzole prolongs survival by several months, mainly in those with difficulty swallowing. The drug also extends the time before a client needs ventilation support. Riluzole does not reverse the damage already done to motor neurons, and clients taking the drug must be monitored for liver damage and other possible side effects.

Diet

A regular diet adapted to provide soft, easily chewed food is maintained as long as the client can swallow. Tube feeding is required to prevent aspiration as chewing and swallowing difficulties arise.

Activity

Ambulation and other activities are encouraged as long as possible.

Other Therapies

Physical and occupational therapy are used to maintain ROM and independence as much as possible. Speech therapy promotes maintenance of communication skills. Mental health counseling assists individual and family coping with the fatal disease.

NURSING MANAGEMENT

Encourage independence as long as possible. Assist with personal hygiene and getting in and out of bed. Provide good skin care, turn client often, keep the bed dry, and use pressure-relieving devices. Position client upright for meals and offer soft, solid foods. When gastrostomy feedings are needed, teach client or family how to administer them.

NURSING PROCESS

ASSESSMENT

Subjective Data

Subjective data gathered include the client's and family's emotional status and knowledge status. The client may also indicate chewing or swallowing difficulties as well as dyspnea and fatigue.

Objective Data

Objective assessment includes evaluation of muscle weakness, muscle atrophy, spasticity of upper extremities, flaccid paralysis, difficulty chewing and swallowing, and respiratory status.

Nursing diagnoses for a client with ALS include the following:

NURSING DIAGNOSES	PLANNING/OUTCOMES	NURSING INTERVENTIONS
*Impaired **Physical** Mobility* related to muscle atrophy, weakness, and spasticity	The client will maintain the highest possible functional ability within limitations of the disease.	Provide active and passive ROM at least twice daily. Use assistive devices to prevent contractures, for ambulation, and for muscle strengthening.

Nursing diagnoses for a client with ALS include the following: (Continued)

NURSING DIAGNOSES	PLANNING/OUTCOMES	NURSING INTERVENTIONS
		Assess breath sounds for presence of congestion; skin for pressure areas; and legs for thrombophlebitis. Turn every 2 hours.
*Impaired Verbal **C**ommunication* related to weakness of muscles used for speech	The client will communicate verbally or through an alternate communication method as speech muscles deteriorate.	Prolong verbal communication with speech therapy interventions consisting of voice projection and speech devices. Develop alternate methods of communicating prior to the loss of verbal skills, e.g., eye-blinking for "yes" and "no"; communication boards, if any arm movement remains; and computer programs can be used.
*Ineffective **B**reathing Pattern* related to weakness of respiratory muscles and to fatigue	The client will maintain an adequate PaO_2 level.	Assess breathing patterns frequently and observe for aspiration and the loss of the swallow reflex. Assess breath sounds every 4 to 8 hours, depending on the progress of the disease. Provide good pulmonary hygiene to prevent aspiration and pneumonia by liquefying secretions and suctioning. Turn from side to side to allow oral secretions to drain from mouth; suction oral pharynx, as necessary. Provide ventilation support, as ordered.
***P**owerlessness* related to loss of control over life; physical dependence; and presence of a fatal disease	The client will inform significant others of wishes while still able to communicate, so as to maintain some control over decisions.	Explore client and family emotional status and coping abilities. Allow client to verbalize feelings while still able to communicate and make decisions in daily care. Promote discussion of client's wishes with family, health care team, and legal representative while client is still able to speak. Provide client education about the disease process, support groups, and counseling to provide support.

Evaluation*:* Evaluate each outcome to determine how it has been met by the client.

ALZHEIMER'S DISEASE

Alzheimer's disease (AD) is a progressive, degenerative neurological disease wherein brain cells are destroyed. The cerebral cortex atrophies, and neuron loss and changes within the brain cells occur. The neurons of the frontal and medial temporal lobes are affected, with resultant biochemical and structural changes. Characteristic physiologic changes are neurofibrillary tangles and amyloid plaques (deposits of protein), which interfere with the cells' ability to transmit impulses. These changes are found in the association areas and scattered throughout the cortex. The hippocampus, that part of the limbic system responsible for learning, memory, and emotions, is affected. The cells most affected are neurons that use acetylcholine as the neurotransmitter. The size of the brain and the

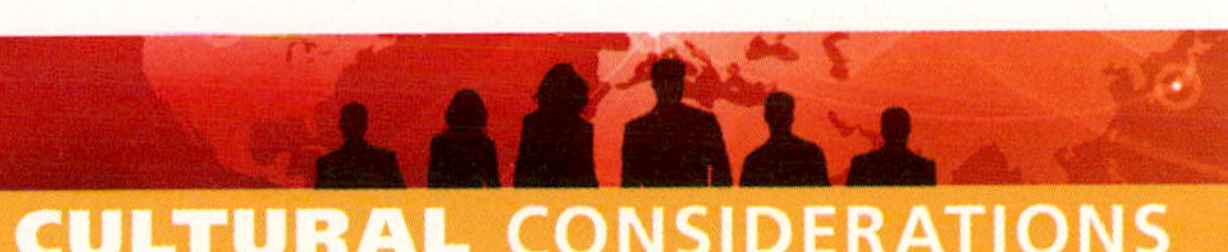

CULTURAL CONSIDERATIONS

African Americans show a greater incidence rate of AD than the Caucasian population. Latinos appear to develop the symptoms almost 7 years earlier on average than non-Latino Americans (Alzheimer's Association, 2008).

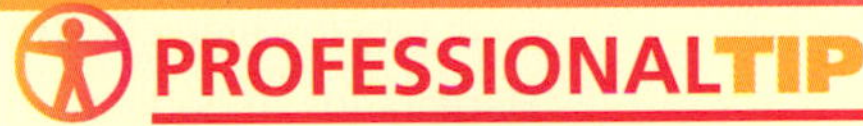

PROFESSIONAL TIP

Sniff Test to Diagnose AD

A new way to diagnose AD, PD, and other neurodegenerative disorders may be through evaluating the client's sense of smell. Measuring how deeply clients inhale a strong or unpleasant odor may be an early warning of brain dysfunction. A device known as a Sniff Magnitude test may be able to identify one of the earliest symptoms of some neurodegenerative diseases, the loss of the sense of smell. Clients with a normal sense of smell take only a small inhalation before detecting strong or unpleasant odors, while those with a damaged sense of smell will inhalation longer and deeper. The test is portable and can be administered to clients with decreased intellectual and language abilities (Hally, 2007; Frank, Gesteland, Bailie, Rybalsky, Seiden, & Dulay, 2006).

amount of acetylcholine both decrease. An increased amount of aluminum is found in the brain tissue on autopsy (Hickey, 2008; Smeltzer, Bare, Hinkle, & Cheever, 2008).

The cause of AD is unknown. Identified risk factors are advanced age, female gender, head injury, a history of thyroid disorders, and chromosomal abnormalities. More than five million Americans have AD, a 10% increase from the last official tally in 2002, and a number expected to more than triple by 2050 as the elderly population increases (Alzheimer's Association, 2008).

Diagnosis is difficult because of the variety in clinical manifestations and the lack of a test specific to AD. Diagnosis is thus based on the clinical picture and the exclusion of other conditions that cause similar clinical patterns, such as overmedication, metabolic disorders, depression, thyroid imbalance, or brain tumors. Neuropsychological tests measuring memory, problem solving, attention, counting, and language assist physicians in diagnosing AD (Alzheimer's Disease Education and Referral Center, 2002). A CT scan may show evidence of brain atrophy, and a PET scan will show changes in the metabolism of the cerebral cortex.

The stages of AD are scaled from early to late. Different authors identify from three to six stages of the disease. The time frame for each stage varies from person to person. Table 41-6 lists clinical manifestations of early, middle, and late stages of AD.

In late stages of the disease, an EEG may indicate general slowing of brain waves. Definitive diagnosis is determined on autopsy with a brain biopsy. Although generally a disease of older people, AD occurs in people ages 40 to 50.

The personal freedom of the family caring for a member who has AD becomes more limited as the disease progresses. Many clients with advanced AD cannot be left alone. Respite care is important for the physical and mental health of the caregiver. With respite care, someone else (e.g., another family member, a friend, or a hired professional licensed

TABLE 41-6 Stages of Alzheimer's Disease

STAGE	CLINICAL MANIFESTATIONS
Stage 1: Early	Forgetfulness, often subtle and masked by client Indecisiveness Increasing self-centeredness; decreasing interest in others, environment, social activities Difficulty in learning new information Slowed reaction time Beginnings of compromised performance at home and at work
Stage 2: Middle	Progressing forgetfulness, inability to remember names of family members or close friends Tendency to lose things Confusion Fearfulness Easily induced frustration and irritability; sometimes, angry outbursts Repetitive storytelling Beginnings of communication problems (inability to remember words, apparent aphasia) Inability to follow simple directions Difficulty in calculating numbers Beginnings of getting lost in familiar places Evasive or anxious interactions with others Physical activity (pacing, wandering) Changes in sleep–rest cycle (with frequent activity at night) Changes in eating patterns (possible constant hunger or none at all) Neglect of ADL and personal hygiene, changes in bowel and bladder continence, and dressing difficulties Inability to maintain safety without supervision Losses of social behaviors Paranoia
Stage 3: Late	Inability to communicate Inability to eat Incontinence (urine and feces) Inability to recognize family or friends Confinement to bed Total dependence relative to care

COURTESY OF DELMAR CENGAGE LEARNING

COMMUNITY/HOME HEALTH CARE

Safe Environment for the Client with AD

- Keep furniture in the same place.
- Orient client to surroundings and reorient as necessary.
- Keep floors free of clutter.
- Provide adequate lighting.
- Monitor temperature of hot water and food.
- Maintain monitoring system to prevent outside wandering.
- Prevent access to sharp items such as knives and razors; hot items such as coffee pot and heaters; poisonous solutions such as cleaning supplies, paints, medications, and insecticides; and hazardous items such as power tools, guns, and electric fans.

practical/vocational nurse or registered nurse) comes in to care for the client with Alzheimer's while the primary caregiver gets away for a time. Respite care should be provided on a routine basis, such as every 2 or 3 weeks or as often as is feasible.

Medical–Surgical Management

There is no curative treatment for AD. Management of the client is geared toward controlling undesirable symptoms and behaviors.

Pharmacological

No drug can stop the progression of AD. Cholinesterase inhibitors (galantamine hydrobromide [Razadyne], rivastigmine tartrate [Exelon], and donepezil hydrocholoride [Aricept]) slow the progression of the disease and enhance cognition in early to middle stage AD. N-methyl-D-asparate (NMDA) Receptor Antagonist, memantine hydrocholoride (Namenda), delays progression of symptoms in moderate-to-severe AD. Other medications treat symptoms such as anxiety, depression, and insomnia.

CRITICAL THINKING

Parkinson's and Alzheimer's

What are the similarities between Parkinson's disease and AD?

What distinguishes Parkinson's disease from AD?

Diet

A high-fiber diet is used to prevent constipation. A high-calorie diet is needed for hyperactive clients. Frequent feedings of high nutritive value are preferable to three meals a day.

Nursing Management

Maintain a safe, structured environment and a consistent daily schedule for the client. Develop memory aids and cues to help the client remember. Support family in adjusting to the client's altered cognitive ability.

NURSING PROCESS

Assessment

Subjective Data

Data about sleeping and eating habits is collected. Each client is assessed for individual signs and symptoms. The client is an expert at hiding these deficits in the early stages of the disease. A family interview is helpful in ascertaining health and personal history.

Objective Data

An objective neurological examination with particular attention to memory loss and gradual loss of thought processes and impaired judgment is important. Eating patterns, bowel and bladder control, aggressiveness, depression, ambulation, agitation, restlessness, sleep patterns, vision, and hearing are assessed. The client's ability to provide self-care, manage finances, drive, prepare meals, use the telephone, perform housekeeping, communicate needs, and perceive the environment also are assessed. Attention is directed to assessing the support system, the family caregiver, support groups, and availability of respite care for the caregiver. The care of the caregiver is often the focus of nursing care of the AD client.

Nursing diagnoses for the client with Alzheimer's include the following:

NURSING DIAGNOSES	PLANNING/OUTCOMES	NURSING INTERVENTIONS
Risk for Injury related to inability to perceive danger in the environment, confusion, impaired judgment, and weakness	The client will not experience injury.	Assess client's ability to perceive environmental hazards. Teach family to provide a safe home environment. Maintain a safe environment: eliminate clutter, position furniture/equipment in same place, monitor temperature of hot water and food, maintain monitoring system to prevent wandering into adverse climate or into traffic, provide adequate lighting, orient client and family to surroundings and reorient as necessary. Ensure that the client wears well-fitting, tied shoes to reduce risk of falls.

(*Continues*)

Nursing diagnoses for the client with Alzheimer's include the following: (Continued)

NURSING DIAGNOSES	PLANNING/OUTCOMES	NURSING INTERVENTIONS
*Disturbed **T**hought Processes* related to neuron degeneration, sleep deprivation	The client will maintain optimal cognitive ability.	Assess for cognitive, memory, and communication deficits. Develop memory aids and cues to help client remember. Maintain a consistent environment and daily schedule. Approach client in a quiet, nonthreatening manner. Do not confront client with reality if it will only upset and agitate him. For example, do not tell a 90-year-old client who wants his mother that she is dead. Attend to nonverbal cues for unmet needs (e.g., pacing, grimacing, crying, agitation). The client may be hungry, have a full bladder, or be unable to ask to be repositioned. Obtain a photo of client that can be recognized by the client. A current photo of client may appear as a stranger to the client, but a photo of the client at age 20 or 30 may be remembered. Give simple, single instructions.
*Disturbed **S**leep Pattern* related to disorientation or irritability	The client will sleep 4 to 5 hours each night.	Advise the client to avoid caffeine. Maintain a quiet environment. Provide comfort measures. Provide a night light. Increase daytime activities to tolerance, and use exercise to tire client.

Evaluation: Evaluate each outcome to determine how it has been met by the client.

CRITICAL THINKING

Alzheimer's Disease

V. A. is a 73-year-old male client diagnosed 5 years ago with AD. He has been married for 52 years and owns a hardware store now managed by his son. Spanish is his native language, but he is fluent in English. At this time he is having significant word-finding difficulties and is unable to name common objects in both English and Spanish. He requires his wife's assistance to eat, bathe, toilet, dress, and take medications. He is able to walk independently. Until 2 weeks ago, his wife drove him to the hardware store daily, where he would interact with customers and restock nails, screws, and other small items. The last day at the store, though, he wandered out when his son was occupied with customers and became lost. He was found by the police 2 miles from the store. His son now wants V.A. placed in a nursing home, but his wife feels that he should remain at home until he "no longer knows who I am."

1. Identify V.A.'s stage of Alzheimer's disease and explain the rationale.
2. Identify safety issues and appropriate nursing interventions.
3. How can the nurse help the family reach consensus on appropriate placement and care for V.A.?

GUILLAIN-BARRÉ SYNDROME

Guillain-Barré syndrome (GBS) is an acute inflammatory process involving the motor and sensory neurons of the peripheral nervous system. The cause of Guillain-Barré syndrome is not known, but most cases are preceded by a nonspecific infection. There may be an autoimmune or viral basis for this syndrome. Both spinal and cranial motor nerves are involved. The demyelination process begins in distal nerves and ascends symmetrically. Remyelination occurs from proximal to distal (Hickey, 2008).

Clinical manifestations occur in differing patterns but include motor weakness and areflexia, or absence of reflexes. Characteristically, motor weakness begins in the legs and progresses up the body. Respiratory failure results from loss of respiratory muscle function. Cranial nerve involvement results in facial muscle deficits, difficulty in swallowing, and autonomic dysfunctions. Autonomic functions possibly affected are cardiac rhythm, blood pressure regulation, gastrointestinal mobility, and urine elimination.

Sensory involvement causes paresthesia and pain in the hands and feet. The pain progresses up the body and may interfere with sleep.

The three stages of Guillain-Barré syndrome are acute onset, lasting 1 to 3 weeks, the plateau period, lasting several days to 2 weeks, and the recovery phase, which involves remyelination and may last up to 2 years.

Diagnosis is based on the clinical picture of a recent viral infection and motor and possibly sensory deficits, along with characteristic diagnostic results. These results include both an elevated protein level in CSF without elevation of red blood cells or white blood cells and EMG showing slowed nerve conduction velocity of paralyzed muscles.

Medical–Surgical Management

Medical

The goal of medical management is prevention and treatment of complications such as immobility, infection, and respiratory failure.

Plasma exchanges decrease the severity and duration of symptoms. Plasmapheresis is performed in severe cases. Complete plasma exchange removes the antibodies affecting the myelin sheath. Three to four exchanges 1 to 2 days apart are initiated within the first 2 weeks of diagnosis of Guillain-Barré. Plasmapheresis also is used late in the disease process for continued demyelination or lack of progress in remyelination. Mechanical ventilatory support may be required. Blood gas monitoring is used to assess respiratory function.

Surgical

Those who develop respiratory failure require a tracheostomy along with mechanical ventilation.

 Pharmacological

Steroids, such as adrenocorticotropic hormone (ACTH) and prednisone (Detasone), and immunosuppressive agents, such as azathioprine (Imuran) or cyclophosphamide (Cytoxan), slow the demyelination process. Low doses of anticoagulants, such as heparin, prevent thrombophlebitis.

Diet

A balanced diet is necessary to prevent tissue and muscle breakdown and to promote healing. If severe paralysis is present, a gastrostomy tube is used to provide adequate nutrition.

Activity

Physical therapy maintains range of motion and muscle strength. Occupational therapy activities teach the client to maintain optional self-care within the limitation of the disease process. Pool therapy, or exercising in a swimming pool, maintains and strengthens muscles.

Nursing Management

Monitor vital signs, LOC, pulse oximetry, ABGs, and for ascending sensory loss, which precedes motor loss. Turn client frequently and encourage coughing and deep breathing. Provide skin care to prevent skin breakdown and position client to prevent contractures. Perform passive ROM exercises. Apply antiembolism stockings and assess Homans' sign. Provide eye and mouth care every 4 hours if there is facial paralysis. Monitor I&O and encourage adequate fluid intake. Offer prune juice and high-fiber diet to prevent constipation.

NURSING PROCESS

Assessment

Subjective Data

Subjective data include client statements about return of sensation, pain, respiratory function, and knowledge.

Objective Data

Assessment includes the status of motor and sensory functions, which are monitored continuously in the acute phase of the illness. Monitor progression of loss of function from distal to proximal with particular emphasis on respiratory status. Decreased depth and quality of respirations and diminished breath sounds may be found. Monitor status of autonomic functions by assessing blood pressure, cardiac rhythm, urinary elimination, and bowel sounds. Assessment for complications of immobility includes breath sounds, signs of thrombophlebitis, loss of ROM, skin condition, and temperature.

Nursing diagnoses for a client with Guillain-Barré syndrome include the following:

NURSING DIAGNOSES	PLANNING/OUTCOMES	NURSING INTERVENTIONS
*Ineffective **Breathing** Pattern* related to loss of respiratory muscle function	The client will be adequately ventilated.	Monitor respiratory status of client by assessing breath sounds, respiratory rate, and respiratory quality. Position client to facilitate maximal expansion of the chest wall for optimal breathing. Monitor oxygenation by assessing skin color, mental status, pulse oximeter readings, and blood gas values. Administer oxygen as ordered. Report failing respiratory status to the physician. Provide mechanical ventilation for respiratory failure.
*Impaired **Physical** Mobility* related to progressive loss of motor function	The client will avoid complications of immobility (pneumonia, thrombophlebitis, pressure areas, and loss of ROM).	Monitor status of motor and sensory functions in an ongoing fashion. Have client turn, deep breathe, and cough every 2 hours. Suction client as necessary. Perform respiratory assessment for diminished breath sounds or congestion. Monitor vital signs (blood pressure, pulse, respiration, and temperature) every 4 to 8 hours. Assess for calf tenderness, redness, or increased warmth. Monitor for positive Homans' sign, indicative of deep vein thrombosis.

(*Continues*)

Nursing diagnoses for a client with Guillain-Barré syndrome include the following: (Continued)

NURSING DIAGNOSES	PLANNING/OUTCOMES	NURSING INTERVENTIONS
		Perform ROM to lower extremities every 2 to 4 hours. Use PlexiPulse boots, which are intermittent-pumping boots that promote return blood flow from the lower extremities. Administer low doses of heparin or other anticoagulants as prescribed. Apply antiembolism stockings or alternating compression devices. Assess condition of skin for pressure areas. Massage client's back and pressure points with lotion three times a day. Use specialty mattress. Assist client to sitting position in wheelchair two to three times daily. Progress to ambulation as motor function returns. Apply high-topped shoes to keep feet in correct alignment.
*Dressing/Grooming **S**elf-care Deficit* related to decreased motor function	The client will have self-care needs met.	Encourage self-care within the limitations of the neurological deficits. Provide daily care needs that client is unable to perform. Maintain muscle strength and ROM with physical therapy. Provide ROM to all extremities three to four times daily. Initiate rehabilitation following acute phase of illness with strengthening exercises, occupational therapy, and getting client out of bed several times per day to build strength and endurance.

Evaluation: Evaluate each outcome to determine how it has been met by the client.

HEADACHE

Headache, or **cephalalgia**, the condition of pain in the head, is caused by stimulation of pain-sensitive structures in the cranium, head, or neck. Headaches are symptoms rather than a disease.

The pain-sensitive areas of the intracranial structure include the peripheral nerves, cerebral vasculature, and parts of the dura mater. The external supporting structures of the skin, muscles, and nasal passages are also sensitive to pain. The skull, brain tissue, and most of the meninges are insensitive to pain.

More than 45 million people in the United States each year have chronic, recurring headaches (National Headache Foundation, 2002). Headaches are generally classified as either primary or secondary.

PRIMARY HEADACHES

Primary headaches are not caused by an underlying medical condition. They include tension-type, migraine, and cluster headaches (AHS, 2007) (Table 41-7).

Tension-Type Headache

The most common type of headache is the tension type (ACHE, 2007). The ache is steady rather than throbbing, affects both sides of the head, and occurs frequently, sometimes daily.

Migraine Headaches

Up to 18% of women experience migraine headaches each year, compared to 6% of men (AHS, 2007). Migraine headaches are vascular and recurrent. The initial vasoconstriction causes neurological symptoms or an aura before the vasodilation that causes the headache. The aura is a visual disturbance typically consisting of brightly colored or blinking lights or a pattern moving across the field of vision. When only the aura occurs, and there is no pain in the head, the migraine is termed "silent." Migraines generally are a throbbing on one side of the head. Other symptoms include irritability, anorexia, nausea, vomiting, and photophobia. Some migraine headaches are triggered by certain foods or chemicals.

Cluster Headaches

A cluster headache develops around or behind one eye and is very severe. Generally, it awakens the person from sleep. The affected eye may tear and the nose becomes congested on the same side. These headaches occur in clusters daily for weeks or months, and then disappear for a year or more. Most cluster headaches occur in men. Alcohol often triggers attacks.

SECONDARY HEADACHES

Secondary headaches are the result of pathological conditions such as aneurysm, brain tumor, or inflamed cranial nerves.

TABLE 41-7 Primary Headache Patterns

TYPE	AURA	PAIN	TYPICAL PATTERN	DURATION
Tension	None	Steady ache	Usually begins gradually in frontal or temporal areas; affects both sides of the head; occur frequently, maybe daily	Hours
Classic Migraine	Duration of 15 to 30 minutes; sensory, usually visual (bright spots, zig-zag lines), unilateral or bilateral numbness or tingling in lips, face, or hand; difficulty thinking; confusion or drowsiness; sometimes preceded by premonition 24 hours before	Throbbing, intense; unilateral; tenderness in scalp; muscle contractions in neck and scalp followed by feelings of exhaustion	Periodic, recurrent; usually begins on awakening; begins in childhood or early adolescence; tends to be familial; nausea and vomiting typical; sensitivity to light and sound	Hours to days
Cluster	None	Intense throbbing; unilateral pain in orbitotemporal area	Causes awakening two to three times during the night; accompanied by watering eyes, nasal congestion, runny nose, facial flushing over the throbbing area; after cluster headaches for days, weeks, or months may be free of symptoms for a year or more; same side of head usually involved; usually in men	30 minutes to 2 hours

COURTESY OF DELMAR CENGAGE LEARNING

The headache is caused by compression, inflammation, or hypoxia of pain-sensitive structures.

MEDICAL–SURGICAL MANAGEMENT

Medical

Medical management is based on the underlying cause of the headache. A thorough history of headache pattern, dietary pattern, and coping pattern is essential. Underlying pathology of brain tumor, aneurysm, and infection is ruled out. If pathology is identified, secondary headache is diagnosed and, therefore, treatment is based on findings. If no cause is found, management of primary headache is based on symptoms.

Surgical

Surgical management includes repair of an aneurysm or resection of a brain tumor.

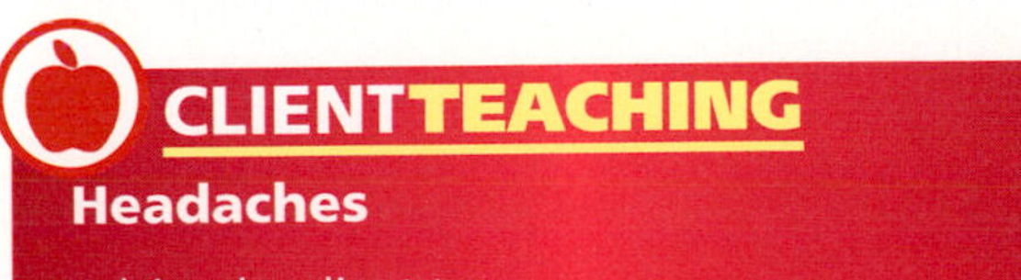

CLIENT TEACHING

Headaches

Advise the client to:

- Keep a diary of headache history to ascertain pattern.
- Avoid foods that trigger headache.
- Reduce salt intake.
- Practice relaxation techniques.

Pharmacological

Management is either abortive, to stop the headache, or prophylactic, to prevent reoccurrence or to decrease frequency of headaches. Abortive therapy for migraine headaches includes naproxen (Aleve), ibuprofen (Advil), sumatriptan (Imitrex), rizatriptan (Maxalt), zolmitriptan (Zomig), naratriptan (Amerge), almotriptan (Axert), and older drugs like cafergot, containing ergotamine and caffeine (McGuire, 2002). Promethazine hydrochloride (Phenergan) controls nausea and vomiting.

Prophylactic treatment includes the beta-blockers propranolol hydrochloride (Inderal) and methysergide maleate (Sansert), which prevent dilation of the blood vessels and interrupt the serotonin mechanism. Clonidine hydrochloride (Catapres) directly affects the ability of the blood vessels to constrict or dilate. Tricyclic antidepressants, such as amitriptyline hydrochloride (Elavil), block the uptake of serotonin.

Diet

A strict food diary is kept to identify precipitating foods. After all suspect foods are eliminated from the diet, skin testing for allergies is performed. Introduction of suspect foods is done one at a time to identify triggering foods. Alcohol, cured meats containing nitrates, aged cheeses, monosodium glutamate (MSG), citrus fruits, chocolate, and red wines are common precipitating foods.

Activity

Activities that precipitate headaches are identified and eliminated if possible. Stressful situations are frequently precipitating agents. Biofeedback, relaxation techniques, stress reduction, and development of coping mechanisms are useful in reducing the occurrence of headaches caused by stress and tension.

Nursing Management

Nursing interventions focus on relieving pain and assisting the client in managing the pain. Identifying methods of decreasing pain, such as effective use of medications and managing the environment to minimize stimulation from light, noise, and activity, are also nursing priorities.

Assist the client to develop a plan for accomplishing daily activities when incapacitated by a headache. Teach the client to keep a diary of headache history to determine patterns in headache development. Assist the client in changing lifestyle to decrease the incidence of headaches by minimizing stress, avoiding certain foods, reducing salt intake during premenstrual time frame, and using relaxation techniques.

TRIGEMINAL NEURALGIA (TIC DOULOUREUX)

Trigeminal neuralgia is a condition of cranial nerve V and is characterized by abrupt paroxysms of pain and facial muscle contractions. **Neuralgia** is nerve pain. The pain follows one of the three branches of the trigeminal nerve: the ophthalmic, maxillary, or mandibular. The last two branches are most commonly affected (Figure 41-21).

The etiology of trigeminal neuralgia is not known, but injury, dental caries, dental work, and anatomic position of the nerves have been identified as possible causes. Pain begins when trigger points are stimulated, causing periods of intense pain and facial twitching lasting from seconds to minutes. These periods may last several weeks to months. Periods of remission interspersed with exacerbations occur with increasing frequency with advancing age (Hickey, 2008).

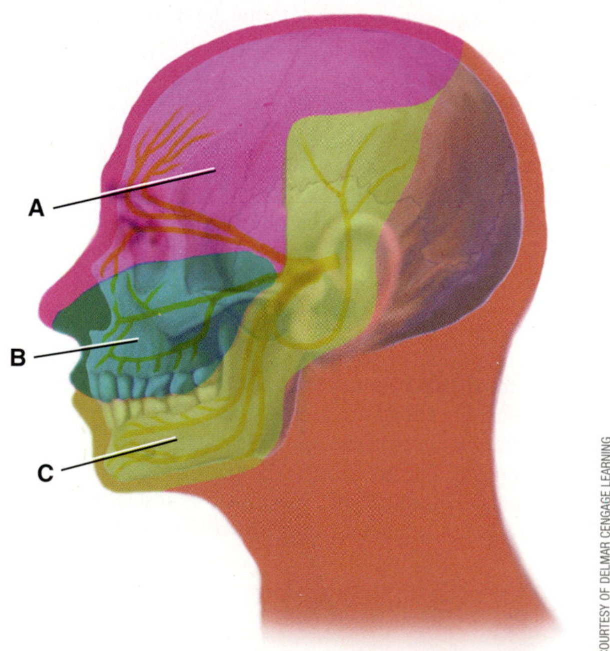

Figure 41-21 Areas of Face Innervated by the Trigeminal Nerve (CN-1); *A*, Ophthalmic; *B*, Maxillary; *C*, Mandibular

CLIENT TEACHING

Dental Work on the Client with Trigeminal Neuralgia

The client with trigeminal neuralgia should:

- Plan to have dental work done during a period of remission.
- Inform the dentist of the condition.
- Maintain good dental hygiene, especially during remission.

Medical–Surgical Management

Drug therapy, nerve blocks, and surgery are treatment modalities for trigeminal neuralgia.

Surgical

Surgical approaches to relieve pain include percutaneous electrocoagulation with radio frequency. This procedure affects the pain-sensory fibers but causes little damage to the touch, proprioception, and motor fibers. Longer-term relief or permanent relief may be obtained.

Pharmacological

Phenytoin (Dilantin) and carbamazepine (Tegretol) are used to shorten the length of the paroxysmal pain. Nerve blocks using alcohol and phenol injections into the nerve provide temporary relief for 8 to 16 months.

Nursing Management

Goals of nursing interventions are relief of pain, prevention of injury, prevention of self-care deficits, and promotion of social interaction. The client with trigeminal neuralgia frequently experiences such severe pain that grooming, talking, and eating are avoided. It is especially important to provide good oral hygiene if the client is on phenytoin (Dilantin) because the medication causes hyperplasia of the gums. Teach the client to identify both the trigger points that stimulate the pain and ways to avoid those areas without neglecting daily needs.

The client who has had surgery may have lost the mechanisms that protect the eye from injury, and is taught not to touch his eye and to observe for redness of the eye and conjunctiva. Following surgery, the client may not feel pain caused by dental caries, so routine visits to the dentist for oral examination are needed.

ENCEPHALITIS, MENINGITIS

Encephalitis is inflammation of the brain. **Meningitis** is inflammation of the meninges. The most common cause of encephalitis or meningitis is a virus. Bacteria, fungi, or parasites also are causative factors. Meningococcal meningitis is highly contagious. Contacts of the client are identified and prophylactic medication is recommended. The virus or other causative agent enters the brain either through the bloodstream as a direct extension of trauma or by nerve pathways.

The inflammatory process causes demyelination of white matter and degeneration of neurons. Cerebral edema, hemorrhage, and necrosis of brain tissue also occur. Clinical manifestations vary depending on the causative agent, area of involvement, and degree of damage to nerve tissue. Fever, headache, nuchal rigidity, photophobia, irritability, lethargy, nausea, and vomiting are typical signs and symptoms. As the disease progresses, level of consciousness decreases and other neurological dysfunctions occur, including motor weakness, aphasia, seizures, behavioral changes, or even death. A lumbar puncture is performed to test CSF for the causative agent, presence of white blood cells or red blood cells, and elevated protein level. A complete blood count identifies the presence of viral or bacterial infection.

Medical–Surgical Management

Medical

Treatment is supportive and based on presenting symptoms. The aim of treatment is to prevent or decrease increased intracranial pressure and to minimize neurological deficits. Intravenous fluids are given to rehydrate the client. Clients are placed in isolation until the cause of meningitis can be determined.

Pharmacological

Antibiotics or antiinfectives are administered in massive doses as appropriate for the causative agent. They are given intravenously or intrathecally into the spinal canal. Most viral agents do not respond to antibiotics or antiinfectives. Glucocorticosteroids are administered to prevent cerebral edema. Osmotic diuretics may be used to reduce cerebral edema. To prevent seizures, anticonvulsants are often ordered. Antipyretics are often given to reduce fever.

Diet

Optimal nutritional status is maintained to promote response to the infection.

Activity

A quiet environment with minimal stimulation from noise, light, or client activity is maintained. Routine turning, ROM exercises, pulmonary hygiene, and skin care are required to prevent the complications of immobility.

Nursing Management

In the acute stage, monitor the client for changes in neurological status, especially for changes in level of consciousness and for signs of increasing intracranial pressure. A quiet environment decreases external stimulation. Observe the client for seizure activity and protect from injury. Comfort measures such as oral hygiene, tepid baths, and administration of analgesics for relief of headaches are offered.

HUNTINGTON'S DISEASE

Huntington's disease (HD) is a chronic, progressive hereditary disease of the nervous system. It is characterized by a progressive involuntary choreiform movement and progressive dementia.

The cells of the basal ganglia, which control movement, die prematurely. Cells in the cerebral cortex also die, interfering with thought processes, memory, perception, and judgment. Age of onset is usually 35 to 45 years, with death occurring 10 to 15 years following onset of symptoms (Smeltzer, Bare, Hinkle, & Cheever, 2008). Each child of a person with Huntington's disease has a 50% chance of inheriting the fatal gene. Everyone who has the gene will develop the disease (HDSA, 2002). However, there is no cure for this devastating progressive disease.

Clinical manifestations are **chorea**, abnormal involuntary, purposeless movements of all musculature of the body. Facial tic, grimacing, difficulty in chewing and swallowing, speech impairment, disorganized gait, and bowel and bladder incontinence also occur. Mental or intellectual impairment progresses to dementia. The client may experience paranoia, hallucinations, or delusions. Emotions are labile, from outbursts of anger to profound depression, apathy, or euphoria. A ravenous appetite is usually present, but because of the constant movement, the client is often emaciated and exhausted. Death usually results from heart failure, pneumonia, infection, or choking (HDSA, 2002).

The entire family experiences this disease in an emotional, physical, social, and financial way. Supportive care is required as the family progresses through life with a loved one with Huntington's disease. Because of the hereditary factor, genetic counseling is suggested.

Medical–Surgical Management

Pharmacological

A medication that decreases choreiform movement is the benzodiazepine, clonazepam (Klonopin). Do not stop clonazepam abruptly but taper off medication to avoid symptoms of withdrawal, especially if client has epilepsy. Assess client for excessive fatigue. Antidepressants, such as desipramine hydrochloride (Norpramin) and fluoxetine hydrochloride (Prozac), and antipsychotics, such as fluphenazine hydrochloride (Prolixin), are used for emotional disturbances. Many people do better with minimal medication (HDSA, 2001).

Diet

The diet must be high in calories to provide for the high energy needs caused by the continuous movement. Chewing and swallowing difficulties necessitate foods that are easy to chew or foods cut into small pieces to prevent choking.

Activity

Ambulation is maintained as long as possible. A safe environment is maintained to prevent injury from falls or from sharp objects. Driving is usually restricted when choreiform movement or impaired judgment interferes with the ability to drive safely.

Nursing Management

Nursing interventions include a holistic approach to the client's care. Collaboration with the social worker, the chaplain, the physician, and the mental health worker is necessary.

Teach the client and family about the disease process, the progress of the disease, and the genetic factors involved.

Safety factors are considered. Fall prevention measures, such as removing throw rugs and small objects from the floor, and injury prevention measures, such as removing sharp or dangerous objects such as guns and knives from the home, are implemented. The hazard of choking also is addressed, by teaching the family to cut the client's food into small pieces, to serve soft foods, and by teaching the Heimlich maneuver.

GILLES DE LA TOURETTE'S SYNDROME

Gilles de la Tourette's syndrome is a neurological movement disorder that also has prominent behavioral manifestations. Clinical manifestations include motor tics and involuntary repetitive movements of the mouth, face, head, or neck muscles. The trunk and extremities may also be involved. Motor tics take the form of forceful eye blinking or toe touching. Vocal tics or repetitive involuntary vocalizations take the form of sniffing, grunting, throat clearing, or **coprolalia** (involuntary and inappropriate swearing). Other complex motor and vocal tics that also are present include copropraxia, involuntary and effectively appropriate use of obscene gestures; echolalia, involuntary repetition of the speech of others; and palilia, involuntary repetition of the person's own speech. The obsessive–compulsive symptoms of repetitive handwashing or checking rituals also are exhibited. Attention deficit hyperactivity disorder (ADHD) and obsessive–compulsive disorders may also coexist with Tourette's syndrome.

Onset is before age 18 years, with males being more commonly affected than females. Tourette's is an inherited disorder, with the affected individual having a 50% chance of passing the gene on to children.

MEDICAL–SURGICAL MANAGEMENT

Pharmacological

Tics are controlled with clonadine (Catapres), haloperidol (Haldol), or primozide (Orap). Coexisting ADHD is controlled with clonidine (Catapres), methylphenidate (Ritalin), or pemoline (Cylert). Clomypramine (Anafranil) or fluoxetine (Prozac) are used to keep obsessive–compulsive behaviors under control (Kurlan, 1998). Acetaminophen (Tylenol) may help the discomfort of muscle spasms.

Other Therapies

As they age, clients learn to suppress tics in social situations. Psychotherapy and family counseling are beneficial in coping with social stigma and adjustment problems.

NURSING MANAGEMENT

The client and the family with Tourette's syndrome need a great deal of emotional support and benefit from knowing about the availability of support groups for clients with Tourette's syndrome. The nurse instructs the client about the disease process and personal and behavioral expectations. Behavioral modification techniques are generally effective; the nurse must know which modification techniques are being used and must follow through with consistent responses.

CASE STUDY

D.O., a 76-year-old retired farmer, was admitted to the emergency department with left-sided hemiplegia, difficulty swallowing, and inability to speak. He was awake and watching the staff upon admission. He moved his right arm to indicate that M.O. was his wife but was unable to speak or form sounds. M.O. stated that her husband was working in the garden, picking tomatoes and cucumbers, when he fell to the ground 30 minutes before admission. The department room nurse administered oxygen through nasal cannula at 2 liters per minute and obtained vital signs. His blood pressure was 182/110 mm Hg, pulse was 88 beats per minute, respirations were 20 breaths per minute, and temperature was 100.5°F. The emergency department physician ordered an MRI scan of the head, a complete blood count, and prothrombin time (PT). The MRI indicated that D.O. experienced a CVA caused by bleeding into the brain.

The following questions will guide your development of a nursing care plan for the case study.

1. List clinical manifestations other than the symptoms D.O. experienced that can occur with a CVA.
2. List subjective and objective data that a nurse would obtain.
3. Identify three individualized nursing diagnoses and goals for D.O.
4. D.O. is transferred to a general medical unit for 3 days, and then is transferred to a rehabilitation center for intensive therapy. What pertinent nursing actions should a nurse perform in caring for D.O. in the acute setting and the rehabilitation setting related to:
   - Mobility
   - Safety
   - Elimination
   - Skin integrity
   - Comfort and rest
5. What teaching will D.O. need before discharge from the rehabilitation facility?
6. List at least three client outcomes for D.O.

SUMMARY

- The nervous system controls all bodily functions, from movement to thinking to processing information to autonomic responses.
- The frontal lobe of the cerebrum specializes in emotional attitudes and responses, formation of thought processes, motor function, judgment, personality, and inhibitions.
- The parietal lobe of the cerebrum is a purely sensory region for interpretation of all senses except smell; the purpose is to analyze sensations, including pain, touch, and temperature, from receptors in the skin.
- The temporal lobe of the cerebrum houses Wernicke's area, the primary auditory association area, where words that are heard are interpreted. Memory is also a function of the temporal lobe, especially memories that are highly detailed or involve multiple sensations.
- A special interpretive area located at the junction of the temporal, parietal, and occipital lobes integrates somatic, auditory, and visual sensory interpretations.
- The occipital lobe of the cerebrum is responsible for visual interpretation and visual association.
- Disorders of the nervous system cause complex dysfunctions; the nurse uses assessment skills and quickly recognizes changes in condition.
- Teaching about injury prevention and the effects and prognosis of the disorder are required to meet the physical and psychosocial needs of the client and family.
- Many neurological disorders potentiate injury. Nursing care includes providing the client and family with necessary safety information.
- To maintain and restore functional ability, rehabilitation is initiated from the first contact with the client.

REVIEW QUESTIONS

1. The most important indicator of change in neurological status is:
   1. level of consciousness.
   2. pupil reaction.
   3. vital signs.
   4. motor function.
2. Assessment of intellectual function requires that the nurse:
   1. have knowledge of the client's previous ability to function.
   2. administer a written test to determine the client's IQ level.
   3. utilize auscultation, percussion, and palpation skills.
   4. observe the client's behavior, posture, and facial expression.
3. Contusion of the brain is a (an):
   1. shaking of the brain.
   2. bleeding into the brain tissue.
   3. open head injury.
   4. bruising of the brain.
4. Benign brain tumors can be:
   1. more anxiety producing than are malignant tumors.
   2. more life threatening than are malignant tumors.
   3. treated with radiation therapy.
   4. the cause of increased intracranial pressure.
5. A nurse is teaching A.W., a 24-year-old client with Guillain-Barré syndrome, about her condition. What statement does the nurse include in her teaching?
   1. The nerve degeneration continues to slowly progress in this chronic degenerative nerve disease.
   2. The disease is an acute inflammatory process with most clients regaining complete function.
   3. Respiratory failure requiring chronic ventilatory support may occur.
   4. Motor function deficit will occur, but sensation will remain.
6. The client's wife asks the nurse what she thinks of memory training and reality orientation for a client with Stage 2 Alzheimer's disease. The nurse responds that those interventions should be used with caution because:
   1. reality is painful.
   2. they are very costly.
   3. they can accelerate the disease process.
   4. they might trigger anger and agitation.
7. A nurse is caring for a client with amyotrophic lateral sclerosis (ALS) who has the following symptoms. What symptom requires a prompt nursing intervention?
   1. Loss of bowel and urine control.
   2. Confusion.
   3. Tonic-clonic seizures.
   4. Shallow respirations.
8. What client response indicates he understands the nurse's instructions about taking carbidopa-levodopa (Sinemet)?
   1. "I will slowly rise from a sitting position to standing position."
   2. "I will limit my fluids to 1000 milliliters a day."
   3. "I will reduce my medication dosage by half when my symptoms improve."
   4. "I will have a diet high in protein and vitamin B_6 since I am taking Sinemet."
9. A nurse completes an assessment on her client. She finds that the client opens his eyes when she enters the room; answers questions but has incorrect answers about time, place, and events; and raises

right hand when requested. According to the Glasgow Coma Scale, what score does the nurse give the client?
   1. 3
   2. 6
   3. 12
   4. 14

10. What are expected findings when the nurse assesses the client's trigeminal nerve? (Select all that apply.)
   1. Eye moves smoothly upward and outward.
   2. Eye blinks rapidly when cotton ball sweeps across cornea.
   3. Client tastes sweet sensation when given a piece of candy.
   4. Jaw moves symmetrical and overcomes resistance.
   5. Gag reflect is intact.
   6. Client feels cotton ball when swiped across cheek.

REFERENCES/SUGGESTED READINGS

Agnew, T. (2006). Nurses out of step with Parkinson's patients. *Nursing Older People, 18*(6), 8–9.

Alzheimer's Association. (2002). Facts: About Alzheimer's disease. Retrieved from http://www.alz.org/Resource Center/FactSheets/FSAlzheimerdisease.pdf

Alzheimer's Disease Education and Referral Center. (2002). Alzheimer's disease fact sheet. Retrieved from http://www.alzheimers.org/pubs/adfact.html

Alzheimer's Organization. (2008). Alzheimer's disease prevalence rates rise to more than 5 million in the United States. Retrieved July 19, 2008 from http://www.alz.org/news_and_events_rates_rise.asp

American Headache Society (AHS). (2007). Types of headaches. Retrieved June 5, 2009 from http://www.achenet.org/education/patients/TypesofHeadaches.asp

Andersen, G. (1998). DX dementia: But what kind? *RN, 61*(6), 26–30.

Backer, J. (2006). The symptom experience of patients with Parkinson's disease. *Journal of Neuroscience Nursing, 38*(1), 51–57.

Barker, E. (1999). Brain attack! A call to action. *RN, 62*(5), 54–57.

Barker, E. (2001). What's your patient's stroke risk? *Nursing2001, 31*(4), 32hn1–32hn5.

Barker, E., & Saulino, M. (2002). First-ever guidelines for spinal cord injuries. *RN, 65*(10), 32–37.

Beare, P. & Myers, J. (Eds.). (1998). *Principles and practice of adult health nursing* (3rd ed.). St. Louis, MO: Mosby.

Best, J. (2001). Cauda equina syndrome. *Nursing2001, 31*(4), 43.

Bond, C. (2002). Traumatic brain injury: Help for the family. *RN, 65*(11), 60–66.

Bulechek, G., Butcher, H., McCloskey, J., & Dochterman, J., eds. (2008). *Nursing Interventions Classification (NIC)* (5th ed.). St. Louis, MO: Mosby/Elsevier.

Bunting-Perry, L. (2006). Palliative care in Parkinson's disease: Implications for neuroscience nursing. *Journal Neuroscience Nursing, 38*(2), 106–113.

Costa, M. (1998). Clinical snapshot: Trigeminal neuralgia. *AJN, 98*(6), 42–43.

Crigger, N., & Forbes, W. (1997). Assessing neurologic function in older patients. *AJN, 97*(3), 37–40.

Cross, C. (2002). Spotting concussions in children and in adults. *RN, 65*(7), 72.

Finesilver, C. (2003). Multiple sclerosis. *RN, 66*(4), 36–43.

Frank, R., Gesteland, R., Bailie, J., Rybalsky, K., Seiden, A., & Dulay, M. (2006). Characterization of the sniff magnitude test. *Archives of Otolaryngol Head Neck Surgery, 132*(5), 532–536.

Galvan, T. (2001). Dysphagia: Going down and staying down. *AJN, 101*(1), 37–42.

Gendreau-Webb, R. (2001). Acute ischemic stroke. *Nursing2001, 31*(11), 120.

Gray-Vickrey, P. (2002). Advances in Alzheimer's disease. *Nursing2002, 32*(11), 64.

Gumm, S. (2000). Straight talk about MS. *Nursing2000, 30*(1), 50–51.

Hally, Z. (2007). Simple sniff test could diagnose Alzheimer's and Parkinson's disease. Retrieved June 5, 2009 from http://www.associatedcontent.com/article/202499/simple_sniff_test_could_daignose_alzheimer?cat=5

Halper, J., & Holland, N. (1998a). Meeting the challenge of multiple sclerosis (Part I). *AJN, 98*(10), 26–31.

Halper, J., & Holland, N. (1998b). Meeting the challenge of multiple sclerosis (Part II). *AJN, 98*(11), 39–46.

Hickey, J. (2008). *The clinical practice of neurological and neurosurgical nursing* (6th ed.). Philadelphia: Lippincott Williams & Wilkins.

Hilgers, J. (2003). Comforting a confused patient. *Nursing2003, 33*(1), 48–50.

Hilton, G. (2001). Acute head injury: Distinguishing subdural from epidural hematoma. *AJN, 101*(9), 51–52.

Huntington's Disease Society of America (HDSA). (2002). *Huntington's disease*. Retrieved from http://www.hdsa.org/edu/HD_booklet.htm

Huston, C. (1998). Emergency! Cervical spine injury. *AJN, 98*(6), 33.

Huston, C., & Boelman, R. (1995). Autonomic dysreflexia. *AJN, 95*(6), 55.

Kurlan, R. (1998). Current pharmacology of Tourette's syndrome. Bayside, NY: Tourette Syndrome Association. Retrieved from http://www.2mgh.harvard.edu/lsa/medsci/medicationsanddosages.html

Lewis, A. (1999). Neurologic emergency! *Nursing99, 29*(10), 54–56.

Lower, J. (2002). Facing neuro assessment fearlessly. *Nursing2002, 32*(2), 58–64.

Lower, J. (2003). Using pain to assess neurologic response. *Nursing2003, 33*(6), 56–57.

MayoClinic.com. (2008). Brain tumor. Retrieved June 2, 2009 from http://www.mayoclinci.com/helath/brain-tumor/DS00281/METHOD=print&DSECTION-all

McCance, K., & Huether, S. (2001). *Pathophysiology: The biological basis for disease in adults and children* (4th ed.). St. Louis, MO: Mosby.

McGuire, L. (2002). How to treat a migraine. *Nursing2002, 32*(12), 76–77.

McNamara, P. (2009). Parkinson's disease: Diet in early stages of PD. Retrieved June 4, 2009 from http://parkinsons.about.com/od/livingwithpd/a/foods_to_eat.htm?p=1

Monlus-Swift, C. (2002). Neurological disorders. In P. L. Swearingen (Ed.), *Manual of medical–surgical nursing care: Nursing interventions and collaborative management* (5th ed.). St. Louis, MO: Mosby.

Moorhead, S., Johnson, M., Maas, M., & Swanson, E. (2007). *Nursing Outcomes Classification (NOC)* (4th ed.). St. Louis, MO: Mosby.

Morgan, J., & Sethi, K. (2005). Treatment of early Parkinson's disease. In M. Ebadi & R.E. Pfeiffer (Eds.), *Parkinson's disease* (pp. 839–849). New York: CRC Press.

Mower-Wade, D., Cavanaugh, M., & Bush, D. (2001). Protecting a patient with ruptured cerebral aneurysm. *Nursing2001, 31*(2), 52–57.

Nadler-Moodie, M., & Wilson, M. (1998). Latest approaches in Alzheimer's care. *RN, 61*(7), 42–46.

National Headache Foundation (NHF). (2002). Fact sheet. Retrieved from http://www.headaches.org/consumer/generalinfo/factsheet.html

National Institute of Neurological Disorders and Stroke. (2006). Hope through research. Retrieved July 17, 2008 from http://www.ninds.nih.gov/disorders/parkinsons_disease/detail_parkinsons_disease.htm#120463159

National Multiple Sclerosis Society (NMSS). (2003). *What is multiple sclerosis?* Retrieved from http://www.nationalmssociety.org/What%20is%20MS.asp

National Parkinson's Foundation. (2000). Parkinson's and B_6: What's the connection. Retrieved July 20, 2008 from http://www.parkinson.org/NETCOMMUNITY/Page.aspx?pid=458&srcid=377

National Parkinson Foundation. (2008). About Parkinson disease. Retrieved July 17, 2008 from http://www.parkinson.org?NETCOMMUNITY/Page.aspx?pid=225&srcid=210

National Stroke Association (NSA). (1999). *Stroke prevention guidelines.* Retrieved from http://www.stroke.org/pages/ prev_guide.cfm

National Stroke Association (NSA). (2002a). *Stroke in America campaign.* Retrieved from http://www.stroke.org/pages/america_main.cfm

National Stroke Association (NSA). (2002b). *Stroke statistics.* Retrieved from http://www.stroke.org/brain_stat.cfm

National Stroke Association (NSA). (2002c). *Stroke: What it is.* Retrieved from http://www.stroke.org/whats.cfm

National Stroke Association (NSA). (2008). Talk about TIA! Retrieved June 3, 2009 at http://www.stroke.org/site/PageNavigator/HOME

National Stroke Association (NSA). (2009a). Stroke 101. Retrieved June 3, 2009 at http://www.stroke.org/site/DocServer/STROKE_101_Fact_Sheet.pdf?docID=454

National Stroke Association (NSA). (2009b). Stroke risk factors. Retrieved June 3, 2009 from http://www.stroke.org/site/PageServer?pagename=RISK

North American Nursing Diagnosis Association International. (2010). *NANDA-I nursing diagnoses: Definitions and classification 2009–2011.* Ames, IA: Wiley-Blackwell.

O'Hanlon-Nichols, T. (1999). Neurologic assessment. *AJN, 99*(6), 44–50.

Parini, S. (2001). 8 faces of meningitis. *Nursing2001, 31*(8), 51–53.

Parkinson's Disease Foundation (PDF). (2002). *Parkinson's disease.* Retrieved from http://www.pdf.org/aboutdisease/overview.html

Parkinson's Disease Foundation.(2008). Ten frequently asked questions about Parkinson's disease. Retrieved July 19, 2008 from http://www.pdf.org/Publications/factsheets/PDF_Fact_Sheet_1.0_Final.pdf

Pullen, R. (2003). Protecting your patient during a seizure. *Nursing2003, 33*(4), 78.

Rudick, R. (1997). New approaches to multiple sclerosis. *Health News,* 3(17), 1–2. Waltham, MA: Massachusetts Medical Society.

Samuels, M. (Ed.). (2004). *Manual of neurological therapeutics* (7th ed.). Philadelphia: Lippincott Williams & Wilkins.

Santa Rosa County Citizen Service Center. (2009) Blood clots/stroke–They now have a fourth indicator, the tongue. Retrieved June 3, 2009 from http://www.santarosa.fl.gov/hr/documents/identiyastroke.pdf

Schweiger, J. (1999). Alzheimer's disease. *Nursing99, 29*(6), 34–41.

Smeltzer, S., Bare, B., Hinkle, J., & Cheever, K. (2008). *Brunner & Suddarth's textbook of medical-surgical nursing* (11th ed.). Philadelphia: Lippincott Williams & Wilkins.

Smith, L. (2002). Steady the course of Parkinson's disease. *Nursing2002, 32*(3), 43–45.

Son, G., Therrien, B., & Whall, A. (2002). Implicit memory and familiarity among elders with dementia. *Journal of Nursing Scholarship, 34*(3), 263–267.

Spinal Cord Injury Information Network. (2009). Facts and figures at a glance. Retrieved June 4, 2009 from http://www.spinalcord.uab.edu/show.asp?durki=119513&site=4716&return=19775

Taggart, H.(1998). Multiple sclerosis update. *Orthopaedic Nursing (March/April),* 23–29.

The American Association of Neurological Surgeons & The Congress of Neurological Surgeons. (2002). Guidelines for the management of acute cervical spine and spinal cord injuries. *Neurosurgery, 50*(3), S1.

Thomure, A. (2006). Helping your patient manage Parkinson's disease. *Nursing 2006, 6*(8), 20–21.

Urden, L., Stacy, K., & Lough, M. (2009). *Critical care nursing: Diagnosis and management* (6th ed.). St. Louis: Mosby.

Weintraub, D., & Stern, M. (2005). Psychiatric complications in Parkinson's disease. *American Journal of Geriatric Psychiatry, 13,* 844–851.

Williams, M., Wood H., & Waxman, J. (2002). How to assess swallowing after a stroke. *Nursing2002, 32*(8), 32hn5–32hn6.

Wilson, R., Mendes de Leon, C., Barnes, L., et al. (2002). Participation in cognitively stimulating activities and risk of incident Alzheimer's disease. *JAMA, 287*(6), 742.

RESOURCES

Alzheimer's Association, http://www.alz.org

American Academy of Neurology, http://www.aan.com

American Association of Spinal Cord Injury Professionals, http://nurses.ascipro.org

American Headache Society, http://www.achenet.org/

American Spinal Injury Association, http://www.asia-spinal injury.org

Brain Injury Association of America, http://www.biausa.org

Coma/Traumatic Brain Injury Recovery Association, Inc., http://www.comarecovery.org

Epilepsy Foundation of America, http://www.epilepsyfoundation.org/

Guillain-Barré Syndrome/Chronic Inflammatory Demyelinating Polyneuropathy Foundation International, http://www.gbs-cidp.org/

Huntington's Disease Society of America, http://www.hdsa.org/

National Headache Foundation, http://www.headaches.org

National Institute of Neurological Disorders and Stroke, http://www.ninds.nih.gov

National Multiple Sclerosis Society, http://www.nationalmssociety.org/index.aspx

National Parkinson's Foundation, Inc., http://www.parkinson.org

National Spinal Cord Injury Association, http://www.spinalcord.org

National Stroke Association, http://www.stroke.org

Parkinson's Disease Foundation, http://www.pdf.org

Tourette Syndrome Association, Inc., http://www.tsa-usa.org

CHAPTER 42
Sensory System

MAKING THE CONNECTION

Refer to the following chapters to increase your understanding of the sensory system:

Basic Nursing

- ***Communication***
- ***End-of-Life Care***
- ***Wellness Concepts***
- ***Assessment***
- ***Pain Management***
- ***Diagnostic Tests***

Adult Health Nursing

- ***Surgery***
- ***Neurological System***
- ***The Older Adult***

Intermediate Procedures

- ***Administering Eye and Ear Medications***

LEARNING OBJECTIVES

Upon completion of this chapter, you should be able to:

- Define key terms.
- Compare and differentiate common disorders of the special senses.
- Identify the structure and function of the major parts of the eye and ear.
- Explain the purpose of the common diagnostic tests for sensory problems.
- List the nursing assessments and common nursing diagnoses related to sensory impairment.
- Assist in planning nursing care for clients with sensory disorders.
- List some of the common sensory aids for the visual and hearing impaired.

KEY TERMS

affect
afferent nerve pathway
arousal
astigmatism
awareness
cerumen
chalazion
cognition
conductive hearing loss
conjunctivitis
consciousness
disorientation
efferent nerve pathway
hallucination
hyperopia
illusion
judgment
keratitis
myopia
nystagmus
orientation
perception
presbycusis
presbyopia
sensation
sensorineural hearing loss
sensory deficit
sensory deprivation
sensory overload
sensory perception
strabismus
stye
tinnitus
vertigo

INTRODUCTION

From the moment we wake in the morning until we fall asleep at night, we are inundated with information from the outside world through our senses. We depend on visual and auditory alarms to keep us from harm. This chapter reviews the structure and function, identifies appropriate nursing diagnoses, and presents the medical and nursing management for hearing and vision with some discussion of taste, smell, and touch.

SENSATION, PERCEPTION, AND COGNITION

Sensation is the ability to receive and process stimuli through the sensory organs. There are two types of stimuli: external and internal. External stimuli are received and processed through the senses of sight (visual), hearing (auditory), smell (olfactory), taste (gustatory), and touch (tactile). Internal stimuli are received and processed through kinesthetic (an awareness of the position of the body) and visceral (feelings originating from large organs within the body) modes.

Perception is the ability to experience, recognize, organize, and interpret sensory stimuli. **Sensory perception** is the ability to receive sensory impressions and, through cortical association, relate the stimuli to past experiences and form an impression of the nature of the stimulus.

Perception is closely associated with **cognition**, the intellectual ability to think. The processes of organizing and interpreting stimuli depend on a person's level of intellectual functioning. Cognition includes the elements of memory, judgment, and orientation. The well-being of an individual depends on the functions of sensation, perception, and cognition because the person fully experiences and interacts with the environment through these mechanisms.

Sensory, perceptual, and cognitive alterations are either temporary or progressive in their manifestations and result from disease or trauma. Whatever the status or cause of the alterations, these conditions usually lead to social isolation and increased dependence on others. In addition, impairment in sensory, perceptual, and cognitive functions place the individual at risk for injury to self or others.

ANATOMY AND PHYSIOLOGY REVIEW

Sensation, perception, and cognition are neurological functions. The nervous system is composed of two major subsystems: the central nervous system (CNS) and the peripheral nervous system (PNS), which consists of the somatic and autonomic nervous systems. The CNS and PNS act in unison to accomplish three purposes: (1) collection of stimuli from the receptors at the end of the peripheral nerves; (2) transportation of the stimuli to the brain for integration and cognition processing; and (3) conduction of responses to the stimuli from the brain to responsive motor centers in the body.

Sensory perception involves the function of both the cranial and peripheral nerves. The cranial nerves arise from the brain and govern the movement and function of various muscles and nerves throughout the body. The peripheral nerves connect the CNS to other parts of the body.

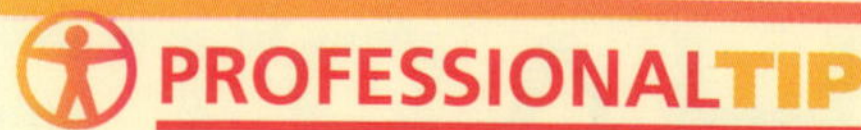

CNS Deficits and Illness

Specific conditions, such as diabetes mellitus and atherosclerosis, can impair neurosensory pathways and result in deficits in sensation, perception, and cognition. Diseases of the CNS can result in loss of sensory function and paralysis.

COMPONENTS OF SENSATION AND PERCEPTION

The sensory system is a complex network that consists of **afferent nerve pathways** (ascending pathways that transmit sensory impulses to the brain), **efferent nerve pathways** (descending pathways that send sensory impulses from the brain), the spinal cord, the brainstem, and the cerebrum.

COMPONENTS OF COGNITION

Cognition includes the cerebral functions of memory, affect, judgment, perception, and language. In order for these higher functions to occur, consciousness must be present.

Consciousness

Consciousness is a state of awareness of self, others, and the surrounding environment. It affects both cognitive (intellectual) and affective (emotional) functions. An alert individual (one who is aware of self and stimuli) is able to perceive reality accurately and to base behavior on those perceptions. The components of consciousness provide a foundation for behavior and emotional expression, thereby contributing to the uniqueness of each individual's personality. Consciousness may be altered by various metabolic, traumatic, or other factors, such as the pharmacological actions of drugs that affect mental status. The primary components of consciousness are arousal and awareness, both of which must be present before higher cognitive functioning occurs.

Arousal The degree of **arousal** (state of wakefulness and alertness) is indicated by a person's general response and reaction to the environment. People exhibit arousal by behaving in an alert and aware manner and by experiencing periods of wakefulness. The degree of an individual's arousal is indicated by the general response and reaction to the environment. Impaired arousal can exist when a sleep pattern deficit is

PROFESSIONALTIP

Effects of Medications on Sensation

Certain medications have the potential to alter or depress the neurosensory system. For example, sedatives and narcotics alter the perception of sensory stimuli. Medications such as analgesics alter the level of consciousness.

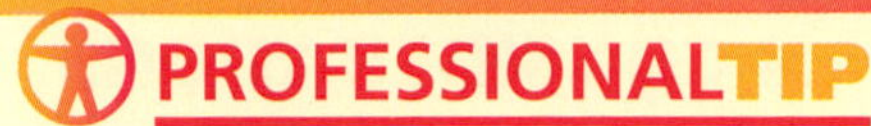

Remote Memory

Remote memory is accurately assessed only when client responses about past events can be validated, either by others or by written account.

experienced. There may be an inability to take advantage of opportunities for activity because of inadequate periods of rest.

Awareness Awareness is the capacity to perceive sensory impressions and react appropriately through thoughts and actions. An essential element in awareness is **orientation** (perception of self in relation to the surrounding environment). When awareness is impaired, orientation to time is frequently the first area affected. The degree of disorientation is worse when the individual loses awareness of place, self (person), and purpose/situation.

Memory

There are three types of memory: immediate, recent, and remote. Immediate memory is the retention of information for a specified and usually short period of time. The recall of a telephone number long enough to dial it is an example of immediate memory. Recent memory is the ability to recall events that have occurred over the past 24 hours, such as remembering the foods eaten for dinner the previous night. Remote memory is the retention of experiences that occurred during earlier periods of life, such as an adult's memories of childhood or school days. The ability to learn depends on remote memory.

Affect

Affect (expression of mood or feeling) is an important component of cognition in that variations of mood can affect one's thinking ability. For example, a client with a flat affect caused by depression may have difficulty sustaining concentration or attention.

Judgment

Judgment is the ability to compare or evaluate alternatives to arrive at a conclusion based on sound reasoning and supported by evidence. Judgment is closely related to reality testing and depends on effective cognitive functioning. Behaviors indicating impaired judgment include impulsiveness, unrealistic decision making, and inadequate problem-solving ability.

Perception

Perceptions are considered in the context of the individual's awareness of reality. Misperceptions of reality can occur in the form of an **illusion** (an inaccurate perception or misinterpretation of sensory stimuli) or a **hallucination** (a sensory perception that occurs in the absence of external stimuli and is not based on reality).

Clients who are anxious and fearful or who are on therapeutic regimens involving the use of certain medications may experience misperceptions of environmental stimuli. For example, a postoperative client, after receiving analgesic medication for pain, may see the belt from his bathrobe lying on the floor and become terrified because he thinks there is a snake in the room. Once the nurse determines that the client is experiencing an illusion, appropriate reassurance and reality orientation is implemented to reduce the client's anxiety.

Language

Language is one of the most complex of cognitive functions, involving not only the spoken word but also reading, writing, and comprehension. Characteristics of speech are fluency (ability to talk in a steady manner), prosody (melody of speech that conveys meaning through changes in the tempo, rhythm, and intonation), and content.

ASSESSMENT

When caring for clients with sensory, perceptual, and cognitive alterations, the nurse obtains a health history and performs a physical examination to identify existing or potential problems in this area of functioning. The physical examination focuses specifically on the client's ability to hear, see, taste, smell, and touch. For hearing (auditory): Ask about hearing problems, ability to distinguish sounds, buzzing or ringing noises, recent changes in hearing ability, and use of a hearing aid. For seeing (visual): Ask about blurred vision, double vision, blind spots, photosensitivity, rainbows or halos around objects, difficulty seeing far or near, family history of visual problems, use of glasses or contact lenses, and date of last eye examination. For tasting (gustatory): Ask about changes in tasting ability or appetite and ability to differentiate sweet, sour, salty, and bitter tastes. For smelling (olfactory): Ask about changes in the ability to smell and the ability to distinguish common smells. For touch (tactile): Ask about ability to feel temperature changes and pain perception in extremities and the presence of unusual sensations in extremities (tingling or numbness). Refer to the neurologic system chapter for assessment of cranial nerves.

When assessing clients for sensory, perceptual, and cognitive alterations, the level of consciousness (LOC) also is evaluated. Refer to the neurologic system chapter for the Glasgow Coma Scale, developed to assess LOC objectively.

SAFETY

Sensory Impairments

Vision—Risk of tripping, falling

Hearing—Lack of awareness of warning sounds such as automobile horns, sirens, smoke alarms

Olfactory—Inability to perceive warning odors such as burning food, escaping gas

Gustatory—Inability to recognize spoiled or contaminated food or beverages

Tactile—Lack of awareness of excessive pressure on a body part; at risk for exposure to extreme temperatures (frostbite, burns)

The Ear

The human ear is divided into three main anatomical components: the outer ear, middle ear, and inner ear (Figure 42-1). Each part plays a major role in hearing. Similar to other paired organs in the body, dysfunction of part or all of one ear does not affect the function of the other.

Outer Ear

The outer ear is composed of the auricle (pinna), a cartilaginous flap on the temporal sides of the head, and the external ear canal, or external auditory meatus. The outer ear is responsible for collecting, conducting, and amplifying sound waves. The auricle directs sounds through the external ear canal to the tympanic membrane (eardrum). This canal is lined with ceruminous glands that secrete **cerumen** (ear wax), a yellowish brown protective substance that guards against certain bacteria and small insects, and traps dust and debris that may damage the inner ear. Normally, the cerumen works its way out of the ear as we eat, chew, or speak; however, cerumen can build up and actually cause significant hearing loss in the affected ear.

The tympanic membrane (TM) serves as a boundary between the outer and middle ear. As sound waves vibrate against the membrane, the motion is transmitted to the bones of the inner ear. In an acute ear infection, fluid fills the middle ear, creating significant pressure on the tympanic membrane.

Middle Ear

The three bones of the middle ear are collectively referred to as the ossicles and include the *malleus* (hammer), *incus* (anvil), and *stapes* (stirrup), so named because they resemble the tools of a blacksmith's trade. The malleus is attached to the upper, inner portion of the tympanic membrane. The head of the malleus connects with the incus, which then joins the stapes. The flat oval bone of the stapes, called the footplate, rests on the oval window (part of the inner ear). The vibration created by sound waves passes through the outer ear canal to the tympanic membrane and then to these three bones.

The eustachian tube opens into the pharynx from the middle ear. It is approximately 3 to 4 cm long, and its primary function is to equalize pressure on both sides of the eardrum by providing a path (via the nasal passages) to relieve the pressure. In addition to pressure equalization, the functions of the middle ear include amplification of the sound waves and stimulation of the oval window to move the fluids of the inner ear.

LIFE SPAN CONSIDERATIONS

Sensory Changes in the Elderly

- When the eye lens yellows and becomes cloudy, the ability to discern colors, especially greens and blues, is impaired.
- The elderly need more light to see because the pupils become smaller, letting in less light.
- It takes the elderly longer to accommodate (adjust) to darkness and glare.
- Tear production decreases with age, predisposing to dry eye syndrome and corneal irritation.
- The most common hearing loss is sensorineural, which can be helped by a hearing aid.
- Taste sensation may be dulled with age.

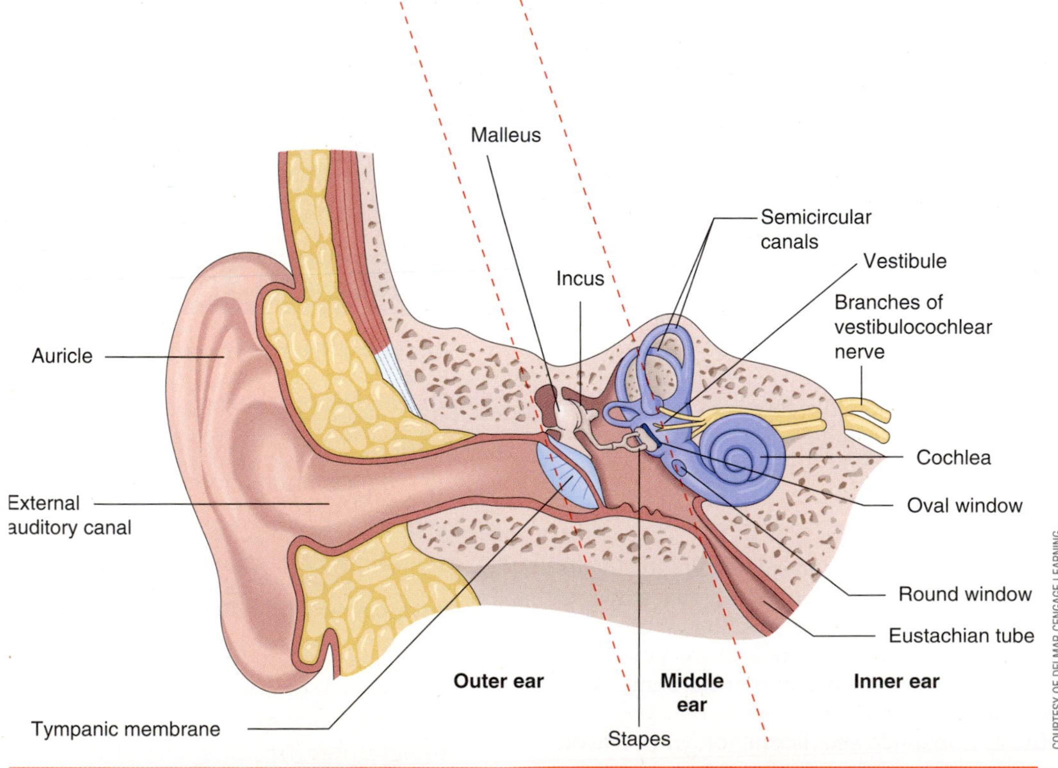

Figure 42-1 Structures of the Ear

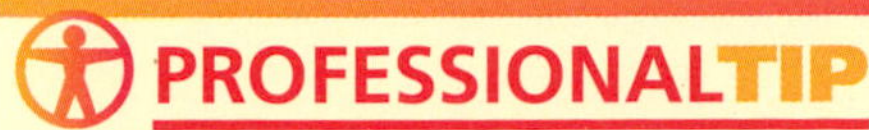

Tympanic Membrane

The tympanic membrane is normally concave on otoscopic exam, so a convex or bulging tympanic membrane is an important sign of an acute infectious process.

Inner Ear

The inner ear has two main functions: hearing and equilibrium. It consists of a complex series of interconnected, fluid-filled chambers and tubes called the labyrinth. It is divided into three main parts: the semicircular canals, the vestibule, and the cochlea, all located in the temporal bone. The semicircular canals, which function in providing the sense of balance, open into the vestibule. The vestibule is the central chamber of the inner ear. The cochlea is a snail-shaped structure that contains the auditory organ for the sense of hearing.

Vibration of the stapes creates pressure and causes the nerves to respond to different sounds and initiate neural responses that are sent along the auditory nerve (cranial nerve VIII) to the brain. Thus mechanical information is translated into nerve impulses and sent to the brain, which translates the sound into meaningful impressions and language.

The Eye

The eyes are a pair of spherical organs located in bony orbital cavities in the front of the skull. They are the sensory receptor organs of the visual system that transduce light from the environment into electrical impulses, which the optic nerve (cranial nerve II) then transmits to the brain, where they are interpreted as the sensation of vision. The adult eyeball measures about 1 inch in diameter. Of its total surface area, only the anterior one-sixth is exposed. The remainder is recessed and protected by the bony orbit into which it fits. Anatomically, the eye is divided into three separate coats, or "tunics": the outer fibrous tunic, the middle vascular tunic, and the inner nervous tunic.

Fibrous Tunic

The fibrous tunic is the outer coat of the eyeball and is composed posteriorly of the sclera and anteriorly of the transparent cornea. The sclera, or "white of the eye," is leathery, white, and relatively thick and is composed of connective tissue. The cornea, or "window of the eye," is a continuation of the sclera and forms a transparent rounded bulge through which light passes.

Vascular Tunic

The vascular tunic is the eye's middle layer and is composed of three portions: the posterior choroid, the anterior ciliary body, and the iris. Collectively, these three structures are called the uveal tract. The choroid carries the blood vessels for the eyeball and contains a large amount of pigment, thus preventing internal reflection of light. Around the edge of the cornea the choroid forms the ciliary body, a thickened structure containing smooth muscle. A thin diaphragm of mostly connective tissue and smooth muscle fibers with an opening in the center is attached around the anterior margin of the ciliary body. The muscles of the ciliary body serve to change the shape of the lens, allowing changes in the focal distance of the eye. The third portion of the vascular tunic is known as the iris and contains the pigment responsible for the color of the eye. The hole in the iris is the pupil, which permits light to enter the eye. Some of the smooth muscle fibers in the iris encircle the pupil and others radiate from it. Contraction of the radial muscle dilates the pupil and contraction of the circular muscle constricts the pupil. By their control of pupil diameter, these muscles regulate the amount of light entering the eye.

Nervous Tunic

The third and innermost tunic of the eye, the retina, translates light waves into neural impulses. An extremely complex structure, the retina contains several layers of nerve cells and their processes, including two types of receptors, the rods for vision in dim light, and the cones for daytime or color vision. Cones are most densely concentrated in the central fovea, a small depression in the center of the macula lutea. The macula lutea, or yellow spot, is in the central part of the retina. The fovea is the area of sharpest vision because the highest concentration of cones is located there. Rods are absent from the fovea and macula, but they increase in density toward the periphery of the retina. The optic disk, where the optic nerve exits the eye, is a weak spot in the fundus (posterior wall) of the eye because it is not reinforced by the sclera. The optic disk is also called the blind spot because it lacks photoreceptors and light focused on it is not detected.

The interior of the eyeball contains an anterior and posterior chamber separated by the lens. The anterior chamber is filled with a watery fluid, called the aqueous humor, that maintains intraocular pressure, provides nourishment, and helps maintain the shape of the eyeball. The posterior chamber is filled with a jelly-like substance, called the vitreous humor, that maintains the spherical shape of the eye and supports the inner structures. Both substances are transparent, thus allowing light to pass through the eye to the retina (Figure 42-2).

The lens, located in the anterior chamber of the eye, is a transparent biconvex crystalline body enclosed in an elastic capsule held by suspensory ligaments. The shape of the lens changes to focus the image.

External Structures

The eyeball is protected from the external world by the eyelid, which contains a thin protective layer of epithelium, the conjunctiva (Figure 42-3). The conjunctiva covers the anterior portion of the eyeball and lines the eyelid. Projecting from the border of each eyelid is a row of eyelashes that protect the eye from foreign particles. The lacrimal gland produces a secretion called tears that contains a lysozyme, muramidase, to destroy pathogens.

COMMON DIAGNOSTIC TESTS

Commonly used diagnostic tests for clients with problems in hearing and vision are listed in Table 42-1.

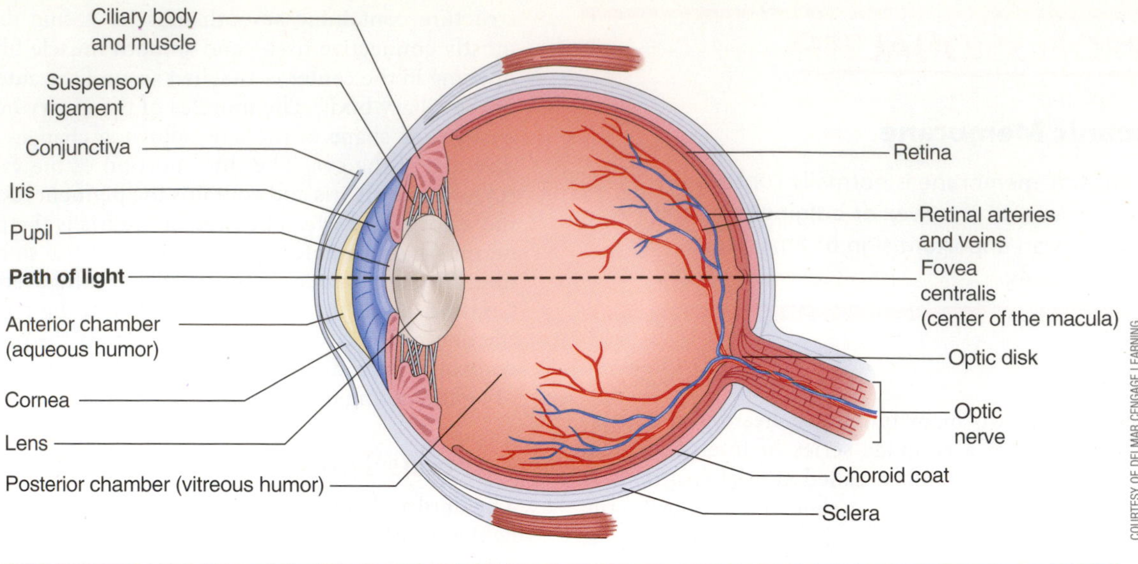

FIGURE 42-2 Lateral View of the Interior Eyeball

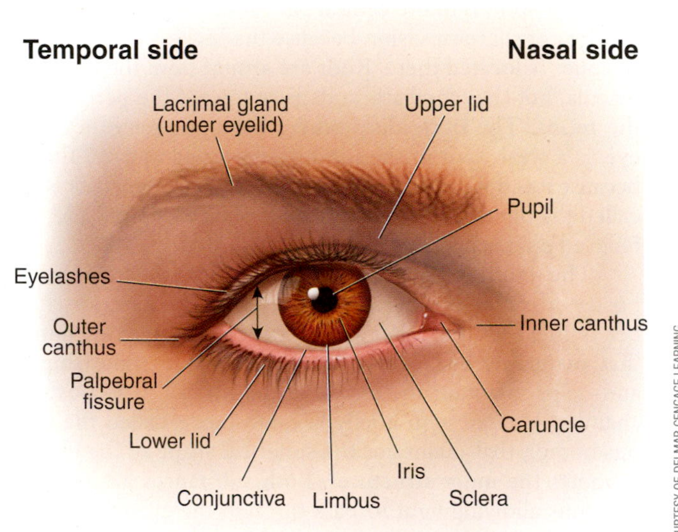

FIGURE 42-3 External View of the Right Eye

TABLE 42-1 Common Diagnostic Tests for Sensory Alterations

- Weber test (tuning fork)
- Rinne test (tuning fork)
- Audiometric testing (audiogram)
- Speech audiometry (Spondee threshold)
- Caloric test
- Brainstem auditory evoked response (ErA and BAER)
- Tympanometry
- Computed tomography (CT)
- Magnetic resonance imaging (MRI)
- Romberg test
- Otoscopic exam
- Past-point testing
- Color vision tests
- Tonometry
- Slit lamp examination
- Perimetry
- Visual acuity
- Electroretinogram (ERG)
- Ocular ultrasonography
- Ophthalmoscopic examination
- Orbital computerized tomography
- Fluoresce in angiography

COURTESY OF DELMAR CENGAGE LEARNING

SENSORY, PERCEPTUAL, AND COGNITIVE ALTERATIONS

An individual usually experiences discomfort and/or anxiety when subjected to a change in the type or amount of incoming stimuli. A person can become confused as a result of either overstimulation or understimulation. According to the individual's ability to process the stimuli, confusion (or disorientation) may occur. **Disorientation** is a mentally confused state in which the person's awareness of time, place, self, and/or situation is impaired. When awareness of these four factors is accurate, a person is said to be "oriented × 4."

A person admitted to a health-care agency experiences stimuli that are different from those usually encountered. A change in environment can overwhelm one's ability to perceive and interpret sensory input. As a result, the treatment setting becomes a stressor that negatively affects sensory, perceptual, and cognitive functions. If one or more of the factors just discussed causes an alteration in sensation, perception, or cognition, the client experiences problems with perceiving and interpreting stimuli. These problems are manifested by three types of alterations: sensory deficit, sensory deprivation, and sensory overload.

SENSORY DEFICIT

A **sensory deficit** is a change in the perception of sensory stimuli. This deficit affects all five senses. Examples of sensory deficit are vision and hearing losses such as those caused by cataracts, glaucoma, and presbycusis (steady loss of hearing acuity that occurs with aging).

The client's response to these losses usually depends on the time of onset and the severity of the condition. If the problem occurs suddenly and without warning, the client has difficulty adjusting to the loss of sensory and perceptual function. If these alterations occur gradually, the client may be able to accommodate the change and actually compensate for it by strengthening one or more of the other senses.

The effects of hospitalization or intensive medical treatments exacerbate the problems related to sensory deficit. For example, a client with acute hearing loss can feel alone and vulnerable. Clients with sensory deficit are at serious risk of experiencing either sensory deprivation or sensory overload.

SENSORY DEPRIVATION

Sensory deprivation is a state of reduced sensory input from the internal or external environment, manifested by alterations in sensory perception. Individuals experience sensory deprivation as a result of illness, trauma, or isolation. A person experiencing sensory deprivation misinterprets the limited stimuli with a resultant impairment of thoughts and feelings. Factors that contribute to sensory deprivation include:

- Visual or auditory impairments that limit or prohibit perception of stimuli
- Drugs that produce a sedative effect on the CNS and interfere with the interpretation of stimuli
- Trauma that results in brain damage and decreased cognitive function
- Isolation (either physical or social) that results in a nonstimulating environment

Some contributing factors (such as brain damage or blindness) result in chronic sensory deprivation. Other factors lead to acute, transient states of deprivation (such as receiving analgesic medications).

Individuals who are sensory-deprived may exhibit any of the following characteristics:

- Inability to concentrate
- Poor memory
- Impaired problem-solving ability
- Confusion
- Irritability
- Emotional lability (mood swings)
- Hallucinations
- Depression
- Boredom and apathy
- Drowsiness

SENSORY OVERLOAD

Sensory overload is a state of excessive and sustained multisensory stimulation manifested by behavior change and perceptual distortion. The individual experiencing this alteration is unable to process the amount or intensity of stimuli received. Factors contributing to sensory overload are:

- Pain originating from a heightened quality or quantity of internal stimuli
- Invasive procedures that result in an increased amount of external stimuli
- Activity-filled, busy environment that contributes to the amount of stimuli perceived
- Medications that stimulate the CNS and prohibit the client from ignoring selective stimuli
- Presence of strangers (both health care professionals and others) who contribute to the quantity of stimuli
- Diseases that affect the CNS and maximize the perception of stimuli

DISORDERS OF THE EAR

Disorders of the ear include impaired hearing, Ménière's disease, otosclerosis, acoustic neuroma, otitis media, otitis externa, and mastoiditis.

IMPAIRED HEARING

According to a study by Agrawal, Platz, and Niparko (2008), an estimated 55 million Americans have high-frequency hearing loss. Men were 5.5 times more likely to have hearing loss than women (Crosta, 2008). It can be seriously debilitating by limiting the ability to socialize and work, or respond to the telephone or alarms, yet relatively few individuals who experience impaired hearing actually seek help. Some may deny the problem and others may feel that a hearing aid is a sign of old age. Family members are often the first to be aware of a hearing deficit.

Types of Hearing Loss

Hearing loss is generally categorized in two ways: conductive and sensorineural. Mixed hearing loss, both conductive and

> **LIFE SPAN CONSIDERATIONS**
>
> **Effects of Aging**
>
> Sensory, perceptual, and cognitive function begin to diminish with aging. Decreased visual or auditory senses or impairments in memory are experienced. These changes can have a profound effect on a client's self-esteem and response to life.

CULTURAL CONSIDERATIONS

Hearing Loss

Caucasian and Mexican-American men had the greatest incidence of both high-frequency hearing loss and hearing loss in both ears. African-American clients were 70% less likely to have hearing loss than Caucasian clients. Hearing loss is preventable by reducing risk factors and by screening for hearing loss in young adulthood, especially in Caucasian and Mexican-American men (Agrawal, Platz, & Niparko, 2008).

sensorineural, is possible but far less likely. Either may occur at birth (congenital), develop later in life, be genetic, or be caused by injury or trauma.

Conductive hearing loss indicates an inability of the sound waves to reach the inner ear. This is caused by cerumen buildup or blockage, perforated tympanic membrane, or fixation of one or all of the ossicles.

In **sensorineural hearing loss**, the inner ear or cochlear portion of cranial nerve VIII is abnormal or diseased. A tumor, infection, trauma, or exposure to loud noises may cause destruction of the nerve and result in sensorineural hearing loss.

Sensorineural hearing loss associated with aging is termed **presbycusis**. Higher frequency sounds such as women's voices become especially difficult to hear, and distinguishing words may be a problem. People with sensorineural hearing loss can be helped by hearing aids or cochlear implants (Ruben, 2007).

Behaviors Indicating Hearing Loss

A hearing impairment is a serious disorder that is often debilitating and embarrassing to the client. Hearing is part of the communication process, so the inability to hear may cause the person to do or say the wrong thing in response to a question or command. Persons with hearing impairment may withdraw from conversation or seem indifferent to their surroundings or to those around them.

Alterations in hearing are often manifested by changes in speech habits and patterns. Individuals with hearing impairments may not notice the changes in their own speech pattern until someone constantly asks them to repeat themselves or to speak clearly. Indifference and withdrawal are common behaviors in response to hearing loss. If left undiagnosed and untreated, the person may truly regress, become unhappy, lonely, and possibly even paranoid. Some individuals overcompensate for the hearing loss by becoming very loud and aggressive.

Research on hearing impairment has created many devices to aid speech and sound discrimination. Early diagnosis, treatment, and rehabilitation are essential to help hearing-impaired persons enjoy and appreciate the world in which they live.

Hearing Aids/Assistive Devices

Hearing aids today come in a variety of designs and sizes. Some are quite small and tinted to a person's skin color so as to be virtually unnoticeable. Some are worn in the ear, behind the ear, or are part of eyeglasses frames. Persons with bilateral hearing loss may need *binaural* (worn in both ears) hearing aids.

A hearing aid converts environmental sound and speech into electronic signals that are amplified and converted to acoustic signals. It makes speech and sound louder but not necessarily clearer. Depending on the extent of hearing impairment and preference, the client may need to experiment with several different types of hearing aids. In addition, speech therapy, lip reading, and auditory training may be necessary to help discriminate speech and develop better listening skills.

Many other assistive hearing devices are available for the hearing impaired. Numerous television programs are closed-caption. Advanced technology allows telecommunication through a device called the Telecommunication Device for the Deaf (TDD), also called TTY Typewriter, which sends a printed message onto a small screen. Both sender and receiver must have the typewriter/telephone device. Many hospitals have these to comply with ADA requirements.

Alarm clocks offer strobe lights or vibrators to awaken clients. State-of-the-art receivers give instant access to radio, television, computer, and stereos to enhance receiving and listening systems. For travelers, complete kits are available to provide ready access for smoke alarm, clock, TDD, and door-knock alert in hotels or inns.

Hearing guide dogs are also available. The animals are specially trained to meet the needs of the hearing impaired. At home, the dog responds to alarms, knocking on doors, and babies crying. In public, the dog takes a position between owner and a potential threat. Special identifiers, such as a collar for the dog and ID card for the owner, are available. The dogs are trained to go wherever their master goes, including restaurants, grocery stores, and on public transportation.

PROFESSIONALTIP

Hearing Specialists

An audiologist evaluates hearing and determines the extent and type of hearing loss, and provides nonmedical treatment such as fitting hearing aids, advice about assistive listening devices, and communication/aural rehabilitative training. An otolaryngologist (ear, nose, and throat physician) provides medical evaluation of hearing disorders and medical and surgical interventions. A hearing aid specialist is licensed to dispense hearing aids but is not a medical doctor.

Medical–Surgical Management

Medical

The type of hearing loss and underlying etiology determines the best medical or surgical management. The client undergoes a complete physical examination as well as thorough diagnostic hearing tests to determine the etiology. The client and doctor together decide on the best course of therapy.

Surgical

The cochlear implant is a possible treatment for persons with profound deafness. In this procedure, a receiver/stimulator is implanted in the skull and a group of electrodes are planted in front of the round window in the inner ear. The client wears a microphone near the ear that picks up and translates sound into electrical signals. These signals are then transmitted to the brain via the cochlear implant and cranial nerve VIII.

Nursing Management

If the client uses a sign language interpreter, arrange for one to assist with communication. Writing notes, using a TDD, or a computer may be helpful. Approach the client and elicit the client's attention by waving. Make sure all personnel know the client is hearing impaired as well as the client's preferred method of communication. The publication *Pictograms for Hospital Communication* is available from the U.S. Department of Justice.

NURSING PROCESS

Assessment

Subjective Data

Ask the client to describe the initial onset of symptoms and possible familial traits, recent infections of the ears, nose, or upper respiratory system. Determine recent trauma and past surgery as well as medical history such as diabetes, heart disease, or cancer. Ask about allergies to food, drugs, or environmental factors, associated symptoms such as **tinnitus** (ringing sound in the ear), **vertigo** (dizziness), nausea, and vomiting. The client's work history may reveal exposure to loud noises.

Objective Data

Listen closely to the client and note any deterioration of speech, slurring, or dropping of word endings. Document current and recent medications used.

Inspect the outer ear for abnormalities, lesions, or cerumen. Palpate the mastoid process, neck, jaw, and temporal regions of the head for swelling or tenderness to touch. Note the degree of hearing loss as reported by the client and compare it to the diagnostic tests such as the speech audiogram. The client's perception of hearing loss may be significantly different from the diagnostic findings.

A nursing diagnosis for a client with impaired hearing is:

NURSING DIAGNOSES	PLANNING/OUTCOMES	NURSING INTERVENTIONS
Social Isolation related to hearing impairment	The client will participate in conversations and other social situations.	Take time to engage client in conversation. Make sure you have the client's attention and be at eye level. Speak slowly and distinctly. Give the client time to respond. Provide the client and family members written information regarding the availability, variety, and quality of assistive hearing devices. Encourage client to participate in social situations.

Evaluation: Evaluate each outcome to determine how it has been met by the client.

MÉNIÈRE'S DISEASE

Ménière's disease, also known as endolymphatic hydrops, is a state of hearing loss characterized by tinnitus and vertigo. Although the exact etiology is unknown, it is thought to be an excessive accumulation of endolymph in the cochlear duct and possible leakage of endolymph into the perilymph caused by increased capillary permeability. Mixing of the two fluids chemically alters the homeostasis of the perilymph and endolymph and could be responsible for the symptoms associated with Ménière's disease.

The major symptoms are the classic triad of vertigo, tinnitus, and unilateral fluctuating hearing loss. The vertigo is often associated with nausea and vomiting. Tinnitus may either be a preceding aura or occur simultaneously with the vertigo. Initially, tinnitus is intermittent, but as the disease progresses, it may be a constant, low-pitched roaring sound. The fluctuating, unilateral hearing loss becomes more profound with each attack.

The symptoms are frequently at their worst during the first attack, which may last from a few minutes to six hours. **Nystagmus**, repetitive and involuntary movement of the eyeballs, and diaphoresis may occur during an attack. Subsequent attacks are less severe, but over time may involve both ears and cause permanent bilateral hearing loss. Clients report many different precipitating events, such as stress, weather changes, menstruation, or pregnancy, and various dietary influences, including caffeine, alcohol, and salt. Smoking has also been implicated.

Medical–Surgical Management

Medical

Medical management is the preferred treatment and most helpful to 80% to 85% of persons with this disease. Diagnosis is not difficult and is usually made based on the client's report of symptoms. Diagnosis may also be confirmed with caloric stimulation (although this test is primarily conducted on comatose clients) and magnetic resonance imaging to rule out a tumor. Medical management is symptomatic.

Surgical

Surgical intervention is needed only when the attacks are frequent and debilitating, or when the disease severely affects the quality of life and the ability for self-care. Surgical treatment includes endolymphatic, subarachnoid shunt placement to drain excessive endolymph. With this procedure, hearing is preserved in 60% to 70% of the clients. With a vestibular neurectomy, the vestibular portion of cranial nerve VIII is severed; hearing is preserved in 90% of clients having this procedure. In surgical destruction of the labyrinth, hearing is destroyed but the incapacitating vertigo is completely relieved.

> **PROFESSIONALTIP**
>
> **Assisting the Hearing-Impaired Client**
>
> - Speak slowly and distinctly after getting the client's attention.
> - Face the client and sit or stand to be at eye level with the client.
> - Use short, simple sentences and give the client time to respond. Repeat or rephrase if necessary.
> - Use written materials when possible to communicate information.
> - Keep a notepad and pen or pencil available to write down new or unfamiliar words and concepts.
> - If sign language is the client's preferred method of communication, locate a person who understands sign language.
> - If the client wears a hearing aid, make sure that the battery is functional, it is turned on, and is adjusted to a comfortable level.

Pharmacological

Several medications are useful to help control the symptoms, such as antihistamines, antiemetics, benzodiazepines, diuretics, tranquilizers, vasoactive agents, and oral niacin. The medications are prescribed for long-term use or at the onset of symptoms. Because the cause of Ménière's disease is unknown, there is no cure.

Diet

Dietary interventions include strict salt restriction and avoidance of those foods or beverages that precipitate or aggravate an attack. Examples are beer, wine, soda, salty food or snacks, chocolate, and caffeinated coffee and tea.

Activity

Activity is not limited except during or after an attack, when clients require prolonged bed rest and restriction of activities that are unsafe, such as driving or operating heavy equipment.

Nursing Management

Advise client against reading and use of glaring lights. Instruct client to avoid sudden position changes and have assistance when getting out of bed or ambulating. Keep side rails up and the call light within the client's reach.

NURSING PROCESS

Assessment

Subjective Data

The history begins with identifying significant contributory data. Ask the client to describe the initial onset of symptoms including, but not limited to, the classic triad of tinnitus, vertigo, and fluctuating unilateral hearing loss.

Relate questions to recent viral illness; upper respiratory infections; past medical, surgical, and dental history; and any problems related to the neck and face. Document food, drug, or environmental allergies. Record current or recent long-term medications. Identify the client's occupation and hobbies that contribute to hearing loss.

Objective Data

A thorough physical examination includes looking at the ear for abnormalities, lesions and cerumen blockage, or unusual drainage. Palpate the neck, jaw, and mastoid process for possible lymph node enlargement and tenderness. The nurse assists with the otologic examination as needed. Audiologic testing determines unilateral or bilateral hearing loss.

Nursing diagnoses for a client with Ménière's disease include the following:

NURSING DIAGNOSES	PLANNING/OUTCOMES	NURSING INTERVENTIONS
Activity Intolerance related to severe vertigo	The client will be able to tolerate activities of daily living.	Provide adequate periods of bed rest. Provide assistance with ambulation and encourage increased activity as tolerated. Keep the room dim and quiet when possible. Avoid jarring the bed and caution client to avoid sudden movements. Administer antiemetic before symptoms become too severe.
Deficient Knowledge related to abrupt onset and unknown progression of the disease	The client will verbalize understanding of the disease process and potential precipitating factors and how to manage or control the symptoms.	Assess the client's current knowledge of the disease process. Review the disease process and underlying etiology of Ménière's disease with the client. Ask the client to identify possible precipitating factors such as stress or dietary habits. Discuss health promotion programs for stress management and healthy cooking classes. Suggest consultations with dietary and social services. Review follow-up appointments, medications, dietary management, activity, and rest parameters. Evaluate client's readiness to discuss progressive hearing loss and current assistive hearing devices available.
Risk for Injury related to vertigo	The client will not fall or be injured because of vertigo.	Keep side rails up. Teach client to move or turn slowly. Instruct client to sit or lie down when vertigo occurs. Reiterate need to call for assistance when ambulating. Keep call bell within client's reach. Administer medications for vertigo prior to worsening of symptoms. Avoid glaring, bright lights.

Evaluation: Evaluate each outcome to determine how it has been met by the client.

CRITICAL THINKING

Hearing Impaired

How can nurses assist the hearing impaired during a hospitalization?

OTOSCLEROSIS

Otosclerosis, the most common conductive hearing loss, is secondary to a pathologic change of the bones in the middle ear. The exact cause is unknown. The ossicles are normally hard, but over time and without warning, the bone becomes softened, spongy, highly vascular, and partially or totally fixed. This fixation reduces or prevents transmission of source waves to inner ear fluids. Although all three bones may be affected, the stapes, which must vibrate on the oval window in order to transmit sound waves, is most commonly afflicted.

Otosclerosis is more common in adults, more often in women, and it is familial in some cases. The primary clinical manifestations are subtle changes in hearing and low-pitched tinnitus. It becomes more difficult to distinguish a whisper, or to hear in crowded places or understand conversation. Individuals affected by otosclerosis often blame others for speaking too softly or mumbling. Frequently, rather than asking others to speak up or to repeat themselves, the person will be irritable and withdrawn.

Diagnostic testing begins with the Weber and Rinne tuning fork tests. In addition, audiometric testing should be performed. Schwartz's sign, a pink blush, is seen on otoscopic examination. Tympanometry shows stiffness in the sound conduction system.

Medical–Surgical Management

Medical

Treatment for otosclerosis is limited to three options. The individual may choose to do nothing and obtain periodic audiometry to evaluate progression of the disease. The second choice is to use a hearing aid, and the third choice is surgical management with an outpatient procedure known as a stapedectomy.

Surgical

A stapedectomy is the preferred surgical technique for improving hearing loss caused by otosclerosis. A stapedectomy is done under local or general anesthesia and routinely requires a surgical incision in the posterior ear canal, removal of the stapes, and implantation of a plastic prosthesis. Laser stapedectomy is performed through the ear canal without an incision. The stapes tendon is vaporized, chards are removed with delicate micro instruments, and an opening is made allowing the surgeon to implant a prosthetic piston. This restores normal vibration against the inner ear.

Nursing Management

Postoperatively, instruct the client to turn or move slowly, not to blow the nose for 10 days, to avoid lifting for 1 month, and if sneezing occurs, to keep the mouth open. Administer antibiotics as ordered. Advise the client that hearing is decreased for 3 to 4 weeks until gel-foam packing dissolves.

NURSING PROCESS

Assessment

Subjective Data

A careful history discovers possible hereditary traits or acquired disease. Ask about recent infections of the ears, nose, or upper respiratory system, and also about past surgery, trauma, or other illnesses such as diabetes, heart disease, or cancer. Identify associated symptoms, such as dizziness, tinnitus, vertigo, and nausea.

Note allergies to foods, drugs, or any environmental factors, such as exposure to loud noises. Record current and recent medications, especially those known to be ototoxic.

Objective Data

Objective data include a thorough physical examination. Inspect the outer ear for abnormalities, lesions, or impacted ear wax and palpate the mastoid process, neck, jaw, and temporal regions of the head for pain or swelling. Assess the degree of hearing loss. The client may experience vomiting.

Nursing diagnoses for the client with otosclerosis include the following:

NURSING DIAGNOSES	PLANNING/OUTCOMES	NURSING INTERVENTIONS
***A**nxiety* related to decrease or loss in hearing	The client will show evidence of reduced anxiety and verbalize understanding of the disease process and treatment regimen.	Encourage the client to explore feelings of anxiety and to ask questions to clarify concerns. Provide honest and realistic feedback. Collaborate with the physician to provide thorough and clear explanations of the disease process, treatment options, and anticipated results.
*Risk for **I**njury* related to vertigo	The client will not fall or be injured because of vertigo.	Keep side rails up. Reiterate need to call for assistance when ambulating and keep call bell within client's reach. Instruct the client to move or turn slowly. Administer medications for vertigo prior to worsening of symptoms. Keep room well lit when client is ambulating.
*Deficient **K**nowledge* related to activities after surgery	The client will demonstrate the ability to change dressing correctly and verbalize knowledge of self-care and follow-up.	Teach client how and when to perform dressing change and have client demonstrate the procedure. Instruct client to avoid pressure changes (such as flying in an unpressurized aircraft), avoid heavy lifting (60 lbs) for 1 month, avoid nose blowing for 10 days, and if sneezing occurs, keep mouth open. Advise client to keep water out of the ear and keep the ear exposed to air as much as possible for one month. There will be some drainage which is initially red, then pink, and then brownish. Tell client to report any greenish, yellowish, or foul-smelling drainage.

Nursing diagnoses for the client with otosclerosis include the following: (Continued)

NURSING DIAGNOSES	PLANNING/OUTCOMES	NURSING INTERVENTIONS
		Instruct client to take all antibiotics as prescribed and complete the full course of treatment. Advise client there should be very little pain or discomfort but if there is, take prescribed analgesics and notify doctor if pain is prolonged or intense. Warn client that hearing is decreased for 3 to 4 weeks after surgery until gel-foam packing dissolves. Inform client that audiometric testing will be conducted 1 month after surgery. Instruct client to schedule an appointment with the physician in 1 month but call physician if uncontrolled pain is experienced or a malodorous, greenish discharge comes from the ear.

Evaluation: Evaluate each outcome to determine how it has been met by the client.

ACOUSTIC NEUROMA

Acoustic neuroma is a slow-growing and usually benign tumor of the vestibular portion of the inner ear (cranial nerve VIII). Detection at the onset of symptoms is essential and is accomplished with magnetic resonance imaging. Presenting symptoms of dizziness, tinnitus, and hearing loss are common to many dysfunctions of the ear, and the possibility of acoustic neuroma must not be overlooked.

Clients who present with dizziness, tinnitus, and hearing loss have a complete workup for auditory and vestibular (balance) function. Facial weakness is caused by compression of the tumor on cranial nerve VII. Cranial nerve V may also be affected as the tumor grows, causing paresthesia of the face and loss of the corneal reflex. Large neuromas cause increased intracranial pressure, papilledema, vomiting, and headache.

MEDICAL–SURGICAL MANAGEMENT

Treatment is almost always surgical excision of the tumor. Although antihistamines may reduce the dizziness, pharmacologic treatment is only temporary until diagnostic tests are completed and surgery is planned.

NURSING MANAGEMENT

Assist client to express feelings about progressive hearing loss and the changes in activities of daily living, employment, and quality of life issues. Note the family's feelings and ability to cope. Perform postoperative care as ordered.

NURSING PROCESS

ASSESSMENT

Subjective Data

Obtain through the client history signs and symptoms and all contributing data.

Objective Data

Obtain with the physical examination a complete cranial nerve evaluation performed by the physician or audiologist to determine the extent of cranial nerve involvement.

A nursing diagnosis for a client with acoustic neuroma is:

NURSING DIAGNOSES	PLANNING/OUTCOMES	NURSING INTERVENTIONS
*Anticipatory **G**rieving* related to diminished quality of life, loss of ability for self-care, or possible loss of life	The client will express feelings of grief and demonstrate adaptive coping mechanisms.	Assist the client to express feelings about progressive hearing loss and changes in activities of daily living, employment, and quality of life issues. Collaborate with physician and other members of the health care team to provide thorough and clear explanations of the disease process, treatment options, and anticipated results.

(Continues)

A nursing diagnosis for a client with acoustic neuroma is: (Continued)

NURSING DIAGNOSES	PLANNING/OUTCOMES	NURSING INTERVENTIONS
		Observe the client's coping styles. Support those that the client finds helpful and explore other coping mechanisms that may prove useful in time (e.g., hobbies and other diversional activities, prayer, reading, and so on).
		Include the family in all interventions that the client desires. Examine the family's feelings and ability to cope.
		Consult social services, pastoral care, or other hospital and community resources when appropriate.

Evaluation: Evaluate each outcome to determine how it has been met by the client.

OTITIS MEDIA

Otitis media is an inflammation of the middle ear and a common cause of conductive hearing loss, although usually temporary. Symptoms include ear pain, fever, redness of auricle and ear canal, and sometimes enlarged lymph nodes over the mastoid process, parotids, and upper neck. Otitis media occurs more frequently in children than in adults.

Fluid accumulates behind the eardrum because of blockage of the eustachian tube. This is secondary to an upper respiratory infection, allergies, or acute bacterial infection. On physical examination, the tympanic membrane is retracted, normal, or bulging. A pneumatic otoscope allows the practitioner to blow soft puffs of air against the tympanic membrane to assess movement. A stiff, nonmoving, or bulging tympanic membrane indicates inflammation or fluid accumulation in the middle ear (Figure 42-4A-C). Visualization of the normal landmarks may be obscured. The Rinne tuning fork test and audiometry confirm a conductive hearing loss.

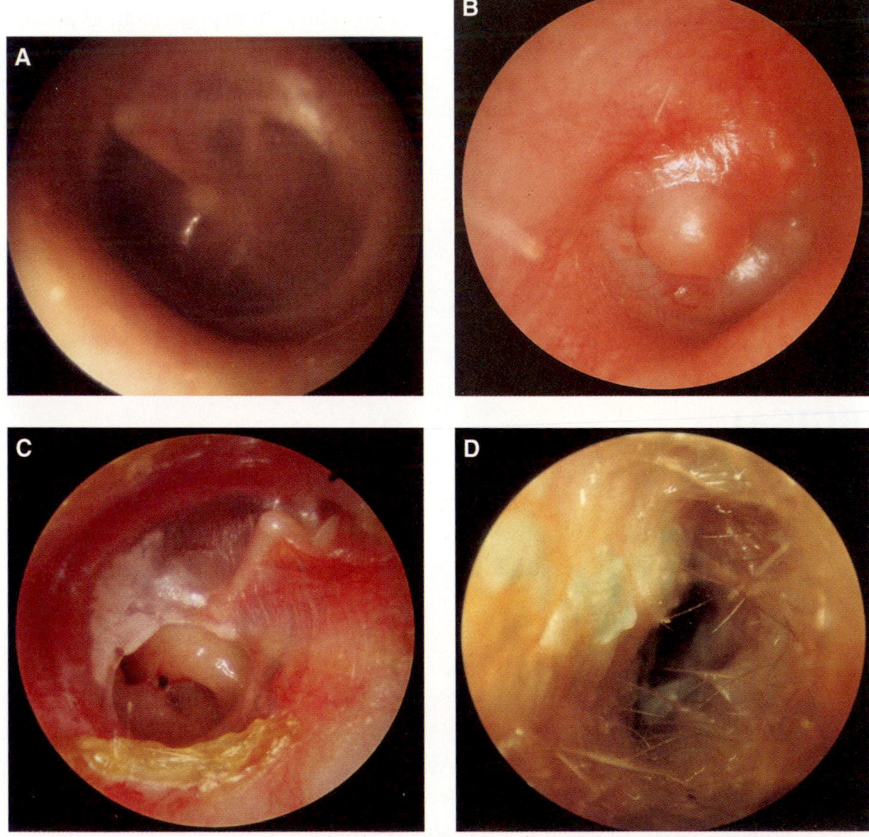

FIGURE 42-4 *A*, Normal Tympanic Membrane; *B*, Bulging Tympanic Membrane; *C*, Tympanic Membrane Perforation; *D*, Acute Otitis Externa (*Images A and C courtesy of Dr. Andrew B. Silva, Pediatric Otolaryngology; images B and D courtesy of Bruce Black, MD, Brisbane, Australia.*)

CRITICAL THINKING

Hearing Impairment

What modifications would need to be made in the life of a person who could suddenly no longer hear?

Medical–Surgical Management

Medical

Topical heat and systemic analgesics may be used to control pain. The client should lie on the affected side to facilitate drainage.

Surgical

Surgical management may be necessary for diagnostic or therapeutic reasons. A myringotomy may be performed, in which an incision is made in the eardrum and fluid is aspirated. A polyethylene tube may be placed in the eardrum to equalize pressure and allow drainage of fluid.

A tympanoplasty may be needed if the tympanic membrane is ruptured. If there is a large tympanic membrane perforation, the malleus, which is connected to the tympanic membrane, or other ossicles may be damaged. Ossicular chain reconstruction typically refers to the removal of the actual bones and replacement with a plastic prosthesis. The prosthesis and the tympanic membrane reconstruction often result in a significant improvement in hearing.

Pharmacological

Medications used include decongestants, such as pseudoephedrine hydrochloride (Sudafed); antihistamines, such as diphenhydramine hydrochloride (Benadryl); and systemic antibiotics, such as ampicillin (Omnipen).

Activity

Activity is not restricted unless surgical management is indicated.

Nursing Management

After myringotomy, maintain drainage flow. Sterile cotton may be loosely placed in the external ear to absorb drainage. Change cotton whenever it is damp. Perform hand hygiene before and after ear care. Monitor vital signs. Warn client against blowing nose or getting ear wet when bathing. Encourage client to complete prescribed antibiotics.

NURSING PROCESS

Assessment

Subjective Data

Ask about the onset, duration, and severity of pain and what home remedies have been used. Hearing loss and/or tinnitus and a deep throbbing pain in the ear may be reported.

Objective Data

A watery or yellow discharge may be seen. It may have a foul odor. The client may have a fever.

A nursing diagnosis for a client with otitis media is:

NURSING DIAGNOSES	PLANNING/OUTCOMES	NURSING INTERVENTIONS
*Acute **Pain*** related to inflammation in the middle ear	The client will experience pain relief.	Administer antibiotics and analgesics as ordered. Teach client and family the importance of administering medications as ordered and to complete full course of prescription. Apply heating pad, set on low, for 20 minutes every 2 hours. Do not use on small children. Teach client if pain is unrelieved in 48 hours, to contact physician.

Evaluation: Evaluate each outcome to determine how it has been met by the client.

OTITIS EXTERNA

Otitis externa, or "swimmer's ear," typically involves a bacterial infection of the external ear canal skin. The canal skin becomes red and edematous. If the swelling is severe enough, it will block the ear passage and cause a mild conductive hearing loss (Figure 42-4D). Also, in most cases, there is a discharge. If the discharge is copious and the canal size is constricted, a mild conductive hearing loss results.

MASTOIDITIS

Mastoiditis (inflammation of the mastoid) is most often the direct result of chronic or recurrent bacterial otitis media. The recurrent infection may find its way into the bone and structures surrounding the middle ear and, if left untreated, causes severe damage, sensorineural deafness, facial weakness, brain abscess, and meningitis. Symptoms include earache, fever, headache, and malaise. Antibiotics are given for a trial period. If symptoms do not resolve, surgical intervention such as mastoidectomy or meatoplasty may be necessary.

DISORDERS OF THE EYE

Disorders of the eye include cataracts, glaucoma, retinal detachment, infections, refractive errors, injuries, impaired vision, and macular degeneration.

CATARACTS

A cataract is a disorder that causes the lens or its capsule to lose its transparency and/or become opaque (Figure 42-5). The lens is normally clear and transparent and allows light to pass through to the retina. As clouding develops, visual impairment occurs. Cataracts usually affect both eyes; however, the degree of visual impairment is often different in each eye.

Cataracts are typically associated with aging; however, they may be congenital, caused by severe eye injury, or secondary to certain systemic diseases, such as metabolic problems (diabetes mellitus) and chronic eye disease (uveitis). Ophthalmoscopic examination is the primary method of evaluation.

MEDICAL–SURGICAL MANAGEMENT

Surgical

The only treatment for a cataract is surgical removal of the lens; however, the mere finding of a cataract is not an indication for surgery. Surgery is indicated when significant vision loss has occurred. The lens are removed by the intracapsular or extracapsular approach. During the intracapsular cataract extraction, the ophthalmologist removes the lens within its capsule.

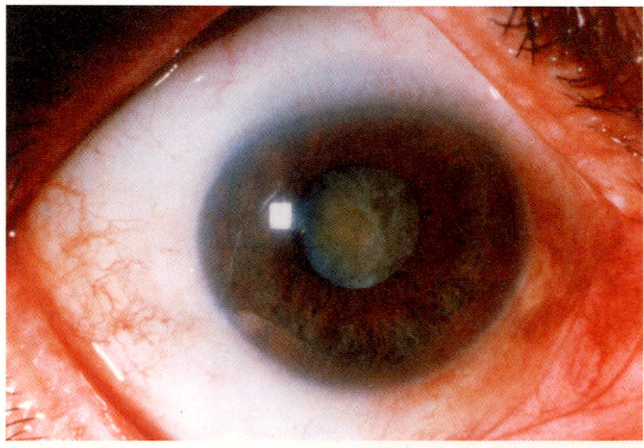

FIGURE 42-5 A cataract results in the loss of transparency of the lens of the eye. (*Courtesy of the National Eye Institute, Bethesda, MD.*)

> **PROFESSIONAL TIP**
>
> **Eye Specialists**
>
> An ophthalmologist is a medical doctor who specializes in the diagnosis and treatment, medical and surgical, of diseases of the eye, visual disorders, and eye injuries. An optometrist is a doctor of optometry and is licensed to examine, diagnose, manage and treat vision problems, diseases, and other abnormalities of the eyes and related structures.

Extracapsular cataract extraction is the procedure most commonly used (Figure 42-6). The ophthalmologist removes the anterior portion of the capsule and then expresses, or removes, the lens. An intraocular lens (IOL) is generally implanted. Glasses or special contact lenses also are used.

Most eye surgery is done on an outpatient basis under local anesthesia. General anesthesia is used at the client's request and for clients who are extremely anxious, deaf, or mentally retarded. A tranquilizer such as diazepam (Valium) or midazolam (Versed) is often given to reduce anxiety when receiving injections on the face and around the eye.

Preoperatively, the client can receive several types of eye medications to prepare the eye for surgery: mydriatic (makes pupil dilate) and cycloplegic (paralyzes ciliary muscle) eyedrops, antibiotic eyedrops as a prophylaxis against infection, and an intravenous infusion of an agent

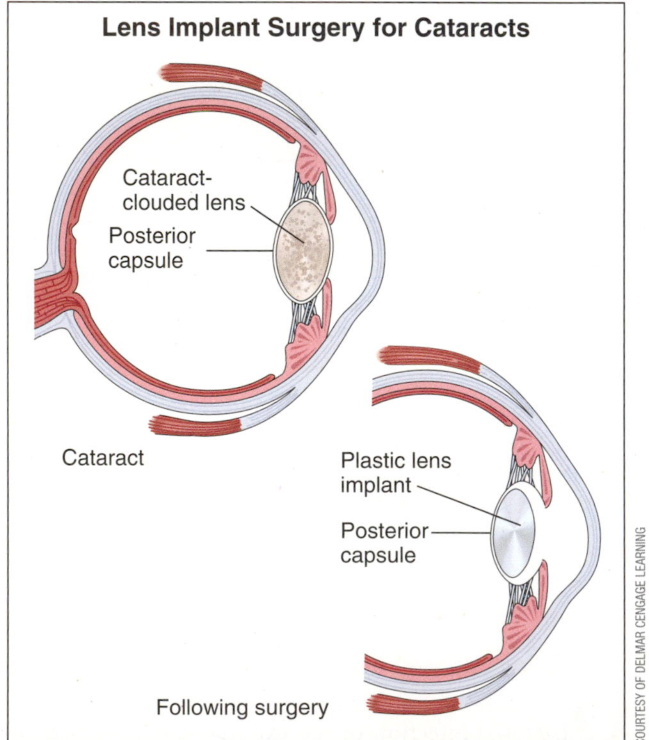

FIGURE 42-6 To correct cataracts with an extracapsular extraction, the lens is removed, the posterior lens capsule is left intact, and a plastic IOL is placed.

to lower intraocular pressure (mannitol or a carbonic anhydrase inhibitor).

After the anesthesia wears off, the client is discharged. The client is instructed to have a driver available for the trip home. Driving is restricted for a few days.

Postoperatively, the client has a patch over the eye. The patch is removed and reapplied on the first postoperative day, when miotic (makes pupil contract) eye drops are begun. Mild discomfort and scratchiness are expected. Atropine sulfate eyedrops and cold compresses are ordered to relieve these discomforts.

Nursing Management

Assist with ambulation because depth perception has changed. Maintain eye patch on affected eye. Advise client to sleep with eye patch on as ordered. Teach client or family to administer eyedrops and ointments. Client should avoid heavy lifting, straining during defecation, and vigorous coughing and sneezing. Dark glasses will relieve glare. Encourage client to keep all follow-up appointments.

NURSING PROCESS

Assessment

Subjective Data

A general medical history as well as a history of symptoms is obtained. Symptoms may include haziness, cloudiness, blurred vision, double vision, altered color perception, and glare when looking at lights, especially with night driving. Fear of losing one's eyesight is very devastating. There is often a great deal of anxiety when the client seeks an eye examination.

Objective Data

Upon inspection of the eye, the usual black pupil appears clouded, progressing to a milky white appearance, which is a characteristic finding of a mature cataract and indicates significant vision loss.

Nursing diagnoses for a client with cataracts include the following:

NURSING DIAGNOSES	PLANNING/OUTCOMES	NURSING INTERVENTIONS
*Disturbed **Sensory** Perception (Visual)* related to ocular lens opacity	The client will demonstrate improved ability to process visual stimuli and communicate visual limitations.	Assess and document baseline visual acuity. Elicit functional description of what the client can and cannot see.
*Risk for **Injury*** related to difficulty in processing visual images and altered depth perception	The client will avoid activities associated with increased potential for injury.	Teach the client to change position slowly. Teach the client to avoid reaching for objects to maintain stability when ambulating, as depth perception is altered.
*Impaired **Home** Maintenance* related to age, limited vision or activity restrictions imposed by surgery	The client will perform self-care activities in home environment.	Discuss the client's ability to meet self-care needs and activities of daily living. Evaluate how the client's current functional abilities are affected by activity restrictions and postoperative care needs. Help the client decide on a realistic site for postoperative care needs.

Evaluation: Evaluate each outcome to determine how it has been met by the client.

GLAUCOMA

Glaucoma is a disorder characterized by an abnormally high pressure of fluid inside the eyeball (intraocular pressure, IOP). The aqueous humor does not return into the bloodstream through the canal of Schlemm as quickly as it is formed. The fluid accumulates and, by compressing the lens into the vitreous humor, puts pressure on the neurons of the retina. If the pressure continues over a long period, it destroys the neurons and brings about blindness.

There are two primary forms of glaucoma: open-angle glaucoma and closed-angle glaucoma. In open-angle glaucoma (chronic simple glaucoma) there is a gradual rise in IOP, a slowly progressive loss of peripheral vision, and, if not controlled, a late loss of central vision and ultimate blindness. This is the most prevalent form of glaucoma and is usually bilateral. Closed-angle glaucoma (acute glaucoma) is characterized by attacks of suddenly increased IOP, exhibited clinically by a bulging iris, which is an emergency situation. Closed-angle glaucoma is usually unilateral with severe pain and loss of vision caused by acute obstruction of aqueous humor drainage within the eye.

Secondary glaucoma results from ocular or systemic disorders that elevate the IOP. These disorders indirectly disrupt the activity of the structures involved in circulation and/or reabsorption of aqueous humor. This can happen suddenly and without warning.

CLIENT TEACHING

Glaucoma Care

- Continue the use of eye medications as ordered.
- Continue to receive medical supervision for observation of intraocular pressure to ensure control of the disorder.
- Avoid exertion, stooping, heavy lifting, or wearing constrictive clothing because these actions increase intra-ocular pressure.

Medical–Surgical Management

Medical

Medical management for glaucoma is focused on drug therapy, and the main objective is to reduce intraocular pressure. Two mechanisms for reducing this pressure are (1) physically constricting the pupil so that the ciliary muscle is contracted, which allows better circulation of the aqueous humor to the site of absorption, and (2) inhibiting the production of aqueous humor.

Surgical

Surgical intervention to facilitate drainage of the aqueous humor is called an iridectomy. A surgical incision is made through the cornea to remove a portion of the iris to facilitate aqueous drainage.

A laser also is used to treat various eye disorders. In open-angle glaucoma, a laser is used to create multiple scars around the trabecular meshwork (a supporting or anchoring strand that allows increased outflow of aqueous humor), thereby reducing intraocular pressure. In closed-angle glaucoma, laser energy is used to create a hole in the periphery of the iris, creating an opening between the anterior and posterior chambers for aqueous drainage.

 Pharmacological

Drugs that enhance pupillary constriction are commonly used to treat glaucoma. Miotics and cholinesterase inhibitors such as pilocarpine hydrochloride (Isopto Carpine), carbachol (Carbacel), and demecarium bromide (Humorsol) are frequently used.

Beta-adrenergics such as timolol maleate (Timoptic Solution) are the drugs of choice for decreasing IOP. When used as eyedrops, beta-adrenergics reduce aqueous humor production without pupil constriction.

Carbonic anhydrase inhibitors, such as acetazolamide (Diamox), reduce production of aqueous humor to help maintain a lowered IOP. Side effects reported are numbness, weakness, tingling of extremities, and rashes. Adrenergics such as epinephrine bitartrate (Epitrate) also reduce aqueous humor production. Osmotic agents such as mannitol and glycerin (Osmoglyn) are administered systemically to the client with closed-angle glaucoma in an emergency as an effort to decrease IOP. The high osmolarity of these agents draws fluid into the intravascular space, which lowers the IOP.

Nursing Management

Administer medications as ordered. Stress client compliance with prescribed medication therapy. Encourage glaucoma screening for all persons older than age 35, especially if there is a family history of glaucoma.

NURSING PROCESS

Assessment

Subjective Data

Obtain a history, noting the presence of risk factors: positive family history (believed to be linked in open-angle glaucoma), eye tumor, intraocular hemorrhage, intraocular inflammation, or contusion of the eye from trauma during cataract surgery.

Symptoms of open-angle glaucoma include gradual loss of peripheral vision, eye pain, difficulty adjusting to darkness, halos around lights, and an inability to detect color. For closed-angle glaucoma, symptoms include sudden onset of severe pain in the eye often accompanied by headache, nausea, vomiting, malaise, rainbow halos around lights, and blurred vision.

Objective Data

Assessment reveals acute increased intraocular pressure (21 to 32 mm Hg) as measured with a tonometer (normal range is 12 to 22 mm Hg).

A nursing diagnosis for a client with glaucoma is:

NURSING DIAGNOSES	PLANNING/OUTCOMES	NURSING INTERVENTIONS
*Acute **Pain*** related to closed-angle glaucoma	The client will verbalize relief from discomfort.	Administer prescribed ophthalmic agent for glaucoma. Notify physician of the following: hypotension, urinary output less than 240 mL for 8 hours, no relief in eye pain within 30 minutes of drug therapy, and continual diminishing visual acuity. Monitor blood pressure, pulse, and respiration every 4 hours if not receiving osmotic agent intravenously and every 2 hours if receiving intravenous osmotic agent.

A nursing diagnosis for a client with glaucoma is: (Continued)

NURSING DIAGNOSES	PLANNING/OUTCOMES	NURSING INTERVENTIONS
		Monitor degree of eye pain every 30 minutes. Monitor intake and output every 8 hours while receiving intravenous osmotic agent. Monitor visual acuity before each instillation of prescribed ophthalmic agent by asking if objects are clear or blurred and if the client can read printed material held at arm's length. Remind the client that miotics may cause blurred vision for 1 to 2 hours after use and that adaptation to dark environments is difficult because of the pupillary constriction.

Evaluation: Evaluate each outcome to determine how it has been met by the client.

RETINAL DETACHMENT

In retinal detachment, the retina separates from the choroid (Figure 42-7). Partial separation becomes complete, if untreated, with the subsequent total loss of vision. A tear or hole in the retina can extend the separation as vitreous humor seeps through the opening and separates the retina from the choroid. The cause of retinal detachment is from severe trauma to the eye or from intraocular disorders such as cataract extraction, perforating injuries, or severe **myopia** (nearsightedness). This condition is painless because there are no pain receptors in the retina.

MEDICAL–SURGICAL MANAGEMENT

Medical

Early corrective intervention to reattach the retina uses one of several techniques. Two procedures are used to create an inflammatory reaction that, once healing and scarring occur, results in the retina reattaching to the choroid. Freezing (cryopexy) is an intensely cold probe applied to the scleral surface directly over the hole in the retina. Laser photocoagulation also seals tears or holes in the retina.

Surgical

A surgical procedure called scleral buckling is sometimes used. This operation reduces the scleral surface and allows contact between the choroid and retina.

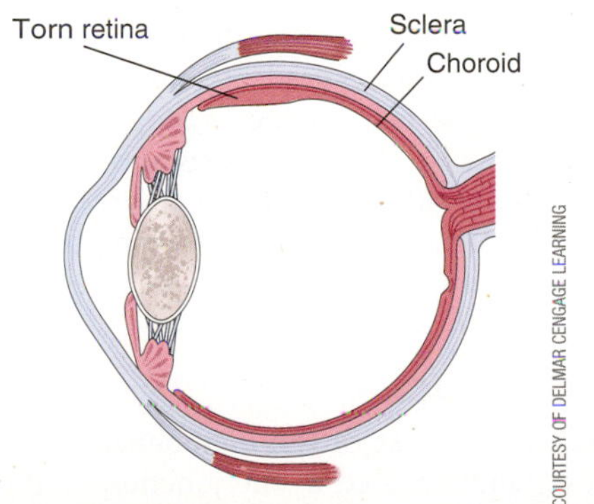

FIGURE 42-7 Retinal Detachment

Pneumatic retinopexy is used for an uncomplicated detachment. A small amount of fluid is withdrawn from the anterior chamber and an expandable gas is injected into the posterior chamber. The gas pushes against the retinal tear and seals it off. The fluid under the retinal tear is absorbed and the gas is released from the eye over several weeks (Mayo Clinic, 2008).

Sometimes when the surgeon cannot see the retinal tear because of vitreous cloudiness or retinal scarring that prevents a pneumatic retinopexy or scleral buckling, sections of the vitreous are removed (vitrectomy). Delicate instruments are inserted into the eye through incisions in the sclera. The surgeon removes scar tissue from the vitreous and infuses a salt solution into the eye to maintain the normal pressure and shape. A scleral buckling may be performed after the vitrectomy, and the posterior chamber is filled with air, gas, or silicone oil to hold the retina against the inside of the eye (Mayo Clinic, 2008).

Pharmacological

Cycloplegic-mydriatic and antiinfective eyedrops are often ordered following the attachment procedure.

Activity

Bed rest and a patch on one or both eyes restricts activity. If air is injected into the vitreous humor, the client either lies prone or sits forward with the unaffected eye upward.

NURSING MANAGEMENT

Explain surgery routines. *Preoperative*: Level of activity—ocular rest, which includes bilateral eye patching and bed rest to facilitate settling of the retina and prevent detachment from worsening. The affected eye is maximally dilated before surgery to permit adequate visualization of the fundus. *Intraoperative*: Client must lie still during surgery or give surgeon warning if needs to cough or change position. Face covered with drapes. Air and oxygen provided. Monitoring, including frequent blood pressure measurements. *Postoperative*: Positioning (supine with a small pillow under the head), bilateral eye patches, activity restrictions, and need to call for assistance with ambulation until stable and vision is adequate.

NURSING PROCESS

Assessment

Subjective Data

Obtain a medical history for presence of causative factors: trauma, recent cataract surgery, eye tumor, severe myopia, uveitis. The client may describe sudden flashes of light (photopsia), floating spots (caused by bleeding into the vitreous cavity), blurred vision that becomes progressively worse, or complaints of a sensation of a veil in the line of sight.

Objective Data

Ophthalmoscopic examination visualizes the detachment. An ultrasound is ordered if blood restricts ophthalmoscopic vision of the retina.

Nursing diagnoses for a client with retinal detachment include the following:

NURSING DIAGNOSES	PLANNING/OUTCOMES	NURSING INTERVENTIONS
Anxiety related to sensory visual impairment and lack of understanding about treatment	The client will demonstrate reduction of emotional stress, fear, and depression; and an acceptance of surgery	Assess degree and duration of visual impairment. Encourage conversation to determine client's concerns, feelings, and level of understanding. Answer questions, offer support, and assist client to devise methods for coping. Orient client to new surroundings. Explain interventions clearly. Announce yourself with each interaction; interpret unfamiliar sounds; use touch to assist with verbal communication. Encourage to carry out ADLs as ability allows. Order finger foods for those who cannot see well enough or do not have the coping skills to use implements. Encourage participation of family or significant others in client care. Encourage participation in social and diversional activities as allowed (visitor, radio, audio tapes, television, crafts, games).
*Risk for **Injury*** related to visual impairment or knowledge deficit	The client will not have injury caused by visual impairment.	Assist client when able to ambulate postoperatively until stable and has adequate vision or coping skills (remember that clients with bilateral eye patches are unable to see). Assist client in arranging environment and do not rearrange furnishings without reorienting client. Discuss importance of wearing metal shield or glasses as ordered. Apply no pressure to the affected eye. Use proper procedure to administer eye medications.

Evaluation: Evaluate each outcome to determine how it has been met by the client.

INFECTIONS

Infections of the eye include keratitis, stye, chalazion, and conjunctivitis.

Keratitis

Keratitis is inflammation of the cornea that may be caused by infection, irritation, injury, or allergies. Symptoms associated with keratitis include severe eye pain, red watering eye, photophobia, sometimes reduced vision, and sometimes rash (e.g., herpes simplex, herpes zoster, or rosacea).

Treatment of keratitis includes optical anesthetics to relieve pain and mydriatics to dilate the pupil. Dark glasses should be worn to relieve the photophobia. Antibiotic solutions are prescribed for the specific type of infection.

Stye

A **stye** is also referred to as a hordeolum. It is a pustular inflammation of an eyelash follicle or sebaceous gland on the lid margin commonly caused by staphylococcal organisms. Symptoms include pain, redness, and swelling of a specific area of the eyelid. Treatment consists of warm compresses and topical antibiotic ointments. More severe cases may require incision and drainage. Once the pus drains, the pain is relieved and healing begins.

Chalazion

A **chalazion** is a cyst of the meibomian glands, which are sebaceous glands located at the junction of the conjunctiva and inner eyelid margins (Figure 42-8A). The hard cyst is filled with fatty material from the chronically obstructed

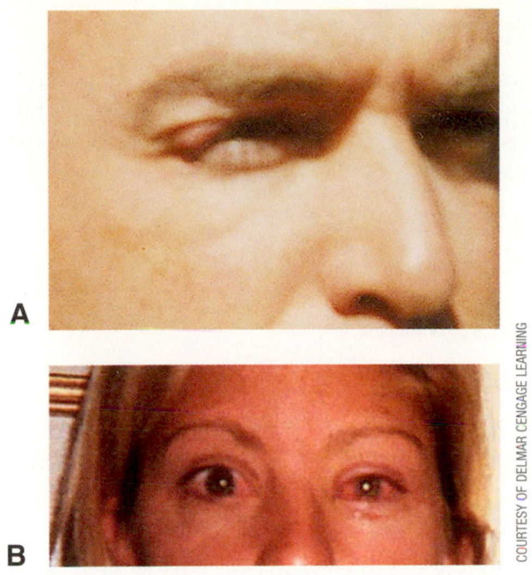

FIGURE 42-8 *A,* Chalazion; *B,* Bacterial Conjunctivitis

meibomian glands. The inherent feature of a chalazion is painless localized swelling that develops over a period of weeks. Treatment usually involves surgical excision if the cyst is large, becomes infected, or interferes with vision or closure of the eyelids. The cyst remains when the inflammation subsides.

CONJUNCTIVITIS (PINK EYE)

Conjunctivitis is an inflammation of the conjunctiva (a membrane that lines the inside of the eyelids and covers the cornea) that results from invasion by bacterial, viral, or rickettsial organisms, allergens, or irritants (Figure 42-8B). Symptoms include burning and itching of eyes, discharge, swelling, pain, and redness. Treatment consists of applying warm compresses using saline or boric acid solution and instilling antibiotic or antiviral ointments. When caused by allergens, treatment includes avoiding the allergen, taking antihistamines, or being desensitized.

Conjunctivitis is contagious. Proper hand hygiene is essential for the nurse and client. Gloves are worn when applying compresses or instilling ointment. The client's linen is disinfected to prevent spread of the infection.

REFRACTIVE ERRORS

Refraction is the deflection or bending of light rays when they pass from a medium of one density to a medium of another density. In the case of the eye, light waves pass through the air (less dense) into the fluids of the eye (more dense) and are brought to focus on the retina.

Refractive errors result in changes in visual acuity or vision that is not 20/20. Refractive errors include **myopia** (nearsightedness), **hyperopia** (farsightedness), **astigmatism** (asymmetric focus of light rays on the retina), **presbyopia** (inability of the lens to change curvature in order to focus on near objects), and **strabismus** (inability of the eyes to focus in the same direction) (Figure 42-9).

With myopia, parallel light rays come to focus in front of the retina because the refractive system is too strong or the eyeball is elongated. Near vision is normal, but distant vision is poor.

With hyperopia, parallel light rays come to focus behind the retina because the refractive system is too weak or the eyeball is flattened. Vision beyond 20 feet is normal, but near vision is poor. Figure 42-10 illustrates where light rays focus for myopia and hyperopia.

Astigmatism is a visual defect caused by unequal curvatures of the refractive surfaces of the eye. Light rays from a point do not come to focus on the retina, resulting in visual distortion.

Presbyopia is the loss of elasticity of the lens of the eye caused by aging that causes the near point of vision to recede.

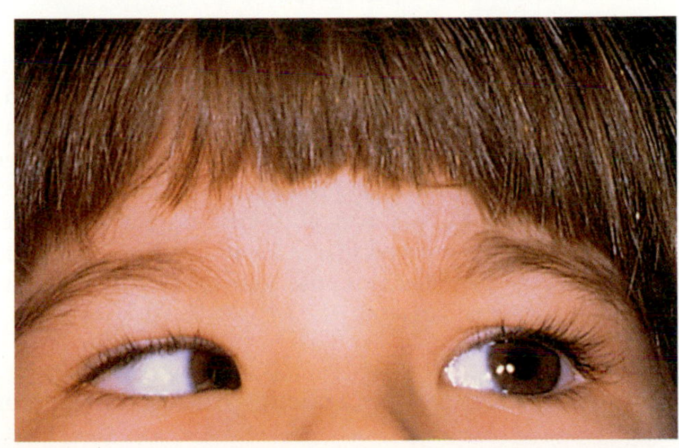

FIGURE 42-9 Strabismus (*Courtesy of the Armed Forces Institute of Pathology*)

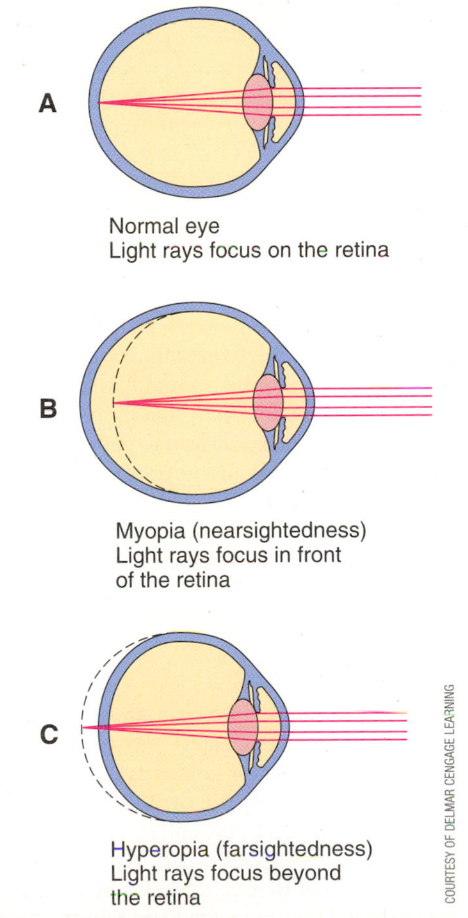

FIGURE 42-10 Refraction; *A,* Normal Eye; *B,* Myopia; *C,* Hyperopia

The eye loses the ability to accommodate to near objects but remains accommodated for far objects.

Strabismus occurs when one eye is constantly deviated to the side.

Medical–Surgical Management

Medical

Refractory errors are corrected by prescription glasses or contact lenses. The corrective lenses bend light rays to compensate for a client's refractive error.

Surgical

Radial keratotomy is a surgical procedure used to correct myopia and astigmatism. Under local anesthesia, incisions that resemble the spokes of a wheel are made in the cornea. After the cuts are made, pressure in the anterior chamber of the eye reshapes the cornea to a normal or near-normal curvature. Both LASIK (laser-assisted in-situ keratomileusis) and PRK (photo-refractive keratectomy) use laser to correct nearsightedness and astigmatism.

Nursing Management

Reassure client that refraction testing is painless and that dilating eyedrops are instilled. Advise client that it takes time to adjust to new glasses and not to wear old glasses after getting new ones.

NURSING PROCESS

Assessment

Subjective Data

Obtain a general medical history as well as a history of symptoms. Symptoms include blurred vision, headache, or eye fatigue.

Objective Data

The client is asked to view an eye chart while lenses of different strengths are systematically placed in front of the eye. The client is asked if the lenses sharpen or blur vision. The power or strength of the lens necessary to permit focusing of the image on the retina is expressed in measurements called diopters.

A nursing diagnosis for a client with refractive errors is:

NURSING DIAGNOSES	PLANNING/OUTCOMES	NURSING INTERVENTIONS
Anxiety related to impaired vision and having to wear glasses or contact lenses	The client will accept wearing glasses or contact lenses.	Allow client to discuss impact of wearing glasses or contact lenses. Encourage client to wear the glasses or contact lenses as prescribed.

Evaluation: Evaluate each outcome to determine how it has been met by the client.

INJURY

Injury to the eye or periorbital area results from a variety of things, such as chemical sprays, tree branches, slingshots, BB guns, flying debris from lawn mowers, and fireworks. Both children and adults are susceptible to eye injuries, and the importance of protecting the eyes cannot be overemphasized. Injuries to the eyes require immediate attention by an ophthalmologist. Even a few hours' delay in treatment may lead to permanent damage.

Corneal abrasion is the disruption of cells and the loss of the superficial epithelium. The outer surface is easily separated from the underlying layers and is injured or destroyed by exposure (lack of moisture), chemical irritants that dissolve in the protective tear film, and abrasion from foreign bodies.

SAFETY

Avoiding Eye Injury

The eyes are easily protected from injury by wearing protective goggles when performing tasks that are potentially hazardous to the eyes. Those who wear contact lenses should follow the manufacturer's recommendations for wearing them during certain activities, such as swimming or when sleeping.

Foreign Bodies

Foreign bodies in the conjunctiva or on the cornea cause excessive tearing and redness. The safest way to remove a foreign object from the conjunctiva or cornea is to flush sterile saline starting from the sclera across the cornea (Primary Care Ophthalmology, 2004). Foreign bodies often become embedded in the conjunctiva under the upper eyelid. The lid must be everted and the client instructed to look up to facilitate inspection and removal. If the particle is not located and removed, sterile fluorescein drops or strips are instilled to visualize minute foreign bodies that are not readily visible with the naked eye.

Chemical Burns

Emergency treatment of chemical burns to the conjunctiva or cornea includes immediate lavage of the eye with tap water and referral to an emergency room or ophthalmologist. In the emergency room, a specially made lid speculum is placed directly on the eyeball and connected to a minimum of 1 liter of isotonic saline solution for irrigation. A topical anesthetic may be instilled to minimize pain during irrigation. No attempt is made to neutralize the chemical because the heat generated by the chemical reaction may cause further injury. Both eyes are then patched to allow more comfort.

IMPAIRED VISION

The term *blindness* evokes an image of total darkness and is used for many legal purposes when central visual acuity is 20/200 or less with corrective lenses, in the better eye. Those who have visual acuity between 20/70 and 20/200 in the better eye, with the use of glasses, are often referred to as partially sighted.

The aids that follow are designed to make the most of the available vision (those in italics can also be used by persons who are blind): magnifying glasses; hand and stand magnifiers; telescopes; large-print books, newspapers, magazines; talking books; *Braille* books; closed-circuit television, which produces highly magnified images; *tactually marked watches and clocks; tactually modified tabletop games*; enlarged telephone dials, kitchen implements, tools, medication devices; talking clocks, timers, scales, calculators, computers; *text scanner, which converts text to audio mode or Braille*; speech synthesizer; flashlight eye sonar devices; canes, laser canes, and seeing eye dogs.

MACULAR DEGENERATION

Macular degeneration is atrophy or deterioration of the macula, the point on the retina where light rays meet as they are focused by the cornea and lens of the eye. The person loses central vision but still has peripheral vision.

The most common form of macular degeneration is associated with the aging process and is called age-related macular degeneration. Other forms of this disorder include exudative (wet) macular degeneration (sudden growth of new blood vessels in the area of the macula) and injury, infection, or inflammation that damages the macula.

Medical–Surgical Management

Medical

The treatment of age-related macular degeneration is geared toward assisting the client to maximize the use of the remaining vision. The loss of central vision interferes with the client's ability to read, write, recognize safety hazards, and drive.

Management of clients with exudative macular degeneration is geared toward halting the initiating process and identifying further changes in visual perception. Fluid and blood may resorb in a small percentage of clients with exudative degeneration. Laser therapy to seal the leaking blood vessels in or near the macula may also limit the extent of the damage.

CRITICAL THINKING

Visual Impairment

What modifications have to be made in the life of a person who can no longer see?

Nursing Management

Provide a safe environment. Announce your presence when entering the client's room and let the client know when you are leaving. Make sure all personnel know of the client's decreased vision. Respond to the client's call light quickly.

NURSING PROCESS

Assessment

Subjective Data

Obtain a general medical history and a history of symptoms. Symptoms include blurred vision, disturbance in color vision (colors become dim), difficulty in reading or doing close work, distortion of objects (especially those with lines), and an empty area within the central field of vision.

Objective Data

Note coping mechanisms such as turning the head to use peripheral vision.

A nursing diagnosis for the client with macular degeneration is:

NURSING DIAGNOSES	PLANNING/OUTCOMES	NURSING INTERVENTIONS
Disturbed **S***ensory Perception (Visual)* related to macular degeneration	The client will discuss the impact of vision loss on lifestyle and use adaptive measures.	Allow client to express feelings about vision loss such as its impact on lifestyle. Convey a willingness to listen, but do not pressure client to talk.
		Provide a safe environment by removing excess furniture or equipment from client's surroundings.
		Orient client to surroundings and show how to use call light.
		Provide reality orientation if client is confused or disoriented.
		Always introduce yourself or announce your presence upon entering the client's room; let client know when you are leaving.
		Provide sensory stimulation by using tactile, auditory, and gustatory stimuli to help compensate for vision loss.
		Suggest large-print books, talking books, audiotapes, or radio as preferred by client.
		Give clear, concise explanations of treatments and procedures but avoid information overload.

(*Continues*)

A nursing diagnosis for the client with macular degeneration is: (Continued)

NURSING DIAGNOSES	PLANNING/OUTCOMES	NURSING INTERVENTIONS
		Make sure that health care personnel are aware of client's vision loss. Record information on the client's chart or post in room.
		Respond to call light quickly.
		Provide continuity by assigning same staff members to care for client when possible.
		Refer to appropriate community resources.

Evaluation: Evaluate each outcome to determine how it has been met by the client.

SAMPLE NURSING CARE PLAN

The Client with Macular Degeneration

J.R. is a 60-year-old high school Latin teacher. He describes having blurred vision in both eyes with a gradual loss of vision in only the right eye. He has trouble reading and is afraid to drive because he can no longer recognize safety hazards. He denies having pain. He also relates having fallen several times recently at home while going up and down the stairs. The family practitioner referred him to an ophthalmologist, who diagnosed J.R. as having macular degeneration in the right eye.

NURSING DIAGNOSIS 1 *Disturbed* ***S****ensory Perception (Visual)* related to macular degeneration as evidenced by his inability to recognize safety hazards when driving

Nursing Outcomes Classification (NOC)
Vision Compensation Behavior

Nursing Interventions Classification (NIC)
Environmental Management
Communication Enhancement: Visual Deficit

PLANNING/OUTCOMES	INTERVENTION	RATIONALE
J.R. will discuss impact of vision loss on lifestyle.	Encourage J.R. to express feelings about vision loss.	Aids in the acceptance of vision loss.
	Convey a willingness to listen, and discuss J.R.'s current ability to meet self-care needs and activities of daily living.	Determines J.R.'s awareness of his limitations.
	Educate J.R. in alternative ways of coping with vision loss; care of such adaptive devices as eyeglasses, magnifying glass, and contact lenses.	Client will be better able to cope with vision loss.
	Refer to appropriate community resources.	Helps J.R. and his family cope better with his vision loss.

EVALUATION

J.R. discussed the effects of vision loss on his lifestyle and contacted a local agency that provides assistance to the visually impaired.

NURSING DIAGNOSIS 2 *Risk for* ***I****njury* related to difficulty in processing visual images and altered depth perception as evidenced by recent falls

Nursing Outcomes Classification (NOC)
Risk Control: Visual Impairment

Nursing Interventions Classification (NIC)
Teaching: Disease Process
Fall Prevention

SAMPLE NURSING CARE PLAN (Continued)

PLANNING/OUTCOMES	NURSING INTERVENTIONS	RATIONALE
J.R. will not experience injury or visual compromise resulting from a fall.	Advise J.R. that depth perception is changed with macular degeneration.	Information promotes understanding.
	Teach J.R. to avoid reaching for objects for stability when ambulating.	Objects may not be where they are perceived. Excessive reaching alters the center of gravity which can precipitate a fall.
	Advise J.R. to go up and down steps one at a time.	Enhances the sense of balance.

EVALUATION

J.R. has not fallen in 2 weeks.

NURSING DIAGNOSIS

*Impaired **Home** Maintenance* related to limited vision, as evidenced by recent falls at home

NOC: Family Functioning
NIC: Home Maintenance Assistance, Environmental Management: Safety

CLIENT GOAL

J.R. will develop a plan for self-care in the desired living environment.

NURSING INTERVENTIONS

1. Inform J.R. about required self-care activities: personal care, eyedrop instillation, activities permitted, activity restrictions, medications, and how to monitor for complications.
2. Assist J.R. to determine which activities will require assistance.
3. Evaluate sources of assistance: friends/family, home health care (skilled nursing care), or home-care aids.
4. Critique the safety of J.R.'s home: location of telephone, emergency plan, presence of loose rugs or carpets.

SCIENTIFIC RATIONALES

1. Knowing what self-care activities are needed helps J.R. plan for his care at home.
2. Helps J.R. to plan for his care at home.
3. Determines availability of assistance.
4. Changes are made to make J. R.'s home safer.

EVALUATION

Has J.R. developed a plan to care for himself at home?

OTHER SENSES

Other senses include taste, smell, and touch.

TASTE

The sense of taste (gustation) serves as a protector from rotten or putrid food and provides delightful sensations of creamy chocolate, crunchy carrots, chewy taffy, and fruitful pies. Taste sensors are most efficient at room temperature and respond only to substances in solution. The taste buds are located in four areas of the tongue that sense sweet, salt, bitter, and sour (as shown in Figure 42-11).

Taste sensations are altered secondary to neurological disorders or trauma. Assess clients who complain of food not "tasting good" for possible causes, including dietary habits, medication use, smoking and caffeine use, as well as olfactory disturbances. The sense of taste works very closely with the sense of smell for identification of the taste sensations.

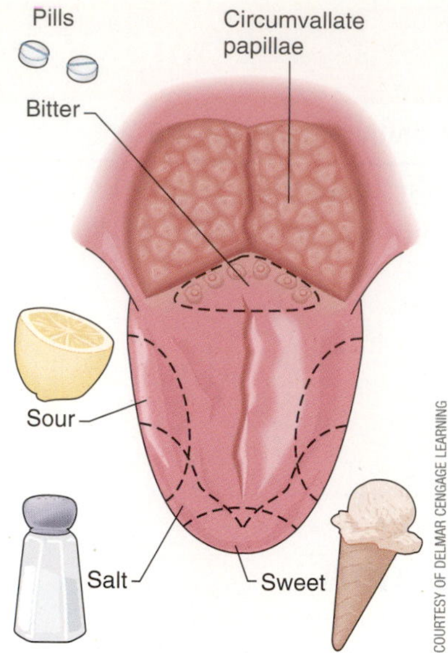

FIGURE 42-11 Taste Regions of the Tongue

SMELL

The sense of smell (olfaction) also serves as a guardian from danger. An individual's nose warns of impending danger from gas leaks, smoke, fires, rancid meat or fish, and sour dairy products. Body odors and halitosis are clues for personal hygiene and dental care.

Disorders of the olfactory sense often go unnoticed. Tests such as the University of Pennsylvania Smell Identification Test (UPSIT) allow self-testing of smelling deficiencies. Early identification of the loss of the sense of smell offers clues to alterations in dietary habits, weight loss or gain, anorexia, malnourishment, and changes in daily habits, such as bathing and brushing teeth. The receptors for the sense of smell are located in the roof of the nasal cavity. If these cells are damaged, the sense of smell is impaired. The body cannot regenerate the olfactory cells.

TOUCH

The sense of touch (tactile) includes sensations pertaining to the skin. The tactile receptors are located throughout the integumentary system. Cutaneous sensations of touch, pressure, vibration, cold, heat, and pain are examples. Clients who are unable to sense temperature variations are taught cautionary measures when applying heat or cold therapies, preparing bath water, cooking, or exposing self to hot or cold climates and environmental temperatures.

Clients with reduced or loss of tactile sensation risk injury when their condition confines them to bed. They are unable to sense pressure on bony prominences or the need to change position. The nurse's role in reducing or preventing impairment of skin integrity is crucial. Timely positioning, securing tubes or devices away from the client's body, and using products to minimize skin breakdown are a few of the interventions vital to excellent client care.

LIFE SPAN CONSIDERATIONS

Aging and Taste Sensation

The ability to taste sweetness remains as one ages, but the ability to taste bitterness declines.

CASE STUDY

K.R. is a 34-year-old nurse who was diagnosed with a right ear hearing impairment during a routine physical examination. She admitted to her doctor that she noticed she would only use her left ear to talk on the phone and that she had particular difficulty hearing her family or friends in a crowded restaurant or other public settings. She also noted that her husband asked her why she played the television so loud, yet if he turned it down to his normal hearing level, she could not hear it clearly. Her physician ordered an audiogram, which showed a conductive hearing loss of 40% secondary to otosclerosis. Hearing in her left ear was normal.

K.R.'s doctor gave her three medical treatment options:

1. Do nothing and monitor her hearing impairment by audiogram every 6 months. If it were to worsen, other options would be considered.
2. Be fitted with a hearing aid.
3. Have a surgical procedure to correct the hearing loss.

CASE STUDY (Continued)

K.R. agreed to have surgery. She thought she would be too self-conscious to wear a hearing aid, after all she was only 34, but she simply could not ignore the problem by doing nothing. K.R. was scheduled for same-day surgery.

The following questions will guide your development of a nursing care plan for the case study.

1. How is a conductive hearing loss differentiated from a sensorineural hearing loss?
2. What does an audiogram reveal? What special things should K.R. know before she has the audiogram?
3. Describe the surgical procedure that will most likely be used to correct the conductive hearing loss.
4. What will the nurse teach K.R. before her surgery about the procedure and expected postoperative course?
5. List four individualized nursing diagnoses and expected outcomes for K.R., and nursing interventions for each diagnosis.
6. Describe the expected discharge instructions that K.R. must know related to diet, medications, activity restrictions, and follow-up care.

SUMMARY

- Hearing loss is conductive, sensorineural, or a combination of the two. It may also be congenital.
- Ménière's disease is a result of excessive accumulation of endolymph, causing severe vertigo, dizziness, and hearing loss. Treatment is primarily symptomatic.
- Otosclerosis is a conductive hearing loss that is treated medically with the use of a hearing aid or surgically with a stapedectomy.
- Otitis media is inflammation of the middle ear. Treatment usually includes antibiotics, decongestants, and possibly a myringotomy.
- Cataract surgery is indicated when significant vision loss has occurred.
- Untreated retinal detachment results in total loss of vision.
- Many resources are available for the hearing impaired through community and national agencies.
- The senses of taste, smell, and touch are essential to our enjoyment of life and serve to protect us from danger or harm.

REVIEW QUESTIONS

1. In a conductive hearing loss:
   1. the endolymph may cross the capillary membrane and mix with the perilymph, resulting in severe vertigo.
   2. the ossicles of the middle ear fracture, resulting in a tear of the eighth cranial nerve.
   3. sound waves are not transmitted through the ear canal to inner ear fluid.
   4. a tumor in the inner ear blocks the flow of fluid through the bony and membranous labyrinths.
2. A possible nursing diagnosis for a client with Ménière's disease is:
   1. activity intolerance related to impaired hearing.
   2. knowledge deficit related to surgical shunt placement to drain excessive endolymph.
   3. communication, impaired, verbal, related to tinnitus.
   4. risk for injury related to vertigo.
3. Chemical burns of the eye are initially treated with:
   1. local anesthetics and antibacterial drops for 24 to 36 hours.
   2. hot compresses applied at 15-minute intervals.
   3. flushing of the lids, conjunctiva, and cornea with water.
   4. cleansing of the conjunctiva with a small, cotton-tipped applicator.
4. A clinical symptom of a detached retina is:
   1. an increase in tearing.
   2. an area of vague vision.
   3. momentary flashes of light.
   4. pain in the eye.
5. Macular degeneration is characterized by:
   1. purulent periorbital drainage.
   2. pupil dilation.
   3. loss of central vision.
   4. ptosis (droopy lid).
6. A client presents to the emergency room with symptoms of seeing several floaters with flashes of light in the affected eye and having blurred vision. The nurse recognizes these as symptoms of:
   1. macular degeneration, and it is not an emergency.
   2. glaucoma, and it is not an emergency.
   3. a cataract, and it is not an emergency.
   4. a retinal detachment, and it is an emergency.
7. A teenager arrives at the clinic with an inflamed conjunctiva of the right eye that burns and itches, is swollen and reddened, and has a discharge. The nursing interventions include: (Select all that apply.)
   1. washing his hands after examining the client's eye.
   2. teaching the client to wash her hands frequently and especially after touching her eye.
   3. teaching the client that conjunctivitis is contagious.

4. instilling an antibiotic in the eye without wearing gloves because he is going to wash his hands after the instillation.
5. teaching the client to wash linens to prevent spreading the conjunctivitis to others.
6. teaching the client to apply ice to the affected eye.

8. Nursing interventions for a client with glaucoma include: (Select all that apply.)
   1. applying warm compresses and topical antibiotic ointment.
   2. administering prescribed ophthalmic agent.
   3. teaching the client to avoid reaching for objects to maintain stability when ambulating, as depth perception is altered.
   4. monitoring blood pressure, pulse, and respiration every 4 hours if not receiving osmotic agent intravenously.
   5. reminding the client that miotics may cause blurred vision for 1 to 2 hours after use.
   6. immediately lavaging the eye with saline solution.

9. The nurse completed teaching postoperative stapedectomy care to a client. The nurse knows the client needs some reteaching when he states:
   1. "I will turn and move slowly."
   2. "I will sneeze with my mouth closed."
   3. "I will report any greenish, yellowish, or foul-smelling drainage."
   4. "I will keep water out of my ear and keep it exposed to air as much as possible."

10. Which of the following is an appropriate nursing diagnosis for a gradual hearing impaired client who is 80- years-old?
   1. *Activity Intolerance* related to severe vertigo.
   2. *Deficit **K**nowledge* related to abrupt onset and unknown progression of the disease.
   3. *Social **I**solation* related to hearing impairment.
   4. *Acute **P**ain* related to inflammation in the middle ear.

REFERENCES/SUGGESTED READINGS

Agrawal, Y., Platz, E., & Niparko, J. (2008). Prevalence of hearing loss and differences by demographic characteristics among US adults: Data from the national health and nutrition examination survey, 1999–2004. *Archives of Internal Medicine, 168*(14), pp. 1522–1530.

American Speech-Language-Hearing Association. (2002). Types of hearing loss. Retrieved December 27, 2004 from www.asha.org/hearing/disorders/types/cfm

Barnie, D. (2002). Restoring vision in older patients. *RN, 65*(1), 30–35.

Bulechek, G., Butcher, H., McCloskey, J., & Dochterman, J., eds. (2008). *Nursing Interventions Classification (NIC)* (5th ed.). St. Louis, MO: Mosby/Elsevier.

Crosta, P. (2008). Hearing loss affects millions of US adults. Medical News Today. Retrieved August 3, 2008 from http:www/medicalnewstoday.com/printerfriendlynews.php?newsid=116360

Cavendish, R. (1998). Clinical snapshot: Hearing loss. *AJN, 98*(8), 50–51.

Dana, R. (1998, January 27). Dry eye syndrome. *Health News 1*, 3.

Daniels, R. (2009). *Delmar's guide to laboratory and diagnostic tests* (2nd ed). Clifton Park, NY: Delmar Cengage Learning.

Estes, M. (2010). *Health assessment & physical examination* (4th ed.). Clifton Park, NY: Delmar Cengage Learning.

Kearney, K. (1997). Retinal detachment. *AJN, 97*(8), 50.

Lucas, L., & Matthews-Flint, L. (2001). Sound advice about hearing aids. *Nursing2001, 31*(2), 59–61.

McConnell, E. (2001a). Instilling ear drops. *Nursing2001, 31*(4), 17.

McConnell, E. (2001b). Myths & Facts . . . about macular degeneration. *Nursing2001, 31*(8), 30.

McConnell, E. (2002). How to converse with a hearing-impaired patient. *Nursing2002, 32*(8), 20.

Mayo Clinic. (2008). Retinal detachment. Retrieved August 3, 2009 from http://mayoclinic.com/health/retinal-detachment/DS00254/METHOD=print&DSECTION=all

Moorhead, S., Johnson, M., Maas, M., & Swanson, E. (2007). *Nursing Outcomes Classification (NOC)* (4th ed). St. Louis, MO: Elsevier - Health Sciences Division.

National Institute on Deafness and Other Communication Disorders. (2002). Cochlear implants. Retrieved October 4, 2004 from www.nidcd.nih.gov/health/pubs_hb/coch.htm

North American Nursing Diagnosis Association International. (2010). *NANDA-I nursing diagnoses: Definitions and classification 2009–2011.* Ames, IA: Wiley-Blackwell.

Primary Care Ophthalmology. (2004). Foreign body removal. Retrieved August 3, 2009 from http://www.med.uottawa.ca/procedures/slamp/body_removal.htm

Ralph, S. & Taylor, C. (2007). *Sparks and Taylor's nursing diagnosis reference manual* (7th ed.). Philadelphia: Lippincott Williams & Wilkins.

Ramponi, D. (2000). Go with the flow during an eye emergency. *Nursing2000, 30*(8), 54–56.

Ramponi, D. (2001). Contact lens removal. *Nursing2001, 31*(8), 56–57.

Ruben, R. (2007). Hearing loss and deafness. Retrieved August 3, 2009 from http://www.merck.com/mmhe/sec19/ch218/ch218a.html

Shelp, S. (1997). Your patient is deaf, now what? *RN, 60*(2), 37–40.

Smeltzer, S., Bare, B., Hinkle, J., & Cheever, K. (2008). *Brunner and Suddarth's textbook of medical surgical nursing* (11th ed.). Philadelphia: Lippincott Williams & Wilkins.

Sommer, S., & Sommer, N. (2002). When your patient is hearing impaired. *RN, 65*(12), 28–32.

Spencer, J. (1998, February 17). Coping with hearing loss. *Health News 2*, 1–2.

Spratto, G., & Woods, A. (2008). *2009 Delmar's (nurses drug handbook).* Clifton Park, NY: Delmar Cengage Learning.

Tupper, S. (1999). When the inner ear is out of balance. *RN, 62*(11), 36–40.

Walbecker, J. (1997). Knowing the signs. *RN, 60*(2), 40–41.

RESOURCES

Alexander Graham Bell Association for the Deaf, http://www.agbell.org

American Academy of Ophthalmology Head and Neck Surgery, http://www.aao.org

American Academy of Otolaryngology, http://www.entnet.org

American Council of the Blind, http://acb.org

American Foundation for the Blind, Inc., http://www.afb.org

American Speech-Language-Hearing Association, http://www.asha.org

American Tinnitus Association, http://www.ata.org

Better Hearing Institute, http://www.betterhearing.org/

Guide Dogs for the Blind, http://www.guidedogs.com

Guide Dog Users, Inc., http://www.gdui.org

Guiding Eyes for the Blind, http://www.guidingeyes.org

Hearing Loss Association of America, http://www.hearingloss.org/

International Hearing Dog Inc., http://www.hearinglossweb.com

Leader Dogs for the Blind, http://www.leaderdog.org/

Lion's Club International, http://www.lionsclubs.org

Prevent Blindness America, http://www.preventblindness.org

National Association for the Deaf, http://www.nad.org

National Association for Visually Handicapped, http://www.navh.org

Recording for the Blind & Dyslexic, Inc., http://www.rfbd.org

Self Help for the Hard of Hearing, http://www.shhh.org

The Vision Council/The Better Vision Institute, http://www.thevisioncouncil.org/bvi/

University of Ottawa – Canada's University, http://www.med.uottawa.ca

CHAPTER 43
Endocrine System

MAKING THE CONNECTION

Refer to the following chapters to increase your understanding of the endocrine system:

Basic Nursing

- ***Wellness Concepts***
- ***Fluid, Electrolyte, and Acid–Base Balance***
- ***Assessment***
- ***Diagnostic Tests***

Adult Health Nursing

- ***Oncology***
- ***Cardiovascular System***
- ***Hematologic and Lymphatic Systems***
- ***Urinary System***
- ***Musculoskeletal System***
- ***Neurological System***
- ***Sensory System***
- ***Reproductive System***
- ***Integumentary System***
- ***Immune System***
- ***The Older Adult***

Basic Procedures

- ***Measuring Intake and Output***

Intermediate Procedures

- ***Withdrawing Medication from a Vial***
- ***Administering a Subcutaneous Injection***
- ***Performing a Skin Puncture***

LEARNING OBJECTIVES

Upon completion of this chapter, you should be able to:

- Define key terms.
- Identify and locate the endocrine glands and list function(s) and hormone(s) secreted by each.
- Differentiate between type 1 and type 2 diabetes in terms of pathophysiology, presenting symptoms and treatment.
- Discuss the roles of diet and exercise in the management of diabetes mellitus.
- Identify signs, causes, and treatment of acute complications of hypoglycemia, diabetic ketoacidosis, and hyperosmolar hyperglycemic nonketotic syndrome.
- Discuss the major long-term complications of diabetes.
- Discuss rationale for the pituitary gland being traditionally called the "master" gland.

- Compare symptoms of the disease process resulting from a hyper- or hyposecretion of an endocrine gland.
- Discuss assessment techniques for a client suspected of having an endocrine disorder.
- Formulate a nursing care plan for the client with an endocrine disorder.

KEY TERMS

agranulocytosis
autosomal
Chvostek's sign
cretinism
dawn phenomenon
endocrine
exophthalmos
glucagon
glycosuria
goiter
gynecomastia
hirsutism
hormone
hyperglycemia
hypoglycemia
hypovolemia
iatrogenic
insulin
ketonuria
lipodystrophy
myxedema
paroxysmal
polydipsia
polyphagia
polyuria
Somogyi phenomenon
tetany
Trousseau's sign

INTRODUCTION

The endocrine system provides the same general functions as the nervous system: communication and control; however, the endocrine system is generally slower and has longer-lasting control over the various body activities and functions. It exerts this control through the secretion of hormones that circulate through the blood. A malfunction of any part of the endocrine system can result in a shift of homeostasis with far-reaching systemic reactions.

Assessment of the endocrine system is difficult. Not only are the components not in direct contact, but only the thyroid gland is close enough to the body surface for direct physical assessment. Still, the nurse needs to be familiar with the normal functioning of the endocrine system. In assessing the client for endocrine dysfunction, the nurse must note negative findings as well as positive ones. Assessment includes results of diagnostic tests as well as any precipitating or aggravating factors.

ANATOMY AND PHYSIOLOGY REVIEW

The endocrine system is unique in that it is composed of a group of various glands scattered throughout the body. The glands of the body have either exocrine or endocrine functions. Exocrine glands, including sweat glands and lacrimal glands, are responsible for secreting substances directly into ducts that lead to the target area. The term **endocrine** (*endo*—within, *crin*—secrete) indicates that the secretions formed by these glands directly enter the blood or lymph circulation, rather than being transported via tubes or ducts. These secretions, called **hormones**, are chemical substances that initiate or regulate activity of another organ, system, or gland in another part of the body. The level of hormone in the blood is regulated by the homeostasis mechanism called *negative feedback*. If the blood level for a specific hormone falls below normal, negative feedback causes the specific endocrine gland to produce more of the hormone, which when increased to the normal level causes a decrease in production.

The glands discussed in this chapter that make up the endocrine system are the pancreas, pituitary, hypothalamus, thyroid, parathyroid, and adrenals (Figure 43-1). Several endocrine glands such as the pineal, thymus, ovaries, and testes are of great importance; however, they are discussed in other chapters in connection with the organ system in which they function.

The pancreas lies horizontally behind the stomach at the level of the first and second lumbar vertebrae. The head of the pancreas is attached to the duodenum with the tail reaching to the spleen. It has both exocrine and endocrine functions.

The pituitary gland consists of an anterior and a posterior lobe. It has traditionally been called the "master" gland because so many of its secretions influence other endocrine glands and body systems. It is attached to the hypothalamus by a stalk called the *infundibulum*. The hypothalamus is located in the lower portion of the brain and produces secretions

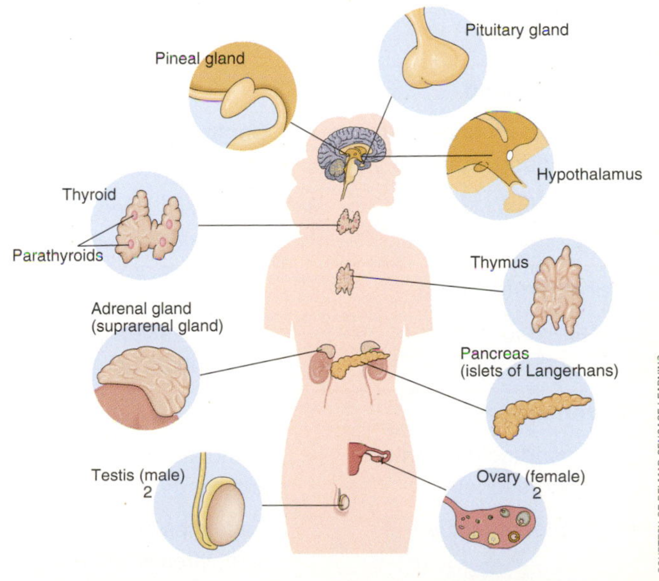

FIGURE 43-1 Structures of the Endocrine System

influencing the production and release of the anterior pituitary hormones as well as the posterior pituitary hormones. Both the pituitary and hypothalamus are located in the head. The pituitary, about the size of a pea, is located in the sella turcica, a small depression in the sphenoid bone. Refer to Table 43-1 for specific endocrine hormones and functions.

The thyroid gland is butterfly-shaped and lies in the neck. It consists of two lobes—one on each side of the trachea connected by an isthmus. The gland sits saddle-like starting on the anterior surface of the trachea just below the larynx and surrounds it partway. The thyroid gland stores iodine. The thyroid gland produces thyroid hormones including thyroxine, which is the most abundant, and triiodothyronine. It regulates the metabolic rate for carbohydrates, protein, and fats.

There are usually four parathyroid glands. Two glands are embedded in the posterior portion of each thyroid lobe.

TABLE 43-1 Endocrine Glands and Hormones

HORMONE	FUNCTION
Pancreas	
Glucagon	Released by alpha cells to increase the blood glucose level
Insulin	Released by beta cells to decrease blood sugar
Somatostatin	Inhibits secretion of insulin, glucagon, and growth hormone (GH) from the anterior pituitary and gastrin from the stomach
Anterior Pituitary	
Thyroid-stimulating hormone (TSH)	Stimulates thyroid growth and secretion of the thyroid hormone
Adrenocorticotropic hormone (ACTH)	Stimulates the growth and secretion of glucocorticoids from the adrenal cortex
Follicle-stimulating hormone (FSH)	Stimulates ovarian follicle to mature and produce estrogen; in the male, stimulates sperm production
Luteinizing hormone (LH)	Acts with FSH to stimulate estrogen production; causes ovulation; stimulates progesterone production by corpus luteum; in male, stimulates testes to produce testosterone
Melanocyte-stimulating hormone (MSH)	Causes increase in synthesis and spread of melanin (pigment) in skin
Growth hormone (GH)	Stimulates growth by stimulating the epiphyseal plates of long bones and by increasing protein production
Prolactin or lactogenic hormone	Stimulates breast development during pregnancy and milk secretion after delivery of baby
Posterior Pituitary	
Antidiuretic hormone (ADH)	Stimulates water retention by kidneys to decrease urine secretion
Oxytocin	Stimulates uterine contractions; causes breast to release milk into ducts
Thyroid Gland	
Thyroid hormone (thyroxine T_4 and triiodothyronine T_3)	Controls metabolic rate of all cells; aids in carbohydrate, fat, and protein metabolism Both released in response to TSH
Calcitonin	When stimulated, decreases blood calcium (Ca) by promoting excretion of Ca and phosphorus by the kidneys; also decreases bone resorption by maintaining adequate Ca levels
Parathyroid Gland	
Parathyroid hormone	When stimulated, increases blood calcium concentration by promoting resorption of Ca and phosphorus from the bones; by increasing blood calcium levels, bone formation is decreased
Adrenal Cortex	
Glucocorticoids (cortisol, hydrocortisone)	Stimulates gluconeogenesis and increases blood glucose; antiinflammatory; antiimmunity; antiallergy; aids in the metabolism of carbohydrates, fats, and proteins
Mineralocorticoids	Regulates electrolyte and fluid homeostasis by increasing sodium and water reabsorption; stimulates K excretion in the kidneys
Sex hormones (androgen)	Stimulates sexual drive in females; in males, negligible effect

TABLE 43-1 Endocrine Glands and Hormones (Continued)

HORMONE	FUNCTION
Adrenal Medulla	
Epinephrine (adrenalin)	Prolongs and intensifies sympathetic nervous response to stress, resulting in increased heart rate, constriction of blood vessels, dilation of bronchioles, and hyperglycemia
Norepinephrine	Prolongs and intensifies sympathetic nervous response to stress, resulting in increased heart rate, constriction of blood vessels, dilation of bronchioles, and hyperglycemia

COURTESY OF DELMAR CENGAGE LEARNING

They produce parathyroid hormone, parathormone, which regulates the concentration of blood calcium and phosphorus.

The adrenal, or suprarenal, glands are located on top of each kidney. The adrenal cortex secretes mineralocorticoids including aldosterone, glucocorticoids including cortisol, and androgens, which are sex hormones. The adrenal medulla secretes epinephrine or adrenalin and norepinephrine or noradrenalin, which help the body function under stress.

It is important to understand the normal function of the endocrine glands and hormones. Most endocrine disorders are a result of either overactivity or underactivity of these glands.

COMMON DIAGNOSTIC TESTS

Commonly used diagnostic tests for clients with symptoms of endocrine system disorders are listed in Table 43-2.

DIABETES MELLITUS

Nearly 23.6 million Americans or approximately 7.8% of the American population have diabetes mellitus. Of the 23.6 million people, almost 1 in 4 cases are undiagnosed (CDC, 2007). Diabetes mellitus (DM) is a disorder of metabolism. When we eat, most of the food we eat is broken down by digestive juices. Of the food we eat, 100% of carbohydrate and approximately 58% of protein and 10% of fat is broken down to glucose. For the glucose to get into the cells, insulin must be present (Figure 43-2).

Insulin is a hormone produced and secreted by the beta cells of the islets of Langerhans in the pancreas. Insulin stimulates the active transport of glucose into muscle and adipose tissue cells, making it available for cell use. For glucose to cross the cell membrane, insulin must connect with a receptor on

TABLE 43-2 Common Diagnostic Tests for Endocrine System Disorders

Pancreas Diagnostic Tests

- Blood glucose, Fasting blood sugar (FBS)
- 2-hour postprandial glucose (2hPPG) or 2-hour postprandial blood sugar (2hPPBS)
- Glucose tolerance test (GTT)

Pituitary Gland Diagnostic Tests

- Adrenocorticotropic hormone (ACTH), Corticotropin
- Antidiuretic hormone (ADH), Vasopressin
- Follicle-stimulating hormone (FSH)
- Growth hormone (GH), Human GH (HGH), Somatotropin hormone (SH)
- Growth hormone (GH) stimulation test, GH provocation test, Insulin tolerance test (ITT), Arginine test
- Luteinizing hormone (LH) assay
- Prolactin level (PRL)
- Thyrotropin-releasing hormone (TRH) test, Thyrotropin-releasing factor (TRF) test
- Urine specific gravity
- Long bone x-rays
- Sella turcica x-ray
- Computed tomography of head (CT scan of head), Computerized axial transverse tomography (CATT)

Thyroid Gland Diagnostic Tests

- Antithyroid microsomal antibody, Antimicrosomal antibody, Microsomal antibody, Thyroid autoantibody, Thyroid antimicrosomal antibody
- Calcitonin, HCT, Thyrocalcitonin
- Serum-free triiodothyronine (T_3)
- Thyroid-stimulating hormone (TSH), Thyrotropin
- Thyroid-stimulating hormone (TSH) stimulation test
- Thyroxine index free, FTI, FT_4 Index
- Thyroxine, T_4, Thyroxine screen
- Triiodothyronine, T_3 radioimmunoassay, T_3 by RIA
- Radioactive iodine uptake (RAIU), Iodine uptake test, ^{131}I uptake
- Thyroid scan, Thyroid scintiscan
- Thyroid ultrasound, Thyroid echogram, Thyroid sonogram
- Thyroid biopsy

Parathyroid Gland Diagnostic Tests

- Parathyroid hormone (PTH), Parathormone
- Calcium, total/ionized Ca^{++}
- Phosphorus

(Continues)

TABLE 43-2 Common Diagnostic Tests for Endocrine System Disorders (Continued)

Adrenal Glands Diagnostic Tests	
Adrenocorticotropic hormone (ACTH) stimulation test, Cortisol stimulation test, Cosyntropin test	17-Hydroxycorticosteroids (17-OHCS)
Cortisol, Hydrocortisone	17-Ketosteroids (17-KS)
Dexamethasone suppression test (DST), Prolonged/rapid DST, Cortisol suppression test, ACTH suppression test	Urine cortisol, Hydrocortisone
Plasma renin assay, Plasma renin activity (PRA)	Vanillylmandelic acid (VMA) and catecholamines, VMA and epinephrine, Norepinephrine, Metanephrine, Normetanephrine, Dopamine
Progesterone assay	Adrenal angiography, Adrenal arteriogram
Aldosterone assay	Adrenal venography
	Computed tomography of adrenals (CT scan of adrenals)

COURTESY OF DELMAR CENGAGE LEARNING

the cell membrane. Some clients with diabetes mellitus have enough insulin but too few functioning receptor sites. Others have inadequate or no insulin production. Blood glucose can always be used by the brain and kidneys. Insulin is not needed for glucose to enter brain cells or cells of the glomeruli.

The amount of glucose in the blood regulates the rate of insulin secretion. When a meal is eaten, the blood glucose elevates and the beta cells of the islets of Langerhans release insulin. As the blood glucose level drops, insulin secretion diminishes. It is important to note that during times of fasting (overnight or between meals), a low level of insulin continues to be secreted along with **glucagon**. Glucagon secreted by the alpha cells of the pancreas stimulates release of glucose by the liver. The balance and interactions of insulin and glucagon maintain a constant serum glucose level.

Other functions of insulin include:

- Promoting conversion of glucose to glycogen for storage in the liver and inhibiting conversion of glycogen to glucose
- Promoting conversion of fatty acids into fat that can be stored as adipose tissue and preventing breakdown of adipose tissue and conversion of fat to ketone bodies
- Stimulating protein synthesis within tissues and inhibiting the breakdown of protein into amino acids

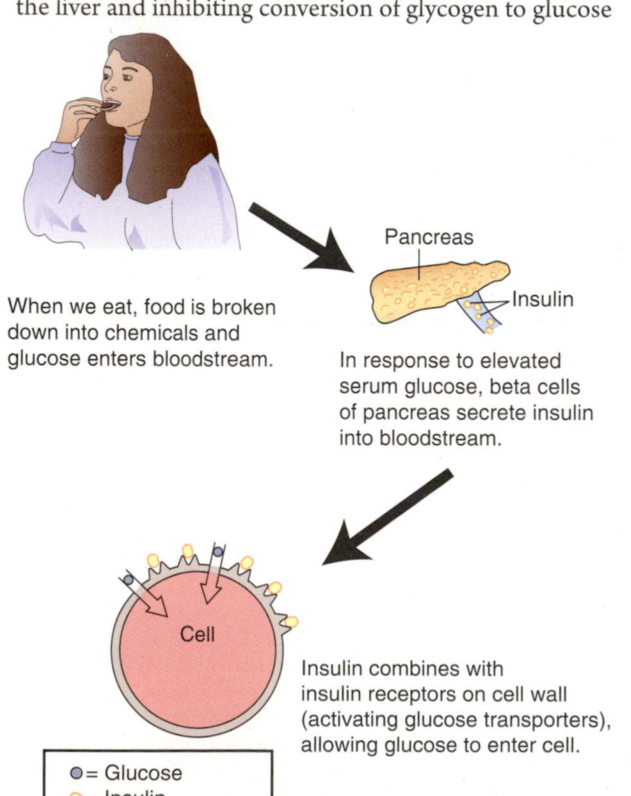

When we eat, food is broken down into chemicals and glucose enters bloodstream.
Pancreas
Insulin
In response to elevated serum glucose, beta cells of pancreas secrete insulin into bloodstream.
Cell
Insulin combines with insulin receptors on cell wall (activating glucose transporters), allowing glucose to enter cell.
= Glucose
= Insulin
= Insulin receptors
COURTESY OF DELMAR CENGAGE LEARNING

FIGURE 43-2 How Insulin Works

In summary, insulin actively promotes those processes that lower the blood glucose level and inhibits those processes that raise the blood glucose level. A deficiency of insulin results in **hyperglycemia**, or elevated blood glucose. Excess insulin results in **hypoglycemia** (low blood glucose). Diabetes mellitus is actually a group of disorders characterized by chronic hyperglycemia.

DIAGNOSIS AND CLASSIFICATION

The Expert Committee on the Diagnosis and Classification of Diabetes Mellitus (1997) presented to the American Diabetes Association (ADA) new criteria for diagnosis and new classifications for diabetes, which the ADA approved.

DIAGNOSIS

The Committee identified two precursors to diabetes, screening criteria, and diagnostic criteria.

The two precursors identified are:

1. Impaired glucose tolerance (IGT)—a glucose level of 140 to 199 mg/dL 2 hours after a glucose load
2. Impaired fasting glucose (IFG)—a fasting glucose of 110 to 125 mg/dL

The criteria for who should be screened for diabetes include:

1. Anyone age 45 and older
2. Anyone, regardless of age, with one of the following risk factors:
   - Obesity (body mass index of 27 or greater)
   - Immediate family member with diabetes
   - Member of high-risk ethnic group (African American, Hispanic American, some Native American groups)
   - Having a baby weighing more than 9 pounds
   - History of gestational diabetes mellitus (GDM)
   - Hypertension
   - High-density lipoprotein level of 35 mg/dL or less, or a triglyceride level of 250 mg/dL or more
   - Have either of the two precursors of diabetes

The diagnostic criteria identify when a physician can make a diagnosis of diabetes. The situations are:

- A random blood glucose of 200 mg/dL or greater with the classic symptoms of polyuria, polydipsia, and unexplained weight loss
  or
- A fasting blood sugar of 126 mg/dL or greater
  or
- The 2-hour sample of the oral glucose tolerance test is 200 mg/dL or greater using a load of 75 grams of anhydrous glucose
- In the absence of a definitive diagnosis, the testing should be repeated on an alternative date.

The committee also recommended not using glycosylated hemoglobin (HA1C) to diagnose diabetes since terminology is confusing, and many methods of measuring glycosylated hemoglobin are used. Glycosylated hemoglobin (HA1C) is primarily used to evaluate the effectiveness of the client's adherence to the treatment regimen.

Classification

Etiology, not insulin use, is used to classify diabetes into four categories: type 1 diabetes, type 2 diabetes, other specific types, and gestational diabetes mellitus.

Type 1 Diabetes

There are two forms of diabetes resulting from pancreatic beta-cell destruction or a primary defect in beta-cell function, resulting in no release of insulin and ineffective glucose transport. There is usually an absolute insulin deficiency so the clients are insulin-dependent. The two subdivisions of type 1 diabetes are:

- *Immune-mediated*—the body's immune system destroys the beta cells. These beta cells are the body's only mechanism to produce insulin to help control blood glucose levels. The rate of this destruction is usually higher in children than in adults. Children and adolescents may rapidly develop ketoacidosis. Adults seldom develop ketoacidosis unless they have an infection or other stressor. This is what used to be called insulin-dependent diabetes mellitus (IDDM), or juvenile-onset diabetes.
- *Idiopathic*—no evidence of autoimmunity; the individual just does not produce insulin and is prone to ketoacidosis.

In the absence of insulin, glucose from food eaten cannot be used or stored and remains in the bloodstream, resulting in hyperglycemia. In addition, glucose production from the liver goes unchecked, further elevating the blood glucose level.

As the blood glucose rises, the kidney begins to excrete excess glucose in the urine (**glycosuria**). Glucose eliminated in the urine pulls excessive amounts of water with it (osmotic diuresis), resulting in fluid volume deficit and producing symptoms of excessive thirst (**polydipsia**) and increased urination (**polyuria**).

Insulin deficiency also results in impaired metabolism of fats and proteins. Because of the impaired glucose, fat, and protein metabolism and the inability to store glucose, clients frequently experience protein wasting, weight loss, and increased hunger (**polyphagia**).

Metabolism of fat stores for energy leads to production of acid by-products called ketones, which can be detected in the urine (**ketonuria**). As ketones accumulate, the associated decrease in pH leads to metabolic acidosis, or more specifically a condition known as diabetic ketoacidosis, discussed later in this chapter.

Type 2 Diabetes

Type 2 diabetes mellitus initially begins with insulin resistance, where the cells are not able to use the insulin properly. Then, as the disease progresses, the pancreas gradually loses its ability to produce adequate quantities of insulin. Most of these clients are obese. When weight is lost, insulin resistance diminishes but reappears if the client regains weight. A strong family history of diabetes is often evident. Many clients do not require insulin, but eventually one-third will need insulin to maintain a normal glucose level. This is what used to be called noninsulin-dependent diabetes mellitus (NIDDM), or adult-onset diabetes.

Hyperglycemia results when the pancreas cannot match the body's need for insulin and/or when the number of insulin receptor sites are decreased or altered. Although available insulin may be insufficient to meet the body's metabolic needs and prevent hyperglycemia, there is a sufficient amount of insulin to prevent fat breakdown for energy and the resulting ketoacidosis. Extremely elevated glucose in the type 2 diabetic will result in development of hyperosmolar hyperglycemic nonketotic syndrome (HHNS), discussed later in this chapter. Table 43-3 compares the clinical manifestations of type 1 and type 2 diabetes.

Other Specific Types

This section includes conditions such as beta-cell genetic defects, endocrinopathies, and drug- or chemical-induced diabetes. These are in a separate category because there are different disease etiologies.

Gestational Diabetes Mellitus

Occurring during pregnancy, this may be controlled either with or without insulin. Generally, the client's glucose tolerance

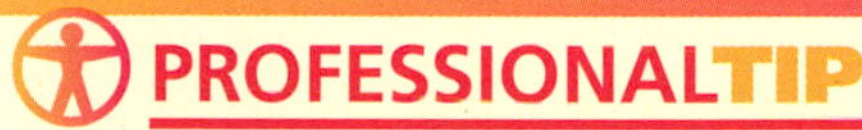

Diabetes

According to the Centers for Disease Control and Prevention (CDC, 2007), 17.9 million Americans are diagnosed as having diabetes mellitus. Another 5.7 million are estimated to be undiagnosed. Diabetes was the seventh-leading cause of death in the United States in 2006 and is associated with many serious complications (CDC, 2007). Diabetes is the leading cause of new blindness among adults and accounts for 44% of new cases of renal failure. The risk of heart disease and stroke is 2-4 times greater in clients with diabetes mellitus.

Diabetes is seen in all age groups and races. About 33% of clients with diabetes are older than age 60. African American, Hispanic, and some Native American populations have a higher incidence of diabetes than the white population (CDC, 2002a).

Direct and indirect medical costs (disability, lost work, health care costs) have risen to $174 billion annually (CDC, 2007).

TABLE 43-3 Comparison of the Clinical Manifestations of Type 1 Diabetes and Type 2 Diabetes

	TYPE 1 DIABETES	TYPE 2 DIABETES
Etiology	Autoimmune	Genetic susceptibility associated; usually associated with obesity.
Age of onset	Rare before age 1	Incidence increases with age
Percent of diabetics	5%–10%	90%–95%
Onset	Abrupt, rapid	Gradual, over years
Body weight at onset	Normal or thin	80% are overweight
Insulin production	None	Less than normal, normal, or greater than normal
Insulin injection	Always	Necessary for approximately 30%
Ketosis	Occurs mainly in children and adolescents	Unlikely
Management	Insulin, diet, exercise	Diet and weight loss, exercise, possibly oral hypoglycemics or insulin

COURTESY OF DELMAR CENGAGE LEARNING

returns to normal after the infant's birth. The client should be rechecked 6 weeks after the birth to see if the diabetes persists.

CONTRIBUTING FACTORS

Persons with a family history of diabetes are at greater risk for developing diabetes. Other factors associated with diabetes include obesity, lack of exercise, aging, and ethnicity. The most powerful risk factor for type 2 diabetes is obesity. For persons with a family history of type 2 diabetes, maintenance of an ideal body weight may delay or prevent the onset of diabetes. Aging can also be considered a contributing factor.

It is known that members of certain racial groups are more likely to develop diabetes. In the United States, there is a greater chance of developing type 2 diabetes for Hispanics, Latinos, certain Native American populations, African Americans, and Asian/Pacific Islanders. Other groups at risk for development of diabetes include those with a history of gestational diabetes or impaired glucose tolerance (IGT).

MEDICAL–SURGICAL MANAGEMENT

Medical

There is no known cure for diabetes. The goal of therapeutic management is aimed at the control of blood sugar and the prevention and early detection of the complications associated with diabetes. Diabetes is considered under control if the client maintains ideal body weight and enjoys good health, preprandial glucose levels are less than 140 mg/dL, and postprandial glucose levels do not rise above 180 mg/dL.

Treatment plans vary and are individualized for each client. Control of blood glucose generally involves a balance of a dietary prescription, an exercise plan, and medications. Ultimately, the client is the manager of the treatment plan and, therefore, must be very well informed about diabetes and involved in all aspects of care planning and decision making.

Since the advent of home glucose monitoring devices, urine testing for glucose is rarely used. Testing urine for ketone (product of fatty acid oxidation) production, however, continues to be recommended when the blood glucose level is consistently higher than 240 mg/dL or when any symptoms of ketoacidosis are present.

The client with type 1 diabetes will always require administration of insulin to lower the glucose level and prevent complications of diabetes. Diet and exercise regimens are also important to control the glucose level and maintain health.

Dietary management is the cornerstone of treatment for the person with type 2 diabetes. As the obese person loses weight, the body's insulin requirements decrease, resulting in improved glucose tolerance. Exercise plays an important role in losing weight and lowering the blood glucose level. Type 2 diabetes not controlled by diet and exercise may necessitate administration of medications. Oral hypoglycemic agents or parenteral administration of insulin may be required for optimal control.

Surgical

Pancreas transplantations have been performed and have successfully eliminated the need for exogenous insulin in some clients. At present, pancreas transplants are being performed primarily on clients with type 1 diabetes who also need kidney or other organ transplants because the serious side effects of the antirejection medications do not justify a pancreas transplant alone. Pancreatic islet cell transplants are also being done experimentally with limited success but hold much promise for the future.

Pharmacological

Various pharmacological treatments that are used in the management of type 1 and type 2 diabetes are discussed in the following text.

Insulin Persons with type 1 diabetes always require insulin administration. Persons with type 2 diabetes may not initially require insulin, but it may become necessary as endogenous insulin production decreases or during times of stress or illness.

COMMUNITY/HOME HEALTH CARE

Glucose Monitoring

The availability and use of home glucose monitoring equipment to evaluate serum (blood) glucose has revolutionized self-care for the diabetic client. Also called "fingerstick blood glucose" (FSBG), self-monitoring of blood glucose (SMBG) can be done quickly using capillary blood that provides fairly accurate reading of the current blood glucose. Most often, the glucose level is checked before meals and at bedtime so the client can adjust the treatment plan accordingly. Self-monitoring of blood glucose is recommended for all clients requiring insulin or those with a widely fluctuating glucose level. Symptoms of hypoglycemia at any time warrant immediate evaluation of the blood glucose level.

Historically, insulin has been obtained from beef or pork pancreas. Today, biosynthetic human insulin is used almost exclusively, but some clients still use pork or beef insulin. Human insulin is purer, more effective, and has a much lower incidence of causing insulin allergies and resistance. Insulin is available in very short-, short-, fast-, intermediate-, and long-acting forms that can be injected separately or mixed in the same syringe. Premixed insulins are also available. See Table 43-4 for descriptions of types of insulins and their actions. Insulin is routinely administered subcutaneously. Regular insulin (short-acting) may be administered intravenously when immediate response is desired, as in treatment of greatly elevated glucose levels occurring with diabetic ketoacidosis (DKA) or HHNS. Regular insulin is the *only* insulin that can be given intravenously (IV).

The strength of insulin correlates to the number of units of insulin per cubic centimeter. The most common concentrations of insulin used today are U-50 and U-100 insulin (50 and 100 units of insulin per 1 mL, respectively). U-500 insulin is available for clients who require very high doses.

Insulin should always be measured in an insulin syringe, which is marked in units (Figure 43-3). When mixing two types of insulin in the same syringe, it is important that the regular (clear, short-acting) insulin be drawn up first. The

TABLE 43-4 Types of Insulin and Their Actions

		ACTION IN HOURS			
TYPES OF INSULIN	APPEARANCE	ONSET	PEAK	DURATION	NURSING INTERVENTIONS
Very short-acting					
Insulin lispro (Humalog)	Clear	¼	1–1½	5 or less	Eat meals 5 to 10 minutes after injection. Glulisine (Apidra) can be taken 15 minutes before or 20 minutes after the start of a meal. Medication can be mixed with NPH insulin.
Insulin aspart (Novolog)	Clear	¼	1–3	3–5	
Glulisine (Apidra)	Clear	⅓	½–1½	3–4	
Short-acting					
Humulin R	Clear	½–1	2–4	6–8	Available in U-100 and U-500 strengths. Eat meal 15 minutes following injection.
Intermediate-acting					
Humulin N	Cloudy	1–1½	4–12	Up to 24	Roll insulin vial between palms of hands to equally distribute.
Humulin L	Cloudy	1–2½	7–15	22	
Long-acting					
Humulin U	Cloudy	4–8	10–30	36+	Usually given once a day. Cannot be mixed with any other insulin preparations.
Insulin glargine (Lantus)	Clear	1	None	up to 24	
Detemir (Levimir)	Clear	1	None	24	
Premixed					
Humulin N/Reg	Cloudy	½–1	4–8	24	Roll insulin vial between palms of hands to equally distribute. Do not mix with any other insulin preparations. With Humalog 75/25, eat meal within 5 to 10 minutes of injection.
Humulin 70/30	Cloudy	½–60	Varies	10–16	
Humulin 50/50	Cloudy	½–1	Varies	10–16	
Humalog mix 75/25	Cloudy	¼	Varies	10–16	

COURTESY OF DELMAR CENGAGE LEARNING

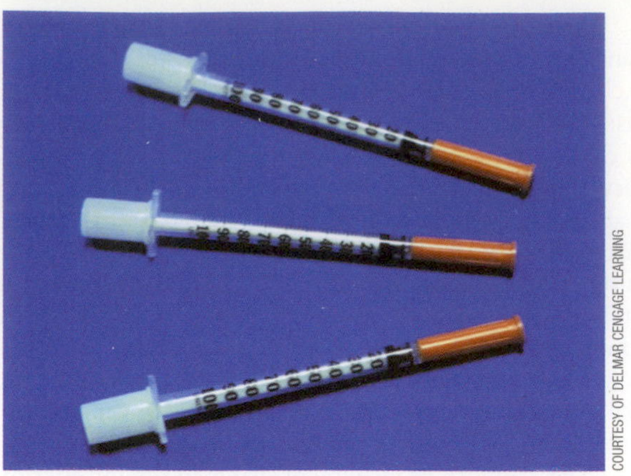

FIGURE 43-3 Insulin syringes are used to administer insulin subcutaneously.

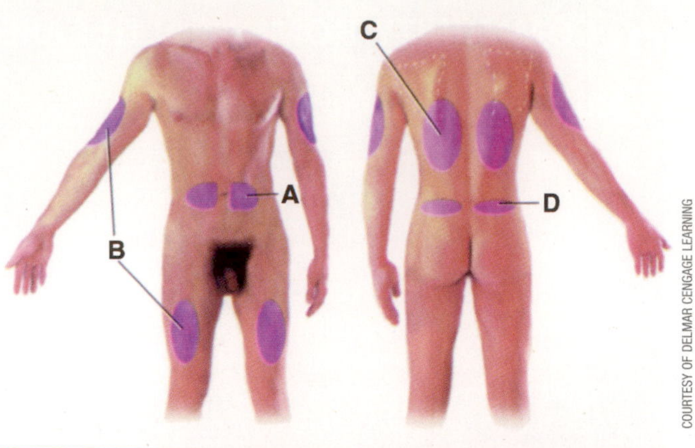

FIGURE 43-4 Subcutaneous Injection Sites; *A*, Abdomen; *B*, Lateral and Anterior Aspects of the Upper Arm and Thigh; *C*, Scapular Area of Back; *D*, Upper Ventrodorsal Gluteal Area

policy of many health care institutions requires that two nurses check insulin dosages before administration. Even if the facility does not have such a policy, checking the insulin dosage with another nurse will help protect against an adverse reaction resulting from error.

Insulin dosages are individually determined, usually requiring two or more injections per day and involving a combination of a short-acting and a longer-acting insulin. Various regimens of insulin administration can be used, each with its own advantages and disadvantages. In general, the more complex the regimen, the more normal the blood glucose level throughout the day. Clients can be taught to use the results of their self-monitoring blood glucose to adjust their insulin doses, allowing more flexibility in their meals and schedules. Recent studies strongly support the theory that intensive insulin regimens that tightly control the blood glucose level delay the onset and progression of complications of diabetic retinopathy, nephropathy, and neuropathy.

Sliding-Scale Insulin During times of surgery, illness, or stress, clients may have their glucose level managed with an insulin sliding scale in lieu of their regular regimen of insulin or oral hypoglycemics. A sliding scale determines insulin dosage based on fingerstick blood glucose level. Regular lispro (Humalog) or aspart (Novolog) insulin may be used, and a dose is administered every 4 or 6 hours based on the blood glucose level. The sliding scale allows for much flexibility and ensures frequent monitoring of and response to changes in the client's glucose level. An example sliding scale might be as follows:

- 4 units of Humulin R Insulin for glucose 151–200 mg/dL
- 6 units of Humulin R Insulin for glucose 201–250 mg/dL
- 8 units of Humulin R Insulin for glucose 251–300 mg/dL
- 10 units of Humulin R Insulin for glucose 301–350 mg/dL
- Call physician for glucose >350 mg/dL

Insulin Injections Insulin injections are administered into the subcutaneous tissue. If an inch of skin can be pinched, the needle is injected at a 90-degree angle, otherwise, at a 45-degree angle. The five main areas for injection are the abdomen, arms, thighs, hips, and subscapular regions (Figure 43-4). Factors affecting absorption should be considered when selecting an injection site. Absorption occurs most quickly in the abdomen, followed by the arms, thighs, hips, and subscapular regions.

Rotation of sites for injection has traditionally been recommended to prevent **lipodystrophy** (atrophy or hypertrophy in the subcutaneous fat). More recently, some authorities are recommending that the abdomen, which provides the most predictable absorption of insulin, be used exclusively for insulin administration.

If sites other than the abdomen are used, site rotation needs to be done systematically to prevent erratic absorption. Failure to rotate injection sites may cause a complication known as lipodystrophy; a change in the subcutaneous fat that decreases the absorption of the insulin. One system of rotation is to always use the same area of injection the same time each day (e.g., always using the abdomen in the morning and the thigh in the afternoon). Another system of rotation is to use all available injection sites in one area before moving to another.

Exercise will increase the rate of absorption, so diabetics planning to exercise should not inject insulin into the areas to be exercised.

Vials of insulin not being used should be refrigerated to prevent loss of potency. Vials in use may be kept at room temperature to decrease local irritation at the injection site, which can occur when cold insulin is used. When mixing a short-acting and a longer-acting insulin in the same syringe, the regular (clear) should always be drawn up into the syringe first, followed by the longer-acting (cloudy) insulin. Figure 43-5 illustrates mixing and administering insulin. It is recommended that insulin syringes be used only once and then discarded.

The visually and/or neurologically impaired diabetic client may benefit from assistive devices available to facilitate drawing up the insulin and administering it. Clients dependent on others for drawing up their insulin may benefit from prefilled syringes, which are considered stable for up to 3 weeks when stored in the refrigerator.

The nurse should keep in mind that the most important factor in the administration of insulin is consistency in technique. Also, simplification of the procedure may have a major impact on a client's ability to comply and to maintain independence. It is important that the nurse understand the basic principles of insulin administration and thereby remain flexible when teaching new clients or assessing the skills of experienced clients.

Insulin Pumps A portable insulin infusion pump delivers insulin continuously through a subcutaneous needle, usually anchored in the abdomen. A continuous, or basal, rate of regular

1. Cleanse the rubber stopper on both vials with an alcohol wipe, then inject the amount of air equal to the dose of the intermediate-acting insulin into the N vial.

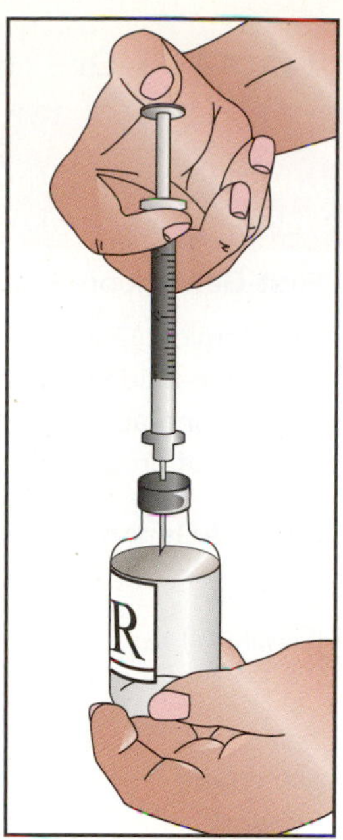

2. Inject the amount of air equal to the dose of the rapid-acting insulin into the R vial.

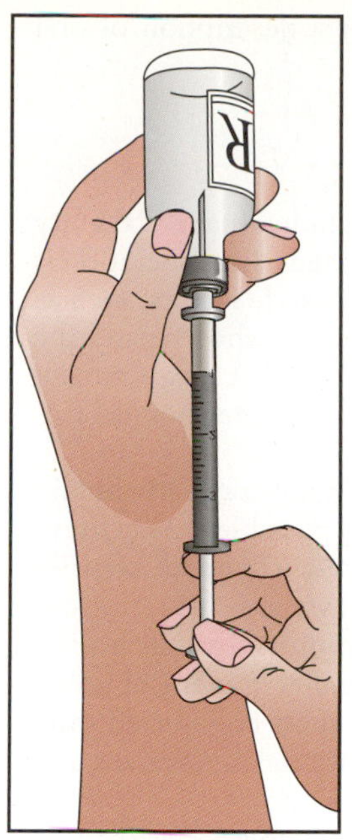

3. Withdraw the correct amount of rapid-acting insulin.

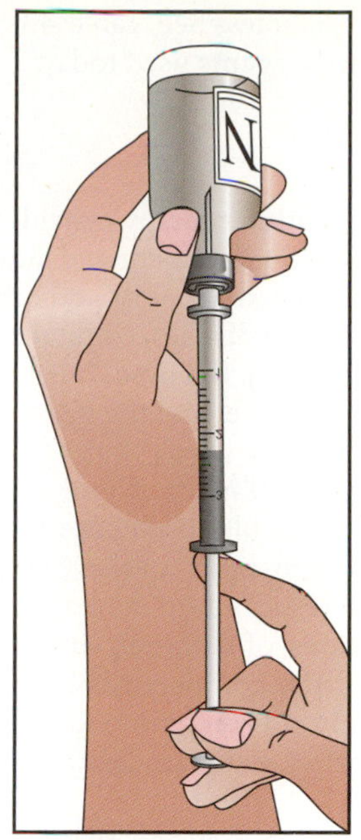

4. Withdraw the correct amount of intermediate-acting insulin by pulling the plunger down to the unit mark that equals the dose of rapid-acting insulin plus the dose of intermediate-acting insulin. The insulins mix immediately in the syringe. If too much intermediate-acting insulin is withdrawn, the entire contents of the syringe must be discarded.

COURTESY OF DELMAR CENGAGE LEARNING

FIGURE 43-5 How to Mix Insulin

aspart (Novolog) or lispro (Humalog) insulin is programmed and delivered to closely imitate the body's natural insulin secretion. Additional boluses can be manually administered to coordinate with meal times. The injection site is changed every 48 to 72 hours. The use of the insulin pump prevents multiple injections and allows flexibility in meal size and time. Use of the pump requires a motivated and educated client because intensive self-monitoring of blood glucose is essential.

Complications of Insulin Therapy Complications of insulin therapy include hypoglycemia (discussed later in this chapter), insulin resistance (requiring >200 units/day), lipodystrophy, Somogyi phenomenon, and the dawn phenomenon. Lipodystrophy can be minimized by using human insulin, using room temperature insulin, and by rotating sites of insulin injection.

The **Somogyi phenomenon** occurs when a rapid decrease in blood glucose (hypoglycemia) causes the release of glucose-elevating hormones (epinephrine, cortisol, glucagon). The hypoglycemia usually occurs during the night but manifests as an elevated glucose in the morning and may be inadvertently treated with an increase in insulin dosage. The Somogyi phenomenon can be diagnosed by checking the blood glucose during the night at about 3:00 a.m. Adjusting the insulin regimen to avoid the peaking of insulin during the night will correct this effect.

The **dawn phenomenon** is an early morning glucose elevation produced by the release of growth hormone. The release of the growth hormone decreases the peripheral uptake of the glucose resulting in elevated morning glucose levels. Administering the evening insulin dose at a later time will coordinate the insulin peak with the hormone release.

Oral Hypoglycemic Agents Oral hypoglycemic agents are used to treat persons with type 2 diabetes who are not controlled with exercise and diet. These agents are meant to supplement diet and exercise, not replace them. Oral hypoglycemics are not insulin and work by other mechanisms.

Sulfonylurea is the original class of oral hypoglycemic medications used for diabetes therapy. The sulfonylureas work primarily by increasing the ability of the islet cells of the pancreas to excrete insulin. To a lesser degree, they increase the cells' sensitivity to insulin and decrease glucose production by the liver.

Metformin (Glucophage), a biguanide, does not increase insulin release but works by making existing insulin more effective at the cellular level. Metformin decreases the amount of glucose produced by the liver. Muscle tissues become more sensitive to insulin and improve glucose absorption. Metformin may be given alone or in combination with other oral hypoglycemics. In some clients, Glucophage works more effectively if given with some dose of Diabeta. Because it does not stimulate increased insulin release, metformin is not associated with episodes of hypoglycemia. The major side effects of metformin are gastrointestinal and include anorexia, nausea, abdominal discomfort, and diarrhea.

Oral hypoglycemics require some production of insulin by the pancreas and, therefore, are not useful in the treatment of type 1 diabetes. See Table 43-5 for a description of oral hypoglycemic agents used today.

Diet

Medical nutrition therapy provides an individualized dietary prescription to meet client and family needs. Consideration is given to usual eating habits and other lifestyle factors, such as dietary likes and dislikes, cultural influences, who prepares the meals, and family finances. It is important that meals remain a social experience, and the person with diabetes not feel isolated or different.

The goals of medical nutrition therapy are (1) maintain as near-normal blood glucose level as possible, (2) achieve optimal serum lipid levels, (3) provide adequate calories to maintain or attain a reasonable weight, (4) prevent complications of diabetes, and (5) improve overall health. Because of the complexity of individualizing medical nutrition therapy, it is recommended that clients be referred early to a registered dietician (RD) for nutritional assessment and education.

Diabetes is a strong risk factor for atherosclerosis and cardiovascular disease. Therefore, reducing serum lipid levels is a goal of medical nutrition therapy. To reduce the risk of cardiovascular disease, the ADA recommendations incorporate a reduction in saturated fat and cholesterol consumption.

It is recommended that individuals taking insulin or oral hypoglycemic agents eat at consistent times synchronized with the actions of the medications used. Distribution of calories over 24 hours, with regular meals and snacks, helps prevent extreme highs and lows in blood glucose.

Consistent-Carbohydrate Meal Plan Current ADA nutrition guidelines suggest using a "consistent-carbohydrate meal plan." The client eats an individually prescribed amount of carbohydrates at each meal or snack. Carbohydrates determine premeal insulin requirements more than the amount of protein or fat in the meal, and they have the greatest effect on the postprandial blood glucose level. Protein and fat intake must be watched to avoid weight gain and increased serum lipid levels.

Protein intake of both animal and vegetable sources should make up 15% to 20% of the daily calorie intake. Cholesterol intake should not exceed 300 mg per day (Bartels, 2004). If nephropathy is present, protein should be 10% of the daily calorie intake.

Total fat intake depends on the goals set by the client and health care provider for desired levels of glucose, lipid, and weight. If lipid level is normal, 30% or less of calories should come from fat with less than 10% from saturated fat. If weight loss is a primary issue, reduction in fat intake is an efficient way to reduce calorie intake. When lipid level is a problem, a decrease of saturated fat intake to less than 7% of the total calories, total fat to less than 30% of total calories, and cholesterol to less than 300 mg per day is recommended.

The remainder of the calorie intake comes from carbohydrates. The amount consumed is more important than the source of the carbohydrate.

Persons with diabetes should follow the same precautions regarding the use of alcohol as applied to the general public. Alcohol may increase the risk for hypoglycemia in people treated with insulin or sulfonylureas, such as acetohexamide (Dymelor), chlorpropamide (Diabinese), or tolazamide (Tolinase).

TABLE 43-5 Oral Hypoglycemics

GENERIC (BRAND)	USUAL DOSE	ONSET TIME (HOURS)	DURATION (HOURS)
First-Generation Sulfonylureas			
Tolbutamide (Orinase), tolazamide, (Tolinase), and chlorpropamide (Diabinese) are seldom used because of their long action, higher incidence of adverse effects, and risk of drug interactions (Cincinnati & Veliko, 2001).			
Second-Generation Sulfonylureas			
glipizide (Glucatrol)	2.5–40 mg single or divided dose	1–1½	10–16
glimepride (Amaryl)	1–4 mg single dose	1	24
glyburide (Diabeta, Micronase)	1.25–20 mg single or divided dose	2–4	24
Biguanides			
metformin HCl (Glucophage)	500–2,500 mg two or three divided doses	24–48	6–12
Alpha-Glucosidase Inhibitors			
acarbose (Precose)	25–100 mg with meals (tid)	1	No data
miglitol (Glyset)	25–100 mg with meals (tid)	2–3	4–6
Thiazolidenediones			
rosiglitazone maleate (Avandia)	4 mg daily	1	
Combinations			
glyburide and metformin HCl (Glucovance)	1.25 mg/250 mg 2.5 mg/500 mg once or twice a day		
rosiglitazone maleate and metformin HCl (Avandamet)	1 mg/500 mg 2 mg/500 mg 4 mg/500 mg		

COURTESY OF DELMAR CENGAGE LEARNING

Activity

The beneficial effects of regular exercise for the diabetic are multiple. Exercise decreases the blood glucose by increasing the uptake of glucose by muscles and improving insulin usage. Exercise also increases circulation, improves cardiovascular status, decreases stress, and assists with weight loss.

Before starting an exercise program, the person with diabetes should have a complete physical and review the exercise plan with the physician or primary health care provider. Regular daily exercise rather than sporadic exercise should be encouraged.

Persons with diabetes need to correlate exercise with their blood glucose, taking care to avoid periods of hypoglycemia or exercising when blood glucose is too high. Exercise potentiates the action of insulin, resulting in lower insulin requirements and an increased risk of hypoglycemia during and after exercise. On the other hand, in the person with diabetes who is insulin-deficient, exercise may cause a further rise in blood glucose and rapid development of ketosis. Diabetics should not exercise at the peak of insulin activity, when their blood glucose is greater than 250 mg/dL, or if they have ketones in their urine.

Health Promotion

The diabetic educator plays a pivotal role in assisting the diabetic client/family to understand diabetes and the necessary lifestyle changes. Some teaching is unique to an individual client and is done one-to-one, whereas some teaching applies to all clients with diabetes and is often done in a class setting. This also allows clients with diabetes to meet each other and share concerns, information, and ideas that have worked for them.

The diabetic educator nurse is part of a team, including the client/family, physician, dietician, and pharmacist, who all work together to help the client understand and comply with the treatment plan.

Sick-Day Management It is important that persons with diabetes have a plan for managing their diabetes in the event of illness. It is important that they continue taking their insulin or oral hypoglycemic medication when they are experiencing illness because illness and fever can increase blood glucose and the need for insulin. Some persons with diabetes who do not normally take short-acting insulin may require it during times of fever or illness. Blood glucose should be monitored 4 to 6 times per day (Figure 43-6), and urine should be checked for ketones. Blood glucose greater than 300 mg/dL or ketones in the urine should be reported to the physician.

If the client cannot ingest the planned meal, carbohydrates in the form of soft foods and liquids can be substituted. Extreme nausea and vomiting or diarrhea should be reported to the physician because extreme fluid loss can be dangerous. Clients with type 1 diabetes who are unable to retain fluids may need to be hospitalized to avoid ketoacidosis.

Acute Complications of Diabetes

There are three major acute complications of diabetes related to blood glucose imbalance: hypoglycemia, diabetic ketoacidosis (DKA), and HHNS (Table 43-6).

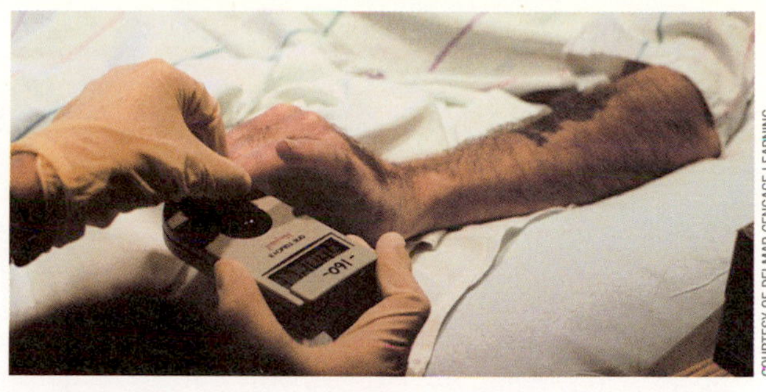
COURTESY OF DELMAR CENGAGE LEARNING

Figure 43-6 The nurse measures a client's blood glucose level.

Hypoglycemia (Insulin Reaction)

Hypoglycemia (low blood glucose) occurs when a client's glucose level decreases to less than 70 mg/dL, with the most severe reactions occurring when it decreases to less than 50 mg/dL. Hypoglycemia can occur any time of the day, but most often will occur before meals or when insulin action is peaking. Factors that can contribute to the development of a hypoglycemic reaction are skipping meals or eating late, unplanned exercise, and administration of excess insulin.

Hypoglycemic symptoms can occur suddenly and unexpectedly and vary from client to client. The cardinal rule is: *Always believe clients who tell you they are having an insulin reaction.* Most persons with diabetes have had hypoglycemic reactions before, so they know the symptoms that precede an insulin reaction. Hypoglycemia unawareness occurs when the client experiences an inability to recognize the warning symptoms of hypoglycemia. It is usually a complication of type 1 diabetes but can occur in type 2.

When a hypoglycemic reaction is suspected, the nurse must respond immediately according to the institution's protocol. Treatment involves assessing the client, checking blood glucose level, and administering glucose in the most appropriate form. Daniels (2007) recommends providing

LIFE SPAN CONSIDERATIONS

Hybrid or Mixed Diabetes

Usually a child or teenager develops either type 1 or type 2 diabetes. Some teenagers have elements of both kinds of diabetes. This phenomenon is referred to as "hybrid" or "mixed" diabetes. Given the fact that more children and teenagers are becoming overweight and obese, it is not surprising that these age groups have elements of both types of diabetes. Youth with "hybrid" or "mixed" diabetes typically have:

- insulin resistance associated with obesity and type 2 diabetes, and
- antibodies against the pancreatic islet cells that are associated with autoimmunity and type 1 diabetes.

(National Diabetes Education Program, 2008; Lorenz & Silverstein, 2005)

CLIENT TEACHING

Guidelines for Exercising

- Try to exercise at the same time and in the same amount each day.
- Test blood glucose level before, during, and after exercise.
- Do not inject insulin into a limb that you will be exercising.
- Do not exercise at the peak of insulin activity.
- Do not exercise before meals unless trying to lower blood glucose level.
- Do not exercise with a blood glucose level over 250 mg/dL or with ketones in the urine. This indicates severe insulin deficiency and may predispose to hyperglycemia.
- Eat a snack (15 g of carbohydrates) before or during exercise if appropriate, based on blood glucose level.
- Always carry a source of carbohydrates and emergency cash, if away from home, in case hypoglycemia occurs while exercising.
- Always carry personal and medical alert identification.
- Watch for post-exercise hypoglycemia. Individuals who have more than usual exercise during the day should increase their carbohydrate intake and test their glucose during the night to detect nocturnal hypoglycemia. (Hypoglycemia can occur 8 to 15 hours after exercise.)

CLIENT TEACHING

Fingersticks

- Use shallow skin penetration, just to get enough blood for the meter.
- Rotate sites; use sides of fingertips and thumb.
- Use alcohol sparingly or wash hands with warm soapy water before fingerstick *instead* of using alcohol. The warm water brings more blood into the fingers.
- Apply firm pressure *directly* over the puncture for 10 to 15 seconds; if area is still bleeding, apply pressure until it stops.

the client with 10–15 grams of simple carbohydrates, for example 8 oz of low-fat milk or 4 oz of fruit juice. The client taking acarbose (Precose), which slows digestion and absorption of most carbohydrates—including hard candies and many fruit juices—but not glucose, will not have the rapid response to fruit juice or sugar that other clients will have. Hypoglycemic reactions can be fatal, *so leaving the client untreated is more dangerous than causing mild hyperglycemia with overtreatment*. Figure 43-7 provides a sample hypoglycemic protocol.

Persons with diabetes and their families must know the symptoms and treatment for hypoglycemia. Hypoglycemic episodes can be prevented by following a regular pattern of eating, exercise, and insulin administration. Between-meal and bedtime snacks can be used to cover times of peak insulin action. Additional food should be eaten when engaging in greater than usual exercise. Blood glucose level should be checked at the first suspicion of hypoglycemia. All clients should wear an identification bracelet or tag indicating that they have diabetes because hypoglycemic reactions can occur unexpectedly.

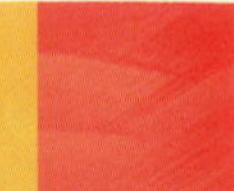

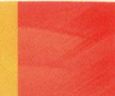

TABLE 43-6 Symptoms of Acute Complications of Diabetes

Symptoms of Hypoglycemia (Insulin Reaction)

Mild hypoglycemia
- Diaphoresis; cold, clammy skin
- Palpitations
- Pallor
- Tremors
- Excess hunger
- Anxious but alert

Moderate hypoglycemia
- Confusion, vertigo
- Behavior changes
- Slurred speech
- Irritability
- Paresthesia

Severe hypoglycemia
- Seizures
- Loss of consciousness
- Shallow respirations
- Nursing Alert: Severe hypoglycemia is a medical emergency. Administer some form of glucose immediately.

Symptoms of Diabetic Ketoacidosis (DKA)
- Same as HHNS plus symptoms of acidosis:
  - "Fruity" odor to breath
  - Kussmaul's respirations (deep, nonlabored)

Symptoms of Hyperosmolar Hyperglycemic Nonketotic Syndrome (HHNS)
- Polyuria
- Polydipsia
- Skin hot, dry, decreased turgor
- Dehydration—hypotension, increased pulse
- Blurred vision
- Weakness
- Mental status changes, confusion to coma

COURTESY OF DELMAR CENGAGE LEARNING

Diabetic Ketoacidosis

Diabetic ketoacidosis (DKA) is one of the most serious complications of hyperglycemia. Glucose is a hyperosmolar

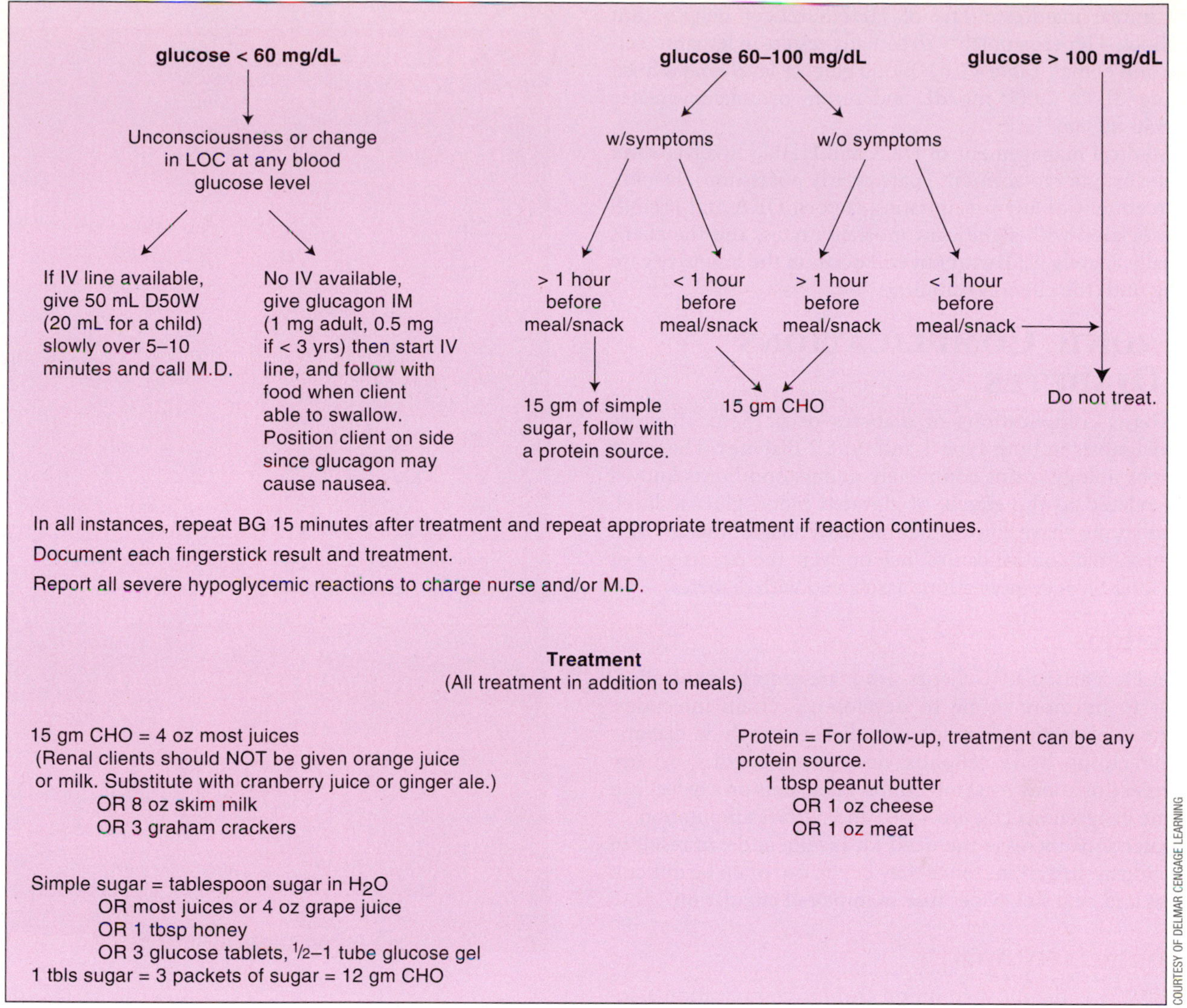

FIGURE 43-7 Sample Hypoglycemic Protocol

substance drawing fluid out of the cell and into the circulation, where it is excreted by the kidneys. This oncotic diuresis results in polyuria (increased urine output), dehydration, and electrolyte imbalances. Increased fat metabolism results in accumulation of ketones, resulting in metabolic acidosis. Surgery, stress, or illness may trigger DKA, which usually develops in clients with immune-mediated type 1 diabetes, although it can occur in clients with type 2 diabetes. The client with undiagnosed immune-mediated type 1 diabetes may also present with DKA.

The onset of DKA may be gradual or sudden. Classic symptoms of hyperglycemia (polyuria, polyphagia, polydipsia) usually precede DKA. Other symptoms include nausea and vomiting, abdominal pain from acidosis, headache, weakness, fatigue, and blurred vision. Assessment may reveal hot, flushed skin and signs of hypovolemia or shock. Acidosis will produce signs of hyperpnea (Kussmaul's breathing), fruity odor to breath from respiratory elimination of acetone, and decreased level of consciousness ranging from lethargy to coma.

Laboratory values will reveal blood glucose from 300 mg/dL to 800 mg/dL and metabolic acidosis. Urine will be positive for glucose and ketones.

Treatment regimen must be initiated immediately with clients experiencing DKA. Fluid replacement consists of NS intravenously to improve blood pressure. Regular insulin may be provided intravenously to assist in decreasing the blood glucose levels. Potassium replacement is also necessary to prevent any additional complication associated with fluid replacement (Daniels, 2007).

Hyperosmolar Hyperglycemic Nonketotic Syndrome

HHNS occurs when there is insufficient insulin to prevent hyperglycemia but enough insulin to prevent ketoacidosis. HHNS occurs in persons with type 2 diabetes. Because symptoms of acidosis do not occur, no symptoms may be noticed until the glucose level is dangerously high.

HHNS occurs most often in the elderly client with undiagnosed type 2 diabetes. HHNS can also occur in the poorly controlled client and is usually precipitated by illness or another stressor. The onset of symptoms of HHNS is lower than DKA, often taking days to weeks to display clinical symptoms.

Clinical manifestations of HHNS reflect dehydration and shock. Hyperosmolality eventually results in lethargy, seizures, and coma (Table 43-6). Blood glucose level ranges from 600 mg/dL to 2,000 mg/dL and serum osmolality greater than 350 mOsm/L.

Medical management of DKA and HHNS involves fluid and electrolyte replacement (particularly potassium), insulin, and treatment of any precipitating factors. DKA and HHNS are associated with significant mortality rates, and the client is usually acutely ill. Treatment will occur in the intensive care setting until the client is stabilized.

Chronic Complications of Diabetes

Long-term complications of diabetes occur 5 to 10 years after diagnosis in both type 1 and type 2 diabetes. The exact pathophysiology is not completely understood but is known to be related to the effects of elevated blood glucose level. Recent studies have shown that intensive insulin therapy and tight glycemic control can reduce or delay the occurrence of many long-term complications associated with diabetes.

Infections

Diabetics, particularly clients who are poorly controlled, appear to be more prone to developing certain infections. Infections of particular concern to diabetics include diabetic foot infections, boils, cellulitis, necrotizing fasciitis, urinary tract infections, and yeast infections. Small cuts on the feet can become gangrenous (Figure 43-8) and require amputation.

Infections increase the need for insulin and can result in ketoacidosis. Infections, once they occur, can often be difficult to treat and heal slowly because of impaired circulation.

Diabetic Neuropathy

Neuropathy is the most common chronic complication associated with diabetes. The incidence of neuropathy increases with age and duration of disease and is related to elevated blood glucose level. Neuropathy can affect all types of nerves, but the two most common types of diabetic neuropathy are peripheral neuropathy and autonomic neuropathy.

Peripheral neuropathy causes paresthesias and burning sensations, primarily in the lower extremities. Decreased sensations of pain and temperature coupled with decreased peripheral circulation place the client at risk for undetected foot injury.

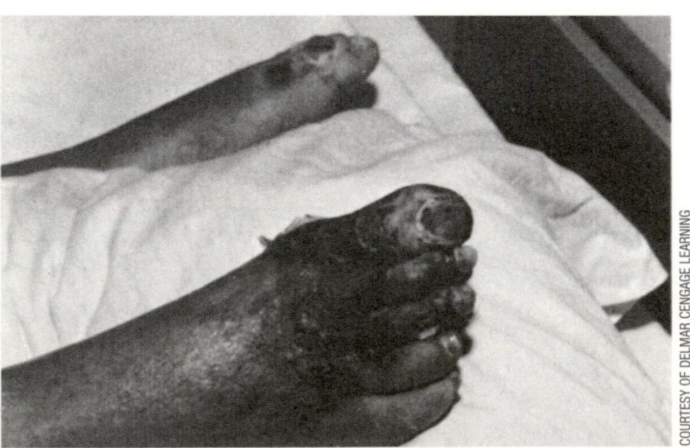

COURTESY OF DELMAR CENGAGE LEARNING

FIGURE 43-8 Gangrene of the toes and foot as a result of an infection often means eventual amputation.

CLIENT TEACHING

Guidelines to Healthy Feet

- Wash feet daily and dry them carefully, especially between the toes.
- Inspect feet and between toes for blisters, cuts, and infections. Use a mirror to see the bottoms of the feet. If your vision is impaired, have a family member examine your feet. Remember, because of decreased feeling in your feet, you may have an infection and not know it.
- Avoid activities that restrict blood flow to the feet, especially smoking and sitting with legs crossed.
- Wear shoes that are comfortable, well-fitting, and closed toed. Wear new shoes for short intervals until broken in. Do not walk barefoot.
- Prevent cuts and irritations. Always wear stockings. Look inside shoes for rough edges, nail points, foreign objects.
- Avoid temperature extremes. Test bath water with hands before getting in. Do not use water bottles or heating pads on feet.
- See your physician regularly and make sure that your feet are examined each visit.
- When toenails are trimmed, cut them straight across. When corns or calluses are present, see a physician or podiatrist. *Do not* cut them yourself.

Autonomic neuropathy can affect almost any organ system, including gastrointestinal (delayed gastric emptying, constipation, diarrhea), urinary (retention, neurogenic bladder), and reproductive (male impotence).

Nephropathy (Chronic Renal Failure)

Diabetic nephropathy develops slowly over many years, progressing eventually to kidney failure. Elevated blood glucose level causes a decrease in the glomerular filtration rate resulting in fluid retention. Prolonged injury to the nephron may eventually lead to renal failure. Controlling hypertension and blood glucose level is the key to delaying renal damage. Good hydration before and diuresis following any dye study is valuable in preventing renal damage. Diligent monitoring of a

LIFE SPAN CONSIDERATIONS

Diabetic Neuropathy

Advancing age is the strongest risk factor regardless of disease duration and blood sugar control.

client's urinary output is essential. Clients may be required to adhere to a low protein, low salt diet.

Retinopathy

Changes in the small vessels of the retina result in diabetic retinopathy, which is a major cause of blindness among persons with diabetes (Figure 43-9). Because of the insidious onset of type 2 diabetes, retinopathy is often present at diagnosis. The severity and progression of retinopathy appear to be closely related to glucose and blood pressure control. Persons with diabetes also develop cataracts at an earlier age. Although most clients develop some degree of retinopathy, most do not develop visual impairment. To facilitate early detection, diabetics should have ophthalmologic evaluations every 6 to 12 months.

Vascular Changes

Diabetes is an independent risk factor for atherosclerotic vessel disease. Atherosclerotic changes that occur in persons with diabetes are similar to those that occur in nondiabetics, but they occur at earlier ages and progress at a more rapid rate.

Cardiovascular Hypertension is twice as common in persons with diabetes and is an important factor in the progression of retinopathy, nephropathy, and vascular (large vessel) disease. The incidence of coronary artery disease, angina, and myocardial infarction is higher when compared to the nondiabetic population. Cerebral vascular disease and cerebral vascular accident are also more common in persons with diabetes. Therapies aimed at lowering risk factors and effects of atherosclerosis include weight control, low-fat diet, treatment of hypertension and hyperlipidemia, regular exercise, and control of blood glucose level.

Peripheral Vascular Disease Peripheral vascular disease occurs most commonly in diabetics with hypertension or hyperlipidemia and in diabetics who smoke. Diabetics have two to three times the incidence of occlusive peripheral arterial disease when compared to the nondiabetic population. Diabetes is present in more than half of persons experiencing nontraumatic lower extremity amputations.

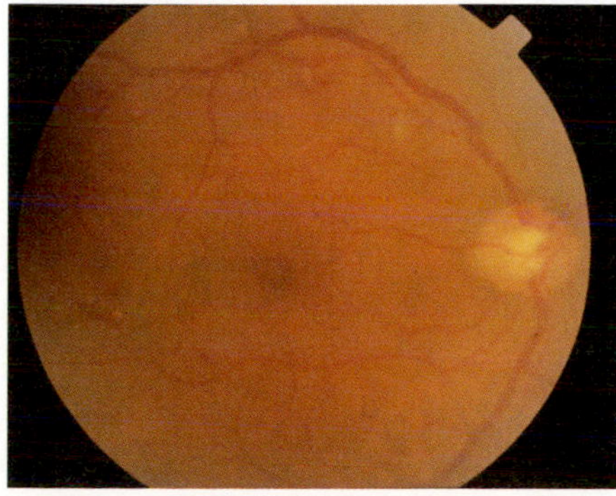

FIGURE 43-9 Microaneurysms in Diabetic Retinopathy (*Courtesy of Salim I. Butrus, M.D., Senior Attending, Department of Opthalmology, Washington Hospital Center, Washington, D.C., and Associate Clinical Professor, Georgetown University Medical Center, Washington, D.C.*)

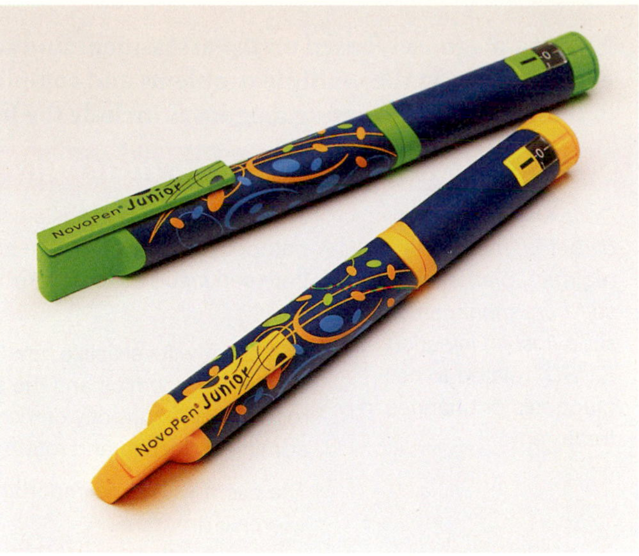

FIGURE 43-10 NovoPen Junior insulin pens are used by younger children and adolescents. (*Courtesy of Novo Nordisk.*)

NURSING MANAGEMENT

Monitor vital signs and serum electrolytes. Record I&O, administer fluids as ordered, and encourage oral fluid intake. Teach client about diabetes, use of insulin or oral hypoglycemics, methods of insulin administration (syringe, pen injector [Figure 43-10], and pump), relationship of exercise to diabetes management, and how to perform SMBG. Provide a list of symptoms and treatment for hypoglycemia.

NURSING PROCESS

ASSESSMENT

Subjective Data

This includes assessment of the health history, family history, diet, activity regimen, and the understanding of the disease and medical therapies. The client may describe fatigue, weakness, weight changes, mental status changes, polyuria, polyphagia, polydipsia, numbness or tingling of the extremities, blurred vision, and increased appetite.

Objective Data

Objective data should focus on the symptoms of diabetes, the common acute and chronic complications, and the results of diagnostic tests. There may be dependent redness or cyanosis of the lower extremities as well as the absence of hair. A fasting

CLIENT TEACHING

Retinopathy Prevention

- Refrain from straining to have a bowel movement.
- Use stool softener or laxative.
- Avoid postures that lower the head.
- Avoid lifting weight above shoulders.

Nursing diagnoses, based on the assessment findings, may be varied and extensive due to the multiple problems and complications caused by diabetes mellitus. Nursing diagnoses include the following:

NURSING DIAGNOSES	PLANNING/OUTCOMES	NURSING INTERVENTIONS
*Deficient **K**nowledge diabetes, medical regimen, diet, exercise, self-care management skills (insulin injection, SMBG)* related to new diagnosis or changes in treatment	The client will relate basic understanding of pathophysiology of diabetes, and relationship between insulin and hyper-/hypoglycemia.	Teach client about diabetes and the use of insulin to prevent hyper-/hypoglycemia or assist client to enroll in a formal diabetic education program.
	The client will verbalize how/when to take oral hypoglycemics and the side effects to report or will correctly demonstrate how to administer insulin and rotate sites.	Teach client about oral hypoglycemics or insulin, whichever the client will be using.
	The client will relate importance of an exercise program.	Discuss how exercise is related to diabetes management.
	The client will describe the relationship between dietary management and glycemic control; choose foods that comply with diet prescription.	Discuss how dietary management is related to the control of blood glucose and provide an exchange list of foods.
	The client will correctly demonstrate how to use SMBG to determine blood glucose level.	Teach client how to perform SMBG and have client return demonstration.
	The client will verbalize symptoms and treatment of hypoglycemia.	Provide client with a list of symptoms and treatment for hypoglycemia.
*Risk for Deficient **F**luid Volume* related to hyperglycemia, polyuria, and dehydration	The client will exhibit normal skin turgor, moist mucous membranes, and maintain oral fluid intake of 2,500–3,000 mL/day.	Measure client's intake and output, administer intravenous fluids as ordered, and encourage oral fluids.
	The client will have vital signs within normal limits.	Monitor vital signs and serum electrolytes.
*Imbalanced **N**utrition: Less than Body Requirements* related to imbalance between insulin, diet, and activity	The client will have weight within normal range for height and age.	Refer client to dietician to adjust dietary intake in order to maintain weight in normal range.

Evaluation: Evaluate each outcome to determine how it has been met by the client.

glucose level greater than 126 mg/dL or a nonfasting (random) level greater than 200 mg/dL on two separate occasions is diagnostic of diabetes.

PITUITARY DISORDERS

Hyperpituitarism and hypopituitarism are discussed in this section.

HYPERPITUITARISM

Hyperpituitarism is most commonly diagnosed between the second and fourth decade of life but can appear in infancy and childhood. Although other pituitary hormones may be affected, the most common are the GH and antidiuretic hormone.

Excess secretion of GH produces different changes depending on the client's age when it occurs. When the excess secretion occurs in childhood before the epiphyses close, gigantism is the result; in adults, acromegaly is the result.

Syndrome of inappropriate antidiuretic hormone and pituitary tumors are also discussed.

GIGANTISM

Gigantism affects infants and children, causing proportional overgrowth of all body tissues. By the time these children reach adulthood, they may be more than 8 feet tall.

Hyperplasia of the anterior pituitary is usually the cause of GH oversecretion. The oversecretion of GH is often caused by benign tumors of the pituitary gland. Clients with gigantism do not have the strength their size implies. Additional signs and symptoms often experienced by clients with gigantism include delayed puberty, double vision, increased sweating, large hands and feet with thick fingers and toes, and weakness.

Medical–Surgical Management

Medical

Irradiation of the anterior pituitary may be the treatment chosen. The child must then be observed for heart failure, hypertension, thickened bones, osteoporosis, and delayed sexual development.

Surgical

If the cause is a tumor, surgery may be performed to remove the tumor (explained under the section "Acromegaly"). If surgery cannot completely remove the tumor, medication management including somatostatin analogs may be used.

Pharmacological

When the pituitary is either destroyed by irradiation or removed by surgery, pituitary hormone replacement is necessary.

Nursing Management

Monitor children's growth for early identification of a problem. Be understanding and emphasize the positive aspects of being tall.

NURSING PROCESS

Assessment

Subjective Data

Listening to the child's description of the disease process may provide insight into the child's emotional responses.

Objective Data

Frequent measurements of growth indicate a more rapid rate of growth than expected.

ACROMEGALY

Acromegaly affects nearly 60 of every 1 million Americans (NIDDK, 2008a). Because acromegaly occurs after epiphyseal closure of bones, there is bone thickening with transverse growth and tissue enlargement. This occurs between 30 and 50 years of age. Photographs over years will reveal a progressive enlargement of the face and hands.

Acromegaly involves a gradual onset of clinical manifestations, including visual defects from pressure of the pituitary tumor on the optic nerve, soft tissue swelling, or hypertrophy of the face and extremities. The cartilaginous and connective tissue overgrowths result in a characteristic hulking appearance with thickened ears and nose, and marked projection of the jaw. The jaw can appear enlarged and the tongue may also thicken. The paranasal sinuses can become enlarged. Also laryngeal hypertrophy can occur. The client has thick fingers with tips that appear "tufted" (shaped like arrowheads on x-rays). The client exhibits a characteristic moist, weak, doughy handshake. The heart, liver, and spleen may enlarge. Some other characteristics are diaphoresis (profuse perspiration), oily or leathery skin, fatigue, heat intolerance, weight gain, headache, joint pain, hirsutism (excessive hairiness especially in females), and sleep disturbance. The client may experience decreased libido or impotence, oligomenorrhea (scanty or infrequent menstruation), and infertility.

The client's history and clinical manifestations along with cranial x-rays and a CT scan make a diagnosis of acromegaly. Serum GH level is elevated.

Prognosis depends on the causative factor, hyperplasia or a tumor; however, there is generally a reduced life span. Diabetes mellitus, hypertension, and a higher risk of cardiovascular disease are the most serious health consequences (NIDDK, 2009).

Medical–Surgical Management

Medical

Medical treatment consists of either medication that affects the GH or irradiation of the pituitary gland. Proton beam therapy uses a very low dose of radiation and is much less destructive to nearby tissue than conventional radiation therapy.

Surgical

Surgical treatment for hyperpituitarism is to remove the pituitary gland. Two surgical approaches to remove the pituitary are transfrontal or transsphenoid hypophysectomy. The transfrontal approach is rarely used because it has a high risk of mortality as well as permanent loss of smell and taste and causes severe diabetes insipidus. The transsphenoid approach (Figure 43-11) involves an incision in the superior maxillary gingiva. Surgery may be the treatment of choice or used after attempting medical treatment.

Postoperatively, nasal packing should be checked for clear, colorless drainage. If it occurs, the drainage must be documented and reported to the physician. If this drainage is suspected of being cerebrospinal fluid, it should be checked for glucose, which is found in cerebrospinal fluid. The nurse should observe for meningitis infection, which includes elevated leukocytes, sudden temperature elevation, or complaint of headache or nuchal rigidity. Analgesics are administered as needed. The client should avoid activities such as coughing,

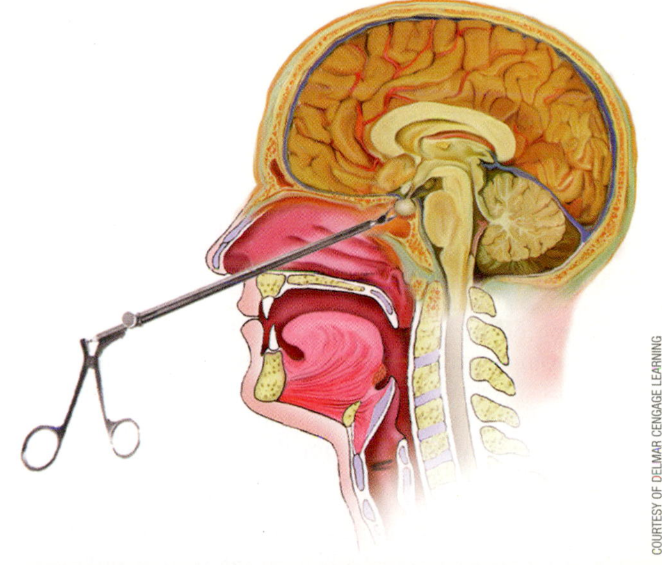

Figure 43-11 Transsphenoidal Approach to Hypophysectomy

straining, vomiting, or sneezing. The client should be encouraged to use an incentive spirometer instead of coughing. The client should not brush teeth for 2 weeks to avoid problems with the incision. Mouthwash can be used. The client should be instructed to avoid lifting and bending at the waist for 2 to 3 months after surgery.

Pharmacological

Two drugs may be prescribed for acromegaly. Bromocriptine mesylate (Parlodel) is a nonhormonal drug that activates dopamine receptors to inhibit the release of the GH and prolactin. Bromocriptine mesylate (Parlodel) should be given with food to decrease gastric upset. Because this drug can cause drowsiness or dizziness, the client should be instructed to avoid activities that require mental alertness. If the client is on oral contraceptives, alternate contraceptive measures should also be used because bromocriptine can stimulate ovulation.

The other drug, octreotide acetate (Sandostatin), inhibits the GH. Although octreotide is given by injection, it can still cause gastric distress. The injections should be given between meals and at bedtime. Clients with diabetes mellitus should closely monitor their blood sugar level.

Nursing Management

Be supportive. Show respect and acceptance. Assess ability to perform ADLs. Provide soft diet and encourage client to thoroughly chew food and drink fluids often.

NURSING PROCESS

Assessment

Subjective Data

Obtain a thorough nursing history, asking about vision impairment, headache, muscular weakness, menstrual irregularities, fatigue, sleep pattern changes, and sexual and psychological disturbances.

Objective Data

Objective data includes gait changes, vital sign changes (tachycardia or hypotension, which may indicate congestive heart failure), dyspnea, thick oily skin, and a deepening of the voice. The jaw is enlarged and projected, so the client may have difficulty in chewing.

Nursing diagnoses for a client with gigantism or acromegaly include the following:

NURSING DIAGNOSES	PLANNING/OUTCOMES	NURSING INTERVENTIONS
*Risk for Disproportionate **G**rowth* related to increased level of GH	The client will comply with treatment to minimize hyperpituitarism and stop excessive growth with treatment.	Assist client with activities of daily living and range-of-motion exercises. Administer medications as ordered. Remind client to carry medications on person.
*Disturbed **B**ody Image* related to irreversible physical changes	The client will acknowledge physical changes, express positive feelings about self, and exhibit ability to cope with altered body.	Encourage client to verbalize feelings. Assist client in setting achievable short-term goals. Offer emotional support and help client to develop coping strategies. Show respect and acceptance of the client as a person. Provide a positive but realistic assessment of the situation. Refer to professional counseling as needed. Provide education to client and family members concerning disease process.

Evaluation: Evaluate each outcome to determine how it has been met by the client.

SYNDROME OF INAPPROPRIATE ANTIDIURETIC HORMONE

Syndrome of inappropriate antidiuretic hormone (SIADH) results from an excess of ADH. The posterior pituitary gland continues to release ADH, causing the kidneys to reabsorb excess water, which decreases urine output and increases fluid volume. The most common cause is oat-cell lung cancer (NIH, 2007). Other causes are lymphoid pancreatic, duodenal, thymus, and prostate cancer; central nervous system trauma; infection; chronic obstructive pulmonary disease; acute respiratory failure; mechanical ventilation; and medications such as antineoplastic agents, tricyclic antidepressants, anesthetics, thiazides, and opioids.

The client will have hyponatremia (<130 mEq/L), water retention, weight gain, concentrated urine (urine osmolality >1,200 mOsm/L; specific gravity >1.020), muscle cramps, and weakness. The low osmolality of the blood allows fluid to leak out of vessels and causes brain swelling. If untreated, lethargy, seizures, coma, and death will result.

Medical–Surgical Management

Medical

The underlying disorder must be treated or medications stopped that may be contributing to SIADH. Fluid restriction will be implemented to prevent further hemodilution. Serious hyponatremia (<120 mEq/L) usually is treated with intravenous administration of 3% NaCl. The serum sodium level should be increased by 12 mEq/L or less per day. If the Na level is increased too rapidly, the client may experience fluid volume overload and congestive heart failure.

Pharmacological

Furosemide (Lasix) is given to increase urine output, while demeclocycline hydrochloride (Declomycin) and fludrocortisone (Florinef) are given to enhance sodium retention.

Diet

Fluid restriction is determined by the serum sodium level. Fluid restrictions of 1–1.5 liters/day are often implemented for the client with SIADH (Goh, 2004).

Nursing Management

Assess client's hydration and neurologic status every 3 to 4 hours. Provide a safe environment for the client. Accurately record I&O. Auscultate lungs every 2 to 4 hours. Explain why fluid intake is restricted. Weigh client daily. Provide frequent mouth care and apply lubricant to lips.

NURSING PROCESS

Assessment

Subjective Data

The client may describe muscle cramps, weakness, anorexia, nausea, and headache.

Objective Data

The client will have weight gain and fluid intake greater than output, may be irritable and disoriented, become progressively lethargic, and have seizures and diminished or absent deep tendon reflexes. Serum sodium and osmolality will be decreased. Urine osmolality and specific gravity will be increased.

Nursing diagnoses for a client with SIADH include the following:

NURSING DIAGNOSES	PLANNING/OUTCOMES	NURSING INTERVENTIONS
*Excess **Fluid** Volume* related to decreased urine output	The client will have increased urine output.	Assess client's weight daily on same scale at same time and vital signs. Accurately record I&O. Maintain fluid restrictions. Monitor laboratory reports, including Na, serum osmolality, urine Na, and urine osmolality. Administer medications as ordered.
*Impaired **Oral** Mucous Membrane* related to restriction of fluid intake	The client will have moist, intact oral mucous membranes.	Provide frequent oral care, avoiding alcohol-based mouth washes and lemon-glycerine swabs. Allow client to rinse mouth with water, but not swallow any. Provide lubricant for client's lips. Allow client to choose fluids and times to drink them.

Evaluation: Evaluate each outcome to determine how it has been met by the client.

PITUITARY TUMORS

Pituitary tumors more often affect the anterior pituitary rather than the posterior portion. Adenomas of the pituitary, which are rarely malignant, replace glandular tissue and enlarge the sella turcica. The cause is unknown, but there may be a predisposition toward tumor formation from an inherited **autosomal** dominant trait, meaning it is a dominant characteristic carried on any chromosome other than the one determining sex.

Clinical manifestations frequently start with a headache unrelated to stress or other factors. The next obvious manifestation is visual problems caused by the tumor putting pressure on the optic nerve. Others include personality changes, dementia, amenorrhea, impotence, lethargy, and weakness. The client may complain of cold intolerance, increased fatigue, constipation, and may have seizures. Although the tumor is not malignant, damage is done by tumor invasion of normal tissue.

Treatment is removal of the tumor. Complications of pituitary tumors are endocrine abnormalities if there is no replacement therapy after removal of the tumor. If the hypothalamus is compressed, diabetes insipidus can result. If the tumor has eroded the base of the skull, the client may have rhinorrhea (thin watery nasal discharge). Prognosis depends on the extent of invasion. In most cases, the tumor causes excessive secretion of the anterior pituitary hormones. Diagnostic testing includes dexamethasone suppression test, urine cortisol, FSH, LH, free T_4, TSH, and MRI of the head.

Medical–Surgical Management

Medical

Medical treatment of a pituitary tumor often includes radiation therapy. This can be used for small tumors or if the client is a poor surgical risk. Radiation can also be used after surgery to shrink tissue remaining after surgical excision. Another alternative to surgery is cryohypophysectomy. This involves freezing the area with a probe inserted via the transsphenoidal approach.

Surgical

Large tumors, especially those impinging on the optic nerve, are generally removed by using the transfrontal approach. Smaller tumors can be resected via the transsphenoidal approach.

Pharmacological

Permanent hormone imbalances frequently result from surgical removal of the tumor. Consequently, long term hormone replacement therapy is necessary.

Nursing Management

Provide a safe, clutter-free environment. Keep a call light within the client's reach. Provide periods of rest after activity. Adjust room temperature for client's comfort or provide extra blankets. The client will be in ICU for several days if surgery is performed.

After a transphenoid approach to removal of the tumor, prohibit the client from sneezing, coughing or brushing the teeth. Monitor dressing for clear leakage which may indicate CSF leakage.

NURSING PROCESS

Assessment

Subjective Data

Obtain a thorough client history and assess for manifestations of a tumor, such as visual problems, headache, impotence, lethargy, cold intolerance, fatigue, or constipation. The family may provide insight into any personality changes.

Objective Data

Assess the client for tilting of the head to compensate for visual disturbances, axillary and pubic hair loss, a waxy appearance to the skin, and few wrinkles.

Nursing diagnoses for a client with a pituitary tumor include the following:

NURSING DIAGNOSES	PLANNING/OUTCOMES	NURSING INTERVENTIONS
***F**atigue* related to decreased ACTH and TSH levels	The client will verbalize an understanding of the relationship between fatigue, the disease, and activity level, and express feeling of increasing energy as treatment progresses.	Explain relationship between pituitary tumor, fatigue, and activity level. Suggest alternating periods of activity with periods of rest. Administer medications as ordered. Encourage completion of all treatments.
*Disturbed **S**ensory Perception (Visual)* related to altered sensory reception, transmission, and/or integration due to pressure on optic nerve by the pituitary tumor	The client will use adaptive devices and appropriate resources to compensate for visual changes, and regain normal vision with treatment.	Provide information about adaptive devices and resources for visual changes. Provide a safe clutter-free environment. Make certain that the bed is in the low position and the call signal is in reach of the client. Use side rails as needed.

Evaluation: Evaluate each outcome to determine how it has been met by the client.

HYPOPITUITARISM

Hypopituitarism is a complex syndrome marked by metabolic dysfunction, sexual immaturity, and growth retardation when it occurs in childhood; Simmonds' disease and diabetes insipidus are examples of hypopituitarism. The most common cause of hypopituitarism is a tumor. Other causes are congenital defects (hypoplasia or aplasia), pituitary infarction (from postpartum hemorrhage), pituitary surgery or irradiation, or chemical agents. Hypopituitarism can be primary (meaning there is no known cause) or secondary. Secondary hypopituitarism can be a result of a deficiency of hypothalamic-releasing hormones. This deficiency can be idiopathic (without a known cause) or a result of infection, trauma, or tumor.

Clinical manifestations develop slowly and generally are not apparent until 75% of the pituitary is destroyed. Specific manifestations will vary with the specific hormone that is deficient.

Deficiency of the GH results in dwarfism, which becomes apparent by 6 months of age as the infant exhibits growth retardation, with chubbiness in the lower trunk and a short stature. As it progresses, secondary tooth eruption is delayed, and later there is a delay in puberty. Growth continues at about half the normal rate until the child reaches about 4 feet in height. Body proportions are normal, as is mental development. Frequently in adulthood, sex organs may not develop normally unless treated with hormones. Clients experience an accelerated pattern of aging, resulting in the life span being shortened by as much as 20 years. If the deficiency occurs in adults, manifestations are not as apparent. There are subtle signs such as wrinkles near the mouth and eyes.

Deficiencies of follicle-stimulating hormone and LH cause differences in clinical manifestations between female and male clients. In the female, symptoms include amenorrhea, dyspareunia, infertility, decreased libido, breast atrophy, sparse or absent axillary and pubic hair, and dry skin. In the male, symptoms include weakness, impotence, decreased libido, decreased muscle strength, testicular softening and shrinkage, and retarded secondary sexual hair growth.

In a child, a deficiency of TSH will result in severe growth retardation even with treatment. Other deficiency manifestations include cold intolerance; constipation; increased or decreased menstrual flow; lethargy; dry, pale puffy skin, and bradycardia. Thought processes may also be slowed.

A deficiency of adrenocorticotrophic hormone (ACTH) results in fatigue, nausea, vomiting, anorexia, weight loss, and depigmentation of the skin and nipples. Vital signs taken during periods of stress would show fever and hypotension.

Prolactin deficiency results in absent postpartum lactation, amenorrhea, and sparse or absent axillary and pubic hair. There may also be manifestations of thyroid or adrenal cortex failure.

Findings of hypopituitarism depend on the specific hormone, client's age, and severity of condition when detected. X-rays of the wrist determine bone age, and a skull series will rule out a pituitary tumor. Total failure of the pituitary without treatment is fatal; however, prognosis is good with treatment by the appropriate hormone(s). Treatment is primarily replacement therapy for the deficient hormone(s).

SIMMONDS' DISEASE

Simmonds' disease is defined as a total absence of all pituitary secretions. This is also called *panhypopituitarism*. This disease results from surgery, infection, injury, or tumor. It may also occur after a difficult labor in childbirth because of thrombosis formation during or after delivery.

Clinical manifestations, which vary in intensity, include extreme weight loss, general debility, lethargy, pallor, dry yellowish skin, loss of libido, amenorrhea, and intolerance to cold. The disease leads to loss of axillary and pubic hair and atrophy of genitalia and breasts. It progresses to bradycardia (slow pulse), hypotension, premature wrinkling of the skin, and atrophy of the thyroid and adrenal glands.

Treatment consists of administration of ACTH, TSH, or thyroid, adrenal, and sex hormones for a lifetime.

DIABETES INSIPIDUS

Diabetes insipidus (DI) is a deficiency of ADH, causing a metabolic disorder characterized by severe polyuria and polydipsia. Diabetes insipidus generally starts in childhood or early adulthood, with a median onset of 21 years. It affects males more often than females. Although a deficiency of ADH is the most common cause (central), diabetes insipidus can also be caused by failure of the kidneys to respond to ADH (nephrogenic), a defect in or damage to the thirst mechanism (dipsogenic), or during pregnancy (gestational) (NIDDK, 2008b).

Neurogenic diabetes insipidus may be caused by injury or ischemia to the hypothalamus or pituitary gland, CNS infections, head injuries, neurosurgery, or sickle-cell disease. Nephrogenic diabetes insipidus may be caused by pyelonephritis, chronic renal failure, polycystic disease, or medications such as lithium carbonate (Carbolith), amphotericin B (Fungizone), furosemide (Lasix), or ethycrynic acid (Edecrin). Dipsogenic diabetes insipidus results in an extreme increase in thirst and then fluid intake, which suppresses ADH secretion, increasing urine output. Often dypsogenic DI is caused by damage to the hypothalamus. Gestational diabetes insipidus is caused by a placenta enzyme that destroys ADH in the mother (NIDDK, 2008b).

Clinical manifestations have an abrupt onset. The client experiences extreme polyuria of 4–16 L of dilute urine daily. In some cases, there can be up to 30 L of urine per day. Serum osmolality is >295 mOsm/L and urine osmolality is <150 mOsm/L. Urine specific gravity is <1.005 and serum sodium is 145–150 mEq/L. The client has extreme thirst, preferring cold beverages. Even though there is an extraordinary volume of fluid intake, weight is lost. Other manifestations include dizziness, weakness, bed wetting, constipation, nocturia, and fatigue that may be a result of inadequate rest because of frequent nighttime voiding and excess thirst. Diagnostic tests used to diagnose DI include measurement of ADH, MRI (brain), a trail of DDAVP (synthetic ADH), and water deprivation test.

Complications of untreated diabetes insipidus are **hypovolemia** (abnormally low circulatory blood volume), circulatory collapse, unconsciousness, and central nervous system damage. Prolonged urine flow can cause chronic urinary system conditions such as bladder distension, enlarged calyces, and hydronephrosis.

Prognosis is generally good with fluid replacement in uncomplicated cases. Prognosis also depends on the underlying cause of diabetes insipidus.

MEDICAL–SURGICAL MANAGEMENT

Pharmacological

In addition to intravenous fluids, several medications can be used to treat diabetes insipidus. For neurogenic and gestational diabetes insipidus, desmopressin acetate (DDAVP), a synthetic antidiuretic hormone that can be given parenterally or nasally, is the drug of choice. Also, vasopressin (Pitressin Synthetic) may be given parenterally or nasally. Make certain that the nasal passage is clear before administering the medication. Monitor intake and output and assess for hypovolemia and electrolyte imbalance. The client should drink fluids or water only when thirsty (NIDDK, 2008b).

For nephrogenic diabetes insipidus, a diuretic such as hydrochlorothiazide (HydroDiuril) may be given alone or with amiloride (NIDDK, 2008b).

NURSING MANAGEMENT

Carefully and accurately monitor and record the client's I&O. Assess skin turgor and condition of oral mucous membranes. Weigh client daily. Oral fluids are often restricted and provided only in amounts equal to the client's urine output. Assess skin on each shift. Apply moisturizing lotion to skin. Provide eggcrate mattress or sheepskin.

NURSING PROCESS

ASSESSMENT

Subjective Data

Obtain a thorough client history, including severity of thirst, weakness, fatigue, lethargy, bed wetting, dizziness, constipation, and nocturia.

Objective Data

Assess for weight loss, constipation, and signs of fluid volume deficit, such as dry skin and mucous membranes, fever, dyspnea, and poor skin turgor. Check urine for color, amount, and specific gravity. Assess weight daily. Figure 43-12 illustrates the comparison of assessment findings between SIADH and DI.

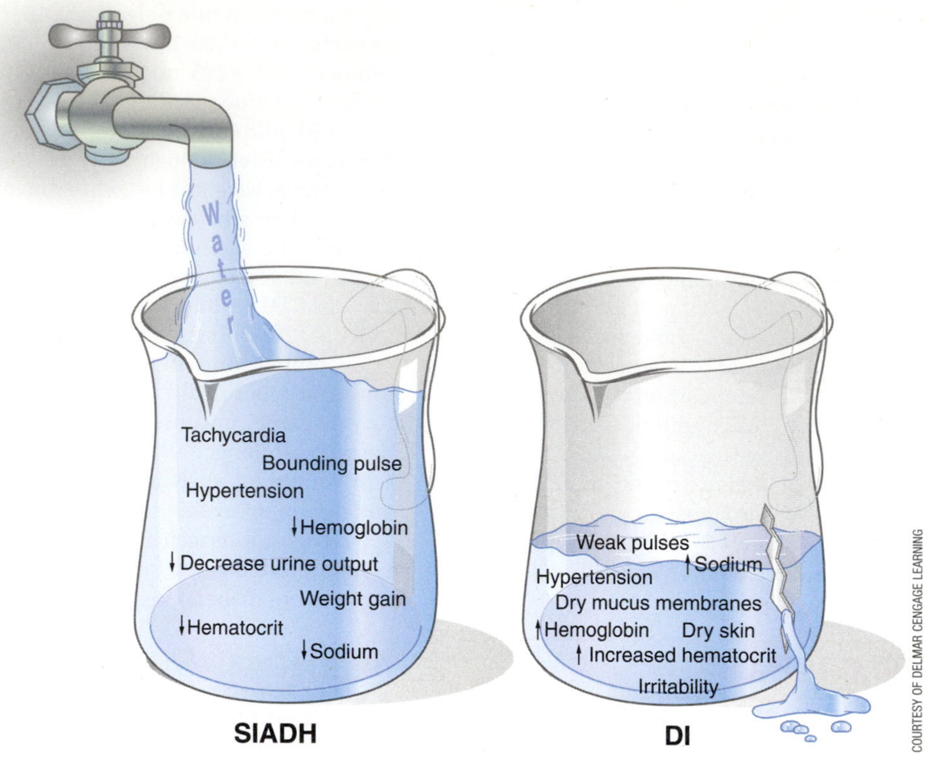

FIGURE 43-12 Comparison of Assessment Findings between SIADH and DI

Nursing diagnoses for a client with diabetes insipidus include the following:

NURSING DIAGNOSES	PLANNING/OUTCOMES	NURSING INTERVENTIONS
*Risk for Imbalanced **F**luid Volume* related to polyuria	The client will have sufficient fluid intake to prevent dehydration.	Provide easy access to bedpan/bathroom. Answer call signal promptly. Monitor the client for dizziness and weakness. Record client intake and output. Teach client and family how to record intake and output. Provide fluids as ordered to cover output. Monitor weight daily. Use same scale, same amount of clothing, at the same time daily. Provide oral care. Use a soft toothbrush, mild mouthwash, and lubricant for the lips. Assess condition of oral mucous membranes. Administer medications via intranasal or subcutaneous routes.
*Risk for Impaired **S**kin Integrity* related to altered hydration	The client will maintain skin integrity.	Assess skin, especially pressure points, 3 times a day. Apply moisturizing lotion to skin. Prevent pressure on skin by turning or ambulating client. Use egg-crate mattress or sheepskin. Encourage adequate intake of fluids, protein, vitamin C, and calories. Monitor for incontinence and nocturia. Thoroughly clean and dry area following episodes of incontinence.

Evaluation: Evaluate each outcome to determine how it has been met by the client.

THYROID DISORDERS

Worldwide, a deficiency of iodine is the most likely cause of thyroid disorders; however, in countries where iodine in food is plentiful, autoimmune thyroid disease is the most common thyroid disorder (Walpert, 1998). The thyroid gland is a butterfly shaped gland located anteriorly to the trachea. The purpose of the thyroid gland is to produce, store, and release hormones into the bloodstream. The hormones, T_3 and T_4, are responsible for the regulation of body metabolism (brain development, breathing, heart rate, temperature, and the nervous system) (NIDDK, 2008c). The production of T_3 and T_4 is regulated by the release of TSH from the anterior pituitary gland. Thyroid disorders are classified as hyperthyroidism, hypothyroidism, tumors, cancer, or goiter.

HYPERTHYROIDISM

Hyperthyroidism is a collective term for a condition marked by increased thyroid activity and overproduction of thyroid hormones thyroxine (T_4) and triiodothyronine (T_3). The thyroid gland may be enlarged. Different forms of hyperthyroidism are Graves' disease, Basedow's disease, Parry's disease, or thyrotoxicosis. Graves' disease is the most common cause of hyperthyroidism and occurs more frequently in women over age 20 (NIH, 2009).

In this autoimmune disorder, the immune system triggers the formation of thyroid-stimulating immunoglobulins (TSIs). The TSIs bind with TSH receptors, causing an overproduction of thyroid hormone.

Clinical manifestations include two obvious physical changes. The thyroid, palpated for asymmetry and size, may be enlarged 3 to 4 times its normal size. The enlargement of the thyroid gland is called **goiter**. This is generally a result of overactivity of the thyroid gland. The accumulation of orbital fluid behind the eyeball, forcing it to protrude, is called **exophthalmos**. This occurs in about half the cases of hyperthyroidism. It produces a characteristic stare.

The increased thyroid hormone production causes an increased metabolic rate. This leads to weight loss despite increased appetite, fatigue, poor tolerance to heat, and profuse perspiration. The client is very nervous, restless, irritable, has difficulty concentrating, is emotionally labile, has mood swings, possible personality changes, and sleep disturbances. The client may have fine tremors of the fingers and tongue, shaky handwriting, clumsiness, trouble climbing stairs, or dyspnea on exertion and possibly at rest. The skin is warm and moist with a velvety texture. The skin may be a characteristic salmon color. The hair is fine and soft with premature graying and increased hair loss. The nails appear fragile with distal nail separation from the nail bed (onycholysis). There may be general or local muscle atrophy and acropachy (soft tissue swelling with underlying bone changes where new bone forms). There is a tachycardia with bounding pulse up to 160 beats per minute and down to 80 beats per minute during sleep. Pulse pressure is widened. There can be muscular weakness and atrophy; osteoporosis; paralysis; vitiligo, milky-white patches on the skin surrounded by areas of normal pigmentation; decreased libido; impaired fertility; and **gynecomastia** (abnormal enlargement of one or both breasts in males).

> ### LIFE SPAN CONSIDERATIONS
>
> **Hyperthyroid Complications**
>
> The older client in particular develops cardiovascular problems such as arrhythmias (atrial fibrillation), cardiac insufficiency leading to cardiac decompensation, and resistance to the usual dose of digoxin.

Diagnostic tests generally include TSH, T_3, T_4, radioactive iodine uptake, and a thyroid scan.

One major complication is thyrotoxic crisis, also called *thyroid storm*. This is a medical emergency that can lead to cardiac, hepatic, or renal failure. Undiagnosed or inadequately treated hyperthyroid clients often experience thyroid storm. Thyroid storm can be precipitated by stressful situations such as surgery, infection, or trauma. Less common causes are cerebrovascular accident (CVA), myocardial infarction, sudden discontinuing of antithyroid medications, subtotal thyroidectomy with excess intake of synthetic thyroid hormone, toxemia, or diabetic ketoacidosis. Any of these events can lead to overproduction of thyroid hormone, causing an increase in systemic adrenergic activity. This causes an overproduction of epinephrine and severe hypermetabolism, leading to rapid cardiac, gastrointestinal, and sympathetic nervous system decompensation. The client will rapidly exhibit severe clinical manifestations of hyperthyroidism, including extreme high fever, restlessness, agitation, coma, heart failure, and angina.

If the nurse suspects that the client is experiencing thyrotoxic crisis, inform the physician immediately. The client will be transferred to intensive care for closer monitoring of vital signs, EKG pattern, and cardiopulmonary status. Priority treatment includes respiratory support and hemodynamic stability. Antithyroid therapy is initiated immediately. Adrenergic blocking agents are administered to decrease the sympathetic nervous system stimulation. The client's temperature is monitored and cooling measures initiated as needed. Acetaminophen is administered to lower the temperature, but aspirin is not given because it can increase the free T_4 level. Supportive care is given until the client is out of the thyrotoxic crisis.

MEDICAL–SURGICAL MANAGEMENT

Medical

The goal of managing hyperthyroidism is to decrease excessive thyroid hormone production. With treatment to decrease the thyroid production of the thyroid's hormone, the prognosis is good. The client can live a normal life. There can be a combination of treatment methods. The first method is to administer antithyroid medications. This is usually a temporary solution.

Radiation therapy of the thyroid gland could be external radiation to the neck; however, the more accepted method is the oral administration of radioactive iodine, either liquid or capsule, that targets the thyroid tissue. Radioactive iodine acts on the thyroid tissue to destroy thyroid cells, potentially leading to hypothyroidism (NIDDK, 2008c). It is most commonly used for women past the reproductive years or clients not planning to have children. The client of reproductive age must sign an informed consent form because small amounts of the radioactive iodine could lodge in the gonads.

Antithyroid medications are stopped 4 to 7 days before treatment. The physician must know if the client is receiving amiodarone hydrochloride (Cordarone), an antiarrhythmic, because it contains large amounts of iodine. The oral ^{131}I should not be given to the client with severe vomiting or diarrhea.

A single dose of oral ^{131}I will destroy some iodine concentrating cells that produce the thyroxine. Clinical manifestations decrease in about 3 weeks, with the full effect in about 3 months. Some clients require a second or third dose.

The client usually resumes the thyroid hormone antagonist 3 to 5 days after ^{131}I therapy until the physician determines the thyroid to be atrophic (decreased in size). The client may continue to take propranolol hydrochloride (Inderal) for tachycardia, tremor, and diaphoresis. Continued monitoring of thyroid hormone blood levels and physical condition is necessary.

The most common complication is hypothyroidism, which occurs about 2 to 4 months after treatment. The client is then placed on thyroid replacement therapy, generally for life.

Surgical

Generally just a portion of the thyroid gland is removed, but a total thyroidectomy may be performed. This is the most expensive option and has the most risks. A thyroidectomy may also be done for respiratory obstruction by a goiter or thyroid cancer. If a partial thyroidectomy is done, the remaining thyroid tissue should provide adequate amounts of thyroid hormones. If a complete thyroidectomy is done, the client will require thyroid hormone replacement for life.

Clients usually take propylthiouracil (PTU) for 4 to 6 weeks before surgery and iodine preparations may be prescribed 10 to 14 days before surgery to decrease thyroid vascularity and decrease bleeding. Depending on the symptoms, the client may also be taking propranolol hydrochloride (Inderal). Thyroid function tests and an EKG are performed before surgery to provide baseline information. Informed consent must be obtained.

Preoperatively, the client should be told about activities after surgery. There will be a neck incision, generally with some type of drain. The client may experience a sore throat and hoarseness. The client is kept in high-Fowler's position to promote venous drainage. The client should support the head with a hand when moving the head to prevent strain on the incision. Respiratory problems may occur, such as tracheal collapse, tracheal mucous accumulation, or laryngeal or local tissue edema. Laryngeal spasms may occur following injury to the parathyroid glands resulting in hypocalcemia and tetany. *A tracheotomy tray or endotracheal tubes and insertion tray are kept readily available at the client's bedside in case of a respiratory emergency.*

Because the thyroid is so vascular, the dressing must be checked frequently for drainage, especially at the back of the neck. If there is a drain, approximately 50 mL of drainage is expected the first day. If there is no drainage, the drain must be checked for kinks or obstruction. Voice rest is encouraged for 48 hours, with voice checks every 2 to 4 hours as ordered to make certain there is no laryngeal nerve damage.

Because the parathyroid glands could be accidentally removed during the thyroidectomy, the client's blood calcium level is monitored. The client is checked for Chvostek's sign or Trousseau's sign. (These are discussed under hypoparathyroidism.) Analgesics are administered as needed.

Complications of thyroidectomy are respiratory distress and hemorrhage. There can be damage to the laryngeal nerves, affecting the voice. Manipulation of the thyroid gland during surgery can cause a release of large amounts of thyroid hormone causing thyroid storm, which is rare but may occur. Thyroid crisis usually occurs within the first 12 hours postoperative. Hyperthyroid signs and symptoms are exaggerated, plus the client may vomit, have severe hypertension and tachycardia, and sometimes have hyperthermia up to 106°F (41°C). The client may develop congestive heart failure and die. The client must be advised that tetany can occur up to 10 days after surgery. **Tetany** is sharp flexion of the wrist and ankle joints, muscle twitchings, or cramps caused by decreased blood calcium level.

Pharmacological

Antithyroid therapy is used for children, younger adults, pregnant females, the client who refuses surgery, or clients after surgery. The goal of pharmaceutical management includes the client reaching a euthroid state (Daniels, 2007). Several drugs can be used for antithyroid therapy. PTU is used frequently, especially in cases of thyroid storm. It reduces the production of the thyroid hormones. It should be given with food. The client must be instructed to avoid foods high in iodine such as shellfish and iodized salt. Over-the-counter preparations must be checked to see if they contain iodine. This drug requires several weeks to exert the full effect, and it may be administered up to 2 years. This drug may cause **agranulocytosis** (a decreased number of granulocytes), so it is important to report signs and symptoms of infection immediately to the physician.

Methimazole (Tapazole) is another antithyroid preparation that interferes with thyroid hormone synthesis. It has a more rapid onset than PTU; however, it does not have as much consistency in effect. It should be administered at evenly spaced intervals with food to prevent gastric upset. This drug can also cause agranulocytosis, particularly in the client older than age 40.

Iodide preparations may be given to the client with hyperthyroidism. Because iodides inhibit the release of thyroid hormones rather than the synthesis, they take effect in 2 days. Two common preparations are saturated solution potassium iodide (SSKI) and a solution of iodine and potassium iodide that is called Lugol's solution. When iodide preparations are administered orally, they should be mixed with milk, juice, or water and given after meals to decrease gastric upset. Drinking the preparations through a straw will decrease discoloration of the

SAFETY

Radioactive Iodine

No pregnant nurse should care for the client. The client should expectorate carefully for the first day because the saliva is radioactive. The client should drink plenty of fluids for 2 days to help circulate and eliminate the radioactive iodine. The toilet should be flushed twice after each use for at least 2 days or throughout the hospitalization. Disposable eating utensils should be used by the client. Close contact with children or pregnant females should be avoided for a week after the administration. Females should avoid pregnancy for 6 months after treatment.

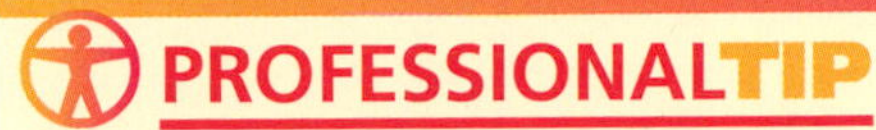

Hypersensitivity to Iodides

The first signs of hypersensitivity reactions caused by iodides are irritation and swollen eyelids.

teeth. These drugs are contraindicated in the client with acute bronchitis or a known hypersensitivity to iodine and shellfish.

Clients may be prescribed propranolol hydrochloride (Inderal) to counteract tachycardia and peripheral effects of hyperthyroidism. Clients should not smoke while taking this medication. Abrupt withdrawal of the drug can cause hypertension, myocardial ischemia, or cardiac arrhythmias. Clients should rise slowly from a sitting or lying position in order to prevent orthostatic hypotension.

Topical medications such as isotonic eyedrops may be ordered to protect the eyes of the client with exophthalmos. Care must be taken that the eyes are not injured or infected, including the use of tinted eye glasses, artificial tears, ointments and protective shields. Some physicians may order high doses of corticosteroids to help reduce exophthalmos.

During a thyrotoxic crisis, antithyroid drugs are given. Other medications that may be used are propranolol, corticosteroids, and iodine preparations. Individual client needs could indicate a need for vitamins, nutrients, fluids, or sedation.

Diet

Because the client has a greatly increased metabolic rate as well as weight loss, diet is important. The client may require between 4,000 to 6,000 calories per day. There is a need for increased protein, vitamins (especially vitamins B and C), and minerals. In addition to 3 meals per day, the client needs additional meals or snacks. Fluids should be encouraged, but caffeine should be avoided. Clients also may experience extreme fatigue due to the increased metabolism.

Nursing Management

Provide a high-calorie diet and snacks throughout the day. Encourage fluids, but avoid caffeine. Keep client's skin dry and clean and change gown and linens as needed. Preoperatively, teach the client how to support his head while turning or rising to a sitting or standing position. Inform client that "voice rest" may be enforced for 48 hours and provide paper and pencil for writing notes.

Postoperatively, keep bed in semi-Fowler's position with head and shoulders supported by pillows. Keep suction equipment and tracheotomy tray in the client's room. Monitor vital signs. Inspect dressing, sides and back of neck, and shoulders frequently for bleeding. Watch for signs of internal bleeding (apprehension, restlessness, increased pulse, decreased blood pressure, and fullness feeling in the neck). Watch for signs of tetany and for signs of edema in the operative area.

NURSING PROCESS

Assessment

Subjective Data

Obtain a thorough client history and ask about the ability to concentrate, nervousness, insomnia, jitteriness, excitability, emotional lability, dysphagia, weight loss, personality changes, or sleep disturbances.

Objective Data

Assess for rapid pulse, elevated blood pressure, warm skin, elevated temperature, diaphoresis, or hand tremors. Female clients may cease to menstruate. Hair is fine and soft.

Nursing diagnoses for a client with hyperthyroidism include the following:

NURSING DIAGNOSES	PLANNING/OUTCOMES	NURSING INTERVENTIONS
Preoperative		
*Imbalanced **N**utrition: Less than Body Requirements* related to increased metabolism	The client will eat a nutritionally balanced diet with enough calories to prevent weight loss.	Monitor weight daily. Use same scale, same amount of clothing, at the same time daily. Encourage 6 meals per day with adequate protein, carbohydrate, and caloric intake. Arrange a consultation with the dietitian to assist in determining the client's increased nutritional needs. Encourage client to eat a well-balanced diet. Provide snacks throughout the day. Complete pre-albumin test to determine protein reserve.
*Risk for **I**njury* related to exophthalmos	The client's eyes will not be injured from exophthalmos.	Administer isotonic solutions or eye lubricants to keep the eye moist. At night, elevate head of the bed which may assist in keeping the eyelids closed, or cover the eyes with eye guards to prevent drying.

(Continues)

Nursing diagnoses for a client with hyperthyroidism include the following: (Continued)

NURSING DIAGNOSES	PLANNING/OUTCOMES	NURSING INTERVENTIONS
		Suggest to client that dark or tinted wraparound glasses may protect the eyes from wind and airborne particles.
Postoperative *Impaired **S**wallowing* related to mechanical obstruction (edema)	The client will have diminished problems with swallowing.	Ensure gag, cough, and swallowing reflexes are present before offering oral fluids. Maintain client in Fowler's position when drinking or eating. Encourage client to drink slowly and chew thoroughly.
*Ineffective **A**irway Clearance* related to edema and pain	The client will be able to clear airway.	Keep intubation and tracheostomy kits readily available. Keep suctioning equipment ready. Administer analgesic as ordered. Complete respiratory assessment frequently and monitor for respiratory distress and laryngeal spasms.

Evaluation: Evaluate each outcome to determine how it has been met by the client.

SAMPLE NURSING CARE PLAN

The Client with Hyperthyroidism

A.J., 33 years old, has returned to her physician's office to find out results of her tests for hyperthyroidism. She continues to have multiple complaints. "I have lost 15 pounds in the last month despite eating all the time. I am restless and can't sleep. I feel jittery and irritable. My family says my moods change so rapidly they don't know what to expect from me. I feel so hot most of the time and sweat a lot."

During assessment, the client appears flushed and her eyes protrude slightly. Her vital signs are temperature 100.6°F orally, pulse 120 beats/min, respiration 26 breaths/min, and blood pressure 140/88 mm Hg, which are slightly elevated from her previous office visit. Test results confirm the presence of hyperthyroidism.

NURSING DIAGNOSIS 1 *Imbalanced **N**utrition: Less than Body Requirements* related to increased metabolism as evidenced by weight loss despite eating

Nursing Outcomes Classification (NOC)
Nutritional Status: Food & Fluid Intake
Nutritional Status: Nutrient Intake

Nursing Interventions Classification (NIC)
Fluid Management
Nutrition Management

PLANNING/OUTCOMES	NURSING INTERVENTIONS	RATIONALE
A.J. will eat a nutritionally balanced diet with enough calories to prevent weight loss.	Monitor amount of food ingested and caloric intake.	Provides data to determine if diet is adequate to prevent weight loss.
	Monitor weight daily.	Determines weight gains or losses.
	Provide a diet high in calories, protein, and carbohydrates.	Maintains or increases weight while preventing muscle mass breakdown.
	Advise A.J. to avoid highly seasoned or fibrous foods or foods causing flatulence.	Prevents increased peristalsis resulting in diarrhea.

SAMPLE NURSING CARE PLAN (Continued)

PLANNING/OUTCOMES	NURSING INTERVENTIONS	RATIONALE
	Provide small frequent meals spread over waking hours, up to 6 meals per day.	Provides calories without extremely large meals.
	Obtain nutritional consult as needed.	Ensures nutritional status.

EVALUATION

A.J. gained or maintained weight.

NURSING DIAGNOSIS 2 *Hyperthermia* related to increased metabolic rate as evidenced by complaints of feeling hot, flushing, and elevated temperature

Nursing Outcomes Classification (NOC)
Hydration
Thermoregulation

Nursing Interventions Classification (NIC)
Fluid Management

PLANNING/OUTCOMES	NURSING INTERVENTIONS	RATIONALE
A.J.'s body temperature will be within normal range.	Assess for elevated temperature, heat intolerance, and diaphoresis.	Indicates increased heat production from increased metabolic rate.
	Provide a well-ventilated room with temperature control.	Promotes comfort if heat intolerant.
	Suggest wearing cool, loose-fitting, lightweight clothing.	Provides comfort and prevents overheating.
	Provide frequent bathing and changes in linens or clothing.	Promotes comfort if diaphoretic.
	Provide fluids up to 3 L per day.	Replaces fluid if diaphoretic.

EVALUATION

A.J. maintained her temperature in a normal range.

NURSING DIAGNOSIS 3 *Risk for Impaired Skin Integrity* related to diaphoresis as evidenced by excessive sweating

Nursing Outcomes Classification (NOC)
Nutritional Status
Tissue Integrity: Skin & Mucous Membranes

Nursing Interventions Classification (NIC)
Fluid/Electrolyte Management
Nutrition Management

PLANNING/OUTCOMES	NURSING INTERVENTIONS	RATIONALE
A.J.'s skin will remain intact and free of injury.	Complete Braden Scale.	Indentifies risk level of skin breakdown.
	Assess skin for flushing and moisture.	Indicates heat intolerance.
	Assess skin for redness, especially bony prominences.	Indicates potential for breakdown.
	Keep skin clean and dry.	Prevents skin breakdown.

EVALUATION

A.J. maintained intact skin without impairment.

HYPOTHYROIDISM

Hypothyroidism is a condition in which the metabolic processes are decreased because of a deficiency of thyroid hormones. It is termed primary if the problem arises from a dysfunction solely of the thyroid. It is secondary if the thyroid gland is not stimulated to produce normally or if the target cells fail to respond to normal thyroid functioning. This condition is more common in females than males. There is a significant increase in incidence between the ages of 30 to 60. Hypothyroid conditions include cretinism, myxedema, and Hashimoto's thyroiditis.

CRETINISM

A congenital condition with decreased thyroid hormone production causes defective physical development and mental retardation. This is called **cretinism** and occurs in about 1 of 3,000 live births (NIH, 2007). Female clients are two times more likely to be affected than male clients. The child generally has a large head, short limbs, puffy eyes, thick and protruding tongue, excessively dry skin, and a lack of coordination. If untreated, the child will be permanently dwarfed, mentally retarded, and sterile. This condition is rare in the United States and is diagnosed by the T_4, serum TSH, x-ray of long bones, and thyroid scan.

MYXEDEMA

Myxedema is the term for severe hypothyroidism in adults. A variety of abnormalities lead to decreased thyroid hormone production. The obvious ones are thyroid gland surgery such as thyroidectomy or irradiation of the thyroid gland. Some other causes are chronic autoimmune Hashimoto's thyroiditis, inflammatory conditions (sarcoidosis), pituitary failure to produce TSH, or hypothalamus failure to produce thyrotropin-releasing hormone. There may be an inability to synthesize thyroid hormones related to iodine deficiency (rarely from general diet deficiency) or as a result of taking antithyroid medications.

Clinical manifestations are vague and varied, developing slowly over a period of time, but are primarily related to the reduced metabolic rate. These include an energy loss, fatigue, forgetfulness, sensitivity to cold, unexplained weight gain, hypoventilation, and constipation. As the condition progresses, manifestations include reduced libido, menorrhagia, paresthesias, joint stiffness, and muscle cramping. There is a characteristic alteration in overall appearance and behavior, including decreased mental stability and a thick and dry tongue, causing hoarseness and slow, slurred speech. The skin is flaky and inelastic, and feels cool, dry, rough, and doughy. There is edema of the face, hands, and feet. The hair is dry and sparse, with patchy hair loss including loss of the outer third of the eyebrow. The nails are thick and brittle with visible transverse and longitudinal grooves. The pulse is weak and bradycardic because of the decreased pumping strength of the heart. The thyroid gland may be so small that it may not be palpated unless there is a goiter. The blood pressure is generally lower than normal for the client.

Diagnostic tests generally include TSH, T_3, T_4, radioactive iodine uptake, and a thyroid scan.

Complications affect almost every system. Cardiovascular complications include ischemic heart disease, poor peripheral circulation, enlarged heart, or pleural or pericardial effusion. Gastrointestinal complications include adynamic colon (decreased functioning of the colon), megacolon (massive and abnormal dilation of the colon), or intestinal obstruction. Other complications include conductive or sensorineural deafness, psychiatric disorders, carpal tunnel syndrome, or impotence or infertility. Prognosis depends on the organs involved, duration, and severity of condition.

Myxedema coma or hypothyroid crisis is a rare but serious complication of extreme hypothyroidism. It is life threatening, with symptoms of unresponsiveness, hypothermia, decreased respirations, low blood pressure, and low blood sugar. It has a gradual onset but is triggered by severe stress such as infection, exposure to cold, or trauma. Abrupt withdrawal of thyroid medication or the use of narcotics, sedatives, or anesthetics can also cause myxedema coma. If myxedema coma occurs, it must be reported to the physician immediately. The client is moved to the ICU, where intubation and mechanical ventilation are instituted. The client is monitored closely for vital signs, EKG changes, and cardiopulmonary status. Wrapping the client in blankets will warm the client, but a warming blanket should not be used because it could cause peripheral vasodilation and shock. Thyroid medications and possibly corticosteroids are administered. Supportive care is given until the client comes out of the myxedema coma. Myxedema coma is often fatal.

MEDICAL–SURGICAL MANAGEMENT

Pharmacological

Thyroid replacement therapy is lifelong. Thyroid (Armour Thyroid) is a natural form, whereas levothyroxine sodium (Levothroid, Synthroid) is a synthetic. The physician orders thyroid hormone to begin slowly and increases the dosage every 2 to 3 weeks until the desired response is achieved. Medication should be administered 1 hour prior to or 2 hours after meals to improve absorption. The medication should be given in the morning to prevent insomnia.

If the client has diabetes mellitus, insulin or oral hypoglycemic dosage might have to be adjusted. The blood sugar level must be monitored closely. If the client is on anticoagulant therapy, thyroid potentiates the anticoagulant action. The client should be taught to watch for excessive bleeding or bruising. Digitalis preparations are also potentiated by thyroid.

Because hypothyroidism impairs the metabolic rate, the client may have difficulty metabolizing medications. The client may have an increased sensitivity to hypnotics, sedatives, or opiates. Dosage may have to be adjusted appropriately. Synthesis of the thyroid hormone can be impaired by drugs such as lithium carbonate (Lithotabs) or aminoglutethimide (Cytadren).

Diet

The client is instructed to avoid foods high in iodine and foods that interfere with thyroid hormone replacement, such as dried kelp, shellfish, iodized salt, saltwater fish, cabbage, turnips, pears, and peaches. The diet is designed for weight loss and to combat constipation. A high-fiber, high-protein, low-calorie diet is given. Sodium is decreased to prevent fluid retention. A dietary consultation for meal planning and a list of foods to avoid is provided to the client.

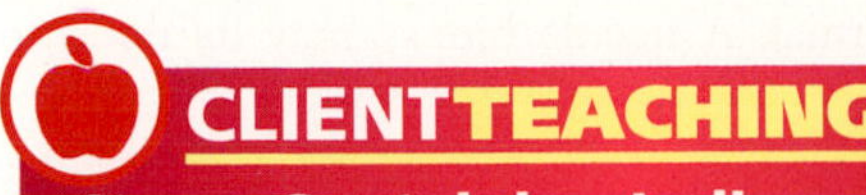

Items Containing Iodine

Check the labels on multivitamins, dentrifices, and nonprescription medications; they may contain iodine.

Nursing Management

Monitor vital signs, heart sounds, lung sounds, I&O, weight, and check for edema. Prevent client fatigue by providing rest periods between activities. Provide a high-fiber diet and encourage intake of oral fluids. Administer stool softener, bulk laxative, or enema as ordered.

NURSING PROCESS

Assessment

Subjective Data

Obtain a thorough client history, asking about lethargy, depression, irritability, impaired memory, and slowing of thought processes. The client may describe speech and hearing problems, anorexia, decreased libido, constipation, cold intolerance, and changes in menstruation.

Objective Data

Assess for hearing and speech deficits, thin hair, dry and thickened skin, enlarged facial features, masklike expression, low and hoarse voice, bradycardia, decreased blood pressure and respirations, and exercise intolerance.

Nursing diagnoses for a client with myxedema include the following:

NURSING DIAGNOSES	PLANNING/OUTCOMES	NURSING INTERVENTIONS
Activity Intolerance related to decreased metabolic and energy level	The client will express understanding to increase activity level gradually. The client will maintain blood pressure, pulse, and respirations within normal limits when active. The client will regain normal activity levels.	Assist client to gradually increase activity level but encourage rest between activities to avoid fatigue and decrease cardiac oxygen demands. Measure client's legs correctly so antiembolic hose, which help venous return, will fit properly when worn. Reposition client every 2 hours and encourage client to continue activity when normal activity level is achieved. Assess blood pressure, pulse, and respirations frequently and inform physician of abnormal results.
Ineffective Tissue Perfusion (Cardiopulmonary) related to decreased cardiac output	The client will not have chest pain at rest. The client will have a normal heart rate and rhythm. The client will avoid ischemic EKG changes. The client will maintain adequate cardiopulmonary perfusion.	Assess for chest pain and advise client to report any episodes of angina immediately. Monitor client's vital signs. Monitor cardiac status through EKG and assessment of heart and lung sounds plus checking for edema. Restrict fluid and sodium during the time of cardiac decompensation as ordered. Monitor intake and output and weight.
Constipation related to decreased motility of the gastrointestinal tract	The client will have regular bowel movements.	Provide high-fiber diet. Encourage intake of oral fluids. Assess frequency and character of stool. Administer stool softener, bulk laxative, or enema as ordered.

Evaluation: Evaluate each outcome to determine how it has been met by the client.

HASHIMOTO'S THYROIDITIS

Hashimoto's thyroiditis, the most common cause of hypothyroidism, is an autoimmune disease characterized by the production of antiperoxidase antibodies, which destroy an essential enzyme necessary for production of T_3 and T_4. The disease occurs more often in females than in males, between the ages of 30 and 50, and shows a marked hereditary pattern. There is an increased incidence in clients with Down syndrome and Turner's syndrome.

Clinical manifestations include a thyroid that is enlarged and has a lumpy surface. Generally, the goiter is asymptomatic, but it could cause dysphagia and a feeling of local pressure. The thymus gland is also enlarged. Other clinical manifestations are similar to hypothyroidism.

Treatment of Hashimoto's thyroiditis is similar to that of hypothyroidism. Thyroid hormone replacement is used. This chronic disorder can be treated but not cured. The client will be on lifetime thyroid hormone replacement.

THYROID TUMORS

There are several neoplasms of the thyroid gland. The benign thyroid cyst and adenoma are firm, encapsulated, noninvasive, slowly growing neoplasms of unknown etiology. Diagnosis of benign neoplasms is done by needle biopsy. These growths tend to be nonfunctioning (not affecting the functioning of the thyroid gland), so there is no treatment other than continued monitoring. If the adenoma is functioning (increasing the functioning of the thyroid gland), then it is treated by radioactive iodine or surgery.

CANCER OF THE THYROID

Cancer of the thyroid is rare and occurs in all age groups. Individuals who have had radiation therapy to the neck are more susceptible. There are four major types of thyroid cancer:

- Papillary carcinoma is the most common type. It can affect any age but is more common in females of childbearing age. It is well-differentiated, grows slowly, is usually contained, and does not spread beyond the adjacent lymph nodes. Cure rate after thyroidectomy is excellent.
- Follicular carcinoma metastasizes to the regional lymph nodes and spreads through the blood vessels to the bone, liver, and lungs. It has a very low cure rate.
- Medullary carcinoma is a solid carcinoma associated with pheochromocytoma. These tumors often secrete calcitonin, adrenocorticotropic hormone, serotonin, and prostaglandins. It is curable if detected before signs and symptoms occur. Without treatment, it grows rapidly, metastasizing to the bones, liver, and kidneys.
- Anaplastic or undifferentiated carcinoma resists radiation. It is almost never curable by resection. It metastasizes rapidly, generally causing death by invasion of the trachea and adjacent structures. It generally affects individuals older than age 60.

There are several risk factors, such as radiation exposure, especially in those children and adolescents who received radiation therapy to treat severe cases of acne vulgaris, or to shrink enlarged tonsils, adenoids, and thymus tissue; prolonged secretion of TSH resulting from radiation or heredity; familial disposition; or chronic goiter.

The first clinical manifestation is a painless lump. As it enlarges, it destroys the thyroid, which leads to clinical manifestations of hypothyroidism. Although rare, the tumor could trigger excessive thyroid hormone production, causing the client to display the clinical manifestations of hyperthyroidism. There can be dysphagia, hoarseness, and vocal stridor. There may be a detectable, disfiguring thyroid mass with a firm nodule on palpation.

The thyroid scan shows a "cold" nodule (decreased uptake of ^{131}I) for papillary carcinoma. Follicular carcinoma and benign adenomas show a "hot" nodule. Thyroid function tests are usually normal. A needle biopsy may be done to confirm diagnosis.

MEDICAL–SURGICAL MANAGEMENT

Surgical

All carcinomas can be treated with surgery (discussed previously). Radioactive iodine or external radiation therapy may also be used. Radioiodine ablation may be used to destroy any remaining thyroid tissue. Response of the tumor will depend on early diagnosis and treatment. These methods of treatment may be used individually or in combination. Client care is the same as for hyperthyroidism.

Pharmacological

Exogenous thyroid hormone may suppress thyroid activity. To increase tolerance to surgery or radiation therapy, the physician may prescribe simultaneous exogenous thyroid hormone and adrenergic blocker such as propranolol hydrochloride (Inderal). If there is widespread metastasis, the cancers will be treated with neoplastic chemotherapy.

NURSING MANAGEMENT

The nurse monitors the client's level of anxiety and encourages the client to discuss feelings about the diagnosis and possible surgery. The nurse also assists the client in identifying previously successful coping methods and teaches new coping methods if needed. After surgical intervention, the nurse must monitor the client for signs and symptoms of airway obstruction. Clients will also require education regarding long-term medical management of the disease.

GOITER

A goiter is an enlargement of the thyroid unrelated to inflammation or neoplasm. There are three types of goiter. One type is a diffuse toxic goiter found in hyperthyroidism. The body's immune system creates an antibody known as thyroid-stimulating immunoglobin that mimics TSH, creating an overproduction of thyroid hormone. This type of goiter may be moderate to massively enlarged. The consistency varies from soft to firm and rubbery. It generally feels smooth. It is often associated with exophthalmos.

Another type of goiter is a simple nontoxic goiter. It develops when the thyroid is unable to use iodine properly or in response to a low iodine level in the blood. These goiters are more common in females. They develop during times of great metabolic demands such as adolescence or pregnancy. A deficiency of iodine can cause goiter formation. Clinical manifestations depend on the size of the goiter. There is an obvious enlargement of the thyroid gland. A large goiter can compress the esophagus or trachea, causing dysphagia, a choking sensation, or respiratory difficulty. If the goiter impairs venous return from the head and neck, the client may experience dizziness and syncope.

Diagnosis is based on history, clinical manifestations, and results of thyroid function tests. T_3 is generally very low. Treatment concentrates on the underlying cause and may involve thyroid hormone replacement therapy, iodine supplements, or increasing dietary iodine sources. Surgery is done when respiration or swallowing is impaired or for cosmetic effect.

The third type of goiter is the nodular goiter. It is similar to the simple goiter except that palpation reveals multiple nodules causing the enlargement. It is found frequently in females older than 40. It usually is asymptomatic. Treatment varies with the client's age and clinical manifestations.

PARATHYROID DISORDERS

Disorders discussed include hyperparathyroidism and hypoparathyroidism.

HYPERPARATHYROIDISM

Hyperparathyroidism is a condition resulting from overactivity of one or more of the parathyroid glands. It results in increased secretion of parathyroid hormone (PTH), which causes calcium to leave the bones and accumulate in the blood. This cannot be compensated by renal excretion or uptake into the soft tissues. It occurs twice as often in postmenopausal females than males. It occurs frequently between the ages of 35 and 65. Hypercalcemia may also be caused by excessive intake of thiazide diuretics, vitamin D, or calcium supplements.

X-rays will show skeletal decalcification. Blood PTH and alkaline phosphate levels are increased. Serum calcium level is elevated. As the result of calcium loss from the bones, a bone density test may be completed to assess the risk for fractures.

Hyperparathyroidism is termed primary if there is an enlargement of one or more of the parathyroid glands, increasing secretion of PTH and thus increasing the blood calcium level. The most common cause is adenoma, but other primary causes include genetics, multiple endocrine neoplasms, or hyperplasia.

The condition is termed secondary if there is excess compensatory production of PTH stemming from a hypocalcemia-producing abnormality other than the parathyroid gland. Some of these abnormalities are rickets, chronic renal failure, vitamin D deficiency, or osteomalacia caused by laxative abuse or phenytoin (Dilantin).

Many clients are asymptomatic; however, there are several clinical manifestations. The client may have polyuria, chronic low-back pain, bone tenderness, or renal calculi. The client may also experience nausea, vomiting, anorexia, constipation, lethargy, or drowsiness. There can be changes in level of consciousness, disorientation, stupor, coma, or personality changes with a loss of initiative and memory. There may be marked muscle weakness and atrophy especially of the legs, joint hyperextensibility, long bone skeletal deformity, or hyporeflexia.

Without treatment, there can be permanent damage to the skeleton or kidneys. There can be bone and articular problems including pathologic fractures. Renal complications include colic, nephrolithiasis, urinary tract infection, and renal insufficiency leading to chronic renal failure. Other complications may be stone formation in various organs, cardiac or vascular problems, or central nervous system changes.

MEDICAL–SURGICAL MANAGEMENT

Medical

Medical management is aimed at decreasing overactivity of the parathyroid glands. This may be accomplished by medication or surgery. If there is severe renal involvement, the client may require dialysis.

Surgical

Primary hyperparathyroidism can be treated by surgical removal of three and one-half of the four parathyroid glands. Surgery can relieve bone pain in 3 days but may not reverse renal damage.

Preoperative care includes explanations, encouraging fluids, limiting calcium intake, and administering medications to lower the blood calcium level.

Postoperative care involves administration of magnesium or phosphate. The client may receive calcium supplements for several days. The nursing care is similar to that provided to the client with thyroidectomy (refer to hyperthyroidism). A major complication is airway obstruction.

Pharmacological

Pharmacological treatment is aimed toward correcting secondary hyperparathyroidism, which involves treating the underlying cause. Because hypercalcemia is a major manifestation, medications are geared to decrease the calcium level in the blood. This includes the use of diuretics such as furosemide (Lasix) and ethacrynic acid (Edecrin).

Other drugs that decrease the calcium level in the blood are calcitonin-human (Cibacalcin), plicamycin (Mithracin), and magnesium- or phosphate-based drugs. Phosphate-based drugs lower the calcium level based on the inverse relationship between phosphorus and calcium.

NURSING MANAGEMENT

Preoperatively, encourage oral fluid intake, monitor I&O, strain urine for calculi, and offer cranberry juice to acidify the urine. Postoperatively, carefully monitor I&O, and assess for signs of hypocalcemia (tetany, cardiac dysrhythmias, and carpopedal spasms). Teach client the principles of good body mechanics. Reassure client that bone pain will gradually disappear. Encourage mild exercise as ordered.

NURSING PROCESS

ASSESSMENT

Subjective Data

Obtain a thorough client history and ask about muscle weakness, apathy, nausea, mental status, and pain (low back or renal). Ask about increased calcium intake, either dietary or supplements.

Objective Data

Note fatigue, drowsiness, anorexia, constipation, personality changes, renal colic, skeletal deformity, output, hematuria, vomiting, weight loss, hypertension, bradycardia, or dysrhythmias.

Nursing diagnoses for a client with hyperparathyroidism include the following:

NURSING DIAGNOSES	PLANNING/OUTCOMES	NURSING INTERVENTIONS
Activity Intolerance related to generalized weakness caused by neuromuscular dysfunction	The client will regain and maintain normal muscle mass and strength, maintain maximum joint range of motion, and perform self-care activity as tolerated.	Alternate rest and activity periods. Assist client with prescribed, individualized activities. Assist client to identify factors that increase or decrease activity intolerance. Encourage client to perform self-care.
*Acute **Pain*** related to musculoskeletal changes resulting from persistently increased serum calcium level	The client will express relief after analgesics, use comfort measures to decrease pain, and be pain-free when serum calcium level reaches normal.	Administer analgesics as ordered. Provide comfort measures for bone pain, and include turning and repositioning every 2 hours. Assess pain level and compare to serum calcium level. Assess environment for hazards and eliminate them. Assist the client to ambulate. Maintain the bed in a low position with side rails up and call light in reach. Lift and move the client gently to prevent pathologic fractures. Provide a safe environment to prevent injuries associated with pain and weakness.

Evaluation: Evaluate each outcome to determine how it has been met by the client.

HYPOPARATHYROIDISM

Hypoparathyroidism is a condition resulting from a deficiency of PTH secretion by the parathyroids or the decreased action of peripheral PTH. Because the parathyroids normally regulate the serum calcium level, hypoparathyroidism will result in a decreased serum calcium level. PTH normally maintains the serum calcium level by increasing bone resorption and gastric reabsorption. It also maintains the inverse relationship between calcium and phosphorus levels. Hypoparathyroidism can be acute or chronic.

If hypoparathyroidism is idiopathic, it may be the result of an autoimmune disorder or congenital absence of parathyroid glands. Acquired hypoparathyroidism is generally irreversible. The most common cause is accidental removal of the parathyroid glands during thyroid or other neck surgery. It can also result from ischemic infarction during surgery, sarcoidosis, tuberculosis, neoplasms, trauma, or massive thyroid irradiation. Reversible hypoparathyroidism can result from hypomagnesemia-induced impairment of hormone synthesis, suppression of normal gland function because of hypercalcemia, or delayed maturation of the parathyroid glands.

The characteristic sign of hypoparathyroidism is tetany, which is muscle spasms and tremors caused by a lack of calcium. Other clinical manifestations include dry skin, brittle hair, alopecia (loss of hair or baldness), and loss of eyelashes and fingernails. The teeth are stained, cracked, and decayed because of weak enamel. The client may have altered level of consciousness, neuromuscular irritability, tingling and twitching of the face and hands, and increased deep tendon reflexes. There may be personality changes or EKG changes.

Two diagnostic assessment tests can be performed. One is the **Chvostek's sign**, which is an abnormal spasm of the facial muscles in response to a light tapping of the facial nerve. The other test is **Trousseau's sign**, which is a carpal spasm caused by inflating a blood pressure cuff above the client's systolic pressure and leaving it in place for 3 minutes (Figure 43-13).

Expected test results include decreased serum calcium, increased urinary calcium, increased serum phosphorus, and decreased urinary phosphorus.

Complications are related to long-standing hypocalcemia, which leads to decreased heart contractility leading to cardiac failure. There can be cataract formation or papillary edema from increased intracranial pressure. There may be bone deformity. In cases of severe tetany, the client can experience laryngospasm, respiratory stridor, anoxia, paralysis of vocal cords, and death.

MEDICAL–SURGICAL MANAGEMENT

Pharmacological

Calcium gluconate or calcium chloride may be given intravenously. Give very slowly because it is very irritating to the vessel wall. Too-rapid IV calcium infusion can cause cardiac arrest. Additional complications from IV administration of calcium gluconate include seizure activity and laryngeal spasms. After the initial IV dose, calcium may be given orally.

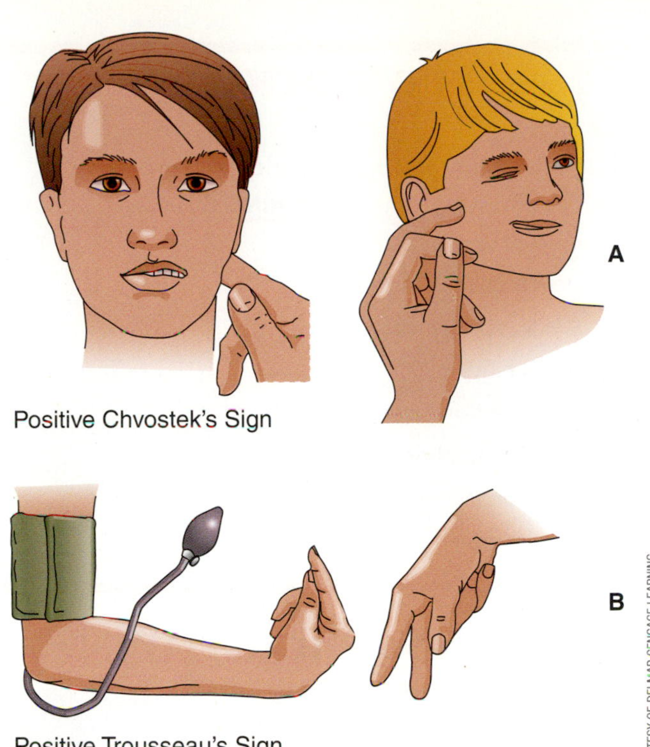

FIGURE 43-13 Signs of Hypocalcemia and Hypoparathyroidism; *A*, Chvostek's Sign; *B*, Trousseau's Sign

Unless the hypoparathyroidism is reversible, the client will require lifelong calcium replacement. Vitamin D may also be given to assist in the absorption of calcium. The calcium supplements should be given 1 to 1½ hours after meals to increase absorption. If the client cannot swallow the large tablets, they can be dissolved in hot water and the suspension cooled before administering to the client. The best sources of calcium are from the diet. The client needs to take calcium as ordered and not abruptly stop taking it. The client must be advised that calcium may cause digitalis toxicity. Cimetidine (Tagamet) interferes with normal parathyroid functioning.

Diet

The diet should be high in calcium and low in phosphorus-containing foods. Because many foods that are high in calcium are also high in phosphorus, the client should be given a list of foods that are high in calcium but lower in phosphorus. Foods on this list include vegetables such as asparagus, broccoli, collards, and tomatoes; fruits such as apricots, bananas, cantaloupe, and many berries; and other foods such as kidney beans, lima beans, and brown sugar. Foods that have a high phosphorus content and should be avoided include most legumes, nuts, cheeses, and seafood.

NURSING MANAGEMENT

Monitor vital signs and for signs of hypercalcemia (anorexia, vomiting, disorientation, abdominal pain, and weakness). Assess for respiratory distress. Provide a diet high in calcium-containing foods. Emphasize the importance of having the blood level of calcium and phosphorus checked.

NURSING PROCESS

ASSESSMENT

Subjective Data

Obtain a thorough client history, asking the client about recent surgery or irradiation, use of alcohol, numbness or tingling of the skin, anxiety, headache, irritability, depression, or nausea.

Objective Data

Assess for dysphagia, level of consciouisness changes, laryngeal spasm, stridor, cyanosis, dysrhythmias, Chvostek's sign, and Trousseau's sign.

Nursing diagnoses for a client with hypoparathyroidism include the following:

NURSING DIAGNOSES	PLANNING/OUTCOMES	NURSING INTERVENTIONS
*Risk for **I**njury* related to calcium deficiency	The client will not exhibit signs and symptoms of tetany, and will prevent injury from hypocalcemia.	Monitor Chvostek's and Trousseau's signs, serum calcium and phosphorus levels, as well as EKG changes. Keep tracheotomy tray readily available and maintain seizure precautions. Support client while walking to prevent injury. Monitor client taking digoxin for toxicity.
*Imbalanced **N**utrition: Less than Body Requirements* related to calcium intake	The client will have adequate calcium intake.	Provide diet with calcium-rich foods. Give calcium replacement as ordered. The client who is taking digoxin must be monitored for toxicity. Give calcium supplement 1 to 1½ hours before or after meals to increase absorption.

Evaluation: Evaluate each outcome to determine how it has been met by the client.

ADRENAL DISORDERS

Disorders in this category include Cushing's disease/syndrome, Addison's disease, and pheochromocytoma.

CUSHING'S DISEASE SYNDROME (ADRENAL HYPERFUNCTION)

Cushing's *disease*, primary adrenal hyperfunction, is the result of increased pituitary secretion of ACTH, which causes an increased production of cortisol by the adrenal cortex. Cortisol, a stress hormone, regulates the body's metabolism of carbohydrates, fats, and proteins. Cushing's *syndrome* refers to symptoms of cortisol excess caused by other factors. One cause is a corticotropin-producing tumor in another organ, such as oat-cell carcinoma of the lung (secondary adrenal hyperfunction). The most common cause of Cushing's syndrome is prolonged use of glucocorticoid or corticotropin medications for chronic inflammatory disorders such as chronic obstructive pulmonary disease, Crohn's disease, and rheumatoid arthritis. This is **iatrogenic** (caused by treatment or diagnostic procedures) adrenal hyperfunction.

Cushing's syndrome occurs in females more than males, generally between 30 and 50 years of age.

Classic clinical manifestations are adiposity of the face, neck, and trunk, which give rise to the moon-shaped face and buffalo hump. Others include purple striae on the abdomen, hirsutism, and thin extremities caused by muscle wasting. Boys exhibit an early onset of puberty, whereas girls exhibit development of masculine characteristics. The client may complain of fatigue, muscle weakness, weight gain, sleep disturbances, water retention, amenorrhea, decreased libido, irritability, and emotional lability. There could be petechiae, ecchymoses, decreased wound healing, or swollen ankles.

There are multiple complications of Cushing's syndrome, most of which are produced by the stimulating and catabolic effects of cortisol. There can be increased calcium resorption from the bone, leading to osteoporosis and pathologic fractures. It can cause increased hepatic gluconeogenesis and insulin resistance, causing glucose intolerance and diabetes mellitus. The client may have frequent infections and slowed wound healing. There is a suppressed inflammatory response that can mask severe infections. The client may have decreased ability to handle stress, which can lead to psychological problems from mood swings to psychosis. Other complications include hypertension, ischemic heart disease, congestive heart failure, menstrual disturbances, and sexual dysfunction.

Plasma cortisol level is elevated. Plasma ACTH level may be elevated or low. Adrenalangiography is done for adrenal tumor. Twenty-four-hour urine tests for 17-ketosteroids, 17-hydroxysteroids, and free cortisol are elevated. A dexamethasone suppression test may also be completed. If the client's blood and urine cortisol levels do not decrease, then Cushing's disease is suspected.

Prognosis depends on early diagnosis, identifying the underlying cause, and effective treatment. Without treatment, about half of these clients will die within 5 years.

MEMORY TRICK

The following is a memory trick to remember the signs and symptoms of **CUSHING'S** Disease:

- **C** = Cortisol
- **U** = Unusually high ACTH
- **S** = Sleep disturbances
- **H** = Hirsutism
- **I** = Infection
- **N** = Non-healing wounds
- **G** = Gain weight
- **S** = Striae

MEDICAL–SURGICAL MANAGEMENT

Medical

The major goal is to restore hormone balance. Treatment is based on the causative factor. This is accomplished primarily by medications. If there is adrenal cancer, the client may have either radiation therapy to the adrenal gland or surgery on either the pituitary gland or the adrenal glands, or all three treatments.

Surgical

If the underlying cause of Cushing's syndrome is related to the pituitary gland, the client may have a hypophysectomy done. (Refer to hypophysectomy in the section on hyperpituitarism.)

For an adrenal tumor, an adrenalectomy is performed to decrease the high levels of circulating cortisol. This could be unilateral or bilateral. During the first 24 to 48 hours after surgery, the client is observed closely for hemorrhage and shock. Vital signs and urine output are monitored. Glucocorticoids are administered with changing dosage until a maintenance dose is established. The client's blood glucose level must be monitored, especially for hypoglycemia.

COMMUNITY/HOME HEALTH CARE

Cushing's Syndrome

- Carry Medic Alert tag, indicating Cushing's syndrome.
- Avoid extreme temperature changes, activities that could result in trauma, and people with infections.
- Wash hands often and protect skin with good care.
- Maintain medication regimen.
- Notify physician if weakness, fainting, fever, nausea, or vomiting occur.

Pharmacological

Aminoglutethimide (Cytadren) inhibits synthesis of adrenal steroids. It can cause dizziness or drowsiness. The client should be instructed to avoid activities requiring mental alertness or manual dexterity.

Ketoconazole (Nizoral), while classified as an antifungal, inhibits adrenal steroidogenesis and is used to treat Cushing's syndrome.

Mitotane (Lysodren) directly suppresses the activity of the adrenal cortex. This cytotoxic agent is generally used for inoperable adrenal cortex cancer. It is given for at least 3 months. The client should avoid situations that cause injury or exposure to infections.

If the client had pituitary or adrenal surgery, cortisol therapy may be given before and after surgery to decrease physical stress. The client may need to adhere to lifetime treatment with steroids. The client should take the drug with food or antacids to decrease gastric distress. Two-thirds dose of the steroids should be taken in the morning, with the remaining one-third in the early evening to mimic the body's diurnal schedule. Steroids can lead to osteoporosis and the possibility of pathologic fractures. Females should be warned that steroid use can interfere with oral contraceptive effectiveness. There may be an adverse effect on the male's sperm production and count.

The client with diabetes mellitus may have to adjust insulin dosage because the steroids can affect the glucose level. Steroids can mask severe infections and cause some immunosuppression. Wounds are slower to heal. The client should be instructed to contact a physician before using over-the-counter preparations. The client should not abruptly discontinue the steroid drug; dosage must be tapered before discontinuing.

Diet

The diet should be high in protein and potassium but low in sodium. Foods high in protein include eggs, milk, whole grains, legumes, and meat; however, milk, cheeses, and whole grains are also high in sodium, depending on processing. Many foods high in potassium are also low in sodium. These foods are legumes; fruits such as figs, oranges, bananas, prunes, and raisins; and vegetables such as avocado, potato, and spinach. The client should be advised to read labels for sodium content. Processed foods and many preservatives have high sodium content and should be avoided. Reduced carbohydrates and calories help control hyperglycemia.

NURSING MANAGEMENT

Encourage client to turn frequently and ambulate to prevent pressure on bony prominences. Gently handle client to prevent ecchymosis. Provide elbow and heel protectors and an egg-crate mattress. Provide rest periods during personal hygiene activities.

NURSING PROCESS

ASSESSMENT

Subjective Data

Obtain a thorough client history, asking about the use of steroids, stress, methods of coping with stress, irritability, depression, mood swings, loss of libido, and the possibility of suicide.

Objective Data

Assess for thin and fragile skin, petechiae, ecchymoses, delayed wound healing, weight gain, increased abdominal girth, thin extremities with muscle wasting, purple striae, hyperglycemia, and hypokalemia. Women may have **hirsutism** (excessive body hair in a masculine distribution), deepening of the voice, and menstrual irregularities.

Nursing diagnoses for a client with Cushing's syndrome include the following:

NURSING DIAGNOSES	PLANNING/OUTCOMES	NURSING INTERVENTIONS
*Disturbed **Body** Image* related to changes in physical appearance	The client will verbalize feelings about changed appearance.	Encourage client to verbalize feelings about changed body image. Offer emotional support and a positive realistic assessment of the condition.
*Risk for **Infection*** related to suppressed inflammatory response from excessive corticosteroid production	The client will take precautions to avoid or decrease exposure to infection.	Advise client to avoid people with infections. Provide a private room with reverse or protective isolation as indicated. Monitor client's vital signs, intake and output, and weight.

Evaluation: Evaluate each outcome to determine how it has been met by the client.

ADDISON'S DISEASE (ADRENAL HYPOFUNCTION)

Addison's disease, primary hypofunctioning of the adrenals, involves decreased functioning of the adrenal cortex and its secretions—mineralocorticoids, glucocorticoids, and androgens. It can also be called *adrenal hypofunction* or *insufficiency*. It is fairly uncommon, occurring in 5 per 100,000 people in the United States (Daniels, 2007). Although it affects all ages and both sexes, it is less common among the elderly.

Addison's disease occurs when more than 90% of the adrenal gland is destroyed. It is an autoimmune disease in response to conditions such as tuberculosis, histoplasmosis, HIV, and meningococcal pneumonia. It can be caused by bilateral adrenalectomy, hemorrhage into the adrenal gland related to anticoagulant therapy, or cancer of the adrenal gland. It is termed secondary if it results from decreased pituitary or hypothalamus function or abrupt withdrawal of long-term steroid therapy.

A classical clinical manifestation of Addison's disease is a bronze coloration of the skin resembling a deep suntan, especially in the creases on the hands, elbows, and knees. There may be some areas of vitiligo. The client may complain of fatigue, muscle weakness, lightheadedness upon rising, weight loss, and craving for salty foods. The client may have decreased tolerance even to minor stress. The client is anxious, irritable, and may become confused. The pulse may be weak and irregular. There is hypotension and a variety of gastrointestinal complaints. The client is also at risk for orthostatic hypotension.

The acute form is called adrenal crisis. It may occur when there is trauma, surgery, other physiologic stress, or abrupt withdrawal of steroids. The clinical manifestations are the same, only more severe with a rapid onset. The crisis requires immediate treatment. The client will be placed on intravenous therapy and IV administration of hydrocortisone (Cortef, Hydrocortone). Measures to maintain a stable blood pressure and normal water and sodium levels are instituted. EKG monitoring is needed to assess for complications associated with elevated K and Ca levels. After the crisis, the client will be placed on a maintenance dose of hydrocortisone.

Expected test results include low serum sodium, high serum potassium, low serum glucose, low cortisol and aldosterone serum levels, and decreased urinary 17-ketosteroid and 17-hydroxysteroid levels.

Medical–Surgical Management

Medical

Treatment is geared toward prompt restoration of fluid and electrolyte balance and replacement of deficient adrenal hormones.

Pharmacological

The client will require lifetime maintenance of steroids. Administration of glucocorticoids such as hydrocortisone (Hydrocortone) and mineralocorticoids such as fludrocortisone acetate (Florinef) are given two-thirds of the daily dose in the morning and one-third in the evening. In times of stress, the dose may need to be doubled or tripled.

Diet

The diet should be high in sodium and low in potassium. It should contain adequate calories and protein. If the client is anorexic, six small meals may increase caloric intake. A late afternoon or evening snack should be available if the client's blood glucose level drops.

Nursing Management

Carefully assess the client's circulatory status. Weigh client daily. Accurately record I&O. Monitor vital signs and skin turgor. Provide a private room and screen visitors for infections. Teach importance of taking medications as prescribed, wearing a Medic Alert bracelet, reporting any illness to the physician, and having regular checkups. A kit including injectable hydrocortisone should be available when oral intake is not feasible.

NURSING PROCESS

Assessment

Subjective Data

Obtain a thorough client history, asking about recent synthetic steroid use, adrenal surgery, infection, salt craving, nausea, weakness, vertigo, headache, disorientation, emotional status, anxiety, and apprehension.

Objective Data

Assess for postural hypotension, inability to perform normal activities, syncope, dark pigmented areas on skin and mucous membrane, weight loss, vomiting, diarrhea, and very low or very high temperature.

Nursing diagnoses for a client with Addison's disease include the following:

NURSING DIAGNOSES	PLANNING/OUTCOMES	NURSING INTERVENTIONS
*Deficient **Fluid Volume*** related to low sodium level, vomiting, diarrhea, and increased renal losses	The client will regain normal fluid and electrolyte balance.	Monitor client's vital signs, level of consciousness, intake and output, and weight. Administer IV fluids as ordered and encourage fluid intake.
*Risk for **Infection*** related to suppressed inflammatory response	The client will maintain normal temperature and leukocyte count and differential, and use precautions to avoid or reduce risks of infection.	Monitor temperature every 4 hours unless elevated, then every 2 hours. Provide a private room with reverse or protective isolation as needed. Screen personnel and visitors for infection. Teach proper hand hygiene. Monitor laboratory test results for WBC and differential.

Evaluation: Evaluate each outcome to determine how it has been met by the client.

LIFE SPAN CONSIDERATIONS

Pheochromocytoma

Pheochromocytoma is frequently diagnosed during pregnancy when the enlarged uterus puts pressure on the tumor, causing more frequent attacks. The attacks could prove fatal to both mother and fetus. Although there is an increased risk of spontaneous abortion, most fetal deaths occur during labor or immediately after delivery.

PHEOCHROMOCYTOMA

Pheochromocytoma, sometimes known as *chromaffin cell tumor*, is a rare disease characterized by **paroxysmal** (a symptom that begins and ends abruptly) or sustained hypertension caused by excessive secretion of epinephrine and norepinephrine. The excessive secretion of epinephrine and norepinephrine stimulates the sympathetic nervous system leading to hypertension and tachycardia. Some medical experts estimate that about 0.5% of clients newly diagnosed with hypertension have pheochromocytoma. Although the tumor is generally benign, it can be malignant in 5% to 10% of the cases. It affects all races and both sexes. It is most common in women ages 20 to 50 years.

It is caused by a chromaffin cell tumor of the adrenal medulla, more commonly on the right side. Extraadrenal pheochromocytomas can also occur. Epinephrine overproduction occurs with the adrenal pheochromocytoma; however, norepinephrine overproduction is associated with both adrenal and extraadrenal pheochromocytoma. It is associated with a family history of pheochromocytoma or endocrine gland cancer. It is considered to be inherited on the autosomal-dominant gene in about 5% of the cases.

The classic triad of clinical manifestations is hypertension with diastolic pressure above 115 mm Hg, unrelenting headache, and profuse diaphoresis. Other clinical manifestations include palpitations, visual disturbances, nausea, or vomiting. These attacks may be triggered by activities or conditions that displace the abdominal contents, such as heavy lifting, exercise, bladder distention, or pregnancy. Severe attacks can be precipitated by administration of opiates, histamine, glucagon, and corticotropin. Some attacks may have no precipitating factor. Some other clinical manifestations are mild to moderate weight loss caused by increased metabolism and orthostatic hypotension when rising to an upright position. The client will have tachycardia. The actual tumor is rarely palpable; however, palpation could trigger a hypertensive attack.

The complications are similar to those of severe and persistent hypertension. These complications are stroke, retinopathy, heart disease, or irreversible kidney disease. The client with pheochromocytoma has an increased risk of severe complications or death during invasive diagnostic tests or surgery.

Although pheochromocytoma can be potentially fatal, the prognosis is good with treatment. About 90% of the clients are cured.

Medical–Surgical Management

Surgical

The treatment of choice is surgical removal of the tumor. Sometimes the adrenal gland is also removed. The blood pressure is monitored closely during the immediate postoperative period. The client may have hypotension, but hypertension is more common. About 10% of the clients are not candidates for surgery. They are treated with medications to lower the blood pressure.

Pharmacological

During acute hypertensive attacks, the drugs of choice are phentolamine mesylate (Regitine) or nitroprusside sodium (Nipride). Phentolamine mesylate (Regitine) and phenoxybenzamine HCl (Dibenzyline) are alpha-adrenergic blocking agents. They are used to control hypertension before surgery or when surgery is contraindicated. The client should be warned about orthostatic hypotension and rise slowly from a supine position to an upright position. The client should not take over-the-counter drugs or alcohol.

Nitroprusside sodium (Nipride, Nitropress) acts on the vascular smooth muscle to cause peripheral vasodilation. The drug is given in an intravenous infusion. An electronic infusion device must be used to monitor the infusion rate. The client's blood pressure is used to titrate the infusion rate per the physician's orders.

Metyrosine (Demser) is used to block catecholamine synthesis. This drug must be continued for life if the tumor is inoperable. Ongoing medications include adrenergic blockers such as propranolol hydrochloride (Inderal), atenolol (Tenormin), prazosin HCl (Minipress), labetalol HCl (Normodyne), or nifedipine (Procardia), a calcium channel blocker. The client's blood pressure must be monitored frequently to determine the effectiveness of the medication.

Propranolol hydrochloride (Inderal) should not be stopped abruptly. The client should not smoke while taking this medication. Atenolol (Tenormin) may enhance the client's sensitivity to cold. Prazosin HCl (Minipress) should be taken on an empty stomach. The initial dose should be given at bedtime. The client should not use cough, cold, or allergy medications without the physician's knowledge. If the client is given parenteral labetalol HCl (Normodyne, Trandate), the client should remain supine for 3 hours to decrease the possibility of orthostatic hypotension. Nifedipine (Adalat, Procardia) should be protected from light and moisture and stored at room temperature. Over-the-counter medications should not be taken.

Diet

The diet should be high in protein with adequate calories. Stimulating foods such as aged cheeses and yogurt; caffeine-containing beverages such as coffee, tea, and soft drinks; and beer and red wine should be avoided (Smeltzer & Bare, 2006).

Nursing Management

The nurse should ask about heat intolerance, severe headaches during hypertensive crisis, anxiety, trouble sleeping, palpitations, nervousness, dizziness, paresthesias, and nausea. The client is assessed for dyspnea, tremors, diaphoresis, glycosuria, hyperglycemia, or dilated pupils. Frequently assess blood pressure, pulse, and respirations for elevations, and observe for signs of anxiety.

CASE STUDY

A.F., a 44-year-old African-American man, is admitted to the medical unit from his physician's office. He reports that he has lost 18 pounds over the last month and has been very tired. He also reports symptoms of thirst, frequent urination, and blurred vision. His vital signs are blood pressure 166/92 mm Hg, pulse 88 beats/min, respiration 16 breaths/min, and temperature 99.2°F. Physical assessment reveals hot, dry, flushed skin. Laboratory exams reveal a blood glucose 490 mg/dL and urine negative for ketones. A.F. is a truck driver and leads a fairly sedentary lifestyle. History reveals that he is usually 30 to 35 pounds overweight but has otherwise been in good health. He reports that his mother died from diabetes and renal failure, and an older brother was diagnosed as having type 2 diabetes 3 years ago.

The following questions will guide your development of a nursing care plan for this case study:

1. List physical symptoms that A.F. is experiencing that are suggestive of diabetes.
2. On the basis of the client's history and laboratory values, would you expect A.F. to be diagnosed with type 1 or type 2 diabetes?
3. Which nursing diagnoses would you identify as priorities for A.F. right now? List two.
4. A.F. is treated with IV fluids and insulin sliding scale until his blood glucose is stabilized. Describe what an insulin sliding scale is, and when it is used.
5. A 2,000-calorie ADA diet is ordered for A.F. He does not care to eat the apple that came on his breakfast tray and asks if he can exchange it for another serving of scrambled eggs. How would you respond to Mr. Carnes?
6. A.F. is being discharged and will continue to attend diabetic education classes at a local diabetic treatment center. Assuming A.F. is to continue on a diabetic diet and will be receiving mixed insulin injections, list the pertinent information A.F. will need to know about his disease and therapies related to:
    - Diabetes and symptoms of hyperglycemia
    - Role of exercise
    - Effects of diet
    - Self-monitoring blood glucose
    - Insulin injections/technique
    - Symptoms of hypoglycemia
    - Sick-day care
    - Long-term complications

SUMMARY

- The endocrine system is composed of glands at various body locations producing secretions (hormones) that directly enter the blood or lymph circulation.
- The endocrine system provides slower and longer-lasting control over various body activities and functions.
- A malfunction of any part of the endocrine system can result in a shift of homeostasis with far-reaching systemic reactions.
- Assessment of the endocrine system can be challenging because the glands are scattered. Negative findings are as important as positive findings.
- Diabetes is a complex chronic disease with multiple acute and chronic complications. It is a systemic disease caused by an imbalance between insulin supply and demand.
- A coordinated program of exercise, diet, and medications is used to achieve diabetic control. Persons with type 1 diabetes always require insulin therapy in addition to dietary control and an exercise program. Persons with type 2 diabetes are managed through diet and exercise and may or may not require oral hypoglycemic agents or insulin.
- The goal of diabetes management is enabling the diabetic to manage the disease by maintaining a blood glucose level within an acceptable range and thereby minimizing the incidence of acute and chronic complications.
- Regardless of disorder, the client should wear a Medic Alert bracelet and be aware that the treatment generally lasts a lifetime.

REVIEW QUESTIONS

1. A client tells the nurse that she is surprised that she developed diabetes at 40 years of age. The nurse knows that the development of diabetes in middle-aged people is most directly the result of:
    1. atherosclerosis.
    2. eating too much sugar.
    3. obesity.
    4. viral infection.

2. Which of the following principles is used when planning for a client with diabetes who is to undergo surgery?
   1. All insulin is withheld until surgery is over and the client is eating.
   2. Insulin or oral hypoglycemics are given as usual.
   3. Sliding-scale insulin is used to regulate glucose levels during the operative period.
   4. Hyperglycemia poses the most serious danger to the client during surgery.
3. Which of the following nursing diagnoses would be most appropriate for the client with diabetes insipidus?
   1. Alteration in growth and development related to increased growth hormone production.
   2. Alteration in thought processes related to decreased neurologic function.
   3. Fluid volume deficit related to polyuria.
   4. Hypothermia related to decreased metabolic rate.
4. Meticulous skin care is especially important for the client with hyperthyroidism because of:
   1. diaphoresis from heat intolerance.
   2. edema from sodium and water retention.
   3. poor nutrition due to nausea and vomiting.
   4. pressure from immobility due to paralysis.
5. The nurse is caring for a client immediately after surgery for a complete thyroidectomy. Which of the following signs/symptoms would alert the nurse to a life threatening complication of the surgery?
   1. Urine output of 30 mL/hour.
   2. Laryngeal stridor.
   3. Neck stiffness.
   4. Sinus tachycardia 110 beats/min.
6. Which of the following statements made by a client indicates the need for further teaching regarding foot care associated with diabetes mellitus?
   1. "I will contact my podiatrist to have callouses and corns removed."
   2. "I will use a mirror to inspect my feet for bruises, cuts, and abrasions."
   3. "Walking barefoot is advised. It will improve the circulation in my feet."
   4. "I will check the temperature of my bath water before entering the tub."
7. A client with SIADH has been admitted to the hospital. Which of the lab values listed below is congruent with this diagnosis?
   1. Serum Na 124 meq/L.
   2. Urine osmolality <300 mOsm/L.
   3. Urine specific gravity 1.010.
   4. Hemoglobin A1C 4.7.
8. Which of the following nursing diagnoses would the nurse plan to institute on a client suffering from SIADH?
   1. *Fluid* **V***olume Excess* related to decreased urine output.
   2. *Ineffective* **C***oping Mechanism* related to disease process progression.
   3. *Risk for* **H***yperthermia* related to alteration in temperature regulation control.
   4. *Fluid* **V***olume Deficit* related to excessive urine output.
9. A client with suspected Addison's disease is admitted to the hospital. Which diagnostic tests indicate a positive diagnosis of Addison's disease?
   1. Elevated blood sugar.
   2. Decreased cortisol.
   3. Decreased potassium.
   4. Elevated sodium.
10. Which of the following nursing diagnoses would the nurse question when caring for a client with Cushing's disease?
    1. *Risk for Disturbed* **B***ody Image* related to disease process.
    2. *Risk for* **I***nfection* related to immunological changes.
    3. *Risk for* **I***njury* related to muscle weakness and wasting.
    4. *Risk for Deficient* **F***luid Volume* related to excessive excretion of water and sodium.

REFERENCES/SUGGESTED READINGS

Alexander, I. (2008). *PDR nurses drug handbook.* Clifton Park, NY: Delmar Cengage Learning.

American Diabetes Association. (2009). Diagnosis and classification of diabetes mellitus. *Diabetes Care 32,* S62–S67.

American Thyroid Association. (2004). Severe mental impairment and poor physiological status predict mortality in patients with myxedema coma. Retreived from www.thyroid.org/patients/notes/july4/04_07_28.html

Anthony, M. (2003). Hypoglycemia. *Nursing2003, 33*(2), 88.

Bacoka, J. (2001). Thyroid storm. *Nursing2001, 31*(12), 88.

Bartels, D. (2004). Adherence to oral therapy for type 2 diabetes: Opportunities for enhancing glycemic control. *Journal of American Academy of Nurse Practitioners, 16*(1), 8–16.

Bartol, T. (2002). Putting a patient with diabetes in the driver's seat. *Nursing2002, 32*(2), 53–55.

Bulechek, G., Butcher, H., McCloskey, J., & Dochterman, J., eds. (2008). *Nursing Interventions Classification (NIC)* (5th ed.). St. Louis, MO: Mosby/Elsevier.

Caffrey, R. (2003). Are all syringes created equal? *AJN, 103*(6), 46–49.

Cameron, B. (2002). Making diabetes management routine. *AJN, 102*(2), 26–32.

Centers for Disease Control and Prevention. (2007). National diabetes fact sheet, 2007. Retrieved May 2009 from http://www.cdc.gov/diabetes/pubs/general.htm

Centers for Disease Control and Prevention. (2008). Frequently asked questions: Groups especially affected by diabetes. Retrieved August 2, 2009 from http://www.cdc.gov/diabetes/faq/groups.htm#9

Cincinnati, R., & Veliko, J. (2001). Oral medications. *RN, 64*(8), 30–36.

Clarke, K. (2002). No needles needed. *Nursing2002, 32*(5), 49–51.
Cypress, M. (2001). Acute complications. *RN, 64*(4), 26–31.
Daniels, R. (2009). *Delmar's guide to laboratory and diagnostic tests* (2nd ed.) Clifton Park, NY: Delmar Cengage Learning.
Diabetes Insipidus Foundation Inc. (2003–Update 2006). Available from http://www.diabetesinsipidus.org/whatisdi.htm
Estes, M. E. Z. (2010). *Health assessment & physical examination* (4th ed.). Clifton Park, NY: Delmar Cengage Learning.
Fain, J. (2001). Lowering the boom on hyperglycemia. *Nursing2001, 31*(8), 49–50.
Fain, J. (2003). Pump up your knowledge of insulin pumps. *Nursing2003, 33*(6), 51–53.
Flood, L., & Constance, A. (2002). Diabetes & exercise safety. *AJN, 102*(6), 47–55.
Goh, K (2004). Management of hyponatremia. *American Family Physician*, 69(10), 2387–94, 2303–5, 2480.
Goldberg, J. (2001). Nutrition and exercise. *RN, 64*(7), 34–39.
Halpin-Landry, J., & Goldsmith, S. (1999). Feet first: Diabetes care. *AJN, 99*(2), 26–33.
Hardman, L., & Young, F. (2001). Combating hyperosmolar hyperglycemic nonketotic syndrome. *Nursing2001, 31*(3), 32hn1–32hn4.
Holcomb, S. (2003). Detecting thyroid disease, part 1. *Nursing2003, 33*(8), 32cc1–32cc4.
Ignatavicius, D., & Workman, L. (2006). *Medical surgical nursing – critical thinking for collaborative care* (5th ed.). St. Louis, MO: Saunders/Elsevier.
LeMone, P., & Burke, K. (2008). *Medical-surgical nursing: Critical thinking in client care* (4th ed.). New York, NY: Prentice Hall.
Lorenz, R., & Silverstein, J. (2005). *Managing insulin requirements at school*. Retrieved August 2, 2009 from http://ndep.nih.gov/media/SNN_March_2005.pdf
Malchiodi, L. (2002). Thyroid storm. *AJN, 102*(5), 33–35.
McCance, K., & Huether, S. (2005). *Pathophysiology: The biologic basis for disease in adults and children* (5th ed.). St. Louis, MO: Mosby.
McConnell, E. (2002). Myths & facts . . . about Addison's disease. *Nursing2002, 32*(8), 79.
McConnell, E. (2003). Myths & facts . . . about diabetes insipidus. *Nursing2003, 33*(6), 84.
Melmed, S., Kleinberg, D., et al. (2008) *Williams textbook of endocrinology* (11th ed.). Philadelphia, PA: Saunders/Elsevier
Moorhead, S., Johnson, M., Maas, M., & Swanson, E. (2007). *Nursing Outcomes Classification (NOC)* (4th ed.). St. Louis, MO: Mosby.
National Cancer Institute. (2009). Retrieved from http://www.cancer.gov/cancertopics/pdq/treatment/pheochromocytoma/patient
National Diabetes Education Program. (2008). Overview of diabetes in children and adolescents. Retrieved August 2, 2009 from http://ndep.nih.gov/media/diabetes/youth/youth_FS.htm#Diabetes
National Institutes of Health. (2009). Graves disease. Retrieved August 3, 2009 from http://www.nlm.nih.gov/medlineplus/ency/article/000358.htm
National Institution of Diabetes and Digestive and Kidney Diseases (NIDDK). (2008a). Acromegaly. Retrieved from http://www.nlm.nih.gov/medlineplus/encyc/article/00321.htm
National Institution of Diabetes and Digestive and Kidney Diseases (NIDDK). (2008b). Diabetes insipidus. Retrieved October 18, 2009 from http://www.nlm.nih.gov/medlineplus/ency/article/000377.htm
National Institution of Diabetes and Digestive and Kidney Diseases (NIDDK). (2008c). Hyperthyroidism. Retrieved from http://www.nlm.nih.gov/hyperthyroidism.htm
National Institution of Diabetes and Digestive and Kidney Diseases (NIDDK). (2008d). Hypoparathyroidism. Retrieved from http://www.nlm.nih.gov/medlineplus/encyc/article/00385.htm
National Institution of Diabetes and Digestive and Kidney Diseases (NIDDK). (2008e). Pheochromocytoma. Retrieved from http://www.nlm.nih.gov/medlineplus/pheochromocytoma.htm
Norris, J. (senior ed.). (1998). *Handbook of medical–surgical nursing* (2d ed.). Springhouse, PA: Springhouse Corp.
North American Nursing Diagnosis Association International. (2010). *NANDA-I nursing diagnoses: Definitions and classification* 2009–2011. Ames, IA: Wiley-Blackwell.
Olohan, K., & Zappitelli, D. (2003). The insulin pump. *AJN, 103*(4), 48–56.
Plummer, E. (2001). Chronic complications. *RN, 64*(5), 34–40.
Robertson, C. (2001). The untold story of disease progression. *RN, 64*(3), 60–64.
Ruiz, E. (2001). Type 2 disease in children. *RN, 64*(10), 44–48.
Sachse, D. (2001). Acromegaly. *AJN, 101*(1), 69–77.
Sammer, C. (2001). How should you respond to hypoglycemia? *Nursing2001, 31*(7), 48–50.
Schori-Ahmed, D. (2003). Thyroid disease, *RN, 66*(6), 38–43.
Seley, J. (2003). Giving the fingers a rest. *AJN, 103*(3), 73–77.
Shelly, A. (2002). Elderly patients with diabetes. *AJN, 102*(2), 15–16.
Smeltzer, S., & Bare, B. (2006). *Brunner & Suddarth's textbook of medical–surgical nursing* (11th ed.). Philadelphia: Lippincott Williams & Wilkins.
Spratto, G., & Woods, A. (2009). *2009 PDR nurse's drug handbook*. Clifton Park, NY: Delmar Cengage Learning.
Strowig, S., (2001). Insulin therapy. *RN*, 64(9), 38–44.
The Expert Committee on the Diagnosis and Classification of Diabetes Mellitus. (1997). Report of the expert committee on the diagnosis and classification of diabetes mellitus. *Diabetes Care, 20*(7), 1183–1197.
Thibodeau, G., & Patton, K. (2009). *The human body in health & disease* (4th ed.). St. Louis, MO: Mosby.
Tkacs, N. (2002). Hypoglycemia unawareness. *AJN, 102*(2), 34–39.
U.S. Department of Health and Human Services, National Center for Chronic Disease Control and Prevention, Division of Diabetes Translation. (1992). *Diabetes in the United States: A strategy for prevention*. Washington, DC: U.S. Public Health Service.
Valentine, V. (2002). Using a laser to make a point. *Nursing2002, 32*(10), 56–57.
Watts, S., Anselmo, J., & Smith, M. (2003). Combating hypoglycemia in the hospital and at home. *Nursing2003, 33*(3), 32hn1–32hn5.
Williams, J. (2001). We make foot exams a priority. *RN, 64*(5), 40–41.

RESOURCES

American Association of Diabetes Educators, http://www.aadenet.org
American Diabetes Association, http://www.diabetes.org
American Dietetic Association, http://www.eatright.org
Juvenile Diabetes Foundation International, http:// www.jdrf.org
National Institutes of Health, http://www.nih.gov/science/campus
National Organization for Rare Disorders, Inc. (NORD), http://www.rarediseases.org
The Diabetes Insipidus Foundation, Inc., http://www.diabetesinsipidus.org

UNIT 13 Nursing Care of the Client: Reproductive and Sexual Health

CHAPTER 44
Reproductive System

MAKING THE CONNECTION

Refer to the following chapters to increase your understanding of the female and male reproductive systems:

Basic Nursing
- ***Wellness Concepts***
- ***Fluid, Electrolyte, and Acid–Base Balance***
- ***Assessment***
- ***Diagnostic Tests***

Adult Health Nursing
- ***Oncology***
- ***Cardiovascular System***
- ***Urinary System***
- ***Endocrine System***
- ***Sexually Transmitted Infections***
- ***The Older Adult***

Basic Procedures
- ***Urine Collection—Closed Drainage System***

Intermediate Procedures
- ***Irrigating a Urinary Catheter***

LEARNING OBJECTIVES

Upon completion of this chapter, you should be able to:

- Define key terms.
- Identify the anatomy of the reproductive systems.
- Describe the hormonal mechanisms that regulate the reproductive functions, including the menstrual cycle.
- Interpret diagnostic tests for disorders of the reproductive systems.
- List the changes in the reproductive systems that occur with aging.
- Discuss common problems of the reproductive system.
- Differentiate between impotence and infertility.
- Discuss contraceptive methods, including actions, side effects, and client teaching.
- Utilize the nursing process to develop a care plan for a client with a reproductive system disorder.

KEY TERMS

abortion
amenorrhea
contraception
cystocele
dysmenorrhea
dyspareunia
endometriosis
hematuria
hesitancy
impotence
infertility
menopause
menorrhagia
metrorrhagia
nocturia
oligomenorrhea
orchiectomy
polymenorrhea
postvoid residual
priapism
prolapsed uterus
rectocele
spermatogenesis
stent
tenesmus
urethrocele
urethrostomy
vasectomy

INTRODUCTION

Through modern technology, current medical and nursing knowledge, and health education programs, laypersons have access to much information about their bodies and their reproductive systems. Yet, individuals continue to be seriously affected by health disorders. In some instances they may lack knowledge of how to detect signs and symptoms of these disorders. Often, they simply delay routine medical examinations or avoid seeking medical treatment. In addition, individuals may have difficulty discussing symptoms related to their reproductive system.

Routine health care must be maintained and early diagnosis made in order to reduce the incidence and seriousness of reproductive health disorders. These goals can be facilitated with skilled nursing assessment and client education.

For most people, the reproductive system functions without problems throughout life. For others, minor and major disorders require treatment. Some of the problems are related to alterations in structure; others are related more to altered physiology of the reproductive system. This chapter discusses disorders of the reproductive systems by applying the steps of the nursing process.

ANATOMY AND PHYSIOLOGY REVIEW

The female and male reproductive systems consist of external and internal structures and organs.

EXTERNAL FEMALE STRUCTURES

The area known as the vulva includes the external female structures, such as the mons pubis, labia majora, labia minora, and clitoris. The Bartholin glands and Skene's glands, located proximal to the vaginal opening, produce and secrete lubricating fluids. The labia majora and minora serve as protective barriers for the softer internal structures. The clitoris, located proximal to the mons pubis and superior to the urinary meatus, plays a role in sexual arousal in the female and is considered analogous to the male penis. During foreplay, the clitoris engorges and stimulates orgasm or climax in the female. It is covered by a small hood called the prepuce. The perineum is the distal portion of the vulva, located below the vaginal opening and superior to the anus.

The breasts are also a part of the external female reproductive system (Figure 44-1). Their external structures include the nipple, areola, and Montgomery tubercles. The nipples have several openings, or ducts, that lead from the lactiferous glands inside the breast. Milk is ejected through the ducts when the infant sucks on the breast. The areola, or the darker area around the nipple, becomes darker in response to the increased hormone levels during pregnancy. Small, mole-like, raised areas around the areola are the Montgomery tubercles. These glands produce a lubricant that keeps the nipple soft and supple.

INTERNAL FEMALE STRUCTURES

The vagina is an elastic, tube-like structure leading from the outside of the female body to the cervix. Approximately 2 to 3 inches long, it contains many rugae that allow it to stretch during intercourse and also permit the passage of the baby during delivery. The pH environment of the vagina is normally acidic, providing protection from microorganisms that could cause infections.

The uterus is a 3-inch-long, 2-inch-wide, 1-inch-thick hollow, muscular structure, as seen in Figure 44-2. The top is the fundus, the middle is the body (corpus), and the lower

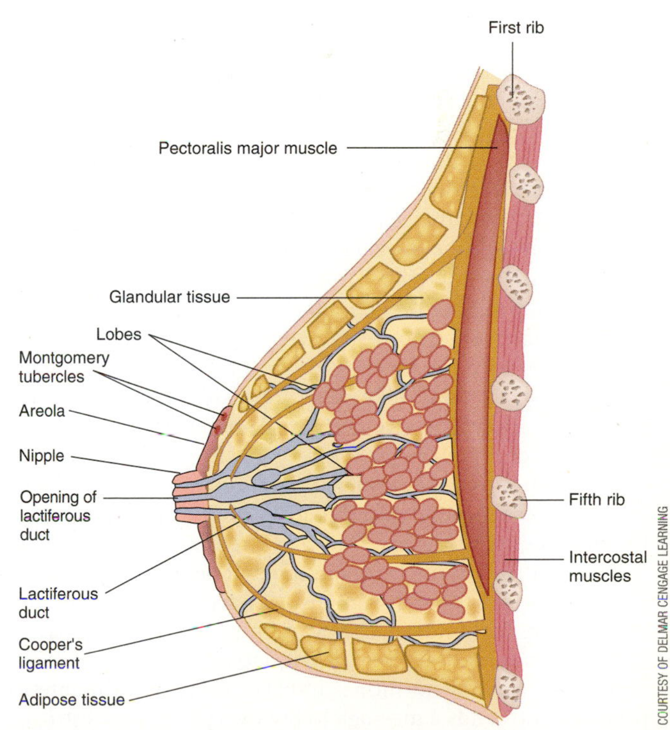

FIGURE 44-1 Cross Section of the Female Breast

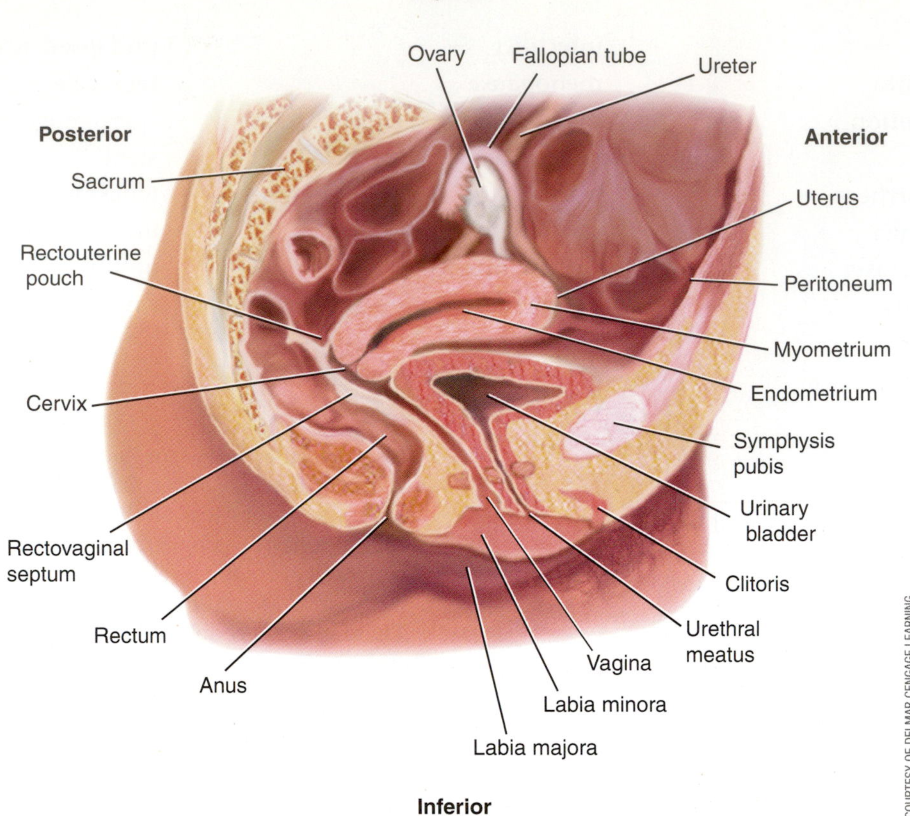

FIGURE 44-2 The Female Reproductive System

portion is the cervix. Four sets of ligaments hold the uterus in its normal anteverted (forward) position and permit it the freedom to grow and move during pregnancy. The uterus has three distinct layers. The innermost layer is the endometrium, which sloughs with menstruation each month. The middle layer is the myometrium, which is constructed of many muscle fibers that are interwoven for strength, stretch, and contractility. The outer layer is the perimetrium, which is an external serous membrane covering.

The fallopian tubes are connected to the uterus on either side. They are continuous with the mucous membrane lining of the endometrium on the inside. Billions of cilia line each fallopian tube and make a sweeping motion toward the uterus, especially at the time of ovulation. This sweeping action moves the ovum along the path toward the uterus. The movement may also impede the progress of the sperm, which must swim upstream against the downward current produced by the cilia.

The cervix is the lower portion of the uterus and extends into the vaginal vault. Like the vagina, the cervix has muscle layers that allow it to stretch to a diameter of at least 10 cm (about 4 inches) during delivery.

An almond-shaped ovary, about 2 inches long and 1 inch wide, is located within the broad ligament on either side of the uterus, just below the fimbriae, the fingerlike projections at the distal end of the fallopian tubes. The ovaries contain all of the ova (eggs) that a woman will have from puberty until menopause. Each month, the ovary responds to hormonal signals from the anterior pituitary gland to ripen one or more ova. Follicle-stimulating hormone (FSH) is released by the anterior pituitary and sends a message to the ovary to release estrogen, which causes the ovum to ripen and enlarge. The entire first part of the cycle is known as the proliferative phase.

Luteinizing hormone (LH) is then released. LH triggers a chain of events that stimulates the ovary to release the ovum. This point in the menstrual cycle is called ovulation. Another hormone, progesterone, causes the glands and blood vessels of the endometrial lining to grow and thicken in preparation for implantation of a fertilized ovum. If fertilization does not occur, the progesterone level decreases, the endometrium sloughs off, and the woman experiences menstruation. If fertilization does occur, the progesterone level remains elevated to ensure the optimal environment for implantation of the zygote about 6 to 8 days after fertilization. Figure 44-3 illustrates the menstrual cycle.

MALE REPRODUCTIVE STRUCTURES

The male reproductive organs and associated structures are illustrated in Figure 44-4. The scrotum is a fleshy structure suspended below the perineum, anterior to the anus. It is divided into two parts, each of which contains a testis, an epididymis, and a portion of the spermatic cord (vas deferens). The left side of the scrotum is usually lower than the right because the left spermatic cord is often longer.

The testes, two smooth, oval endocrine glands, are suspended in the scrotum. This location helps maintain proper temperature and also protects the testes from trauma. Certain cells of the epithelium lining the seminiferous tubules of the testes produce half a billion sperm each day (**spermatogenesis**). They also secrete the androgenic (causing masculinization) hormone testosterone. Spermatogenesis is regulated by follicle-stimulating hormone (FSH), produced by the anterior pituitary gland. The production of testosterone

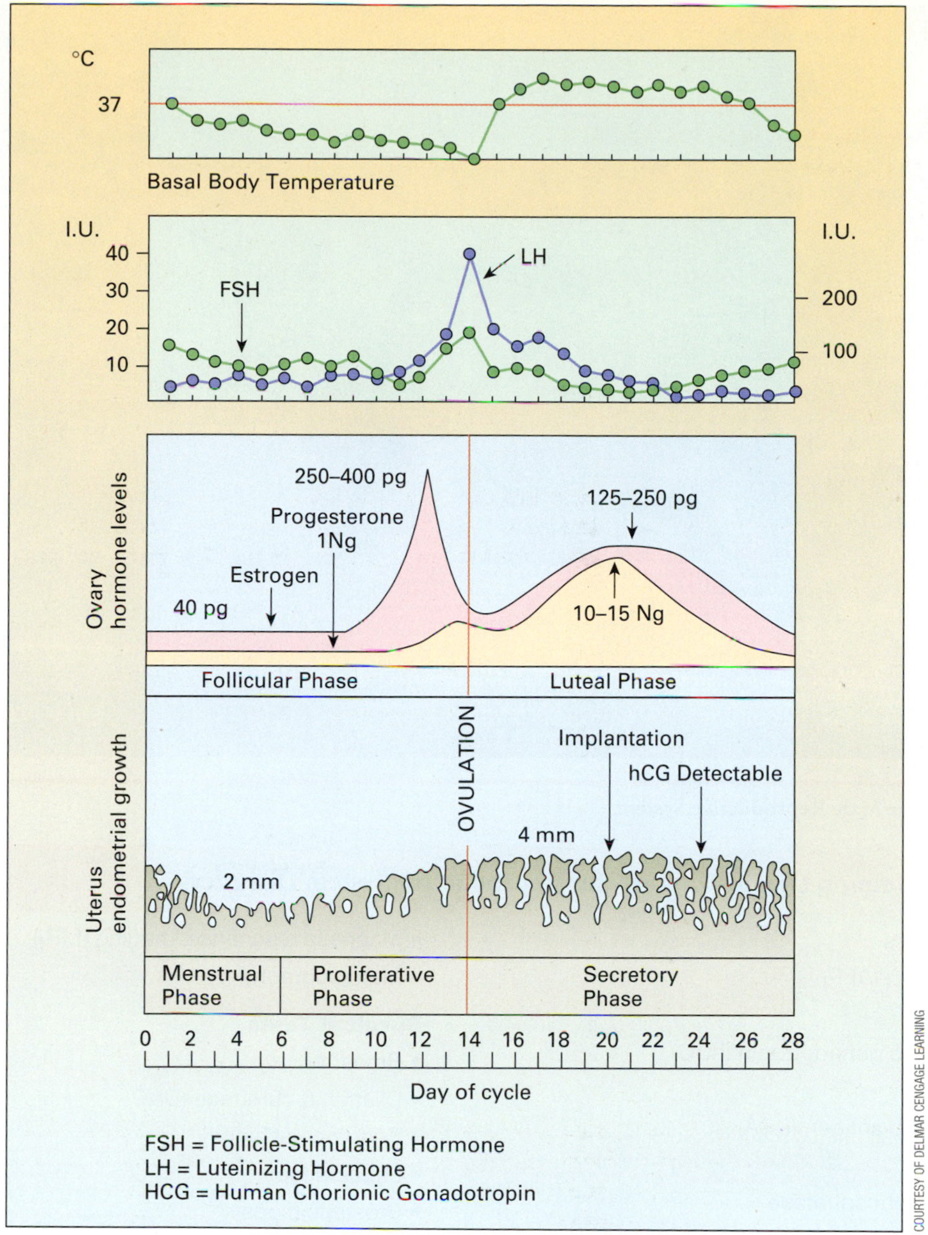

FIGURE 44-3 Cyclic Changes Associated with the Menstrual Cycle

is regulated by luteinizing hormone (LH), also produced by the anterior pituitary gland. After the sperm mature in the epididymis, they travel through the vas (ductus) deferens, a long tube attached to the epididymis. The vas deferens, along with associated nerves and blood vessels, forms the spermatic cord.

The vas deferens travels up and around the bladder and carries sperm from the epididymis to the seminal vesicle, a small pouch that produces secretions that, when mixed with sperm and prostatic fluid, form semen.

The prostate is an encapsulated gland that encircles the proximal portion of the urethra. The prostatic fossa, a depression on the cranial border of the prostate, allows entry of the ejaculatory ducts. Within the prostate is a cluster of 30 to 50 tubuloalveolar glands that secrete prostatic fluid. The prostate gland is of clinical significance because as men age, it is a common site for malignant disease or benign enlargement that can cause urethral obstruction.

The penis is a cylindrical organ through which urine is passed and semen is ejaculated. Half of the penis is located within the body. The external half of the penis is flaccid, unless the male is sexually aroused, at which time it becomes erect because of engorgement with blood. A fold of skin, the prepuce, surrounds the tip of the penis in the uncircumcised male.

COMMON DIAGNOSTIC TESTS

Commonly used diagnostic tests for clients with symptoms of reproductive system disorders are listed in Table 44-1.

INFLAMMATORY DISORDERS

Inflammatory disorders discussed include pelvic inflammatory disease, endometriosis, vaginitis, toxic shock syndrome, and epididymitis/orchitis/prostatitis.

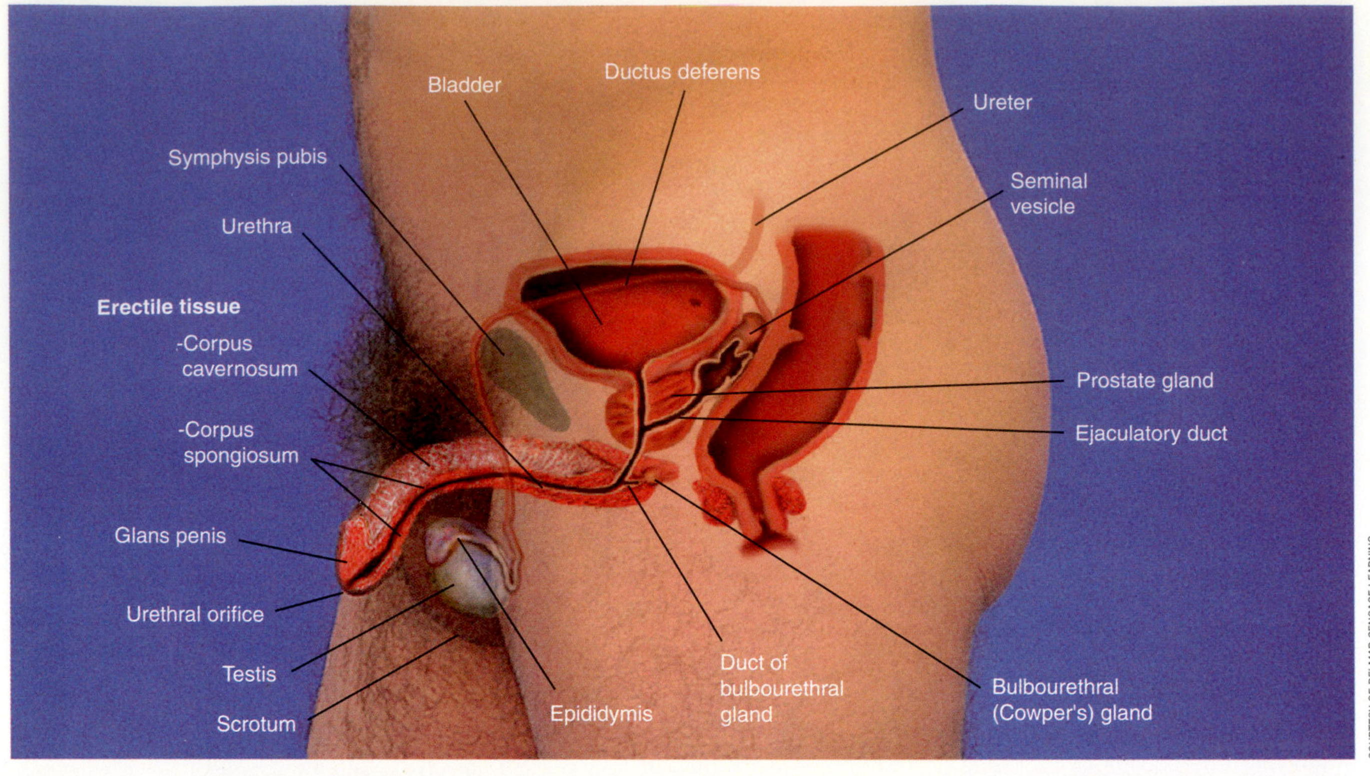

FIGURE 44-4 The Male Reproductive System

TABLE 44-1 Common Diagnostic Tests for Reproductive System Disorders

Laboratory Tests

- Alpha-fetoprotein (AFP)
- Cultures
- Human chorionic gonadotropin (hCG)
- Pap smear
- Prostate-specific antigen (PSA)
- Prostatic smear
- Serum alkaline phosphatase
- Serum calcium
- Semen analysis
- Segmented bacteriologic localization culture

Radiologic Tests

- Computed tomography (CT) scan
- Dynamic infusion cavernosometry and cavernosography (DICC)
- Hysterosalpingogram
- Magnetic resonance imaging (MRI)
- Mammography

Surgical Tests

- Breast biopsy
- Dilation & curettage (D&C)
- Endometrial biopsy
- Laparoscopy
- Prostatic biopsy
- Testicular biopsy

Other Tests

- Colposcopy
- Nocturnal tumescence penile monitoring
- Pelvic examination
- Schiller test
- Ultrasound

COURTESY OF DELMAR CENGAGE LEARNING

PELVIC INFLAMMATORY DISEASE

Pelvic inflammatory disease (PID) is an inflammatory process involving pathogenic invasion of the uterus, fallopian tubes (salpingitis), and ovaries (oophoritis), along with vascular and supporting structures within the pelvis. Pathogenic microorganisms such as chlamydia, gonococcus, streptococcus, staphylococcus, and herpes simplex virus II, may cause PID. The CDC estimates that each year more than 1 million American women will experience an episode of acute PID, and more than 100,000 women will become infertile as a result (CDC, 2008). Infections are usually ascending by nature; that is, the pathogens are introduced into the reproductive system from outside and travel upward from the vagina to the fallopian tubes and then out into the pelvis. Risk factors associated with the incidence of PID include multiple sexual partners, frequent intercourse, IUDs (intrauterine contraceptive devices), douching, and childbirth.

The symptoms of PID include a low-grade fever, pelvic pain, abdominal pain, a "bearing down" backache, a foul-smelling vaginal discharge, nausea and vomiting, abnormal uterine bleeding, **dysmenorrhea** (painful menstruation), **dyspareunia** (painful intercourse), and intense pelvic tenderness upon examination. Peritonitis or pelvic abscesses may develop as complications of PID if the pathogens spread into the pelvic cavity. Future **infertility** (inability or diminished ability to produce offspring) can be related to scarring and strictures of the fallopian tubes, which develop from the chronic inflammatory process within the pelvis. These problems have been associated with ectopic pregnancies because the fertilized ovum becomes trapped inside the fallopian tube before it can complete its trip to the uterus.

PID is often diagnosed during a pelvic examination. Vaginal and cervical cultures are obtained at the time of the exam to determine the causative agent. A pelvic ultrasound may be ordered to rule out other causes of pelvic pain. Instruct the client on the purpose of the procedures and any special preparations that may be required, such as having a full bladder.

MEDICAL–SURGICAL MANAGEMENT

Medical

The client who is not acutely ill from PID may be treated as an outpatient at home with oral antibiotics and bed rest, unless the infection is herpes simplex virus II. Clients with herpes simplex II infections may require more intensive care in the hospital with IV antibiotic therapy. The physician may also order medicated vaginal suppositories for the vaginal discharge. The acutely ill client may require hospitalization for IV antibiotic therapy.

Surgical

If the inflammation is extensive, or if medical treatment is not successful, the client may require a hysterectomy.

Pharmacological

Antibiotics used may include doxycycline monohydrate (Vibramycin), metronidazole (Flagyl), cefoxitin (Mefoxin), clindamycin (Cleocin), and gentamicin (Garamycin). IV fluids are frequently administered to promote adequate hydration, and analgesics are given for pain management.

Activity

During hospitalization, the client is placed on bed rest with bathroom privileges. A semi-Fowler's position is preferred because it will facilitate drainage of the pelvis. If vaginal suppositories are used, the client should lie in a supine position for 30 minutes.

> **CLIENT TEACHING**
>
> **Inserting Vaginal Suppositories**
>
> - Have the client wash her hands, then cleanse the vulva with a mild soap and warm water to remove any external discharge.
> - Client should lie down in a supine position with her knees flexed.
> - With one hand, the client can separate the labia and gently insert the suppository high inside the vagina.
> - The client should remain supine for a minimum of 30 minutes to ensure adequate absorption of the medication through the vaginal mucosa.

NURSING MANAGEMENT

Support the client with a nonjudgmental attitude. Maintain client in semi-Fowler's position to facilitate drainage. Monitor vital signs and I&O. Teach client proper pericare, hygiene, and hand hygiene. Administer antibiotic therapy as ordered.

NURSING PROCESS

ASSESSMENT

Subjective Data

Obtain information about the client's sexual activity, including the number of partners. Unprotected intercourse is the most frequent method of entry for the microorganisms that cause PID. Also include the client's history of **contraception** (measures taken to prevent pregnancy), previous vaginal infections and treatments, obstetrical history, and normal hygiene practices such as douching and tampon use. Description of nagging pelvic pain and a low-grade fever are often expressed.

Objective Data

Assess for an elevated temperature, flushed, dry skin, the presence of a malodorous vaginal discharge, and positive vaginal or cervical cultures.

Nursing diagnoses for a client with pelvic inflammatory disease include the following:

NURSING DIAGNOSES	PLANNING/OUTCOMES	NURSING INTERVENTIONS
*Acute **Pain*** related to inflammation of the pelvic structures caused by invasion of pathogens	Using a pain rating scale of 0 to 10, the client will report that her pain has decreased.	Assess client's pain level every 4 hours, noting the location, duration, sensation, intensity, and factors that increase or decrease the pain. Administer analgesics as ordered.

(*Continues*)

Nursing diagnoses for a client with pelvic inflammatory disease include the following: (Continued)

NURSING DIAGNOSES	PLANNING/OUTCOMES	NURSING INTERVENTIONS
*Deficient **K**nowledge* related to the etiology of the pelvic inflammatory process, treatment regimen, self-care, and preventive measures	The client will follow prescribed treatment regimen, self-care, and preventive measures.	If suppositories are ordered, instruct the client in the proper method of insertion. Provide instructions to the client and partner (if available) about the causes of PID and ways to prevent the inflammation. Teach proper pericare and hygiene, especially hand hygiene before and after changing sanitary pads. Change sanitary pads every 3 to 4 hours. Encourage client to make time for rest periods during the acute phase of the inflammation and to avoid strenuous activities such as straining or heavy lifting. Instruct client about pelvic rest, which includes no douching, tampons, or intercourse. Recommend that the client wear underpants with a cotton crotch. Teach client to cleanse the perineal area from front to back after each voiding or bowel movement. Discuss and encourage the use of safe sexual practices and the use of barrier contraceptives to prevent recurrence of PID symptoms. Encourage client to make follow-up appointment.
	The client will contact her health care provider for follow-up and if her symptoms persist, worsen, or return.	Encourage client to notify the NP or physician at the first sign of PID symptoms. Recommend that the client monitor her own temperature, upon discharge, twice daily for 2 weeks and notify the physician or nurse practitioner (NP) if the temperature increases or remains elevated.
***H**yperthermia* related to physiologic responses to the inflammatory or infectious process	The client's temperature will return to normal range after the initiation of therapy.	Monitor client's vital signs every 4 hours. Administer antipyretic and antibiotic as ordered by the physician.

Evaluation: Evaluate each outcome to determine how it has been met by the client.

ENDOMETRIOSIS

Endometriosis is the growth of endometrial tissue, the normal lining of the uterus, outside of the uterus within the pelvic cavity. It occurs most frequently in women 30 years and older and tends to be familial. It predominantly affects Caucasian females who have not given birth and is most common among the higher socioeconomic population. Endometriosis has been called the "career woman's disorder," because it is often diagnosed in the late twenties or thirties when the working woman makes plans for childbearing.

The endometrial tissue implants itself on other pelvic structures (Figure 44-5). Two of the most common areas for endometrial implants are the pouch of Douglas and the ovaries. The tissue implants respond to the monthly hormonal changes in the same way as the endometrial tissue inside the uterus does. Bleeding of the implants during the menses results in the formation of adhesions and scar tissue. The endometriosis appears as brownish or black "powder burns" or larger lesions. If the endometriosis becomes encapsulated in an ovarian cyst it is called a "chocolate cyst."

The disease appears to be progressive and has a tendency to be recurrent. Some women with minimal endometriosis experience severe monthly symptoms, such as lower backache, painful intercourse, a feeling of heaviness on the pelvis, and spotting. Other women have a more extensive disease but have minimal symptoms. Thus the amount of endometriosis present may or may not be correlated with the severity of the client's symptoms.

Endometriosis is one cause of female infertility because of the amount of scar tissue and adhesions around the pelvic organs, ligaments, and fallopian tubes. Pregnancy inhibits the growth and bleeding of the endometrial implants because ovulation and menstruation are suppressed.

MEDICAL–SURGICAL MANAGEMENT

Medical

Endometriosis may be tentatively diagnosed by palpation of endometrial implants within the pelvis or a pelvic ultrasound

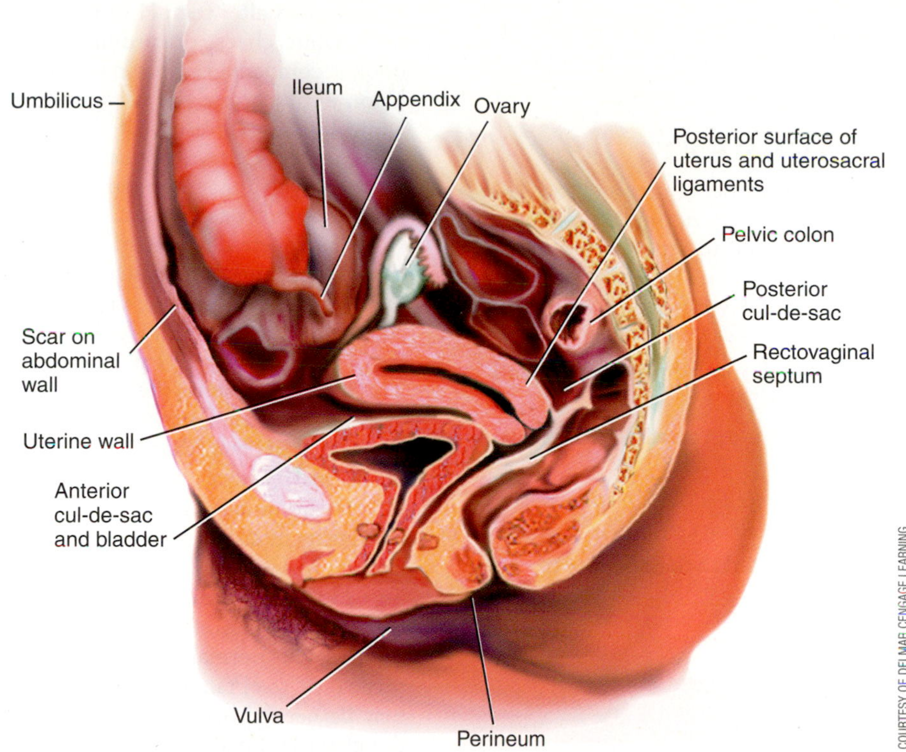

FIGURE 44-5 Common Areas of Endometriosis

may be ordered. To confirm the diagnosis, laparoscopy, performed under general anesthesia is the best method of diagnosis by direct visualization of the pelvic structures. Consideration for treatment depends on the client's age and desire for future childbearing. Sometimes pregnancy relieves the symptoms even after delivery.

Surgical

The older multigravida who is experiencing severe, debilitating symptoms that affect her lifestyle and normal functions, role, or activity may desire a hysterectomy. If the lesions are large or extensive, a laparotomy may be performed for adequate removal; however, if the implants are small and scattered, laparoscopic cauterization or laser ablation may be most desirable. Lysis of pelvic adhesions is performed at the same time.

Pharmacological

The goals of pharmacological therapy are to suppress ovulation and menstruation, reduce symptoms, and cause the implants to shrink. Medications used in the treatment of endometriosis must effectively suppress the monthly hypothalamic-pituitary-ovarian hormonal stimulation of ovulation. Some medications act on the body as "pseudopregnancy" agents that produce anovulation, breast tenderness, nausea, weight gain, and hirsutism. Other hormonal therapies cause a temporary medically induced menopause state. Hormonal treatments include contraceptives (pills, patches, vaginal rings), medroxyprogesterone (Depo-Provera), gonadotropin-releasing hormone (Gn-RH) agonists and antagonists, and aromatase inhibitors (CDC, 2008). Nafarelin acetate (Synarel) is a nasally administered gonadotropin analog that inhibits cyclic hormone release. Danazol (Danocrine) is an androgen hormone that must be taken continuously for at least 6 to 8 months. This medication inhibits the release of gonadotropin. The resulting **amenorrhea** (absence of menstruation) will suppress the growth of the endometrial tissue and is used in moderate to severe cases of endometriosis. Occasionally, Danocrine is given after surgical removal or cauterization of the endometriosis to relieve symptoms from residual disease.

All medications used to treat endometriosis cause mild to moderate side effects that may affect the client's desire to take them or her compliance with continuous usage. Examples of problems that may be experienced include oily skin, fluid retention, weight gain, acne, hot flashes, metrorrhagia, mastalgia, depression, and masculization.

NURSING PROCESS

ASSESSMENT

Subjective Data

Obtain a description of the pelvic pain, which increases at the time of menstruation. The client may voice concerns about dyspareunia, pelvic discomfort with intercourse. This may result in marital tension if the client avoids sexual intimacy to reduce her pain. Be alert to what the client says as well as what is left unsaid. The client may describe prolonged, excessive menstrual periods that are getting closer and closer together. Another sign, although not as significant, is pain with defecation during the menstrual period.

Also note the onset of menses, regularity of cycles, and any changes that client has noted in the frequency, comfort, duration, and amount of menstrual flow. Note the onset of the client's symptoms in relationship to the menstrual cycle, the severity as reported by the client, any alterations in lifestyle related to the pain or other symptoms, and the client's future plans for childbearing.

Objective Data

The nurse's role is usually focused on collecting subjective data from the client interview and assisting the physician during actual procedures.

Nursing Management

Encourage the client to express her concerns and fears. Teach the client about prescribed medications. Emphasize the importance of regular checkups and to report any abnormal vaginal bleeding.

Nursing diagnoses for a client with endometriosis may include the following:

- *Acute **Pain*** related to bleeding from endometrial implants in the pelvic cavity
- ***Anxiety*** related to treatment options, possible side effects, and infertility
- *Ineffective **Sexuality** Patterns*, or ***Sexual** Dysfunction*, related to altered body function or structure (painful intercourse)
- *Situational Low **Self**-Esteem*, related to the inability to conceive

VAGINITIS

Several common types of vaginitis are caused by bacteria, protozoa, viruses, and yeasts. The vaginal mucosa is normally protected by an acid mantle. The acidic (pH less than 5.0) environment inhibits the growth of many pathogenic microorganisms. Because the vaginal opening is close to the external environment, microorganisms have an opportunity to invade the reproductive tract. Some organisms that cause vaginitis are transmitted to the female from the male partner during sexual contact. Natural protective barriers may vary with the fluctuating hormonal levels during the woman's monthly cycle because the hormones affect the vaginal pH. At ovulation, the vaginal pH becomes slightly less acidic because of the high level of estrogen. Times when the woman's system has a lower estrogen level, such as immediately after the menses and after menopause, are times when there is a higher risk for infection because the epithelium is less active, no glycogen is present, and the pH may be as high as 7.0.

Diagnosis is made after performing a vaginal examination and obtaining a cervical culture and a sample of the vaginal discharge. When the client contacts the physician or nurse practitioner to report symptoms of vaginitis, the nurse should instruct her to avoid douching or using tampons before being examined because douching will wash away the discharge needed to be examined and tampons will absorb it.

Common types of vaginitis include candidiasis caused by *Candida albicans* (yeast infection), trichomoniasis caused by *Trichomonas vaginalis* (a protozoan), *Gardnerella vaginalis* (a bacterium), and *Chlamydia trachomatis* (a parasite). Other causes of vaginitis may include streptococcus, staphylococcus, gonococcus, and herpes simplex II. Usually the symptoms depend on the causative agent. The client's description of her symptoms along with the examination of the discharge help confirm the diagnosis. Most infections have a characteristic discharge and irritation with burning or itching that may be internal, external, or both.

Predisposing factors for candidiasis, also called monilia, may include obesity, diabetes, pregnancy, oral contraceptives, antibiotics, bubble baths, and frequent douching. Many of these factors alter the pH of the vagina. Symptoms include a thick, white, cheesy or curd-like discharge with a musty, sweet odor, accompanied by vaginal or vulvar itching and irritation. Upon examination, the vaginal mucosa will have patches of white discharge present. If the patches are scraped off, the tissue underneath will appear reddened and may bleed. Externally, the vulva may be reddened and edematous. The client may have scratches from attempting to ease the itching.

The preferred treatment is vaginal application of antifungal creams or suppositories such as miconazole (Monistat), clotrimazole (Mycelex-G, Gyne-Lotrimin), or nystatin (Mycostatin). Alternative therapies include douching with white vinegar solution (1 tablespoon per 1 pint of water) twice a day for a week. This treatment restores the acid balance of the vagina and washes away the *Candida albicans*. Eating cultured yogurt with active acidophilus or applying the yogurt directly to the labia helps restore the normal bacteria and protective mechanisms in the vagina.

Trichomoniasis is frequently passed from partner to partner during intercourse. A copious green-yellow, foul-smelling, frothy vaginal discharge is characteristic. It may produce itching or external burning and irritation. Metronidazole (Flagyl) should be taken orally by both partners.

Flagyl is normally contraindicated in the first trimester of pregnancy, so obtaining a menstrual history or a pregnancy test may be needed before administering this medication. Inform the client and her partner to avoid any alcohol intake during therapy. Flagyl causes a strong antabuse-like effect, which results in severe nausea and vomiting. Clients should read labels on over-the-counter medications being taken concurrently with the Flagyl because many preparations contain alcohol bases.

Instruct the client and her partner to abstain from intercourse during therapy and to finish all of the medication.

Gardnerella vaginalis often produces a gray-white vaginal discharge with a strong fishy odor or is asymptomatic. If itching or burning is present, it may suggest another microorganism. For the treatment of *Gardnerella*, and other bacterial vaginitis, the physician may order Flagyl or an oral antibiotic such as tetracycline hydrochloride (Achromycin) or ampicillin (Omnipen). Sulfa-based creams such as Sultrin, Triple Sulfa, and AVC may be used vaginally in conjunction with the oral medications once or twice a day for 6 to 14 days to completely treat this type of infection.

Chlamydial vaginitis infections are often asymptomatic but have been associated with infertility problems. A culture of vaginal secretions is necessary to specifically identify the organism. The treatment is usually oral antibiotics for at least 7 days. A repeat culture is recommended following treatment to ensure that the parasites have been eradicated.

CLIENT TEACHING

Ways to Decrease Risk of Vaginitis

- Wear cotton-crotch underwear.
- Avoid sitting in a wet bathing suit in warm weather for long periods.
- Seek prompt medical attention at the first signs of infection.
- Eat an 8-oz container of yogurt with active cultures daily while taking antibiotics.

Postmenopausal vaginitis (atrophic) is caused by a decreased level of estrogen in the vaginal tissue. The client may describe painful intercourse (dyspareunia), itching, burning, or irritation. Estrogen replacement therapy often relieves the symptoms of this type of vaginitis. The medication may be administered orally, vaginally, or by transdermal patch.

NURSING PROCESS

ASSESSMENT

Subjective Data

Obtain information from the client regarding the nature of her symptoms, the onset, menstrual history, contraceptive methods, recent or current use of antibiotics or other medications, recent illness, diabetes mellitus, sexual history, pregnancy history, usual hygiene practices such as douching, deodorant sprays, bubble baths, wearing of pantyhose, type of underwear, and use of deodorized tampons or pads.

Objective Data

Observe the vaginal discharge and note any odor. Vaginal or vulvar irritation and possible scratches may be seen.

NURSING MANAGEMENT

Emphasize the significance of hand hygiene before and after applying vaginal medications. Notify client that her sexual partner should also be treated.

Nursing diagnoses for a client with vaginitis, regardless of the etiology, include the following:

- *Acute **Pain***, related to irritation, excoriation, or ulceration of vaginal tissue
- *Deficient **Knowledge***, related to the origin of the infection, prevention, and treatment options
- *Impaired **Tissue** Integrity*, related to the presence of vaginal discharge, itching, or irritation
- ***Sexual** Dysfunction*, related to discomfort during intercourse or fear of transmitting the infection to the sexual partner
- *Risk for Impaired **Skin** Integrity*, related to internal and external irritation from discharge and itching

TOXIC SHOCK SYNDROME

Toxic shock syndrome (TSS) is a rare, life-threatening condition most often associated with *Staphylococcus aureus*, which enters the bloodstream. Toxins produced by group A *streptococcus* have also been associated with causing TSS. A strong relationship has been found between the use of tampons (especially superabsorbent) during menstruation and the onset of TSS symptoms. It has been hypothesized that the fibers from the tampon lower the level of magnesium in the woman's body and, therefore, produce a favorable environment for the growth of pathogenic microorganisms. The condition was first diagnosed in the mid-1970s, and the incidence increased throughout the 1980s. A high percentage of women who are affected by TSS are younger than age 30. TSS can also occur in nonmenstruating women, men, and children.

The client presents with a sudden high temperature of 102°F or greater, vomiting, diarrhea, progressive hypotension, and flulike symptoms of malaise, muscle soreness, sore throat, and headache (Neighbors & Tannehill-Jones, 2006). There may be a macular erythematous (flat, red) rash followed in 1 to 2 weeks by peeling of the palms and soles. Disorientation may occur from the release of toxins and dehydration. Symptoms of TSS develop suddenly and can be fatal.

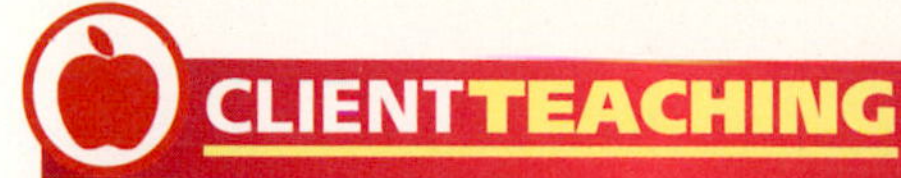

TSS and Tampon Use

Instruct client to avoid tampon use for several cycles. If she chooses to use tampons in the future, they should be changed every 2 to 3 hours. Avoid the superabsorbent types.

MEDICAL–SURGICAL MANAGEMENT

Medical

Blood, urine, genitourinary, and throat cultures may be obtained and are usually negative except for *Staphylococcus aureus*. The goals of treatment are focused on controlling the falling blood pressure, replacing fluid volume, halting the infectious process, and maintaining adequate ventilation efforts. IV fluids are administered per the physician's order. The client may require mechanical ventilation and CPAP (continuous positive airway pressure). Dialysis may be needed if kidney failure occurs.

Pharmacological

Broad-spectrum antibiotic therapy is recommended. Culture and sensitivity tests will indicate which type of antibiotic is best. Examples include dicloxacillin sodium (Dynapen), clexacillin sodium (Tegopen), nafcillin sodium (Nafcil), and methicillin sodium (Staphcillin). The medication regimen is continued for at least 2 weeks to ensure control of the pathogens.

Activity

Bed rest is usually prescribed.

NURSING MANAGEMENT

Maintain client on prescribed bed rest. Administer antipyretics and antibiotics as ordered. Monitor vital signs, I&O, and skin turgor. Encourage oral fluid intake.

NURSING PROCESS

ASSESSMENT

Subjective Data

Obtain information on recent use of tampons, length of time tampon is left in before changing, use of contraceptive sponges, sore throat, headache, myalgia, and fatigue.

Objective Data

Assess erythematous rash, edema, peeling of palms and soles, hypotension, fever, level of consciousness, nonpurulent conjunctivitis, and hyperemia of vagina and oropharynx.

Nursing diagnoses for a client with toxic shock syndrome include the following:

NURSING DIAGNOSES	PLANNING/OUTCOMES	NURSING INTERVENTIONS
Hyperthermia related to inflammatory process	The client will have normal-range temperature within 48 hours.	Administer antipyretics as ordered. Give cooling sponge bath. Encourage oral fluids as tolerated. Monitor body temperature.
Deficient Fluid Volume related to diarrhea, vomiting, fever, and decreased intake	The client will have normal fluid and electrolyte balance within 24 hours.	Administer intravenous fluids as ordered. Encourage oral fluids if client is not vomiting. Monitor I&O. Monitor blood pressure. Administer antiemetic and antidiarrheal medications as ordered. Assess skin turgor and mucous membranes.
Risk for Impaired Skin Integrity related to dehydration and effects of circulating toxins	The client will maintain skin integrity.	Encourage or assist with position change every 2 hours. Provide or assist with personal hygiene, especially after diarrhea. Assess bony prominences for reddened areas.

Evaluation: Evaluate each outcome to determine how it has been met by the client.

EPIDIDYMITIS/ORCHITIS/ PROSTATITIS

Epididymitis can be a sterile or nonsterile inflammation of the epididymis. A sterile inflammation is caused by direct injury or reflux of urine down the vas deferens. Urinary reflux that is related to strain exerted by a male while his bladder is full can be caused by lifting heavy objects or doing strenuous exercises. Nonsterile inflammation may occur as a complication of gonorrhea, chlamydia, mumps, tuberculosis, prostatitis, or urethritis. Prolonged use of an indwelling catheter or an invasive procedure can also lead to nonsterile inflammation.

Signs and symptoms of epididymitis include sudden severe scrotal pain, warmth, redness and swelling, testicular tenderness usually on one side that worsens when having a bowel movement, dysuria, pyuria, chills, fever, penile discharge, and blood in the semen. Treatment includes bed rest, antibiotics, scrotal support (Figure 44-6), and ice compresses to the area. Bilateral epididymitis can cause sterility. Untreated epididymitis leads quickly to testicular tissue necrosis, septicemia, and death.

Orchitis is an inflammation of the testes that most often occurs as a complication of a bloodborne infection originating in the epididymis. Other causes of orchitis include gonorrhea, trauma, surgical manipulation, and tuberculosis and mumps that occur after puberty. In most instances, both testes are involved, and often sterility results. In orchitis, unilateral involvement does not cause sterility. Signs and symptoms of orchitis include sudden scrotal pain with pain radiating to the inguinal canal, scrotal edema, chills, fever, nausea, and vomiting. Treatment includes bed rest, scrotal support, and ice to the area.

Prostatitis, an inflammation of the prostate, is a common complication of urethritis caused by chlamydia or gonorrhea. Infecting organisms may reach the genital tract by direct spread through the urethra or may be borne by blood or lymph. The condition may be acute or chronic, with the chronic form leading to development of fibrotic tissue. This fibrotic tissue causes the prostate to harden, so prostatitis may be difficult to differentiate from prostate cancer. It may take 3 to 6 months for the granulomatous form to resolve. Signs and symptoms of prostatitis include perineal pain, fever, dysuria, and urethral discharge.

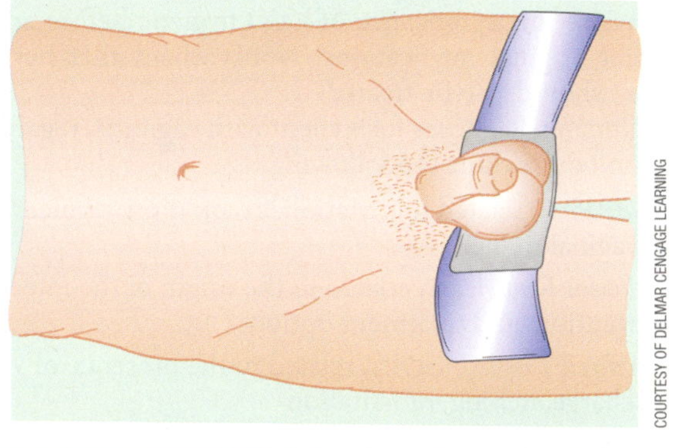

FIGURE 44-6 Bellevue Bridge for Scrotal Support

MEDICAL–SURGICAL MANAGEMENT

Medical

When it is suspected that the client currently has urethritis, he should not be catheterized. The infection spreads rapidly to the genital organs because of the trauma of catheterization and the possible spread of bacteria from the nonsterile distal part of the urethra. The physician may order that segmented bacteriologic localization cultures be obtained.

Pharmacological

Treatment of epididymitis and orchitis includes antibiotics and injection of procaine around the spermatic cord.

Pharmacological treatment of prostatitis includes antibiotics, analgesics, and stool softeners.

Activity

Treatment of prostatitis includes bed rest. While the client is in bed, his scrotum should be elevated and cold packs applied to the area. Encourage the client to drink a large amount of fluids and use sitz baths for comfort. These interventions are used to reduce inflammation, swelling, and discomfort. Periodic digital massage of the prostate by the physician increases the flow of infected prostatic secretions.

Nursing Management

Monitor vital signs, especially temperature and I&O. Encourage intake of oral fluids. Objectively assess client's pain and administer analgesics as ordered. Maintain client on bed rest. Keep scrotum elevated when the client is in bed and have client use an athletic support when ambulatory. Apply cold pack under scrotum as ordered.

NURSING PROCESS

Assessment

Subjective Data

Ask the client about the presence of urethral discharge or dysuria as well as the nature and location of the pain. A description of pain may include arthralgia, low-back pain, and myalgia. A positive history of recent bacterial or viral infection is of special significance. Ongoing nursing assessment includes monitoring of pain, using a pain scale to objectify data. Ask the client if he is experiencing nausea, because this could be a sign that his condition is deteriorating. Assess the client's educational and emotional needs because he may be worrying needlessly about possible sterility or impotence.

Objective Data

Assess vital signs, especially temperature. An increase in temperature may be an indication that the client's condition is worsening. Scrotal edema and purulent urethral discharge may be present. Monitor intake and output. Ask about constipation.

Nursing diagnoses for the male client with an inflammatory disorder include the following:

NURSING DIAGNOSES	PLANNING/OUTCOMES	NURSING INTERVENTIONS
*Risk for **Injury*** related to worsening of the inflammatory process	The client will not experience worsening of his condition.	Monitor client's vital signs, especially his temperature. Report hyperthermia, hypotension, nausea, and tachycardia to the physician immediately.
*Deficient **Fluid** Volume* related to nausea and vomiting	The client will maintain fluid balance.	Monitor client's I&O. Encourage him to drink plenty of fluids when not nauseated.
*Acute **Pain*** related to Inflammation	Using a pain scale of 0 to 10, the client will report pain has decreased to 2 or less within 48 hours after treatment initiation.	Assess client's pain level every 4 hours. Administer analgesics as ordered. Encourage client to maintain bed rest. Provide diversional activities to increase compliance. Encourage client with prostatitis to take a sitz bath, but never the client with epididymitis or orchitis as local heat may increase destruction of sperm cells. Fill a plastic glove with crushed ice and place it under the scrotum when heat is contraindicated. Remove the ice for short intervals every hour to prevent ice burns.
Anxiety related to concerns about possible sterility or impotence	The client will verbalize decreased anxiety.	Reassure client that with proper treatment, sterility and impotence are not likely complications of prostatitis.

Evaluation: Evaluate each outcome to determine how it has been met by the client.

BENIGN NEOPLASMS

Benign neoplasms include fibrocystic breast changes, fibroid tumors, and benign prostatic hyperplasia.

FIBROCYSTIC BREAST CHANGES

Fibrocystic breasts (formerly called fibrocystic breast disease) contain lumpy, nodular, glandular tissue. Fibrocystic breast changes are common between 30 and 50 years of age and occur in more than half of women at some point in their lifetime. Many cases will subside after menopause. The incidence of the potential for developing breast cancer is increased 3 to 4 times with fibrocystic breast changes. There appears to be a familial tendency toward the development of breast cancer.

Lumps may occur as single or multiple cysts that are frequently fluid-filled. It is difficult to differentiate fibrocystic tissue changes from other breast lesions because the dense fibrocystic areas may mask areas of breast cancer. Figure 44-7 shows the differences among cysts, fibroadenomas, and carcinomas of the breast.

The pathophysiology of a fibrocystic breast is found in the formation of fibrous tissue caused by hyperplasia of the epithelial cells in the breast lobules and ducts. The proliferation of the fibrous tissue deviates from the expected normal cyclic response to female hormone shifts during the menstrual cycle.

Routine mammograms provide baseline information and differentiate the palpable breast lumps between benign and malignant types. A computer-directed biopsy may also be performed.

Women should be taught breast self-examination (BSE) as adolescents and encouraged to practice it at the end of each menstrual cycle, when it is easier to palpate the breast tissue. Figure 44-8 provides specific information on how to perform a BSE.

A yellow-greenish, sticky discharge from the nipple is occasionally present with fibrocystic breasts. A Pap smear may be done on the discharge to rule out the presence of malignant cells. Note the presence of any breast discharge and report it to the health care provider as soon as possible. The physician or nurse practitioner (NP) may perform a biopsy or aspiration of the abnormal areas in the office. If fluid is obtained from the area, it is sent to pathology for examination. If no fluid is obtained, it may be a solid cyst or tumor, and biopsy may be required.

In the office, a breast biopsy may be performed with a local anesthetic. If there is any question of malignancy, or if the physician suspects that the lesion will be malignant on the basis of the mammography report, the biopsy may be performed in the hospital under general anesthetic so that additional tissue may be removed if necessary. A frozen section may be obtained and sent to the laboratory for a preliminary examination to rule out a malignant lesion.

Medical–Surgical Management

Surgical

Aspiration or surgical excision may be indicated for diagnostic or therapeutic reasons. The cystic tissue may be aspirated with a small-gauge needle and syringe. The nurse prepares the client for the procedure and assists the doctor or NP with the procedure. The nurse assists the client into a supine position on the examination table and sets up the equipment and instruments needed. The area to be biopsied is cleansed. Upon completion of the aspiration or biopsy, the nurse labels the specimen and sends it to the pathology department.

If the areas of fibrocystic tissue are extensive and have not responded to conservative treatments and methods, or if the risk of cancer is high, the tissue may be excised completely. Removal of fibrocystic tissue does not guarantee that the client will not develop breast cancer in the remaining tissue, and she must continue to perform monthly BSE.

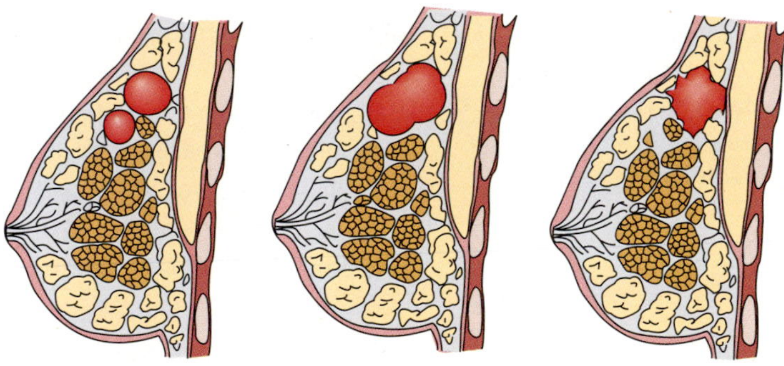

	GROSS CYST	FIBROADENOMA	CARCINOMA
Age	30–50; diminishes after menopause	Puberty to menopause; peaks between ages 20–30	Most common after 50 years
Shape	Round	Round, lobular, or ovoid	Irregular, stellate, or crab-like
Consistency	Soft to firm	Usually firm	Firm to hard
Discreteness	Well defined	Well defined	Not clearly defined
Number	Single or grouped	Most often single	Usually single
Mobility	Mobile	Very mobile	May be mobile or fixed to skin, underlying tissue, or chest wall
Tenderness	Tender	Nontender	Usually nontender
Erythema	No erythema	No erythema	May be present
Retraction/dimpling	Not present	Not present	Often present

COURTESY OF DELMAR CENGAGE LEARNING

FIGURE 44-7 Characteristics of Common Breast Masses

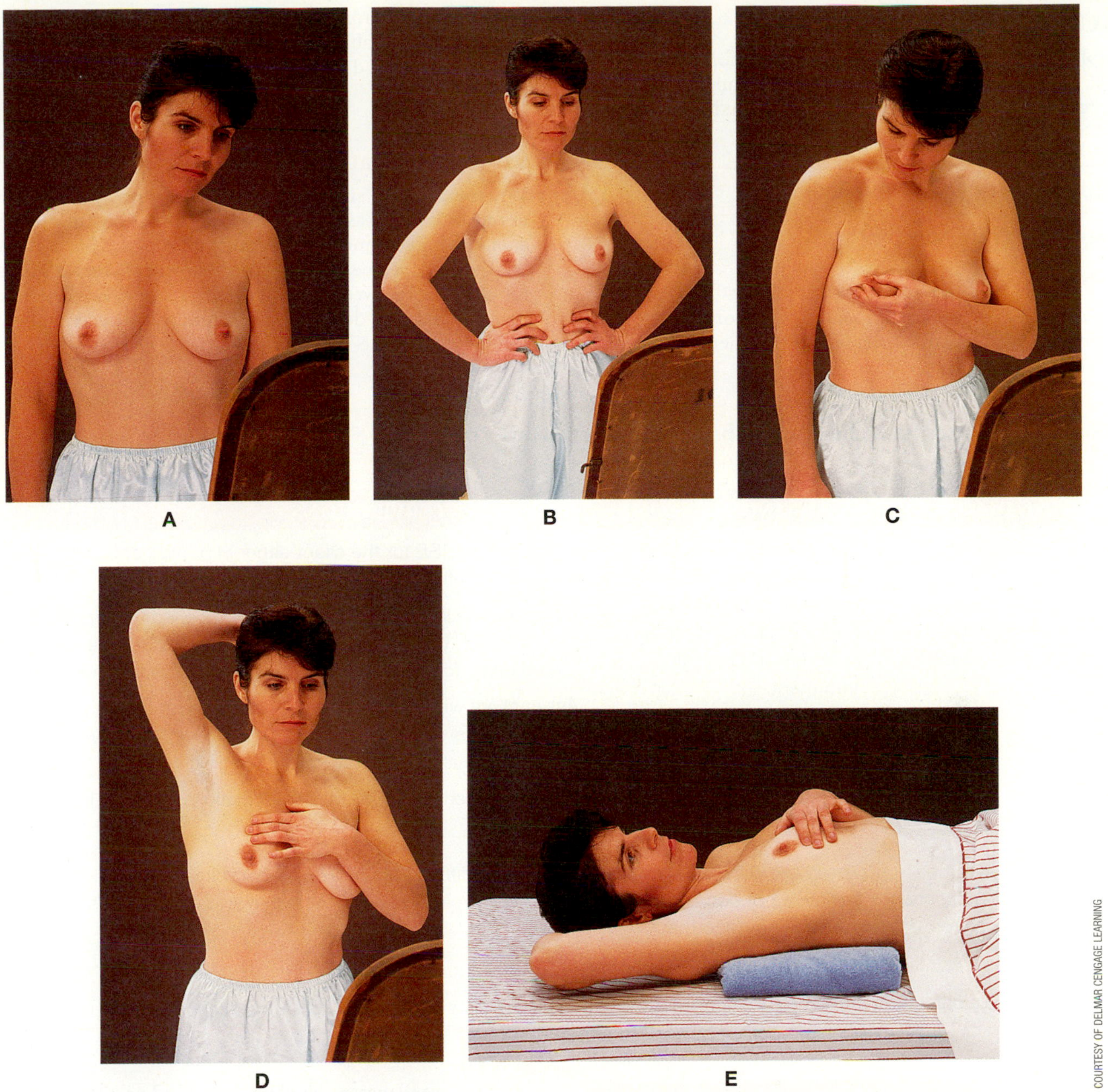

A B C

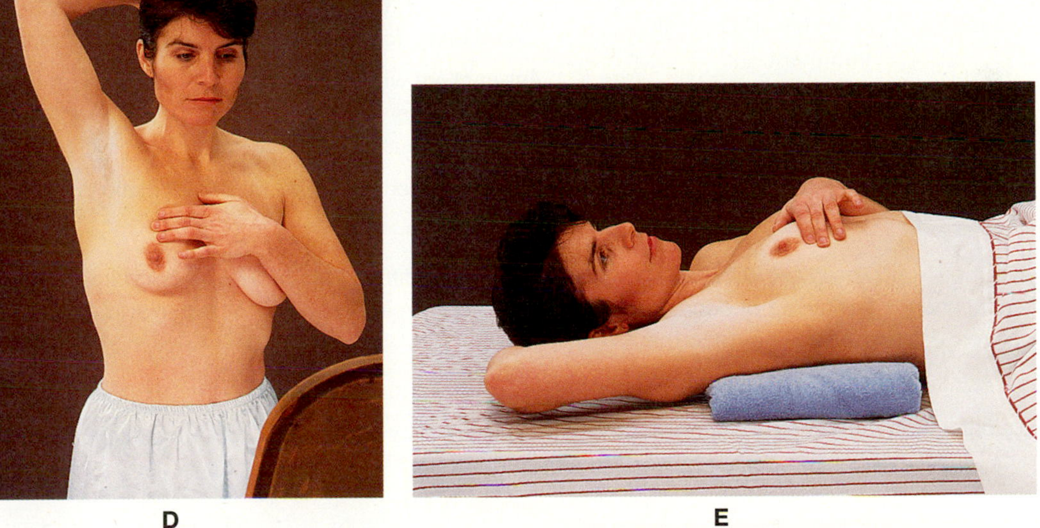

D E

COURTESY OF DELMAR CENGAGE LEARNING

FIGURE 44-8 Performing a Breast Self-Examination; *A,* Standing in front of mirror, check breasts for puckering, dimpling, scaliness, or discharge from nipples; *B,* Clasp hands behind head and press hands forward, watching for changes in the shape or contour of breasts. Press hands on hips and bend toward mirror while pulling shoulders and elbows forward (shown); *C,* Gently squeeze each nipple, looking for discharge; *D,* Raise one arm and use fingers of other hand to check breast for lumps or masses under skin. Use a pattern of motion (circular, up-and-down, etc.) to cover entire breast; *E,* Repeat "D" while lying flat on back with one arm over head and a towel under the shoulder.

CRITICAL THINKING

Breast Self-Examination

How would you teach a client to do a breast self-examination? Make a teaching plan.

Pharmacological

Some physicians recommend up to 600 units of vitamin E daily. It is believed that the vitamin supplement helps break down the fibrocystic tissue because it reacts with the polyunsaturated fats in the cell membrane. It may also have some effect on the balance of female hormones.

Diet

Most health care providers recommend limiting or completely eliminating caffeine-containing products from the woman's diet. This would include teas, colas, coffee, and chocolate. These products are all available in caffeine-free forms. Dietary fat should be decreased to less than 20% of total calories (Mayo Clinic, 2008b).

Nursing Management

Emphasize the importance of the client performing BSE one week following menses and having a mammogram as appropriate for age and risk factors. Teach the client how to perform BSE and to wear a firm, supportive bra.

NURSING PROCESS

Assessment

Subjective Data

The client may report that the lumps are more tender as she approaches her menstrual period and that there is a greenish, sticky discharge from one or both breasts. Inquire about the client's dietary habits, especially caffeine intake, frequency of BSE, and the date of the most recent mammogram, if applicable.

Objective Data

When examined, single or multiple lumps may be palpated in one or both breasts. The lumps are not always discrete but should be freely movable. Because fibrocystic breast lumps are more tender near the menses, the client should be seen for an exam the week after her menstrual period. The tissue contains less fluid during that time and palpation is easier and less uncomfortable.

Nursing diagnoses for a client with fibrocystic breast changes include the following:

NURSING DIAGNOSES	PLANNING/OUTCOMES	NURSING INTERVENTIONS
*Deficient **K**nowledge* related to the cause of fibrocystic breast changes and method of breast self-examination	The client will verbalize and demonstrate her understanding of the cause of fibrocystic breast changes and her role in treatment.	Demonstrate BSE for the client either in person or by video with a follow-up return demonstration by the client. Observe the client as she performs the BSE so that immediate feedback can be given. Explain the best timing for the BSE and the rationale for performing the procedure after the menses. Assist client with mammogram. Encourage mammography at regular intervals dependent upon the client's age and risk factors. Teach the client about dietary modifications, such as limiting caffeine.
***A**nxiety* related to the underlying potential and risk of breast cancer	The client will display behaviors of decreased anxiety related to the potential for breast cancer.	Explain the differences between malignant breast lesions and fibrocystic breast changes to help alleviate the client's anxiety.

Evaluation: Evaluate each outcome to determine how it has been met by the client.

FIBROID TUMORS

Fibroids (leiomyomas) are benign tumors that grow in or on the uterus. A higher incidence is seen with nulliparous women and those who are more than 35 years old. The fibroids may appear below the serosal membrane or the mucosa. An early symptom is often **menorrhagia**, an excessively heavy menstrual flow. Later, the client may experience increasing pelvic pressure as the tumors grow, along with dysmenorrhea, abdominal enlargement, and constipation. Growth of the fibroids is usually slow but can be stimulated by estrogen. During pregnancy, when the estrogen and progesterone levels increase dramatically, the tumors grow much faster. Concern arises for the fetus when the fibroids begin to enlarge and crowd the uterus. Overcrowding may compress the fetus or initiate the onset of preterm labor. With either situation, the pregnancy must be monitored carefully.

A medical diagnosis of uterine fibroids may initially be based on the client's symptoms and the findings of the pelvic examination. If on palpation the uterus feels like an irregular mass or several masses, a pelvic ultrasound or a laparoscopy is ordered to confirm the diagnosis.

Medical–Surgical Management

Medical

The physician may opt to wait and observe the growth pattern of the fibroids before advising the client to have surgery. This

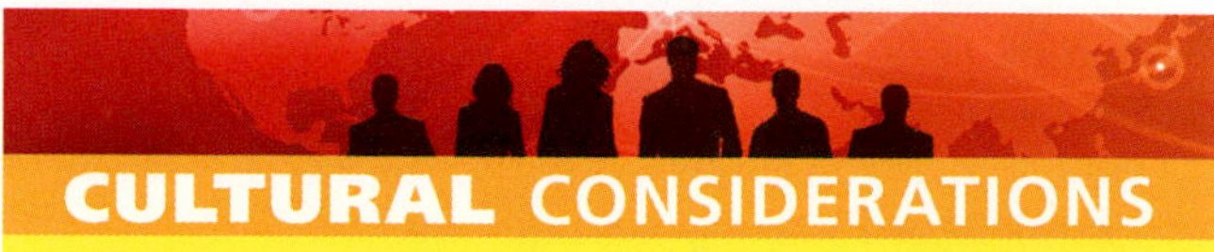

CULTURAL CONSIDERATIONS

Fibroid Tumors

Fibroid tumors are most prevalent in African-American and Mediterranean clients with dark skin.

"wait-and-see" attitude may be swayed by the significance of the client's symptoms, size of the fibroids, amount of discomfort the client is experiencing, and amount of menorrhagia and/or **metrorrhagia**, vaginal bleeding between menstrual periods. Reexamination is encouraged at least every 6 months.

Surgical

If the menorrhagia is significant with each menstrual cycle, a dilation and curettage (D&C) may be performed to determine the exact etiology of the bleeding. A myomectomy, a surgical procedure to remove the tumor, may be performed if the client desires future pregnancies. In the case of severe menorrhagia, with a dropping hemoglobin level or multiple tumors, the physician may recommend a hysterectomy as the option of choice.

Diet

A diet with many sources of iron helps prevent iron-deficiency anemia, which may result from the extra blood loss.

Nursing Management

Monitor vital signs and hemoglobin level. Assess client's blood loss for amount, color, and clots. Objectively assess pain with a 0 to 10 scale and administer analgesics as ordered. Encourage a diet high in iron-containing foods to prevent iron-deficiency anemia.

NURSING PROCESS

Assessment

Subjective Data

Obtain the client's description of menstrual flow, dysmenorrhea, and/or pelvic pain and pressure. The client may also report difficulty fitting into clothes because of abdominal enlargement, constipation, or urinary frequency or urgency.

Objective Data

Count the number of sanitary pads the client saturates in an hour; observe the presence or absence of clots in the blood, a hemoglobin level of less than 12 mg/dL, and the client's pale skin color. Her blood pressure may be slightly lower than normal and her pulse may be increased as a compensatory mechanism.

Nursing diagnoses for a client with fibroids include the following:

NURSING DIAGNOSES	PLANNING/OUTCOMES	NURSING INTERVENTIONS
*Risk for Deficient **Fluid** Volume* related to excessive blood losses	The client will have a hemoglobin above 12 mg/dL and will maintain fluid balance.	Assess client's blood loss for amount, color, and clots. Provide an accurate count of the saturated sanitary pads, along with the length of time taken to saturate a pad. Monitor vital signs at least every 4 hours, or more frequently if the client is having active blood loss. Monitor laboratory reports for Hgb level.
*Acute **Pain*** related to pressure on pelvic structures caused by growing tumors and cramping during the menses	The client will verbalize less discomfort and pelvic pressure.	Assess pain on 0 (least) to 10 (most) pain scale and note location, onset, and duration. Administer analgesics as ordered.

Evaluation: Evaluate each outcome to determine how it has been met by the client.

BENIGN PROSTATIC HYPERPLASIA

Benign prostatic hyperplasia (BPH) is a progressive adenomatous enlargement of the prostate gland that occurs with aging. More than 50% of men older than age 60 and 90% of men older than age 70 have some symptoms of BPH (National Institutes of Health, 2006). Although this disorder is not harmful, the urinary outlet obstruction that may be associated with the disorder is a problem.

Because the urethra is encircled by the prostate, common early symptoms of BPH are related to partial or complete obstruction of the urethra. Early symptoms include **hesitancy** (difficulty initiating the urinary stream), decreased force of stream, urinary frequency, and **nocturia** (awakening at night to void). However, a temporary reduction of these symptoms may occur as the bladder muscles hypertrophy in response to the increased work they must do to force the urinary stream past the obstruction.

Although this bladder muscle compensatory response may temporarily reduce symptoms, eventually the muscle decompensates, becoming noncompliant and hypotonic. This decompensation leads to atony of the mucous membranes between the muscle bands, which causes stagnant urine to collect in the small compartments (cellules) of the membranes. In addition, the man is unable to completely empty the bladder when voiding (**postvoid residual**). Because these changes in urinary function promote urinary alkalosis by increasing the urine pH, a perfect environment for bacterial growth is created. This bacterial growth can cause a urinary tract infection (UTI), which may eventually lead to kidney damage.

Medical–Surgical Management

Medical

The physician performs a digital rectal examination (DRE) to identify any enlargement of the lateral lobes or nodular lumps on the surface of the prostate gland. Diagnostic tests ordered to learn more about the client's condition may include a prostate-specific antigen (PSA), blood test, post-void bladder scan, cystoscopy, rectal ultrasonography, and prostate biopsy. The physician will carefully monitor the client's condition to detect any exacerbation of symptoms such as increased hesitancy, urgency, hematuria, or repeated UTI.

Many alternatives to surgical treatment of BPH have been introduced over the past several years, including balloon dilation of the prostate, a prostate urethral **stent**, as shown in Figure 44-9, and thermotherapy. Balloon dilation of the prostate during an endoscopic examination breaks the prostatic capsule and facilitates decompression of the prostate. A stent is material that is used to hold tissue in place or, in this instance, to provide support to the urethra, which is being compressed by the prostate. An alternative to a transurethral resection of the prostate (TURP) is a thermotherapy transurethral microwave procedure (TUMP) (Daniels, Nosek, & Nicoll, 2007). This outpatient procedure does not correct the problem of incomplete bladder emptying, but does reduce urinary flow symptoms. Another minimally invasive procedure is the transurethral needle ablation (TUNA) system that delivers low-level radiofrequency energy via twin needles to burn away enlarged prostate tissue and improve urine flow with fewer side effects than the TURP (NIH, 2006).

Surgical

The traditional surgical intervention for 90% of all prostate surgeries for BPH is a TURP. This surgery is performed via a resectoscope, an instrument that includes a cutting and cauterization device (Figure 44-10). The client receives either a general or a spinal anesthetic, and the resectoscope is passed through the urethra to remove small pieces of prostate tissue while controlling bleeding. The bladder is continuously irrigated with normal saline or another solution during the procedure. This irrigation is continued during the postoperative period to reduce clot formation that can interfere with urinary drainage.

The traditional surgical alternative to a TURP is open surgery. A suprapubic resection (Figure 44-11), in which the prostate is removed from around the urethra via the bladder, is performed when the prostate mass is large. In a retropubic prostatectomy, the bladder is not opened but instead is retracted and prostatic tissue is removed through an incision in the anterior prostatic capsule. Both of these alternatives involve an abdominal incision. In a perineal prostatectomy, a perineal incision is made and the prostatic tissue is removed through an incision in the posterior prostatic capsule.

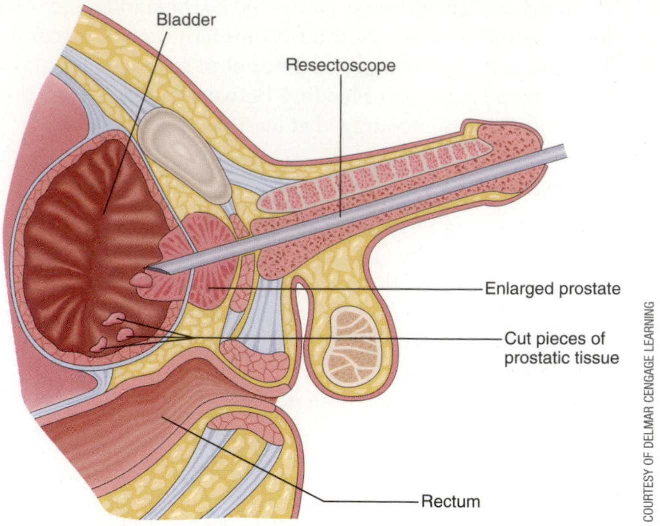

Figure 44-10 Transurethral Resection of the Prostate Gland via Resectoscope

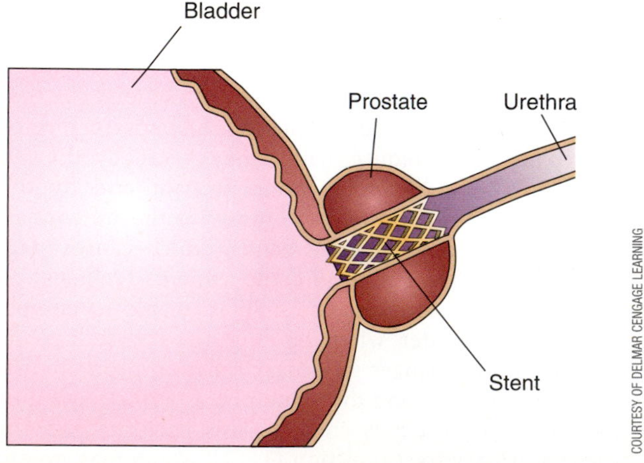

Figure 44-9 Urethral Stent

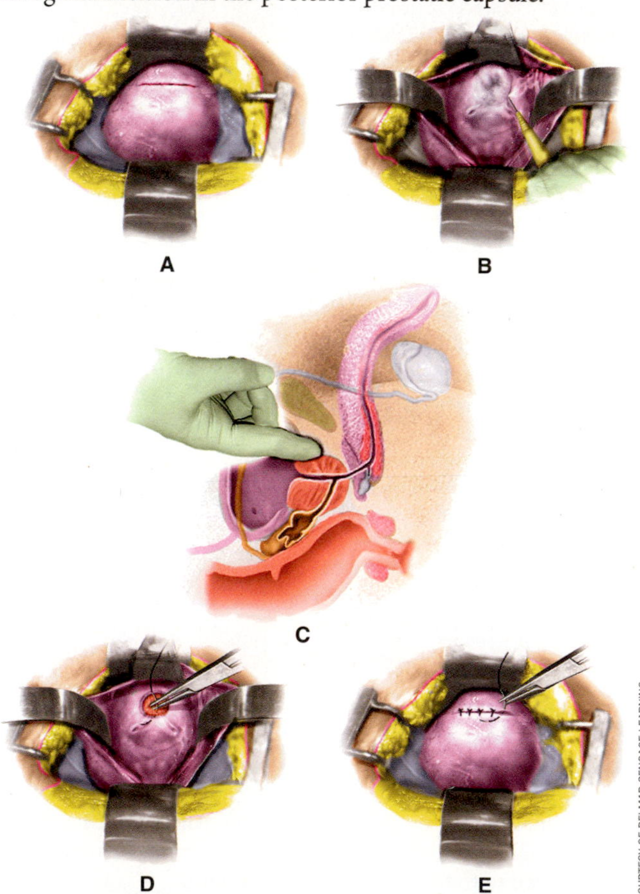

Figure 44-11 Suprapubic Prostatectomy; *A*, Bladder Exposed through Low Transverse Incision; *B*, Bladder Entered; *C*, Blunt Dissection of Prostate; *D*, Prostate Fossa Sutured to Bladder Mucosa

Although these traditional surgeries successfully relieve bladder obstruction, they are costly, and postoperative complications can endanger or seriously affect the quality of a man's life. These complications include hemorrhage, water intoxication, infection, thrombosis, damage to surrounding structures, sexual dysfunction, and urinary incontinence.

Laser prostatectomy is based on thermal action. The transurethral ultrasound-guided laser-induced prostatectomy (TULIP) is performed with a probe that is passed transurethrally into the prostatic urethra. While the adjacent prostate area is visualized by ultrasound, the laser energy is directed at the prostate tissue, resulting in tissue necrosis and sloughing. The client is less likely to experience water intoxication because this surgical method allows blood vessels to seal rapidly, keeping irrigant fluid from being forced into the circulation.

Pharmacological

Finasteride (Proscar) can shrink the prostate in some men. Alpha blockers relax the smooth muscles along the urinary tract without compromising normal urinary control reflexes. Examples are terazosin hydrochloride (Hytrin), doxazosin mesylate (Cardura), alfuzosin (Uroxatral), and tamsulosin Hcl (Flomax). They are also used to treat hypertension, so the side effect of orthostatic hypotension is possible. Belladonna and opium (B & O) suppositories are used to reduce postoperative bladder spasms, and narcotic analgesics are used to relieve postoperative pain.

Nursing Management

When inserting a Foley catheter, remove no more than 1,000 mL initially. Provide preoperative care as ordered. Monitor and accurately record I&O to prevent water intoxication; monitor vital signs and color of urine. Provide routine postoperative care. After catheter removal, encourage client to void with the first urge to prevent increased bladder pressure.

NURSING PROCESS

Assessment

Subjective Data

Ask the client about the presence of urinary frequency, hesitancy, dribbling, number of times he gets up at night to void, and the force of the urinary stream. In addition to a careful general medical history, any information pertaining to a history of chronic urinary tract infections needs to be noted.

Postoperative nursing assessment includes assessing for pain (on a 0 to 10 scale) related to bladder spasms. The client's emotional needs should also be assessed, especially for anticipatory grieving, body image disturbance, anxiety, incontinence, or concerns about alteration in sexuality patterns or possible sexual dysfunction. Observe for client behavioral or verbal cues indicating a need for further information or reassurance about his condition and treatment.

Objective Data

Monitor vital signs but *avoid* the use of a rectal thermometer. A bright red urine color persisting for more than a few hours after surgery may be a sign of hemorrhage. Report hemorrhage, hyperthermia, hypotension (low blood pressure), and tachycardia to the physician immediately.

After a TURP, the client will have a three-way Foley catheter and continuous bladder irrigation for at least 24 hours. Accurately record I&O to ensure that the client has adequate oral intake to promote urinary flow and reduce the infection risk. *In measuring output, the amount of irrigant must be subtracted from the total output in order to determine the actual urinary output.* After the catheter is removed, assess the client for postvoid residual and incontinence. Palpate the abdomen for bladder distention, check the bed linens and clothing for signs of incontinence, and ask the client if he is experiencing loss of urinary control.

Assess for water intoxication, which may be the result of absorbing irrigating fluid in addition to the IV fluids. The most common early symptoms of water intoxication are changes in the client's mental status. These may be manifested by agitation, confusion, and, later, convulsions. The client may also have a slow bounding pulse with an increase in systolic and decrease in diastolic blood pressure.

A suprapubic or retropubic prostatectomy does not require a three-way Foley. Instead, the client will have a urethral catheter, a tissue drain from the prostatic fossa, and an abdominal dressing. Assess for incisional pain and do a dressing check. Especially check the linens underneath the client's back for drainage.

Nursing diagnoses for a postoperative client having a TURP for benign prostatic hyperplasia include the following:

NURSING DIAGNOSES	PLANNING/OUTCOMES	NURSING INTERVENTIONS
*Acute **Pain*** related to bladder spasms or incision	The client will state that pain has decreased.	Assess for pain using a pain scale every 2 to 4 hours. Maintain traction on the urethral catheter by anchoring the catheter to the leg with tape, ensuring that accidental additional traction will not occur with leg movement. Monitor for signs of bladder spasm pain such as facial grimacing, nonflow of irrigating solution into bladder, and urinating around the catheter. Administer analgesics and antispasmodics as ordered. Teach deep breathing, relaxation techniques.

(*Continues*)

Nursing diagnoses for a postoperative client having a TURP for benign prostatic hyperplasia include the following: (Continued)

NURSING DIAGNOSES	PLANNING/OUTCOMES	NURSING INTERVENTIONS
*Risk for Imbalanced **F**luid Volume* related to postoperative irrigation	The client will not experience water intoxication.	Accurately record I&O including irrigation fluid. Monitor for changes in the client's behavior, especially confusion and agitation, which may be the first signs of cerebral edema. Monitor for hypertension, bradycardia, weakness, and seizures.
*Stress or Urge Urinary **I**ncontinence* related to poor sphincter control after catheter removal after surgery	The client will achieve urinary control after removal of the catheter.	Educate the client that temporary urinary incontinence frequently occurs after surgery, and reassure him that this is normal. Teach the client perineal exercises that will help him regain urinary control. These exercises consist of tightening and relaxing gluteal muscles and are to be used each time the client urinates.
***S**exual Dysfunction* related to surgery	The client will regain sexual function postoperatively.	Monitor client's statements to determine if he has any misunderstanding of the surgery and sexual function. Instruct client to avoid sexual intercourse until physician approval is given and that it may take time for his previous level of sexual function to return. Encourage client to use a variety of forms of sexual expression, such as kissing, stroking, and cuddling. Provide client with opportunities to voice his feelings and ask questions. Teach client that it is normal and not harmful if his urine has a milky appearance due to retrograde ejaculation.

Evaluation: Evaluate each outcome to determine how it has been met by the client.

MALIGNANT NEOPLASM

Malignant neoplasms include breast, cervical, endometrial, ovarian, prostate, testicular, and penile cancers.

BREAST CANCER

Breast cancer is the second major cause of cancer death among women. Statistics indicate that 1 woman in 8 will develop breast cancer some time during her life. The American Cancer Society (ACS) estimates that 192,370 new cases were diagnosed in the United States in 2009. The 5-year survival rate is 98% for localized stage and 89% for all stages combined (ACS, 2008). Older adult women (older than 61) have twice the incidence of breast cancer as do younger women. Less than 1% of all breast cancers occur in men; in 2008, approximately 1,990 new cases of breast cancer were diagnosed in men (ACS, 2008).

The key to cure is early detection by physical examination, mammography, and BSE. A new painless mass or lump is the most common presenting symptom.

Because it is so uncommon, breast cancer in men is all the more dangerous. Late diagnosis is quite common; therefore, males need to be educated in the technique of and encouraged to perform BSE. Signs and symptoms of breast cancer include breast masses, lumps, thickening, and generalized swelling of part of a breast; skin dimpling, redness, scaliness, and irritation; nipple pain, retraction (Figure 44-12), or discharge other than breast milk.

Women at greatest risk for developing breast cancer are those who:

- Had a mother or sibling with breast cancer
- Never had children or had their first child after the age of 30
- Never breast-fed
- Have a history of fibrocystic breast changes
- Started menstruating before age 10
- Are obese
- Consume a high-fat diet and a moderate amount of alcohol

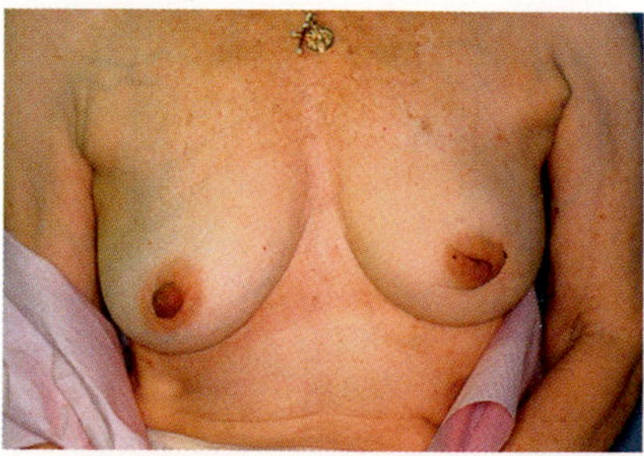

FIGURE 44-12 Nipple Retraction of Left Breast (*Courtesy of Steven M. Lynch, MD.*)

- Smoke
- Experienced a late menopause
- Are physically inactive
- Take postmenopausal hormone therapy
- Have had previous chest radiation to treat different cancer

A woman generally presents at the health-care office after the discovery of a lump in her breast. If she has been performing BE routinely each month, she is likely to be familiar with even minute changes in her breast tissue. Breast cancers often occur in the upper, outer quadrant of the breast and may extend into the tail of the breast and spread upward into the axilla (Figure 44-13). It is important to teach clients to examine the axillary region as well as the breast during BSE (Figure 44-8).

Women also seek medical advice because they notice a discharge from the breast, dimpling of the skin, retraction of the nipple, pain, a unilateral change in breast size, or an orange-peel appearance (peau d'orange) of the skin (Figure 44-14). Dimpling and puckering are usually associated with the breast tissue or tumor attaching to the skin or the underlying muscle mass, which does not permit movement. The nurse should not be misled by the client's report of a tender lump or mass and assume it is fibrocystic breast changes. All new or enlarged lumps or masses in the breast require immediate assessment.

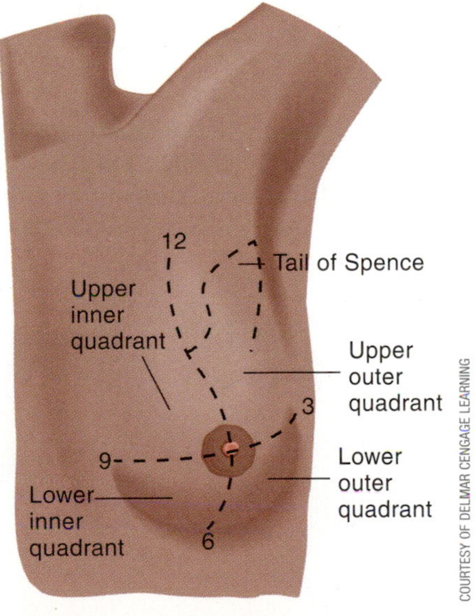

FIGURE 44-13 Quadrants of the Left Breast

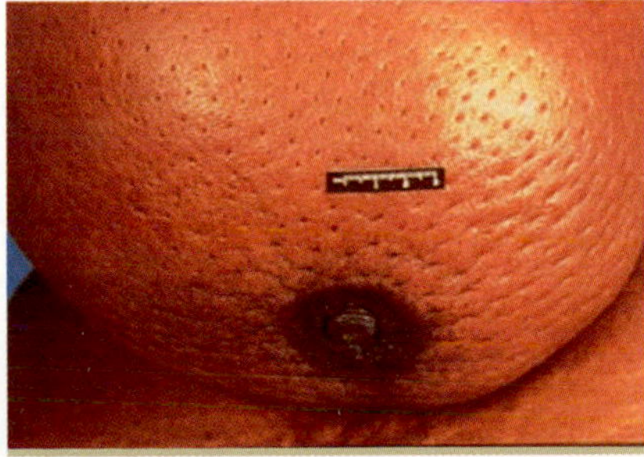

FIGURE 44-14 Peau d' Orange (*Courtesy of Dr. S. Eva Singletary, University of Texas, M.D. Anderson Cancer Center.*)

MEMORY TRICK
Staging Breast Cancer

Using a staging system provides a standardized method for health care providers to summarize how far the breast cancer has spread. The most common system used is the American Joint Committee on Cancer's **TNM** system. This staging system classifies cancers based on their **T**, **N**, and **M** stages:

T = Tumor (the size and how far has it spread within the breast and to nearby organs)

N = Nodes (spread to lymph nodes)

M = Metastasis (spread to distant organs)

(American Cancer Society, 2009b)

The presence of tiny, palpable clusters of calcium, or "microclusters," may be an early sign of breast cancer. These should be followed closely with mammography every 6 to 12 months to detect subtle changes in shape or size.

The American Cancer Society (2009) recommends that women ages 20 to 39 perform BSE each month and have a clinical breast examination every 3 years. For women age 40 and older, BSE should be performed monthly, a clinical examination every year, and a mammogram every year.

Mammography may be performed by the stereotactic computer-guided technique. This advanced method allows needle biopsies to be taken at the same time if necessary. The physician or nurse practitioner may recommend this method after an initial mammogram has shown suspicious areas. This technique is less costly than excisional biopsy and can be performed with little discomfort to the client. The client is placed in a prone position on the special examination table with the breast hanging down through the opening in the table. The operator moves the position of the table to visualize the entire breast area via computerized guidance.

After the breast has been biopsied and the tissue has been examined by the pathologist, if a malignancy is confirmed, the client may be advised to proceed with surgical removal (lumpectomy or mastectomy) of the affected tissue. Figure 44-15 shows the staging of breast cancer.

MEDICAL–SURGICAL MANAGEMENT

Medical

Radiation and chemotherapy are used as adjuvant therapy, but surgery is the primary treatment. Other types of treatment for breast cancer include targeted therapy, immunotherapy, photodynamic therapy, gene therapy, hyperthermia, and antiangiogenesis therapy. For more information about these treatments go to the American Cancer Society website at www.cancer.org.

Surgical

There is an abundance of lymphatic vessels proximal to the breast. Malignant cells can thus escape into the general lymphatic

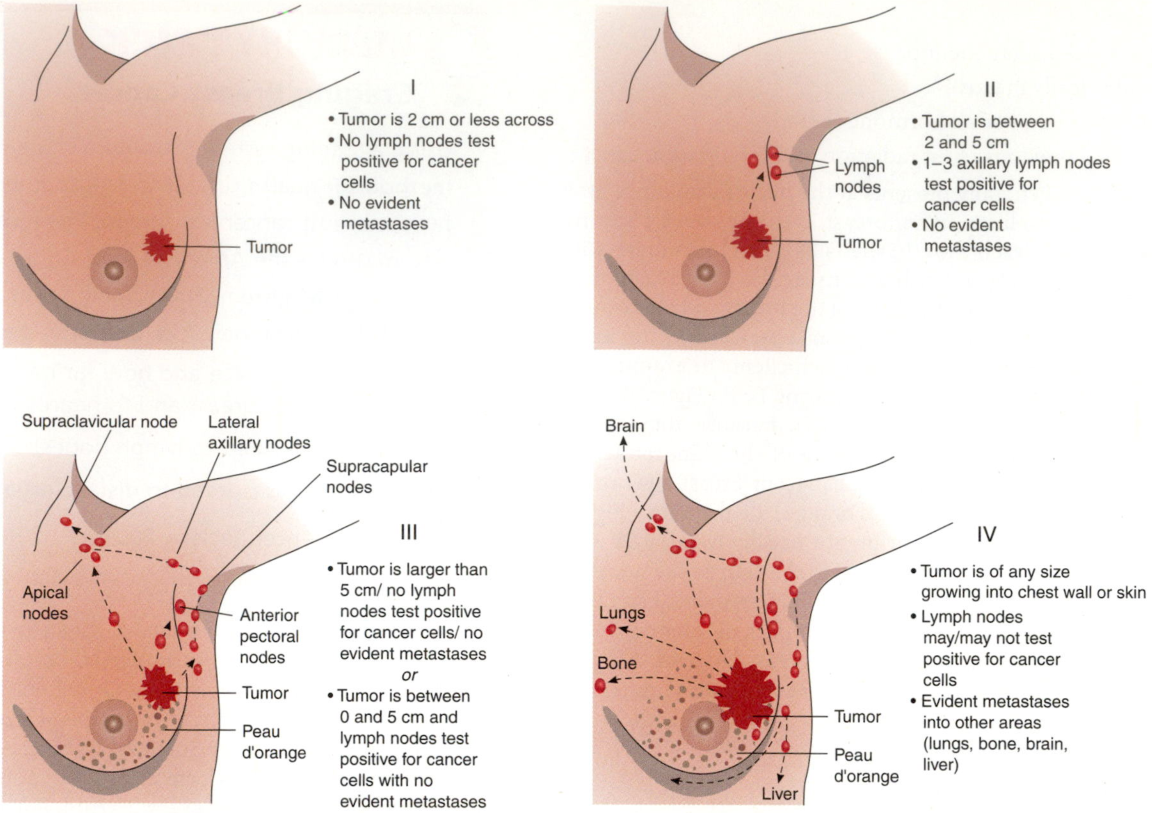

I

- Tumor is 2 cm or less across
- No lymph nodes test positive for cancer cells
- No evident metastases

Tumor

II

- Tumor is between 2 and 5 cm
- 1–3 axillary lymph nodes test positive for cancer cells
- No evident metastases

Lymph nodes

Tumor

III

- Tumor is larger than 5 cm/ no lymph nodes test positive for cancer cells/ no evident metastases

or

- Tumor is between 0 and 5 cm and lymph nodes test positive for cancer cells with no evident metastases

Supraclavicular node

Lateral axillary nodes

Supracapular nodes

Apical nodes

Anterior pectoral nodes

Tumor

Peau d'orange

IV

- Tumor is of any size growing into chest wall or skin
- Lymph nodes may/may not test positive for cancer cells
- Evident metastases into other areas (lungs, bone, brain, liver)

Brain

Lungs

Bone

Tumor

Peau d'orange

Liver

COURTESY OF DELMAR CENGAGE LEARNING

FIGURE 44-15 Breast Cancer Staging

system and be spread throughout the body. A lumpectomy is surgical removal of the cancerous mass. A simple mastectomy removes the tumor mass and only a small portion of the adjacent tissue. In the modified mastectomy, the entire breast tissue and nearby lymph nodes are removed; the muscles of the chest wall are left relatively intact (Figure 44-16A). With the radical mastectomy, the entire breast, lymph nodes, and underlying pectoralis muscle are removed (Figure 44-16B). Figure 44-17 shows the various options in the surgical management of breast cancer. The greater the extent of the surgical removal, the longer the client's recovery process and the greater the need for rehabilitation in using the upper extremity on the affected side.

The more lymph nodes that are removed, the greater the chance the client will have lymphedema, an accumulation of lymph in soft tissue. An elastic sleeve may be worn for compression, and range-of-motion (ROM) exercises may reduce edema. A sodium-restricted diet may be ordered.

Reconstructive surgery after a mastectomy may be determined by the amount of breast tissue and muscle remaining after the initial procedure, the position of the mastectomy scar, and the probability of recurrent breast cancer. Breast reconstruction can help the client deal with the disfigurement that results from the mastectomy.

The client's desire for reconstruction and her psychological status play an important role in determining the personal value of additional surgery. In the United States particularly, the breast is associated with childbearing and female sexuality. It may be difficult for the client to express her concerns to her partner regarding her sexuality and desirability after the mastectomy. She may have difficulty facing the physical alteration immediately after surgery and for some time after. The nurse with good interpersonal communication skills can help the client identify and verbalize her feelings of loss, thus promoting the psychological healing process and acceptance of altered body image.

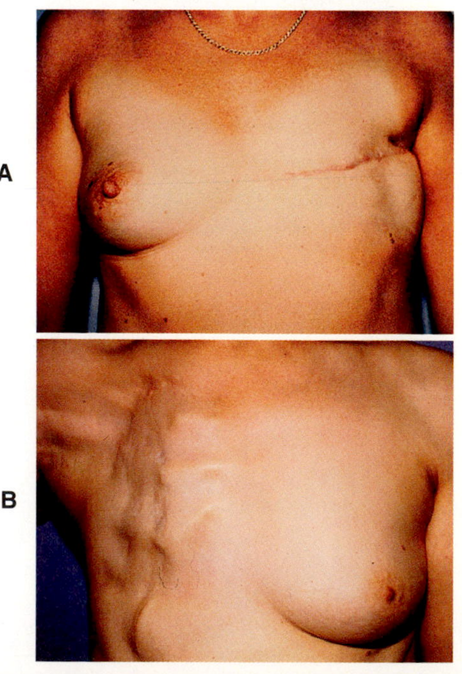

FIGURE 44-16 Mastectomy Clients; *A*, Modified Radical; *B*, Radical (*Courtesy of Steven M. Lynch, MD.*)

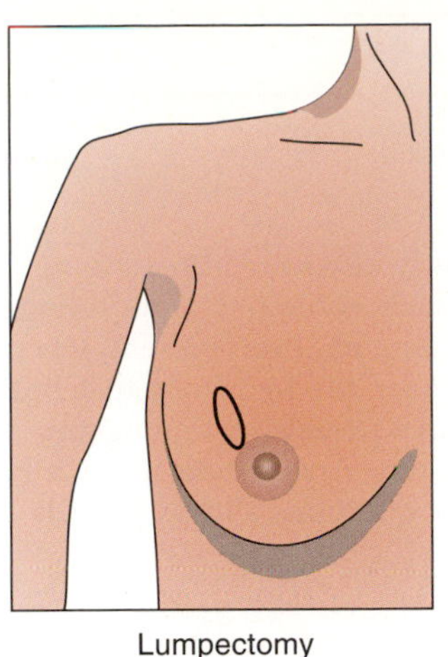

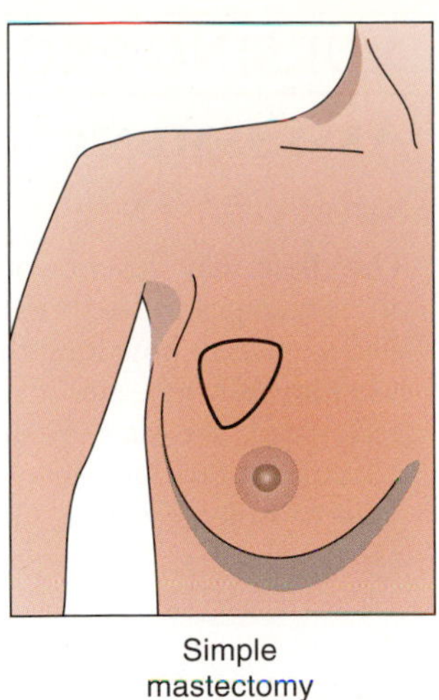

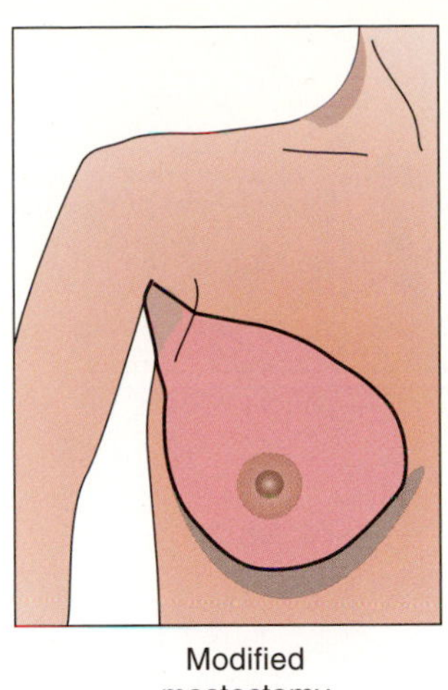

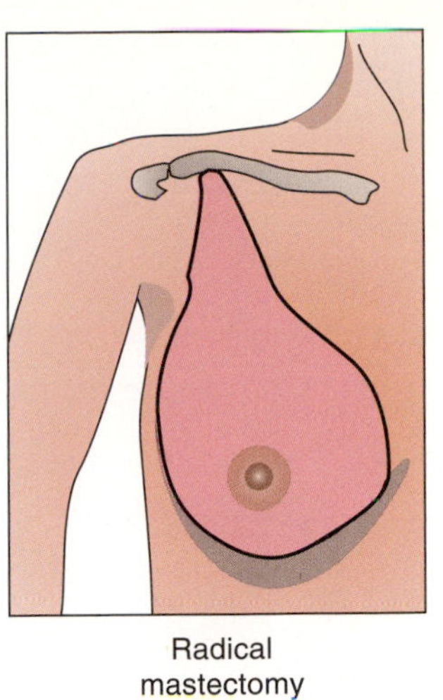

COURTESY OF DELMAR CENGAGE LEARNING

FIGURE 44-17 Surgical Options for Breast Cancer

Breast prostheses constructed to look and feel like real breast tissue are available. The prosthesis fits into a special pocket inside the brassiere. Some types are available for swimsuits and strapless tops. The construction of the prosthesis varies from sponge rubber to fluid- or air-filled.

Volunteers from the local cancer society often visit new mastectomy clients to assist them in the physical and psychological transition and adjustment after breast surgery.

Pharmacological

Some of the agents used to treat breast cancer include antineoplastic drugs such as antiestrogens: megastrol acetate (Megace), and tamoxifen (Nolvadex). Additional agents include androgens for postmenopausal clients includes testolactone (Teslac) or rotating combinations of chemotherapy agents such as cyclophosphamide (Cytoxan), an alkylating agent, doxorubicin hydrochloride (Adriamycin), an antitumor antibiotic; 5-fluorouracil (Adrucil) and methotrexate sodium (Rheumatrex); antimetabolites; and prednisone (Orasone), a glucocorticoid via intravenous or oral routes. These drugs may be used before or after surgery. These antineoplastic agents act in several ways to either inhibit cellular growth or interfere with DNA replication. A laboratory test called tissue assay determines if estrogen or progesterone stimulates the cancer cells to grow. If the cancerous growth is stimulated by estrogen, antiestrogen drugs are used to treat the breast cancer. When the tumors are not estrogen-dependent, estrogen is used as a chemotherapy agent to treat breast cancers. Examples of two estrogen medications are diethylstilbestrol diphosphate (Stilphostrol) and ethinyl estradiol (Estinyl).

Paclitaxel (Taxol) has demonstrated positive results in clinical trials with breast cancer therapies. It acts by prohibiting cell replication. One of the benefits of this agent is that it causes milder nausea than many of the other chemotherapy agents that are used. It has the potential to cause severe anaphylactic reactions resulting from a histamine release. To avoid this problem, the client should be medicated with the following medications before Taxol infusion therapy: a corticosteroid such as dexamethasone (Decadron), a histamine blocker such as cimetidine (Tagamet), and an antihistamine diphenhydramine hydrochloride (Benadryl).

COMMUNITY/HOME HEALTH CARE

After a Mastectomy

- Avoid carrying items in the affected arm or wearing purse straps over the affected shoulder.
- Have vaccinations, blood pressure, and lab tests or blood drawn on the unaffected side only.
- Obtain immediate medical attention for all injuries and infections of the affected side to prevent complications.

Tamoxifen (Nolvadex) is used in certain high-risk women to reduce the incidence of breast cancer (Spratto & Woods, 2009).

Other Therapies

Breast tissue and lymphatic regions may be radiated before or after surgical excision of the tumor. This treatment may be done prophylactically to prevent the metastasis of malignant cells to other areas, or it may be done as a palliative measure to maintain the client's comfort. Figure 44-18 illustrates brachytherapy, the use of radioactive implants (needles, seeds, wires, or catheters) at the site of breast cancer.

Nursing Management

Encourage all clients to perform BSE and have a mammogram and clinical evaluation as recommended. Actively listen to client's fears and concerns and reinforce the information from the physician or nurse practitioner. Provide routine preoperative care. Identify the client's support system. Encourage client to contact the local American Cancer Society and Reach to Recovery support groups.

Postoperative care includes monitoring vital signs, drains, and dressing, and for signs of hemorrhage or shock. Encourage client to turn, cough, and deep breathe. If arm is not restricted by the dressing, elevate it with the hand highest to encourage fluid flow through the venous and lymph routes.

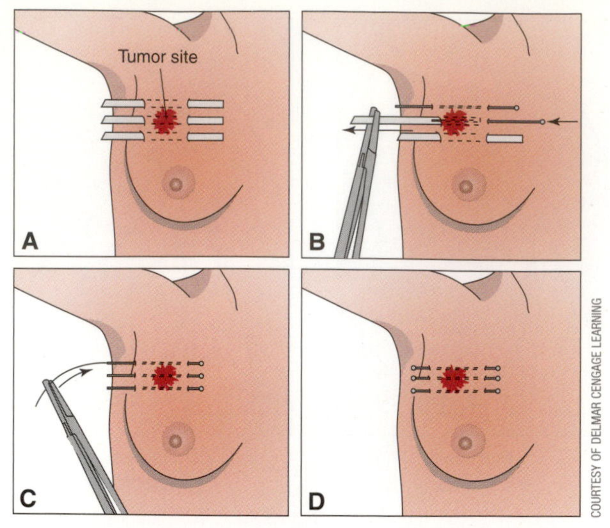

FIGURE 44-18 Brachytherapy for Treatment of Breast Cancer; *A,* Hollow Metal Needles are Placed at Site; *B,* Hollow Plastic Catheters Replace Metal Needles; *C,* Radioactive Material is Placed in Catheters, with Metal Buttons Holding the Catheters in Place; *D,* Radioactive Implants Remain in Place for Treatment

NURSING PROCESS

ASSESSMENT

Subjective Data

The client may describe a newly discovered breast lump and other changes in the breast, such as dimpling, puckering, or discharge. Ask how long the lump has been present, whether it is movable, whether it is tender, the frequency that BSE is performed, the date of the most recent mammogram, and current medications being taken. Assess pain using a pain scale to objectify data. Other questions should include the risk factors.

Objective Data

Assess vital signs and weight and review the report of the last mammogram. Examine the breasts for lumps and discharge from the nipples. During the postoperative phase, assess the client's vital signs and incisional site. Monitor client's statements and behaviors to determine emotional status.

Nursing diagnoses for a client with breast cancer include the following:

NURSING DIAGNOSES	PLANNING/OUTCOMES	NURSING INTERVENTIONS
Fear related to breast cancer, possible metastasis, surgery, and disfigurement	The client will express fears. The client will state one positive method of coping.	Encourage client to express specific feelings of fear. Take extra time to clarify or explain procedures and treatments. Provide written information along with verbal information. Encourage support of family members and significant others, and a preoperative visit by a member of the cancer society, Reach to Recovery, and local support group.
*Disturbed **B**ody Image* related to removal of the breast	The client will discuss her feelings related to the loss of her breast and demonstrate acceptance of the change in physical appearance.	Remain attentive to signals from the client indicating readiness to look at the surgical site and encourage doing so when readiness is displayed. Be alert for client's comments regarding body changes. Encourage client recommended for chemotherapy to obtain a wig before therapy begins. Approximately 80% of clients undergoing chemotherapy will experience hair loss, and, if the client becomes accustomed to wearing a wig before hair begins to fall out, the client may feel more comfortable later. Inform client that she may have decreased sensation and lymphatic fluid retention in the arm on the affected side. Teach client to keep arm on affected side elevated above the level of the heart to promote lymph drainage, and to wear a properly fitting elastic compression sleeve on the affected arm that will help reduce the lymphedema. Anticipate the client's need to grieve the loss of her breast. Encourage use of rehabilitation services (Reach to Recovery).

Nursing diagnoses for a client with breast cancer include the following: (Continued)

NURSING DIAGNOSES	PLANNING/OUTCOMES	NURSING INTERVENTIONS
*Ineffective **B**reathing Pattern* related to the proximity of the surgical incision to respiratory muscles and pain with respiratory effort	The client's breath sounds will remain clear to auscultation. The client will effectively cough and deep breathe every 2 hours.	Preoperatively, teach the client how to turn, cough, and deep breathe. Postoperatively, assess the client's breath sounds, rate, and quality of respirations every 4 hours. Monitor O_2 saturation with pulse oximeter. Encourage deep breathing or the use of incentive spirometry every hour. Provide O_2 as needed. Medicate the client or encourage use of the PCA pump before performing exercises or deep breathing.
***S**elf-Care Deficit* related to limited use and range of motion on the affected side and postoperative discomforts	The client will gradually regain ROM and provide self-care.	Begin passive range-of-motion exercises on the first or second postoperative day as ordered. Demonstrate postoperative exercises for the affected arm or request a consult from the physical therapy department. Observe the client as exercises are performed and reinforce correct performance. Encourage active ROM as soon as ordered by the physician to strengthen the operative side. This may be difficult at first due to tissue soreness from surgery. Encourage client to provide self-care as much as able.

Evaluation: Evaluate each outcome to determine how it has been met by the client.

SAMPLE NURSING CARE PLAN

The Client with Breast Cancer

C.W., age 57, is married, with two children ages 24 and 22. During a bath, she noted a small, movable lump in her right breast, grew concerned, and went to see her health-care provider. Family history is significant for fibrocystic breast disease and breast cancer on the maternal side (mother, aunt, sister). Personal history: onset of menses at age 10 with regular 28-day cycle, 5-day flow. She is 5 feet 5 inches tall and weighs 175 pounds. Her history is negative for alcohol use, but she smokes one to one-and-a-half packs of cigarettes daily. She did not breastfeed the children. Her last mammogram was 15 years ago. BSE is not practiced routinely. States: "I'm not sure just how to do the exam anyway."

Physical examination reveals a pea-sized lump in the upper right quadrant of the right breast and multiple clusters of lumps throughout each breast. Dimpling is present superior to the nipple. No nipple discharge was noted. The remainder of the exam was unremarkable. Vital signs were within normal limits. A mammogram revealed a suspicious mass, and a biopsy performed using stereotactic visualization was positive for cancer cells. A modified mastectomy was performed the next day with biopsies of adjacent lymph nodes. Six of ten nodes were also positive.

The morning after surgery, C.W. displayed behaviors that the nurse interpreted as anxiety. She confided in the nurse that she was afraid she was going to die, as her mother had, from the cancer. C.W. had a large chest pressure dressing with two Jackson-Pratt drains in place. She stated that she was glad she had the PCA pump to take care of the pain.

(Continues)

SAMPLE NURSING CARE PLAN (Continued)

NURSING DIAGNOSIS 1 *Bathing/Hygiene and Dressing/Grooming **S**elf-Care Deficit*, related to temporary altered function of arm as evidenced by large chest pressure dressing and two drains in place

Nursing Outcomes Classification (NOC)
Self-Care: Activities of Daily Living (ADLs)
Comfort Level

Nursing Interventions Classification (NIC)
Self-Care Assistance: Bathing/Hygiene
Self-Care Assistance: Dressing/Grooming
Pain Management

PLANNING/OUTCOMES	NURSING INTERVENTIONS	RATIONALE
C.W. will meet her daily hygiene needs before discharge.	Assess C.W.'s ability to use affected arm to perform ADLs.	Provides baseline information of C.W.'s abilities and limitations.
	Provide assistance as needed to complete hygiene tasks, such as bathing and grooming.	Assisting with tasks and encouraging C.W. to participate will facilitate the return of function and self-esteem.
	Encourage gradual resumption of activities as C.W. indicates readiness.	Empowers C.W. to help perform her own care, validating her self-image and worth, and she will regain strength and maintain the mobility of the extremity.

EVALUATION

C.W.'s hygiene needs were met.

NURSING DIAGNOSIS 2 ***F**ear*, related to removal of the breast as evidenced by her fear of dying as her mother had

Nursing Outcomes Classification (NOC)
Anxiety Control
Coping

Nursing Interventions Classification (NIC)
Anxiety Reduction
Coping Enhancement

PLANNING/OUTCOMES	NURSING INTERVENTIONS	RATIONALE
C.W. will have less fear about breast removal.	Encourage C.W. and family to verbalize their feelings and concerns related to the diagnosis and treatment.	Relieves fear, and perceptions that differ from that of the health-care worker are identified.
	Assess C.W.'s normal or previously used coping behaviors.	Enables the nurse to help C.W. use or change coping behaviors.
	Involve C.W. and her family in care planning.	Makes them more likely to feel a part of the team rather than simply accepting a passive "client role."

EVALUATION

C.W. verbalized having less fear about the removal of her breast.

SAMPLE NURSING CARE PLAN (Continued)

NURSING DIAGNOSIS 3 *Acute **Pain**,* related to surgical manipulation of tissues and excision of tissue as evidenced by client statement that she was glad she had the PCA pump to take care of the pain

Nursing Outcomes Classification (NOC)	Nursing Interventions Classification (NIC)
Symptom Severity	*Pain Management*
Pain Level	*Patient-Controlled Analgesia (PCA) Assistance*

PLANNING/OUTCOMES	NURSING INTERVENTIONS	RATIONALE
C.W. will verbalize that pain is controlled.	Assess C.W.'s pain level and response to analgesia every 2 hours.	Alerts the nurse to increasing pain and C.W.'s tolerance of the pain medication.
	Instruct C.W. how to use the PCA pump.	Allows C.W. control over analgesia and provides consistent pain relief.
	Evaluate the effectiveness of analgesia every 2 hours.	Allows the nurse to identify any untoward effects and effectiveness of the medication.
	Reposition C.W. every 2 hours.	Helps improve vascular flow and relieves pressure on bony prominences.
	Elevate the right arm on pillows.	Decreases edema and discomfort due to pressure on nerves in the area.

EVALUATION

C.W. reports pain is controlled at less than 2 on a 1 to 10 scale.

CERVICAL CANCER

An abnormal condition of the cervix known as dysplasia may be an early sign of developing cervical cancer. Dysplasia is a change in the size and shape of the cervical cells, and it is classified as mild, moderate, or severe. An abnormal Papanicolaou (Pap) smear may be the first indication of a problem.

Cervical cancer is the most preventable gynecological cancer. Sexual habits constitute a major factor in the development of cancer of the cervix. Sexually transmitted infection, particularly the human papillomavirus (HPV), is a particularly significant factor (ACS, 2009c). Other factors associated with cervical cancer include smoking, long-term use of oral contraceptives, immunosuppression, multiple pregnancies, family history, diet low in fruits and vegetables, obesity, a history of multiple sexual partners and maternal use of diethylstilbestrol (DES) during pregnancy. The most common sign of cervical cancer is abnormal bleeding, which progresses from a thin, watery, blood-tinged discharge to frank bleeding. Contact bleeding may also occur after intercourse. Advanced disease is indicated by odor, pain in the lower back and groin, difficulty in voiding, hematuria, and rectal bleeding. The Pap smear is the key to early detection. Promotion of regular pelvic exams and education regarding risk are essential.

Although cervical cancer can occur at any age, it occurs most frequently in women between 30 and 50 years of age. It is insidious because it is asymptomatic. Cervical cancer has a high cure rate in the early stages, and it is easily detected by the routine annual Pap smear. The overall 5-year survival rate is 74% (ACS, 2009c). The two main types of cervical cancer are squamous-cell carcinoma (80% to 90%) and adenocarcinoma (10% to 20%) (ACS, 2009c).

The nurse should immediately bring any abnormal Pap smear results to the attention of the physician or nurse practitioner so the client can be notified and the appropriate follow-up treatment initiated. A repeat Pap smear may be indicated after treatment with a vaginal antibiotic cream, or a colposcopy may be performed.

Staging of the cancer progresses from I to IV (Figure 44-19). Carcinoma *in situ* (CIS) means that the cancerous cells remain within the cervix and have not yet spread to adjacent areas. The greater the number on the staging table, the more the cancer has metastasized to other structures.

MEDICAL–SURGICAL MANAGEMENT

Surgical

Treatment modalities may include conization, a surgical excision of a cone-shaped section of the abnormal cervical tissues.

STAGING SYSTEM FOR CANCER OF THE CERVIX	
Stage	Characteristics
I	• Carcinoma is strictly confined to cervix (extension to corpus should be disregarded)
IA	• Preclinical carcinoma
IA1	• Minimal microscopically evident stromal invasion
IA2	• Microscopic lesions no more than 5 mm depth measured from base of epithelium surface or glandular from which it originates, and horizontal spread not to exceed 7 mm
IB	• All other cases of stage I; occult cancer should be marked "occ"
II	• Carcinoma extends beyond cervix but has not extended to pelvic wall; it involves vagina, but not as far as lower third
IIA	• No obvious parametrical involvement
IIB	• Obvious parametrical involvement
III	• Carcinoma has extended to pelvic wall; on rectal examination, there is no cancer-free space between tumor and pelvic wall; tumor involves lower third of vagina; all cases with hydronephrosis or nonfunctioning kidney should be included, unless they are known to be due to another cause
IIIA	• No extension to pelvic wall, but involvement of lower third of vagina
IIIB	• Extension to pelvic wall, or hydronephrosis or nonfunctioning kidney due to tumor
IV	• Carcinoma has extended beyond true pelvis or has clinically involved mucosa of bladder or rectum
IVA	• Spread of growth to adjacent pelvic organs
IVB	• Spread to distant organs (lungs, liver)

COURTESY OF DELMAR CENGAGE LEARNING

FIGURE 44-19 Cervical Cancer Screening

This procedure is desirable if the client is of childbearing age and wants children in the future.

Laser surgery, cryosurgery (freezing of the cells with liquid nitrogen), or cauterization (burning) may be performed as alternative methods of treatment if the cervical lesions are easily visible for the procedure. A total hysterectomy or radical pelvic surgery may be required to eradicate the cancer. If the spread of the disease has become too extensive, treatment will be directed toward palliative measures.

Other Therapies

The physician may recommend the use of radium implants or radiation therapy before the surgical excision of the cervix. The nurse must be cautious in providing nursing care for the client with radium implants. Pregnant nurses or female nurses of childbearing age should not care for this client or spend extended periods at the bedside. Direct client care should be organized to optimize time spent at the bedside. A sign should be hung on the door to indicate that radiation is being used in the room and provide a warning for visitors to limit their visit time. With the implants in place, the client will remain on complete bed rest.

In addition, chemotherapy may be utilized as an adjunct therapy to help shrink the tumor or slow its growth.

Nursing Management

Provide therapeutic emotional support to the client to help her cope with the diagnosis. After surgery, monitor vital signs and I&O. Encourage client to ambulate as ordered and to turn, cough, deep breathe, and use a spirometer. Assist with active and passive ROM exercises. Provide careful catheter care.

NURSING PROCESS

Assessment

Subjective Data

The client may describe postcoital bleeding (bleeding after intercourse) or spotting between menstrual periods or after menopause and, occasionally, a foul-smelling vaginal discharge. As the disease progresses, she may describe increased or bloody discharge, weight loss, and pain that radiates down the lower back and legs.

Objective Data

Objective data may include the presence and appearance of a vaginal discharge. The cervix may appear eroded or raw and may bleed easily when touched with a cotton-tipped applicator or Pap scraper. Necrotic tissue may be present and cause a foul odor. Pap smear results can indicate dyplasia. Tissue samples obtained through colposcopic examination may show cellular changes. In advanced disease, weight loss and anemia may be present. Laparotomy may be performed to stage the disease and along with other laboratory and diagnostic testing to identify metastases, which are most likely to occur in the rectum, vagina, bladder, and pelvis.

Nursing diagnoses for a client with cervical cancer include the following:

NURSING DIAGNOSES	PLANNING/OUTCOMES	NURSING INTERVENTIONS
Anxiety related to unknown outcome and possible treatments	The client will verbalize having less anxiety about treatment and possible outcome.	Be aware of the client's emotional state throughout the course of care and use effective interpersonal communication to facilitate the client's acceptance of her condition and the treatments. Explain diagnostic tests and procedures to client to decrease her anxiety. Provide therapeutic emotional support to client to help her cope with feelings.
Sexual Dysfunction related to vaginal bleeding, discomfort, and procedures	The client will return to normal sexual function after recovery from treatment for cervical cancer.	Inform client that she may experience dyspareunia related to vaginal dryness after radiation therapy. Instruct client to use a water-soluble lubricant during intercourse or to use lubricated condoms to decrease irritation. Listen to client's concerns.
Impaired Urinary Elimination related to sensory motor impairment from radiation effects	The client will regain normal urinary elimination.	Assess the function of the Foley catheter to ensure patency and drainage. Provide careful catheter care. Promote urination when catheter is removed. Record I&O, including color of urine. Encourage the client to drink fluids to flush the kidneys and decrease risk of UTI.

Evaluation: Evaluate each outcome to determine how it has been met by the client.

ENDOMETRIAL CANCER

Postmenopausal women are at the greatest risk for endometrial cancer, especially if they have taken estrogen replacement therapy for several years (usually more than 5 years). Research has shown that unopposed estrogen stimulation of the endometrial lining has a strong relationship with the development of endometrial cancer. During the normal menstrual cycle, estrogen and progesterone rise and fall. These hormonal fluctuations affect the stimulation of the endometrial tissue to grow and be sloughed off. Without the progesterone effects, the endometrial tissue is not sloughed off at regular intervals and may undergo cellular changes, leading to a high risk for endometrial dysplasia or cancer. For this reason, many physicians and nurse practitioners have recommended estrogen-progesterone therapy for clients who experience menopausal symptoms.

In summer 2002, the data and safety monitoring board for the Women's Health Initiative study of estrogen/progestin recommended stopping the trial because of an increased risk of invasive breast cancer (Fletcher & Colditz, 2002). It is recommended that long-term use of this combination be stopped.

Other risk factors associated with endometrial cancer may include never having borne a child, being Caucasian, being middle class, never having had sexual intercourse, use of oral contraceptives, total number of menstrual cycles, use of tamoxifen, obesity, diabetes, and family history.

Cancer of the endometrium usually does not produce symptoms until it becomes relatively advanced. Routine Pap smear and pelvic examinations are inadequate for early diagnosis. An endometrial biopsy, which examines the tissue from the uterine lining under a microscope, is the best diagnostic tool to identify cellular changes. This may be done on an annual basis when the client has a routine examination. The medical follow-up treatment plan depends on the biopsy results. D&C has a potential for spreading the cancer cells to adjacent tissues because the malignant cells may escape into the bloodstream at the time of the procedure. This is not usually a problem with the biopsy because the amount of tissue removed is so small and blood loss is minimal. A D&C is also more expensive, higher risk, and requires some type of anesthesia.

MEDICAL–SURGICAL MANAGEMENT

Treatments for endometrial cancer may range from radiation, radium implants, chemotherapy, or surgery to a combination of any of the above. The choices of treatment are related to the staging of the cancer.

PROFESSIONALTIP

Radiation Exposure Risk

Because of the risk of radiation exposure to the caregiver from the radiation implant device, keep procedures that require exposure to the client's perineal area at a minimum.

Medical

Intravenous fluid administration will be implemented to replace fluids lost by the excessive bleeding. A blood transfusion may be ordered for a low hemoglobin. A hemoglobin above 10 gm/dL is preferred before surgical intervention. The physician may order whole blood or packed red blood cells to increase the hemoglobin rapidly.

Surgical

Surgery for endometrial or cervical cancer includes hysterectomy. A total hysterectomy is removal of the cervix and the uterus. In a subtotal hysterectomy, only the uterus is removed and the cervix remains. A radical or pan hysterectomy includes removal of the ovaries, cervix, uterus, fallopian tubes, pelvic lymph nodes, and part of the vagina. Vaginal hysterectomy procedures have been refined with the laparoscopic approach so that many clients are released from the hospital within 24 to 36 hours postoperatively. If the cancer has spread beyond the uterus into the pelvic region, an abdominal hysterectomy may be the best approach for visualization during surgery. The physician may recommend a course of radiation therapy after surgery.

Pharmacological

Drug therapy includes the use of the chemotherapy agents doxorubicin (Adriamycin), cisplatin, carboplatin, and paclitaxel (Taxol). Two or more drugs may be combined for treatment such as cisplatin and doxorubicin. Side effects of chemotherapy depend on the drug taken, the amount, and the length of time the client has been taking the drug.

Other Therapies

There is a tendency for endometrial cancer to confine itself to the uterus, which increases the client's 5-year survival prognosis. Endometrial cancer also usually responds well to the therapies available at this time, including radiation. Radiation may be delivered to the pelvic region via external sources, or it may be delivered via intracavitary devices or implants with radium or cesium. There is a potential danger for injury to adjacent pelvic structures during radiation therapy. The nurse should be alert for signs of complications, such as bleeding from the rectum, moderate to severe abdominal pain, constipation, or diarrhea.

Nursing Management

One of the earliest symptoms reported by many clients is vaginal bleeding. For the postmenopausal client, it is imperative that all bleeding be investigated immediately unless it is from hormonally induced periods. Late in the progression of the cancer, the client may experience symptoms similar to those discussed with cervical cancer. Pain is often associated with the spread of cancer to adjacent organs and is considered a late sign.

Objective data may be collected from the client's physical exam findings, biopsy reports, and a history of hormone replacement therapy with or without the estrogen-progesterone combination.

OVARIAN CANCER

Ovarian cancer most often originates in the epithelial tissue of the ovary, and, like cervical and endometrial cancer, does not produce symptoms until it is in an advanced, inoperable stage. It is sometimes called "the silent killer." Its symptoms are vague and may be ignored for a long time before the client seeks medical attention. According to Lehman (2007), the first national consensus statement on ovarian cancer symptoms was issued and recognizes that the symptoms of bloating, abdominal or pelvic pain, difficult eating, feeling full quickly, and urinary urgency or frequency are more likely to occur in woman with ovarian cancer than women in the general population (Lehman, 2007).

Ovarian cancer causes more deaths than does any other gynecological cancer, an estimated 14,600 in 2009 (ACS, 2009d; Lehman, 2007). The incidence is greatest in women between 45 and 65 years of age. Nulliparity (never having borne a child), smoking, alcohol use, infertility, and a high-fat diet are factors that place the client at higher risk for developing ovarian cancer. Metastasis occurs in more than 75% of cases before diagnosis, and often the cancer has spread beyond the pelvis. The colon is the most frequent site of ovarian cancer metastasis, then the stomach, and diaphragm.

Unfortunately, medical research has not yet developed an early diagnostic or screening tool to detect ovarian cancer. It is believed, however, that there is an increased risk of ovarian cancer for clients with breast cancer and vice versa. A family history of two or more female relatives with breast or ovarian cancer provides a sound rationale for more frequent breast and pelvic examinations. Often, the physician or NP palpates an ovarian mass on a routine bimanual examination. This finding is cause for further investigation by pelvic ultrasound or CT scan to determine the size, character, and consistency (solid or fluid-filled) of the mass and whether other pelvic structures are involved. Some experts believe that there is a link between the occurrence of ovarian cysts and the development of ovarian cancers in certain women.

General diagnostic studies, such as a lower GI series, chest x-ray, intravenous pyelogram (IVP), transvaginal ultrasound, and laparoscopy may be useful in determining the extent of the primary and secondary lesions. A blood test, CA-125 assay, measures a tumor marker CA-125 that is often higher than normal in women with ovarian cancer (Lehman, 2007). If the client develops peritoneal fluid or ascites as the cancer progresses, it may be removed by paracentesis for cytologic examination.

Recurrent disease is common and may occur in 2 years or less. Continued medical surveillance is recommended every 2 months for a period of 2 years for the earliest possible detection of new lesions. The 5-year survival rate is 45% (ACS, 2009d).

Medical–Surgical Management

Surgical

Surgical excision of the ovary is rarely successful because of the extensiveness of the disease. A total abdominal hysterectomy with a bilateral salpingo-oophorectomy or omentectomy is performed for most stages of the disease. Most often, a combination of radiation, chemotherapy, immunotherapy, and surgery produces the best results, even if they are only palliative for the client. The client must be actively involved and informed of her treatment options as well as her prognosis to enable her to make sound choices in the treatments chosen.

Pharmacological

Chemotherapy drugs that are used with ovarian cancer treatment include cyclophosphamide (Cytoxan), doxorubicin hydrochloride (Adriamycin), mitomycin (Mutamycin), cisplatin (Platinol), paclitaxel (Taxol) and carboplatin. For intravenous chemotherapy, carboplatin is preferred over cisplatin due to being as effective and having less side effects (ACS, 2009d). In 2006, the National Cancer Institute encouraged physicians to use a combined approach of intraperitoneal (IP) chemotherapy in addition to intravenous chemotherapy (Lehman, 2007). Intraperitoneal chemotherapy administers paclitaxel (Taxol) or cisplatin (Platinol) directly into the client's abdominal cavity. This technique can add a year to the lives of women with advanced stages of ovarian cancer. Combination chemotherapy is the standard approach for treatment of ovarian cancer. These may be administered by regional or intraarterial perfusion techniques. These percutaneous modes direct the drugs to the lesion's vascular supply. If the cancer has not metastasized, a regimen of chemotherapy using a single drug, such as Cytoxan, may be administered over the course of 5 days and repeated again at regular intervals over the course of a year. A combination of the chemotherapy agents, used in a rotating series, is often more effective for reproductive cancers in advanced stages. For example, the client would receive one drug over the course of 5 days, then switch to another drug for 5 days, and then a third drug for 5 days. This series may be repeated over the year in a similar pattern to that used with a single agent.

Sometimes two or three different medications are necessary to achieve pain control. Intravenous medications are often given by a PCA pump with continuous low-dose narcotics. This method seems more effective for the client than IV bolus doses every 4 hours. Medications may also be given slow IV push (an RN procedure), orally in tablets or liquids, intramuscularly, or by transdermal patches (Duragesic). A liquid mixture of syrup, cocaine, morphine, alcohol, flavoring, and water called "Brompton's mixture, elixir, or cocktail" may be ordered. The client may drink up to 20 mL every 3 to 4 hours for pain relief. Most of these methods of narcotic administration are equally effective and may be used in the home care or hospice setting. Other types of medication that may be given include tranquilizers, antiemetics, and laxatives.

Nursing Management

Accurately measure the client's legs to ensure the proper fit of antiembolic stockings. Provide comfort measures of back rub and position change. Teach client about skin care if receiving radiation. Assess bowel sounds and for abdominal distention. Maintain an accurate I&O record.

NURSING PROCESS

Assessment

Subjective Data

The client may describe fatigue, malaise, diarrhea or constipation, pelvic pressure, frequency of urination, loss of appetite, nausea, weight gain or loss, vaginal bleeding or spotting with intercourse, a foul-smelling vaginal discharge, and pain in the lower back. The list of symptoms is very vague and could be related to many reproductive and nonreproductive disorders.

Objective Data

Objective data pertinent to all cancers of the pelvic reproductive organs may include information from the client's previous health history, reproductive history (onset of menses, pregnancies, contraceptive methods, infections, hormonal replacement therapy, and surgeries), the discovery of a palpable mass during a bimanual examination, an abnormal appearance of the cervix or adjacent tissues, abnormal Pap smear results greater than Class II dysplasia, abnormal cervical or endometrial biopsies, increased abdominal girth, or the presence of ascites and pleural effusion.

Diagnostic tests and laboratory studies may include all or some of the following: Pap smear, pelvic ultrasound, chest x-ray, IVP, kidney/ureters/bladder x-ray (KUB), CBC with differential, blood chemistry studies, bleeding and clotting time, endometrial biopsy, cervical biopsy, D&C tissue specimens, Schiller's test and colposcopy, laparoscopy, barium enema, and bone scan.

Nursing diagnoses for a client with endometrial or ovarian cancer include the following:

NURSING DIAGNOSES	PLANNING/OUTCOMES	NURSING INTERVENTIONS
Preoperative:		
Fear related to tentative diagnoses, pending surgical procedures, cancer treatment and its side effects, incapacitating or extended illness with resulting dependence, and possible death	The client will verbalize fears and have behaviors consistent with reduced fear before and after surgery.	Facilitate client's expression of fear by encouraging the client's open discussion of her concerns. Be alert for nonverbal cues as well. Arrange a consultation with a social worker or chaplain, if appropriate.
*Chronic **Pain*** related to the spread of cancer throughout the pelvis and adjacent structures	The client will have pain controlled at a level that allows continual functioning in her activities of daily living as long as possible.	Administer analgesics as ordered. Provide comfort measures, such as position changes and back rub.

(*Continues*)

Nursing diagnoses for a client with endometrial or ovarian cancer include the following: (Continued)

NURSING DIAGNOSES	PLANNING/OUTCOMES	NURSING INTERVENTIONS
Postoperative:		
*Impaired **S**kin Integrity* related to surgical interventions, radiation, and chemotherapy side effects	The client's skin integrity will be maintained.	Provide client with proper skin-care instructions during and after radiation therapy that may include avoiding soaps, creams, powder, deodorants, and other substances around the incision that may irritate the skin; not washing off the radiation markings; and avoiding tight clothing around the area. Teach client to look for signs of reactions to radiation therapy, such as tenderness, flushed color (like a sunburn), delayed wound healing, and itching. Perform daily cleansing of the incisional area with water only. If client is on complete bed rest due to radium implant therapy, provide a complete bedbath as well as morning and bedtime skin care. Organize time near the client's bedside to brief periods to avoid overexposure to radiation. Wear rubber gloves when disposing of soiled materials. Put soiled dressings in a biohazard waste container.
*Impaired **U**rinary Elimination, **B**owel Incontinence, or **C**onstipation* related to the proximity of surgical site to bowel and bladder, spread of cancer to adjacent structures, manipulation of organs during surgery, administration of narcotic analgesics, lack of activity, and changes in dietary intake	The client will have adequate bowel and bladder function during the postoperative period.	Explain dietary modifications designed to reduce residue. The diet should be limited in dairy products, raw fruits, grains, and vegetables. Meats must be well cooked and possibly ground. If client is not receiving radium implant therapy, weigh her daily on the same scale at the same time of the day. Review client's normal elimination patterns from the baseline assessment data to help identify early changes in bowel or bladder elimination. Forewarn client of radiation enteritis and cystitis, and common tissue responses to radiation therapy. Instruct her to report symptoms, such as diarrhea, cramping, frequency, urgency, and dysuria. Assess bowel sounds and abdominal distention at least every 4 to 8 hours. Carefully monitor the client's urinary pattern and maintain an accurate intake and output record. Observe urine and stool for color, consistency, amount, and the presence of blood. Monitor client for other gastrointestinal problems, such as nausea, vomiting, and **tenesmus** (spasmodic contraction of the anal or bladder sphincter, causing pain and a persistent urge to empty the bowel or bladder).
*Impaired Physical **M**obility* related to intracavity radiation	The client will not develop deep vein thrombosis.	Accurately measure client's legs to ensure the proper fit of the hose. Apply thigh-high antiembolic stockings (TEDS) as ordered. Assist client to ambulate when allowed.

Evaluation: Evaluate each outcome to determine how it has been met by the client.

PROSTATE CANCER

Prostate cancer is the second leading cause of cancer deaths in men. According to 2009 estimates by the ACS, 192,280 new cases were diagnosed. Survival rate for all cases is nearly 100%. Incidence increases with age, as 70% of all prostate cancers are diagnosed in men older than age 65. Improved detection methods have greatly increased the number of individuals having positive outcomes. Diagnostic tests that may be performed are measurement of serum prostate-specific antigen (PSA), transrectal ultrasonic examination, DRE, and prostatic biopsy. Studies indicate that the PSA alone for routine screening is not especially useful. The American Cancer Society (2009f) recommends a yearly PSA level and digital rectal examination to screen for prostate cancer in men age 50 and older with a life expectancy of more than 10 years.

Most prostatic cancers are adenocarcinomas, slow-growing tumors that spread through the lymphatics. Early symptoms include dysuria, a weak urinary stream, and increased urinary frequency. Later symptoms are related to complete urethral obstruction or hematuria. Blood in the urine (**hematuria**), which can lead to anemia, occurs because of the rupture of blood vessels that have been overstretched.

MEDICAL–SURGICAL MANAGEMENT

Treatment depends on the extent of the disease and the age of the client.

Medical

Radiation is the traditional alternative to surgical removal of the malignant prostate gland; however, radiation may fail to eradicate the tumor or may lead to diarrhea, bowel obstruction, lymphocele formation, edema of the extremities, pulmonary embolism, wound infections, infection, impotence, incontinence, or radiation cystitis. An alternate successful radiation treatment option for early-stage prostate cancer is transrectal assisted radioactive seed implant. With the use of ultrasound, the physician is able to precisely position the rice-sized radioactive seeds inside the malignant prostate gland.

Surgical

Surgical treatment of prostatic cancer involves removal of the entire prostate gland, including the capsule and adjacent tissue. The urethra is then anastomosed to the bladder neck. Sometimes the perineal approach is used, but the usual approach is retropubic prostatectomy. Since 2003, a newer approach is the robotic-assisted laparoscopic radical prostatectomy using a robotic interface called the "da Vinci" system. The surgeon sits at a panel controlling the robotic arms to perform the operation through small incisions in the client's abdomen. This method has shown less blood loss and shorter recovery time than the standard radical prostatectomy.

Because of the proximity of the bladder sphincters to the prostate gland, urinary incontinence may be a complication. Other complications include sexual dysfunction and the universal surgical risks of hemorrhage, infection, thrombosis, and strictures. Removal of the testes (**orchiectomy**) may also be done as a palliative measure to help eliminate the androgenic effect that promotes tumor growth.

Cryosurgery (freezing) was used in the 1960s but abandoned because of tissue sloughing and fistula development. With the advent of the transrectal ultrasound and the transurethral warming device, cryosurgery is again a viable alternative.

> **PROFESSIONALTIP**
>
> **Risk Factors for Prostate Cancer**
>
> - Advancing age (more than 55 years)
> - First-degree relative with prostate cancer
> - African American heritage
> - High level of serum testosterone (Estes, 2010)

The ultrasound allows the surgeon to selectively freeze prostate gland tissue while the temperature of the prostatic urethra is kept at 44°C by irrigation with heated water. This approach is an option for those who cannot tolerate more extensive surgery, have a localized tumor, or do not have successful radiation treatment. It can be performed more than once, involves a shorter hospital stay, and produces fewer side effects.

Pharmacological

Hormonal agents such as diethylstilbestrol (DES), luteinizing hormone releasing hormone agonist (LHRH) leuprolide acetate (Lupron), and nonsteroidal antiandrogens flutamide (Eulexin) may be used in the management of advanced prostate cancer. Chemotherapy drugs used to treat prostate cancer include paclitaxel (Taxol), carboplatin (Paraplatin), mitoxantrone (Novantrone), and vinblastine (Velban). A combination of prednisone and docetaxel (Taxotere) is used in clients with advanced prostate cancer.

NURSING MANAGEMENT

Encourage all male clients older than age 40 to have an annual rectal examination of the prostate and a PSA serum level. Monitor vital signs (*no rectal temperature*), urinary output, and fluid intake. Assess urine for signs of bleeding. Objectively assess for pain and administer analgesics as ordered. Keep perineal area clean and dry.

NURSING PROCESS

ASSESSMENT

Subjective Data

The client may seek care for BPH, which often accompanies cancer of the prostate. He may describe back pain or sciatica, frequency, dysuria, or nocturia.

Objective Data

Complete a physical assessment, including palpation of the abdomen and skin assessment. Palpate the abdomen to determine if there is any bladder distention. Skin assessment is important because the client is at risk for skin breakdown. There may or may not be hematuria present. Vital signs, the incisional site, and intake and output must all be assessed. Report hyperthermia, hypotension, tachycardia, or increased incisional drainage to the physician immediately.

A catheter is used postoperatively to maintain urinary drainage and as a splint for the urethral anastomosis rather than for hemostasis, so there are minimal bladder spasms. Monitor catheter patency by assessing the drainage for color, amount, and presence of clots. If the tubing is not draining freely, reposition or milk it. Call the physician if these measures fail to restore patency. During the first week of the postoperative period, monitor the client for fecal incontinence related to relaxation of the perineal sphincter. This complication occurs when the perineal surgical approach is used because the incision is made between the scrotum and the rectum.

Nursing diagnoses for a client (postoperative) with prostate cancer include the following:

NURSING DIAGNOSES	PLANNING/OUTCOMES	NURSING INTERVENTIONS
Urinary Retention related to urethral obstruction, secondary to urethral anastomosis.	The client will not experience urinary retention.	Monitor the client's urinary output, noting the amount, color, and presence of clots. The urine should not appear bright red for more than a few hours postoperatively, after which time it should be dark red. Reposition or milk the catheter tubing if not patent. If these interventions fail, notify the physician. Monitor the client's intake, encouraging a fluid intake of 2,500 to 3,000 mL/day.
Bowel Incontinence related to loss of rectal sphincter control becauseof perineal incision	The client will achieve rectal sphincter control.	Teach the client that temporary fecal incontinence frequently occurs after a perineal incision. Teach the client perineal exercises that will help him regain bowel control. Avoid the use of rectal thermometers, rectal examinations, and enemas.
Risk for Impaired Skin Integrity related to incontinence	The client will not experience skin breakdown.	Keep the client clean and dry, especially if he is experiencing fecal or urinary incontinence and reposition every 2 hours.

Evaluation: Evaluate each outcome to determine how it has been met by the client.

TESTICULAR CANCER

Although testicular cancer accounts for only 1% of all cancer in men, it is the most common cancer in young men between the ages of 15 and 35. According to the ACS (2009g), advances in treatment have made the 5-year survival rate 96%. The etiology is unknown, but the incidence is highest in men with undescended testicles and those whose mothers had taken hormones during pregnancy. A small, hard, painless lump is usually the first symptom noted.

Because early diagnosis of testicular cancer is so essential for a positive surgical outcome, men need to be taught how to perform a testicular self-examination (TSE) and be encouraged to routinely perform that examination (Figure 44-20).

TSE is performed as follows:

- Perform TSE after a bath or shower when scrotum is warm and most relaxed.
- Grasp testis with both hands and palpate gently between thumbs and forefingers.
- The testis should feel smooth, egg-shaped, and firm to the touch.
- The epididymis, located behind the testis, should feel like a soft tube.
- Any abnormal lumps or changes in the testes should be reported to a physician.

MEDICAL–SURGICAL MANAGEMENT

Medical

Testicular ultrasound is used to study the testes for enlargement or lesions. In addition to a testicular ultrasound, the client may have a blood test for alpha-fetoprotein (AFP) and human chorionic gonadotropin (hCG). These proteins are called tumor markers, and when elevated levels are present in the blood it suggests testicular cancer.

Surgical

Biopsy of the testis is contraindicated because of the increased potential for metastases. Surgical removal of the testis, spermatic cord, and inguinal canal contents, with examination of the nodes, is indicated for testicular cancers. If unilateral removal of a testis is indicated, the remaining healthy testis will continue to maintain sperm and androgen production.

Pharmacological

Although chemotherapy and radiation are used as adjuvant treatments, radical inguinal orchiectomy remains the primary intervention. Combination chemotherapy with cisplatin (Platinol), vinblastine sulfate (Velban), and bleomycin sulfate (Blenoxane) is effective.

CRITICAL THINKING

Testicular Self-Examination

How would you teach a client to do a testicular self-examination? Make a teaching plan.

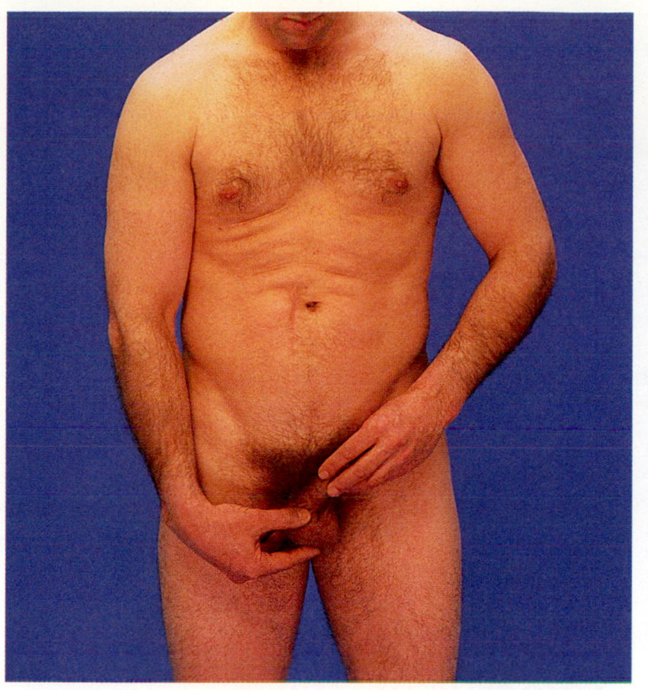
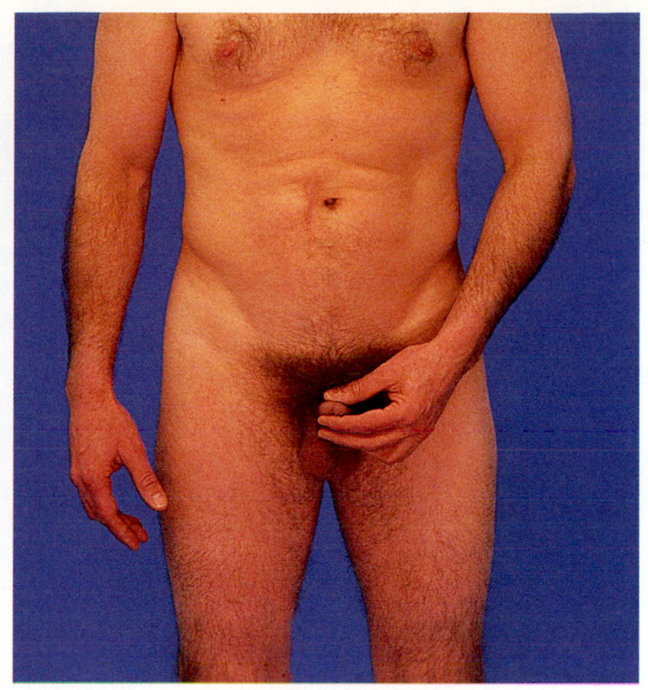

COURTESY OF DELMAR CENGAGE LEARNING

FIGURE 44-20 Performing a Testicular Self-Examination

NURSING MANAGEMENT

Encourage all male clients older than age 15 to perform testicular self-examination monthly. Cancer is suspected in a testicle that is hard. Postoperatively, monitor vital signs and incisional drainage. Maintain strict asepsis when changing dressings. Provide opportunities for the client to voice fears and concerns.

NURSING PROCESS

ASSESSMENT

Subjective Data

The client may describe a feeling of heaviness in the scrotum and may mention weight loss. During the postoperative phase, the client needs to be assessed for pain, using a pain scale to objectify data. Assess his emotional and educational needs. Monitor his behaviors and statements for signs of anxiety or depression.

Objective Data

A physical examination should include palpation of the abdomen and assessment of the scrotum. Positive findings in the scrotum include a firm, painless mass in the testis and an enlarged scrotum. Because gynecomastia (breast enlargement) is another symptom of testicular cancer, the client's breast tissue should be assessed for enlargement.

Nursing diagnoses for the client with testicular cancer include the following:

NURSING DIAGNOSES	PLANNING/OUTCOMES	NURSING INTERVENTIONS
*Risk for **I**njury* due to infection and hemorrhage related to surgery	The client will experience minimal bleeding and avoid infection.	Monitor the client's vital signs and incisional drainage. Report hyperthermia, tachycardia, hypotension, increased incisional drainage, and swelling or redness around the incision to the physician immediately. Maintain strict asepsis when handling wound dressings.
*Disturbed **B**ody Image* related to surgery	The client will maintain or regain a positive body image.	Provide client with opportunities to voice concerns and ask questions. Monitor the client for statements and behaviors that indicate concern about loss of masculinity. Educate client that unilateral removal of a testis will not cause him to be sterile or demasculinized. Suggest sexual counseling if he does not appear to be resolving these issues. Sperm may be frozen before treatment.

(*Continues*)

Nursing diagnoses for the client with testicular cancer include the following: (Continued)

NURSING DIAGNOSES	PLANNING/OUTCOMES	NURSING INTERVENTIONS
*Deficient **K**nowledge* related to surgery and post operative care	The client will demonstrate understanding of postoperative activity restrictions and medical follow-up.	Teach the client that he needs to be on bed rest for 12 to 24 hours postoperatively. Instruct the client to wear tight-fitting underwear or an athletic supporter when ambulating and to avoid heavy lifting for 4 to 6 weeks.

Evaluation: Evaluate each outcome to determine how it has been met by the client.

PENILE CANCER

Penile cancer is rare and has a high correlation with poor hygiene and delayed or no circumcision. The bacteria harbored in the foreskin of the uncircumcised male are irritants to the glans penis and the prepuce. The chronic nature of this irritation is thought to be carcinogenic. Males with a history of sexually transmitted infections (STIs) are also predisposed to developing penile cancer. Symptoms of penile cancer include a painless, nodular growth on the foreskin, fatigue, and weight loss. Metastases are common in the inguinal nodes and adjacent organs.

Medical–Surgical Management

Medical

The primary penile cancer treatment is surgery. Treatment with radiation alone is ineffective, and chemotherapy alone is used only for palliative treatment of penile cancer with deep, distant metastases; however, the client may receive adjuvant therapy with either radiation or chemotherapy.

Surgical

If the tumor is not extensive and no metastases are involved, the remaining penis should be long enough for the client to void standing and avoid soiling himself. If a penectomy is necessary, a perineal urethrostomy may be created.

Nursing Management

Provide emotional support if penectomy is required. Monitor vital signs and I&O. Elevate the scrotum to prevent edema. Objectively assess pain and administer analgesics as ordered.

NURSING PROCESS

Assessment

Subjective Data

Although the tumor is painless, ask the client if he is experiencing any pain, to rule out other possible diagnoses. Also ask about fatigue or weight loss. Preoperatively, assess the client for emotional and educational needs. Ask questions that can determine his understanding of the surgical procedure and the need for counseling. Postoperative assessment includes monitoring for pain and using a pain scale to objectify data.

Objective Data

The client's physical assessment should include inspection of the penis for the presence of painless, nodular growths. During the postoperative phase, monitor vital signs, incisional site, and intake and output. Hypotension, tachycardia, excessive incisional drainage, redness or swelling around the incision, or bright red or low urinary output could be signs of complications.

Nursing diagnoses for a client with penile cancer include the following:

NURSING DIAGNOSES	PLANNING/OUTCOMES	NURSING INTERVENTIONS
*Risk for **I**njury* due to infection and hemorrhage related to surgery	The client will experience minimal bleeding and avoid infection.	Monitor client's vital signs and incisional drainage. Report hyperthermia, tachycardia, hypotension, increased incisional drainage, and swelling or redness around the incision to the physician immediately. Maintain strict asepsis when handling wound dressings.
***A**nxiety* related to surgery	The client will discuss anxieties.	Provide client with information about the operative procedure, postoperative and discharge care. When available, a video may be used to present this information, with the nurse being available to answer the client's questions.

Nursing diagnoses for a client with penile cancer include the following: (Continued)

NURSING DIAGNOSES	PLANNING/OUTCOMES	NURSING INTERVENTIONS
*Ineffective **S**exuality Patterns* related to the altered body function or structure	The client will maintain satisfactory sexuality patterns postoperatively.	Recommend the client to seek sexual counseling for both himself and his partner if he is unable to maintain normal sexuality patterns.

Evaluation: Evaluate each outcome to determine how it has been met by the client.

MENSTRUAL DISORDERS

Abnormalities of menstruation may be associated with an increase or decrease in secretion from any of the following glands: hypothalamus, pituitary, ovaries, adrenals, and thyroid. The normal menstrual pattern is controlled by a series of hormonal negative feedback mechanisms. The average menstrual cycle occurs every 28 to 30 days when the endometrial lining of the uterus sloughs off in the absence of a fertilized ovum.

DYSMENORRHEA

Painful menstruation, dysmenorrhea, also called "menstrual cramps," is more common in nulliparous women and in women who are not having intercourse. The exact pathophysiology is unknown, but it may be related to endocrine secretions such as prostaglandin F, which causes uterine cramping, irritation, and contractions. Other causes may include uterine anatomical anomalies, chronic illness, or psychological factors.

The primary symptom is pelvic pain before or at the onset of menses that may be caused by spasms of the uterus, cervical stenosis, uterine fibroids, emotional factors, endometriosis, pelvic inflammatory disease, or the presence of an intrauterine contraceptive device (IUD). The client may also state that the pain radiates across the lower back and downward into the legs.

The condition is diagnosed on the basis of the client's complaints and description of the timing of the onset of symptoms. Obtain information pertaining to the menstrual history and general health status of the client. A thorough physical exam is performed by the physician, including a bimanual exam to rule out other possible causes. A pelvic ultrasound may be ordered.

One effective preventive intervention may begin before the young woman begins menstruation. A positive parental attitude toward the onset of menstruation can aid the young girl in adjusting to the physiologic and psychological changes that occur with puberty.

Some medications are effective in the treatment of dysmenorrhea. Analgesics such as acetaminophen (Tylenol) and ibuprofen (Motrin) are useful in relieving pain. Oral contraceptives have been used for some clients to inhibit ovulation, which appears to be an associated cause. Prostaglandin inhibitors such as naproxen sodium (Aleve) and mefenamic acid (Ponstel) are useful if taken at the earliest sign of discomfort.

AMENORRHEA

Amenorrhea, the absence of menstruation, may be primary or secondary. Primary amenorrhea is defined as the absence of menstruation by the age of 16. Possible causes are related to anatomical or genetic abnormalities (Turner's syndrome). The treatment depends on the cause. Secondary amenorrhea is defined as the absence of menstruation after 6 months of regular periods or after 12 months of irregular periods. Several etiologies are possible for secondary amenorrhea, including anatomic abnormalities, nutritional deficits (anorexia nervosa), excessive exercise with significant decreases in body fat, endocrine dysfunction, emotional disturbances, side effects of medications, pregnancy, and lactation.

Diagnosis is based on the length of menstruation absence. A complete physical examination is performed, including a pelvic examination to rule out many other factors. A pregnancy test will be one of the first tests ordered, to rule out pregnancy. A progestin challenge test may be administered in an attempt to force the body to respond hormonally. Medroxyprogesterone acetate (Depo-Provera) is taken orally for 5 to 10 days as ordered by the physician. When the medication is finished, the client should have a menstrual period within 3 or 4 days. A menstrual flow after taking the medication may be an indicator that the client has not been ovulating. If no bleeding occurs, further investigation may be necessary to uncover other causes. Hormonal imbalances, microscopic pituitary tumors, and nutritional deficits are common etiologies of secondary amenorrhea. A microscopic pituitary tumor will cause an elevation in the prolactin level and result in anovulation and amenorrhea. A serum prolactin level should be ordered, especially if the client has noticed any breast discharge. Normal prolactin level should not exceed 15 ng/dL. With pituitary tumors, the prolactin level may exceed 400 ng/dL. In these cases, the drug of choice is bromocriptine mesylate (Parlodel), which had been used in the past to suppress lactation in mothers who did not breastfeed their newborns. A careful examination of the client is needed before administration of Parlodel because of an increased potential for cardiovascular problems associated with this medication. Because of this risk, the medication is no longer used for the postpartum client to suppress milk production. Other medical or surgical interventions depend on the cause of the amenorrhea.

OTHER DISORDERS

Other menstrual disorders include menorrhagia and metrorrhagia. Both types of abnormal bleeding can be problematic for the client and require further investigation. **Polymenorrhea** is a term used to describe short menstrual cycles of less than 21 days in length. The causes are similar to those of the other menstrual disorders. **Oligomenorrhea**, is a diminished menstrual flow, but it is not classified as amenorrhea. It may be associated with low-dose oral contraceptives that inhibit the growth of the endometrium and result in minimal tissue sloughing at the end of the cycle. Other causes may be metabolic or hormonal. Again, treatment is specific to the etiology.

For conditions associated with heavy bleeding or bleeding between periods, a dilation and curettage (D&C) may be performed. In this case, the procedure may be diagnostic and therapeutic. Tissue removed from the uterus is examined microscopically and histologically to evaluate its stage in the menstrual cycle. A hysterectomy may be indicated if abnormalities are discovered or if the bleeding is so excessive that the client is significantly compromised. The client may require a blood transfusion to correct low hemoglobin and hematocrit levels before any other procedures are performed. Supplemental iron generally is prescribed by the physician to also help correct the deficiency.

NURSING PROCESS

Assessment

Subjective Data

Ask the client about the onset of the bleeding and its relationship to the timing of her normal menstruation, the color of the bleeding, amount, number of pads saturated, presence of clots, and presence of pain with the bleeding. A history of current medications, contraception, and the possibility of pregnancy are additional data needed. Explore any preexisting health problems that could affect bleeding and clotting times, as well as life stressors.

Objective Data

Assessment of vital signs may indicate hypertension and tachycardia. Monitor laboratory test results.

Nursing Management

Acknowledge the client's feelings about the problem. Explain diagnostic tests and procedures. Encourage good nutrition, good posture, and exercise. Emphasize the importance of follow-up care.

Possible nursing diagnoses for a client with any of the menstrual disorders discussed in this section may include:

- *Acute **Pain*** related to uterine cramping or heavy bleeding
- *Decreased **Cardiac** Output* related to excessive blood loss
- ***Fatigue*** related to decreased hemoglobin and hematocrit levels
- *Disturbed **Body** Image* related to the absence of menstruation

PREMENSTRUAL SYNDROME

One-third to one-half of women between 20 and 50 years of age experience some of the symptoms known as premenstrual syndrome (PMS). Once, this condition was thought by many physicians to be a psychological problem of women; however, recent research has supported data that many physiologic as well as psychological factors are involved. PMS often occurs during the secretory phase of the menstrual cycle, after ovulation. Risk factors associated with the development of PMS include age (older than 30), multiple life stressors, inappropriate nutritional status, a previous reaction to or side effects from oral contraceptive use, a sedentary lifestyle, marital status, a history of preeclampsia in pregnancy, and multiparity.

More than 150 symptoms have been reported that have been related to PMS. These include weight gain, bloating, irritability, edema, headache, mood swings, inability to concentrate, food cravings, acne, and numerous others. For many women, the PMS symptoms are merely a monthly nuisance, but for others, the symptoms are so incapacitating that they cannot function in their normal roles or responsibilities. The onset of symptoms is usually 7 to 10 days before the menstrual period starts; symptoms end after the menstrual flow begins.

Research has correlated hormonal imbalances of estrogen, progesterone, ACTH, and androgens with the symptoms of PMS. The presence of prostaglandin F in the tissue may also be a cause of some of the symptoms. Prostaglandins are associated with many inflammatory responses in the tissues.

The first step in identifying PMS is a physical examination to rule out other possible disorders of the reproductive system. The client may be asked to keep a monthly calendar of symptoms to see if there are patterns in severity, type, or onset. Blood tests may be ordered to assess estrogen and progesterone levels, as well as checking the glucose level. Low blood glucose level has been associated with irritability that sometimes accompanies PMS symptoms. The client should receive counseling, if needed, to facilitate coping with life stressors that may be complicating the complexity of the PMS symptoms.

Medical–Surgical Management

Pharmacological

Some physicians and NPs recommend medication such as acetaminophen (Tylenol), naproxen (Naprosyn), mefenamic acid (Ponstel), and ibuprofen (Advil) for the relief of minor discomforts of PMS. Several PMS symptoms are thought to be related to a low progesterone level. For some clients, the use of progesterone suppositories or oral progesterone to supplement their own production during the secretory phase of the menstrual cycle has been useful. Selective serotonin reuptake inhibitors used to treat and relieve PMS symptoms include citalopram hydrobromide (Celexa), fluvoxamine maleate (Luvox), fluoxetine hydrochloride (Prozac), sertraline hydrochloride (Zoloft), escitalopram oxalate (Lexapro), and paroxetine hydrochloride (Paxil) (Daniels, Nosek, & Nicoll, 2007).

Diet

A thorough diet history should be included in the assessment data collected. Certain nutritional deficits or cravings have been linked to the worsening of PMS. Items such as sugar, salt, caffeine, and chocolate are in this category. Many studies have shown that limiting intake of these substances may be helpful. Caffeinated beverages may increase anxiety, irritability, and deplete vitamin B stores in the body. Dairy products interfere with the absorption of magnesium, which helps stabilize the mood. Chocolates have been related to increased sugar cravings, mood swings, fluid retention, and increased vitamin B demands. Oranges and other fruits or vegetables that are highly acidic may worsen PMS. Foods that are recommended are whole grains, nuts, pasta, legumes, root vegetables, fruits such as apples and pears, poultry, and seafood. A good vitamin supplement rich in vitamin B-complex, calcium, magnesium, and zinc should be taken daily, especially during the PMS period. Herbal tea formulas have shown some promise as alternative methods of relieving PMS.

Activity

A regular exercise routine, coupled with the use of stress-management techniques such as deep breathing and relaxation exercises, help the client cope with the increased sense of anxiety or irritability that may accompany PMS. Meditation, positive affirmation, visualization, and imagery may be helpful, as well as acupressure, neurolymphatic or neurovascular massage, and yoga.

Nursing Management

Encourage client to keep a monthly PMS calendar of events. Recommend that the client limit sodium, sugar, alcohol, caffeine, nicotine, and refined carbohydrate intake, and increase calcium intake to reduce PMS symptoms (Daniels, Nosek, & Nicoll, 2007).

NURSING PROCESS

Assessment

Subjective Data

Ask the client to describe her symptoms and the impact on her lifestyle. Many times, clients will seek medical attention for their PMS symptoms when the emotional impact has caused friction in the home, marriage, work, or family environment. Symptoms described may include weight gain, bloating, irritability, headache, mood swings, inability to concentrate, or food cravings. Ask the client to relate symptoms to time of menstrual cycle.

Objective Data

Assess the client for weight gain and edema. Review laboratory test results.

Nursing diagnoses for a client with premenstrual syndrome include the following:

NURSING DIAGNOSES	PLANNING/OUTCOMES	NURSING INTERVENTIONS
*Excess **F**luid Volume* related to hormonal imbalance and increased sodium or sugar intake	The client's intake and output will be balanced, and edema will be decreased.	Educate client that a certain amount of fluid retention is normal before the onset of the menstrual period and cannot be avoided, but by limiting sodium and sugar intake, she may be able to influence the amount of fluid retained.
***H**ealth-Seeking Behaviors*, related to finding methods to cope with symptoms of PMS	The client will develop effective health-promotion skills to increase coping with PMS symptoms or to decrease symptom severity or frequency.	Teach client how to keep a monthly PMS calendar of events. Discuss prescribed medications with the client, including the dosage, expected effects, and side effects. Discuss relationship of foods to PMS.

Evaluation: Evaluate each outcome to determine how it has been met by the client.

MENOPAUSE

Menopause, or climacteric, is the cessation of menstruation. It may occur as a natural hormonal decline or it may be surgically induced by removal of the uterus and ovaries. Many people think of menopause as the "change of life" and accept it as part of aging. Most women will begin to experience signs and symptoms of approaching menopause around 50 years of age; however, the range of onset is from 45 to 60 years old. During this perimenopause transition, menstrual cycles become further apart and the flow decreases. The onset is usually gradual, and it may take more than a year before the woman has completely ceased menstruation. Reproductive capability is also lost with menopause. For some women this is a sad time perceived as the loss of womanhood; for others it is a welcome relief. Postmenopause is considered the time period one year after the last menstrual cycle and lasts the rest of a woman's lifetime.

The decreasing level of ovarian hormone production affects women in a variety of ways, more than just the end of menstruation. There may be a relaxation of the pelvic support structures, loss of skin turgor and elasticity, and thinning of the hair on the head, axilla, and pubic regions. Other signs of decreasing hormones (estrogen and progesterone) are vaginal dryness, thinning of the vaginal mucosa, weight gain, dry skin, and stress incontinence. The estrogen level plays an important protective role in maintaining an adequate calcium balance in the bones and preventing coronary artery disease. Without calcium, bones become brittle, and there is an increased risk of fractures and osteoporosis. A baseline bone density study may be recommended before menopause.

Some women experience psychological responses to menopause, such as mild to moderate depression, nervousness, and insomnia. Consultation with a psychologist, minister, or counselor may be useful in facilitating the transition through this period for some women.

Women may also experience mild to moderate periods of profuse perspiration called "hot flashes." These usually move from the waist upward. They are caused by the decreased estrogen level and its effect on the hypothalamus. The sensation may last from 30 seconds to 10 minutes. It appears that many different things can trigger a hot flash—drinking hot beverages, eating spicy foods, smoking, and consuming caffeine and alcohol.

Medical–Surgical Management

Pharmacological

For some women, estrogen replacement therapy is recommended, especially if they are experiencing moderately uncomfortable symptoms. Estrogen replacement therapy (ERT) may help decrease some symptoms, such as insomnia, hot flashes, mood swings, and lack of concentration. Estrogen elevates the high-density lipoproteins (healthy ones) and lowers the low-density lipoproteins (unhealthy) in the circulation. Estrogen may be administered orally, as a transdermal patch, or as a vaginal cream. Conjugated estrogen (Premarin), estradiol (Estrace), and synthetic conjugated estrogens Cenestin and Enjuvia are examples of oral estrogens available. Estrogen creams or water-soluble gels such as Lubrifax or K-Y may be used to combat the vaginal dryness and resulting dyspareunia (The North American Menopause Society, 2009).

Diet

Provide the client with instructions regarding the importance of an adequate daily intake of calcium-rich products, such as dairy products. Many low-fat, high-calcium products are available if the client has a concern about weight gain. Calcium supplements may also be taken in a tablet form. The woman should consult her health care provider before adding a calcium supplement because too much calcium increases the risk for other health problems. Herbal teas, vitamin E, magnesium, and primrose oil have been used as alternative methods to alleviate or decrease hot flashes and promote relaxation for some women.

Activity

One important way that the client can decrease the potential for calcium loss from weight-bearing bones is to exercise. A planned 30-minute program performed at least 3 times per week is adequate to maintain bone density. Exercises such as walking or swimming are excellent. Swimming provides good non–weight-bearing activity and promotes active movement of all extremities. Biking is a good exercise to maintain joint mobility in the lower extremities, but it does not require the use of the same muscle groups as walking.

Nursing Management

Encourage the client to exercise regularly, especially walking. Explain nutritional requirements for vitamins and calcium. Advise the client to try water-soluble gels for vaginal dryness and body lotion to prevent dry skin.

NURSING PROCESS

Assessment

Subjective Data

The client may describe decreasing regularity of menstruation or hot flashes. Obtain information from the client about gynecological and obstetrical history, including menstruation. It is helpful to know when the client began experiencing symptoms in predicting the length of time they may continue.

Objective Data

These include a physical examination and Pap smear. The results of the Pap smear can indicate if there is less estrogen present in the cervical tissue than normal.

Nursing diagnoses for a client experiencing menopausal symptoms include the following:

NURSING DIAGNOSES	PLANNING/OUTCOMES	NURSING INTERVENTIONS
Health-Seeking Behaviors related to perceived physiological and psychologic impact of decreased estrogen	The client will develop effective health promotion skills to increase coping with menopausal symptoms or to decrease symptom severity or frequency.	Encourage client to continue to see her health care provider for annual Pap smears and breast examinations. Explain nutritional requirements for vitamins and calcium that increase with menopause. Encourage client to begin a regular exercise program that includes weight-bearing activities such as walking to prevent loss of calcium from the bones.
Impaired Tissue Integrity related to vaginal dryness and dry skin	The client will maintain skin integrity, and vagina will not be dry.	Recommend that the client try estrogen creams or water-soluble gels such as Lubrifax or K-Y to combat the vaginal dryness and resulting dyspareunia. Encourage client to use body lotion to prevent dry skin.
Decisional Conflict related to taking supplemental estrogen therapy	The client will make informed decisions about taking supplemental estrogen.	Discuss the advantages and disadvantages of estrogen replacement therapy with the client. Remind client that if she has a uterus and takes hormonal replacements, she will continue to have monthly menstrual cycles.

Evaluation: Evaluate each outcome to determine how it has been met by the client.

STRUCTURAL DISORDERS

Structural anomalies are separated into female and male disorders.

CYSTOCELE, URETHROCELE, RECTOCELE, PROLAPSED UTERUS

Cystocele, urethrocele, rectocele, and prolapsed uterus are often associated with relaxation of the pelvic muscles that support the uterus, bladder, and rectum. A **cystocele** is a downward displacement of the bladder into the anterior vaginal wall. A **urethrocele** is a downward displacement of the urethra into the vagina, and a **rectocele** is an anterior displacement of the rectum into the posterior vaginal wall. **Prolapsed uterus** is a downward displacement of the uterus into the vagina (Figure 44-21). Possible causes for the four conditions are multiple pregnancies, third- or fourth-degree perineal lacerations with childbirth, and age-related weakening of the pelvic muscles.

A prolapsed uterus is often accompanied by a cystocele and/or rectocele. With a first-degree prolapse, the cervix is visible at the vaginal introitus, or opening, without straining. With a second-degree prolapse, the cervix extends beyond the vaginal opening to the perineum. With a third-degree prolapse, the uterus protrudes outside of the vagina. This severe condition is called *procidentia uteri.*

MEDICAL–SURGICAL MANAGEMENT

Medical and surgical interventions for the treatment of each of these conditions are focused on relief of discomfort and restoration of the structure and function of the pelvic organs.

Medical

The pessary is a small molded plastic or rubber apparatus that fits into the vagina behind the pubic bone and in front of the rectum. Its function is to provide an artificial or mechanical support for the uterus. Pessaries are not uncomfortable and should not be felt by the client if properly fitted and in the correct position. The client should be taught how to insert and remove the pessary so it can be cleaned. The pessary may be washed in warm, soapy water once every 1 to 2 weeks. Prolonged use of a mechanical device such as a pessary may result in vaginal necrosis and ulceration. Periodic examination by a health care professional is recommended.

Surgical

Surgery for a prolapsed uterus may require a hysterectomy. If the prolapse is accompanied by a cystocele or rectocele, an A&P repair may also be performed. An A&P repair (anterior/posterior colporrhaphy) may be performed vaginally to replace the bladder, urethra, or rectum in the correct anatomic position. Another procedure, the Marshall-Marchette-Krantz, may be performed to attach the bladder to the inferior surface of the pubic bone. Postoperatively, the client may be sent home with an indwelling Foley catheter because of the potential inability to void. This is a common postoperative situation that usually resolves itself spontaneously within 1 or 2 weeks after discharge.

Activity

The Kegel exercise is performed by tightening and releasing the perineal muscles. An important muscle group, called the "levators," helps lift and support the organs inside the pelvis.

CLIENT TEACHING

Kegel Exercises

- Suggest that the client practice when she has a full bladder. If she can successfully start and stop the flow of urine from the bladder, she is identifying and using the correct muscle groups.
- The muscles should be tightened and held for 5 to 10 seconds and then released slowly.
- Repeat the exercises at least 10 times.
- Kegel exercise can be practiced anytime and anyplace.
- A secondary benefit of increasing the strength and contractility of the pelvic and perineal muscles is seen in an improvement in pelvic sensations for both partners during intercourse.

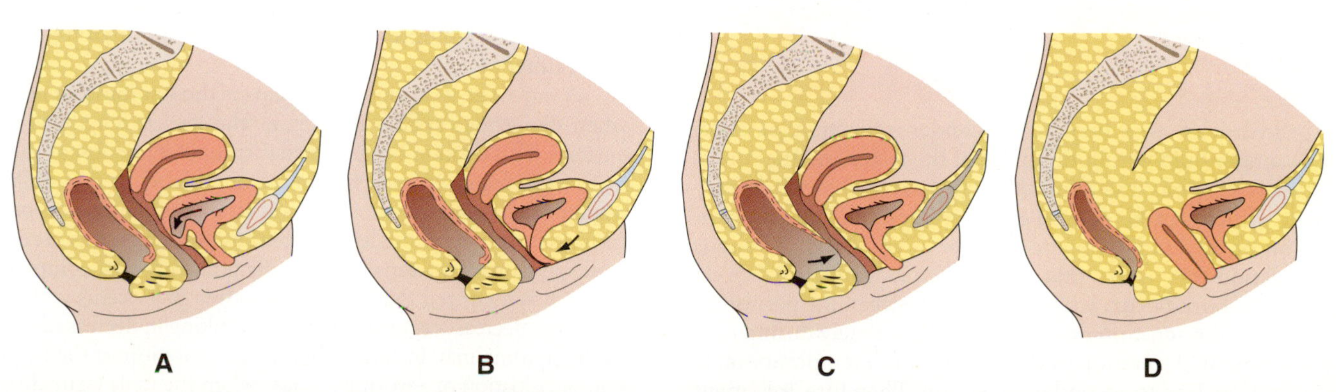

FIGURE 44-21 *A,* Cystocele; *B,* Urethrocele; *C,* Rectocele; *D,* Uterine Prolapse

Nursing Management

Teach client Kegel exercise and encourage daily practice. Describe to the client how a high-fiber diet and drinking plenty of fluids will help prevent constipation. Postoperatively, monitor vital signs and I&O. Cleanse perineal area following surgical asepsis. Encourage early ambulation.

NURSING PROCESS

Assessment

Subjective Data

The client often describes stress incontinence, a loss of urine when she coughs, sneezes, laughs, or jumps. She may describe it as "a leaky bladder." She may notice that her panties are damp or that she dribbles urine. Many women complain of frequent urination in small quantities with a feeling of urgency without burning or dysuria. The client may notice constipation or a sense of bearing-down pressure in the pelvis with a rectocele. Many of these symptoms will decrease or subside completely when lying down. Ask about the client's childbearing history, onset of current symptoms, and any other pertinent gynecological data.

Objective Data

These include the visualization of a bulging of the bladder, urethra, or rectum into the vagina. The bulging increases when the client is asked to bear down. Urinalysis results should be evaluated.

Nursing diagnoses for a female client with a structural disorder of the reproductive system include the following:

NURSING DIAGNOSES	PLANNING/OUTCOMES	NURSING INTERVENTIONS
*Stress Urinary **I**ncontinence* related to relaxation of the pelvic muscles	The client will have less stress incontinence.	Teach the client Kegel exercise and encourage daily practice. Encourage client to empty bladder frequently.
***C**onstipation* related to relaxation of the anterior rectal wall into the vagina and decreased function	The client will not have constipation.	Encourage client to defecate at same time each day. Encourage client to eat high-fiber foods, drink plenty of fluids, and exercise regularly.
*Risk for **I**nfection* related to exposure of internal tissues to external environmental factors	The client will be free of signs and symptoms of infection.	Monitor client's vital signs. Encourage client to practice proper personal hygiene and wear clean undergarments daily.
***S**exual Dysfunction* related to discomforts with intercourse	The client will have a fulfilling sexual relationship without discomfort.	Be sensitive to client cues related to her sexual concerns. Help the client set realistic goals during her recovery period to facilitate a new outlook on her relationship. Encourage client to openly discuss her feelings with her partner.

Evaluation: Evaluate each outcome to determine how it has been met by the client.

HYDROCELE, SPERMATOCELE, VARICOCELE, TORSION OF THE SPERMATIC CORD

A hydrocele is a benign, nontender collection of clear, amber fluid within the space of the testes and the tunica vaginalis or along the spermatic cord. Scrotal swelling may result, which can be painful if it develops suddenly. Inflammation of the epididymis or testis or a lymphatic or venous obstruction may cause this condition. Congenital hydrocele in the newborn occurs when the canal between the peritoneal cavity and the scrotum does not close completely during fetal development. Aspiration of the fluid is only a temporary measure and can lead to secondary infection. Therefore, treatment for the condition is surgery.

A spermatocele is a benign nontender cyst of either the epididymis or the rete testis. It contains milky fluid and sperm. Usually, this condition is painless and does not require medical treatment.

A varicocele is dilation of the veins of the scrotum that occurs when the venous system that drains the testicle lengthens and enlarges. This dilation occurs when incompetent or absent valves in the spermatic venous system permit blood to accumulate, resulting in increased hydrostatic pressure. This condition is most commonly found on the left side because of the increased retrograde pressure of the renal vein, the length, and fewer competent valves. It is theorized that the hyperthermia that occurs with this condition decreases spermatogenesis, resulting in decreased fertility. Symptoms may include a bluish discoloration of the scrotal skin or palpation of a wormlike mass when the male bears down. This condition seldom requires treatment.

Torsion of the spermatic cord occurs when the vascular pedicle of the testis twists, resulting in partial or complete venous occlusion. The three forms of this disorder are (1) rotation of the spermatic cord, (2) torsion of a testicular appendage, or (3) torsion of the spermatic cord and epididymis. Testicular torsion may be related to recent trauma, and the onset of symptoms often occurs suddenly. Symptoms of testicular torsion may include abdominal and scrotal pain, scrotal edema, nausea and vomiting, and, possibly, a slight fever. The pain caused by testicular torsion is not relieved by bed rest or scrotal support.

Medical–Surgical Management

Medical/surgical management of male structural disorders is specific to the condition. In some newborns, a hydrocele may resolve without medical intervention. Clients of all ages may have aspiration performed to reduce the swelling caused by fluid or a hematoma; however, this solution is usually only temporary, and surgical removal of the sac provides the only permanent solution to the problem. Although a spermatocele usually does not require treatment, sometimes surgical aspiration or excision is necessary.

Because a common complication of a varicocele is male infertility, ligation of the spermatic vein may be performed if infertility is a concern. Sometimes this does not resolve infertility problems because varicoceles may recur after surgery. When fertility is not a concern, the varicocele may be treated simply with scrotal support.

Torsion of the spermatic cord is one disorder that does require immediate surgery to perform surgical detorsion (untwisting) and suturing of the testicle to the scrotum.

Nursing Management

Maintain the client on bed rest with scrotal support and ice to the area. Objectively assess the client's pain and administer analgesics as ordered. Monitor vital signs, incisional drainage, and dressing. Use strict asepsis when changing dressings.

NURSING PROCESS

Assessment

Subjective Data

Ask the client about the type and location of his pain and related symptoms such as alteration in urinary patterns, warmth, fatigue, nausea, or vomiting. Assess the client's knowledge of his condition, treatment, follow-up care, and the implications of sterility and impotence to the client's life.

Objective Data

Inspect and palpate the genitals to detect the presence of scrotal swelling, testicular enlargement, scrotal immobility, redness, and warmth of the scrotum. Large varicoceles may be visible through the scrotal skin as a bluish discoloration.

Nursing diagnoses for a male client with a structural disorder of the reproductive system may include the following:

NURSING DIAGNOSES	PLANNING/OUTCOMES	NURSING INTERVENTIONS
*Risk for **Injury*** related to inflammation and hemorrhage	The client will experience minimal bleeding and avoid infection.	Monitor client's vital signs and incisional drainage. Maintain strict asepsis when handling wound dressings. Report hyperthermia, tachycardia, hypotension, increased incisional drainage, and swelling or redness around the incision to the physician immediately.
*Deficient **Knowledge*** related to the condition and possible complications	The client will demonstrate understanding of the possible complications of his condition.	Monitor statements made by the client to determine if there is any misunderstanding about how the surgery will affect his masculinity and fertility. Provide client with opportunities to voice his feelings and ask questions.

Evaluation: Evaluate each outcome to determine how it has been met by the client.

FUNCTIONAL DISORDERS AND CONCERNS

Included in this category are impotence, infertility, and contraception.

IMPOTENCE

Impotence is defined as the inability of an adult male to have an erection firm enough or to maintain it long enough to complete sexual intercourse. There are three types of impotence: functional, atonic, and anatomic. Psychological factors that lead to concerns about sexual performance may contribute to functional impotence. These factors include aging and difficulty with communication or relationships.

Atonic impotence may be the result of medications such as antihypertensives, sedatives, antidepressants, or tranquilizers. For example, antihypertensives lower blood pressure in all arteries of the body, and reduction of the blood pressure to penile arteries may lead to failure of the penis to fill sufficiently to achieve erection. The use of alcohol, cocaine, and nicotine can also decrease potency. Disease processes leading to atonic

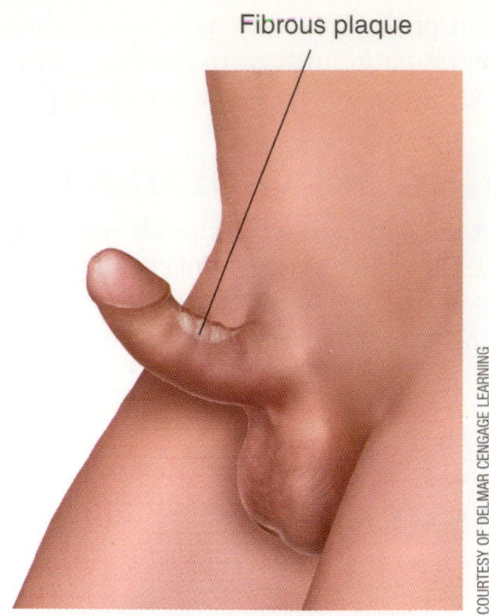

FIGURE 44-22 Dorsal Curvature of the Penis in Peyronie's Disease Caused by Fibrous Plaque

impotence include diabetes and vascular and neurological disorders. Diabetic clients are at increased risk for impotence because of their tendency to develop atherosclerosis and autonomic neuropathy. Vascular and neurological disorders include atherosclerosis, hypertension, spinal cord injuries, and multiple sclerosis. End-stage renal disease and chronic obstructive pulmonary disorders can also decrease potency.

Peyronie's disease is the development of nonelastic, fibrous tissue just beneath the penile skin, leading to anatomic impotence. The resulting loss of elasticity leads to a decreased ability of the penis to fill with and store blood during an erection. Peyronie's disease often causes the penis to bend upward, possibly leading to pain and an inability to penetrate the vagina (Figure 44-22).

Medical–Surgical Management

Medical

The first step in treating impotence is to determine whether the client's lifestyle is a factor. Further assessment may include nocturnal penile tumescence monitoring or dynamic infusion cavernosometry and cavernosography (DICC). Treatment will be based on the assessment findings and test results. Treatment may include changes in lifestyle to reduce the need for medications, manage stress, lose weight, and exercise. These changes often help improve the client's physical health, self-image, and attitude about his ability to function sexually.

External devices can be used to promote an erection. A vacuum constriction device (VCD) may be used to increase the blood supply to the penis, causing engorgement and rigidity. The client inserts his penis into a plastic cylinder and squeezes a pump to withdraw the air from the cylinder, creating a vacuum that draws blood into the penis. Once an erection has been achieved in this manner, a rubber ring is moved from the bottom of the cylinder to the base of the penis. This permits the blood to be safely trapped in the penis for up to one-half hour. Advantages of the VCD over surgical intervention are less expense and fewer complications.

Surgical

Surgical interventions for impotency include revascularization and penile implants. For clients with impotence related to blocked arteries, revascularization is done to bypass blocked arteries and remove veins that are causing excessive drainage. For clients who are not candidates for revascularization, penile prostheses are another option. One type is a semirigid implant, which is a silicone cylinder that may be flexible or inflexible. Another type is a hydraulic implant that has a cylinder that can be inflated by squeezing a pump located in the scrotum or at the end of the penis. Because of its ability to fill and empty, the hydraulic implant, unlike the silicone implant, which is always semirigid, most closely mimics flaccidity and erection. The disadvantages of surgical interventions are expense and postoperative complications, the most serious being postoperative infection.

Pharmacological

Medications that promote erections are sildenafil citrate (Viagra), vardenafil hydrochloride (Levitra), and tadalafil (Cialis), which belong to a class of drugs called phosphodiesterase (PDE) inhibitors. These drugs should not be used by men for whom sexual activity is not advisable because of underlying cardiovascular problems (Spratto & Woods, 2009). One side effect of drug therapy is prolonged erection that does not occur in response to sexual stimulation (**priapism**). Oral neurotransmitters have been used with variable success, and sublingual apomorphine shows some promise as an erectogenic agent. When administered sublingually rather than subcutaneously, as was done in the past, there are fewer side effects. Self-injections of vasodilators or other drugs may result in serious complications.

NURSING PROCESS

Assessment

Subjective Data

The client may describe a history of illicit and prescribed drug use, and alcohol consumption. Previous diagnoses, lifestyle, sexual functioning, and family disorders must be explored. Assess the client's emotional and educational needs to determine whether anxiety about sexual performance or lack of knowledge are contributing factors to impotence.

Objective Data

If the client has surgery, the nurse needs to monitor vital signs, incisional site, and I&O.

Nursing Management

Teach client how to take prescribed medications. If an implant has been inserted, teach client the signs of infection such as tenderness, fever, and dysuria.

Nursing diagnoses for a client who is impotent may include the following:

- *Sexual Dysfunction* related to altered body function or structure
- *Ineffective Sexuality Patterns* related to altered body function or structure
- *Disturbed Body Image* related to impotence
- *Deficient Knowledge* related to impotence

INFERTILITY

Approximately one in every eight couples experiences infertility, the inability to produce offspring. Infertility may be primary or secondary. In primary infertility, the couple have never achieved a pregnancy or have never carried a pregnancy to viability. Secondary infertility involves problems that arise after the couple has had a successful pregnancy. Many factors may be investigated as causes of infertility in both female and male clients. Forty percent of infertility factors are female-related, 40% are male-related, and 20% are a combination of multiple factors that involve both partners. The more factors that are involved, the more difficult the infertility resolution.

The etiology of infertility may be related to anatomic or endocrine problems. The female anatomic or structural abnormalities may include blocked passages through the cervix or fallopian tubes caused by failed development or by past infections, such as PID, or STIs. Uterine and cervical abnormalities may also occur. The cervix may be too narrow or closed, and sperm are unable to navigate through the passage. The uterus may have a partial or complete septum inside that limits the internal cavity space. Immune problems involve the development of antibodies by the woman's system to the male's sperm. These antibodies may be present in the cervical mucus and kill the sperm on contact. Hyposecretion or hypersecretion of FSH, LH, estrogen, or progesterone have been associated with infertility.

The causes of infertility in males include varicoceles, cryptorchidism, impaired sperm, insufficient number of sperm, and hormonal imbalance. The use of hot tubs, saunas, tight underwear, and laptop computers may decrease the sperm count.

The first step in treating an infertile couple is to obtain a history of sexual practices. In addition, detailed health histories need to be obtained and physical examinations performed.

A basic infertility workup may be initiated when the client has been unable to conceive after 6 to 12 months of unprotected intercourse. One simple, noninvasive procedure is the use of a basal body temperature chart. The chart is kept for a minimum of 3 months and then reviewed for normal ovulatory fluctuations in the basal temperature. During the first half of the menstrual cycle, the body temperature may remain below 98°F. At ovulation, there is often a slight decrease in the temperature for a 24-hour period. This is the optimal period of fertility. After ovulation, the woman's basal body temperature should go above 98°F and remain in that range for a period of 14 days. The length of the luteal phase (secretory phase) of the cycle following ovulation is a critical factor in some infertility disorders. Variations in the temperature chart may indicate that the client has had an anovulatory cycle or has a shortened luteal phase. Because the fertilized ovum does not implant in the endometrium until 6 to 8 days after conception, the luteal phase is critical to maintain the blood-rich lining long enough for implantation to occur. A low progesterone level during the luteal phase may result in spontaneous **abortion** (ending a pregnancy before the age of viability) of the fertilized ovum before implantation. Diagnostic tests that may be ordered include the following:

- Endometrial biopsy to detect tissue responses during both phases of the enstrual cycle
- Semen analysis, including sperm count, motility, and morphology
- Testicular biopsy (done when sperm are absent from the semen) to ascertain the presence of sperm
- Endocrine imbalance testing, which measures pituitary, gonadotropin, testosterone, estrogen, and progesterone levels
- Male–female interaction studies (Huhner test) to determine motility and number of sperm 2 to 4 hours after intercourse
- Laparoscopy to discover conditions such as endometriosis, adhesions, or scar tissue that potentially immobilize the fimbriae or polycystic ovarian disease (Stein-Leventhal syndrome)

MEDICAL–SURGICAL MANAGEMENT

There is no one treatment for infertility problems. The goal of treatment is successful achievement of a pregnancy that is carried to full term and produces a healthy offspring.

Medical

Infertility treatment may include artificial insemination with either the partner's sperm or donor sperm. This method is particularly useful if the male partner has a low sperm count, abnormal sperm, or no sperm production. With the procedure, the semen is placed directly into the cervix or uterus with a small flexible catheter and a syringe.

Surgical

Assisted reproductive technology (ART) has revolutionized infertility treatment. It is fertility treatment in which the eggs are surgically removed and combined with sperm in the laboratory and then returned to the woman's body. One method is *in vitro* fertilization. This may be by GIFT (gamete-intra-fallopian transfer) or ZIFT (zygote-intra-fallopian transfer). With the GIFT technique, the female partner receives monthly cyclic hormone injections that cause ova to ripen. The hormones may cause more than one ovum to ripen during each cycle, which enhances the possibility that more than one ovum will be fertilized and implanted in the uterus. A semen specimen is collected from the male partner 1 to 2 hours before the GIFT procedure and the sperm placed into a special catheter. The ripened ovum is obtained from the female via laparoscopy or ultrasound aspiration and is loaded into the catheter in a sequential manner with the sperm and then injected through the fimbrial end of the fallopian tube, also by laparoscopy. This procedure takes approximately 1 hour to complete. Pregnancy is confirmed within 7 to 10 days with a blood hormonal test (Beta hCG) or an ultrasound, or both.

The ZIFT procedure is similar to GIFT; however, several ova are obtained just before ovulation and are placed in a special fluid for several hours while the sperm are prepared. The ova and sperm are then carefully mixed and closely observed for 2 to 3 days. The fertilized ova (now zygotes) are transferred into the fallopian tube or into the uterine cavity. Another name for the ZIFT procedure is IVF-ER (in vitro fertilization and embryo replacement), which more clearly defines what actually occurs.

Both GIFT and ZIFT are relatively expensive procedures and may or may not be covered by health insurance. For many couples, these are final efforts to conceive.

Pharmacological

Several medications are used in the treatment of infertility disorders, and most are focused on hormone imbalances or deficiencies. Clomiphene citrate (Clomid) stimulates release of follicle-stimulating hormone (FSH) and luteinizing hormone (LH), and is used to induce ovulation. Clomid is administered orally beginning on the fifth day of the menstrual cycle. If ovulation does not occur, the dosage will be increased for 5 days in the next cycle. If ovulation does not occur by the time the dose has been increased 4 or 5 times, it may be considered a Clomid failure. There is some chance of multiple gestation while the client is taking Clomid, and she should be so informed. Most often it is a twin pregnancy, but occasionally triplets may be conceived.

Menotropins (Pergonal) mimics FSH and LH, causing follicular growth and maturation. It is administered by intramuscular injection. Although Pergonal is an expensive drug, it has been shown to increase the possibility for ovulation in clients who have not responded to other medications.

Human chorionic gonadotropin (Pregnyl) may also be administered with the Clomid or Pergonal therapy to help maintain the endometrial lining for implantation. It stimulates the production of progesterone from the ovary until the fertilized ovum implants and the placenta begins to function. Progesterone suppositories may be used vaginally two times per day to help correct a luteal phase defect by lengthening the time from ovulation until the onset of the menses or through implantation and pregnancy. Some clients continue with the progesterone suppositories throughout the first few weeks of the pregnancy to ensure that the endometrium remains intact. If the sperm count or motility is low, testosterone or thyroid extracts may be prescribed.

Health Promotion

Seeking prompt medical treatment for infections that involve the reproductive system is an essential means of preventing infertility problems, especially with STIs and PID. PID causes scarring of the outside of the fallopian tubes, and gonorrhea can result in scarring or strictures of the internal fallopian tube. Either cause can result in an ectopic pregnancy when the fertilized ovum cannot pass through the tube.

Other considerations may include wise choices in contraceptive methods. The use of oral contraceptives has been associated with primary and secondary infertility caused by decreased pituitary function. This condition may resolve spontaneously, or medications may be required to stimulate ovulation in order to conceive.

Multiple sexual partners have also been associated with an increased risk of sexually transmitted disease, infections, and cervical cancer.

CONTRACEPTION

Contraception, or prevention of pregnancy, has been accomplished by many methods over the centuries. In weighing the options, safety, ease of use, effectiveness, and cost should be considered. Both partners' wishes should be considered in this decision-making process.

Contraception may be accomplished by natural means or medical interventions. This section of the chapter discusses a basic overview of the types of contraceptive methods currently available, the advantages and disadvantages, the effectiveness of each kind, the mechanisms by which they work, and the client education that should accompany the methods (Table 44-2).

NATURAL METHOD

Natural methods of contraception may include what is called the "rhythm method." During the woman's fertile period of the month, usually lasting 7 days (3 days before ovulation to 3 days after), the couple should abstain from intercourse. The determination of the fertile period is based on the time of ovulation. Sperm can live up to 72 hours after ejaculation, and it is possible for sperm to still be in the cervix or uterus if the couple had intercourse 3 days before ovulation. The couple may also decide to maintain a basal body temperature chart to more accurately

Table 44-2 Contraception Methods: Effectiveness and Concerns

METHOD	EFFECTIVENESS RATE	RISKS	POSSIBLE SIDE EFFECTS	OTHER ADVANTAGES
Abstinence	100%	None known	Psychological reactions	Prevents infections including HIV
Hormonal				
Oral contraceptives	97%	Cardiovascular complications such as stroke, blood clots, high blood pressure, and heart attacks with the higher-dose combined oral contraceptive	Possible nausea, headaches, dizziness, spotting, weight gain, breast tenderness, chloasma, cramping	Protects against PID, decreases risk of ovarian and endometrial cancer, decreases menstrual blood loss and dysmenorrhea (cramps), decreases benign breast disease, regulates irregular menses, protects bone density, decreases risk of atherosclerosis, lessens the risk of rheumatoid arthritis, decreases uterine fibroids, and decreases ovarian cysts
Depo-Provera	98%	Pulmonary embolism	Headache, depression, hypertension, edema, nausea	Effective to treat obstructive sleep apnea
Lunelle	99%	None known	Breast tenderness, weight gain	None known

Table 44-2 Contraception Methods: Effectiveness and Concerns (Continued)

METHOD	EFFECTIVENESS RATE	RISKS	POSSIBLE SIDE EFFECTS	OTHER ADVANTAGES
Mirena	99.8%	None known	Headache, acne, breast tenderness first few months	Decreases menstrual blood loss, may protect against endometrial cancer
Transdermal patch	99%	None known	Skin reaction at application site	None known
Vaginal ring	97%	None known	Vaginal infections or irritation, headache, weight gain, nausea	None known
Nonhormonal				
IUD	94%	Pelvic inflammatory disease, uterine perforation, anemia	Menstrual cramping, spotting, increased bleeding	None known
Barriers				
Diaphragm Cervical cap Spermicide	84% 73–92% 79%	Mechanical irritation, vaginal infections, toxic shock syndrome	Pelvic pressure, cervical erosion, vaginal discharges if left in too long	Protects to some degree against sexually transmitted infections
Condoms	86%	None known	Decreased sensation, allergy to latex, less spontaneity in lovemaking	Protects against sexually transmitted infections, including AIDS; delays premature ejaculation
Sterilization				
Female Male	99.6% 99.8%	Infection	Pain at surgical site, psychological reaction with subsequent regret	None known

COURTESY OF DELMAR CENGAGE LEARNING

pinpoint ovulation each month. Another method to determine the approaching ovulation is to monitor the stretchiness of the cervical mucus. This is called "spinnbarkeit." As the woman nears ovulation, estrogen causes the cervical mucus to become clear, thin, and stretchy. This type of mucus provides a favorable environment for the sperm and helps their motility toward the ova. Immediately after ovulation, the cervical mucus becomes hostile to sperm. It becomes thick, cloudy, and more acidic. It also loses its stretchiness. Kits are available for purchase from the local drug store or pharmacy that react to chemicals in the cervical mucus and predict the time of ovulation. The kits are inexpensive and simple to use, much like home pregnancy tests.

HORMONAL METHODS

The many forms of hormonal contraceptives are discussed following.

Oral Contraceptives

The "pill" has been available as a contraceptive method for many years. Since its earliest form, it has been refined and the level of hormones reduced. Oral contraceptives work by suppressing ovulation. In a sense, the body thinks it is pregnant when the pill is used. Some oral contraceptives contain estrogen and progesterone; others contain only progestins.

In response to the pseudopregnancy state, the client may experience mild side effects and discomforts often associated with pregnancy such as nausea, headache, breast tenderness, or weight gain. Major side effects from oral contraceptives may include cardiovascular accidents or thrombophlebitis.

There is approximately a 1 in 200 chance of becoming pregnant while taking the oral contraceptive. If the woman thinks that she might be pregnant, she should stop the pill immediately and contact her physician. When the woman and her partner decide that it is time for a pregnancy, she should discontinue the oral contraceptive for at least 2 to 3 cycles before having unprotected intercourse. This "rest period" will lessen the possibility that pill effects will remain in her system and will allow her body to return to its own natural rhythm. Some women find that they experience primary or secondary infertility problems after being on the pill for several years because of pituitary suppression. The remedy is often fertility drugs such as clomiphene citrate (Clomid). Women who have never established a regular pattern of menstruation may not be good candidates for oral contraceptives, except as being used to regulate the cycle by artificial means. Other clients who should not take oral contraceptives include women with a history of hypertension, diabetes, cardiovascular disease, or thrombophlebitis. Some physicians may consider oral contraceptives in the newer low-dose combinations for clients who were previously in this high-risk group.

Depo-Provera

The medroxyprogesterone acetate (Depo-Provera) injection is administered intramuscularly (IM) every 12 weeks. It works like oral contraceptives to suppress ovulation. The client may experience breakthrough bleeding after the first injection, but this is not an indication that the hormone is not working. It usually requires about 3 weeks after the first injection before the contraceptive is effective, so the client should be advised to use a barrier contraceptive method during that period. The client must receive the injections at regular intervals to ensure effectiveness. Depo-Provera is a good option for the client who is approaching her forties or who smokes because it contains only progestins, which decreases the risk of cardiovascular problems.

Lunelle

The combination of estradiol cypionate and medroxyprogesterone acetate (Lunelle) is administered by IM injection every 28 to 30 days. It suppresses ovulation, thickens cervical mucus, and thins the endometrial lining. Monthly clinic visits are necessary, or the client must learn self-injection (Akert, 2003).

Mirena

Mirena, a levonorgestrol-releasing intrauterine system device, is placed in the uterus, providing contraception for 5 years. The small, soft T-shaped polyethylene frame has a hormone reservoir on the vertical stem that slowly releases the hormone. Cervical mucus thickens, sperm migration is inhibited, and endometrial growth is reduced. Mirena must be placed and removed by a health care provider (Akert, 2003).

Transdermal Patch

This first contraceptive patch, called OrthoEvra, contains norelgestromin and ethinyl estradiol. A new patch is applied every 7 days for 3 weeks. No patch is worn for the fourth week. Skin reactions are possible at the application site. The patch adheres during exercise, swimming, and hot tub/whirlpool use. It may not be as effective if the client weighs more than 198 pounds (Akert, 2003).

Vaginal Ring

The NuvaRing contains etonogestrel and ethinyl estradiol in a nonbiodegradable, flexible, transparent ring and provides constant delivery of hormones. It is inserted into the vagina and left for 3 weeks and then removed for 1 week. Precise ring position is not critical (Akert, 2003).

NONHORMONAL METHODS

Intrauterine Device

The intrauterine device (IUD) has been used for many years and has undergone several changes. The IUD is a T-shaped device wrapped with copper wire, which acts like a spermicide. The intrauterine device is recommended for women who have had children because the cervix has been dilated. This allows for easier insertion of the device. The IUD is inserted or removed by a clinician while the client is having her period because there is slight dilation of the cervix at that time. A string attached to the distal end of the device hangs out of the cervix into the vagina. The client is instructed to check the string each month after the menstrual period to make sure the device has not been expelled. Some women with an IUD experience more dysmenorrhea and a heavier menstrual flow. The IUD lasts 10 years. Fertility returns immediately upon removal.

Barriers

Methods of barrier contraception include male and female condoms, the diaphragm, and the cervical cap. Barrier devices work by blocking the pathway of the sperm through the cervix into the uterus. This type of contraceptive requires some preplanning on the part of one or both of the partners and may reduce the spontaneity of the sex act.

Spermicides

Spermicides contain a chemical, nonoxynol-9, that kills sperm on contact. If used alone, spermicidal agents have a lower efficacy rate than if used with a condom. The nurse should advise the couple to use a spermicidal gel, foam suppository, or film in addition to another barrier method for the greatest effectiveness. Foam should not be used with the diaphragm because it can result in deterioration of the latex. These agents must be placed in the vagina at least 15 minutes before intercourse to promote the spermicidal reaction. This method is safe and inexpensive but requires a high level of compliance each time or the effectiveness of the method drops significantly.

STERILIZATION METHOD

Sterilization is considered a permanent and very effective method of contraception. In a rare incident, a woman will become pregnant after a tubal ligation or after her partner has had a vasectomy. The female procedure interrupts the pathway through the fallopian tube. Sterilization may be performed on an outpatient basis in a surgical clinic or the outpatient department at the hospital. The tubal ligation is done under a general or epidural anesthetic with laparoscopy. The procedure takes about 30 to 60 minutes. The abdomen is distended with a gas to permit better visualization of the pelvic structures during the procedure.

The male sterilization, **vasectomy** (surgical resection of the vas deferens), is usually performed with local anesthesia on an outpatient basis. Rest, with ice to the scrotum, for 4 hours should follow. The client should not engage in strenuous activity or exercise for 1 week.

It may take up to 6 weeks for the semen to be clear of sperm. The client is instructed to return to the clinic for a sperm count after 20 ejaculations. If he is sexually active, during those ejaculations he should use a condom or some other form of contraception. At 6 months, a sperm count should be repeated and then monitored annually thereafter.

The female sterilization is more expensive and, because it requires more anesthesia, carries a slightly higher risk than the male procedure.

Refined microsurgical techniques have made it possible to reverse sterilization procedures. The reversals are not always successful, and the couple need to consider the odds of success before venturing into the expense of this type of surgery.

CASE STUDY

M.A. is a 70-year-old Caucasian man with a diagnosis of benign prostatic hyperplasia. Before his hospital admission for a TURP, he had been in good health. He returned from surgery 3 hours ago with a three-way Foley catheter and continuous bladder irrigation. His vital signs 1 hour ago were as follows: temperature 98.9°F, apical pulse 68, blood pressure 130/84, and respirations 18. When the nurse enters his room to take another set of vitals, M.A. is restless and moaning and has cool, moist skin; his catheter is not draining properly. His pulse is now 120 and blood pressure is 88/50. The nurse calls the physician to report the change in M.A.'s condition. The physician orders a STAT hematocrit and a bleeding and clotting time. An increase in the IV fluid drip rate is also ordered. The doctor is planning to arrive at the hospital within the next hour.

The following questions will guide your development of a nursing care plan for the case study.

1. List symptoms and clinical manifestations, other than M.A.'s, that a client may experience after a TURP.
2. List reasons why the doctor has ordered the STAT blood work and the IV changes.
3. List other diagnostic tests that may have been ordered for M.A.
4. Mentally do a head-to-toe or functional assessment on M.A. List subjective and objective data a nurse would want to obtain.
5. Write three individualized nursing diagnoses and goals for M.A.
6. Upon assessing M.A., the doctor decides to inject additional fluid into the balloon that anchors the indwelling catheter and apply increased traction to the catheter. List pertinent nursing actions a nurse would do following these medical interventions.
    - Medications
    - Comfort/rest
    - Cardiac output
    - Intake and output
    - Activity
    - Teaching
7. List resources within the medical center and the local area that could assist M.A. with his postoperative recovery.
8. List teaching that M.A. will need before his discharge.
9. List at least three successful outcomes for M.A.

SUMMARY

- Potential complications from PID may include sterility or infertility from scarring of fallopian tubes.
- Toxic shock syndrome occurs during the menses, and a strong correlation exists between the onset and use of super-absorbent tampons.
- Common male reproductive system inflammatory disorders include epididymitis, orchitis, and prostatitis. Bilateral epididymitis and orchitis can lead to sterility. Treatment includes antibiotic therapy.
- A BSE is an important method for detecting breast changes and should be practiced each month. Breast cancer is the most common female cancer in the United States.
- Benign prostatic hyperplasia is a common disorder in males older than age 50. Early symptoms include hesitancy, decreased force of stream, urinary frequency, and nocturia.
- Cervical cancer is most common in women with multiple sexual partners.
- Endometrial cancer often produces symptoms only after it is widespread. Any unusual vaginal bleeding should be investigated, especially if it occurs after menopause.
- Male cancers related to the reproductive system involve the prostate, testes, breast, and penis. Emphasis should be placed on testicular self-examination and regular physical examinations in order to facilitate early diagnosis and treatment.
- Menstrual disorders are often associated with hormonal imbalances, increased or decreased function of the endocrine glands, or neoplasms.
- Menopause is a normal, gradual decline in the ovarian production of female hormones that occurs around age 50.
- Infertility affects at least 1 in every 8 couples in the United States and is caused by hormonal imbalances and structural or physiologic abnormalities in both male and female clients.
- Women who smoke and are older than age 40 are at greater risk for major complications while using oral contraceptives. Major health risks include cardiovascular accidents and deep vein thrombosis.
- Impotence may be caused by emotional or physical factors. Treatment includes counseling, medications, circulatory aids, and surgery.

REVIEW QUESTIONS

1. A postoperative prostatectomy client has a three-way indwelling catheter for continuous bladder irrigation. During second shift, 2,700 mL of irrigation solution was instilled. At the end of the shift, 3,250 mL of fluid was drained from the catheter collection bag. The total urine output for the shift is:
   1. 6,250 mL
   2. 3,250 mL
   3. 2,700 mL
   4. 550 mL
2. A client complains of pain and discomfort in the lower abdominal area after a suprapubic prostatectomy. The initial nursing action should be to:
   1. administer the intravenous antibiotic as ordered.
   2. inspect the drainage tube for occlusion.
   3. increase the intravenous rate.
   4. administer oxygen at 2 liter per minute per nasal cannula.
3. The nurse is teaching a female client about fibrocystic breast changes. Which of the following should be included in the teaching plan?
   1. Breast self-examination should not be performed because it will aggravate fibrocystic breasts.
   2. Caffeine and sodium intake should be limited.
   3. Wearing a bra will increase breast discomfort.
   4. Take hot showers to promote comfort.
4. The nurse is teaching a 20-year-old man how to perform a testicular self-examination. Which of the following is an abnormal finding?
   1. The right testes is larger than the left testes.
   2. The testes are slightly sensitive to compression.
   3. The testes are oval shape and movable.
   4. The left testes hangs lower than the right testes.
5. A client has been informed that her sister has been diagnosed with ovarian cancer. The client asks the nurse if she is at risk of developing this type of cancer. The nurse informs the client that risk factors associated with ovarian cancer include: (Select all that apply.)
   1. nulliparity.
   2. infertility.
   3. low-fat diet.
   4. smoking.
   5. family history.
   6. multiparity.
6. The nurse is teaching a female client about breast self-examination (BSE). Which of the following statements indicates that the client correctly understands when she should perform a BSE?
   1. "I should perform a BSE a few days before my menstrual period begins."
   2. "During the time I am ovulating is when I should do a BSE."
   3. "I should do a BSE right after my menstrual period."
   4. "I can perform a BSE anytime of the month."
7. Which nursing intervention must be included in a care plan for a 12-day post radical mastectomy client?
   1. Maintain NPO status for 24 hours.
   2. Place client on complete bed rest for 24 hours.
   3. Place commode at bedside.
   4. Elevate operative arm for 24 hours.
8. A 21-year-old female client makes an appointment with her physician to ask about beginning oral contraceptives. Which of the following questions asked by the nurse would determine if oral contraceptives are an appropriate method of contraception for this client?
   1. "Have you ever had a blood clot or deep vein thrombosis?"
   2. "Do you exercise every day?"
   3. "Are you married?"
   4. "Have you been pregnant before?"
9. What information should be included in a teaching plan for a women's health program to raise awareness of toxic shock syndrome? (Select all that apply.)
   1. Most often caused by Streptococcus group A.
   2. Hypothermia occurs due to inflammatory process.
   3. There is a strong relationship with the use of tampons.
   4. A macular erythematous rash may develop.
   5. Bed rest is usually prescribed.
   6. Hypertensive crisis is a common complication.
10. A 45-year-old male client asks the nurse why he is experiencing impotence since he started taking antihypertensive medication. The best response from the nurse is:
    1. "Antihypertensive medication lowers blood pressure to penile arteries leading to failure of the penis to fill sufficiently to achieve erection."
    2. "You should not be experiencing impotence and need to notify your physician immediately."
    3. "Impotence is only a temporary side effect and will go away within 3 weeks of taking the medication."
    4. "Antihypertensive medication only causes impotence in diabetic men that smoke."

REFERENCES/SUGGESTED READINGS

Akert, J. (2003). A new generation of contraceptives. *RN, 66*(2), 54–61.

American Cancer Society (ACS). (2003). Cancer facts & figures—2003. Retrieved from http://www.cancer.org/downloads/ STT/CFF2003DUSSecured.pdf

American Cancer Society. (2008). Breast cancer. Retrieved August 9, 2009 from http://www.cancer.org/downloads/PRO/BreastCancer.pdf

American Cancer Society. (2009a). Cancer statistics 2009 a presentation from the American Cancer Society. Retrieved August 9, 2009 from http://www.cancer.org/docroot/PRO/content/PRO_1_1_Cancer_Statistics_2009_Presentation.asp

American Cancer Society. (2009b). Detailed guide: Breast cancer—how is breast cancer staged? Retrieved August 9, 2009 from http://www.cancer.org/docroot/CRI/content/CRI_2_4_3X_How_is_breast_cancer_staged_5.asp?sitearea=

American Cancer Society. (2009c). Detailed guide: Cervical cancer—what is cervical cancer? Retrieved August 9, 2009 from http://www.cancer.org/docroot/CRI/content/CRI_2_4_1X_What_is_cervical_cancer_8.asp?sitearea=

American Cancer Society. (2009d). Detailed guide: Ovarian cancer—chemotherapy. Retrieved August 9, 2009 from http://www.cancer.org/docroot/CRI/content/CRI_2_4_4X_Chemotherapy_33.asp?rnav=cri

American Cancer Society. (2009e). Detailed guide: Prostate cancer—chemotherapy. Retrieved August 9, 2009 from http://www.cancer.org/docroot/CRI/content/CRI_2_4_4X_Chemotherapy_36.asp?rnav=cri

American Cancer Society. (2009f). Detailed guide: Prostate cancer—what are the key statistics about prostate cancer? Retrieved August 9, 2009 from http://www.cancer.org/docroot/CRI/content/CRI_2_4_1X_What_are_the_key_statistics_for_prostate_cancer_36.asp?rnav=cri

American Cancer Society. (2009g). Detailed guide: Testicular cancer—what are the key statistics about testicular cancer? Retrieved August 9, 2009 from http://www.cancer.org/docroot/CRI/content/CRI_2_4_1X_What_are_the_key_statistics_for_testicular_cancer_41.asp?sitearea=

Arbique, D., Carter, S., & Van Sell, S. (2008). Endometriosis can evade diagnosis. *RN, 71*(9), 28–32.

Aschenbrenner, D. (2006). Over-the-counter access to emergency contraception. *American Journal of Nursing, 106*(11), 34–36.

Baird, S., Donehower, M., Stalsbroten, V., & Ades, T. (Eds.). (1997). *A cancer source book for nurses* (7th ed.). Atlanta: American Cancer Society.

Carroll, C. (2006). Sorting out breast biopsy options. *Nursing2006, 36*(3), 70–71.

Centers for Disease Control and Prevention. (2008). Pelvic inflammatory disease—CDC fact sheet. Retrieved August 8, 2009 from http://www.cdc.gov/std/PID/STDFact-PID.htm#What

Choma, K. (2003). ASC-US HPV testing. *AJN, 103*(2), 42–50.

Conversations with Colleagues. (2003). Endometriosis sufferers risk other diseases. *AWHONN Lifelines, 6*(6), 502–504.

Crandall, L. (1997). Menopause made easier. *RN, 60*(7), 46–50.

D'Arcy, Y. (2002). What is postmastectomy pain syndrome? *Nursing2002, 32*(11), 17.

Daniels, R. (2010). *Delmar's guide to laboratory and diagnostic tests* (2nd ed.). Clifton Park, NY: Delmar Cengage Learning.

Daniels, R., Nosek, L. & Nicoll, L. (2007). *Contemporary medical-surgical nursing*. Clifton Park, NY: Delmar Cengage Learning.

Dell, D. (2001). Regaining range of motion after breast surgery. *Nursing2001, 31*(10), 50–52.

Estes, M. (2010). *Health assessment & physical examination.* (4th ed.). Clifton Park, NY: Delmar Cengage Learning.

Ficorelli, C., & Weeks, B. (2006). Facing up to prostate cancer. *Nursing2006, 36*(5), 66–68.

Fink, J. (2003). Beyond the shock of an abnormal Pap. *RN, 66*(6), 56–61.

Fletcher, S., & Colditz, G. (2003). Editorial: Failure of estrogen plus progestin therapy for prevention. *Journal of the American Medical Association, 288*(3). Available from http://jama.ama-assn.org/issues/v288n3/ffull/jed20042.html

Fu, M., Ridner, S., & Armor, J. (2009). Post-breast cancer lymphedema. *American Journal of Nursing, 109*(7), 48–54.

Gordon, S., Brenden, J., Wyble, J., & Ivey, C. (1997). When the Dx is penile cancer. *RN, 60*(3), 41–44.

Harris, L. (2002). Ovarian cancer: Screening for early detection. *AJN, 102*(10), 46–52.

Held-Warmkessel, J. (2002). Prostate cancer. *Nursing2002, 32*(12), 36–42.

Hurley, M. (2007). More evidence that race affects breast cancer survival. *RN*, 70(4).

Hutti, M. (2003). New & emerging contraceptive methods. *AWHONN Lifelines*, 7(1), 32–39.

Katz, A. (2007a). 'Not tonight, dear': The elusive female libido. *American Journal of Nursing*, 107(12), 32–34.

Katz, A. (2007b). When sex hurts: Menopause-related dyspareunia. *American Journal of Nursing*, 107(7), 34–39.

Katz, A. (2009). Fertility preservation in young cancer patients. *American Journal of Nursing*, 109(4), 44–47.

Kessenich, C. (1999). Myths & facts about menopause. *Nursing99, 29*(4), 67.

Kring, D. (2003). Benign prostatic hyperplasia. *Nursing2003, 33*(5), 44–45.

Lehman, M. (2007). Ovarian cancer it whispers so listen. *RN*, 70(10), 28–32.

Machia, J. (2002). Breast cancer: Risk, prevention, & tamoxifen. *AJN, 101*(4), 26–34.

Marchbanks, P., McDonald, J., Wilson, H., et al. (2002). Oral contraceptives and the risk of breast cancer. *New England Journal of Medicine, 346*(26), 2025.

Marieb, E. (2003). *Human anatomy and physiology* (6th ed.). Redwood City, CA: Benjamin/Cummings.

Martini, F. (2002). *Fundamentals of anatomy & physiology* (6th ed.). Englewood Cliffs, NJ: Prentice Hall.

Mayo Clinic. (2008a). Endometriosis treatments and drugs. Retrieved August 8, 2009 from http://www.mayoclinic.com/health/endometriosis/DS00289/DSECTION=treatments-and-drugs

Mayo Clinic. (2008b). Fibrocystic breasts lifestyle and home remedies. Retrieved August 8, 2009 from http://www.mayoclinic.com/health/fibrocystic-breasts/DS01070/DSECTION=lifestyle-and-home-remedies

McDaniel, C. (2007). Uterine fibroid embolism: the less invasive alternative. *Nursing2007, 37*(7), 26–27.

Miller, K. (1999). Testicular torsion. *AJN 99*(6), 33.

Moorhead, S., Johnson, M., Maas, M., & Swanson, E. (2007). *Nursing Outcomes Classification (NOC)* (4th ed.). St. Louis, MO: Mosby.

National Cancer Institute (NCI). (2002a). What you need to know about breast cancer (NIH Publication No. 00-1556). Retrieved from http://www.nci.nihl.gov/cancerinfo/wyntk/ breast

National Cancer Institute (NCI). (2002b). What you need to know about cancer of the cervix (NIH Publication No. 95-2047). Retrieved from http://www.nci.nih.gov/cancerinfo/wyntk/cervix

National Cancer Institute (NCI). (2002c). What you need to know about cancer of the uterus (NIH Publication No. 01-1562). Retrieved from http://www.nci.nih.gov/cancerinfo/ wyntk/uterus

National Cancer Institute (NCI). (2002d). What you need to know about ovarian cancer (NIH Publication No. 00-1561). Retrieved from http://www.nci.nih.gov/cancerinfo/wyntk/ovary

National Institute of Diabetes, and Digestive and Kidney Disease (NIDDK). (2002). Prostate enlargement: Benign prostatic hyperplasia. Retrieved from http://www.niddk.nih.gov/ health/ urolog/pubs/prostate/index.htm

National Institutes of Health. (2006). Prostate enlargement: benign prostatic hyperplasia. Retrieved August 8, 2009 from http://kidney .niddk.nih.gov/kudiseases/pubs/prostateenlargement/index.htm

Neighbors, M., & Tannehill-Jones, R. (2006). *Human disease* (2nd ed). Clifton Park, NY: Delmar Cengage Learning.

North American Nursing Diagnosis Association International. (2010). *NANDA-I nursing diagnoses: Definitions and classification 2009–2011*. Ames, IA: Wiley-Blackwell.

Otto, S. (2001). *Oncology nursing* (4th ed.). St. Louis, MO: Mosby–Year Book.

Pasacreta, J., Jacobs, L., & Cataldo, J. (2002). Genetic testing for breast and ovarian cancer risk: The psychosocial issues. *AJN, 102*(12), 40–47.

Pickar, G., & Abernethy Pickar, A. (2008). *Dosage calculations* (8th ed.). Clifton Park, NY: Delmar Cengage Learning.

Resnick, B., & Belcher, A. (2002). Breast reconstruction. *AJN, 102*(4), 26–33.

Rizzo, D. (2010). *Fundamentals of anatomy & physiology* (3rd ed). Clifton Park, NY: Delmar Cengage Learning.

Sarvis, C. (2003). When lymphedema takes hold. *RN, 66*(9), 32–36.

Spratto, G., & Woods, A. (2009). *2009 PDR nurse's drug handbook*. Clifton Park, NY: Delmar Cengage Learning.

The North American Menopause Society. (2009). Hormone products for postmenopausal use in the United States and Canada. Retrieved August 9, 2009 from http://www.menopause.org/htcharts.pdf

U. S. Food and Drug Administration (FDA). (2002). Update on advisory for Norplant contraception kits. Retrieved from http//:www.fda.gov/medwatch/safety/2002/norplant.htm

Wallace, M. (2008). Assessment of sexual health in older adults using the PLISSIT model to talk about sex. *American Journal of Nursing, 108*(7), 52–60.

Walter, L., Bertenthal, D., et al. (2006). PSA screening among elderly men with limited life expectancies. *Journal of American Medical Association, 296*(19), 2336.

Workman, L. (2002). Breast cancer. *Nursing2002, 32*(10), 58–63.

Wynd, C. (2002). Testicular self-examination in young adult men. *Journal of Nursing Scholarship, 34*(3), 251–255.

Zaccognini, M. (1999). Prostate cancer, *AJN, 99*(4), 34–35.

Zuckerman, D. (2002). The breast cancer information gap. *RN, 65*(2), 39–41.

RESOURCES

American Association of Sex Educators, Counselors, and Therapists, http://www.aasect.org

American Cancer Society, Inc., http://www.cancer.org

American College of Obstetricians and Gynecologists (ACOG), http://www.acog.org

American Society of Reproductive Medicine, http://www.asrm.org

Association of Women's Health, Obstetric, and Neonatal Nurses (AWHONN), http://www.awhonn.org

Breast Cancer Network of Strength, http://www.networkofstrength.org

National Cancer Institute (NCI), http://www.cancer.gov

National Ovarian Cancer Coalition, http://www.ovarian.org

North American Menopause Society (NAMS), http://www.menopause.org

Older Women's League, http://www.owl-national.org

Ovarian Cancer National Alliance, http://www.ovariancancer.org

RESOLVE: The National Infertility Association, http://www.resolve.org

CHAPTER 45
Sexually Transmitted Infections

MAKING THE CONNECTION

Refer to the following chapters to increase your understanding of sexually transmitted infections:

Basic Nursing
- ***Life Span Development***
- ***Infection Control/Asepsis***
- ***Diagnostic Tests***

Adult Health Nursing
- ***Reproductive System***
- ***Immune System***

LEARNING OBJECTIVES

Upon completion of this chapter, you should be able to:

- Define key terms.
- List the most prevalent STIs, including causative agents.
- Describe currently used methods of prevention of STIs.
- Describe signs and symptoms, diagnostic aids, and treatment of the common STIs.
- Utilize the nursing process to plan the care of a client with an STI.
- Demonstrate the ability to teach self-care and reinfection prevention measures to the client with an STI.

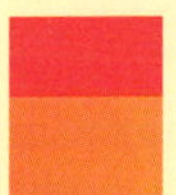

KEY TERMS

abstinence
asymptomatic
chancre
exposure
incidence
incubation period

INTRODUCTION

Sexually transmitted infections (STIs) are transmitted or passed from one person to another primarily through sexual contact. The STIs covered in this chapter are chlamydia, gonorrhea, syphilis, genital herpes, cytomegalovirus, genital warts, trichomoniasis, and hepatitis B. Acquired immunodeficiency syndrome (AIDS) is not solely an STI, although sexual activity is one of the primary modes of transmission. AIDS is discussed in detail in Chapter 47 and will be briefly discussed here.

The **incidence** (frequency of disease occurrence) of STIs has been increasing worldwide, with chlamydia and gonorrhea being the most widespread STIs today. Syphilis has been described as an STI for centuries. An estimated 19 million Americans are diagnosed annually with an STI (CDC, 2007). Almost half of the newly diagnosed infections are among young people who are 15 to 24 years of age. Chlamydia remains to be the most commonly reported STI with approximately 2.8 million new cases infecting Americans every year. Gonorrhea is the second most commonly reported STI in the United States, infecting an estimated 700,000 people (Mayo Clinic, 2009a). Syphilis, although less common than either chlamydia or gonorrhea, has seen a 17.5% increase from 2006 to 2007 in the United States (CDC, 2007a).

The development of antibiotic treatment for STIs in the 1940s caused a dramatic decrease in the prevalence of STIs, and for awhile, it was predicted that STIs would be eradicated completely. However, a variety of factors have contributed to the dramatic increase of STIs, such as casual sex, asymptomatic carriers of the disease, the use of nonbarrier methods of birth control, and lack of knowledge of methods of preventing STIs.

Another factor that has contributed to the vast increase in STIs in recent years is the increased consumption of alcohol and the use of illegal drugs. The sharing of needles among intravenous (IV) drug abusers is a factor in the increased incidence of STIs, as is the lessening of inhibitions that occurs with drug and alcohol abuse. The trading of sex for drugs is also a factor in the spread of STIs.

Inadequate reporting of STIs may also cause statistics to be inaccurate. There is no uniformity in reporting requirements for STIs. Regulations differ from state to state and from disease to disease. Health-care providers are required to report new cases of chlamydia, gonorrhea, syphilis, and hepatitis to state health departments and the CDC (Freedom Network, 2009). The Centers for Disease Control and Prevention (CDC) keeps statistics on reportable diseases.

Public education regarding the causes, methods of transmission, and methods of prevention of STIs is the most important weapon in the battle against STIs. Although many STIs caused by bacterial infection are curable with modern antibiotics, the viruses are not. The CDC (2007a) estimates that STIs cost the U.S. health-care system $15.3 billion annually.

Because sexual activity is beginning at earlier ages today, sex education, including information about STIs, is being presented in elementary schools. Many schools have comprehensive education programs already in place to teach about STIs and recommendations to prevent the spread of STIs. Television, especially educational programs, has been helpful in informing the public of the dangers of having sex without protection against STIs.

Many messages have been disseminated to the general public regarding the best methods of prevention of STIs. The only 100% effective method of prevention of STIs is **abstinence** (refraining from sexual intercourse or mucous membrane–to–mucous membrane contact altogether). Couples who are mutually monogamous are also not at risk, unless one of them was previously infected. The popularity of the birth control pill has decreased consistent condom use. Most current methods of birth control are not effective in preventing the transmission of STIs. Only a barrier method, such as the latex condom, has been effective in preventing the spread of STIs, although even this method provides only safer sex, not completely safe sex.

Once the diagnosis of an STI is made, identification of all sexual contacts is important. Many people are reluctant to be candid regarding sexual activity and sexual contacts because this is an area of life considered to be extremely private. One of the most difficult aspects in dealing with STIs is that many of the diseases are asymptomatic, especially in women. These asymptomatic partners can both transmit the disease to new partners and/or reinfect a treated partner, if they are not identified and treated.

An overview of the STIs covered in this chapter is presented in Table 45-1.

ANATOMY AND PHYSIOLOGY REVIEW

The major system affected by STIs is the reproductive system. Males are generally more symptomatic than females and will seek health care more readily because the signs of disease on the external genitalia are more visible. In females, the sex organs are internal; females, therefore, are more likely to have complications and increased severity of symptoms by the time the disease is identified.

In addition to the reproductive system, any area of sexual contact, such as oral and rectal areas, may also exhibit signs and symptoms of the disease process.

COMMON DIAGNOSTIC TESTS

Commonly used diagnostic tests for clients with symptoms of STIs are listed in Table 45-2.

CHLAMYDIA

Chlamydia is caused by a spherical bacterial organism known as *Chlamydia trachomatis*. Outside the body, the organism has difficulty surviving, but inside the body, chlamydia reproduces rapidly. The mode of transmission in chlamydia must be through intimate body contact because the organism is so fragile that it cannot survive long when outside of the body.

Because nearly 50% of chlamydia infections are **asymptomatic**, having no symptoms at all, it is known as the "silent STI" and usually goes untreated (Freedom Network, 2009). If left untreated, chlamydial infections cause tissue inflammation, ulceration, and scar tissue formation in both women and men. Salpingitis (inflammation of the fallopian tubes) or pelvic inflammatory disease (PID) can lead to scarring of the delicate fallopian tubes, ectopic pregnancy, or even infertility.

TABLE 45-1 Sexually Transmitted Infections: An Overview

DISEASE	CHARACTERISTICS	NURSING IMPLICATIONS
Chlamydia	Asymptomatic or may experience purulent discharge Painful urination Urethral discharge *Note:* If untreated, pelvic inflammatory disease (PID) can develop	Instruct client to notify sexual partner(s) of past 2 months of their need for treatment. Instruct client to avoid sexual activity or to use condoms until both client and partner(s) are symptom free. Provide instruction regarding medications prescribed.
Cytomegalovirus (CMV) (Human herpesvirus type 5 [HHV-5])	Often asymptomatic, occasionally fever, fatigue, and weakness Generally acquired during childhood or adolescence 50% to 80% of adults have antibodies to CMV by age 40	Implicated in some spontaneous abortions or mental retardation. Congenital infection produces cytomegalic inclusion disease. May be life threatening in a client with a poorly functioning immune system.
Genital Herpes: Herpes Simplex Virus 2 (HSV-2) (Human herpes-virus type 2 [HHV-2])	Vesicles on penis, vagina, labia, perineum, or anus Can progress to painful ulceration Lesions may last up to 6 weeks Recurrence common *Note:* May be asymptomatic	Refer sexual partner(s) for examination. Teach that virus can be transmitted even when the person experiences no symptoms. Instruct in use of condoms. Teach females of the need for annual Pap smears. Provide instruction regarding medications prescribed.
Gonorrhea	*Male:* Urethritis (inflammation of the urethra) Purulent discharge Urinary frequency Epididymitis (inflammation of the epididymis) *Female:* Often asymptomatic May lead to PID or salpingitis (inflammation of the fallopian tube) Can occlude the fallopian tubes, resulting in sterility	Instruct client to return if symptoms persist. Sexual partner(s) of past 60 days must be assessed. Instruct client to avoid sexual activity until symptoms subside in both client and partner(s). Provide instruction regarding medications prescribed.
Hepatitis B Virus (HBV)	Varies greatly from asymptomatic state, to severe hepatitis, to cancer	Partner(s) should receive medical prophylaxis within 14 days after exposure. For client and partner(s), recommend three-dose immunization series when this episode has abated.
Genital Warts (Human Papillomavirus) (HPV)	Fleshy, cauliflower-like growth on genitalia	Inform and treat sexual partner(s). Provide instruction regarding medications prescribed.

(*Continues*)

TABLE 45-1 Sexually Transmitted Infections: An Overview (Continued)

DISEASE	CHARACTERISTICS	NURSING IMPLICATIONS
Syphilis	Disease consists of four stages with distinct manifestations as follows:	Interview client to identify sexual contacts.
	Primary:	
	A painless papule on penis, vagina, or cervix (chancre)	All those exposed to the disease should be given penicillin or other antibiotic if allergic to penicillin.
	Usually negative serologic blood test	
	Highly infectious during this stage	
	Secondary:	
	Rash, especially prevalent on palms and soles	Educate client and sexual contacts about the disease.
	Low-grade fever	Provide instruction regarding medications prescribed.
	Sore throat	
	Headache	
	Early latency:	
	Possible infectious lesions, otherwise asymptomatic	Counsel and educate client.
	Reactive serologic tests	
	Late latency:	
	Possible lesions in central nervous and cardiovascular systems	Counsel and educate client.
	Noninfectious except to fetus of pregnant woman	
Trichomoniasis	Petechial lesions	Treat sexual partners simultaneously with metronidazole (Flagyl).
	Profuse urethral or vaginal discharge that is foul smelling, yellow, and foamy	Provide instruction regarding medication prescribed.

COURTESY OF DELMAR CENGAGE LEARNING

When symptoms of chlamydia appear in men, they include dysuria; watery white, cloudy discharge from the urethra; and testicular pain and swelling. Women may have grayish white mucopurulent vaginal drainage, bleeding between periods, dysuria, low abdominal pain, and bleeding or pain during or after sexual intercourse.

MEDICAL–SURGICAL MANAGEMENT

Pharmacological

The treatment of choice is doxycycline (Vibramycin). If compliance with an extended period of drug therapy is thought to be a problem, azithromycin (Zithromax) can be given orally in a single dose. Pregnant women may be treated with erythromycin estolate (Ilosone) or amoxicillin (Amoxil), but they should be cultured again after treatment is completed to confirm the absence of chlamydial infection. Retesting is not required after treatment with doxycycline or azithromycin. It is important that all sexual partners are tested and treated for chlamydia because reinfection is probable if only one partner is treated.

Health Promotion

Persons who have more than one sexual partner, especially women less than 25 years old, should regularly be tested for chlamydial infection even when there are no symptoms. The current use of male latex condoms during sexual intercourse may help reduce transmission.

GONORRHEA

Gonorrheal infections are often seen in combination with chlamydia. Gonorrhea is a serious bacterial infection, caused by the gram-negative bacterial organism *Neisseria gonorrhea*. In 2007, more than 350,000 cases occurred in the United States (CDC, 2007a). The organism multiplies

TABLE 45-2 Common Diagnostic Tests for STIs

Blood Tests
- Enzyme immunoassay (EIA) (rapid test)
- Western Blot
- Venereal Disease Research Laboratories (VDRL)
- Rapid plasma reagin (RPR)
- Fluorescent treponemal antibody-absorption test (FTA-ABS)
- Reiter test
- Antigen test for HSV

Culture
- Tissue: Male urethra, female endocervix
- Discharge—swab test
- Tzanck
- Nucleic Acid Amplification Test (NAAT)

Urine
- Urine specimen
- NAAT

Other
- Dark field examination of wart screenings
- Microscopic examination
- OSOM Trichomonas rapid test
- Immunofloresence testing

COURTESY OF DELMAR CENGAGE LEARNING

quickly in warm, moist areas of the body, including the oral cavity, reproductive tract, and rectum. Mouth-to-mouth kissing does not transmit gonorrhea. It is spread during sexual intercourse—vaginal, oral, and anal. The cervix is the usual site of infection in women. The disease progresses in much the same manner as chlamydia and can cause many of the same complications, such as infertility from salpingitis and PID.

Symptoms of infection may occur within 2 to 10 days after **exposure** (contact with an infected person or agent). Men are more likely to exhibit symptoms such as white, yellow, or green thick discharge from the tip of the penis (Figure 45-1), swelling of the testicles and prostate gland, dysuria, and anal irritation and discharge. Many women are asymptomatic, but the remainder may have pain or burning on urination and/or a yellow or bloody vaginal discharge.

If a woman is infected with gonorrhea when she gives birth, the infection may be transmitted to the newborn's eyes as the baby travels through the birth canal. In the United States, all infants are treated with an antibiotic ophthalmic

CLIENT TEACHING

Proper Use of Condoms

No method of barrier birth control works perfectly to protect against STIs. Therefore, the client should be educated regarding the proper use of both male and female condoms.

- Aside from abstinence, condoms provide the most protection against STIs by preventing mucous membrane contact.
- Clients should be advised to use condoms for every sexual encounter.
- Latex sheaths are available to prevent oral-genital mucous membrane contact.
- The client should be instructed to store condoms in a cool, dry place, away from sunlight.
- A new condom must be used for each sexual encounter; condoms cannot be reused.
- Proper condom disposal includes holding the condom at the base of the penile shaft after ejaculation so that the condom does not slip out of place.

CRITICAL THINKING

Chlamydia Treatment

1. Your client has been prescribed doxycycline for treatment of chlamydia. What precautions will the nurse include with the prescription?
2. The client asks you if she needs to continue taking the medication even though she no longer has any STI symptoms. What will the nurse tell her?
3. The client asks if she can continue to engage in sexual activity with her boyfriend while she is taking the antibiotic. What will the nurse recommend?

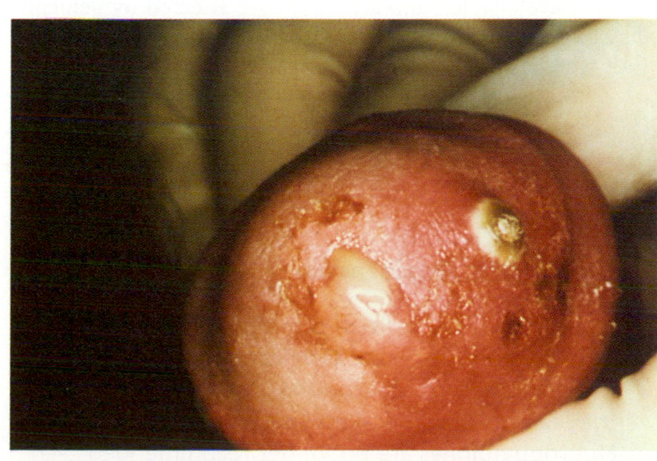

FIGURE 45-1 Male clients with gonorrhea exhibit purulent discharge from the penis. (*Courtesy of Centers for Disease Control and Prevention.*)

CLIENT TEACHING

Reducing Your Risk

- Practice abstinence or mutual monogamy.
- The best method is to use latex condoms at the beginning of vaginal and/or anal sex until there is no longer skin contact.
- Water-based spermicides are not recommended for the prevention of gonorrhea.
- Recent studies have shown that nonoxynol-9 is not effective in preventing gonorrhea (American Social Health Association [ASHA], 2009).
- Do not share sex toys.
- You cannot catch gonorrhea from sharing toilet seats or sharing towels.
- Several barrier methods can be used to reduce the risk of transmission of gonorrhea during oral sex.
  - A nonlubricated condom can be used for mouth-to-penis contact.
  - A dental dam or food plastic wrap can be used during mouth-to vulva/vaginal or oral-anal (rimming) contact.

(ASHA, 2009; Freedom Network, 2009)

ointment at birth to prevent the gonorrheal-induced eye infection known as ophthalmia neonatorum.

Medical–Surgical Management

Once the presence of gonorrhea has been confirmed, both partners should be treated with a course of antibiotic therapy. Penicillin used to be the drug of choice when treating gonorrhea, but because penicillin has been so widely used against many types of infection, some strains of *Neisseria gonorrhea* have adapted and are no longer affected by penicillin. The current practice is to treat all cases of gonorrhea as though they were resistant to the traditional drug therapies.

PROFESSIONAL TIP

Antibiotic Resistance

In 2007, the CDC revised its gonorrhea treatment guidelines based on data indicating widespread drug resistance to fluoroquinolones, which were the leading antibiotic class to treat gonorrhea. Fluoroquinolones are no longer recommended to treat gonorrhea. Cephalosporins are now the antibiotic choice for treatment.

CULTURAL CONSIDERATIONS

Gonorrhea

Traditionally, ethnic minorities in the United States have had greater rates of reported gonorrhea and other STIs—in part, a reflection of limited access to quality health care. African-American subjects are most widely affected by gonorrhea, with a rate of infection approximately 19 times greater than that of Caucasian subjects. American Indians/Alaska Natives had the second highest gonorrhea rate in 2007, followed by Hispanics. Asians/Pacific Islanders had the lowest rates of gonorrhea (CDC, 2007b).

Pharmacological

A variety of antibiotics are effective against gonorrhea. One of the most effective therapies includes a single dose of ciprofloxacin (Cipro), followed by a 7-day course of oral doxycycline (Vibramycin). Because almost half of all clients with gonorrhea also have chlamydia, doxycycline (Vibramycin) is an appropriate choice of drug therapy because it combats both infections effectively. For pregnant clients, or those younger than 16 years of age, an injection of ceftriaxone sodium (Rocephlin), followed by oral erythromycin estolate (Ilosone), is recommended. Follow-up cultures to determine the success of the course of treatment are recommended when the treatment has been completed.

SYPHILIS

Syphilis, an STI that was almost eradicated after the discovery of antibiotic therapy in the 1940s, is on the upswing again, with 11,466 cases reported in 2007, a 15.2 % increase from 2006 (CDC, 2007a). The causative organism of syphilis is a spirochete, a spiral-shaped bacterium known as *Treponema pallidum*, which was first identified in 1905. Transmission of syphilis is either through sexual contact or congenitally (mother to child). Syphilis is often seen with human immunodeficiency virus (HIV) infection, just as chlamydia is often seen with gonorrhea.

Syphilis has four stages. In primary stage syphilis, the **incubation period**, time between exposure to an infectious disease and the first appearance of symptoms, can be 10 to 90 days with the development of a chancre usually occurring within 2 to 6 weeks. A **chancre** is a clean, painless ulcer that usually is present at the site of body contact (Figure 45-2). There is usually just one chancre present, but multiple chancres have been known to occur. Chancres may occur on the internal genitalia of women (e.g., the cervix) and thus not be noticed. The chancre will heal within a few weeks, even without treatment, and either leave a thin scar or none at all. If not identified and treated, about one-third will progress to secondary syphilis.

In secondary syphilis, the client has a skin rash of penny-sized brown sores that appear approximately 3 to 6 weeks after the chancre. The rash may be on all or any part of the body but almost always involves the palms of the hands and the soles of

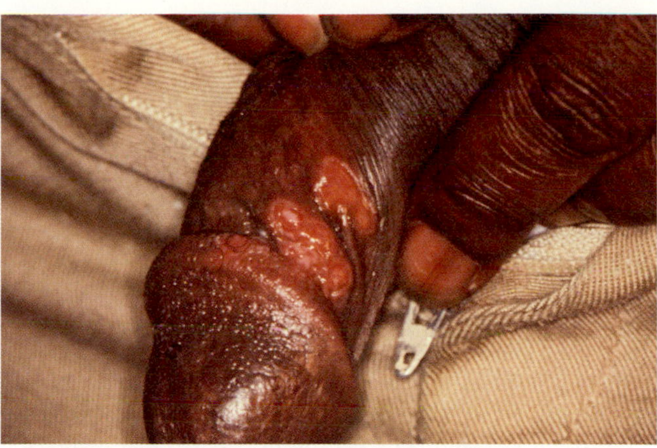

FIGURE 45-2 The primary stage of syphilis is usually marked by the appearance of a single sore called a chancre. (*Courtesy of Centers for Disease Control and Prevention.*)

the feet. Active bacteria are in the sores, so any contact, sexual or nonsexual, with the broken skin of the infected person may spread the infection. The rash heals within several months. Other symptoms, such as low-grade fever, fatigue, headache, sore throat, and generalized lymph node swelling, may occur. Occasionally, a wart-like growth known as condyloma latum may be present in the genital area of both men and women. Because this growth is so close in appearance to the condylomata acuminata of human papillomavirus infection, it may be confused with genital warts. Symptoms of secondary syphilis may come and go for 1 or 2 years. Because many of these symptoms are also common to many other diseases, syphilis has often been called "the great imitator."

When not treated, syphilis enters into a latent period when no symptoms are present and the disease is no longer contagious. Only approximately one-third of those clients with secondary syphilis will develop the symptoms of tertiary syphilis, that is, when the bacteria damages the heart, eyes, brain, nervous system, bones, joints, or any other part of the body. Tertiary syphilis can last for years or decades and may result in heart disease, blindness, neurologic problems, and death.

Medical–Surgical Management

Pharmacological

Since the time that syphilis was first treated with antibiotic therapy, penicillin has remained the drug of choice because no cases of penicillin-resistant syphilis have been identified. All types of penicillin are effective, but penicillin G benzathine (Bicillin L-A) is often preferred. Antimicrobial therapy will destroy Treponema pallidum at any stage, but any damage done to body organs is irreversible. If the client has a demonstrated allergy to penicillin, alternative medications may be administered, such as doxycycline (Vibramycin), tetracycline HCl (Achromycin V), or erythromycin estolate (Ilosone). For pregnant women who are allergic to penicillin, erythromycin is recommended as the best alternative therapy.

Clients being treated for syphilis must have periodic blood tests to ensure that the infecting agent has been completely destroyed.

MEMORY TRICK

RASH

A useful memory trick to use when assessing a client for signs and symptoms of syphilis is **RASH**:

- **R** = Rash (on palms and soles)
- **A** = A painless papule (on penis, vagina, or cervix)
- **S** = Sore throat
- **H** = Headache

CLIENT TEACHING

Testing for Syphilis

- According to the CDC (2007a), regular screening of men who have sex with men (MSM), is an important step toward preventing the spread of syphilis.
- Pregnant women being screened at their first prenatal visit is critical in protecting infants from congenital syphilis complications such as blindness.

GENITAL HERPES

Genital herpes affects an estimated 45 million persons in the United States. (1 out of 5 adolescents and adults) (CDC, 2009). It is caused by the human herpesvirus type 2, commonly called the herpes simplex virus (HSV-2). HSV-1 commonly causes sores on the lips (fever blisters, cold sores). HSV-2 causes genital sores. Either can infect the other area following oral-genital sex. Genital herpes is usually acquired through sexual contact with an infected person. That person may or may not be aware of having genital herpes.

When symptoms occur in the first episode, they usually appear in 2 to 10 days after infection and last an average of 2 to 3 weeks. Itching or burning sensations; pain in the genital area, legs, or buttocks; vaginal discharge; or abdominal pressure are the early symptoms. Within a few days, lesions (sores) appear at the infection site (perianal area), in the vagina or on the cervix of women, or in the urethra of women and men.

Small red bumps appear first, change into blisters (Figure 45-3), and then become open sores that crust over in a few days. Other symptoms with the first episode may include fever, muscle aches, headache, dysuria, vaginal discharge, and swollen glands in the groin.

With the first episode, the virus travels through the sensory nerves and remains inactive in nerve cells until the virus travels back to the skin, causing a recurrence. The frequency of recurrences vary greatly (some only 1 or 2 a year), but new sores may or may not be apparent. Symptoms are usually milder than the first episode and last approximately 1 week.

The most accurate method of diagnosis is a viral culture, which takes several days. A blood test detecting HSV antibodies only indicates that the person has been infected at some time.

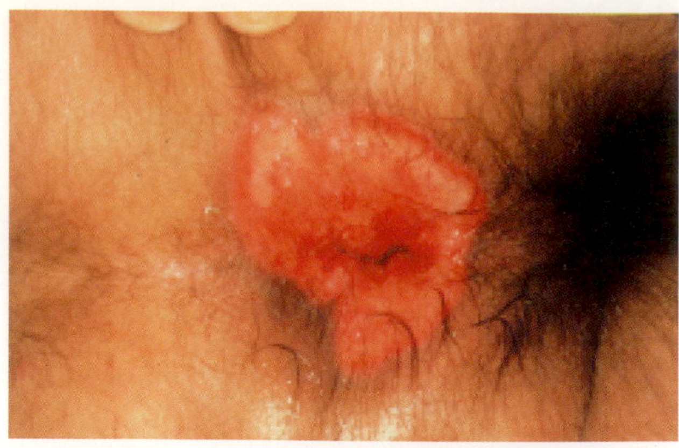

FIGURE 45-3 Chronic Mucocutaneous Perianal Herpes Infection (*Courtesy of Centers for Disease Control and Prevention.*)

MEDICAL–SURGICAL MANAGEMENT

Pharmacological

There is no known cure for the herpes simplex virus at this time. Treatment has been geared toward alleviating symptoms of the disease. Acyclovir (Zovirax) has been used in the treatment of herpes. A topical form may be applied to the lesions; the drug may also be taken orally to shorten the duration of the lesions in a primary outbreak. When taken daily, it prevents most recurrences. Famciclovir (Famivir) and valacyclovir (Valtrex) treat later episodes and prevent recurrences.

Cleansing the area of the lesions with mild soap and water, hydrogen peroxide, or Burow's solution often helps reduce the discomfort of the lesions and decrease the chance of secondary infections. The area should be blown dry with a hairdryer, and then the dry skin may be dusted with a cornstarch powder, which aids in decreasing client discomfort.

CYTOMEGALOVIRUS

Another virus in the herpes virus family is cytomegalovirus (CMV). Unlike the more commonly recognized herpes viruses, CMV rarely produces noticeable clinical symptoms.

CMV is primarily transmitted from person to person through contact with body fluids such as saliva, breast milk, urine, and blood. The virus has been identified in semen, vaginal fluids, and cervical mucus, so it can be spread by sexual contact. CMV is incurable; people are infected for life. The inactive virus may reactivate from time to time.

Most people acquire CMV during childhood or adolescence through contact with saliva and respiratory secretions and will not notice any symptoms. Occasionally, a client will present with fever, fatigue, and weakness. These symptoms may persist for several weeks and may lead to a tentative diagnosis of infectious mononucleosis, although the sore throat and swollen lymph nodes of "mono" are not present with CMV.

CMV has been implicated in some complications of pregnancy, such as spontaneous abortion or mental retardation of the neonate. Congenital infection of an infant produces cytomegalic inclusion disease that ranges from an asymptomatic condition to a severely debilitating condition that may even result in death. The central nervous system damage to the infant may be profound, although it rarely occurs. An estimated 8,000 children each year will suffer permanent disabilities caused by CMV such as mental retardation, blindness, deafness, or epilepsy (CDC, 2008a). CMV can also become a life-threatening illness in a client who has a poorly functioning immune system, such as a client with AIDS.

There is no antiviral agent specifically utilized for this disorder because most of the population will not have any symptoms.

> **PROFESSIONALTIP**
>
> **Client Support**
>
> The client may need emotional support, since the diagnosis of herpes means lifelong management. The disease will not be cured after a course of antiviral medication, and the client must thoroughly understand this fact. The client may be referred to a counselor or to a support group such as HELP at the Herpes Resource Center (ASHA, 2009a).

HUMAN PAPILLOMAVIRUS/ GENITAL WARTS

Another virus that is sexually transmitted is the human papillomavirus (HPV), which causes genital warts, also called condylomata acuminata. Genital warts may occur in the urogenital, perineal, or anal areas and may be either external or internal. The population at risk seems to be teenage girls or young women in their twenties. In the United States, it is estimated that there are approximately 25,000 new cases of HPV identified every year, and at least 20 million people are already infected (National Institutes of Health, 2008). The incubation period for genital warts appears to be approximately 1 to 2 months but may be up to 6 months. Unlike genital herpes, genital warts are usually painless, soft fleshy growths appearing most commonly in the genital area. Sometimes many warts may grow together to form a large cauliflower-shaped growth (Figure 45-4).

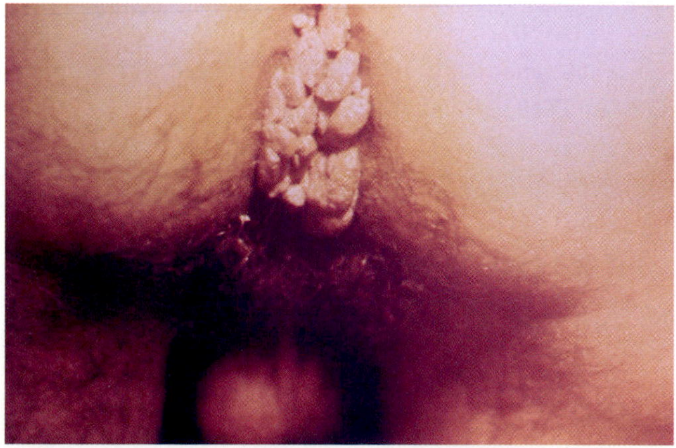

FIGURE 45-4 Genital warts (*Condylomata acuminate*) are caused by human papillomavirus (HPV), which presents as bumps or warts on the genitalia and within the perineal region. (*Courtesy of Centers for Disease Control and Prevention.*)

The greatest health threat that HPV poses to a female client is the potential development of cervical cancer. Although there are more than 100 different types of HPV, only 30 types are spread through sexual contact, and some of these can cause cervical cancer. Cigarette smoking has been linked to the development of cancerous cervical changes in women with HPV. Women who have HPV should be advised not to smoke. HPV appears to play a role in the development of cervical cancer, along with many other factors. An abnormal Pap test may be the first indication of HPV.

Genital warts are less common in men. If seen, they are usually on the tip of the penis or anal area.

Medical–Surgical Management

Because genital warts are caused by a virus, there is no cure for the disease. The focus is on preventing the spread of the disease to sexual partners and reducing the possibility of cancer. Use of a condom during sexual intercourse may provide some protection. Once the genital warts disappear, the disease may lie dormant for many years until there is a recurrence of the outbreak.

Surgical

The warts may be removed under local anesthesia. This is especially recommended if the warts have formed a large, fleshy cauliflower-like growth. Freezing the warts off with cryosurgery, surgical use of extreme cold, is the treatment of choice for small warts. The warts may also be removed with laser surgery or cauterized. Whatever treatment is recommended, it must be remembered that the treatment will not cure HPV, but only provide a palliative effect. The warts may recur after any treatment.

Pharmacological

A topical solution of podophyllum resin (Poddoen) may be applied to the genital warts. It is only recommended for treatment of one or two lesions at a time because it can be toxic if applied to too large an area at one time. Most people report experiencing a good deal of pain from the treatment. After the solution has been in contact with the genital warts for a period of 4 to 6 hours, it is then washed off with soap and water. If not thoroughly washed off, podophyllum may cause chemical burns that heal very slowly and are very painful. This therapy must not be used on a diabetic client, a client with poor circulation, or a pregnant client.

A cream, imiquimod (Aldara), is applied before bedtime and washed off in the morning. It can be used 3 times a week for 16 weeks or less.

Health Promotion

There is currently a vaccine (Gardasil) available that can protect females from the four types of HPV that cause the majority of cervical cancers and genital warts. The vaccine is recommended for females 11 to 26 years of age. The immunization schedule for the vaccine includes a series of three intramuscular injections. There are no vaccines available at this time for males. Studies are currently being conducted to find out if the vaccine is safe for females and effective in males.

AIDS

AIDS, or acquired immunodeficiency syndrome, is not truly an STI, but it needs to be discussed briefly here because sexual contact is one of the primary modes of its transmission. AIDS is the end stage of the disease process caused by the human immunodeficiency virus (HIV) (Chapter 47). Similar to the viruses previously discussed in this chapter, AIDS is not curable. Unlike the other viruses, herpes genitalis and genital warts, AIDS is ultimately fatal. AIDS results in a severe disorder of the body's immune system, leading to an inability of the body to fight off disease.

Persons at risk are those who have multiple sexual partners, IV drug users who share needles, and persons with hemophilia. There are three basic modes of transmission: sexual, bloodborne, and from mother to baby either prenatally, during the birth process, or when breastfeeding. When first identified in 1981, HIV infection was primarily found among homosexual men, but by 1990, the disease was moving into heterosexual populations with great rapidity. By the mid-1990s, cases of AIDS were occurring more frequently among women than among men. The greatest growth in AIDS rates among women occurred in African-American and Hispanic women. Teenagers also have one of the fastest growing rates of HIV infection.

The CDC's HIV/AIDS surveillance system is the nation's source for current information and statistics, tracking the epidemic, and collecting, analyzing, interpreting, and evaluating data regarding HIV/AIDS. The CDC also conducts research studies to find new treatment options and potential vaccines (Figure 45-5). It is estimated that 1.1 million

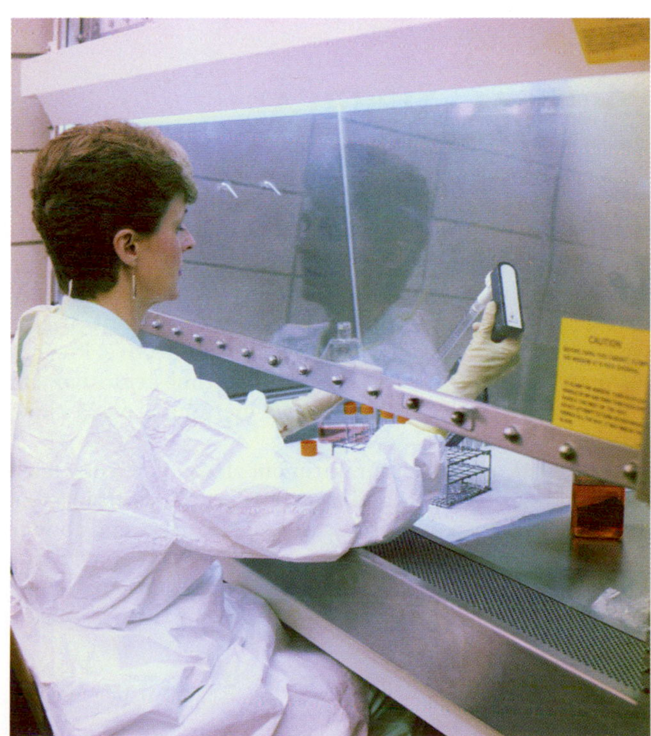

Figure 45-5 Since the beginning of the AIDS epidemic, the CDC has been at the forefront of HIV investigation and lab research. (*Courtesy of Centers for Disease Control and Prevention.*)

Americans are living with HIV and 33.2 million persons worldwide. Two-thirds of HIV infections are in sub-Saharan Africa (CDC, 2008c; WHO, 2009).

TRICHOMONIASIS

Trichomoniasis is caused by a parasitic protozoan called *Trichomonas vaginalis*. Trichomoniasis is a very common STI with an incidence of approximately 8 million new cases a year (CDC, 2008b). It is seen frequently in combination with gonorrhea. The most common method of transmission is sexual, although the protozoa can survive for a period of time in water, so other modes of transmission are possible.

The incubation period after initial exposure to trichomoniasis ranges from approximately 4 to 20 days. About 25% of women infected with trichomoniasis will have no symptoms, and men almost never have symptoms. In these clients, the *Trichomonas* organisms may remain dormant for years without becoming an active infection. Precipitating factors that may encourage the growth of *Trichomonas* include pregnancy, sexual intercourse, menstruation, or illness. Vulval and vaginal pruritus are the most common symptoms, with a vaginal discharge of a frothy, copious yellow-green mucus. Only 10% of women will present with the classic symptoms of a *Trichomonas* infection: severe itching of the vulva, redness, swelling of the vulva, pain on intercourse and urination, urinary frequency, a grayish, malodorous discharge, and the appearance of a "strawberry cervix" caused by hemorrhages with accompanying papules and vesicles. Men most often have a watery, whitish discharge and difficult or painful urination, but they may also have urethritis and an accompanying inflammation. In men, *Trichomonas* in the dormant state are usually harbored in the prostate or urethra.

MEDICAL–SURGICAL MANAGEMENT

Pharmacological

Both partners should be treated with metronidazole (Flagyl or Protostat) given either orally in a single dose or for a period of approximately 1 week. Metronidazole is effective against both protozoal and bacterial infections. If given vaginally, metronidazole (Flagyl) is not as effective. Pregnant women are usually treated after the first trimester to avoid the possibility of birth defects, because metronidazole is known to cross the placenta.

Adverse effects occur in about 10% of clients taking metronidazole (Flagyl) and usually affect the gastrointestinal system in the form of nausea, vomiting, diarrhea, and abdominal cramping. CNS effects such as headache or dizziness may also be seen.

> **CLIENT TEACHING**
>
> **Metronidazole (Flagyl or Protostat)**
>
> No alcohol should be consumed when taking this drug because it causes severe nausea and vomiting, flushing, palpitations, abdominal cramps, and headache (Cleveland Clinic, 2009).

HEPATITIS B

Hepatitis B, caused by the hepatitis B virus, is now recognized as an STI. Today, it is primarily transmitted through direct contact with blood, vaginal secretions, and semen. In 2006, approximately 46,000 people were newly infected with HBV. An estimated 800,000 to 1.4 million Americans have chronic HBV infection (CDC, 2008e).

Clients with hepatitis B experience inflammation of the liver, anorexia, vague abdominal discomfort, nausea, vomiting, fatigue, and jaundice. Fever may be mild or absent. Symptoms may progress to chronic liver disease, hepatic cancer, hepatic failure, and death.

MEDICAL–SURGICAL MANAGEMENT

Medical

There is no specific treatment for acute HBV infection. Treatment is based on relieving symptoms. Several antiviral medications are available to treat chronic HBV infection including adefovir dipivoxil (Hepsera), peginterferon (Pegasys), lamivudine (Epivir), and entecavir (Baraclude). Interferon, another antiviral agent, helps to stop the replication of HBV.

Health Promotion

Hepatitis B has two single-antigen vaccines and three combination vaccines currently available for administration in the United States. The immunization schedule most commonly followed consists of a series of three intramuscular injections. Recommendations for immunization include all newborns, health-care workers, and high-risk groups of all ages (CDC, 2008e).

NURSING MANAGEMENT

Follow proper hand hygiene technique. Teach the client hand hygiene to be followed after using the bathroom and every time the penis, vagina, or perineal areas are touched. Provide nonjudgmental support to all clients. Encourage clients to notify past and present sexual partners of the diagnosis and the need to seek medical care. Advise client to wear loose-fitting clothes and cotton underwear for comfort.

NURSING PROCESS

The following is a general nursing process for the client with an STI.

ASSESSMENT

Subjective Data

Data to be gathered from a client who presents with a suspected STI are very similar, regardless of the actual STI. A thorough history must be obtained. A relaxed, nonjudgmental attitude will help to elicit accurate information from the client. Confidentiality and privacy are extremely important

CRITICAL THINKING

Multiple Sexual Partners

What should a client who has multiple sexual partners be taught about STIs? Make a teaching plan while keeping in mind the sensitivity of the information to be shared and the client's receptivity.

when dealing with both the history and physical examination for STIs. Gather pertinent information regarding the client's sexual orientation (homosexual, heterosexual, bisexual), any prior treatment for an STI, and the number of sexual partners that the client has had in the last 6 months.

Ask women about symptoms such as vulval or vaginal itching, vaginal discharge, pain or discomfort, skin rashes or pruritus, and any changes in the menstrual periods or other abnormal bleeding. Question men regarding the presence of symptoms such as pain or burning on urination, abnormal penile discharges, skin rashes or itching, or lesions on external genitalia. Ask both men and women about urinary frequency or discomfort and systemic symptoms such as fatigue, malaise, or sore throat. Ask homosexual men about rectal symptoms such as abnormal discharge, itching, lesions, or pain on defecation (Table 45-3).

Objective Data

Carefully assess the reproductive, gastrointestinal, and integumentary systems. Determine the presence or absence of skin rashes or lesions and abnormal discharges. Females need a speculum examination of the vagina and cervix to closely observe internal organs for changes consistent with STIs. Examine the rectal area to look for any abnormal discharge, lesions, or tenderness. Palpate inguinal lymph nodes to look for signs of infection.

LIFE SPAN CONSIDERATIONS

Sexual Activity in Older Adults

Many young nurses find it difficult to think of older adults as sexual beings. As the "baby boomers" age, however, they are becoming very assertive about living life to the fullest, which includes continuing to enjoy an active sex life. An older adult who is single may still be sexually active and engage in high-risk sexual activities. A tactful, respectful approach will allow the nurse to obtain an accurate sexual history if symptoms seem to indicate the likelihood of an STI.

TABLE 45-3 Health History Questions: STIs

Questions for Women and Men

- Can you share with me your sexual orientation (homosexual, heterosexual, bisexual)?
- Have you been diagnosed with an STI in the past?
- If so, which STI(s) have you been diagnosed with?
- Have you been diagnosed with more than one STI? If so, which disease(s)?
- How many sexual partners have you had in the past 6 months?
- How many sexual partners have you had since you became sexually active?
- Do you have any skin rashes or itching? If so, where on your body?
- Does it burn or hurt when you urinate?
- Are you urinating more frequently than usual?
- Have you been more tired than usual?
- Do you have a sore throat?
- Have you had any sores or lesions on your lips, tongue, or in your mouth?
- Have you noticed any anal discharge or tenderness?

Questions for Women

- Have you experienced vaginal itching? Vaginal pain or discomfort?
- Are you experiencing any changes in your menstrual cycle?
- Do you have any abnormal vaginal bleeding or discharge?

Questions for Men

- Do you have any sores or lesions in your pubic area?
- Do you have any sores or lesions on your penis?
- Are you experiencing any discharge from the tip of your penis?
- Are your testicles swollen or tender?

COURTESY OF DELMAR CENGAGE LEARNING

Nursing diagnoses for the client with an STI include the following:

NURSING DIAGNOSES	PLANNING/OUTCOMES	NURSING INTERVENTIONS
Anxiety related to unknown procedures, embarrassment, or other factors (relates to nearly every client who presents with an STI)	The client will verbalize a lack of knowledge and embarrassment.	Provide a relaxed, nonjudgmental attitude which will aid in reducing client anxiety. Listen actively to both the spoken and unspoken concerns of the client. The nurse must examine own attitudes toward STIs and the clients who suffer from them.
Deficient Knowledge related to mode of transmission of the STI, prevention methods, and risk for spread of the STI	The client will accurately discuss the mode of transmission of an STI and list appropriate measures to avoid reinfection or future infection.	Teach mode of transmission, prevention of further infection, and risk for spread. Take time to make sure the client has a thorough understanding of all necessary aspects of the disease.
Risk for Infection related to incomplete treatment or lack of precautions with untreated, infected partners	The client will state the need for having all sexual partners notified and treated. The client will state understanding of the treatment regimen and of the importance of completing treatment. The client will explain appropriate use of latex condoms, including how and when to apply and remove the device.	Discuss the need for all sexual partners to be notified and treated. Discuss the importance of completing treatment regimen. Teach the importance of abstaining from sexual intercourse until the infection is resolved, or of using appropriate measures, such as latex condoms, to prevent reinfection.

Evaluation: Evaluate each outcome to determine how it has been met by the client.

SAMPLE NURSING CARE PLAN

The Client with Genital Herpes

J.B. is a single woman in her middle twenties who has been coming to the clinic for annual Pap smears and birth control for several years. She is a well-nourished, healthy-appearing young woman of medium height. She rescheduled her annual Pap smear to come into the clinic early because she noticed a cluster of small blisters on the inside of her left thigh that also involves the labia majora. She also reports that she has just gotten the flu as evidenced by headache, fever, and general achiness.

J.B. has used birth control pills in the past and reports satisfaction with this method of birth control. She reports that she and her new boyfriend became intimate about 2 weeks ago, so she wants to renew her birth control pill prescription. She also states that intercourse has been uncomfortable since the appearance of the lesions and that she does not feel comfortable with sexual activity while the lesions are present because they make her feel "ugly."

The assessment determines the presence of a cluster of small blisters as well as swollen, tender inguinal lymph nodes. A Tzanck smear test is obtained. J.B.'s test results come back positive for genital herpes.

NURSING DIAGNOSIS 1 *Ineffective Sexuality Pattern* related to lesions as evidenced by her comment that intercourse has been uncomfortable since the appearance of the lesions

Nursing Outcomes Classification (NOC)
Psychosocial Adjustment: Life Change

Nursing Interventions Classification (NIC)
Sexual Counseling

SAMPLE NURSING CARE PLAN (Continued)

PLANNING/OUTCOMES	NURSING INTERVENTIONS	RATIONALE
J.B. will express her feelings about potential changes in her sexual behavior before leaving the clinic.	Provide a nonjudgmental atmosphere to encourage J.B. to express her feelings about this perceived change in her sexual identity.	Demonstrates the caregiver's positive feelings toward J.B. and concerns she may have regarding her future sexuality.
	Provide privacy and an uninterrupted amount of time to talk with J.B.	Shows respect and conveys reassurance in discussing sexuality issues and concerns with her.
	Provide accurate information to J.B. about genital herpes and include literature or videos for her to share with her boyfriend.	Helps J.B. focus on specific, necessary information and encourages her to ask questions.
	Offer the names of local support groups such as HELP (Herpetics Engaged in Living Productively) or other support persons who can provide information and group support to J.B.	Provides J.B. with resources for support once she has returned home and the reality of her diagnosis has set in.

EVALUATION

J.B. states that she is still in shock but thinks that she will be able to deal with her diagnosis. She also states that she will call back to the clinic in a few days with more questions after she has assimilated some of the information.

NURSING DIAGNOSIS 2 *Anxiety* related to threatened sexual identity, as evidenced by her comment that she is not comfortable with sexual activity while the lesions are present because they make her feel "ugly"

Nursing Outcomes Classification (NOC)
Acceptance: Health Status

Nursing Interventions Classification (NIC)
Teaching: Individual

PLANNING/OUTCOMES	NURSING INTERVENTIONS	RATIONALE
J.B. will be able to express feelings of anxiety and identify support systems to help her cope with these feelings before leaving the clinic.	Explain any procedures clearly and concisely before performing them.	Helps alleviate anxiety.
	Listen attentively to concerns or expressions of anxiety from J.B.	Helps identify anxious behaviors and source of her anxiety.
	Include J.B. in as many decisions related to her care and follow-up as is possible.	May reduce her feelings of anxiety and gives her some control.

EVALUATION

J.B. expresses feelings of anxiety about the diagnosis. States she has a cousin with herpes whom she will use as a resource person. Also states that she has a secure relationship with her boyfriend and will talk to him about herpes. Agrees to call the clinic for any further support or information that she may need.

(Continues)

SAMPLE NURSING CARE PLAN (Continued)

NURSING DIAGNOSIS 3 *Risk for Infection* related to break in skin integrity as evidenced by the presence of blisters

Nursing Outcomes Classification (NOC)
Risk Control: Sexually Transmitted Infections (STI)

Nursing Interventions Classification (NIC)
Teaching: Disease Process
Teaching: Sexuality

PLANNING/OUTCOMES	NURSING INTERVENTIONS	RATIONALE
J.B.'s herpes blisters will heal without secondary infection within 10 days.	Wear gloves when examining perineal area and when handling exudate from herpes lesions.	Prevents secondary infection in herpes blisters from caregiver's hands and protects caregiver when dealing with wound exudate.
	Teach J.B. how to wash hands very thoroughly after using the toilet or handling the area around the herpes lesions.	Prevents spread of herpes infection from genital area to other areas of J.B.'s body or to another person.
	Instruct J.B. in the importance of keeping the herpes lesions clean and dry until they heal.	Helps prevent the occurrence of a secondary infection that may delay healing for up to 6 weeks.
	Instruct J.B. to wear cotton underwear and loose-fitting clothing during herpes outbreaks.	Provides air circulation to promote healing and reduce further local irritation.

EVALUATION

J.B. has been taught to keep blisters clean and dry and states that she will contact the clinic if the lesions develop any signs of a secondary infection. She makes an appointment to return to the clinic in 10 days for a follow-up evaluation.

CASE STUDY

N.L., a 17-year-old student, has come to your clinic seeking treatment. N.L. is complaining of pain and burning on urination, as well as pain during intercourse. She states that she is infrequently sexually active with her 17-year-old boyfriend and is also seeking a form of birth control. She has not used any form of birth control in the past and neither has her boyfriend. She also complains of a yellowish vaginal discharge and has been wearing a panty liner to deal with this. Upon examination, N.L. complains of some abdominal tenderness but denies that she has had any tenderness before this time. N.L. is screened for chlamydia and gonorrhea. She denies having had sex with any other partners but does admit that she and her boyfriend had a fight and broke up temporarily about a month ago. They went back together about a week later. She does not know if he had any other sexual contacts during their period of separation. N.L. is concerned that she has contracted an STI and states, "I'll die of embarrassment!"

The following questions will guide your development of a nursing care plan for the case study.

1. What other information should be elicited from N.L.?
2. What other STIs will N.L. most likely be tested for in addition to chlamydia and gonorrhea?
3. Write three nursing diagnoses and goals for N.L.
4. List the medications that N.L. will be most likely to receive to treat a chlamydial infection.
5. List some complications that N.L. may experience if she does not receive treatment for an active chlamydial or gonorrheal infection.
6. What information will you include when you counsel N.L. regarding sexual activity and forms of birth control? (See the chapter on Reproductive Systems for additional information.)

SUMMARY

- STIs are among the most common infections occurring in the United States today.
- Despite massive education efforts, the number of new STI cases identified each year continues to grow.
- Early, intensive education regarding STIs is being used to help combat the high incidence of STIs, which virtually are an epidemic among young, urban-dwelling populations.
- Many STIs, such as gonorrhea, syphilis, and chlamydia, are treatable with antibiotics, but many others are caused by viruses and are not curable.
- Identification of groups at risk for STIs and appropriate prevention teaching are the most effective weapons in the ongoing battle against STIs.

REVIEW QUESTIONS

1. A female client comes to the health clinic because her boyfriend was recently diagnosed with chlamydia. She asks the nurse what would have happened to her if she had not found out and had gone without treatment. The nurse explains to her that lack of treatment could result in:
   1. development of a chancre.
   2. heart disease and blindness.
   3. scar tissue formation.
   4. nervous system damage.
2. A nursing diagnosis for a client with an STI is *Risk for Infection related to incomplete treatment and lack of precautions with an infected partner*. Which of the following are desired outcomes for the client? (Select all that apply.)
   1. The client will state the need for having all sexual partners notified and treated.
   2. The client will maintain adequate tissue perfusion as manifested by stable vital signs.
   3. The client will maintain adequate fluid balance.
   4. The client will state understanding of the treatment regimen and of the importance of completing treatment.
   5. The client will explain appropriate use of condoms, including how and when to apply and remove the device.
   6. The client will maintain skin integrity and vagina will not be dry.
3. A male client informs the nurse that his girlfriend is being treated for cytomegalovirus (CMV). What common symptoms of cytomegalovirus (CMV) will the nurse assess for in a male client?
   1. Urethritis, purulent drainage, and epididymitis.
   2. Often asymptomatic, occasionally fever, fatigue, and weakness.
   3. Fleshy cauliflower like growth on genitalia.
   4. Rash on palms and soles.
4. A 29-year-old male client is diagnosed with gonorrhea. Which of the following treatments are included in his plan of care? (Select all that apply.)
   1. A single dose of ciprofloxacin (Cipro) followed by a 7-day course of oral doxycycline (Vibramycin).
   2. Follow-up cultures to determine the success of the course of treatment.
   3. An injection of ceftriaxone sodium (Rocephin) followed by oral erythromycin estolate (Ilosone).
   4. Abstain from mouth-to-mouth kissing.
   5. An antibiotic ophthalmic ointment is administered in both eyes.
   6. Administer mild analgesics as ordered to minimize dysuria.
5. A 22-year-old male has recently been diagnosed with syphilis and presents with a skin rash, sore throat, headache, and small papules on the tip of his penis. The nursing assessment data indicates that the client is in which stage of syphilis?
   1. Primary.
   2. Secondary.
   3. Tertiary.
   4. Latent.
6. The nurse is teaching a classroom of college students the proper use of condoms to protect against STIs. Which of the following statements made by a student indicates that further teaching is needed?
   1. "I always wear a condom and use a water based lubricant when having sex with my girlfriend."
   2. "I never reuse a condom."
   3. "I keep extra condoms in the glove compartment of my car so I am always prepared."
   4. "I prefer lambskin condoms because they fit the best."
7. The nurse knows that which of the following is the best method for reducing the risk of acquiring an STI?
   1. Always wear a condom during sexual intercourse.
   2. Do not share sex toys.
   3. Use a barrier method when engaging in oral sex.
   4. Abstinence.
8. The client has been diagnosed with trichomonas and is prescribed the medication Flagyl for treatment. Which of the following is the most important information for the nurse to teach the client regarding the administration of Flagyl?
   1. Do not drink alcoholic beverages while taking this medication.
   2. Take with food.
   3. Do not drink grapefruit juice while taking this medication.
   4. Do not take use an antacid one hour before or after taking the medication.

9. When conducting a health history, which of the following questions is inappropriate to ask a client suspected of having an STI?
   1. Have you been diagnosed with a STI in the past?
   2. How many sexual partners have you had in the past 6 months?
   3. Have you noticed any anal discharge or tenderness?
   4. Why didn't you use a condom when having sex with your partner?
10. A 45-year-old male client has been recently diagnosed with chlamydia. His wife is in the room and asks the nurse why she has to be tested and treated as well, since she does not have any symptoms. The best explanation by the nurse is:
    1. "It is important that all sexual partners be tested and treated, because reinfection can occur if only one partner is treated."
    2. "The doctor requires that spouses be tested and treated even if they do not have any symptoms."
    3. "Because chlamydia is a silent disease with no symptoms."
    4. "It is something that all doctors require."

REFERENCES/SUGGESTED READINGS

American Social Health Association (ASHA). (2009). Gonorrhea: questions & answers. Retrieved January 17, 2009 from http://www.ashastd.org/learn/learn_gonorrhea.cfm

American Social Health Association (ASHA). (2009a). Herpes resource center: overview. Retrieved January 17, 2009 from http://www.ashastd.org/herpes/herpes_aboutcenter.cfm

Apoola, A. & Radcliffe, K. (2004). Antiviral treatment of genital herpes. *International Journal of STD & AIDS, 15*(7), 429–433.

Ballard, R. & Morse, S. (2003). Chancroid. In: *Atlas of sexually transmitted diseases and AIDS* (3rd ed.). Edinburgh: Mosby.

Baseman, J. & Koutsky, L. (2005). The epidemiology of human papillomavirus infections. *Journal of Clinical Virology, 32*(Suppl. 1), S16–S24.

Bulechek, G., Butcher, H., McCloskey, J., & Dochterman, J., eds. (2008). *Nursing Interventions Classification (NIC)* (5th ed.). St. Louis, MO: Mosby/Elsevier.

Centers for Disease Control and Prevention. (2007a). Trends in reportable sexually transmitted disease in the United States, 2007: national surveillance data for chlamydia, gonorrhea, and syphilis. Retrieved January 17, 2009 from http://www.cdc.gov/std/stats07/trends.htm

Centers for Disease Control and Prevention. (2007b). Sexually transmitted disease surveillance, 2007: gonorrhea. Retrieved January 17, 2009 from http://www.cdc.gov/std/stats07/gonorrhea.htm

Centers for Disease Control and Prevention. (2008a). About CMV: general information. Retrieved July 8, 2009 from http://www.cdc.gov/cmv/facts.htm

Centers for Disease Control and Prevention. (2008b). Division of parasitic diseases: trichomonas infection fact sheet. Retrieved January 18, 2009 from http://www.cdc.gov/ncidod/dpd/parasites/trichomonas/factsht_trichomonas.htm

Centers for Disease Control and Prevention. (2008c). HIV transmission rates in the United States. Retrieved January 18, 2009 from http://www.cdc.gov/hiv/topics/surveillance/resources/factsheets/transmission.htm

Centers for Disease Control and Prevention. (2008d). Vaccines and Preventable Diseases: HPV vaccination. Retrieved January 17, 2009 from http://www.cdc.gov/vaccines/vpd-vac/hpv/default.htm

Centers for Disease Control and Prevention. (2008e). Viral hepatitis: FAQs for health professionals. Retrieved January 17, 2009 from http://www.cdc.gov/hepatitis/HBV/HBVfaq.htm#overview

Centers for Disease Control and Prevention. (2009). Genital herpes—CDC fact sheet. Retrieved January 17, 2009 from http://www.cdc.gov/std/Herpes/STDFact-Herpes.htm

Cleveland Clinic. (2009). Sexually transmitted diseases: an overview. Retrieved January 18, 2009 from my.clevelandclinic.org/disorders/Sexually_Transmitted_Disease_STD/hic_Sexually_Transmitted_Diseases_An_Overview.aspx

Daniels, R. (2010). *Delmar's guide to laboratory and diagnostic tests* (2nd ed.). Clifton Park, NY: Delmar Cengage Learning.

Ehreth, J. (2005). The economics of vaccination from a global perspective: present and future. 2-3 December, 2004, Vaccines: all things considered. *Expert Rev. Vaccines, 4*, 19–21.

Estes, M. (2010). *Health assessment & physical examination* (4th ed.). Clifton Park, NY: Delmar Cengage Learning.

Freedom Network. (2009). Facts about STD. Retrieved January 17, 2009 from http://std-gov.org/

Keck, J. (2005). Ulcerative lesions. *Clinical Family Practice, 7*(1), 13–30.

Mayo Clinic. (2009a). Gonorrhea: definition. Retrieved January 16, 2009 from http://www.mayoclinic.com/print/gonorrhea/DS00180/DSECTION=all&method=print

Mayo Clinic. (2009b). HIV/AIDS. Retrieved January 18, 2009 from http://www.who.int/features/qa/71/en/index.html

Moorhead, S., Johnson, M., Maas, M., & Swanson, E. (2007). *Nursing Outcomes Classification (NOC)* (4th ed.). St. Louis, MO: Mosby.

National Institutes of Health. (2008). U.S. reported 25,000 cases of HPV-related cancers annually. Retrieved January 18, 2009 from http://www.nlm.nih.gov/medlineplus/news/fullstory_71187.html

National Institutes of Health. (2009). Sexually transmitted diseases. Retrieved January 18, 2009 from http://www.nlm.nih.gov/medlineplus/sexuallytransmitteddiseases.html

North American Nursing Diagnosis Association International. (2010). *NANDA-I nursing diagnoses: Definitions and classification 2009–2011*. Ames, IA: Wiley-Blackwell.

Ohio Department of Health. (2007). Genital warts. Retrieved January 18, 2009 from http://www.odh.ohio.gov/pdf/idcm/genwart.pdf

Roden, R., Ling, M., & Wu, T. (2004). Vaccination to prevent and treat cervical cancer. *Human Pathology, 35*, 971–982.

Rural Center for AIDS/STD Prevention. (2006). Rural methamphetamine use and HIV/STD risk. Fact sheet No. 18. Retrieved January 15, 2009 from http://www.indiana.edu/~aids/factsheets18.pdf

Spratto, G., & Woods, A. (2009). *2009 edition Delmar nurse's drug handbook*. Clifton Park, NY: Delmar Cengage Learning.

World Health Organization (WHO). (2009). HIV surveillance, estimates, monitoring and evaluation. Retrieved July 8, 2009 from http://www.who.int/hiv/topics/me/en/index.html

RESOURCES

American College of Obstetricians and Gynecologists (ACOG), http://www.acog.org

American Public Health Association (APHA), http://www.apha.org

American Social Health Association (ASHA), http://www.ashastd.org

Centers for Disease Control and Prevention (CDC), http://www.cdc.gov

National Foundation for Infectious Diseases, http://www.nfid.org

National Institute of Allergy and Infectious Diseases, http://www.niaid. nih.gov

Planned Parenthood Federation of America, Inc., http://www.plannedparenthood.org

U.S. Department of Health and Human Services (USDHHS), http://www.hhs.gov

World Health Organization (WHO), http://www.who.int

UNIT 14 Nursing Care of the Client: Body Defenses

CHAPTER 46

Integumentary System

MAKING THE CONNECTION

Refer to the following chapters to increase your understanding of the integumentary system:

Basic Nursing
- ***Fluid, Electrolyte, and Acid–Base Balance***
- ***Assessment***
- ***Diagnostic Tests***

Adult Health Nursing
- ***Oncology***
- ***Immune System***
- ***The Older Adult***

Basic Procedures
- ***Bathing a Client in Bed***
- ***Giving a Back Rub***
- ***Shaving a Client***

Intermediate Procedures
- ***Application of Heat and Cold***
- ***Applying a Wet to Damp Dressing***
- ***Culturing a Wound***
- ***Irrigating a Wound***

Advanced Procedures
- ***Removing Skin Sutures and Staples***

LEARNING OBJECTIVES

Upon completion of this chapter, you should be able to:

- Define key terms.
- Describe common disorders of the integumentary system.
- Relate the pathophysiology of each skin disorder.
- Discuss the common diagnostic tests used to differentiate skin disorders.
- State the usual treatment for each skin disorder.
- Assess the nursing care needs of a client with a disorder of the integument.
- Plan and implement effective nursing care.

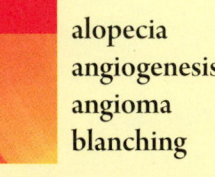

KEY TERMS

alopecia
angiogenesis
angioma
blanching
cyanosis
debride
ecchymosis
erythema
eschar
exudate
friction
granulation tissue

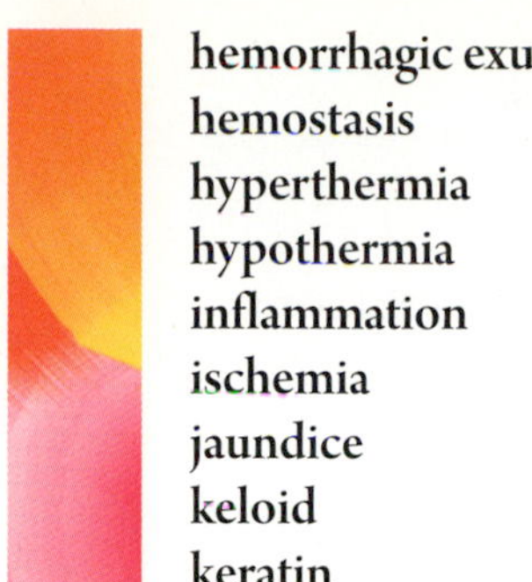

- hemorrhagic exudate
- hemostasis
- hyperthermia
- hypothermia
- inflammation
- ischemia
- jaundice
- keloid
- keratin
- lipoma
- melanin
- nevi
- pallor
- petechiae
- purulent exudate
- sanguineous exudate
- sebaceous cyst
- sebum
- serosanguineous exudate
- serous exudate
- shearing
- telangiectasia
- vitiligo
- wound

INTRODUCTION

As an old adage asserts, the health of the skin mirrors the health of the body. Many systemic diseases have skin manifestations. Psychological stress can affect the condition of the skin, and skin rashes can be a complication of drug therapy. As the largest and the most visible system in the body, the integumentary system (skin, hair, scalp, nails, and mucous membranes) is vulnerable to injury and susceptible to several primary diseases. Although the outward appearance of the skin is important for psychological well-being, the healthy, intact status of the skin is also essential for physiologic well-being. Maintaining this status of the integumentary system is, therefore, an important independent nursing function. The focus of this chapter is to describe common skin disorders, identify the usual treatment modalities for these disorders, and discuss measures that nurses can implement to provide effective nursing care for clients with disorders of the integument.

ANATOMY AND PHYSIOLOGY REVIEW

As the external covering of the body, the skin performs the vital function of protecting internal body structures from harmful microorganisms and substances. The skin is continuous with mucous membranes at external body openings of the respiratory tract, the digestive system, and the urogenital tract. As appendages of the skin, the hair and nails also have protective functions. In addition to its vital protective role, the skin also plays other roles in the normal functioning of the human organism. These roles include participating in the regulation of body temperature, functioning as a sensory organ, helping to maintain fluid and electrolyte balance, producing vitamin D, and excreting certain waste products from the body.

Structure of the Skin

The skin is composed of three layers: the epidermis, the dermis, and the subcutaneous fatty tissue (Figure 46-1).

Epidermis

The epidermis is a layer of squamous epithelial cells. Most of the cells are keratinocytes that produce a tough, fibrous protein called **keratin**. As new cells are produced in the deep layers of the epidermis, old cells are pushed to the surface of the skin. As these cells move from the deeper epidermal layers to the surface, they undergo a process of keratinization in which they become filled with keratin, thus hardening the outer layer of epidermal cells. The keratin creates a barrier that repels bacteria and foreign matter and is impermeable to most substances. The epidermal cells on the palms of the hands and soles of the feet, areas of the body subjected to increased friction and pressure, contain larger amounts of keratin, resulting in thickened skin and callouses.

The epidermis also contains specialized cells called melanocytes. These cells produce **melanin**, the pigment that gives the skin its color. The more melanin present, the darker the skin color. Exposure to ultraviolet light (sun) causes an increase in the production of melanin, which darkens (tans) the skin and provides some protection against the harmful effects of suntanning. Moles and birthmarks (**nevi**), pigmented areas in the skin, are aggregations of melanocytes. In **vitiligo**, melanocytes are destroyed, causing milk-white patches of depigmented skin surrounded by normal skin.

Dermis

The dermis is dense, irregular connective tissue composed of collagen and elastic fibers, blood and lymph vessels, nerves, sweat and sebaceous glands, and hair roots. The sebaceous glands secrete an oily substance called **sebum** that lubricates the skin, helping to keep it soft and pliable. Sweat (eccrine) glands are found in the skin over most of the body surface. Another type of sweat gland, apocrine glands, is concentrated in the axillae, anal region, scrotum, and labia majora. These glands secrete an organic substance that is odorless at first but is quickly metabolized by skin bacteria, causing the characteristic odor commonly referred to as body odor (Tate, 2008). Intradermal injections, such as the TB skin test, are given in the dermis.

Subcutaneous Tissue

The subcutaneous tissue is primarily connective and adipose (fatty) tissue. Here the skin is anchored to muscles and bones. An individual's nutritional status and genetic makeup dictate the amount of subcutaneous tissue present. Emaciated persons have very little subcutaneous tissue, whereas obese persons may have several inches of subcutaneous tissue. The amount of subcutaneous tissue is an important factor in body temperature regulation.

Functions of the Skin

Understanding the functions of the skin and contiguous mucous membranes guides the nurse in planning and implementing appropriate nursing care. Because intact, healthy skin and mucous membranes serve as the first line of defense against

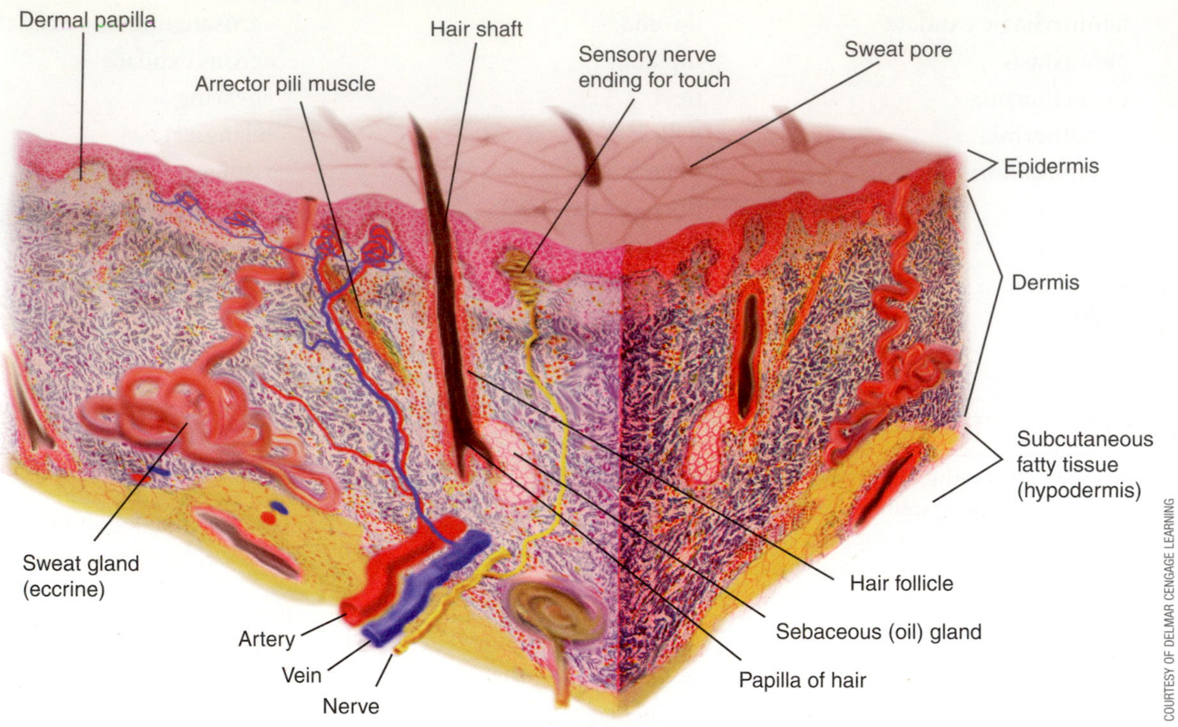

FIGURE 46-1 Cross Section of the Skin

harmful agents, *maintaining skin integrity is one of the most important independent functions of the nurse.* Nursing interventions such as providing daily hygiene care and regularly turning and repositioning dependent clients are aimed at preventing skin breakdown.

Protection

The first and most important function of the skin is protection. As long as the skin is intact and healthy, it is a barrier against microorganisms and numerous substances that could be harmful to the individual. Not only is the skin a barrier to keep harmful substances out, it is also a barrier to keep essential substances such as water and electrolytes inside the body. It also cushions internal organs.

Temperature Regulation

The body produces heat as a result of metabolism of food. Exercise, fever, or a hot environment can raise body temperature. Through several mechanisms, the skin can either release or conserve body heat to maintain normal body temperature. Radiation is the primary means of heat loss. As body heat increases, arterioles in the dermis dilate, bringing body heat to the skin surface. By the process of radiation, waves of heat from uncovered body surfaces are released to the environment. Layering clothes in winter, for example, helps prevent excess loss of body heat by radiation. Heat is also lost by conduction. In conduction, heat is transferred from warmer surfaces to cooler ones. Placing a cool washcloth on a client's forehead is an example of using the principle of conduction. The washcloth becomes warmer, the forehead cooler. Evaporation is another way in which excess body heat is lost. As moisture on the skin—either from perspiration or from a tepid sponge bath—dries, the body is cooled. To conserve (prevent excess loss) body heat, arterioles in the dermis contract to decrease the flow of blood to the skin surface, thus decreasing heat lost by radiation. The phenomenon of "goose flesh" is another method of conserving body heat. Tiny hairs standing on end create a layer of air insulation decreasing loss of body heat to the environment.

Sensory Perception

The skin contains receptors for pain, touch, pressure, and temperature. The sensory receptors pick up information to help protect the body from environmental dangers as well as provide sensations of comfort and pleasure. The brain then processes the information and causes a response.

Fluid and Electrolyte Balance

The skin helps maintain the stability of the internal environment by preventing loss of body fluids and electrolytes and by preventing subcutaneous tissues from drying out. Skin damage, such as that occurring with severe burns, results in rapid loss of large quantities of fluid and electrolytes. This can lead to shock, circulatory collapse, and death.

Structure and Function of Hair

Hair is composed of dead epidermal cells that begin to grow and divide in the base of the hair follicle. As the cells are pushed toward the skin surface, they become keratinized and die. Hair color is genetically determined.

Scalp hair grows for 2 to 5 years, then the follicle becomes inactive. When the growth cycle begins again, a new hair is produced and the old hair is pushed out. Approximately 50 hairs are lost each day. Sustained hair loss of more than 100 hairs each day usually indicates that something is wrong.

There are 5 million hairs covering the entire human body except for the lips, palmar and plantar surfaces, nipples, and the glans penis. The amount and texture of hair vary with age, sex, race, and body part.

Hair on the head protects the scalp from the ultraviolet rays from the sun and cushions blows to the head. Eyelashes help prevent foreign particles from entering the eyes just as the hairs in the nostrils and external ear canals help keep particles from entering the nose and ears.

Structure and Function of Nails

Nail production occurs in the nail root, an epithelial fold that cannot be seen from the surface (Figure 46-2). The nail plate covers the nail bed. The blood vessels under the nail bed give the nails their pink color.

The nails protect the ends of the fingers and toes.

Structure and Function of Mucous Membranes

Mucous membranes have epithelium overlying a layer of loose connective tissue. Specialized cells within the mucous membrane secrete mucus.

The cavities and tubes that open to the outside of the body are lined with mucous membranes. These include the oral and nasal cavities and the tubes of the respiratory, gastrointestinal, urinary, and reproductive systems. Mucous membranes perform absorptive or secretory functions depending on their placement.

Effects of Aging

With advancing years, the blood flow to the skin is reduced. The skin becomes thinner and is more easily injured. Older skin breaks down easily from prolonged pressure. The long-accepted rule of thumb is to turn clients every 2 hours, but for the ill older client, every 2 hours may not be often enough. *Significant skin damage can occur in just 1 hour of unrelieved pressure.* Preventing skin breakdown in the elderly client depends on an accurate assessment of both the client's skin condition and mobility status.

Loss of subcutaneous tissue causes skin sagging and wrinkling. The activity of sebaceous and sweat glands diminishes, resulting in dry skin and a decreased ability to adapt to changes in environmental temperature. Extremes in temperature pose hazards for older adults. In very hot weather, they are susceptible to **hyperthermia**, a condition in which the core body temperature reaches 106°F (41.1°C). In hyperthermia, the hypothalamus no longer functions appropriately. Sweating stops, the skin becomes dry and flushed, and the person becomes confused and eventually comatose. Each summer many elderly persons die from the effects of hyperthermia. Winter puts older adults at risk for **hypothermia**, a condition in which the core body temperature drops below 95°F (35°C). The hypothermic client may become confused and disoriented. As the core body temperature continues to drop, the person becomes comatose. Each winter some older adults die from severe hypothermia (Tate, 2008).

On the hands and face, melanocytes increase in number, causing the age spots commonly seen in older adults. Gray hair occurs from a lack of melanin production. Skin exposed to sunlight ages faster.

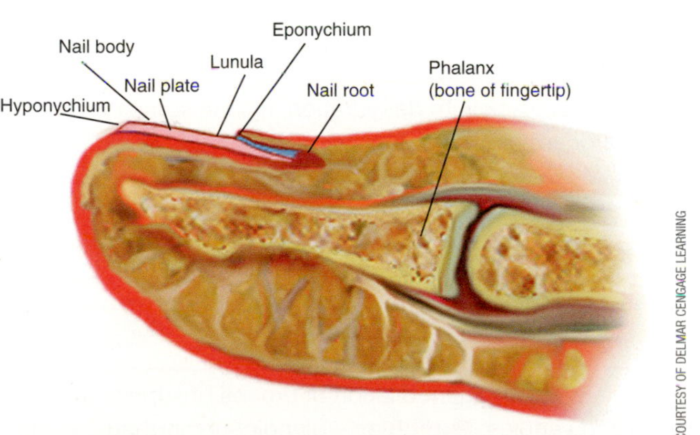

Figure 46-2 Structures of the Fingernail

LIFE SPAN CONSIDERATIONS

Effects of Aging on the Skin

- Skin vascularity and the number of sweat and sebaceous glands decrease, affecting thermoregulation.
- Inflammatory response and pain perception diminish, increasing the risk of adverse effects from noxious stimuli.
- A thinning epidermis and prolonged wound healing make the elderly more prone to injury and skin infections.
- Skin cancer is more common among the elderly.
- Use of skin lotions containing alcohol can cause drying of the skin, increasing the risk of injury. Moisture-enhancing products should be used instead.

ASSESSMENT

Assessing clients with disorders of the integument includes obtaining a health history and performing a physical assessment of the skin, hair, nails, and mucous membranes. The nurse's assessment skills, along with an understanding of the anatomy and physiology of the integumentary system, ensure a complete, factual database from which to plan and implement appropriate nursing care. Box 46-1 contains a list of questions to ask and observations to make in obtaining a health history.

Assessment of Skin

Seven parameters should be examined when performing a physical assessment of the skin. They are integrity, color, temperature and moisture, texture, turgor and mobility, sensation, and vascularity. Table 46-1 outlines these parameters with the normal and abnormal findings. Inspection and palpation are the two assessment techniques used when examining the skin. Good lighting is essential for accurate assessment.

Any skin lesions should be identified according to type and described regarding color, size, and location. Describe the amount, color, odor, and appearance of any drainage that might be present. Document assessment findings clearly, concisely,

BOX 46-1: QUESTIONS TO ASK AND OBSERVATIONS TO MAKE WHEN COLLECTING DATA

Subjective Data

- When did you first notice this problem?
- Where did the first symptom appear?
- What did the rash/lesion look like when it first appeared?
- Describe what happened in the days/weeks after the first symptom appeared.
- Are the symptoms worse at any particular time? Season?
- Have you experienced any itching or burning sensations?
- Are the lesions painful?
- What do you think might have caused this problem?
- Have you ever had a skin problem like this before?
- Has anyone in your family ever had a problem like this?
- What have you been doing to treat this problem?
- What kind of skin care products do you normally use?
- Have you changed any of your usual products/habits/routines?
- Is there anything else you would like to tell me about this problem?

Objective Data

- Check vital signs.
- Inspect color and integrity of skin.
- Observe skin for rashes, lesions, moles, calluses, tattoos, scars, and piercings.
- Inspect skin folds and creases.
- Inspect skin for edema.
- Observe for signs of bleeding and ecchymosis.
- Observe hair distribution, quality, and texture.
- Inspect scalp for dryness and lesions.
- Inspect nail curvature, color, thickness.
- Palpate skin for temperature, moisture, and texture.
- Assess skin turgor.
- Palpate the skin for pitting edema.
- Note any skin odor.
- Report diagnostic test results.

TABLE 46-1 Skin Assessment Parameters

PARAMETER	NORMAL	ABNORMAL
Integrity	Skin intact; no diseased or injured tissue	Broken skin; open areas such as fissures, ulcers, excoriations. Rash or lesions such as papules, nodules, vesicles, pustules, wheals, scales (Figures 46-3 and 46-4).
Color	Varies with skin type and race: pink, tanned, olive, brown	**Pallor**—pale skin, especially in face, conjunctiva, nail beds, and oral mucous membranes. **Cyanosis**—bluish discoloration noticed in lips, earlobes, and nail beds. **Jaundice**—a yellowing of the skin, mucous membranes, and sclera. **Erythema**—reddish hue to the skin as in sunburn and inflammation or increased blood flow.
Temperature and moisture	Usually warm and dry, depending on environmental temperature	Cool, cold, moist, clammy, or warmer than normal
Texture	Smooth, soft. Thickness varies in different areas.	Loose, wrinkled, rough, thickened, thin, oily, flaking, scaling
Turgor and mobility	An assessment of skin hydration. Normally skin moves freely. A pinched fold of skin returns immediately to normal position (Figure 46-5).	Taut with edema; slack with dehydration; rigid in some diseases such as scleroderma
Sensation	Distinguishes hot and cold, sharp and dull	Numbness, tingling, insensitive to pressure and sharp objects
Vascularity	Clear; no discoloration	**Telangiectasia**—permanent dilation of groups of superficial capillaries and venules. **Petechiae**—pinpoint hemorrhagic spots. **Ecchymosis**—large, irregular, hemorrhagic areas (Figure 46-6).

COURTESY OF DELMAR CENGAGE LEARNING

NONPALPABLE

A

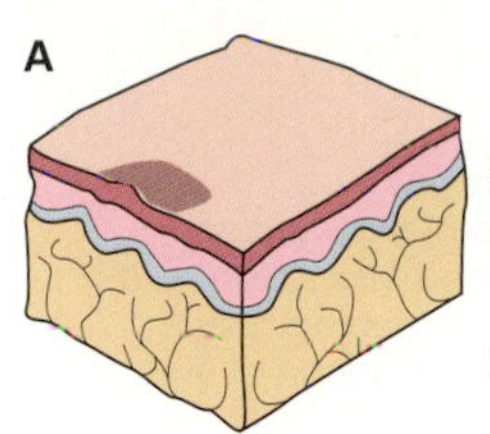

Macule:
Localized changes in skin color of less than 1 cm in diameter
Example:
Freckle

B

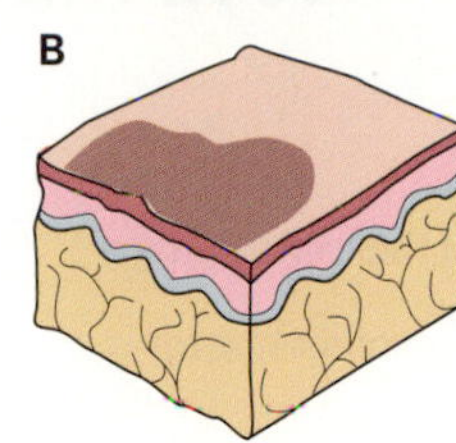

Patch:
Localized changes in skin color of greater than 1 cm in diameter
Example:
Vitiligo, stage 1 of pressure ulcer

PALPABLE

C

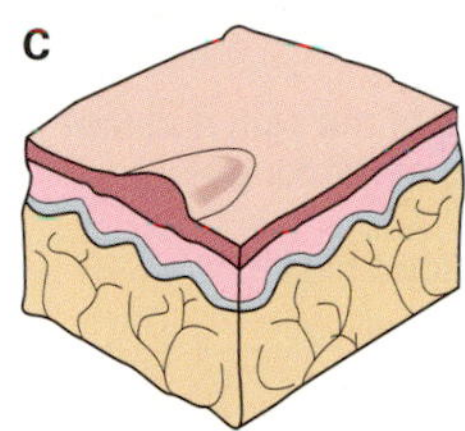

Papule:
Solid, elevated lesion less than 0.5 cm in diameter
Example:
Warts, elevated nevi, seborrheic keratosis

D

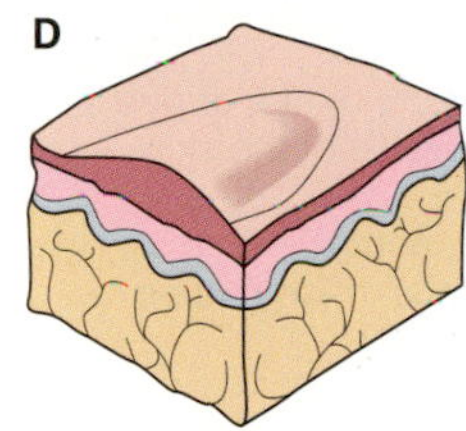

Plaque:
Solid, elevated lesion greater than 0.5 cm in diameter
Example:
Psoriasis, eczema

E

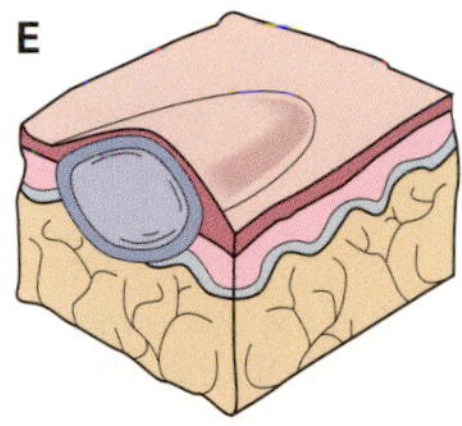

Nodules:
Solid and elevated; however, they extend deeper than papules into the dermis or subcutaneous tissues, 0.5–2 cm
Example:
Lipoma, erythema nodosum, cyst, melamoma, hemangioma

F

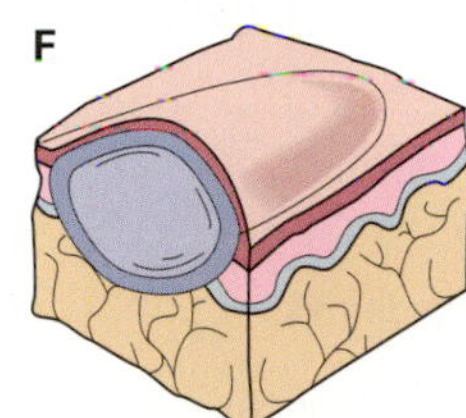

Tumor:
The same as a nodule only greater than 2 cm

Example:
Carcinoma (such as advanced breast carcinoma); **not** basal cell or squamous cell of the skin

G

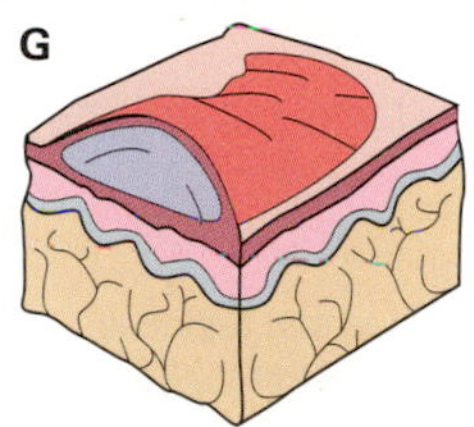

Wheal:
Localized edema in the epidermis causing irregular elevation that may be red or pale
Example:
Insect bite, hive, angioedema

FLUID-FILLED CAVITIES WITHIN THE SKIN

H

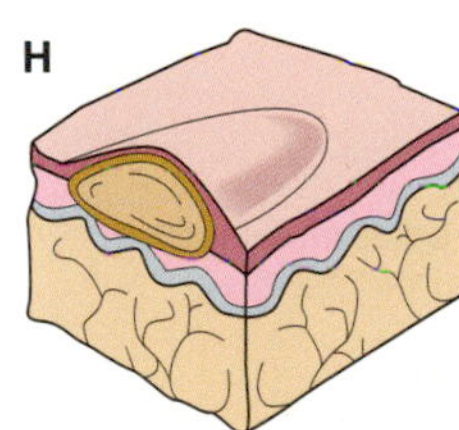

Vesicle:
Accumulation of fluid between the upper layers of the skin; elevated mass containing serous fluid; less than 0.5 cm
Example:
Herpes simplex, herpes zoster, chickenpox, scabies

I

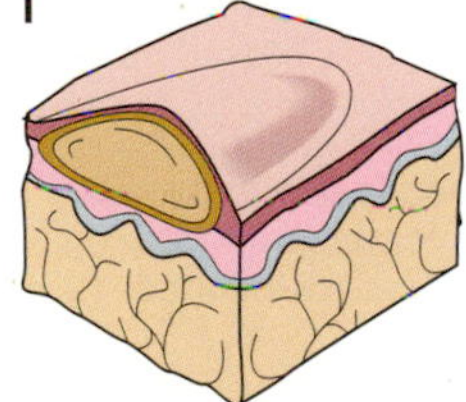

Bullae:
Same as a vesicle only greater than 0.5 cm
Example:
Contact dermatitis, large second-degree burns, bullous impetigo, pemphigus

J

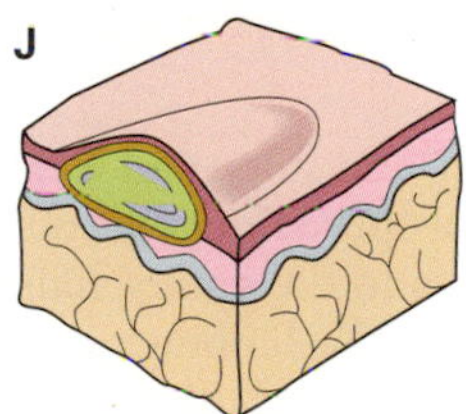

Pustule:
Vesicle or bullae that becomes filled with pus, usually described as less than 0.5 cm in diameter
Example:
Acne, impetigo, furuncles, carbuncles, folliculitis

K

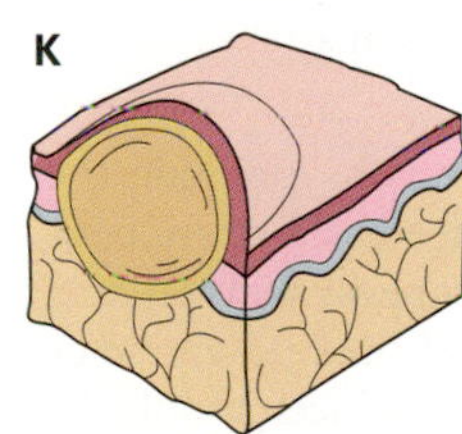

Cyst:
Encapsulated fluid-filled or semi-solid mass in the subcutaneous tissue or dermis
Example:
Sebaceous cyst, epidermoid cyst

COURTESY OF DELMAR CENGAGE LEARNING

FIGURE 46-3 Types of Primary Skin Lesions

ABOVE THE SKIN SURFACE

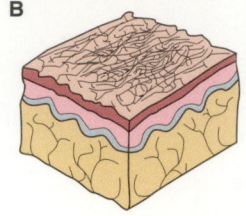

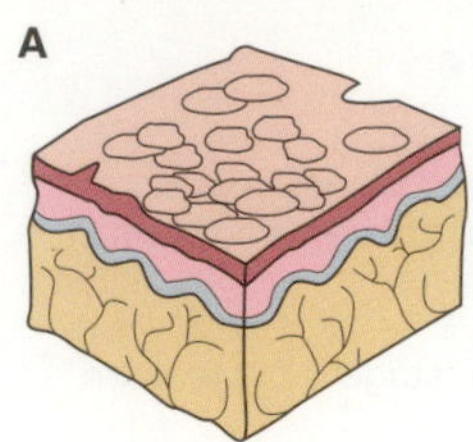

B
Lichenification:
Layers of skin become thickened and rough as a result of rubbing over a prolonged period of time
Example:
Chronic contact dermatitis

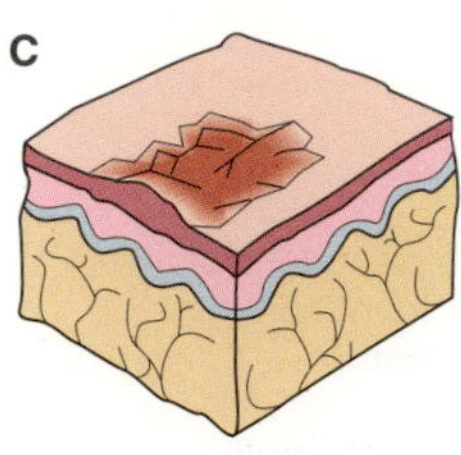

C
Crust:
Dried serum, blood, or pus on the surface of the skin
Example:
Impetigo, acute eczematous inflammation

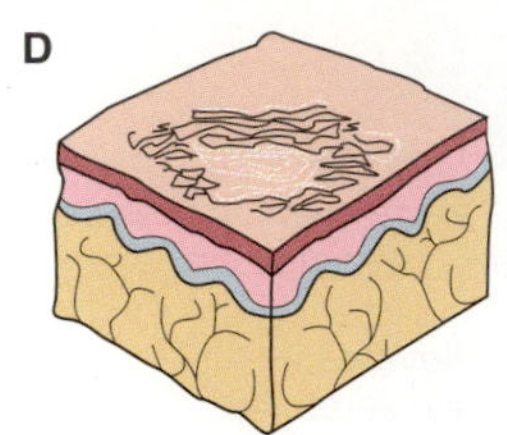

BELOW THE SKIN SURFACE

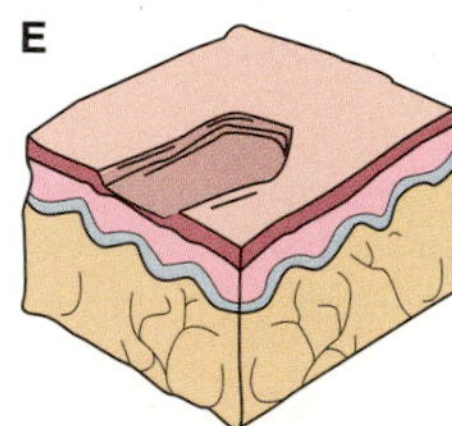

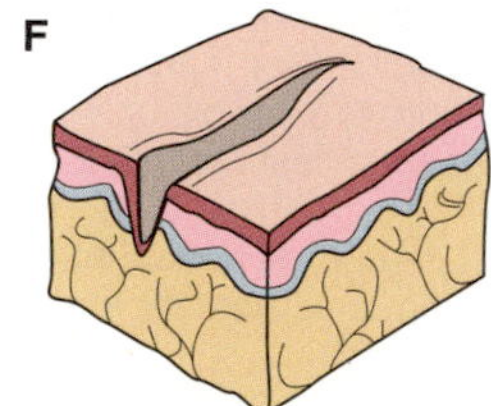

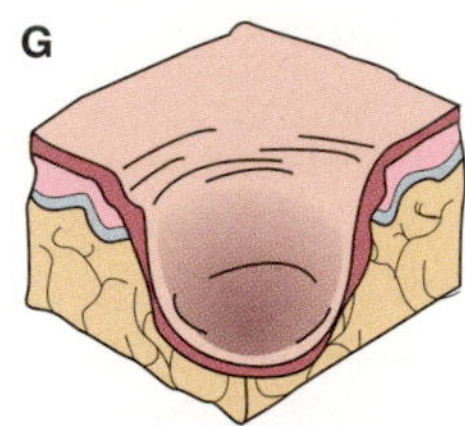

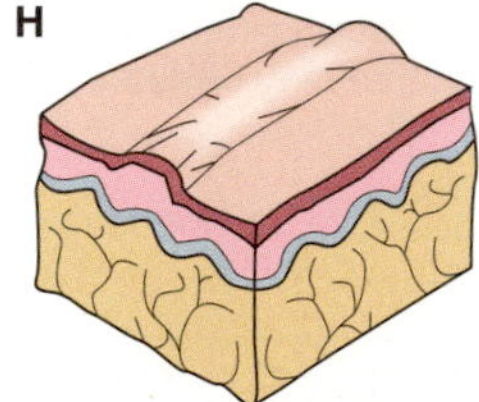

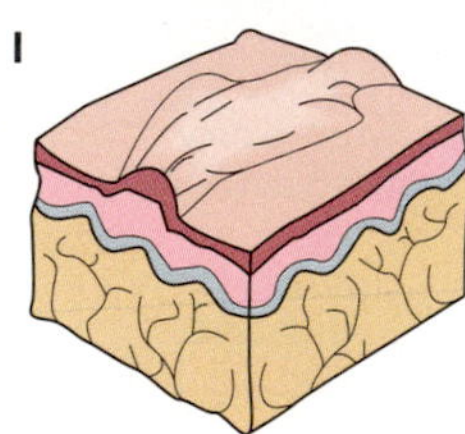

I
Keloid:
Enlarging of a scar past wound edges due to excess collagen formation (more prevalent in dark skinned persons)
Example:
Burn scar

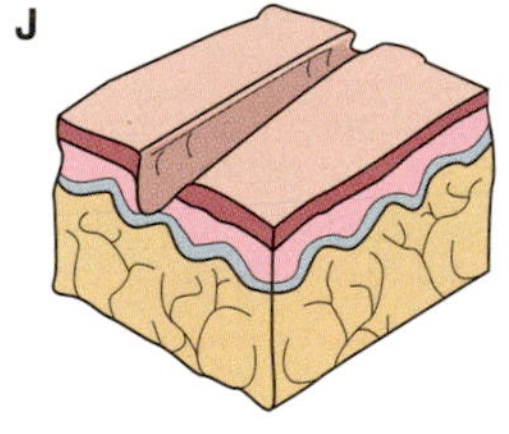

COURTESY OF DELMAR CENGAGE LEARNING

FIGURE 46-4 Types of Secondary Skin Lesions

and completely. The intent of nursing care is to maintain the integrity of intact skin and to restore damaged skin or mucous membranes to an intact state. Aging changes skin texture, moisture, and mobility, requiring increased nursing vigilance to maintain skin integrity. Daily hygiene products should be selected to meet the client's individual skin care needs.

Assessment of Hair, Nails, and Mucous Membranes

Hair should be smooth, shiny, and resilient. Excess hair loss can result from drugs, radiation, dietary or hormonal factors, stress, and high fever.

Nails should be pink, smooth, and shiny and feel firm yet flexible when palpated. An angle of approximately 160° should be present between the nail body and the eponychium. Early clubbing is a nail angle of at least 180°. Clubbing occurs when long-standing hypoxia is present, particularly with cyanotic heart disease and advanced chronic obstructed pulmonary disease. Koilonychia, also known as "spoon nails," is a sign of iron deficiency anemia, malnutrition, or trauma of the nail bed. The nails are thin and concave. Beau's lines are white lines across the nail seen with acute severe illness, malnutrition, or trauma. Paronychia is an infection of the nail caused by bacteria or *Candida albicans* (Figure 46-7).

Mucous membranes normally appear pink and moist.

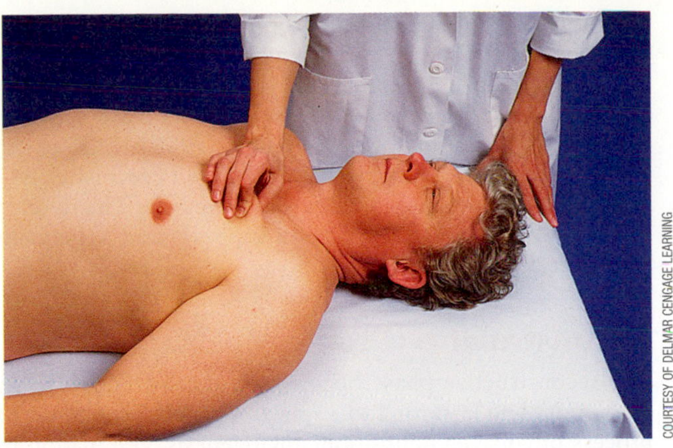

FIGURE 46-5 Assessment of Skin Turgor

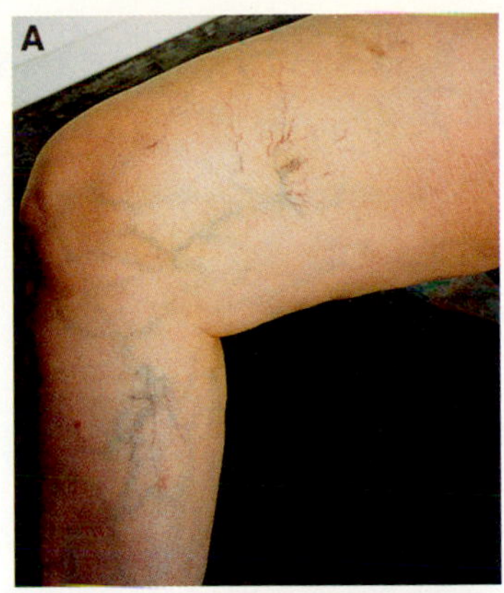

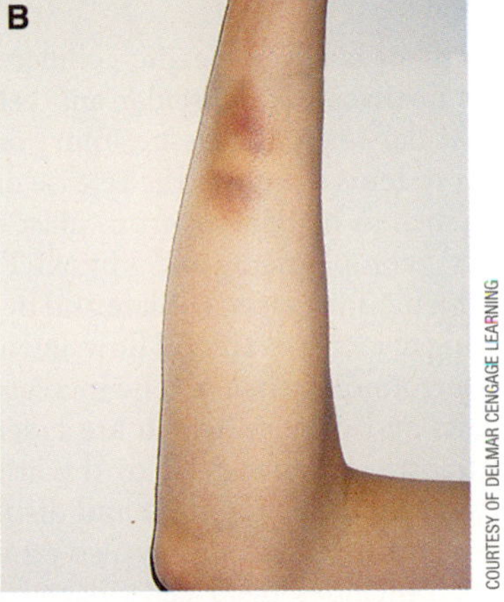

FIGURE 46-6 *A*, Telangiectasis (Spider Veins); *B*, Ecchymosis (Bruise)

COMMON DIAGNOSTIC TESTS

Commonly used diagnostic tests for clients with integumentary disorders are listed in Table 46-2.

WOUNDS

A disruption in the integrity of body tissue is called a **wound**.

Physiology of Wound Healing

When an injury is sustained, a complex set of responses is set into motion, and the body begins a three-phase process of wound healing. Understanding these physiological responses will assist the nurse in caring for clients with impaired skin integrity and promoting optimal wound healing.

Defensive (Inflammatory) Phase

The defensive phase occurs immediately after injury and lasts about 3 to 4 days. The major events that occur in this phase are hemostasis and inflammation. **Hemostasis**, or cessation of bleeding, occurs by vasoconstriction of large blood vessels in the affected area. Platelets, activated by the injury, aggregate to form a platelet plug and stop the bleeding. Activation of the clotting cascade results in the eventual formation of fibrin and a fibrinous meshwork, which further entraps platelets and other cells. The result is fibrin clot formation, which provides initial wound closure, prevents excessive loss of blood and body fluids, and inhibits contamination of the wound by microorganisms.

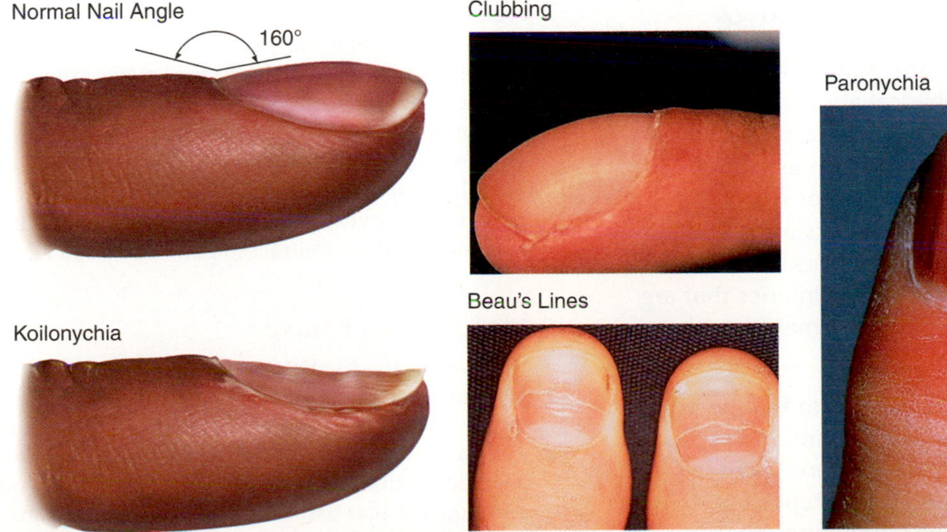

FIGURE 46-7 Nail Variations (*Photos of clubbing and Beau's line courtesy of Robert A. Silverman, MD, Clinical Associate Professor, Department of Pediatrics, Georgetown University; all other images courtesy of Delmar Cengage Learning.*)

TABLE 46-2 Common Diagnostic Tests for Integumentary Disorders

Biopsy (punch, incisional, excisional, shave)
Patch testing
Tzanck smear
Immunofluorescence (IF testing)
Wood's light examination
Skin scrapings
Culture and sensitivity

COURTESY OF DELMAR CENGAGE LEARNING

Inflammation is a nonspecific cellular response to tissue injury and involves both vascular and cellular responses. During the vascular response, tissue injury and activation of plasma protein systems stimulate the release of various chemical mediators, such as histamine (from mast cells), serotonin (from platelets), complement, and kinins. These vasoactive substances cause blood vessels to dilate and become more permeable, resulting in increased blood flow and leakage of serous fluid into the surrounding tissues. The increased blood supply carries nutrients and oxygen, which are essential for wound healing, and transports leukocytes to the area to participate in phagocytosis, or the envelopment and disposal of microorganisms. The increased blood supply also removes the "debris of battle," which includes dead cells, bacteria, and **exudate** (material, fluid, and cells slowly discharged from cells or blood vessels). The area is red, edematous, and warm to touch, and it has varying amounts of exudate.

During the cellular response, leukocytes move out of the blood vessel into the interstitial space. Neutrophils are the first cells to arrive at the injured site and begin phagocytosis. They subsequently die and are replaced by macrophages, which arise from blood monocytes. Macrophages perform the same function as neutrophils but remain for a longer time. In addition to being the primary phagocyte of debridement, macrophages are important cells in wound healing because they secrete several factors, including fibroblast activating factor (FAF) and angiogenesis factor (AGF). FAF attracts fibroblasts, which form collagen or collagen precursors. AGF stimulates the formation of new blood vessels. The development of this new microcirculation supports and sustains the wound and the healing process.

PROFESSIONALTIP

Possible Signs of Physical Abuse

Areas of ecchymosis are one sign of trauma that could be the result of physical abuse. Injuries noted at the base of the skull or on the face, buttocks, breasts, abdomen, or any area such as the top of the back that the client could not reach, are suspicious for abuse. Unusual marks on the skin such as cigarette burns and belt buckle or bite marks may also be signs of abuse. Injuries that are inconsistent with the client's story may also be the result of abuse.

Institutional policies generally relate to reporting and to whom to report when the situation of possible physical abuse is encountered. This is usually based on state laws about reporting physical abuse. Nurses must know the reporting laws of the state in which they are employed.

Reconstructive (Proliferative) Phase

The reconstructive phase begins on the third or fourth day after injury and lasts for 2 to 3 weeks. This phase contains the process of collagen deposition, angiogenesis, granulation tissue development, and wound contraction.

Fibroblasts, normally found in connective tissue, migrate into the wound because of various cellular mediators. They are the most important cells in this phase because they synthesize and secrete collagen. Collagen is the most abundant protein in the body and is the material of tissue repair. Initially, collagen is gel-like, but within several months it cross-links to form collagen fibrils and adds tensile strength to the wound. As the wound gains strength, the risk of wound separation or rupture is less likely. The wound can resist normal stress such as tension or twisting after 15 to 20 days. During this time, a raised "healing ridge" may be visible under the injury or suture line.

Angiogenesis (formation of new blood vessels) begins within hours after the injury. The endothelial cells in preexisting vessels begin to produce enzymes that break down the basement membrane. The membrane opens, and new endothelial cells build a new vessel. These capillaries grow across the wound, increasing blood flow, which increases the supply of nutrients and oxygen needed for wound healing.

Repair begins as granulation tissue, or new tissue, grows inward from surrounding healthy connective tissue. Granulation tissue is filled with new capillaries that are fragile and bleed easily, thus giving the healing area a red, translucent, granular appearance. As granulation tissue is formed, epithelialization, or growth of epithelial tissue, begins. Epithelial cells migrate into the wound from the wound margins. Eventually, the migrating cells contact similar cells that have migrated from the outer edges. Contact stops migration. The cells then begin to differentiate into the various cells that comprise the different layers of epidermis.

Wound contraction is the final step of the reconstructive phase of wound healing. Contraction is noticeable 6 to 12 days after injury and is necessary for closure of all wounds. The edges of the wound are drawn together by the action of myofibroblasts, specialized cells that contain bundles of parallel fibers in their cytoplasm. These myofibroblasts bridge across a wound and then contract to pull the wound closed.

Maturation Phase

Maturation, the final stage of healing, begins about the 21st day and may continue for up to 2 years or more, depending on the depth and extent of the wound. During this phase, the scar tissue is remodeled (reshaped or reconstructed by collagen deposition and lysis and debridement of wound edges). Although the scar tissue continues to gain strength, it remains weaker than the tissue it replaces. Capillaries eventually disappear, leaving an avascular scar (a scar that is white because it lacks a blood supply).

Types of Healing

Tissue may heal by one of three methods, which are characterized by the degree of tissue loss. *Primary intention* healing occurs in wounds that have minimal tissue loss and edges that are well-approximated (closed). If there are no complications, such as infection, necrosis, or abnormal scar formation, wound healing occurs with minimal granulation tissue and scarring.

Secondary intention healing is seen in wounds with extensive tissue loss and wounds in which the edges cannot be approximated. The wound is left open, and granulation tissue gradually fills in the deficit. Repair time is longer, tissue replacement and scarring are greater, and the susceptibility to infection is increased because of the lack of an epidermal barrier to microorganisms.

Tertiary intention healing, also known as delayed or secondary closure, is indicated when primary closure of a wound is undesirable. Conditions in which healing by tertiary intention may occur include poor circulation or infection. Suturing of the wound is delayed until the problems resolve and more favorable conditions exist for wound healing.

Kinds of Wound Drainage

Chemical mediators released during the inflammatory response cause vascular changes and exudation of fluid and cells from blood vessels into tissues. Exudates may vary in composition, but all have similar functions. These functions include the following:

- Dilution of toxins produced by bacteria and dying cells
- Transport of leukocytes and plasma proteins, including antibodies, to the site
- Transport of bacterial toxins, dead cells, debris, and other products of inflammation away from the site

The nature and amount of exudate vary depending on the tissue involved, the intensity and duration of the inflammation, and the presence and type of microorganisms.

Serous exudate is composed primarily of serum (the clear portion of blood), is watery in appearance, and has a low protein level. This type of exudate is seen with mild inflammation, resulting in minimal capillary permeability changes and minimal protein molecule escape (e.g., seen in blister formation after a burn).

Purulent exudate is also called pus. It generally occurs with severe inflammation accompanied by infection. Purulent exudate is thicker than serous exudate because of the presence of leukocytes (particularly neutrophils), liquefied dead tissue debris, and dead and living bacteria. The process of pus formation is called suppuration, and bacteria that produce pus are referred to as pyogenic bacteria. Purulent exudates may vary in color (e.g., yellow, green, brown) depending on the causative organism.

Hemorrhagic exudate or **sanguineous exudate** has a large component of red blood cells (RBCs) because of capillary damage, which allows RBCs to escape. This type of exudate is usually present with severe inflammation. The color of the exudate (bright red versus dark red) reflects whether the bleeding is fresh or old.

Mixed types of exudates may also be seen, depending on the type of wound. For example, a **serosanguineous exudate** is clear with some blood tinge and is seen with surgical incisions.

Factors Affecting Wound Healing

Wound healing depends on multiple influences, both intrinsic and extrinsic. Wounds may fail to heal or may require a longer healing period when unfavorable conditions exist. Factors that may negatively influence healing include age, oxygenation, smoking, drug therapy, and diseases such as diabetes. Such factors reduce local blood supply and impair wound healing. Nutrition and diet can also affect the healing process.

Hemorrhage

Some bleeding from a wound is normal during and immediately after initial trauma and surgery, but hemostasis usually occurs within a few minutes. Hemorrhage is abnormal and may indicate a slipped surgical suture, a dislodged clot, or erosion of a blood vessel. Swelling in the area around the wound or affected body part and the presence of sanguineous, bloody, drainage from the surgical drain may indicate internal bleeding. Other evidence of bleeding may include the signs and symptoms seen in hypovolemic shock (decreased blood pressure, rapid thready pulse, increased respiratory rate, diaphoresis, restlessness, and cool clammy skin). A hematoma (localized collection of blood underneath the tissues) may also be seen and appears as a reddish-blue swelling or mass. External hemorrhaging is detected when the surgical dressing becomes saturated with sanguineous drainage. It is also important to assess the linen under the client's wound site because it is possible for the blood to seep out from under the sides of the dressing and pool under the client. The risk for hemorrhage is greatest during the first 24 to 48 hours after surgery.

Infection

Bacterial wound contamination is one of the most common causes of altered wound healing. A wound can become infected with microorganisms preoperatively, intraoperatively, or postoperatively. During the preoperative period, the wound may become exposed to pathogens because of the manner in which the wound was inflicted, such as in traumatic injuries. Nicks or abrasions created during preoperative shaving may also be a source of pathogens. The risk for intraoperative exposure to pathogens increases when the respiratory, gastrointestinal, genitourinary, and oropharyngeal tracts are opened.

If the amount of bacteria in the wound is sufficient or the client's immune defenses are compromised, clinical infection may result and become apparent 2 to 11 days postoperatively. Infection slows healing by prolonging the inflammatory phase of healing, competing for nutrients, and producing chemicals and enzymes that are damaging to the tissues.

Wound Classification

Many different classification systems are used to describe wounds. These systems describe either how the wound was acquired, how clean it is, or which tissue layers are involved. A classification system will assist the nurse in planning wound care management. The following are commonly used classification systems.

Cause of Wound

Intentional wounds occur during treatment or therapy. These wounds are usually made under aseptic conditions. Examples include surgical incisions and venipunctures.

Unintentional wounds are unanticipated and are often the result of trauma or an accident. These wounds are created in an unsterile environment and therefore pose a greater risk of infection.

Cleanliness of Wound

This classification system ranks the wound according to its contamination by bacteria and risk for infection (Brunicardi, Anderson, Billiar, & Dunn, 2005).

- *Clean wounds* are intentional wounds that were created under conditions in which no inflammation was encountered and the respiratory, alimentary, genitourinary, and oropharyngeal tracts were not entered.
- *Clean-contaminated wounds* are intentional wounds that were created by entry into the alimentary, respiratory, genitourinary, or oropharyngeal tract under controlled conditions.
- *Contaminated wounds* are open, traumatic wounds or intentional wounds in which there was a major break in aseptic technique, spillage from the gastrointestinal tract, or incision into infected urinary or biliary tracts. These wounds have acute nonpurulent inflammation present.
- *Dirty and infected wounds* are traumatic wounds with retained dead tissue or foreign material or intentional wounds created in situations where purulent drainage was present.

Depth of Wound

The third classification system is based on the depth of the wound, taking into account the skin layers involved.

- *Superficial wounds* are confined to the epidermis layer, which comprises the four outermost layers of skin.
- *Partial-thickness wounds* involve the epidermis and part of the dermis, which is the layer of skin beneath the epidermis.
- *Full-thickness wounds* involve the entire epidermis and dermis. Deeper structures such as fascia, muscle, and bone may be involved.

Assessment

Nurses are confronted with wounds that are extremely diverse. The wound may have occurred traumatically just before the client presents to the emergency room, or the wound may be a slow-healing chronic ulcer. Approach wound assessment systematically, evaluating the wound's stage in the healing process. Show sensitivity to the client's pain and tolerance levels during assessment and always follow Standard Precautions to prevent transfer of pathogens. Following are some basic criteria for wound assessment.

Location

Assessment begins with a description of the anatomical location of the wound (e.g., "5-inch suture line on the right lower quadrant of the abdomen"). This task often becomes difficult if the client has multiple wounds close to each other, as is common in burn or multiple-trauma victims. Use of a skin documentation form that incorporates drawings of the body allows the nurse to number the location of the various wounds and then describe them.

Size

The length (head to toe), width (side to side), and depth of a wound are measured in centimeters. Single-use measurement guides (tape measures) often come with dressing supplies. To determine the depth of a wound, a sterile cotton swab, moistened with 0.9% saline solution, is inserted into the deepest point of the wound and marked at the skin surface level. Then the swab can be measured and the wound depth in centimeters documented. Tunneling, also called undermining, can be measured by using a cotton swab to gently probe the wound margins. If tunneling is noted, the location and depth are documented. For clarity in describing the location of the tunneling, the hands of the clock can be used as a guide, with 12 o'clock pointing at the client's head. Example: "Tunneling occurs at 1 o'clock and its depth is 2 cm."

General Appearance and Drainage

A general description of the color of the wound and surrounding area helps determine the wound's present phase of healing. Gently palpate the edges of the wound for swelling, and document the amount, color, location, odor, and consistency of any drainage.

Pain

Document and notify the physician of any pain or tenderness at the wound site. Pain may indicate infection or bleeding. It is normal to experience pain in a surgical incision wound for approximately 3 days. Report any sudden increase in pain accompanied by changes in the appearance of the wound to the physician immediately.

Laboratory Data

Cultures of wound drainage are used to determine the presence of infection and the identity of the causative organism. The sensitivity results list the antibiotics that will effectively treat the infection. An elevated WBC count indicates an infectious process. A decreased leukocyte count may indicate that the client is at increased risk for developing an infection related to decreased defense mechanisms. Albumin is a measure of the client's protein reserves; if the albumin is decreased, the client will have decreased resources of protein for wound healing.

Nursing Diagnoses

Nursing diagnoses for clients with wounds focus on prevention of complications and promotion of the healing process through proper wound care and client teaching. Following are NANDA-approved nursing diagnoses with a partial list of related factors:

- *Impaired **T**issue Integrity* related to surgical incision, pressure, shearing forces, decreased blood flow, immobility, mechanical irritants
- *Risk for **I**nfection* related to malnutrition, decreased defense mechanisms
- *Acute **P**ain* related to inflammation, infection
- *Disturbed **B**ody Image* related to changes in body appearance secondary to scars, drains, removal of body parts
- *Deficient **K**nowledge (Wound Care)* related to lack of exposure to information, misinterpretation, lack of interest in learning

Planning/Outcome Identification

After identifying the nursing diagnoses, establish targeted outcomes for wound healing based on the client's identified needs and individualized to the client's condition. Changes in the health care delivery system have brought about early discharge from the hospital, so clients are often sent home with wounds that need continued care; the goals for clients with wounds generally focus on promoting wound healing, preventing infection, and educating the client.

Implementation

Nursing interventions to promote wound healing and prevent infection include emergency measures to maintain homeostasis (state of internal constancy of the body), and cleansing and dressing of the wound.

Emergency Measures

Assess the type and extent of injury that the client has sustained. If hemorrhage is detected, apply sterile dressings and pressure to stop the bleeding, and notify the physician immediately. Always implement Standard Precautions. Monitor the client's vital signs frequently.

When dehiscence or evisceration occurs, instruct the client to remain quiet and avoid coughing or straining. Position the client to prevent further stress on the wound. Use sterile dressings, such as ABD pads soaked with sterile normal saline, to cover the wound and internal contents. This reduces the risk of bacterial contamination and drying of the viscera. Notify the surgeon immediately and prepare the client for surgical repair of the area.

Cleansing the Wound

The goal of cleansing the wound is to remove debris and bacteria from the wound bed with as little trauma to the healthy granulation tissue as possible. Choice of cleansing agent depends on the physician's prescription as well as agency protocol. It is recommended that isotonic solutions such as normal saline or lactated Ringer's be used to preserve healthy tissue.

> **PROFESSIONALTIP**
>
> **Wound Cleansing**
>
> Following are the major principles to keep in mind when cleansing a wound:
>
> - Use Standard Precautions at all times.
> - When using a swab or gauze to cleanse a wound, work from the clean area out toward the dirtier area. For example, when cleaning a surgical incision, start over the incision line, and swab downward from top to bottom. Change the swab and proceed again on either side of the incision, using a new swab each time.
> - When irrigating a wound, warm the solution to room temperature, preferably to body temperature, to prevent lowering of the tissue temperature. Be sure to allow the irrigant to flow from the cleanest area to the contaminated area to avoid spreading pathogens.

Dressing the Wound

A dressing serves several purposes:

1. To protect the wound from bacterial contamination
2. To promote homeostasis
3. To provide a moist environment to enhance epithelialization
4. To support healing by absorbing drainage
5. To enhance debridement of the wound
6. To provide thermal insulation of the wound
7. To provide splinting or support of the wound site
8. To shield the client from seeing the wound when perceived as unpleasant

Keeping these purposes in mind, determine an appropriate dressing for the client's wound. There are thousands of different wound care products on the market. The physician may prescribe a specific dressing, or follow agency policy. Remember that dressing plans must be modified as the wound changes.

Monitoring Drainage of Wounds

During the inflammatory response, exudates develop within a wound. When excessive drainage accumulates in the wound bed, tissue healing is delayed. If the outer surface is allowed to heal while the drainage remains entrapped within the wound, infection and abscess may form. To facilitate drainage of any excess fluid, the physician may insert a tube or drain.

Other Therapies

Negative-pressure wound therapy, also called vacuum-assisted closure (VAC), increases healing rates. It supports the wound-healing efforts of the body by increasing cellular proliferation, reducing edema around the wound, and providing a moist, protected wound bed.

Biodebridement or maggot debridement therapy (MDT) is mainly used for chronic wounds. Maggots ingest and digest bacteria and dead tissue, thus they debride and disinfect the wound. This decreases wound odor. Maggots excrete a variety of substances, such as calcium carbonate and urea that promotes granulation tissue formation. The Food and Drug Administration regulates MDT since only certain types of maggots are therapeutic. The first intentional use occurred during the Civil War (Hunter, Langemo, Thompson, Hanson, & Anderson, 2009). Unintentional use can occur if flies are allowed to land on open wounds.

Electrical stimulation helps speed healing by increasing capillary density and perfusion, improving wound oxygenation, and encouraging fibroblast activity and granulation. Placement of the electrodes varies with the stage of healing. A physical therapist determines electrode placement and polarity (Ramadan & Zyada, 2008).

Evaluation

Evaluate the client's achievement of the goals established during the planning phase to achieve or maintain skin integrity. Goals for clients with wounds generally focus on wound healing, prevention of infection, and client education. If the goals are not achieved, examine the nursing interventions and strategies that were employed and revise the nursing care plan accordingly. Review techniques and procedures, especially those performed by the client or other caregivers in the client's support system.

BURNS

Burns are among the most devastating injuries an individual can suffer. Burns can be painful and disfiguring, requiring long hospitalizations. Many are fatal. Most burns occur in the home and are preventable. Often, the burn injury is the result of the individual's own action. Feelings of anger and guilt can complicate recovery. Often, the individual suffers self-image disturbances, and family relationships can be strained.

MAJOR CAUSES

There are many different causes for burns to the skin. A major source of burn injury for all ages is overexposure to the sun. Most burn injuries to adults are associated with cigarette smoking and cooking. The elderly are more likely to spill hot liquid on themselves or catch their clothes on fire as they cook or smoke. Young children are especially prone to burn injuries from spilling scalding liquids on themselves and playing with matches or cigarette lighters. Industrial accidents account for a significant number of burn injuries in young adults.

SEVERITY

Burns are classified according to the depth of the burn and the extent of skin surface involved. First- and second-degree burns are partial-thickness (within the epidermis/dermis) burns. First-degree burns involve only the epidermis. The skin is hot, red, and painful. Sunburn is an example of a first-degree burn. First-degree burns heal in about a week without scarring. Second-degree burns damage the dermis and the epidermis. The skin is red, hot, and painful; blisters form and tissue around the burn is edematous. An example of a second-degree burn is spilling boiling water on the skin. Usually, second-degree burns heal in about 2 weeks without scarring; however, if deep layers of the dermis are involved, healing might take months and scarring can occur. Second-degree burns involving deep layers of the dermis may appear white, tan, or red in color.

When the dermis and epidermis are completely destroyed and deeper tissues are involved, burns are classified as full-thickness burns. Third-degree and fourth-degree burns are full-thickness burns. In third-degree burns all dermal structures are destroyed and cannot be regenerated. Subcutaneous tissue is also damaged. Full-thickness burns can be white, tan, brown, black, charred, or bright red in color. Fourth-degree burns, which extend to the underlying muscles and bones, appear white to black or charred with dark networks of thrombosed capillaries visible inside the wound. Fourth-degree burns result from fires, explosions, and nuclear radiation. Figure 46-8 depicts the various layers of skin involved in burn injuries.

Severely burned individuals generally have both partial-thickness and full-thickness burns. Whereas first- and second-degree burns are painful, third- and fourth-degree burns are not painful because sensory nerve endings are destroyed. The client, however, will still be in severe pain. Body movement causes pain in areas of first- and second-degree burns that often surround the full-thickness burns. Skin can regenerate

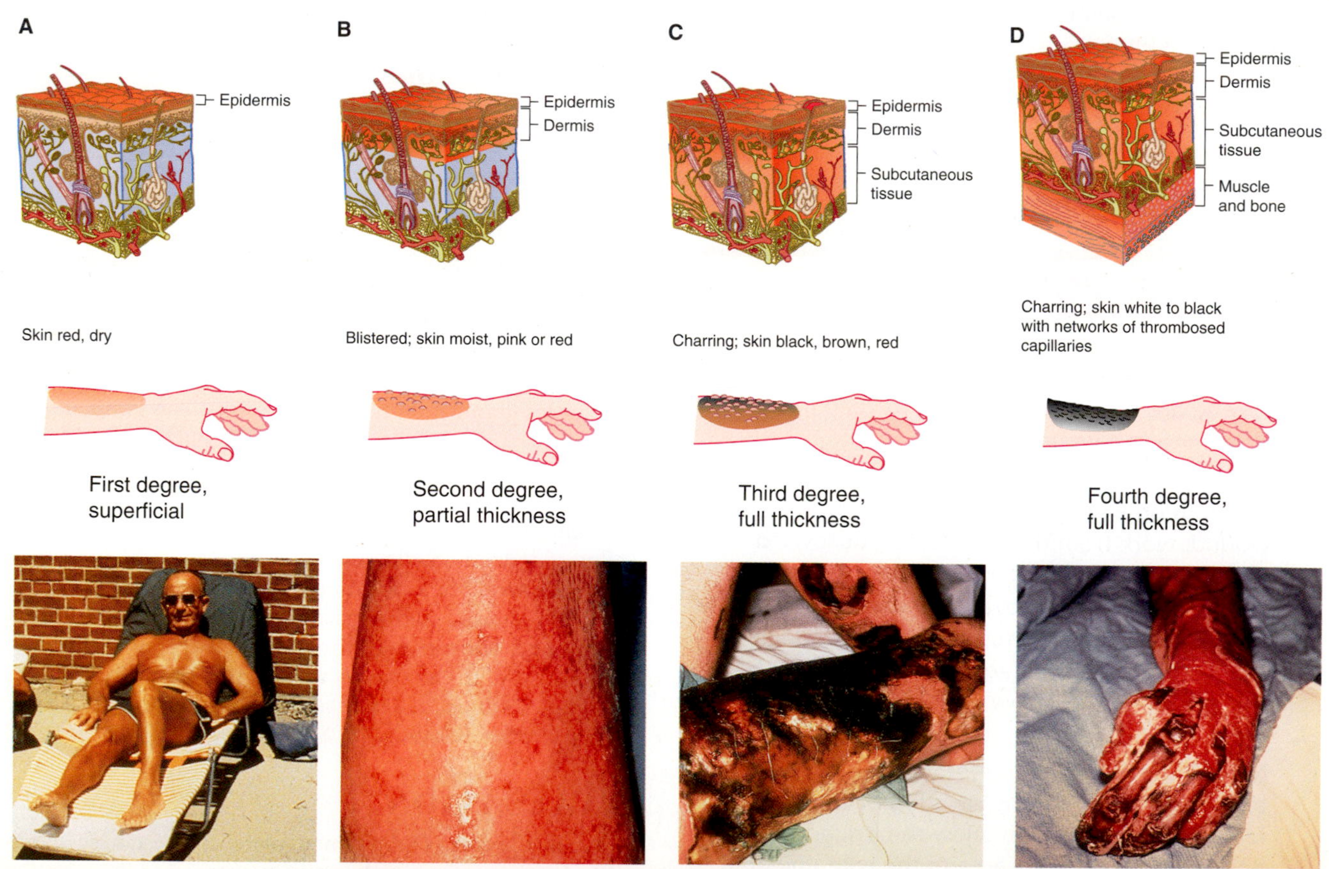

FIGURE 46-8 Skin Layers Involved in Burn Injuries; *A*, First-Degree Burn; *B*, Second-Degree Burn; *C*, Third-Degree Burn; *D*, Fourth-Degree Burn (*Photos courtesy of the Phoenix Society of Burn Survivors, Inc.*)

only from the edges of full-thickness burns. Scarring is inevitable. Skin grafting is necessary to promote healing because the section of skin destroyed by the burn cannot regenerate itself.

Prognosis in burn cases depends on the severity of the burn, the surface area of the body burned, and the preinjury health status of the individual. Local tissue injury response from burns becomes systemic when more than 20 percent of the body is involved. These clients have an increased susceptibility to multiple organ failure and sepsis. The most frequent burn related problem is inhalation injury, and it has the most significant effect on survival (Grunwald & Warren, 2008). Elderly burn victims whose physiologic reserves are already reduced as an effect of aging will have an extended recovery period and a greater risk of complications.

For years, documenting the extent of burn injuries was done by using the Rule-of-Nines method to estimate the body surface area burned for adults. The body is divided into areas that are about 9% (or multiples of 9%). The head comprises 9% (4.5% anterior and 4.5% posterior). Each arm is 9% (4.5% anterior and 4.5% posterior). The anterior trunk and posterior trunk are each 18%. Each leg is 18% (9% anterior and 9% posterior). The genitalia comprise the remaining 1%.

More recently, Milner (2001), inventor of the "Burn Wheel" (Figure 46-9), incorporated a chart similar to the Rule-of-Nines. His chart has a specific percentage for the upper and lower parts of the arms and legs and for the hands and feet, making a more accurate assessment. One side is for infants and children; the other side is for adults.

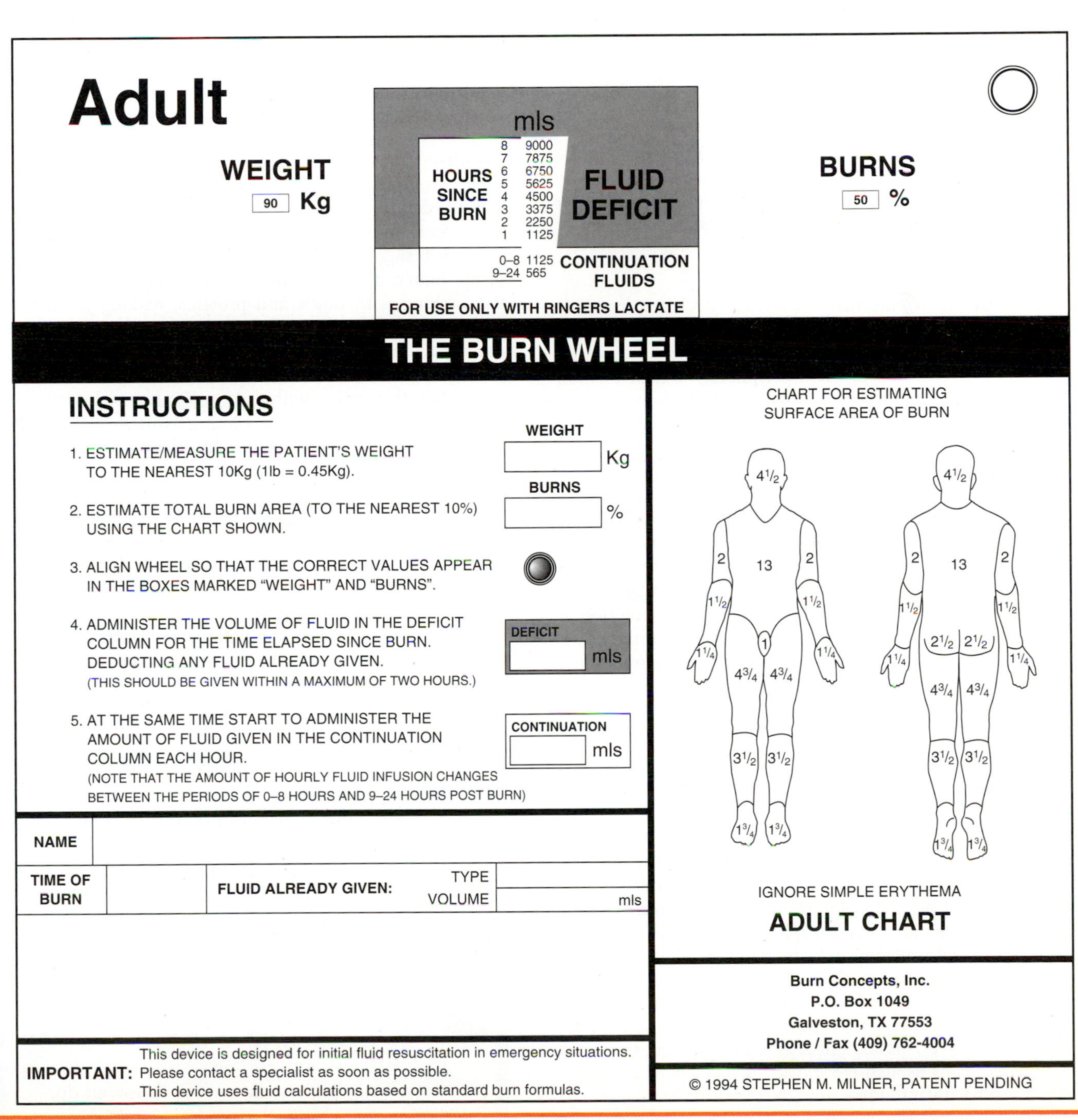

FIGURE 46-9 Burn Wheel (*Invented by Stephen M. Milner.*)

COMPLICATIONS

Destruction of the skin renders it unable to fulfill its functions. Vast amounts of internal fluids and electrolytes are lost. The ability to maintain body temperature is altered, and the individual is susceptible to serious infections. Initially, the complications that are the most life threatening are respiratory failure and massive loss of body fluids.

Smoke Inhalation and Carbon Monoxide Poisoning

Heat and smoke can cause serious damage to the respiratory tract. Signs and symptoms of potential respiratory tract damage include facial burns, singed nasal hairs, changes in voice, difficulty breathing, wheezing, coughing, and carbon-tinged sputum (National Institutes of Health, 2008a). Inhaling heat and smoke in a closed-space fire causes airway inflammation and edema of the respiratory mucosa. The carbon-monoxide that is inhaled along with the heat and smoke attaches to hemoglobin, forming the compound carboxyhemoglobin. A high level of carboxyhemoglobin in the blood means that oxygen is not being delivered to vital body tissues. The client may be stuporous because of cerebral anoxia. Keeping an open airway and administering 100% humidified oxygen are essential for treating these two conditions. Intubation is often necessary.

Shock

Severely burned clients may experience both hypovolemic shock (a life-threatening condition caused by massive loss of blood and circulating fluids) and neurogenic shock (a form of shock that occurs when peripheral vascular dilation occurs causing hypotension). Fluids and electrolytes must be replaced as fast as they are being lost. Tremendous amounts of fluids are lost through the burn wounds themselves as well as into surrounding tissues in the form of edema. The fluid loss shock that results can lead to circulatory collapse and renal shutdown. The Burn Wheel was developed for use in hospitals and emergency departments (EDs) because the first 24 hours after a burn injury are crucial (Milner, 2001). The Burn Wheel uses the client's weight (in g) along with the percentage of area burned to identify the amount of Ringer's lactate solution to be given IV within 2 hours and the amount to be continued for 24 hours. Use of the wheel takes seconds to determine fluid replacement, whereas remembering and figuring formulae may take much longer and mistakes can be easily made. At least two large-bore venous catheters are used to give large volumes of fluid rapidly.

Infection

Once the client has been stabilized, infection poses a serious risk. *Staphylococcus aureus*, an ever-present organism in the environment, is a common cause of infections. Of grave concern is an infection caused by methicillin-resistant *Staphylococcus aureus* (MRSA) because this strain of staphylococcus is resistant to all antibiotics except vancomycin hydrochloride (Vancocin). This antibiotic has serious side effects, especially to the otic nerve and to the liver, and is used only when other antibiotics fail.

All persons coming into contact with the burn client must wear gowns, gloves, masks, and caps to help prevent the introduction of organisms such as *S. aureus*, *Pseudomonas aeruginosa*, or coliform bacilli, into burn wounds. Sterile technique is used for wound care and dressing changes. Care in special burn units reduces the chance of infection because of stringent infection control precautions and a carefully controlled environment.

MEDICAL–SURGICAL MANAGEMENT

Medical

Immediate Care Initially, medical management of the client involves keeping an open airway, maintaining an adequate level of oxygenation, replacing body fluids and electrolytes, monitoring kidney function, controlling pain, and protecting the burns with sterile dressings to minimize the loss of body temperature and the risk of infection. In cases of severe burns, the client usually requires endotracheal intubation and administration of 100% humidified oxygen. A multiport central venous catheter or two large-bore peripheral venous catheters are needed for fluid and electrolyte replacement. A Foley catheter is inserted and urine output measured hourly to help monitor kidney function.

Pain is controlled with small intravenous doses of morphine. Emotional and psychological trauma can intensify pain perception. The client will be anxious about survival, physical appearance, and the effect this injury will have on the family. Prophylactically, the client is given tetanus toxoid.

Stabilized Care Once the client's condition has been stabilized, care focuses on promoting healing, preventing complications, controlling pain, and restoring function. Preventing infection is an important priority. Burn wounds may require daily cleansing and dressing changes. Because of the nature of the injury, burn wounds contain a large amount of dead tissue along with fluids and proteins, making them highly susceptible to infection even with the best of care. Antibiotics and strict aseptic technique are essential. The dead tissue of full-thickness burns forms a dry, dark leathery **eschar** (a scab of denatured protein) within 48 to 72 hours. Infection can often begin under the eschar, causing tissue sloughing. Loose eschar must be **debrided** before skin grafting can occur. Debriding, removing dead and damaged tissue or foreign material within the burn wound, can sometimes be done mechanically by hydrotherapy. Burn wounds may require surgical debridement. The base of the wound must be free of infection and necrotic tissue before it can be covered with skin grafts.

Use of specialty beds, such as fluidized or alternating air-filled mattresses, minimizes pressure on skin surfaces, thus promoting comfort. Limiting movement and maintaining normal body alignment with the use of splints can also help alleviate client discomfort.

Surgical

Skin grafts cover the burn wound to promote healing. Four types of skin grafts might be used:

1. Autograft—the client's own skin that is removed from an unburned area and applied to the wound
2. Homograft—skin obtained from a cadaver within 6 to 24 hours after death

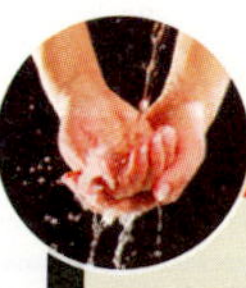

INFECTION CONTROL

Debridement

Strict aseptic techniques must be followed during burn debridement procedures.

3. Heterograft—skin obtained from an animal, such as a pig
4. Synthetic skin substitute—a manmade product that has properties similar to skin (Fritsch & Yurko, 2003)

Homografts, heterografts, and synthetic skin substitutes are temporary grafts that facilitate healing. These grafts prevent water, electrolyte, and protein loss. They decrease pain and allow more freedom of movement for the client. When the client's condition is stable and the wound beds have healthy **granulation tissue** (delicate connective tissue consisting of fibroblasts, collagen, and capillaries), permanent closure of the burn wounds is done with autographs. Granulation tissue is red and provides a base for healing (Tate, 2008).

Autografts are taken from areas of healthy skin. They may be either split-thickness grafts or full-thickness grafts. Split-thickness grafts include the epidermis and part of the dermis. They are not so deep as to prevent regeneration of skin at the donor site.

The application of pressure dressings during the rehabilitative phase reduces the development of hypertrophic scarring, a condition in which the scar becomes elevated and has a "Swiss cheese" appearance. Pressure dressings, which may be elastic wraps, stockinettes, or custom-made pressure garments, must be worn constantly and are to be removed only for daily hygiene care. Full maturation of the burn scar may take 1 to 2 years. As the physical wounds heal, so do the emotional and psychological wounds. The client's ability to cope with daily stresses and resume social and work activities typically coincides with the physical healing process.

Pharmacological

Dressing changes, wound debridement, as well as any movement or manipulation, are extremely painful for clients. Many clients become extremely anxious, fearing pain as well as permanent disfiguration and loss of function. Intravenous narcotics, usually morphine, may be administered 10 to 15 minutes before procedures. By decreasing anxiety and fear, daily doses of psychotropic drugs can enhance the effectiveness of pain medications and help the client cope with the prospect of long-term rehabilitation.

Treatment of the burn wound with topical agents can decrease infection and promote healing. Common topical agents used are mafenide acetate (Sulfamylon); silver sulfadiazine (Silvadene); povidone-iodine (Betadine); nitrofurazone (Furacin); and antibiotic agents such as neomycin sulfate (Myciguent), bacitracin (Baciguent), and gentamicin sulfate (Garamycin). Mafenide acetate (Sulfamylon) can penetrate thick eschar and is effective against gram-negative and gram-positive organisms, including *P. aeruginosa*. Silver sulfadiazine (Silvadene) is effective against many gram-positive and gram-negative organisms as well as *Candida* organisms. It is painless and somewhat soothing but may cause a skin rash. Povidone-iodine (Betadine) has broad-spectrum microbial action against a wide variety of bacteria, fungi, yeasts, viruses, and protozoa. Application of povidone-iodine (Betadine) to large open areas could lead to elevated serum iodine levels. Nitrofurazone (Furacin) has broad-spectrum activity and is effective against *S. aureus*. It is not absorbed systemically and has a low incidence of sensitivity.

Antibiotic ointments are used to decrease infection. Neomycin sulfate (Myciguent) and gentamicin sulfate (Garamycin) can be absorbed systemically and have serious side effects of ototoxicity and nephrotoxicity. Bacitracin (Baciguent) has minimal antimicrobial activity, but it is especially useful to prevent drying of the wound. Topical agents must be applied in a thin layer with a sterile glove. The wound may be left open to air or covered with a gauze dressing, depending on the properties of the medication and the physician's orders. Application of these medications can be painful because of manipulation of the burned tissue. Administration of pain medication may be necessary before providing wound care. The surrounding skin should be assessed for any allergic rashes.

Diet

After experiencing a moderate to severe burn, the client's need for calories and protein increases. Actual protein loss occurs with the burn injury itself, and some protein is metabolized to meet the increased energy requirements brought on by stress. For tissue repair and healing, daily protein needs of the client increase significantly. Twice the normal caloric requirement may be needed to meet the body's energy needs. Supplemental vitamins and minerals are given.

Initially, the client's daily nutritional needs may be met with total parenteral nutrition (TPN) because of a paralytic ileus and gastric dilation. Following a severe burn, decreased enteric circulation leads to slowed or stopped peristalsis. Food and fluids cannot be given orally or by tube feeding until peristalsis is restored. Hearing active bowel sounds is one indication of peristaltic activity in the bowel. Immobility, stress, and the negative nitrogen balance brought on by protein catabolism depress appetite. Curling's ulcer may develop. Meeting the client's nutritional needs can be a challenge. Six to eight small feedings daily and high-protein milkshakes or protein supplements can help meet daily nutritional needs. Involving the family in bringing in favorite foods can also stimulate the client's appetite.

INFECTION CONTROL

Skin Grafts

Follow strict aseptic care of both the donor sites and the newly grafted burn wounds to prevent infection.

PROFESSIONALTIP

Serving Meals

Serve foods attractively and put an occasional small "surprise" on the tray (e.g., a flower, a small, brightly colored seasonal decoration, a funny card) so that the client will look forward to meals.

CRITICAL THINKING

Burns and Self-Image

How might a person's self-image be affected when the person has burns on the face, arms, or legs?

LIFE SPAN CONSIDERATIONS

Burn Injuries in the Elderly

- Normal physiologic changes that occur with aging delay recovery and put the older adult at greater risk for complications following a burn injury.
- As a person ages, the physiologic reserves of organ systems decrease.
- While the older person may have adequate pulmonary and cardiac functions at rest, the stress of a severe burn can leave the body unable to cope with demands for increased oxygen and increased cardiac output.
- Renal changes that occur with aging, such as decreased renal blood flow, fewer nephrons, and a decreased glomerular filtration rate, put the older adult at higher risk for kidney failure after a severe burn.
- With loss of subcutaneous tissue and decreased secretion of sebum, the older person's skin is normally more fragile.
- Circulation, especially in the lower extremities, may already be compromised, so healing will be delayed.
- Skin-grafting procedures may not be successful because of impaired circulation and impaired tissue nutrition.

Activity

Contractures, among the most serious complications of severe burns, can be prevented with a program of positioning, splinting, exercising, and ambulating. When repositioning, the client's body must be kept in correct alignment. Use pillows to keep limbs in alignment and splints on limbs to prevent contractures or to immobilize joints following skin grafting. Range-of-motion exercises maintain joint mobility. Whenever possible, encourage active rather than passive range-of-motion exercises. Active exercise increases circulation, maintains joint flexibility, and improves muscle tone. As the client recovers, activities of daily living can be increased and ambulation can be initiated.

Nursing Management

Immediate care includes establishing an airway and administering oxygen. (The physician often inserts an endotracheal tube). Initiate IV fluid therapy with Ringer's lactate solution. Insert a Foley catheter and monitor output, which should be 30 to 50 mL per hour. Administer analgesic IV as ordered. Monitor vital signs, noting respiratory pattern, effort, and breath sounds. Assess pulse oximetry, client's color, and level of consciousness. Accurately record I&O. Monitor client's laboratory results, especially electrolytes.

When the client is stabilized, continue monitoring vital signs, I&O, respiratory pattern, daily weight, and for pain. Strictly follow Standard Precautions. Monitor wounds for signs of infection. Assess mental status. If client is on TPN or enteral tube feedings, monitor client's reaction to feedings. Assess abdomen for bowel sounds. Use pillows and splints, if ordered, to keep client's body in good alignment and turn and reposition every 2 hours. Perform passive ROM exercises when able. Explain the healing process to the client and family. Provide opportunities for the client to express feelings. Listen actively. Encourage the client to look at the wounds to see evidence of healing. Maintain an open, honest approach with the client and family. Assist client and family to prepare for discharge.

NURSING PROCESS

Assessment

Subjective Data

Observe for emotional reactions such as anger, self-consciousness, embarrassment, or isolation. Clients with burns are likely to be frightened and anxious. Feelings of guilt, anger, and depression are also common following burns. Ask the client to describe the pain according to location, intensity, and duration, and also to rate the pain on a scale of 0 to 10. Hypoxia or fluid and electrolyte imbalances can cause confusion, disorientation, and decreased level of consciousness. The client may be nauseated.

Objective Data

Assess vital signs, level of consciousness, and breath sounds. If the client has a productive cough, the amount, consistency, and color of sputum should be noted. Black/gray sputum indicates smoke inhalation. Clients with smoke inhalation may also have crackles, wheezing, or diminished breath sounds. Observe burn wounds for signs of infection such as redness, swelling, purulent drainage, and a foul odor. Measure urine output hourly. Monitor intake and output and daily weight. Routinely check for bowel sounds. As rehabilitation progresses, continue to assess wounds for signs of healing, such as a moist, clean, red wound base and decrease in the size of the wound. Note the client's mobility status and degree of involvement in care. Assess daily dietary intake. Monitor laboratory test results for the following:

- Red blood cell count and hemoglobin level give information about the body's ability to meet oxygen demands of body tissues and organs.
- Creatinine and blood urea nitrogen as well as urine specific gravity give information about kidney function.
- Total protein and albumin levels yield information about the ability to maintain the volume of circulating fluid as well as information about nutritional status.
- White blood cell count indicates the presence of infection and the body's ability to fight it.
- Wound culture and sensitivity data indicate the specific organisms causing infection and the specific antibiotics effective against these organisms.
- Electrolytes yield information about the homeostasis of body fluids. Alterations in pH and electrolyte levels affect cell function in every body tissue, particularly vital body organs such as the heart and cerebrum.

Nursing diagnoses for a client with a burn injury include the following. Initially, the greatest dangers to the client will be:

NURSING DIAGNOSES	PLANNING/OUTCOMES	NURSING INTERVENTIONS
*Impaired **G**as Exchange* related to edema and inflammation of the respiratory tract	The client will achieve a regular respiratory pattern and oxygen saturation level >90%.	Monitor the client's vital signs every 4 hours if stable; otherwise, every 1 to 2 hours. Listen to breath sounds, especially noting respiratory pattern and effort. If the client is on continuous oximetry, note the oxygen saturation reading each time vital signs are assessed. Assess the client's color and level of consciousness. Document assessments and keep the physician informed about the client's condition. Elevate the head of the bed 30 degrees to facilitate full chest expansion with each breath.
*Deficient **F**luid Volume* related to increased capillary permeability with loss of large amounts of fluid through open burn wounds	The client will maintain electrolytes within normal limits and an hourly urine output >30 mL per hour.	Administer intravenous fluids at the ordered rate. Monitor for signs and symptoms of fluid overload such as shortness of breath, crackles auscultated in lung bases, changes in heart rate and/or heart sounds, changes in blood pressure, increased anxiety, or changes in mental status. Measure urine output hourly, report outputs below 30 mL to the physician. Record intake and output. Involve the client and family in keeping a bedside record of fluid intake. Weigh client daily, preferably before breakfast, and in the same type of clothing each day. When the client can tolerate oral fluids, set a fluid intake goal for each shift (e.g., 1,200 mL during the day; 800 mL during the evening; 500 mL during the night). Explain to the client and family the reasons for a high fluid intake. Involve family members in helping the client achieve the fluid maintenance goal. Keep fluids available at the bedside, including, within dietary restrictions, the client's favorite fluids. Monitor for signs and symptoms of electrolyte imbalances such as increased muscle weakness, muscle cramps, cardiac arrhythmias, fatigue, nausea, dizziness. Monitor the client's laboratory results.

Evaluation: Evaluate each outcome to determine how it has been met by the client.

During the stabilization and recovery period after a burn, the nursing diagnoses include the following:

NURSING DIAGNOSES	PLANNING/OUTCOMES	NURSING INTERVENTIONS
*Risk for **I**nfection* related to risk factors of tissue destruction and inadequate primary defenses	The client's burn wounds will exhibit signs of healing without serious or life-threatening infections.	Wash hands with an antibacterial skin cleanser before and after gloving. Wear clean gloves when giving client care. Wear an isolation gown over your uniform when giving client care. Whenever the client's wounds are exposed, wear gown, cap, mask, and sterile gloves. Use sterile technique for wound care and dressing changes. Monitor wound daily for signs of infection: redness, swelling, purulent drainage, pain.

(*Continues*)

During the stabilization and recovery period after a burn, the nursing diagnoses include the following: (Continued)

NURSING DIAGNOSES	PLANNING/OUTCOMES	NURSING INTERVENTIONS
		Assess for signs of systemic infections. Observe for increased pulse and respirations, decreased blood pressure, fever, and any changes in mentation such as disorientation and delirium. Note urinary output and assess for hypoactive bowel sounds. Monitor the client's white blood cell count. Assist client with personal hygiene, and keep noninjured areas of the body clean.
*Acute **Pain** related to* physical injury	The client will verbalize that pain is controlled at a tolerable level.	Assess for pain every 2 to 4 hours by asking client to rate pain level on a scale of 0 to 10. Observe for nonverbal signs of pain such as grimacing or crying. Administer pain medications as ordered, especially prior to wound care or exercise and mobilization activities. Monitor and document response to medications. Implement comfort and diversional measures: a. Reposition client; use pillows or foam supports to keep all body parts in good alignment. b. Teach client to use progressive relaxation exercises or to use guided imagery. c. Encourage the client to use diversionary activities of his choice such as television or music, or place him so that he can see into the hallway.
*Imbalanced **Nutrition**: Less than Body Requirements*, related to increased caloric requirements and difficulty ingesting sufficient quantities of food	The client will ingest sufficient calories daily to meet increased metabolic needs.	If the client is currently on TPN or enteral tube feedings, administer the ordered nutrients at the correct rate and closely monitor the client's reaction. When oral intake is tolerated, encourage the client to eat 90% to 100% of daily diet. Provide oral hygiene before meals to stimulate salivation and eliminate any bad taste in the client's mouth. Give 6 to 8 small feedings daily of the client's favorite foods within dietary restrictions and encourage family members to bring in home-prepared foods and to eat with the client. When permitted, encourage the client to sit up in a chair for each meal. Plan care so that painful procedures are not done immediately before meals. A rest period of 20 to 30 minutes before meals helps the client feel more like eating. Determine the time of day when the client feels most like eating and does indeed eat most of the meal, and serve the highest calorie/protein nutrients at that time.
*Impaired Physical **Mobility*** related to pain and decreased muscle strength	The client will participate in daily activity to maintain joint mobility and prevent contractures.	Perform passive ROM exercises 4 times a day by supporting the limb above and below the joint and performing exercises slowly and smoothly. As the client is able, have him perform active ROM exercises every 3 to 4 hours. Turn and reposition the client every 2 hours. Use small pillows and foam supports to keep the client's body in good alignment.

During the stabilization and recovery period after a burn, the nursing diagnoses include the following: (Continued)

NURSING DIAGNOSES	PLANNING/OUTCOMES	NURSING INTERVENTIONS
		Use splints as ordered by the physician to keep hands, wrists, feet, and ankles in natural alignment and explain the reason for these activities to the client. As healing and rehabilitation progress, encourage progressive ambulation and self-care activities. Gradually guide and assist the client to resume activities of daily living (ADLs). Encourage family members to participate in ADLs and provide positive reinforcement as the client becomes involved in his care.
*Disturbed **B**ody Image* related to change in physical appearance with loss of body tissues or body parts	The client will state realistic expectations for recovery and participate in rehabilitation.	Provide time for the client to express feelings (fear, anger, frustration, regret, and depression are commonly expressed by clients with burns) and practice active listening. Explain the healing process to the client. Give the client daily updates on the degree of wound healing and on his progress in rehabilitation. Encourage the client to look at the wounds to see evidence of healing. Stress that wound healing following serious burn injuries proceeds slowly and that complete healing with improved skin appearance may take a year or more.
*Interrupted **F**amily Processes* related to the shift in health status of a family member	The client and family members will verbalize feelings to nurses and each other and will participate in client care.	Involve family members in the client's care and encourage daily visits. Encourage family members to express their fears and concerns, especially any feelings of anger, blame, or guilt. Guide family members in recognizing and reflecting to the client small, step-by-step progress that is made. Maintain an honest, open approach with the client and family but do not give false reassurance. Collaborate with counselor, social worker, and chaplain to help the client and family cope with the condition. Assist the family to appraise the situation and plan for discharge. What is at stake? What is realistic for the future? What can they expect during the rehabilitation phase? What are their choices? Where can they get help?

Evaluation: Evaluate each outcome to determine how it has been met by the client.

NEOPLASMS: MALIGNANT

Skin cancer is one of the most common malignant neoplasms in the United States and is the most preventable cancer. In 2009, the American Cancer Society estimates more than one million new diagnoses of basal cell carcinoma (approximately 800,000–900,000) and squamous cell carcinoma (approximately 200,000–300,000) in the United States (American Cancer Society [ACS], 2008a). Approximately 68,720 new diagnoses of melanomas are expected to occur in 2009 (ACS, 2008b). These are the three most common skin cancers.

Skin lymphoma is another type of malignancy. Exposure to the sun is the leading cause of skin cancer. Skin damage from sun exposure is cumulative. The ability of skin to tan is not fully developed until the teenage years, meaning that most of the long-term skin damage from sun exposure occurs during childhood. By age 20, most adults have already experienced significant skin damage; however, it takes 10 to 20 years before unprotected sunbathing results in skin cancer.

BASAL CELL CARCINOMA

Basal cell carcinoma, the most frequent type of skin cancer, arises from the basal cell layer of the epidermis. Prolonged sun exposure, poor tanning ability, and previous therapy with x-rays for facial acne are risk factors for basal cell carcinoma (Figure 46-10). Metastasis is rare.

It is generally found on the face and upper torso, and is scaly in appearance. As the disease develops, it extends into the dermis and may form an open ulcer. Surgical removal cures this type of cancer.

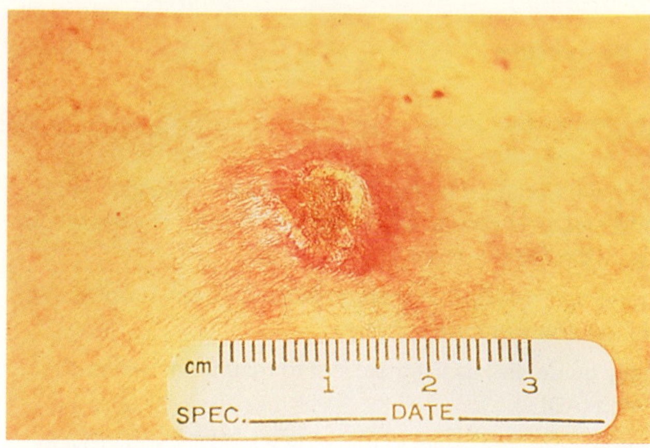

FIGURE 46-10 Basal Cell Carcinoma (*Courtesy of Robert A. Silverman, MD, Clinical Associate Professor, Department of Pediatrics, Georgetown University.*)

SQUAMOUS CELL CARCINOMA

Squamous cell carcinoma appears as a nodular lesion in the epidermis. It is much less common than basal cell carcinoma. Risk factors include prolonged sun exposure and exposure to gamma radiation and x-rays. The sun-exposed lower lip is a common site for squamous cell carcinoma. Without treatment, it can extend into the dermis and ultimately metastasize to other body tissues, causing death (Figure 46-11). Treatment, for squamous cell carcinoma may be by excision of lesion, electrodesiccation (cautery) and curettage (scraping of lesion), cryosurgery (freezing with liquid nitrogen), Mohs surgery (a microscopic surgical procedure of removing layers of cancerous tissue with very high rates of success), radiation therapy, lymph node dissection, and/or chemotherapy (ACS, 2008c).

MALIGNANT MELANOMA

In malignant melanoma, atypical melanocytes are present in both the dermis and epidermis. Malignant melanoma is the most serious of the three types of skin cancers and may begin in a preexisting mole (nevus). These moles have an irregular shape. Contrasted to normal moles, they are larger than 6 mm in diameter and do not have a uniform color (see ABCD rule). Malignant melanoma can metastasize to every organ in the body through the bloodstream and lymphatic system.

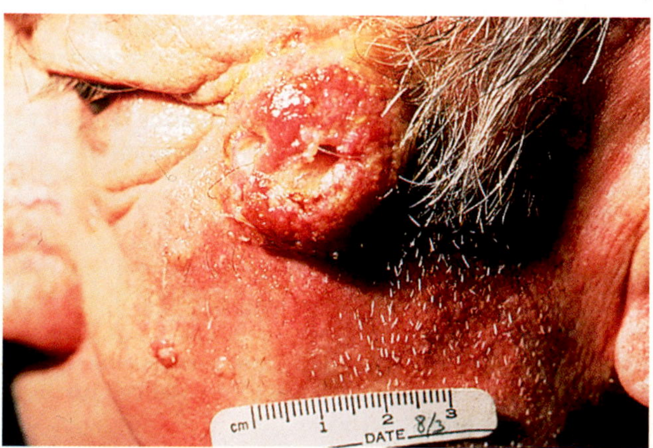

FIGURE 46-11 Squamous Cell Carcinoma (*Courtesy of Robert A. Silverman, MD, Clinical Associate Professor, Department of Pediatrics, Georgetown University.*)

MEMORY TRICK

ABCD rule: Usual warning signs for melanoma

A = ASYMMETRICAL – Both halves of the mole or birthmark do not match.

B = BORDER – Borders are irregular, blurred, or. notched

C = COLOR – Color is uneven, in different shades of black, brown, or red, white or blue.

D = DIAMETER – Diameter is greater than 6 mm (¼ inch).

The most significant warning sign is a mole or birthmark that is changing in size, shape, or color over time (ACS, 2009e).

Melanoma is more common in fair-skinned individuals and occurs most often on the trunk of males and the lower legs on females, but can occur on any area of the body and in all skin tones. Malignant melanomas can arise from a mole that has been present for a client's entire life as well as from skin independent of mole existence. Any mole that looks significantly different from other moles present on the body whether or not it has always been present should be examined carefully, photographed, followed, and/or biopsied.

The incidence of malignant melanoma is increasing in the United States as a result of increased sun exposure and use of artificial ultraviolet light (tanning lights/beds). Clearly, the best hope of preventing skin cancer lies in education. Limiting sun exposure (and artificial ultraviolet light) and using sunscreen at least SPF 15 on exposed skin markedly reduce damage from ultraviolet rays and ultimately decrease the risk of skin cancer. Figure 46-12 shows lentigo malignant melanoma.

CUTANEOUS T-CELL LYMPHOMA

Cutaneous T-cell lymphoma is also known as mycosis fungoides and skin lymphoma. It is a malignant disease involving T-helper cells that has both skin manifestations and multiple organ system manifestations. In the early stages, it resembles psoriasis or seborrheic dermatitis. Later, fissures and skin ulcers develop. Pruritus can be severe. Even if the skin condition can be improved with topical steroids and chemotherapeutic agents, the disease is ultimately fatal because of the involvement of vital organ systems. Clients with AIDS can develop cutaneous T-cell lymphoma.

MEDICAL–SURGICAL MANAGEMENT

Surgical

Treatment is determined by the size of the lesion, the type of neoplasm, and the stage of the disease. The primary treatment is surgery: a simple excision or a wide excision (removing skin in a large area around the lesion), amputation if on fingers or toes, and/or lymph node dissection if lymph nodes are enlarged or a sentinel node biopsy confirms the presence of malignant cells. If indicated, chemotherapy may be used either systemically or directly into the affected extremity. By injecting chemo into an artery of the affected limb, high doses are targeted to the tumor

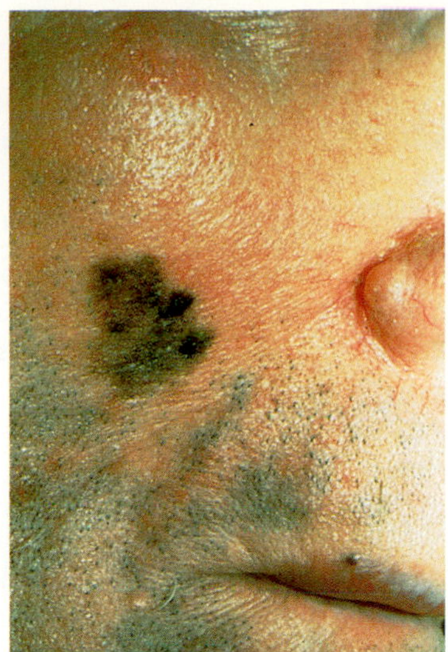

FIGURE 46-12 Lentigo Malignant Melanoma (*Courtesy of Robert A. Silverman, MD, Clinical Associate Professor, Department of Pediatrics, Georgetown University.*)

area without affecting the entire body. Radiation therapy may also be used (ACS, 2009d). With early detection, melanoma can be successfully treated, but presently there is no cure with advanced melanoma. Melanomas have a rapid rate of metastasis.

NURSING MANAGEMENT

Careful assessment of the client's skin can reveal suspicious skin lesions. Clients with blue eyes, fair complexion, blonde or red hair, and freckles have the greatest risk. Clients who have had one skin cancer are likely to have more. Early referral and prompt care can ensure a good prognosis. Because most skin cancers are treated by excision, client teaching and follow-up care focus on proper wound care to promote healing and prevent infection. Many clients will experience body image disturbance; the nurse can help the client cope with this. All other nursing care should be focused on prevention.

NEOPLASMS: NONMALIGNANT

Benign tumors of the skin include a variety of lesions such as skin tags, lipomas, keloids, sebaceous cysts, nevi (moles), and angiomas. In general, they do not require medical or nursing intervention except for cosmetic reasons or unless they are subject to continual irritation that might predispose to a break in skin integrity and infection. **Lipomas** (benign, fatty tumors) or **sebaceous cysts** (distended sebaceous glands filled with sebum) might cause pressure on surrounding nerves or interfere with normal body function. In these instances they would be surgically removed. A **keloid** is abnormal growth of scar tissue that is elevated, rounded, and firm with irregular, clawlike margins. Surgical removal is not always successful; healing following surgery can again result in a keloid. Steroids or radiation have been helpful in some conditions. **Angiomas**, commonly known as birthmarks, are vascular tumors involving skin and subcutaneous tissue. They can be raised, bright red nodular lesions (strawberry birthmarks) or dark red/purple patches (port-wine angiomas). Cosmetics can be used to camouflage them. Laser treatments are being used on some angiomas with some success.

INFECTIOUS DISORDERS OF THE SKIN

Given an accessible portal of entry and decreased host resistance, virulent organisms can invade the skin, causing inflammation, infection, itching, and pain. Bacteria, viruses, fungi, or parasites can cause infectious disorders of the skin (Figure 46-13). Treating the client's disease is only one aspect

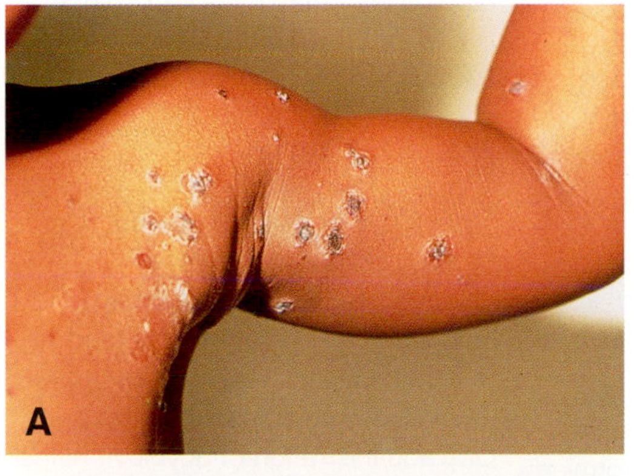

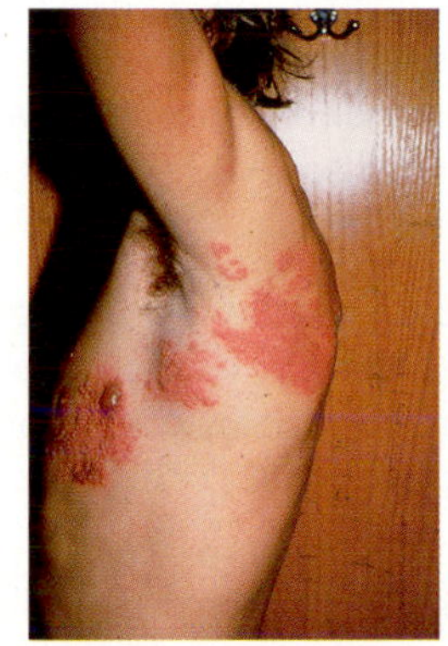

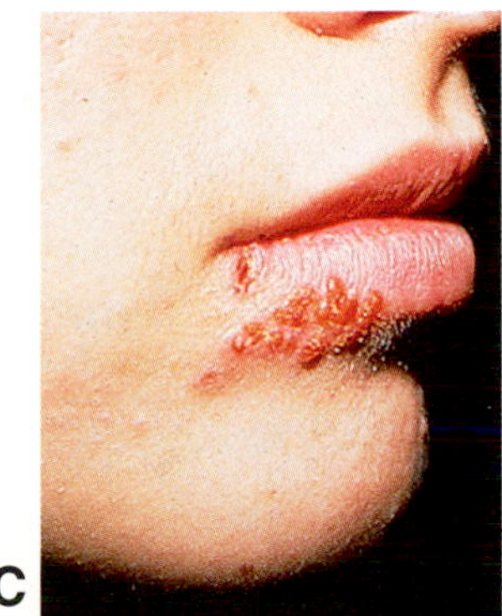

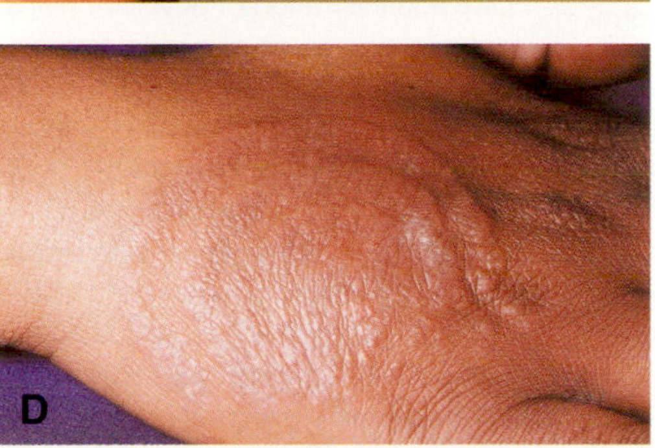

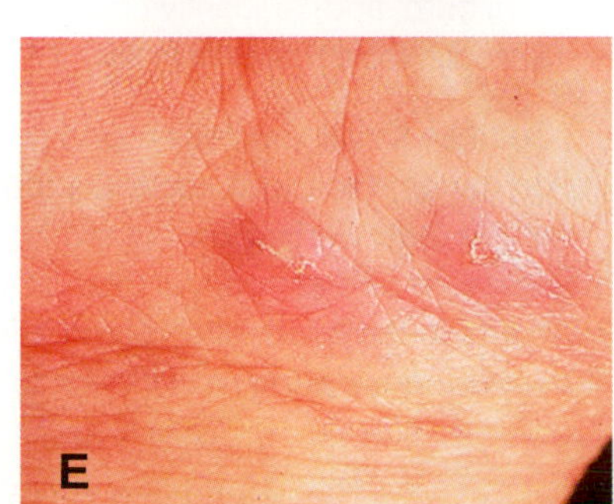

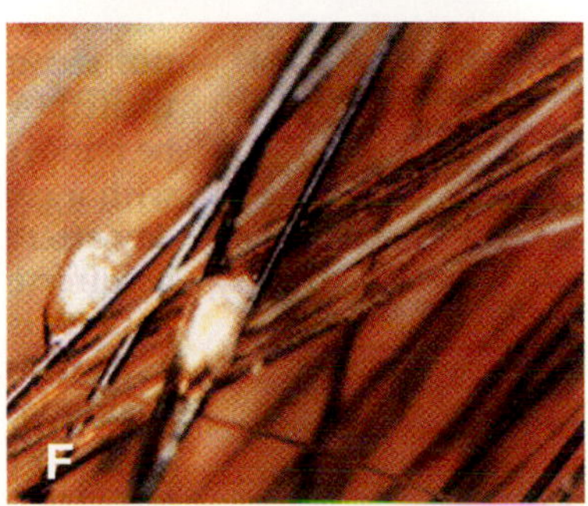

FIGURE 46-13 Infectious Disorders of the Skin; *A*, Impetigo Contagiosa; *B*, Herpes Zoster (Shingles); *C*, Herpes Simplex Type 1; *D*, Tinea Corporis (Ringworm); *E*, Scabies; *F*, Pediculosis (Head Lice) (*Images A, B, C, D and E courtesy of Robert A. Silverman, MD, Clinical Associate Professor, Department of Pediatrics, Georgetown University; image F courtesy of Hogil Pharmaceutical Corporation.*)

TABLE 46-3 Infectious Disorders of the Skin

DISEASE	ORGANISM	CLINICAL MANIFESTATIONS	MANAGEMENT
Bacterial Infections			
Impetigo contagiosa	*Staphylococcus aureus*	Begins as a small vesicle; becomes weeping lesion; forms a light brown crust. Usually on the face and upper trunk (Figure 46-13A). More common in children. More common in spring and fall. Poor hygiene coupled with warm weather facilitates the spread of the disease.	Cleanse the affected area at least 3 times a day. Apply an antibiotic ointment. Occasionally, systemic antibiotics are needed.
Carbuncle	*Staphylococcus aureus*	Begins as infected hair follicles in the dermis. Symptoms are redness, swelling, pain. Yellow cores of pus develop. Carbuncles usually occur on the nape of the neck and upper back. Obese or malnourished persons with poor hygiene as well as diabetics are most susceptible to carbuncles.	Warm, moist soaks may help "bring the boil to a head." Once the carbuncle ruptures or is incised and drained, pain subsides. Carbuncles tend to recur. The *Staphylococcus* organism may be resistant to topical antibiotics. Systemic antibiotics may be needed.
Viral Infections			
Herpes zoster (shingles)	V-Z (varicella-zoster)	Clusters of small vesicles over the course of a peripheral sensory nerve. Two-thirds of clients have lesions just in the thoracic region. Lesions can occur over the trigeminal nerve, affecting the face, scalp, and eyes (Figure 46-13B). Crusts develop in several days. Symptoms are mild to severe pain, itching, fever, malaise. In older adults, pain can last for months or years. Persons who have not had chickenpox risk contracting the disease if they care for herpes zoster clients with open lesions. Persons who previously had chickenpox, but developed only partial immunity to it, may still be susceptible to herpes zoster.	Acyclovir (Zovirax), valacyclovir (Valtrex), or famciclovir (Famvir) may be given to clients in severe pain or to immunosuppressed clients. Analgesics help control the pain. Narcotic analgesics are prescribed for severe pain. Antipruritic topical medications decrease the itching. Shingles (herpes zoster) vaccine is recommended for adults 60 and older even if they have had shingles in the past (Harvard Health Letter, 2008).
Herpes simplex, Type 1 (fever blisters, cold sores) Type 2 (genital)	*Herpes simplex virus*	Type 1—a cluster of vesicles on an erythematous base occurring most commonly at the corners of the mouth (Figure 46-13C) or at the edge of the nostrils. Type 2—lesions in the vagina or cervix of a woman or on the penis of a man. The lesions itch, burn, and frequently break open, forming a crust. Healing occurs in about 10 days.	Topical use of antiviral agents such as acyclovir decreases discomfort. Even with treatment, cold sores and fever blisters tend to recur, especially with fever, upper respiratory infections, and stress. Oral administration of acyclovir helps prevent recurrence of genital herpes.
Warts	Human papillomavirus	Seen as small, painless round papules on hands, face, and neck. On the bottom of the feet, warts grow inward from the pressure and are painful (plantar warts). Warts in the anogenital region itch. Genital warts increase the risk of cervical cancer.	No treatment is indicated for painless warts; they tend to disappear eventually. Plantar warts may be removed by cryosurgery or with locally applied chemicals such as nitric acid. Warts are not highly contagious from person to person but may be spread on the person's own body by rubbing or scratching. Genital warts are spread by sexual intercourse.

(*Continues*)

TABLE 46-3 Infectious Disorders of the Skin (Continued)

DISEASE	ORGANISM	CLINICAL MANIFESTATIONS	MANAGEMENT
Fungal Infections			
Tinea (ringworm) Tinea capitis (ringworm of the scalp) Tinea corporis (ringworm of the body) Tinea cruris (jock itch) Tinea pedis (athlete's foot)	*Microsporum audouini*	Tinea is a superficial infection of the skin called ringworm because of its circumscribed appearance, typically round, and reddened with slight scaling (Figure 46-13D). Lesions of tinea corporis have a pale center. Itching is common with tinea cruris. Itching and burning occur with tinea pedis. Tinea is spread easily. Jock itch and athlete's foot are more common among men than women.	Treat mild infections with a topical antifungal drug such as miconazole nitrate (Micatin) or tolnaftate (Aftate). Severe infections are treated with oral administration of griseofulvin microsize (Grisactin).
Parasitic Infections			
Scabies	*Sarcoptes scabiei* (female itch mite)	The itch mite burrows under the skin, lays eggs, and deposits fecal material. Short, dark-red wavy lines may be seen on hands, wrists, elbows, axillary folds, nipples, waistline, and gluteal folds (Figure 46-13E). Pruritis is severe and can persist for up to 3 months after treatment. Scratching leads to secondary infection. Scabies is spread by prolonged contact and is frequently seen in several members of a family.	Apply the scabicide, lindane (Kwell), topically to the entire body at bedtime so that the medication remains on the skin 8 to 12 hours. Treat all family members even if they do not have symptoms. Wash all underclothing and bed and bath linens in hot water and dry in dryer. Change linens daily. Items that cannot be washed should be dry cleaned.
Pediculosis (lice)	*Pediculus capitis* (head lice) *Pediculus corporis* (body lice) *Phthirus Pubis* (pubic lice)	Eggs, or nits, of pediculosis capitis attach themselves firmly to a hair shaft on the head or in a beard (Figure 46-13F). Nits have a gray, pearly appearance. The pubic louse resembles a tiny crab that attaches itself to pubic hair. Body lice live in the seams of clothing. The bite of the louse causes severe pruritis. Scratching leads to secondary infection.	Lindane (Kwell) is applied topically to the hair as a shampoo or to the body as a cream or lotion. Repeat the treatment again in 8 to 10 days. Wash or dry clean clothing and linens. Disinfect combs and brushes. Vacuum carpets and furniture; then spray with a pediculicide. All nits must be removed to prevent reinfection.

COURTESY OF DELMAR CENGAGE LEARNING

of the treatment plan; preventing the spread of infection is the other. Table 46-3 outlines several disease conditions and identifies the organism responsible, clinical manifestations, and the management for each disorder.

Nursing Management

Teach the client and family about preventing the spread of infection. Follow Standard Precautions. Stress the importance of not scratching lesions. Provide emotional support to client and family. Encourage expression of feelings.

NURSING PROCESS

Assessment

Subjective Data

Ask the client how long the problem has existed, if there is any itching or pain, and what treatment has been used. Clients with infectious disorders of the skin may feel shame or embarrassment because of stigmas attached to some of these conditions, so also note the client's mood.

Objective Data

A complete skin assessment is performed, describing the size, appearance, and distribution of all lesions, as well as any drainage, itching, odor, or pain present.

CRITICAL THINKING

Preventing Spread of Skin Infections

How can the spread of skin infections be prevented? Prepare a teaching plan for a client with a skin infection.

CLIENT TEACHING

Herpes Zoster

- Take the full course of prescribed medications.
- Use topical measures along with NSAIDs for pain management.
- Avoid persons who have not had chickenpox, especially pregnant women, so they do not get chickenpox.
- When dark crusts form over pustules, the client is no longer contagious.
- In older adults, pain may last for months or years.

Nursing diagnoses for a client with an infectious disorder of the skin include the following:

NURSING DIAGNOSES	PLANNING/OUTCOMES	NURSING INTERVENTIONS
*Impaired **S**kin Integrity* related to invasion of skin structures by pathogenic organisms	The client will regain skin integrity.	Wear gloves when caring for the client with skin lesions. Cleanse the skin thoroughly, but gently. In the case of bacterial infections or lesions with secondary infections, use an antibacterial soap. Gently remove crusts, scales, and traces of old medication before applying fresh creams or lotions. Administer prescribed medications; apply creams and lotions; then monitor their effectiveness. Explain what you are doing and why.
*Acute **P**ain*, related to itching, burning, and infection	The client will report less pain.	Instruct client to keep the environmental temperature cool because warmth increases itching; also cleanse skin lesions with tepid water, not hot. Stress the importance of not scratching the lesions.
*Disturbed **B**ody Image* related to unsightly skin lesions and embarrassment	The client will verbalize a positive body image.	Encourage client to ask questions and to talk about feelings. Provide positive reinforcement as the client learns to care for the skin lesions. When possible, suggest ways to camouflage the lesions or minimize their appearance. When there is no danger of spreading the infection, encourage client to participate in social and work activities.

Evaluation: Evaluate each outcome to determine how it has been met by the client.

SAMPLE NURSING CARE PLAN

The Client with Scabies

E.E., 68, has had a skin rash for the past 2 weeks. The dark red lesions occur mainly on her hands, wrists, and elbows, around her nipples, at her waistline, and in her gluteal folds. The itching has become increasingly intense. She states that she has been scratching the lesions, sometimes until they are open and bleeding. Upon examination, some of the lesions are open with small amounts of serosanguineous drainage. Other lesions are scabbed. She lives with her daughter and two teenaged granddaughters. Because the lesions were getting steadily worse, her daughter finally convinced her to seek medical attention. She was horrified when the doctor told her that she had scabies. She had always associated "the itch" with "dirty people who didn't take care of themselves."

NURSING DIAGNOSIS 1 *Impaired **S**kin Integrity* related to scratching scabies lesions as evidenced by open lesions draining serosanguineous fluid, scabbed lesions, and client statements of scratching the lesions until they bleed

(*Continues*)

SAMPLE NURSING CARE PLAN (Continued)

Nursing Outcomes Classification (NOC)
Tissue Integrity: Skin & Mucous Membranes
Self-Care: Hygiene

Nursing Interventions Classification (NIC)
Skin Care: Topical Treatments
Skin Surveillance

PLANNING/OUTCOMES	NURSING INTERVENTIONS	RATIONALE
E.E. will follow the prescribed treatment protocol to promote healing of skin lesions and regain skin integrity.	Instruct E.E. to cleanse lesions carefully using an antibacterial soap and tepid water. The lesions can be cleaned 1 to 3 times daily.	Reduces the number of microorganisms present and decreases the risk of infection. Tepid water does not intensify itching as hot water does.
	Teach E.E. to apply antipruritic lotions as prescribed by the doctor after cleansing the skin.	Lotions applied just after bathing help to retain skin moisture.
	Instruct E.E. to keep fingernails short with smooth edges.	Less likely to break the skin if the client scratches.
	Teach E.E. to press itching lesions, and not to scratch them.	Stimulates nerve endings and reduces the sensation of itching. Prevents breaks in the skin, which would be portals of entry for microorganisms.
	Explain that itching can persist up to 3 months following treatment with the scabicide but persistent itching does not mean that treatment was ineffective.	Skin reaction to the toxins and secretions of the itch mite can persist for up to 3 months after the itch mites are killed by the scabicide.
	Keep room temperature between 68° and 72°F and humidity constant at 30% to 35%.	Itching is intensified in hot, humid environments.

EVALUATION

E.E.'s lesions are still red, but none are open and draining. Some lesions are still scabbed. No new open lesions have developed. E.E. states that the recommended measures "help," but that the itching is still "pretty bad." Goal of promoting healing of skin lesions is being met. Encourage E.E. to continue outlined protocols. Reassure her that itching will gradually subside as healing progresses.

NURSING DIAGNOSIS 2 *Deficient Knowledge (infection control measures),* related to lack of familiarity with treatment and prevention protocols as evidenced by client's inability to recognize the skin lesions as infectious and by statements about scabies happening only to people with poor hygiene

Nursing Outcomes Classification (NOC)
Knowledge: Infection Control

Nursing Interventions Classification (NIC)
Teaching: Disease Process
Teaching: Prescribed Medication

PLANNING/OUTCOMES	NURSING INTERVENTIONS	RATIONALE
E.E. will apply the scabicide correctly and state ways to avoid spreading infection to others.	Assess E.E's knowledge of scabies, its treatment regimen and infection control measures. Ask specific questions.	Provides a frame of reference for the client, helping her relate new information and integrate it into her behavior.

(*Continues*)

SAMPLE NURSING CARE PLAN (Continued)

PLANNING/OUTCOMES	NURSING INTERVENTIONS	RATIONALE
	Explain that scabies is transmitted by skin-to-skin contact or by contact with articles freshly contaminated by infected persons, and affects persons of all social, economic, and age levels.	Teaching that does not "talk down" to the client communicates respect.
	Stress the importance of following treatment protocol exactly. Review salient points such as (1) shower before applying the scabicide; (2) apply the scabicide to the entire body surface, including skin without scabies lesions; and (3) apply the scabicide at bedtime so that the medication remains on the skin 8 to 12 hours.	Failure to apply the scabicide as directed and/or failure to leave the lotion on the skin for the prescribed length of time will not kill the itch mite.
	Give E.E. step-by-step written instructions.	Enhances compliance with the treatment regimen.
	Instruct E.E. to wash hands under warm running water with plenty of soap (preferably an antibacterial soap) for at least 10 seconds after touching lesions and clean carefully under fingernails while washing hands.	Thorough handwashing is the single most effective means of preventing the spread of infection. Large numbers of bacteria reside under the fingernails.
	Advise E.E. not to share washcloths, towels, clothing, pillows, or bed linens with other family members.	Disease-causing microorganisms can be spread to well individuals indirectly when their skin comes into contact with contaminated items.
	Instruct E.E. to wash underclothing and bed and bath linens in detergent and hot water and dry outside in sunlight or in a dryer on the hot setting.	Soap reduces surface tension. When fat or protein substances that shield organisms are broken down, the organisms are exposed to the killing effects of heat. Prolonged exposure to heat or ultraviolet rays from direct sunlight kills microorganisms.
	Advise E.E. to shower daily, use an antibacterial soap, rinse thoroughly, and dry carefully, especially in skin folds and between toes, using a towel and washcloth only once before laundering it.	Reduces the number of microorganisms on the skin. Moisture encourages the growth of microorganisms. Laundering the towel and washcloth after only one use prevents the indirect transfer of the itch mite.

(Continues)

SAMPLE NURSING CARE PLAN (Continued)

PLANNING/OUTCOMES	NURSING INTERVENTIONS	RATIONALE
	Assess lesions daily for signs of healing. Report any signs and symptoms of infection in secondary lesions such as redness, swelling, pain, drainage (describe characteristics of the drainage) to the physician or clinic.	Increases the probability of effective treatment with fewer complications.
	Teach E.E. and family members the early signs and symptoms of scabies infection, such as any reddened papules with wavy, threadlike lines visible on the skin around the papules and severe itching, especially at night.	Early recognition and treatment of scabies can minimize the severity of the infection.
	Instruct them to assess their skin daily.	A daily examination allows treatment to begin as soon as the problem is identified.

EVALUATION

E.E. and her family did apply the scabicide as prescribed. The client can describe how scabies are transmitted but continues to express fear that she will give "this awful thing to somebody." Goal of correctly applying scabicide met. Although E.E. can state how scabies are transmitted, she still has doubts; hence, the goal of stating ways to avoid spreading the infection to others has only been partially met. Reinforce that even though red skin lesions are still visible, the itch mites were killed by treatment and cannot be transmitted to others even if the client does shake hands, hug, or touch someone else.

NURSING DIAGNOSIS 3 *Disturbed **B**ody Image* related to unsightly lesions and embarrassment as evidenced by distribution of lesions on exposed skin areas and client statements of being horrified about the diagnosis and associating scabies with "dirty people"

Nursing Outcomes Classification (NOC)
Body Image

Nursing Interventions Classification (NIC)
Anxiety Reduction
Mutual Goal Setting

PLANNING/OUTCOMES	NURSING INTERVENTIONS	RATIONALE
E.E. will assume self-care of lesions.	Explain that by using the scabicide, lindane (Kwell), as directed and by following measures to prevent secondary infection of the scabies lesions, she can expect complete healing of the lesions without any visible scars within a few weeks.	Reassurance that scabies can be cured enhances the client's self-image.
E.E. will maintain relationships with family and friends.	Encourage E.E. to express her feelings about herself and her opinions about scabies.	Brings feelings and opinions out into the open where they can be dealt with appropriately.

(*Continues*)

SAMPLE NURSING CARE PLAN (Continued)

PLANNING/OUTCOMES	NURSING INTERVENTIONS	RATIONALE
	Provide information to correct any misconceptions she might have.	Accurate information dispels misconceptions.
	Encourage E.E. to verbalize the perceptions she has about her family's and friends' feelings about persons with scabies.	A person perceiving derogatory opinions of her is likely to socially isolate herself from them.
	Be alert to verbal and nonverbal messages.	Nonverbal messages give insight into the client's real feelings. Identifying and discussing feelings can lead to behavioral changes.
	Reassure her that she will not infect friends and family members by sitting beside them or being in the same room with them for prolonged periods.	The client will be unlikely to avoid friends or make disparaging remarks about herself when she realizes that she is not a danger to them.
	Share with E.E. that wearing long-sleeved cotton blouses or dresses will hide most of the visible lesions.	Makes the client less self-conscious and embarrassed. Cotton fabric allows good air circulation. Cool skin itches less.

EVALUATION

The client has assumed self-care responsibilities. She does interact with her family but emphasizes that she "doesn't want to get too close to them until these things are completely gone." She has refused to go to church, social gatherings, or activities outside of the house.

Goal has been partially met in that the client does follow proper procedures when caring for her skin lesions, but goal has not been met in so far as maintaining relationships is concerned. Encourage the client to talk about her feelings, particularly feelings of embarrassment. Point out to her the evidence that her lesions are healing. Emphasize that symptoms of intense itching, worsening of present skin lesions, and signs of more skin lesions would be present if the itch mites were alive and still spreading. Encourage her to go on at least one outing with her family during the coming week. Reevaluate in 1 week.

INFLAMMATORY DISORDERS OF THE SKIN

Included in this category are dermatitis and psoriasis.

DERMATITIS

By definition, dermatitis is an inflammatory condition of the skin. In current usage, eczema has almost become synonymous with dermatitis, although eczema tends to be used most often to refer to chronic forms of dermatitis. Most clients with dermatitis are treated as outpatients. Patch testing may identify a specific allergen that is causing the dermatitis. Avoiding the allergenic substance may prevent future dermatitis. In some cases, application of a topical corticosteroid is all that is needed. Other types of this inflammatory disorder include contact dermatitis and exfoliative dermatitis.

ECZEMA

Eczema is an atopic dermatitis often associated with allergic rhinitis and asthma. It is a chronic superficial inflammation that evolves into pruritic, red, weeping, crusted lesions (Estes, 2010). See Figure 46-14. Mostly infants get eczema, but older children and adults may have it. The common allergens are chocolate, orange juice, wheat, and eggs. Heredity is a major factor. Elimination of dietary substances is used to identify the client's allergen(s). Tiny cracks in the skin allow body fluid to escape, so skin hydration is the major treatment.

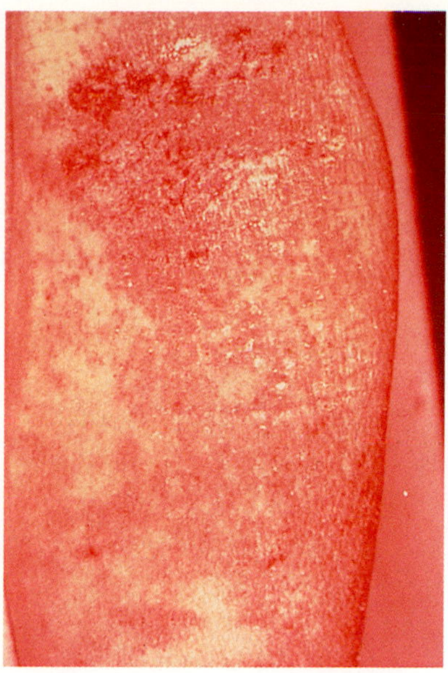

FIGURE 46-14 Eczema (*Courtesy of Centers for Disease Control and Prevention.*)

NURSING MANAGEMENT

Nursing management is directed toward promoting healing, providing comfort, preventing infection, and fostering a positive attitude to help the client cope with an altered body image. Nursing diagnoses may include *Impaired **S**kin Integrity; Risk for **I**nfection; Acute **P**ain*; and *Disturbed **B**ody Image.*

Affected areas are soaked in warm water for 15 to 20 minutes and then an occlusive ointment is applied, as directed, to retain the water. Following a bath or shower, pat the skin dry and immediately apply the occlusive ointment. Wet dressings may be ordered to maximize skin hydration. Moisturizing lotions such as Curel or Lubriderm may be used as the lesions heal. Client teaching is focused on identifying and avoiding substances that cause dermatitis, care for the lesions, how to prevent infection, and how to cope with the conditions.

CONTACT DERMATITIS

In contact dermatitis the skin reacts to external irritants such as (1) allergens like cosmetics, (2) harsh chemical substances like detergents or insecticides, (3) metals such as nickel, (4) mechanical irritation from wool or glass fibers, and (5) body substances like urine or feces. Symptoms include pruritus, burning, and erythema. Often, a maculopapular rash or a combination of papules and vesicles develops. Scratching the lesions may spread the dermatitis as well as lead to secondary infections of the skin (Figure 46-15).

Treatment of symptoms may include a corticosteroid ointment and an oral antihistamine such as diphenhydramine hydrochloride (Benadryl).

> ### LIFE SPAN CONSIDERATIONS
> **Skin Integrity in the Older Adult**
>
> The thinning and drying of the skin due to aging makes older adults more susceptible to irritants that cause dermatitis. Restoring skin integrity in older adults takes longer and requires persistent nursing effort.

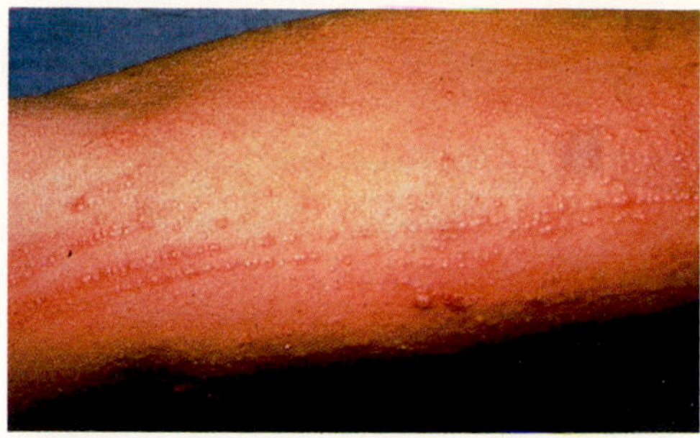

FIGURE 46-15 Allergic Contact Dermatitis from Poison Oak: Note Linear Pattern to Lesions (*Courtesy of Centers for Disease Control and Prevention.*)

NURSING MANAGEMENT

Assist the client in identifying the causative allergen. Use aseptic technique when caring for open lesions. Apply dressings wet with Burow's solution as ordered. Advise the client that a cool, moist environment reduces pruritis.

DERMATITIS VENENATA AND MEDICAMENTOSA

Dermatitis venenata is a specific type of contact dermatitis when the allergen is from a plant (e.g., poison ivy, poison oak). The first exposure sensitizes the client's body to form antigens against the allergen. Later exposures lead to inflammation, pruritis, edema, and vesicle formation.

Dermatitis medicamentosa is a skin reaction to a medication (e.g., penicillin, codeine). Symptoms range from mild to severe erythema and vesicle formation. Respiratory distress may occur.

NURSING MANAGEMENT

For dermatitis venenata, wash the affected area immediately. Calamine lotion relieves the pruritis. Corticosteroids may be needed for more severe cases to decrease inflammation and itching.

For dermatitis medicamentosa, notify the physician immediately so the medication can be discontinued and treatment of symptoms initiated. Advise the client to wear a Medic Alert bracelet or necklace and to notify all health care members of the allergy.

EXFOLIATIVE DERMATITIS

In exfoliative dermatitis, inflammation of the skin gradually worsens. Localized symptoms include erythema, severe pruritus, extensive scaling, and skin sloughing. Exfoliative dermatitis affects the entire body, not just the skin. Systemic symptoms include chills, fever, and malaise. With the loss of

LIFE SPAN CONSIDERATIONS

Exfoliative Dermatitis

Older adults have a greater risk of fatal complications from exfoliative dermatitis. As body systems age, they are less able to respond quickly and effectively to the stress of illness.

large areas of skin surface, the individual has difficulty maintaining body temperature, loses body fluids and electrolytes, and is susceptible to infection.

In most cases, the cause of exfoliative dermatitis is unknown. Severe reactions to drugs such as penicillin may sometimes cause exfoliative dermatitis. It may also be associated with other types of dermatitis or lymphoma. Exfoliative dermatitis can be fatal, primarily because of overwhelming systemic infections and/or massive loss of body fluids and electrolytes.

Nursing Management

When clients are hospitalized with exfoliative dermatitis, management is directed toward maintaining fluid balance, preventing infection, decreasing inflammation, and promoting comfort. The client requires intravenous fluids to maintain the volume of circulating fluid, corticosteroids to decrease inflammation, and antibiotics to treat infection. Medicated baths, topical steroids, and mild analgesics may be prescribed to ease the pruritus.

PSORIASIS

Psoriasis, a chronic, inflammatory, noninfectious autoimmune disease of the skin, affects about 7.5 million Americans, especially young adults. Psoriasis is more prevalent in Caucasians. The parts of the body most commonly affected are the scalp, elbows, palms, knees, lower back, and soles of the feet (National Psoriasis Foundation, 2009) (Figure 46-16). The exact cause of psoriasis is unknown, although a genetic component may be involved. Emotional stress, infections, trauma, and seasonal and hormonal changes trigger exacerbations of psoriasis. It may improve for a while only to recur. This process of subsiding and recurring continues throughout the client's life. Psoriasis is not curable. In psoriasis, the process of keratinization has gone awry. Instead of producing cells that provide a natural barrier against harmful substances and microorganisms, abnormal keratinization causes large, red patches covered with thick silvery scales in the outermost layer of the epidermis (Tate, 2008). If these scales are scraped away, bleeding occurs. When fingernails are affected, pitting and yellow discoloration is seen.

Medical–Surgical Management

Medical

Treatment is directed toward slowing down the rate of cell formation in the epidermis or toward altering the abnormal process of keratinization. Treatment regimens can be effective in reducing the scaling and itching. The client must recognize that psoriasis can only be controlled, not cured. Furthermore, the client must be committed to lifetime therapy.

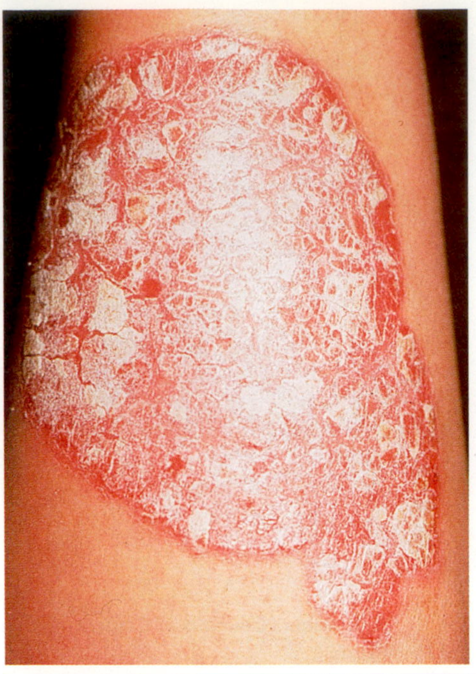

FIGURE 46-16 Psoriasis (*Courtesy of Robert A. Silverman, MD, Clinical Associate Professor, Department of Pediatrics, Georgetown University.*)

Pharmacological

Keratolytic agents such as salicylic acid preparations and coal tar preparations are applied topically to the lesions. Corticosteroids may also be used to reduce inflammation. Ultraviolet light and methotrexate (Mexate) inhibit DNA synthesis in the epidermal cells, thus slowing the rate of cell division and the process of abnormal keratinization. Because of its toxicity to the liver, methotrexate is used only in severe cases of psoriasis that do not respond to any other form of treatment. The Goeckerman regimen, which combines the use of coal tar and ultraviolet light, is one of the oldest effective treatments available but is not offered in many centers in the United States (American Academy of Dermatology [AAD], 2007).

Photochemotherapy is used for severe psoriasis. Photochemotherapy (psorafen and ultraviolet A-range, or PUVA) combines the use of psorafen with ultraviolet A light waves. Psorafen is a photosensitizing agent that reacts with ultraviolet A light waves to markedly reduce DNA synthesis, thereby slowing cell division in psoriasis lesions and relieving symptoms. PUVA is effective in approximately 85% of cases, but approximately 25 treatments occur over several months before clearing of psoriasis occurs. Continued treatments are needed to maintain control over this disease (AAD, 2007).

Etretinate (Tegison), a compound related to retinoic acid vitamin A, is used in severe psoriasis not amenable to other therapies. It may be used alone or in combination with ultraviolet A light waves. Etretinate has numerous adverse effects, including liver damage and severe birth defects. The client must be monitored closely. Women of childbearing age must use effective contraception during treatment and for at least 1 month after treatment.

Alternative therapies, such as aloe vera, may decrease itching, scaling, redness and inflammation. Capsaicin cream may lessen itching, and Omega 3 fatty acids (fish oil) may reduce inflammation. These treatments are considered safe to use (Mayo Clinic, 2009).

Nursing Management

Assist the client to understand and comply with the treatment. Teach the client proper hand hygiene. Listen to the client's feelings and frustrations.

NURSING PROCESS

Assessment

Subjective Data

Psoriasis lesions are generally very visible and likely to make the client feel self-conscious and uncomfortable. Many clients tend to suffer self-esteem and body image disturbances, and sometimes depression, because psoriasis requires lifelong treatment. The treatment can be time-consuming, bothersome, and, from the client's point of view, not completely effective. Encourage the client to verbalize feelings. Ask about itching, burning, and discomfort, as well as the client's mood.

Objective Data

Check the skin carefully, noting the distribution, size, and appearance of lesions. Note signs of infection such as redness, swelling, pain, or drainage.

Nursing diagnoses for a client with psoriasis include the following:

NURSING DIAGNOSES	PLANNING/OUTCOMES	NURSING INTERVENTIONS
*Deficient **K**nowledge* related to psoriasis and its treatment	The client will discuss condition and adhere to treatment.	Help client gain an understanding of psoriasis and comply with the treatment regimen. Support and encourage the client. Explain the purpose of each medication.
*Risk for **I**nfection* related to open lesions	The client will not get an infection.	Teach client how to prevent infections by proper hand hygiene and not scratching the lesions.
*Disturbed **B**ody Image* related to scaly lesions	The client will identify positive attributes about self.	Listen actively and encourage client to express feelings and frustrations. Reinforce positive behavior.
*Situational Low **S**elf-Esteem* related to appearance	The client will demonstrate behaviors that promote self-esteem.	Guide client in identifying effective coping techniques. Help client focus on personal attributes that contribute to effective functioning and a positive self-image. Encourage work and social interactions.

Evaluation: Evaluate each outcome to determine how it has been met by the client.

ULCERS

The two most common types of ulcers of the skin are venous ulcers and pressure ulcers.

VENOUS ULCERS

Poor venous circulation, especially in lower extremities, can lead to a condition known as stasis dermatitis (Figure 46-17). The skin changes in texture, turgor, and color. The skin develops a brownish discoloration and a brawny induration—that is, skin in the affected area becomes dry and looks rough; subcutaneous tissue atrophies; and it loses its usual resiliency and feels hard to the touch. Body hair is lost in this area. Pruritus is common. Scratching or small injuries can lead to ulcer formation because of the poor circulation.

Venous ulcers begin as small, tender, inflamed areas above the ankle. Any slight trauma to the area causes an open area that develops into an ulcer. Some edema surrounds the ulcer, which can easily become infected, most often with *Staphylococcus* or *Streptococcus*. Healing is very slow. In an effort to decrease venous congestion and improve circulation, varicose veins, if present, may be removed. Ulcers that do not heal may require surgery. If diagnostic testing reveals adequate circulation, skin grafting will result in the healing of large venous ulcers. In cases that do not respond to treatment, the affected leg has to be amputated.

Medical–Surgical Management

Medical

Vacuum-assisted closure (VAC) therapy may be used for chronic open wounds such as venous ulcers. Applying negative pressure to the wound is painless for the client. The negative pressure stretches or distorts the cells, causing the epithelial cells to multiply rapidly and form granulation tissue. As the vacuum pulls fluid from the surrounding tissues, reducing edema that compressed blood vessels, blood flow to the wound is improved.

Elevation and compression are the keys to reducing edema of the leg and improving blood return to the heart. This

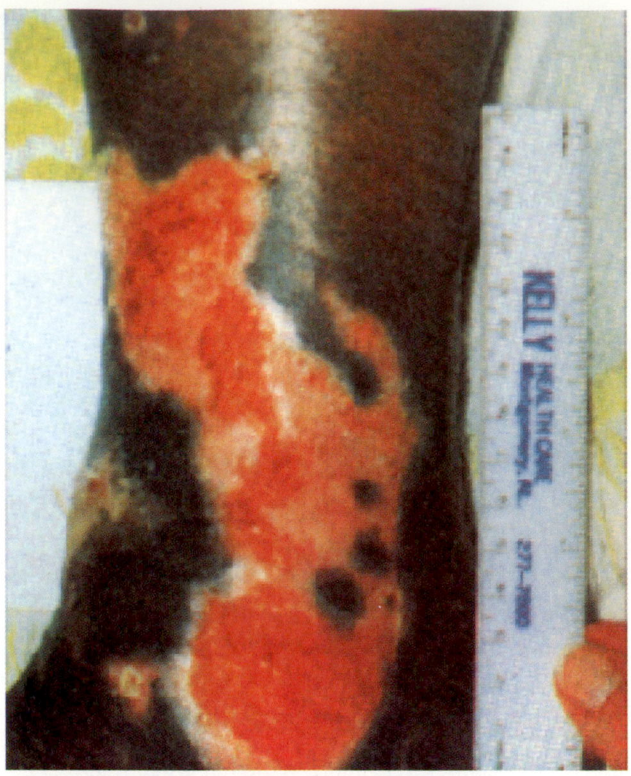

FIGURE 46-17 Venous Stasis Ulcer (*Courtesy of Carrington Laboratories, Inc., Irving, TX.*)

reduces venous hypertension and helps the venous ulcer heal. The legs should be elevated 7 inches above the heart at night and for several hours during the day. Many types of compression therapy products are available, including Unna's boot, elastic wraps, intermittent pneumatic or sequential compression stockings, compression pumps, and sustained graduated compression using an elastic, multilayered bandage system.

Pharmacological

For healing to occur, the ulcer must have adequate circulation and be free of infection and necrotic tissue. Usually, antibiotics are prescribed. Enzyme preparations such as fibrinolysin and desoxyribonuclease (ELASE) or wet-to-dry dressings may be used to debride the ulcer. Normal saline is the solution most often used in wet-to-dry dressings because it is not irritating to healthy tissue.

Diet

A diet high in protein and vitamin C is needed for tissue regeneration. If the client is anemic, lean meats, whole grains, and green, leafy vegetables should be encouraged.

NURSING MANAGEMENT

Maintain peripheral tissue perfusion by encouraging the client to elevate legs when sitting, wear support hose, and not cross legs. Promote comfort by encouraging the client to keep legs elevated, cleansing the venous ulcer as prescribed, and keeping the area covered as ordered. Promote wound healing by reviewing the client's diet and encouraging foods high in iron, protein, and vitamin C.

NURSING PROCESS

ASSESSMENT

Subjective Data

Ask the client to describe any pain and rate its severity on a scale of 0 to 10. Note whether the pain is worse with the leg in a dependent position or when the client is standing. Document measures used to relieve the pain. Note if the skin around the ulcer itches, the length of time the client had the ulcer before seeking care, and any palliative measures tried.

Objective Data

Describe the size and location of the ulcer, as well as the appearance of the ulcer and surrounding skin. Observe for necrotic tissue inside the ulcer. It may be yellow and look like thin strands of fibers. The base of the ulcer may have a dark red, "beefy" appearance. Document the color and appearance of the extremity in both a dependent and an elevated position as well as any drainage, including its odor and characteristics. Edema may be present, and the lower extremity may appear swollen. Hardened and indurated tissue may surround the ulcer. Tissue farther away from the ulcer may "pit" with firm pressure. Assess peripheral pulses.

Nursing diagnoses for a client with a venous ulcer include the following:

NURSING DIAGNOSES	PLANNING/OUTCOMES	NURSING INTERVENTIONS
Ineffective ***Tissue*** *Perfusion (Peripheral)* related to edema and pooling of venous blood	Client will follow prescribed measures to improve peripheral circulation.	Assess for edema. Encourage client to elevate legs while sitting or when in bed and to avoid standing for more than a few minutes at a time. Advise client to wear elastic stockings when walking and that new stockings should be purchased every few months because continual wear and laundering tend to decrease the elasticity of the stockings. Instruct not to sit with legs crossed. Note the client's hemoglobin level because anemic clients will have difficulty meeting tissue demands for oxygen.

Nursing diagnoses for a client with a venous ulcer include the following: (Continued)

NURSING DIAGNOSES	PLANNING/OUTCOMES	NURSING INTERVENTIONS
Chronic ***Pain*** related to exposed sensory nerve endings and edema	Client will report decreased pain after implementing recommended measures.	Assess for pain. Encourage client to elevate legs. Cleanse ulcer with prescribed solutions. Keep ulcer covered with prescribed medications and dressings.
Risk for ***Infection*** related to poorly nourished tissue in and around the ulcer and to nonintact skin	Client will describe and implement measures to minimize the risk of infection.	Assess the ulcer daily for signs of healing. Assess the client's ability to care for the ulcer physically and financially. Review diet with the client and instruct in food choices as needed. Encourage foods high in iron such as fortified cereal, lean meats, whole grains, and leafy green vegetables.

Evaluation: Evaluate each outcome to determine how it has been met by the client.

PRESSURE ULCERS

Pressure ulcers, also known as bedsores or decubitus ulcers, are localized areas of tissue necrosis that tend to develop when soft tissue is compressed between a bony prominence and an external surface such as a mattress or chair seat for a prolonged period. Pressure ulcers are caused by **ischemia**, a local and temporary decrease in blood supply, and commonly occur in areas subject to high pressure from body weight on bony prominences.

PHYSIOLOGY OF PRESSURE ULCERS

A pressure ulcer occurs when pressure on the skin is sufficient to cause collapse of blood vessels in the area. Ischemia and redness can occur at the site within 1 hour; when pressure continues for more than 2 hours, necrosis (tissue death) may occur in the involved area. Bony prominences such as the occipital skull, pinna of ears, sacrum, ischial tuberosities, trochanter area of hips, ankles, and heels are the areas most likely to develop a pressure ulcer.

Other forces acting in conjunction with pressure contribute to pressure ulcer formation. **Shearing** is the force exerted against the skin by movement or repositioning. The skin and subcutaneous tissue tend to adhere to the bed surface and remain stationary while deeper underlying tissues pull away and slide in the direction of movement. This action results in stretching and tearing of blood vessels, reduced blood flow, and necrosis.

Friction is the force of two surfaces moving across one another. When a client moves or is pulled up in bed, rubbing of the skin against the sheets creates friction. Friction can remove the superficial layers of the skin, making it more prone to breakdown.

The reduction of blood flow causes **blanching** (white color) of the skin when pressure is applied. When pressure is relieved, the skin takes on a brighter color (reactive hyperemia) because of vasodilation, the body's normal compensatory response to the absence of blood flow. If this area blanches with fingertip pressure or if the redness disappears within an hour, no tissue damage is anticipated. If, however, the redness persists and no blanching occurs, then tissue damage is present.

Pressure ulcers are staged to classify the degree of tissue damage (Figure 46-18). The National Pressure Ulcer Advisory Panel (NPUAP, 2008) recommends the following staging system:

- *Suspected Deep Tissue Injury*: Discolored intact skin, either maroon or purple, caused by shear or pressure resulting in soft tissue damage to underlying tissue. This localized area may be warmer or cooler, firmer or boggy in comparison to surrounding tissue.
- *Stage I*: Nonblanchable erythema of intact skin; the heralding lesion of skin ulceration. No blanching may be noticeable in darkly pigmented skin. A change in color usually occurs in comparison to surrounding tissue.
- *Stage II*: Partial-thickness skin loss involving epidermis, dermis, or both. The ulcer is superficial and presents clinically as an abrasion, blister, or shallow crater.
- *Stage III*: Full-thickness skin loss involving damage or necrosis of subcutaneous tissue that may extend down to, but not through, underlying fascia. The ulcer presents clinically as a deep crater with or without undermining and tunneling.
- *Stage IV*: Full-thickness skin loss with extensive destruction, tissue necrosis, or damage to muscle, bone, or supporting structures. Undermining and tunneling may also be associated with stage IV pressure ulcers.
- *Unstageable*: A full-thickness tissue loss where slough (yellow, gray or tan) or eschar (black or brown) covers the base of the wound bed. This ulcer is unstageable until debridement of the slough and/or eschar occurs.

The NPUAP (1999) has developed an assessment tool, Pressure Ulcer Scale for Healing (PUSH Tool). It uses three parameters: the surface area of the wound, amount of exudate, and type of tissue present in the wound. The scores for each parameter are added together and plotted to show wound healing or worsening. This PUSH Tool is available on the Internet (www.npuap.org/push3-0.htm).

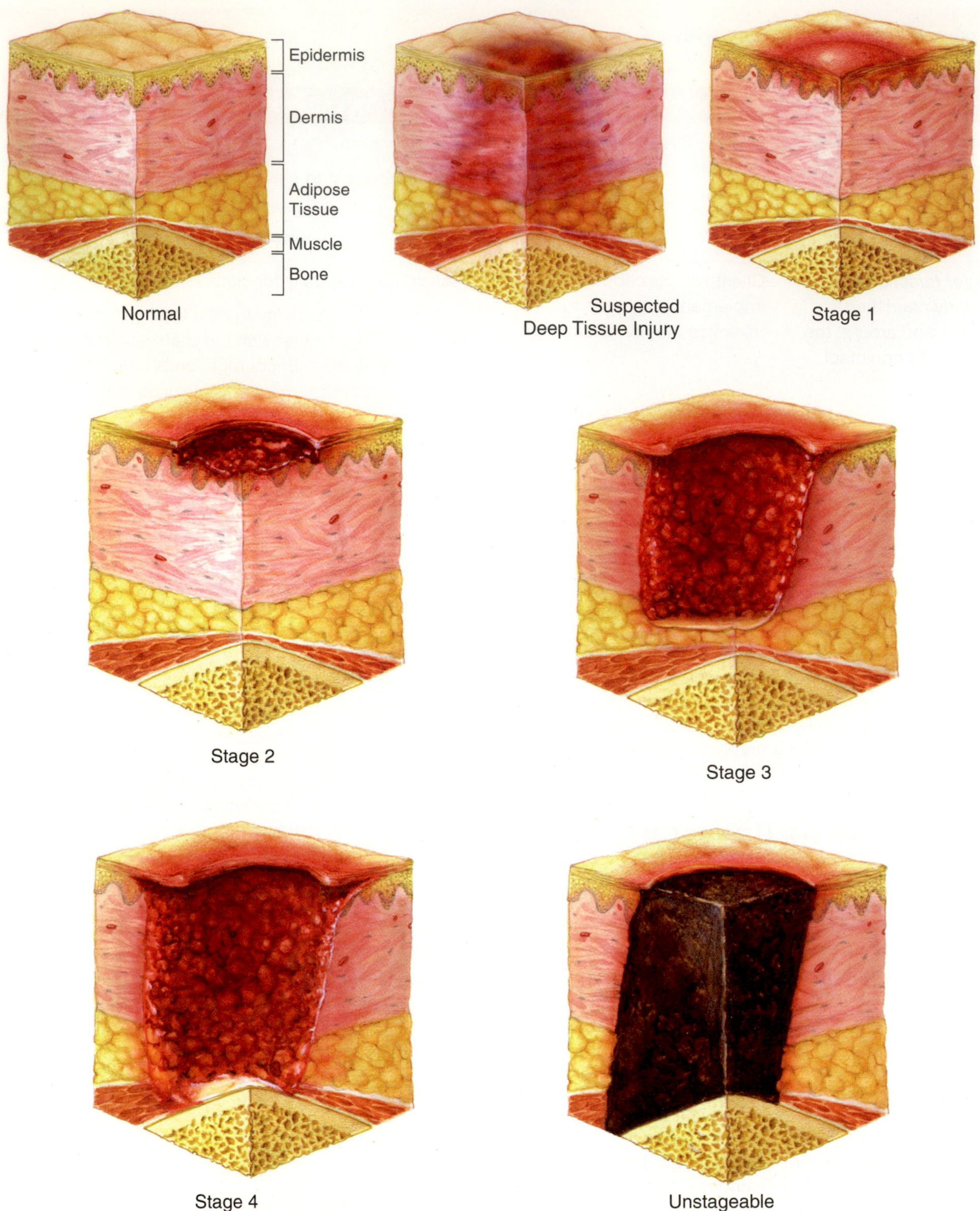

FIGURE 46-18 Pressure Ulcers (*Courtesy of the NPUAP. Reproduction of the National Pressure Ulcer Advisory Panel [NPUAP] materials in this document does not imply endorsement by the NPUAP of any products, organizatons, companies, or any statements made by any organization or company.*)

The Braden Scale for Predicting Pressure Sore Risk (Table 46-4) is a research-based tool that estimates risk level for pressure ulcers and predicts those clients who are most likely to develop pressure ulcers.

Risk Factors for Pressure Ulcers

Pressure ulcers can be prevented if at-risk individuals are identified and the specific factors placing them at risk are reduced or eliminated. More than 2.5 million clients each year have pressure ulcers, and most of these clients are in their 70s and 80s (Institute for Healthcare Improvement, 2008). Both intrinsic and extrinsic factors may influence tissue response to pressure. Intrinsic factors include impaired immobility, incontinence, nutritional status, and altered level of consciousness. Extrinsic factors include pressure, shearing, friction, and moisture. Any condition that decreases tissue perfusion, such

TABLE 46-4 Braden Scale for Predicting Pressure Sore Risk

Patient's Name ______		Evaluator's Name ______		Date of Assessment				
SENSORY PERCEPTION ability to respond meaningfully to pressure-related discomfort	**1. Completely Limited** Unresponsive (does not moan, flinch, or grasp) to painful stimuli, due to diminished level of consciousness or sedation OR has limited ability to feel pain over most of body.	**2. Very Limited** Responds only to painful stimuli. Cannot communicate discomfort except by moaning or restlessness OR has a sensory impairment which limits the ability to feel pain or discomfort over ½ of body.	**3. Slightly Limited** Responds to verbal commands, but cannot always communicate discomfort or the need to be turned OR has some sensory impairment which limits ability to feel pain or discomfort in 1 or 2 extremities.	**4. No Impairment** Responds to verbal commands. Has no sensory deficit which would limit ability to feel or voice pain or discomfort.				
MOISTURE degree to which skin is exposed to moisture	**1. Constantly Moist** Skin is kept moist almost constantly by perspiration, urine, etc. Dampness is detected every time patient is moved or turned.	**2. Very Moist** Skin is often, but not always moist. Linen must be changed at least once a shift.	**3. Occasionally Moist** Skin is occasionally moist, requiring an extra linen change approximately once a day.	**4. Rarely Moist** Skin is usually dry, linen only requires changing at routine intervals.				
ACTIVITY degree of physical activity	**1. Bedfast** Confined to bed.	**2. Chairfast** Ability to walk severely limited or non-existent. Cannot bear own weight and/or must be assisted into chair or wheelchair.	**3. Walks Occasionally** Walks occasionally during day, but for very short distances, with or without assistance. Spends majority of each shift in bed or chair.	**4. Walks Frequently** Walks outside room at least twice a day and inside room at least once every two hours during waking hours.				
MOBILITY ability to change and control body position	**1. Completely Immobile** Does not make even slight changes in body or extremity position without assistance.	**2. Very Limited** Makes occasional slight changes in body or extremity position but unable to make frequent or significant changes independently.	**3. Slightly Limited** Makes frequent though slight changes in body or extremity position independently.	**4. No Limitation** Makes major and frequent changes in position without assistance.				

(*Continues*)

Table 46-4 Braden Scale for Predicting Pressure Sore Risk (Continued)

NUTRITION usual food intake pattern	**1. Very Poor** Never eats a complete meal. Rarely eats more than ⅓ of any food offered. Eats 2 servings or less of protein (meat or dairy products) per day. Takes fluids poorly. Does not take a liquid dietary supplement OR is NPO and/or maintained on clear liquids or IVs for more than 5 days.	**2. Probably Inadequate** Rarely eats a complete meal and generally eats only about ½ of any food offered. Protein intake includes only 3 servings of meat or dairy products per day. Occasionally will take a dietary supplement OR receives less than optimum amount of liquid diet or tube feeding.	**3. Adequate** Eats over ½ of most meals. Eats a total of 4 servings of protein (meat, dairy products) per day. Occasionally will refuse a meal, but will usually take a supplement when offered OR is on a tube feeding or TPN regimen which probably meets most nutritional needs.	**4. Excellent** Eats most of every meal. Never refuses a meal. Usually eats a total of 4 or more servings of meat and dairy products. Occasionally eats between meals. Does not require supplementation.				
FRICTION & SHEAR	**1. Problem** Requires moderate to maximum assistance in moving. Complete lifting without sliding against sheets is impossible. Frequently slides down in bed or chair, requiring frequent repositioning with maximum assistance. Spasticity, contractures or agitation leads to almost constant friction.	**2. Potential Problem** Moves feebly or requires minimum assistance. During a move, skin probably slides to some extent against sheets, chair, restraints, or other devices. Maintains relatively good position in chair or bed most of the time but occasionally slides down.	**3. No Apparent Problem** Moves in bed and in chair independently and has sufficient muscle strength to lift up completely during move. Maintains good position in bed or chair.					
				Total Score				

© Copyright Barbara Braden and Nancy Bergstrom, 1988. All rights reserved.

as edema, anemia, or atherosclerosis, also increases the risk. Other factors are decreased mental status, diminished sensation, and age-related changes.

Individuals should be assessed for pressure ulcer risk on admission to acute care hospitals and at least every 48 hours, long-term care facilities at least daily, and home health care at every RN visit.

Medical–Surgical Management

Medical

Follow sterile technique in the care of all pressure ulcers to prevent secondary infection. Cleanse the wound with normal saline or a noncytotoxic wound cleaner at each dressing change. Such agents as povodine-iodine, iodophor, sodium hypochlorite, hydrogen peroxide, or acetic acid should not be used because they can damage the cells. A 35-mL syringe with a 19-gauge needle or angiocatheter provides enough pressure to cleanse the wound and enhance wound healing without causing trauma to the tissue.

Debridement must be done as needed. Topical enzyme agents may be applied or a mechanical method of wet-to-dry dressings, or hydrotherapy, may be used. Refer to the discussion of VAC therapy in the section on venous ulcers; this therapy can also be used for pressure ulcers.

There are many commercial products available for treatment and dressing of pressure ulcers. Whichever products the physician prescribes, everyone should be taught how to use them and have a commitment to use them properly.

Support Surfaces and Beds A variety of support surfaces and beds are available to support the entire body and evenly distribute pressure. These devices help reduce pressure, but they are no substitute for frequent positioning.

In addition to pressure reduction or relief, many support surfaces reduce shear and friction and control moisture. Pressure-reducing support surfaces include overlays filled with foam, gel, or water.

- *Egg-crate mattress*: The egg-crate mattress is composed of thick foam with a unique, egg-crate design. The purposes of the egg-crate mattress include minimizing pressure and shearing force. The open design of the mattress surface allows air to circulate to dissipate heat and moisture. Egg-crate foam is also used as wheelchair cushions, heel-ankle protectors, wrist restraint cushioning pads, and ulnar protectors.
- *Air-filled mattresses*: The air-filled mattress is placed over the mattress of the hospital bed for weight redistribution. Varieties of air-filled mattresses include some with a pump and alternating bands of inflation and deflation and some that are inflated continuously with air. Mattresses are covered with a sheet for client comfort. These types of mattresses are frequently used in long-term care situations.
- *Clinitron® bed*: A Clinitron® bed (Figure 46-19) is a specialized bed that has a mattress filled with small glass sand particles. Moisture from urine, stool, or drainage flows through the mattress, preventing moisture exposure to the skin. Because warm air is circulating through the mattress, the accumulation of moisture next to the skin is inhibited. The mattress aids in positioning the client because it is constructed to mold against the client's body.
- *Kin Air bed*: A Kin Air bed, another type of specialized bed, has a mattress of air-inflated pillows divided in sections for the head, back, seat, legs, and feet. The pressure can be adjusted in each of the sections for the client's specific needs. Air flows from the mattress to eliminate moisture. The bed frame can be adjusted for various positions such as Fowler's, Trendelenburg, prone, or supine. A trapeze can be connected to the bed frame (Figure 46-20).
- *Roto Kinetic bed*: A Roto Kinetic bed is a specialized bed that rocks slowly from side to side, thus relieving pressure areas and countering the effects of immobility. The client is placed on the mattress, with dividers between the legs and dividers between the trunk and arms. Clients can be maintained in traction while on this bed.

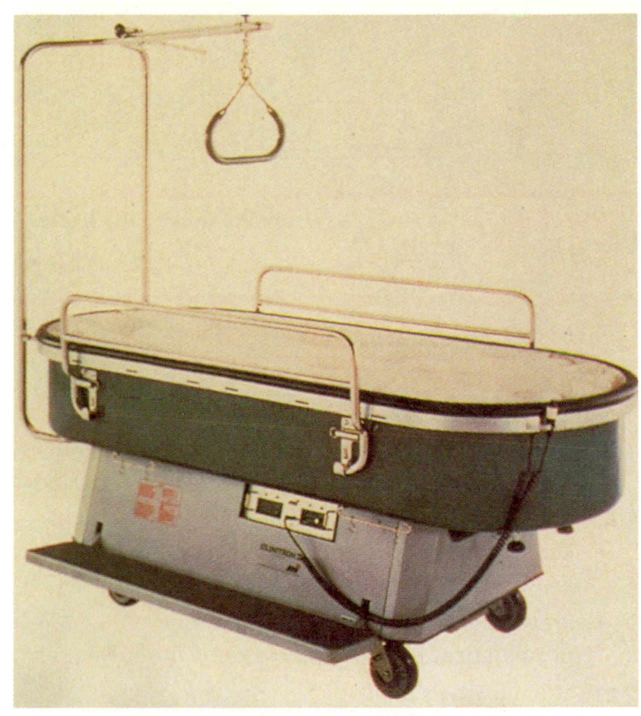

FIGURE 46-19 Clinitron® Air-Fluidized Therapy Unit Model C11 (*Courtesy of Hill-Rom, Batesville, IN.*)

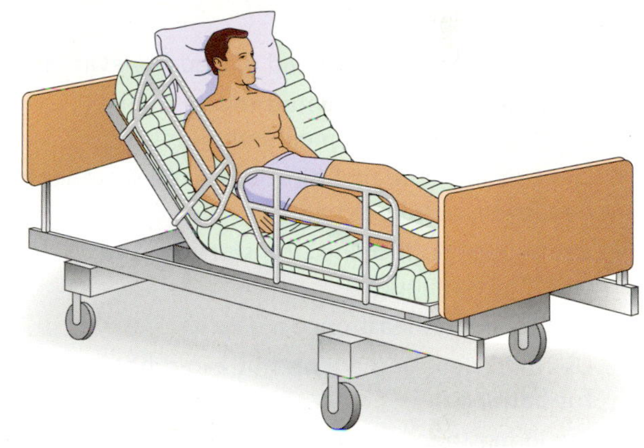

FIGURE 46-20 Kin Air Bed

Regardless of the type of surface or bed on which the client is lying, the 30-degree side-lying position prevents pressure on the sacrum and trochanters. This position is illustrated in Figure 46-21.

Surgical

Occasionally, surgical debridement may be necessary.

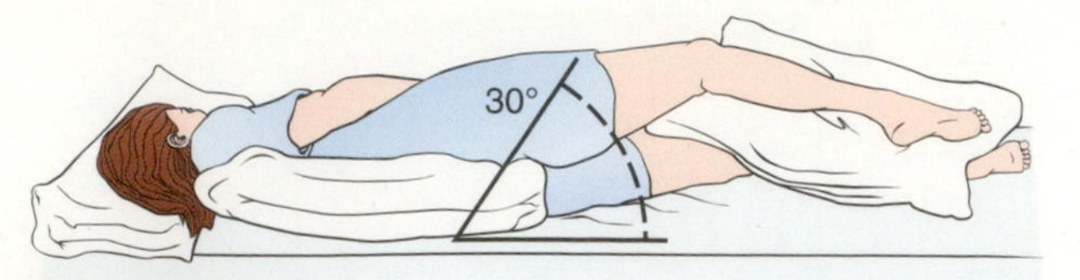

COURTESY OF DELMAR CENGAGE LEARNING

FIGURE 46-21 Avoiding Pressure Points with the 30-Degree Lateral Position

PROFESSIONALTIP

Preventing Pressure Ulcers

- Establish written repositioning/turning schedule for clients, including those on pressure-reducing support surfaces.
- Use 30-degree position when side-lying position is used.
- Prevent direct contact between bony prominences by using pillows and foam wedges.
- Use a lifting sheet.
- Encourage clients in wheelchairs to shift their weight every 15 minutes.
- Raise heels off the bed with pillow lengthwise to support legs.
- Use knee gatch when head of bed is elevated.
- Keep head of bed elevated to less than 30 degrees except at mealtimes.
- Limit sitting time to 1 hour at a time whether in bed, chair, or wheelchair.
- Use proper positioning, transferring, and turning techniques.
- Inspect skin at least once a day.
- Use mild cleansing agent, but avoid hot water for bathing.
- Avoid massage over bony prominences.
- Use moisturizer on skin.
- Use protective barrier on skin if client is incontinent.
- Cleanse skin at time of soiling and at routine intervals.

Pharmacological

Vitamin and mineral supplements may be ordered. Antibiotics may also be ordered.

Diet

Eating a well-balanced diet should be encouraged, including 2 half-cup servings of orange juice or other juice high in vitamin C and 6 ounces of a high-protein drink. Adequate calories, protein, vitamins, and minerals, especially vitamin C and zinc, improve wound healing and prevents tissue breakdown. Offering small, frequent feedings enhances nutritional needs.

Activity

Active ROM exercises should be performed, if possible. If not, passive ROM exercises should be performed with the client several times a day.

NURSING MANAGEMENT

Assess skin several times a day. Keep linens clean, dry, and free from wrinkles. Provide daily bath and skin care when the client is incontinent of bowel or bladder. Encourage adequate fluid intake, a well-balanced diet, and active or passive ROM exercises. Turn client at least every 2 hours. Use the 30-degree lateral position to avoid pressure on the sacrum and trochanters. Position client on unaffected areas and protect skin as ordered. Monitor vital signs, especially temperature.

NURSING PROCESS

ASSESSMENT

Subjective Data

Statements such as, "I'm tired of lying on my side"; "I wish I could move more"; or "my hips (back, heels, and so on) are sore" may be expressed.

Objective Data

Symptoms may include any of the risk factors already mentioned; shiny, erythematous area; small blisters or erosions or ulcerations. Check for reddened areas and blanching of those areas.

Nursing diagnoses for a client at risk for pressure ulcers or who has a pressure ulcer include the following:

NURSING DIAGNOSES	PLANNING/OUTCOMES	NURSING INTERVENTIONS
*Risk for Impaired **S**kin Integrity* related to immobility	The client will maintain skin integrity.	Assess skin 3 times a day for pressure areas. Provide daily bath and skin care as needed for incontinence of urine or stool. Use mild cleansing agents with warm water, use moisturizing lotion, and minimize exposure to cold and low humidity.

Nursing diagnoses for a client at risk for pressure ulcers or who has a pressure ulcer include the following: (Continued)

NURSING DIAGNOSES	PLANNING/OUTCOMES	NURSING INTERVENTIONS
		Avoid massage over bony prominences. Keep bed linen clean, dry, and free from wrinkles. Encourage adequate fluid intake and a well-balanced diet, including 2 half-cup servings of orange juice or other juice high in vitamin C, and 6 ounces of a high-protein drink. Encourage active ROM exercises or provide passive ROM exercises. Turn and reposition client at least every 2 hours. If reddened area does not blanch when you press it, turn the client more often. Use the 30-degree lateral position to avoid pressure on the sacrum and trochanters. Use pressure-reducing surfaces. Do not use donut-shaped cushions; they put pressure around the pressure ulcer.
*Impaired **S**kin Integrity* related to pressure ulcer formation	The client will show healing of pressure ulcer.	Assess skin daily, identifying the stage of pressure ulcer development (size, color, odor, and exudate). Continue all preventive nursing interventions. Position client on unaffected areas. Protect skin surface and affected area as per facility protocol or as ordered. Monitor temperature. Administer antibiotics as ordered.
*Disturbed **B**ody Image* related to trauma or injury (pressure ulcer)	The client will make a positive statement about body image.	Encourage client to discuss meaning of pressure ulcer to the client. Provide information as requested by client.
***A**nxiety* related to threat to or change in health status (pressure ulcer)	The client will discuss concerns about pressure ulcer with caregivers.	Schedule time to be with client, other than care times. Encourage client to discuss fears and concerns. Provide information as requested by client.

Evaluation: Evaluate each outcome to determine how it has been met by the client.

ALOPECIA

Alopecia, which is partial or complete baldness or loss of hair, can be caused by illness, malnutrition, effects of certain drugs such as those used in cancer therapy, hormonal imbalances, heredity, or diseases that affect the scalp.

There are many types of alopecia, ranging from head or beard hair loss to loss of all hair over the entire body. Treatment depends on the cause. Hair transplants may be performed on the head, but this is very expensive. In some clients, minoxidil (Rogaine) can promote hair growth, but hair growth stops when the drug is stopped. This is also very expensive.

CASE STUDY

M.M., age 68, noticed that the skin on the outside of her left lower leg just above the ankle was changing in color and texture. The skin felt rigid and did not move as easily as skin on the upper part of her leg did. Itching was becoming a problem. Inadvertently, she would scratch the area, sometimes causing small excoriations. One day she bumped her leg against the rough edge of the outside steps as she was going into the house. The cut was only an inch long and was not very deep. Over the next few weeks, she noticed that instead of healing, it was getting bigger and was becoming quite painful. The skin around the wound was red and swollen. The yellow drainage coming from the wound had a bad smell. She had never had this kind of problem before. She did have varicose veins in that leg, and while she knew that she was uncomfortable if she was standing for long periods, she did not think the problem was serious. When she went to the doctor, he diagnosed a venous stasis ulcer and cultured the drainage. He ordered the following treatment:

1. Cefaclor (Ceclor) 500 mg p.o. every 8 hours for 2 weeks (culture of the wound identified *Staphylococcus aureus*)
2. Wet-to-dry dressings with normal saline solution. Change every 8 hours.
3. Bed rest with left leg elevated. May have bathroom privileges and be up for meals.

The doctor explained that he would be ordering an Unna's boot after the wound was debrided and the infection controlled so that she could be ambulatory, but that even after the Unna's boot was applied, he would want her to have rest periods during the day with her leg elevated. M.M. thought she could learn to change the dressings, but she expressed doubt that she could stay in bed most of the time. She was used to being up and active and getting her work done each day.

The following questions will guide your development of a nursing care plan for the case study.

1. List the clinical manifestations of a venous stasis ulcer.
2. What is the usual medical treatment?
3. List the subjective and objective assessment data that the nurse should obtain from M.M.
4. Write two to four individualized nursing diagnoses to address these problems.
5. What will be the goals (expected outcomes) of nursing treatment?
6. List appropriate nursing actions for each diagnosis. Include basic nursing care measures. Be specific about client education needs. Address nutrition and pharmacologic implications. Give a rationale for each action.
7. Describe how to evaluate goal achievement for M.M.

SUMMARY

- Maintaining intact skin and mucous membranes to protect internal body structures from harmful substances and from invasion by microorganisms is an important independent nursing responsibility.
- Burns are devastating, traumatic injuries that can often be prevented.
- In general, skin cancers can be prevented by avoiding excessive sun exposure.
- Treatment of benign skin tumors such as nevi, lipomas, keloids, sebaceous cysts, and angiomas depends on the kind of tumor and its location.
- Psoriasis is a chronic skin condition that can be treated but not cured.
- Skin infections caused by bacteria, viruses, fungi, or parasites are effectively treated with medications and supportive nursing care.
- Dermatitis, an inflammation of the skin, can have many causes.
- Eczema is a term that is often used for chronic forms of dermatitis.
- Venous ulcers are more common in older persons, heal slowly, and often recur following a slight injury.
- Alopecia, or baldness, can be caused by illness, drugs, hormonal imbalances, or heredity.

REVIEW QUESTIONS

1. A client is brought into the emergency room with facial burns, singed nasal hairs, and change in voice. The client states he is having pain of a 7 on a 0–10 pain scale in the facial area and he appears anxious. Based on these clinical findings, what is the most important initial nursing intervention?
   1. Attempt to calm client.
   2. Maintain an adequate level of oxygenation.
   3. Protect burns with a sterile dressing.
   4. Administer pain medication.
2. The nurse charted that the client's skin was loose, wrinkled, and thin with mild scaling. The nurse was describing:
   1. integrity.
   2. texture.
   3. turgor and mobility.
   4. vascularity.
3. An effective nursing intervention related to the care of open burn wounds that require daily dressing changes would be:
   1. keep the head of the bed elevated 30 degrees with all four side rails up.
   2. set a fluid intake goal of 2,500 mL/24 hours (1,200 mL during the day; 950 mL during the evening; 350 mL during the night).
   3. wear a cap, gown, mask, and sterile gloves when providing wound care.
   4. weigh daily, preferably before breakfast, and in the same type of clothing each day.

4. The client has lesions on his scalp and on his arms near his elbows. The lesions appear as red patches covered with thick silvery scales. The most likely cause of these lesions is:
   1. herpes zoster (shingles).
   2. pemphigus vulgaris.
   3. psoriasis.
   4. tinea (ringworm).
5. A nursing care plan for a client with an infectious disorder of the skin would include interventions to teach the client:
   1. how to avoid spreading the infection to others.
   2. how to do range-of-motion exercises to maintain joint flexibility.
   3. ways to conserve energy.
   4. which foods are most likely to cause allergic reactions.
6. The nursing care plan of a client at risk for impaired skin integrity is likely to include:
   1. turning and repositioning client every 4 hours.
   2. massaging bony prominences.
   3. using a donut-shaped cushion around the pressure ulcer.
   4. using the 30-degree lateral positioning when turning client.
7. The nurse is assessing a client's dressing after an abdominal surgery. The nurse notices clear with some blood-tinged drainage on the dressing. The nurse would document the drainage to be:
   1. purulent exudates.
   2. serosanguineous exudates.
   3. serous exudates.
   4. sanguineous exudates.
8. When admitting a new client, the nurse performs a physical assessment of the client's skin. What parameters will the nurse assess? (Select all that apply.)
   1. Integrity and color.
   2. Temperature and moisture.
   3. Texture and vascularity.
   4. Culture and sensitivity.
   5. Turgor and mobility.
   6. Sensation.
9. A 75-year-old man comes to the outpatient clinic. He has long-standing severe chronic obstructive pulmonary disease. He is short of breath at rest with oxygen at 3 yes L? per minute via nasal cannula. When inspecting his nail beds, you would expect his nail angle to be:
   1. greater than 160 degrees.
   2. less than 140 degrees.
   3. less than 90 degrees.
   4. greater than 90 degrees.
10. The nurse is teaching a client's wife about preventing pressure ulcers. Which statement best demonstrates that the wife correctly understands the risk factors for pressure ulcers?
    1. "I need to assess the skin once a week for redness or open areas."
    2. "If my husband is wearing Depends®, they will absorb his urine incontinence, so I will need to change his Depends only when saturated."
    3. "He has his favorite foods, so as long as he is eating, I will not need to worry."
    4. "I will try to encourage him to change positions frequently during the day."

REFERENCES/SUGGESTED READINGS

American Academy of Dermatology (AAD). (2007). Psoriasis & psoriatic arthritis. Retrieved May 20, 2009 from http://www.aad.org/public/publications/pamphlets/common_psoriasis.html

American Cancer Society (ACS). (2008a). What are the key statistics about squamous and basal cell skin cancer? Retrieved May 22, 2009 from www.cancer.org/docroot/CRI/content/CRI_2_4_1X_What_are_the_key_statistics_for_skin_cancer_51.asp?sitearea=cri

American Cancer Society (ACS). (2008b). What are the risk factors of melanoma? Retrieved May 22, 2009 from www.cancer.org/docroot/CRI/content/CRI_2_4_2X_What_are_the_risk_factors_for_melanoma_50.asp?rnav=cri

American Cancer Society (ACS). (2008c). What are the key statistics about melanomas? Retrieved May 20, 2009 from www.cancer.org/docroot/CRI/content/CRI_2_4_1X_What_are_the_key_statistics_for_melanoma_50.asp?sitearea=

American Cancer Society (ACS). (2008d). Treating squamous cell carcinoma. Retrieved May 25, 2009 from www.cancer.org/docroot/CRI_2_4_4X_Treatment_of_Squamous_Cell_Carcinoma_51.asp?sitearea=

American Cancer Society (ACS). (2008e). Skin (pressure) sores. Retrieved May 20, 2009 from http://www.cancer.org/docroot/MBC?content/MBC_2_3X_Skin_Pressure_Sores.asp

American Cancer Society (ACS). (2009a). How is melanoma skin cancer treated? Retrieved May 25, 2009 from www.cancer.org/docroot/CRI/content/CRI_2_2_4X_How_Is_Melanoma_Skin_Cancer_Treated_50.asp?rnav=cri

American Cancer Society (ACS). (2009b). *The ABCD rule for early detection of melanoma*. Retrieved May 25, 2009 from www.cancer.org/docroot/SPC/content/SPC_1_ABCD_Mole_Check_Tips.asp

Bolton, L. (2008). Compression in venous ulcer management. *Journal of Wound, Ostomy & Continence Nursing, 35*(1), 40–49.

Brunicardi, F., Anderson, D., Billiar, T., & Dunn, D. (2005). *Schwartz's principles of surgery* (8th ed.). New York: McGraw-Hill.

Bulechek, G., Butcher, H., McCloskey, J., & Dochterman, J., eds. (2008). *Nursing Interventions Classification* (*NIC*) (5th ed.). St. Louis, MO: Mosby/Elsevier.

Daniels, R. (2010). *Delmar's guide to laboratory and diagnostic tests, (2nd ed.).* Clifton Park, NY: Delmar Cengage Learning.

Davidson, M. (2002). Sharpen your wound assessment skills. *Nursing2002, 32*(10), 32hn1–32hn4.

Drisdelle, R. (2003). Maggot debridement therapy: A living cure. *Nursing2003, 33*(6), 17.

Estes, M. (2010). *Health assessment & physical examination* (4th ed). Clifton Park, NY: Delmar Cengage Learning.

Goldsmith, J. (2003). Nit-Picking. *AJN, 103*(9), 22–23.

Grunwald, T., & Garner, W. (2008). Acute burns. *Plastic and Reconstructive Surgery: Journal of the American Society of Plastic Surgeons, 121*(5), 311e–319e.

Harvard Health Letter. (2008). Should you get the shingles vaccine? *33*(12), 6–7.

Hayes, J. (2003). Are you assessing for melanoma? *RN, 66*(2), 36–40.

Hess, C. (2003a). Managing a patient with a venous ulcer. *Nursing2003, 33*(4), 73–74.

Hess, C. (2003b). Treating a fungal rash. *Nursing2003, 33*(9), 20–22.

Hill, M. (1998). Nursing management of adults with skin disorders. In P. G. Beare & J. L. Myers (Eds.), *Principles and practice of adult health nursing* (3rd ed., pp. 2089–2115). St. Louis, MO: Mosby.

Hilton, G. (2001). Thermal burns. *AJN, 101*(11), 32–34.

Hunter, S., Langemo, D., Thompson, P., Hanson, D., & Anderson, J. (2009). Maggot therapy for wound management. *Advances in Skin & Wound Care, 22*(1), 25–27.

Institute for Healthcare Improvement. (2008). The 5 million lives campaign. getting started kit: prevent pressure ulcers how-to-guide. Retrieved May 31, 2009 from www.ihi.org/IHI/Programs/Campaign

Kloth, L. (2002). How to use electrical stimulation for wound healing. *Nursing2002, 32*(12), 17.

Leukemia-Lymphoma Society. (2006). Skin lymphoma. Retrieved May 20, 2009 from www.leukemia-lymphoma.org/all_mat_toc .adp?item_id=9846

Magnan, M. & Maklebust. J. (2009). The nursing process and pressure ulcer prevention: Making the connection. *Advances in Skin & Wound Care, 22*(2), 83–92.

Martin, S. (2001). There's what in the wound? *RN, 64*(2), 44–47.

Martini, F., & Bartholomew. E. (2008). *Essentials of anatomy and physiology* (4th ed.). Englewood Cliffs, NJ: Prentice-Hall.

Mayo Clinic. (2009). Psoriasis. Retrieved May 27, 2009 from www.mayoclinic.com/health/psoriasis/DS00193? DSECTION=treatments-and-drugs

McCain, D., & Sutherland, S. (1998). Skin grafts for patients with burns. *AJN, 98*(7), 34–39.

Mendez-Eastman, S. (1998). When wounds won't heal. *RN, 61*(1), 20–23.

Mendez-Eastman, S. (2002). New treatment for an old problem: Negative-pressure wound therapy. *Nursing2002, 32*(5), 58–63.

Milner, S., Mottar, R., & Smith, C. (2001). The burn wheel. *AJN, 101*(11), 35–37.

Moorhead, S., Johnson, M., Maas, M., & Swanson, E. (2007). *Nursing Outcomes Classification (NOC)* (4th ed.). St. Louis, MO: Mosby.

Moses, M. (2003). A simple matter of grooming. *AJN, 103*(9), 11.

National Institutes of Health (NIH). (2008). Burns. Retrieved May 25, 2009 from http://www.nlm.nih.gov/medlineplus/ency/imagepages/1078.htm

National Institutes of Health (NIH). (2009). Psoriasis. Retrieved May 20, 2009 from www.nlm.nih.gov/medlineplus/psoriasis.html

National Pressure Ulcer Advisary Panal (NPUAP). (1998). PUSH Tool Version 3.0. Retrieved May 20 2009, from http://www.npuap.org/push3-0.htm

National Psoriasis Foundation. (2009). About psoriasis. Retrieved May 27, 2009 from http://www.psoriasis.org/netcommunity/learn_statistics

North American Nursing Diagnosis Association International. (2010). *NANDA-I nursing diagnoses: Definitions and classification 2009–2011.* Ames, IA: Wiley-Blackwell.

Ramadan, A., & Zyada, R. (2008). Effect of low-intensity direct current on the healing of chronic wounds: A literature review. *Journal of Wound Care, 17*(7), 292–296.

Regojo, P. (2003). Burn care basics. *Nursing2003, 33*(3), 50–53.

Roy, D., & Stotts, N. (2002). Targeting cellulitis. *Nursing2002, 32*(12), 46–47.

Sarvis, C. (2007). Calling on NERDS for critically colonized wounds. *Nursing2007, 37*(5), 26–27.

Schweon, S., & Novatnack, E. (2002). What's causing that itch? *RN, 65*(8), 43–46.

Smeltzer, S., Bare, B., Hinkle, J., & Cheever, K. (2008). *Brunner & Suddarth's textbook of medicalsurgical nursing* (11th ed.). Philadelphia, PA: Lippincott Williams & Wilkins.

Spratto, G., & Woods, A. (2008). *2009 Edition Delmar nurse's drug handbook.* Clifton Park, NJ: Delmar Cengage Learning.

Tate, P. (2008). *Seelay's principles of anatomy & physiology.* New York: McGraw-Hill.

Thompson, J. (2003). Maximizing your pressure ulcer care. *Travel Nursing Today, a supplement to RN,* (April 2003), 16–24.

Wiebelhaus, P., & Hansen, S. (2001a). Another choice for burn victims. *RN, 64*(9), 34–37.

Wiebelhaus, P., & Hansen, S. (2001b). What you should know about burn emergencies. *Nursing2001, 31*(1), 36–41.

Zulkowski, K., & Ratliff, C. (2006). Perineal dermatitis or pressure ulcer: How can you tell? *Nursing2006, 36*(12), 22–23.

RESOURCES

American Burn Association, http://www.ameriburn.org

American Hair Loss Council, http://www.ahlc.org

Dermatology Foundation, http://www.dermfnd.org

National Burn Victim Foundation, http://www.nbvf.org

National Decubitus Foundation, http://www.decubitus.org

National Pressure Ulcer Advisory Panel (NPUAP), http://www.npuap.org

National Psoriasis Foundation, http://www.psoriasis.org

Skin Cancer Foundation, http://www.skincancer.org

Wound Healing Society, http://www.woundheal.org

Wound, Ostomy and Continence Nurses Society, http://www.wocn.org

CHAPTER 47
Immune System

MAKING THE CONNECTION

Refer to the following chapters to increase your understanding of immune system disorders:

Basic Nursing

- ***Legal and Ethical Responsibilities***
- ***Communication***
- ***Wellness Concepts***
- ***Infection Control/Asepsis***
- ***Standard Precautions and Isolation***
- ***Fluid, Electrolyte, and Acid-Base Balance***
- ***Assessment***
- ***Pain Management***
- ***Diagnostic Tests***

Adult Health Nursing

- ***Oncology***
- ***Respiratory System***
- ***Cardiovascular System***
- ***Hematologic and Lymphatic Systems***
- ***Gastrointestinal System***
- ***Musculoskeletal System***
- ***Neurologic System***
- ***Sexually Transmitted Infections***
- ***Integumentary System***
- ***Substance Abuse***

Basic Procedures

- ***Hand Hygiene***
- ***Use of Protective Equipment***
- ***Initiating Strict Isolation Precautions***

LEARNING OBJECTIVES

Upon completion of this chapter, you should be able to:

- Define key terms.
- Identify three allergic reactions with a systemic response.
- Describe symptoms of anaphylaxis and appropriate first aid.
- Recall common diagnostic tests used to evaluate immunological functioning.
- Discuss the medical–surgical management of clients with immunological disorders.
- Relate signs and symptoms of complications clients with immunological disorders could experience.
- Explain the modes of transmission of HIV.
- Identify methods of risk reduction of HIV for health care workers.
- Use the nursing process to plan the care of clients with immune system disorders.

KEY TERMS

acquired immunodeficiency syndrome (AIDS)
allergen
allogeneic
anaphylaxis
angioedema
antibody
antigen
autoimmune disorder
autologous
cellular immunity
diplopia
enzyme-linked immunosorbent assay (ELISA)
exacerbation
histamine
human immunodeficiency virus (HIV)
human leukocyte antigen
humoral immunity
hypersensitivity
immune response
immunity
immunotherapy
opportunistic infection
ptosis
remission
seroconversion
urticaria
viral load test
Western blot test

INTRODUCTION

Immunity is the body's ability to protect itself from foreign agents or organisms. This occurs through the complex interaction of the tissues within the immune system. Constant surveillance of cells within the body occurs to differentiate self from nonself. Those identified as nonself are then neutralized or destroyed. Dead or damaged cells are eliminated and homeostasis is maintained. When alterations in the system develop, immunological conditions develop. They may be hypersensitivity responses, such as allergies; immunological deficiencies, such as those associated with corticosteroid medications; or **autoimmune disorders**, where the body identifies its own cells as foreign and activates mechanisms to destroy them. Rheumatoid arthritis, systemic lupus erythematosus, and myasthenia gravis are examples of autoimmune disorders. Immunosuppressive disorders suppress the body's natural immune response to an antigen. Kaposi's sarcoma and non-Hodgkin's lymphoma are examples of immunosuppressive disorders.

ANATOMY AND PHYSIOLOGY REVIEW

The human body has a variety of natural physical and chemical mechanisms that enhance immunological functioning. The skin, eyelashes, cilia in the nose and respiratory system, gastric acidity, intestinal mucosa, and pH of vaginal mucosa all act to protect against invading organisms. In addition, all body tissues are linked together via lymphatic ducts and blood vessels to the organs and cells of the immune system.

ORGANS OF THE IMMUNE SYSTEM

The organs of the immune system are classified as primary or peripheral lymphoid organs. Primary lymphoid organs are bone marrow and the thymus gland. Within bone marrow, stem cells, the parent cells for all blood cells, are produced. Peripheral lymphoid organs are lymph nodes, spleen, tonsils, appendix, Peyer's patches of the small intestines, and the liver. Lymph nodes, located throughout the body, connected by an elaborate ductal system, filter lymphatic fluid, removing destroyed matter. Enlargement of lymphoid organs indicates an infectious or malignant process is occurring. The spleen serves as a reservoir for macrophages, lymphocytes, and plasma cells. The tonsils, appendix, and Peyer's patches also contain plasma cells and lymphocytes. The Kupffer cells of the liver house monocytes that ingest and destroy foreign organisms in hepatic circulation.

CELLS OF THE IMMUNE SYSTEM

Leukocytes, white blood cells (WBCs), are vital components of the immune system. They are formed mostly in the bone marrow and partially in the lymph tissue. After formation, they are transported to different parts of the body, where they fight infectious organisms. There are five types of WBCs normally found in the blood: neutrophils, eosinophils, basophils, monocytes, and lymphocytes. Adults have between 4,000 and 11,000 WBCs/mm^3 of blood. Each type is a percentage of the total number of WBCs (Table 47-1).

Those cells with granules in the cytoplasm are called *granulocytes*, while those lacking them are called *agranulocytes* (Figure 47-1). Eosinophils, neutrophils, and basophils are granular leukocytes. Monocytes and lymphocytes are agranular leukocytes. Each has its own unique function. Eosinophils come into play during allergic reactions or parasitic invasions. Neutrophils are useful in ingesting bacteria (Figure 47-2). Basophils secrete **histamine**, a substance released during allergic reactions, and heparin. Monocytes travel to the sites of invading organisms and transform into macrophages, capable of ingesting large quantities of microorganisms and damaged cells, a process known as *phagocytosis*. They also secrete Interleuken-1, which stimulates the activation of specific lymphocytes. Granulocytes, also called *polymorphonuclear leukocytes*, make up the greatest number of WBCs.

TABLE 47-1 Percentages of Different WBC Types

WBC Type	Percentage
Neutrophils	55%–70%
Eosinophils	1%–4%
Basophils	0%–2%
Monocytes	2%–8%
Lymphocytes	20%–40%

COURTESY OF DELMAR CENGAGE LEARNING

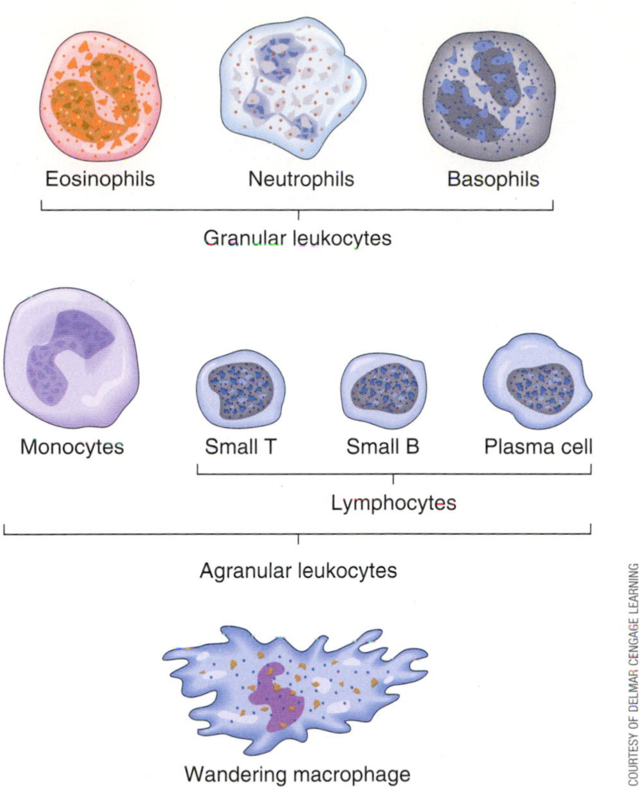

FIGURE 47-1 Cells of the Immune System

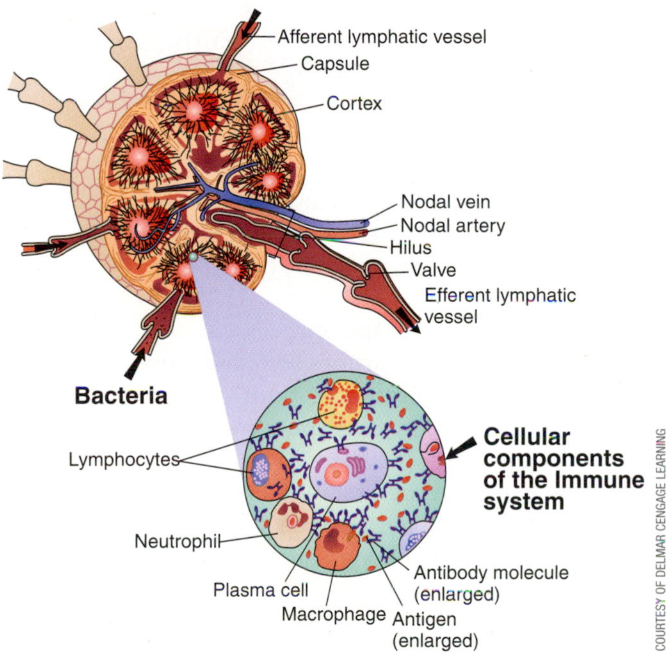

FIGURE 47-2 Bacteria and Common Cellular Components of the Immune System

TABLE 47-2 Humoral and Cellular Responses

HUMORAL RESPONSE (B-CELL RESPONSE)	CELLULAR RESPONSE (T-CELL RESPONSE)
• B-lymphocytes stimulate plasma cells, which manufacture antibodies in response to an antigen and release them into the bloodstream. • Predominant role in response to: Bacteria and some viral infections Allergic reactions Autoimmune diseases	• Plasma cells are transformed into special T-lymphocyte cells, which detect, attack, and destroy invading antigens. • Predominant role in response to: Viral and some bacterial infections Delayed hypersensitivity (TB testing) Transplant rejection Graft-versus-host disease Fungal and parasitic infections Detection and destruction of tumor cells

COURTESY OF DELMAR CENGAGE LEARNING

B-lymphocytes (or B-cells) and T-lymphocytes (or T-cells) play a vital role in the immune response. B-cells are responsible for **humoral immunity** (antibody-mediated defenses), or immunity dominated by antibodies (Table 47-2). They stimulate plasma cells to secrete **antibodies** (proteins that react with antigens to neutralize or destroy them) in response to **antigens** (any substance identified by the body as nonself). Antibodies are also called *immunoglobulins.* IgA, IgD, IgE, IgG, and IgM are common antibodies found in plasma. When an antibody-antigen reaction occurs, the complement system, a complex sequential immunological process, is activated. This system is composed of plasma proteins made in the liver. They alter cell membranes in the antibody-antigen reaction, facilitating the cellular breakdown of the invading antigen, and attract macrophages and granulocytes to the antibody-antigen reaction site. When a B-cell identifies an antigen, it places the characteristics of that antigen in a memory bank. B-cells also produce "memory cells" capable of identifying the antigen, if and when it is introduced to the body again.

T-cells are responsible for cellular immunity (cell-mediated defenses), a type of acquired immunity involving T-cell lymphocytes (Table 47-2). With T-cell–mediated immunity, large numbers of activated lymphocytes are formed specifically to destroy the foreign agent. T cells include helper cells (CD4), suppressor cells (CD8), and killer (cytotoxic) cells. CD4 and CD8 are molecules on the T-helper and T-suppressor cells and are important in understanding how HIV attacks the immune system.

Human immunodeficiency virus (HIV) infection affects the immune system and the brain. In the immune system, the main characteristic of HIV infection is progressive depletion of the CD4-T helper cells. The normal ratio of T-helper cells to T-suppressor cells (CD4:CD8 ratio) is 2:1. As immunodeficiency worsens, it is not uncommon for the CD4:CD8 ratio to fall to as low as 0:1. The altered T-helper cells cause malfunction of the B-cells and macrophages, which leads to collapse of the immune system. HIV also affects the CD4

TABLE 47-3 Comparison of Natural and Acquired Immunity

	ACQUIRED IMMUNITY	
NATURAL IMMUNITY	ACTIVE ACQUIRED IMMUNITY	PASSIVE ACQUIRED IMMUNITY
• Innate immunity • Present at birth • Includes physical and chemical barriers to invading antigens	• Long-term immunity • Antibodies develop as a result of exposure to a disease or vaccine • Antibodies neutralize future invasions of the same antigen	• Temporary immunity • Antibodies obtained from an animal or another human who has been exposed to an antigen • Examples are gamma-globulin or antiserum

COURTESY OF DELMAR CENGAGE LEARNING

molecule present on microglial cells in the brain, causing memory loss and other brain dysfunctions.

HIV is a retrovirus. Retroviruses use RNA to make DNA copies that then become part of the genetic material of the human cell. These viruses are called retroviruses because this is a reversal of the usual DNA-to-RNA transcription of genetic information.

TYPES OF IMMUNITY

There are two types of immunity: natural (innate) and acquired (adaptive) (Table 47-3). One is born with natural immunity; it is species specific. For example, humans have an innate resistance to distemper, whereas dogs never develop measles or syphilis. Acquired immunity develops after birth and may be active or passive. Active acquired immunity is the result of exposure to the disease or its vaccine. As a result, the body develops antibodies and memory cells for the causative microorganism. A repeated exposure results in rapid activation of these components of the immune system and annihilation of the invading agent. Passive acquired immunity utilizes antibodies produced by another human being or an animal. Injection of these immunoglobulins temporarily prevents development of the disease after exposure. Transmission of antibodies through fetal circulation is an example of passive acquired immunity.

FACTORS INFLUENCING IMMUNITY

Although the exact physiological mechanisms involved are unknown, it has been well documented that several factors influence the **immune response** (body's reaction to substances identified as nonself, neutralization of antigen). These include age, sex, nutritional status, stress, and treatment modalities. As one ages, the immune system becomes less effective. Sex hormones affect immunity; estrogen enhances immunological functioning, while androgen suppresses it. Therefore, women are especially prone to autoimmune diseases, whereas men are more prone to immunosuppressive disorders. Poor nutritional status and emotional stress lead to increased susceptibility to infections. Radiation therapy and a variety of medications, such as corticosteroids and chemotherapeutic agents, suppress the immune system.

ASSESSMENT

Physical assessment of the immune system involves the entire body. The skin and mucous membranes are evaluated for urticaria, inflammation, or bleeding. Superficial head, neck, supraclavicular, axilla, and inguinal lymph nodes are inspected and palpated for redness, tenderness, or swelling. Elevated temperature may indicate infection. Joints must be evaluated for possible tenderness, swelling, or limited range of motion. Changes in the rate and rhythm of respirations, presence of a cough, or abnormal lung sounds may indicate immunological conditions. Cardiovascular status, including rate, rhythm, arrhythmias, and peripheral vascular circulation, must be assessed. Enlarged liver or spleen and gastrointestinal conditions, such as nausea, vomiting, or diarrhea, may have an immunological basis. Alterations in vision, hearing, urinary habits, and neurological function may occur.

BOX 47.1: QUESTIONS TO ASK AND OBSERVATIONS TO MAKE WHEN COLLECTING DATA

Subjective Data

Have you had a history of infections?
Have you experienced a loss of appetite?
How would you describe your diet?
Do you have food, seasonal, or medication allergies?
If so, how are they treated?
Describe allergic reactions you have experienced?
Are your immunizations current?
When was the last time you were tested for tuberculosis?
Have you been tired more than usual?
How would you describe the stress in your life?
Are you currently taking immunosuppressive medication?

Objective Data

Nasal stuffiness
Sneezing
Watery discharge from the nose
Skin rash or hives
Puffy swollen eyelids
Difficulty breathing
Fever
Increased pulse and respirations
Enlargement and tenderness of lymph nodes
Weight loss

TABLE 47-4 Common Diagnostic Tests for Immune System Disorders

- Antinuclear antibodies (ANA)
- Complement assay (Total complement, C3 and C4)
- C-reactive protein test (CRP)
- CD4 T-cells
- Enzyme-linked immunosorbent assay (ELISA)
- Erythrocyte sedimentation rate (ESR or Sed Rate Test)
- Human leukocyte antigen DW4 (HLA-DW4)
- Lupus erythematosus test (LE Prep)
- Polymerase chain reaction (PCR)
- Red blood cell count (RBC count)
- Rheumatoid factor (RF)
- Total white blood cell count
    - Differential count
    - Neutrophils
        - —Segs (mature neutrophils)
        - —Bands (immature neutrophils)
    - Eosinophils
    - Basophils
    - Lymphocytes
    - Monocytes
- Western blot

COURTESY OF DELMAR CENGAGE LEARNING

COMMON DIAGNOSTIC TESTS

Commonly used diagnostic tests for clients with symptoms of immune system disorders are listed in Table 47-4.

HYPERSENSITIVE IMMUNE RESPONSE

Hypersensitive immune responses include allergies, anaphylaxis, transfusion reactions, transplant rejection, and latex allergy.

ALLERGIES

Allergic disorders are the result of **hypersensitivity** (excessive reaction to a stimulus) of the immune system to **allergens** (a type of antigen commonly found in the environment). Allergens may be inhaled, injected, ingested, or contacted. There are four types of hypersensitivity reactions based on how tissue is injured.

Type I reactions occur immediately upon exposure to a specific antigen. Upon first exposure to an allergen, IgE antibodies are produced. They adhere to mast cells. When a subsequent exposure occurs, these cells attach to the antigen and activate the release of chemical mediators, such as histamine, bradykinin, and serotonin. These chemicals cause vasodilation, enhanced capillary permeability, and bronchoconstriction (Figure 47-3).

Allergic response

First exposure

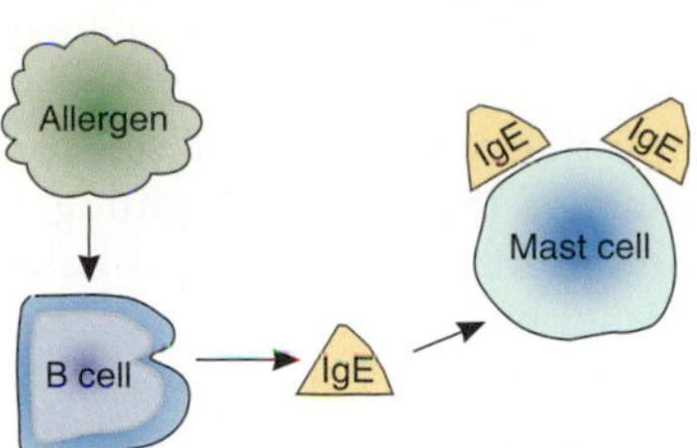

Second or subsequent exposure

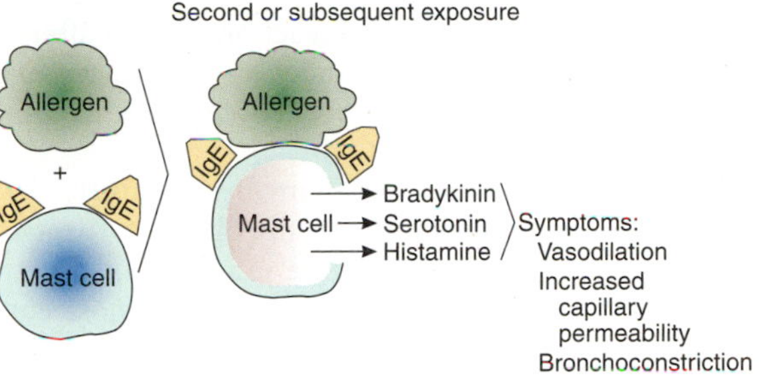

COURTESY OF DELMAR CENGAGE LEARNING

FIGURE 47-3 Allergic Response

The most common Type I reactions include allergic rhinitis, urticaria, and angioedema. Anaphylaxis is the most severe and is covered separately.

Allergic rhinitis, also known as *hay fever* or *pollinosis*, is a common allergy in our society caused by airborne allergens such as pollen, mold, animal dander, dust, and ragweed. Symptoms include nasal congestion; thin, clear, watery discharge; sneezing; itching; swelling; and redness of the eyes. Headaches and ear infections may also develop. Approximately 12.2 million office visits to health care providers each year are for allergic rhinitis (Centers for Disease Control and Prevention, 2008e).

Urticaria (hives) are raised pruritic, red, nontender wheals on the skin. They are usually on the trunk and on the areas of the extremities closest to the trunk.

Angioedema, edema of subcutaneous layers and mucous membranes, is painless and only slightly pruritic.

Drug and food allergies are also Type I hypersensitivity. Any drug potentially may cause a drug reaction, but common ones include penicillin, cephalosporins, codeine, pain medications, vaccines, and local anesthetics. Reactions vary from mild to severe. Usually, symptoms do not occur until the client has taken several doses of the medication, although they can occur at first exposure. The most common reaction is the sudden development of a bright red, itchy rash, often appearing initially on the trunk or arms. Occasionally, a client may develop an anaphylactic reaction.

Although individuals may be allergic to any edible substance, certain foods, such as milk, shellfish, eggs, wheat, and nuts, are common allergens. According to the CDC (2008a), 4 of every 100 children in the United States have a food allergy. Diarrhea is a result of immunological reaction in the intestinal mucosa. Headache, nausea, vomiting, rash, itching, and wheezing may also develop.

Type II reactions are the destruction of cells or substances with antigens attached that either immunoglobulin G (IgG) or immunoglobulin M (IgM) senses as being foreign. Antibodies cause either lysis of the cells or accelerated phagocytosis. Hemolytic transfusion reactions are this type of reaction. Transfusion reactions are discussed in detail later.

Type III reaction involves IgG immune antigen-antibody complexes. It is a local reaction evident after several hours that may change from red skin to hemorrhage and tissue necrosis. Occasionally, this is noted after penicillin or sulfonamide use.

Type IV is a delayed reaction involving sensitized T-lymphocytes coming in contact with the allergen. Contact dermatitis and transplant rejection are examples of this type of reaction. Poison ivy and poison oak are the most common causes of contact dermatitis. Latex rubber is a more recently discovered cause of contact dermatitis or occasionally a Type I (anaphylactic) reaction. Transplant rejection and latex allergy are covered separately.

MEDICAL–SURGICAL MANAGEMENT

Medical

Medical management of clients experiencing an allergic response (reaction to allergen) includes drug therapy to treat symptoms and identification of precipitating agents. Allergen **immunotherapy** (treatment to suppress or enhance immunological functioning) involves repeated injections of the diluted allergen. Decreased levels of histamine are released upon subsequent exposure to the allergen. Venom can be used to treat allergies to bees, wasps, yellowjackets, and hornets.

Pharmacological

Several medications are employed to treat the symptoms of an allergic response. Antihistamines counteract the effects of histamine. They may be taken orally, topically, or intravenously, depending on the type of allergic response and urgency for treatment. Nasal decongestants help relieve respiratory symptoms. Topical corticosteroids effectively relieve inflammation associated with contact dermatitis and dermatitis medicamentosa. Oral or injectable forms of corticosteroids may be used either alone or in combination with antihistamines and nasal decongestants.

Skin testing by a physician can determine the specific causative allergen.

Diet

Individuals who are allergic to certain foods should be taught to check food labels carefully, be aware of how food is prepared, and not eat any product that could lead to a reaction. This includes restaurant foods and foods prepared in another person's home.

LIFE SPAN CONSIDERATIONS

Allergy to Foods

- Food allergies have increased among children in the United States during the past 10 years by 18%.
- Boys and girls have similar rates of food allergies.
- Children younger than the age of 5 have a greater rate of reported food allergies than children between the ages of 5 to 17 years.
- Children with food allergies are two to four times more likely to have other related conditions such as asthma, compares with children without food allergies.

(CDC, 2008a)

Activity

Avoidance of the causative allergen prevents allergic reactions. Activities should be centered around this, if at all possible. For instance, individuals who are allergic to pollen may need to stay in air-conditioned environments on those days when the pollen count is extremely high.

NURSING MANAGEMENT

Teach the client that with allergic rhinitis to stay indoors when airborne allergens are present in great numbers. Ask about pets in the house. Encourage the client to read labels if there are food allergies and to inform all health care personnel if there are drug allergies. Assist the client to plan lifestyle changes to avoid exposure to allergens. Emphasize the importance of following the medication regimen prescribed. Figure 47-4 outlines the differences between a cold and an airborne allergy.

NURSING PROCESS

ASSESSMENT

Subjective Data

Take detailed, comprehensive client history, including information about previous allergic reactions, foods eaten or medications taken recently, and contact with environmental pollutants or anything not normally encountered. The client may describe having nausea, pruritus, and being uneasy.

Objective Data

Assess gastrointestinal and respiratory functioning, cardiovascular and neurological status, and the presence of urticaria, angioedema, sneezing, excessive nasal secretions, diarrhea, wheezes, cough, or hypotension.

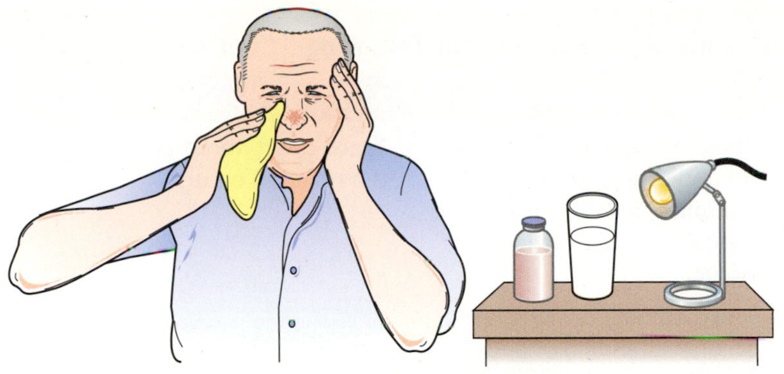

Is It a Cold or an Allergy?

Symptoms	Cold	Airborne Allergy
Cough	Common	Sometimes
General Aches, Pains	Slight	Never
Fatique, Weakness	Sometimes	Sometimes
Itchy Eyes	Rare or Never	Common
Sneezing	Usual	Usual
Sore Throat	Common	Sometimes
Runny Nose	Common	Common
Stuffy Nose	Common	Common
Fever	Rare	Never
Duration	3 to 14 days	Weeks (for example, 6 weeks for ragweed or grass pollen seasons)
Treatment	Antihistamines Decongestants Nonsteroidal anti-inflammatory medicines	Antihistamines Nasal steroids Decongestants
Prevention	Wash your hands often with soap and water Avoid close contact with anyone with a cold	Avoid those things that you are allergic to such as pollen, house dust mites, mold, pet dander, cockroaches
Complications	Sinus infection Middle ear infection Asthma	Sinus infection Asthma

FIGURE 47-4 Differences Between a Cold and an Airborne Allergy (*National Institute of Allergy and Infectious Diseases. (2008). http://www3.naid.nih.gov/topics/allergicDiseases/PDF/ColdAllergy.pdf.*)

Nursing diagnoses for clients with allergies include the following:

NURSING DIAGNOSES	PLANNING/OUTCOMES	NURSING INTERVENTIONS
Risk for Injury, related to an allergic reaction	The client will identify factors that increase the potential of a reaction.	Assist client in identifying those factors that increase the potential for a reaction.
Health-Seeking Behaviors related to causative allergen, therapeutic modalities, and/or preventive measures	The client will relate methods to avoid exposure to allergens.	Assist client in planning lifestyle changes that will help in avoiding exposure to allergens.

(*Continues*)

Nursing diagnoses for clients with allergies include the following: (Continued)

NURSING DIAGNOSES	PLANNING/OUTCOMES	NURSING INTERVENTIONS
Deficient Knowledge related to lack of information about allergens, treatment, or preventive measures	The client will demonstrate an understanding of and compliance with therapeutic modalities if a reaction occurs. The client will demonstrate an understanding of and compliance with preventive measures to avoid subsequent allergic reactions.	Teach client about allergy treatments and what to do if a reaction occurs.

Evaluation: Evaluate each outcome to determine how it has been met by the client.

ANAPHYLACTIC REACTION

Anaphylaxis is a type I systemic reaction to allergens and is the most serious type of allergic reaction. It occurs in individuals who are extremely sensitive to an allergen. Symptoms develop suddenly and can progress to severe levels within minutes. Usually, the faster the reaction, the worse it is. Foods, drugs, hormones, insect bites, blood, and vaccines all are associated with anaphylactic reactions. Shellfish, eggs, nuts, berries, and chocolates are the most common foods involved. According to the National Institute of Allergy and Infectious Diseases (2008a), peanut and tree nut allergies are the leading causes of anaphylaxis in the United States. Any medication has the potential of causing a reaction, but antibiotics (especially penicillin), insulin, muscle relaxants, and x-ray dyes are the most frequent precipitating agents. Bee, wasp, hornet, and snake bites may also cause anaphylactic reactions. According to Golden (2007), anaphylaxis to insect bites occurs in 3% of adults and can be fatal on the first reaction.

Anaphylactic reactions may be life-threatening. Symptoms involve the skin, GI tract, and cardiovascular and respiratory systems. Clients experience peripheral tingling, flushing, fullness in the mouth, throat/nasal congestion, tearing and swelling around the eyes, itching, cough, laryngeal edema, bronchospasms, severe dyspnea, vasodilation, and cyanosis. If untreated, these catastrophic effects lead to respiratory failure, severe hypotension, anaphylactic shock, and death. Therefore, it is crucial that symptoms be identified early and treatment initiated immediately because death can occur in minutes.

CLIENT TEACHING

Severe Allergies

- Advise clients with severe allergies to wear a Medic Alert tag.
- Encourage clients who are allergic to insect stings to carry an emergency anaphylactic kit containing epinephrine at all times.

CASE STUDY

Allergic Reaction

A client is stung by a bee and experiences an allergic reaction with severe shortness of breath. The client is transported to the local emergency department.

Answer the following questions and state the rationale for your answer.

1. Briefly describe the role of B-cells and T-helper lymphocytes in immune physiology.
2. What role does the antigen play in an immune response?
3. What is the difference between an "allergen" and an "antigen"?

MEDICAL–SURGICAL MANAGEMENT

Medical

Medical management centers around establishing an intravenous line, administering fluids and emergency drugs, and maintaining an airway. Provide oxygen via a nonrebreather oxygen mask. In severe cases, endotracheal intubation or a tracheotomy may be required.

Pharmacological

Epinephrine is administered subcutaneously as soon as symptoms develop to dilate bronchioles, increase heart contractions, and constrict blood vessels. Antihistamines, such as diphenhydramine hydrochloride (Benadryl), block the effects of histamine in bronchioles, blood vessels, and the GI tract. Corticosteroids are given for their anti-inflammatory effect. Vasopressors, such as norepinephrine bitartrate (Levophed) or dopamine hydrochloride (Intropin), may be needed to increase blood pressure. If bronchoconstriction and spasms are severe, albuterol (Proventil), metaproterenol sulfate (Alupent), and/or aminophylline (Aminophyllin) may be administered.

Diet

Clients will be NPO until normal respiratory and circulatory function have been restored.

Activity

Clients will remain on bed rest until vital signs are stable and normal breathing patterns have been restored. Those experiencing severe anaphylactic responses are generally transferred to intensive care units for continued treatment and observation.

Nursing Management

Monitor vital signs frequently as well as I&O. Administer IV fluids and medications as ordered. Teach client and family the importance of providing the name of the causative agent and a description of the reaction when asked about allergies.

NURSING PROCESS

Assessment

Subjective Data

Client history may reveal a previous anaphylaxis reaction. The client may describe feelings of uneasiness, anxiety, weakness, itching, dizziness, nausea, peripheral tingling, and a generalized warm sensation throughout the body.

Objective Data

Because anaphylaxis is a sudden, unexpected event, be aware that variations in a client's cardiovascular and respiratory status may be signs of an impending anaphylactic reaction. The first symptoms are sweating, sneezing, tachycardia, hypotension, dysrhythmias, cyanosis, edema of tongue and larynx, wheezing, bronchospasms, vascular collapse, and cardiac arrest. Regularly assessing client's vital signs and cardiovascular, respiratory, and neurological status will detect changes before the severe signs of respiratory distress and impending shock develop.

Nursing diagnoses for clients with anaphylaxis include the following:

NURSING DIAGNOSES	PLANNING/OUTCOMES	NURSING INTERVENTIONS
Ineffective Tissue Perfusion, related to increased capillary permeability and vasodilation	The client will have adequate tissue perfusion.	Monitor vital signs frequently. Place client in Trendelenburg position for hypotension. Monitor I&O. Administer IV fluids and medications as ordered.
Ineffective Breathing Pattern related to bronchoconstriction, laryngeal edema, and increased secretions	The client will have effective breathing patterns.	Monitor vital signs. Maintain patent airway. Suction secretions as needed. Administer oxygen and medications as ordered.
Deficient Knowledge related to causative allergen, therapeutic modalities, and/or preventive measures	The client will relate causative allergen, therapeutic modalities, and preventive measures.	Teach client and family importance of avoiding allergen and symptoms of anaphylactic reactions. Teach client to provide the name of the causative agent and a description of reaction experienced when asked about allergies. Document allergy on all medical records.

Evaluation: Evaluate each outcome to determine how it has been met by the client.

TRANSFUSION REACTIONS

Blood components, such as whole blood, packed or frozen red blood cells (RBCs), leukocytes, platelets, and plasma, may be administered to clients when their own bodies are incapable of manufacturing them at a rate required to maintain vascular homeostasis. Any client receiving blood products that are **allogeneic**, or from a donor of the same species, may develop a transfusion reaction. For this reason, some clients are arranging to have their own blood collected, saved, and available for infusion, if needed, during or following elective surgeries. This is known as an **autologous** blood transfusion. Immunological reactions do not develop with this type of blood transfusion.

There are five types of transfusion reactions: febrile nonhemolytic, allergic urticarial, delayed hemolytic, acute hemolytic, and anaphylactic. Febrile nonhemolytic reactions are the most common and occur in clients who have had previous blood transfusions as a result of an antibody-antigen reaction to WBCs. Symptoms may develop soon after the infusion has started or up to 5 to 6 hours after completion. Fever is the classic symptom and may be accompanied by chills, nausea, headache, hypotension, and respiratory problems. Clients who have allergic urticarial reactions develop a skin rash during or within 1 hour following the transfusion. A delayed hemolytic reaction may occur days to weeks following the transfusion. The client's hemoglobin level falls because of incompatibility of RBC antigens. This type of reaction is often misdiagnosed and thought to be related to the condition that created the need for blood replacement rather than a transfusion reaction. An acute hemolytic reaction is potentially a life-threatening situation. Symptoms, resulting from the incompatibility of ABO

CRITICAL THINKING

Donor Blood Transfusion

What are the pros and cons of receiving a blood transfusion from a donor?

groups, usually occur during the first 15 minutes of administration, but can develop anytime during the transfusion. Clients complain of chills, nausea, and back pain. Fever, drop in blood pressure (hypotension), vomiting, hematuria, or oliguria may be observed. As the condition progresses, chest pain, dyspnea, anuria, and shock develop. Anaphylactic reactions, although rare, are also life-threatening. Symptoms of acute gastrointestinal malfunctioning and cardiovascular and respiratory collapse develop moments after the transfusion has started.

MEDICAL–SURGICAL MANAGEMENT

Medical

Medical management of clients experiencing a blood transfusion reaction depends on the type of reaction. Treatment of a febrile nonhemolytic reaction includes stopping the blood, infusing normal saline, and treating the symptoms. For clients experiencing an allergic urticarial reaction, the transfusion should be slowed and an antihistamine administered. Delayed hemolytic reactions often go undetected and untreated. Both acute hemolytic reactions and anaphylactic reactions are medical emergencies. The transfusion must be stopped immediately. Normal saline and emergency drugs are given intravenously.

Pharmacological

If a febrile nonhemolytic or allergic urticarial reaction occurs, diphenhydramine hydrochloride (Benadryl) and a corticosteroid (hydrocortisone or prednisone) are administered to counteract the immunological response. Antipyretics are ordered to control fever. For life-threatening conditions, emergency medications are employed. (Refer back to Anaphylactic Reaction.)

Diet

Clients should not be fed if a reaction is occurring, especially if respiratory symptoms have developed, because aspiration could occur.

Activity

Clients should remain in bed until symptoms of the reaction have subsided.

NURSING MANAGEMENT

Follow agency protocol for use and administration of blood products. Assess vital signs before administration of blood products and at 15-minute intervals four times. Stay with the client for at least the first 15 minutes of administration. When reaction occurs, stop transfusion, but keep saline going for IV access if needed. Notify physician immediately.

NURSING PROCESS

ASSESSMENT

Subjective Data

Occasionally, clients verbalize the feeling of something "not being right" or "something strange is going on in my body" before actual symptoms become apparent. They may have itching, headache, or low-back pain.

Objective Data

Assess for any signs of a transfusion reaction, such as fever, chills, or respiratory problems.

A nursing diagnosis for clients with transfusion reactions is:

NURSING DIAGNOSES	PLANNING/OUTCOMES	NURSING INTERVENTIONS
Risk for Injury related to infusion of allogeneic blood components	The client will not have injury from infusion of allogeneic blood products.	Follow protocol for blood products and administration. Check client's identification and blood product with another nurse. If a reaction occurs, stop transfusion immediately, then call the physician. Administer medications as ordered. Send blood tubing and a urine specimen to the lab for analysis. Monitor and document client's condition. Teach client who has a blood transfusion reaction to inform health care providers whenever questioned about allergies.

Evaluation: Evaluate each outcome to determine how it has been met by the client.

TRANSPLANT REJECTION

In 2005, more than 163,000 organ transplants were performed in the United States (Department of Health and Human Services, 2007). The success of these procedures is directly related to matching antibodies and antigens of the donor and recipient and to the effectiveness of immunosuppressive medications in preventing rejection. Immunosuppressive medications make the client prone to the development of infections and cancers. Clients must have a regular medical checkup, including cancer screening tests.

Medical–Surgical Management

Medical

Although blood components are the most common type of tissue transplants, today it is possible to transplant bone marrow, corneal tissue, skin, kidneys, pancreas, hearts, livers, and lungs. Bone marrow and blood components often employ autologous donations. Allogeneic donations may be from living related donors or living nonrelated donors. Cadaveric donations are harvested from individuals after they are pronounced clinically dead. It is important to match ABO blood groups and **human leukocyte antigen** (antigens present in human blood) to prevent rejection when allogeneic and cadaveric donors are used.

Pharmacological

A combination of immunosuppressive medications is used to hinder rejection. Steroids such as prednisone (Deltasone) and methylprednisolone sodium succinate (Solu-Medrol) decrease the inflammatory response. Cyclosporine (Sandimmune), antithymocyte globulin (equine), ATG (Atgam), and tacrolimus (Prograf) inhibit T-cells. Azathioprine (Imuran) inhibits purine synthesis. Muromonab-CD3 (Orthoclone, OKT 3) prevents acute rejection in kidney transplant clients. Clients taking immunosuppressive medications are especially prone to developing infections. Antibiotics may be prescribed prophylactically.

Steroids cause fluid and sodium retention, low potassium level, elevated blood pressure, moon face, muscle wasting, elevated glucose level, impaired wound healing, mood swings, and masculinization in women. Cyclosporine may be toxic to the kidneys and liver. Imuran may cause hair loss and lower platelet level. OKT 3 also causes fluid retention.

Activity

Activity depends on the type of transplant. Clients who receive a major organ, such as a heart, lung, pancreas, or liver, are placed in reverse isolation in the hospital setting for at least 2 weeks. They are carefully observed for signs of rejection. Exposure to others is limited. Before discharge, they are taught to avoid contact with anyone who may have an infection and to wear a mask whenever out in public.

Nursing Management

Monitor vital signs, fluid balance, nutritional status, mental status, and cardiovascular and respiratory functioning. Prevent contact with anyone who may have an infection. Teach client and family proper hand hygiene. Emphasize the importance of taking all medications as prescribed.

NURSING PROCESS

Assessment

Subjective Data

Client history may reveal fear of possible transplant rejection. The client generally describes tenderness at the transplant site.

Objective Data

After transplantation, carefully monitor clients' vital signs, nutritional status, fluid balance, urinary output, mental status, and respiratory and cardiovascular functioning. Weigh client daily. Check wound sites frequently. Signs of rejection include fever, weight gain, and swelling or tenderness at the transplant site.

Nursing diagnoses for clients with organ transplants include the following:

NURSING DIAGNOSES	PLANNING/OUTCOMES	NURSING INTERVENTIONS
Fear related to possible transplant rejection.	The client will relate less fear regarding rejection.	Allow client to verbalize concerns and develop realistic expectations. Set aside time to sit down and talk to client.
Deficient Knowledge related to home care following transplantation	The client will discuss signs and symptoms of rejection. The client will demonstrate an understanding of the side effects of immunosuppressive drugs and lifestyle changes to adapt to their effects.	Teach client and family about signs of rejection and infection. Teach client and family ramifications of taking immunosuppressive medications. Teach client to watch for side effects and report them to physician.

(Continues)

Nursing diagnoses for clients with organ transplants include the following: (Continued)

NURSING DIAGNOSES	PLANNING/OUTCOMES	NURSING INTERVENTIONS
Risk for Infection related to immunosuppressive medications	The client will demonstrate appropriate wound care. The client will be free of infection.	Teach client and family appropriate wound care and proper hand hygiene. Teach client importance of taking antibiotics as ordered, wearing a mask whenever out in public, and regular checkups, including cancer screening tests.

Evaluation: Evaluate each outcome to determine how it has been met by the client.

LATEX ALLERGY

Since 1987, when universal precautions (now called Standard Precautions) were mandated, exposure to latex by health care workers has dramatically increased. Today, between 8% and 17% of health care workers and less than 1% of the general population are sensitized to natural rubber latex (American Latex Allergy Association, 2009).

The latex proteins can enter the body through the skin and mucous membranes, intravascularly, and by inhalation. The cornstarch powder on gloves absorbs the latex proteins and becomes airborne when the gloves are put on or taken off. From the air, the latex proteins may be inhaled or may be in contact with the skin and mucous membranes. Anyone, client or health care worker, who after exposure to latex develops red, watery, itchy eyes; sinus or nasal irritation; hives; shortness of breath; dry cough; wheezing; chest tightness; or flushing, tachycardia, and hypotension should be suspected of latex allergy.

Latex allergy has the potential to induce a life-threatening anaphylactic reaction with repeated exposure; avoidance of latex products is of utmost importance. Synthetic versions of products are often available. An individual product may be "latex free," but an environment is "latex safe" only when all items of latex that might come in contact with the allergic individual are removed.

CLIENT TEACHING

Latex Safety

- Clients with latex allergy are at risk for cross-reactivity to banana, avocado, chestnuts, kiwi, and passion fruit (NIAID, 2003).
- Clients with spina bifida, or who need multiple surgeries, have a risk of nearly 50% of developing allergies to latex (American Academy of Allergy Asthma & Immunology, 2007). These clients need to avoid exposure to latex products such as gloves, band-aids, rubber bands, condoms, and latex birthday balloons.
- Health care workers and others whose job requires wearing latex gloves have nearly a 10% risk of developing a latex allergy (American Academy of Allergy Asthma & Immunology, 2007).
- Clients with latex allergy are instructed to avoid all latex products, including the powder/dust from inside latex gloves.

SAFETY

Latex Allergy

A Medic Alert tag stating "latex allergy" should be worn by any individual with a latex allergy.

AUTOIMMUNE DISEASES

Disorders in this category include rheumatoid arthritis, systemic lupus erythematosus, and myasthenia gravis.

RHEUMATOID ARTHRITIS

Rheumatoid arthritis (RA) is a chronic, systemic autoimmune disease characterized by joint stiffness. It affects 1.3 million people in the United States, and occurs in women two to three times more often than men (Arthritis Foundation, 2009e). Rheumatoid arthritis can affect anyone, including children, and onset usually occurs between 30 to 50 years of age. Clients with the genetic marker HLA-DR4 may have an increased risk of developing rheumatoid arthritis (Arthritis Foundation, 2009f).

The cause of RA is unknown, but there seems to be a genetic predisposition (susceptibility) in many, but not all, persons affected. It is believed that something must trigger the disease process such as a virus, bacterium, hormonal factors, or stress. The person's immune system attacks the cells inside the joint(s), producing substances that act as antigens. Immune complexes are formed within the joint, causing inflammation, swelling, and increased synovial fluid. As this chronic, systemic condition progresses, surrounding cartilage, tendons, and ligaments become involved. Thickening of synovial tissue eventually leads to calcification of the joint, joint pain, limited mobility, and deformity.

It is believed that the damage to the bones begins within the first two years of the onset of RA. Early diagnosis and aggressive treatment are important to control the disease. Usually, the joints of the hand and wrist are affected initially. As the disease progresses, shoulder, elbow, hip, knee, ankle, and cervical spine joints become affected. The pattern of joint involvement is symmetrical (i.e., if a joint is affected on the right side of the body, the same joint will also be affected on the left side) (Arthritis Foundation, 2009). Other areas of the body where connective tissue is present may also be involved, such as blood vessels, lining of the lungs, and pericordial sac.

Clients experience periods of **remission**, a decrease or absence of symptoms, and **exacerbations**, an increase in symptoms. Both physical and emotional stressors lead to increased symptomatology. This means that simple tasks such as answering the telephone or buttoning clothes may become very challenging.

Medical–Surgical Management

Medical

Medical management centers around reducing inflammation, relieving pain, slowing down or a stopping joint damage, and promoting general health. Therapeutic regimen includes medications, exercise, rest, hot and cold applications, and stress management. Currently researchers are working on developing and testing a vaccine for the prevention of rheumatoid arthritis (Arthritis Foundation, 2009a).

Surgical

Hip, knee, and finger joints may be surgically replaced. Refer to the Musculoskeletal System chapter for a discussion of joint replacement.

Pharmacological

Nonsteroidal anti-inflammatory drugs (NSAIDs) and salicylates have the potential to relieve symptoms such as joint pain, stiffness, and swelling but do not control the disease. Disease-modifying antirheumatic drugs (DMARDs) have the potential to modify the disease and should be given early in the disease to control progression. The commonly used DMARDs include prednisone (Deltasone), gold salts, and sulfasalazine (Azulfidine EN-Tabs) (Table 47-5). Aggressive treatment includes disease-modifying antirheumatic drugs such as methotrexate, hydroxychloroquine (Plaquenil), sulfasalazine (Azulfidine), a biologic agent such as etanercept (Enbrel), or adalimumab (Humira), or a combination of both a biologic and a DMARD (Arthritis Foundation, 2009b). Because of the large doses required to control inflammation and the long-term use because of the chronicity of this condition, side effects often develop. In severe cases, azathioprine (Imuran), hydroxychloroquine sulfate (Plaquenil Sulfate), D-penicillamine (Depen), or methotrexate sodium (Rheumatrex) may be used. These medications also have serious side effects. Minocycline, an antibiotic, is increasingly being used to treat rheumatoid arthritis. Researchers have been investigating the use of the antimalarial drug, hydrochloroquine in protecting clients with RA from developing diabetes (Arthritis Foundation, 2009b).

Diet

Clients should eat a nutritious, well-balanced diet. Poorly nourished individuals are prone to infections. For clients with RA, an infection results in exacerbation of symptoms. Foods high in iron are encouraged when RBCs are low.

Activity

Because joint mobility is a major problem, occupational and physical therapists are part of the therapeutic team. Range-of-motion exercises, resting splints, and assistive devices such as canes and hand rails are often employed to promote mobility.

Nursing Management

Encourage the client to practice relaxation techniques and take a warm shower to relieve joint stiffness and pain. Emphasize the importance of doing ROM exercises several times a day and to have planned rest periods. Teach the client to use assistive devices such as handrails, tools to pick up objects, raised toilet seat, walker, or cane.

Table 47-5 Medications Used to Treat Rheumatoid Arthritis

DRUG	USE/ACTIONS	SIDE EFFECTS	NURSING CONSIDERATIONS
Salicylates			
• aspirin	Inhibit prostaglandin synthesis resulting in decreased pain. (Analgesia) antipyretic and anti-inflammatory effects.	GI upset, tinnitus, easy bruising, nausea, prolonged bleeding time.	Instruct client to take with food or take enteric coated aspirin and to report ringing in ears. Do not give to clients on oral anticoagulants. Assess for bleeding/bruising.
Nonsteroidal Anti-inflammatory Drugs (NSAIDs)			
• ibuprofen (Motrin, Rufen) • naproxen (Naprosyn) • phenylbutazone (Butazolidin) • nabumetone (Relafen)	Inhibit prostaglandin synthesis. Reduce joint swelling stiffness. Analgesic and antipyretic properties.	GI irritation, nausea, vomiting, heartburn. GI bleeding and ulceration, dizziness, headache, liver toxicity.	Administer with food. May prolong bleeding time, may require frequent blood count.

(*Continues*)

TABLE 47-5 Medications Used to Treat Rheumatoid Arthritis (Continued)

DRUG	USE/ACTIONS	SIDE EFFECTS	NURSING CONSIDERATIONS
Indole Analogues			
• indomethacin (Indocin) • sulindac (Clinoril)	Analgesic anti-inflammatory effect.	Gastric bleeding, headaches, dizziness, psychiatric disturbances.	Administer with food. Instruct client to report any bleeding (tarry stools, hematemesis). Avoid giving aspirin.
Corticosteroids			
• prednisone (Deltasone)	Decreases inflammation.	GI irritation, muscle weakness, fluid retention, moon face, muscle wasting, impaired wound healing.	Administer with food. Weigh daily. Monitor BP, sleep pattern, and serum potassium.
Antimalarials			
• hydroxychloroquine sulfate (Plaquenil Sulfate)	Not a drug of choice.	Visual disturbances, nightmares, skin lesions, nausea, diarrhea, low blood count.	Monitor CBC and liver function tests. Discontinue after 6 months if no beneficial effects noted.
Gold Salts			
• auranofin (Ridaura)	Anti-inflammatory effect.	Diarrhea, nausea, vomiting, jaundice.	Remind client to keep all physician appointments. Beneficial effects may take 3 months to appear.
Chelating Agent			
• penicillamine (Depen)	Palliative when other medications have failed.	Bone marrow depression, fever, rashes, blood dyscrasias, liver toxicity.	Give on empty stomach. Have epinephrine 1;1,000 handy for anaphylaxis. Fluids to 3,000 mL/day to prevent renal failure.
Sulfonamide			
• sulfasalazine (Azulfidine EN-TABS)	For clients who do not respond well to NSAIDs.	Anorexia, headache, nausea, vomiting, gastric distress, reversible oligospermia.	Give with food. May discolor urine or skin yellow-orange. Take at least 2–3 L/day of water. May increase sensitivity to sun.
Immunomodulator			
• adalimumab (Humira)	Decreases inflammation and inhibits progression of structural damage.	Increased risk for infections, redness and pain, itching, swelling and/or bruising at the injection site.	Drug must be refrigerated but not frozen. Comes in pre-filled syringes and is injected into the abdomen, upper arm, or thigh.
• etanercept (Enbrel)	Delays structural damage and improves physical function.	Redness and pain, itching, swelling and/or bruising at the injection site.	Comes in pre-filled syringe or pen device. The needle cover contains latex; do not handle if sensitive to latex. Drug must be refrigerated and allowed to come to room temperature before administration.
Immunosuppressant			
• azathioprine (Imuran)	For clients that are nonresponsive to conventional therapy.	Bone marrow depression, loss of appetite, liver problems, low blood counts, unusual tiredness or weakness.	Take with food. Improvement may take 6 to 12 weeks.

TABLE 47-5 Medications Used to Treat Rheumatoid Arthritis (Continued)

DRUG	USE/ACTIONS	SIDE EFFECTS	NURSING CONSIDERATIONS
Antibiotic			
• minocycline (Minocin)	Increasingly being used for clients that do not respond to conventional therapy.	Cramps or burning of the stomach, diarrhea, darkening of the skin, dizziness, light-headed or unsteadiness, liver problems, and sun sensitivity.	Take on an empty stomach.
Antimetabolite			
• methotrexate (Rheumatrex, Trexall)	For clients that do not respond well to NSAIDS.	Bone marrow depression, increased sun sensitivity, hair loss, liver problems, low blood counts, mouth sores, yeast infections.	Take tablets at bedtime with an antacid to minimize GI upset. Monitor CBC and liver function tests.

COURTESY OF DELMAR CENGAGE LEARNING

NURSING PROCESS

ASSESSMENT

Subjective Data

Client history frequently reveals a gradual development of symptoms, beginning initially with early-morning stiffness and pain in finger joints. Eventually, other joints become involved. Fatigue, weight loss, temperature elevation, and anemia develop, along with malaise, loss of appetite, fatigue, and muscle weakness. Obtain information about periods of remissions and exacerbations as well as the client's understanding of and compliance with the treatment regimen.

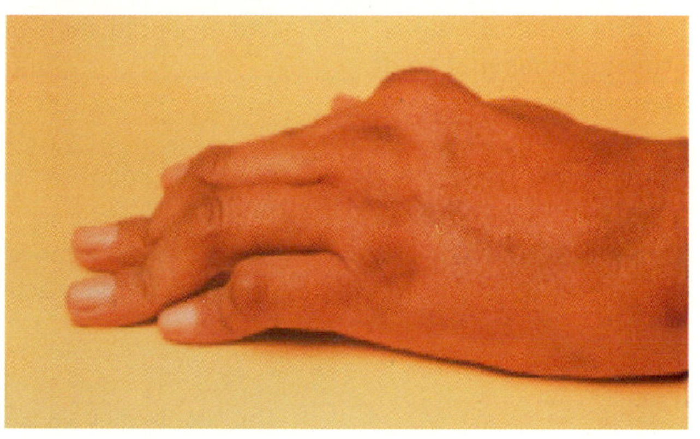

FIGURE 47-5 Arthritic Hands (*Courtesy of the Arthritis Foundation.*)

Objective Data

Assessment of the hands may reveal the classic deformities associated with RA: boutonniere deformity (fixed flexion of the proximal interphalangeal joint and hyperextension of the distal interphalangeal joint), ulnar drift (deviation of the fingers to the ulnar side of the hand), and swan-neck deformity (fixed flexion of the distal interphalangeal joint and hyperextension of the proximal interphalangeal joint). Figure 47-5 illustrates these changes in the hands.

Skin may show the presence of ulcers, caused by vasculitis, and moveable, subcutaneous skin nodes, known as *rheumatoid nodules*. Eye tissue may be inflamed. Reduction in tear and saliva production can occur, causing dryness of the eyes, mouth, and mucous membranes. This is known as Sjögren's syndrome. The client may have weight loss and an elevated temperature.

X-rays demonstrate the amount and degree of deformity. No specific laboratory test confirms a diagnosis of RA, although alterations in the following may occur: RBCs decrease (anemia) as the disease progresses, elevation of WBCs, erythrocyte sedimentation rate (ESR), antinuclear antibodies (ANAs), C-reactive proteins, and platelet count. The rheumatoid factor (RF) is present in about 75% of adult clients with RA (Daniels, 2010).

Nursing diagnoses for clients with rheumatoid arthritis include the following:

NURSING DIAGNOSES	PLANNING/OUTCOMES	NURSING INTERVENTIONS
Chronic Pain related to swollen, inflamed joints	The client will relate appropriate use of anti-inflammatory medications. The client will relate methods to decrease pain.	Teach client about prescribed analgesics and anti-inflammatory medications. Encourage client to practice relaxation techniques and take warm shower to relieve early morning joint stiffness and pain. Use hot and cold packs to decrease muscle spasms. Teach client proper body alignment and to avoid using pillows under the knees, which leads to pooling of blood in the feet.

(*Continues*)

Nursing diagnoses for clients with rheumatoid arthritis include the following: (Continued)

NURSING DIAGNOSES	PLANNING/OUTCOMES	NURSING INTERVENTIONS
Impaired Physical Mobility related to edema, and joint immobility	The client will demonstrate measures to maintain joint mobility.	Teach hospitalized clients to use the overhead trapeze when moving in bed and to change position frequently.
	The client will demonstrate use of adaptive devices.	Assist with ROM exercises and maintain planned rest periods.
		Teach client use of assistive devices, such as handrests, tools to pick up objects, or three-legged canes, as needed.
		Check with occupational and physical therapists for available equipment. Assist client to use handrails in tub, shower, and toilet; raised toilet seat; and rubber-tipped walker or cane.
Bathing/Dressing/Grooming Self-care Deficit related to joint inflammation or deformity	The client will bathe, dress, and groom to abilities.	Encourage client to stop and rest when tired.
		Teach self-care using assistive devices, as required. Recommend shoes with Velcro® closures.
		Assist with routine plan for ADLs.
Fatigue related to chronic inflammatory process	The client will state less fatigue.	Explain that fatigue is a common symptom of autoimmune disorders. Plan rest periods between activities.
	The client will establish priorities for daily activities.	Allow the client to express feelings about altered lifestyle.
		Inform client of community services such as Meals on Wheels.
	The client will balance daily activities with periods of rest.	Help identify activities client should perform and what can be delegated. Instruct client to record level of fatigue and activities performed on an hourly basis for 24 hours. One method uses 0 to 10 scale (0 = not tired, peppy; 10 = totally exhausted).
		Help plan important tasks during high-energy periods and distribute difficult ones throughout the week.

Evaluation: Evaluate each outcome to determine how it has been met by the client.

SYSTEMIC LUPUS ERYTHEMATOSUS

Systemic lupus erythematosus (SLE) is a chronic, progressive, incurable autoimmune disease affecting multiple body organs. It is characterized by periods of exacerbation (flares) and remission. SLE occurs most commonly in women during their childbearing years and is 2 to 3 times more common in African-American women (Lupus Foundation of America, 2009). In clients with SLE, abnormal B-lymphocyte cells produce autoantibodies that destroy body cells. Immune complexes are formed and circulate in serum, causing inflammation and tissue damage in the skin, brain, kidney, lung, heart, or joints. Production of these autoantibodies is influenced by genetic predisposition, medications, infections, stress, and sunlight (ultraviolet light rays).

No single test is conclusive for a diagnosis. The American College of Rheumatology has established criteria for SLE. These criteria include a malar rash (over cheeks); discoid rash; photosensitivity; oral ulcers; arthritis; serositis (pleuritis or pericarditis); excessive protein or cellular casts in the urine; seizures or psychosis; hemolytic anemia, or leukopenia, or lymphopenia, or thrombocytopenia; and positive for LE cells, or anti-DNA antibody, or anti-Sm, or a false-positive syphilis test. If four or more of these criteria are present, a client is diagnosed with SLE.

MEDICAL–SURGICAL MANAGEMENT

Medical

Medical treatment is aimed at decreasing tissue inflammation and destruction. A knowledgeable client can assist in controlling the disease process through stress management, rest, exercise, taking medications as prescribed, and immediately reporting symptoms to the health care provider. During acute

CLIENT TEACHING

Systemic Lupus Erythematosus

- Get adequate rest.
- Use stress-reduction techniques such as visualization, guided imagery, meditation, or yoga.
- Avoid exposure to sunlight; use sunscreen.
- Involve family and friends in care.
- Report fever, chills, anorexia, or symptom worsening to health care provider immediately.
- Never just stop taking medications.
- Contact the Lupus Foundation of America, Inc., for information and support (see Resources at the end of chapter).

exacerbations, plasmapheresis may be used. This treatment modality involves removal of the client's plasma, processing it through a special machine to eliminate various cellular elements, and reinfusing the cleansed plasma. In SLE, autoantibodies are removed.

Because clients with SLE are prone to a variety of complications, they are carefully monitored for renal, cardiac, pulmonary, hematological, and neurological damage. A large percentage of SLE clients eventually develop renal failure, requiring dialysis to maintain life.

Pharmacological

NSAIDs are used for muscle and joint pain. The lowest possible dose of corticosteroid is used to suppress immune system activity. During periods of exacerbations, higher doses may be required. Prolonged use of these medications leads to multiple side effects. Hydroxychloroquine sulfate (Plaquenil sulfate), an antimalarial agent, is used. Although the exact mechanism involved is unknown, it does work effectively in decreasing joint and skin problems. It can lead to the development of retinal toxicity; therefore, clients should have yearly eye exams. Cyclophosphamide (Cytoxan) or azathioprine (Imuran) may be used for severe SLE.

Diet

Clients on corticosteroids are prone to developing hypernatremia, hyperglycemia, hypokalemia, and fluid retention. Diet should be low in sodium and glucose and high in potassium. Excessive fluid intake should be discouraged.

PROFESSIONAL TIP

RA and SLE

Clients with RA and SLE have common nursing diagnoses of fatigue and impaired mobility. Clients with SLE have an additional risk for infection if WBC count is low.

CRITICAL THINKING

Lifestyle Implications

What are the lifestyle implications of being diagnosed with a chronic disease such as rheumatoid arthritis or systemic lupus erythematosus?

Activity

Clients should be encouraged to sleep at least 8 hours a night and rest periodically during the day. Regular exercise helps prevent muscle weakness and fatigue.

Nursing Management

Teach the client the importance of avoiding direct sunlight and the use of protective clothing and sunscreen (SPF 15 or higher). Encourage the client to balance rest and activity and to eat a balanced diet with reduced sodium. Emphasize the signs of exacerbation (rash, fever, cough, or increased joint and muscle pain) and early signs of infection. Provide emotional, psychosocial, and spiritual support.

NURSING PROCESS

ASSESSMENT

Subjective Data

Ask when the disease began, what symptoms have developed, and how they have been treated. Note information about medications the client is taking and side effects, activity level, and degree of fatigue. Determine client's understanding of the disease process, how lifestyle has changed, and how effectively client is coping. The client may describe having malaise, photosensitivity, pain in joints, irregular menses, irritability, confusion, or hallucinations.

Objective Data

Most common findings include joint swelling and pain, fever, swollen glands, nausea, vomiting, anorexia, hypertension, respiratory and cardiac infections, renal involvement, enlarged liver and spleen, and skin lesions, especially the classic "butterfly" rash. Figure 47-6 shows

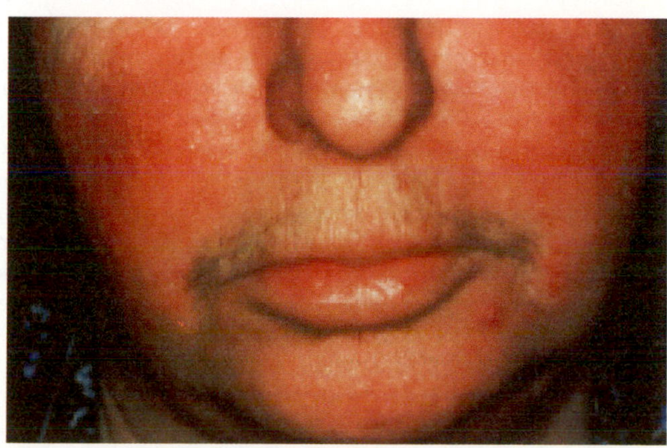

FIGURE 47-6 Butterfly Rash (*Courtesy of the American Academy of Dermatology.*)

an individual with a "butterfly" rash. If exposed to the cold, Raynaud's phenomenon (intermittent attacks of diminished blood supply to fingers, toes, ears, and nose) may develop.

Laboratory tests frequently reveal serum antinuclear antibodies (ANA) and anti-DNA antibodies. Lupus erythematosus cells (LE cells) are present in most clients. Anemia, leukopenia, and thrombocytopenia are evident.

Nursing diagnoses for a client with SLE include the following:

NURSING DIAGNOSES	PLANNING/OUTCOMES	NURSING INTERVENTIONS
Impaired Skin Integrity related to presence of butterfly rash, skin lesions, Raynaud's phenomenon, and/or oral ulcers	The client will participate in a plan to promote wound healing.	Teach client to clean and dry area prior to application of topical corticosteroids. Warn client that sunlight and ultraviolet rays increase symptoms and tanning sessions are contraindicated. Encourage client to wear protective clothing, sunscreen of at least SPF 15, and sunglasses. In cold weather, client should wear a hat and gloves. Encourage client in regular oral care to promote healing of mouth sores.
Deficient Knowledge related to adapting lifestyle with treatment and prevention of complications	The client will describe disease process, factors contributing to symptoms, and regimen for control.	Teach client effects of disease and methods to control complications. Teach stress management techniques. Allow client to vent feelings. Help client plan methods to adapt lifestyle. Encourage client to visit the physician on a regular basis to monitor for early symptoms of major organ involvement. Advise client to have regular eye exam if taking Plaquenil Sulfate. Inform client of community support groups available through the Lupus Foundation of America, Inc. (see Resources).

Evaluation: Evaluate each outcome to determine how it has been met by the client.

MYASTHENIA GRAVIS

Myasthenia gravis (MG) is an autoimmune disease characterized by extreme muscle weakness and fatigue caused by the body's inability to transmit nerve impulses to voluntary muscles. It is thought that clients with MG develop antibodies that act to decrease the number and effectiveness of acetylcholine receptor sites at neuromuscular junctions. Voluntary muscles are most commonly involved, especially those innervated by cranial nerves. Muscle weakness increases during periods of activity and improves after a period of rest.

Severity of symptoms varies. In mild conditions known as Group I ocular myasthenia, only the eye muscles are involved. As severity increases, symptoms of Group II generalized myasthenia develop: Facial, neck, skeletal, and respiratory muscles become affected. The thymus gland is enlarged in most clients. Anti-ACh receptor antibodies are produced in this organ. MG affects men more frequently than women, with the onset of symptoms after age 50. Periods of remission and exacerbation occur, usually during the first few years.

There are three possible complications: respiratory distress, myasthenic crisis, and cholinergic crisis. Clients need to be carefully monitored for early signs of respiratory distress, such as dyspnea, tachypnea, tachycardia, and diaphoresis.

Myasthenia crisis is an acute emergency characterized by increased muscle weakness; difficulty swallowing, chewing, or talking; and respiratory distress. It occurs in newly diagnosed clients who are not responding to anticholinesterase medications following infections, surgery, or delivery of a child.

Cholinergic crisis is the result of an overdose of anticholinesterase medications. Physical symptoms of both myasthenia crisis and cholinergic crisis are the same. An edrophonium chloride (Tensilon) test is used to differentiate between the two. Tensilon is administered intravenously; symptoms of clients experiencing a myasthenia crisis will be relieved within seconds, whereas clients in cholinergic crisis will show no response. Atropine is administered to counteract the effects of excessive amounts of anticholinesterase drugs. The treatment goal for both is restoration of normal respiratory functioning and alleviation of symptoms.

Medical–Surgical Management

Medical

Medical management involves the use of anticholinesterase medications and plasmapheresis, which removes anti-ACh receptor antibodies. Because it affords only temporary relief of symptoms, it is used primarily for clients in acute crisis who are not responding to drug therapy or before a thymectomy. A client's relief of symptoms is a good indicator of how successful surgery might be.

Surgical

Surgical removal of the thymus gland has shown the best results in young people early in the course of the disease. In some people, the weakness may completely disappear, but it varies with each client.

Pharmacological

Anticholinesterase medications, such as pyridostigmine bromide (Mestinon), neostigmine bromide (Prostigmin), and ambenonium chloride (Mytelase), are prescribed early in the course of the disease and act to increase acetylcholine at the neuromuscular junction. Dosages need to be individually determined. Early side effects of overdosage include nausea, abdominal cramping, vomiting, diarrhea, increased saliva, diaphoresis, and low pulse rate. Variation may occur in muscle group responses for the same client. Steroids may slow down the immunological response.

Diet

Clients need to be encouraged to eat a snack before taking anticholinesterase medications to avoid GI irritation. If the client's ability to chew and swallow is affected, food should be chopped, mashed, or pureed. A commercial thickener can be added to liquids to reduce the risk of aspiration. Sit upright when eating and do not talk.

PROFESSIONALTIP

Myasthenia Gravis

Clients with myasthenia gravis experience problems similar to those with RA and SLE (e.g., fatigue and impaired physical mobility). Although the cause, in this case, is weakness of voluntary muscles, client goals and nursing interventions are the same.

Activity

Symptoms of MG increase with exercise. Clients should avoid excessive muscular activity and should rest periodically throughout the day. ROM exercises, braces, splints, and walkers assist in keeping the client independent.

Nursing Management

Teach the client airway protective techniques (e.g., double swallowing, chin tuck). Encourage the client to change daily activity pattern for minimal energy expenditure, and to do ROM exercises to help maintain muscle function. Emphasize the need to see the physician at the first sign of an upper respiratory infection. Advise client to avoid crowds during cold and flu season and anyone known to have either.

NURSING PROCESS

Assessment

Subjective Data

Client describes muscle weakness, fatigue, and possibly difficulty chewing or swallowing.

Objective Data

Assess muscle groups affecting the eyes, face, neck, and chest, looking for **diplopia** (double vision), **ptosis** (drooping upper eyelids), and facial symmetry. Note chewing or swallowing problems and weakness in arm and legs muscles as well as muscles used for breathing. Assess vocal tones and breath sounds.

ACh receptor antibody and LE cell tests are often positive. X-rays and CT scans of the thymus gland are used to detect enlargement. Electromyogram (EMG) determines the extent of muscle damage.

Nursing diagnoses for a client with MG include the following:

NURSING DIAGNOSES	PLANNING/OUTCOMES	NURSING INTERVENTIONS
Ineffective Breathing Pattern related to muscle weakness	The client will have normal respiratory rate and rhythm and normal breath sounds bilaterally.	Monitor client's respiratory rate and rhythm and breath sounds frequently. Administer oxygen as ordered. Notify physician immediately if respiratory problem develops. Elevate head of client's bed.

(*Continues*)

Nursing diagnoses for a client with MG include the following: (Continued)

NURSING DIAGNOSES	PLANNING/OUTCOMES	NURSING INTERVENTIONS
Risk for Aspiration related to impaired swallowing	The client will not experience aspiration.	Have client eat in a sitting position or with head of the bed elevated. Teach client to chew food well and swallow only small bites. Request a special diet of thickened, soft foods. Suction oral secretions as required. Teach client to suction secretions as needed.
Deficient Knowledge related to disease process and understanding of methods to control disease and prevent complications	The client will describe disease process, factors contributing to symptoms, and regimen for control. The client will practice health behaviors needed to manage the effects of MG and methods to prevent complications.	Teach client stress management techniques and methods to avoid infections. Teach clients to take medications at regularly scheduled times to maintain appropriate level. Encourage client to wear a Medic Alert bracelet indicating the name and dosage of medications being taken. Refer to the Myasthenia Gravis Foundation for information and support groups (see Resources).

Evaluation: Evaluate each outcome to determine how it has been met by the client.

SAMPLE NURSING CARE PLAN

The Client with Myasthenia Gravis

M.H., a 29-year-old mother of two preschool children, was diagnosed with myasthenia gravis 2 years ago. Initially, she had double vision and drooping eyelids, but after beginning a course of pyridostigmine bromide (Mestinon), she went into remission. Recently, she has been experiencing facial, neck, and chest muscle weakness and is now admitted to the hospital for evaluation. Occasionally, she has difficulty swallowing and breathing. Her thymus gland is enlarged. She has asked the nurse to teach her some strategies for managing this chronic illness.

NURSING DIAGNOSIS 1 *Ineffective Breathing Pattern* related to respiratory muscle fatigue as evidenced by facial, neck, and chest weakness

Nursing Outcomes Classification (NOC)
Respiratory Status: Ventilation

Nursing Interventions Classification (NIC)
Airway Management
Energy Management
Neurologic Monitoring

PLANNING/OUTCOMES	NURSING INTERVENTIONS	RATIONALE
M.H.'s respiratory rate and rhythm and breath sounds will remain within normal limits.	Assess M.H.'s breathing patterns q2h.	Detects early signs of respiratory distress.
	Ask M.H. to notify the nurse immediately if she has any breathing difficulties.	May be reluctant to call the nurse and needs to be encouraged to do so.
	Notify physician immediately if respiratory problems develop.	Physician must determine the cause and if a tracheostomy is needed.

SAMPLE NURSING CARE PLAN (Continued)

EVALUATION

M.H.'s respiratory rate and rhythm have remained within normal limits.

NURSING DIAGNOSIS 2 *Risk for Aspiration* related to impaired swallowing as evidenced by difficulty swallowing

Nursing Outcomes Classification (NOC)
Neurological Status
Respiratory Status: Ventilation

Nursing Interventions Classification (NIC)
Aspiration Precautions
Neurologic Monitoring

PLANNING/OUTCOMES	NURSING INTERVENTIONS	RATIONALE
M.H. will not experience aspiration.	Position M.H. to eat in a sitting position.	Promotes passage of food into the stomach.
	Teach M.H. the importance of thoroughly chewing food, and swallowing only small bites.	Can cause aspiration.
	Have oral suctioning equipment at the bedside.	Readily available if required.

EVALUATION

M.H. has not aspirated. She makes a point of always sitting up when eating.

NURSING DIAGNOSIS 3 *Deficient Knowledge*, related to disease process and understanding of methods to control effects of myasthenia gravis and prevent complications as evidenced by verbalization of need for future teaching

Nursing Outcomes Classification (NOC)
Knowledge: Disease Process
Knowledge: Energy Conservation

Nursing Interventions Classification (NIC)
Teaching: Disease Process
Teaching: Individual

PLANNING/OUTCOMES	NURSING INTERVENTIONS	RATIONALE
M.H. will practice health behaviors needed to manage the effects of MG and prevent complications.	Assess M.H.'s prior knowledge of MG and methods of controlling the effects of prescribed medications and preventing complications.	Provides a basis for planning teaching.
	Include M.H.'s family members in teaching sessions.	Fosters implementation of regimen at home.
	Teach M.H. and family members basic information about MG, the actions of anticholinesterase medication, the need to take it on a regular basis with a snack, side effects of overdose, and the importance of notifying the physician of any signs of respiratory problems or infection.	Information about one's disease, medications, and when to notify the physician is essential knowledge the client and family members need to effectively manage this chronic illness.

(*Continues*)

SAMPLE NURSING CARE PLAN (Continued)

PLANNING/OUTCOMES	NURSING INTERVENTIONS	RATIONALE
	Encourage M.H. to wear a Medic Alert bracelet, which lists here name, diagnoses, and dosage of prescribed medications.	Provides accurate information to medical personnel in case of an emergency.
	Provide M.H. with the address and telephone number of the Myasthenia Gravis Foundation and encourage her to contact them for additional information and support.	Facilitates future attainment of knowledge and possible involvement with a support group.

EVALUATION

M.H. and her husband related information about MG, action and side effects of Mestinon, signs and symptoms to watch for, and when to notify the physician. She has obtained a Medic Alert bracelet and has contacted the MG Foundation. She plans to attend the next local chapter meeting.

INADEQUATE IMMUNOLOGICAL RESPONSE

This category includes HIV/AIDS; pulmonary, gastrointestinal, oral, gynecological, and central nervous system opportunistic infections; and opportunistic malignancies.

HIV/AIDS

Although allergies are hypersensitive immune responses, and autoimmune diseases literally have the body attacking itself, acquired immunodeficiency syndrome (AIDS) is a disease that causes an inadequate immunological response by the body. The human immunodeficiency virus (HIV) may be acquired anytime after conception.

The **human immunodeficiency virus (HIV)**, a retrovirus that causes **acquired immunodeficiency syndrome (AIDS)**, was first reported in the United States in 1981. AIDS is a progressively fatal disease that destroys the immune system and the body's ability to fight infection. By the end of 2007, it was estimated that 33 million people in the world were living with HIV/AIDS (World Health Organization [WHO], 2008a). In the United States, 1,051,875 cases of AIDS had been reported by the end of 2007, and as many as 1,106,400 may be infected with HIV (CDC, 2008d).

Following exposure to HIV and an incubation period of 2 to 4 weeks, some individuals, but not all, will experience flulike symptoms such as fever, sweats, headache, myalgia, neuralgia, sore throat, GI distress, and photophobia (Figure 47-7). Many persons, if tested at this time, will test negative because antibodies may not yet be present in the blood. In 2 or 3 weeks, these symptoms disappear. Infected individuals are very infectious during this period, with large quantities of HIV present in genital secretions.

Most individuals will remain symptom free for years (10 or more), but some may begin to have symptoms in a few months. During this "asymptomatic" period, HIV is multiplying, infecting, and killing the CD4 T-cells of the immune system.

A variety of symptoms become evident as the CD4 T-cells disappear. Lymph nodes enlarged for more than 3 months are one of the first symptoms. Others may include weight loss, lack of energy, fevers and sweats, persistent skin rashes or flaky skin, persistent or frequent oral or vaginal yeast infections, PID that does not respond to treatment, and short-term memory loss. Oral, genital, or anal herpes infection or shingles may also develop.

When the CD4 T-cell count is less than 200 cells/mm^3 (healthy persons have 1,000 or more CD4 cells/mm^3) and

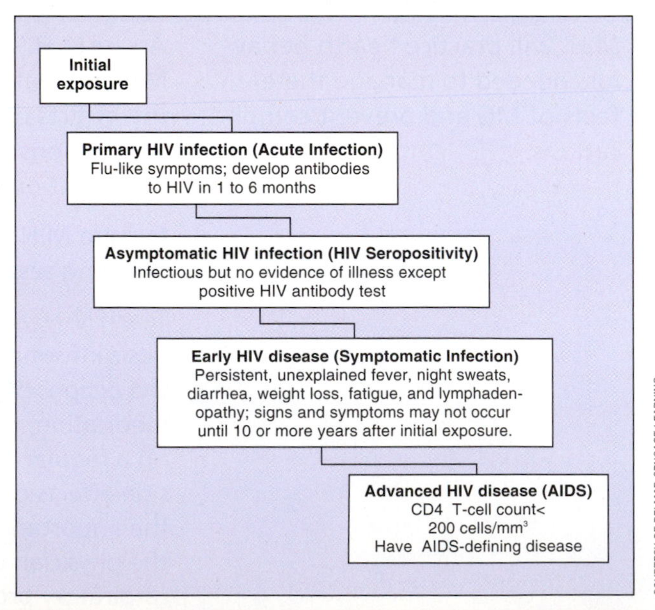

FIGURE 47-7 Continuum of HIV Disease

PROFESSIONALTIP

Prevention for Health Care Workers

Health care workers are at risk for contracting HIV because of being near blood, semen, vaginal fluids, and placentas. The health care worker needs to follow standard precautions and wear gloves at all times when in contact with these fluids. The health care worker should wear goggles and a gown if there is potential of HIV contaminated fluids spraying or splashing into their eyes or on their clothes.

the individual has 1 or more of the 26 clinical conditions that affect persons with advanced HIV disease, the individual is considered to have AIDS. Most of the AIDS-defining conditions are **opportunistic infections** (infections in persons with a defective immune system that rarely cause harm in healthy individuals). Tuberculosis is the most common life-threatening opportunistic infection affecting people living with HIV/AIDS (WHO, 2008b). It kills nearly 250,000 people living with HIV each year, and is the leading cause of death among HIV-infected people living in Africa (WHO, 2008b).

The **enzyme-linked immunosorbent assay (ELISA)** is the basic screening test to detect antibodies to HIV. A positive test result is always retested to rule out false-positive results and/or technician error. A confirmatory test, the **Western blot** test, is always employed when the ELISA test is positive. Results of both the ELISA and Western blot taken together have an extremely high accuracy rate.

Obtaining a signed informed consent for testing is often a nursing responsibility. Most states mandate a consent form solely for HIV testing. Some states allow verbal consent and a statement of the client's consent signed by the health care provider.

The FDA has approved the OraQuick Rapid HIV-1 Antibody Test, which provides results with over 99.3% accuracy in 20 minutes (FDA, 2004).

Demographics of AIDS in the United States

Demographics are viewed in terms of clients' age, gender, and race.

Age

AIDS mainly affects people during the most productive years of their life. As of 2007, the age group with the highest number of new HIV diagnoses (219, 601 cases) was persons between the ages of 35-39 (CDC, 2009).The estimated number of new cases of AIDS among individuals younger than 13 in the United States fell from 954 in 1992 to 28 in 2007 (CDC, 2009).

Gender

Trends in HIV-related mortality reflect changes in the demographic patterns of the HIV epidemic. Although more men than women are infected with HIV, the number of AIDS cases in women in the United States has increased from 7% in 1985 to 25% in 2001. By the end of 2005, the proportion had decreased to 23% (CDC, 2008c).

Race

Of the new AIDS cases reported in the United States in 2005:

- African Americans accounted for 71.3/100,000 population.
- Hispanic Americans accounted for 27.8/100,000 population.
- Caucasians accounted for 8.8/100,000 population.
- American Indian/Alaska Natives accounted for 10.4/100,000 population.
- Asian American/Pacific Islanders accounted for 7.4/100,000 population (CDC, 2008)

The HIV/AIDS epidemic is growing most rapidly among some minority populations (see Figure 47-8) and is a leading cause of death of African-American men ages 25 to 44 (CDC, 2009b).

Modes of Transmission

There are many way to become infected with HIV. The virus may be found in blood, semen, vaginal secretions, and breast milk of infected individuals. There is no evidence that HIV is spread through sweat, tears, urine, or feces. The saliva of infected individuals has the virus, but there is no evidence that it is spread to others through kissing. The risk of infection from "deep kissing" and oral sex is unknown. Tissue transplantation (including artificial insemination), blood transfusion, and needlesticks are high-risk situations but are relatively rare methods of transmission in the United States today. Having another sexually transmitted infection such as chlamydia, genital herpes, syphilis, or gonorrhea seems to make an individual more susceptible to becoming infected with HIV during sexual intercourse with an infected partner. Theoretically, HIV is present in sufficient quantities in amniotic fluid, cerebrospinal fluid, pleural fluid, peritoneal fluid, and pericardial fluid whereby infection could occur with exchange of these body fluids, particularly in health care settings where contact with these fluids may occur. Behaviors associated with increased risk of sexual transmission of HIV by infected persons include unprotected sexual intercourse, multiple sex partners, failure to disclose HIV status, and trading sex for money or drugs.

LIFE SPAN CONSIDERATIONS

Life Span Considerations

Mark Cichocki (2007) wrote in an article for amazon.com titled *HIV and the Older Adult—A Growing Population*, that there is a myth regarding the population aged 50 years and older not having sex. This age group is sexually active, contracting HIV, and needs to be assessed closely and asked the same questions as the other population age groups as to their sexual behaviors. The 50 years of age and older population also need to be educated about HIV, and how it is contracted to help reduce the risk of transmission.

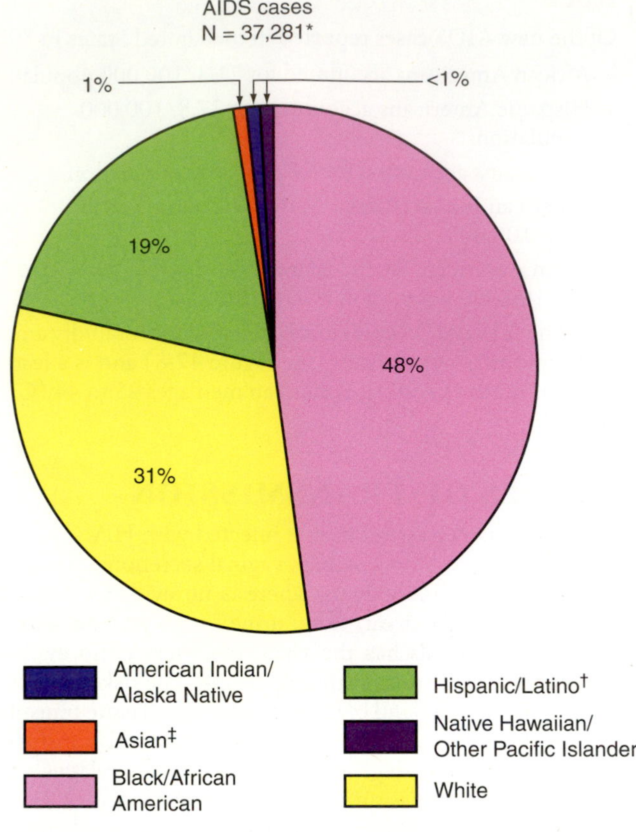

FIGURE 47-8 **Percentages of AIDS Cases by Race/Ethnicity in 2007** (*Centers for Dieseas Control and Prevention, 2009b, Atlanta, GA.*)

Transmission of HIV can also take place by having contact with infected blood or sharing needles or syringes; it may also transmit from mother to fetus during pregnancy or birth.

Sexual intercourse (anal, oral, vaginal) without using a condom is the most frequently reported risk behavior for infection with HIV. Injection-drug use is the second most frequently reported risk behavior for infection with HIV. When HIV seropositive women take zidovudine (AZT) during pregnancy and labor and zidovudine is given to the newborn, perinatal transmission is significantly reduced.

Medical–Surgical Management

Medical

The goal of care is to keep the disease from progressing for as long as possible. The client's chance of disease progression can now be monitored by a viral load test that measures copies of HIV RNA. The approved **viral load test** is the Amplicor HIV-1 Monitor test, better known as the *polymerase chain*

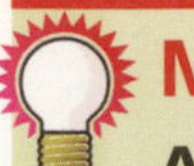

MEMORY TRICK

ABCs of HIV/AIDS Prevention

To protect oneself from acquiring HIV/AIDS, remember these **ABC**s:

A = Abstinence

B = Be Faithful

C = Condoms

(CDC, 2008)

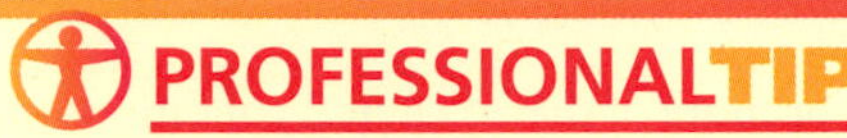

HIV Testing

Although physicians are responsible for client counseling, the nurse must know the information to be able to answer questions and clarify the client's knowledge. Pretest counseling should include the following:

- Ask why the client believes the test should be done.
- Explain the meaning of a positive or negative test result and the possibility of a false-negative result.
- Discuss risk reduction and ways to modify behavior.
- Share state reporting requirements.
- Ensure confidentiality of test results.
- Explain that there is often stress related to test results and possible reactions to learning the results, such as depression or anxiety.
- Discuss the potential negative social consequences of positive results.
- Assist the client in making a decision about testing.
- Arrange a return appointment for the client to receive test results.

Post-test counseling should include the following:

- Review the test results with the client.
- Assess the client's understanding of the test results.
- Allow the client to express feelings about the test results.
- Review routes of HIV transmission.
- Assess the client's psychological condition including the risk for suicide.
- Assess the client's risk behavior and strategies for reducing risk.
- Provide information about support groups and national/ local resources.

reaction (PCR) test.* It can be used to see if individuals with HIV are at risk for getting sick, for checking the effects of drugs taken by individuals with HIV to see if they are working against the virus, and to distinguish the difference between actual HIV infection in a newborn and maternally acquired antibodies. The "ultra-sensitive" PCR test can measure as few as 50 copies/mL of HIV RNA. There is no "safe" level of viral load. The risk is less, but HIV can be passed to another person if the viral load is undetectable.

Pharmacological

The goal of anti-HIV treatment is to keep the viral load as low as possible for as long as possible, ideally below what the viral load test can detect. Currently available antiretroviral drugs do not cure HIV/AIDS. Treatment is usually begun at the time of **seroconversion** (evidence of antibody formation in response to disease or vaccine). In high-risk occupational exposures, treatment may be started immediately.

One group of drugs, called *nucleoside analog reverse transcriptase inhibitors* (NRTIs), interrupt HIV's life cycle at an early stage. The spread of HIV in the body may be slowed and the onset of opportunistic infections may be delayed by NRTIs, but these drugs do not prevent HIV transmission to other individuals. This group includes zidovudine (Retrovir), formerly known as AZT, zalcitabine (Hivid), didanosine (Videx), stavudine (Zerit), lamivudine (Epivir), and abacavir (Ziagen). A combination of zidovudine and lamivudine (Combivir) is available. Zidovudine (Retrovir) may cause depletion of red or white blood cells. If this depletion is severe, the drug must be discontinued. Painful nerve damage and pancreatitis may be caused by didanosine (Videx).

Non-nucleoside reverse transcriptase inhibitors (NNRTIs) are available to be used only in combination with other antiretroviral drugs. These include delavirdine (Rescriptor), nevirapine (Viramune), and efavirenz (Sustiva).

The protease inhibitors interrupt HIV's life cycle at a later step. These include ritonavir (Norvir), saquinavir mesylate (Fortovase, Invirase), indinavir sulfate (Crixivan), and nelfinavir mesylate (Viracept). Nausea, diarrhea, and other GI symptoms are common side effects of protease inhibitors.

HIV can become resistant to any of three drugs, so combination treatments are necessary to effectively suppress the virus. When NRTIs and protease inhibitors are combined, it is referred to as highly active antiretroviral therapy or HAART. Researchers credit HAART with significantly reducing the number of AIDS deaths in the United States. Current guidelines recommend drug therapy for any client with symptomatic HIV disease (evidence of opportunistic infections or tumors). For asymptomatic HIV-positive clients, drug therapy is recommended if:

- Viral load test results are greater than 500 copies/mL,

or

- The client's CD4 T-cell count is under 500 cells/mm^3.

Health Promotion

The CDC and the Occupational Safety and Health Administration (OSHA) have developed Standard Precautions to reduce the risk of health care personnel exposure to blood and body fluids. Personal protective equipment should be worn while caring for all clients when there is a reasonable likelihood of contact with any blood or body fluids.

CRITICAL THINKING

HIV and Lifestyle

How might a person's lifestyle change after receiving a diagnosis of being HIV positive?

PULMONARY OPPORTUNISTIC INFECTIONS

Conditions discussed following include *pneumocystis carinii* pneumonia, histoplasmosis, and tuberculosis.

PNEUMOCYSTIS CARINII PNEUMONIA

Pneumocystis carinii pneumonia (PCP) is the most common serious infection among HIV-infected individuals. PCP can be prevented and treated, yet it also can be fatal. A marked decrease in the number of AIDS clients diagnosed with PCP is a result of initiation of prophylactic treatment when the CD4 T-cell count is 200 or less/mm^3. Although *Pneumocystis carinii* is found primarily in the lungs, it has also been reported in the adrenal glands, bone marrow, skin, thyroid, kidneys, and spleen of persons with AIDS.

Clinical signs and symptoms include fever, dyspnea, nonproductive cough, and crackles. Initial diagnosis is made by chest x-ray, which shows diffuse infiltrates. Fiber-optic bronchoscopy is the procedure of choice to obtain a definitive diagnosis. During the bronchoscopy, sputum is obtained to demonstrate the presence of the organism.

Current standard treatment for PCP includes either intravenous pentamidine isethionate (Pneumopent, Pentam 300) or sulfamethoxazole-trimethoprim (Bactrim, Septra), given orally or intravenously. Oral sulfamethoxazole-trimethoprim is the treatment of choice; however, approximately one-third of people with AIDS eventually develop hypersensitivity reactions and must switch to pentamidine for primary therapy. Prophylaxis against PCP is a therapeutic necessity for all persons infected with HIV when the CD4 T-cell count is 200 or less. Primary prophylaxis refers to therapy for those considered at risk for PCP based on the CD4 count to prevent infection with PCP. Secondary prophylaxis refers to therapy to prevent recurrences in clients who have already had PCP. Current guidelines recommend either oral sulfamethoxazole-trimethoprim or aerosolized pentamidine for prophylaxis. For those allergic to sulfamethoxazole-trimethoprim, pentamidine diluted in sterile water administered by a Respigard II nebulizer can be used.

HISTOPLASMOSIS

Histoplasmosis is an infection caused by the fungus *Histoplasma capsulatum.* The fungus has been isolated in bird droppings, dirt from chicken coops, and caves. The spores from the fungus are introduced into the body by inhalation. Histoplasmosis is not specific to the lung. In most clients with HIV disease, histoplasmosis is disseminated (spread out).

Histoplasmosis should be suspected if the person presents with fever of uncertain origin, cough, and malaise.

The diagnosis is confirmed by culture or biopsy of the bone marrow, blood, lymph nodes, lungs, or skin. Initial treatment of histoplasmosis is usually IV amphotericin B. Oral ketoconazole (Nizoral) can be used for maintenance therapy. Prophylaxis against recurrence of histoplasmosis is provided by itraconazole (Sporanox).

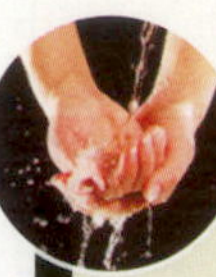

INFECTION CONTROL

TB

A densely woven, snug-fitting mask (N95 particulate respirator) should be worn by all persons in contact with the person who has TB until the person has received treatment for 2 to 3 weeks. Persons with TB should also be taught to cover their mouths while coughing and should wear a particulate respirator when they are out of their room for tests.

TUBERCULOSIS

Mycobacterium tuberculosis, an acid-fast aerobic bacterium, is the cause of tuberculosis (TB). It is spread through airborne particles and enters the body by inhalation. The particles usually lodge in the apex of the lungs; however, one-half to two-thirds of cases of HIV-associated or AIDS-associated TB involve organs outside the lungs as well.

Clinical manifestations include fever, night sweats, cough, and weight loss. People with AIDS will commonly present with a productive cough and pleuritic pain. Diagnosis is made by a combination of tests: skin testing with purified protein derivative (PPD); examination and culture of sputum, urine, and other fluids; x-rays; and other tests such as IVP.

The most common test for exposure to TB is the Mantoux skin test, which consists of injecting 0.1 mL of (PPD) intradermally. A negative reaction does not rule out infection. HIV-positive clients with a CD4 count lower than 200/mm3 may no longer have an immune response to the PPD. The chest x-ray may reveal middle and lower lobe infiltrates. A sputum specimen is smeared and stained with an acid-fast stain, then examined under the microscope for acid-fast bacillus (AFB). Other body fluids such as urine, blood, and stool may also be tested for AFB.

The risk of transmission of TB to health care workers is highest during and immediately after procedures that induce coughing. In the home and health care setting, cough-inducing procedures should be performed only in well-ventilated areas.

Because of the upsurge of multidrug-resistant TB (MDR-TB), the CDC recommends treating with multiple medications. Treatment is provided in two phases. In the initial treatment phase, the client receives isoniazid (Laniazid), rifampin (Rifadin), pyrazinamide, and ethambutol Hcl (Myambutol) or streptomycin sulfate for 2 to 6 months, depending on whether *Mycobacterium tuberculosis* is identified outside the lungs. In the continuation phase, treatment with two to four of the medications used in the initial phase is indicated for 4 to 6 months longer.

Nursing Management

Monitor vital signs and laboratory test results. Encourage fluid intake of 2.5 to 3 L per day. Administer oxygen and medications as ordered. Encourage the use of an incentive spirometer, unless contraindicated. Reposition client at least every 2 hours. Plan for client rest periods during the day.

NURSING PROCESS

Assessment

Subjective Data

Assess the client's ability to dress, bathe, ambulate, and so on. Note the client's perception of breathlessness.

Objective Data

Assess the client's respiratory rate, depth, and breath sounds. Note cough (productive or nonproductive), cyanosis, dyspnea, use of accessory muscles, and fever. Monitor arterial blood gas (ABG) results for decreased PaO2, increased PaCO2, and decreased pH.

Nursing diagnoses for the HIV-positive client with pulmonary disorders include the following:

NURSING DIAGNOSES	PLANNING/OUTCOMES	NURSING INTERVENTIONS
Ineffective Airway Clearance related to chronic, unrelieved cough, pain, or viscous secretions	The client will mobilize secretions effectively.	Administer 2.5–3 L of fluid per day (oral or IV) to decrease thick secretions and medications as ordered to suppress cough and decrease pain. Reposition client every 2 hours and PRN.
Impaired Gas Exchange related to inadequate ventilation/oxygenation	The client will maintain an SaO_2 > 90%.	Administer oxygen as ordered. Encourage use of incentive spirometer, if not contraindicated.

Nursing diagnoses for the HIV-positive client with pulmonary disorders include the following: (Continued)

NURSING DIAGNOSES	PLANNING/OUTCOMES	NURSING INTERVENTIONS
Ineffective Breathing Pattern related to fatigue	The client will pace activities to minimize fatigue.	Plan care to allow rest periods.

Evaluation: Evaluate each outcome to determine how it has been met by the client.

GASTROINTESTINAL OPPORTUNISTIC INFECTIONS

Disorders discussed following include *Mycobacterium avium* complex, cytomegalovirus, cryptosporidiosis, hepatitis, and HIV-wasting syndrome.

MYCOBACTERIUM AVIUM COMPLEX

Mycobacterium avium and *Mycobacterium intracellulare* are two closely related mycobacteria that are grouped together and called *Mycobacterium avium* complex (MAC). The source of exposure to MAC for humans is contaminated water, although it has been isolated from soil, dust, sediments, and aerosols. In persons with AIDS, MAC involvement of the bowel is usually extensive, suggesting that the gastrointestinal tract may be the site of initial infection, with spread to other organs after that. The microorganism can fill the bone marrow and lymph nodes.

The most common symptoms of MAC include chronic fever, malaise, anemia, weight loss, diarrhea, and abdominal pain. Often the client will appear cachectic because of malabsorption. Because the symptoms are nonspecific, MAC is often difficult to distinguish from other AIDS-related infections. MAC is usually disseminated at the time of diagnosis. Diagnosis is made by tissue biopsy and cultures of the lung, bone marrow, lymph nodes, liver, or blood.

Treatment for MAC infection may include one or more of the following medications: clarithromycin (Biaxin Filmtabs) to treat disseminated MAC; and a combination of amikacin sulfate (Amikin), azithromycin (Zithromax), ciprofloxacin hydrochloride (Cipro), cycloserine (Seromycin), and ethionamide (Trecator-SC). For persons with AIDS who have a CD4 count of less than 75/mm^3, rifabutin (Mycobutin) is recommended for prevention of disseminated MAC.

CYTOMEGALOVIRUS

Cytomegalovirus (CMV) belongs to the herpes virus group. Thus it shares the same phenomena of latency and reactivation. The virus lies dormant in tissues waiting to be reactivated in the immunocompromised client. The potential for infection with CMV is increased during two periods: the perinatal period through the preschool years, and later during the sexually active years.

CMV causes disease by destroying the brain, lung, retina, and liver, CMV infection has been identified in all parts of the gastrointestinal tract from the oral cavity to the perianal area. CMV can be life-threatening for persons with suppressed immune systems. Persons with HIV infection or AIDS may develop severe infections, including CMV retinitis that can lead to blindness.

Signs and symptoms of CMV include weight loss, fever, diarrhea, and malaise. The diagnosis of CMV is based on microscopic identification of CMV from specific organs such as the brain, lung, liver, or adrenal gland. Ganciclovir sodium (Cytovene) is the drug of choice for treating individuals infected with CMV. Maintenance therapy is required to prevent relapse. Intravenous foscarnet sodium (Foscavir) has been approved as an alternative therapy.

CRYPTOSPORIDIOSIS

Cryptosporidium, a protozoan causing cryptosporidiosis, usually infects the epithelial cells that line the digestive tract. Transmission is often by the fecal-oral route, but can be spread from animal to person as well as person to person. *Cryptosporidium* can also be spread by ingesting contaminated food and water.

Clinical signs and symptoms include profuse watery diarrhea. Abdominal pain, serious weight loss, abdominal cramping, anorexia, low-grade fever, dehydration, electrolyte imbalance, and malaise may also be present. Diagnosis is made by identifying the organism in fresh stool specimens.

There is no effective treatment for cryptosporidiosis. Antidiarrheals such as diphenoxylate hydrochloride with atropine sulfate (Lomotil), loperamide hydrochloride (Imodium), and opium tincture (Paregoric) should be given on a programmed schedule rather than PRN. Treatment is palliative and focused toward the symptoms. This includes fluid and electrolyte replacement (orally if possible), analgesics, and occasionally the use of total parenteral nutrition (TPN). Anticryptosporidial agents are under investigation. Protecting the integrity of the client's perianal skin is extremely important. A low-residue, high-protein, high-calorie diet helps maintain nutritional status.

HEPATITIS

Only hepatitis B virus (HBV), hepatitis C virus (HCV), and hepatitis D virus (HDV) are commonly seen with HIV infection. All three viruses have been associated with chronic infection and have similar transmission and risk factors. Risk factors include exposure to blood or blood products, exposure to contaminated needles and syringes, and multiple sexual contacts.

Signs and symptoms include malaise, weakness, anorexia, nausea, vomiting, and right upper quadrant pain. Abnormalities in bilirubin and hepatic enzymes may also occur. Diagnosis is made by serologic assays identifying antigens and antibodies.

Interferon has been approved for treatment of chronic HBV and HCV and is being investigated for the treatment of HDV. Response to therapy varies but is decreased with HIV infection.

HIV-WASTING SYNDROME

HIV-wasting syndrome is defined as unexplained weight loss of more than 10% of body weight accompanied by weakness, chronic diarrhea, and fever in those infected with HIV. Weight loss and malnutrition are related to reduced food intake, malabsorption of nutrients, and altered metabolism of nutrients. Some of the factors related to reduced intake include anorexia, oral or esophageal lesions, nausea, neurologic or psychiatric conditions, fatigue, inadequate finances, and side effects of medications. Nutritional malabsorption is related to injury of the small intestine caused by opportunistic infections or by HIV infection of the cells in the gastrointestinal tract. Opportunistic infections produce fever that depletes the body's energy stores and causes weight loss.

Signs and symptoms of HIV-wasting syndrome are anorexia, diarrhea, nausea, vomiting, changes in taste and smell, aphthous ulcers of mouth and esophagus, and abdominal pain.

Symptom control is the major focus for HIV-wasting syndrome. Medications to control nausea and vomiting should be given routinely, not PRN. Treatment of anorexia includes megestrol acetate (Megace) or dronabinol (Marinol). Antimotility drugs such as loperamide hydrochloride (Imodium), luminal acting agents such as kaolin and pectin mixture (Kaopectate) and hormonal agents such as octreotide acetate (Sandostatin) are used to treat diarrhea. This makes eating much easier. Oral nutritional supplements are most frequently used for weight loss. TPN is usually considered a final option except in cases of severe malnutrition, because of the risk and expense involved.

Nursing Management

Monitor stools for blood, fat, and undigested food. Keep perirectal area clean and protect with ointment as ordered. Have a schedule for turning the client. Encourage the client to drink fluids between meals and to use hard candy or chewing gum to stimulate saliva production. Monitor laboratory test results. Provide a prescribed diet in small frequent meals at room temperature. Assist with oral hygiene before and after meals. Weigh client daily. Administer antiemetics and antidiarrheals as ordered.

NURSING PROCESS

Assessment

Subjective Data

Ask the client about bowel habits and what causes and relieves diarrhea. Inquire about alcohol consumption because excessive alcohol intake depletes B vitamins and provides no nutrition. Note activities that cause fatigue. Discuss food likes/dislikes, food intolerances, and food intake for the previous 3 days.

Objective Data

Assess the client's skin integrity, including temperature, moisture, color, vascularity, texture, lesions, areas of excoriation, and wound healing. Note fever, weight, and daily nutritional intake. Monitor laboratory values of nutritional status, including serum albumin, total protein, hemoglobin, and hematocrit, as well as stool specimens for ova and parasites.

Nursing diagnoses for the HIV-positive client with gastrointestinal disorders include the following:

NURSING DIAGNOSES	PLANNING/OUTCOMES	NURSING INTERVENTIONS
Deficient Fluid Volume related to nausea, vomiting, diarrhea, or inadequate oral intake	The client will have normal skin turgor and decreased frequency and amount of stools.	Suggest client use hard candy or chewing gum to stimulate saliva production if mouth is dry. Encourage client to drink liquids between (not with) meals. Monitor and record intake and output. Monitor client for evidence of electrolyte imbalance (hypokalemia, hypochloremia, confusion, muscle weakness).
Imbalanced Nutrition: Less than Body Requirements related to anorexia, dysphagia, malabsorption, or side effects of medications	The client will eat 75% of prescribed diet and maintain current weight.	Provide the prescribed diet (usually low-residue, high-calorie, high-protein) in small frequent meals at room temperature. Provide oral hygiene before and after meals to enhance taste sensation.
		Offer commercially prepared nutritional supplements between meals. Weigh client daily. Administer supplemental vitamins and minerals as prescribed.

Nursing diagnoses for the HIV-positive client with gastrointestinal disorders include the following: (Continued)

NURSING DIAGNOSES	PLANNING/OUTCOMES	NURSING INTERVENTIONS
		Administer antiemetics and antidiarrheals as ordered. Teach client to keep a food diary and a log of exacerbation and remission of signs and symptoms.
Risk for Impaired Skin Integrity related to diarrhea, malnutrition, decreased mobility	The client will maintain skin integrity.	Monitor stool for presence of blood, fat, undigested food and stool cultures for evidence of new infections. Protect the perirectal area by keeping it clean and using compounds such as Aloe Vesta cream. Avoid prolonged pressure on bony prominences by a scheduled turning plan. If nonambulatory, provide client with a pressure relief mattress. Use soft sheets on the bed and avoid wrinkles. Teach client to use nondrying soaps and to pat skin dry.
Evaluation: Evaluate each outcome to determine how it has been met by the client.		

ORAL OPPORTUNISTIC INFECTIONS

Candidiasis and leukoplakia are discussed following.

ORAL AND ESOPHAGEAL CANDIDIASIS

Oral candidiasis (thrush) is a fungal infection caused by *Candida albicans* (Figure 47-9), and usually only appears if CD4 levels fall below 300 (Mayo Clinic, 2007). Many clients complain of an unpleasant taste or mouth dryness. Other clinical signs and symptoms include creamy, white oral plaques and mucosal tenderness. When the white oral plaques are wiped off, they leave an erythematous or even bleeding mucosal lesions. Esophageal candidiasis, an AIDS-defining disease, causes dysphagia and painful swallowing.

These symptoms may interfere with the client's eating, nutrition, and weight. Diagnosis is established by the presence of the characteristic lesions in the oral cavity. Microscopic examination of oral or esophageal lesions reveals budding yeast cells.

Treatment for esophageal candidiasis is oral fluconazole (Diflucan). Oral candidiasis is treated with nystatin suspension (Mycostatin) and clotrimazole (Mycelex Troches). Another medication used to treat candidiasis is ketoconazole (Nizoral). Amphotericin B (Amphotericin B) is used to treat disseminated candida infection. The antiulcer drug sucralfate (Carafate) may be used as a slurry to relieve mouth pain before eating.

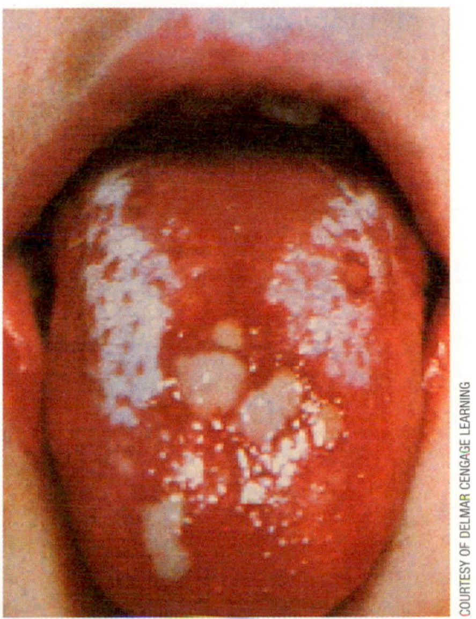
COURTESY OF DELMAR CENGAGE LEARNING

FIGURE 47-9 Oral Candidiasis (Thrush)

ORAL HAIRY LEUKOPLAKIA

Oral hairy leukoplakia (OHL) usually appears as a white patch on the lateral borders of the tongue as shown in Figure 47-10. It is caused by the Epstein-Barr virus. The lesions are rarely in other areas of the mouth and are different in appearance from candidiasis. The irregular surface of the lesion appears as projections that resemble hairs and cannot be scraped off. Diagnosis is made by visual inspection of the lesion. OHL is not usually bothersome to the client and may regress spontaneously. No treatment is necessary for most cases of OHL; however, oral acyclovir (Zovirax) may be given to selected clients.

NURSING MANAGEMENT

Assess oral cavity frequently. Assist with oral hygiene before and after meals. Administer prescribed medications. Teach

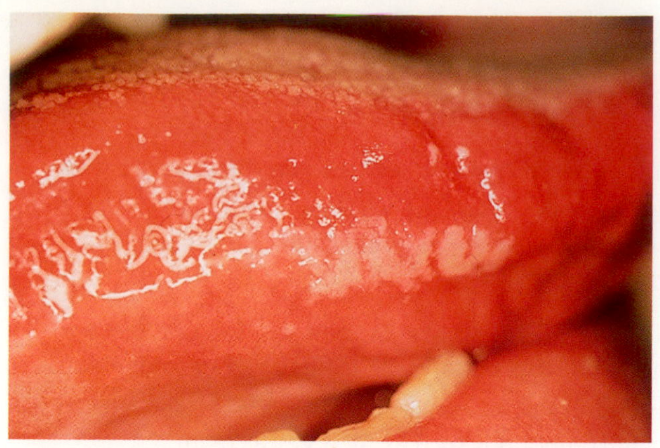

FIGURE 47-10 Oral Hairy Leukoplakia (*Courtesy of Dr. Joseph Konzelman, School of Dentistry, Medical College of Georgia.*)

client to avoid mouthwashes containing alcohol or glycerine because they are very drying.

NURSING PROCESS

ASSESSMENT

Subjective Data

Assess the client's symptoms and oral hygiene habits. Ask about recent nutritional intake, use of alcohol and tobacco, and current medications.

Objective Data

Assess the client's lips, tongue, and buccal mucosal surfaces for lesions, white cheesy patches, and bleeding. Note any difficulty swallowing.

A nursing diagnosis for an HIV-positive client with oral manifestations is:

NURSING DIAGNOSES	PLANNING/OUTCOMES	NURSING INTERVENTIONS
*Impaired **O**ral Mucous Membrane* related to oral lesions	The client will be free from oral lesions.	Administer prescribed medications. Frequently assess the oral cavity. Provide oral hygiene with a small soft toothbrush before and after meals. Instruct client to avoid commercial mouthwashes containing alcohol or glycerine.

Evaluation: Evaluate each outcome to determine how it has been met by the client.

GYNECOLOGICAL OPPORTUNISTIC INFECTIONS

Gynecological infections discussed include vaginal candidiasis and cervical intraepithelial neoplasia.

VAGINAL CANDIDIASIS

Vaginal candidiasis is a fungal infection caused by *Candida albicans*. It is the most common initial infection occurring in HIV-infected women. Clinical manifestations include a white, clumped-appearing vaginal discharge, vaginal wall inflammation, and vaginal itching. Diagnosis is made by microscopic identification of yeast.

Most cases of vaginal candidiasis are treated with topical antifungal agents such as clotrimazole (Gyne-Lotrimin). For clients who do not respond to treatment with clotrimazole, ketoconazole (Nizoral) or fluconazole (Diflucan) is recommended.

CERVICAL INTRAEPITHELIAL NEOPLASIA

Women infected with HIV have a much higher incidence of cervical intraepithelial neoplasia (CIN) than women who are not infected. CIN and cancer of the cervix are considered to be on a continuum of abnormal cervical cells, ranging from mild abnormality (Grade I) to severe abnormality and cancer Grade III). CIN in HIV-infected women progresses more rapidly and is less responsive to standard treatments than in noninfected women. Factors related to increased risk of CIN in HIV-positive women include a decreased number of CD4 T-cells and infection with human papilloma virus (HPV). It is thought that HIV activates HPV, causing cellular abnormalities.

The early stages of CIN have no symptoms. Clinical manifestations of cervical cancer include painless postcoital bleeding and blood-tinged vaginal discharge. As CIN progresses, back pain, abdominal or pelvic pain, weight loss, anorexia, and leg edema caused by obstruction of lymph nodes may occur. Initial diagnosis is made by Pap smear to determine the presence of abnormal cells. Clients with abnormal Pap smears are referred for cervical biopsy and colposcopy.

Treatment for CIN includes laser therapy, conization, and hysterectomy. Treatment for invasive cervical cancer depends on the stage of the disease and may include chemotherapy, surgery, and radiation.

NURSING MANAGEMENT

Encourage the client to have a Pap test every 6 months, to keep vaginal area clean and dry, and to wear loose-fitting cotton underwear. Inquire about bleeding following sexual intercourse, pelvic and abdominal pain, and vaginal itching or discharge.

NURSING PROCESS

ASSESSMENT

Subjective Data

Assess the client's history of symptoms, and ask the client about bleeding after intercourse, abdominal and pelvic pain, and vaginal itching or discharge.

Objective Data

Assess vaginal discharge for white or blood-tinged secretions. Note weight loss and edema.

Nursing diagnoses for a female HIV-positive client with gynecological manifestations include the following:

NURSING DIAGNOSES	PLANNING/OUTCOMES	NURSING INTERVENTIONS
Impaired Tissue Integrity related to vaginal mucosal lesions	The client will be free of vaginal infections.	Teach the client to have Pap smears every 6 months. Assess the frequency and consistency of vaginal discharge. Teach client to keep the vaginal area clean and dry and to wear loose-fitting cotton underwear to prevent irritation.
Disturbed Body Image related to chronic vaginal infections or surgery, radiation, or removal of cervix	The client will verbalize feelings and concerns about body image.	Encourage client to verbalize feelings and concerns about body image. Refer client to a support group for women with HIV.

Evaluation: Evaluate each outcome to determine how it has been met by the client.

CENTRAL NERVOUS SYSTEM OPPORTUNISTIC INFECTIONS

Disorders covered include AIDS dementia complex, toxoplasmosis, and cryptococcosis.

AIDS DEMENTIA COMPLEX

The most common central nervous system complication in persons with AIDS is AIDS dementia complex (ADC). This disorder is chronic and progressive, with cognitive, motor, and behavioral dysfunction. ADC is caused by infection of glial cells in the brain with HIV. Signs and symptoms are sometimes vague during the initial stages of ADC. Early signs include poor concentration, forgetfulness, loss of balance, leg weakness, apathy, and social withdrawal. Clients with advanced ADC may exhibit psychotic behaviors and delirium and progress to a catatonic-like state with minimal responsiveness to the environment.

Diagnosis is made by neurological testing of cognitive, motor, and behavioral functioning. Other diagnostic tests include brain imaging to look for cerebral atrophy. Cerebrospinal fluid analysis can show elevated proteins and will exclude other pathogens. Clients treated with zidovudine (Retrovir) have shown a delay in disease progression in asymptomatic HIV-infected clients (FDA, 2003).

TOXOPLASMOSIS

Toxoplasmosis is caused by the protozoan *Toxoplasma gondii*. Cats and other animals serve as a reservoir for this organism. It is spread to humans by ingestion of oocytes found in contaminated water, soil, or food, especially raw or undercooked meat. After entering the body, *Toxoplasma gondii* reproduces and spreads via the blood or lymph system. A person with an intact immune system may have no symptoms or mild symptoms, and the organism may remain dormant for years. In the immunocompromised person, the infection may be reactivated (secondary) or occur with the ingestion of oocytes from contaminated sources. Clinical signs and symptoms may be vague and nonspecific, or range from a mild headache, fever, and lethargy to poor coordination, seizures, and coma. Diagnosis is made by identification of a lesion through brain imaging (computerized tomography or magnetic resonance imaging), presence of serum antibodies to *Toxoplasma gondii*, and recent onset of a neurologic abnormality.

The treatment of choice is oral pyrimethamine (Daraprim) and sulfadiazine (Microsulfon). Lifelong suppressive therapy of pyrimethamine plus sulfadiazine and leukovorin calcium (Wellcovorin) is needed.

CRYPTOCOCCOSIS

Cryptococcosis is a fungal infection caused by *Cryptococcus neoformans*. Cryptococcosis is one of the most life-threatening fungal infections in clients with AIDS (National Institutes of Health, 2008). The organism is acquired in the environment, usually from bird droppings. In the noncompromised host, the fungus is inhaled and contained in the lungs. In the immunocompromised host with AIDS, *Cryptococcus neoformans* can be disseminated, remain in the lungs, or infect the brain and meninges. Clinical manifestations include fever, headache, nausea and vomiting, dizziness, photophobia, mental status changes, seizures, and a stiff neck. Detection of cryptococcal antigen in cerebrospinal fluid, urine, or blood can be used for diagnosis. If untreated, this condition is fatal.

Treatment for acute cryptococcal infections includes intravenous amphotericin B (Fungizone Intravenous) to be given for at least 2 weeks, followed by fluconazole (Diflucan) for 10 to 12 weeks. Once treatment for acute infection is complete, lifelong suppressive therapy with oral fluconazole daily is recommended.

Nursing Management

Monitor client for forgetfulness, poor concentration, loss of balance, leg weakness, social withdrawal, apathy, stiff neck, seizures, nausea, and headache. Assess vital signs. Provide cues for orientation (e.g., calendar, clock) and a structured environment and activities for social interaction.

NURSING PROCESS

Assessment

Subjective Data

Ask the client about forgetfulness, missing appointments, ability to complete activities of daily living, and if there have been any recent falls or accidents. Ask the client's family and significant others about behavior changes such as social withdrawal or unusual behavior.

Objective Data

Assess the client for subtle mental status changes such as poor concentration and inability to remember instructions or previous conversations. Assess the client for motor impairment such as dropping things, poor coordination, or changes in writing ability. Assess the client's ability to remember usual medication schedule. Observe the environment for safety.

Nursing diagnoses for an HIV-positive client with central nervous system manifestations include the following:

NURSING DIAGNOSES	PLANNING/OUTCOMES	NURSING INTERVENTIONS
Disturbed Thought Processes related to mental status changes	The client will maintain cognitive functioning.	Assess client's mental and neurologic status and emotional, cognitive, and motor skills. Provide cues for orientation (clock, calendar). Monitor client for adherence to medical regimen.
Social Isolation related to alteration in mental status	The client will have contact and interact with significant others.	Encourage family and significant others to visit client. Provide structured activities and environment for social interaction. Encourage client to verbalize feelings and concerns.

Evaluation: Evaluate each outcome to determine how it has been met by the client.

OPPORTUNISTIC MALIGNANCIES

Kaposi's sarcoma and non-Hodgkin's lymphoma are discussed.

KAPOSI'S SARCOMA

Kaposi's sarcoma (KS) is a vascular malignancy that can occur any place in the body, including internal organs. The first lesions often appear subtly on the face or in the oral cavity. The more immunosuppressed the person is, the more aggressive the spread of KS. Clinical manifestations of KS are red to purple lesions, which are painless, nonblanching, and palpable (Figure 47-11). These lesions are sometimes mistaken for bruises. Edema in the face, penis, scrotum, and legs can occur as a result of blockages in the lymphatic system. KS can also be found in the GI tract and lungs. Diagnosis is made by tissue biopsy.

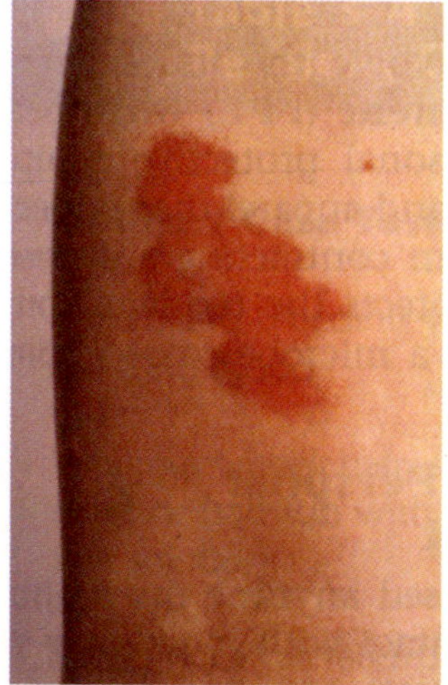

FIGURE 47-11 Kaposi's Sarcoma (*Courtesy of Daniel J. Barbaro, MD, Fort Worth, TX.*)

Treatment involves a variety of options depending on whether the lesions are local or systemic. Radiation therapy, intralesional therapy with interferon alpha 2a or 2b (Roferon A, Intron A) or vinblastine sulfate (Velban), laser therapy, and cryotherapy are used on single or isolated KS lesions. For clients with advanced widespread symptomatic disease, single or combination chemotherapeutic regimens include vinblastine sulfate (Velban), vincristine sulfate (Oncovin), etoposide (VePesid), bleomycin sulfate (Blenoxane), doxorubicin Hcl (Rubex), and mitoxantrone Hcl (Novantrone).

NON-HODGKIN'S LYMPHOMA

Lymphomas are malignant tumors of the immune system. B-cells are the origin of malignancy for most clients with AIDS-related non-Hodgkin's lymphoma (NHL). Clinical manifestations are nonspecific and may include fever, night sweats, and weight loss. Confusion, lethargy, and memory loss may be present in persons with CNS involvement.

Diagnosis of NHL is complicated because of the nonspecific symptoms. Examination of tissue is the recommended diagnostic procedure. There is no standard treatment of NHL. Individualized treatment may include a combination of chemotherapy, antiretroviral agents, prophylaxis against opportunistic infections, and colony-stimulating factors to enhance bone marrow production of blood cells; however, in many clients with advanced HIV disease, treatment of NHL is withheld because it is not tolerated well and may even lead to earlier death.

Nursing Management

Assess client for fever, night sweats, weight loss, confusion, lethargy, memory loss, and ability to perform ADLs. Emphasize no scratching of skin lesions, not using drying soaps, and making sure clothing and linens are thoroughly rinsed of detergent. Encourage significant others to participate in the client's care. Provide access to clergy, social worker, or HIV counselor.

NURSING PROCESS

Assessment

Subjective Data

Ask the client about frequency, onset, and persistence of current symptoms. Note the effect of current symptoms on ability to perform activities of daily living and relationships with others, as well as the effect of treatment plan on quality of life.

Objective Data

Assess skin lesions. Document increased frequency, intensity, or recurrence of nonspecific symptoms, including fever, night sweats, and weight loss.

Nursing diagnoses for an HIV-positive client with a malignancy include the following:

NURSING DIAGNOSES	PLANNING/OUTCOMES	NURSING INTERVENTIONS
Risk for Impaired Skin Integrity related to lesions or treatment	The client will maintain skin integrity.	Teach client to avoid scratching skin lesions, to avoid drying soaps, and to make sure clothing and linen have been thoroughly rinsed of detergent.
Social Isolation related to change in appearance	The client will maintain usual social interactions and identify factors that enhance quality of life.	Facilitate the client's interaction with others. Keep client and significant others aware of treatment plan. Encourage significant others to participate in the care of the client. Encourage physical closeness between the client and significant others. Provide client with access to clergy, social worker, or HIV counselor. Encourage the client to join a support group or obtain peer support. Assist client in identifying positive coping strategies.

Evaluation: Evaluate each outcome to determine how it has been met by the client.

CASE STUDY

J.H., a 37-year-old man, suspects that he is HIV positive. He enters the medical unit with chronic symptoms such as fever, night sweats, diarrhea, weight loss, shortness of breath, and a nonproductive cough. On the initial assessment, he is alert and oriented, color is pale, temperature 100.6°F, pulse 92, respirations 36, and blood pressure 140/70. He has generalized lymphadenopathy. His height is 5′11″, and his weight is 125 pounds. J.H. states that he is not currently taking any medications, although he is "familiar" with the drug zidovudine (Retrovir).

The following questions will guide your development of a nursing care plan for the case study.

1. List symptoms/clinical manifestations, other than J.H., that a client may experience when HIV-positive.
2. List two reasons zidovudine (Retrovir) may be initiated for J.H.

(*Continues*)

CASE STUDY (Continued)

3. List two diagnostic tests that will confirm the diagnosis of HIV.
4. List subjective and objective data the nurse would want to obtain about J.H.
5. Write three individual nursing diagnoses and goals for J.H.
6. List pertinent nursing actions the nurse would perform in caring for J.H. related to:
   hydration
   fatigue
   nutrition
   oxygenation
   medications
7. List resources that could assist J.H. with his diagnosis.
8. List teaching J.H. will need before leaving the medical unit.

SUMMARY

- The immune system identifies substances as self or nonself and protects the body by neutralizing or destroying foreign organisms.
- Immunity to a disease is either natural or acquired.
- Age, sex, nutritional status, medications, and stress influence the immune response.
- Clients receiving blood transfusions must be carefully monitored, especially during the first half-hour, for signs of a reaction.
- Anaphylactic reactions, which may occur as a result of exposure to foods, medications, blood, or insect bites, can potentially be life-threatening.
- Organ transplant clients must understand the implications of taking immunosuppressive medications.
- Clients with rheumatoid arthritis must be taught methods of adapting to the effects of synovial joint inflammation, immobility, and deformity.
- Systemic lupus erythematosus affects multiple body systems.
- Clients with myasthenia gravis experience extreme muscle weakness and fatigue and must be carefully monitored for signs of respiratory distress, and myasthenic or cholinergic crisis.
- Diagnosis of HIV/AIDS is made by the ELISA and Western blot test. These tests determine the presence of antibodies to HIV, not the virus itself.
- *Pneumocystis carinii* pneumonia is the most common opportunistic infection associated with HIV.
- Oral candidiasis can be painful and interfere with the client's nutritional status.
- AIDS dementia complex is a progressive disorder with cognitive, motor, and behavioral dysfunction.

REVIEW QUESTIONS

1. A client has just been diagnosed with syphilis and has an order for 1,000,000 units of penicillin IM. She has no history of allergies to medications. She has never had penicillin. When giving her the injection in the right upper outer quadrant of her buttocks, you note a tattoo. Several minutes after receiving the injection, she tells you she feels anxious and weak. You note she is diaphoretic, scratching her forearm, and is breathing faster than normal. Based upon this assessment data, you would conclude:
   1. she is embarrassed because you saw her tattoo.
   2. she is probably anxious since you know she has a sexually transmitted disease.
   3. her syphilis is getting worse.
   4. these are early signs of an anaphylactic reaction.

2. Which of the following statements shows that the client understands a diagnosis of HIV positive?
   1. "Being HIV positive means that I have AIDs."
   2. "Since I am only HIV positive, I cannot infect others."
   3. "Because I am HIV positive, I have the virus that causes AIDS."
   4. "I became infected by donating blood."

3. The nurse is caring for a client who is experiencing diarrhea and weight loss. Which of the following nursing interventions is appropriate for him?
   1. Encourage fluids with meals.
   2. Substitute a milk shake for lunch.
   3. Offer small, frequent meals.
   4. Suggest he eat more sweets.

4. The nurse is caring for a client who asks when zidovudine (Retrovir) is normally started. Which of the following would be the nurse's correct response?
   1. When the client becomes symptomatic.
   2. When CD4 level reaches 500/mm3.
   3. After the client's first opportunistic infection.
   4. As soon as the client is diagnosed as HIV positive.
5. The nurse is discussing transmission of HIV with a client. Which of the following statements indicates that the client needs more education?
   1. "I should not share needles with anyone."
   2. "I can spread the virus through sexual contact."
   3. "I can no longer donate blood."
   4. "I should not hug or kiss anyone."
6. The nurse enters the room of an HIV client who cannot remember where he is. What is the first priority for the nurse to implement?
   1. Call the physician.
   2. Perform a neurological assessment on the client.
   3. Tell the client where he is.
   4. Give the client his medication that is due at this time.
7. The client tells the nurse, "I am going to quit taking my HIV medication because I have no symptoms and the medication makes me very nauseated" What would be the best response from the nurse?
   1. "I agree with you and I will not give you your medication."
   2. "Let me ask the physician first to see what he thinks."
   3. "Taking the medication with food will help with the nausea."
   4. "I am going to continue to give you your medications, it is up to you if you decide to take the medications or not."
8. A client diagnosed with AIDS spends most of his day sitting at a window. The nurse wants the client to implement a physical activity plan. The nurse knows that the purpose of this plan is to:
   1. Help the client discuss the problems creating his depression.
   2. Help reduce the client's risk for obesity.
   3. Encourage socialization.
   4. Increase the client's appetite.
9. A client is admitted to the hospital with a diagnosis of AIDS and is being treated for Kaposi's sarcoma. Which client would be an appropriate roommate for this client?
   1. A client who just had abdominal surgery.
   2. A client that has pneumonia.
   3. A client that has lymphoma.
   4. A client that has Kaposi's sarcoma.
10. Which client is at highest risk for developing an infection?
   1. A 16-year-old student who plays football on the high school team.
   2. A 34-year-old pregnant school teacher.
   3. A 45-year-old homemaker who smokes two packages of cigarettes daily.
   4. A 73-year-old retired banker who lives in an assisted living facility.

REFERENCES/SUGGESTED READINGS

American Academy of Allergy Asthma & Immunology (AAAAI). (2007). Tips to remember: latex allergy. [Online] Retrieved April 26, 2009, from www.aaaai.org/patients/publicedmat/tips/latexallergy.stm

American Latex Allergy Association. (2009). Latex allergy statistics. [Online] Retrieved April 26, 2009, from www.latexallergyresources.org/topics/LatexAllergyStatistics.cfm

Arthritis Foundation. (2009a). *Arthritis today: a vaccine for rheumatoid arthritis.* [Online] Retrieved April 26, 2009, from www.arthritistoday.org/conditions/rheumatoid-arthritis/news-and-research/rheumatoid-arthritis-vaccine.php

Arthritis Foundation. (2009b). Arthritis today: antimalarial drug may help rheumatoid arthritis and diabetes. [Online] Retrieved April 26, 2009, from www.arthritistoday.org/conditions/rheumatoid-arthritis/news-and-research/antimalarial-drug.php

Arthritis Foundation. (2009c). *Arthritis today: how rheumatoid arthritis is diagnosed.* [Online] Retrieved April 26, 2009, from www.arthritistoday.org/conditions/rheumatoid-arthritis/all-about-ra/diagnosing-ra.php

Arthritis Foundation. (2009d). Arthritis today: how to treat rheumatoid arthritis. [Online] Retrieved April 26, 2009, from www.arthritistoday.org/conditions/rheumatoid-arthritis/ra-treatment/how-to-treat-ra.php

Arthritis Foundation. (2009e). Rheumatoid arthritis what is it? [Online] Retrieved April 27, 2009, from www.arthritis.org/disease-center.php?disease_id=31

Arthritis Foundation. (2009f). Rheumatoid arthritis: who is at risk? [Online] Retrieved April 27, 2009, from www.arthritis.org/disease-center.php?disease_id=31&df=whos_at_risk

Arnold, L. (2001). Living with AIDS. *Nursing2001*, 31(10), 53.

Barroso, J. (2002). HIV-related fatigue. *AJN*, 102(5), 83–86.

Bradley-Springer, L. (2001). HIV prevention: what works? *AJN*, 101(6), 45–50.

Bulechek, G., Butcher, H., McCloskey, J., & Dochterman, J., eds. (2008). *Nursing Interventions Classification (NIC)* (5th ed.). St. Louis, MO: Mosby/Elsevier.

Bursaw, M., Keenan, K., & Ehrhart, M. (2001). HIV update. *Nursing2001*, 31(2), 62–63.

Carroll, P. (2001). Anaphylaxis. *RN*, 64(12), 45–49.

Centers for Disease Control and Prevention. (2006). Revised recommendations for HIV testing of adults, adolescents, and pregnant women in health-care settings. *Morbidity and Mortality Weekly Report*, 55(RR14), 1–17.

Centers for Disease Control and Prevention. (2008). Basic information. [Online] Retrieved May 3, 2009, from www.cdc.gov/hiv/topics/basic/index.htm

Centers for Disease Control and Prevention. (2008a). Food allergy among U.S. children: trends in prevalence and hospitalizations. [Online] Retrieved April 26, 2009, from www.cdc.gov/nchs/data/databriefs/db10.htm

Centers for Disease Control and Prevention. (2008b). HIV/AIDS among American Indians and Alaska Natives. [Online] Retrieved April 29, 2009, from www.cdc.gov/hiv/resources/factsheets/aian.htm

Centers for Disease Control and Prevention. (2008c). HIV/AIDS among women. [Online] Retrieved April 29, 2009, from www.cdc.gov/hiv/topics/women/resources/factsheets/women.htm

Centers for Disease Control and Prevention. (2008d). HIV prevalence estimates-United States, 2006. *Morbidity and Mortality Weekly Report*, *57*(39), 1073–1076.

Centers for Disease Control and Prevention. (2008e). National ambulatory medical care survey: 2006 summary. [Online] Retrieved April 26, 2009, from www.cdc.gov/nchs/data/nhsr/nhsr003.pdf

Centers for Disease Control and Prevention. (2009). Basic statistics. [Online] Retrieved May 3, 2009, from www.cdc.gov/hiv/topics/surveillance/basic.htm#aidsage

Centers for Disease Control and Prevention. (2009a). Guidelines for prevention and treatment of opportunistic infections in HIV-infected adults and adolescents. *Morbidity and Mortality Weekly Report*, *58*(RR-4), 1–207.

Centers for Disease Control and Prevention. (2009b). HIV/AIDS surveillance by race/ethnicity (through 2007). [Online] Retrieved April 27, 2009, from www.cdc.gov/hiv/topics/surveillance/resources/slides/race-ethnicity/index.htm

Cichocki, M. (2007). HIV and the older adult—a growing population. [Online] Retrieved May 17, 2008 from http://aids.about.com/cs/aidsfactsheets/a/seniors.htm

Cohen, S. (2001). Myths & facts…about latex allergy. *Nursing2001*, 31(2), 76.

Coyne, P., Lyne, M., & Watson, A. (2002). Symptom management in people with AIDS. *AJN*, 102(9), 48–55.

Daniels, R., Nosek, L., & Nicoll, L. (2007). Contemporary medical-surgical nursing. Clifton Park, NY: Delmar Cengage Learning.

Daniels, R. (2010). *Delmar's guide to laboratory and diagnostic tests (2nd ed.).* Clifton Park, NY: Delmar Cengage Learning.

D'Arcy, Y. (2002). How to treat arthritis pain. *Nursing 2002*, 32(7), 30–31.

Daughtry, L., Bankston, J., & Deshotels, J. (2002). HIV meds: keeping trouble at bay. *RN*, 65(2), 31–35.

Department of Health and Human Services. (2007). OPTN/SRTR annual report: transplant data 1997-2006, chapter 1, trends in organ donation and transplantation in the United States, 1997-2006. [Online] Retrieved April 26, 2009, from www.ustransplant.org/annual_reports/current/chapter_i_AR_cd.htm?cp=2

Estes, M. (2010). *Health assessment & physical examination* (4nd ed.). Clifton Park, NY: Delmar Cengage Learning.

Food and Drug Administration (FDA). (2003). Retrovir. [Online] Retrieved May 3, 2009, from www.fda.gov/medwatch/SAFETY/2003/03Oct_PI/Retrovir_PI.pdf

Food and Drug Administration (FDA). (2004). OraQuick ADVANCE Rapid HIV-1/2 antibody test. [Online] Retrieved May 3, 2009, from www.fda.gov/cber/pma/p01004716.htm

Golden, D. (2007). Insect sting anaphylaxis. [Online] Retrieved April 26, 2009, from www.pubmedcentral.nih.gov/articlerender.fcgi?artid=1961691.

Goldrick, B. (2005). Emerging infections: infection in the older adult. *American Journal of Nursing, 105*(6), 31–34.

Halzemer, W. (2002). HIV and AIDS: the symptom experience. *AJN*, 102(4), 48–52.

Jones, S. (2001). Taking HAART: How to support patients with HIV/AIDS. *Nursing2001*, 31(2), 36–41.

Jurewicz, M. (2000). Anaphylaxis: When the body overreacts. *Nursing2000*, 30(7), 58.

Lenehan, G. (2002). Latex allergy: Separating fact from fiction. *Nursing2002, 32*(3), 58–63.

Lenehan, G. (2003). Latex allergy. *Nursing2003*, 33(6), 54–55.

Litton, K. (2003). Defenses gone awry: lupus. *RN*, *66*(3), 53–59.

Lupus Foundation of America (LFA). (2009a). How lupus affects the body. [Online] Retrieved April 27, 2009, from www.lupus.org/webmodules/webarticlesnet/templates/new_learnaffects.aspx?articleid=2268&zoneid=526

Lupus Foundation of America (LFA). (2009b). Living with lupus. [Online] Retrieved April 27, 2009, from www.lupus.org/webmodules/webarticlesnet/templates/new_learnliving.aspx?articleid=2252&zoneid=527

Lupus Foundation of America (LFA). (2009c). Medications to treat lupus symptoms. [Online] Retrieved April 27, 2009, from www.lupus.org/webmodules/webarticlesnet/templates/new_learntreating.aspx?articleid=2246&zoneid=525

Lupus Foundation of America (LFA). (2009d). What is lupus. [Online] Retrieved April 27, 2009, from www.lupus.org/webmodules/webarticlesnet/templates/new_learnunderstanding.aspx?articleid=2232&zoneid=523

Mayo Clinic. (2007). *Oral thrush*. [Online] Retrieved May 3, 2009, from www.mayoclinic.com/print/oral-thrush/DS00408/DSECTION=all&METHOD=print

Moorhead, S., Johnson, M., Maas, M., & Swanson, E. (2007). *Nursing Outcomes Classification (NOC)* (4th ed.). St. Louis, MO: Mosby.

National Institute for Occupational Safety and Health (2009). Latex allergy a prevention guide. [Online] Retrieved April 26, 2009, from www.cdc.gov/niosh/98-113.html

National Institute of Allergy and Infectious Diseases (NIAID). (2003). Current trends in allergic reactions: a multidisciplinary approach to patient management. [Online] Retrieved April 26, 2009, from www3.niaid.nih.gov/about/organization/dait/PDF/Allergic_Reactions.pdf

National Institute of Allergy and Infectious Diseases (NIAID). (2008a). Food allergy: living with food allergies. [Online] Retrieved April 26, 2009, from www3.niaid.nih.gov/topics/foodAllergy/living.htm

National Institute of Allergy and Infectious Diseases (NIAID). (2008b). Is it a cold or an allergy? [Online] Retrieved April 26, 2009, from www3.niaid.nih.gov/topics/allergicDiseases/PDF/ColdAllergy.pdf

National Institutes of Health. (2008). Cryptococcosis. [Online] Retrieved May 3, 2009, from www.nlm.nih.gov/medlineplus/ency/article/001328.htm

Putnam, J., & May, K. (2001). Relief for patients with severe allergies. *RN*, 64(6), 26–30.

Spratto, G., & Woods, A. (2009). *2009 PDR nurses' drug handbook*. Clifton Park, NY: Delmar Cengage Learning.

Trzcianowska, H., & Mortensen, E. (2001). HIV and AIDS: Separating fact from fiction. AJN, 101(6), 53–59.

Veronesi, J. (2003). Rheumatoid arthritis. *RN*, *66*(8), 46–52.

World Health Organization (2008a). Global summary of the AIDS epidemic, December 2007. [Online] Retrieved April 27, 2009, from www.who.int/hiv/data/2008_global_summary_AIDS_ep.png

World Health Organization (2008b). HIV/AIDS. [Online] Retrieved April 27, 2009, from www.who.int/features/qa/71/en/index.html

World Health Organization (2009). *TB/HIV facts 2009*. [Online] Retrieved April 27, 2009, from www.who.int/tb/challenges/hiv/factsheet_hivtb_2009.pdf

Yee, C. (2002). Getting a grip on myasthenia gravis. *Nursing2002*, 32(1), 32hn1–32hn4.

RESOURCES

The American Academy of Allergy, Asthma, and Immunology, http:// www.aaaai.org

American Association of Blood Banks, http:// www.aabb.org

American College of Rheumatology, http:// www.rheumatology.org

American Latex Allergy Association, http:// www.latexallergyresources.org

Arthritis Foundation, http:// www.arthritis.org

Association of Nurses in AIDS Care, http:// www.anacnet.org

Asthma and Allergy Foundation of America, http:// www.aafa.org

CDC National STD & AIDS Hotlines, 800-232-4636

Lupus Foundation of America, Inc., http:// www.lupus.org

Myasthenia Gravis Foundation of America, http:// www.myasthenia.org

National Institute of Arthritis and Musculoskeletal and Skin Diseases (NIAMS), http:// www.niams.nih.gov

United Network for Organ Sharing, http:// www.unos.org

UNIT 15 Nursing Care of the Client: Physical and Mental Integrity

CHAPTER 48
Mental Illness

MAKING THE CONNECTION

Refer to the following chapters to increase your understanding of mental illness:

Basic Nursing
- ***Communication***
- ***Stress, Adaptation, and Anxiety***
- ***Wellness Concepts***
- ***Self-Concept***

Adult Health Nursing
- ***Immune System***
- ***Substance Abuse***
- ***The Older Adult***

LEARNING OBJECTIVES

Upon completion of this chapter, you should be able to:
- Define key terms.
- Identify and describe the components of a therapeutic nurse–client relationship.
- Cite nursing interventions for working with clients who are angry, aggressive, homicidal, and/or suicidal.
- Detail nursing interventions for working with clients who are experiencing anxiety.
- Identify and explain the potential side effects associated with antianxiety medications.
- Recount nursing interventions for working with clients who are depressed.
- Identify and explain the potential side effects associated with antidepressant medications.
- Detail nursing interventions for working with clients who have schizophrenia.
- Identify and explain the potential side effects associated with antipsychotic medications.
- Detail nursing interventions for working with clients who have bipolar disorder.
- Identify and explain the potential side effects associated with mood stabilizers.
- Cite nursing interventions for working with clients who have attention-deficit/hyperactivity disorder.
- Recount nursing interventions for working with clients who have been neglected or abused or who have been exposed to domestic violence.
- Discuss nursing interventions for working with clients who have an eating disorder.

KEY TERMS

abuse
actively suicidal
affect
anger-control assistance
anxiety
anxiolytic
auditory hallucination
brief dynamic therapy
cognitive-behavior therapy
command hallucination
crisis
cycling
delusion
depression
domestic violence
electroconvulsive therapy (ECT)
empathy
euphoric
flashback
genuineness
hallucination
hypervigilant
hypomania
mania
mental disorder
mental illness
mood
neglect
paradoxical reaction
physically aggressive
pressured speech
psychoanalysis
psychosis
psychotherapy
rapport
respect
seclusion
serum lithium level
startle response
suicidal ideation
tolerance
trust
verbally aggressive
visual hallucination
word salad

INTRODUCTION

Because they will encounter clients who are emotionally disturbed and/or mentally ill, it is imperative that nurses understand and feel comfortable working with such individuals—not just on psychiatric units, but in all types of circumstances and settings. This chapter is designed to give LP/VNs a beginning knowledge base regarding mental health and illness and to better prepare them for working with individuals who are in a state of crisis or who have emotional needs and/or psychiatric problems.

As the nurse becomes more knowledgeable about mental illness, opportunities arise to increase self-awareness and to examine any personal experiences, preconceived ideas, or prejudices that might negatively affect the nurse's ability to work effectively with clients. For example, the nurse who has unresolved issues regarding sexuality or becomes embarrassed when discussing sexuality will probably be uncomfortable talking about the potential problems in sexual functioning secondary to antidepressant therapy. Examining personal ideas and prejudices before working with clients will facilitate a positive nurse–client relationship.

MENTAL HEALTH AND ILLNESS

In general, people are considered mentally healthy when they possess knowledge of themselves; meet their basic needs; assume responsibility for their behavior; have learned to integrate thoughts, feelings, and actions; can successfully resolve conflicts; maintain relationships; communicate directly with others; respect others; and adapt to change. **Mental illness** occurs when an individual is not able to view self clearly or has a distorted view of self; is unable to maintain satisfying personal relationships; and is unable to adapt to the environment (Frisch & Frisch, 2010). The American Psychiatric Association defines **mental disorder** as "clinically significant behavior or psychological syndrome or pattern that occurs in an individual and is associated with present distress (i.e., negative response to stimuli that are perceived as threatening) or disability (i.e., impairment in one or more important areas of functioning) or with a significantly increased risk of suffering, death, pain, disability, or an important loss of freedom."

One of the ways to conceptualize psychiatric disorders is to think of a continuum, with mental health being situated at one end and mental illness at the other (Figure 48-1). Between these two extremes lie a variety of psychiatric disorders ranging in nature from mild to severe. The fourth edition of the *Diagnostic and Statistical Manual of Mental Disorders* (better known as the DSM-IV) (American Psychiatric Association [APA], 2000) is the reference tool used to identify and establish psychiatric diagnoses. The psychiatrist is the individual most often involved in this process, although other mental health care practitioners may give input and make recommendations for diagnoses.

One of the primary roles of the nurse in working with clients who have mental illness is that of teaching. The nurse is responsible not only for teaching clients about their illnesses, including the probable courses of their given disorders, but also for adequately preparing and educating the client's family. The nurse is usually the first individual to have contact with the family and is most often the one with whom family members maintain consistent contact. Because of the highly personal and sensitive nature of mental disorders, the concept of confidentiality, the nondisclosure of the identity of or personal information about an individual, is vitally important in psychiatric nursing.

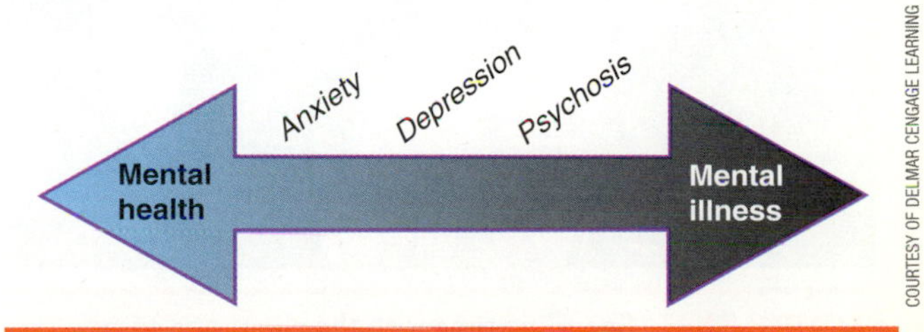

COURTESY OF DELMAR CENGAGE LEARNING

FIGURE 48-1 Mental Health Continuum

RELATIONSHIP DEVELOPMENT

Psychiatric nursing differs from some of the other fields of nursing in that the primary skill the nurse employs is what is referred to as "the therapeutic use of self." Many theorists such as Rogers and Peplau have been instrumental in identifying and exploring the factors that significantly influence the development of therapeutic relationships. Townsend (2008) identifies five components necessary to the development of a therapeutic working relationship and of particular importance in the therapeutic nurse–client relationship. These five components are trust, rapport, respect, genuineness, and empathy.

TRUST

Trust is the ability to rely on an individual's character and ability. Trust must be present for help to be given and received. A therapeutic relationship is firmly rooted in trust. Three major activities facilitate the development of trust: consistency, respect, and honesty. Consistency includes following through on plans, adhering to the schedule, being straightforward with no hidden motives, and seeking extra time for client interaction. Respect includes addressing clients the way they wish to be addressed (e.g., Mr., Mrs., Ms., first name), listening to the clients, and providing clear explanations. Honesty includes keeping promises and maintaining confidentiality. Being consistently trustworthy is an expression of the nurse's personal integrity and builds the foundation for nursing effectiveness (Figure 48-2).

Many clients with emotional and/or psychiatric problems have great difficulty trusting and having confidence that others will be good to their word. They may have been lied to or hurt in the past, and this makes it difficult for them to trust again, even with health care professionals who are trying to help them. It is very important, therefore, that the nurse fulfill any promise made to the client.

RAPPORT

Rapport is a bond or connection between two people that is based on mutual trust. Such a bond does not just happen spontaneously; it is planned by the nurse, who purposefully implements behaviors that promote trust. The nurse sets the tone of the relationship by creating an atmosphere wherein the client feels free to express feelings. When seeking to develop trust, the nurse acts in a manner that indicates recognition of the client as a unique individual and reinforces that individuality. Such actions, which serve to humanize the client, are therapeutic. To establish rapport, the nurse must show that the client is important. Actions are implemented to boost the level of the client's self-esteem. Nonverbal interventions are of utmost importance in helping establish rapport. Interacting with family and significant others is also helpful in establishing rapport with the client. Recognizing the importance of the family and its influence on the healing process allows the nurse to bond with those who will encourage and support the client during recovery.

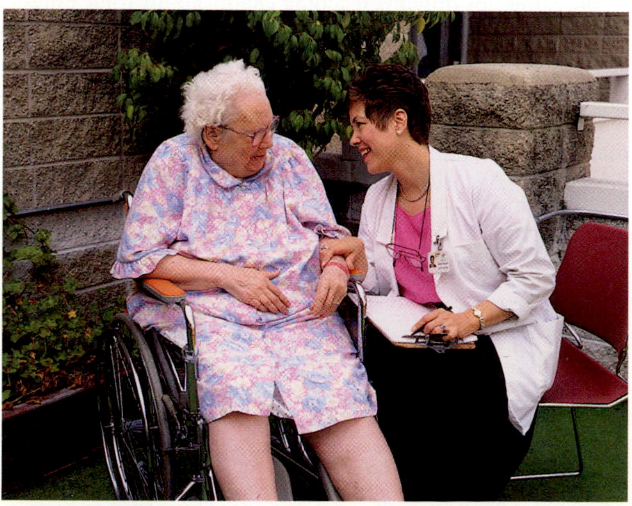

COURTESY OF DELMAR CENGAGE LEARNING

FIGURE 48-2 Spending time with the client one-to-one helps promote a trusting relationship.

RESPECT

Respect is the acceptance of an individual as is, in a nonjudgmental manner. The concept of respect is an integral component of the nurse–client relationship. Respect means caring for clients whose vvalue system may differ greatly from that of the nurse. To show respect, the nurse must not react with shock, surprise, or disapproval toward a client's lifestyle, dress, or behaviors. The nurse respects the client's choices and actions yet sets limits on unhealthy or undesirable behavior.

GENUINENESS

Genuineness (sincerity) is an attribute easily perceived by the client and can be the most significant aspect of the nurse–client relationship. Nurses are often concerned about whether they will say the right thing to a client; though saying the right thing is important, more important is that the nurse be honest and genuine in communications with the client.

EMPATHY

Empathy (the ability to perceive and relate to another's personal experience) is an important quality necessary to successful nurse–client interactions. The empathic nurse understands that the client's perception of the situation is real to him. By perceiving the client's understanding of her own needs, the nurse is better able to assist the client in determining what will work best. Empathy enables the nurse to assist the client to become a fully participating partner in treatment, rather than a passive recipient of care. Through empathy, the nurse validates the experiences of the client (Figure 48-3).

THE CLIENT EXPERIENCING A CRISIS

In psychological terms, a **crisis** is a stressor that forces an individual to respond and/or adapt in some way. Emotions may intensify during a crisis situation or serious illness, and any situation or illness can potentially become a crisis if the stressors are severe enough. The understanding of crisis is particularly important in psychiatric and mental health nursing. A crisis taxes the individual's coping resources, and each person responds differently to seemingly identical situations. Crisis requires that an individual call on all of her personal skills as well as on the outside social and familial supports that she has built through her life (Frisch & Frisch, 2010). Each individual has personality strengths, interpersonal networks, and socioeconomic resources that offer some protection against the threat of crisis. When any (or all) of these protections are weak, however, a person's

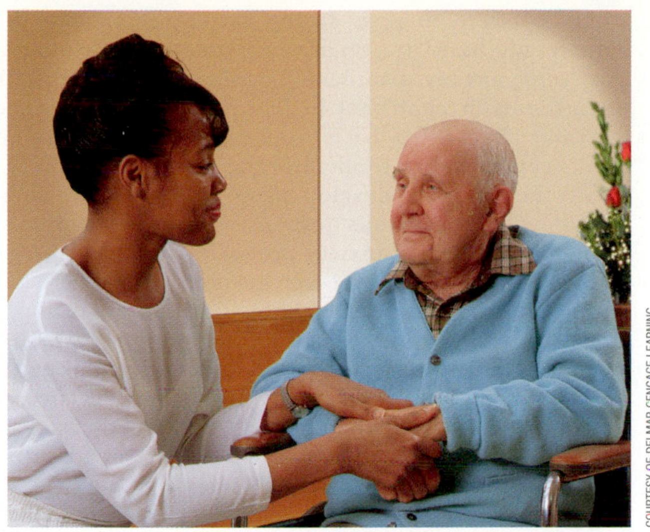

FIGURE 48-3 **Through empathic listening, the nurse can reach an understanding of the client's experience and help the client see the positive aspects of the experience.**

response to crisis may be dysfunctional, and the result may be one or more symptoms of mental illness. Although theories differ in their definitions of crisis and stress, it is generally accepted that most psychiatric problems result from or are strongly influenced by the interaction of stress and overwhelmed coping mechanisms (Frisch & Frisch, 2010). The client experiencing crisis may be anxious, angry, aggressive, homicidal, suicidal, psychotic, or any combination of these.

ANXIETY

Anxiety is a state wherein a person feels a strong sense of dread frequently accompanied by physical symptoms of increased heart and respiratory rates and elevated blood pressure in the absence of a specific source or reason for these emotions or responses. Nurses frequently encounter clients and family members who are anxious because of alterations in or threats to health and physical well-being. Peplau (1963) identifies four escalating stages of anxiety beginning with mild anxiety, moving to moderate anxiety, followed by severe anxiety, and, finally, to the stage of panic, if not effectively treated. Intervention can occur at any point along the continuum, preferably before the stages of severe anxiety or panic are reached.

MILD ANXIETY

The mildly anxious client is beginning to experience some of the signs and symptoms of anxiety, such as irritability and restlessness; however, the person is still able to concentrate and focus on the task at hand. In fact, *mild* anxiety can actually benefit an individual as far as enhancing performance ability (Townsend, 2008).

MODERATE ANXIETY

The individual with moderate anxiety experiences additional physiologic and cognitive symptoms. Blood pressure, pulse, and respirations increase, and the client becomes diaphoretic. The moderately anxious individual begins to have difficulty concentrating or learning new material. This is important to recognize before teaching a client about a medication or test, or performing a procedure. Before teaching can be effective, the client must be assisted in lowering the level of anxiety (Townsend, 2008).

SEVERE ANXIETY

Severely anxious clients are significantly impaired in several areas. Their ability to cognitively process material may drastically diminish, they may experience tunnel vision, their focus may become very limited, and the physiologic symptoms of anxiety become much more pronounced. Clients at this high level of anxiety are often very fearful and may be irrational in their thought processes (Townsend, 2008).

PANIC

The individual experiencing panic may begin to manifest symptoms of **psychosis** (losing touch with reality), such as **delusions** (false beliefs that misrepresent reality) and/or **hallucinations** (perceptions that something is present when it is not, e.g., hearing voices that are not really there). The individual with this level of anxiety requires constant reassurance and continuous assessment for suicide risk and maladaptive coping behaviors (Antai-Otong, 2008).

ANXIETY DISORDERS

Some of the most common psychiatric diagnoses related to anxiety are Generalized Anxiety Disorder, Panic Disorder, Obsessive-Compulsive Disorder, and Post-Traumatic Stress Disorder. It is estimated that 40 million adult Americans have an anxiety disorder (Anxiety Disorders Association of America [ADAA], 2009a).

GENERALIZED ANXIETY DISORDER

The client with Generalized Anxiety Disorder (GAD) exhibits symptoms of excessive anxiety, chronic worry, or dread. Clients usually realize that their symptoms are out of proportion to any real threat. The symptoms include three or more of the following: restlessness, easy fatigue, difficulty concentrating, irritability, trembling, muscle tension, abdominal upsets, and sleep disturbance. For anxiety to be termed excessive, clients must experience symptoms frequently over a period of 6 months or more (ADAA, 2009b).

PANIC DISORDER

Panic Disorder is diagnosed when the client experiences at least two panic attacks followed by at least 1 month's concern about having another panic attack (ADAA, 2009d). These attacks begin abruptly and peak within 10 minutes and are characterized by a set of any four of the following symptoms: palpitations or rapid heart rate, sweating, trembling, shortness of breath, sensation of choking, chest pain, nausea, dizziness, fear of losing control, fear of dying, numbness or tingling, chills or hot flushes, and some sense of altered reality. The client has a strong desire to run away or escape from the situation that triggered the attack. In some individuals, the attack is brought about by specific stimuli or a particular setting, for example the dentist's office. In others, the attacks come on "out of the blue."

OBSESSIVE-COMPULSIVE DISORDER

In Obsessive-Compulsive Disorder (OCD), the individual has persistent, recurring thoughts or impulses (obsessions) that are intrusive or inappropriate, causing anxiety or fears leading the individual to perform repetitive behaviors or rituals (compulsions) to neutralize the anxiety caused by the obsession. The obsessions and/or compulsions may take up at least several hours a day and interfere with the individual's normal routine, occupation, social activities, or relationships (ADAA, 2009c).

POST-TRAUMATIC STRESS DISORDER

Clients suffering from Post-Traumatic Stress Disorder (PTSD) have experienced a serious trauma. Being severely beaten or emotionally, physically, or sexually abused or living through or witnessing a catastrophic event or natural disaster such as a flood, earthquake, hurricane, war, or plane crash might lead to PTSD. The response to the trauma must have been one of fear or helplessness, and the event is persistently reexperienced through recurrent recollections, dreams, or hallucinatory-like flashbacks. Individuals with this disorder have symptoms for more than 1 month and exhibit impairment of social functioning, anxiety symptoms, avoidance of stimuli associated with the trauma, and a general numbness. More than 7.7 million Americans are diagnosed with PTSD (ADAA, 2009e).

MEDICAL–SURGICAL MANAGEMENT

Medical

Psychotherapy (the treatment of mental and emotional disorders through psychological rather than physical methods) continues to be widely used in the treatment of anxiety disorders. Psychotherapy can be viewed as falling into two general categories: those therapies based on helping individuals achieve insight into *why* they feel anxiety and those that emphasize behavioral means of controlling the anxiety.

Psychotherapy based on insight into symptoms may sometimes be valuable, especially for highly motivated individuals whose symptoms are not disabling. **Psychoanalysis** (therapy focused on uncovering unconscious memories and processes) is among the best known of the insight therapies and has been widely employed to assist persons with anxiety.

In contrast, there is strong empirical evidence that behaviorally based treatments are effective in treating at least some anxiety disorders. Cognitive-behavior therapy often results in significant benefit for persons experiencing panic attacks. **Cognitive-behavior therapy** assumes that clients can learn to identify the common stimuli that create their anxiety, develop plans to respond to those stimuli with nonanxious responses, and problem solve when unanticipated anxiety-provoking situations arise. Although insight is very much involved in this process, it is not insight into deep psychological causes, as in psychoanalysis, but rather, practical, commonsense problem solving. Treatment appears both to be effective during the relatively brief course of therapy and to remain effective for some months after therapy finishes. Sometimes medical and psychological follow-up are important to ensure satisfactory improvement.

A new treatment method for PTSD is eye-movement desensitization and reprocessing (EMDR). This method involves asking a client to imagine a traumatic event or anxiety provoking occurrence and processing the traumatic event in a non-threatening manner. Special training is necessary to perform EMDR (Antai-Otong, 2008).

Pharmacological

The drugs of choice for treating clients with anxiety are usually the **anxiolytics** or antianxiety agents (Table 48-1). Some of the antianxiety medications such as alprazolam (Xanax) and lorazepam (Ativan) may also be helpful in alleviating the symptoms of anxiety, nervousness, and sleeplessness frequently associated with panic disorder and PTSD.

Most of these medications can be used on either a routine or as-needed (PRN) basis and belong to the family of benzodiazepines. Onset of action for the benzodiazepines usually occurs within 30 minutes after oral administration, and most individuals respond favorably to these medications; that is, a reduction or cessation of the symptoms of anxiety is experienced.

Clients should be warned about the potential risk of addiction associated with antianxiety medications. These particular medications should be used with extreme caution because long-term use can lead to an increased **tolerance**, acquired resistance to the effects of the drug. Tolerance results in the need to increase the frequency and amount of medication in order to achieve the same benefit. Over time, this may cause a dependency on the medication, actually creating another serious problem for the client. Therefore, the antianxiety agents are usually indicated for short-term management of anxiety rather than for long-term use. The benefits of a particular medication for the client must always be weighed against the possible risk of addiction, particularly if long-term use is or may be indicated. The *one exception* is buspirone hydrochloride (BuSpar), a nonbenzodiazepine antianxiety medication, which does not appear to have any addictive potential; however, the therapeutic effectiveness of BuSpar is not reached for approximately 7 to 10 days; thus, although it can be given as a regularly scheduled antianxiety agent, BuSpar has absolutely no value as a PRN medication. When initiating therapy with BuSpar, another antianxiety medication such as alprazolam (Xanax) or lorazepam (Ativan) may be given concurrently until the therapeutic level is reached; then the other medication can be gradually decreased.

TABLE 48-1 Antianxiety Medications

GENERIC NAME	TRADE NAME	TYPE	POTENTIAL SIDE EFFECTS
aprazolam	Xanax	Benzodiazepine	Dizziness, drowsiness, lethargy, physical and psychological dependence, tolerance
buspirone hydrochloride	BuSpar	Nonbenzodiazepine	Blurred vision, chest pain, clamminess, dizziness, drowsiness, excitement, fatigue, headache, insomnia, nasal congestion, numbness, myalgia, nausea, nervousness, palpitations, paresthesia, skin rashes, sore throat, syncope, tachycardia, tinnitus, incoordination, weakness
clonazepam	Klonopin	Benzodiazepine	Ataxia, behavioral changes, drowsiness, physical and psychological dependence, tolerance
diazepam	Valium	Benzodiazepine	Dizziness, drowsiness, fatigue, hypotension, hypertension, CV collapse, dependence, tolerance
lorazepam	Ativan	Benzodiazepine	Agranulocytosis, CV collapse, dizziness, drowsiness, lethargy

Data from *Delmar Nurses's Drug Handbook 2010 Edition*, by G. Spratto and A. Woods, 2010, Clifton Park, NY: Delmar Cengage Learning.

Activity

The anxious client's activity level may be negatively affected by both the anxiety disorder and the side effects of the prescribed medication. The side effects of sedation and drowsiness can pose safety hazards for certain activities and must be emphasized to the client.

NURSING MANAGEMENT

Remain with the client while fear level and/or anxiety level is high and speak in a calm, soothing voice. Reassure the client that she is in a safe place. Explore with the client what things are relaxing and calming. Teach the client relaxation exercises. Encourage participation in recreation or sports activities.

Do not touch the client with PTSD without permission. If the client is confused or disoriented, orient the client to reality.

MEMORYTRICK

CALM

A memory trick to remember nursing management methods for anxiety is **CALM**:

C = Cognitive-behavior therapy

A = Anxiolytic medication management

L = Learn methods to reduce/control anxiety

M = Maintain a safe, calm environment

NURSING PROCESS

ASSESSMENT

Subjective Data

Clients experiencing anxiety report problems concentrating, and fear that something dreadful is about to happen. They may verbalize an overwhelming feeling of impending doom. They may also report that the anxiety is very frightening to them and that they are afraid of losing control. Table 48-2 lists questions that may help in identifying a client's anxiety.

Clients with PTSD may describe unwanted memories of an event, express suicidal ideation, or express fantasies of retaliation toward the identified source of trauma. The client with PTSD may describe feeling extremely fearful and "on guard" at all times and may report having **flashbacks** (reliving of the original trauma as if currently experiencing it) along with recurrent dreams and/or nightmares.

Objective Data

Changes in vital signs, such as an increase in blood pressure, pulse, and respirations, as well as restlessness, irritability, pacing, and agitation may become more pronounced as anxiety level increases.

Clients with PTSD may exhibit an exaggerated **startle response** (overreaction to minor sounds or noises), or they may be **hypervigilant** (constantly scanning the environment for potentially dangerous situations). Clients with PTSD may react with survival responses appropriate for the trauma they survived. For example, abused children may seek to placate adults and female incest victims may become flirtatious or seductive with men.

TABLE 48-2 Asking Clients about Symptoms of Anxiety Disorders

Following are questions that have proven useful in eliciting information from clients about symptoms of anxiety disorders. You may find that you prefer to word these questions somewhat differently, but the important thing is to ask them. Many clients experience anxiety symptoms for years before a doctor, nurse, or psychologist takes the time to ask about these symptoms.

Generalized Anxiety Disorder	Do you find yourself worrying frequently about a number of different things, such as the way things are going for you at home, work, or school? Do you find yourself feeling anxious or tense much of the time without any obvious reason?
Panic Disorder	Have you ever experienced sudden, intense fear for no reason? Have you found yourself experiencing intense physical symptoms of chest pain, shortness of breath, dizziness, or sweating, along with a sense that something terrible or life threatening was happening to you?
Post-Traumatic Stress Disorder	Have you ever had a particularly traumatic experience such as witnessing or experiencing violence or a catastrophic event (such as a flood or fire)? Have you ever found yourself reexperiencing a violent or catastrophic event through dreams or waking "flashbacks"?

From *Psychiatric Mental Health Nursing*, by N. Frisch and L. Frisch (4th ed.). 2010, Clifton Park, NY: Delmar Cengage Learning.

Nursing diagnoses for the client with anxiety include the following:

NURSING DIAGNOSES	PLANNING/OUTCOMES	NURSING INTERVENTIONS
Anxiety related to a subjective sense of uneasiness and tension	The client will learn how to demonstrate and utilize new and more effective methods of managing anxiety.	Teach the client relaxation exercises. Explore with the client those things that are calming and relaxing. Encourage physical movement or participation in some type of recreational or sporting activity to release excess energy.
Fear related to a specific object (e.g., hospitals)	The client will report feeling less fearful.	Remain with the client while level of fear is high. Talk to the client in a calm, soothing voice. Reassure the client that he is in a safe place.
Post-Trauma Syndrome related to anxiety felt following a significant life-threatening event	The client will experience a decrease in frequency and intensity of symptoms.	Orient the client to reality, if the client is confused, disoriented, or experiencing flashbacks. Do not touch the client without permission. Teach the client, family, and significant others about the symptoms of PTSD, including flashbacks, amnesia, memory loss, and nightmares.

Evaluation: Evaluate each outcome to determine how it has been met by the client.

DEPRESSION

Depression is the state wherein an individual experiences feelings of extreme sadness, hopelessness, and helplessness. Several symptoms may be seen with depression, which can range anywhere from mild to severe and be manifested in many different ways.

It involves an imbalance of neurotransmitters and is treatable. The direct cause of depression is unclear; however, changes in body chemistry caused by experiencing a traumatic event, hormonal changes, altered health habits, presence of another illness, or substance abuse can bring on depression (Depression and Bipolar Support Alliance [DBSA], 2007).

Symptoms of depression include prolonged sadness; significant changes in appetite and sleep patterns; irritability, agitation, anxiety, worry; pessimism; loss of energy; feelings of guilt, worthlessness; inability to concentrate; inability to take pleasure in former interests; unexplained aches and pains; and recurring thoughts of death or suicide. Adult Americans of all ages, races, ethnic groups, and social class experience depression every day. According to the

PROFESSIONALTIP

Achieving a State of Relaxation

Clients who are anxious and feeling overwhelmed will often require assistance in achieving a state of relaxation. Help the client identify activities that are relaxing, such as listening to favorite music, watching television, reading a book, playing a game, drawing a picture, working a puzzle, or whatever is calming to the client. Teach the client a variety of stress-management techniques such as deep-breathing exercises, progressive deep-muscle relaxation, and guided imagery. All of these can assist the client in reaching a greater state of relaxation. Explore with the client the possibility of enrolling in a course such as Tai Chi. In addition to providing physical activity, it assists the client in achieving a state of balance and an increasing ability to focus.

CRITICAL THINKING

Anxiety

A client shares with you that she is feeling anxious and cannot stop worrying about who will take care of her cat, how she will afford her health care, and she is anxiously waiting for her lab results.

1. Which client concern do you think should be addressed first?
2. How will you handle this situation?

Substance Abuse and Mental Health Services Administration (SAMHSA) (2008), 16.5 million adult Americans had at least one major depressive episode (MDE) between the years 2006-2007. Clients can experience mild, moderate, or severe depression with varying degrees of symptomatology.

MILD DEPRESSION

Individuals with mild depression may notice a difference in the way they are feeling and their ability to function in certain situations, but they may not be able to identify the problem at this point in time. Although they are still able to function and carry on their daily routines, doing so may put quite a strain on them both physically and mentally.

MODERATE DEPRESSION

Moderate depression interferes with the individual's life in a variety of ways. A decrease in the ability to perform on the job may be noticed. Relationships are affected as the individual becomes increasingly withdrawn and isolated and disinterested in things that previously were pleasurable, such as hobbies and leisure-time activities. Interventions performed at this stage are most effective in arresting the depression before the individual's mental health deteriorates any further.

PROFESSIONALTIP

Flashbacks

The client experiencing a flashback is usually not aware of current surroundings and often does not recognize familiar individuals. For the duration of the flashback, the client is actually reexperiencing and reliving the original trauma once again. For this reason, it is extremely important to never touch a client during a flashback, as the client may perceive you as dangerous and react to you as if you are trying to inflict harm. Talk to the client in a soft, calm voice and gently let the client know who you are, where the client is, and what is happening.

SEVERE DEPRESSION

When depression progresses to a severe state, the individual becomes seriously impaired. The individual with severe depression may experience psychosis, or a loss of contact with reality, in addition to the symptoms of depression.

DEPRESSION DISORDERS

Some of the psychiatric diagnoses associated with depression include Major Depressive Disorder and Dysthymic Disorder.

MAJOR DEPRESSIVE DISORDER

To qualify for the diagnosis of Major Depressive Disorder, *DSM-IV* requires the presence of at least one major depressive episode that (1) lasts at least 2 weeks, (2) represents a change from previous functioning, and (3) causes some impairment in a person's social or occupational functioning. Five or more symptoms of depression must also be present. One of these symptoms *must* be either depressed mood or loss of interest in previously enjoyable activities. The other four symptoms may include changes in appetite or weight; sleep disturbance (usually trouble staying asleep); fatigue or loss of energy; feelings of worthlessness or guilt; difficulty concentrating, thinking, or making decisions; or recurrent thoughts of death or suicide.

Some individuals, particularly adolescents, exhibit irritability or crankiness rather than sadness. Family members or close friends will notice a change in the individual, most commonly a social withdrawal and a neglect of activities that previously brought the person pleasure.

Major depressive episodes frequently develop over a few days or weeks, and without treatment commonly last longer than 6 months (Frisch & Frisch, 2010).

DYSTHYMIC DISORDER

Whereas the essence of Major Depressive Disorder is discrete episodes of depression, persons with Dysthymic Disorder feel depressed nearly all of the time. The *DSM-IV* criteria for Dysthymic Disorder include "depressed mood for most of the day, for more days than not . . . for at least 2 years." A person with Dysthymic Disorder must also have at least two of the following symptoms: appetite disturbance, sleep disturbance, fatigue, low self-esteem, poor concentration or difficulty making decisions, and feelings of hopelessness. As with Major Depressive Disorder, the symptoms must cause clinically significant distress or impairment in social or occupational functioning. Dysthymic Disorder is somewhat rarer than Major Depressive Disorder, occurring during a lifetime in approximately 6% of persons (Frisch & Frisch, 2010).

MEDICAL–SURGICAL MANAGEMENT

Medical

Psychotherapy refers to any of more than 250 types of largely verbal techniques designed to help individuals surmount psychological stresses including depression. Psychotherapy based on psychoanalytic interventions emphasizes helping clients gain insight into the causes of their depression. This approach is long term and requires much motivation on the part of the client to invest considerable time, effort, and money (Frisch & Frisch, 2010).

Brief dynamic therapy focuses on core conflicts from personality and living situations. The goal is to resolve depressive symptoms by improving these conflicts and resolving stresses. The therapist in this approach takes an active role to direct sessions toward resolution of conflicts. Techniques of confrontation and interpretation of behaviors and events are frequently used. Conflicts, their meanings, and individuals' choices are emphasized. This type of therapy can be done either with individuals or in a group format.

Cognitive therapy focuses on removing symptoms by identifying and correcting perceptual biases in clients' thinking and correcting unrecognized assumptions. The therapy concentrates on changing negative thoughts and behaviors into alternatives that do not sustain depression.

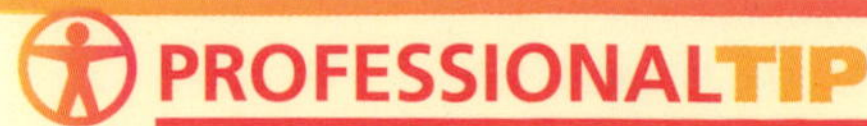

Journaling

Suggest to depressed clients that they keep personal journals in which they write down their thoughts and feelings. Putting thoughts and emotions down on paper may help clarify issues relating to depression and is an excellent way of venting or releasing pent-up feelings.

Electroconvulsive therapy (ECT) is used for clients with severe depression who have not responded to medications. The client under anesthesia is treated with pulses of electrical energy sufficient to cause a brief convulsion or seizure. Muscle-depolarizing agents are also given so that no actual convulsive movements occur; the primary effect of ECT is on the brain. Studies show that clients do not find the actual ECT treatment frightening, painful, or unpleasant. Although deaths have occurred from ECT, particularly in elderly clients or those with heart disease, the risk is quite low. Side effects depend on the specific technique used but are mostly limited to memory deficits (Frisch & Frisch, 2010).

Pharmacological

The main classification of medications usually prescribed for treatment of depression is the antidepressants. Within this classification are several groups, including the tetracyclic and atypical antidepressants (Table 48-3), the selective serotonin reuptake inhibitors (SSRIs) (Table 48-4), the tricyclic antidepressants (Table 48-5), and the monoamine oxidase inhibitors (MAOIs) (Table 48-6). These antidepressant families have unique properties, as do the individual medications within each. Many of these medications must be taken at bedtime. It is a nursing responsibility to adequately educate the client and family about the prescribed medications.

Diet

The client experiencing depression often has a disturbance in eating patterns. Some individuals will not be hungry and will

TABLE 48-3 Tetracyclic and Atypical Antidepressants

GENERIC NAME	TRADE NAME	TYPE	POTENTIAL SIDE EFFECTS
mirtazapine	Remeron	Tetracyclic	Agranulocytosis, drowsiness, dry mouth, nausea, suicidal ideation
nefazodone hydrochloride	Serzone	Antidepressant	Constipation, dizziness, dry mouth, insomnia, nausea, weight loss
venlafaxine hydrochloride	Effexor	Antidepressant	Abnormal dreams, altered taste, anorexia, constipation, diarrhea, dizziness, dry mouth, dyspepsia, headache, nausea, nervousness, paresthesia, rectal hemorrhage, rhinitis, seizures, sexual dysfunction, visual disturbances, vaginal/uterine hemorrhage, weakness, weight loss

Data from *Delmar Nurses's Drug Handbook 2010 Edition*, by G. Spratto and A. Woods, 2010, Clifton Park, NY: Delmar Cengage Learning.

eat very little or sometimes not at all, whereas others will overeat. A nutritional assessment should be done as part of the health history obtained by the nurse, and if any significant problem areas are identified, a dietary consult may be indicated.

When a client is started on antidepressant therapy, the client and family must be educated regarding any special dietary needs, depending on the type of medication prescribed. The client receiving SSRI therapy may experience an initial loss of appetite during the first part of therapy, because of the gastrointestinal (GI) side effects frequently associated with these medications (Table 48-4). Anorectic clients or those at risk for weight loss must be closely monitored. The client receiving MAOI therapy must be especially alert to the dietary restrictions associated with this particular type of medication (Table 48-6).

Table 48-4 Selective Serotonin Reuptake Inhibitors (SSRIs)

GENERIC NAME	TRADE NAME	POTENTIAL SIDE EFFECTS
fluoxetine hydrochloride	Prozac	Headache, abnormal dreams, anxiety, diarrhea, drowsiness, excessive sweating, insomnia, nervousness, palpitations, pruritus, seizures, tremors, visual disturbances, weight loss
fluvoxamine maleate	Luvox	Constipation, convulsions, impotence, dry mouth, drowsiness, dyspepsia, headache, heart failure, insomnia, MI, nausea, nervousness, weakness
paroxetine hydrochloride	Paxil	Anxiety, constipation, diarrhea, dizziness, drowsiness, dry mouth, ejaculatory disturbance, headache, insomnia, nausea, seizures, sweating, weakness, tremors
sertraline hydrochloride	Zoloft	Diarrhea, dizziness, drowsiness, dry mouth, fatigue, headache, increased sweating, insomnia, nausea, palpitations, sexual dysfunction, tremors, vomiting when given with pimozide (Orap) raises pimozide concentration by about 40% (FDA, 2002)

Data from *Delmar Nurses's Drug Handbook 2010 Edition*, by G. Spratto and A. Woods, 2010, Clifton Park, NY: Delmar Cengage Learning.

Table 48-5 Tricyclic Antidepressants

GENERIC NAME	TRADE NAME	POTENTIAL SIDE EFFECTS
amitriptyline hydrochloride	Elavil	Arrhythmia, blurred vision, constipation, dry eyes, dry mouth, heart block, hypotension, lethargy, MI, sedation, stroke
imipramine hydrochloride	Tofranil	Arrhythmia, blurred vision, constipation, drowsiness, dry eyes, dry mouth, fatigue, hypotension, seizures, urinary retention

Data from *Delmar Nurses's Drug Handbook 2010 Edition*, by G. Spratto and A. Woods, 2010, Clifton Park, NY: Delmar Cengage Learning.

Table 48-6 Monoamine Oxidase Inhibitors (MAOIs)

GENERIC NAME	TRADE NAME	POTENTIAL SIDE EFFECTS
isocarboxazid	Marplan	Arrhythmia, blurred vision, diarrhea, dizziness, headache, orthostatic hypotension, insomnia, restlessness, seizures, weakness; these medications usually have the side-effect of lowering blood pressure. A potentially fatal hypertensive crisis can result when MAOIs are taken in combination with certain foods and drugs such as broad beans, certain cheeses (e.g., brie, cheddar), liver, caffeine, figs, dry sausage (pepperoni), tea, yogurt, amphetamine, cocaine, dopa, and many OTC cold products, hay fever medications, and nasal decongestants.
phenelzine sulfate	Nardil	
tranylcypromine sulfate	Parnate	

Data from *Delmar Nurses's Drug Handbook 2010 Edition*, by G. Spratto and A. Woods, 2010, Clifton Park, NY: Delmar Cengage Learning.

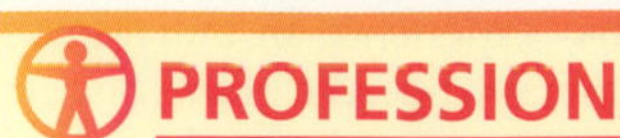

PROFESSIONAL TIP

Antidepressant Therapy

Before initiating antidepressant therapy, a baseline electrocardiogram (EKG) is needed to determine whether any preexisting underlying cardiac problems are present. If the client develops cardiac difficulties during antidepressant therapy, another EKG is obtained and compared to the original to assist in ascertaining whether the antidepressant exacerbated the cardiac condition.

CLIENT TEACHING

Tricyclic Antidepressants

Be sure to instruct each client taking a tricyclic antidepressant medication in the following:

- Do not drink alcohol while on the medication.
- Do not take any other medications unless prescribed by your physician.
- Drowsiness and sedation may impair the ability to drive and operate heavy machinery.
- Some of the side effects may diminish in intensity once your body adjusts to the medication.
- Do not stop taking the medications without physician approval.
- Increase fluid intake to assist in combating dry mouth and constipation.
- Sugarless candy and gum can help decrease the side effect of dry mouth.
- Increase dietary fiber to decrease the side effect of constipation.
- Rise slowly from a lying position to prevent dizziness and a sudden drop in blood pressure.

CLIENT TEACHING

Potential Adverse Drug–Drug Reactions with MAOIs

A serious drug–drug reaction can occur when an MAOI is taken concurrently with certain other medications. The combination of an MAOI and some common prescription or OTC medications can result in a hypertensive crisis that is often fatal. Some of the most dangerous reactive medications include meperidine (Demerol), stimulants, decongestants, and weight-reduction aids.

CLIENT TEACHING

Tetracyclic and SSRI Antidepressants

Be sure to instruct each client taking a tetracyclic, atypical, or SSRI antidepressant medication in the following:

- Take the medication *only* as directed by your physician.
- Do not take the medication unless prescribed by your physician.
- Do not take fluoxetine (Prozac), paroxetine (Paxil), or sertraline (Zoloft) on an empty stomach.
- Mirtazapine (Remeron) does not need to be taken with food.
- Ability to drive and/or operate heavy machinery may be impaired while taking the medication.
- Do not drink alcohol while taking the medication.
- If female, advise your physician if you are breastfeeding, suspect you are pregnant, or are planning a pregnancy while taking the medication.
- Wear sunscreen and protective clothing while outdoors, as fluoxetine (Prozac), paroxetine (Paxil), and sertraline (Zoloft) increase susceptibility to sunburn.
- The medications may cause drowsiness.
- If taking fluoxetine (Prozac), mirtazapine (Remeron), or nefazodone (Serzone), rise slowly from a lying position to prevent dizziness and a sudden drop in blood pressure.
- Utilize good oral hygiene in conjunction with sugarless candy or gum to minimize the discomforting side effect of dry mouth associated with fluoxetine (Prozac), mirtazapine (Remeron), nefazodone (Serzone), paroxetine (Paxil), and sertraline (Zoloft).
- Monitor weight, as mirtazapine (Remeron) may cause an increase in appetite.
- Do not take any over-the-counter (OTC) cold medications with mirtazapine (Remeron).
- If taking mirtazapine (Remeron), inform your physician of the medication regimen prior to surgery.
- If taking venlafaxine (Effexor), fluvoxamine (Luvox), or nefazodone (Serzone), inform your physician if signs of allergic reaction occur.

CLIENT TEACHING

MAOIs

Be sure to instruct each client taking an MAOI antidepressant medication in the following:

- *Do not take any other medications, including OTC medications*, unless prescribed by your physician.
- Take the medication exactly as prescribed.
- Do not drink alcohol while on the medication.
- Rise slowly from a lying position to prevent dizziness and a sudden drop in blood pressure.
- *Avoid all foods containing tyramine*, including alcoholic beverages, especially beer and wine; aged cheeses; avocados; bananas; caffeine; chocolate; and smoked or pickled meats (such as salami, pepperoni, smoked fish, and summer sausage).

CRITICAL THINKING

Coworker Depression

What actions would you take if you felt a coworker was suffering from depression?

Activity

Clients experiencing depression often experience a significant decrease in level of activity and report feeling tired and lethargic. Clients experiencing depression will often require encouragement to engage in any type of physical activity.

NURSING MANAGEMENT

Spend time with the client one-on-one to build rapport and develop a therapeutic relationship. Encourage the client to initiate conversation and interact with others. Guide the client to bathe, groom, and wear clean clothes. Praise the client verbally for conversing and interacting with others and for taking care of hygiene and grooming.

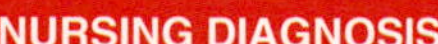

NURSING DIAGNOSIS

Social Isolation related to inadequate resources, impaired or inadequate personal relationships

CLIENT GOAL

The client will increase social interactions

NURSING INTERVENTIONS

1. Encourage client to join local organizations or volunteer.
2. Encourage client to surround themselves with people with the same interests and goals.
3. Encourage client to avoid negative relations.

SCIENTIFIC RATIONALES

1. Client can control the amount of social interactions with others, and it encourages social relationships.
2. This provides support and positive reinforcement.
3. Negative situations may lead to social withdrawal.

EVALUATION

The client has joined the local ladies axillary that volunteers services at the community hospital once a week.

CONCEPT CARE MAP 48-1

NURSING PROCESS

ASSESSMENT

Subjective Data

The client may verbalize overwhelming feelings of sadness, thoughts of suicide, a loss of interest and pleasure in activities that were previously enjoyable, and problems with memory, recall, and concentration. In addition, a decreased libido, extreme lethargy, and having insufficient energy to complete activities of daily living (ADLs) and needed tasks may be reported. The depressed client who has become increasingly withdrawn and socially isolated may experience problems in intimate, personal, and social relationships.

Objective Data

The client may manifest a noticeable decline in personal hygiene and grooming, possibly because of a lack of energy and an inability to perform even the simplest of tasks. Weight loss resulting from the client's failure to eat may also be noted.

Nursing diagnoses for the client with depression include the following:

NURSING DIAGNOSES	PLANNING/OUTCOMES	NURSING INTERVENTIONS
***S**ocial Isolation* related to inability to engage in satisfying personal relationships	The client will increase the number of interactions with other individuals.	Build rapport and develop therapeutic relationship with client. Spend time with client individually. Encourage client to initiate conversation and interact with others. Verbally praise client for increasing interactions and initiating conversation.
*Bathing/Dressing and Feeding **S**elf-care Deficit* related to lack of concern or regard toward self	The client will attend to own basic health care needs.	Encourage client to bathe and wear clean clothes. Teach client the importance of balanced nutrition. Praise client for each activity done on own.

Evaluation: Evaluate each outcome to determine how it has been met by the client.

THE CLIENT WHO IS POTENTIALLY VIOLENT

In today's society, violence has become increasingly common and widespread. The media routinely and graphically reports the numerous violent crimes and acts that occur on a daily basis. Nurses may come face to face with angry clients and their families and significant others and, perhaps, even angry colleagues. When confronted by someone who is angry, the natural reaction is to respond in a like manner or, perhaps, to feel intimidated. In such difficult situations, it is important to maintain objectivity and not get "hooked" into the client's anger and respond in an inappropriate manner.

Nurses may encounter clients who are **verbally aggressive** (prone to saying things in a loud and/or intimidating manner), **physically aggressive** (prone to threatening or actually harming someone), or a combination of the two. Mind-altering substances such as alcohol and phencyclidine (PCP) often increase the risk of aggression. **Anger-control assistance** is defined as a nursing intervention aimed at facilitation of the expression of anger in an adaptive and nonviolent manner. Anger control includes establishing a basic level of trust and rapport with the client and using a calm and reassuring manner. The nurse should use every means possible to learn from the client (or his family/friends) those situations that are likely to bring on anger, and should encourage the client to inform the nursing staff when he is feeling tension. Although the nurse has a responsibility to help the client learn to deal with his anger, she also has a clear duty to assess for inappropriate aggression and to intervene before such aggression is expressed.

Some of the techniques used in anger control include limiting access to frustrating situations, providing physical outlets for expression of anger or tension (such as punching bags, large motor activities [sports], and anger journals), and ensuring that a client for whom anger is a problem is given enough personal space that he does not have to feel encroached upon by others when he is unable to tolerate environmental stimuli.

HOMICIDAL INTENT

The client who is homicidal is planning or threatening to harm or kill another individual or individuals. It is the responsibility of health care personnel to attempt to ascertain the seriousness of the intent; that is, whether the individual is actually threatening someone else or just "blowing off steam." Once aware of an individual's threat or intent to harm someone else, the nurse must inform the individual(s) at risk of the potential for harm and/or notify the proper authorities and enlist their help. The first step in such a situation is to contact the supervisor and offer an accurate appraisal of the situation.

SUICIDAL INTENT

Purposefully taking one's own life, or suicide, is the ultimate form of self-destruction. Clients who are suicidal often feel overwhelmed by life events and decide that the only relief will come from ending their own lives. Intense feelings of fear, loss, anger, or despair can drive individuals to commit suicide, and the effects of an attempted or completed suicide can be devastating

PROFESSIONAL TIP

Assessing for Risk of Violence

- Be aware of those clients with past history of violence and poor impulse control.
- Observe the client's body language: Notice changes in behavior, words, or dress.
- Assess for aggressive behaviors, increasing tension, clenched fists, loud or angry tone of voice, narrowed eyes, and pacing.
- Remember that hostility tends to be contagious. Do not reciprocate with anger and hostility!

and long lasting. Nurses must learn to recognize the danger signs of clients at risk for suicide and know the appropriate interventions to help clients preserve their health and dignity.

Suicide is the eleventh leading cause of death in the United States, claiming more than 32,000 lives each year (CDC, 2008a). The populations at greatest risk are individuals with diagnosed mood disorders such as Major Depressive Disorder, elders, and those with serious or life-threatening medical illnesses such as cancer or human immunodeficiency virus.

SUICIDAL IDEATIONS

The client experiencing **suicidal ideations** has thoughts of hurting or killing himself but may or may not be planning to act on these thoughts. It is important to understand the difference between thoughts and actions; that is, having a thought does not necessarily mean that the behavior will follow. When confronted with a client's verbalization of possible suicide, however, it is always wise to take the client's expression of intent seriously. Because suicide is a leading cause of death in the United States, nurses must know how to evaluate a client for the likelihood of a completed suicide. It is critical to thoroughly assess the client and attempt to accurately ascertain the degree of danger the client is experiencing. Once this is done, take the precautions necessary to maintain the client's safety (Table 48-7).

ACTIVELY SUICIDAL

The **actively suicidal** client is intent on hurting or killing himself and is in imminent danger of doing so. This situation requires immediate and appropriate action to protect the client from potentially fatal self-destructive behavior. If the client is in a supervised setting, it is the nurse's responsibility to maintain the safety of the client and to inform other staff members of the client's suicidal intentions. The client at risk for self-inflicted injury must be monitored closely (per institutional policy and the frequency as ordered by the physician).

The frequency of client observation is determined by the degree of suicide risk and is written as a specific order from the physician. Observations of the client are documented. Some clients must be checked a minimum of once every 15 minutes. Other clients may require more frequent observation and monitoring. If the client is *actively* suicidal and/or homicidal and is indicating an imminent intent to harm self or others, a specific staff member will be assigned to that client at all times on a one-to-one basis.

All pertinent observations such as verbalizations and behaviors that indicate self-harm potential should be documented in the client's record. Any changes in the client's condition should be reported immediately to the physician. The conversation

Table 48-7 Assessment of Risk for Suicide

The following areas are to be assessed in all potentially suicidal clients:	
1. Does the client have a *plan* to commit suicide?	
Example: Client plans to "end it all" after wife leaves for work on a Monday.	***Rationale:*** Some clients may be experiencing thoughts of wishing they were dead or killing themselves, but may not have a plan for doing so. *The client who has a plan for committing suicide is at increased risk.*
2. How *specific* is the plan to commit suicide?	
Example: Client states he plans to overdose on sleeping pills.	***Rationale:*** *A specific plan increases the risk of completing a suicide.*
3. Does the client have access to the *means* to commit suicide?	
Example: Client states he will use his spouse's sleeping pills to overdose.	***Rationale:*** *Easy availability of the means to kill oneself increases the risk of suicide.*
4. How *lethal* is the intended means to commit suicide?	
Example: Client states he will "blow his brains out" with a gun.	***Rationale:*** Some means of suicide are more likely to result in a completed suicide. *Gunshots are the most common cause of completed suicide.* The lethality of guns makes the potential for a successful intervention very slim. Intervention in light of means that are less lethal may yield a more favorable outcome (e.g., overdose, cutting of wrists).

COURTESY OF DELMAR CENGAGE LEARNING

with the doctor, as well as any new orders or changes in orders, must also be documented in the client's record.

Medical–Surgical Management

Medical

The client who is severely agitated, aggressive, actively suicidal, and/or homicidal and who is exhibiting or threatening violent acts may need to be restrained or placed in seclusion in order to be safely contained. The physical holding of someone or use of mechanical restraints severely restricts movement and can constitute a violation of the client's rights unless sufficient clinical justification exists. Thus, all of the client's comments and behaviors plus any nursing interventions must be documented in the client record per agency policy. This documentation provides the necessary justification for the use of restraints or seclusion. In addition, the physician must write a specific, time-limited order that spells out the reason restraints or seclusion was indicated for use with the client.

Physical Restraints Physical restraints, usually leather straps, are used to immobilize a person who is clearly dangerous to self or others and who poses sufficient risk of harm. Physical restraints may be applied only under the direction and supervision of a registered nurse (RN) and must comply with state laws regarding their use. In almost all cases, there must be a physician's order to apply the restraints, and there must be clearly documented evidence that the restraints were needed. Some of the observable behaviors indicating that restraints are necessary include increased motor activity, verbal and/or physical threats, overresponsiveness to stimuli, and actual physical assault (Frisch & Frisch, 2010).

Seclusion Seclusion is the process of confining a client to a single room. The room may be locked or unlocked, and it may or may not have furnishings. The purpose of seclusion is to provide security, to remove the client from a situation of escalating anger and violence, or to remove the client who is hypersensitive to environmental stimuli from the stimulation of a hospital unit. Seclusion, like the use of physical restraints, can be used only when all other avenues for control have been exhausted. The client must be told what is happening and why. He must not be left alone; a staff member should be assigned to observe the client, usually from the doorway. Seclusion is an enforced "time-out," where the client is removed from the situation only long enough to allow him to calm down, regain a sense of control, and then reenter the unit.

Therapy Psychotherapy is often indicated and initially may focus on personal and social conditions that bring about and/or perpetuate suicidal thoughts. Cognitive-behavioral therapy may be particularly useful, as may techniques to deal with frustration and anger. Substance use and abuse are often involved and may require separate outpatient or inpatient interventions.

> **PROFESSIONALTIP**
>
> **Providing a Safe Environment**
>
> When a client verbalizes an intention to inflict self-harm, measures must be taken to ensure the client's safety. One way is to provide and maintain a safe, secure environment for the client. This may require a change in items allowed in the client's surroundings and living space. For example, a pencil or pen could be used as a dangerous weapon; an empty soda can could be used to deeply cut the wrists or to seriously injure someone else; and the broken glass from a bottle of make-up could cause great harm. These and all other potentially dangerous items must be removed from the client's immediate area.

Pharmacological

The severely agitated, aggressive, suicidal, and/or homicidal client who is violent or threatening violence may require a medication with strong anxiolytic (antianxiety) and/or sedative properties, such as one of the antianxiety agents or a sedative-hypnotic (Table 48-1). Additionally, the suicidal client who is depressed may be evaluated for treatment with one of the many available antidepressants such as fluoxetine hydrochloride (Prozac), sertraline hydrochloride (Zoloft), paroxetine hydrochloride (Paxil), fluvoxamine maleate (Luvox), mirtazapine (Remeron), or one of the many others (Tables 48-3, 48-4, 48-5, and 48-6).

Diet

Foods are not restricted because a client is severely agitated, aggressive, actively suicidal, and/or homicidal, but may be restricted depending on the medications being taken. The food tray should be inspected for any potentially dangerous objects such as glassware or silverware. Even plasticware can be broken in such a way as to yield a very dangerous weapon for hurting self or others.

Activity

The activity level of the client who is severely agitated, aggressive, actively suicidal, and/or homicidal may need to be restricted for a period of time in order to maintain the client's safety and the safety of others.

Nursing Management

Assess the client for suicidal thoughts. If the client has a specific plan, evaluate the degree of risk for the client and contact the physician. Assess the environment for potentially dangerous items. Increase the level of client observation.

NURSING PROCESS

Assessment

Subjective Data

The client may argue, yell, curse, and make numerous verbal threats in a loud voice. The suicidal client may indicate intentions verbally, nonverbally, or a combination of the two. The client contemplating suicide may verbalize his thoughts either directly or indirectly. A direct statement may be something as straightforward as "I am planning to kill myself." An indirect

PROFESSIONALTIP

No-Suicide Contract

Obtaining a "No-Suicide Contract" from the client is one way to help reduce the risk of suicide attempts. There are several guidelines to follow in working through this process:

- Ask the client whether he is able to make a promise *to himself* that he will not do anything to harm himself. ***Rationale:*** It is important for the client to make the contract with himself, because if the contract is made with someone else, such as a nurse, and the client later becomes angry or upset with that person, he may then harm himself in order to "get back" at that person.
- If the client is unable to commit to the No-Suicide Contract for the rest of his life, work with him on establishing a time frame to which he can commit, for example, 1 week, 24 hours, 8 hours, or some other time frame. Always meet with the client at the end of the allotted time frame and review/renew the contract at that time. ***Rationale:*** The suicidal individual may feel overwhelmed at the thought of promising *never* to harm himself, but may be able to sincerely commit for a shorter length of time.
- Ask the client whether he is able to maintain the No-Suicide Contract *no matter what happens*. ***Rationale:*** Some clients will leave a way out of the contract. For example, the suicidal client may outwardly make a promise to not commit suicide but inwardly think "unless something really bad happens, like if my wife leaves me." If the wife then files for a divorce, the client may feel that he has "permission" to kill himself. Adding the *no matter what happens* clause blocks off this avenue of escape from the contract.
- Ask the client whether he can make a promise to himself that if thoughts of suicide return, he will talk to someone before taking any action. ***Rationale:*** If the client talks to someone regarding his thoughts of suicide *before* he attempts suicide, a successful intervention and suicide prevention are more likely.
- Assist the client in developing a detailed plan of action regarding those persons he will contact in the event that he again experiences suicidal thoughts. Include names and phone numbers of all significant and supportive individuals. ***Rationale:*** During a crisis, the suicidal individual is not able to think rationally and will behave and act in an impulsive manner. Having a well-developed plan of action increases the likelihood that the suicidal individual can follow these guidelines.
- At the bottom of the list, put the name and phone number of the local suicide crisis hotline and/or local emergency number (911). ***Rationale:*** Including these numbers ensures that there will always be someone available for the suicidal client to talk to 24 hours a day, 7 days a week, 365 days a year.
- Assist the client in putting the No-Suicide Contract in writing and in his own words. Give the client the original and put a copy in the client's chart. ***Rationale:*** When the contract is in writing and the client has a copy, he will be more likely to follow through with his promise to not commit suicide.

statement might be "I'm not going to be around here anymore" or "Everyone will be better off without me."

Objective Data

The client may exhibit restlessness, pacing, and "poor impulse control"; may be physically intimidating; and may use or try to use items in the environment, such as books, furniture, or a coffee pot, as weapons. A nonverbal signal of possible intentions of suicide may be seen in the client who begins making arrangements for people and pets to be taken care of, putting personal affairs in order, and giving away personal possessions, especially treasured items.

Nursing diagnoses for the client who is severely agitated, aggressive, actively suicidal, and/or homicidal include the following:

NURSING DIAGNOSES	PLANNING/OUTCOMES	NURSING INTERVENTIONS
Risk for Self-Directed Violence related to risk factors such as mental health, emotional status, or suicidal plan	The client will not harm self.	Assess for the presence of suicidal thoughts and whether a specific plan is present. Evaluate the degree of risk associated with the client's verbalization of suicide intent. Contact the attending physician or psychiatrist and inform of the client's intentions and current condition.

(*Continues*)

Nursing diagnoses for the client who is severely agitated, aggressive, actively suicidal, and/or homicidal include the following: (Continued)

NURSING DIAGNOSES	PLANNING/OUTCOMES	NURSING INTERVENTIONS
		Assess and evaluate the client's surroundings and environment for any potentially dangerous items or objects that could be used for self-harm. Remove or secure any potentially harmful items. Increase the level of observation so that the client is frequently monitored. Assist the client in developing a No-suicide Contract.
Risk for Other-Directed Violence related to risk factors such as history of violence against others, suicidal behavior, impulsivity	The client will not harm anyone.	Assess for the presence of homicidal ideations. If the client is verbalizing a plan to harm someone, immediately notify the proper authorities so they can alert this individual.

Evaluation: Evaluate each outcome to determine how it has been met by the client.

SAMPLE NURSING CARE PLAN

The Suicidal Client with Major Depression

A.J. is a 27-year-old woman who was brought to the emergency department of a county hospital by ambulance after a serious suicide attempt via ingesting a bottle of insecticide. After being treated in the emergency room, she spent 2 days in the intensive care unit (ICU) and then was transferred to a locked adult inpatient psychiatric unit for evaluation and treatment. A.J. reports she became suicidal following the recent ending of a 4-year relationship with her boyfriend and decided to take her life because she felt "completely hopeless," that "there was nothing left to live for," that "no one would miss her" if she were dead, that she "would never be loved," and that she "could never be happy again." Before the suicide attempt, A.J. reports that she had not been eating, had only been sleeping 1 to 2 hours per night, and had been crying almost continuously throughout the day. Since admission to the psychiatric unit, A.J. has been started on sertraline (Zoloft).

NURSING DIAGNOSIS 1 *Risk for Self-Directed Violence* related to recent loss, feelings of abandonment, and impulsive behavior as evidenced by suicide attempt of drinking bottle of insecticide, verbalizations that "there was nothing left to live for" and that "no one would miss her" if she were dead

Nursing Outcomes Classification (NOC)
Depression Level
Suicide Self-Restraint

Nursing Interventions Classification (NIC)
Self-Esteem Enhancement
Coping Enhancement

PLANNING/OUTCOMES	NURSING INTERVENTIONS	RATIONALE
A.J. will verbalize that she is no longer at risk of harming herself.	Assist A.J. in developing a No-Suicide Contract. Obtain in writing if possible, make a copy for her chart, and give her the original.	May help deter self-destructive behavior in the future.
	Explore with A.J. factors that contributed to her becoming suicidal.	Can be the first step in preventing another attempt.

SAMPLE NURSING CARE PLAN (Continued)

PLANNING/OUTCOMES	NURSING INTERVENTIONS	RATIONALE
	Encourage A.J. to verbalize her feelings related to the recent break-up and to explore any unresolved past issues that this loss might have triggered.	Current feelings of loss and abandonment are often magnified and intensified by unresolved past situations and circumstances that were never effectively handled.
	Explore with A.J. her usual methods of coping with stressful situations and whether these have been effective for her.	Can lead to a better understanding of those behaviors that must be changed.
	Assist A.J. in identifying and then developing stress-management methods as alternatives to attempting suicide.	Assists the client in recognizing alternate methods of managing stressful situations.
	Assist A.J. in developing a suicide-prevention plan and in identifying supportive individuals and resources that she can turn to in the event that she begins to again have suicidal thoughts.	Plans to prevent suicide must be developed ahead of time, because individuals contemplating suicide are impulsive and unable to problem solve or think clearly. They may, however, be able to follow through with a previously defined plan of action.
	Teach A.J. about possible side effects associated with sertraline (Zoloft), such as nausea and GI upset, and encourage her to have something to eat prior to taking this medication.	Medication education is an integral part of treatment.
	Emphasize the importance of taking this medication as prescribed and not stopping the medication on her own, even if she starts to feel better and thinks that she no longer needs it.	If medications are discontinued prematurely, symptoms usually reappear and are often much more serious.
	Encourage A.J. to keep a journal to reflect on her thoughts and feelings.	Writing in a journal can be a safe and effective method of identifying, expressing, and releasing feelings and emotions.
	Encourage A.J. to keep follow-up appointments for medication to monitor progress.	Recommended to evaluate effectiveness and to monitor for any side effects.
	Assist A.J. in setting up an appointment for outpatient counseling/therapy upon discharge per recommendation from the treatment team. Encourage A.J. to keep counseling appointments.	Recommended after a suicide attempt in order to address the underlying issues and to prevent future attempts.

(*Continues*)

SAMPLE NURSING CARE PLAN (Continued)

EVALUATION

At the time of discharge from the adult inpatient psychiatric unit, A.J. was no longer actively suicidal or intent upon harming herself. She still had occasional suicidal ideations; however, she did not feel compelled to act on them. She had made a promise to herself that she would never try to kill herself again no matter what happened, and that if those thoughts returned, she would find someone to talk to before she did anything. She also had developed a written list of friends and relatives she could call if she again experienced thoughts of suicide.

NURSING DIAGNOSIS 2 *Hopelessness* related to feelings of loss about her life and future as evidenced by verbalizations of feeling: "completely hopeless," that she "would never be loved," and that she "could never be happy again"

Nursing Outcomes Classification (NOC)
Depression Control
Mood Equilibrium

Nursing Interventions Classification (NIC)
Suicide Prevention
Patient Contracting

PLANNING/OUTCOMES	NURSING INTERVENTIONS	RATIONALE
A.J. will be less hopeless as indicated by verbalizations of plans for her future	Develop a therapeutic nurse–client relationship with A.J. using the components of trust, rapport, respect, genuineness, and empathy.	Fosters the development of a therapeutic nurse–client relationship.
	Encourage A.J. to become involved in activities on the unit, for example, interacting with staff and other clients and attending and participating in therapy groups and recreational activities.	Helps distract the mind from a preoccupation with losses, overwhelming feelings of depression, and suicidal ideations.
	Provide things for A.J. to do when she is feeling down, for example, go for a walk with the staff, read a newspaper or book, or play a game.	Provides time to allow for something to shift for her, to see the situation as not so utterly and permanently hopeless or for her to begin to feel better and think differently once she has started responding to medication.
	Assist A.J. in identifying the irrational beliefs or thoughts that she is having, for example, when she says no one will ever love or want her again.	Changing the way a person thinks by replacing irrational thoughts with rational or healthier ones, will change the way the person feels.

EVALUATION

A.J. continued to have fleeting thoughts of hopelessness as far as ever having another significant relationship or being in love again; however, she now was beginning to catch herself and could identify these thoughts as being irrational and negative in nature and not helpful to her in any way.

THE CLIENT WHO IS PSYCHOTIC

Psychosis is a state wherein an individual loses the ability to recognize reality. A psychotic person may experience hallucinations, wherein he hears voices or sees images of persons or things that others cannot see or hear. A psychotic person is frequently unable to care for basic needs of safety, security, nutrition, and so on. Such an individual is hospitalized for his own safety and to initiate treatment (usually involving some form of medication) to bring the symptoms under control. A psychotic person may slip into and out of reality.

Psychosis can be a component of several illnesses, including Schizophrenia and Bipolar Disorder.

SCHIZOPHRENIA

The client with schizophrenia can be very difficult to understand and treat because the symptoms of schizophrenia can be confusing and frightening to caregivers. Clients with schizophrenia frequently have belief systems that have become distorted, so that they hold firmly to false ideas or delusions, even when presented with evidence to the contrary. When confronted with an opposing belief system, they may become even more entrenched in their mistaken views and begin to believe others are "against them," when, in fact, they are not. This makes them even more paranoid and suspicious, adding to their already distorted views of reality. As a result, these individuals are often struggling to determine the difference between that which is real and that which is unreal or delusional.

Hallucinations can occur in relation to any of the five senses (hearing, sight, touch, taste, and smell), but the most common types of hallucinations are auditory and visual. Individuals experiencing **auditory hallucinations** hear someone talking to them, when, in reality, no one is. The voice may be that of someone the individual recognizes, or the voice may be unknown to the person. If the voice or voices are comforting, the individual will be very resistant to "giving them up." Most of the time, however, the voices are derogatory in nature, telling the person that there is something wrong with him.

The individual experiencing a **visual hallucination** perceives or sees someone or something that is not actually there. Depending on the nature of the hallucination and whether the individual perceives it as threatening, the situation can be very frightening.

The most serious type of hallucination is referred to as the **command hallucination**, which occurs when the voice or voices tell the individual to harm himself or someone else. For example, the voices may tell the individual to jump off a bridge or building, step in front of a moving motor vehicle, or take an overdose of medication. These hallucinations are extremely dangerous because the demands are so strong that the individual is very likely to act on them.

MEDICAL–SURGICAL MANAGEMENT

Medical

At this time, there is no cure for schizophrenia; however, it is possible for some clients with schizophrenia to lead functional lives with minimally debilitating symptoms through psychosocial treatments.

The goals of psychosocial treatment can be divided into three categories: clinical and family support services, rehabilitative services, and humanitarian aid/public safety. Clinical support involves outpatient management and family/community services. Rehabilitation involves increasing clients' capacities, both for social interactions and for productive activity (including gainful employment, when feasible). Humanitarian interventions are those efforts that maximize an individual's independence and quality of life within the bounds of the mental disability. Public safety involves balancing personal liberty with the recognition that some social control may be needed to prevent harm, both to the individual and to society.

Pharmacological

The most commonly prescribed classification of medications for the client experiencing schizophrenia is the antipsychotics (Tables 48-8 and 48-9). This group of medications is given to reduce the signs and symptoms of psychosis, with a long-term goal of the client eventually being symptom free. If this is not possible, the goal is to reduce symptoms to a manageable level.

Because several side effects are associated with the antipsychotics, client teaching is an important part of the nurse's role. In addition to common side effects, some antipsychotic medications also have the potential for causing adverse reactions such as extrapyramidal symptoms (EPS), tardive dyskinesia (TD), and neuroleptic malignant syndrome (NMS).

One of the most important factors in symptom management for schizophrenia is medication compliance. In most cases, individuals who are schizophrenic must take some type of antipsychotic medication for the remainder of their lives. Clients suffering from schizophrenia are often extremely resistant to taking their medications as prescribed and usually require multiple repeat hospitalizations for stabilization. Multiple reasons exist for noncompliance, one being the client's denial of the diagnosis or the illness or of the seriousness of the illness. As a result of denial, the individual with schizophrenia resists taking medication, because to the client, taking medication equates to acceptance of having a serious mental disorder. Clients may

> **CLIENT TEACHING**
>
> **Schizophrenia**
>
> Family involvement is important for all clients, but it is especially critical for the client with schizophrenia. Because the client may be too ill or confused to be trusted to take medications reliably, it becomes the responsibility of family members to help ensure medication compliance. Most hospital readmissions for the client with schizophrenia are a result of noncompliance with the prescribed medication regimen. If the family understands the important role psychotropic medications can play in preventing decompensation (a return of the psychiatric symptoms) and subsequent hospital readmission, the client has a much better chance of remaining stabilized.

Table 48-8 Atypical Antipsychotics

GENERIC NAME	TRADE NAME	POTENTIAL SIDE EFFECTS
clozapine	Clozaril	Agranulocytosis, angina, constipation, dizziness, orthostatic hypotension, increased salivation, leukopenia, NMS, drowsiness, seizures, tachycardia, weight gain
olanzapine	Zyprexa	Agitation, acute renal failure, amblyopia, constipation, CVA, dizziness, dry mouth, headache, NMS, orthostatic hypotension, restlessness, rhinitis, sedation, seizures, tachycardia, TD, tremors, weakness, weight gain
quetiapine fumarate	Seroquel	Dizziness, headache, NMS, seizures, TD, weight gain
risperidone	Risperdal	Acute renal failure, constipation, cough, decreased libido, diarrhea, dizziness, dry mouth, dysmenorrhea/menorrhagia, headache, increased dreams, increased sleep duration, insomnia, itching/skin rash, MI, nausea, NMS, pharyngitis, rhinitis, sedation, visual disturbances

Data from *Delmar Nurse's Drug Handbook 2010 Edition*, by G. Spratto and A. Woods, 2010, Clifton Park, NY: Delmar Cengage Learning.

Table 48-9 Phenothiazines (Antipsychotics)

GENERIC NAME	TRADE NAME	POTENTIAL SIDE EFFECTS
chlorpromazine, hydrochloride	Thorazine	Agranulocytosis, blurred vision, constipation, dry eyes, dry mouth, hypotension, laryngeal edema, NMS, photosensitivity, sedation, TD
fluphenazine hydrochloride	Prolixin	Agranulocytosis, EPS, photosensitivity, TD
thioridazine hydro-chloride	Mellaril	Agranulocytosis, blurred vision, constipation, dry eyes, dry mouth, hypotension, NMS, photosensitivity, sedation, TD

Data from *Delmar Nurse's Drug Handbook 2010 Edition*, by G. Spratto and A. Woods, 2010, Clifton Park, NY: Delmar Cengage Learning.

CLIENT TEACHING

Adverse Reactions to Antipsychotic Medications

- *Extrapyramidal side effects:* a common adverse reaction of some antipsychotic medications (especially the older ones) involving muscle rigidity and involuntary muscle movements; reversible if the dose is lowered or an anti-Parkinson agent is administered
- *Tardive dyskinesia:* irreversible reaction to antipsychotics (usually associated with high doses over a long period) consisting of involuntary muscle and body movements
- *Neuroleptic malignant syndrome:* a rare and potentially fatal reaction to antipsychotic medications characterized by a very high fever, severe muscle stiffness, and changes in sensorium progressing to coma

also become noncompliant after a period of time on medication; once they start to feel better, they think the medication is no longer needed and stop taking it. After a short time of being off the prescribed medication, however, most individuals with schizophrenia will experience a return or significant worsening of their previous symptoms.

Probably the most common reason for medication noncompliance, however, is the number of troublesome side effects and potentially dangerous adverse reactions historically associated with antipsychotic medications. Fortunately, newer antipsychotic medications are now available that have fewer side effects and are much better tolerated. Even with the advent of these newer and more effective medications, however, many individuals are unable to benefit from them because of the high cost and the difficulties sometimes associated with accessing these medications.

Diet

Some of the antipsychotics such as clozapine (Clozaril), olanzapine (Zyprexa), quetiapine fumerate (Seroquel), and risperidone (Risperdal) can cause weight gain over time. For the individual who has schizophrenia and its multiple

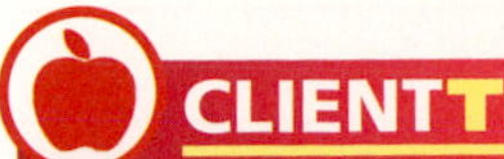

CLIENT TEACHING

Phenothiazines

Be sure to instruct each client taking a phenothiazine medication in the following:

- Do not drink alcohol while on the medication.
- Do not take any other medications unless prescribed by your physician.
- Do not stop taking the medication abruptly.
- The ability to drive and/or operate heavy machinery may be impaired while taking the medication.
- Be aware of possible side effects of the medication.
- Increase fluid intake to minimize the side effects of dry mouth and constipation.
- Increase dietary fiber to minimize the side effect of constipation.
- Rise slowly from a lying position to prevent dizziness and a sudden drop in blood pressure.
- These medications are contraindicated during pregnancy and lactation. Female clients should advise their physicians immediately if they are either pregnant or planning to become pregnant.
- Wear sunscreen and protective clothing while outdoors, as the medication increases susceptibility to sunburn.
- Some of the side effects may diminish in intensity after an initial period of adjustment.
- The medication may increase your risk of developing EPS, TD, and NMS.

associated problems, weight gain can constitute yet one more stressor. Teaching for the client who is at risk for gaining weight must therefore emphasize the importance of being cognizant of and conservative with regard to caloric and fat intake, avoiding a sedentary lifestyle, and increasing physical activity.

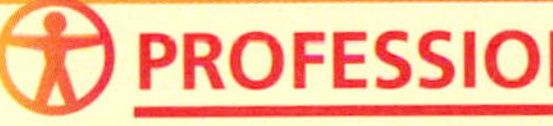

PROFESSIONAL TIP

Refrain from Making Judgments

Changing the words we use may help the client and family feel less defensive and may open the door for more effective communication. One example of an often-used term that carries negative connotations is *noncompliance*. Ward-Collins (1998) encourages nurses to consider using another term such as *nonadherence*, which does not carry the same degree of negative connotations.

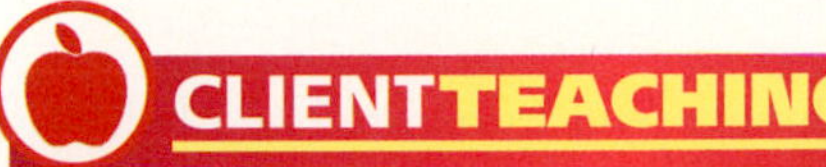

CLIENT TEACHING

Atypical Antipsychotics

Be sure to instruct each client taking an atypical antipsychotic medication in the following:

- Do not drink alcohol while taking the medication.
- Do not take any other medications, prescription or OTC, unless prescribed by your physician.
- Do not stop taking the medication without authorization from your physician.
- Do not stop taking the medication abruptly.
- The ability to drive and/or operate heavy machinery may be impaired while taking the medication.
- Rise slowly from a lying position to prevent dizziness and a sudden drop in blood pressure.
- The medication is contraindicated during pregnancy and lactation. Reliable contraception should be utilized while taking the medication. Female clients should advise their physicians immediately if they suspect they are either pregnant or planning to become pregnant.
- Be aware of the potential side effects of the medications.
- Notify your physician immediately of unexplained fever, sore throat, bleeding, bruising, or petechiae.
- Wear sunscreen and protective clothing while outdoors, as olanzapine (Zyprexa) and risperidone (Risperdal) increase susceptibility to sunburn.
- Avoid temperature extremes if taking olanzapine (Zyprexa), quetiapine fumerate (Seroquel), or risperidone (Risperdal), as the body's ability to regulate internal temperature is affected by these medications.
- Utilize good oral hygiene in conjunction with sugarless candy or gum to minimize the discomforting side effect of dry mouth associated most frequently with clozapine (Clozaril) and olanzapine (Zyprexa).
- Beware of associated risks including EPS, NMS, and a high risk of agranulocytosis and seizures with clozapine (Clozaril); EPS, TD, and NMS with olanzapine (Zyprexa), quetiapine (Seroquel), and risperidone (Risperdal); and seizures with olanzapine (Zyprexa) and quetiapine fumerate (Seroquel).
- Treatment with clozapine (Clozaril) requires weekly white blood cell (WBC) monitoring to assess for onset of agranulocytosis. Medication is dispensed in 7-day increments to maintain policy compliance and prevent this potentially life-threatening occurrence.

Activity

Clients with schizophrenia tend to be tired and lethargic, probably because of multiple factors including the disease process and, possibly, the sedative properties associated with some of the antipsychotics, especially some of the older ones such as chlorpromazine (Thorazine) and thioridazine (Mellaril).

NURSING MANAGEMENT

Carefully observe the client's behavior. Listen to the client but neither agree nor disagree with what the client is saying. Accurately document what is seen and heard. Include the family in client care. Encourage the client to perform ADLs.

NURSING PROCESS

ASSESSMENT

Subjective Data

The client may be very frightened, confused, and have disorganized thought processes, using a nonsensical combination of words that is meaningless to others (**word salad**), talk out loud even when no one is present, or respond to internal stimulation or hallucinations.

Objective Data

The client may be isolated, withdrawn, experience great difficulty in any type of social interaction or situation, and stay in bed and sleep. Thus, the client may require a great deal of assistance and encouragement to perform ADLs and complete basic hygiene needs.

Nursing diagnoses for the client with schizophrenia include the following:

NURSING DIAGNOSES	PLANNING/OUTCOMES	NURSING INTERVENTIONS
*Disturbed **S**ensory Perception (Visual, Auditory)* related to altered sensory perception	The client will experience a decrease in the intensity and frequency of symptoms.	Assess for the presence of hallucinations. Assist the client in beginning to exert some control over the hallucinations. Educate the client about ways to decrease the intensity and power of the hallucinations.
*Deficient **K**nowledge* related to medication therapy	The client will verbalize an understanding of the disorder and the ongoing need for medications.	Educate the client and family about the disorder of Schizophrenia, the need for antipsychotic medications, and the importance of continuing the prescribed medication regimen.

Evaluation: Evaluate each outcome to determine how it has been met by the client.

BIPOLAR DISORDER

Bipolar Disorder (previously known as manic–depressive disorder) is characterized by wide fluctuations in **mood** (the way an individual reports feeling, e.g., depressed, elated, happy, sad) and **affect** (the objective or outward manifestation of the way an individual is feeling). Nearly 6 million Americans have bipolar disorder (DBSA, 2009). Bipolar disorders are a personal and public health concern with as many as 19 % of bipolar individuals dying from suicide, and bipolar disorder ranking sixth as a leading cause of disability in the United States (Antai-Otong, 2008). In addition to having a wide range of both affect and mood, the individual with bipolar disorder may experience fluctuations between depression and **mania** (extremely elevated mood with accompanying agitated behavior). The client with bipolar disorder may experience these fluctuations in mood and affect in varying degrees and over varying time frames. For example, an individual may experience changes in mood and affect every few years, at certain times of the year, every few months, every few weeks, or even every few days. The alterations in mood between depression and mania are often referred to as cycling. Individuals who suffer what is known as rapid cycling may experience multiple swings between depression and mania in the same day. There are also several degrees of both depression and mania that the individual can experience. As is the case with depression, an individual can experience mild, moderate, or severe mania. The degrees of mania range on a continuum from **hypomania** (a mild form of mania without significant impairment) to severe or delirious mania (DBSA, 2006).

An individual in the depressed phase of bipolar disorder will manifest the same signs and symptoms as an individual with depression. The client in the manic phase of bipolar disorder may be very irritable and agitated and can be intimidating toward others, both verbally and physically. The client exhibiting manic behavior is often hyperactive, unable to sit down or remain still, and may display a **euphoric** (being elated out of context to the situation) affect and mood. Once in the manic phase of illness, clients will often exhibit behaviors incongruent with their usual personalities. For example, the manic client may dress in a flamboyant and provocative manner; spend money and buy things in a very lavish fashion; and become sexually promiscuous and engage in risky behaviors that would otherwise be out of character. After a while, the client may experience a great deal of conflict in social, familial, and personal relationships. It often becomes the responsibility of a significant other or family member to seek professional assistance for the individual. This already difficult situation is compounded by the fact that the client

Table 48-10 Mood Stabilitzer: Antimanic

GENERIC NAME	TRADE NAME	POTENTIAL SIDE EFFECTS	SIGNS AND SYMPTOMS OF TOXICITY
lithium carbonate	Eskalith, Lithonate	Abdominal pain, acneiform eruption, anorexia, arrhythmia, bloating, diarrhea, dizziness, drowsiness, EKG changes, fatigue, folliculitis, GI upset, headache, hypothyroidism, impaired memory, irritability, leukocytosis, muscle weakness, nausea, polyuria, seizures, tinnitus, tremors	Ataxia, change in level of orientation, confusion, diarrhea, drowsiness, excessive urination, lack of coordination, muscle weakness, tremors, vomiting

Data from *Delmar Nurse's Drug Handbook 2010 Edition,* by G. Spratto and A. Woods, 2010, Clifton Park, NY: Delmar Cengage Learning.

in the manic phase of bipolar disorder is frequently in denial about the illness, does not perceive the erratic behavior as problematic, and enjoys the "high" created by the disorder. As a result, the individual often refuses any type of help, and the family may be required to seek involuntary hospitalization in order to obtain the much-needed treatment.

Medical–Surgical Management

Medical

The severely agitated client in the manic phase of bipolar disorder may need to be secluded and/or restrained in order to protect against self-inflicted injury and/or the risk of injury to others.

Psychotherapy may be helpful to the client experiencing bipolar disorder, but it is not recommended as the only intervention. These clients typically require some type of medication management for the remainder of their lives in order to function adequately.

Pharmacological

The drug of choice for treatment of bipolar disorder is lithium carbonate (Lithonate) (Table 48-10). Lithium is a naturally occurring salt that has proven highly effective for many individuals in managing the severe mood swings associated with bipolar disorder. Lithium is referred to as a "mood stabilizer," meaning that it helps level or even out the wide mood swings associated with the disorder; however, some individuals either cannot tolerate lithium therapy or become resistant to its therapeutic effectiveness after a period of time. Fortunately, some other medications are often prescribed for clients who cannot take lithium. These include the anticonvulsants valproic acid (Depakene) and carbamazepine (Tegretol) (Table 48-11) and the anxiolytic/anticonvulsant clonazepam (Klonopin).

Lithium has a very narrow range of therapeutic effectiveness. The amount of lithium the individual has available and whether this level is appropriate is measured by a blood test called serum lithium level. The acceptable therapeutic range for the **serum lithium level** is 0.4 to 1.0 mEq/L; however, the value may vary slightly depending on the laboratory that is performing the test (Spratto & Woods, 2008). A lithium level that is too low will not produce any benefit, and one that is too high may be toxic, or poisonous. It is therefore critical that the serum lithium level be obtained every 5 days until the client is stabilized on the medication. Blood should then be drawn monthly for as long as the client is taking the medication (Spratto & Woods, 2008). Before initiating lithium therapy, a 24-hour urine creatinine clearance test is done to evaluate the functioning of the kidneys and their ability to adequately excrete the lithium.

Diet

Because lithium is a salt that is chemically similar to sodium chloride (table salt), lithium and sodium compete for

Table 48-11 Mood Stabilizers: Anticonvulsants

GENERIC NAME	TRADE NAME	POTENTIAL SIDE EFFECTS
carbamazepine	Tegretol	Agranulocytosis, aplastic anemia, ataxia, drowsiness, drug-induced hepatitis, thrombocytopenia
valproic acid	Depakene	Depression, dizziness, indigestion, hepatotoxicity, leukopenia, nausea, thrombocytopenia, vomiting, weight gain

Data from *Delmar Nurse's Drug Handbook 2010 Edition*, by G. Spratto and A. Woods, 2010, Clifton Park, NY: Delmar Cengage Learning.

LIFE SPAN CONSIDERATIONS

Lithium Use in Older Adults

Because older adults have a reduced creatinine clearance, they are at greater risk for developing toxicity while taking lithium. Use caution in the older adult because lithium is more toxic to the central nervous system. The older adult may also develop a lithium-induced goiter and hypothyroidism (Spratto & Woods, 2010).

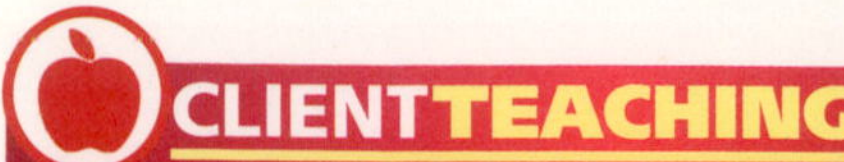

CLIENT TEACHING
Lithium

Be sure to instruct each client taking lithium in the following:

- Do not drink alcohol while taking this medication.
- Do not take any other medications, prescribed or OTC, unless authorized by your physician.
- Do not stop taking this medication without authorization from your physician.
- Female clients should utilize a reliable form of contraception while taking this medication. Immediately inform your physician if pregnancy is suspected.
- Drink 2,000 to 3,000 mL of fluid (10–12 glasses) per day.
- Maintain a consistent level of salt in the diet.
- The ability to drive or operate heavy machinery may be impaired while on this medication.
- Serum lithium level must be checked at scheduled intervals throughout therapy.
- Be aware of signs and symptoms of lithium toxicity.

absorption at receptor sites. This relationship is inversely proportional; thus, any changes in the body's sodium level will directly affect lithium level. Adequate fluid intake is very important for the client on lithium therapy. It is recommended that the client taking lithium consume a minimum of 2,000 to 3,000 mL of water per day. Because of the stimulating effects of caffeine, clients taking lithium should avoid any beverages containing caffeine.

Activity

The balance of sodium chloride to lithium can also be affected by the client's level of activity. An increase in activity, especially in hot and/or humid conditions when excessive perspiration is likely, can deplete the client's sodium level, thereby causing a drastic increase in lithium level and, potentially, lithium toxicity. A sudden increase in a client's activity level requires close monitoring and replacement of both fluid and electrolytes in order to prevent a sudden increase in the lithium level.

CLIENT TEACHING
Anticonvulsants

Be sure to instruct each client taking an anticonvulsant medication in the following:

- Do not drink alcohol while taking the medication.
- Do not take any other medications, prescribed or OTC, unless authorized by your physician.
- Take the medication exactly as prescribed.
- Do not stop taking the medication without authorization from your physician.
- Do not stop taking the medication abruptly.
- The medications are contraindicated during pregnancy and lactation. Female clients should advise their physicians immediately if they are either pregnant or planning to become pregnant.
- Carbamazepine (Tegretol) can impair the effectiveness of hormonal forms of contraception. Female clients should practice an alternate form of birth control while on this medication.
- The ability to drive or operate heavy machinery may be impaired while on the medication.
- Laboratory tests monitoring complete blood count (CBC), platelet count, bleeding time, and hepatic functioning must be performed periodically throughout therapy.
- Notify your physician immediately of unexplained fever, sore throat, bleeding, bruising, or petechiae.
- Serum level must be checked at scheduled intervals throughout therapy.

Nursing Management

Include the family in client education about the disease process, illness progression, medications, and importance

CASE STUDY

Bipolar Disorder

A 28-year-old male client is admitted to the psychiatric unit with a diagnosis of Bipolar Disorder. He is unable to sleep, in constant motion, very talkative, exaggerating and glamorizing life events, and inappropriately talking about sexual promiscuity to other clients.

1. The client is exhibiting which phase of bipolar disorder?
2. The drug of choice for treatment of bipolar disorder is?
3. List two types of treatment for bipolar disorder.

of taking the medications as prescribed (even if the client's condition improves dramatically). Emphasize the need to keep follow-up appointments and to have lab work done for lithium level. Encourage the family to help the client maintain a regular eating and sleeping schedule.

NURSING PROCESS

ASSESSMENT

Subjective Data

The client may deny having a problem or may view the problem as residing in other people. The client may also be quite loud, flamboyant, and grandiose in verbalizations and manifest very quick and **pressured speech** (rapid, intense speech).

Objective Data

The client may be sleeping very little or not at all and may not be eating or drinking, if in the manic phase. The client may at times be very irritable, agitated, quick to anger, and, possibly, violent. Clients with bipolar disorder often have extreme difficulty in interpersonal and social relationships because they have no personal boundaries. They may also be invasive and intrusive in their interactions with others, both verbally and physically.

Nursing diagnoses for the client with bipolar disorder include the following:

NURSING DIAGNOSES	PLANNING/OUTCOMES	NURSING INTERVENTIONS
*Disturbed **S**leep Pattern* related to sensory alterations	The client will sleep 6 hours per night.	Provide a quiet, peaceful environment. Decrease external stimulation and environmental distractions. Teach client relaxation exercises.
***N**oncompliance (medication and treatment regimen)* related to health beliefs	The client will demonstrate increased compliance with medication and treatment.	Educate the client and family about the disease process and the progression of the illness over time, prescribed medication, indications for use, dosage, times, and any possible side effects or untoward reactions, and the importance of taking the medication as prescribed. Teach the client to continue taking medication and to not miss doses *even if the condition improves dramatically.*

Evaluation: Evaluate each outcome to determine how it has been met by the client.

THE CLIENT REQUIRING SPECIAL CONSIDERATION

Several disorders require special attention and consideration on the part of the nurse. These include disorders commonly associated with childhood and adolescence and with individuals who have been violated in some manner, such as via neglect and/or abuse.

ATTENTION-DEFICIT/HYPERACTIVITY DISORDER

The *DSM-IV* identifies 18 diagnostic criteria for Attention-Deficit/Hyperactivity Disorder (ADHD) that fall under the categories of *inattention*, *hyperactivity*, and *impulsivity* (APA, 2000). There are three varieties of Attention-Deficit/Hyperactivity Disorder listed in the DSM-IV: Attention-Deficit/Hyperactivity Disorder, Predominantly Hyperactive-Impulsive Type; Attention-Deficit/Hyperactivity Disorder, Predominantly Inattentive Type; and Attention-Deficit/Hyperactivity Disorder, Combined Type. The child with ADHD may exhibit one or more of these behaviors in any combination (inattention, hyperactivity, and impulsivity). The problematic behaviors associated with these disorders vary in severity for each individual. Once thought to be a disorder only of childhood, it is now known that ADHD may continue well into adulthood. Individuals with ADHD are extremely sensitive to their environments and surroundings and respond immediately to any type of stimuli or distraction that most individuals would not even notice.

PROFESSIONALTIP

Token-Economy System

A token-economy system is a form of behavior modification used to shape a client's behavior over time. The client receives a "token" (poker chips work well) each time an appropriate or desired behavior is exhibited. In the classroom, the desired behavior might be working 15 minutes on a math assignment; at home, it might be picking up dirty clothes from the floor. Receiving the token is a form of positive reinforcement for the client and provides immediate gratification. At the end of a designated period, the client may "cash in" earned tokens for a prize (game, puzzle) or a special privilege (going to get an ice cream). The cashing in of tokens emphasizes the concept of delayed gratification, which in turn teaches patience.

PREDOMINANTLY HYPERACTIVE-IMPULSIVE TYPE

Hyperactivity is the hallmark feature of Predominantly Hyperactive-Impulsive Type ADHD, which is usually diagnosed in childhood when the symptoms first manifest. The pediatric client with ADHD may be referred for evaluation and treatment by parents or teachers because of impulsive and disruptive behavior in the classroom and/or at home. In many cases, there seems to be a familial or possible genetic link, as seen in health histories, which often reveal a parent or immediate family member as having had a similar problem as a child.

PREDOMINANTLY INATTENTIVE TYPE

In some children with ADHD predominantly inattentive type, the symptom of hyperactivity is not always present. The children have problems primarily with attention span. The inattentive child cannot maintain attention on one task, does not appear to listen when spoken to, and is easily distracted and forgetful.

COMBINED TYPE

Children with ADHD of the combined type exhibit symptoms of hyperactivity, impulsivity, and inattention. The characteristics must typically be exhibited for a period of at least 6 months in order to qualify for the diagnosis.

MEDICAL–SURGICAL MANAGEMENT

Medical

Counseling and therapy are often recommended to the client and family to assist in managing the child. The parents will require assistance in developing an effective behavior-modification program, such as a token-economy system that rewards desired behaviors, to help manage some of the child's problematic behaviors.

> **LIFE SPAN CONSIDERATIONS**
>
> **ADHD**
>
> In the past, it was believed that most children would outgrow ADHD. Today, it is known that symptoms of ADHD can continue into adulthood (Antai-Otong, 2008).

Pharmacological

The central nervous system (CNS) stimulants, which include methylphenidate hydrochloride (Ritalin), pemoline (Cylert), dextroamphetamine sulfate (Dexedrine), and amphetamine sulfate (Adderall), are usually prescribed to treat ADHD (Table 48-12). When one of the CNS stimulants is given to someone with ADHD, however, it has the opposite effect, or **paradoxical reaction**. Thus, instead of making someone with ADHD more hyperactive, it actually helps calm him. Because most of the symptoms of the child with ADHD, such as hyperactivity and the inability to concentrate and remain on task, are manifested in the classroom, any improvement will likely first be noted in this setting. When a child begins a new medication, it is vitally important that the family communicate openly with the child's teacher to ensure close monitoring of the child's response to medication. The child with ADHD who has been hyperactive, unable to stay on task, or complete assignments before receiving medication may now be less disruptive in the classroom and better able to remain on task and complete assignments. In addition, the medication can be a useful adjunct to facilitate the child's ability to develop and strengthen internal mechanisms for improving behavior.

Table 48-12 Central Nervous System Stimulants

GENERIC NAME	TRADE NAME	POTENTIAL SIDE EFFECTS
dextroamphetamine sulfate	Dexedrine	Anorexia, headache, hyperactivity, hypertension, insomnia, palpitations, physical and psychological dependence, restlessness, tachycardia, tolerance, tremors, urticaria, weight loss
amphetamine sulfate	Adderall	Anorexia, hyperactivity, insomnia, palpitations, physical and psychological dependence, restlessness, tachycardia, tremors
methylphenidate hydrochloride	Ritalin	Anemia, anorexia, hyperactivity, hypertension, insomnia, leukopenia, physical and psychological dependence, restlessness, skin rash, suppression of weight gain, tolerance, tremors
pemoline	Cylert	Insomnia, anorexia, aplastic anemia, decreased growth, drug-induced hepatitis, nausea, physical or psychological dependence, seizures, stomachache, tolerance, weight loss
atomoxetine hydrochloride	Strattera	Fatigue, decreased appetite, aggression, nausea, vomiting, postural hypotension

Data from *Delmar Nurse's Drug Handbook 2010 Edition*, by G. Spratto and A. Woods, 2010, Clifton Park, NY: Delmar Cengage Learning.

Teaching the client and family about the prescribed medication is very important, as there are some common side effects associated with the CNS stimulants, such as insomnia. To help decrease the risk of insomnia, these medications are usually given in the morning at breakfast, and if more is needed, another dose is given again at lunchtime. In some cases, a late-afternoon dose may be needed after school; however, this decision must be made very cautiously, because the later in the day that the dose is given, the greater the risk of insomnia that night for the child.

The client on CNS stimulants must be monitored for any vocal or motor tics, which might indicate the development of Tourette's syndrome. The CNS stimulant should be discontinued immediately if these symptoms are noted.

Diet

One potential problem associated with the CNS stimulants is that of decreased appetite, which can become serious if the child begins losing weight as a side effect of the medication. If this occurs, the medication may be given immediately after a meal to decrease the chance of appetite suppression. The family can adjust the timing and amount of food intake, such as eating larger meals later in the day, when the effects of the medication have worn off, or having a larger snack in the evening before bedtime.

The role and importance of diet in the management of ADHD continues to be highly controversial; however, some data supports the restriction of certain foods as an effective method of managing this disorder. Foods that contain sugar and caffeine are sometimes recommended to be excluded from the diet of the child with ADHD. The theory behind this recommendation is that sugar and caffeine tend to energize and increase any child's activity level, and in the case of some children with ADHD, this effect seems to be even more accentuated. Another controversial issue surrounding the significance of diet is that of food sensitivities and allergies. Food allergies sometimes manifest in symptoms such as irritability and hyperactivity, which may then be confused or misdiagnosed as ADHD.

Activity

The child with ADHD will usually respond best to a highly structured environment, which includes clear expectations and firm, consistent limits as well as appropriate consequences for unruly and disruptive behaviors. For example, a "time-out" may be used when the child must be temporarily removed from a setting or the environment.

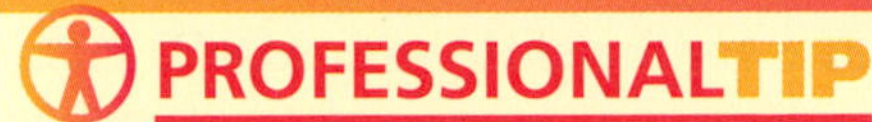

CNS-Stimulant Abuse

Another consideration often overlooked in terms of the CNS stimulants is the risk for abuse because of the strong addictive potential of these medications. Not only is the client with ADHD at risk for abusing these medications, but sometimes the client "shares" prescribed medication with schoolmates and friends interested in drug experimentation. Another problem that may be encountered is abuse of the prescribed medication by a family member with a substance-abuse problem.

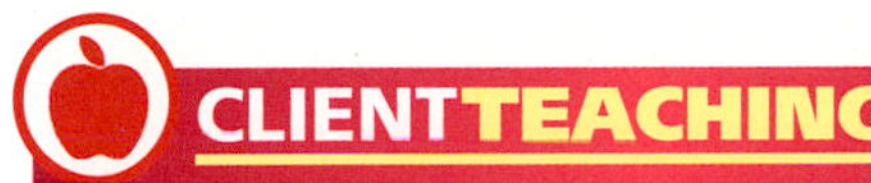

CNS Stimulants

For each client taking a CNS-stimulant medication, instruct the client or, if the client is too young to understand or reliably carry out the instructions, the client's caregivers in the following:

- Take the medication only as prescribed.
- Do not take any other medications without physician approval.
- Be alert for decreased appetite and adjust meals and mealtimes accordingly.
- Do not take any doses after 5 p.m. because doing so will increase the risk of insomnia.
- Obtain periodic liver function tests if taking pemoline (Cylert).
- Obtain periodic CBC, platelet count, and differential if taking methylphenidate (Ritalin).
- Limit caffeine intake.

Nursing Management

Monitor growth (height and weight) and development. Explain to the client what comprise acceptable behaviors. Provide positive reinforcement for appropriate behavior. Teach the client and family about prescribed medications.

NURSING PROCESS

Assessment

Subjective Data

The child or adolescent frequently verbalizes feeling "bad" about being unable to control hyperactive and disruptive behaviors and feeling like a failure, especially in the classroom. After only a single dose of medication, however, the child sometimes states a noticeable difference in the ability to remain centered and focused.

Objective Data

Although usually described as being hyperactive, unable to concentrate, unable to focus, and unable to remain on task, children with ADHD may sometimes be able to concentrate and remain quite attentive and focused. This usually happens in situations that the child enjoys and sometimes in situations that are new to the child. It can be quite frustrating for parents to bring in their child for an evaluation or screening, only to have the child not exhibit any of the usual problematic behaviors. The knowledgeable practitioner or evaluator will be aware of what is happening and will obtain the necessary information from the parental report of the child's health history.

Nursing diagnoses for the child with ADHD include the following:

NURSING DIAGNOSES	PLANNING/OUTCOMES	NURSING INTERVENTIONS
*Deficient **K**nowledge (medications and disease process)* related to new diagnosis of disorder and treatment regimen	The child and parents will verbalize an increased understanding of the disorder. The child and parents will verbalize an understanding about the role medications can play in treatment.	Educate the child and family about the disorder, including signs and symptoms, about the medication, including indications for use, dosages, when to take the medication, possible side effects, and the benefits that can be expected with the particular medication. Emphasize the importance of taking the medication as prescribed.
*Impaired **S**ocial Interaction* related to unaccepted social behaviors	The child will demonstrate an increase in appropriate peer interactions.	Explain to the child those behaviors that are acceptable. Observe the child in social situations with peers. Provide positive reinforcement for demonstration of appropriate behaviors. Immediately intervene when unacceptable behaviors are observed.

Evaluation: Evaluate each outcome to determine how it has been met by the client.

NEGLECT AND/OR ABUSE

There are many types of **neglect** (a situation wherein a basic need of the client is not being provided) and **abuse** (an incident involving some type of violation to the client). Neglect can be quite evident, such as a lack of adequate food, clothing, or shelter, or less tangible, such as emotional neglect or an absence of nurturing. Abuse can be physical, emotional, psychological, financial, or sexual in nature, or any combination of these. Abuse can also take the form of **domestic violence**, which is aggression and violence involving family members. Neglect and abuse often go hand in hand.

A client experiencing neglect or abuse is usually dependent on another individual for the meeting of basic care and needs. In many neglectful or abusive situations, the clients are vulnerable individuals such as children, adolescents, or elders. Others who are neglected or abused include individuals with some type of illness or incapacitation. Neglect and abuse can take many shapes and forms, ranging anywhere from mild cases to situations so severe that death is the end result.

ELDER ABUSE AND NEGLECT

Elder abuse became nationally recognized in 1981 after the House Select Committee on Aging issued its landmark report *Elder Abuse: An Examination of a Hidden Problem.* The committee found that elder abuse was simply "alien to the American ideal." Because it is such a difficult concept to come to grips with, even abused elders are reluctant to admit that their loved ones have abused them.

The committee defined the following types of elder abuse: physical, passive physical, financial, psychological, sexual, and violation of rights. There is no federal legislation to protect elders from abuse, neglect, or exploitation. All 50 states, including the District of Columbia, have some form of elder abuse prevention laws (AoA, 2003). Adult abuse and protection laws are based on the legal premise that society (represented by the state) has the authority to act in a parental capacity for persons who are unable to care for and protect themselves and thus prevent them from suffering from abuse, neglect, or exploitation by those responsible for their care or from self-abuse (Frisch & Frisch, 2010). The purposes of adult protection service laws are to facilitate the identification of functionally impaired elders who are being abused, neglected, or exploited by others; to encourage expeditious reporting; and to extend protective services while protecting the rights of the abused. In most states, the adult protective services (APS) agency is the principal agency designated to receive and investigate allegations of elder abuse and neglect. In most jurisdictions, the county departments of social services maintain the APS unit.

The National Elder Abuse Incidence Study of 1996 found that almost 450,000 persons age 60 and older experienced abuse and/or neglect in domestic settings. Only 16% were reported to APS; that is, less than 1 of 5 cases were reported. Persons age 80 and older were abused and neglected two to three times their proportion of the elderly population.

LIFE SPAN CONSIDERATIONS

Teen Dating Violence

Teen dating violence is a serious public health concern in the United States. Three common types of dating violence are physical, emotional, and sexual. Approximately 10% of students report being physically hurt by a boyfriend or girlfriend in the past 12 months (CDC, 2008b).

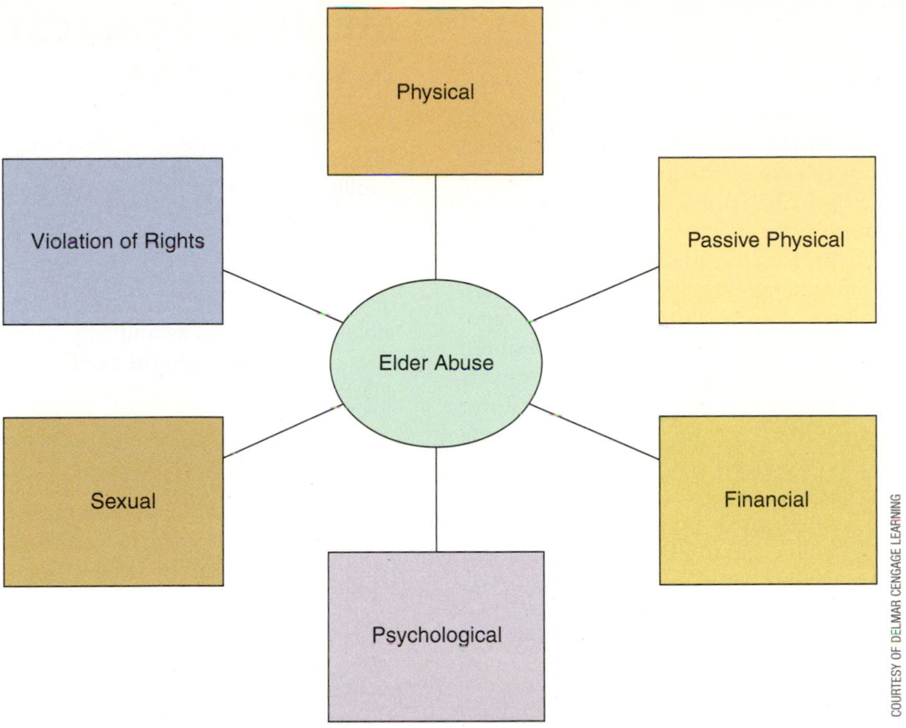

FIGURE 48-4 Types of Elder Abuse

DOMESTIC VIOLENCE

Domestic violence is a pattern of controlling behavior and assaults, including physical, sexual, and psychological attacks and economic control, that adolescents and adults use against their intimate partners. It is common and lethal, affecting people of all ages, cultures, religions, sexual orientations, educational backgrounds, and income levels.

Domestic violence occurs in relationships where conflict is the continuous result of power inequality between partners. One of the partners is afraid of and harmed by the other. In all cultures, the perpetrators are most often men and the victims are most often women (National Coalition Against Domestic Violence [NCADV], 2005).

In all states, domestic violence is a crime, but the laws in each state are a little different. The nurse is responsible for knowing the laws, especially mandatory reporting, about domestic violence in the state of employment. Each state has a coalition against domestic violence, which are valuable resources. The National Domestic Violence Hotline is 800-799-7233 (SAFE).

CRITICAL THINKING

Domestic Violence

What are your feelings about domestic violence? How would you react to a client who was a victim of domestic violence? Would you be able to respond appropriately? What if the client refuses your attempt to assist her to leave the abusive situation?

PROFESSIONALTIP

Caring for the Abused Client

When questioning clients about the possibility of interpersonal violence or sexual assault, the nurse must quickly develop a rapport and create an environment indicating that personal experiences are acceptable topics to discuss. This allows them the opportunity to express their fears and concerns. This can be done by:

- Treating them with dignity and concern.
- Giving priority to them over nonemergency clients.
- Placing them in quiet and private areas.
- Not leaving them alone.
- Speaking quietly and in a nonjudgmental manner.
- Using active and empathic listening skills.
- Not acting shocked or surprised at the details of their experiences.
- Reassuring them that the abuse was not their fault.
- Explaining any delays in treatment.
- Asking permission to call family members, friends, or in the case of rape, rape crisis advocates.
- Providing information about community resources.

RAPE

Rape is a legal term, not a medical entity. It is a crime of violence. Rapists use sexual violence to dominate and degrade their victims and to express their own anger. It is not an act of lust or an overzealous release of passion done to satisfy a sexual urge (Frisch & Frisch, 2010).

There are three basic types of rape: (1) rape by a person known to the survivor, for example, father, former and current friends (date rape), neighbors, partner or separated partner, dissatisfied clients of prostitutes; (2) gang rape; and (3) stranger-to-stranger rape. The latter, which women fear the most, follows an identifiable pattern. Such rapists look for women who are vulnerable, even though they differ on defining who is vulnerable. They might attempt to rape elders, people who are developmentally, physically, or mentally challenged, or intoxicated people. They might look for environments that are easy to enter and relatively safe (e.g., women's bedrooms) and where they will not be interrupted. They often select their victims long before they approach them and repeat the same pattern of victim selection over and over again. All types of rape can be an emotionally terrorizing experience for the survivors.

PROFESSIONALTIP

Interviewing the Survivor of Abuse or Violence

The type of questions will depend on the type of violence and whether survivors have told you they have been abused. If they have told you they have been abused, you must ask specific questions about the abuse. If they have not, you must ask more open-ended questions to allow them to disclose sensitive information. Generally speaking:

- Inform the client that it is necessary to ask some very personal questions.
- Use language appropriate for the age and developmental level of the survivor.
- Use conversational language or street language.
- Keep questions simple, nonthreatening, and direct.
- Pose questions in a manner that permits brief answers.
- Indicate sensitivity to and acceptance of the client's state of confusion.
- Avoid using leading statements that can distort the client's report.
- Do not criticize the client's family.
- Do not promise not to report the abuse; indicate that you are required by law to report the abuse.

MEDICAL–SURGICAL MANAGEMENT

Medical

Planning care for survivors of neglect and abuse and their families requires input from the clients and a survey of their resources to ensure that care is in line with their expectations and commitments. Nursing interventions directed at primary prevention of interpersonal violence are those that reduce or control the causative factors associated with interpersonal violence and sexual assaults. By identifying families at risk for abuse, nurses can help the family plan efforts to modify those risk factors.

Health Promotion

Primary prevention includes empowering survivors of abuse by helping them learn to care for and protect themselves from the imposition by others. For example, children can be taught in health care settings or schools those things to do if they are being abused. It also includes changing the family's perceptions of violence as an acceptable mode of conflict resolution.

Provide anticipatory guidance. For example, by anticipating the challenges of toddlerhood, acknowledge that this can be a difficult period for parents and provide practical advice about constructive discipline. Teach college freshmen about date rape and to avoid vulnerable situations. Encourage families with dependent elderly members to use respite care services and day care programs. Such support and anticipatory guidance can enhance the family's and client's competence and diminish the likelihood of violence or abuse.

NURSING MANAGEMENT

Know the mandatory reporting laws in your state of employment. When assessing clients, ask about bruises, scars, and burns when seen. Provide anticipatory guidance for challenging events in a client's family life that will enhance the family's competence and diminish the probability of abuse or violence.

NURSING PROCESS

ASSESSMENT

Subjective Data

There is no comprehensive assessment tool that offers conclusive evidence that neglect, abuse, or violence has occurred. Act like detectives when assessing clients, given that clients or their abusers will rarely admit to abuse or violence. Make direct observations of the client and family members (e.g., Does the child seem afraid of the caregiver? Does the caregiver hit the child?). These observations are clues that more probing is necessary.

To properly assess survivors of abuse, the symptoms that are commonly seen in interpersonal violence and sexual assaults and the common characteristics of the abusers must be known. Many of the symptoms are subjective, so the health care team must piece together the evidence to ascertain whether interpersonal violence has occurred or clients are at risk for violence. Psychological abuse is a particularly difficult area to assess because emotional relationships are very culture bound, and words and emotions that may be harmful in one family are not necessarily so in another family.

Objective Data

A more extensive examination is warranted when the history or behavioral symptoms indicate interpersonal abuse. Clients need to have physical examinations to assess the extent of their injuries and to collect forensic evidence to prove who assaulted them. A traumagram, or body map (a drawing of the front and back of a nude human figure), is generally used to mark the location of all visible injuries. Each state has legally mandated procedures for collecting evidentiary material, and it is a nursing responsibility to be sure that the legal "chain of evidence" pertaining to collection of forensic samples is unbroken. The medical record should document the injuries and nursing and medical treatment that may serve as legal evidence of the client's condition.

Nursing diagnoses for the client experiencing neglect or abuse include the following:

NURSING DIAGNOSES	PLANNING/OUTCOMES	NURSING INTERVENTIONS
*Interrupted **Family** Processes* related to neglect	The client will not experience any further Neglect.	Provide support for the client. Document the evidence of neglect with which the client presents via written observations, laboratory reports, and/or pictures, if indicated. Report the case of neglect to the proper authorities: police, child protective services (CPS), APS, and any others that might be indicated.
Fear related to abuse	The client will verbalize being less fearful.	Reassure the client that the client is in a safe place and that you are there to help in any way that you can. Provide emotional support to the client in a nonjudgmental manner.
*Risk for **Injury*** related to abusive home life	The client will not experience any further injury or abuse.	Address the client's safety needs and attempt to assess whether abuse is occurring. If you suspect that abuse is occurring notify your supervisor so the proper authorities can be notified (Ladebauche, 1997).

Evaluation: Evaluate each outcome to determine how it has been met by the client.

EATING DISORDERS

Eating disorders include anorexia nervosa and bulimia nervosa. Anorexia nervosa is characterized by self-imposed starvation by restricting caloric intake and compulsive exercising. Bulimia nervosa is characterized by periods of binge eating of up to 10,000 calories at one time followed by self-induced vomiting and other forms of purging such as laxative and diuretic abuse. In bulimia nervosa, the client's weight is normal or above normal. In anorexia nervosa, body weight is low and keeps getting lower. Most clients with these disorders are female and younger than age 30.

Complications can be serious and include cardiac abnormalities such as bradycardia, hypotension, arrhythmias, CHF, and cardiovascular collapse; oral and esophageal erosions and dental caries from vomiting; renal abnormalities that affect the kidney's ability to filter urine; skin rashes from malnutrition; and bruising from vomiting.

Clients with anorexia nervosa tend to be high achievers, perfectionists, have a distorted body image in that they see themselves as fat, and are rigid and ritualistic.

Bulimia nervosa occurs more frequently than anorexia nervosa, with clients experiencing a fear of not being able to stop eating. Clients often experience guilt and depression after a binge.

Medical–Surgical Management

Diet

During severe cases, clients may be admitted for enforced feeding, including the placement of a feeding tube or TPN, IV fluid rehydration, and electrolyte replacement. Clients need to be monitored for refeeding complications such as pancreatitis and gastric dilation. Small quantities are given at first, and very gradually the amount is increased.

Other Therapies

Treatment is primarily psychiatric, involving the client and family, and is typically done on an outpatient basis.

Nursing Management

Monitor weight, calorie intake, I&O, and exercise program. Assess behavior around mealtime. Administer IV fluid and electrolyte replacement. Check vital signs and laboratory test results.

NURSING PROCESS

ASSESSMENT

Subjective Data

Clients with either anorexia nervosa or bulimia nervosa may verbalize feelings of helplessness and being out of control, and may exhibit low self-esteem. They may also have overprotective parents. Clients with anorexia nervosa may also describe bad dreams and cold intolerance.

Objective Data

Clients with anorexia nervosa are underweight, usually lost over a short period of time, reluctant to eat with others, move food around the plate without eating it, hypotensive, have heart irregularities, and altered thinking patterns.

Clients with bulimia nervosa have normal weight, tooth erosions and dental caries, puffy face, callused knuckles, broken blood vessels in the eyes and face, reluctance to eat with others, and going to the bathroom immediately after eating.

Laboratory analysis will include a CBC, which may show low Hgb, Hct, and platelets; electrolytes, which may show low sodium, potassium, and chloride; an SMA-22 that shows low protein, phosphate, and magnesium; and elevated BUN.

Nursing diagnoses for a hospitalized client with anorexia nervosa or bulimia nervosa include the following:

NURSING DIAGNOSES	PLANNING/OUTCOMES	NURSING INTERVENTIONS
*Imbalanced **N**utrition: Less than Body Requirements* related to psychological restriction of food intake, excessive activity	The client will demonstrate increased consumption of nutrients as evidenced by weight gain daily and improved laboratory values.	Weigh daily. Monitor calorie intake. Monitor I&O every shift. Administer IV rehydration, electrolyte replacement, and TPN or tube feedings as ordered. Monitor behavior at and around meal time, such as going to the bathroom right after eating. Monitor exercise patterns.
*Risk for Deficient **F**luid Volume* related to inadequate intake of liquids, self-induced vomiting, laxative and diuretic use	The client's intake and output will be approximately equal by the fourth hospital day. The client's electrolytes will be within normal limits, by the third hospital day. The client's fluid intake will be at least 2,000 mL per day.	Monitor I&O every shift and bowel movements for diarrhea (a sign of continued laxative abuse). Monitor laboratory reports for electrolyte levels as ordered. Administer IV fluid and electrolyte replacement as ordered.
*Ineffective **C**oping (Individual)* related tomaturational crisis andattempting to control environment	The client will verbalize feelings regarding disease process and hospitalization, by discharge. The client will identify current coping strategies, by discharge. The client will identify personal strengths, by discharge.	Provide opportunities for the client to express feelings regarding hospitalization. Encourage client to identify coping mechanisms and strengths. Give positive feedback regarding identified personal strengths.

Evaluation: Evaluate each outcome to determine how it has been met by the client.

SUMMARY

- The components of a therapeutic nurse–client relationship include trust, rapport, respect, genuineness, and empathy.
- An individual's anxiety level may range anywhere from mild to panic level.
- The nurse often encounters clients and/or family members who are angry, aggressive, homicidal, and/or suicidal in the midst of a crisis situation.
- The depressed individual must be evaluated for risk of suicide.
- The individual with schizophrenia may be out of touch with reality and influenced by delusions and/or hallucinations.
- Individuals with bipolar disorder may experience wide mood swings ranging from depression to mania.
- Neglect and abuse can occur among any age group.
- Anorexia nervosa and bulimia nervosa are psychological disorders affecting mostly women. Severe nutritional imbalances can occur leading to serious effects on the cardiovascular system.

REVIEW QUESTIONS

1. The client who is experiencing severe or panic level anxiety should:
   1. be left alone to calm down.
   2. be taught new information.
   3. never be left alone.
   4. be given an antidepressant immediately.
2. A nurse who is aware of a client's plan to kill someone else should:
   1. do nothing; it is not her responsibility.
   2. contact the physician and alert the proper authorities.
   3. discourage the client from following through with the plan.
   4. continue preparing the client for discharge per orders in the chart.
3. Components of a therapeutic nurse–client relationship include: (Select all that apply.)
   1. genuineness.
   2. rapport.
   3. independence.
   4. trust.
   5. mild anxiety.
   6. respect.
4. A client experiencing panic level anxiety informs the nurse that she is hearing the voice of her deceased husband and wants it to stop. The most appropriate nursing action is to:
   1. provide constant reassurance, monitoring, and supervision.
   2. apply wrist restraints.
   3. place all four bed side rails up.
   4. medicate the client with a sedative and supervise for safety.
5. The nurse notices that a client on your unit is giving away prized personal possessions to his family and friends. This action is indicative of:
   1. a client that is schizophrenic.
   2. a client that is contemplating suicide.
   3. a client that is experiencing excessive anxiety.
   4. an anorexic client that is recovering.
6. A client has an order for Paxil 12.5 mg one tablet every morning. Which of the following client statements indicates that further teaching is needed?
   1. "I should take the medication on an empty stomach."
   2. "Paxil can cause drowsiness."
   3. "I cannot drink alcohol while taking Paxil."
   4. "I should put on sunscreen when outside because I will be more susceptible to sunburn."
7. The nurse is assessing a client admitted to the psychiatric unit with a diagnosis of Bipolar Disorder The nurse can expect the client to exhibit all but which of the following behaviors?
   1. Conflict in relationships.
   2. Sexual promiscuousness.
   3. Euphoria.
   4. Drug seeking behavior.
8. Before the administration of MAOI antidepressant medication to a client with depression symptoms, it is imperative for the nurse to teach the client which of the following?
   1. It is safe to drink alcohol while taking this medication.
   2. Over the counter medications can be taken with MAOIs.
   3. Avoid all foods containing tyramine.
   4. MAOIs do not affect blood pressure.
9. A 45-year-old female client is diagnosed with depression. An appropriate nursing intervention for working with this client is:
   1. to allow plenty of alone time to think through issues.
   2. to provide at least 14 hours of sleep time each day.
   3. to encourage her to engage in any type of physical activity.
   4. to do her activities of daily living for her since she cannot.
10. The nurse is assessing a client admitted with schizophrenia. The nurse can expect to observe which of the following signs and symptoms?
    1. Able to care for basic needs.
    2. Alert and oriented.
    3. Speech clear and appropriate.
    4. Delusional.

REFERENCES/SUGGESTED READINGS

American Psychiatric Association. (APA). (2000). *Diagnostic and statistical manual of mental disorders (4th ed.)*. (DSM-IV-TR [text-revision]) Washington, DC: Author.

Antai-Otong, D. (2008). *Psychiatric nursing, biological & behavioral concepts*. Clifton Park, NY: Delmar Cengage Learning.

Anxiety Disorders Association of America (ADAA). (2009a). Brief overview of anxiety disorders. [Online] Retrieved May 18, 2009, from www.adaa.org/GettingHelp/Briefoverview.asp

Anxiety Disorders Association of America (ADAA). (2009b). Generalized anxiety disorder (GAD). [Online] Retrieved May 18, 2009, from www.adaa.org/GettingHelp/AnxietyDisorders/GAD.asp

Anxiety Disorders Association of America (ADAA). (2009c). Obsessive-compulsive disorder (OCD). [Online] Retrieved May 18, 2009, from www.adaa.org/GettingHelp/AnxietyDisorders/OCD.asp

Anxiety Disorders Association of America (ADAA). (2009d). Panic disorder (panic attack). [Online] Retrieved May 18, 2009, from www.adaa.org/GettingHelp/AnxietyDisorders/Panicattack.asp

Anxiety Disorders Association of America (ADAA). (2009e). Posttraumatic stress disorder (PTSD). [Online] Retrieved May 18, 2009, from www.adaa.org/GettingHelp/AnxietyDisorders/PTSD.asp

Berlinger, J. (2002). Domestic violence: How you can make a difference. *Nursing*2001, 31(8), 58–63.

Bulechek, G., Butcher, H., McCloskey, J., & Dochterman, J., eds. (2008). *Nursing Inteventions Classification (NIC)* (5th ed.). St. Louis, MO: Mosby/Elsevier.

Centers for Disease Prevention and Control (CDC). (2008a). Suicide-datasheet. [Online] Retrieved May 19, 2009, from http://www.cdc.gov/ViolencePrevention/pdf/Suicide-DataSheet-a.pdf

Centers for Disease Prevention and Control (CDC). (2008b). Youth risk behavioral surveillance – United States, 2007. *Morbidity and Mortality Weekly Report, 57*(No. SS #4).

Daniels, R. (2010). *Delmar's guide to laboratory and diagnostic tests* (2nd ed.). Clifton Park, NY: Delmar Cengage Learning.

Depression and Bipolar Support Alliance (DBSA). (2006). *Types of bipolar disorder.* [Online] Retrieved May 19, 2009, from www.dbsalliance.org/site/PageServer?pagename=about_bipolar_types

Depression and Bipolar Support Alliance (DBSA). (2007). Depression and other illnesses. [Online] Retrieved May 18, 2009, from www.dbsalliance.org/site/PageServer?pagename=about_depression_otherillnesses

Depression and Bipolar Support Alliance (DBSA). (2009). Bipolar disorder. [Online] Retrieved May 19, 2009, from www.dbsalliance.org/site/PageServer?pagename=about_bipolar_overview

Ferri, R., Sofer, D., & Zolot, J. (2003). Depression in America, *AJN, 103*(9), 17.

Frisch, N., & Frisch, L. (2010). *Psychiatric mental health nursing.* (4th ed.). Clifton Park, NY: Delmar Cengage Learning.

Gale, G. (2002). A useful screening tool. *RN, 65*(9), 41–43.

Koschel, M. (2003). Is it child abuse? *AJN, 103*(4), 45–46.

McGlotten, S. (2003). Attempted suicide. *Nursing*2003, 33(4), 96.

Moorhead, S., Johnson, M., Maas, M., & Swanson, E. (2007). *Nursing Outcomes Classification (NOC)* (4th ed.). St. Louis, MO: Mosby.

Morris, R. (1998). Elder abuse: What the law requires. *RN, 61*(8), 52–53.

National Coalition against Domestic Violence (NCADV). (2005). The Problem. [Online]. Retrieved from www.ncadv.org/problem/what.htm

North American Nursing Diagnosis Association International. (2010). *NANDA-I nursing diagnoses: Definitions and classification 2009–2011. Ames, IA: Wiley-Blackwell.*

Orbanic, S. (2002). Understanding bulimia. *AJN, 101*(3), 35–41.

Peplau, H. (1962). Interpersonal techniques: The crux of psychiatric nursing. *AJN, 62*(6), 50–54.

Peplau, H. (1963). A working definition of anxiety. In S. Burd & M. Marshall (Eds.), *Some clinical approaches to psychiatric nursing.* New York: Macmillan.

Peplau, H. (1991). *Interpersonal relations in nursing.* New York: Springer.

Richardson, B. (2007). *Clinical decision making, case studies in psychiatric nursing.* Clifton Park, NY: Delmar Cengage Learning.

Rother, L. (2003). Electroconvulsive therapy sheds its shocking image. *Nursing2003, 33*(3), 48–49.

Ryan, B. (2003). Do you suspect child abuse? *RN, 66*(9), 73–77.

Spratto, G., & Woods, A. (2010). *Delmar nurse's drug handbook 2010 edition.* Clifton Park, NY: Delmar Cengage Learning.

Substance Abuse and Mental Health Services Administration (SAMHSA). (2008). Results from the 2007 national survey on drug use and health: national findings. [Online] Retrieved May 19, 2009, from www.oas.samhsa.gov/NSDUH/2k7nsduh/2k7results.cfm#8.1

Townsend, M. (2008). *Psychiatric mental health nursing: Concepts of care in evidence-based practice* (6th ed.). Philadelphia: F. A. Davis.

Townsend, M. (2009). *Nursing diagnoses in psychiatric nursing: Care plans and psychotropic medications* (7th ed.). Philadelphia: F. A. Davis.

U. S. Food and Drug Administration. MedWatch. (2002). Zoloft (sertraline hydrochloride). [Online]. Retrieved from www.fda.gov/medwatch/SAFETY/2002/safety02.htm#zoloft

U. S. House of Representatives, Select Committee on Aging (1981, April 3). *Elder Abuse (an examination of a hidden problem)* (Comm. Pub. No. 97–277). Washington, DC: U. S. Government Printing Office.

U. S. Preventive Services Task Force (2002). Screening for depression: Recommendations and rationale. *Annals of Internal Medicine,* 136(10), 760.

United States Code Annotated, Title 42, The Public Health and Welfare, Chapter 67, Child Abuse Prevention and Treatment and Adoption Reform; Subchapter 1, Child Abuse Prevention and Treatment; Definitions; Title II, Victims of Child Abuse Act of 1990; Subtitle D, Federal Victims' Protection and Rights; Section 226, Child Abuse Reporting. St. Paul, MN: West.

Vernarec, E. (2002). The hidden threat to our nation's kids. *RN,* 65(9), 36–40.

Woods, A. (2003). Depression. *Nursing2003,* 33(3), 54–55.

RESOURCES

Administration on Aging (AoA), http://www.aoa.gov

American Anorexia/Bulimia Association, http://www.aabainc.org

American Psychiatric Association, http://www.psych.org

American Psychiatric Nurses Association, http://www.apna.org

Anxiety Disorders Association of America, http://www.adaa.org

Depression and Bipolar Support Alliance, http://www.dbsalliance.org

Family Violence Prevention Fund (FVPF), http://www.endabuse.org

National Alliance for Research on Schizophrenia and Depression (NARSAD), http://www.narsad.org

National Alliance for the Mentally Ill (NAMI), http://www.nami.org

National Association of Anorexia Nervosa and Associated Disorders, http://www.anad.org

National Center on Elder Abuse, http://www.ncea.aoa.gov

National Coalition against Domestic Violence (NCADV), http://www.ncadv.org

National Domestic Violence Hotline, http://www.ndvh.org

National Eating Disorders Association, http://www.nationaleatingdisorders.org

National Institute of Mental Health, http://www.nimh.nih.gov

Parents Anonymous, The National Organization, http://www.parentsanonymous.org

Recovery, Inc.: The Association of Nervous and Former Mental Patients, http://www.recovery-inc.com

Victims of Incest Can Emerge Survivors (VOICES), http://www.healthywomen.org

CHAPTER 49
Substance Abuse

MAKING THE CONNECTION

Refer to the following chapters to increase your understanding of substance abuse:

Basic Nursing
- ***Legal and Ethical Responsibilities***
- ***Life Span Development***
- ***Wellness Concepts***
- ***Assessment***

Adult Health Nursing
- ***Respiratory System***
- ***Gastrointestinal System***
- ***Sexually Transmitted Infections***
- ***The Older Adult***

LEARNING OBJECTIVES

Upon completion of this chapter, you should be able to:

- Define key terms.
- Differentiate among dependence, abuse, and intoxication.
- Describe issues related to drug testing.
- Discuss substances frequently abused.
- Use assessment skills to identify possible substance abuse.
- Describe nursing interventions in working with substance abusers.
- Describe stages of alcoholism and the impact on the individual, family, and society.
- Discuss medications frequently used in the treatment of substance abuse.
- Describe an impaired nurse.
- Identify goals of programs for impaired nurses.

KEY TERMS

abuse
addiction
behavioral tolerance
codependent
confabulation
cross-tolerance
dependence
detoxification
hallucination
intoxication
Johnsonian intervention
misuse
opisthotonos
relapse
reverse tolerance
substance
synesthesia
teratogenic
tolerance
withdrawal

INTRODUCTION

Substance use has taken place for many centuries. It is not a new problem for society. A **substance** is a drug, legal or illegal, that may cause physical or mental impairment. With the great increase in world population, there are more people involved in substance abuse. Today's speed of travel and communication has facilitated the broad distribution of substances.

Many street drugs are "cut" (mixed) with substances that should not be consumed, such as talcum powder, rodent exterminating powder, or even strychnine. The purity (strength) of the drug is then not known and overdose easily occurs. Fatalities can occur from the substance with which the drug is cut.

In the United States, substance disorders affect males and females, all ethnic groups, and persons of all levels of education and income. From the newborn to the elderly, all ages can be affected.

Substance disorders may be classified as intoxication, abuse, or dependence (addiction); definitions are based on the criteria presented in the *American Psychiatric Association's Diagnostic and Statistical Manual of Mental Disorders*, fourth edition (DSM-IV). The reversible effect on the central nervous system (CNS) soon after the use of a substance is termed **intoxication**. **Abuse** is the misuse, excessive, or improper use of a substance, the abstinence of which does not cause withdrawal symptoms. **Dependence (addiction)** is reliance on a substance to such a degree that abstinence causes functional impairment, physical withdrawal symptoms, and/or a psychological craving for the substance.

According to the National Institute on Drug Abuse (NIDA, 2008h), substances interfere with normal brain function, inducing powerful feelings of pleasure and having long-term effects on brain metabolism and activity. At some point, changes in the brain turn substance abuse into addiction, a chronic, relapsing illness. Table 49-1 shows diagnostic criteria for abuse and dependence.

HISTORICAL PERSPECTIVES

Nearly 6,500 years ago, ancient Egyptians used opium for pain relief. Later they used it for recreation when they discovered it provided anxiety relief, a pleasurable experience, and an escape from reality. Drug problems began in the United States with the Civil War in 1861. Wounded soldiers were given their own supply of morphine. Its use was uncontrolled. Dependence-producing drugs such as cocaine, heroin, and morphine were given freely to clients by doctors. Patent medicines, many containing alcohol, cocaine, and heroin, were said to cure almost any ailment a person might have.

The Pure Food and Drug Act of 1906, requiring accurate labeling of drugs, was the first measure designed to control drugs in the United States. In 1914, The Harrison Act made the use of certain narcotics illegal. Physicians then became unwilling to give individuals these drugs, and drug use actually increased as those persons already using drugs turned to illegal markets for a supply. In 1919, Congress passed the 19th Amendment to the Constitution declaring the making and selling of alcohol illegal. Prohibition lasted until 1933, when the 19th Amendment was finally repealed because it had not controlled drunkenness or alcoholism as it was intended.

Many medical, law enforcement, and legislative efforts in the 1930s slowed narcotic abuse and addiction. Then marijuana flooded the market. The Marijuana Tax Act of 1937 was intended to raise revenue, identify the persons involved in its use, and discourage the recreational use of marijuana. Marijuana was removed in 1941 from the official list of drugs U.S. physicians could prescribe. World War II disrupted supply routes of drugs from Asia and Europe, and large-scale drug use disappeared in the United States.

The 1960s, saw drug use move into the mainstream of life in the United States. Drugs were used as a form of relaxation. The Comprehensive Drug Abuse Prevention and Control Act was passed in 1970; it is commonly referred to as the Controlled Substance Act. This act regulates the manufacture, distribution, and dispensing of controlled substances. To enforce the provisions of this act, the Drug Enforcement Administration (DEA) was organized.

There are five classifications or schedules of controlled substances. The categories are based on the drugs' potential to cause psychological and/or physical dependence, and also on their potential for abuse. Table 49-2 identifies and explains the five schedules.

In the 1980s, marijuana and other drug use declined, especially among high school students. Cocaine and its derivative, crack, were the new drugs of choice. The increased supply hooked many people into heavy drug use. The early 1990s saw an increase in the use of all substances. Adolescent illicit drug use is decreasing for almost all of the specific types of drugs. Combined data for 8th, 10th, and 12th graders show an overall decline in illicit drug use by 24% between 2001 and 2007 (NIDA, 2008g).

FACTORS RELATED TO SUBSTANCE ABUSE

Many factors interact to influence a person's substance abuse. Many people who have stopped substance abuse **relapse** (return to a previous behavior or condition) because of these same factors. These factors may be categorized as individual, family, lifestyle, environmental, and developmental.

Individual Factors

Genetic factors are being researched as a possible reason for a person's susceptibility to substance abuse. Research suggests that variations in the intensity of the flow of neurotransmitters may cause certain individuals to be more susceptible to addiction. The personality traits of sensation seeking and being impulsive may make it easier for the person to experiment with substances.

Family Patterns

Substance abuse, especially in the adolescent, seems to be related to family relationships. Close family relationships, with the parents involved in their children's activities, appear to discourage substance abuse. Families with positive relationships between parents and children generally have less use of illicit drugs. Parent–child interactions that show a lack of closeness, lack of involvement in the children's activities, lack of or inconsistent discipline, and low aspirations for the children's education contribute to the prediction of substance abuse by the children.

Families of adolescent substance abusers generally have negative communication patterns. That is, there is a lack

TABLE 49-1 Diagnostic Criteria for Substance Dependence and Abuse

SUBSTANCE DEPENDENCE

A maladaptive pattern of substance use, leading to clinically significant impairment or distress, as manifested by three (or more) of the following, occurring at any time in the same 12-month period:

(1) tolerance, as defined by either of the following:
  (a) a need for markedly increased amounts of the substance to achieve intoxication or desired effect
  (b) markedly diminished effect with continued use of the same amount of the substance
(2) withdrawal, as manifested by either of the following:
  (a) the characteristic withdrawal syndrome for the substance (refer to Criteria A and B of the criteria sets for Withdrawal from the specific substances)
  (b) the same (or a closely related) substance is taken to relieve or avoid withdrawal symptoms
(3) the substance is often taken in larger amounts or over a longer period than was intended
(4) there is a persistent desire or unsuccessful efforts to cut down or control substance use
(5) a great deal of time is spent in activities necessary to obtain the substance (e.g., visiting multiple doctors or driving long distances), use the substance (e.g., chain-smoking), or recover from its effects
(6) important social, occupational, or recreational activities are given up or reduced because of substance use
(7) the substance use is continued despite knowledge of having a persistent or recurrent physical or psychological problem that is likely to have been caused or exacerbated by the substance (e.g., current cocaine use despite recognition of cocaine-induced depression, or continued drinking despite recognition that an ulcer was made worse by alcohol consumption)

SUBSTANCE ABUSE

A. A maladaptive pattern of substance use leading to clinically significant impairment or distress, as manifested by one (or more) of the following, occurring within a 12-month period:
  (1) recurrent substance use resulting in a failure to fulfill major role obligations at work, school, or home (e.g., repeated absences or poor work performance related to substance use; substance-related absences, suspensions, or expulsions from school; neglect of children or household)
  (2) recurrent substance use in situations in which it is physically hazardous (e.g., driving an automobile or operating a machine when impaired by substance use)
  (3) recurrent substance-related legal problems (e.g., arrests for substance-related disorderly conduct)
  (4) continued substance use despite having persistent or recurrent social or interpersonal problems caused, or exacerbated by the effects of the substance (e.g., arguments with spouse about consequences of intoxication, physical fights)

B. The symptoms have never met the criteria for Substance Dependence for this class of substance.

Reprinted with permission from the *Diagnostic and Statistical Manual of Mental Disorders*, Fourth Edition. Copyright 2000 American Psychiatric Association.

TABLE 49-2 Schedules of Controlled Substances

Schedule I (C-I)	High abuse and dependence potential. No accepted medical use in the United States. Includes heroin, mescaline, LSD, marijuana, and other hallucinogens and certain opiates. Can be obtained legally for limited research programs.
Schedule II (C-II)	High abuse and dependence potential. Have currently accepted medical use. Includes narcotics, barbiturates, and amphetamines. Obtained only with physician's prescription, nonrefillable.
Schedule III (C-III)	Less abuse potential, moderate dependence likely. Includes nonbarbiturate sedatives and some narcotics in limited doses. Prescription refills good for 6 months. Fewer controls than for Schedule II.
Schedule IV (C-IV)	Even less abuse potential, limited dependence likely. Includes some sedatives and antianxiety agents and nonnarcotic analgesics.
Schedule V (C-V)	Limited abuse potential. Includes cough medicines containing codeine and antidiarrheals. May be sold over-the-counter in pharmacies to persons over 18 years old. A record is kept of the buyer's name.

COURTESY OF DELMAR CENGAGE LEARNING

of praise and a great deal of blaming and criticism. Often there are unreal expectations of the children by the parents, inconsistent or unclear behavioral limits, and a pattern of self-medication by family members.

Lifestyle

All dimensions of a person's life that influence how that person lives are termed *lifestyle*. First is the physical dimension, which includes food, clothing, shelter, and health care. The second is the social dimension, which includes friends, organizations, and activities with others. Third is the intellectual/emotional dimension, including education, parental support of education, self-esteem, and how the individual is treated by others. The fourth dimension is spiritual and includes a belief in a "higher being," caring and compassion for others, and being in touch with the inner self. Substance use, abuse, or dependence may be the coping mechanism used by an individual who has problems in any dimension of lifestyle.

Environmental Factors

Many environmental factors may encourage or predispose an individual to substance abuse. The social environment in which persons find themselves, the groups, clubs, gangs, sororities, fraternities, and other organizations influence the acceptance or rejection of substance abuse. Stresses in a person's life, including accidents, disabilities, illnesses, stressful family relations, frequent job changes, divorce, death, or precarious financial conditions may be too much for that person to handle. The maladaptive coping of substance abuse offers temporary relief. Because the symptoms of the stressors are reduced, substance abuse is reinforced.

Social traditions, especially in the use of alcohol, may open the door for abuse in certain individuals. Examples of these social traditions are having wine with meals, making toasts at weddings and other celebrations, serving "holiday cheer," and going to "happy hour." For some individuals, these situations may predispose them to alcohol abuse or dependence.

Peer activities, especially during adolescence, may result in substance abuse. Even adults often feel they must go along with certain activities, such as drinks after work or cocktail hour, to get ahead in their careers.

Some occupations, like health care, seem to be more associated with substance problems than others. Physicians and nurses, particularly, have access to many substances that can be abused.

Developmental Factors

Many individuals have not had good role models in their lives. They have not learned to identify with others and do not understand that their behavior affects others. Not learning the skills and attitudes of problem solving leaves individuals unable to apply personal resources to situations, and escape seems the only answer. Substances provide that escape.

Learning the intrapersonal skills of self-discipline, self-control, and self-assessment helps the individual cope with tension and stress. These skills also work to prevent dishonesty with self, inability to defer gratification, and low self-esteem. A lack of interpersonal skills results in dishonesty with others, resistance to feedback, and inability to share feelings and give or accept help. Not learning to take responsibility or adapt one's behavior to a situation results in irresponsibility, not accepting the consequences of behavior, and seeing oneself as a victim of circumstances. Individuals who do not view themselves as empowered may choose substance use as a means of gratification.

PREVENTION

Prevention of substance abuse must be a proactive process to empower people to constructively confront stressful situations in adaptive ways. There are three levels of prevention. *Primary prevention* focuses on preventing the initial use or preventing further uses that may lead to abuse or dependence. This is usually aimed at school-age children. Children need to hear the message that drugs are not good for them. Education about substances and their effects must also emphasize personal, social, and health risks. Children need role models to teach them how to cope with life without drugs, to resist social and peer pressure, and to make effective decisions.

Secondary prevention focuses on preventing ongoing use from becoming a situation of abuse or dependence. If abuse is already evident, the focus is to return the client to a state of abstinence or at least reduced use.

Tertiary prevention focuses on returning the client to a drug-free state. If this is not possible, the goal is then to prevent physical and psychosocial problems from getting worse.

DIAGNOSTIC TESTING

Clients who have a problem with substance abuse or dependence often have abnormal liver function tests and electrolyte levels. Diagnostic criteria for specific substance-related disorders can be found in DSM-IV.

Tests may be done with either a blood or urine specimen. A positive test indicates only that the person has been exposed to the substance. It does not indicate abuse, addiction, or intoxication (except alcohol). Positive screening tests should be confirmed by a more specific test using a different process. Drugs for which tests can be done include alcohol, benzodiazepines, barbiturates, cocaine, crack, amphetamines, opiates, synthetic narcotic analgesics, marijuana, and PCP.

Urine is usually the body fluid tested because it is easily obtained and tested. When obtaining a urine specimen for drug screening, the client should be observed to prevent adulteration of the specimen by the client, such as substituting another person's drug-free urine. A "chain of custody" is maintained by having each person who handles the specimen sign an attached paper until the specimen has been tested.

Detection of a substance depends on the amount used and the time since last used. Most substances are detectable for less than 7 days. Chronic marijuana use, however, may be detected for up to 30 days. Barbiturates, amphetamines, and opiates are detectable for less than 2 days and alcohol less than 1 day. A false negative may result if the client's drug level falls below the threshold of sensitivity for the test.

Positive results for reasons other than substance abuse can occur. This is called a false positive. Poppy seeds may give a positive result for opiates for up to 60 hours after ingestion. Using a Vicks® inhaler or over-the-counter diet aids may give a positive result for amphetamines. The client should be asked about the use of these items.

Breath specimens can be used to determine alcohol levels. Law enforcement officials do this with the breathalyzer tests.

If hair is not cut, hair analysis can detect cocaine and heroin use for up to a year or more after the person has used the drug. Testing meconium (first stools) from a newborn can detect illicit drug use by the mother during pregnancy.

TREATMENT/RECOVERY

Treatment depends on many factors, including the amount and frequency of substance use, age, health, diet, and overall lifestyle of the individual. Infection from the use of unsterile needles and/or tissue or organ damage caused by the substance used, such as lung damage from smoking crack or marijuana or using inhalants, will also require treatment.

Recovery requires abstinence along with intrapersonal and interpersonal changes. Most individuals need professional treatment and participation in a self-help program. There are four areas of recovery: physical recovery, psychological and behavioral recovery, social and family recovery, and spiritual recovery.

Physical recovery means eliminating the substance from the body. This is termed **detoxification**. If the client cannot stop using the substance or if withdrawal symptoms are present, admission to a detoxification unit is usually necessary. After detoxification, treatment must focus on restoring the client's physical health and dealing with the cravings for the substance now removed from the client's body. It helps if environmental cues such as drug paraphernalia and alcohol bottles or cans are removed.

Psychological and behavioral recovery becomes evident when the client no longer denies the problem and accepts the inability to consistently control the substance abuse. The client will have developed a desire for abstinence and accepted the need for long-term recovery and support. Emotional stability will be restored when the client learns to cope with uncomfortable emotional states without the use of the abused substance.

Social and family recovery occurs when the client no longer denies the impact on the family and makes amends to family members and significant others who have been negatively affected by the substance abuse. The client works to improve family relationships and develops a recovery support system. Also, the client learns to resist social pressures to use alcohol or other drugs and participates in healthy leisure-time activities. The client's family should also attend a program for recovery. If a client returns to a dysfunctional family, it may be difficult for the client to maintain recovery.

Spiritual recovery is attained when the client has resolved the feelings of guilt and shame and developed a meaning for life and a relationship with a higher power.

SUBSTANCE USE PATTERNS

Patterns of substance use have changed throughout the years. Coffee (caffeine) and cigarettes (nicotine) are legal in our society and widely used. Although many people still drink coffee, more are using decaffeinated coffee. Cigarette use has decreased in the older population as the addictive nature and negative effects of nicotine have become more evident; however, cigarette use has increased in the adolescent population.

The substance of choice is alcohol, which is legal and easily obtained. Many high school seniors have been drunk and some are already regular drinkers. There are still more alcoholic men than women, but the number of identified women alcoholics is increasing.

CRITICAL THINKING

Attitude toward Substance Abusers

What is your attitude toward substance abusers? How would you respond to a client who is a substance abuser? Discuss with your classmates.

Elderly persons are more commonly addicted to prescription medications, especially minor tranquilizers and sleeping pills. Alcohol may be used by the elderly to soothe feelings of isolation and loneliness. Depression and paranoia may be misidentified as senility rather than a problem with alcohol.

Moderate consumption of alcohol may have been influenced by Mothers Against Drunk Driving (MADD) and Students Against Destructive Decisions (SADD) (founded as Students Against Driving Drunk). Laws that make bars and individuals liable if they let guests leave and drive while drunk, called social host laws, and famous people like Betty Ford and Liza Minelli sharing with the public their illness and recovery, are other influences.

The National Institute on Drug Abuse (2008h) report on the ongoing study of illicit drug use among 8th-, 10th-, and 12th-grade students shows a decrease in use.

CNS DEPRESSANTS

Central nervous system depressants usually decrease the heart and respiratory rates as well as voluntary muscle responses. Substances in this category include alcohol, benzodiazepines, and marijuana.

ALCOHOL

Low doses of alcohol depress areas of the brain that are inhibitory, causing diminished self-control and impaired judgment. Continued alcohol ingestion may cause unconsciousness and even death. According to the National Institute on Alcohol Abuse and Alcoholism (NIAAA) (2006), 39.5% of all traffic crash fatalities were alcohol related.

The active ingredient in alcoholic beverages is ethanol. Depending on the alcoholic beverage consumed, varying amounts of ethanol are ingested (Figure 49-1). It is metabolized at an average rate of 10 mL/hr. Table 49-3 shows the alcohol content in some beverages.

One ounce of alcohol provides 200 Kcal but no other nutrients. It is not converted to glycogen. The blood alcohol level depends on the size of the person, the amount ingested, and the time since ingestion. Most states have set the legal limit for blood alcohol while driving a motor vehicle at 0.08%, but driving skills are affected at a much lower level.

INCIDENCE

Several national surveys have found that approximately two-thirds of the population has more than an occasional drink. Men are likely to drink more frequently and in greater quantity than women. Some alcoholics drink little or nothing in public or with friends. They are "at home" or "hidden" alcoholics and

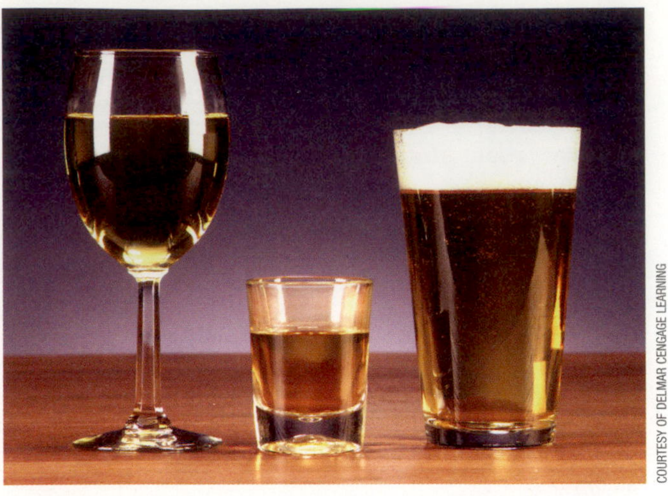
COURTESY OF DELMAR CENGAGE LEARNING

FIGURE 49-1 Each of these drinks contains approximately the same level of alcohol.

are more likely to be women. It often takes a family quite awhile to realize that one of its members has an alcohol problem.

The individual with an alcohol problem often learns **behavioral tolerance**, a compensatory adjustment made by an individual under the influence of a particular substance. The person under the influence of alcohol learns how to compensate for the deterioration of motor performance and speech.

SIGNS AND SYMPTOMS

The ingestion of alcohol causes a feeling of euphoria, relaxation of skeletal muscles, changes in mental activity such as altered judgment, and reduced self-control. It has a diuretic effect that, in heavy drinkers, may cause increased loss of electrolytes, especially potassium, magnesium, and zinc. An increased level of alcohol depresses the cardiovascular and respiratory systems and produces a toxic effect on the intestinal mucosa, resulting in decreased absorption of thiamine, folic acid, and vitamin B_{12}. Excess long-term consumption of alcohol often results in a severe lack of nutrient intake.

Psychosocial aspects include memory blackouts, secretive drinking, rationalization of drinking behavior, trouble with family and employer, loss of outside interests, neglect of food intake, impaired thinking, and moral deterioration. **Confabulation**, making up information to fill in memory gaps, is used by individuals abusing or depending on alcohol. Alcohol may be detected in the blood for 6 to 10 hours after ingestion.

POTENTIAL FOR ADDICTION

The potential for addiction is high. Alcohol is not a scheduled or controlled drug.

TABLE 49-3 Alcohol Content in Selected Beverages

BEVERAGE	PERCENT ALCOHOL	EQUIVALENT AMOUNTS
Beer	4	12 ounces
Wine cooler	4	12 ounces
Wine	14	4 ounces
Hard liquor	40	1½ ounces

COURTESY OF DELMAR CENGAGE LEARNING

ASSOCIATED PROBLEMS/ DISORDERS

Excessive and prolonged alcohol intake can affect numerous body systems.

Liver Deterioration

Chronic alcohol abuse causes three distinct diseases of the liver: *fatty liver*, an accumulation of triglycerides in the liver caused by obesity, excessive alcohol consumption, and certain drugs; *alcoholic hepatitis*, an acute toxic liver injury from excess alcohol consumption; and *cirrhosis*, a chronic degenerative liver disease that can be caused by alcohol consumption. Fatty liver is reversible, but alcoholic hepatitis and cirrhosis are not. Liver cells will not function once the scar tissue of cirrhosis develops. In 2005, 45.9% of deaths from cirrhosis of the liver were related to alcohol consumption (NIAAA, 2008a). Esophageal varices are associated with cirrhosis and could cause death if they bleed.

Gastrointestinal Disturbances

Alcohol damages the lining of the stomach and esophagus by irritating the mucosa and causing inflammation or ulcer formation. Aspirin with alcohol can result in greater irritation and bleeding in the gastrointestinal (GI) tract. Gastric pain, vomiting, and diarrhea are common in alcohol abuse and are often what brings the individual to the health care system.

Pancreatitis

An alcoholic has a higher risk of developing pancreatitis than an abstainer. Severe pancreatitis can result in death.

Wernicke's Encephalopathy

This inflammatory hemorrhagic and degenerative condition of the brain is caused by a thiamine deficiency. It is characterized by delirium, memory loss, unsteady gait, a sense of apprehension, and an altered level of consciousness. Thiamine intake improves the situation.

Korsakoff's Psychosis

Disorientation, amnesia, insomnia, hallucinations, and peripheral neuropathologies characterize this psychosis. Both thiamine and B_{12} deficiencies contribute to the degeneration of the brain and peripheral nervous system. Frequently, there is bilateral foot drop and pain. Thiamine and B_{12} intake may improve the situation.

Cardiovascular Disturbances

Moderate amounts of alcohol cause cutaneous vasodilation (flushed skin). This causes rapid heat loss, and the core temperature may drop to a dangerous level. Blood pressure decreases with intoxicating doses of alcohol. There may be irregularities in cardiac rhythm. Hematologic alterations such as bone marrow depression, anemia, leukopenia, or thrombocytopenia may also occur.

Fetal Alcohol Syndrome

Fetal alcohol syndrome (FAS) is caused by the **teratogenic** (causing abnormal development of the embryo) effects of alcohol related to the amount of alcohol ingested and the stage of pregnancy when the alcohol is ingested. Even a small amount of alcohol can be detrimental and have lifelong consequences for the infant. For a diagnosis of FAS, the infant must meet these criteria:

- Prenatal and/or postnatal growth retardation (weight, length, or head circumference below the 10th percentile)
- CNS involvement (signs of neurologic abnormality, developmental delay, or intellectual impairment)
- Craniofacial anomalies, at least two of the following (microcephaly or head circumference below 3rd percentile, microophthalmia or short palpebral fissure, poorly developed philtrum, thin upper lip, or flattening of maxillary area)

If only some of the FAS criteria are met, it is called fetal alcohol effects (FAE). The only treatment for FAS or FAE is prevention. Women who are pregnant or are trying to get pregnant should abstain from alcohol consumption.

Withdrawal

Withdrawal refers to the symptoms produced when a substance on which an individual has dependence is no longer used by that individual. Alcohol withdrawal syndrome (AWS) appears when the blood alcohol concentration of the alcoholic decreases. The onset of symptoms usually occurs 6 to 12 hours after drinking stops and may last up to 8 days. Chronologically, how long the drinking has occurred and the amount of alcohol consistently consumed are factors in the severity of the withdrawal symptoms. Figure 49-2 shows alcohol withdrawal patterns.

Alcohol withdrawal has three stages:

- *Stage 1* (minor withdrawal) includes restlessness, anxiety, sleeping problems, agitation, and tremors; other signs include low-grade fever, tachycardia, diaphoresis, and hypertension.
- *Stage 2* (major withdrawal) includes stage 1 signs and symptoms plus visual and auditory hallucinations, whole-body tremors, pulse >100 beats/min, diastolic BP >100 mm Hg, pronounced diaphoresis, and possibly vomiting.
- *Stage 3* (delirium tremens) includes a temperature >37.8°C (100°F); disorientation to time, place, and person; global confusion; and inability to recognize familiar objects or persons. This is a medical emergency with a mortality rate of 1% to 5% (Kasser, Geller, Howell, & Wartenberg, 2004).

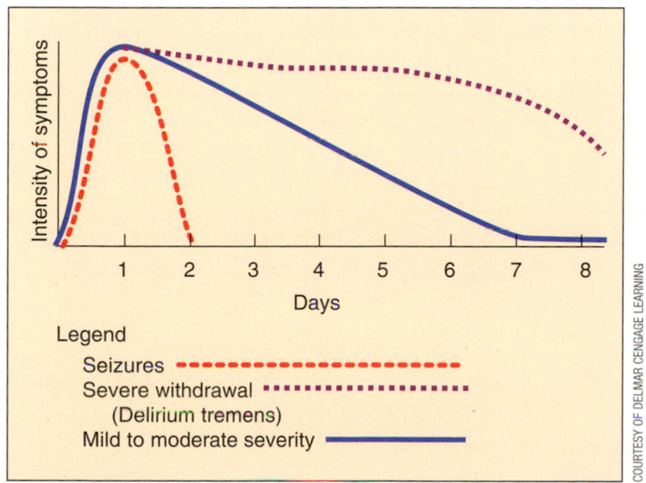

FIGURE 49-2 Alcohol Withdrawal Patterns

> **CRITICAL THINKING**
>
> **Alcohol Withdrawal**
>
> A client, who is going through alcohol withdrawal and is on the appropriate medication protocol, is not clear mentally and is becoming very agitated. What would you investigate and how would you communicate your findings to the physician?

If alcohol abuse continues, symptoms of subsequent withdrawals are generally more severe. It is recommended that withdrawal be medically monitored to decrease the chance of fatality.

Treatment/Rehabilitation

Many treatment programs are based in hospital or residential treatment centers. These are generally called inpatient programs and last 30 days. Many insurance companies are encouraging clients to participate in lower-cost outpatient programs. Currently, there is no evidence that inpatient programs are more effective than outpatient programs.

Many outpatient programs have both day and evening sessions so clients can maintain their usual occupations. The programs usually consist of a 4-week intensive session with follow-up sessions for 6 to 24 months. The first part of either type of treatment program is detoxification.

Detoxification

The goal of detoxification (DETOX) is to halt or control the neuronal overactivity that occurs when the alcohol level is reduced or alcohol is no longer present in the client's body. This is done by substituting a pharmacologically similar drug and gradually reducing the dose given. The benzodiazepine drugs, chlordiazepoxide (Librium), diazepam (Valium), lorazepam (Ativan), and clorazepate dipotassium (Tranxene), are the most commonly used.

During DETOX, other problems such as malnutrition, vitamin deficiencies (B vitamins, especially thiamine), dehydration, and potassium and magnesium deficiencies must also be treated. A client with hypoglycemia should be given thiamine before administering dextrose to prevent Wernicke's encephalopathy. Ignoring these problems complicates the management of detoxification.

Psychological Intervention

The classic psychological intervention technique was originally described by Johnson in 1973 (Johnson, 1990 & 2001). Although several modifications have been published and used since then, the technique is still used and is known as **Johnsonian intervention**, which is a confrontational approach to a client with a substance problem that lessens the chance of denial and encourages treatment before the client "hits bottom." The client's significant others (spouse, teenage or older children, one or two close friends, possibly employer) meet with a professional addiction counselor. This group rehearses so that they may present a united front when confronting the client. They present specific examples of painful or embarrassing behaviors by the client while intoxicated that caused problems and concerns. It is difficult for the client to maintain denial in this situation. Then the group encourages the client to accept professional help. If the client refuses help, each individual of the group must plan to minimize codependent behavior in the future. This technique can also be used for substances other than alcohol. Examples of confrontations may be found in Johnson's books (1989, 1990, 2001). Codependency is discussed later in the chapter.

Education

The abuse of or dependence on alcohol is a maladaptive way to cope with life stressors. Learning basic life skills to improve personal competence and provide adaptive coping mechanisms helps the individual resist the use of alcohol.

One adaptive coping mechanism is exercise. Assist clients to become active in an exercise program and encourage them to participate. Exercise helps relieve feelings of stress and promotes feelings of well-being.

Teach clients about the Food Guide Pyramid for an adequate, balanced diet. Most alcoholics have, in the past, received most of their calories from alcohol. They must now learn how to maintain health by eating nutritious foods.

The interaction of alcohol with other drugs should also be taught. Some effects can be life-threatening. Table 49-4 shows the interaction of alcohol with some classifications of drugs.

Self-Help Groups

Alcoholics Anonymous (AA), begun in 1935, is the model for other self-help groups such as AL-ANON for adults, AL-ATEEN for teenage children, and AL-ATOT for younger children in the family of an alcoholic. The holistic approach of AA to the individual with alcohol problems is described in the Twelve Steps (Table 49-5).

Disulfiram

Disulfiram (Antabuse) may be given to some alcohol abusers as a deterrent to drinking. It inhibits the enzyme needed to metabolize alcohol (NIAAA, 2008b). Drinking alcohol with disulfiram in the body causes flushing of the neck and face, blurred vision, nausea, vertigo, anxiety, palpitations, tachycardia, and hypotension. Clients must be instructed not to use cologne, mouthwash, aftershave, over-the-counter cold preparations, cough syrups, vitamin-mineral tonics, as well as candies, sauces, and foods made with alcohol. These items will cause the same reaction as if the person took a drink of alcohol.

Therapy should not be started until at least 12 hours after the last drink of alcohol. The effects of disulfiram with alcohol can occur for 6 to 12 days after taking the disulfiram. As with any drug, there are side effects such as drowsiness, fatigue, and impotence. Garlic-like breath occurs frequently and is sometimes used as an indicator of compliance in taking

TABLE 49-4 Alcohol Interaction with Other Drugs

DRUG CLASSIFICATIONS WITH EXAMPLES	INTERACTION
Narcotic analgesics • meperidine hydrochloride (Demerol) • morphine sulfate (Morphine) • proproxyphene HCl (Darvon) • hydromorphone HCl (Dilaudid)	• Loss of effective breathing (respiratory arrest) • Can be fatal
Nonnarcotic analgesics • aspirin • acetaminophen (Tylenol)	• Stomach and intestinal bleeding • Liver damage
Anticoagulants • warfarin sodium (Coumadin, Panwarfin) • dicumarol	• Increases drugs' ability to stop blood clotting • May cause life-threatening or fatal hemorrhage
Antihypertensives • reserpine (Serpasil) • methyldopa (Aldomet)	• Orthostatic hypotension
Antimicrobials • metronidazole (Flagyl) • cefotetan disodium (Cefotan) • rifampin (Rifadin)	• Possible disulfiram-like reaction, nausea, cramps, vomiting, headache, flushing or hepatotoxicity
CNS stimulants • most diet pills • dextroamphetamine sulfate (Dexedrine) • caffeine (No Doz) • methylphenidate HCl (Ritalin)	• May reverse depressant effect of alcohol and give a false sense of security

TABLE 49-4 Alcohol Interaction with Other Drugs (Continued)

DRUG CLASSIFICATIONS WITH EXAMPLES	INTERACTION
Diuretics • chlorothiazide (Diuril) • furosemide (Lasix)	• May reduce blood pressure and cause dizziness
Antidepressants • imipramine HCl (Tofranil) • desipramine HCl (Pertofrane) • perphenazine and amitriptyline HCl (Triavil)	• Reduces CNS functioning • Chianti wine may cause hypertensive crisis
Antihistamines • Most cold remedies • pseudoephedrine HCl and triprolidine HCl (Actifed) • chlorpheniramine maleate and acetaminophen (Couricidin)	• Increased calming effect • Person becomes very drowsy • Driving is hazardous
Antipsychotics • thioridazine HCl (Mellaril) • chlorpromazine HCl (Thorazine)	• Added CNS depression and impairs voluntary movements • Causes respiratory depression • Can be fatal
Sedative-hypnotics • glutethimine (Doriden) • pentobarbital (Nembutal)	• Reduces CNS functioning • Sometimes causes coma and respiratory arrest • Can be fatal
Antianxiety agents • diazepam (Valium) • chlordiazepoxide (Librium)	• Reduces CNS functioning • Decreased alertness and judgment • Can lead to household and driving accidents

COURTESY OF DELMAR CENGAGE LEARNING

TABLE 49-5 Alcoholics Anonymous

1. We admitted we were powerless over alcohol—that our lives had become unmanageable.
2. Came to believe that a Power greater than ourselves could restore us to sanity.
3. Made a decision to turn our will and our lives over to the care of God *as we understood Him*.
4. Made a searching and fearless moral inventory of ourselves.
5. Admitted to God, to ourselves and to another human being the exact nature of our wrongs.
6. Were entirely ready to have God remove all these defects of character.
7. Humbly asked Him to remove our shortcomings.
8. Made a list of all persons we had harmed, and became willing to make amends to them all.
9. Made direct amends to such people wherever possible, except when to do so would injure them or others.
10. Continued to take personal inventory and when we were wrong promptly admitted it.
11. Sought through prayer and meditation to improve our conscious contact with God, *as we understood Him*, praying only for knowledge of His will for us and the power to carry that out.
12. Having had a spiritual awakening as the result of these steps, we tried to carry this message to alcoholics, and to practice these principles in all our affairs.

The Twelve Steps are reprinted with permission of Alcoholics Anonymous World Services, Inc. (A.A.) Permission to reprint the Twelve Steps does not mean that A.A. has reviewed or approved the contents of this publication, nor that A.A. agrees with the views expressed herein. A.A. is a program of recovery from alcoholism only. Use of the Twelve Steps in connection with programs and activities that are patterned after A.A., but address other problems, or in any other non-A.A. context, does not imply otherwise.

the disulfiram. Disulfiram is contraindicated in clients with cardiovascular disease, hypothyroidism, suicide ideation, and in clients receiving antihypertensives or monoamine oxidase inhibitors (MAOI).

BENZODIAZEPINES AND OTHER SEDATIVE-HYPNOTICS

With the introduction in 1961 of chlordiazepoxide (Librium), the benzodiazepines have replaced most of the short-acting barbiturates and other nonbarbiturate sedative-hypnotics that were in use before that time. Examples of benzodiazepines include diazepam (Valium), secobarbital (Seconal), paraldehyde (Paral), and flunitrazepam (Rohypnol). Rohypnol when mixed with alcohol can incapacitate and prevent the person from resisting sexual assault or remembering what she experiences under the effects of the drug. It is known as the "date rape drug" (NIDA, 2008b). Street names include roofies, tranks, ludes, and barbs.

INCIDENCE

Benzodiazepines are not commonly used as recreational drugs but are widely prescribed and are thus available for abuse. Statistics are not available because some clinicians still deny that addiction to these drugs occurs. Withdrawal symptoms are subtle and delayed, and the symptoms are not always connected to the benzodiazepines.

Barbiturates and other sedative-hypnotics are more abused but less prescribed. These are available on the illegal market.

SIGNS AND SYMPTOMS

Benzodiazepines in low doses produce drowsiness or sedation. Larger doses produce sleep, but surgical anesthesia cannot be induced. Respirations are not depressed, and there is little effect on the cardiovascular system unless extremely large doses are taken. Then a decrease in systolic blood pressure and an increase in heart rate may result. Side effects may include motor incoordination, ataxia, increased hostility or rage, confusion, metallic-like aftertaste, headache, and blurred vision. **Tolerance** (a decreased sensitivity to subsequent doses of the same substance; an increased dose of a substance is needed to produce the same desired effect) to other benzodiazepines and **cross-tolerance** (a decreased sensitivity to other substances in the same category) to other CNS depressants occur with chronic use. In some clients, particularly pediatric, geriatric, or autistic, a paradoxical reaction can occur. They show excessive movement, increased talkativeness, agitation, violent behavior, and physical assault instead of the expected calming effect (Bramness, J., Skurtveit, S., & Morland, J., 2006, Mancuso, C.E., Tanzi, M.G., & Gabay, M., 2004).

Barbiturates depress all areas of the CNS, some selectively according to the dosage. They do not reduce pain. Respirations are depressed but not significantly when therapeutic doses are taken. When a barbiturate is given to a client in pain, excitement rather than sedation may occur. Side effects may include drowsiness, residual effects on motor skills, and especially in the elderly, excitement, irritability, or delirium. An overdose of barbiturates causes decreased respirations, rapid and weak pulse, cyanosis, coma, and sometimes respiratory paralysis. Tolerance results from chronic use or abuse. Benzodiazepines may be detected for 1 to 6 weeks.

POTENTIAL FOR ADDICTION

The potential for addiction is high for all of these substances. Benzodiazepines are schedule IV drugs; barbiturates may be either schedule II, III, or IV drugs; and methaqualone is a schedule I drug.

WITHDRAWAL

Symptoms of withdrawal for benzodiazepines, which may not manifest for a week or more, include cramping, sweating, disorientation, confusion, tremors, depression, hallucinations, and paranoia. Barbiturate withdrawal symptoms include anxiety, weakness, anorexia, insomnia, tremors, delirium, and seizures that occur within 72 hours of the last use. Withdrawal reactions related to other sedative-hypnotics include nausea, headache, cramping, toxic psychosis, insomnia, and convulsions.

The withdrawal pattern is the same as for alcohol.

TREATMENT/REHABILITATION

Ideally, treatment for benzodiazepine abuse is a gradual reduction in the amount taken until the client is no longer taking any. A cross-tolerant drug such as phenobarbital is sometimes given to control symptoms and then its dosage is reduced. Hospital treatment is likely to be needed. Treatment for barbiturate and other sedative-hypnotics overdose or withdrawal is symptomatic.

Rehabilitation that focuses on teaching clients alternative methods of coping with the anxiety and stressors in their lives is necessary. Supportive individual psychotherapy or a self-help recovery group is almost always advisable. The goal is to assist the client to identify the consequences of the behavior and to understand the risks of relapse.

MARIJUANA (CANNABIS)

Marijuana is the most common type of cannabis used. It is composed of dried leaves, stems, and flowers of the plant *Cannabis sativa* and can be smoked or added to food. Hash or hashish is a potent concentrate of the resin from the flowers. Hash oil is extremely concentrated, made by boiling hashish in a solvent and filtering out the solid matter. Street names include grass, pot, reefer, smoke, weed, and Mary Jane. "Blunts" are cigars emptied of tobacco and refilled with marijuana. It is the most commonly used illicit drug in the United States (NIDA, 2009d). Often, it is the "gateway" drug leading to the abuse of other drugs.

INCIDENCE

Use in the United States began in the early 1900s, peaked in the period 1978 to 1980, and has steadily decreased since. According to Johnston, O'Malley, and Buchman (1991, 1998, 2008a, and 2008b), the prevalence of marijuana use by high school seniors increased from 20% in the class of 1969 to 60.4% in the class of 1979 and decreased to 50.2% in the class of 1987 and decreased again to 40.7 percent in the class of 1990. Use increased between 1990 and 1997 but declined in 1998 to 49%. A National Institute on Drug Abuse study (NIDA, 2007) showed that 10.3% of 8th, 24.6% of 10th, and 31.7% of 12th graders had abused marijuana at least once in 2006. The 2007 National Survey of Drug Use and Health (Substance Abuse and Mental Health Services Administration (SAMHSA, 2008) showed that of the 2.7 million Americans aged 12 or older who used illicit drugs for the first time within the past 12 months, 56.2% reported that their first drug was marijuana (Figure 49-3).

Signs and Symptoms

Short-term effects of marijuana use include memory and learning problems; distorted perception; difficulty in thinking and problem solving; loss of coordination; and increased heart rate, anxiety, and panic attacks. Long-term use produces changes in the brain that make a person more at risk of becoming addicted to alcohol and cocaine. Long-term effects of marijuana use may lead to lung cancer, impairment of the immune system, and a greater risk of getting lung infections (NIDA, 2009d). A **reverse tolerance** can develop whereby a smaller amount of marijuana will elicit the desired psychic effects. Marijuana may be detected in urine for up to 3 to 30 days depending on how much and how long it has been used.

Potential for Addiction

The potential for psychological addiction is moderate. More than 290,000 persons seek treatment each year for their primary marijuana addiction (NIDA, 2009d). Marijuana is a schedule I drug.

Associated Problems/Disorders

Critical skills related to attention, learning, and memory are impaired in heavy marijuana users even 24 hours after the last use. Also, persons who use marijuana tend to be more accepting of deviant behavior, have more aggression and delinquent behavior, act more rebellious, and have poorer relationships with parents.

Withdrawal

Nausea, myalgia, restlessness, irritability, nervousness, insomnia, and depression may appear after ceasing marijuana use. Symptoms may not appear for up to 1 week after the last use.

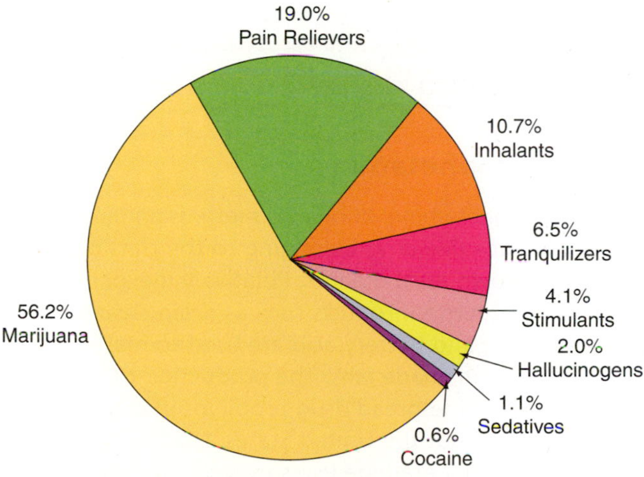

FIGURE 49-3 Specific Drug Used When Initiating Illicit Drug Use among Persons Aged 12 or Older *(Results from the 2007 National Survey on Drug Use and Health: National Findings, Department of Health and Human Services, Substance Abuse and Mental Health Services Administration [SAMHSA] [2008].)*

Treatment/Rehabilitation

Treatment focuses on relapse prevention and the development of new coping mechanisms, ways of living, and means of having fun without drugs. Weekly group therapy sessions to maintain a commitment to abstinence and enhance interpersonal skills are often used. Participation in a self-help group is encouraged.

CNS STIMULANTS

Drugs that stimulate the CNS include cocaine, amphetamines, caffeine, nicotine, and methylphenidate hydrochloride (Ritalin). They increase cortical alertness and electrical activity in the brain and spinal cord. There is tachycardia and an increase in blood pressure.

COCAINE

Cocaine is extracted from the leaves of the coca plant, *Erythroxylum coca*. It may be heated and the fumes inhaled. This is termed *free-basing*. As a white powder, cocaine is snorted by inhaling it through the nose or heated to a liquid state and injected intravenously. Crack is a crystallized form of cocaine that is melted in a water pipe and smoked. Street names include coke, crack, flake, rocks, snow, "C," and blow.

Incidence

Cocaine abuse and dependence was the major illicit drug problem for the United States in the 1980s. The introduction of crack dramatically increased cocaine abuse among the poor. Crack is low cost and gives an intense "high." It is estimated that 1.6 million Americans are dependent on or abuse cocaine (SAMHSA, 2008).

Signs and Symptoms

The immediate reaction, less than 10 seconds, is an intense euphoria that lasts 10 to 15 minutes. This short response time leads people to repeatedly use cocaine trying to maintain the euphoria.

The heart rate increases, blood pressure goes up, pupils dilate, peripheral blood vessels constrict, and temperature increases. Normal pleasures are magnified, anxiety decreases, self-confidence increases, social inhibitions are reduced, communication is facilitated, and sexual feelings are enhanced. Other psychological effects are inability to concentrate, insomnia, reduced sense of humor, antisocial behavior, hallucinations, and compulsive behavior.

An overdose may occur with the first use because there is little quality control of drug strength in the street drug culture. A client with an overdose may have arrhythmias, tremors, convulsions, respiratory failure, cardiovascular collapse, and death. Cocaine may be detected for up to 2 to 3 days in urine and for up to several months to years in hair.

Potential for Addiction

The potential for addiction is high. Cocaine is a schedule II drug.

Associated Problems/ Disorders

Many types of heart disease are linked to cocaine use, especially ventricular fibrillation, heart attack, and hypertension. When cocaine is snorted regularly, respiratory problems occur, including loss of sense of smell, nosebleeds, hoarseness, and respiratory failure.

When cocaine is taken with alcohol, the two drugs are converted in the body to cocaethylene, which is more toxic than either drug alone (NIDA, 2008a).

Withdrawal

The crash, a period of exhaustion, occurs with symptoms of depression, anxiety, and a great need for sleep. The depression may be to the point of suicidal behavior. The client has no energy, shows little interest in the surroundings, and seems to have little ability to experience pleasure. These symptoms are the most intense during the first 3 days but continue for 1 to 4 months. An intense craving for cocaine is felt, including dreaming about cocaine. Then there is a period of less intense craving for cocaine called extinction, which may last months or even years. Withdrawal does not result in a medical emergency as seen with alcohol.

Treatment/Rehabilitation

Treatment is aimed at reducing the craving and managing the severe depression. Careful monitoring of the client is necessary to identify and prevent actions aimed at carrying out the idea of suicide. An individual with a history of cocaine usage has an intense craving for cocaine and a strong denial that cocaine is addicting. This creates a problem in engaging an individual in treatment. Inpatient programs are necessary for some clients with cocaine dependence, whereas other clients can be effectively treated in outpatient programs.

Medications

Bromocriptine mesylate (Parlodel) in small doses seems to reduce the withdrawal symptoms. Amantadine hydrochloride (Symmetrel) also has some success in treating cocaine withdrawal. Desipramine hydrochloride (Pertofrane) seems to reduce the craving for cocaine.

Education

Individual or group therapy should focus on helping the client feel pleasure again, improve energy level, and reduce cocaine craving. Peer support groups and self-help groups, such as Cocaine Anonymous, may be very effective. Random and regular urine testing is an external support to promote abstinence.

AMPHETAMINES

Amphetamines (also called uppers, speed, bennies) include dextroamphetamine sulfate (Dexedrine), amphetamine sulfate (Amphetamine), and methamphetamine hydrochloride (Desoxyn). Medically they are used to treat attention deficit hyperactivity disorder (ADHD), narcolepsy, and obesity.

Incidence

Amphetamines have been abused since the early 1930s. World War II greatly increased use and abuse when military personnel used amphetamines to decrease fatigue and increase alertness. Today, abuse ranges from truck drivers and college students who want to ward off sleep and increase alertness to the heavy abuser who injects or smokes homemade methamphetamine, known as meth, chalk, ice, crystal, crank, and glass. An estimated 10.4 million people in the United States have tried methamphetamine at some time (NIDA, 2005b).

Signs and Symptoms

Besides suppressing fatigue and increasing alertness, amphetamines enhance psychomotor performance, induce a temporary state of well-being, and give an instantaneous euphoria. Like cocaine, after several days the person becomes exhausted and lapses into a long period of sleep and depression (crash). The action of amphetamines lasts much longer than that of cocaine, and there is a greater potential for adverse reactions and severe toxicity (Figure 49-4).

High abuse doses may cause insomnia, tachycardia, headache, arrhythmias, hypertension followed by hypotension, nausea, vomiting, cramping, diarrhea, hyperreflexia, convulsions, and death. The psychological effect is termed *amphetamine psychosis* and closely resembles paranoid schizophrenia. Symptoms include paranoid ideation, confusion, compulsive behaviors, and visual and auditory hallucinations. Tolerance does develop. Amphetamines may be detected for up to 2 days.

Potential for Addiction

The potential for addiction is high. Amphetamines are schedule II drugs.

Associated Problems/ Disorders

Cardiovascular problems occur, including irregular and rapid heartbeat; hypertension; and irreversible, stroke-producing

> **PROFESSIONALTIP**
>
> **Methamphetamine**
>
> Methamphetamine, known as meth, is an illegal highly addictive drug belonging to the class of drugs known as stimulants. Relatively inexpensive over the counter products such as drain cleaner, antifreeze, and battery acid are used to make meth in homemade labs. The production of meth has led to widespread drug problems in communities throughout the United States. Nurses can identify methamphetamine users by signs of excited speech, agitation, decreased appetite, weight loss, nausea, vomiting, diarrhea, increased physical activity and energy level, dilated pupils, hypertension, angina, dyspnea, and hyperthermia.

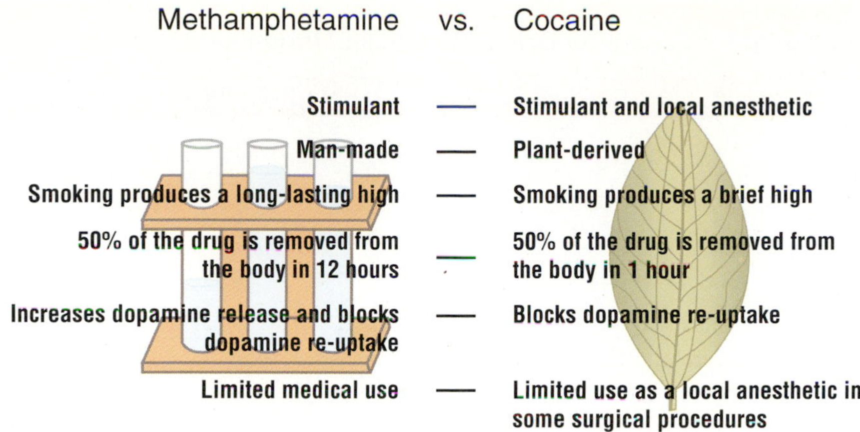

Methamphetamine vs. Cocaine
Stimulant — Stimulant and local anesthetic
Man-made — Plant-derived
Smoking produces a long-lasting high — Smoking produces a brief high
50% of the drug is removed from the body in 12 hours — 50% of the drug is removed from the body in 1 hour
Increases dopamine release and blocks dopamine re-uptake — Blocks dopamine re-uptake
Limited medical use — Limited use as a local anesthetic in some surgical procedures

FIGURE 49-4 **Basic Differences between Methamphetamine and Cocaine** (*Adapted from Research Report Series—Methamphetamine Abuse and Addiction, National Institute on Drug Abuse, 2008.*)

damage to small blood vessels in the brain (NIDA, 2008j). Injecting the drug may damage blood vessels and cause skin abscesses, and if injection equipment is shared, there is an increased risk of HIV/AIDS and hepatitis B and C transmission.

WITHDRAWAL

Symptoms of withdrawal include apathy, fatigue, irritability, depression, disorientation, anxiety, paranoia, aggression, and an intense craving for the drug.

TREATMENT/REHABILITATION

Urinary acidifiers, such as ascorbic acid (vitamin C), increase the excretion of amphetamines. Diazepam (Valium) is given for sedation to ease the withdrawal crash. Bromocriptine mesylate (Parlodel) or levodopa (Dopar) may help decrease the craving. A quiet environment is also helpful.

Behavioral therapy is used to help the client recognize and accept the need to stop using amphetamines. Supportive individual or group therapy, and especially self-help groups, aids the client to stay abstinent and in treatment.

CAFFEINE

Caffeine is found in coffee, tea, cola beverages, energy drinks, cocoa, chocolate, and some nonprescription drugs (Table 49-6).

INCIDENCE

Caffeine is probably the best known and most frequently used and abused CNS stimulant.

SIGNS AND SYMPTOMS

Caffeine causes relaxation of smooth muscles in blood vessels and bronchi, diuresis, an increased gastric acid secretion, suppression of appetite, increased feeling of energy, and constriction of cerebral blood vessels. An increased level of caffeine intake causes jitteriness, restlessness, nervousness, excitement, flushed face, palpitations, and nausea.

POTENTIAL FOR ADDICTION

The potential for addiction is moderate. Caffeine is not a scheduled drug.

WITHDRAWAL

Withdrawal produces headache, irritability, and tremulousness.

TREATMENT/REHABILITATION

A gradual reduction of caffeine intake can reduce or eliminate the withdrawal symptoms. The client can then drink decaffeinated coffee and tea and caffeine-free soft drinks. The intake of cocoa and chocolate should be greatly reduced or eliminated. Caffeine can be avoided by reading labels and not using nonprescription products that contain caffeine.

NICOTINE

Nicotine is found in tobacco in a 1% to 2% concentration. There is no therapeutic use for nicotine. Smoking and other uses of tobacco have been in and out of favor several times during the past five centuries. This century has seen the greatest degree of abuse. Reasons for this increase are related to the mass production of tobacco products, mass advertising campaigns, and the psychological dependence produced by nicotine. Tobacco, even when used in moderation, will likely produce disease and death. Tobacco kills more than 430,000 U.S. citizens and 5 million persons worldwide each year (World Health Organization (WHO, 2008), Centers for Disease Control and Prevention (CDC, 2008c).

INCIDENCE

In the United States 19.8% of the population, (43.4 million people) are current cigarette smokers (CDC, 2008a). Among high school students, 20% were current smokers in 2007 (CDC, 2008b).

SIGNS AND SYMPTOMS

Nicotine causes decreased skeletal muscle tone, decreased sensitivity of some receptor sites (pain, heat, taste buds),

Table 49-6 Caffeine Content of Common Drinks, Foods, and Products

SUBSTANCE	SERVING SIZE	CAFFEINE CONTENT (MILLIGRAMS)
Coffee		
Brewed, drip method	8 oz.	65–150
Instant	8 oz.	60–130
Decaffeinated	8 oz.	2–9
Espresso	1 oz.	30–64
Starbucks Cafe Latte	16 oz.	150
Starbucks Coffee Grande	16 oz.	330
Tea		
Brewed	8 oz.	20–110
Instant	8 oz.	10–35
Green tea, brewed	8 oz.	30–50
Canned or bottled	8–12 oz.	10–75
Lipton Brisk Iced Tea, lemon flavored	12 oz.	10
Nestea, sweetened or unsweetened	12 oz.	17
Snapple Iced Tea	16 oz.	18
Soft Drinks		
Mountain Dew (Regular & Diet)	12 oz.	54
Mello Yellow	12 oz.	53
Diet Coke	12 oz.	47
Sunkist Orange	12 oz.	41
Pepsi	12 oz.	38
Coca-Cola	12 oz.	35
Diet Pepsi	12 oz.	35
Sprite	12 oz.	0
Sports/Energy Drinks		
Spike Shooter	8.4 oz.	300
No Name (formerly known as Cocaine)	8.4 oz.	280
Monster Energy	16 oz.	160
Rockstar	16 oz.	160
Full Throttle	16 oz.	144
Red Bull	8.3 oz.	76
Vault	8 oz.	47
Foods & Products		
Milk chocolate candy bar	1–1.5 oz	2–10
Dark chocolate candy bar	1–1.5 oz.	5–35
Hot cocoa	8 oz.	2–10
Jolt Caffeinated Gum	1 stick	33
Foosh Energy Mints	1 mint	100
Coffee ice cream	8 oz.	8–85
NoDoz Maximum Strength	1 tablet	200
Vivarin	1 tablet	200
Excedrin Extra Strength	2 tablets	130

Data from Johns Hopkins University School of Medicine, Johns Hopkins Bayview Campus, Behavioral Biology Research Center, 2009, www.caffeinedependence.org/caffeine_dependence.html#sources; Mayo Clinic, 2007, *How much caffeine is in your daily habit?* Retrieved from http://www.mayoclinic.com/health/caffeine/AN01211/METHOD=print; Center for Science in the Public Interest, 2007, *Caffeine content of food and drugs.* Retrieved from http://www.cspinet.org/new/cafchart.htm

LIFE SPAN CONSIDERATIONS

Smoking

- Menopause generally occurs earlier in women who smoke.
- The older smoker is often less motivated to quit because of the feeling that "I've survived this long."

reduced appetite, vasoconstriction, decreased body temperature, and increased blood pressure. Tolerance develops so the daily intake must increase to continue the desired effect.

Potential for Addiction

The potential for addiction is high. Even first-time users can become dependent within weeks of their initial use. Nicotine is not a scheduled drug.

Associated Problems/ Disorders

Other ingredients in the smoke (tar, carbon monoxide, and incompletely burned waste products) are largely responsible for the negative health consequences.

Respiratory

Chronic obstructive pulmonary disease is caused by the many changes tobacco use makes in the respiratory system. Smokers are more prone to developing pneumonia, and asthma is exacerbated by smoking. Chronic exposure to smoke inhalation gives children higher rates of otitis media and respiratory illnesses.

Cardiovascular

Ischemic heart disease is twice as likely to develop in a smoker than in a nonsmoker. Cerebrovascular accidents and peripheral vascular disease are strongly associated with smoking. Cessation of smoking, about 10 years, reduces the risks for these three vascular diseases to the nonsmoker's level.

Cancer

Many cancers—oral, pharyngeal, laryngeal, esophageal, lung, pancreatic, kidney, and bladder—are strongly associated with tobacco. Secondhand smoke causes lung cancer in nonsmoking adults. Tobacco use is by far the most important risk factor in lung cancer development (American Cancer Society, 2007).

Withdrawal

Short-term effects of nicotine withdrawal include nausea, diarrhea, headache, drowsiness, insomnia, irritability, and poor concentration. Increased appetite along with an intense craving for tobacco may persist for 6 months or longer.

Treatment/Rehabilitation

Nicotine replacement therapy by patch, nasal spray, inhaler, or gum helps individuals break the habit. It is important that the client not smoke while using the patch. Serious adverse effects may be experienced with a high serum nicotine level. It can be toxic. Later, a gradual withdrawal of the nicotine patch can be accomplished. The first non-nicotine prescription drug to treat nicotine addiction, bupropion (Zyban), was approved by the Food and Drug Administration in 1996.

An exercise program will help with stress management and minimize possible weight gain. Relaxation techniques will also reduce stress. Support by family and significant others for the person quitting tobacco use may help the process. A lack of support may greatly increase the difficulty of quitting for the individual. The rate of relapse is highest in the first few weeks and diminishes considerably after 3 months.

METHYLPHENIDATE HYDROCHLORIDE (RITALIN)

Currently, there is an increase in the use (misuse and overuse) of Ritalin that is becoming a growing problem. Ritalin is an accepted treatment for children with attention deficit hyperactivity disorder (ADHD). Although Ritalin is a CNS stimulant, there is a paradoxical calming effect on children with ADHD. Many children are being given Ritalin without thorough testing to eliminate other causes of attention deficit. These children have the potential for dependence. Ritalin is also used for narcolepsy. It can be detected for 1 to 2 days and is a schedule II drug.

HALLUCINOGENS

Hallucinogens refers to a group of naturally occurring and synthetic agents that produce essentially the same mind-altering effects.

Psilocybin and psilocin are naturally occurring organic compounds found in some mushrooms that grow in the United States and Mexico. These mushrooms have been used for centuries in southern Mexico, primarily in religious ceremonies. Fresh or dried mushrooms, sometimes mixed with food, are ingested orally.

Dimethyltryptamine (DMT) and diethyltryptamine (DET) are found in tropical plant leaves and seeds. For centuries they have been dried and powdered and used as snuff. They are not orally active. Sometimes the powder is added to tobacco or marijuana.

There are several amphetamine-like hallucinogens. Probably the two best known are 2,5 dimethyl-4-ethylamphetamine (DOM) and methylene-dioxyamphetamine (MDMA, ecstasy), which are chemically manufactured compounds. These are usually taken orally but may be injected intravenously or inhaled.

LYSERGIC ACID DIETHYLAMIDE

Lysergic acid diethylamide (LSD), a manufactured chemical compound, is perhaps the most widely known and used hallucinogen. In the past, LSD has been used as a legitimate medication and in research. In the 1960s, when its abuse became so widespread, the manufacturer refused to supply it for research. It had already been discontinued as a useful medication. It is generally taken orally but can be injected intravenously.

Incidence

The use of hallucinogens declined throughout the 1980s. In the early 1990s, LSD made a comeback. The 1990 and 1991 annual survey of high school seniors found that for the first time since 1976, more seniors had used LSD than cocaine in the previous 12 months. The 1998 survey showed a slight downward movement in LSD use. The 2007 survey showed that in 2006 more than 23 million Americans aged 12 or older had used LSD in their lifetime (SAMHSA, 2008). Other names for LSD are acid, blotter, and microdot.

Signs and Symptoms

The functioning of both the peripheral nervous system and the central nervous system is altered by LSD. Physical effects include hypertension, increased temperature, sweating, loss of appetite, dilated pupils, and dry mouth. Time and distance are distorted, rational judgment is impaired, and visual **hallucinations** (perceiving things that are not really there) and delusions along with **synesthesia** (hearing colors and seeing sounds) occur. A state of either euphoria or depression is experienced. The depression with feelings of anxiety, panic, or suicidal tendencies is termed a "bad trip." Flashbacks occur suddenly days or years after LSD use. Their occurrence and frequency are unpredictable but seem to happen in times of high stress. LSD may be detected up to 8 hours after use.

Potential for Addiction

LSD is not considered an addictive drug, but it does produce tolerance. It is a schedule I drug.

Associated Problems/Disorders

Personality changes occur with LSD use and may happen after a single LSD experience. Acceptable social behaviors seem to diminish with use.

Withdrawal

There is no withdrawal seen.

Treatment/Rehabilitation

A person on a "bad trip" should be carefully watched to prevent self-injury. Reassurance, support, and "talking down" should be done in a quiet, pleasant manner. The person should be encouraged to sit up or walk. Closing the eyes intensifies the "bad trip." The person should be reminded that the drug is causing the effects, which will soon go away.

After cessation of chronic LSD use, long-term psychotherapy is usually required to determine what needs were fulfilled by the use of this drug. A 12-step program and family assistance are usually necessary to reinforce the decision to remain abstinent. If the client is upset by flashbacks or the fear of flashbacks, an anxiolytic drug such as diazepam (Valium) may be ordered.

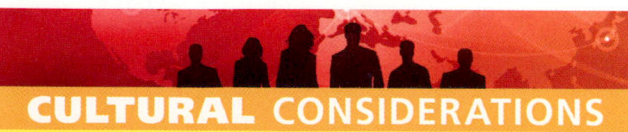

CULTURAL CONSIDERATIONS

Mescaline

Mescaline is the active ingredient in peyote cactus found growing in the southwestern United States and Mexico. It is the only legally used hallucinogen. Members of the Native American Church of the United States may use it for religious purposes. It is ingested orally. A cross-tolerance to LSD and psilocybin occurs.

PHENCYCLIDINE

Phencyclidine (PCP) was made for use as an anesthetic agent, but it produced such adverse reactions that it was withdrawn from clinical trials; however, it can easily be manufactured in an unsophisticated laboratory from simple materials. The degree of purity varies widely. It is often found as a contaminant in other street drugs. The anesthetic is used in veterinary medicine.

Incidence

PCP is primarily used by adolescents and young adults, with the first use between the ages of 13 and 15 years. Approximately 12.8% of those between the ages of 12 and 17 years had used PCP in 1979. The use decreased to 2.4% in 1992 and increased to 3.9% in 1997. In 2006, *The National Survey on Drug Use and Health* reported that 6.6 million persons aged 12 or older had used PCP in their lifetime (SAMHSA, 2008). The *Monitoring the Future Survey* showed that in 2007, 2.1% of high school seniors had tried PCP (NIDA, 2007). Other names for PCP are angel dust, ozone, wack, and rocket fuel. Marijuana combined with PCP is called killer joints or crystal super grass.

Signs and Symptoms

There are usually four phases, with the symptoms dose related. Acute toxicity is characterized by visual disturbances, auditory hallucinations, combativeness, catatonia, convulsions, and coma, and lasts about 3 days. The toxic psychosis phase has visual and auditory hallucinations, agitation, paranoid delusions, and disturbed judgment, and lasts about 7 days. The third phase has psychotic episodes, including thought disorders, paranoid ideation, and affect disorders much like schizophrenia and lasts a month or more. Depression is the fourth phase that may end in suicide. The use of other street drugs may alleviate the depression. Behavior is highly unpredictable. Death can occur from respiratory depression. For 2 to 8 days, PCP can be detected.

Potential for Addiction

Even chronic use does not produce physical dependence. Psychological dependence does develop as evidenced by a craving for PCP. It is a schedule I and II drug.

Associated Problems/Disorders

Seizures are a common occurrence with PCP. Hypertension and hyperthermia must be treated before they become a crisis situation. **Opisthotonos**, a complete arching of the body with only the head and feet on the bed, usually is relieved as the blood level of PCP decreases. Cardiac arrhythmias may need interventions by a cardiologist. Acute renal failure may result from the use of PCP. Strokes also have been reported.

Withdrawal

PCP is fat soluble and its effects are felt weeks after the last use as it is gradually released from the fatty tissue into the circulation.

Treatment/Rehabilitation

Treatment should begin in an inpatient setting because of the high risk of suicide. The goal is to keep the client from resuming drug use. Sedatives may be used, and urinary acidifiers such as ascorbic acid may be given to increase excretion of PCP. Minimal confrontation should be used in a nonthreatening, nonstimulating, supportive environment. No effort should be made to "talk down" or calm the individual. Diazepam (Valium) may be ordered.

Vocational counseling and training may enhance self-esteem. Body awareness, yoga, and progressive relaxation help the client focus and improve attention span and concentration. Participation in a self-help group such as Narcotics Anonymous (NA) should be encouraged, although initial involvement is usually minimal.

OPIOIDS

Opioids is a term used to refer to naturally occurring opiates, semisynthetic opiates, synthetic opiates, and agonist-antagonists. Table 49-7 provides examples of these opioids. Heroin is the most abused and the most rapid acting of the opioids (NIDA, 2008i).

Table 49-7 Opioids

TYPE	EXAMPLE
Natural Opiates	morphine sulfate codeine sulfate
Semisynthetic Opiates	heroin hydromorphone hydrochloride (Dilaudid) oxymorphone hydrochloride (Numorphan) oxycodone (in Percodan) hydrocodone (in Hycodan)
Synthetic Opiates	meperidine hydrochloride (Demerol) methadone hydrochloride (Dolophine) propoxyphene (Darvon)
Agonist-Antagonists	pentazocine (Talwin) nalbuphine hydrochloride (Nubain) butorphanol tartrate (Stadol)

COURTESY OF DELMAR CENGAGE LEARNING

Incidence

Kleber (1999) described the 1990s as the decade of heroin. Cocaine addicts switched to heroin. Heroin was easily available, the purity was higher than in decades, and it could now be sniffed or smoked instead of injected (NIDA, 2008i). In 2006, 560,000 Americans age 12 and older had abused heroin at least once in the year before being surveyed (SAMHSA, 2008). Other names for heroin are horse, smack, "H," skag, and junk.

Signs and Symptoms

All of these drugs affect the CNS, causing mental changes, euphoria, drowsiness, analgesia, constricted pupils, and depressed respirations (Figure 49-5). These changes become more pronounced as the dose is increased.

Opioids increase stomach tone, decrease intestinal peristalsis, and increase the tone of the anal sphincter. This all adds up to constipation. Prolonged drug use may result in a fecal impaction.

Peripheral blood vessels are dilated by opioids, and orthostatic hypotension frequently occurs. The work of the heart is not changed by opioids, so they are frequently used to treat the severe pain of a myocardial infarction.

Tolerance may develop to one or more of the effects of opioids but not to others. For example, morphine addicts will always have pinpoint pupils even when the euphoric effects are not experienced. Tolerance to one opioid usually means tolerance to other opioids as well. Withdrawal symptoms from one opioid can be suppressed by using another opioid.

Potential for Addiction

The potential for addiction is high. Heroin is a schedule I drug; methadone, schedule II; morphine, schedule II or III; and codeine and opium are schedule II, III, or IV.

The Short-Term Effects of Opiates

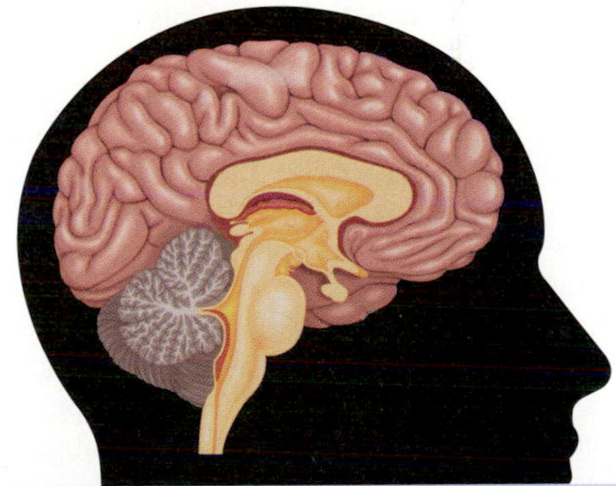

- Opiates can depress breathing by changing neurochemical activity in the brain stem, where automatic body functions are controlled.
- Opiates can change the limbic system, which controls emotions, to increase feelings of pleasure.
- Opiates can block pain messages transmitted through the spinal cord from the body.

Figure 49-5 Opiates act on many places in the brain and spinal cord. (*From Research Report Series—Heroin Abuse and Addiction, National Institute on Drug Abuse, 2008.*)

CRITICAL THINKING

Narcotic Addiction

A client who has had a series of abdominal surgeries with recurrent infections told his wife that he is afraid that he is becoming addicted to narcotics, but he does not want anyone to know. The wife confides in you and asks for advice. How would you respond to the wife?

Associated Problems/Disorders

Chronic heroin injection may cause scarred and collapsed veins, bacterial infections of heart valves and blood vessels, abscesses, and liver or kidney disease. Pneumonia may result from the respiratory-depressing effect of heroin. Additives to street heroin may clog blood vessels or cause immune reactions, leading to arthritis or other rheumatologic conditions. Sharing injection equipment can lead to infections of hepatitis B and C, HIV, and other blood-borne viruses, which can be passed on to sexual partners and children.

Withdrawal

Withdrawal symptoms depend on drug purity, dose, and route of administration. Withdrawal is characterized by a rebound excitability of those functions that had been depressed. Symptoms include stomach cramps, nausea, vomiting, diarrhea, diaphoresis, hypertension, aching of bones and muscles, lacrimation, rhinorrhea, cold flashes with goose bumps, yawning, mydriasis, anxiety, irritability, restlessness, and sometimes paranoia, violence, fear, or depersonalization.

Morphine withdrawal symptoms begin within 8 to 12 hours after the last dose, and the acute phase is over in about 10 to 14 days. Figure 49-6 illustrates the signs and symptoms of morphine withdrawal. This is the basic pattern of withdrawal for all opioids.

Codeine withdrawal symptoms may be a little less severe than those of morphine withdrawal. Dilaudid and heroin withdrawal may begin slightly earlier than morphine withdrawal. Meperidine (Demerol) withdrawal begins within 3 hours and peaks in 8 to 12 hours. Propoxyphene (Darvon) withdrawal is considerably milder.

Methadone withdrawal is slower to develop and lasts longer. Symptoms may not occur for 1 to 2 days, with acute symptoms lasting 2 to 3 weeks but not disappearing until 6 weeks after abstinence begins. Symptoms of fatigue, sluggishness, and irritability may last up to 6 months.

Withdrawal from the agonist-antagonists begins in 6 to 8 hours and is usually over in 8 days. The symptoms are the same as for morphine only in a milder form.

Treatment/Rehabilitation

Initial treatment is symptomatic and supportive of vital functions until the acute phase is over.

Detoxification

Several methods currently used for opioid detoxification are methadone, LAAM, and naltrexone.

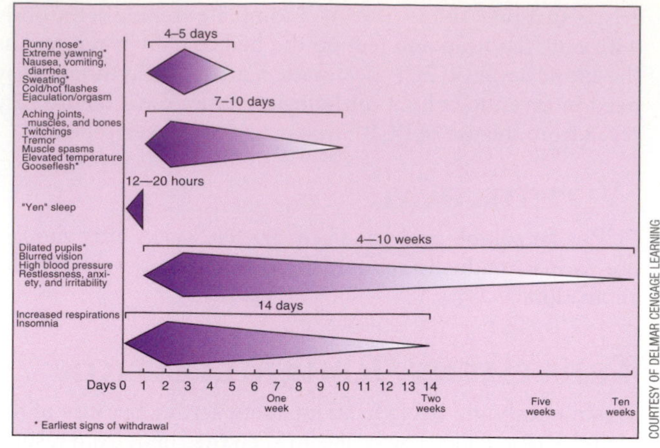

COURTESY OF DELMAR CENGAGE LEARNING

FIGURE 49-6 Duration of Morphine Withdrawal Signs and Symptoms (Basic Pattern for All Opioids)

Methadone Methadone is given and the dose adjusted to keep withdrawal symptoms under control. The daily dose is gradually reduced over a period of 3 to 6 months. Routine and random urine testing is usually done to ensure no other drug use.

Levo-alpha-acetyl-methadol Levo-alpha-acetyl-methadol (LAAM) is a synthetic opiate, like methadone, used to treat heroin addiction. It blocks the effects of heroin for up to 72 hours, so it need be taken only 3 times a week.

Naltrexone Naltrexone (ReVia) blocks the effects of morphine, heroin, and other opiates. Its effects last for 1 to 3 days, depending on the dose. The pleasurable effects of heroin are blocked, making it useful to treat highly motivated individuals. It is also used to prevent relapse in former opiate addicts.

Counseling/Self-Help Groups

Individual and/or group counseling must go hand in hand with the detoxification to help the client learn new methods of coping with life's stresses. Participation in Narcotics Anonymous (NA) helps the client maintain abstinence from drugs.

Behavioral Therapy

Contingency management therapy employs a voucher system. Clients earn "points" for having negative drug tests. These can be exchanged for items encouraging healthy living.

INHALANTS

Inhalants are inexpensive and easy to obtain. Examples are toluene (glues), gasoline, kerosene, isopropyl alcohol, lacquer thinner, acetone, benzene, naptha, carbon tetrachloride, fluorocarbons (aerosol propellants), correction fluid, and nitrous oxide. They are rapidly absorbed into the brain and stored in body fat. Common names for inhalants are whippets, poppers, and snappers.

Incidence

In 1997, 21% of 8th graders, 18.3% of 10th graders, and 16.1% of 12th graders reported using inhalants at least once. By 2002, 15.2% of 8th graders, 13.5% of 10th graders, and

11.7% of 13th graders reported using inhalants at least once. The Monitoring the Future Study (NIDA, 2005a) revealed that 17.3% of 8th graders have abused inhalants. Several National Surveys have reported that more than 22.9 million Americans have abused inhalants at least once in their lives (NIDA, 2005a). Inhalants are not scheduled drugs.

Signs and Symptoms

The desired effect of euphoria is followed by nausea, headache, and amnesia. Other effects of using inhalants include dizziness, unsteady gait, slurred speech, auditory and visual hallucinations, drowsiness, hypotension, heightened sexual response caused by profound vasodilation, stupor, unconsciousness, and coma. Heavy use can lead to hypoxia, multiple organ damage, and death. Airway freezing and/or laryngospasm can be caused by nitrous oxide.

Behaviors that may indicate inhalant abuse include decreased school performance; loss of interest in extracurricular, family, and social activities; and the onset of legal problems.

Potential for Addiction

The potential for addiction is high for psychological dependence only.

Associated Problems/Disorders

Chronic pulmonary irritation and/or chemical pneumonitis may be caused by the use of inhalants. Toluene may cause renal tubular acidosis, hearing loss, and brain damage. Fluorocarbons sensitize the myocardium to catacholemines and may cause arrhythmias.

Withdrawal

There are no withdrawal symptoms.

Treatment/Rehabilitation

Initial treatment is to provide oxygen and respiratory support. Participation in a traditional chemical dependency program is often needed. An adolescent 12-step group is very helpful. Individual and family counseling are essential.

Ecstasy

Ecstasy, also called MDMA (3,4-methylenedioxymethamphetamine), is a complex drug having similarities to methamphetamine, a stimulant, and mescaline, a hallucinogen (NIDA, 2008f). It produces stimulant effects and distorted time and perception rather than true hallucinations. Street names include "X", "E", "XTC", Adam, hug, beans, clarity, lover's speed, and love drug. Ecstasy tablets also often contain one or more of the following: caffeine, methamphetamine, dextromethorphan, ephedrine, or cocaine.

Incidence

Americans using ecstasy for the first time increased from 615,000 in 2005 to 860,000 in 2006. Most of these new users were 18 or older (SAMHSA, 2008).

Signs and Symptoms

Ecstasy provides an enhanced sense of pleasure and self-confidence; feelings of peacefulness, acceptance, and closeness with others; and increased energy. Research has shown that ecstasy can lead to disruptions in body temperature and cardiovascular regulation. It also damages the nerves in the brain's serotonin system and appears to produce long-term deficits in memory and cognition (NIDA, 2001b). It appears that the more ecstasy taken, the greater the deficit (NIDA, 2001a).

Potential for Addiction

The potential for addiction is currently being researched by clinical studies. For some people, studies have found that ecstasy can be addictive (NIDA, 2008f).

Associated Problems/Disorders

MDMA interferes with the metabolism of other drugs, including some that may be in the tablet with the ecstasy.

Anabolic Steroids

Anabolic steroids are synthetic derivatives of testosterone. They cause both androgenic (masculinizing) and anabolic (tissue-building) effects. Most people use anabolic steroids for their anabolic effects. Medically, they are used in the treatment of some anemias and in some cancer therapies. The use of anabolic steroids is banned by the International Olympic Committee and the National Collegiate Athletic Association.

Incidence

Primary users are athletes seeking to improve their performance. Other people use anabolic steroids to improve their physical appearance. In 2000, 3% of 8th graders, 3.5% of 10th graders, and 2.5% of 12th graders had used anabolic steroids. The *2007 Monitoring the Future Study* (NIDA, 2009e) reported that 0.8% of 8th, 1.1% of 10th, and 1.4% of 12th graders had abused anabolic steroids at least once in the year prior to being surveyed.

PROFESSIONALTIP

Club Drugs

Club drugs are being used by young adults at all-night parties such as "raves" or "trances," dance clubs, and bars. MDMA (Ecstasy), GHB, Rohypnol, ketamine, methamphetamine, and LSD are some of the club or party drugs. These drugs can cause serious health problems. Used in combination with alcohol, the drugs are even more dangerous (NIDA, 2009b).

Signs and Symptoms

The commonly perceived effects of anabolic steroids are an increase in skeletal muscle mass, enhanced physical performance of the skeletal muscles, and improved athletic ability; however, there is no conclusive evidence that these perceived effects are medically accurate.

Potential for Addiction

The potential for addiction is moderate. Anabolic steroids are schedule III drugs.

Associated Problems/ Disorders

Other effects found when anabolic steroids are used include hepatocellular damage, cholestasis, hepatoadenoma, hepatocarcinoma, acne, hirsutism, male-pattern baldness, a deepening of the voice, increased cholesterol level, increased blood pressure, decreased glucose tolerance, mood swings, aggressiveness, depression, psychosis, and hepatitis or HIV infection if needles are shared. In males, there is also testicular atrophy, oligospermia, impotence, prostatic hypertrophy, prostatic carcinoma, and gynecomastia. In females, there is also amenorrhea, clitoromegaly, uterine atrophy, breast atrophy, facial hair growth, and teratogenicity.

These effects seem to be reversible when the anabolic steroids are no longer taken, except for the male-pattern baldness, liver tumors, and gynecomastia in males and clitoral enlargement, virilization, and male-pattern baldness in females. The increased aggressiveness and euphoria are probably beneficial during athletic competitions but otherwise may cause severe social problems.

Withdrawal

Symptoms of withdrawal include lethargy, abdominal muscle cramps, constipation, headache, and depression.

Treatment/Rehabilitation

Treatment of withdrawal focuses on providing symptom relief for the client and counseling to build self-esteem and self-confidence in abilities without the use of anabolic steroids.

NURSING PROCESS

Nursing care is an essential component of the multidisciplinary approach to substance abuse treatment.

Assessment

The subjective and objective data given are related to substance abuse and dependence in general.

Subjective Data

The client will often describe being very relaxed; feeling wonderful; or having a headache, fatigue, depression, sleep disturbance, suppression of appetite, dizziness, hallucinations, paranoia, anxiety, emotional lability, memory loss, heightened sexual desire (with early use), or loss of sexual desire (with continued use). Problems in various areas of life are common, such as frequent job changes; marital conflict, separation and/or divorce; work-related accidents, lateness, absenteeism; and legal problems, including arrest for driving while intoxicated. The client may describe having falls or fights and financial problems. Normal diet pattern and the presence of any disease conditions should be noted.

The client should be asked health history questions regarding substance abuse (Table 49-8). The information received from the client may not always be accurate. Validation with the family or significant other is helpful.

Objective Data

Neglect of health and personal care is often evident. The client may have dental caries, bad breath, gingivitis, unkempt appearance, and be undernourished or malnourished. If substances have been inhaled, there may be irritation and bleeding of the nasal mucosa, destruction of the nasal mucosa and cartilaginous structures, or depression of respirations. If substances have been injected intravenously, there will be scarring of veins (needle marks, track marks), possibly skin infections, enlarged lymph nodes, and hematomas.

Table 49-8 Obtaining a Client History of Substance Abuse Problems

How often do you use drugs/alcohol?
How much do you usually use?
Have you ever used drugs/alcohol more than you use them now? When?
Under what circumstances?
What substance did you last use?
Has anyone ever told you to cut back or quit using drugs/alcohol?
Have you tried?
Have you or are you having interpersonal, occupational, physical, psychological or legal problems due to drugs/alcohol?

COURTESY OF DELMAR CENGAGE LEARNING

MEMORY TRICK

Substance Abuse Client Assessment

An easy memory trick for general assessment findings for a client participating in substance abuse is **DRUGS**:

- **D** = Depression
- **R** = Reduced self-control
- **U** = Unkept appearance
- **G** = Gives excuses (for absenteeism, memory loss, etc.)
- **S** = Sleep disturbance

The client may appear older than the stated age and have a chronic cough producing brown to black sputum, dilated or pinpoint pupils, tremors, slurred speech, lack of coordination, frequent episodes of sexually transmitted diseases, jaundice, or vomiting. There may be tachycardia, hypertension, ascites, or petechiae.

Nursing Diagnoses

NANDA-International (2009) nursing diagnoses for a client with substance abuse or dependence may include the following:

- *Imbalanced **N**utrition: Less than Body Requirements*
- ***S**elf-Care Deficits*
- *Risk for **I**njury*
- *Disturbed **S**leep Pattern*
- ***A**ctivity Intolerance*
- *Impaired Physical **M**obility*
- *Disturbed **S**ensory Perception*
- *Impaired Verbal **C**ommunication*
- *Risk for **I**nfection*
- *Excess or Deficient **F**luid Volume*
- *Disturbed **T**hought Processes*
- *Ineffective **C**oping*
- *Situational Low **S**elf-Esteem*
- *Risk for **V**iolence (Other-Directed or Self-Directed)*
- ***A**nxiety*
- *Impaired **S**ocial Interaction*
- ***H**opelessness*
- ***P**owerlessness*
- *Compromised Family **C**oping*
- *Defensive **C**oping*
- *Self-**N**eglect*

Planning/Outcome Identification

There are several overall goals for the care of a client with a substance abuse problem. The client will do the following:

1. Abstain from using psychoactive substances
2. Adhere to the treatment plan
3. Make lifestyle changes to maintain abstinence
4. Engage in behaviors that foster good health

Possible outcomes from Nursing Outcomes Classification (NOC) include:

- Distorted Thought Control
- Risk Control: Alcohol Use
- Risk Control: Drug Use

Nursing Interventions

Nursing interventions include active listening, providing care in a nonjudgmental manner, teaching health promotion, and referral to self-help groups or individual counseling. Other nursing interventions must be specific for the goals and nursing diagnoses identified for the individual client. Examples might include the following:

1. Provide a well-balanced diet. Monitor intake and results of lab tests. Assess for GI bleeding.
2. Assist with personal hygiene. Encourage self-care.
3. Administer medications as ordered to decrease or prevent symptoms of withdrawal. Keep call light in client's reach. Keep siderails up.
4. Provide warm milk at bedtime. Plan with client a time for bed. Encourage use of relaxation techniques. Reassure client that insomnia will improve.
5. Encourage client to do active ROM exercises.
6. Assist client to turn in bed. Assist client to ambulate as able. Answer call light promptly.
7. Do not argue with a client having hallucinations. Remind client of day, time, and place.
8. Monitor the client's nonverbal communication.
9. Encourage good personal hygiene. Inspect skin for integrity.
10. Administer antibiotics as ordered. Monitor vital signs, I&O, and results of diagnostic testing.
11. Administer vitamins as ordered. Provide cues as needed. Encourage adequate diet intake.
12. Assess coping patterns to identify strengths and weaknesses. Actively listen to client. Refer to appropriate community agencies.
13. Assist client to identify areas of low self-esteem. Encourage client participation in group therapy. Refer to individual counseling as needed.
14. Monitor client closely. Use restraints as ordered. Keep bed in low position and side rails up.
15. Introduce client to other recovering persons. Encourage client to participate in self-help group.
16. Provide spiritual support if asked.
17. Involve client in decision making when possible. Give positive reinforcement for abstinence.
18. Encourage family to participate in treatment program.

LIFE SPAN CONSIDERATIONS

Substance Misuse or Abuse

In the older adult:

- Misuse (using a legal drug for something other than intended or exceeding the recommended dose of a drug) is more common than abuse or dependence.
- Substances that decrease respirations can increase the frequency of mental confusion.
- Decreased coordination from alcohol or other substances is associated with falling more often and fracturing the wrist, back, and hips.
- Chronic medical conditions can be made worse from even minimal use of alcohol or other drugs because these substances can change the effect of prescribed medications.
- Unrealistic expectations of retirement may lead to use of mood-altering substances to relieve depression and boredom.

Possible interventions from Nursing Interventions Classification (NIC) include:

- Delusion Management
- Hallucination Management
- Anxiety Reduction
- Delirium Management
- Mood Management

Evaluation

Each goal must be evaluated to determine how it has been met by the client and modified as necessary.

CODEPENDENCY

Codependency was first recognized by those working with families of alcoholics. It is a learned pattern of feeling and behaving, a problem with relationships. In healthy relationships, people share love, concern, and respect for each other. There is equal give-and-take. This is termed *interdependence*. In unhealthy relationships, people are often out of touch with their own needs and feelings. They may be unwilling or unable to take care of themselves and have little self-esteem. Only by fulfilling the expectations of others do they feel good about themselves. This is termed *codependence*. **Codependent** persons live based on what others think of them. They always try to meet the needs of others, demand love from others, and manipulate and control the lives of others.

Serious family problems like addictions, abuse, family secrets, or other major stresses cause confusion and put a family at risk. Codependent behavior thrives when fear, guilt, blame, and low self-esteem become evident. When family members do not relate to each other in positive ways or when their interactions do not provide a healthy environment, the family is called *dysfunctional*. Many children grow up in dysfunctional families and learn to be codependent.

Codependency tends to run in families. Parents cannot teach their children how to cope in healthy ways if they do not know how themselves. Without intervention or a conscious change by the individual, a pattern of codependent behavior will continue in other relationships.

Characteristics

Persons who are codependent have specific characteristics or traits. They have low self-esteem, never feel they are good enough, and often feel shame. Emotions are denied. They are out of touch with their own feelings and deny their own needs. Their smile is phony much of the time. Problems with communication become evident as they have trouble expressing their needs and feelings. Often they say the opposite to hide their true feelings. They expect others to read their minds. Relationship problems occur because they are afraid of being hurt or that others might learn of their secret feelings and reject them. They cannot risk loving and losing. Relationships are desired, but walls are always put up.

Codependent persons live through others. They are people pleasers who would rather give than take. The approval of others means they are okay. They think they can fix others. The feeling of powerlessness occurs because they give power to others by looking to them for approval. They go to extremes. For a while they will try very hard for approval, and then they will not try at all or they will keep negative feelings inside with a smile on their face and then blow up over some little thing. Table 49-9 lists some characteristics of the codependent person.

Table 49-9 Characteristics of the Codependent Person

Caretaking	"I always give to others. No one gives to me."
Obsession	"I can't stop worrying about problems."
Denial	"I pretend I don't have problems."
Poor communication	"No one understands me."
Lack of trust	"I don't trust myself."
Anger	"I resent feeling controlled and manipulated."

From *Mental Health Concepts* (5th ed.), by C. Waughfield, 2002, Clifton Park, NY: Delmar Cengage Learning. Copyright 2002 by Delmar Cengage Learning. Adapted with permission.

Treatment

Professional help is usually necessary to change codependent behavior. The goal of treatment is to help the codependent person feel happy and good about himself or herself. Therapy sessions focus on identifying and reconnecting with the true self, dealing with feelings, learning how to communicate feelings, learning to trust, setting boundaries for relationships, and taking charge of their own life.

THE IMPAIRED NURSE

Most states now have peer assistance programs to help nurses who are impaired by either alcohol or other substances. Substance abuse and dependence are greater problems among nurses than among the general public because nurses have access to many controlled substances. The impaired nurse often requests to give medications, makes medication errors, and "wastes" drugs frequently. This nurse may wear long sleeves and spend an extraordinary amount of time in the bathroom.

Peer assistance programs first appeared in 1980. They have been formed through the state nursing association or the state board of nursing, or through joint effort of both. The goals of the peer assistance programs are to assist the impaired nurse to receive treatment; protect the public from impaired nurses; help the recovering nurse reenter the nursing workforce in a planned, safe manner; and monitor the nurse's recovery for a time. The state board of nursing may restrict access to controlled substances for the recovering nurse for some period.

PROFESSIONALTIP

The Impaired Nurse

One of the reasons that nurses either lose their license or have it suspended is due to either alcohol use or drug diversion. As nurses, giving medications is a large part of our responsibility. Unless we have developed positive self care skills, it may be tempting to use drugs to cope. Most nursing programs have a professional development course in which this issue is addressed. If it is not addressed in your program, review your Board of Nursing Nurse Practice Act. Many states have treatment programs specifically for nurses.

CRITICAL THINKING

Drug Testing

Should drug testing of all health-care workers be required? How would you feel if you were requested to comply?

Before the peer assistance programs, impaired nurses were generally just dismissed from employment. Then they would find employment at another health care agency where substance abuse or dependence would continue. This pattern often went on for years.

As the name implies, peer assistance programs are staffed with nurses to help nurses. Many of the staff are volunteers who work in psychiatric nursing or substance abuse centers or who are themselves recovering from substance abuse. It is best not to cover up for a colleague with a substance abuse problem; rather, the nurse should report the situation to a supervisor, who can arrange for the nurse to receive help. Some boards of nursing will discipline a nurse for failing to report a fellow nurse who is abusing drugs.

CASE STUDY

Z.G., age 19, quit school 3 years ago. He has a part-time job at a fast-food place but has been tardy or absent quite often lately. Sometimes he is easy to get along with, and sometimes he is aggressive and difficult. His mother, with whom he lives, says he is a good boy and does not give her any trouble. Z.G. was brought to the emergency room by a friend after he passed out. His temperature is 99°F, respirations 10, and pupils are pinpoint. There are track marks on both arms.

The following activities will guide your development of a nursing care plan for the case study.

1. List signs and symptoms, other than Z.G.'s, that a client may experience as a heroin addict.
2. List diagnostic tests that may be ordered.
3. List subjective and objective data the nurse should obtain.
4. Write three individualized nursing diagnoses and goals for Z.G.
5. List resources within the medical center and local area that could assist Z.G.
6. Describe the use of methadone in heroin addiction.
7. List teaching that Z.G. will need as a part of his rehabilitation.

Nursing diagnoses for a client with substance abuse or dependency include the following:

NURSING DIAGNOSES	PLANNING/OUTCOMES	NURSING INTERVENTIONS
*Imbalanced **N**utrition: Less than Body Requirements* related to chemical dependency	The client will maintain body mass and weight within range determined by health care provider.	Teach client required nutritional needs and provide written information. Measure body mass and weigh client daily. Monitor intake for nutritional content and calories. Monitor lab values.

(*Continues*)

Nursing diagnoses for a client with substance abuse or dependency include the following: (Continued)

NURSING DIAGNOSES	PLANNING/OUTCOMES	NURSING INTERVENTIONS
*Risk for **Injury*** related to physical and mental alterations resulting from alcohol and/or drug abuse	The client will avoid physical injury.	Provide a safe environment. Identify factors that affect the client's safety needs, degree of intoxication, and/or changes in mental status. Encourage and assist client to develop risk control strategies.
*Self-**Neglect*** related to substance abuse.	The client will demonstrate adequate personal hygiene.	Provide a supportive nonjudgmental environment. Teach the client the importance of daily personal hygiene. Provide hygiene supplies if needed (shampoo, soap, toothbrush, toothpaste, comb, deodorant, etc.).
Evaluation: Evaluate each outcome to determine how it has been met by the client.		

SUMMARY

- Substance abuse and dependence have been problems for centuries.
- Factors related to substance abuse include individual, family patterns, lifestyle, environmental, and developmental factors.
- A false-positive result on a drug screening test may be caused by ingestion of poppy seeds, use of a Vicks® inhaler, or use of over-the-counter diet aids.
- Detoxification is the first step in the treatment and rehabilitation of a substance abuser.
- Street drugs vary in strength and purity. Higher-priced drugs are often mixed with drugs that are cheaper or easier to obtain.
- Neglect of health and personal care are often evident in substance abuse and dependence.
- Nurses have a higher incidence of substance abuse and dependence than the general public.
- Most states have peer assistance programs for impaired nurses.

REVIEW QUESTIONS

1. A client is brought to the emergency room with pin point pupils, shallow breathing, and cyanosis of nail beds and oral mucosa. Based on these clinical findings what is the most important initial nursing intervention?
   1. Administer medication to reverse the action of the stimulant medication.
   2. Offer fluids to reduce dehydration.
   3. Maintain an open airway.
   4. Explain all procedures to the client.
2. A client with a history of methamphetamine dependence is brought to the primary care clinic with suspected overdose. Which of the following assessments will the nurse be able to make?
   1. Pinpoint pupils, hypothermia, elevated blood pressure.
   2. Decreased respirations, low blood pressure, constricted pupils.
   3. Clammy skin, dilated pupils, slow pulse, and low blood pressure.
   4. Dilated pupils, agitation, visual hallucinations, and elevated blood pressure.
3. The nursing care plan of a client in moderate to severe stage of alcohol withdrawal is likely to include:
   1. providing environmental stimulation.
   2. expecting the client to participate in self-care activities.
   3. administering intravenous fluids and anti-anxiety medications.
   4. administering antipsychotic medications.
4. A 30-year-old client is brought to the emergency room by a police officer after his family calls 911 and reports that the client uses methamphetamine. His vital signs are blood pressure 170/100 mm Hg, pulse 92 beats/min, and respirations 32 breaths/min.

He is uncooperative with dilated pupils, mild diaphoresis, and paranoia. On the basis of his presentation, what is the most important nursing intervention?
1. Ensure personal safety.
2. Administer an IM antipsychotic agent.
3. Establish rapport by taking him by the hand.
4. Administer an IM benzodiazepine.

5. A 16-year-old client informs the nurse that she has been drinking alcohol and smoking cigarettes several times a week for the past year. The most appropriate response from the nurse would be:
1. "How many people know this?"
2. "Why do you drink and smoke?"
3. "May I ask you a couple of questions about this?"
4. "You need to stop this behavior immediately!"

6. A 32-year-old client informs the nurse that she experiences headaches and shakiness on the weekends, but not during the work week. The nurse knows that this can be a symptom of caffeine:
1. Tolerance
2. Withdrawal
3. Reverse Tolerance
4. Relapse

7. Parents of a 14-year-old teenager suspect that their son is using inhalants to "get high". The parents should observe their son for signs and symptoms of inhalant abuse that include: (Select all that apply.)
1. euphoria.
2. increased school performance.
3. dizziness.
4. amnesia.
5. increased interest in social activities.
6. headache.

8. The nurse is caring for a client that has been admitted to the hospital for morphine addiction. Which of the following symptoms will the client experience during morphine withdrawal?
1. Runny nose, nausea, yawning.
2. Constipation, diaphoresis, tremors.
3. Hypotension, irritability, lacrimation.
4. Nausea, vomiting, hypotension.

9. The health-care provider has prescribed methadone for a morphine addicted client as part of their treatment plan. Which of the following statements made by the client regarding methadone indicates that further teaching is needed by the nurse?
1. The daily dose is gradually reduced over a period of 1 to 2 weeks.
2. Routine and random urine testing is usually done to ensure no other drug use.
3. Methadone is given and the dose adjusted to keep withdrawal symptoms under control.
4. Counseling with the detoxification helps the client learn new methods of coping with stress.

10. A nurse suspects that one of her coworkers is stealing narcotics from the medication cart. Which of the following is the most appropriate action for the nurse to take?
1. Inform the supervisor immediately.
2. Confront the coworker.
3. Search the coworker's locker.
4. Ask the other coworkers if they have witnessed anything.

REFERENCES/SUGGESTED READING

Alcoholics Anonymous. (1939). *Alcoholics anonymous.* New York: Alcoholics Anonymous World Services.

American Cancer Society. (2007). *Lung cancer.* Retrieved April 5, 2009 from www.cancer.org/downloads/PRO/LungCancer.pdf

Antai-Otong, D. (2009). Manuscript submitted for publication. Arlington, Texas.

Bayard, M., McIntyre, J., Hill, K., & Woodside, J. (2004). Alcohol withdrawal syndrome. *American Family Physician, 69*(6), 1443–1450.

Bramness, J., Skurtveit, S., & Morland, J. (2006). Flunitrazepam: psychomotor impairment, agitation, and paradoxical reactions. *Forensic Science International, 159*(2), 83–91.

Bulechek, G., Butcher, H., McCloskey, J., & Dochterman, J., eds. (2008). *Nursing Interventions Classification (NIC)* (5th ed.). St. Louis, MO: Mosby/Elsevier.

Centers for Disease Control and Prevention (CDC). (2008a). Cigarette smoking among adults—United States, 2007. *Morbidity and Mortality Weekly Report, 57*(45), 1221–1226.

Centers for Disease Control and Prevention (CDC). (2008b). Cigarette use among high school students- United States, 1991-2007. *Morbidity and Mortality Weekly Report, 57*(25), 689–691.

Centers for Disease Control and Prevention (CDC). (2008c). Smoking attribute mortality, years of potential life lost, and productivity losses—United States, 2000–2004. *Morbidity and Mortality Weekly Report, 57*(45), 1226–1228.

Griffiths, R. Juliano, L. & Chausmer, A. (2003). Caffeine pharmacology and clinical effects. In: Graham, A., Schultz, T., Mayo-Smith, M., Ries, R., & Wilford, B. *Principles of addiction medicine* (3rd ed.), 193–224.

Hitchens, E. (2009). Manuscript submitted for publication. Seattle Pacific University, Seattle, Washington.

Johnson, V. (1989). *Intervention: How to help someone who doesn't want help.* New York: New American Library.

Johnson, V. (1990). *I'll quit tomorrow: A practical guide to alcoholism treatment.* San Francisco: Harper San Francisco.

Johnson, V. (2001). *I'll quit tomorrow: a practical guide to alcoholism treatment: revised edition.* New York: HarperCollins

Johnston, L., O'Malley, P., & Bachman, J. (1991). *Drug use among American high school seniors, college students and young adults 1975–1990.* Rockville, MD: National Institute on Drug Abuse, U.S. Department of Health and Human Services, Alcohol Drug Abuse, and Mental Health Administration.

Johnston, L., O'Malley, P., & Bachman, J. (1998). Drug use by American young people begins to turn downward. Retrieved from www.isr.umich.edu/src/mtf

Johnston, L., O'Malley, P., Bachman, J., & Schulenberg, J. (2008a). *Monitoring the future national survey results on drug use, 1975-2007: Volume I, secondary school students.* NIH Publication No. 08-6418A, pp. 707, Bethesda, MD: National Institute on Drug Abuse.

Johnston, L., O'Malley, P., Bachman, J., & Schulenberg, J. (2008b). *Monitoring the future national survey results on drug use, 1975-2007: Volume II, college students and adults ages 19-45.* NIH Publication No. 08-6418A, pp. 707, Bethesda, MD: National Institute on Drug Abuse.

Kasser, C., Geller, A., Howell, E., & Wartenberg, A. (2004). Detoxification: principles and protocols. American Society of Addiction Medicine. Retrieved April 5, 2009 from http://www.asam.org/publ/detoxification.htm

Mancuso, C., Tanzi, M., & Gabay, M. (2007). Paradoxical reactions to benzodiazepines: literature review and treatment options. *Pharmacotherapy, 24*(9), 1177–1185.

Moorhead, S., Johnson, M., Maas, M., & Swanson, E. (2007). *Nursing Outcomes Classification (NOC)* (3rd ed.). St. Louis, MO: Mosby.

National Institute on Alcohol Abuse and Alcoholism (NIAAA). (2006). Trends in alcohol-related fatal traffic crashes, United States, 1982–2004. Retrieved April 5, 2009 from http://pubs.niaaa.nih.gov/publications/surveillance76/fars04.htm

National Institute on Alcohol Abuse and Alcoholism (NIAAA). (2008a). Liver cirrhosis mortality in the United States, 1970–2005. Retrieved April 5, 2009 from http://pubs.niaaa.nih.gov/publications/surveillance83/Cirr05.htm

National Institute on Alcohol Abuse and Alcoholism (NIAAA). (2008b). Alcohol alert. Retrieved April 5, 2009 from http://pubs.niaaa.nih.gov/publications/AA76/AA76.htm

National Institute on Drug Abuse (NIDA). (2005a). Research report series—inhalant abuse. Retrieved April 5, 2009 from www.drugabuse.gov/ResearchReports/Inhalants/Inhalants.html

National Institute on Drug Abuse (NIDA). (2005b). Research report series—methamphetamine abuse and addiction. Retrieved April 5, 2009 from www.nida.nih.gov/ResearchReports/methamph/methamph2.html#scope

National Institute on Drug Abuse (NIDA). (2007). Monitoring the future study. Retrieved April 5, 2009 from www.monitoringthefuture.org/

National Institute on Drug Abuse (NIDA). (2008a). Frequently asked questions of NIDA's drug facts chat day. Retrieved April 5, 2009 from www.drugabuse.gov/chat/chatfaqs308.html

National Institute on Drug Abuse (NIDA). (2008b). NIDA infofacts: club drugs (GHB, ketamine, and rohypnol). Retrieved April 5, 2009 from www.nida.nih.gov/infofacts/clubdrugs.html

National Institute on Drug Abuse (NIDA). (2008c). NIDA infofacts: crack and cocaine. Retrieved April 5, 2009 from www.nida.nih.gov/infofacts/cocaine.html

National Institute on Drug Abuse (NIDA). (2008d). NIDA infofacts: heroin Retrieved April 5, 2009 from www.nida.nih.gov/infofacts/heroin.html

National Institute on Drug Abuse (NIDA). (2008e). NIDA infofacts: inhalants. Retrieved April 5, 2009 from www.drugabuse.gov/infofacts/inhalants.html

National Institute on Drug Abuse (NIDA). (2008f). NIDA infofacts: MDMA (ecstasy). Retrieved April 5, 2009 from www.drugabuse.gov/infofacts/ecstasy.html

National Institute on Drug Abuse (NIDA). (2008g). NIDA infofacts: nationwide trends. Retrieved April 5, 2009 from www.drugabuse.gov/infofacts/nationtrends.html

National Institute on Drug Abuse (NIDA). (2008h). NIDA infofacts: understanding drug abuse and addiction. Retrieved April 5, 2009 from www.drugabuse.gov/infofacts/understand.html

National Institute on Drug Abuse (NIDA). (2008i). Research report series—heroin abuse and addiction. Retrieved April 5, 2009 from www.nida.nih.gov/ResearchReports/Heroin/heroin2.html#what

National Institute on Drug Abuse (NIDA). (2008j). Research report series—methamphetamine abuse and addiction. Retrieved April 5, 2009 from www.nida.nih.gov/ResearchReports/methamph/methamph3.html#long

National Institute on Drug Abuse (NIDA). (2009a). Heroin. Retrieved April 5, 2009 from www.nida.nih.gov/DrugPages/Heroin.html

National Institute on Drug Abuse (NIDA). (2009b). Important information and resources on club drugs. Retrieved July 2, 2009 from http://www.clubdrugs.gov/

National Institute on Drug Abuse (NIDA). (2009c). Inhalants. Retrieved April 6, 2009 from www.drugabuse.gov/DrugPages/Inhalants.html

National Institute on Drug Abuse (NIDA). (2009d). Marijuana. Retrieved April 5, 2009 from www.nida.nih.gov/DrugPages/Marijuana.html

National Institute on Drug Abuse (NIDA). (2009e). Marijuana: facts for teens. Retrieved April 5, 2009 from www.nida.nih.gov/MarijBroch/teenpg9-10.html

National Institute on Drug Abuse (NIDA). (2009f). Steroids (anabolic). Retrieved April 5, 2009 from www.drugabuse.gov/DrugPages/Steroids.html

North American Nursing Diagnosis Association International. (2010). *NANDA-I nursing diagnoses: Definitions and classification 2009-2011.* Ames, IA: Wiley-Blackwell.

Santomier, J., & Hogan, P. (1992). Health implications of alcohol and other drug use. In M. Naegle (Ed.), *Substance abuse education in nursing* (Vol. 1). New York: National League for Nursing.

Spratto, G., & Woods, A. (2009). *2009 PDR Nurses' drug handbook.* Clifton Park, NY: Delmar Cengage Learning.

Substance Abuse and Mental Health Services Administration (SAMHSA). (2008). Results from the 2007 national survey on drug use and health: national findings. Retrieved April 6, 2009 from oas.samhsa.gov/NSDUH/2k7NSDUH/2k7results.cfm#Ch5

Waughfield, C. (2002). *Mental health concepts* (5th ed.). Clifton Park, NY: Delmar Cengage Learning.

World Health Organization (WHO). (2008). WHO report on the global tobacco epidemic, 2008. Retrieved April 5, 2009 from www.cdc.gov/tobacco/data_statistics/fact_sheets/fast_facts/index.htm

RESOURCES

Al-Anon Family Group, http://www.al-anon.org

Alcoholics Anonymous (AA), http://www.aa.org

American Council for Drug Education, http://www.acde.org

Codependents Anonymous (CODA), http://www.codependents.org

Drug Abuse Resistance Education (DARE), Local Police Department, http://www.dare-america.com

Drug Enforcement Administration (DEA), http://www.usdoj.gov/dea

Families Anonymous, (Families of Substance Abusers), http://www.familiesanonymous.org

Mothers Against Drunk Driving (MADD), http://www.madd.org

Narcotics Anonymous (NA), http://www.na.org

National Clearinghouse for Alcohol and Drug Information, http://www.health.org

National Council on Alcoholism and Drug Dependence, http://www.ncadd.org

Students Against Destructive Decisions (Founded as Students Against Driving Drunk), http://www.saddonline.com

UNIT 16 Nursing Care of the Client: Older Adult

CHAPTER 50
The Older Adult

MAKING THE CONNECTION

Refer to the following chapters to increase your understanding of the older adult:

Basic Nursing
- ***Communication***
- ***Life Span Development***
- ***Fluid, Electrolyte, and Acid–Base Balance***

Adult Health Nursing
- ***Surgery***
- ***Respiratory System***
- ***Cardiovascular System***
- ***Gastrointestinal System***
- ***Urinary System***
- ***Musculoskeletal System***
- ***Neurological System***
- ***Sensory System***
- ***Endocrine System***
- ***Reproductive Systems***
- ***Integumentary System***
- ***Mental Illness***
- ***Substance Abuse***

LEARNING OBJECTIVES

Upon completion of this chapter, you should be able to:

- Define key terms.
- Describe stereotypes associated with older adults.
- Discuss the biological and psychosocial theories of aging.
- Cite the normal physiologic changes that occur with aging.
- List the normal functional changes that occur with aging.
- Describe key factors of optimal health maintenance in the aging adult.
- Identify funding and policy changes that have influenced older-adult care.
- Identify common disorders related to aging.
- Detail nursing interventions for each disorder.
- Discuss areas wherein the nurse can advocate for older adults on the individual, community, state, and national levels.

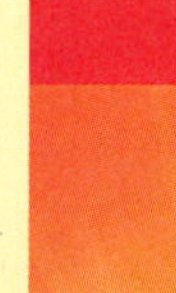

KEY TERMS

activities of daily living
ageism
delirium
dementia
gerontological nursing
gerontologist
gerontology
polypharmacy

INTRODUCTION

Gerontology is the study of the effects of normal aging and age-related diseases on human beings. It is a general term used by all health care and social services disciplines. Aging (senescence) is a complex phenomenon that occurs on a continuum, beginning with birth and continuing throughout the life span.

The phrase *older adult* is very subjective and has historically meant persons who are 65 years of age and older. However, there is a great deal of debate among **gerontologists** (gerontological specialists in advanced-practice nursing, geriatric psychiatry, medicine, and social services) as to whether this specific age delineation should continue to be used. The practice of using 65 years of age as a dividing line for social welfare benefits began in the 1880s when Otto von Bismark randomly selected that age for benefits in Germany. It should be noted that there was no standardized clinical basis for establishing this age as the dividing line between young and old. Longer average life-expectancy rates (84 years for both sexes, 82.4 years for men, and 85.3 years for women) (AoA, 2009b) along with a decrease in the average number of children per family since the late 1960s have changed U.S. demographics. As a result, there is a great need to support and strengthen independence among older adults, and to value and use their life experiences in the areas of career, family, and community.

Retirement age is now less consistently determined by a mandatory age limit. Rather, retirement frequently is offered when the employee meets a formula of combined age and years of service. Since the 1990s, benefit penalties have been imposed on Social Security beneficiaries up to 70 years of age and who continue to earn incomes over a minimum amount. This was changed in April 2000 when the Senior Citizens' Freedom to Work Act of 2000 was signed into law by the president. This eliminates the Social Security retirement earnings test in and after the month in which a person is 65 years of age (the current full retirement age) (Social Security Administration [SSA], 2000).

Currently, the clinical delineation of an older adult is still someone who is 65 years of age or older; older-old adults are defined as those individuals 85 years of age or older. In 1900, there were a total of 3.1 million individuals older than age 65 in the United States; by 1996, there were 33.2 million, 3.8 million of whom were older than age 85 years (AARP, 1998). In 2001, there were 4.2 million people aged 85 and older in the United States (NCOA, 2002). It is projected that by the year 2030, the number of older individuals in the United States will reach 72.1 million (Figure 50-1)(AoA, 2009a). The most rapid increase is expected to occur in the years 2010–2030, when the "baby boomers" reach age 65.

The future will also place demands on those who were born from the late 1950s to the late 1960s. Many in this age group chose to focus first on career, delaying marriage and childrearing until in their thirties. They have thus been labeled "the sandwich generation" to denote the challenges they will face in meeting social and financial responsibilities later in life as they work to provide for children entering college and for aging parents and, sometimes, grandparents and, in a few instances, great-grandparents.

This chapter presents an overview of influences on the older adult, including the social impacts of aging. Also examined are theories of aging; myths and realities of aging; health promotion and aging; physiologic and functional changes that normally occur with aging; and some common disorders of aging along with nursing interventions to assist clients to achieve optimal outcomes related to those disorders.

As caregivers for older adults, nurses and other members of the health care team must understand the budgetary and policy decisions that can affect the care they will provide to their clients. Thus, this chapter concludes with a short discussion on health care financing for older adult care in the 21st century.

GERONTOLOGICAL NURSING

The acceptance of **gerontological nursing** as a separate nursing specialty that addresses and advocates for the special care needs of older adults has not been realized without a struggle. In 1961, gerontological nursing attained national recognition with the creation of its own division of nursing within the American Nurses Association (ANA). Nurses in the United States who were aware of the trends toward an aging population realized the importance of taking such a step. The charter members of the Division of Gerontological Nursing deserve a great deal of credit for their vision and commitment to developing gerontology education and recognizing the special nursing care needs of older adults. The major topics addressed in the expanding scope of practice for gerontological nursing included:

- The historical evolution of gerontological nursing practice based on population statistics
- The way that ageism in U.S. society has affected the profession of nursing, the health care delivery system, and the care of older adults
- Nursing education and care of older adults with a perspective derived from studies of the attitudes and interests of nursing personnel and nursing students
- The delineation of various aspects of nursing care of older adults, including clinical practice based on the ANA Standards of Nursing Practice; select theories of nursing applied to the care of older adults; and the expanding scope of gerontological nursing, in general, and the roles of clinical nurse specialists and geriatric nurse practitioners, in particular
- Trends in gerontological nursing and long-term care

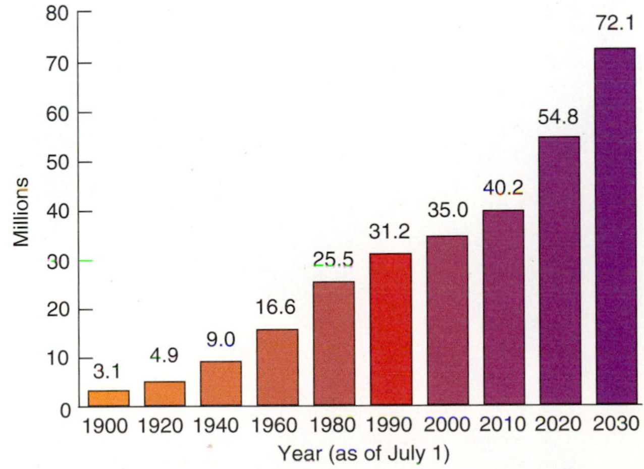

FIGURE 50-1 Number of Persons Older Than Age 65: 1900–2030 (*Data from Administration on Aging [AOA], 2009a.*)

The battle continues against stereotyping older adults, both in the health professions and in the community at large. Health professionals, in particular, must be diligent in avoiding age prejudice. Stereotypes can influence interactions between older adults and caregivers. The caregiver may treat the older adult as a child in an old body. This approach is demeaning to older adults and strips them of their self-esteem and dignity. Clients with cognitive or expressive deficits cannot always process questions or comments quickly or follow through with responses. Nurses and caregivers must never make the mistake of believing that clients do not understand verbal and, especially, nonverbal messages. Older adults are a diverse group; they deserve respect and, through their memories and life examples, can teach a great deal to younger persons about life and survival and coping skills. Learning from clients and their families and assisting clients to find activities that enhance the quality of life (regardless of state of health) make caring for older adults a rewarding and satisfying experience.

Aging is universal, progressive, and irreversible, and eventually leads to death. The aging process itself, however, is very individualized and is independent of chronological age. The way an individual ages is influenced by genetics, lifestyle, availability and quality of health services, cultural beliefs, and socioeconomic status. Certain physiologic changes are expected with aging (Figure 50-2), although there exists considerable variation in the time of onset, rate, and degree of these changes. In order to render effective and compassionate care to older clients, nurses working in gerontology must be familiar with the normal processes as well as the common disorders of aging.

THEORIES OF AGING

At this time, no single theory of aging has been universally accepted by practitioners in gerontology. Aging is a complex issue that takes into account the psychosocial, cultural, and experiential aspects of living. Several biological theories of aging have been proposed to explain the physiologic and functional changes that are observed in older adults. Psychosocial theories of aging strive to explain the behaviors and social interactions of older adults. These theories are summarized in Table 50-1. Also, as more knowledge is garnered from scientific studies (e.g., the study of the impact on cells of auto-oxidization by free radicals and the study of dietary chemical exposure) and gene sequencing efforts (e.g., the human genome project), it is likely that the biological theories of aging will change as well.

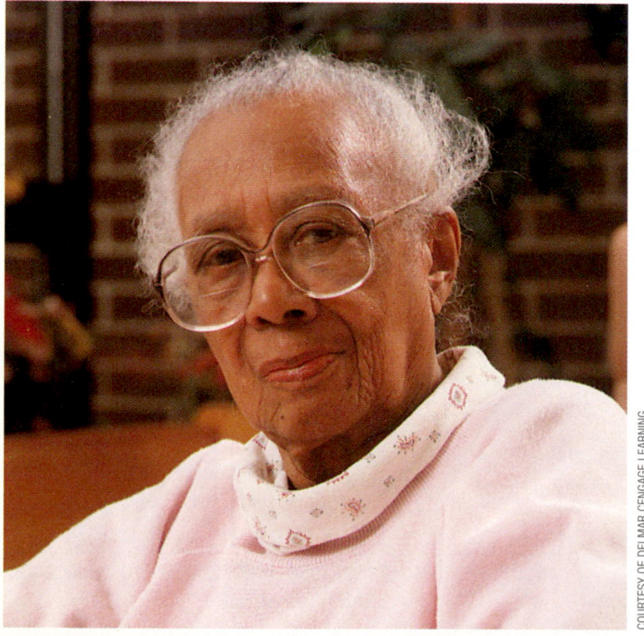

COURTESY OF DELMAR CENGAGE LEARNING

FIGURE 50-2 The aging process is a normal and natural part of growth and development.

MYTHS AND REALITIES OF AGING

Myths are fictitious ideas. Myths about the older adult are abundant and do not reflect the reality of the aging population. **Ageism** is the stereotyping of older adults based upon myths. Some common ageism myths based in part on data from the National Institute on Aging (2009), the U.S. Census Bureau, and *A Profile of Older Americans* developed by the American Association of Retired Persons (AARP) in 1998 are:

Myth: Senility is an expected result of aging.

Reality: Senility is an outdated term once used to refer to any form of dementia that occurred in older people. Dementia is a result of disease, can affect adults of all ages, and is not a natural consequence of aging. Although some slight declines are noted in short-term memory from the age of 40 on, most people adjust through the use of memory aids such as lists and calendars. Although long-term memory can remain somewhat intact long into a dementia disease process, there is slower retrieval of information. Thus, nurses and caregivers find that interventions such as reminiscence, memory photo books, and activities that draw on the client's long-practiced skills provide positive client outcomes.

Myth: Incontinence is an expected result of aging.

Reality: Incontinence is not an expected outcome of aging and, in most cases, can be reversed through assessment and treatment. Incontinence may be caused by infection, disease, injury, and certain types of medication. The challenge is that many people are embarrassed to discuss this problem with family or primary providers. Also, in long-term care settings, both the belief in this myth and the historically low staffing levels have served to dissuade clinical efforts at providing the needed nursing interventions (prompted voiding; consistent, nonhurried,

CULTURAL CONSIDERATIONS

Aging

It is important to assess the older client's spiritual/religious beliefs, traditions, and culture because they can influence the client's health beliefs and health practices. When assessing a client of a different culture, show respect by using the client's full name.

TABLE 50-1 Theories of Aging

Biological Theories	
Title	**Major Premise**
Somatic mutation theory	Radiation or miscoding of enzymes causes changes in the DNA. Changes associated with aging are the result of decreased function and efficiency of the cells and organs.
Programmed aging theory	The life span is programmed within the cells. This genetic clock determines the speed at which the person ages and eventually dies.
Cross-linkage, or collagen theory	Collagen is the principal component of connective tissue and is also found in the skin, bones, muscles, lungs, and heart. Chemical reactions between collagen and cross-linking molecules cause loss of flexibility, resulting in diminished functional mobility.
Immunity theory	The thymus becomes smaller with age. The ability to produce T-cell differentiation decreases. This impairs immunologic functions and results in increased incidence of infections, neoplasms, and autoimmune disorders.
Stress theory	Stress throughout the lifetime causes structural and chemical changes in the body. These changes eventually cause irreversible tissue damage.
Psychosocial Theories	
Title	**Major Premise**
Activity theory	Roles and responsibilities change throughout the lifetime. Life satisfaction depends on maintaining an involvement with life by developing new interests, hobbies, roles, and relationships.
Disengagement theory	There is decreased interaction between the older person and others in his social system. The disengagement is inevitable, mutual, and acceptable to both the individual and society.
Continuity theory	Successful methods used throughout life for adjusting and adapting to life events are repeated. Characteristic traits, habits, values, associations, and goals remain stable throughout the lifetime, regardless of life changes.

COURTESY OF DELMAR CENGAGE LEARNING

timed voiding) to reverse urinary incontinence. In settings where care is provided to older adults, lack of funding, lack of policy support and education, and inconsistent enforcement of adequate staffing levels have often had a negative impact on client health outcomes. By developing urinary incontinence treatment programs, care facilities could improve clinical outcomes for clients and also reduce health-care costs.

Myth: Older adults are no longer interested in sexuality or sexual activity.

Reality: Sexuality is a lifelong need. Older adults can be and are sexually active, regardless of age. Although a slowing response time is a normal part of aging, many older adults want and lead a satisfying sex life, and persons of both genders are capable of orgasm into old age. Despite interest and desire, physiologic or psychological problems and medication side effects may present barriers to intercourse. In such situations, sexuality without coitus can provide older adults with love and intimacy. Just as small babies can fail to thrive without human touch (hugs, nurturing, companionship, valuing of the individual), so can older adults fail to thrive without these same human interactions and support (Figure 50-3).

A national survey by NCOA in 1998 revealed that half of those age 60 and older were sexually active. Approximately 72% of those were as satisfied or more satisfied with their sex lives compared to when they were in their forties (NCOA, 2001).

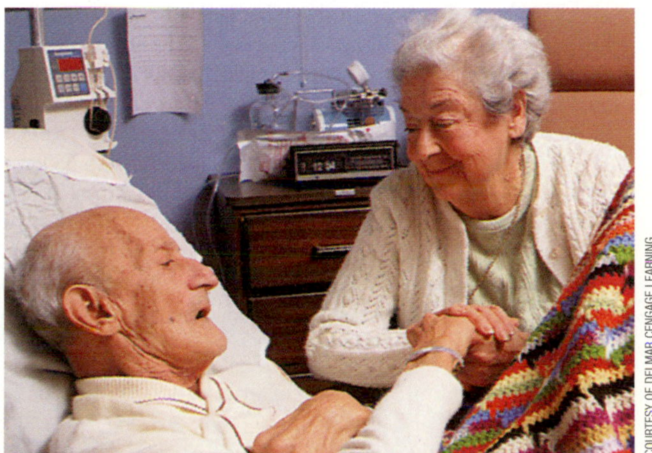

COURTESY OF DELMAR CENGAGE LEARNING

FIGURE 50-3 Individuals of all ages benefit from intimacy and companionship.

The medication sildenafil citrate (Viagra) has proven beneficial to many older couples as they work to meet their sexual health needs. The debate over the acceptance and funding of this medication for erectile dysfunction sheds light on just how far U.S. society still has to go in debunking this myth and replacing it with the truth that normal human sexuality needs continue throughout the life span.

Myth: Most people spend the last years of their lives in nursing homes.

Reality: According to NCOA (2002), in 2000, only 4.5% of those older than age 65 lived in nursing homes. The percentage rises steeply with age, however (1.1% of those 65 to 74 years of age, 4.7% of those 75 to 84 years of age, and 18% of those older than 85 years of age). For many, that stay will involve rehabilitation after surgery, a fracture, or stroke before returning home after a short hospital stay. The late 1990s saw a growing interest in the use of alternative care options for older adults (retirement communities, assisted-living centers, group homes, respite care, and partial hospitalization/adult day programs); however, most older adults continue to live in communities with varying levels of assistive services or support as they age. The projected trends in long-term care needs are for continued use of alternate settings that will support interventions to meet residents' physical, psychosocial, cultural, spiritual, cognitive, and mental health needs.

Traditionally, older adults in long-term care facilities have been taken from home environments where they have likely experienced the highest level of independence they have had in their lifetimes (to choose when to get up, eat, go to bed, and the like), and have been placed in settings where very few, if any, choices, including care decisions, are made based on their preferences. Gerontological nurses have an ongoing responsibility to help re-create the way care is provided and to advocate for older clients in long-term care facilities. Nurse leaders must learn to think in new ways about how to work with older clients and their families.

Myth: All older adults are financially impoverished.

Reality: Income range varies among those older than 65 years of age, just as it does among those in younger groups; however, the high costs of medications does disproportionately affect those older than age 65, who are more likely to have one or more chronic conditions that require management with medication. In the past, lack of reimbursement for preventive assessment, treatments, and medications led many older adults to go without medications or to delay care until they were too ill to wait any longer. This resulted in increased use of acute care services in hospitals.

In 2001, families headed by persons older than 65 years of age had a median income of $33,938 (AoA, 2002). The challenge for most older adults below the median (especially older women, who often have lower retirement incomes) is that most of their assets are tied up in the family home or in other nonliquid holdings. Thus, when an acute illness strikes, there is little financial reserve to help cover costs.

CRITICAL THINKING

Myths/Stereotypes

A health team member makes an ageist remark to one of your older adult friends. How would you respond using a therapeutic communication technique?

HEALTH AND AGING

Like all age groups, older adults can do much to adopt a healthy lifestyle that will enhance their remaining years.

ACTIVITIES OF DAILY LIVING

Being well groomed enhances the self-esteem of all older adults. Adaptive devices and techniques are available for those who need assistance with the **activities of daily living** (ADLs), basic care activities that include mobility, bathing, hygiene, grooming, dressing, eating, and toileting.

Mobility

Many assistive devices are available to help the older client maintain mobility and independence. Handrails can decrease the risk of falls while the person is walking; they are also useful in the tub and, when used in conjunction with a plastic riser, can help the older adult get on and off the toilet safely.

Bathing

Skin dryness increases with aging; thus, it may be preferable for older adults to bathe or shower only two to three times per week and to take sponge baths in between. A gentle soap should be used sparingly for the bath, after which a moisturizing lotion should be applied. The individual or caregiver should be instructed to inspect the skin during bathing for any indication of skin breakdown, lumps, or changes in moles.

With aging, oil secretion decreases in the scalp, and hair can thus become dry. Shampooing one or two times per week is usually adequate for most older adults, and a simplified hairstyle may be helpful to those with limited mobility in the arms. The use of mild shampoos and conditioners can also enhance hair texture.

PROFESSIONALTIP

Activities of Daily Living

Additional safety measures to consider during ADL include:

- Filing nails instead of cutting because brittle nails may split
- Avoiding perfumed bathing products due to their potential irritating effects
- Showering (preferred) instead of taking a tub bath because it is easier to step into a shower stall than into a tub, the easier availability of shower chairs and hand bars that make it more accessable and safer than stepping into a tub, and clean water is constantly circulating over the client during the shower procedure

Hygiene

Fingernails may become more brittle with aging. Keeping the client's fingernails clean and short can prevent accidental injury or scratches to fragile older skin. Impaired circulation is common among older adults, so special attention should be given to care of the feet and lower extremities. Because toenails frequently become thick and tougher with aging, soaking the feet before trimming the toenails may ease the task. For clients with circulation or skin integrity problems of the feet and toes or for clients with diabetes, a referral to a podiatrist should be made for nail trimming. During bathing, monitor the client's feet for discomfort; inflammation; broken skin; color changes such as redness, pallor, or cyanosis (blue or purple discoloration resulting from lack of circulation); heat or coldness; cracking between toes; and corns or calluses.

The need for adequate oral care does not diminish with aging. Dental problems can result in poor eating habits and inadequate nutrition. Inadequate brushing and dental checkups can lead to gingivitis (bleeding and edematous gums), which, if left untreated, can progress to periodontal disease that can destroy connective tissue, alveolar bone, and periodontal ligaments. Monitor clients for proper oral care. Yoneyama et al. (2002) reports that nursing home residents who received oral hygiene after each meal and professional cleaning once a week were two times less likely to get pneumonia and two times less likely to die from it. For those clients with dentures, inspect the dentures for cleanliness and proper fit. Clients with dentures must brush the dentures and the gums regularly with a soft brush and a mild cleanser. It is helpful to label dentures with the client's name to facilitate identification of the dentures in the event that the client is admitted to a hospital or an assistive care setting.

Grooming

Good grooming is important in promoting the older client's self-esteem and confidence. Keeping the hair neat and tidy, choosing attractive clothing and jewelry, and making decisions about makeup and other personal care practices will all contribute to the older client's sense of well-being and independence (Figure 50-4).

Male clients may feel much better with a clean-shaven face. Infection-control principles demand that each razor (either electric or blade) be used for only one individual and

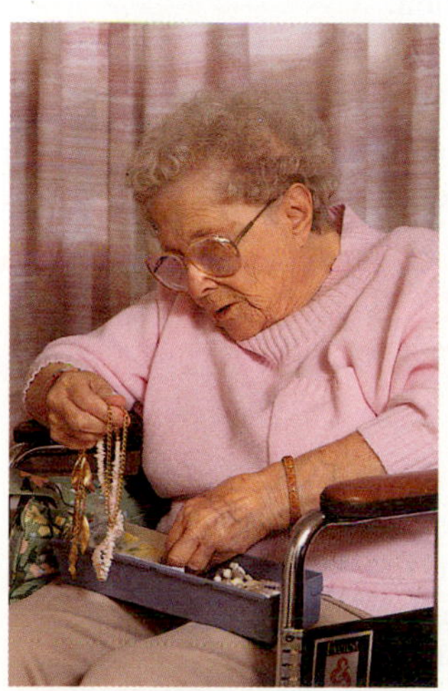

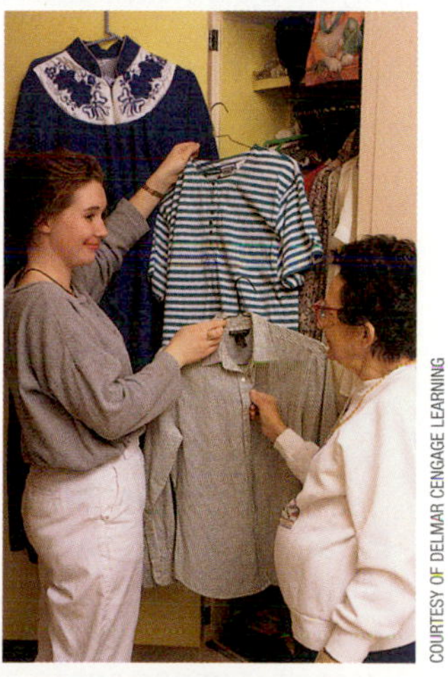

COURTESY OF DELMAR CENGAGE LEARNING

FIGURE 50-4 Good grooming for the older adult includes choosing personal items such as jewelry and clothing.

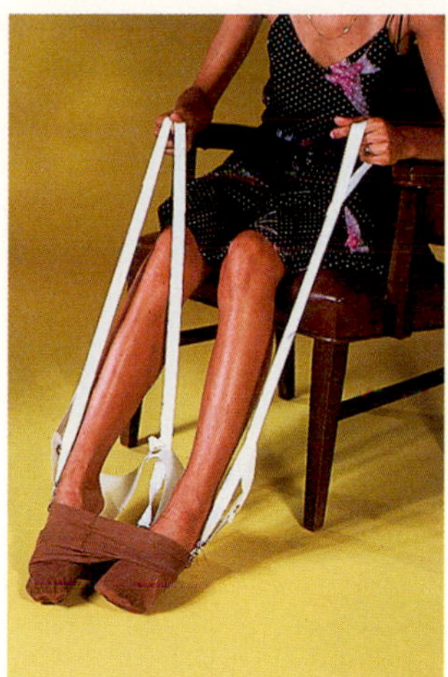

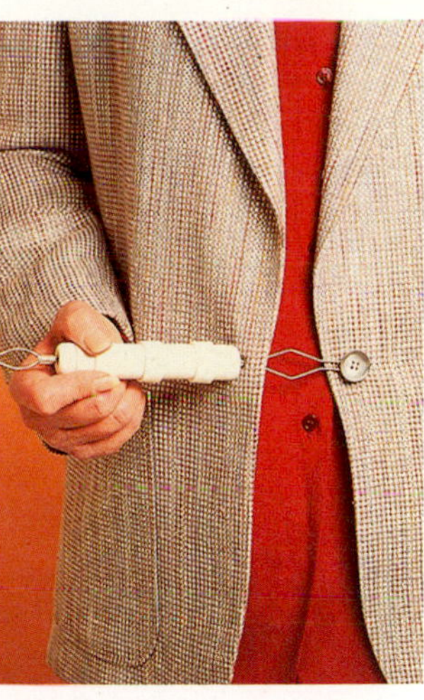

FIGURE 50-5 Assistive devices such as these for pantyhose and getting dressed are available to help older adults dress independently. (*Courtesy of Maddak, Inc.*)

that that razor be marked with the client's name. Women may also require attention to facial hair, as estrogen levels decrease after menopause. It is not uncommon for older women to notice hairs on the chin or upper lip that were not there in younger days. Also, both men and women are likely to notice graying and diminished hair on legs, underarms, and pubic areas as they age.

Dressing

Dressing may be difficult for clients who have restricted joint movement, paralysis, or limited endurance because of health problems. Many choices are available to ease dressing, such as elastic waists, Velcro fasteners, and assistive reaching and dressing devices (Figure 50-5).

Eating

Many older adults are able to maintain the ability to self-feed, thereby promoting independence and self-esteem. Neurological and musculoskeletal alterations may, however, affect the ability to self-feed. Dysphagia, or difficulty swallowing, may place the older client at increased risk of choking. A mouth check is advisable until it is known that the client is safely swallowing. Diminished taste sensation affects the desire to eat. Adding seasonings and herbs to food may improve the taste. Encourage client to eat dessert after consuming nutrient dense foods.

Toileting

Toileting habits also change with aging. Bowel elimination problems can often be prevented as clients age by:

- Ensuring adequate fiber intake (whole grains, fresh fruit)
- Ensuring adequate fluid intake (minimum 1500 mL/day)
- Ensuring regular daily exercise (prescribed by physician)
- Developing regular elimination habits

For the client in the hospital or a long-term care facility, it is helpful to:

- Maintain previously effective habits such as drinking warm liquids upon arising
- Assist the client to the toilet approximately 30 minutes after eating, to take advantage of the gastrocolic reflex

> **PROFESSIONALTIP**
>
> **Bowel Patterns in Older Adults**
>
> It is extremely important that caregivers of older adults monitor bowel patterns. Long periods of constipation (>2 to 3 days) should alert caregivers to the need for interventions to minimize the likelihood of bowel impaction, which can ultimately be life threatening if left untreated. Evacuation aids such as laxatives, lubricants, stool softeners, and enemas all have side effects and should thus be avoided if at all possible. Dietary changes or an exercise regimen should be introduced first.

As a result of the physical changes that occur with aging, increased frequency of urination may be noted in older adults of both genders. It is not uncommon for older adults to self-limit fluid intake because of a fear of incontinence. This habit is unhealthy and should be discouraged. Assess cases of incontinence to determine the cause and type, so that appropriate interventions and treatment can be implemented. Timing the use of prescribed diuretics in the morning rather than the evening can prevent the increased need for urination at night, which is especially helpful to older clients who are being treated for congestive heart failure (CHF).

Exercise

What was once accepted as the normal deterioration of old age is now considered the result of disuse through sitting and bed rest. Research indicates that high-intensity, progressive resistance training can improve muscle strength and muscle size in frail older adult clients. Walking and all other maneuvers required for ADLs are also beneficial. Individually plan exercise programs taking into consideration the older person's:

- General health status (Figure 50-6)
- Physiologic disorders (if present)
- Preference for solidarity or group activity
- Physical environment
- Financial status

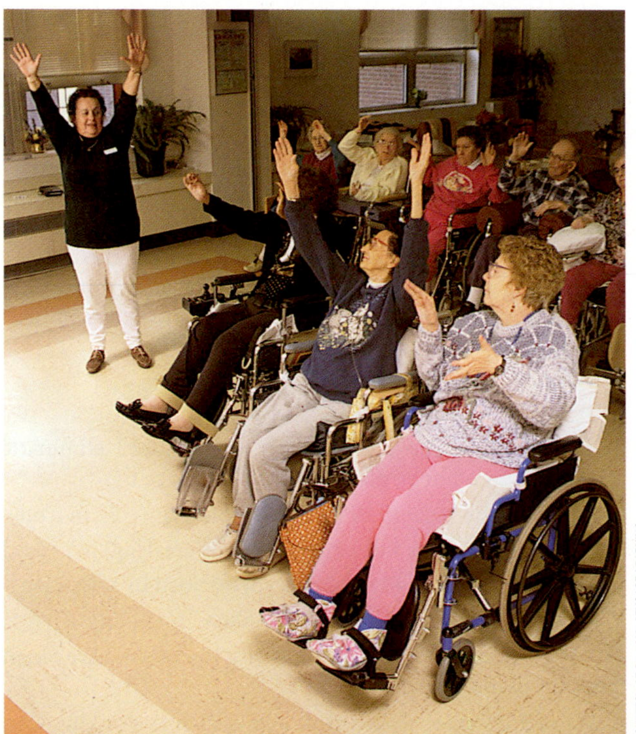

COURTESY OF DELMAR CENGAGE LEARNING

Figure 50-6 Exercise is important to all clients and should be tailored to interests and ability levels.

Nutrition

For many older adults, cultural heritage, religious rites, ethnic practices, and family traditions are linked to food. The physiologic, psychological, sociological, and economic changes of aging may compromise nutritional status. Older adults must follow a balanced diet, often with lowered intakes of sugar, caffeine, and sodium. There are no universally accepted dietary guidelines specific to older adults. A dietitian can determine the needed food intake for a specific individual by taking into account the individual's height, ideal weight, activity level, and disease processes.

Older adults need 1,000 mg to 1,500 mg of calcium per day for both men and women. Calcium supplements should also contain vitamin D to provide for optimal metabolism by the body. Calcium supplements should not be taken at the same time as enteric coated medications because drugs containing calcium dissolve enteric coatings, thus leading to gastric irritation (Shepler, Grogan, & Pater, 2006). The need for additional supplements depends on the older individual's nutritional status and ability to maintain an adequate diet. Growing discussion supports the needs for adequate protein intake, to maintain both skin integrity and bone density, and moderate carbohydrate intake because carbohydrates metabolize to sugars.

It is important to know about community services designed to help older clients meet their nutritional needs. Such services include grocery transportation and delivery services, homebound meals (e.g., Meals On Wheels), group meals at senior food sites, and the Food Stamp program. Nurses and caregivers should also realize that socialization and companionship are necessary components of adequate dietary intake, and should ensure that these areas are addressed as part of any food-assistance intervention.

Psychosocial Considerations

Older adults, like all individuals, have psychosocial and cognitive needs for lifelong learning. Many colleges have

> **PROFESSIONALTIP**
>
> **Iron**
>
> When iron is prescribed for an older adult, encourage taking with foods and fluids containing vitamin C to assist with iron absorption. A common side effect when taking iron is constipation. Clients may stop taking iron because of this problem. Therefore, it is important to ask clients about the constipating factor when reviewing their medications.

developed education program options for older adult students (often at no tuition), and employers are beginning to recruit older workers for part-time positions (recognizing their historically good work ethic and experience). Many older adults continue to volunteer countless hours each year, offering to help meet the social service needs of their communities. These efforts can result in feelings of productivity and self-worth for the older adult. Mental activity and emotional involvement are as necessary to the overall well-being as is physical activity. Older clients can benefit from building on their long-practiced skills to develop interesting and stimulating activities or hobbies. Such activities may be of an individual or group nature. Socialization with people of all age groups can help not only the older participants, but also the young and middle-aged participants, by illustrating that aging is not a disease but rather, a rich and natural part of the life process.

Strengths

Older adults generally have experienced many losses over the years. Some losses are slight and require only minor adaptation, whereas others may significantly affect the person. Physiologic changes or disease processes may result in losses, causing impairments in:

- Communication
- Vision and learning
- Mobility
- Cognition
- Psychosocial skills

If the impairment is severe, the individual could lose some degree of independence, and adaptations may be required. Furthermore, losses can cascade for the older client, as one loss contributes to another. For example, if an older adult with diabetes were to lose her driver's license because of impaired vision related to diabetic retinopathy, socialization might be restricted, which in turn might increase her feelings of loneliness and diminished self-esteem. If, however, her spouse provides caregiving and transportation, these adaptations might allow her to remain active socially while still living in her home. If her spouse later dies, and her health continues to decline, a move to an assisted-living facility may become necessary, if other community adaptations are unavailable. She would then be faced with adapting to the loss of both her home and her spouse.

Health-care professionals should remember that persons who have lived for many years are survivors and can adapt to life changes better if they are allowed to use their existing strengths. They are often much stronger and more ingenious and enterprising than they are given credit for. Identify the strengths of each individual (including past coping skills) and use them when planning care and assisting the older client to find new ways to adapt and maintain optimal independence in a new setting.

Health Promotion and Disease Prevention

Older adults must be alerted to ways of preventing disease and reducing risks. Being knowledgeable about self-care and participating in screening tests are important for health maintenance. For older men, an annual prostate examination and a prostate specific antigen (PSA) level lab test, which can detect prostate cancer in the early stages, are recommended every 1 to 2 years. For older women, the annual mammogram may be delayed by the physician depending on the client's risk factors. If a client's Pap smears have been negative (normal) for 5 consecutive years, they can be done less often. Men and women older than age 50 should have a yearly stool test for occult blood performed. A colonoscopy may be recommended to monitor for colon cancer. Teach clients habits for healthy living and inform them of signs and symptoms that require medical investigation. Older clients who have been exposed to environmental chemicals, tobacco, or extensive alcohol use over many years often experience serious health consequences as they reach older age. Older clients of any age can benefit from healthy lifestyles and from disease-prevention interventions, such as being inoculated yearly against influenza and every 5 years against pneumonia, assessment of tuberculosis (TB) status, and adequate safe food and clean water intake.

In many cases, by the time a person reaches 65 to 70 years of age, that person has been prescribed medication to address at least one ongoing (chronic) medical problem (e.g., hypertension, heart disease, diabetes, allergies, gastrointestinal disorders). The challenge many older adults face is that side effects from one medication are often treated with another prescription medication. If the client then goes to different doctors, these doctors may prescribe even more medications to address the same or other health concerns. This is called **polypharmacy**, or the problem of clients taking numerous prescription and over-the-counter medications for the same or various disease processes, with unknown consequences from the resulting combinations of chemical compounds and cumulative side effects. In many settings, primary care providers, nurses, clinical pharmacists, and social workers collaborate to assist the older client and the family to oversee the client's medication management and other health needs.

Among the biggest challenges facing older clients are shorter hospitalization stays and reduced time with physicians in the physician's offices. There is less time to ensure that the follow-up services the client will need are understood and in place and less time to educate client and family about medication regimens, including timing and possible interactions with other prescription and over-the-counter drugs or herbal remedies that the client may also be taking. The nurse, as part of the interdisciplinary team, plays a vital role as client advocate when ensuring that older clients have the teaching, services, and follow-up care they need. Figure 50-7 is a concept map that discusses safe nursing considerations when administering a medication to an older adult.

PHYSIOLOGIC CHANGES ASSOCIATED WITH AGING

Although the aging process brings with it many physiologic changes, it should be remembered that aging and disease are not synonymous. Whereas the physiologic changes of aging

CRITICAL THINKING

Polypharmacy

You are caring for a client who is suffering from the effects of polypharmacy. What interventions will you discuss with this client to prevent future polypharmacy problems?

PROFESSIONALTIP

Identifying Strengths of Older Adults as Part of Assessment

Assessment should include the identification of strengths as well as problems. Strengths are utilized to achieve or maintain optimal physical, mental, and emotional function. All of the following can be considered strengths:

- Cognitive health
- Freedom from or successful adaptation to deficits or impairments
- A history of healthy lifestyle with regard to diet, sleep, stress management, exercise, and chemical abuse (none)
- Adequate functional ability to carry out ADL
- Freedom from incapacitating physical discomfort and pain
- A physically safe living environment
- Feelings of security in present environment
- Realistic knowledge about capabilities
- Pattern of avoiding dangerous situations and unnecessary risks
- Compliance with health care regimen
- Capability with regard to managing own environment
- An intact support system
- Satisfying relationships with others
- Opportunities for sexual expression
- Access to transportation
- Adequate functional mobility
- Successful adaptation to life changes and crises
- History of relinquishing roles as phases of life require and replacing them with satisfying new roles
- A pattern of successful mourning for losses
- Participation in groups: religious, spiritual, community, hobbies
- Membership in family whose members respect each other and are willing to give and receive help when necessary
- Successful problem-solving skills
- Willingness to seek information to improve situation
- Evidence of initiative and self-confidence in abilities and judgment
- Participation in self-care by making decisions and accepting responsibility for decisions
- Acceptance of that which cannot be changed
- Successful use of assertive skills
- Ability to find comfort and strength in spiritual and religious practices
- Appreciation for aging, with demonstrative embrace of the positive aspects and adaptation to the negative aspects
- Participation in healthy reminiscing; evidence of few regrets about life past
- Appreciation for nature, art, music, hobbies, and activities
- A sense of humor

described in the following sections are normal for most people, the medical disorders described are not considered normal. Older adults age at different rates. The following aging changes for each system may not occur until late in the aging process.

Respiratory System

The following respiratory changes result from the aging process:

- Calcification of the rib cage and less flexible respiratory muscles may lead to a barrel chest and decreased vital capacity of the lungs.
- Decrease in functional capacity results in dyspnea on exertion or stress; usual activity does not affect breathing.
- Decreased ciliary action and a less effective cough mechanism increase the risk for lung infection.
- The alveoli thicken and decrease in number and size, causing less effective gas exchange (decreased oxygen saturation) and, in individuals who also have chronic lung disease, intensifying respiratory deficits.
- Structural changes in the skeleton, such as kyphosis (seen in clients with osteoporosis as an often asymmetrical convex curve of the spine) can decrease diaphragmatic expansion. Kyphosis in older clients can lead to a need for small, more frequent meals to balance nutritional requirements and respiratory function because of the restriction of adequate space for expansion and contraction of the diaphragm. It can also create skin integrity risks because the bony prominences of the client's back press against the backs of chairs.

Common respiratory disorders related to aging include the following:

- Respiratory tract infection (RTI)
- Chronic obstructive pulmonary disease (COPD)
- Pulmonary tuberculosis (TB)

Nursing Management: Respiratory Tract Infections

1. Encourage discussing the pneumovaccine with the primary care provider.
2. Encourage obtaining annual influenza vaccine.
3. Assist the client to assume a position of comfort and assist with medications and respiratory treatments, as ordered.

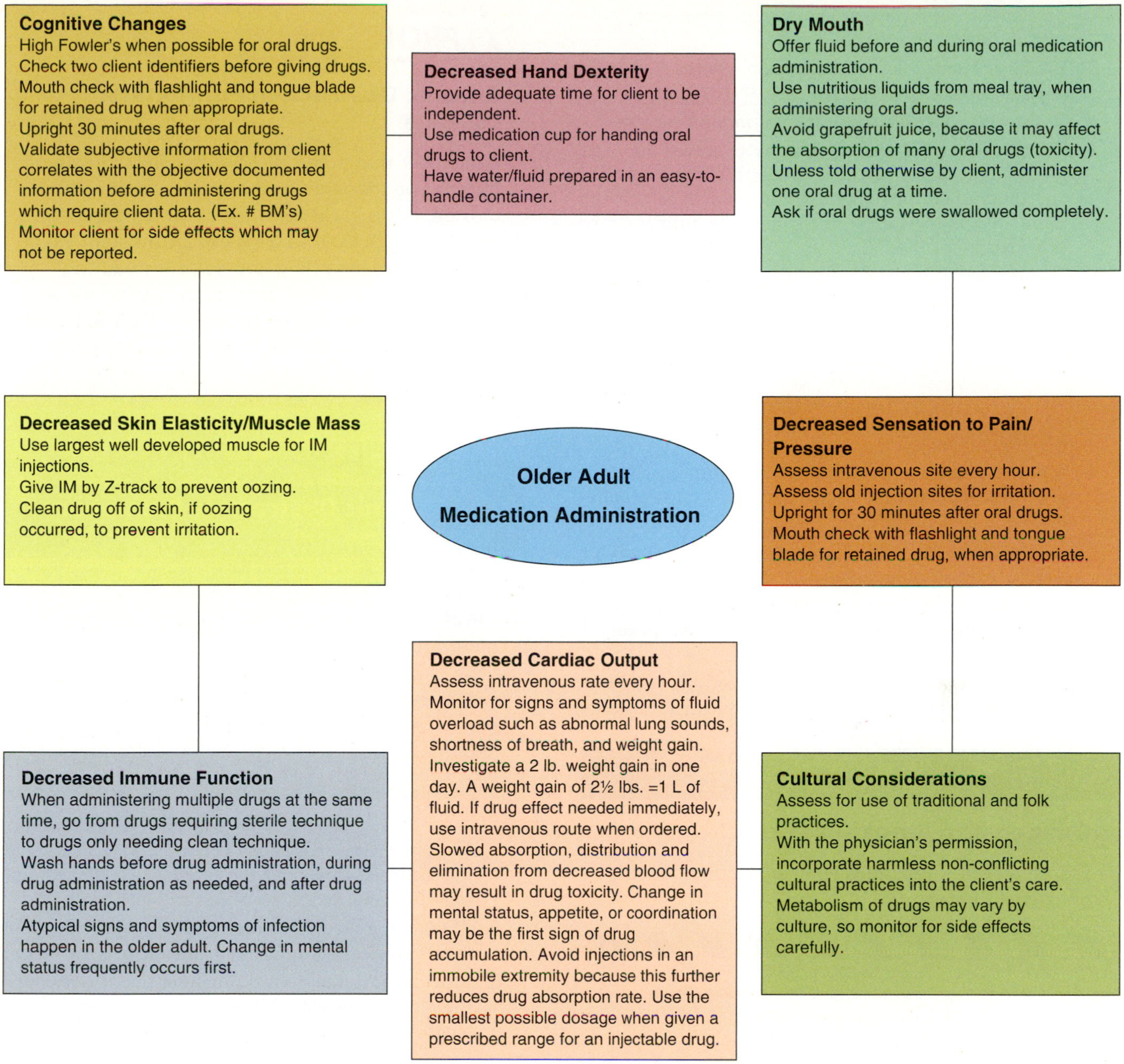

Cognitive Changes
High Fowler's when possible for oral drugs.
Check two client identifiers before giving drugs.
Mouth check with flashlight and tongue blade for retained drug when appropriate.
Upright 30 minutes after oral drugs.
Validate subjective information from client correlates with the objective documented information before administering drugs which require client data. (Ex. # BM's)
Monitor client for side effects which may not be reported.

Decreased Hand Dexterity
Provide adequate time for client to be independent.
Use medication cup for handing oral drugs to client.
Have water/fluid prepared in an easy-to-handle container.

Dry Mouth
Offer fluid before and during oral medication administration.
Use nutritious liquids from meal tray, when administering oral drugs.
Avoid grapefruit juice, because it may affect the absorption of many oral drugs (toxicity).
Unless told otherwise by client, administer one oral drug at a time.
Ask if oral drugs were swallowed completely.

Decreased Skin Elasticity/Muscle Mass
Use largest well developed muscle for IM injections.
Give IM by Z-track to prevent oozing.
Clean drug off of skin, if oozing occurred, to prevent irritation.

Older Adult Medication Administration

Decreased Sensation to Pain/ Pressure
Assess intravenous site every hour.
Assess old injection sites for irritation.
Upright for 30 minutes after oral drugs.
Mouth check with flashlight and tongue blade for retained drug, when appropriate.

Decreased Immune Function
When administering multiple drugs at the same time, go from drugs requiring sterile technique to drugs only needing clean technique.
Wash hands before drug administration, during drug administration as needed, and after drug administration.
Atypical signs and symptoms of infection happen in the older adult. Change in mental status frequently occurs first.

Decreased Cardiac Output
Assess intravenous rate every hour.
Monitor for signs and symptoms of fluid overload such as abnormal lung sounds, shortness of breath, and weight gain.
Investigate a 2 lb. weight gain in one day. A weight gain of 2½ lbs. =1 L of fluid. If drug effect needed immediately, use intravenous route when ordered.
Slowed absorption, distribution and elimination from decreased blood flow may result in drug toxicity. Change in mental status, appetite, or coordination may be the first sign of drug accumulation. Avoid injections in an immobile extremity because this further reduces drug absorption rate. Use the smallest possible dosage when given a prescribed range for an injectable drug.

Cultural Considerations
Assess for use of traditional and folk practices.
With the physician's permission, incorporate harmless non-conflicting cultural practices into the client's care.
Metabolism of drugs may vary by culture, so monitor for side effects carefully.

COURTESY OF DELMAR CENGAGE LEARNING

FIGURE 50-7 Concept Map: Safe Administration of Medication to an Older Adult

4. Avoid distention of bowel, bladder, or stomach, any of which can increase breathing discomfort.
5. Allow adequate time for nursing care.
6. Administer humidified oxygen therapy, as prescribed.
7. Administer analgesics and antipyretics, as prescribed.
8. Assess for signs of dehydration and ensure that fluids are accessible to the client, unless contraindicated.
9. Review diagnostic data and monitor lung sounds and intake and output every 8 hours or as needed given changes in the client's condition. Weigh the client daily, assessing for fluid retention.
10. Monitor for any signs of respiratory distress (cyanosis of lips, mucous membranes, or nailbeds) and obtain pulse-oximetry readings, as needed.

Nursing Management: Chronic Obstructive Pulmonary Disease

1. Assist the client to a position of comfort.
2. Teach the client to use pursed-lip breathing to avoid hyperventilation when short of breath.
3. Teach the client diaphragmatic breathing for use when active.
4. Teach proper use of inhalers. Steroid inhalers should be used first, with a full 60-second wait between puffs; after waiting 5 minutes, any bronchodilator inhalers that are prescribed should then be used, also with a 60-second wait between puffs.
5. Teach the client to cough and clear the airway.

6. Administer chest physiotherapy (e.g., percussion, postural drainage), if prescribed.
7. Establish a schedule for ambulation, gradually increasing the distance ambulated.
8. Assist with active assistive range-of-motion exercises.
9. Monitor for signs and symptoms of infections (e.g., fever, blood-tinged or thick, greenish colored sputum, and diminished lung sounds) and immediately report same to the registered nurse and the primary care provider.
10. Monitor breathing and pulse rate and administer oxygen, if necessary, during periods of increased activity.
11. Suggest smoking cessation programs, if the client is a smoker.

Nursing Management: Pulmonary Tuberculosis

1. Monitor clients for TB status and for symptoms including fever, night sweats, weight loss, and cough producing blood-tinged sputum.
2. Inform the client, family, and caregivers of the need for adequate isolation techniques.
3. Evaluate the client's risk for infection with the human immunodeficiency virus (HIV) and related pneumocystic pneumonia.
4. Monitor that the client's psychosocial needs are being adequately met while the disease is being pharmacologically addressed with medications like isoniazid (Laniazid). Tell the client and family that the entire course of medication must be completed.
5. Monitor the client's nutrition intake and provide supplements as necessary to maintain adequate body weight.
6. Provide for rest periods throughout the day. Encourage the older client with TB to monitor activity level and length of visits by family so as not to become overtired.

SAFETY

Oxygen and Smoking

Ensure that no smoking is allowed around clients on oxygen therapy.

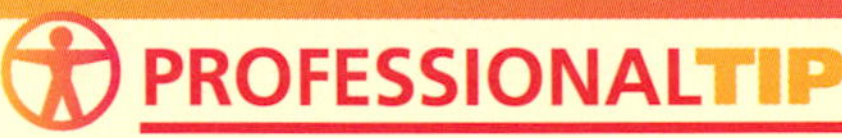

PROFESSIONALTIP

TB in the Older Adult

Older adults can be vulnerable to TB because of:

- An ineffective cough reflex and the resulting inability to clear the lungs.
- An altered immune system and a reduced response to extrinsic antigens. Not only are older adults at increased risk of infection via a new contagion, but older clients who contracted TB years ago and have been in remission since can experience reexacerbation. The risk of reexacerbation increases in cases where the initial infection was remote and healed (encapsulated) such that the immune system's memory of the T cells has been lost. Facilities where health care is provided to older clients and to immune-compromised clients thus must regularly assess the TB status of both their clients and their employees.

PROFESSIONALTIP

Chronic Obstructive Pulmonary Disease

Remember that in the client with COPD, breathing may not be triggered by a higher level of carbon dioxide as it is in clients without COPD, because the client with COPD always has a consistently high CO_2 level. The breathing impulse is instead triggered by a low level of oxygen. Increasing the oxygen level by more than 1 to 2 L/h in the client with COPD can shut down the trigger to breathe, and can put the client in respiratory failure.

CRITICAL THINKING

Chronic Obstructive Pulmonary Disease

A 69-year-old client with COPD was given some stressful news by a relative 1 hour ago. Now, the client reports that he can't breathe. He wants his nasal oxygen turned up. What physical respiratory assessment data will you collect? List the interventions that you will perform to assist the client to breathe easier.

Cardiovascular System

The following cardiovascular changes result from the aging process:

- Left ventricle and heart valves become fibrotic leading to decreased cardiac output and slowed recovery time.

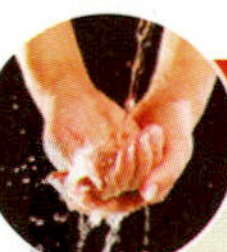

INFECTION CONTROL

TB

Remember that TB is spread through droplets when a client sneezes or coughs (direct and indirect contact). Consult the infection-control nurse on the client's interdisciplinary team and work to protect the client and others from transmission of *Mycobacterium tuberculosis* and other infections.

The heart requires more time to return to a normal rate after a rate increase in response to activity.

- The heart rate slows. Dysrhythmias are more common.
- Blood flow to all organs decreases. The brain and coronary arteries continue to receive a larger volume than do other organs.
- Arterial elasticity decreases (arteriosclerosis), causing increased peripheral resistance and, in turn, a rise in systolic blood pressure and a slight rise in diastolic blood pressure.
- Veins dilate, and superficial vessels become more prominent.

Common cardiovascular disorders related to aging include the following:

- Peripheral vascular disease (PVD)
- Hypertension
- Chronic CHF

Nursing Management: Peripheral Vascular Disease

1. Assess the lower extremities, including the peripheral pulses, for signs of arterial or venous insufficiency, such as cool pale skin and decreased sensation.
2. Evaluate lifestyle factors that may aggravate or advance atherosclerosis, such as a high-carbohydrate, high-fat diet and little exercise.
3. Teach the client about the disease, including treatment, medication actions and side effects, and signs of thrombosis.
4. Educate the client and caregivers about the care and inspection of the lower extremities.
5. Provide instructions on interventions specific to the client's type of PVD (arterial or venous).

Nursing Management: Hypertension

1. Evaluate food intake patterns, especially of cholesterol, fats, sodium, and carbohydrates. Make recommendations based on findings.
2. Evaluate for fluid retention. Weigh the client daily. Investigate a weight gain of 2 lbs. in one day.
3. Recommend a smoking-cessation program, if necessary.
4. Teach the client the importance of avoiding alcohol use.
5. Recommend and facilitate a consistent and appropriate exercise program.
6. Discuss the relationship of stress to hypertension and provide resources from which the client can learn relaxation techniques.
7. Provide information on medications and the importance of taking daily blood pressure medications as prescribed, regardless of health status on any given day.
8. Arrange for and encourage regular blood pressure checks and teach the client or significant others proper use of blood pressure equipment, if applicable.

Nursing Management: Chronic Congestive Heart Failure

1. Frequently monitor serum digitalis level and monitor for any signs of digoxin toxicity, for which older clients are at increased risk because of the decreased rate of renal clearance of the drug. Withhold the digoxin and immediately contact the registered nurse and the physician if abnormal serum level or signs and symptoms of toxicity are present.
2. Take the apical pulse for a full 1 minute before administering digoxin. Withhold the medication if the apical pulse is below 60, and consult the registered nurse and the physician if this or any other significant changes in vital signs are noted.
3. Monitor the client's blood pressure and lung sounds.
4. Monitor electrolyte levels, blood urea nitrogen (BUN), and creatinine level to observe system changes including decreased kidney efficiency.
5. Monitor for signs of fluid retention such as intake and output (output too small), weight gain, shortness of breath, coughing, and edema.
6. Encourage alternating periods of activity with periods of rest.
7. Encourage the client to maintain a level of exercise/physical activity appropriate to physical condition.
8. Teach the client and family about the safe use of the prescribed medications.
9. For clients on diuretics, which deplete potassium, monitor fluid intake and level of potassium, ensuring adequacy of each. Encourage administration of diuretics early in the day, unless contraindicated, to prevent increased urination at night.

CLIENT TEACHING

Digoxin Toxicity

Possible signs and symptoms of digoxin toxicity include the following:

- Disturbances in cardiac rhythms
- Fatigue
- Listlessness
- Anorexia
- Nausea
- Visual disturbances (halos around lights)
- Shaking
- Unsteady gait
- Confusion

Gastrointestinal System

The following gastrointestinal changes result from the aging process:

- Tooth enamel thins.
- Periodontal disease rate increases.
- Taste buds decrease in number and sense of smell decreases. Saliva production diminishes leading to a dry mouth.
- Effectiveness of the gag reflex lessens, resulting in an increased risk of choking.
- Esophageal peristalsis slows, and the effectiveness of the esophageal sphincter lessens, causing delayed entry of food into the stomach and increasing the risk of aspiration.

- Hiatal hernia may occur.
- Gastric emptying slows. Food remains in the stomach longer, decreasing the capacity of the stomach.
- Peristalsis and nerve sensation of the large intestine decreases, contributing to constipation.
- The incidence of diverticulosis increases with age.
- Liver size decreases after age 70.
- Liver enzymes decrease, slowing drug metabolism and the detoxification process.
- Emptying of the gallbladder lessens in efficiency, resulting in thickened bile, increased cholesterol content, and increased incidence of gallstones.

Common gastrointestinal disorders related to aging include the following:

- Over-/undernutrition
- Constipation
- Dehydration
- Dental disorders

Nursing Management: Over-/Undernutrition

1. Assess nutritional status.
2. Provide nutritional instruction based on assessment findings.
3. Recommend and discuss community nutrition programs (e.g., Meals On Wheels, senior center food sites, food pantries, and Food Stamp program).
4. Small, frequent meals may be more tolerable.
5. Maintain client in upright position for several hours after each meal to reduce the risk of aspiration.

Nursing Management: Constipation

1. Assess food and fluid intake.
2. Make recommendations based on assessment findings (e.g., increase fiber intake, increase fluid intake).
3. Discuss the relationship of exercise to bowel activity.
4. Discuss the importance of routine for regular bowel elimination.
5. Teach the importance of avoiding the overuse of laxatives. Frequent use leads to dependency.
6. Monitor adequate bowel elimination and provide interventions (e.g., prune juice, senna bars, milk of magnesia, as ordered) to assist the client in returning to a normal bowel elimination routine.

Nursing Management: Dehydration

1. Identify the reason for dehydration (e.g., inadequate fluid intake or excessive fluid output).
2. Identify the reason and corresponding interventions for inadequate fluid intake:
   - Fluids are inaccessible because of the client's physical limitations: offer fluids on a regular basis throughout the day.
   - The client dislikes water or other available fluids: identify fluid choices.
   - The client restricts fluids because of a fear of incontinence: explain the relationship of decreased fluid intake to bladder infections and arrange for assistance, as needed, for toileting.
3. Identify the reasons for any excessive fluid output and treat accordingly.

Nursing Management: Dental Disorders

1. Teach the oral hygiene procedures of brushing and flossing, and facilitate and encourage brushing of the teeth and gums and flossing of the teeth, as tolerated.
2. Inspect the mouth regularly for signs of dental disorders.
3. Encourage fluids to assist with salivary secretions and reduction of bacterial growth.
4. Advise regular dental checkups.

PROFESSIONALTIP

Determining Alterations in Nutrition

- Height and weight: Record actual body weight, usual body weight, and ideal body weight. If usual weight has varied significantly from the ideal for several years, the use of height/weight tables may be meaningless. Compare actual body weight to usual body weight to determine present status.
- Review laboratory values: hematocrit, hemoglobin, total iron-binding capacity, total protein, BUN.
- Determine whether client is on a weight-loss diet.
- Determine whether client was edematous when initially weighed and has lost weight with treatment.
- Evaluate cognitive status. Cognitively impaired clients may be unaware of hunger or be unable to attend to the task of eating.
- In clients with central nervous system damage, evaluate the presence of sensory–perceptual deficits that interfere with eating.
- Evaluate ability to pick up utensils and glasses and to get items from table to mouth.
- Evaluate dental/oral status: status of teeth/dentures, gums, presence of oral dryness (xerostomia).
- Determine presence of impaired swallowing.
- Determine whether client has distaste for certain food groups.
- Assess knowledge in regard to nutrition and food purchase and preparation.
- Determine whether client is taking medications that interfere with taste or food absorption.
- Determine whether financial status interferes with food purchasing.
- Evaluate for history of compulsive eating.

COMMUNITY/HOME HEALTH CARE

Nutritional Status

Evaluate the following when assessing a client's nutritional status in the home:

- Ability to shop for and prepare meals
- Mealtime environment, for unpleasant odors, noises, and visual stimuli
- Table setting, for appealing table cover, centerpiece, colorful dishes
- Appropriateness of food storage system (cabinets, refrigerator, freezer)

URINARY SYSTEM

The following urinary changes result from the aging process:

- Nephrons in the kidneys decrease in number and function, resulting in decreased filtration and gradual decrease in excretory and reabsorption functions of the renal tubules.
- Glomerular filtration rate decreases, resulting in decreased renal clearance of drugs. By age 75, renal blood flow typically diminishes by 40% (Shepler, Grogan, & Pater, 2006).
- Blood urea nitrogen increases. The creatinine clearance test is a better indicator than is BUN of renal function in older adults.
- Sodium-conserving ability diminishes.
- Bladder capacity decreases, causing increased frequency of urination, including nocturia.
- Renal function increases when the older client lies down, sometimes causing a need to void shortly after going to bed.
- Bladder and perineal muscles weaken, resulting in the inability to empty the bladder and predisposing the older client to cystitis.
- Incidence of stress incontinence increases in older females.
- The prostate may enlarge in older males, causing urinary frequency or dribbling.

Common urinary disorders related to aging include the following:

- Incontinence
- Urinary tract infections (UTIs)

Nursing Management: Incontinence

1. Complete an assessment for bladder management (Figure 50-8).
2. Identify the type of incontinence present (Table 50-2).
3. Implement an appropriate bladder management program (Table 50-3).
4. Frequently monitor for skin impairment.
5. Offer absorbent incontinent pads or briefs that draw the moisture away from the skin.
6. Teach all caregivers, the client, and the family the importance both of adequate cleansing of the genital area (proper retraction, cleansing, and replacement of the foreskin in the uncircumcised male and proper cleansing of the skin folds of the female), legs, and back and of the use of clean linens, to ensure that the client's skin is kept clean and dry. Apply a moisture barrier cream as needed to prevent skin maceration from excessive exposure to moisture.
7. Teach and employ effective infection-control techniques (e.g., wipe and clean [from front to back only] after toileting and when bathing).
8. Instruct client to avoid bladder irritants such as caffeine, spicy foods, and alcohol.

To be completed and reviewed every 90 days or as frequently as needed based on outcome and response.

CLIENT__________________ Adm No. _________ Date____________ Diagnoses_______________ Birthdate_______

Bladder function: History of infection or other urinary problem.____________________________ Urinalysis: Date_________

Protein___ Glucose__ Ketones__ RBC__ WBC__ Bacteria__ Crystals__ Sp.Gr.__ Culture: Date_____ Result_______

Treatment________

BUN___ Ser.Creatinine___ Tot.Pro.___ FBS___ To be completed after 2-week assessment period.

Frequency of voiding______ Average amount______ Is client aware of need to void?____ Urgency?____ Dribbling?____

Incontinence preceded by laughing, sneezing_____

Medications affecting bladder function/continence____

Mental status: Short-term memory__________ Orientation__________ Able to express self__________

Able to follow directions__________ Reaction to incontinence__________

Hydration baseline: Daily average fluid intake: Days______ Eve.______ Night______

Mobility/self-care skills: Ambulatory/self______ Cane______ Walker______ Requires assist of one or two______

Weight-bearing______ Propels self by w/c______ Transfers self______ Requires assistance______

Can manage clothing______ Cleanses self after toileting______ Washes hands______

COURTESY OF DELMAR CENGAGE LEARNING

FIGURE 50-8 Assessment for Bladder Management

TABLE 50-2 Types of Urinary Incontinence

TYPE	CHARACTERISTICS
Functional	Bladder emptying is unpredictable but complete. Incontinence is related to impairment of cognitive, physical, or psychological functioning or to environmental barriers.
Urge	Incontinence occurs immediately after the sensation to void is perceived.
Reflex	Incontinence is related to neurogenic bladder and central nervous system or spinal cord injury. Bladder fills, and uninhibited bladder contractions cause loss of urine.
Stress	Increased abdominal pressure is higher than urethral resistance. Stress associated with coughing or laughing causes incontinence.
Total	Unpredictable, unvoluntary, continuous loss of urine.

COURTESY OF DELMAR CENGAGE LEARNING

9. Encourage referral to discuss medical options (in addition to nursing interventions) for treatment of incontinence.
10. Allow the client to voice concerns over incontinence and assist to overcome any adverse effects on psychosocial functioning.

Nursing Management: Urinary Tract Infections

NOTE: Older persons frequently do not present with the usual signs and symptoms of urinary tract infections. Falling or signs of acute confusion (more than usual) often are the major clinical manifestations.

1. Monitor fluid intake and output. Increase intake unless contraindicated. Offer cranberry juice frequently, per ordered diet.
2. Teach and encourage client to empty the bladder every 3 to 4 hours.
3. Encourage the client to take all medication as prescribed.
4. Use proper infection-control techniques to minimize the risk of infection, including maintaining sterile technique for any urinary catheterization procedure (for urinalysis, assessment for bladder retention, or insertion of indwelling catheter), to prevent unnecessary introduction of bacteria into the bladder.
5. Teach female clients to wipe from front to back only; cleanse thoroughly after bowel movements; avoid bubble baths, colored toilet paper, douches, and vaginal sprays; and wear underwear made from cotton rather than synthetic fibers.
6. Teach the client and caregivers that hematuria (blood in the urine) and fever indicate the need for immediate assessment and intervention, as these signs and symptoms can signify a potentially serious infection or condition. Any signs and symptoms of bladder infection should be immediately reported to the registered nurse and the physician.

MUSCULOSKELETAL SYSTEM

The following musculoskeletal changes result from the aging process:

- Muscle mass and elasticity diminish, resulting in decreased strength, endurance, coordination, and increased reaction time.
- Bone demineralization (osteoporosis) occurs, causing skeletal instability and shrinkage of intervertebral discs.

TABLE 50-3 Bladder Management Techniques

PROGRAM	DESCRIPTION
Kegel exercises	Used for stress incontinence in cognitively alert persons. Exercises strengthen pelvic floor musculature.
Scheduled toileting	Client is on a fixed schedule of toileting—usually every 2 hours. Technique can be used to facilitate voiding and emptying of the bladder.
Habit training	Client is toileted according to individual pattern of voiding. Several days must be spent assessing pattern.
Bladder retraining	Restores normal pattern of voiding/continence. Requires accurate assessment before establishing schedule with progressive shortening or lengthening of toileting intervals. Client must be cognitively alert.
Prompted voiding	Client is prompted to toilet at regular intervals and is given social reinforcement for appropriate toileting behavior.

COURTESY OF DELMAR CENGAGE LEARNING

The flexibility of the spine lessens, and spinal curvature (kyphosis) often occurs. Height may decrease 1 to 4 inches throughout the aging process.

- Joints undergo degenerative changes, resulting in pain, stiffness, and loss of range of motion.

Common musculoskeletal system disorders related to aging include the following:

- Osteoporosis
- Osteoarthritis
- Fractured hip

Nursing Management: Osteoporosis

1. Make dietary recommendations to ensure adequate intake of calcium, protein, and vitamin D.
2. Recommend a smoking cessation program, if necessary.
3. Teach the client the importance of avoiding alcohol.
4. Encourage the client to take a calcium supplement in conjunction with vitamin D, as ordered by the client's primary care provider.
5. Recommend consultation with the primary care provider regarding bone-density testing and to discuss estrogen replacement therapy (ERT) options for females or the use of medications like alendronate sodium (Fosamax) and ibandronate (Boniva) to address bone density loss associated with osteoporosis.
6. Teach the client, family, and caregivers about measures to reduce the risk of falling and sustaining fractures.
7. Recommend evaluation (x-ray) for the presence of stress, or compression, fractures of the spine in cases of severe back pain that occurs with or without a fall. In clients with osteoporosis, these fractures can occur more easily because the vertebrae are compacted by shrinkage of the intervertebral spaces as a consequence of aging.
8. Provide adequate pain control for back pain or other musculoskeletal discomfort.
9. Monitor for adequate dietary intake of calories and fluids and for effective elimination patterns.
10. Teach, encourage, and assist clients to establish exercise programs appropriate to their capabilities. Especially promote exercise programs that include walking or other weight-bearing activities, as tolerated.

Nursing Management: Osteoarthritis

1. Suggest a schedule for alternating periods of activity and rest.
2. Recommend a weight-reduction plan, if necessary, to eliminate extra strain on affected joints.
3. Teach, assist, and encourage the client to establish an exercise program that emphasizes gentle stretching and movement of all joints. For those clients who are more independent, exercise programs in warm water can have positive outcomes.
4. Provide adequate pain control. Teach clients and caregivers to monitor for gastrointestinal distress related to arthritis medications such as nonsteroidal anti-inflammatory drugs (NSAIDs) and to be aware that enteric-coated medications cannot be crushed because they are designed to protect the stomach by dissolving in the duodenum.
5. Encourage the client to seek ongoing evaluation by the physician, as new arthritis medications such as celecoxib (Celebrex) are continually being developed and trialed.

Nursing Management: Fractured Hip

NOTE: Nursing interventions may vary depending on whether the older client has an open reduction/internal fixation fracture (ORIF) or total hip arthroplasty (THA).

1. Maintain postoperative positioning as appropriate to the client's form of treatment.
2. Provide adequate pain control before physical therapy and on an ongoing basis throughout the recovery process.
3. Prevent complications, including skin breakdown, RTIs, infections at the surgical site, and dislocation of the prosthesis or internal fixation device.
4. Facilitate and monitor with the registered nurse the client's consistent use of antiembolism stockings as ordered and the administration of anticoagulant medications and the related monitoring of lab values, to decrease the risk of pulmonary embolism (which can be a significant risk to older clients after hip fracture and/or hip replacement).
5. Teach the client about fall prevention. Evaluate the client's environment (home, room, bathroom) for safety with regard to mobility and make recommendations for rectifying any threats to safety.

Neurological System

The following neurological changes result from the aging process:

- Neurons in the brain decrease in number, resulting in decreased production of neurotransmitters and, thus, reduced synaptic transmission.

CRITICAL THINKING

Home Safety

Your 65-year-old grandmother tells you that she is planning to build a new home. She has been researching and gathering information about safety measures to include in her new home for people over age 60. She wants reassurance that her money is going to be well spent and asks you what are important safety measures to consider. Share pertinent information about the following along with rationale.

1. Location of home (country versus town)
2. One- versus two-story home
3. Paint colors to use
4. Gas versus electric appliances and heat
5. Type of door knobs for opening doors
6. Type and location of alarms
7. Location of lighting
8. Location for grab bars/railing
9. Type of flooring

PROFESSIONALTIP

Neurological System in the Older Adult

In the absence of pathology, intellect and capacity for learning remain unchanged with aging.

- Cerebral blood flow and oxygen utilization decrease.
- Time required to carry out motor and sensory tasks requiring speed, coordination, balance, and fine-motor hand movements increases. Incidence of slight tremors is common.
- Short-term memory may somewhat diminish without much change in long-term memory.
- Night sleep disturbances occur because of more frequent and longer wakeful periods.
- Deep-tendon reflexes decrease, although reflexes at the knees remain fairly intact.

Many disorders that affect the neurological system are not unique to older adults; however, the risk of acquiring one of these disorders increases with age. One of the most common diagnoses among older adults in long-term care facilities is dementia, particularly one form of dementia called Alzheimer's disease (AD). **Dementia** is an organic brain pathology characterized by losses in intellectual functioning. The clinical manifestations associated with dementia are never considered normal aging changes.

It is important for care providers to assess the length of onset of confusion or cognitive changes in the client. Generally, dementia describes declines that have a slow onset of greater than 6 months, whereas **delirium** (or acute confusion) describes cognitive changes that have a shorter onset of 6 months or less. Acute confusion can occur independently or as an exacerbation of a current dementia-related disorder in the client. Acute confusion can result from many stresses such as infections, medication side effects, drug interactions, metabolic imbalances, dehydration, or injuries from falls (e.g., subdural hematomas). Elimination of the causative factor can often turn the acute confusion around in a relatively short period to the preexacerbation level of functioning, unless further pathology to the brain has occurred.

PROFESSIONALTIP

Mental Health in the Older Adult

Mood disorders including depression, bipolar disorder, anxiety disorders, late-onset psychosis, sleep disorders, substance abuse, schizophrenia (chronic and late-onset), and other psychiatric diseases certainly occur among older clients and often go unaddressed or are ineffectively treated. Appropriate assessment, treatment, and clinical management of these clients require effective interdisciplinary teams comprising a geriatric psychiatrist; a neurologist; a clinical nurse specialist specializing in gerontology and mental health; a licensed social worker; a clinical pharmacist; other multidisciplinary team members (including direct care nurses and staff and activity therapists); and the client's family and, whenever possible, the client.

Nursing Management: Alzheimer's Disease

1. Before diagnosis, encourage a medical and psychological diagnostic workup including a mental status examination.
2. Facilitate orientation in the early stages of the disease with calendars, lists, and consistent schedules.
3. Arrange an environment that is therapeutic, consistent, calm, and safe and that alternates rest with activities that require the use of long-practiced skills.
4. Encourage and facilitate access for the client and family to support groups where they can independently share their feelings and concerns and have questions addressed.
5. When assistance is needed with ADLs, implement consistent routines with consistent caregivers but allow for delay of care if needed because of client stress or irritability. Encourage independence of the client while assisting with ADLs (e.g., offer a warm washcloth for client to wash the face and assist with those ADLs that the client cannot complete without assistance).
6. Monitor general health status. Treat any underlying medical problems. Provide adequate pain control, as needed, and monitor for lack of sleep to minimize the risk of violent behavior. Observe for the client's better times of the day, and plan activities or interventions accordingly.
7. Build a trusting relationship with the client. Use clear, simple directions and treat clients with respect and as individuals, building on their strengths and their unique interests and histories. Doing so demonstrates appreciation for the individual and can help build the client's self-esteem.
8. Be aware that as much is communicated to the AD client through the caregiver's nonverbal behavior and tone and volume of voice as is communicated through actual words. A calm attitude allows the client time to process and retrieve information when spoken to or asked a question.
9. Support the client's mobility within a safe environment, recognizing that as the disease progresses, baseline wandering often increases as a coping skill, whereas verbal communication often decreases. Beanbag chairs, low mattresses, bed and chair alarms, positional (antisliding) wedges for chairs, merry walkers that support independent mobility, and assisted-ambulation programs to build leg strength are all therapeutic interventions for AD clients as the disease progresses and represent preferable alternatives to the use of restraints.

10. Monitor for changes in baseline behaviors and for intensity of wandering, pacing, and lethargy, as these often indicate underlying infections, metabolic imbalances, or stress. Encourage clients to alternate periods of activity and rest.

Nursing Management: Depression

1. Assess for signs of a physical basis for any fatigue (e.g., infection, pain, altered nutritional status, or shortness of breath upon exertion).
2. Administer treatment for underlying physiologic problems, if applicable.
3. If symptoms persist, encourage the client to have a medical diagnostic workup with a geriatric psychiatrist, if such a workup has not yet been done.
4. Monitor for verbal or nonverbal signs of suicidal thoughts/intent. Determine whether the client has a plan.
5. Provide one-on-one supervision of the client as needed and assure the client that the caregiver will keep him safe. If appropriate for the client, seek an agreement that he will not try to harm himself.
6. Administer antidepressant medication as ordered. Provide client and family education regarding medication, including length of time before therapeutic results should occur, and potential side effects. Report immediately to the registered nurse and primary care provider any extrapyramidal side effects (e.g., tremors, drooling, pin rolling of the fingers, shuffling gait) that are observed.
7. If the client is not assessed as being at risk for suicide but is isolating in his room, establish small goals with the client (e.g., coming out of the room and sitting safely in the hallway with the nurse for 5 minutes two times per day and for meals). Advance to more challenging goals as the client demonstrates increased tolerance for social interaction.
8. Facilitate the client's reintegration into a healthy support system and provide small community group time for the client to share his views.

Nursing Management: Transient Ischemic Attack

1. Assess for risk factors for stroke and for the existence of any previous carotid vascular tests for potential narrowing, stenosis, or blockage.
2. Provide client and family education explaining the relationship between risk factors and TIA and stroke.
3. Provide teaching to assist in reducing risk factors.
4. Monitor orthostatic blood pressure and encourage clients to change positions slowly to decrease the risk of falling.

Sensory Changes

The following sensory changes in vision and hearing result from the aging process.

Vision

- With aging, the lens becomes less pliable and less able to increase its curvature in order to focus on near objects, causing presbyopia (trouble seeing objects up close) and decreased accommodation. The lens also yellows, causing distorted color perceptions, with greens and blues washing out and warm colors such as reds and oranges becoming more distinct. The incidence of cataracts also increases (Figure 50-9).

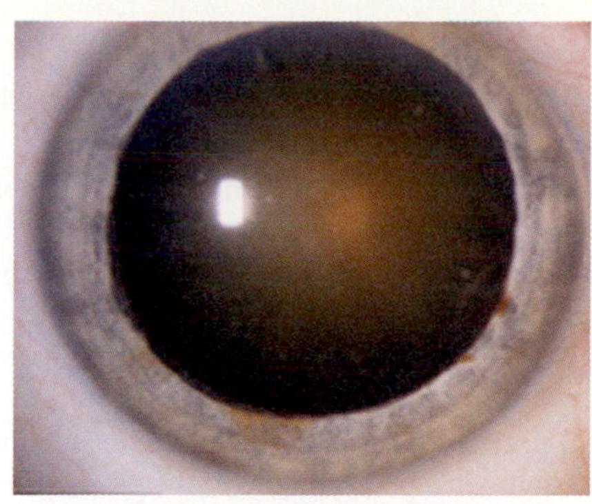

FIGURE 50-9 Cataract (*Courtesy of Salim L. Butrus, MD, Senior Attending, Department of Opthalmology, Washington Hospital Center, Washington, D.C., and Associate Clinical Professor, Georgetown University Medical Center, Washington, D.C.*)

- Accommodation of pupil size decreases, resulting in both decreased adjustment to changes in lighting and decreased ability to tolerate glare. For instance, high-gloss tile floors in hallways can appear like hills and valleys to older clients, especially those with perceptual deficits; this may increase anxiety and safety risks.
- Vitreous humor changes in consistency, causing blurred vision. Changes in the anterior chamber may increase the pressure of the aqueous humor, resulting in glaucoma.
- Lacrimal glands secrete less fluids, causing dryness and itching. Entropion or ectropion (turning of the eye inward) or ectropion (turning of the eye outward) occasionally occurs in older clients. These conditions can not only impact vision, but can also increase the risk of infection caused by dryness and ineffective blinking. In these conditions, obtaining an order for artificial tears, lacrilube, and eye drop treatments for dryness or infection may be necessary.
- Arcus senilus, a hazy grayish yellow ring around the cornea may develop, but it does not affect vision.

INFECTION CONTROL

Eye Care

To decrease infection risks, all caregivers should wash from the nose outward when washing clients' eyes.

Common vision disorders related to aging include the following:

- Presbyopia
- Cataract
- Glaucoma
- Age-related macular degeneration

Nursing Management: Visual Impairment

1. Teach visually impaired clients adaptive techniques for ADL, such as extra lighting.
2. Recommend regular examination by an ophthalmologist.
3. Provide preoperative and postoperative care and teaching to clients undergoing cataract surgery, including lifting and bending restrictions as well as measures to prevent infection.
4. Teach proper eye drop administration techniques to all clients who are prescribed eye drops, including holding the drop in the eye with the lid closed for 30 seconds after administration and lacrimal pressure for 1 minute when appropriate.
5. Ensure that older clients have their glasses on when needed to decrease perceptual and spatial deficits.

Teach clients that to have a better chance of keeping their vision they should not smoke, maintain a healthy weight, control blood pressure, and eat a healthy diet rich in fish and green leafy vegetables (Covell, Graziano, Rich, & Tobin, 2007).

HEARING

- As aging occurs, the pinna becomes less flexible, the hair cells in the inner ear stiffen and atrophy, and cerumen (earwax) increases.
- The number of neurons in the cochlea decrease, and the blood supply lessens, causing the cochlea and the ossicles to degenerate.
- Presbycusis, the impairment of hearing in older adults, is often accompanied by a loss of tone discrimination. High-frequency tones are lost first; thus, keeping the voice low and calm and decreasing any background noise can improve the client's comprehension of the caregiver's message.

Nursing Management: Hearing Impairment

1. Assess for ear pain, drainage, inflammation, abnormalities, surgeries, perforations, impacted cerumen.
2. Evaluate medication regimen and assess for ototoxicity, if medication history reveals such a risk.
3. Recommend hearing testing by an audiologist, if the previous assessments are negative.
4. Monitor the care and use of a hearing aid by the older client with unilateral or bilateral aids (Figure 50-10). Provide teaching and assistance as needed for cleaning the hearing aid(s) and replacing batteries.
5. Instruct caregivers and family about the communication and socialization needs of the client. For some older clients, either the use of a small erasable board to augment verbal questions or communication with written text represents a therapeutic intervention for hearing impairment. If writing dexterity or ability is also impaired, a story board that has pictures indicating the client's needs (e.g., bathroom, food, rest) can assist the client to independently communicate needs to caregivers.
6. The consonants f, g, s, and t may become difficult to understand as the client ages. Rephrase sentences and questions when the client has difficulty with interpreting communication.

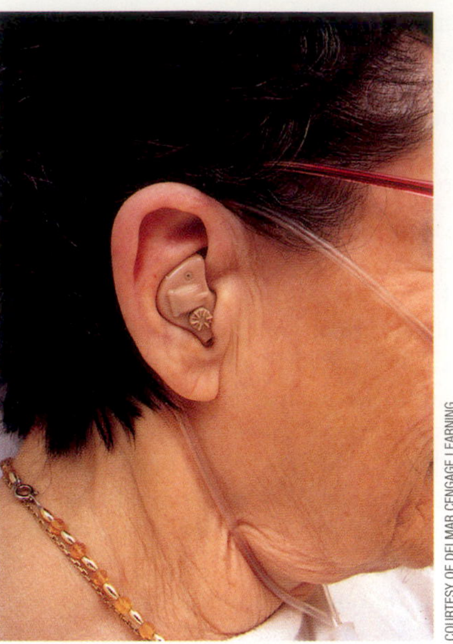

FIGURE 50-10 The use of hearing aids helps to compensate for hearing loss experienced by some clients.

CRITICAL THINKING

Driving Safety

An 80-year-old client is contemplating giving up automobile driving. What physical changes have occurred with aging that make it more difficult to drive safely? If the client decides to continue driving, what safety measures would you recommend?

PROFESSIONALTIP

New Technology for the Older Adult

Massachusetts Institute of Technology's (MIT) AgeLab designs new ideas to improve the quality of life for older adults and those who care for them. Health innovations that AgeLab is researching or has developed include: the Home Health Station, an intelligent cardiopulmonary decisions system that uses telemedicine at home to provide a "checkup a day" for managing chronic illnesses such as CHF and diabetes; the Smart Personal Advisor that uses the older adult's diet information to provide guidance when grocery shopping; Pill Pets, an electronic pill pet that uses emotions and play to remind the older adult to take their medication; Digital Danskins for older adults that integrate biosensors to monitor health conditions and chronic diseases; and the "Aware Car," a Volvo XC90 designed with cameras and sensors that provide the older adult driver with information to promote safe driving. To view additional technology being created by MIT for the aging population visit http://web.mit.edu/agelab/index.shtml (MIT, 2009).

SAMPLE NURSING CARE PLAN

The Client with Alzheimer's Disease (AD)

J.R., 64 years old, was admitted to the Alzheimer's unit of a long-term care facility. Last month, J.R. was visiting her daughter in another state and wandered away from the daughter's home. J.R. was found 60 miles away, unharmed but completely disoriented and agitated. J.R. had worked as a nursing assistant before she retired. She is a widow and has two children in the same community where the nursing home is located, in addition to the daughter who she was visiting in another state. Unless reminded, J.R. does not shower or change clothes. She awakens at least once each night and asks for breakfast.

NURSING DIAGNOSIS 1 *Disturbed Thought Processes* related to progressive dementia as evidenced by disorientation to time and place, loss of short-term memory, inability to concentrate, and periods of agitation

Nursing Outcomes Classification (NOC)
Memory
Cognitive Ability
Cognitive Orientation

Nursing Interventions Classification (NIC)
Dementia Management
Environmental Management

PLANNING/OUTCOMES	NURSING INTERVENTIONS	RATIONALE
J.R. will remain calm and will not experience agitation and anxiety as a result of her disorientation and memory loss.	Provide J.R. with clues for orientation: "Good morning, J.R. My name is Jean, and I will help you today." Avoid putting her on the spot.	Helps J.R. cope with her environment.
	Place a large sign on J.R.'s door with her name printed in large letters.	Helps her find her room.
	Have family bring in snapshots and photos taken in past years.	Stimulates reminiscing and allows her to recall happy times.
	Avoid changing J.R.'s room. Always put items back in the same place.	Consistency reduces frustration.
	Consult with activities staff in planning self-expressive, non-fail activities that require little concentration (e.g., painting with nontoxic paints, modeling with nontoxic clay).	Prevents boredom, which can lead to irritation.
	If J.R. is resistant to care, provide clear, simple, nonthreatening instructions and delay care as needed until she is calmer.	Often, delaying care for even 10 to 15 minutes when resistance is encountered improves client outcomes.

EVALUATION

J.R. remained calm and showed no signs of agitation or anxiety.

NURSING DIAGNOSIS 2 *Risk for Injury* related to risk factors of mode of transportation and cognitive and affective factors as evidenced by wandering behavior, impaired judgment, and disorientation

Nursing Outcomes Classification (NOC)
Safety Behavior: Personal
Safety Behavior: Home Physical Environment

Nursing Interventions Classification (NIC)
Pain Management
Dementia Management

(Continues)

SAMPLE NURSING CARE PLAN (Continued)

PLANNING/OUTCOMES	NURSING INTERVENTIONS	RATIONALE
J.R. will remain free of injury while retaining as much independence and freedom as possible.	Keep only nonpoisonous plants on the unit. Arrange furniture so that walkways are open. Pad sharp corners of tables and chests. Cover electrical outlets and hot radiators. Place electrical cords and telephone wires out of reach.	Does not recognize unsafe acts or conditions due to loss of impulse control and loss of judgment. Does not comprehend cause and effect.
	Provide assurance during fire drills.	Agitation increases especially when noise level is increased.

EVALUATION

J.R. has experienced no injury.

NURSING DIAGNOSIS 3 *Bathing/Hygiene and Dressing/Grooming* ***S****elf-Care Deficit* related to perceptual or cognitive impairment (memory loss and sensory–perceptual deficits) as evidenced by needing a reminder to shower and change clothes

Nursing Outcomes Classification (NOC)

Self-Care: Bathing
Self-Care: Hygiene
Self-Care: Dressing
Self-Care: Grooming

Nursing Interventions Classification (NIC)

Self-Care Assistance: Dressing/Grooming
Self-Care Assistance: Bathing/Hygiene

PLANNING/OUTCOMES	NURSING INTERVENTIONS	RATIONALE
J.R. will complete ADLs with minimal assistance now and with increasing assistance as the disease progresses.	Use verbal cues and hand-over-hand assistance with ADLs. Instruct staff to avoid doing tasks that J.R. can do by herself. Watch for signs of frustration and irritation and intervene when appropriate.	Minimizes the need for assistance, thereby increasing feelings of self-esteem.
	Ask family to bring in clothing that is easy to manipulate. Set clothing out in the order it is to be put on.	Allows J.R. to be more independent.
	Consider tub baths rather than showers. Provide privacy, check the temperature of the bathroom, and do not leave the client alone.	Showers may be threatening or confusing to persons with Alzheimer's disease. Tub baths are more relaxing.

EVALUATION

J.R. participates in ADLs.

NURSING DIAGNOSIS 4 *Disturbed* ***S****leep Pattern* related to disorientation as evidenced by wakefulness at night

Nursing Outcomes Classification (NOC)

Information Processing
Mood Equilibrium

Nursing Interventions Classification (NIC)

Sleep Enhancement
Simple Massage

SAMPLE NURSING CARE PLAN (Continued)

PLANNING/OUTCOMES	NURSING INTERVENTIONS	RATIONALE
J.R. will experience fewer periods of wakefulness during the night. If she awakens, she will remain calm and free of agitation.	Avoid stimulating activities prior to bedtime. Establish a consistent bedtime routine. Take J.R. to the bathroom and allow sufficient time for complete bladder emptying.	Overstimulation before bedtime may increase anxiety, preventing sleep. A consistent bedtime routine is helpful.
	Help J.R. with a sponge bath and with oral care; give her a back rub using warm lotion and slow, smooth strokes.	Provides relaxation.
	Provide a light snack of a warm, noncaffeinated beverage and a plain, easily digested cracker, cookie, or a piece of toast. Be patient and do not rush her.	Hunger or overeating can interfere with sleep.
	Question family concerning previous bedtime routines and sleeping habits.	Allows same routine to be followed.
	Repeat bedtime routine when J.R. awakens during night.	Makes J.R. think it is time to go to bed.
	Encourage a short nap early in the afternoon.	Sleep pattern disturbances may result from overfatigue.
	Avoid the use of sleeping medications.	Prevents confusion, disorientation, and restlessness.

EVALUATION

J.R. sleeps through the night several times a week.

Endocrine System

The following endocrine changes result from the aging process:

- Alterations occur in both the reception and the production of hormones.
- Release of insulin by the beta cells of the pancreas slows, causing an increase in blood sugar.
- Thyroid changes may lead to decreased T_4 and hypothyroidism.

The most common endocrine disorder related to aging is diabetes mellitus type 2.

Nursing Management: Diabetes Mellitus Type 2

1. Arrange for a consultation with a dietitian to assess nutritional status and to provide food-management instruction.
2. Teach the client, family members, or caregivers (as appropriate) the procedure for blood glucose monitoring specific to the equipment the client will be using.
3. Develop a personal exercise program with the client based on the client's physical condition, mental status, resources, and interests.
4. Provide information on prescribed oral hypoglycemic medications.
5. Teach the causes, signs, and treatment of hypoglycemia and hyperglycemia.
6. Educate on self-care and on careful monitoring of the extremities and of sores on the skin to minimize threats to skin integrity.
7. Encourage the client to wear shoes and to have nails trimmed by a podiatrist, if unable to safely perform self-care.

Reproductive System: Female

The following reproductive changes result from the aging process:

- Estrogen production decreases with the onset of menopause.
- Ovaries, uterus, and cervix decrease in size.

- The vagina shortens, narrows, and becomes less elastic, and the vaginal lining thins. Secretions decrease and become more alkaline, resulting in increased incidence of atrophic vaginitis. These changes may result in dyspareunia (discomfort during coitus), which can often be rectified with the use of a water-based lubricant. As at any age, protected intercourse (safe sex) through the use of a latex condom should be advised with new partners.
- Supporting musculature of the reproductive organs weakens, increasing the risk of uterine prolapse.
- Breast tissue diminishes and nipple erection lessens during sexual arousal.
- Libido and the need for intimacy and companionship in older women remain unchanged (Figure 50-11).

Common female reproductive system disorders related to aging include the following:

- Breast cancer (the risk of which increases with age)
- Altered sexuality patterns related to physiologic changes, medications, changes in body image, or psychosocial changes such as the loss of a significant other or a move to a setting that provides some level of assistive care (i.e., group home, assisted living center, or care facility)

Nursing Management: Female Reproductive System Disorders

1. Teach and encourage monthly breast self-exams and yearly mammograms for early detection and treatment of disorders.
2. Establish rapport and encourage the client to verbalize feelings and concerns related to sexuality, body image, and self-esteem.
3. Complete a sexual history and recommend interventions based on findings. Support the client's needs for companionship and intimacy throughout the life span.
4. Recommend that a bone density scan (Dexa-Scan) be discussed with the client's primary care provider to allow for early detection and treatment of osteoporosis.
5. Encourage annual gynecological examinations with the client's primary care provider.

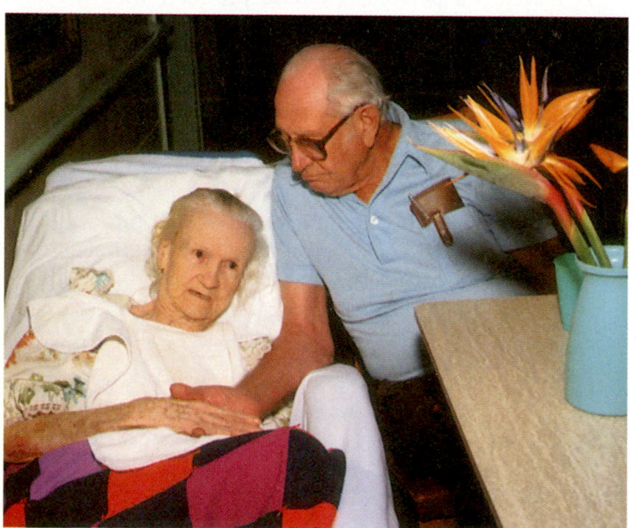

COURTESY OF DELMAR CENGAGE LEARNING

FIGURE 50-11 Sexuality and companionship remain important throughout the life span.

Reproductive System: Male

The following reproductive changes result from the aging process:

- Testosterone production decreases, resulting in decreased size of the testicles.
- Sperm count and viscosity of seminal fluid decrease.
- Although more time is required to obtain erection, the older man often finds that he and his partner can enjoy longer periods of lovemaking (greater control) before ejaculation. As at any age, protected intercourse (safe sex) through the use of a latex condom should be advised with new partners.
- The prostate gland may enlarge.
- Impotency may occur. Medications and other medical interventions have been successful in reversing impotency problems in many older males. A thorough evaluation by the primary care provider and a urologist can provide clients with available options given health status and current medication regimen.
- Libido and the need for intimacy and companionship remain unchanged in older males.

Common male reproductive disorders related to aging include the following:

- Altered sexuality patterns related to physiologic changes, medications, changes in body image, or psychosocial changes such as the loss of a significant other or a move to a setting that provides some level of assistive care (i.e., group home, assisted living center, or care facility)
- Benign prostatic hypertrophy (BPH)

Nursing Management: Male Reproductive System Disorders

1. Establish rapport and encourage the client to verbalize feelings and concerns related to sexuality, body image, and self-esteem.
2. Complete a sexual history and recommend interventions based on findings. Support the client's needs for companionship and intimacy throughout the life span.
3. Provide client and family education regarding the signs and symptoms of prostate disorders (e.g., difficulty in starting the urine stream, a smaller urine stream, frequent urination, frequent nighttime awakening for the purpose of urinating, or, in severe cases, the failure or inability to urinate).
4. Teach and encourage monthly testicular self-exam and yearly digital rectal examinations of the prostate gland by a primary care provider. The benefits of a PSA lab test performed every 1 to 2 years to facilitate early detection and treatment of prostate cancer are being researched and debated.

Integumentary System

The following integumentary changes result from the normal aging process:

- Subcutaneous tissue and elastin fibers diminish, causing the skin to become thinner, less elastic, and wrinkled.
- Ability of melanocytes to produce even pigmentation diminishes, resulting in hyperpigmentation or liver spots, typically on the hands and wrists (Figure 50-12).

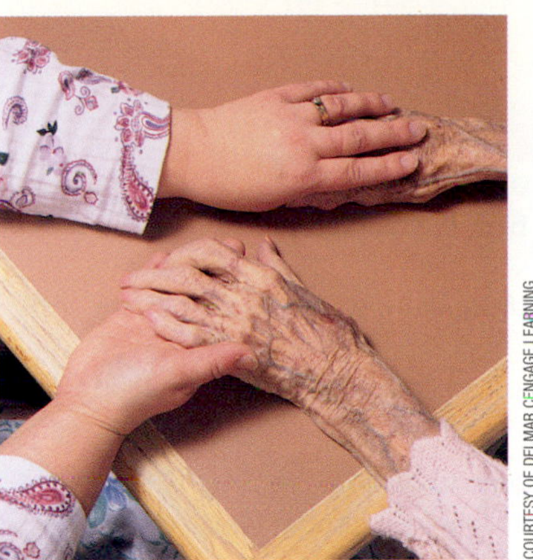
COURTESY OF DELMAR CENGAGE LEARNING

FIGURE 50-12 Hyperpigmentation is a normal result of the aging process.

- Eccrine, apocrine, and sebaceous glands decrease in size, number, and function, resulting in diminished secretions and moisturization and, thus, pruritis.
- Body temperature regulation diminishes because of decreased perspiration and, many times, decreased circulation, placing the older adult at risk for hypo- and hyperthermia.
- Capillary blood flow decreases, resulting in slower wound healing.
- Blood flow decreases, especially to lower extremities.
- Vascular fragility causes senile purpura.
- Cutaneous sensitivity to pressure, touch, pain, and temperature decreases.
- Melanin production decreases, causing gray-white hair.
- Scalp, pubic, and axillary hair thin, and women display increased facial hair on the upper lip and chin.
- Nail growth slows, nails become more brittle, and longitudinal nail ridges form.

Common integumentary disorders related to aging include the following:

- Pressure ulcers (alteration in skin integrity)
- Herpes zoster (shingles)
- Skin cancer (included because the risk of skin cancer increases with age)

Nursing Management: Alteration in Skin Integrity

1. Perform a pressure ulcer risk assessment upon the client's admission to the health care setting (Figure 50-13).
2. Implement pressure ulcer prevention protocol for clients at risk for pressure ulcer formation. It is important to consider and document pressure-relieving interventions for all surfaces that the client will sit or lay on during the course of the day (Table 50-4).
3. Encourage adequate intake of protein and fluids to help ensure good skin integrity.
4. Dress clients in long sleeves and slacks, when appropriate, to protect fragile skin and provide warmth.
5. Assess skin turgor on sternum or forehead due to loss of skin elasticity.
6. Monitor client for exaggerated drug effects due to age related thinning of skin, potentially causing faster absorption of topical medications (Shepler, Grogan, & Pater, 2006).

Date of assessment: _____ Nurse: ____________________

Pressure ulcer present on admission: No ____ Yes ____ Stage ____

A score of 11 or more places a client at risk for pressure ulcer formation. Preventive protocol should be established.

Activity		**Total**	**Level of Consciousness**		**Total**
Ambulant without assistance	0		Alert	0	
Ambulant with assistance	2		Slow verbal response	1	
Chairfast	4		Responds to verbal or painful stimuli	2	
Bedfast	6	____	Absence of response to stimuli	3	____
Mobility—Range of Motion			**Nutritional Status**		
Full range of motion	0		Good (eats 75% or more of required intake)	0	
Moves with minimal assistance	2		Fair (eats less than 75% of required intake)	1	
Moves with moderate assistance	4		Poor (minimal intake, consistent weight loss)	2	
Immobile	6	____	Unable/refuses to eat/drink, emaciated	3	____
Skin Condition			**Incontinence—Bladder**		
Hydrated and intact	0		None	0	
Rashes or abrasions	2		Occasional (fewer than 2/24 hours)	1	
Decreased turgor, dry	4		Usually (more than 2/24 hours)	2	
Edema, erythema, pressure ulcers	6	____	Total (no control)	3	____
Predisposing Disease Process			**Incontinence—Bowel**		
No involvement	0		None	0	
Chronic, stable	1		Occasional (formed stool)	1	
Acute or chronic, unstable	2		Usually (semi-formed stool)	2	
Terminal	3	____	Total (no control, loose stool)	3	____

COURTESY OF DELMAR CENGAGE LEARNING

FIGURE 50-13 Pressure Ulcer Risk Assessment

TABLE 50-4 Protocol for Clients at Risk for Pressure Ulcers

OBJECTIVE	INTERVENTIONS
Relieve pressure	• Establish positioning schedule. • Place pressure relieving mattress on bed, cushions on chair. • Teach client wheelchair exercises. • Stand and/or ambulate client in chair frequently. • Use wheelchair for transporting only. • Allow client to sit on bedpan, commode, or toilet for only brief periods. • Check areas of pressure under casts, braces, splints, slings, prostheses.
Relieve friction and shearing	• Use turning sheet for positioning in bed and chair. • Keep head of bed lower than 30 degrees unless contraindicated. • Use supportive devices to prevent sliding in chairs. • Use appropriate transfer techniques. • Do not use powder on skin. • Place bed cradle under top covers.
Prevent moisture/maceration	• Implement scheduled toileting or bladder retraining program. • Use absorbent incontinent briefs or pads. • Check incontinent clients frequently. Wash and rinse thoroughly. Apply moisture barrier. • Avoid use of plastic/rubber sheets, protectors.
Prevent spasticity and contractures	• Avoid quick, rough movements. • Do range-of-motion exercises at least twice daily. • Assess for synergy patterns when positioning. • Administer oral antispasmodics if ordered.
Maintain hydration/nutritional status	• Assess nutritional status. • Investigate causes of anorexia. • Correct underlying nutritional deficits. • Encourage additional fluids, unless contraindicated. • Give high protein supplement, if necessary. • Monitor weight weekly.
Continue with routine skin care. Do skin checks with each position change.	

COURTESY OF DELMAR CENGAGE LEARNING

INFECTION CONTROL

Skin Integrity

It is a nursing responsibility to educate caregivers (including other staff members, as necessary) about the need to thoroughly wash and dry the client's perineal area and to keep linens and clothing clean and dry, especially when incontinence is a problem. Such education may also include instruction on maintaining client privacy; properly retracting, cleansing, and repositioning the foreskin of an uncircumcised older male client; and proper cleansing of the skin folds of a female client's perineal area. Clients and caregivers should also be instructed to cleanse front to back only and to not rinse and reuse washcloths again or use them on other body areas. These simple hygiene and infection-control guidelines can help maintain the client's skin integrity and can also prevent unnecessary infections.

Nursing Management: Herpes Zoster

1. Treat the pain.
2. Treat the ulcer with medications (e.g., acyclovir [Zovirax] topical cream), as ordered, to reduce the length of time of the outbreak.
3. Develop a plan to ensure continuity in meeting the client's psychosocial needs, and allow the client time to share concerns.

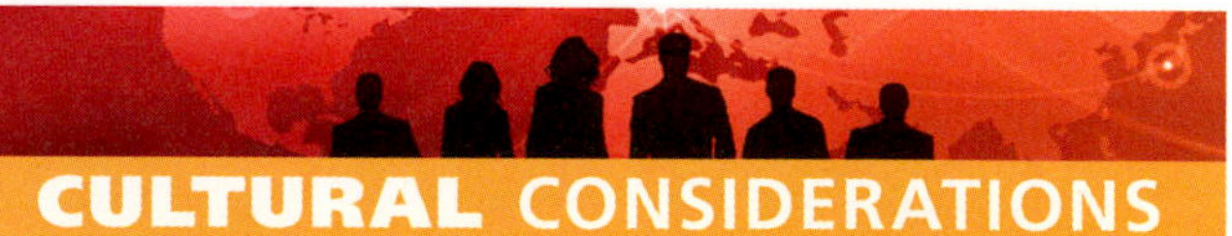

CULTURAL CONSIDERATIONS

Pain Assessment

Overt signs of pain may not be expressed by some cultures or sexes. Older adults may not sense pain until the condition has become severe. Therefore, a thorough pain assessment is crucial for effective pain management.

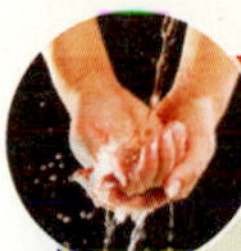

INFECTION CONTROL

Herpes Zoster

Prevent cross-infection from drainage from the vesicular eruptions by practicing proper hand hygiene and implementing appropriate isolation procedures, especially if the client is in the hospital or another health care facility.

Nursing Management: Skin Cancer

1. Teach clients and caregivers both cancer prevention methods and skin self-examination to detect lesions early. Early detection and treatment of skin cancers are essential to optimal client outcomes.
2. Provide information in both verbal and written form and in collaboration with the client's multidisciplinary team regarding treatment (surgery, chemotherapy, radiation, and other options).
3. Monitor for signs of infection at the lesion site.
4. Ensure that the client's psychological, psychosocial, spiritual, and dietary needs are also addressed.

FINANCING OLDER ADULT CARE

Since the 1960s, the U.S. Congress has developed and implemented a series of national entitlement programs to help ensure adequate income, housing, and access to medical care for older Americans. As the number of older clients (those older than age 65, particularly those older than age 85) continues to rise, caregivers and advocates for older-adult care should strive to understand the budgetary policies that have influenced and continue to influence the U.S. health care delivery system.

Medicare

Medicare (Title XVIII) is a nationwide health insurance program for Americans who are 65 years of age or older, for persons who are eligible for Social Security disability payments for longer than 2 years, and for certain workers and dependents who need kidney transplants or dialysis. The Health Care Financing Administration (HCFA) was the federal agency in charge of administering the Medicare program. Since July 2001, the HCFA is now the Centers for Medicare and Medicaid Services (CMS). More than the name has changed. Now there is an increased emphasis on responsiveness to beneficiaries and providers, and quality improvement (CMS, 2001).

The program was enacted as part of the Social Security Act of 1965 and became effective on June 1, 1966. It consists of two separate but coordinated programs: hospital insurance (called Part A) and medical insurance (called Part B), which covers physician's services, outpatient services, some medical supplies, and some skilled nursing and home health services. Medicare provides basic protection for the cost of health care but does not cover all expenses. Among the expenses *not* covered by Medicare for older Americans are those associated with the following:

- Acupuncture
- Chiropractic services (some exceptions)
- Cosmetic surgery
- Dental care and dentures (few exceptions)
- Eye exams (routine) and eye glasses
- Foot care (routine)
- Hearing aids
- Laboratory tests (screening)
- Long-term care
- Orthopedic shoes (few exceptions)
- Physical exams (routine)
- Prescription drugs (few exceptions)
- Travel (healthcare while traveling outside the United States) (Medicare, 2009a)

In the late 1990s, many insurance policies were available to supplement at varying levels the benefits paid by Medicare. This led many older clients to "stack" insurance policies or to buy numerous overlapping policies for fear of being underinsured. The insurance industry and Congress worked together to outlaw stacking of Medicare supplement policies.

Although there has been some improvement in insurance coverage for preventive screening tests such as mammograms, the lack of reimbursement for prescription drugs continues to significantly burden older Americans, many of whom must choose between costly medications and food.

On January 1, 2006, a new prescription drug coverage program began for persons older than 65 with Medicare regardless of income or health (CMS, 2009c). This program is referred to as Medicare Part D. This is insurance that should cover half of the cost of needed medications for the older adult. Medicare reports that 33% of persons covered by Medicare will meet the qualifying factors for extra help so that almost all of the medication costs for this group will be covered.

According to Kurtzman and Buerhaus (2008), the CMS, in an effect to refine Medicare's prospective payment system and improve quality care, implemented a new payment rule known as CMS-1533-FC to eliminate additional Medicare payments for eight preventable hospital-acquired conditions. The eight conditions include pressure ulcers, preventable injuries, catheter associated UTI's, vascular catheter associated infections, surgical site infections, air emboli, blood incompatibility reactions, and objects mistakenly left inside surgical clients.

In 2009, Medicare estimates coverage for items and services for more than 43 million beneficiaries (CMS, 2009b).

Medicaid

The Medicaid program was also enacted as part of the Social Security Act of 1966 and is often referred to as Title XIX. This program, which is federally funded but state operated and administered, provides medical benefits to certain indigent, or low-income, Americans. Nursing home bills represent a staggering burden for many older Americans who require nursing care. In 1995, nursing home bills averaged $22,000 per person per year, and projections showed that two-thirds of older adults who lived alone would run out of savings after 13 weeks in a nursing home (Gallo, Paveza, Fulmer, 2003). Medicaid takes into account government-determined poverty levels when providing benefits, with coverage being extended to persons who are at certain percentages of the poverty level (e.g., 200% of poverty level, 150% of poverty level, and 100% of poverty level). Long-term care facilities serve both private-pay clients (those whose expenses are paid by themselves, their families, or their long-term care insurance policies) and Title XIX- (Medicaid-) funded clients. Medicaid coverage for long-term care is not available until a person's assets have been depleted to a certain set level. Older-adult care advocates continue their efforts to protect the assets of the spouse who is able to stay in the family home after the other spouse must be placed in a nursing home.

To some in the United States, the debate over Social Security, Medicare, and Medicaid financing is viewed as someone else's priority; however, the moral responsibility for providing access to quality services and care for our country's older adults is shared by all Americans. Older-adult care services should be developed to promote independence yet should provide assistance when needed.

Omnibus Budget Reconciliation Act

The Omnibus Budget Reconciliation Act (OBRA), first enacted in 1987 and reenacted in 1990, sought to ensure quality services for older Americans. The act included guidelines for services that were required to be made available to seniors and promoted the rights of seniors. As was the case with all health care costs, however, older-adult care costs continued to rise in the United States, and discussions and proposed legislation for financial reforms intensified.

Balanced Budget Act of 1997

Among the most significant influences on the financing of older-adult care is the Balanced Budget Act (BBA) of 1997. The BBA replaced cost-based reimbursement for care provided in skilled nursing facilities (SNFs) with a prospective payment system (PPS) based on client assessment within a resource utilization group system (RUGS). Reimbursement for home health services also shifted to a PPS.

The BBA also states that discharge from hospitals to SNFs or home care for 10 common but as yet unpublished diagnosis-related groups (DRGs) is to be considered as a transfer for payment purposes. Medicare's goal was to make a single blended payment that combined the traditional hospital DRG payment and the payment for postacute care services to be shared by the providers.

The intended implications for practice included reduced reimbursement to some SNFs, fewer discharges from hospitals to independent facilities for subacute care or home care, and, thus, encouraged the creation of integrated delivery systems and managed care. In reality, however, it has become more difficult to find placement in SNFs for clients with complex needs because the new reimbursement system simply does not fund all of their health care needs.

These reimbursement and regulatory changes surely represent only the beginning of such efforts to balance resources and need as the U.S. population continues to age. Certainly, significant work lies ahead for advocates of quality older-adult care in the United States and the world. Nurses will play a vital role in the ensuing debates, for they will see firsthand the positive and negative outcomes of their clients.

CRITICAL THINKING

Nurse Advocate

How can you, as a nurse, advocate for your older clients?

CASE STUDY

N.O., a 72-year-old man, was admitted to a skilled care facility for rehabilitation after an open reduction/internal fixation of the right hip. N.O. had fallen while going up the stairs of his home, suffering an intertrochanteric, comminuted fracture of the right femur. He has no recollection of what caused him to fall. He is married and, until his surgery, was working part time as a school-crossing guard. While in the hospital, N.O. exhibited mental status changes, including disorientation and confusion. His wife reports that he never had this problem before the surgery. He is continent of bowel and bladder. N.O. was in relatively good health until the fall. He and his wife agree that he should return home after rehabilitation is complete.

The following questions will guide your development of a nursing care plan for the case study.

1. Identify specific admission assessments that would be required for N.O. because of his age and condition.
2. Identify complications for which N.O. is at risk.
3. List interventions to prevent each complication.
4. Cite possible reasons for N.O.'s fall.
5. Describe methods for assessing N.O.'s mental status.
6. Describe possible reasons for his altered mental status.
7. Write three individualized nursing diagnoses and goals for N.O.
8. List nursing actions related to altered mental status.
9. List four successful outcomes for N.O.
10. Develop a teaching plan for N.O.
11. List the community resources N.O. may need after discharge.

SUMMARY

- The older adult population is rapidly growing.
- Although many stereotypes and myths are associated with aging, older adults are in fact very diverse in their characteristics.
- Health maintenance is as important for older adults as it is for younger persons. A healthy lifestyle can enhance the quality of life.
- Many changes are associated with aging. The disorders commonly seen among older adults are often the results of pathology and are thus not considered a normal part of aging; however, the risk of acquiring these disorders increases with age.
- Nurses knowledgeable about aging can plan interventions that will prevent complications for which older adults are at risk.
- Nurses have a responsibility to advocate for their older clients. Nurses should be active legislatively and should work collaboratively to develop older-adult care services that are affordable, provide equal access for all older Americans, and promote optimal wellness and independence.

REVIEW QUESTIONS

1. The senior citizens center has requested a nurse to speak to its members on the effects of aging. Which statement would be included in the presentation?
   1. All people eventually become senile if they live long enough.
   2. People lose interest in sex as they age.
   3. Most older adults are financially impoverished.
   4. Incontinence is not an expected or normal change of aging.
2. A student nurse is reading a book on the theories of aging. You know the student understands the programmed aging theory if the student states that:
   1. "Stress causes structural and chemical changes in the body, which, in turn, cause aging."
   2. "A genetic clock determines the speed at which people age."
   3. "Changes in collagen are the cause of aging."
   4. "The decreasing ability to produce T-cell differentiation causes aging."
3. The nurse is reviewing preventive respiratory tract infection care with an older adult client. A preventive instruction would include:
   1. obtaining an influenza vaccine each year.
   2. staying inside throughout the winter.
   3. avoiding exercise.
   4. limiting fluid intake.
4. The family of an older adult client is requesting information about the appropriate amount of exercise needed to maintain musculoskeletal function in their family member. As a nurse you would explain that:
   1. weight-bearing exercise is not recommended for older adults.
   2. high-intensity resistance training can improve muscle strength in older adults.
   3. muscle deterioration in older adults is to be expected.
   4. walking is the only healthy exercise for older adults.
5. While assisting an older client during bathing, the client asks "What is causing all of my skin problems?" How should the nurse respond?
   1. "The increased glandular secretions cause pruritus."
   2. "The increased capillary blood flow reduces body temperature."
   3. "The melanin production results in loss of hair."
   4. "The increased vascular fragility leads to ecchymosis."
6. The nurse assesses bilateral ectropion and presbycusis on an older client. As care is being planned, the nurse should:
   1. refer the client to a dermatologist and otologist for treatment.
   2. ask the nursing technician to obtain a walker for the client.
   3. provide additional fluids and extra protein in the client's diet.
   4. use a low-pitched voice to give the client directions while instilling artificial tears into his eyes.
7. The nurse is preparing medications for a newly admitted client. The medication sheet states the client is 95 years old. Which of the following age-related changes would the nurse expect to find which will increase the risk for drug toxicity?
   1. Faint pedal pulses and low body temperature.
   2. Loss of bone density and decreased blood flow.
   3. Urinary incontinence and thoracic rigidity.
   4. Dry skin and decreased heart conduction time.
8. An older adult nursing home client frequently repeats his World War II stories. The nursing assistant complains she is tired of hearing about his war stories. How should the nurse respond?
   1. "Yes, I'm tired of hearing about those war stories, too."
   2. "Reminiscing is good to help maintain long-term memory and self esteem."

3. "Whenever he starts to repeat another war story, change the subject."
4. "Just pretend you're listening to the war stories, so you won't hurt his feelings."

9. Your older adult client complains he feels bloated. Upon reading the chart, you note he has gained 2.5 pounds since yesterday. This 2.5 pounds would be equivalent to approximately how many milliliters of body fluid?
   1. 1000 mL
   2. 800 mL
   3. 600 mL
   4. 400 mL

10. A family member of a client with dementia asks the nurse the difference between delirium and dementia. The best response would be:
    1. dementia is a reversible confusion which is treatable.
    2. delirium is a chronic confusion with remissions and exacerbations.
    3. dementia is a slow progressive confusion which is irreversible.
    4. delirium is an acute confusion which is irreversible.

REFERENCES/SUGGESTED READING

Administration on Aging (AoA). (2001). The Administration on Aging and the Older American's Act. Retrieved from www.aoa.dhhs.gov/aoa/pages/aoafact.html

Administration on Aging (AoA). (2002). Income and poverty among the elderly. Retrieved from http://www.aoa.gov

Administration on Aging (AoA). (2009a). A profile of older Americans: 2008: Future growth. Retrieved August 4, 2009 from http://www.aoa.gov/AoARoot/Aging_Statistics/Profile/2008/4.aspx

Administration on Aging (AoA). (2009b). A profile of older Americans: 2008: The older population. Retrieved August 4, 2009 from http://www.aoa.gov/AoARoot/Aging_Statistics/Profile/2008/3.aspx

American Association of Retired Persons (AARP). (1998). *A profile of older Americans.* Washington, DC: Department of Health and Human Services.

Andersen, C. (1999). *Antecedents, correlates, and impact of violent behaviors in the elderly VA client.* Unpublished thesis, University of Iowa, Iowa City, IA.

Andersen, C. (1998). *Nursing student to nursing leader: The critical path to leadership development.* Clifton Park, NY: Delmar Cengage Learning.

Bendix, J. (2009). Exploiting the elderly. *RN,* 72(3), 42–46.

Bray, B., Van Sell, S., & Miller-Anderson, M. (2007). Stress incontinence: It's no laughing matter. *RN,* 70(4), 25–29.

Bulechek, G., Butcher, H., McCloskey, J., & Dochterman, J., eds. (2008). *Nursing Interventions Classification (NIC)* (5th ed.). St. Louis, MO: Mosby/Elsevier.

Covell, C., Graziano, J., Rich, D., & Tobin, K. (2007). New outlook for age-related macular degeneration. *Nursing2007,* 37(3), 22–24.

Centers for Medicare & Medicaid Services (CMS). (2002). Medicare aged and disabled enrollees by type of coverage. Retrieved from http://cms.hhs.gov/statistics/enrollment/natltrends/hi_smi.asp

Centers for Medicare & Medicaid Services (CMS). (2003). Medicare Part B physicians supplier data. Retrieved from http://cms.hhs.gov/data/betos/cy2001.asp

Centers for Medicare and Medicaid Services (CMS). (2009a). Medicare & you *2009.* Retrieved August 7, 2009 from http://www.medicare.gov/Publications/Pubs/pdf/10050.pdf

Centers for Medicare and Medicaid Services (CMS). (2009b). Medicare coverage – general information overview. Retrieved August 7, 2009 from http://www.cms.hhs.gov/CoverageGenInfo/

Centers for Medicare and Medicaid Services (CMS). (2009c). Now Medicare covers more than ever. Retrieved August 7, 2009 from http://www.cms.hhs.gov/AIAN/Downloads/CMS-11142-N.pdf

Collins, J. (2002). Helping an older patient eat well to stay well. *Nursing2002, 32*(11), 32hn6–32hn8.

Dowling-Castronovo, A., & Specht, J. (2009). Assessment of transient urinary incontinence in older adults. *American Journal of Nursing, 109*(2), 62–71.

Estes, M. (2010). *Health assessment & physical examination* (4th ed.). Clifton Park, NY: Delmar Cengage Learning.

Flaherty, E. (2008). Using pain-rating scales with older adults. *American Journal of Nursing,* 108(6), 40–47.

Gallo, J., Paveza, G., & Fulmer, T. (2005). *Handbook of geriatric assessment.* Gaithersburg, MD: Jones & Bartlett.

Hamilton, S. (2001). Detecting dehydration & malnutrition in the elderly. *Nursing2001, 31*(12), 56–57.

Hogstel, M. (Ed.). (2001). *Gerontology: Nursing care of the older adult.* Clifton Park, NY: Delmar Cengage Learning.

Kimbell, S. (2001). Before the fall: Keeping your patient on his feet. *Nursing2001, 31*(8), 44–45.

Kurtzman, E., & Buerhaus, P. (2008). New Medicare payment rules: Danger or opportunity for nursing? *American Journal of Nursing, 108*(6), 30–35.

Logue, R. (2002). Self-medication and the elderly: How technology can help. *AJN, 102*(7), 51–55.

Manno, M., & Hayes, D. (2006). How medication reconciliation saves lives. *Nursing 2006, 36*(3), 63–64.

Massachusetts Institute of Technology (MIT). (2009). Innovations. Retrieved August 4, 2009 from http://web.mit.edu/agelab/index.shtml

Mezey, M., Mitty, & E. (2006). The teaching nursing home: Models for training clinicians in geriatrics. *American Journal of Nursing, 106*(10), 72.

Moorhead, S., Johnson, M., Maas, M., & Swanson, E. (2007). *Nursing Outcomes Classification (NOC)* (4th ed.). St. Louis, MO: Mosby.

Napoli, M. (2009). The marketing of osteoporosis. *American Journal of Nursing, 109*(4), 58–61.

National Council on Aging (NCOA) (2002). Facts about older Americans. Retrieved from http://www.ncoa.org/content.cfm5sectionID.106

National Institute on Aging. (2009). What's your aging IQ? Retrieved August 4, 2009 from http://www.niapublications.org/quiz/index.php

Peskin, B. (1999). *Beyond the zone.* Houston, TX: Noble.

Sharts-Hopko, N., & Glynn-Milley, C. (2009). Primary open-angle glaucoma. *American Journal of Nursing, 109*(2), 40–47.

Shepler, S., Grogan, T., & Pater, K. (2006). Keep your older patients out of medication trouble. *Nursing2006, 36*(9), 44–47.

Social Security Administration (SSA). (2000). The president signs the "Senior Citizens' Freedom to Work Act of 2000." Retrieved from www.ssa.gov/legislation/legis_bulletin_040700.html

Steffen, K. (2003). When your trauma patient is over 65. *Nursing2003, 33*(4), 53–56.

Stein, A. (2003). Aging is more than skin deep. *Nursing2003, 33*(2), 32hn7–32hn8.

Stockdell, R., & Amella, E. (2008). The Edinburgh feeding evaluation in dementia scale. *American Journal of Nursing, 108*(8), 46–53.

Victor, K. (2001). Properly assessing pain in the elderly. *RN,* 64(5), 45–49.

Wallhagen, M., Pettengill, E., & Whiteside, M. (2006). Sensory impairment in older adults: Part 1: Hearing loss. *American Journal of Nursing, 106*(10), 40–48.

Wilkinson, J. (1999). *A family caregiver's guide to planning and decision making for the elderly.* Minneapolis, MN: Fairview Press.

RESOURCES

Administration on Aging (AoA), http://www.aoa.gov

American Association for Geriatric Psychiatry, http://www.aagpgpa.org

American Association of Retired Persons (AARP), http://www.aarp.org

American Geriatrics Society, http://www.americangeriatrics.org

American Nurses Association (ANA), Council on Gerontological Nursing Practice, http://www.nursingworld.org

National Council on Aging (NCOA), http://www.ncoa.org

UNIT 17 Nursing Care of the Client: Health Care in the Community

CHAPTER 51

Ambulatory, Restorative, and Palliative Care in Community Settings

MAKING THE CONNECTION

Refer to the following chapters to increase your understanding of nursing care within ambulatory/urgent, rehabilitative/restorative, home health, long-term, palliative, and hospice care settings:

Basic Nursing

- ***Legal and Ethical Responsibilities***
- ***Arenas of Care***
- ***Communication***
- ***Client Teaching***
- ***Nursing Process/Documentation/Informatics***
- ***Life Span Development***
- ***Cultural Considerations***
- ***Stress, Adaptation, and Anxiety***
- ***End-of-Life Care***
- ***Wellness Concepts***
- ***Complementary/Alternative Therapies***
- ***Assessment***
- ***Pain Management***

Adult Health Nursing

- ***The Older Adult***

LEARNING OBJECTIVES

Upon completion of this chapter, you should be able to:

- Define key terms.
- List reasons for a significant change in the growth of nonacute care services.
- Describe the differences between Medicaid and Medicare.
- Explain the role of the licensed practical nurse/vocational nurse (LPN/VN) as a member of the interdisciplinary health care team in various health care settings.
- Discuss the types of clients that would benefit from participation in a rehabilitation/restorative care program.
- Explain the responsibilities of the LPN/VN in ambulatory care, rehabilitation/restorative care nursing, nursing in long-term care, in-home care, and hospice.

KEY TERMS

adult day care
age-appropriate care
ambulatory care
assisted living
disability
extended care facility (ECF)
handicap
hospice
impairment
long-term care
managed care
minimum data set (MDS)
Outcomes and Assessment Information Set (OASIS)
palliative care
rehabilitation
reportable conditions
respite care
restorative care
telehealth
urgent care center

INTRODUCTION

There has been a strong emergence in the past decade of nonacute health care services. The growth of these services is a reflection of changes occurring in health care within the United States. These changes resulted in a vast increase in ambulatory/urgent care services, rehabilitation/restorative care, home health, long-term care, and hospice. There is an intermingling of services and settings under each of these categories of care. Restorative care, for example, may be provided in an acute care setting, in a rehabilitation hospital, in a long-term care facility, in an extended care facility with rehabilitation units, or in the client's home. Although many of the clients requiring these services are elderly, there is an increasing number of services specializing in pediatric care.

AMBULATORY AND URGENT CARE SETTINGS

The tremendous changes in the delivery of health care during the past several decades are expected to continue (Cicatiello, 2000). These changes have a direct impact on the environment where nurses practice. Decreasing reimbursement rates for health care are creating a competitive climate for physicians and other health care providers. Direct marketing of pharmaceuticals and renewed interest in alternative therapy is changing the expectations of people who seek health care solutions. U.S. populations are shifting, and the immigration of people to this country from other parts of the world requires increasingly complex ability on the part of nurses to communicate and interact effectively.

Providing care outside of a hospital is less costly for clients, their employers, and their insurers. Changes in healthcare policies and reimbursement rates during the past several decades have resulted in shorter hospital stays. That means that clients are being discharged before their need for medical and nursing interventions are completely resolved, which increases the need for outpatient follow-up.

AMBULATORY CARE SETTINGS

Ambulatory care settings are facilities where diagnosis, treatment, preventive care, and even restorative care are provided for clients on an outpatient basis. The client is able to walk in, receive care, and return home. The average American visits an ambulatory care center 4 times per year (National Center for Health Statistics, 2008). This number is increasing because the aging population increasingly requires the treatment and monitoring of chronic diseases. Ambulatory care settings are the primary site for health care delivery in this country.

Many types of ambulatory care exist and include health care provided at physician's offices, urgent care centers, and hospital emergency departments. Family practice clinic care is provided to clients of all ages and at all points on the health and wellness continuum. Specialty centers provide services such as family planning, ambulatory surgery, and oncology care. Other facilities provide care to a specific group of clients, for example primary care centers for Veterans and Indian Health Service. There are also specialty clinics (orthopedic, dermatologic, or urologic centers) defined by their providers.

Some clinics categorize clients according to their disease processes. There are nurse-run clinics for anticoagulation therapy, diabetes management, and hypertension. At these clinics, specially trained registered nurses coordinate care, provide educational services, and make treatment recommendations as a delegated medical function.

Another cost-saving effort is the development of **managed care**, a system where a case management individual or team controls what specialists the client sees, as well as the frequency or duration of that specialty care. Within these systems, primary care clinics often serve as gatekeepers for clients, who must receive an initial evaluation by their provider before receiving a referral for specialty services. Although managed care reduces unnecessary health care expenditures, it is a source of frustration for clients who perceive it as a loss of control and independence.

CARE PROVIDED IN AMBULATORY/URGENT CARE CENTERS

Traditionally, medical clinics provided preventive, wellness, and illness family-centered care, where the client forms a relationship with the same provider or group of providers over time. Changing health care needs brought about **urgent care centers**, facilities designed for the effective and efficient treatment of acute illnesses and injuries. At an urgent care center, clients receive many of the same services they receive at a traditional medical clinic. Clients do not require an appointment, they do not see the same provider consistently, and they are usually seen either in the order of arrival or the order of acuity. An urgent care center is fast paced similar to a hospital emergency department and serves the needs of an increasingly busy, mobile population. Clients with severe trauma or who have life-threatening conditions, such as chest pain or respiratory distress, typically are rerouted to a hospital emergency room, where appropriate interventions are provided.

An innovation in health care delivery is the development of nonemergent clinics that are cropping up to provide rapid care for minor illnesses. These clinics are located in shopping malls and grocery stores and provide care to clients who are in a hurry. They are often staffed by advanced practice nurses who specialize in providing treatment for non-complicated cases while offering client convenience.

Ambulatory Care Nurses

Within the ambulatory care setting, one may find nurses at every educational level, including practical, associate degree, baccalaureate degree, and advanced practice nurses. It is vital for the ambulatory care nurse to have strong interpersonal communication skills and a high level of maturity to function effectively as part of the health care team.

The focus of the visit may be as simple as routine blood work or a complex procedure or treatment. In most cases, clients return home after receiving care within a relatively short time. Within this timeframe, the nurse collects pertinent data and assesses the client quickly and efficiently, as shown in Figure 51-1. The nurse provides **age-appropriate care**, taking into consideration the client's physical, mental, emotional, and spiritual developmental level. Health care is adapting to reflect the needs of society despite soaring costs, limited reimbursement, and an increasingly diverse and aging population.

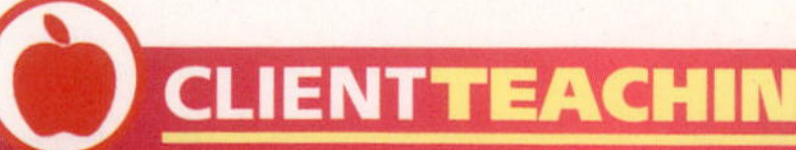

CLIENT TEACHING

Client Teaching in an Ambulatory Care Setting

The nurse in an ambulatory care setting relinquishes control over much of the treatment the client ultimately receives versus the care received in a hospital setting and understands that thorough and appropriate client education is vital to ensure adequate understanding of, and compliance with, medical treatment. For example, the nurse cannot be sure that the client will fill his prescription and, if he does fill it, that the medication will be taken as ordered or for the length of time indicated. The nurse accepts the responsibility of providing education to the client to ensure this result. The nurse customizes education to the client's age, socioeconomic status, educational and cognitive level, and health status.

LEGAL ISSUES

As our society changes and technology continues to take a more important position in the workplace, nurses are faced with extraordinary ethical and legal challenges. All nurses receive education to help them understand the challenges and make wise decisions in their practice. Whether nurses are practicing in a hospital, clinic, long-term care facility, or in the client's home, they must be prepared to act within safe and legal parameters. In the ambulatory care setting, the legal issues that most likely occur center on confidentiality, obtaining consent to treat, care of a minor, and reportable conditions.

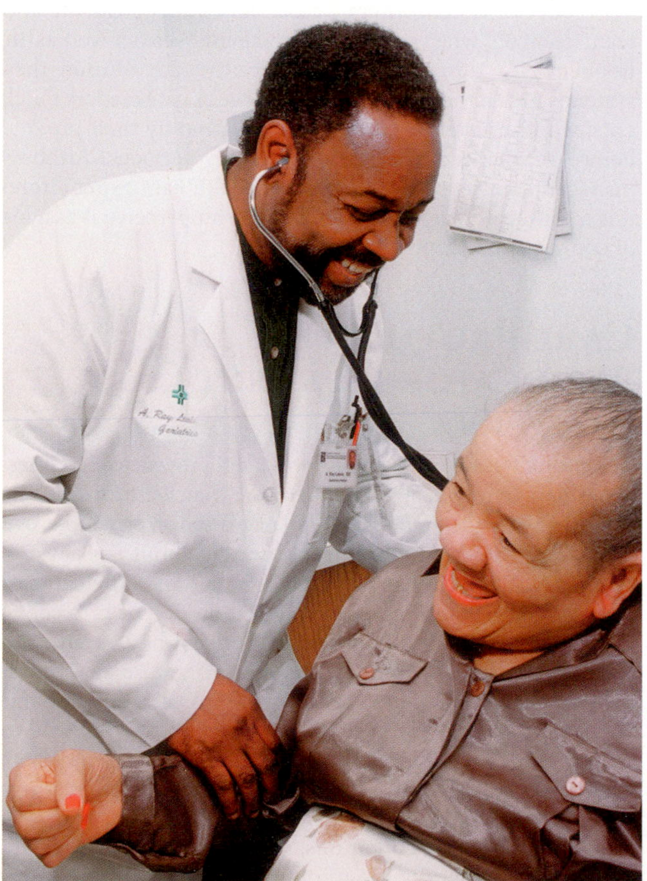

COURTESY OF DELMAR CENGAGE LEARNING

Figure 51-1 A nurse is collecting pertinent data from a client in an ambulatory care center.

Confidentiality

Protecting client's medical confidentiality is part of a nurse's ethical responsibility. In 1996, the Health Insurance Portability and Accountability Act, or HIPAA, became law. This legislation was enacted with several purposes—to simplify health care administration, to assure the portability of insurance coverage for pre-existing conditions, and to provide standardization of electronic billing and claims settlement.

HIPAA requirements mandate that access to protected health information is limited only to those who are authorized to receive that information and who need the information to provide care. The law also requires that adequate security measures are in place to safeguard protected health information

PROFESSIONAL TIP

Workload Stress

Work management is one of the biggest stressors of nurses working in an ambulatory care setting. According to Swan and Griffin (2005), nursing workload measurement is influenced by the number of clients who present for care, the characteristics of the clients, and the characteristics of the nursing role. Ambulatory care settings require the nurse to work quickly and efficiently to provide care and teaching to clients.

CRITICAL THINKING

HIPPA

L.W. is a nurse in a busy obstetrical/gynecological clinic. Another nurse has just completed care of a client and cleaned the examination room. As L.W. enters the room with a new client, she sees that the nurse left the previous client's chart open on the computer screen in clear view of the new client and herself.

1. What should L.W. do to protect the privacy of the previous client?
2. What measures can be taken to prevent this potential HIPPA violation from occurring again?

where it is stored or used (Futch & Phillips, 2003). This legislation has provided uniformity from facility to facility and from state to state in the management and protection of client health information. All individuals who are involved in the procuring or storing of medical information, or those who may come across medical information in their work, are required to receive HIPPA training on an annual basis.

Consent to Treat

When selected invasive procedures are performed in an office setting, it is necessary to obtain a consent form signed by the client. The information the client receives before signing is provided by the physician and includes possible procedure risks as well as the benefits. The nurse's role is to witness the client's signature and provide any necessary clarification or explanation after the physician provides the basic information.

Treatment of a Minor

Another legal issue that may arise in an ambulatory care setting concerns the care of a minor. Two frequently asked questions are whether the minor receives treatment when a parent or legal guardian is not present and whether the minor's medical information is released to parents. This comes into question particularly with an older child, most often in the areas of mental health and reproductive health. Legislation regarding these issues varies from state to state, and it is important for nurses to know the statutes in the state where they practice to meet legal requirements.

The nurse encounters ethical issues regarding the care of a vulnerable adult, such as a person who is developmentally challenged. In most cases, there is a guardian appointed to provide support to the vulnerable adult and serve as their advocate in a medical setting.

Reportable Conditions

The nurse notes **reportable conditions**, diseases or injuries that the government requires to be reported to the appropriate authority or agency, and the protocol to follow in reporting these conditions. Reportable conditions include suspected abuse and/or neglect, sexually transmitted infections (i.e., STIs), and certain other contagious illnesses that could threaten the health of the general public. These fall under state regulation and vary from state to state.

CRITICAL THINKING

Teenage Ambulatory Care Client

T.G., age 16, presents to the clinic unaccompanied by a parent. T.G. wants the health care provider to give her oral contraceptives. She tells the nurse, "My boyfriend and I are having sex. I cannot talk to my parents about it because they would be very upset with me. I am old enough to make my own decisions and I do not want to have an unplanned pregnancy. Please let me talk to the doctor." The nurse knows that the state where they practice requires parental consent for a minor child to receive non-emergent medical care.

1. What should the nurse tell T.G.?
2. If the nurse believes that T.G. has the right to contraceptive care without parental consent, how does the nurse resolve the conflict between ethical beliefs and legal requirements?

REHABILITATION/RESTORATIVE CARE

Rehabilitation and restorative care are used interchangeably. The goal of **rehabilitation** (rehab) is to assist individuals in reaching their optimal physical, mental, and psychosocial functioning level. This goal is accomplished by preventing complications, modifying the effects of the disability, and increasing independence. **Restorative care** is an organized, methodical interdisciplinary program that thoroughly evaluates the client's feelings, thoughts, lifestyle, and physical abilities with the goal of restoring and maintaining each individual's performance potential. An emphasis is on improving the client's self esteem by having them manage as much self care as possible by focusing on potential rather than limitations (Resnick & Fleishell, 2002) (See Figure 51-2). For the restorative staff to know the functional level of an individual, the team uses measurement instruments or tools to assess the functional status. The functional areas assessed are called activities of daily living (ADL). These include bathing, grooming, eating, toileting, and dressing. Also assessed are instrumental activities of daily living (IADL). These tasks include meal preparation, shopping, management of money, taking medication, and housekeeping. Restorative care is concerned with increasing the client's ability to complete basic ADL and IADL (See Figure 51-3).

Minimum Data Set

The **minimum data set (MDS)** is an assessment tool for assessing resident's physical, psychological, and psychosocial functioning in a Medicare and Medicaid-certified, long-term care facility. Refer to Box 51-1 for an example of an MDS

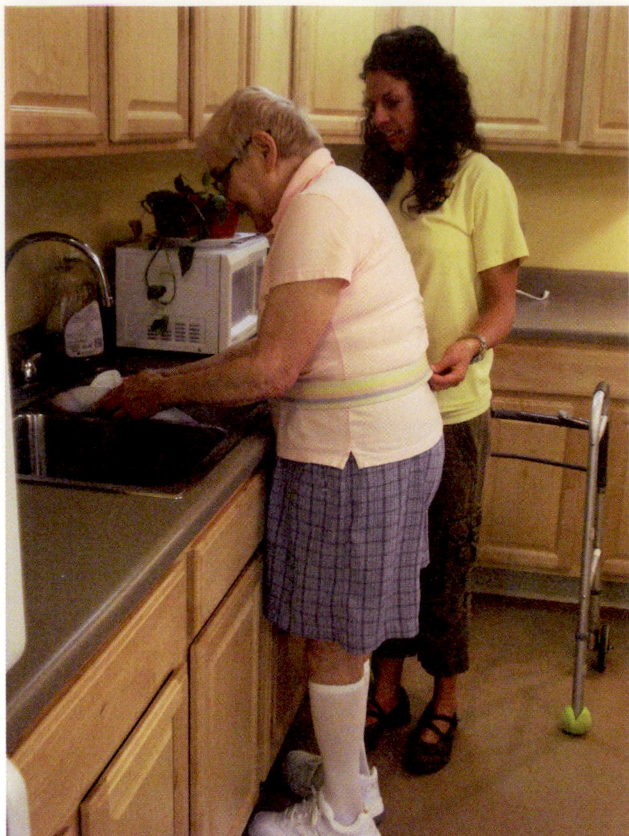

FIGURE 51-2 **An occupational therapist teaches ADL to a client. The kitchen is in a rehabilitation unit.** (*Courtesy of Kingston Residence of Fort Wayne, Fort Wayne, IN.*)

areas of assessment. Medicare and Medicaid use the MDS as a reimbursement tool. The MDS is completed upon the resident's admission to the extended care facility and at regular time intervals set by federal policy. After reviewing the MDS data, the interdisciplinary team (MDS coordinator, director of nursing, dietitian, activities director, social worker, and director of therapy departments) completes a care plan to assist the resident in reaching their full potential while living in the facility.

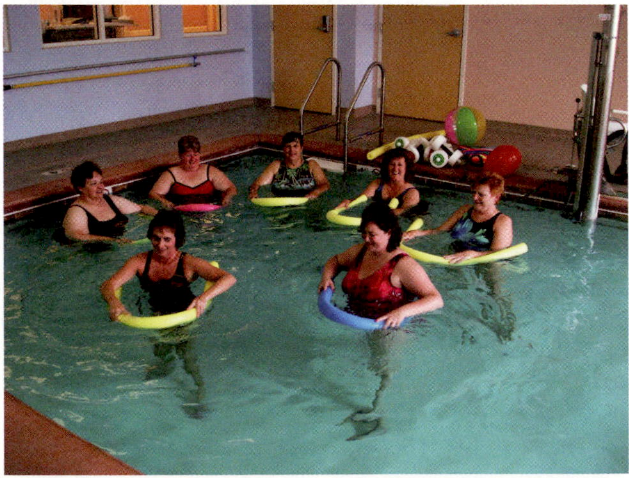

FIGURE 51-3 **Pool therapy in a rehabilitation unit assists individuals in reaching their optimal physical, mental, and psychosocial functioning level.** (*Courtesy of Kingston Residence of Fort Wayne, Fort Wayne, IN.*)

BOX 51-1 MDS ASSESSMENT AREAS

Cognitive patterns
Communication/hearing patterns
Vision patterns
Mood and behavior patterns
Psychosocial well-being
Physical functioning and structural problems
Continence in last 14 days
Disease diagnoses
Health conditions
Oral/nutritional status
Oral/dental status
Skin condition
Activity patterns
Medications
Special treatments and procedures
Discharge potential and overall status
Therapy supplement

Interdisciplinary Health Care Team

The interdisciplinary health care team, as shown in Table 51-1, is an essential component to any restorative care process. The client and family are the focus of the team and are encouraged to participate in the planning of care. The degree of family participation is determined by the client. The professional members of the team are selected based on the needs of the client (See Figure 51-4).

Roles of the Interdisciplinary Health Care Team

The interdisciplinary health care team assesses, maintains, and evaluates the abilities of individuals in need of functional therapy. The physical therapist develops a specific exercise program to improve or maintain physical mobility, function, and strength as shown in Figure 51-5. The occupational therapist assesses individuals to regain or maintain their ADLs. Occupational therapy includes the use of assistive devices to reach a needed item, or

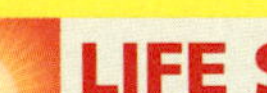

LIFE SPAN CONSIDERATIONS

Pneumonia and Urinary Tract Infections in the Elderly

A study by Lim and Macfarlane (2001) showed that those who are elderly and in long-term care display more functional impairment when they have pneumonia than the same populace in the community. Clients with urinary tract infections who are asymptomatic also have decreased functional abilities. An MDS assessment effectively reveals the declined function level in elderly clients with pneumonia and urinary tract infections (Goldrick, 2005).

TABLE 51-1 Interdisciplinary Health Care Team Roles

TEAM MEMBER	ROLE
Nurse	See text for description of roles
Physician or physiatrist	Prescribe medical and pharmacological treatment
Physical therapist	Muscle and joint training
Occupational therapist	Fine muscle training, self-care skills
Nutritionist	Assess for caloric intake
Speech therapist	Swallow evaluations, speech retraining
Psychologist	Test for cognitive, emotional, and psychological function; counseling for grief, loss, and depression
Social worker	Evaluate need for financial resources, community resources; counseling family issues
Visiting nurse	Evaluation of home setting; assess, teach, and coordinate home care
Vocational counselor	Vocational retraining, adaptation of work setting
Recreational therapist	Provides socialization opportunities; teaches how to adapt to community
Respiratory therapist	Treatment of respiratory or ventilatory equipment problems
Clergy	Spiritual counseling
Clinical nurse specialist	Case management

From *Nursing Fundamentals: Caring and Clinical Decision Making* (2nd ed.), by R. Daniels, R. Grendell, & F. Wilkins, 2010, Clifton Park, NY: Delmar Cengage Learning.

pull up socks, or move a leg after a stroke or knee replacement. The speech therapist is the professional who assesses disabilities involving speech, communication whether spoken or written, and swallowing ability. All of these individuals are professionally trained to complete these tasks.

The social worker is a professionally trained individual who assists in the admissions process. Resident and family questions or concerns are usually addressed by a social worker in an extended care facility.

A pharmacist reviews the resident's medications monthly and oversees that the facility is meeting federal state regulations. If the resident's physician does not serve the facility, a medical director provides medical care to the resident and also to any residents in need of a physician while in the extended care facility. Depending on the facility, a dentist, podiatrist, and psychologist are available every month to every three months as needed.

Each discipline completes an assessment and pools this information at the care planning conference so that a consensus among members, including the client and family, are reached. The team process avoids both duplication of services and fragmented care. A holistic approach is used so that the client's physical, mental, and psychosocial needs are identified (Wenckus, 1995).

Role of the LPN/VN

Restorative nursing is a specialty practice and requires specialized knowledge, skills, and attitudes. A sound knowledge base in anatomy and physiology of the neurological, musculoskeletal, gastrointestinal, and urological systems is a prerequisite. The nurse has excellent clinical skills in the areas of therapeutic positioning, range of joint motion exercises, transfers, ambulation, and ADLs, as shown in Figure 51-6. The nurse is responsible for planning measures to prevent complications such as impaired skin integrity and contractures and to implement interventions for dysphagia, incontinence, and other identified problems.

The nurse is a member of the interdisciplinary team and functions as caregiver, counselor, coordinator of care, and client advocate (Mauk, 2007). The nurse seeks to understand the roles and responsibilities and to interrelate with each discipline. There is a steady demand for restorative nurses in all settings.

Nurses are advocates for the older adults and their families in the health care system. The nurse is aware of the residents needs and refers them to the appropriate health care service. The nurse continues to work alongside the health care services to reinforce the older adult's optimal health promotion and wellness.

Functional Assessment and Evaluation for Rehabilitation/Restoration

Terms such as disability, impairment, and handicap describe functional levels. **Disability** is an individual's lack of ability to complete an activity in the normal manner. **Impairment** refers to an abnormal psychological or physiologic behavior or an anatomic loss, such as a loss of a limb (Eliopoulos, 2005). According to the Self-identification of Handicap form, **handicap** means the physical or mental inability to complete a role in one or more major ADL (U.S. Office of Personnel Management, 1987).

Clients who need restorative care are screened before admission to a program. Assessments are completed by health care professionals whose services may be required by the client (Figure 51-7). The purpose of screening is to select the best setting for services. Criteria for admission to a program usually require that the client be:

- Medically stable
- Able to learn
- Able to sit supported for at least one hour a day and to actively participate in the program

Interdisciplinary programs may stipulate that the client has disabilities in 2 or more areas of function:

- Mobility
- Performance of ADL

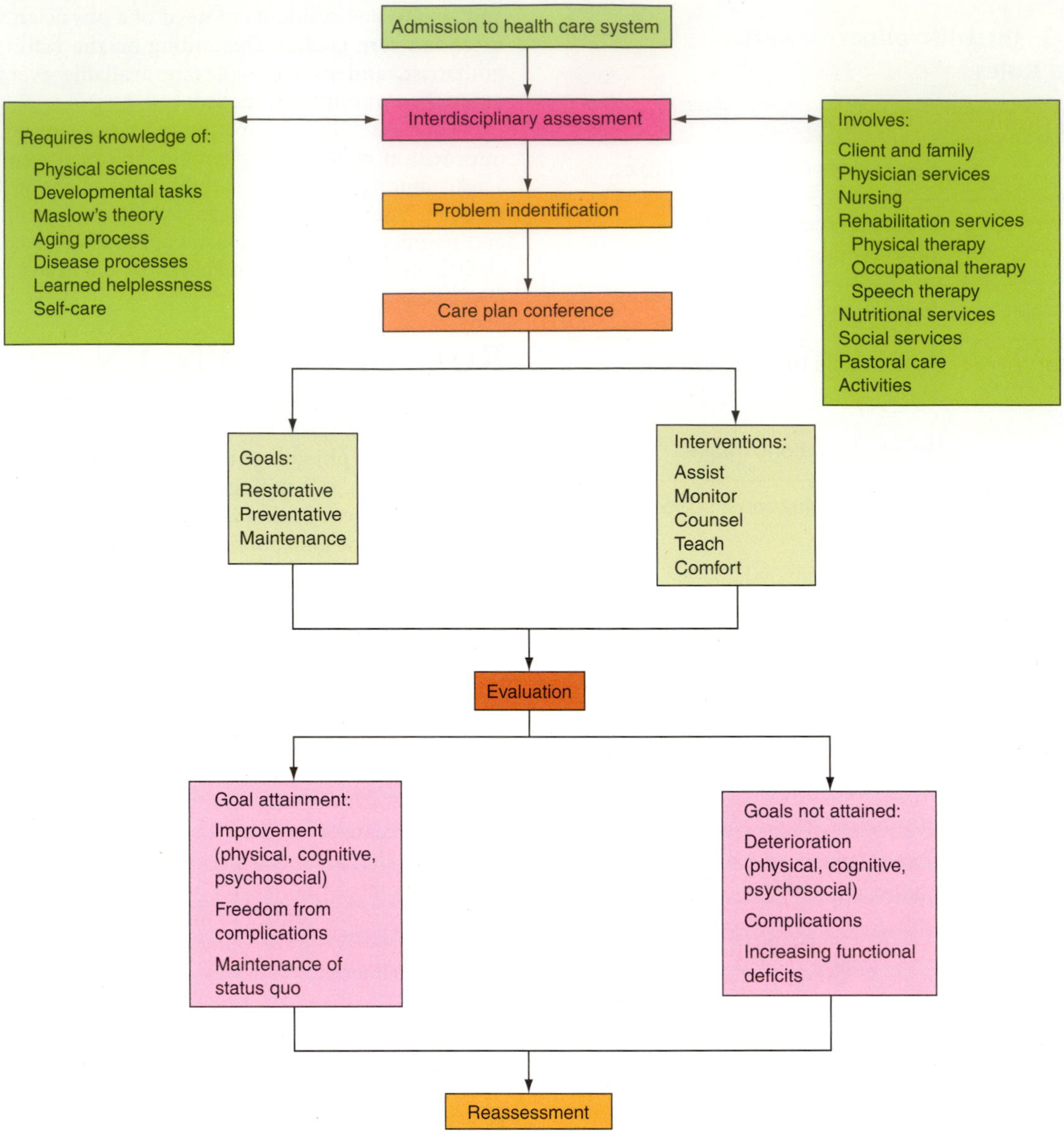

Admission to health care system

Interdisciplinary assessment

Requires knowledge of:
- Physical sciences
- Developmental tasks
- Maslow's theory
- Aging process
- Disease processes
- Learned helplessness
- Self-care

Involves:
- Client and family
- Physician services
- Nursing
- Rehabilitation services
  - Physical therapy
  - Occupational therapy
  - Speech therapy
- Nutritional services
- Social services
- Pastoral care
- Activities

Problem indentification

Care plan conference

Goals:
- Restorative
- Preventative
- Maintenance

Interventions:
- Assist
- Monitor
- Counsel
- Teach
- Comfort

Evaluation

Goal attainment:
- Improvement (physical, cognitive, psychosocial)
- Freedom from complications
- Maintenance of status quo

Goals not attained:
- Deterioration (physical, cognitive, psychosocial)
- Complications
- Increasing functional deficits

Reassessment

COURTESY OF DELMAR CENGAGE LEARNING

FIGURE 51-4 The Interdisciplinary Health Care Team Process

- Bowel and bladder control
- Cognition
- Emotional function
- Pain management
- Swallowing
- Communication

There are a number of standardized assessment instruments that are designed to evaluate motor function, cognition, speech and language, mobility, and the client's performance of ADLs.

ASSESSMENT OF ABILITIES

The Uniform Data System for Medical Rehabilitation (UDS) was developed by a grant from the U.S. Department of Education, National Institute on Disability and Rehabilitation Research. The UDS offers a uniform method to document a client's disability and medical rehabilitation, thereby providing a database of disability rehabilitation in more than 1,400 facilities with more than 13 million clients for standardized

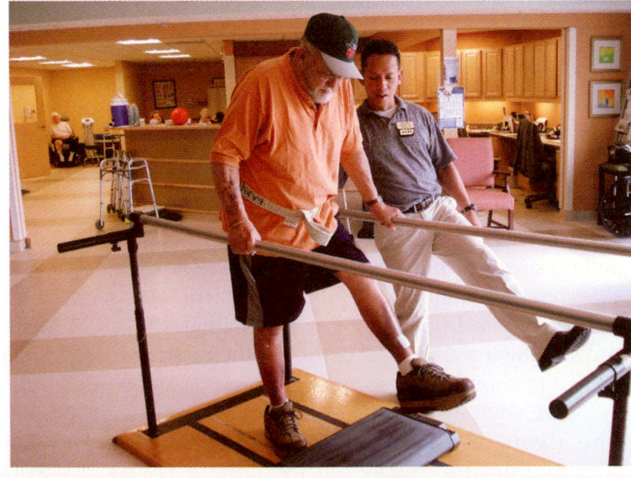

FIGURE 51-5 The physical therapist assists a client with a specific exercise program to improve or maintain physical mobility, function, and strength. (*Courtesy of Kingston Residence of Fort Wayne, Fort Wayne, IN.*)

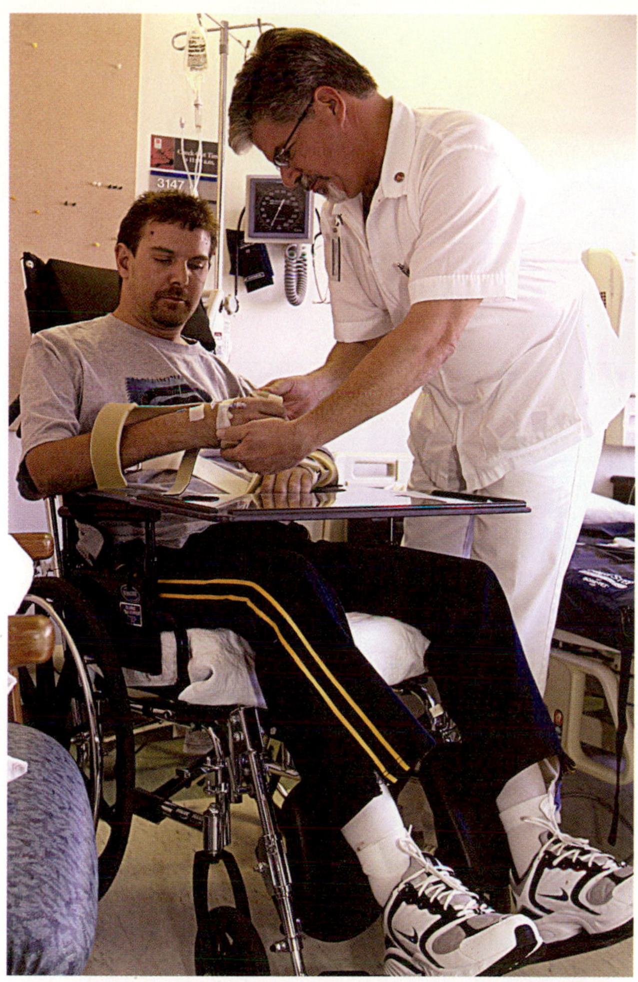

FIGURE 51-6 A nurse applies a splint to the arm of a rehabilitation client. (*Courtesy of Association of Rehabilitation Nurses.*)

rehabilitation comparison. The UDS measures impairment (function), disability (activity), and handicap (role).

There are several functional measurement tools to assess functional status. Three functional measurement tools are discussed in this chapter: Functional Independence Measure (FIM), Functional Assessment Measure (FAM), and the Barthel Index. The FIM and the FAM are more commonly used for the UDS.

Functional Independence Measure and Functional Assessment Measure

The FIM is an assessment tool that assesses cognitive and motor function status in relation to the amount of assistance needed to complete ADLs or IADL. Specific areas covered include independence in cognition problem solving, memory, communication, and social interaction. It also assesses physical independence in self care, control of bowel and bladder, transfers, and ambulation. The FIM is a widely used evaluation tool to review resident progress and rehabilitation/restorative outcomes.

The FAM assesses cognitive, behavioral, communication, and community functioning. The FAM is designed to use with the FIM (FIM+FAM) to provide a more comprehensive view of the rehabilitation client.

Barthel Index

The Barthel Index is a functional measurement tool that measures a person's level of independence in areas of self care and mobility. It is used in restorative care areas to predict length of stay and the amount of assisted care needed to complete ADL. The Barthel Index is included in the FIM and PULSES profile tools and only takes 5 minutes to complete.

These functional measurement tools assist in the objective documentation of changes that occur over time. With these tools, professionals recognize changes as they occur and promote optimal functional independence, which is the goal of restorative care.

Rehabilitation/Restorative Care Settings

Rehabilitation/restorative care settings are found in hospitals, extended care facilities with rehabilitation units, and rehabilitation hospitals as stand-alone facilities. Private rooms in hospitals and rehabilitation units are now the norm.

Special Beds

For residents with integumentary needs, whether they are the result of poor nutrition or poor circulation, there are special beds to aid in protecting the skin from breakdown. Pressure-relieving support surfaces, including special beds, mattresses, and mattress overlays, are available to support the body in bed. Special air-fluidized beds flow pressurized air through the oversized mattress to relieve pressure areas. A similar bed is a low-air-loss bed that works on the same principle of relieving pressure areas. Ring cushions (donuts) are not recommended because they cause fluid congestion and edema. None of these devices replace timely repositioning and assessing for skin breakdown on at risk residents. Repositioning the body decreases pressure point areas, and using positioning devices to raise vulnerable areas prone to pressure decreases skin breakdown. Pillows and foam wedges are placed between bony areas and under heels to relieve pressure points from the mattress. Avoid shearing force when moving residents in bed.

Urinary Devices

Incontinence causes skin tissue breakdown, and keeping the skin dry prevents skin breakdown. In the past, indwelling catheters were used. But years of research have proven that indwelling catheters cause urinary tract infections and are not used as frequently. For men, condom catheters are fit over the penis and drained into a leg bag. Other devices for men are urinary devices that act as an artificial sphincter for control of urinary incontinence. The male incontinence clamp attaches to the penis to restrict incontinence.

For women, there are medical devices to treat incontinence. One such device is a urethral insert, which is used in times of predictable incontinence, such as when taking part in an activity like running. The disposable device is a small tampon-like plug that inserts into the urethra to prevent leaking urine. These devices require a prescription and are not meant for everyday use. Another female urinary device is a pessary that is a stiff ring inserted into the vagina that holds up a prolapsed bladder or uterus to prevent leakage of urine. The device is worn all day and removed for cleaning on a regular basis.

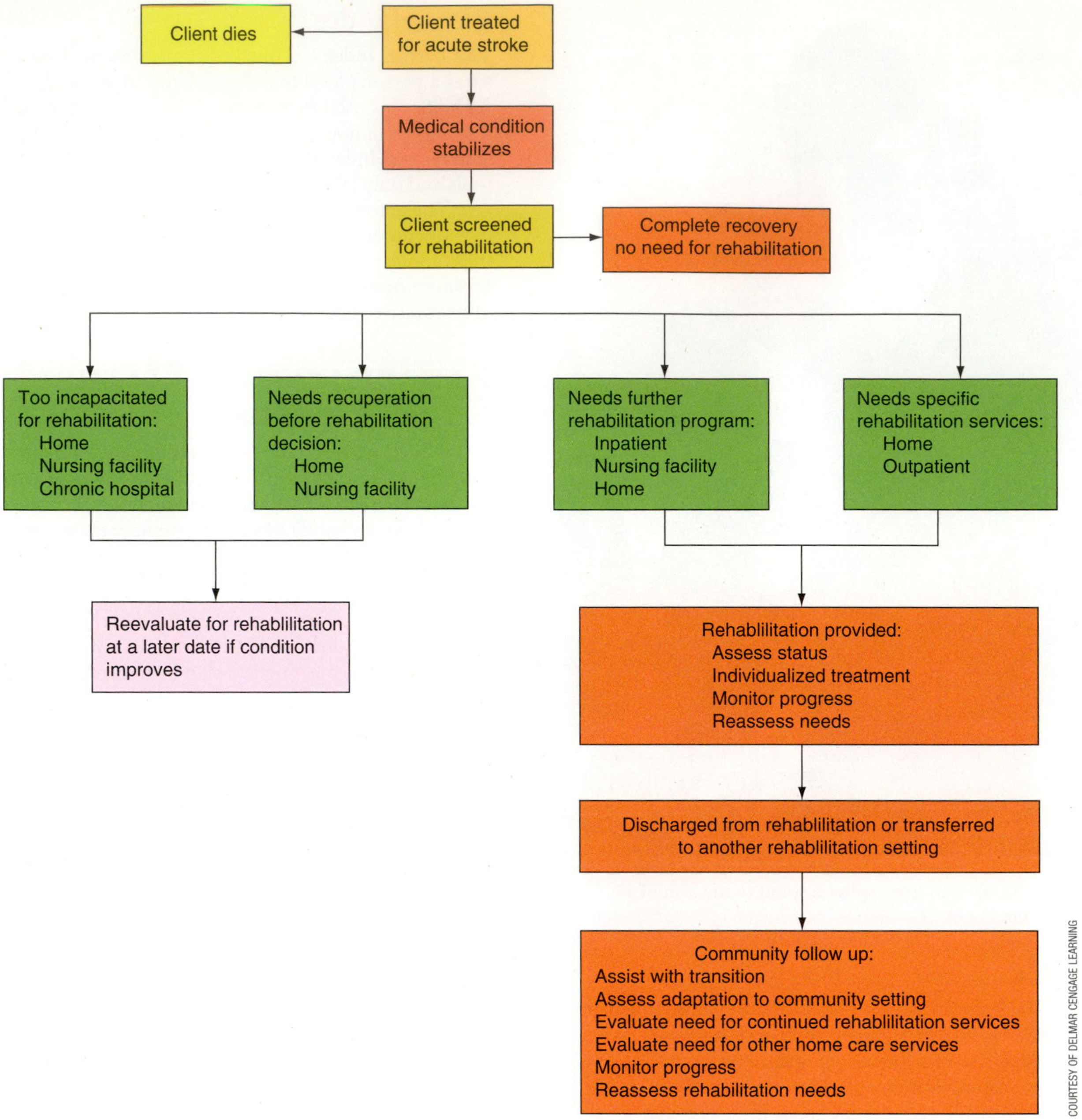

Client dies

Client treated for acute stroke

Medical condition stabilizes

Client screened for rehabilitation

Complete recovery no need for rehabilitation

Too incapacitated for rehabilitation:
Home
Nursing facility
Chronic hospital

Needs recuperation before rehabilitation decision:
Home
Nursing facility

Needs further rehabilitation program:
Inpatient
Nursing facility
Home

Needs specific rehabilitation services:
Home
Outpatient

Reevaluate for rehablilitation at a later date if condition improves

Rehablilitation provided:
Assess status
Individualized treatment
Monitor progress
Reassess needs

Discharged from rehablilitation or transferred to another rehablilitation setting

Community follow up:
Assist with transition
Assess adaptation to community setting
Evaluate need for continued rehablilitation services
Evaluate need for other home care services
Monitor progress
Reassess rehabilitation needs

COURTESY OF DELMAR CENGAGE LEARNING

FIGURE 51-7 Assessing Potential Stroke Rehabilitation

HOME HEALTH CARE

Home care encompasses a number of services delivered to persons in their homes and is one of the fastest-growing segments of health care delivery. Clients are receiving intravenous therapy, ventilator care, parenteral nutrition, and chemotherapy at home. Many agencies have nurse specialists on staff for complicated cases involving care required for wounds, intravenous therapy, diabetes, and cardiac or respiratory problems.

Medicare-certified agencies provide intermittent care to persons meeting the criteria for care. A registered nurse calls on the client a specified number of times each week to assess the client's condition, supervise the work of LPN/VNs and nonlicensed staff, and deliver skilled nursing care. Nursing assistants are assigned to give personal care; check vital signs; and do positioning, transfers, and passive range-of-motion exercises. In addition to nursing staff, the agency provides therapists and social workers to serve their clients. These services are time-limited by Medicare and are not reimbursable if the client is not deemed to require skilled care.

CRITICAL THINKING

Choosing Housing for a Family Member

How could a nurse assist an individual in evaluating an extended care facility for a family member?

TYPES OF HOME-BASED CARE

There are two types of home-based care. One type is professional and the other is technical.

Professional

The professional division is based on scientific theory and principles bound by legal and professional standards and guidelines with licensed and certified employees. Employees offering skilled services are nurses, therapists, social workers, and nursing assistants. Other additional services offered are homemaker assistance, meal preparation, cleaning, sitter services, and transportation to physician offices. **Respite care** provides the caregiver with a short break from providing care. This short break may be a period of hours, days, or even weeks.

Technical

The technical division is driven by products sold for profit, following guidelines for reimbursement of payment. Included in the technical division would be the home medical equipment services or durable medical equipment that provides hospital beds, wheelchairs, scooters, walkers, oxygen, and related equipment. Also included in this division is the intravenous or home-infusion service that supplies the client with intravenous equipment. Personnel from the home-infusion service either teach the caregiver how to run the equipment or teach the client how to administer the infusion. Therapies include tube feedings, hyperalimentation, antibiotics, blood or blood products, analgesics, or antineoplastics. Reimbursement payment is determined by insurance companies, managed care companies, and Medicare.

Home Visit Outcomes

In 1999, Medicare reimbursement requirements were mandated for home health agencies to validate client outcomes, quality improvement, and client satisfaction of care. An outcomes measurable tool called **Outcomes and Assessment Information Set (OASIS)** was developed and implemented to determine the care given and reimbursement required. OASIS data are reported to the Centers for Medicare and Medicaid Services. Each home health care agency uses this system to review the agencies' data results and compare their outcomes and client satisfaction to other similar agencies. Other home health care agencies, although not required by Medicare, use the Outcome Based Quality Improvement System to improve client outcomes.

Trends in Home Care

Home health care has evolved into a more technologic nursing care. Care within the home now includes apnea monitors, electrocardiographs, ventilators, parenteral nutrition, intravenous therapy, chemotherapy, chest tubes, and skeletal traction. Client x-rays are taken by mobile x-ray machines. The advanced technology provides client care without clients leaving their homes.

Telehealth

Telehealth is electronic information services that offer increased client and family participation. The nurse and client use interactive videos, telephone cardiac rate monitoring with EKG readout, digital subscriber lines, and internet transmission of data. Photos of client's wounds are viewed with an in-home computerized, two-way viewing screen. Home health care nurses use hand-held or laptop computers that hold the assessment and plan of care for each home care client. Most home health care facilities use an electronic clinical documentation system. The Centers for Medicare and Medicaid Services developed a computerized plan of care (Form 485) that is compatible with the home health care electronic system. Nurses electronically document their client assessments and delivery of nursing care on Form 485. The data are downloaded to the main frame computer in the main office for nurse managers to coordinate client care day or night. Through advanced technology, a nurse prioritizes the needs of the clients, implements a tighter control of nursing case management, and decreases the cost of health care.

Role of the Home Health Nurse

It is vital that the home health care nurse is experienced and knowledgeable in various disease processes seen in clients within the home setting. The nurse works alone, draws on previous experience, and knows when to call on or direct the client to community resources to meet the health needs of the client. The nurse has fine tuned assessment skills along with technological knowledge to use different equipment. The nurse manages home cases by using the federal government assessment and plan of care forms necessary for reimbursement. Communication techniques are crucial between all of the health team members.

Role of the LPN/VN

Although the role of the LPN is expanding, in 2006, 56,610 LPNs were working in home health care. This means that 7.5% of all employed LPNs worked in home care (Bureau of Labor Statistics, 2007). The responsibilities of the LPN/VN vary among agencies. All nurses working in home care must have excellent assessment skills and a keen ability to identify actual and potential problems. Teaching the client and family is a major responsibility for the home health nurse. Communication skills are essential as the nurse provides care to the client and meets the needs of the client's family (See Figure 51-8). The client with a chronic health problem will have ongoing needs after the home health care is discontinued. The home health nurse continually seeks out community resources to use in caring for clients. Clients and their family caregivers are taught the following:

The disease process

- Complications that may occur
- How to prevent the complications
- Signs and symptoms of the complications
- How to reduce risk factors such as dietary changes and exercise programs

Medications

- Actions of medications
- Special administration guidelines such as timing related to meals
- Side effects

Special skills

- Drawing up and administering insulin or other injectables
- Using a blood glucose monitor
- Changing dressings
- Monitoring vital signs

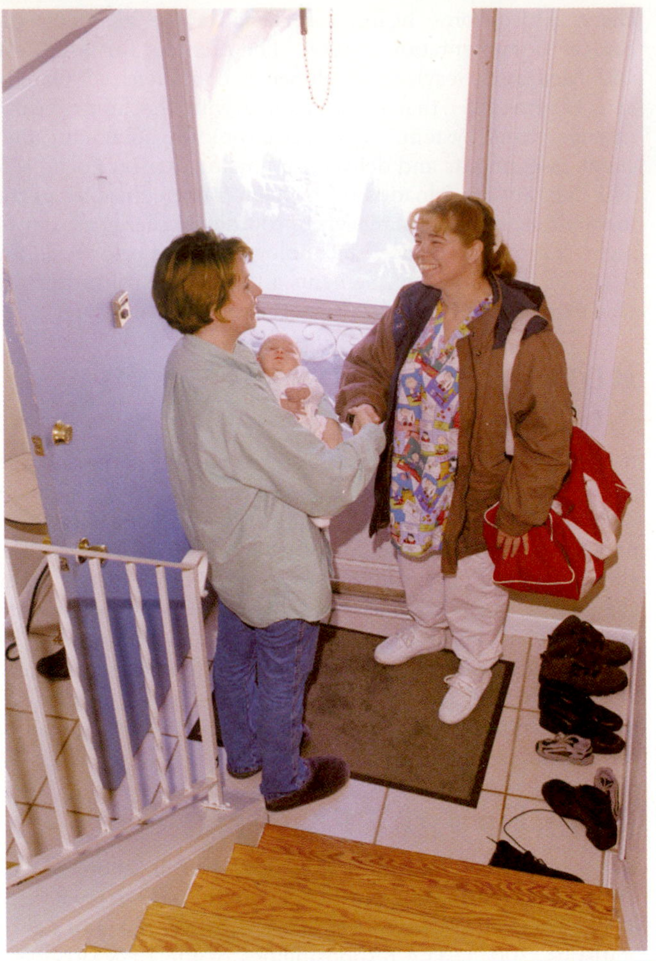

COURTESY OF DELMAR CENGAGE LEARNING

FIGURE 51-8 A home health nurse provides care to the client and meets the needs of the client's family.

- Using special client care equipment, adaptive devices, and assistive devices

Documentation and communication

- How to keep records for nurse or physician visit; for example, blood glucose, blood pressure, and weight
- Communication with health care providers
- How and when to contact the home health nurse
- How and when to contact the physician
- How and when to contact emergency services

FUTURE OF HOME HEALTH CARE

Home health care has met the challenges of changes in the past with OASIS and reimbursement requirements of Medicare. It is imperative that home health care agencies and nurses continue to use evidence-based research to implement improvements to client care that is cost effective and ensures quality of healthcare.

ASSISTED LIVING

Assisted living combines housing and services for persons who require assistance with ADLs. Nursing care is usually provided for an additional fee. These are persons who cannot live alone but who do not need 24-hour care. It is a less restrictive environment than a long-term care facility and maintains the individual's independence and freedom of choice. This level of care may be offered in a freestanding facility or as a section of a long-term care facility. A monthly fee is charged and covers rent, utilities, housekeeping services, meals, transportation, health promotion, exercise programs, and assistance with ADL. There are an estimated 36,000 assisted living residences in the United States, with more than 1 million residents (Assisted Living Federation of America, 2009).

ADULT DAY CARE

Adult day care centers are located in a separate unit of a long-term care facility, in a private home, or are freestanding. They provide a variety of services in a protective setting for adults who are unable to stay alone but who do not need 24-hour care. The centers are generally open from 7:00 A.M. to 6:00 P.M., 5 days a week, and serve two or three meals in a day. A daily or hourly fee is charged with an additional charge for meals. Services are limited to socialization or may be comprehensive, offering modest restorative care services and nursing care. Adult day care is often used by working persons who have a spouse or a parent living with them who cannot be left alone.

RESPITE CARE

Respite care is offered by adult day care centers, long-term care facilities, or in private homes. It is intended to provide a break to caregivers and is used a few hours a week, for an occasional weekend, or for longer vacations. Planned activities, meals, and supervision are included in respite care services.

LONG-TERM CARE

Long-term care refers to a spectrum of services provided to individuals who have an ongoing need for health care. Long-term care has traditionally meant a community-based nursing home licensed for skilled or intermediate care. Although there is a great demand for this type of care, there is also a market for other levels of health care.

LONG-TERM CARE FACILITIES

Long-term care facilities provide services to individuals who are not acutely ill, have continuing health care needs, and cannot function independently at home. They are licensed for either intermediate care or skilled nursing care. Intermediate care facilities are not certified for reimbursement from Medicare but may be certified for Medicaid funding. Skilled nursing facilities are eligible for certification by both Medicare and Medicaid, but not all facilities choose to become certified. These facilities were formerly called nursing homes, rest homes, or convalescent centers. The term **extended care facility (ECF)** refers to any facility that provides care for a long period of time. It has no concrete definition and could refer to either an intermediate or skilled nursing facility. Facilities in every state that receive any government funds from any source are required by law to be in compliance with the Omnibus Budget Reconciliation Act of 1987 (OBRA) regulations. The Act requires that residents be free from all unneeded drugs and chemical restraints (psychotropic drugs).

A restorative philosophy of care provides direction for the interdisciplinary team. Emphasis is placed on assisting the client (usually called resident) to attain and maintain the highest level of physical, mental, and psychosocial function. A holistic approach is used, and families are important members of the care team. A large number of facilities have special units devoted to the care of residents with specific problems. These units care for persons with Alzheimer's disease, diabetes, respiratory disorders, wounds, and other conditions.

Long-term care or extended care facilities are available for older adults in need of nursing care 24 hours a day. The older adult receives assistance with ADLs, nursing supervision, and activities to keep the mind stimulated. Physical, speech, and occupational therapy are offered to assist the older adult. Also offered are three nutritious meals planned by a dietitian to meet the physician's orders, along with snacks for the older adult. The nursing staff includes registered nurses, LPNs, and certified nursing assistants 24 hours a day. Housekeeping services are available to keep the older adult's room and linens clean. An activity coordinator and social service personnel are included in the extended care facility staff. This could be one or two people based on the number of beds in the extended care facility. Added client expenses include medications, outside physician costs, various therapies, personal care items, and laundry services.

Reimbursement

Federal and state reimbursement is determined by the resident's functional abilities and services used while in the facility. The facility is reimbursed for a certain amount of money for expenses by Medicare and Medicaid. Each year, the Medicare/Medicaid facility is reviewed by state and/or federal personnel to ensure that the facility is meeting expected standards of care. If not, and if the infractions are severe enough, the facility is fined and/or loses Medicare/Medicaid funding. Facilities have closed their doors based on poor results. Every facility has to post these state/federal findings within the facility for the public.

Discharge

Client discharge planning begins at the time of admission and is included in the care plan. By placing the information on the care plan, all long-term care personnel know the same information and goals for a satisfactory outcome.

EXTENDED CARE FACILITIES

Extended care facilities are designed to provide different services to meet specific client needs. The basic extended care facility offers 24-hour supervised nursing care with a certified nursing aide to assist with ADLs. The next level is skilled nursing care. This level offers services of registered nurses and licensed practical nurses 24 hours a day that includes treatments, administration of medications, and procedures. Skilled care services include professionals in physical, speech, occupational, and respiratory therapies. Subacute care offers the same services as skilled care but is more focused on residents with acute or chronic illness or injury. Some extended care facilities are designed for special needs children and for older adults with special needs, such as Alzheimer's/dementia units. Senior communities offer living options to meet the older adults' needs such as totally independent apartments or condos, assisted-living areas, and skilled nursing care facilities.

Holistic Nursing in Extended Care

Holistic nursing reaches beyond treating diseases and meets the needs of the total person by nourishing the biological, psychological, social, and spiritual parts of a person. The holistic view promotes health and wellness.

As the body changes through the aging process and has acute and chronic health problems, the effect on the wellness of the body, mind, and spirit is diminished. Wellness develops from maintaining a positive purpose in life and an inner spiritual wholeness. Nurses change health outcomes as the result of their knowledge in the sciences and humanities. In caring for the older adult, nursing plays a significant role in assisting the older adult to find their balance of health promotion and wellness (See Figure 51-9).

Routines and Treatments

In an extended care facility, holistic gerontological nursing care goals are to: (1) enhance the older adult's growth to wholeness; (2) encourage improvement and learning from an acute or chronic disease; (3) optimize the quality of life during a terminal illness or disability; and (4) ensure comfort, peace, dignity and integrity in death (Eliopoulos 2005).

Activities

The enjoyment of life does not have to end when an older adult enters an extended care facility. An older adult can continue to find purpose in life. This time in life provides the individual with the freedom to reflect on life's work experiences,

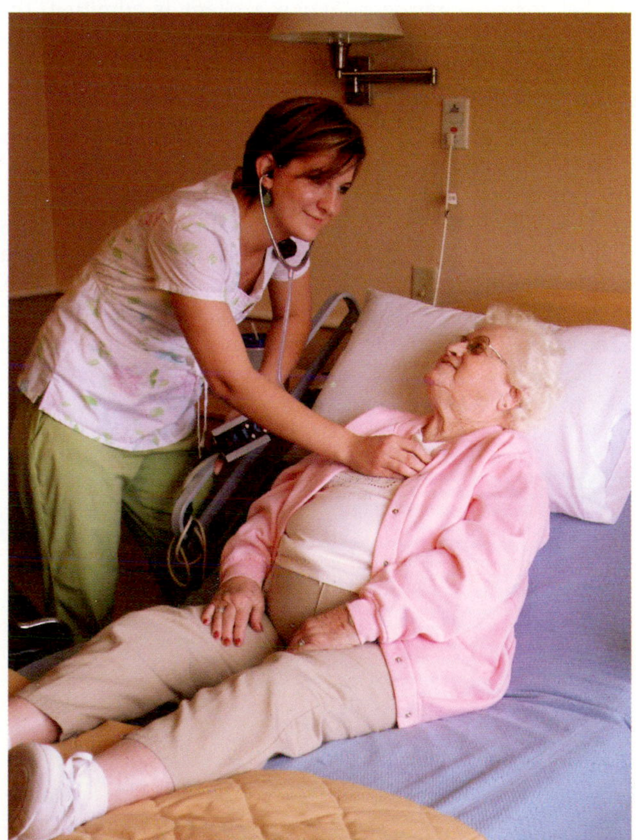

FIGURE 51-9 A nurse provides quality care to a client in an extended care facility. (*Courtesy of Kingston Residence of Fort Wayne, Fort Wayne, IN.*)

family life, future goals, spiritual renewal, and social interactions. Taking part in extended care facility activities can assist in these pursuits.

The activity department is staffed with professionally trained personnel to create activities that meet the needs of each older adult. Some of the outside activities include trips to malls, picnics that include the family, gardening, shopping, and attending local concerts. Some of the indoor activities include musical activities; perhaps a local organ or piano talent, a choir, dances, or parties that may include a juke box. Christmas dinner with the resident's family, woodworking projects, pet therapy, craft making, exercise groups, bingo, Bible study, and cooking are other activities that are offered. Religious services of various beliefs are arranged by the activity department. The activity department can also assist in scheduling a visit to the beautician or barber. Individual activities such as the use of audio taped books are arranged when a resident is unable to leave the room. Monthly activities are posted so residents anticipate the event and participate as desired. Activities provide a social gathering and stimulation for the mind along with physical activity.

Dietary

There are several meals planned by a dietitian in an extended care facility. The dietitian consultant reviews each resident's intake of meals by percentage, fluid intake, and laboratory test values to avoid nutrition deficiencies and dehydration. The dietician then makes recommendations to the extended care facility's dietary manager and the director of nursing. Meal planning and dietary services are reviewed annually by the state government review board and, if necessary, the federal review board. It is the physician who determines and orders the diet for each resident. When a client is admitted, the dietary staff reviews personal food preferences.

Financial Issues

Private funds, Medicare, Medicaid, long-term care insurance, and supplemental security income cover the cost of extended care. Private funds are mostly used for independent and assistive living options. Assistive living facilities in some states accept Medicaid. Medicaid is a federal and state program that assists individuals and families who need financial assistance. Medicaid services vary from state to state; this is called a Medicaid waiver. The Medicaid rates are agreed on by the supplier of services and Medicaid and are accepted as full payment. Refer to Box 51-2 for expenses covered by Medicaid.

CRITICAL THINKING

Social Isolation

Social isolation is a common psychological problem for clients who are admitted to rehabilitative or restorative facilities.

1. How can the nurse reduce the client's social isolation while in the rehabilitation/restorative care hospital?
2. What other disciplines within the rehabilitation/restorative care hospital reduce the client's social isolation?
3. In what ways can the nurse involve the family to resolve the client's social isolation?

BOX 51-2 SERVICES COVERED FOR THE OLDER ADULT BY MEDICAID

- Outpatient/inpatient hospital
- Laboratory
- Radiology
- Medical expenses
- Surgery expenses
- Dental care exams
- Home health care
- Extended care facility
- Physician expenses
- Family nurse practitioner services

Medicare is a federal health insurance program for persons 65 years of age and older or disabled individuals, regardless of the income. There are two parts to Medicare: Part A and Part B. Part A is considered hospital insurance. Part A covers an extended care facility if the resident requires skilled care after a hospital stay of 3 days within a 30-day time limit for 100 days. Medicare covers home health and hospice care if the illness is terminal within 6 months. Medicare also covers hospital services such as laboratory, pharmacy, radiology, surgical operations, critical care, rehabilitation/restorative care, extended stays, and meals. Part B is a supplementary medical insurance plan and covers physician services, and non-physician services such as flu vaccinations and some therapies.

Long-term care insurance is paid monthly before the need of service to offset the cost of long-term care. Policies vary on what services are covered and type of facility.

Supplemental Security Income is not the same as social security but is similar in that the government supplies a monthly check to a disabled person or one with a financial need at age 65 and older. To receive Supplemental Security Income, a person has to have little or no income.

Veterans with a health condition can receive medical care or rehabilitation/restorative care in a veterans' affairs hospital or an extended care facility approved by the state to serve veterans. If the health condition is service related, the long-term care is provided as needed in an approved extended care facility.

PALLIATIVE CARE AND HOSPICE

Clients with chronic diseases or diseases that are not responsive to a cure are candidates for **palliative care**. Palliative care addresses the complications of the illness rather than the prognosis. Palliative care is separate from hospice care and is effective if started early in the disease process rather than at the end stages of the disease. Palliative care relieves symptoms of the disease and assists the family in setting and reaching goals, addressing and resolving conflict, and putting meaning to the dynamics of the illness and dying experience (Ferrell & Coyle, 2002). The illness affects the entire life of the client and family.

The interdisciplinary team works through multiple obstacles, such as client symptoms, family miscommunications, family members' grief, and cultural barriers to provide quality care. Nurses play a vital role as the client and family rely on them to meet their needs. Clients have countless emotions that nurses acknowledge and address such as anxiety,

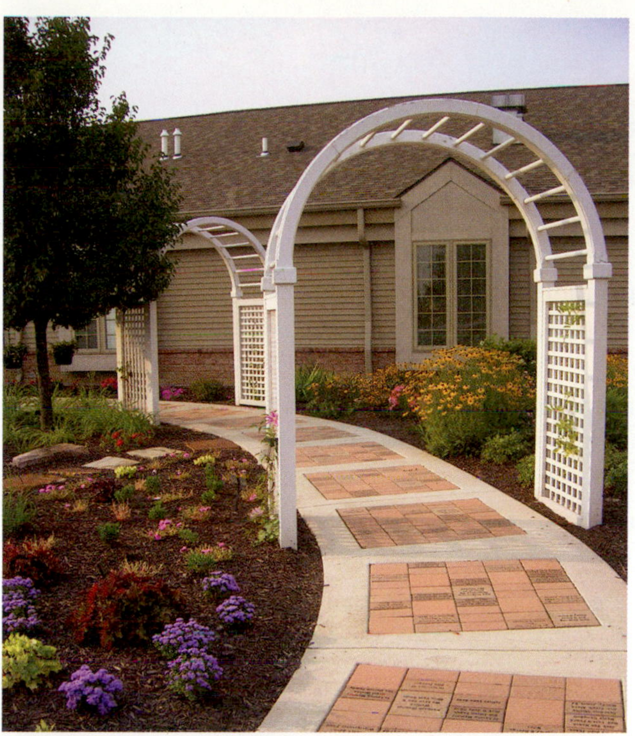

FIGURE 51-10 A garden is a place of solace for a hospice client and family. (*Courtesy of Visiting Nurse and Hospice Home, Fort Wayne, IN.*)

depression, sadness, loneliness, hopelessness, and anger (See Figure 51-10). The palliative and hospice nurses not only attend to physical conditions but must be perceptive in handling psychological, psychosocial, and spiritual needs. The nurse acknowledges the client and family members' emotions and guides the client and family in gaining a sense of control and focusing on positive aspects of life.

Hospice provides care to the client and family through the dying process and assists the family in the grief process. Hospice provides pain relief for the client, focuses on the family during the loss of their loved one, and supports the family as they work through their grief (Ferrell & Coyle, 2002). End-of-life care is care provided in the last few weeks of life.

Medicare covers the cost of hospice if the client is eligible for Medicare Part A. The criteria for Medicare Part A is that the physician or hospice medical director states the client has 6 months or less to live, the client signs a paper choosing hospice care rather than curative care, and the client signs a paper to enter a Medicare-certified hospice program (Ferrell & Coyle, 2002).

BOX 51-3 HOSPICE SERVICES COVERED BY MEDICARE

- Physician and nursing care
- Home health aide care
- House keeping services
- Physical, occupational, and speech therapy
- Counseling services
- Pastoral services
- Assistance with transportation, shopping, or other chores
- Bereavement support
- Medical equipment and supplies
- Pain medication (no prescription costs more than $5)
- Five days of respite care for caregiver

(Scala-Foley M, Caruso J, Archer D, & Reinhard S, 2004; Medicare.com, 2008)

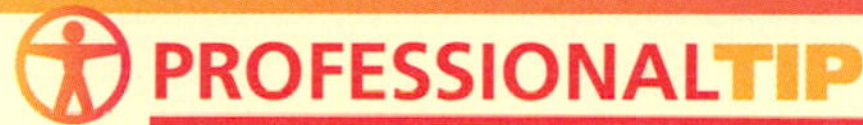

PROFESSIONALTIP

Questions about Medicare Hospice Benefits

The State Health Insurance Assistance Program (SHIP) answers question regarding Medicare coverage of Hospice benefits. The phone number is 800-MEDICARE or the website is www.medicare.gov (search for "Helpful Contacts"). Clients or nurses can call SHIP for any Medicare hospice benefit questions.

SAMPLE NURSING CARE PLAN

The Stroke Client

R.A. has had an altered state of wellness caused by a recede stroke and is living at the local restorative care hospital. She is distrustful of the new surroundings and is feeling socially isolated from her friends and family. She has left-sided paralysis and is scheduled for daily physical therapy to regain her strength and mobility. She walks with a cane.

NURSING DIAGNOSIS 1 *Impaired Physical Mobility* related to decreased strength and endurance as evidenced by paralysis of left arm and leg and inability to walk without a cane

Nursing Outcomes Classification (NOC)
Ambulation: Walking

Nursing Interventions Classification (NIC)
Exercise Therapy: Joint Mobility
Exercise Promotion: Strength Training
Exercise Therapy: Ambulation
Teaching: Prescribed Activity: Exercise
Teaching: Safety

SAMPLE NURSING CARE PLAN (Continued)

PLANNING/OUTCOMES	NURSING INTERVENTIONS	RATIONALE
R.A. will regain strength in left arm and leg and walk independently with a cane within 6 weeks.	Maintain the left arm and leg in natural alignment.	Prevents contractures and maintains proper alignment for future use.
	Place pillows to support left arm and leg in proper alignment.	Prevents pressure on body surfaces and maintains extremities in proper alignment for future use.
	Assist with ambulation frequently and gradually extend ambulation time frames.	Client gains strength in extremities and improves ambulation skills with cane.
	Teach safe crutch walking.	Teaches client correct use of cane when ambulating to prevent falls.
	Encourage use of left arm and leg for self-care activities.	Improves client's self esteem and improves self care.
	Encourage arm and leg exercises.	Client increases strength in affected arm and leg.

EVALUATION

At the end of 6 weeks, R.A. has full range of motion against gravity and flexes both arm and leg against resistance. R.A. walks independently with cane and relates ambulating safety precautions to the nurse.

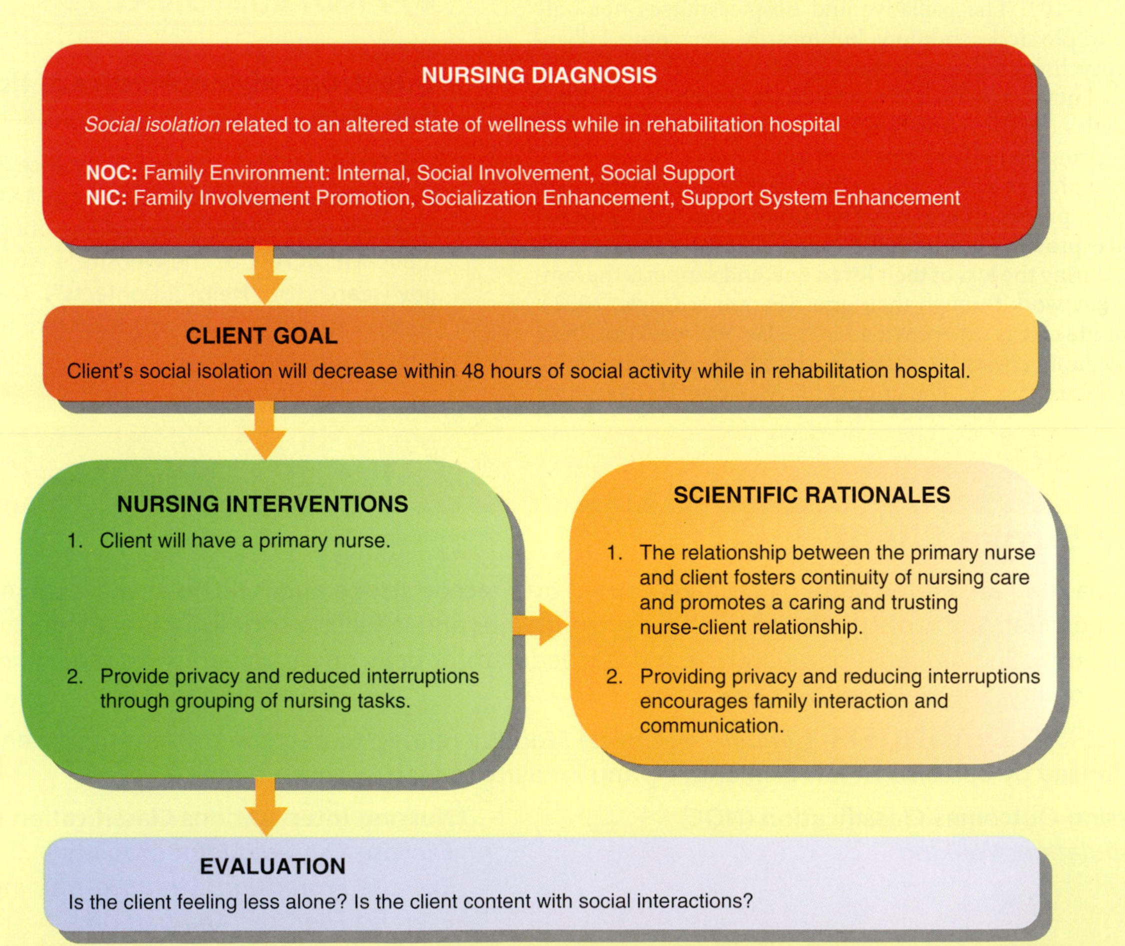

NURSING DIAGNOSIS
Social isolation related to an altered state of wellness while in rehabilitation hospital
NOC: Family Environment: Internal, Social Involvement, Social Support
NIC: Family Involvement Promotion, Socialization Enhancement, Support System Enhancement
CLIENT GOAL
Client's social isolation will decrease within 48 hours of social activity while in rehabilitation hospital.
NURSING INTERVENTIONS
1. Client will have a primary nurse.
2. Provide privacy and reduced interruptions through grouping of nursing tasks.
SCIENTIFIC RATIONALES
1. The relationship between the primary nurse and client fosters continuity of nursing care and promotes a caring and trusting nurse-client relationship.
2. Providing privacy and reducing interruptions encourages family interaction and communication.
EVALUATION
Is the client feeling less alone? Is the client content with social interactions?

CONCEPT CARE MAP 51-1

CASE STUDY

E.J., 72 years old, was admitted to Community Hospital for a left below-knee amputation. E.J. was an insulin-dependent diabetic for 35 years. The amputation followed a long and unsuccessful period of treatment for venous stasis ulcers. E.J. was transferred from the hospital to a rehabilitation hospital on her fourth postoperative day. After 2 weeks at the rehabilitation hospital, she was transferred to a skilled care facility near her home for additional restorative care and regulation of the diabetes. She is now ready to be discharged to her home. E.J. has a prosthesis and is able to ambulate with a walker. She performs her ADL with minimal assistance. She was on a sliding scale and blood glucose monitoring 4 times a day while in the long-term care facility. Her physician has now placed her on insulin twice a day with daily blood glucose checks. Her vision is somewhat impaired due to the diabetes. E.J. lives alone in a one-story home in a sage residential area. The discharge planner at the skilled care facility has arranged continuing care for E.J. through a local home health agency.

The following questions guide your development of a nursing care plan for the case study.

1. Identify the assessment factors that are most important in planning E.J.'s care.
2. List the nursing diagnoses that are applicable to E.J.'s assessment.
3. Describe the complications for which E.J. is at risk.
4. Describe nursing interventions for preventing the complications.
5. What specific actions would you take to prevent a recurrence of venous stasis ulcers?
6. What additional community services does E.J. need?
7. What nursing services (frequency of nurse visits, services from a nursing assistant, other home health services) would you plan to meet her needs? What services would each person provide?
8. Describe the outcomes you expect for E.J.?

SUMMARY

- Ambulatory care provides the nurse with opportunities to work with clients of all ages across the health continuum.
- Ambulatory care nurses require a high degree of skill in communication and client education.
- The goal of rehabilitation/restorative care is to assist individuals in reaching their optimal physical, mental, and psychosocial functioning level.
- The interdisciplinary health care team assesses, maintains, and evaluates the abilities of individuals in need of functional therapy.
- The minimum data set (MDS) is an assessment tool for assessing resident's physical, psychological, and psychosocial functioning in a Medicare and Medicaid-certified long term care facility.
- Long-term care facilities provide services to individuals who are not acutely ill, have continuing health care needs, and cannot function independently at home.
- Home Health Care requires the nurse to be technologically competent.
- The home health care nurse refers clients to community resources.
- The home health care nurse possesses knowledge of the various federal government forms and data systems necessary to carry out the position and ensure planned outcomes and quality of care to client.
- Palliative care relieves symptoms of the disease and assists the family in setting and reaching goals, addressing and resolving conflict, and putting meaning to the dynamics of the illness and dying experience.
- Hospice provides pain relief for the client, focuses on the family during the loss of their loved one, and supports the family as they work through their grief.

REVIEW QUESTIONS

1. A reason for the growth in nonacute health care services is: (Select all that apply.)
   1. the diminishing supply of physicians.
   2. an increase in the number of hospitals in the country.
   3. direct marketing of pharmaceuticals.
   4. the increase in Medicare reimbursement.
   5. the population shifts in the United States.
   6. the increased interest in alternative therapy.

2. Medicare is a reimbursement system for health care providers that:
   1. is based upon the client's personal financial resources.
   2. is available to persons 65 years of age and older or who have been disabled for 2 or more years.
   3. pays the full cost of all medical care.
   4. is managed by each state.

3. What client would be the most likely to benefit from rehabilitation/restorative care services?
   1. J.B., 64 years old, had a stroke, is responsive and stable.
   2. M.C., 89 years old, has Alzheimer's disease in the fourth stage.
   3. M.Z., 26 years old, is recovering from pneumonia.
   4. R. K., 56 years old, has terminal cancer of the lung.
4. As a member of the interdisciplinary health care team, the LPN/VN: (Select all that apply.)
   1. participates in the planning of client care.
   2. plans the appropriate diet for clients.
   3. teaches the new amputee how to walk with a prosthesis.
   4. advocates the needs of the client.
   5. provides alternative methods of communication for the client with recent stroke.
   6. understands the roles and responsibilities of each discipline.
5. In the home health care setting, it is essential that the LPN/VN possess skills in: (Select all that apply.)
   1. total parenteral nutrition.
   2. respiratory therapy treatments.
   3. data collection.
   4. planning and providing speech therapy.
   5. medication administration.
   6. client teaching.
6. In a long-term care facility, the LPN/VN serves as the:
   1. charge nurse of a unit.
   2. director of nursing.
   3. clinical nurse specialist.
   4. social worker.
7. The Minimum Data Set is a government tool to assess: (Select all that apply.)
   1. a functional need.
   2. psychosocial need.
   3. medical needs.
   4. discharge planning.
   5. psychological patterns.
   6. effect of medications.
8. What main factor determines the choice of housing for the older adult?
   1. The facility's floor plan.
   2. Dietary menu.
   3. Functional perimeters.
   4. Activity program.
9. The OASIS
   1. is used to assess a client's physical, psychological, and psychosocial functioning.
   2. is a computerized plan of care that is compatible with the home health care electronic system.
   3. provides a uniform method to document a client's disability and medical rehabilitation.
   4. is used to review the agencies' data results and measures home health care outcomes.
10. A client was just admitted to the rehabilitation unit. The nurse's restorative care goal for the client is to:
    1. restore health.
    2. assist in reaching optimal functional level.
    3. send residents home after two weeks of therapy.
    4. restore only ADLs.

REFERENCES/SUGGESTED READING

American Academy of Pediatrics. (2006). AAP Immunization Initiatives. Retrieved on October 10, 2007 from http://www.cispimmunize.org/aap/aap_main.html

Assisted Living Federation of America. (ALFA). (1999). What is assisted living? Retrieved from http://www.alfa.org

Assisted Living Federation of America (ALFA). (2009). About ALFA. Retrieved on May 31, 2009 from http://www.alfa.org/alfa/About_ALFA.asp?SnID=1173654858

Baker, L., Reifsteck, S., & Mann, W. (2003). Connected: Communication skills for nurses using the electronic medical record. *Nursing Economics, 21*(2), 85–88.

Bartz, K. (1999) The orientation experiences of urgent care nurses: Sources of learning. *Journal for Nurses in Staff Development, 15*(5), 210–216.

Bergman-Evans, B. (2004). Beyond the basics: Effects of the Eden alternative model on quality of life issues. *Journal of Gerontological Nursing, 30*(6), 27–34.

Brain Injury Resource Foundation. (2009). Bi assessment tools. Retrieved on May, 23, 2009 from http://www.birf.info/home/bi-tools/tests/fam.html

Bureau of Labor Statistics. (2007). National Employment Matrix, employment by industry, occupation, and percent distribution, 2006 and projected 2016. Retrieved on May 22, 2009 from ftp://ftp.bls.gov/pub/special.requests/ep/ind-occ.matrix/occ_pdf/occ_29-2061.pdf

Cameron, M. (2002). Older persons' ethical problems involving health. *Nursing Ethics, 9*(5), 537–556.

Castle, N. (2003). Searching for and selecting a nursing facility. *Medical Care Research and Review, 60*(2), 223–247.

Center for Disease Control. (2006). Clinical laboratory improvement amendments. Retrieved on October 10. 2007 from http://www.phppo.cdc.gov/clia/regs/subpart_a.aspx#493.15

Center for Disease Control. (2006). Healthy people—tracking the nation's health. Retrieved on October 12, 2007 from http://www.cdc.gov/nchs/hphome.htm#Healthy%20People%202010

Center to Improve Care of the Dying. (2006). Functional status. Retrieved on October 13, 2007 from http://www.gwu.edu/-cicd/toolkit/function.htm

Centers for Medicare and Medicaid Services. (2009). Long term care minimum data set (MDS). Retrieved on May 26, 2009 from http://www.cms.hhs.gov/IdentifiableDataFiles/10_LongTermCareMinimumDataSetMDS.asp

Cherlin, A. (1996) *Public and private families, and introduction*. New York, NY: McGraw Hill.

Cicatiello, J. (2000). A perspective of health care in the past insights and challenges for a health care system in the new millennium. *Nursing Administration Quarterly, 25*(1), 18–29.

Cusack, G., Jones-Wells, A., & Chisholm, L. (2004). Patient Intensity in an Ambulatory Oncology Research Center: A Step Forward for the Field of Ambulatory Care. *Nursing Economics, 22*(2), 58–63.

Department of Health and Human Services. (2006). HIPPA—general information. Retrieved on October 11, 2007 from http://www.cms.hhs.gov/HIPAAGenInfo/

Eliopoulos, C. (2005). *Gerontological nursing* (6th ed.). Philadelphia: Lippincott Williams & Wilkins.

Ferrell, B., & Coyle, N. (2002). An overview of palliative nursing care. *American Journal of Nursing, 102*(5), 26–31.

Futch, C., & Phillips, R. (2003) The mega issues of ambulatory care nursing. *Nursing Economics, 21*(3), 140–142.

Galarneau, L. (1993). An interdisciplinary approach to mobility and safety education for caregivers and stroke patients. *Rehabilitation Nursing, 18*(6), 395–398.

Glosner, G. (1995). How subacute care fills the gap. *Nursing95, 25*(3), 51.

Goldrick, B. (2005). Emerging infections: Infection in the older adult. *American Journal of Nursing, 105*(6), 31–34.

Hammons, T., Piland, N., Small, S., Hatlie, M., & Burstin, H. (2003) Ambulatory patient safety: What we know and need to know. *Journal of Ambulatory Care Management, 26*(1), 63–82.

Hawkins, D. (2001). *Migrant health issues: Introduction.* Buda, TX: National Center for Farmworker Health, Inc.

Health Resources and Services Administration (HSRA). (2009). Telehealth. Retrieved on May 24, 2009 from http://www.hrsa.gov/telehealth/

Hogstel, M. (2001). *Gerontology: Nursing Care of the Older Adult.* Albany, NY: Delmar Cengage Learning.

Hsu, C. (2006). The greening of aging. *US News & World Report, 140*(23), 48–52.

Illinois State University. (2006). Dr. William H. Thomas to Deliver Expanding Teaching Nursing Home Lecture on April 11. US Fed News Service, Including US State News. Washington, DC, March 28.

Indiana Health Facilities Rules. (1997). *Comprehensive care facilities. Resident's Rights.* 401 IAC 16.2-3.1.

Kimball, B., & O'Neil, E. (2002). Healthcare's human crisis: The American nursing shortage. The Robert Wood Johnson Foundation, Retrieved on October 14, 2007 from http://www.rwjf.org

Kolbe, L. (2005). A framework for school health programs in the 21st century. *Journal of School Health, 75*, 6.

Lasky, W. (1995). Assisted living: A brand new world. *Nursing Homes, 44*(7), 40–41.

Levac, K. (2002). Putting outcomes in practice in physician offices. *Journal of Nursing Care Quality, 71*(1), 51–62.

Lincoln Hospital. (2006). Long term care. Retrieved on October 10, 2007 from http://www.lincolnhospital.org/long_term_care.html

Lim, W., & Macfarlane, J. (2001). A prospective comparison of nursing home acquired pneumonia with community acquired pneumonia. *European Respiratory Journal, 18*(2), 362–368.

Male Incontinence Clamp. (2006). Retrieved from http://www.ppstop.com/

Mauk, K. (2007). *Specialty practice of rehabilitation nursing: A core curriculum* (5th ed.). Rehabilitation Nursing Foundation of the Association.

Maurer, F., & Smith, C. (2005). *Community/public health nursing practice: Health for families and populations* (3rd ed). St Louis, MO: Elsevier Saunders.

Mayo Clinic. (2006). Urinary incontinence: Treatment. Retrieved on November 10, 2007 from http://www.mayoclinic.com/health/urinary-incontinence/DS00404/DSECTION=8

Medicare.com. (2008). Hospice care. Retrieved August 5, 2009 from http://www.medicare.com/assisted-living/hospice-care.html?ht=

Meng, M. (1995). Starting an adult day care center. *Provider, 21*(12), 38–40.

National Center for Health Statistics. (2008). Americans make nearly four medical visits a year on average. Retrieved on May 24, 2009 from http://www.cdc.gov/nchs/pressroom/08newsreleases/visitstodoctor.htm

National Coalition for the Homeless: *How many people experience homelessness? Fact Sheet #3,* Washington DC, 1998a, NCH.

National Library of Medicare. (2006). AHCPR supported clinical practice guidelines: Treatment of pressure ulcers-managing tissue loads. Retrieved on November 11, 2007 from http://www.ncbi.nlm.nih.gov/book/bv.fcgi?rid=hstat2.section.5420

Nursing Homes and Senior Citizen Care. (1990). OBRA regulations and chemical restraints. (Omnibus budget Reconciliation Act of 1987). Retrieved on May 31, 2009 from http://www.accessmylibrary.com/comsite5/bin/aml_land_tt.pl?purchase_type=ITM&ite

O'Neill, P. (2002). *Caring for the older adult: A health promotion perspective.* Philadelphia: W.B. Saunders Company.

Parve, J. (2004) Remove vaccination barriers for children 12 to 24 months. *The Nurse Practitioner, 29*(4), 35–38.

Resnick, B., & Fleishell, A. (2002). Developing a restorative care program. *American Journal of Nursing, 102*(7), 91–95.

Saucier Lundy, K., & Janes, S. (2003). Essentials of community-based nursing. Jones and Bartlett Publishers. Retrieved on November 2, 2007 from http://communitynursing.jbpub.com/essentials/powerpoint.cfm

Scala-Foley, M., Caruso, J., Archer, D., & Reinhard, S. (2004). Making sense of Medicare: Medicare's hospice benefits. *American Journal of Nursing, 104*(9), 66–67.

Schim, S., Thornburg, P., & Kravutske, M. (2001). Time, task, and talents in ambulatory care nursing. *Journal of Nursing Administration, 31*(6), 311–315.

Senior Housing Net. (2006a). Assisted living. Retrieved on October 10, 2007 from http://www.seniorhousingnet.com/seniors/kyo/assisted_living.jhtml

Senior Housing Net. (2006b). Independent living. Retrieved on October 10, 2007 from http://www.seniorhousingnet.com/seniors/kyo/ind_living.jhtml

Senior Housing Net. (2006c). Nursing homes. Retrieved on October 10, 2007 from http://www.seniorhousingnet.com/seniors/kyo/nursing_home.jhtml

Senior Housing Net. (2006d). Payment options. Retrieved on October 10, 2007 from http://www.seniorhousingnet.com/seniors/finance_pay/plan/payment_options.jhtml

Smith, K. (2006). Appreciation of holistic nursing. *Journal of Holistic Nursing, 24*(2), 139.

Stanhope, M., & Lancaster, J. (2004). *Community & public health nursing* (6th ed). St Louis, MO: CV Mosby.

Symm, B., Averitt, M., Forjuoh, S., & Preece, C. (2006). Effects of using free sample medications on the prescribing practices of family physicians. *Journal of the American Board of Family Medicine, 19,* 443–449.

Swan, B., & Griffin, K. (2005). Measuring nursing workload in ambulatory care. *Nursing Economics, 23*(5), 253–260.

Uniform Data System for Medical Rehabilitation. (2009). The functional assessment specialists. Amherst, NY: Uniform Data System for Medical Rehabilitation. Retrieved on May 28, 2909 from http://www.udsmr.org/WebModules/UDSMR/Com_About.aspx

U.S. Office of Personnel Management. (1987). Self-identification of handicap. Retrieved May 23, 2009 from http://www.opm.gov/forms/pdfimage/sf256.pdf

Venes, D. (2005). *Taber's cyclopedic medical dictionary.* Philadelphia: F.A. Davis Company.

Walsh, G. (1995). How subacute care fills the gap. *Nursing95, 25*(3), 51.

Wellness Letter. (August 2006). Wellness guide to dietary supplements. Retrieved on October 15, 2007 from http://wellnessletter.com/html/ds/dsCalcium.php

Wenckus, E. (1995). Working for an interdisciplinary team. *The Nursing Spectrum, 8*(6), 11–12.

Wesley. (2006a). Assistive living. Retrieved on October 10, 2007 from http://www.wesleyhealth.com/Assistive-living-c29.html

Wesley. (2006b). Independent living. Retrieved on November 2, 2007 from http://www.wesleyhealth.com/Independent-living-c3.html

Wright, J. (2000). The Functional Assessment Measure. The Center for Outcome Measurement in Brain Injury. Retrieved on May 23, 2009 from http://www.birf.info/home/bi-tools/tests/fam.html

RESOURCES

Association of Rehabilitation Nurses, http://www.rehabnurse.org/

Brain Injury Resource Foundation, http://www.birf.info

City of Hope Pain/Palliative Care Resource Center, http://prc.coh.org

End-of-Life Nursing Education Consortium (ELNEC), http://www.aacn.nche.edu/elnec

Last Acts, http://www.lastacts.org

National Institute on Disability and Rehabilitation Research (NIDRR), http://www.ed.gov

American Association of Neuroscience Nurses (NNF), http://www.aann.org

UNIT 18 Applications

CHAPTER 52
Responding to Emergencies

MAKING THE CONNECTION

Refer to the following chapters to increase your understanding of emergency situations:

Basic Nursing

- ***Holistic Care***
- ***Legal and Ethical Responsibilities***
- ***Bioterrorism***

Adult Health Nursing

- ***Respiratory System***
- ***Cardiovascular System***
- ***Gastrointestinal System***
- ***Urinary System***
- ***Musculoskeletal System***
- ***Neurological System***
- ***Sensory System***
- ***Reproductive Systems***
- ***Integumentary System***
- ***Mental Illness***
- ***Substance Abuse***

LEARNING OBJECTIVES

Upon completion of this chapter, you should be able to:

- Define key terms.
- Describe the emergency medical services.
- Explain the role of the nurse in emergency situations.
- List personnel needed to respond to an in-hospital emergency.
- Discuss the steps in assessing an emergency client.
- Cite the different levels of triage.

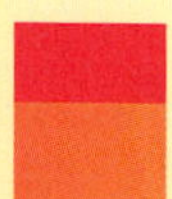

KEY TERMS

chain of custody
disaster
emergency
emergency medical technician (EMT)
emergency nursing
Glasgow Coma Scale
paramedic
shock
trauma
triage

INTRODUCTION

An **emergency** can be defined as a medical or surgical condition requiring immediate or timely intervention to prevent permanent disability or death. Emergency nursing has developed rapidly over the years in response to the changing environment and expectations of the community. Many advancements in emergency care is attributed to the military. To manage vast numbers of injured soldiers, the military developed a systematic method of treating and responding to **trauma** (wound or injury). Casualties caused by wartime situations created the need for advancements in the care of large numbers of clients with injuries, wounds, and illness. Methods of caring for multiple clients were developed and implemented as a result of military influence.

In the United States, trauma is the number one killer of those younger than age 43 and the fourth leading cause of death overall (The American Association for the Surgery of Trauma, 2007). Motor vehicle collisions kill more than 43,000 people each year, with almost 5 million car crash victims cared for in emergency departments (EDs) (The American Association for the Surgery of Trauma, 2007; CDC, 2009).

Emergency nursing is the care of clients who require emergency intervention. The emergency nurse must be capable of rapid assessment and history taking and immediate intervention formulation and implementation utilizing the nursing process. This role carries great responsibility. Throughout the assessment and care of the client, the emergency nurse plans and teaches prevention and health promotion, as well as rapidly develops rapport with the client and family, including assisting with emotional needs. Clinical knowledge, communication, client teaching, and empathy skills are essential to effective emergency care. Although LP/VNs are seldom hired for EDs, they may float or help during emergency situations; therefore, a brief overview of emergency nursing is justified.

A **disaster** is a situation or event of greater magnitude than an emergency that has unforeseen, serious, or immediate threats to public health. They are *natural* events such as large fires, earthquakes, floods, hurricanes, or tornadoes; or *human-made* events such as war, terrorism, or overwhelming contamination of the environment (Gebbie & Qureshi, 2002).

EMERGENCY/DISASTER PREPAREDNESS

To prepare for emergencies or disasters, it is necessary to identify *who* needs to know *how* to do *what*. To this end, Gebbie and Qureshi (2002) have outlined the following core competencies for nurses that were modeled after the CDC's core emergency preparedness competencies for public health workers:

- *Describe* the agency's role in responding to a range of emergencies that might arise.
- *Describe* the chain of command in emergency response.
- *Identify* and locate the agency's emergency response plan (or the pertinent portion of it).
- *Describe* emergency response functions or roles and *demonstrate* them in regularly performed drills.
- *Demonstrate* the use of equipment (including personal protective equipment) and the skills required in emergency response during regular drills.
- *Demonstrate* the correct operation of all equipment used for emergency communication.
- *Describe* communication roles in emergency response within your agency, with news media, with the general public, and with personal contacts.
- *Identify* the limits of your own knowledge, skills, and authority and identify key system resources for referring matters that exceed these limits.
- *Apply* creative problem-solving skills and flexible thinking to the situation, within the confines of your role, and evaluate the effectiveness of all actions taken.
- *Recognize* deviations from the norm that might indicate an emergency and describe appropriate action.
- *Participate* in continuing education to maintain up-to-date knowledge in relevant areas.
- *Participate* in evaluating every drill or response and identify necessary changes to the plan.

CRITICAL THINKING

Stress

Describe factors that contribute to stress in an emergency room setting.

What can nurses do to effectively reduce stress when working in a stressful environment?

APPROACHES TO EMERGENCY CARE

There are three general approaches to emergency care: hospital triage, disaster triage, and the emergency medical services. To care for the emergent client, one first determines the severity of illness.

HOSPITAL TRIAGE

Each hospital with an ED has an established "triage" system in effect. **Triage** refers to classification of clients to determine priority of need and proper place of treatment. Triage is typically used in the ED to establish priorities and levels of care needed by the clients. Although clients and their families

PROFESSIONALTIP

Golden Rules of Emergency Care

1. Establish the safety of the scene.
2. Remove the client from danger.
3. Establish airway, breathing, and circulation.
4. Manage shock.
5. Attend to eye injuries.
6. Treat skin injuries.
7. Call for help.

INFECTION CONTROL

Mouth-to-Mouth Resuscitation

When delivering care to any client, the nurse is careful to practice Standard Precautions. Direct mouth-to-mouth breathing should not be administered; instead, use of a bag-valve-mask for resuscitation is more effective in both protecting the health care worker and the client from possible infection and in administering respirations.

define emergency according to their perceptions, it is the triage nurse's responsibility to sort and prioritize the clients as they arrive in the ED.

The simplest method of triaging clients is to use the American Heart Association's basic life support principles: Airway, Breathing, and Circulation (ABCs). By using this method, clients with airway problems are immediately assessed and become a top priority of care. If any of the ABCs are not functioning, either the Heimlich maneuver or cardiopulmonary resuscitation (CPR) is initiated.

Most hospitals have a triage system established to provide expedient care to those requiring it first. Although the term *emergency department* implies emergency care, the client using this department does not always require immediate care. In 2000, there were 108 million visits to hospital EDs (McMahon, 2003). The most commonly used triage classifications are emergent, urgent, and nonurgent and are recognized by the Emergency Nurses Association (McMahon, 2003) (Table 52-1). Emergent clients require immediate care in order to sustain life or limb. Examples of emergent conditions include foreign bodies in the eye, shortness of breath, impending birth, and cardiopulmonary arrest. Urgent clients require care within 1 to 2 hours to prevent worsening of their conditions. Examples of urgent situations include acute abdominal pain and compound fractures. For nonurgent clients, care can be delayed without the risk of permanent consequences. Contusions and sprains are examples of nonurgent complaints.

TABLE 52-1 Triage Categories

CATEGORY/ PRIORITY	CLIENT NEEDS	EXAMPLES
Emergent	Immediate intervention is required to sustain life or limb.	Cardiac arrest Multiple trauma
Urgent	Care is required within 1 to 2 hours to prevent deterioration of condition.	Compound fractures Persistent vomiting and diarrhea
Nonurgent	Care may be delayed without risk of permanent sequelae.	Contusions Minor sprains and fractures

Developed from Military Standard Operating Procedure (SOP) for General Hospitals.

COURTESY OF DELMAR CENGAGE LEARNING

DISASTER TRIAGE AND MASS CASUALTY INCIDENTS

Disaster or mass casualty incident triage systems represent a second approach to emergency care. In the event of a mass casualty incident (MCI), where there are more victims than care providers, these systems are used. The disaster may be a natural occurrence like a tornado, hurricane, or flood, or human-made, such as a train accident, chemical spill, or terrorism. In the event of an MCI, an Incident Command System is established to provide safe and orderly management. Given the possibility of large numbers of casualties as a result of disasters, different approaches to triaging from that of the hospital system may be used. Another similar system developed for pre-hospital providers is the START (Simple Triage and Rapid Treatment) system, where the victims are rapidly color coded based on respirations, perfusion, and mental status (Figure 52-1). A victim is given a red tag if immediate treatment is needed, such as shock or a severe head injury, and is at risk for death. Yellow tags are given to victims who have serious injuries but their respirations are <30 per minute, the capillary refill is <2 seconds, and they can follow simple commands. A yellow tag indicates the victim can receive delayed treatment. Green tags are given to victims with minor injuries. The treatment for these victims is reassurance and transportation to a facility when other clients with more urgent needs have been transferred. A navy tag is given to victims who are dead or whose injuries are so severe they will die soon (BCEMS Web, 2009).

Most communities have disaster/mass casualty committees or an emergency management agency (EMA) director. These committees include all hospitals, the emergency medical services (EMS) system, and citizens needed to alert the community of an impending or real disaster.

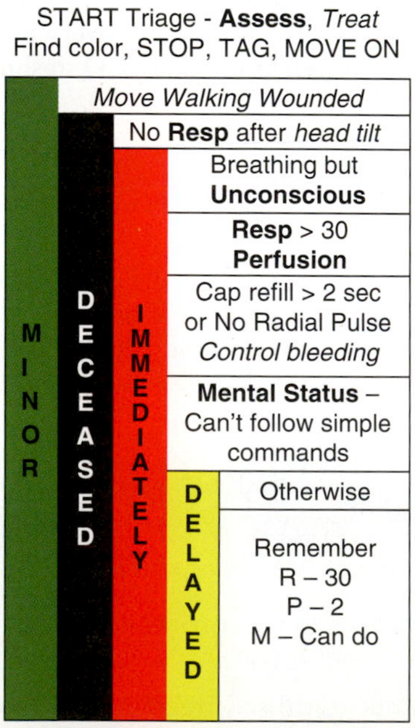

START Triage - **Assess**, *Treat*
Find color, STOP, TAG, MOVE ON

MINOR: *Move Walking Wounded*
DECEASED: No **Resp** after *head tilt*
IMMEDIATELY: Breathing but **Unconscious**; **Resp** > 30 **Perfusion**; Cap refill > 2 sec or No Radial Pulse *Control bleeding*; **Mental Status** – Can't follow simple commands
DELAYED: Otherwise
Remember R – 30 P – 2 M – Can do

FIGURE 52-1 START Triage (*Courtesy of Critical Illness and Trauma Foundation, Inc.*)

Emergency Medical Services

Before admission to the ED, the client usually is cared for by a first responder or an **emergency medical technician (EMT)**. An EMT-B (Basic) is a health care professional trained to provide basic lifesaving measures before arrival at the hospital. An EMT-P (**Paramedic**) is a more specialized health care professional educated to provide advance life support to the client requiring emergency interventions (Figure 52-2). Both are part of the EMS and are essential to prehospital care of the emergency client.

Principles of first aid, developed for emergency medicine, are part of the triage process and include what are referred to as the golden rules of emergency care. The first of these rules cautions the health care worker to assess the physical environment for self-protection. That is, safety at the scene must be established before rescue is attempted (Figure 52-3). The next rule is to remove the client from danger, such as that presented by passing vehicles. These first two rules typically apply to emergencies occurring outside of an institutional setting.

Once the safety at the emergency scene and of the client have been established, assessment turns to the ABCDs of emergency care—airway, breathing, circulation, and disability. Obtain and maintain an open *airway*. Assess *breathing* and provide resuscitative breathing as needed. *Circulation* includes starting CPR to restore cardiac output, assessing and controlling bleeding, and assessing and treating possible shock. Care for a potential central nervous system *disability* by assessing neurological status using the Glasgow Coma Scale and apply a neck collar for any head or neck injury (Integrated Publishing: Medical, 2009). Eye and skin injuries are evaluated next.

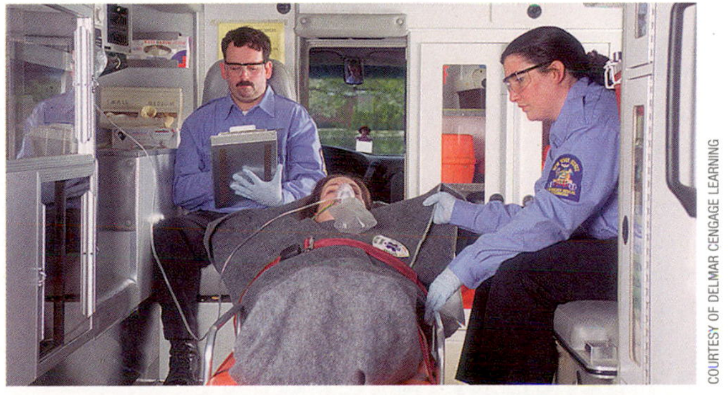

FIGURE 52-2 **EMTs and paramedics are often the first to arrive at an emergency scene.**

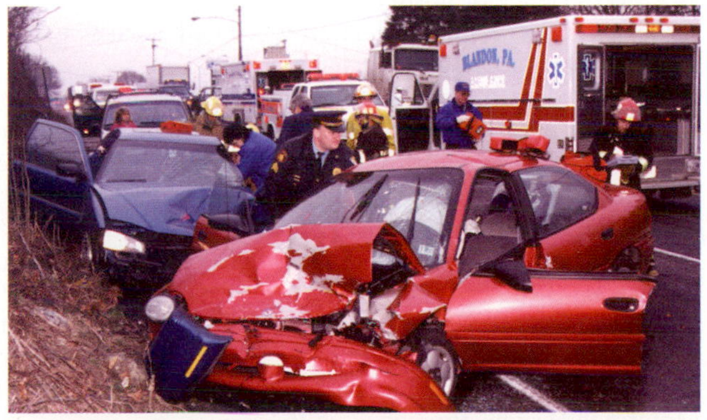

FIGURE 52-3 **Establishing the safety of the scene is the first priority in emergency care, as in this scene of a motor vehicle accident, where rescue workers may be in danger from oncoming vehicles. (*Courtesy of David J. Reimer, Sr.*)**

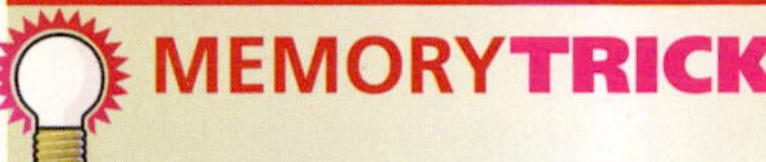

MEMORYTRICK

Use the **ABCD**s of emergency care when assessing a client in a prehospital setting:

A = Airway — Establish a patent airway.

B = Breathing — Provide ventilation; use resuscitation measures as needed.

C = Circulation — Restore and maintain circulation by restoring cardiac output, controlling bleeding, and providing adequate fluid volume.

D = Disability — Assess for and prevent neurological disability by using the Glasgow Coma Scale.

SHOCK

Shock is a condition of profound hemodynamic and metabolic disturbance characterized by inadequate tissue perfusion (the body's inability to meet tissue demand for oxygen) (Table 52-2). Shock can result from trauma, injury, or insult. Recognizing and immediately treating shock are critical to the client's survival. There are four major types of shock: hypovolemic shock, cardiogenic shock, distributive shock, and obstructive shock (Chavez & Brewer, 2002).

Hypovolemic shock is usually easily recognized. It results from severe fluid volume depletion through vomiting, dehydration, diarrhea, or blood loss. Severe external bleeding may be obvious, but internal bleeding, such as that from a gastric ulcer, is not readily observable.

Cardiogenic shock may be caused by several different heart conditions that result in loss of the contractile property of the heart muscle. The most common of these is acute myocardial infarction (heart attack). Severe heart failure and certain arrhythmias may also cause shock.

There are three types of distributive shock: septic, anaphylatic, and neurogenic. In all of these, shock results from vasodilation and an abnormal fluid distribution within the circulatory system.

Septic shock is usually caused by overwhelming infection. Certain organisms may cause severe reactions, resulting in collapse of the circulatory system. Toxic shock syndrome, gram-negative shock, and urogenic shock are types of septic shock.

Anaphylactic shock is a severe allergic reaction to a toxin to which a client has been exposed. Causes of anaphylactic reaction include insect bites and certain medications.

Neurogenic shock is the body's response to extreme pain or trauma to the spinal cord. As with the other forms of shock, it results in inadequate supply of oxygen, electrolytes, and other essential chemicals to the tissues.

Obstructive shock is the result of indirect pump failure that leads to decreased cardiac function and reduced circulation. Conditions causing obstructive shock include pulmonary

TABLE 52-2 Types of Shock

TYPE	CAUSES	SIGNS AND SYMPTOMS	TREATMENT
Hypovolemic	Hemorrhage,* burns	Increased heart rate; hypotension, cold, clammy skin; profound thirst	Replace fluids
Cardiogenic	Myocardial infarction*	Increased heart rate; hypotension; cold, clammy skin	Initiate drug therapy for myocardial infarction; replace fluids; consider possible emergency coronary bypass surgery
Septic	Overwhelming infection	Hot, dry, flushed skin; hypotension; increased heart rate	Locate source of infection and treat with broad-spectrum antibiotic; replace fluids
Anaphylactic	Medications,* insect bites or stings, foods	Throat edema in conjunction with increasing difficulty breathing; hypotension; increased heart rate	Manage ABCs; administer epinephrine (Adrenalin); administer diphenhydramine hydrochloride (Benadryl)
Neurogenic	Spinal cord injury, head trauma	Slowed heart rate; hypotension	Replace fluids, administer drugs to increase blood pressure and heart rate
Obstructive	Arterial stenosis, pulmonary embolism, pulmonary hypertension, cardiac tamponade	Increased heart rate, dyspnea	Treat underlying cause

*Most common cause

COURTESY OF DELMAR CENGAGE LEARNING

embolism, pulmonary hypertension, arterial stenosis, and cardiac tamponade.

In all types of shock, diminished blood flow causes the signs and symptoms. There is usually no clinical evidence of shock in the *early stage*. There may be an increase in heart rate (above client's baseline), restlessness, and the client may have a sense of impending doom. In the *compensatory stage*, respirations and heart rate increase; pulses may be weak; urinary output decreases; skin is cold and clammy, mottled, and pale; pupils dilate; bowel sounds are hypoactive, and there is hyperglycemia. Interventions at this stage reduce the possibility of permanent damage. If shock advances to the *progressive stage*, the client's condition noticeably deteriorates. The pulse may be too rapid to count, blood pressure falls below 80 mm Hg, peripheral pulses disappear, there is metabolic acidosis, peripheral edema, pulmonary crackles and wheezes are heard, and the client may be unresponsive. In the *refractory stage*, there is too much cell death and tissue damage from inadequate oxygenation. The client does not respond to treatment. Multiple organ failure occurs, which generally results in death.

MEDICAL–SURGICAL MANAGEMENT

Medical

Management of shock is supportive in nature during initial resuscitation. The immediate priority is maintenance of the ABCs. Active bleeding should then be stopped. Blood is administered in the event of major blood loss. After the client is stabilized, the underlying cause of shock is identified and treated.

Pharmacological

Initial treatment involves the administration of oxygen and the insertion of two large-bore intravenous (IV) lines. Intravenous lines are instituted to establish lifelines through which life saving drugs and fluids are administered. Fluid resuscitation and oxygen delivery are critical to management of the client in shock. Medications, including epinephrine, are administered to improve circulation.

NURSING MANAGEMENT

The focus is to identify the type of shock and initiate interventions as soon as possible. For hypovolemic shock, the treatment goal is to restore volume. Administer IV solutions such as Ringer's lactate or normal saline, or packed red blood cells, serum albumin, plasma, or dextran as ordered. Excessive fluids dilute clotting factors and worsen bleeding.

For cardiogenic shock, treatment focuses on improving myocardial function. Medications for hypotension are frequently ordered. Provide oxygen. Monitor the client's respiratory and cardiac status.

Septic shock is the most common type of distributive shock. Administer IV antibiotics and fluids as ordered. Monitor vital signs.

Clients in neurogenic shock generally have hypotension, bradycardia, hypothermia, and dry warm skin. Administer medications as ordered for hypotension and bradycardia. Monitor vital signs. Provide warmth.

For clients in anaphylactic shock, talk with family (or client if able) to identify the cause. After assessing ABCs, administer IV fluids, epinephrine, and antihistamines as ordered. Monitor vital signs.

Obstructive shock is managed by identifying the source of the obstruction and treating it. Administer fluids cautiously. Seldom are diuretics used.

NURSING PROCESS

Assessment

Subjective Data

Determine whether the client is responsive and able to respond to questions or is unconscious. When the client is alert and stabilized, assessment includes obtaining a history of the events leading to the injury or illness, including any food consumed or medication taken and any unusual event (such as a bee sting) that precipitated the shock state. Ask the client to describe any pain with regard to intensity, location, and duration.

Objective Data

Immediate assessment involves evaluating the ABCs. Take vital signs, because many clients in shock will present with hypotension, tachycardia, tachypnea, and pale, diaphoretic, clammy skin.

Nursing diagnoses for a client in shock include the following:

NURSING DIAGNOSES	PLANNING/OUTCOMES	NURSING INTERVENTIONS
*Risk for Deficient **Fluid** Volume* related to acute blood loss/vomiting/ diarrhea	The client will maintain adequate fluid balance.	Initiate and maintain fluid replacement with two large-bore IV access lines. Administer blood as ordered.
*Ineffective **Tissue** Perfusion* related to decreased oxygen-carrying hemoglobin secondary to blood loss and fluid depletion	The client will maintain adequate tissue perfusion as manifested by stable vital signs.	Assess vital signs at least every 30 minutes. Administer oxygen per physician order.
*Anticipatory **Grieving*** related to grave nature of illness/ injury	The client will cope with illness/ injury by cooperating with care provided by health care workers and will discuss outcomes with nurse and family.	Communicate with client and family. Explain all interventions as they occur, to decrease acute anxiety. Allow client and family to express their fears and worries about the situation. Answer questions about care.

Evaluation: Evaluate each outcome to determine how it has been met by the client.

CARDIOPULMONARY EMERGENCIES

Cardiopulmonary emergencies are those emergencies that jeopardize the function of the heart and lungs. These emergencies can result from trauma or illness. Cardiopulmonary emergencies such as drowning, foreign body obstruction of the airway, chest trauma, and chest pain are grouped together, because the effects, medical management, and nursing priorities are similar.

Near-drowning episodes occur most frequently in the summer. Many clients will suffer other related injuries associated with drowning, such as head and spinal cord injuries (Table 52-3).

Foreign-body obstruction of the airway most commonly occurs in the larger, right main bronchus. The most common source of airway obstruction is the tongue. Other sources of airway obstruction include hot dogs, candy, steak, and coins (especially in children).

Penetrating or blunt trauma to the chest can cause multiple injuries. Penetrating injuries are insults that puncture the chest, such as gunshot or knife wounds. Blunt trauma is more likely caused by falls or by forceful contact with a blunt object, such as a baseball bat or steering wheel. Injuries associated with pneumothorax include cardiac tamponade, fractured ribs, fractured sternum, and flail chest.

Table 52-3 Freshwater versus Saltwater Near-Drowning

TYPE	CLIENT SYMPTOMS	PATHOPHYSIOLOGY	SIGNS
Freshwater	Fatigue, anxiety, difficulty breathing, fear	Water in lungs causes changes in surfactant, which in turn causes alveolar collapse.	Hypoxia, collapsed alveoli
Saltwater	Fatigue, anxiety, difficulty breathing, fear, rales, rhonchi	Hypertonic salt water pulls fluid into the alveoli.	Hypoxia, pulmonary edema

COURTESY OF DELMAR CENGAGE LEARNING

One of the most common complaints evaluated in the ED is chest pain. Those clients presenting with the symptom of chest pain must be clearly and carefully evaluated. Chest pain has a multitude of potential causes and can be frightening to the client until the cause is confirmed.

MEDICAL–SURGICAL MANAGEMENT

Medical

Management of all cardiopulmonary emergencies is directed at maintaining the ABCs. If indicated, intubation is part of resuscitation in cardiopulmonary emergencies. Establishment of an IV line is essential for medical management, because the line provides access for administration of lifesaving medications.

After resuscitation is achieved, other treatment modalities are instituted. Obtain chest x-rays, electrocardiograms (EKGs), and blood tests. Initiate pain control. Morphine sulfate is the drug of choice for clients with these types of emergencies, because morphine decreases both pain and anxiety in the client, which, in turn, leads to improved breathing.

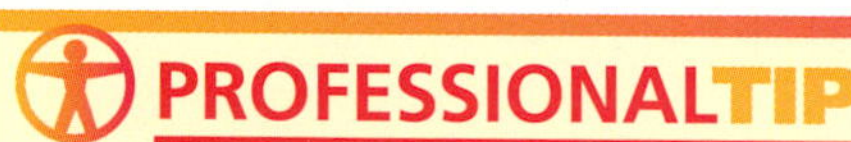

Flail Chest

A flail chest is defined as instability in the chest wall. This condition is caused by fracture of three or more ribs in two or more places. With a flail chest, breathing is unique: The flail segment moves inward during inspiration and outward during expiration. This is called paradoxical breathing.

Pharmacological

With the near-drowning client, mannitol (Osmitrol) and furosemide (Lasix) are occasionally indicated in the event of fluid overload. Pain medication is essential for the client with chest injury, because hypoventilation may occur as a result of the pain associated with deep breathing. Pain control is also essential for the client experiencing chest pain. Pain medications vary from sublingual nitroglycerine to IV morphine sulfate.

Activity

Most clients with cardiopulmonary emergencies are initially confined to bed and must frequently be rolled from side to side. Encourage deep breathing and coughing to prevent stasis of fluid and development of pneumonia.

NURSING MANAGEMENT

Initiate CPR if indicated. Remain with the client to reduce anxiety. Administer pain medication as ordered. Suction as necessary to keep airway patent. Monitor vital signs and lung sounds. Encourage turning and deep breathing.

NURSING PROCESS

ASSESSMENT

Subjective Data

Evaluate for restlessness, an early sign of hypoxia. Note pain description. Other areas to include in assessment are fatigue, anxiety, and level of consciousness. Ability to give a brief history of events before the cardiopulmonary emergency is evaluated.

Objective Data

Immediately assess airway and breathing. Note any cough, stridor, cyanosis, or inability to talk. Initial vital signs are essential for a baseline.

Nursing diagnoses for a client with a cardiopulmonary emergency include the following:

NURSING DIAGNOSES	PLANNING/OUTCOMES	NURSING INTERVENTIONS
*Ineffective **Airway** Clearance* related to accumulation of fluid and blood in the airway and to the client's inability to cough	Client's lungs will be clear bilaterally to auscultation.	Maintain airway and breathing with suctioning, if secretions accumulate. Turn client frequently to mobilize secretions. Encourage deep breathing and coughing. Listen to lungs hourly, or more frequently, to evaluate secretions and suctioning.
*Ineffective **Breathing** Pattern* related to injury to the chest and inability to fully expand the lungs	Client will regain spontaneous respiration within normal rate range and pattern.	Initiate CPR, if indicated. Administer pain medications as ordered to ease the work of breathing. Note response to pain medications. Remain with the client during episodes of respiratory distress, because being left alone at these times escalates both the anxiety and breathing problems. Explain all procedures.

Evaluation: Evaluate each outcome to determine how it has been met by the client.

NEUROLOGICAL/ NEUROSURGICAL EMERGENCIES

Head injuries are the most common type of neurological trauma. Spinal cord trauma can also occur as a result of injuries sustained in a head injury. Head trauma most often results from motor vehicle collisions (MVCs) (Figure 21-4). Head injuries vary from very minor contusions to major head trauma.

Clients experiencing any altered level of consciousness (LOC) are admitted to the health care system for prompt evaluation and care. Cerebrovascular accidents (CVA), also called strokes or "brain attacks," occur in different areas of the brain when it becomes starved for oxygen or hypoxic. These events are caused by a blood clot (ischemic stroke) or a bleeding blood vessel (hemorrhagic stroke), which causes symptoms ranging from mild confusion or a slight lip droop to total unresponsiveness. Establishing the exact time of onset, if possible, is extremely important for prompt and effective treatment. CVAs, or "brain attacks," require the same initial consideration given to myocardial infarctions, or "heart attacks."

Another common event causing an altered LOC is low blood sugar (hypoglycemia). The client appears lethargic, intoxicated and combative, or comatose. Prompt restoration of adequate blood glucose levels and supplemental oxygen support are critical to protect the brain from further insult. Other medical emergencies that cause an altered LOC include carbon monoxide poisoning, drug overdose, severe infections, and electrolyte imbalances.

MEDICAL–SURGICAL MANAGEMENT

Medical

As with all trauma, management is aimed at maintaining the ABCs. In addition, if head, neck, or spinal cord trauma is suspected, the client is placed on a backboard, with the head and neck immobilized. Blood alcohol level is determined. Intravenous access is initiated early in the resuscitation phase. Radiological examination is necessary to determine the extent of damage. If the client does not have spontaneous respirations, the injury has probably occurred at C-4 or above, meaning that the client will not be able to independently maintain respirations. The client is continuously monitored for increased intracranial pressure. Early signs of increased intracranial pressure include a headache; later signs include widened pulse pressure, dilated pupils, and spontaneous emesis without warning. Hiccups are an ominous sign and thus are reported immediately. Use of the **Glasgow Coma Scale**, a neurological screening test that measures a client's best verbal, motor, and eye response to stimuli, is indicated (Figure 52-5).

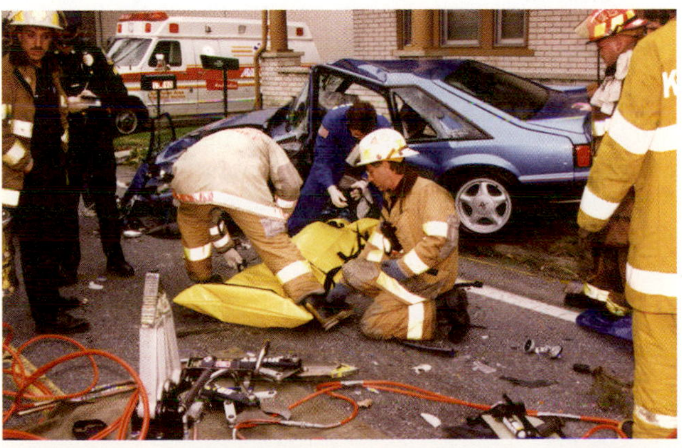

FIGURE 52-4 MVCs are the most common cause of head trauma. (*Courtesy of David J. Reimer, Sr.*)

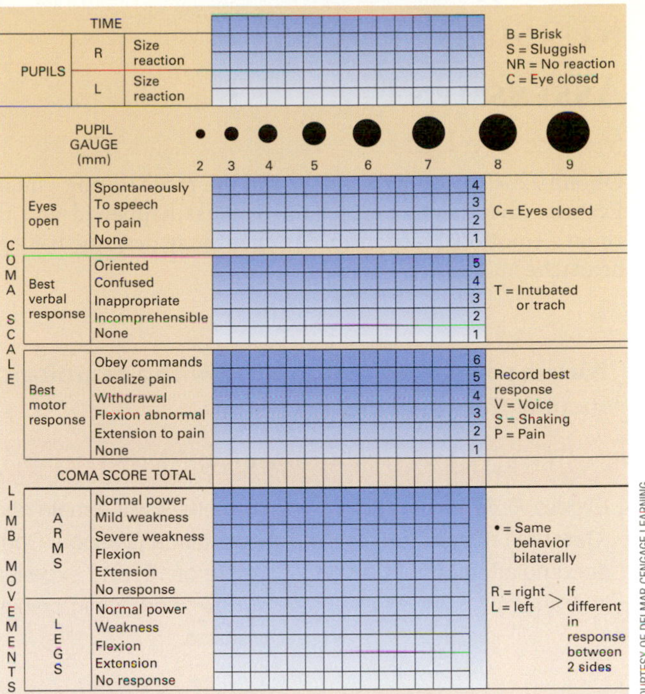

FIGURE 52-5 Neurological Flow Sheet, Including Glasgow Coma Scale

Pharmacological

Increased cranial pressure and buildup of carbon dioxide complicate the client's condition; oxygen most often alleviates the resultant complications. Thus, administer oxygen immediately. Pain management is accomplished through IV access.

Activity

Clients with head injuries are placed in semi-Fowler's position to decrease edema and intracranial pressure.

NURSING MANAGEMENT

Immediately administer oxygen as ordered. Monitor vital signs. Assess Glasgow Coma Scale score. Maintain the client in a semi-Fowler's position or as ordered. Orient to date and time as needed.

CRITICAL THINKING

Motor Vehicle Crash

You come upon an MVC involving several vehicles and no emergency response vehicles have yet arrived. What steps can you take to secure the accident site and aid the victims until emergency services arrive?

NURSING PROCESS

ASSESSMENT

Subjective Data

Obtain a history of the accident and the mechanism of injury. Evaluate the client's perception of what happened and the client's emotional response. The client may describe having a headache and difficulty seeing.

Objective Data

Assess the client's vital signs and Glasgow Coma Scale level. Note cerebrospinal fluid leaks, such as clear fluid coming from the nares or ear. Document the client's unequal pupillary response, trouble making self understood, or difficulty swallowing.

Nursing diagnoses for the client with a neurological/neurosurgical emergency include the following:

NURSING DIAGNOSES	PLANNING/OUTCOMES	NURSING INTERVENTIONS
*Excess **F**luid Volume (Cerebral)* related to accumulation of fluid/blood in cranium	The client will remain conscious, maintain a Glasgow Coma Scale score of 15, and experience no further increase in cranial fluid volume.	Monitor intracranial pressure. Maintain the client in semi-Fowler's position. Document vital signs hourly. Assess Glasgow Coma Scale level and record hourly. Administer oxygen.
*Impaired Verbal **C**ommunication* related to injury to speech center	The client will be able to communicate with the nurse and family.	Orient the client frequently to date and time. Explain all nursing interventions. Modify communication methods, such as use of a message board, depending on the client needs. Encourage client to verbalize feelings about condition; offer support.

Evaluation: Evaluate each outcome to determine how it has been met by the client.

ABDOMINAL EMERGENCIES

Abdominal emergencies are diverse in nature. Trauma to the upper body and torso can result in multiple abdominal injuries, from a simple contusion and bruising to a ruptured spleen. Clients presenting to the ED with complaints of abdominal pain require careful evaluation. Illnesses causing abdominal pain range from gastroenteritis to gastrointestinal bleeding.

Abdominal injuries can result from blunt or penetrating trauma. It is important to determine the mechanism of injury, because certain causes, such as MVCs, often result in multisystem trauma. Blunt trauma, for instance from falling on the abdomen, usually results in injury to internal organs, such as the kidneys or spleen. Penetrating injuries such as gunshot wounds can affect any internal organ. Hemorrhage is a potential complication of both types of trauma.

MEDICAL–SURGICAL MANAGEMENT

Medical

Initial management of abdominal emergencies is IV access with large-bore catheters. Oxygen is administered immediately, and standard protocol calls for managing the ABCs. Blood products or plasma expanders are administered in the event of large-volume blood loss. Insertion of a nasogastric tube decompresses the stomach. A peritoneal lavage may be performed to check for blood in the abdominal cavity of clients with abdominal trauma. Presence of blood indicates a need for immediate surgical intervention. A computed tomography (CT) scan of the abdomen may be indicated as well. Blood work is drawn, and a urinalysis is done. Hematuria is evaluated, and x-rays may be indicated.

Pharmacological

If the client is in severe pain and has been evaluated, narcotics are indicated.

NURSING MANAGEMENT

Administer oxygen and follow agency protocol for managing ABCs. Initiate IV access. Administer analgesics as ordered. Monitor vital signs, bowel sounds, and abdominal girth. Administer medications and ambulate as allowed.

PROFESSIONALTIP

Open Abdominal Wound

If loops of intestines are exposed to outside air, cover with sterile saline-soaked gauze.

NURSING PROCESS

Assessment

Subjective Data

Ask about the location, duration, severity, and radiation of pain. Obtain history of nausea, vomiting, and diarrhea. Note the times of the client's last meal, bowel movement, and urination.

Objective Data

Assess vital signs, active bleeding, abdominal girth, and weight. Inspect the abdomen for bruises, edema, and wounds.

Nursing diagnoses for the client with an abdominal emergency include the following:

NURSING DIAGNOSES	PLANNING/OUTCOMES	NURSING INTERVENTIONS
*Deficient **F**luid Volume* related to active bleeding	The client will stabilize, and vital signs and fluid balance will return to normal.	Establish IV access with at least two large-bore catheters. Monitor vital signs frequently, at least hourly. Evaluate abdominal girth and bowel sounds hourly.
*Risk for **I**nfection* related to penetrating injury	The client will not experience an elevated temperature or show signs and symptoms of infection.	Administer antibiotics as ordered to reduce the risk of infection. Monitor temperature at least every 2 hours. Change saturated dressings as needed. Note amount and quality of any drainage.
***A**ctivity Intolerance* related to pain and bleeding	The client will ambulate with assistance the evening of or 1 day after surgical correction.	Turn client hourly from side to side. Assist client to ambulate when able to prevent stasis of fluid and to diminish the risk of infection.

Evaluation: Evaluate each outcome to determine how it has been met by the client.

GENITOURINARY EMERGENCIES

Rape is a legal term and is not considered a medical condition. It is defined as sexual penetration of a forceful and threatening nature with a nonconsenting person. Included under this legal term is penetration of persons who are unable to consent because of intoxication or mental illness. *Alleged sexual assault* is the terminology used by most centers for rape survivors. Because of the many legal implications and the fact that there are not only physical symptoms, but also long-lasting psychological consequences of sexual assault, accurate and methodical care must be given to the survivors of sexual assault. Most communities have hospitals designated to care for rape survivors. These facilities are staffed with registered nurses and doctors familiar with the medical, psychological, and legal issues particular to caring for the client who has experienced a sexual assault. Many facilities now have a Sexual Assault Nurse Examiner (SANE). These nurses are trained in collecting and accurately documenting the forensic evidence needed to protect the rights of the victim.

Straddle injuries are another type of genitourinary emergency. These injuries occur when a client falls while straddling an object, such as a fence or metal bar, thereby injuring the perineum. Though not a very common injury, it is imperative to assess the client and promptly initiate treatment. These injuries can occur with multiple traumas or as a single injury.

Medical–Surgical Management

Medical

As with all emergencies, the ABCs must be managed first. Intravenous access is established, and blood and urine specimens are obtained. Rape crisis intervention is essential for the sexual assault victim. Those with straddle injuries are evaluated for fractures. If blood is seen at the external urethral meatus, a urethral tear is suspected, and catheterization is avoided because it will further damage the urethra. Radiological examination is done to confirm injury.

Surgical

Certain injuries such as urethral or vaginal tears may require surgical repair.

Pharmacological

Douching and bathing for the sexual assault survivor is delayed until all specimens are collected and all examinations are performed. For the sexual assault client, antibiotics are usually prescribed for possible sexually transmitted infection. Blood tests for baseline human immunodeficiency virus (HIV) and acquired immunodeficiency syndrome (AIDS) and a pregnancy test are usually part of the protocol. In addition, a "morning after" pill, such as diethylstilbestrol diphosphate (DES), may be prescribed in the event of a possible pregnancy.

PROFESSIONALTIP

Chain of Custody

Care is taken in handling the clothing and belongings of a survivor of sexual assault, as these items may become valuable in legal proceedings. For purposes of potential future litigation, it is thus imperative to maintain a strict **chain of custody** of evidence. The chain of custody is the documentation of the transfer of evidence from one worker to the next in a secure fashion. This means that to follow the rape protocol, each person handling the client's clothing or lab work must sign the document used by the facility to indicate receipt and release of items. The fewer the names on the chain, the more secure the integrity of evidence.

Diet

The client is designated nothing by mouth (NPO) in case of the need to go to immediate surgery. Fluids can be given intravenously.

Activity

The sexual assault survivor returns to full activity as soon as able, although counseling may be needed before the client regains the desire to resume activities of daily living. Those with straddle injuries need bed rest and careful observation until testing is complete. Clients are taught to resume sexual activities only when they feel physically and emotionally ready.

Nursing Management

Manage the ABCs and establish IV access. Obtain blood and urine specimens. Monitor output and test urine for blood. Make a list of the client's clothing worn during the assault and keep the clothing for evidence in case of legal proceedings. Instruct client to delay bathing or douching until all examinations are completed and all specimens are collected.

NURSING PROCESS

Assessment

Subjective Data

Obtain a description of the rape or assault. A history of menstrual cycles, including date of last menstrual period, is vital in determining the potential for pregnancy.

Objective Data

Assess all bruises, scrapes, or abrasions caused by the assault. Make a list of the client's clothing worn during the assault, and keep the clothing for evidence in case of legal proceedings.

Nursing diagnoses for the client with genitourinary emergencies include the following:

NURSING DIAGNOSES	PLANNING/OUTCOMES	NURSING INTERVENTIONS
*Impaired **U**rinary Elimination* related to break in urethra	Client will void clear urine before discharge and will regain normal pre-injury elimination patterns.	Closely monitor output. Test urine for blood using dipstick. Note and report hematuria. Offer bladder retraining and encourage client to resume pre-assault elimination patterns.
*Risk for **I**nfection (Sexually Transmitted Infection)* related to alleged sexual assault	Client will have negative outcomes on all lab specimens obtained.	Obtain all specimens as ordered. Teach the client how and when to obtain further specimens, as needed. Keep the client informed about all test results.
***R**ape-Trauma Syndrome* related to alleged sexual assault and violence of event	Client will state awareness of help groups for therapy and follow-up care.	Maintain open and nonjudgmental communication with the client. Call rape crisis center for immediate referral and assistance for the client. Refer the client to crisis help per community offerings. Teach the client that the trauma does not resolve overnight and that help is available at all times.

Evaluation: Evaluate each outcome to determine how it has been met by the client.

OCULAR EMERGENCIES

Most eye emergencies are urgent to emergent in nature. Foreign bodies can cause damage to vision very rapidly, and thus they require immediate attention. Clients with objects impaled in the eye must be immediately evaluated by an ophthalmologist. An eyeball may be avulsed, or forcibly torn out of its socket, either by blunt or penetrating trauma; such an injury requires immediate referral to and treatment by an ophthalmologist. Retinal detachment is a surgical emergency, as it is one of the leading causes of accidental blindness.

Medical–Surgical Management

Medical

The primary goal of care is restoring the health of the eye. The foreign body or impaled object is removed as soon as the client's condition allows and the effects on the eye of removal of the object have been determined. The client's eye is protected until definitive treatment is provided. Protective dressings are needed. In the event of ocular avulsion, the eyeball is protected with a warm saline dressing. Because both eyes move together, patching of the opposite eye decreases movement of the affected eye, allowing it to heal more quickly.

Surgical

Immediate surgical intervention is needed for retinal detachment.

Pharmacological

As a prophylactic measure, all eye trauma is treated with an antibiotic eye medication.

Diet

There are no modifications to the diet of the client with a foreign body in the eye. Clients with avulsed eyes are kept NPO in case immediate surgical intervention is needed.

Activity

Because sensory and depth perceptions may be altered when one eye is patched, activity is limited initially. Clients are maintained in semi-Fowler's position to prevent or alleviate intraocular edema.

Nursing Management

Maintain the client in semi-Fowler's position. Instill eye medications and apply an eye patch (sometimes both eyes are patched to decrease eye movement). Assist the client to ambulate while wearing an eye patch.

NURSING PROCESS

Assessment

Subjective Data

Obtain both the client's perception of what happened to the eye and a history of the accident, including the time it occurred. Document care given to an avulsed eye, such as placement in a plastic bag with water.

Objective Data

Assessment includes visual acuity testing and observation of tearing and/or redness of the eye.

Nursing diagnoses for the client with an ocular emergency include the following:

NURSING DIAGNOSES	PLANNING/OUTCOMES	NURSING INTERVENTIONS
*Disturbed **S**ensory Perception (Visual)* related to impaired vision	The client will regain partial preinjury vision.	Maintain the client in semi-Fowler's position in cases of ocular avulsion or retinal detachment. Assist the client to walk while wearing an eye patch and discuss problems that may be encountered and ways to accommodate decreased vision. Ask the client to name one resource person to assist with decreased vision at home.
*Risk for **I**nfection* related to trauma caused by foreign body	The client will not develop ocular infection.	Instill initial eye medication and apply initial eye patch for the client. Teach the client to instill eye medication and apply eye patch. Instruct the client to immediately report any visual changes or drainage. Be alert and listen to the client's concerns.

Evaluation: Evaluate each outcome to determine how it has been met by the client.

MUSCULOSKELETAL EMERGENCIES

Musculoskeletal emergencies can vary from simple muscle strains to major trauma. A muscle strain is the overstretching of a muscle. A sprain is defined as a twisting of the joint with partial rupture of ligaments, which can cause injury to surrounding tissue. Sprains often occur in the wrist and ankle. A dislocation is the displacement of a bone from its joint. The most common sites of dislocation are the fingers and toes. A fracture is a break in the continuity of a bone. In the event of a long-bone fracture, care also is given to the cardiopulmonary system: Fat emboli from the fracture site can develop and cause severe respiratory problems if they settle in the pulmonary system.

Medical–Surgical Management

Medical

Initial treatment of simple strains and sprains are managed by use of the "RICE" formula, meaning rest, ice, compression, and elevation. Fractures are immediately immobilized, with attention to body areas proximal to the fracture. Radiological examination is indicated to validate the diagnosis. Dislocations are immediately reduced. Many fractures and dislocations are reduced in the ED by the use of procedural sedation. Tetanus toxoid is given to any client with an open injury.

Surgical

Some fractures require immediate surgical intervention. Most open, compound fractures fall into this category. Debridement is often indicated, because most fractures are trauma related, and dirt and other matter imbed in the wound.

Pharmacological

Pain control is a major consideration in relation to musculoskeletal system injuries. Reduction and immobilization often significantly decrease pain. Those clients with minor sprains and strains respond well to anti-inflammatory medications such as ibuprofen (Advil, Motrin) and other nonsteroidal anti-inflammatory drugs (NSAIDs). Those with major or multiple fractures initially require narcotic relief.

Diet

Clients with sprains, strains, and simple fractures do not need special diets. Those with major fractures and trauma are kept NPO pending surgical intervention.

Activity

Depending on the site of the fracture, activity may be limited because of casting or immobilization. To help strengthen the muscles and minimize atrophy in cases of immobilization, teach the client to contract and release those muscles immobilized in the casting.

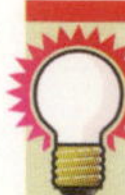

MEMORYTRICK

Treatment for Strains and Sprains

Remember **RICE** when treating a strain or sprain:

R = Rest

I = Ice

C = Compression

E = Elevation

Nursing Management

Immobilize the affected part. Administer analgesic as ordered. Elevate the injured area. Apply ice packs, as ordered. Assess pulse, skin color, capillary refill, ability to move fingers or toes, and sensation in the injured area.

NURSING PROCESS

Assessment

Subjective Data

The client will initially verbalize intense pain, tingling, and loss of use of the injured part.

Objective Data

Obvious deformities, edema, cool skin, and decreased capillary refill are present on the affected part. Note breaks in the skin and visual bone fragments.

Nursing diagnoses for the client with a musculoskeletal emergency include the following:

NURSING DIAGNOSES	PLANNING/OUTCOMES	NURSING INTERVENTIONS
*Acute **Pain** related to traumatic fracture/dislocation*	The client's pain will decrease with immobilization and pain medications.	Administer pain medications as ordered. Immobilize affected body part. Elevate injured extremity. Apply ice packs as directed. Listen attentively to the client's concerns and verbalizations of pain.
*Ineffective Tissue **Perfusion*** related to edema and fracture/dislocation	The client's pulses will be equal bilaterally, and capillary refill will be less than 2 seconds at the affected site.	Assess the client's pulse, skin color, capillary refill, and ability to move the fingers and toes every 30 minutes. Ask the client about sensation in the injured body part. Instruct the client to move the toes and fingers. Apply an elastic bandage for compression in cases of a sprain.
*Impaired Physical **Mobility*** related to limitations of pain and immobilization of fracture/dislocation	The client will demonstrate the ability to mobilize with cast or other assistive devices.	Teach the client to care for the cast. Teach the client exercises to minimize muscle atrophy and crutch walking, if needed.

Evaluation: Evaluate each outcome to determine how it has been met by the client.

SOFT-TISSUE EMERGENCIES

Minor abrasions, lacerations, puncture wounds, contusions, bites of all varieties (human, insect, animal, and snake), and burn injuries fall into the category of soft-tissue injuries. Although most such injuries do not require emergency care, some are more severe than others, and some are potentially fatal. Clients will seek medical attention for these injuries because of fear.

MEDICAL–SURGICAL MANAGEMENT

Medical

Skin emergencies require prompt intervention. All injuries must be cleansed or debrided. Infection is a major consideration, and prophylactic treatment must therefore be initiated immediately. If a laceration is large, suturing is necessary. Bites, unless extremely large, are usually not sutured because of the increased risk of infection presented by suturing these lacerations, which provide an excellent growth medium for bacteria. Burns sometimes are treated in an ED, with follow-up care provided at home. The application of cool water decreases the pain associated with minor burns. The burn is carefully debrided with the use of running cool water and then an antiseptic solution is applied. Because burns are painful, debridement is performed after administration of pain medication. A silver sulfadiazine (Silvadene) dressing is usually applied after debridement.

Major burns may require client resuscitation with rapid EMS transport to a burn center. Initially, the ABCs are established. "Packaging" the client for transport to a burn unit usually involves insertion of at least two large-bore IV lines, insertion of a nasogastric tube, intubation, Foley catheterization, sterile wrapping, and temperature regulation/monitoring.

Snakebites do not always result in envenomation (poisoning). A rubber band (not a tourniquet) above the site is the best intervention to control rapid spreading of the venom. Most snakebites occur in the foot, so a rubber band is easy to apply. In managing snakebites, it is best to establish the ABCs and, once the type of snake is identified, start antivenom treatment as necessary.

> **PROFESSIONALTIP**
>
> **Animal Bites**
>
> Many states require that all instances of clients seeking treatment in an ED for animal bites be reported to animal control officials. Know your state reporting rules and regulations.

Pharmacological

All clients with soft-tissue injuries, including those with burns, must be current with regard to immunizations, especially the diphtheria and tetanus (Td) immunizations. Pain medication is given to alleviate pain related to lacerations, bites, and burns. Topical antibiotic agents are applied to all injuries. Silver sulfadiazine (Silvadene) is the most widely used topical agent for burn injuries. Systemic antibiotics are often included in the treatment regimen.

Activity

Movement may be somewhat limited depending on the location of injury. Because muscle weakness and atrophy occur rapidly, physical therapy is initiated immediately for immobilized clients.

NURSING MANAGEMENT

Determine the client's immunization status. Use aseptic technique when cleansing soft-tissue injuries. Administer analgesic, immunization(s), and antibiotic as ordered. Encourage the client to keep the wound and dressing dry and clean, but instruct how to remove and change the dressing when dirty or wet.

NURSING PROCESS

ASSESSMENT

Subjective Data

Elicit the client's report of the injury. Evaluate and document the client's level of pain.

Objective Data

Obtain vital signs. Assess the wound or damaged area with regard to depth, location, and size (in centimeters). In the event of a bite, note the location and source of the bite.

> **PROFESSIONALTIP**
>
> **Snakebites**
>
> In the event of snakebite, it is essential to note the location of the fang marks and the distance (in centimeters) between the marks. Doing so helps determine the size of the snake and, thus, the likelihood of envenomation, as smaller, younger snakes typically have not yet learned to control the amount of venom released.

Nursing diagnoses for the client with a soft-tissue injury include the following:

NURSING DIAGNOSES	PLANNING/OUTCOMES	NURSING INTERVENTIONS
*Impaired **S**kin Integrity* related to break/wound in skin	The client's wound will heal.	Prepare client for cleansing and possible suturing of wound. Assist with possible suturing.
*Risk for **I**nfection* related to imbedded dirt/bacteria in the wound	The client's wound will heal without evidence of infection.	Cleanse wound thoroughly with soap and water. Administer tetanus intramuscularly (IM) if ordered. Teach the client to keep the wound and sutures dry and clean. Apply a topical antibiotic and clean dressing, if indicated. Teach the client to remove and change the dressing if it becomes dirty or wet. Tell the client to return for additional care if wound becomes red, edematous, or painful or exhibits purulent discharge.

Evaluation: Evaluate each outcome to determine how it has been met by the client.

SAMPLE NURSING CARE PLAN

The Client with a Soft-Tissue Injury

E.H., a 23-year-old Hispanic rancher, was brought to the ED after an accident at his ranch. He was riding his horse and fixing fences. The horse threw E.H. over its head and stomped E.H.'s left upper abdomen with its right forefoot. E.H., who states that he has never been hurt or previously admitted in the hospital, presents with a large, 6-centimeter-by-3-centimeter and 2-centimeter in depth, jagged laceration imbedded with dirt and other foreign material. There are no other associated injuries. A large pressure bandage that is saturated with bright-red blood is controlling the bleeding.

NURSING DIAGNOSIS 1 *Deficient Fluid Volume* related to active bleeding from traumatic abdominal laceration as evidenced by a large, jagged laceration measuring 6 centimeters by 3 centimeters and a large, bulky, saturated dressing

Nursing Outcomes Classification (NOC)
Fluid Balance
Hydration

Nursing Interventions Classification (NIC)
Wound Care
Fluid Monitoring

PLANNING/OUTCOMES	NURSING INTERVENTIONS	RATIONALE
E.H. will lose no more blood.	Apply clean pressure dressing.	Controls amount of bleeding.
	Prepare E.H. for suturing of the laceration.	Provides E.H. with knowledge of what is to happen.
	Monitor vital signs.	Identifies the client is going into shock from blood loss. Increased pulse and respiration and hypotension require immediate attention and intervention.

EVALUATION

E.H.'s wound was sutured. The dressing applied after suturing is clean and dry and showed no further evidence of bleeding at discharge.

SAMPLE NURSING CARE PLAN (Continued)

NURSING DIAGNOSIS 2 *Impaired Skin Integrity* related to abdominal injury as evidenced by a jagged laceration measuring 6 centimeters by 3 centimeters and 2 centimeters in depth

Nursing Outcomes Classification (NOC)
Tissue Integrity: Skin and Mucous Membranes
Wound Healing: Primary Intention

Nursing Interventions Classification (NIC)
Wound Care
Infection Protection

PLANNING/OUTCOMES	NURSING INTERVENTIONS	RATIONALE
E.H. will have regained skin integrity with sutures.	Prepare sterile environment for suturing.	Prevents additional bacteria from contaminating the wound.
	Assist physician with suturing of E.H.'s wound.	The nurse is responsible for assisting the physician, who is suturing.

EVALUATION

E.H. had intact skin integrity, with 22 sutures in place.

NURSING DIAGNOSIS 3 *Risk for Infection* related to laceration as evidenced by dirt and other foreign material imbedded in abdominal wound

Nursing Outcomes Classification (NOC)
Treatment Behavior: Illness or Injury
Immune Status

Nursing Interventions Classification (NIC)
Immunization/Vaccination Management
Infection Protection

PLANNING/OUTCOMES	NURSING INTERVENTIONS	RATIONALE
E.H.'s wound will not become infected.	Administer tetanus booster.	All wounds require that the client be current with regard to tetanus booster.
	Cleanse E.H.'s wound thoroughly after local anesthesia has been administered.	Wound is cleansed with the least discomfort to E.H.
	Remove as much dirt and foreign material as possible.	Prevents inflammation and infection at the wound site.
	Cleanse sutured wound and demonstrate care to E.H.	Removes old blood and other debris from the suturing. Teaches E.H. how to cleanse wound at home.
	Give E.H. explicit directions regarding taking oral antibiotics after discharge.	It is imperative that E.H. takes the full course of the antibiotics to prevent infection.
	Teach E.H. to care for wound.	Provides E.H. with knowledge to remove the dressing when it becomes wet or dirty and apply a new and clean dressing.
	Teach E.H. the signs and symptoms that require a return visit to the doctor (redness, inflammation, increased pain, purulent drainage).	Provides E.H. with knowledge to identify if the wound becomes infected.

(*Continues*)

SAMPLE NURSING CARE PLAN (Continued)

EVALUATION

E.H. was given a tetanus booster because he remembered having received his last at the age of 15. He verbalized the need to take the complete course of antibiotics when he went home.

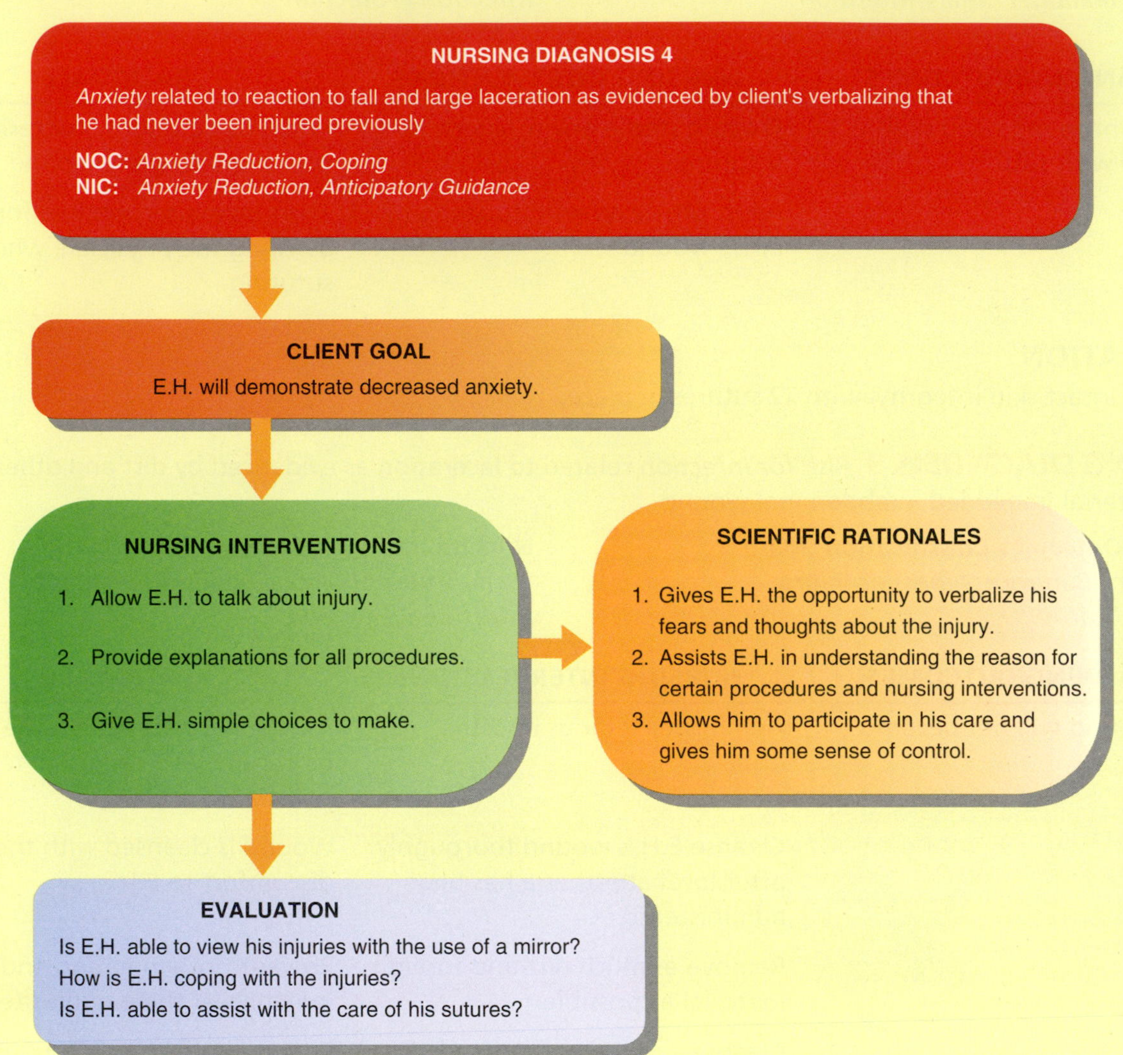

NURSING DIAGNOSIS 4
Anxiety related to reaction to fall and large laceration as evidenced by client's verbalizing that he had never been injured previously
NOC: Anxiety Reduction, Coping
NIC: Anxiety Reduction, Anticipatory Guidance
CLIENT GOAL
E.H. will demonstrate decreased anxiety.
NURSING INTERVENTIONS
1. Allow E.H. to talk about injury.
2. Provide explanations for all procedures.
3. Give E.H. simple choices to make.
SCIENTIFIC RATIONALES
1. Gives E.H. the opportunity to verbalize his fears and thoughts about the injury.
2. Assists E.H. in understanding the reason for certain procedures and nursing interventions.
3. Allows him to participate in his care and gives him some sense of control.
EVALUATION
Is E.H. able to view his injuries with the use of a mirror?
How is E.H. coping with the injuries?
Is E.H. able to assist with the care of his sutures?

POISONING AND DRUG OVERDOSES

Poisoning or drug overdose, whether accidental or intentional, is treated as an emergency. Poison is defined as any substance that causes harm to the body and may be tasteless, odorless, or colorless. There are many types of poisonings and drug overdoses with several different entry routes. Ingested poisonings are most common. The nurse obtains a clear history of the route of entry: inhalation, ingestion, topical, or injection. Poison exposure is difficult to diagnose and accurate identification of the substance is the most important aspect of safe and effective treatment. Poison control centers are the best source of antidote information for the client suffering from poisoning or drug overdose. The nationwide Poison Help Hotline (1-800-222-1222) is staffed 24 hours a day, 7 days a week, in the event of a poison related emergency, to help identify potential poisons and serve as a resource for medical treatment. In addition to treating for poisoning or drug overdose, evaluate the client for any associated injuries, such as lacerations from a fall.

Medical–Surgical Management

Medical

The ABCs are still the number one client priority. Oxygen is immediately initiated and IV access established. In addition, institute cardiac monitoring and obtain blood and urine samples for toxicology screening. Once the client is stabilized with adequate breathing, a protected airway, and sufficient perfusion of the brain and organs, try to identify the substance to minimize or reverse the effects. Treatments for ingestion include client monitoring and gastric lavage. Treatments for exposure include flushing the affected area or treating as a soft tissue injury.

Pharmacological

If the substance has been ingested, and institutional protocol dictates, administer activated charcoal. Give clients who have ingested caustic products copious amounts of water to dilute the substance. Sometimes the health care provider orders reversal agents, antidotes, and medications with complex nomograms and regimens of multiple labs to track blood concentrations.

In the event of accidental ingestion of pills or medication, the client may not be aware that over the counter (OTC) drugs, herbs or vitamins can cause serious side effects in combination with prescription drugs. When interviewing the client, review all forms of oral medication and supplements. Elderly clients sometimes see multiple physicians and receive medications of which other prescribing physicians are unaware. The nurse utilizes resources and teaches the clients to identify and eliminate these safety hazards.

Diet

The client who has overdosed is typically kept NPO until cleared by the health-care provider.

Nursing Management

Assess ABCs, initiate IV access, and administer oxygen. Begin cardiac monitoring. Obtain blood and urine samples. Keep client NPO. Obtain a history of the entire incident. Maintain a calm, supportive, nonjudgmental environment with the client and family while administering the prescribed treatment regimen. Continually monitor the client for changes in mental status or vital signs. Insure that the client and/or family receive adequate instruction regarding the use of OTC medications or supplements.

> **PROFESSIONAL TIP**
>
> **Interviewing a Client of Intentional Drug Overdose**
>
> The nurse requests additional family members to leave the room during the interview so the client is more free to answer questions. A client of intentional drug overdose may be reluctant to reveal what was taken. Ask the client or family to see the pill bottles if they are available. Look at the date the prescription was filled and then calculate how many pills should be in the bottle. If an excessive number of pills are missing from a bottle, it is considered suspect for intentional drug overdose. Admission to taking any form of pill or drug is recorded and evaluated.

NURSING PROCESS

Assessment

Subjective Data

Ask about the timing and the route of overdose. Evaluate mental status to establish whether the exposure was intentional. Document other incidences related to an overdose, such as an altercation with a loved one.

Objective Data

The client's vital signs are critical for baseline data. Try to identify the substance involved, as well as the amount.

Nursing diagnoses for the client with an overdose include the following:

NURSING DIAGNOSES	PLANNING/OUTCOMES	NURSING INTERVENTIONS
*Risk for **P**oisoning* related to ingestion of toxin	The client will recover with no residual effects of poisoning.	Manage the ABCs and stabilize the client. Monitor baseline laboratory work and ECG. Administer antidotes to toxins. Document the client's response.
*Risk for Self-Directed **V**iolence* related to harmful ingestion of toxic substance	The client will not harm self and will participate in help groups to work through issues.	Encourage the client to share reasons for overdose. Maintain a supportive, calm, reassuring environment for the client. If overdose was accidental, discuss exposure to toxin and ways to avoid exposure in the future. Teach varying methods of coping. Refer to help groups.

(*Continues*)

Nursing diagnoses for the client with an overdose include the following: (Continued)

NURSING DIAGNOSES	PLANNING/OUTCOMES	NURSING INTERVENTIONS
Interrupted ***Family*** *Processes* related to ingestion of harmful toxin	Client will begin to discuss problems with family.	Encourage client and family to discuss their problems openly and supportively and assist them in identifying different methods of coping. Encourage family counseling.

Evaluation: Evaluate each outcome to determine how it has been met by the client.

ENVIRONMENTAL/ TEMPERATURE EMERGENCIES

Exposure to extremes of heat and cold can be potentially life threatening. Severe cold, or hypothermia, occurs in very cold weather and from prolonged submersion in cold water. Heart rate and metabolic rate fall, and cardiac arrest may follow. Frostbite is another potentially dangerous result of exposure to cold (Table 52-4). The most common sites of frostbite are the fingers, toes, ears, and nose. Initially, frostbite causes paleness and numbness to the affected areas. If exposure continues, frostbite can progress to blistering and loss of feeling. The client may lose voluntary control over the affected body part. Rewarming in an emergency setting is imperative.

Extreme heat also causes potentially serious problems, especially in very young or elderly clients. As temperature rises, the body's ability to cool lessens. Table 52-5 compares heat injuries.

Table 52-4 Degrees of Frostbite Severity

DEGREE	SYMPTOMS	TREATMENT
Mild	Skin is cold to touch, pale, tingling, and numb, with a prickly sensation	Use blankets, warm clothing to warm cold flesh
Moderate	Affects deeper body tissue; skin appears waxy and is puffy to touch and itchy and burning with pain	Use gloves, blankets, warm clothing to warm cold flesh, observe closely for deeper injuries
Severe	Blistering, damage to all layers of soft tissue; flesh appears lifeless and is hard to the touch; no pain sensation in or ability to move frozen area	Initiate emergency rewarming in an ED using warm-water baths at 40.6°C (105°F); observe carefully for increased edema

COURTESY OF DELMAR CENGAGE LEARNING

Table 52-5 Comparison of Heat Injuries

TYPE	SYMPTOMS	TREATMENT
Heat cramps	Muscle cramps in arms, legs, and abdomen	Move client to cool, shady area. Slowly administer copious amounts of water. Reevaluate.
Heat exhaustion	Diaphoresis, with pale, moist, cool skin, headache, weakness, dizziness; muscle cramps, nausea, chills, tachypnea, confusion, tingling of hands and feet	Move client to cool, shady area. Loosen/remove constrictive clothing. Pour water over client; place client near fan. Encourage client to slowly drink water. Elevate client's legs. Reevaluate.
Heat stroke (a medical emergency)	Red, flushed, hot, dry skin; no diaphoresis	Reduce client's body temperature by removing client's clothing and pouring cool water over client. Start two large-bore IV lines. Use fan to cool client. Place client on cardiac monitor. Elevate client's legs. Assess client's vital signs, especially core (rectal) temperature. Check for neurological signs (confused, combative, disoriented). Check client's core (rectal) temperature frequently.

Developed from U.S. Army Training Support Command Protocols.

Medical–Surgical Management

Medical

For those exposed to extreme cold, rewarming is essential to resuscitation. The body's core (rectal) temperature is taken. Gradual warming is initiated using warm blankets, warmed oxygen, warmed IV fluids, warmed nasogastric tubes, and, in extreme instances, warmed enemas. Resuscitation should continue until the body has reached a core temperature of at least 34.4°C (94°F).

For frostbite, rewarming of the exposed body part is indicated. If the frostbite is severe, rapid rewarming is essential. This involves placing the frozen area in warm-water baths not exceeding 40.6°C (105°F). Tetanus is administered. Acute pain is treated with analgesics.

For heat injuries, rapidly reducing the body's temperature is vital. Supplemental oxygen may be administered. Pouring cool water over the client, chilling IV fluids, and fanning the client accelerates the cooling process.

Pharmacological

For heat and cold injuries, establishment of at least two large-bore IV lines is essential. Supplemental oxygen should be administered. Replacement of fluid and electrolytes is essential.

Diet

In the event of heat injuries, fluids, especially water, should be encouraged, if the client is able.

Nursing Management

Initiate CPR if needed. Monitor vital signs. Establish IV access. Provide oxygen and administer fluid and electrolytes as ordered. Warm or cool body as indicated. Monitor cardiac response.

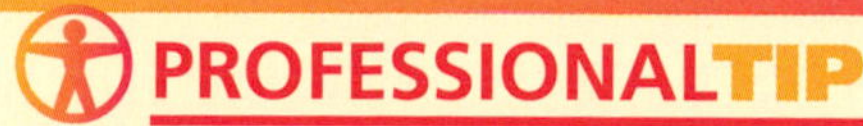

Frostbite

Do not massage or rub frostbite injuries because doing so can increase the severity of damage to tissue. Caffeine, alcohol, and smoking are avoided because they decrease circulation to the damaged tissue.

NURSING PROCESS

Assessment

Subjective Data

Ask the client to give a history of the heat/cold injury, if able, and any current medications taken.

Objective Data

Measure and document core (rectal) body temperature and vital signs. Record the client's skin color and temperature. Initiate cardiac monitoring to track any cardiac response to the heat or cold stress to the body. Evaluate pupillary response because neurological problems may result from the heat/cold injury.

Nursing diagnoses for the client with a temperature/environmental injury include the following:

NURSING DIAGNOSES	PLANNING/OUTCOMES	NURSING INTERVENTIONS
Hypothermia related to exposure to cold environment/long submersion in cold water	The client will regain normal core body temperature.	Administer supplemental oxygen. Monitor cardiac response carefully. If CPR is in progress, continue until the client's core temperature reaches 94°F and cardiac status is evaluated. Administer warmed IV fluids. Place warmed blankets on the client.
Hyperthermia related to environmental exposure to heat	The client will regain normal core body temperature.	Remove the client's clothing. Pour cool water over the client. Use large fan to cool the client. Administer chilled IV fluids and supplemental oxygen. Initiate cardiac monitoring. Evaluate client's neurological status with reference to orientation to time, person, and place. Measure core temperature every 30 minutes to assess progress.

Evaluation: Evaluate each outcome to determine how it has been met by the client.

MULTIPLE-SYSTEM TRAUMA

Multiple-system trauma is injury sustained in more than one body system. During the initial care of the emergent client, the mechanism of injury is determined. Blunt injuries and penetrating trauma are most likely to result in multiple-system involvement.

Medical–Surgical Management

Medical

Immediate management of the ABCs is imperative. Bleeding is stopped by the use of pressure applied to the wound. Two to four large-bore IV lines are started. Remove all clothing for visualization of bleeding and injuries. Obtain blood and urine specimens. Radiographic studies are performed. A tetanus booster also be administered.

Nursing Management

Assess and manage ABCs. Establish IV access. Remove the client's clothing for visualization of injuries. Obtain blood and urine specimens. Assess level of consciousness. Monitor vital signs and neurological status.

CRITICAL THINKING

Multiple-System Trauma

Under what circumstances might a client present with multiple-system trauma? How would you proceed with the assessment of such a client? What immediate actions would the nurse take to maintain the stability of this client?

NURSING PROCESS

Assessment

Subjective Data

Assess for level of consciousness and orientation to time, person, and place. Evaluate verbalizations of pain. Ask the client for an account of the accident.

Objective Data

Airway, breathing, and circulation are immediately assessed. Assess vital signs and neurological status by use of the Glasgow Coma Scale. Assess and control active bleeding.

Nursing diagnoses for the client with multiple-system trauma include the following:

NURSING DIAGNOSES	PLANNING/OUTCOMES	NURSING INTERVENTIONS
Impaired Spontaneous Ventilation related to major trauma and severe hypotension	The client will breathe without assistive devices.	Maintain open airway. Initiate rescue breathing. Ventilate per CPR protocol. Assist with insertion of endotracheal tube. Maintain pulse oximetry reading at 94% to 99%. Start multiple large-bore IV lines.
Powerlessness related to the inability to sustain life without emergency interventions	The client will survive the emergency and within several hours be able to indicate simple choices about care.	Explain all nursing/medical interventions to client. Provide emotional and physiological support to client and family as much as possible throughout resuscitation. Allow the client to make simple choices about care.

Evaluation: Evaluate each outcome to determine how it has been met by the client.

TERRORISM

Terrorist acts can appear in many forms; the events of September 11, 2001, is one example. Nuclear, chemical, and biological terrorism are other forms.

NUCLEAR TERRORISM

According to Kilpatrick (2002), the threat of nuclear terrorism is real. One example is the use of a radiation dispersal device (RDD), a so-called dirty bomb, which has nuclear waste in a conventional bomb. Another example is an attack on a domestic nuclear weapon facility. The effects of either example would be severe and widespread.

The source of radiation on contaminated clients is on the body or clothing, or has been ingested, or absorbed through a skin opening. The amount of radiation absorbed determines the effects on the client. Absorbed radiation, now measured by the gray (Gy), is equal to 100 Rads (old measurement) (Kilpatrick, 2002). When less than 0.75 Gy are absorbed, clients are not likely to have any symptoms, clients with 8 Gy would die, and 30 Gy is always fatal. The Occupational Safety and Health Administration (OSHA) requires that hospitals have an emergency plan for treating clients contaminated with radioactive substances. A decontamination area is set up in or near the ED.

The client who absorbs more than 0.75 Gy can develop acute radiation syndrome (ARS). Symptoms of ARS depend on the dose of radiation and include:

- *Hematopoietic.* Deficiency of WBCs and platelets leading to bleeding, anemia, infections, impaired wound healing, and immunodeficiency
- *Gastrointestinal.* Loss of mucosal barrier and cells lining intestines leading to fluid and electrolyte loss, vomiting, diarrhea, loss of normal flora, and sepsis
- *Cerebrovascular/CNS.* Cerebral edema, hyperpyrexia, hypotension, confusion, and disorientation
- *Skin.* Loss of epidermis and possibly dermis

Signs and symptoms in one or more of these areas appear immediately after exposure. This is the *prodromal phase.* In a day or so, all symptoms generally disappear for a few days to a few weeks. This is the *latent phase.* Next is the *illness phase,* in which the signs and symptoms reappear and intensify. After the peak of the illness phase, the client either begins to recover or dies from infection or other complications.

CHEMICAL TERRORISM

Several types of agents can be used in chemical terrorism, including nerve agents, pulmonary agents, cyanide agents, vesicant agents, and incapacitating agents. All clients exposed to chemical agents must be decontaminated.

Nerve Agents

Nerve agents include taubin (GA), sarin (GB), sonan, cyclosarin (GF), and one called VX (Armstrong, 2003; Yergler, 2002; Reilly & Deason, 2003). These are the most toxic of chemical agents and cause death within minutes. Clinical effects depend on dose and route of exposure, i.e., inhalation, skin contact, or ingestion. Inhalation is the most dangerous. These agents cause acetylcholine to accumulate either by preventing its breakdown or by desensitizing the receptor sites.

Symptoms range from increased saliva production, chest pressure, rhinorrhea, and vomiting to muscle weakness, incontinence, and convulsions. Symptoms may take up to 18 hours to appear with low exposure.

The antidotes are atropine and pralidoxime (2-PAM). Seizures are treated with diazepam (Valium).

Pulmonary Agents

Pulmonary agents include chlorine (CL), phosgene (CG), diphosgene (DP), and chloropicrin (PS). These agents, when inhaled, destroy the alveoli and capillary bed, resulting in pulmonary edema. There may be a 2- to 24-hour latent period before pulmonary edema occurs. The fluid in the lungs leads to hypovolemia and hypotension (Armstrong, 2002; Reilly & Deason, 2003).

Cyanide Agents

Hydrogen cyanide (AC) and cyanogen chloride (CR), which forms cyanide when metabolized, can be either ingested or inhaled. Cyanide prevents the transfer of oxygen from the blood to tissues. A client in severe respiratory distress but not cyanotic probably was exposed to cyanide. It has a pungent odor like bitter almonds or peaches. Death occurs in 5 to 10 minutes when exposed to a high concentration. Amyl nitrite is the antidote (Reilly & Deason, 2003).

Vesicant Agents

Sulfur mustard (HD), lewisite (L), and phosgene oxime (CX) are in the vesicant group. Phosgene oxime causes skin lesions not vesicles, as do the other two. These agents are more lethal than pulmonary agents and cyanide agents because they can remain in the environment for weeks, providing a continuing source of exposure to populations. Sulfur mustard smells like mustard or garlic, lewisite smells like geraniums, and phosgene oxime has a peppery smell.

All three agents affect the skin, eyes, and airway. Sulfur mustard, in large quantities, damages the bone marrow. Lewisite is immediately irritating, causing vesicles that progress to severe tissue necrosis and sloughing. Symptoms from sulfur mustard exposure appear in 4 to 8 hours, but cellular damage begins in 2 minutes (Reilly & Deason, 2003; Armstrong, 2002). Supportive care is primary treatment.

Incapacitating Agents

BZ, a glycolate anticholinergic compound, and Agent 15, a BZ "copy" made by Iraq, impair rather than kill or seriously injure victims (Armstrong, 2002). The effects are understimulation of organs similar to those of high doses of atropine. Hyperthermia, hallucinations, illusions, and erratic behavior are the greatest risks. The antidote is physostigmine sulfate (Eserine sulfate) or physostigmine salicylate (Antilirium).

BIOTERRORISM

Bioterrorism is deliberate releasing of pathogenic microorganisms such as viruses, bacteria, fungi, or toxins into a community. Many biologic agents are easily made and disseminated and can potentially injure or kill many people. The CDC has categorized these agents into three categories (Persell et al., 2002).

- *Category A* agents are easily disseminated or transmitted, have a high mortality, cause public panic, and require special public health management.
- *Category B* agents usually spread through water and food, have moderate morbidity and low mortality.
- *Category C* agents have not yet been weaponized (put into a form for mass destruction) but cause high morbidity and mortality.

The category A agents are the ones considered most likely to be used in a bioterrorism attack. Included are anthrax, smallpox, plague, botulism, viral hemorrhagic fevers (VHF), and tularemia. Many of these diseases begin with flu-like symptoms and are difficult to identify early. Knowledge about these diseases, careful observation for the sudden appearance of a disease or symptoms occurring at an unusual time, and some critical thinking may help identify a bioterrorist attack. An example is if many people suddenly have flu symptoms in the middle of summer (Steinhauer, 2002).

Anthrax

Anthrax is caused by *Bacillus anthracis.* It may manifest as a cutaneous, inhalation, or gastrointestinal disease. Cutaneous anthrax develops when spores enter a break in the skin. A pruritic macule or papule becomes vesicular and then forms a black, depressed scab. It is completely curable with treatment. Inhalation anthrax has an incubation period of up to 60 days. Mild flulike symptoms improve for 1 to 2 days and are followed by acute, severe dyspnea; stridor; and cyanosis. Gastrointestinal anthrax is unlikely because aerosolizing anthrax is easier than sabotaging food supplies.

Use Standard Precautions. No isolation is necessary. Treatment recommendations include ciprofloxacin (Cipro) or doxycycline calcium (Vibramycin, Monodox) given orally for cutaneous anthrax. These two drugs are initially given IV for inhalation anthrax along with one or two other antimicrobials, such as rifamin (Rifadin), vancomycin HCl (Vancocin), imipenem (Primaxin), penicillin, ampicillin, clindomycin HCl (Clocin), or clarithromycin (Biaxin) (Steinhauer, 2002). Later, clients are given the medications orally.

Smallpox

Smallpox, caused by variola virus, is easily transmitted from person to person by direct contact or inhalation of respiratory droplets. It has an incubation period of 7 to 19 days and is most contagious during the first week. This disease produces lesions in a body area in the same level of development. They progress from macules to vesicles to pustules and then scabs. Smallpox can be transmitted until all scabs fall off. This is unlike chicken pox, which has some lesions at each level of development in a body area at the same time.

Vaccination after exposure may decrease disease severity if given within 3 to 4 days of exposure. Standard Precautions, as well as isolation, airborne, and contact precautions, must be observed. Treatment is supportive with adequate hydration. All laundry and wastes must be autoclaved before washing or incinerating (Persell et al., 2002).

Plague

Plague, also called "black death," is caused by *Yersinia pastis.* When it is transmitted from an infected rodent to humans by an infected flea bite, it is called bubonic plague. Transmission from an infected individual to an uninfected individual by inhalation of respiratory droplets is called pneumonic plague. Terrorists would probably aerosolize the bacteria to cause pneumonic plague. Respiratory symptoms are the main manifestation.

The incubation period for pneumonic plague is 1 to 6 days. Clients must be treated with antibiotics within 24 hours of the first symptoms. Recommended antibiotics are streptomycin IM or gentamicin sulfate (Garamycin). For postexposure prophylaxis, doxycycline calcium (Vibramycin), ciprofloxacin (Cipro), or tetracycline HCl (Sumycin, Tetracyn) may be used.

Standard Precautions including gown, gloves, mask, and eye protection are used. Droplet precautions are followed for the first 48 hours of antibiotic therapy and until clinical improvement occurs.

Botulism

Botulism is caused by a toxin made by *Clostridium botulinum,* which paralyzes muscles. The toxin, one of the most poisonous substances known, is usually food borne. Terrorists would probably aerosolize the toxin for inhalation. The absorbed toxin irreversibly blocks cholinergic synapses, resulting in bilateral descending paralysis. There is no elevation of temperature, and clients retain complete cognitive functioning, although they may appear comatose.

Standard Precautions are used. Passive immunization with botulinum antitoxin may be used if botulism is recognized early. Care is supportive and may involve intensive care.

Viral Hemorrhagic Fevers

VHF includes Ebola, Lassa, Marburg, Crimean-Congo, Argentine, Yellow fever, and Dengue fever. Fever onset is sudden with signs and symptoms of circulatory compromise. All are infectious by aerosol except for Dengue fever. Ebola, Marburg, Lassa, and Crimean-Congo can be spread from person to person, especially during later stages of the disease.

Isolation in a negative-pressure room is recommended. Caregivers use a personal respirator, gown, gloves, face shield, and shoe and head covers. Care is supportive. There is no treatment or proven cure.

Tularemia

Tularemia, caused by *Francisella tularensis,* is not nearly as deadly as anthrax or plague. Inhalation of the bacteria is the likely route used in bioterrorist acts. Terrorists are believed to have developed antibiotic-resistant strains, so the number of fatalities could be high (Persell et al., 2002). There are currently no methods of rapid identification.

Standard Precautions are followed. For small outbreaks, parenteral therapy with either streptomycin or gentamicin sulfate (Garamycin) is recommended. When there are large outbreaks or for postexposure prophylaxis, oral doxycycline calcium (Vibramycin) or ciprofloxacin (Cipro) are the drugs of choice. Refer to Table 52-6 for isolation guidelines for biological agents.

LEGAL ISSUES

Emergency medicine allows medical personnel to care for clients without obtaining informed consent. In life-threatening and emergency situations, consent is implied. In addition, the Good Samaritan Law, one of the laws and regulations enforced for the benefit of both the caregiver and the client, provides protection against malpractice to persons who stop at the scene of an accident and render care. It should be noted, however, that the Good Samaritan Law offers protection only to those who provide safe and appropriate care; it does not protect those charged with gross negligence or willful misconduct.

There are other legal issues specific to emergency care. Several injuries/illnesses are reported to proper authorities. For instance, most states require that police be notified of MVCs, assaults, or rape. Likewise, animal control authorities require that animal bite reports be filed to facilitate follow-up on the possibility of rabies.

DEATH IN THE EMERGENCY DEPARTMENT

Death can occur in the ED at any time as a result of trauma, sudden illness, or even extended illness. This creates a delicate situation, because the death is usually unexpected. Family members may have a difficult time dealing with sudden death. If their loved one is being resuscitated in the ED, there is little time for health care personnel to comfort the family because the personnel are very busy providing care to the client. In the event of sudden death, the family is usually in a state of shock and will need further assistance to cope with the death of their loved one. Special support groups are available for this assistance and are contacted for the family.

TABLE 52-6 Isolation Guidelines for Biological Agents

	Bacterial Agents	Anthrax	Brucellosis	Cholera	Glanders	Bubonic plague	Pneumonic plague	Tularemia	Q fever	***Viruses***	Smallpox	Venez. equine encephalitis	Viral hemorrhagic fever	***Biological Toxins***	Botulism	Ricin
Isolation Precautions																
Standard precautions for all aspects of patient care		X	X	X	X	X	X	X	X		X	X	X		X	X
Contact precautions (gown and gloves; wash hands after each patient encounter)			X[c]	X[a]	X[a]						X		X			
Airborne precautions (negative pressure room and N-95 masks for all individuals entering the room)											X		X[b]			
Droplet precautions (surgical mask)							X									
Patient Placement																
No restrictions		X	X	X	X			X	X			X			X	X
Cohort like patients when private room unavailable				X[c]	X[a]	X	X				X		X			
Private room				X[c]	X[a]	X[a]	X				X		X			
Negative pressure											X		X[b]			
Door closed at all times											X		X[b]			
Patient Transport																
No restrictions		X	X	X	X	X		X	X			X			X	X
Limit movement to essential medical purposes only				X[c]	X[a]	X[a]	X[a]				X[a]		X			
Place mask on patient to minimize dispersal of droplets							X[a]				X[a]		X[b]			
Discontinuation of Isolation																
48 hours of appropriate antibiotic and clinical improvement							X									
Until all scabs separate											X					
Until skin decontamination completed (1 hour contact time)																
Duration of illness				X[c]	X[a]	X[a]							X			

[a] Contact precautions needed only if the patient has skin involvement (bubonic plague: draining bubo) or until decontamination of skin is complete.

[b] A surgical mask and eye protection should be worn if you come within three feet of patient. Airborne precautions are needed if patient has cough, vomiting, diarrhea, or hemorrhage.

[c] Contact precautions needed only if the patient is diapered or incontinent.

Adapted by R. Daniels, L. H. Nicoll, & L. J. Nosek, 2007, from Biological weapons and emergency preparedness, Part I, by R. Stilp, 2004. Retrieved June 27, 2006, from nsweb.nursingspectrum.com

CASE STUDY

J.D. fell from a fishing boat into deep, cold water. He was wearing a life vest and was rescued within 10 minutes, at which time he was immediately dried, placed in a blanket, and brought to the ED. He is alert and oriented to person, time, and place, but is shivering uncontrollably and pale in color. His core temperature is 93°F.

The following questions will guide your development of a nursing care plan for the case study.

1. List the assessments according to the priority of performance.
2. Identify the priority nursing diagnoses for J.D.
3. List nursing interventions according to the priority of performance.
4. Identify the treatment outcomes for J.D.

SUMMARY

- Clients in shock need immediate assessment and intervention.
- Rapid assessment and observation of ABCs is essential in treating all cardiovascular emergencies.
- Evaluation of abdominal emergencies include taking a history of the onset of pain because this is critical to outcome and survival.
- Ocular emergencies can be a threat to vision and thus require immediate assessment and treatment.
- Musculoskeletal and soft-tissue injuries are painful but manageable with rapid assessment and treatment.
- In cases of poisoning or drug overdoses, the ABCs are first established, then the agent to which the client was exposed is immediately identified so that prompt treatment is initiated.
- Major trauma is a life-threatening and unexpected occurrence for both client and loved ones.
- Terrorism is a viable threat and emergency nurses need to be knowledgeable about possible biological, chemical and nuclear exposure agents, symptoms of exposed victims, and nursing interventions for each situation.
- Nurses must be aware of the legal issues related to emergency care, such as Good Samaritan Laws and mandated reporting.

REVIEW QUESTIONS

1. Triage is a system of:
   1. identifying clients by disease.
   2. prioritizing client care.
   3. counting clients waiting for care.
   4. medical diagnosing.

2. A client with a small branch sticking out of the right midchest arrives at the ED during a hurricane. There is bubbling and oozing at the site. Medical personnel should first:
   1. remove the branch and save it.
   2. administer pain medication to the client.
   3. start the ABCs of CPR.
   4. stop the bleeding and take vital signs.

3. An example of a nonurgent client is one with:
   1. CPR in progress.
   2. fractures of both legs.
   3. heat stroke.
   4. a sprained ankle.

4. The ambulance brings a client with a large, bleeding laceration of the upper leg to the ED. Vital signs are as follows: blood pressure 78/62 mm Hg, pulse 112 beats/min, and respirations 26 breaths/min. A priority nursing diagnosis is:
   1. *Deficient **F**luid Volume.*
   2. *Risk for **A**spiration.*
   3. *Risk for **I**nfection.*
   4. *Disturbed **B**ody Image.*

5. Interventions for a client in shock include:
   1. pain control and assessment of vital signs.
   2. administration of oxygen and IV fluids.
   3. insertion of a nasogastric tube.
   4. calling the physician.

6. For which client should the nurse provide care first?
   1. A client who needs her dressing changed.
   2. A client who needs to be suctioned.
   3. A client who needs to be medicated for incisional pain.
   4. A client who is incontinent and needs to be cleaned.

7. An adult suffered a diving accident and is brought in by an ambulance intubated and on a backboard with a cervical collar. What is the nurse's first action when the client arrives at the hospital?
   1. Take the client's vital signs.
   2. Check the lungs for equal breath sounds bilaterally.

3. Insert a large bore IV line according to physician orders.
4. Perform a neurologic check using the Glasgow Coma Scale.

8. An adult is brought in by ambulance after a motor vehicle crash. He is unconscious and on a backboard, with his neck immobilized. He is bleeding profusely from a large gash on his right thigh. What is the nurse's second priority action in caring for the client?
   1. Stop the bleeding.
   2. Check the airway.
   3. Connect the client to a cardiac monitor.
   4. Cleanse the wound.
9. A client is brought to the emergency room after taking an overdose of several different types of pills. What choice is the last priority for the nurse?
   1. Check the airway.
   2. Connect the client to the cardiac monitor.
   3. Identify the pills the client swallowed.
   4. Lavage the stomach contents according to physician orders.
10. What symptoms are third in the sequence of signs and symptoms of nuclear exposure?
   1. Signs and symptoms reappear and intensify.
   2. After the peak of the symptoms, the client begins to recover.
   3. Signs and symptoms appear immediately after exposure.
   4. Symptoms disappear for a few day or weeks.

REFERENCES/SUGGESTED READINGS

American Heart Association. (1997). *Advanced cardiac life support*. Dallas, TX: Author.

Arbour, R. (1998). Aggressive management of intracranial dynamics. *Critical Care Nurse, 18*, 30–40.

Armstrong, J. (1998). Bombs and other blasts. *RN, 61*(11), 26–29.

Armstrong, J. (2002). Chemical warfare. *RN, 65*(4), 32–39.

BCEMS Web. (2009). START. Retrieved July 24, 2009 from http://emsstaff.buncombecounty.org/inhousetraining/start/start_overview2.htm

Blank-Reid, C. (1999). Strangulation. *RN, 62*(2), 32–35.

Bowen, T., & Bellamy, R. (Eds.). (1998). *Emergency war surgery*. United States Department of Defense. Washington, DC: United States Government Printing Office.

Bulechek, G., Butcher, H., McCloskey, J., & Dochterman, J., eds. (2008). *Nursing Interventions Classification (NIC)* (5th ed.). St. Louis, MO: Mosby/Elsevier.

Carroll, P. (1999). Chest injuries. *RN, 62*(1), 36–43.

Centers for Disease Control and Prevention (CDC). (2009). Motor vehicle safety. Retrieved July 24, 2009 from http://www.cdc.gov/Motorvehiclesafety/index.html

Chavez, J., & Brewer, C. (2002). Stopping the shock slide. *RN, 65*(9), 30–34.

Coleman, E. (2001). Anthrax. *AJN, 101*(12), 48–52.

Coleman, E. (2002). Tularemia. *AJN, 102*(6), 65–69.

Coleman, E., & Yergler, M. (2002). Botulism. *AJN, 102*(9), 44–47.

Critical Illness and Trauma Foundation, Inc. (2001). START. Retrieved July 24, 2009 from http://www.citmt.org/start/flowchart.htm#Simplified

Daniels R., Nosek, L., & Nicoll, L. (2007). *Contemporary medical-surgical nursing*. Clifton Park, NY: Delmar Cengage Learning.

Easter, A. (2002). Ebola. *AJN*, 102(12), 49–52.

Estes, M. (2010). *Health assessment & physical examination* (4th ed.). Clifton Park, NY: Delmar Cengage Learning.

Gebbie, K., & Qureshi, K. (2002). Emergency and disaster preparedness: Core competencies for nurses. *AJN, 102*(1), 46–51.

Harrison, T., Gustafson, E., & Dixon, J. (2003). Radiologic emergency: Protecting schoolchildren & the public. *AJN, 103*(5), 41–48.

Hayes, L. (2000). Poison emergency. *Nursing2000, 30*(9), 34–39.

Huston, C. (2001). Dog bite. *Nursing2001, 31*(7), 88.

Integrated Publishing: Medical. (2009). Primary survery. Retrieved July 27, 2009 from http://www.tpub.com/content/medical/14295/css/14295_144.htm

Kilpatrick, J. (2002). Nuclear attacks. *RN, 65*(5), 46–51.

Laskowski-Jones, L. (2000a). Responding to summer emergencies. *Nursing2000, 30*(5), 34–39.

Laskowski-Jones, L. (2000b). Responding to winter emergencies. *Nursing2000, 30*(1), 34–39.

Laskowski-Jones, L. (2002). Responding to an out-of-hospital emergency. *Nursing2002, 32*(9), 36–42.

Lewis, A. (1999). Neurologic emergency. *Nursing99, 29*(10), 54–56.

McMahon, M. (2003). ED triage. *AJN, 102*(3), 61–63.

Moorhead, S., Johnson, M., Maas, M., & Swanson, E. (2007). *Nursing Outcomes Classification (NOC)* (4th ed). St. Louis, MO: Mosby.

National Association of Emergency Medical Technicians. (2006). PHTLS. Basic and advanced pre-hospital trauma life-support (6th ed.). St. Louis, MO: Mosby/JEMS.

North American Nursing Diagnosis Association International. (2010). *NANDA-I nursing diagnoses: Definitions and classification 2009–2011*. Ames, IA: Wiley-Blackwell.

Persell, D., Arangie, P., Young, C., Stokes, E., Payne, W., Skorga, P., & Gilbert-Palmer, D. (2002). Preparing for bioterrorism. *Nursing2002, 32*(2), 36–43.

Pettinicchi, T. (1998). Lightning strike. *Nursing98, 28*(7), 33.

Quinn, S. (1998). ED triage. *RN, 61*(9), 53–60.

Ramponi, D. (2000). Go with the flow during an eye emergency. *Nursing2000, 30*(8), 54–56.

Rebmann, T., Carrico, R., & English, J. (2002). Are you prepared for a bioterrorist attack? *Nursing2002, 32*(9), 32hn1–32hn6.

Reilly, C., & Deason, D. (2002). Plague: A naturally occurring bacterial species can be weaponized *AJN, 102*(11), 47–50.

Reilly, C., & Deason, D. (2002). Smallpox: Eradicated more than 20 years ago, this killer is again causing concern. Will you know it when you see it? *AJN, 102*(2), 51–55.

Reilly, C., & Deason, D. (2003). How would you respond to a chemical release? *Nursing2003, 33*(1), 36–42.

Ruffolo, D. (2002). Hypothermia in trauma. *RN, 65*(2), 46–51.

Schulmerich, S. (1999). When nature turns up the heat. *RN, 62*(8), 35–38.

Sibley, C. (2002). Smallpox: Vaccination revisited. *AJN, 102*(9), 26–32.

Siwula, C. (2003). Managing pediatric emergencies. *Nursing2003, 33*(2), 48–51.

Sommers, M. (1998). Missed injuries. *RN, 61*(10), 28–31.

Spratto, G., & Woods, A. (2009). *2009 PDR nurses' drug handbook.* Clifton Park, NY: Delmar Cengage Learning.

Stacy, P. (1998). On-scene care. *RN, 61*(9), 50–52.

Steffen, K. (2003). When your trauma patient is over 65. *Nursing2003, 33*(4), 53–56.

Steinhauer, R. (2002). Bioterrorism. *RN, 65*(3), 48–54.

Talbert, S., & Talbert, P. (1998). Flight nursing: Summary of strategies for managing severe traumatic brain injury during early posttraumatic phase. *Journal of Emergency Nursing, 24,* 254–257.

The American Association for the Surgery of Trauma. (2007). Introduction. Retrieved July 24, 2009 from http://www.aast.org/TraumaFacts/dynamic.aspx?id=964

TRAUMA! (1998). *RN, 61*(9), 49.

Veenema, T. (2002). The smallpox vaccine debate. *AJN, 102*(9), 33–38.

Veenema, T., & Daram, P. (2003). Radiation. *AJN 103*(5), 32–40.

Wiebelhaus, P., & Hansen, S. (2001). Burn emergencies. *Nursing2001, 31*(1), 36-41.

Woods, A. (2002). New threat from an ancient microbe: Anthrax. *Nursing2002, 32*(1), 44–45.

Yergler, M. (2002). Nerve gas attack. *AJN, 102*(7), 57–60.

RESOURCES

Agency for Toxic Substances and Disease Registry, http://www.atsdr.cdc.gov

American Association of Critical Care Nurses (AACN), http://www.aacn.org

American Association of Poison Control Centers, http://www.aapcc.org/DNN/

American Red Cross, http://www.redcross.org

Centers for Disease Control and Prevention, http://www.cdc.gov

Emergency Nurses Association (ENA), http://www.ena.org

International Nursing Coalition for Mass Casualty Education, http://www.nursing.vanderbilt.edu

Johns Hopkins University, Center for Civilian Biodefense Strategies, http://www.jhu.edu/

Oak Ridge Institute for Science and Education, Radiation Emergency Assistance Center/Training Site, http://www.orau.gov/reacts

Salvation Army USA National Headquarters, http://www.salvationarmyusa.org

U. S. Food and Drug Administration, http://www.fda.gov

CHAPTER 53
Integration

MAKING THE CONNECTION

Through careful study of Adult Health Nursing, a knowledge base is developed in preparation for the critical thinking exercises in this chapter. Each critical thinking exercise begins with an index of the body systems relevant to the case study. Refer back to these chapters as needed while working through the case study.

LEARNING OBJECTIVES

Upon completion of this chapter, you should be able to:

- Integrate how a condition affects several body systems and causes multiple clinical problems.

INTRODUCTION

The format of this chapter is different than previous chapters. Multiple system disease processes are presented in a case study format. Answering the case study questions enhances problem-solving techniques and critical thinking skills. Information learned in previous chapters is integrated into the case studies to develop a holistic view of the disease as it affects multiple systems. The student examines the interweaving of pathophysiology causing the disease process and develops the nursing process for the disease. An example is diabetes that affects other body systems such as the integumentary, nervous, musculoskeletal, cardiac, vascular, blood, gastrointestinal, urinary, and reproductive.

Read the case study, and then analyze how the condition affects other body systems. It may be helpful to first outline the condition presented in the case study by making a grid of the signs and symptoms, pathophysiology, diagnostic studies, and nursing interventions. Refer to the grid when answering the questions (see Table 53-1).

The case study questions can be completed alone, in a study group, or in a classroom setting. When completed, share the answers and charts with the entire group to enhance everyone's learning experience. Remember, each student or group of students arrives at the answers or present the answers in a different manner. The process followed is less important than the opportunity to integrate all aspects of the

TABLE 53-1 Grid for Reviewing the Case Study Disease

DISEASE	
Pathophysiology	
Incidence/Risk factors	
Diagnostic tests	
Signs and symptoms	
Nursing interventions	

COURTESY OF DELMAR CENGAGE LEARNING

condition and use critical thinking skills, as long as sound, logical nursing judgment is utilized in obtaining an appropriate answer. This is an opportunity to think creatively and freely.

SYSTEMS REVIEWED IN DIABETES MELLITUS MULTISYSTEM CASE STUDY

- Cardiovascular system
- Urinary system
- Neurological system
- Sensory system
- Endocrine system
- Reproductive systems
- Integumentary system

DIABETES MELLITUS CASE STUDY

M.B., a 46-year-old insurance salesman, is admitted to the hospital with the diagnosis of diabetes type 1.

- List the etiological risk factors for diabetes type 1.
- Brainstorm subjective and objective data that would be included in the assessment of M.B.
- Develop a patho-flow diagram identifying the symptoms M.B. may have been experiencing on admission and relate the pathophysiology of diabetes to the symptoms (see the examples of a patho-flow diagram in Figure 53-1 and an interrelationship chart in Figure 53-2).
- What diagnostic tests could the physician have ordered to confirm the diagnosis of diabetes?
- Relate the possible results of the diagnostic tests to the pathophysiological cause of the results on the patho-flow diagram.
- If M.B. had been diagnosed with diabetes type 2, how would the pathophysiology and nursing care vary?

A couple of days after M.B. was diagnosed with diabetes, he said to the nurse, "One of my friends at work said there are a lot of future problems with diabetes. I am concerned about this. What are some of the problems? What can I do to keep these problems from occurring?"

- What would be appropriate responses of the nurse?
- List local resources or support groups where M.B. and his family could be referred.

The discharge teaching included insulin administration, diet, exercise, foot care, and eye exams.

- What is important to include in the discharge teaching regarding:
  - insulin administration
  - diet
  - exercise
  - foot care
  - eye exams
- Develop a care plan for M.B.

Eight years after M.B. was diagnosed with diabetes, he had a routine physical examination. At that time his blood pressure (BP) was 174/96. The physician monitored the

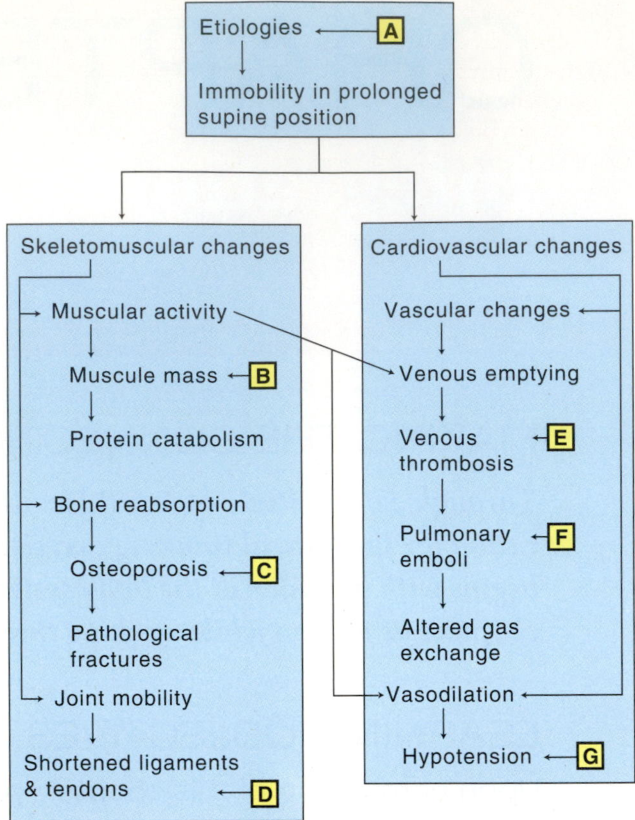

FIGURE 53-1 An example of a patho-flow diagram of skeletomuscular and cardiovascular changes caused by immobility. Complete the following instructions corresponding to the letters located at specific points along the pathophysiologic sequence of events. *A,* List the risk conditions that may lead to immobility. *B,* Name the assessment data at this point. *C,* List the interventions that would minimize calcium loss. *D,* Name the outcome criteria associated with effective nursing interventions at this point. *E,* State the assessment data at this point. *F,* List the interventions that may prevent the development of this complication. *G,* List the nursing interventions to minimize this consequence. (*Courtesy of the* Journal of Nursing Education.)

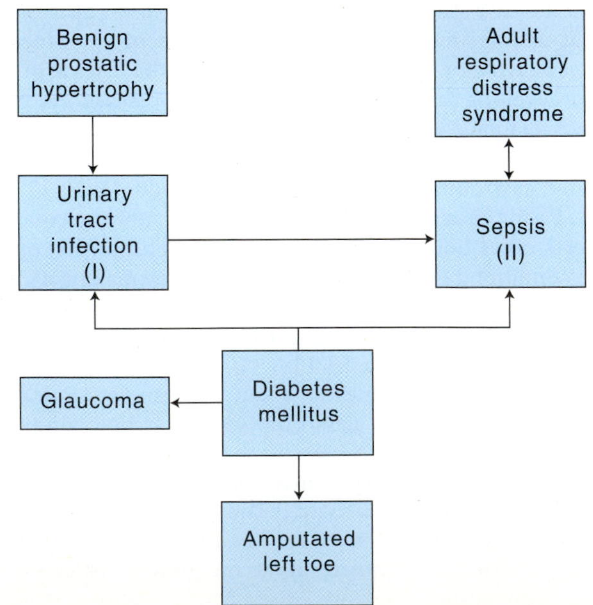

FIGURE 53-2 Interrelationships of Conditions and Symptoms (*Courtesy of the* Journal of Nursing Education.)

BP for 3 weeks and then placed M.B. on enalapril maleate (Vasotec). His urine had a trace of albumin.

- What common complication of diabetes could be occurring to cause M.B. to have hypertension? Explain the pathophysiology of the complication.
- What is the action of Vasotec in lowering BP?
- What is the rationale for placing M.B. on enalapril maleate (Vasotec) rather than propranolol hydrochloride (Inderal), verapamil (Calan), or clonidine hydrochloride (Catapres)?
- What other complications could have a circulatory etiology?
- What could be the possible long-term renal complication from diabetes mellitus?
- Explain the pathophysiology of renal complications as they relate to diabetes. Relate these to the patho-flow diagram previously developed.

One evening, M.B. was massaging his foot while watching television. He noticed an ulcerated area between his third and fourth toe.

- State possible reasons M.B. may not have felt pain from the ulcerated area. Relate these to the patho-flow diagram previously developed.

During a yearly physical, M.B. relates difficulty obtaining an erection.

- Explain the rationale for this complication.
- What nursing interventions are appropriate at this time?

In later years, M.B. may experience some symptoms from autonomic neuropathies.

- List symptoms that may occur and relate the symptoms to the pathophysiological etiology.

SYSTEMS REVIEWED IN CIRRHOSIS MULTISYSTEM CASE STUDY

- Respiratory system
- Cardiovascular system
- Hematologic and lymphatic systems
- Gastrointestinal system
- Urinary system
- Musculoskeletal system
- Neurological system
- Endocrine system
- Integumentary system

CIRRHOSIS CASE STUDY

B.W., a 60-year-old male client, is admitted to the hospital with hematemesis. He has a history of alcohol abuse. B.W.'s wife and two daughters accompany him. B.W. is 5'10" tall and weighs 140 lbs. His vital signs are temperature (T) 98.2°F, apical pulse (AP) 98 and slightly irregular, respiration (R) 24 breaths/min, and BP 152/88. He is lethargic, confused, and jaundiced. When the nurse assesses his lung sounds, she hears pulmonary crackles in all lobes. His abdominal girth measures 44 inches. His wife states he has not gone to the bathroom all morning. He has +3 edema in his feet and ankles. B.W.'s primary diagnosis is hematemesis with a secondary diagnosis of cirrhosis.

- Brainstorm other subjective and objective data that are important to include in the assessment of B.W.
- Relate the pathophysiology of cirrhosis to the assessed symptoms and other symptoms B.W. may have experienced. Develop a patho-flow chart relating the symptoms to the pathological cause.
- List diagnostic tests that would be appropriate for the health care provider to order for B.W. What abnormal laboratory results would be typical of cirrhosis?
- Relate the possible results of the diagnostic tests to the developed patho-flow chart.
- Besides alcohol abuse, what are some other causes of cirrhosis?
- List complications of cirrhosis caused by chronic alcohol abuse.
- Explain the pathophysiology of portal hypertension as it relates to cirrhosis. Relate these to the patho-flow chart previously developed.
- List diuretics that may be ordered for B.W. to decrease the ascites.
- How does the action of lactulose (Cephulac) lower the level of ammonia in the blood?
- What other complications result from portal hypertension?
- Explain the rationale for the complication of pleural effusion.
- Identify possible nursing diagnoses for B.W.
- What nursing interventions would be appropriate at this time?
- Develop a care plan for B.W.
- If B.W.'s condition improved and he was scheduled for discharge, what is important to include in the discharge teaching regarding:
  - bleeding tendencies
  - exercise
  - nutrition
  - skin care
- Develop diet instructions for B.W. according to various cultural influences.
- List local resources/support groups where B.W. and his family could be referred.

B.W.'s daughter says, "I wish Dad would have quit drinking years ago. I was always embarrassed by his behavior when he had too much to drink. His life could have had so much potential."

- What would be appropriate therapeutic responses of the nurse?

SYSTEMS REVIEWED IN HYPERTENSION, CONGESTIVE HEART FAILURE, AND CHRONIC RENAL FAILURE MULTISYSTEM CASE STUDY

- Respiratory system
- Cardiovascular system
- Hematologic and lymphatic systems

- Gastrointestinal system
- Urinary system
- Musculoskeletal system
- Neurological system
- Endocrine system
- Reproductive systems
- Integumentary system
- Immune system

HYPERTENSION, CONGESTIVE HEART FAILURE, AND CHRONIC RENAL FAILURE CASE STUDY

M.B has a 20-year history of hypertension. She has been noncompliant in taking her antihypertensive medications that were prescribed by her physician. She recently developed symptoms of congestive heart failure and renal failure.

- Brainstorm some reasons for M.B.'s noncompliance.
- Name some medications that may have been prescribed to treat M.B.'s hypertension. List the advantage and disadvantage of each medication.
- Using Table 39-4, Effects of Chronic Renal Failure by Body System, develop a concept map showing the relationship of hypertension to the effects of renal failure on each listed system.
- What is the relationship between hypertension, increased peripheral resistance, cardiac hypertrophy, and congestive heart failure?
- What is the relationship of blood pressure (hypotension and hypertension) and renal failure?
- What is the relationship between the heart's decreasing ability to pump blood through the blood vessels and pulmonary edema?
- Explain the relationship between fluid in the alveoli and dyspnea.
- Physiologically, what is occurring in M.B.'s body to cause an increased rate of respiration?
- List laboratory results that would indicate that M.B. is developing chronic renal failure.
- List symptoms that would indicate M.B. is developing chronic renal failure.
- List subjective and objective data for which the nurse would assess for symptoms of chronic renal failure.
- List laboratory results that would indicate that M.B. is developing congestive heart failure.
- List symptoms that would indicate M.B. is developing congestive heart failure. Give the cause/etiology for each symptom.
- List subjective and objective data for which the nurse would assess for symptoms of congestive heart failure.
- Identify possible nursing diagnoses for M.B.
- List nursing interventions and give rationale for each intervention.

M.B.'s abdomen is distended, and she has lost her appetite for the last 2 days. She has had hiccups constantly for 2 hours. She says, "I am so tired of these hiccups. Why am I having them?"

- Explain to M.B. the cause for her hiccups.
- What are some medical and nursing interventions to relieve the distress of constant hiccups?

SYSTEMS REVIEWED IN PARKINSON DISEASE CASE STUDY

- Respiratory system
- Gastrointestinal system
- Urinary system
- Musculoskeletal system
- Neurological system
- Sensory system
- Integumentary system

PARKINSON DISEASE CASE STUDY

P.K. is a 76-year-old man who was exposed to several chemicals during his farming career. For the last 7 years, he has walked with his arms flexed, leaning forward with his head bowed. Recently, he has had difficulty rising from a chair and balancing himself when he walks. He fell twice when doing odd jobs around the house. He started making a "to-do list" because he has difficulty remembering. He goes to the store for three items but returns with only two. His wife noticed that he has a slight tremor in his hand when he eats and often rolls his forefinger and thumb together in a circular motion.

- Use deductive reasoning and identify P.K.'s possible diagnosis.
- With these symptoms, what diagnostic tests may the doctor order?

P.K. shared his symptoms with his family physician. After some tests were completed and results of referrals to specialists were returned, the physician told P.K. he was suspecting Parkinson disease. P.K. said, "Tell me about Parkinson disease."

- Relate what a nurse could teach P.K. about Parkinson disease.
- List objective and subjective data needed to make an appropriate and thorough assessment on P.K.
- List etiological causes of Parkinson disease. What possible etiological factors does P.K. have?
- Explain the function of dopamine, a neurotransmitter, to the symptoms displayed in a client with Parkinson disease.
- List drugs that interfere in the synthesis and storage of dopamine.
- List the signs and symptoms of Parkinson disease. Think of a client with Parkinson disease, and relate his or her symptoms to the textbook symptoms.
- Develop a patho-flow map or concept map relating the pathophysiology of Parkinson disease to the systems that could be affected and the typical symptoms of that system.
- List drugs that P.K. may receive to control symptoms of Parkinson disease. List the symptoms and side effects that need monitoring with each of the drugs listed.

P.K. is becoming more rigid, having difficulty swallowing food, falling frequently, reaching for items to assist in ambulating, experiencing frequent incontinence, complaining of his eyes itching, and having severe memory loss. His voice has become soft, and his speech is slurred.

- List P.K.'s autonomic symptoms.
- Develop diet instructions for P.K. and his wife.
- What possible surgical procedures could be done to relieve P.K.'s symptoms.
- Develop a nursing care plan for P.K. listing nursing diagnoses, goals, and nursing interventions to address each symptom.
- Using the Internet, research new therapies for Parkinson disease, and share them with other students.

After a year, P.K. is unable to walk and is lifted from his bed to his wheelchair. He is unable to verbally communicate. He no longer has bladder control. When he was fed his lunch, he started coughing and perhaps aspirated some food.

- List appropriate subjective and objective data needed in a nursing assessment.
- Reevaluate the previously developed nursing care plan and revise appropriately.

SYSTEMS REVIEWED IN HEMATOLOGIC DISORDER MULTISYSTEM CASE STUDY

- Respiratory system
- Cardiovascular system
- Hematologic system
- Lymphatic system
- Gastrointestinal system
- Urinary system
- Musculoskeletal system
- Neurological system
- Integumentary system

HEMATOLOGIC DISORDER CASE STUDY

J.D., a 69-year-old man, visits the health care clinic. When seen by the health-care provider, he states he has had a cold for 4 weeks and cannot seem to get over it. He also mentions that the bones in his legs are "hurting." The nurse notes on his chart that he has a productive cough and nasal drainage. He states he is tired all the time and cannot seem to get rested. His skin is pale, and he became short of breath walking from the waiting room to the exam room. His vital signs are T 100.2°F, P 92 beats/min, R 22 breaths/min, SaO_2 90, and weight is 140 lbs, a decrease of 10 pounds since his last visit 3 months ago. During his physical exam the health care provider notes two open sores in J. D's mouth, petechiae on his lower extremities, an ecchymosed spot on his right lower arm, and swollen lymph nodes in his neck and groin.

- From the listed symptoms, what do you suspect is J.D.'s diagnosis?
- What diagnostic tests are appropriate for the health care provider to order for J.D.?

The health care provider ordered a complete blood count (CBC), fibrin degradation fragment, and activated partial thromboplastin time (APTT) for J.D. The results of the CBC are hemoglobin (Hgb) 13.0 g/dL, hematocrit (HCT) 40%, white blood cells (WBCs) 75,000, red blood cells (RBCs) 3.5 M/mL, platelets 130 K/mL. The fibrin degradation fragment is 25 mg/mL, and the APTT is 45 sec.

- Complete the lab values chart and compare normal lab values with J.D.'s results.

CBC TEST	NORMAL VALUES	J.D.'S RESULTS
Hgb		13.0 g/dL
HCT		40%
WBC		75 K/mL
RBC		3.5 M/mL
Platelet count		130 K/mL
Fibrin degradation fragment		25 mg/mL
APTT		45 sec

- What hematologic diagnosis does J.D.'s lab results suggest?
- What lab results, either ones ordered or not ordered, rule out thrombocytopenia, myeloma, Hodgkin disease, and non-Hodgkin's lymphoma?
- According to your data-gathering skills, what is the next confirmative diagnostic test the health care provider would order?

The health-care provider orders a chest x-ray and a skeletal bone x-ray. With J.D.'s potential diagnosis, what do you think the x-rays will reveal?

The health-care provider completes a bone biopsy on J.D. and the results confirm the diagnosis of leukemia. The health care provider determines that J.D. has AML.

- What other symptoms could J.D. have with AML?
- Normally increased WBCs fight off an infection. Explain the reason the increased WBCs are not able to fight the bacteria causing J.D.'s infection.
- J.D. has bone pain. Explain the pathophysiology of the bone pain.
- J.D. has dyspnea with slight exertion. Explain the pathophysiology of the dyspnea.
- The health-care provider places J.D. on a bland, high-protein, high-carbohydrate diet. Following the health care provider's orders, develop a nutritious diet for J.D. for 3 days.
- What are the treatment options for J.D.?
- What type of chemotherapy is used for AML?
- Explain the steps of bone marrow transplantation.
- J.D.'s gums are bleeding. What nursing assessments and nursing interventions are appropriate at this time?
- What nursing interventions are taken when starting or removing J.D.'s IV?

After the chemotherapy treatments, J.D.'s condition goes into remission for 3 months. Then, he starts having headaches, and blurred vision. He recently fell when rising from a chair.

- What do these symptoms indicate?
- What safety precautions should the nurse take since these symptoms occurred?

- What nursing assessment and nursing interventions are appropriate at this time?
- J.D. states "I know the leukemia is active again. Are there any other treatments I can have?"
- What other treatment options does J.D. have?
- What are some possible therapeutic responses from the nurse?
- Develop a concept map relating the different body systems to the possible symptoms and to the pathophysiology causing the symptoms. Then map nursing interventions for each symptom.

SUMMARY

This may be the first time anatomy and physiology were related to a disease process, or understanding was gained as to why clients have particular symptoms with a specific disease or condition. Ill clients rarely have only one problem but several inter-related problems. These exercises provide an opportunity to think through situations before they are encountered in a clinical situation. The case studies asked pertinent questions, evaluated clinical situations, and allowed the student to make clinical decisions, much the way it is done in the clinical environment. Analyzing and synthesizing skills were used to work through these questions. Perhaps a renewed interest and amazement at the complexity of the body was gained while discovering the inter-relatedness of the body systems. Hopefully, these integration exercises and the critical thinking experience are catalysts to becoming a proficient, critical thinking nurse.

SECTION III
Maternal & Pediatric Nursing

UNIT 19 Nursing Care of the Client: Childbearing

CHAPTER 54
Prenatal Care

MAKING THE CONNECTION

Refer to the following chapters to increase your understanding of prenatal care:

Basic Nursing
- ***Basic Nutrition***

Adult Health Nursing
- ***Reproductive Systems***

LEARNING OBJECTIVES

Upon completion of this chapter, you should be able to:

- Define key terms.
- Discuss historical factors affecting pregnancy and childbirth.
- Describe fetal development from conception to birth.
- Identify the physical and psychological maternal changes during pregnancy.
- Describe the assessments performed at each prenatal visit.
- Discuss the nutritional needs of a woman during pregnancy.
- List the discomforts of pregnancy and one way a client might alleviate each.
- Use the nursing process to plan care for a pregnant client.

KEY TERMS

abortion
age of viability
amenorrhea
amnion
anticipatory guidance
ballottement
blastocyst
Braxton-Hicks contractions
Chadwick's sign
chloasma
chorion
coitus
colostrum
copulation
cotyledon
couvade
decidua
ductus arteriosus
ductus venosus
fertilization
foramen ovale
fundus
funic souffle
Goodell's sign
GP/TPAL
gravida
Hegar's sign
implantation
lanugo
Leopold's maneuvers
linea nigra
meconium
morula

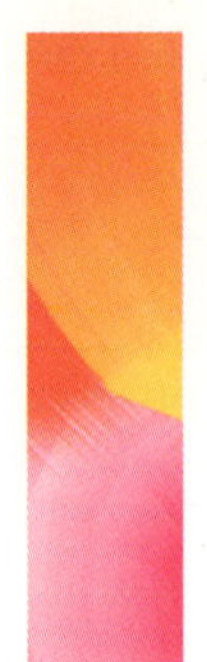

- multigravida
- multipara
- nesting
- nulligravida
- nullipara
- para
- physiologic anemia of pregnancy
- pica
- placenta
- polyhydramnios
- postterm
- prenatal care
- preterm
- primigravida
- primipara
- pseudocyesis
- psychoprophylaxis
- quickening
- striae gravidarum
- supine hypotensive syndrome
- teratogen
- term
- umbilical cord
- uterine souffle
- vernix caseosa
- Wharton's jelly
- zygote

INTRODUCTION

For centuries, birth was part of family life and took place at home. Women learned about pregnancy and childbirth by asking female family members or friends and by being present when other women gave birth. In the United States in 1900, more than 90% of births were in the home.

In 1908, the American Red Cross and the Maternity Center Association offered the first formal programs for prenatal education. These early classes taught women about pregnancy, nutrition, and health care during pregnancy. By the 1950s, the classes included preparation for birth. In 1960, the American Society for Psychoprophylaxis in Obstetrics (ASPO/Lamaze) and the International Childbirth Education Association (ICEA) were founded. They both promote the idea that birth is a healthy process and that parents should have choices about the process.

In 1969, the Nurses Association of the American College of Obstetricians and Gynecologists (NAACOG) was formed with a goal of improving the health of women and newborn infants. The organization was renamed the Association of Women's Health, Obstetric and Neonatal Nurses (AWHONN) in 1993. The National Certification Corporation (NCC) is a not-for-profit organization that has provided a nationally accredited certification program for nurses and other health care professionals in obstetric, gynecologic and neonatal specialties since 1975.

Today, many couples postpone pregnancy to obtain advanced education or establish careers; they may expect to participate in every aspect of the pregnancy, including decision making, and are much more informed than in the past of the educational offerings available. Today's nurse must have a firm understanding of the physical and psychological changes brought about by pregnancy, as well as the application of the nursing process in meeting the needs of the childbearing family.

PRECONCEPTION EDUCATION AND CARE

It has long been known that prenatal education and care identifies and reduces some problems in pregnancy and improves many outcomes. Yet, in 2004, the United States ranked 29th in the world in infant mortality, tied with Poland and Slovakia (CDC, 2008). More perinatal health experts are recognizing that a healthy pregnancy begins before conception.

Preconception education and care are focused on helping a couple prepare to conceive and identifying their reproductive risks before conception. The main goal is to protect the fetus during embryogenesis. Unhealthy habits can harm the fetus before the mother knows she is pregnant. Adopting a healthy lifestyle before pregnancy means eating a low-fat, high-fiber diet rich in vegetables and fruits; exercising at least 3 times a week; and getting to within 15 pounds of one's ideal weight. To prevent neural tube defects, all women who could possibly become pregnant should have an intake of 400 mcg of folic acid from a vitamin supplement and/or fortified foods and eat a healthful diet (Hasenau & Covington, 2002). Another goal is to help the couple identify genetic factors that may affect a pregnancy.

Immunizations and Disease Status

Immunization status is confirmed, and needed immunizations, especially rubella and hepatitis B, are administered before pregnancy. Tests are completed for infectious diseases such as syphilis, hepatitis B, HIV, Chlamydia, gonorrhea, human papilloma virus and herpes simplex. Some states also test for group B streptococcus. These diseases are treated to minimize adverse effects on the mother and fetus. Chronic diseases such as hypertension, cardiac disease, diabetes, epilepsy, thyroid dysfunction, asthma, renal disease, and phenylketonuria should be under control for the best outcome of pregnancy.

Medications

Known teratogens to avoid are warfarin (Coumadin), gold salts, isotretinoin (Accutane), valproic acid (Depakene), lithium (Eskalith), diazepam (Valium), phenytoin (Dilantin), tetracycline, diethylstilbestrol, DES (stilphostrol), live-virus vaccines, and folic acid antagonists. Taking any medication, either over-the-counter (OTC) or prescription, should first be discussed with the health care provider. It is best to have the system cleared of medications before conception, if possible.

Smoking, Alcohol, and Illicit Drugs

Smoking, alcohol, and illicit drugs all have negative effects on pregnancy. Smoking is associated with major complications for pregnancy and low-birth-weight infants. Nearly 12% of pregnant women report drinking while pregnant, although there is no safe level of alcohol use in pregnancy (ACOG, 2008). Use of illicit drugs can lead to any number of fetal anomalies or disorders. The newborn can experience withdrawal symptoms depending on what substance the mother uses, the amount taken, and when taken relative to the birth of the infant. Health care providers may screen for substance abuse during pregnancy and encourage women to discontinue use of these substances before and throughout pregnancy. Nurses caring for substance-abusing women should understand addiction and develop compassionate, trusting relationships with the client. As this can be challenging to health care providers, there should be a support system for the nurses as well (Morton & Cohen Konrad, 2009).

Genetic Risk Factors

A review of family history helps identify genetic risk factors (De Sevo, 2009). If any are identified, encourage the couple to have genetic counseling. Genetic services are used preconceptually to determine the risk to a fetus of a particular disorder that has appeared in either parent's family, by individuals believed to be at risk for a genetic disorder but who have no symptoms, and by individuals who have clinical findings indicative of a genetic disorder.

Paternal Considerations

A lower birth weight, mean deficit of 88 g, has been found in the infants of fathers who smoked and whose mothers did not (Martinez et al., 1994). Also, smoking affects spermatogenesis and sperm mobility. Male exposure to occupational chemicals has been associated with spontaneous abortion, stillbirth, preterm delivery, and small-for-gestational-age babies (Robaire & Hales, 1993). Because spermatogenesis is continuous in that a new supply of sperm is generated every 12 weeks, men can avoid smoking and exposure to occupational chemicals for the period when the couple is planning a pregnancy, and thus eliminate their effects.

CRITICAL THINKING

Pregnant Drug Addict or Alcoholic

What are your feelings about caring for a pregnant drug addict or alcoholic?

What approach might you use in providing their care?

CULTURAL CONSIDERATIONS

Childbearing

Caring for a pregnant client from another culture can be a very rewarding experience for the nurse who takes time to learn and who shows sensitivity and respect toward cultural differences. Journal articles describe the childbirth practices of other cultures, such as those listed in the suggested readings at the end of the chapter.

PREGNANCY

Pregnancy refers to the condition of carrying an offspring within the body. It is a form of reproduction that unites the cells of two individuals to form a unique new individual who embodies characteristics of both parents.

Fertilization

Pregnancy typically begins as a result of **coitus** or **copulation**, which is the sexual act that delivers sperm to the cervix by ejaculation of an erect penis. Sperm entering the vagina by other means such as artificial insemination may also result in fertilization. **Fertilization** or conception occurs when a sperm and ovum unite. This union generally occurs in the distal third of the fallopian tube. The fertilized ovum is now called a **zygote**.

The gender of the zygote is determined at the time of fertilization. When the ovum and sperm each contribute an X chromosome, the result is a female. When the ovum contributes an X chromosome and the sperm a Y chromosome, the result is a male.

Cell division occurs as the zygote travels the fallopian tube to the uterus. It takes 3 to 4 days of cell division, or mitosis, for the zygote to become a **morula**, which resembles a mulberry. The morula entering the uterus is now called a **blastocyst**. The cells have differentiated into an inner mass of embryonic cells, which becomes the embryo, and an outer layer called the trophoblast, which is involved in implantation, hormone secretion, and membrane and placental formation (Figure 54-1).

Multiple pregnancy occurs when more than one fetus develops at the same time. When twins result from two ova being fertilized by two sperm, the twins are fraternal or dizygotic. They are nonidentical and may be two males, two females, or one male and one female.

If one ovum is fertilized by one sperm and the inner cell mass of the blastocyst splits in two to form two embryos, the twins are identical or monozygotic. They may be two males or two females. The genetic makeup is identical in each fetus (Figure 54-2).

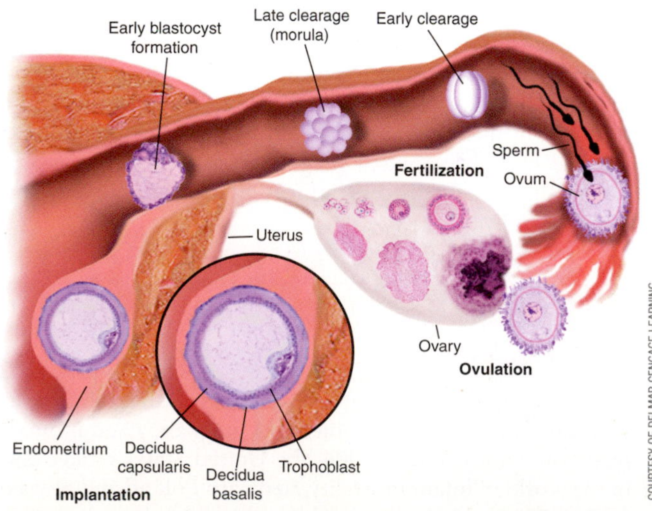

Figure 54-1 Ovulation, Fertilization, and Implantation

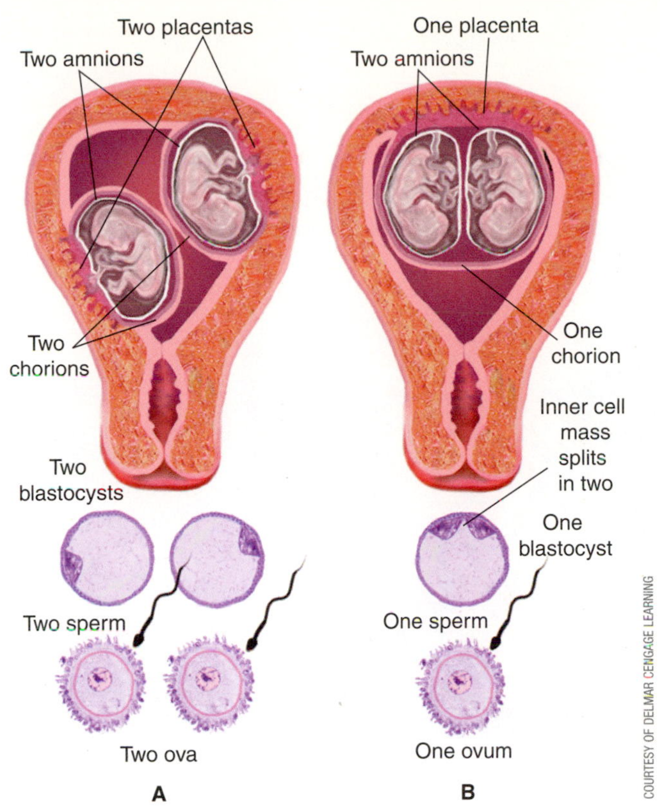

FIGURE 54-2 **Formation of Twins; *A*, Fraternal (nonidentical); *B*, Identical**

IMPLANTATION

About 7 days after ovulation or 5 days after fertilization, the trophoblast burrows into the endometrium, usually in the upper part of the uterus. This process is called **implantation**, or embedding of the fertilized egg into the uterine lining. The endometrium is now called the **decidua**. The trophoblast puts out villi, fingerlike projections, to anchor the blastocyst.

The outer fetal membrane is the **chorion**, formed from the trophoblast. The chorionic villi degenerate, except for those attached to the uterine wall, which become the maternal side of the placenta. The inner membrane (fetal side), the **amnion**, originates in the blastocyst during the early stages of development. The amnion expands as the fetus grows until it slightly adheres to the chorion. These two fetal membranes form the amniotic sac or bag of water (BOW).

AMNIOTIC FLUID

The amniotic fluid is formed by the secretions from the amniotic cells, lungs and skin of the fetus, and fetal urine. It is 98% water, but also contains glucose, protein, sodium, urea, creatinine, **lanugo** (fine hair covering body of fetus), and **vernix caseosa** (white, creamy covering on the fetus's body). Amniotic fluid is slightly alkaline. Approximately every 3 hours, the fluid is replaced. The amnionic cells and the fetus urinating and swallowing regulate the secretion and reabsorption of the fluid.

The amniotic fluid has several important functions in that it:

- Equalizes the pressure around the fetus
- Cushions the fetus from external compression
- Provides a constant temperature and fluid for the fetus to swallow
- Allows freedom of movement for the fetus
- Lubricates the membranes and the fetus

The yolk sac develops as a second cavity in the blastocyst. It forms primitive red blood cells until the liver is able to take over the process in about 6 weeks. Gradually, the yolk sac is incorporated into the umbilical cord.

PLACENTA AND UMBILICAL CORD

The chorionic villi at the base of the implanted fertilized ovum and the decidua basalis, the endometrium at the site of implantation, form the placenta. The **placenta** is a membranous vascular organ connecting the fetus to the mother, which produces hormones to sustain a pregnancy, supplies the fetus with oxygen and food, and transports waste products out of the fetal system. The development of the placenta, stimulated by progesterone secreted by the corpus luteum, begins about the third week following fertilization. The placenta is fully functional by the 12th week.

There is a maternal side to the placenta and a fetal side. The maternal side is irregular and is divided into subdivisions called **cotyledons**. It resembles liver both in color and texture. The fetal side is covered by the amnion, so it is smooth and shiny.

The chorionic villi contain blood vessels that join to form larger and larger vessels, eventually becoming the umbilical cord. The **umbilical cord**, a structure that connects the fetus to the placenta, has two arteries and one vein. It is surrounded and protected by a thick substance called **Wharton's jelly** and covered by the amnion. The two umbilical arteries carry deoxygenated blood from the fetus to the placenta, where carbon dioxide and other waste products are eliminated. The one umbilical vein carries oxygenated blood to the fetus along with nutrients, hormones, antibodies, and whatever drugs or toxic substances the mother may have in her body. This is one instance in which arteries carry deoxygenated blood and a vein transports oxygenated blood. Generally, the cord is attached to the center of the placenta, but it can be attached any place on the placenta.

The circulatory systems of the mother and fetus are separate. Maternal blood enters the intervillous spaces of the placenta. Fetal blood is in the vessels of the chorionic villi. Thus the cells of the fetal blood vessels and the chorion keep maternal blood and fetal blood separate (Figure 54-3).

Functions of the Placenta

The placenta has three major functions: transport, endocrine, and metabolic. All are necessary to maintain the pregnancy and promote normal fetal growth and development. The placenta provides the respiratory and excretory functions for the fetus as well as providing nutrition to the fetus.

Transport There are several mechanisms by which the placenta transports substances.

- Some substances move by diffusion from an area of higher concentration to an area of lower concentration. Those substances transported by this mechanism are oxygen, carbon dioxide, carbon monoxide, water, electrolytes, fat-soluble vitamins, anesthetic gases, and drugs.
- Facilitated diffusion uses a carrier system to move molecules more rapidly than simple diffusion. Some glucose and oxygen are transported by this method.

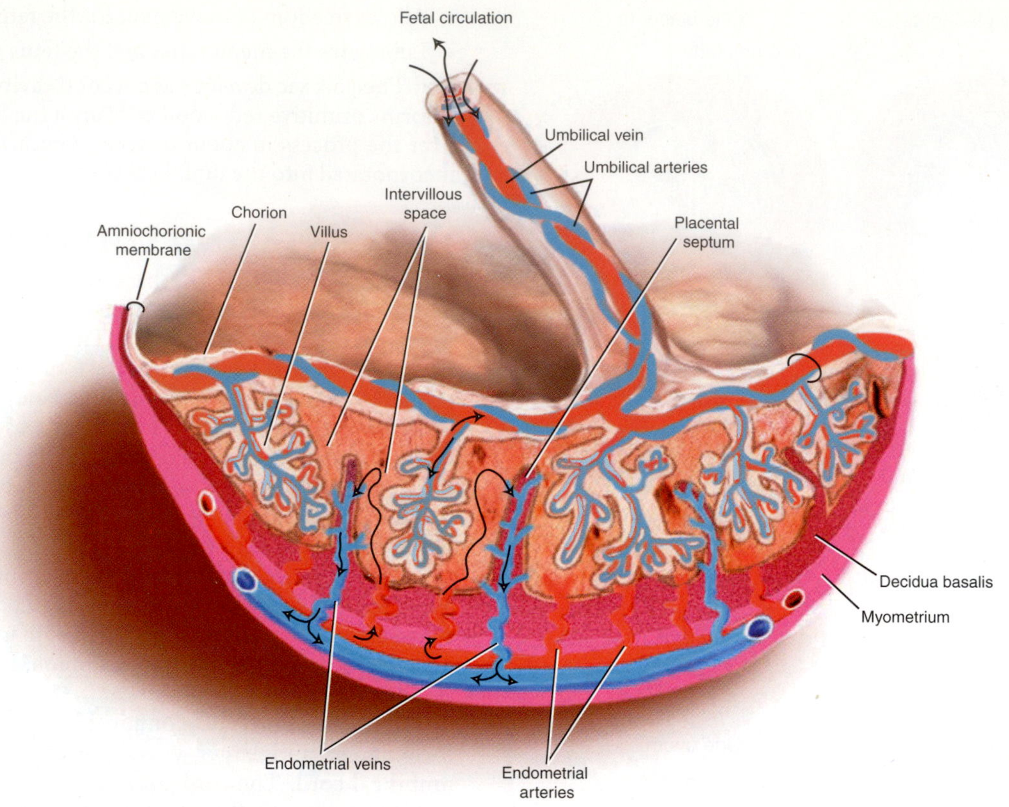

FIGURE 54-3 Placental Circulation

- Active transport allows molecules to move from an area of lower concentration to an area of higher concentration. Substances moved across the placenta by active transport are amino acids, glucose, iron, calcium, iodine, and water-soluble vitamins.
- Pinocytosis transfers larger molecules such as albumin, globulins, antibodies, and viruses through cell membranes.
- Osmotic pressure and hydrostatic pressure move most of the water.

Very large molecules such as insulin, heparin, IgM, and blood cells do not move across the placenta unless there is a tear in the placenta.

Endocrine The placenta secretes five hormones that are essential to pregnancy: human chorionic gonadotropin (hCG), which is the basis for pregnancy tests; human placental lactogen (hPL); estrogen; progesterone; and relaxin.

The trophoblast secretes hCG during early pregnancy. The hCG prevents involution of the corpus luteum and stimulates it to continue producing progesterone and estrogen for 11 to 12 weeks. Eight to ten days after fertilization, hCG is present in maternal blood serum; a few days after the missed menstrual period, hCG is found in maternal urine. After 11 weeks, the placenta is producing enough estrogen and progesterone to maintain the pregnancy.

Human placental lactogen makes a sufficient supply of protein, glucose, and minerals available to the fetus by stimulating changes in maternal metabolism. Human placental lactogen is an insulin antagonist, thus decreasing maternal metabolism of glucose. It also ensures that the mother's body is prepared for lactation.

The placenta secretes primarily the estrogen estriol. Estrogen stimulates development of uterine and breast tissues in the mother. It also increases vascularity and vasodilation in the villous capillaries.

After 11 weeks of pregnancy, the placenta takes over the production of progesterone from the corpus luteum. Progesterone, a smooth muscle relaxant, prevents uterine contractions by decreasing its contractility. It also maintains the endometrium.

Relaxin causes changes in collagen. The connective tissue of the symphysis pubis and sacroiliac joints are softened and become slightly flexible.

Metabolic The placenta produces fatty acids, glycogen, and cholesterol for fetal use and hormone production. The enzymes required for fetoplacental transfer are also produced by the placenta. It breaks down epinephrine and histamine and stores glycogen and iron.

FETAL DEVELOPMENT

Fetal development is divided into three stages. The pre-embryonic or germinal stage is the first 14 days after fertilization. The second stage, the embryonic stage, is from the beginning of the third week (day 15) through week eight. The fetal stage is from week 9 until 38 to 40 weeks or full term.

Development occurs in a systematic manner from head to toe (cephalo-caudal), from proximal to distal (close to body–farthest from body), and from general to specific. This means that the head develops before the arms and the arms develop before the legs; the arms and legs develop before the fingers and toes; and the fetus moves its arms before grasping with the hands.

Fetal development is sometimes described in general terms of trimester. The first trimester is the first 12 weeks, second trimester weeks 13 through 27, and third trimester weeks 28 to 40.

Pregnancy generally lasts 10 lunar (28-day) months, 40 weeks, or 280 days. It is calculated from the first day of the mother's last menstrual period (LMP). Table 54-1 identifies

Table 54-1 Stages of Fetal Development

STAGE	FETAL DEVELOPMENT
Preembryonic or Germinal Stage	
Weeks 1 and 2	Rapid cell division and differentiation. Germinal layers form.
Embryonic Stage	
Week 3	Primitive nervous system, eyes, ears, red blood cells present. Heart begins to beat day 21.
Week 4 Wt 0.4 g L 4–6 mm (crown–rump, C–R)	Half the size of a pea. Brain differentiates. GI tract begins to form. Limb buds appear.
Week 5 L6–8 mm (C–R)	Cranial nerves present. Muscles have innervation.
Week 6 L 10–14 mm (C–R)	Fetal circulation established. Liver produces red blood cells. Central autonomic nervous system forms. Primitive kidneys form. Lung buds present. Cartilage forms. Primitive skeleton forms. Muscles differentiate.
Week 7 L 22–28 mm (C–R)	Eyelids form. Palate and tongue form. Stomach formed. Diaphragm formed. Arms, legs move.
Week 8 Wt 2 g L 3 cm (1.5 in) (C–R)	Resembles human being. Eyes moved to face front. Heart development complete. Hands and feet well formed. Bone cells begin replacing cartilage. All body organs have begun forming.
Fetal Stage	
Week 9	Finger and toe nails form. Eyelids fuse shut.
Week 10 Wt 14 g (1/2 oz) L 5–6 cm (2 in) crown-heel (C–H)	Head growth slows. Islets of Langerhans differentiated. Bone marrow forms, RBCs produced. Bladder sac forms Kidneys make urine.
Week 11	Tooth buds appear. Liver secretes bile. Urinary system functions. Insulin forms in pancreas.
Week 12 Wt 45 g (1.5 oz) L 9 cm (3.5 in) (C–R) 11.5 cm (4.5 in) (C–H)	Lungs take shape. Palate fuses. Heart beat heard with Doppler. Ossification established. Swallowing reflex present. External genitalia, male or female distinguished.
Second Trimester	
Week 16 Wt 200 g (7 oz) L 13.5 cm (5.5 in) (C–R) 15 cm (6 in) (C–H)	Meconium forms in bowels. Scalp hair appears. Frequent fetal movement. Skin thin, pink. Sensitive to light. 200 mL amniotic fluid. (Amniocentesis possible.)
Week 20 Wt 435 g (15 oz) L 19 cm (7.5 in) (C–R) 25 cm (10 in) (C–H)	Myelination of spinal cord begins. Peristalsis begins. Lanugo covers body. Vernix caseosa covers body. Brown fat deposits begun. Sucks and swallows amniotic fluid. Heart beat heard with fetoscope. Hands can grasp. Regular schedule of sucking, kicking, and sleeping.
Week 24 Wt 780 g (1 lb, 12 oz) L 23 cm (9 in) (C–R) 28 cm (11 in) (C–H)	Alveoli present in lungs, begin producing surfactant. Eyes completely formed. Eyelashes and eyebrows appear. Many reflexes appear. Chance of survival if born.

(*Continues*)

Table 54-1 Stages of Fetal Development (Continued)

STAGE	FETAL DEVELOPMENT	STAGE	FETAL DEVELOPMENT
Third Trimester Week 28 Wt 1200 g (2 lb, 10 oz) L 28 cm (11 in) (C–R) 35 cm (14 in) (C–H)	Subcutaneous fat deposits begun. Lanugo begins to disappear. Nails appear. Eyelids open and close. Testes begin to descend.	Week 36 Wt 2,500–2,750 g (5 lb, 8 oz) L 35 cm (14 in) (C–R) 48 cm (19 in) (C–H)	A few creases on soles of feet. Skin less wrinkled. Fingernails reach fingertips. Sleep-wake cycle fairly definite. Transfer of maternal antibodies.
Week 32 Wt 2,000 g (4 lb, 6.5 oz) L 31 cm (12 in) (C–R) 41 cm (16 in) (C–H)	More reflexes present. CNS directs rhythmic breathing movements. CNS partially controls body temperature. Begins storing iron, calcium, phosphorus. Ratio of the lung surfactants lecithin and sphingomyelin (L/S) is 1.2:2.	Week 38	L/S ratio 2:1
		Week 40 Wt 3,000–3,600 g (6 lb, 10 oz-7 lb, 15 oz) L 50 cm (20 in) (C–H)	Lanugo only on shoulders and upper back. Creases cover sole. Vernix mainly in folds of skin. Ear cartilage firm. Less active, limited space. Ready to be born.

COURTESY OF DELMAR CENGAGE LEARNING

stages of fetal development and gives the weight and length (crown-rump length, or C-R) or crown-heel (C-H) beginning in week 4.

System Development

All systems in the fetus have begun forming by the eighth week. They grow, develop, and mature at different rates, and some do not mature until years after birth.

Cardiovascular System

With the primitive heart beginning to beat on the 21st day after conception, the cardiovascular system is the first to function in the embryo. Most congenital malformations of the heart and great vessels develop during the sixth to eighth weeks.

Fetal Circulation Fetal circulation has several unique features. Oxygenated blood comes from the placenta and enters the fetus, at the umbilicus, through the umbilical vein. It divides at the liver with a small branch going to the liver and the other branch, the **ductus venosus**, entering the inferior vena cava. The blood is now partially deoxygenated by the blood coming from the lower part of the fetus's body.

This blood enters the right atrium and moves through the **foramen ovale** (a flap opening in the atrial septum that allows only right-to-left movement of blood) to the left atrium and then to the left ventricle. A small portion of this blood passes into the right ventricle. The left ventricle pumps the blood out through the aorta.

Blood entering the right atrium from the superior vena cava flows to the right ventricle. It is pumped out through the pulmonary arteries. Most of this blood goes into the aorta through the **ductus arteriosus**, a fetal vessel connecting the pulmonary trunk to the aorta. Normally this closes at birth. A small amount of blood goes to the lungs to nourish the lung tissue.

The aorta and its branches supply blood to the rest of the body. The two umbilical arteries branch from the internal iliac arteries and return blood to the placenta to be oxygenated. Figure 54-4 shows fetal circulation.

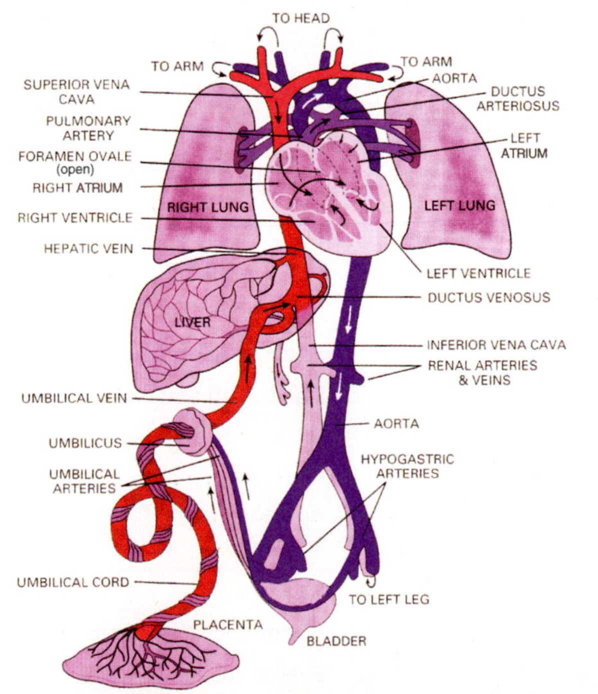

COURTESY OF DELMAR CENGAGE LEARNING

Figure 54-4 Fetal Circulation. Red is arterial (oxygenated) blood, light purple is venous (unoxygenated) blood, and dark purple is mixed arterial-venous blood.

Hematologic Development The formation of blood goes along with cardiovascular development. About day 14, primitive blood cells are formed in the yolk sac. It is the fifth week of gestation before the fetal liver begins hematopoiesis.

Fetal hemoglobin (Hgb F), found only during gestation and the early neonatal period, has a great attraction for oxygen. This ensures an adequate oxygen supply. Blood type is genetically determined at conception.

Gastrointestinal System

During the fourth week of gestation, the gastrointestinal tract begins forming. The fetus begins swallowing amniotic fluid by the 20th week, but there is no coordination of the swallow and suck reflexes until 34 weeks or later.

Meconium (fecal material stored in the fetal intestines) begins to form about week 16; however, there should not be passage of meconium in utero. If the fetus encounters hypoxic stress, the anal sphincter may relax and meconium may be passed, causing meconium staining of the amniotic fluid.

Musculoskeletal System

Limb buds appear late in the fourth week and development is complete by the eighth week. Growth of the skeleton is determined by genetics and maternal supply of calcium and phosphorus. Cartilage is noted about 5 weeks and ossification begins about 12 weeks but is not completed until after puberty.

By the end of the 12th week, skeletal muscles begin involuntary movements. Skeletal muscle development depends on an adequate volume of amniotic fluid to allow plenty of fetal movement.

Genitourinary System

Kidneys begin forming at about 3 weeks and pass through several changes. Around 12 weeks, they begin to produce a hypotonic urine. The placenta and the maternal kidneys are still responsible for fetal waste removal. All the nephrons are in the kidneys at birth.

The reproductive system develops at the same time as the urinary system. Testes can be seen in the abdomen by 7 weeks and begin descending to the scrotum about 30 weeks. The ovaries develop in the abdomen and stay in the pelvic cavity. All of the ova a female will ever have are in the ovaries at birth. Visual determination of fetal gender can be made through ultrasound by the end of week 12.

Integumentary System

The skin protects the underlying tissues. Vernix caseosa protects the skin, with the amount present decreasing as the pregnancy progresses. Creases form on the palms, fingers, and soles during week 11, with permanent designs formed by week 17. Skin color is genetically determined.

Lanugo appears during week 20 and slowly disappears; most is gone by birth. Tooth buds for the deciduous (baby) teeth appear during week 6 while tooth buds for permanent teeth do not appear until week 10. Second and third permanent molar tooth buds do not appear until after birth.

Mammary glands develop during the 6th week.

Respiratory System

Lung buds begin forming during week 6, with bronchi forming by week 16. Primitive lungs are formed by 23 weeks, but there are not enough alveoli for sufficient gas exchange. Surfactant production begins between weeks 20 and 24. Surfactant reduces the surface tension of the fluid lining the alveoli in the lungs, thus facilitating breathing by keeping the alveoli from collapsing with expiration. Surfactant production matures between weeks 35 and 37. The **age of viability**, or gestational age at which a fetus could live outside the uterus, is considered to be 20 weeks. Adequate lung functioning also depends on surfactant production and neurologic maturation.

Immunologic System

Between the 12th and 15th weeks, immune capability begins developing. It functions very minimally because the fetus lives in a sterile environment. The fetus produces small amounts of the immunoglobins IgG, IgA, and IgE before 20 weeks. IgG provides the most immunity. Maternal IgG is actively transported across the placenta to provide passive immunity against many infectious diseases. Blood group antibodies are a type of IgG. They can move across the placenta by active transport and cause hemolytic disease of the newborn.

Factors Affecting Fetal Development

Many factors influence fetal development, especially during the first trimester. Even before the mother knows she is pregnant, factors are affecting embryonic development. One of the very first is the quality of the sperm and the ovum and the genetic code. **Teratogens** (any agent, such as radiation, drugs, viruses, or other microorganisms, capable of causing abnormal fetal development) exert the greatest influence on cells undergoing the most rapid growth. Each organ has a period when teratogenic agents or other insults can cause physical and functional defects.

A well-provided maternal environment is also important. Maternal malnutrition, acute and chronic diseases, drugs, alcohol, and smoking all can exert potentially harmful effects on the fetus before birth.

MATERNAL PHYSIOLOGICAL CHANGES OF PREGNANCY

Many physiological changes take place when a woman is pregnant. Every system of the mother's body undergoes some change during pregnancy.

Reproductive System

The most obvious physiological changes occur in the reproductive system.

Uterus

The most dramatic change occurs in the size of the uterus. Before pregnancy, it is a small, pear-shaped, thick-walled, muscular organ weighing 60 g (2 oz). At the end of pregnancy, it is a large, thin-walled organ weighing 1,000 g (2 lb). Its capacity has increased from 10 mL to 5 L. The uterus enlarges mainly by hypertrophy of the muscle cells stimulated by estrogen and the growing fetus. There are three layers of smooth (involuntary)

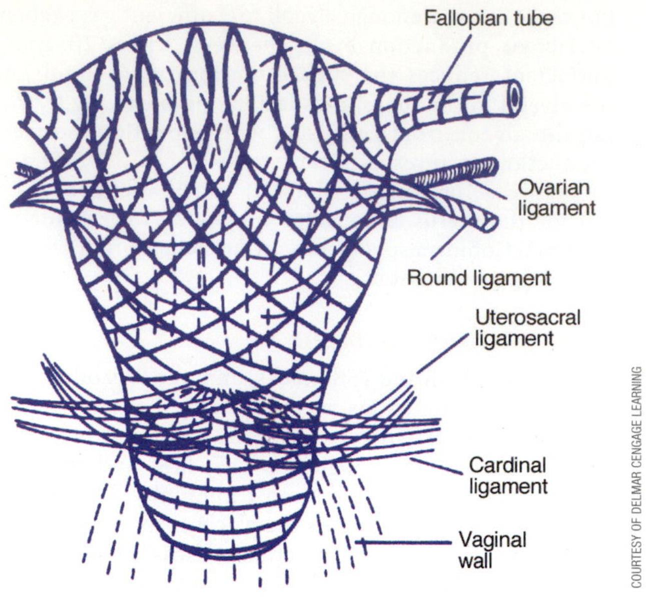

FIGURE 54-5 Muscle Layers of the Uterus

muscles in the uterus (Figure 54-5). The outer layer is made of longitudinal muscles. The muscle fibers of the middle layer are interlaced in a figure eight pattern. Circular fibers that form sphincters at the openings of the fallopian tubes and at the internal os of the cervix make up the inner layer of uterine muscle. This configuration of muscle layers allows the uterus to expand evenly in all directions during pregnancy. One-sixth of the mother's blood volume is in the vascular system of the uterus by the end of pregnancy.

Irregular uterine contractions occur throughout pregnancy. About 16 weeks or later, the mother may become aware of these **Braxton-Hicks contractions**. These generally painless contractions assist in uterine and placental circulation. Pain is an individual perceptual experience. A softening of the uterine isthmus about the sixth week of pregnancy, noted during a pelvic exam, is called **Hegar's sign**.

Cervix

The cervix increases in cell number by the influence of estrogen. It secretes a thick, sticky mucus that forms a plug in the cervix. This plug prevents microorganisms from entering through the vagina. During labor, as the cervix dilates, this mucus plug is expelled. **Goodell's sign** (softening of the cervix) and **Chadwick's sign** (a purplish-blue color of the cervix and vagina caused by the increased vascularity) are both noted at about 8 weeks.

Ovaries

Follicles do not mature and ovulation does not occur during pregnancy. The corpus luteum produces progesterone and estrogen for about 12 weeks, at which time the placenta takes over the production.

Vagina

Estrogen causes a loosening of connective tissue and an increase in vaginal secretions. The acidic secretions prevent bacterial infections. The increased level of glycogen in cells may enhance growth of organisms such as *Trichomonas vaginalis* or *Candida albicans.*

Breasts

In addition to breast enlargement from hormonal influence, the nipples become more erect, the areolas darken, and Montgomery's tubercles enlarge. **Colostrum**, an antibody-rich yellow fluid, is secreted by the breasts during the last trimester and first 2–3 days after birth, and gradually changes to milk a few days after delivery.

Cardiovascular System

Blood flow increases to the uterus and kidneys, where the workload is increased. The pulse increases by 10 to 15 beats/minute by the end of pregnancy. Cardiac output increases 30% to 50% early in pregnancy. Blood pressure decreases, is lowest during the second trimester, and increases gradually to near the prepregnant level during the third trimester. This occurs because of the progesterone's relaxing effect on the smooth muscles.

Stasis of blood in the lower extremities, caused by the enlarged uterus interfering with return blood flow, may lead to dependent edema and varicose veins of the legs, vulva, or rectum.

Supine hypotensive syndrome, also known as vena caval syndrome, occurs when the mother lies supine. The enlarged, heavy uterus presses on the inferior vena cava, causing a reduced blood flow back to the right atrium (Figure 54-6). The mother experiences dizziness, clammy-pale skin, nausea, and a lowering of her blood pressure. This decreases placental perfusion, which can affect fetal reserve. The situation is relieved when the mother lies on her side.

Maternal blood volume increases 30% to 50%, reaching its peak at about 30 weeks. There is some increase in red blood cells, but most of the increase is plasma. This hemodilution is manifested by a lower hematocrit (34% to 40%) and is termed **physiologic anemia of pregnancy**.

The white blood cell count begins to increase by about 8 weeks and may reach 18,000/mm^3 by the time of delivery. Platelets, fibrin, fibrinogen, and coagulation factors VII, IX, and X increase. This increase with possible venous stasis in late pregnancy increases the risk of venous thrombosis.

Respiratory System

Progesterone decreases airway resistance, allowing an increase in oxygen consumption. The depth of respirations increases,

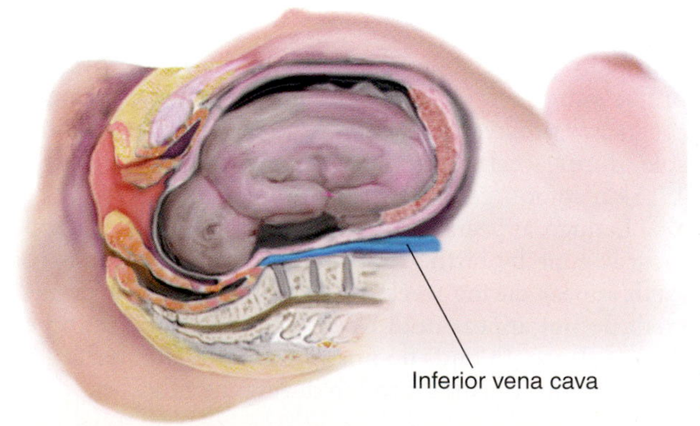

FIGURE 54-6 Supine Hypotensive Syndrome. Enlarged uterus presses on vena cava when mother is supine. Side-lying position relieves pressure.

causing a mild respiratory alkalosis, which is compensated by increased renal secretion of bicarbonate (Littleton & Engebretson, 2002). The enlarging uterus presses upward on the diaphragm. The rib cage flares and the chest circumference expands to keep the intrathoracic volume the same as when not pregnant. Estrogen causes edema and vascular congestion of the nasal mucosa.

Musculoskeletal System

The relaxation of the pelvic joints in preparation for delivery is caused by relaxin. As pregnancy progresses, the mother's center of gravity gradually changes because of the increased size and weight of the uterus anteriorly. To compensate, the mother increases the curve of the lumbosacral spine (lordosis), which frequently results in a low backache, and may cause the woman to have a waddling gait. Figure 54-7 illustrates this change throughout pregnancy.

Gastrointestinal System

Nausea and/or vomiting, known as "morning sickness," are common in early pregnancy but usually disappear by 12 weeks. The smooth muscle relaxation effect of progesterone results in delayed gastric emptying and decreased peristalsis. The enlarging uterus displaces the stomach and intestines. All of these changes contribute to constipation. Relaxation of the cardiac sphincter allows reflux of acidic gastric contents into the esophagus, giving the mother heartburn.

Urinary System

Urinary frequency occurs in the first trimester as the enlarging uterus presses on the bladder and in the third trimester as the fetus settles into the pelvis and presses on the bladder. Progesterone causes the ureters to relax and dilate. Glomerular filtration rate (GFR) begins rising in the second trimester. Tubular reabsorption also increases.

Glycosuria (excretion of glucose in the urine) develops if the kidneys are unable to reabsorb all of the glucose filtered by the glomeruli. Any amount more than a trace of glucose in the urine is investigated.

Integumentary System

Several skin pigment changes generally occur during pregnancy. The nipples, areola, vulva, and perineal area darken. **Linea nigra** is a pigmented line on the abdomen from umbilicus to symphysis pubis. **Chloasma**, also called "mask of pregnancy," is a darkening of the skin of the forehead and around the eyes. It is generally more pronounced in dark-haired women. **Striae gravidarum**, or "stretch marks," are reddish streaks frequently found on the abdomen, thighs, buttocks, and breasts. They are the result of separation of the underlying connective tissue of the skin (Figure 54-8). As the skin stretches, the client may experience itching.

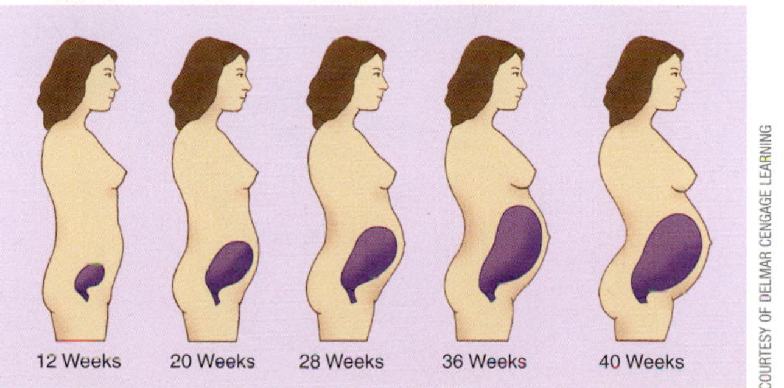

Figure 54-7 Lordosis increases throughout pregnancy.

Endocrine System

The anterior pituitary hormone prolactin is responsible for initial milk production. The posterior pituitary hormone oxytocin causes uterine contractions and the ejection of milk from the breasts (let-down reflex) after delivery.

The placental hormones, especially hPL, are insulin antagonists, so a greater insulin production is required. This puts an increased stress on the islets of Langerhans in the pancreas to put out more insulin. A woman with a marginally functioning pancreas may show signs of gestational diabetes in the latter half of pregnancy.

A slight increase in the size of the thyroid often occurs, as well as an increase in its capacity to bind thyroxine. Maternal thyroxine is important for fetal neural development throughout pregnancy, especially during the first trimester. This results in a higher level of serum protein-bound iodine (PBI).

Metabolism

The metabolic rate of the mother increases during pregnancy as the demands of the growing fetus increase. The mother must meet her own and the fetus's nutritional needs.

SIGNS OF PREGNANCY

The many physiological changes that a woman experiences during pregnancy are categorized as presumptive, probable, or positive signs of pregnancy.

Presumptive Signs

Changes that the woman experiences and reports are termed presumptive or subjective signs. They may be caused by other conditions, so are not diagnostic of pregnancy. Presumptive signs include:

- **Amenorrhea** (absence of menses), usually the first sign that a woman notices causing her to think she is pregnant.
- Nausea and vomiting, often referred to as "morning sickness," but can occur any time of the day. This sign usually disappears by 12 weeks of pregnancy.

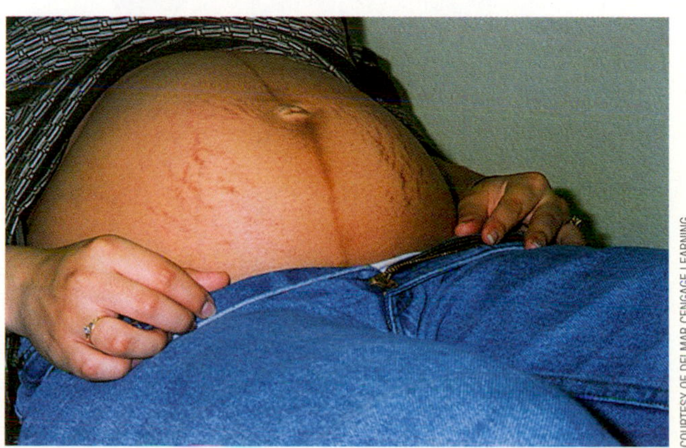

Figure 54-8 Linea Nigra and Striae Gravidarum

- Breast changes, tenderness, or tingling.
- Urinary frequency, as the growing uterus presses against the bladder, giving the woman the sensation of needing to urinate.
- Excessive fatigue, often noted after the first missed menstrual period. It may last for several months.
- Abdominal enlargement usually noticed by the woman, generally after 12 weeks.
- **Quickening**, perception of fetal movement by the mother, usually between 16 and 20 weeks. It begins as a fluttering sensation and gradually gets stronger and more frequent.

A positive diagnosis of pregnancy is usually made before these last two signs are noted by the woman; however, there is a condition called **pseudocyesis** or false pregnancy, in which the woman believes so strongly that she is pregnant that she appears to have all the early presumptive signs of pregnancy.

Probable Signs

The examiner can identify these objective changes, but since they can be caused by conditions other than pregnancy, they are not diagnostic of pregnancy.

Pelvic Signs

Goodell's sign (softening of the cervix), Hegar's sign (softening of the uterine isthmus), and Chadwick's sign (purplish discoloration of the vagina, cervix, and vulva) can be identified by the examiner during the first 12 weeks of pregnancy.

Uterine enlargement is identified after the eighth week of pregnancy. The fundus is palpable just above the symphysis at 12 weeks and at the umbilicus at 20 weeks (Figure 54-9). If these uterine enlargement milestones are reached earlier, multiple pregnancy, or **polyhydramnios**, excessive amniotic fluid, is suspected.

Braxton-Hicks Contractions

After the 28th week, these contractions can be felt by the examiner and also by the client.

Increased Pigmentation

The nipples and areola darken. Linea nigra may appear on the abdomen, chloasma may mark the face, and striae gravidarum may be noticed on the breasts and abdomen.

Ballottement

During the fourth or fifth month, if the fetus is pushed upward through the vagina or abdomen, the floating fetus rebounds against the examiner's fingers; this is known as **ballottement** (Figure 54-10).

Pregnancy Test

The basis for a pregnancy test is the presence of hCG in either the urine or blood of the woman. A test of the blood is positive 8 days after conception, and a test of the urine is positive 10 to 14 days after conception.

Positive Signs

A positive sign of pregnancy proves conclusively that the woman is pregnant. No other condition can cause these signs to appear. There are only three positive signs of pregnancy: hearing the fetal heartbeat, visualization of the fetus, and the examiner feeling fetal movement.

Hearing the Fetal Heartbeat

The fetal heartbeat can be detected at 10 to 12 weeks using the Doppler ultrasound method (Figure 54-11).

When auscultating the abdomen over the uterus, a soft, blowing sound may be heard. The sound occurring at the same rate as the mother's pulse is called the **uterine souffle**, caused by the blood pulsating through the uterus and placenta. The sound occurring at the same rate as the fetal heart rate is called the **funic souffle**, caused by blood pulsating through the umbilical cord.

Visualization of the Fetus

An abdominal ultrasound examination can detect a pregnancy by the sixth week after the last menstrual period (LMP). An endovaginal ultrasound examination, using a vaginal probe, can detect a gestational sac 10 days after implantation.

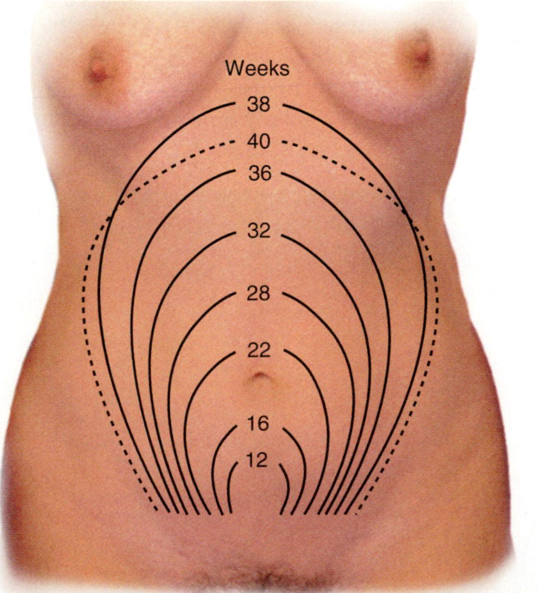

FIGURE 54-9 Fundal Height Milestones

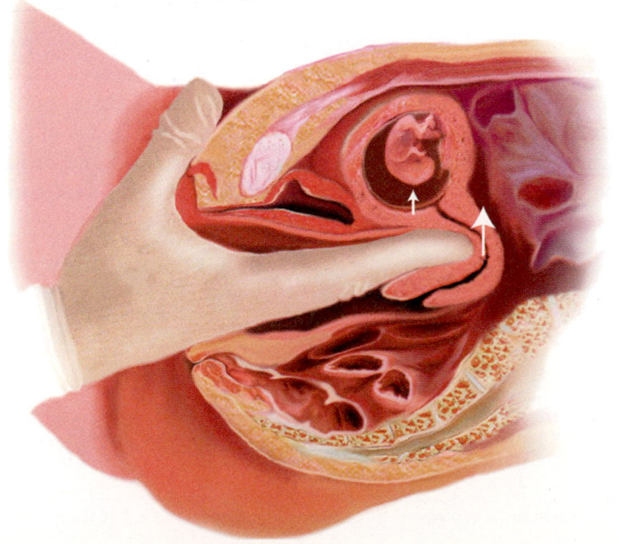

FIGURE 54-10 Ballottement

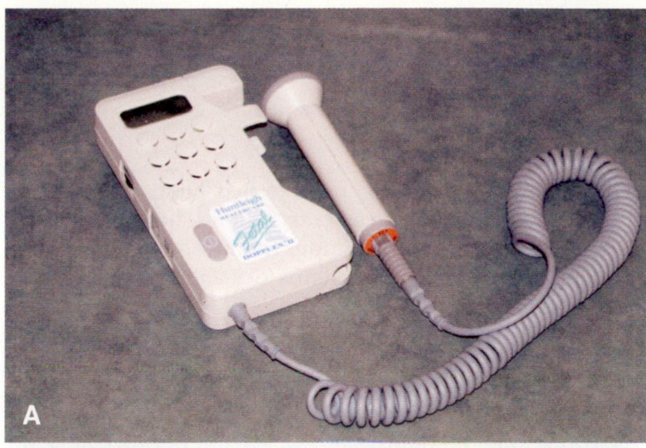

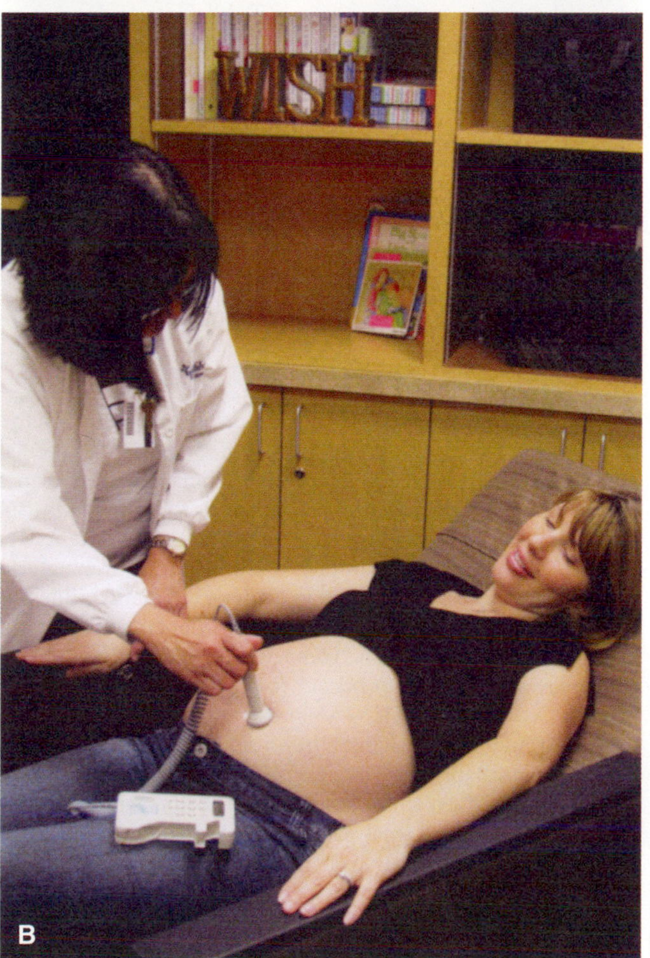

PHOTOS COURTESY OF DELMAR CENGAGE LEARNING

FIGURE 54-11 ***A,* Fetal Doppler; *B,* Fetal Doppler in Use**

Examiner Feeling Fetal Movement

Fetal movement felt by the examiner, not the mother, is a positive sign of pregnancy.

PSYCHOLOGICAL ADAPTATION TO PREGNANCY

Pregnancy is often viewed as a developmental stage having its own developmental tasks. Both the expectant mother and father deal with significant changes and major psychosocial adjustment.

Developmental Tasks

Four major developmental tasks are identified for pregnancy. They are pregnancy validation, fetal embodiment, fetal distinction, and role transition. These developmental tasks are met in this order. The rate at which they are met varies. According to Malnory (1996), completion of the developmental tasks is critical to positive parenting.

Pregnancy Validation

During the first trimester, the pregnant woman's task is to validate and accept the pregnancy. Until the woman meets this task, she cannot meet the rest of the developmental tasks. Even when pregnancy is planned, there are normal feelings of ambivalence and disbelief about the pregnancy. Many women become introspective or have mood swings caused by hormone fluctuations.

Fetal Embodiment

Fetal embodiment occurs as the mother incorporates the growing fetus into her body image. The physical changes she is experiencing, especially the growing uterus, help her meet this task. She feels that the fetus is a part of her. Self-involvement, depression, or regressive behavior are signs of difficulty in meeting this task.

Fetal Distinction

When fetal movement is felt, it becomes easier for the mother to think of the fetus as a separate being. She may daydream about what the baby will be like and think about the kind of mother she wants to be.

Role Transition

The last trimester is a time of preparation. Many expectant parents attend childbirth classes to learn about and prepare for labor, delivery, infant care, and self-care. Preparing a nursery, buying baby clothes, and selecting a day care are all ways of preparing for the infant's arrival. Role transition also includes parents exploring together the meaning of fathering and mothering, learning parenting skills, the amazing skills of a newborn for interactions, and the physical maturing and behavioral changes of the first 12 months of life. Another aspect is learning to enjoy watching the other parent interact with the newborn.

At the end of pregnancy, many mothers experience a surge of energy and see to it that the entire household is organized for the coming of the infant. This is called **nesting**. All of these preparations assist the pregnant woman in the transition to her new role of mother.

Partners' Tasks

Fathers and other partners must meet the same developmental tasks as the expectant mother but in a more abstract way. Accepting the fact that they (as a couple) are pregnant and announcing it to family and friends meets the first task. The partner may also have ambivalent feelings about the pregnancy. By accepting the changes in the pregnant partner, both physical and psychological, the task of fetal embodiment is met. Fetal distinction is generally met when the partner hears the fetal heartbeat and feels the fetus moving. Role transition is met in virtually the same way as is done by the pregnant woman.

Factors Affecting Psychological Response

Factors that contribute to a woman's psychological response to her pregnancy include body image, financial situation, cultural expectations, emotional security, and support from significant others.

Body Image

The mother's body image, or perception of her own body, may change in several areas. The noticeable changes in body shape and the speed with which those changes occur may be very threatening to some women. Some women feel "fat" and "ugly" when they are pregnant, and others feel "so good" and "beautiful" when they are pregnant.

The physical discomforts of pregnancy may cause the mother to feel a lack of control over her own body. For example, urinary frequency or urinary incontinence may increase negative feelings about the pregnancy.

Pregnant women often feel restricted in their physical activities. As long as there is no problem with the pregnancy, encourage the mother to continue regular activities, keeping in mind that moderation is the key.

Financial Situation

A poor financial situation may cause anxiety about paying bills, buying needed items for infant care, or having enough and proper foods for good nutrition. Financial consideration may also be a significant concern for the expectant mother's partner.

Cultural Expectations

Cultural expectations of the family may cause conflicts for the pregnant woman and her partner if their ideas are different from their families' expectations. Conflicts occur if the cultural expectations of the mother are different from the cultural expectations of the father or partner.

Emotional Security

A pregnant woman's satisfaction with herself and her life situation has an impact on how she responds to being pregnant. If the woman is secure in her feelings about herself and her perceived abilities as a mother, the pregnancy is more likely to be enjoyable. A pregnancy that was planned or long anticipated will likely be received with joy and excitement, whereas an unexpected or unwanted pregnancy may be met with fear, dread, or uncertainty.

Support from Significant Others

It is important for the nurse and the expectant mother to take into consideration the psychological responses of significant others, namely, the father/partner, siblings, and grandparents.

Father/Partner The expectant father or partner must shift thinking from being a person without children to a person with a child. He may feel left out, neglected, or resent the attention focused on the expectant mother.

Couvade is the development of physical symptoms by the expectant father such as fatigue, depression, headache, backache, and nausea. Longobucco and Freston (1989) found that men who show couvade have greater paternal role preparation.

Siblings A new baby may be seen by siblings as a threat to their relationship with the parents. Siblings should be included in the pregnancy and preparations for the new baby on an age-appropriate basis. Feeling the fetus kick and hearing the heartbeat often are helpful activities for siblings. Parents must be sure to maintain some special time just for the siblings. Many areas have classes for siblings to help them understand what is happening in their lives.

Grandparents Grandparents are usually the first ones told about the pregnancy. It is often difficult for grandparents to know how much to become involved in the process. Some grandparents feel they are not ready or are too young to become grandparents.

Practices of childbearing and childrearing often change greatly from one generation to another. Some areas have classes to provide information to grandparents about these changes.

PRENATAL EDUCATION AND CARE

Prenatal care (care of a woman during pregnancy, before labor) is credited with the reduction of perinatal mortality over the last 50 years. The earlier prenatal care is begun, the better. This provides an opportunity for the health care provider to obtain baseline data on physical assessments and laboratory test results. Women who do not seek prenatal care in a timely fashion often have an underlying mental illness or substance abuse problem, or may be in denial of their pregnancy (Hatters Friedman, Heneghan, & Rosenthal, 2009). Cost may also be a major barrier to prenatal care.

Anticipatory guidance (providing information, teaching, or guidance to a client in anticipation of an expected event) is probably the most important aspect of prenatal care. It is based on the assessment of mother and fetus and knowledge of the normal process of pregnancy and possible complications.

Prenatal Care

The goals of prenatal care are as follows:

- A healthy, prepared mother having minimal discomforts
- Identification of potential problems or complications as early as possible
- Safe delivery of a healthy infant
- A prepared father or partner who participates as much or as little as the couple desires
- Prepared siblings and grandparents

Initial Visit

A comfortable environment, open communication, and the nurse's attitude will help put the woman at ease during the initial prenatal visit. The first visit is often quite lengthy. A complete history is recorded to identify factors that may

CULTURAL CONSIDERATIONS

Beliefs Influencing Pregnancy

Some cultural practices may not always be observed by a client, but some general practices that have cultural influences include the following:

- Muslim women are to keep hair, body, arms to the wrist, and legs to the ankles covered at all times. Also, a Muslim woman may not be alone in the presence of a man other than her husband or a male relative, including during a physical examination (Hutchinson & Baqi-Aziz, 1994).
- Korean women defer to elders, especially the mother-in-law, for care decisions (Schneiderman, 1996).
- Native American women should not look at a deformed, injured, or blind person, or the baby will have the same defect (Cesario, 2001).
- Orthodox Jewish women must keep their hair covered at all times except in the presence of their husbands. They may wear wigs or scarves. Men may not touch any woman except his wife, so he may not shake hands. The nurse may nod rather than offer to shake hands. A husband is not allowed to touch his wife when she is in *niddah*, whenever she is pregnant, menstruating, or nursing and there is blood from the vagina. Thus, he is unable to touch her or pass her anything when she is in labor (Zauderer C, 2009).
- Mexican women consider pregnancy a "hot" state and will avoid cold liquids, fearing they will cause an imbalance resulting in illness or miscarriage (Holtz C. 2008).
- Guatemalan women believe that a pregnant woman and her unborn child are physically and spiritually weak and may be vulnerable to illnesses and evil forces (Callister & Vega, 1998).
- In Malawi, Africa, the father determines family size and the timing of the pregnancies (Gennaro et al., 1998).

negatively affect the pregnancy, and a physical examination is performed. If the woman did not seek preconception care, all of the topics covered in that section would then be discussed at the first prenatal visit. Important terms used in describing a pregnant client are provided in Table 54-2.

Initial History The history provides the health care provider with the client's past and present health. Figure 54-12 shows a sample health history summary.

Estimating Duration of Pregnancy Every family wants to know the "due date," the estimated date when the infant is to be born. The estimated date of birth (EDB) or estimated date of delivery (EDD) is 40 weeks from the first day of the woman's LMP. Many women do not keep track of their menstrual periods, or have irregular periods; but an EDB can be identified based on other factors such as uterine size, date of quickening, date when the fetal heartbeat is heard, and ultrasound fetal measurements.

TABLE 54-2 Terms Used in Describing a Pregnant Client

Abortion Loss of pregnancy before the age of viability (20 weeks gestation)

GP/TPAL Gravida, para/term, preterm, abortions, living

Examples: Mary Jo is G2 P1/T2 P0 A0 L2; second pregnancy, one delivery/two infants at term (twins), both living.

Susan is G4 P2/T1 P1 A1 L2; fourth pregnancy, two deliveries/one term infant, one preterm infant, one abortion, two living children.

Gravida Pregnancy, regardless of duration, includes present pregnancy

Para Delivery (birth) after 20 weeks' gestation, whether infant born alive or dead or number of infants born

Preterm Delivery after 20 weeks' gestation but before 38 weeks (full term)

Term A pregnancy between 38 and 42 weeks' gestation

Nulligravida Never been pregnant

Primigravida Pregnant for first time

Multigravida Pregnant two or more times

Nullipara Never having delivered an infant after 20 weeks' gestation

Primipara Has delivered once after 20 weeks' gestation

Multipara Has delivered twice or more after 20 weeks' gestation

Postterm Delivery after 42 weeks' gestation

COURTESY OF DELMAR CENGAGE LEARNING

Naegele's Rule Naegele's rule is the most common method of calculating the EDB. The rule is: Take the date of the first day of the last menstrual period, subtract 3 months, and add 7 days. For instance, if the LMP was June 28, the calculation would be as follows:

Month		Day
6	(June)	28
−3	months	+7 days
3	(March)	35

Because there are 31 days in March, the EDB moves forward to April 4.

Gestation Calculator A gestation calculator, in the shape of either a chart or a wheel, allows a quick EDB calculation. The wheel generally provides other information also, such as fetal weight and body length for each week (Figure 54-13).

Fundal Height Fundal height generally indicates gestational age through the second trimester (refer back to Figure 54-9).

Hollister

Patient's Name ____
ID. No. ____

Health History Summary

Hollister Maternal/Newborn Record System — Page 1 of 2
To order call: 1.800.323.4060 — Re-order No. 5700

Demographic Data

Date of Birth ____ Age ____ Language ☐ English ☐ ____ Interpreter ☐ None ☐ ____
Religion ☐ N/A ☐ ____ Race/Ethnicity ____
Marital Status S M SEP D W Father of Baby's Name ____

	Education	Occupation	Full	Part	Self	Unemp	Work Tel No	Home Tel No
Patient			☐	☐	☐	☐		
Father of Baby			☐	☐	☐	☐		

Allergies/Sensitivities

Medication ☐ None ☐ ____
Other ☐ None ☐ ____

Primary/Referring Physician

Menstrual History

Menarche ____ yrs Interval ____ days Length ____ days Abnormalities ☐ None
LMP ___/___/___ Certain ☐ Yes ☐ No Normal ☐ Yes ☐ No
Positive Pregnancy Test ___/___/___ ☐ Blood ☐ Urine

EDD By Dates ___/___/___ By Ultrasound ___/___/___ Date of Ultrasound ___/___/___

Pregnancy History

Gravida	Full Term	Premature	Spontaneous Ab	Induced Ab	Ectopic	Multiple Births	Live

No	Month/ Year	Infant Sex	Weight at Birth	Wks Gest	Hours In Labor	Type of Delivery	Anesthesia	Comments/Complications
1								
2								
3								
4								
5								
6								
7								

Medical History

(Patient / Family)

Check and detail positive findings below. Use reference numbers.

Obstetric
1. Anemia ☐
2. Fetal/Neonatal Death or Anomaly ☐ ☐
3. Gestational Diabetes ☐
4. Hemorrhage ☐
5. Hyperemesis ☐
6. Incompetent Cervix ☐
7. Intrauterine Growth Retardation ☐
8. Isoimmunization ☐
9. Polyhydramnios ☐
10. Postpartum Depression ☐
11. Pregnancy Induced Hypertension ☐ ☐
12. Preterm Labor or Birth ☐
13. PROM-Chorioamnionitis ☐
14. Rhogam Given ☐
15. RH Neg ☐

Gynecologic
16. Contraceptive Use ☐
17. Abnormal PAP ☐
18. Fibroids ☐
19. GYN Surgery ☐

Gynecologic (Cont'd.)
20. Infertility ☐
21. In Utero Exposure to DES ☐
22. Uterine/Cervical Anomaly ☐

Sexually Transmitted Diseases
23. Chlamydia ☐
24. Gonorrhea ☐
25. Herpes (HSV) ☐
26. Syphilis ☐

Vaginal/Genital Infections
27. Trichomonas ☐
28. Condylomata ☐
29. Candidiasis ☐

Other Infections
30. Toxoplasmosis ☐
31. Group B Streptococcus ☐
32. Rubella ☐
33. Varicella ☐
34. Cytomegalovirus (CMV) ☐
35. AIDS (HIV) ☐
36. Hepatitis (type ____) ☐

Hollister

Patient's Name ____
ID. No. ____

Health History Summary

Hollister Maternal/Newborn Record System — Page 2 of 2
To order call: 1.800.323.4060 — Re-order No. 5700

(Patient / Family)

Check and detail positive findings below. Use reference numbers.

Cardiovascular
37. Heart Disease ☐ ☐
38. Rheumatic Fever ☐
39. Mitral Valve Prolapse ☐
40. Chronic Hypertension ☐ ☐
41. Varicosities Thrombophlebitis ☐ ☐
42. Previous Pulmonary Embolism ☐
43. Blood Disorders ☐ ☐
44. Anemia/ Hemoglobinopathy ☐ ☐
45. Blood Transfusions ☐

Pulmonary
46. Asthma ☐
47. Tuberculosis ☐ ☐
48. Chronic Obstructive Pulmonary Disease ☐ ☐

Endocrine
49. Diabetes ☐ ☐
50. Thyroid Dysfunction ☐ ☐
51. Maternal PKU ☐
52. Endocrinopathy ☐ ☐
53. Gastrointestinal ☐
54. Liver Disease ☐

Renal Disease
55. Cystitis ☐
56. Pyelonephritis ☐
57. Asymptomatic Bacteriuria ☐
58. Chonic Renal Disease ☐ ☐
59. Neurologic/ Seizure Disorder ☐ ☐
60. Autoimmune Disease ☐ ☐
61. Cancer ☐ ☐
62. Other ____ ☐

Other
63. Psychiatric Disease ☐ ☐
64. Physical Abuse or Neglect ☐ ☐
65. Emotional Abuse or Neglect ☐ ☐
66. Addiction (Drug, Alcohol, Nicotine) ☐ ☐
67. Major Accidents ☐
68. Surgery ☐
69. Anesthetic Complications ☐
70. Non-Surgical Hospitalization ☐
71. Other ____ ☐
72. No Known Disease/Problems ____ ☐

Genetic History

(Patient / Father of Baby / Family)

73. Age ≥ 35 (♀) ≥ 50 (♂) ☐ ☐
74. Cerebral Palsy ☐ ☐ ☐
75. Cleft Lip/Palate ☐ ☐ ☐
76. Congenital Anomalies ☐ ☐ ☐
77. Congenital Heart Disease ☐ ☐ ☐
78. Consanguinity ☐ ☐ ☐
79. Cystic Fibrosis ☐ ☐ ☐
80. Down's Syndrome ☐ ☐ ☐
81. Hemophilia ☐ ☐ ☐
82. Huntington's Chorea ☐ ☐ ☐
83. Mental Retardation ☐ ☐ ☐
84. Muscular Dystrophy ☐ ☐ ☐
85. Neural Tube Defect ☐ ☐ ☐
86. Sickle Cell Disease or Trait ☐ ☐ ☐
87. Tay-Sachs Disease ☐ ☐ ☐
88. Test for Fragile X ☐ ☐ ☐
89. Thalassemia A or B ☐ ☐ ☐
90. Other ____ ☐ ☐ ☐
91. Other ____ ☐ ☐ ☐
92. Other ____ ☐ ☐ ☐

Historical Risk Status

☐ No Risk Factors Noted
☐ At Risk (Identify)

Signature ____

FIGURE 54-12 Representative Health History Forms (*Permission to use this copyrighted material has been granted by the owner, Hollister Incorporated.*)

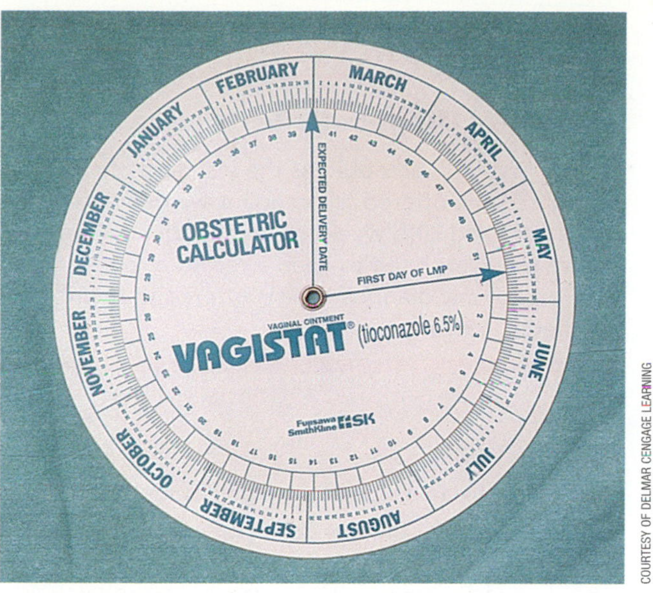

COURTESY OF DELMAR CENGAGE LEARNING

FIGURE 54-13 **Gestation Calculation Wheel. Place arrow labeled *first day of LMP* on that date. Read date at arrow labeled *expected delivery date.***

The **fundus** (top of the uterus) is measured in centimeters from the top of the pubic symphysis to the top of the uterine fundus (McDonald's method). This is fairly accurate between 18 and 30 weeks' gestation. The fundal height, for example, is generally 20 cm (at the umbilicus) at 20 weeks' gestation and 25 cm at 25 weeks' gestation in the average-height woman. Evaluating the visit-to-visit fundal height measurements provides a general pattern of fetal growth. A sudden increase may indicate twins or hydramnios (excessive amount of amniotic fluid), whereas a smaller increase may indicate growth restriction (Figure 54-14).

Other Indicators Additional assessments that indicate the gestational week of pregnancy include ultrasound, fetal heartbeat, and quickening.

- *Ultrasound*: Five to six weeks after the LMP, an ultrasound can detect a gestational sac. It shows fetal heartbeat activity at 9 to 10 weeks' gestation. By 12 to 13 weeks, the biparietal diameter (BPD), or distance between the parietal bones of the fetal skull, can be measured.

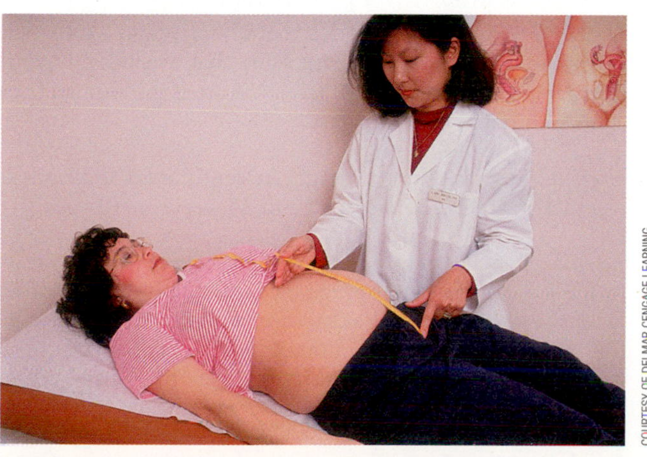

COURTESY OF DELMAR CENGAGE LEARNING

FIGURE 54-14 **Measuring Fundal Height**

- *Fetal Heartbeat*: The fetal heartbeat is generally heard by 10 to 12 weeks with the fetal Doppler but may be heard as early as 8 weeks' gestation. It is usually 18 to 20 weeks before the fetal heartbeat can be heard with a fetoscope.
- *Quickening*: Fetal movement is usually felt by the mother at about 20 weeks' gestation. Women identify these movements as early as 16 weeks or as late as 22 weeks. Typically, the woman will detect this movement earlier with a second pregnancy than with a first.

Physical Examination The physical examination begins with measuring the client's height and weight and vital signs. A head-to-toe examination is performed by the health care provider. Special attention is given to the assessment of the heart, lungs, pelvis, breasts, and nipples. Figure 54-15 shows an initial pregnancy profile form, and Figure 54-16 shows a prenatal flow record.

The pelvic examination is performed last. The external genitalia are examined for scars, lesions, or infection. A Pap smear for cervical cancer and a specimen of cervical mucous for gonorrhea are usually obtained. A bimanual examination is performed to determine uterine changes (Figure 54-17) and pelvic size to estimate adequacy of the pelvic opening for delivery.

Pelvic size is estimated by the examiner during the manual examination. The diagonal conjugate (distance from the lower border of the pubic symphysis to the sacral promontory) is an estimate of the pelvic inlet. It is generally 11.5 cm. The anteroposterior diameter (9.5 to 11.5 cm), measured from the lower border of the pubic symphysis to the tip of the sacrum, is an estimate of the pelvic outlet.

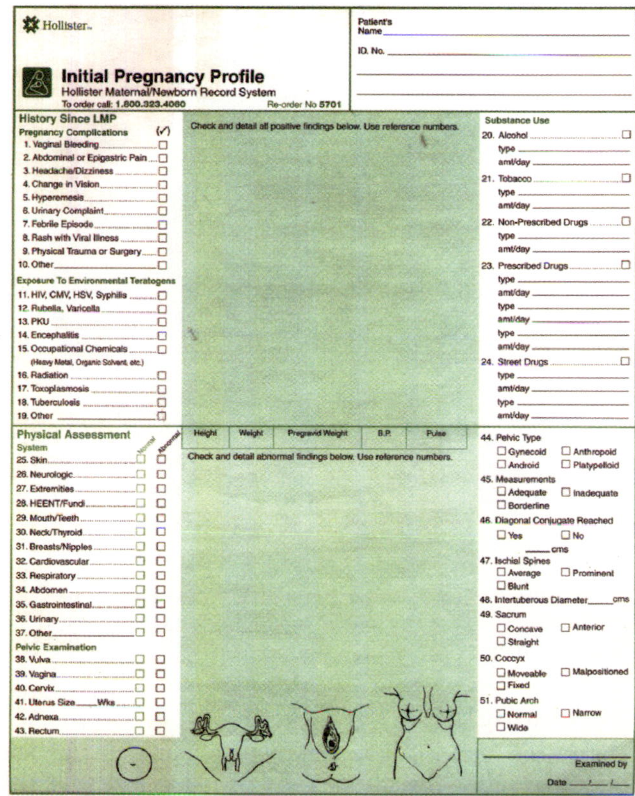

Hollister

Initial Pregnancy Profile
Hollister Maternal/Newborn Record System
To order call: 1.800.323.4060 Re-order No 5701

Patient's Name ______
ID. No. ______

History Since LMP

Pregnancy Complications (✓)
1. Vaginal Bleeding ☐
2. Abdominal or Epigastric Pain ☐
3. Headache/Dizziness ☐
4. Change in Vision ☐
5. Hyperemesis ☐
6. Urinary Complaint ☐
7. Febrile Episode ☐
8. Rash with Viral Illness ☐
9. Physical Trauma or Surgery ☐
10. Other ______ ☐

Exposure To Environmental Teratogens
11. HIV, CMV, HSV, Syphilis ☐
12. Rubella, Varicella ☐
13. PKU ☐
14. Encephalitis ☐
15. Occupational Chemicals ☐ (Heavy Metal, Organic Solvent, etc.)
16. Radiation ☐
17. Toxoplasmosis ☐
18. Tuberculosis ☐
19. Other ______ ☐

Check and detail all positive findings below. Use reference numbers.

Substance Use
20. Alcohol ☐ type ______ amt/day ______
21. Tobacco ☐ type ______ amt/day ______
22. Non-Prescribed Drugs ☐ type ______ amt/day ______
23. Prescribed Drugs ☐ type ______ amt/day ______ type ______ amt/day ______ type ______ amt/day ______
24. Street Drugs ☐ type ______ amt/day ______ type ______ amt/day ______

Physical Assessment

Height	Weight	Pregravid Weight	B.P.	Pulse

Check and detail abnormal findings below. Use reference numbers.

System (Normal / Abnormal)
25. Skin ☐ ☐
26. Neurologic ☐ ☐
27. Extremities ☐ ☐
28. HEENT/Fundi ☐ ☐
29. Mouth/Teeth ☐ ☐
30. Neck/Thyroid ☐ ☐
31. Breasts/Nipples ☐ ☐
32. Cardiovascular ☐ ☐
33. Respiratory ☐ ☐
34. Abdomen ☐ ☐
35. Gastrointestinal ☐ ☐
36. Urinary ☐ ☐
37. Other ______ ☐ ☐

Pelvic Examination
38. Vulva ☐ ☐
39. Vagina ☐ ☐
40. Cervix ☐ ☐
41. Uterus Size ____ Wks ☐ ☐
42. Adnexa ☐ ☐
43. Rectum ☐ ☐

44. Pelvic Type ☐ Gynecoid ☐ Anthropoid ☐ Android ☐ Platypelloid
45. Measurements ☐ Adequate ☐ Inadequate ☐ Borderline
46. Diagonal Conjugate Reached ☐ Yes ☐ No ____ cms
47. Ischial Spines ☐ Average ☐ Prominent ☐ Blunt
48. Intertuberous Diameter ____ cms
49. Sacrum ☐ Concave ☐ Anterior ☐ Straight
50. Coccyx ☐ Moveable ☐ Malpositioned ☐ Fixed
51. Pubic Arch ☐ Normal ☐ Narrow ☐ Wide

Examined by ______
Date ___/___/___

FIGURE 54-15 **Representative Initial Pregnancy Profile** ***(Permission to use this copyrighted material has been granted by the owner, Hollister Incorporated.)***

Hollister™

Prenatal Flow Record
Hollister Maternal/Newborn Record System
To order call: 1.800.323.4060 Re-order No. 5703

Patient's Name ____
ID. No. ____

Medication Allergy/Sensitivity ☐ None (Identify) ____

Meds Prescribed | Indication | Start Date | Stop Date
1.–6. ____

Tests Recommended | Date Explained to Patient | Patient Accepted/Declined
☐ CVS ☐ Amniocentesis

Problems/Risks Identified ☐ None | Date Identified | Date Resolved
1.–8. ____

LMP __/__/__ EDD __/__/__
Confirmed By: Yes No Date-Variation
Ultrasound ☐ ☐
Repeat Ultrasound ☐ ☐

Initial Prenatal Screens				Additional Lab Results		
D=Declined			N/A=Not Applicable			
Date: __/__/__		Test	Result	Test	Date	Result
Hgb/Hct		PPD		MSAFP (15-20 Wks)	/	
Platelets				Triple Marker (15-20 Wks)	/	
Blood type/Rh		Glucose Challenge		Glucose Challenge (24-28 Wks)	/	
Rh Antibody		Urinalysis Micro/Culture		Rh Antibody (28 Wks)	/	
Sickle Cell Trait		Toxicology		Hgb/Hct (28 Wks)	/	
Thalassemia		Pap Test		Hgb/Hct (36 Wks)	/	
Tay-Sachs Trait		Gonorrhea		RPR (36 Wks)	/	
Toxoplasmosis		Chlamydia		HBsAG (36 Wks)	/	
VDRL/RPR		HSV		HIV (36 Wks)	/	
Rubella Titer		GBS		Gonorrhea (36 Wks)	/	
CMV				Chlamydia (36 Wks)	/	
HBsAG				GBS (36 Wks)	/	
HIV						

G | T | Pt | A | L
Age
Visit date
19 __

Fetal: FHR | Fundal Height | Weeks Gestation (est) (date/size) | Fetal Movement +=Active 0=Absent ↑ Diminished | Weight this Visit Pregravid | Urine (protein/sugar)

Maternal Physical: Blood Pressure Base Line __/__ | Edema | Preterm Risk Factors: Uterine Contractions 0=None +=Reg I=Irreg | Pain/Pressure 0=Absent +=Present | Vaginal Discharge 0=None M=Mucous W=White B=Bloody | Cervix (pos. dil. length)

Pediatric Provider ____ ☐ Breast ☐ Bottle
Inits | Signature
Return Visit | Init.
Provider's Signature

FIGURE 54-16 Representative Prenatal Flow Record (*Permission to use this copyrighted material has been granted by the owner, Hollister Incorporated.*)

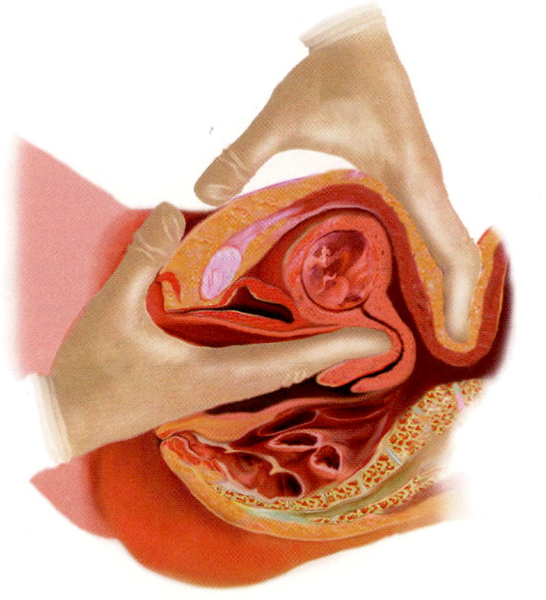

COURTESY OF DELMAR CENGAGE LEARNING

FIGURE 54-17 Bimanual Examination to Determine Uterine Changes

Screening Tests

During the first visit, screening tests are performed to determine the mother's health and to have baseline data with which to compare subsequent test results. Other screening tests are gestational age dependent and are ordered at a later time in pregnancy. Tests may vary for a specific client but generally include those listed in Table 54-3.

> **PROFESSIONALTIP**
>
> ### Prenatal Diagnostic Tests
>
> "AFP testing is accepted as the standard of care and must be offered to pregnant women between the 16th and 20th weeks of pregnancy. . . . [H]ealth care providers need to keep a record of patients' refusal of any diagnostic tests offered to them" (Rhodes, 1995).

Return Visits

Return visits for an uncomplicated pregnancy generally are:

- Every 4 weeks for the first 28 weeks
- Every 2 weeks during weeks 29 to 36
- Every week, after 36 weeks, until birth of infant

Subjective Data The following subjective data should be collected at each return visit:

- How the client is feeling
- Any discomforts, concerns, or questions the client may have
- Any body changes noticed by the client
- How developmental tasks are being met

At an early return visit, the mother's expectations for childbirth should be discussed. Closer to the EDB, preparations for the baby should also be covered.

Objective Data On each return visit, the following objective data should be collected and compared with data collected on previous visits and to prepregnant data, if known.

Blood Pressure Any increase of 30 mm Hg systolic or 15 mm Hg diastolic from one visit to the next is reported to the health care provider. If there is no previous BP to compare to, a blood pressure of 140/90 or greater is reported.

Weight Total weight gain in a normal-weighted woman should be approximately 25 to 35 pounds, distributed as follows:

- Weeks 1 to 12: 2 to 4 pounds
- Weeks 13 to 40: 1 pound/week

The ACOG recommends that underweight women gain 28–40 pounds during pregnancy and that overweight women gain 15–25 pounds. Weight gain is more if the woman is carrying multiples.

Uterine Size The fundal height in centimeters indicates the weeks of gestation between 18 and 30 weeks.

Edema A small amount of dependent edema is often present in the last few weeks of pregnancy. Edema of the hands and face is reported to the health care provider. Sometimes it is difficult to detect small amounts of edema in the hands, so ask the client if her rings are tighter or if she has had to remove her rings.

Fetal Position Assessment of fetal position is performed using **Leopold's maneuvers**, a series of specific palpations

TABLE 54-3 Screening Tests in Pregnancy

TEST	RESULTS
Initial visit	
Complete Blood Count	
RBC	3.75 million/mm^3 due to hemodilution.
WBC	Rises to 18,000/mm^3 by late pregnancy. Mostly an increase in neutrophils.
Hemoglobin (Hgb)	May decrease to 11.5g/dL later in pregnancy due to hemodilution. Repeat at 28 and 36 weeks.
Hematocrit (Hct)	33% lowest acceptable, due to hemodilution.
Blood Type	A, B, AB, or O
Rh factor	Positive or negative. If negative, do indirect Coomb's test. Check father's Rh.
Coomb's Test	Should remain negative. Retest Rh negative women at 28 weeks.
Rubella Titer (HAI)	>1:10 indicates immunity. <1:10, immunize after birth of infant.
Blood Glucose	Should be 70–110 mg/dL. Retest at 24 and 32 weeks.
VDRL or RPR (Syphilis)	Should be negative.
Cervical/Vaginal Culture Gonorrhea Chlamydia Group B *Streptococcus*	Should be negative.
Hepatitis B Surface	Positive indicates either active hepatitis or carrier state.
Antigen (HB_sAg)	
Antibody Titer HB_sAg	Positive indicates immunity to hepatitis.
HIV (many states mandate that it be offered)	Should be negative.
Tuberculosis Skin tests: Mantoux or Tine	Should be negative. If positive, do chest x-ray.
Urinalysis Color, specific Gravity, pH, ketones, albumin, glucose	Same as nonpregnant. Repeat at 28 weeks. Trace of glycosuria may occur in pregnancy.
Subsequent visits	
Alpha-fetoprotein (AFP)	Check with laboratory for normal range for each week of gestation. If elevated, may have neural tube defects. If decreased, may have Down syndrome.
Glucose tolerance test/glucose challenge test	Completed near 28 weeks' gestation to determine the client's ability to metabolize glucose. Normal values are less than 130 or 140, depending upon the reference used by the laboratory.

COURTESY OF DELMAR CENGAGE LEARNING

of the pregnant uterus to determine fetal position and presentation. The client is placed in the supine position with knees bent, and the examiner stands at the client's right side facing her head.

- First, the examiner palpates to determine which fetal part is in the fundus. Generally, it is the breech (buttocks).
- Second, the examiner moves hands to the sides of the uterus and determines on which side of the mother the fetal back is located.
- Third, the examiner's right hand is placed above the symphysis pubis to note whether the head or breech is near the pubic symphysis (this should correlate with the first maneuver).
- Fourth, the examiner changes position to face the client's feet, and palpates the sides of the abdomen to determine on which side the cephalic prominence presents (Figure 54-18).

Fetal Heartbeat After Leopold's maneuvers have determined fetal position, the fetal heartbeat is assessed over the location of the fetal back. The rate should be 110 to 160 beats/minute. The rate is recorded, indicating the abdominal quadrant in which the heartbeat was noted.

Laboratory Tests At each visit, a urine sample is tested with a dipstick for protein, glucose, and ketones. If the results are positive for any of these three, the health care provider is notified.

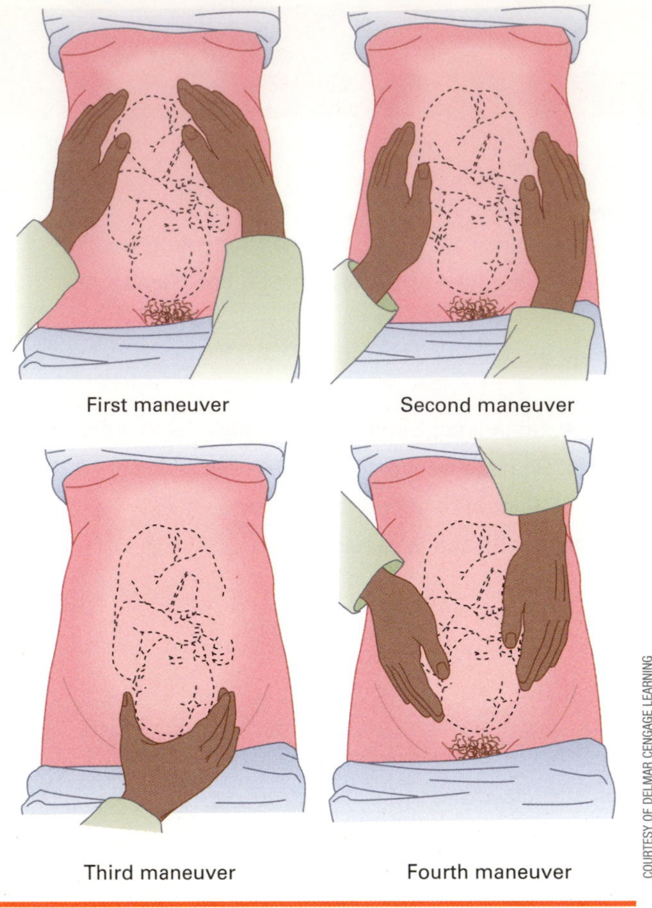

FIGURE 54-18 Leopold's Maneuvers

ANTICIPATORY GUIDANCE

Many of the nursing interventions during pregnancy are anticipatory guidance (teaching). The order in which topics are covered and the time frame when topics are covered may vary from client to client, depending on when prenatal care was begun and if there are any complications.

Environmental Hazards

Any chemicals, metals, anesthetic agents, antineoplastic and viral drugs, and x-ray examinations should be avoided. Excessive heat from saunas, hot tubs, or exercise in hot, humid weather should be avoided to prevent maternal hyperthermia (core temperature above 38.9°C/102°F). This has been associated with neural tube defects. Rogers and Davis (1995) report that the time needed to reach this core temperature is 15 minutes in a 39°C (102.2°F) tub and 10 minutes in a 41.1°C (106°F) tub.

Discomforts of Pregnancy

The physiological changes in pregnancy often cause discomforts to the woman. Table 54-4 identifies the common discomforts of pregnancy, possible causes, and interventions the client can try to alleviate or reduce the discomfort.

Warning Signs

The client is taught to immediately report to the health care provider the warning signs listed in Table 54-5. They may indicate complications of pregnancy. Generally, the sooner interventions are begun, the better the outcome.

TABLE 54-4 Discomforts of Pregnancy

DISCOMFORT	CAUSE	CLIENT INTERVENTIONS
Nausea/vomiting	Elevated hCG level Decreased gastric emptying time due to progesterone Ambivalence about pregnancy Fatigue	Limit fluid intake at meals and upon waking. Eat crackers or toast upon waking. Eat small amounts more frequently. Avoid fried, spicy, odorous, or gas-forming foods.
Heartburn (pyrosis)	Gastric reflux—cardiac sphincter relaxed due to progesterone	Avoid overeating. Eat small, frequent meals. Avoid greasy foods. Sit up for 1 hour after eating. Take antacid only with health care provider's approval.
Urinary frequency	Pressure of uterus on bladder (early and late in pregnancy) Urinary tract infection	Empty bladder when urge is felt. Do not restrict fluid intake. Avoid fluids containing caffeine.
Breast tenderness	Effect of estrogen and progesterone	Wear well-fitting, supportive bra.
Flatulence	Relaxation of GI tract due to progesterone	Eat small meals. Omit gas-forming foods from diet. Have regular elimination.

TABLE 54-4 Discomforts of Pregnancy (Continued)

DISCOMFORT	CAUSE	CLIENT INTERVENTIONS
Constipation	Bowel sluggishness due to progesterone Pressure of uterus on bowel Decreased activity and fluid intake Inadequate fiber in diet Iron supplement	Have regular schedule for bowel movement. Increase activity and fluid intake. Increase fiber in diet (raisins, prunes, fresh fruits and vegetables).
Hemorrhoids	Constipation Straining to have bowel movement Pressure of gravid (pregnant) uterus on veins Prolonged standing	Prevent constipation (see above). Apply ice packs. Use topical anesthetic ointments. Take sitz bath. Gently push hemorrhoids back into rectum.
Ankle edema	Prolonged standing or sitting Sodium and water retention from hormonal influence Increased capillary permeability	Dorsiflex feet when prolonged standing or sitting necessary. Elevate legs when sitting or resting. Increase number of rest periods.
Varicose veins (legs)	Increased blood volume Congenital predisposition to weak vascular walls Relaxation of vessel walls due to progesterone Inactivity Poor muscle tone Prolonged standing Obesity	Rest with feet and legs elevated. Avoid crossing legs, standing still, garters and restrictive clothing. Wear support hose.
Backache	Relaxation of joints due to estrogen and relaxin Exaggerated lordosis from change in center of gravity Wearing high-heeled shoes Excessive weight Fatigue Poor body mechanics	Get adequate rest. Use proper posture. Use proper body mechanics. Wear low-heeled shoes.
Dyspnea	Supine hypotensive syndrome Decreased lung capacity from pressure of uterus on diaphragm	Lie on either side. Sleep in semi-Fowler's position. Maintain proper posture.
Leg cramps	Calcium/phosphorus imbalance Pointing toes Fatigue or muscle strain Pressure of gravid uterus impairs circulation to legs	Evaluate diet for adequate calcium and phosphorus intake. Pull toes up toward knees. Rest with legs elevated.
Dizziness and Fainting	Supine hypotensive syndrome Sudden change of position Standing for long period in warm area Hyperventilation Hypoglycemia Anemia	Lie on either side, not on back. Arise slowly. Avoid standing in warm area. Practice slow, deep respirations. Drink orange juice for fast-acting sugar.

(*Continues*)

TABLE 54-4 Discomforts of Pregnancy (Continued)

DISCOMFORT	CAUSE	CLIENT INTERVENTIONS
Bleeding gums, nasal stuffiness, and epistaxis	Increased estrogen level Increased blood volume Lack of vitamin C	Avoid use of decongestants. Use cool vaporizer or humidifier. Use saline nasal spray several times a day. Drink orange juice. Have dental checkup.
Vaginal discharge	Increased estrogen causes more cervical Mucous	Bathe or shower daily. Avoid douching. Wear absorbent cotton underwear.
Itchy skin	Tissue stretching Soap use Dehydration	Use lotion on skin. Change soap, rinse well. Drink more fluids.
Mood swings	Hormonal changes Inadequate rest Inadequate diet Ambivalence about pregnancy	Get more rest. Eat balanced diet. Express fears, feelings, and concerns.

COURTESY OF DELMAR CENGAGE LEARNING

TABLE 54-5 Warning Signs during Pregnancy

WARNING SIGN	POSSIBLE CAUSE
Vaginal bleeding (any), "bloody show"	Abortion (miscarriage), placenta previa, placenta abruptio, lesions of cervix or vagina
Sudden gush of fluid from vagina	Rupture of membranes
Persistent vomiting	Hyperemesis gravidarum, infection
Severe, continuous headache	Hypertension, preeclampsia
Swelling of face, hands, legs, feet when arising in morning	Preeclampsia
Visual disturbances: blurring, double vision, flashes of light, spots before eyes	Hypertension, preeclampsia
Dizziness	Hypertension, preeclampsia
Fever over 100°F (37.8°C) and chills	Infection
Pain in abdomen or cramping	Ectopic pregnancy, abortion (miscarriage), placenta abruptio, labor
Epigastric pain	Preeclampsia
Irritating vaginal discharge	Vaginal infection
Dysuria	Urinary tract infection
Oliguria	Dehydration, renal impairment
Noticeable reduction or absence of fetal movement	Fetal distress, fetal death

COURTESY OF DELMAR CENGAGE LEARNING

Nutrition

There is very little change needed in the diet of a pregnant woman if she is already following the food guide pyramid. A woman eating a balanced, adequate diet needs to add only 300 kcalories a day to her diet when pregnant and 500 kcalories a day when breastfeeding. The addition of two milk servings and one meat serving will meet the 300 kcalorie increase as well as the increased need for calcium and protein.

Many health care providers have their pregnant clients take a multivitamin with calcium and iron to ensure an

CLIENT TEACHING

Pregnancy and Fluid Intake

A pregnant woman should drink at least 8 to 10 (8 oz) glasses of fluids each day. At least 4 to 6 of these should be water.

adequate intake of these essential nutrients. Folic acid in the multivitamin prevents neural tube defects, calcium is needed for bone and teeth, and iron prevents anemia in mother and fetus. On the basis of a nutritional assessment, suggestions can be made to the client for a more adequate dietary intake, taking into account personal and cultural preferences.

Some pregnant women eat substances that are not considered edible and have no nutritive value. This is called **pica**. Eating ice, freezer frost, clay, soil or starch may interfere with the absorption of nutrients, cause constipation and most commonly cause iron deficiency anemia in the mother. Pica may be related to the mother's cultural beliefs. Kenyan woman believe eating soil increases fertility and reproductive success. Pica is underreported due to women's embarrassment in discussing the practice (Mills, 2007).

Factors that place a woman at risk for nutritional inadequacy during pregnancy include:

- Adolescence, due to demands for own growth and pregnancy; possible poor dietary habits; and possibility of trying to hide pregnancy
- Inadequate nutritional intake
- Pica
- Low income
- Smoking, alcohol, or drug use
- Short interval between pregnancies—no time to replenish nutrient stores
- Medical conditions such as diabetes or kidney problems
- Depression

Self-Care

Physical care during pregnancy generally involves minor adjustments in or moderation of normal habits.

Breast Care

Proper support of the breasts is important during pregnancy whether the woman is planning to breast-feed or bottle-feed her baby. A properly fitted maternity or nursing bra promotes comfort, retains breast shape, and prevents back strain if breasts are very large.

Cleanliness of the breasts is very important. Washing with water is sufficient because soap removes the natural lubricant provided by Montgomery's tubercles, causing drying and possible cracking of the nipples. If leakage is experienced, a nursing pad can be worn inside the bra, and the pregnant woman encouraged to rub the fluid into the nipple to lubricate the skin. Air-drying the nipples after leaking will also promote breast health.

Personal Hygiene

Daily bathing is important because the pregnant woman generally has increased perspiration and vaginal mucous. Either a tub bath or shower may be taken, depending on the woman's preference and facilities available. Later in pregnancy, a tub bath may require that the mother have help in getting out of the tub. Douching should not be done because it changes the pH of the vagina and alters the normal flora.

CLIENT TEACHING

Exercises for Pregnancy

Specific exercises are taught to clients to strengthen muscle tone in preparation for birth.

- The pelvic tilt reduces back strain and strengthens the abdominal muscles. Figure 54-19 illustrates how to perform the pelvic tilt in both a standing and kneeling position. Exhale, roll the hips and buttocks forward, hold for a count of five, then inhale and relax.
- Abdominal muscle tightening with every breath increases abdominal muscle tone. This can be done anywhere in any position. While slowly taking in a deep breath, expand the abdomen. Then exhale slowly while pulling the abdomen in until the muscles are completely contracted. Relax a few seconds and repeat the exercise.
- Kegel's exercises strengthen and tighten the perineal muscles. Tighten these muscles and pull them up toward the vagina as if trying to stop urination midstream. This exercise also can be done anytime, anyplace.
- The tailor sit (cross-legged sit) stretches the inner thigh muscles; adding arm reaches stretches the sides and upper body and helps relieve upper backache. Sit cross-legged and stretch one arm high over head, then release and exhale and repeat on the other side. Figure 54-20 illustrates the tailor sit and arm reaches.

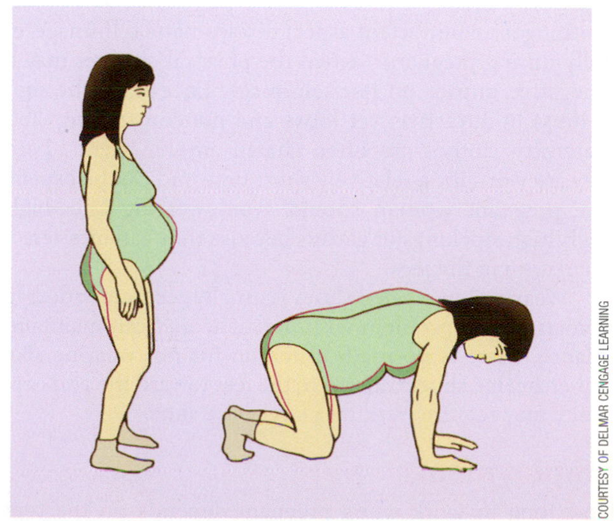
COURTESY OF DELMAR CENGAGE LEARNING

FIGURE 54-19 Pelvic Tilt

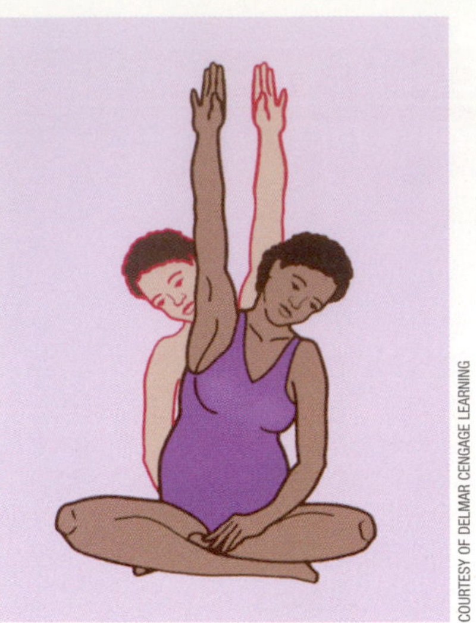

FIGURE 54-20 Tailor Sit and Arm Reaches

Activity/Rest

The pregnant woman should have some type of regular physical activity. Walking, swimming, and cycling are perhaps the best activities for most women. Women who routinely participate in exercise before pregnancy should continue and nonexercising women should begin exercising. Fatigue should be avoided. Exercise during pregnancy could reduce the risk of cesarean birth (Bungum, Peaslee, Jackson, & Perez, 2000). They should avoid hyperthermia and drink plenty of water before and after exercise to prevent dehydration. Exercise is contraindicated during pregnancy when the following are present: pregnancy-induced hypertension, preterm rupture of membranes, preterm labor during a prior or present pregnancy, incompetent cervix, persistent second or third trimester bleeding, or fetal growth restriction (Bungum et al., 2000).

Adequate rest is important for the pregnant woman. It is a challenge to find rest time during the day, especially for women who work outside the home or have small children. More sleep is needed, especially during the first and last trimester. Most women experience significant sleep problems throughout pregnancy (Mindell & Jacobson, 2000).

Clothing

Clothing is an important aspect of a woman's self-image, especially during pregnancy when the physical changes may have a negative impact on her self-image. Encourage the mother to dress in attractive, yet loose and nonconstricting clothes. Maternity clothes are often shared among friends because they are worn for a relatively short time and can be expensive. The pregnant woman should avoid wearing knee-high or thigh-high stockings or garters because they interfere with circulation in the legs.

Wearing low-heeled shoes is usually recommended. If the woman has no problem with backache *and* can maintain her balance, there is no medical reason for not wearing slightly higher-heeled shoes. Edema in the feet toward the end of pregnancy may require wearing a larger size shoe.

Employment

How long to work when pregnant depends on the type of work done by the woman and how the pregnancy is progressing. The major factors to consider are whether there are teratogenic hazards in the work environment, if the woman is subject to physical strain or overfatigue, and if there are obstetrical or medical complications of the pregnancy. Rest periods should be available during the workday.

Travel

Unless there are obstetrical or medical complications, travel is not restricted. When traveling by car, the pregnant client is encouraged to stop every 2 hours and walk around for 10 minutes or so. It is imperative always to wear the seat belt, both lap and shoulder, and to keep the lap belt snug below the abdomen. Possible bladder trauma, in case of an accident, is decreased by keeping the bladder empty. Travel by air is best for long trips. Many airlines and cruise ships will not accept passengers past a certain week of pregnancy.

Dental Care

Regular oral hygiene should continue during pregnancy, and dental care can be performed. The woman should inform her dentist that she is pregnant. If possible, x-rays are delayed until after the infant is born. If x-rays must be done, a lead apron must be used.

Sexual Activity

There is no reason to limit sexual activity in a healthy pregnancy. Only when the woman has a history of preterm labor, there is bleeding, or the membranes have ruptured is sexual intercourse contraindicated. As always, barrier protection should be used to prevent sexually transmitted diseases.

The expectant woman's sexual desire may decrease during the first trimester because of fatigue, nausea/vomiting, and breast tenderness. Often, during the second trimester, when the discomforts have lessened, she has greater sexual satisfaction than when not pregnant. By the third trimester, the discomforts of fatigue, dyspnea, urinary frequency, and painful pelvic ligaments may decrease her sexual desire.

After the fourth month, the woman should not lie flat on her back during intercourse because of supine hypotensive syndrome. A pillow can be placed under her right hip to displace the uterus or an alternate position used.

Men may find a change in their desire too. This may be related to their feelings about their partner's changing appearance, concern about hurting her or the fetus, and having sexual intercourse with a pregnant woman.

CHILDBIRTH EDUCATION

Many health care providers recommend that their clients attend a prepared childbirth class. Several persons are recognized for developing childbirth education programs. The three most commonly known are Dick-Read, Bradley, and Lamaze.

In the 1930s, Dr Grantly Dick-Read believed women experience fear during childbirth because they do not understand what is happening in their bodies. This causes tension, which causes the woman to perceive pain more intensely. Later, Dr Robert Bradley stressed that labor is a normal process and felt that the partner support is most important. Dr Fernand Lamaze introduced the childbirth preparation method called **psychoprophylaxis**, teaching mental and physical preparation for childbirth. Further research is needed to conclude that other methods of relaxation and stress reduction, such as acupuncture, hypnotherapy and yoga produce positive outcomes (Beddoe & Lee, 2008).

Most childbirth education today combines these principles, teaching mothers and their support persons basic physiology of labor and how to relax to promote a safe and most comfortable delivery. Included is information regarding controlled breathing, contraction and relaxation of isolated muscles, guided imagery, counter pressure to the back for pain relief, positioning for comfort, use of massage and others. There are also classes teaching care of the newborn, infant massage, CPR, sibling rivalry and grandparenting.

Some women employ a doula to assist with birth or in the postpartum period. The term doula is a Greek term meaning "a woman who serves." Doulas are specially trained birth companions who provide information and emotional support during pregnancy, birth and in the postpartum period. Certification programs exist as well as professional organizations (DONA.org, 2009).

NURSING PROCESS

The nurse's role centers on helping the client maintain a healthy pregnancy and preparing the client for childbirth and delivery.

Assessment

The information presented in this chapter encompasses the possible subjective data and objective data that may be gathered about a specific client.

Nursing Diagnoses

Nursing diagnoses applicable to a pregnant client may include:

- ***A**ctivity Intolerance*
- ***A**nxiety*
- *Disturbed **B**ody Image*
- *Ineffective **B**reathing Pattern*
- ***C**onstipation*
- *Ineffective **C**oping*
- *Readiness for Enhanced Family **C**oping*
- ***F**atigue*
- ***F**ear*
- *Deficient **F**luid Volume*
- *Excess **F**luid Volume*
- *Ineffective **H**ealth Maintenance*
- ***H**ealth Seeking Behaviors* (specify)
- *Risk for **I**njury*
- *Deficient **K**nowledge* (specify)
- *Impaired Physical **M**obility*
- ***N**oncompliance*
- *Imbalanced **N**utrition: Less Than Body Requirements*
- *Disturbed **S**leep Pattern*
- ***S**exual Dysfunction*

Planning/Outcome Identification

Set appropriate goals with the client and her family to meet needs as identified by the nursing diagnoses.

Nursing Interventions

Nursing interventions are individualized and specific for the client based on the assessment, nursing diagnoses, and goals. Nursing interventions for prenatal care are focused on teaching the client and providing anticipatory guidance.

Evaluation

Each goal is evaluated to determine how it has been met by the client.

SAMPLE NURSING CARE PLAN

Prenatal Care

P.S., age 23, first pregnancy, states she has been nauseated and has not eaten for about 3 weeks, feels very tired all the time, takes a nap after work, and then has trouble sleeping because she has to go to the bathroom frequently. Her LMP was 6 weeks ago, menstrual periods have always been regular every 28 days. She smokes 1 pack/day and drinks beer on the weekends. She does not like to cook, so most meals are eaten out. She has lost 3 pounds in the last month. She is unmarried, lives alone, and did not plan to get pregnant.

NURSING DIAGNOSIS 1 *Knowledge Deficit (Self-Care in Pregnancy)* related to inexperience as evidenced by eating, drinking, and smoking habits

Nursing Outcomes Classification (NOC)
Knowledge: Pregnancy

Nursing Interventions Classification (NIC)
Prenatal Care

PLANNING/OUTCOMES	NURSING INTERVENTIONS	RATIONALE
P.S. will competently care for herself during pregnancy.	Teach physiology of pregnancy, discomforts of pregnancy, things she can do to relieve the discomforts, self-care aspects, and fetal development.	Provides reasons for P.S. to take care of herself.

(*Continues*)

SAMPLE NURSING CARE PLAN (Continued)

PLANNING/OUTCOMES	NURSING INTERVENTIONS	RATIONALE
	Gather more data about her work environment and psychosocial aspects of nutrition, smoking, and drinking.	Provides data for additional teaching regarding self-care.

EVALUATION

P.S. states that she now understands the changes pregnancy makes in her body.

NURSING DIAGNOSIS 2 *Imbalanced Nutrition: Less than Body Requirements* related to inadequate food intake as evidenced by nausea and weight loss

Nursing Outcomes Classification (NOC)
Nutritional Status: Energy
Nutritional Status: Nutrient Intake

Nursing Interventions Classification (NIC)
Nutrition Management
Teaching: Individual

PLANNING/OUTCOMES	NURSING INTERVENTIONS	RATIONALE
P.S. will have sufficient nutritional intake during pregnancy	Have P.S. keep a food diary for 3 days.	To determine current eating habits.
	Assess P.S.'s knowledge of healthy eating habits and her food and drink preferences.	To determine her knowledge base and to incorporate her preferences into her dietary plan.
	Teach basic nutrition, food guide pyramid, and nutritional needs during pregnancy.	May encourage changes in P.S.'s eating pattern.

EVALUATION

P.S. follows the food guide pyramid most of the time and is drinking 4 glasses of milk a day.

NURSING DIAGNOSIS 3 *Risk for Injury* related to teratogenic substances as evidenced by smoking and alcohol consumption

Nursing Outcomes Classification (NOC)
Risk Control: Tobacco Use
Risk Control: Alcohol
Risk Control: Unintended Pregnancy

Nursing Interventions Classification (NIC)
Teaching: Individual
Risk Identification: Childbearing Family

PLANNING/OUTCOMES	NURSING INTERVENTIONS	RATIONALE
P.S. will stop smoking and drinking alcohol.	Assess when P.S. is most likely to smoke cigarettes or drink alcohol.	May find behaviors/situations that P.S. can avoid to prevent craving cigarettes and alcohol.
	Refer to smoking-cessation programs.	To provide needed support while trying to quit.
	Teach effects of smoking and alcohol on fetal development.	May encourage P.S. to abstain from both.

EVALUATION

P.S. has cut her smoking in half and only drinks one beer on the weekend.

CASE STUDY

B.W., age 30, and J.W., age 30, have been married 4 years. B.W.'s LMP was 12 weeks ago, but her menstrual periods have always been very irregular. She is tired all the time and nauseated every day, her clothes are very tight around her waist, and her abdomen is protruding.

The following questions will guide your development of a nursing care plan for the case study.

1. What other data would you collect about B.W.?
2. What diagnostic tests would you anticipate the health care provider performing or ordering?
3. What anticipatory guidance would be appropriate for B.W.?
4. When should B.W. return for a checkup?

SUMMARY

- Ideally, planning for pregnancy begins before conception.
- Fetal development proceeds in an orderly and predictable manner.
- Prenatal care involves all aspects of the couple's life.
- A complete history for a pregnant client includes her own medical and obstetrical history, family history, and the fetus's father's history.
- Nutrition increase for pregnancy is 300 kcalories/day. Two extra glasses of milk and one extra serving of meat meets this need and supplies the extra calcium and protein needed.
- Anticipatory guidance comprises the majority of nursing interventions when caring for a pregnant client.

REVIEW QUESTIONS

1. A woman arrives for her first prenatal visit. Her history reveals three pregnancies, including one spontaneous abortion. Her 2-year-old son was born at 36 weeks. The nurse accurately records which of the following into the medical record?
   1. G3 P2 T1 P1 A1 L1
   2. G3 P1 T0 P1 A1 L1
   3. G3 P1 T1 P0 A1 L1
   4. G2 P1 T0 P1 A1 L1
2. The pregnant client states her last menstrual period began on July 8th. Using Naegele's Rule, her due date would be identified as:
   1. April 15.
   2. October 15.
   3. October 1.
   4. April 1.
3. A client weighs 178 pounds at her 26 week prenatal visit. Her pre-pregnancy weight was162 pounds. Which is correct regarding her weight gain?
   1. She has gained too little weight.
   2. She has gained too much weight.
   3. She has gained the appropriate amount of weight.
   4. She is too early to determine appropriate weight gain.
4. A client in her first trimester complains of nausea and vomiting occurring nearly every morning. The nurse appropriately explains the reason for her symptoms when she says:
   1. "Estrogen increases vascularity, which causes pressure on the stomach from surrounding organs."
   2. "Progesterone promotes smooth muscle relaxation, causing food to stay in the stomach longer than when she is not pregnant."
   3. "Hormones cause changes in the gastric lining, resulting in increased acid production in the stomach."
   4. "The effects of estrogen cause the cardiac sphincter to relax, resulting in acid reflux, nausea and vomiting."
5. A nurse preceptor asks the novice nurse to tell her about the purpose of amniotic fluid. The preceptor knows the novice nurse needs further instruction when she says the amniotic fluid:
   1. provides a constant temperature for the fetus.
   2. allows the fetus to swallow and urinate.
   3. increases the pressure around the fetus.
   4. allows the fetus to move more freely.
6. Which statement indicates the nurse understands the treatment of supine hypotension?
   1. Have the client breathe into a paper bag slowly.
   2. Give the client a bolus of intravenous fluids over one hour.
   3. Check the client's blood pressure lying, sitting and standing.
   4. Have the client turn to either side to relieve symptoms.
7. A 34-week pregnant woman is at the mall, buying items for her nursery. She stops and smiles as she

watches a mother talking to her own baby. The client is most likely experiencing which developmental task of pregnancy?

1. Fetal embodiment.
2. Pregnancy validation.
3. Role transition.
4. Fetal distinction.

8. The client is fourteen weeks pregnant at her second prenatal visit. During her assessment, the health care provider measures her fundal height at 17cm. She suspects the client has:

1. a twin gestation.
2. gained more weight than expected.
3. a baby with congenital anomalies.
4. an ectopic pregnancy.

9. A Korean woman is admitted to the labor and delivery unit in active labor. During the admission assessment, she lets her mother answer all of the questions. The nurse understands that the client:

1. is mentally limited and doesn't understand the questions.
2. does not speak English as well as her mother.
3. does not feel comfortable in the hospital setting.
4. is following her own cultural standards.

10. A nurse is instructing a client in ways to minimize heartburn in pregnancy. She knows the client understands her teaching when she says: (Select all that apply.)

1. "I will eat small, frequent meals."
2. "I will lie down for one hour after meals."
3. "I should take a laxative each evening."
4. "I should avoid gassy foods."
5. "I should contact my physician before taking an antacid."
6. "I should avoid fatty foods."

REFERENCES/SUGGESTED READINGS

American College of Obstetrics & Gynecology. (2005). ACOG Updates Definitive Guide to Pregnancy. Retrieved March 9, 2009, from ACOG News Release Web site, http://www.acog.org.

American College of Obstetrics & Gynecology. (2008). Alcohol and Pregnancy: Know the Facts. Retrieved March 9, 2009, from ACOG News Release Web site, http://www.acog.org.

American College of Obstetrics & Gynecology. (2008). All Patients Should be Asked About Alcohol and Drug Abuse. Retrieved March 9, 2009, from ACOG News Release Web site, http://www.acog.org.

American College of Obstetrics & Gynecology. (2008). Pregnant Women Reminded to Get Flu Vaccine. Retrieved March 9, 2009, from ACOG News Release Web site http://www.acog.org.

Allard-Hendren, R. (2000). Alcohol use and adolescent pregnancy. *MCN, 25*(3), 159–162.

Beckmann, C., Buford, T., & Witt, J. (2000). Perceived barriers to prenatal care services. *MCN, 25*(1), 43–46.

Beddoe, A., & Lee, K. (2008). Mind-body interventions during pregnancy. *Journal of Obstetric Gynecologic and Neonatal Nursing, 37*(2), 165–175.

Brucker, M., & Reedy, N. (2000). Nurse-midwifery: Yesterday, today, and tomorrow. *MCN, 25*(6), 322–326.

Bryan, A. (2000). Enhancing parent-child interaction with a prenatal couple intervention. *MCN, 25*(3), 139–144.

Bulechek, G., Butcher, H., McCloskey, J., & Dochterman, J., eds. (2008). *Nursing Interventions Classification (NIC)* (5th ed.). St. Louis, MO: Mosby/Elsevier.

Bungum, T., Peaslee, D., Jackson, A., & Perez, M. (2000). Exercise during pregnancy and type of delivery in nulliparae. *JOGNN, 29*(1), 258–264.

Callister, L., & Vega, R. (1998). Giving birth: Guatemalan women's voices. *JOGNN, 27*(3), 289–295.

Cesario, S. (2001). Care of the Native American woman: Strategies for practice, education, and research. *JOGNN, 30*(1), 13–19.

Cordero, S. (2003). Assessing fetal heart sounds. *Nursing2003, 33*(10), 54–55.

De Sevo, M. (2009). Unlocking the Clues of Family Health History, the Importance of Creating a Pedigree. *Nursing for Women's Health, 11*(3), 122–131.

Dick-Read, G. (1933). *Natural childbirth*. London: Heinemann.

Dick-Read, G. (1944). *Childbirth without fear*. New York: Harper & Row.

Dickason, E., Silverman, B., & Kaplan J. (1998). *Maternal-infant nursing care* (3rd ed.). St. Louis, MO: Mosby-Year Book.

Freda, M. (1998). Confronting the myths. *MCN, 23*(2), 107.

Gennaro, S., Kamwendo, L., Mbweza, E., & Kershbaumer, R. (1998). Childbearing in Malawi, Africa. *JOGNN, 27*(2), 191–196.

Giarelli, E. (2001). A legal look at genetic testing. *RN, 64*(10), 73–75.

Hall, S. (2002). Amniotomy: Necessary intervention or bad habit. *AWHONN Lifelines, 5*(6), 10–13.

Hasenau, S., & Covington, C. (2002). Neural tube defects: Prevention and folic acid. *MCN, 27*(2), 87–91.

Hatters Friedman, S., Heneghan, A., & Rosenthal, M. (2009). Characteristics of Women Who Do Not Seek Prenatal Care and Implications for Prevention. *Journal of Obstetric, Gynecologic & Neonatal Nursing, 38*(2), 174–181.

Holtz, C. (2008). *Global health care: issues and policies* (p. 459). Boston: Jones and Bartlett.

Howard, J., & Berbiglia, V. (1997). Caring for childbearing Korean women. *JOGNN, 26*(6), 665–671.

Hutchinson, M., & Baqi-Aziz, M. (1994). Nursing care of the childbearing Muslim family. *JOGNN, 23*(9), 767–771.

Jones, S. (1996). Genetics: Changing health care in the 21st century. *JOGNN, 25*(9), 777–783.

Ladewig, P., Moberly, S., Olds, S., & London, M. (2001). Contemporary *maternal-newborn nursing care* (5th ed.). Menlo Park, CA: Addison-Wesley Longman.

Lamaze, F. (1965). *Painless childbirth*. New York: Dimon & Schuster.

Littleton, L., & Engebretson, J. (2002). *Maternal, neonatal, and women's health nursing*. Clifton Park, NY: Delmar Cengage Learning.

Longobucco, D., & Freston, M. (1989). Relation of somatic symptoms to degree of paternal-role preparation of first-time expectant fathers. *JOGNN, 18*, 482.

Malnory, M. (1996). Developmental care of the pregnant couple. *JOGNN, 25*(6), 525–532.

Martinez, F., Wright, A., & Taussig, L. (1994, Sept.). The effect of paternal smoking on the birthweight of newborns whose mothers did not smoke. The Health Medical Associates. *Am J Public Health, 84*, 1489–1491.

Matthews, T. (1998). Smoking during pregnancy 1990-1996. *National Vital Statistics Reports, 47*(10), 1–12.

Mills, M. (2007). Craving more than food, the implications of pica. *Nursing for Women's Health*, 11(3), 266–273.

Mindell, J., & Jacobson, B. (2000). Sleep disturbances during pregnancy. *JOGNN, 29*(6), 590–597.

Moorhead, S., Johnson, M., & Maas, M. (2007). Nursing *Outcomes Classification (NOC)* (4th ed.). St. Louis, MO: Mosby.

Morton, J., and Choen Knorad, S. (2009). Introducing a caring/relational framework for building relationships with addicted mothers. *Journal of Obstetric, Gynecologic & Neonatal Nursing, 38*(2), 206–213.

Nasso, J. (1997). Planning for pregnancy—A preconception health program. *MCN, 22*(3), 142–146.

North American Nursing Diagnosis Association International. (2010). *NANDA-I nursing diagnoses: Definitions & classification 2009–2011.* Ames, IA: Wiley-Blackwell.

Pletsch, P., Morgan, S., & Pieper, A. (2003). Context & beliefs about smoking & smoking cessation. *MCN, 28*(5), 320–325.

Reifsnider, E., & Gill, S. (2000). Nutrition for childbearing years. *JOGNN, 29*(1), 43–55.

Remich, M. (1997). Promoting a healthy pregnancy. In E. Q. Younkin & M. S. Davis (Eds.), *Women's health: A primary care clinical guide* (2d ed.). Norwalk, CT: Appleton & Lange.

Rentschler, D. (2003). Pregnant adolescent's perspectives of pregnancy. *MCN, 28*(6), 377–383.

Rhodes, A. (1995). Liability for failure to offer prenatal AFP testing. *MCN, 20*(3), 169.

Robaire, B., & Hales, B. (1993, August). Paternal exposure to chemicals before conception. *BMI, 307*, 341–342.

Rogers, J., & Davis, B. (1995). How risky are hot tubs and saunas for pregnant women? *MCN, 20*(3), 137–140.

Rossner, S. (1998). Obesity and pregnancy. In G. Bray, C. Bouchard, & W. James (Eds.). *Handbook of obesity* (pp. 575–590). New York: Marcel Dekker.

Schneiderman, J. (1996). Postpartum nursing for Korean mothers. *MCN, 21*(3), 155–158.

Simpson, K., & Creehan, P. (2001). *AWHONN perinatal nursing* (2nd ed.). Philadelphia: Lippincott Williams & Wilkins.

Todd, S., LaSala, K., & Neil-Urbon, S. (2001). An integrated approach to prenatal smoking cessation interventions. *MCN, 26*(4), 185–190.

Wisborg, K., Kesmodel, U., Bech B., et al. (2003). Maternal consumption of coffee during pregnancy and stillbirth and infant death in first year of life: Prospective study. *British Medical Journal, 326*(7386), 420.

Zauderer, C. (2009). Maternity Care for Orthodox Jewish Couples, Implications for Nurses in the Obstetric Setting. *Nursing for Women's Health, 13*(2), 112–120.

RESOURCES

American Dietetic Association, http://www.eatright.org

Association of Women's Health, Obstetric, and Neonatal Nurses (AWHONN), http://www.awhonn.org

Center for Disease Control and Prevention (CDC), National Center for Health Statistics, http://www.cdc.gov/nchs

DONA International, http://www.dona.org

Food and Nutrition Information Center, http://www.nal.usda.gov

International Childbirth Education Association (ICEA), http://www.icea.org

Lamaze International, http://www.lamaze.org

March of Dimes, http://www.modimes.org

National Certification Corporation (NCC), http://www.nccwebsite.org

CHAPTER 55
Complications of Pregnancy

MAKING THE CONNECTION

Refer to the following chapters to increase your understanding of the complications of pregnancy:

Basic Nursing
- ***End-of-Life Care***

Adult Health Nursing
- ***Cardiovascular System***
- ***Hematologic and Lymphatic Systems***
- ***Endocrine System***
- ***Sexually Transmitted Infections***
- ***Substance Abuse***

Maternal & Pediatric Nursing
- ***Prenatal Care***
- ***The Birth Process***

Basic Procedures
- ***Hand Hygiene***
- ***Use of Protective Equipment***
- ***Taking Blood Pressure***
- ***Measuring Intake and Output***

Intermediate Procedures
- ***Surgical Asepsis: Preparing and Maintaining a Sterile Field***
- ***Performing Open Gloving***
- ***Performing Urinary Catheterization: Female***

LEARNING OBJECTIVES

Upon completion of this chapter, you should be able to:

- Define key terms.
- Explain medical and nursing interventions for a client with hyperemesis gravidarum.
- Compare and contrast the etiology, medical–surgical management, and nursing care for the bleeding situations in pregnancy.
- Describe the development, medical–surgical management, and nursing care of a client with gestational hypertension.
- Describe the nursing care for a client with a chronic medical problem: diabetes, hypertension, heart disease, maternal PKU.
- Discuss the effects of infection on a pregnant woman and her fetus and ways of preventing the infections.
- Compare and contrast the etiology, medical–surgical management, nursing care, and effect on the fetus of Rh incompatibility and ABO incompatibility.

- Explain the effects of multiple pregnancies on the mother, fetuses, and family.
- Describe the effects of addiction on the mother and fetus.
- Summarize the needs of a woman in preterm labor.

KEY TERMS

abortion
abruptio placenta
amniocentesis
biophysical profile
early deceleration
eclampsia
ectopic pregnancy
euglycemia
HELLP syndrome
hydatidiform mole
hydramnios
hyperemesis gravidarum
incompetent cervix
kernicterus
late deceleration
macrosomia
miscarriage
modified biophysical profile
oligohydramnios
placenta previa
preeclampsia
surfactant
tocolysis
variable deceleration

INTRODUCTION

It is truly impressive that most pregnancies have no complications. For those clients who do have complications, it can be a very frightening and guilt-ridden situation. Regular prenatal care is the best way to identify clients who have high-risk factors. These clients are assessed and monitored more closely, and signs and symptoms of complications are detected as early as possible. Medical–surgical management and effective nursing care can then be implemented. Many of the high-risk factors in pregnancy are listed in Table 55-1.

This chapter covers the common complications of pregnancy including etiology, medical–surgical management, and the nursing process.

ASSESSMENT OF FETAL WELL-BEING

When complications arise in a pregnancy, more intense and specific assessments of the fetus are required.

PROFESSIONALTIP

Ultrasound

After more than 40 years of use, no studies have confirmed harmful effects from ultrasound use in pregnancy. The Power Doppler or pulsed Doppler emits more power signals than the 2-D ultrasound scan or flow velocity waveform Doppler. Therefore, cautious use of the pulsed Doppler is recommended in the first trimester until safety is proven (Woo, 2009).

ULTRASOUND

Two-dimensional (2D) ultrasound allows visualization of the uterine contents. The fetal assessments described in the Prenatal Care chapter are also used. High-frequency, inaudible sound waves are directed toward the uterus. The

TABLE 55-1 High-Risk Factors in Pregnancy

GENERAL	OBSTETRICAL	MEDICAL	OTHER
Age (under 15 or over 35 years)	Previous problems	Chronic diseases	Smoking
Unmarried	Abortion	Diabetes	Drug abuse
Low socioeconomic group, little education	Excessive size of infant	Hypertension	Alcohol abuse
Prenatal care begun 27 weeks or later	Cesarean birth	Sickle-cell anemia	Nutritional deficit
	Preterm/Postterm birth	Thyroid disease	Obesity
	Incompetent cervix	Sexually transmitted infection	
	Abnormal fetal presentation	Cervical neoplasia	
	Rh negative and sensitized	Urinary tract infection	
	Preeclampsia	Neurological problem	
	Multiple pregnancy	Psychiatric problem	

COURTESY OF DELMAR CENGAGE LEARNING

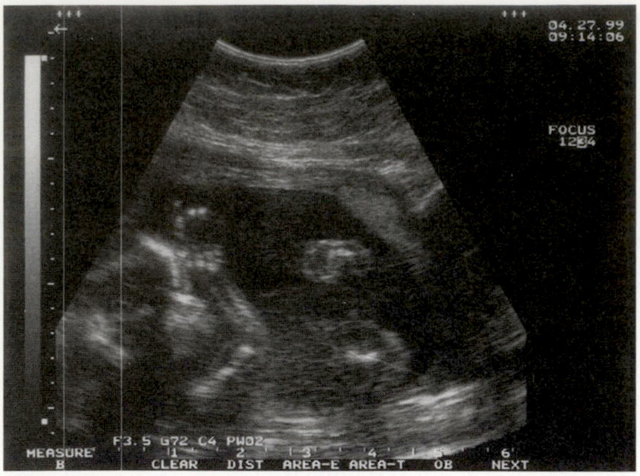

COURTESY OF DELMAR CENGAGE LEARNING

FIGURE 55-1 Ultrasound provides a visual image of uterine contents.

sound waves reflected back are converted into a visual image (Figure 55-1).

Ultrasound provides the following information.

First Trimester

- Early positive diagnosis of pregnancy about 5 or 6 weeks after LMP.
- Identification of more than one fetus.
- Observation of cardiac activity at 21 days and respiratory movements about 11th week of gestation.
- Diagnosis of an ectopic pregnancy.
- Diagnosis of a molar pregnancy.
- Visualization of ultrasonic "soft" markers indicating chromosomal abnormalities (Woo, 2009).

Second and Third Trimester

- Location of pockets of amniotic fluid for retrieval of fluid for testing.
- Measurement of biparietal diameter, femur length, overall length (crown-heel and crown-rump), gestational age, and intrauterine growth restriction (IUGR), formerly intrauterine growth retardation.
- Detection of some fetal anomalies, especially anencephaly and hydrocephalus.
- Detection of amniotic fluid volume, including hydramnios, also known as polyhydramnios, (excessive amniotic fluid) or **oligohydramnios** (deficiency of amniotic fluid), either of which is frequently associated with fetal anomalies.
- Identification of amniotic fluid pockets; a vertical pocket of 2 cm is associated with normal fetal status.
- Location of the placenta, which is necessary before an amniocentesis and to determine placenta abnormalities.
- Determination of fetal position and presentation.
- Detection of fetal death; fetal heart beating is not visualized, and the bones in the fetal head separate.
- Evaluation of cervical length.

Three- and four-dimensional (3-D and 4-D) ultrasound is currently used to improve visualization of fetal anatomic structures and to promote parental bonding. Pictures are obtained with sound waves similar to 2-D, but 3-D images are more life-like in appearance. 4-D ultrasounds are 3-D images shown in rapid succession to view the image as if it is moving. 2-D ultrasound is the standard, and benefits of 3- and 4-D images will be determined with more research (Lee & Simpson, 2007; NIH, 2009).

Transabdominal Ultrasound

The mother is asked to have a full bladder when the ultrasound is performed. This allows the other structures to be assessed in relation to the bladder. The transducer is moved slowly over the abdomen while the client lies on her back. This position may cause shortness of breath or supine hypotension syndrome. The procedure takes about 20 to 30 minutes.

Transvaginal Ultrasound

During a transvaginal ultrasound or endovaginal ultrasound, a probe is inserted into the vagina and placed close to the structures being imaged. This produces a clearer image. The client is in the lithotomy position and has an empty bladder. These scans assist with early detection of ectopic pregnancies, fetal abnormalities in the first trimester, and diagnosing congenital anomalies in the second trimester (Woo, 2009).

Nonstress Test

A nonstress test (NST) assesses the well being of the fetus by recording the fetal heart rate (FHR) and determining increased heart rate with fetal movement. Fetal movement indicates a well oxygenated fetus with a healthy central and autonomic nervous system. An NST requires an electronic fetal monitor to record fetal movement and FHR accelerations (short-term increases in FHR caused by fetal movement). Specific equipment may vary. The mother reclines in a chair or in bed in semi-Fowler's or side-lying position. This noninvasive test is used every day or once weekly as needed after 30 weeks gestation in high-risk clients (Figure 55-2).

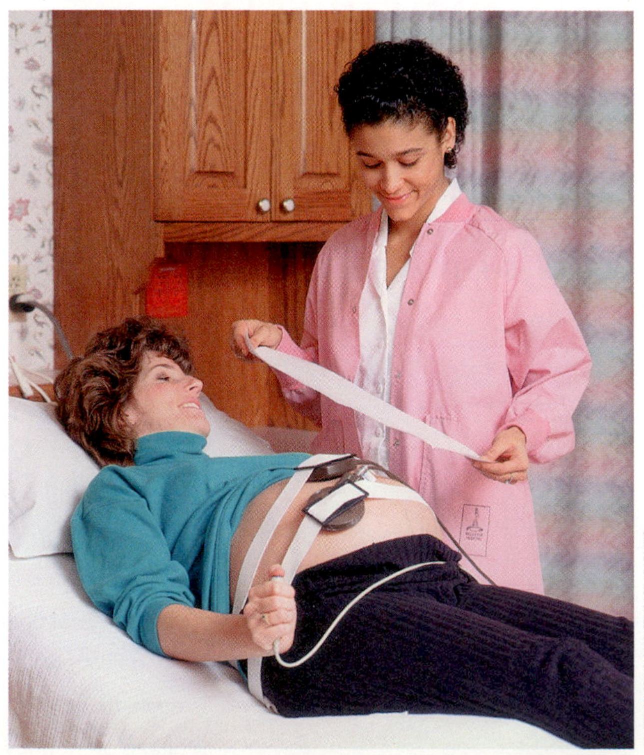

COURTESY OF DELMAR CENGAGE LEARNING

FIGURE 55-2 Nonstress Test (NST) to Assess Fetal Well-Being

The test is reactive if there are two accelerations of 15 beats/min, lasting 15 seconds in a 20-minute period. This indicates that the fetus has adequate oxygenation and an intact central nervous system.

The test is nonreactive if the criteria for reactive are not met. This may indicate that the fetus is asleep or there are problems with fetal oxygenation, and the health care provider is notified. A repeat NST or additional testing is ordered to determine fetal status.

An unsatisfactory test is identified if there is inadequate fetal activity or the data cannot be interpreted. If decelerations of the FHR are noted, the health care provider is notified promptly.

Vibroacoustic Stimulation Test

The vibroacoustic stimulation (VAS) test, also called the fetal acoustic stimulation test (FAST) is used in conjunction with the NST. A small, battery-operated device is placed on the mother's abdomen over the fetal head. A low-frequency vibration and a buzzing sound are emitted from the device to stimulate the fetus who had a nonreactive NST. The sounds emitted last no more than 3 seconds and are repeated every minute if no accelerations occur.

Biophysical Profile

The fetal **biophysical profile** (BPP) assesses five biophysical variables: fetal breathing movement, fetal movements of body or limbs, fetal tone (extension/flexion of extremities), amniotic fluid volume, and reactive NST (Table 55-2). The first four are assessed by ultrasound. A score of 8 or more shows probable fetal well-being.

Table 55-2 Biophysical Profile

	SCORE 2	SCORE 0
Fetal breathing	One or more episodes lasting 30 seconds in 30 minutes	Not present or not lasting 30 seconds
Fetal movement	Three or more body/limb movements in 30 minutes	Two or fewer body/limb movements in 30 minutes
Fetal tone	One or more episodes of active flexion/extension	Slow extension with return to partial flexion, or movement absent
Fluid assessment	One or more pockets of amniotic fluid 1 cm in two perpendicular planes	No pocket, or no pocket 1 cm in two perpendicular planes
Fetal reaction	Reactive NST	Nonreactive NST

COURTESY OF DELMAR CENGAGE LEARNING

Modified Biophysical Profile

The **modified biophysical profile** (MBPP) assesses only two of the variables of the BPP; the NST and the amniotic fluid volume. The MBPP indicates positive fetal well-being if the NST is reactive and the amniotic fluid volume is greater than 5 cm. If either of these two assessments is abnormal, the complete BPP is completed. The MBPP saves time and decreases the cost of fetal surveillance.

Fetal Movements

From the time of quickening (16 to 20 weeks), fetal movement is reassuring to the mother. Counting fetal movement daily provides evidence that the fetus is not having difficulty.

One method is to count fetal movements for 10 minutes three times a day. Another, which is the Cardiff method, requires the mother to count fetal movements at the same time each day until 10 movements are felt. The start and stop times are recorded.

The health care provider should be contacted if there are:

- fewer than 10 movements in 12 hours
- no movements for 8 hours
- sudden violent movements followed by reduced movements

Biochemical Assessments

Three tests include maternal serum alpha-fetoprotein, estriol, and human placental lactogen.

Maternal Serum Alpha-Fetoprotein

Maternal serum alpha-fetoprotein (MSAFP) identifies some birth defects and chromosomal anomalies during the antepartum period. AFP is found in maternal serum about 7 weeks' gestation and rises steadily until the last trimester. Women should have the test between 16 and 18 weeks' gestation. Because there is a normal range for each week of pregnancy, a correct gestational age is important to the interpretation of the test.

If the MSAFP level is high, it indicates a fetal open neural tube defect, multiple gestation, Rh isoimmunization, maternal diabetes mellitus, or fetal distress and death. If the MSAFP level is low, the fetus may have Down syndrome or there may be a maternal hypertensive state.

Estriol

Maternal estriol level indicates fetoplacental function. Essential precursors from the fetal adrenal glands are converted by the placenta to estriol. The level in maternal serum and urine usually increases throughout pregnancy, so there must be a series of tests throughout pregnancy. Gradual increase in the maternal estriol level indicates that the fetal adrenal glands and the placenta are functioning normally.

Human Placental Lactogen

Human placental lactogen (hPL) increases throughout pregnancy correlating with increased fetal weight.

Amniocentesis

Amniocentesis is a procedure in which a needle is inserted through the abdomen into the amniotic sac. Amniotic fluid

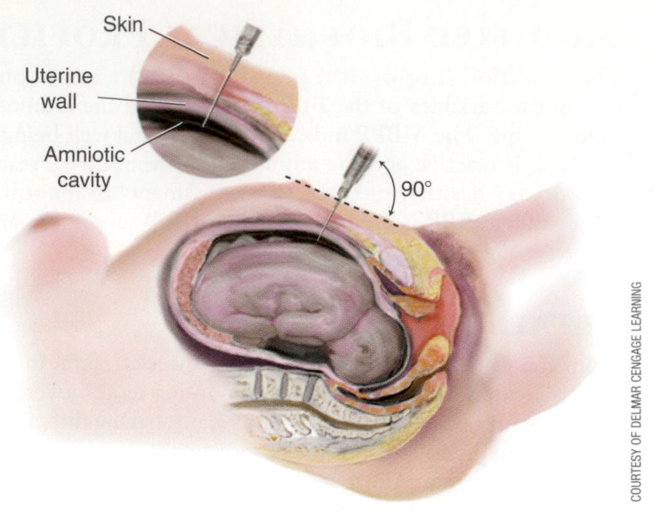

FIGURE 55-3 **Amniocentesis: 15 to 20 mL of amniotic fluid is withdrawn for study.**

is withdrawn and sent to the laboratory for testing. At 14 to 16 weeks' gestation, an amniocentesis may be performed for diagnosis of genetic diseases or birth defects if the mother is older than 35 or either parent has a family history of genetic disease (Figure 55-3).

Later in pregnancy, amniocentesis is most often used to determine fetal lung maturity. In a high-risk pregnancy when preterm delivery of the fetus is a possibility, the physician will often try to maintain the pregnancy until the lungs are mature.

An ultrasound is used to determine the location of pockets of fluid so the fetus, placenta, and cord are not damaged. The nurse assists the physician performing the amniocentesis and provides emotional support to the client.

Tests on Amniotic Fluid

Both the fluid and the cells in the amniotic fluid are used for testing. The fluid should be clear, colorless, and may have flecks of vernix caseosa floating in it.

Lecithin/Sphingomyelin Ratio **Surfactant** is phospholipids in the lungs that lower surface tension and stabilize the alveoli so they do not collapse on exhalation. The ratio of two phospholipids, which are components of surfactant, lecithin and sphingomyelin (L/S ratio), determines the maturity of the lungs.

▼ SAFETY ▼

Amniocentesis

- Wash hands.
- Wear goggles or face mask, splash apron, and disposable gloves.
- Label specimen clearly so laboratory personnel can use appropriate precautions.
- Wash hands after removal of gloves.

Early in pregnancy, the lecithin level is low and the sphingomyelin level is high. At about 32 weeks' gestation, this relationship begins to change. By 35 weeks' gestation, the lecithin level is twice as high as the level of sphingomyelin. An L/S ratio of 2:1 is considered indicative of lung maturity.

Some conditions may accelerate lung maturation, such as severe pregnancy-induced hypertension (PIH), chronic maternal hypertension, or prolonged rupture of membranes. Diabetes and Rh isoimmunization seem to delay fetal lung maturity.

Phosphatidylglycerol Another phospholipid in surfactant, phosphatidylglycerol (PG), appears in the amniotic fluid when the lungs are mature, about 35 weeks' gestation.

Bilirubin In clients with Rh incompatibility, there is bilirubin in the amniotic fluid. The level of bilirubin corresponds to the degree of fetal anemia.

Sex Determination The sex of the fetus can be accurately determined by cell studies. This is important in sex-linked genetic abnormalities.

Chorionic Villi Sampling

In chorionic villi sampling (CVS), samples of chorionic villi from the developing placenta are obtained to assess for the same genetic disorders as in amniocentesis. CVS is performed between 8 and 10 weeks' gestation. Either a vaginal or abdominal approach is used (Figure 55-4).

Contraction Stress Test

A contraction stress test (CST) evaluates the respiratory function of the placenta. During a uterine contraction, blood flow to the intervillous spaces is momentarily reduced, thus decreasing oxygen available to the fetus. A healthy fetus tolerates this well. Fetal hypoxia, myocardial depression, and a decrease in FHR occur if the placenta's reserve is not sufficient.

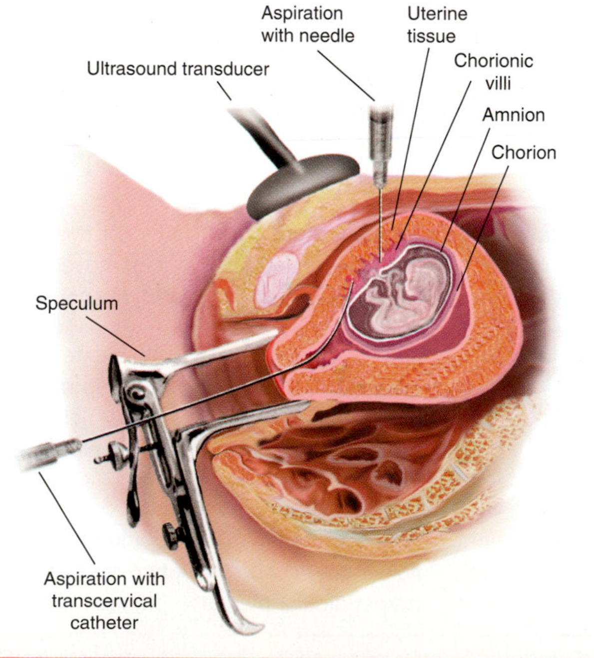

FIGURE 55-4 **Chorionic Villi Sampling (Performed between 8 and 10 Weeks' Gestation)**

This test is used with clients who have heart disease, hypertension, gestational hypertension, sickle-cell anemia, previous stillbirths, Rh sensitization, or a nonreactive NST. It is most often performed on the client with diabetes (chronic or gestational).

The vascular changes that take place in diabetes also affect the placenta. Vascular changes in the placenta cause placental insufficiency, so the fetus will not tolerate a CST well. Contraindications for use of this test are placenta previa, abruptio placenta, premature rupture of membranes, a history of preterm labor, or previous cesarean birth.

The uterine contractions are induced by either intravenous oxytocin or breast self-stimulation. An electronic fetal monitor provides continuous information of the FHR and uterine contractions. The FHR is observed for decelerations with the contractions. A 15-minute baseline recording on the fetal monitor is obtained before contractions are stimulated. Intravenous oxytocin is given piggyback to another IV so it can be stopped when necessary. When three uterine contractions lasting 40 to 60 seconds occur in 10 minutes, the oxytocin is stopped. If three late decelerations occur, the oxytocin is stopped.

For nipple stimulation, warm washcloths are applied to the breasts and/or one nipple is manually rolled by the client. When three uterine contractions lasting 40 to 60 seconds occur in 10 minutes, the stimulation is discontinued. If a decrease in FHR occurs with a contraction, the nipple stimulation is stopped.

A negative CST with no late decelerations indicates the fetus is well-oxygenated. The fetus is able to tolerate the hypoxia of uterine contractions. A CST with late decelerations that occur with at least 50% of contractions is considered a positive CST, which indicates fetoplacental exchange may be compromised. The CST is more invasive and time consuming, so the BPP or MBPP is the preferred method of determining fetal well-being.

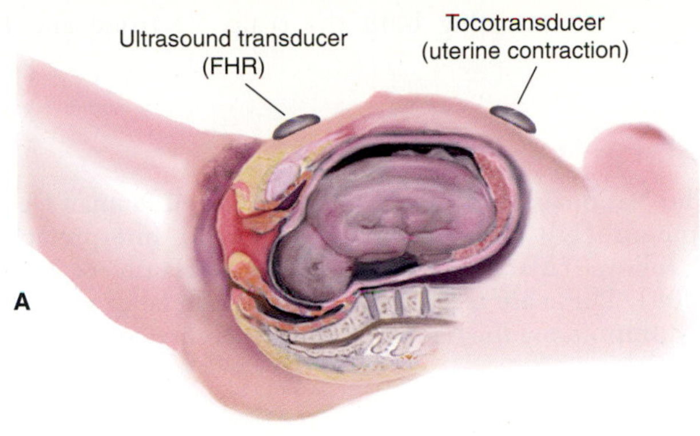

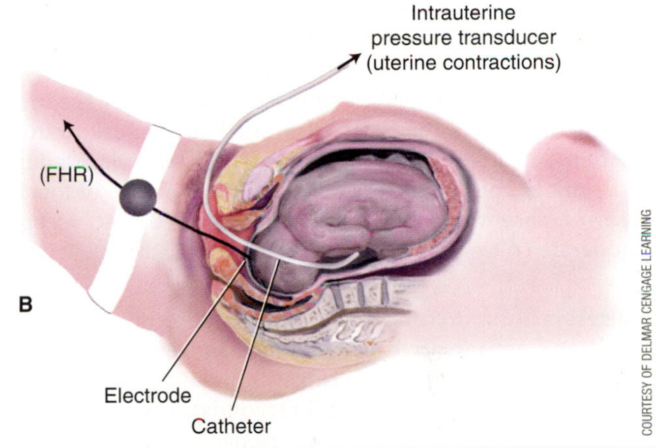

FIGURE 55-5 **Fetal Monitoring: *A,* External (indirect). The top transducer picks up the fetal heart tones and transmits the signal as an electrical impulse to the monitor where they are recorded; *B,* Internal (direct). The EKG electrode on the fetus's scalp picks up the fetal heart tones and the intrauterine catheter picks up uterine contractions.**

Electronic Fetal Monitoring

Electronic fetal monitoring (EFM) provides a visual record of the FHR in relation to the uterine contractions. It allows early detection of fetal distress and abnormal uterine activity. High-risk clients and clients with a problem in their pregnancy are candidates for EFM. Most birthing places routinely have all clients on EFM.

External (Indirect) Monitoring

A tocodynamometer (tocotransducer) that records uterine activity is placed on the mother's abdomen, on the fundus of the uterus. The least amount of tissue is between the dynamometer and fundus at this location so activity is recorded more accurately. With this device, contraction frequency, the amount of time between the beginning of one contraction to the beginning of the next contraction, is determined. The nurse palpates the client's abdomen during a contraction to determine the contraction strength.

An ultrasound transducer that records the FHR is placed over the maternal abdomen in a location where the fetal heart is heard. When the head is the presenting part, the fetal heart is usually best heard just below the umbilicus on one side or the other. With this device, sound waves are bounced off the fetal heart and picked up and displayed as a rate by the monitor. FHR baseline and periodic/nonperiodic changes of the FHR are determined. Elastic bands are placed around the maternal abdomen to hold the transducers in place (Figure 55-5A).

Internal (Direct) Monitoring

This is a more reliable method then external monitoring. An EKG electrode to directly monitor FHR is attached to the fetal presenting part (head) (Figure 55-5B). For this to be initiated, the membranes must be ruptured, the cervix must be dilated at least 2 cm, the presenting part must be down against the cervix, and the presenting part must be known. Only a person specially trained for this procedure should perform it.

Either the external tocodynamometer or an intrauterine catheter may be used to assess uterine contractions. A thin, flexible polyethylene catheter filled with sterile, distilled water is inserted into the amniotic fluid in the uterus. Other catheters used are solid and flexible. In either case, the catheter is inserted between the fetus and the uterine wall into a pocket of amniotic fluid.

The increased pressure on the fluid during a contraction is translated into an electrical signal. This provides reliable information about the contractions. Sterile technique is used when inserting both the scalp electrode and the catheter.

Interpretations

The National Institute of Child Health and Human Development (NICHD) recommended EFM interpretations as follows (Macones, Hankins, Spong, Hauth, & Moore, 2008). These are recommended for use in labor and delivery units across the nation to achieve a more consistent use of terms.

Baseline Rate Baseline rate is the average FHR during a 10-minute period. The normal rate is 110 to 160 beats/minute. A rate greater than 160 beats/minute is tachycardia, and a rate below 110 beats/minute is bradycardia.

Baseline Variability Variability is determined by the irregular fluctuations of the FHR, quantified as the peak to trough amplitude noted in beats per minute (bpm) that occurs during a 10-minute period. These are classified into one of four categories: absent (no difference), minimal (> 0 to </=5 bpm), moderate (6 to </=25 bpm) or marked (>25 bpm).

Accelerations Accelerations are short-term increases in FHR and are usually caused by fetal movement. There is a change in FHR that is a visible abrupt increase: (onset of acceleration to peak less than 30 seconds) by at least 15 bpm, lasting at least 15 seconds. The presence of accelerations indicates the fetus has a pH of at least 7.2, which is normal. The fetus is not in an acidotic state.

Early Deceleration **Early decelerations** are gradual reductions in FHR that begin early with the contraction and typically mirror the contraction. Head compression during contractions causes a decrease in cerebral blood flow, which stimulates a vagal response and causes the heart rate to decrease. The decreased heart rate displays on the monitor as an early deceleration. As pressure is relieved, the FHR returns to normal by the end of the contraction. No intervention is required (Figure 55-6).

Late Deceleration **Late decelerations** are reductions in FHR that begin at or after the peak of the contraction and increase to the baseline level after the contraction has ceased, caused by uteroplacental insufficiency. When a timing discrepancy exists and early versus late decelerations are in question, the nadir (the lowest point) of the deceleration and the peak of the contraction will differentiate early from late. Oxygen administered to the mother may be started. Late decelerations should be reported to the health care provider (Figure 55-6).

Variable Deceleration **Variable decelerations** are abrupt reductions in FHR that have no relationship to contractions of the uterus. They occur when compression of the umbilical cord reduces blood flow between fetus and placenta. A change in the mother's position may take pressure off the cord. When pressure is relieved, the FHR abruptly returns to the baseline. These should also be reported immediately (Figure 55-6).

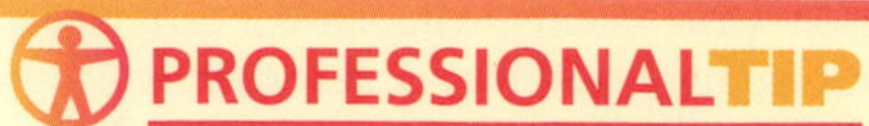

Electronic Fetal Monitoring

The NICHD agreed upon 3 categories of FHR patterns to help guide obstetrical health care providers in providing consistent care in relation to the pattern observed. The categories are listed as follows (Macones, Hankins, Spong, Hauth, & Moore, 2008).

Category I – **Normal** There is no acidosis and there are no interventions necessary.

FHR baseline rate is 110 to 160 bpm

Moderate variability

Absence of variable or late decelerations

Presence or absence of accelerations or early decelerations

Category II – **Indeterminate** In this category, patterns from categories I or III are not found. These patterns do not indicate compromised acid-base balance but necessitate close observation and reevaluation. Health care providers may perform fetal scalp stimulation (gentle rubbing of the presenting part to elicit an acceleration) to determine if fetal oxygenation has been compromised. Other actions may be indicated if there is no positive response.

Category III – **Abnormal** In this category, any one of the following FHR patterns in the absence of FHR variability indicate probable abnormal fetal acid-base balance.

Recurrent late decelerations

Recurrent variable decelerations

Bradycardia

Also considered abnormal is the sinusoidal pattern. This is a wavy pattern of regular variability occurring at 3-5 cycles per minute with an amplitude of 5 to 40 bpm. This pattern resembles a "sine wave" and may indicate a serious condition in the fetus, such as anemia.

Category III patterns require that the health care provider be present to determine timing and mode of delivery. The cause of the pattern is determined, if possible, and the following measures are implemented to correct the problem. These interventions may also be used in Category II patterns that do not respond to scalp stimulation with an acceleration.

Change maternal position

Increase the rate of the mainline intravenous infusion

Administer oxygen to the mother

Discontinue oxytocin if infusing

Resolve maternal hypotension

If the interventions do not improve fetal status, delivery is immediate.

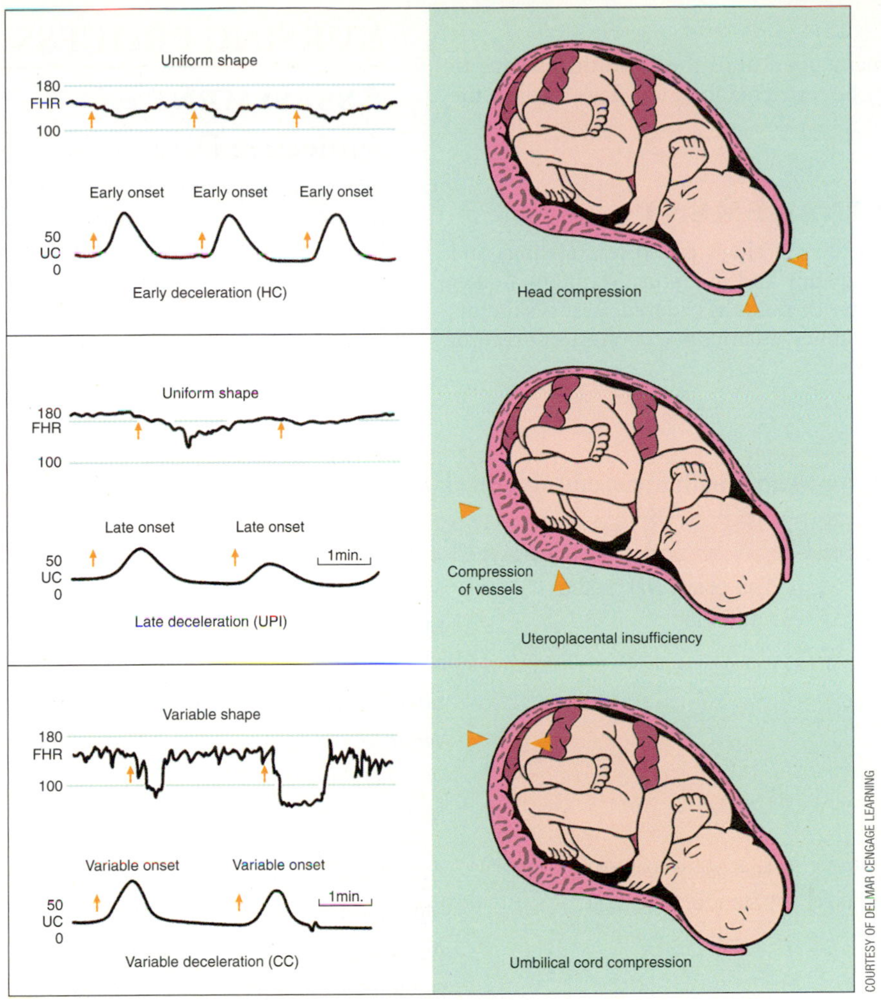

FIGURE 55-6 Fetal Heart Rate Patterns from Continuous Electronic Fetal Monitoring

HYPEREMESIS GRAVIDARUM

Hyperemesis gravidarum is a severe form of nausea and vomiting occurring during pregnancy that usually persists beyond the first trimester. The cause is unknown but may be related to an increased estrogen level, gonadotropin production, or trophoblastic activity. Psychological factors may also be involved. The excessive secretion of saliva (ptyalism) may contribute to the feeling of nausea. The nausea and vomiting does not subside at about 12 weeks' gestation as does "morning sickness." If untreated, the vomiting causes nutritional deficiencies and dehydration.

Dehydration leads to fluid and electrolyte imbalance and alkalosis from the loss of hydrochloric acid. As the situation becomes worse, the client experiences tachycardia and may have hypovolemia, hypotension, an increase in hematocrit and blood urea nitrogen (BUN), and a decrease in urine output.

The starvation situation causes protein and vitamin deficiencies. Cardiac functioning may be disrupted by severe potassium loss. Untreated, the client may experience metabolic changes or death. Embryonic or fetal death may occur.

The treatment goals are to control vomiting, correct dehydration, restore electrolyte balance, and maintain adequate nutrition.

MEDICAL–SURGICAL MANAGEMENT

Medical

The client is usually hospitalized and intravenous fluids containing glucose, vitamins, and electrolytes are started immediately. IV therapy is continued until all vomiting has stopped for 48 hours. Psychotherapy may be recommended.

Pharmacological

A sedative may be given, but medications are kept to a minimum because of potential teratogenic (harmful) effects to the fetus.

Diet

The client is kept NPO until all vomiting has stopped for 48 hours. Small amounts of dry foods are then offered with slow progression to a regular diet. If the client is unable to eat without vomiting, total parenteral nutrition may be initiated through a peripherally inserted central catheter (i.e., PICC) or other IV access.

Activity

Bed rest is usually maintained until the condition begins to improve. Visitors may be restricted for a few days to allow the client to rest.

Nursing Management

Provide opportunities for the client to express feelings and perceptions of the pregnancy and the fetus. Maintain a quiet environment. Administer IV fluids as ordered. Assess skin turgor and mucous membranes. Maintain accurate I&O record. Ensure good oral hygiene.

NURSING PROCESS

Assessment

Subjective Data

Especially important is the client's emotional state and her feelings about the pregnancy, the fetus, and her mate. Ask what triggers her nausea and vomiting.

Objective Data

Check the amount and character of all emesis, intake and output, and FHR. Note signs of jaundice and vaginal bleeding.

Nursing diagnoses for a client with hyperemesis gravidarum include the following:

NURSING DIAGNOSES	PLANNING/OUTCOMES	NURSING INTERVENTIONS
*Imbalanced **N**utrition: Less than Body Requirements* related to persistent vomiting	The client will cease vomiting.	Maintain relaxed, quiet environment. Monitor amount and character of all emesis, and maintain accurate I&O record. Ensure good oral hygiene after each vomiting episode. When vomiting stops, provide dry foods, then bland foods and oral fluids as ordered. Maintain cheerful, optimistic attitude.
*Deficient **F**luid Volume* related to decreased fluid intake and excessive fluid loss	The client will have fluid balance.	Administer IV fluids as ordered. Monitor laboratory reports for electrolyte levels. Assess skin turgor and mucous membranes. Provide small amounts of oral fluids when tolerated. Maintain accurate I&O record.
***F**ear* related to fetal well-being	The client will discuss fears with health caregivers.	Provide opportunities for client to express concerns. Show acceptance of client's perceptions. Assist client to identify personal strengths. Listen to the client's concerns. Help client identify sources of support.

Evaluation: Evaluate each outcome to determine how it has been met by the client.

BLEEDING

Bleeding disorders include abortion, ectopic pregnancy, hydatidiform mole, placenta previa, abruptio placenta, and disseminated intravascular coagulation.

ABORTION

Abortion is the spontaneous (natural) or induced (elective) termination of a pregnancy before viability of the fetus. A fetus is considered viable at 20 weeks' gestation. With medical intervention, a fetus between 20 and 24 weeks' gestation may survive. Some states have defined viability as 20 weeks' gestation and a weight of 500 g.

A spontaneous abortion is often called a **miscarriage**. Spontaneous abortions may be related to chromosomal abnormalities, faulty implantation, teratogenic substances, placental abnormalities, incompetent cervix, chronic maternal diseases, maternal infections, and endocrine imbalances. Clinically, spontaneous abortions are classified as:

- *Threatened*: Unexplained bleeding and cramping. The cervix is closed and membranes are intact (Figure 55-7A).
- *Inevitable*: Increased bleeding and cramping. The cervix begins to dilate and the membranes may rupture (Figure 55-7B).
- *Incomplete*: Some of the products of conception are expelled. Most often the placenta is not expelled. Bleeding is heavy and cramping severe (Figure 55-7C).
- *Complete*: All products of conception are expelled.

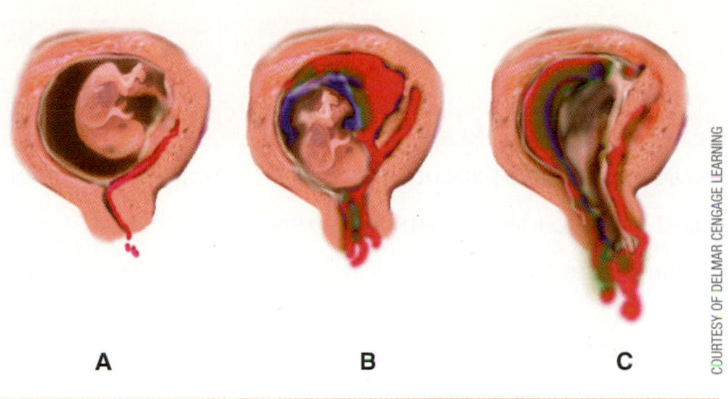

FIGURE 55-7 Types of Spontaneous Abortions; *A*, Threatened; *B*, Inevitable; *C*, Incomplete

- *Missed*: Embryo or fetus dies but is retained. The cervix is closed. If the fetus is not expelled within 6 weeks, disseminated intravascular coagulation (DIC) may develop.
- *Recurrent spontaneous*: Any of the above occurring in three consecutive pregnancies. Most commonly, the cervix begins to dilate in the second trimester. This is called an **incompetent cervix**.

MEDICAL–SURGICAL MANAGEMENT

Medical

For threatened abortion, the client is usually told to limit activities for 24 to 48 hours. If the bleeding is going to stop, it will usually do so in 48 hours. If the bleeding stops, the client is advised to avoid stress, fatigue, strenuous activity, and sexual intercourse. Having one or two rest periods during the day is also recommended until the pregnancy seems to be progressing normally.

Surgical

A client with an inevitable or incomplete abortion generally is hospitalized to remove the products of conception from the uterus. A dilation and curettage (D & C) or suction evacuation is performed. Depending on the amount of blood loss, the client may be given blood transfusions.

When the products of conception, in a missed abortion, are not expelled in 4 to 6 weeks, the client is hospitalized. For 12 weeks' gestation or less, a D & C is performed. If more than 12 weeks' gestation, induction of labor with oxytocin may be used.

PROFESSIONALTIP

Spontaneous Abortion

The client who has a miscarriage may experience a wide spectrum of emotions from shock, disbelief, and guilt, to anger and despair. She may have difficulty managing these feelings as well as responding to the reactions of her partner, family, and friends. The nurse can assist by answering the woman's questions, allowing her to express her emotions, and respecting her need to grieve.

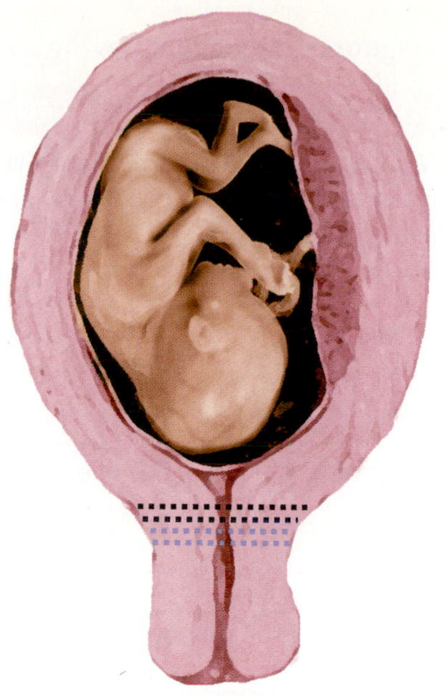

FIGURE 55-8 Shirodkar or McDonald Procedure. Purse-string sutures keep the cervix closed in an incompetent cervix.

When recurrent spontaneous abortions are caused by an incompetent cervix, a treatment option is surgical cerclage (Shirodkar or McDonald procedure, Figure 55-8). The cervix is stitched with a heavy suture in a purse-string fashion at the level of the internal os at about 13 to 17 weeks' gestation. The difference between the Shirodkar and the McDonald method is the height on the cervix and method of suture placement. The Shirodkar suture can be left in for future pregnancies and a cesarean birth planned, or the suture may be removed at term and a vaginal birth occurs (Trofatter, 2009). If the mother goes into labor or the membranes rupture, she must call her health-care provider and go to the hospital immediately.

NURSING MANAGEMENT

Frequently assess the amount of bleeding, presence of clots, and any expelled tissue. Provide a calm environment and actively listen to the client. Provide information about the situation and prepare client for procedures and treatments.

NURSING PROCESS

ASSESSMENT

Subjective Data

The client may describe abdominal cramping and vaginal bleeding, and may have feelings of fear and guilt.

Objective Data

Note the amount of bleeding, presence of clots, and any tissue expelled. Expelled tissue is sent to pathology as ordered for analysis. Vital signs may indicate excessive blood loss (hypovolemia). Assess location, quality, and intensity of pain.

Nursing diagnoses for a client having an abortion include the following:

NURSING DIAGNOSES	PLANNING/OUTCOMES	NURSING INTERVENTIONS
*Situational Low **S**elf-esteem* related to feelings of guilt for doing something to cause abortion	The client will maintain usual level of self-esteem.	Provide information about causes of a spontaneous abortion. Assist client to identify personal strengths. Actively listen to the client.
*Aute **P**ain* related to contractions (cramping) of uterine muscle	The client will describe having less pain.	Administer analgesic as ordered. Monitor effect of analgesic.
***F**ear* related to potential loss of pregnancy	The client will discuss fear with family.	Provide opportunities for the client to express fears. Help client identify sources of support. Show acceptance of client's perceptions.

Evaluation: Evaluate each outcome to determine how it has been met by the client.

SAMPLE NURSING CARE PLAN

The Client Having a Spontaneous Abortion

P.C., age 25, G4, P3, T2, P1, A0, L3, is admitted to the hospital with some bleeding and cramping. She states, "I'm scared, I don't understand what's happening." Vital signs are BP 108/66, T 98.6, P 86, R 24. Her skin is cool. At her first prenatal visit, 3 weeks ago, the fetus was 12 weeks' gestation. Crying, she says, "I don't know what I did to cause this to happen."

Two hours later, P.C.'s cramping is severe and the bleeding heavy, bright red. Vital signs are BP 88/60, P 100, and R 28. Her skin is cold and clammy.

NURSING DIAGNOSIS 1 *Deficient **F**luid Volume* related to heavy bleeding as evidenced by hypotension and decreased pulse pressure

Nursing Outcomes Classification (NOC)
Fluid Balance

Nursing Interventions Classification (NIC)
Fluid Monitoring

PLANNING/OUTCOMES	NURSING INTERVENTIONS	RATIONALE
P.C. will have vital signs return to baseline values.	Administer IV fluids and/or blood as ordered.	Replaces fluid volume lost by bleeding.
	Monitor P.C.'s vital signs every 15 minutes or less.	Clinical indicators of fluid volume.
	Save all vaginal pads and clots or tissue passed for physician to see.	Allows physician to estimate blood loss and identify any tissue passed.
	Administer analgesic as ordered.	Relieving pain will make P.C. more comfortable.
	Prepare P.C. for surgery as ordered.	Most likely, a D & C will be performed.

EVALUATION

After a D & C, P.C.'s vital signs returned to baseline values.

NURSING DIAGNOSIS 2 ***A**nxiety* related to changes in her pregnancy as evidenced by statement "I'm scared, I don't understand what's happening."

Nursing Outcomes Classification (NOC)
Anxiety Reduction
Coping

Nursing Interventions Classification (NIC)
Anxiety Reduction

(*Continues*)

SAMPLE NURSING CARE PLAN (Continued)

PLANNING/OUTCOMES	NURSING INTERVENTIONS	RATIONALE
P.C. will verbalize her feelings about bleeding and cramping while pregnant.	Speak slowly and calmly to P.C.	Conveys calmness and sense of security.
	Evaluate P.C.'s understanding of what is happening and possible treatment options.	Provides information for educational needs.
	Involve spouse/significant other in discussion.	Gives family information and a feeling of control.
	Be direct and focus on the specific topic.	Anxiety decreases ability to concentrate.
	Help P.C. identify coping methods used in the past.	Reviewing past coping mechanisms helps P.C. find effective coping mechanisms to use now.

EVALUATION

P.C. shared feelings of fear and guilt about the bleeding and cramping.

NURSING DIAGNOSIS 3

*Anticipatory **G**rieving* related to probable loss of pregnancy as evidenced by crying and statement "I don't know what I did to cause this to happen."

NOC: *Coping, Family Coping, Grief Resolution*
NIC: *Family Support, Grief Work Facilitation, Coping Enhancement, Emotional Support*

CLIENT GOAL

P.C. will verbalize what losing a pregnancy means to her.

NURSING INTERVENTIONS

1. Allow P.C. to express her feelings.
2. Assess P.C.'s coping skills.
3. Assist P.C.'s to identify personal resources and strengths.
4. Provide privacy for P.C. and her family.
5. Refer to local pregnancy loss support group.

SCIENTIFIC RATIONALES

1. Releases energy and is calming.
2. Coping skills may need reinforcing or adapting.
3. Promotes integrity of self.
4. Allows them a chance to discuss the situation and make plans.
5. Referral assists family to find encouragement and support from others.

EVALUATION

Have P.C.'s vital signs returned to baseline values?
Is P.C. expressing her feelings about losing the pregnancy?

ECTOPIC PREGNANCY

An **ectopic pregnancy** occurs when a fertilized ovum implants outside the uterine cavity. The most common site is in the fallopian tube. This generally happens when the fertilized ovum is unable to move through the tube. Figure 55-9 illustrates other possible sites of implantation in an ectopic pregnancy.

In the United States, an ectopic pregnancy occurs in 2% of all pregnancies (Sepilian & Wood, 2009). Risk factors include pelvic inflammatory disease, in utero exposure to diethylstilbestrol (DES), sexually transmitted infections, pharmacologic treatment of infertility, endometriosis, smoking, advanced maternal age, and prior abdominal surgery (Sepilian & Wood, 2009).

The pregnancy appears normal at first with the usual signs and symptoms, including the presence of hCG in the blood and urine. Symptoms of ectopic pregnancy begin gradually about 3 to 5 weeks after the first missed menstrual period. Pain is noted as the fallopian tube stretches with the growing embryo. The tube finally ruptures (a severe pain occurs) and bleeds into the peritoneal cavity. Some vaginal bleeding may be apparent. The client may rapidly show signs of hypovolemic shock. The signs of shock are out of proportion to the apparent blood loss. Ectopic pregnancy is nearly always fatal to the embryo.

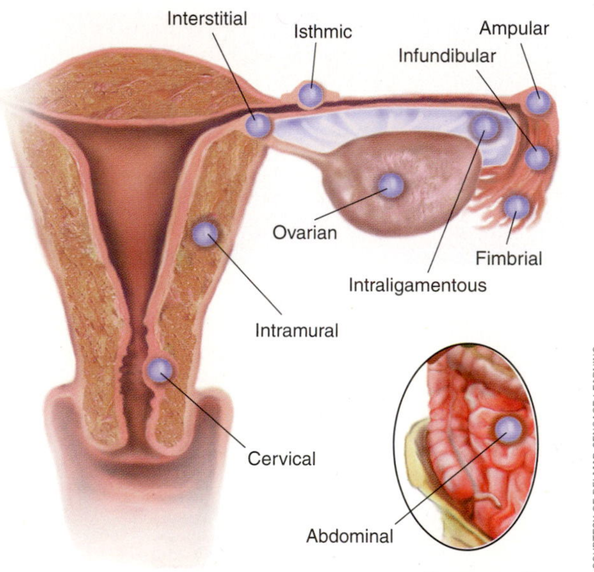

FIGURE 55-9 Possible Sites of Implantation in Ectopic Pregnancy

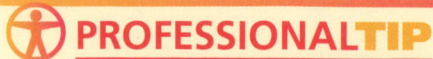

PROFESSIONAL TIP

Treatment Alternative for Ectopic Pregnancy

A viable alternative to surgery that is just as successful as laparoscopic salpingostomy is now available. Methotrexate (Mexate, Folex) works by interfering with DNA synthesis and cell multiplication. The actively proliferating trophoblastic tissue is sensitive to methotrexate.

Women who desire future fertility and have an unruptured ectopic pregnancy 3.5 cm or less in size and have no symptoms of bleeding are candidates for methotrexate therapy. The treatment is a single dose of methotrexate (Mexate, Folex) 50 mg/m^2 IM in a single injection or as a divided dose injected into each hip.

Potential drug side effects are photosensitivity, nausea and vomiting, stomatitis, gastris, diarrhea, and dizziness. Effects to expect from methotrexate treatment are increased abdominal pain 2 to 3 days after the injection, an increase in bhCG for 1 to 3 days, and vaginal bleeding or spotting.

Stress the importance of follow-up visits with the health care provider until the weekly monitored levels of bhCG levels are not present. If the client is Rh negative, administer Rh immune globulin (RhoGAM) (Sepilian & Wood, 2009).

MEMORY TRICK

To remember the 3 classic symptoms of an ectopic pregnancy, recall **VAP**:

V = Vaginal bleeding

A = Amenorrhea

P = Pain

(Sepilian & Wood, 2009)

MEDICAL–SURGICAL MANAGEMENT

Medical

The menstrual history is reviewed and a pelvic examination performed to identify abnormal pelvic masses and tenderness. Severe pain occurs when the cervix is moved. A transvaginal ultrasound is also done. Serial testing of hCG shows a slower increase than in a normal pregnancy, in which the hCG level doubles every 48 to 72 hours. A serum progesterone level of 25 ng/mL strongly suggests a normal pregnancy, whereas a level of 5 ng/mL or less indicates a nonviable pregnancy. A level between 5 ng/mL and 25 ng/mL is uncertain, and a transvaginal ultrasound is needed.

Surgical

Rapid surgical treatment is generally necessary to remove the products of conception and to control bleeding. Laparotomy is seldom used unless the client has orthostatic hypotension, tachycardia, or a falling hematocrit.

Laparoscopic salpingostomy or salpingectomy are preferred. The procedure of choice is salpingostomy when future fertility is desired (Sepilian & Wood, 2009). If the fallopian tube is badly damaged, a salpingectomy is performed. The ovary is left in place if not damaged. Blood transfusions are often required.

Pharmacological

Methotrexate (Mexate, Folex) may be given to resolve an ectopic pregnancy.

Diet

If the client has surgery, she will be NPO before and after surgery.

Activity

The client is usually on bed rest until the situation is resolved.

Nursing Management

Administer analgesics as ordered. Provide information about an ectopic pregnancy. Actively listen to client. Encourage client to express feelings. Monitor vital signs. Prepare for surgery as ordered and begin preoperative teaching.

NURSING PROCESS

Assessment

Subjective Data

The client describes amenorrhea, nausea, breast tenderness, and a dull ache on one side that has increasingly become more severe. When the tube ruptures, the client will describe a single excruciating pain in the abdomen and may also have referred shoulder pain.

Objective Data

Some vaginal bleeding may be apparent. Laboratory reports may show a low hemoglobin and hematocrit, a rising leukocyte level, and a slowly rising hCG level. The red blood count (RBC) count is low and sedimentation rate elevated. The abdomen may be rigid and tender. Vital signs may indicate hypovolemic shock.

Nursing diagnoses for a client with an ectopic pregnancy include the following:

NURSING DIAGNOSES	PLANNING/OUTCOMES	NURSING INTERVENTIONS
*Anticipatory **G**rieving* related to the loss of the pregnancy	The client will understand that grieving may last several months.	Encourage client and family to talk about their feelings. Allow them privacy to grieve. Listen actively to concerns about this and future pregnancies. Provide information about causes of ectopic pregnancy. Refer to other professionals for help as needed.
*Impaired **T**issue Integrity* related to the rupture of a fallopian tube	The client will regain tissue integrity of the fallopian tube or it will be removed.	Prepare client for surgery as ordered. Begin preoperative teaching.
*Acute **P**ain* related to tubal rupture and blood in the abdomen	The client will express less pain.	Administer analgesics as ordered and evaluate its effectiveness. Provide information about cause of pain.

Evaluation: Evaluate each outcome to determine how it has been met by the client.

HYDATIDIFORM MOLE

Hydatidiform mole (trophoblastic disease), or molar pregnancy, is an abnormality of the placenta. The chorionic villi become fluid-filled, grapelike clusters; the trophoblastic tissue proliferates; and there is no viable embryo. In effect, the fertilized ovum dies and the chorion develops into vesicles. There is a possibility of developing choriocarcinoma (malignant, metastaic, potentially fatal trophoblastic disease).

Two types of hydatidiform moles are the complete and the partial. The complete mole has only paternal genetic material. There is no embryonic tissue, only the fluid-filled cystic villi. A large amount of hCG is produced because the chorionic villi are proliferating. The classic signs are bleeding (usually brownish but may be red), uterine enlargement greater than would be expected for the gestation, and no fetal heart tones (FHT) heard (Figure 55-10). If any of the grapelike clusters are passed, it is diagnostic. There is greater potential of developing a choriocarcinoma with the complete than the partial mole.

The partial mole has only focal areas of the fluid-filled cystic villi; some chorionic villi are formed normally. There is a fetus with multiple chromosomal anomalies and little chance for survival. A partial mole may not be recognized until

PROFESSIONAL TIP

Classic Symptoms of Hydatidiform Mole

No FHT with other signs of pregnancy
Increased elevation of hCG
Brownish vaginal bleeding that may also be bright red
Discharge of fluid-filled vesicles

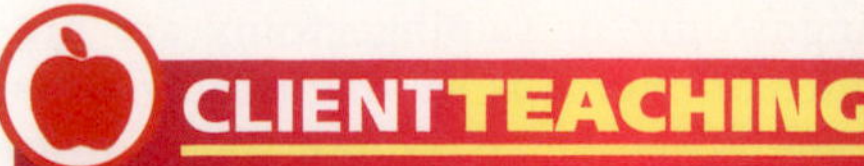

CLIENT TEACHING

Methotrexate

- There is a risk of photosensitivity when taking methotrexate (Mexate, Folex) to reduce hCG levels after treatment for hydatidiform mole.
- Clients should avoid sun exposure while taking this medication.

the products of conception are examined after a spontaneous abortion.

The client may experience hyperemesis gravidarum because of the higher serum hCG level. If symptoms of pregnancy-induced hypertension appear before 24 weeks' gestation, a molar pregnancy is very probable. The primary diagnostic tool is ultrasound.

Medical–Surgical Management

Medical

After surgery to remove the mole, the client must be followed for 1 to 2 years. The care includes chest x-rays to detect metastases, physical examinations with a pelvic examination, and regular (usually weekly) laboratory measurement of hCG level. The client is advised not to become pregnant during the follow-up time.

Surgical

The desire of the client for future fertility influences the surgical procedure used to empty the uterus. A D & C may be performed, but it is difficult to make certain that no fragment of the molar pregnancy is left in the uterus. A hysterotomy, cutting the uterus open (like cesarean birth), allows visual determination that the uterus is completely emptied. If the client is older and no future pregnancy is desired or there is excessive bleeding, a hysterectomy is performed.

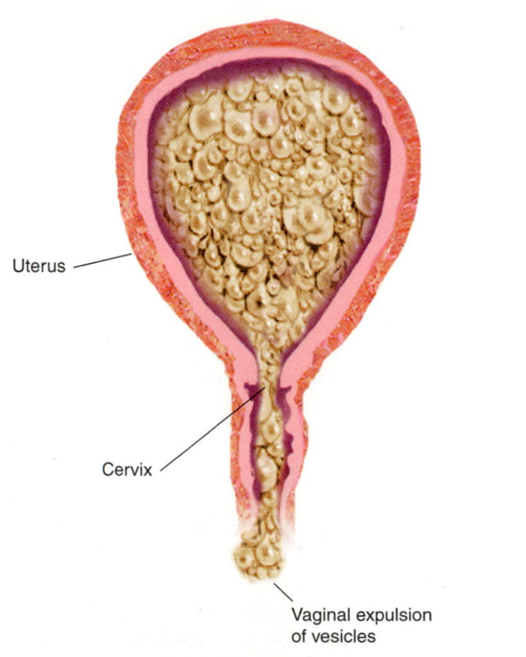

FIGURE 55-10 Hydatidiform Mole

Pharmacological

If the hCG level remains high or rises after the uterus is evacuated, methotrexate (Mexate, Folex) is given. Oxytocin is given to keep the uterus contracted to control bleeding. Typed and cross-matched blood must be available.

Activity

Bed rest is maintained until after surgery, then ambulation is progressively increased.

Nursing Management

Monitor vaginal bleeding. Assess uterine size and FHT (none heard). Prepare for ultrasound. Prepare for surgery as ordered.

NURSING PROCESS

Assessment

Subjective Data

The client may describe severe nausea and vomiting and may have some brownish vaginal discharge.

Objective Data

There is vaginal bleeding, usually brownish but may be bright red. Uterine enlargement is greater than expected for gestational age. Ultrasound reveals a characteristic molar pattern. The client may have symptoms of gestational hypertension (BP 140/90 mm Hg or an increase of 30/15, proteinuria, and edema measured by sudden weight gain). The lack of FHTs when the client has other signs of pregnancy is a classic symptom of a hydatidiform mole. The client has very low levels of serum alpha-fetoprotein.

Nursing diagnoses for a client with hydatidiform mole include the following:

NURSING DIAGNOSES	PLANNING/OUTCOMES	NURSING INTERVENTIONS
Fear related to the possible development of choriocarcinoma	The client will discuss fears with health care provider or other professional.	Provide opportunities for client to express fears. Help client identify sources of support. Refer to other professionals as needed.
Deficient Knowledge related to lack of understanding for regular monitoring of hCG level and delaying pregnancy	The client will discuss reasons for regular monitoring of hCG level and reasons for delaying pregnancy.	Explain that the hCG level indicates whether choriocarcinoma is developing. Provide reasons for delaying another pregnancy. Allow client to express feelings about regular laboratory testing of blood.

Evaluation: Evaluate each outcome to determine how it has been met by the client.

PLACENTA PREVIA

Placenta previa occurs when implantation is in the lower uterine segment with the placenta lying over or very near the internal cervical os, the opening into the uterus (Figure 55-11). The cause is unknown, but predisposing factors may be multiparity, uterine scarring from D & C or cesarean birth, endometritis, maternal advancing age, and smoking.

The classic symptom is *painless bleeding* in the last half of pregnancy. There may be occasional bright red spotting or intermittent gushes of blood. Rarely is bleeding continuous. The uterus is relaxed and not tender. Bleeding is unrelated to maternal activity. Placenta previa is classified in three ways:

- *Low-lying or Marginal*: Placenta is near the internal cervical os but does not cover any part of the opening
- *Partial*: Placenta covers part of internal cervical os opening
- *Complete or Total*: Placenta completely covers internal cervical os opening

Toward the last part of pregnancy, the cervix effaces (thins). This movement of the cervix pulls away from the placenta, and the exposed placental sinuses begin to bleed. The earlier this happens, the more serious the situation.

EFFECTS ON THE FETUS/NEONATE

The gestational age of the fetus and the amount of bleeding determine the effects on the fetus/neonate. During profuse bleeding, the fetus may suffer from hypoxia. After delivery, the neonate is assessed to see whether the bleeding resulted in anemia.

MEDICAL–SURGICAL MANAGEMENT

Medical

The goal is to maintain the pregnancy until the fetus is mature enough to survive outside the uterus. Fetal maturity is assessed by checking the lecithin/sphingomyelin ratio for lung maturity. The mother is usually hospitalized. Hemoglobin and hematocrit (H & H) is usually determined every 12 hours. The laboratory will type and cross-match, and two units of blood is kept on call in the event of severe blood loss.

Diagnosis is made with an ultrasound. Once the diagnosis is made, no vaginal examinations are performed because of the risk of causing more bleeding by disturbing the placenta. If an ultrasound is unavailable, vaginal bleeding profuse, and the pregnancy near term, the health care provider may examine the client vaginally. This is done in the delivery room with a setup for both a vaginal delivery and a cesarean delivery. An IV is started in case the client starts bleeding profusely. Urinary output decreases as the bleeding increases.

Surgical

If the maternal situation becomes worse or there are signs of fetal distress, a cesarean birth is begun immediately.

Pharmacological

In an attempt to accelerate fetal lung maturity, a drug such as betamethasone (Celestone) may be given to the mother.

Activity

The client is on bed rest with bathroom privileges as long as no bleeding occurs. If the client has bathroom privileges, place a graduated container or commode "hat" in the toilet

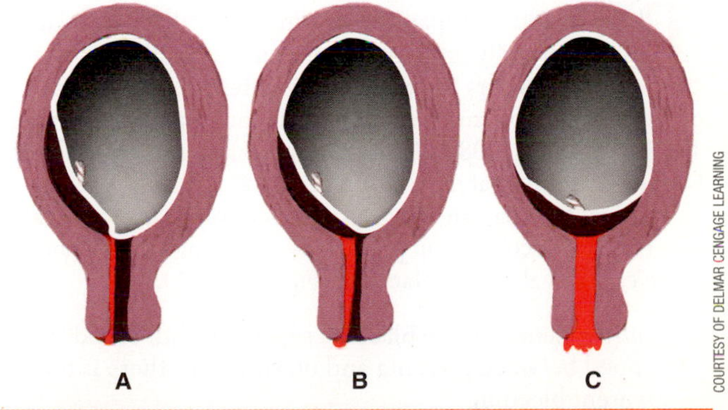

FIGURE 55-11 Placenta Previa; *A*, Low Implantation (Marginal); *B*, Partial Placenta Previa; *C*, Total Placenta Previa

to collect urine and any products of conception passed by the woman. If bleeding begins, the client is on complete bed rest.

Nursing Management

Maintain the client on bed rest. Monitor vital signs and FHR. Prepare for ultrasound. Maintain a calm environment.

CRITICAL THINKING

Placenta Previa

A client is admitted with a placenta previa.

1. What assessments does the nurse do to monitor for blood loss?
2. What is the most important assessment the nurse does throughout the labor process?

Assess for uterine contractions. Administer IV solutions as ordered. Monitor urinary output. Be prepared for a possible C-section.

NURSING PROCESS

Assessment

Subjective Data

The client describes painless bleeding.

Objective Data

Vaginal bleeding may range from spotting to profuse bleeding. The uterus remains soft and relaxes fully between contractions if labor begins. FHR generally remains stable unless bleeding is profuse and maternal shock occurs.

Nursing diagnoses for a client with placenta previa include the following:

NURSING DIAGNOSES	PLANNING/OUTCOMES	NURSING INTERVENTIONS
*Deficient **F**luid Volume* related to blood loss	The client will maintain perfusion to placenta and vital organs.	Observe, report, and record blood loss (count and/or weigh pads). Monitor client's vital signs, FHR, I&O, and laboratory reports. Maintain comfortable environment to prevent diaphoresis. Inspect skin for pallor, cyanosis, clamminess, and coldness. Encourage client to maintain fluid intake.
*Impaired **G**as Exchange, Fetal* related to decreased maternal blood volume and hypotension	FHR will remain within normal limits.	Monitor FHR, baseline variability, and decelerations. Observe amniotic fluid for meconium. Instruct client in positions to promote placental perfusion. Administer IV fluids to mother to promote placental perfusion.

Evaluation: Evaluate each outcome to determine how it has been met by the client.

ABRUPTIO PLACENTA

The premature separation from the wall of the uterus of a normally implanted placenta is called **abruptio placenta**. It occurs spontaneously after the 20th week of gestation in approximately 1% of all pregnancies (Bougere, 1998; Deering, 2008). The cause is unknown. Contributing factors include maternal hypertension, multiple pregnancy, abdominal trauma, smoking, use of alcohol, or use of cocaine. Generally, it occurs late in pregnancy or during labor. There are three types of abruptio placenta (Figure 55-12).

- *Central*: Center of the placenta separates with blood trapped between placenta and uterine wall; there is no apparent bleeding
- *Marginal*: Edge of placenta separates and bright red bleeding is apparent vaginally

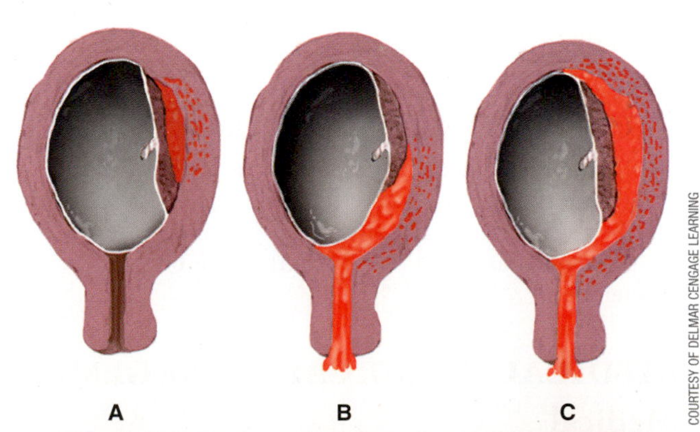

FIGURE 55-12 Abruptio Placenta; *A*, Central Abruption, Concealed Hemorrhage; *B*, Marginal Abruption, External Hemorrhage; *C*, Complete Abruption, External Hemorrhage (Could also Be Concealed)

TABLE 55-3 Comparison of Placenta Previa and Abruptio Placenta

CONDITION	BLEEDING	ABDOMEN	PAIN	BP
Placenta Previa	Bright red	No rigidity	None	Depends on amount of bleeding
Abruptio Placenta				
Central	None	Rigid	Acute	Decreased
Marginal	Dark red	No rigidity	Uterine tenderness	Decreased
Complete	Profuse or concealed	Rigid	Acute	Shock

COURTESY OF DELMAR CENGAGE LEARNING

- *Complete*: Entire placenta separates with profuse bleeding apparent vaginally or concealed

A central abruption may progress to a complete abruption. In central and complete, blood invades the uterine muscle (bruising called *Couvelaire uterus*), causing a rigid, painful abdomen. After delivery, the uterus contracts poorly and the client may require a hysterectomy to control the bleeding. The damage to the uterine muscle and the retroplacental clotting can cause a large release of thromboplastin. This can trigger the development of disseminated intravascular coagulation (DIC). Maternal mortality is relatively low. Problems after the delivery depend on the severity of the bleeding. Table 55-3 compares placenta previa and the various types of abruptio placenta.

Effects on the Fetus/Neonate

Perinatal mortality occurs in 0.12% (1:830) of pregnancies (Deering, 2008). The outcome depends on fetal maturity and severity of the abruption. Preterm labor, hypoxia, and anemia are the most serious complications. Irreversible brain damage or fetal death occurs if hypoxia is not reversed quickly.

Medical–Surgical Management

Medical

Intravenous fluids, generally lactated Ringer's solution, are given to prevent or reverse hypovolemia. Laboratory tests to evaluate client's status and the clotting mechanism are ordered: H & H, platelet count, fibrinogen level, fibrin split products, thrombin time, prothrombin time, partial thromboplastin time, and bleeding time. Also, a type and cross-match for three to four units of blood or packed cells is requested (Bougere, 1998). If the mother is Rh negative, she is checked for Rh sensitization. An indwelling urinary catheter is inserted.

If separation is small and the pregnancy near term, induction of labor and vaginal delivery may be possible. If labor is not progressing, a cesarean birth is performed. If separation is moderate or severe, a cesarean birth is performed as soon as possible.

Surgical

Cesarean delivery is performed in many cases to prevent fetal demise. A hysterectomy may be required to control hemorrhage.

Pharmacological

Rh immune globulin (RhoGAM) is given to the nonsensitized Rh-negative mother. Cryoprecipitate or plasma is given to treat hypofibrinogenemia. Analgesics are given as ordered.

Diet

No special diet or restrictions are required, although the client will be NPO if surgery is necessary.

Activity

The client will remain on bed rest until the situation is resolved.

Nursing Management

Monitor the client's bleeding, pain, vital signs, FHR, and fetal activity. Administer blood products or blood as ordered. Provide oxygen as ordered. If a cesarean delivery is to be performed, prepare the client for surgery. Maintain the client on bed rest. Accurately record I&O and insert indwelling urinary catheter as ordered. Have client lie on her side (left preferred) but not on her back.

NURSING PROCESS

Assessment

Subjective Data

The client may describe moderate to severe pain in the abdomen. Fetal movement may become hyperactive and then may cease.

Objective Data

Vaginal bleeding is assessed. External fetal monitor will show uteroplacental insufficiency, baseline changes, late decelerations, and reduced variability. The contraction pattern will change and the resting tone will increase. Vital signs show indications of shock.

Nursing diagnoses for a client with abruptio placenta include the following:

NURSING DIAGNOSES	PLANNING/OUTCOMES	NURSING INTERVENTIONS
*Impaired **G**as Exchange, Fetal* related to altered uteroplacenta oxygen transfer due to placental separation	The fetus will have a normal baseline FHR, variability with no decelerations.	Observe external fetal monitor for decelerations, decreased baseline variability, and FHR. Provide oxygen to mother via mask. Have mother lie on left side.
***A**nxiety* related to vaginal bleeding and possible fetal loss	The client will be able to verbalize feelings about bleeding and possible loss of pregnancy.	Explain pathophysiology of bleeding and status of fetus. Encourage client and family to talk about their feelings. Allow them some privacy to grieve. Contact minister, priest, or rabbi as requested by the client.
*Acute **P**ain* related to retroplacental bleeding and possibly contractions	The client will verbalize an understanding of the cause of the pain.	Provide simple explanation for cause of pain. Encourage and assist client to relax. Prepare for cesarean delivery.
*Deficient **F**luid Volume* related to blood loss	The client will regain fluid balance.	Monitor vital signs and assess for cold, clammy, cyanotic skin. Administer IV fluids as ordered and accurately record I&O. Evaluate client's state of consciousness.

Evaluation: Evaluate each outcome to determine how it has been met by the client.

DISSEMINATED INTRAVASCULAR COAGULATION

Disseminated intravascular coagulation (DIC) is an overstimulation of the normal clotting process. Rapid, massive fibrin formation causes small thrombi to form throughout the circulatory system, depleting the clotting factors and platelets. Generalized bleeding may then occur, leading to anemia or ischemia to vital organs because of the clots in the blood vessels.

DIC occurs as a complication of a primary problem. It is not only a complication of obstetrical situations, but also of many medical–surgical situations such as neoplasms, blood transfusion reaction, traumas, and infections. Men can also experience DIC. Obstetrical problems that may precipitate DIC include abruptio placenta, placenta previa, hydatidiform mole, gestational hypertension, retained products of conception, amniotic fluid embolism, and infections.

Effects on the Fetus/Neonate

The primary problem may require immediate delivery of the fetus, even if preterm. The fetus may experience hypoxia to varying degrees. Fetal death can occur.

Medical–Surgical Management

Medical

Symptom onset is sudden. The client may have spontaneous bleeding from the gums, nose, or any orifice. The client may experience dyspnea or chest pain and become very restless and cyanotic with frothy, blood-tinged mucus. A catheter is anchored to monitor urinary output and to observe for hematuria. The mother may have tachycardia and diaphoresis.

The underlying cause must be identified and corrected. If the fetus is not yet born, delivery should be facilitated. Diagnostic tests are hemoglobin, hematocrit, fibrinogen level, fibrin split, or degradation products, platelet count, prothrombin time, and partial thromboplastin time. The laboratory tests reveal a prolonged PT and PTT, a decreased platelet count and fibrinogen level, and fibrin split products are present. Administer intravenous fluids to replace fluid loss from bleeding and to maintain an output of 30 mL/hr.

Pharmacological

Intravenous administration of blood, fibrinogen, or cryoprecipitate is begun. Heparin given by continuous-infusion pump inhibits thrombin activity and thus prevents formation of microemboli. There is no effect on already existing clots. Oxygen therapy is often begun.

Nursing Management

Closely monitor all clients with an obstetrical problem that may precipitate DIC for sudden onset of dyspnea or chest pain, restlessness, cyanosis, and spitting frothy blood-tinged mucus. Maintain a calm, positive manner. Administer IV fluids, blood, or other substance to help restore normal clotting. Give heparin as ordered. Provide oxygen as ordered. Place the client in a semi-Fowlers side-lying position to increase blood flow to the uterus. Continuously monitor vital signs, lung sounds, and fetus (if not yet delivered) with an electronic fetal monitor. Monitor urinary output for an output of a least 30 mL/hr.

NURSING PROCESS

ASSESSMENT

Subjective Data

The client may describe dyspnea or chest pain.

Objective Data

The client may be extremely restless or cyanotic and be expectorating blood-tinged frothy mucus. Bleeding gums, epistaxis (nose bleed), hematuria, petechiae under the blood pressure cuff around the client's arm, or bleeding from injection sites may also be present.

Nursing diagnoses for a pregnant client with DIC include the following:

NURSING DIAGNOSES	PLANNING/OUTCOMES	NURSING INTERVENTIONS
Anxiety related to the sudden change in health status	The client will express understanding of what is happening to her and will feel less anxious.	Maintain a calm, positive manner. Explain to client what is happening, procedures, and treatment to be implemented. Remain with client. Allow client to express her anxiety. Answer client's questions.
Impaired Gas Exchange related to reduced oxygen-carrying capacity and ischemia of lung tissue	The client will maintain adequate gas exchange to prevent tissue death.	Administer O_2 by mask. Place the client in a semi-Fowlers side-lying position. Administer IV fluids, blood, or other substance to help restore a normal clotting mechanism. Administer heparin and provide oxygen as ordered. Monitor lung sounds and respiratory rate. If fetus not yet delivered, monitor continuously with electronic fetal monitor.

Evaluation: Evaluate each outcome to determine how it has been met by the client.

GESTATIONAL HYPERTENSION

Gestational hypertension, also known as pregnancy-induced hypertension, is the most common hypertensive disorder in pregnancy that appears after 20 weeks' gestation. The classic symptoms are hypertension, edema, and proteinuria. It is seen most often in primigravidas, especially those younger than 20 or older than 35 years of age, who are in the lower socioeconomic group and have poor nutritional status. Diabetes, multiple pregnancy, or a family history of gestational hypertension also increase a client's risk.

Peripheral arteriole vasoconstriction and vasospasm lead to increased blood pressure and decreased perfusion of the uterus and placenta. Blood vessels are constricted and there is less circulating blood volume. Renal blood flow is decreased as well as the glomerular filtration rate. Wide spread vasospasm may cause capillary damage and leakage. If this occurs in the kidneys, proteinuria results. Cerebral edema causes headaches and visual disturbances. Deep tendon reflexes become hyperactive. The liver enlarges, putting pressure on the liver capsule, which causes epigastric pain. The condition may progress to **eclampsia**, or convulsions.

Despite decades of research, the cause remains unknown. It was previously called *toxemia* because it was thought that a toxin was produced in a pregnant woman's body. This term is no longer used. The only cure is delivery of the baby. Gestational hypertension may progress from mild to severe **preeclampsia** to eclampsia.

EFFECTS ON THE FETUS/NEONATE

Abruptio placenta and placental infarction may occur. IUGR may occur as well as acute hypoxia and intrauterine death. A preterm infant may be born either because of spontaneous labor or obstetrical intervention.

CRITICAL THINKING

Noncompliance

How would you counsel a client with severe gestational hypertension who tells you that she just cannot stay in bed and gets up when no one is around?

Mild Preeclampsia

In mild preeclampsia, the blood pressure is 140/90 mm Hg *or* increases 30 mm Hg systolic *or* 15 mm Hg diastolic over the client's baseline blood pressure on two occasions at least 6 hours apart. For example, a client with a baseline BP of 92/64 would be considered hypertensive at 122/80. Thus it is very important to have a baseline BP early in pregnancy.

Edema (1+) may be noted in the face and hands. It is objectively defined as weight gain of more than 1 pound per week.

Proteinuria shows as 1+ (300 mg/L) or 2+ (1 g/L) albumin on a dipstick in 24 hours. Proteinuria is usually the last of the three classic symptoms to appear.

Severe Preeclampsia

Blood pressure increases to 160/110 mm hg or higher on two occasions 6 hours apart in severe preeclampsia. Generalized edema is easily noted in the face, hands, sacral area, lower extremities, and abdomen. Weight gain may be more than 2 pounds/week.

Urinary albumin is 3+ or 4+ on dipstick. Urine output may drop to less than 500 mL/24 hours. Hematocrit, uric acid, and serum creatinine levels are elevated. The client may exhibit other symptoms such as continuous headache, blurred vision, scotomata (spots before the eyes), nausea, vomiting, irritability, hyperreflexia, cerebral disturbances, pulmonary edema, dyspnea, cyanosis, and epigastric pain. Epigastric pain indicates the condition is worsening and is often the last symptom identified before the client moves into eclampsia.

Eclampsia

The grand mal seizure experienced by the client has a tonic phase (pronounced muscular contractions) and a clonic phase (alternate contraction and relaxation of muscles). Then the client slips into a coma lasting from minutes to hours. With no treatment, the seizure/coma sequence may be repeated one or more times and death may follow.

Seizure activity may trigger uterine contractions, but the client in a coma is unaware of them and unable to let anyone know.

CLIENT TEACHING

Home Management of Mild Preeclampsia

- Bed rest is essential.
- Lie on either side but not on the back.
- Reduce anxiety.
- Take medications as prescribed.
- Eat a high-protein, moderate-sodium diet.
- Keep all prenatal appointments (may be two per week).
- Report immediately headache, visual disturbances, edema of face or hands, severe nausea and vomiting, and epigastric pain.

HELLP Syndrome

HELLP syndrome is a complication of preeclampsia/eclampsia that includes liver damage. The syndrome occurs in 20% of women with gestational hypertension (Ruddy & Kearney, 2000). It is characterized by hemolysis, elevated liver enzymes, and low platelet count (See Memory Trick: HELLP).

HELLP syndrome is a multisystem condition with widespread coagulation abnormalities characterized by weak vessel tone, vasospasm, and a coagulation defect. The exact pathophysiology of HELLP syndrome is unknown, but there seems to be an underlying activation of the coagulation cascade/mechanism (clot formation process). HELLP is a complication of gestational hypertension, but there is no common factor that causes HELLP except for the final group of symptoms that causes endothelial damage in small vessels and platelet activation within the vessels. RBCs are damaged and break as they pass through the damaged endothelium. With the activation of the platelets in the clotting mechanism, thromboxane A and serotonin are released, leading to vasospasm and platelet agglutination (clumping). Vasospasms, triggered from the clotting mechanism, force RBCs through the fibrin mesh formed by the clotting mechanism potentially causing the destruction of the RBCs (hemolysis). The RBC lyses produces a large drop in hematocrit (Padden, 1999).

Hemorrhaging occurs in the liver and the clotting mechanism stimulates the formation of microemboli in the vessels of the liver, causing ischemia. The damaged liver tissue causes the elevated liver enzymes (AST and ALT). Thrombocytopenia (low platelet count) of less than 100,000/mm^3 results as the platelets are depleted attempting to control the hemorrhaging or by being trapped in the fibrin mesh (Padden, 1999).

Weak vessel tone leads to capillary leakage causing edema and pulmonary edema (Sibai & Stella, 2009).

The client presents with malaise, epigastric pain, nausea and vomiting, and headache usually in the third trimester. They also may have right upper quadrant tenderness, edema, hypertension, and proteinuria. With these last 4 symptoms, a

MEMORY TRICK

HELLP is characterized by **h**emolysis, **e**levated **l**iver enzymes, and **l**ow **p**latelet count:

H = Hemolysis – caused when intra-arterial lesions develop as a result of vasopasm, causing platelets to aggregate and a fibrin network to form. The RBCs are forced through the fibrin network and lysed, resulting in a large drop in hematocrit.

E = Elevated.

L = Liver enzymes – may be caused by microemboli in the vessels of the liver, causing ischemia.

L = Low.

P = Platelet count – results when the platelets are entrapped at the intra-arterial lesions.

complete blood count and liver functions are done to confirm the diagnosis of HELLP syndrome.

A low platelet count and a positive D-dimer test are the most reliable indicators to diagnose HELLP syndrome. If the platelet count drops below 40,000 per mm3, the client is prone to hemorrhaging. If the client has severe right upper quadrant pain, neck pain, or shoulder pain, the health care provider orders a liver scan to assess for a liver hematoma or liver rupture.

The main treatment is seizure prophylaxis, blood pressure control in clients with hypertension, and prompt delivery of the fetus. The administration of corticosteroids (dexamethasone [Decadron]) is controversial. Magnesium sulfate is given intravenously to prevent seizures and is titrated according to urine output and magnesium blood level. If magnesium toxicity occurs, calcium gluconate is given intravenously. A hypertensive crisis is treated with nitroprusside (Nipride). HELLP laboratory tests worsen after delivery but begin to return to normal by the third to fourth day postpartum.

Medical–Surgical Management

Medical

The goals of treatment are to lower blood pressure, prevent convulsions, and deliver a healthy baby.

A client with mild preeclampsia may be allowed to stay home but is advised to stay in bed, lying on either side. This increases renal and placental blood flow. The client generally feels well, so education is very important to improve compliance with the plan of care.

Laboratory tests may include hematocrit, platelet count, electrolytes, liver function (AST and ALT), estriol level, 24-hour urine for protein and creatinine, and serum creatinine.

Surgical

If the mother's condition continues to deteriorate or the environment within the uterus becomes harmful to fetal well-being, a cesarean birth may be necessary.

Pharmacological

Magnesium sulfate ($MgSO_4$) is a central nervous system depressant that decreases the possibility of convulsions. It also relaxes smooth muscles and may decrease blood pressure to some degree. $MgSO_4$ is given intravenously. It is excreted by the kidneys and may reach a toxic level if the client has impaired renal function. Magnesium sulfate toxicity may lead to cardiac arrest. Common side effects are flushing, sweating, hypotension, bradycardia, respiratory depression, hypothermia, muscle weakness, constipation, nausea, and vomiting. An indwelling catheter is generally inserted to accurately measure output.

Calcium gluconate, the antidote for $MgSO_4$ must be kept in a syringe at the bedside ready to be given if signs of magnesium toxicity are noted. $MgSO_4$ is usually given for 24 to 48 hours after delivery to ensure that convulsions do not occur.

An antihypertensive drug may be given. Hydralazine (Apresoline) is the drug of choice except for clients with cardiac dysfunctions, who are given labetalol hydrochloride (Normodyne, Trandate).

A sedative such as phenobarbital or diazepam (Valium) may be given to help the client rest quietly.

PROFESSIONALTIP

Magnesium Sulfate Administration

- Respirations must be at least 14 per minute.
- Deep tendon reflexes must be kept at normal response. The deep tendon reflex is obtained by giving a brisk tap with the blunt end of a reflex hammer to the patellar tendon just below the patella. The reflex response is a contraction of the quadriceps muscle and an extension of the lower leg. The reflex is graded as 0 - no response, 1+ - sluggish, 2+ - normal, 3+ - brisk, or 4+ - hyperreflexic.
- Urine output must be at least 30 mL/hr.
- Serum magnesium level must be monitored (therapeutic level 4.0 to 8.0 mEq/dL).

Oxytocin may be given to induce labor. It may be given along with magnesium sulfate.

Diet

A well-balanced, high-protein, moderate-sodium diet is provided. Excessively salty foods are not eaten, but sodium restriction is no longer recommended. If the client is nauseated or there are signs of impending convulsions, the diet is withheld.

Activity

The client is on bed rest, lying preferably on the left side but not on the back.

Nursing Management

Frequently monitor vital signs and FHT. Assess for edema (hands and face), proteinuria, headache, blurred vision, irritability, hyperreflexia (deep tendon reflexes), dyspnea, cyanosis, nausea, and epigastric pain. Involve client and family in decisions when possible. Assist client and family to identify sources of support. Encourage the client to express feelings about her situation. Assess for toxicity when magnesium sulfate is administered. Keep environmental stimuli at a minimum.

NURSING PROCESS

Assessment

Subjective Data

Ask the client about headache, visual disturbances, epigastric pain, swelling of hands and face, nausea, and dyspnea.

Objective Data

Check vital signs and weight and compare to previous figures, and check urine for protein. Edema may be found in the face, hands, sacral area, lower extremities, or abdomen. Check laboratory reports of electrolytes, platelet count, liver enzymes, and hematocrit. Monitor I&O.

Nursing diagnoses for a client with gestational hypertension include the following:

NURSING DIAGNOSES	PLANNING/OUTCOMES	NURSING INTERVENTIONS
*Interrupted **F**amily Processes* related to illness and bed rest or hospitalization of mother	The family will work together to maintain family functioning.	Involve client and family in decisions when possible. Encourage client and family to verbalize feelings about situation. Encourage family to visit client as client's condition allows. Assist family in discussions regarding how they will manage the household while the client is hospitalized or on bed rest at home. Help client and family identify sources of support. Refer to social service or local community resources as necessary.
*Deficient **K**nowledge* related to lack of information about gestational hypertension, its treatment, and implications for mother and baby	The client will verbalize an understanding of gestational hypertension, its treatment, and implications for herself and her baby.	Teach symptoms of gestational hypertension, importance of following care guidelines, and what to report to the health care provider. Explain the purpose and importance of each aspect of the plan of care. Encourage client to express feelings about her situation.
*Deficient **F**luid Volume* related to shift in fluids from intravascular to interstitial	The client will maintain intravascular fluid volume.	Assess BP and FHT every 1 to 4 hours. Weigh daily. Maintain client on bed rest, lying on side, especially the left side. Assess for edema. Accurately record I&O. Test urine for protein as ordered. Monitor laboratory test results.

Evaluation: Evaluate each outcome to determine how it has been met by the client.

CHRONIC MEDICAL PROBLEMS

Conditions in this section include diabetes mellitus, chronic hypertension, heart disease, and maternal phenylketonuria.

DIABETES MELLITUS

Diabetic clients who wish to become pregnant should have their diabetes well under control before conception. Gestational diabetes mellitus (GDM) is an abnormal glucose metabolism that appears only during pregnancy. Many women with GDM will have diabetes later in life. Whether the mother has chronic diabetes or GDM, the effects during pregnancy are the same.

Pregnancy and Carbohydrate Metabolism

Insulin production is increased in early pregnancy because of the stimulation of the mother's pancreas by the increased levels of estrogen, progesterone, and other hormones. The tissue response to insulin is also increased along with increased storage of glycogen in the liver and muscles. An increased resistance to insulin develops in the last half of pregnancy because of hPL (an insulin antagonist), prolactin, and elevated levels of cortisol and placental enzymes called insulinases, which destroy insulin. This diabetogenic effect of pregnancy occurs after about 20 weeks' gestation. The result is a catabolic state after a meal is absorbed and also during the night. Fat, at this time, is more readily metabolized, and ketones may be found in the mother's urine. Glucose from the mother provides the growing fetus with energy, thus putting stress on the balance of glucose production and utilization. Diabetes already present is more difficult to control. In cases in which the pancreas has little insulin reserve, gestational diabetes occurs.

Effects of Pregnancy on Diabetes

The insulin requirements change throughout pregnancy. The need for insulin may decrease during the first trimester. The risk of hypoglycemia or hyperinsulinemia is increased if nausea and vomiting are present. Placental maturation and the increasing production of hPL cause the insulin requirements to rise during the second trimester, and they may even be four times higher by the end of pregnancy. After the placenta is passed, removing the source of hPL, there is generally an immediate decrease in the amount of insulin required.

There is a physiological decrease in the renal threshold for glucose. The risk of ketoacidosis is greater during pregnancy, as is an acceleration of vascular disease.

Effects of Diabetes on Pregnancy

Pregnancy in a diabetic client has a higher risk of complications than for a nondiabetic client. If vascular changes already exist, the chance for gestational hypertension is greater.

Hydramnios, an excessive amount of amniotic fluid, may occur. This may lead to preterm labor or premature rupture of the membranes.

Hyperglycemia can result in ketoacidosis caused by increased fat metabolism. Often, ketoacidosis develops slowly, but it can result in maternal and fetal death if untreated. Maternal complications are directly related to the degree of blood glucose control.

Effects on the Fetus/Neonate

Macrosomia, excessive fetal growth, results from maternal hyperglycemia. The hyperglycemia stimulates fetal insulin production to utilize the available glucose. After birth, there is no more maternal glucose, but the fetal pancreas continues to produce a high level of insulin. In 2 to 4 hours, the neonate is hypoglycemic. Fetal insulin production gradually decreases to an appropriate level.

IUGR may result when the mother has vascular changes, which also occur in the placenta. This decreases perfusion of the placenta, and the fetus does not receive adequate amounts of nutrients.

A high fetal insulin level inhibits the production of surfactant in the lungs, making the possibility of respiratory distress syndrome very high. The decreased ability of maternal glycosylated hemoglobin (hemoglobin with glucose attached) to release oxygen causes the fetus to have polycythemia (excessive number of red blood cells). Polycythemia is a direct cause of hyperbilirubinemia in the infant because the immature liver is unable to metabolize the increased amount of bilirubin.

Congenital anomalies are several times higher in diabetic pregnancies and may be caused by hyperglycemia in early pregnancy. Many anomalies involve the heart, central nervous system, and skeletal system.

Medical–Surgical Management

Medical

The goals of care are to maintain **euglycemia** (normal blood glucose level) between 70 mg/dL and 105 mg/dL, and to have a healthy mother and baby. The client is usually followed by both her endocrinologist and obstetrician.

Clients are taught to monitor their blood glucose level and give themselves insulin according to a sliding scale. For clients with GDM, this may be very difficult because diabetes is new to them.

Fetal status is evaluated throughout the pregnancy. AFP screening is performed because diabetic pregnancies have an increased risk of fetal neural tube defects. Gestational age is established by ultrasound at about 18 weeks' gestation and repeated every 4 to 6 weeks to monitor fetal growth and assess for congenital abnormalities. The mother monitors fetal activity daily beginning about 28 weeks' gestation. An NST is scheduled weekly beginning also at about 28 weeks. A BPP may be performed at about 32 weeks and may be scheduled weekly. According to research, insulin lispo (Humalog) does not cross the placenta at low dose concentrations (Holcberg, Tsadkin-Tamir, Sapir, Wiznizer, Segal, Polacheck, & Ben Zvi, 2004). The American Diabetes Association (2009) also states insulin does not cross the placenta to the fetus (ADA, 2009).

Many clients with diabetes are hospitalized several times during the pregnancy. The timing of birth is based mainly on fetal well-being but should never be past 40 weeks' gestation. The L/S ratio and presence of PG in the amniotic fluid is usually checked about 38 weeks or earlier if indicated by fetal status.

Surgical

If fetal well-being is deteriorating, a cesarean birth is often performed.

Pharmacological

To monitor fetal well-being, humalin is generally used because it is unlikely to cause an allergic reaction. Insulin is given, most commonly, by multiple injections. This may be scheduled twice a day or four to six times per day after a blood glucose check. Some oral hypoglycemics should be discontinued, with the physician's knowledge, when the client plans to become pregnant, or immediately when she becomes pregnant, to prevent teratogenic effects on the fetus. Glyburide (Diabeta, Micronase) is an oral hypoglycemic that is often administered safely during pregnancy.

Diet

Pregnant women increase their caloric intake about 300 kcal/day (35 to 40 kcal/Kg/day of ideal weight is recommended). Total kilocalories for the day are divided among three meals and three snacks. The bedtime snack, eaten as late as possible, has complex carbohydrates and protein to prevent hypoglycemia during the night. There should be no more than 10 hours between the bedtime snack and breakfast. A dietician assists the pregnant diabetic client with meal plans based on food preferences, lifestyle, and culture.

Activity

Activity is maintained throughout pregnancy unless contraindicated by complications. Activity level is taken into account when the diet and insulin are prescribed.

Nursing Management

Listen actively to the client. Answer questions and provide support. Teach glucose monitoring and insulin self-injection as needed. Monitor fetal status through results of AFP screening, ultrasound, NST, BPP, and amniocentesis. Emphasize the importance of keeping all scheduled prenatal visits and testing appointments.

NURSING PROCESS

ASSESSMENT

Subjective Data

Ask questions regarding a family history of diabetes, congenital abnormalities, neonatal deaths, or unexplained stillbirths. At each prenatal visit, ask about diet, activity, and medication compliance. After 28 weeks, record maternal evaluation of fetal activity.

Objective Data

Check blood sugar per fingerstick as ordered, and also measure vital signs and weight. Evaluate NST results and results of laboratory tests. Note signs of infection.

Nursing diagnoses for a client with diabetes during pregnancy include the following:

NURSING DIAGNOSES	PLANNING/OUTCOMES	NURSING INTERVENTIONS
*Deficient **K**nowledge* related to disease process of diabetes, control of diabetes, and implications for pregnancy	The client will verbalize an understanding of the disease process of diabetes, control of diabetes, and implications for the pregnancy.	Present to or review with the client the pathophysiology of diabetes and clarify client misconceptions. Teach how to monitor blood glucose level, the desired range, and importance of good control. Teach self-administration of insulin (if applicable) to client and significant other. Review effects of diabetes on client and fetus. Teach danger signs and whom to notify. Refer to diabetic support group in the community. Refer to dietitian for diet instructions.
*Risk for **I**njury, Fetus* related to decreased uteroplacental functioning	The client will verbalize an understanding of the various antepartal tests and what to expect during the procedures.	Teach client the possible effects of inadequate glucose control and uteroplacental functioning. Explain purpose of periodic ultrasound, fetal activity record, weekly NST, amniocentesis for L/S ratio and PG level, and biophysical profile.
***N**oncompliance* related to need for close monitoring and extra prenatal visits	The client will perform blood glucose testing on schedule and attend all scheduled prenatal visits.	Review the importance of maintaining euglycemia. Assist client in making a chart on which to record results of blood glucose testing. Review importance of attending all scheduled prenatal visits. Schedule prenatal visits when most convenient for the client.

Evaluation: Evaluate each outcome to determine how it has been met by the client.

CHRONIC HYPERTENSION

Chronic hypertension is a BP of 140/90 mm Hg or higher before pregnancy or before the 20th week of gestation that lasts longer than 6 weeks after delivery. A diastolic pressure of more than 80 mm Hg in the second trimester may indicate chronic hypertension.

A client with untreated or poorly controlled hypertension may show signs of hypertensive vascular disease such as arteriosclerosis and retinal hemorrhage. Renal, disease may be present. The placenta may have infarcts, and placenta abruptio may occur.

EFFECTS ON THE FETUS/NEONATE

A placenta with infarcts has reduced perfusion. This may cause IUGR and fetal hypoxia.

GESTATIONAL HYPERTENSION SUPERIMPOSED ON CHRONIC HYPERTENSION

Clients who have moderate-to-severe chronic hypertension are most at risk to develop gestational hypertension. In these women, gestational hypertension develops rapidly and moves to a crisis state faster than in women without chronic hypertension. More stillbirths, abruptio placenta, and severe renal failure are found in clients with chronic hypertension. These clients are hospitalized for medical management and nursing care.

MEDICAL–SURGICAL MANAGEMENT

Medical

The goals of care are to prevent development of preeclampsia and to ensure a healthy fetus. Prenatal visits are generally scheduled every 2 weeks. An ultrasound is performed early to establish, or verify, the EDB. Around 22 and 32 weeks' gestation, an ultrasound checks for IUGR. If renal disease is suspected, creatinine clearance is determined early and repeated every 2 months.

Pharmacological

Antihypertensive medication, such as methyldopa (Aldomet), nifedipine (Procardia), or labetalol (Trandate) is continued throughout the pregnancy. Dosage is adjusted according to maternal needs.

Diet

A well-balanced diet providing 1.5 g/kg/day of protein is recommended. Salt intake should remain as it was before pregnancy.

Activity

Daily rest periods, with the client preferably lying on her left side (never on the back), are important to maintain adequate perfusion to the placenta and relieve dependent edema.

Nursing Management

Provide information about hypertension and how it may affect a pregnancy. Answer client's questions. Encourage client to plan rest periods (lying on the side) throughout the day. Emphasize the importance of keeping all scheduled prenatal visits and testing appointments.

NURSING PROCESS

Assessment

Subjective Data

Most clients have no symptoms of hypertension until it becomes severe. Then headaches or visual disturbances may occur.

Objective Data

Blood pressure will be 140/90 mm Hg or higher.

Nursing diagnoses for a pregnant client with chronic hypertension include the following:

NURSING DIAGNOSES	PLANNING/OUTCOMES	NURSING INTERVENTIONS
*Risk for **I**njury, Fetus* related to placental infarcts and poor placental perfusion	The client will verbalize an understanding of possible placental changes leading to fetal injury and interventions to prevent this.	Teach client the possible placental changes related to hypertension. Assist client to plan for rest periods throughout the day. Administer antihypertensive medications as ordered.
*Deficient **K**nowledge* related to disease process and effects on pregnancy	The client will verbalize an understanding of the disease process and effects on pregnancy.	Provide the client with information about the disease process and how pregnancy may be affected. Allow opportunity for client to ask questions.

Evaluation: Evaluate each outcome to determine how it has been met by the client.

HEART DISEASE

The normal physiological increase in blood volume that peaks about 28 to 32 weeks' gestation, and the increased cardiac output and heart rate, may cause problems in the client with heart disease. The heart compensates at first by tachycardia, and ventricular dilation and hypertrophy. When these mechanisms fail, the heart is no longer able to compensate and congestive heart failure occurs.

The results of having had rheumatic fever often restrict cardiac output and cause pulmonary congestion. The effects of congenital heart disease on pregnancy depend on the specific defect. Hypertension may cause cardiac insufficiency.

Effects on the Fetus/Neonate

IUGR and hypoxia may occur.

Medical–Surgical Management

Medical

Many clients are cared for by both their cardiologist and obstetrician. Early diagnosis and ongoing management is assessed by the use of chest x-rays, auscultation of heart sounds, EKG, echocardiogram, and sometimes cardiac catheterization. Prenatal care appointments may be increased to two or three per week between 28 and 32 weeks' gestation, when blood volume is highest. Sometimes hospitalization is necessary.

Pharmacological

Antibiotics are often used as a prophylaxis for all pregnant women with heart disease. Enoxaparin sodium (Lovenex) may be used if coagulation problems develop because enoxaparin sodium does not cross the placenta. Thiazide diuretics and furosemide (Lasix) may be used for congestive heart failure.

Diet

The diet should be high in iron and protein but low in sodium. Adequate kilocalories for normal weight gain should be provided.

Activity

Physical activity is restricted depending on the client's symptoms. Eight to 10 hours of sleep and frequent rest periods throughout the day are important. The side-lying position is best to prevent compression of the inferior vena cava.

Nursing Management

Monitor vital signs, lung and heart sounds, and FHT. Emphasize the importance of keeping all scheduled prenatal visits and testing appointments. Encourage the client to eat a diet high in iron and protein, but low in sodium. Stress importance of side lying during daytime rest periods and during the night. Assist client to identify a support system to help with household chores.

NURSING PROCESS

Assessment

Subjective Data

Ask about activity level, amount of rest, increasing fatigue with activity, dyspnea, palpitations, cough, and anxiety. Inquire about the availability of household help and her support system, to ascertain the client's ability to rest and relax.

Objective Data

These data include weight gain (fluid retention), edema, vital signs, signs of infection, anemia, heart murmurs, or crackles in the lungs.

Nursing diagnoses for a pregnant client with heart disease include the following:

NURSING DIAGNOSES	PLANNING/OUTCOMES	NURSING INTERVENTIONS
Impaired Gas Exchange related to pulmonary edema	The client will maintain adequate gas exchange.	Monitor and accurately record I&O. Assess vital signs frequently. Administer medications as ordered.
Activity Intolerance related to generalized decreased perfusion	The client will be able to tolerate some activity.	Assess activity tolerance frequently. Promote activity level established by the physician. Discuss activity limitations and the need for sleep and rest periods.
Fear related to effects of maternal cardiac condition on fetal well-being	The client will express her fears about fetal well-being.	Provide information on how fetal well-being may be affected by maternal cardiac condition. Listen to the client express her fears about fetal well-being.

Evaluation: Evaluate each outcome to determine how it has been met by the client.

MATERNAL PHENYLKETONURIA

Phenylketonuria (PKU) is an inborn error of metabolism in which there is a deficiency of the enzyme necessary to metabolize the amino acid phenylalanine. It is genetically inherited by a recessive gene. Accumulation of this amino acid and its metabolites leads to irreversible brain damage.

Since 1967, all newborns in the United States have had a screening blood test for PKU. The infants diagnosed with PKU were put on a phenylalanine-free diet. For years, it was thought that the child treated with a phenylalanine-free diet outgrew the problem by about age 9. Research has shown that dietary therapy throughout childhood and adolescence preserves intelligence. Some researchers recommend lifelong dietary therapy (Saal, Braddock, Bull, Enns, Gruen, Mendelsohn, & Saul, 2008). According to research, the best outcomes of pregnancy occur when the woman with PKU maintains a phenylalanine level between 2 and 6 mg/dL before conception, or at least by 8 weeks of gestation, and continuing throughout pregnancy (Koch, Azen, Friedman, et al, 2003).

Effects on the Fetus/Neonate

A poorly regulated maternal phenylalanine level causes an increase in the incidence of IUGR, mental retardation, microcephaly, and heart defects.

Medical–Surgical Management

Medical

The mother's blood phenylalanine level is checked every 2 to 4 weeks during the first half of pregnancy. It is checked every week in the last half of pregnancy.

Research indicates that the restricted intake of protein in the phenylalanine-free diet results in lower blood levels of iron and zinc (Acosta, 1996). Therefore, the iron and zinc blood levels are also checked every week in the last half of pregnancy. Low levels of iron may lead to anemia.

Diet

A very expensive modified protein supplement is used before and during pregnancy. Fruits, vegetables, fats, and some low-protein cereals make up the rest of the diet.

Nursing Management

Encourage client to maintain a phenylalanine-free diet and to have her blood level checked throughout the pregnancy. Refer the client to dietary and genetic counseling.

INFECTIONS

Any infection is a risk factor during pregnancy and should be diagnosed and treated promptly. Untreated infections may cause abortion, congenital anomalies, fetal infections, IUGR, preterm labor, mental retardation, or death.

TORCH GROUP

The TORCH group of congenital (passed from the mother to her fetus) infections include toxoplasmosis, rubella, cytomegalovirus, and herpesvirus type 2. The TORCH panel is a laboratory test used to screen for infections in the TORCH group (AACC, 2009).

TOXOPLASMOSIS

Toxoplasmosis is caused by the protozoan *Toxoplasma gondii*. This disease goes almost unnoticed by adults because the symptoms are mild, vague, and flu-like. The organism may be ingested by eating undercooked, raw, or cured meat or by contact with contaminated soil or cat litter (Hokelek, 2009). Maternal toxoplasmosis before pregnancy seems to offer protection against fetal infection.

Effects on the Fetus/Neonate

There is an increased incidence of abortion, preterm birth, stillbirth, and neonatal death if the mother contracts toxoplasmosis when she is pregnant. The time, within the pregnancy that a mother has the primary infection, determines the severity of symptoms in the fetus (Rorman, Zamir, Rilkis, Ben-David, 2006). Damage to the fetus is generally more severe if the disease is acquired before 20 weeks' gestation. The neonate may have microcephaly, hydrocephaly, and convulsions. Many infants die soon after birth. Those who survive may be blind, deaf, or severely retarded.

Medical–Surgical Management

Medical

The goals are to identify the pregnant client at risk and treat the disease promptly when diagnosed. The incubation period is 10 days. Tests that confirm the diagnosis of congenital toxoplasmosis is T cell proliferation and CD25 expression (Ciardelli, Meroni, Avanzini, Bollani, Tinelli, Garofoli, Gasparoni, & Stronati, 2008).

Pharmacological

The client is treated with sulfadiazine (Microsulfon) or pyrimethamine (Daraprim). Spiramycin (Rovamycine) may also be used to treat toxoplasmosis (Hokelek, 2009).

Diet

No raw or partially cooked meats are eaten. Fruits and vegetables are washed before they are eaten.

Activity

Gloves are worn when gardening because contact with soil is a significant risk factor. Travel outside the United States, Canada, and Europe is also a significant risk factor (Hokelek, 2009).

Nursing Management

Encourage the client to eat only well-done meats, to wash all fruits and vegetables before eating them, and to wear gloves when gardening.

CRITICAL THINKING

Toxoplasmosis

In Figure 55-13, the, pregnant woman is keeping the cat indoors and feeding it "canned" food. If the cat were an outside cat eating birds and rodents, it could acquire the parasite, *Toxoplasmia gondii*. The pregnant woman would be placing herself at risk for Toxoplasmosis and potentially causing harm to her unborn child. The cat is also kept off of any countertops where food is prepared. What other precautions should she take in caring for her cat?

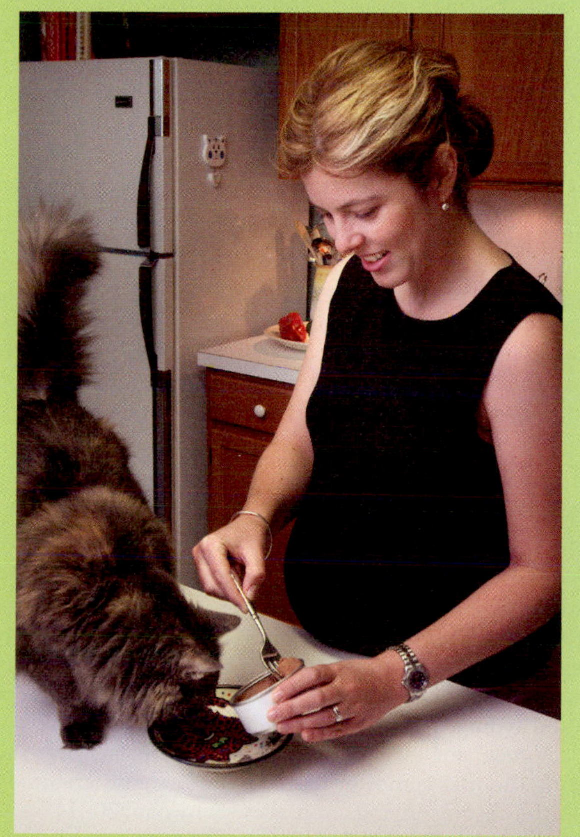

Figure 55-13 Preventing Toxoplasmosis (*Courtesy of the CDC/Photo by James Gathany.*)

NURSING PROCESS

Assessment

Subjective Data

The client may have no symptoms or may have malaise and/or myalgia.

Objective Data

A rash may be evident as well as splenomegaly and enlarged cervical lymph nodes.

Nursing diagnoses for a pregnant client with toxoplasmosis include the following:

NURSING DIAGNOSES	PLANNING/OUTCOMES	NURSING INTERVENTIONS
*Deficient **K**nowledge* related to lack of knowledge about toxoplasmosis disease process	The client will verbalize an understanding of toxoplasmosis disease process.	Provide information about toxoplasmosis, incubation period, how acquired, and ways to prevent it. Allow time for client to ask questions and clarify misconceptions.
*Anticipatory **G**rieving* related to effects of toxoplasmosis on fetus/ neonate	The client will express feelings about possible effects on fetus/ neonate.	Encourage client to discuss feelings about possible effects of toxoplasmosis on her fetus. Provide a private place for client and family to discuss the situation.

Evaluation: Evaluate each outcome to determine how it has been met by the client.

RUBELLA

Rubella, German measles, and 3-day measles are all names for the same disease. After an incubation period of 14 to 21 days, a maculopapular rash appears and then vanishes in 3 days. Rubella is highly contagious and is spread by airborne droplets.

Effects on the Fetus/Neonate

The earlier in pregnancy the infection occurs, the more severe the fetal effects. Congenital rubella syndrome occurs in many of the infections that occur before 8 weeks' gestation. It is characterized by cataracts, deafness, and patent ductus arteriosus. The infant may also have IUGR, mental retardation, and hyperbilirubinemia. Sometimes a petechial rash may be seen. These infants are infectious and may shed the virus for months.

Medical–Surgical Management

Medical

Prevention is the best cure. The prenatal laboratory screening includes the hemagglutination inhibition. A titer of 1:16 or greater signifies immunity, while a titer of less than 1:8 signifies a susceptibility to rubella. The client who is susceptible should avoid exposure to rubella while pregnant.

A pregnant woman who becomes infected with rubella during the first trimester has a 90% chance of fetal infection with the accompanying anomalies (Schweon, 2001).

Pharmacological

All children should be immunized with the live attenuated vaccine by age 1. Susceptible pregnant women should be immunized very soon after delivery, and they should avoid becoming pregnant at least for 1 month after immunization to avoid the chance of infecting a fetus.

Nursing Management

Identify clients who are susceptible to rubella and provide information about avoiding exposure while pregnant. Encourage susceptible clients to receive the immunization very soon after delivery and then delay another pregnancy at least for 1 month. Encourage parents to have infants receive all immunizations as scheduled.

RhoGAM may prevent the effectiveness of the measles, mumps, and Rubella vaccine (MMR) if the two medications are administered at the same time. Therefore, the client returns to the health care providers' office in 2 months for a blood test to check for immunity against rubella. The MMR vaccine administration is repeated if the client has no immunity to rubella (Hamilton Health Sciences, 2008).

NURSING PROCESS

Assessment

Subjective Data

There may be no symptoms or the client may describe muscle aches and joint pain.

Objective Data

Temperature may be slightly elevated, and a maculopapular rash and lymphadenopathy may be present.

Nursing diagnoses for a pregnant client with rubella include the following:

NURSING DIAGNOSES	PLANNING/OUTCOMES	NURSING INTERVENTIONS
*Ineffective **H**ealth Maintenance* related to lack of knowledge about her need for rubella immunization before becoming pregnant	The client will receive rubella vaccine soon after delivery.	Provide information about the implications of rubella when the hemagglutination inhibition results are known. Provide information about rubella immunization. Answer client questions and clarify any misunderstandings.
*Interrupted **F**amily Processes* related to the probability of fetal anomalies caused by maternal rubella	The client and family will verbalize understanding of the probability of fetal anomalies.	Discuss with client and family the probability and types of fetal anomalies that generally occur with maternal rubella. Provide a private place for client and family to discuss the situation. Answer questions and clarify misconceptions.

Evaluation: Evaluate each outcome to determine how it has been met by the client.

CYTOMEGALOVIRUS

Cytomegalovirus (CMV) is a member of the herpesvirus group. More than half of all adults have antibodies for CMV, which is found in saliva, breast milk, cervical mucus, urine, and semen. It spreads by close contact. It is asymptomatic in adults and children but can affect the fetus in utero or during delivery.

Effects on the Fetus/Neonate

The fetus may have extensive damage leading to fetal death; however, the fetus may survive with hydrocephaly, microcephaly, mental retardation, cerebral palsy, or with no noticeable damage. An infected newborn is usually small for gestational age (SGA). Mental retardation, auditory deficits, or learning disabilities may not be immediately apparent.

Medical–Surgical Management

Medical

Diagnosis is made when CMV is found in the maternal urine and an elevated IgM level with CMV antibodies identified in the blood. There is no treatment for the mother or neonate.

HERPES GENITALIS (HERPES SIMPLEX VIRUS TYPE 2)

Genital herpes is one of the three most common sexually transmitted infections with approximately 22% of pregnant women having HSV-2 (Perozzi, Zalice, Howard, Skariot, 2007). Herpes simplex virus type 2 (HSV-2) causes painful, vesicular genital lesions. The lesions appear within a few hours to 20 days after exposure. The primary episode is the most severe. Women who have their first infection close to the time of delivery have a greater chance of transmitting the infection to the neonate during a vaginal birth. After the membranes rupture, the virus ascends from active lesions to the fetus, or the fetus comes in contact with the lesions during a vaginal delivery. HSV-2 is not found in breast milk, so the mother may breast-feed.

Effects on the Fetus/Neonate

When there is an active HSV-2 infection in the first trimester, about one-half will end in spontaneous abortion or stillbirth. Most infected infants have no symptoms at birth. Symptoms of poor feeding, jaundice, and seizures develop after a 2- to 12-day incubation period. Many of these infants will also have the vesicular lesions.

Medical–Surgical Management

Medical

Diagnosis is made by culturing active lesions. Treatment is mainly to relieve pain. When no lesions are visible at the time of delivery, a vaginal birth is acceptable. Pregnancy is one of many causes of recurrence. There is no known cure.

Surgical

When active lesions are visible at the time of delivery, a cesarean birth is best to prevent fetal contact with the lesions (virus).

Pharmacological

Antiviral therapy for HSV-2 is acyclovir (Zovirax), famciclovir (Famvir), and valacyclovir hydrochloride (Valtrex). The use of acyclovir has been studied in pregnant women and does not increase birth defects or harm the neonate (Brown, Gardella, Wald, Morrow, & Corey, 2005). The use of acyclovir in the third trimester has decreased symptoms and viral shedding, thus decreasing the need for cesarean births (Watts, Brown, Money, Selke, Huang, Sacks, et al., 2003). Burow's solution may relieve discomfort.

Nursing Management

Inquire whether client has ever had a herpes infection. Provide information regarding possible effect on the fetus/neonate, preventing spread of infection, and how to care for active lesions.

NURSING PROCESS

Assessment

Subjective Data

Ask whether the client or her partner have ever had a herpes infection. Client may describe pain and discomfort from the lesions if she has a herpes infection.

Objective Data

Lesions may be seen when infection is active. A cervical culture may indicate presence or absence of the virus.

Nursing diagnoses for the pregnant client with HSV-2 infection include the following:

NURSING DIAGNOSES	PLANNING/OUTCOMES	NURSING INTERVENTIONS
*Acute **P**ain* related to local, open vulvar lesions	The client will describe a decrease in pain after treatment is begun.	Administer medications as ordered. Suggest a sitz bath several times a day followed by air-drying of the vulva and wearing cotton underwear.
*Ineffective **S**exuality Patterns* related to unwillingness to engage in sexual intercourse	The client will maintain sexuality patterns.	Provide client with information about disease process, and the method of transmission. Refer client to community resources. Encourage client to engage in forms of sexual expression that do not involve genital contact.
*Ineffective **C**oping* related to depression about risk to fetus if herpes lesions are present at birth	The client will verbalize an understanding about how decision is made regarding the type of delivery when herpes lesions are present.	Provide client with information about the factors relative to type of delivery performed. Encourage client to have appropriate cultures run as recommended by her health care provider. Encourage client to report any changes that may indicate a recurrence of lesions.

Evaluation: Evaluate each outcome to determine how it has been met by the client.

HIV/AIDS

Weight gain or even maintenance of weight during pregnancy is a challenge for an HIV-infected client. Counseling is provided regarding optimum nutrition, exercise, rest, and sleep.

Pregnancy is considered to be a somewhat immunosuppressive state and may theoretically speed up the process of going from being HIV positive to an AIDS diagnosis.

Effects on the Fetus/Neonate

HIV may be transmitted to the fetus through the placenta, at the time of birth when exposed to maternal blood and vaginal secretions, or through breast milk. Infants often have a positive antibody titer for as long as 15 months after birth because of the transfer of maternal antibodies. Those infants who are not infected with HIV will seroconvert to a negative antibody titer.

Medical–Surgical Management

Medical

There is no cure for HIV or AIDS. Routine prenatal testing includes a CD 4 lymphocyte count and serologic testing for changes indicating that AIDS is progressing. NST and ultrasound are performed at 32 weeks' gestation. NST is continued weekly, and ultrasound is performed every few weeks to monitor for fetal status.

Diet

Nutritional counseling and support regarding food handling, food preparation, and diet choices is often necessary.

Nursing Management

Follow Standard Precautions at all times. Discuss how HIV/AIDS affects the pregnancy. Encourage an adequate food intake for fetal development. Emphasize the importance of attending all scheduled prenatal visits and testing appointments.

NURSING PROCESS

Assessment

Subjective Data

The client may be asymptomatic or may describe having fatigue, malaise, loss of appetite, or diarrhea.

Objective Data

Signs of anemia, cell-mediated immunodeficiency, progressive weight loss, lymphadenopathy, and neurologic dysfunction may be present. Purplish lesions may also be noted during assessment.

Nursing diagnoses for a pregnant client who has HIV/AIDS include the following:

NURSING DIAGNOSES	PLANNING/OUTCOMES	NURSING INTERVENTIONS
Risk for ***I****nfection* related to altered immune status	The client will not develop infections during pregnancy.	Use Standard Precautions at all times. Monitor client for signs of infection (fever, cough, sore throat). Teach client to report changes that may indicate infection. Teach client to avoid large crowds or known cases of infectious diseases.
F*ear* related to outcome of pregnancy and disease	The client will verbalize fears about her pregnancy and HIV/AIDS.	Discuss HIV/AIDS disease process and how it can affect pregnancy and fetus. Provide opportunities for client to ask questions and clarify misconceptions. Assess client's support system and refer to community resources.
Imbalanced ***N****utrition: Less than Body Requirements* related to lack of appetite	The client will maintain weight or gain weight.	Monitor client's weight. Obtain 24-hour diet recall from client. Provide information about nutritional needs. Assist client in planning a high-protein, high-calorie diet.

Evaluation: Evaluate each outcome to determine how it has been met by the client.

OTHER INFECTIONS

Maternal infections may result in spontaneous abortion, a preterm infant, or an infected infant. Table 55-4 provides a summary of other infections affecting pregnancy.

HEMOLYTIC DISEASES

There are two types of hemolytic diseases: Rh incompatibility and ABO incompatibility. Rh incompatibility can be devastating to the fetus, but it can be prevented. ABO incompatibility is naturally occurring and much less severe, but it cannot be prevented.

RH INCOMPATIBILITY

Rh incompatibility can happen only when the mother is Rh negative and the fetus is Rh positive. That is, the mother does not have the Rh factor and the fetus does have the Rh factor. In this case, the father is Rh positive for the fetus to be Rh positive. If the father is Rh negative, there is no problem because the fetus will also be Rh negative.

The placenta keeps the mother's blood and the fetus's blood separated. In cases of ectopic pregnancy, abortion, infection of the placenta, abruptio placenta, birth, or at the time of placental separation, small tears occur in the placenta and fetal blood enters maternal circulation. The mother is then sensitized by the fetal Rh-positive blood. She also is sensitized by having a transfusion of Rh-positive blood, even the smallest amount.

Fetal (Rh-positive) blood in maternal (Rh-negative) circulation stimulates maternal production of Rh antibodies. The Rh antibodies, like many other antibodies, pass through the placenta and destroy fetal RBCs (Figure 55-14). Because this usually occurs at the time of birth, the first infant is usually not affected.

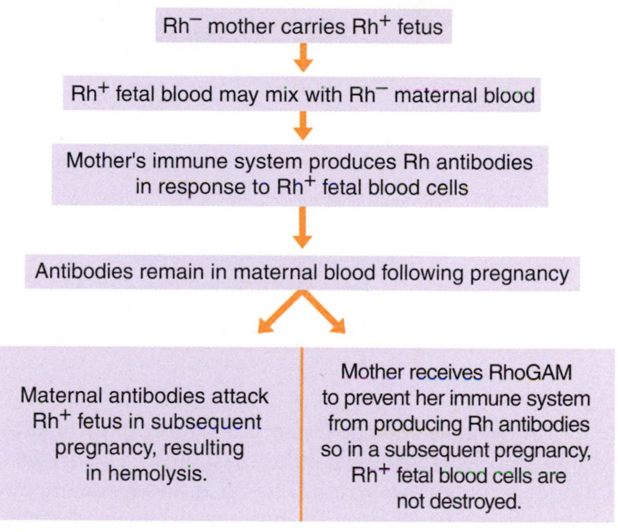

FIGURE 55-14 Rh Sensitization and Prevention

EFFECTS ON THE FETUS/NEONATE

If a placental tear occurred and there was no treatment, the next Rh-positive fetus will have red blood cells destroyed by the maternal Rh antibodies. This causes anemia, which in turn causes fetal edema (hydrops fetalis).

The next step is congestive heart failure and severe jaundice, which can cause neurologic damage called **kernicterus**. This entire syndrome, the most severe of the two hemolytic diseases of the newborn, is called erythroblastosis fetalis.

MEDICAL–SURGICAL MANAGEMENT

Medical

One of the screening tests performed at the first prenatal visit determines the mother's Rh factor. When the mother is found

Table 55-4 Selected Infections and Pregnancy

INFECTION	TREATMENT	MATERNAL EFFECTS	FETAL EFFECTS
Sexually Transmitted			
Syphilis	penicillin G benzathin (Bicillin L-A) or doxycycline (Vibramycin) Sexual partner should also be treated	Chancre, slight fever, malaise Progresses through secondary and tertiary stages if untreated	Spontaneous abortion, stillbirth, congenital syphilis, sniffling, peeling of soles and palms
Gonorrhea	ceftriaxone (Rocephin) plus erythromycin (Erythrocin Lactobionate) Partners must be treated	Often no symptoms; may have purulent vaginal discharge, dysuria, or urinary frequency	Ophthalmia neonatorum
Chlamydia	erthromycin ethyl succinate (ABO-Erythro-ES)	Often no symptoms; may have purulent or thin vaginal discharge, burning on urination, preterm labor	Conjunctivitis, chlamydial pneumonia, fetal death
Condylomata acuminata (venereal warts)	Cryosurgery, laser surgery, electrocautery, or trichloroacetic acid	Soft, grayish, raised lesions	Laryngeal papillomatosis if infection is present at birth
Hepatitis B (HBV)	Supportive; vaccine available	Often no symptoms	Most become carriers
Vaginal Infections			
Monilia	miconazole (Monistat), clotrimazole (Gyne-Lotrimin)	Thick, white, cheesy discharge Itching, dysuria	Thrush
Trichomoniasis	clotrimazole (Gyne-Lotrimin) in early pregnancy, metronidazole (Flagyl)	Foamy, green-gray discharge, prutitus	
Urinary Tract Infection			
Cystitis	Oral sulfonamides in early pregnancy, nitrofurantoin (Furadantin) in late pregnancy	Dysuria, urgency, low-grade fever; if not treated, may result in acute pyelonephritis	Hyperbilirubinemia if sulfonamides taken in last few weeks of pregnancy

to be Rh negative and the father is Rh positive or unknown, additional tests are run. An indirect Coombs' test detects Rh antibodies in maternal serum. The Rh antibody titer monitors what is happening when an Rh-negative woman is carrying an Rh-positive fetus. A rising titer indicates the need for immediate intervention.

Ultrasound is performed at about 15 weeks to determine gestational age. It is repeated several times throughout the pregnancy to measure fetal growth, assess fetal heart size, and check for hydramnios.

Amniocentesis may also be performed several times to determine the bilirubin (product of RBC breakdown) level and lung maturity. A fetal intrauterine blood transfusion may be indicated to maintain the fetus in the uterus until the lungs are more mature. The fetus is given Rh-negative erythrocytes to replace those destroyed by the Rh-positive antibodies. The erythrocytes are put into the peritoneal cavity, where they are absorbed. Rh-positive antibodies will not harm the Rh-negative blood given to the fetus.

Pharmacological

RhoGAM is given to an Rh-negative mother who is not sensitized (has a negative indirect Coombs' and antibody titer) and whose Rh-positive infant has no antibodies on the infant's RBCs (negative direct Coombs'). RhoGAM must be administered within 72 hours of the infant's birth. It prevents the mother's body from making the Rh antibodies by providing temporary passive immunity.

It is recommended that RhoGAM be given at 28 weeks' gestation and after the delivery. RhoGAM is also given to an Rh-negative woman after an abortion (spontaneous or induced), an ectopic pregnancy, and amniocentesis. It is never given to an Rh-positive woman.

Nursing Management

Ensure that the client's Rh factor is known. If the client is Rh-negative and the father is Rh-positive or unknown, ensure that the client keeps all appointments to have her Rh antibody titer checked. At 28 weeks' gestation and after the delivery, administer RhoGAM as ordered.

ABO INCOMPATIBILITY

In ABO incompatibility, the way in which a tear in the placenta may occur and fetal and maternal blood mix is the

TABLE 55-5 Possible Combinations for ABO Incompatibility

MOTHER	FETUS
A	B
B	A
O	A, B, AB

COURTESY OF DELMAR CENGAGE LEARNING

same as for Rh incompatibility. In this situation, the problem occurs when maternal blood enters fetal circulation. Possible combinations for ABO incompatibility are given in Table 55-5. The most common type of ABO incompatibility occurs when the mother is type O and the fetus is either type A, B, or AB. The mother's plasma naturally contains anti-A and anti-B antibodies. These antibodies have a weaker hemolytic effect than Rh antibodies, and they only affect mature RBCs. The number of antibodies is limited to the amount of maternal blood that entered fetal circulation. There is not a continuous supply of antibodies. Because ABO incompatibility is naturally occurring, it may affect the fetus of the first pregnancy. The affected newborn will have a positive direct Coombs' and will become jaundiced in the first 3 days of life.

NURSING MANAGEMENT

Ensure that the client's blood type is known. Observe the newborn for jaundice within the first 3 days of life.

MULTIPLE PREGNANCY

The twin birth rate has increased 42% since 1990 (CDC, 2007). Women having children after 30 years of age have a higher risk of delivering multiples than younger women. The use of fertility stimulating drugs and assisted reproductive technology (infertility treatment) has increased a woman's chance of carrying multiple fetuses.

A multiple pregnancy is suspected when the fundal height is greater than expected for the weeks of gestation. An ultrasound will verify two or more fetuses. Two or more heartbeats that differ by 10 bpm may be heard. The alpha fetoprotein level may be elevated. The first trimester proceeds much the same as with a single fetus except that maternal blood volume has a greater increase. Some women have more severe nausea and vomiting as well as shortness of breath on exertion, dyspnea, and backache.

As the uterus grows, there is greater pressure on and displacement of the internal organs. Pressure on the ureters causes urinary stasis and possible infection. Digestive problems and constipation is more disturbing, dependent edema more marked, and varicose veins more prominent. Gestational hypertension is more frequent than with a single fetus.

EFFECTS ON THE FETUS/NEONATE

Each fetus may have a decreased intrauterine growth rate (low birthweight). There is a greater risk of fetal anomalies, abnormal presentations, and preterm birth. Perinatal mortality is much greater for twins than for a single fetus.

MEDICAL–SURGICAL MANAGEMENT

Medical

The goals are to promote normal fetal development for all fetuses and to prevent delivery of preterm infants. Prenatal visits are more frequent, and serial ultrasounds assess the growth of each fetus. NST and BPP testing usually begin about 30 weeks' gestation and are repeated as indicated by fetal condition.

Surgical

The method of birth may not be determined until the mother is in labor. Depending on complications that may occur, a cesarean birth may be required.

Pharmacological

A prenatal vitamin/mineral preparation is doubly important with a multiple pregnancy. An extra calcium supplement and folic acid is required.

Diet

A well-balanced diet of 4,000 kcal with 135 g of protein is recommended. A weight gain of 40 to 50 pounds is acceptable, with 15 to 20 pounds being gained by 20 weeks' gestation.

Activity

Frequent rest periods are planned during the day. Resting in the side-lying position increases uteroplacental blood flow. The legs and feet are elevated to reduce edema. Good posture is maintained and good body mechanics used when lifting or moving objects.

NURSING MANAGEMENT

Actively listen to the client. Provide anticipatory guidance regarding the discomforts of pregnancy because they may be more intense with a multiple pregnancy. Encourage keeping scheduled prenatal visits and testing appointments. Emphasize the importance of taking the prescribed prenatal vitamin/mineral supplements and eating a well-balanced, high-protein diet. Assist the client to plan for rest periods in the side-lying position.

SUBSTANCE ABUSE

Drugs commonly abused include tobacco, alcohol, cocaine, crack, marijuana, methamphetamine, and heroin. The use of any of these substances is a threat to pregnancy. Substance abusers may not seek prenatal care, or they seek prenatal care very late in pregnancy. Most substance abusers do not voluntarily admit their addiction. These mothers may have an increased rate of gestational hypertension, abruptio placenta, poor nutrition, and sexually transmitted infections. They often use available money for the drug habit instead of food.

EFFECTS ON THE FETUS/NEONATE

Maternal smoking causes placenta previa, abruption placenta, premature rupture of membranes, premature birth, intrauterine growth restriction, and sudden death syndrome (Andres & Day, 2000). Alcohol may result in fetal alcohol syndrome, which manifests as both physical and mental abnormalities. Cocaine/crack increases the risk for IUGR, short body length, small head circumference, preterm birth, irritability, and low Apgar scores (an assessment of infant at 1 and 5 minutes after birth). Marijuana causes fine tremors and irritability. Methamphetamine causes low birth weight, microencephaly, premature birth, and heart defects (March of Dimes, 2009). Heroin increases the risk for IUGR, hypoxia, preterm birth, irritability, and meconium aspiration. Irritability and poor consolability may interfere with maternal–infant bonding and attachment and increase the risk of infant abuse and neglect.

Medical–Surgical Management

Medical

When a client is known or discovered to be a substance abuser, a multidisciplinary approach is best to manage the medical, legal, and socioeconomic considerations, and provide a safe labor and delivery. The client may require hospitalization for detoxification. "Cold turkey" withdrawal is not recommended during pregnancy because of possible fetal risks. Urine and blood screening is performed regularly.

Nursing Management

Maintain a calm, nonjudgmental manner. Actively listen to the client. Provide information and care as needed. Know the state laws regarding prenatal drug use, as some states require a referral to child protective services.

> **CRITICAL THINKING**
>
> **Substance Abuse**
>
> How would you handle the situation if you knew a client was a substance abuser, but she would not tell anyone at the prenatal clinic?

NURSING PROCESS

Assessment

Subjective Data

Ask questions about the use of caffeine, tobacco, and over-the-counter drugs, and then about alcohol use and drug use. The client may have altered perceptions, so validation through other sources, if possible, is desirable.

Objective Data

Assess for irritability, psychomotor problems, poor nutrition, and possible infections.

Nursing diagnoses for a pregnant client who is a substance abuser include the following:

NURSING DIAGNOSES	PLANNING/OUTCOMES	NURSING INTERVENTIONS
*Imbalanced **N**utrition: Less than Body Requirements* related to inadequate intake of food	The client will gain appropriate weight during pregnancy.	Refer client to WIC (women, infant, and children) nutrition program. Monitor weight gain. Collect 24-hour diet recall from client. Explain the rationale for a nutritious diet, listing foods the client could eat for her health and the fetus. Assist the client to plan meals.
*Deficient **K**nowledge* related to not understanding how substance abuse affects the fetus	The client will verbalize how substance abuse can affect the fetus.	Explain how substance abuse affects the fetus. Provide written materials regarding effects of the client's drug of choice on the fetal development. Allow time for client questions and for clarification of misconceptions.
*Risk for **I**nfection* related to use of dirty needles and syringes	The client will not have an infection from dirty needles and syringes.	Explain how client may pick up an infection from dirty needles and syringes. Refer client to community resources where clean syringes and needles are available. Refer client to drug counseling program.

Evaluation: Evaluate each outcome to determine how it has been met by the client.

PRETERM LABOR

Preterm labor is labor that begins after viability but before 37 weeks' gestation. The causes of preterm labor may be maternal, fetal, or placental. Maternal factors that may cause preterm labor include gestational hypertension, diabetes, heart or renal disease, an incompetent cervix, premature rupture of membranes, and maternal infection. Fetal factors include fetal infection, multiple pregnancy, and hydramnios. Placental factors are placenta previa and abruptio placenta.

EFFECTS ON THE FETUS/NEONATE

Preterm labor may produce a neonate who is not able to cope well with extrauterine life.

MEDICAL–SURGICAL MANAGEMENT

Medical

Preterm labor is confirmed by documented uterine contractions, ruptured membranes, and cervical dilation and effacement. No attempt is made to stop labor if any of the following conditions exist: the cervix dilated 4 cm or more, severe gestational hypertension, prolonged rupture of membranes, hemorrhage, abruptio placenta, fetal complications, or fetal death.

Pharmacological

The process of stopping labor with medications is called **tocolysis**. The drugs used in an attempt to stop preterm labor are called *tocolytics*. Tocolytics include beta-adrenergic agonists, magnesium sulfate, calcium-channel blockers, and prostaglandin inhibitors.

Ritodrine hydrochloride (Yutopar) is a beta-adrenergic agonist that inhibits contractility of the uterus. Maternal pulse, BP, lung sounds, and FHR must be closely monitored.

Terbutaline sulfate (Brethine) is also a beta-adrenergic agonist that relaxes the uterine muscle. It is used frequently, although the Food and Drug Administration has not approved it for tocolysis.

Magnesium sulfate ($MgSO_4$) has fewer side effects than the beta-adrenergic agonists and is being used more in preterm labor. A loading dose is given and then continued at the lowest rate necessary to maintain a noncontracting uterus. Tocolysis is usually maintained with a maternal serum level of 5 to 8 mg/dL.

> **PROFESSIONAL TIP**
>
> **Progesterone**
>
> Progesterone may not delay preterm birth by decreasing uterine contractility but may reduce preterm birth by preventing the softening of the cervix (Bernstein, 2008).

Nifedipine (Procardia) and nicardipine hydrochloride (Cardene), calcium channel blockers, are used to delay delivery. Indomethacin (Indocin), sulindac (Clinoril), and ketorolac tromethamine (Toradol), prostaglandin inhibitors, also delay delivery.

A research study by Murphy and MACS Collaborative Group (2007) recommended that women who are at risk for preterm delivery be given a single injection of corticosteroids to enhance fetal lung maturity. Weekly injections gave no better results.

NURSING MANAGEMENT

Explain all treatments and procedures and keep the client informed of responses to them. Allow client time to ask questions. Monitor vital signs, FHT, and contractions. Administer medications as ordered.

NURSING PROCESS

ASSESSMENT

Subjective Data

Client may describe having contractions or that "my water broke." The client expresses concern about what is happening.

Objective Data

Contractions may be documented, cervix dilating and effacing, or membranes ruptured. The client may experience tension, restlessness, or vital sign changes.

Nursing diagnoses for a client in preterm labor include the following:

NURSING DIAGNOSES	PLANNING/OUTCOMES	NURSING INTERVENTIONS
Anxiety related to perception of what is happening and not having time to prepare for labor	The client will express less anxiety about being in preterm labor.	Explain what is happening to client and all tests and procedures before beginning them. Spend time with client so she can express her anxieties and ask questions. Keep client informed about how the preterm labor is responding to treatment.
Deficient Knowledge related to lack of information about preterm labor causes, determination, and treatment	The client will verbalize an understanding about preterm labor and treatments.	Explain what preterm labor is, possible/probable causes, and treatment. Allow client time to ask questions. Clarify any misunderstandings.

(*Continues*)

Nursing diagnoses for a client in preterm labor include the following: (Continued)

NURSING DIAGNOSES	PLANNING/OUTCOMES	NURSING INTERVENTIONS
Fear related to risk for fetus	The client will express her fears for fetal welfare.	Encourage client to express fears related to fetal well-being. Keep client informed about fetal status. Encourage family to spend time with client.

Evaluation: Evaluate each outcome to determine how it has been met by the client.

CASE STUDY

Part A: M.J., age 32, is G 3, P 2, T 1, P 1, A 0, L 2. The children are ages 1-1/2, and 3. B.J., her husband, works 8 to 5. She is 32 weeks' gestation. Her BP has been 104/68 mm Hg at her prenatal visits. Today, her BP is 136/84. She has gained 6-1/2 pounds in the 4 weeks since her last visit. There is edema in both feet.

Part B: Two weeks later, M.J.'s BP is 140/90 mm Hg, and she has gained 4 more pounds. She states that she had to take her rings off because they were too tight. The physician admits her to the hospital with orders for bed rest in side-lying position, $MgSO_4$ IV drip, and a high-protein diet.

Part C: The electronic fetal monitor shows a sustained increase in the baseline FHR. M.J.'s deep tendon reflexes are very reactive.

The following questions will guide your development of a nursing care plan for the case study:

Part A:

1. What other assessments should be made?
2. What advice would you anticipate the physician giving M.J.?
3. How can you assist M.J. to implement the physician's advice?

Part B:

4. What are the goals for M.J.'s care?
5. What nursing assessments must now be obtained?
6. What diagnostic tests might be ordered?

Part C:

7. Identify three nursing diagnoses and goals for M.J.
8. Identify nursing interventions for each nursing diagnosis.

SUMMARY

- High-risk factors can often be identified early in prenatal care.
- Continuing prenatal care allows for signs of complications to be identified as early as possible.
- Many procedures and tests are available to assess fetal well-being.
- When bleeding occurs in pregnancy, mothers often feel guilty that they may have done something to cause the bleeding.
- Mothers with chronic medical conditions are often cared for by both the medical physician and the obstetrician during pregnancy.
- Complications of pregnancy add to the emotional and financial stress for the client and family.

REVIEW QUESTIONS

1. J.S. is a 16-year-old primigravida at 38 weeks, whose membranes ruptured spontaneously. Her chart indicates that she was seen by a physician for the first time 2 weeks ago. She is having contractions 10 to 12 minutes apart. The assessment finding indicating a high-risk pregnancy is:

1. lack of prenatal care and age.
2. she is not considered high risk.
3. the membranes rupturing spontaneously.
4. the contractions being 10 to 12 minutes apart.

2. The maturity of which organ is based on the ratio of lecithin to sphingomyelin?
   1. Placenta.
   2. Fetal lungs.
   3. Acini glands.
   4. Fetal kidneys.
3. In planning the care of a client with DIC, the nurse would include:
   1. giving coagulants.
   2. turning every 2 hours.
   3. watching for signs of bleeding.
   4. massaging the fundus frequently.
4. A pregnant client is receiving magnesium sulfate. The nurse observes that the client's respirations are 8 and her patellar reflexes have decreased. The nurse recognizes that these observations should be:
   1. considered to be the desired result.
   2. recorded and monitored to see if they continue.
   3. brought to the attention of the charge nurse immediately.
   4. considered as an indication that a higher dose of medication is needed.
5. A pregnant woman's blood is found to be Rh negative. Which of the following must be true for Rh incompatibility to be possible?
   1. Father's blood is found to be Rh positive.
   2. Father's blood is found to be Rh negative.
   3. Mother does not develop a secondary anemia during pregnancy.
   4. Mother has at least 2 blood transfusions during pregnancy.
6. A client is admitted at 18 weeks' gestation with a probable diagnosis of hydatidiform mole. For the nursing diagnosis, Fear related to the possible development of choriocarcinoma, which of these nursing interventions is appropriate?
   1. Educate the client regarding the need for weekly blood tests.
   2. Explain the need for follow-up physical examinations and chest x-rays.
   3. Stress the importance of delaying another pregnancy until her baby is one year old.
   4. Allow the client to express her feelings and refer her to support sources.
7. A client at 28 weeks' gestation is Rh negative. The nurse determines that the client understands what the nurse has taught her about Rh sensitization when the client states:
   1. "I know I can never have another child."
   2. "I may have to have a shot after delivery if my baby's blood type is Rh positive."
   3. "I will have to have an injection once per month until the baby is born."
   4. "I'm glad I won't have to receive RhoGam if I have another child."
8. A nurse is monitoring a pregnant client with gestational hypertension who is at risk for preeclampsia. The nurse asks the client about subjective signs of preeclampsia, which include:
   1. headache and scomato.
   2. nausea and weight gain of 3 pounds in the last week.
   3. epigastric pain and hypertension.
   4. hypertension and proteinuria.
9. A nurse is assigned to a client with abruption placenta who is experiencing vaginal bleeding. The nurse collects data from the client, knowing that abruption placenta is often accompanied by which additional finding?
   1. A soft abdomen.
   2. No complaints of abdominal pain.
   3. Lack of uterine contractions.
   4. A rigid, board-like abdomen.
10. A client is admitted to the labor suite complaining of painless vaginal bleeding. The nurse assists with the examination of the client, knowing that a routine procedure contraindicated with this client's situation is:
    1. Leopold's maneuvers.
    2. external electronic fetal monitoring.
    3. a manual pelvic examination.
    4. hemoglobin and hematocrit evaluation.

REFERENCES/SUGGESTED READINGS

Acosta, P. (1996). Nutrition studies in treated infants and children with phenylketonuria: Vitamins, minerals, trace elements. *European Journal of Pediatrics, 155*(1), S136–S139.

Acosta, P., & Wright, L. (1992). Nurses' role in preventing birth defects in offspring of women with phenylketonuria. *JOGNN, 21*(4), 270.

American Association for Clinical Chemistry (AACC). (2009). Pregnancy and prenatal testing. Retrieved August 21, 2009 from http://www.labtestonline.org/understanding/wellness/pre_torch.html

American Diabetes Association (ADA). (2009). Gestational diabetes. Retrieved August 20, 2009 from http://www.diabetes.org/gestational-diabetes.jsp

Andres, R, & Day, M. (2000). Perinatal complications associated with maternal tobacco use. *Seminars in Fetal and Neonatal, 5*(3), 231–241.

Atassi, K., & Harris, M. (2001). Disseminated intravascular coagulation. *Nursing2001, 31*(3), 64.

Barton, J. B., & Sibai, B. M. (2001). HELLP syndrome. In B. M. Sibai (Ed.). *Hypertensive disorders in women*. Philadelphia: W. B. Saunders.

Berstein, P. (2008). Highlights of the 2008 annual clinical meeting of the society of maternal-fetal medicine. Retrieved August 22, 2009 from http://www.medscape.com/viewarticle/570338_print

Bougere, M. (1998). Action stat: Abruptio placenta. *Nursing98, 28*(2), 47.

Brown, Z., Gardella, C., Wald, A., Morrow, R., & Corey, L. (2005). Genital herpes complicating pregnancy. *Obstetrics and Gynecology, 106*, 845–856.

Bulechek, G., Butcher, H., McCloskey, J., & Dochterman, J., eds. (2008). *Nursing Interventions Classification (NIC)* (5th ed.). St. Louis, MO: Mosby/Elsevier.

Carpenter, T. (2003). Is it morning sickness or something worse? *RN, 66*(10), 34–37.

Centers for Disease Control and Prevention (CDC). (2007). *Births: Final data for 2005. National Vital Statistics Reports (NVSS), 56*(6), 1–104. Retrieved August 22, 2009 from http://www.cdc.gov/nchs/data/nvsr/nvsr56/nvsr56_06.pdf

Ciardelli, L., Meroni, V., Avanzini, A., Bollani, L., Tinelli, C., Garofoli, F., Gasparoni, A., & Stronati, M. (2008). Early and accurate diagnosis of congenital toxoplasmosis. *The Pediatric Infectious DiseaseJournal, 27*, 125–129.

Cook, A., Gilbert, R., Buffolano, W., Zufferey, J., Petersen, E., et al. (2000). Sources of toxoplasma infection in pregnant women: European multicentre case-control study. European Research Network on Congenital Toxoplasmosis. *BMJ, 321*(7254), 142–147.

Davidson, M., London, M., & Ladewig, P. (2008). *Old's maternal-newborn nursing and women's health across the lifespan* (8th ed.). Upper Saddle River, NJ: Pearson Prentice Hall.

Deering, S. (2008). Abruptio placentae. Retrieved August 20, 2009 from http://emedicince.medscape.com/article/252810-overview

Dickason, E., Silverman, B., & Kaplan J. (1998). *Maternal-infant nursing care* (3rd ed.). St. Louis: MO: Mosby–Year Book.

Farrell, M. (2003). Improving the care of women with gestational diabetes. *MCN, 28*(5), 301–305.

Feig, D., Briggs, G., & Koren, G. (2007). Oral antidiabetic agents in pregnancy and lactation: a paradigm shift? *The Annuals of Pharmacotherapy, 41*(7), 1174–1180.

Friedman, S.A., Lubarsky, S.L., & Lim, K.H. (2001). Mild gestational hypertension and preeclampsia. In B. M. Sibai (Ed.). *Hypertensive disorders in women*. Philadelphia: W. B. Saunders.

Guinn, D., Atkinson, M. ., Sullivan, L., Lee, M., MacGregor, S., et al. (2001). Single vs weekly courses of antenatal corticosteroids for women at risk of preterm delivery: A randomized controlled trial. *JAMA, 286*(13), 1581–1587.

Hamilton Health Sciences. (2008). Are you immune to rubella? Retrieved August 21, 2009 from http://www.hhsc.ca/documents/Patient%20Education/Rubella-th.pdf

Harvey, C. (1997). A look at electronic fetal monitoring update; the new terms. *Lifelines, 1*(6), 49–51.

Hokelek, M. 2009. Toxoplasmosis. Retrieved August 21, 2009 from http://emedicine.medscape.com/article/229969-print

Holcberg, G., Tsadkin-Tamir, M., Sapir, O., Wiznizer, A., Segal, D., et al. (2004). Transfer of insulin lispro across the human placenta. *European Journal of Obstetrics and Gynecology and Reproductive Biology, 115*(1), 117–118.

Irgens, J.U., Reisaeter, L. Irgens, L.M., & Lie, R.T. (2001). Long-term mortality of mothers and fathers after preeclampsia: Population-based cohort study. *BMJ, 323*(7323), 1213–1217.

Katz, V., Farmer, R., & Kuller, J. (2000). Preeclampsia into eclampsia: Towards a new paradigm. *American Journal of Obstetrics & Gynecology, 182*(6), 1389–1396.

Koch, R., Azen, C., Friedman, E., Hanley, W., Kevy, H., et al. (2003). Research design, organization, and sample characteristics of the maternal PKU collaborative study. *Pediatrics, 112*(6), 1519–1522.

Lachat, M., Scott, C., & Refl, M. (2006). HIV and pregnancy: Considerations for nursing practice. *The American Journal of Maternal Child Nursing, 31*(4), 233–241.

Ladewig, P., Moberly, S., Olds, L., & London, M. (2001). *Contemporary maternal-newborn nursing care* (5th ed.). Menlo Park, CA: Addison-Wesley.

Lee, Y., & Simpson, L. (2007). Major fetal structural malformations: The role of new imaging modalities. *American Journal of Medical Genetics Part C (Seminars in Medical Genetics), 145C*, 33–44.

Littleton, L., & Engebretson, J. (2004). *Maternity nursing care*. Clifton Park, NY: Delmar Cengage Learning.

Lu, J., & Nightengale, C. (2000). Magnesium sulfate in eclampsia and preeclampsia: Pharmokinetic principles. *Clinical Pharmacology, 38*(4), 305–314.

Macones, G., Hankins, G., Spong, C., Hauth, J., & Moore, T. (2008). The 2008 National Institute of Child Health and Human Development Research Workshop Report on electronic fetal heart rate monitoring. *Obstetrics and Gynecology, 112*, 661–666.

Mandeville, L.K., & Troiano, N.H. (1999). *High risk and critical care intrapartum nursing* (2nd ed.). Philadelphia: Lippincott Williams & Wilkins.

March of Dimes. (2009). Illicit drug use during pregnancy. Retrieved August 22, 2009 from http://www.marchofdimes.com/professionals/14332_1169.asp#head3

Minnick-Smith, K., & Cook, F. (1997). Current treatment options for ectopic pregnancy. *MCN, 22*(1), 21–25.

Montgomery, K. (2003). Health promotion for pregnant adolescents. *Lifelines, 7*(5), 432–444.

Moorhead, S., Johnson, M., Maas, M., & Swanson, E. (2007). *Nursing outcomes classification (NOC)* (4th ed). St. Louis, MO: Elsevier–Health Sciences Division.

Morgan, E. (2002). Eclampsia. *Nursing2002, 32*(3), 104.

Murphy, K., & MACS Collaborative Group. (2007). Multiple courses of antenatal corticosteroids for preterm birth study. *American Journal of Obstetrics and Gynecology, 197*, S2.

National Heart, Lung, and Blood Institute. (2000). *Working group report on high blood pressure in pregnancy*. Washington, DC: National Institutes of Health.

National Institute of Child Health and Human Development Research Planning Workshop. (1997). Electronic fetal heart rate monitoring: Research guidelines for interpretation. *American Journal of Obstetrics and Gynecology, 177*, 1385–1390.

National Institutes of Health (NIH). (2009). Use of 3D/4D Ultrasound in the Evaluation of Fetal Anomalies. Retrieved August 17, 2009 from http://clinicaltrials.gov/ct2/show/NCT00826917

Neal, J. (2001). RhD isoimmunization and current management modalities. *JOGNN, 30*(6), 589–606.

Neuman, M., & Graf, C. (2003). Pregnancy after age 35: Are these women at high risk? *Lifelines, 7*(5), 422–430.

NICHD (1997). Electronic fetal heart monitoring: Research guidelines for interpretation. The National Institute of Child Health and Human Development Research Planning Workshop. *JOGNN, 26*(6), 635–640.

Nick, J. (2003). Deep tendon reflexes: The what, why, where, and how of tapping. *JOGNN, 32*(3), 297–306.

North American Nursing Diagnosis Association International. (2010). *NANDA-I nursing diagnoses: Definitions and classification 2009–2011.* Ames, IA: Wiley-Blackwell.

Padden, M. (1999). HELLP syndrome: Recognition and pernatal management. *American Family Physician*. Retrieved August 22, 2009 from http://www.aafp.org/afp/990901ap/829.html

Perozzi, K., Zalice, K., Howard, V., & Skariot, L. (2007). What you need to know to care for your pregnant patient. *The American Journal of Maternal Child Nursing, 32*(6), 345–352.

Reis, P., Sander, C., & Pearlman, M. (2000). Abruptio placentae after auto accidents: A case control study. *Journal of Reproductive Medicine, 45*(1), 6–10.

Rorman, E., Zamir, C., Rilkis, I., & Ben-David, H. (2006). Congenital toxoplasmosisprenatal aspects of Toxoplasma gondii infection. *Reproductive Toxicology, 21*(4), 458–472.

Ruddy, L. (2000). Preeclampsia. *AJN, 100*(8), 45–46.

Ruddy, L., & Kearney, K. (2000). Preeclampsia. *American Journal of Nursing, 100*(8), 45–46.

Saal, H., Braddock, S., Bull, M., Enns, G., Gruen, J., et al. (2008). Maternal phenylketonuria. *Pediatrics, 122*, 445–449.

Schweon, S. (2001). Protecting yourself during pregnancy. Nursing2001, 31(3), 72.

Sepilian, V., & Wood, E. (2009). Ectopic pregnancy. Retrieved August 18, 2009 from http://emedicine.medscape.com/article/258768-print

Sibai, B., & Stella, C. (2009). Diagnosis and management of atypical preeclampsia-eclampsia. *American Journal of Obstetrics and Gynecology, 200*, 481.e1–481.e7.

Simpson, K., & Creehan, P. (2007). *AWHONN's Perinatal nursing: Co-published with AWHONN* (3rd ed.). Philadelphia: Lippincott Williams & Wilkins.

Spratto, G., & Woods, A. (2008). *2009 PDR for nursing*. Clifton Park, NY: Delmar Cengage Learning.

Tenore, J. (2000). Ectopic pregnancy. *American Family Physician, 61*(4), 1080–1088.

Trofatter, K. (2009). Cervical incompetence and cerclage-8-Shirodkar vs McDonald cerclage. Retrieved August 18, 2009 from http://www.healthline.com/blogs/pregnancy_childbirth/2008/09/cervical-incompetence-and-cerclage-8.html

Urbanski, T., Higgins, P., Murray, M., & Joffe, G. (1996). Caring for a woman with a hydatidiform mole and coexisting pregnancy. *MCN, 21*(2), 85–89.

Watts, D., Brown, Z., Money, D., Selke, S., Huang, M., Sacks, S., & Corey, L. (2003). A double-blind, randomized, placebo-controlled trial of acyclovir in late pregnancy for the reduction of herpes simplex virus shedding and cesarean delivery. *American Journal of Obstetrics and Gynecology, 188*, 836–843.

Woo, J. (2009). Obstetric ultrasound: A comprehensive guide to ultrasound scans in pregnancy. Retrieved August 15, 2009 from http://www.ob-ultrasound.net/

RESOURCES

Association of Women's Health, Obstetric, and Neonatal Nurses (AWHONN), http:// www.awhonn.org

National Organization of Mothers of Twins Clubs, Inc. (NOMOTC), http://www.nomotc.org

The Society of Obstetricians and Gynaecologists of Canada (SOGC), http://www.sogc.org

CHAPTER 56
The Birth Process

MAKING THE CONNECTION

Refer to the following chapters to increase your understanding of the birth process:

Basic Nursing
- ***Assessment***
- ***Pain Management***

Adult Health Nursing
- ***Anesthesia***

Maternal & Pediatric Nursing
- ***Prenatal Care***
- ***Complications of Pregnancy***

LEARNING OBJECTIVES

Upon completion of this chapter, you should be able to:

- Explain key terms.
- Describe possible causes of labor.
- Identify premonitory signs of labor.
- Differentiate between true labor and false labor.
- Discuss the maternal systemic responses to labor.
- Identify the variables that affect the progress of labor.
- Explain the four stages of labor.
- Describe the mechanisms of labor.
- Show nursing actions necessary when admitting a woman to the labor unit.
- Demonstrate the specific assessments used when caring for a woman in labor: fetopelvic relationships, fetal assessment, contractions, Leopold's maneuvers, vaginal examination.
- Explain possible nursing diagnoses and nursing interventions for a client during labor and delivery.
- Identify the most common complications of labor—dystocia and fetal distress.
- Identify possible medical—surgical interventions for labor: cesarean birth, induction and augmentation of labor, amniotomy, episiotomy, forceps, vacuum extractor, and analgesia/anesthesia.
- Provide care for a client during labor and delivery.

KEY TERMS

acme
amniotomy
augmentation of labor
bloody show
Braxton Hicks contractions
cardinal movements
cephalopelvic disproportion (CPD)
cervical dilation
cesarean birth
crowning
decrement
duration
dysfunctional labor
dystocia
effacement
engagement
episiotomy
external version
false labor
Ferguson's reflex
fetal attitude
fetal lie
fetal position
fetal presentation
fontanelle
forceps
frequency
fundus
increment
induction of labor
intensity
interval
lightening
macrosomic
molding
nuchal cord
precipitate birth
precipitate labor
presenting part
preterm birth
preterm labor
prolapsed cord
pudendal block
restitution
rupture of membranes (ROM)
station
suture
tocolytic agent
uterine retraction

INTRODUCTION

The past decade has brought great changes in birthing practices. For hospital births, the concept of labor, delivery, recovery, postpartum (LDRP) rooms has given the expecting couple a more homelike environment, and the mother is not moved from the labor room to the delivery room, to the recovery room, to the postpartum room during the birthing process (Figure 56-1). Family and friends, even the baby's siblings, may be present in the LDRP room during the birth process.

Community birthing centers and other settings offer alternatives for the laboring couple. Many clients attend childbirth classes and have in mind a birthing plan or expectations of what they anticipate the birthing process will be like.

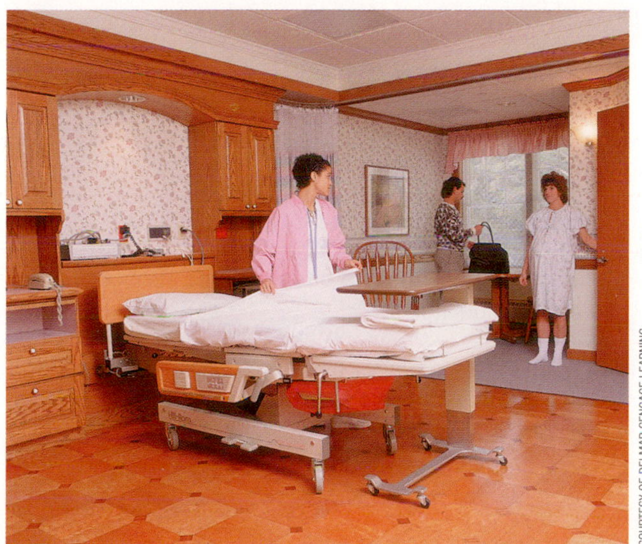

FIGURE 56-1 **The LDRP concept allows the laboring couple to remain in the same room throughout the birth experience.**

Some clients hire a midwife or doula to assist them through the process of labor, birth, and postpartum. Midwives are classified as either a certified midwife (CM) or a certified nurse-midwife (CNM) depending on their education and training. Midwives provide health care to women throughout the life span (American College of Nurse-Midwives, 2009). The CNM is trained to independently manage the care of low-risk pregnancy, birth, and postpartum care for healthy woman and newborns.

Doulas are trained and experienced childbirth support persons who continuously attend to the physical, emotional, and informational needs of the laboring woman and family through the entire birthing process. According to the Doulas of North America International (2009) when a doula attends the birth, the labor is shorter with fewer complications, and the infants are healthier and breastfeed more easily. The doula is an adjunct and can be an asset to the health care team (London, Ladewig, Ball, & Bindler, 2007).

This chapter outlines the birth process, from the onset of labor through the birth of the infant.

ONSET OF LABOR

For 38 to 40 weeks, the pregnancy has been advancing and the fetus developing. Now, as the fetus reaches maturity, the birth process begins. Researchers are still trying to determine exactly what causes the onset of true labor; however, there are two theories relative to why labor begins.

THEORIES REGARDING ONSET OF LABOR

The mechanical theory is based on the principle that as a hollow organ in the body becomes filled and distended, the organ tends to empty itself. Examples of this phenomenon are the bladder and sigmoid colon. This mechanism alone is not enough to fully explain the onset of labor because a woman can have a full-term 6 ½ lb baby with one pregnancy and full-term twins each weighing 5-½ lb with the next pregnancy.

The hormonal theory of the onset of labor relates to the changes in maternal progesterone and estrogen levels, the maternal production of oxytocin and prostaglandin, and the increase in fetal production of cortisol. There seems to be a highly integrated relationship among these hormones.

As the pregnancy nears its end, the placental production of progesterone decreases, thus decreasing the relaxing effect of progesterone on the uterus. The estrogen level rises, causing an increased sensitivity of the myometrium to oxytocin. Oxytocin, now produced by the mother's posterior pituitary gland, stimulates uterine contractions. As the pregnancy nears 40 weeks of gestation, the uterus becomes more sensitive to oxytocin. Fetal cortisol production increases as the pregnancy nears term. It is believed to decrease the placental production of progesterone and stimulate the precursors of prostaglandin.

Premonitory Signs of Labor

Several signs indicate that labor will soon begin. The signs are lightening, Braxton Hicks contractions, cervical changes, bloody show, rupture of membranes, gastrointestinal disturbance, and a sudden burst of energy.

Lightening

Lightening is the descent of the fetus into the pelvis. This may occur as early as 2 weeks before labor begins in the primigravida client but may not occur until a multigravida client is already in labor. The downward movement of the fetus and thus the uterus makes the upper part of the abdomen flatter. This relieves pressure on the diaphragm, allowing the mother to breathe easier, but she may experience:

- Leg cramps from pressure now on pelvic nerves.
- Urinary frequency from pressure now on the bladder.
- Increased venous stasis from pressure now on the veins, resulting in edema of the lower extremities.
- Increased vaginal secretions.

Braxton Hicks Contractions

Braxton Hicks contractions are irregular, intermittent contractions felt by the pregnant woman toward the end of pregnancy. The tightening sensation in the abdomen may become fairly regular and uncomfortable. The woman may go to the care provider's office or the hospital thinking she is in labor. If the cervix is not dilated and then the contractions stop, this is called **false labor**. Table 56-1 compares false labor and true labor.

Cervical Changes

At about 34 weeks of gestation, because of the changing ratio of estrogen to progesterone and the production of prostaglandin, the cervix begins to "mature" or "ripen." That is, the cervix becomes softer and spongier. **Effacement**, thinning and shortening of the cervix, may begin, especially when the woman is a primigravida. Cervical changes of dilation and effacement progress during labor to allow delivery of the fetus.

Bloody Show

Bloody show consists of cervical secretion, blood-tinged mucus, and the mucous plug that blocked the cervix during pregnancy. Labor often begins within 24 to 48 hours after the bloody show is noticed; however, a vaginal examination that includes cervical manipulation may result in a blood-tinged discharge. This may be confused with bloody show.

Rupture of Membranes

Rupture of membranes (ROM), the rupture of the amniotic sac, usually occurs after labor has begun; however, in about 12% of women, the amniotic membranes rupture

Table 56-1 Comparison of False Labor and True Labor

FALSE LABOR	TRUE LABOR
Contractions often irregular but may be regular for a short time (1 to 2 hours).	Contractions occur at regular intervals.
Interval between contractions stays the same.	Interval between contractions gradually shortens.
Contraction intensity and duration remain the same.	Contractions increase in intensity and duration.
Contractions frequently stop when the client ambulates or changes position.	Contractions continue and often become stronger when the client ambulates.
Contractions eventually cease with controlled breathing, relaxation techniques, comfort measures, or hydration.	Contractions are usually not stopped with controlled breathing, other relaxation techniques, sedation, comfort measures, or hydration.
Cervix may soften but does not efface or dilate.	Cervix softens, effaces, and dilates.
Contractions felt above navel.	Contractions felt in lower back and radiate to abdomen.
No change in cervical dilation and effacement.	Produces cervical dilation and effacement.

COURTESY OF DELMAR CENGAGE LEARNING

before the onset of labor (London, Ladewig, Ball, & Bindler, 2007). Spontaneous rupture of membranes (SROM) occurs naturally with a gush of amniotic fluid out of the vagina. Artificial rupture of membranes (AROM) is a procedure known as an amniotomy (discussed later in chapter) in which a physician or certified nurse-midwife uses an amnihook instrument to rupture the amniotic membranes. If **engagement** (when the widest diameter of the fetal presenting part [head] enters the inlet to the true pelvis) has not yet occurred, there exists the danger that the umbilical cord will wash out with the amniotic fluid (prolapsed cord).

If labor does not begin spontaneously within 12 to 24 hours after the membranes rupture and the pregnancy is near term, labor is often induced to avoid infection.

It is sometimes difficult for the woman to determine whether the membranes have ruptured or whether urine has escaped from her bladder. A simple test with nitrazine paper is helpful. When moistened in the discharge, the nitrazine paper will turn a deep blue (react) if the discharge is amniotic fluid; the paper will usually not react if the membranes are still intact. The health-care provider may also test for "ferning." When amniotic fluid is placed on a microscope slide, it dries in the shape of fern leaves. Newer testing devices for detecting rupture of the amniotic membrane in pregnant women include the Amnisure and Amnioswab. Both of these testing methods are convenient swab screenings that are rapid and less invasive.

Gastrointestinal Disturbance

Some women report having one or more of the following near the time of labor: indigestion, nausea, vomiting, and diarrhea. They may experience a 1- to 3-pound weight loss.

Sudden Burst of Energy

Approximately 24 to 48 hours before labor begins, some women will have a sudden burst of energy. The reason for this is unknown. The prospective mother should be careful not to tire herself. She will need the energy when labor begins. Encourage the client to eat frequent small nutritious meals during this time.

MATERNAL SYSTEMIC RESPONSES TO LABOR

Knowing how the various systems of the mother's body respond to labor is important when making assessments and performing nursing interventions.

Cardiovascular System

Cardiac output increases because 300 to 500 mL of blood is squeezed from the uterus into maternal circulation with each contraction (London, et al., 2007). The client's blood pressure increases during the first and second stages of labor due to contractions. Blood pressure is highest during a contraction, so blood pressure should be taken *between* contractions. Anxiety and pain may also make the blood pressure increase. Women in labor may experience supine hypotensive syndrome, or decreased blood pressure when in a supine position due to the vessels being compressed by the fetal weight (Leifer, 2008).

Respiratory System

Oxygen consumption during labor is equal to that of moderate to strenuous exercise. As long as the respiratory center is not depressed by medication, the increased respiratory rate continues with oxygen consumption almost double the normal amount. If the mother develops hypoxia or acidosis, the fetus may be compromised. Hyperventilation may decrease the level of carbon dioxide in the mother's blood.

Renal System

When engagement occurs, the bladder, now an abdominal organ, is pushed forward and upward. A distended bladder may impede fetal descent. Pressure from the presenting part, especially during a contraction, may cause edema of the tissues because of impaired blood and lymph drainage (Cunningham, Leveno, Gilstrap, Bloom, Hauth, & Wenstrom, 2005). Urinary flow is decreased, especially when the woman is supine, because the uterus compresses the ureters. Often there is a lessened urge to void, so the client must be encouraged to do so.

Gastrointestinal System

During labor, peristalsis and absorption decrease. Gastric emptying time is prolonged and gastric contents increase in acidity (Blackburn, 2007). The client in labor should not eat solid food because there is always a possibility of an obstetrical emergency requiring surgery. Eating solid food would increase the risk of aspirating vomitus. The absorption of liquid is unchanged during labor. The lips and mouth become dry as a result of mouth breathing.

Fluid and Electrolyte Balance

Because of the muscular activity of labor, the mother's body temperature increases and she perspires profusely. The normal increase in respiratory rate and the tendency of women in labor to hyperventilate both cause an increase in fluid loss. The hyperventilation also affects electrolyte balance. To prevent dehydration, it is routine for intravenous fluids such as lactated ringers to be administered to women during labor and delivery.

Immune System

The white blood count (WBC) increases, sometimes up to 25,000/mm^3, during labor and stays elevated during the early postpartum period. The natural increase makes it difficult to identify any infectious process the woman may have.

Integumentary System

The vagina and perineum have a great ability to stretch. The degree of stretching varies with each client; however, minute tears may occur in the vagina and/or perineum during the birth of the baby.

Musculoskeletal System

The marked increase in muscle activity during labor is accompanied by increased body temperature, diaphoresis, fatigue, and some proteinuria (1+) (Lowdermilk & Perry,

> **PROFESSIONAL TIP**
>
> **Mother to Infant HIV Transmission**
>
> A mother can pass HIV to her infant during pregnancy, childbirth delivery, or through breast milk. According to the CDC (2007), mother-to-infant transmission is the most common way that children become infected with HIV. Antiretroviral medications work well to stop the transmission of HIV if the mother takes these drugs before and during childbirth and if the newborn is given the drugs after birth. Without breastfeeding or treatment, approximately 25% of pregnant women with HIV will transmit HIV to the infant. By following this protocol of antiviral medication administration, mother-to-infant HIV transmission is reduced from 25% to less than 2% (CDC, 2007).

2006). The relaxation of pelvic joints, caused by the influence of relaxin, may result in backache. Leg cramps also may be experienced.

Neurological System

The client may be euphoric at the beginning of labor. This often changes to seriousness and then to amnesia between contractions during the second stage of labor. Endogenous endorphins (a morphine-like chemical produced naturally by the body) increase the client's pain threshold and have a sedative effect. Pressure on the perineum, by the fetus descending through the birth canal, causes physiologic anesthesia in the perineal tissues.

Pain

The discomfort and pain of labor and birth are individual, subjective, very personal, and have a wide range of expression. Visceral pain usually predominates the first stage of labor, with the stimuli originating in the uterus, cervix, adnexa, and pelvic ligaments. With fetal descent increasing during the late first stage and beginning second stage of labor, the traction and distention on the pelvic structures around the vagina are the primary stimuli for pain. The distention of the perineum is the stimulus for pain during the remainder of the second stage of labor and is transmitted primarily by the pudendal nerves. Figure 56-2 illustrates the intensity and distribution of discomfort during various stages of labor. Stages of labor are discussed later in this chapter.

The softness of pelvic tissues in parous women (women who have delivered at least one child) seems to cause less nociceptive stimuli than in nulliparous women (women who have never delivered a child) during the first stage of labor; however, during the second stage of labor, parous women have increased nociceptive stimuli because of the speed and the intensity of fetal descent. As with pain from any other cause, individuals respond in ways that are acceptable in their culture. Health-care providers must be sensitive to the fact that expression of pain is rooted in cultural heritage.

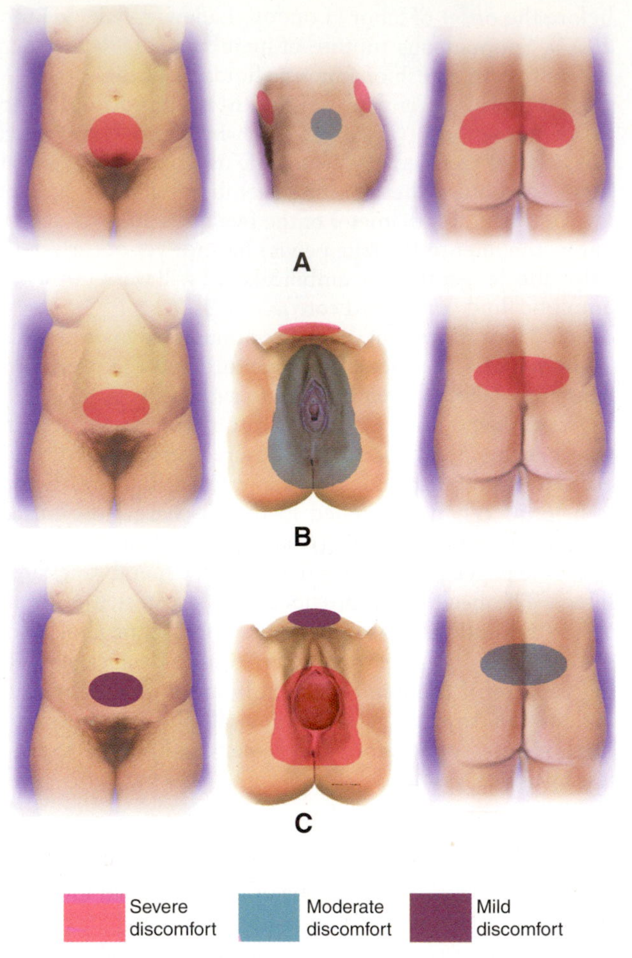

FIGURE 56-2 **Intensity and Distribution of Discomfort during Various Stages of Labor; *A*, First Stage; *B*, Early Second Stage; *C*, Late Second Stage and Birth**

VARIABLES AFFECTING LABOR

There are five major variables that affect labor. They are known as the five Ps: passageway, passenger, position, powers, and psychological response.

Passageway

The passageway consists of the bony pelvis, uterus, cervix, vagina, and perineum.

Pelvis

The size and shape of the true pelvis must be adequate for the fetal head to pass through for a vaginal birth. The CNM/physician uses several methods to determine the adequacy of the true pelvis, such as:

- *Palpation*—Internally, the bony prominences are felt; externally, the distance between the ischial tuberosities is measured and then the distance between the ischial spines estimated.
- *Ultrasound*—An ultrasound is used to estimate pelvic adequacy as well as fetal growth, multiple pregnancy, placenta location, and **fetal presentation**.
- *Pelvimetry*—X-ray of the pelvis is seldom performed during pregnancy because of the radiation involved.

Uterus

The upper part of the uterus (fundus) becomes thicker with contractions and the lower section becomes thinner, forming a tube.

Cervix

The uterine contractions put pressure on the fetus, which in turn puts pressure on the cervix, causing the cervix to efface and dilate. The cervix must dilate and efface sufficiently for the fetus to descend into the vagina.

Vagina

The vagina sustains many changes throughout pregnancy. Various hormones cause an increase in vascularity, loosening of connective tissue, and hypertrophy of the smooth muscle cells. These changes allow the vagina to stretch enough for the fetus to pass through.

Perineum

The pressure of the fetus on the perineum causes stretching and thinning of the perineum.

PASSENGER

The size of the fetus as well as the fetal attitude, fetal lie, fetal presentation, and fetal position affects how easily the fetus can advance through the passage.

Size

The largest part of the fetal body is usually the head. Because the bones of the fetal skull are not fused, the bones can move, sometimes even overlap, as the fetus moves through the mother's bony pelvis. The shaping of the fetal head to adapt to the mother's pelvis during labor is called **molding**.

The major bones of the skull are two frontal bones, two temporal bones, two parietal bones, and the occiput. The bones are joined by thin, fibrous, membrane-covered spaces called **sutures**. Where the sutures meet, there are larger membranous areas called **fontanelles** (Figure 56-3). The largest is the diamond-shaped anterior fontanelle. The posterior fontanelle is triangular and smaller. The care providers can palpate the two fontanelles and the suture connecting them through the cervix and determine fetal position.

Fetal Attitude

Fetal attitude is the relationship of fetal body parts to one another. The ideal attitude of the fetus at term is flexion, with the head flexed onto the chest, the arms flexed over the chest, and the hips and knees flexed on the abdomen. If any part of the fetus is extended, especially the head or the legs, labor is usually more difficult. The attitude is then called extension.

Fetal Lie

The relationship of the cephalocaudal (head to foot) axis of the fetus to the cephalocaudal axis of the mother is called the **fetal lie**. When the fetal cephalocaudal axis is parallel to the mother's, it is called a longitudinal lie. When the fetal cephalocaudal axis is at a right angle to the mother's, it is called a transverse lie (Figure 56-4).

Fetal Presentation

Fetal presentation is determined by the fetal lie and the part of the fetus that enters the pelvis first. The part of the fetus in contact with the cervix is called the **presenting part**. The most common type of presentation is cephalic (head), in 95% of deliveries, with breech (buttocks) being 4%, and shoulder 1% of deliveries (Leifer, 2008) (Figure 56-5).

Cephalic Presentations Cephalic presentations may be further differentiated by the part of the head entering the pelvis first. They may be:

- Vertex—with the occiput as the presenting part
- Brow—with the sinciput as the presenting part
- Face—with the face as the presenting part

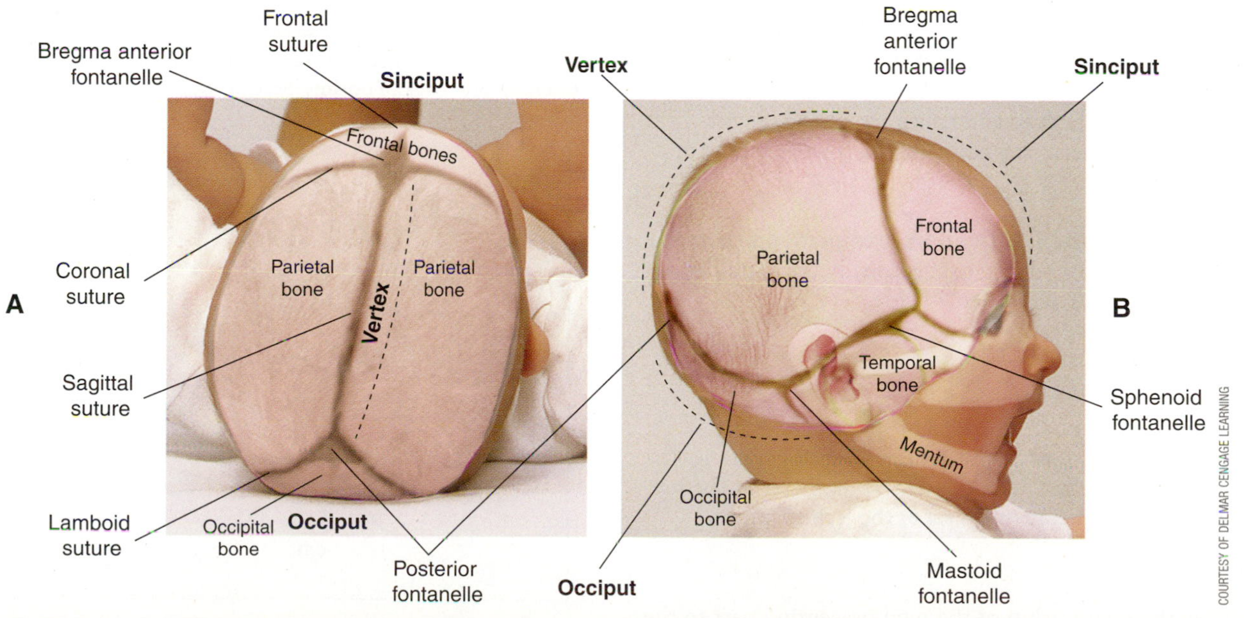

FIGURE 56-3 Fetal Skull—Sutures and Fontanelles; *A*, Superior View; *B*, Lateral View

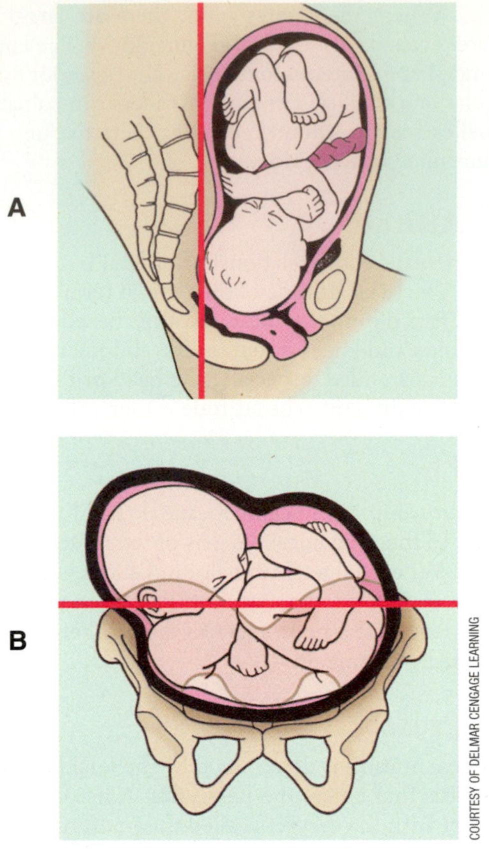

FIGURE 56-4 **Fetal Attitude and Fetal Lie; *A,* Fetal Attitude Flexion, Fetal Lie Longitudinal; *B,* Fetal Attitude Flexion, Fetal Lie Transverse**

Breech Presentations Breech presentations are differentiated by the attitude of the fetus's legs. The various breech presentations are as follows:

- *Complete breech*: Hips and knees are flexed on the abdomen in an attitude of flexion, with the buttocks as the presenting part
- *Frank breech*: The hips are flexed, but the knees are extended with the buttocks as the presenting part
- *Footling breech*: The hips and knees are extended with the foot as the presenting part (may be single footling or double footling)

Shoulder Presentation A shoulder presentation occurs in a transverse lie. The presenting part is usually the shoulder but may be the arm, back, abdomen, or side.

POSITION

Engagement

Engagement is fixation of the fetal presenting part in the maternal true pelvis in which the widest diameter of the presenting part is at or below the level of the ischial spines.

Station

Station is the relationship of the fetal presenting part to the ischial spines. It is measured in centimeters above (−) or below (+) the ischial spines (Figure 56-6).

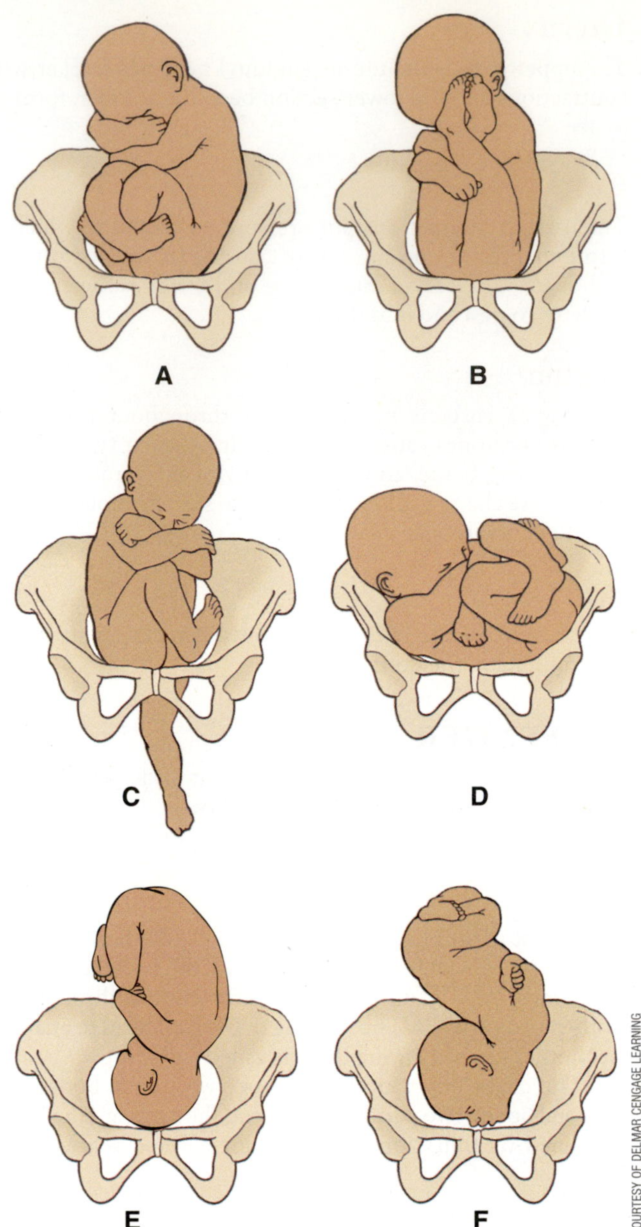

FIGURE 56-5 **Fetal Presentation; *A,* Complete breech; *B,* Frank breech; *C,* Footling breech; *D,* Shoulder; *E,* Vertex; *F,* Face**

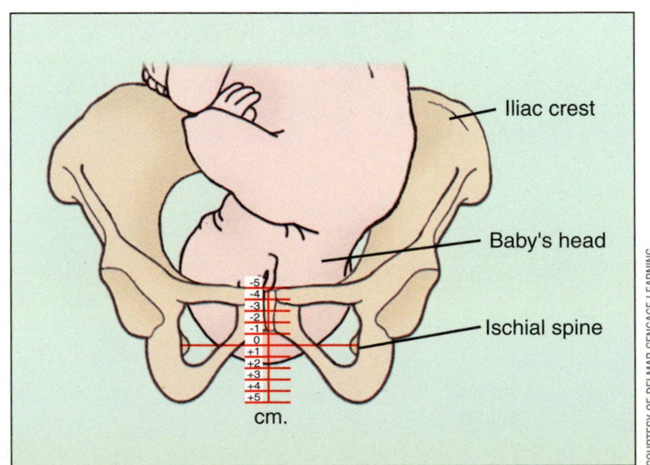

FIGURE 56-6 **Station: Relationship of the fetal presenting part to the ischial spines. The station illustrated is +2.**

Fetal Position

Fetal position refers to the relationship of the identified landmark on the presenting part of the four quadrants of the mother's pelvis (Figure 56-7). The identified landmarks on various presenting parts are shown in Table 56-2.

The brow presentation does not have an identified landmark. The brow usually changes either to a vertex or face presentation. Although the shoulder presentation cannot be delivered vaginally, there is still a landmark designated for it, which is SC (scapula).

There are six possible positions for each presenting part as follows:

- Right occiput anterior (ROA) mentum (RMA) sacrum (RSA)
- Right occiput transverse (ROT) mentum (RMT) sacrum (RST)
- Right occiput posterior (ROP) mentum (RMP) sacrum (RSP)
- Left occiput anterior (LOA) mentum (LMA) sacrum (LSA)
- Left occiput transverse (LOT) mentum (LMT) sacrum (LST)
- Left occiput posterior (LOP) mentum (LMP) sacrum (LSP)

Figure 56-8 illustrates the six positions of a vertex presentation. The same six positions apply to the face and breech presentations. The most common position is LOA, which is considered to be the most favorable for the welfare of both mother and baby.

Powers

The primary power during labor is the involuntary contractions of the uterus, which cause cervical effacement and dilatation during the first stage of labor. The secondary power is the voluntary use of the abdominal muscles by the mother to push or "bear-down" during the second stage of labor to expel the fetus.

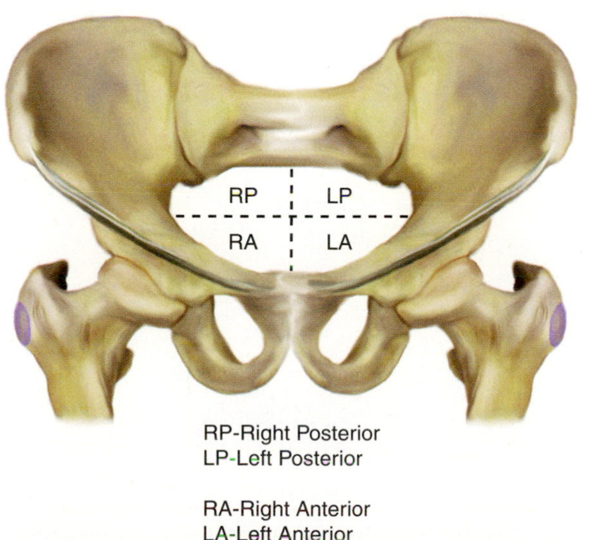

Figure 56-7 Pelvic Quadrants

Table 56-2 Identified Landmarks on Various Presenting Part

PRESENTING PART	IDENTIFIED LANDMARK
Vertex	Occiput (O)
Face	Mentum (M)
Breech (all)	Sacrum (S)

COURTESY OF DELMAR CENGAGE LEARNING

Uterine Contractions

The smooth muscle of the uterus has the ability to contract and relax rhythmically. The relaxation period between contractions allows the muscles and the mother to rest. Uterine relaxation also restores uteroplacental circulation, which is important to fetal oxygenation and effective circulation in the uterus. Contractions begin in the **fundus**, top of the uterus, and spread over the uterus in about 15 seconds (Leifer, 2008).

The muscle fibers of the uterus have the unique property of remaining permanently shortened to a small degree after

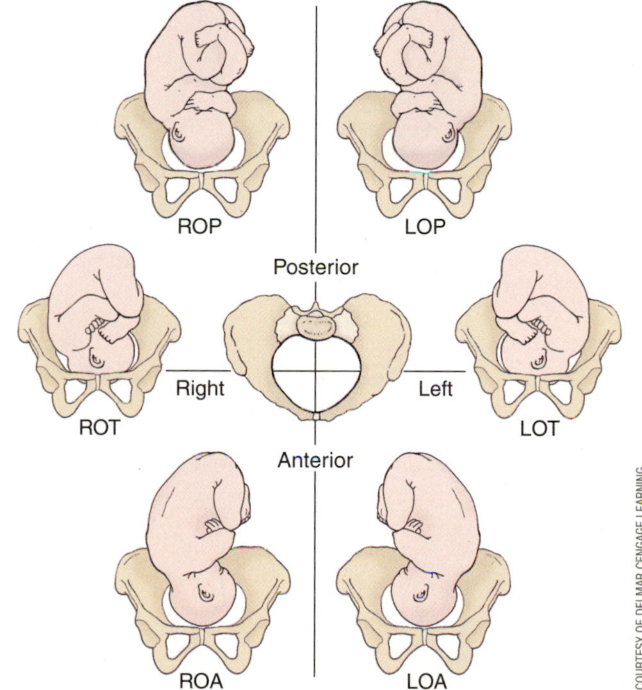

Figure 56-8 Various Positions of a Vertex Presentation

> **PROFESSIONALTIP**
>
> **Fetal Positions**
>
> - The right or left and anterior, posterior, or transverse always refer to the mother's pelvis.
> - The middle word or letter refers to the identified landmark on the fetus, either occiput, mentum, or sacrum.

each contraction. This is called **uterine retraction**. The shortening of the muscle fibers results in a gradual decrease in the uterine cavity size and a thickening of the muscle in the fundus. As the muscle fibers in the fundus retract, the lower uterine segment is pulled up. These two actions efface and dilate the cervix (Figure 56-9).

Each contraction has three phases:

1. **Increment:** increasing intensity of a contraction
2. **Acme:** peak of a contraction
3. **Decrement:** decreasing intensity of a contraction

Contractions are described in terms of frequency, duration, and intensity. **Frequency** is the time from the beginning of one contraction to the beginning of the next contraction. It includes one contraction and one resting period between contractions (**interval**). **Duration** is the length of one contraction, from the beginning of the increment to the conclusion of the decrement. **Intensity** is the strength of the contraction at the acme. Figure 56-10A illustrates these aspects of a contraction while B shows the mother's abdomen before and during a contraction.

The duration of a contraction should not be longer than 90 seconds nor should the interval be less than 60 seconds. The uterus should completely relax between contractions. Contractions lasting longer than 90 seconds reduce uterine and placental circulation because of the prolonged compression of the blood vessels. This in turn compromises the fetus.

Contractions are affected by the mother's position. When the mother lies on her back, the contractions are often more frequent but have less intensity. When she lies on her side, the contractions are usually less frequent but have greater intensity. Thus, a side-lying position improves progress in labor. Lying on the side also prevents supine hypotension syndrome in the mother and improves oxygenation of the uterus, placenta, and fetus because the heavy uterus is not compressing the inferior vena cava.

Maternal Pushing Efforts

Once the cervix has dilated completely, it is time for the fetus to navigate through the remaining mechanisms of labor. The accepted procedure has been for the mother to take a deep breath at the beginning of a contraction, hold her breath, and voluntarily push in a Valsalva-type bearing down throughout a contraction. This pushing technique is directed by the nurses and/or the CNM/physician.

The spontaneous onset of the urge to bear down is triggered when the presenting part reaches the pelvic floor where stretch receptors in the posterior vagina cause the release of oxytocin, which spontaneously increases the pushing sensation. This spontaneous, involuntary urge to bear down is known as **Ferguson's reflex**.

Psychological Response

Psychological response refers to the mother's attitude toward labor and her preparation for labor. The mother's attitude toward labor is shaped by her experiences and expectations. Culture shapes values about and responses to childbirth.

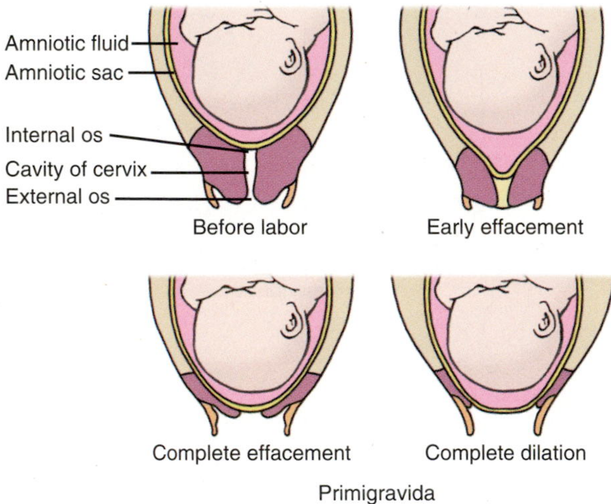

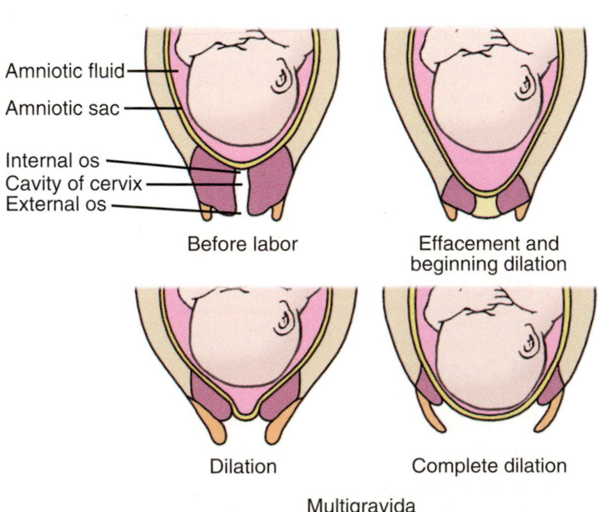

COURTESY OF DELMAR CENGAGE LEARNING

FIGURE 56-9 **Examples of Effacement and Dilation; *A*, Primigravida; *B*, Multigravida**

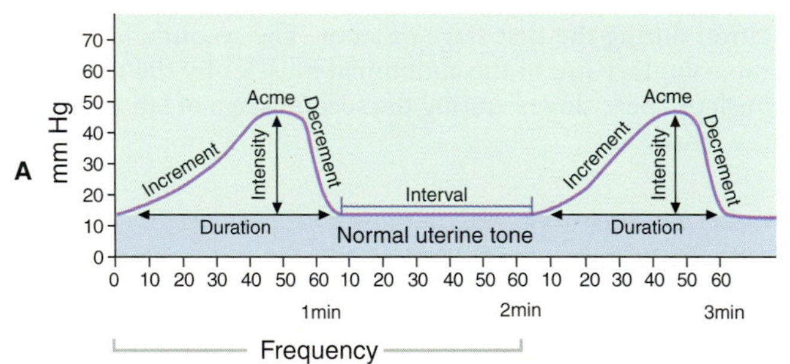

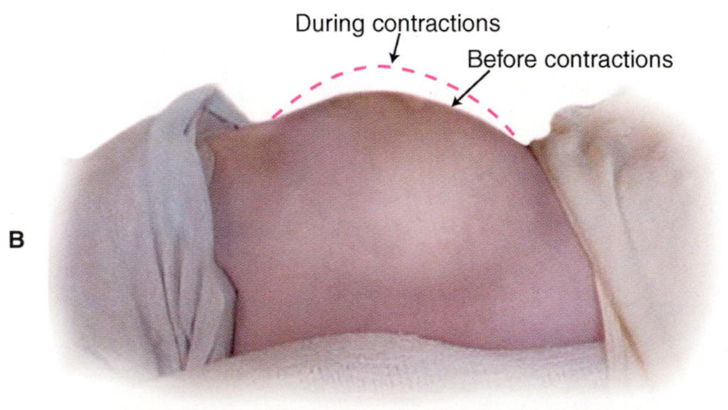

COURTESY OF DELMAR CENGAGE LEARNING

FIGURE 56-10 ***A*, Aspects of a Contraction (frequency 2 minutes, duration 60 seconds, intensity moderate); *B*, Abdominal Contour Before and During a Contraction**

It provides the mother with ideas about how to behave during labor and how to interact with her baby.

Anxiety or fear causes the mother's body to secrete catecholamines, which can suppress uterine contractions and restrict placental blood flow. Relaxation increases the progress of labor. Childbirth preparation classes enhance the mother's ability to work with her body rather than working against it. When a woman has realistic expectations about childbirth, she is more likely to have a positive experience.

STAGES OF LABOR

For many years, labor was divided into three stages. In each of these three stages, specific events can be identified. A fourth stage has been acknowledged as being critical to the birth process: the recovery period after the birth of the baby. This chapter discusses four stages of labor. Table 56-3 presents an overview of the average duration of the first two stages. Stages 1 and 2 vary in average length for primigravida clients and multigravida clients. Stages 3 and 4 are approximately the same length for all clients and are not included in this table.

First Stage: Dilation and Effacement

The first stage of labor begins with the onset of regular contractions and ends when **cervical dilation**, the enlargement of the cervical opening (os), is complete (10 cm). This is usually the longest stage of labor and is divided into three phases: latent, active, and transition.

Latent Phase

The latent phase of the first stage of labor ends when the cervix is dilated 3 cm and is the longest phase. Contractions occur every 10 to 20 minutes. The duration of the contractions lasts 15 to 30 seconds. The contraction intensity begins as mild and gradually becomes moderate.

The client is usually alert and often talkative. She is often relieved that labor has started yet anxious about what is ahead of her. This is a good time to review the client's preparations for labor and expectations of how labor and delivery will be handled (e.g., medications, persons present). Any needed teaching, especially breathing techniques, should be undertaken at this time. If the membranes have not ruptured, many women prefer to walk during this time.

Active Phase

The active phase of the first stage of labor begins when the cervix is dilated 4 cm and ends when the cervix is dilated 8 cm. Contractions occur every 3 to 5 minutes with a duration of 30 to 60 seconds. They are of moderate intensity, progressing to strong. Clients perceive varying degrees of discomfort. The client now focuses more on the breathing techniques during contractions and is less talkative.

Transition Phase

The transition phase of the first stage of labor begins when the cervix is dilated 8 cm and ends when the cervix is dilated 10 cm. Contractions occur every 2 to 3 minutes with a duration of 60 to 90 seconds. There is little rest for the client between contractions. The intensity of the contractions is strong. The client usually needs to be reminded to focus, relax, and breathe with each contraction. She is very aware of the increasing intensity of the contractions, may become very restless, and may fear being left alone. Requests for medication often accompany statements like "I can't take it anymore." Following are characteristics of the transition phase:

- Restlessness
- Hyperventilation
- Bewilderment and sometimes anger
- Difficulty following directions
- Focus on self
- Irritability
- Statements like "Don't touch me"
- Nausea, occasionally vomiting
- Very warm feeling
- Perspiration on upper lip
- Increasing rectal pressure

Second Stage: Birth of Baby

The second stage of labor begins when cervical dilation is complete (10 cm) and ends with the birth of the baby. Contractions continue at a frequency of every 1 to 2 minutes, duration of 60 to 90 seconds, and strong intensity. Now that the

Table 56-3 Average Length of Labor Stages 1 and 2

	FIRST STAGE			
CHARACTERISTIC	LATENT PHASE	ACTIVE PHASE	TRANSITION PHASE	SECOND STAGE
Primigravida	8 to 20 hours	6 hours	2 hours	1 hour
Multigravida	5-14 hours	4 hours	1 hour	15 minutes
Cervical dilation	0 to 3 cm	4 to 8 cm	8 to 10 cm	10 cm (full dilation)
Contractions				
Frequency	10 to 20 minutes	3 to 5 minutes	2 to 3 minutes	1 to 2 minutes
Duration	15 to 30 seconds	30 to 60 seconds	60 to 90 seconds	60 to 90 seconds
Intensity	Mild progressing to moderate	Moderate progressing to strong	Strong	Strong

COURTESY OF DELMAR CENGAGE LEARNING

SAFETY

Use of Stirrups during Birth

Clients who are delivering in a modified lithotomy position may have their feet placed in stirrups to open the pelvis and facilitate access to the perineum.

- Stirrup height and lower leg length must be adjusted for each client.
- Both legs must be raised into the stirrups at the same time to prevent strain on the pelvic ligaments.

cervix is completely dilated, the mother can actively assist in the descent of the fetus by contracting the abdominal muscles and bearing down with each contraction. This active participation in the process often gives her a sense of control.

As the fetal head descends, it puts pressure on the pelvic nerves and the mother has a greater desire to push. Pressure from the fetal head makes the perineum bulge, then flatten and move anteriorly. With each contraction, the labia begin to separate and the baby's head is seen, but the head recedes between contractions. When the largest diameter of the fetal head is past the vulva (head can be seen between contractions), **crowning** has occurred and the birth is imminent (Figure 56-11). At this time, an **episiotomy**, an incision in the perineum to facilitate passage of the baby, may be performed (Figure 56-12). Routine episiotomies are no longer considered necessary, but in some cases, it is still warranted (CDC, 2008). The health-care provider may recommend an episiotomy if the baby is in an abnormal position, needs to be delivered quickly, or it appears that extensive vaginal tearing is going to occur. A few more contractions will push the head out, and a few more will deliver the body.

As the fetus moves through the pelvis and birth canal, several changes in position must occur. This series of movements is collectively called the mechanisms of labor or **cardinal movements**.

Mechanisms of Labor

The mechanisms of labor are engagement, descent, flexion, internal rotation, extension, external rotation, and expulsion

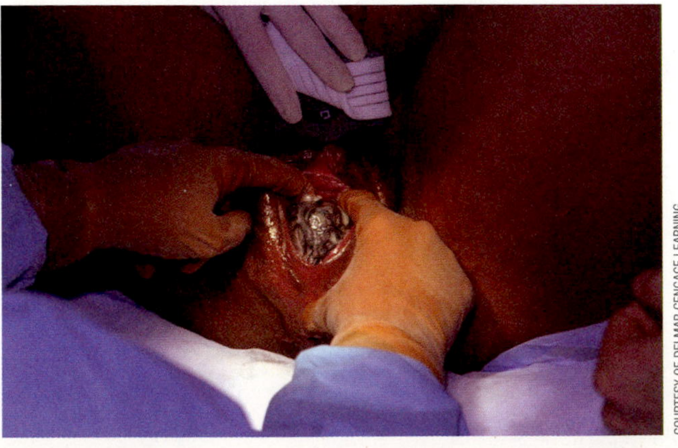

FIGURE 56-11 Crowning

CLIENT TEACHING

Effective Pushing in Upright or Squatting Position

The mother can push more effectively if she:

- Flexes her chin on her chest and bends over her uterus.
- With elbows *bent*, pulls on her flexed knees.
- Exhales and vocalizes when pushing.

(Figure 56-13). The first three generally occur during the first stage of labor.

Engagement As explained earlier, engagement occurs when the presenting part of the fetus (usually head) fully enters the true pelvis. It generally happens before labor begins in primigravidas and after labor begins in multigravidas.

Descent Descent begins with engagement and continues with each contraction throughout the labor process.

Flexion The fetal head is bent forward as it meets resistance during descent, causing the chin to rest on the sternum. This allows the narrowest part of the head to enter the pelvic outlet.

Inernal Rotation Internal rotation takes place mainly during the second stage of labor. The head rotates so the occiput is next to the symphysis pubis.

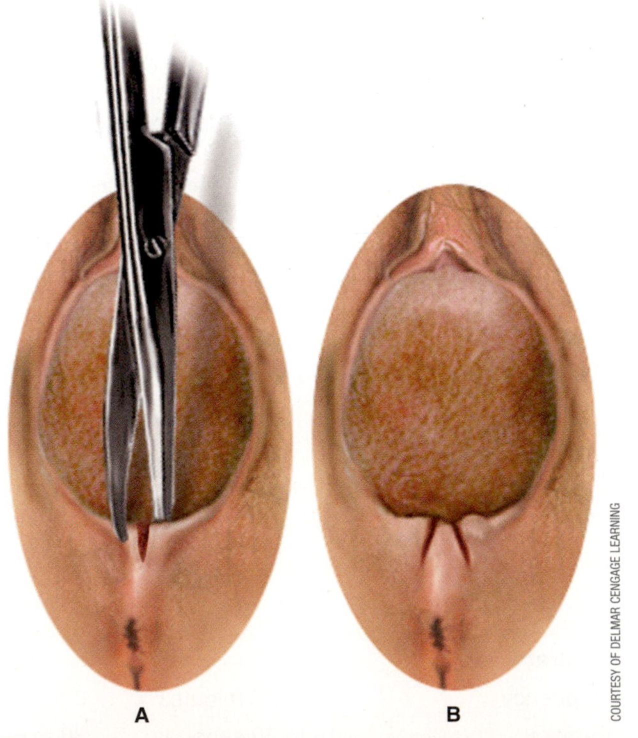

FIGURE 56-12 Episiotomy; *A*, Midline, Most Common, Directly toward Anus; *B*, Right and Left Mediolateral, Diagonal Cut toward the Side to Prevent Tearing into the Rectum

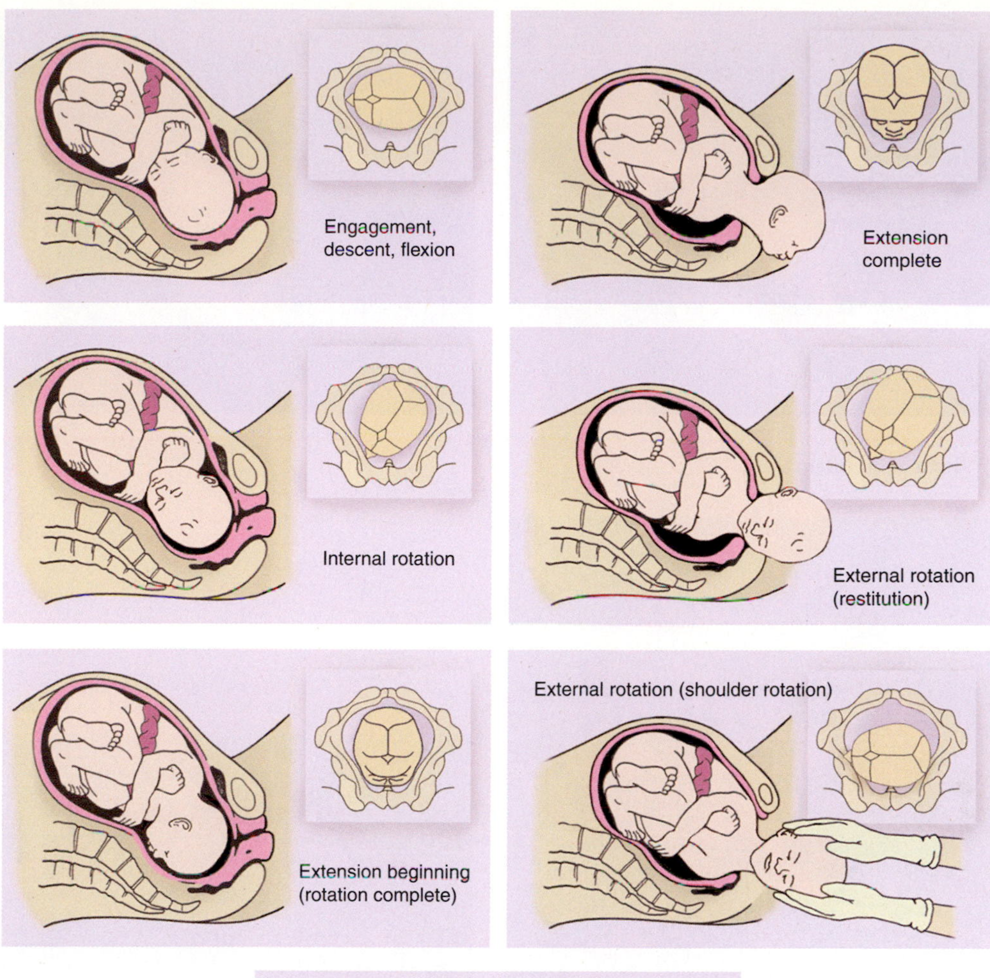

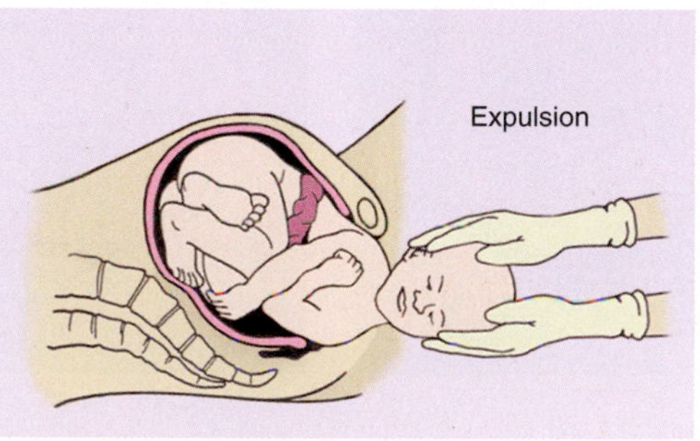

COURTESY OF DELMAR CENGAGE LEARNING

FIGURE 56-13 Mechanisms of Labor

Extension As the fetal head continues to descend, the occiput pivots under the symphysis pubis and the fetal head becomes extended and pushes upward out of the vagina. The head is actually born at this time.

Restitution and External Rotation Once the head has emerged, it rotates back to be in normal alignment with the shoulders. This is called **restitution**. Fetal position in the uterus can be identified by observing this turning of the head. The shoulders now rotate to be in an anteroposterior position under the symphysis pubis.

Expulsion The health-care provider assisting with the birth applies gentle downward pressure on the baby's head to allow the anterior shoulder to emerge. Then the baby's head is gently raised so the posterior shoulder can be delivered. The rest of the baby's body then just slides out. This is called expulsion (Figure 56-14).

THIRD STAGE: DELIVERY OF PLACENTA

The third stage of labor begins with the birth of the baby and ends with the delivery of the placenta. This should occur in 5 to 30 minutes. After the baby is born, the uterus continues contracting, decreasing its capacity and thereby reducing the surface area of placental attachment. The reduced surface area causes the placenta to separate from the uterine wall. As it separates, bleeding occurs, causing the formation of a retroplacental (behind the placenta) hematoma. This hematoma facilitates the separation process. The membranes are peeled from the uterine wall as the placenta slides into the vagina.

Signs that the placenta has separated should be observed about 5 to 10 minutes after the birth of the baby. These signs are:

- Globular shape of the uterus.

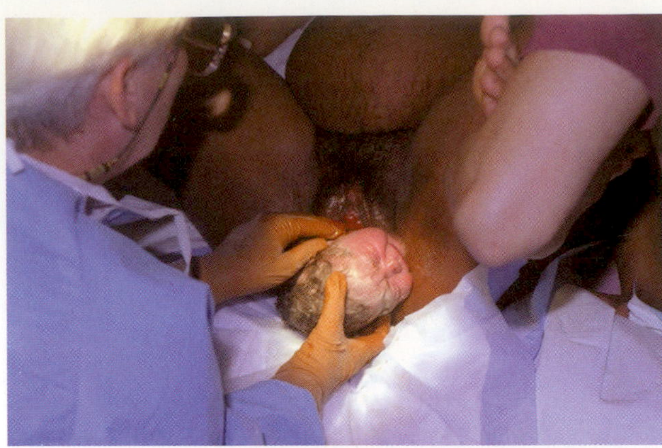

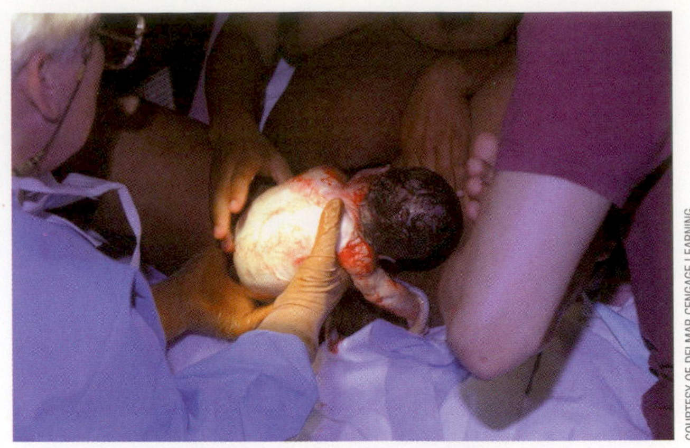

COURTESY OF DELMAR CENGAGE LEARNING

FIGURE 56-14 Birth of an Infant

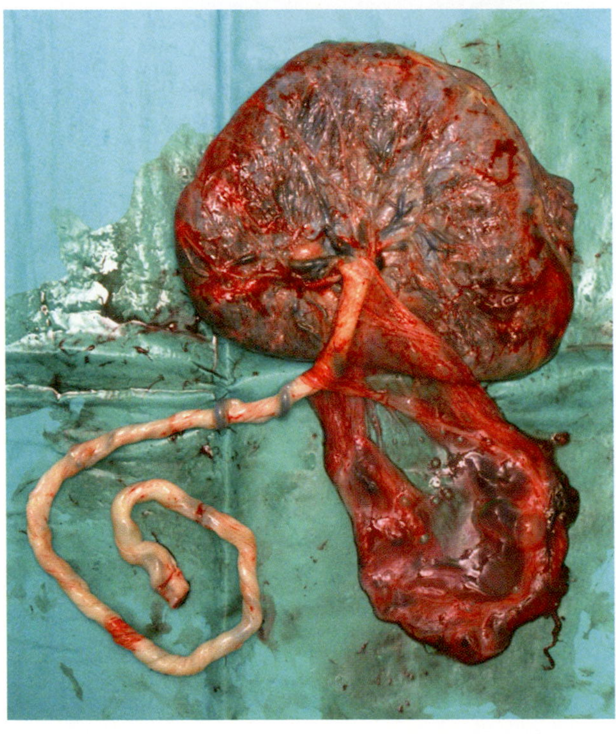

A

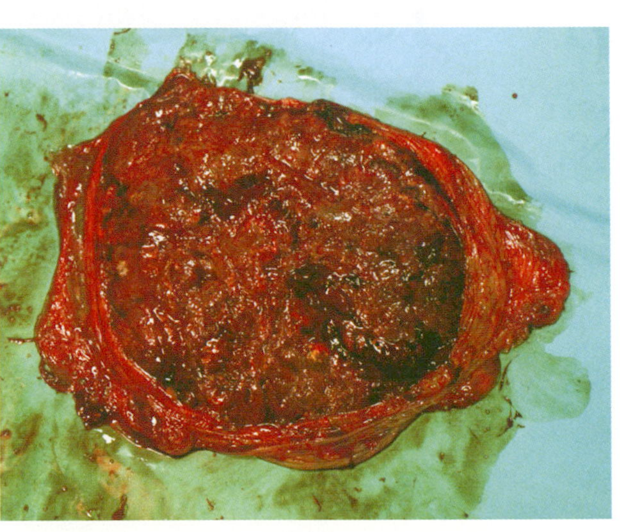

B

COURTESY OF DELMAR CENGAGE LEARNING

FIGURE 56-15 *A,* Fetal Side (note empty amniotic sac); *B,* Maternal Side

- Gush of blood from the vagina.
- More of the cord protrudes from the vagina (is visible).

When these signs of placental separation have appeared, the client is asked to push one last time to deliver the placenta. Figure 56-15 shows a placenta.

The birthing facility disposes of the placenta after the delivery. Occasionally, a client may request to have the placenta to uphold cultural expectations.

FOURTH STAGE: RECOVERY

The fourth stage of labor is the first 4 hours after the birth of the baby when the mother's body begins its physiological readjustments. Blood loss is usually between 250 mL and 500 mL. There is a moderate decrease in the systolic and diastolic blood pressure and an increase in pulse rate. The uterus should remain contracted to control bleeding and be positioned in the midline of the abdomen about level with the umbilicus.

The new mother may be very hungry and thirsty. A shaking chill may be experienced in response to the ending of the physical work of labor. The bladder may be hypotonic due either to trauma during the second stage of labor and/or to decreased sensation from anesthesia. This may result in urinary retention. Mother–infant bonding is important in this stage.

CRITICAL THINKING

Care Throughout Labor

How and why does the care of the client change as she moves through the phases and stages of labor?

PROFESSIONALTIP

Prenatal Care and Childbirth Classes

- The client who has not had prenatal care or has not attended childbirth classes deserves the same care, support, and respect as the client who has had prenatal care and is prepared for childbirth.
- Nurses must be careful not to be judgmental toward clients who have not participated in prenatal care or childbirth classes.

CULTURAL CONSIDERATIONS

Client Beliefs

Most people believe that their own cultural beliefs are the best. The birth experience is given meaning by the client's cultural beliefs and practices. Incorporate cultural practices into care as much as possible as long as they are not detrimental to mother or fetus.

ADMISSION OF CLIENT IN LABOR

Admission of a client in labor may be different for each person. Although there are standard nursing assessments and interventions for a woman in labor, each client must be cared for individually based on her particular situation. The priorities of establishing a nurse– client relationship and assessing the condition of mother and fetus may be undertaken in a sequential order or may need to be performed simultaneously.

It is important to determine which stage of labor the mother may be in at the time of admission. A few specific questions might include the following:

- When did your labor begin?
- How frequent are the contractions and how long do they last?
- Have the membranes ruptured? (Has your water broken?)
- What time did the membranes rupture?
- What was the color was the fluid?
- How many times have you been pregnant?
- How long were your other labors (if this is not the first pregnancy)?

Depending on the answers to these questions, a determination is made about how to proceed with the admission. When a woman is admitted in early labor, time can be taken to establish the nurse–client relationship by:

- Making the woman and her partner or family feel welcome
- Determining their expectations about the birth (did they attend childbirth classes?)
- Determining if a birth plan has been developed

Hollister

Obstetric Admitting Record
Hollister Maternal/Newborn Record System — Page 1 of 2
To order call: 1.800.323.4060 — Re-order No. 5710

Basic Admission Data Date ___/___/___ Time ______
☐ Ambulatory ☐ Stretcher ☐ Oriented to Unit
☐ Wheelchair ☐ Transfer From ______ ☐ Safety/Security
G | T | Pt | A | L | LMP / / | EDD / / | Wks | EDD By Fetal Assessment / /
Race/Ethnicity ______ Age ______
Advance Directives ☐ None ☐ Living Will ☐ Medical Power of Attorney
Organ Donor ☐ Yes ☐ No
Last Oral Intake
Fluids ___/___/___ Time ______
Solids ___/___/___ Time ______
Medications ☐ None
Type/Dose | Last Taken | With Patient No Yes | Disposition
MD/CNM | Tel No | Support Person/Relationship | Tel No

Allergies/Sensitivities ☐ None
☐ Medication ______
☐ Other ______
Reasons for Admission
☐ Onset of Labor
☐ Induction of Labor
☐ Spontaneous Abortion
☐ Cesarean Section ☐ Primary ☐ Repeat (reason for primary ______)
☐ Tubal Ligation
☐ Vaginal Bleeding
☐ ROM ☐ Premature ☐ Prolonged
☐ Preterm Labor
Detail Reasons for Admission ______
Observation Evaluation
☐ Fetal Status ☐ Ultrasound ☐ Amniocentesis ☐ NST ☐ CST
☐ Medical Complications
☐ Obstetric Complications
Personal Effects | Item | Disposition: With Patient | With Support Person | Other (Describe)

Patient Triage Data ☐ See Triage Record
Contractions ☐ None ☐ Palpation ☐ Tocotransducer
Frequency ______ Duration ______ Intensity ______
Began on ___/___/___ Time ______
Membranes ☐ Intact ☐ Bulging
☐ Ruptured (Date ___/___/___ Time ______)
☐ Nitrazine test (☐ pos ☐ neg) ☐ Sterile Speculum Exam
☐ Fern test (☐ pos ☐ neg) (findings ______)
Fluid ☐ Clear ☐ Bloody ☐ Meconium Stained ☐ Foul Odor ☐ No Foul Odor ☐ None Observed
Vaginal Bleeding ☐ None ☐ Normal Show ☐ Bleeding (Describe ______)
Cervical Exam By ______
Station ______ Effacement ______ Dilatation ______ cms
Presentation ☐ Vertex ☐ Face/Brow ☐ Breech (type ______) ☐ Transverse Lie ☐ Compound ☐ Unknown

Physical Assessment
Height | Wt Pregrav/Grav | Temp | Pulse | Resp | BP
System (Normal / Abnormal) — Detail Abnormal Findings
HEENT, Neurologic, Skin, Breasts, Extremities, Cardiovascular, Respiratory, Abdomen, Gastrointestinal, Urinary, Genitalia
Initial Problems Identified ☐ None | Plan
1. 2. 3.

Fetal Evaluation Data Multiple Gestation ☐ No ☐ Yes
Fundal Height ______ cms
Fetal Weight (est.) ______
FHR ______
☐ Fetoscope ☐ Fetal Monitor ☐ Doppler ☐ Other ______
Presentation | Position: 1. 2. 3.

Specimens Obtained (Check all that apply)

Urine Test	Time	Results	Blood Test	Time	Results
☐ Urinalysis			☐ Hgb		
☐ C + S			☐ Hct		
☐ Glucose			☐ VDRL/RPR		
☐ Albumin			☐ Type/Screen		
☐ Ketones			☐		
☐ pH			Cervical Culture		
☐ Blood			☐ GBS		
☐ Toxicology			☐		

Admitting Signature | Date/Time | Examiner Signature | Date/Time

Hollister

Obstetric Admitting Record
Hollister Maternal/Newborn Record System — Page 2 of 2
To order call: 1.800.323.4060 — Re-order No. 5710

Significant Prenatal Data
Prenatal Records Available on Admission ☐ No ☐ Yes Source ______
First Visit by 13 Wks ☐ Yes ☐ No
Regular Care ☐ Yes ☐ No
Prenatal Classes ☐ Yes ☐ No
Pediatric Provider
Lab Findings ☐ None: Blood Type & Rh, Rubella Titer, Serology, HBsAg, HIV, GBS
Fetal Assessment Tests ☐ None: Date | Test | Result
Problems Identified ☐ None — Active / Resolved: 1. 2. 3. 4.
Hospitalizations ☐ None: 1. / / Reason ______ 2. / / Reason ______
General Health ☐ Healthy
☐ Recent Exposure to Communicable Disease Type/Date ______ ___/___/___
☐ Illness (≤ 14 days prior to admission) Type/Treatment ______
☐ Chronic Condition Type ______
Nutritional Status ☐ Well-nourished ☐ Malnourished ☐ Obese
☐ Special Diet ______
Eating Disorder ☐ None ☐ Identify ______
Nutritional Problems ☐ None ☐ Identify ______
Plans for Birth and Hospital Stay ☐ Birth Plan Attached
Support Person Present in L&D ☐ No ☐ Yes ______
Other Family Members in L&D ☐ No ☐ Yes ______
Anesthesia ☐ None ☐ Local ☐ Epidural ☐ Spinal ☐ General
Delivery Site/Position ______
Personal Requests ______
Adoption ☐ No ☐ Yes Contact with Infant ☐ No ☐ Yes
Adoption Contact ______
Feeding Preference ☐ Breast ☐ Bottle
☐ Tubal Ligation Authorization Signed ☐ Yes ☐ No
☐ Circumcision Authorization Signed ☐ Yes ☐ No

Psychosocial Data ☐ See Prenatal Records
Emotional Status ☐ Happy ☐ Ambivalent ☐ Concerned ☐ Depressed ☐ Angry ☐ Other ______
Communication Barriers ☐ None
☐ Language ☐ Interpreter ______
☐ Vision ☐ Reading ☐ Writing ☐ Hearing
☐ Speech ☐ Other ______
Support System
Marital Status: S M Sep D W Father involved ☐ Yes ☐ No
Other Support ☐ None ☐ ______
Occupation ______ Education ______
Religion ☐ N/A ☐ ______
Personal/Cultural/Religious Customs Affecting Care and/or Learning ☐ None ☐ Identify ______
Basic Needs Met (Yes / No) If No, Explain: Food, Clothing, Housing, Transportation, Finances
Life Stress (No / Yes) If Yes, Explain: Physical Abuse, Emotional Abuse
Life Stress(Cont.) (No / Yes) If Yes, Explain: Major Change, Self Care Needs, Serious Illness, Other ______
Substance Use (No / Yes) If Yes, amt/day, last use: Tobacco, Alcohol, Prescribed Drugs, Illicit Drugs
Educational Needs — Mother | Support Person | Comments: Stages/Phases of Labor, Coping Techniques, Infant Feeding, Infant Care, ______
Preferred Learning Methods (Yes / No): One-on-One Instruction, Group Instruction, Written Information, Audio/Visual Information, Demonstration/Practice, Other ______

Discharge Planning Data Planned Length of Stay ______ Days
Home Setting (Yes / No): Heat, running water, refrigeration; Infant Care Supplies/Car Seat; Phone in home; Transportation available; Adult assistance available
Referrals ☐ RN Case Manager ☐ Utilization Review ☐ Other ☐ Home Care RN ☐ Social Service ☐ Nutritionist/Dietician ☐ Pediatric Provider
MD/CNM notified by ______ Date ___/___/___ Time ______
Admitting Signature ______ Date ___/___/___ Time ______

FIGURE 56-16 Representative Obstetric Admitting Record (*Permission to use this copyright material has been granted by the owner, Hollister Incorporated.*)

- Identifying cultural values and preferences related to the birth process

Initial Assessment

After the nurse–client relationship has been established on admission, more specific assessments are made. Figure 56-16 shows a sample obstetric admitting record. Many facilities are changing to electronic client records. These records may be initiated in the health-care provider's office and are transferred to the nursing unit upon admission to the hospital. A copy of the prenatal record is generally sent to the birthing facility and is added to the client's record when she is admitted. Information can be obtained from the prenatal record. Clients who have not received prenatal care will need a more extensive assessment.

A physical examination is performed, including the following:

- Vital signs.
- Auscultation of heart and lungs.
- Leopold's maneuvers (described in Prenatal Care chapter) to determine fetal lie and presentation.
- Fetal heart rate (FHR) (described in Prenatal Care chapter), continuous electronic fetal monitoring may be used during the birthing process (described in Complications of Pregnancy chapter).
- Contractions for frequency, duration, and intensity.
- Nitrazine test, ferning test, Amnisure, or Aminoswab test if mother is not sure whether the membranes have ruptured.
- Vaginal examination (Figure 56-17) to determine cervical effacement and dilation, fetal position, and station; usually done by the registered nurse (RN) or CNM/physician.
- Inspection for signs of edema of face, hands, legs, and sacrum.

The FHR may be heard in various places on the mother's abdomen depending on the position of the fetus (Figure 56-18).

Contractions are assessed by placing the fingers of one hand on the fundus of the uterus, and using light pressure to

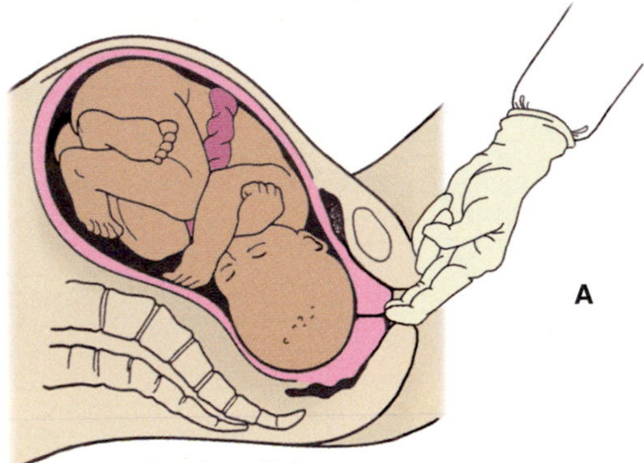

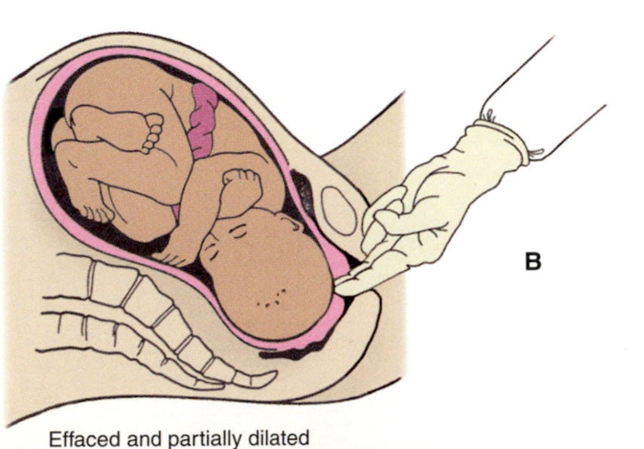

Figure 56-17 Vaginal Examination; *A*, 50% Effaced, No Dilation; *B*, 100% Effaced, Partly Dilated

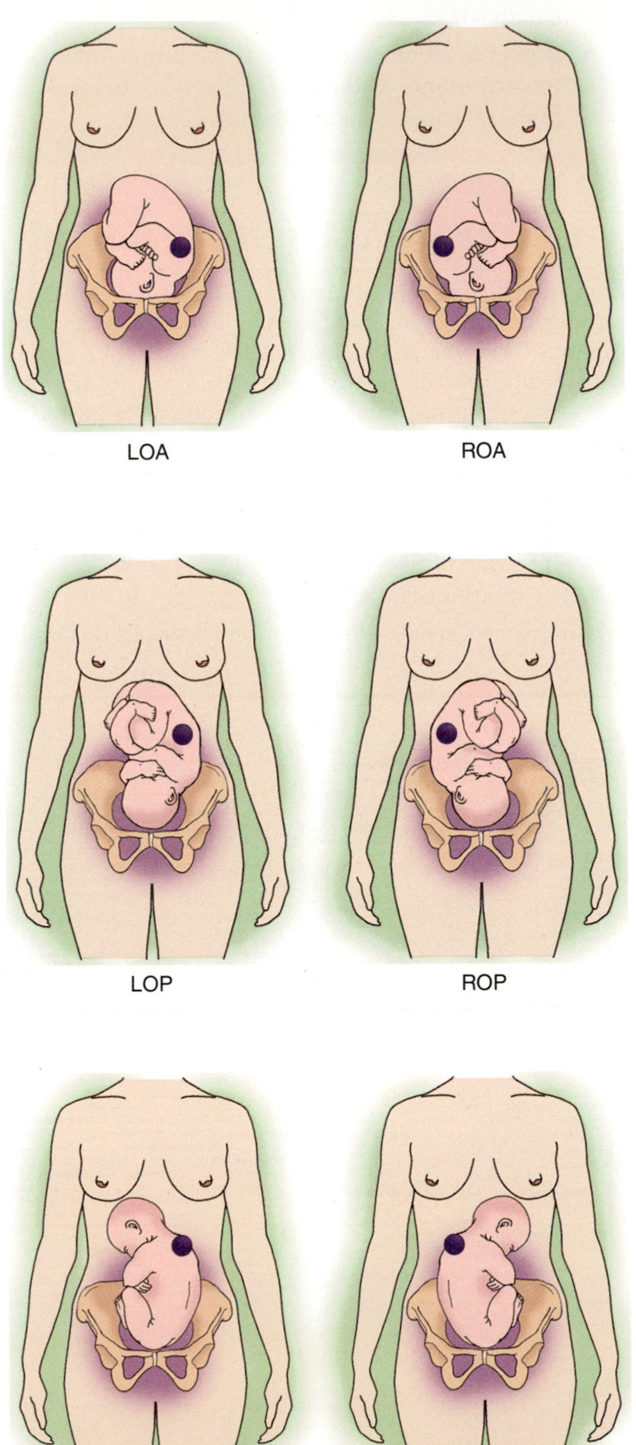

Figure 56-18 Based on Leopold's maneuvers, FHR will best be heard in the marked areas for the various positions.

INFECTION CONTROL

Standard Precautions

- Disposable gloves should be worn any time hands might come in contact with amniotic fluid, blood, bloody show, urine, or feces.
- Wear a splash apron and eye covering (goggles or face mask) when the splashing of body fluids is possible.
- Wash hands before putting on gloves and immediately after removing them.

keep the fingers still. Contractions begin in the fundus and spread down the uterus. The person assessing the contractions can feel the tightening of the uterus before the mother is aware of it.

At least three contractions in a row should be assessed. The time each contraction begins and ends and the time lapse between contractions should be noted. The intensity can be estimated by how easily the uterus can be indented during a contraction.

- *Mild contraction*: Uterus is easily indented with the fingertips; feels like the tip of the nose.
- *Moderate contraction*: Uterus is more difficult to indent with the fingertips; feels similar to the chin.
- *Strong contraction*: Uterus unable to be indented with the fingertips; feels like the forehead.

PROFESSIONALTIP

Intrapartum Care for Obese Women

Obesity in pregnant women during the intrapartum period can challenge nursing management. Special nursing care and preparation during birthing for obese clients includes:

- Maintaining a nonjudgmental attitude.
- Assessing the client for underlying medical conditions.
- Coordinating multidisciplinary care involving CNM/physicians, anesthesia providers, and nursing staff.
- Determining if the unit's furniture and equipment are appropriate and safe for obese clients.
- Evaluating equipment for size and weight limits (beds, operating tables, commodes, blood pressure cuffs, gowns, walkers, scales, wheel chairs, transfer devices, external fetal monitoring equipment and belts, and intermittent pneumatic compression devices).
- Assessing availability of extra staff nurses to assist in moving and positioning of client during certain procedures (amniotomy, analgesia, and pushing).

(James & Maher, 2009)

NURSING PROCESS

The nurse is an important member of the team that helps the mother successfully progress through the birth experience.

Assessment

The nurse's role begins with a thorough assessment of the laboring woman and her progress.

Subjective Data

Subjective data to be gathered throughout labor and birth of the infant include the comfort of the mother, her ability to cope, and her desire to urinate or defecate.

Objective Data

Objective data include vital signs; FHR; frequency, duration, interval, and intensity of contractions; fetopelvic relationships, including fetal attitude, fetal lie, fetal presentation, and station; condition of membranes; maternal behavior, including tone of voice and facial expressions; and maternal verbalizations. Table 56-4 provides suggested time frames for selected assessments.

Nursing Diagnoses

Many different nursing diagnoses may be appropriate for a client during labor and the birthing process. Selected nursing diagnoses appropriate for the first three stages of labor are listed.

- ***A**nxiety*
- *Impaired Verbal **C**ommunication*
- *Ineffective **C**oping*
- *Interrupted **F**amily Processes*
- ***F**atigue*
- ***F**ear*
- *Risk for Deficient **F**luid Volume*
- ***G**as Exchange Impaired (fetal)*
- *Risk for **I**nfection*
- *Risk for **I**njury*
- *Deficient **K**nowledge*
- *Acute **P**ain*

PROFESSIONALTIP

Station

- It is often a challenge to remember the notations of station.
- Remember, plus (+) is what is desired; the presenting part is below the level of the ischial spines. Minus (–) means the presenting part is not yet to the level of the ischial spines.

TABLE 56-4 Suggested Time Frames for Selected Assessments

ASSESSMENT	LATENT PHASE	ACTIVE PHASE	TRANSITION PHASE	SECOND STAGE
BP, P, R	every 1 h	every 1 h	every 30 min	every 5 min
Temperature	every 4 h	every 4 h	every 4 h	
(if ROM)	every 2 h	every 2 h	every 2 h	
FHR	every 1 h	every 30 min	every 15 min	every 15 min
Contractions	every 1 h	every 30 min	every 15 min	continuously

COURTESY OF DELMAR CENGAGE LEARNING

- *Impaired **P**hysical Mobility*
- ***S**ocial Isolation*
- *Impaired **U**rinary Elimination*

Planning/Outcome Identification

Based on the client's expectations of labor and the birthing process and the assessments performed by the facility staff, the planning and goals can be mutually set by the client and the nurse. Examples of possible goals may include that the client will:

- Demonstrate expected progress through labor
- Express satisfaction with the assistance provided by her support person and facility staff
- Maintain adequate hydration with oral and/or IV intake
- Void at least every 2 hours to prevent bladder distention
- Actively participate in the labor process
- Not experience any injury during the labor and birthing process

Nursing Interventions

Nursing interventions focus on continuing assessment of labor progress and fetal well-being, providing maternal physical care, assisting the client and her support person, and providing or assisting with pharmacologic comfort measures.

Continuing Assessment of Labor and Fetal Well-Being

Continuing assessment of labor progress and fetal well-being is performed as previously discussed. Any changes outside the normally expected changes must be reported immediately. Some facilities use continuous electronic fetal monitoring on all clients; however, the nurse should still personally assess and time contractions and listen to the FHR at regular intervals. Figure 56-19 presents a sample labor in progress record.

Providing Maternal Physical Care

Maternal physical care includes comfort measures, hygiene measures, ambulation and position, food and fluid intake, and elimination.

Comfort Measures Many comfort measures can be used with the client in labor. Some may work with one client and not the next, or may work for a while with one client and then she will not want that comfort measure used any more. Comfort measures include the following:

- Offer the client fluids and ice chips as ordered per institutional policy
- Provide oral care
- Assist the client with frequent position changes, encouraging side-lying or upright positions
- Encourage voluntary relaxation of specific muscle groups and the use of effleurage
- Suggest the use of a cold washcloth on the forehead or nape of the neck
- Provide encouragement and praise
- Keep the client informed of progress
- Palpate for bladder distention and encourage urination every 2 hours
- Give a back rub or apply counterpressure to the sacrococcygeal area
- Assist the client in walking and using a shower or Jacuzzi.
- Offer the client analgesics as ordered
- Offer the client complementary therapies such as aromatherapy, massage, use of birth balls, hydrotherapy, and music therapy (Zwelling, Johnson, & Allen, 2006)

Hygiene Measures If showers or jacuzzis are available and are not contraindicated for the client, their use should be offered to the client. The discomfort of labor is often reduced by these measures. Bed linens should be kept clean and dry. Linen savers should be changed frequently.

Ambulation and Position Ambulation may increase uterine activity, provide distraction from the discomforts of labor, and enhance maternal control of the situation. The client should be encouraged to walk only if the membranes are still intact, the presenting part is engaged after ROM, and if she has not had pain medication.

The side-lying position promotes utero-placental blood flow (and thus fetal oxygenation) and renal blood flow. If the client wants to lie on her back, a pillow can be placed under one hip to keep the uterus from compressing the aorta and vena cava. Both the squatting position and the hands-and-knees position seem to facilitate an occiput posterior fetal position to rotate to an anterior position.

Food and Fluid Intake Clear liquids and ice chips are usually all that is offered to clients in labor. Because regional anesthesia has almost replaced general anesthesia in childbirth, the risk of aspiration is also almost eliminated, and the practice of giving clear liquids only is being challenged (Lowdermilk & Perry, 2006).

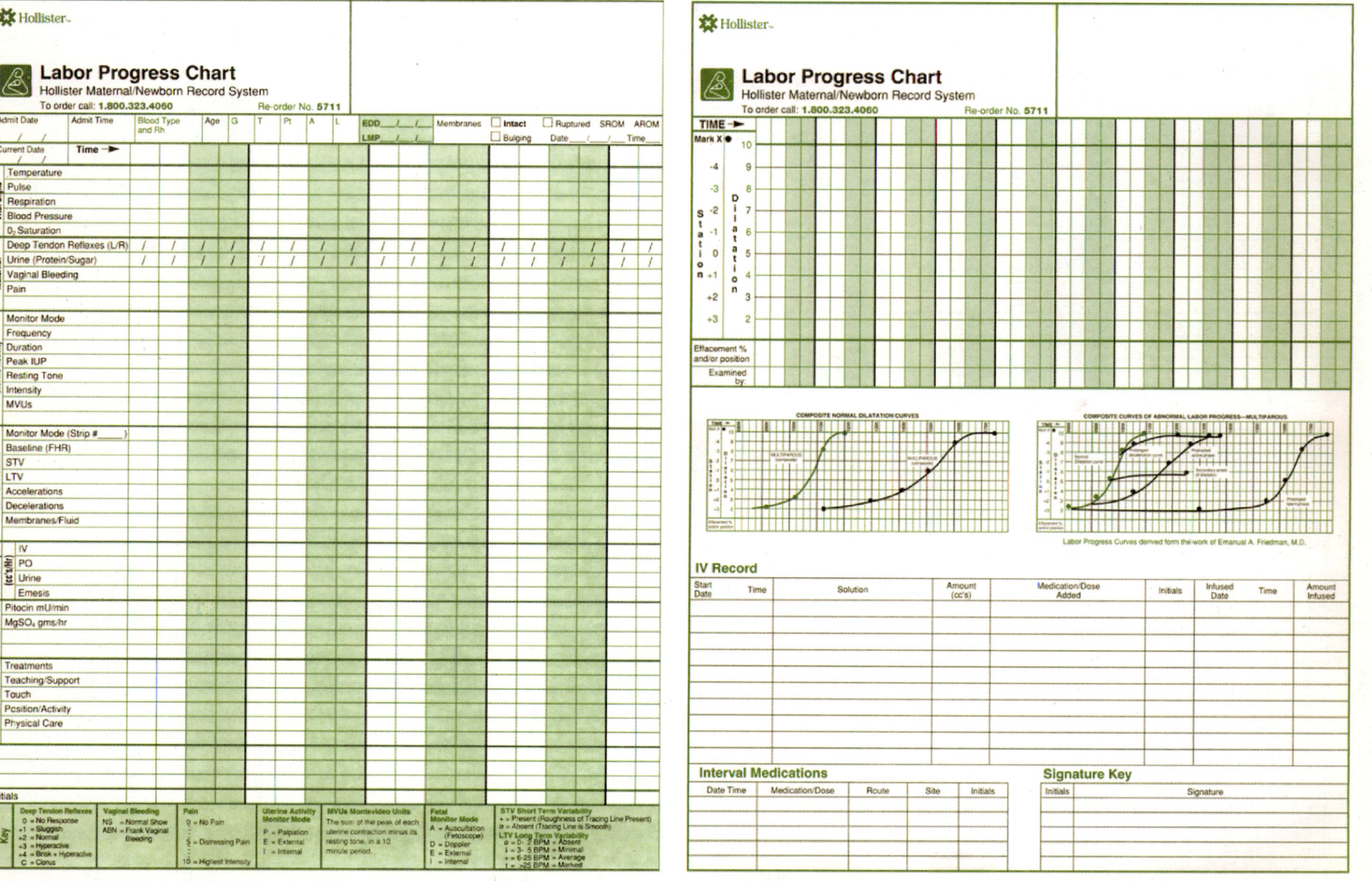

Hollister

Labor Progress Chart
Hollister Maternal/Newborn Record System
To order call: 1.800.323.4060 Re-order No. 5711

Admit Date / /	Admit Time	Blood Type and Rh	Age	G	T	Pt	A	L	EDD / / LMP / /	Membranes	☐ Intact ☐ Bulging	☐ Ruptured Date / /	SROM	AROM Time

	Current Date / / — Time ➔
Vital Signs	Temperature
	Pulse
	Respiration
	Blood Pressure
	O_2 Saturation
Maternal	Deep Tendon Reflexes (L/R)
	Urine (Protein/Sugar)
	Vaginal Bleeding
	Pain
Uterine Activity	Monitor Mode
	Frequency
	Duration
	Peak IUP
	Resting Tone
	Intensity
	MVUs
Fetal Assessment	Monitor Mode (Strip #____)
	Baseline (FHR)
	STV
	LTV
	Accelerations
	Decelerations
	Membranes/Fluid
Intake/Output (cc's/Hr)	IV
	PO
	Urine
	Emesis
Cont Meds	Pitocin mU/min
	$MgSO_4$ gms/hr
Intervention	Treatments
	Teaching/Support
	Touch
	Position/Activity
	Physical Care
	Initials

Abbreviations/Key

Deep Tendon Reflexes	Vaginal Bleeding	Pain	Uterine Activity Monitor Mode	MVUs Montevideo Units	Fetal Monitor Mode	STV Short Term Variability
0 = No Response +1 = Sluggish +2 = Normal +3 = Hyperactive +4 = Brisk + Hyperactive C = Clonus	NS = Normal Show ABN = Frank Vaginal Bleeding	0 = No Pain 5 = Distressing Pain 10 = Highest Intensity	P = Palpation E = External I = Internal	The sum of the peak of each uterine contraction minus its resting tone, in a 10 minute period.	A = Auscultation (Fetoscope) D = Doppler E = External I = Internal	+ = Present (Roughness of Tracing Line Present) ø = Absent (Tracing Line is Smooth) LTV Long Term Variability ø = 0- 2 BPM = Absent ↓ = 3- 5 BPM = Minimal + = 6-25 BPM = Average ↑ = >25 BPM = Marked

Hollister

Labor Progress Chart
Hollister Maternal/Newborn Record System
To order call: 1.800.323.4060 Re-order No. 5711

TIME ➔ Mark X ●	Station	Dilatation
		10
	-4	9
	-3	8
	-2	7
	-1	6
	0	5
	+1	4
	+2	3
	+3	2
Effacement % and/or position		
Examined by:		

IV Record

Start Date	Time	Solution	Amount (cc's)	Medication/Dose Added	Initials	Infused Date	Time	Amount Infused

Interval Medications

Date Time	Medication/Dose	Route	Site	Initials

Signature Key

Initials	Signature

FIGURE 56-19 Representative Labor Progress Record (*Permission to use this copyright material has been granted by the owner, Hollister Incorporated.*)

In some facilities, IV fluids are started on every client. It is very important to keep an accurate I&O when IV fluids are infusing because of the danger of hypervolemia.

Elimination The client should be encouraged to void every 2 hours. A distended bladder may impede descent of the presenting part, cause undue discomfort, and lead to bladder atony after the birth.

If allowed, getting up to go to the bathroom may be the easiest for the client. Sitting on a bedpan at the edge of the bed with feet on a chair may be the next best option.

Catheterization may be required if the client cannot void and the bladder is distended. The vulva and perineum must be thoroughly cleaned to remove any amniotic fluid and bloody show before catheterization. If the catheter cannot be inserted, the presenting part is probably compressing the urethra. The procedure must be discontinued and the CNM/physician notified.

Because of the decrease in intestinal motility, most women do not have a bowel movement during labor; however, the pushing and birth of the infant during the second stage of labor may cause some stool to be expelled from the rectum. This should be cleaned immediately and the client reassured that this is a normal and expected outcome.

Assisting Client and Support Person

The support person many times is the father, but it may be another woman or man. The person the mother has chosen to be the support person should be treated with the same respect as the mother, regardless of the relationship to the mother or the fetus.

The client who has participated in childbirth preparation classes with a support person already has some skills and a plan for coping with labor and birth. The nurse should determine what that plan is and assist, as needed, in carrying out that plan.

The client and support person who have not attended childbirth preparation classes should be taught the various techniques of coping with labor during the latent phase of labor. The nurse may actually provide more of the supportive care in this situation.

Breathing Techniques Three different breathing patterns are used. The first pattern is used until it is no longer effective, then the next pattern is used. Each breathing pattern begins and ends with a deep cleansing breath, with inhalation through the nose and exhalation through pursed lips, moving only the chest. The breathing techniques:

- Provide adequate oxygenation of mother and fetus
- Provide a focus of attention
- Decrease anxiety
- Increase mental and physical relaxation

These breathing patterns are used only during a uterine contraction. Between contractions, breathing returns to the woman's regular breathing pattern. The client is encouraged to rest between contractions.

Slow, Deep Chest Breathing For this pattern, the client takes a cleansing breath, then inhales through the nose and exhales through pursed lips, 6 to 9 breaths per minute. At the end of the contraction, she takes another cleansing breath. It takes concentration to breathe this slowly.

Shallow Breathing A cleansing breath is taken first. The client inhales and exhales through the mouth about 4 times every 5 seconds. This may be increased to 2 breaths per second, usually at the peak of a contraction. The client should take another deep cleansing breath at the end of the contraction.

Pant-Blow Breathing The pant-blow breathing is generally used when the contractions become very intense. This pattern is very similar to the shallow breathing except that every three or four breaths a forceful exhalation (blow) is made through pursed lips. A cleansing breath is taken at the beginning and end of the contraction. It takes great concentration to maintain this pattern during a contraction.

All clients should be kept informed of their progress in labor. Positive feedback to the client and support person regarding how they are coping with the labor process is also important.

If siblings are to be present for labor and the birth, another person should be there to watch over the children and provide them with explanations, diversions, and comfort as needed. Neither the support person nor the nurses should be responsible for the children. Their focus should be on the client.

Providing Pharmacological Comfort Measures

The nonpharmacological comfort measures may be all that is needed for some women in labor. For other women, the increasing discomfort interferes with their ability to relax, use the breathing techniques appropriately, and maintain a sense of control. Pharmacological comfort measures include systemic medications, regional blocks, and general anesthesia.

Systemic Medications Systemic medications should be administered only if:

- The client is willing to receive them and her vital signs are stable.
- The fetus is at term, exhibits regular movement, has a FHR between 110 and 160 with no late or variable decelerations and average variability.
- Contractions are well established with the cervix dilated at least 4 to 5 cm in a nullipara or 3 to 4 cm in a multipara, the presenting part is engaged, and no complications are identified.

Effect on the fetus depends on the dosage given, timing and route of administration, and the pharmacokinetics of the drug. The intravenous (IV) route is generally preferred over the intramuscular (IM) route because the drug's effect is faster and more reliable. Table 56-5 lists drugs commonly used for pain management during labor.

CRITICAL THINKING

Pushing in Labor

A client gravida 1 para 0 in labor is 7 cm dilated, station +1, and says that she wants to push. Her grandmother told her that she would have to push hard to have a baby, so the client wants to push and get it over with. How should the nurse respond?

TABLE 56-5 Pain-Management Drugs Commonly Used During Labor

DRUG	ROUTE	ONSET	PEAK EFFECT	LASTING
Narcotic Analgesics				
meperidine	IV	30 sec	5 to 10 min	2 to 4 hr
(Demerol)	IM	10 to 15 min	40 to 50 min	2 to 4 hr
fentanyl citrate	IV	1 to 2 min	3 to 5 min	1/2 to 1 hr
(Sulimaze)	IM	7 to 10 min	20 to 30 min	1 to 2 hr
Narcotic Agonist-Antagonists				
nalbuphine hydrochloride	IV	2 to 3 min	30 min	3 to 4 hr
(Nubain)	IM	15 min	60 min	3 to 6 hr
butorphanol tartrate	IV	2 to 3 min	½ to 1 hr	2 to 4 hr
(Stadol)	IM	10 to 30 min	½ to 1 hr	3 to 4 hr
pentazocine lactate	IV	2 to 3 min	15 to 30 min	2 to 3 hr
(Talwin)	IM	15 to 20 min	30 to 60 min	2 to 3 hr
Narcotic Antagonist				
Naloxone	IV	1 to 2 min	unknown	depends on dose
(Narcan)	IM	2 to 5 min	unknown	longer than IV
Analgesic Potentiators				
promethazine hydrochloride	IV	3 to 5 min	unknown	12 hr
(Phenergan)	IM	20 min	unknown	12 hr
hydroxyzine hydrochloride Z-track (Atarax, Vistaril)	IM only	unknown	unknown	4 to 6 hr

COURTESY OF DELMAR CENGAGE LEARNING

Regional Blocks Several types of regional blocks may be used during labor and/or birth, including epidural block, intrathecal block, local infiltration, and pudendal block.

Epidural Block An epidural block may be used for pain control during labor and birth. It may be a continuous or intermittent infusion of a local anesthetic drug through a catheter placed in the epidural space. A very small dose of fentanyl (Sublimaze) or sufentanil (Sufenta) is often added to the local anesthetic drug for faster and longer-lasting relief of pain. Advantages are good pain control, yet the client can participate in the birth process and interact with her infant and support person. Disadvantages may include maternal hypotension, bladder distention, epidural catheter migration, nausea and vomiting, pruritis, and delayed respiratory depression.

PROFESSIONALTIP

Pain-Relief Medications

Before receiving a medication, the client should understand the following:

- Type of medication
- Route of administration
- Expected effects of the medication
- Possible side effects of the medication
- Implications for the fetus/neonate
- Safety measures to be followed (e.g., stay in bed, have siderails up)
- Duration of effects of the medication

Intrathecal Block Intrathecal injection of an opioid analgesic such as fentanyl (Sublimaze), sufentanil (Sufenta), or morphine (Duramorph) is a pain management option for labor. A much smaller dose than is given systemically is injected into the subarachnoid space. Advantages are rapid onset yet no sedation, no hypotensive effect, and no motor block, so the client may walk during labor. Disadvantages may include the short duration of action so that the client may require another injection and the inadequate relief of pain in late labor and during birth so that another pain relief measure is required.

Local Infiltration Local infiltration anesthesia of the perineum is achieved by injecting a local anesthetic into the perineum. This is used just before the time of birth in preparation for performing an episiotomy, suturing a laceration, or when a pudendal block cannot be performed. Local anesthetics such as procaine hydrochloride (Novocain), chloroprocaine hydrochloride (Nesacaine), and tetracaine hydrochloride (Pontocaine), which metabolize rapidly, and bupivacaine hydrochloride (Marcaine), lidocaine hydrochloride (Xylocaine), and mepivacaine hydrochloride (Carbocaine), which are more powerful and longer-acting, are often used. Advantages are that the procedure is technically uncomplicated and

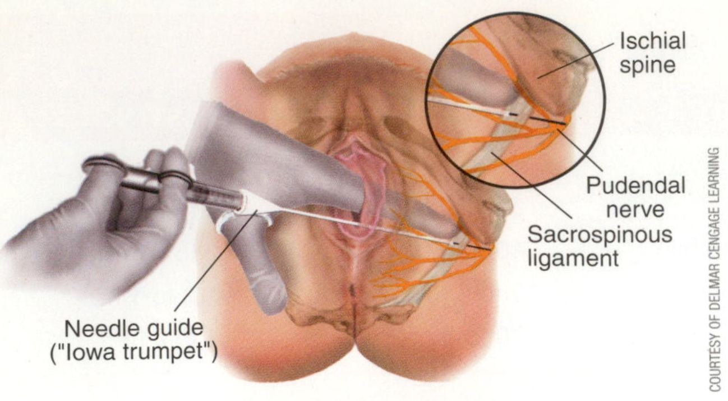

FIGURE 56-20 Pudendal block provides anesthesia to the perineum, external genitalia, and lower vagina.

practically free of complications. A disadvantage is that a large amount of local anesthetic may be required.

Pudendal Block A **pudendal block** is not commonly used today. It is the injection of a local anesthetic into the pudendal nerve to provide perineal, external genitalia, and lower vaginal anesthesia (Figure 56-20). The pudendal block may be performed during the transition phase of the first stage or the second stage of labor. The advantage is that there are no changes in maternal vital signs or the FHR. Disadvantages may include rectal puncture, sciatic nerve block, or a hematoma.

General Anesthesia Because general anesthesia involves loss of consciousness, it is rarely used in vaginal births. It is used for cesarean births only in extreme emergency situations. The greatest danger is fetal depression because most general anesthetics reach the fetus in about 2 minutes.

PROFESSIONALTIP

Meperidine (Demerol) Use in Labor

When meperidine (Demerol) is given IM during labor, the birth of the infant should ideally occur in less than 1 hour after administration or more than 4 hours after administration (time of peak affect) to minimize respiratory depression of the neonate.

PROFESSIONALTIP

Narcotic Agonist-Antagonists and Narcotic Antagonists Administration

The drugs nalbuphine hydrochloride (Nubain), butorphanol tartrate (Stadol), pentazocine lactate (Talwin), and naloxone (Narcan) should not be given to substance-dependent clients because these drugs may precipitate withdrawal symptoms.

RISKS OF LABOR AND BIRTH

Most labors and births proceed as expected; however, there are complications that may be anticipated and some that happen unexpectedly. The most common risks—preterm labor and birth, premature rupture of membranes, dystocia, abnormal duration of labor, and prolapsed cord—are discussed.

PRETERM LABOR AND BIRTH

Preterm labor is the onset of regular contractions of the uterus that cause cervical changes between 20 and 37 weeks of gestation. **Preterm birth** is a birth that takes place before the end of the 37th week of gestation. Only about half of the time can a precipitating cause be identified. The single most important factor predisposing to preterm labor and birth is having already had a preterm birth. Other factors often associated with preterm labor and birth include premature rupture of the membranes (PROM), multiple gestation, bacterial vaginosis, intraamniotic infection, bleeding, and uterine/cervical abnormalities.

Most women in preterm labor are admitted to the hospital for further evaluation. A urine specimen is examined for evidence of a urinary tract infection. Cervical or vaginal secretions are obtained during a sterile speculum examination to culture for Chlamydia trachomatis, group B streptococcus, or gonococcus infections.

If contractions are continuing and cervical changes are occurring, tocolytic agents may be prescribed. **Tocolytic agents** are medications that inhibit contractions. The most commonly used are terbutaline (Breathine) and magnesium sulfate. A corticosteroid may also be given to accelerate fetal lung maturation. There is greater fetal benefit if at least 24 hours elapse between the first dose and the birth.

If contractions subside and cervical dilation and effacement remain the same, the client may be discharged with instructions to limit activities and medication to prevent labor.

PREMATURE RUPTURE OF MEMBRANES

When the membranes rupture before labor begins, it is called premature rupture of membranes (PROM). This is the most common cause of preterm labor. Contractions usually begin

LIFE SPAN CONSIDERATIONS

Risks of Labor and Birth

- Adolescents (younger than age 15) have a greater risk of preterm labor, prolonged labor, and dystocia related to the small size of the pelvis because they have not yet reached bone growth maturity, which results in cephalopelvic disproportion (CPD).
- Mature women (older than age 35) have a greater risk of preterm labor, longer labor, cesarean birth, and dystocia related to fetal anomalies.

(Lowdermilk & Perry, 2006)

within 24 hours when the client is at term. In pregnancies of 28 to 34 weeks' gestation, labor may not start for a week or more. If the amniotic membranes rupture before labor begins in a client who is less than 37 weeks gestation, it is called preterm premature rupture of membranes (PPROM). African American mothers are more at risk for occurrence and reoccurrence of PPROM than Caucasian mothers, with the greatest risk at less than 28 weeks gestation (Shen, DeFranco, Stamilio, Chang, & Muglia, 2008).

In most cases of PROM, the cause is unknown. New evidence suggests that a contributing factor to preterm delivery is intrauterine infection (Hutzal, Boyle, Kenyon, Nash, Winsor, Taylor, & Kirpalani, 2008).

Besides preterm labor and birth, PROM can result in prolapse of the cord and intrauterine infection. A positive identification of amniotic fluid is made by observation of amniotic fluid escape from the cervix during a sterile speculum examination, a positive nitrazine test, a positive Amnisure or Amnioswab test, or the presence of ferning when the fluid is viewed under a microscope. The client may be hospitalized until after the birth of the infant, or if there are no signs of infections or fetal distress, she may be sent home. If hospitalized, continuing assessments include maternal vital signs; FHR; fetal movements; vaginal discharge for odor, color, and amount; and palpation of the uterus for tenderness.

COMMUNITY/HOME HEALTH CARE

Preterm Labor

- Follow instructions regarding activity limitation.
- Monitor uterine contractions 2 to 3 times a day for 30 minutes to 1 hour.
- Count fetal movements as instructed.
- Practice relaxation techniques.
- Drink 8 to 10 (8 oz) glasses of fluids each day.
- Empty bladder frequently.
- Avoid smoking, alcohol, and nontherapeutic drugs.
- Limit caffeine intake (colas, coffee, tea, chocolate).
- Avoid activities that can stimulate labor (e.g., nipple stimulation, any sexual activity that causes orgasm).
- Take medications as prescribed.
- Keep appointments with CNM/physician.

COMMUNITY/HOME HEALTH CARE

Premature Rupture of Membranes

- Stay in bed, lying on either side, except to go to the bathroom (or as instructed).
- Take temperature every 4 hours when awake.
- Count fetal movements daily (report if less than 4 in 1 hour or an abnormal increase).
- Be aware of uterine contractions; if frequency is less than 10 minutes, notify CNM/physician.
- Use good perineal hygiene (e.g., wipe from front to back).
- Report any foul-smelling vaginal discharge or uterine tenderness.
- Take showers or sponge baths, not a tub bath.
- Avoid breast stimulation, sexual stimulation, and sexual intercourse.

DYSTOCIA

Dystocia is a long, difficult, or abnormal labor caused by any of the five major variables (5 Ps) that affect labor. The following may be causes:

- Dysfunctional labor: ineffective contractions or maternal pushing efforts (powers).
- Pelvic structure variations (passageway).
- Fetal variations: anomalies, abnormal presentation, very large size, or number of fetuses (passenger).
- Mother's responses: related to preparation for childbirth, past experiences, culture, and support persons (psychological response).
- Engagement of the presenting part, station, and fetal position (position).

Dysfunctional Labor

Dysfunctional labor is a labor with problems of the contractions or with maternal bearing-down efforts. The contractions may be hypertonic or hypotonic.

Hypertonic Uterine Contractions Hypertonic uterine contractions, usually occurring in the latent phase of labor, are very frequent and uncoordinated and have an increased resting tone. The mother has discomfort out of proportion to the intensity of the contractions, which do not dilate or efface the cervix. The excessive pain results from anoxia of the uterine muscle cells. A prolonged latent phase is generally the result.

The client may become fatigued and dehydrated and may express fear that she is losing control with the lack of progress. The fetus may experience distress because the hypertonic contractions and increased resting tone of the uterus interfere with uteroplacental blood flow. The increased and prolonged pressure on the fetal head may cause excessive molding, caput succedaneum, or cephalhematoma (discussed in Newborn chapter).

Bed rest and analgesics such as morphine sulfate or meperidine hydrochloride (Demerol) are given to relieve pain, promote relaxation, and induce sleep. When the client awakens, uterine contractions are often normal and labor proceeds.

Hypotonic Uterine Contractions Hypotonic uterine contractions, also called uterine inertia, usually occur in the active phase of labor. After normal progress through the latent phase of labor, the contractions become weak and inefficient in the active phase and may even cease. Common causes are cephalopelvic disproportion (CPD) (discussed later), malposition of the fetus, an overstretched uterus from multiple fetuses, a fetus of very large body size, hydramnios, or grandmultiparity (having delivered more than six infants).

The risks for the mother include intrauterine infection, especially if the membranes are ruptured and labor is prolonged; postpartum hemorrhage caused by inefficient uterine contractions after birth; exhaustion; and decreased coping ability. The fetus may experience distress because of the length of labor and sepsis from maternal pathogens ascending the birth canal.

An ultrasound is usually performed to rule out CPD. If all factors are normal, one or more measures for augmentation of (increasing) labor are instituted, including ambulation, amniotomy, nipple stimulation, and oxytocin infusion (discussed later).

Amniotomy An **amniotomy**, artificial rupture of membranes (AROM), is performed by the CNM/physician. Several linen savers and a folded bath towel are placed under the client to absorb the amniotic fluid. A disposable plastic hook (amnihook) is generally used (Figure 56-21). A vaginal examination is performed to determine dilation, effacement, presenting part, and station, and FHR is assessed to determine fetal well-being. If the presenting part is not engaged or if the presentation is not cephalic, the risk of a prolapsed cord is high and the amniotomy is generally not performed.

After an amniotomy, the FHR must be assessed for 1 full minute. A monitor pattern that is nonreassuring or has any significant changes must be promptly reported to the CNM/physician. Amniotic fluid odor, color, and quantity are documented. The fluid should be clear (sometimes flecks of vernix are present) with a mild odor. Greenish meconium-stained fluid may indicate placental insufficiency. Foul-smelling fluid or fluid with a strong odor with a cloudy appearance or yellow color often indicates chorioamnionitis. Maternal temperature should be taken every hour after ROM and any elevation above 38°C (100.4°F) reported to the CNM/physician.

Maternal Bearing-Down Efforts Analgesia and/or anesthesia may block Ferguson's reflex and thus decrease the effectiveness of maternal bearing down. Lack of sleep, a long labor, inadequate hydration, and maternal position may also have an adverse effect on the mother's bearing-down efforts.

Pelvic Structure Variations

A woman with a small or abnormally shaped pelvis may experience a long and difficult labor. Only about 50% of women have the pelvic shape (gynecoid) most conducive to labor, fetal descent, and birth (Murray et al., 2001).

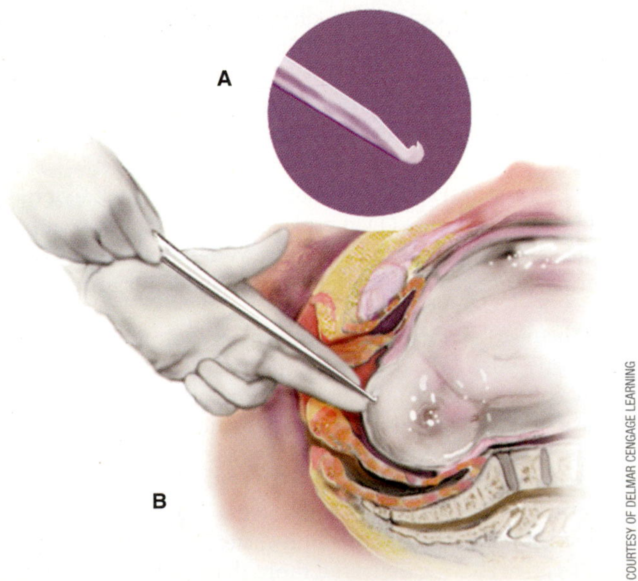

FIGURE 56-21 ***A*, Disposable Plastic Hook to Rupture Membranes: *B*, Technique for Rupturing Membranes**

A distended bladder reduces the space available in the pelvis and is an obstruction to fetal descent. This greatly increases the client's discomfort. Other, less common obstructions are uterine fibroids or pelvic cysts.

Fetal Variations

Variations of the fetus that may cause dystocia include the following:

- Anomalies
- Abnormal presentation or position
- Size
- Number of fetuses

Anomalies Fetal anomalies such as hydrocephalus may prevent descent of the fetus. Anomalies are often discovered by an ultrasound during pregnancy. If a vaginal birth is not advisable or not possible, a cesarean birth is scheduled.

Abnormal Presentation or Position A cephalic presentation other than vertex makes a larger diameter of the fetal head move through the birth canal. Labor generally takes longer and is more difficult.

In a breech presentation, cervical effacement and dilatation are often slower because the buttocks are softer than the head and do not put firm pressure on the cervix to aid in dilation. Following are risks to the fetus born in a breech presentation:

- Prolapsed cord
- Cord compression
- Aspiration of fluids in the vagina
- Head becoming stuck

External version (manipulation of the fetus through the mother's abdomen to a presentation facilitating birth) may be tried to change the presentation to cephalic.

It is not always possible to change the presentation of the fetus. Figure 56-22 illustrates the birth of a fetus in a complete breech presentation.

A position of occiput posterior or occiput transverse can contribute to dysfunctional labor. Labor is generally longer and causes more discomfort because the head has farther to rotate during internal rotation. Many women describe severe back pain and have leg pain on the side where the head is positioned. A change in the mother's position may promote rotation of the fetal head. When the mother's abdomen is dependent to her spine, as in the hands-and-knees position, fetal rotation is encouraged (Figure 56-23).

Size An infant weighing more than 4,000 g (8.8 lb) is said to be **macrosomic**—having a very large body size. This may cause problems for a vaginal birth. As long as the mother's pelvis is of a size and shape to accommodate an infant this size, there is no problem. When the fetal head will not fit through the mother's pelvis, it is called **cephalopelvic disproportion (CPD)**. The cause can be either fetal or maternal. The fetal head may be abnormally large and the mother's pelvis of normal size and shape, or the fetal head may be of average size and the mother's pelvis small or abnormally shaped. Whatever the cause, a cesarean birth is required.

Number of Fetuses When more than one fetus is present, the uterus is overdistended. One or more of the fetuses may be

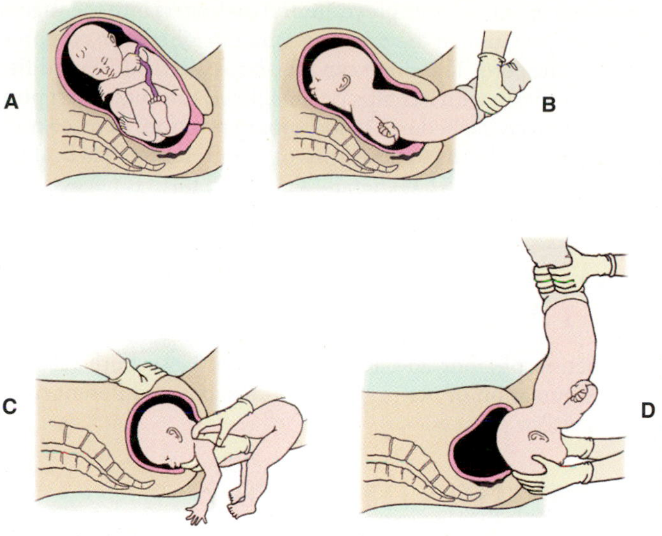

FIGURE 56-22 Birth of Fetus in Complete Breech Presentation; *A,* Descent and Internal Rotation; *B,* Extension of Fetal Back Under Symphysis (Towel on Legs Used for Traction); *C,* CNM/Physician Maintains Head Flexion by Putting Pressure on Lower Face with Fingers of Left Hand (Suprapubic Pressure is Applied by Assistant to Keep Fetal Head Flexed); *D,* Assistant Holds Fetal Legs with Towel while CNM/Physician Assists the Face and Head Over the Perineum

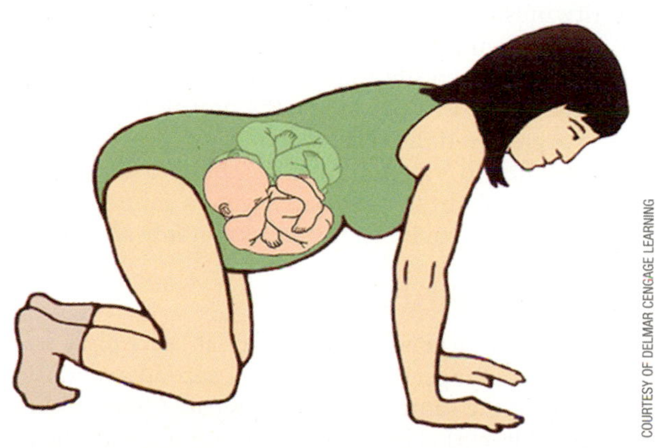

FIGURE 56-23 Fetus tends to rotate from occiput posterior to occiput anterior when mother is in a hands-and-knees position.

in a presentation less desirable than vertex. Twins often have a cesarean birth, and when there are three or more fetuses, birth is almost always cesarean.

Mother's Responses

The mother's perception of labor is more important than her actual experience in labor. Tales from family and friends, a bad experience with a previous labor, and cultural expectations can add to the stress of labor. Excessive or prolonged stress experienced by the woman in labor may interfere with the progress of labor in several ways:

- Secretion of catecholamines (epinephrine and norepinephrine) by the adrenal glands in response to stress inhibits uterine contractions and decreases blood supply to the uterus and placenta while increasing blood supply to the skeletal muscles.
- Tense abdominal and pelvic muscles make contractions less effective.
- Contractions working against tense abdominal muscles increase pain, which adds stress to the situation and makes the mother more anxious.

The nurse can help allay the client's fears by offering encouragement, answering her questions honestly, and offering tips on how to make labor more successful. For instance, the nurse might suggest a change of position to a squatting bar to aid in fetal descent, or may offer a mirror so the mother can see the baby crown and be encouraged by her progress.

Abnormal Duration of Labor

Labor may be prolonged or abnormally short (precipitate).

Prolonged Labor

Many of the conditions previously discussed, such as hypotonic uterine contractions, CPD, abnormal fetal presentations or positions, or early use of analgesics may cause prolonged labor. Labor progress in either the first or second stage may be prolonged or arrested (stopped). The plotting of cervical dilation on a labor graph, as found in Figure 56-19, helps in identifying these situations. Once the cause of the prolonged labor is identified, the CNM/physician can take steps to remedy the situation. A possible course of action might be induction of labor, a forceps- or vacuum-assisted birth, or cesarean birth (all discussed later).

When the active phase of the first stage of labor lasts more than15 hours, the risk of fetal death increases (Lowdermilk & Perry, 2006). With prolonged labor, maternal morbidity and mortality may result from infection, uterine rupture, serious dehydration, and postpartum hemorrhage.

Precipitate Labor/Precipitate Birth

A labor lasting less than 3 hours from the onset of contractions to the birth of the infant is considered a **precipitate labor.** Although a precipitate labor may end with a precipitate birth, they are not the same. Possible maternal complications during a precipitate labor include a loss of coping ability; an increased risk of uterine rupture; lacerations of the cervix, vagina, and perineum; and postpartum hemorrhage. Possible fetal complications include hypoxia, distress, and cerebral trauma.

A **precipitate birth** is a birth occurring suddenly and unexpectedly without a CNM/physician to assist. When a client says "the baby's coming" or words to that effect, the health care provider should always inspect to see whether she is correct. Most of the time a large part of the fetal head is visible, if not already crowning. In this situation the nurse should do the following:

- Stay with the mother.
- Call for assistance or send support person to get assistance. Other staff members can notify the CNM/ physician.
- Remain calm and reassure mother.
- Open emergency birth pack.
- If time permits, scrub hands, put on sterile gloves, and place sterile drape under mother's buttocks.
- As the head crowns, instruct mother to pant.
- If membranes are still intact, tear the sac, allowing amniotic fluid to flow out.
- Apply gentle pressure to the fetal head with one hand to prevent it from popping out. *Do not hold the head back with force enough to prevent it from being born.*

- With the mother still panting, check at the back of the fetal head for the umbilical cord. If there is a **nuchal cord** (umbilical cord around the neck) and it is loose enough, slip the cord over the baby's head. If it is too tight, place two clamps on the cord, cut the cord between the clamps, and unwind the cord from the neck.
- Suction the baby's mouth and throat first and then the nose to prevent the infant from aspirating amniotic fluid.
- With one hand on each side of the head, push gently downward until the anterior shoulder comes under the symphysis. Then gently raise the baby's head so the posterior shoulder is born.
- Ask the mother to push gently to assist in the birth of the rest of the infant's body.
- Hold the infant at the level of the uterus, being careful not to drop the slippery infant.
- Again, suction the mouth, throat, and nose of the infant.
- Dry the infant to prevent heat loss and place the infant on the mother's abdomen. Cover with a dry blanket.
- If not already completed, clamp the cord in two places and cut it between the two.
- Document on the birth record the fetal position, nuchal cord, time of birth, Apgar scores (addressed later in this chapter) at 1 and 5 minutes after birth, gender, time and method of placental expulsion, and mother's condition.

Prolapsed Cord

When the umbilical cord lies below the presenting part of the fetus, it is termed a **prolapsed cord**. Prolapse of the cord may occur anytime and may be hidden (occult, not visible) or visible (Figure 56-24). It most commonly occurs with ROM, either spontaneous rupture of membranes (SROM) or AROM, as the cord washes down with the amniotic fluid.

A cord below the presenting part is compressed between the fetus and the mother's pelvis, resulting in decreased blood flow to the fetus. The fetus will have bradycardia with variable decelerations during uterine contractions. Contributing factors include a long cord (greater than 100 cm or 40 in), unengaged presenting part, breech presentation, or transverse lie.

When a prolapsed cord is identified, pressure on the cord must be relieved immediately. The provider must call for assistance, don a sterile glove, insert two fingers into the vagina, and put pressure on the presenting part to relieve the compression of the cord. The client can then be assisted into a modified Sims' position with her hips up on pillows, the knee-chest position, or place the bed in Trendelenburg position. In these positions, gravity keeps the pressure of the presenting part off the cord (Figure 56-25). Generally a cesarean birth is necessary.

INDUCTION/AUGMENTATION OF LABOR

Induction of labor and augmentation of labor both relate to the stimulation of uterine contractions, but at different times in the labor process.

Induction of Labor

Induction of labor is the stimulation of uterine contractions *before* they begin spontaneously for the purpose of birthing an infant. Both chemical and mechanical methods can be used to induce labor. The most common methods used in the United States are intravenous oxytocin and amniotomy. Induction of labor is considered in situations of preexisting maternal disease, maternal diabetes mellitus, gestational hypertension (PIH), preeclampsia/eclampsia, PROM, intrauterine fetal growth restriction, postterm pregnancy, fetal demise, and chorioamniotis (Moleti, 2009). Fetal maturity, especially lung maturity, must also be considered. Contraindications to induction are the same as those to spontaneous labor and vaginal birth (e.g., hydrocephaly, transverse lie).

If the cervix is "ripe" (soft), the probability of induction success is greater. If the cervix is not "ripe," prostaglandins are often used first to "ripen" the cervix. Dinoprostone (Prepidil) is often used, and the next day oxytocin infusion is begun. Frequently, oxytocin infusion and amniotomy are both used.

Oxytocin Infusion

A primary IV infusion of 1,000 mL of an electrolyte solution (e.g., lactated Ringer's) is started. A secondary infusion of 1,000 mL of the same solution is prepared with 20 units of oxytocin (Pitocin). The secondary infusion (with the oxytocin) is regulated by an infusion pump. The rate is very slow

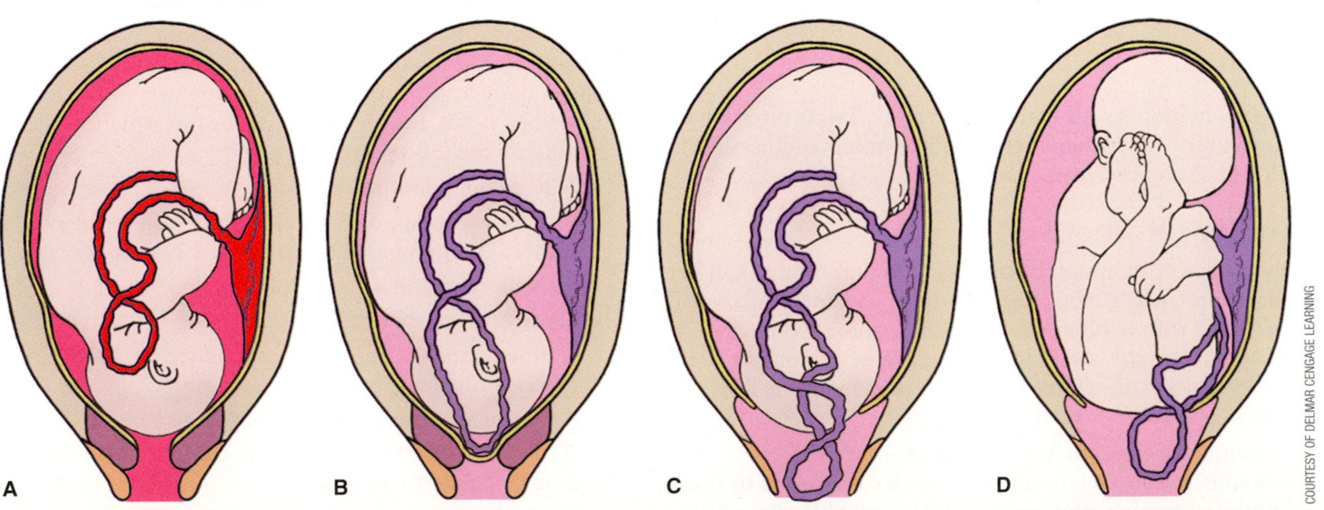

Figure 56-24 Prolapsed Cord; *A*, Hidden (Occult, Not Visible); *B*, Prolapse with Membranes Still Intact; *C*, Cord May Be Seen in Vagina; *D*, Breech with Prolapsed Cord

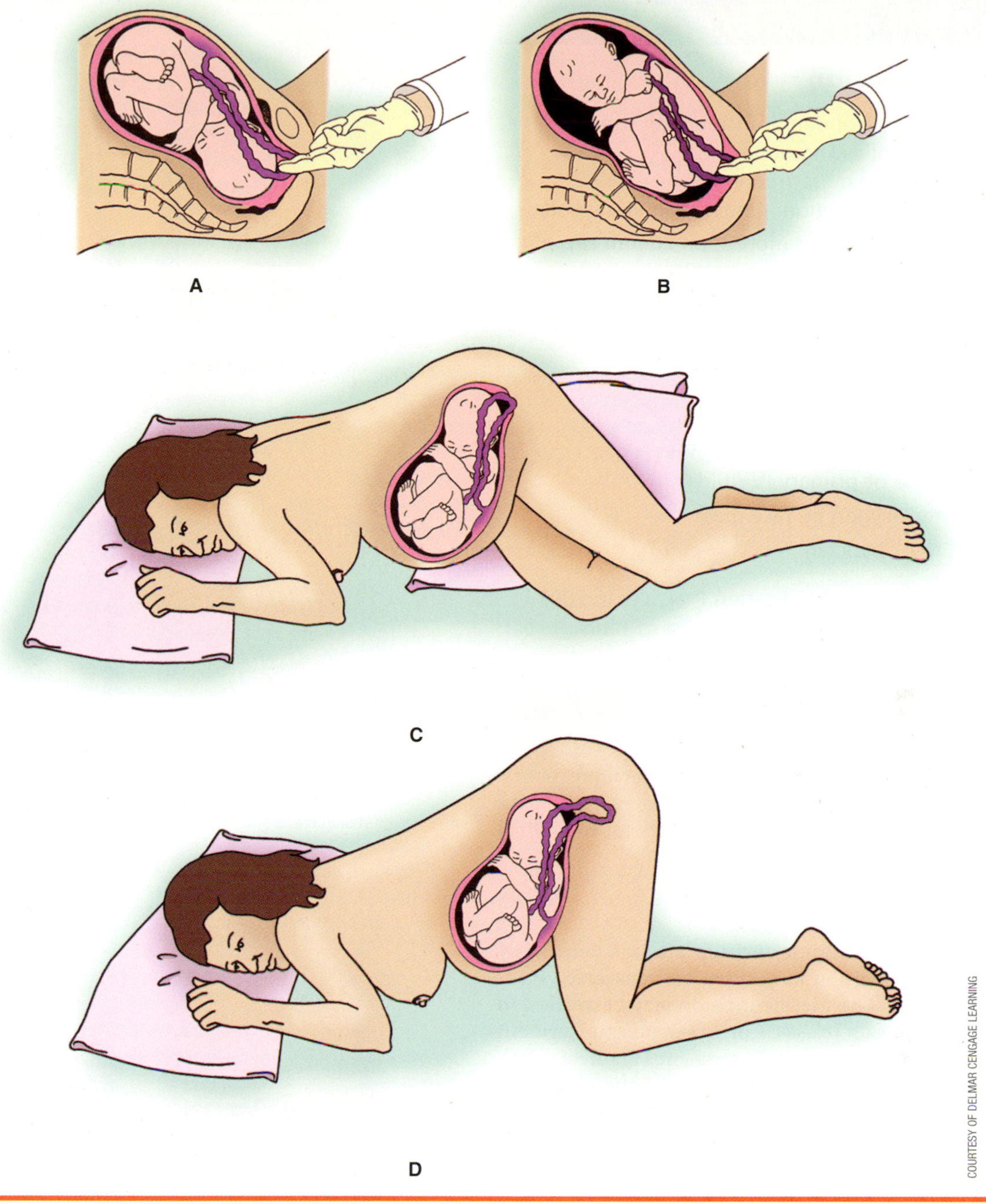

FIGURE 56-25 Examiner's fingers relieve pressure on prolapsed cord in *A,* vertex presentation and *B,* breech presentation. Gravity relieves pressure on prolapsed cord with mother in *C,* modified Sim's position and *D,* knee-chest position.

at the beginning with very small increases at regular intervals according to agency protocol or CNM/physician orders. The goal is to have contractions with a frequency 2 to 3 minutes, duration less than 80 to 90 seconds, and moderate intensity (Clark, Simpson, Knox, & Garite, 2009).

A fetal monitor is used to provide continuous data about FHR and contractions. Before each increase of the infusion rate, assessments of maternal blood pressure and pulse, FHR (bradycardia or decelerations), and contractions should be made and documented. An intake and output record is maintained throughout the induction process.

Augmentation of Labor

Augmentation of labor is the stimulation of uterine contractions *after* spontaneously beginning but the progress of labor is unsatisfactory. Intravenous oxytocin is used in the same manner as for induction of labor.

OBSTETRIC PROCEDURES

Sometimes a special obstetric procedure is needed to assist with the birth of an infant. These procedures are cesarean birth, forceps-assisted birth, and vacuum-assisted birth.

Cesarean Birth

Cesarean birth is the birth of an infant through an incision in the abdomen and uterus. Indications for cesarean birth include placenta previa, placenta abruptio, CPD, prolapsed cord, breech presentation, active genital herpes, dystocia,

SAFETY

Oxytocin Infusion

Discontinue the secondary infusion with the oxytocin if the following occur:

- Contractions are more frequent than every 2 minutes or the duration is more than 90 seconds.
- Uterine resting tone is more than 20 mm Hg.
- Fetal monitor shows:
  repeated late decelerations
  prolonged decelerations
  no variability

And then:

- Keep mother in side-lying position.
- Increase rate of primary IV fluid.
- Administer oxygen by face mask.
- Notify CNM/physician.

The Institute for Safe Medication Practices in 2007 added intravenous oxytocin to the list of high-alert medications (Simpson & Knox, 2009).

gestational hypertension, hydrocephaly, multifetal pregnancy, and repeat cesarean birth. Globally, the rate of cesarean births is escalating, and birthing is becoming surgery for more than ⅓ of pregnant women (Callister, 2008).

Incisions

The skin incision and uterine incision are not necessarily the same. The skin incision may either be transverse (Pfannenstiel) or vertical. The uterine incision may be vertical in either the upper uterus (classic) or lower uterine segment or transverse in the lower uterine segment (Figure 56-26). Which incisions are used are determined by the client and physician depending on the time factor, reason for the cesarean birth, client's desire for future pregnancies, and physician preference.

Anesthesia

Regional block, epidural, or spinal anesthesia are the most popular because the mother is awake and aware of the birth of her infant. When time is of the essence or when an epidural or spinal cannot be used, general anesthetic is used.

Scheduled or Unscheduled Cesarean Birth

A cesarean birth may either be scheduled or unscheduled.

Scheduled Cesarean Birth A cesarean birth is scheduled if it is to be a repeat cesarean birth, if labor is contraindicated (e.g., complete placenta previa, hydrocephaly), or if labor cannot be induced and birth is necessary. These clients have some time to prepare for the cesarean birth.

Unscheduled Cesarean Birth Unscheduled cesarean births are usually the result of some difficulty in the labor process. Besides concern about the situation causing the need for a cesarean birth, the client and her support person often experience a sense of failure at not being able to have the baby "normally." The client is generally tired from the labor process and forgets or misunderstands any explanations given. After the infant's birth, it is important for the client to review with the nurse the events before the cesarean birth to ensure the client's understanding of what happened.

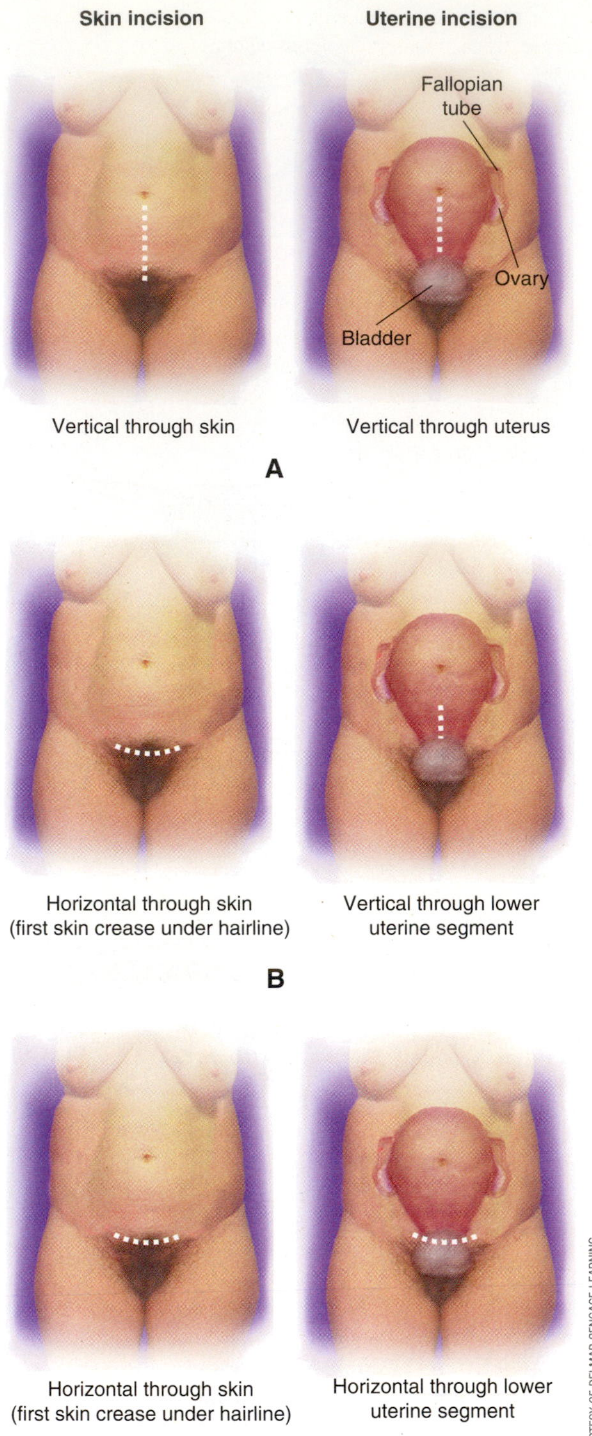

FIGURE 56-26 Cesarean Birth—Skin and Uterine Incisions; *A,* Classic, Vertical Skin Incision with High Uterine Incision; Seldom used Except in Emergency Situation; *B,* Horizontal Skin Incision with Low Vertical Uterine Incision; *C,* Horizontal Skin Incision with Horizontal Uterine Incision

Preoperative procedures must be performed quickly. Generally, a urinary catheter is inserted to keep the bladder empty; an abdominal-mons surgical shave prep is completed; abdomen is scrubbed with a solution such as betadine; intravenous fluids are started (if not already running); blood and urine tests are ordered; and, if time is available, preoperative teaching may be instituted. The support person is encouraged to remain with the mother even in surgery to provide emotional support.

When the mother is awake during the cesarean birth, she is involved in seeing and holding her infant just as in a vaginal birth, unless infant resuscitation is required. A pediatrician is usually present to care for the infant. It is extremely important to keep the mother informed about what is happening. Some facilities allow the mother to breastfeed the newborn on the operating table after delivery.

Vaginal Birth after Cesarean

When the reason for the initial cesarean birth is a nonrecurring situation such as placenta previa, prolapsed cord, or breech presentation, the client may be able to have a vaginal birth with the next pregnancy. If a low transverse uterine incision was made for the cesarean birth, a trial of labor is often recommended. If a classic uterine incision was made in the uterus, a trial of labor is contraindicated because the possibility of uterine rupture is very great. The possibility of a vaginal birth after cesarean (VBAC) is discussed throughout the pregnancy with the obstetrician.

Forceps-Assisted Birth

Forceps are metal instruments used on the fetal head to provide traction or to provide a method of rotating the fetal head to an occiput-anterior position. There are several types of forceps. Some forceps have fenestrated (open) blades and some solid blades, but they all have a locking mechanism that prevents the blades from compressing the fetal skull (Figure 56-27).

Forceps may be applied as:

- *Outlet forceps*—when head is crowning (Figure 56-28).
- *Low forceps*—when head is at +2 station or lower but not yet crowning.
- *Midforceps*—when head is engaged but above +2 stations.

Indications

Any situation that threatens the mother or fetus that can be relieved by a vaginal birth is an indication for forceps use. Examples are an exhausted mother or one who has heart disease and a fetus in distress, in arrested rotation, or breech position (after coming head).

Application of Forceps

Before forceps are applied, the cervix must be completely dilated, membranes must be ruptured, and position and station of the fetal head must be known. The FHR must be checked, reported, and recorded *before* forceps are applied and again *after* forceps are applied to make sure the cord is not being compressed by the forceps. It may help the mother to understand about the forceps if it is explained that the forceps blades fit around the baby's head like two teaspoons fit around an egg (Lowdermilk & Perry, 2006). Traction is applied to the forceps only during contractions. Rotation is performed between contractions.

After the birth of the infant, the mother must be assessed for vaginal and cervical lacerations, hematoma, and bruising. The newborn infant may have facial bruising or edema.

Vacuum-Assisted Birth

A cup connected to suction is placed over the occiput on the fetal head. After the suction (negative pressure) is attained, traction downward and outward is applied during contractions (Figure 56-29). Indications are the same as for forceps-assisted birth.

Maternal risks include vaginal and rectal lacerations. Fetal risks include cephalhematoma, brachial plexus palsy, retinal and intracranial hemorrhage, and hyperbilirubinemia.

IMMEDIATE INFANT/ MOTHER CARE

During the first 20 to 30 minutes after the infant's birth, specific care is given to the infant and the mother.

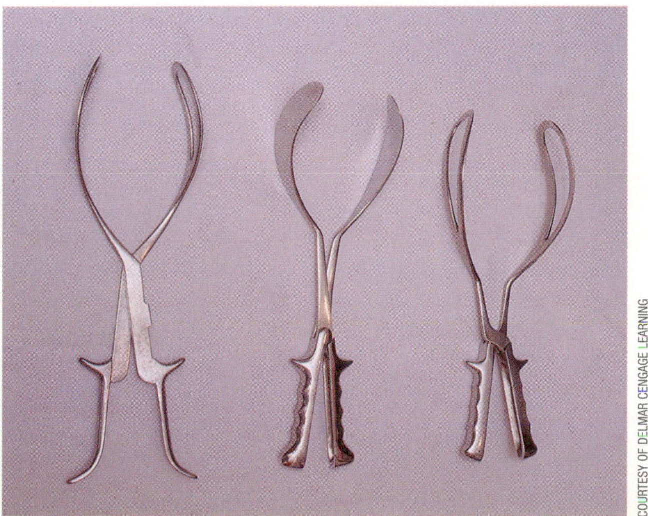

Figure 56-27 Types of Forceps

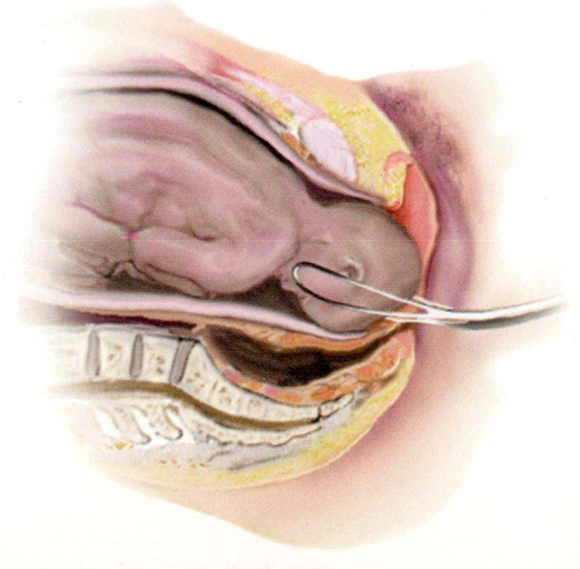

Figure 56-28 Outlet Forceps. Traction is applied downward and outward during contractions.

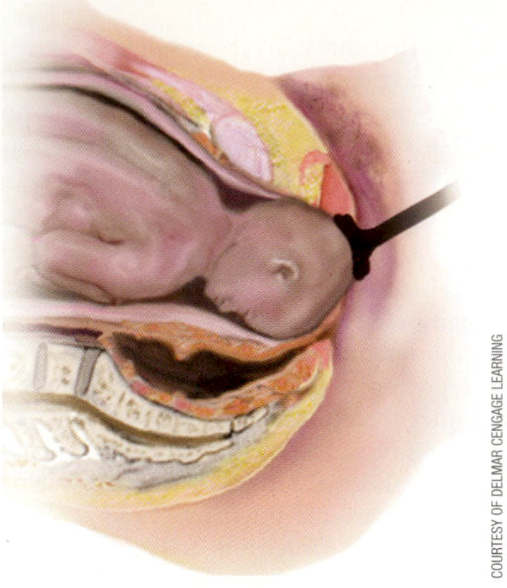

COURTESY OF DELMAR CENGAGE LEARNING

FIGURE 56-29 Vacuum-Assisted Birth

CARE OF THE INFANT

Following are the immediate needs of the newborn infant:

- A—airway
- B—breathing
- C—circulation
- W—warmth

Infants born by cesarean delivery are at greater risk for respiratory distress because they do not receive the "vaginal squeeze" that aids in expelling amniotic fluid from the lungs.

Identification of the infant is the top priority after the immediate needs are met.

Airway

The CNM/physician suctions secretions from the mouth and nose of the infant at the time of birth. Shortly thereafter, the infant takes the first breath and may begin to cry. The mouth and nose of the infant are suctioned by the nurse as needed to maintain an open airway. The bulb syringe must be compressed before inserting into the mouth or nose of infant.

Breathing/Circulation

The infant's cardiopulmonary adaptation to extrauterine life is assessed by using the Apgar score (Table 56-6).

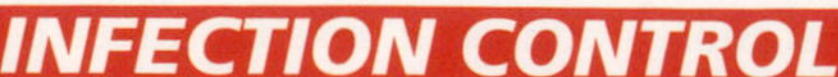

INFECTION CONTROL

Standard Precautions

Disposable gloves should be worn when:

- Caring for the newborn until after the infant has received the initial bath
- Assessing the amount of lochia and the perineum
- Cleansing the perineum

Each of the five items are assessed at 1 and 5 minutes after birth, providing a quick evaluation of how the heart and lungs are adapting. The five items to be assessed are arranged in priority from most important (heart rate) to least important (color). The infant is given a score, from 0 to 2, for each item. The five scores are then totaled.

The Apgar score indicates how the infant is transitioning at 1 and 5 minutes. Caregivers should not wait for Apgar scores to determine the next step in neonatal resuscitation. When the Apgar score is less than 6, it is an indication that the neonate is in distress. A nurse or physician who is skilled in neonatal resuscitation must take action to assist the newborn in their transition process. It must be determined whether and when the mother received a narcotic for pain management during labor. Naloxone (Narcan) may be administered if the mother received a narcotic during labor.

Warmth

The infant must be dried to prevent heat loss by evaporation. A prewarmed radiant warmer is used while giving initial care. Skin-to-skin contact with a parent can also be used to provide warmth. A stockinette cap on the infant's *dry head* also helps prevent heat loss.

Identification

A set of four identification bands, two long and two short, imprinted with the same number are used. The mother's name, sex of infant, time of birth, and CNM/physician's name are written on each band. The two small bands are put on the infant (both ankles or a wrist and an ankle).

TABLE 56-6 APGAR Score

	SCORE		
ITEM ASSESSED	0	1	2
Heart rate	Absent	Slow (<100)	Over 100
Respiratory rate	Absent	Slow, weak cry	Good cry
Muscle tone	Flaccid	Some flexion of extremities	Well flexed
Reflex irritability	No response	Grimace	Cry, cough, or sneeze
Color	Blue, pale	Body pink, extremities blue	Completely pink (light skinned); absence of cyanosis (dark skinned)

COURTESY OF DELMAR CENGAGE LEARNING

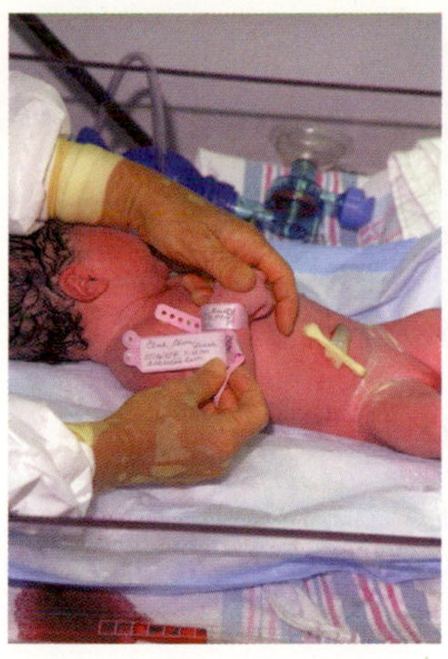
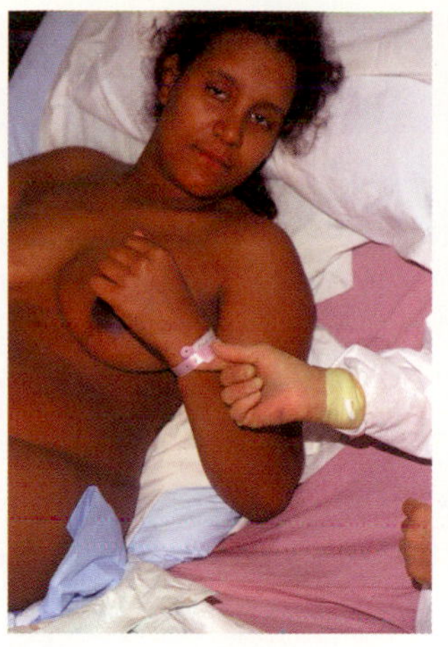
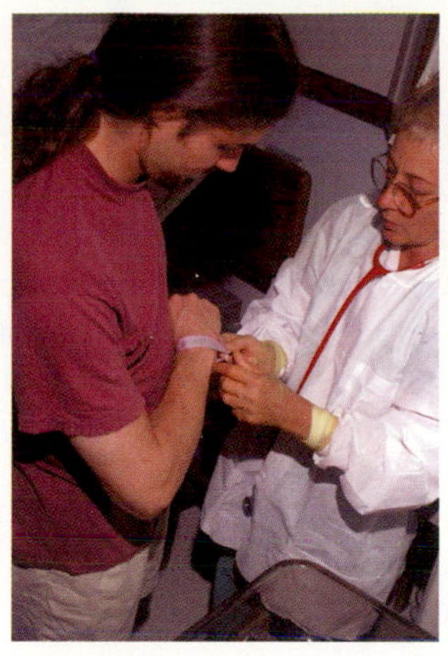
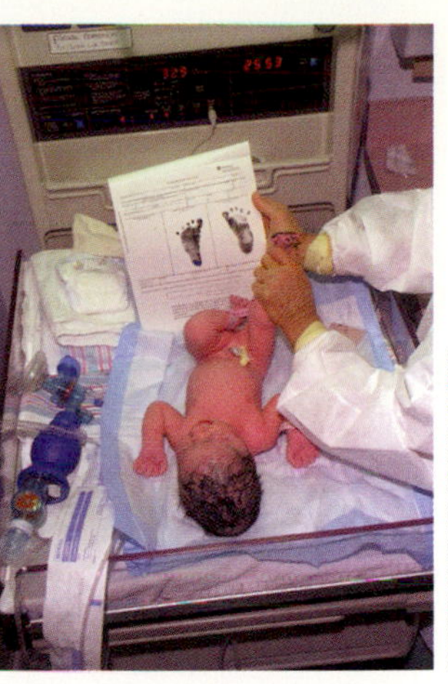

COURTESY OF DELMAR CENGAGE LEARNING

FIGURE 56-30 **Matching identification bands are placed on infant, mother, and partner; infant is foot printed.**

The bands must fit the infant snugly but not too tightly (Figure 56-30).

A long band is applied to the mother's wrist. The other long band is usually applied to the father's wrist or other person serving as primary support. In multiple births, the mother and father have a band for each infant. Barcode technology on wrist and ankle bands is currently being used in some hospitals for newborn and mother identification. A small two-dimensional barcode fits perfectly on a newborn's identification band and can be scanned through an Isolette (McCartney, 2008).

Most hospitals also footprint the newborn infant and either fingerprint or thumbprint the mother. The soles of the infant's feet must be dried and any vernix caseosa removed before footprinting.

CARE OF THE MOTHER

If an oxytocic medication is to be given when the placenta is delivered, the blood pressure is taken both before and after the medication is administered. Maternal blood pressure is monitored every 5 to 15 minutes. The oxytocic medication may increase the BP. Excessive blood loss will cause the BP to fall.

The fundus of the uterus is palpated for firmness. It should be firm, about the size of a grapefruit, in the midline, below the umbilicus. The proper method of palpating the uterus is illustrated in Figure 56-31.

After the CNM/physician has completed repairing the episiotomy (if one was made) and/or any lacerations, the perineum is washed with warm, sterile water and dried with a sterile towel. Maternity vaginal pads are then applied.

The mother may remain in the same bed (LDRP) or be moved to a recovery room bed. If the client is cold and begins to shiver, she should be covered with a warmed blanket, and a second blanket placed over it.

Mother, infant, and father or other support person are allowed time together to further the bonding and attachment process.

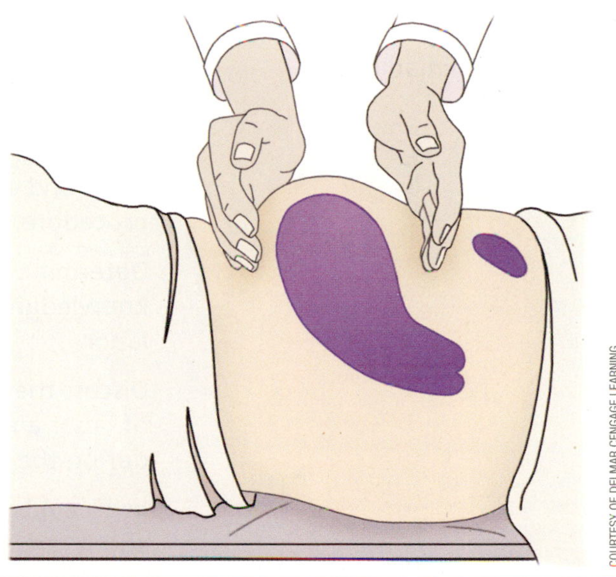

COURTESY OF DELMAR CENGAGE LEARNING

FIGURE 56-31 **Palpation of Uterus after Delivery of Placenta**

SAFETY

Removing Legs from Stirrups

If legs were in stirrups during the birth:

- Two persons are needed to remove them.
- Each person places one hand under the knee and one under the heel (the mother generally has little control over leg movement).
- At the same time, both legs are lowered to the bed.
- If the legs are numb, they may be bicycled to aid circulation return.

SAMPLE NURSING CARE PLAN

The Client in Labor

A.L., a 23-year-old gravida 1, para 0, is admitted in early labor. Her cervix is dilated 3 cm and is completely effaced. The fetus is at station 0. Contractions are every 5 minutes, duration 50 seconds, and of mild intensity. Her husband, J.L., is with her. They attend only the first two of the six childbirth preparation classes due to J.L.'s work schedule. A.L. is tightly holding J.L.'s hand. Her voice is quivering as she says, "My water just broke. I'm scared. I don't know if I can do this. I've never done this before."

NURSING DIAGNOSIS 1 *Anxiety* related to the situational crisis of labor and the birthing process at evidenced by gravida 1, para 0, attended only first 2 childbirth classes, voice quivering, statement that she is scared and doesn't know if she can do this

Nursing Outcomes Classification (NOC)
Anxiety Control
Coping

Nursing Interventions Classification (NIC)
Anxiety Reduction
Coping Enhancement

PLANNING/OUTCOMES	NURSING INTERVENTIONS	RATIONALE
A.L. will express less anxiety within an hour.	Maintain calm and confident manner.	Provides verbal and nonverbal message that labor is a normal process.
	Orient A.L. and J.L. to birthing room and explain admission procedure.	Allays feelings of anxiety regarding unfamiliar environment.
	Determine A.L.'s and J.L.'s knowledge and expectation of labor.	Establishes a baseline for intervention and enhances their sense of control.
	Discuss the expected progress of labor and what will happen during the process.	Lessens anxiety associated with the unknown.
	Involve A.L. and J.L. in decisions about care and share information on progress of labor.	Increases their sense of control.
	Involve J.L. in the care of A.L.	Strengthens A.L.'s ability to cope.

EVALUATION

A.L. states that she feels a little better and is now gently holding J.L.'s hand.

NURSING DIAGNOSIS 2 *Risk for Infection* related to rupture of membranes as evidenced by statement "My water just broke."

Nursing Outcomes Classification (NOC)
Treatment Behavior: Illness or Injury

Nursing Interventions Classification (NIC)
Infection Protection
Labor Induction

PLANNING/OUTCOMES	NURSING INTERVENTIONS	RATIONALE
A.L. will show no evidence of infection.	Assess amniotic fluid's color, odor, amount, and presence of meconium.	May indicate intrauterine infection or fetal distress.

SAMPLE NURSING CARE PLAN (Continued)

PLANNING/OUTCOMES	NURSING INTERVENTIONS	RATIONALE
	Monitor maternal vital signs and the FHR.	Evaluates for signs of infection and fetal distress.
	Maintain Standard Precautions by following good hand hygiene, wearing gloves when providing perineal care to A.L., and using aseptic technique when indicated.	Prevents spread of microorganisms.

EVALUATION

There are no signs of intrauterine infection or fetal distress.

A.L.'s vital signs are normal: T 98.6°F, P 84, R 20, and BP 114/70 mm Hg. FHR is 138. A.L. reports back pain. Contractions are now every 3 to 4 minutes, duration 60 seconds, and of moderate intensity. The cervix is dilated 5 cm with station +1.

NURSING DIAGNOSIS 3 *Acute Pain* related to increasing frequency, duration, and intensity as evidenced by contraction assessment

Nursing Outcomes Classification (NOC)
Pain Level
Pain: Disruptive Effects

Nursing Interventions Classification (NIC)
Pain Management
Anxiety Reduction

PLANNING/OUTCOMES	NURSING INTERVENTIONS	RATIONALE
A.L. will be able to cope with the discomfort.	Encourage A.L. to change position frequently (every 30 minutes), using such positions as leaning forward when sitting or standing, side-lying, and hands and knees.	Shifts weight of fetus away from the back, relieving back pain; relieves strain and constant pressure; and helps fetus descend through pelvis.
	Instruct A.L. and J.L. to use focused breathing, effleurage, massage, sacral pressure, and conscious relaxation.	Increases relaxation and counteracts some of the discomfort.
	Offer the use of shower, jacuzzi, or hydrotherapy.	Increases ability to relax. Heat interferes with transmission of pain impulses.
	Palpate for distended bladder and encourage regular voiding (at least every 2 hours).	Prevents discomfort and the impediment of fetal descent.
	Share with A.L. and J.L. about the progress in labor.	Increases willingness to continue when A.L. knows efforts are having desired results.
	Provide comfort measures such as oral care; ice chips; and cool, damp cloth to head or neck, and change damp gown and bed linens.	Relieves discomforts of dry mouth, diaphoresis, and leaking amniotic fluid.

(Continues)

SAMPLE NURSING CARE PLAN (Continued)

PLANNING/OUTCOMES	NURSING INTERVENTIONS	RATIONALE
	Inform A.L. about the pharmacologic pain relief measures available to her.	Gives A.L. a sense of control when she can choose when to use medication for pain.
	Administer pain medication as ordered.	Provides pain relief and increases the ability to relax.

EVALUATION

A.L. is able to handle the discomfort with J.L.'s help with focused breathing and by applying counterpressure to her back.

NURSING DIAGNOSIS 4 *Risk for Impaired **U**rinary Elimination*, related to sensory impairment as evidenced by progress of labor, station 11

Nursing Outcomes Classification (NOC)
Neurological Status: Autonomic

Nursing Interventions Classification (NIC)
Urinary Catheterization

PLANNING/OUTCOMES	NURSING INTERVENTIONS	RATIONALE
A.L.'s bladder will not exhibit signs of distention.	Palpate A.L.'s bladder at least every 2 hours.	Identifies a full bladder when A.L. is unable to feel the urge to void.
	Encourage frequent voiding; catheterize if necessary.	Avoids bladder distention that may impede descent of fetus and result in trauma to bladder.

EVALUATION

A.L. voids every 2 hours.

A.L.'s cervix is now 8 cm dilated, station is +2. Contractions are every 2 to 3 minutes, duration 70 seconds, and strong intensity. She is very uncomfortable, requests the pain medication, and says, "I can't take it anymore." J.L. is concerned and asks, "Is she alright?" FHR and maternal vital signs remain close to the admission assessment. A.L. is given meperidine (Demerol) 50 mg IV. She is now resting well between contractions. In 30 minutes A.L.'s cervix is completely dilated, station is +3. She pushes spontaneously several times during each contraction. When she pushes her back stiffens, her arms push on the bed, and she holds her breath. A.L. prefers a semi-Fowler's position.

NURSING DIAGNOSIS 5 *Deficient **K**nowledge (effective pushing technique)* related to lack of exposure to information since only attended first 2 prenatal classes, as evidenced by posture during pushing and breath holding

Nursing Outcomes Classification (NOC)
Knowledge: Labor and Delivery

Nursing Interventions Classification (NIC)
Teaching: Individual

PLANNING/OUTCOMES	NURSING INTERVENTIONS	RATIONALE
A.L. will push more effectively after instructions.	Teach A.L. techniques to push more effectively.	Makes pushing more effective.
	During each contraction, A.L. should do the following:	
	• Sit upright or squat	• Takes advantage of gravity; squatting slightly enlarges the pelvic outlet

SAMPLE NURSING CARE PLAN (Continued)

PLANNING/OUTCOMES	NURSING INTERVENTIONS	RATIONALE
	• Flex chin on chest and curl over uterus	• Directs force of push into pelvis
	• *With elbows bent*, pull on her flexed knees	• Provides more force to push
	• Exhale and vocalize when she pushes	• Prevents Valsalva maneuver, which causes a decrease in palcenta blood flow and thus oxygenation to the fetus
	Observe A.L.'s perineum for crowning.	Keeps everyone informed of progress.
	Allow A.L. to rest between contractions (no unnecessary talking).	Allows A.L. to gain strength for next contraction.

EVALUATION

In 30 minutes A.L. and J.L. have a 6 lb 10 oz (3,005 g) baby girl. The baby's Apgar scores are 8 at 1 minute and 9 at 5 minutes.

CASE STUDY

P.K., a 30-year-old gravida 4, para 3, has been in labor 3 hours. Her cervix is 7 cm dilated, station is –1. The fetus is in a vertex presentation, LOA position. When the membranes rupture during a strong contraction, the umbilical cord prolapses from the vagina, and the head is making the perineum bulge. P.K. begins to cry and asks, "What is happening? I feel something hanging out of me."

The following questions will guide your development of a nursing care plan for the case study.

1. What are the first actions the nurse should take?
2. What assessments should be made?
3. Identify two nursing diagnoses and goals for P.K.
4. Identify appropriate nursing interventions for the diagnoses.

SUMMARY

- There are two theories relative to why labor begins: the mechanical theory and the hormonal theory.
- Signs of impending labor are lightening, Braxton Hicks contractions, cervical softening, bloody show, rupture of membranes, and a sudden burst of energy.
- The five major variables that affect labor are known as the 5 Ps: passageway, passenger, position, powers, and psychological response.
- Labor is divided into four stages, which include first stage (dilation and effacement), second stage (birth of baby), third stage (delivery of placenta), and fourth stage (recovery).
- The mechanisms of labor describe how the fetus moves through the maternal pelvis and birth canal.
- There are many cultural aspects of labor and birth for the nurse to consider when caring for a client from another culture.
- Standard Precautions must be kept in mind when caring for a client during labor and birth because of the many opportunities for contact with body fluids and blood.
- Contractions are assessed for frequency, duration, interval, and intensity.
- Pain management is an important nursing intervention with both nonpharmacological and pharmacological measures.
- The most common risks of labor and birth are preterm labor and birth, premature rupture of membranes, dystocia, abnormal duration of labor, and prolapsed cord.
- Obstetric procedures that may be required to assist with the birth of an infant are cesarean birth, forceps-assisted birth, and vacuum-assisted birth.

REVIEW QUESTIONS

1. Which of the following measures should the nurse take when supporting a prepared couple during labor?
   1. Verbally encouraging them.
   2. Staying with them all the time.
   3. Taking FHR after each contraction.
   4. Leaving them alone to do "their own thing."
2. It is important for the nurse caring for a client in labor to make sure the bladder is kept empty because a full bladder may:
   1. cause glucosuria.
   2. cause proteinuria.
   3. impede the progress of labor.
   4. make the mother's back ache more.
3. After rupture of the membranes, the most appropriate action for the nurse is to:
   1. listen to the FHR.
   2. remove the wet linen.
   3. time the contractions.
   4. report the color and odor of the fluid.
4. A client is admitted for induction of labor with an oxytocic drug. She is 2 weeks past her EDB. Which of the following findings, if present, would it be essential to report to the CNM/physician before the oxytocic infusion is started?
   1. Low back ache.
   2. Regular contractions of 60 seconds' duration.
   3. Irregular contractions of 20 seconds' duration.
   4. An increase in blood pressure from 122/80 to 130/84 mm Hg.
5. A client is having a precipitate birth. The most appropriate nursing action is to:
   1. stay with her and call for help.
   2. quickly move her to the delivery room.
   3. carefully monitor the FHR and contractions.
   4 assist her to change her position and breathe deeply.
6. The client's membranes have just ruptured. The nurse's initial action is to:
   1. listen to the FHR.
   2. remove the wet linen.
   3. time the contractions.
   4. report the color and odor of the amniotic fluid.
7. A client comes to the hospital at 38 weeks gestation thinking she is in labor, but after several hours of observation, she is sent home. The student nurse asks how she can tell the difference between true and false labor. Which of the following responses should the nurse indicate will occur in true labor?
   1. A sudden burst of energy.
   2. Discomfort with uterine contractions.
   3. Bloody show with a vaginal exam.
   4. Cervical dilation.
8. A client is admitted to the labor and delivery unit stating she has not felt her baby move in several hours. Which of the following is the nurse's initial assessment?
   1. Cervical dilation and effacement.
   2. Status of amniotic membranes.
   3. Contraction pattern.
   4. Fetal heart rate.
9. The client is 5 cm dilated and is having back pain. She is asked to rest on her hands and knees because this position:
   1. keeps her from being bored in one position.
   2. prevents pressure sores from developing during labor.
   3. may rotate the fetus from occiput posterior to anterior.
   4. better allows the nurse to determine cervical dilation.
10. The nurse is assessing whether or not the client's membranes are ruptured. Which of the following findings would indicate her water has broken?
    1. The nitrazine tape turns green.
    2. There is clear fluid on the client's peripad.
    3. The client says her water broke.
    4. There is ferning on the microscope slide.

REFERENCES/SUGGESTED READINGS

Adams, E., & Bianchi, A. (2008). A practical approach to labor support. *Journal of Obstetric, Gynecological, & Neonatal Nursing, 37*, 106–115.

Ahmed, S. (1994, December). *Culturally sensitive caregiving for Pakistani women.* Lecture presented at the Medical College of Virginia Hospitals, Richmond, VA.

American College of Nurse-Midwives. (2009). Become a midwife. Retrieved August 19, 2009, from http://www.midwife.org/become_midwife.cfm.

Bergstrom, L., Seidel, J., Skellman-Hull, L., & Roberts, J. (1997). "I gotta push. Please let me push!": Social interactions during the change from first to second stage labor. *Birth, 24*, 173–180.

Blackburn, S. (2003). *Maternal, fetal, and neonatal physiology.* Philadelphia: W. B. Saunders.

Bulechek, G., Butcher, H., McCloskey, J., & Dochterman, J., eds. (2008). *Nursing Interventions Classification (NIC)* (5th ed.). St. Louis, MO: Mosby/Elsevier.

Burst, H. (2004). *Varney's midwifery* (4th ed). Sudberry, MA: Jones & Barlett.

Callister, L. (2008). Cesarean birth rates: global trends. *MCN: The American Journal of Maternal/Child Nursing*, 33(2), 129.

Callister, L., & Vega, R. (1998). Giving birth: Guatemalan women's voices. *JOGNN, 27*(3), 289–295.

Centers for Disease Control and Prevention. (2007). Pregnancy and childbirth. Retrieved August 20, 2009, from http://www.cdc.gov/hiv/topics/perinatal/.

Centers for Disease and Prevention. (2008). Episiotomy: can you deliver a baby without one? Retrieved August 20, 2009, from http://www.mayoclinic.com/health/episiotomy/HO00064.

Cesario, S. (2001). Care of the Native American woman: Strategies for practice, education, and research. *JOGNN, 30*(1), 13–19.

Chapman, L. (2000). Expectant fathers and labor epidurals. *MCN, 25*(3), 133–138.

Clark, S., Simpson, K., Knox, E., & Garite, T. (2009). Oxytocin: new perspectives on an old drug. *American Journal of Obstetrics & Gynecology*, 200, 35–37.

Cunningham, F., Leveno, K., Gilstrap, L., Bloom, S., Hauth, J., & Wenstrom, K. D. (2005). *Williams obstetrics* (22nd ed). New York, NY: McGraw-Hill.

D'Arcy, Y. (1999). Managing discomfort with a walking epidural. *Nursing99, 29*(6), 22.

DeSeve, M. (1997). Keeping the faith: Jewish traditions in pregnancy & childbirth. *Lifelines, 1*(4), 46–49.

Dickason, L., Silverman, B., & Kaplan, J. (1998). *Maternal–infant nursing care* (3rd ed.). St. Louis, MO: Mosby–Year Book.

Doulas of North America International. (2009). What is a doula? Retrieved August 19, 2009, from http://www.dona.org/mothers/index.php.

Dwyer, D., & Swayze, S. (2002). Problems after vacuum-assisted childbirth. *Nursing2002, 32*(1), 74.

Ferri, R., & Sofer, D. (2003). Do vaginal births need a good push? *AJN, 103*(4), 19.

Gennaro, S., Kamwendo, L., Mbweza, E., & Kershbaumer, R. (1998). Childbearing in Malawi, Africa. *JOGNN, 27*(2), 191–196.

Gilbert, E., & Harmon, J. (1998). *Manual of high risk pregnancy and delivery* (2nd ed.). St. Louis, MO: Mosby–Year Book.

Howard, J., & Berbiglia, V. (1997). Caring for childbearing Korean women. *JOGNN, 26*(6), 665–671.

Hutchinson, M., & Baqi-Aziz, M. (1994). Nursing care of the childbearing Muslim family. *JOGNN, 23*(9), 767–771.

Hutzal, C., Boyle, E., Kenyon, S., Nash, J., Winsor, S., Taylor, D., & Kirpalani, H. (2008). Use of antibiotics for the treatment of preterm parturition and prevention of neonatal morbidity: a metaanalysis. *American Journal of Obstetrics & Gynecology, 199*(6), 115–121.

James, D., & Maher, M. (2009). Caring for the extremely obese woman during pregnancy and birth. *MCN: The American Journal of Maternal/Child Nursing, 34*(1), 24–30.

Jordan, B. (1978). *Birth in four cultures*. St. Albans: Eden Press Women's Publications.

Lambert, P. (2003). Laboring Lessons. *AWHONN Lifelines, 7*(2), 184.

Leifer, G. (2008). *Maternity nursing: an introductory text* (10th ed). St. Louis, MO: Saunders Elsevier.

Littleton, L., & Engebretson, J. (2002). *Maternal, neonatal, and women's health nursing*. Clifton Park, NY: Delmar Cengage Learning.

London, M., Ladewig, P., Ball, J., & Bindler, R. (2007). *Maternal & child nursing care* (2nd ed). Upper Saddle River, NJ: Pearson Education, Inc.

Lowdermilk, D., & Perry, S. (2006). *Maternity nursing* (7th ed.). St. Louis, MO: Mosby–Year Book.

Lowe, N. (1996). The pain and discomfort of labor and birth. *JOGNN, 25*(1), 82–92.

Martin, P., & Leaton, M. (2001). Amniotic fluid embolism. *AJN, 101*(3), 43–44.

Mattson, S. (1995). Culturally sensitive perinatal care for Southeast Asians. *JOGNN, 24*(4), 335–341.

McCartney, P. (1998a). The birth ball—Are you using it in your practice setting? *MCN, 23*(4), 218.

McCartney, P. (1998b). Caring for women with epidurals using the "laboring down" technique. *MCN, 23*(5), 274.

McCartney, P. (2008). Newborn identification and barcodes. *MCN: The American Journal of Maternal/Child Nursing, 33*(2), 128.

Moleti, C. (2009). Trends and controversies in labor induction. *MCN: The American Journal of Maternal/Child Nursing, 34*(1), 41–47.

Moorhead, S., Johnson, M., Maas, M., & Swanson, E. (2008). *Nursing Outcomes Classification (NOC)* (4th ed.). St. Louis, MO: Elsevier-Health Sciences Division.

Murray, S., McKinney, E., & Gorrie, T. (2001). *Foundations of maternal–newborn nursing* (3rd ed.). Philadelphia, W. B. Saunders.

North American Nursing Diagnosis Association International. (2010). *NANDA-I nursing diagnoses: Definitions and classification 2009–2011*. Ames, IA: Wiley-Blackwell.

O'Brian, W.F., & Cefalo, R.C. (1996). Labor and delivery. In S. G. Gabbe, J. R. Niehyl, & J. L. Simpson (Eds.). *Obstetrics: Normal and problem pregnancies* (3rd ed.). New York: Churchill Livingstone.

Payant, L., Davies, B., Graham, I., Peterson, W., & Clinch, J. (2008). Nurses' intentions to provide continuous labor support to women. *Journal of Obstetric, Gynecological, & Neonatal Nursing, 37*, 405–414.

Perez, P., & Herrick, L. (1998). Doulas: Exploring their roles with parents, hospitals & nurses. *Lifelines, 2*(2), 54.

Petersen, L., & Besuner, P. (1997). Pushing techniques during labor: Issues and controversies. *JOGNN, 26*(6), 719–726.

Romano, A., & Lothian, J. (2008). Promoting, protecting, and supporting normal birth: a look at the evidence. *Journal of Obstetric, Gynecological, & Neonatal Nursing, 37*, 94–105.

Schneiderman, J. (1998). Rituals of placenta disposal. *MCN, 23*(3), 142–143.

Scott-Ramos, I. (1995, January). *Culturally sensitive care giving for Latino women*. Lecture presented at the Medical College of Virginia Hospitals. Richmond, VA.

Sharts-Hopko, N. (1995). Birth in the Japanese context. *JOGNN, 24*(4), 343–351.

Shen, T., DeFranco, E., Stamilio, D., Chang, J., & Muglia, L. (2008). A population-based study of race-specific risk for preterm premature rupture of membranes. *American Journal of Obstetrics & Gynecology, 199*, 373–375.

Shrestha, N. (2007). Nuchal cord and perinatal outcome. *Kathmandu University Medical Journal, 5*(19), 360–363.

Simpson, K., & Creehan, P. (2001). *AWHONN perinatal nursing* (2nd ed.). Philadelphia: Lippincott Williams & Wilkins.

Simpson, K., & Knox, G. (2009). Oxytocin as a high-alert medication: implications for perinatal patient safety. *MCN: The American Journal of Maternal/Child Nursing, 34*(1), 8–15.

Stark, M., Rudell, B., & Haus, G. (2008). Observing position and movements in hydrotherapy: a pilot study. *Journal of Obstetric, Gynecological, & Neonatal Nursing, 37*, 116–122.

Stremler, R., Halpren, S., Weston, J., Yee, J., & Hodnett, E. (2009). Hands-and-knees positioning during labor with epidural analgesic. *Journal of Obstetric, Gynecological, & Neonatal Nursing, 38*, 391–398.

Suplee, P., Dawley, K., & Bloch, J. (2007). Tailoring peripartum nursing care for women of advanced maternal age. *Journal of Obstetric, Gynecological, & Neonatal Nursing*, 36, 616–623.

Tennyson, M. (2000). Labor at 20,000 feet. *AJN, 100*(9), 49–52.

Usta, M., Merier, B.M., & Sibai, B.M. (1999). Current obstetrical practice & umbilical cord prolapse. *AWHONN Lifelines, 5*(6), 10–13.

Weber, S. (1996). Cultural aspects of pain in childbearing women. *JOGNN, 25*(1), 67–72.

World Health Organization. (2008). Adolescent pregnancy fact sheet. Retrieved August 20, 2009, from http://www.who.int/making_pregnancy_safer/events/2008/mdg5/adolescent_preg.pdf.

World Health Organization. (2008). Maternal mortality fact sheet. Retrieved August 20, 2009, from http://www.who.int/making_pregnancy_safer/events/2008/mdg5/factsheet_maternal_mortality.pdf.

Zwelling, E. (2008). The emergence of high-tech birthing. *Journal of Obstetric, Gynecological, & Neonatal Nursing, 37*, 85–93.

Zwelling, E., Johnson, K., & Allen, J. (2006). How to implement complementary therapies for laboring women. *MCN: The American Journal of Maternal/Child Nursing, 31*(6), 364–370.

RESOURCES

American College of Nurse-Midwives (ACNM), http://www.midwife.org

American College of Obstetricians and Gynecologists (ACOG), http://www.acog.com

Association of Women's Health, Obstetric, and Neonatal Nurses (AWHONN), http://www.awhonn.org

Childbirth Graphics, http://www.childbirthgraphics.com

Doulas of North America (DONA) International, http://www.dona.org

InterNational Association of Parents & Professionals for Safe Alternatives in Childbirth (NAPSAC), http://www.napsac.org

Midwives Alliance of North America, http://www.mana.org

National Association of Childbearing Centers, http://www.BirthCenters.org

CHAPTER 57
Postpartum Care

MAKING THE CONNECTION

Refer to the following chapters to increase your understanding of postpartum care:

Basic Nursing

- ***Communication***
- ***Client Teaching***
- ***Infection Control/ Asepsis***
- ***Pain Management***

Adult Health Nursing

- ***Reproductive System***

Maternal & Pediatric Nursing

- ***Prenatal Care***
- ***Complications of Pregnancy***
- ***The Birth Process***

LEARNING OBJECTIVES

Upon completion of this chapter, you should be able to:

- Define key terms.
- Describe the various aspects of family adaptation.
- Discuss the mother's physiologic changes after the birth of her baby.
- Describe the expected and unexpected emotional/behavioral changes in the new mother.
- Demonstrate the postpartum assessments for every new mother and the additional assessments for a mother who has had a cesarean birth.
- Discuss the possible postpartum complications of hemorrhage and puerperal infection, including endometritis, mastitis, and thrombophlebitis.
- Explain the advantages and disadvantages of the various methods of family planning.
- Plan and provide the care of a woman who has had a baby.

KEY TERMS

afterpains
attachment
bonding
claiming process
colostrum
disseminated intravascular coagulation (DIC)
dyspareunia
engorgement
engrossment
entrainment
involution
let-down reflex
lochia
mastitis
metritis
neonate
oophoritis
postpartum blues
postpartum depression (PPD)
postpartum hemorrhage
postpartum psychosis
puerperal (postpartum) infection
puerperium
salpingitis
subinvolution
thrombophlebitis

INTRODUCTION

Postpartum period, or **puerperium**, is the term for the first 6 weeks after the birth of an infant. During this time, the mother and family will experience many changes, including changes in the structure and function of a family. The mother and, if she has one, her partner begin to establish a relationship with their newborn infant and adjust their lives to include the newborn. The mother and partner must also redefine their own relationship. If there are siblings, they must adjust to their new place in the family structure and the newborn's claim on the time and love of the parents.

Many factors influence family adaptation, including previous experience with a newborn and the convenience of a support system. Previously, postpartum care was focused on the mother and newborn, but now the father or partner, siblings, and sometimes grandparents are included. This chapter explores the events of the postpartum period, including the various ways a family adapts to the newborn; the physiologic and psychosocial changes the mother experiences; preparation for discharge; health promotion; postcesarean section care; and possible postpartum complications.

FAMILY ADAPTATION

Family roles and relationships must be reorganized with the birth of a baby. Bonding and attachment are the terms used to describe this process of becoming acquainted with the **neonate** (a newborn from birth to 28 days of life). The terms bonding and attachment are often used interchangeably, although they do have different meanings.

Bonding refers to a rapid process of attachment, parent to child only, taking place during the sensitive period—the first 30 to 60 minutes after the birth. The bonding is enhanced when parent and infant touch and interact with each other (Figure 57-1). Immediately after birth, the neonate generally is in a quiet, alert state and is ready for bonding and closeness. It is very important that the nurse facilitate quiet time for mother and her new infant. This might mean that the nurse may have to delay bathing the infant so mom has adequate time to bond. It is a good time to initiate breastfeeding.

Attachment, a long-term process that begins during pregnancy and intensifies during the postpartum period, establishes an enduring bond between parent and child and develops through reciprocal (parent-to-child and child-to-parent) behaviors. Becoming acquainted with the neonate is an important part of attachment. Touching, exploring, talking to, and using eye contact are all methods used to become acquainted.

The family identifies the infant's "likeness" to and the infant's "differences" from family members, and then the infant's unique qualities. This is often referred to as the **claiming process**.

Mother's Adaptation to Neonate

A mother's touch changes as she moves through a discovery phase with her infant. The mother usually begins by using her fingertips to explore her infant's face, fingers, and toes. This is called finger-tipping. The mother may then change to using her palm to stroke her infant's back, chest, arms, and legs. The mother uses her arms to enfold and bring her infant close to her body (Figure 57-2). She may smooth her infant's hair and rub her cheek on the infant's cheek or head. A parent's intense interest and preoccupation in the newborn is termed **engrossment**.

Most mothers speak in a high-pitched voice spontaneously to their infants, seeming to know intuitively that infants respond to higher-pitched voices. Soon after birth, infants can distinguish their mother's voice from others.

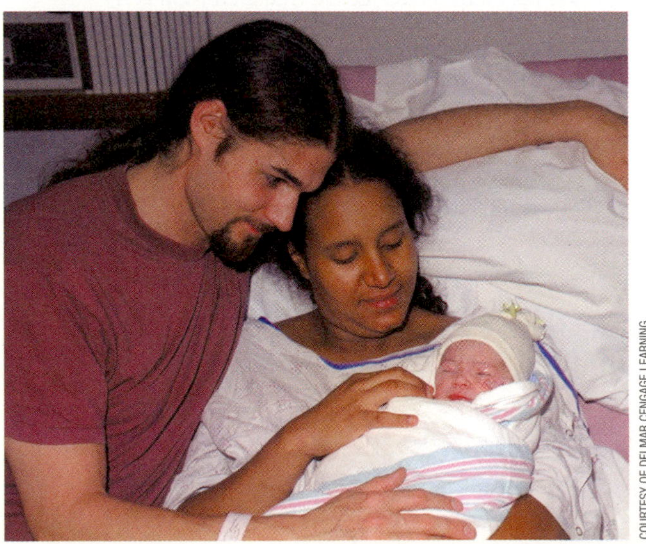

COURTESY OF DELMAR CENGAGE LEARNING

Figure 57-1 Bonding Between Parents and Infant after the Birth

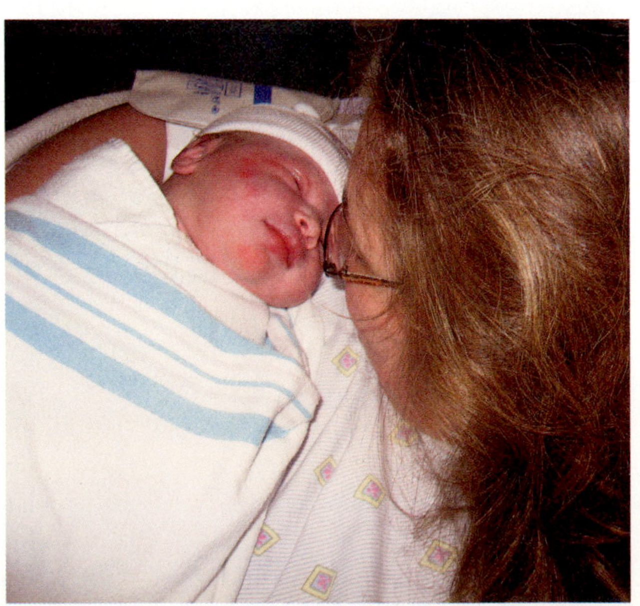

COURTESY OF DELMAR CENGAGE LEARNING

Figure 57-2 Mother Enfolding and Cuddling Her Infant

CULTURAL CONSIDERATIONS

Touching an Infant

Nurses should be aware that in some cultures (Southeast Asian, Vietnamese, Cambodian, and Laotian), it is considered offensive to pat an infant on the head because the head is viewed as a sacred place where the soul resides (Mattson, 1995).

Father/Partner's Adaptation to Neonate—Nurse's Role in Assessing with Adaptation

A father or partner may also exhibit engrossment and display an intense interest in how the baby looks and responds (Figure 57-3). The father also has a desire to touch and hold his baby.

Research has shown that, for fathers and partners, variables other than being an active participant in the birth process are important in developing attachment to the newborn. They include the father or partner's relationship with his own parents, relationship with the infant's mother, and previous experience with children.

Montigny & Lacharité (2003) found that a father's interaction in the immediate postpartum period can have an effect on the ability to bond with their newborns. The study also found that nurses played a big role in this process. The fathers in the study gave specific examples of situations that helped in the bonding experience with their new infant, "obtaining a response from nurses in regard to father's emotional and physical needs" (333). Fathers also stated that being able to talk with the nurse and "sharing needs, preoccupations, and worries with nurses" helped them feel involved in the infant process. A few things that were noted as having a negative effect on paternal bonding were nurses who humiliated new fathers when they were helping to care for their new infant and nurses who gave contradictory information to new fathers on infant care.

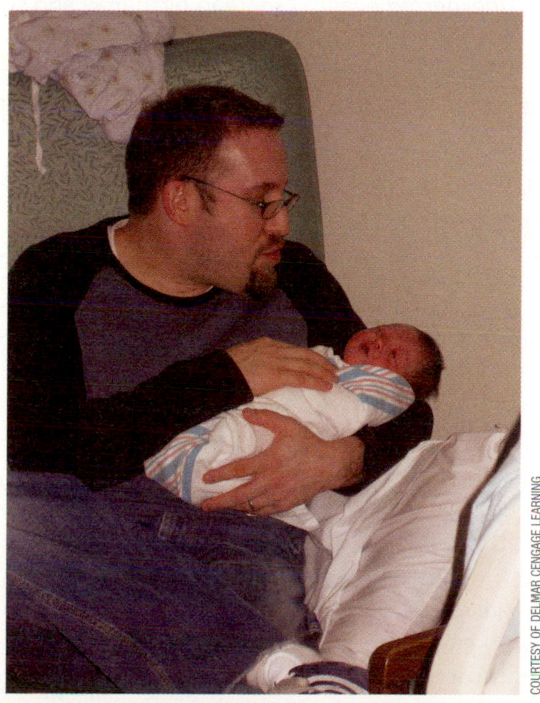

COURTESY OF DELMAR CENGAGE LEARNING

FIGURE 57-3 Father Displaying Engrossment

LIFE SPAN CONSIDERATIONS

Neonates' Reciprocal Behaviors

Neonates have the ability to:

- Make eye contact and move eyes to follow parent's face.
- Engage in intense, prolonged mutual gazing.
- Grasp parent's finger and hold on.
- Move in rhythm to the parent's voice. This is called **entrainment**.

Studies have shown that the infant's vision goes from the mother's breast to her face. For bottle feeding infants, it is from the crook of the mothers arm to her face. Encourage the mother to look at her infant and talk to the infant while the infant is feeding (Staff, 2008).

The study also looked at the level of involvement of the father in the postpartum period and found the following results:

- Fathers who were less involved reported very few incidents positive or negative in the postpartum period.
- Fathers who were moderately involved reported the highest number of negative incidents and reported that the highlight of their experience was feeding their infant.
- The fathers who were highly involved in the postpartum period were most likely to report positive interactions between new infant, spouse, and staff.
- The highly involved fathers were interested in all aspects of infant care and took an active role in learning (Montigny & Lacharité, 2003).

It is important for the nurse to recognize the important role that the father/partner has in the postpartum period. The nurse should understand that by helping to facilitate positive experiences for the new father they may help build stronger family bonds in the future.

Siblings' Adaptation to Neonate

The response of a sibling to the birth of a new sister or brother depends on the age and developmental level of the older sibling. The adaptation is probably most difficult for toddlers, who often view the new baby as competition, someone who takes the parent's time and love. Negative behavioral changes may occur in the toddler, such as a return to thumb sucking or bed wetting; sleep problems; or hostility toward the mother, especially when she is caring for the new baby. Positive behavioral changes may be increased independence and taking an interest in the care of the newborn.

Parents' attitudes toward the newborn and their preparation of the siblings for the new arrival guide the older children's reactions. Parents can include each child in the care of the baby according to their capabilities. For example, toddlers may be able to bring a clean diaper to the parent; preschoolers may help prepare for the baby's bath; and older children may hold, carry, or feed the baby (Figure 57-4). Parents need to ensure that siblings are not left out. In addition to allowing the sibling to help with the new baby, parents should provide quality time with the older children.

Grandparents' Adaptation to Neonate

Grandparents go through a transition to grandparenthood just as parents go through a transition to parenthood. Practices and attitudes about childbirth and childrearing change from one generation to another, as do the roles of men and women. The extent to which grandparents understand and accept the current practices and attitudes affects their relationship with their children and how supportive they may be (Figure 57-5). It is important for the nurse to take into consideration that some pregnancies are not always a joyous occasion in some families, especially in the case of a teenage pregnancy. As the nurse, you should encourage the new grandparent to hold the baby and help the family with any resources that they might need.

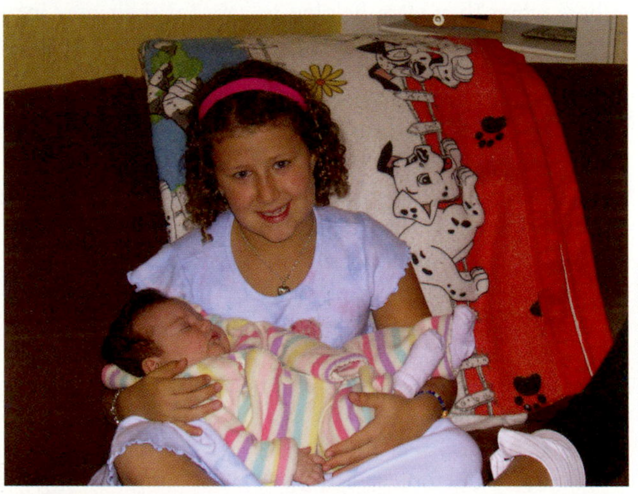

COURTESY OF DELMAR CENGAGE LEARNING

Figure 57-4 An older sibling can help hold the baby.

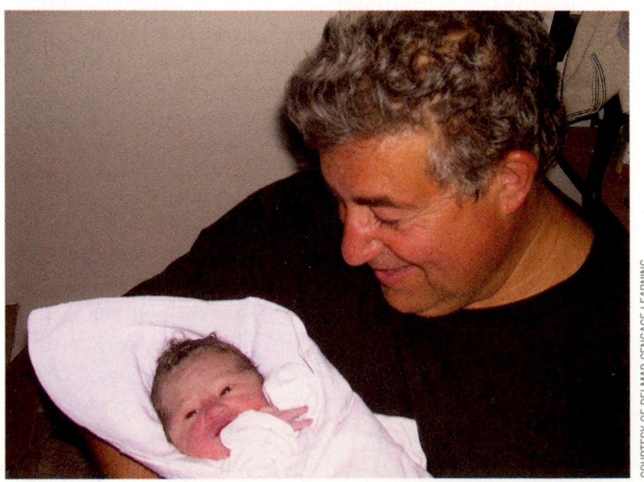

COURTESY OF DELMAR CENGAGE LEARNING

Figure 57-5 Grandparent Enjoying New Grandchild

PROFESSIONALTIP

Factors Affecting Family Adaptation

Many factors affect family adaptation to the newborn:

- *Parental fatigue*: Not being able to sleep uninterrupted through the night may affect the caregivers' energy level.
- *Previous experience with a newborn*: First-time parents and parents with children will progress at different rates through the attachment process.
- *Parental expectations of the newborn*: The newborn's appearance, gender, and behaviors in relation to parental expectations may influence the attachment process.
- *Knowledge of and confidence in providing for newborn needs*: Parents have varying levels of experience in feeding, consoling, and providing care in general to newborns.
- *Temperament of the newborn*: Some infants are calm, easily consoled, and cuddly, whereas others are irritable, difficult to console, and do not like cuddling.
- *Temperament of parents*: Anxious, insecure, excitable parents have more difficulties than calm, secure, less anxious parents.
- *Age of parents*: Teenage, middle-age, and older parents will all react differently to the new family structure based on their life experiences.
- *Available support system*: Help with household tasks and help and encouragement with infant care can ease family adaptation to the newborn.
- *Unexpected events*: Cesarean birth may add stress and increase recovery time, therefore limiting time and energies available for newborn care.

MATERNAL PHYSIOLOGIC CHANGES

Many of the physiologic changes postpartum (following birth) are a reversal of the changes in the various body systems that occurred during pregnancy. The initiation of lactation and reestablishment of normal menstrual cycles also occur.

Reproductive System

Changes occur in the uterus, cervix, vagina, and perineum.

Uterus

Involution is the return of the uterus to its prepregnancy size and condition. There are three processes involved in involution:

- *Muscle fiber contraction*: With the uterus now empty, it firmly contracts to control bleeding from the area of placental attachment; the muscle fibers gradually regain their former size and shape.

CULTURAL CONSIDERATIONS

Lochia

Cultural norms may affect interpretation of postpartum events. For instance, women in Malawi, Africa, are considered "dirty" as long as they have a lochia discharge; sexual intercourse is therefore prohibited for 6 months after birth (Gennaro, Kamwendo, Mbweza, & Kershbaumer, 1998). In Judaism, husbands may not touch their wives during the postpartum period, as the wives are considered unclean when they are bleeding. The nurse should recognize this and assist by passing the newborn back and forth between parents if they are in the room.

- *Catabolism*: The enlarged muscle cells of the uterus experience catabolic changes in protein cytoplasm that reduce the size of each cell. Catabolic products are excreted as nitrogenous wastes in the urine.
- *Regeneration*: The endometrium is regenerated within 2 to 3 weeks, except for the placental site, which is healed and regenerated by approximately 6 weeks.

Uterine Fundal Descent Immediately after the birth, the uterus is about the size of a grapefruit, with the fundus about halfway between the umbilicus and symphysis pubis. The fundus then rises to the umbilicus and stays there about 12 hours. Then the fundus descends about 1 cm, 1 finger breadth, each day for about 10 days, when it is once again in the pelvis and unable to be palpated abdominally (Figure 57-6). A full bladder will push the uterus upward.

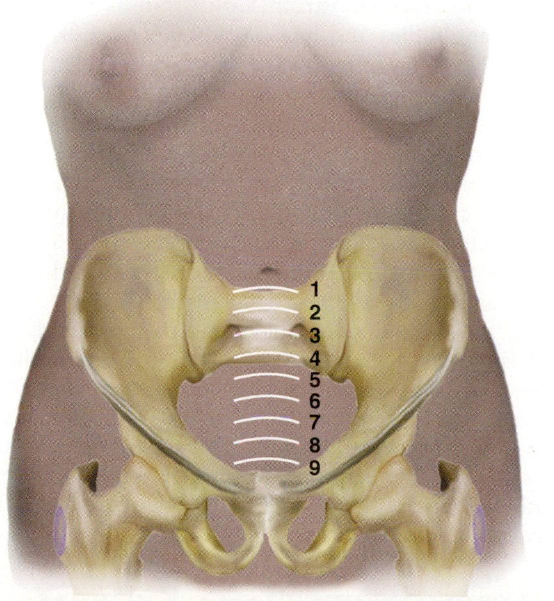

FIGURE 57-6 Uterine Involution. Uterine fundal descent is approximately 1 cm/day.

PROFESSIONAL TIP

Postpartum Vaginal Bleeding

- All vaginal bleeding in the postpartum period is not necessarily lochia. Lochia usually trickles from the vagina, although a gush of bright red blood may result when the fundus is massaged or when blood pooled in the vagina is expelled when the mother stands up.
- Ambulation and breastfeeding usually increases the amount of lochia.
- If blood spurts from the vagina or the amount is excessive when the uterus is firmly contracted, suspect cervical or vaginal tears.

Even a slow trickle of blood should be cause for further investigation in the postpartum period. Some postpartum hemorrhages start out very slowly. It is important to teach clients the difference in normal lochia flow versus a hemorrhage. A good time for teaching is the first time the client ambulates to the bathroom for pericare.

The contracting uterus may be a source of discomfort for some women after the infant's birth, especially for multiparas and those who are breastfeeding. Breastfeeding stimulates the release of oxytocin from the posterior pituitary, which stimulates strong uterine contractions as well as the "let-down" reflex. These contractions are known as **afterpains**.

Lochia **Lochia** is the uterine/vaginal discharge after childbirth. It is initially bright red, then changes to a pink or pinkish brown, and then to a yellowish white. The odor of lochia is like a normal menstrual flow. A foul odor indicates infection.

For the first 3 days, the lochia is mostly blood with small pieces of decidua and mucus. This is called lochia rubra. About the 4th day, the amount decreases and the color changes to a pink or pinkish brown called lochia serosa. It is mostly a serous exudate with cervical mucus, erythrocytes, and leukocytes. After the 10th day, the erythrocyte level decreases and the discharge becomes yellowish white, lochia alba. Now the lochia consists of leukocytes, epithelial cells, decidua, mucus, serum, and bacteria. This discharge may last for 6 weeks or more (Lowdermilk & Perry, 2007).

Cervix

Within 18 hours after birth, the cervix has become firm, has shortened, and has regained its form (Lowdermilk & Perry, 2007). By the end of 2 weeks, the cervical os (cervical opening) is closed, but after delivery, the opening appears as a horizontal slit. The cervical os of a nulliparous woman is round or oval, but a parous woman's cervical os is a horizontal slit.

Vagina and Perineum

The vagina was greatly stretched during labor. It takes 6 weeks for the vagina to complete involution and regain the contour it had before pregnancy. It never does regain the size it had before pregnancy. The vaginal mucosa is atrophic in lactating women, at least until menstruation returns. The reduced level of estrogen causes a decrease in vaginal lubrication, which may cause **dyspareunia**, or coital discomfort.

The stretching and thinning of the perineum during labor may cause edema and bruising of the perineum after the birth. Many women have an episiotomy (surgical incision of the perineum) before the infant's birth. Lacerations of the perineum also may occur. Both lacerations and episiotomies are classified according to the tissues involved and will take time to heal:

First degree: skin and mucous membrane.

Second degree: skin, mucous membrane, and muscle.

Third degree: skin, mucous membrane, muscle, and anal sphincter.

Fourth degree: skin, mucous membrane, muscle, anal sphincter, and rectal mucosa.

Even when the episiotomy or laceration is small, it can cause a great deal of discomfort because the muscles of the perineum are used when sitting, stooping, bending, squatting, walking, and defecating.

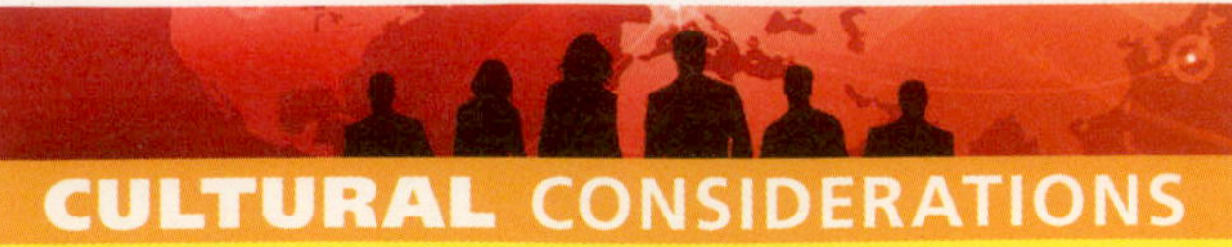

CULTURAL CONSIDERATIONS

Breastfeeding

- Some Hispanic, Southeast Asian, Vietnamese, Cambodian, and Laotian women may choose not to breastfeed until the milk comes in (Mattson, 1995).
- Rural Indian women discard the colostrum because they think it harms the child's health. The child is not breastfeed until the milk comes in (Bandyonpadhyay, 2009).
- Many women will breastfeed until the child is 2 years old, based on cultural practices and expectations (Hutchinson & Baqi-Aziz, 1994).
- African-American women have the lowest rate of breastfeeding at 6 months of age in the postpartum period, currently ranking at 52.9% (Oyeku, 2003). It is important for the nurse to encourage breastfeeding initiation if wanted in the postpartum period.

Endocrine System

After the expulsion of the placenta, the levels of the placental hormones estrogen, progesterone, human placental lactogen (hPL), human chorionic gonadotropin (hCG), and relaxin rapidly decline. The decrease in hPL, estrogen, and cortisol causes a reversal of the diabetogenic effect of pregnancy. This rapid change necessitates frequent assessment of the diabetic mother's blood glucose level.

Lactation

The rapid decrease of the estrogen and progesterone levels allows the prolactin to initiate milk production within 2 to 3 days after the infant's birth. Oxytocin, a posterior pituitary hormone, causes the milk to be expressed from the alveoli into the lactiferous ducts. This is called "let down." The **let-down reflex** is a neurohormonal reflex; that is, either neuro (the mind) or the hormone (oxytocin) may initiate "let down." A breastfeeding mother hearing a baby cry or thinking about feeding her infant often stimulates the let-down reflex, and milk will drip from the nipples (neuro). The release of oxytocin in response to the infant's sucking also stimulates the let-down reflex (hormonal). Many women describe a tingling/burning feeling in the breasts when the milk is "let down."

Menstrual Cycle

There is a great difference when ovulation and menstruation are reestablished based on whether the mother is breastfeeding or not breastfeeding. The level of follicle-stimulating hormone (FSH) is the same in both breastfeeding and nonbreastfeeding mothers. It is believed that the increased level of prolactin in breastfeeding mothers causes the ovaries to not respond to the FSH and ovulation does not occur (Bowes, 2001). The prolactin level remains high in breastfeeding women for approximately 6 weeks. The prolactin level is influenced by three factors: frequency and duration of feedings, supplemental feedings, and possibly the strength of the infant's sucking (Lowdermilk & Perry, 2007). In nonbreastfeeding mothers, the prolactin level returns to the prepregnant level within 2 weeks.

Ovulation in nonbreastfeeding mothers takes place as early as 27 days after the birth and usually has resumed by 2 months (Bowes, 2001). Most nonbreastfeeding mothers resume menstruating within 3 months after the birth.

The average time for ovulation to take place in breastfeeding mothers is approximately 190 days (Bowes, 2001). The return of ovulation and menstruation in breastfeeding mothers is determined, to a large measure, by the breastfeeding pattern. This underscores the fact that breastfeeding is not a reliable form of birth control.

Breasts

During the last few weeks of pregnancy, the breasts begin to fill with a fluid called colostrum. **Colostrum** is a yellowish fluid rich in antibodies and high in protein. As milk production begins, 2 to 3 days after birth, the breasts feel firm, warm, and may be tender. This lasts about 48 hours. By day 3 or 4 after the birth, **engorgement** may occur; the breasts become quite distended (swollen), tender, and warm. This is caused mainly by vasocongestion, especially of the veins and lymphatics.

The changes in the breasts after the birth of a baby are partly determined by whether the mother is breastfeeding or not. For the nursing mother, frequent breastfeeding sessions encourage milk production and sustain lactation.

If the mother does not intend to breastfeed, although milk is present it should not be expressed because this causes more milk to be produced. Engorgement spontaneously disappears and discomfort decreases in 24 to 48 hours if the breasts are not emptied of milk. If breastfeeding is never begun or is stopped, lactation ceases within a week. Encourage the mother to wear a tight-fitting sports bra to help with the pain during this period.

Gastrointestinal System

Most new mothers are hungry and thirsty after giving birth because of the energy expended during labor. Following

CULTURAL CONSIDERATIONS

Foods in the Postpartum Period

A nurse must be sensitive to the fact that a new mother's food choices and preferences may have cultural or ethnic foundations. For instance:

- Women of Southeast Asia are taught that any food or drink must be hot in temperature for at least 1 month. Foods are mainly rice and boiled chicken (Davis, 2001).
- Muslim women may request a vegetarian or kosher diet following childbirth (Hutchinson & Baqi-Aziz, 1994).
- Rural Indian women avoid high-fiber foods, acidic foods, cold foods of foods considered hot and cold. Instead, they eat milk, ghee, butter and some types of fish. Garlic is believed to cause uterine contraction (Bandyopadhyay, 2009).

recovery from any analgesia or anesthesia the mother may have received, she may request extra food.

Mothers may encounter difficulty in having a bowel movement after giving birth. There are several reasons, including:

- Peristalsis has been decreased by the effects of the increased progesterone level during pregnancy; this may take several days to become normal again.
- Prelabor diarrhea.
- Lack of food during labor.
- Dehydration.
- Perineal trauma, episiotomy repair, or hemorrhoids.
- Mother's anticipation of discomfort.
- Certain pain medications can cause constipation.

Cardiovascular System

The increase in blood volume during pregnancy allows a significant loss of blood without any ill effects to the mother. In a vaginal birth, blood loss averages 500 mL, whereas a cesarean birth averages a 1,000 mL blood loss.

Vital Signs

The new mother's temperature may increase to 100.4°F (38°C) during the first 24 hours because of dehydration during labor and the trauma of delivery. After 24 hours, the temperature returns to normal, although it may rise again when milk production begins.

The pulse, which increased during pregnancy, remains elevated or may even rise for up to 24 to 48 hours, but it should not exceed 100 beats per minute. Periods of bradycardia may also be experienced. The pulse returns to the prepregnant rate in approximately 8 weeks (Bowes, 2001).

The diaphragm descends when the uterus is emptied, making respirations much easier. In 6 to 8 weeks, respiratory function returns to the prepregnant rate. The blood pressure may have a small increase in both the systolic and diastolic aspects that lasts about 4 days (Bowes, 2001). The rapid decrease in intra-abdominal pressure after birth results in visceral blood vessel dilation, which may cause orthostatic hypotension.

Cardiac Output

Cardiac output that increased during pregnancy, may increase even higher for up to 60 minutes following delivery. This increase occurs following both vaginal and cesarean births (Bowes, 2001). Cardiac output remains elevated for at least 48 hours, and then rapidly decreases in the first 2 weeks postpartum. The return of cardiac output to the prepregnancy level takes about 24 weeks (Simpson & Creehan, 2007).

Blood Volume

The changes in blood volume are rapid and dramatic. Three physiologic changes protect from excessive blood loss:

- Loss of the uteroplacental circulation (when the placenta is expelled) reduces the maternal vascular bed by 10% to 15%.
- Stimulus for vasodilation is removed with the loss of placental endocrine function.
- Movement of extravascular water, stored during pregnancy, into the blood vessels increases blood volume.

The excess plasma volume is eliminated from the body by both diuresis and diaphoresis. Diuresis (excessive urine excretion) results from a decrease in aldosterone, which was increased during pregnancy. It is not uncommon for a new mother to have a urinary output of 3,000 mL per day for 2 to 3 days (Murray, McKinney, & Gorrie, 2005). Diaphoresis (profuse perspiration), while not clinically significant relative to fluid elimination, may be uncomfortable for the mother, especially if she is not expecting it to occur. It often occurs at night for 2 to 3 nights after delivery.

Blood Values

The white blood cell count, which increased slightly during pregnancy (to 12,000/mm^3), now increases to 20,000 or even 30,000/mm^3 during the first 10 to 12 days after the infant's birth (Cunningham, Grant, Leveno, Gilstrap, & Cox, 2005). The neutrophil level increases the most for protection against invading organisms.

The large loss of plasma volume during the first 3 days after the birth results in a rise in both the hemoglobin and hematocrit levels by the seventh day, unless excessive blood loss has occurred.

Coagulation

The increased levels of clotting factors and fibrinogen during pregnancy remain elevated for a few days as protection against postpartum hemorrhage. Thus, there is an increased risk for thrombus (clot) formation. Mothers having varicose veins, a cesarean birth, or a history of thrombophlebitis are at greater risk for thrombus formation.

Varicosities

Varices of the legs, anus (hemorrhoids), and vulvar area empty rapidly immediately after the birth. For clients who have residual hemorrhoids, try to encourage them to eat a diet high in fiber. Diets that are high in fiber will make softer stool, which will reduce straining and pressure on the hemorrhoids. Sitz baths offer a client temporary relief of hemorrhoid symptoms such as pressure, pain, and itching (Harvard.edu, 2008).

Urinary System

Physical changes take place in the structures of the urinary system; there are also chemical changes in the urine.

Physical Changes

The hypotonia of the bladder and dilation of the ureters during pregnancy take approximately 2 to 8 weeks to return to the prepregnant state (Cunningham et al., 2005). Also, the bladder, urethra, and tissue around the urinary meatus may have been traumatized and become edematous during labor and birth, which may result in difficulty in urination.

The mother may have a problem with overdistention and incomplete emptying of the bladder and residual retention of urine because the diuresis causes the bladder to fill quickly. Those mothers who received a regional anesthesia are especially at risk for bladder distention and difficulty voiding until the anesthesia wears off.

Postpartum hemorrhage and urinary tract infection are two complications related to urinary retention and bladder overdistention. Urinary stasis provides the bacteria with enough time to multiply and cause an infection. A full bladder displaces the uterus up and to the side, resulting in uterine atony (inability of the uterus to contract). This is the primary cause of excessive bleeding. Adequate emptying of the bladder helps the bladder regain its tone in 5 to 7 days after the birth (Lowdermilk & Perry, 2003).

Chemical Changes

The catabolic processes of uterine involution cause a mild proteinuria for 1 to 2 days in approximately 50% of new mothers (Simpson & Creehan, 2007). Ketonuria and elevated blood urea nitrogen (BUN) may also be present.

Musculoskeletal System

The musculoskeletal changes that occur during pregnancy are reversed during the postpartum period.

Joints, Ligaments, and Cartilage

As the level of the hormone relaxin decreases, the ligaments and cartilage, especially of the pelvis, begin to revert to their prepregnant positions. Hip or joint pain may be noticed as these changes take place. Joints, cartilage, and ligaments are stabilized by 6 to 8 weeks after the birth.

All joints return to their normal prepregnant state, except those in the feet. The new mother may discover a permanent increase in her shoe size (Lowdermilk & Perry, 2007).

Abdominal Muscles

Many new mothers, when they stand up, are dismayed when the abdominal muscles protrude, giving a still-pregnant appearance. It usually takes 6 weeks for the abdominal muscles to return almost to their prepregnant state (Lowdermilk & Perry, 2007). Previous muscle tone, proper exercise, and the amount of adipose tissue all influence the return of muscle tone.

Integumentary System

The level of melanocyte-stimulating hormone (MSH) declines rapidly after the birth, and the areas of hyperpigmentation begin to lighten in color. In some women, however, the linea nigra and the darkened nipple areola may remain dark. Most of the skin's elasticity returns, but some striae may still be visible as small or large silver streaks on the breasts, abdomen, buttocks, or thighs.

Spider angiomas (nevi) and palmar erythema usually fade with the decrease in the estrogen level. In some women, however, they do stay.

Any fine hair appearing during pregnancy usually disappears; however, any coarse or bristly hair appearing during pregnancy may remain.

Neurologic System

Any pregnancy-induced neurologic discomforts usually lessen after birth (Lowdermilk & Perry, 2003); however, fatigue, afterpains, muscle aches, episiotomy or abdominal incision pain, and breast engorgement all may create maternal discomfort. If the mother received an analgesic or anesthesia, she may experience a temporary loss of feeling in her legs and dizziness.

The mother who has a headache must be carefully assessed. If the mother had a regional anesthesia (epidural or spinal), the headache may be caused by a leakage of cerebrospinal fluid into the extradural space during needle placement; this is known as a spinal headache. This headache is generally more severe when the mother sits or stands and is relieved when she lies down. If the mother has blurred vision, photophobia, and abdominal pain with a headache, it may indicate that she is developing pregnancy-induced hypertension (PIH), or if she had PIH during pregnancy, that it is getting worse.

Weight Loss

Immediate weight loss is the sum of the infant's weight, placenta, amniotic fluid, and blood loss. Typically, this is approximately 13 lbs. During the next 6 weeks, an additional 8 to 9 lbs is lost as the result of diuresis, diaphoresis, and the involution of the reproductive organs. It takes most mothers approximately 6 months to return to their prepregnant weight, and some may take an entire year. The energy required for breastfeeding may assist in the weight-loss process.

MATERNAL PSYCHOSOCIAL CHANGES

Both expected and unexpected emotional/behavioral changes may be encountered. The effects of early discharge must also be considered.

Expected Changes

Expected emotional/behavioral changes include those restorative/adaptive phases described by Reva Rubin, postpartum "blues," and those related to a cesarean birth.

Rubin's Restorative/Adaptive Phases

Rubin (1961) described three phases of maternal restoration/adaptation: *taking-in*, *taking-hold*, and *letting-go*.

Taking-In Phase This phase is focused mainly on the mother's need for food, fluid, and sleep. The mother's behavior is passive as she takes in the physical care and attention from others. She depends on others to meet her needs. Rubin (1961) described this as the phase of nurturing and protective care lasting 2 to 3 days. Studies by Ament (1990) and Wrasper (1996) confirmed the behavior described by Rubin but noted that the behavior was present only during the first 24 hours after birth.

Integration of the labor and birth experience into reality is the major task of the mother at this time. It is important for her to discuss the details of the labor and birth, especially with the nurse(s) who cared for her. She is thus able to clarify details about her experience that she may not remember because of the effects of medication or the natural sleep and amnesia between contractions, especially in the second stage of labor. By describing to family and friends the birth experience, the mother realizes that the pregnancy is past and the infant is now a separate individual.

The father or partner may also experience a taking-in phase as he is congratulated on the birth of the infant. Family members often treat him in a special way.

Taking-Hold Phase In the taking-hold phase, the mother becomes more independent as she takes an interest in and responsibility for her own physical care. Her focus shifts to the care of her infant. She welcomes opportunities to learn about the behavior of infants and to practice caring for her infant. Martell (1996) and Wrasper (1996) believe that childbirth preparation classes, pain management practices, early newborn contact, rooming-in, and early discharge enhance taking-hold behaviors. Because most mothers are discharged during this phase, which lasts approximately 10 days, continued coping with the physical and emotional/behavioral changes at home is required.

The father or partner's interest in infant behaviors and care is similar to the mother's in the taking-hold phase. He may also be anxious but is usually willing to learn.

Letting-Go Phase If this is a first baby, the mother and father/partner must give up the role and carefree lifestyle of being only a couple. They are now a couple with a child. The expected birth experience may not have been realized. For example, a planned vaginal birth with no anesthesia may have changed to a cesarean birth and/or use of regional anesthesia. The parents must let go of the planned experience and accept what really happened.

For some mothers and/or fathers, the newborn infant does not fit the expected baby they dreamed of and talked about during pregnancy. They may be disappointed in the gender, size, or other characteristics of the infant. Now they must let go of their expectations and accept the reality of their infant.

The mother and father let go of their role of "expecting" and move forward as a unit with a new member. They establish a lifestyle that includes the child and their role as parents. Time must be made for sharing adult activities and interests.

COMMUNITY/HOME HEALTH CARE

Coping with Taking-Hold Phase

- Acknowledge parents' anxiety about caretaking abilities.
- Provide information about infant behaviors.
- Allow parents to provide infant care (nurse should not take over) even if performed awkwardly.
- Praise parents' caregiving efforts.
- Provide parents with a contact and phone number in the event they have questions.

Postpartum Blues

Postpartum blues or "baby blues" is a mild, transient condition of emotional lability and crying for no apparent reason that affects women who have just given birth and lasts about 2 weeks. Other symptoms include fatigue, anxiety, restlessness, let-down feeling, headache, and sadness. The etiology is unknown. This is a self-limiting situation that begins about 3 days, peaks about 5 days, and disappears approximately 10 days after birth.

Cesarean Birth

When a cesarean birth is an emergency (unplanned), the taking-in phase may last longer because these mothers also need to accept and understand the events that made the cesarean birth necessary. It is important for the nurse to understand that these mothers are surgical clients requiring immediate physical care to restore or maintain physiologic health. When pain, bleeding, and incision care are under control, the nurse can help the mother understand the birth and incorporate the experience into her reality.

Some mothers have feelings of frustration, anger, low self-esteem, or disappointment that they could not have their baby the "normal way" (vaginal birth). At the same time, they are relieved, happy, and filled with gratitude that the infant had a safe birth and is healthy. It may be a time of many, often opposing, emotions. The nurse offers encouragement and support to the client and her family. The nurse helps the patient understand that she did not fail just because her birth did not go as planned. The client needs to talk through the birth again and again to help gain a better understanding of the situation. The nurse demonstrates patience and tries to help the client reach a level of comfort with the situation.

UNEXPECTED CHANGES

Unexpected emotional/behavioral changes include postpartum depression, postpartum psychosis, and reaction to an infant with problems.

Postpartum Depression

Postpartum depression (PPD) is similar to postpartum blues but is more serious, intense, and persistent. Approximately 12% of new mothers experience a syndrome more severe than postpartum blues (Lowdermilk & Perry, 2007). PPD may be mild, moderate, or severe, with symptoms becoming more numerous and intense as the severity increases.

The mother with mild PPD cares lovingly for her infant but is unable to feel the love. She may express feelings of irritability, guilt, shame, unworthiness, and a sense of loss of self. Symptoms persist past the first few weeks after the infant's birth.

Moderate PPD is characterized by spontaneous crying, insomnia or hypersomnia, fatigue, decreased concentration, and sometimes food cravings.

With severe PPD, the irritability of the mother may explode into violent outbursts or uncontrollable crying often directed toward significant others. She often will not discuss her symptoms or negative feelings toward the infant, which may include disinterest, annoyance with care demands, or even thoughts of harming the infant.

Psychotherapy and pharmacological interventions are generally required. Sometimes, hospitalization is necessary.

Postpartum Psychosis

Postpartum psychosis is the most dangerous form of depression in a new mother. Postpartum psychosis occurs in 1 to 2/1000 births usually within the first 2 to 4 weeks after delivery but can happen as early as 2 to 3 days postpartum. The psychosis is marked by "paranoid, grandiose, or bizarre delusions, mood swings, confused thinking, and grossly disorganized behavior that represent a dramatic change from her previous functioning" (Sit, Rothchild, & Wisner, 2006). Postpartum psychosis is the least common form of postpartum depression, affecting approximately 10 to 13% of new mothers as compared with the 50 to 75% who are affected by milder forms of depression/baby blues.

Postpartum psychosis is a medical emergency. Many women will require a psychiatric evaluation and, in many cases, hospitalization, until they are no longer a threat to themselves or others. The initial medical evaluation will include "thorough history, physical examination, and laboratory investigations" (Sit, Rothchild, & Wisner, 2006). It is very important for the nurse to educate new mothers and their families about the signs and symptoms of postpartum depression so it can be caught early and treated.

Infant with a Problem

It may be difficult for the mother and/or father to bond with and attach to an infant born preterm or with physical or functional anomalies (Figure 57-7). The parents may have feelings of guilt that they, somehow, caused the infant's problem. Either or both of the parents may not be able to accept an infant who does not look like a normal, healthy infant. When one parent's reaction to the infant with a problem is opposite that of the other's, there may be a terrific strain on their relationship.

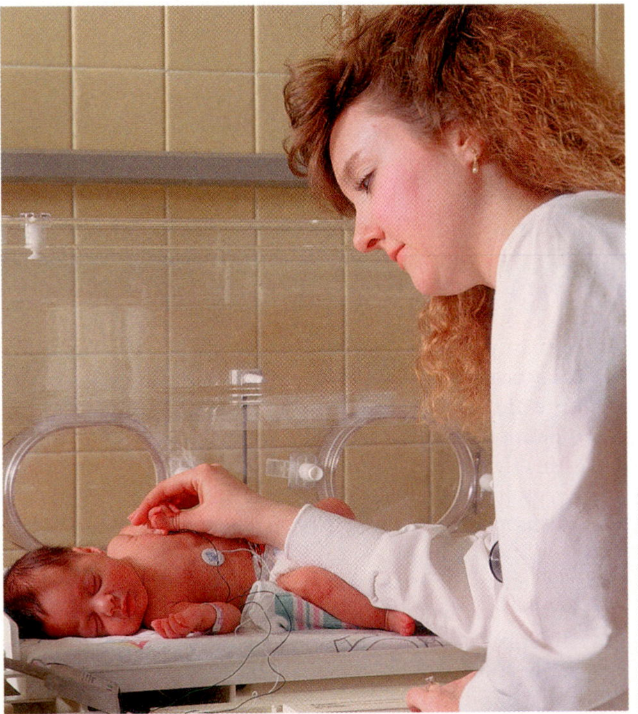

COURTESY OF DELMAR CENGAGE LEARNING

FIGURE 57-7 Parents of an infant who requires special medical care should be encouraged to spend as much time with their child as possible.

DISCHARGE

In an effort to reduce health care costs and meet consumer demand for a more family-centered experience with less medical intervention, the short hospital stay came into existence. In the 1950s, most new mothers remained in the hospital 5 days for a vaginal birth and 7 days for a cesarean birth. The stays were gradually reduced to 3 days for a vaginal birth and 5 days for a cesarean birth. For several years in the early 1990s, third-party payers (health plans and insurance companies) mandated discharge within 24 hours for a vaginal birth and 72 hours or less for a cesarean birth.

Health-care professionals became concerned about client (mother and infant) safety because many problems do not show up in the first 24 hours after birth. The time for assessing bonding/attachment and parenting behaviors was almost eliminated. Parents were barely acquainted with their infant and client teaching about newborn care, and identifying health problems such as dehydration, jaundice, and breastfeeding difficulties had to be rushed.

The federal government passed the Newborns' and Mothers' Health Protection Act of 1996, which requires all health plans to allow a stay of 48 hours following vaginal birth and 96 hours following a cesarean birth (Health Care Financing Administration, 2002). Self-insured health plans must comply with this act. Group insurance plans and individual insurance may not have to comply if the client lives in a state having a law with certain protections for hospital stays after childbirth. More than 40 states and the District of Columbia have such laws (Health Care Financing Administration, 2002).

Follow-up home care is being used in many areas. This may be a telephone call or two to see how the mother and infant are doing, or it may include actual home visits. Research has shown that women who receive follow-up care at home by phone or in person did better overall in the postpartum period. Unfortunately, the United States lags behind in this area. This area of more efficient postpartum care is part of a nationwide initiative to improve care of women and children in this period (Chang, Fowles, & Walker, 2006).

INFECTION CONTROL

Standard Precautions in Postpartum Care

Gloves should be worn when:

- Assessing the breasts if there is leakage of colostrum or milk
- Handling used breast pads
- Assessing lochia and the perineum
- Changing peripads or chux
- Handling anything on which there is lochia (bed linen, towels, washcloth, clothing, peripads, chux)

CLIENT TEACHING

Breast Assessment

- Explain the characteristics of the breast and what to expect depending on whether the mother is breastfeeding or not.
- Describe how to recognize problems such as mastitis and nipple fissures or cracks.

NURSING PROCESS

ASSESSMENT

Assessments specific to the first few days postpartum include breasts, uterus, bladder, bowel, lochia, and episiotomy; vital signs; lower extremities and Homans' sign; bonding/attachment; parenting; activity; comfort; and self-care. These assessments are usually performed, at least once a shift, until the mother is discharged. A sample initial postpartum profile sheet is shown in Figure 57-8.

Subjective Data

Ask the mother whether the milk has come in or whether there is any breast discomfort; whether the bladder feels empty after urination; whether the mother is able to pass gas rectally or has the urge to have a bowel movement; whether any clots are passed vaginally and when the peripad was last changed; whether there is dizziness when getting up; whether contractions are felt during breastfeeding; or whether there is discomfort or pain, especially in the perineal area.

Objective Data

Breasts

Note the size and shape of the breasts and any abnormalities or reddened areas. The breasts should be gently palpated for softness, firmness, engorgement, warmth, or tenderness. Check the nipples for cracks, fissures, soreness, and inversion.

Uterus

Palpate the abdomen to find the top (fundus) of the uterus by pressing in and down with the side of one hand, and placing the other hand above the symphysis to support the uterus. The size, consistency, and placement (midline or off to one side) of the uterus is noted. It should be firm (not boggy) and in the midline. Each day it should descend approximately 1 cm (1 finger breadth). Fundal descent is documented in relation to the umbilicus (Figure 57-9).

CLIENT TEACHING

Assessing the Fundus

- Explain why it is important for the uterus to be firmly contracted.
- Demonstrate how to palpate the uterine fundus.
- Demonstrate the way to gently massage the fundus.

Hollister™

Initial Postpartum Profile
Hollister Maternal/Newborn Record System
To order call: **1.800.323.4060** Re-order No **5714**

Admit Data
Date ___/___/___ Time ______
Admitted From
☐ Recovery Care ☐ Home ☐ ______
Via ☐ Wheelchair ☐ Stretcher ☐ ______
Oriented to Unit
☐ Safety/Security ☐ Television
☐ Room ☐ Meals/Kitchen
☐ Call Light ☐ Visiting Hours
☐ Bed Control ☐ ______
☐ Telephone
Planned LOS ______
Signature ______

Maternal Data G | T | Pt | A | L
Medication Allergy/Sensitivity ☐ **None**
(Identify) ______
Del ______ Time ______
☐ Vaginal ☐ Cesarean ☐ VBAC ☐ Tubal
Incision (type) ______
Anesthesia ______
Blood Type/Rh ______
Hepatitus Immune ☐ Yes ☐ No
Rubella Immune ☐ Yes ☐ No
Intrapartal Problems Identified ☐ **None**
1. ______
2. ______

Infant Data ☐ Male ☐ Female
ID/Band No. ______ Name ______
Condition ☐ **Live/Normal**
☐ Live/Compromised
☐ Fetal/Neonatal Death
Feeding ☐ Breast ☐ Bottle
Blood Type/Rh ______
Location ☐ With Mother ☐ Nursery
☐ ______
Intrapartal Problems Identified ☐ **None**
1. ______
2. ______
3. ______

Psychological Assessment Date ___/___/___ Time ______
Mother's General Comments (Feelings, Body Image, Self Concept): ______
Mother Appears ☐ Happy ☐ Ambivalent ☐ Concerned ☐ Depressed ☐ Angry ☐ Other ______
Review of Labor and Birth: Missing Pieces ☐ **No** ☐ Yes Identify ______

Physical Assessment Temp | Pulse | Resp | BP
Date ___/___/___ Time ______
General Health ☐ **Good** ☐ Significant History ______
Breath Sounds ☐ **Normal** ☐ Abnormal ______

Breasts ☐ Nursing ☐ Non-Nursing
Discharge ☐ None ☐ Colostrum ☐ Other ______
Support Bra ☐ No
☐ Yes Fit ☐ Tight ☐ Loose ☐ Appropriate
If Nursing, Nipple Type
☐ Everted ☐ Inverted ☐ Flat

Abdomen
Diastasis Recti ☐ **Absent** ☐ Present (width) ______
Incision ☐ **None** ☐ Present(color, discharge, approximation) ______

Reproductive Tract
Fundus (consistency, height, position) ______
Lochia Peri Pad in place ______ Hrs
Pad Saturation (amt) ______
Clots ☐ **No** ☐ Yes
Odor ☐ Fleshy ☐ Foul
Perineum ☐ **Intact** ☐ Laceration ☐ Episiotomy
(type) ______
Condition: **Redness** ______
Ecchymosis ______
Edema ______
Discharge ______
Approximation ______

Elimination Pattern
Urinary Tract
Void ☐ No ☐ Yes (Time ______ Amount ______)
Bladder Distention ☐ No ☐ Yes
Catheter ☐ No ☐ Yes
☐ Straight (Time ______ Amount ______)
☐ Foley to CD
Specimen Obtained ☐ **None** ☐ UA ☐ C+S
Gastrointestinal Tract
Bowel Sounds ☐ Absent ☐ Present + ______
Hemorrhoids ☐ No ☐ Yes
Pattern ☐ Normal ☐ Diarrhea
☐ Constipation (Laxative Use ______)

Lower Extremities
Varicosities ☐ Absent ☐ Present, location ______
Signs of Thrombophlebitis ☐ No ☐ Yes
Redness ______
Swelling ______
Warmth ______
Pain ______
Positive Homans' Sign ☐ R ☐ L
Edema ☐ No ☐ Yes ______
DTRs (R) ☐ 0 ☐ +1 ☐ +2 ☐ +3 ☐ +4 Clonus ☐ No ☐ Yes ______
DTRs (L) ☐ 0 ☐ +1 ☐ +2 ☐ +3 ☐ +4 Clonus ☐ No ☐ Yes ______

Pain

	No	Yes	
Headache	☐	☐	______
Breasts	☐	☐	______
Back	☐	☐	______
Abdominal Cramping	☐	☐	______
Perineum	☐	☐	______
Hemorrhoid	☐	☐	______
Legs	☐	☐	______
Other	☐	☐	______

Hollister™

Initial Postpartum Profile
Hollister Maternal/Newborn Record System
To order call: **1.800.323.4060** Re-order No **5714**

Attachment Assessment

	Yes	No	
Accepts Sex of Infant	☐	☐	______
Calls Infant By Name	☐	☐	______
Comments on Appearance of Infant	☐	☐	______
Looks at Infant	☐	☐	______
Touches Infant	☐	☐	______
Smiles at Infant	☐	☐	______

Problems Identified ☐ **None**
☐ Identify

Signature ______ Date ___/___/___

FIGURE 57-8 **Representative Initial Postpartum Profile** (*Permission to use this copyrighted material has been granted by the owner, Hollister Incorporated.*)

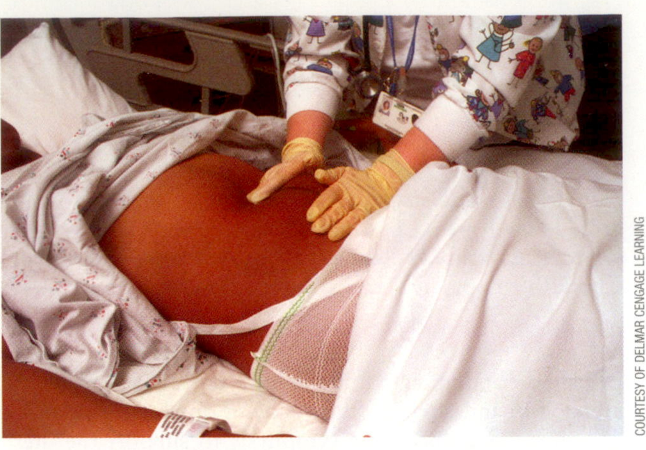

FIGURE 57-9 The nurse supports the uterus with her left hand held beneath it while palpating the uterus to determine if it is firm or boggy and its position, midline, or displaced.

MEMORY TRICK

Postpartum Assessment

Remember **BUBBLE** for the order of the Post-Partum Assessment:

B = Breasts

U = Uterus

B = Bowels

B = Bladder

L = Lochia

E = Episiotomy/laceration/C-section incision

CLIENT TEACHING

Bladder and Bowel Elimination

Encourage the new mother to:

- Drink plenty of fluids.
- Ambulate frequently and use the bathroom, not a bedpan.
- Eat a well-balanced diet with increased fiber and fluids.
- Promptly answer nature's call to urinate or defecate.

Bladder

When the abdomen is palpated for the uterine fundus, the bladder can also be palpated for distention. A full, distended bladder is very often the cause for the fundus to be higher than it should be and to be positioned off to one side (not in the midline) (Figure 57-10). An intake and output (I&O) record is kept during the first 24 hours, at least, to assist in identifying urine retention.

CLIENT TEACHING

Lochia Assessment

- Describe the expected changes in the color and amount of lochia.
- Advise the mother that if the lochia changes from serosa back to rubra, she is either doing too much heavy work or the uterus is not firmly contracted. The mother should check fundal firmness and rest for a while.
- Instruct mother to notify her certified nurse-midwife (CNM)/physician if clots are passed or if the lochia has an unusual or unpleasant odor.

Bowels

Inspect the abdomen for distention and auscultate for the presence of bowel sounds. The client's labor record should be reviewed to check whether she received an enema. The anus can be inspected when the episiotomy is checked. Make sure to check for hemorrhoids at this point.

Lochia

Ask the mother to lie on her back with knees flexed so the peripad can be lowered in the front. Lochia is assessed for color, amount, odor, and presence of clots. Then, ask the mother to turn to her side to see whether any lochia has pooled under her buttocks.

Amount It is difficult to estimate the amount of lochia on a perineal pad. Luegenbiehl, Brophy, Artigue, Phillips, and Flack (1990) identified a method to estimate the amount of lochia discharged in 1 hour (Figure 57-11).

The mother who has had a cesarean birth will have less lochia after the first 24 hours than a mother who had

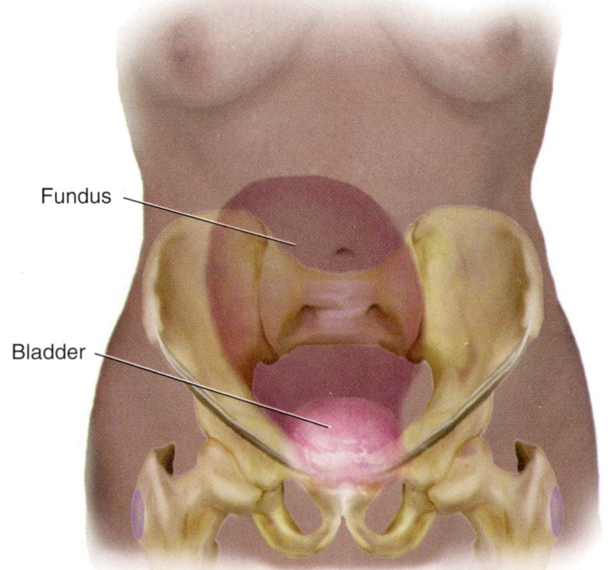

FIGURE 57-10 A full bladder displaces the uterus and prevents its contractions.

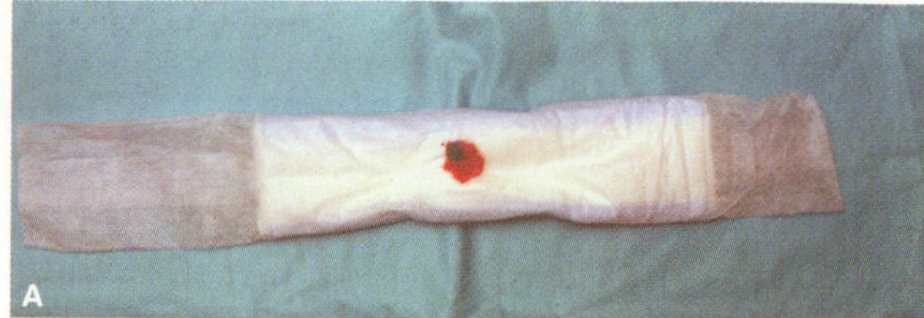

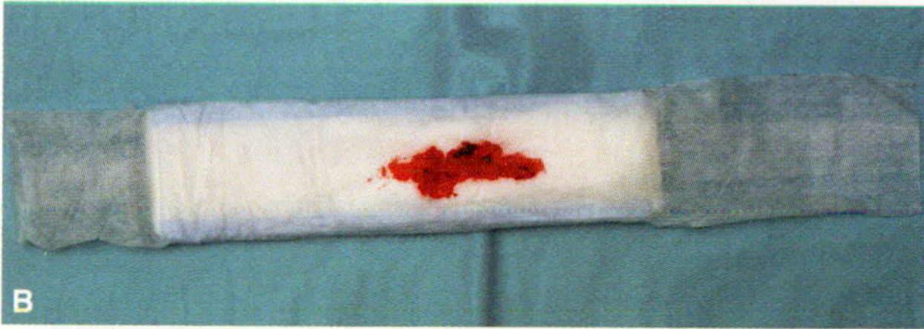

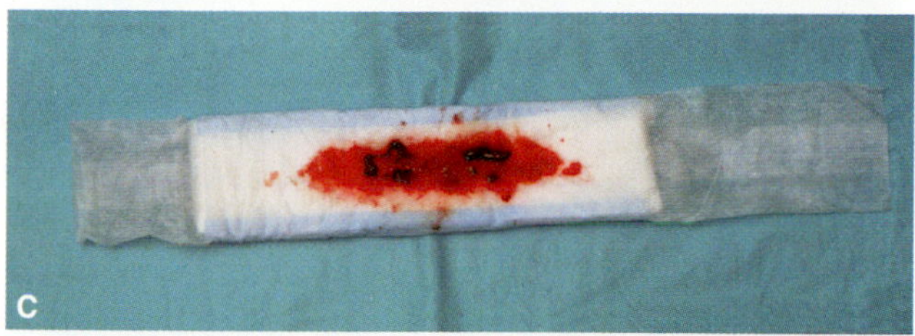

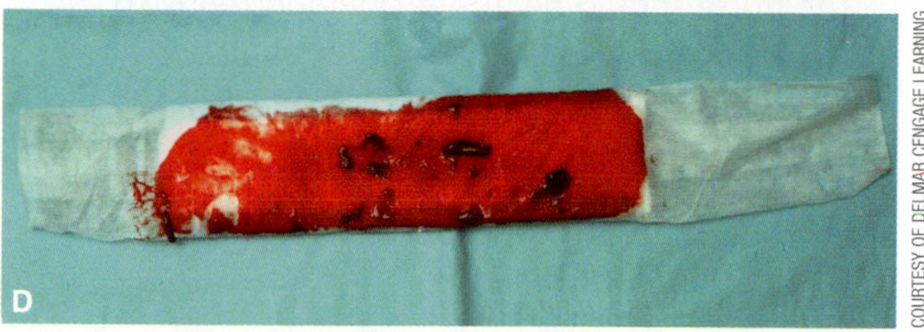

COURTESY OF DELMAR CENGAGE LEARNING

FIGURE 57-11 An assessment of lochia is based on the amount of blood saturation on a peripad. *A*, Scant: 2-inch stain (10 mL); *B*, Small: 4-inch stain (10-25 mL); *C*, Moderate: 6-inch stain (25-50 mL); *D*, Large: >6-inch stain (50-80 mL).

a vaginal birth. The lochia also usually changes from rubra to serosa sooner because the inside of the uterus is wiped with sponges during a cesarean birth, removing some of the endometrium.

Odor Lochia has a nonoffensive odor. If the lochia has a foul odor, an infection is present and the certified nurse-midwife (CNM)/physician must be notified at once.

Presence of Clots A few small clots, which occur when blood pools in the vagina, are normal. Passing many or large clots is not normal and requires further investigation. Any clot that is larger than the size of an egg should be cause for further investigation and assessment by the nurse.

Episiotomy

Assess the episiotomy with the mother in Sims' position (Figure 57-12). This can be done when the mother is on her side for lochia assessment. With a gloved hand, very gently raise the upper buttock just enough to see the episiotomy. Changes in the episiotomy should be noted. See Memory Trick for episiotomy assessment.

With the client in the same position, gently touch the external labia and note whether this causes pain. The labia should also be inspected for ecchymosis and edema. The anus can be inspected for hemorrhoids.

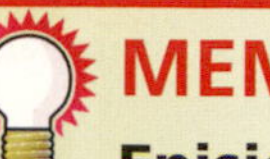

MEMORY TRICK

Episiotomy Assessment

When assessing a client's episiotomy, remember to assess the 5 items that are recalled by the **REEDA** mnemonic:

R = Redness—inflammation
E = Ecchymosis—bruising
E = Edema—swelling
D = Discharge—from incision
A = Approximation of suture line (Davidson, 1974).

CLIENT TEACHING

Techniques to Decrease Episiotomy Discomfort

Instruct mother to:

- Tighten her buttocks and perineum before sitting to prevent pulling on the episiotomy and perineal area, and to release the tightening after being seated.
- Rest several times a day with feet elevated.
- Practice the Kegel exercise many times a day to increase circulation to the perineal area and to strengthen the perineal muscles.
- Use peri-bottle when urinating to relieve pain and ease in lochia cleansing.

Vital Signs

Assess vital signs every 15 minutes for the first 1 to 2 hours after birth. If no problems are identified, vital signs may then be checked every 8 hours.

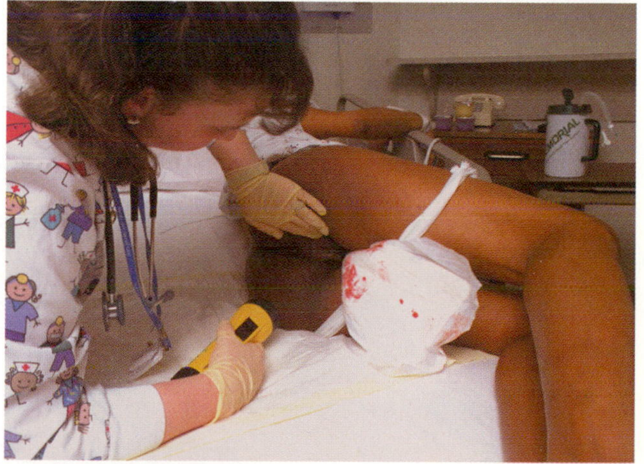

COURTESY OF DELMAR CENGAGE LEARNING

FIGURE 57-12 The episiotomy is assessed with the mother lying on her side. The upper buttock is raised gently, just enough to see the episotomy. The anal area can be assessed for hemorrhoids at the same time.

Temperature Temperature may increase to 100.4°F (38°C) during the first 24 hours. After the first 24 hours, a temperature over 100.4°F suggests an infection.

Pulse After the first hour after the birth, the mother's pulse rate may decrease to 50 to 70 beats/minute for 6 to 8 days. An elevated pulse may indicate excessive blood loss, infection, anxiety, or pain.

Blood Pressure Blood pressure should remain consistent with the baseline during pregnancy. An increase suggests PIH, whereas a decrease may indicate excessive bleeding.

Lower Extremities and Homans' Sign

Examine the mother's legs for signs of thrombophlebitis such as redness, heat, edema, and tenderness. Palpate the pedal pulses. Perform the assessment for Homans' sign.

To assess for Homans' sign, support the client's leg under the knee while sharply dorsiflexing the foot (Figure 57-13). Homans' sign is positive if the client experiences calf discomfort when the foot is dorsiflexed and negative if the client does not experience discomfort in the calf. When Homans' sign is positive, it must be reported at once to the CNM/physician because it may indicate thrombophlebitis.

Bonding/Attachment

Assess the interaction of the mother with her infant for the expected behaviors of bonding and beginning attachment. The manner in which the mother holds, examines, and speaks to the infant is important. For instance, the mother who cradles her infant, gazes at her infant's face, and speaks in a pleasant manner to the infant is exhibiting signs of bonding and attachment.

Parenting

Assess the skill with which the mother cares for her infant. For example, observe feeding, diapering, bathing, and consoling skills to determine whether additional teaching is required.

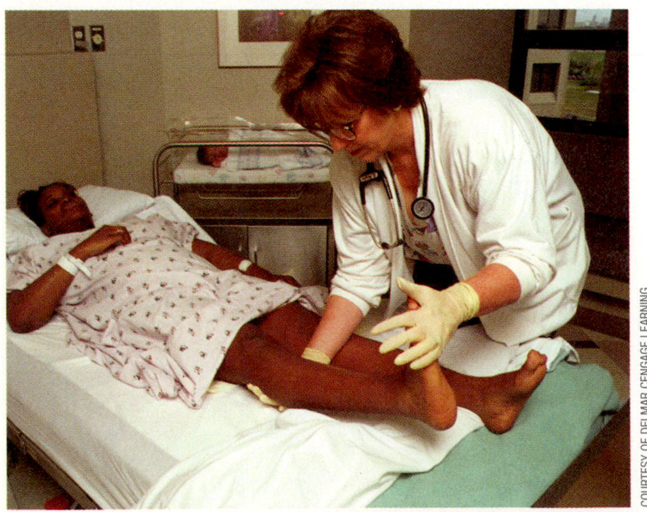

COURTESY OF DELMAR CENGAGE LEARNING

FIGURE 57-13 **Homans' Sign Assessment. Discomfort experienced in the calf when the foot is sharply dorsiflexed is considered positive and may indicate thrombophlebitis.**

CULTURAL CONSIDERATIONS

Rest

Expectations of maternal activity during the postpartum period may be influenced by cultural norms. For example:

- Korean women rest an average of 21 days following birth (Howard & Berbiglia, 1997).
- Southeast Asian, Vietnamese, Cambodian, and Laotian women stay in bed without a pillow and keep warm for 2 days (Mattson, 1995).

SAFETY

First Ambulation

The first time a new mother gets out of bed, the nurse should be at her side and ready to assist in case the mother becomes lightheaded, weak, or dizzy. Encourage client to sit at the side of the bed for a few moments before ambulating. Leave bathroom door slightly ajar and stay within close proximity to client in case she begins to feel faint.

Activity

Determine that the mother is ambulating, that is, getting up to go to the bathroom and frequently walking around. Many complications such as thromboses, emboli, and hypostatic pneumonia occur when the mother is in bed for extended periods.

Rest is just as important as activity. The mother expended a great deal of energy during labor and birth. Care should be planned so the mother has some uninterrupted periods of rest.

Comfort

Comfort is essential to rest. Many new mothers never say anything about discomforts because they are so excited and pleased with their new infant. Be alert to any behavioral signs of discomfort. Most discomfort is related to perineal pain or afterpains.

Self-Care

Assessment of self-care includes the mother's knowledge of how to care for herself and also whether she actually performs the care. Self-care includes showering, perineal care, checking the fundus, breast care, and rest. Support the client's recovery by encouraging her to bathe, toilet, and feed herself independently.

Nursing diagnoses for a postpartum mother include the following:

NURSING DIAGNOSES	PLANNING/OUTCOMES	NURSING INTERVENTIONS
*Urinary **R**etention* related to sensory motor impairment from bladder trauma during labor and birth as evidenced by client being unable to urinate after delivery	The client will have appropriate urinary elimination (no bladder distention).	Monitor intake for adequate amount. Assess for bladder distention every 2 to 4 hours. Assist client to bathroom for elimination. Pour warm water over vulvar area or run water in the sink to stimulate urination. Catheterize, if necessary, as ordered.
*Risk for **I**nfection* related to episiotomy	The client will have no signs of infection.	Assess episiotomy for redness and swelling. Teach mother pericare: wash hands, remove peripad from front to back, pour warm water over perineum, pat dry from front to back, apply clean peripad front first then toward the back, wash hands. Advise client to change peripad every 2 to 4 hours and every time she goes to the bathroom.
*Acute **P**ain* related to episiotomy, engorged breasts, or involution of the uterus	The client will state that discomfort has decreased.	*Episiotomy* Assess perineum for edema. Apply ice pack for 20 minutes; remove for at least 10 minutes before reapplying. Assist mother with Sitz bath as ordered, and watch for dizziness, floating feeling, or difficulty hearing (signs of possible fainting). Apply Dermoplast spray or Americain spray (topical anesthetics) to perineum after a sitz bath or pericare, as ordered. Emphasize the need to wash hands before and after any care of the episiotomy. Teach mother to squeeze buttocks together before sitting, release after sitting. Encourage mother to practice Kegel exercise 4 or 5 times a day. Administer analgesic as ordered. Avoid using rectal suppositories for clients with 3rd- or 4th-degree episiotomy. *Engorged Breasts* (not breastfeeding) Encourage mother to wear a well-fitting supportive bra, removing it only for showers, to suppress lactation. Provide ice pack to axillary area and side of breast for 20 minutes 4 times a day to suppress lactation. Advise mother to avoid any stimulation to breast; stand with back to shower so warm water does not hit breasts. Administer analgesic as ordered. *Engorged Breasts* (breastfeeding) Encourage the mother to feed her infant approximately every 2 hours; empty (until soft) one breast; then feed from second breast or pump to soften. Administer antiinflammatory pain medication as ordered. Apply ice pack between feedings for 15 minutes on and 45 minutes off as ordered. *Involution of Uterus* (afterpains) Assess fundus for firmness and position.

(*Continues*)

Nursing diagnoses for a postpartum mother include the following: (Continued)

NURSING DIAGNOSES	PLANNING/OUTCOMES	NURSING INTERVENTIONS
		Determine when mother has pain. Explain, if mother is breastfeeding, that the oxytocin released in response to breastfeeding causes the uterus to contract. The discomfort lasts only a few minutes at the beginning of each breastfeeding session for the first 4 to 6 days. Administer analgesic as ordered.

Evaluation: Evaluate each outcome to determine how it has been met by the client.

HEALTH PROMOTION

The mother's record must be checked to determine the mother's need for Rh immune globulin (RhoGAM) and rubella immunization. When required, these two items protect the fetuses of future pregnancies.

Rh Immune Globulin

Rh immune globulin (RhoGAM) is given within 72 hours after birth to prevent sensitization of Rh-negative mothers who gave birth to Rh-positive infants. The RhoGAM promotes lysis of fetal Rh-positive red blood cells before the mother's body is able to form antibodies against them.

Rubella Immunization

It is recommended that all women who have not had rubella or who have a 1:8 rubella titer be given rubella vaccine in the immediate postpartum period. This will prevent fetal anomalies in future pregnancies if the mother is exposed to rubella. Breastfeeding is not a contraindication to receiving the immunization. Because the vaccine may be teratogenic, pregnancy must be avoided for 2 to 3 months

CESAREAN BIRTH

All of the assessments just discussed are also performed on a mother who has had a cesarean birth. In addition, postoperative assessments are performed, including incision, respirations and breath sounds, abdomen and bowel sounds, fluid intake, urine output, and the degree of pain.

Incision

Inspect the dressing for intactness and any bleeding or discharge. After the dressing is removed, assess the incision for signs of infection such as redness, heat, pain, or edema and the suture line for approximation.

> **PROFESSIONALTIP**
>
> **Rh Immune Globulin (RhoGAM) Administration**
>
> Rho-GAM is considered a blood product. Some patients with cultural aversions to blood products might refuse administration. Since this is a blood product, two nurses must check labs and orders before administration.

Respirations and Breath Sounds

If the mother received narcotics either epidurally or with patient-controlled analgesia (PCA), assess respirations frequently because narcotics depress the respiratory center. Assess respiratory rate and depth every 15 minutes for the first hour, every 30 minutes for the next 4 to 5 hours, and every hour for the remainder of the first 24 hours. Some institutions may use an apnea monitor. Auscultate breath sounds at each respiratory check to identify whether secretions are beginning to pool in the bronchioles. Assess the client's efforts of turning (changing position), coughing, deep breathing, and use of the incentive spirometer.

Abdomen and Bowel Sounds

In addition to the incision, assess the abdomen for softness or distention. Auscultate bowel sounds until peristalsis is noted in all four quadrants. Ask the mother whether she has been able to pass any flatus (gas) rectally.

Fluid Intake

Frequently assess the flow rate of intravenous fluids as well as the site. Record the amount of intravenous fluid and any oral fluid intake.

Urine Output

A Foley catheter is generally inserted into the bladder before the cesarean birth. Assess and record the amount of urine output as well as the clarity and color. Make sure that client is eliminating at least 30 mL/hour. If urine output is less than 30 mL, notify the attending physician.

Pain

Most new mothers who have a vaginal birth are eager to interact with their newborn infant. This is no different following a cesarean birth; however, these mothers will need to be taught how to hold and carry the infant in a way that will not disturb or irritate their incisions. The mothers may not want pain medication because they want to stay awake with and enjoy their infants.

Breastfeeding mothers who have had a cesarean birth may also not admit to having pain because they are concerned that pain medication will be present in the breast milk. Pain medication is generally required for 24 to 48 hours following a cesarean birth. These mothers are taught to support the baby with a pillow to avoid incisional pain while nursing.

SAMPLE NURSING CARE PLAN

The Postpartum Client

S.V. and her husband, J.V, have just participated in the birth of their first child, a daughter, weighing 6 lbs, 8 oz, and measuring 21 inches long. A small episiotomy was made. J.V. has "always wanted a son" and is "disappointed about having a daughter." He looks at the infant but does not touch her or speak to her.

S.V. is exhausted from the labor and birth, says she is too tired to hold the baby and wants only to sleep. Her vital signs are within normal range, and the uterus tends to relax. Within 1-1/2 hours, she has saturated three peripads. A bulge is noted above the symphysis. S.V. is unable to urinate at this time.

NURSING DIAGNOSIS 1 *Risk for Deficient **F**luid Volume* related to early postpartum hemorrhage as evidenced by saturating three peripads in 1-1/2 hours

Nursing Outcomes Classification (NOC)
Fluid Balance

Nursing Interventions Classification (NIC)
Fluid Monitoring

PLANNING/OUTCOMES	NURSING INTERVENTIONS	RATIONALE
S.V.'s fluid volume will be maintained by reducing the amount of lochia discharge.	Palpate and monitor fundal height, location, and consistency.	Determines status of uterus (firm or boggy) and height and location relative to umbilicus.
	For boggy uterus, gently massage and assess muscle tone.	Promotes uterine contraction and increases uterine tone.
	Monitor lochia (amount and color), time peripad changed, and degree of peripad saturation.	Evaluates the amount of lochia.
	Assess for bladder fullness and encourage voiding.	A full bladder interferes with contracting of the uterus.
	Monitor intake and output.	Identifies potential need to urinate.
	Monitor vital signs, skin temperature, and color.	Detects signs of shock.
	Administer oxytocic agent as ordered.	Promotes uterine contraction.
	Explain involution process to S.V. and teach her to check and gently massage her uterus.	Involves S.V. in self-care.

EVALUATION

S.V.'s fluid volume is maintained. S.V. is voiding adequately, allowing the uterus to contract and the amount of lochia to decrease.

NURSING DIAGNOSIS 2 *Risk for Impaired **P**arenting* related to not gender desired as evidenced by J.V. expressing a desire for a son, showing seeming disappointment with a daughter, not touching or speaking to the infant, and S.V. saying she is too tired to hold the baby

Nursing Outcomes Classification (NOC)
Parent–Infant Attachment

Nursing Interventions Classification (NIC)
Parenting Promotion

(*Continues*)

SAMPLE NURSING CARE PLAN (Continued)

PLANNING/OUTCOMES	NURSING INTERVENTIONS	RATIONALE
S.V. and J.V. will demonstrate bonding and attachment behaviors with their daughter.	Assist S.V. in holding her daughter.	Emphasizes holding infant as important.
	Point out unique characteristics about the infant (e.g., dimple in right cheek, long fingers).	Helps S.V. and J.V. get acquainted with their daughter.
	Ask S.V. and J.V. who the infant looks like.	Assists S.V. and J.V. in identifying family characteristics.
	Model bonding and attachment behaviors for S.V. and J.V. such as talking to infant, finger-tipping, and examining infant.	Shows S.V. and J.V. how to interact with their daughter.
	Describe infant's behavior and explain that the infant can see and hear her parents.	Enables S.V. and J.V. to understand their infant and her abilities.

EVALUATION

S.V. follows nurse's example and strokes the infant's head and face with her fingertips and talks to her. J.V. touches the infant's fingers but does not watch her intently or for longer than a few seconds.

NURSING DIAGNOSIS 3 ***Urinary Retention*** related to sensory motor function impairment as evidenced by client's inability to urinate after delivery, as well as a bulge above the pubic symphysis, indicating bladder distention

Nursing Outcomes Classification (NOC)
Urinary Elimination

Nursing Interventions Classification (NIC)
Urinary Elimination Management
Urinary Catheterization

PLANNING/OUTCOMES	NURSING INTERVENTIONS	RATIONALE
S.V. will have regular urinary elimination with no bladder distention.	Palpate bulge above symphysis while asking S.V. whether bladder feels full.	Confirms that bulge is a full bladder.
	Assist S.V. to the bathroom or onto bedpan if she is unable to ambulate.	Allows S.V. to empty her bladder.
	Run water in sink, place S.V.'s hands in warm water, or pour water over her perineum.	Stimulates urination.
	Administer analgesic as ordered if S.V. has vulvar/perineal discomfort and is afraid to void.	Relieves discomfort; may help S.V. relax and void.
	Catheterize if necessary, as ordered.	Empties bladder, allowing uterus to contract and promoting comfort.

SAMPLE NURSING CARE PLAN (Continued)

EVALUATION

S.V. empties her bladder when assisted to the bathroom.

NURSING DIAGNOSIS 4 *Risk for Infection* related to tissue destruction at episiotomy site and increased environmental exposure to pathogens as evidenced by inflammation and drainage at episiotomy site

Nursing Outcomes Classification (NOC)
Infection Status
Primary Intention

Nursing Interventions Classification (NIC)
Infection Protection
Incision Site Care
Health Education

PLANNING/OUTCOMES	NURSING INTERVENTIONS	RATIONALE
S.V. will have no evidence of infection.	Follow Standard Precautions, especially good hand hygiene before and after providing care, and wear gloves when contact with lochia or urine is possible.	Prevents spread of infection.
	Use strict aseptic technique when inserting a catheter or starting an intravenous infusion.	Reduces the risk of a nosocomial infection.
	Monitor vital signs.	If elevated, may indicate an infection.
	Monitor for loss of appetite, malaise, and chills.	May indicate infection.
	Assess episiotomy for redness, edema, drainage, and pain; and lochia for a foul odor.	Indicates infection.
	Teach S.V. proper perineal care.	Keeps perineum clean and prevents contamination of episiotomy by anal organisms.

EVALUATION

S.V. has no signs of infection.

COMPLICATIONS

The most common complications of childbirth are postpartum hemorrhage, infection, thromboembolic conditions, and disseminated intravascular coagulation.

POSTPARTUM HEMORRHAGE

Postpartum hemorrhage is defined as a blood loss of more than 500 mL after the third stage of labor or 1,000 mL after a cesarean birth. The hemorrhage is identified as either early, within the first 24 hours, or late, generally occurring 1 to 2 weeks after the birth, but may occur up to 6 weeks after the birth.

A postpartum hemorrhage can occur rapidly and may not be recognized until the client is in moderate to severe shock (Table 57-1).

EARLY POSTPARTUM HEMORRHAGE

Early postpartum hemorrhage has several possible causes: uterine atony, retained placental fragments, lacerations of the birth canal, and hematomas. Predisposing factors for postpartum hemorrhage include the following:

- Overdistention of the uterus (large infant, multiple gestation, or hydramnios)
- Grandmultiparity (more than 5)
- Precipitate labor or birth

TABLE 57-1 Hemorrhagic Shock

	BP	PULSE	RESP	SKIN	URINE OUTPUT	BLOOD LOSS	LEVEL OF CONSCIOUSNESS
Mild	Normal or increased	Increased becoming weaker	Increased deep	Cool, pale	Normal 30 mL/hr	500–900 mL	Alert, oriented, anxious
Moderate	Systolic 60–90	Tachycardia becoming irregular	Tachypnea becoming shallow	Cool, pale, moist	Decreased 10–22 mL/hr	1,200–1,500 mL	Oriented, increasing anxiety, restless
Severe	Systolic <60	120–160 irregular	30–50 shallow	Cool, clammy	Oliguric <10 mL/hr	1,800–2,100 mL	Lethargic
Very Severe	May not be detected	May be absent	>50	Cyanotic	Oliguria to anuria	>2,400 mL	Slipping into unconsciousness

COURTESY OF DELMAR CENGAGE LEARNING

- Prolonged labor
- Use of forceps or vacuum extractor
- Use of tocolytic drugs
- Use of oxytocin to augment or induce labor
- Cesarean birth
- Manual removal of the placenta
- Clotting disorders

UTERINE ATONY

Uterine atony is a lack of muscle tone in the uterus. The uterus feels soft and boggy. Hemorrhage from uterine atony is usually a steady flow. Blood pressure and pulse changes may not occur until the blood loss is severe because during pregnancy there is an increase in blood volume.

RETAINED PLACENTAL FRAGMENTS

Occasionally, small pieces of the placenta may not be expelled. These pieces prevent the uterus from contracting effectively, and bleeding continues.

LACERATIONS OF THE BIRTH CANAL

Factors predisposing a woman to lacerations of the birth canal include the following:

- Nulliparity
- Forceps-assisted or vacuum-assisted birth
- Precipitous birth
- Macrosomia
- Epidural anesthesia

Lacerations may occur in the perineum, vagina, cervix, or around the urethral meatus. Most lacerations are identified and repaired by the CNM/physician immediately following the birth. Occasionally, a laceration is overlooked and bright red bleeding persists when the uterus is firmly contracted. It is at this point that the nurse should suspect a laceration and notify the attending CNM/physician.

HEMATOMA

A hematoma forms when there is bleeding into the tissues; there is no external laceration. Spontaneous or forceps-assisted births may result in hematoma formation. The most common sites are the vulva, vagina, and retroperitoneal area (Figure 57-14). A hematoma is a bluish-purple mass that produces deep, severe, unrelenting pain and a feeling of great pressure. When the uterus is firmly contracted, the amount of lochia is within normal limits, and the mother has a falling blood pressure or tachycardia and persistently describes severe pain, suspect a hematoma.

LATE POSTPARTUM HEMORRHAGE

A late postpartum hemorrhage usually occurs 1 to 2 weeks after the birth because of **subinvolution** (incomplete return of the uterus to its prepregnant size and consistency) or retained placental fragments. Clots may form around the retained placental fragments immediately postpartum, thus keeping lochia

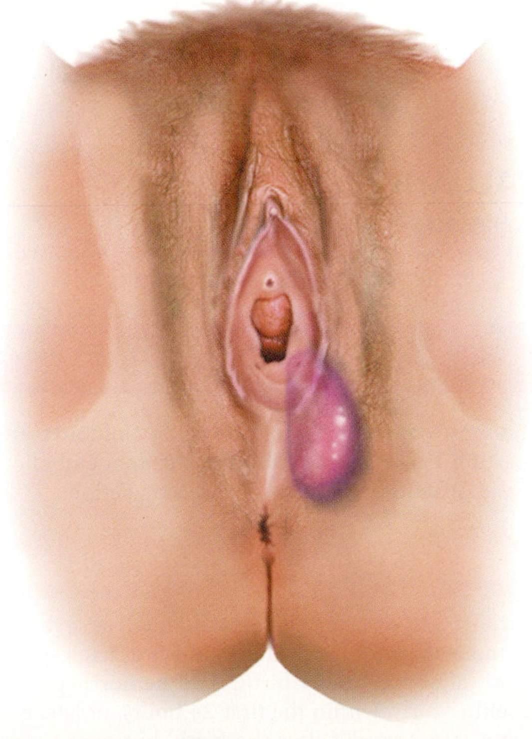

COURTESY OF DELMAR CENGAGE LEARNING

FIGURE 57-14 Hematoma of the Vulva

within normal limits. Several days later, when the clots slough, excessive bleeding occurs. There is usually no warning of a late postpartum hemorrhage. This should be viewed as a medical emergency. The nurse teaches clients prior to discharge the signs and symptoms of a late postpartum hemorrhage.

Medical–Surgical Management

Medical

The CNM/physician carefully palpates the uterus to make sure it is contracting after the birth. A thorough examination of the birth canal for lacerations or hematomas is also undertaken. A sonogram may be used to determine the presence of retained placental fragments.

Surgical

Cunningham et al. (2005) report that curettage, formerly the usual treatment, is now believed to cause more bleeding because of trauma to the placental site. It now is performed when other methods have failed to control the bleeding.

Surgical evacuation of a large hematoma or one increasing in size may be necessary to attain hemostasis. The bleeding vessel is identified and ligated (tied).

Pharmacological

Oxytocin (Pitocin), methylergonovine maleate (Methergine), misoprostol (Cytotec), or prostaglandins may be given to contract the uterus. Methylergonovine maleate (Methergine) should not be given to a client with an elevated blood pressure. The strong contractions produced by these medications often loosen the retained placental fragments, which are then discharged with the lochia. Antibiotics are often used prophylactically to prevent infection. Blood transfusion or replacement of coagulation factors may be necessary depending on the amount of blood lost.

CRITICAL THINKING

Contracted Uterus and Heavy Lochia

A client with a well-contracted uterus is having an extremely heavy lochia discharge. What assessments does the nurse make? What nursing care should be provided?

PROFESSIONALTIP

Factors That Predispose a Postpartum Client to Hemorrhage:

If the postpartum client has any of these predisposing factors, carefully assess for hemorrhage.

- Low platelets count
- A history of bleeding
- A history of alcohol abuse
- Taking any herbal or homeopathic remedies
- Taking any aspirin or NSAIDs
- Obese or suffering from poor nutrition

Catastrophic Intraoperative Hemorrhage, by D. Gallup, 2005, June, *OBG Management*, 54–61.

Activity

The mother is usually kept in bed until the bleeding is under control.

Nursing Management

Monitor vital signs; urine output; uterine height, firmness, and position; blood loss; and level of consciousness. Assess bladder for distension. Save all peripads, linen, and linen savers for estimate of blood loss.

For a hematoma, apply ice, assess pain using pain scale, and continue assessing the hematoma size.

NURSING PROCESS

Assessment

Subjective Data

The mother may either describe feeling like a lot of blood is coming from her vagina or a severe pain in the vulvar or perineal area.

Objective Data

Palpate the fundus for size, consistency, and position. Check how long the peripad has been in place, how much lochia is present, and whether the bladder is distended. Vital signs will probably be within the normal range.

Nursing diagnoses for a client with a postpartum hemorrhage include the following:

NURSING DIAGNOSES	PLANNING/OUTCOMES	NURSING INTERVENTIONS
Risk for *Imbalanced Fluid Volume* related to significant blood loss from uterine atony, as evidenced by client's fundus displaced from	The client will maintain adequate fluid volume.	Assess vital signs and the bladder for distention. Assess fundal height, firmness, and location as per agency protocol. If client has predisposing factors for postpartum hemorrhage, assess more frequently. Assess lochia amount and color and relate to firmness of fundus. Notify CNM/physician about excessive bleeding.

(*Continues*)

Nursing diagnoses for a client with a postpartum hemorrhage include the following: (Continued)

NURSING DIAGNOSES	PLANNING/OUTCOMES	NURSING INTERVENTIONS
midline and unable to maintain a firm fundus on palpation		Maintain mother on bed rest. Call for assistance; one nurse to monitor vital signs while a second nurse monitors fundus and lochia. Save all peripads, linen, and linen savers for more accurate estimate of blood loss. Document all assessments, interventions, and each time CNM/physician is notified. Administer medications as ordered.
*Acute **Pain*** related to tissue damage from hematoma formation, as evidenced by client crying during peri care when RN was assessing the hematoma area	The client will describe having less pain.	Apply ice pack to hematoma. Continue assessment of hematoma size. Assess client's pain using 0 to 10 pain scale (0 = no pain, 10 = most pain). Notify CNM/physician of hematoma and pain assessment. Administer medications as ordered. Document all assessments, interventions, and each time CNM/physician is notified.

Evaluation: Evaluate each outcome to determine how it has been met by the client.

INFECTIONS

Puerperal (postpartum) infection is an infection after childbirth occurring between the birth and 6 weeks postpartum. It is defined as a temperature of 38°C (100.4°F) or more on two separate occasions, after the first 24 hours, on any two of the first 10 postpartum days (Bowes, 1996).

Because all parts of the reproductive tract are connected to each other, it is easy for organisms to move from the vagina through the cervix, to the uterus, through the fallopian tubes, and out to the ovaries and peritoneal cavity. The increased blood supply to the reproductive tract during pregnancy provides more avenues for invading bacteria to be spread throughout the body with the possibility of causing a life-threatening septicemia.

Amniotic fluid and lochia are alkaline, so during labor and in the postpartum period, the normal acidity of the vagina is reduced, which encourages bacterial growth. Predisposing factors include the frequency of vaginal examinations during labor, the length of time membranes had been ruptured, and the length of labor. The growing rates of cesarean sections in the United States have been a major concern and risk factor for postpartum infection. Research has shown that women who underwent labor before having a cesarean birth were at greater risk for postpartum infection (Tharpe, 2008)

It is currently recommended that a prophylactic antibiotic be given to the mother having a cesarean birth after the cord is clamped. This prevents masking or partial treatment of any neonatal infections (Normand & Damato, 2001). The use of prophylactic antibiotics after a caesarean delivery has been noted to reduce postpartum infection by up to 75% (Tharpe, 2008).

It is seldom necessary to keep the baby separated from the mother during maternal infection because they generally share the same organisms. Someone should be available to care for the infant because the mother is usually tired and does not have the energy to fully care for her infant.

Common postpartum infections are wound infection, metritis, mastitis, and urinary tract infection. Predisposing factors for puerperal infection are listed in Table 57-2.

WOUND INFECTION

The break in the skin from lacerations, episiotomies, and surgical incisions from cesarean birth provides an easy portal of entry for bacteria. Localized signs of infection (redness, warmth, edema, and tenderness) are assessed at the skin break, which, if untreated, will develop into generalized signs of infection, including an elevated temperature and malaise. Wound edges may separate and drainage may be evident.

METRITIS

Metritis, inflammation of the uterus, includes both endometritis (inflammation of the inside of the uterus, or endometrium) and parametritis (inflammation of the outside of the uterus, or parametrium, including the connective tissue of the broad ligaments). The usual causes are the organisms that normally inhabit the vagina and cervix. This infection easily spreads through the fallopian tubes (**salpingitis**) to the

TABLE 57-2 Predisposing Factors for Postpartum Infection

PREDISPOSING FACTORS	DESCRIPTION/ EXPLANATION
Antepartum	
Medical conditions	
• Diabetes • Alcoholism • Drug abuse • Anemia • Poor nutrition/ malnutrition • Immunosuppression	Ability to defend against any infection is decreased
History of previous infections	Possibly more vulnerable to infections
Intrapartum	
Prolonged rupture of membranes	Provides direct access to interior of uterus
Chorioamnionitis	Organisms already in uterus
Prolonged labor	More time for bacteria to multiply
Excessive number of vaginal examinations	Increases opportunity for organisms from outside source or vagina to be introduced into the uterus
Internal fetal monitoring	Provides opportunity for introduction of organisms
Bladder catheterization	Possible introduction of organisms into bladder
Episiotomy, lacerations, and cesarean birth	Provide portals of entry for organisms
Postpartum	
Retained placental fragments	Good medium for bacterial growth
Hematoma	Makes tissues more susceptible
Hemorrhage	Infection-fighting components of blood are lost

COURTESY OF DELMAR CENGAGE LEARNING

ovaries (**oophoritis**). The client may not appear ill except for chills and fever spikes (Ernest & Mead, 1998).

MASTITIS

Mastitis is inflammation of the breast, generally during breastfeeding. The usual cause is *Staphylococcus aureus* but may also be *Candida albicans*. Symptoms appear between 2 and 4 weeks after birth. There is usually a crack or fissure in the nipple for the portal of entry. Nipple soreness may result in shorter breastfeeding times, allowing milk stasis, which is a good medium for bacterial growth.

URINARY TRACT INFECTION

Approximately 2% to 4% of new mothers will have a urinary tract infection (UTI) (Murray et al., 2005). Trauma to the bladder and urethra during labor and birth, urinary stasis after the birth, and catheterization all contribute to the development of a UTI.

MEDICAL–SURGICAL MANAGEMENT

Medical

The goal of treatment is to confine the infection and prevent it from spreading systemically.

A culture of drainage from a wound, the uterine cavity, or urine is performed to identify the causative agent of the infection. Breastfeeding should continue during an infection unless the antibiotic used is contraindicated during lactation. Even with mastitis, breastfeeding should continue; emptying the breast at regular intervals is beneficial. If an abscess forms and ruptures into the breast ducts, the breast should be pumped and the milk discarded. Breastfeeding should continue with the unaffected breast.

Surgical

Some sutures may be removed from the episiotomy, laceration repair, or abdominal incision to allow for drainage. If an abscess forms in mastitis, it may require an incision to allow drainage.

Pharmacological

As soon as a culture is taken, a broad-spectrum antibiotic is usually administered pending the results of the culture.

- *Wound infection*: Iodoform gauze may be placed in the open incision. An analgesic may be necessary.
- *Metritis*: Intravenous administration of antibiotics may be required initially. An antipyretic is given to reduce fever, and methylergonovine maleate (Methergine) is given to increase lochia drainage and promote involution.
- *Mastitis*: Early antibiotic therapy usually prevents abscess formation. An analgesic may be necessary.

Diet

A diet high in protein and vitamin C is needed for wound healing. Fluid intake should be increased to 3,000 mL/day for mothers with a urinary tract infection. Maintaining the increased fluid intake necessary for breastfeeding is essential even when the mother has mastitis.

Activity

Extra rest periods are necessary for all new mothers with an infection. This is especially important for mothers with metritis and mastitis, who should ambulate only enough for their own self-care initially. While in bed, the mother with metritis should be in Fowler's position to aid in lochial drainage from the uterus.

Health Promotion

Strict aseptic technique during labor and birth as well as frequent hand hygiene by those providing care to the mother are major factors in preventing postpartum infections.

Nursing Management

Monitor vital signs and assess pain level. Perform a BUBBLE assessment at least every shift. Administer medications as ordered. Encourage client to stay in bed to rest and to increase fluid intake. Maintain client with metritis in the Fowler's position. Assist client to feed and interact with her infant.

NURSING PROCESS

Assessment

Subjective Data

The mother may describe nausea, fatigue, malaise, pelvic pain or heaviness, leg tenderness, or breast tenderness.

Objective Data

The objective data may include fever; chills; foul-smelling lochia; redness, edema, drainage, or wound separation; dysuria, frequency, or urgency; cracked nipple; and redness and edema of the breast.

Nursing diagnoses for a client with a postpartum infection include the following:

NURSING DIAGNOSES	PLANNING/OUTCOMES	NURSING INTERVENTIONS
*Deficient **Knowledge*** related to unfamiliarity with information resources about the etiology, management, as well as the prevention of postpartum infection as evidenced by client's inaccurate follow through of instruction given by RN.	The client will follow the management plan for her infection.	Teach client how changes after birth predispose to infection. Explain the specific management for client's infection. Answer client's questions.
*Acute **Pain*** related to wound infection, metritis, mastitis, or urinary tract infection, as evidenced by client reporting her pain as greater than 2/10 on the pain scale on assessment.	The client will describe less discomfort.	Administer analgesics and antibiotics as ordered. Continue assessing degree of pain using 0 to 10 pain scale (0 = no pain, 10 = worst pain).
*Interrupted **Family** Processes* related to shift in health status of family member (mother)	The family will make adjustments for the mother's infection.	Assist family in understanding mother's limitations. Help family identify resources, people that assist with care, until the mother is well.

Evaluation: Evaluate each outcome to determine how it has been met by the client.

THROMBOEMBOLIC CONDITIONS

Thrombophlebitis refers to the formation of a clot in an inflamed vein. Superficial thrombophlebitis is more common when the mother had preexisting varicose veins. Deep vein thrombosis (DVT) may or may not be related to vein inflammation and is seen more in women with a history of thromboses. Pulmonary embolism may be a complication of DVT. Septic pelvic thrombophlebitis is more commonly found in a mother with metritis as the inflammation spreads to the pelvic veins.

The incidence of thromboembolic conditions has decreased since early ambulation has become a standard practice after childbirth (Lowdermilk & Perry, 2007). Venous stasis and hypercoagulation, which are present during pregnancy, are the major causes. Other risk factors include maternal age older than 35, cesarean birth, prolonged time in stirrups during second stage of labor, obesity, smoking, and a history of varicosities or venous thromboses.

Medical–Surgical Management

Medical

Thrombophlebitis is usually managed with rest, elevation of the affected leg, and local application of heat. Elastic stockings are fitted for use when the mother is able to ambulate. Doppler ultrasound is an accurate diagnostic test for DVT. The mother who is receiving a broad-spectrum antibiotic for metritis and whose symptoms are not diminishing should be suspected of having septic pelvic thrombophlebitis.

Pharmacological

An analgesic is given to relieve discomfort. Antibiotics are often given if the mother has a fever. DVT and septic pelvic thrombophlebitis are usually treated with intravenous heparin for 5 to 7 days. During this time, warfarin sodium (Coumadin) is begun and is usually continued for several months.

Activity

Follow the CNM/physicians orders for all thromboembolic conditions. When the mother is allowed to ambulate, she must wear elastic stockings. In thrombophlebitis and DVT, the affected leg is elevated until symptoms decrease.

Health Promotion

Instruct the client to avoid prolonged standing or sitting. Legs are not to be crossed when sitting. Encourage walking to increase venous return. Pad stirrups and properly adjust for correct support and to prevent pressure on the legs.

Nursing Management

Maintain client in postion ordered by CNM/physician. Elevate the affected leg. Measure legs for elastic stockings for client to wear when able to ambulate. Administer medications as ordered. Teach client to avoid prolonged sitting or standing and to never cross her legs.

NURSING PROCESS

Assessment

Subjective Data

The mother may describe discomfort or pain in the leg affected with superficial thrombophlebitis or DVT and a fullness/heaviness or pain in the pelvis if septic pelvic thrombosis occurs.

Objective Data

Signs of superficial thrombophlebitis include redness, warmth, and swelling where the vein is inflamed. Deep vein thrombosis may manifest as edema and calf pain. A positive Homans' sign may be present, but may also be caused by a strained muscle or improper use of stirrups during the birth. The classic sign of septic pelvic thrombophlebitis is fever of unknown origin. When it is untreated, tachycardia, ileus, and an elevated white count develop.

A nursing diagnosis for clients with thromboembolic conditions may be:

NURSING DIAGNOSIS	PLANNING/OUTCOME	NURSING INTERVENTIONS
Ineffective Peripheral Tissue Perfusion related to mechanical reduction of venous blood flow as evidenced by positive Homans' Sign and pain on palpation of client's calf	The client will maintain adequate tissue perfusion.	Ensure affected leg is properly elevated. Apply heat to affected leg, as ordered. Measure client for antiembolic stockings and teach proper application when able to ambulate. Encourage fluid intake to prevent dehydration. Administer analgesics, antibiotics, heparin, and Coumadin as ordered. Assess for signs of pulmonary embolism (chest pain and dyspnea) and evidence of bleeding (i.e., petechiae, bruising, nosebleed, hematoma) related to heparin therapy. Emphasize importance of having prothrombin time checked while taking warfarin sodium (Coumadin). Keep protamine sulfate, the heparin antagonist, readily available.

Evaluation: Evaluate each outcome to determine how it has been met by the client.

DISSEMINATED INTRAVASCULAR COAGULATION

Disseminated intravascular coagulation (DIC) is an abnormal stimulation of the clotting mechanism, which consumes clotting factors, causing small clots throughout the vascular system and widespread bleeding internally, externally, or both. This results in platelet and clotting factor depletion. DIC may result from a missed abortion, abruptio placenta, amniotic fluid embolism, severe preeclampsia, hemorrhage, and a dead fetus. It is a complication of a preexisting problem.

Correction of the underlying cause is the main aspect of medical management. Blood replacement products including whole blood, packed red cells, or cryoprecipitate may be administered. Nursing care includes continued assessment for signs of bleeding and of complications from the blood products. Intake and output is recorded; urinary output must be maintained at more than 30 mL/hour.

CASE STUDY

R.L. and his wife, M.L, had a second son yesterday, their third child. The baby weighed 8 lbs, 10 oz, the largest of their three children. The labor lasted 5 hours. An episiotomy was performed this time but had not been for the previous births.

M.L. is having problems walking to the bathroom and says she feels faint and dizzy when she stands up. She talks constantly about the pain from the episiotomy. A bruised, edematous area is noted beside the episiotomy. Analgesics provide little relief. Plans were to breastfeed this infant as she had the first two. Today she does not want to feed the baby because she "hurts too much."

The following questions will guide your development of a nursing care plan for this case study.

1. What assessments should be made?
2. Identify three nursing diagnoses for M.L.
3. Identify planning/goals for M.L.
4. List nursing interventions to help M.L. meet the goals.
5. How can the effectiveness of this plan be evaluated?

SUMMARY

- The first 6 weeks after the birth of an infant is called the puerperium or postpartum period.
- Mothers, fathers, siblings, and grandparents all make special adaptations for the neonate.
- During the postpartum period, most of the physiologic changes of pregnancy are reversed and the mother's body returns to its prepregnant state.
- Immediate weight loss of the mother is 13 lbs with an additional 8- to 9-lb loss during the first 6 weeks postpartum.
- Rubin describes three phases of maternal restoration/adaptation—taking in, taking hold, and letting go.
- Unexpected emotional/behavioral changes include postpartum depression, postpartum psychosis, and reaction to an infant with problems.
- Specific assessments for the first few days postpartum include BUBBLE (breasts, uterus, bladder, bowel, lochia, and episiotomy), vital signs, Homans' sign, bonding/attachment, parenting, activity, comfort, and self-care.

REVIEW QUESTIONS

1. Client R.H. is 3 days postpartum and needs RhoGam. Before administering the injection, what should the nurse do?
   1. Check the orders and lab result to make sure that the Coomb's test was negative.
   2. Make sure the infant is Rh negative.
   3. Prepare a sub-q injection for the shot.
   4. Prepare to give the injection to the infant.
2. The nurse is checking a client after a scheduled cesarean delivery. On palpation of the fundus, the RN notices that the fundus is deviated to the right, firm, and with moderate lochial flow. What would be the nurse's first response to the situation?
   1. Administer 20 units of pitocin IM.
   2. Call the CNM/physician.
   3. Palpate the bladder and ask the client when she last voided.
   4. Insert a straight catheter into the client.
3. What is the best position to assess a postpartum woman's fundus?
   1. On her right side.
   2. Semi-Fowler position.
   3. Supine with knees slightly flexed.
   4. In a chair, with feet elevated.
4. A nurse is working triage in a busy labor and delivery unit when a patient calls, stating that "she is alone in her house and wants to harm herself and her new baby." The nurse's first response should be?
   1. "Let me help you schedule an appointment to see the doctor."
   2. Keep the client on the phone and call for police assistance to her house.
   3. Reassure the patient that she will be okay if she just gets some sleep.
   4. Have the patient drive herself to the emergency room.
5. The nurse is teaching a non-breastfeeding mother about breast care. The nurse knows that more teaching is needed when the client responds with the following statement:
   1. "I will make sure I wear a tight-fitting bra when my breast milk comes in."
   2. "I will express my milk to help it dry up."
   3. "I will avoid hot water on my breasts until my breast milk dries up."
   4. "I will use ice packs to help relieve the pain of engorgement."

6. The nurse observes passive and dependent behaviors displayed by a postpartum client. According to Reva Rubin, the client is in the:
   1. taking-in phase.
   2. letting-go phase.
   3. taking-hold phase.
   4. transitional phase.
7. A client has excessive vaginal bleeding after delivery. The assessment reveals a soft, boggy uterus located above the level of the umbilicus and displaced to the right side. The first action of the nurse should be to:
   1. notify the CNM/physician.
   2. massage the fundus and take vital signs.
   3. initiate measures that encourage voiding.
   4. put the client flat, take vital signs, and notify the CNM/physician.
8. A new mother tells the nurse that she is afraid of her baby and that she doubts she will be able to love the baby. The most appropriate action for the nurse would be to:
   1. tell the client she will learn fast.
   2. tell the client what a beautiful baby she has.
   3. encourage the client to talk about her feelings.
   4. have a psychiatrist visit the client immediately.
9. A client has excessive vaginal bleeding following the birth. The nurse should suspect a cervical or vaginal tear if the client assessment reveals:
   1. acute pelvic pain.
   2. a hard, contracted uterus.
   3. an elevation of blood pressure.
   4. a firmly contracted uterus with blood spurting from the vagina.
10. A client wants to know when she can begin breastfeeding and is anxious for her milk to start. The best response of the nurse would be:
    1. "Ask your CNM/physician."
    2. "Your baby will be brought to you at the next feeding time. Your milk will start right after that."
    3. "We encourage you to breastfeed as soon as you wish. Your milk will probably "come in" in about 3 days."
    4. "The baby can breastfeed anytime after birth. After your colostrum is gone (3 to 4 days), your milk will come in (5 to 6 days)."

REFERENCES/SUGGESTED READINGS

Albright, A. (1993). Postpartum depression: An overview. *Journal of Counseling Development 71*(3), 316.

Ament, L. (1990). Maternal tasks of the puerperium reidentified. *JOGNN, 19*(4), 330.

American Academy of Pediatrics (AP) & American College of Obstetricians and Gynecologists (ACOG). (1977). *Guidelines for perinatal care* (3rd ed.). Elk Grove Village, IL: American Academy of Pediatrics.

Bandyopadhyay, M. (2009). Impact of ritual pollution on lactation and breastfeeding practices in rural West Bengal, India. *International Breastfeeding Journal, 4(10)*, 1186/1746-4358-4-2.

Beck, C., & Gable, R. (2001). Further validation of the Postpartum Depression Screening Scale. *Nursing Research, 50*(3), 155.

Beeber, L. (2002). The pinks and the blues. *AJN, 102*(11), 91–97.

Berger, D., & Loveland-Cook, C. (1998). Postpartum teaching priorities: The viewpoints of nurses and mothers. *JOGNN, 27*(2), 161–168.

Bowes, W. (2001). Postpartum care. In S. Gabbe, J. Niebyl, & J. Simpson (Eds.), *Obstetrics: Normal and problem pregnancies* (4th ed.). New York: Churchill Livingstone.

Brown, S., & Johnson, B. (1998). Enhancing early discharge with home. follow-up. A pilot project. *JOGNN*, 27(1), 33–38.

Bulechek, G., Butcher, H., McCloskey, J., & Dochterman, J., eds. (2008). *Nursing Interventions Classification (NIC)* (5th ed.). St. Louis, MO: Mosby/Elsevier.

Burroughs, A., & Leifer, G. (2007). *Maternity nursing* (10th ed.). Philadelphia: W. B. Saunders.

Callister, L., & Vega, R. (1998). Giving birth: Guatemalan women's voices. *JOGNN, 27*(3), 289–295.

Cesario, S. (2001). Care of the Native American woman: Strategies for practice, education, and research. *JOGNN, 30*(1), 13–19.

Cheng, C., Fowles, E., & Walker, L. (2006). Postpartum Maternal Health Care in the United States. *The Journal of Perinatal Education, 15* (3), 34-42.

Cunningham, F., Grant, N., Leveno, K., Gilstrap, L., & Cox, S. (2005). *William's obstetrics* (22nd ed.). Norwalk, CT: Appleton & Lange.

Davis, R. (2001). The postpartum experience for Southeast Asian women in the United States. *MCN, 26*(4), 208–213.

Davidson, N. (1974). REEDA: Evaluating postpartum healing. *Journal of Nurse Midwifery*, 19(2), 6-8.

Ernest, J., & Mead, P. (1998). Postpartum endometritis. *Contemporary OB/GYN, 43*(1), 33–38.

Ferguson, S., & Engelhard, C. (1996). Maternity length of stay and public policy: Issues and implications. *Journal of Pediatric Nursing, 11*(6), 392.

Ferketich, S., & Mercer, R. (1995). Paternal–infant attachment of experienced and inexperienced fathers during infancy. *Nursing Research, 44*(1), 31–37.

Gallup, D. (2005, June). Catastrophic Intraoperative Hemorrhage. *OBG Management*, 54–61.

Gennaro, S., Kamwendo, L., Mbweza, E., & Kershbaumer, R. (1998). Childbearing in Malawi, Africa. *JOGNN, 27*(2), 191–196.

Green, S., & Adams, W. (1993). Chronic psychiatric illness and pregnancy: Nursing implications. *Journal of Perinatal, Neonatal Nursing, 7*(3), 7–18.

Ha, L. (1994, December). *Culturally sensitive caregiving for Vietnamese women*. Lecture presented at the Medical College of Virginia Hospitals, Richmond, VA.

Harvard's Women's Health Page. (2008, June). Retrieved July 2, 2009, from Harvard Health: https://www.health.harvard.edu/newsweek/Hemorrhoids_and_what_to_do_about_them.htm

Havens, D., & Hannan, C. (1996). Legislation to mandate maternal and newborn length of stay. *Journal of Pediatric Health Care, 10*(3), 141.

Health Care Financing Administration (2002). The Newborns' and Mothers' Health Protection Act of 1996. [Online]. Retrieved from http://www.hcfa.gov/medicaid/hipaa/content/nmhpa.asp

Higgins, P. (2000). Postpartum complications. In S. Mattson & J. E. Smith (Eds.). *Core curriculum for maternal-newborn nursing* (2nd ed.). Philadelphia: W. B. Saunders.

Howard, J., & Berbiglia, V. (1997). Caring for childbearing Korean women. *JOGNN, 26*(6), 665–671.

Hutchinson, M., & Baqi-Aziz, M. (1994). Nursing care of the childbearing Muslim family. *JOGNN, 23*(9), 767–771.

Johnson & Johnson (1996). *Compendium of postpartum care.* Skillman, NJ: Johnson & Johnson Consumer Products.

Kim-Godwin, Y. (2003). Postpartum beliefs & practices among non-western cultures. *MCN, 28*(2), 74–78.

Ladewig, P., Moberly, S., Olds, S., & London, M. (2009). *Contemporary maternal-newborn nursing care* (7th ed.). Menlo Park, CA: Addison-Wesley.

Leifer, G. (2007). *Maternity nursing: An introductory text (Burroughs)* (10th ed). Philadelphia: W.B. Saunders.

Littleton, L., & Engebretson, J. (2002). *Maternal, neonatal, and women's health nursing.* Clifton Park, NY: Delmar Cengage Learning.

Lowdermilk, D., & Perry, S. (2007). *Maternity and women's health care* (9th ed.). St. Louis, Missouri: Mosby Elsever.

Luegenbiehl, D., Brophy, G., Artigue, G., Phillips, K., & Flack, R. (1990). Standardized assessment of blood loss. *MCN, 15*(4), 241–244.

Martell, L. (1996). Is Rubin's "taking-in" and "taking-hold" a useful paradigm? *Health Care Women International 17*(1), 1.

Mattson, S. (1995). Culturally sensitive perinatal care for Southeast Asians. *JOGNN, 24*(4), 335–341.

Montigny, F., & Lacharité, C. (2005). Father's perceptions of the imediate postpartal period. *JOGNN, 33* (3), 328–339.

Moorhead, S., Johnson, M., Maas, M., & Swanson, E. (2007). *Nursing Outcomes Classifications (NOC)* (4th ed). St. Louis, MO: Elsevier–Health Sciences Division.

Murray, S., McKinney, E., & Gorrie, T. (2005). *Foundations of maternal–newborn nursing* (4th ed.). Philadelphia: W. B. Saunders.

Neal, J. (2001). RhD isoimmunization and current management modalities. *JOGNN, 309*(6), 589–606.

Normand, M., & Damato, E. (2001). Postcesarean infection. *JOGNN, 30*(6), 642–647.

North American Nursing Diagnosis Association International. (2010). *NANDA-I nursing diagnoses: Definitions and classification 2009–2011.* Ames, IA: Wiley-Blackwell.

Oyeku, S. (2003). *A Closer Look at Racial/Ethnic Disparities in Breastfeeding.* Boston: Harvard Pediatric Health Services.

Placksin, S. (2000). *Mothering the new mother: Women's feelings and needs after childbirth. A support and resource guide.* New York: Newmark Press.

Rubin, R. (1961). Puerperal change. *Nursing Outlook, 9*(12), 743–755.

Ruchala, P., & Halstead, L. (1994). The postpartum experience of low-risk women: A time of adjustment and change. *MCN, 22*(3), 83.

Savoia, M.. (1999). Bacterial, fungal, and parasitic disease during pregnancy. In G. Burrow, T. Duffy, & R. Kersey (Eds.). *Medical complications during pregnancy* (5th ed.). Philadelphia: W. B. Saunders.

Schneiderman, J. (1996). Postpartum nursing for Korean mothers. *MCN, 21*(3), 155–158.

Sharts-Hopko, N. (1995). Birth in the Japanese context. *JOGNN, 24*(4), 343–351.

Simpson, K., & Creehan, P. (2007). *AWHONN perinatal nursing* (3rd ed.). Philadelphia, Lippincott Williams & Wilkins.

Sit, D., Rothschild, A., & Wisner, K. (2006). A Review of Postpartum Psychosis. *Journal of Women's Health, 15* (4), 352–368.

Smith-Hanrahan, C., & Deblois, D. (1995). Postpartum early discharge. *Clinical Nursing Research, 4*(1), 50.

Spratto, G., & Woods, A. (2008). *PDR nurse's drug handbook.* Clifton Park, NY: Delmar Cengage Learning.

Squires, A. (2003). Documenting surgical incision site care. *Nursing2003, 33*(1), 74.

Staff, M. (2008, January). Infant and toddler health. Retrieved July 2, 2009, from Mayo Clinic: http://www.mayoclinic.com/health/infant-development/PR00061/NSECTIONGROUP=2

Tharpe, N. (2008). Postpregnancy Genital tract and Wound Infections. *Journal of Midwifery and Women's Health, 53*(3), 236–246.

Troy, N. (2003). Is the significance of postpartum fatigue being overlooked in the lives of women? *MCN, 28*(4), 252–257.

Visness, C., Kennedy, K., & Ramos, R. (1997). The duration and character of postpartum bleeding among breast-feeding women. *Obstetrics and Gynecology, 89*(2), 159.

Wilkerson, N. (1996). Appraisal of early discharge programs. *Journal of Perinatal Education, 5*(2), 1.

Wrasper, C. (1996). Discharge and timing and Rubin's concept of puerperal change. *Journal of Perinatal Education, 5*(2), 13.

Zlatnik, F. (1999). The normal and abnormal puerperlium. In J.R. Scott, P.J. Di Saia, C.B. Hammond, & W.N. Spellacy (Eds.), *Danforths' obstetrics and gynecology* (8th ed.). Philadelphia: Lippincott Williams & Wilkins.

RESOURCES

Association of Women's Health, Obstetric and Neonatal Nurses (AWHONN), http://www.awhonn.org

Depression After Delivery (DAD), Inc., http://www.depressionafterdelivery.com

Health Science Consortium, http://www.healthsciencesconsortium.com/

Hollister, Inc., http://www.hollister.com

International Lactation Consultant Association (ILCA), http://www.ilca.org

Johnson & Johnson Consumer Products, Inc., http://www.JNJ.com

Postpartum Support International, http://www.postpartum.net

CHAPTER 58
Newborn Care

MAKING THE CONNECTION

Refer to the following chapters to increase your understanding of newborn care:

Basic Nursing
- ***Life Span Development***

Maternal & Pediatric Nursing
- ***Complications of Pregnancy***
- ***The Birth Process***
- ***Postpartum Care***
- ***Basics of Pediatric Care***
- ***Infants with Special Needs: Birth to 12 Months***

Basic Procedures
- ***Hand Hygiene***
- ***Use of Protective Equipment***
- ***Taking a Temperature***
- ***Taking a Pulse***
- ***Counting Respirations***
- ***Performing Cardiopulmonary Resuscitation (Infant)***

Intermediate Procedures
- ***Administering an Intramuscular Injection***
- ***Administering Oxygen Therapy***
- ***Performing a Skin Puncture***

LEARNING OBJECTIVES

- Define key terms.
- Describe the immediate needs of the newborn.
- Discuss what initiates breathing in the newborn.
- Describe the newborn's methods of heat production and heat retention.
- Identify the four ways heat is lost and nursing interventions to prevent heat loss.
- Describe the immediate care of the newborn.
- Discuss the Apgar score and how it is used.
- Describe the physical characteristics of the newborn.
- Identify the common variations in the newborn.
- Elicit the newborn's reflexes.
- Determine the gestational age of a newborn.
- Discuss the newborn's nutritional needs and how they can be met by breastfeeding and bottle feeding.

- Identify common problems the newborn may encounter and nursing interventions for each.
- Plan the care and then care for a newborn.

KEY TERMS

acrocyanosis
appropriate for gestational age
caput succedaneum
cephalhematoma
circumcision
cold stress
conduction
convection
cryptorchidism
Down syndrome
epispadias
Epstein's pearls
erythema toxicum neonatorum
evaporation
foremilk
hallux varus
hindmilk
hydrocele
hyperbilirubinemia
hypospadias
kernicterus
lanugo
large for gestational age
meconium
meningocele
milia
molding
mongolian spots
myelomeningocele
neonatal transition
neutral thermal environment
nevus flammeus
nevus vascularis
nonshivering thermogenesis
ophthalmia neonatorum
phimosis
polydactyly
pseudomenstruation
radiation
small for gestational age
spina bifida occulta
syndactyly
talipes equinovarus (clubfoot)
telangiectactic nevi
thermogenesis
thermoregulation
vernix caseosa
witch's milk

INTRODUCTION

At the time of birth, the newborn must quickly make changes in the respiratory system to allow gas exchange to take place in the lungs and also make changes in the circulatory system to support the change to respiratory gas exchange. These profound, vital changes are critical to maintaining extrauterine life. The first few hours after birth wherein the newborn makes these changes and stabilizes respiratory and circulatory functions is called the **neonatal transition** period (Figure 58-1). Other body systems also make changes in their functioning over a longer period, although they are not crucial to the immediate survival of the infant.

Nurses are instrumental in assisting the newborn and mother through the neonatal transition period.

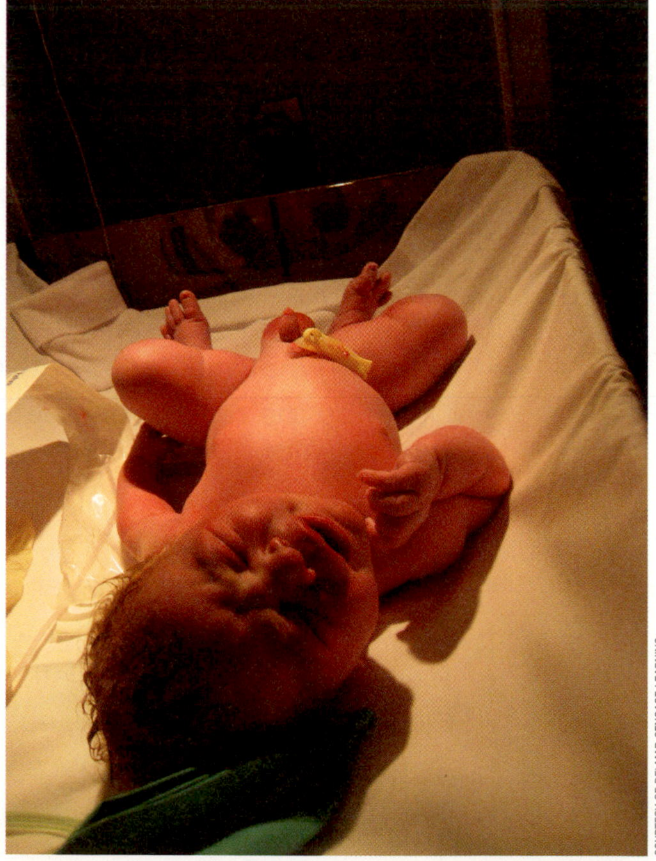

COURTESY OF DELMAR CENGAGE LEARNING

FIGURE 58-1 The first few hours after birth are called the neonatal transition period, during which the infant experiences profound changes.

IMMEDIATE NEEDS OF THE NEWBORN

The immediate needs of the newborn are airway, breathing, circulation, and warmth.

AIRWAY

A clear airway is necessary for adequate gas exchange.

BREATHING

In utero, the fetus relied on the placenta and the mother's respirations for gas exchange; however, fetal breathing movements, from approximately 11 weeks' gestation, help develop the chest wall muscles and the diaphragm (Ladewig, Moberly, Olds, & London, 2005). By approximately 35 weeks' gestation, the surfactant produced by the alveoli is sufficient in

PROFESSIONALTIP

Healthy People 2010

Healthy People 2010 includes initiatives to help people have good health and live longer lives. The following are the initiatives geared toward healthy mothers and their children:

- Increase the percentage of healthy full-term infants who are put down to sleep on their backs.
- Increase the proportion of mothers who breastfeed their babies.
- Ensure appropriate newborn bloodspot screening, follow up testing, and referral to services. (Healthy People 2010, 2009)

amount (L/S ratio 2:1) to allow the alveoli to remain partially expanded when the newborn begins to breathe at birth.

For the lungs to function, two changes must happen:

- Pulmonary ventilation must be established with lung expansion at the first breath.
- Pulmonary circulation must greatly increase.

The initiation of breathing is influenced by four factors—physical, chemical, thermal, and sensory—which work together.

Physical Factors

The physical (sometimes called mechanical) factors include the compression of the fetal chest as it moves through the birth canal, which squeezes fluid from the lungs and increases intrathoracic pressure; and the chest wall recoil, which occurs as the newborn's trunk emerges. The chest recoil creates negative intrathoracic pressure, which causes a small amount of air to replace the fluid that was squeezed out of the lungs and some of the lung fluid to move across the alveolar membranes into the interstitial tissue of the lungs. Each breath allows more air into the alveoli and more fluid into the interstitial tissue. Because the protein concentration is higher in the capillaries, the interstitial fluid is drawn into them. All of the alveolar fluid is absorbed within the first day after birth.

Chemical Factors

When the cord is clamped, placental gas exchange ceases, causing an increase in $PaCO_2$ and a decrease in PaO_2 and pH (a transitory asphyxia). These changes stimulate the carotid and aortic chemoreceptors, which send impulses to the respiratory center in the medulla, which in turn stimulates respirations. A brief period of asphyxia stimulates respirations, whereas prolonged asphyxia is a central nervous system (CNS) respiratory depressant.

Thermal Factors

The change in temperature from the intrauterine environment to the extrauterine environment, a decrease of more than 20°F, is also a stimulus to breathing. The colder temperature stimulates the skin nerve endings and the newborn breathes as a response. Cold stress and respiratory depression result from excessive cooling of the newborn.

Sensory Factors

The comfortable, relatively quiet uterine environment is left behind for an environment full of sensory stimuli. The auditory and visual stimuli associated with birth, along with the tactile stimulation of being handled, assist in the initiation of respirations.

Circulation

Several circulatory changes are necessary for the successful change from fetal circulation to neonatal circulation. These changes involve the pulmonary blood vessels, ductus arteriosus, foramen ovale, and ductus venosus.

Pulmonary Blood Vessels

The dilation of these blood vessels begins with the first breath taken by the newborn. This results in lower pulmonary resistance, which allows the blood to freely circulate through the lungs to be oxygenated.

Ductus Arteriosus

Within minutes after birth, the ductus arteriosus has a reversal of blood flow caused by the increased pressure in the aorta and the increase of oxygen in the blood. This results in more blood flowing through the pulmonary arteries for oxygenation. Closure of the ductus arteriosus is complete within 24 hours and is permanent in 3 to 4 weeks.

Foramen Ovale

The foramen ovale closes within minutes after birth because of the higher pressure in the left atrium than in the right atrium. The increased blood flow in the lungs decreases pressure in the right atrium, and the return of blood from the lungs increases the pressure in the left atrium. Closure of the foramen ovale is permanent in approximately 3 months.

Ductus Venosus

When the cord is clamped, the blood ceases flowing through the umbilical vein to the ductus venosus and into the inferior vena cava. Blood now flows through the liver and is filtered as in adult circulation.

Warmth

At birth the newborn must begin **thermoregulation**, maintenance of body temperature. Three factors are instrumental in thermoregulation: heat production, heat retention, and heat loss.

Heat Production

The newborn produces heat (**thermogenesis**) through general metabolism, muscular activity, and nonshivering thermogenesis (unique to the newborn). Newborns rarely shiver as adults do to increase heat production. Shivering seen in a newborn indicates that the metabolic rate has already doubled (Ladewig et al., 2005).

When the infant is in a cool environment and requires more heat, the metabolic rate increases, producing more heat. The newborn may cry and have muscular activity when cold, but there is no voluntary control of muscular activity.

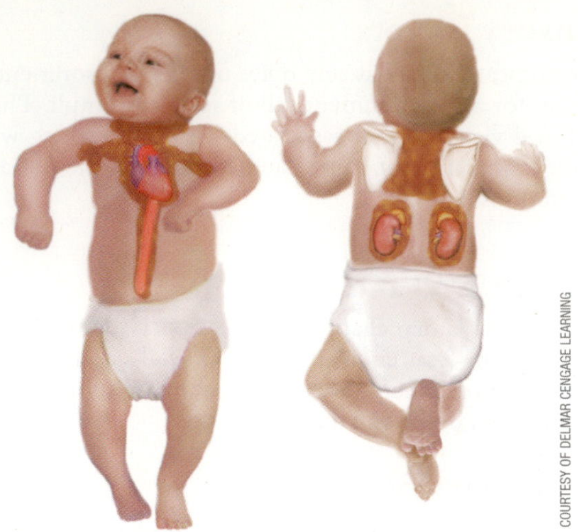

FIGURE 58-2 Brown fat distribution in the newborn.

If the infant's temperature is not adequately raised through increased metabolism, **nonshivering thermogenesis**, the metabolism of brown fat, begins. Brown fat is a special fat found only in newborns. It appears at about 26 to 30 weeks of gestation and increases until 2 to 5 weeks of age (unless depleted by cold stress). The fat is highly vascularized, which gives it the brown color. The brown fat is located at the back of the neck, between the scapula, around the kidneys and adrenals, in the axilla, and around the heart and abdominal aorta (Figure 58-2). Once the brown fat has been metabolized, the infant no longer has this method of heat production available.

Heat Retention

Newborns retain heat by staying in a flexed position. This reduces the area of skin exposed to the environmental temperature, thus decreasing heat loss. They also use the mechanism of peripheral vasoconstriction to retain heat.

Heat Loss

The newborn has thin skin with blood vessels close to the surface and little subcutaneous fat to prevent heat loss. Heat moves from the warm internal areas to the cooler skin surface and then to the surrounding environment. Excessive heat loss is called **cold stress**. An increase in metabolism leads to a significant increase in the need for oxygen. When oxygen is used for metabolism (heat production), the infant may experience hypoxia. There may not be enough oxygen for the metabolic rate to increase, and the newborn will not be able to maintain body temperature. Prolonged cold stress causes respiratory difficulties and a decrease in surfactant production. Less surfactant hinders lung expansion, which in turn leads to more respiratory distress. Decreased blood oxygen may cause vasoconstriction of the pulmonary vessels with a return to fetal circulation patterns, which further increases respiratory distress.

The glucose necessary for increased metabolism is made available when glycogen stores are converted to glucose. If the glycogen is depleted, hypoglycemia results.

Brown fat metabolism results in the release of fatty acids. Continuous brown fat metabolism, when the newborn is in a cold stress situation for a considerable time, results in metabolic acidosis, which can be life-threatening. Excess fatty acids in the blood interfere with bilirubin transportation to the liver, which increases the risk of jaundice.

PROFESSIONALTIP

Effects of Cold Stress

- Oxygen need increased
- Respiratory distress
- Surfactant production decreased
- Hypoglycemia
- Metabolic acidosis
- Jaundice

There are four methods by which the newborn loses heat: conduction, convection, evaporation, and radiation.

Conduction **Conduction** is the loss of heat by direct contact with a cooler object. When a newborn is touched by cold hands or a cold stethoscope or is placed on a cold surface such as a scale, heat is lost. Heat loss can be prevented by warming objects touching the newborn. If a newborn is wrapped in a warmed blanket or placed against the mother's warm skin, heat will be lost by the blanket or mother's skin to the cooler newborn and the newborn is warmed.

Convection **Convection** is the loss of heat by the movement of air. When air moves (air currents), heat is transferred to the air. Air currents from an open door or window, air conditioning, or from people moving around increase heat loss. A radiant warmer is often used for the newborn immediately after birth to prevent heat loss by convection (Figure 58-3).

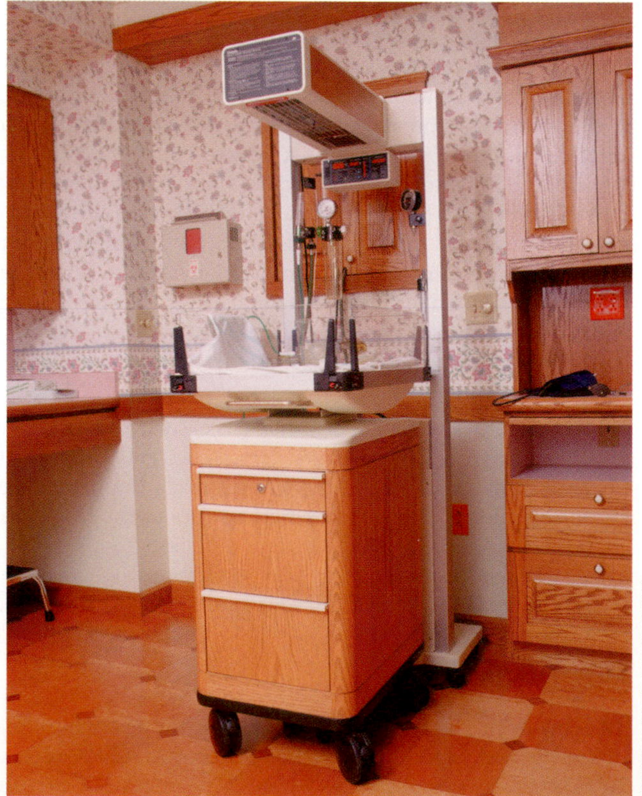

FIGURE 58-3 A radiant warmer keeps the air surrounding the newborn warm, preventing heat loss by convection.

> **SAFETY**
>
> **Newborns and Standard Precautions**
>
> Penny-MacGillivray (1996) explains that blood and amniotic fluid, once believed to be sterile, are now considered contaminated with blood-borne pathogens. All newborns are now also considered contaminated until the first bath has removed all blood and amniotic fluid from the infant's body. The nurse performing the assessment and giving the first bath *must wear gloves*.

Heat loss in the newborn can be prevented by wrapping the infant in a blanket and placing a stocking cap on the head and by keeping the newborn out of any drafts.

Evaporation **Evaporation** is the loss of heat when water is changed to a vapor. When a wet body dries, heat is lost, such as a newborn wet with amniotic fluid or during a bath. The insensible water loss from the skin and respiratory tract also results in heat loss. Heat loss can be prevented by immediately drying the newborn at birth and after receiving a bath, and by changing wet clothing and diapers promptly.

Radiation **Radiation** is the loss of heat by transfer to cooler objects nearby, but not through direct contact. An infant placed near a cold window loses heat by radiation to the sides of the crib and the window. If the walls of an incubator are cold, the infant loses heat. Heat loss can be prevented by keeping cribs and incubators away from cold windows.

IMMEDIATE CARE OF THE NEWBORN

The immediate care of the newborn includes obtaining the Apgar score, resuscitation (if needed), providing a neutral thermal environment, proper identification of the infant, parent/infant bonding, and prophylactic care.

Apgar Score

The Apgar score, which assesses the infant's cardiopulmonary adaptations to extrauterine life, is given immediately after the delivery. The Apgar scores are assigned by the nurse caring for the infant. More information on Apgar scoring can be found in the Birth Process chapter.

Resuscitation

Resuscitation is begun if no respirations are initiated by the infant. The LP/VN may be asked to use a bulb syringe to suction mucus from the infant's oropharynx, gently rub the infant's back for stimulation, or provide oxygen. More intense resuscitation would typically be performed by an RN or physician who have gone through a Neonatal Resuscitation Program (NRP).

Neutral Thermal Environment

A **neutral thermal environment** is an environment in which the newborn can maintain internal body temperature with minimal oxygen consumption and metabolism. In this environment, the newborn's body does not have to focus on temperature maintenance but can focus on growth and development.

Identification

Proper identification of the newborn is vital. The identification bands must be checked and compared to the mother's band each time the baby is brought into the mother's room. No infant should ever leave the hospital without having their bands checked against the mother's bands. One band will usually be kept in the infant's hospital records when the infant is discharged. The process of applying the identification bands is discussed in the Birth Process chapter.

Parent/Infant Bonding

Interaction between the parents and infant should be promoted as soon as the infant is stable. The nurse assists the parents in holding their baby or to give them permission to examine the infant. This is a good time for the nurse to answer any questions that the parents might have.

Prophylactic Care

Prophylactic care includes the administration of vitamin K and hepatitis B vaccine, instillation of an antibiotic ophthalmic ointment, and umbilical cord care.

Vitamin K

At birth, newborns lack vitamin K, which is necessary for the clotting process. Vitamin K is synthesized in the intestine and requires food and normal intestinal flora for the process. Because the intestines are sterile at birth, no vitamin K can be produced for several days. An intramuscular (IM) injection of vitamin K, phytonadione (aquaMEPHYTON), is generally given within the first hour after birth to prevent hemorrhagic disorders. A normal newborn is able to produce vitamin K by the eighth day (Lowdermilk & Perry, 2007).

Hepatitis B Vaccination

The Centers for Disease Control and Prevention (CDC), along with the Advisory Committee on Immunization Practices (ACIP), the American Academy of Pediatrics (AAP), and the American Academy of Family Physicians (AAFP), recommend giving the first dose of hepatitis B (Hep B) vaccine within 12 hours of birth. Infants whose mothers have hepatitis B should also receive hepatitis B immune globulin (HBIG) at the same time, but at a different site than the vaccine. The HBIG provides passive immunity until the newborn develops antibodies. In many agencies, the parents must give written permission for the infant to receive the hepatitis B vaccine. Parents who do not wish to vaccinate their infant should sign a refusal of treatment after the infant is born. Many parents will opt to have their pediatrician vaccinate the infant at their one week visit.

Eye Prophylaxis

In the United States, it is mandatory to instill a prophylactic agent in the eyes of all neonates to prevent **ophthalmia neonatorum**. This is an inflammation of the newborn's eyes that results from passing through the birth canal when a gonorrheal or chlamydial infection is present. The medication used for prophylaxis varies with agency protocol but is generally erythromycin (Ilotycin Ophthalmic Ointment) or tetracycline (Achromycin Ophthalmic Ointment) (Lowdermilk & Perry, 2007). Silver nitrate 1% is now seldom used because it protects only against gonorrheal infection and not chlamydial infection. To promote parent/infant eye contact, bonding, and attachment, some agencies delay the eye prophylaxis for an hour or so.

Umbilical Cord Care

Umbilical cord care is similar to caring for an open sore or wound. In the past, agencies used triple blue dye, alcohol, or an erythromycin solution to clean the cord. Keeping the cord dry and clean is the best way to promote healing and prevent infection of the cord. Early signs of infection to inspect for at the cord and the skin at the base include purulent drainage, pus, active bleeding from the site, infant showing signs of pain, and redness and irritation at site. Make sure parents are informed that the infant should not be fully bathed until the cord falls off. The prevention of or early identification of any hemorrhage or infection is the goal of care.

SAFETY

Cord Hemorrhage

- When bleeding from the cord is noted, check the clamp and apply a second clamp on the body side of the first one.
- If the bleeding does not stop immediately, notify the health care provider.

PHYSICAL CHARACTERISTICS OF THE NEWBORN

The newborn infant is not just a miniature adult. Identification of the physical characteristics and common variations of the newborn found in the infant are documented. This provides a basis for nursing diagnoses and care. Agencies generally have a form to follow such as the one shown in Figure 58-4. This form incorporates data about the mother, the delivery, Apgar score, and gestational age along with the physical assessment of the infant.

Weight and Length

Most full-term newborns weigh between 2,500 g and 4,000 g or approximately 5 lb, 8 oz to 8 lb, 13 oz. Newborns lose 5% to

Initial Newborn Profile
Hollister Maternal/Newborn Record System
To order call: 1.800.323.4060 Re-order No. 5720

Admit Data Date __/__/__ Date ____
ID/Band No. ____ Name ____
Admitted By ____
Medications ☐ None ☐ See Delivery Data

Date	Time	Medication	Dose	Route Site	Inits
		Eye Prophylaxis Erythromycin			
		Vitamin K			

Newborn Data ☐ male ☐ Female ☐ Breast ☐ Bottle
Birthdate __/__/__ Time ____
Place of Birth ☐ Hospital ☐ ____
☐ Vertex ☐ Breech ☐ Vaginal ☐ Cesarean
Delivered by ____
Apgar ____ 1min ____ 5min ____ 10min
Cord Blood pH ____ Type/Rh ____ Coombs ____
Intrapartum Problems Identified ☐ None
1. ____
2. ____
3. ____

Maternal Data G T Pt A L
Name ____ Age ____
Record No. ____ Room No. ____
Blood Type/Rh ____ Antibody + -

Screens	Neg	Pos	Comments
STD	☐	☐	
Urine Tox	☐	☐	
Hepatitis B	☐	☐	
	☐	☐	
	☐	☐	

Measurements/Gestational Age Assessment
See Delivery Data
☐ Weight ____ lbs ____ gms
☐ Length ____ cms ____ ins
☐ Head Circ ____ cms ____ ins
☐ Chest Circ ____ cms ____ ins
☐ Abd Cric ____ cms ____ ins
Gest Age by Dates ____ Wks
Gest Age by Exam ____ Wks
☐ Preterm
☐ Term
☐ Postterm
☐ SGA ☐ AGA ☐ LGA

Physical Assessment
Date __/__/__ Time ____ Age ____ hrs
Temp ____ Pulse Rate/Rhythm ____ Resp ____ BP ☐ Not done ☐ ____
Head/Neck — Detail Abnormal Findings

1. Fontanels	Level	Bulging	Depressed
Anterior	☐	☐	☐
Posterior	☐	☐	☐

2. Sutures ☐ Open ☐ Closed ☐ Overriding
3. Variations ☐ None ☐ Molding ☐ Caput ☐ Cephalhematoma
4. Lacerations ☐ No ☐ Yes

	Normal	Abnormal
5. Face	☐	☐
6. Eyes	☐	☐
7. Ears	☐	☐
8. Nose	☐	☐
9. Mouth	☐	☐
10. Neck	☐	☐
Chest		
11. Breath sounds	☐	☐
12. Thorax	☐	☐
13. Clavicles	☐	☐
Cardiovascular		
14. Heart sounds	☐	☐
15. Pulses	☐	☐
Abdomen		
16. Structure	☐	☐
17. Bowel sounds	☐	☐
18. Cord	☐	☐
19. Liver	☐	☐
20. Spleen	☐	☐
21. Kidneys	☐	☐
Genitalia		
22. Female	☐	☐
23. Male	☐	☐
Musculoskeletal		
24. Tone	☐	☐
25. Extremities	☐	☐
26. Hips	☐	☐
27. Spine	☐	☐
Neurologic		
28. Reflexes	☐	☐
29. Cry	☐	☐

Detail Abnormal Findings

Skin
30. Condition ☐ Smooth ☐ Dry ☐ Peeling ☐ Vernix ☐ Mec Stain
31. Color ☐ Pink ☐ Ruddy ☐ Pale ☐ Mottled ☐ Cyanotic ☐ Jaundice (time noted ____)
32. Variations (i.e. rash, lesion, birthmark) ____

Elimination
33. Bowel Anus Patent ☐ Yes ☐ No ____
First Meconium (date, time) ____
34. Urine First Void (date, time) ____

Problems identified ☐ None
1. ____
2. ____
3. ____

Comments/Plan

Hollister Incorporated, 2000 Hollister Drive, Libertyville, Illinois 60048

Newborn Risk Indicators

Observable at birth	Within 24 hrs. postpartum
☐ **No risk factors noted**	☐ **No risk factors noted**
☐ Abnormal presentation	☐ Abdominal presentation
☐ Multiple birth	☐ Vomiting
☐ Low birth rate	☐ Failure to pass meconium (if skin not stained)
☐ Resuscitation at birth	☐ Melena
☐ 1 min. Apgar <5	☐ Apneic episodes (>20 seconds)
☐ 5 min. Apgar <7	☐ Tachypnea (transient)
☐ Placental Abnormalities	☐ See-saw breathing
☐ Two cord vessels	☐ Cyanosis
☐ Difficult catheterization	☐ Petechiae/Ecchymoses
☐ > 20 ml. of gastric aspirate	☐ Jaundice
☐ Small mandible with cleft palate	☐ Pallor
☐ Grunting	☐ Plethora
☐ Deep retractions	☐ Fever
☐ Imperforate anus	☐ Hypothermia
☐ Pallor	☐ Arrhythmias
☐ Jaundice	☐ Murmur
☐ Plethora	☐ Lethargy
☐ Convulsions	☐ Tremors (jitters)
☐ Decreased tone	☐ Convulsions
☐ Congenial malformations	
☐ ____	☐ ____
☐ ____	☐ ____
☐ ____	☐ ____

Signature

FIGURE 58-4 Initial Newborn Profile with Newborn Risk Indicators (*Permission to use this copyright material has been granted by the owner, Hollister Incorporated.*)

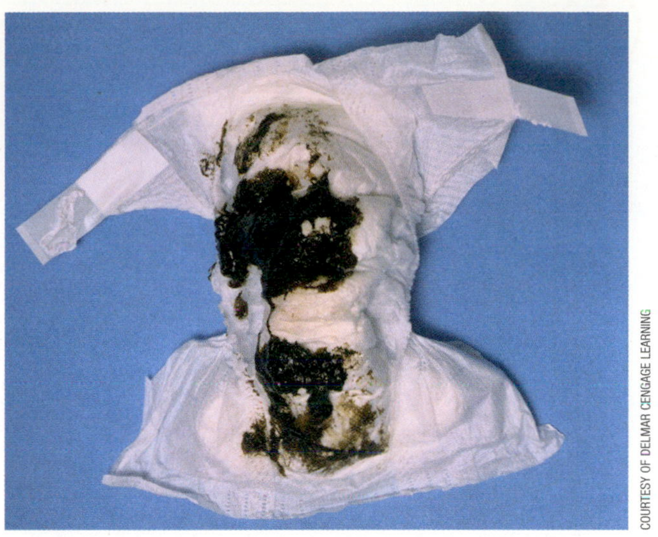

FIGURE 58-5 Meconium Stool

10% of their body weight in the first 3 to 4 days. This is a result of small fluid intake, volume of **meconium** (first bowel movements of newborn, black and tarry) (Figure 58-5), and urination. Birth weight is generally regained by 10 days of age.

Their head-to-heel length is 48 cm to 53 cm (approximately 19 in. to 21 in.), and crown-to-rump length is 31 cm to 35 cm (approximately 12 in. to 14 in.) or approximately equal to the head circumference.

VITAL SIGNS

The axillary temperature should be between 36.5°C and 37.2°C (97.6°F and 98.9°F). A continuous skin probe is best for small newborns or those in a radiant warmer. Normal skin temperature is 36°C to 36.5°C (96.8°F to 97.6°F). Crying may slightly increase temperature.

The apical heart rate is 120 to 160 beats per minute. When the newborn is sleeping, the heart rate decreases, and when crying, the heart rate increases.

Respirations are 30 to 60 breaths per minute. As with the heart rate, sleep decreases respirations and crying increases respirations.

Blood pressure ranges between 60 and 80 mm Hg systolic and 40 and 45 mm Hg diastolic. By 10 days of age, it is 100/50 mm Hg. Activity and crying will increase the newborn's blood pressure.

GENERAL APPEARANCE

Full-term newborns have a flexed posture. The head is flexed, the arms are flexed on the chest, and the legs are flexed on the abdomen.

Skin

At birth, the skin is red, puffy, and smooth. Some **vernix caseosa** (a white, creamy substance) may thinly cover the skin, with large amounts found in body creases. **Lanugo** (fine, downy hair) may still be seen on the forehead and shoulders, or it may all have disappeared. **Acrocyanosis**, blue coloring of the hands and feet, is generally present for several hours until the cardiopulmonary changes have stabilized and fully oxygenated blood has reached the hands and feet. Edema may be present around the eyes, face, dorsa of hands, legs, feet, and labia or scrotum.

Head

The head circumference, measured over the most prominent part of the occiput and just above the eyebrows, is between 33 cm and 35 cm (approximately 13 in. to 14 in.). There are two fontanelles, one anterior and one posterior. The anterior fontanelle is largest, diamond shaped, and closes by 18 months of age. The posterior fontanelle is triangular in shape and closes about 2 months after birth. The fontanelles should be soft and flat.

Eyes

Eye color varies, being either slate gray, blue, or brown. Permanent eye color is usually established by 3 months of age. The eyelids are usually edematous, and there are no tears.

Ears

The ears are soft, pliable, and recoil swiftly when bent and released. Ear placement should be so the top of the ear is in line with the outer canthus of the eye (Figure 58-6).

Neck

The neck is short, thick, and usually has several skin folds.

Chest

Chest circumference is 30.5 cm to 33 cm (approximately 12 in. to 13 in.). It is measured directly over the nipple line and lower edge of the scapulas. The chest circumference is 2 cm to 3 cm smaller than the head circumference. The diameters front to back and side to side are equal (Figure 58-7).

Abdomen

The abdomen is cylindrical in shape. The bluish-white umbilical cord protrudes from the center.

Genitalia

The labia are usually edematous with vernix caseosa between the labia.

If the testes are descended, the scrotum is large, pendulous, and edematous; if the testes are not descended, the scrotum is small. In either case, the scrotum is covered with rugae. The newborn with dark skin has a deeply pigmented scrotum. The newborn should urinate within 24 hours.

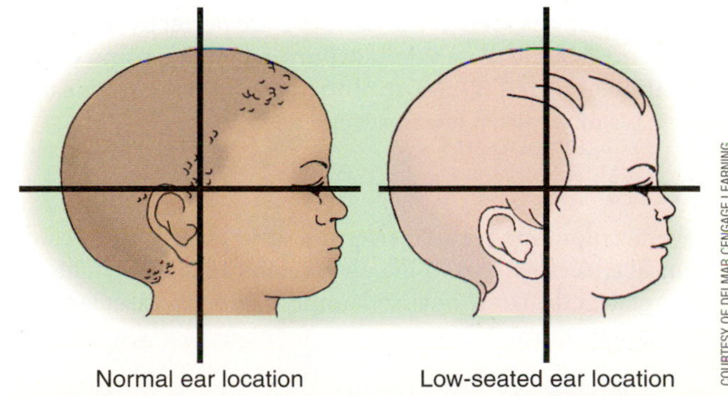

FIGURE 58-6 Ear Placement. Top of ear should be in line with the outer canthus of the eye.

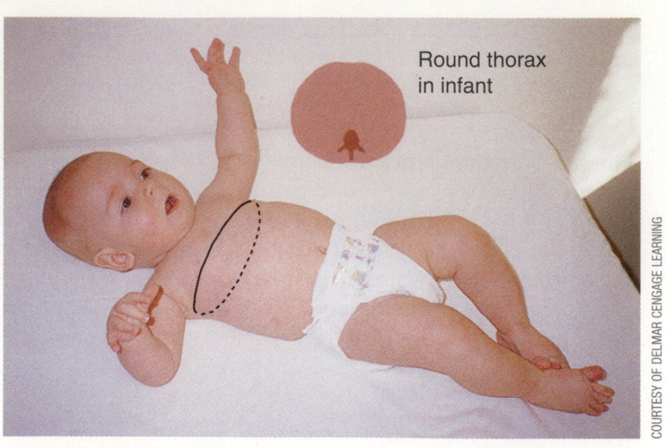

COURTESY OF DELMAR CENGAGE LEARNING

FIGURE 58-7 **Newborn chest is round, having the same diameter front to back and side to side.**

SAFETY

Disposable Paper Tape Measure

When a measurement has been completed, either roll the infant off the paper tape measure or lift the newborn and remove the paper tape measure. Never pull the tape measure out from under the newborn; a paper cut on the newborn's body may result.

Back

The spine is intact with no openings, masses, or prominent curves. Tufts of hair on the spinal area should be reported for evaluation.

Extremities

The extremities are usually flexed, have a full range of motion, and are symmetrical. Ten fingers and ten toes are present, with creases visible on the anterior two-thirds of the sole of the foot.

COMMON VARIATIONS IN THE NEWBORN

Many variations seen in the newborn are perfectly normal and cause no trouble. Any one newborn may have some of these variations but not all. Most of these variations disappear in a few days or weeks, a few in several years.

SKIN

Several colorations or skin eruptions may be present, including jaundice, ecchymoses, milia, erythema toxicum neonatorum, telangiectactic nevi, nevus flammeus, nevus vascularis, and mongolian spots.

Jaundice

Jaundice occurring *after* the first 24 hours of life is related to the normal destruction of the excess red blood cells (RBCs) in the newborn. With direct oxygenation of the blood in the newborn's lungs, the extra RBCs of the fetus are no longer needed. The infant's immature liver is often unable to conjugate all of the bilirubin released by the destroyed RBCs, and this is evident as jaundice. The jaundice usually peaks at 72 hours and then disappears in a couple of weeks. Jaundice appearing *within* the first 24 hours of life is discussed later in this chapter.

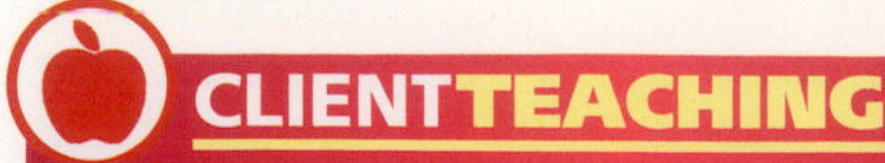

CLIENT TEACHING

Milia

Milia are not whiteheads and should never be squeezed.

Ecchymosis

Areas of ecchymosis (bruising) may be evident after a difficult delivery. Petechiae may also be present.

Milia

Milia are white, pinhead-size, distended sebaceous glands on the cheeks, nose, chin, and occasionally on the trunk. After a few weeks of bathing, they usually disappear.

Erythema Toxicum Neonatorum

Erythema toxicum neonatorum is a pink rash with firm, yellow-white papules or pustules found on the chest, abdomen, back, and buttocks of some newborns. It only appears in the neonatal period and the pathophysiology is unknown. It may appear 24 to 48 hours after birth and dissapears in a few days without any treatment.

Telangiectactic Nevi

Telangiectactic nevi ("stork-bites") are birthmarks of dilated capillaries that blanch with pressure. They may appear on the eyelids, nose, occipital area, or nape of the neck and fade between 1 and 2 years of age.

Nevus Flammeus

Nevus flammeus (port-wine stain) is a large reddish-purple birthmark usually found on the face or neck that does not blanch with pressure. It is not raised above the skin. This does not spontaneously disappear but may be lightened with special laser treatments.

Nevus Vascularis

Nevus vascularis (strawberry mark) is a birthmark of enlarged superficial blood vessels. They are elevated, red, and of variable

PROFESSIONALTIP

Mongolian Spots

Carefully document the presence of mongolian spots on the newborn's record. This may prevent charges of child abuse being filed later against the parents or caregivers.

size and shape. They are most often found on the head, face, neck, and arms. By school age, they have generally disappeared.

Mongolian Spots

Mongolian spots are deep blue areas of coloration, usually in the sacral region, at birth. They are seen mainly in infants of African, Asian, American Indian, Hispanic, and Southern European descent.

HEAD

Three common variations in newborns involve the head: molding, caput succedaneum, and cephalhematoma.

Molding

Molding is the shaping of the fetal head to adapt to the mother's pelvis during labor. In 2 to 3 days the cranial bones typically return to their proper placement (Figure 58-8).

Caput Succedaneum

Caput succedaneum, edema of the newborn's scalp that is present at birth, may cross suture lines and is caused by head compression against the cervix (Figure 58-9A). The edema disappears in 2 to 3 days. No treatment is needed.

Cephalhematoma

Cephalhematoma is a collection of blood between the periosteum and the skull of a newborn. It appears several hours to a day after birth, does not cross suture lines, and is caused by the rupturing of the periosteal bridging veins because of friction and pressure during labor and delivery (Figure 58-9B). It is usually the largest on the second or third day and spontaneously reabsorbs in 3 to 6 weeks. Table 58-1 compares caput succedaneum and cephalhematoma.

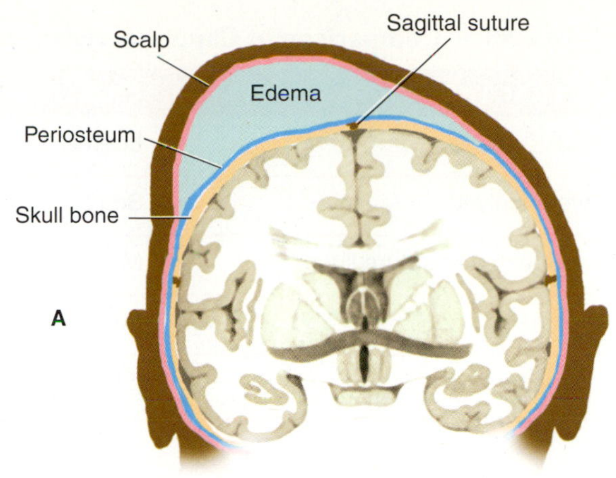

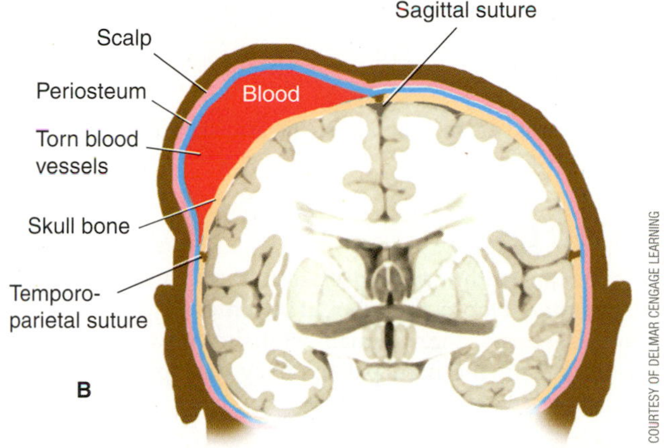

FIGURE 58-9 *A,* Caput Succedaneum; *B,* Cephalhematoma

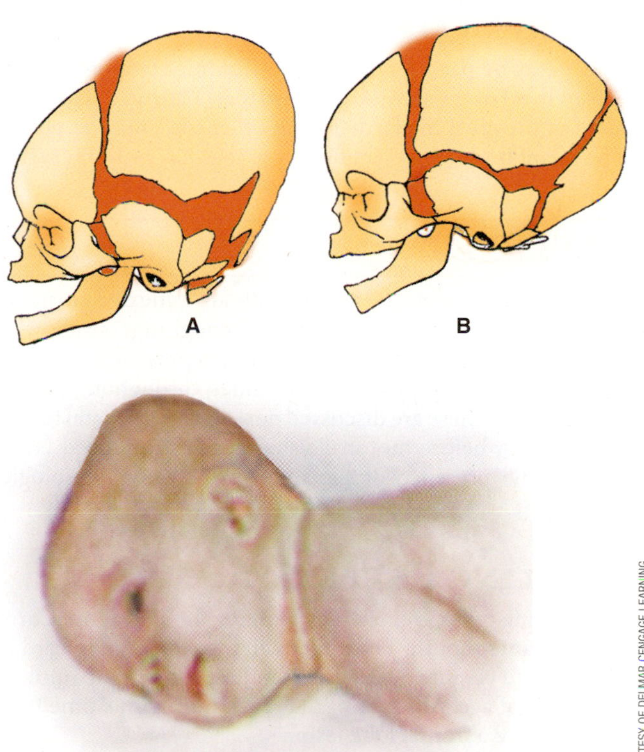

FIGURE 58-8 Molding; *A,* Movement of the Cranial Bones during Labor; *B,* Cranial Bones Return to their Proper Placement in 2 to 3 Days; *C,* Infant Exhibiting Molding

EYES

The newborn's eyes may show signs of strabismus, which is caused by poor neuromuscular control. This usually disappears in 3 to 4 months. Subconjunctival hemorrhages are present in approximately 10% of newborns (Ladewig et al., 2005). Change in vascular tension or ocular pressure during birth

PROFESSIONALTIP

Newborn Skin Variations

Many of the newborn skin variations can be surprising and upsetting to new parents. The nurse should educate the parents and help them understand that several of these skin variations are common and that often they will disappear over time without any interventions.

TABLE 58-1 Comparison of Caput Succedaneum and Cephalhematoma

CHARACTERISTIC	CAPUT SUCCEDANEUM	CEPHALHEMATOMA
Fluid	Edema	Blood
Layer involved	Scalp	Between periosteum and skull
Relationship to suture lines	May cross suture lines	Does not cross suture lines
Appears	Present at birth	First or second day
Disappears	2 to 3 days	3 to 6 weeks

COURTESY OF DELMAR CENGAGE LEARNING

causes these hemorrhages. They last for a few weeks and do not impair vision.

Ears

The ears may be of irregular shape and size. The pinna may be flat against the head.

Mouth

Precocious teeth may be present at birth in the center of the lower gum. If loose, they should be removed to prevent aspiration. **Epstein's pearls**, small, whitish-yellow epithelial cysts, are found on the hard palate. They disappear within a few weeks.

Chest

Many newborns, both male and female, have engorged breasts as a result of maternal hormones. This occurs by the third day and may last 2 weeks. The nipples may secrete a whitish fluid, often called "**witch's milk**." Witch's milk is a term for any milk that comes from the breast of someone who is not lactating. This phenomena is only seen in full term infants.

Genitalia

There are several variations in the female and male genitalia.

MEMORY TRICK

Caput Succedaneum

R U
O T
S U
S R
E E
S S

If you can remember that this collection of fluids crosses the suture lines you will automatically know that the Cephalhematoma does not.

Female

Pseudomenstruation, a blood-tinged mucous discharge from the vagina, may be evident in the first week after birth. It is caused by the withdrawal of maternal hormones. A vaginal tag or hymenal tag may be present but will disappear in a few weeks.

Male

Hypospadias, placement of the urinary meatus on the underside of the penis, may be present. **Phimosis**, when the opening in the foreskin is so small that it cannot be pulled back over the glans, may interfere with urination. **Cryptorchidism**, failure of one or both testes to descend, may be evident. **Hydrocele**, fluid around the testes in the scrotum, usually disappears without any treatment. **Epispadias** is the placement of the urinary meatus on the top of the penis.

Extremities

There may be partial **syndactyly** (fusion of two or more fingers or toes) of the second and third toes. **Hallux varus**, placement of the great toe farther from other toes, may be present. The infant born with extra fingers or toes has **polydactyly**.

REFLEXES

Many of the newborn's movements are reflexive in nature. Some reflexes, such as sneezing, coughing, swallowing, blinking, yawning, and hiccupping, are present throughout life. Others disappear at various times throughout the first 2 years of life; these are discussed next. These neonatal reflexes must be lost before motor development can proceed (Estes, 2010). The presence of the reflexes indicates neurological integrity.

Rooting Reflex

The rooting reflex is elicited by stroking the skin at one corner of the infant's mouth. The infant will turn the head toward the side stroked (Figure 58-10). This reflex is present up until 3 or 4 months of age. Absence of the reflex during this time frame may indicate a frontal lobe lesion.

Sucking Reflex

Touching the newborn's lips elicits the sucking reflex (Figure 58-11). This reflex occurs until approximately 10 months of

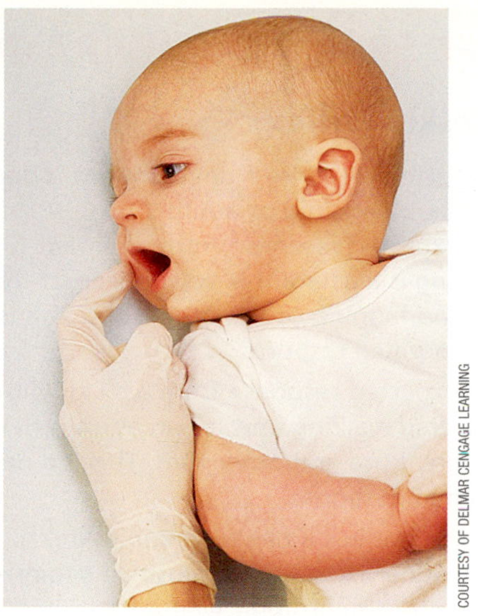

FIGURE 58-10 Rooting Reflex

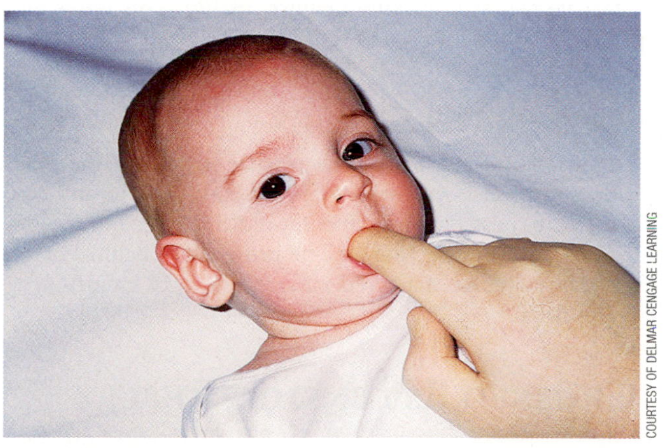

FIGURE 58-11 Sucking Reflex

age. Preterm infants or an infant who is breastfed by a mother taking barbiturates will not exhibit the sucking reflex because of central nervous system depression.

EXTRUSION REFLEX

When the tip of the tongue is touched or depressed, the infant will force the tongue outward. This reflex disappears at approximately 4 months of age. Feeding an infant food with a spoon before 4 months of age is difficult because of the extrusion reflex.

PALMAR GRASP REFLEX

When a finger is placed across the palm, the infant's fingers flex and grasp the examiner's finger (Figure 58-12). If the palmar grasp reflex is present after 4 months of age, frontal lobe lesions are suspected.

PLANTAR GRASP REFLEX

When the infant's leg is held in one hand, and the plantar surface of the foot is touched below the toes with the other hand, the infant's toes will curl downward (Figure 58-13).

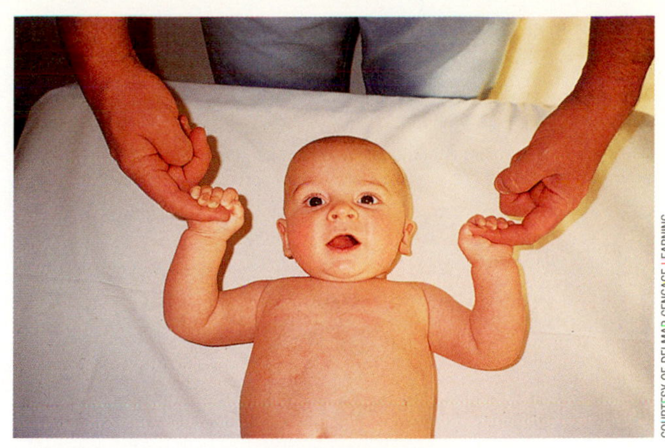

FIGURE 58-12 Palmar Grasp Reflex

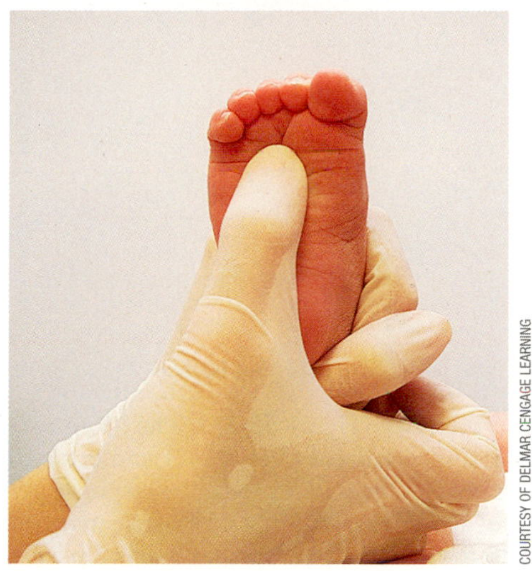

FIGURE 58-13 Plantar Grasp Reflex

This reflex lasts until 8 months of age. If the plantar grasp reflex is absent on one foot, an obstructive lesion is suspected. Absence of the reflex in both feet is seen with neurological alterations such as cerebral palsy.

TONIC NECK REFLEX

The tonic neck reflex is sometimes referred to as the "fencing" reflex because of the position assumed by the infant. This reflex is elicited by placing the infant supine and rotating the head to one side. The arm and leg on the side to which the jaw is turned will extend and the opposite arm and leg will flex (Figure 58-14). Sometimes, this reflex may not be displayed until 6 to 8 weeks of age. If it is still seen after 6 months of age, cerebral damage is suspected.

MORO REFLEX

The Moro reflex is sometimes called the startle reflex. It is elicited either by holding the newborn in a semisitting position and then allowing the head to fall backward to an angle of 30°, or having the infant lying on a flat surface and then hitting the surface to startle the infant. The response by the infant less than 4 months of age is to quickly extend and abduct the arms with the fingers fanning out. The thumb and forefinger form a "C" followed by adduction of the arms in an embracing motion. A slight tremor may be noted. The legs may also

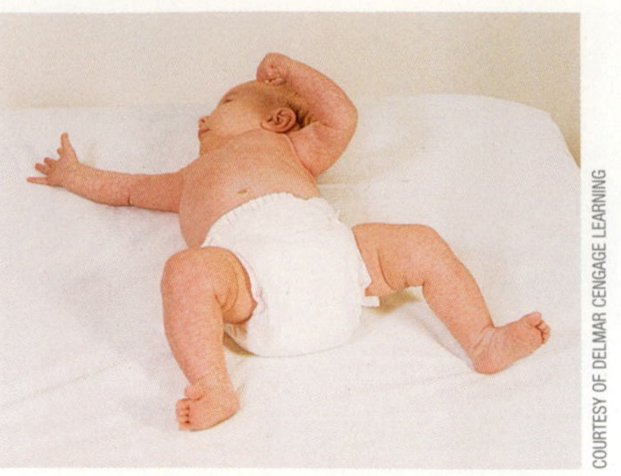

FIGURE 58-14 Tonic Neck Reflex

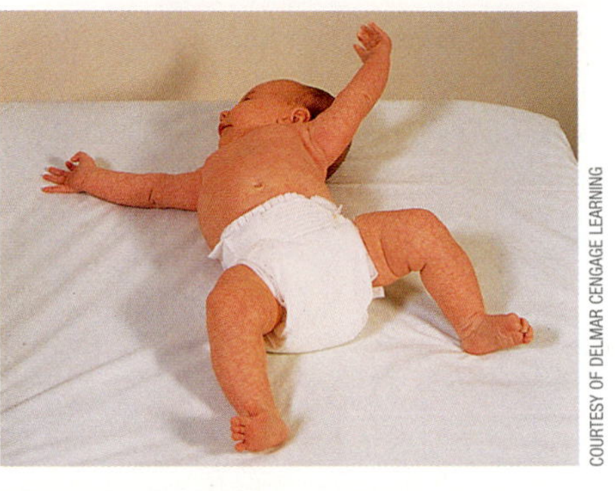

FIGURE 58-15 Moro (Startle) Reflex

extend and then flex (Figure 58-15). The Moro reflex is present at birth and disappears between 4 and 6 months of age. Possible brain damage is indicated if the response persists after 6 months of age. An asymmetrical response may be caused by an injury to the clavicle, humerus, or brachial plexus.

Gallant Reflex

The Gallant reflex is elicited with the infant lying prone with the hands under the abdomen. The infant's skin is stroked along one side of the spine; the infant's shoulders and pelvis turn toward the stimulated side (Figure 58-16). A spinal cord lesion is suspected if there is no response from an infant younger than 2 months of age. This reflex is present from birth to age 2 months.

Stepping Reflex

To elicit the stepping reflex, the newborn is held under the arms with the feet placed on a firm surface. The infant will lift alternate feet as if walking (Figure 58-17). This reflex disappears at about 3 months of age.

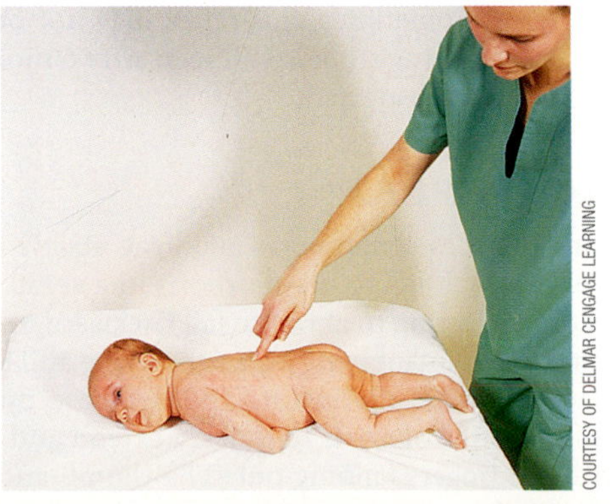

FIGURE 58-16 Gallant Reflex

LIFE SPAN CONSIDERATIONS

Babinski's Reflex

The expected response from an infant is opposite that of an older child or adult.

- The expected response from an infant (until walking is mastered) is dorsiflexion of the great toe and fanning of the other toes. This is a positive (normal) response.
- The expected response from a child who has mastered walking and for an adult is flexion of the great toe and other toes. This is a negative (normal) response.
- If an infant has a negative Babinski response or an older person has a positive Babinski response, a neurologic evaluation is required.

Babinski's Reflex

To elicit Babinski's reflex, the plantar surface of the infant's foot is stroked from the lateral heel area upward and across under the toes. The great toe should dorsiflex and the other toes fan out (Figure 58-18). The presence of Babinski's reflex after the infant has mastered walking (12 to 18 months of age) is abnormal.

Crossed Extension Reflex

The crossed extension reflex is elicited with the infant supine by holding one leg extended with the knee pressed down and stimulating the bottom of that foot. The other leg should flex, adduct, and then extend as if trying to push away the stimulus. This reflex should be present during the first 4 weeks of life.

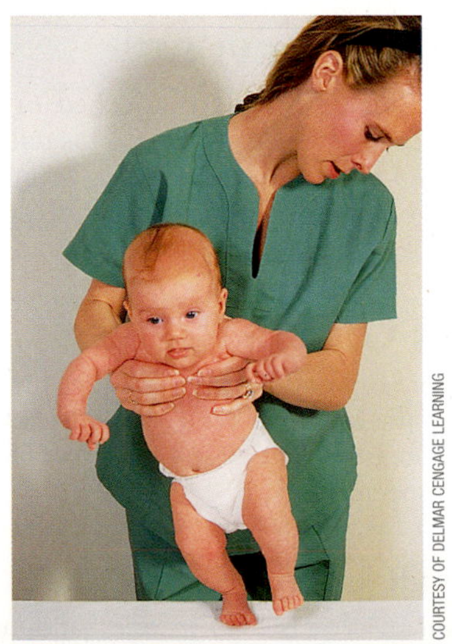

FIGURE 58-17 Stepping Reflex

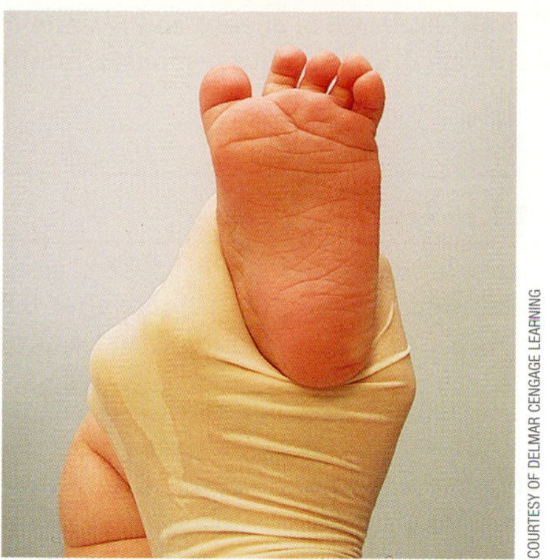

FIGURE 58-18 Babinski's Reflex

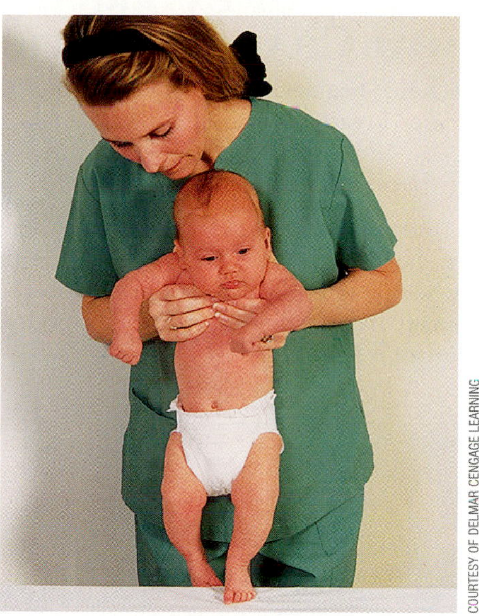

FIGURE 58-19 Placing Reflex

Placing Reflex

To elicit the placing reflex, the infant is held under the arms from behind then brought to a standing position, touching the dorsum of one foot on the edge of the table. The tested leg will flex and lift onto the table (Figure 58-19). It is abnormal for there to be no response. An infant born in a breech presentation or one with paralysis or cerebral cortex difficulties may not respond to this stimulus.

BEHAVIORAL CHARACTERISTICS

During the first 6 to 10 hours after birth, the infant has a fairly predictable pattern of behavior called the periods of reactivity. Following that, the infant will exhibit various behavioral states, divided into sleeping and waking phases.

Periods of Reactivity

Two periods of reactivity occur during the first few hours of life, separated by a period of sleep.

> **PROFESSIONALTIP**
>
> **Stepping Reflex and Placing Reflex**
>
> While fairly similar, the stepping and placing reflexes are two different reflexes and should not be tested at the same time.

First Period of Reactivity

During the first period of reactivity, the first 30 minutes after birth, the newborn is awake, alert, and active. It is a prime time for parent/infant interaction. The newborn may act hungry, with a strong sucking reflex evident. If the mother plans to breastfeed, this is the ideal time for her to begin. During this period, the newborn's heart rate and respirations are rapid, and bowel sounds are seldom heard.

Sleep Period

The newborn enters a sleep period that usually lasts from 2 to 4 hours. This is a time of deep sleep, from which it is difficult to awaken the newborn. The heart and respiratory rates return to baseline and bowel sounds become audible.

Second Period of Reactivity

The second period of reactivity lasts from 4 to 6 hours. The newborn is once again awake and alert. Physiologic responses vary. The heart and respiratory rates increase, yet there may be periods of apnea, which may cause the heart rate to decrease. During these fluctuations, the newborn may become mottled or slightly cyanotic.

The newborn may gag, spit up, or choke as gastric and respiratory mucus increases. Close observation is a must during this period of activity so that appropriate interventions may be taken to maintain a clear airway for the infant.

The first meconium stool is often passed as the gastrointestinal tract becomes more active. The first voiding may now occur. The newborn may begin rooting, sucking, and swallowing, indicating a readiness for feeding.

Behavioral States

Brazelton (1995) identified that newborns have different states of being. He categorized them as sleep states and alert states.

Sleep States

Two sleep states have been identified for the newborn: quiet sleep and active sleep. At term, a newborn changes from one sleep state to the other approximately every 45 to 50 minutes during sleep. Of the total amount of sleep, 45% to 50% is active sleep, 35% to 45% is quiet sleep, and 10% is shifting between the two sleep states (Ladewig et al., 2005).

Quiet Sleep State In quiet sleep, the eyes are closed and there are no eye movements. Respirations are regular, quiet, and slower than in any other state. The heart rate is 100 to 120 beats per minute. There are startles or jerky movements at regular intervals. Stimuli in the environment are not likely to cause a change in the newborn's state.

Active Sleep State During active sleep, respirations are rapid and irregular and sucking movements may be observed.

The infant stretches, moves extremities, makes faces, and may fuss briefly. Rapid eye movements (REM) occur. Environmental stimuli may startle the infant, who may then go back to sleep or awaken.

Alert States

There are four alert states: drowsy, quiet alert, active alert, and crying.

Drowsy State The transition between sleep and awake is called the drowsy state. The eyes open and then slowly close, as if unable to stay open. When open, the eyes appear glazed and unfocused. From this state, the infant may go back to sleep or awaken.

Quiet Alert State In the quiet alert state, the infant focuses on people or objects, responds with intense gazing, and seems very interested in the immediate environment. Body movements are minimal. When the infant is in the quiet alert state, it is a good time to enhance bonding. Parents should be made aware of this so they can take advantage of this opportunity.

Active Alert State The infant is often fussy and restless in the active alert state, with more rapid and irregular respirations. The awareness of discomfort from hunger or cold is more intense. Motor activity is quite frequent. The infant is less focused on visual stimuli than in the quiet alert state.

Crying State Crying is generally accompanied by jerky motor activity. Crying serves as a distraction from disturbing stimuli, allows a discharge of energy, and is a method of communication to elicit appropriate responses from parents or caregivers.

GESTATIONAL AGE

According to Alexander and Allen (1996), gestational age must be determined in the first 4 hours after birth so that age-related problems can be identified and appropriate care initiated.

The New Ballard Score is the most commonly used tool (Figure 58-20). It has two elements: external physical characteristics and neuromuscular maturity. If the findings of neuromuscular maturity are not in line with the findings of the external physical characteristics, a second assessment should be performed within 24 hours.

Assessment of External Physical Characteristics

The nurse should begin with resting posture, then skin, lanugo, plantar creases, breast, eye/ear, and then genitals.

Resting Posture

Although resting posture is a characteristic of neuromuscular maturity, it should be assessed first. The posture the newborn assumes when lying undisturbed is to be assessed. The very preterm infant has no flexion of the extremities, while the full-term infant is fully flexed.

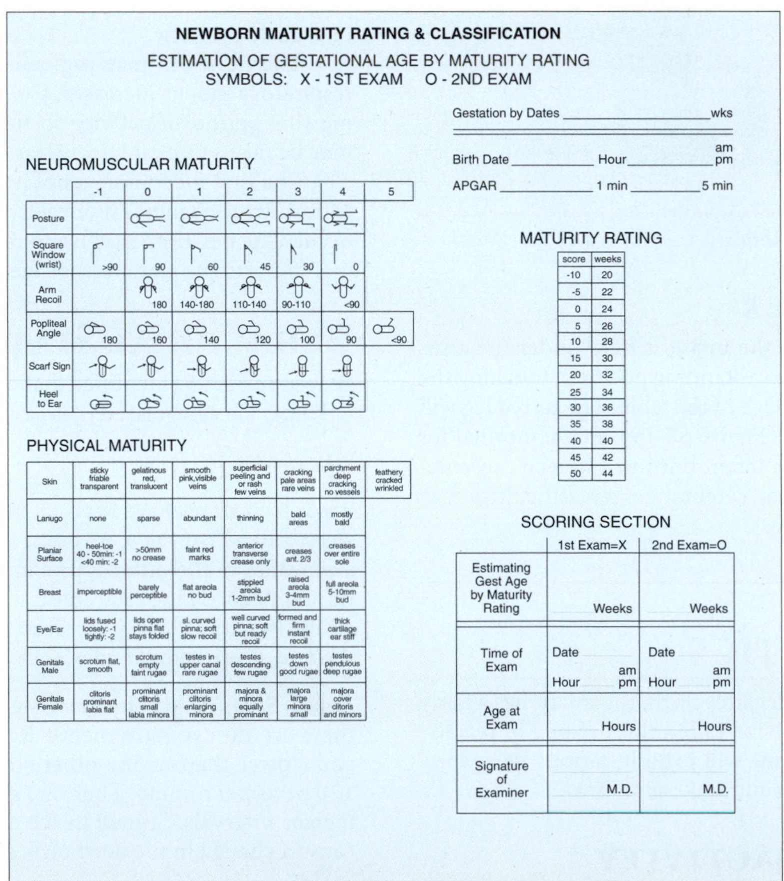

NEWBORN MATURITY RATING & CLASSIFICATION

ESTIMATION OF GESTATIONAL AGE BY MATURITY RATING

SYMBOLS: X - 1ST EXAM O - 2ND EXAM

NEUROMUSCULAR MATURITY

	-1	0	1	2	3	4	5
Posture							
Square Window (wrist)	>90	90	60	45	30	0	
Arm Recoil		180	140-180	110-140	90-110	<90	
Popliteal Angle	180	160	140	120	100	90	<90
Scarf Sign							
Heel to Ear							

PHYSICAL MATURITY

Skin	sticky friable transparent	gelatinous red, translucent	smooth pink, visible veins	superficial peeling and or rash few veins	cracking pale areas rare veins	parchment deep cracking no vessels	feathery cracked wrinkled
Lanugo	none	sparse	abundant	thinning	bald areas	mostly bald	
Planiar Surface	heel-toe 40 - 50min: -1 <40 min: -2	>50mm no crease	faint red marks	anterior transverse crease only	creases ant. 2/3	creases over entire sole	
Breast	imperceptible	barely perceptible	flat areola no bud	stippled areola 1-2mm bud	raised areola 3-4mm bud	full areola 5-10mm bud	
Eye/Ear	lids fused loosely: -1 tightly: -2	lids open pinna flat stays folded	sl. curved pinna; soft slow recoil	well curved pinna; soft but ready recoil	formed and firm instant recoil	thick cartilage ear stiff	
Genitals Male	scrotum flat, smooth	scrotum empty faint rugae	testes in upper canal rare rugae	testes descending few rugae	testes down good rugae	testes pendulous deep rugae	
Genitals Female	clitoris prominant labia flat	prominant clitoris small labia minora	prominant clitoris enlarging minora	majora & minora equally prominant	majora large minora small	majora cover clitoris and minors	

Gestation by Dates ______ wks

Birth Date ______ Hour ______ am pm

APGAR ______ 1 min ______ 5 min

MATURITY RATING

score	weeks
-10	20
-5	22
0	24
5	26
10	28
15	30
20	32
25	34
30	36
35	38
40	40
45	42
50	44

SCORING SECTION

	1st Exam=X	2nd Exam=O
Estimating Gest Age by Maturity Rating	Weeks	Weeks
Time of Exam	Date Hour am pm	Date Hour am pm
Age at Exam	Hours	Hours
Signature of Examiner	M.D.	M.D.

FIGURE 58-20 New Ballard Score (*Courtesy of Mead Johnson Nutritionals.*)

Skin

The skin of a preterm infant is very transparent and thin. As gestation progresses, the veins disappear from view as subcutaneous fat is deposited. Vernix caseosa disappears near term but may remain in the creases. There may be some cracking and peeling of the skin, especially around the ankles and feet. As the skin loses moisture after birth, peeling is more apparent.

Lanugo

Lanugo is most abundant between 28 and 30 weeks' gestation. It disappears as the gestational age increases, first disappearing from the face, then the extremities and trunk. A small amount may remain on the shoulders, ears, and sides of the forehead at full term.

Plantar Creases

During the first 12 hours of life, the plantar creases are reliable signs of gestational age. Sole creases develop from the top (under toes) beginning about 32 weeks of gestation. The creases cover two-thirds of the sole by 37 weeks and cover the sole at 40 weeks' gestation.

Breast

The size of the breast bud tissue is measured by placing the forefinger and middle finger on each side of the breast tissue and measuring between the fingers. At term, the breast bud tissue should be 1 cm. This procedure should be performed gently to prevent tissue damage.

Eye/Ear

The eyelids are fused until 26 to 28 weeks of gestation. The upper pinna begins to curve over at about 33 to 34 weeks of gestation. The curving over continues until it is complete at 39 to 40 weeks of gestation.

The infant at less than 32 weeks of gestation has almost no ear cartilage. When folded, the ear remains folded. By 36 weeks, there is enough cartilage for the ear to slowly return to its original state when folded. The ear of a full-term infant springs back quickly when folded.

Male Genitals

The male genitals are evaluated for descent of the testes, presence of rugae on the scrotum, and scrotal size. The testes are formed in the abdomen, move into the inguinal canal at 30 weeks of gestation, then into the upper scrotum by 37 weeks of gestation, and are fully descended by full term. Before 36 weeks, there are few rugae on the scrotum. By 38 weeks, rugae have formed on the anterior part of the scrotum and cover the scrotum by 40 weeks of gestation. The scrotum is large and pendulous by 40 weeks.

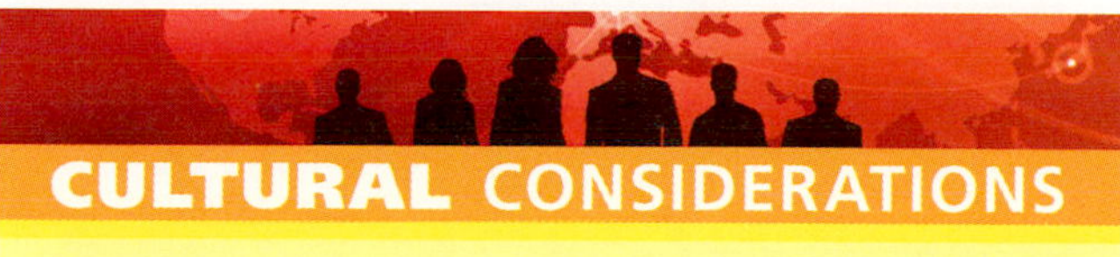

CULTURAL CONSIDERATIONS

Lanugo

There may be more lanugo on infants with dark skin coloring than on fair-skinned infants with light-colored hair.

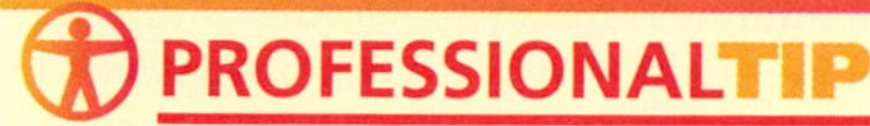

PROFESSIONALTIP

Ears

When caring for an infant of 32 weeks' gestation or less, be sure the infant's ears are flat to the head and not bent over. Lying on a bent ear can impair circulation to the ear.

Female Genitals

Deposits of subcutaneous fat related to nutritional status as well as gestational age determine the appearance of the female genitals. The clitoris and labia minora seem large in comparison to the labia majora, which are small and widely separated at 30 to 32 weeks of gestation. By 36 to 38 weeks of gestation, the clitoris is mostly covered by the labia majora. By 40 weeks of gestation, the labia majora covers the labia minora and clitoris.

Neuromuscular Maturity

The five remaining neuromuscular characteristics to be evaluated are square window, arm recoil, popliteal angle, scarf sign, and heel to ear.

Square Window

The square window sign is elicited by bending the wrist so the palm is as flat against the arm as possible. If the angle between the palm and arm is 90 degrees and looks like a square window, the gestational age is 32 weeks or less and receives a score of 0. If the angle is greater than 90 degrees, the score is −1. The angle becomes smaller the more mature the infant is, until the palm can fold flat against the arm in a full-term newborn.

Arm Recoil

The infant's arms are held with the elbows fully flexed for 5 seconds. Then the arms are pulled straight down at the infant's sides and quickly released. The elbows of a full-term newborn, when released, rapidly recoil and have an angle less than 90 degrees. That infant is given a score of 4. Very preterm infants may not move their arms (no recoil) and receive a score of 0.

Popliteal Angle

The popliteal angle is measured when the thigh is flexed on the abdomen, the hips remain flat on the table, and the lower leg is straightened just until met by resistance. Then the angle behind the knee is scored. When the leg can be fully extended, a score of −1 is given, but if the popliteal angle is less than 90 degrees, a score of 5 is given.

Scarf Sign

The newborn's arm is drawn across the body toward the opposite shoulder until resistance is felt. The shoulder of the arm being tested should remain on the table. The relation of the elbow to the infant's midline is noted for scoring. If the elbow does not reach near the midline, it is a score of 4. When the elbow goes across and beyond the infant's body, a score of −1 is given.

Heel to Ear

With the hips remaining on the surface of the table, the newborn's foot is moved toward the ear on the same side. When resistance is felt, foot position relative to the ear and the degree of knee extension is noted. The preterm infant's leg will remain straight and the foot will be near the ear. The more mature the infant, the more resistance will be felt and more flexion will be noted.

Gestational Age Relationship to Intrauterine Growth

There is a normal range of birth weight for each week of gestation as well as for length, head circumference, and intrauterine weight–length ratio (Figure 58-21). Birth weight is classified as follows:

- **Large for gestational age (LGA)**: Infant's weight falls above the 90th percentile for gestational age.
- **Appropriate for gestational age (AGA)**: Infant's weight falls between the 90th and 10th percentile for gestational age.
- **Small for gestational age (SGA)**: Infant's weight falls below the 10th percentile for gestational age.

The correlation of the infant's measurements for length and head circumference also documents the infant's level of maturity and appropriate classification of LGA, AGA, or SGA.

All of these determinations assist caregivers to expect possible physiologic complications, and together with the results of a physical assessment are the basis for preparing an appropriate care plan for the infant.

SLEEPING POSITION

In 1992, the American Academy of Pediatrics (AAP) recommended that babies be put to sleep on their back to prevent sudden infant death syndrome (SIDS). Since the AAP started their program "back to sleep" and suggested that parents allow infants to use a pacifier when sleeping, the incidence of SIDS has greatly decreased. Another easily prevented and treated condition, positional plagiocephaly, has increased. The recommendation for back sleeping still stands. Both conditions

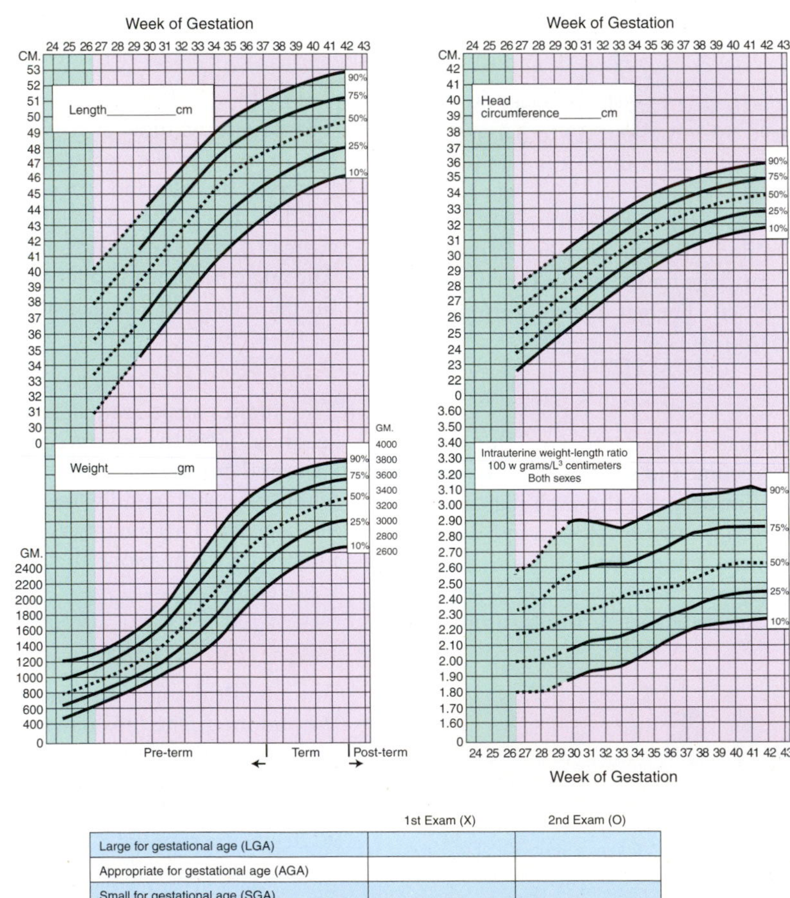

	1st Exam (X)	2nd Exam (O)
Large for gestational age (LGA)		
Appropriate for gestational age (AGA)		
Small for gestational age (SGA)		
Age at Exam	hrs	hrs
Signature of Examiner	M.D.	M.D.

Figure 58-21 Intrauterine Growth Grids (*Courtesy of Mead Johnson Nutritionals.*)

are discussed in the chapter on Infant with Special Needs: Birth to 12 Months.

FIRST BATH AND CORD CARE

The infant's first bath, and the type of bath for the next 10 days to 2 weeks, is a sponge bath. Newborns are not generally given a tub bath until after the cord has fallen off and healing is complete. Placing the infant under a radiant warmer during the bath helps prevent heat loss. Follow agency protocol for the order of the bath.

Nurses giving the first bath to newborns must wear gloves to comply with Standard Precautions regarding contact with blood or body fluids. A study by Varda and Behnke (2000) found that bathing could be done safely as soon as 1 hour after birth if the newborn's condition is stable and appropriate care is provided. Bathing newborns at 1 hour could decrease exposure of the family and health care providers to blood-borne pathogens (Varda & Behnke, 2000).

Wipe each eye with either a separate cotton ball or a separate place on a washcloth. The eyes are wiped from the inner to outer canthus. The entire face is washed. All of the creases of the ears are cleaned with a corner of a washcloth; a cotton-tipped applicator should never be used in the ears.

Using gauze squares and the approved soap, firmly wash the head to remove all blood and body fluids. Infants with a large amount of hair may require the use of a comb to remove all traces of substances in the hair. A second washing and rinsing of the head may be necessary. The head must be well dried when finished.

Soap or a cleansing agent is used on the rest of the body according to agency protocol. Creases must have special attention to be sure that all traces of blood and the majority of vernix caseosa are removed. The skin should be well rinsed to reduce the drying or potential irritating effect of the soap or cleansing agent (Lund et al., 1999). When completely washed and rinsed, the infant is dried and wrapped in a dry, warm blanket.

The infant may remain in the radiant warmer on dry linens or may be dressed, wrapped in a blanket with a hat on the head, and placed in a regular crib and covered with another blanket. Within 30 minutes to 1 hour, the infant's temperature should be checked. Some infants maintain body temperature better than others. It is important to check the infant's temperature often and according to agency protocol so that when the infant is at an appropriate temperature he can leave the radiant warmer and be taken to his mother to feed.

CULTURAL CONSIDERATIONS

Umbilical Cord

In Malawi, Africa, infants are kept indoors and are not named until the umbilical cord falls off, typically within the first 2 weeks (Gennaro, Kamwendo, Mbweza, & Kershbaumer, 1998).

CULTURAL CONSIDERATIONS

Infant Care

Nurses must be aware of different cultural practices in order to provide sensitive care. A few examples include:

- Korean tradition is to consider a newborn 1 year old at the time of birth.
- Korean parents will often tightly wrap a newborn in a blanket to prevent possible harm from the wind (Howard & Berbiglia, 1997).
- Japanese parents often choose to immerse the infant for a bath before the cord is healed (Sharts-Hopko, 1995).
- Muslim fathers traditionally call praise to Allah in the newborn's right ear before cleansing the infant.
- Most infants of Muslim parents are not named until they are 7 days old (Hutchinson & Baqi-Aziz, 1994).
- Babies of Southeast Asian parents are kept swaddled for the first few days (Mattson, 1995).
- Jewish male infants are not to be named until the eigth day of life when they have their circumcision.

The cord should be cleaned, at least daily, with alcohol. The diaper should be folded under to allow the cord to dry and prevent urine from getting on the cord.

CIRCUMCISION

Circumcision is the surgical removal of the prepuce (foreskin), which covers the glans penis. In 1999, the American Academy of Pediatrics made a policy statement on circumcision that "data are not sufficient to recommend routine neonatal circumcision. . . . If a decision for circumcision is made, procedural analgesia should be provided" (AAP, 1999). Circumcision is considered an elective procedure for which parents must give written consent. Only full-term, healthy newborns should be circumcised.

PROCEDURE

The infant is placed on a circumcision board just before the procedure begins (Figure 58-22). Because infants prefer a flexed position, being placed on a circumcision board is frustrating to the newborn. Crying often begins at this point, before the procedure is started.

The best pain relief is provided by a penile nerve root block (Lenhart, Lenhart, Reid, & Chong, 1997; Pasero, 2001). A pacifier with 20% sucrose provides comfort and has been shown to be analgesic (Pasero, 2001). The physician

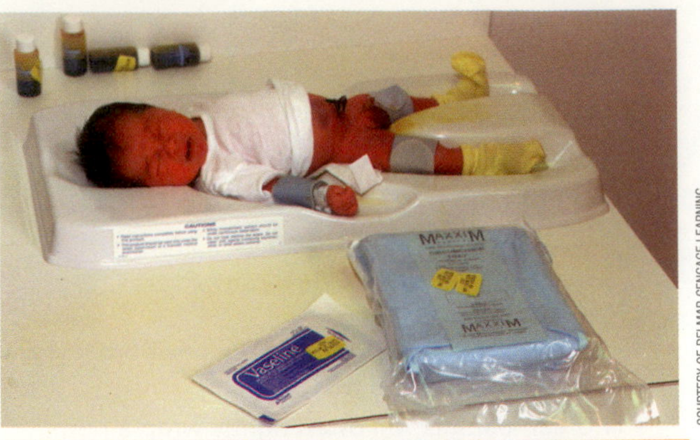

COURTESY OF DELMAR CENGAGE LEARNING

FIGURE 58-22 **Circumcision Board. The infant is restrained just before the procedure begins.**

then makes a slit in the prepuce and then uses either a Gomco (Yellen) clamp (Figure 58-23) or Plastibell (Figure 58-24) to control bleeding when the prepuce is cut off. After a circumcision with the Gomco clamp, A+D ointment or petroleum jelly is put on the penis to prevent the diaper from sticking to the site. At each diaper change, new ointment is applied for at least 24 to 48 hours.

NURSING MANAGEMENT

The nurse ensures that the circumcision permit has been signed by a parent. Equipment and supplies are set up, and the infant is placed on the circumcision board with diaper removed. Most infants are not fed for 2 to 4 hours before the procedure to prevent regurgitation. The nurse administers

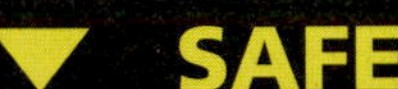

SAFETY

Gomco (Yellen) Clamp

Inspect the clamp before use for inadequate closure or corrosion. Check the marks on component parts to make sure they match.

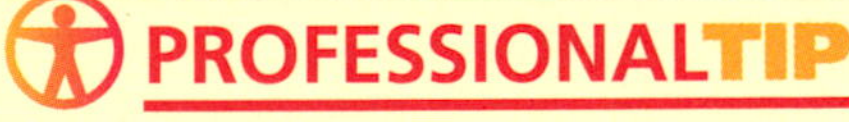

PROFESSIONALTIP

Reasons for and against Circumcision

For:

- Religious rite.
- Prevent need for procedure later in life.
- May reduce urinary tract infections, penile cancer, and sexually transmitted diseases.

Against:

- Procedure is painful.
- Possibility of hemorrhage, infection, or adhesions.

(Kaufman, Clark & Castro, 2001)

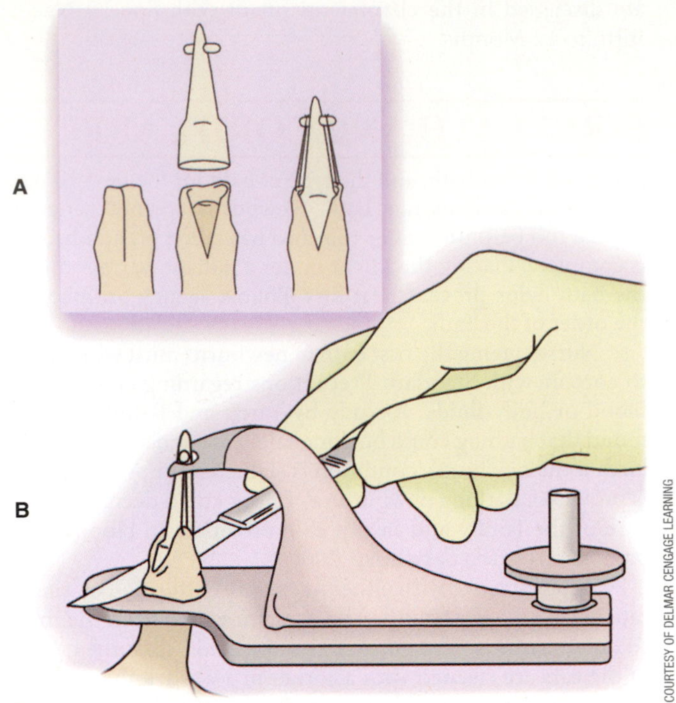

COURTESY OF DELMAR CENGAGE LEARNING

FIGURE 58-23 **Gomgo (Yellen) Clamp Used for Circumcision; *A,* After slit is made in prepuce, the cone is placed over the glans and the prepuce is pulled up around the cone; *B,* The cone is placed in the clamp, which is tightened to obliterate the blood vessels. This prevents bleeding. The prepuce is cut away and the clamp is removed in 3 to 5 minutes.**

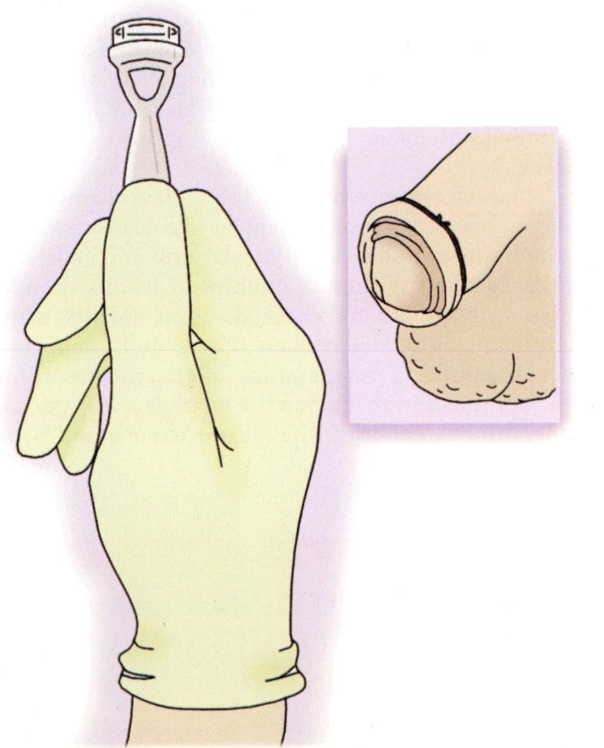

COURTESY OF DELMAR CENGAGE LEARNING

FIGURE 58-24 **Plastibell Used for Circumcision. The plastibell is placed over the glans after a slit is made in the prepuce. A suture is tied around the ring. This prevents bleeding when the prepuce is cut away. The handle is removed, leaving the ring to fall off in 5 to 8 days, after healing.**

SAFETY

Circumcision Procedure

Many infants often spit up or vomit during the procedure when they get upset. Keep a bulb syringe nearby in case the infant requires suctioning.

ordered pain medication for the infant 20 to 30 minutes before the procedure.

During the procedure, comfort the infant by talking to the infant, playing a tape of soft music or intrauterine sounds, or lightly stroking the infant. The infant should be kept warm during the circumcision procedure with a well-placed heat lamp. After the procedure, hold the infant to provide comfort. Care following a circumcision includes checking hourly for 12 hours to see if any bleeding is occurring and that the infant is voiding.

If the infant goes home within the first 12 hours after circumcision, bleeding must be minimal and the infant must have voided. Ensure that the parents know how to care for the circumcision and that they have the physician's telephone number.

NUTRITION

Feeding the newborn is an important aspect of parenting. Nurses assisting in the choice of a feeding method must have knowledge of the newborn's nutritional needs. The American Academy of Pediatrics recommends breast milk for at least 12 months (AAP, 1997).

COMMUNITY/HOME HEALTH CARE

Circumcision

- Wash hands before touching penis.
- Continue checking circumcision hourly until 12 hours after procedure.
- If bleeding, apply gentle pressure with sterile 4 × 4 gauze. If bleeding does not stop, call physician.
- Check that infant has a wet diaper 6 to 10 times in 24 hours.
- Change diaper frequently. Use warm water to gently clean penis and reapply A + D ointment or petroleum jelly after each change, except when Plastibell is used.
- Check for redness, swelling, or discharge, which are signs of infection.
- Provide comfort by holding and talking soothingly to infant.

CULTURAL CONSIDERATIONS

Circumcision

- Jewish parents have a special religious ceremony on the eighth day after birth when the infant is circumcised and named.
- Muslim parents practice circumcision as a religious rite.
- In the United States, circumcision is generally culturally accepted.
- In European countries, circumcision is performed infrequently.

CRITICAL THINKING

Routine Circumcision

Your personal belief is that newborn circumcision should not be performed routinely. You are assigned to assist with a routine circumcision. How will you handle this situation?

Nutritional Needs of Newborn

The full-term newborn needs a sufficient intake of calories to meet energy and growth requirements. There should be adequate carbohydrates and fats for energy so that proteins can be used for growth. A newborn requires 110 to 120 kcal/kg (50 to 55 kcal/lb) each day to meet these needs.

This equates to approximately 20 oz of breast milk or formula each day. Newborns lose weight the first few days of life partly because their intake of calories is less than their requirement. One reason is that the newborn's stomach capacity is only 20 mL (30 mL = 1 oz). This capacity increases rapidly, so that by 7 days of age the infant may consume 2 to 3 oz at each feeding. The infant regains birth weight by age 10 days.

Breast Milk and Infant Formula Composition

The compositions of breast milk and infant formula are different.

Breast Milk

Breast milk is biologically designed to meet the needs of human infants. Its composition changes to meet the changing nutritional and immunologic needs of the infant. Breast milk is easily digested.

The colostrum (first few days) is rich in immunoglobulins to protect the newborn's gastrointestinal tract from infection. Colostrum helps establish normal intestinal flora and has a laxative effect that assists in the passage of meconium.

In 2 weeks, mature milk is being produced. It contains sufficient nutrients to meet the infant's needs and has 20 kcal/oz. Breast stimulation and removal of milk from the breast stimulates the secretion of prolactin by the anterior pituitary of the mother. Prolactin increases milk production. As the demand becomes greater (infant feeding longer and more frequently), the milk supply increases.

The mother's diet makes little difference in the proportions of carbohydrates, protein, and most minerals in her breast milk, but fat content and the amount of vitamins are affected. The breastfeeding mother must eat a well-balanced diet to provide the most nutritious milk for her infant and to maintain her own health and energy level. An extra 500 calories per day is needed to support breastfeeding.

Infant Formula

Many infant formulas are modified to match the components in breast milk as nearly as possible. Most formulas are modified cow's milk. Protein is reduced, saturated fat is removed and replaced with vegetable fats, and vitamins and some minerals are added. Soy formulas are used for infants with allergies or who do not tolerate cow's milk–based formula. Nutramigen is a protein hydrolysate formula made from cow's milk but treated to be hypoallergenic. Nutramigen typically is used only when all other formulas have failed as it can be very costly for the parents.

Special formulas are made to meet special needs of some infants. Preterm infants need more calories but less quantity; these formulas provide 24 kcal/oz. Other formulas are modified to be low in the amino acid phenylalanine for infants with phenylketonuria (PKU), who cannot digest phenylalanine.

Feeding Method

Nutrition is provided for the newborn either through breastfeeding or bottle feeding. Whichever method the parents choose, nurses must support and assist the parents to make the experience meaningful. Some of the advantages and disadvantages of breastfeeding and bottle feeding are identified in Table 58-2.

Other factors besides the advantages and disadvantages of breastfeeding and bottle feeding enter into the decision of how to feed the newborn. These factors include support offered by the infant's father; support by other family members; the need to work outside the home by the mother; and age, educational level, and income level of the parents.

When the mother is breastfeeding (8 to 12 times a day at first), she is focused on the infant. Various tasks around the home may need to be left undone or the father will need to do them. Support from other family members may be based on how other family members have chosen to feed their infants.

Table 58-2 Breastfeeding/Bottle Feeding, Advantages and Disadvantages

	BREASTFEEDING	BOTTLE FEEDING
Advantages	Nonallergenic Meets infant's specific nutritional needs Immunologic properties help prevent infections Easily digested Constipation unlikely (Figure 58-25) Overfeeding less likely Convenient, always available No formula or bottles to buy No formula and bottles to prepare Oxytocin release helps involution Mother more likely to eat well-balanced diet May help with mother's weight loss Enhances mother/infant attachment through skin-to-skin contact Infant determines amount	Father or others may feed infant day or night Feed less frequently (3 to 4 hours) Amount of milk taken at each feeding known Easier to go back to work Caregiver determines amount
Disadvantages	Feed more frequently (2 to 3 hours) More frequent diaper changes Amount of milk taken at each feeding unknown Medications taken by mother present in milk Discomfort of some mothers to nurse in public Expense of pumping and storing milk for periods when mother is unavailable (such as work hours)	Expense of formula, bottles ($50 to $200 per month) Washing bottles Fixing and refrigerating formula Carrying bottles on outings May cause constipation

COURTESY OF DELMAR CENGAGE LEARNING

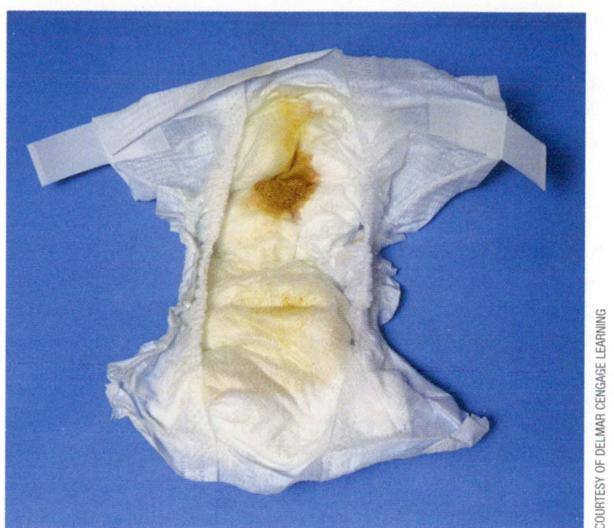

FIGURE 58-25 Stool of a Breastfed Infant

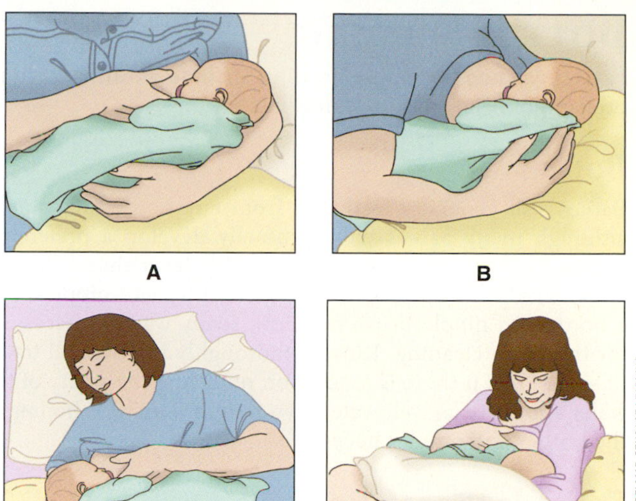

FIGURE 58-26 Positions for Feeding Infant; *A*, Cradling, used for Breast and Bottle Feeding; *B*, Football Hold; *C*, Lying Down; *D*, Across Lap

BREASTFEEDING

Many factors influence breastfeeding, including positions for feeding, latching on, and length of feeding.

Positions for Feeding

The infant should be held with the head slightly higher than the rest of the body. The cradle hold, with the infant's head in the bend of the mother's elbow and the arm supporting the infant's body, is probably the most common. It can be used whether breastfeeding or bottle feeding. Other positions that are particularly adaptable to breastfeeding are the football hold, side-lying position, and across-the-lap position (Figure 58-26). The mother's free hand should be in a "C" position, supporting the underside of her breast with the fingers.

Latching On

The mother should use the infant's rooting reflex to allow proper positioning of the nipple in the infant's mouth. Brushing the nipple against the infant's lower lip will cause the infant to open the mouth. When the mouth is wide open and the tongue is down, the mother quickly brings the infant closer to the breast so the infant can latch on to the nipple and areola. When properly positioned, the tongue is on top of the lower gum and under the breast, with the lips flared outward. When the infant is properly latched on, the suction is strong. To remove the infant from the breast, the mother should insert a finger into the corner of the infant's mouth between the gums to break the suction and quickly remove the breast. The nipple should never be simply pulled out from the infant's mouth because this will cause the mother pain and may also result in tissue damage to the nipple.

Length of Feeding

Feeding length varies with each mother/infant unit; however, the feeding should be long enough to remove all of the **foremilk**, the watery first milk from the breast, which is high in lactose, like skim milk, and is effective in quenching thirst. This allows the infant to receive the **hindmilk**, which is higher in fat content, leads to weight gain, and is more satisfying.

The average time for a feeding session is approximately 30 minutes. It is more important to know when the infant is finished feeding than to go by the clock. When an infant is satisfied, the sucking and swallowing will be much slower and the breast will be soft. The infant may fall asleep and release the nipple.

The first breast should be emptied (very soft) before moving the infant to the other breast. At the next feeding, the breast used last at the previous feeding should be used first. This ensures that each breast is emptied at least at every other feeding. As the infant grows and requires more milk, both breasts may be emptied at each feeding.

CLIENT TEACHING

Timing of Feedings

Feedings should be given when the infant is hungry (demand feeding) rather than on a fixed schedule. The infant is ready to eat when wide awake, sucking on hands, rooting, and slightly fussy. New mothers are encouraged to feed on demand as this will help their milk supply build. Some breastfeeding mothers fear that they will overfeed or spoil their infant if they are fed on demand. Teach the mother that this is acceptable and that they should continue to observe the infant for hunger clues and then feed them.

CRITICAL THINKING

Breastfeeding

Your client is trying to breastfeed her second child. With her first child, she gave up in three weeks because of cracked, sore nipples. What factors may affect her success or failure? What nursing interventions should be planned and implemented?

Bottle Feeding

Factors related to bottle feeding include bottles, formula preparation, and amount of feeding.

Bottles

Babies will generally feed well from any bottle and nipple, although many babies will eventually develop a preference and may refuse a new type of nipple. Whatever choice the parents make will be fine. Washing the bottles and nipples with a bottle and nipple brush in warm, soapy water is necessary for thorough cleaning. Rinsing thoroughly removes all traces of soap. Only if there is a question regarding the safety of the water supply (e.g., well water on a farm or ranch) is boiling of the bottles and nipples necessary.

Formula Preparation

Formulas are available in three forms: ready to feed, concentrated, and powdered. The latter two require addition of water. The choice of formula is generally left up to the parents. There is a great difference in price, so the choice may be made based on finances. Mixing of formula must be accurate to provide the 20 kcal/oz.

Amount of Feeding

Most newborns begin by drinking 7.5 mL to 15 mL (1/4 to 1/2 oz) at a feeding but gradually increase to approximately 90 mL to 120 mL (3 to 4 oz) at each feeding in 2 weeks. The infant's appetite will generally increase during growth spurts at 2 weeks, 6 to 9 weeks, and 3 to 6 months, so the amount of formula should be increased by 30 mL (1 oz) in each bottle to meet this need.

Burping

All infants require burping, whether breastfed or bottle fed. Burping is needed to expel the air swallowed when the infant sucks. Some infants swallow more air than others and require more frequent burping.

To facilitate burping, the infant can be held upright on the feeder's shoulder, in a sitting position on the feeder's lap with the head and chest supported with one hand, or prone across the feeder's lap (Figure 58-27). The other hand is used to gently pat or rub the infant's back.

Burping should be done generally about halfway through the feeding for bottle feeding and when changing breasts for breastfeeding. Parents soon learn the infant's cues regarding the need to be burped.

Pacifiers

Many parents are anxious to comfort their new baby. This usually means offering the infant a pacifier to help sooth them. The best practice is to wait at least 4 to 6 weeks to prevent nipple confusion and ensure that the infant has a solid feeding relationship with either breast or bottle.

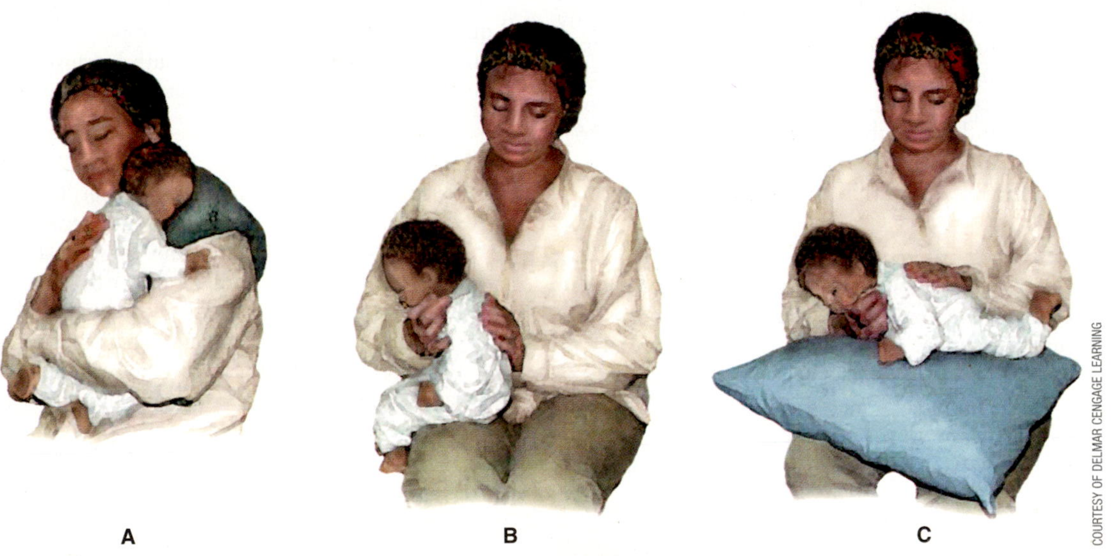

COURTESY OF DELMAR CENGAGE LEARNING

FIGURE 58-27 Burping positions: *A*, Supported on the shoulder; *B*, Upright on the lap; *C*, Face down across the lap.

SAMPLE NURSING CARE PLAN

Newborn Infant

S.S., born at 36 weeks' gestation, weighs 6 pounds 3 ounces and is 19 inches long. Her Apgar score was 8 at 1 minute and 9 at 5 minutes. Axillary temperature is 96.5°F (35.8°C), respirations 56, and apical pulse 148. The parents are very excited about S.S., their first child. S.S. is very sleepy and is not breastfeeding well.

NURSING DIAGNOSIS 1 *Ineffective Thermoregulation* related to immaturity as evidenced by birth at 36 weeks' gestation

SAMPLE NURSING CARE PLAN (Continued)

Nursing Outcomes Classification (NOC)
Thermoregulation: Neonate

Nursing Interventions Classification (NIC)
Temperature Regulation

PLANNING/OUTCOMES	NURSING INTERVENTIONS	RATIONALE
S.S.'s temperature will be between 97.5°F (36.4°C) and 98.9°F (37.2°C).	Keep S.S. adequately clothed and covered.	Maintains her temperature.
	Maintain ambient room temperature between 77.2°F (25.1°C) and 78.1°F (25.6°C).	Is optimum environmental temperature.
	Keep S.S. away from air conditioning vents, drafts, and fans.	Prevents heat loss by convection.
	Use warm water when bathing S.S., wrap her in a towel, and dry her quickly. Dry her head thoroughly and put a cap on her head.	Prevents heat loss by evaporation.
	Cover scales and examination area before S.S. is laid down.	Prevents heat loss by conduction.
	Keep S.S.'s crib away from outside windows.	Prevents heat loss by radiation.
	Teach S.S.'s parents how to maintain a neutral thermal environment for S.S.	Prevents S.S. from using her brown fat too fast.

EVALUATION

S.S.'s temperature is 97.8°F.

NURSING DIAGNOSIS 2 *Risk for Infection* related to risk factor of inadequate primary defenses as evidenced by cut umbilical cord and immature immune system

Nursing Outcomes Classification (NOC)
Infection Status, Wound Healing, Immune Status

Nursing Interventions Classification (NIC)
Infection Control, Wound Care

PLANNING/OUTCOMES	NURSING INTERVENTIONS	RATIONALE
S.S. will have no signs of infection of the eyes, diaper area, or umbilical cord.	Use good hand hygiene technique (caregivers and parents) before and after caring for S.S.	Prevents spread of infection.
	Provide prescribed eye prophylaxis and keep eyes clean.	Prevents infection.
	Keep diaper area clean and dry.	Prevents skin irritation and infection.
	Place diaper below the umbilical cord.	Allows cord to dry and heal.

EVALUATION

S.S. shows no signs of infection.

(*Continues*)

SAMPLE NURSING CARE PLAN (Continued)

NURSING DIAGNOSIS 3 *Imbalanced **N**utrition, Less than Body Requirements* related to infants prematurity and limited nutritional intake as evidenced by infant remaining sleepy and not breastfeeding well during feedings

Nursing Outcomes Classification (NOC)
Nutritional Status

Nursing Interventions Classification (NIC)
Nutrition Management, Nutrition Monitoring

PLANNING/OUTCOMES	NURSING INTERVENTIONS	RATIONALE
S.S. will lose only 5 to 10 ounces of weight during the first 3 days.	Assist mother in breastfeeding S.S.	Provides support for first time breastfeeding.
	Demonstrate use of rooting reflex to ensure proper latch on.	Uses natural response of infant for proper position of mouth and tongue.
	Explain that S.S. will suck in spurts.	Assists mother in knowing that S.S. has not finished breastfeeding when she rests.
	Explain that the breast has foremilk and hindmilk (needed for growth), so breasts must be emptied.	Ensures that mother will allow S.S. to empty one breast before changing to the other breast.

EVALUATION
S.S. lost 7 ounces during the first 3 days.

PROBLEMS OF THE NEWBORN

Problems of the newborn identified either at birth or before discharge include hyperbilirubinemia, respiratory distress, cleft lip/palate, hydrocephalus, spina bifida, Down syndrome, and talipes equinovarus. Newborn problems may also occur when the mother is diabetic, HIV positive, or a substance abuser. Phenylketonuria must be tested for as soon as possible so treatment can begin immediately.

HYPERBILIRUBINEMIA

Hyperbilirubinemia, an excess of bilirubin in the blood, may be related to physiologic jaundice or pathologic jaundice. Physiologic jaundice does not appear until after 24 hours of age and is more commonly seen after the infant has gone home. It is discussed in the Infants with Special Needs: Birth to 12 Months chapter.

Pathologic jaundice appears in the first 24 hours and may lead to **kernicterus** (deposits of bilirubin causing yellow staining in the brain, especially the basal ganglia, cerebellum, and hippocampus). The exact level of total bilirubin when kernicterus occurs is not known but may occur at 20 mg/dL in full-term infants and at a lower level in preterm neonates. Kernicterus is a chronic and clinically permanent result of bilirubin toxcity. Preterm infants are at a greater risk of developing kernicterus, and the most common cause is Rh incompatibility and severe dehydration (AAP, 2004).

MEDICAL–SURGICAL MANAGEMENT

Medical

Phototherapy is the most common treatment for jaundice. The "bili" lights are special flourescent lamps (in the blue-light spectrum) placed over the infant. Only a diaper and an eye covering are on the infant to expose the most skin surface to the light. A fiber-optic phototherapy blanket and the BiliBed® with the Bilicombi™ blanket (Figure 58-28) have been designed to provide phototherapy without the eyes needing to be covered. Because the infant is covered, thermal regulation is no longer a problem, and interaction with the parents can take place. The infant may experience frequent, green, loose stools as the bilirubin is excreted.

Surgical

If the bilirubin level cannot be reduced quickly or maintained below 12 mg/dL with phototherapy treatment, exchange transfusion is necessary. Blood type O, Rh-negative blood is used. During this procedure, 5 mL to 10 mL of blood are removed from the infant and replaced with a like amount of donor blood. This is a very slow process. Complications of hypervolemia, hypovolemia, infection, cardiac arrhythmias, and air embolism may occur.

This procedure is seldom necessary today because of the widespread use of RhoGAM to prevent Rh incompatibility.

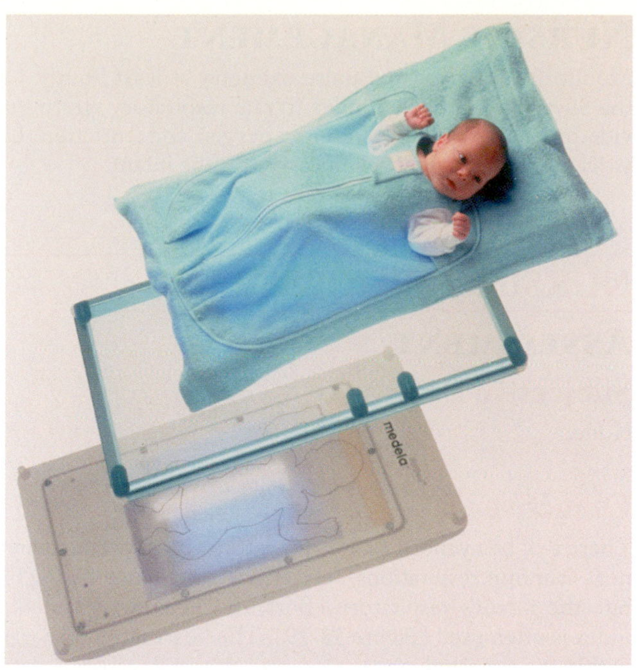

FIGURE 58-28 Bilibed® with Bilicombi™ Blanket (*Photo courtesy of Medela, Inc.*)

Diet

Fluid intake is increased to assist in elimination of the bilirubin through the urine.

Nursing Management

Review record to identify factors predisposing the infant to jaundice. Assess infant for jaundice every 4 hours. Encourage adequate amount taken at each feeding. Breastfeeding mothers should feed their infants at least 8 to 12 times a day for the first several days after delivery. Make sure to keep diaper area clean and protected. The American Academy of Pediatrics (2004), recommends against supplementations with extra fluids such as water or dextrose with water, as they will not prevent or lower the bilirubin levels.

NURSING PROCESS

Assessment

Subjective Data

None.

Objective Data

Prenatal and perinatal records are reviewed to identify factors predisposing to jaundice. Jaundice in light-skinned infants is assessed by blanching the skin (pressing firmly with the thumb) over a bony prominence such as the forehead, nose, or sternum. When the thumb is removed, the area has a yellowish appearance before normal color returns if jaundice is present. In darker-skinned infants, the infant's oral mucosa, posterior aspect of the hard palate, or conjunctival sacs will have a yellow coloring when jaundice is present.

Nursing diagnoses for an infant with hyperbilirubinemia include the following:

NURSING DIAGNOSES	PLANNING/OUTCOMES	NURSING INTERVENTIONS
*Risk for Deficient **F**luid Volume* related to increased insensible water loss and frequent loose stools secondary to phototherapy	The infant's intake will be at least 100 to 150 mL/kg/day.	Encourage adequate feedings of infant by mother.
*Risk for **N**eonatal Jaundice* related to abnormal weight loss (>7% to 8% in breastfeeding newborn; 15% in term infant) as evidenced by infant experiencing difficulty in establishing a consistent breastfeeding pattern	The infant will maintain a 2% to 3% in weight prior to discharge.	Assist in proper latch on technique. Instruct parents on weighing wet diapers to help ensure appropriate intake.
*Risk for Impaired **S**kin Integrity* related to frequent loose stools secondary to phototherapy	The infant's diaper area will maintain skin integrity.	Check diaper frequently and change as soon as soiled. Apply A+D ointment or petroleum jelly to diaper area after cleansing.

Evaluation: Evaluate each outcome to determine how it has been met by the client.

RESPIRATORY DISTRESS

Two types of respiratory distress may occur in a newborn: respiratory distress syndrome (RDS) and transient tachypnea of the newborn (TTN).

Respiratory distress syndrome is associated with preterm infants and surfactant deficiency. Verma (1995) describes respiratory distress syndrome as caused by alterations in surfactant quantity, composition, function, or production. These infants have hypoxia, respiratory acidosis, and metabolic acidosis.

Transient tachypnea of the newborn is found mainly in AGA and near-term infants (Ladewig et al., 2005). Either intrauterine or intrapartum asphyxia has been experienced by these infants. This results in the newborn's failure to clear the airway of lung fluid and mucus or aspiration of amniotic fluid. No respiratory difficulties are experienced at birth, but shortly after birth, the newborn may have flaring of the nares and expiratory grunting. By 6 hours of age, tachypnea is noted, with respirations as high as 100 to 140 breaths per minute.

Medical–Surgical Management

Medical

The goal is to determine which type of respiratory distress is affecting the newborn and begin treatment. For RDS, the goals of treatment are maintenance of adequate oxygenation and ventilation and correction of the respiratory and metabolic acidosis. Mild RDS is often treated only with increased, humidified oxygen concentration. Infants with moderate RDS may require continuous positive airway pressure (CPAP). Mechanical ventilation is required for severe RDS. The oxygen needs of infants with RDS increase over the first 48 hours.

Infants with TTN generally require ambient oxygen of 30% to 50% initially. This need for increased oxygen generally decreases over the first 48 hours. Treatment is usually required only for 4 days.

Nursing Management

Monitor respirations and pulse oximetry at least hourly. Use the Silverman-Anderson index to rate respiratory effort. Provide oxygen as ordered. Monitor oxygen concentration. Use strict aseptic technique when caring for the infant.

NURSING PROCESS

Assessment

Subjective Data

None.

Objective Data

There will be cyanosis pallor or mottling of the skin, tachypnea, grunting respirations, retractions, and nasal flaring. To rate the infant's respiratory effort, the Silverman-Anderson index is often used (Figure 58-29). The heart rate is generally within the expected range.

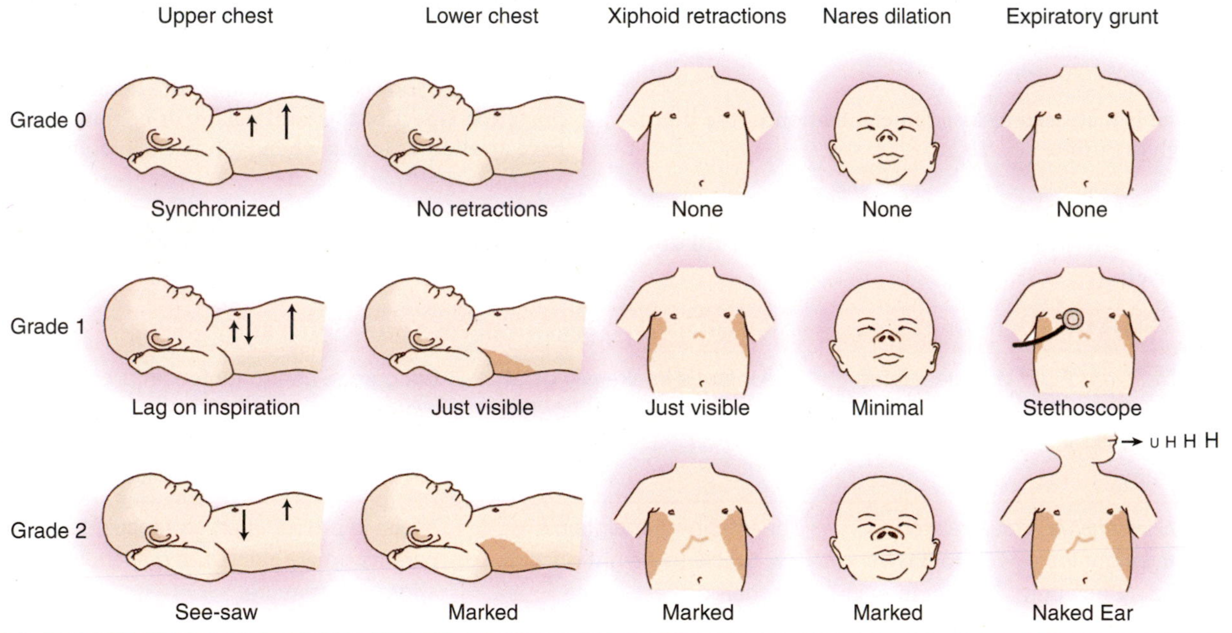

FIGURE 58-29 Silverman-Anderson Index (*Reproduced with permission from* Pediatrics *17:1-10. Copyright 1956.*)

Nursing diagnoses for an infant with respiratory distress include the following:

NURSING DIAGNOSES	PLANNING/OUTCOMES	NURSING INTERVENTIONS
Respiratory Distress related to premature infant lung maturity	The infant will maintain optimum lung function as evidenced by pulse oximetry within normal limits 98% or higher.	Monitor arterial blood gases. Administer oxygen as ordered. Assess infant for periods of apnea. Monitor infant's skin and reposition as needed. Monitor for nasal flaring.
Risk for Infection related to invasive procedures	The infant will show no signs or symptoms of infection at the procedure site.	Assess procedure site for signs of infection (redness, swelling, color, size, and odor).

Nursing diagnoses for an infant with respiratory distress include the following: (Continued)

NURSING DIAGNOSES	PLANNING/OUTCOMES	NURSING INTERVENTIONS
		Monitor infant's temperature hourly. Maintain strict aseptic technique when caring for infant. Review all lab work and report status changes.

Evaluation: Evaluate each outcome to determine how it has been met by the client.

CLEFT LIP/PALATE

The immediate concern with cleft lip/palate (Figure 58-30) is the problem of feeding the infant. The size of the cleft and whether the palate is also involved determine the difficulty of feeding. Special nipples and feeding devices are available. Hold the infant in an upright sitting position when feeding. Burp frequently because these infants swallow more air than usual. When sleeping, keep the infant in a side-lying position.

Parents of an infant with any congenital anomaly need support from the nurse as they learn to care for an infant with special needs. The nurse must role model interacting with the infant. Complete coverage is found in the Infants with Special Needs: Birth to 12 Months chapter.

HYDROCEPHALUS

Hydrocephalus, excess cerebrospinal fluid in the cerebral ventricles, causes the infant's head to be enlarged. Head circumference is measured daily, fontanelles checked to see whether they are flat or bulging, and the infant's position changed frequently. The infant usually cannot move the head. Complete coverage is found in the Infant with Special Needs: Birth to 12 Months chapter.

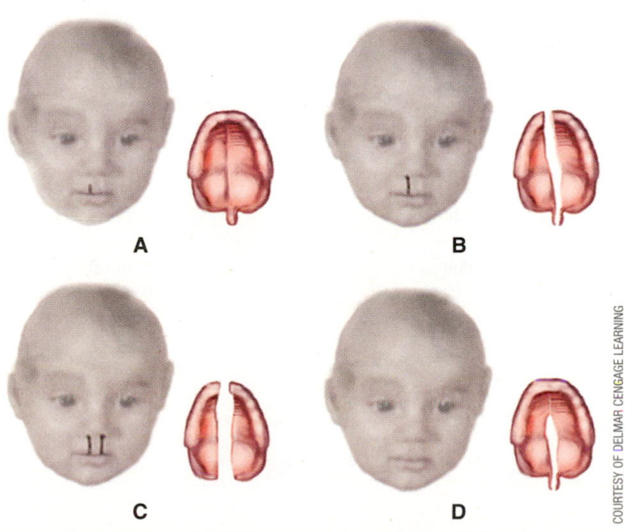

FIGURE 58-30 Types of Cleft Lip/Palate; *A*, Small Notch in Lip, Palate Normal; *B*, Cleft Lip and Cleft Palate; *C*, Bilateral Cleft Lip and Cleft Palate; *D*, Lip Normal, Cleft Palate

SPINA BIFIDA

There are three types of spina bifida (neural tube defects): spina bifida occulta, meningocele, and myelomeningocele (Figure 58-31). **Spina bifida occulta** is a failure of the vertebral arch to close. There is a dimple on the back, which may have a tuft of hair in it. No care is required.

A **meningocele** is a saclike protrusion along the vertebral column filled with cerebrospinal fluid and meninges. Surgery is required to repair the defect, but there are no long-term effects.

A **myelomeningocele** is a saclike protrusion along the vertebral column filled with spinal fluid, meninges, nerve roots, and spinal cord. Because of the nerve root and spinal cord involvement, there will be paralysis at some level after surgical repair.

The saclike protrusions must be kept covered with sterile saline dressings, and the infant handled carefully when changing position from side to side. The sac must be kept free from contamination by urine and stool. Head circumference is measured and fontanelles checked for bulging on each shift because hydrocephalus often develops. Complete coverage of myelomeningocele is found in the Infant with Special Needs: Birth to 12 Months chapter.

DOWN SYNDROME

Down syndrome is caused by a chromosomal abnormality, also called trisomy 21. Routine care is provided in the newborn period. Complete coverage is found in the Infant with Special Needs: Birth to 12 Months chapter.

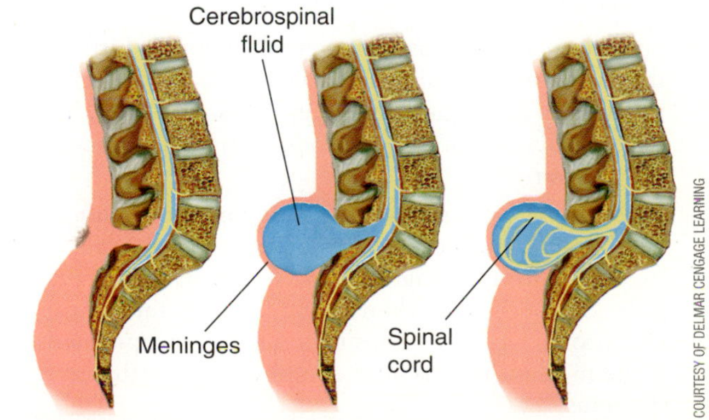

FIGURE 58-31 Types of Spina Bifida; *A*, Spina Bifida Occulta; *B*, Meningocele; *C*, Myelomeningocele

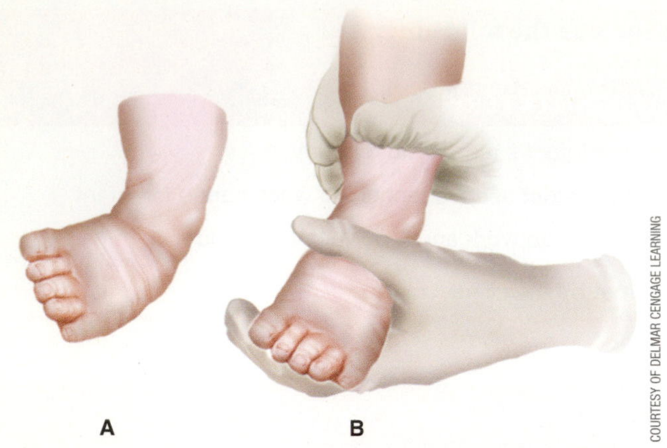

FIGURE 58-32 ***A,*** **Talipes Equinovarus (clubfoot);** ***B,*** **Foot Moves to Midline; Positional, not Clubfoot**

TALIPES EQUINOVARUS

Talipes equinovarus, also called clubfoot, is a congenital deformity in which the foot and ankle are twisted inward and cannot be moved to a midline position (Figure 58-32). The foot or feet of some infants appear to turn inward, but if they can be moved to the midline, the cause is intrauterine position. Range-of-motion exercises will often correct this problem.

Infants with true clubfoot may have a cast on before going home. Complete coverage is found in the Infant with Special Needs: Birth to 12 Months chapter.

INFANT OF A DIABETIC MOTHER

The infant of a diabetic mother (IDM) requires close observation the first few hours to several days after birth. If the mother has vascular complications with the diabetes, the infant is generally SGA. If the mother has gestational diabetes or diabetes without vascular changes, the infant is generally LGA, especially if the diabetes has not been well-controlled. The large size is the result of fat deposits and increased size of all organs except the brain. The IDM has less total body water, especially in the extracellular spaces. The following are complications seen most often in the IDM:

- *Hypoglycemia*: The loss of maternal glucose at birth and the high level of insulin produced by the infant decrease the infant's blood glucose within hours after birth. It takes a period of time for insulin production to be reduced in the newborn.
- *Respiratory distress*: Insulin is antagonistic to the cortisol-induced stimulation of lecithin (phospholipid necessary for lung maturation) synthesis. This results in less-mature lungs than would be expected for the gestational age. This does not seem to be a problem if the mother has vascular complications with her diabetes.
- *Hyperbilirubinemia*: Hepatic immaturity and a decreased extracellular fluid volume, which increases hematocrit, may be the cause of the hyperbilirubinemia seen 48 to 72 hours after birth (Ladewig et al., 2005). Any bruises from a difficult delivery may also be a cause.
- *Birth trauma*: The large size of many IDMs predisposes them to trauma during labor and delivery.
- *Congenital birth defects*: Birth defects may include patent ductus arteriosus, ventricular septal defect, transposition of the great vessels, small left colon syndrome, and sacral agenesis.

MEDICAL–SURGICAL MANAGEMENT

Medical

Blood glucose monitoring is performed hourly during the first 4 to 6 hours of life and then every 4 hours for 24 hours, or per agency protocol. Blood is generally obtained by heelstick (Figure 58-33).

Pharmacological

An intravenous infusion of glucose may be necessary if early feeding does not keep the blood glucose at 45 mg/dL or above.

Diet

A feeding of 5% glucose water may be given soon after birth, followed in 1 hour by a breast or formula feeding, which is continued on a regular basis.

NURSING MANAGEMENT

Monitor blood glucose level as ordered. Ensure timely feedings. Administer glucose orally or IV as ordered. Prevent cold stress. Hold and comfort the infant after heelsticks.

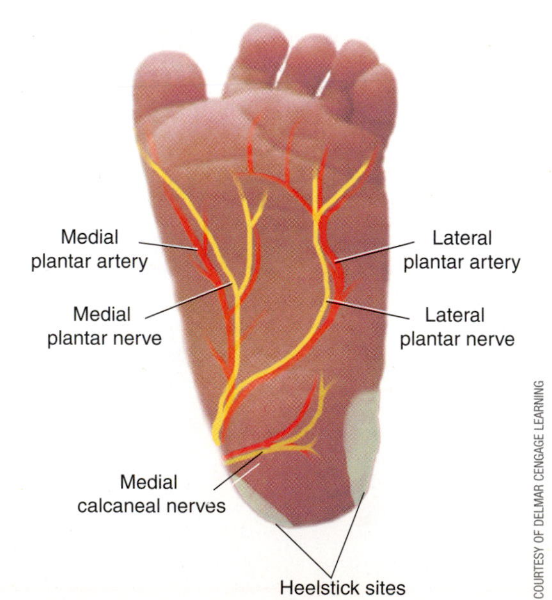

FIGURE 58-33 **Shaded areas shown are heelstick sites.**

NURSING PROCESS

Assessment

Subjective Data

None.

Objective Data

Blood glucose screening of less than 45 mg/dL should be verified by laboratory analysis. The infant may show signs of jitteriness or tremors. Diaphoresis, although uncommon for a newborn, may occur with hypoglycemia. Poor muscle tone, low temperature, and rapid respirations may also be noted.

Nursing diagnoses for an infant with hypoglycemia include the following:

NURSING DIAGNOSES	PLANNING/OUTCOMES	NURSING INTERVENTIONS
*Imbalanced **Nutrition**: Less than Body Requirements* related to increased glucose use secondary to being IDM	The infant will maintain an adequate glucose level.	Initiate feedings as soon as possible. Prepare dextrose solution IV if infant is unable to take PO fluids. Weigh infant every day at the same time for adequate weight checks. Monitor infant's temperature and the temperature in the isolette to maintain warm environment and to prevent cold stress, which could increase the glucose levels. Monitor lab work and report any changes. Ensure timely infant feedings. Monitor blood glucose level according to protocol. Prevent cold stress and identify other stressors (hypoxia, sepsis, RDS) that increase glucose use.
*Acute **Pain*** related to physical injury of heelsticks for glucose monitoring	The infant will decrease crying after each heelstick.	Warm infant's heel before heelstick to increase blood flow to the area. Properly perform heelstick to avoid nerves and arteries. Hold and comfort infant after heelstick procedure.

Evaluation: Evaluate each outcome to determine how it has been met by the client.

INFANT OF AN HIV-POSITIVE MOTHER

The transmission rate of HIV infection from mother to infant is 28% to 35% (Merenstein, Adams, & Weisman, 2006). This transmission may occur through the placenta at various gestational ages, through maternal blood and secretions during labor and birth, and through breast milk after the birth (Fanaroff & Martin, 2005).

Every infant born to an HIV-seropositive mother will have HIV antibodies that have crossed the placenta from the mother. By 8 to 15 months of age, uninfected infants have lost the maternal antibodies; but the infected infants have begun to develop their own antibodies and remain HIV seropositive (Fanaroff & Martin, 2005).

At birth, the HIV-infected infant typically has no symptoms. The appearance of an opportunistic disease between 3 and 6 months of age may alert caregivers to the presence of HIV infection. Lymphoid interstitial pneumonitis is considered a criterion for diagnosis (Fanaroff & Martin, 2005). As a basis for care, all infants of HIV-positive mothers must be presumed to be HIV positive.

Breastfeeding is not recommended. HIV-positive women that breastfeed their infants increase the risk of trasmission by 15% to 40%. HIV transmission occurs most often in the first few months of the infants life. In the United States, the rate of transmission has been significantly reduced due to medications and formula that are available for HIV-positive mothers (Amman, 2009).

INFANT OF A SUBSTANCE-ABUSING MOTHER

The infant of a substance-abusing mother (ISAM) is a substance abuser at birth. When the umbilical cord is cut at birth, the newborn experiences withdrawal. The severity of withdrawal symptoms depends on the substance(s) abused by the mother and the time and amount of the last dose. The symptoms may occur within the first 24 to 48 hours after birth or not until 4 or 5 days of age. Alcohol withdrawal symptoms often appear within 6 to 12 hours after birth or at least within the first 3 days. Infant alcohol dependence is physiologic. It may be very difficult for the substance-abusing mother to care for her infant initially and/or long term.

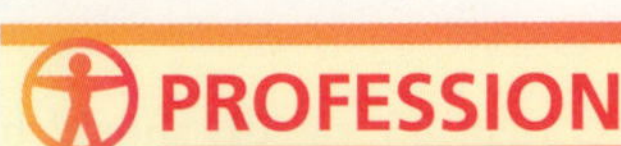

Narcotic Antagonists

The use of naloxone (Narcan) is contraindicated for infants born to narcotic abusers. It may cause severe signs and symptoms of narcotic withdrawal, especially seizures.

Complications commonly found in an ISAM include withdrawal, respiratory distress, jaundice, behavior problems, congenital anomalies, and growth retardation. Infants of alcohol-dependent mothers may also have fetal alcohol syndrome (FAS). Narcon (Naxalone), an opiod antagonist, is pulled for delivery whenever the client has tested positive for drugs on admission. Narcan is used when a mother has had a narcotic during delivery for pain relief.

MEDICAL–SURGICAL MANAGEMENT

Medical

Treatment is focused on management of the previously mentioned complications that may be present. Approximately 50% of these infants experience withdrawal symptoms severe enough to require treatment.

Pharmacological

Phenobarbital or tincture of opium may be used to control drug withdrawal symptoms. Phenobarbital or diazepam (Valium) may be used to control seizures in the alcohol-dependent infant.

Diet

Formula supplying 24 kcal/oz is recommended for the infant who experiences vomiting and diarrhea or who is excessively active.

NURSING MANAGEMENT

Monitor the infant's temperature, weight, skin turgor, and fontanells. Maintain strict intake and output. Provide small, frequent feedings. Provide a quiet environment and keep stimulation at a minimum. Administer medications as ordered. Role model interacting with the infant and encourage the mother to do so. Make referrals as necessary to social agencies and infant development programs.

NURSING PROCESS

ASSESSMENT

Subjective Data

None.

Objective Data

The drug-dependent infant may experience hyperactivity, persistent high-pitched shrill cry, tremors, seizures, tachypnea, fever, disorganized sucking and swallowing, vomiting, diarrhea, stuffy nose, yawning, sneezing, and sweating. The alcohol-dependent infant may or may not have FAS, which includes mental retardation, hyperactivity, growth deficiency, distinctive facial abnormalities, and other congenital anomalies. This infant may also experience tremors, seizures, inconsolable crying, abdominal distention, great activity, and exaggerated rooting and sucking.

Nursing diagnoses for an infant experiencing withdrawal include the following:

NURSING DIAGNOSES	PLANNING/OUTCOMES	NURSING INTERVENTIONS
*Imbalanced **N**utrition: Less than Body Requirements* related to disorganized sucking and swallowing, vomiting, diarrhea, and hyperactivity	The infant will not lose excessive weight (more than 10% of birth weight).	Monitor infant's temperature so environment can be adjusted to maintain normal infant temperature. Provide small frequent feedings. Administer medications as ordered. Position infant on the side to avoid possible aspiration. Maintain strict intake and output. Weigh infant every 8 hours. Monitor for signs of dehydration (sunken fontanel, dry mucous membranes, poor skin turgor, weight loss).
*Risk for **I**njury* related to effects of substancewithdrawal (seizures, hyperactivity)	The infant will not exhibit signs of seizures.	Administer medications as ordered. Decrease environmental activity. Plan care to necessitate minimum stimulation. Wrap infant snugly. Monitor activity level.

Nursing diagnoses for an infant experiencing withdrawal include the following: (Continued)

NURSING DIAGNOSES	PLANNING/OUTCOMES	NURSING INTERVENTIONS
*Risk for Impaired **P**arenting* related to substance abuse and difficult temperament of the infant	The parent will show signs of bonding/attachment and an interest in infant care.	Explain effects of maternal substance abuse on infant and the process of withdrawal. Role model interacting with the infant. Encourage mother to interact with her infant. Explain and demonstrate infant care procedures, especially how to avoid excess stimulation of the infant. Make referrals to social agencies and infant development programs.

Evaluation: Evaluate each outcome to determine how it has been met by the client.

PHENYLKETONURIA

Most states require neonatal screening for the genetic disease phenylketonuria (PKU), an inborn error of metabolism in which the infant has a deficiency of the enzyme required to digest the amino acid phenylalanine. The infant must ingest an ample amount of phenylalanine, found in both breast milk and regular infant formulas, for the PKU test to be reliable. The test is performed at least 24 hours after the initial breast or formula feeding.

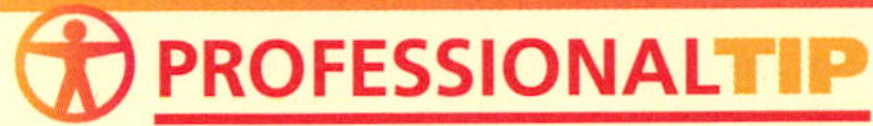

PKU

The time of the first breast or formula feeding is to be documented so at least 24 hours passes before the heelstick for the PKU test is performed.

An infant with PKU must be put on a diet low in phenylalanine, preferably by 1 month of age. Infant formulas that are very low in phenylalanine are available. Without screening and diet modification, severe mental retardation results. Even with neonatal PKU screening, many affected children have some intellectual impairment (Lowdermilk & Perry, 2007).

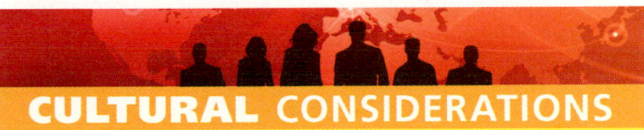

CULTURAL CONSIDERATIONS

Phenylketonuria

The highest incidence of PKU is found in the white populations of Northern Europe and the United States; it is less common in populations of African, Chinese, and Japanese descent (Hardelid & Etal, 2008).

CASE STUDY

Baby boy H.R., a full-term newborn, is 36 hours old. He has type B, Rh-positive blood and his mother has type O, Rh-positive blood. There is a small cephalhematoma on the right parietal bone. Routine assessment identified the appearance of jaundice when the skin was blanched on his forehead. His bilirubin level was 2 mg/dL on the cord blood and 4 mg/dL at 24 hours of age.

The following questions will guide your development of a nursing care plan for the case study.

1. What factors may be causing the jaundice?
2. What orders would you anticipate the physician would write?
3. What are the critical levels of bilirubin?
4. Phototherapy is begun using "bili" lights. What assessments and precautions must be taken when these lights are used?
5. Identify two possible nursing diagnoses and a goal for each for baby boy H.R.
6. Describe nursing interventions for meeting the goals.
7. How can the goals be evaluated?

SUMMARY

- The immediate needs of the newborn are airway, breathing, circulation, and warmth.
- The initiation of breathing is related to physical, chemical, thermal, and sensory factors.
- Circulatory changes include the closing of the three fetal structures: the ductus arteriosus, foramen ovale, and the ductus venosus.
- Nonshivering thermogenesis, metabolism of brown fat, is the newborn's unique method of heat production.
- Infants lose heat through conduction, convection, evaporation, and radiation.
- The immediate care of the newborn includes obtaining the Apgar score, resuscitation (if required), providing a neutral thermal environment, identification, parent/infant bonding, and prophylactic care.
- Common variations of the newborn must be carefully documented, especially mongolian spots, to possibly prevent parents from being charged with child abuse.
- Neurologic integrity can be assessed through the many reflexes of the newborn. Most of these reflexes disappear during the first 2 years of life.
- Six states of being have been identified for the newborn: quiet sleep, active sleep, drowsy, quiet alert, active alert, and crying.
- Gestational age can be determined by assessing six physical characteristics and six neuromuscular maturity characteristics.
- Infants are considered contaminated with blood-borne pathogens until after the first bath.
- Problems of the newborn include hyperbilirubinemia, respiratory distress, cleft lip/palate, hydrocephalus, spina bifida, Down syndrome, talipes equinovarus, and phenylketonuria.
- Infants need special care when the mother is a diabetic, HIV positive, or a substance abuser.

REVIEW QUESTIONS

1. Which of the following is the result of a metabolic error in the newborn?
   1. Leukemia.
   2. Patent ductus arteriosus.
   3. Phenylketonuria.
   4. Pyloric stenosis.
2. A nurse working in the special care nursery admits a 35 4/7 newborn. Given the infants prematurity, the nurse would want to monitor for which of the following conditions?
   1. Hypothermia.
   2. Hyperthermia.
   3. Hyperglycemia.
   4. Tachycardia.
3. A nurse is teaching new parents safety positions for their new baby to sleep in. The nurse knows that the parents understand the teaching when they make which of following statements.
   1. "We will place our baby on her stomach to sleep."
   2. "We will place our baby on her back to sleep."
   3. "We will place our baby on her pillow to sleep."
   4. "We will place our baby under the covers to sleep."
4. A new mother calls the nurse and states, "My baby has been sleeping for the past 3 hours and does not want to wake up to feed, I am so worried" The mother has just given birth 5 hours ago. Which explanation by the nurse would be the most appropriate to put the new mother at ease?
   1. "I would be worried too. How about we wake the baby up together."
   2. "Let me go get a bottle warmed up and see what I can do."
   3. "Do not worry; your baby is going through a sleep period. You should try to get some rest."
   4. "I will call the pediatrician's office right away to see what they can do."
5. A newborn male is scheduled for a circumcision. Which of the following is essential for the nurse to teach the parents after the procedure is over?
   1. Apply Emla cream to the penis for pain relief.
   2. Give Tylenol every 4 to 6 hours round the clock.
   3. Apply A+D ointment and gauze to the penis with every diaper change for the first 24 hours.
   4. Withhold feedings for 4 hours after the procedure.
6. The nurse is aware that survival of a newborn infant depends primarily on:
   1. the infant's regulation of body temperature.
   2. prompt expansion of the lungs and the establishment of gaseous exchange.
   3. the infant's energy provided from materials obtained from the environment.
   4. the rise in the infant's arterial oxygen tension and a rapid fall in carbon dioxide tension.
7. When assisting the establishment of respirations in a newborn, which of these actions should the nurse do first?
   1. Tie the cord.
   2. Provide continuous oxygen.
   3. Use a resuscitation machine.
   4. Remove mucus from the mouth, throat, and nose.

8. The nurse dries a newborn infant as soon after birth as possible, primarily to help:
   1. stimulate the infant's circulatory system.
   2. avoid excess heat loss from the infant's body.
   3. remove organisms from the infant's skin acquired during birth.
   4. remove the amniotic fluid so the infant is not so slippery.
9. A new mother asks the nurse about the bluish area on her infant's buttocks. The nurse's response is based on knowledge that this discoloration:
   1. is called mongolian spots.
   2. may need to be removed surgically.
   3. is a birthmark that the infant will have for life.
   4. should be checked about twice a year for precancerous cells.
10. The nurse is aware that the most generally accepted theory of the cause of physiologic jaundice is that it results from:
   1. dehydration fever.
   2. congenital obliteration of the bile ducts.
   3. rapid destruction of excess red blood cells.
   4. antibodies caused by the Rh negative factor in the maternal blood.

REFERENCES/SUGGESTED READINGS

Alexander, G. & Allen, M. (1996). Conceptualization, measurement, and use of gestational age: I. clinical and public health practice. *Journal of Perinatology, 16*(1), 53.

Alexander, I., & Reuters, T. (2009). *PDR nurse's drug handbook 2010.* Montvale, NJ: Physicians' Desk Reference.

Allard-Hendren, R. (2000). Alcohol use and adolescent pregnancy. *MCN, 25*(3), 159–162.

American Academy of Pediatrics (AAP). Committee on Pediatrics and Committee on Genetics (1996). Newborn screening fact sheets. *Pediatrics, 98*(3), 473.

American Academy of Pediatrics (AAP). Work Group on Breastfeeding (1997). Breastfeeding and the use of human milk. *Pediatrics, 100*(6), 1035.

American Academy of Pediatrics. (1999). Task force on circumcision. Circumcision policy statement. *Pediatrics, 103*(3), 686–693.

American Academy of Pediatrics. (2004). Management of hyperbilirubinemia in the newborn infant 35 or more weeks of gestation. *Pediatrics, 114*, 297–316.

Ammann, A. (2009). Global stratagies for HIV prevention. Retrieved July 2, 2009, from http://www.globalstrategies.org/new_documents/resources/PMTCToverviewweb06.pdf.

Armentrout, D., & Huseby, V. (2003). Polycythemia in the newborn. *MCN, 28*(4), 234–240.

Ballard, J. Khoury, J. Wedig, K., Wang, L., Eilers-Walsman, B. & Lipp, R. (1991). New Ballard Score, expanded to include extremely premature infants. *Journal of Pediatrics, 19*(3), 417–423.

Behrman, R. Kliegman, R. & Jenson, H. (Eds.). (2007). *Nelson's textbook of pediatrics* (18th ed.). Philadelphia: W. B. Saunders.

Blackwell, W. (2009). In H. Herdman, Ed., *Nursing Diagnosis 2009–2011.* Iowa: Blackwell.

Blecher, M. (2001). Cutting to the point on circumcision. Retrieved from: http://www.webmd.com/content/article/3609.220.

Brazelton, T. & Nagent, J. (1995). *Neonatal behavioral assessment scale* (3rd ed.). London: Cambridge University Press.

Bulechek, G., Butcher, H., McCloskey, J., & Dochterman, J., eds. (2008). *Nursing Interventions Classification (NIC)* (5th ed.). St. Louis, MO: Mosby/Elsevier.

Burroughs, A., & Leifer, G. (2001). *Maternity nursing* (8th ed.). Philadelphia: W.B. Saunders.

Callister, L., & Vega, R. (1998). Giving birth: Guatemalan women's voices. *JOGNN, 27*(3), 289–295.

Choudhry, U. (1997). Traditional practices of women from India: Pregnancy, childbirth, and newborn care. *JOGNN, 26*(5), 533–539.

Clinical Rounds. (2002). Why circumcision helps protect against infection. *Nursing2002, 32*(10), 33–34.

Estes, M. (2010). *Health assessment & physical examination* (4th ed.). Clifton Park, NY: Delmar Cengage Learning.

Fanaroff, A., & Martin, R. (2005). *Neonatal-perinatal medicine: Diseases of the fetus and infant* (7th ed.). St. Louis, MO: Mosby–Year Book.

Gennaro, S., Kamwendo, L., Mbweza, E., & Kershbaumer, R. (1998). Childbearing in Malawi, Africa. *JOGNN, 27*(2), 191–196.

Hardelid, P., Cortina-Borja, M., Munro, A., Jones, H., Cleary, M., Champion, M., et al. (2008). The birth prevalence of PKU in populations of European, South Asian and Sub-Saharan African Ancestry. *Annals of Human Genetics, 72*, 65–71.

Healthy People 2010. (2009, July). Retrieved July 2, 2009, from http://www.healthypeople.gov/Document/HTML/Volume2/16MICH.htm#_Toc494699664.

Howard, J., & Berbiglia, V. (1997). Caring for childbearing Korean women. *JOGNN, 26*(6), 665–671.

Hutchinson, M., & Baqi-Aziz, M. (1994). Nursing care of the childbearing Muslim family. *JOGNN, 23*(9), 767–771.

Kaufman, M., Clark, J., & Castro, C. (2001). Neonatal circumcision: Benefits, risks, and family teaching. *MCN, 26*(4), 197–201.

Ladewig, P., Moberly, S., Olds, S., & London, M. (2005). *Contemporary maternal–newborn nursing care* (6th ed.). Menlo Park: CA: Addison-Wesley.

Lenhart, J. Lenhart, N. Reid, A., & Chong, B. (1997). Local anesthesia for circumcision: Which techniques are more effective? *Journal of the American Board of Family Practice, 10*(1), 13–19.

Letko, M. (1996). Understanding the Apgar score. *JOGNN, 25*(4), 299.

Littleton, L., & Engebretson, J. (2002). *Maternal, neonatal, and women's health nursing.* Clifton Park, NY: Delmar Cengage Learning.

Lowdermilk, D., & Perry, S. (2007). *Maternity and women's health care* (9th ed.). St. Louis, Missouri: Mosby Elsever.

Lund, C., Kuller, J., Lane, A., Lott, J., & Raines, D. (1999). Neonatal skin care: The scientific basis for practice. *JOGNN, 28*(3), 241–254.

Matsuura, T., Callister, L., & Schwartz, R. (2003). First-time mothers' views of breastfeeding support from nurses. *MCN, 28*(1), 10–15.

Mattson, S. (1995). Culturally sensitive perinatal care for Southeast Asians. *JOGNN, 24*(4), 335–341.

McCaffery, M. (2002). Circumcision: Is a local anesthetic appropriate? *Nursing2002, 32*(4), 24.

Merenstein, G., Adams, K., & Weisman, L. (2006). Infections in the neonate. In G. Merenstein & S. Gardner (Eds.), *Handbook of neonatal intensive care* (6th ed.). St. Louis, MO: Mosby–Year Book.

Moorhead, S., Johnson, M., Maas, M., & Swanson, E. (2007). *Nursing Outcomes Classification* (NOC) (4th ed.). St. Louis, MO: Elsevier-Health Sciences Division.

Murray, S., McKinney, E., & Gorrie, T. (2002). *Foundations of maternal–newborn nursing* (3rd ed.). Philadelphia: W. B. Saunders.

North American Nursing Diagnosis Association International. (2010). *NANDA-I nursing diagnoses: Definitions and classification 2009–2011.* Ames, IA: Wiley-Blackwell.

Pasero, C. (2001). Circumcision requires anesthesia and analgesia. *American Journal of Nursing, 101*(9), 22–23.

Penny-MacGillivray, T. (1996). A newborn's first bath: When. *JOGNN, 25*(6), 481.

Queenan, J. (2001). Positional plagiocephaly (flattened head). Retrieved from: http://kidshealth.org/parent/general/ sleep/positional _plagiocephaly.html.

Reifsnider, E., & Gill, S. (2000). Nutrition for the childbearing years. *JOGNN, 29*(1), 43–55.

Schneiderman, J. (1996). Postpartum nursing for Korean mothers. *MCN, 21*(3), 155–158.

Sharts-Hopko, N. (1995). Birth in the Japanese context. *JOGNN, 24*(4), 343–351.

Simpson, K., & Creehan, P. (2007). *AWHONN perinatal nursing* (3rd ed.). Philadelphia: Lippincott Williams & Wilkins.

Swayze, S. (1999). Clamping down on circumcision. *Nursing99, 29*(9), 73.

Task Force on Sudden Infant Death Syndrome. (2005). *Pediatrics, 116*(5), 1245–1255.

Thoyre, S. (2003). Technique for feeding preterm infants. *AJN, 103*(9), 69–73.

Tiedje, L., Schiffman, R., Omar, M., Wright, J., Buzzitta, C., McCann, A., & Metzger, S. (2002). An ecological approach to breastfeeding. *MCN, 27*(3), 154–161.

Varda, K., & Behnke, R. (2000). The effect of timing of initial bath on newborn's temperature. *JOGNN, 29*(1), 27–32.

Verma, R. (1995). Respiratory distress syndrome of the newborn infant. *Obstetric Gynecologic Survey, 50*(7), 542.

Workman, E. (2001). Guiding parents through the death of their infant. JOGNN, 30(6), 569–573.

York, R., Bhuttarowas, P., & Brown, L. (1999). The development of nursing in Thailand. *MCN, 24*(3), 145–150.

RESOURCES

Association of Women's Health, Obstetric and Neonatal Nurses AWHONN, http://www.awhonn.org

International Lactation Consultant Association (ILCA), http://www.ilca.org

LaLeche League International, http://www.llli.org

Women, Infants, and Children (WIC), http://www.fns.usda.gov/wic

UNIT 20 Nursing Care of the Client: Childrearing

CHAPTER 59
Basics of Pediatric Care

MAKING THE CONNECTION

Refer to the following chapters to increase your understanding of pediatric care:

Basic Nursing
- ***Legal and Ethical Responsibilities***
- ***Life Span Development***
- ***Cultural Considerations***
- ***End-of-Life Care***
- ***Wellness Concepts***
- ***Medication Administration and IV Therapy***
- ***Pain Management***

Adult Health Nursing
- ***Anesthesia***
- ***Surgery***

Maternal & Pediatric Nursing
- ***Infants with Special Needs: Birth to 12 Months***
- ***Common Problems: 1 to 18 Years***

LEARNING OBJECTIVES

Upon completion of this chapter, you should be able to:

- Define key terms.
- Discuss the role of the nurse in preparing a child and family for hospitalization.
- Explain the role of the nurse in admission and discharge of the pediatric client.
- Prepare children at different developmental stages for procedures.
- Discuss various methods for assessing basic needs and planning daily care.
- Safely perform supportive pediatric procedures.
- Identify the child's concept of death at various developmental stages.
- Describe common responses (child, family, siblings, nurses) to a dying child.
- Discuss sources of support for the dying child.

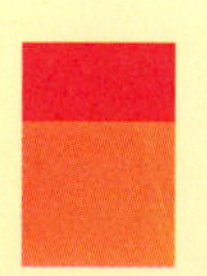

KEY TERMS

assent
child life specialist
emancipated minor
family-centered care
rooming-in

INTRODUCTION

Nursing care of children centers on promoting, maintaining, and restoring the health of the child and family. While families are very important to all clients in the health-care area, caregivers are essential to the care and nurturing of the pediatric client. For this reason, when providing care to children, inclusion of the family is essential. **Family-centered care** recognizes the family as the constant in a child's life. Family-centered care describes a philosophy of care recognizing the centrality of the family in the child's life and including the family's contribution and involvement in the plan of care and its delivery. An additional factor that impacts the health care of children is their rapidly evolving growth and development.

Children differ from adults in their physical, emotional, and cognitive responses. Physical, emotional, and cognitive immaturity affects the child's response to comprehension of and reaction to illness or injury. For that reason, a child's developmental level always is assessed and care plans based on that level. Nursing care of children covers the neonatal period (birth to 28 days), infancy (1 month to 1 year), toddlerhood (12 months to 3 years), preschool age (3 to 6 years), school age (6 to 10 years), preadolescence (10 to 12 years), and adolescence (13 to 20 years). For more detailed information on physical, emotional, cognitive, and moral development, refer to the lifespan development chapter.

Trends in health care, leading to shorter hospital stays, provision of care in the home, outpatient surgery, and managed care, have changed the settings in which children and their caregivers receive care. These settings include the home, school-based and outpatient clinics, 24-hour observation and outpatient surgery areas, emergency rooms, rehabilitative care, hospitals, and intensive care units. Nurses must be able to rapidly assess, plan, implement, and evaluate care in these diverse settings.

Although any illness of a child is a major stressor for a family, it can also result in a positive experience. Nurses can maximize the client/family/nurse contact by fostering parent–child relationships, providing educational opportunities, promoting self-mastery, and providing socialization.

This chapter discusses preparing the child and family for hospitalization, pediatric procedures, and dealing with the dying child.

PREPARING THE CHILD AND FAMILY FOR HOSPITALIZATION

Foremost in the preparation of children for hospitalization on any unit is preparing the family. If the family is well informed about and understands the child's illness, confidence in their medical recommendations, and the support of understanding nurses, then they are more likely to be able to assist in preparing the child for the hospital experience. Hospitalization may be planned or unexpected. When the hospitalization is planned, the caregivers and child have time to prepare for the event. Many hospitals and agencies concerned with the care of the young child provide age-appropriate materials to assist caregivers and children to prepare for the experience of hospitalization. These materials include tours of the hospital with dress-up in surgical attire and playing with equipment, photographs and videotapes, health fairs to explain procedures, and books and films to explain in age-appropriate terms of what to expect. Adolescents require different approaches in preparation for hospitalization; they not only learn from written materials, models, and films but also benefit from peers who have experienced the same procedures. Allowing them to ask questions of health-care workers without their caregivers being present is also beneficial.

When hospitalization is unexpected, it is of utmost importance that children be given opportunities to explore their new surroundings and encouraged to view hospitalization as an adventure that they can handle. The nurse treats all children and their caregivers with respect, listening attentively, with an open-mind, in a nonjudgmental way.

Many hospitals have **child life specialists**, who are health-care professionals with extensive knowledge of psychology and early childhood development, trained to prepare the child and caregivers for hospitalization, surgery, and procedures. Their goals include maintaining normalcy, minimizing psychological trauma, and promoting optimal development of the child and family. A collaborative effort between the nurse, the child life specialist, and other health-care providers ensures the best possible hospital experience for the child and family.

Many hospitals provide various educational programs such as an open house for well children and preadmission orientation. These programs are designed to orient the child and family to the environment and procedures and may incorporate such learning activities as audiovisuals, art, puppets, tours, and role-play.

The preparation of the child and family should be guided by consideration of the child's developmental level. Caregivers of infants and toddlers must be reassured of their important role as primary care providers, even during hospitalization (Figure 59-1). Caregivers are encouraged to make the necessary arrangements that will allow them to room-in with the hospitalized child. **Rooming-in** is the practice of staying with a hospitalized client (child) 24 hours a day to provide care and comfort to that child. It may also be the method of choice when caregivers need to learn and practice specialized treatments that they will be performing at home for the child.

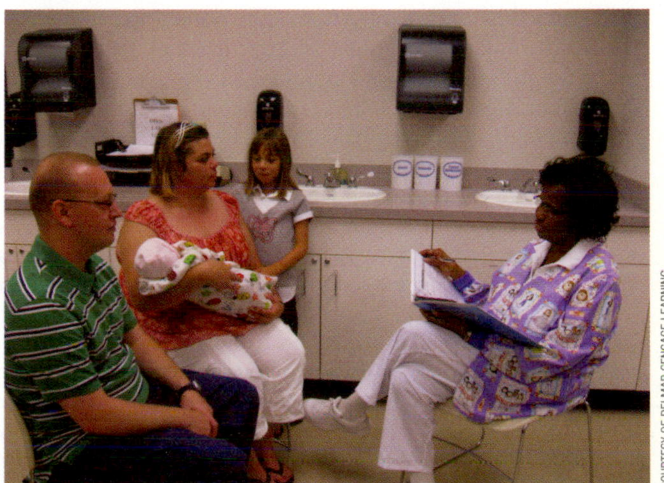

COURTESY OF DELMAR CENGAGE LEARNING

FIGURE 59-1 The nurse helps prepare the caregivers for an infant's hospitalization.

CLIENT TEACHING

Sample Teaching Materials for Children Requiring Hospitalization

Videotapes

- *Special kids, special dads: Fathers of children with disabilities* (James May, Video), Association for the Care of Children's Health.
- *Super asthma kids: We take control* (Through Our Eyes Productions, Video), Association for the Care of Children's Health.
- *Operation sneek-a-peek.* (Donna Kaufman, video). Aquarius Health Care Videos.

Books

- *Becky's Story*. Baznick, Donna. Association for the Care of Children's Health.
- *Curious George goes to the hospital.* M. Rey & H.A. Rey. Houghton Mifflin Company.
- *The moon balloon*. Drescher, J. Association for the Care of Children's Health.
- *Fuzzy and Frankie*. Murray, S. Association for the Care of Children's Health.

Booklets

- *Your child in the hospital: A practical guide for caregivers* (2nd ed.). N. Keene & R. Prentice, 2004. Parent Center Guides.

Admission

In the past, most care provided to ill children was in the hospital setting. The current trend is to use community-based areas such as clinics, free-standing surgical units, schools, and the home. Children admitted to the hospital are more acutely ill, yet the time spent in the facility often is shorter. Nursing's role in the care of pediatric clients is changing and expanding. In planning care for children, prevention is a key component as well as teaching for the child and family. The nurse is frequently the first person who sees the child and family when they enter the health-care system. The nurse's ability to assess the child and family for physical, psychosocial, cultural, spiritual, and growth and developmental factors sets the stage for the plan of care.

The plan of care begins with admission to the health care facility. The completion of admission information includes previous data regarding the child and family as well as information regarding peers and play patterns, eating patterns, sleeping patterns, school history, normal activity patterns, fears, comfort measures, habits, primary language spoken, language development and level of understanding, usual reaction to pain, special routines, and perception of caregivers regarding prior or present hospitalizations. In addition, an assessment of basic needs and daily care planning information is obtained. Most healthcare facilities have policies and procedures for admission. Many institutions have a form for caregivers to complete regarding the child's routines, previous illnesses, current medications, and specific adaptations needed for the child and family. This form is usually signed by the parent and kept in the medical record. Although the agency may have a set policy for admission, the routine may need to be altered based on the needs of the child and family. For example, a fearful child in pain may need to have pain medication and support before being interviewed. Always focus on the needs of the client and family in order to support and assist in mobilizing coping mechanisms rather than data gathering.

The initial assessment determines the need for immediate care. After the family and child are made comfortable or stabilized, a more thorough physical assessment and health history is obtained. The standard data collected are history of the client, allergies, nutritional intake, sleep, elimination, psychosocial information, spiritual and cultural factors, and the initial physical assessment. Data collected at the time of admission are used to identify nursing diagnoses and to establish a plan of care; these are placed in the child's medical record. Figure 59-2 shows an example of a pediatric admission form.

Many agencies have standardized care plans based on the most common problems identified by the assessment. These care plans are also placed on the medical records and are the basis of care. In addition to standardized care plans, many agencies are developing clinical paths or care paths for specific disease states. These tools assist the health care providers in giving care based on protocols that result in more rapid recovery, prevention of complications, reduction of length of stay, and cost-containing care for the client and family.

Protection/Safety

Situations may arise during hospitalization that may jeopardize the safety and well-being of the child. Be ever mindful of who has custody of the child, and screen visitors if there are threats to the child's safety. Issues of custody, disputes among family members, and kidnapping of children are no longer remote problems for hospital personnel. Security measures have been put in place on pediatric units with visible identification of caregivers, approved visitors, and personnel. Many units utilize electronic surveillance for visitors and monitoring devices for hospitalized children.

Informed consent of the legal guardian is obtained at the time of admission for general treatment, including procedures such as IV insertions, specimen collection, and medication and oxygen administration. Separate informed consents of the legal guardian must be obtained for procedures such as lumbar punctures, chest tube insertion, and bone marrow aspirations. Federal guidelines state that children older than 7 years of age have the right to give **assent** (the child's voluntary agreement to participate in a research project or to accept treatment) for treatment and research procedures. In most states, clients older than 18 years of age can legally give informed consent. In addition, most states allow some exceptions for parental consent in cases involving emancipated minors. An **emancipated minor** is a child who has the legal competency of an adult because of circumstances involving marriage, divorce, parenting a child, living independently without caregivers, or enlistment in the armed services.

Choking and falls are also areas of concern with hospitalized children. To avoid choking, the environment must be free of objects that could be placed in the mouth and possibly occlude the airway (e.g., broken balloons, syringe caps, toys, food). An adult should always be present when a young child

ADMISSION FORM PART 1 OF 2
PARENT / PATIENT INFORMATION

Dear Parent,
We want to work with you to individually plan the care which your child will receive. You can help us by completing this form. The information will help us learn about your child's illness or condition and about his/her general health. If you have any questions or if you do not want to answer any or all of the questions, please return the form to the nurse. Your nurse will review your answers and together we will develop a plan for your child's care.
Thank you for your cooperation.

The DCH Nursing Staff

GENERAL INFORMATION

Primary language ______ Interpreter ______
Where will you be staying during your child's hospitalization? ______
Whom should we call in case of emergency, NAME: ______ RELATIONSHIP: ______
in case you are not available: Phone, days ______ Phone, nights ______
What do you expect to happen during this hospitalization? ______
What childhood disease has your child had? ☐ measles; ☐ chicken pox; ☐ mumps; ☐ rubella;
Has your child been exposed to any of these within the past two weeks? ☐ Yes ☐ No
Do you have child's **immunization** card? ☐ Yes ☐ No
Are your child's **immunizations** current? ☐ Yes ☐ No Check those which your child has had.
DPT ☐ 2 mo. ☐ 4 mo. ☐ 6 mo. ☐ 15 mo. ☐ 4-6 yrs. OPV ☐ 2 mo. ☐ 4 mo. ☐ 15-18 mo. ☐ 4-6 yrs
HIB ☐ 2 mo. ☐ 4 mo. ☐ 6 mo. ☐ 12-15 mo. MMR ☐ 15 mo. ☐ 11-12 yrs
Td ☐ 14-16 yrs. Hepatitis ☐ Birth ☐ 1-2 mo. ☐ 6-18 mo.
What is your child's grade in school? ______ TB Skin Test ______ Boosters ______
(Patient only) Do you...smoke? ☐ No ☐ Yes... ______ packs/day ...use alcohol? ☐ No ☐ Yes... ______
Previous hospitalization ______
Where? ______ Why? ______

Parent/Guardian: present ☐ Not available ☐ Telephone interview ☐

DISCHARGE PLANNING INFORMATION

Have you been receiving help from any agencies? ☐ Yes ☐ No
☐ Home Health ☐ Visiting Nurse ☐ WIC ☐ AFDC ☐ CIDCS ☐ Early Childhood Intervention
If you need help with your child at home, who can assist you? ______
Does your child require any special equipment or supplies in his/her daily home care? ☐ Yes ☐ No
(apnea monitor, oxygen, suction, etc....) ______
What information do you need regarding your child's illness and/or hospitalization? ______

IF YOU NEED HELP ARRANGING FOR POSTHOSPITAL SERVICES INFORM YOUR PHYSICIAN OR NURSE THAT YOU WOULD LIKE TO TALK TO A PROFESSIONAL STAFF MEMBER WHO HANDLES DISCHARGE PLANNING.

MEDICATION HISTORY

In this section, please list for each medication your child takes, the dose, how often taken, the time of the last dose, and you/your child's understanding of the reason the drug has been prescribed. If there are problems taking the drug, please describe those also. While your child is in the hospital, ALL medications will be provided. If you have brought medications with you, please do not leave them. Please take them home. Thank you.

Medication	Dose	Frequency	Last Taken	Purpose/Problems Taking

Allergies: Not known ☐ Medications ______ Foods ______ Other: ______

DRISCOLL CHILDREN'S HOSPITAL
CHILDREN'S MEDICAL CENTER OF SOUTH TEXAS

ADMISSION ASSESSMENT

For the following questions, please check your answer – yes or no – and use the space provided to describe or provide more information.

NUTRITIONAL METABOLIC

YES NO
☐ ☐ Use a pacifier, bottle, cup, special nipple, feeding tube? ______
Type of diet? ______
☐ ☐ Take formula? Type ______ Amount? ______ How often? ______
☐ ☐ Has your child had any recent weight change? Loss ______ Gain ______
☐ ☐ Any changes in appetite or thirst? ______
☐ ☐ Any difficulties with eating, or swallowing food? ______
☐ ☐ When did child last eat or drink? ______

ELIMINATION

☐ ☐ Is child potty trained? Special words ______
☐ ☐ Diapers? Type ______ Size ______
☐ ☐ Has your child experienced any changes or difficulties with urination? ______
☐ ☐ Does your child have a history of bed wetting? ______
☐ ☐ Does your child often have diarrhea or constipation? ______
☐ ☐ Are laxatives or other aids used for regularity? ______

ACTIVITY EXERCISE

☐ ☐ Does your child have preferred play activities? ______
☐ ☐ Does your child tire easily with play? ______
☐ ☐ Does your child have appliances or need assistance for walking or mobility? (walker, wheelchair) ______
Briefly describe your child's usual daily routine: ______

COGNITIVE-PERCEPTUAL

YES NO
☐ ☐ Does your child have any difficulty hearing? Use a hearing aid? ______ Type: ______
☐ ☐ Does your child have any difficulty seeing/ When were the eyes last checked? ______ Wear glasses? ______
☐ ☐ Does your child sometimes have difficulty learning? ______
What is the easiest way for him/her to learn? (books, film watching, demonstrations) ______
What do you do special to comfort your child when having pain/discomfort? ______

COPING-STRESS

☐ ☐ Are there any recent changes in family life that may affect this hospitalization? ______
☐ ☐ How have your child/you and your family responded to these changes? ______
☐ ☐ Are there other children in family? ______ Ages ______
☐ ☐ Do you have family or friends in the Corpus Christi area? ______
Whom do you define as your family or support system? ______
☐ ☐ Being in the hospital is stressful for many people. Is there anything we can do to make it easier for you or for your child?

ORIENTED TO
☐ Phone; ☐ Bed; ☐ Call light/Intercom; ☐ Parent bed/regulations (Recliners up by 8 a.m.) ☐ Patient Rights & Responsibilities
☐ Playroom; ☐ Mealtimes; ☐ Smoking policy; ☐ IV, VS routine, a.m. wts. ☐ Visitation Limits/hrs. ☐ Intake & Output Monitored
☐ Care of valuables; ☐ Side rails; ☐ TV; ☐ Isolation; ☐ ID Band ☐ Car seat for discharge ☐ Save diapers
☐ Bear Questionnaires ☐ No electrical appliances
Oriented by: ______

Parent Signature: ______ Date: ______ Time: ______

FIGURE 59-2 Pediatric Admission Form (*Courtesy of Driscoll Children's Hospital, Corpus Christi, TX.*)

(*Continues*)

ADMISSION FORM PART 2 OF 2

TO BE COMPLETED BY ADMITTING NURSE. Attn. Physician/Time Notified ________ by ____

Arrival to RM ________ Date ________ Time ________ Resident ________ by ____

Brief History ________

GENERAL APPEARANCE: ________

NEUROLOGICAL: Responds to: ☐ Verbal ☐ Pain ☐ Nonresponsive

Gait: ☐ N/A ☐ Walks ☐ Unable to stand ☐ Uncoordinated LOC: ☐ Lethargic ☐ Semi-Comatose ☐ Comatose ☐ Alert

Movement: ☐ Coordinated ☐ Voluntary ☐ Involuntary; Speech ________ Head Circ ____

Anterior Fontanel ________

Seizures ________ Pupil Scale: (mm) 1 2 3 4 5 6 7 8

Developmental level: ________

CARDIO VASCULAR: HR ____

Apical pulse: rhythm ________ Peripheral pulses: RA ____ RL ____ LA ____ LL ____ BP ____

Clubbing: ________ Nailbed Color ________ Capillary Refill ________

Comments: ________

RESPIRATORY: ________ Temp. ____

Breath Sounds: ☐ Clear ☐ Crackles ☐ Wheezing ☐ Coarse ☐ Diminished ________ RR ____

Retractions: ☐ None ☐ Substernal ☐ Intercostal ☐ Subcostal ________ Chest Circ ____

Effort: ☐ Shallow ☐ Deep ☐ Labored ☐ Unlabored; Cough ________ Sputum ________

Chest Symmetry ________ Comments: ________

GASTRO-INTESTINAL:

Abdomen: ☐ Soft ☐ Tender ☐ Nontender ☐ Rigid ☐ Distended; Last B.M. ________ Wt ____

Bowel Sounds: ☐ Active ☐ Hyperactive ☐ Hypoactive; Appetite ________ Ht ____

Tubes: ☐ OG ☐ NG ☐ GT ☐ JT ________ Abd girth ____

Comments: ________

GYNECOLOGICAL: ☐ No abnormalities reported ☐ Sexually active; LMP ________

Discharge ________ Lesions ________ Comments: ________

GENITOURINARY: Urine color ________ Amt. ____ Odor ____ Discharge ________

Incontinent ________ Last void ________

Comments: ________

MUSCULO-SKELETAL:

☐ Moves all extremities ☐ Limited ROM; Swelling ________

Contractures ________ Edema ________ Prosthetic devices ________

Comments: ________

INTEGUMENTARY: (on figure in box, note location of any items with the appropriate letter and check the box by the letter)

☐ Skin intact ☐ Warm ☐ Cool ☐ Cold ☐ Moist ☐ Dry; Color: ☐ Pale ☐ Pink ☐ Jaundiced ☐ Cyanotic ☐ Mottled

Turgor ________ Masses/Size ________ IV site, condition, fluids ________

Wounds/Dressings ________

Comments: ________

☐ B - Bruise
☐ D - Decubitus
☐ L - Laceration
☐ R - Rash
☐ S - Scar

Nursing Process/Plan of care initiated ________ Nurse initials

Allergies: Not Known ________ Medications ________

Foods ________ Environmental ________

R.N. ________ Date/Time ________

FIGURE 59-2 *Continued*

is eating. Other safety concerns in the hospital setting include machinery (e.g., IV pumps and equipment, needles). Doors to treatment rooms, staircases, supply closets, and rooms containing extra equipment need to be equipped with locks preventing access by children.

Side rails on cribs must be up at all times. If a toddler is able to climb over the rails, a safety cover is placed over the crib, or a regular bed is used. Never turn your back to a child or reach for materials when the side rail is down if the child is not properly secured.

Pediatric Clients Experiencing Surgery

The child and family experience with surgery may be an elective procedure, planned in advance, or the result of an emergency with little time for planning. When possible, preadmission visits are an excellent way to prepare the child and family for surgery. Sessions are scheduled within the week before admission. Table 59-1 contains suggestions for hospital preparation and surgery that are appropriate for planned procedures. As with any preparation, a multidisciplinary approach that includes caregivers, nursing staff, child

PROFESSIONALTIP

ID Bands

It is very important for all clients to have a hospital identification (ID) band on at all times (Figure 59-3). It is equally important that all health-care providers check the band for proper client identification before performing any procedure. The nurse replaces an ID band on any child that does not have a band before performing treatments.

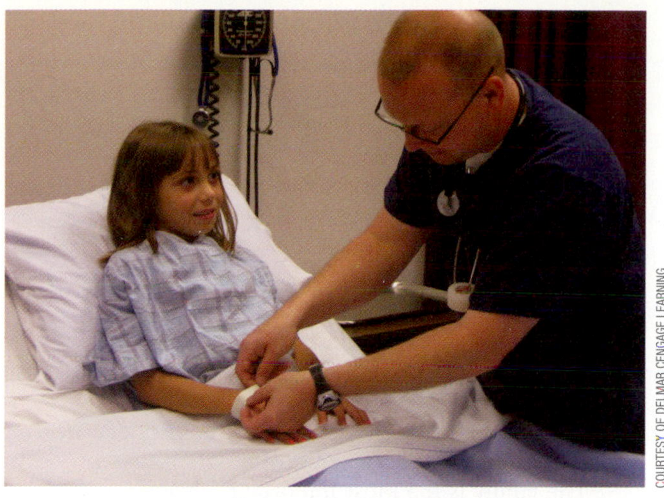

COURTESY OF DELMAR CENGAGE LEARNING

FIGURE 59-3 All hospitalized children will have an ID band.

life specialists, medical staff, and other involved professionals is best.

Preparation for surgery includes both psychosocial and physical preparation. The purpose of preoperative preparation is to reduce fear and anxiety associated with the surgical procedure and the surrounding environment. Play can facilitate preparation for hospitalization. Visits to units before the experience can familiarize the child and family with sights, sounds, smells, and equipment. Anatomically correct dolls and puppets, drawings, and models can be used to teach the child and family about the procedures. Through play, the child experiences the use of equipment to take vital signs and become familiar with other health-care interventions.

The nurse reassures the child that she will be transported to the operating room accompanied by caregivers and that her caregivers will be there when she wakes up. Inform caregivers of the expected length of the surgery and inform them of the child's status throughout the procedure. The child and caregivers feel more secure if one nurse is designated to be the contact before, during, and after surgery.

Many hospitals and surgical units allow and encourage caregivers to be present during anesthesia induction. The presence of caregivers and familiar objects such as blankets and toys in the presurgical area decreases the child's and caregivers' anxiety. Decreased anxiety lessens the need for premedication for the child. Some common induction techniques for young children include concealing the breathing circuit in a play phone, behind a pacifier, or within a stuffed animal, and providing a choice of flavored gases (e.g., watermelon, grape, chocolate).

TABLE 59-1 Nursing Responsibilities to the Child Having Surgery

PREPARATION FOR SURGERY	AGE CONSIDERATIONS
Psychological	
Explain surgery.	*Infant:* Allow infant to remain on caregiver's lap as long as possible.
Prepare for separation from family.	*Toddler:* Use dolls, puppets, play hospital.
Conduct preadmission visit.	*Preschooler:* Use books, videos, art. Assure toddlers and preschoolers that the surgery is not their fault and is not a punishment.
	School-age Child: Offer brief explanations with supporting visuals.
	Adolescent: Involve in the procedure planning and decision making.
Physical	
Discontinue food and drink after specified time.	*Infant:* Explain to caregivers only.
Monitor fluid level (child has less fluid within body and can become dehydrated quickly).	*Toddler:* Explain 3 days in advance.
Perform specific preparation for procedure.	*Preschooler:* Prepare formally no more than 1 week in advance.
Ensure that consent form is signed by guardian.	*School-age Child:* Videos and tours.
Administer preoperative medication.	*Adolescent:* Provide detailed information and encourage questioning.
Postoperative Care	
Make preparations for return of child.	*Infant:* Maintain body warmth. Monitor intake and output.
Obtain vital signs.	*Toddler and Preschooler:* Give favorite animal or try to provide comfort.
Assess pain level.	*School-age Child:* Ask about comfort and preferred distraction activities.
Inspect operative site.	*All children:* Presence of caregivers on return to postoperative area and in child's room is important. Know the manifestations of pain and medicate as needed.
Check dressings for bleeding or other drainage.	*Adolescent:* Provide privacy
Check bowel and bladder function.	
Observe for signs of shock, dehydration, infection.	

COURTESY OF DELMAR CENGAGE LEARNING

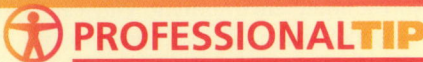

PROFESSIONALTIP

Emancipated Minor

Emancipation laws vary from state to state, with some states not officially recognizing any form of emancipation.

During the postoperative period, the child is monitored for bleeding, pain level, and pulmonary and circulatory status. When the child awakens, it is important that the caregivers be present to calm and comfort the child. Comfort objects from home such as favorite toys may assist the child in feeling at ease. Use pain medication as necessary. Most health-care facilities have instructions to follow for general and specific surgical procedures.

The child may be discharged home or admitted to an inpatient unit for further care. Because children recuperate more quickly in a familiar environment, they are discharged as soon as is safely possible following surgery. Discharge planning ideally is initiated at admission. The ability of the caregivers to provide adequate care at home determines the extent of education provided before discharge and the involvement of a home health agency after discharge.

Discharge/Discharge Planning

Use a multidisciplinary approach that includes the social service department, home care agencies, rehabilitation therapists, and the family to plan for equipment, procedures, and other home care needs. Discharge plans begin with admission of the child. Many agencies have a discharge planning nurse who coordinates the plans for home care. The nurse working with the client and family takes part in the planning and communicates frequently with the discharge nurse regarding information about the client and family.

Make the caregivers aware that behavioral changes often occur after hospitalization. These changes are most evident in children 6 months to 6 years of age. The changes may include fear or anxiety about sleeping and separation, regression, withdrawal, aggression, and demanding behavior.

Assessment of the family's ability to manage the child's care and the ability of the home environment to support the care needed by the child is important. Early planning gives the health-care providers and family time to investigate financial support by agencies such as Medicaid and private insurance. If the child is school-aged, involve the school district to plan for continued education. This may require special assessment by the school system and a plan of educational care developed to include home tutors, specialized services such as speech therapists and occupational therapists, and/or transportation to school with specialized medical care delivered at the school.

Caregivers may need to learn special or rehabilitative procedures for the child's care. Demonstrate, explain, and observe as the caregivers assume the care they will be responsible for at home. The education provided and the caregivers' ability to perform care are discussed with the public health nurse, home health nurse, or individual who will be managing the home care program. Assist caregivers in exploring options for relief from the child's care, such as respite care, relatives, church groups, or lists of caregivers with ability to give specialized care.

COMMUNITY/HOME HEALTH CARE

Tips for Discharge

- Assess needs and resources.
- Plan for comprehensive care.
- Provide clear, concise written instructions.
- Link client with service provider.
- Coordinate services.
- Advocate for appropriate services.

The family is the most important advocate and spokesperson for the child. When a child needs long-term care, the family will need the services of many agencies and numerous health-care personnel. To coordinate health care and to prevent gaps and overlaps, one person is identified as the case manager. The parent may decide to act as the child's case manager with support and education from discharge planners.

Discharge documentation includes the condition and behavior at discharge, instructions given to caretaker, the mode of transportation, time of discharge, and who accompanied the child.

PEDIATRIC PROCEDURES

In preparing the child and family for procedures performed either at home or in an agency, consider the child's growth and development, cognitive abilities, and physical and psychosocial factors. The nurse performs the procedures effectively and efficiently with the least amount of discomfort to the client and family. The following procedures are common to the care of children. While they are similar to procedures performed on adults, they also may differ in several ways. Be knowledgeable about variations in preparation, equipment, positioning, and specific steps when performing procedures on children.

Physical Assessment

Physical assessments for the child are similar to those for the adult with a few differences. Measurements of physical size are significant in evaluating a child's health status. Deviation from the established norms may indicate a significant health problem.

Growth Measurements

Growth measurements for children are recorded at each well-child visit as well as visits for disease episodes. Take

CRITICAL THINKING

Preoperative Plan

Prepare a preoperative plan for a 3-year-old Hispanic male client undergoing surgery for an inguinal hernia. What developmental, cultural, and physiological considerations for the child and his family should be included?

measurements correctly and accurately. Values for growth parameters are placed on percentile charts and evaluated with those of the general population. In general, percentiles from 5% to 95% are considered within normal ranges. All growth evaluations take into consideration a child's genetic predisposition. As well as genetic concerns, ethnic and socioeconomic background may influence growth norms. It is unknown whether the differences within the ethnic and socioeconomic backgrounds are from the cultural norms or the result of nutritional differences.

The growth charts most commonly used in the United States are those from the National Center for Health Statistics (NCHS) and are available for boys and girls of different ages. There are growth charts available for children 2 to 3 based on whether their height is measured in a lying or standing position. Lying position is referred to as recumbent, and height while standing is referred to as stature. Most children younger than age 2 are measured in a recumbent position, and children older than 2 are measured in a standing position.

Children Younger Than Two Years of Age Growth measurements for children younger than 2 differ in the procedure and types of measurements taken. Typical measurements taken for the child younger than 2 are length; weight; and head, chest, and abdominal circumferences.

Length Measurement of length is taken with the child in a supine position. The method for children younger than 2 is as follows:

1. Use a paper sheet to lay the infant in a recumbent (lying down) position. Extend the infant's body.
2. Ensure that the infant's head is in midline and legs are extended. Gently grasp knees and push toward table to fully extend legs (Figure 59-4).
3. Place a mark on the paper at the crown of the infant's head.
4. Extend the leg and place a mark on the paper at the base of the heel (toes pointing upward).
5. If a measuring board is used, place the infant's head against the board and extend the legs, placing the heels of the feet on the footboard.
6. Measure the distance between the two marks or on the measuring board.
7. Record the length.

Weight Infants are weighed on a platform scale. They may be placed in either a sitting or supine position, depending on their ability to sit unsupported. Before weighing the infant, make sure the scale is cleaned, a paper cover is placed on the

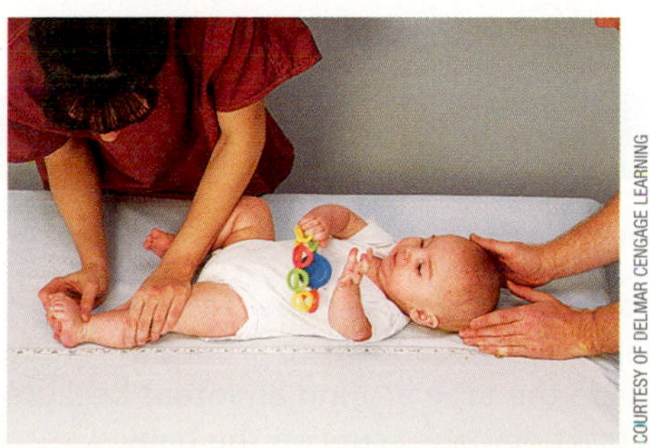
COURTESY OF DELMAR CENGAGE LEARNING

FIGURE 59-4 Measuring Recumbent Length of an Infant

PROFESSIONALTIP

General Instructions for All Pediatric Procedures

Preprocedure

Check physician's orders.
Review procedure in agency procedure manual.
Gather equipment and assistance if necessary.
Introduce yourself and assistants to child and caregivers.
Identify child by name band or approved identification method.
Give instructions and explanation to the child and parent and ask if there are any questions.
If parent is going to hold child, demonstrate exactly what you want done. Make sure the parent feels secure about assisting with the procedure. Make sure you know the agency policy regarding caregivers assisting with procedures by holding the child.
Wash your hands.
Don protective clothing if necessary.

During the Procedure

Maintain privacy.
Tell the child exactly what is expected of her, never threaten or tell a child you will have to "hold him/her down."
Have someone assist you if necessary and if it will facilitate the procedure being completed more quickly.
Maintain a conversation with parent and child, explaining what you are doing, in a calm soothing voice.
Keep the child and parent informed of the procedure's progress.
Tell the child when the procedure is nearly complete.

Support of Child and Family

Offer ways of coping with pain or discomfort (imagery, music). Give permission to cry.
Use developmentally appropriate words.
Give child as much choice over the procedure as possible.

PROFESSIONALTIP

Growth

Growth is a continuous and uneven process, and the most important point for monitoring the growth of children is comparison over time.

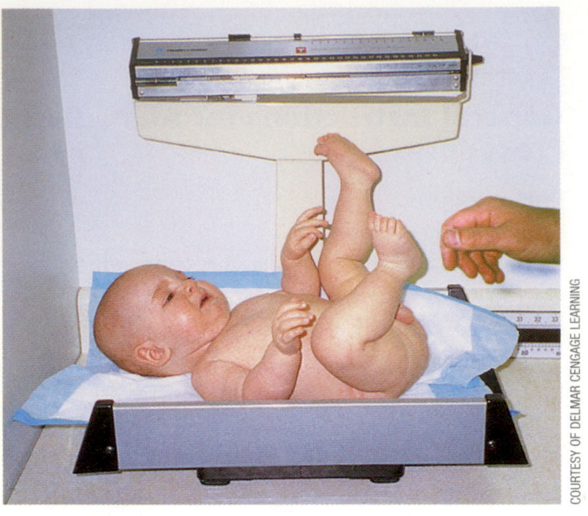

COURTESY OF DELMAR CENGAGE LEARNING

FIGURE 59-5 Measuring Weight of an Infant

scale, and the room is warm. The nurse balances the scale before weighing the infant. The method for weighing is as follows:

1. Place the nude child on the scale, making sure never to turn your back to the child on the scale. Hold your hand over the infant but do not touch the infant while obtaining the weight (Figure 59-5).
2. Measure to the nearest 10 grams or 2 ounces and record the weight.

Head Circumference During the first year or two of life, head circumference is measured as an important indication of brain growth. The method for obtaining head circumference is as follows:

1. Measure the head at its greatest circumference.
2. Wrap a measuring tape around the infant's head, placing it above the brows, the pinna of the ears, and around the occipital prominence. Make sure the tape is flat against the skin.
3. Record the circumference.

Chest Circumference The chest circumference is often measured during the first year of life as an indicator of adequate growth. During the first year, head circumference is greater than chest circumference; after age 1, chest circumference exceeds head circumference. The method for obtaining chest circumference is as follows:

1. Measure the chest at its greatest circumference.
2. Wrap a measuring tape around the infant's chest, placing it under the axilla and over the nipple line (Figure 59-6).
3. Measure between inspiration and expiration.
4. Record the circumference.

Abdominal Circumference The abdominal circumference is obtained on very young or preterm infants to detect abdominal distention. The method for measuring abdominal circumference is as follows:

1. Measure the abdomen at its point of greatest girth.
2. Place a paper tape around the infant's abdomen at the umbilicus.
3. Record the circumference.

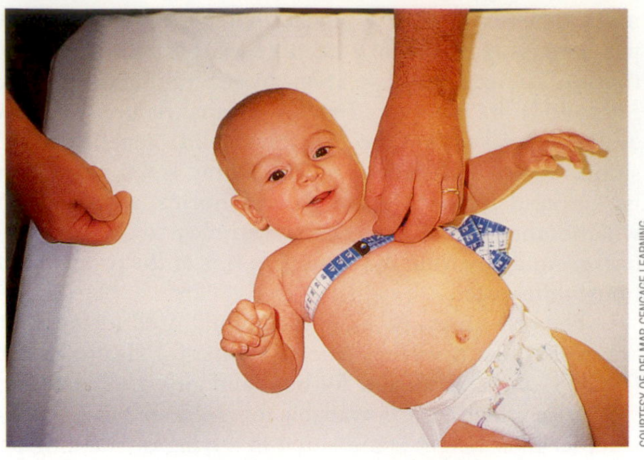

COURTESY OF DELMAR CENGAGE LEARNING

FIGURE 59-6 Measuring Chest Circumference of an Infant

Children Older Than Two Years of Age Typical measurements taken on children older than 2 years of age include height and weight.

Height After the age of 2 or 3, height is measured with the child standing upright. Remove the child's shoes before the measurement is taken, and have the child stand upright, with the back to the wall or scale. Ask the child to stand very straight with head in midline and shoulders, buttocks, and heels touching the wall or the attachment to a balance scale. The method for measuring height is as follows:

1. On the balance scale, lower the ruler device until it touches the top of the child's head (Figure 59-7).
   Take the measurement.
2. If measuring the child against a wall, place a flat edge such as a ruler on top of the child's head. Make a mark on the wall; measure from the floor to the mark.
3. Record the height.

Weight After a child can stand and balance well, weight is taken on a standing scale. Standing scales are digital or balance. Remove shoes for all children. Toddlers are weighed in their underclothes, older children are weighed in street clothes with heavy jackets removed. The method for weighing is as follows:

1. Keep the room warm and ensure privacy.
2. Balance the scale before asking the child to step on it.
3. Place child in center of scale and, with a balance scale, move the weights until the scale is balanced.
4. On digital scale, have child stand in center of scale and take reading.
5. Measure to the nearest 100 grams or 1/4 pound and record the weight.

SAFETY

Paper Tape Measures

Use care when placing paper tape measures. Place under the infant and wrap around carefully. Do not slide the tape around an infant because this may result in paper cuts on the baby.

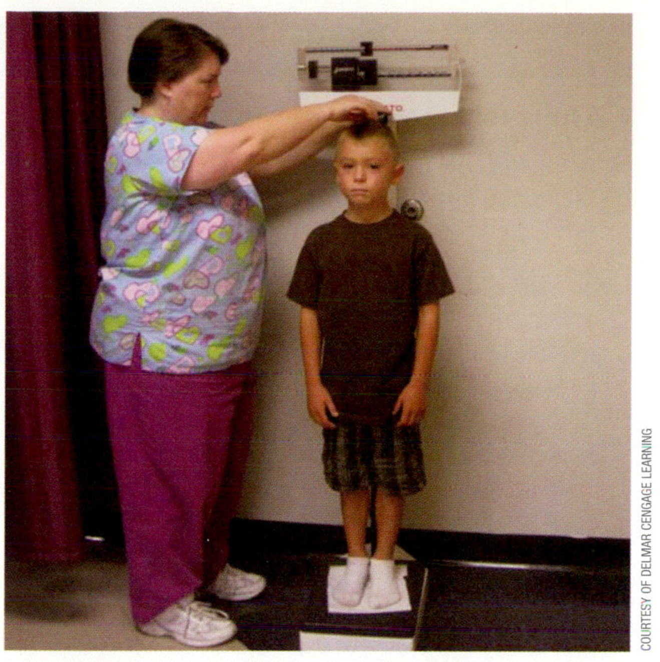
COURTESY OF DELMAR CENGAGE LEARNING

FIGURE 59-7 Measuring Height of a Child

Vital Signs

Assessment of vital signs (temperature, pulse, respiratory rate, and blood pressure) is an important method for measuring and monitoring vital body functioning. In children, vital signs may change quickly and will provide the basis for decisions regarding care. Table 59-2 describes normal vital signs by age.

Body Temperature Temperature assessment is a simple, objective, inexpensive, and reliable indicator of illness and is part of the pediatric assessment. Currently, there are three types of thermometers utilized in pediatric agencies: electronic, digital, and tympanic membrane. The electronic and tympanic membrane thermometers are the most common types utilized in acute care agencies. Another type of thermometer known as a thermograph (plastic strips or dots) is used for screening only. Each agency will have guidelines to follow in taking temperatures.

Four routes are utilized for obtaining temperatures: axillary, oral, rectal, and tympanic. Axillary temperatures are usually taken on newborns, preterm infants, and infants and children younger than 3 years of age. The thermometer is placed in the axilla and the child's arm pressed close to the body for a minimum of 5 minutes if it is a mercury device or until the electronic thermometer registers.

An oral temperature may be taken in most children 6 years of age or older, including adolescents; the procedure is the same as for adults.

Because of the risk of complications, rectal temperatures are taken only when no other route is available (Betz & Sowden, 2008). The child is positioned supine, prone, or side-lying, and a well-lubricated thermometer is inserted no more than a maximum of 2.5 cm for 3 to 5 minutes. Rectal temperatures are contraindicated on preterm infants, immunosuppressed children, and children with rectal surgery or gastrointestional disorders (i.e., diarrhea and any bleeding disorder).

Tympanic temperature measurement is more quickly and easily obtained. The procedure appears to be less upsetting to children and is easy to learn by caregivers for home care. Tympanic temperatures and rectal temperatures appear to strongly correlate. Technique is very important in using the tympanic thermometer. Position of the thermometer enhances the accuracy of the reading. The ear canal must be straightened as when using an otoscope. With the ear tugged correctly and the probe tip pointing at the midpoint between the eyebrow and the sideburn on the opposite side of the face, more accurate temperature readings are obtained. Size of the probe also influences temperature. Using appropriately sized ear probes for children increases the accuracy of the reading.

TABLE 59-2 Normal Vital Signs by Age

AGE	TEMPERATURE	PULSE RATE	RESPIRATORY RATE	BLOOD PRESSURE
Newborn	98.8–99°F	100–170	30–50	Systolic: 65–95 Diastolic: 30–60
6 months–1 year	97.5–98.6°F	80–130	20–40	Systolic: 65–115 Diastolic: 42–80
3 years	97.5–98.6°F	80–120	20–30	Systolic: 72–122 Diastolic: 46–84
6 years	97.5–98.6°F	70–115	16–22	Systolic: 85–115 Diastolic: 48–64
10–14 years	97.5–98.6°F	60–110	14–20	Systolic: 93–137 Diastolic: 46–71
14–19 years	97.5–98.6°F	60–100	12–20	Systolic: 99–140 Diastolic: 51–80

COURTESY OF DELMAR CENGAGE LEARNING

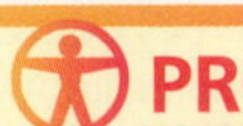
PROFESSIONALTIP

Measuring Temperature

Regardless of the type of thermometer used, the child's temperature should be measured at the same site and with the same type of device to maintain consistency and allow for reliable comparison and tracking of temperatures over time.

The method for taking a temperature is as follows:

1. Prepare the child and family for the procedure and assure them that little discomfort will arise from the procedure.
2. Select the appropriate method for obtaining the temperature measurement based on the child's age and condition.
3. Provide an explanation of the procedure to the child and family.
4. Assist the child into a position of comfort. The child may remain on the parent's lap if preferred.
5. Wash hands.
6. Don gloves and use Standard Precautions.
7. Obtain the child's temperature using method chosen.
8. Offer praise to the child for cooperating.
9. Document and report core temperatures of less than 36°C (96.8°F) or greater than 38.5°C (101.4°F) or specified parameters for individual child.
10. Reassess the child's temperature every one-half to 1 hour, or per instructions.
11. Document method of temperature assessment, measurement obtained, and any resulting action.

Heart Rate or Pulse For children younger than age 2 and those having irregular heart rhythms or congenital heart disease, apical pulse is the preferred site. Radial pulse is taken for children older than 3 years of age unless contraindicated. The method for taking a heart rate/pulse is as follows:

1. To count the pulse rate, place the stethoscope on the anterior chest at the fifth intercostal space in a midclavicular position (Figure 59-8).
2. Count the rate for 1 full minute.

CLIENTTEACHING

Temperature Measurement

The nurse teaches the caregivers how to take their child's temperature at home. Demonstrate how it is done and then observe the parent in performing. Make sure the parent is comfortable with the procedure and is able to read the thermometer accurately. Digital thermometers are easy to read because the temperature is displayed on a small screen on the thermometer; they may be used to take oral, axillary, and rectal temperatures.

SAFETY

Thermometers

Regardless of the device utilized for temperature taking, do not lay it down in the child's bed for safety and for infection control reasons.

3. Note whether the rhythm is regular or irregular.
4. Note whether the pulse is normal, bounding, or thready.
5. Compare the distal and proximal pulses for strength.
6. Pulse rates may be checked at sites other than the apex of the heart, for example, the carotid, brachial, radial, femoral, and dorsal pedis sites.
7. Record rate, quality, and rhythm.

Respiratory Rate The rate, depth, and ease of respiration are observed in the child. Respiratory rate will vary by age of the child. Therefore, the nurse counts the respiratory rate for 1 full minute because it is irregular. It is best if the child is unaware that respirations are being counted. The method for obtaining a respiratory rate is as follows:

1. Children's respirations are diaphragmatic, so observe abdominal movement to count respirations.
2. Count respirations before obtaining temperature or pulse rates (expect abdominal respirations to be irregular).
3. Count for 1 full minute.
4. Record rate, quality, and rhythm.

Blood Pressure Blood pressure measurement for the child is basically the same as for an adult. The size of the cuff is determined by the size of the child's arm or leg. To obtain an accurate blood pressure, the bladder of the cuff encircles 80% of the limb in which the BP is measured. If the bladder is too small, the pressure will be falsely high; if it is too large, the pressure will be falsely low. Blood pressure may be taken on the upper or lower extremities. General instructions for BP measurement are as follows:

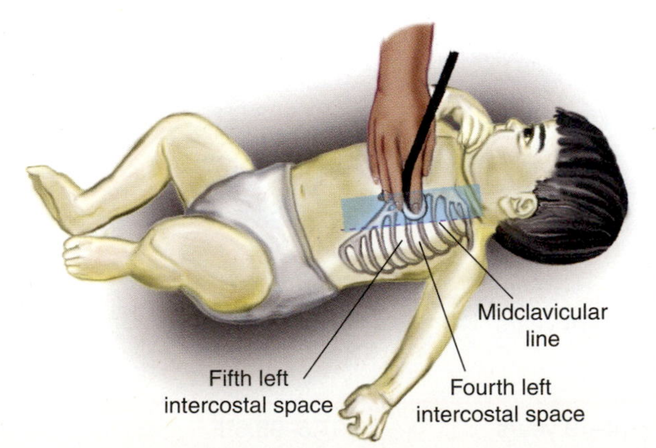

COURTESY OF DELMAR CENGAGE LEARNING

FIGURE 59-8 Apical Pulse Position for Infant and Child

CLIENT TEACHING

Measuring Pulse Rate

Teach caregivers that have children taking medication, such as digoxin, how to take a pulse rate on their child before administering the drug. The nurse demonstrates the method of taking the pulse and observes the caregivers as they take the pulse on their child. Teach the caregivers the acceptable pulse range for their child as well as the method of obtaining the pulse.

Electronic Monitoring:

1. Place the cuff around the desired extremity.
2. Activate the equipment according to the manufacturer's recommendations.
3. Stabilize limb during inflation and deflation because movement sometimes interferes with the device's ability to measure the blood pressure accurately.
4. For some devices, the first reading is a priming reading and the second reading is considered the true blood pressure reading. Refer to manual.
5. Record the reading.

Manual Cuff:

1. Position limb at level of heart.
2. Rapidly inflate cuff to about 20 mm Hg above point at which radial pulse disappears.
3. Release cuff pressure at a rate of about 2 to 3 mm Hg per second during auscultation of artery.
4. Record systolic value as onset of a clear tapping sound.
5. Record diastolic pressure as disappearance of all sounds. Record systolic, diastolic pressures, limb used, position, cuff size, and method.

Developmental Assessment

Developmental assessment for the growing child is an important measure. A tool that is frequently used for the child younger than 6 years of age is the Denver Developmental Screening Test II (DDST-2). The test is composed of four sections: personal–social, fine motor-adaptive, language, and gross motor. Of the 125 items on the test, responses can be obtained by observing the child, asking the parent, and having the child perform a task.

Inform the parent that the DDST-2 is not an I.Q. (intelligence quotient) test but a helpful measure of the child's growth and development. The parent and child are made comfortable in the testing environment. Age-appropriate communication and approaches are directed toward the child (e.g., very young children may prefer to sit on parent's lap). The child is then evaluated on a series of tasks, and rated on each with a "P" for pass, "F" for refuse, and "NO" for no opportunity. A caution is given when the child fails to perform an item that has been achieved by 75% to 90% of children of the same age. A delay indicates the child's inability to perform a task that would be expected to be mastered by children in the developmental stage just before the child's current developmental stage. A suspect test is one with one or more delays and/or two or more cautions.

Current illness, lack of sleep, anxiety, chronic disability, or sensory deficits can affect a child's performance. If these factors can explain a child's failure to successfully complete the DDST-2, then the test may be readministered in 1 month, providing resolution of the problem has occurred. If a developmental delay exists, early detection can lead to intervention and possible resolution.

Child Safety Devices

Restraints are rarely used in the pediatric unit. Some alternatives are having a person sit with the child, using diversion with the child, and using some behavior modification techniques. IVs, dressings, or other equipment is hidden from the child's view by taping a washcloth over an IV site or covering a dressing with a gown. If the child does not see the IV, dressing, or other equipment; he may forget about the item of interest.

The Joint Commission provides guidelines for the use of restraints that provide for the self-respect and safety of the client (The Joint Commission, 2009). The use of a restraint requires a physician's order stating the reason the restraint is needed and how long it will be left in place.

Specimen Collection

Specimens are collected from children the same as adults with a few modifications. Children require more specific explanations and directions in an age-appropriate format. Explain any sensation that may be felt. Regardless of the type of specimen collected, the nurse follows Standard Precautions.

Urine

A urine sample is obtained to assess for infection and to determine levels of blood, protein, glucose, acetone, bilirubin, drugs, hormones, metals, and electrolytes excreted by the kidneys. Urine also is assessed for concentration/specific gravity, pH, and other substances.

A collection bag is used to obtain a clean-catch urine sample from an infant and non-toilet-trained children. Intermittent catheterization is used when obtaining a specimen for culture to decrease the risk of contamination (Bekeris et al., 2008). Older children, after being given clear instructions, are usually capable of collecting their own urine. Usually, 5–10 mL of urine is adequate.

The method of obtaining a urine sample for the infant is as follows:

1. Remove the diaper and clean the skin around the meatus; allow to dry thoroughly.
2. Attach the bag with the adhesive tabs, for girls, around the labia, and for boys, around the scrotum (Figure 59-9).
3. Make sure the seal is tight to prevent leakage.
4. Check the bag frequently for urine.
5. To remove the bag, pull away gently from the skin using moistened cotton balls to assist in releasing the adhesive.
6. Pour into container and cap tightly.
7. Double bag the specimen and then send it to the lab immediately.
8. Document color, amount, clarity, and lab tests requested.

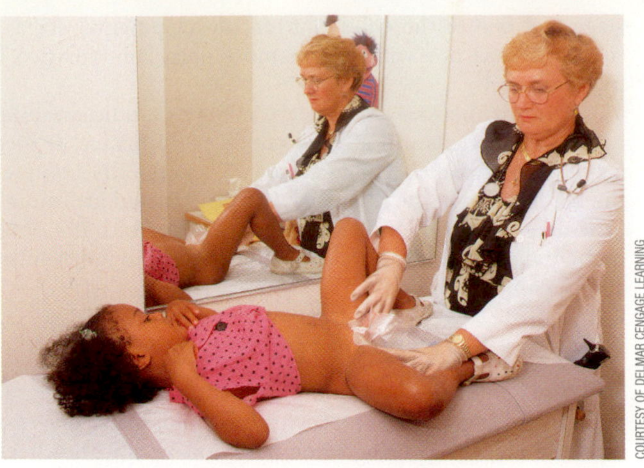

FIGURE 59-9 Applying a Urine Collection Bag to a Child

A clean-catch sample for a male older child is collected in the following manner:

1. Instruct the older child to clean the head of his penis (after retracting the foreskin, if not circumcised) three times, each time using a different towelette, moving from the urethral meatus outward.
2. Have the child urinate into the toilet and, while urinating, collect urine in the sterile container. Have the child remove the container before stopping the flow of urine.
3. Proceed as above.

A clean-catch sample for a female older child is collected in the following manner:

1. Instruct the child to sit back on the toilet as far as possible with her legs apart. Have her spread her labia with her fingers and wipe each side with a separate towelette using a front-to-back stroke. Tell the child to use a third wipe to clean the meatus, repeating the front-to-back motion.
2. Have the child urinate into the toilet and, while urinating, collect urine in the sterile container. Have the child remove the container before stopping the flow of urine.
3. Proceed as above.

Stool

Stool specimens are used in pediatric clients to check for the presence of fat, blood, bacteria, parasites, or reducing substances. If the stool specimen is needed from an infant or incontinent child, scrape it from the diaper and place in the appropriate container. If the child is potty-trained, use a bedpan or container to collect the specimen. Record the time the specimen is obtained, color, consistency, any odor, and disposition.

Blood

Blood specimens are obtained from children by accessing veins of the hand or antecubital space, heelsticks, and femoral and jugular venipunctures. Collection of blood is very distressing to young children because of their lack of discrete body boundaries and the pain involved. The use of EMLA, a topical anesthetic cream, can reduce the discomfort of the needle penetrating the skin. EMLA contains lidocaine-prilocaine 5% and can be used to decrease pain associated with selected procedures: venipuncture, lumbar puncture, suture removal, immunizations, bone marrow aspiration, and removal of foreign bodies. EMLA is not approved for infants because of lack of testing and is not placed on skin that is broken. The cream is applied to the site liberally with an occlusive dressing and left in place 60 minutes before the procedure. The duration of the anesthesia is at least 2 and not more than 5 hours. Permission to use EMLA varies by institution; some may require a physician's order, and others allow the nurse to use it without an order. Children still may fear the needlestick; however, when the stick is not painful, they are more content. Venipunctures that are the same as those in adults are not covered in this section.

Jugular Venipuncture Jugular and femoral venipunctures are performed by a physician, with the nurse assisting and monitoring the child. The blood specimen is obtained from the large superficial external jugular vein. The nurse assists the physician by doing the following:

1. Place child in mummy restraint (possibly just hold child's arms).
2. Position child with head and shoulders extended over the edge of a table or small pillow with neck area hyperextended (Figure 59-10).
3. Take care that circulation and breathing during the procedure are not impaired.
4. Make sure that the nose and mouth are not covered by the restrainer's hand.
5. Document in the chart the amount of blood drawn, the site, condition of the site, and the type of dressing applied.

Femoral Venipuncture The nurse assists the physician by doing the following:

1. Place child in modified mummy restraint with legs exposed.
2. Position child's legs in a froglike position to provide extensive exposure of the groin area (Figure 59-11).
3. Restrain legs in frog position with hands while controlling the child's arm and body movements with downward and inward pressure of forearms.

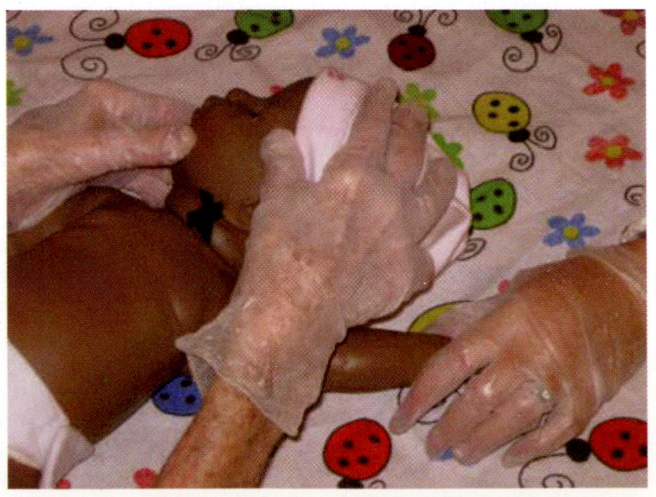

FIGURE 59-10 Positioning for Jugular Venipuncture

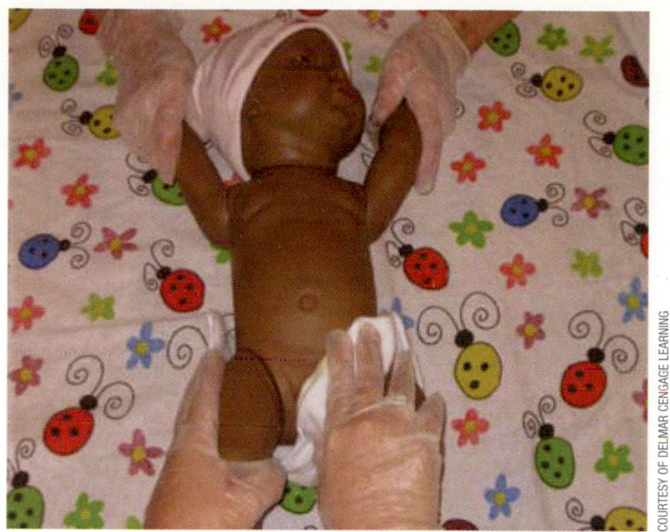

FIGURE 59-11 Positioning for Femoral Venipuncture

4. Cover genitalia to avoid contamination if the child urinates.
5. Document in chart amount of blood drawn, site, condition of the site, and type of dressing applied.

Lumbar Puncture

Lumbar puncture (spinal tap) requires the infant or child to be held perfectly still. It is desirable to have an experienced staff member hold the child for the procedure. Lumbar puncture is performed as follows:

1. Place infant in sitting or side-lying position (neonates) with modified head extension to decrease respiratory distress during procedure.
2. Immobilize arms and legs with nurse's hands.
3. Observe child for difficulty in breathing.
4. Place child on side with back close to or extended over the edge of examining table, head flexed, and knees drawn up toward the chest.
5. Reach over the top of the child and place one arm behind child's neck and the other behind the knees (Figure 59-12).

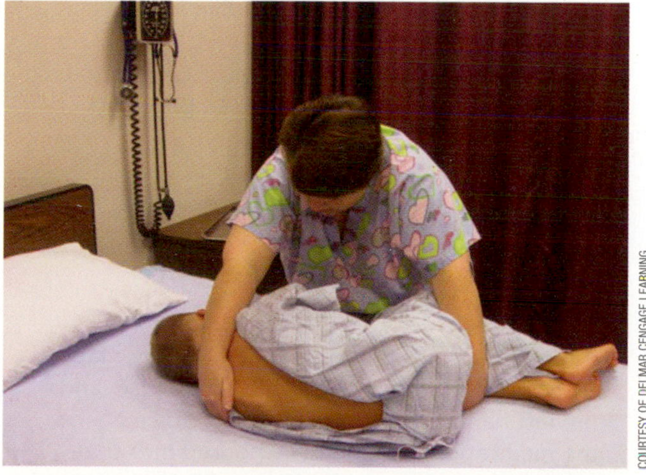

FIGURE 59-12 Positioning for Lumbar Puncture

6. Stabilize this position by clasping own hands in front of the child's abdomen.
7. Observe carefully for compromise in circulatory or respiratory systems. The restrainer's body should not cover the nose and mouth of the child.
8. Document number of attempts to obtain spinal fluid, number of cc's to lab, lab tests requested, color and consistency of spinal fluid, and response of child to procedure.

INTAKE AND OUTPUT

Most children in acute care agencies will be on intake and output, which is critical for children with the following conditions:

- Anyone receiving IV fluids or TPN
- Major surgery
- Prematurity
- Renal disease or dysfunction
- Congestive heart failure
- Heart disease or anomalies
- Endocrine disorders
- Gastrointestinal disorders
- Shock
- Burns
- Taking medications such as digoxin (Lanoxin), furosemide (Lasix), or corticosteriods
- Neurological conditions

To measure output for infants, the nurse should:

1. Weigh the diaper before placing it on the infant and then again when wet. For each mg the diaper weighs, record 1 mL of urine. *Caution*: For those diapers that protect against wetness, the accuracy may be distorted because of the absorbent material embedded in the diaper.
2. A urine bag with adhesive may be placed on the child and the urine collected measured in this way. This is not usually done because of the irritation of the adhesive over time.

For toddlers and older children, measure urine and stool output in a bedpan or other container. All intake is measured and recorded on the intake and output sheet. If caregivers are present, instruct them to measure and record fluids taken in and those eliminated. Record all fluids from IVs and other sources. Measure drainage from stomas, colostomies, fistulas, and emesis and record.

ADMINISTRATION OF MEDICATIONS

Administration of medications to infants and children presents a number of adaptations. The medication dosage is determined by the physician; however, the nurse observes the five rights of medication administration. Explain all procedures or treatments to the child and caregivers based on the child's developmental stage and the level of understanding of both parties. The nurse gives explanations truthfully, using nonthreatening words. All questions posed by the caregivers and child are answered before giving the medication.

Approaches to Pediatric Clients

Children's reactions to medication administration are affected by developmental characteristics such as physical skills and

LIFE SPAN CONSIDERATIONS

Medication Administration in Children

Suggestions to facilitate successful medication administration in infants and children:

- Be honest with the child.
- Allow the child choices when possible.
- Provide distraction when appropriate.
- Praise the child for doing her best.
- Expect success; use a positive approach.
- Allow the child opportunity to express feelings.
- Involve the child in order to gain cooperation.
- Provide a developmentally appropriate explanation.
- Do not use basic foods such as milk to disguise medication.
- Spend some time with the child after administering the medication.

cognitive understanding, environmental influences, past experiences, cultural influences, parental responses, current relationship with the nurse, and perception of the present situation.

Calculating Dosages for Children

Standardized doses of medication for children do not exist. The most common method of determining medication amounts is based on the child's weight. This method of determining the medication amount is more reliable because it allows for a more precise dose based on weight (see example in Professional Tip box). Medication doses also may be calculated by body surface area (BSA, mg/m^2). The formula to calculate dosage using surface area is:

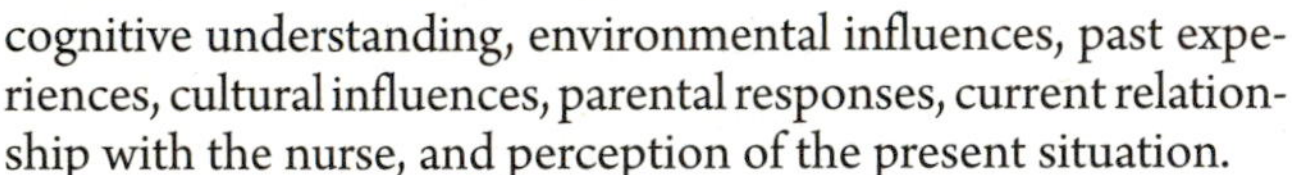

$$\text{Approximate dose} = \frac{\text{BSA of child (m}^2\text{)}}{1.7} \times \text{Adult dose}$$

Oral Medications

The oral route of medication is the preferred method of administering medication to a child. Oral medications may come in liquids, pills, tablets, and caplets. Pediatric medications are frequently in a liquid suspension that tastes "good" and is colorful. Many medications have an unpleasant after-taste. Become aware of medications that are bitter or unpleasant and methods to decrease the unpleasant taste such as numbing the tongue before administration by giving a flavored ice popsicle or small ice cube. The method for administering oral medication to a child is as follows:

1. Select appropriate vehicle (e.g., calibrated cup, syringe, dropper, measuring spoon, nipple)
2. Prepare medication
3. Measure into appropriate vehicle
4. Avoid mixing medications with essential food items such as milk, formula, etc. (The child may later refuse the essential food item because of the association with medication.)
5. Administer the medication, employing safety precautions in identification and administration

Specific instructions for administering oral medications to infants are as follows:

1. Hold infant in semi-reclining position
2. Place syringe, measuring spoon, or dropper with medication in mouth well back on the tongue or to the side of the tongue
3. Administer slowly and wait for the child to swallow to reduce likelihood of choking or aspiration
4. Allow infant to suck medication placed in nipple

Specific instructions for administering oral medications to the older infant or toddler are as follows:

1. Explain in developmentally appropriate terms what you are going to do
2. Allow the child to sit on your lap or the parent's lap in a sitting or modified supine position
3. Use mild or partial restraint
4. Administer the medication slowly with a syringe or small medicine cup
5. Never force actively resistive children because of the danger of aspiration; postpone 20 to 30 minutes and offer medication again

Specific instructions for administering oral medications to a preschool child are as follows:

1. Use a straightforward approach
2. For a reluctant child, use the following:
    - Simple persuasion (e.g., "When you take your medicine, we can go to the playroom.")
    - Reinforcement, such as stickers or other rewards for compliance

PROFESSIONALTIP

Dosage Calculations for Children

The recommended dose of ampicillin is 50–100 mg/kg/day in equally divided doses every 6 hours. For a child weighing 5 kg, the dose would be 250–500 mg divided by 4, or 63–125 mg every 6 hours.

PROFESSIONALTIP

Resistant Child

If the nurse holds the small child on his/her lap with the child's right arm behind the nurse, and the left hand firmly grasped by the nurse's hand, the medication can be slowly poured into the mouth of a resisting child (Figure 59-13).

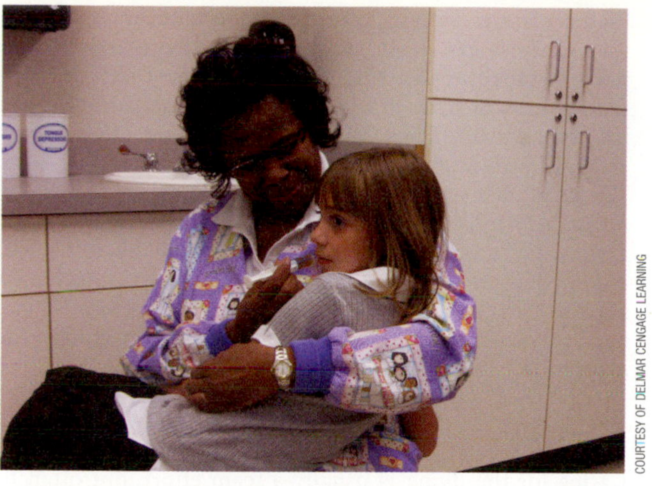
COURTESY OF DELMAR CENGAGE LEARNING

FIGURE 59-13 Administering Oral Medication to a Child

CRITICAL THINKING

Needle Threats

A child who has received multiple intramuscular injections has a real fear of the "needle." The caregivers threaten the child that if he does not do what they say, the nurse will come and give him a "needle." How would you approach the caregivers? What interventions would assist the child to lessen his fear and regain control?

Intramuscular Injections

Intramuscular injections are used for pediatric clients but avoided when possible because of physical discomfort and psychological distress (Potts & Mandleco, 2007). Medications given by the intramuscular route include immunizations, antibiotics, and other drugs. Preparation of the child is important as injections can be painful and a source of stress to children (Carter-Templeton & McCoy, 2008). The task for nurses is to support the child while administering the medication quickly, safely, and with the least amount of pain and stress to the child. Pain perception is lessened with a distraction such as the child blowing bubbles or the skin being stroked around the injection site before and during the injection (Sparks, 2001).

Otic Medications

Otic medication is used frequently in children who have ear infections. Because of pain associated with cold coming in contact with the tympanic membrane, warm all otic medications to room temperature before administering. The child should receive an age-appropriate explanation regarding what will be felt and heard and what can be done to help. Assistance in restraining a young child may be needed.

Position the child on the side with the affected ear up, and clean any discharge with a clean gauze pad. Brace the administering hand above the ear on the head. To instill the solution in a child younger than 3 years of age, pull the pinna of the ear back and down; for an older child, the pinna is pulled back and up. After instillation, the tragus of the ear is massaged to ensure the drops reach the tympanic membrane. If ordered, place cotton loosely into the ear canal to allow for drainage.

Intravenous Medications

Children in acute care settings frequently receive intravenous (IV) medications. Children who have poor absorption as a result of dehydration, malabsorption syndromes, shock, and those in need of a high concentration of the drug quickly would receive IV fluids and medication. Children needing continuous pain relief benefit from IV medication administration. Advantages of IV medications are the immediate effect and the ability to control blood levels of the drugs used. Disadvantages are the same: side effects occur very quickly, and the drug may be very harmful to the veins. Once the drug is administered into the bloodstream, further control is limited.

All drugs given by IV route require a specified minimum dilution and specific rate of flow. It is difficult to control the IV flow rate in children by gravity. Children are at risk for fluid overload when IV rates are not controlled; therefore, all children receiving IV fluids or medications should receive those fluids through a volumetric infusion pump. IV medication may be delivered as a continuous infusion or intermittently. Syringe pumps are used in many agencies to deliver small amounts of medication.

Nursing care of the client receiving IV fluids and/or medication includes site assessment every hour for signs and symptoms of infiltration. Site assessment includes color of the site, tension of the skin, and skin temperature. When administering IV fluids and medications to the pediatric client, know the following:

- Type of fluid.
- Compatibility of medication and IV solutions.
- Recommended dilution of the drug.
- Recommended time frame for administration.
- Amount of flush needed.
- Any precautions to observe before administration (e.g., for aminophylline [Aminophyllin], take apical pulse before administering).
- Side effects of the drug.

THE DYING CHILD

Care of the dying child presents one of the greatest challenges to nurses. It involves sensitive, gentle physical care and comfort measures for the child as well as continuing emotional support for the family and caregivers.

Child

Children's understanding of death parallels their cognitive and psychosocial development. Preverbal infants and toddlers have no clear concept of death. Children between the ages of 3 and 5 may view death as a kind of sleep that is interchangeable with life. Because of their concrete thinking, school-age children begin developing the concept of death as final. Adolescents have a maturing understanding of death. In addition to their developmental level, children are greatly influenced by their life experiences and the attitudes of those around them.

Children can sense when they are seriously ill. They may realize they are dying because of the effects of disease and treatments on their body. The child usually experiences fear of death, of dying alone, and of pain. Nursing interventions include promoting socialization with family and peers, providing avenues for self-expression (i.e., drawings, fantasy play, storytelling), dealing directly with the child's questions, and allowing the death to occur in peace and with dignity.

Caregivers

When death is expected, the family begins a mourning process called anticipatory grieving. Manifestations of this process include denial, anger, and depression. It is important to acknowledge the caregivers' feelings, encourage expression, and guide them through the gradual process to reorganization. Spouses may need additional support when they are at different levels of grieving to prevent a sense of loneliness and isolation.

Explore options with the family concerning the child's care. The child and family have a right to request termination of treatment and to determine the care setting.

Caregivers who are caring for their dying child usually fear what the death will be like, not being present at the death, and pain the child will experience. The family needs to be encouraged to talk to the child about dying. Families need help to focus on the time that remains with the child. Openness and honesty allow the health-care providers and the family to provide effective care, to avoid misunderstandings, to see that the child and the family resolve problems, and to share their love.

Siblings

The nurse must recognize that each family member will handle the grief process in a different and personal way. Like their caregivers, siblings may experience anticipatory grief in the form of anger, denial, or fear. They may resent the attention given to the dying child. Siblings may fear that they caused their brother or sister to become ill or that the same thing will happen to them. They may need help in adapting to their caregivers' distraction, grief, and increased protectiveness. The death of a sibling can affect a child's ability to make and maintain friendships (Hinds, Schum, Baker, & Wolfe, 2005). Encourage caregivers to include siblings in the care of the dying child, in discussions about dying, and in the funeral. Like the dying child and the grieving caregivers, siblings need acknowledgment of their feelings and opportunities for expression.

Nurse

Caring for the dying is usually a team effort, but often the nurse is the coordinator of the care. Working effectively with dying children and their families requires confidence, empathy, and competence in addition to attention to managing personal stress. Nurses who are comfortable with their own mortality can help make the remainder of the child's life more meaningful and the family's mourning experience more healing.

Nurses experience reactions to caring for dying children including denial, anger, depression, guilt, and ambivalent feelings. Nurses may even cry in the presence of the child and the family. Learning to care for the dying involves talking with other professionals, sharing concerns, comforting each other in stressful times, maintaining good general health, using distancing techniques, and focusing on the positive aspects of the caregiver role.

Sources of Support

Hospice care may be an option for the dying child. Hospice services provide palliative care for the dying to live life to the fullest without pain, with choices of dignity, and with family support including follow-up care after death. Self-help groups such as Compassionate Friends, an international organization for bereaved caregivers and siblings, are available in many communities.

CASE STUDY

T.C., a 5-year-old client with an inoperable abdominal tumor, lives with her caregivers and a 7-year-old sister, M.C. The decision has been made to discontinue chemotherapy. T.C. has been involved in decisions about her care throughout her illness. When asked about her condition, she states, "I'm very sick and I'm not getting better." T.C. spends much of her time curled in a fetal position with her favorite toy, a tattered rag doll named Dolly. T.C. refuses physical exams and pills and gets little sleep because of her pain.

The following questions will guide your development of a nursing care plan for the case study.

1. List subjective and objective data a nurse would want to know about T.C. and her family.
2. List three nursing diagnoses and goals for T.C.
3. What would you expect a 5-year-old client to understand about death?
4. List affective nursing interventions for T.C. and her family?
5. List three successful outcomes for T.C. and her family.

SUMMARY

- Even though hospitalization places great stress on children and their families, it can be a positive growth experience for the child.
- Teaching children and their families what to expect and explaining what is going to happen before, during, and after procedures helps reduce anxiety.
- Children's developmental stage and cognitive ability influence the preparation for treatments and procedures.
- Children must be protected from hazards that can cause harm to them.
- The child's stage of development, cognitive ability, and life experiences contribute to the child's understanding of death.

REVIEW QUESTIONS

1. The major stressor of hospitalization for infants and young children is:
   1. pain.
   2. bodily injury.
   3. loss of control.
   4. separation anxiety.
2. Because of their stage of development, preschoolers may view hospitalization as:
   1. abuse.
   2. rejection.
   3. punishment.
   4. abandonment.
3. Before drawing blood on a 9-year-old client, the nurse tells the child:
   1. a Band-Aid will not be necessary.
   2. the procedure will not be painful.
   3. not to worry about the tight tourniquet.
   4. the body will produce more blood to replace what is being taken.
4. An appropriate method for administering oral medication to a small child is to mix it with:
   1. milk.
   2. food from the child's plate.
   3. a large amount of water.
   4. sweet-tasting food or syrup.
5. The physician orders Demerol 10 mg for pain after an infant has surgery. The stock medication is 50 mg/mL. The nurse would administer:
   1. 5.0 mL
   2. 0.5 mL
   3. 2.0 mL
   4. 0.2 mL
6. The nurse would expect the normal pulse range of a school age child to be:
   1. 70–115
   2. 90–120
   3. 60–110
   4. 80–130
7. When administering medications to children, what strategies does the nurse include to facilitate the process? (Select all that apply.)
   1. Give the child choices when possible.
   2. Do not use foods such as milk to disguise medications.
   3. Praise the child when possible.
   4. Do not let the child know that they are taking medication.
   5. Leave the medication with the parent to decrease anxiety.
   6. Explain medication procedure according to child's developmental stage.
8. Additional assessments done with the pediatric client that differ from an adult client include: (Select all that apply.)
   1. blood pressure.
   2. pulse.
   3. weight.
   4. head circumference.
   5. abdominal circumference.
   6. height.
9. The sibling of a terminally ill child may experience all of the following except:
   1. fear.
   2. anxiety.
   3. denial.
   4. acceptance.
10. The nurse understands that which of the following affects a child's ability to understand death: (Select all that apply.)
    1. developmental stage.
    2. cognitive ability.
    3. pain.
    4. life experiences.
    5. ability to express feelings.
    6. age-appropriate explanations.

REFERENCES/SUGGESTED READINGS

Alam, M., Coulter, J., Pacheco, J., Correia, J., Ribeiro, M., Coelho, M., et al. (2005). Comparison of urine contamination rates using three different methods of collection: Clean-catch, cotton wool pad and urine bag. *Annals of Tropical Paediatrics, 25*(1), 29–34.

Allen, L. (2008). Dosage form design and development. *Clinical Therapeutics, 30*(11), 2102–2111.

Ball, J., & Bindler, R. (2000). *Pediatric nursing* (2nd ed.). Norwalk, CT: Appleton & Lange.

Ball, J., & Bindler, R. (2007). *Pediatric Nursing*, (4th ed.). Upper Saddle River, NJ: Pearson.

Bekeris, L., Jones, B., Walsh, M., & Wagar, E. (2008). Urine culture contamination: A college of American pathologists Q-probes study of 127 labora. *Archives of Pathology & Laboratory Medicine, 132*(6), 913–917.

Betz, C., & Sowden, L. (2008). *Mosby's Pediatric Nursing Reference* (6th ed.). St. Louis, MO: Mosby.

Carter-Templeton, H., & McCoy, T. (2008). Are we on the same page?: A comparison of intramuscular injection Explanations in Nursing Fundamental Texts. *MEDSURG Nursing, 17*(4), 237–240.

Cooper, L., Gooding, J., Gallagher, J., Sternesky, L., Ledsky, R., & Berns, S. (2007). Impact of a family-centered care initiative on NICU care, staff and families. *Journal of Perinatology, 27*, 32–37.

Eland, J., & Anderson, J. (1977). The experience of pain in children. In A. Jacox (Ed.), *Pain: A sourcebook for nurses and other health professionals*. Philadelphia: Lippincott Williams & Wilkins.

Estes, M. (2010). *Health assessment & physical examination* (4th ed.). Clifton Park, NY: Delmar Cengage Learning.

Gedaly-Duff, V., & Burns, C. (1992). Reducing children's pain-distress associated with injection using cold: A pilot study. *Journal of the American Academy of Nurse Practitioners, 4*(3), 95–99.

Hinds, P., Schum, L., Baker, J., & Wolfe, J. (2005). Key factors affecting dying children and their families. *Journal of Palliative Medicine, 8*, 70–78.

Hockenberry, M., & Wilson, D. (2008). *Wong's essentials of pediatric care* (8th ed.). St. Louis, MO: Mosby.

Hockenberry, M., Wilson, D., & Barrera, P. (2006). Implementing evidence-based nursing practice in a pediatric hospital. *Pediatric Nursing, 32*(4), 371–377.

Hughes, R., & Edgerton, E. (2005). First, do no harm: Reducing pediatric medication errors. *American Journal of Nursing, 105*(5), 79–92.

James, S., Ashwill, J., & Droske, S. (2002). *Nursing care of children: Principles and practice* (2nd ed.). Philadelphia: W. B. Saunders.

Johnston, A., Bullock, C., Graham, J., Reilly, M., Rocha, C., Hoopes, J., et al. (2006). Implementation and case-study results of potentially better practices for family-centered care: The family-centered care map. *Pediatrics, 118*, 108–114.

Jones, H., Kleber, C., Eckert, G., & Mahon, B. (2003). Comparison of rectal temperature measured by digital vs. mercury glass thermometer in infants under two months old. *Clinical Pediatrics, 42*(4), 357.

Kliegman, R., Jenson, H., & Behrman, R. (2000). *Nelson textbook of pediatrics* (16th ed.). Philadelphia: W. B. Saunders.

Leifer, G. (2006). *Introduction to maternity and pediatric nursing* (5th ed.). Philadelphia: W.B. Saunders.

Moldow, D., & Martinson, I. *Home care for seriously ill children: A manual for caregivers.* Children's Hospice International, 901 N. Washington Street, 7th Floor, Alexandria, VA 22314, (800) 24-CHILD.

Morgan, D. (2009). Caring for dying children: Assessing the needs of the pediatric palliative care nurse. *Pediatric Nursing, 35*(2), 86–90.

Newton, M. (2000). Family-centered care: Current realities in parent-participation. *Pediatric Nursing, 26*(2), 164–168.

North American Nursing Diagnosis Association International. (2010). *NANDA-I nursing diagnoses: Definitions and classification 2009–2011.* Ames, IA: Wiley-Blackwell.

Parson, A., & White, J. (2008). Learning from reflection on intramuscular injections. *Nursing Standard, 22*(17), 35–40.

Potts, N., & Mandleco, B. (2007). *Pediatric nursing: Caring for children and their families* (2nd ed.). Clifton Park, NY: Delmar Cengage Learning.

Timby, B., & Harrison, L. (2005). *Fundamental Skills and Concepts in Patient Care* (8th ed.). Philadelphia: Lippincott.

The Joint Commission. (2009). The Joint Commission 2009 requirements that support effective communication, cultural competence, and patient-centered care hospital accreditation program (HAP) (Standard PC.03.02.03, Standard PC.03.02.05, & Standard PC.03.02.07). Retrieved November 25, 2009 from http://www.jointcommission.org/NR/rdonlyres/B48B39E3-107D-495A-9032-24C3EBD96176/0/PDF32009HAPSupportingStds.pdf

RESOURCES

Association for the Care of Children's Health,
http://www.acch.org

Children's Hospice International,
http://www.chionline.org

Compassionate Friends, Inc.,
http://www.compassionatefriends.org/index.html

National Father's Network,
http://www.fathersnetwork.org

Sibling Support Project,
http://www.chmc.org/departmt/sibsupp

CHAPTER 60
Infants with Special Needs: Birth to 12 Months

MAKING THE CONNECTION

Refer to the following chapters to increase your understanding of infants with special needs:

Basic Nursing

- ***Life Span Development***
- ***Cultural Considerations***
- ***End-of-Life Care***
- ***Fluid, Electrolyte, and Acid–Base Balance***
- ***Assessment***
- ***Pain Management***

Adult Health Nursing

- ***Anesthesia***
- ***Surgery***
- ***Respiratory System***
- ***Cardiovascular System***
- ***Hematologic and Lymphatic Systems***
- ***Gastrointestinal System***
- ***Urinary System***
- ***Musculoskeletal System***
- ***Neurological System***
- ***Sensory System***
- ***Integumentary System***
- ***Immune System***

Maternal & Pediatric Nursing

- ***Basics of Pediatric Care***

LEARNING OBJECTIVES

Upon completion of this chapter, you should be able to:

- Define key terms.
- Differentiate the most common respiratory conditions affecting infants.
- Describe nursing care for infants with circulatory conditions.
- Discuss nursing considerations for infants with digestive conditions.
- Explain the evaluative techniques used for infants suspected of having musculoskeletal alterations.
- Differentiate among the skin disorders most commonly seen in infants.
- Explain the causes and effects of nervous system disorders seen in infants.
- Describe nursing care for infants with genitourinary conditions.
- Outline teaching strategies for caregivers of infants with visual and hearing impairments and cognitive disorders.

- Implement nursing interventions for infants who have been abused.
- Describe teaching guidelines for families of infants who have unsafe environments.

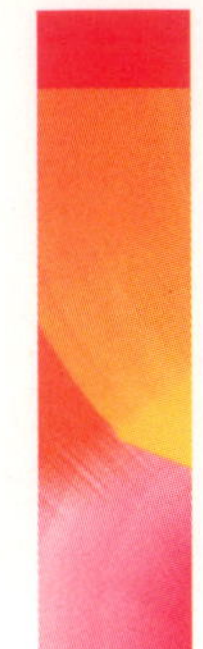

KEY TERMS

abduction
antipyretic
atresia
child abuse
circumoral cyanosis
colic
dislocation
dysplasia
erythematous
hypotonia
intussusception
jaundice
kernicterus
lecithin
meconium ileus
meningitis
milia
mongolian spots
multifactorial inheritance
myelomeningocele
myringotomy
projectile vomiting
pruritus
stridor

INTRODUCTION

The immaturity of all body systems leaves infants vulnerable to numerous illnesses and disorders. Most health problems during infancy are caused by respiratory and gastrointestinal infections or congenital anomalies. Although infants can become ill rapidly, they usually recover quickly. This chapter describes common conditions and illnesses affecting all systems of the infant, typical medical and surgical management, and nursing care of infants.

RESPIRATORY SYSTEM

In the normal infant, breathing is quiet and shallow with variations in rate and rhythm. Respiratory movement is primarily abdominal. Respirations should be counted for 1 full minute while watching the rise and fall of the abdomen. The normal rate ranges from 30 to 50 breaths per minute. A persistent rate greater than 60 breaths per minute is an important sign of respiratory distress.

The child's respiratory tract is constantly changing and growing during the first 12 years of life. Differences between the respiratory tract of the adult and the infant contribute to the greater potential for obstruction, aspiration, infection, and airway resistance in the child (Table 60-1). In the infant, the most common respiratory disorders include otitis media, laryngotracheobronchitis, pneumonia, respiratory distress syndrome, cystic fibrosis, and sudden infant death syndrome.

TABLE 60-1 Respiratory Tract Characteristics in Infants

FINDINGS IN CHILDREN	SIGNIFICANCE
Small nares, oral cavity, and nasopharynx; large tongue	Increases risk for obstruction
Obligatory nose breathers (<6 months) due to immature neurological function	Increases risk for obstruction
Rapid growth of lymph tissue	Increases risk for obstruction with infection
Larynx and glottis high in neck	Increases risk for aspiration
Large amount of soft tissues and loose, poorly anchored mucous membranes; long floppy epiglottis	Increases risk for obstruction with infection
Fewer functional airway muscles	Increases risk for aspiration
Immature cartilages that may collapse when neck is flexed	Increases risk for obstruction
Short neck resulting in structures being closer together	Increases risk for infection
Short, narrow airway	Increases risk for obstruction and aspiration; increases airway resistance/respiratory effort
Bifurcation of trachea at the third thoracic space	Increases risk for infection and aspiration
Immature intercostal muscles and cartilaginous ribs; primarily diaphragmatic breathers	Increases respiratory effort
Eustachian tube shorter, wider, and straighter	Increases risk for infection

COURTESY OF DELMAR CENGAGE LEARNING

OTITIS MEDIA

Otitis media, an inflammation of the middle ear, can occur unilaterally or bilaterally. The eustachian tubes, which allow for drainage from the middle ear to the nasopharynx, are shorter, wider, and more horizontal in infants than in adults (Figure 60-1). As a result, drainage is frequently impaired, resulting in retention of secretions and air in the middle ear. This positioning also facilitates the movement of bacteria up the eustachian tube from the pharynx into the middle ear. An upper respiratory infection often precedes the development of otitis media in infants. *Streptococcus pneumoniae, Haemophilus influenzae,* and *Moxarella catarrhalis* are the most common causative agents of otitis media in infants (AAP 2004; Ramakrishnan et al., 2007).

The onset of signs and symptoms in otitis media is usually rapid and abrupt (AAP, 2004; Ramakrishnan et al., 2007). Infants with otitis media may be irritable, pull at the infected ear, or have diarrhea, vomiting, fever, and hearing loss. Upon inspection, the ear drum will be red, bulging, and nonmobile. Prolonged otitis media may result in sensorineural and/or conductive hearing loss, which is further discussed in the hearing impairment section of this chapter.

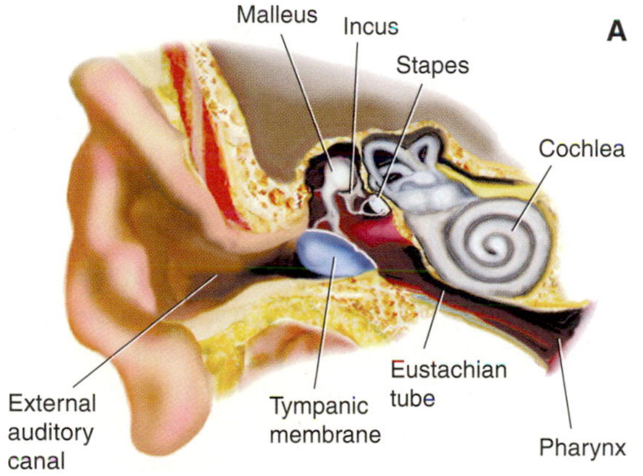

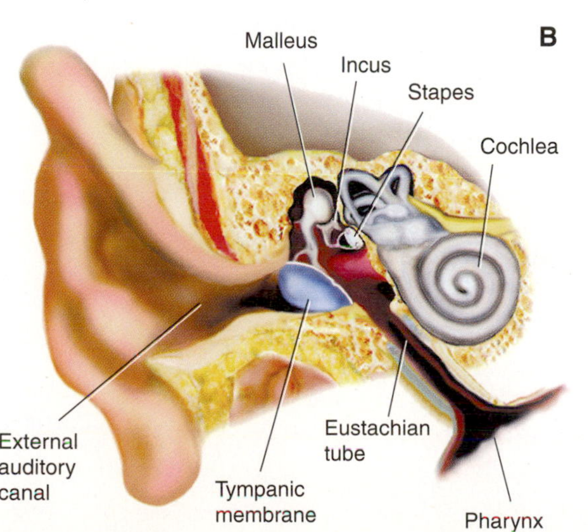

COURTESY OF DELMAR CENGAGE LEARNING

FIGURE 60-1 Eustachian Tubes; *A*, Infant; *B*, Adult

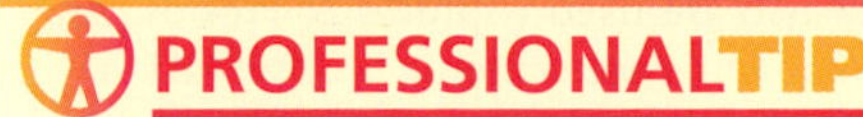

PROFESSIONAL TIP

Pertussis

Incidence

Bacterial infection of the respiratory tract
Caused by *Bordatella pertussis*
Transmitted through aerosolized droplets of respiratory secretions
5,000 to 7,000 cases reported each year

Clinical Manifestations

Nasal congestion
Runny nose
Mild sore throat
Minimal or no fever
Mild dry, intermittent cough (initially)
Paroxysmal spasms of severe coughing, whooping
Posttussive vomiting

Treatment

Erythromycin, clarithromycin, and azithromycin are the preferred antibiotics for infants ≥1 month.
For infants <1 month, azithomycin is preferred.

Nursing considerations

Vaccinate with diphtheria, tetanus, and acellular pertussis (DTaP) vaccine at ages 2, 4, 6, 15 to 18 months, and 4 to 6 years.
Protect children that are too young to have completed the primary vaccination series.

MEDICAL–SURGICAL MANAGEMENT

Medical

Medical treatment focuses on elimination of the infection and follow-up evaluation to determine the extent of hearing loss, if any.

Surgical

If infections recur, **myringotomy** (surgical incision of the eardrum) may be performed and tympanoplasty tubes inserted to drain the fluid from the middle ear.

Pharmacological

Treatment usually includes antibiotics, **antipyretics** (drug used to reduce an abnormally high temperature), and analgesics. Considerations when deciding which antibiotic to administer include compliance of caregivers in giving the medication, the child's willingness to take oral medications, and the pain involved with injections. The most common used antibiotic is amoxicillin (Amoxil) at 80 to 90 mg/kg/day for 10 days. Amoxicillin (Amoxil) is a safe, low-cost antibiotic, that when used in sufficient doses kills susceptible bacteria and has an acceptable taste to the child (AAP, 2004; Ramakrishnan et al., 2007). Another commonly used antibiotic is cefaclor (Ceclor), and newer antibiotics such as cefixime (Suprax) and loracarbef (Lorabid) also are used (Spratto & Woods, 2009). Another option for managing otitis media is observation without the use of antibiotics. This option is for select children based on their age (> 6 months), illness severity, and assurance of follow-up. This option involves treating the child only for pain and waiting 48 to 72 hours to reassess for improvement. If there is no improvement then antibiotic therapy is initiated (AAP, 2004; Spiro et al., 2006).

Nursing Management

The primary nursing concerns are relieving fever and pain and teaching the caregivers about signs and symptoms, management, and prevention of otitis media. Acetaminophen (Tylenol) or ibuprofen (Motrin) may be used to reduce fever. In addition to analgesic administration, pain may be minimized by applying a heating pad on the low setting or an ice pack compress to the affected ear. Lying on the affected side will facilitate drainage, if the eardrum has ruptured or myringotomy has been performed. Providing liquids and soft foods may minimize pain caused by chewing.

Teach caregivers to have the infant examined at the first sign of a possible ear infection. Early possible signs of infection include hearing difficulties, pulling or rubbing of the ears, and irritability.

If antibiotics are prescribed, it is imperative that the child be given all of the medication. Failure to adhere to prescribed treatment may lead to the need for additional antibiotics, hearing loss, potential speech and language problems, and antibiotic resistance.

Prevention of otitis media involves ensuring proper positioning during feeding. Infants who are bottle-fed should be held with the head slightly elevated to prevent formula from draining into the middle ear through the wide eustachian tube. Breastfed infants receive immunoglobulin A contained in the breast milk. Immunizations are also preventive (Burns et al., 2008).

Providing a smoke-free environment is another important element of prevention. Inform parents of the relationship between environmental tobacco smoke and otitis media in young children. Passive smoking has been associated with an increase in blocked eustachian tubes, which can lead to nasopharyngeal congestion and upper respiratory infections (Burns et al., 2008).

LARYNGOTRACHEOBRONCHITIS

Laryngotracheobronchitis (LTB), the most common type of croup, is a viral illness that causes swelling (narrowing) of the upper airway (Figure 60-2).

Initial symptoms include inspiratory **stridor** (a high-pitched, harsh sound), a "barking" cough, and hoarseness. The child may have a persistent, low-grade fever and a history of profuse nasal drainage with increased respiratory effort for several days.

Medical–Surgical Management

Medical

Treatment is focused on maintaining a patent airway and improving respiratory effort by creating a highly humid, cool-mist environment.

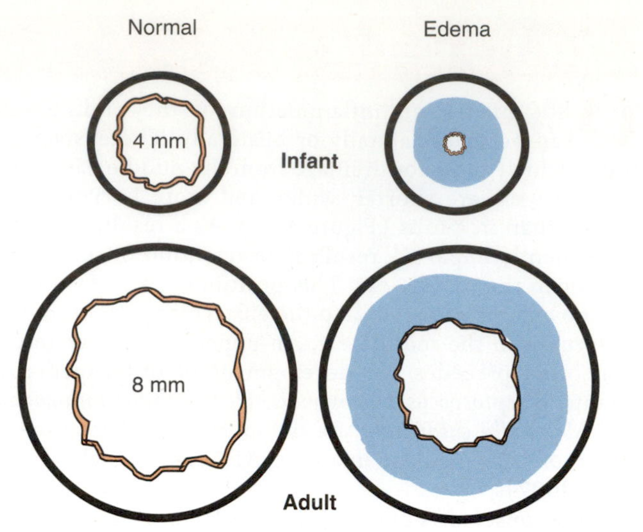

FIGURE 60-2 Effect of edema on airway resistance in the infant versus the adult: Whereas 1 mm of circumferential edema (on right) can cause a 75% decrease in the cross-sectional area of an infant's airway, it only causes a 44% decrease in the adult's.

Pharmacological

Use of medications such as bronchodilators, corticosteroids, and sedatives is controversial because of potential side effects. In severe cases caused by respiratory syncytial virus (RSV), ribavirin (Virazole), an aerosoled antiviral agent, may be used.

> **PROFESSIONALTIP**
>
> **Throat Procedures**
>
> Procedures involving the throat (e.g., cultures and visual inspection) can cause laryngospasm and airway obstruction and should therefore be avoided when children present with symptoms such as inspiratory stridor, a barking cough, or hoarseness.

> **COMMUNITY/HOME HEALTH CARE**
>
> **Managing LTB at Home**
>
> - Observe for early signs of respiratory distress, such as stridor at rest; lower rib retractions; difficulty swallowing; absence of cough; agitation; respiration >50; flaring nares
> - Maintain high humidity with cool-air vaporizer, 10 to 15 minutes in the bathroom with steam from a hot shower, cool air through a window
> - Hydrate with cool, noncarbonated, nonacidic beverages of choice; ice pops; gelatin; small pieces of ice
> - Provide rest by holding, rocking, soothing, and staying calm

Nursing Management

Children with mild croup (no stridor at rest, mild retractions, no cyanosis, and restlessness only when disturbed) are managed at home. Teach caregivers how to monitor for signs of respiratory distress and ways to maintain high humidity and hydration. Instruct caregivers to not give the child red-colored drinks because it may be difficult to differentiate between the food coloring and blood in the client's vomit or stool.

Care for the hospitalized infant includes a mist hood or tent with oxygen and, if the child is refusing oral fluids or respirations are greater than 60 breaths per minute, intravenous (IV) therapy. Infants may be held with the mist blowing in the face if being in the tent causes distress. Caregivers should remain with the child and provide routine care throughout hospitalization in an effort to keep the infant calm, quiet, and in the tent. The presence of favorite toys and items from home can also be comforting to the infant. It is important to keep linens and clothes dry and the child in a comfortable position (usually semireclined in an infant seat placed under the tent). If oxygen is administered, the concentration delivered is regulated to maintain arterial saturation > 95% (according to pulse oximetry).

As with home care, monitoring for early signs of impending airway obstruction is paramount. Intubation equipment should be readily available at all times.

PNEUMONIA

An inflammation of the bronchioles and alveolar spaces of the lungs, pneumonia is most commonly caused by RSV in infants. Pneumonia is often preceded by an upper respiratory infection. Viral infections render the infant more susceptible to secondary bacterial invasion. Pneumococcal pneumonia is the most common form of bacterial pneumonia found in infants.

Onset is usually abrupt, with rapidly increasing fever, flaring nostrils, **circumoral cyanosis** (bluish discoloration surrounding the mouth), chest retractions, pulse rate of 140 to 180 beats per minute, respiratory rate of 60 to 80 breaths per minute, and nonproductive cough. Chest x-rays and secretion cultures are used to confirm the diagnosis.

Medical–Surgical Management

Medical

Treatment involves oxygen and cool-mist administration, chest physiotherapy, postural drainage, hydration, caregiver support, antipyretics, and antibiotics (if causative agent is bacterial) such as penicillin and macrolides (erythromycin, azithromycin, and clarithromycin) (Klugman & Lonks, 2005).

Nursing Management

Assess lung sounds, monitor respiratory status, prevent further infection, and promote safety. Monitor hydration by accurate intake and output (I&O) measurement and assessment of skin turgor and anterior fontanel. Use a bulb syringe to suction the nose and nasopharynx as needed and before feeding. Saline nose drops may aid in clearing passages. Change the infant's position frequently to prevent both stasis of secretions in the lungs and secretion drainage into the eustachian tubes. Encourage caregivers to be active participants in their infant's routine daily care.

RESPIRATORY DISTRESS SYNDROME

Preterm infants often have respiratory distress syndrome (RDS) because the lungs are deficient in surfactant, a substance that reduces surface tension inside the air sacs. The lungs collapse after each breath, greatly reducing the infant's supply of oxygen. This, in turn, damages the lung cells, contributing to the formation of hyaline membrane. This membrane blocks gas exchange in the alveoli. Infants born at 28 weeks' gestation or less are most at risk for developing respiratory distress syndrome (Hermansen & Lorah, 2007).

Clinical manifestations include tachypnea (70 to 120 breaths per minute in children), retractions, grunting, crackles, pallor, cyanosis, slow capillary refill, hypothermia, peripheral edema, flaccid muscle tone, gastrointestinal (GI) shutdown, jaundice, and acidosis. Chest radiographs confirm the diagnosis.

The first 96 hours are critical to the recovery of infants with RDS. Complications of RDS include complications of oxygen administration; intraventricular hemorrhage; bronchopulmonary dysplasia (BPD); and necrotizing enterocolitis.

Medical–Surgical Management

Medical

Treatment includes administration of surfactant through the endotracheal tube immediately at or soon after birth. In addition, continuous positive airway pressure (CPAP) helps keep the lungs partially expanded until they begin producing surfactant (approximately 5 days).

Health Promotion

Attempts may be made to prevent the occurrence of RDS. Surfactant may be administered to at-risk infants before the development of RDS. If preterm delivery is expected, **lecithin**, the major component of surfactant, may be measured to determine lung maturity. If insufficient lecithin is present, the mother may be given a glucocorticosteroid (betamethasone) that crosses the placenta and causes the infant's lungs to produce surfactant within 72 hours.

Nursing Management

Closely monitor respirations, eliminate unnecessary physical stimulation and metabolic demands, and establish a positive relationship with the caregivers. Place the infant in a warmer under an oxygen hood or with mechanical ventilation.

CYSTIC FIBROSIS

Cystic fibrosis (CF), a major dysfunction of all exocrine glands, primarily affects the lungs, pancreas, liver, and reproductive organs. Characteristics of this disease include increased viscosity of mucous gland secretions, elevated sweat electrolytes, increased organic and enzymatic constituents of saliva, and abnormalities in autonomic nervous system function. This disease is transmitted as an autosomal-recessive trait, meaning that both parents must be carriers (Table 60-2). Therefore, it is common that infants with CF also have siblings with CF.

Most children show evidence of the disease by 1 year of age. The earliest manifestation of CF is **meconium ileus** (impacted feces in the newborn, causing bowel obstruction).

TABLE 60-2 Autosomal-Recessive Inheritance

	GAMETES	MOTHER (CARRIER: HAS TRAIT) A	a
Father (Carrier: Has Trait)	A	AA (no disease/ trait)	**Aa** (has trait)
	a	**Aa** (has trait)	**aa** (has disease)

COURTESY OF DELMAR CENGAGE LEARNING

Intussusception (telescoping of the bowel) may be another sign of the disorder. Rectal prolapse is a common problem resulting from difficulty passing the sticky, thick, fatty stools. These GI problems result from the lack of pancreatic enzymes. Most children have difficulty gaining and maintaining weight, despite a voracious appetite. Failure to thrive is common in these infants. Pulmonary complications, such as chronic moist, productive cough and frequent infections, are present in most children with CF due to their inability to clear mucoid secretions. Many children develop barrel chests and clubbed fingers because of the chronic lack of oxygen. Fertility is low in females and males are usually sterile (Burns et al., 2008).

Caregivers frequently report that their infants taste like salt when they kiss them. This common manifestation is a result of the elevated sweat electrolytes. Diagnosis is confirmed with the sweat chloride test. Results greater than 60 mEq/L of chloride are considered positive for CF (Burns et al., 2008).

Although CF is a life-threatening illness, families must be encouraged to focus on positive outcomes. The life expectancy continues to rise, and the search for improved treatments continues. In 2008, the median predicted age of survival for children affected with CF rose to 37.4 years, up from 32 in 2000.

MEDICAL–SURGICAL MANAGEMENT

Medical

Treatment focuses on managing pulmonary complications, ensuring adequate nutrition, and assisting the child and family in adapting to a chronic disorder. Chest physiotherapy (CPT, postural drainage) is usually performed one to three times per day to maintain patent airways.

Pharmacological

Aerosol treatments and antibiotic therapy may be used as indicated. Commercially prepared pancreatic enzymes are given with meals and snacks to aid digestion and absorption of fats and proteins.

VX (a chemical derivative of existing lead compounds) is a new protein repair therapy that may interact directly with the cystic fibrosis transmembrane regulator (CFTR) protein, the product of the CF gene. It appears to repair the faulty protein, thereby curing the basic CF defect. Clinical studies of this new drug began in August 1998. Researchers are evaluating the safety and pharmacodynamics of oral doses of VX during phase 3 clinical trials starting in 2009 (Cystic Fibrosis Foundation, 2009).

Diet

Well-balanced, high-caloric diets should be maintained because children with CF often absorb only 50% of ingested foods.

NURSING MANAGEMENT

Monitor respiratory status, adventitious lung sounds, cough, stools, abdominal distension, and weight. Assess growth and development, hydration, and nutrition. Administer oxygen and medications as ordered. Encourage physical activity. Teach family skills needed to follow the prescribed therapeutic plan.

NURSING PROCESS

ASSESSMENT

Subjective Data

Assess the child and caregivers for indications of anxiety and fear. Interview the caregiver about activities or events leading up to the crisis, effects of illness on day-to-day functioning, previous hospitalizations, and knowledge about the condition.

Objective Data

Physical assessment focuses on respiratory status, growth and development, hydration, and nutrition. Observe for adventitious lung sounds, cough, finger clubbing, barrel chest, frequency and nature of stools, abdominal distention, weight loss, fatigue, and pallor. Routinely plot height and weight on a growth chart, and assess developmental level using the Denver II test.

Nursing diagnoses for the infant with CF include the following:

NURSING DIAGNOSES	PLANNING/OUTCOMES	NURSING INTERVENTIONS
Ineffective Airway Clearance related to thick, tenacious secretions	The client will maintain a clear airway.	Initiate aerosol therapy, CPT, and breathing exercises as prescribed; schedule at least 1 hour before or after meals. Administer oxygen as prescribed and monitor closely for level of consciousness. Calculate and maintain required fluid intake. Observe for signs of infection. Assess respiratory status frequently. Administer antibiotics as prescribed.

Nursing diagnoses for the infant with CF include the following: (Continued)

NURSING DIAGNOSES	PLANNING/OUTCOMES	NURSING INTERVENTIONS
*Delayed **Growth** and Development* related to inability to digest nutrients and possible loss of appetite	The client will exhibit signs of adequate growth and development.	Ensure high-caloric intake. Administer prescribed pancreatic enzymes with meals and snacks. Offer small, frequent feedings if appetite poor. Monitor weight and height (plot on growth chart). Assess developmental level (e.g., with the Denver II test). Encourage physical activity limited only by the child's endurance.
***Fear** (family)* related to long-term care and prognosis	The family will verbalize knowledge of disease and demonstrate proper techniques for care. The family will verbalize lessened fears and anxiety. The family will utilize available support systems and community resources.	Teach the family the importance of carrying out prescribed therapeutic plan. Teach the family skills for carrying out prescribed therapeutic plan. Provide numbers for CF Foundation and community resources. Encourage expression of feelings and concerns. Refer the family for genetic counseling.

Evaluation: Evaluate each outcome to determine how it has been met by the client.

SUDDEN INFANT DEATH SYNDROME

Sudden infant death syndrome (SIDS), commonly called "crib death," is the sudden, unexpected death of an apparently healthy infant in whom the postmortem fails to reveal an adequate cause. It is the leading cause of death in infants older than 1 month of age, peaking between 2 and 30 months of age (AAP, 2005). Although numerous theories have been proposed regarding the cause of SIDS (including airway obstruction, abnormal cardiorespiratory control, and hyperactive airway reflexes), no single cause has been identified.

In 1994 the American Academy of Pediatrics (AAP) implemented the "Back to Sleep" campaign, recommending that infants be laid down for sleep in a supine position (AAP, 2005). Since then, the incidence of SIDS has dramatically decreased. Other modifiable risk factors to focus on are sleeping on a soft surface, maternal smoking, bed sharing, and overheating (AAP, 2005). Hersheberger (Dowshen, Hersheberger & Rutherford, 2001) states: "Parents need to know that SIDS is not caused by vomiting and choking or other minor illnesses. It is not caused by vaccines or other immunizations."

Typically, the infant is found huddled in the corner of a disheveled bed, with blankets over the head. Frothy, blood-tinged fluid fills the mouth and nose, and the infant may be lying face down in the secretions. The diaper is wet and full of stool. The hands may be clenched.

Nursing Management

Provide empathic support to the family. Ask caregivers only factual questions, with no suggestion of responsibility. It is vital to reassure them that death caused by SIDS is not predictable or completely preventable. Inform the caregiver that an autopsy must be performed to confirm the diagnosis of SIDS. Encourage them to hold their child and say "good-bye." If the mother was breastfeeding, provide information about abrupt discontinuation of lactation. Refer to the SIDS Foundation.

Ideally, the family will receive a visit from a competent, qualified professional as soon after the death as possible. Areas needing to be discussed include expression of feelings, coping mechanisms, siblings' reactions, and birth of a subsequent child.

CARDIOVASCULAR SYSTEM

Indications that the heart is functioning normally include warm skin, pink mucous membranes, easily palpated pulses, symmetrical chest, normal growth and development, and high activity tolerance. Upon auscultation of a healthy heart at the point of maximum intensity (PMI), two sounds (S1 ["lub"] and S2 ["dub"]) are heard. Heart sounds should be clear and distinct, regular and even. The rate should be the same as the radial pulse. In many children, a *sinus arrhythmia*, wherein the heart rate increases on inspiration and decreases on expiration, is considered normal.

During fetal life, the lungs are inactive and require only a small amount of blood to nourish their tissues. Blood is circulated through the umbilical arteries to the placenta, where waste products and carbon dioxide are exchanged for oxygen and nutrients. The blood is then returned to the fetus through the umbilical vein.

At birth, the umbilical cord is cut, and the infant's own independent system is established. The ductus arteriosus, the foramen ovale, and the ductus venosus are no longer needed. They normally close and atrophy during the first several weeks after birth. Figure 60-3 illustrates the circulatory patterns of the healthy prenatal and postnatal heart.

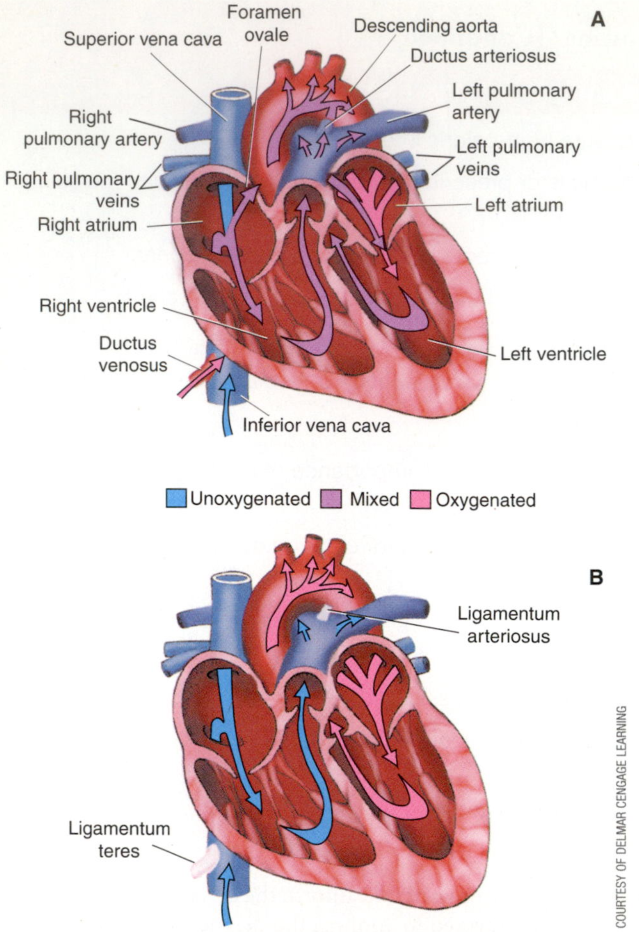

FIGURE 60-3 **Circulation of the Heart; *A*, Prenatal; *B*, Postnatal**

COURTESY OF DELMAR CENGAGE LEARNING

Congenital cardiovascular defects range from mild to severe. They may be detected immediately at birth or may not be detected for several months.

CONGENITAL CARDIOVASCULAR DEFECTS

Congenital cardiovascular defects are among the leading causes of death during the first year of life (American Heart Association, 2009). Errors in formation of the heart or great vessels can occur prenatally, and persistence of fetal circulation can occur postnatally. Cardiovascular defects are best categorized according to blood flow patterns: (1) increased pulmonary blood flow, (2) decreased pulmonary blood flow, (3) obstructed blood flow out of the heart, or (4) mixed blood flow. Four of the most common cardiovascular defects in infants are listed in Table 60-3. Congenital heart disease is considered to be of **multifactorial inheritance**, a combination of genetic and environmental factors.

Rubella in the mother during the first trimester of pregnancy is a common cause of heart defects in infants. Other possible maternal causes include alcoholism, irradiation, ingestion of drugs, diabetes, malnutrition, and being more than 40 years of age. Heredity is seldom a contributing factor.

Infants with severe cardiovascular defects may be born with obvious distress caused by hypoxia. Those with less serious defects may compensate and appear to be healthy at birth. Heart murmurs and delayed growth and development observed later may call attention to problems. Infants with severe defects will often manifest signs and symptoms of CHF, such as fatigability; orthopnea; failure to thrive;

TABLE 60-3 Common Cardiovascular Defects in Infants

	VENTRICULAR SEPTAL DEFECT (VSD)	ATRIAL SEPTAL DEFECT (ASD)	PATENT DUCTUS ARTERIOSUS (PDA)	TETRALOGY OF FALLOT (TOF)
Description	Opening between ventricles	Opening between atria; incompetent foramen ovale	Failure of fetal ductus arteriosus to close postnatally	Four defects: (VSD), pulmonic stenosis, overriding aorta, and right ventricular hypertrophy
Blood Flow Pattern	↑Pulmonary flow, left-to-right shunting	↑Pulmonary flow; left-to-right shunting	↑Pulmonary flow, left-to-right shunting	↓Pulmonary flow; right-to-left shunting
Manifestations	↑Respiratory infections; normal growth and development; congestive heart failure (CHF), if defect large	Usually asymptomatic, possible dysrhythmias, CHF if defect large	Usually asymptomatic, CHF possible, machinery-like murmur	Hypoxia, murmur, delayed growth and development
Treatment	Surgical correction by 2 years of age; prognosis dependent on extent of defect	Surgical correction by 6 years of age; excellent prognosis	Possiblity indomethacin (Indocin) administration to premature babies; surgical correction by 2 years; excellent prognosis	Surgical correction by 1 year of age

COURTESY OF DELMAR CENGAGE LEARNING

pale, mottled, or cyanotic skin; hoarse or weak cry; tachycardia; and signs of respiratory distress, such as rate > 60 breaths per minute, costal retractions, orthopnea, wheezing, and coughing.

Medical–Surgical Management

Surgical

Surgical intervention to repair a defect may be postponed until the child develops CHF. Generally, the older the infant, the better the surgical outcome. Refer to Table 60-3 for treatments of common heart defects.

Pharmacological

Digoxin (Lanoxin) is the drug most often used to improve the heart's contractility and increase its output. Furosemide (Lasix) is the most commonly used diuretic. Because most diuretics cause potassium loss, serum potassium level is monitored, and potassium supplements may be ordered. Oxygen therapy and fluid management are also part of the treatment plan.

Diet

When infants experience significant dyspnea while feeding, special feeding techniques are needed, such as providing small, frequent feedings and softer nipples. Some infants need higher caloric formulas and diets to meet nutritional needs. Gavage feedings may be required if the infant becomes fatigued before taking an adequate amount of formula.

Nursing Management

Assess cardiac and respiratory function. Monitor behavioral patterns and growth and development. Administer oxygen and medications as ordered. Accurately record I&O. Weigh daily. Provide high-calorie feedings. If infant tires easily when eating, implement gavage feedings.

NURSING PROCESS

Assessment

Subjective Data

Take a history of the child's previous hospitalizations and assess the caregiver's knowledge about the condition. Note the caregiver anxiety level, coping strategies, and economic status.

Objective Data

Assess the child's behavioral patterns, cardiac and respiratory function, fluid status, and growth and development. Obtain a detailed history of onset of symptoms and a typical day's activity schedule.

Nursing diagnoses for the infant with a heart defect include the following:

NURSING DIAGNOSES	PLANNING/OUTCOMES	NURSING INTERVENTIONS
*Decreased **Cardiac** Output* related to structural defect	The client will demonstrate sufficient cardiac output to meet metabolic demands.	Administer digoxin as prescribed. Monitor vital signs (including apical pulse for 1 minute), potassium level, urine output, cardiac rhythm, activity tolerance. Assess for signs of digoxin toxicity (vomiting, anorexia, dysrhythmias, bradycardia [pulse rate < 90 to 110]), peripheral perfusion. Provide periods of rest each hour.
*Ineffective **Breathing** Pattern* related to pulmonary congestion	The client will breathe effortlessly at rest.	Keep the client in semi-Fowler's position (i.e., use infant seat). Administer humidified oxygen as prescribed, assess respiratory rate and effort, color, and oxygen saturation. Employ comfort measures (e.g., holding, rocking, presence of caregivers). Respond quickly to crying.
*Excess **Fluid** Volume* related to fluid accumulation	The client will experience decreased edema.	Administer diuretics as prescribed. Measure I&O. Weigh daily (same time and scale). Assess skin for edema, breakdown. Turn every 2 hours and elevate edematous extremities. Monitor electrolytes.

(*Continues*)

Nursing diagnoses for the infant with a heart defect include the following: (Continued)

NURSING DIAGNOSES	PLANNING/OUTCOMES	NURSING INTERVENTIONS
*Imbalanced **N**utrition: Less than Body Requirements* related to fatigue and dyspnea	The client will demonstrate normal weight gain for age.	Give small, frequent, high-caloric feedings. Use soft nipple with large hole. Implement gavage feeding, if the infant tires before taking prescribed amount of formula. Make feeding time as stress free as possible. Hold the infant when bottle-feeding (preferably by primary caregiver).
*Delayed **G**rowth and Development* related to low energy level	The client will meet developmental milestones for age.	Encourage age-appropriate activities, stimulation, and socialization. Allow the child to set own pace.
*Interrupted **F**amily Processes* related to child with life-threatening illness/condition	The family will receive needed support.	Teach the family as needed about medication administration, signs and symptoms of CHF and when to report, feeding techniques, and appropriate activities for the child. Refer the family to appropriate community resources.

Evaluation: Evaluate each outcome to determine how it has been met by the client.

HEMATOLOGIC AND LYMPHATIC SYSTEMS

The hematologic system regulates, directly or indirectly, the functions of all body tissues and organs. Some of the most common disorders occurring in infants include hyperbilirubinemia, iron-deficiency anemia, and sickle-cell anemia (SCA).

HYPERBILIRUBINEMIA

Hyperbilirubinemia, often referred to as jaundice, is a common occurrence in neonates. **Jaundice** is the yellow discoloration of the skin, sclera, mucous membranes, and body fluids resulting from excess bilirubin and deposition of bile pigments. Physiologically, hemoglobin is broken down by the liver into iron, protein, and bilirubin. The bilirubin binds to albumin and is transported to the liver, where it is conjugated. Conjugated bilirubin is then eliminated through the intestines. Neonates have an intestinal enzyme that can convert the conjugated bilirubin back to unconjugated bilirubin, which can be reabsorbed into the bloodstream. This process can contribute significantly to the amount of bilirubin that the immature liver must break down. As the bilirubin level rises, some of the excess bilirubin is deposited in body tissues, resulting in a temporary yellow discoloration of the skin and sclera. A high level of bilirubin can penetrate and damage brain cells, causing severe neural symptoms (**kernicterus**). Hyperbilirubinemia develops during the first few days of life, with a greater incidence in preterm infants.

PROFESSIONALTIP

Stress at Feeding Time

Ways to decrease stress at feeding time include the following:

- Decrease the noise level.
- Hold the infant while sitting in a rocker.
- Assess the infant's readiness to eat. (Infant is calm, demonstrates rooting, latches onto nipple eagerly, opens mouth voluntarily, looks at caregiver.)

MEDICAL–SURGICAL MANAGEMENT

Medical

The main objective of treatment is to reduce the amount of unconjugated bilirubin and aid in the conversion of bilirubin to a form that can be excreted by the body (urobilinogen). Full-term infants with jaundice may benefit from early and frequent breastfeeding (every 2 hours) (Moerschel et al., 2008). Otherwise, treatment usually begins with a phototherapy light, called a bililight, or a fiber-optic blanket. This light causes a chemical reaction in the skin and converts unconjugated bilirubin to a form that can be excreted by the body (lumirubin). Therapy is usually continual, with short breaks for feeding and holding. Phototherapy may be done at home because it is less expensive than treatment in the hospital and the caregivers will not have to be separated from their newborn.

Pharmacological

If the bilirubin level responds slowly to phototherapy, phenobarbital is sometimes given to enhance both the liver enzyme action and bilirubin excretion. Breastfed infants should continue nursing (8 to 12 times per day) whether or not phototherapy is required. Increasing the frequency of breastfeeding aids in the removal of bilirubin from the gastrointestinal tract. In cases where the mother's milk supply is inadequate, substituting formula for breastfeeding or incorporating it as a supplement may help decrease bilirubin levels. Ideally, breastfeeding should not be interrupted. (AAP, 2004; Moerschel et al., 2008).

NURSING MANAGEMENT

Frequently assess for jaundice. Encourage frequent feedings. Maintain phototherapy as prescribed. Teach caregivers to do phototherapy at home.

NURSING PROCESS

ASSESSMENT

Subjective Data

Assess perinatal risk factors such as familial history of hyperbilirubinemia and induced delivery.

Objective Data

Assess for jaundice by applying light pressure to the skin over either the tip of the nose or the sternum in natural daylight. For dark-skinned infants, observe the sclera, conjunctiva, and oral mucosa for a yellow color. Bruising, petechiae, and pallor are also suggestive of hyperbilirubenemia.

Nursing diagnoses for the infant with hyperbilirubinemia include the following:

NURSING DIAGNOSES	PLANNING/OUTCOMES	NURSING INTERVENTIONS
Risk for Deficient ***Fluid*** *Volume* related to insensible losses	The client will maintain fluid balance.	Assess skin for signs of dehydration (i.e., dry mouth, sleepiness, decreased urine output). Calculate needed fluid intake to compensate for losses. Monitor I&O.
Risk for Impaired ***Skin*** *Integrity* related to use of phototherapy	The client's skin will remain intact.	Assess skin for breakdown. Monitor temperature every 2 to 4 hours. Keep skin clean and dry, do not apply any oils or lotions.
Interrupted ***Family*** *Processes* related to situational crisis	The family will receive needed support.	Encourage bonding by removing eye shields and allowing the caregivers to hold/feed the infant. Teach the importance of eye shields under light. Support the breastfeeding mother. Encourage pumping the breasts if feeding must be stopped temporarily. Keep the caregivers informed.

Evaluation: Evaluate each outcome to determine how it has been met by the client.

IRON-DEFICIENCY ANEMIA

The incidence of iron-deficiency anemia is usually related to the infant's consuming large amounts of milk and foods that do not contain supplemental iron. These babies are often overweight because of excessive intake of cow's milk, which is a poor source of iron. In addition, cow's milk can cause loss of blood in the stool.

Because full-term infants have iron stores from fetal circulation that usually last for 5 to 6 months, iron-deficiency anemia usually surfaces between 9 and 24 months of age. Clinical manifestations may include extreme pallor (porcelain-like in fair-skinned infants), tachycardia, lethargy, irritability, and below-normal hemoglobin, hematocrit, and iron levels.

MEDICAL–SURGICAL MANAGEMENT

Pharmacological

Iron therapy is usually prescribed and continued for 3 months after hemoglobin and hematocrit levels return to normal. An increase in hemoglobin level can be expected within 4 to 30 days. Ascorbic acid may also be prescribed in an attempt to facilitate iron absorption. Intramuscular (IM) or IV injections may be necessary if the level does not improve after 1 month of oral iron. Transfusions are indicated only for the most severe cases.

Diet

Long-term therapy is directed at increasing the dietary intake of iron and continuing the use of iron-fortified formula until

PROFESSIONALTIP

WIC

The federal supplemental food program called Women, Infants, and Children (WIC) is an excellent resource for nutritious food for low-income families with pregnant, postpartum, or lactating women and children up to 5 years of age. In addition to food, this program provides nutritional education and screening.

12 months of age. At 4 to 6 months of age, iron-fortified cereal can be used (Burns et al., 2008).

Nursing Management

Prevent anemia by educating the caregivers about administration of iron. It is important to explore any misconceptions caregivers may have, such as "milk is a perfect food" and "excessive weight gain equates to a healthy child and good mothering."

Encourage foods rich in iron, such as dried beans, iron-fortified cereals, apricots, prunes, egg yolks, and dark-green, leafy vegetables. Infants should remain on iron-fortified formulas until 12 months of age.

Instruct caregivers in the proper administration of oral iron. When administering IM preparations, no more than 1 mL should be given deep into the muscle using the Z-track method to prevent staining of tissues and to minimize irritation.

SICKLE-CELL ANEMIA

Sickle-cell anemia is a genetic disorder characterized by the production of abnormal hemoglobin and resulting in red blood cells (RBCs) taking on a "sickle" shape (Figure 60-4). Because of the presence of fetal hemoglobin, clinical symptoms usually do not appear until 6 months of age. Episodes of sickling may be triggered by infection, dehydration, hypoxia, trauma, or general physical or

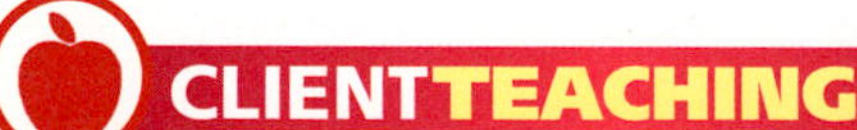

CLIENTTEACHING

Administration of Iron to Infants

When instructing caregivers in the administration of iron to infants, teach to:

- Administer with citrus fruit or juice in order to increase its absorption.
- Administer through a straw or medicine dropper placed at the back of the mouth, to decrease staining of the teeth.
- Brush or wipe the infant's teeth after administration.
- Expect dark, black stools.

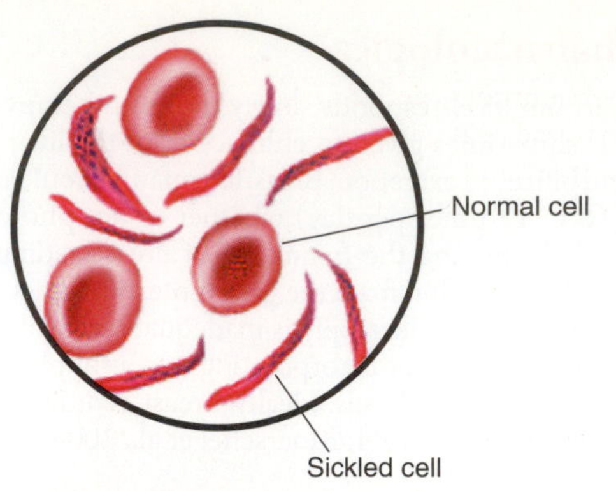

COURTESY OF DELMAR CENGAGE LEARNING

FIGURE 60-4 Sickling Cells

emotional stress resulting in impaired circulation and increased RBC destruction.

The most common symptoms of SCA include abdominal pain (caused by sludging in the spleen and leading to its enlargement), fever, severe leg pain, and hot, swollen joints. In addition, growth retardation, chronic anemia, and increased susceptibility to infection may be experienced. This disease occurs primarily among African Americans and is transmitted as an autosomal-recessive trait wherein both parents are carriers (refer back to Table 60-2).

Medical–Surgical Management

Medical

Between episodes, the goal is to prevent crises with adequate hydration (1,500 to 3,000 mL per day). During crises, treatment may include bed rest, oxygen, analgesics (morphine), and fluids.

Pharmacological

Children with this disease must be immunized with influenza, pneumococcal, meningococcal, and hepatitis B vaccines because of increased susceptibility to infection and the likelihood of transfusion therapy. Prophylactic oral penicillin is often prescribed twice a day until age 5 or 6, and a daily supplement of folic acid is taken (Mayo Clinic, 2009).

MEMORYTRICK

Sickle-Cell Anemia

When a client is experiencing a sickle-cell crisis, remember the 5 As:

A = Administer analgesics

A = Administer antibiotics

A = Administer oxygen

A = Administer fluids

A = Apply heat to affected area

Health Promotion

Avoid high altitudes, poorly pressurized airplanes, and exposure to extreme heat or cold. Maintaining hydration is of paramount importance. Neonatal screening, early intervention, prophylactic antibiotics, and parent education have allowed children with SCA to live into adulthood.

Nursing Management

Encourage continuous adequate hydration and immunizations. Prevent exposure to extreme heat or cold. Provide caregiver education. Monitor growth and development. When in crisis, administer analgesics, antibiotics, oxygen, and fluids as ordered. Apply heat to affected area.

NURSING PROCESS

Assessment

Subjective Data

Interview the caregivers about activities or events leading up to the crisis, a history of child's health, and previous episodes. Evaluate the caregivers level of knowledge about the condition.

Objective Data

Assess all areas and systems that can be affected by circulatory obstruction, such as vital signs, vision, hearing, growth and development, and the respiratory, GI, renal, neurological, and musculoskeletal systems.

Nursing diagnoses for the infant with sickle-cell anemia include the following:

NURSING DIAGNOSES	PLANNING/OUTCOMES	NURSING INTERVENTIONS
*Ineffective **Tissue** Perfusion* related to vaso-occlusion and anemia	The client will maintain oxygen saturation levels at 95% or greater.	Administer oxygen as prescribed. Monitor oxygen saturation, capillary refill, and respiratory status. Maintain the client in a position of comfort (semi- to high-Fowler's). Administer packed RBCs as prescribed.
*Acute **Pain*** related to vaso-occlusion and tissue ischemia	The client will be pain free.	Apply heat to affected area; avoid cold compresses. Administer analgesics as prescribed (preferably morphine) and assess effectiveness by assessing behavior and vital signs. Reassure the caregivers that opioids are appropriate, high doses may be needed, and addiction is rare. Position the client carefully and handle gently.
*Risk for **Infection*** related to splenic malfunction	The client will be infection-free.	Provide one to one and one-half daily fluid requirement as determined by body weight. Provide daily food requirements as determined by body weight and length. Administer antibiotics as prescribed. Ensure that the infant avoids contact with known sources of infection. Ensure that immunizations are up-to-date.
*Deficient **Knowledge** (family)* related to cause and treatment of disease	The family will verbalize an understanding of the risk factors and ways to minimize them.	Teach need for one to one and one-half times daily fluid requirement. Teach importance of hand hygiene and avoiding known sources of infection. Reinforce importance of up-to-date immunizations for the infant. Teach to shield the infant from overexertion, emotional stress, and low-oxygen environments. Teach early intervention for any sign of infection (e.g., temperature of 101.5°F or greater) or dehydration (weight loss, dry skin and mucous membranes, sunken fontanel). Teach medication administration as ordered.

(*Continues*)

Nursing diagnoses for the infant with sickle-cell anemia include the following: (Continued)

NURSING DIAGNOSES	PLANNING/OUTCOMES	NURSING INTERVENTIONS
Interrupted Family Processes related to child with chronic condition	The family will adjust to lifelong, potentially fatal hereditary disease.	Explain procedures and planned treatments. Allow the family to provide care in the hospital. Provide information about appropriate developmental activities. Encourage the family to talk about feelings and concerns. Stress positive outcomes (e.g., that most of the time, children are asymptomatic and can participate in appropriate activities without restrictions). Provide information regarding transmission of the condition; refer for genetic counseling. Provide numbers for American Sickle Cell Anemia Association and available support groups.

Evaluation: Evaluate each outcome to determine how it has been met by the client.

GASTROINTESTINAL SYSTEM

Infants have minimal saliva, no voluntary control of swallowing, a small stomach, rapid intestinal motility, a relaxed cardiac sphincter, deficiency of enzymes in the duodenum, and immature liver function. This accounts for the numerous GI problems that occur during the first 12 months of life, such as vomiting, diarrhea, **colic** (sudden, recurrent bouts of abdominal pain), and failure to thrive. In addition, because the immune system is also immature, the infant is highly susceptible to infection. Congenital defects resulting in **atresia** (absence or closure of a body orifice), malposition, nonclosure, or other abnormalities can occur in any area of the GI tract. Any GI problem, whether a lack of nutrients, an infection, or a congenital disorder, can quickly affect other parts of the body and ultimately affect general health and growth and development. The GI disorders discussed following include thrush, acute gastroenteritis, colic, failure to thrive, cleft lip/palate, esophageal atresia with tracheoesophageal fistula, pyloric stenosis, Hirschsprung's disease, gastroesophageal reflux, and intussusception.

THRUSH

Thrush (moniliasis, candidiasis) is an oral fungal infection that is transmitted from the vaginal canal of an infected mother to the newborn. Other contributing factors include poor hand hygiene by care providers, inadequate washing of bottles and nipples, and antibiotic therapy. Thrush is characterized by painless, white patches that look like curdled milk on the oral mucosa (Figure 60-5). Bottle-fed infants are at greater risk of developing thrush than breastfed infants.

Medical–Surgical Management

Pharmacological

Topical nystatin (Mycostatin) is the most commonly used treatment for thrush. It is applied to the oral mucosa four times per day with an applicator or a gloved finger and then swallowed (Su et al., 2008). Rinse the mouth before medicating. In addition, if infants are breastfed, apply the medication to the breasts.

Nursing Management

Teach caregivers proper hand hygiene. Boiling bottles, pacifiers, and nipples for 20 minutes will kill the spores.

ACUTE GASTROENTERITIS

Acute gastroenteritis (AGE) is an inflammation of the stomach and intestines that may be accompanied by diarrhea and vomiting. This common condition may be caused by malnutrition, lactose intolerance, chronic conditions, or infections by viruses, bacteria, and parasites.

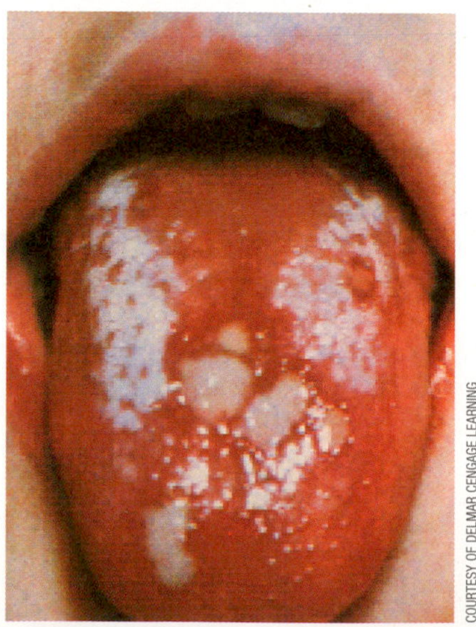
COURTESY OF DELMAR CENGAGE LEARNING

Figure 60-5 Thrush

The infant with AGE will have an increased number of green, liquid stools tinged with mucus or blood. In addition, symptoms of fluid and electrolyte imbalance, cramping, extreme irritability, and vomiting may be exhibited. Depending on age and nutritional status and on the severity and duration of the diarrhea, the infant may become severely dehydrated and gravely ill.

Medical–Surgical Management

Medical

Regaining and maintaining fluid balance is paramount. Use oral rehydrating fluids such as Pedialyte and Lytren for mild dehydration. For severe dehydration, IV solutions are needed to replace fluids and electrolytes. Antibiotics may be prescribed if bacterial infection is indicated from stool cultures.

Diet

Once rehydration is attained, the usual diet is continued. Research has indicated that early reintroduction of normal nutrients is desirable, and delayed introduction of food may be harmful in terms of nutritional status and duration of illness. Breastfed infants should continue on supplemental oral rehydrating solutions throughout the illness. If formula feedings are not tolerated, suggest lactose-free formulas. Complex carbohydrates, lean meats, fruits, and vegetables are well tolerated. Foods high in simple sugars such as carbonated soft drinks, juice, and gelatin should be avoided (MMWR, 2003).

Nursing Management

Assess for dehydration. Monitor I&O and electrolyte levels. Administer fluids and electrolytes as ordered. Provide clear fluids and oral rehydrating solutions every 30 minutes. Follow proper hand hygiene and teach to caregivers. Keep diaper area clean and apply a barrier ointment.

NURSING PROCESS

Assessment

Subjective Data

Question caregivers regarding probable etiologic agents such as introduction of new food; exposure to infectious agents; travel to an area where the infectious agent is endemic; contact with foods that might be contaminated; crowded, dirty living conditions; and contact with pets that are known to be sources of enteric infections, such as pet turtles. Obtain allergy, drug, health, and diet histories.

Objective Data

Assessing for dehydration is paramount for infants with AGE (Table 60-4). Assess the diaper area for skin breakdown resulting from repeated contact with diarrheal stools.

INFECTION CONTROL

Diaper Hygiene

- Change diapers as soon as they are soiled.
- Wear gloves when changing diapers.
- Fold the used diaper with soiled area to the inside and immediately place the diaper in a covered receptacle.
- Cleanse the skin and dispose of wipes along with the diaper.
- Remove gloves after disposal of wipes.
- Rediaper.
- Wash hands immediately after rediapering is complete.
- Store soiled clothing, cloth diapers, and washcloths in a covered receptacle.
- Cleanse surface of changing area.

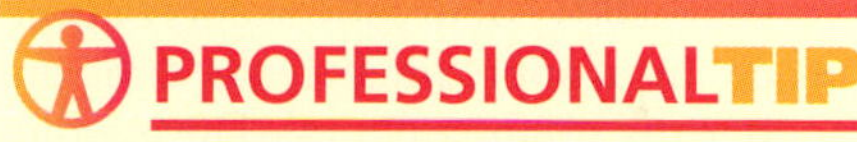

Potassium Administration

Potassium is excreted by the kidneys. If kidney function is impaired, potassium can build up in the body and can lead to arrhythmias and become life-threatening. Therefore, urine output must be established prior to administering potassium.

Table 60-4 Assessing Dehydration

SIGNS AND SYMPTOMS	MILD	MODERATE	SEVERE
Weight loss	<3%	3–9%	>9%
Skin turgor	Taut	Tenting	Tenting
Skin color	Pale	Grey	Mottled
Mucous membranes	Slightly dry, pale	Very dry, grey	Parched
Urine output	Decreased	Absent	Absent
Blood pressure	Normal	Normal	Decreased
Pulse	Normal or increased	Increased	Increased/thready
Fontanelle	Flat	Depressed	Sunken

COURTESY OF DELMAR CENGAGE LEARNING

Nursing diagnoses for the infant with AGE include the following:

NURSING DIAGNOSES	PLANNING/OUTCOMES	NURSING INTERVENTIONS
*Deficient **F**luid Volume* related to excessive GI losses	The client will be adequately hydrated (specify).	Monitor I&O and notify physician if output <1 mL/kg/h. Assess weight daily and compare with previous weights. Assess for degree of hydration. Monitor electrolyte levels. Administer fluids and electrolytes as prescribed. Encourage clear liquids and oral rehydrating solutions (Pedialyte, Lytren) in small doses every 30 minutes until rehydrated; after rehydration, alternate with water, breast milk, or half-strength formula, as needed.
*Risk for **I**nfection* related to GI infection	The client and family will be infection free.	Teach proper hand hygiene and diaper hygiene to care providers. Wear gloves when handling diapers.
*Risk for Impaired **S**kin Integrity* related to frequent contact with diarrheal stools	The client's skin will remain intact.	Change diapers every 2 hours, as needed. Cleanse skin with mild soap (Dove) and water. Apply barrier (A&D Ointment).

Evaluation: Evaluate each outcome to determine how it has been met by the client.

COLIC

Colic is a sudden, periodic attack of abdominal pain and cramping that is defined as "crying for more than three hours per day, for more than three days per week, and for longer than three weeks in an infant who is well-fed and otherwise healthy" (Roberts et al., 2004). It usually occurs between birth and 3 months of age and at approximately the same time each day (late afternoon, early evening hours). During these episodes, the infant is generally inconsolable, which may interfere with caregiver–child attachment and family relations.

The child is usually eager to eat and is growing appropriately. There is no known cause of colic; however, speculation points to overfeeding, overly rapid feeding, improper burping, the swallowing of large amounts of air, and emotional stress between parent and child (Hockenberry et al., 2006).

MEDICAL–SURGICAL MANAGEMENT

Medical

Sensitivity to formula, food allergies, peritoneal infection, and intestinal obstruction must be ruled out as specific causes of the distress. If sensitivity to formula is suspected, another brand of formula may be substituted. In the case of breastfeeding mothers, avoid dairy products, onions, cabbage, and dry beans for several days in an attempt to relieve the infant's symptoms.

Pharmacological

Sedatives, antispasmodics, antihistamines, and antiflatulents are sometimes recommended in an attempt to relieve symptoms.

NURSING MANAGEMENT

Assessing circumstances surrounding the colicky event, exploring techniques to relieve symptoms, and supporting

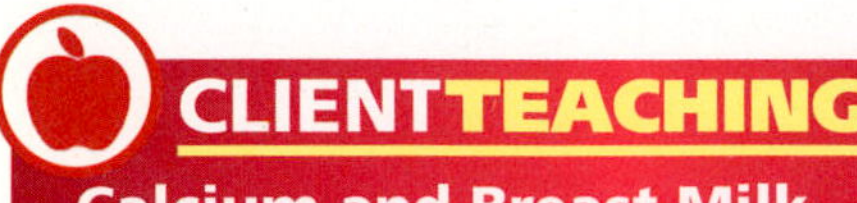

CLIENT TEACHING

Calcium and Breast Milk

If the breastfeeding mother maintains a milk-free diet for more than several days, she must take calcium supplements in order to maintain the calcium content of the breast milk.

CLIENT TEACHING

Suggestions for Alleviating Colic

- Provide rhythmic movement, such as rocking, swinging, and riding in the car.
- Alternate positions, such as placing the infant face down across the lap.
- Reduce environmental stimuli, especially during feedings.
- Provide a variety of tactile stimulation, such as rubbing the head or abdomen or placing prone on a warm heating pad.
- Provide small, frequent feedings.
- Burp during and after feedings.
- Respond immediately to crying.
- Provide background or "white" noise (vacuum cleaner, hair dryer) or play music.

caregivers during the colicky period are the primary nursing goals. Observe the feeding technique in order to assess the parent's sensitivity and response to the infant's cues of distress and evaluate the clarity of the infant's cues and the infant's responsiveness to the parent.

Reassure caregivers that colic usually resolves by 3 months of age and does not indicate poor or inadequate parenting. Encourage them to talk about their feelings toward the infant and any insecurities they may feel.

FAILURE TO THRIVE

Failure to thrive (FTT) is the label applied to infants who fail to gain weight and who show signs of delayed development. There are two categories of FTT: organic, which is caused by a physical defect or condition; and nonorganic, which is the result of psychosocial factors such as an impaired parent–child relationship. Manifestations of FTT include sustained growth failure (below the fifth percentile on the standardized growth chart), developmental delays in all areas, and poor feeding and sleeping patterns.

Medical–Surgical Management

Medical

If FTT is the result of a physical defect or condition, the condition is treated. Regardless of the cause, the primary goals are to provide adequate nutrition, promote growth and development, and assist caregivers in developing the skills needed to nurture their infant.

Health Promotion

In most cases of nonorganic FTT, a multidisciplinary health care team is needed to deal with the physical, psychosocial, mental, and emotional problems that may be occurring in the family. If the entire family is to become healthy, each member must be helped to change.

Nursing Management

Monitor weight gain and development. Provide adequate nutrition. Assist caregivers to develop nurturing skills.

NURSING PROCESS

Assessment

Subjective Data

Focus on the infant's routine, respiratory status, and diet history. Assess the family for depression, substance abuse, mental retardation, and psychosis as well as socioeconomic level, education, social isolation, stress factors, and support systems.

Objective Data

Focus on signs of malnutrition (skin, hair, nails, mucous membranes, energy level, developmental milestones) and on parent–infant interactions (parent's cues, infant's cues, and synchrony).

Nursing diagnoses for the infant with FTT include the following:

NURSING DIAGNOSES	PLANNING/OUTCOMES	NURSING INTERVENTIONS
*Imbalanced **N**utrition: Less than Body Requirements* related to insufficient intake of calories and/or impaired parent/child interaction	The client will demonstrate growth curve above the 5th percentile.	Provide consistent nursing staff and develop a structured routine. Feed the infant on demand and increase intake as tolerated. Monitor I&O. Weigh daily. Encourage caregiver involvement in care, demonstrate and model appropriate care techniques, praise positive attempts at care, and provide for rooming-in. Use a variety of methods to teach child care to the caregivers.
*Risk for **D**elayed Development* related to inadequate stimulation	The client will attain age-appropriate developmental milestones.	Begin a program of play that stimulates interest and responsiveness. Teach the caregivers ways to play and interact with the infant and to cuddle the infant.

Evaluation: Evaluate each outcome to determine how it has been met by the client.

CLEFT LIP/PALATE

The most common facial malformations are cleft lip and cleft palate. They may occur separately or together. Failure of the palates and/or lip to fuse is evident at birth. The defect may occur unilaterally on either side or bilaterally and with varying degrees of severity. The cause is unclear, but some genetic component seems likely.

Clinical manifestations include nasal, lip, and palate distortions. The child born with a cleft palate and intact lip does not manifest the external disfigurement so potentially distressing to caregivers, but the physical problems are more serious. The infant with a cleft palate is at risk for aspiration,

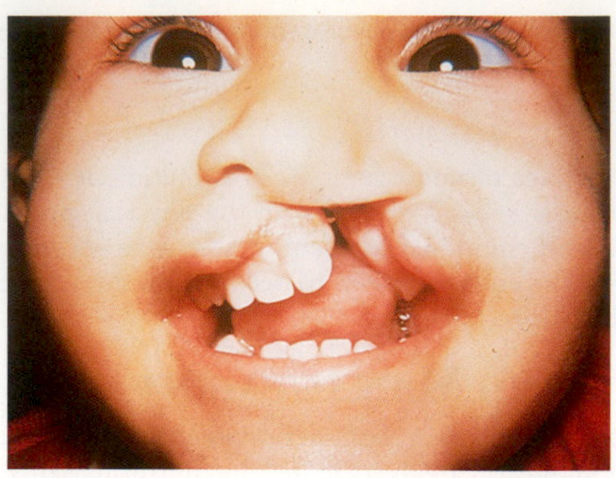

FIGURE 60-6 Older Child with Unrepaired Cleft Lip (*Courtesy of Dr. Joseph Konzelman, School of Dentistry, Medical College of Georgia.*)

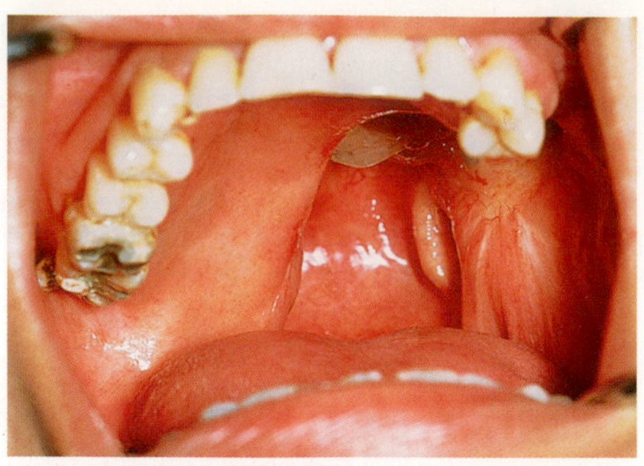

FIGURE 60-7 Older Child with Unrepaired Cleft Palate (*Courtesy of Dr. Joseph Konzelman, School of Dentistry, Medical College of Georgia.*)

feeding difficulties, and respiratory infections (Figures 60-6 and 60-7).

MEDICAL–SURGICAL MANAGEMENT

Medical

Care is directed toward closing the defects, maintaining adequate nutrition, preventing complications, and fostering normal growth and development of the child. Total care may involve many specialists, including pediatricians, nurses, plastic surgeons, orthodontists, prosthodontists, otolaryngologists, speech therapists, and psychiatrists. The extent of multidisciplinary care depends on the severity of the defect. Infants with cleft lip and palate are prone to recurrent otitis media, which will likely be treated with antibiotics.

Surgical

Closure of the lip precedes that of the palate, usually at 6 to 12 weeks of age. The palate is usually closed surgically at 12 to 18 months of age to facilitate speech development.

Health Promotion

Maternal use of multivitamin supplements containing folic acid around the time of conception has been reported to reduce the risk of cleft malformations by up to 50% (Bailey & Berry, 2005).

NURSING MANAGEMENT

Encourage caregivers to hold and interact with their infant and to participate in the care of the infant. Provide feedings as ordered using assistive devices. Keep infant in upright position for feeding. Burp frequently.

NURSING PROCESS

ASSESSMENT

Subjective Data

Assess immediately the emotional impact of the birth of an infant with a facial deformity. Assess the caregivers acceptance of the child periodically, at various appointments and hospital admissions.

Objective Data

Cleft lip and palate are observable at birth. A cleft palate is palpable with the finger. Document the degree of involvement. Evaluate the ability to suck, swallow, breathe, and handle secretions.

Nursing diagnoses for the infant with cleft lip or palate include the following:

NURSING DIAGNOSES	PLANNING/OUTCOMES	NURSING INTERVENTIONS
*Compromised Family **C**oping* related to birth of infant with visible and/or structural defect	The family will bond with the infant.	Encourage the caregivers to hold the infant. Point out positive attributes of the infant (e.g., hair, eyes, alertness); convey attitude of acceptance of the infant and family. Explain expected outcomes of surgical repair; show pictures of repaired children. Allow expression of feelings. Assess the caregivers' knowledge, degree of anxiety, level of discomfort, interpersonal relationships. Explore reactions of extended family. Encourage the caregivers to participate in care of the infant. Refer to support groups and to other families in similar situations.

Nursing diagnoses for the infant with cleft lip or palate include the following: (Continued)

NURSING DIAGNOSES	PLANNING/OUTCOMES	NURSING INTERVENTIONS
*Imbalanced **N**utrition: Less than Body Requirements* related to infant's inability to form an adequate seal when sucking on the nipple	The infant will maintain a growth curve above the 5th percentile.	Provide 100 to 150 cal/kg/d and 100 to 130 mL/kg/d. Assess output daily. Weigh daily. Observe for respiratory impairment (i.e., for adventitious breath sounds, increased respiratory rate). Facilitate breastfeeding; refer for ongoing support (e.g., to La Leche League). Position the infant in an upright or semi-sitting position for feeding. Use effective assistive devices (e.g., longer, softer nipples; feeders). Feed small amounts slowly, allowing ample time for sucking and swallowing; burp after 15 to 30 mL. Initiate nasogastric feeding if infant is unable to ingest sufficient calories by mouth. Teach caregivers the proper placement and use of nasogastric tube.
*Impaired **T**issue Integrity* related to surgical correction of cleft	The client's tissue will heal with minimal scarring.	Position the infant on side or back. Use elbow restraints for 7 to 10 days as needed and teach proper application to caregivers. Medicate for pain around-the-clock for at least 24 hours postoperatively. Provide developmentally appropriate activities (e.g., music, mobiles, holding) to distract the infant's attention from the incision site. Do not use pacifiers, spoons, or straws for 7 to 10 days postoperatively. Progress to a soft diet appropriate for age and as ordered and tolerated within 48 hours.
*Risk for **I**nfection* related to surgical procedure and accumulation of formula and secretions in oral cavity	The client's surgical site will be free of infection.	Assess vital signs and oral cavity every 2 hours. Cleanse suture line with normal saline or sterile water, as ordered. Give 5 to 15 mL water after each feeding to cleanse the mouth. Apply antibiotic cream as ordered. Ensure hand hygiene by all care providers. Include caregivers in care and prepare for home care.

Evaluation: Evaluate each outcome to determine how it has been met by the client.

ESOPHAGEAL ATRESIA WITH TRACHEOESOPHAGEAL FISTULA

Esophageal atresia and tracheoesophageal fistula are rare malformations that may occur alone or in combination and represent a failure of the esophagus to develop as a continuous passage (atresia) to the stomach and/or an unnatural connection between the esophagus and the trachea (fistula) (Figure 60-8). The cause is unknown.

Manifestations include excessive salivation, drooling, coughing, choking when feeding, and cyanosis. A history of polyhydramnios (excessive production of amniotic fluid) during the prenatal period is common.

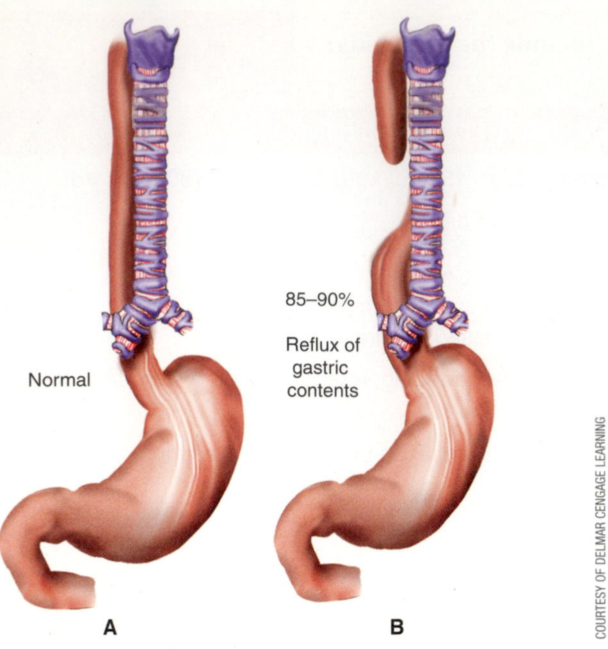

FIGURE 60-8 Esophagus; *A*, Normal; *B*, Atresia/Fistula

Medical–Surgical Management

Medical

The primary goal is prevention and treatment of aspiration pneumonia. The infant will be designated NPO and administered IV fluids. Removal of secretions from the mouth and esophagus requires frequent or continuous suctioning through a nasogastric tube (NGT). Antibiotics are prescribed for any developing pneumonia.

Surgical

These defects represent a critical neonatal surgical emergency. Surgical correction may be accomplished in several stages depending on the size and condition of the infant and the extent of the defect. If closure of the gap requires staged repair, a gastrostomy tube will be placed for feeding. The prognosis is usually good with surgery.

Nursing Management

Nursing responsibility for detection of this malformation begins immediately after birth. Assess the newborn for color, amount of saliva, ability to swallow, respiratory distress, and abdominal distention. A maternal history of polyhydramnios necessitates assessment for the defect with insertion of an NGT. Do not initiate feedings until the infant has been assessed. When the defect is diagnosed, prepare the infant and the family for immediate surgery. Postoperative care is the same as that provided to any high-risk newborn.

PYLORIC STENOSIS

Pyloric stenosis is a common disorder that occurs when the circular muscle surrounding the pylorus hypertrophies and blocks gastric emptying (Figure 60-9). It is rarely diagnosed before the third week of life. Manifestations include **projectile vomiting** (ejection of stomach contents up to 3 feet), ravenous hunger, hyperactive bowel sounds, irritability, FTT, decreased number and volume of stools, an olive-shaped mass in the right upper quadrant, and visible peristaltic waves.

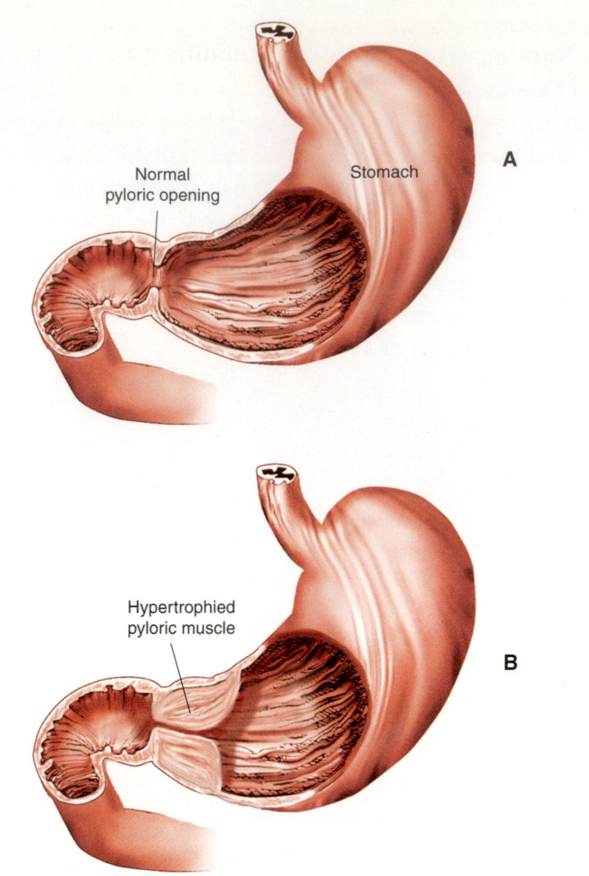

FIGURE 60-9 Stomach; *A*, Normal Opening; *B*, Pyloric Stenosis

Medical–Surgical Management

Medical

Diagnosis is usually made before malnutrition, dehydration, and alkalosis are severe. It is unusual for the infant to require IV fluid therapy before surgery.

Surgical

The defect usually is discovered early and repaired immediately. Most infants recover rapidly and completely with surgery.

Nursing Management

Recognize the signs and symptoms early. Pre- and postoperative care are the same as for any GI surgical client. Infants are allowed to resume feedings 4 to 6 hours postoperatively and may be discharged within 24 hours.

HIRSCHSPRUNG'S DISEASE/ MEGACOLON

Hirschsprung's disease is a congenital anomaly manifested as a partial or complete mechanical obstruction resulting from inadequate motility of part of the colon. There is an absence of parasympathetic ganglion cells and, thus, of peristalsis within the muscular wall of the distal colon and the rectum. As a result, the affected portion of the bowel narrows, and the portion directly above the affected area becomes greatly dilated and fills with feces and gas (Figure 60-10). Failure of the newborn to have a stool during the first 24 to 48 hours may indicate this defect. Older infants may have constipation or ribbonlike stools and an enlarged, distended abdomen.

Medical–Surgical Management

Medical

For the child with a mild defect, management may involve dietary modification, stool softeners, and isotonic irrigations until the child is toilet trained. Most infants with Hirschsprung's require surgical intervention.

Surgical

Surgical intervention involves removal of the aganglionic bowel and creation of a temporary colostomy. Resection and colostomy closure are performed after the child reaches 10 kg.

Nursing Management

Assess the newborn for passage of stool during the first 24 to 48 hours and observe for signs of constipation and for malformed stools throughout infancy. Assess all infants with Hirschsprung's for weight gain, nutritional intake, and bowel habits. Teach caregivers both to ensure regular bowel habits with daily saline irrigations and a balanced diet and to observe for signs of fluid and electrolyte imbalances, such as dry mucous membranes and increased thirst.

Postoperative care may include reduction of anxiety and preparation for home care of the colostomy.

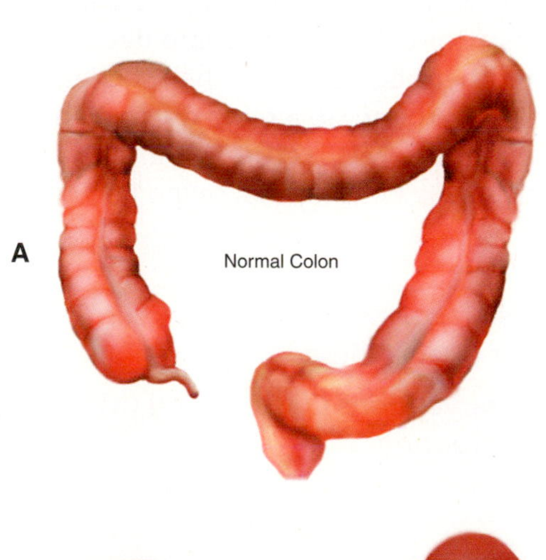

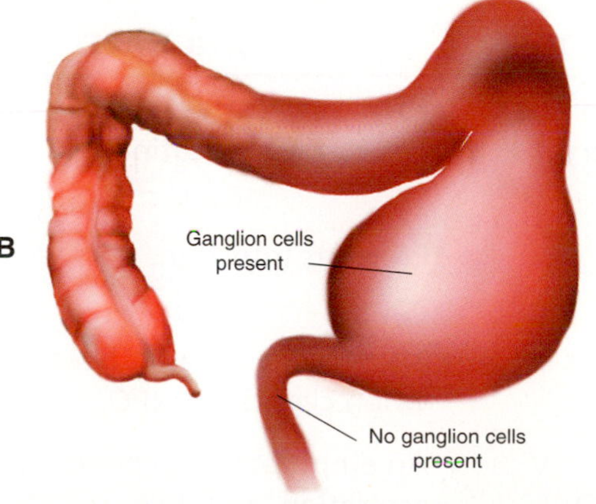

Figure 60-10 Colon; *A*, Normal; *B*, Hirshprung's Disease/ Megacolon

Gastroesophageal Reflux

Gastroesophageal reflux (GER) is the return of stomach contents into the esophagus caused by an immature sphincter. Manifestations such as hunger, irritability, FTT, vomiting, and frequent upper respiratory infections usually occur during the first 6 weeks of life.

Most infants have mild reflux and generally improve without surgical intervention by 1 year of age. Severe cases of GER that do not respond to therapy can result in esophageal strictures, respiratory distress, and FTT.

Medical–Surgical Management

Medical

Gastroesophageal reflux often resolves with dietary modifications, medication, and positioning. Small, frequent feedings and frequent burping are measures for minimizing reflux. Thickening formula with cereal (1 to 3 teaspoons of cereal for each ounce of formula) may be recommended if FTT persists.

Placing the infant prone and with the head elevated 30 degrees is generally thought to be the most effective positioning for reducing the frequency of reflux (Orenstein, Izadnia & Khan, 1999). Positioning in an infant seat may cause increased intra-abdominal pressure and is not recommended.

Surgical

Severe cases of GER that do not respond to medical interventions may be treated with a surgical procedure called fundoplication, which involves loosely wrapping the gastric fundus around the lower esophagus.

Pharmacological

Medications such as cimetidine (Tagamet), ranitidine (Zantac), or famotidine (Pepcid) may be effective in reducing gastric acid content.

Nursing Management

Recognize signs and symptoms of GER and educate caregivers regarding home care, including feeding, positioning, and medications. Pre- and postoperative care will be needed if the defect is surgically repaired.

Intussusception

Intussusception is a disorder characterized by the telescoping of one portion of the bowel (usually the ileum) into a distal portion (usually the ascending colon). A previously healthy infant who develops intussusception will suddenly become pale, cry out sharply, and draw up the legs in a severe colicky spasm of pain. Such episodes last for several minutes and recur within 20 minutes. Vomiting and passage of "currant-jelly stools" (containing bloody mucus) also occur; however, these symptoms are present in fewer than 50% of infants with this condition (Kuppermann, O'Dea, Pincherry, & Hoecker, 2000). Symptoms of shock, such as increased heart rate and changes in level of consciousness, appear quickly. If the intussusception is detected and reduced within 24 hours, morbidity is minimal. Complications such as perforation, peritonitis, and sepsis can occur (Applegate, 2005).

Medical–Surgical Management

Medical

Initial treatment involves hydrostatic reduction with barium or air enema at the time of diagnosis. Air enema is considered more successful at reduction and has significantly higher reduction rates when compared with liquid enemas; 82% versus 68% (Applegate, 2005).

Surgical

If hydrostatic reduction fails or bowel damage is visualized during x-ray, surgical repair is done immediately. Surgery may consist of manual reduction of the telescoping, resection and anastomosis, or, possibly, colostomy, if the intestine is gangrenous.

Nursing Management

Recognize early the signs and symptoms of intussusception (e.g., abrupt onset of colicky pain and vomiting with currant-jelly stools). Help caregivers visualize telescoping by pressing the finger of an inflated rubber glove into the glove; pressing on the glove will then demonstrate hydrostatic reduction as the finger is pushed back to its normal position.

SAMPLE NURSING CARE PLAN

The Infant Client with Abdominal Surgery

Eight-month-old N.W. was brought to the emergency room by his mother and father, who stated that he was perfectly fine until approximately 4 hours ago, when he refused to eat lunch or take his bottle. He wanted to be held and became increasingly irritable. He began alternating between inconsolable crying and being quiet and limp. Physical examination revealed a palpable abdominal mass and passage of currant-jelly stool. Barium enema confirmed the diagnosis of intussusception, but attempts to reduce the blockage were unsuccessful. N.W. was admitted and prepared for surgery. N.W. weighs 8.8 kg and is maintaining a normal growth curve at the 50th percentile. He has attained all appropriate developmental milestones. This is N.W.'s first illness and hospitalization. His mother begins to cry when she learns of the impending surgery and says, "What did I do wrong?" When the surgery is over, the doctor reports that N.W. has a temporary colostomy that will be closed in a few months. N.W. returns from surgery with a nasogastric tube and a urinary catheter in place and with dextrose 5% with normal saline being administered by IV at 40 mL per hour.

NURSING DIAGNOSIS 1 *Risk for Injury* related to physical risk factors as evidenced by surgical procedure, loss of fluids, altered nutrition, and chemical risk factor of anesthesia

Nursing Outcomes Classification (NOC)
Risk Control

Nursing Interventions Classification (NIC)
Surgical Precautions
Post-Anesthesia Care

PLANNING/OUTCOMES	NURSING INTERVENTIONS	RATIONALE
N.W. will be free of injury, infection, and complications.	Assess vital signs, skin, hydration, and respiratory status every 4 hours.	Facilitates early detection of signs of complications.
	Administer antibiotics as prescribed.	Prevents infection.
N.W. will demonstrate required fluid I&O.	Provide mouth care at least every 4 hours.	Mucous membranes become dry when clients are NPO.
	Maintain NPO and monitor IV as prescribed, and record I&O.	An empty stomach prevents aspiration, and fluids maintain hydration.

SAMPLE NURSING CARE PLAN (Continued)

PLANNING/OUTCOMES	NURSING INTERVENTIONS	RATIONALE
	Assess bowel sounds every 2 hours.	Active bowel sounds indicate ability to tolerate food.
N.W. will maintain growth curve at 50th percentile.	When diet is ordered, offer small sips of water and advance as tolerated.	Small, frequent feedings decrease vomiting.

EVALUATION

Surgical site is infection free and shows signs of healing. Mucous membranes are moist. Fluid requirements are maintained. Client loses less than 5% of admission weight.

NURSING DIAGNOSIS 2 *Acute **P**ain* related to physical injury as evidenced by surgical procedure

Nursing Outcomes Classification (NOC)
Pain Level

Nursing Interventions Classification (NIC)
Post-Anesthesia Care
Pain Management

PLANNING/OUTCOMES	NURSING INTERVENTIONS	RATIONALE
N.W. will be pain free.	Administer pain medications every 3 to 4 hours as prescribed and around-the-clock.	If child is able to sleep and rest, recovery is faster.
	Position for comfort; allow caregivers to hold and comfort.	
	Lubricate nostrils, if nasogatric tube present.	
	Perform procedures such as dressing changes and respiratory therapy after analgesia.	

EVALUATION

Child sleeps quietly and shows no signs of restlessness.

NURSING DIAGNOSIS 3 ***A**nxiety (parental)* related to hospitalization, colostomy, and home care as evidenced by parental reaction and questioning

Nursing Outcomes Classification (NOC)
Coping
Acceptance: Health Status

Nursing Interventions Classification (NIC)
Coping Enhancement
Anticipatory Guidance

PLANNING/OUTCOMES	NURSING INTERVENTIONS	RATIONALE
N.W.'s parents will understand etiology, pathology, and treatment of illness.	Encourage expression of feelings.	Maintain positive family interaction during hospitalization.
	Explain procedures, keep informed of progress, and answer questions.	Facilitates development of rapport with the family.

(Continues)

SAMPLE NURSING CARE PLAN (Continued)

PLANNING/OUTCOMES	NURSING INTERVENTIONS	RATIONALE
N.W.'s parents will provide comfort to their child.	Encourage parental presence and give positive reinforcement to client and family for cooperation and participation in care.	Active participation facilitates coping and decreases anxiety.
N.W.'s parents will demonstrate proper techniques for home care procedures.	Teach parents to provide colostomy care, dressing changes, fluids, nutrition, and growth-fostering activities.	Provides parents with skills required to care for N.W. at home.
	Refer to appropriate community resources.	Decreases parents' anxiety and ensures proper care is provided.

EVALUATION

Family care providers demonstrate skill and knowledge in caring for their child's needs. Parents verbalize decreased anxiety and return demonstrations of colostomy care and dressing changes.

MUSCULOSKELETAL SYSTEM

The musculoskeletal system provides protection to vital organs, supports weight, stores minerals, and supplies RBCs. Disorders may be congenital or acquired and require short- or long-term care. Most alterations of the arms and legs are mild variations of normal posturing, but some are severe anomalies. The two most common congenital skeletal defects are clubfoot and dislocated hip.

CONGENITAL TALIPES EQUINOVARUS (CLUB FOOT)

The equinovarus foot has a clublike appearance with the entire foot inverted, the heel drawn up, and the forefoot adducted (Figure 60-11). It can occur as a single anomaly or in connection with other defects such as **myelomeningocele** (a saclike protrusion situated along the vertebral column and filled with spinal fluid, meninges, nerve roots, and spinal cord). Club foot is apparent at birth and may be bilateral or unilateral. The degree of malformation and likelihood for complete correction varies. Even with correction, recurrence is common.

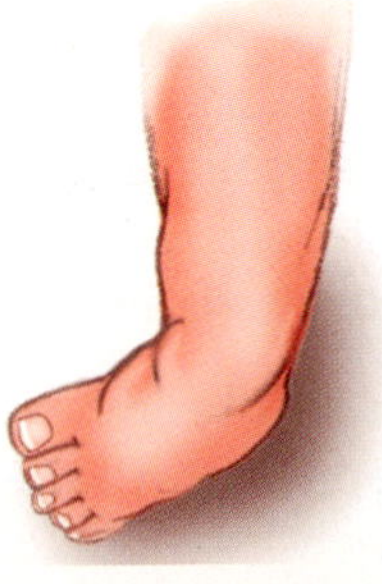

COURTESY OF DELMAR CENGAGE LEARNING

FIGURE 60-11 Club Foot

MEDICAL–SURGICAL MANAGEMENT

Medical

Correction is usually started during the neonatal period with manipulation and casting of the foot. The long leg cast is changed every few days for the first few weeks and then every week or two for several months. Correction is confirmed by x-ray. Following casting, a splint with shoes attached is used for several months to maintain correction.

Surgical

Children who do not respond to nonsurgical treatment within 3 to 6 months need surgical correction. Following surgery, a

CLIENT TEACHING

Cast Care

Instruct caregivers in the following regarding cast care:

- Casts must be changed as prescribed to maintain growth and comfort.
- Wet casts should be handled with the palms (to prevent indentations).
- Hair dryers should not be used to facilitate drying of the cast.
- Plaster of Paris casts should dry within 10 to 72 hours, depending on the size.
- Dry casts should be felt for "hot spots" and observed for visible stains due to drainage, which may indicate skin breakdown.
- Signs of swelling should be noted and reported immediately.
- Toes should be warm, pink, and moving.

cast is applied with the knee in a flexed position. After 6 to 12 weeks, casting is discontinued, and corrective shoes or bracing may be prescribed. Even with aggressive therapy, the foot is seldom entirely normal, and atrophy of the calf is common.

Nursing Management

Assess and explore the caregivers' feelings about their less-than-perfect newborn, the caregivers knowledge about the defect, treatment, and need for long-term care. Nursing responsibilities include teaching the caregivers cast care, monitoring for complications, encouraging compliance with long-term follow-up, and facilitating normal development.

DEVELOPMENTAL DYSPLASIA OF THE HIP

Developmental **dysplasia** (abnormal development) of the hip (DDH) refers to a variety of conditions wherein the femoral head and the acetabulum are improperly aligned. These conditions include **dislocation** (displacement of the bone from its normal position in a joint), subluxation (partial dislocation), and acetabular dysplasia. These conditions can be congenital, but in some children, they develop after birth.

Manifestations include limited **abduction** (lateral movement away from body) of the affected hip, asymmetry of the gluteal and thigh fat folds, and telescoping or pistoning of the thigh. The walking infant may manifest minimal to pronounced variations in gait, with lurching toward the affected side. The longer the disorder goes untreated, the more pronounced the clinical manifestations become and the worse the prognosis.

Medical–Surgical Management

Early screening, detection, and treatment enable most affected children to attain normal hip function.

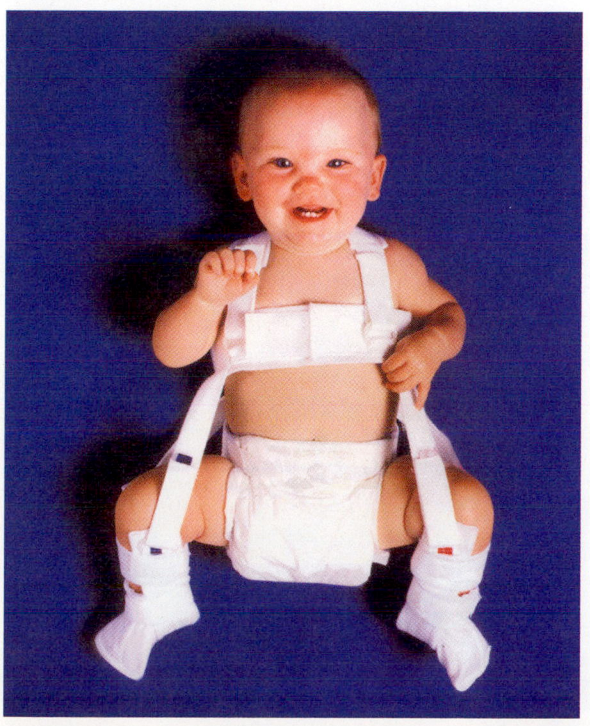

Figure 60-12 A Pavlik harness is used to treat an infant with developmental dysplasia of the hip. (*Courtesy Wheaton Brace Co., Carol Tream, IL.*)

Medical

For young infants, the Pavlik harness is used to maintain flexion, abduction, and external rotation (Figure 60-12). This harness is highly effective when used as prescribed. A hip spica cast may be necessary when the harness is ineffective. Older infants may require traction for weeks, either at home or in the hospital.

Surgical

The older infant may require closed reduction under anesthesia and/or open reduction followed by a hip spica cast.

Nursing Management

Teach caregivers how to use the Pavlik harness. If cast is necessary, teach caregivers cast care.

NURSING PROCESS

Assessment

Subjective Data

The nurse is alerted to the possibility of DDH when the infant has a history of being delivered by cesarean section or frank breech, is large for gestational age, or is a twin.

Objective Data

During the newborn assessment and routine nurturing activities, inspect the infant for limited abduction of the hip, a wide perineum, and unequal gluteal folds (Figure 60-13). The walking infant is assessed for a limp or an unusual gait.

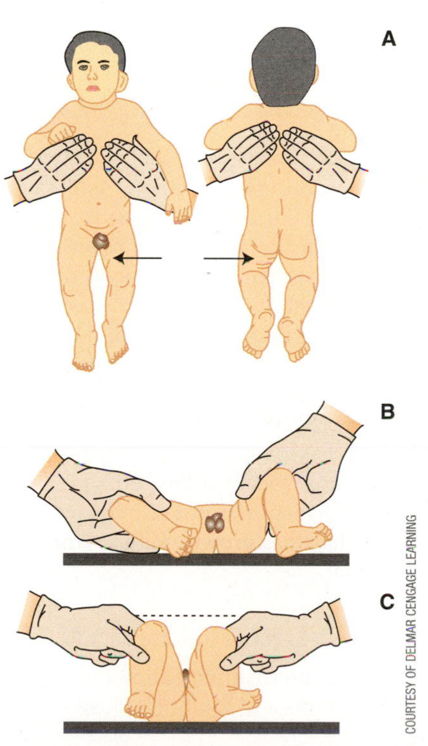

Figure 60-13 Assessing for DDH; *A,* Thighs and gluteal folds will show asymmetry. *B,* Flexion will show limited hip abduction. *C,* Knee height will show uneven level caused by shortened femur.

Nursing diagnoses for the infant with DDH include the following:

NURSING DIAGNOSES	PLANNING/OUTCOMES	NURSING INTERVENTIONS
Anxiety (parental) related to having a less-than-perfect child and to the need to provide complex long-term care	The parents will verbalize feelings about their child and the condition. The parents will carry out prescribed therapy and provide daily care with confidence.	Explore the parents' feelings about their less-than-perfect newborn and their knowledge about the defect, treatment, and need for long-term care. Teach the parents about harness use (e.g., the hips should be flexed without being tight, the harness should be worn 23 hours per day). Explore options for the safe transport of the infant (e.g., use of a special car seat, adaptation of stroller).
*Risk for Impaired **S**kin Integrity* related to devices	The client's skin will remain intact.	Teach the parents to assess the infant's skin for irritation and to change the infant's position every 2 to 4 hours. Teach the parents ways of protecting the infant's skin from the brace (e.g., using a shirt that snaps at the crotch, long socks under the harness). Teach the parents to change diapers without removing the harness. Teach the parents to bathe the infant daily during the 1 hour that the harness is off.
*Delayed **G**rowth and Development* related to immobility and difficulty in positioning	The client will attain milestones appropriate for age and limitations.	Teach the parents to provide activities that stimulate the infant's upper extremities and all five senses (e.g., blocks, musical toys, balls, bright mobiles) and to interact with the infant. Teach the parents methods of holding, nursing, feeding, and cuddling the infant when the harness is in use. Instruct the parents to include the infant in family activities and outings.

Evaluation: Evaluate each outcome to determine how it has been met by the client.

POSITIONAL PLAGIOCEPHALY

Positional plagiocephaly, also called flattened head syndrome, is a condition in which one side or the back of an infant's head is flattened. This can be caused when the infant is put to sleep in the same position repeatedly or by neck muscle problems. Queenan (2001) reports that the number of positional plagiocephaly cases increased six-fold from 1992 to 1994. These were the first two years following the American Academy of Pediatrics' (AAP) "Back to Sleep" promotion for infants to sleep on their backs to prevent sudden infant death syndrome (SIDS). SIDS has decreased, but positional plagiocephaly, which has an excellent corrective prognosis when treated early, has dramatically increased.

This head deformation is not self-correcting. Sometimes, after the infant's hair has grown, mild asymmetrical features may appear normal.

Medical–Surgical Management

Early identification and treatment allows time for reshaping of the head before sutures and fontanels close.

Medical

When this positional deformity is detected, infants are generally placed in a light-weight plastic helmet or band, which redirects symmetrical growth of the infant's head (Figure 60-14).

Nursing Management

Prevention is the key through caregiver teaching. Caregivers should be taught to alternate the infant's head position during sleep (one sleep period with the right side of the head touching the mattress and the next sleep period the left). The infant is supine to sleep. Infants should not be left in an infant carrier,

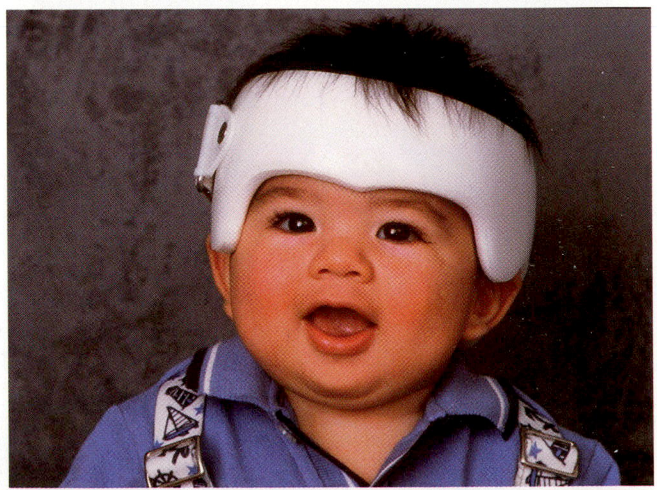

FIGURE 60-14 Child in DOC (Dynamic Orthotic Cranioplasy) Band for Positional Plagiocephaly (*Courtesy of Cranial Technologies, Inc.*)

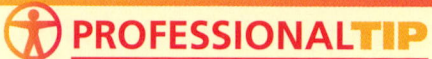

car seat, or swing for extended periods. Providing as much "tummy time" as possible when the infant is awake and supervised gives the back of the infant's head a rest and reduces the risk of developing positional plagiocephaly. This tummy position also strengthens neck muscles and arms and encourages learning and discovery of the world around.

INTEGUMENTARY SYSTEM

Normally, infants have soft, smooth, dry, cool, taut, elastic skin. Color is evenly distributed but may display variations such as freckles, **mongolian spots** (large patches of bluish skin on the buttocks of dark-skinned infants), small hemangiomas called "stork bites" (on eyelids or back of the neck), and **milia** (pearly white cysts on the face). Most of these blemishes disappear within months and require no treatment.

The infant's skin is immature and, thus, susceptible to disorders. The most frequently seen skin disorders include milia rubra, diaper dermatitis, seborrheic dermatitis, and atopic dermatitis.

MILIA RUBRA

Milia rubra, also known as prickly heat, is most noticeable on the folds of the skin, chest, and neck. This rash appears as pinhead-sized **erythematous** (reddishness of the skin) papules. It commonly occurs when infants are febrile or overdressed in summer heat. Infants may be irritable because of itching.

NURSING MANAGEMENT

Treatment is primarily preventive. Teach caregivers to avoid bundling infants in hot weather. Tepid baths may help alleviate itching.

DIAPER DERMATITIS

Diaper dermatitis, also called diaper rash, is characterized by erythema (redness), edema, vesicles, papules, and scaling on the perineum, genitals, buttocks, and skin folds. It is caused by repetitive exposure to an irritant such as urine, feces, soap, detergent, ointment, friction, or infection resulting from bacteria or yeast (*Candida albicans*) (Figure 60-15). The incidence is generally reported to be greater among bottle-fed than among breastfed infants (Hockenberry et al., 2006).

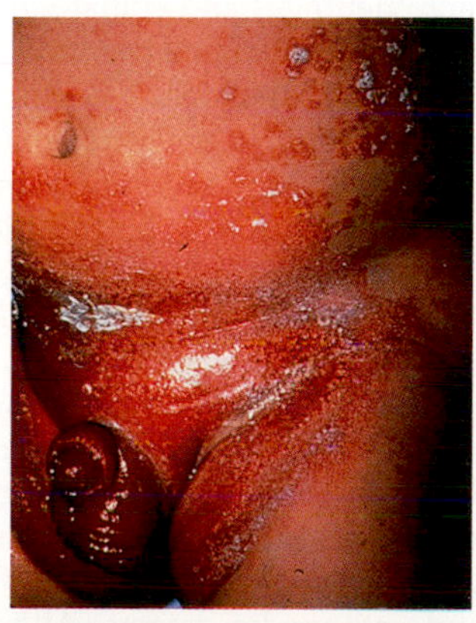

FIGURE 60-15 Candidiasis (*Courtesy of the Centers for Disease Control and Prevention.*)

> **PROFESSIONALTIP**
>
> **Mongolian Spots**
>
> It is important for nurses to be aware that blemishes such as mongolian spots are common in dark-skinned infants up to 24 months of age and, thus, should not be mistaken for signs of child abuse.

NURSING MANAGEMENT

To prevent diaper rash, teach care providers to change diapers frequently and keep the infant's skin clean and dry. Use of disposable diapers and exposure of healthy skin to air, not heat, will help keep the skin dry. Ointments such as zinc oxide or petrolatum may be used to protect inflamed skin. Nystatin (Mycostatin) ointment or cream may be applied to treat *Candida*.

SEBORRHEIC DERMATITIS

Seborrheic dermatitis, also called cradle cap, is characterized by yellowish, scaly, or crusted patches on the scalp of infants up to 3 months of age (Figure 60-16). It typically results from excessive sebaceous gland activity.

NURSING MANAGEMENT

Teach caregivers that cradle cap is not caused by poor hygiene but, rather, by increased sebum production by the scalp. It will eventually disappear, although children with dry skin may continue to have flakes on the scalp. A mild shampoo or mineral oil may be left on the scalp for a few minutes to help soften and loosen the crust. Then rinse and comb the hair with a fine-toothed comb to loosen and remove the crust. In most cases, no further treatment is needed. The crusting can usually be prevented by washing the infant's head with a washcloth and using a fine-toothed comb.

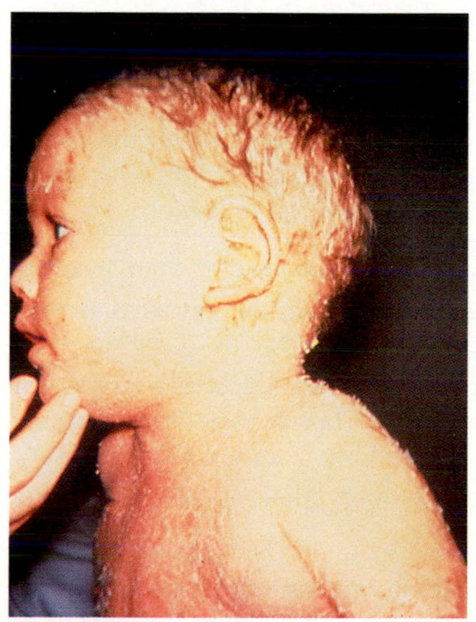

FIGURE 60-16 Seborrheic Dermatitis (*Courtesy of the Center for Disease Control and Prevention.*)

LIFE SPAN CONSIDERATIONS

Dressing Infants

Caregivers should be advised to dress infants as they themselves are dressed, being careful not to overdress the infant.

ATOPIC DERMATITIS

Atopic dermatitis, also called eczema, is a chronic, superficial inflammatory skin disorder characterized by intense **pruritus** (severe itching). It is considered to be at least in part an allergic reaction to irritants (wool, nylon, plastics, detergents, perspiration, cosmetics, and perfumed lotions and soaps) and allergens (dust, pollens, and foods). A strong family history of eczema, asthma, food allergies, or allergic rhinitis usually predisposes a child to eczema. The disorder is uncommon among breastfed infants before other foods are added to the diet.

Papules and vesicles usually begin forming on the cheeks and spread to the arms and legs and then to the trunk. Exudate and crust are often present.

Infantile eczema usually resolves by the age of 3 years; however, infants who have eczema tend to develop hay fever or asthma later in life.

Medical–Surgical Management

Medical

Treatment is aimed at relieving pruritus, hydrating skin, reducing inflammation, and preventing secondary infections. Baths and compresses may provide temporary relief.

Pharmacological

A variety of lotions, oral antihistamines, topical corticosteroids, and antibiotics may be prescribed.

PROFESSIONALTIP

Controlling Allergens

When teaching caregivers about the need to decrease allergens in the child's environment, the nurse should stress the following:

- "Smoking outside" rather than "not smoking"
- "Keeping pets outside" rather than "getting rid of pets"
- "Removing as much dust as possible from the child's room" rather than "removing as much dust as possible from the entire house"
- Consider using an air purifier or air-filtering machine

Providing alternatives to the ideal situation may empower caregivers to set more realistic goals for improving their child's environment.

Diet

A diet including a milk substitute such as soy formula, a vitamin supplement, and foods known to be hypoallergenic may be instituted to rule out offending foods. If the child's skin improves, foods are added back into the diet one at a time at intervals of approximately 1 week. The effects are then noted and any allergenic foods eliminated from the child's diet.

Health Promotion

Guidelines for preventing eczema include practicing breastfeeding; prohibiting cow's milk, eggs, fish, corn, citrus, peanuts, nuts, and chocolate for the first 12 months of life; and delaying introduction of solid foods until 6 months of age. Environmental control of dust, mold, animals, and cigarette smoke is also recommended.

Nursing Management

The major nursing goals are to soothe and relieve pruritus, maintain skin integrity, provide adequate nutrition and fluids, offer sensory stimulation, and teach the family about the condition. Caregivers may feel apprehensive or repulsed by their infant's appearance. They need to be encouraged to express their feelings but be assured that eczema, while potentially distressing, is a temporary condition.

NEUROLOGICAL SYSTEM

By the fourth week of gestation, the neural tube has closed, and the brain and the spinal cord have begun to form. By the second month of gestation, the brain is the most prominent part of the body. It grows rapidly and continues to grow through the fifth year of life. As myelinization of the peripheral nerves progresses, so do the child's coordination and fine motor abilities. The primitive reflexes (Moro, grasp, and rooting) disappear by 12 months of age. Alterations discussed following are spina bifida, hydrocephalus, febrile convulsions, **meningitis** (inflammation of the meninges), and cerebral palsy.

SPINA BIFIDA

Spina bifida is a neural tube defect wherein incomplete closure of the vertebrae and neural tube results in an opening through which meninges and spinal cord may protrude. Although the cause remains undetermined, genetic predisposition, maternal folic acid deficiency during pregnancy, and environmental factors such as pollution may be implicated. The severity of the defect can vary, with manifestations ranging from a dimple or small tuft of hair (which may be overlooked at birth) to a large, saclike protrusion anywhere along the lumbar or sacral area (Figure 60-17). The most severe form is myelomeningocele. The degree of neurological impairment depends on the location of the defect on the spinal cord and the size of the defect. The child may be asymptomatic or display neurological impairments varying from mild sensory loss to complete paralysis below the lesion. Associated defects may include hydrocephalus (present in 90% of clients) and genitourinary and orthopedic defects. Although these children often require lifelong therapy and care, many ultimately go on to live independently and become productive adults.

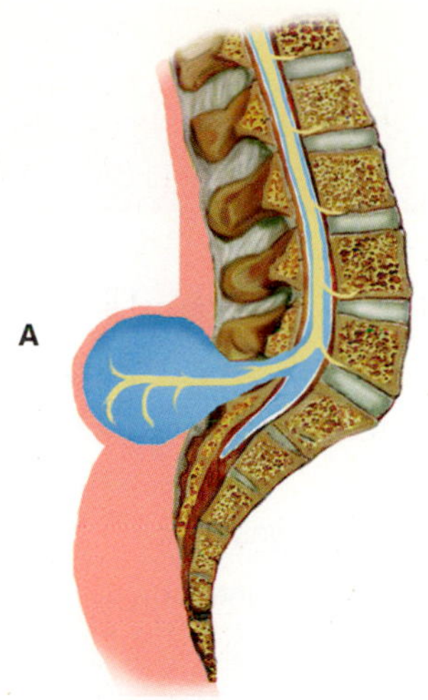

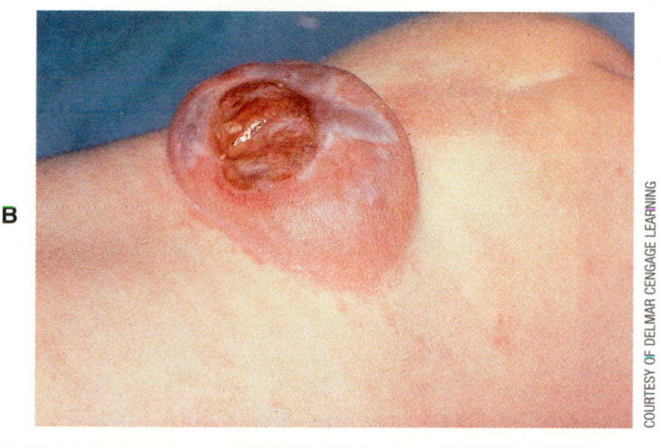

COURTESY OF DELMAR CENGAGE LEARNING

FIGURE 60-17 ***A,*** **Illustration of Myelomeningocele;** ***B,*** **Myeleomeningocele**

MEDICAL–SURGICAL MANAGEMENT

Medical

Specialists such as neurologists, neurosurgeons, orthopedic specialists, pediatricians, urologists, and physical therapists may be needed to provide surgical repair and follow-up treatment.

Surgical

Surgery is required to close the defect but may not be performed immediately after birth. Waiting several days gives the family time to adjust to the initial shock and become involved in the decision-making process. Immediate closure reduces the risk of infection and allows for easier handling of the infant, which, in turn, facilitates earlier bonding.

NURSING MANAGEMENT

Preoperatively, monitor vital signs, neurological status, and behavior. Maintain infant in a prone position. Keep sac covered with moist, warm, sterile dressings and change every 2 hours. Administer medications as ordered.

Postoperatively, monitor vital signs, I&O, and provide prescribed wound care. Teach caregivers intermittent catheterization to keep infant's bladder empty until incision heals. Teach caregivers how to elicit sucking and to feed and cuddle infant, signs of increased intracranial pressure, and signs of constipation. Refer to Spina Bifida Association.

NURSING PROCESS

ASSESSMENT

Subjective Data

Assess the caregivers' feelings about their less-than-perfect newborn and their knowledge about the defect, the treatment, and the need for long-term care.

Objective Data

At birth, assess the intactness of the membranous sac. Assess neurological impairment by noting movement of the extremities; reflexes; anal reflex; urinary output; vital signs; fontanelles; and head circumference.

Nursing diagnoses for the infant with spina bifida include the following:

NURSING DIAGNOSES	PLANNING/OUTCOMES	NURSING INTERVENTIONS
Anxiety (parental) related to having a less-than-perfect child and to the need to provide complex long-term care	The caregivers will verbalize their feelings about the child and condition. The caregivers will carry out prescribed therapy and provide daily care with confidence.	Explore the caregivers' feelings about their less-than-perfect newborn and their knowledge about the defect, the treatment, and the need for long-term care. Teach the caregivers ways to elicit sucking and to feed and cuddle the infant. Teach the caregivers to assess for signs of constipation, such as abdominal distention, vomiting, and poor feeding. Teach the caregivers to recognize signs of increased intracranial pressure, such as irritability, restlessness, and vomiting. Explore options for mobility, such as splints, a walker, or a wheelchair. Refer caregivers to the Spina Bifida Association and to local resources and support groups.

(Continues)

Nursing diagnoses for the infant with spina bifida include the following: (Continued)

NURSING DIAGNOSES	PLANNING/OUTCOMES	NURSING INTERVENTIONS
*Risk for **I**nfection* related to vulnerability of the sac, the surgical procedure, and the lack of bowel and bladder control	The client will be infection free.	***Preoperative:*** Monitor the infant's vital signs, neurological status, and behavior. Administer prophylactic antibiotics, as ordered. Keep the sac covered with a moist, warm, sterile dressing and change every 2 hours. Maintain the infant in the prone position. Protect the sac from fecal contamination. ***Postoperative:*** Provide prescribed wound care. Instruct the caregivers in the use of intermittent, clean catheterization to keep bladder empty.
*Delayed **G**rowth and Development* related to immobility	The client will attain milestones appropriate for age and limitations.	Teach the caregivers to provide activities that stimulate the infant's upper extremities and all five senses and to interact with the infant. Instruct the caregivers to include the infant in family activities and outings. Explore options for education and vocational training as the child grows older.

Evaluation: Evaluate each outcome to determine how it has been met by the client.

HYDROCEPHALUS

In hydrocephalus, the balance between the rate of cerebrospinal fluid (CSF) formation and absorption is disturbed. This disturbance may result from an obstruction in the circulation of CSF or from defective absorption. Hydrocephalus may be recognized at birth or weeks or months later. The condition may be congenital or occur as the result of a neoplasm, a head injury, or an infection.

Manifestations include an excessively large head at birth or rapid head growth along with widening cranial sutures. As pressure increases, the anterior fontanel becomes tense and bulges, and the eyes appear to be pushed downward, with the sclera visible above the iris ("sunset eyes"). Because of the increase in intracranial pressure, the infant may display irritability, restlessness, a high-pitched cry, vomiting, seizure, and change in level of consciousness.

MEDICAL–SURGICAL MANAGEMENT

Surgical

Surgical intervention is the only effective means of relieving brain pressure and preventing further damage to the brain tissue. Surgery involves removing the obstruction or inserting a shunting device that bypasses the point of obstruction and drains the excess CSF into a body cavity, usually the peritoneum.

NURSING MANAGEMENT

Monitor vital signs, head circumference, and neurological signs. Prevent infections, provide loving care to the child and support to the caregivers, and increase the family's knowledge about the condition. Set realistic growth and development goals. Many infants with hydrocephalus are able to ultimately live independently and become productive adults despite associated neurological disabilities.

FEBRILE CONVULSIONS

A convulsion or seizure involves involuntary muscle contraction and relaxation. Seizures may be a symptom of a wide variety of disorders. In infants and children, febrile seizures usually accompany such infections as otitis media, upper respiratory infections, and meningitis. Clinical manifestations include sudden occurrence, body stiffening, and loss of consciousness followed by quick, jerking movements of the arms, legs, and facial muscles. Breathing may be irregular, and swallowing ability may be absent.

Febrile seizures usually occur early in the course of a high fever. Usually, only one seizure occurs, and it will last less than 3 minutes. Febrile seizures carry little risk of neurological damage.

MEDICAL–SURGICAL MANAGEMENT

Pharmacological

Most febrile seizures stop before the infant can be taken for medical attention. If the seizure continues, diazepam (Valium) is the drug of choice. Antipyretics such as acetaminophen (Tylenol) or ibuprofen (Motrin) may be used to reduce the infant's fever.

Nursing Management

Focus on teaching caregivers about febrile seizures and treating a fever. caregivers are naturally extremely anxious when their child has experienced a seizure, especially the first time. Reassure the caregivers that febrile seizures are not life threatening, do not cause neurological damage, are common in children younger than 5 years of age who are experiencing infection, usually do not recur, and usually last less than 3 minutes.

MENINGITIS

The most common infection of the central nervous system (CNS) in infants is meningitis. The three main types of causative organisms are bacterial, tubercular, and viral. Meningitis may also occur as the result of complications of neurosurgery, trauma, systemic infection, or sinus or ear infection. Bacterial meningitis is the most common and serves as the focus of this discussion.

Clinical manifestations may occur suddenly or gradually and include neurological symptoms such as a high-pitched cry, fever, seizures, irritability, as well as vomiting, a bulging anterior fontanel, and poor feeding. Early diagnosis and treatment are essential for uncomplicated recovery.

Medical–Surgical Management

Medical

Meningitis is a medical emergency. A spinal tap (lumbar puncture) is performed promptly whenever symptoms are present and before administration of antibiotics. The causative organism usually can be ascertained from stained smears of the spinal fluid. Appropriate IV antibiotics are prescribed for bacterial meningitis. The infant is isolated from other clients for at least 24 hours.

Health Promotion

Current immunization schedules include the *Haemophilus influenzae* type b conjugate vaccine (HbCV). The incidence of *H. influenza* type B (Hib) has greatly decreased since the advent of this immunization.

Nursing Management

After assisting with the spinal tap and starting the IV, complete the history and physical. It is important to note any food and fluid intake, nausea, vomiting, or loss of appetite, as well as recent immunizations, illnesses, surgery, and injuries and previous lumbar puncture.

Perform a complete neurological assessment and an evaluation of head circumference. Examine the fontanelles for bulging.

Maintain in isolation for at least 24 hours, administer antibiotics, monitor neurological status every 4 hours, maintain fluid balance, establish trust with the caregivers and infant, teach the caregivers about the disease and ways to care for their infant, and refer close contacts for possible prophylactic treatment.

CLIENT TEACHING

Tips for Treating a Fever

Teach caregivers to care for their febrile infant by:

- Administering acetaminophen or ibuprophen, but never aspirin
- Providing more clothing if the child is too cold and less clothing if the child is too warm, to prevent shivering
- Applying cool, moist compresses to the forehead 1 hour after administering an antipyretic
- Encouraging fluid intake (e.g., water, juice, ice, popsicles)

CEREBRAL PALSY

Cerebral palsy (CP) is a nonprogressive motor disorder resulting from damage to the motor centers of the brain. This damage can occur during the prenatal, perinatal, or postnatal period.

Manifestations of CP vary in severity and may include delayed gross motor development (e.g., persistent head lag), alterations in muscle tone (e.g., body stiffness), abnormal motor performance (e.g., uncoordinated or involuntary movements), and reflex abnormalities (e.g., persistent tonic neck). In addition, the child may experience seizures, impaired vision and hearing, difficulty swallowing and speaking, and subnormal learning and reasoning. Less-severe cases of CP may not be diagnosed until 2 years of age.

Medical–Surgical Management

Medical

A multidisciplinary team including the family, pediatricians, neurologists, surgeons, nurses, nutritionists, therapists, social workers, and special education teachers is necessary to assist the child in developing maximum potential.

Surgical

Surgical intervention such as lengthening the Achilles' tendon and releasing the hamstrings may be necessary to improve ambulation.

Nursing Management

Encourage caregivers to stimulate and interact with their infant and participate in an infant-stimulation program. Refer to nutritionist, occupational therapist, and speech therapist as needed.

NURSING PROCESS

Assessment

Subjective Data

A history of conditions such as maternal diabetes, ABO or Rh incompatibilities, rubella in the first trimester, prematurity, prolonged labor, and postnatal infections or trauma may predispose an infant to brain damage and CP.

Objective Data

Further observe the infant who feeds poorly and is rigid, tense, or hypotonic. Assess for developmental delays with an instrument such as the Denver II test.

Nursing diagnoses for the infant with CP include the following:

NURSING DIAGNOSES	PLANNING/OUTCOMES	NURSING INTERVENTIONS
*Imbalanced **N**utrition: Less than Body Requirements* related to difficulty chewing and swallowing and to increased muscle activity	The client will maintain a normal growth curve above the fifth percentile on the growth chart.	Encourage active swallowing by maintenance of a flexed sitting position, with the arms brought forward. Provide jaw stabilization from the front or side of the face. Provide a flexible feeding schedule with frequent, small feedings. Encourage use of adaptive utensils and foods to stimulate self-care (e.g., finger foods, foods that stick to utensils, spoon with padded handle). Refer to a nutritionist and an occupational therapist, as needed.
*Delayed **G**rowth and Development* related to neuromuscular impairment	The client will achieve maximum potential.	Teach the caregivers to stimulate the infant and to interact on the infant's functional level. Encourage early intervention and participation in infant-stimulation programs.
*Impaired Physical **M**obility* related to spasticity and muscle weakness	The client will attain mobility via assistive devices.	Refer to a physical therapist, as needed. Evaluate the need for special equipment. Ensure adequate rest. Perform prescribed range-of-motion and stretching exercises. Provide preoperative and postoperative care for the infant who requires corrective surgery. Select toys and activities that improve motor activity (e.g., place a desired toy such that the child must reach).
*Impaired Verbal **C**ommunication* related to neuromuscular impairment and difficulty with articulation	The client will develop methods of communication.	Refer to a speech therapist, as needed. Encourage the use of flash cards, articles, pictures, talking boards, a computer with a voice synthesizer. Encourage jaw-stabilization methods (as with feeding) to facilitate speech.

Evaluation: Evaluate each outcome to determine how it has been met by the client.

GENITOURINARY SYSTEM

During infancy, the kidneys are less able to concentrate urine, and output per kilogram of body weight is higher than that of an adult. Bladder capacity increases with age, from 20 to 50 mL at birth to 700 mL in adulthood, and the infant's urethra is shorter than the adult's. In addition, infants lack bladder control because of insufficient nerve development.

Most external defects of the genitourinary (GU) tract are not life threatening in the physical sense but may present social problems with lifelong implications for the child and family. More severe disorders such as exstrophy of the bladder and ambiguous genitalia lead to concerns about penis size, appearance of the genitalia, altered elimination, potential ability to procreate, and rejection by peers. These children and their caregivers need emotional support in order to adjust to these permanent alterations. Hypospadias, hydrocele, cryptorchidism, vesicoureteral reflux, and Wilms' tumor are the most common types of urinary alterations.

HYPOSPADIAS

Hypospadias is a condition wherein the urethral opening is on the ventral (under) surface of the penis (Figure 60-18). It is often associated with undescended testes and inguinal hernia and is visible on inspection at birth.

Medical–Surgical Management

Surgical

Hypospadias is surgically corrected during the first year of life. The infant is not circumcised at birth because the foreskin may be used to correct the defect.

Nursing Management

Focus on preparing caregivers for the surgical procedure and for postoperative and home care. Assure caregivers that normal urination will be restored and that sexual function will

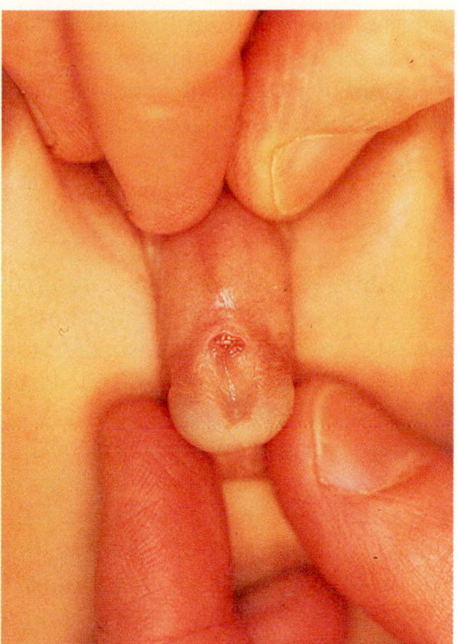

FIGURE 60-18 Hypospadias (*Courtesy of Dr. James Mandell, Chief Surgeon, Urology, Albany Medical College, Albany, NY.*)

not be impeded. Tell them that the penis may never appear perfectly normal, even after the surgery. The infant may go home with a catheter in place until healing is complete. Teach caregivers proper catheterization technique and have them demonstrate catheter care before discharge.

HYDROCELE

Hydrocele is the result of the processus vaginalis failing to close, which allows fluid to enter the scrotum. The scrotum contains a palpable, round, nontender mass. This defect is often associated with inguinal hernia.

MEDICAL–SURGICAL MANAGEMENT

Medical

Most hydroceles will close by 1 year of age without intervention.

Surgical

If spontaneous closure does not occur by 1 year of age, surgical intervention may be done on an outpatient basis.

NURSING MANAGEMENT

Preoperative preparation and postoperative care are the focus of the nurse. Postoperatively, focus on pain management, infection control, and activity restriction. Alert caregivers to the potential for temporary swelling and discoloration of the scrotum.

CRYPTORCHIDISM

Cryptorchidism is a condition wherein one or both testes do not descend into the scrotal sac. One or both sides of the scrotum appear to be smaller than normal. When palpated, the scrotal sac is empty. This defect is often associated with inguinal hernia.

COMMUNITY/HOME HEALTH CARE

Infant with External GU Defect Repair

Pain Management

- Medicate for pain as prescribed for 24 to 48 hours postoperatively.
- Protect the site by double diapering.

Infection Control

- Wash hands before and after diapering.
- Carefully and thoroughly cleanse any area soiled with stool or urine.
- Watch for signs of infection, such as fever, irritability, drainage, and redness.
- Increase fluid intake.

Activity Restriction

- Do not allow the infant to play on riding toys.
- Do not allow the infant to straddle the caregiver's hip when being carried.

MEDICAL–SURGICAL MANAGEMENT

Medical

The testes usually descend spontaneously by 1 year of age. If the testes have not descended after 1 year, hormone therapy may be prescribed.

Surgical

Surgical correction, if required, is performed by 3 years of age to prevent sterility.

NURSING MANAGEMENT

Preoperative preparation and postoperative care are the primary nursing concerns. Postoperative care focuses on pain management, infection control, and activity restriction.

VESICOURETERAL REFLUX

Vesicoureteral reflux refers to the backflow of urine from the bladder into the ureters and, possibly, the kidneys. Reflux can result from abnormal insertion of the ureters into the bladder or from a urinary tract infection (UTI). The primary manifestation of vesicoureteral reflux is recurrent UTIs. Specific clues of a UTI in the infant include poor feeding; vomiting; and failure to gain weight. A UTI is confirmed by detection of bacteria in the urine. Early diagnosis with radiological studies is important to prevent renal injury.

MEDICAL–SURGICAL MANAGEMENT

Medical

The primary concern is preventing UTIs. Low-dose prophylactic antibiotic therapy is prescribed until the reflux is resolved. In addition, urine cultures, cystograms, and blood studies are necessary to monitor for UTI and kidney function. Less-severe refluxes will resolve spontaneously.

Surgical

Surgical reimplantation of the ureter(s) into the bladder may be necessary if UTIs persist.

Nursing Management

Nursing care includes treatment and prevention of UTIs (see the Urinary System chapter). Help caregivers understand that medical treatment may be needed for years and that compliance as well as follow-up is important. If surgery is required, provide pre- and postoperative care.

WILMS' TUMOR

Wilms' tumor (nephroblastoma) is found in the kidney region and is one of the most common early childhood cancers. The tumor arises from bits of embryonic tissue remaining after birth. The etiology is unknown, but Wilms' tumor is associated with other anomalies such as GU defects, microcephaly, and mental retardation. The most common manifestations are an abdominal mass located to one side of the midline, abdominal pain, malaise, anemia, and fever.

Medical–Surgical Management

Surgical

Surgical removal of the involved kidney and lymph node is the treatment of choice. Chemotherapy and radiation may be used pre- and postoperatively, depending on the stage and size of the tumor.

Nursing Management

If a mass is felt in a child's abdomen, stop palpation immediately because it is possible to dislodge cells and spread the tumor. Focus on pre- and postoperative care, chemotherapy administration, and caregiver support.

COGNITIVE AND SENSORY SYSTEMS

Cognitive and sensory impairments result in a variety of lifelong challenges for infants and their families. Nursing care focuses on assessment of the degree of impairment and on appropriate interventions for individual and caregiver adaptation. Some of the most common cognitive and sensory impairments occurring in infants include Down syndrome and visual and hearing impairments.

> **PROFESSIONAL TIP**
>
> **Wilms' Tumor**
>
> If a client has a Wilms' tumor, a sign stating, "Do not palpate the abdomen" should be posted at the head of the bed. Palpating the abdomen can dislodge cells and spread the tumor.

DOWN SYNDROME

Down syndrome is a chromosomal anomaly resulting in moderate to severe mental retardation. Evidence supports trisomy 21 (an extra chromosome); translocation of chromosomes 15, 21, and 22; and advanced parental age as possible causes of Down syndrome.

Manifestations include a variety of facial and body abnormalities and intellectual, language, and social alterations. Typically, the child with Down syndrome has upward- and outward-slanted (almond-shaped) eyes; a depressed nasal bridge; a protruding tongue; small, short, low-set ears; a short, broad neck; transverse palmar crease; broad, short hands with stubby fingers; a protruding abdomen; **hypotonia** (lax muscle tone); and a blunted affect (Figure 60-19). Numerous medical conditions may be associated with Down syndrome, including cardiac anomalies, GI defects, endocrine disorders, and leukemia.

> **CLIENT TEACHING**
>
> **Feeding the Infant with Down Syndrome**
>
> - The tongue thrust represents a physiologic response rather than a refusal to eat.
> - Use a long, straight-handled spoon to place food to the back and side of the mouth.
> - Refeed food that is thrust out of the mouth.
> - Increase fluids and fiber to prevent constipation.
> - Monitor height and weight by plotting on a growth chart each month.

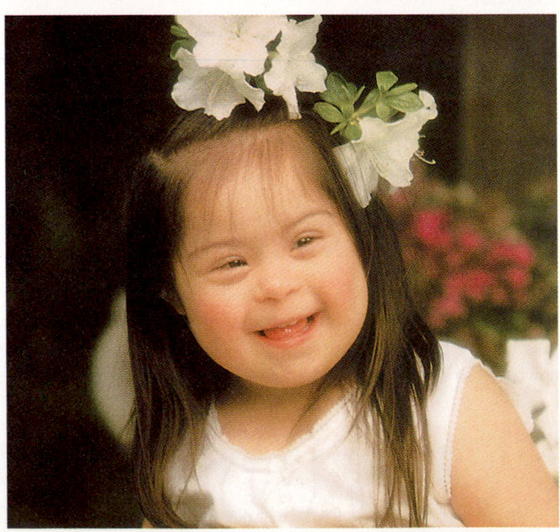

FIGURE 60-19 Young Girl with Down Syndrome (*Courtesy of Down Right Beautiful 1996 Calendar, Marijane Scott, Marijane's Designer Portraits.*)

Medical–Surgical Management

Medical

A multidisciplinary team of health care providers may be needed to assist the child with Down syndrome to reach personal maximum potential. During the first year, the focus is on monitoring for GI and cardiac disorders. Between the second and fourth years, medical emphasis is on sleep and behavioral difficulties, thyroid screening, and visual and dental assessment. Frequent infections are a common problem.

Surgical

Surgery may be required for correction of associated cardiac and GI anomalies.

Health Promotion

Prenatal diagnosis of Down syndrome is possible through genetic testing, alpha-fetoprotein (AFP) level, or amniotic fluid samples. As a result of increased prenatal diagnosis, approximately 40% of fetuses with Down syndrome in women older than 35 years of age are now electively terminated (James et al., 2002). Therefore, the number of children born with Down syndrome is decreasing. For people born with Down syndrome, life expectancy has increased dramatically in recent decades from 25-years-of-age in 1983 to 60-years-of-age today.

Nursing Management

Assist caregivers to identify positive features and behaviors of infant. Emphasize that the infant needs play, discipline, and social interactions like every infant. Encourage the caregivers to teach the child socially acceptable behaviors and to express their own fears and concerns.

NURSING PROCESS

Assessment

Subjective Data

At birth, it is especially important to elicit the family's health history, the results of amniocentesis (if done), and parental ages. As the infant grows, thoroughly evaluate interaction between the child and caregivers, the caregiver's coping abilities, and the degree to which the child is thriving.

Objective Data

During the initial physical examination at birth, assess for the unique features that indicate Down syndrome. As the child grows, assessment of developmental milestones will indicate delays in all areas (language, social, and motor).

Nursing diagnoses for the infant with Down syndrome include the following:

NURSING DIAGNOSES	PLANNING/OUTCOMES	NURSING INTERVENTIONS
***S**ocial Isolation* related to fear of and embarrassment about the child's behavior or appearance	The family will achieve optimal socialization.	Assist in identifying positive features and behaviors in the infant. Emphasize that the infant needs play, discipline, and social interaction, as does any infant. Encourage the family to teach the child socially acceptable behaviors (e.g., manners and appropriate touch). Encourage the family to express feelings and concerns. Refer the family to support groups.
*Delayed **G**rowth and Development* related to poor sucking abilities and anomalies	The client will maintain a normal growth curve above the fifth percentile.	Explore options for ensuring optimal fluid and calorie intake (e.g., adaptive utensils). Encourage self-feeding, when age appropriate. Maintain routine. Refer to dietitian, as needed.

Evaluation: Evaluate each outcome to determine how it has been met by the client.

VISUAL IMPAIRMENT

The eye is not fully developed until approximately 10 to 12 years of age. Visual acuity normally increases from a range of 20/50 to 20/80 at birth to a range of 20/20 to 20/30 by age 5 years.

Visual impairments are classified as follows: sighted with eye problems, partially sighted (20/70 to 20/200), and legally blind (20/200 or less). Refractory errors are the most common type of childhood visual disorders.

Strabismus (crossed eye) is caused by lack of coordination of the extraocular muscles. When both eyes are unable to focus simultaneously, the brain suppresses the image from the deviating eye to prevent double vision (diplopia). Amblyopia (blindness from disuse) can develop if strabismus is not treated early. If untreated amblyopia occurs in a child younger than 4 years of age, permanent loss of vision in the deviated eye may result.

Manifestations of visual impairment may include failure to follow an object or to react to bright light, excessive rubbing of the eyes, squinting, tilting of the head, and crossed eyes (after 6 months of age). Visual impairments may be caused by perinatal and postnatal infections; conditions such as sickle-cell disease, juvenile rheumatoid arthritis, glaucoma, cataracts, and retinoblastoma; and injuries.

Medical–Surgical Management

Medical

Most visual disorders are treated with corrective lenses. Strabismus may require patching of the stronger eye to increase visual stimulation of the weaker eye. The earlier the treatment, the better the chances of normal development and function and adequate vision.

Surgical

Surgical intervention is required for glaucoma, cataracts, and, sometimes, strabismus.

Nursing Management

Early detection and referral are crucial in preventing childhood visual impairment. At birth, assess response to visual stimuli, ability to fixate and follow an object to midline, and ability to make eye contact. At 3 months of age, assess the infant for ability to follow moving objects. Crossed eyes after 6 months of age warrants further evaluation. Make referrals to available associations and support groups as needed (see the Resources listed at the end of this chapter).

Provide preoperative and postoperative care when surgical intervention is required. Educate the caregivers about the condition, the prescribed treatment, home care, and follow-up.

HEARING IMPAIRMENT

At birth, the ear is completely developed. Hearing impairments range from mild to profound and include deaf as well as hard of hearing. Hearing loss is divided into four categories. Conductive (middle-ear hearing loss) is the most common type of hearing impairment and results from interference of transmission of sound to the middle ear. It is usually caused by otitis media. Sensorineural hearing loss (nerve deafness) involves damage to the inner-ear structures and/or auditory nerves. Mixed hearing loss is a combination of conductive and sensorineural loss. It is usually caused by recurrent otitis media. Central hearing loss results from damage to the conduction system between the brainstem and the cerebral cortex.

Infants at risk for hearing loss include those with prenatal, perinatal, and postnatal conditions including a family history of hearing impairments; malformations; low birthweight; asphyxia; infection; CP; Down syndrome; or a history of being administered ototoxic drugs.

Manifestations of hearing impairment in the infant include failure to startle or awaken to a loud sound, to turn the head to sound by 4 months of age, and to babble by 3 months of age. As the child with a hearing impairment matures, language skills are affected, and the child may be perceived as having cognitive as well as behavioral problems.

CRITICAL THINKING

Altered Sensory Functioning

What can nurses do to decrease the incidence of alterations in sensory function among children?

Medical–Surgical Management

Medical

Treatment depends on the cause and type of loss. Antibiotics are prescribed for otitis media, which is the most common cause of conduction loss. Sensorineural loss is usually irreversible. Hearing aids or cochlear implants may be recommended.

Surgical

Insertion of tympanostomy tubes for chronic otitis media is controversial.

Nursing Management

Detection and prevention are the most important goals for the nurse. Assess all children for hearing acuity at birth, at well-child visits, and whenever there is a complaint specific to the ears. Developmental assessments reveal language delays in infants and children with hearing impairments. When delays are noted, refer the child for further evaluation.

CHILD ABUSE

Child abuse is any intentional act of physical neglect or physical, emotional, or sexual abuse committed by a person responsible for the care of a child. In 2007, an estimated 794,000 children were victims of maltreatment, and there were an estimated 1,760 child fatalities, with children younger than 1 year accounting for 42.2% of fatalities. Young children are more vulnerable due to their dependency on care givers, small size, and inability to defend themselves. One or both parents are usually responsible for child abuse or neglect fatalities. Fatalities from physical abuse are most often perpetrated by fathers and mothers and commonly result from neglect (USDHHS, 2009).

PHYSICAL NEGLECT

Physical neglect is failure to provide the adequate hygiene, health care, nutrition, love, nurturing, and supervision required for an infant's normal growth and development. Clinical manifestations of physical neglect in the infant may include inadequate weight gain, dental caries, poor hygiene, and lack of immunizations.

PHYSICAL ABUSE

Physical punishment that leaves marks, causes injury, or threatens the child's physical or emotional well-being is considered physical abuse. Typical clinical manifestations of physical abuse include bruises on the abdomen, buttocks, genitalia, thighs, and mouth; bruises with distinctive outlines indicative of such things as hangers, belt buckles, hands, teeth, and sticks; bone fractures at various stages of healing; spiral fractures; cerebral edema or hemorrhage; and burns (e.g., from immersion of feet in hot water or from cigarettes). The child may appear sad and forlorn or may actively seek to please.

Predisposing factors to physical abuse include characteristics of the caregiver, child, and environment. Caregivers who abuse their children may have been severely punished as children, have difficulty controlling aggressive impulses, be socially isolated, and have few supportive relationships. Children at greatest risk for abuse are those who are premature, illegitimate, unwanted, brain damaged, hyperactive, physically disabled, or "difficult" (James et al., 2002; Hockenberry et al., 2006). A stressful environment caused by divorce, poverty, unemployment, poor housing, frequent relocation, and drug addiction may contribute to physical abuse; however, abuse occurs at all educational, social, and economic levels.

A more unusual type of abuse is Munchausen syndrome by proxy, also known as pediatric symptom falsification or child abuse. This occurs when a caregiver (usually the mother) causes injury to a child that involves unnecessary and harmful or potentially harmful medical care. Nursing and support staff can frequently help the physician make the right diagnosis by reporting their observations and experiences with the child and caregivers. Videotape surveillance has been recommended to help facilitate capturing a caregiver's misbehavior. Videotaping can help confirm or exclude symptoms reported by the caregiver (Stirling, 2007).

EMOTIONAL ABUSE

Emotional abuse includes acts or omissions by the caregiver that could cause serious behavioral, cognitive, emotional, or mental disorders. Emotional abuse may involve shaming, ridiculing, embarrassing, or insulting the child and destruction of the child's personal property. Clinical manifestations in the emotionally abused child may include developmental delays, failure to thrive, disruptive behavior, extreme behavior (withdrawal, aggression), unusual fearfulness, obsessions, and suicide attempts.

SEXUAL ABUSE

Sexual abuse is the exploitation of a child for the sexual gratification of an adult. Common forms of sexual abuse are oral–genital contact, fondling and caressing of the genitals, intercourse (vaginal or anal), rape, sodomy, and prostitution. Possible clinical manifestations in the infant include vaginal discharge; blood-stained diapers; genital redness, pain, itching, or bruising; lax rectal tone; difficulty sitting; and UTIs.

MEDICAL–SURGICAL MANAGEMENT

Medical

Diagnosis of abuse is based on a careful history and thorough physical examination. Injuries are treated as needed. All health care providers are legally required to report any suspected child abuse to the local child protective agency.

NURSING MANAGEMENT

Monitor for inadequate weight gain; lack of immunizations; poor hygiene; bruises; bone fractures at different stages of healing; cerebral edema or hemorrhage; burns; developmental delays; failure to thrive; disruptive behavior; unusual fearfulness; vaginal discharge; blood-stained diaper; genital redness, pain, itching, or bruising; difficulty sitting; and UTIs. Assess child's history and physical examination, parent–infant interactions, child's response to surroundings and strangers, and developmental level.

Report all cases of suspected child abuse to the local child protective agency.

NURSING PROCESS

ASSESSMENT

Subjective Data

Obtain information about caregiver concerns; a general family history; and a specific child history. Begin with nonthreatening topics to demonstrate concern before asking about suspected abuse. Document verbatim details about the way the injuries occurred and use quotation marks.

Objective Data

Physical assessment and documentation must be thorough. Use figure diagrams to document skin injuries. Inconsistencies between what reportedly happened and the extent of injuries constitute a strong indicator of child abuse.

Nursing diagnoses for the abused child include the following:

NURSING DIAGNOSES	PLANNING/OUTCOMES	NURSING INTERVENTIONS
Risk for Injury related to family history of abuse/neglect	The client will be free from abuse/neglect.	Use a nonthreatening, nonjudgmental manner when interacting with the caregivers. Assess and document the child's history and physical examination results, family history, caregiver–child interactions, the child's response to surroundings and strangers, and the child's developmental level. Report all cases of suspected child abuse. Assist in removing the child from the unsafe environment. Refer the family to social services, as needed.

(Continues)

Nursing diagnoses for the abused child include the following: (Continued)

NURSING DIAGNOSES	PLANNING/OUTCOMES	NURSING INTERVENTIONS
*Impaired **P**arenting* related to lack of knowledge	The family will respond to the child's needs appropriately.	Assess the family's strengths, weaknesses, coping mechanisms, and support systems. Assess the caregivers' expectations of the child, choice and use of comfort measures, responses to the child, and general knowledge about the child. Discuss the parenting that the caregivers received as children. Provide information regarding normal growth and development, nutrition, well-child care, and nurturing. Role-model when interacting with the child. Encourage the caregivers to participate in the child's care. Reinforce positive behaviors on the part of the caregivers. Assist the family in identifying stressors and options for decreasing stress. Refer the parents to a support group such as Parents Anonymous.

Evaluation: Evaluate each outcome to determine how it has been met by the client.

ENVIRONMENTAL SAFETY

As infants develop and become mobile explorers, environmental safety becomes a major concern for all caregivers. An important role of the nurse is to educate caregivers regarding maintaining a safe environment and administering appropriate aid in the event of an accident. Common environmental safety hazards include poisoning, trauma, suffocation, and drowning.

POISONING

Poisonous substances can be found everywhere. Commonly ingested substances include cosmetics and other personal care products, medicines, cleaning products, plants, gasoline, toys, lead-based paint, and other miscellaneous foreign substances.

Medical–Surgical Management

Medical

The poison control center should be called initially and immediately to ascertain whether the child should be treated at home or taken to a treatment center. When the exact substance and amount are unknown, take the child to a treatment center, where complications can be anticipated and life support provided, if needed.

Vomiting is usually initiated immediately to the conscious child, unless the ingested substance is corrosive or highly irritating. Corrosives and irritants can cause further damage to mucous membranes of the esophagus and pharynx if vomited.

When emesis is contraindicated, gastric lavage is used to evacuate the stomach contents. In addition, activated charcoal may be administered to prevent further absorption of the poison.

Pharmacological

Activated charcoal may be administered orally or through an orogastric tube to absorb the poison and remove it from the body. Activated charcoal may be mixed with a cathartic such as magnesium sulfate (Epsom salts). An antiemetic is sometimes needed.

Magnesium sulfate may be prescribed to promote rapid elimination, thereby decreasing absorption of the poison. Mixing magnesium sulfate with a sweet liquid may enhance its palatability. Results should occur within 2 to 4 hours.

Nursing Management

Focus on poison prevention as well as on care of the poisoned child. Educate the public about ways to decrease the incidence of poisonings through printed materials such as checklists for poison proofing a home and illustrated first-aid guidelines. Consciousness-raising efforts should be included in each plan of care. Remind caregivers of the importance of keeping the phone number of the poison control center on the phone.

When confronted with a poisoning incident, focus on maintaining vital functions, preventing continued absorption of the poison, preventing complications related to the poisoning and treatment, reducing fear, and educating the caregiver about poison prevention. Once the child's condition is stabilized, exposure to the poison must be terminated. Substances should be removed from the mouth, first manually and then by a sip of water; from the eye with a continuous flush of normal saline; and from the skin by removing contaminated clothing and washing the skin with soap and water.

Once exposure is terminated, identify the substance and consult the poison control center. Procedures to induce vomiting and prevent absorption are initiated as directed by the poison control center.

CLIENT TEACHING

Poison Prevention

Advise caregivers of the following poison prevention measures:

- Keep all medicines and household cleaners in original containers with childproof caps and out of reach of children.
- Do not treat medicine like candy *or* candy like medicine.
- Read labels carefully before using medicines and household cleaners.
- Attach the poison control center's phone number to the phone.
- Prevent children from chewing or ingesting plants.
- Be aware of those things at a child's eye level by crawling around the house on hands and knees.
- Regularly wet-mop floors and wet-wipe window components because household dust is a major source of lead (from chipping paint in houses built before 1960).
- Caregivers should wet-mop floors and wet-wipe horizontal surfaces every 2 to 3 weeks.
- Windowsills and wells can contain high levels of leaded dust. They should be kept clean. If feasible, windows should be shut to prevent abrasion of painted surfaces or opened from the top sash.
- Avoid using traditional home remedies that may contain lead.
- Avoid eating candies imported from Mexico because they may be cooked in cookware that contains lead.
- Avoid using containers, cookware, or tableware to store or cook foods or liquids that are not shown to be lead-free.
- Remove recalled toys and toy jewelry immediately from children.
- Toys that have been made in other countries and then imported into the United States (mostly from China) or antique toys and collectibles passed down through generations put children at risk for lead exposure.
- Lead may be found in the paint used on toys or in the plastic used to make toys. Lead is used in plastic toys to stabilize molecules from heat. When the plastic is exposed to substances such as sunlight, air, and detergents, the chemical bond between the lead and plastics breaks down and forms a dust that can then be inhaled or consumed by children.

Source: http://www.cdc.gov/nceh/lead/tips.htm

CLIENT TEACHING

Tips for Maintaining a Safe Environment throughout Infancy

At 4 months, infants begin to roll and become very active:

- Keep crib side rails all the way up.
- Do not leave the infant unattended on raised areas such as beds, sofas, changing tables; instead, place on the floor or in a playpen.
- Use walkers away from the stairs.
- Never leave the infant unattended in the tub.
- Place car seat in the center of the back seat and facing backward until the infant weighs 20 pounds or is 12 months old. *Always use a car seat.*

At 6 months, infants begin to crawl, reach, and put things in their mouths:

- Keep the floor swept and be alert for small objects that may be put in the mouth.
- Put gates at the tops and bottoms of stairways.
- Keep bathroom doors closed.
- Dress the infant in clothing that allows freedom of movement.
- Do not leave the infant unattended in highchair.
- Keep cords and plastic bags out of the infant's reach.

At 8 months, infants begin to pull up and walk around furniture:

- Ensure that furniture both inside and outside the house is sturdy enough for the infant to pull self to standing.
- Eliminate containers of water inside and outside the house.
- Avoid dressing the infant in socks without shoes.

At 10 to 12 months, infants may begin to walk:

- Keep exterior doors secure.
- Secure gates around swimming pools.
- Keep appliance doors closed at all times.
- Place the infant weighing more than 20 pounds in a front-facing car seat.

TRAUMA

Falls and motor vehicle injuries are the most common causes of trauma in infants. Medical–surgical management is dictated by the location and extent of the injury.

NURSING MANAGEMENT

Preventing trauma or injuries is of utmost importance. Caregivers must stay aware of their infant's abilities as the infant grows and develops and be prepared to provide a safe environment. Every time a nurse encounters a caregiver, provide developmentally appropriate safety information and reminders. Stress car seat safety.

SUFFOCATION/DROWNING

Suffocation occurs when air exchange is hindered by covering the mouth or nose, applying pressure to the throat and chest, or excluding air (e.g., via refrigerator entrapment).

Drowning can occur in only inches of water. Drowning is a great concern when an infant is in the tub.

Nursing Management

Educate parents and care providers. Safe cribs have no more than 2 3/8 inch space between the slats, and the crib mattress fits snugly against the slats. The crib is placed out of reach of windows and other furniture that may have cords or strings that could entrap or strangle a child. Other objects that may contribute to suffocation are electrical cords, toys with strings, plastic bags, pieces of balloons, crib mobiles, pieces of hard food, and restraining straps.

Drowning may occur in toilets, buckets of water, tubs, and pools. Remind caregivers that an infant or young child will not roll from the back to the stomach when the child's face is covered with water and that infants are top heavy and do not have the strength to pull themselves out of a bucket if they fall in head first.

CASE STUDY

J.F. is a 10-month-old female who was brought to the clinic by her grandmother. The grandmother reports that J.F. is irritable, refuses to eat, and does not want to be rocked or cuddled. J.F.'s temperature is 102°F. She had been treated for an upper respiratory infection 10 days ago. A spinal tap indicates that J.F. has meningitis. An IV is started, and antibiotics are administered.

The following questions will guide your development of a nursing care plan for the case study.

1. List subjective and objective data a nurse should obtain about J.F.
2. List three nursing diagnoses and goals for J.F.
3. List three successful outcomes for J.F.
4. How can the spread of this infection be prevented?
5. What must be included in discharge planning if J.F.'s recovery is uneventful?

SUMMARY

- The most common skin disorders of infancy are diaper rash, eczema, and cradle cap.
- The immaturity of the respiratory system creates hazards for the healthy infant and places the compromised infant at even greater risk of infection.
- Sudden infant death syndrome is the leading cause of death among infants.
- Signs of congenital heart disease in the infant include poor weight gain, poor feeding habits, fatigue, and respiratory infections.
- Iron-deficiency anemia can be prevented largely by teaching caregivers the importance of providing iron-fortified formula to infants until the age of 12 months.
- Possible signs of GI obstruction in the infant include abdominal pain, nausea and vomiting, abdominal distention, and decreased stool output.
- Treatment of colic may involve a change in feeding practices, correction of a stressful environment, and support of the caregivers.
- The most common defects of the GU tract include cryptorchidism, hydrocele, and hypospadias.
- The nursing goals when caring for infants with musculoskeletal impairments focus on preventing both skin breakdown and developmental delays.
- Infants become feverish quickly and must be observed for febrile seizures and protected from injury.
- Routine immunization of infants against *H. Influenzae* type B infection has reduced the incidence of bacterial meningitis.
- Developmental assessment will reveal language and social delays in infants with hearing and visual impairments.
- Inconsistencies between what reportedly happened and the extent of injuries constitute a strong indicator of child abuse.

REVIEW QUESTIONS

1. The mother of a newborn infant tells the nurse, "He seems to be breathing hard and makes a grunting noise. Is he ok?" The nurse determines that:
   1. the infant must be assessed immediately.
   2. the infant needs oxygen.
   3. the infant is experiencing difficulty transitioning to post-natal life.
   4. the infant is exhibiting normal newborn behavior.

2. An infant diagnosed with ventricular septal defect (VSD) is being discharged to home. The nurse is doing discharge teaching to the mother and explains that when feeding the infant, the mother should:
   1. stimulate the infant to keep his attention.
   2. give large feeds to decrease the amount of time handling the infant.
   3. provide small, frequent, high-caloric feedings.
   4. allow infant to feed lying down.
3. An 8-month-old African-American infant has just been diagnosed with SCA. The nurse determines the parents need further teaching when they state:
   1. "We will keep him well hydrated."
   2. "He will not be immunized."
   3. "We will avoid high altitudes."
   4. "We will avoid extreme temperatures."
4. A nurse is teaching a child safety class at a child day care facility. What is the most important information that the nurse can provide to the child care providers on poisonings?
   1. Strategies to prevent poisonings.
   2. Keeping the child care center clean.
   3. Care of the poisoned child.
   4. Having the phone number to the poison control center readily available.
5. An infant is admitted to the hospital to be tested for Wilms' tumor. Upon assessment, the nurse palpates a mass in the infant's abdomen. The nurse should:
   1. continue palpating the abdomen to accurately document this finding.
   2. auscultate breath sounds and document findings in the chart.
   3. stop palpating immediately and document findings in the chart.
   4. check the infant's blood sugar and document findings in the chart.
6. An appropriate nursing assessment of an infant with spina bifida includes all of the following, except:
   1. head circumference.
   2. checking reflexes.
   3. palpating fontanelles.
   4. abdominal girth.
7. The nurse at a pediatric clinic is teaching the father of a 6-month-old infant diagnosed with atopic dermatitis about home care for the child. The nurse knows the father needs more education when he states:
   1. "I will smoke outside."
   2. "I will keep pets outside."
   3. "I will remove as much dust as possible from his room."
   4. "I will only use perfumed lotions and soaps."
8. A 5-month-old infant girl is being seen at the clinic for gastroesophageal reflux. The nurse teaches the parents strategies to help control and prevent gastroesophageal reflux. Select all of the strategies that apply:
   1. place the infant in a thirty-degree prone position.
   2. provide infant with small, frequent feeds.
   3. thicken formula with cereal.
   4. position in an infant seat to put pressure on the abdomen.
   5. administer orange juice as tolerated.
   6. lay infant on back after feeding.
9. The nurse is providing education regarding use of the Pavlik harness to a family with an infant with developmental dysplasia of the hip (DDH). The nurse has provided accurate information if she tells them:
   1. take off the harness to change diapers.
   2. the harness can be on only 8 to 12 hours a day.
   3. the infant does not have to wear the harness in the car seat.
   4. bathe the infant during the 1 hour the harness is off.
10. The nurse performing a physical assessment notices marks on the client's right leg. What is the most appropriate nursing action?
    1. Tell the mother the marks look like she spanked the infant.
    2. Report this case to the local child protective agency.
    3. Ask the mother how the injury occurred.
    4. Discuss different parenting styles and techniques with the mother.

REFERENCES/SUGGESTED READINGS

American Academy of Pediatrics, Task Force on Sudden Infant Death Syndrome. (2005). The changing concept of sudden infant death syndrome: Diagnostic coding shifts, controversies regarding the sleeping environment, and new variables to consider in reducing risk. *Pediatrics, 116(5)*, 1245–1255.

American Academy of Pediatrics and American Academy of Family Physicians. Subcommittee on Management of Acute Otitis Media. (2004). Diagnosis and management of acute otitis media. *Pediatrics, 113(5)*, 1451–1465.

American Academy of Pediatrics. Subcommittee on Hyperbilirubinemia. (2004). Management of hyperbilirubinemia in the newborn infant 35 or more weeks of gestation. *Pediatrics, 114(1)*, 297–316.

American Academy of Pediatrics. Committee on Injury, Violence, and Poison Prevention. (2003). Poison treatment in the home. *Pediatrics, 112(5)*, 1182–1185.

American Heart Association. (2009). *Congenital cardiovascular defects: statistics*. Retrieved July 10, 2009, from http://216.185.112.5/presenter.jhtml?identifier=4576.

Anderson, R., Kochanek, K., & Murphy, S. (1997). Report of final mortality statistics, 1995. *Monthly Vital Statistics Report 4511* (Suppl. 2). Hyattsville, MD: National Center for Health Statistics.

Applegate, K. (2005). Clinically suspected intussusception in children: Evidence-based review and self-assessment module. *American Journal of Roentgenology, 185*, S175–S183.

Bailey, L., & Berry, R. (2005). Folic acid supplementation and the occurrence of congenital heart defects, orofacial clefts, multiple births, and miscarriage. *American Journal of Clinical Nutrition, 81*(5), 1213–1217.

Ball, J., & Bindler, R. (2007). *Pediatric nursing* (4th ed.). Norwalk, CT: Appleton & Lange.

Barker, E., Sauline, M., & Caristo, A. (2002). Spina bifida. *RN, 65*(12), 33–38.

Bulechek, G., Butcher, H., McCloskey, J., & Dochterman, J. (2007). *Nursing Interventions Classification (NIC)* (5th ed.). St. Louis, MO: Mosby-Elsevier.

Burns, C., Dunn, A., Brady, M., Starr, N., & Blosser, C. (2008). *Pediatric primary care: A handbook for nurse practitioners.* (4th ed.) St. Louis, MO: W.B. Saunders.

Castiglia, P. (1998). Trisomy 21 syndrome: Is there anything new? *Journal of Pediatric Health Care, 12*(1), 35–37.

Centers for Disease Control and Prevention. (2003). Managing acute gastroenteritis among children: Oral rehydration, maintenance, and nutritional therapy. *MMWR 52*(No. RR-16), 1–17.

Clinical Rounds. (2002). SIDS linked to *E. coli. Nursing2002, 32*(7), 34–45.

Cystic Fibrosis Foundation. (2009). *CFTR modulation*. Retrieved from http://www.cff.org/research/DrugDevelopmentPipeline/.

Dowshen, S., Hersheberger, M., & Rutherford, K. (2001). *SIDS: Sudden and silent.* Retrieved August 13, 2009, from http://kidshealth. org/parent/general/sleep/sids.html.

Duncan, B., Ey, J., Holberg, C., Wright, A., Martinez, F., & Taussig, L. M. (1993). Exclusive breast-feeding for at least 4 months protects against otitis media. *Pediatrics 91*(5), 867–872.

Eisenhauer, L., Nichols, L., Spencer, R., & Bergan, F. (1998). *Clinical pharmacology and nursing management* (5th ed.). Philadelphia: Lippincott.

Ellmers, K., & Criddle, L. (2002). Cystic fibrosis. *RN, 65*(9), 61–66.

Estes, M. (2010). *Health assessment & physical examination* (4th ed). Clifton Park, NY: Delmar Cengage Learning.

Finesilver, C. (2002). Down syndrome. *RN, 65*(11), 43–48.

Gartner, L., & Greer, F. (2003). Prevention of rickets and vitamin D deficiency: New guidelines for vitamin D intake. *Pediatrics, 111*(4Pt1), 908.

Godshall, M. (2003). Caring for families of chronically ill kids. *RN, 66*(2), 30–34.

Gorman, K. (1999). Sickle cell disease. *AJN, 99*(3), 38–43.

Hermansen, C., & Lorah, K. (2007). Respiratory distress in the newborn. *American Family Physician, 76*(7), 987–994.

Hockenberry, M., & Wilson, D. (2008). *Wong's nursing care of infants and children* (8th ed.). St. Louis, MO: Mosby.

James, S., Ashwill, J., & Jackson, C. (2007). *Nursing care of children: Principles and practice* (3rd ed.). Philadelphia: W. B. Saunders.

Kaditis, A., & Wald, E. (1998). Viral croup: Current diagnosis and treatment. Pediatric *Infectious Disease Journal, 17*(9), 827–834.

Kamarakrishnan, K., Sparks, R., & Berryhill, W. (2007). Diagnosis and treatment of otitis media. *American Family Physician, 76*(11), 1650–1658.

Kitchens, G. (1995). Relationship of environmental tobacco smoke to otitis media in young children. *Laryngoscope. 105*(5, Part 2), 1–3.

Kline, A. (2003). Pinpointing the cause of pediatric respiratory distress. *Nursing2003, 33*(9), 58–63.

Kuppermann, N., O'Dea, T., Pinchney, L., & Hoecher, C. (2000). Predictors of intussusception in young children. *Archives of Pediatric and Adolescent Medicine, 154*, 250–255.

Marks, M. (1998). *Broadribb's introductory pediatric nursing* (5th ed.). Philadelphia: J. B. Lippincott Williams & Wilkins.

Mayo Clinic. (2009). *Sickle cell anemia*. Retrieved from http://www.mayoclinic.com/health/sickle-cell-anemia/DS00324/DSECTION=lifestyle-and-home-remedies.

Meekins, E. (2002). Would you recognize this pediatric disorder? *RN, 65*(4), 26–30.

Mera, K., & Hackley, B. (2003). Childhood vaccines: How safe are they? *AJN, 103*(2), 79–88.

Miles, M. (2003). Support for parents during a child's hospitalization. *AJN, 103*(2), 62–64.

Moerschel, S. K., Cianciaruso, L. B., & Tracy, L. R. (2008). A practical approach to neonatal jaundice. *American Family Physicians, 77*(9), 1255–1262.

Moorhead, S., Johnson, M., Maas, M., & Swanson, E. (2007). *Nursing Outcomes Classification (NOC)* (4th ed.). St. Louis, MO: Elsevier-Health Sciences Division.

North American Nursing Diagnosis Association International. (2010). *NANDA-I nursing diagnoses: Definitions and classification 2009–2011*. Ames, IA: Wiley-Blackwell.

Orenstein, S., Izadnia, F., & Khan, S. (1999). Gastroesophageal reflux disease in children. *Gastroenterology Clinics of North America, 28*(4), 947–969.

Queenan, J. (2001). *Positional plagiocephaly (flattened head)*. Retrieved August 10, 2009, from http://kidshealth.org/parent/general/sleep/positional_plagiocephaly.html.

Roberts, D., Ostapchuk, M., & O'Brien, J. (2004). Infantile colic. *American Family Physician, 70*(4), 735–740.

Sassen, M., Brand, R., & Grote, J. (1997). Risk factors for otitis media with effusion in children 0 to 2 years of age. *American Journal of Otolaryngology 18*(5), 324–330.

Schuman, A. (1997). Disposable diapers? Definitely! *Contemporary Pediatrics, 14*(11), 131–139.

Simmerman, J., & Mauzy, C. (2001). Finally! Babies can get this vaccine. *RN, 64*(7), 28–32.

Spiro, D., Tay, K., Arnold, D., Dziura, J., Baker, M., & Shapiro, E. (2006). Wait-and-see prescription for the treatment of acute otitis media: A randomized controlled trial. *JAMA, 296*(10), 1235–1241.

Spratto, G., & Woods, A. (2009). *2009 PDR nurses' drug handbook*. Clifton Park, NY: Delmar Cengage Learning.

Su, C., Gaskie, S., & Jamieson, B. (2008). What is the best treatment for oral thrush in healthy infants? *The Journal of Family Practice, 57*(7), 484–485.

Swanson, E., Johnson, M., Moorhead, S., & Maas, M. (2007). *Nursing Outcomes Classification (NOC)* (4th ed.). St. Louis, MO: Mosby.

Tinkle, M. (2002). Cystic fibrosis carrier screening. *AWHONN Lifelines, 6*(2), 134–139.

Tully, S., Bar-Haim, Y., & Bradley, R. (1995). Abnormal tympanography after supine bottle feeding. *Journal of Pediatrics, 1995*(126), S105–S111.

Van Riper, M. (2003). A change of plans. *AJN, 103*(6), 71–74.

Wahlgren, D., Hovell, M., Meltzer, S., Hofstetter, C., & Zakarian, J. (1997). Reduction of environmental tobacco smoke exposure in asthmatic children: A 2 year follow-up. *Chest, 111*(1), 81–88.

White, K., Munro, C., & Pickler, R. (1995). Therapeutic implications of recent advances in cystic fibrosis. *MCN, 20*(6), 58–64.

Wittmann-Price, R., & Pope, K. (2002). Universal newborn hearing screening. *AJN, 102*(11), 71–77.

Yetman, R., & Coody, D. (1997). Failure to thrive: A clinical guideline. *Journal of Pediatric Health Care, 11*(3), 134–137.

Zorb, S. (2002). Transplantation offers hope. *RN, 65*(9), 66–68.

RESOURCES

American Cleft Palate–Craniofacial Association, http://www.acpa-cpf.org
American Lung Association, http://www.lungusa.org
American Sickle-Cell Anemia Association, http://www.ascaa.org
American SIDS Institute, http://www.sids.org
American Society for Deaf Children, http://www.deafchildren.org
American Speech-Language-Hearing Association, http://www.asha.org
Automotive Safety for Children Program, http://www.preventinjury.org
Cystic Fibrosis Foundation, http://www.cff.org
Hydrocephalus Association, http://www.hydroassoc.org
Kids Health, Nemours Foundation, http://www.kidshealth.org, www.nemours.org
La Leche League International, http://www.llli.org
National Down Syndrome Society, http://www.ndss.org
Sickle Cell Disease Association of America, http://www.sicklecelldisease.org
Spina Bifida Association of America, http://www.sbaa.org
United Cerebral Palsy National, http://www.ucpa.org
Women, Infants and Children (WIC), http://www.fns.usda.gov/wic

CHAPTER 61
Common Problems: 1 to 18 Years

MAKING THE CONNECTION

Refer to the following chapters to increase your understanding of common pediatric problems:

Basic Nursing
- ***Life Span Development***
- ***Cultural Considerations***
- ***Stress, Adaptation, and Anxiety***
- ***End-of-Life Care***
- ***Wellness Concepts***
- ***Self-Concept***
- ***Basic Nutrition***
- ***Safety/Hygiene***
- ***Fluid, Electrolyte, and Acid–Base Balance***
- ***Assessment***
- ***Pain Management***

Adult Health Nursing
- ***Anesthesia***
- ***Surgery***
- ***Oncology***
- ***Respiratory System***
- ***Cardiovascular System***
- ***Hematologic and Lymphatic Systems***
- ***Gastrointestinal System***
- ***Urinary System***
- ***Musculoskeletal System***
- ***Neurological System***
- ***Endocrine System***
- ***Integumentary System***
- ***Immune System***
- ***Mental Illness***

Maternal & Pediatric Nursing
- ***Basics of Pediatric Care***

LEARNING OBJECTIVES

Upon completion of this chapter, you should be able to:

- Define key terms.
- Discuss the common disorders of the integumentary system in children.
- Differentiate the pathophysiology, common diagnostic tests, treatment, and nursing care for skin conditions in children as compared to adults.
- Differentiate the etiology, medical–surgical management, and nursing care for respiratory conditions in children as compared to adults.
- Describe the causes, assessment, and management of rheumatic fever in children.

- Differentiate the pathophysiology, common diagnostic tests, treatment, and nursing care for digestive conditions in children as compared to adults.
- Differentiate the etiology, medical–surgical management, and nursing care for genitourinary conditions in children as compared to adults.
- Discuss communicable and infectious diseases of childhood, including their causative agents, transmission, incubation periods, contagious periods, prevention, signs and symptoms, treatment, and nursing care.
- Differentiate the etiology, medical–surgical management, and nursing care for orthopedic conditions in children as compared to adults.
- Briefly describe behavioral problems in children, including symptoms, treatment, and nursing care.
- Plan care for a child with any of the common pediatric disorders.

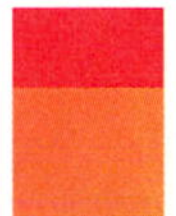

KEY TERMS

acanthosis nigricans
comedones
encopresis
epistaxis
Gowers' sign
rhinorrhea

INTRODUCTION

Pediatric nursing focuses on protecting children from illness and injury as well as assisting them to attain optimal levels of functioning, regardless of health status. The pediatric nurse must understand the phases of a child's growth and development (refer to the Life Span Development chapter) and be sensitive to the importance of family interactions. This chapter focuses on common childhood conditions and illnesses affecting all systems of the body; the typical medical and surgical management for these conditions; and nursing management of the child and caregivers.

RESPIRATORY SYSTEM

Disorders of the respiratory system that occur most often in children include upper-respiratory infections, allergic rhinitis, tonsillitis, asthma, and foreign-body aspiration.

UPPER-RESPIRATORY INFECTIONS

Common upper-respiratory infections include nasopharyngitis (the common cold), pharyngitis, and influenza. Nasopharyngitis is usually credited with being the most common childhood respiratory illness. These disorders are generally responsive to supportive therapies, and symptoms typically improve within 3 days. Clinical manifestations, etiology, and management of these common upper-respiratory disorders are presented in Table 61-1.

Nursing Management

Maintaining fluid intake, providing comfort measures, and preventing spread of infection are the main goals of care for the child with an upper-respiratory infection. The child should not be forced to eat if appetite is decreased. An appropriate diet may include cool, bland fluids and soft foods such as gelatin, soup, mashed potatoes, puddings, hot cereals, and flavored ice pops. Teach caregivers to observe for urinary output and for moist mucous membranes as signs of adequate hydration.

Comfort measures may include warm salt-water gargles (1/4 tsp salt per 8 oz glass of water) and warm or cool compresses applied to the throat. Nasal decongestion may be relieved with normal saline drops before feedings and at bedtime. A cool-mist humidifier at the bedside may also relieve symptoms.

It is important that caregivers know how both to take a child's temperature and to safely administer nonsalicylate antipyretics, such as acetaminophen (Tylenol). Salicylates, such as aspirin, are not used because of the associated risk of Reye's syndrome.

Teach caregivers and children methods for preventing the spread of infection, such as conscientious hand hygiene, proper disposal of tissues, and covering of the nose and mouth when coughing and sneezing. Also avoid contact with infectious persons. Preventing the spread of infection is especially challenging in school and crowded living environments. Children in day care centers have a higher rate of infection than do children who spend their days in the home.

Untreated streptococcal infections may lead to complications such as rheumatic fever, meningitis, and glomerulonephritis. Emphasize to the caregivers of children with pharyngitis caused by streptococcal infection ("strep throat") the importance of completing the course of prescribed antibiotics.

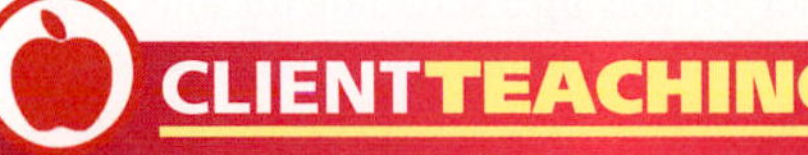

CLIENT TEACHING

Administering Normal Saline Drops

1. Instill two drops.
2. Wait 5 minutes.
3. Instill two more drops.
4. Drops should not be used for more than 3 days.

TABLE 61-1 Distinguishing Characteristics of Common Upper Respiratory Infections

	NASOPHARYNGITIS	PHARYNGITIS	INFLUENZA
Manifestations	**Rhinorrhea** (watery nasal discharge), congestion, sneezing, fever, cough, sore throat, muscular aches, and possibly, enlarged lymph nodes	Sore throat; erythema and inflammation of the pharynx and tonsils; fever; enlarged, tender cervical lymph nodes Viral: gradual onset, hoarseness, cough, rhinitis, malaise Bacterial: abdominal pain, vomiting, headache	Chills, fever, flushed face, myalgia (pain in muscles), cough, rhinitis, headache, sore throat, photophobia, conjunctivitis
Etiology	Viral	Viral (80%) or bacterial (20%)	Influenza virus
Incidence	Typically 6 to 9 colds per year, most commonly in the fall and spring	Most common among 4 to 7-year-old children	Highest among school-age children
Management	Rest, fluids, nonsalicylate antipyretics, oral decongestants, sterile saline nose drops	Rest; fluids; nonsalicylate antipyretics or ibuprofen; warm salt-water gargles; cool, bland liquids; antibiotics for streptococcal infections	Rest, fluids, nonsalicylate Antipyretics

COURTESY OF DELMAR CENGAGE LEARNING

ALLERGIC RHINITIS

Allergic rhinitis ("hay fever") is an inflammatory disorder of the nasal mucosa. Most often, it is a seasonal, recurrent response to allergens such as animal dander, house dust, pollens, and molds. Manifestations include **rhinorrhea**, postnasal drip, sneezing, allergic conjunctivitis, sniffing, itchy nose and palate, dark circles under the eyes, and the "allergic salute" (transverse nasal crease that results from repeatedly pushing nose upward and backward to relieve itching).

MEDICAL–SURGICAL MANAGEMENT

Pharmacological

Antihistamines, decongestants, and bronchodilators may be given to relieve symptoms of congestion and difficulty with breathing. Topical intranasal corticosteroids are quite effective in children who do not respond to antihistamines and decongestants. Systemic corticosteroids may be used in extreme cases. Immunotherapy or desensitization to allergens may be initiated if antihistamines and decongestants are not effective in relieving symptoms or are needed chronically. Desensitization is performed for those allergens that produce a positive reaction on skin testing. The allergist sets up a schedule for injections in gradually increasing doses until a maintenance dose is reached. Desensitization is considered to be a safe procedure with considerable benefit for some children. Severe reactions are uncommon. During immunotherapy, children must be observed for signs of anaphylaxis for 30 minutes after each injection.

Health Promotion

The treatment of choice is to eliminate the allergen from the child's environment. Recommendations for limiting the child's exposure to allergens include avoiding wool and down; using dust-proof covers on bedding; removing carpets, draperies, and blinds from the child's room, if not the whole house; keeping humidity lower than 50%; keeping pets outside; and using air filters.

NURSING MANAGEMENT

Focus on therapeutic management of the disease. After identification of the allergens, assist the caregivers with allergy proofing the home and administering medications.

Drowsiness, dry mouth, and excitability are side effects of some antihistamines. Combining an antihistamine and decongestant may prevent drowsiness.

TONSILLITIS

Tonsillitis, a common illness among children, is an inflammation of the tonsils (two masses of lymphoid tissue located at the back of the mouth), resulting from pharyngitis.

PROFESSIONALTIP

Throat Culture

The only reliable means of determining whether pharyngitis is viral or bacterial is with a throat culture. The nurse is most often the person who performs a throat smear for culture, which requires a physician's order. The applicator is swabbed across the tonsils, the posterior edge of the soft palate, and the uvula.

Tonsils filter and protect the respiratory and alimentary tracts from infection. They normally enlarge progressively between 2 and 10 years of age and reduce during preadolescence. If the tonsils become enlarged from infection, they can interfere with breathing and swallowing and cause partial deafness. Clinical manifestations of tonsillitis include recurrent sore throat; enlarged, bright-red tonsils; mouth breathing; halitosis; nasal speech; fever; difficulty swallowing; and snoring.

Medical–Surgical Management

Surgical

Tonsillectomy may be warranted in cases of abscesses, upper airway obstruction, and obstructive sleep apnea. Adenoidectomy (removal of lymphoid tissue in the nasal pharynx) is performed in cases of recurrent otitis media with Eustachian tube obstruction or for persistent nasal or airway obstruction. If tonsillectomy can be postponed until 4 or 5 years of age, the apparent need often will have disappeared.

Pharmacological

Medical treatment includes analgesics for pain, antipyretics for fever, and antibiotics for streptococcal infections.

Nursing Management

Prepare child for surgery. Use dolls or puppets to assist the child in expressing fears and concerns and acting out the pending experience.

Postoperatively, monitor vital signs, intake and output (I&O), and for signs of blood loss. Maintain child in prone or side-lying position. Encourage intake of cool or cold clear liquids when child is fully awake. Administer analgesic as ordered. Educate child and caregivers to avoid red or brown liquids, using straws, coughing or blowing nose to decrease the risk of spontaneous hemorrhage.

NURSING PROCESS

Assessment

Subjective Data

Be sensitive to the child's and caregiver's level of anxiety and offer opportunities for expression of concerns. The use of puppets, dolls, and other materials may be an effective way to allow the child to act out the pending surgical experience and to express concerns and fears.

Objective Data

Presurgical assessments such as complete blood count (CBC), clotting time, and urinalysis are usually done on an outpatient basis.

Upon admission on the day of surgery, review vital signs and laboratory results for abnormalities, and assess the child for signs of infection (fever, elevated white blood count [WBC], and redness and exudate of the throat). Observe the child's mouth for loose teeth that could be aspirated during anesthesia.

Postoperatively, monitor vital signs and observe for hemorrhage, ability to swallow, and dehydration. The most obvious signs of bleeding from the surgical site are restlessness or anxiety, frequent swallowing, and rapid pulse. Each time vital signs are taken, use a flashlight to observe the pharynx for bleeding.

Nursing diagnoses for the child after a tonsillectomy include the following:

NURSING DIAGNOSES	PLANNING/OUTCOMES	NURSING INTERVENTIONS
*Risk for **A**spiration* related to unswallowed saliva and postoperative bleeding	The child's airway will remain patent.	Maintain the child in a prone or side-lying position. Monitor vital signs every 15 minutes for 1 hour and hourly for the next 4 hours. Ensure availability of suction equipment. Do not give oral fluids until the child is completely awake. Avoid hot liquids, irritating foods, and use of straws. Instruct the child to avoid coughing and clearing the throat; encourage the child to expectorate secretions into a tissue.
*Deficient Risk for **F**luid Volume* related to excessive loss through blood loss and decreased oral intake	The child will maintain appropriate fluid intake and demonstrate no signs and symptoms of dehydration.	Observe for signs of blood loss, such as frequent swallowing, elevated pulse and respirations, pallor, restlessness and anxiety; report to physician immediately. Maintain intravenous (IV) fluids until the child is taking oral fluids. Encourage intake of cold or cool liquids such as ice pops (no red or brown), noncitric juices, gelatin (no red), and ice chips; introduce milk products only after clear liquids are tolerated. Record hourly I&O, daily weight.

(Continues)

Nursing diagnoses for the child after a tonsillectomy include the following: (Continued)

NURSING DIAGNOSES	PLANNING/OUTCOMES	NURSING INTERVENTIONS
*Acute **Pain** related to* surgical procedure	The child will have pain relief (<3 on a scale of 1 to 10).	Provide nonaspirin analgesic every 4 hours for at least the first 24 hours after surgery. Use age-appropriate pain assessment tools. Encourage the caregivers to stay at the child's bedside to provide reassurance and comfort.
*Deficient **Knowledge*** (*parents*) related to unfamiliarity with information for discharge care	The caregivers will verbalize an understanding of discharge care.	Instruct the caregivers to: • Watch for signs of hemorrhage especially between the fifth and tenth postoperative days. • Watch for signs of infection (persistent earache, temperature over 102°F). • Call physician if bleeding or signs of infection occurs. • Encourage liquids and soft foods as tolerated for 10 days. • Avoid rough, scratchy foods for 3 weeks. • Maintain pain control with nonaspirin analgesics every 4 hours as needed during first week. • Restrict the child's activity to quiet play for 10 days (i.e., no school or vigorous exercise). • Expect the throat to be white in appearance and the mouth odor to be bad for the first week. • Bring child for follow-up visit in 1 to 2 weeks.

Evaluation: Evaluate each outcome to determine how it has been met by the client.

ASTHMA

Asthma, a reactive airway disease (RAD), is defined as narrowing or obstruction of the airway triggered by stimuli (such as cold air, smoke, viral infection, exercise, stress, drugs, or allergens) and inflammation that leads to mucosal edema and mucus hypersecretion. Asthma is the leading cause of school absenteeism and the most common admitting diagnosis in children's hospitals (Boychuk et al., 2006). Clinical manifestations of asthmatic attacks or episodes include a dry, hacking cough; wheezing; and difficulty breathing. The child may need to sit up to breathe. Attacks may last for hours or days. Thick, tenacious mucus may be expectorated after a coughing episode. In children with repeated acute exacerbations, barrel chest and the use of accessory muscles of respiration are common findings. Chronic asthmatics are usually small according to the standard growth charts. In some cases, episodes no longer occur after puberty, and growth usually catches up in adolescence. A definitive diagnosis of asthma can be made when the airway obstruction (indicated by pulmonary function tests) is reversed with bronchodilators.

> **PROFESSIONALTIP**
>
> **Theophylline**
>
> The margin of safety is narrow with theophylline. Early adverse effects include tachycardia, irritability, restlessness, insomnia, headache, vomiting, and diarrhea.

MEDICAL–SURGICAL MANAGEMENT

Medical

Medical treatment is aimed at preventing airway damage resulting from repeated and severe episodes of asthma. Care is focused on early recognition and treatment of episodes, identification and elimination of allergens, and education of the child and caregivers. Allergy proofing the home along with skin testing followed by desensitization are methods used to control allergens (refer to the section on Allergic Rhinitis).

Educate families about the disease, including ways to prevent attacks; early signs of episodes; drug therapy; appropriate exercise; and chest physiotherapy (CPT), if needed. Early symptoms include increasing cough at night, in the early morning, or in conjunction with activity; respiratory retractions; and wheezing. Using a peak flowmeter is an objective way to measure airway obstruction: families must learn how both to use this device and to record the results.

Pharmacological

A combination of bronchodilators, short-acting inhaled beta-2 agonists, and anti-inflammatory agents is used to treat asthma. Short-acting bronchodilators, such as beta-2 agonists, are used to treat mild intermittent asthma in children. Short-acting inhaled beta-2 agonists are used with acute symptoms in mild persistent asthma. Long acting bronchodilators, salmeterol xinafoate (Serevent Diskus) and formoterol fumarate (Foradil), are used with moderate and severe persistent asthma. The drugs of choice for long-term mild persistent asthma are inhaled corticosteroids, inhaled antiasthmatics (cromolyn sodium [Crolom] and nedocromil sodium [Tilade]), or oral antiasthmatics (leukotriene modifiers—montelukast sodium [Singulair]) (Spratto & Woods, 2009).

The most commonly prescribed bronchodilator is albuterol (Ventolin). These drugs cause relaxation of bronchial smooth muscle and inhibit the release of mediators from mast cells. Small doses by inhalation are the most effective mode of administration. Bronchodilators may be taken together by inhalation and be given parenterally for additional effect. Repetitive use may mask increasing airway inflammation and hyper-responsiveness. Correct use of the metered-dose inhaler (MDI) is important for maintaining control of asthma symptoms.

Theophylline (Theo-Dur) is the oldest effective bronchodilator. It requires continuous oral or IV administration and is most therapeutic when the serum level measures 10–20 mcg/mL. Educate child and caregivers to monitor for signs of toxicity which include: headache, tachycardia, abdominal pain, and hypotension (Leifer, 2006).

Anti-inflammatory drugs of choice include cromolyn sodium (Crolom) and corticosteroids such as prednisone (Deltasone). Cromolyn is an antiasthmatic, mast cell stabilizer that prevents asthma symptoms by blocking the release of mast cell mediators. Once symptoms start, however, cromolyn is ineffective. Adverse effects associated with cromolyn are airway irritation with mild cough and a bad taste. Corticosteroids effectively reduce mucosal edema and potentiate the effect of bronchodilators. Steroids may be given in inhaled form to reduce the oral dose required and to decrease systemic effects that accompany oral administration. Long-term use of oral steroids is reserved for chronic asthma that has not responded to other drugs. Adverse side effects of long-term oral therapy include Cushing's syndrome, growth suppression, osteoporosis, glaucoma, cataracts, peptic ulcer, hyperglycemia, and decreased resistance to infection (Lenhardt et al., 2006).

CRITICAL THINKING

Smoking and Asthma

What teaching would you provide to a caregiver who smokes around a child who has asthma?

Activity

Children with asthma should not be automatically restricted from physical activity. With adequate treatment, a child with asthma can participate in most physical activities. Sports that do not require sustained exertion, such as gymnastics, baseball, and weight lifting, are well tolerated. Swimming is frequently recommended as an ideal sport because the air is humidified, and breathing increases end expiratory pressure.

SAMPLE NURSING CARE PLAN

The Child with Asthma

M.O., a 5-year-old girl, was admitted to the emergency department (ED) with severe coughing, fever, and difficulty breathing. Crackles and wheezing were evident in all fields upon auscultation. Vital signs were temperature, 102°F; pulse, 160; and respirations, 40. Pulse oximetry was 90%. Her parents had given her Tylenol for what they thought was a "cold." When her condition worsened during the night, they brought her to the ED. M.O. has no history of asthma but has eczema. She has just started kindergarten. Her parents are extremely distraught and are asking many questions. M.O. cries every time anyone enters the room.

NURSING DIAGNOSIS 1 *Ineffective **A**irway Clearance* related to secretions in the bronchi and exudate in the alveoli as evidenced by difficulty breathing, crackles, and wheezing

Nursing Outcomes Classification (NOC)
Respiratory Status

Nursing Interventions Classification (NIC)
Airway Suctioning
Cough Enhancement
Positioning

PLANNING/OUTCOMES	NURSING INTERVENTIONS	RATIONALE
M.O. will have effective airway clearance.	Monitor vital signs, auscultate breath sounds, assess respiratory effort and rate, assess skin color every 15 to 30 minutes, arterial blood gases (ABGs), pulse oximetry, and pulmonary function tests results.	Subtle changes may serve as an early warning of increased airway obstruction.

(*Continues*)

SAMPLE NURSING CARE PLAN (Continued)

PLANNING/OUTCOMES	NURSING INTERVENTIONS	RATIONALE
	Administer oxygen at the ordered flow rate (if chronic asthmatic, not to exceed 2 L/min).	Decreases hypoxia. Administration of oxygen to a child with chronic carbon dioxide retention may cause respiratory depression.
	Position the child upright or for comfort.	Enhances lung expansion.
	Ensure availability of suction equipment and tracheostomy tray.	Condition can deteriorate rapidly.
	Provide at least 1,600 mL fluids (IV/PO)/24 hours.	Liquefies secretions and replaces insensible fluid losses.
	Initiate nothing-by-mouth (NPO) status during periods of severe respiratory distress.	Oral fluid intake during periods of distress can cause aspiration.
	Administer ordered medications and assess for therapeutic effect.	Bronchodilators and steroids open airways and decrease edema.
	Assess breath sounds before and after CPT.	Theophylline level of >30 can cause serious complication.
	Encourage child to cough and deep breathe by blowing bubbles through a wand.	CPT, coughing, and deep breathing help loosen/eliminate secretions.

EVALUATION

M.O.'s airway is clear.

NURSING DIAGNOSIS 2 ***A****nxiety* related to threat to or change in health status as evidenced by respiratory distress and hospitalization

Nursing Outcomes Classification (NOC)
Coping
Anxiety Reduction

Nursing Interventions Classification (NIC)
Anxiety Reduction
Anticipatory Guidance

PLANNING/OUTCOMES	NURSING INTERVENTIONS	RATIONALE
M.O. and her caregivers will demonstrate no signs of anxiety.	Maintain a calm, quiet environment and a reassuring manner.	Decreases oxygen demand and the work of breathing.
	Encourage therapeutic play.	Builds rapport and trust.
	Keep the caregivers informed of procedures, treatments, and condition of their child.	Builds rapport and trust. Calming the parents can help calm the child.

EVALUATION

M.O.'s anxiety level is decreased and her respiration rate is decreased. The parents participate in M.O.'s care.

SAMPLE NURSING CARE PLAN (Continued)

NURSING DIAGNOSIS 3 *Deficient Knowledge* related to disease process as evidenced by many questions

Nursing Outcomes Classification (NOC)	Nursing Interventions Classification (NIC)
Knowledge Deficit: Disease Process	*Teaching: Disease Process*
Knowledge Deficit: Treatment Regimen	*Teaching: Prescribed Medication*

PLANNING/OUTCOMES	NURSING INTERVENTIONS	RATIONALE
M.O.'s parents will verbalize accurate knowledge about asthma.	Teach parents about the disease, its triggers, and prescribed medications and treatment.	Understanding increases compliance with treatment.
	Assess the parents' knowledge about triggers, precipitating factors (such as colds), and allergen control.	Triggers may have been assessed. Knowledge of allergen control may decrease the likelihood of future episodes.
	Teach the importance of taking medications as prescribed.	Maintains therapeutic levels.
	Teach the importance of exercise and ways to choose appropriate activities based on the child's condition.	Promotes pulmonary and cardiovascular health, enhances self-esteem, and offers peer interaction.

EVALUATION

M.O. verbalizes knowledge about disease and treatment in age appropriate terms. M.O.'s caregivers verbalize accurate knowledge about the disease and its treatment.

FOREIGN-BODY ASPIRATION

Foreign-body aspiration is the inhalation of any object into the respiratory tract. Commonly aspirated items among children include nuts, grapes, popcorn, hard candy, dried beans, bones, coins, parts of toys, screws, and balloons. Aspiration may occur at any age but is most common between the ages of 6 months and 4 years. Clinical manifestations may include spasmodic coughing, respiratory distress, or gagging in the absence of fever or other symptoms of illness.

Medical–Surgical Management

Medical

Removal of foreign bodies from the respiratory tract is done by direct laryngoscopy or bronchoscopy. After the procedure, the child remains hospitalized for observation of laryngeal edema and respiratory distress. Cool mist is provided and antibiotic therapy ordered if appropriate.

Health Promotion

It is important that caregivers and child care providers remain watchful as the child gains increased locomotor and manipulative skills and becomes more curious about the environment.

Nursing Management

After the object has been removed, the main focus of care is prevention. Assess the caregivers' knowledge of safety in relation to the child's developmental level. Encourage parents/caregivers to keep cylindric, spheric, and pliable objects smaller than 1 and 1/4 inches out of children's reach. In addition, supervise children when eating, and cut food into small, irregular pieces.

CARDIOVASCULAR SYSTEM

A major threat to the child's cardiovascular system is rheumatic fever, which may lead to permanent heart damage and disability.

RHEUMATIC FEVER

Rheumatic fever is a chronic childhood disease affecting the heart, joints, lungs, and brain. It results from an autoimmune response to untreated group A *beta-hemolytic streptococcus* infections. Clinical manifestations are classified as minor and major. Minor clinical manifestations include fever, listlessness, anorexia, pallor, weight loss, and vague muscle, joint, or abdominal pain. Major clinical manifestations include polyarthritis, chorea (spasmodic twitchings), carditis, erythema marginatum (red skin lesions), and subcutaneous nodules. An elevated antistreptolysin-O (ASO) titer and an anti-DNAse B (both tests indicate a recent streptococcal infection) are common among children with rheumatic fever. The child may have a late complication of chorea known as Sydenham's chorea, perhaps years after the initial rheumatic fever. Chorea is caused inflammatory changes in the neurons of the central nervous system. The child with chorea has purposeless, rapid, involuntary movements of the extremities and trunk of the body (Potts & Mandleco, 2007).

Medical–Surgical Management

Medical

Diagnosis is made by evaluating presenting signs and symptoms and laboratory test results. A throat culture determines whether the infection is active. Erythrocyte sedimentation rate (ESR), C-reactive protein, and leukocyte count are elevated in the presence of inflammatory processes. An antistreptolysin O-titer (ASO) and anti-DNAse B indicate a previous streptococcal infection. These two tests together confirm the diagnosis of rheumatic fever up to 92% (Potts & Mandleco, 2007). Chest x-ray, electrocardiogram, and echocardiogram may demonstrate evidence of carditis.

The goals of medical management are to treat any existing strep infection, prevent recurrences and heart damage, and alleviate pain and fever. Bed rest is prescribed for the child with carditis until ESR and heart rate are within normal limits.

Pharmacological

Penicillin, salicylates, and corticosteroids are used to treat rheumatic fever. Long-term administration (as long as 5 years) of penicillin helps prevent the recurrence of rheumatic heart disease. Salicylates relieve pain, reduce inflammation of polyarthritis, and reduce fever. Corticosteroids are used in the presence of carditis. Residual heart disease (congestive heart failure) is treated as needed with digitalis and diuretics. Anticonvulsants may be prescribed to alleviate severe chorea.

Diet

A low-sodium diet may be prescribed in the presence of congestive heart failure. The intake and output is monitored to prevent dehydration or overhydration.

Activity

Bed rest is essential to reduce the workload of the heart. The length of bed rest can range from weeks to months depending on the cardiac status. Position the child for comfort and to prevent pressure areas and skin breakdown. A bed cradle may be used to relieve pressure on joints. Ensure safety and protect from falls; keep environment free from bright lights.

Health Promotion

Continual health supervision for children is the key to prevention of rheumatic fever and resulting heart disease. It is important that children with upper respiratory infections be evaluated for group A *beta-hemolytic streptococcus* and treated with penicillin as prescribed. Prophylactic antibiotics are required prior to any invasive procedure to prevent endocarditis.

Nursing Management

Maintain child on bed rest. Alternately apply heat and cold to affected joints. Provide distractions such as guided imagery, relaxation, board games, movies, books, or puzzles. Stress importance of evaluating children with upper-respiratory infections and taking penicillin as prescribed even if symptoms disappear.

NURSING PROCESS

Assessment

Subjective Data

Initially, determine whether any family members or caregivers have had a sore throat or unexplained fever within the past 2 months. Find out when symptoms began; what, if any, treatment was obtained; and if an antibiotic was prescribed, whether it was taken as directed.

Objective Data

Monitor the child for cardiac complications such as abnormal vital signs, shortness of breath, edema, and precordial pain. Assess joints for tenderness, small lumps, and rapid, purposeless movements. Use age-appropriate tools to assess pain.

Nursing diagnoses for the child with rheumatic fever include the following:

NURSING DIAGNOSES	PLANNING/OUTCOMES	NURSING INTERVENTIONS
*Acute **Pain*** related to inflamed joints	The child will rate pain ≤3 on a 0 to 10 scale.	Alternate applying heat and cold to affected joints. Reposition the child every 2 hours, handle joints gently. Provide distraction such as guided imagery and relaxation.
***Activity** Intolerance* related to shortness of breath and pain	The child will tolerate restricted activities.	Limit activities to bed and chair, with bathroom privileges, and meals at the table. Include rest periods alternated with activities such as board games, computer use, movies, puzzles, books, art, and crafts.

Nursing diagnoses for the child with rheumatic fever include the following: (Continued)

NURSING DIAGNOSES	PLANNING/OUTCOMES	NURSING INTERVENTIONS
*Risk for **Injury*** related to weakness and chorea	Child will be injury free.	If the child is experiencing chorea, the mattress may need to be placed on the floor and the child may require assistance going up and down stairs. Seizure precautions are taken. Teach the importance of evaluating children with upper respiratory infections for streptococcus, and treating with penicillin.
*Deficient **Knowledge*** related to medication administration	The child and caregiver will understand the importance of antibiotic therapy in preventing recurrence of the disease and further heart damage.	Stress the importance of taking penicillin as prescribed even if symptoms disappear.

Evaluation: Evaluate each outcome to determine how it has been met by the client.

HEMATOLOGIC AND LYMPHATIC SYSTEMS

Leukemia, idiopathic thrombocytopenic purpura, and hemophilia are blood disorders that commonly occur during childhood.

LEUKEMIA

Leukemia, the most common childhood cancer, is the uncontrolled production of lymphocytes (immature white blood cells). The most common form of leukemia is acute lymphocytic leukemia (ALL). The prognosis has been improving dramatically because of vigorous therapy, but there is concern related to adverse effects of the therapy. Clinical manifestations, the results of neutropenia and decreased red blood cells (RBCs) and platelets, include pallor, weakness, fever, excessive bruising, petechiae, purpura, bone or joint pain, and abdominal pain.

Medical–Surgical Management

Medical

In addition to the child's history, symptoms, and laboratory studies, bone marrow aspiration is done to confirm the diagnosis of leukemia. The goals of medical intervention are to eradicate the leukemic cells via chemotherapy and to provide supportive care during treatment.

Surgical

Bone marrow transplant may be recommended after the second remission.

Pharmacological

A combination of chemotherapy drugs is administered through a subclavian catheter and/or intrathecally to bring about remission. Treatment may last 2 to 3 years. After 30 days of initial treatment, remission can be verified via bone marrow aspiration and lumbar puncture. If remission occurs, the prognosis is good. For the child who suffers a relapse, different drugs are used in an attempt to reinduce a remission. Relapses decrease the probability of survival.

Nursing Management

Assess the emotional status of the child and the caregivers and identify areas of concern. A plan is made to assist them in working through and resolving their feelings and fears. Explore how the child and caregivers are coping with the illness as well as the treatment.

IDIOPATHIC THROMBOCYTOPENIC PURPURA

Idiopathic thrombocytopenic purpura (ITP) is a blood disorder associated with a deficit of platelets in the circulatory system. An autoimmune disorder often preceded by a viral infection, ITP may be acute and self-limiting or be chronic and require therapy. The peak age of occurrence is 2 to 4 years. Manifestations include bruising and petechiae.

Medical–Surgical Management

Medical

Diagnostic evaluation involves gathering a history of viral illness, information about any medications, and a CBC, which will be normal except for a low platelet level. If the history and CBC suggest ITP, bone marrow aspiration may be done to rule out oncological disorders. Most cases are self-limiting, with the platelet count returning to normal within 6 months without therapy. Platelet transfusions may be necessary for the child with chronic ITP if active, uncontrolled bleeding occurs.

PROFESSIONALTIP

Life-Threatening Illness

The following questions can be used in assessing the feelings and fears associated with the diagnosis of life-threatening illness:

- Has the child and/or caregivers been associated with hospitals, nurses, and doctors in the past? If yes, what were the positive and negative aspects of the experience?
- Do the caregivers know anyone diagnosed with a life-threatening illness? If yes, what happened to that person?
- Are there concerns about the child's future? The family or caregiver's future?

Surgical

When drugs no longer control the thrombocytopenia in a child with chronic ITP, a splenectomy may be indicated. Splenectomy is usually not performed before 5 years of age because of the immaturity of the child's immune system.

Pharmacological

Steroids and immune globulin are given to block the autoimmune destruction of platelets.

Nursing Management

Encourage the curtailing of physical activities and sports until condition is resolved. Observe for signs of bleeding. Advise to use soft-bristled toothbrush. Assist parents/caregivers to establish a safe, age-appropriate home environment. Teach the child's caregiver the signs and symptoms of infection.

NURSING PROCESS

Assessment

Subjective Data

Caregivers may bring the child to the doctor because of a "red rash" or bruising. The child's activity level may be reported to be normal.

Objective Data

Observe for further bleeding (e.g., epistaxis, hematuria, blood in stools) and level of consciousness.

Nursing diagnoses for the child with ITP include the following:

NURSING DIAGNOSES	PLANNING/OUTCOMES	NURSING INTERVENTIONS
*Risk for **I**njury* related to low platelet count	The child will be free of injury.	Have the child curtail physical activities and sports until platelets return to normal. Encourage the use of a soft-bristled toothbrush to minimize gum bleeding. Observe for signs of bleeding. Flush the catheter with saline to confirm proper placement of an IV line.
*Deficient **K**nowledge (parents)* related to disorder and treatment	The caregivers will verbalize an understanding of the disorder and treatment.	Teach the caregivers that ITP should subside within 6 months. Teach the caregivers side effects of steroids, such as edema, insomnia, mood changes, poor healing, peptic ulcers, and growth retardation. Establish a safe, age-appropriate home environment (e.g., pad table corners, crib rails, and knees and elbows to decrease injury). Instruct caregivers to use nonaspirin analgesics and antipyretics. Evaluate the child's platelet count weekly.
*Risk for **I**nfection* related to chronic use of steroids and/or splenectomy	The child will be free of infection.	Teach the caregivers the signs and symptoms of infection. Administer pneumococcus vaccine and/or daily antibiotics, if the child has a splenectomy.

Evaluation: Evaluate each outcome to determine how it has been met by the client.

HEMOPHILIA

Neonatal bleeding from the umbilical cord or circumcision site may be an early manifestation of severe hemophilia. Mild hemophilia may not be detected until the toddler becomes mobile, and unusual bruising and bleeding occur from small injuries.

Nursing interventions center on prevention and teaching. Regular physical exercise strengthens muscles and

CRITICAL THINKING

Fluid Volume Deficit

What is the priority data to gather when assessing a child for fluid volume deficit? Why?

joints and may decrease the number of bleeding episodes. The infusion of recombinant factor VIII concentrates is the treatment for hemophilia. Recombinant factor concentrates are an effective treatment for hemophilia and prevent the exposure to HIV or hepatitis that previous transfusions caused.

GASTROINTESTINAL SYSTEM

Gastrointestinal disorders in children interfere with nutrition and fluid and electrolyte balance and have the potential for impairing growth. Common GI disorders of childhood include constipation and parasitic infections.

CONSTIPATION

Constipation is the infrequent or difficult passage of hard, dry stools. It is most common during the toddler and preschool years because of the child's (and caregivers') efforts at toilet training. School-age children may experience constipation as a result of busy schedules, hesitation to use unfamiliar bathrooms, and limited bathroom privileges. Other potential causes of constipation include lack of fresh fruit and vegetables and grains in the diet, dehydration, lack of exercise, emotional stress, certain drugs, pain from passage of hard stool, excessive milk intake, and a variety of GI tract and systemic disorders and spinal lesions.

CLIENT TEACHING

Guidelines for Preventing Constipation in Children

For toddlers and preschool children:

- Increase cereal, fruit, vegetable, and fluid intake.
- Encourage sitting on the toilet for 5 to 10 minutes after breakfast and after dinner.

For school-age children:

- Allow 1 hour to finish breakfast before leaving for school to allow sufficient time for bathroom use.
- Encourage children to take responsibility for including cereals, fruits, vegetables, and fluids in their diets.
- Encourage children to exercise daily.
- Decrease the anxiety of children by taking time each day to communicate about their day's activities, concerns, and fears.

Chronic constipation causes an enlarged rectum, which impairs sphincter control, resulting in **encopresis** (the passage of watery colonic contents around a hard fecal mass). Predisposing factors for encopresis include inadequate or inconsistent toilet training or psychological stress such as that related to starting school or the birth of a sibling. Clinical manifestations of constipation include abdominal pain and cramping without distention; palpable, movable fecal mass and a large amount of stool inside rectum; diarrhea; malaise; anorexia; and headache.

MEDICAL–SURGICAL MANAGEMENT

Medical

Abdominal x-rays may reveal a rectum enlarged with stool and gas. The impaction is removed with enemas.

Pharmacological

Stool softeners or laxatives may be prescribed in an effort to retrain the rectum after the impaction has been removed. Mineral oil may be prescribed to decrease the pain of defecation.

Diet

Increasing water and fiber intake and limiting milk intake will often decrease constipation and promote defecation.

Health Promotion

Counseling may be part of the treatment plan, if there is no evidence of physiologic disorders. Establishing and maintaining regular toileting habits, drinking fluids, eating a high-fiber diet, and participating in regular exercise will also help prevent constipation.

NURSING MANAGEMENT

Focus on teaching caregivers about normal bowel patterns in children and the importance of diet and exercise in maintaining those patterns. Assess the child's diet history and elicit a description of bowel patterns to provide clues to the cause of constipation. Dietary changes may be all that is required to resolve constipation.

Requiring the child to sit on the toilet for 10 minutes approximately 30 minutes after meals encourages regular bowel habits. Caution caregivers about the overuse of laxatives, stool softeners, and enemas. Use of mineral oil may cause soiling from leakage, which should not be mistaken for encopresis.

INTESTINAL PARASITIC INFECTIONS

Common parasitic infections include giardiasis (a protozoan) and helminths (i.e., pinworms, roundworms, hookworms; see Figures 61-1, 61-2, 61-3, and 61-4). Children are more commonly infected than adults because they frequently put their hands in their mouths. Temperate climates, crowded conditions (i.e., day care centers, schools), untreated water, and poor hygiene practices may contribute to outbreaks of parasitic infections. Appearance, mode of transmission,

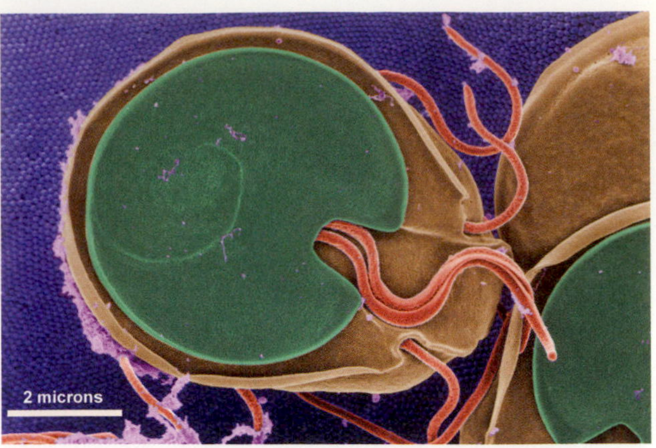

FIGURE 61-1 Scanning electron micrograph (SEM) of a *Giardia muris* trophozoite that had settled atop the mucosal surface of a rat's intestine. The protozoan Giardia causes the diarrheal disease called giardiasis. (*Courtesy of the Centers for Disease Control and Prevention/Photo by Dr. Stan Erlandsen.*)

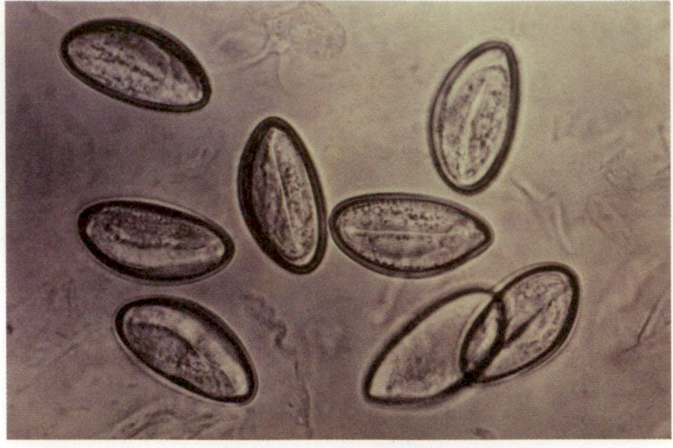

FIGURE 61-2 Human pinworm eggs, captured on cellulose tape. (*Courtesy of the Centers for Disease Control and Prevention.*)

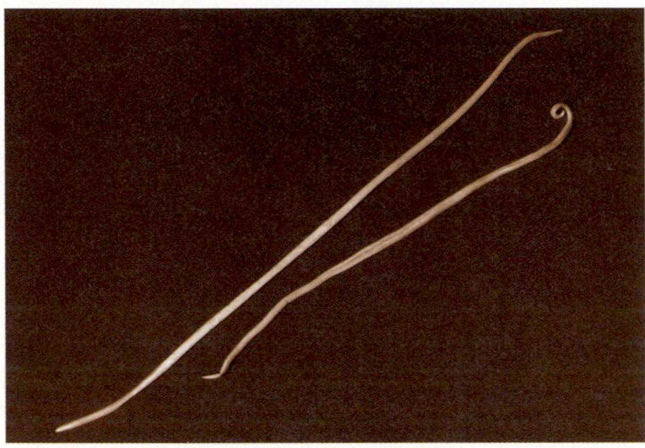

FIGURE 61-3 A 1960 photograph of two roundworms. The larger of the two is the female while the normally smaller male is on the right. Adult worms live in the lumen of the small intestine. Adult roundworms can live for 1 to 2 years and adult female worms can grow over 12 inches in length. (*Courtesy of the Centers for Disease Control and Prevention.*)

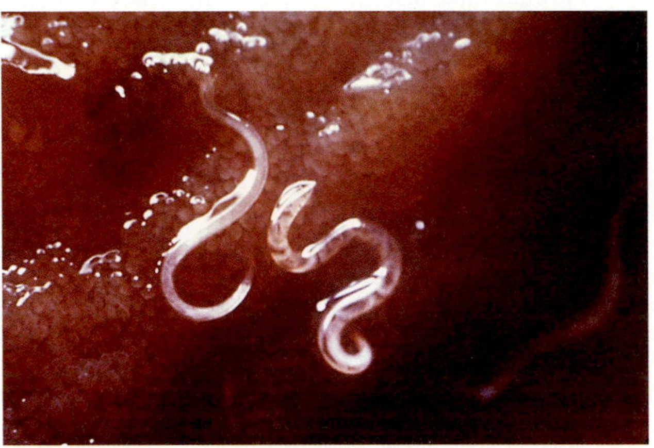

FIGURE 61-4 A photographic enlargement showing hookworms attached to the intestinal mucosa. Barely visible larvae penetrate the skin, are carried to the lungs, go through the respiratory tract to the mouth, are swallowed, and eventually reach the small intestine. This journey takes about a week. (*Courtesy of the Centers for Disease Control and Prevention.*)

and clinical manifestations vary, depending on the parasite (Table 61-2).

MEDICAL–SURGICAL MANAGEMENT

Medical

Identification of a parasitic infection is done with a fecal smear or a microscopic examination. Pinworms may be diagnosed by using cellophane tape to capture eggs from around the anus and then examining them under a microscope.

Pharmacological

Helminths are treated with oral anthelmintic medications such as pyrantel pamoate (Antiminth) or mebendazole (Vermox). Medication should be repeated 2 to 3 weeks later to eliminate any parasites that may hatch after the initial treatment. All family members and caregivers should also be treated.

CLIENT TEACHING

Preventing Parasitic Infestations

- Care providers should wash hands thoroughly after changing diapers.
- Dispose of soiled diapers in trash receptacles.
- Teach children to wash their hands and fingernails after using the toilet and before eating.
- Wash bedding and undergarments in hot water.
- Regularly use cleaning agents containing bleach in bathrooms.
- Wash all raw fruits and vegetables before eating.
- Cover sandboxes when not in use.
- Avoid swimming pools that allow diapered children.
- Wear shoes outside.

TABLE 61-2 Common Intestinal Parasites

	APPEARANCE	MODE OF TRANSMISSION	CLINICAL MANIFESTATIONS
Giardiasis	Microscopic	Ingested cysts Person to person Untreated water Contaminated food Animals Soil Feces	Diarrhea Weight loss Abdominal cramping
Pinworm	White, threadlike worm	Person to person Ingested or inhaled eggs	Itching around the anus Irritability Distractibility
Roundworm	Pink worm, 9 to 12 inches in length	Eggs passed from hand to mouth (may migrate to liver and lungs)	Abdominal pain, distention, or obstruction Vomiting Jaundice Pneumonitis
Hookworm	Microscopic	Skin penetration by contact with contaminated soil (may migrate to lungs)	Dermatitis Anemia Pneumonitis Malnutrition

COURTESY OF DELMAR CENGAGE LEARNING

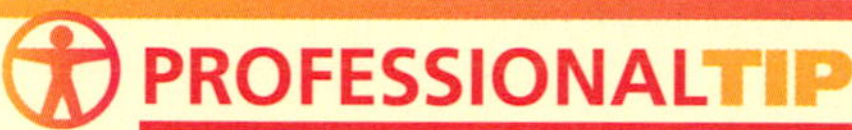

Quinacrine Hydrochloride (Atabrine HCl)

To disguise the bitter taste of quinacrine tablets, pulverize and mix with jam or honey.

COMMUNITY/HOME HEALTH CARE

Instructions for the Tape Test for Pinworms

Perform the test early in the morning, before the child awakens:

1. Wind the tape around the end of a tongue blade, sticky side out.
2. Spread the child's buttocks and press the tape against the anus, rolling the blade from side to side.
3. Place the tongue blade in a glass jar or plastic bag.
4. Take to the lab for microscopic examination. If a glass slide is available, remove the tape from the tongue blade and place it smoothly on the slide, sticky side down.

Metronidazole (Flagyl) or quinacrine hydrochloride (Atabrine HCl) are effective in treating giardiasis. Alert child care providers to the possibility of a yellow discoloration to the skin for the child on quinacrine hydrochloride (Atabrine HCl).

Diet

A well-balanced diet with additional protein and iron may be prescribed for the child with hookworms. These nutrients may be depleted from blood loss and malnutrition.

Health Promotion

Attention to meticulous sanitary practices is essential.

NURSING MANAGEMENT

Assist with collection of specimens, treatment of infections, and prevention of reinfection. Collect stool specimens from diapers, potty chairs, or a toilet covered with clear plastic wrap. Use a tongue blade to place the specimen into the designated and properly labeled container. Provide caregivers with detailed instructions for performing the tape test (see the accompanying Community/Home Health Care box). Provide education regarding the course of treatment and home care.

ENDOCRINE SYSTEM

A common endocrine disorder in children is type 1, formerly called insulin-dependent, diabetes. The management of diabetes in children presents some unique challenges because of their physical immaturity and dependence on caregivers for care. Stabilizing insulin needs during puberty requires vigilant monitoring of the glucose level and regulating diet, insulin, and exercise. The lifestyle of the entire family or caregivers must change in order to effectively treat the child with diabetes. Family members and caregivers should be familiar with and adhere to the prescribed regimen. Most school-age children are ready and able to learn to give their own injections and should be encouraged to do so.

An increasing number of children, up to 45% of those with diabetes, have type 2 diabetes (American Diabetes Association, 2006). Most of these children are overweight or obese. Testing for type 2 diabetes in children is shown in Table 61-3. They are usually treated initially with nutrition therapy and an exercise program. Eventually, most will require drug therapy. Most pediatric diabetologists use oral agents for children with type 2 diabetes (American Diabetes Association, 2006). For medical–surgical management and nursing management of the child with endocrine disorders, see the endocrine system chapter.

MUSCULOSKELETAL SYSTEM

Maximizing bone mass in childhood reduces the impact of bone loss related to aging. It is also a critical time for developing lifestyle habits important to maintaining good bone health such as proper nutrition and physical activity (NIH, 2000).

Common musculoskeletal disorders in children include scoliosis, Legg-Calvé-Perthes disease, muscular dystrophy, juvenile arthritis, and fractures.

SCOLIOSIS

Scoliosis, the most common spinal deformity in children, involves lateral curvature greater than 20 degrees, spinal rotation, rib asymmetry, and thoracic hypokyphosis (Figure 61-5). It occurs most frequently in prepubescent girls and is usually not caused by any other injury or disease.

Clinical manifestations include visible curve of the spine, posterior rib hump when bending forward, asymmetrical rib cage, and uneven shoulder or pelvic heights. Caregivers may notice that the child's clothes do not fit properly (e.g., uneven hems).

TABLE 61-3 Recommendations for Testing Children for Type 2 Diabetes

Overweight: BMI greater than 85th percentile for age and sex, weight for height greater than 85th percentile, or weight greater than 120% of ideal for height

plus

Any two of the following risk factors:

- Family history of type 2 diabetes in first- or second-degree relative
- Being Native American, African American, Hispanic, or Asian/Pacific Islander
- Show signs of insulin resistance or conditions associated with insulin resistance such as **acanthosis nigricans**, a velvety hyperpigmented patch on back of neck, in axilla, or antecubital area; hypertension; dyslipidemia, or polycystic ovarian syndrome (PCOS)

Age for Testing: At age 10 years or at onset of puberty, whichever occurs first, and then every 2 years

Test: Fasting plasma glucose (FPG) preferred

From American Diabetes Association. (2006). Type 2 diabetes in children and adolescents. *Diabetes Care, 22*(12), 381. [Online]. Available: www.diabetes.org

LIFE SPAN CONSIDERATIONS

Backpacks

A child should be able to stand up straight and maintain good posture when carrying a backpack. Therefore:

- Backpacks should be positioned above the child's buttocks.
- Both straps should be used instead of just one.
- The backpack should not be overloaded so the child has to lean forward when carrying it.

From Nemours. (2002). School backpacks: How they affect your child's general health. Retrieved December 23, 2003 from www.nemours.org/no/news/releases/2002/020206_ backpack_study.html

MEDICAL–SURGICAL MANAGEMENT

Medical

The goal of medical treatment is to stop the curvature of the spine. Early detection and treatment of scoliosis are essential to successful management. The treatment regimen depends on the degree and progression of the curvature and the reaction of the child and caregivers. Children with mild curvatures

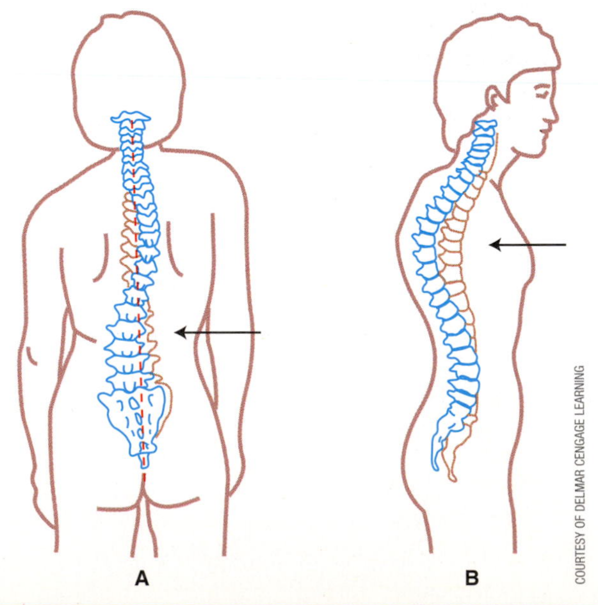

FIGURE 61-5 ***A,* Scoliosis; *B,* Kyphosis**

may simply be monitored throughout the growth cycle. Electrical stimulation, bracing, and exercise may be prescribed for children with mild to moderate curvatures.

Surgical

Surgical intervention may be required for children with curvatures greater than 40 degrees. The goal of surgery is to correct the curvature of the spine with internal fixation and instrumentation.

Nursing Management

Involve child in the plan of care. Encourage child to perform exercises as prescribed. Provide suggestions to protect bony prominences when wearing a brace.

Postoperatively, assess extremities for color, capillary refill, warmth, sensation, and movement. Log roll the child every 2 hours. Monitor vital signs, for bowel distention, and urinary retention. Assess pain level and provide analgesics as ordered. Teach caregivers about wound care. Discuss restrictions on activity. Emphasize importance of keeping follow-up appointments.

NURSING PROCESS

Assessment

Subjective Data

Initially, the child may complain of a sore back, improperly fitting clothing, or a slight limp. When being treated with a brace, assess the child for problems related to self-esteem and body image. Ask the child and caregivers to report on the degree of compliance with the prescribed regimen. If the child requires surgery, assess feelings and fears of the child and the family.

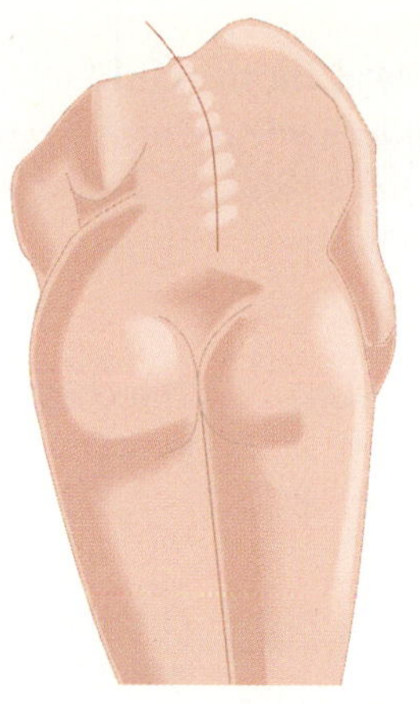

COURTESY OF DELMAR CENGAGE LEARNING

Figure 61-6 Scoliosis screening reveals a rib hump and curved spine.

Objective Data

Screening for scoliosis is an important role of the nurse. Assess children 10 years of age and older. With clothes removed, observe the back for uneven shoulders and hips, prominent shoulder blade on one side, and curved spine. While bending at the waist and touching the toes, assess the child's back for a rib hump and curved spine (Figure 61-6).

When a brace is in place, continue monitoring the degree of curvature and assess the skin at pressure points for irritation. Progression of the curve may indicate either noncompliance with the prescribed treatment or the need for more aggressive therapy.

Postoperatively, the child is assessed for neurological status, pain, fluid balance, bleeding, and bowel and bladder function. Mobility and nutrition are quickly resumed if there are no complications.

Nursing diagnoses for the child with scoliosis include the following:

NURSING DIAGNOSES	PLANNING/OUTCOMES	NURSING INTERVENTIONS
*Deficient **K**nowledge (parents and child)* related to lack of information about scoliosis, including treatment and surgery	The child and caregiver will verbalize an understanding of and comply with the medical regimen.	Identify the child's and caregiver's knowledge level and areas of concern. Inform the child and caregiver that the brace must be worn for prescribed hours per day for recommended length of time. Inform the child and caregiver that use of brace may eliminate need for surgery. If surgery is necessary, prepare the child and caregiver for the need to log roll the child and the need for the child to cough and have them demonstrate preoperatively.
*Disturbed **B**ody Image* related to deformity, bracing, and surgical scar	The child will talk about feelings. The child will demonstrate self-confidence.	Involve the child in the plan of care. Provide the child with opportunities to ventilate feelings about being different. Encourage the child to talk about experiences with friends. Help the child select clothing that is stylish yet loose enough to fit over the brace. Help the child focus on positive body features (e.g., hair, complexion).

(*Continues*)

Nursing diagnoses for the child with scoliosis include the following: (Continued)

NURSING DIAGNOSES	PLANNING/OUTCOMES	NURSING INTERVENTIONS
		Help the child select activities that will enhance abilities. Provide the child with privacy during hospitalization.
*Risk for Impaired **S**kin Integrity* related to wearing of a brace	The child's skin will remain intact.	Have the child wear a knit cotton shirt under the brace. Place a protective pad over bony prominences. Report reddened areas so that the brace can be adjusted.
*Impaired Physical **M**obility* related to restricted movement (brace/surgery)	The child will adjust to restricted movement.	Perform exercises as prescribed. Instruct the child in how to move with the brace (i.e., climb stairs; get in and out of a vehicle, chair, desk, and bed).
*Risk for **I**njury* related to neurovascular deficit secondary to instrumentation	The child will regain all body functions postoperatively.	Assess all extremities for color, capillary refill, warmth, sensation, and motion. Monitor signs of bowel distention and urinary retention. Maintain body alignment by logrolling every 2 hours and rolling from a side-lying position to a sitting position. Assist with early ambulation postoperatively.
*Acute **P**ain* related to operative procedure	The child will experience pain reduction to an acceptable level.	Assess pain level postoperatively, using pain scale. Provide prescribed analgesics around the clock for the first 24 to 48 hours. Explore alternate means of relieving pain (e.g., dim lights, music). Assess and document the child's response to relief measures.
*Deficient **K**nowledge (parent and child)* related to home care	The child and caregiver will successfully manage postoperative treatment at home.	Teach proper wound care. Discuss the importance of a well-balanced diet in maintaining healthy bones. Discuss activity restrictions (e.g., lifting no more than 10 pounds) and the length of time they will be in place. Have the child demonstrate moving without twisting or bending at the waist. Emphasize the importance of keeping follow-up appointments.

Evaluation: Evaluate each outcome to determine how it has been met by the client.

LEGG-CALVÉ-PERTHES DISEASE

Legg-Calvé-Perthes disease is necrosis of the head of the femur. The disease occurs most commonly in Caucasian boys between the ages of 4 and 8 years. The cause is unknown. Clinical manifestations include hip and knee soreness or stiffness, painful limp, and quadriceps muscle atrophy.

MEDICAL–SURGICAL MANAGEMENT

Medical

Diagnosis is made by x-ray. The goal of treatment is to maintain the shape of the femoral head and reduce the risk of permanent stiffness and degenerative arthritis. Methods used to accomplish this goal include traction, bracing, and surgery.

Initially, the child is hospitalized for non–weight-bearing range-of-motion exercises and bed rest. If there is no improvement within 10 days, alternate methods of treatment are usually begun.

Nonsurgical intervention may involve traction followed by the use of a non–weight-bearing abduction brace to position the femoral head in the acetabulum. Exercises maintain muscle integrity during the time that the child is required to wear the brace, for as long as 1 to 3 years.

Surgical

Surgical intervention is often the treatment of choice because it reduces treatment time and eliminates compliance problems.

The child is usually able to resume normal activities in 3 to 4 months.

NURSING MANAGEMENT

Maintaining mobility and educating the child and caregivers are the primary nursing goals. Encourage the caregivers and child to adhere to treatment plans and keep follow-up visits. Demonstrate proper application of the abduction brace. Perform skin assessments daily. Encourage the child to maintain muscle integrity via prescribed exercises. Involvement in activities such as horseback riding and swimming may be permitted.

DUCHENNE MUSCULAR DYSTROPHY

Duchenne muscular dystrophy (DMD) is an x-linked, recessive, hereditary, progressive, degenerative disease of the muscles. The disease occurs almost exclusively among males and is carried by females. Clinical manifestations include delayed motor development, difficulty standing or walking, progressive muscle weakness, increasing abnormalities in gait and posture, lordosis, pelvic waddling, frequent falling, **Gowers' sign** (walking the hands up legs to move from a sitting to a standing position), and a flat affect and smile. The disease continues into adolescence and young adulthood, when the child usually succumbs to respiratory failure. Children with DMD rarely live beyond 20 years of age. Complications include obesity, contractures, respiratory infections, and cardiac failure. Diagnosis is confirmed by serum enzyme assay, muscle biopsy, and electromyography.

MEDICAL–SURGICAL MANAGEMENT

Medical

Initially, therapeutic management is aimed at maintaining ambulation and independence for as long as possible with bracing and physical therapy. Later, therapy is directed at maximizing sitting capabilities, respiratory function, and self-care. Genetic counseling is recommended for caregivers, female siblings, and maternal aunts and their female offspring.

Surgical

Contractures may be released surgically in order to keep the child as mobile as possible.

NURSING MANAGEMENT

Monitor children when there is a family history of muscular dystrophy. Encourage physical therapy exercise regimen and use of adaptive devices. Focus on the things the child can do.

NURSING PROCESS

ASSESSMENT

Subjective Data

When there is a family history of muscular dystrophy, monitor the child carefully. Assess both the family or caregivers' ability to cope with a chronic, debilitating illness and the support systems available.

Objective Data

Routinely monitor the child for mobility, self-care abilities, weight gain, and infections.

Nursing diagnoses for the child with DMD include the following:

NURSING DIAGNOSES	PLANNING/OUTCOMES	NURSING INTERVENTIONS
Impaired Physical ***M****obility* related to progressive muscle wasting and contractures	The child will remain physically active.	Reinforce physical therapy exercise regimen. Encourage activity (e.g., school attendance, swimming). Encourage the use of adaptive equipment as needed (e.g., a back brace).
S*elf-Care Deficit (all)* related to progressive weakness	The child will be able to perform activities of daily living (ADLs) as long as possible.	Instruct the caregivers in ways to adapt the home as needed (e.g., grab bars, overhead sling, raised toilet, wheelchair access). Focus on those things the child can do to prevent frustration. Maintain the child's independence as long as possible (e.g., via an electric wheelchair and portable phone).
Compromised ***C****oping, Family* related to increased demands of care, financial burdens, and needs of other children	The caregivers coping will be effective with the disease process.	Refer the caregivers to resource and support groups. Assist the family or caregivers in anticipating needs and coordinating services. Encourage involvement of extended family and friends. Encourage the family and caregivers to express feelings.

Evaluation: Evaluate each outcome to determine how it has been met by the client.

JUVENILE ARTHRITIS

Juvenile arthritis (JA) is a systemic, multisystem disorder that affects the body's connective tissue; it is also known as an autoimmune inflammatory disease. There are many different forms of the disease, including juvenile rheumatoid arthritis.

Clinical manifestations include joint swelling accompanied by limited range of motion; pain; tenderness; and inflammation lasting longer than 6 weeks. Complications include blindness and disability. Prognosis is generally good with early detection and treatment.

Medical–Surgical Management

Medical

The goal of treatment is to maintain mobility and preserve joint function. The therapeutic regimen includes drugs, physical therapy, and/or surgery.

Surgical

Depending on the severity of the disease, surgery may be necessary to release contractures, correct leg-length discrepancies, and replace joints.

Pharmacological

Drug therapy includes aspirin, nonsteroidal anti-inflammatory drugs such as ibuprofen (Motrin) and naproxen (Naprosyn), slower-acting antirheumatic drugs such as gold sodium thiomalate (Myochrysine), and penicillamine (Cuprimine). Cytotoxic drugs may be used for severe disease that does not respond to other drugs. Corticosteroids may be used sparingly when the disease is life threatening.

Nursing Management

Refer to the Immune System chapter.

FRACTURES

Fractures in children tend to be less complicated and heal more quickly than do those in adults. The bones most commonly fractured in children include the clavicle, femur, tibia, humerus, wrist, and fingers. Fractures in the area of the epiphyseal plate (growth plate) can cause permanent damage and severely impair growth. Greenstick fractures are common among young children because of incomplete ossification. Evidence of old fractures in a young child suggests possible child abuse, whereas fractures in infants may indicate osteogenesis imperfecta (brittle bone disease).

Treatment usually involves realignment and immobilization using traction or closed manipulation and casting.

Refer to the Musculoskeletal System chapter for medical management and the nursing process.

> **COMMUNITY/HOME HEALTH CARE**
>
> **Juvenile Arthritis**
>
> Home treatment for juvenile rheumatoid arthritis may include the following:
>
> - Exercise, such as swimming and bicycling, to maximize muscle strength and range of motion
> - Splints, positioning, and application of heat and cold to provide comfort during painful episodes

IMMUNE SYSTEM

Infectious or communicable diseases are not life threatening to most children; however, children with immature or compromised immune systems are at greater risk of developing severe and even fatal complications as the result of communicable diseases.

COMMUNICABLE DISEASES

A communicable disease is an illness that is directly or indirectly transmitted from one person to another. Infants and young children are more susceptible to infectious diseases because their immune systems are not fully developed until 6 years of age, and their hygiene habits (e.g., covering the mouth when coughing) are lacking. Selected communicable diseases, along with causal agent, transmission mode, communicable period, incubation period, clinical manifestations, potential complications, treatment, and immunity conferment are listed in Table 61-4.

Nursing Management

Immunization is critical to the health of children. One of the goals of the U.S. government is to immunize 90% of children ages 15 to 35 months by the year 2010 (Healthy People 2010, 2000). Conscientious nurses and health care providers familiarize themselves with immunization schedules and the various frequent revisions to these schedules. The Advisory Committee on Immunization Practices (ACIP) of the U.S. Public Health Service Centers for Disease Control (CDC) and the American Academy of Pediatrics (AAP) Committee on Infectious Diseases are responsible for recommendations regarding vaccinations. Changes in recommendations are published in the *Morbidity and Mortality Weekly Report* for the ACIP and in *Pediatrics* for the AAP.

Recognize barriers to immunizations and educate caregivers about vaccine safety, administration, precautions, and contraindications. Barriers to immunization include long waiting lines, appointment-only systems, inaccessible clinic sites, and inability to speak English. The nurse takes every opportunity to immunize children whenever children enter any health care facility.

Federal law requires health care providers to provide general information about immunizations before administration. This general information includes nature, prevalence, and risks of the disease; type of immunization product to be used; the expected benefits and the risk of side effects of the vaccine; and the need for accurate immunization records. If possible, provide this lengthy information before the immunization appointment so that families have time to read and understand the information and to ask questions. Otherwise, the health care provider must inform parents at the time of administration. Document informed consent of the parent(s).

Table 61-4 Select Common Communicable Diseases

DISEASE (CAUSAL AGENT)	TRANSMISSION MODE AND COMMUNICABLE PERIOD	INCUBATION PERIOD	CLINICAL MANIFESTATIONS AND POTENTIAL COMPLICATIONS	TREATMENT AND IMMUNITY CONFERMENT
Chicken pox (varicella-zoster virus, Figure 61-7)	*Transmission mode*: direct contact, respiratory droplet, airborne particles *Communicable period*: 1 day before lesions appear until all lesions crust over	10–21 days	*Clinical manifestations*: fever, malaise, irritability, and a rash that begins as macules and progresses to fluid-filled papules to crusted lesions. *Potential complications*: Reye's syndrome, skin infections, encephalitis	*Treatment*: antihistamines, baths, and lotions for itching *Immunity conferment*: natural or with vaccine; may reactivate in adults as herpes zoster
Diphtheria (*Corynebacterium diphtheriae*)	*Transmission mode*: direct contact, contact with contaminated articles, or consumption of unpasteurized milk *Communicable period:* 2 to 4 weeks in presence of antibiotic treatment, months without treatment	2–5 days	*Clinical manifestations*: fever, cough, pharyngitis, anorexia, membranous lesion on tonsils, pharynx, or larynx *Potential complications*: neuritis, carditis, congestive heart failure, respiratory failure	*Treatment*: Isolation, antitoxin, antibiotics, and analgesics *Immunity conferment*: diphtheria, tetanus, and acellular pertussis (DTaP) vaccine; passive immunity conferred by maternal antibodies
Erythema infectiosum, or Fifth disease (Parvovirus B19, Figure 61-8)	*Transmission mode*: contact with respiratory secretions and blood *Communicable period*: unknown	4–20 days	*Clinical manifestations*: fiery-red cheeks ("slapped face" appearance); erythematous, maculopapular, lacy rash on trunk then limbs *Potential complications*: none	*Treatment*: *Supportive* *Immunity conferment*: no vaccine
Hepatitis B, or serum hepatitis (hepatitis B virus [HBV])	*Transmission mode*: blood, secretions, prenatally, perinatally, sexual contact *Communicable period*: throughout clinical course	50–180 days	*Transmission mode*: mild flulike symptoms, jaundice in adolescents *Potential complications*: Liver failure	*Treatment*: supportive care *Immunity conferment*: hepatitis B vaccine (Hep B)

(*Continues*)

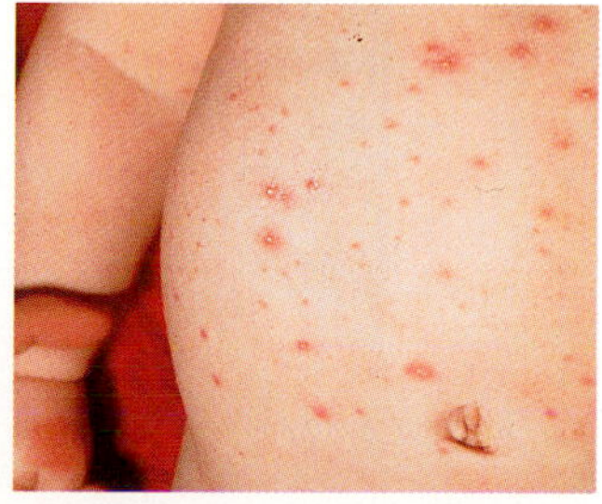

Figure 61-7 Varicella (*Courtesy of Robert A. Silverman, M.D., Clinical Associate Professor, Department of Pediatrics, Georgetown University.*)

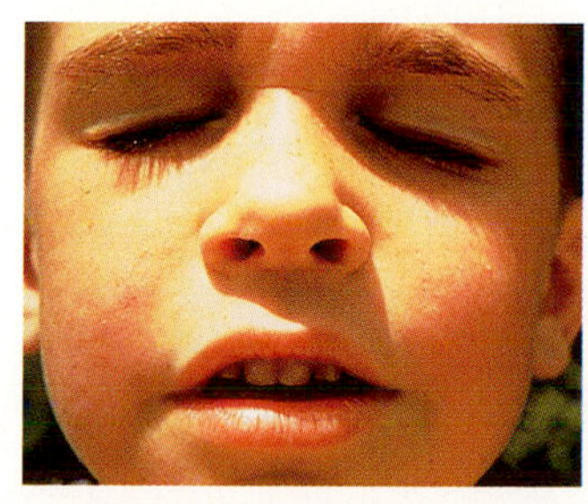

Figure 61-8 "Slapped Face" in Erythema Infectiousum (Fifth Disease) (*Courtesy of the Centers for Disease Control and Prevention.*)

TABLE 61-4 Select Common Communicable Diseases (Continued)

DISEASE (CAUSAL AGENT)	TRANSMISSION MODE AND COMMUNICABLE PERIOD	INCUBATION PERIOD	CLINICAL MANIFESTATIONS AND POTENTIAL COMPLICATIONS	TREATMENT AND IMMUNITY CONFERMENT
Measles, or rubeola (measles virus, Figure 61-9)	*Transmission mode*: direct or indirect contact with respiratory droplets *Communicable period*: 4 days before to 5 days after appearance of rash	10–21 days	*Clinical manifestations*: fever, runny nose, cough, enlarged lymph nodes, Koplik's spots (small, red spots with blue-white centers on oral mucosa, Figure 61-10), photophobia, maculopapular rash from hairline over entire body *Potential complications*: otitis media, pneumonia, encephalitis, airway obstruction	*Treatment*: supportive care *Immunity conferment*: measles, mumps, rubella (MMR) vaccine *Active*: from infection with causative agent
Mononucleosis (Epstein-Barr virus)	*Transmission mode*: direct contact with saliva; blood transfusions; most common in adolescents and young adults *Communicable period*: unknown	30–50 days	*Clinical manifestations*: fever, pharyngitis, fatigue, sore throat, enlarged lymph nodes *Potential complications*: splenic rupture, hepatitis, meningitis, encephalitis, Guillain-Barré syndrome	*Treatment*: supportive care, antipyretics, analgesics *Immunity conferment*: no vaccine
Mumps, or parotitis *(paramyxovirus)*	*Transmission mode*: direct or indirect contact with saliva *Communicable period*: 7 days before swelling until 2 to 3 days after swelling subsides	14–21 days	*Clinical manifestations*: fever, headache, malaise, anorexia, "earache" aggravated by chewing, enlarged parotid gland (Figure 61-11) *Potential complications*: orchitis, meningoen-cephalitis, hearing loss	*Treatment*: supportive care, antipyretics, analgesics *Immunity conferment*: MMR vaccine, natural; passive: mumps immune globulin

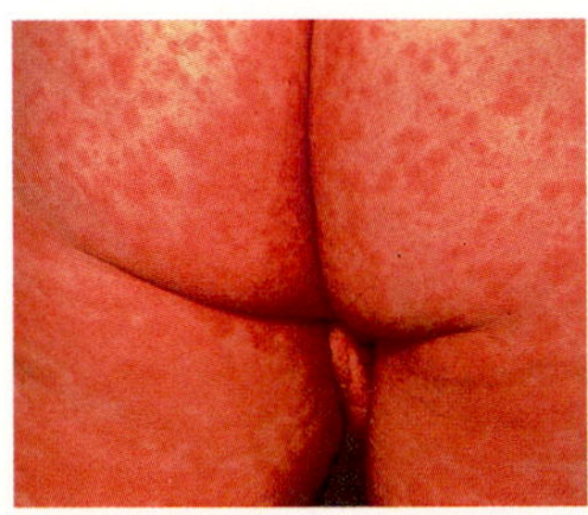

FIGURE 61-9 Rubeola/Measles (*Courtesy of the Centers for Disease Control and Prevention.*)

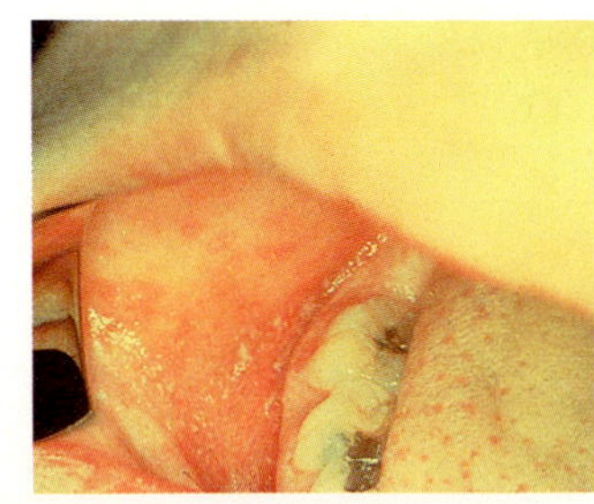

FIGURE 61-10 Koplik's Spots in Rubeloa (*Courtesy of the Centers for Disease Control and Prevention.*)

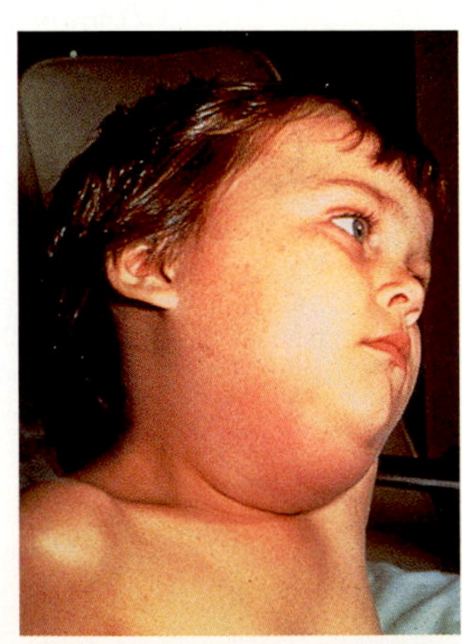

FIGURE 61-11 Mumps (*Courtesy of the Centers for Disease Control and Prevention.*)

Table 61-4 Select Common Communicable Diseases (Continued)

DISEASE (CAUSAL AGENT)	TRANSMISSION MODE AND COMMUNICABLE PERIOD	INCUBATION PERIOD	CLINICAL MANIFESTATIONS AND POTENTIAL COMPLICATIONS	TREATMENT AND IMMUNITY CONFERMENT
Pertussis, or whooping cough (*Bordetella pertussis*)	*Transmission mode*: direct contact or respiratory droplets *Communicable period*: 1 week after exposure until 4 to 6 weeks	5–21 days	*Clinical manifestations*: upper respiratory symptoms progressing to severe paroxysmal cough with inspiratory whoop *Potential complications*: pneumonia, otitis media, hemorrhage, convulsions	*Treatment*: antibiotics, supportive care with high humidity *Immunity conferment*: DTaP vaccine; *active*: from infection with causative agent
Poliomyelitis, or infantile paralysis (poliovirus types I, II, III)	*Transmission mode*: fecal–oral, respiratory droplets *Communicable period*: unknown prior to symptoms, 1 week after symptoms for respiratory contact, up to 6 weeks for fecal contact	5–14 days	*Clinical manifestations*: fever, headache, abdominal pain, stiff neck, pain and tenderness in lower extremities, paralysis *Potential complications*: permanent paralysis, respiratory arrest	*Treatment*: supportive, rehabilitative care *Immunity conferment*: poliovirus vaccine (inactivated) [IPV] or live oral [OPV]; *active*: immunity against a specific strain conferred by disease
Roseola, or exanthema subitum (herpesvirus type 6, Figure 61-12)	*Transmission mode*: unknown; appears between 6 months and 2 years of age *Communicable period*: unknown	Unknown	*Clinical manifestations*: rose-pink, nonpruitic maulopapules on trunk then face, neck, and limbs that fade on pressure *Potential complications*: febrile seizures	*Treatment:* antipyretics, supportive care *Immunity conferment*: no vaccine

(*Continues*)

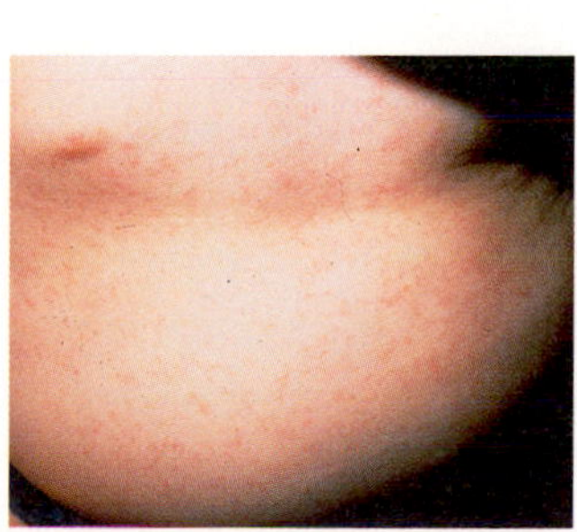

Figure 61-12 Roseola (*Courtesy of Robert A. Silverman, MD, Clinical Associate Professor, Department of Pediatrics, Georgetown University.*)

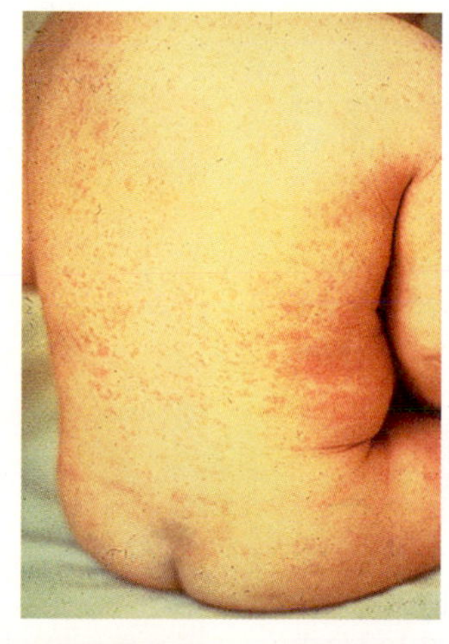

Figure 61-13 Rubella (German Measles/3-Day Measles) (*Courtesy of the Centers for Disease Control and Prevention.*)

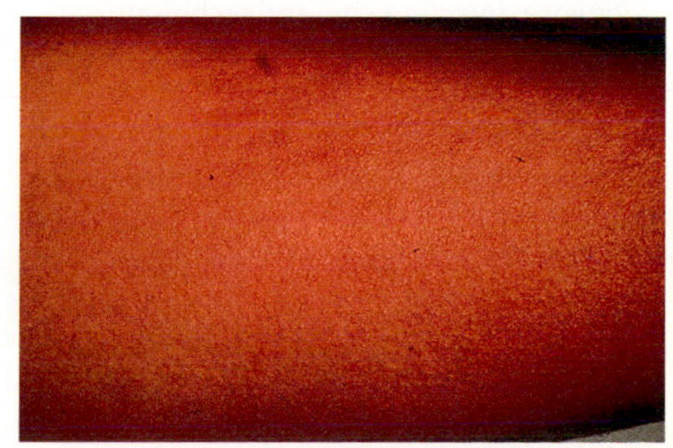

Figure 61-14 Scarlet Fever (*Courtesy of the Centers for Disease Control and Prevention.*)

Table 61-4 Select Common Communicable Diseases (Continued)

DISEASE (CAUSAL AGENT)	TRANSMISSION MODE AND COMMUNICABLE PERIOD	INCUBATION PERIOD	CLINICAL MANIFESTATIONS AND POTENTIAL COMPLICATIONS	TREATMENT AND IMMUNITY CONFERMENT
Rubella, or German measles, 3-day measles (Rubella virus, Figure 61-13)	*Transmission mode*: airborne, direct contact with droplets, transplacental *Communicable period*: 10 days before symptoms and 15 days after rash appears	14–21 days	*Clinical manifestations*: fever, headache, malaise, runny nose, anorexia, maculopapular rash progressing from head to extremities *Potential complications*: risks for unborn fetus of infected mother; spontaneous abortion, stillbirth, ear, eye, and cardiac anomalies	*Treatment*: supportive care *Immunity conferment*: MMR vaccine
Scarlet fever, or scarlatina (group A *beta-hemolytic streptococci*, Figure 61-14)	*Transmission mode*: airborne respiratory droplets and contaminated articles *Communicable period*: from onset of symptoms until 24 hours after antibiotic therapy is initiated	1–7 days	*Clinical manifestations*: fever, headache, "strawberry tongue," abdominal pain, sore throat, skin on hands and feet peels in sheets after first week *Potential complications*: glomerulonephritis, rheumatic fever	*Treatment:* penicillin, antipyretics, analgesics *Immunity conferment*: no immunity
Tetanus, or lockjaw (*Clostridium tetani*)	*Transmission mode*: direct contact of skin wound with contaminated soil or implements *Communicable period*: not communicable	3–21 days	*Clinical manifestations*: stiffness of neck and jaw, difficulty breathing *Potential complications*: laryngospasm, death	*Treatment*: supportive care *Immunity conferment*: DTaP vaccine: passive: from tetanus antitoxin or immune globulin (TIG)

COURTESY OF DELMAR CENGAGE LEARNING

Be knowledgeable about the safe administration of immunizations. This includes proper storage, reconstitution, sequence, injection site, and technique.

The nurse is responsible for documenting on the child's immunization record the type of vaccine, the date of administration, the manufacturer and lot number, the expiration date, and the administration site. Encourage caregivers to keep and provide immunization records at every health care visit.

INTEGUMENTARY SYSTEM

Because they are visible and often disfiguring, skin disorders can prove emotionally and psychologically stressful for the child and family/caregivers. It is important to teach families and children strategies to maintain healthy skin. Skin disorders may be caused by infections (bacterial, fungal, viral), infestations (pediculosis, scabies), insects, substances (contact dermatitis), acne, and injuries such as burns.

COMMUNITY/HOME HEALTH CARE

Preventing Children from Scratching Lesions

To prevent children from scratching lesions:

- Cut the fingernails short.
- Give cool baths.
- Cover the lesions with clothing, when possible.
- At nighttime, cover the hands with socks or gloves.
- During the day, encourage activities that require use of the hands; administer antihistamines or sedatives as needed to control itching.
- Keep the child cool.

BACTERIAL INFECTIONS

Bacterial infections of the skin are usually caused by staphylococci or streptococci. The two most common skin disorders of childhood resulting from bacterial infections are impetigo and cellulitis.

IMPETIGO

Impetigo, the most common skin infection of childhood, often begins in an area of broken skin, such as that caused by an insect bite or eczema. The face, mouth, hands, neck, and extremities are the most common sites.

Clinical manifestations include primary lesions (macules that change rapidly to form small, thin-walled vesicles with an erythematous halo), secondary lesions (ruptured vesicles covered by a honey-colored crust over an ulcerated base), pruritus, burning, and lymph node enlargement (Figure 61-15). Lesions usually resolve within 2 weeks. Because impetigo is commonly caused by streptococci, rheumatic fever or glomerulonephritis are possible complications.

Medical–Surgical Management

Pharmacological

A topical bactericidal ointment such as polymyxin B sulfate-neomycin (Neosporin) is applied for 5 to 7 days. Children with multiple lesions may require oral antibiotics such as erythromycin (E-Mycin). In extreme and extended situations, parenteral antibiotics may be required.

Nursing Management

The primary nursing goals are to prevent the spread of infection and promote healing. The child with impetigo is treated at home and should not return to school until 2 days after antibiotics are initiated. Emphasize the importance of taking antibiotics as prescribed.

Encourage caregivers to employ preventive hygiene practices such as sleeping alone, bathing daily with antibacterial soap, using a separate towel, washing hands properly, and using separate eating utensils. Wash the lesions gently three times per day with a warm, soapy washcloth. Remove soaked crusts and apply topical bactericidal ointment. A small amount of bleeding after crust removal is common. Leave the lesions uncovered. Teach children to keep their fingers away from the lesions.

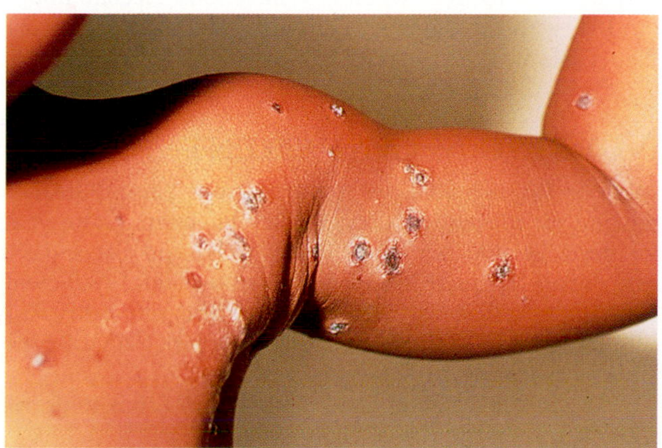

FIGURE 61-15 Impetigo (*Courtesy of Robert A. Silverman, MD, Clinical Associate Professor, Department of Pediatrics, Georgetown University.*)

CELLULITIS

Cellulitis is a bacterial infection of the skin and subcutaneous tissue. The condition usually affects the face (buccal and periorbital regions) or lower extremities. Children with cellulitis have a history of trauma, impetigo, upper-respiratory infections, sinusitis, otitis media, or tooth abscess. Common causative organisms are staphylococci and streptococci. Clinical manifestations include rapid onset of red or lilac color; tender, hot, edematous skin; and enlarged lymph nodes. Possible complications of cellulitis include septic arthritis, osteomyelitis, meningitis, brain abscess, or blindness.

Medical–Surgical Management

Medical

Cellulitis of the extremities is usually treated at home with oral antibiotics and warm compresses. Cellulitis involving the joints or face is extremely serious, requiring hospitalization and IV antibiotics.

Surgical

Incision and drainage of the affected area may be necessary if the condition does not improve with treatment.

Nursing Management

Elevate the affected extremity and immobilize. Apply warm, moist soaks every 4 hours to increase circulation to the affected area, relieve pain, and promote healing. Inform caregivers that failure to administer the entire course of antibiotics as ordered may result in a more serious infection.

FUNGAL INFECTIONS

Fungal infections are named using the term *tinea* (ringworm) followed by the Latin word for the affected part of the body (Table 61-5).

Nursing Management

Adequate teaching is essential for successful treatment of tinea. Apply lotion and cream to the entire lesion and extending to approximately 1 inch beyond the lesion. Take oral medication for the full course of treatment, even if symptoms disappear. Proper hygiene is essential.

VIRAL INFECTIONS

Viral skin infections can produce lesions such as rashes, macules, papules, vesicles, urticaria (hives), and warts. Common communicable diseases of childhood that produce rashes and are preventable through immunizations include rubeola, rubella, and varicella (refer back to Table 61-3). Herpes simplex virus type 1 is a common, contagious skin infection for which there is no cure or prevention.

TABLE 61-5 Common Fungal Infections

INFECTION (SITES)	CLINICAL MANIFESTATIONS	AFFECTED POPULATION	TREATMENT AND PREVENTION
Tinea capitis (scalp)	Erythema, pruritus, scaly scalp with round patches of alopecia	2- to 10-year-old children	*Treatment*: oral griseofulvin (Fulvicin P/G, Grifulvin V) *Prevention:* avoid sharing combs, barber scissors, hats, and towels; avoid direct contact with infected scalp
Tinea corporis (trunk, face, extremities)	Ringlike, scaly plaques measuring 1/2 to 1 inch and having pale centers and red margins	Young boys living in hot, humid climates	*Treatment*: antifungal cream applied three times per day until lesions have been gone for 1 week (usually 2 to 4 weeks). *Prevention:* treat infected pets
Tinea pedis (feet, toes; "athletes foot")	Fissures, red scaly lesions	Adolescents and adults	*Treatment*: daily washing and application of antifungal cream for up to 6 weeks. *Prevention:* avoid contaminated floors, sidewalks, and showers; nylon socks; plastic shoes; closed shoes
Tinea cruris (inner thighs, inguinal area; "jock itch")	Scaly lesions, erythema, pruritus, possible papules or vesicles	Most commonly, athletes and obese individuals	*Treatment:* oral griseofulvin (Fulvicin P/G, Grifulvin V), sitz baths to soothe *Prevention:* wear loose-fitting undergarments to promote dryness

COURTESY OF DELMAR CENGAGE LEARNING

HERPES SIMPLEX VIRUS TYPE 1

Herpes simplex virus type 1 (HSV-1) is an often recurrent infection of the mouth ("cold sore," "fever blister"), throat, eyes, or fingers (Figure 61-16). After initial infection, the virus remains dormant within nerve cells and can be reactivated by fever, stress, trauma, sun exposure, menstruation, or immunosuppression. Children suffering from burns, eczema, diaper rash, or immunosuppression are particularly susceptible to HSV-1. Clinical manifestations include clusters of fluid-filled vesicles; ulcerations; swelling; inflammation; pruritus; and severe pain. Lesions usually dry and crust within 7 to 10 days.

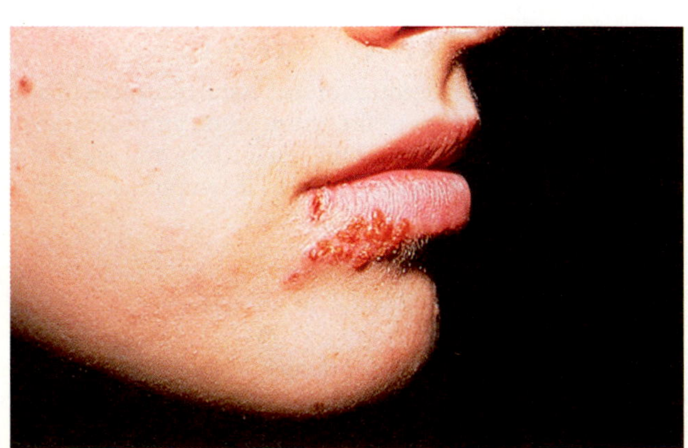

FIGURE 61-16 Herpes Simplex Virus Type 1 (*Courtesy of Robert A. Silverman, MD, Clinical Associate Professor, Department of Pediatrics, Georgetown University.*)

MEDICAL–SURGICAL MANAGEMENT

Medical

Treatment is directed toward relieving symptoms. Usually, children are managed at home by ensuring adequate hydration, pain management, and secondary-infection prevention.

Pharmacological

Oral acyclovir (Zovirax) is given early in the development of the condition and for recurrent infections. Topical acyclovir cream also is used for recurrent infections. Results are best when applied early in the onset of lesions. Antibiotic ointment may be used to treat secondary infections. Acetaminophen (with or without codeine) and topical and mouth-rinse anesthetics may be prescribed for pain relief.

NURSING MANAGEMENT

Monitor for dehydration resulting from painful swallowing and for prevention of secondary infection. Offer frozen ice pops, gelatin, noncitrus juices, milk, and flat sodas to help ensure adequate fluid intake despite painful swallowing. Encourage small, frequent feedings of bland, soft foods. Reassure caregivers that fluids are more important than solid food for the first few days.

Teach child to keep hands away from lesions to prevent spreading it to other areas.

Place the hospitalized child in contact isolation or under drainage and secretion precautions. The child is considered contagious until lesions have fallen off or mucous membrane ulcerations have healed.

COMMUNITY/HOME HEALTH CARE

Caring for the Child with HSV-1

- Wear gloves when suctioning or providing oral care and when handling soiled linens and clothing.
- Practice proper hand hygiene (remembering to wash hands after removing gloves).
- Wash all eating utensils and towels in hot, soapy water.
- Do not eat after the child.
- Prevent the child from putting the fingers in the mouth.
- Use a protective cover such as a sheet when holding and cuddling the child.
- Provide oral fluids that do not irritate the mucous membrane, such as noncitrus juices, flat sodas, milk, and ice pops.
- Provide at least 100 mL (approximately 1/2 cup) /kg/day of fluids for a child weighing less than 20 kg.
- Watch for signs of dehydration, such as dry skin and mucous membranes and decreased urine output (<3 to 4 times per day).
- Administer medications as prescribed.

INFESTATIONS

Infestations are one of the major health problems in schools. Common infestations are pediculosis and scabies.

PEDICULOSIS

Pediculosis (lice) is an infestation that most typically affects the head (capitis), body (corporis), or pubic area (pubis). Pediculosis of the head is the most common infestation seen in children. Lice attach their eggs (nits) to hair shafts close to the scalp. The nits then hatch in approximately 1 week. Clinical manifestations of head lice infestation include "dandruff" (nits) that is not easily removed, severe itching of the scalp, and "bugs" in the hair (usually behind the ears and at the back of the head) (Figure 61-17). Signs and symptoms

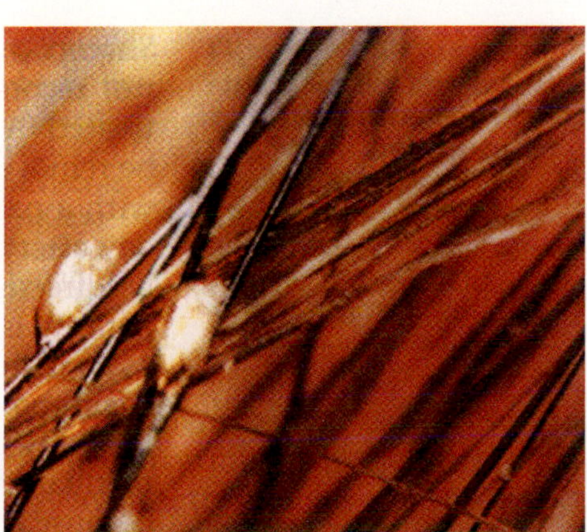

FIGURE 61-17 Nits (*Courtesy of Hogil Pharmaceutical Corporation.*)

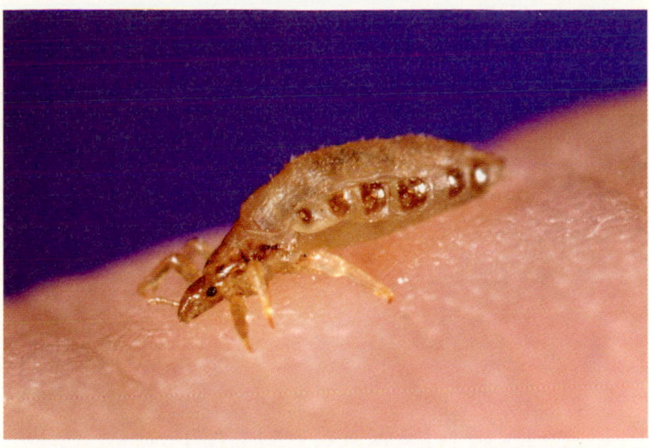

FIGURE 61-18 A female body louse as it was obtaining a blood-meal from a human host, who in this case, happened to be the photographer. Infestation is common, found worldwide, and affects people of all races. Body lice infestations spread rapidly under crowded conditions where hygiene is poor and there is frequent contact among people. (*Courtesy of the Centers for Disease Control and Prevention/provided by Frank Collins, PhD; photo by James Gathany.*)

of body lice infestation include intense pruritus and papular, rose-colored dermatitis in areas under tight-fitting clothing (Figure 61-18). Lice are easily passed from child to child in close-contact situations (e.g., the home, day care centers, and schools) via the sharing of headgear, hair-care products, pillows, blankets, and towels.

MEDICAL–SURGICAL MANAGEMENT

Pharmacological

Several anti-lice products are available (Table 61-6).

PROFESSIONAL TIP

Checking for Lice

Because lice do not transmit from hair to hands, the use of gloves during head checks is neither necessary nor cost effective.

PROFESSIONAL TIP

Manual Removal of Lice

The National Pediculosis Association (NPA) (2009a) advocates early detection and manual removal of nits and lice to prevent the unnecessary use of chemicals. According to the NPA, lindane (Kwell) is the most potentially toxic of all the chemicals available for removing lice and nits. Vacuuming, rather than environmental lice sprays, is a safe and effective way to rid the environment of lice. Lice sprays should not be used in the home or on a child's bedding.

TABLE 61-6 Anti-Lice Products

PRODUCT	TREATMENT	EFFECT
permethrin (Nix)	Apply to shampooed hair, leave on for 10 minutes, and rinse out of hair with water; do not re-shampoo for 24 hours	Safely kills lice and nits with one application
pyrethrins (TripleX, RID)	Apply to hair as directed; repeat treatment in 1 to 2 weeks, if live nits are present	Safely kills lice and nits; product of choice for those under 2 years of age and for pregnant adolescents

COURTESY OF DELMAR CENGAGE LEARNING

NURSING MANAGEMENT

Nursing care for children with pediculosis focuses on screening and education. Encourage caregivers and teachers to incorporate checking for lice into routine daily hygiene. Early detection facilitates immediate removal. There is no need to cut long hair or to shave the child's head, which only draws more attention to the fact that the child is infested.

Teach children that anyone can get lice and that taunting a child who has lice may hurt the child's feelings. Because lice are transmitted from person to person, children should be cautioned about using hair-care products, hats, pillows, blankets, and towels that do not belong to them.

SCABIES

Scabies results from the impregnated "itch mite" burrowing into the epidermis to lay her eggs. Clinical manifestations include intense pruritus and rash (papules, vesicles, and nodules) found most often on the wrists, finger webs, elbows, axillae, feet, ankles, head, neck, abdomen, waist, groin, and buttocks (Figure 61-19). Secondary infections often occur as a result of scratching the lesions.

MEDICAL–SURGICAL MANAGEMENT

Pharmacological

The treatment of choice for scabies is 5% permethrin cream (Elimite, Nix). An oral antihistamine such as diphenhydramine hydrochloride (Benadryl) or hydroxyzine (Atarax) may be prescribed to relieve pruritus.

NURSING MANAGEMENT

Nursing management for the child with scabies focuses on promoting healing, preventing secondary infections, and preventing further transmission of the condition. All persons having direct contact with the child, including care providers and those living in the child's house, should be treated. Itching and rash may endure for 2 to 3 weeks.

COMMUNITY/HOME HEALTH CARE

Guidelines for Managing Infestations

- Wash bedding, clothing, and stuffed animals in hot water and dry in a hot dryer.
- Vacuum carpets, upholstered seats (in the car and house), mattresses, toys, and nonwashable items. According to the NPA (2009a), there is no need to discard the used vacuum bag.
- The NPA (2009a) does not recommend placing toys or other items in plastic bags.
- The NPA (2009a) recommends manually removing the lice and nits with a special lice removing comb that can be boiled if desired.

BITES/STINGS

Animals (usually dogs), spiders, ticks, and insects (e.g., mosquitoes, fleas) account for the many bites and stings suffered by children. Bites and stings generally cause mild discomfort and are simple to treat; however, in some cases, life-threatening situations result.

ANIMAL BITES

Animal bites may result from domestic or wild animals but are most commonly caused by a familiar dog. Children younger than 4 years of age are bitten most frequently because of their height and the associated tendency to be near the dog's face. Dog bites usually occur on the face or extremities and can result in crushing and puncture wounds and lacerations.

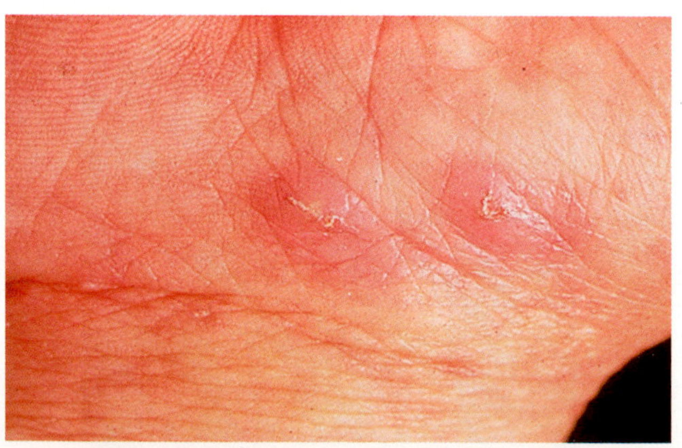

FIGURE 61-19 Scabies (*Courtesy of Robert A. Silverman, MD, Clinical Associate Professor, Department of Pediatrics, Georgetown University.*)

Medical–Surgical Management

Medical

The primary medical concerns for the child who has suffered an animal bite are infections from rabies and tetanus and scarring, especially on the face. Generally, after the wound and surrounding area are thoroughly washed with mild soap and water, a clean dressing is applied.

Pharmacological

If the animal is unvaccinated for rabies, the child will be given a series of immunizations to prevent rabies. Antibiotics may be indicated if the wounds are deep. Tetanus toxoid may be administered, depending on the child's immunization history and the severity of the wound.

Nursing Management

Focus on prevention and wound care. It is important for children to learn "animal safety rules" in order to prevent bites.

Teach caregivers and children to cleanse wounds properly and observe for signs of infection. Encourage parents to keep their child's immunizations up to date. If rabies immunizations are required, parents must understand the importance of returning for the injections on the appropriate days. Report animal bites to the community animal control agency.

SPIDER BITES

Bites from black widow and brown recluse spiders demand medical attention. Characteristically, these spiders are nonagressive, avoid light, and bite only in self-defense. Although both spiders inject toxic venom when they bite, the initial bite may go unnoticed. Within a few hours after the bite, however, manifestations surface such as swollen, painful erythema and systemic reactions. Black widow venom is neurotoxic and may cause dizziness, weakness, abdominal pain, paralysis, seizures, and, possibly, death from shock and renal failure. Brown recluse venom is necrotoxic, with the bite progressing to a necrotic ulcer within 1 to 2 weeks. Systemic reactions may include fever, nausea and vomiting, and joint pain. The recluse bite is not fatal, but the ulcer may take months to heal.

CLIENT TEACHING

Animal Safety Rules

- Stay away from strange or wild animals such as raccoons, skunks, bats, and squirrels.
- Stay away from a dog's face.
- Pet animals by rubbing, stroking, scratching, and patting; never hit, bite, or pinch.
- Allow unfamiliar animals to smell you before attempting to touch them.
- Ask the permission of the owner before petting an animal.
- Never approach an animal while it is eating, sleeping, injured, or tending to its babies.

Medical–Surgical Management

Medical

The child with a black widow spider bite will be hospitalized for supportive care until neurological symptoms subside and renal function is confirmed. The child with a brown recluse bite will require wound care and pain management but will usually not require hospitalization.

Surgical

Skin grafting may be required for large ulcers resulting from the brown recluse spider bite.

Pharmacological

Antivenin (Lactrodectus mactans) is administered to the child with a black widow spider bite, if the child has no allergy to horse serum. In addition, analgesics, muscle relaxants, and tetanus prophylaxis may be required.

There is no antivenin for the brown recluse spider bite. Antibiotics, corticosteroids, analgesics, and tetanus prophylaxis may be prescribed for the time during which the wound is healing.

Nursing Management

Focus on wound care, proper administration of medications, and prevention. Teach caregivers and children to be cautious in areas where spiders are likely to live, such as woodpiles and closets.

TICK BITES

Ticks live in fields and woods. They feed on the blood of mammals (e.g., humans, dogs, livestock, and deer) by embedding their heads into the skin. Tick bites cause pruritic nodules at the site of attachment and, rarely, systemic reactions such as fever, rash, and paralysis. Lyme disease (Figure 61-20) and Rocky Mountain spotted fever are caused by organisms that are transmitted by ticks.

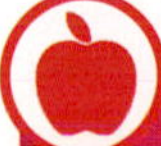

CLIENT TEACHING

Guidelines for Preventing Tick Bites

- When walking in fields or woods, wear long-sleeved shirts, tuck long pants into socks, and use insect repellent. Wearing light colors facilitates finding ticks.
- When returning from a tick-infested area, look for ticks and remove them as soon as possible.
- Bathe dogs with a shampoo containing permethrin.

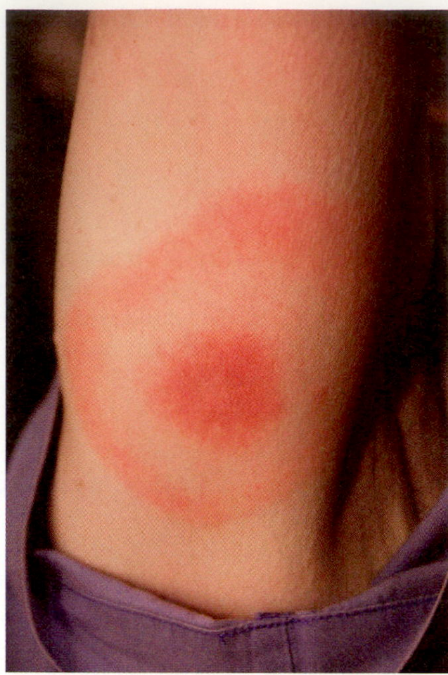

FIGURE 61-20 This "bull's-eye" pattern rash manifested at the site of a tick bite in a client's posterior right upper arm. The client subsequently contracted Lyme disease. Lyme disease patients who are diagnosed early, and receive proper antibiotic treatment, usually recover rapidly and completely. A key component of early diagnosis is recognition of the characteristic Lyme disease bull's-eye rash. (*Courtesy of the Centers for Disease Control and Prevention/photo by James Gathany.*)

NURSING MANAGEMENT

Preventing tick bites and removing embedded ticks are the primary focus. Remove the tick by grasping the tick's body with blunt, angled forceps or tweezers as close to the skin as possible and pulling straight up in an attempt to remove the embedded head along with the body. Do not twist the tick (American Academy of Family Physicians, 2002). Remove any remaining part of the head or attachment secretions from the tick using a sterile needle, and then thoroughly cleanse hands. Cleanse the attachment site and apply an antiseptic solution.

INSECT BITES

Insects such as mosquitoes, flies, fleas, and gnats inject foreign proteins when they penetrate the skin to suck blood. Insect bites usually result in itching, erythema, and a small wheal. The severity of the reaction depends on the degree of the child's hypersensitivity.

MEDICAL–SURGICAL MANAGEMENT

Medical

Medical management focuses on alleviating itching and preventing infection. Baths and cool compresses may relieve itching and prevent scratching, which can lead to bacterial infections.

Pharmacological

Antipruritics and antihistamines may be prescribed to control severe itching and facilitate sleep.

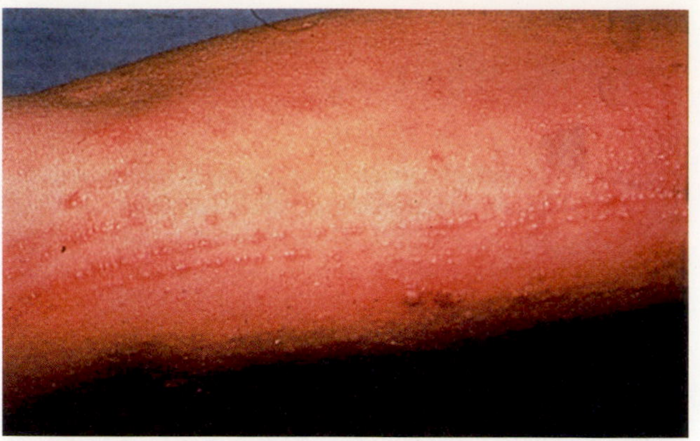

FIGURE 61-21 Contact Dermatitis (*Courtesy of the Centers for Disease Control and Prevention.*)

NURSING MANAGEMENT

Focus on preventing bites, alleviating itching, and preventing infection. Mattresses, carpets, furniture, and pets may require treatment with insecticides.

CONTACT DERMATITIS

Contact dermatitis is an inflammatory reaction of the skin to allergens, such as rubber, dyes, nickel, or poison ivy, or to irritants, such as soaps, wool, urine, or stool. Manifestations of allergic contact dermatitis include tiny, itching, weeping blisters over an area of skin (Figure 61-21). Manifestations of irritant contact dermatitis include localized, dry, inflamed, pruritic skin.

MEDICAL–SURGICAL MANAGEMENT

Medical

Treatment involves discontinuing exposure to the offending agent, washing the skin thoroughly, and applying cool compresses.

Pharmacological

Steroid cream (1%) may be applied in a thin layer several times per day after the application of cool compresses. Oral steroids may be prescribed for severe cases.

NURSING MANAGEMENT

Nursing care is aimed at relieving itching, preventing infection, and identifying and removing offensive substances. In addition to cool compresses, oral antihistamines, antipruritic lotions, and tepid oatmeal baths may relieve itching. Avoid overheating. Teach children to recognize and avoid poison ivy, oak, and sumac.

ACNE

Acne, one of the most common health problems of adolescence, is a noninfectious, inflammatory disease of the skin involving the sebaceous glands and hair follicles (Figure 61-22). Pathophysiologic factors having the greatest

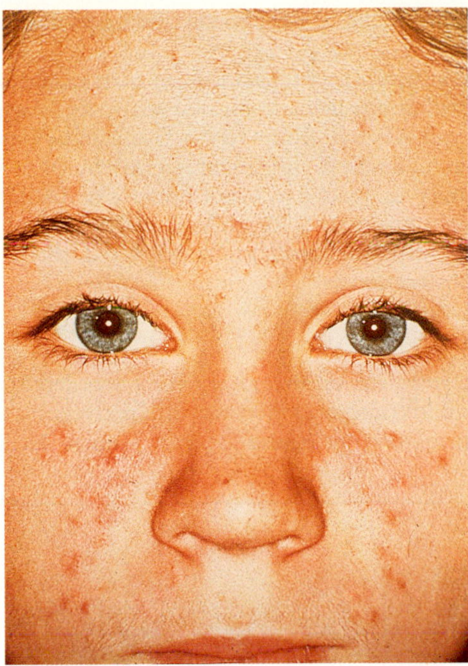

FIGURE 61-22 Acne (*From Acne Vulgaris, by G. Plewig and A. B. Klingman [Eds], 1975, Berlin/Heideberg, Germany; Springer-Verlag. Used with permission.*)

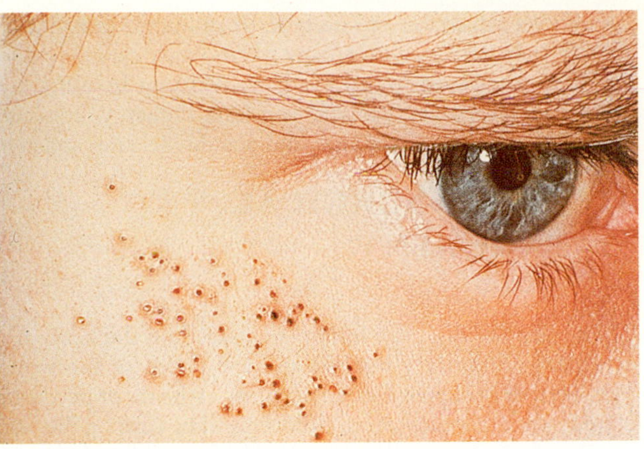

FIGURE 61-23 Open Comedones (*From Acne Vulgaris, by G. Plewig and A. B. Klingman [Eds], 1975, Berlin/Heideberg, Germany; Springer-Verlag. Used with permission.*)

influence on acne development are overproduction of sebum; formation of **comedones**, or whiteheads and blackheads (Figure 61-23); and proliferation of *Propionibacterium acnes* bacteria in the hair follicles.

Manifestations include comedones, papules, pustules, and nodules on the face, neck, back, shoulders, and upper chest. Factors related to the development of acne include elevated hormone levels (especially androgens); predisposition; emotional stress; hot, humid environments; the premenstrual period, in females; and the growth of anaerobic bacteria. The visual lesions of acne, although usually temporary, may be extremely distressing to the adolescent, who is typically very concerned about appearance.

MEDICAL–SURGICAL MANAGEMENT

Pharmacological

Treatment is individualized, depending on the severity and types of lesions. The goal is to decrease sebum production and prevent infection with *P. acnes*. Topical agents benzoyl peroxide (Clearasil, Benoxyl) and tretinoin (Retin-A) are available as cleansers, lotions, creams, sticks, pads, gels, and bars and may be effective for mild cases. Other topical keratolytic agents containing sulfur, resorcinol, or salicylic acid may be prescribed for drying and peeling effects. Topical or oral antibiotics, such as erythromycin and tetracycline preparations, may be administered for infections.

Isotretinoin (Accutane) may be used for nodulocystic acne. Side effects of isotretinoin include dry lips and skin, eye irritation, temporary worsening of acne, **epistaxis** (nosebleed), bleeding and inflammation of the gums, itching, photosensitivity, and joint and muscle pain. In addition, isotretinoin may cause central nervous system, heart, thymus, and craniofacial abnormalities in the fetus.

If isotretinoin is to be prescribed, pregnancy tests are done 2 weeks before initiating, every month during, and 1 month after discontinuing the treatment. All women of childbearing potential are placed on contraception during treatment.

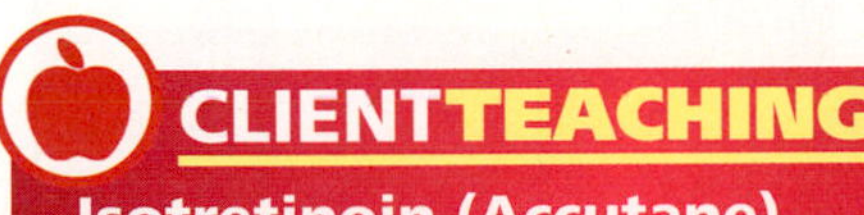

CLIENT TEACHING

Isotretinoin (Accutane)

It is important that adolescent females on isotretinoin who are sexually active use contraceptives 1 month before treatment is started; during treatment; and 1 month after discontinuation of treatment. In addition, children taking isotretinoin should not donate blood during this period.

NURSING MANAGEMENT

A healthy lifestyle, including adequate rest, exercise, and diet, promotes healing of lesions. Be especially sensitive to the adolescent's feelings about the condition, no matter how mild the case may seem.

Educate the adolescent and caregiver about acne and the prescribed treatment. Adolescents are encouraged to take responsibility for implementing the prescribed care.

BURNS

Burns are the second leading cause of injury deaths among children between 1 and 14 years of age (James, Ashwill, & Droske, 2002). Carelessness of adults, the children's curiosity and increasing mobility, and caretakers' failure to adequately supervise children all contribute to the high incidence of burns among children. In addition, burns are a common form of child abuse. Thermal burns (e.g., from scalding liquids, house fires) are most common, followed by chemical (e.g., from touching or ingesting caustic agents) and electrical (e.g., from wires, curling irons, ovens), respectively.

The major manifestations of burns include severe wounds, pain, fluid and nutritional deficits, respiratory complications, and secondary infections. All systems of the burned child are at risk for complications.

Smoke inhalation can be fatal. Toxic fumes from burning plastics, polyurethanes, and many fabrics cause cyanide poisoning. Carbon monoxide and cyanide inhalation have the same signs and symptoms: nausea, vomiting, lethargy, confusion, tachycardia, metabolic acidosis, and possibly seizures and coma.

Medical–Surgical Management

Medical

The severity of the burn injury is assessed on the basis of the percentage of surface burned and the depth of the wound. The Burn Wheel provides an accurate estimate of percentage of body surface area burn in children and by turning the wheel to align the correct values for weight and burns, it provides the amount of fluid resuscitation and continuation needed (Figure 61-24).

The involvement of specific body parts or certain specific burn distributions increase burn severity, regardless of body surface area affected. Burns to the face, hands, feet, perineal area, or anterior chest, and circumferential burns of the thorax or extremity are treated as major because of the potential for functional impairment. Regardless of the amount of tissue destroyed, if smoke inhalation is suspected, there is risk for airway obstruction.

Pharmacological

Tetanus antitoxin or toxoid should be ordered according to the child's immunization status. Intravenous morphine sulfate is the drug of choice for pain control. Analgesics are

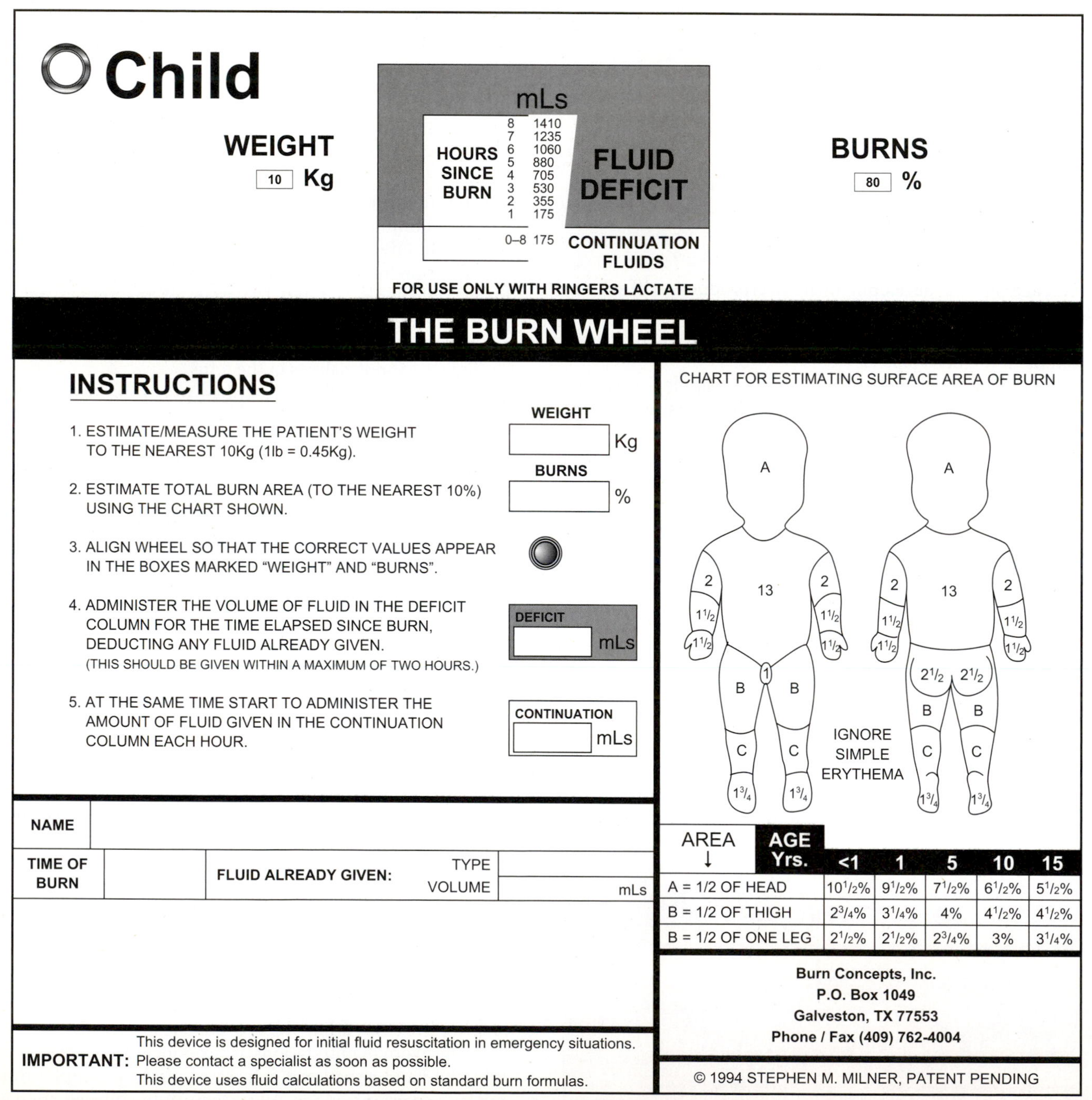

Child

WEIGHT 10 Kg

mLs

HOURS SINCE BURN

Hours	mLs
8	1410
7	1235
6	1060
5	880
4	705
3	530
2	355
1	175
0–8	175

FLUID DEFICIT

CONTINUATION FLUIDS

FOR USE ONLY WITH RINGERS LACTATE

BURNS 80 %

THE BURN WHEEL

INSTRUCTIONS

1. ESTIMATE/MEASURE THE PATIENT'S WEIGHT TO THE NEAREST 10Kg (1lb = 0.45Kg).
2. ESTIMATE TOTAL BURN AREA (TO THE NEAREST 10%) USING THE CHART SHOWN.
3. ALIGN WHEEL SO THAT THE CORRECT VALUES APPEAR IN THE BOXES MARKED "WEIGHT" AND "BURNS".
4. ADMINISTER THE VOLUME OF FLUID IN THE DEFICIT COLUMN FOR THE TIME ELAPSED SINCE BURN, DEDUCTING ANY FLUID ALREADY GIVEN. (THIS SHOULD BE GIVEN WITHIN A MAXIMUM OF TWO HOURS.)
5. AT THE SAME TIME START TO ADMINISTER THE AMOUNT OF FLUID GIVEN IN THE CONTINUATION COLUMN EACH HOUR.

WEIGHT Kg

BURNS %

DEFICIT mLs

CONTINUATION mLs

NAME

TIME OF BURN

FLUID ALREADY GIVEN: TYPE VOLUME mLs

IMPORTANT: This device is designed for initial fluid resuscitation in emergency situations. Please contact a specialist as soon as possible. This device uses fluid calculations based on standard burn formulas.

CHART FOR ESTIMATING SURFACE AREA OF BURN

AREA ↓ / AGE Yrs.	<1	1	5	10	15
A = 1/2 OF HEAD	$10^1/_2$%	$9^1/_2$%	$7^1/_2$%	$6^1/_2$%	$5^1/_2$%
B = 1/2 OF THIGH	$2^3/_4$%	$3^1/_4$%	4%	$4^1/_2$%	$4^1/_2$%
B = 1/2 OF ONE LEG	$2^1/_2$%	$2^1/_2$%	$2^3/_4$%	3%	$3^1/_4$%

Burn Concepts, Inc.
P.O. Box 1049
Galveston, TX 77553
Phone / Fax (409) 762-4004

© 1994 STEPHEN M. MILNER, PATENT PENDING

FIGURE 61-24 The Burn Wheel (invented by Stephen M. Milner)

administered 20 to 30 minutes before dressing changes and debridement to provide the most relief possible. Itching may persist for months and may be relieved with medication.

Health Promotion

Prevention of scarring and contractures is essential for optimal cosmetic and functional recovery. Pressure dressings and suits may need to be worn for more than 1 year to minimize scarring. Physical therapy, initiated at the time of admission and continued until the scars mature, prevents flexion contractures. These treatments add to the child's discomfort.

Nursing Management

Refer to the Integumentary System chapter for information on nursing management of the child who has been burned.

URINARY SYSTEM

Acute poststreptococcal glomerulonephritis, nephrotic syndrome, and enuresis are discussed in the following sections.

ACUTE POSTSTREPTOCOCCAL GLOMERULONEPHRITIS

Glomerulonephritis is an inflammation of the glomeruli of the kidneys. Acute poststreptococcal glomerulonephritis (APSGN) occurs as an immune reaction to streptococcal infection of the throat or skin.

Clinical manifestations of hematuria and periorbital edema usually appear 1 to 3 weeks after a streptococcal infection. Other possible manifestations include decreased urine output, hypertension, fever, and fatigue. The prognosis is excellent.

Medical–Surgical Management

Medical

The diagnosis of APSGN can be made based on history, presenting symptoms, and laboratory results. There is no treatment for APSGN. Medical management focuses on presenting signs and symptoms and the degree of renal dysfunction. Laboratory values usually return to normal within 6 to 12 weeks.

Pharmacological

Hypertension may be treated by limiting sodium and water intake or by administering diuretics or antihypertensives.

Nursing Management

Refer to the Urinary System chapter for information on nursing management of the child with APSGN.

NEPHROTIC SYNDROME

Nephrotic syndrome refers to kidney disorders characterized by proteinuria, hypoalbuminemia, and edema. The most common childhood nephrotic disorder, minimal change nephrotic syndrome (MCNS), results from minimal alterations of the glomerulus. The cause of the alteration is unknown.

Clinical manifestations include pitting edema (periorbital and dependent), anorexia, fatigue, abdominal pain, increased weight, and normal blood pressure. Potential complications include respiratory compromise and peritonitis. Although the child may experience remissions and exacerbations for months, the prognosis in most cases is good.

Medical–Surgical Management

Medical

Diagnosis is made based on clinical presentation, age of the child, massive proteinuria (50 mg/kg/day), and hypoalbuminemia (<27g/L).

Surgical

A kidney biopsy may be done if a lesion other than MCNS is suspected or the child does not respond as expected to pharmacological treatments.

Pharmacological

The use of corticosteroids such as prednisone (Cortan, Deltasone) induces remission in most cases. Corticosteroid therapy usually produces diuresis within 7 to 14 days. After diuresis occurs, prednisone is continued every other day for 3 days per week. Urine is tested daily for protein until protein has been absent from the urine for up to 7 days. The drug dosage is then gradually decreased and discontinued over a 4-week period. Repeat corticosteroid therapy is administered to children who have relapses after drug therapy is discontinued.

Alkylating agents such as cyclophosphamide (Cytoxan) may be used to reduce symptoms and prevent further relapses in children who do not respond adequately to repeated corticosteroid therapy. The risks and benefits of this therapy must be carefully considered.

When the child is in remission, administration of vaccines for pneumococci and flu should be considered because an exacerbation of nephrotic syndrome can occur following an infection.

Diet

A general "no-added-salt" diet is recommended. Offer appealing, small, frequent meals to the child, who typically has a poor appetite.

Nursing Management

Educate the child's caregivers about the disease process. Monitor I&O hourly. Weigh the child daily. Measure abdominal girth and test urine albumin daily. Keep skin clean and dry. Inspect for skin breakdown and turn child every 2 hours. Screen visitors for signs of infection. Follow Standard Precautions carefully.

NURSING PROCESS

Assessment

Subjective Data

Question the caregiver about symptom onset, appetite, urine output, irritability, and signs of fatigue.

Objective Data

Assess daily weight, abdominal girth, vital signs, and skin for pallor, irritation, breakdown, and edema.

Nursing diagnoses for the child with MCNS include the following:

NURSING DIAGNOSES	PLANNING/OUTCOMES	NURSING INTERVENTIONS
*Excess **F**luid Volume* related to compromised regulatory mechanism	The child will maintain fluid balance.	Monitor I&O hourly; report urinary output of <2 mL/kg/hr. Weigh daily. Measure abdominal girth daily at the level of the umbilicus. Test urine albumin daily with reagent strips.
*Risk for Impaired **S**kin Integrity* related to altered circulation	The child's skin will remain intact.	Inspect the child's skin for breakdown. Turn and reposition the child every 2 hours. Keep the child's skin clean and dry. Use a protective mattress (e.g., eggcrate).
*Risk for **I**nfection* related to immunosuppression	The child will remain infection free.	Screen visitors for signs of infection. Practice proper hand hygiene technique. Monitor the child for signs of infection, such as sore throat, cough, fever, abdominal pain. Monitor laboratory values daily.
*Deficient **K**nowledge (parent)* related to treatment regimen	The caregiver will follow through with the prescribed treatment.	Educate the caregivers about the disease process. Instruct the caregivers to test urine for albumin, assess for edema and infection, and administer drugs. Instruct the caregiver to allow a return to ADLs once the child is free of edema.

Evaluation: Evaluate each outcome to determine how it has been met by the client.

ENURESIS

Enuresis is involuntary urination beyond the age when control of urination commonly is acquired. It is not unusual for nocturnal enuresis, or bedwetting, to occur until 8 years of age, because of small bladder capacity and delayed maturation of the neuromuscular system. Most children will outgrow bedwetting without therapeutic intervention.

When enuresis continues to occur beyond the eighth year or recurs in a child who has been dry both day and night for a prolonged period, there may be cause for concern. Possible causes of reoccurring enuresis include urinary tract infections, minor abnormalities of the urinary tract, pinworm infestation, constipation, diabetes, sickle-cell anemia, sexual abuse, stress, and sleep disorders.

Medical–Surgical Management

Medical

Urinalysis and urine culture are done to rule out infection. Other diagnostic studies are performed to rule out all possible causes. Common treatment approaches for enuresis without a physiologic cause include fluid restriction, bladder stretching exercises, behavioral conditioning (e.g., enuresis alarm), and reward systems.

Pharmacological

An anticholinergic such as oxybutynin chloride (Ditropan) may reduce uninhibited bladder contractions. Vasopressins such as desmopressin acetate (DDAVP) nasal spray may reduce nighttime urine output. Antidepressants such as imipramine hydrochloride (Tofranil) may be prescribed.

Other Therapies

If emotional factors are precipitating enuresis, psychosocial support may be an essential part of care. A multidisciplinary team approach is most effective.

PROFESSIONALTIP

Enuresis

It is most important to provide the caregiver and the child with opportunities to ventilate feelings. The caregiver and the child must be active and willing participants in any plan of care that is implemented. Tell caregivers that reprimanding the child will not improve the outcome.

PSYCHOSOCIAL DISORDERS

Psychosocial disorders are responses to stressors. Factors influencing an individual's response to stressors include temperament, developmental level, nature and duration of the stressors, past experiences, and coping and adaptive abilities of the family. Possible manifestations in children include depression, anxiety, encopresis, enuresis, passive–aggressive behavior, and learning problems (James, et al., 2002). Some of the psychosocial disorders of childhood include obesity, anorexia nervosa and bulimia nervosa, autism, attention deficit hyperactivity disorder, and suicide.

OBESITY

Obesity is the excessive accumulation of fat resulting in an increase in body weight to 20% or more above ideal weight. Obesity can be a precursor of cardiovascular disease, hypertension, and diabetes. Factors contributing to obesity include an overconsumption of food; a sedentary lifestyle; a lack of caregiver knowledge regarding nutrition and food preparation; unstructured meals; genetic predisposition; and peer pressure.

CLIENT TEACHING

Caring for the Child Who Is Obese

Share the following ideas with caregivers of obese children.

Nutrition

- Keep a food diary for 1 week; include time, place, type, and amount of food eaten, and the reasons for eating.
- Set a reasonable weight-loss or weight-maintenance goal.
- Establish and maintain regular mealtimes.
- Serve meals at the table only, preferably with the family.
- Serve meals on a small plate in an effort to decrease quantity of food consumed.
- Encourage the child to eat slowly.
- Keep low-calorie snacks on hand.

Exercise

- Get the child involved in regular outside activities.
- Walk instead of ride whenever possible.

Self-Esteem

- Weight the child only one time per week.
- Focus on the child's positive assets.
- Provide positive feedback for positive behavior.

Support

- Establish a group or buddy system.
- Participate in a support group.

The obese child may overeat to compensate for lack of parenteral love and to relieve stress. As a result of obesity, the child may have low self-esteem, poor body image, difficulty in relationships, and recurring bouts of anxiety and depression.

MEDICAL–SURGICAL MANAGEMENT

Medical

Obesity is difficult to treat. Positive outcomes are more likely when the child has a support system, understands the importance of weight reduction, and is actively involved in the plan of care.

Diet

Meals and snacks should consist of small servings of nutritional foods. Teach the caregiver and child ways to select and prepare foods. Incorporate favorite foods into the menu whenever possible.

Activity

Incorporate physical exercise into the child's daily routine.

NURSING MANAGEMENT

Focus on meeting nutritional needs, managing related problems, and promoting self-esteem. Assess weight, exercise, and nutritional intake at predetermined intervals. Provide positive feedback for accomplishments, no matter how small. Discuss and revise goals as needed.

Support groups such as Weight Watchers and Overeaters Anonymous may be helpful. In addition, support groups may be available through schools, summer camps, or children's hospitals. A team approach utilizing a psychiatrist or psychologist, a nutritionist, and a nurse may be appropriate.

ANOREXIA NERVOSA AND BULIMIA NERVOSA

Anorexia nervosa (AN) and bulimia nervosa (BN) are two of the most common eating disorders among children. AN is self-inflicted starvation; BN is binge-eating followed by purging. These disorders usually begin in middle to late adolescence and can last indefinitely, depending on response to treatment. The incidence is highest among Caucasian girls in the higher socioecomonic classes (Hockenberry et al., 2008). Possible causes of these disorders include sensitivity to social pressure for thinness; distorted body image; and longstanding dysfunctional family patterns.

Clinical manifestations include body weight 15% below that expected for age and height, intense fear of gaining weight, dry skin, brittle nails, downy hair on the back and extremities, amenorrhea, constipation, hypothermia, bradycardia, low blood pressure, fluid and electrolyte imbalances, and anemia. Depression, crying spells, feelings of isolation and loneliness, and suicidal thoughts and feelings are common. Clues to frequent vomiting include dental caries, tooth enamel erosion, and throat irritation. Calluses or abrasions may be noted on the back of the hands, from frequent contact with the teeth while inducing vomiting.

Medical–Surgical Management

Medical

The goal of medical treatment is to correct malnutrition and resulting complications. A weight gain of 0.1 to 0.2 kg per day is emphasized until the desired weight is attained. Enteral feedings or total parenteral nutrition (TPN) may be necessary to replace lost fluids, protein, and nutrients.

Pharmacological

Selective serotonin reuptake inhibitors (SSRIs), such as citalopram (Celexa), escitalopram (Lexapro), fluoxetine (Prozac), an sertraline (Zoloft), may decrease binge eating and treat depression (Potts and Mandleco, 2007). SSRIs are also affective with AN.

Other Therapies

Individual and family therapy are used to address dysfunctional family patterns and assist the adolescent in identifying and dealing with self-esteem and body image issues. Treatment is typically long-term.

Nursing Management

Refer to the Mental Illness chapter for possible nursing diagnoses for the client with AN or BN and to the Resources listing at the end of this chapter.

AUTISM

Autism is a complex disorder of brain function involving abnormal emotional, social, and linguistic development. The cause of autism is unknown; however, research suggests it may result from a disturbance in language comprehension, a biochemical problem involving neurotransmitters, or abnormalities in the central nervous system.

Possible clinical manifestations include lack of eye contact, aversion to touch, delayed language development, blank expression, lack of response to verbal stimulation, repetitive behaviors, bizarre body movements, and self-destructive behaviors. Manifestations may vary from mild to severe. The prognosis depends on early detection and the child's response to treatment.

Medical–Surgical Management

Medical

Diagnosis is based on the presence of specific criteria as listed in *the Diagnostic and Statistical Manual of Mental Disorders,* fourth edition (DSM-IV) (American Psychiatric Association, 1994). In addition, a complete physical and neurological examination is necessary to rule out other disorders such as lead poisoning, phenylketonuria, congenital rubella, and measles encephalitis.

Treatment is provided by a multidisciplinary team and focuses on promoting normal development, social interaction, and learning. Behavior-modification techniques are used to reward desirable behaviors and foster positive coping skills.

> **CLIENT TEACHING**
>
> **Modifying Behavior in the Child Who is Autistic**
>
> - Emphasize the child's positive skills.
> - Provide immediate feedback for appropriate behavior.
> - Continue social interactions even when the child is unresponsive.
> - Provide tactile stimulation such as tickling, holding, cuddling, and shaking hands.
> - Teach the child to embrace, kiss, and shake hands.
> - Speak in short sentences.
> - Use a firm but caring approach.
> - Maintain daily routines.

Nursing Management

Focus on early detection, decreasing environmental stimuli, providing supportive care, maintaining a safe environment, and giving caregivers anticipatory guidance. Monitor growth and development, especially language and social skills. When caring for a child with autism, ascertain the child's routines, rituals, and likes and dislikes. Because autistic children do not do well in unfamiliar environments, it is important that they be surrounded by familiar objects. The child may need assistance with self-care. Keep schedules and care providers as consistent as possible. Close supervision is usually required at all times.

Caregivers need a great deal of support to cope with the challenges of having an autistic child. Assist children to reach their maximum potential through enrollment in special education programs and participation in behavior modification. Some children may achieve independence by adulthood. Inform caregivers about local support groups and refer to the Autism Society of America for current information.

ATTENTION DEFICIT HYPERACTIVITY DISORDER

Attention-deficit hyperactivity disorder (ADHD) is a developmental disorder characterized by developmentally inappropriate degrees of inattention, overactivity, and impulsivity. The child is usually diagnosed between the ages of 3 and 6 years. Possible clinical manifestations include poor impulse control, distractibility, fidgeting with hands, squirming in seat, excessive talking, and difficulty following instructions.

Medical–Surgical Management

Medical

Diagnosis may be made based on diagnostic criteria in the *DSM-IV* (American Psychiatric Association, 1994) as well as a complete multidisciplinary evaluation. Treatment focuses on decreasing distractions, modifying behavior (e.g., setting

CLIENT TEACHING

Caring for the Child with ADHD

- Praise positive behavior and set limits.
- Administer medication as prescribed and with meals.
- Give clear, simple instructions and provide frequent reminders to follow instructions.
- Reduce stimuli in the child's environment (e.g., turning off the TV when the child is trying to do homework).
- Allow for a shortened attention span by providing short teaching sessions and activities that allow for mobility.
- Consult with trained professional for behavior-modification therapy.

limits, ensuring consistency, praising accomplishments), and/or initiating pharmacological therapy.

Pharmacological

The most commonly prescribed medications include methylphenidate (Ritalin), pemoline (Cylert), and dextroamphetamine (Dexedrine). These drugs stimulate the area of the child's brain that facilitates concentration. Potential side effects include loss of appetite resulting in delayed growth.

Nursing Management

Focus on improving the child's social interaction and educating the family/caregivers and teachers.

SUICIDE

Suicide is the third-leading cause of death among adolescents. Boys complete suicide four times more often than do girls, but girls attempt suicide five times more often than do boys. Males tend to use lethal methods such as guns, hanging, and jumping from high elevations, whereas girls more often overdose or cut the wrists. Adolescents who have attempted suicide once are at greatest risk for attempting again. Attempted suicide rarely occurs without warning (Centers for Disease Control and Prevention, 1997a).

Clinical manifestations in the suicidal adolescent may include depression, boredom, restlessness, concentration problems, irritability, lethargy, and intentional misbehavior. Children at high risk for committing suicide may be experiencing depression, pregnancy, failure in school, drug use, death of a friend or caregiver, problems with a relationship, sexual abuse, chronic illness, or a broken home.

Medical–Surgical Management

Medical

The child thought to be at high risk for suicide is usually admitted to a psychiatric unit for care. Treatment may include individual, group, and/or family therapy. Negotiating a "No-Suicide" contract is one method that may be used with a suicidal child. In this written and signed contract, the child agrees not to attempt suicide for a negotiated period (e.g., weeks, days, minutes). If at any time the child feels unable to keep the contract, the child agrees to contact help. Children with severe self-abusive behavior may need to be physically or chemically restrained.

Pharmacological

Drugs that may be used for chemical restraint include diphenhydramine hydrochloride (Benadryl), thioridazine hydrochloride (Mellaril), chlorpromazine (Thorazine), and lorazepam (Ativan). The suicidal child may also require antidepressant and/or antipsychotic medications.

Nursing Management

Assess risk factors, behaviors, attitude, how lethal is the proposed method of suicide, coping mechanisms, and support system. Be nonjudgmental and show empathy. Remove potentially harmful objects from the environment. Monitor the high-risk child at all times. Administer medications as prescribed. Encourage individual and group therapy for the entire family and keeping all follow-up appointments.

NURSING PROCESS

Assessment

Subjective Data

Assess the suicidal child for behaviors, attitudes, risk factors, lethality of the proposed method of suicide, coping mechanisms, and support systems.

Objective Data

Observe the child for signs of physical and sexual abuse, self-destructive behaviors, and sudden changes in behavior.

Nursing diagnoses for the child who is suicidal include the following:

NURSING DIAGNOSES	PLANNING/OUTCOMES	NURSING INTERVENTIONS
Risk for Self-directed Violence related to desire to ease emotional pain, solicit attention of others, or avoid responsibility	The child will be less likely to repeat the suicide attempt.	Use a nonjudgmental, empathic approach and a voice and demeanor that are clear, direct, and supportive to discuss feelings and the suicidal event. Remove potentially harmful objects from the environment (e.g., belts, scarves, shoestrings, matches, lighters).

(*Continues*)

Nursing diagnoses for the child who is suicidal include the following: (Continued)

NURSING DIAGNOSES	PLANNING/OUTCOMES	NURSING INTERVENTIONS
		Monitor the high-risk child at all times, even during bathroom use and sleep. Administer prescribed medications. Suggest alternate activities for those times when impulsive behavior occurs. Restrain the child (as ordered) as an act of care, not punishment.
*Interrupted **F**amily Processes* related to relational disturbance or abuse/neglect	The child will feel safe and receive support from others to meet needs.	Encourage individual and group therapy for the entire family to explore personal issues and the need for social support. Assist the caregivers to regain the ability to assist the child and manage the home environment. Foster caregiver–child interaction. Teach the caregivers to monitor the child for sudden changes in behavior. Teach the caregivers and child about medication administration. Encourage the caregivers to keep follow-up appointments.

Evaluation: Evaluate each outcome to determine how it has been met by the client.

CASE STUDY

C.P. is a 14-year-old male. He was diagnosed with DMD at 5 years of age. His older brother also had DMD and died 2 years ago at the age of 16. C.P. lives with his parents and 10-year-old sister, L.P. Associated problems include confinement to a wheelchair; contractures of the hips, knees, and ankles; scoliosis requiring a brace; frequent respiratory infections; and obesity. C.P. attends the ninth grade, is a member of the chess club, and enjoys the youth group at his church.

The following questions will guide your development of a nursing care plan for the case study.

1. List the characteristic progression of DMD.
2. Cite three nursing diagnoses and goals for C.P.
3. Identify interventions to help C.P. and his family address the nursing diagnoses identified in question 2.
4. How might genetic counseling benefit this family?
5. Identify resources available to help C.P. and his family cope with DMD.

SUMMARY

- The most common skin disorders among toddlers and preschoolers are impetigo and dog bites.
- The most common skin disorders among school-age children are pediculosis and scabies.
- The most common skin disorder among adolescents is acne.
- Common respiratory tract infections of childhood include nasopharyngitis, pharyngitis, and influenza.
- Asthma is the leading cause of chronic illness among children.
- Treatment of asthma involves allergen control, drug therapy, controlled exercise, physical therapy, and desensitization.
- Prevention or treatment of group A streptococcal infection in turn prevents rheumatic fever.
- Nursing care of the child with leukemia focuses on preparing the child and family for diagnostic and therapeutic procedures, preventing complications of myelosuppression, managing problems of drug toxicity, and providing emotional support.
- Caregivers of a child with ITP must be able to detect signs of bleeding and know ways to prevent injuries.
- Constipation can be prevented by establishing and maintaining regular toileting habits, drinking fluids, eating a diet high in fiber, and participating in regular exercise.

- Children are more commonly infected with intestinal parasites than are adults because they put their fingers in their mouths more often.
- Obesity can be a precursor to cardiovascular disease, hypertension, and diabetes.
- Acute poststreptococcal glomerulonephritis occurs as an immune reaction to streptococcal infection of the throat or skin.
- Goals for the child with nephrotic syndrome include fluid balance, intact skin, freedom from infection, and compliance with urine testing and drug therapy.
- Goals for children with structural anomalies, such as scoliosis, Legg-Calvé-Perthes disease, and injuries, includes preventing skin breakdown (due to casts and braces) and keeping follow-up appointments.
- Nursing care for the child with DMD focuses on maintaining physical activity, promoting respiratory function, managing weight, and encouraging age-appropriate social activities.
- Nursing care for the child with juvenile rheumatoid arthritis focuses on preventing injury, controlling pain, enhancing mobility, and encouraging age-appropriate activities.
- Nursing goals for the autistic child may include decreasing environmental stimuli, providing supportive care, maintaining a safe environment, and giving caregivers anticipatory guidance.
- Treatment for the child with ADHD focuses on decreasing distractions, modifying behavior, and initiating drug therapy.
- Suicide is the third leading cause of death among adolescents.
- Child abuse can be classified as physical abuse, physical neglect, emotional abuse, or sexual abuse.

REVIEW QUESTIONS

1. Determining the causative agent and administering the proper treatment for skin and throat infections may prevent further complications such as:
   1. leukemia.
   2. mononucleosis.
   3. idiopathic thrombocytopenia purpura.
   4. acute post-streptococcal glomerulonephritis.

2. Children with leukemia are at high risk for infection because of:
   1. decreased lymphocytes.
   2. increased red blood cells.
   3. decreased platelets.
   4. decreased neutrophils.

3. Nursing diagnoses for the child with nephrotic syndrome may include:
   1. *Excess **F**luid Volume* related to fluid retention.
   2. ***P**ain* related to operative procedure.
   3. *Impaired Physical **M**obility* related to use of a brace.
   4. *Disturbed **B**ody Image* related to loss of hair.

4. A clinical manifestation of scoliosis is:
   1. lateral curvature of the spine.
   2. necrosis of the femoral head.
   3. quadriceps muscle atrophy.
   4. Gower's sign.

5. Treatment for the child with ADHD includes:
   1. decreasing distractions.
   2. placing in special education class.
   3. prescribing sedatives.
   4. eating a special diet.

6. The pediatric client is experiencing constipation. This condition occurs most frequently in which of the following ages:
   1. toddler and infants.
   2. pre-school and school-aged.
   3. toddler and school-aged.
   4. toddler and pre-school.

7. The nurse educates the caregiver and child regarding juvenile arthritis. Which statement by the caregivers indicates the need for more education?
   1. It is an autoimmune disorder.
   2. There are only two different forms.
   3. Complications can include blindness.
   4. With early treatment, prognosis is good.

8. A client is experiencing pediculosis. The student nurse knows that this is a condition that requires: (Select all that apply.)
   1. standard precautions when screening.
   2. checking for infestation during daily hygiene.
   3. close-contact situations for lice to be passed from person to person.
   4. cutting long hair to prevent further infestation.
   5. the use of lice sprays on a child's bedding.
   6. the use of lindane (Kwell) for lice removal.

9. The pediatric client who is experiencing burns is at risk for which of the following severe complications: (Select all that apply.)
   1. respiratory complications.
   2. fluid and electrolyte imbalances.
   3. cyanide poisoning.
   4. immobility.
   5. functional impairment.
   6. scarring and contractures.

10. The nurse is caring for a pediatric client who is at risk for suicide. Manifestations include all of the following except:
   1. depression and restlessness.
   2. empathy and boredom.
   3. intentional misbehavior and irritability.
   4. difficulty concentrating and lethargy.

REFERENCES/SUGGESTED READINGS

American Family Physician (AAFP). (2002). Tick removal. Retrieved October 28-2009 from http://www.aafp.org/afp/20020815/643.html

American Psychiatric Association. (2004). *Diagnostic and statistical manual of mental disorders* (6th ed.). Washington, DC: Author.

American Diabetes Association (ADA). (2006). Type 2 diabetes in children and adolescents. *Diabetes Care, 22*(12), 381. Also available at http://www.diabetes.org/ada/Consensus/.

Belson, M., Kingsley, B., & Holmes, A. (2007, January). Risk factors for acute leukemia in children: A review. *Environmental Health Perspectives, 115*(1), 138–145.

Boychuk, R., DeMesa, C., Kiyabu, K., Yamamoto, F., Yamamoto, L., Sanderson, R., et al. (2006). Change in approach and delivery of medical care in children with asthma: Results from a multicenter emergency department educational asthma management program. *Pediatrics, 117*, 145–151.

Bulechek, G., Butcher, H., McCloskey, J., & Dochterman, J., eds. (2008). *Nursing Interventions Classification (NIC)* (5th ed.). St. Louis, MO: Mosby/Elsevier.

Centers for Disease Control and Prevention. (2004a). Status report on the childhood immunization initiative; National, state, and urban area vaccination coverage levels among children aged 19–35 months—United States, 1996. *MMWR, 46*(29), 657–664.

Centers for Disease Control and Prevention. (2004b). Rates of homicide, suicide, and firearm-related death among children—26 industrialized countries. *MMWR, 46*(5), 101–105.

Centers for Disease Control and Prevention. (2006). Update: Vaccine side effects, adverse reactions, contraindications and precautions: Recommendations of the Advisory Committee on Immunization Practices (ACIP). *MMWR, 45*(RR-12), 1–35.

Centers for Disease Control and Prevention. (2008). General recommendations on immunization: Recommendations of the Advisory Committee on Immunization Practices (ACIP), *MMWR, 43*(RR-1), 1–38.

Croom, K., & McCormack, P. (2008, March). Recombinant factor VIIa (Eptacog Alfa): A review of its use in congenital hemophilia with inhibitors, acquired hemophilia, and other congenital bleeding disorders. *BioDrugs, 22*(2), 121.

Eisenhauer, L., Nichols, L., Spencer, R., & Bergan, F. (1998). *Clinical pharmacology & nursing management* (5th ed.). Philadelphia: Lippincott Williams & Wilkins.

Elbein, S., Das, S., Hallman, D., Hanis, C., & Hasstedt, S. (2009, January). Genome-wide linkage and admixture mapping of type 2 diabetes in African American families from the American Diabetes Association GENNID (Genetics of NIDDM) Study Cohort. *Diabetes, 58*(1), 268–267.

Estes, M. (2010). *Health assessment & physical examination* (4th ed.). Clifton Park, NY: Delmar Cengage Learning.

Gradoni, G., & Gradoni, P. (2009, August). Role of an anti-acetonemic diet in reducing the need for tonsillectomy in children with recurrent tonsillitis. *Auris Nasus Larynx, 36*(4), 438–443.

Hayes, L. (2000). Poison emergency? *Nursing2000, 30*(9), 34–39.

Healthy People 2010. (2000). Objectives. Available from http://www.healthypeople.gov/document/html/objectives/14-22.htm.

Herrin, J., & Antoon, A. (2000). Burn injuries. In R. M. Kliegman, S. Jenson, & R. Behrman (Eds.), *Nelson textbook of pediatrics* (16th ed.). Philadelphia: W. B. Saunders.

Hockenberry, M., & Wilson, D. (2008). *Wong's Essentials of Pediatric Care* (8th ed.). St. Louis, MO: Mosby

James, S., Ashwill, J., & Droske, S. (2002). *Nursing care of children: Principles and practice* (2nd ed.). Philadelphia: W. B. Saunders.

Kamienski, M. (2003). Reye syndrome. *AJN, 103*(7), 54–57.

Kliegman, R., Jensen, H., & Behrman, R. (2000). *Nelson's textbook of pediatrics* (16th ed.). Philadelphia: W. B. Saunders.

Kunkel, L., Bachrach, E., Bennett, R., Guyon, J., & Steffen, L. (2006, May). Diagnosis and cell-based therapy for Duchenne muscular dystrophy in humans, mice, and zebrafish. *Journal of Human Genetics, 51*(5), 397–406.

Leifer, G. (2006). *Introduction to Maternity and Pediatric Nursing* (5th ed.). Philadelphia: W.B. Saunders.

Lenhardt, R., Catrambone, C., McDermott, M., Walter, J., Williams, S., & Weiss, K. (2006). Improving pediatric asthma care through surveillance: The Illinois emergency department asthma collaborative. *Pediatrics, 117*, 96–105.

Marks, M. (1998). *Broadribb's introductory pediatric nursing* (5th ed.). Philadelphia: J.B. Lippincott Williams & Wilkins.

Moorhead, S., Johnson, M., Maas, M., & Swanson, E. (2007). *Nursing Outcomes Classification (NOC)* (4th ed.). St. Louis, MO: Mosby.

National Pediculosis Association,® Inc. (2009a) Set the standard. Retrieved October 28, 2009 from http://www.headlice.org/special/doit4 the kids.htm.

National Pediculosis Association,® Inc. (2009b) *The NPA's ten tips for head lice and nit removal.* Retrieved October 28, 2009 from http://www.headlice.org/downloads/tipsremoval.htm.

National Pediculosis Association,® Inc. (2009c) *Treating head lice without toxins.* Retrieved October 28, 2009 from http://www.headlice.org/news/2004/withouttoxins.htm.

Nemours. (2002). School backpacks: How they affect your child's general health. Available from http://www.nemours.org/no/news/releases/2002/020206_backpack_study.html.

North American Nursing Diagnosis Association International. (2010). *NANDA-I nursing diagnoses: Definitions and classification 2009–2011.* Ames, IA: Wiley-Blackwell.

Potts, N., & Mandleco, B. (2007). *Pediatric Nursing: Caring for children and their families* (2nd ed.). Clifton Park, NY: Delmar Cengage Learning.

Ruiz, E. (2001). Type 2 disease in children. *RN, 64*(10), 44–48.

Schultz, T. (2000). Airing differences in pediatric nebulizer therapy. *Nursing2000, 30*(9), 55–57.

Siwula, C. (2003). Managing pediatric emergencies. *Nursing2003, 33*(2), 48–51.

Spratto, G. and Woods, A. (2008). 2009 edition Delmar's nurses drug handbook. Clifton Park, NY: Delmar Cengage Learning.

Thompson, S. (2003). When kids get cancer. *RN, 66*(7), 29–33.

Timby, B., & Harrison, L. (2005). *Fundamental skills and concepts in patient care* (8th ed.). Philadelphia: Lippincott.

VanBoxel, A., & Puhl, P. (2001). Pediatric emergency: Assessing gut pain. *RN, 64*(4), 38–42.

Wong, D., Hockenberry-Eaton, M. (2001). *Wong's essentials of pediatric nursing* (6th ed.). St. Louis, MO: Mosby.

RESOURCES

American Academy of Pediatrics (AAP), http://www.aap.org

American Diabetes Association (ADA), http://www.diabetes.org

Autism Society of America (ASA), http://www.autism-society.org

Centers for Disease Control and Prevention, http://www.cdc.gov

Children with Diabetes, http://www.castleweb.com

Muscular Dystrophy Association of America, http://www.mdausa.org

National Association of Anorexia Nervosa and Associated Disorders, http://www.anad.org

National Association of Pediatric Nurses Associates and Practitioners (NAPNAP), http://www.napnap.org

National Eating Disorders Association, http://www.nationaleatingdisorders.org

National Hemophilia Foundation, http://www.hemophilia.org

The National Pediculosis Association, http://www.headlice.org

National Scoliosis Foundation, Inc., http://www.stepstn.com

Nemours Foundation, http://www.nemours.org

Scoliosis Association, Inc., http://www.scoliosis-assoc.org

APPENDIX A
NANDA-I Nursing Diagnoses 2009–2011

Domain 1

Health Promotion

Ineffective **Health** Maintenance

Ineffective Self **Health** Management

Impaired **Home** Maintenance

Readiness for Enhanced **Immunization** Status

Self **Neglect**

Readiness for Enhanced **Nutrition**

Ineffective Family **Therapeutic** Regimen Management

Readiness for Enhanced **Self Health** Management

Domain 2

Nutrition

Ineffective Infant **Feeding** Pattern

Imbalanced **Nutrition**: Less Than Body Requirements

Imbalanced **Nutrition**: More Than Body Requirements

Risk for Imbalanced **Nutrition**: More Than Body Requirements

Impaired **Swallowing**

Risk for Unstable Blood **Glucose** Level

Neonatal **Jaundice**

Risk for Impaired **Liver** Function

Risk for **Electrolyte** Imbalance

Readiness for Enhanced **Fluid** Balance

Deficient **Fluid** Volume

Excess **Fluid** Volume

Risk for Deficient **Fluid** Volume

Risk for Imbalanced **Fluid** Volume

Domain 3

Elimination and Exchange

Functional Urinary **Incontinence**

Overflow Urinary **Incontinence**

Reflex Urinary **Incontinence**

Stress Urinary **Incontinence**

Urge Urinary **Incontinence**

Risk for Urge urinary **Incontinence**

Impaired **Urinary** Elimination

Readiness for Enhanced **Urinary** Elimination

Urinary Retention

Bowel Incontinence

Constipation

Perceived **Constipation**

Risk for **Constipation**

Diarrhea

Dysfunctional Gastrointenstinal **Motility**

Risk for Dysfunctional Gastrointestinal **Motility**

Impaired **Gas** Exchange

Domain 4

Activity Rest

Insomnia

Disturbed **Sleep** Pattern

Sleep Deprivation

Readiness for Enhanced **Sleep**

Risk for **Disuse** Syndrome

Deficient **Diversional** Activity

Sedentary **Lifestyle**

Impaired Bed **Mobility**

Impaired Physical **Mobility**

Impaired Wheelchair **Mobility**

Delayed **Surgical** Recovery

Impaired **Transfer** Ability

Impaired **Walking**

Disturbed **Energy** Field

Fatigue

Activity Intolerance

Risk for **Activity** Intolerance

Risk for **Bleeding**

Ineffective **Breathing** Pattern

Decreased **Cardiac** Output

Ineffective Peripheral Tissue **Perfusion**

Risk for Decreased Cardiac Tissue **Perfusion**

Risk for Ineffective Cerebral Tissue **Perfusion**

Risk for Ineffective Gastrointestinal

From *NANDA-I Nursing Diagnoses: Definitions & Classification, 2009–2011*, by North American Nursing Diagnosis Association International, 2009. Ames, IA: Wiley-Blackwell. Copyright 2010. Reprinted with permission.

Perfusion
Risk for **Ineffective Renal Perfusion**
Risk for **Shock**
Impaired Spontaneous **Ventilation**
Dysfunctional **Ventilatory** Weaning Response
Readiness for Enhanced **Self-Care**
Bathing **Self-Care** Deficit
Dressing **Self-Care** Deficit
Feeding **Self-Care** Deficit
Toileting **Self-Care** Deficit

Domain 5
Perception/Cognition
Unilateral **Neglect**
Impaired **Environmental** Interpretation Syndrome
Wandering
Disturbed **Sensory** Perception (Specify: Visual, Auditory, Kinesthetic, Gustatory, Tactile, Olfactory)
Acute **Confusion**
Chronic **Confusion**
Risk for Acute **Confusion**
Deficient **Knowledge**
Readiness for Enhanced **Knowledge**
Impaired **Memory**
Readiness for Enhanced **Decision-Making**
Ineffective **Activity** Planning
Impaired Verbal **Communication**
Readiness for Enhanced **Communication**

Domain 6
Self-Perception
Risk for Compromised Human **Dignity**
Hopelessness
Disturbed Personal **Identity**
Risk for **Loneliness**
Readiness for Enhanced **Power**
Powerlessness
Risk for **Powerlessness**
Readiness for Enhanced **Self-Concept**
Situational Low **Self-Esteem**
Chronic Low **Self-Esteem**
Risk for Situational Low **Self-Esteem**
Disturbed **Body** Image

Domain 7
Role Relationships
Caregiver Role Strain
Risk for **Caregiver** Role Strain
Impaired **Parenting**
Readiness for Enhanced **Parenting**
Risk for Impaired **Parenting**
Risk for Impaired **Attachment**
Dysfunctional **Family** Processes
Interrupted **Family** Processes
Readiness for Enhanced **Family** Processes
Effective **Breastfeeding**
Ineffective **Breastfeeding**
Interrupted **Breastfeeding**
Parental Role **Conflict**
Readiness for Enhanced **Relationship**
Ineffective **Role** Performance
Impaired **Social** Interaction

Domain 8
Sexuality
Sexual Dysfunction
Ineffective **Sexuality** Pattern
Readiness for Enhanced **Childbearing** Process
Risk for Disturbed **Maternal/Fetal** Dyad

Domain 9
Coping/Stress Tolerance
Post-Trauma Syndrome
Risk for **Post-Trauma** Syndrome
Rape-Trauma Syndrome
Relocation Stress Syndrome
Risk for **Relocation** Stress Syndrome
Anxiety
Death **Anxiety**
Risk-Prone Health **Behavior**
Compromised Family **Coping**
Defensive **Coping**
Disabled Family **Coping**
Ineffective **Coping**
Ineffective Community **Coping**
Readiness for Enhanced **Coping**
Readiness for Enhanced Community **Coping**
Readiness for Enhanced Family **Coping**
Ineffective **Denial**
Fear
Grieving
Complicated **Grieving**
Risk for Complicated **Grieving**
Impaired Individual **Resilience**
Readiness for Enhanced **Resilience**
Risk for Compromised **Resilience**
Chronic **Sorrow**
Stress Overload

Autonomic Dysreflexia
Risk for **Autonomic** Dysreflexia
Disorganized **Infant** Behavior
Risk for Disorganized **Infant** Behavior
Readiness for Enhanced Organized **Infant** Behavior
Decreased **Intracranial** Adaptive Capacity

Domain 10
Life Principles
Readiness for Enhanced **Hope**
Readiness for Enhanced **Spiritual** Well-Being
Decisional **Conflict**
Moral **Distress**
Noncompliance
Impaired **Religiosity**
Readiness for Enhanced **Religiosity**
Risk for Impaired **Religiosity**
Spiritual Distress
Risk for **Spiritual** Distress

Domain 11
Safety/Protection
Risk for **Infection**
Ineffective **Airway** Clearance
Risk for **Aspiration**
Risk for Sudden Infant **Death** Syndrome
Impaired **Dentition**
Risk for **Falls**
Risk for **Injury**
Risk for Perioperative-Positioning **Injury**
Impaired **Oral** Mucous Membrane
Risk for **Peripheral** Neurovascular Dysfunction
Ineffective **Protection**
Impaired **Skin** Integrity
Risk for Impaired **Skin** Integrity
Risk for **Suffocation**
Impaired **Tissue** Integrity
Risk for **Trauma**
Risk for Vascular **Trauma**
Self-Mutilation
Risk for **Suicide**
Risk for Other-Directed **Violence**
Risk for Self-Directed **Violence**
Contamination
Risk for **Contamination**
Risk for **Poisoning**
Latex **Allergy** Response
Risk for Latex **Allergy** Response
Risk for Imbalanced **Body** Temperature
Hyperthermia
Hypothermia
Ineffective **Thermoregulation**

Domain 12
Comfort
Readiness for Enhanced **Comfort**
Impaired **Comfort**
Nausea
Acute **Pain**
Chronic **Pain**
Social Isolation

Domain 13
Growth/Development
Adult **Failure** to Thrive
Delayed **Growth** and Development
Risk for Disproportionate **Growth**
Risk for Delayed **Development**

APPENDIX B Recommended Immunization Schedules

Recommended Immunization Schedule for Persons Aged 0 Through 6 Years—United States • 2009

For those who fall behind or start late, see the catch-up schedule

Vaccine ▼ Age ▶	Birth	1 month	2 months	4 months	6 months	12 months	15 months	18 months	19–23 months	2–3 years	4–6 years
Hepatitis B[1]	HepB	HepB		*see footnote 1*	HepB						
Rotavirus[2]			RV	RV	*RV*[2]						
Diphtheria, Tetanus, Pertussis[3]			DTaP	DTaP	DTaP	*see footnote 3*	DTaP				DTaP
Haemophilus influenzae type b[4]			Hib	Hib	*Hib*[4]	Hib					
Pneumococcal[5]			PCV	PCV	PCV	PCV				PPSV	
Inactivated Poliovirus			IPV	IPV	IPV						IPV
Influenza[6]					Influenza (Yearly)						
Measles, Mumps, Rubella[7]						MMR		*see footnote 7*			MMR
Varicella[8]						Varicella		*see footnote 8*			Varicella
Hepatitis A[9]						HepA (2 doses)				HepA Series	
Meningococcal[10]										MCV	

Range of recommended ages

Certain high-risk groups

This schedule indicates the recommended ages for routine administration of currently licensed vaccines, as of December 1, 2008, for children aged 0 through 6 years. Any dose not administered at the recommended age should be administered at a subsequent visit, when indicated and feasible. Licensed combination vaccines may be used whenever any component of the combination is indicated and other components are not contraindicated and if approved by the Food and Drug Administration for that dose of the series. Providers should consult the relevant Advisory Committee on Immunization Practices statement for detailed recommendations, including high-risk conditions: http://www.cdc.gov/vaccines/pubs/acip-list.htm. Clinically significant adverse events that follow immunization should be reported to the Vaccine Adverse Event Reporting System (VAERS). Guidance about how to obtain and complete a VAERS form is available at http://www.vaers.hhs.gov or by telephone, 800-822-7967.

1. **Hepatitis B vaccine (HepB).** ***(Minimum age: birth)***
   At birth:
   - Administer monovalent HepB to all newborns before hospital discharge.
   - If mother is hepatitis B surface antigen (HBsAg)-positive, administer HepB and 0.5 mL of hepatitis B immune globulin (HBIG) within 12 hours of birth.
   - If mother's HBsAg status is unknown, administer HepB within 12 hours of birth. Determine mother's HBsAg status as soon as possible and, if HBsAg-positive, administer HBIG (no later than age 1 week).

   After the birth dose:
   - The HepB series should be completed with either monovalent HepB or a combination vaccine containing HepB. The second dose should be administered at age 1 or 2 months. The final dose should be administered no earlier than age 24 weeks.
   - Infants born to HBsAg-positive mothers should be tested for HBsAg and antibody to HBsAg (anti-HBs) after completion of at least 3 doses of the HepB series, at age 9 through 18 months (generally at the next well-child visit).

   4-month dose:
   - Administration of 4 doses of HepB to infants is permissible when combination vaccines containing HepB are administered after the birth dose.
2. **Rotavirus vaccine (RV).** ***(Minimum age: 6 weeks)***
   - Administer the first dose at age 6 through 14 weeks (maximum age: 14 weeks 6 days). Vaccination should not be initiated for infants aged 15 weeks or older (i.e., 15 weeks 0 days or older).
   - Administer the final dose in the series by age 8 months 0 days.
   - If Rotarix® is administered at ages 2 and 4 months, a dose at 6 months is not indicated.
3. **Diphtheria and tetanus toxoids and acellular pertussis vaccine (DTaP).** ***(Minimum age: 6 weeks)***
   - The fourth dose may be administered as early as age 12 months, provided at least 6 months have elapsed since the third dose.
   - Administer the final dose in the series at age 4 through 6 years.
4. ***Haemophilus influenzae* type b conjugate vaccine (Hib).** ***(Minimum age: 6 weeks)***
   - If PRP-OMP (PedvaxHIB® or Comvax® [HepB-Hib]) is administered at ages 2 and 4 months, a dose at age 6 months is not indicated.
   - TriHiBit® (DTaP/Hib) should not be used for doses at ages 2, 4, or 6 months but can be used as the final dose in children aged 12 months or older.
5. **Pneumococcal vaccine.** ***(Minimum age: 6 weeks for pneumococcal conjugate vaccine [PCV]; 2 years for pneumococcal polysaccharide vaccine [PPSV])***
   - PCV is recommended for all children aged younger than 5 years. Administer 1 dose of PCV to all healthy children aged 24 through 59 months who are not completely vaccinated for their age.
   - Administer PPSV to children aged 2 years or older with certain underlying medical conditions (see *MMWR* 2000;49[No. RR-9]), including a cochlear implant.
6. **Influenza vaccine.** ***(Minimum age: 6 months for trivalent inactivated influenza vaccine [TIV]; 2 years for live, attenuated influenza vaccine [LAIV])***
   - Administer annually to children aged 6 months through 18 years.
   - For healthy nonpregnant persons (i.e., those who do not have underlying medical conditions that predispose them to influenza complications) aged 2 through 49 years, either LAIV or TIV may be used.
   - Children receiving TIV should receive 0.25 mL if aged 6 through 35 months or 0.5 mL if aged 3 years or older.
   - Administer 2 doses (separated by at least 4 weeks) to children aged younger than 9 years who are receiving influenza vaccine for the first time or who were vaccinated for the first time during the previous influenza season but only received 1 dose.
7. **Measles, mumps, and rubella vaccine (MMR).** ***(Minimum age: 12 months)***
   - Administer the second dose at age 4 through 6 years. However, the second dose may be administered before age 4, provided at least 28 days have elapsed since the first dose.
8. **Varicella vaccine.** ***(Minimum age: 12 months)***
   - Administer the second dose at age 4 through 6 years. However, the second dose may be administered before age 4, provided at least 3 months have elapsed since the first dose.
   - For children aged 12 months through 12 years the minimum interval between doses is 3 months. However, if the second dose was administered at least 28 days after the first dose, it can be accepted as valid.
9. **Hepatitis A vaccine (HepA).** ***(Minimum age: 12 months)***
   - Administer to all children aged 1 year (i.e., aged 12 through 23 months). Administer 2 doses at least 6 months apart.
   - Children not fully vaccinated by age 2 years can be vaccinated at subsequent visits.
   - HepA also is recommended for children older than 1 year who live in areas where vaccination programs target older children or who are at increased risk of infection. See *MMWR* 2006;55(No. RR-7).
10. **Meningococcal vaccine.** ***(Minimum age: 2 years for meningococcal conjugate vaccine [MCV] and for meningococcal polysaccharide vaccine [MPSV])***
    - Administer MCV to children aged 2 through 10 years with terminal complement component deficiency, anatomic or functional asplenia, and certain other high-risk groups. See *MMWR* 2005;54(No. RR-7).
    - Persons who received MPSV 3 or more years previously and who remain at increased risk for meningococcal disease should be revaccinated with MCV.

The Recommended Immunization Schedules for Persons Aged 0 Through 18 Years are approved by the Advisory Committee on Immunization Practices (www.cdc.gov/vaccines/recs/acip), the American Academy of Pediatrics (http://www.aap.org), and the American Academy of Family Physicians (http://www.aafp.org).

DEPARTMENT OF HEALTH AND HUMAN SERVICES • CENTERS FOR DISEASE CONTROL AND PREVENTION

Recommended Immunization Schedule for Persons Aged 7 Through 18 Years—United States • 2009

For those who fall behind or start late, see the schedule below and the catch-up schedule

Vaccine ▼ Age ▶	7–10 years	11–12 years	13–18 years
Tetanus, Diphtheria, Pertussis[1]	*see footnote 1*	Tdap	Tdap
Human Papillomavirus[2]	*see footnote 2*	HPV (3 doses)	HPV Series
Meningococcal[3]	MCV	MCV	MCV
Influenza[4]	Influenza (Yearly)		
Pneumococcal[5]	PPSV		
Hepatitis A[6]	HepA Series		
Hepatitis B[7]	HepB Series		
Inactivated Poliovirus[8]	IPV Series		
Measles, Mumps, Rubella[9]	MMR Series		
Varicella[10]	Varicella Series		

Range of recommended ages

Catch-up immunization

Certain high-risk groups

This schedule indicates the recommended ages for routine administration of currently licensed vaccines, as of December 1, 2008, for children aged 7 through 18 years. Any dose not administered at the recommended age should be administered at a subsequent visit, when indicated and feasible. Licensed combination vaccines may be used whenever any component of the combination is indicated and other components are not contraindicated and if approved by the Food and Drug Administration for that dose of the series. Providers should consult the relevant Advisory Committee on Immunization Practices statement for detailed recommendations, including high-risk conditions: http://www.cdc.gov/vaccines/pubs/acip-list.htm. Clinically significant adverse events that follow immunization should be reported to the Vaccine Adverse Event Reporting System (VAERS). Guidance about how to obtain and complete a VAERS form is available at http://www.vaers.hhs.gov or by telephone, 800-822-7967.

1. Tetanus and diphtheria toxoids and acellular pertussis vaccine (Tdap). ***(Minimum age: 10 years for BOOSTRIX® and 11 years for ADACEL®)***
- Administer at age 11 or 12 years for those who have completed the recommended childhood DTP/DTaP vaccination series and have not received a tetanus and diphtheria toxoid (Td) booster dose.
- Persons aged 13 through 18 years who have not received Tdap should receive a dose.
- A 5-year interval from the last Td dose is encouraged when Tdap is used as a booster dose; however, a shorter interval may be used if pertussis immunity is needed.

2. Human papillomavirus vaccine (HPV). ***(Minimum age: 9 years)***
- Administer the first dose to females at age 11 or 12 years.
- Administer the second dose 2 months after the first dose and the third dose 6 months after the first dose (at least 24 weeks after the first dose).
- Administer the series to females at age 13 through 18 years if not previously vaccinated.

3. Meningococcal conjugate vaccine (MCV).
- Administer at age 11 or 12 years, or at age 13 through 18 years if not previously vaccinated.
- Administer to previously unvaccinated college freshmen living in a dormitory.
- MCV is recommended for children aged 2 through 10 years with terminal complement component deficiency, anatomic or functional asplenia, and certain other groups at high risk. See *MMWR* 2005;54(No. RR-7).
- Persons who received MPSV 5 or more years previously and remain at increased risk for meningococcal disease should be revaccinated with MCV.

4. Influenza vaccine.
- Administer annually to children aged 6 months through 18 years.
- For healthy nonpregnant persons (i.e., those who do not have underlying medical conditions that predispose them to influenza complications) aged 2 through 49 years, either LAIV or TIV may be used.
- Administer 2 doses (separated by at least 4 weeks) to children aged younger than 9 years who are receiving influenza vaccine for the first time or who were vaccinated for the first time during the previous influenza season but only received 1 dose.

5. Pneumococcal polysaccharide vaccine (PPSV).
- Administer to children with certain underlying medical conditions (see *MMWR* 1997;46[No. RR-8]), including a cochlear implant. A single revaccination should be administered to children with functional or anatomic asplenia or other immunocompromising condition after 5 years.

6. Hepatitis A vaccine (HepA).
- Administer 2 doses at least 6 months apart.
- HepA is recommended for children older than 1 year who live in areas where vaccination programs target older children or who are at increased risk of infection. See *MMWR* 2006;55(No. RR-7).

7. Hepatitis B vaccine (HepB).
- Administer the 3-dose series to those not previously vaccinated.
- A 2-dose series (separated by at least 4 months) of adult formulation Recombivax HB® is licensed for children aged 11 through 15 years.

8. Inactivated poliovirus vaccine (IPV).
- For children who received an all-IPV or all-oral poliovirus (OPV) series, a fourth dose is not necessary if the third dose was administered at age 4 years or older.
- If both OPV and IPV were administered as part of a series, a total of 4 doses should be administered, regardless of the child's current age.

9. Measles, mumps, and rubella vaccine (MMR).
- If not previously vaccinated, administer 2 doses or the second dose for those who have received only 1 dose, with at least 28 days between doses.

10. Varicella vaccine.
- For persons aged 7 through 18 years without evidence of immunity (see *MMWR* 2007;56[No. RR-4]), administer 2 doses if not previously vaccinated or the second dose if they have received only 1 dose.
- For persons aged 7 through 12 years, the minimum interval between doses is 3 months. However, if the second dose was administered at least 28 days after the first dose, it can be accepted as valid.
- For persons aged 13 years and older, the minimum interval between doses is 28 days.

The Recommended Immunization Schedules for Persons Aged 0 Through 18 Years are approved by the Advisory Committee on Immunization Practices (www.cdc.gov/vaccines/recs/acip), the American Academy of Pediatrics (http://www.aap.org), and the American Academy of Family Physicians (http://www.aafp.org).

DEPARTMENT OF HEALTH AND HUMAN SERVICES • CENTERS FOR DISEASE CONTROL AND PREVENTION

Recommended Adult Immunization Schedule

UNITED STATES · 2009

Note: These recommendations *must* be read with the footnotes that follow containing number of doses, intervals between doses, and other important information.

Figure 1. Recommended adult immunization schedule, by vaccine and age group

VACCINE ▼ / AGE GROUP ▶	19–26 years	27–49 years	50–59 years	60–64 years	≥65 years
Tetanus, diphtheria, pertussis (Td/Tdap)[1,*]	Substitute 1-time dose of Tdap for Td booster; then boost with Td every 10 yrs				Td booster every 10 yrs
Human papillomavirus (HPV)[2,*]	3 doses (females)				
Varicella[3,*]	2 doses				
Zoster[4]				1 dose	
Measles, mumps, rubella (MMR)[5,*]	1 or 2 doses		1 dose		
Influenza[6,*]	1 dose annually				
Pneumococcal (polysaccharide)[7,8]	1 or 2 doses				1 dose
Hepatitis A[9,*]	2 doses				
Hepatitis B[10,*]	3 doses				
Meningococcal[11,*]	1 or more doses				

*Covered by the Vaccine Injury Compensation Program.

Legend:
- Yellow: For all persons in this category who meet the age requirements and who lack evidence of immunity (e.g., lack documentation of vaccination or have no evidence of prior infection)
- Purple: Recommended if some other risk factor is present (e.g., on the basis of medical, occupational, lifestyle, or other indications)
- Blank: No recommendation

Report all clinically significant postvaccination reactions to the Vaccine Adverse Event Reporting System (VAERS). Reporting forms and instructions on filing a VAERS report are available at www.vaers.hhs.gov or by telephone, 800-822-7967.

Information on how to file a Vaccine Injury Compensation Program claim is available at www.hrsa.gov/vaccinecompensation or by telephone, 800-338-2382. To file a claim for vaccine injury, contact the U.S. Court of Federal Claims, 717 Madison Place, N.W., Washington, D.C. 20005; telephone, 202-357-6400.

Additional information about the vaccines in this schedule, extent of available data, and contraindications for vaccination is also available at www.cdc.gov/vaccines or from the CDC-INFO Contact Center at 800-CDC-INFO (800-232-4636) in English and Spanish, 24 hours a day, 7 days a week.

Use of trade names and commercial sources is for identification only and does not imply endorsement by the U.S. Department of Health and Human Services.

Figure 2. Vaccines that might be indicated for adults based on medical and other indications

VACCINE ▼ / INDICATION ▶	Pregnancy	Immuno-compromising conditions (excluding human immunodeficiency virus [HIV])[13]	HIV infection[3,12,13] CD4+ T lymphocyte count <200 cells/μL	HIV infection[3,12,13] CD4+ T lymphocyte count ≥200 cells/μL	Diabetes, heart disease, chronic lung disease, chronic alcoholism	Asplenia[12] (including elective splenectomy and terminal complement component deficiencies)	Chronic liver disease	Kidney failure, end-stage renal disease, receipt of hemodialysis	Health-care personnel
Tetanus, diphtheria, pertussis (Td/Tdap)[1,*]	Td	Substitute 1-time dose of Tdap for Td booster; then boost with Td every 10 yrs							
Human papillomavirus (HPV)[2,*]					3 doses for females through age 26 yrs				
Varicella[3,*]	Contraindicated						2 doses		
Zoster[4]	Contraindicated						1 dose		
Measles, mumps, rubella (MMR)[5,*]	Contraindicated						1 or 2 doses		
Influenza[6,*]					1 dose TIV annually				1 dose TIV or LAIV annually
Pneumococcal (polysaccharide)[7,8]						1 or 2 doses			
Hepatitis A[9,*]						2 doses			
Hepatitis B[10,*]						3 doses			
Meningococcal[11,*]						1 or more doses			

*Covered by the Vaccine Injury Compensation Program.

For all persons in this category who meet the age requirements and who lack evidence of immunity (e.g., lack documentation of vaccination or have no evidence of prior infection)

Recommended if some other risk factor is present (e.g., on the basis of medical, occupational, lifestyle, or other indications)

No recommendation

These schedules indicate the recommended age groups and medical indications for which administration of currently licensed vaccines is commonly indicated for adults ages 19 years and older, as of January 1, 2009. Licensed combination vaccines may be used whenever any components of the combination are indicated and when the vaccine's other components are not contraindicated. For detailed recommendations on all vaccines, including those used primarily for travelers or that are issued during the year, consult the manufacturers' package inserts and the complete statements from the Advisory Committee on Immunization Practices (www.cdc.gov/vaccines/pubs/acip-list.htm).

The recommendations in this schedule were approved by the Centers for Disease Control and Prevention's (CDC) Advisory Committee on Immunization Practices (ACIP), the American Academy of Family Physicians (AAFP), the American College of Obstetricians and Gynecologists (ACOG), and the American College of Physicians (ACP).

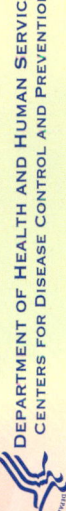

CS200484-A

Footnotes

Recommended Adult Immunization Schedule—UNITED STATES · 2009

For complete statements by the Advisory Committee on Immunization Practices (ACIP), visit www.cdc.gov/vaccines/pubs/ACIP-list.htm.

1. Tetanus, diphtheria, and acellular pertussis (Td/Tdap) vaccination

Tdap should replace a single dose of Td for adults aged 19 through 64 years who have not received a dose of Tdap previously.

Adults with uncertain or incomplete history of primary vaccination series with tetanus and diphtheria toxoid-containing vaccines should begin or complete a primary vaccination series. A primary series for adults is 3 doses of tetanus and diphtheria toxoid-containing vaccines; administer the first 2 doses at least 4 weeks apart and the third dose 6–12 months after the second. However, Tdap can substitute for any one of the doses of Td in the 3-dose primary series. The booster dose of tetanus and diphtheria toxoid-containing vaccine should be administered to adults who have completed a primary series and if the last vaccination was received 10 or more years previously. Tdap or Td vaccine may be used, as indicated.

If a woman is pregnant and received the last Td vaccination 10 or more years previously, administer Td during the second or third trimester. If the woman received the last Td vaccination less than 10 years previously, administer Tdap during the immediate postpartum period. A dose of Tdap is recommended for postpartum women, close contacts of infants aged less than 12 months, and all health-care personnel with direct patient contact if they have not previously received Tdap. An interval as short as 2 years from the last Td is suggested; shorter intervals can be used. Td may be deferred during pregnancy and Tdap substituted in the immediate postpartum period, or Tdap may be administered instead of Td to a pregnant woman after an informed discussion with the woman.

Consult the ACIP statement for recommendations for administering Td as prophylaxis in wound management.

2. Human papillomavirus (HPV) vaccination

HPV vaccination is recommended for all females aged 11 through 26 years (and may begin at 9 years) who have not completed the vaccine series. History of genital warts, abnormal Papanicolaou test, or positive HPV DNA test is not evidence of prior infection with all vaccine HPV types; HPV vaccination is recommended for persons with such histories.

Ideally, vaccine should be administered before potential exposure to HPV through sexual activity; however, females who are sexually active should still be vaccinated consistent with age-based recommendations. Sexually active females who have not been infected with any of the four HPV vaccine types receive the full benefit of the vaccination. Vaccination is less beneficial for females who have already been infected with one or more of the HPV vaccine types.

A complete series consists of 3 doses. The second dose should be administered 2 months after the first dose; the third dose should be administered 6 months after the first dose.

HPV vaccination is not specifically recommended for females with the medical indications described in Figure 2, "Vaccines that might be indicated for adults based on medical and other indications." Because HPV vaccine is not a live-virus vaccine, it may be administered to persons with the medical indications described in Figure 2. However, the immune response and vaccine efficacy might be less for persons with the medical indications described in Figure 2 than in persons who do not have the medical indications described or who are immunocompetent. Health-care personnel are not at increased risk because of occupational exposure, and should be vaccinated consistent with age-based recommendations.

3. Varicella vaccination

All adults without evidence of immunity to varicella should receive 2 doses of single-antigen varicella vaccine if not previously vaccinated or the second dose if they have received only one dose unless they have a medical contraindication. Special consideration should be given to those who 1) have close contact with persons at high risk for severe disease (e.g., health-care personnel and family contacts of persons with immunocompromising conditions) or 2) are at high risk for exposure or transmission (e.g., teachers; child care employees; residents and staff members of institutional settings, including correctional institutions; college students; military personnel; adolescents and adults living in households with children; nonpregnant women of childbearing age; and international travelers).

Evidence of immunity to varicella in adults includes any of the following: 1) documentation of 2 doses of varicella vaccine at least 4 weeks apart; 2) U.S.-born before 1980 (although for health-care personnel and pregnant women, birth before 1980 should not be considered evidence of immunity); 3) history of varicella based on diagnosis or verification of varicella by a health-care provider (for a patient reporting a history of or presenting with an atypical case, a mild case, or both, health-care providers should seek either an epidemiologic link with a typical varicella case or to a laboratory-confirmed case or evidence of laboratory confirmation, if it was performed at the time of acute disease); 4) history of herpes zoster based on health-care provider diagnosis or verification of herpes zoster by a health-care provider; or 5) laboratory evidence of immunity or laboratory confirmation of disease.

Pregnant women should be assessed for evidence of varicella immunity. Women who do not have evidence of immunity should receive the first dose of varicella vaccine upon completion or termination of pregnancy and before discharge from the health-care facility. The second dose should be administered 4–8 weeks after the first dose.

4. Herpes zoster vaccination

A single dose of zoster vaccine is recommended for adults aged 60 years and older regardless of whether they report a prior episode of herpes zoster. Persons with chronic medical conditions may be vaccinated unless their condition constitutes a contraindication.

5. Measles, mumps, rubella (MMR) vaccination

Measles component: Adults born before 1957 generally are considered immune to measles. Adults born during or after 1957 should receive 1 or more doses of MMR unless they have a medical contraindication, documentation of 1 or more doses, history of measles based on health-care provider diagnosis, or laboratory evidence of immunity.

A second dose of MMR is recommended for adults who 1) have been recently exposed to measles or are in an outbreak setting; 2) have been vaccinated previously with killed measles vaccine; 3) have been vaccinated with an unknown type of measles vaccine during 1963–1967; 4) are students in postsecondary educational institutions; 5) work in a health-care facility; or 6) plan to travel internationally.

Mumps component: Adults born before 1957 generally are considered immune to mumps. Adults born during or after 1957 should receive 1 dose of MMR unless they have a medical contraindication, history of mumps based on health-care provider diagnosis, or laboratory evidence of immunity.

A second dose of MMR is recommended for adults who 1) live in a community experiencing a mumps outbreak and are in an affected age group; 2) are students in postsecondary educational institutions; 3) work in a health-care facility; or 4) plan to travel internationally. For unvaccinated health-care personnel born before 1957 who do not have other evidence of mumps immunity, administering 1 dose on a routine basis should be considered and administering a second dose during an outbreak should be strongly considered.

Rubella component: 1 dose of MMR vaccine is recommended for women whose rubella vaccination history is unreliable or who lack laboratory evidence of immunity. For women of childbearing age, regardless of birth year, rubella immunity should be determined and women should be counseled regarding congenital rubella syndrome. Women who do not have evidence of immunity should receive MMR upon completion or termination of pregnancy and before discharge from the health-care facility.

6. Influenza vaccination

Medical indications: Chronic disorders of the cardiovascular or pulmonary systems, including asthma; chronic metabolic diseases, including diabetes mellitus, renal or hepatic dysfunction, hemoglobinopathies, or immunocompromising conditions (including immunocompromising conditions caused by medications or human immunodeficiency virus [HIV]); any condition that compromises respiratory function or the handling of respiratory secretions or that can increase the risk of aspiration (e.g., cognitive dysfunction, spinal cord injury, or seizure disorder or other neuromuscular disorder); and pregnancy during the influenza season. No data exist on the risk for severe or complicated influenza disease among persons with asplenia; however, influenza is a risk factor for secondary bacterial infections that can cause severe disease among persons with asplenia.

Occupational indications: All health-care personnel, including those employed by long-term care and assisted-living facilities, and caregivers of children less than 5 years old.

Other indications: Residents of nursing homes and other long-term care and assisted-living facilities; persons likely to transmit influenza to persons at high risk (e.g., in-home household contacts and caregivers of children aged less than 5 years old, persons 65 years old and older and persons of all ages with high-risk condition[s]); and anyone who would like to decrease their risk of getting influenza. Healthy, nonpregnant adults aged less than 50 years without high-risk medical conditions who are not contacts of severely immunocompromised persons in special care units can receive either intranasally administered live, attenuated influenza vaccine (FluMist®) or inactivated vaccine. Other persons should receive the inactivated vaccine.

7. Pneumococcal polysaccharide (PPSV) vaccination

Medical indications: Chronic lung disease (including asthma); chronic cardiovascular diseases; diabetes mellitus; chronic liver diseases, cirrhosis; chronic alcoholism, chronic renal failure or nephrotic syndrome; functional or anatomic asplenia (e.g., sickle cell disease or splenectomy [if elective splenectomy is planned, vaccinate at least 2 weeks before surgery]); immunocompromising conditions; and cochlear implants and cerebrospinal fluid leaks. Vaccinate as close to HIV diagnosis as possible.

Other indications: Residents of nursing homes or long-term care facilities and persons who smoke cigarettes. Routine use of PPSV is not recommended for Alaska Native or American Indian persons younger than 65 years unless they have underlying medical conditions that are PPSV indications. However, public health authorities may consider recommending PPSV for Alaska Natives and American Indians aged 50 through 64 years who are living in areas in which the risk of invasive pneumococcal disease is increased.

8. Revaccination with PPSV

One-time revaccination after 5 years for persons with chronic renal failure or nephrotic syndrome; functional or anatomic asplenia (e.g., sickle cell disease or splenectomy); and for persons with immunocompromising conditions. For persons aged 65 years and older, one-time revaccination if they were vaccinated 5 or more years previously and were aged less than 65 years at the time of primary vaccination.

9. Hepatitis A vaccination

Medical indications: Persons with chronic liver disease and persons who receive clotting factor concentrates.

Behavioral indications: Men who have sex with men and persons who use illegal drugs.

Occupational indications: Persons working with hepatitis A virus (HAV)-infected primates or with HAV in a research laboratory setting.

Other indications: Persons traveling to or working in countries that have high or intermediate endemicity of hepatitis A (a list of countries is available at wwwn.cdc.gov/travel/contentdiseases.aspx) and any person seeking protection from HAV infection.

Single-antigen vaccine formulations should be administered in a 2-dose schedule at either 0 and 6–12 months (Havrix®), or 0 and 6–18 months (Vaqta®). If the combined hepatitis A and hepatitis B vaccine (Twinrix®) is used, administer 3 doses at 0, 1, and 6 months; alternatively, a 4-dose schedule, administered on days 0, 7 and 21 to 30 followed by a booster dose at month 12 may be used.

10. Hepatitis B vaccination

Medical indications: Persons with end-stage renal disease, including patients receiving hemodialysis; persons with HIV infection; and persons with chronic liver disease.

Occupational indications: Health-care personnel and public-safety workers who are exposed to blood or other potentially infectious body fluids.

Behavioral indications: Sexually active persons who are not in a long-term, mutually monogamous relationship (e.g., persons with more than 1 sex partner during the previous 6 months); persons seeking evaluation or treatment for a sexually transmitted disease (STD); current or recent injection-drug users; and men who have sex with men.

Other indications: Household contacts and sex partners of persons with chronic hepatitis B virus (HBV) infection; clients and staff members of institutions for persons with developmental disabilities; international travelers to countries with high or intermediate prevalence of chronic HBV infection (a list of countries is available at wwwn.cdc.gov/travel/contentdiseases.aspx); and any adult seeking protection from HBV infection.

Hepatitis B vaccination is recommended for all adults in the following settings: STD treatment facilities; HIV testing and treatment facilities; facilities providing drug-abuse treatment and prevention services; health-care settings targeting services to injection-drug users or men who have sex with men; correctional facilities; end-stage renal disease programs and facilities for chronic hemodialysis patients; and institutions and nonresidential daycare facilities for persons with developmental disabilities.

If the combined hepatitis A and hepatitis B vaccine (Twinrix®) is used, administer 3 doses at

0, 1, and 6 months; alternatively, a 4-dose schedule, administered on days 0, 7 and 21 to 30 followed by a booster dose at month 12 may be used.

Special formulation indications: For adult patients receiving hemodialysis or with other immunocompromising conditions, 1 dose of 40 µg/mL (Recombivax HB®) administered on a 3-dose schedule or 2 doses of 20 µg/mL (Engerix-B®) administered simultaneously on a 4-dose schedule at
0, 1, 2 and 6 months.

11. Meningococcal vaccination

Medical indications: Adults with anatomic or functional asplenia, or terminal complement component deficiencies.

Other indications: First-year college students living in dormitories; microbiologists who are routinely exposed to isolates of *Neisseria meningitidis*; military recruits; and persons who travel to or live in countries in which meningococcal disease is hyperendemic or epidemic (e.g., the "meningitis belt" of sub-Saharan Africa during the dry season [December–June]), particularly if their contact with local populations will be prolonged. Vaccination is required by the government of Saudi Arabia for all travelers to Mecca during the annual Hajj.

Meningococcal conjugate (MCV) vaccine is preferred for adults with any of the preceding indications who are aged 55 years or younger, although meningococcal polysaccharide vaccine (MPSV) is an acceptable alternative. Revaccination with MCV after 5 years might be indicated for adults previously vaccinated with MPSV who remain at increased risk for infection (e.g., persons residing in areas in which disease is epidemic).

12. Selected conditions for which *Haemophilus influenzae* type b (Hib) vaccine may be used

Hib vaccine generally is not recommended for persons aged 5 years and older. No efficacy data are available on which to base a recommendation concerning use of Hib vaccine for older children and adults. However, studies suggest good immunogenicity in persons who have sickle cell disease, leukemia, or HIV infection or who have had a splenectomy; administering 1 dose of vaccine to these persons is not contraindicated.

13. Immunocompromising conditions

Inactivated vaccines generally are acceptable (e.g., pneumococcal, meningococcal, and influenza [trivalent inactivated influenza vaccine]), and live vaccines generally are avoided in persons with immune deficiencies or immunocompromising conditions. Information on specific conditions is available at www.cdc.gov/vaccines/pubs/acip-list.htm.

APPENDIX C
Abbreviations, Acronyms, and Symbols

>	greater than
<	less than
ʒ	dram
℥	ounce
♏	minum
ā	before
AAPB	Association of Applied Psychophysiology and Biofeedback
AARP	American Association of Retired Persons
AASM	American Academy of Sleep Medicine
AAT	animal-assisted therapy
AATH	American Association for Therapeutic Humor
ABC	airway, breathing, circulation
ABD	abdominal
ABG	arterial blood gases
ABO	blood types
a.c.	before meals
ACIP	Advisory Committee on Immunization Practices
ACS	American Cancer Society
ACTH	adrenocorticotropic hormone
AD	Alzheimer's disease
AD	right ear
ad lib	freely, as desired
ADA	Americans with Disabilities Act
ADH	antidiuretic hormone
ADLs	activities of daily living
ADN	associate degree nurse (nursing)
AEB	as evidenced by
AFP	alpha-fetoprotein
AHA	American Hospital Association
AHCA	American Health Care Association
AHCPR	Agency for Health Care Policy and Research
AHNA	American Holistic Nurses' Association
AHRQ	Agency for Healthcare Research and Quality
AI	adequate intake
AIDS	acquired immunodeficiency syndrome
AJN	*American Journal of Nursing*
ALFA	Assisted Living Federation of America
ALT	alanine aminotransferase
AMA	against medical advice
AMA	American Medical Association
ANA	American Nurses Association
ANA	antinuclear antibody
AoA	Administration on Aging
AP	anterior/posterior
AP	apical pulse
APIC	Association for Practitioners in Infection Control and Epidemiology
APRN	advance practice registered nurse
APS	Adult Protective Services
APS	American Pain Society
APTT	activated partial thromboplastin time
AROM	active range of motion
AS	left ear
ASA	acetylsalicylic acid
ASO	antireptolysin-O
AST	aspartate aminotransferase
AT	axillary temperature
ATC	around the clock
ATP	adenosine triphosphatase
AU	both ears
B_1	thiamine
B_2	riboflavin
B_6	pyridoxine
B_{12}	cobolomine
BBA	Balanced Budget Act
BE	base excess
bid	twice a day
BMD	bone mineral density
BMI	body mass index
BMR	basal metabolic rate

BP	blood pressure
BPH	benign prostatic hypertrophy
BPM	beats per minute
BSA	body surface area
BSE	breast self-examination
BSI	body substance isolation
BSN	bachelor of science in nursing
BUN	blood urea nitrogen
c	cup
c̄	with
C	Celsius
Ca	calcium
Ca^{++}	calcium ion
$CaCl_2$	calcium chloride
C/A	complementary/alternative
CAD	coronary artery disease
CAI	computer-assisted instruction
CAM	complementary/alternative medicine
C & S	culture and sensitivity
cap	capsule
CARF	Commission on Accreditation of Rehabilitation Facilities
CAT	computed axial tomography
CAT	computerized adaptive testing
CBC	complete blood count
CBD	common bile duct
CBE	charting by exception
cc	cubic centimeter
CCRC	continuing care retirement community
CCU	coronary care unit
CDC	Centers for Disease Control and Prevention
CEA	carcinoembryonic antigen
CEPN-LTC™	Certification Examination for Practical and Vocational Nurses in Long-Term Care
CEU	continuing education unit
CHAP	Community Health Accreditation Program
CHD	coronary heart disease
CHF	congestive heart failure
CHIP	Children's Health Insurance Program
CHO	carbohydrate (carbon, hydrogen, oxygen)
CHON	protein (carbon, hydrogen, oxygen, nitrogen)
CK or CPK	creatine kinase or creatine phosphokinase
Cl	chlorine, chloride
Cl^-	chloride ion
CLTC	certified in long-term care
cm	centimeter
CMS	Centers for Medicare and Medicaid Services
CN	cranial nerve
CNA	certified nursing assistant
CNM	certified nurse midwife
CNO	community nursing organization
CNS	central nervous system
CNS	clinical nurse specialist
Co	cobalt
CO_2	carbon dioxide
CO_2^-	carbon dioxide ion
COBRA	Comprehensive Omnibus Budget Reconciliation Act
COOH	carboxyl group
COPD	chronic obstructive pulmonary disease
CPAP	continuous positive airway pressure
CPNP	Council of Practical Nursing Programs
CPR	cardiopulmonary resuscitation
CPR	computerized patient record
Cr	chromium
CRNA	Certified Registered Nurse Anesthetist
CRP	C-reactive protein
C&S	culture and sensitivity
CSF	cerebrospinal fluid
CSM	circulation, sensation, motion
CT	computed tomography
Cu	copper
CVA	cerebrovascular accident
CVC	central venous catheter
D_5W	dextrose 5% in water
D & C	dilatation and curettage
DAR	document, action, response
dc	discontinue
DDB	Disciplinary Data Bank
DDS	doctor of dental surgery
DEA	Drug Enforcement Agency
DHHS	Department of Health and Human Services
DIC	disseminated intravascular coagulation
DICC	dynamic infusion cavernosometry and cavernosography
dL	deciliter
DMD	doctor of dental medicine
DNA	deoxyribonucleic acid
DNR	do not resuscitate
DO	doctor of osteopathy
DPAHC	durable power of attorney for health care
dr	dram, or ʒ
DRG	diagnosis-related group
DRI	dietary reference intake
DSM-IV	*Diagnostic and Statistical Manual of Mental Disorders,* 4th edition
DST	dexamethasone suppression test
DT	delirium tremens
DTaP	diphtheria, tetanus, acellular pertussis
DTP	diphtheria, tetanus, pertussis
DVT	deep vein thrombosis
EAR	estimated average requirement
ECF	extended care facility
ECF	extracellular fluid
ED	emergency department
EDTA	ethylenediaminetetraacetic acid
EEG	electroencephalograph
EGD	esophagogastroduodenoscopy
EKG (ECG)	electrocardiogram
ELISA	enzyme-linked immunosorbent assay
elix	elixir
EMG	electromyogram
EMLA	eutectic (cream) mixture of local anesthetics
EMS	emergency medical services

EMT	emergency medical technician
EMT-P	emergency medical technician-paramedic
EPA	Environmental Protection Agency
EPO	exclusive provider organization
ER	emergency room
ERCP	endoscopic retrograde cholangiopancreatogram
ERG	electroretinogram
ERT	estrogen replacement therapy
ESR	erythrocyte sedimentation rate
ET	ear (tympanic) temperature
EVAD	explantable venous access device
F	fahrenheit
FAS	fetal alcohol syndrome
FBS	fasting blood sugar
FCA	False Claims Act
FDA	Food and Drug Administration
Fe	iron
$FeSO_4$	iron sulfate
fl	fluid
Fl	fluorine
FOBT	fecal occult blood test
FSH	follicle-stimulating hormone
ft	foot or feet
FVD	fluid volume deficit
g	gram
GAO	General Accounting Office
GAS	general adaptation syndrome
GCS	Glasgow Coma Scale
g/dL	grams per deciliter
GED	general education development
GER	gastroesophageal reflux
GFR	glomerular filtration rate
GGT (GGTP)	gammaglutamy transpeptidase
GH	growth hormone
GHB	glycosylated hemoglobin
GI	gastrointestinal
gr	grain
gtt	drop
GTT	glucose tolerance test
gtt/min	drops per minute
GU	genitourinary
h	hour(s)
H^+	hydrogen ion
H_2CO_3	carbonic acid
H_2O	water
H&H	hemoglobin and hematocrit
HB_sAG	hepatitis B surface antigen
HBV	hepatitis B virus
HCFA	Health Care Financing Administration
hCG	human chorionic gonadotropin
HCl	hydrochloric acid, hydrochloride
HCO_3^-	bicarbonate ion
Hct	hematocrit
HCV	hepatitis C virus
HDL	high density lipoprotein
HDV	hepatitis D virus
Hep B	hepatitis B
HFA	Hospice Foundation of America
Hg	mercury
Hgb	hemoglobin
Hgbs	hemoglobins
HICPAC	Hospital Infection Control Practices Advisory Committee
HIS	hospital information system
HIV	human immunodeficiency virus
HLA	human leukocyte antigen
HMO	health maintenance organization
HPO_4	phosphate
HR	heart rate
HRSA	Health Resources and Services Administration
h.s.	hour of sleep
I	iodine
IADLs	instrumental activities of daily living
I&O	intake and output
IASP	International Association for the Study of Pain
ICF	intermediate care facility
ICF	intracellular fluid
ICN	International Council of Nurses
ICU	intensive care unit
ID	identification
ID	intradermal
IgG	immunoglobulin G
IgM	immunoglobulin M
IHCT	interdisciplinary health care team
IM	intramuscular
in	inch
INR	International Normalized Ratio
I&O	intake and output
IOL	intraocular lens
IOM	Institute of Medicine
ITT	insulin tolerance test
IV	intravenous
IVAD	implantable vascular access device
IVP	intravenous push, intravenous pyelogram
IVPB	intravenous piggyback
JCAHO	Joint Commission on Accreditation of Healthcare Organizations
K	potassium
K^+	potassium ion
kcal	kilocalorie
KCl	potassium chloride
kg	kilogram
KS	ketosteroids
KUB	kidneys/ureters/bladder
KVO	keep vein open
L	liter
LAS	local adaptation syndrome
lb	pound
LDH	lactic dehydrogenase
LDL	low density lipoprotein
LE	lupus erythematosus
LES	lower esophageal sphincter
LFT	liver function test

LH	luteinizing hormone
LLQ	left lower quadrant
LMP	last menstrual period
L/min	liters per minute
LOC	level of consciousness
LP	lumbar puncture
LP/VN	licensed practical/vocational nurse
LPN	licensed practical nurse
LUQ	left upper quadrant
LVN	licensed vocational nurse
m	meter
m^2	square meter
MAO	monoamine oxidase
MAOI	monoamine oxidase inhibitor
MAR	medication administration record
mcg (or μg)	microgram
MD	doctor of medicine
MDI	metered-dose inhaler
MDR	multidrug-resistant
MDR-TB	multidrug-resistant tuberculosis
MDS	minimum data set
mEq	milliequivalent
mEq/L	milliequivalents per liter
mg	milligram
mg/dL	milligrams per deciliter
Mg	magnesium
Mg^{++}	magnesium ion
MgCl	magnesium chloride
$MgSO_4$	magnesium sulfate
MI	myocardial infarction
min	minute
mL	milliliter
mm^3	cubic millimeter
mm Hg	millimeters of mercury
mmol/L	millimoles per liter
MMR	measles, mumps, rubella
Mn	manganese
Mo	molybdenum
MOM	Milk of Magnesia
mOsm/kg	milliosmoles/kilogram
MRI	magnetic resonance imaging
MRSA	methicillin-resistant *staphylococcus aureus*
MS	morphine sulfate
MSDS	material safety data sheet
MUGA	multi-gated acquisition
N_2	nitrogen
Na	sodium
Na^+	sodium ion
Na_2SO_4	sodium sulfate
NaCl	sodium chloride
NA	not applicable
NADSA	National Adult Day Services Associations
NaH_2PO_4	sodium dihydrogen phosphate
Na_2HPO_4	disodium phosphate
NAHC	National Association for Home Care
$NaHCO_3$	sodium bicarbonate
$NaHPO_4$	sodium monohydrogen phosphate
NANDA	North American Nursing Diagnosis Association
NaOH	sodium hydroxide
NAPNE	Natonal Association of Practical Nurse Education
NAPNES	National Association for Practical Nurse Education and Services
NCCAM	National Center for Complementary and Alternative Medicine
NCHS	National Center for Health Statistics
NCLEX®	National Council Licensure Examination
NCLEX-PN®	National Council Licensure Examination—Practical Nurse
NCLEX-RN®	National Council Licensure Examination—Registered Nurse
NCLD	National Center for Learning Disabilities
NCOA	National Council on Aging
NCSBN	National Council of State Boards of Nursing
NCVHS	National Committee on Vital and Health Statistics
NF	*National Formulary*
NFLPN	National Federation of Licensed Practical Nurses, Inc.
NG	nasogastric
NH_2	amino group
NHO	National Hospice Organization
NIA	National Institute on Aging
NIC	Nursing Interventions Classification
NIH	National Institutes of Health
NIOSH	National Institute of Occupational Safety and Health
NIS	nursing information system
NLEA	Nutrition, Labeling, and Education Act
NLN	National League for Nursing
NLNAC	National League for Nursing Accrediting Commission
NMDS	nursing minimum data set
NOC	Nursing Outcomes Classification
NP	nurse practitioner
NPDB	National Practitioner Data Bank
NPO	*nil per os,* Latin for "nothing by mouth"
NREM	non-rapid eye movement
NS	normal saline
NSAID	nonsteroidal anti-inflammatory drug
NSF	National Sleep Foundation
O_2	oxygen
OAM	Office of Alternative Medicine
O&P	ova and parasite
OBRA	Omnibus Budget Reconciliation Act
OD	right eye
OH^-	hydroxyl
OR	operating room
ORIF	open reduction/internal fixation
OS	left eye
OSHA	Occupational Safety and Health Administration
OT	occupational therapist
OT	oral temperature

OTC over-the-counter
OU both eyes
oz ounce
$\bar{p}$ after
P phosphorus
P pulse
PA physician's assistant
PA posterioanterior
$PaCO_2$ partial pressure of carbon dioxide
PaO_2 partial pressure of oxygen
Pap Papanicolaou test
p.c. after meals
PCA patient-controlled analgesia
PCO_2 ($PaCO_2$) partial pressure of carbon dioxide
PCP primary care provider
PCR polymerase chain reaction
PCV pneumococcal conjugate vaccine
PDPH postdural puncture headache
PEG percutaneous endoscopic gastrostomy
PERRLA pupils equal, round, reactive to light and accommodation
PET positron emission tomography
PFT pulmonary function test
pH potential hydrogen
PICC peripherally inserted central catheter
PIE problem, implementation, evaluation
PKU phenylketonuria
PLMS periodic limb movements in sleep
PMI point of maximum intensity
PMR progressive muscle relaxation
PMS premenstrual syndrome
PNI psychoneuroimmunology
PNS peripheral nervous system
po *per os,* Latin for "by mouth"
PO_2 (PaO_2) partial pressure of oxygen
PO_4^{--} phosphate ion
POMR problem-oriented medical record
POR problem-oriented record
PPBS post prandial blood sugar
PPE personal protective equipment
PPG post prandial glucose
PPO preferred provider organization
PPS prospective payment system
PRA plama renin activity
PRL prolactin level
PRN *pro re nata,* Latin for "as required"
PRO peer review organization
PROM passive range of motion
PSA prostate specific antigen
PSDA Patient Self-Determination Act
PSP phenolsulfonphtalein
pt pint
PT physical therapist
PT prothrombin time
PTH parathyroid hormone
PTSD post-traumatic stress disorder
PTT partial thromboplastin time
PVD peripheral vascular disease
q *quaque,* Latin for "every"
qd every day
qh every hour
qid four times a day
qod every other day
qs quantity sufficient
q2h every 2 hours
qt quart
R (Resp) respiration
RAIU radioactive iodine uptake
RAST radio allergosorbent test
RBC red blood count, red blood cell
RD registered dietician
RDA recommended dietary allowance
REM rapid eye movement
RF rheumatoid factor
RLQ right lower quadrant
RLS restless leg syndrome
RN registered nurse
RNA ribonucleic acid
RNFA registered nurse first assistant
ROM range of motion
ROS review of systems
RPCH rural primary care hospital
RPh registered pharmacist
RPR rapid plasma reagin
RR recovery room
RSV respiratory syncytial virus
R/T related to
RT rectal temperature
RT respiratory therapist
RTI respiratory tract infection
RUGS resource utilization group system
RUQ right upper quadrant
RWJF Robert Wood Johnson Foundation
$\bar{s}$ without
S sulfur
SAMe S-adenosylmethionine
SaO_2 oxygen saturation
SBC school-based clinic
SC/SQ subcutaneous
SCHIP State Children's Health Insurance Program
Se selenium
SGOT serum glutamate oxaloacetate transaminase
SGPT serum glutamic pyruvic transaminase
SL sublingual
SNF skilled nursing facility
SOAP subjective data, objective data, assessment, plan
SOAPIE subjective data, objective data, assessment, plan, implementation, evaluation
SOAPIER subjective data, objective data, assessment, plan, implementation, evaluation, revision
SPF sun protection factor
$\bar{s}\bar{s}$ one half
SSA Social Security Administration
STAT *statim,* Latin for "immediately"
STD sexually transmitted disease

supp suppository
susp suspension
SW social worker
T temperature
T_3 triiodothyronine
T_4 thyroxine
tab tablet
TAC tetracaine, adrenaline, cocaine
TB tuberculosis
Tbsp tablespoon
Td tetanus/diphtheria
TDD telecommunication device for the deaf
TEFRA Tax Equity Fiscal Responsibility Act
TENS transcutaneous electrical nerve stimulation
TF tube feeding
THA total hip arthroplasty
TIA transient ischemic attack
TIBC total iron binding capacity
t.i.d. three times a day
TMJ temporomandibular joint
t.o. telephone order
TPN total parenteral nutrition
TPR temperature, pulse, respirations
Tr or tinct tincture
TRH thyrotropin-releasing hormone
TSE testicular self examination
TSH thyroid-stimulating hormone
tsp teaspoon
U unit
U/L unit per liter
UA routine urinalysis
UAP unlicensed assistive personnel
UIS Universal Intellectual Standards
UL upper intake level
UMLS Universal Medical Language System
UNOS United Network for Organ Sharing
U-100 100 units insulin per cc
UPP urethra pressure profile
URQ upper right quadrant
USDHHS United States Department of Health and Human Services
USP *United States Pharmacopeia*
USPHS United States Public Health Service
UTI urinary tract infection
VA Veterans Administration, Veterans Affairs
VAD ventricular assist device, vascular access device
VAS Visual Analog Scale
VDRL venereal disease research laboratory
VLDL very low-density lipoprotein
VMA vanilymandelic acid
VRE vancomycin-resistant enterococci
VS vital signs
WASP white, Anglo-Saxon, Protestant
WBC white blood cell, white blood count
WHO World Health Organization
WNL within normal limits
WPM words per minute
wt weight
YWCA Young Women's Christian Association
Zn Zinc

APPENDIX D
English/Spanish Words and Phrases

Being able to say a few words or phrases in the client's language is one way to show that you care. It lets the client know that you as a nurse are interested in the individual. There are three rules to keep in mind regarding the pronunciation of Spanish words.

- If a word ends in a vowel, or in *n* or *s,* the accent is on the next to the last syllable.
- If the word ends in a consonant other than *n* or *s,* the accent is on the last syllable.
- If the word does not follow these rules, it has a written accent over the vowel of the accented syllable.

Courtesy phrases, names of body parts, and expressions of time and numbers are included in this section for quick reference. The English version will appear first, followed by the Spanish translation and Spanish pronunciation.

Courtesy Phrases

Please	Por favor	Por fah-**vor**
Thank-you	Grácias	**Grah**-the-as
Good morning	Buénos dias	Boo-**ay**-nos **dee**-as
Good afternoon	Buénas tardes	Boo-**ay**-nas **tar**-days
Good evening	Buénas noches	Boo-**ay**-nas **no**-chays
Yes/No	Si/no	See/no
Good	Bien	Be-en
Bad	Mal	Mahl
How many?	¿Cuántos?	¿Coo-**ahn**-tos?
Where?	¿Dónde?	¿**Don**-day?
When?	¿Cuándo?	¿Coo**ahn**-do?

Body Parts

abdomen	el abdomen	el ab-doh-men
ankle	el tobillo	el to-**beel**-lyo
anus	el ano	el **ah**-no
anvil (incus)	el yunque	el **yoon**-kay
appendix	el apéndice	el ah-**pen**-de-thay
aqueous humor	el humor acuoso	el oo-**mor** ah-coo-**o**-so
bladder	la vejiga	lah vay-**nee**-gah
brain	el cerebro	el thay-**ray**-bro
breast	el pecho	el **pay**-cho
buttock	la nalga	lah **nahl**-gah
calf	la pantorrilla	lah pan-tor-**reel**-lyah
cervix	la cerviz	lah ther-**veth**
cheek	la mejilla	lah may-**heel**-lyah

chin	la barbilla	lah bar-**beel**-lyah
choroid	la coroidea	lah co-ro-e-**day**-ah
ciliary body	el cuerpo ciliar	el coo-**err**-po the-le-**ar**
clitoris	el clítoris	el **clee**-to-ris
coccyx	el coxis	el **coc**-sees
conjunctiva	la conjuntiva	lah con-hoon-**tee**vah
cornea	la córnea	lah **cor**-nay-ah
penis	el pene	el **pay**-nay
prostate gland	la próstata	lah **pros**-ta-tah
pupil	la pupila	lah poo-**pee**-lah
rectum	el recto	el **rec**-to
retina	la retina	lah ray-**tee**-nah
sclera	la esclerótica	lah es-clay-**ro**-te-cah
scrotum	el escroto	el es-**cro**-to
seminal vesicle	la vesícula seminal	lah vay-**see**-coo-lah say-me-**nahl**
shoulder	el hombro	el **om**-bro
small intestine	el intestino delgado	el in-tes-**tee**-no del-**gah**-do
spinal cord	la médula espinal	lah **may**-doo-lah es-pe-**nahl**
spleen	el bazo	el **bah**-tho
stirrup (stapes)	el estribo	el es-**tree**-bo
stomach	el estómago	el es-**toh**-mah-go
temple	la sien	lah se-**ayn**
testis	el testículo	el tes-**tee**-coo-lo
thigh	el muslo	el **moos**-lo
thorax	el tórax	el **to**-rax
tongue	la lengua	lah **len**-goo-ah
trachea	la tráquea	lah **trah**-kay-ah
upper extremities	las extremidades superiores	las ex-tray-me-**dahd**-es soo-pay-re-**or**-es
ureter	el uréter	el oo-**ray**-ter
uterus	el útero	el **oo**-tay-ro
vagina	el vagina	lah vah-**hee**-nah
vitreous humor	el humor vítreo	el oo-**mor vee**-tray-o
wrist	la muñeca	lah moo-**nyay**-cah

Expressions of Time, Calendar, and Numbers

after meals	después de comer	des-poo-**es** day co-**merr**
at bedtime	al acostarse	al ah-cos-**tar**-say
before meals	antes de comer	**ahn**-tes day co-**merr**
daily	el diario	el de-**ah**-re-o
date	la fecha	lah **fay**-chah
day	el dia	el **dee**-ah
every hour	a cada hora	ah **cah**-dah **o**-rah
hour (time)	la hora	lah **o**-rah
how often	cada cuánto tiempo	**cah**-dah coo-**ahn**-to te-**em**-po
noon	el mediodia	el may-de-o-**dee**-ah
now	ahora	ah-**o**-rah
once	una vez	**oo**-nah veth
today	hoy	**oh**-e
tomorrow	mañana	mah-**nyah**-nah
tonight	esta noche	**es**-tah **no**-chay
week	la semana	lah say-**mah**-nah
year	año	**a**-nyo
Sunday	el domingo	el do-**meen**-go
Monday	el lunes	el **loo**-nes
Tuesday	el martes	el **mar**-tes
Wednesday	el miércoles	el me-**err**-co-les
Thursday	el jueves	el hoo-**ayves**
Friday	el viernes	el ve-**err**-nes

Saturday	el sábado	el **sah**-bah-do
zero	cero	**thay**-ro
one	uno	**oo**-no
two	dos	dose
three	tres	trays
four	cuatro	coo-**ah**-tro
five	cinco	**theen**-co
six	seis	**say**-ees
seven	siete	se-**ay**-tay
eight	ocho	**o**-cho
nine	nueve	noo-**ay**-vay
ten	diez	de-**eth**

Nursing Care Sentences and Questions

What is your name?
¿Como se llama usted?
¿**Co**-mo say **lyah**-mah oos-**ted?**

I am a student nurse.
Soy estudiente enfermera(o).
Soy es-too-de-**ahn**-tay en-fer-**may**-ra(o).

My name is . . .
Mi nombre es . . .
Mee **nom**-bray es . . .

Do you need a wheelchair?
¿Necesita usted una silla de rueda?
¿Nay-thay-**se**-ta oos-**ted oo**-nah **seel**-lyah day roo-**ay**-dah?

How do you feel?
¿Como se siente?
¿**Co**-mo say se-**ayn**-tah?

When is your family coming?
¿Cuándo viene su familia?
¿Coo-**ahn**-do vee-**en**-nah soo fah-**mee**-le-ah?

This is the call light.
Esta es la luz para llamar a la enfermera.
Es-tah es lah looth **pah**-ra lyah-**mar** a lah en-fer-**may**-ra.

If you need anything, press the button.
Si usted necesita algo, oprima el botón.
See oos-**ted** nay-thay-**se**-ta **ahl**-go o-pre-**ma** el bo-**tone.**

Do not turn without calling the nurse.
No se voltee sin llamar a la enfermera.
No say **vol**-tay seen lyah-**mar** a lah en-fer-**may**-ra.

The side rails on your bed are for your protection.
Los rieles del costado están para su protección.
Los re-**el**-es del cos-**tah**-do es-**tahn pah**-ra soo pro-tec-the-**on.**

Please do not try to lower or climb over the side rail.
Por favor no pretenda bajarlos (barjarlas) o treparse sobre ellos.
Por fah-**vor** no pray-**ten**-dah ba-**har**-los o tray-**par**-say **so**-bray **ayl**-lyos.

The head nurse is . . .
La jefa de enfermeras es . . .
La **hay**-fay day en-fer-**may**-ras es . . .

Do you need more blankets or another pillow?
¿Necesita usted más frazadas u orta almohada?
¿Nay-thay-**si**-ta oos-**ted** mahs frah-**thad**-dahs oo **o**-trah al-mo-**ah**-dah?

You may not smoke in the room.
No se puede fumar en el cuarto.
No say poo-**ay**-day foo-**mar** en el coo-**ar**-to.

Do you want me to turn on (turn off) the lights?
¿Quiere usted que encienda (apague) la luz?
¿Ke-**ay**-ray oos-**ted** day en-the-**en**-dah (a-**pah**-gay) lah looth?

Are you thirsty?
¿Tiene usted sed?
¿Tee-**en**-nah oos-**ted** sayd?

Are you allergic to any medication?
¿Es usted alérgico(a) a alguna medicina?
¿Es oos-**ted** ah-**lehr**-hee-co(a) ah ah-**goo**-nah nay-de-**thee**-nah?

You may take a bath.
Usted puede bañarse.
Oos-**ted** poo-**ay**-day bah-**nyar**-say.

Do not lock the door, please.
No cierre usted la puerta con llave, por favor.
No the-**err**-ray oos-**ted** lah poo-**err**-tah con **lyah**-vay por fah-**vor.**

Call if you feel faint or in need of help.
Llame si usted se siente débil o si necesita ayuda.
Lyah-mah see oos-**ted** say se-**ayn**-tah **day**-bil o see nay-thay-**se**-ta ah-**yoo**-dah.

Call when you have to go to the toilet.
Llame cuando tenga que ir al inodoro.
Lyah-mah coo-**ahn**-do **ten**-gah kay eer al in-o-**do**-ro.

I will give you an enema.
Le pondré una enema.
Lay pon-**dray oo**-nah ay-**nay**-mah.

Turn on your left (right) side.
Voltese a su lado izquierdo (derecho).
Vol-**tay**-say ah soo **lah**-do ith-ke-**er**-do(dah) (day-**ray**-cho[cha]).

Here is an appointment card.
Aqui tiene usted una tarjeta con la información escrito.
Ah-**kee** tee-**en**-nah oos-**ted oo**-nah tar-**hay**-tah con lah in-for-mah-the-**on** es-**cree**-to.

You are going to be discharged (released) today.
A usted le van a dar de alta hoy.
Ah oos-**ted** lay vahn ah dar day **ahl**-tah **oh**-e.

How did this illness begin?
¿Como empezó esta enfermedad?
¿**Co**-mo em-pa-**tho es**-tah en-fer-may-**dahd**?

Is the pain better after the medicine?
¿Siente usted alivio depués de tomar la medicina?
¿Se-**ayn**-tah oos-**ted** al-**lee**-ve-o des-poo-**es** day to-**mar** lah may-de-**thee**-nah?

Where is the pain?
¿Que la duele? (or) Dónde le duele?
¿Kay lah doo-**ay**-le? (or) **Don**-day lay doo-**ay**-le?

Do you have pains in your chest?
¿Tiene usted dolores in el pecho?
¿Tee-**en**-nah oos-**ted** do-**lor**-es en el **pay**-cho?

Are you in pain now?
¿Tiene usted dolores ahora?
¿Tee-**en**-nah oos-**ted** do-**lor**-es ah-**o**-rah?

Is it constant pain or does it come and go?
¿Es un dolor constante o va y vuelve?
¿Es oon do-**lor** cons-**tahn**-tay o vah ee voo-**el**-vah?

Is there anything that makes the pain better?
¿Hay algo que lo alivie?
¿**Ah**-ee **ahl**-go kay lo al-**le**-ve?

Is there anything that makes the pain worse?
¿Hay algo que lo aumente?
¿**Ah**-ee **ahl**-go kay lo ah-oo-**men**-tay?

Where do you feel the pain?
¿Dónde siente usted el dolor?
¿**Don**-day se-**ayn**-tah oos-**ted** el do-**lor**?

Point to where it hurts.
Apunte usted por favor, adonde le duele.
Ah-**poon**-tay oos-**ted** por fah-**vor** ah-**don**-day lay doo-**ay**-le.

Show me where it hurts.
Enséñeme usted donde le duele.
En-**say**-nah-may oos-**ted don**-day lay doo-**ay**-le.

Is the pain sharp or dull?
¿Es agudo o sordo el dolor?
¿Es ah-**goo**-do o **sor**-do el do-**lor**?

Do you know where you are?
¿Sabe usted donde esta?
¿Sah-**bay** oos-**ted don**-day es-**tah**?

You are in the hospital.
Usted está en el hospital.
Oos-**ted** es-**tah** en el os-pee-**tahl**.

You will be okay.
Usted va a estar bien.
Oos-**ted** vah a es-**tar be**-en.

Do you have any drug reactions?
¿Tiene usted alguna sensibilidad a productos químicos?
¿Te-**en**-nah oos-**ted** al-**goo**-nah sen-se-be-le-**dahd** a pro-**dooc**-tos **kee**-me-cos?

Have you seen another doctor or native healer for this problem?
¿Ha visto usted a otro médico o curandero tocante a este problema?
¿Ah **vees**-to oos-**ted** a **o**-tro **may**-de-co o coo-ran-**day**-ro to-**cahn**-tay a **es**-ah pro-**blay**-mah?

Have you vomited?
¿Ha vomitado usted?
¿Ah vo-me-**tah**-do oos-**ted**?

Do you have any difficulty in breathing?
¿Tiene usted alguna dificultad para respirar?
¿Te-**en**-nah oos-**ted** ah-**goo**-nah de-fe-cool-**tahd pah**-ra res-pe-**rar**?

Do you smoke?
¿Fuma usted?
¿Foo-**mar** oos-**ted**?

How many per day?
¿Cuántos al dia?
¿Coo-**ahn**-tos al **dee**-ah?

For how many years?
¿Por cuántos años?
¿por coo-**ahn**-tos **a**-nyos?

Do you awaken in the night because of shortness of breath?
¿Se despierta usted por la noche por falta de respiración?
¿Say des-pee-**err**-tah oos-**ted** por lah **no**-chay por **fahl**-tah day res-pe-rah-the-**on**?

Is any part of your body swollen?
¿Tiene usted alguna parte del cuerpo hinchada?
¿Te-**en**-nah oos-**ted** ah-**goo**-nah **par**-tay del coo-**err**-po in-**chah**-da?

How much water do you drink daily?
¿Cuántos vasos de agua bebe usted diariamente?
¿Coo-**ahn**-tos **vah**-sos day **ah**-goo-ah **bay**-be oos-**ted** de-ah-re-ah-**men**-tay?

Are you nauseated?
¿Tiene náusea?
¿Te-**en**-nah **nah**-oo-say-ah?

Are you going to vomit?
¿Va a vomitar?
¿Vah a vo-me-**tar**?

When was your last bowel movement?
¿Cuánto tiempo hace que evacúa usted?
¿Coo-**ahn**-to te-**em**-po **ah**-the kay ay-vah-**coo**-ah oos-**ted**?

Do you have diarrhea?
¿Tiene usted diarrea?
¿Te-**en**-nah oos-**ted** der-ar-**ray**-ah?

How much do you urinate?
¿Cuánto orina usted?
¿Coo-**ahn**-to o-**re**-nah oos-**ted**?

Did you urinate?
¿Orinó usted?
¿O-re-**no** oos-**ted**?

What color is your urine?
¿De qué color es la orina?
¿Day kay co-**lor** es lah o-**re**-nah?

Call when you have to go to the toilet.
Llame usted cuando tenga que ir al inodoro.
Lyah-mah oos-**ted** coo-**ahn**-do **ten**-gah kay eer al in-o-**do**-ro.

I need a urine specimen from you.
Necesito una muestra de orina de usted.
Nay-thay-**se**-to **oo**-nah moo-**ays**-trah day o-**re**-nah day oos-**ted**.

We will put a tube in your bladder so that you can urinate.
Le pondremos un tubo en la vejiga para que puede orinar.
Lay pon-**dray**-mos un **too**-be en lah vay-**hee**-gah **pah**-rah kay poo-**ay**-day o-re **nar.**

When was your last menstrual period?
¿Cuándo fue se última menstruación?
¿Coo-**ahn**-do foo-**ay** soo **ool**-te-mah mens-troo-ah-the-**on?**

Are you bleeding heavily?
¿Está sangrando mucho?
¿Es-**tah** san-**grahn**-do **moo**-cho?

Take off your clothes, please
Desvístase usted, por favor.
Des-**ves**-tah-say oos-**ted** por-fah-**vor.**

Just relax.
Relaje usted el cuerpo.
Ray-**lah**-he oos-**ted** el coo-**err**-po.

I am going to listen to your chest.
Voy a escucharle el pecho.
Voye a es-coo-**char**-lay el **pay**-cho.

Let me feel your pulse.
Déjeme tomarle el pulso.
Day-ha-me to-**bar**-lay el **pool**-so.

I am going to take your temperature.
Voy a tomarle la temperatura.
Voye a to-**mar**-lay lah tem-pay-rah-**too**-rah.

Lie down, please.
Acuéstese, por favor.
Ah-coo-**es**-tah-say por fah-**vor.**

Do you understand?
¿Me comprende usted?
¿May com-**pren**-day oos-**ted?**

That's right.
Así. Bien.
Ah-**see. Be**-en.

You are doing very well.
Usted va muy bien.
Oos-**ted** vah **moo**-e **be**-en.

Do not take any medicine from home.
No tome usted ninguna medicina traída de su casa.
No **to**-may oos-**ted** nin-**goon**-ay may-de-**thee**-nah trah-**ee**-dah day soo **cah**-sah.

I am going to give you an injection.
Voy a ponerle ana inyección.
Voye a po-**nerr**-lay **oo**-nah in-yec-the-**on.**

Take a sip of water.
Tome usted un traguito de agua.
To-may oos-**ted** un trah-**gee**-to day **ah**-goo-ah.

Very good. That was fine.
Muy bien. Excelente.
Moo-e **be**-en. Ex-thay-**len**-tay.

Don't be nervous.
No se ponga nervioso(a).
No say **pon**-gah ner-ve-**o**-so(ah).

Do you feel dizzy?
¿Se siente vertigo?
¿Say see-**ayn**-tah **verr**-to-go?

Please lie still.
Quédese inmóvil, por favor.
Kay-day-say in-**mo**-veel por fah-**vor.**

You must drink lots of liquids.
Usted debe tomar muchos líquidos.
Oos-**ted day**-bay to-**mar moo**-chos **lee**-ke-dos.

REFERENCES

Kelz, R. K. (1982.) *Conversational Spanish for Medical Personnel.* Clifton Park, NY: Delmar Cengage Learning.

Velazquez de la Cadena, M., Gray, E., & Iribas, J. (1985). *New Revised Velazquez Spanish and English Dictionary.* Clinton, NJ: New Win Publishing, Inc.

GLOSSARY

A

abduction Lateral movement away from the body

ability Competence in an activity

abortion Termination of pregnancy before the age of fetal viability, usually 24 weeks

abruptio placenta Premature separation, from the wall of the uterus, of normally implanted placenta

absorption Passage of a drug from the site of administration into the bloodstream; process whereby the end products of digestion pass through the epithelial membranes in the small and large intestines and into the blood or lymph system

abuse Incident involving some type of violation to the client; misuse, excessive, or improper use of a substance, the absence of which does not cause withdrawal symptoms

acanthosis nigricans A velvety hyperpigmented patch on the back of neck, in axilla, or anticubital area found in children with type 2 diabetes

accreditation Process by which a voluntary, nongovernmental agency or organization appraises and grants accredited status to institutions, programs, services, or any combination of these that meet predetermined structure, process, and outcome criteria

acculturation Process of learning beliefs, norms, and behavioral expectations of a group

acid Any substance that in a solution yields hydrogen ions bearing a positive charge

acidosis Condition characterized by an excessive number of hydrogen ions in a solution

acme Peak of a contraction

acquired immunity Formation of antibodies (memory B cells) to protect against future invasions of an already experienced antigen

acquired immunodeficiency syndrome (AIDS) Progressively fatal disease that destroys the immune system and the body's ability to fight infection; caused by the human immunodeficiency virus (HIV)

acrocyanosis Blue coloring of hands and feet

actively suicidal Descriptor of an individual intent upon hurting or killing him- or herself and who is in imminent danger of doing so

activities of daily living Basic care activities that include mobility, bathing, hygiene, grooming, dressing, eating, and toileting

acupressure Technique of releasing blocked energy within an individual when specific points (tsubas) along the meridians are pressed or massaged by the practitioner's fingers, thumbs, and heel of the hands

acupuncture Technique of application of needles and heat to various points on the body to alter the energy flow

acute pain Has a sudden onset, relatively short duration, mild to severe intensity, with a steady decrease in intensity over several days or weeks

adaptation Ongoing process whereby individuals use various responses to adjust to stressors and change; change resulting from assimilation and accommodation

adaptive energy Inner forces that an individual uses to adapt to stress (phrase coined by Selye)

adaptive measure Measure for coping with stress that requires a minimal amount of energy

addiction Overwhelming preoccupation with obtaining and using a drug for its psychic effects; used interchangeably with dependence

adhesion Internal scar tissue from previous surgeries or disease processes

adjuvant medication Drug used to enhance the analgesic efficacy of opioids, treat concurrent symptoms that exacerbate pain, and provide independent analgesia for specific types of pain

adult day care Centers that provide a variety of services in a protective setting for adults who are unable to stay alone but who do not need 24-hour care; the centers are located in a separate unit of a long-term care facility, in a private home, or are freestanding

adventitious breath sound Abnormal sound, including sibilant wheezes (formerly wheezes), sonorous wheezes (formerly rhonchi), fine and course crackles (formerly rales), pleural friction rubs, and stridor

affect Outward expression of mood or emotions

affective domain Area of learning that involves attitudes, beliefs, and emotions

afferent nerve pathway Ascending spinal cord pathway that transmits sensory impulses to the brain

afferent pain pathway Ascending spinal cord

afterpains Discomfort caused by the contracting uterus after the infant's birth

age appropriate care Nursing care that takes into consideration the client's physical, mental, emotional, and spiritual developmental levels

age of viability Gestational age at which a fetus could live outside the uterus, generally considered to be 24 weeks

agent Entity capable of causing disease

agglutination Clumping together of red blood cells

agglutinin Specific kind of antibody whose interaction with antigens is manifested as agglutination

agglutinogen Any antigenic substance that causes agglutination by the production of agglutinin

agnosia Inability to recognize, either by sight or sound, familiar objects such as a hairbrush

agnostic Individual who believes that the existence of God cannot be proved or disproved

agranulocytosis Acute condition causing a severe reduction in the number of granulocytes (basophils, eosinophils, and neutrophils)

Airborne Precautions Measures taken in addition to Standard Precautions and for clients known to have or suspected of having illnesses spread by airborne droplet nuclei

airborne transmission Transfer of an agent to a susceptible host through droplet nuclei or dust particles suspended in the air

Aldrete Score Scoring system for objectively assessing the physical status of clients recovering from anesthesia; serves as a basis for dismissal from the postanesthesia care unit (PACU) and ambulatory surgery; also known as the postanesthetic recovery score

algor mortis Decrease in body temperature after death, resulting in lack of skin elasticity

alkalosis Condition characterized by an excessive loss of hydrogen ions from a solution

allergen Type of antigen commonly found in the environment

allogeneic From a donor of the same species

alopecia Partial or complete baldness or loss of hair

alternative therapy Therapy used instead of conventional or mainstream medical practices

ambulatory care A facility that provides clients diagnostic treatment, medical treatment, preventive care, and rehabilitative care on an outpatient basis

ambulatory surgery Surgical operation performed under general, regional, or local anesthesia, involving less than 24 hours of hospitalization

amenorrhea Absence of menstruation

amnesia Inability to remember things

amniocentesis Withdrawal of amniotic fluid to obtain a sample for specimen examination

amnion Inner fetal membrane originating in the blastocyst

amniotomy Artificial rupture of the membranes

amphiarthrosis Articulation of slightly movable joints such as the vertebrae

amputation Removal of all or part of an extremity

anabolism Constructive process of metabolism whereby new molecules are synthesized and new tissues are formed, as in growth and repair

analgesia Pain relief without producing anesthesia

analgesic Substance that relieves pain

analyte Substance that is measured

anaphylaxis Type I systemic reaction to allergens

anasarca Generalized edema

anesthesia Absence of normal sensation

anesthesiologist Licensed physician educated and skilled in the delivery of anesthesia who also adds to the knowledge of anesthesia through research or other scholarly pursuits

anesthetist Qualified RN, dentist, or medical doctor who administers anesthetics

aneurysm Weakness in the wall of a blood vessel

anger control assistance Nursing intervention aimed at facilitating the expression of anger in an adaptive and nonviolent manner

angina pectoris Chest pain caused by a narrowing of the coronary arteries

angiocatheter Intracatheter with a metal stylet

angioedema Allergic reaction consisting of edema of subcutaneous tissue, mucous membranes, or viscera

angiogenesis Formation of new blood vessels

angiography Visualization of the vascular structures through the use of fluoroscopy with a contrast medium

angioma Benign vascular tumor involving skin and subcutaneous tissue; most are congenital

anion Ion bearing a negative charge

annulus Valvular ring in the heart
anorexia Loss of appetite
anosognosia Lack of awareness of own neurological deficits
anthrax An acute, infectious disease caused by the bacterium Bacillus anthracis, which has an incubation period of 2-60 days; it is an Important potential agent for bioterrorism
anthropometric measurements Measurements of the size, weight, and proportions of the body
antibody Immunoglobulin produced by the body in response to bacteria, viruses, or other antigenic substances; destroys antigens
anticipatory grief Occurrence of grief before an expected loss actually occurs
anticipatory guidance Information, teaching, and guidance given to a client in anticipation of an expected event
antigen Any substance identified by the body as nonself
antineoplastic Agent that inhibits the growth and reproduction of malignant cells
antioxidant Substance that prevents or inhibits oxidation, a chemical process wherein a substance is joined to oxygen
antipyretic Drug used to reduce an abnormally high temperature
anxiety Subjective response that occurs when a person experiences a real or perceived threat to well-being; a diverse feeling of dread or apprehension
anxiolytic Antianxiety medication
aphasia Absence of speech; often the result of a brain lesion
apheresis Removal of unwanted blood components
appendicitis Inflammation of the vermiform appendix
appropriate for gestational age Infant's weight falls between the 90th and 10th percentile for gestational age
areflexia Absence of reflexes
aromatherapy Therapeutic use of concentrated essences or essential oils extracted from plants and flowers
arousal State of wakefulness and alertness
arterial blood gases Measurement of levels of oxygen, carbon dioxide, pH, partial pressure of oxygen (PO2 or PaO2), partial pressure of carbon dioxide (PCO2 or PaCO2), saturation of oxygen (SaO2), and bicarbonate (HCO3) in arterial blood
arteriography Radiographic study of the vascular system following the injection of a radiopaque dye through a catheter
arteriosclerosis Cardiovascular disease wherein plaque forms on the inside of artery walls, reducing the space for blood flow
arthroplasty Replacement of both articular surfaces within a joint capsule
ascites Abnormal accumulation of fluid in the peritoneal cavity
asepsis Absence of pathogenic microorganisms
aseptic technique Collection of principles used to control and/or prevent the transfer of pathogenic microorganisms from sources within (endogenous) and outside (exogenous) the client
aspiration Procedure performed to withdraw fluid that has abnormally collected or to obtain a specimen; also inhalation of secretion or fluids into the pulmonary system
assent Voluntary agreement to participate in a research project or to accept treatment
assisted living A facility that combines housing and services for persons who require assistance with activities of daily living
asthma Condition characterized by intermittent airway obstruction due to antigen antibody reaction
astigmatism Asymmetric focus of light rays on the retina
ataxia Inability to coordinate voluntary muscle action
atelectasis Collapse of a lung or a portion of a lung
atheist Individual who does not believe in God or any other deity
atherosclerosis Cardiovascular disease of fatty deposits on the inner lining, the tunica intima, of vessel walls
atom Smallest unit of an element that still retains the properties of that element and that cannot be altered by any chemical change
atresia Absence or closure of a body orifice
attachment Long-term process that begins during pregnancy and intensifies during the postpartum period, which establishes an enduring bond between parent and child, and develops through reciprocal (parent-to-child and child-to-parent) behaviors
attitude Manner, feeling, or position toward a person or thing
attribute Characteristic that belongs to an individual
audible wheeze Wheeze that can be heard without the aid of a stethoscope
auditory hallucination Perception by an individual that someone is talking when no one in fact is there
auditory learner Person who learns by processing information through hearing
augmentation of labor Stimulation of uterine contractions after spontaneously beginning but having unsatisfactory progress of labor
aura Peculiar sensation preceding a seizure or migraine; may be a taste, smell, sight, sound, dizziness, or just a "funny feeling"

auscultation Physical examination technique that involves listening to sounds in the body that are created by movement of air or fluid
autoimmune disorder Disease wherein the body identifies its own cells as foreign and activates mechanisms to destroy them
autologous From the same organism (person)
automatism Mechanical, repetitive motor behavior performed unconsciously
autonomic nervous system That part of the peripheral nervous system consisting of the sympathetic and parasympathetic nervous systems and controlling unconscious activities
autonomy Self-direction; ethical principle based on the individual's right to choose and the individual's ability to act on that choice
autopsy Examination of a body after death by a pathologist to determine cause of death
autosomal Pertaining to a condition transmitted by a nonsex chromosome
awareness Capacity to perceive sensory impressions through thoughts and actions
azotemia Nitrogenous wastes present in the blood

B

bacteremia Condition of bacteria in the blood
bactericide Bacteria-killing chemicals; found in tears
ballottement Rebounding of the floating fetus when pushed upward through the vagina or abdomen
bands Immature neutrophils
barium Chalky-white contrast medium
Barrier Precautions Use of personal protective equipment, such as masks, gowns, and gloves, to create a barrier between the person and the microorganisms and thus prevent transmission of the microorganism
basal metabolism Energy needed to maintain essential physiologic functions when a person is at complete rest; the lowest level of energy expenditure
base Substance that when dissociated produces ions that will combine with hydrogen ions
baseline level Lab value that serves as a reference point for future value levels
behavioral tolerance Compensatory adjustments of behavior made under the influence of a particular substance
benign Not progressive; favorable for recovery
bereavement Period of grief that follows the death of a loved one
bioavailability Readiness to produce a drug effect
biofeedback Measures physiologic responses that assist individuals to improve their health by using signals from their own bodies
biologic response modifier Agent that destroys malignant cells by stimulating the body's immune system
biological agent Living organism that invades a host, causing disease
biological clock Internal mechanism in a living organism capable of measuring time
biopsy Excision of a small amount of tissue
bioterrorism the purposeful use of a biological preparation for the purposes of harming, killing large numbers of people, and/or instilling fear in large numbers of people
blanching White color of the skin when pressure is applied
blastic phase Intensified phase of leukemia that resembles an acute phase in which there is an increased production of white blood cells
blastocyst Cluster of cells that will develop into the embryo
bloody show Expulsion of cervical secretions, blood-tinged mucus, and the mucus plug that blocked the cervix during pregnancy
body image Individual's perception of physical self, including appearance, function, and ability
body mass index Measurement used to ascertain whether a person's weight is appropriate for height; calculated by dividing the weight in kilograms by the height in meters squared
body mechanics Use of the body to safely and efficiently move or lift objects
bodymind Inseparable connection and operation of thoughts, feelings, and physiologic functions
bonding Rapid process of attachment, parent to infant, that takes place during the sensitive period, the first 30 to 60 minutes after birth
borborygmi High-pitched, loud, rushing sounds produced by the movement of gas in the liquid contents of the intestine
bradycardia Heart rate less than 60 beats per minute in an adult
bradykinesia Slowness of voluntary movement and speech
bradypnea Respiratory rate of 10 or fewer breaths per minute
Braxton-Hicks contractions Irregular, intermittent contractions felt by the pregnant woman toward the end of pregnancy
breakthrough pain Sudden, acute, temporary pain that is usually precipitated by a treatment, a procedure, or unusual activity of the client
brief dynamic therapy Short-term psychotherapy that focuses on resolving core conflicts deriving from personality and living situations

bronchial sound Loud, high-pitched, hollow-sounding breath sound normally heard over the sternum; longer on expiration than inspiration
bronchiectasis Lung disorder characterized by chronic dilation of the bronchi
bronchitis Inflammation of the bronchial tree accompanied by hypersecretion of mucus
bronchovesicular sound Breath sound normally heard in the area of the scapula and near the sternum; medium in pitched blowing sound, with inspiratory and expiratory phases of equal length
bruxism Grinding of teeth during sleep
buffer Substance that attempts to maintain pH range, or hydrogen ion concentration, in the presence of added acids or bases
burnout State of physical and emotional exhaustion occurring when caregivers use up their adaptive energy
butterfly needle Wing-tipped needle

C

cachectic Being in a state of malnutrition and wasting
cachexia State of malnutrition and protein wasting
calculus Concentration of mineral salts in the body leading to the formation of stone
calorie Amount of heat required to raise the temperature of 1 gram of water 1 degree Celsius
cancer Disease resulting from the uncontrolled growth of cells, which causes malignant cellular tumors
capitated rate Preset fee based on membership rather than services provided; payment system used in managed care
caput succedaneum Edema of the newborn's scalp which is present at birth, may cross suture lines, and is caused by head compression against the cervix
carcinogen Substance that initiates or promotes the development of cancer
carcinoma Cancer occurring in epithelial tissue
cardiac cycle Cycle of an impulse going completely through the conduction system of the heart, and the ventricles contracting
cardiac output Volume of blood pumped per minute by the left ventricle
cardiac tamponade Collection of fluid in the pericardial sac hindering the functioning of the heart
carrier Person who harbors an infectious agent but has no symptoms of disease
caseation Process whereby the center of the primary tubercle formed in the lungs as a result of tuberculosis becomes soft and cheese-like due to decreased perfusion
catabolism Destructive process of metabolism whereby tissues or substances are broken into their component parts
cataplexy Sudden loss of muscle control
catharsis Process of talking out one's feelings; "getting things off the chest" through verbalization
cation Ion bearing a positive charge
cavitation Process whereby a cavity is created in the lung tissue through the liquefaction and rupture of a primary tubercle
ceiling effect Medication dosage beyond which no further analgesia occurs
cellular immunity Type of acquired immunity involving T-cell lymphocytes
Centers for Disease Control & Prevention (CDC) An agency of the federal government that provides for the investigation, identification, prevention, and control of diseases; it plays an important role in preparing for, and disseminating information about, possible terrorist attacks
central line Venous catheter inserted into the superior vena cava through the subclavian or internal or external jugular vein
central nervous system System of the brain and spinal cord
cephalalgia Headache; also known as cephalgia
cephalhematoma Collection of blood between the periosteum and the skull of a newborn; appears several hours to a day after birth, does not cross suture lines, and is caused by the rupturing of the periosteal bridging veins due to friction and pressure during labor and delivery
cephalopelvic disproportion Condition in which the fetal head will not fit through the mother's pelvis
certification Voluntary process that establishes and evaluates standards of care; mandatory for any health care services receiving federal funds
cerumen Earwax
cervical dilatation Enlargement of the cervical opening (os) from 0 to 10 cm (complete dilatation)
cesarean birth Birth of an infant through an incision in the abdomen and uterus
Chadwick's sign Purplish-blue color of the cervix and vagina noted about the eighth week of pregnancy
chain of custody Documentation of the transfer of evidence (of a crime) from one worker to the next in a secure fashion
chain of infection Describes the development of an infectious process
chalazion Cyst of the meibomian glands
chancre Clean, painless, syphilitic primary ulcer appearing 2 to 6 weeks after infection at the site of body contact
change Dynamic process whereby an individual's response to a stressor leads to an alteration in behavior
change agent Person who intentionally creates and implements change

chemical agent Substance that interacts with a host, causing disease
chemical name Precise description of the drug's chemical formula
chemical restraint Medication used to control client behavior
chemical warfare agents Poisonous chemicals and gases that are used to harm or kill a large number of persons; examples of chemical agents include nerve agents, blood agents, choking or vomiting agents, and blister or vesicant agents
Chemical, Biological, Radiological/Nuclear, and Explosive Enhanced Response Force Package A program of the National Guard that responds rapidly, following a call by the governor, and can be at the scene of a disaster, ready to function in 6 hours; it can also include a surgical suite, if needed
chemoreceptor Receptor that monitors the levels of carbon dioxide, oxygen, and pH in the blood
chemotherapy Use of drugs to treat illness, especially cancer
Cheyne-Stokes respirations Breathing characterized by periods of apnea alternating with periods of dyspnea
child abuse Any intentional act of physical, emotional, or sexual abuse or neglect committed by a person responsible for the care of a child
child life specialist Health care professional with extensive knowledge of psychology and early childhood development
chloasma Darkening of the skin of the forehead and around the eyes during pregnancy; also called the "mask of pregnancy"
cholecystitis Inflammation of the gallbladder
cholelithiasis Presence of gallstones or calculi in the gallbladder
cholesterol Sterol produced by the body and used in the synthesis of steroid hormones
chorea Condition characterized by abnormal, involuntary, purposeless movements of all musculature of the body
chorion Outer fetal membrane formed from the trophoblast
chronic acute pain Discomfort that occurs almost daily over a long period, months or years, and may never stop; also known as progressive pain
chronic nonmalignant pain Discomfort that occurs almost daily, has been present for at least 6 months, and ranges from mild to severe in intensity; also known as chronic benign pain
chronic pain Discomfort usually defined as long term (lasting 6 months or longer), persistent, nearly constant, or recurrent pain producing significant negative changes in a person's life
chronobiology Science of studying biorhythms
Chvostek's sign Abnormal spasm of the facial muscles in response to a light tapping of the facial nerve
chyme Acidic, semi-fluid paste found in the gastrointestinal tract
circadian rhythm Biorhythm that cycles on a daily basis
circulating nurse RN responsible and accountable for management of personnel, equipment, supplies, the environment, and communication throughout a surgical procedure
circumcision Surgical removal of the prepuce (foreskin), which covers the glans penis
circumoral cyanosis Bluish discoloration surrounding the mouth
cirrhosis Chronic degenerative changes in the liver cells and thickening of surrounding tissue
claiming process Process whereby a family identifies the infant's "likeness to" and the "differences from" family members, and the infant's unique qualities
clean object Object on which there are microorganisms that are usually not pathogenic
cleansing Removal of soil or organic material from instruments and equipment used in providing client care
client behavior accident Mishap resulting from the client's behavior or actions
clinical Observing and caring for living clients
closed reduction Repair of a fracture done without surgical intervention
coarse crackle Moist, low-pitched crackling and gurgling lung sound of long duration
codependent Description for persons who live based on what others think of them
cognition Intellectual ability to think
cognitive behavior therapy Treatment approach aimed at helping a client identify stimuli that cause the client's anxiety, develop plans to respond to those stimuli in a nonanxious manner, and problem-solve when unanticipated anxiety-provoking situations arise
cognitive domain Area of learning that involves intellectual understanding
cognitive reframing Stress-management technique whereby the individual changes a negative perception of a situation or event to a more positive, less threatening perception
coitus (copulation) Sexual act that delivers sperm to the cervix by ejaculation of the erect penis
cold stress Excessive heat loss
colic Condition of acute abdominal pain
colonization Multiplication of microorganisms on or within a host that does not result in cellular injury
colostomy Opening created anywhere along the large intestine

colostrum Antibody-rich yellow fluid secreted by the breasts during the last trimester of pregnancy and the first 2–3 days after birth; gradually changes to milk

comedone Whitehead or blackhead

command hallucination Perception by an individual of a voice or voices telling the individual to do something, usually to himself and/or someone else

communicable agent Infectious agent transmitted to a client by direct or indirect contact, via vehicle, vector, or airborne route

communicable disease Disease caused by a communicable agent

comorbidity Simultaneous existence of more than one disease process within an individual

complementary therapy Therapy used in conjunction with conventional medical therapies

complete protein Protein containing all nine essential amino acids

complicated grief Grief associated with traumatic death such as death by accident, violence, or homicide; survivors often have more intense emotions than those associated with normal grief

compound Combination of atoms of two or more elements

compromised host Person whose normal body defenses are impaired and is therefore susceptible to infection

computed tomography Radiological scanning of the body with x-ray beams and radiation detectors to transmit data to a computer that transcribes the data into quantitative measurement and multidimensional images of the internal structures

conditioning Teaching a person a behavior until it becomes an automatic response; method of conserving adaptive energy

conduction Loss of heat by direct contact with a cooler object

conductive hearing loss Condition characterized by the inability of sound waves to reach the inner ear

confabulation The making up of information to fill in memory gaps

congruence Agreement between two things

conjunctivitis Inflammation of the conjunctiva

consciousness State of awareness of self, others, and surrounding environment

constipation Condition characterized by hard, infrequent stools that are difficult or painful to pass

Contact Precautions Measures taken in addition to Standard Precautions for clients known to have or suspected of having illnesses easily spread by direct client contact or by contact with fomites

contact transmission Transfer of an agent from an infected person to a host by direct contact with that person, indirect contact with an infected person through a fomite, or close contact with contaminated secretions

contraception Measure taken to prevent pregnancy

contracture Permanent shortening of a muscle

contrast medium Radiopaque substance that facilitates roentgen (x-ray) imaging of the body's internal structures

convalescent stage Time period in which acute symptoms of an infection begin to disappear until the client returns to the previous state of health

convection Loss of heat by the movement of air

copulation Sexual act that delivers sperm to the cervix by ejaculation of the erect penis

cotyledon Subdivision of the maternal side of the placenta

couvade Development of physical symptoms by the expectant father such as fatigue, depression, headache, backache, and nausea

crackle Abnormal breath sound that resembles a popping sound, heard on inhalation and exhalation; not cleared by coughing

crenation Condition wherein cells decrease in size, shrivel and wrinkle, and are no longer functional when in a hypertonic solution

crepitus Grating or crackling sensation or sound

cretinism Congenital lack of thyroid hormones causing defective physical development and mental retardation

crisis Acute state of disorganization that occurs when usual coping mechanisms are no longer adequate; stressor that forces an individual to respond and/or adapt in some way

crisis intervention Specific technique used to help a person regain equilibrium

critical thinking The disciplined intellectual process of applying skillful reasoning, imposing intellectual standards and self-reflective thinking as a guide to a belief or action

cross-tolerance Decreased sensitivity to other substances in the same category

crowning When the largest diameter of the fetal head is past the vulva

cryotherapy Use of cold applications to reduce swelling

cryptorchidism Failure of one or both testes to descend

cultural assimilation Process whereby members of a minority group are absorbed by the dominant culture, taking on characteristics of the dominant culture

cultural diversity Differences among people resulting from ethnic, racial, and cultural variations

culture Integrated, dynamic structure of knowledge, attitudes, behaviors, beliefs, ideas, habits, customs, languages, values, symbols, rituals, and ceremonies that are unique to a particular group of people; growing of microorganisms to identify a pathogen

curative To heal or restore health

curing Ridding one of disease

cutaneous pain Discomfort caused by stimulating the cutaneous nerve endings in the skin

cyanosis Bluish discoloration of the skin and mucous membranes observed in lips, nail beds, and earlobes

cycling Alteration in mood between depression and mania

cystitis Inflammation of the urinary bladder

cystocele Downward displacement of the bladder into the anterior vaginal wall

cytology Study of cells

D

dawn phenomenon Early morning glucose elevation produced by the release of growth hormone

death rattle Noisy respirations in the period preceding death caused by a collection of secretions in the larynx

debride To remove dead or damaged tissue or foreign material from a wound

decerebration Severing of the spinal cord

decidua The endometrium after implantation

decomposition Chemical reaction wherein the bonding between atoms in a molecule is broken and simpler products are formed

decrement Decreasing intensity of a contraction

defense mechanism Unconscious functions protecting the mind from anxiety

deglutition Swallowing of food

dehiscence Complication of wound healing wherein the wound edges separate

dehydration Condition wherein more water is lost from the body than is being replaced

delirium Cognitive changes or acute confusion of rapid onset (less than 6 months)

delusion False belief that misrepresents reality

dementia Organic brain pathology characterized by losses in intellectual functioning and a slow onset (longer than 6 months)

dental caries Cavities

dependence Reliance on a substance to such a degree that abstinence causes functional impairment, physical withdrawal symptoms, and/or psychological craving for the substance; see also addiction

depersonalization Treating an individual as an object rather than as a person

depolarization Contraction of the heart

depression State wherein an individual experiences feelings of extreme sadness, hopelessness, and helplessness

detoxification Elimination of a substance from the body

development Behavioral changes in skills and functional abilities

dialysate Solution used in dialysis, designed to approximate the normal electrolyte structure of plasma and extracellular fluid

dialysis Mechanical means of removing nitrogenous waste from the blood by imitating the function of the nephrons; involves filtration and diffusion of wastes, drugs, and excess electrolytes and/or osmosis of water across a semipermeable membrane into a dialysate solution

diarthrosis Freely movable joint

didactic Systematic presentation of information

diet therapy Treating disease or disorder with special diet

dietary prescription/order Order written by the physician for food, including liquids

differentiation Acquisition of characteristics or functions different from those of the original

diffusion Process whereby a substance moves from an area of higher concentration to an area of lower concentration

digestion Mechanical and chemical processes that convert nutrients into a physically absorbable state

diplopia Double vision

dirty object Object on which there is a high number of microorganisms, some that are potentially pathogenic

disability An individual's lack of ability to complete an activity in the normal manner

disaster A situation or event of greater magnitude than an emergency and that has unforeseen, serious, or immediate threats to public health

disciplined Trained by instruction and exercise

disenfranchised grief Grief not openly acknowledged, socially sanctioned, or publicly shared

disinfectant Chemical solution used to clean inanimate objects

disinfection Elimination of pathogens, with the exception of spores, from inanimate objects

dislocation Injury in which the articular surfaces of a joint are no longer in contact

disorientation State of mental confusion in which awareness of time, place, self, and/or situation is impaired

disseminated intravascular coagulation Abnormal stimulation of the clotting mechanism causing small clots throughout the vascular system and widespread bleeding internally, externally, or both

distraction Technique of focusing attention on stimuli other than pain

distress Subjective experience that occurs when stressors evoke an ineffective response

distribution Movement of drugs from the blood into various tissues and body fluids

diverticula Sac-like protrusion of the intestinal wall that results when the mucosa herniates through the bowel wall

diverticulitis Inflammation of one or more diverticula
diverticulosis Condition in which multiple diverticula are present in the colon
domestic violence Aggression and violence involving family members
dominant culture The group whose values prevail within a given society
Down syndrome Congenital chromosomal abnormality; also called trisomy 21
Droplet Precautions Measures taken in addition to Standard Precautions for clients known to have or suspected of having serious illnesses spread by large particle droplets
drug allergy Hypersensitivity to a drug
drug incompatibility Undesired chemical or physical reaction between a drug and a solution, between a drug and the container or tubing, or between two drugs
drug interaction Effect one drug can have on another drug
drug tolerance Reaction that occurs when the body is accustomed to a specific drug that larger doses are needed to produce the desired therapeutic effects
ductus arteriosus Fetal vessel connecting the pulmonay artery to the aorta
ductus venosus Branch of the umbilical vein that enters the inferior vena cava
duration Length of one contraction, from the beginning of the increment to the conclusion of the decrement
dysarthria Difficult and defective speech due to a dysfunction of the muscles used for speech
dysfunctional grief Persistent pattern of intense grief that does not result in reconciliation of feelings
dysfunctional labor Labor with problems of the contractions or of maternal bearing down
dysmenorrhea Painful menstruation
dyspareunia Painful intercourse
dysphagia Difficulty in swallowing
dysplasia Abnormal development
dyspnea Difficulty breathing as observed by labored or forced respirations through the use of accessory muscles in the chest and neck
dysrhythmia Irregularity in the rate, rhythm, or conduction of the electrical system of the heart
dystocia Long, difficult, or abnormal labor caused by any of the four major variables (4 Ps) that affect labor
dysuria Difficult or painful urination

E

early deceleration Reduction in fetal heart rate that begins early in the contraction and virtually mirrors the uterine contraction
ecchymosis Large, irregular hemorrhagic area on the skin; also called a bruise
eclampsia Convulsion occurring in pregnancy-induced hypertension
ectopic pregnancy Pregnancy in which the fertilized ovum is implanted outside the uterine cavity
edema Detectable accumulation of increased interstitial fluid
effacement Thinning of the cervix
efferent nerve pain pathway Descending spinal cord pathway that transmits sensory impulses from the brain
effluent Liquid output from an ileostomy
electrocardiogram Graphic recording of the heart's electrical activity
electroconvulsive therapy Procedure whereby clients are treated with pulses of electrical energy sufficient to cause brief convulsions or seizures
electroencephalogram Graphic recording of the brain's electrical activity
electrolyte Compound that, when dissolved in water or another solvent, dissociates (separates) into ions (electrically charged particles)
element Basic substance of matter
emancipated minor Child who has the legal competency of an adult because of cicumstances involving marriage, divorce, parenting of a child, living independently without parents, or enlistment in the armed services
embolus Mass, such as a blood clot or an air bubble, that circulates in the bloodstream
embryonic phase Development occuring during the first 2 to 8 weeks after fertilization of a human egg
emergency Medical or surgical condition requiring immediate or timely intervention to prevent permanent disability or death
emergency medical technician (EMT) Health care professional trained to provide basic lifesaving measures prior to arrival at the hospital
emergency nursing Care of clients who require emergency interventions
emotional lability Loss of emotional control
empathy Capacity to understand another person's feelings or perception of a situation
emphysema Lung disease wherein air accumulates in the tissues of the lungs
empowerment A process through which an individual is enabled to change situations, and uses resources, skills, and opportunities to do so
empty calories Calories that provide few nutrients
encephalitis Inflammation of the brain
encoding Laying down tracks in areas of the brain to enhance the ability to recall and use information
encopresis Passage of watery colonic contents around a hard fecal mass

endemic Occurring continuously in a particular population and having low mortality

endocrine Group of cells secreting substances directly into the blood or lymph circulation and affecting another part of the body

endometriosis Growth of endometrial tissue on structures outside of the uterus, within the pelvic cavity

endorphins Group of opiate-like substances produced naturally by the brain that raise the pain threshold, produce sedation and euphoria, and promote a sense of well-being

endoscopy Visualization of a body organ or cavity through a scope

energetic-touch therapy Technique of using the hands to direct or redirect the flow of the body's energy fields and enhance balance within those fields

engagement Condition of the widest diameter of the fetal presenting part (head) entering the inlet to the true pelvis

engorgement Distentions and swelling of the breasts in the first few days following delivery

engrossment Parents' intense interest in and preoccupation with the newborn

enriched Descriptor for food in which nutrients that were removed during processing are added back in

enteral instillation Administration of drugs through a gastrointestinal tube

enteral nutrition Feeding method meaning both the ingestion of food orally and the delivery of nutrients through a gastrointestinal tube, but generally meaning the latter

entrainment Infant's ability to move in rhythm to the parent's voice

enzyme Globular protein produced in the body that catalyzes chemical reactions within the cells

enzyme-linked immunosorbent assay Basic screening test currently used to detect antibodies to HIV

epidemic Infecting many people at the same time and in the same geographic area

epidural analgesia Analgesics administered via a catheter that terminates in the epidural space

episiotomy Incision in the perineum to facilitate passage of the baby

epispadias Placement of the urinary meatus on the top of the penis

epistaxis Hemorrhage of the nares or nostrils; also known as nosebleed

Epstein's pearls Small, whitish-yellow epithelial cysts found on the hard palate

equipment accident Accident resulting from the malfunction or improper use of medical equipment

erythema Redness of the skin due to increased blood flow to the area

erythema toxicum neonatorum Pink rash with firm, yellow-white papules or pustules found on the chest, abdomen, back, and/or buttocks of a newborn

erythematous Characterized by redness of the skin

erythrocytapheresis Procedure that removes abnormal red blood cells and replaces them with healthy ones

erythropoiesis Production of red blood cells and their release by the red bone marrow

eschar Dry, dark, leathery scab composed of denatured protein

ethnicity Cultural group's perception of itself or a group identity

ethnocentrism Assumption of cultural superiority and inability to accept another culture's ways

euglycemia Normal blood glucose level

euphoric Characterized by elation out of context to the situation

eupnea Easy respirations with a rate that is age-appropriate

eustress Stress that results in positive outcomes

evaporation Loss of heat when water is changed to a vapor

evisceration Complication of wound healing characterized by a complete separation of wound edges, accompanied by visceral protrusion

exacerbation Increase in the symptoms of a disease

exclusive provider organization Organization wherein care must be delivered by providers in the plan in order for clients to receive any reimbursement

excretion Elimination of drugs or waste products from the body

Expeditionary Medical Support A total package that includes everything necessary to screen, treat, and release clients to other facilities for longer-term care

exposure Contact with an infected person or agent

extended care facility The term refers to any facility that provides care for a long period of time. It has no concrete definition and could refer to either an intermediate or skilled nursing facility

external respiration Exchange of gases between the atmosphere and the lungs

external version Manipulation of the fetus through the mother's abdomen to a presentation facilitating birth

extracellular fluid Fluid outside of the cells; includes interstitial, intravascular, synovial, cerebrospinal, and serous fluids; aqueous and vitreous humor; and endolymph and perilymph

extravasation Escape of fluid into the surrounding tissue

F

faith Confident belief in the truth, value, or trustworthiness of a person, idea, or thing

false labor Contractions that do not cause the cervix to dilate

family-centered care A philosophy of caring recognizing the centrality of the family in the child's life and including the family's contribution and involvement in the plan of care and its delivery (Potts & Mandleco, 2000)
fasciculation Involuntary twitching of muscle fibers
fat-soluble vitamin Vitamin requiring the presence of fats for its absorption from the gastrointestinal tract into the lymphatic system and for cellular metabolism: vitamins A, D, E, and K
fee for service System in which the health care recipient directly pays the provider for services as they are provided
feedback Response from the receiver of a message so that the sender can verify the message
Ferguson's reflex Spontaneous, involuntary urge to bear down during labor
fertilization Union of an ovum and a sperm
fetal attitude Relationship of fetal body parts to one another, either flexion or extension
fetal biophysical profile Assessment of five variables: fetal breathing movement, fetal movements of body or limbs, fetal tone (flexion/extension of extremities), amniotic fluid volume, and reactive NST
fetal lie Relationship of the cephalocaudal axis of the fetus to the cephalocaudal axis of the mother, either longitudinal or transverse
fetal phase Intrauterine development from 8 weeks to birth
fetal position Relationship of the identified landmark on the presenting part to the four quadrants of the mother's pelvis
fetal presentation Determined by the fetal lie and the part of the fetus that enters the pelvis first
fibrinolysis Process of breaking fibrin apart
fight-or-flight response State wherein the body becomes physiologically ready to defend itself by either fighting or fleeing from the stressor
filtration Process of fluids and the substances dissolved in them being forced through the cell membrane by hydrostatic pressure
fine crackle Dry, high-pitched crackling and popping lung sounds of short duration
first assistant Physician or RN who assists the surgeon to retract tissue, aids in the removal of blood and fluids at the operative site, and assists with homeostasis and wound closure
first responders Persons who have been identified as the first ones to appear at the scene of a disaster or accident; designated first responders include health care workers, emergency medical personnel, police, and firepersons
flashback Rushing of blood back into intravenous tubing when a negative pressure is created on the tubing; reliving of an original trauma as if the individual were currently experiencing it
flora Microorganisms that occur or have adapted to live in a specific environment, such as intestinal, skin, vaginal, or oral flora
flow rate Volume of fluid to infuse over a set period of time
fluoroscopy Immediate, serial images of the body's structure or function
fomite Object contaminated with an infectious agent
fontanelle Membranous area where sutures meet on the fetal skull
foramen ovale Flap opening in the atrial septum that allows only right-to-left movement of blood
forceps Metal instruments used on the fetal head to provide traction or to provide a method of rotating the fetal head to an occiput-anterior position
foremilk Watery first milk from the breast, high in lactose, like skim milk, and effective in quenching thirst
formal teaching Teaching that takes place at a specific time, in a specific place, and on a specific topic
fortified Descriptor for food in which nutrients not naturally occurring in the food are added to it
fracture Break in the continuity of a bone
free radical Unstable molecule that alters genetic codes and triggers the development of cancer growth in cells
frequency Time for the beginning of one contraction to the beginning of the next contraction
friction Force of two surfaces moving against one another
fulguration Procedure to destroy tissue with long, high-frequency electric sparks
fundus Top of the uterus
funic souffle Sound of the blood pulsating through the umbilical cord; rate the same as the fetal heartbeat

G

gastric ulcer Erosion in the stomach
gastritis Inflammation of the stomach mucosa
gate control pain theory Theory that proposes that the cognitive, sensory, emotional, and physiologic components of the body can act together to block an individual's perception of pain
general adaptation syndrome Physiologic response that occurs when a person experiences a stressor
general anesthesia Method of producing unconsciousness; amnesia, motionlessness, muscle relaxation, and complete insensibility to pain
generic name Name assigned by the U.S. Adopted Names Council to the manufacturer who first develops a drug
genogram A way to visualize family members, their birth and death dates, or ages and specific health problems
genuineness Sincerity

germicide Chemical that can be applied to both animate and inanimate objects for the purpose of eliminating pathogens

germinal phase Development beginning with conception and lasting approximately 10 to 14 days

gerontological nursing Specialty within nursing that addresses and advocates for the special care needs of older adults

gerontologist Specialist in gerontology in advanced practice nursing, geriatric psychiatry, medicine, and social services

gerontology Study of the effects of normal aging and age-related diseases on human beings

gingivitis Inflammation of the gums

Glasgow Coma Scale Neurological screening test that measures a client's best verbal, motor, and eye response to stimuli

glucagon Hormone secreted by the alpha cells of the pancreas, which stimulate release of glucose by the liver

gluconeogenesis Conversion of amino acids into glucose

glycogenesis Conversion of glucose into glycogen

glycogenolysis Conversion of glycogen into glucose

glycosuria Presence of excessive glucose in the urine

goiter Enlargement of the thyroid gland

Goodell's sign Softening of the cervix noted about the 8th week of pregnancy

Gower's sign Walking the hands up the legs to get from sitting to standing position (as in Duchenne muscular dystrophy)

granulation tissue Delicate connective tissue consisting of fibroblasts, collagen, and capillaries

graphesthesia Ability to identify letters, numbers, or shapes drawn on the skin

gravida Pregnancy, regardless of duration, including present pregnancy

grief Series of intense psychological and physical responses occuring after a loss; these responses are necessary, normal, natural, and adaptive responses to the loss

growth Measurable changes in the physical size of the body and its parts

gynecomastia Abnormal enlargement of one or both breasts in males

H

half-life Time it takes the body to eliminate half of the blood concentration level of the original dose of medication

halitosis Bad breath

hallucination Sensory perception that occurs in the absence of external stimuli and that is not based on reality

hallux varus Placement of the great toe farther from the other toes

hand hygiene Rubbing together of all surfaces and crevices of the hands using a soap or chemical and water, followed by rinsing in a flowing stream of water

handicap The physical or mental inability to complete a role in one or more major ADL (U.S. Office of Personnel Management, 1987)

healing Process that activates the individual's recovery forces from within; to make whole

healing touch Energy therapy using the hands to clear, energize, and balance the energy field

health According to the World Health Organization, the state of complete physical, mental, and social well-being, not merely the absence of disease or infirmity

health care delivery system Method for providing services to meet the health needs of individuals

health care surrogate law Law enacted by some states that provides a legal means for decision making in the absence of advance directives

health continuum Range of an individual's health, from highest health potential to death

health history Review of the client's functional health patterns prior to the current contact with a health care agency

health maintenance organization Prepaid health plan that provides primary health care services for a preset fee and focuses on cost-effective treatment methods

hearing Act or power of receiving sounds

heart sound Sound heard by auscultating the heart

Heberden's nodes Enlargement and characteristic hypertrophic spurs in the terminal interphalangeal finger joints

Hegar's sign Softening of the uterine isthmus about the 6th week of pregnancy

HELLP syndrome Pregnancy-induced hypertension with liver damage characterized by hemolysis, elevated liver enzymes, and low platelet count

hemarthrosis Bleeding into the joints

hematemesis Vomiting of blood

hematocrit Percentage of red blood cells in a given volume of blood

hematopoiesis Process of blood cell production and development

hematuria Blood in the urine

hemiparesis Weakness of one side of the body

hemiplegia Paralysis of one side of the body

hemolysis Breakdown of red blood cells and the release of hemoglobin

hemopneumothorax Presence of blood and air within the pleural space

hemorrhagic exudate Discharge that has a large component of red blood cells

hemorrhoid Swollen vascular tissue in the rectal area

hemostasis Cessation of bleeding

hemothorax Condition wherein blood accumulates in the pleural space of the lungs

hepatitis Chronic or acute inflammation of the liver
hesitancy Difficulty initiating the urinary stream
hindmilk Follows foremilk, is higher in fat content, leads to weight gain, and is more satisfying
hirsutism Excessive body hair in a masculine distribution
histamine Substance released during allergic reactions
holistic Whole; includes physical, intellectual, sociocultural, psychological, and spiritual aspects as an integrated whole
Homans' sign Test to check for the presence of clots in the leg
homeostasis Balance or equilibrium among the physiologic, psychological, sociocultural, intellectual, and spiritual needs of the body; maintenance of internal environment
homonymous hemianopia Loss of vision in half of the visual field on the same side of both eyes
hope To look forward to with confidence or expectation; a resource clients can use to promote physical, psychological, and spiritual wellness
hormone Substance that initiates or regulates activity of another organ, system, or gland in another part of the body
hospice Humane, compassionate care provided to clients who can no longer benefit from curative treatment and have 6 months or less to live; allows individuals to die with dignity
host Organism that can be affected by an agent
human immunodeficiency virus (HIV) Retrovirus that causes AIDS
human leukocyte antigen Antigen present in human blood
humoral immunity Type of immunity dominated by antibodies
hydatidiform mole Abnormality of the placenta wherein the chorionic villi become fluid filled, grape-like clusters; the trophoblastic tissue proliferates; and there is no viable fetus
hydramnios (polyhydramnios) Excess amount of amniotic fluid
hydrocele Fluid around the testes in the scrotum
hydrostatic pressure Pressure that a fluid exerts against a membrane; also called filtration force
hygiene Study of health and ways of preserving health
hyperbilirubinemia Excess of bilirubin in the blood
hyperemesis gravidarum Excessive vomiting during pregnancy
hypergylcemia Condition wherein the blood glucose level becomes too high as a result of the absence of insulin
hyperopia Farsightedness
hypersensitivity Excessive reaction to a stimulus
hypersomnia Alteration in sleep pattern characterized by excessive sleep, especially in the daytime
hyperthermia Condition in which the core body temperature rises above 106°F
hypertonic solution Solution that has a higher molecular concentration than the cell; also called a hyperosmolar solution
hypertrophy Increase in muscle mass
hyperuricemia Increased uric acid blood level
hyperventilation Breathing characterized by deep, rapid respirations
hypervigilant Condition of constantly scanning the environment for potentially dangerous situations
hypervolemia Increased circulating fluid volume
hypnosis Altered state of consciousness or awareness resembling sleep and during which a person is more receptive to suggestion
hypoglycemia Condition wherein the blood glucose level is exceedingly low
hypomania Mild form of mania without significant impairment
hypospadias Placement of the urinary meatus on the underside of the penis
hypothermia Condition in which the core body temperature drops below 95°F
hypotonia Lax muscle tone
hypotonic solution Solution that has a lower molecular concentration than the cell; also called hypo-osmolar solution
hypoventilation Breathing characterized by shallow respirations
hypovolemia Abnormally low circulatory blood volume
hypoxemia Decreased oxygen level in the blood

I

iatrogenic Caused by treatment or diagnostic procedures
ideal self The person whom the individual would like to be
identity An individual's conscious description of who he or she is
idiopathic Occurring without a known cause
idiosyncratic reaction Very unpredictable response that may be an overresponse, an underresponse, or an atypical response
ileal conduit Implantation of the ureters into a piece of ileum, which is attached to the abdominal wall as a stoma so urine can be removed from the body
ileostomy Opening created in the small intestine at the ileum
illness stage Time period when the client is manifesting specific signs and symptoms of an infectious agent

illusion Inaccurate perception or misinterpretation of sensory stimuli

imagery Relaxation technique of using the imagination to visualize a pleasant, soothing image

immune response Body's reaction to substances identified as nonself

immunity Body's ability to protect itself from foreign agents or organisms

immunization Process of creating immunity or resistance to infection in an individual

immunotherapy Treatment to suppress or enhance immunologic functioning

implantable cardioverter-defibrillator (ICD) Implantable device that senses a dysrythmia and automatically sends an electrical shock directly to the heart to defibrillate it

implantable port Device made of a radiopaque silicone catheter and a plastic or stainless steel injection port with a self-sealing silicone-rubber septum

implantation Embedding of a fertilized egg into the uterine lining

impotence Inability of an adult male to have an erection firm enough or to maintain it long enough to complete sexual intercourse

incidence Frequency of disease occurrence

incompetent cervix Descriptor for when the cervix begins to dilate, usually during the second trimester

incomplete protein Protein with one or more of the essential amino acids missing

increment Increasing intensity of a contraction

incubation period Time between entry of an infectious agent in the host and the onset of symptoms

independent nursing intervention Nursing action initiated by the nurse and do not require direction or an order from another health care professional

induction of labor Stimulation of uterine contractions before contractions begin spontaneously for the purpose of birthing an infant

infancy Development from the end of the first month to the end of the first year of life

infection Invasion and multiplication of pathogenic microorganims in body tissue that results in cellular injury

infectious agent Microorganism that causes cellular injury

infertility Inability or diminished ability to produce offspring

infiltration Seepage of foreign substances into the interstitial tissue, causing swelling and discomfort at the IV site

inflammation Nonspecific cellular response to tissue injury

informal teaching Teaching that takes place anytime, anyplace, and whenever a learning need is identified

informed consent Legal form signed by a competent client and witnessed by another person that grants permission to the client's physician to perform the procedure described by the physician and that demonstrates the client's understanding of the benefits, risks, and possible complications of the procedure, as well as alternate treatment options

ingestion The taking of food into the digestive tract, generally through the mouth

initial planning Development of a preliminary plan of care by the nurse who performs the admission assessment and gathers the comprehensive admission assessment data

insensible water loss Water loss of which the person is not generally aware

insomnia Difficulty in falling asleep initially or in returning to sleep once awakened

inspection Physical examination technique that involves thorough visual observation

insulin Pancreatic hormone that aids in both the diffusion of glucose into the liver and muscle cells, and the synthesis of glycogen

intellectual wellness Ability to function as an independent person capable of making sound decisions

intensity Strength of the contraction at the acme

interdependent nursing intervention Nursing action that is implemented in a collaborative manner with other health care professionals

internal respiration Exchange of oxygen and carbon dioxide at the cellular level

interstitial fluid Fluid in tissue spaces around each cell

interval Resting period between two contractions

intoxication Reversible effect on the central nervous system soon after the use of a substance

intracath Plastic tube for insertion into a vein

intracellular fluid Fluid within the cells

intradermal Injection into the dermis

intramuscular Injection into the muscle

intraoperative phase Time during the surgical experience that begins when the client is transferred to the operating room table and ends when the client is admitted to the postanesthesia care unit

intrathecal analgesia Administration of analgesics into the subarachnoid space

intravascular fluid Fluid consisting of the plasma in the blood vessels and the lymph in the lymphatic system

intravenous Injection into a vein

intravenous therapy Administration of fluids, electrolytes, nutrients, or medications by the venous route

intravesical Within the urinary bladder

intussusception Telescoping of one part of the intestine into another

invasive Accessing the body tissues, organs, or cavities through some type of instrumentation procedure
involution Return of the reproductive organs, especially the uterus, to their pre-pregnancy size and condition
ion Atom bearing an electrical charge
ischemia Oxygen deprivation, usually due to poor perfusion
ischemic pain Discomfort resulting when the blood supply to an area is restricted or cut off completely
isolation Separation from other persons, especially those with infectious diseases
isotonic solution Solution that has the same molecular concentration as does the cell; also called an isosmolar solution
isotopes Atom of the same element that has a different atomic weight (i.e., different numbers of neutrons in the nucleus)
iv push (bolus) The administration of a large dose of medication in a relatively short time, usually 1–30 minutes

J

jaundice Yellow discoloration of the skin, sclera, mucous membranes, and body fluids that occurs when the liver is unable to fully remove bilirubin from the blood
Johnsonian intervention Confrontational approach to a client with a substance problem that lessens the chance of denial and encourages treatment before the client "hits bottom"
judgment Conclusion based on sound reasoning and supported by evidence

K

Kardex A brief worksheet with basic client care information
keloid Abnormal growth of scar tissue that is elevated, rounded, and firm with irregular, clawlike margins
keratin Tough, fibrous protein produced by cells in the epidermis called keratinocytes
keratitis Inflammation of the cornea
kernicterus Severe neurological damage resulting from a high level of bilirubin (jaundice)
Kernig's sign Diagnostic test for inflammation in the nerve roots; the inability to extend the leg when the thigh is flexed against the abdomen
ketone Acidic by-product of fat metabolism
ketonuria Presence of ketones in the urine
ketosis Condition wherein acids called ketones accumulate in the blood and urine, upsetting the acid–base balance
kilocalorie Equivalent to 1,000 calories
kinesthetic learner Person who learns by processing information through touching, feeling, and doing
kwashiorkor Condition resulting when there is a sudden or recent lack of protein-containing foods
kyphosis Increased roundness of the thoracic spinal curve

L

lanugo Fine hair covering the fetus's body
large for gestational age Infant's weight falls above the 90th percentile for gestational age
late deceleration Reduction in fetal heart rate that begins after the uterus has begun contracting and increases to the baseline level after the uterine contraction has ceased
learning Act or process of acquiring knowledge, skill, or both in a particular subject; process of assimilating knowledge resulting in behavior changes
learning disability Heterogenous group of disorders manifested by significant difficulties in the acquisition and use of listening, speaking, reading, writing, reasoning, or mathematical abilities
learning plateau Peak in the effectiveness of teaching and depth of learning
learning style Individual preference for receiving, processing, and assimilating information about a particular subject
lecithin Major component of surfactant
Leopold's maneuvers Series of specific palpations of the pregnant uterus to determine fetal position and presentation
let-down reflex Neurohormonal reflex that causes milk to be expressed from the alveoli into the lactiferous ducts
leukocytosis Increased number of white blood cells
leukopenia Decreased number of white blood cells
licensure Mandatory system of granting licenses according to specified standards
life review Form of reminiscence wherein a client attempts to come to terms with conflict or to gain meaning from life and die peacefully
ligation Application of a band or tie around a structure
lightening Descent of the fetus into the pelvis, causing the uterus to tip forward, relieving pressure on the diaphragm
linea nigra Dark line on the abdomen from umbilicus to symphysis during the pregnancy
lipid Organic compound that is insoluble in water but soluble in organic solvents such as ether and alcohol; also known as fats
lipodystrophy Atrophy or hypertrophy of subcutaneous fat
lipoma Benign tumor consisting of mature fat cells
lipoprotein Blood lipid bound to protein

liquefaction necrosis Death and subsequent change of tissue to a liquid or semi-liquid state; often descriptive of a primary tubercle

listening Interpreting the sounds heard and attaching meaning to them

litholapaxy Procedure involving crushing of a bladder stone and immediate washing out of the fragments through a catheter

lithotripsy Method of crushing a calculus anyplace in the urinary system with ultrasonic waves

liver mortis Bluish-purple discoloration of the skin that is a by-product of red blood cell destruction; it begins within 20 minutes of death

living will Legal document that allows a person to state preferences about the use of life-sustaining measures should he or she be unable to make his or her wishes known

local adaptation syndrome Physiologic response to a stressor (e.g., trauma, illness) affecting a specific part of the body

localized infection Infection limited to a defined area or single organ

lochia Uterine/vaginal discharge after childbirth; initially bright red, then changing to a pink or pinkish brown, then to a yellowish white

locomotor Pertaining to movement or the ability to move

long-term care facility Health care facility that provides services to individuals who are not acutely ill, have continuing health care needs, and cannot function independently at home

long-term care managed care Care that refers to a spectrum of services provided to individuals who have an ongoing need for health care; traditionally a community-based nursing home licensed for skilled or intermediate care

long-term goal Statement that profiles the desired resolution of the nursing diagnosis over a long period of time, usually weeks or months

lordosis Exaggeration of the curvature of the lumbar spine

loss Any situation, either potential, actual, or perceived, wherein a valued object or person is changed or is not accessible to the individual

lumbar puncture Aspiration of cerebrospinal fluid from the subarachnoid space

lung stretch receptor Receptor that monitors the patterns of breathing and prevents overexpansion of the lungs

lymphokine Chemical substance released by sensitized lymphocytes (T cells) and that assists in antigen destruction

lymphoma Tumor of the lymphatic system

M

macrosomia Excessive fetal growth characterized by a fetus weighing more than 4,000 g (8.8 lb.)

magnetic resonance imaging Imaging technique that uses radiowaves and a strong magnetic field to make continuous cross-sectional images of the body

maladaptive measure Measure used to avoid conflict or stress

malignant Becoming progessively worse and often resulting in death

malpractice Negligent acts on the part of a professional; relates to the conduct of a person who is acting in a professional capacity

managed care A cost-saving system where a case management, individual, or team control what specialists the client sees, as well as the frequency or duration of that specialty care

mania Extremely elevated mood with accompanying agitated behavior

marasmus Condition resulting from severe malnutrition; afflicts very young children who lack both energy and protein foods as well as vitamins and minerals

Maslow's hierarchy of needs Theory of behavioral motivation based on needs; includes physiologic, safety and security, love and belonging, self-esteem, and self-actualization needs

mastication Chewing food into fine particles and mixing the food with enzymes in saliva

mastitis Inflammation of the breast, generally during breastfeeding

material principle of justice Rationale for determining those times when there can be unequal allocation of scarce resources

matter Anything that occupies space and possesses mass

maturation Process of becoming fully grown and developed; involves physiologic and behavioral aspects

maturational loss Loss that occurs as a person moves from one developmental stage to another

mechanism of labor Series of movements of the fetus as it passes through the pelvis and birth canal

meconium Fecal material stored in the fetal intestines

meconium ileus Impacted feces in the newborn, causing intestinal obstruction

Medicaid Government title program (XIX) that pays for health services for people who are older, poor, or disabled, and for low-income families with dependent children

medical asepsis Practices that reduce the number, growth, and spread of microorganisms

medical diagnosis Clinical judgment by the physician that identifies or determines a specific disease, condition, or pathological state

medical model Traditional approach to health care wherein the focus is on treatment and cure of disease not prevention
Medicare Amendment (Title XVIII) to the Social Security Act that helps finance the health care of persons over 65 years old and younger persons who are permanently disabled to receive Social Security disability benefits
Medigap insurance Insurance plan for persons with Medicare that pays for health care costs not covered by Medicare
meditation An activity that brings the mind and spirit in focus on the present and provokes a sense of peace and relaxation
melanin Pigment that gives skin its color
melena Stool containing partially broken down blood usually black, sticky, and tar-like
menarche Onset of the first menstrual period
meningitis Inflammation of the meninges
meningocele Saclike protrusion along the vertebral column filled with cerebrospinal fluid and meninges
menopause Cessation of menstruation
menorrhagia Excessively heavy menstrual flow
mental disorder Clinically significant behavior or psychological syndrome or pattern that occurs in an individual and is associated with present distress or disability or with a significantly increased risk of suffering, death, pain, disability, or an important loss of freedom (APA, 1994)
mental illness Condition wherein an individual has a distorted view of self, is unable to maintain satisfying personal relationships, and is unable to adapt to the environment
mentation Ability to concentrate, remember, or think abstractly
metabolic rate Rate of energy utilization in the body
metabolism Sum total of all the biological and chemical processes in the body
metastasis Spread of cancer cells to distant areas of the body by way of the lymph system or bloodstream
metritis Inflammation of the uterus including the endometrium and parametrium
metrorrhagia Vaginal bleeding between menstrual periods
micturition Process of expelling urine from the urinary bladder; also called urination or voiding
middle adulthood Development from the ages of 40 years to 65 years
milia Pearly white cysts on the face
minimum data set An assessment tool for assessing a resident's physical, psychological, and psychosocial functioning in a Medicare and Medicaid-certified long-term care facility
minority group Group of people constituting less than a numerical majority of the population and are often labeled and treated differently from others in the society
miscarriage Spontaneous abortion
misdemeanor Offense that is less serious than a felony and may be punished by a fine or by sentence to a local prison for less than 1 year
misuse Use of a legal substance for which it was not intended, or exceeding the recommended dosage of a drug
mixed agonist-antagonist Compound that blocks opioid effects on one receptor type while producing opioid effects on a second receptor type
mixture Substances combined in no specific way
mnemonic Method to aid in association and recall; a memorable sentence created from the first letters of a list of items to be used to recall the items later
mode of transmission Process of the infectious agent moving from the reservoir or source through the portal of exit to the portal of entry of the susceptible "new" host
modulation Central nervous system pathway that selectively inhibits pain transmission by sending signals back down to the dorsal horn of the spinal cord
molding Shaping of the fetal head to adapt to the mother's pelvis during labor
molecule Atoms of the same element that unite with each other
Mongolian spots Large patches of bluish skin on the buttocks of dark-skinned infants
monounsaturated fatty acid Forms a glycerol ester with a double or triple bond; nuts, fowl, and olive oil
mood Subjective report of the way an individual is feeling
moral maturity Ability to decide for oneself what is "right"
morbidity Illness
mortality Death
morula Mass of cells resembling a mulberry
mourning Period during which grief is expressed and integration and resolution of the loss occur
multigravida Condition of being pregnant two or more times
multipara Condition of having delivered twice or more after 24 weeks' gestation
myelomeningocele Saclike protrusion along the vertebral column that is filled with spinal fluid, meninges, nerve roots, and spinal cord
myocardial infarction Necrosis (death) of the myocardium caused by an obstruction in a coronary artery; commonly known as heart attack
myocarditis Inflammation of the myocardium of the heart

myofascial pain syndrome Group of muscle disorders characterized by pain, muscle spasm, tenderness, stiffness, and limited motion
myopia Nearsightedness
myringotomy Surgical incision of the eardrum
myxedema Severe hypothyroidism in adults

N

narcolepsy Sleep alteration manifested as sudden uncontrollable urges to fall asleep during the daytime
narrative charting Chronological account written in paragraphs describes the client's status, the interventions and treatments, and the client's response to treatments
necrosis Tissue death as the result of disease or injury
neglect Situation wherein a basic need of the client is not being provided
negligence General term referring to careless acts on the part of an individual who is not exercising reasonable or prudent judgment
neonatal stage First 28 days of life following birth
neonatal transition First few hours after birth wherein the newborn makes changes to and stabilizes respiratory and circulatory functions
neonate Newborn from birth to 28 days of life
neoplasm Any abnormal growth of new tissue
nephrotoxic Quality of a substance that causes kidney tissue damage
nerve agents Powerful acetylcholinesterase inhibitors that alter cholinergic synaptic transmission at neuroeffector junctions, at skeletal myoneural junctions and autonomic ganglia, and in the central nervous system
nesting Surge of energy late in pregnancy when the pregnant woman organizes and cleans the house
neuralgia Paroxysmal pain that extends along the course of one or more nerves
neurogenic shock Hypotensive situation resulting from the loss of sympathetic control of vital functions from the brain
neuropeptide Amino acid produced in the brain and other sites in the body that acts as a chemical communicator
neurotransmitter Chemical substance produced by the body that facilitates or inhibits nerve-impulse transmission
neutral thermal environment Environment in which the newborn can maintain internal body temperature with minimal oxygen consumption and metabolism
nevi Pigmented areas in the skin; commonly known as birthmarks or moles
nevus flammeus Large, reddish-purple birthmark usually found on the face or neck and does not blanch with pressure
nevus vascularis Birthmark of enlarged superficial blood vessels, elevated and red in color
nociceptor Receptive neuron for painful sensations
nocturia Awakening at night to void
nocturnal enuresis Incontinence that occurs during sleep
noninvasive Descriptor for procedure wherein the body is not entered with any type of instrument
nonmaleficence Ethical principle based on the obligation to cause no harm to others
nonshivering thermogenesis Metabolism of brown fat; process unique to the newborn
nonverbal communication Body language or a method of sending a message without words
nosocomial infection Infection acquired in the hospital or other health care facility that was not present or incubating at the time of the client's admission
noxious stimulus Underlying pathology that causes pain
nuchal cord Condition of the umbilical cord being wrapped around the baby's neck
nuchal rigidity Pain and rigidity in the neck
nulligravida Condition of never having been pregnant
nullipara Condition of never having delivered an infant after 24 weeks' gestation
nursing The art and science of assisting individuals in learning to care for themselves whenever possible and of caring for them when they are unable to meet their own needs
nursing audit Method of evaluating the quality of care provided to clients
nursing care plan Written guide of strategies to be implemented to help the client achieve optimal health
nursing diagnosis Second step in the nursing process; a clinical judgment about individual, family, or community (aggregate) responses to actual or potential health problems/life processes
nursing intervention Action performed by a nurse that helps the client achieve the results specified by the goals and expected outcomes
nursing interventions classification Standardized language for nursing interventions
nursing minimum data set Elements that should be in clinical records and abstracted for studies on the effectiveness and costs of nursing care
nursing outcomes classification Standardized language for nursing outcomes
nursing practice act Statute that is enacted by the legislature of a state and that outlines the scope of nursing practice in that state

nursing process Systematic method for providing care to clients, consisting of five steps: assessment, diagnosis, outcome identification and planning, implementation, and evaluation
nutrition All of the processes (ingestion, digestion, absorption, metabolism, and elimination) involved in consuming and using food for energy, maintenance, and growth
nystagmus Constant, involuntary movement of the eye in various directions

O

obesity Weight that is 20% or more above the ideal body weight
objective data Observable and measurable data that are obtained through standard assessment techniques performed during the physical examination and through laboratory and diagnostic tests
occult blood Blood in the stool that can be detected only through a microscope or by chemical means
occult blood test (guaiac) Test for microscopic blood done on stool
older adulthood Development occurring from age 65 years until death
oligomenorrhea Decreased menstrual flow
oliguria Diminished production of urine
oncology Study of tumors
ongoing assessment Type of assessment that includes systematic monitoring of specific problems
ongoing planning Updates the client's plan of care
onset of action Time for the body to respond to a drug after administration
oophoritis Inflammation of the ovary
open reduction Surgical procedure that enables the surgeon to reduce (repair) a fracture under direct visualization
ophthalmia neonatorum Inflammation of a newborn's eyes that results from passing through the birth canal when a gonorrheal or chlamydial infection is present
opinion Subjective belief
opisthotonos Complete arching of the body with only the head and feet on the bed
opportunistic infection Infection in persons with a defective immune system that rarely causes harm in healthy individuals
oppression Condition wherein the rules, values, and ideals of one group are imposed on another group
orchiectomy Removal of a testis
orientation Person's awareness of self in relation to person, place, time, and in some cases, situation
orthopedics (orthopaedics) Branch of medicine that deals with the prevention or correction of the disorders and diseases of the musculoskeletal system
orthopnea Difficulty breathing while lying down
orthostatic hypotension Significant decrease in blood pressure that results when a person moves from a lying or sitting (supine) position to a standing position
osmolality Measurement of the total concentration of dissolved particles (solutes) per kilogram of water
osmolarity Concentration of solutes per liter of cellular fluid
osmosis Movement of a solvent, usually water, through a semipermeable membrane, from a region of higher concentration to a region of lower concentration
osmotic pressure Pressure exerted against the cell membrane by the water inside a cell
osteoporosis Increase in the porosity of bone
Outcomes and Assessment Information Set An outcomes measurable tool developed and implemented to determine the care given and reimbursement required; Outcomes and Assessment Information Set (OASIS) data is reported to the Centers for Medicare and Medicaid Services (CMS)
overflow incontinence Leaking of urine when the bladder becomes very full and distended
oxidation Chemical process of combining with oxygen
oxidized Joined with oxygen

P

pain Unpleasant sensory and emotional experience associated with actual or potential tissue damage or described in terms of such
pain threshold Level of intensity at which pain becomes appreciable or perceptible
pain tolerance Level of intensity or duration of pain that a person is willing to endure
palliative care Care that relieves symptoms, such as pain, but does not alter the course of disease
pallor Abnormal paleness of the skin, seen especially in the face, conjunctiva, nail beds, and oral mucous membranes
palpation Physical examination technique that uses the sense of touch to assess texture, temperature, moisture, organ location and size, vibrations and pulsations, swelling, masses, and tenderness
pancreatitis Acute or chronic inflammation of the pancreas
Papanicolaou test Smear method of examining stained exfoliative cells
paracentesis Aspiration of fluid from the abdominal cavity
paradoxical reaction Opposite effect of that which would normally be expected
paramedic Specialized health care professional trained to provide advanced life support to the client requiring emergency interventions

paraplegia Paralysis of lower extremities

parasomnia Disorders that intrude on sleep in very active ways

parenteral Any route other than the oral-gastrointestinal tract

parenteral nutrition Feeding method whereby nutrients bypass the small intestine and enter the blood directly

paresthesia Abnormal sensation such as burning, prickling, or tingling

paroxysmal Descriptor for a symptom that begins and ends abruptly

paroxysmal nocturnal dyspnea Condition of suddenly awakening, sweating, and having difficulty breathing

passive euthanasia Process of working with the client's dying process

patency Being freely opened

pathogen Microorganism that causes disease

pathogenicity Ability of a microorganism to produce disease

patient-controlled analgesia Device that allows the client to control the delivery of intravenous or subcutaneous pain medication in a safe, effective manner through a programmable pump

peak plasma level Highest blood concentration of a single dose of a drug until the elimination rate equals the rate of absorption

peer assistance program Rehabilitation program that provides an impaired nurse with referrals, professional and peer counseling support groups, and assistance and monitoring back into nursing

peptic ulcer Erosion formed in the esophagus, stomach, or duodenum resulting from acid/pepsin imbalance

perception Ability to experience, recognize, organize, and interpret sensory stimuli

percussion Physical examination technique that uses short, tapping strokes on the surface of the skin to create vibrations of underlying organs

perfectionism Overwhelming expectation of being able to get everything done in a flawless manner

perfusion Blood flow through an organ or body part

pericardial friction rub Short, high-pitched squeak heard as two inflamed pericardial surfaces rub together

pericardiocentesis Removal of fluid from the pericardial sac

pericarditis Inflammation of the membrane sac surrounding the heart

perineal care Cleansing of the external genitalia, perineum, and the surrounding area

perioperative Period of time encompassing the preoperative, intraoperative, and postoperative phases of surgery

peripheral nervous system System of the cranial nerves, spinal nerves, and the autonomic nervous system

peripheral resistance Pressure within a vessel that resists the flow of blood such as plaque buildup or vasoconstriction

peristalsis Rhythmic, coordinated, serial contraction of the smooth muscles of the gastrointestinal tract

peritonitis Inflammation of the peritoneum, the membranous covering of the abdomen

permeability Ability of a membrane to permit substances to pass through it

petechiae Pinpoint hemorrhagic spots on the skin

phantom limb pain Neuropathic pain that occurs after amputation with pain sensations referred to an area in the missing portion of the limb

pharmacokinetics Study of the absorption, distribution, metabolism, and excretion of drugs to determine the relationship between the dose of a drug and the drug's concentration in biological fluids

phimosis Condition wherein the opening in the foreskin is so small that it cannot be pulled back over the glans

phlebitis Inflammation in the wall of a vein without clot formation

phlebothrombosis Formation of a clot because of blood pooling in the vessel, trauma to the vessel's endothelial lining, or a coagulation problem with little or no inflammation in the vessel

phlebotomist Individual who performs venipuncture

phlebotomy Removal of blood from a vein

phospholipid Lipid composed of glycerol, fatty acids, and phosphorus; the structural component of cells

physical agent Factor in the environment capable of causing disease in a host

physical restraint Equipment that reduces the client's movement

physical wellness Healthy body that functions at an optimal level

physically aggressive Descriptor of an individual who threatens or actually harms someone

physiologic anemia of pregnancy Condition of having delivered after 24 weeks' gestation, whether infant is born alive or dead or number of infants born

phytochemical Physiologically active compound present in plants in very small amounts that gives plants flavor, odor, and color

pica Practice of eating substances not considered edible and that have no nutritive value, such as laundry starch, dirt, clay, and freezer frost

pie charting Documentation method using the problem, intervention, evaluation (PIE) format

piggyback Addition of an intravenous solution to infuse concurrently with another infusion

placenta Membranous vascular organ connecting the fetus to the mother, which produces hormones to sustain a pregnancy, supplies the fetus with oxygena and food, and transports waste products out of the fetal system

placenta previa Condition in which the placenta forms over or very near the internal cervical os

plague An infectious disease transmitted by a bite of a flea from a rodent (usually a rat) infected with the bacillus Yersinia pestis; plague is a potential agent of bioterrorism

planning Third step of the nursing process; includes both the establishing of guidelines for the proposed course of nursing action to resolve the nursing diagnoses and developing the client's plan of care

plateau Level at which a drug's blood concentration is maintained

pleural effusion Collection of fluid within the pleural cavity

pleural friction rub Abnormal breath sound that is creaky and grating in nature and is heard on inspiration and expiration

pleurisy Condition arising from inflammation of the pleura, or sac, that encases the lung

pneumonia Inflammation of the bronchioles and alveoli accompanied by consolidation, or solidification of exudate, in the lungs

pneumothorax Condition wherein air or gas accumulates in the pleural space of the lungs, causing the lungs to collapse

point-of-care charting Documentation system that allows health care providers to gain immediate access to client information at the bedside

poison Any substance that when taken into the body interferes with normal physiologic functioning; may be inhaled, injected, ingested, or absorbed by the body

polydipsia Excessive thirst

polymenorrhea Menstrual periods that are abnormally frequent, generally less than every 21 days

polyp Abnormal growth of tissue

polyphagia Increased hunger

polypharmacy Problem of clients taking numerous prescription and over-the-counter medications for the same or various disease processes, with unknown consequences from the resulting combinations of chemical compounds and cumulative side-effects

polyunsaturated fatty acid Forms a glycerol ester with many carbons unbonded to hydrogen atoms; fish, corn, sunflower seeds, soybeans, cotton seeds, and safflower oil

polyuria Increased urination

Port-a-Cath Port that has been implanted under the skin with a catheter inserted into the superior vena cava or right atrium through the subclavian or internal jugular vein

portal of entry Route by which an infectious agent enters the host

portal of exit Route by which an infectious agent leaves the reservoir

postictal After a seizure

post-mortem care Care given immediately after death before the body is moved to the mortuary

postoperative phase Time during the surgical experience that begins at the end of the surgical procedure and ends when the client is discharged, not just from the hospital or institution, but from medical care by the surgeon

postpartum blues Mild transient condition of emotional lability and crying for no apparent reason, which affects up to 80% of women who have just given birth, and lasts about 2 weeks

postpartum depression Condition similar to postpartum blues but is more serious, intense, and persistent

postpartum hemorrhage Blood loss of more than 500 mL after the third stage of labor or 1,000 mL following a cesarean birth

postpartum psychosis Condition more severe than postpartum depression and characterized by delusions and thoughts of self-harm or infant harm

postprandial After eating

postterm Delivery after 42 weeks' gestation

post-void residual Urine that remains in the bladder after urination

prayer A type of communication between an individual and spiritual entities

preadolescence Development from the ages of approximately 10 years to 12 years

precipitate birth Birth occurring suddenly and unexpectantly without a CNM/physician present to assist

precipitate labor Labor lasting less than 3 hours from the onset of contractions to the birth of the infant

preeclampsia Phase of pregnancy-induced hypertension prior to convulsions

preferred provider organization Type of managed care model wherein member choice is limited to providers within the system for full reimbursement and other providers for less reimbursement

prenatal care Care of a woman during pregnancy, before labor

prenatal stage Development beginning with conception and ending with birth

preoperative phase Time during the surgical experience that begins when the client decides to have surgery and ends when the client is transferred to the operating table

presbycusis Sensorineural hearing loss associated with aging

presbyopia Inability of the lens of the eye to change curvature to focus near objects
preschool stage Development from the ages of 3 years to 6 years
prescriptive authority Legal recognition of the ability to prescribe medications
presenting part Part of the fetus in contact with the cervix
pressured speech Rapid, intense style of speech
preterm Delivery after 24 weeks' gestation but before 38 weeks (full term)
preterm birth Birth that takes place before the end of the 37th week of gestation
preterm labor Onset of regular contractions of the uterus that cause cervical changes between 20 and 37 weeks' gestation
prevention Obstructing, thwarting, or hindering a disease or illness
priapism Prolonged erection that does not occur in response to sexual stimulation
primary care provider Health care provider whom a client sees first for health care, typically a family practitioner (physician/nurse), internist, or pediatrician
primary health care Client's point of entry into the health care system; includes assessment, diagnosis, treatment, coordination of care, education, prevention services, and surveillance
primary hypertension High blood pressure, the cause of which is unknown; also known as essential hypertension
primary prevention All practices designed to keep health problems from developing
primary source Major provider of information about a client
primary tubercle Nodule that contains tubercle bacilli and forms within lung tissue
primigravida Condition of being pregnant for the first time
primipara Condition of having delivered once after 24 weeks' gestation
privacy The right to be left alone, to choose care based on personal beliefs, to govern body integrity, and to choose when and how sensitive information is shared (Badzek & Gross, 1999)
problem-oriented medical record Documentation method employs a structured, logical format and focuses on the client's problem
process Series of steps or acts that leads to accomplishing some goal or purpose
procrastination Intentionally putting off or delaying something that should be done
prodromal stage Time interval from the onset of nonspecific symptoms until specific symptoms of the infectious process begin to manifest
professional boundaries Limits of the professional relationship that allow for a safe, therapeutic connection between the professional and the client
progressive muscle relaxation Stress-management strategy in which muscles are alternately tensed and relaxed
projectile vomiting Forceful ejection (up to 3 feet) of the contents of the stomach
prolapsed cord Condition in which the umbilical cord lies below the presenting part of the fetus
prolapsed uterus Downward displacement of the uterus into the vagina
prospective payment Predetermined rate paid for each episode of hospitalization based on the client's age and principal diagnosis and the presence or absence of surgery or comorbidity
protocol Series of standing orders or procedures that should be followed under certain specific conditions
proxemics Study of the space between people and its effect on interpersonal behavior
pruritus Severe itching
pseudocyesis False pregnancy
pseudomenstruation Blood-tinged mucus discharge from the vagina of a newborn caused by the withdrawal of maternal hormones
psychoanalysis Therapy focused on uncovering unconscious memories and processes
psychological wellness Enjoyment of creativity, satisfaction of the basic need to love and be loved, understanding of emotions, and ability to maintain control over emotions
psychomotor domain Area of learning that involves performance of motor skills
psychoneuroimmunology Study of the complex relationship among the physical, cognitive, and affective aspects of humans
psychoprophylaxis Mental and physical preparation for childbirth; synonymous with Lamaze
psychosis State wherein an individual has lost the ability to recognize reality
psychotherapy Treatment of mental and emotional disorders through psychological rather than physical methods
ptosis Drooping upper eyelid
puberty Emergence of secondary sex characteristics that signal the beginning of adolescence
public law Law that deals with an individual's relationship to the state
public self What the client thinks others think of him or her
pudendal block Injection of a local anesthetic into the pudendal nerve to provide perineal, external genitalia, and lower vaginal anesthesia

puerperal (postpartum) infection Infection following childbirth occurring between the birth and 6 weeks postpartum
puerperium Term for the first 6 weeks after the birth of an infant
pulse amplitude Measurement of the strength or force exerted by the ejected blood against the arterial wall with each heart contraction
pulse deficit Condition in which the apical pulse rate is greater than the radial pulse rate
pulse rate Indirect measurement of cardiac output obtained by counting the number of peripheral pulse waves over a pulse point
pulse rhythm Regularity of the heartbeat
purpura Reddish-purple patches on the skin indicative of hemorrhage
purulent exudate Discharge resulting from infection; also called pus
pyelonephritis Bacteral infection of the renal pelvis, tubules, and interstitial tissue of one or both kidneys
pyorrhea Periodontal disease
pyuria Pus in the urine

Q

quadriplegia Dysfunction or paralysis of both arms, both legs, and bowel and bladder
quickening Descriptor for when the mother first feels the fetus move, about 16 to 20 weeks' gestation

R

race A group of people with biological similarities
radiation Loss of heat by transfer to cooler near objects, but not through direct contact
radiation sickness An abnormal condition resulting from exposure to ionizing radiation, either purposefully or by accident
radiography Study of x-rays or gamma-ray-exposed film through the action of ionizing radiation
radiotherapy Treatment of cancer with high-energy radiation
rapport Mutual trust established between two people
readiness for learning Evidence of willingness to learn
real self How the individual really thinks about him- or herself
reasoning Use of the elements of thought to solve a problem or settle a question
reconstructive To rebuild or reestablish
rectocele Anterior displacement of the rectum into the posterior vaginal wall
recurrent acute pain Identified by repetitive painful episodes that recur over a prolonged period or throughout a client's lifetime
referred pain Discomfort from the internal organs that is felt in another area of the body
reframing Technique of monitoring negative thoughts and replacing them with positive ones
regional anesthesia Method of temporarily rendering a region of the body insensible to pain
rehabilitation Process or therapy designed to assist individuals to reach their optimal level of physical, mental, and psychosocial functioning
relapse Return to a previous behavior or condition
relaxation technique Method used to decrease anxiety and muscle tension
religion A system of organized beliefs, rituals, and practices with which a person identifies and wishes to be associated
religious support system Group of ministers, priests, nuns, rabbis, shamans, mullahs, or laypersons who are able to meet clients' spiritual needs
REM movement disorder Condition wherein the normal paralysis of REM sleep is absent or incomplete and the sleeper acts out the dream
remission Decrease or absence of symptoms of a disease
renal colic Severe pain in the kidney that radiates to the groin
repolarization Recovery phase of the cardiac muscle
reportable conditions Diseases or injuries that the government requires be reported to the appropriate authority or agency; include suspected abuse and/or neglect, sexually transmitted diseases (STDs), and certain other contagious illnesses that could threaten the health of the general public
reservoir Place where the agent can survive
resident flora Microorganisms that are always present, usually without altering the client's health
residual urine Urine remaining in the bladder after the individual has urinated
respect Acceptance of an individual as is and in a nonjudgmental manner
respiration Process of exchanging oxygen and carbon dioxide
respite care Care and service that provides a break to caregivers and is used for a few hours a week, for an occasional weekend, or for longer periods of time
rest State of mental and physical relaxation and calmness
restitution Rotation of the fetal head back to normal alignment with the shoulders after delivery of the fetal head
restless leg syndrome Condition characterized by uncomfortable sensations of tingling or crawling in the muscles, and twitching, burning, prickling, or deep aching in the foot, calf, or upper leg when at rest

restraint Protective device used to limit the physical activity of a client or to immobilize a client or extremity
resuscitation Support measures implemented to restore consciousness and life
reticulocyte Immature red blood cell
retroperitoneal Behind the peritoneum outside the peritoneal cavity
reverse isolation Barrier protection designed to prevent infection in clients who are severely compromised and highly susceptible to infection; also known as protective isolation
reverse tolerance Phenomenon whereby a smaller amount of substance will elicit the desired psychic effects
review of systems Brief account of any recent signs or symptoms related to any body system
rhinorrhea Watery nasal discharge
Ricin A poison made from the waste products of castor bean processing; a potential agent of bioterrorism because of its ease of dissemination
rigor mortis Natural stiffening of muscles after death; begins about 4 hours after death
risk nursing diagnosis Nursing diagnosis indicating that a problem does not yet exist but that specific risk factors are present; composed of "Risk for" followed by the diagnostic label and a list of the risk factors
role An ascribed or assumed expected behavior in a social position or group
role performance Specific behaviors a person exhibits within each role
rooming-in Practice of staying with the client 24 hours a day to provide care and comfort

S

salpingitis Inflammation of the fallopian tube
salt Product formed when an acid and a base react with each other
sanguineous Bloody drainage from a wound or surgical drain
sarcoma Cancer occurring in connective tissue
Sarin A dangerous man-made nerve agent, first developed as an insecticide that is a potential agent for bioterrorism
satiety Feeling of adequate fullness from food
school-age stage Development from the ages of 6 years to 10 years
sclerotherapy Treatment that involves injecting a chemical into the vein, causing the vein to become sclerosed (hardened) so blood no longer flows through it
sclerotic Hardened tissue
scoliosis Lateral curvature of the spine
scrub nurse RN, LP/VN, or surgical technologist who provides services under the direction of the circulating nurse and who is qualified by training or experience to prepare and maintain the integrity, safety, and efficiency of the sterile field throughout an operation
sebaceous cyst Sebaceous gland filled with sebum
sebum Oily substance secreted by the sebaceous glands of the skin
secondary care Care focused on diagnosis and treatment after the client exhibits symptoms of illness
secondary hypertension High blood pressure occurring as a sequel to a pre-existing disease or injury
secondary prevention Early detection, screening, diagnosis, and intervention, to reduce the consequences of a health problem
sedation Reduction of stress, excitement, or irritability via some central nervous system depression
self-awareness Consciously knowing how the self thinks, feels, believes, and behaves at any specific time
self-care deficit State wherein an individual is not able to perform one or more activities of daily living
self-concept Individual's perception of self; includes self-esteem, body image, and ideal self
self-efficacy Belief in one's ability to succeed in attempts to change behavior
self-esteem A personal opinion of oneself
semipermeable membrane Membrane that allows passage of only certain substances
sensation Ability to receive and process stimuli received through the sensory organs
sensible water loss Water loss of which the person is aware
sensitivity Susceptibility of a pathogen to an antibiotic
sensorineural hearing loss Condition in which the inner ear or cochlear portion of cranial nerve VIII is abnormal or diseased
sensory deficit Change in the perception of sensory stimuli; can affect any of the senses
sensory deprivation State of reduced sensory input from the internal or external environment, manifested by alterations in sensory perception
sensory overload State of excessive and sustained multisensory stimulation manifested by behavior change and perceptual distortion
sensory perception Ability to receive sensory impressions and, through cortical association, relate the stimuli to past experiences and form an impression of the nature of the stimulus
seroconversion Evidence of antibody formation in response to disease or vaccine
serosanguineous exudate Discharge that is clear with some blood tinge; seen with surgical incisions
serous exudate Discharge composed primarily of serum; is watery in appearance and has a low protein level.

serum lithium level Laboratory test done to determine whether the client's lithium level is within a therapeutic range

shaman Folk healer-priest who uses natural and supernatural forces to help others

shearing Force exerted against the skin by movement or repositioning

shift report Report about each client between shifts

shock Condition of profound hemodynamic and metabolic disturbance characterized by inadequate tissue perfusion and inadequate circulation to the vital organs

shroud Covering for the body after death

sibilant wheeze Abnormal breath sound that is high pitched and musical in nature and is heard on inhalation and exhalation

sickle When red blood cells become crescent-shaped and elongated

single point of entry Common feature of HMOs wherein the client is required to enter the health care system through a point designated by the plan

single-payer system Health care delivery model wherein the government is the only entity to reimburse health care costs

situational loss Loss that takes place in response to external events generally beyond the individual's control

slander Words that are communicated verbally to a third party and that harm or injure the personal or professional reputation of another

sleep State of altered consciousness during which a person has minimal physical activity, changes in levels of consciousness, and a slowing of physiologic processes

sleep apnea A period during sleep of not breathing; often associated with heavy snoring

sleep cycle Sequence of sleep beginning with the four stages of NREM sleep, a return to stage 3 and then stage 2 (first phase), followed by the first REM sleep (second phase)

sleep deprivation Prolonged inadequate quality and quantity of sleep

small for gestational age Infant's weight falls below the 10th percentile for gestational age

smallpox (variola) A highly contagious and frequently fatal viral disease, which is a potential agent for a bioterroristic attack; there are two varieties, known as variola major and variola minor

Snellen Chart Chart containing various-sized letters with standardized numbers at the end of each line of letters

sociocultural wellness Ability to appreciate the needs of others and to care about one's environment and the inhabitants of it

somatic nervous system Nerves that connect the central nervous system to the skin and skeletal muscles and control conscious activities

somatic pain Nonlocalized discomfort originating in tendons, ligaments, and nerves

somnambulism Sleepwalking

Somogyi phenomenon In response to hypoglycemia, the release of glucose-elevating hormones (epinephrine, cortisol, glucose), which produces a hyperglycemic state

sonorous wheeze Abnormal breath sound that is low pitched and snoring in nature and is louder on expiration

spermatogenesis Production of sperm

spina bifida occulta Failure of the vertebral arch to close

spinal shock Cessation of motor, sensory, autonomic, and reflex impulses below the level of injury; characterized by flaccid paralysis of all skeletal muscles, loss of spinal reflexes, loss of sensation, and absence of autonomic function below the level of injury

spiritual care Recognition of and assistance toward meeting spiritual needs

spiritual distress A client in this situation may have a troubled, fragmented, or possibly disintegrating spirit

spiritual needs Individual's desire to find purpose and meaning in life, pain, and death

spiritual wellness Inner strength and peace

spirituality The core of a person's being, a higher experience or transcendence of oneself

spore Bacteria in a resistant stage that can withstand unfavorable environments

sprain Injury to ligaments surrounding a joint caused by a sudden twist, wrench, or fall

stable Alert with vital signs within the client's normal range

staff development Delivery of instruction to assist nurses achieve the goals of the employer

standard Level or degree of quality

Standard Precautions Preventive practices to be used in the care of all clients in hospitals regardless of their diagnosis or presumed infection status

standards of practice Guidelines established to direct nursing care

startle response Overreaction to minor sounds or noises

stasis dermatitis Inflammation of the skin due to decreased circulation

station Relationship of the fetal presenting part to the ischial spines

status asthmaticus Persistent, intractable asthma attack

status epilepticus Acute, prolonged episode of seizure activity that lasts at least 30 minutes and may or may not involve loss of consciousness

statutory law Law enacted by legislative bodies

steatorrhea Fatty stool

stent Tiny metal tube with holes in it that prevents a vessel from collapsing and keeps the atherosclerotic plaque pressed against the vessel wall; any material used to hold tissue in place or provide support

stereognosis Ability to recognize an object by feel

stereotyping Belief that all people within the same ethnic, racial, or cultural group act the same way, sharing the same beliefs and attitudes

sterile Without microorganisms

sterile conscience Individual's personal sense of honesty and integrity with regard to adherence to the principles of aseptic technique, including prompt admission and correction of any errors and omissions

sterile field Area surrounding the client and the surgical site that is free from all microorganisms; created by draping of the work area and the client with sterile drape

sterilization Destroying all microorganisms, including spores

stock supply Medications dispensed and labeled in large quantities for storage in the medication room or nursing unit

stoma Surgical opening between a cavity and the surface of the body

stomatitis Inflammation of the oral mucosa

strabismus Inability of the eyes to focus in the same direction

strain Injury to a muscle or tendon due to overuse or overstretching

stress Nonspecific response to any demand made on the body (Selye, 1974)

stress incontinence Leakage of urine when a person does anything that strains the abdomen, such as coughing, laughing, jogging, dancing, sneezing, lifting, making a quick movement, or even walking

stress test Measure of a client's cardiovascular response to exercise

stressor Any situation, event, or agent that produces stress

striae gravidarum Reddish streaks frequently found on the abdomen, thighs, buttocks, and breasts; also called "stretch marks"

stridor High-pitched, harsh sound heard on inspiration when the trachea or larynx is obstructed

stroke volume Volume of blood pumped by the ventricle with each contraction

stye Pustular inflammation of an eyelash follicle or sebaceous gland on the eyelid margin

subacute care Short-term, aggressive care for clients who are out of the acute stage of illness but who still require skilled nursing, monitoring, and ongoing treatment

subcutaneous Injection into the subcutaneous tissue

subinvolution Incomplete return of the uterus to its prepregnant size and consistency

subluxation Partial separation of an articular surface

substance A drug, legal or illegal, that may cause physical or mental impairment

suicidal ideations Thoughts of hurting or killing oneself

supine hypotensive syndrome Lowering of blood pressure in a pregnant woman when lying supine due to compression of the vena cava by the enlarged, heavy uterus

surfactant Phospholipids that are present in the lungs and lower surface tension to prevent collapse of the airways

surgery Treatment of injury, disease, or deformity through invasive operative methods

suture Thin, fibrous, membrane-covered space between skull bones

synarthrosis Immovable joint

syndactyly Fusion of two or more fingers or toes

synergism Result of two or more agents working together to achieve a greater effect than either could produce alone

synthesiasis Hearing colors and seeing sounds

synthesis Chemical reaction when two or more atoms, called reactants, bond and form a more complex molecular product; putting data together in a new way

T

tachycardia Heart rate in excess of 100 beats per minute in an adult

tachypnea Respiratory rate greater than 24 beats per minute

talipes equinovarus A congenital deformity in which the foot and ankle are twisted inward and cannot be moved to a midline position; also known as clubfoot

teaching Active process wherein one individual shares information with another as a means to facilitate learning and thereby promote behavioral changes

teaching strategy Technique to promote learning

teaching–learning process Planned interaction that promotes a behavioral change that is not a result of maturation or coincidence

telangiectasic nevi Birthmarks of dilated capillaries that blanch with pressure; also called stork-bites

telangiestasia Permanent dilation of groups of superficial capillaries and venules; commonly known as "spider veins"

telehealth An electronic information services that offer increased client and family participation; for example, nurse and client use interactive videos, telephone cardiac rate monitoring with EKG readout, digital subscriber lines, and Internet transmission of data

telemedicine An element of telehealth permitting physicians to provide care through a telecommunication system

teleology Ethical theory that states that the value of a situation is determined by its consequences

tenesmus Spasmodic contradiction of the anal or bladder sphincter, causing pain and a persistent urge to empty the bowel or bladder

teratogen Agent such as radiation, drugs, viruses, and other microorganisms capable of causing abnormal fetal development

teratogenic Causing abnormal development of the embryo

teratogenic substance Substance that crosses the placenta and impairs normal growth and development

term Descriptor for a pregnancy between 38 and 42 weeks' gestation

terrorism Instilling fear in large groups of persons by using any product, weapon, or the threat of using a harmful act or substance to kill or injure people

tertiary care Care focused on restoring the client to the state of health that existed before the development of an illness; if unattainable, then care is directed to attaining the optimal level of health possible

tertiary prevention Treatment of an illness or disease after symptoms have appeared, so as to prevent further progression

tetany Sharp flexion of the wrist and ankle joints, involving muscle twitching or cramps

therapeutic communication Communication that is purposeful and goal directed, creating a beneficial outcome for the client

therapeutic massage Application of hand pressure and motion to improve the recipient's well-being

therapeutic procedure accident Accident that occurs during the delivery of medical or nursing interventions

therapeutic touch Technique of assessing alterations in a person's energy fields and using the hands to direct energy to achieve a balanced state

thermogenesis Production of heat

thermoregulation Maintenance of body temperature

thoracentesis Aspiration of fluid from the pleural cavity

thrombocytopenia Decrease in the number of platelets in the blood

thrombophlebitis Formation of a clot due to an inflammation in the wall of the vessel

thrombosis Formation of a clot due to an inflammation in the wall of the vessel

thrombus Formed clot that remains at the site where it formed

time management System to help meet goals through problem solving

tinnitus Ringing sound in the ear

tocolysis Process of stopping labor with medications

tocolytic agent Medication that inhibits uterine contractions

toddler stage Development begins at approximately 12 to 18 months of age, when a child begins to walk, and ends at approximately 3 years of age

tolerance Decreased sensitivity to subsequent doses of the same substance; an increased dose of the substance is needed to produce the same desired effect

tophi Subcutaneous nodules of sodium urate crystals

tort Civil wrong committed by a person against another person or property

tort law Enforcement of duties and rights among individuals and independent of contractual agreements

touch Means of perceiving or experiencing through tactile sensation

toxic effect Reaction that occurs when the body cannot metabolize a drug and the drug accumulates in the blood

trade (brand) name Name assigned to a drug by the pharmaceutical company; always capitalized

transcendence A state of being or existence above and beyond the limits of material experience

transcutaneous electrical nerve stimulation Process of applying a low-voltage electrical current to the skin through cutaneous electrodes

transducer Instrument that converts electrical energy to sound waves

transduction Noxious stimulus that triggers electrical activity in the endings of afferent nerve fibers (nociceptors)

transmission Process whereby the pain impulse travels from the receiving nociceptors to the spinal cord

Transmission-based Precautions Practices designed for clients documented as, or suspected of, being infected with highly transmissible or epidemiologically important pathogens for which additional precautions beyond Standard Precautions are required to interrupt transmission in hospitals

trauma Wound or injury

traumatic imagery Imagining the feelings of horror felt by the victim or reliving the horror of the incident

triage Classification of clients to determine priority of need and proper place of treatment

triglyceride Lipid compound consisting of three fatty acids and a glycerol molecule

trocar Sharply pointed surgical instrument contained in a cannula

Trousseau's sign Carpal spasm caused by inflating a blood pressure cuff above the client's systolic pressure and leaving it in place for 3 minutes

trust Ability to rely on an individual's character and ability

tumor marker Substance found in the serum that indicates the possible presence of malignancy

turgor Normal resiliency of the skin

type and cross-match Laboratory test that identifies the client's blood type (e.g., A or B) and determines the compatibility of the blood between potential donor and recipient

U

ultrasound Use of high-frequency sound waves to visualize deep body structures; also called an echogram or sonogram

umbilical cord Structure that connects the fetus to the placenta

uncomplicated grief Grief reaction normally following a significant loss

unilateral neglect Failure to recognize or care for one side of the body

unit dose form System of packaging and labeling each dose of medication by the pharmacy, usually for a 24-hour period

urethrocele Downward displacement of the urethra into the vagina

urethrostomy Formation of a permanent fistula opening into the urethra

urge incontinence Inability to suppress the sudden urge or need to urinate

urgent care center A facility designed for the effective and efficient treatment of acute illnesses and injuries; clients do not require an appointment, do not see the same provider consistently, and are usually seen in the order of arrival or the order of acuity

urobilinogen Colorless derivative of bilirubin formed by the normal bacterial action of intestinal flora on bilirubin

urticaria Allergic reaction causing raised pruritic, red, nontender wheals on the skin; also called hives

uterine retraction Unique ability of the muscle fibers of the uterus to remain shortened to a small degree after each contraction

uterine souffle Sound of blood pulsating through the uterus and placenta

utility Ethical principle that states that an act must result in the greatest positive benefit for the greatest number of people involved

V

value system Individual's collection of inner beliefs that guides the way the person acts and helps determine the choices the person makes

values Influences on the development of beliefs and attitudes rather than behaviors; a principle, standard, or quality considered worthwhile or desirable

values clarification Process of analyzing one's own values to better understand those things that are truly important

variable deceleration Reduction in fetal heart rate that has no relationship to contractions of the uterus

vasectomy Surgical resection of the vas deferens

venipuncture Puncturing of a vein with a needle to aspirate blood

ventilation Movement of gases into and out of the lungs

veracity Ethical principle based on truthfulness (neither lying nor deceiving others)

verbal communication Using words, either spoken or written, to send a message

verbally aggressive Descriptor of an individual who says things in a loud and/or intimidating manner

vernix caseosa White, creamy substance covering a fetus's body

vertigo Dizziness

vesicant Agent that may produce blisters and tissue necrosis

vesicular sound Soft, breezy, low-pitched sound heard longer on inspiration than expiration resulting from air moving through the smaller airways over the lung periphery, with the exception of the scapular area

villi Finger-like projections that line the small intestine

viral load test Test that measures copies of HIV RNA

visceral pain Discomfort felt in the internal organs

visual hallucination Perception by an individual that something is present when nothing in fact is

visual learner Person who learns by processing information through seeing

vitamin Organic compounds essential to life and health

vitiligo Depigmentation of the skin caused by destruction of melanocytes; appears as milk-white patches on the skin

void Process of urine elimination

volvulus Twisting of a bowel on itself

W

water-soluble vitamin Vitamin that must be ingested daily in normal quantities because it is not stored in the body: vitamins C and B-complex

wellness State of optimal health wherein an individual maximizes human potential, moves toward integration of human functioning, has greater self-awareness and self-satisfaction, and takes responsibility for health
Western blot test Confirmatory test used to detect HIV infection
Wharton's jelly Thick substance surrounding and protecting the vessels of the umbilical cord
whistleblowing Calling public attention to unethical, illegal, or incompetent actions of others
windowing Cutting a hole in a plaster cast to relieve pressure on the skin or a bony area and to permit visualization of the underlying body part
witch's milk A whitish fluid secreted by a newborn's nipples
withdrawal Symptoms produced when a substance on which an individual has dependence is no longer used by that individual
word salad Nonsensical combination of words that is meaningless to others
wound Disruption in the integrity of body tissue

Y

yin and yang Opposing forces that yield health when in balance
young adulthood Development from the ages of 21 years through approximately 40 years

Z

zoonotic disease A disease of animals that is directly transmissible to humans from the primary animal host
zygote Fertilized ovum

INDEX

Page numbers followed by "f" denote fi gures, "t" denote tables, and "b" denote boxes.

A

B

C

D

E

F

G

H

I

J

K

L

M

N

O

Q

R

S

T

U

V

W

X

Z